The Lymphoid Neoplasms

The Lymphoid Neoplasms

Third edition

Edited by

Ian T. Magrath DSc (Med), FRCP, FRCPath
President, International Network for Cancer Treatment and Research,
Adjunct Professor of Pediatrics, Uniformed Services University of the Health Sciences,
International Network for Cancer Treatment and Research,
Brussels, Belgium

Section editors

Kishor Bhatia PhD, FRCPath
Director, AIDS Malignancy Program
OHAM, NCI, NIH
Bethesda, MD
USA

Paolo Boffetta MD, MPH
Head of Environment Section, IARC
Lifestyle and Cancer Group
International Agency for Research on Cancer
Lyon
France

Claire Dearden BSc, MD, FRCP, FRCPath
Consultant Haematologist
Department of Haemato-Oncology
Royal Marsden NHS Foundation Trust and
    Institute of Cancer Research
London
UK

Volker Diehl MD, PhD
Professor of Internal Medicine, Hematology
    and Oncology
Honorary Chairman of German Hodgkin Study
    Group (GHSG)
Former Head of Department I of Internal Medicine
University Hospital Cologne
Cologne
Germany

Randy D. Gascoyne MD, FRCPC
Clinical Professor of Pathology
Department of Pathology and Laboratory Medicine
British Columbia Cancer Agency and
The University of British Columbia
Research Director, Centre for Lymphoid Cancers
Senior Scientist, BC Cancer Research Centre
Vancouver, BC
Canada

Hans Konrad Müller-Hermelink Prof. Dr. Dr. h. c.
Professor and Chairman
Institute of Pathology
University of Würzburg
Würzburg
Germany

Michael Potter MD
Scientist, Emeritus
Laboratory of Cell Biology and Genetics
National Cancer Institute, NIH
Bethesda, MD
USA

Ama Z. S. Rohatiner MD, FRCP
Professor of Haemato-Oncology
Department of Medical Oncology,
St. Bartholomew's Hospital
London
UK

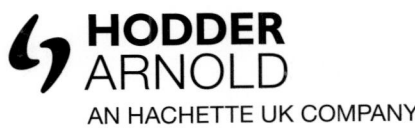

HODDER
ARNOLD
AN HACHETTE UK COMPANY

First published in Great Britain in 2010 by
Hodder Arnold, an imprint of Hodder Education,
an Hachette UK company,
338 Euston Road, London NW1 3BH

http://www.hodderarnold.com

© 2010 Edward Arnold (Publishers) Ltd

Whilst the advice and information in this book are believed to be true
and accurate at the date of going to press, neither the author[s] nor the
publisher can accept any legal responsibility or liability for any errors or
omissions that may be made. In particular, (but without limiting the
generality of the preceding disclaimer) every effort has been made to
check drug dosages; however it is still possible that errors have been
missed. Furthermore, dosage schedules are constantly being revised and
new side-effects recognized. For these reasons the reader is strongly
urged to consult the drug companies' printed instructions before
administering any of the drugs recommended in this book.

British Library Cataloguing in Publication Data
A catalogue record for this book is available from the British Library

Library of Congress Cataloging-in-Publication Data
A catalog record for this book is available from the Library of Congress

ISBN-13   978-0-340-80947-1

1 2 3 4 5 6 7 8 9 10

Commissioning Editor: Gavin Jamieson
Editorial Manager: Francesca Naish
Production Controller: Joanna Walker
Cover Design: Helen Townson

Typeset in 10/12pt Minion by MPS Limited, A Macmillan Company,
Chennai, India
Printed and bound in India by Replika Press

What do you think about this book? Or any other Hodder Arnold
title? Please visit our website: **www.hodderarnold.com**

Dedication

This book is dedicated to the memory of Denis Burkitt (1911–1993) – a man whose curiosity, exceptional powers of observation and unquenchable enthusiasm enabled him to make a number of important discoveries in a small African country, perhaps particularly the possibility of curative cancer chemotherapy in an era when many believed that, at most, drug treatment could only delay the inevitability of death. His discoveries, however, also provided a solid foundation on which many subsequent discoveries could be made by others, including that of Epstein–Barr virus, and the importance of chromosomal translocations involving antigen receptor genes in the pathogenesis of lymphoid neoplasia. Burkitt lymphoma remains a model tumor, the study of which continues to provide new insights into the classification, pathogenesis and treatment of lymphoid neoplasms.

Contents

Contributors

Amal M. Abu-Ghosh, MBBS
Associate Professor of Pediatrics, Department of Pediatrics, Division of Pediatric Hematology/Oncology, Blood and Marrow Transplantation, Lombardi Comprehensive Cancer Center, Georgetown University Medical Center, Washington, DC, USA

Peter Adamson, BSc, MSc
Research Fellow, Department of Health Sciences, University of York, York, UK

Ranjana H. Advani, MD
Associate Professor of Medicine, Division of Oncology, Stanford Cancer Center, Stanford, CA, USA

Anjali S. Advani, MD
Director, Inpatient Leukemia Unit, Assistant Professor, Cleveland Clinic Lerner College of Medicine, Staff, Department of Hematologic Oncology and Blood Disorders, The Cleveland Clinic, Cleveland, OH, USA

Suresh Advani, MD, FICP, FNAMS
Director, Consultant Medical Oncologist, Department of Medical Oncology, Jaslok Hospital and Research Center, Mumbai, India

Claudio Agostinelli, MD, PhD
Department of Haematology and Oncological Sciences 'L. and A. Seràgnoli', Bologna University School of Medicine, Bologna, Italy

Arshad Naveed Ahsanuddin, MD
Hematopathologist, University of Manitoba, Department of Hematopathology, Winnipeg, Manitoba, Canada

Richard F. Ambinder, MD, PhD
Professor, Director, Division of Hematologic Malignancies, Department of Oncology, Johns Hopkins School of Medicine, Baltimore, MD, USA

Peter L. Amlot, MBBS, FRCP
Consultant Immunologist and Oncologist, Department of Immunology, RFUCMS, Royal Free Hospital, London, UK

Nicolas Amoretti, MD
Radiologist, Department of Radiology, CHU L'Archet, Nice, France

James O. Armitage, MD
The Joseph Shapiro Professor of Internal Medicine, Department of Internal Medicine, Section of Oncology-Hematology, University of Nebraska Medical Center, Omaha, NE, USA

John Ashcroft, MA, MB BChir, MRCP (UK), FRCPath, PhD
Consultant Haematologist and Honorary Senior Lecturer, Mid-Yorkshire NHS Trust/University of Leeds Pinderfields Hospital, Wakefield, UK

Andishe Attarbaschi, MD
Associate Professor of Pediatrics, Senior Pediatric Hemato-Oncologist, Department of Pediatric Hematology and Oncology, St Anna Children's Hospital, Vienna, Austria

Rebecca L. Auer, MB, BS, MRCP(UK), FRCPath, PhD
Senior Lecturer in Haematology, Department of Medical Oncology, Bart's and the London School of Medicine, London, UK

Francesco Bacci, MD
Pathologist, Department of Haematology and Oncological Sciences 'L. and A. Seràgnoli', Bologna University School of Medicine, Bologna, Italy

Olga Balagué, MD, PhD
Pathologist, Fellow Supported by Instituto de Salud Carlos III, Department of Pathology, IDIBAPS, Hospital Clinic, University of Barcelona, Barcelona, Spain

Kishor Bhatia, PhD, FRCPath
Director, AIDS Malignancy Program, OHAM, NCI, NIH, Bethesda, MD, USA

Smita Bhatia, MD, MPH
Professor and Chair, Population Sciences, City of Hope National Medical Center, Duarte, CA, USA

Paolo Boffetta, MD, MPH
Deputy Director, The Tisch Cancer Institute, Mount Sinai School of Medicine, New York, NY, USA

Catherine M. Bollard, MBChB, MD, FRACP, FRCPA
Associate Professor of Pediatrics, Medicine and Immunology, Center for Cell and Gene Therapy, Baylor College of Medicine, Houston, TX, USA

Pierre Brousset, MD, PhD
Professor of Pathology, Department of Pathoilogy, CHU Purpan, Toulouse, France

Jean-Noël Bruneton, MD
Professor of Radiology, Department of Radiology, Centre Hospitalier Princesse Grace, Monaco

Cathy Burton, MB BChir, MD, MRCP, FRCPath
Academic Clinical Lecturer, Haemtological Malignancy Diagnostic Service, St James's University Hospital, Leeds, UK

Cristina Campidelli, MD
Pathologist, Department of Haematology and Oncological Sciences 'L. and A. Seràgnoli', Bologna University School of Medicine, Bologna, Italy

Elias Campo, MD
Professor of Anatomic Pathology, Chief, Hematopathology Unit and Department of Pathology, Hospital Clinic, University of Barcelona, Barcelona, Spain

Daniela Capello, PhD
Assistant Professor of Clinical Biochemistry and Molecular Biology, Division of Hematology, Department of Clinical and Experimental Medicine, Amedeo Avogadro University of Eastern Piedmont, Novara, Italy

Jorge A. Carrasquillo, MD
Director, Targeted Radiotherapy Section, Department of Radiology, Nuclear Medicine Division, Memorial-Sloan Kettering Cancer Center, New York, NY, USA

Hetty E. Carraway, MD, MBA
Assistant Professor, Cancer Biology Program and the Division of Hematologic Malignancies, The Sidney Kimmel Comprehensive Cancer Center at Johns Hopkins, Baltimore, MD, USA

Franco Cavalli, MD, FRCP
Associate Professor of Oncology, Medical Director, Oncology Institute of Southern Switzerland (IOSI), Ospedale S. Giovanni, Bellinzona, Switzerland

Nadine Cerf-Bensussan, MD, PhD
Director of Research, INSERM U989, Université Paris Descartes, Paris, France

Soung-Chul Cha, PhD
Assistant Professor, Department of Lymphoma and Myeloma, University of Texas MD Anderson Cancer Center, Houston, TX, USA

John K. C. Chan, MBBS, FRCPath, FRCPA
Consultant, Department of Pathology, Queen Elizabeth Hospital, Hong Kong

Wing C. Chan, MD
Amelia and Austin Vickery Professor of Pathology, Co-Director, Center for Lymphoma and Leukemia Research, University of Nebraska Medical Center, Omaha, NE, USA

Bruce D. Cheson, MD
Professor of Medicine, Head of Hematology, Division of Hematology/Oncology, Georgetown University Hospital, Lombardi Comprehensive Cancer Center, Washington, DC, USA

Wah Cheuk, MBBS, FRCPA
Associate Consultant, Department of Pathology, Queen Elizabeth Hospital, Hong Kong

Patrick Chevallier, MD
Professor of Radiology, Department of Radiology, CHU L'Archet, Nice, France

Yu-Waye Chu, MD
Assistant Clinical Investigator, Experimental Transplantation and Immunology Branch, Center for Cancer Research, National Cancer Institute, Bethesda, MD, USA

Bertrand Coiffier, MD, PhD
Professor of Hematology, Hospices Civils de Lyon, Université Claude Bernard Lyon-1, Lyon, France

Annarita Conconi, MD
Consultant Hematologist, Division of Hematology, Department of Oncology, AOU Maggiore della Carità, Amedeo Avogadro University of Eastern Piedmont, Novara, Italy

Joseph M. Connors, MD
Clinical Professor, Chair, Lymphoma Tumor Group and Clinical Director, Centre for Lymphoid Cancer, University of British Columbia and British Columbia Cancer Agency, Vancouver, British Columbia, Canada

Gordon Cook, MBChB, PhD, FRCP(Glas), FRCPath, FRCPI
Director, BMT, Consultant Haematologist, Department of Haematology, St James's Institute of Oncology, Leeds Teaching Hospitals, Leeds, UK

Finbarr E. Cotter, MB, BS, FRCP(UK), FRCPath, PhD
Chair of Experimental Haematology, Department of Medical Oncology, Bart's and the London School of Medicine, London, UK

Luigino Dal Maso, ScD
Senior Statistician, Unit of Epidemiology and Biostatistics, Centro di Riferimento Oncologico, IRCCS, Aviano, Italy

David J. J. de Gorter, PhD
Research Fellow, Department of Pathology, Academic Medical Center, University of Amsterdam, Amsterdam, The Netherlands

Laurence de Leval, MD, PhD
Professor and Head, Pathology Department, University Institute of Pathology, Lausanne, Switzerland

Claire Dearden, BSc, MD, FRCP, FRCPath
Consultant Haematologist, Department of Haemato-Oncology, Royal Marsden NHS Foundation Trust and Institute of Cancer Research, London, UK

Georges Delsol, MD
Professor of Pathology, Department of Pathology and INSERM U563, CHU Purpan, Toulouse, France

Volker Diehl, MD, PhD
Professor of Internal Medicine, Hematology and Oncology, Honorary Chairman of German Hodgkin Study Group (GHSG), Former Head of Department I of Internal Medicine, University Hospital Cologne, Cologne, Germany

Milton Drachenberg, MD, PhD
Pathologist, Department of Pathology, Medical Director, Hematopathology, Long Beach Memorial Medical Center, Long Beach, CA, USA

ZoAnn E. Dreyer, MD
Associate Professor of Pediatrics, Pediatric Hematology-Oncology, Texas Children's Cancer Center, Texas Children's Hospital, Baylor College of Medicine, Houston, TX, USA

Martin Dreyling, MD, PhD
Professor of Medicine, Hematologist/Oncologist, University Hospital Munich – Grosshadern, Department of Internal Medicine III – Hematology/Oncology, Munich, Germany

Kieron Dunleavy, MD
Investigator/Attending Physician, Center for Cancer Research, National Cancer Institute, Bethesda, MD, USA

Jehan Dupuis, MD
Senior Hematologist, Lymphoid Malignancies Unit, Hôpital Henri Mondor, Créteil, France

Martin J. S. Dyer, MA, PhD, FRCP, FRCPath
Professor of Haemato-Oncology, MRC Toxicology Unit and University of Leicester, Leicester, UK

Estelle Espinos, PhD
Teacher in Molecular Biology/Researcher, CPTP – INSERM U563, CHU Purpan, Toulouse, France

Adnan Ezzat, MBBch, FRCPC, MBA
Consultant Oncologist, King Faisal Specialist Hospital and Research Center, Riyadh, Kingdom of Saudi Arabia

Brunangelo Falini, MD
Professor of Hematology, Institute of Hematology, University of Perugia, Perugia, Italy

Massimo Federico, MD
Professor, Medical Oncology, Department of Oncology and Haematology, Modena Cancer Centre, University of Modena and Reggio Emilia, Modena, Italy

Clodoveo Ferri, MD
Professor of Rheumatology, Chair of Rheumatology, University of Modena and Reggio East, Modena, Italy

Silvia Franceschi, MD
Head, Section of Infections, Head, Infections and Cancer Epidemiology Group, International Agency for Research on Cancer, Lyon, France

Jeremy G. Franklin, PhD
Medical Statistician, German Hodgkin Study Group, and Institute of Medical Statistics, Informatics and Epidemiology, University of Cologne , Germany

Debra L. Friedman, MD, MS
Associate Professor of Pediatrics, E. Bronson Ingram Chair in Pediatric Oncology, Leader, Cancer Control and Prevention Program, Vanderbilt-Ingram Cancer Center, Nashville, TN, USA

Valérie Gaboriau-Routhiau, PhD
Researcher, INSERM U989, Université Paris Descartes, Faculté de Médecine, Paris, INRA UMR1319 MICALIS Jouy-en-Josas, France

Helmut Gadner, MD, FRCP(G)
Professor of Pediatrics, Medical Director and Senior Pediatric Hemato-Oncologist, St Anna Children's Hospital, Vienna, Austria

Gianluca Gaidano, MD, PhD
Professor of Hematology, Director, Division of Hematology, Department of Clinical and Experimental Medicine; Department of Oncology, Azienda Ospedaliero Universitaria Maggiore della Carità, Amedeo Avogadro University of Eastern Piedmont, Novara, Italy

Apar Kishor Ganti, MD
Assistant Professor, Department of Internal Medicine, Omaha VA Medical Center, Department of Internal Medicine, Section of Oncology-Hematology, University of Nebraska Medical Center, Omaha, NE, USA

Randy D. Gascoyne, MD, FRCPC
Clinical Professor of Pathology, Department of Pathology and Laboratory Medicine, British Columbia Cancer Agency and, The University of British Columbia, Research Director, Centre for Lymphoid Cancers, Senior Scientist, BC Cancer Research Centre, Vancouver, BC

Philippe Gaulard, MD
Professor of Pathology, Department of Pathology and INSERM U955, Hôpital Henri Mondor, Créteil, France

Michael Girardi, MD
Associate Professor, Yale University School of Medicine, New Haven, CT, USA

Christian Gisselbrecht, MD
Professor of Haematology, Institut d'Hématologie, Hemato-Oncology Department, Saint Louis Hospital, Paris, France

Marco Giunti, MD
Resident in Rheumatology, Postgraduate Medical School of Rheumatology, Chair of Rheumatology, University of Modena and Reggio East, Modena, Italy

Sylvie Giuriato, PhD
Researcher, CPTP – INSERM U563, Université Toulouse III Paul-Sabatier, Toulouse, France

Earl J. Glusac, MD
Professor, Departments of Pathology and Dermatology, Yale University School of Medicine, New Haven, CT, USA

Ronald E. Gress, MD
Branch Chief, Experimental Transplantation and Immunology Branch, Center for Cancer Research, National Cancer Institute, Bethesda, MD, USA

Anne Grimaud, MD
Radiologist, Department of Radiology, CHU L'Archet, Nice, France

Jeroen E. J. Guikema, PhD
Immunologist, Department of Molecular Genetics and Microbiology, University of Massachusetts Medical School, Worcester, MA, USA

Marina I. Gutiérrez, PhD
Head, Molecular Biology Division, Centro de Estudios Infectológicos, Buenos Aires, Argentina

Martin-Leo Hansmann, MD, PhD
Professor and Chairman of Pathology, Senckenberg Institute of Pathology, Goethe University Frankfurt, Frankfurt, Germany

Eugenia Haralambieva, MD, PhD
Haematopathologist, Institute of Pathology, University of Würzburg, Würzburg, Germany

Nancy Lee Harris, MD
Austen L. Vickery Professor of Pathology, Massachusetts General Hospital and Harvard Medical School, Boston, MA, USA

Sylvia Hartmann, MD
Pathologist, Senckenberg Institute of Pathology, Goethe University Frankfurt, Frankfurt, Germany

Karen Taraszka Hastings, MD, PhD
Assistant Professor, Department of Basic Medical Sciences, University of Arizona College of Medicine, Phoenix, AZ, USA

Antonio M. Hernandez, BSc, MD
Staff Hematopathologist, Ameripath Central Florida, Orlando, FL, USA

Beatriz Herreros, PhD
Lymphoma Group, Molecular Pathology Program, CNIO (Spanish National Cancer Research Center), Madrid, Spain

Helen E. Heslop, MD, MB, ChB
Professor of Medicine and Pediatrics, Dan L Duncan Chair, Center for Cell and Gene Therapy, The Methodist Hospital and Texas Children's Hospital, Baylor College of Medicine, Houston, TX, USA

Wolfgang Hiddemann, MD, PhD
Professor of Medicine, Hematologist/Oncologist, University Hospital Munich – Grosshadern, Department of Internal Medicine III – Hematology/Oncology, Munich, Germany

Richard T. Hoppe, MD, FACR, FASTRO
Henry S. Kaplan-Harry Lebeson Professor in Cancer Biology and Chair, Department of Radiation Oncology, Stanford Cancer Center, Stanford, CA, USA

Ivan D. Horak, MD, FACP
Executive Vice President, Chief Scientific Officer, Enzon Pharmaceuticals, Inc., Piscataway, NJ, USA

Eric D. Hsi, MD
Section Head, Hematopathology, Department of Clinical Pathology, Cleveland Clinic, Cleveland, OH, USA

Mary S. Huang, MD
Pediatric Hematologist-Oncologist, MassGeneral Hospital for Children, Harvard Medical School, Boston, MA, USA

Kazunori Imada, MD, PhD
Chief, Department of Hematology, Kokura Memorial Hospital, Kitakyushu, Japan

Takayuki Ishikawa, MD, PhD
Senior Lecturer, Department of Hematology and Oncology, Faculty of Medicine, Kyoto University, Kyoto, Japan

Andrew Jack, BSc, MB ChB, PhD, FRCPath
Consultant Haematopathologist, Haemtological Malignancy Diagnostic Service, St James's University Hospital, Leeds, UK

Elaine S. Jaffe, MD
Section Chief and Principal Investigator, Hematopathology Section, Laboratory of Pathology, Center for Cancer Research, National Cancer Institute, National Institutes of Health, Bethesda, MD, USA

Reetu Jain, MD
Consultant Medical Oncologist, Department of Medical Oncology, Jaslok Hospital and Research Center, Mumbai, India

Matthew Jenner, MRCP, FRCPath
Consultant Haematologist, Department of Haematology, Southampton General Hospital, Southampton, UK

Matko Kalac, MD
Postdoctoral Research Fellow, NYU Cancer Institute, NYU Langone Medical Center, New York, NY, USA

Judith E. Karp, MD
Professor of Oncology and Medicine, Director, Leukemia Program, Division of Hematologic Malignancies, Johns Hopkins Sidney Kimmel Cancer Center, Baltimore, MD, USA

Ali N. Khan, FRCP, FRCR
Consultant Radiologist and Honorary Professor, North Manchester General Hospital, Pennine Acute NHS Trust, Crumpsall, Manchester, UK

Youn H. Kim, MD
Joanne and Peter Haas Jr. Professor, Director, Multidisciplinary Cutaneous Lymphoma Program, Stanford Cancer Center, Stanford, CA, USA

Yukiko Kitigawa, MD, PhD
Assistant Research Scientist, NYU Cancer Institute, NYU Langone Medical Center, New York, NY, USA

Ulf Klein, PhD
Assistant Professor, Department of Pathology, Department of Microbiology and Immunology, Herbert Irving Comprehensive Cancer Center, Columbia University, New York, NY, USA

Beate Klimm, MD
Assistant Doctor in Internal Medicine, Hematology and Oncology, German Hodgkin Study Group (GHSG), Department I of Internal Medicine , University Hospital Cologne, Cologne, Germany

Philip M. Kluin, MD, PhD
Professor of Pathology, Department of Pathology and Medical Biology, University Medical Center Groningen, Groningen, The Netherlands

Ralf Küppers, PhD
Institute of Cell Biology (Cancer Research), University of Duisburg-Essen, Medical School, Essen, Germany

Larry W. Kwak, MD, PhD
Professor of Medicine, Chair, Department of Lymphoma and Myeloma, The University of Texas MD Anderson Cancer Center, Houston, TX, USA

Yok-Lam Kwong, MD, FRCP, FRCPath
Chair Professor, Department of Medicine, University of Hong Kong, Hong Kong, China

Laurence Lamant, MD, PhD
Professor of Pathology, Department of Pathology and INSERM U563, CHU Purpan , Toulouse, France

Georg Lenz, MD
Assistant Professor, Department of Hematology, Oncology and Tumor Immunology, Molecular Cancer Research Center, Charité – Universitätsmedizin, Berlin, Germany

Raymond Liang, MD, FRCP, FRACP
S.H. Ho Chair; Professor of Haematology and Oncology, Department of Medicine, University of Hong Kong, Hong Kong, China

T. Andrew Lister, MD, FRCP, FRCPath
Professor of Medical Oncology, Department of Medical Oncology, St Bartholomew's Hospital, London, UK

A. Thomas Look, MD
Vice-Chair for Research, Pediatric Oncology Department, Dana-Farber Cancer Institute, Professor of Pediatrics, Harvard Medical School, Boston, MA, USA

Stefano Luminari, MD
Assistant Professor, Medical Oncology, Department of Oncology and Haematology, Modena Cancer Centre, University of Modena and Reggio Emilia, Modena, Italy

Ian C. M. MacLennan, CBE, FMedSci, MB BS, PhD, FRCPath, FRCP
Professor Emeritus of Immunology, University of Birmingham
MRC Centre for Immune Regulation, Birmingham, UK

Irfan Maghfoor, MD
Consultant Oncologist, King Faisal Specialist Hospital and
Research Center, Riyadh, Kingdom of Saudi Arabia

Ian T. Magrath, DSc (Med), FRCP, FRCPath
President, International Network for Cancer Treatment and
Research, Adjunct Professor of Pediatrics, Uniformed Services
University of the Health Sciences, International Network for
Cancer Treatment and Research, Brussels, Belgium

Tak Wah Mak, OC, PhD, DSc, FRSC, FRS
Director, Senior Staff Scientist, University Professor, The Campbell
Family Institute for Breast Cancer Research, Ontario Cancer
Institute at Princess Margaret Hospital, University Health Network,
Department of Medical Biophysics and Immunology, University of
Toronto, Toronto, ON, Canada

Georg Mann, MD
Associate Professor of Pediatrics, Senior Pediatric Hemato-
Oncologist, Department of Pediatric Hematology and Oncology,
St Anna Children's Hospital, Vienna, Austria

Estella Matutes, MD, PhD, FRCPath
Reader and Consultant Haematologist, Haemato-Oncology
Unit, Royal Marsden Hospital/Institute of Cancer Research,
London, UK

Dorothea McAreavey, MD, FRCP, FACC
Staff Clinician, Department of Nuclear Medicine, NIH Clinical
Center, Bethesda, MD, USA

Graham Mead, DM, FRCP, FRCR
Consultant In Medical Oncology, Department of Medical
Oncology, Southampton General Hospital, Southampton, UK

Fabienne Meggetto, PhD
Researcher, CPTP – INSERM U563, Université Toulouse III
Paul-Sabatier, Toulouse, France

Fritz Melchers, PhD
Max Planck Fellow, Max Planck Institute for Infection Biology,
Berlin, Germany, Biozentrum of the Unversity of Basel,
Department of Cell Biology, Basel, Switzerland

Elodie Mohr, PhD
Research Fellow, University of Birmingham MRC Centre for
Immune Regulation, Birmingham, UK

Silvia Montoto, MD
Senior Lecturer, Medical Oncology, CR-UK Medical Oncology Unit,
St Bartholomew's Hospital, Barts and the London School of
Medicine and Dentistry, London, UK

Gareth Morgan, PhD, FRCP, FRCPath
Professor of Haematology and Head of Clinical Unit, Section of
Haemato-Oncology, Institute of Cancer Research and Royal
Marsden Hospital, London, UK

Herbert C. Morse III, MD
Chief, Laboratory of Immunopathology, National Institute of
Allergy and Infectious Diseases, National Institutes of Health,
Bethesda, MD, USA

Nicolas Mounier, MD, PhD
Professor of Medical Oncology, Department of Onco-Hematology,
Hospital l'Archet, Nice, France

Hans Konrad Müller-Hermelink, Prof. Dr. Dr. h. c.
Professor and Chairman, Institute of Pathology, University of
Würzburg, Würzburg, Germany

Kikkeri N. Naresh, MBBS, DCP, MD, FRCPath
Haematopathologist, Department of Histopathology,
Hammersmith Hospital Campus, Imperial College Healthcare
NHS Trust, London, UK

Bharat N. Nathwani, MBBS, MD
Senior Lymphoma Diagnosis Consultant, Cedars Sinai Medical
Center, Department of Pathology, Professor of Pathology,
Department of Pathology, University of Southern California
School of Medicine, Los Angeles, CA, USA

Sattva S. Neelapu, MD
Assistant Professor, Department of Lymphoma and Myeloma,
University of Texas MD Anderson Cancer Center, Houston, TX, USA

Ronald D. Neumann, MD
Chief, Nuclear Medicine Department, Warren Grant Magnusen
Clinical Center, National Institutes of Health, Bethesda, MD, USA

Robert Newton, MBBS, PhD
Reader in Clinical Epidemiology, Department of Health Sciences,
University of York, York, UK

Alexandra Nieters, PhD, MPH
Molecular Epidemiology, Centre of Chronic Immunodeficiency,
Freiburg Medical Center, Freiburg, Germany

Sébastien Novellas, MD
Radiologist, Department of Radiology, CHU L'Archet, Nice, France

Owen A. O'Connor, MD, PhD
Professor of Medicine and Pharmacology, Deputy Director for
Clinical Research and Cancer Treatment, Chief, Division of
Hematologic Malignancies and Medical Oncology, NYU Cancer
Institute, NYU Langone Medical Center, New York, NY, USA

Jennifer O'Neil, PhD
Postdoctoral Fellow, Department of Pediatric Oncology,
Dana-Farber Cancer Institute, Harvard Medical School, Boston,
MA, USA

Steven T. Pals, MD, PhD
Professor of Immuno- and Hematopathology, Department of
Pathology, Academic Medical Center, University of Amsterdam,
Amsterdam, The Netherlands

Luca Paoluzzi, MD
Resident, Greenwich Hospital, Greenwich, CT, USA

Catherine Patte, MD
Paediatric Oncologist, Institut Gustave Roussy, Villejuif, France

Pier Paolo Piccaluga, MD, PhD
Researcher, Department of Haematology and Clinical Oncology
'L. and A. Seràgnoli', Bologna University School of Medicine,
Bologna, Italy

Milena Piccioli, BSc
Department of Haematology and Oncological Sciences 'L. and A.
Seràgnoli', Bologna University School of Medicine, Bologna, Italy

Stefano A. Pileri, MD
Professor of Pathology, Director, Haematopathology Unit, Department of Haematology and Oncological Sciences 'L. and A. Seràgnoli', Bologna University School of Medicine, Bologna, Italy

Alessandro Pileri, MD
Specialist in Dermatology, Fellow, Research Doctorate in Dermatology, Internal Medicine, Aging and Renal Diseases Department, Dermatology Division, Department of Dermatology, Bologna University School of Medicine, Bologna, Italy

Miguel Ángel Piris, MD, PhD
Director of the Molecular Pathology Program at CNIO, CNIO (Spanish National Cancer Research Center), Madrid, Spain

Michael Potter, MD
Scientist, Emeritus, Laboratory of Cell Biology and Genetics, National Cancer Institute, NIH, Bethesda, MD, USA

Hong Qin, MD, PhD
Instructor, Department of Lymphoma and Myeloma, University of Texas MD Anderson Cancer Center, Houston, TX, USA

Zhengxing Qu, PhD
Research Scientist, Enzon Pharmaceuticals, Inc., Piscataway, NJ, USA

Gregory H. Reaman, MD
Chairman, Children's Oncology Group, Professor of Pediatrics and Emeritus, Executive Director, Center for Cancer and Blood Disorders, Children's National Medical Center (CNMC), The George Washington University, School of Medicine and Health Sciences, Washington

Simona Righi, BSc
Biologist, Department of Haematology and Oncological Sciences 'L. and A. Seràgnoli', Bologna University School of Medicine, Bologna, Italy

Ama Z. S. Rohatiner, MD, FRCP
Professor of Haemato-Oncology, Department of Medical Oncology, St. Bartholomew's Hospital, London, UK

Eve Roman, BSc, PhD
Professor of Epidemiology, Department of Health Sciences, University of York, York, UK

Cliona M. Rooney, PhD
Professor Department of Pediatrics, Department of Immunology, Department of Molecular Virology and Microbiology, Center for Cell and Gene Therapy, Baylor College of Medicine, Houston, TX, USA

Angelo Rosolen, MD
Senior Consultant and Laboratory Chief, Department of Pediatrics, Division of Hematology-Oncology, Azienda Ospedaliera-Università di Padova Padua, Italy

Davide Rossi, MD, PhD
Assistant Professor of Hematology, Consultant Hematologist, Division of Hematology, Department of Clinical and Experimental Medicine; Department of Oncology, Azienda Ospedaliero Universitaria Maggiore della Carità, Amedeo Avogadro University of Eastern Piedmon

Maura Rossi, PhD
Researcher, Department of Haematology and Clinical Oncology 'L. and A. Seràgnoli', Bologna University School of Medicine, Bologna, Italy

Elena Sabattini, MD
Pathologist, Department of Haematology and Oncological Sciences 'L. and A. Seràgnoli', Bologna University School of Medicine, Bologna, Italy

Gilles Salles, MD, PhD
Professor of Hematology, Hospices Civils de Lyon, Université Claude Bernard Lyon-1, Lyon, France

Abel Sánchez-Aguilera, PhD
Research Fellow, Division of Hematology/Oncology, Children's Hospital Boston, Boston, MA, USA

John T. Sandlund, MD
Pediatric Oncologist, St Jude's Children's Research Hospital, Memphis, TN, USA

Puja Sapra, PhD
Senior Scientist, Enzon Pharmaceuticals, Inc., Piscataway, NJ, USA

Sebastian J. Sasu, MD
Pathologist, Department of Pathology, Section Head, Hematopathology, St. John's Health Center, Santa Monica, CA, USA

Cindy L. Schwartz, MD
Professor of Pediatrics, Warren Alpert Medical School of Brown University, Director of Pediatric Hematology-Oncology, Hasbro Children's Hospital, Providence, RI, USA

Karine Serre, PhD
Research Fellow, University of Birmingham MRC Centre for Immune Regulation, Birmingham, UK

Aziza T. Shad, MD
Amey Distinguished Professor of Neuro-Oncology and Childhood Cancer, Director, Division of Pediatric Hematology/Oncology, Blood and Marrow Transplantation, Lombardi Comprehensive Cancer Center, Georgetown University Hospital, Washington, DC, USA

Sadhna M. Shankar, MD, MPH
Associate Professor of Pediatrics, George Washington University, Center for Cancer and Blood Disorders, Children's National Medical Center, Washington, DC, USA

Reiner Siebert, Prof. Dr. med.
Professor and Chair of Human Genetics, Director of the Institute of Human Genetics, Institute of Human Genetics, Christian-Albrechts-University Kiel and University Hospital Schleswig-Holstein, Campus Kiel, Kiel, Germany

Christine F. Skibola, PhD
Adjunct Professor, Department of Environmental Health Sciences, School of Public Health, University of California, Berkeley, CA, USA

Brian F. Skinnider, MD, FRCPC
Clinical Assistant Professor, Department of Pathology, Vancouver General Hospital, British Columbia Cancer Agency and University of British Columbia, Vancouver, Canada

Lena Specht, MD, PhD
Professor of Oncology, Chief Oncologist, Associate Professor of Oncology, Departments of Oncology and Haematology, The Finsen Centre, Rigshospitalet, University of Copenhagen, Copenhagen, Denmark

John W. Sweetenham, MD, FRCP
Professor of Medicine, Cleveland Clinic Taussig Cancer Institute, Cleveland, OH, USA

Michael A. Teitell, MD, PhD
Professor and Chief, Division of Pediatric and Neonatal Pathology, David Geffen School of Medicine at UCLA, Los Angeles, CA, USA

Enrico Tiacci, MD
Research Scientist, Institute of Hematology, University of Perugia, Perugia, Italy

Hervé Tilly, MD
Professor of Hematology, Centre Henri Becquerel and University of Rouen, Rouen, France

Olga L. van der Hel, PhD
Epidemiologist, International Agency for Research on Cancer, Lyon, France

David S. Viswanatha, MD
Consultant, Hematopathology, Division of Hematopathology, Department of Laboratory Medicine and Pathology, Mayo Clinic, Rochester, MN, USA

Jerrold M. Ward, DVM, PhD
Diplomate, American College of Veterinary Pathologists, Veterinary Pathologist, Laboratory of Immunopathology, National Institute of Allergy and Infectious Diseases, National Institutes of Health, Rockville, MD, USA

Ronald E. Weiner, PhD
Head, Radiopharmaceutical Research Institute, Australian Nuclear Science and Technology Organization, Menai, NSW, Australia

Howard J. Weinstein, MD
Chief, Pediatric Hematology-Oncology, MassGeneral Hospital for Children, R. Alan Ezekowitz Professor of Pediatrics, Department of Pediatrics, Harvard Medical School, Boston, MA, USA

Lynn D. Wilson, MD, MPH
Professor, Vice Chairman and Clinical Director, Department of Therapeutic Radiology, Yale University School of Medicine, New Haven, CT, USA

Wyndham H. Wilson, MD, PhD
Senior Investigator, Center for Cancer Research, National Cancer Institute, National Institutes of Health, Bethesda, MD, USA

Alison F. Woo, MS
Department of Lymphoma and Myeloma, University of Texas MD Anderson Cancer Center, Houston, TX, USA

Dennis Wright, BSc, MD, FRCPath
Emeritus Professor of Pathology, Department of Pathology, University of Southampton, Southampton General Hospital, Southampton, UK

Jasmine Zain, MD
Director, Bone Marrow Transplant Program, Assistant Professor, Division of Hematologic Malignancies and Medical Oncology, NYU Cancer Institute, NYU Langone Medical Center, New York, NY, USA

Emanuele Zucca, MD
Vice-Head, Research Division, Head, Lymphoma Unit, Oncology Institute of Southern Switzerland (IOSI), Ospedale S. Giovanni, Bellinzona, Switzerland

Preface to the third edition

The third edition of this book differs considerably from the second edition – most obviously with respect to its title, which reflects the fact that the subject matter is no longer confined to the non-Hodgkin lymphomas. There are two main reasons for this. The first is the recognition that the distinction between lymphoid leukemia and lymphoma is artificial, although this was the first distinction made among lymphoid neoplasms at the beginning of the modern era when clinical features and gross pathology were the only diagnostic tools available (histopathology slowly emerged throughout the nineteenth century). It is now clear that the terms leukemia and lymphoma (in the context of lymphoid neoplasia, at least) do not indicate separate disease categories or 'taxons,' (to steal a term more often used in the classification of living organisms). Essentially identical diseases by morphology, immunophenotype and genetic criteria, as described in the pages of this book, may sometimes be manifested as leukemias (involvement of the bone marrow and often peripheral blood by neoplastic cells) and sometimes as lymphoma (i.e., no evidence of such involvement, although this may depend upon the sensitivity of the technique used). Moreover, bone marrow or peripheral blood involvement may be absent at presentation, but emerge prior to therapy or at relapse.

The second reason for the change in the title of the book relates to the term 'non-Hodgkin lymphoma.' It was not until the very late 19th /early 20th century, that the distinction at a microscopic level between Hodgkin's disease and other lymphomas was made. Indeed, the recognition of the 'granulomatous' appearance of some tumors of lymph nodes, if not the first evidence of microscopic heterogeneity, was, initially at least, the most reproducible. The observations of Sternberg and Reed must have given considerable impetus to the emerging era of histological classification but while the microscopic appearance rapidly became the preeminent taxonomic tool, its power to discriminate between specific disease entities improved rather slowly until its dramatic augmentation by the introduction of immunophenotyping and molecular genetic methods such as in situ hybridization (preceded of course by the development of the field of cytogenetics) in the last few decades. Modern techniques, however, also led to the demonstration that Hodgkin lymphoma, like many other lymphoid neoplasms, is derived from the B-lymphocyte lineage. This meant that the obvious histological watershed between Hodgkin lymphoma and all other lymphomas could no longer be considered as of primary importance to classification. Hodgkin lymphoma, like a number of other lymphoid neoplasms of B-cell lineage is of germinal center origin, and although, unlike the vast majority of other B-lineage neoplasms, its tumor cells fail to express surface immunoglobulin and, for the most part, other B cell markers, it represents no more and no less a category than many other neoplasms, such as mantle cell lymphoma or anaplastic large cell lymphoma, both of which, like Hodgkin lymphoma, have several histological and molecular variants. In short, just as leukemia and lymphoma do not define discrete groups of neoplasms, there appears to be no scientific reason for separating lymphomas into Hodgkin and non-Hodgkin subtypes.

It is clear, then, that neither the leukemia/lymphoma, not the Hodgkin/non-Hodgkin lymphoma dichotomies are indicative of basic subdivisions within the broad spectrum of lymphoid neoplasia in the sense that precursor versus mature, or B-cell lineage versus NK/T-cell lineage are. Moreover, in this modern era, when treatment approaches and the prognosis for different categories of lymphoid neoplasms differ so much, there is little value in designating a tumor a non-Hodgkin lymphoma – although in the early days of the development of specific approaches to the radiation therapy of Hodgkin lymphoma a 'two category' classification approach probably was justifiable. Nonetheless, the term 'non-Hodgkin lymphoma' has a lengthy heritage compared to other negatively defined categories such as non-Burkitt's lymphoma, or non-lymphoblastic lymphoma, which may explain why it has taken on the mantle of a legitimate subdivision and remains a widely used term in contrast to the other 'non-lymphomas,' that have largely faded from use. In general, saying what something is not does not constitute a diagnosis (how useful, for example, would the term 'non-reptile' be in biology?) excepting when one is faced with a true dichotomy (e.g., ALK+ and ALK- anaplastic large cell lymphoma). Moreover, the *implication* that a dichotomy exists in the absence of supportive evidence could lead to a negative impact on the construction of a true framework for classification – as, for example, may have been the case with respect to the division of lymphomas into nodular and diffuse subtypes. We should not, of course, be too critical of pioneer taxonomists who, by today's standards, had extremely limited equipment and reagents with which to work. In spite of everything, including the several false conclusions that largely resulted from the speculation that filled the evidentiary vacuum, their persistence in continuously attempting to improve upon existing tools, coupled to insights from other disciplines (especially immunology – see below), eventually laid the foundation upon which modern diagnosis is based. But equally, as improvements in classification are made, we should continue to eliminate terms that have the capacity to mislead, as has been done in the case, for example, of reticulum cell sarcoma and histiocytic lymphoma (although some will always strenuously argue against such a view, presumably for nostalgic reasons). For better or for worse, *The Non-Hodgkin's Lymphomas* has become *The Lymphoid Neoplasms,* and Hodgkin lymphoma has been given no more and no less a position in lymphoma taxonomy than any other entity or group of closely related entities. The new title has had the additional repercussion that the book now includes diseases that were not covered (or only partially covered) in previous editions – particularly those that most frequently present as leukemia (e.g., the acute and chronic lymphoid leukemias), as well as Hodgkin lymphoma itself and plasma cell tumors. The intent has been to ensure as comprehensive a coverage of the neoplastic diseases of lymphoid cells as possible.

A second major change in the book is the inclusion of a section on immunobiology. Lymphoid neoplasms are now known to arise, or at least, to have the phenotype (whether identified by monoclonal antibodies or by molecular profiling of one kind or another), of discrete or closely related lymphocyte populations. Such populations may represent steps in the process of development into mature lymphoid cells (ontogeny), or alternatively, elements of the immune response, although, with occasional exceptions, it remains unknown whether such pathological immune responses (or partial immune responses) have been precipitated by antigen or not. Knowledge of immunological differentiation or activation pathways therefore provides a basis for the understanding of the pathogenesis of lymphoid neoplasia, at least at a cellular level. Coupled to an understanding of both the normal molecular pathways involved in lymphocyte differentiation and activation and the molecular genetic lesions that are present in such pathways in lymphoid neoplasms, we have reached a point in history in which the broad elements of the pathogenetic process (and in some individual neoplasms, rather precise details) are known. While many oncologists may not wish to attempt to understand lymphomas at the level of their immunobiology, being more concerned with the specific diagnosis and predictors of treatment response, an understanding of pathogenesis, which implies knowledge of immunobiology, is not only inherent to the pathology of any given neoplasm, but may provide clues to causation – something which is presently based exclusively on epidemiology but

which may someday be legible in the runes of the molecular lesions. And who knows what new insights into therapy may derive from a sufficient knowledge of molecular pathogenetic pathways? While the inhibition of the expression of a single pathogenetically relevant gene could provide major therapeutic benefit (although a pathogenetic role is not essential for effective targeting), as with combination chemotherapy the best results are likely to be achieved by targeting more than one gene or more than one molecular pathway. In any event, it seems highly likely that the more that is known about pathogenesis, the more opportunities will be identified for developing targeted approaches to therapy.

In the light of these considerations, it is inevitable that the book covers the molecular lesions of lymphoid neoplasms in considerable detail. Histology is now only one of the many characteristics used to define individual neoplasms and their variants. Indeed, based on the new entities included in the latest (2008) WHO classification, we are rapidly moving into an era when molecular characteristics may even take precedence over other taxonomic tools – whether at the level of single genes/proteins (such as ALK in the context of anaplastic large cell lymphoma) or, when molecular profiling data is available, as is increasingly the case, at the level of molecular signatures. An increasingly molecular approach to classification also has advantages in identifying previously unrecognized relationships between neoplasms – e.g., the similarities discerned in the molecular profiles of Hodgkin disease and mediastinal B cell lymphoma – one that makes sense in light of the fact that both neoplasms tend to arise in thymic B cells. Whether or not such insights will have therapeutic value remains to be seen. Unfortunately, molecular approaches to classification do not always result in sharp definitions of entities, in part because lymphoid differentiation pathways must, by their very nature, include what we perceive as intermediate stages, and in part because the pathogenetic molecular abnormalities, while to a considerable extent neoplasm-specific, are not necessarily identical in a given disease, while the same, or a similar, abnormality may be found in different diseases. This is because some of the most basic molecular pathways – those involved with cell proliferation, differentiation and programmed cell death – may be influenced in a broad range of neoplasms, while different lesions in the same molecular pathway, or involvement of partially redundant molecular pathways could lead to similar functional end-points relevant to the neoplastic state. Intermediate or atypical categories will continue to make life difficult for taxonomists, although perhaps less so for therapists who may, increasingly, as targeted therapy takes hold, require the mere presence or absence of a therapeutic target to decide on treatment.

One pragmatic problem faced by this increasingly molecular approach is the problem of gene nomenclature. Genes have often been discovered in more than one laboratory, such that they may have several quite different designations. In addition, the symbols for genes and proteins have undergone significant evolution. Now that international nomenclatures for symbols and gene names, as well as standard procedures for naming new genes have been developed (e.g., by the Human Genome Organization Gene Nomenclature Committee, HGNC) we have attempted to use these internationally recognized symbols and names for genes throughout the book, although acceptance of international nomenclature has not been as high in the scientific community as might be hoped. Inevitably, therefore, some authors have used former names, or aliases for some genes, while new symbols for other genes have yet to be widely accepted and are uncommonly used by anyone. To the extent possible, the editors have converted obsolete names and aliases to approved names, although one major exception to this is the genes involved in regulation of the cell cycle – particularly inhibitors of cell cycle progression. These genes have multiple aliases (alternative symbols) which are still much more widely used than the HUGO approved or official names. CDKN1A, for example, is the approved symbol for a gene officially named cyclin-dependent kinase inhibitor 1A (p21, Cip1) whose multiple aliases include CIP1, P21, p21CIP1, WAF1 and one or two more. The gene whose official symbol is CDKN2A and approved gene name cyclin-dependent kinase inhibitor 2A (melanoma, p16, inhibits CDK4), has many aliases (ARF, p14, p16, p19, INK4a, to name but a few) as well as at least three splice variants coding for separate proteins, two of which are structurally similar (p16 and p19) and inhibit CDK4 kinase, while the third (ARF) contains an alternate first exon, is transcribed from an alternate reading frame, and functions as a stabilizer of p53. Splice variants are designated by the appendices-v1, v2 etc., by HGNC. Sometimes, different genes have been given the same symbols – e.g., both CDKN2A and CDKN2D have been referred to as p19. Given these complexities, it seemed counterproductive to use approved or official symbols for this subset of genes, but rather to stick to the designations used by the authors. Wherever possible, however, we have used the recommended convention that human gene symbols are written in capitalized italic letters, while only the first letter is capitalized in mouse genes (which are also italicized) and capital letters are used for both human and mouse proteins. Punctuation (e.g., hyphenation) is not used. Gene names are neither capitalized nor italicized. Appropriate nomenclature is also followed to the extent possible for *Drosophila* and nematode genes. Readers may wish to refer to the many gene catalogues such as that of the HGNC or the National Center for Biotechnology Entrez gene data base for lists of gene symbols, aliases, names and obsolete terms. In gene catalogues, incidentally, it is standard practice not to write gene symbols in italics.

As in the past, this book is intended for a wide audience, but in spite of its size, it cannot possibly address all relevant topics in great detail. It is designed to provide overviews of each general area, followed by more detailed information on the pathology and clinical characteristics of specific diseases. Although this approach has inevitably resulted in some duplication, it is hoped that it has also led to increased readability of individual chapters and avoided the need for frequent cross referencing. Books, of course, now find themselves in strong competition with electronic media, and suffer from the disadvantage of the rapid pace of advance, particularly in the area of pathogenesis with which standard publishing procedures cannot keep pace. Journals, particularly of the electronic kind, can make new material available in a matter of days or weeks. While standard books cannot compete with this, for the foreseeable future at least, books will continue to have an important role in collecting a large amount of information in a logical sequence and in one place, providing a valuable starting point or conceptual framework – an idea of where we have come from and where we seem to be going – that may be much more difficult to achieve by surfing the internet. For this reason *The Lymphoid Neoplasms* should, even in this electronic era, be of value to a broad range of health professionals as well as to scientists more interested in pathogenesis, but for whom some understanding of the classification, clinical features and even treatment of lymphoid neoplasms is useful.

Finally, a book of this kind cannot possibly be written, or even edited by a single person. Indeed, some 198 authors have contributed to the text, and 9 section editors have taken on responsibility for different areas of the book. Without this large and eminent team, this book could not have come to fruition, and I sincerely thank them all – authors and editors alike – for their dedication and for their exceptional efforts.

Ian T. Magrath
2009

Preface to the second edition

In the several years since the publication of the first edition of this book, there has been considerable progress in attempts to understand the pathobiology of the non-Hodgkin's lymphomas, but rather less tangible success with respect to the therapy of these diseases. Indeed, while the gains in survival rates in the childhood lymphomas of the last decade have been consolidated, little progress has been made in the treatment of adult lymphomas. The apparent advances achieved with so-called 'third-generation regimens' in the diffuse aggressive lymphomas, for example, have been refuted by the results of a randomized clinical trial conducted by the South West Oncology Group in the USA. Whether this difference in results of treatment between children and adults relates primarily to differences in the treatment regimens employed, or to differences in the biology of the diseases, is a question worthy of study. Similarly, the goal of demonstrating cure in the histological categories listed as *low-grade* in the now beleaguered *Working Formulation for Clinical Usage* remains elusive, even with the use of very high dose therapy supported by autologous bone marrow transplantation (ABMT). Perhaps expectations with respect to the value of very high dose therapy have also been too high in the diffuse aggressive lymphomas. While the long-awaited results of the PARMA study have demonstrated, to the satisfaction of most, that this approach is superior to continuation of the dexamethasone, high-dose ara-C, cis-platinum (DHAP) salvage regimen in patients with chemosensitive recurrent disease, the apparent failure of ABMT to date to influence survival rates when moved from second to first remission in patients in poor prognostic categories does not augur well for its overall contribution to the therapy of this subset of lymphomas.

The role of bone marrow transplantation is, in any event, beginning to undergo, if not a revolution, at least a conceptual reformation. The use of repeated infusions of hematopoietic stem cells obtained from peripheral blood for hematopoietic support after high-dose therapy is likely to lead to changes in the chemotherapy regimens traditionally associated with stem cell support. As a result they will probably more closely resemble existing combination regimens, but be much more intensive – a strategy that is strikingly similar to that which has already been used to advantage, without stem cell support, in the pediatric lymphomas. In addition, much more emphasis is being given to the immunotherapeutic elements inherent in allogeneic transplantation, and the use of donor T-cell infusions posttransplant is becoming increasingly common – both as a form of immunotherapy against tumor cells and as a means of preventing some of the complications of immunosuppression, including cytomegalovirus infection and Epstein-Barr virus-associated lymphoproliferative disease. The degree to which these newer approaches will influence treatment results in the non-Hodgkin's lymphomas is a question that may be answered within the next few years.

Advances in treatment are often salutary – previous success slows further progress, for not only is it necessary to ensure that patients receive the best available treatment (however limited such success may be), but the comfort of traditional approaches contrasts starkly with the censure that awaits unsuccessful innovation. Treatment advances will also be slowed if the trend of recent years to emphasize the economic (even business) aspects of health care is continued, with the consequent detrimental influence on clinical research that this will entail. Medicine without research dooms populations to the inadequacies of present knowledge and technology, while the absence of the spirit of enquiry in those who provide health care is likely to lead rapidly to medical mediocrity. This mistake is not a new one. It was made, perhaps for the first time in recorded human history, by the ancient Egyptians, although for a different reason. They considered their once supreme medical knowledge to be of divine origin and therefore already perfect! The present volume represents the antithesis of this philosophy – as evidenced by the marked increase in its size over the first edition. In addition, considerable space has been devoted to pathobiology for, without an understanding of the nature and origins of the non-Hodgkin's lymphomas, we shall remain confronted by the Faustian dilemma that continues to sour our present empirical treatment approaches (the cure is poisonous*), however successful some of them have been.

---

* Es ist so schwer den falschen Weg zu meiden,/ Es liegt in ihr so viel verborgnes Gift,/ Und von der Arzenei ist's kaum zu unterscheiden. (It is so difficult to avoid the wrong path,/ Concealed therein is so much poison,/ And it's scarcely possible to distinguish the poison from the cure.)

Recent advances in our understanding of the non-Hodgkin's lymphomas are reflected in the publication of the new Revised European – American Lymphoma (REAL) classification of lymphoid neoplasms, an event that was received with mixed emotions by pathologists, and which has provided new grounds to bewail the purported obfuscation that pervades lymphoma classification (a bewailing that has continued for more than a century), much of which has been occasioned simply by the multiplicity of classification schemes. Yet as progress is made, new schemes must replace the old. The REAL classification is an attempt on the part of an *ad hoc* assembly of European and American pathologists to identify and characterize as objectively as possible, using immunophenotyping as well as molecular genetics, the individual disease entities that comprise the malignant lymphomas – an endeavor that would appear to be an essential prerequisite to the development of optimal treatment approaches, and further, to move beyond present empiricism into the realm of tumor-targeted therapy. In this respect it is clearly superior to the Working Formulation and is seriously rivaled only by the widely used European scheme, the Kiel classification, which has been modified at intervals throughout the more than 20 years of its existence. Further, as a genuine attempt by pathologists from many countries to reach agreement, the REAL classification could help to eliminate much of the cause for confusion over lymphoma taxonomy.

However, an understanding of lymphoid neoplasia does not stop at diagnosis and treatment. The challenge to relate environmental factors to the derangements of the immune system that precede lymphoma development – either in terms of epidemiological relationships, or better still, in terms of defined molecular genetic pathways – cannot be ignored, for such information could ultimately lead to methods to detect patients or populations at very high risk, and even to prevent lymphoma development. The inherited and acquired immunodeficiency syndromes, with their associated increased risk of lymphoma, provide one model system for understanding changes in the microenvironment that are relevant to lymphomagenesis, but another opportunity – one likely to be even more fruitful in the context of the lymphomas that develop *de novo* – is provided by the vast range of life styles and environments that exist throughout the world. This global laboratory is certainly underutilized, to the detriment of our comprehension of lymphoid neoplasia. It can only be hoped that the recent exponential improvement that has occurred in communications will lead to improved collaboration between industrial and developing nations, with consequent benefits to all.

The present volume, then, is a markedly expanded version of the first edition, and, like the first edition, represents an attempt to summarize our present understanding of the histopathology, immunopathology, molecular genetics, epidemiology, clinical features and treatment of the non-Hodgkin's lymphomas. The book has been extensively revised; most chapters have been completely rewritten and many new chapters have been added. While every effort has been made to make the book as up-to-date as possible, inevitably some new advances will have occurred since going to press. The book should, nevertheless, provide a firm foundation on which such new advances will fall more readily into place and it is to be hoped, for this reason, that it will serve a useful purpose for a number of years. Its contributors have been selected from the most expert and original in their fields and my thanks are due to all of them for their willingness to give so much of their precious time to this project. Any success that the book may enjoy will be entirely due to their efforts, while any imbalance, omissions or other deficiencies are due to my own shortcomings.

Finally, I am inestimably indebted to Laurene Kuhar, whose superlative administrative support has made a daunting task, superimposed on an already overwhelming schedule, manageable.

Ian T. Magrath
1996

Preface to the first edition

The exponential increase in scientific knowledge which has occurred throughout this century has dramatically changed the face of medicine. While the treatment of bacterial infections provides one of the most dramatic success stories, the broad compass of scientific progress can have had no greater impact than it has in the field of cancer.

Modern diagnostic methods include the use of computerized tomography, magnetic resonance imaging, radionuclide scanning, immunophenotyping, cytogenetics and, increasingly, molecular biology. Conventional treatment currently includes an array of the most sophisticated surgical, radiotherapeutic and pharmacological techniques, while experimental therapy is designed to explore the utility of a broad range of 'biological response modifiers' (BRMs), i.e. molecules which have an effect on cell differentiation or proliferation either by influencing host cellular regulatory mechanisms, or by acting directly on tumour cells via pathways which are utilized by normal cells. Such BRMs include monoclonal antibodies and various cytokines such as interleukin-2 and interferons, the latter frequently produced by means of recombinant DNA technology. In the laboratory, progress towards understanding the pathogenesis of cancer has been made with the help of a wide variety of advanced technologies encompassing the fields of biochemistry, immunology and molecular genetics.

One of the groups of tumours which has benefited the most, or, perhaps more accurately, which has provided the most fertile soil for progress, has been the non-Hodgkin's lymphomas. Yet paradoxically, the current therapeutic success which has been achieved with malignant non-Hodgkin's lymphomas is the result of empirical studies carried out over the last 25 years, and so far, little therapeutic benefit has been gained from recent progress in understanding the genetic and biochemical abnormalities of the tumour cell. Similarly, knowledge of the mechanisms of drug-induced cytotoxicity or drug resistance and of the regulation of cellular growth and differentiation has yet to provide tangible benefit to the patient. It seems highly probable, however, that in the near future this burgeoning growth of the science of oncology will have developed to the point where it will begin to have considerable impact upon the management of patients with malignant lymphomas. Moreover, it is likely that therapeutic advances of considerable magnitude will be seen, whereby more specific biochemical targets will be utilized with a resultant increase in therapeutic efficacy and decrease in toxicity. At the same time, we must accept that our present concepts of disease entities are likely to change considerably. New tools will enable us to perceive similarities and differences hitherto unrecognized. Yet the old, as always, will continue to exist beside the new, and the transition will be gradual.

Nomenclature is likely, for the foreseeable future, to continue to be confusing, since it will derive from an increasing number of perspectives and disciplines and, in the absence of international agreement, multiple terms will coexist with varying degrees of synonymity. This process has occurred throughout history, although at markedly different rates in different eras. We live in the most rapidly changing era that mankind has ever experienced, and as such must be more willing than our forebears to give up outmoded concepts, and replace, where necessary, the familiar with the unfamiliar. But this is a small price to pay for the rewards of witnessing, in the course of a professional lifetime, the transition from a purely descriptive morphological view of lymphomas to one which encompasses an understanding of the precise nature of the cell of origin and of the genetic and biochemical changes which lead to malignant behaviour.

This book attempts to convey something of the excitement of the era in which we live, and to deal with the malignant non-Hodgkin's lymphomas, wherever possible, from a biological perspective rather than from a purely clinical and therapeutic one. As a consequence, a large proportion of the book is devoted to the nature of the diseases themselves, and their pathogenesis, representing the foundation upon which future diagnostic and treatment approaches will be built. As such, the practicing oncologist, and even more, the clinical researcher responsible for the design and analysis of clinical trials, will need to become familiar with the broad range of techniques currently available for the characterization of the non-Hodgkin's lymphomas.

Ian T. Magrath
1989

Reference annotation

The reference lists are annotated, where appropriate, to guide readers to key primary papers and major review articles as follows:

- Key primary paper (publication of an important finding relating to the subject matter of the chapter)
- Major review article

We hope that this feature will render extensive lists of references more useful to the reader and will help to encourage self-directed learning among both trainees and practising physicians.

INTRODUCTION

PART 1

INTRODUCTION

Introduction to the lymphoid neoplasms

IAN T MAGRATH

RECOGNITION OF LYMPHOID NEOPLASIA IN THE NINETEENTH CENTURY

The first modern description of lymphoid neoplasia is usually accepted to be that of Thomas Hodgkin in 1832[1] (although some of Hodgkin's cases were, over 100 years later, shown to be tuberculosis). *Hodgkin's disease*, like Virchow's subsequent term *lymphoma*, was initially used to designate swollen lymph nodes of unknown cause (a much broader category than today, given the limited diagnostic tools then available). At that time, the concept of lymphoid neoplasia was poorly developed. This is not surprising. The malignant tumors of lymphocytes, their precursors and their progeny differ in many important respects from other diseases referred to as cancer since they arise from a widely dispersed 'system' comprising more or less organized congregations of lymphoid tissue and free-ranging lymphocytes that migrate through most of the tissues of the body. Thus, the concept of local invasion and blood-borne metastases that works well for most 'solid tumors' is more difficult to apply in the case of lymphoid neoplasms, a high proportion of which, by virtue of the migratory properties of their normal cell counterparts, are widespread from the outset.

Lymphoid tissue is of mesothelial origin, so from an embryological perspective, lymphoid neoplasia is more closely related to the sarcomas than to the carcinomas. Logically, malignant tumors of lymphoid tissue can, therefore, be considered to be *lymphosarcomas* and this term was used for well over a century (although not universally) as one of the general terms for malignant lymphoid neoplasms (see Chapter 2), although obvious leukemias – initially only recognized at post-mortem – were believed to be separate diseases. For unclear reasons, the term lymphosarcoma has fallen by the wayside, to be replaced by Virchow's *lymphoma*, most often in the form *malignant lymphoma*. Many lymphoid neoplasms included in this category, however, such as follicular lymphoma, indolent lymphomas of mucosa-associated lymphoid tissue (MALT), and certain lymphoid neoplasms that merge with chronic inflammatory processes, may have a protracted clinical course, even when widespread.

Leukemia versus lymphoma

The recognition of *leukemia*, another term coined by Virchow on the basis of the white appearance of the blood at post-mortem caused by a very high white blood cell count, led to the distinction in Germany between leukemia and *pseudoleukemia* (i.e. a disease associated with enlarged lymph nodes, but without demonstrable leukemia at post-mortem), and in English-speaking countries, between leukemia and Hodgkin's disease. This was the first major subdivision of lymphoid neoplasms (although leukemias were subsequently shown to include a myeloid cell type), but in the context of our modern understanding of lymphoid neoplasia it has proved to be both an imprecise, and, in retrospect, misleading distinction, although one difficult to exorcize after some 175 years. It arose because of the limited knowledge of physiologic and pathophysiologic processes – even the concept of the cell as the basic unit of life was not proposed until 1839, by Schleiden and Schwann, and it was almost 20 years later that Virchow recognized the importance of the cell – and thus, of microscopy – to an understanding of pathology. Clinical and gross pathologic appearances were only gradually surmounted by microscopy as the primary diagnostic tool, speeded by the development of efficient stains by Ehrlich late in the nineteenth century (see Chapter 2).

In spite of the initial importance given to the separation of leukemia from lymphoma, many lymphoid neoplasms manifest both leukemic (taken here to indicate generalized involvement of the bone marrow, rather than the original concept) and non-leukemic phases, either in different patients or the same patient at different times. Involvement of the bone marrow is frequently present in lymphoid neoplasms, even in those not designated as leukemias, e.g. follicular lymphoma, and can be the presenting manifestation of diseases that more often present as lymphoma, e.g. in Burkitt lymphoma, which, when presenting in the leukemic phase, was included in the L3 category of acute lymphoblastic leukemia (ALL) in the French–American–British cytological classification. It is still generally referred to by pediatric oncologists as acute B cell leukemia – a potentially misleading designation. Thus, the terms leukemia and lymphoma are used somewhat arbitrarily and should not be thought of as distinct groups of diseases – at least, as far as lymphoid neoplasia is concerned. The bone marrow does deserve recognition, however, as the site at which, after birth, lymphoid cells originate from multipotential precursors. But it is also one of the major locations of highly differentiated antibody-producing plasma cells and may be infiltrated in a broad range of lymphoid (and other) neoplasms.

Hodgkin's versus non–Hodgkin's lymphomas

For decades, attempts were made to distinguish between pseudoleukemia and lymphosarcoma, or to subdivide Hodgkin's disease (used in its broader nineteenth-century sense). There were also protracted debates in the medical literature on the likelihood that some diseases (such as pseudoleukemia) may be hyperplastic rather than neoplastic. In the absence of any real understanding of the nature of neoplasia, or of the cell types from which these various 'entities' arose, such debates were largely speculative and entirely inconclusive. It was not until the turn of the century that improved technology and greater use of the microscope led to a second major distinction among lymphoid neoplasms, this time on the basis of histology. Sternberg's and subsequently Reed's recognition of the granulomatous appearance of some lymphomas (Paltauf and Sternberg's term *lymphogranuloma* was an entirely apt description) allowed the term lymphosarcoma to be confined (although by no means was there universal agreement) to all malignant lymphomas other than lymphogranuloma. The latter disease eventually became known as Hodgkin's disease, since Dorothy Reed used this term for the disease in which she, like Sternberg, was able to identify giant cells amid a 'granulomatous' infiltrate, leaving the term 'non-Hodgkin's lymphoma' available as a general term for malignant lymphomas other than Hodgkin's disease – a historical idiosyncrasy that has persisted to the present time. Since these earliest distinctions, the classification of lymphoid neoplasms has evolved in two main ways – either from the identification of entities (not always initially recognized as lymphoid neoplasms) that appeared from their first descriptions to be well defined on the basis of morphology, clinical features or both (e.g. mycosis fungoides, myeloma and follicular lymphoma), or from an increasing ability to distinguish new entities within a category that had been assumed to be homogeneous (e.g. poorly differentiated lymphocytic lymphoma). The latter process, of course, is dependent on both the available tools as well as a conceptual framework for classification.

As Virchow's emphasis on cellular pathology came of age, it became clear that the cellular origins of tumors provided a logical conceptual basis for their understanding. Consequently, histopathology, albeit limited to morphological comparison of the neoplastic lymphoid cells became, and for long remained, the sole approach to classification. Being heavily dependent upon the skill and biases of pathologists, who tended to work in isolation, or at best, small groups, many classification schemes were proposed in the course of the twentieth century, some of which incorporated misconceptions that persisted for decades, e.g. the belief that large cell lymphomas were derived from phagocytic cells (variously referred to as reticulum cells, clasmatocytes or histiocytes).

Defining diseases

Although most cancers can be divided into more and less differentiated subtypes, often with some difficulty in assigning cancers that lie morphologically close to the boundaries, the cellular constituents of epithelial tissue, for example, are much less complex than those of lymphoid tissue such that classifications based on cell types were relatively simple to construct (there are exceptions). Understanding lymphoid neoplasms, i.e. their pathobiology and classification, however, was not possible before the development of a much more complete understanding of the immune system, from which lymphoid neoplasms arise. After perhaps a century of research, the overall organization and microstructure of various elements of the immune system, the ontogeny (development) and function of its cellular components and the regulation of immune responses to a wide range of antigens, particularly those of microorganisms present in the environment, are well enough understood to provide a solid foundation for the classification and diagnosis of lymphoid neoplasms.

NEOPLASIA OF THE IMMUNE SYSTEM

The concept of an immune system, whose primary concern is the maintenance of the integrity of the organism within the ecosystem in which it lives and in the context of the ecosystem that it constitutes, emerged gradually in the late nineteenth and early twentieth centuries *pari passu* with the (then) new discipline of microbiology. A major route of microbial invasion is via mucosal surfaces, yet these same surfaces are colonized with microorganisms that are essential to life, some of which would be pathogens if able to penetrate the mucosa in sufficient numbers. Open wounds provide other entry points while some microorganisms are able to gain direct entry into the bloodstream, e.g. via arthropod vectors that feed on blood. Defenses against invasion via any of these routes, and in the case of the mucosae, without destroying commensal organisms, must be maintained if the individual is to survive. Potential pathogens must be initially contained, then eliminated either by cells or their products (e.g. antibodies).

Prior to the development of a specific primary immune response, which takes time to generate, there is a need for a rapid, frontline response – necessarily nonspecific. This is provided by innate immunity – i.e. that dependent on certain receptors (toll-like receptors or TLR) present on the cell membrane and in the cytoplasm (on the surface of endosomes) of macrophages, mast cells, dendritic cells and natural killer (NK) cells (see Chapter 9). The TLRs recognize various components of bacteria, viruses and parasites, such that they can be deployed immediately after invasion.

The innate immune response also helps trigger the adaptive immune response (i.e. specific for previously encountered microorganisms) by activating antigen-presenting cells (e.g. specialized dendritic cells). In contrast to the low specificity and 'fixed' nature of innate immune responses, adaptive immune responses are generated by lymphocytes that are able to retain long-term memory of the specific antigens to which they have been exposed. Long-term responses are important both for keeping resident pathogens (such as herpesviruses) in check, and for rapid, highly efficient responses to reinvasion by the same organism (antigenically defined) with consequent avoidance of disease, i.e. immunity.

Role of lymphocytes

The immune system was first recognized in the context of phagocytic cells able to engulf particulate material, such as bacteria, which were seen to be dispersed throughout the body. This 'reticuloendothelial' system was subsequently implicated in the production of antibodies which had been discovered initially in the sera of individuals recently infected by tetanus or diphtheria, and which led to the introduction of serotherapy (see Chapter 2). It was not, however, until 1960 that the importance of lymphocytes to adaptive immunity became clear. This resulted from the recognition that lymphocytes were not endstage cells, but rather could be transformed into proliferating blast cells when exposed to certain plant products (e.g. phytohemagglutinin). In the 1970s, the two main lymphocyte lineages were discovered – B lymphocytes (named after cells identified in the bursa of Fabricius of chickens) associated with the production of antibodies and T lymphocytes (thymic-derived) – which could destroy cells expressing foreign antigens on their surface (e.g. derived from intracellular microorganisms). T cells were soon seen to be essential to the regulation of the immune response, and macrophages and dendritic cells to be particularly important in capturing antigens from a wide range of tissues and, after processing them (see below), presenting them to lymphocytes in the context of the major histocompatibility complex (MHC) at the cell surface, usually within the confines of organized lymphoid tissue.

The expression of antigen receptor genes can be considered to be the primary characteristic of lymphocytes (but not natural killer, or NK, cells) since they permit the possibility of specific immune responses to antigens. Consequently, the construction of functional antigen receptor genes is a central component of lymphocyte development (ontogeny). Because antigen-binding domains of antigen receptors (consisting of heavy and light chain proteins in B cells and either α and β, or γ and δ chain proteins in T cells) are constructed through processes involving both recombination between different variable (V), joining (J), and (sometimes) diversity (D) subcomponents during lymphocyte ontogeny, followed, in the case of B cells, by somatic mutation of the so-called hypervariable regions of the antigen-binding domains (this does not appear to occur in T cells) lymphocytes are able to generate highly specific responses to antigens that have never have been encountered before (see immunobiology section). Amplification and cell differentiation necessary to such immune responses takes place in large part in secondary lymphoid tissue, particularly in lymph nodes, spleen, bone marrow and MALT.

Communication between the various cells participating in the immune response takes place either through direct contact between cell-associated ligands and their cognate receptors on other cells, or via chemical messengers or interleukins secreted by lymphocytes, macrophages and dendritic cells – cytokines and chemokines. Cytokines influence the functional properties of cells bearing cognate cytokine receptors by activating intracellular pathways, and thereby governing the migration, differentiation and proliferation of lymphocytes (see Chapters 9 and 15). Chemokines are a subset of cytokines primarily involved with regulating the trafficking of lymphoid (and other) cells, by attracting them to and trapping them in specific locations – again, through binding to specific cell-associated receptors.

Lymphocyte ontogeny and immune responses

Lymphocytes arise from multipotential hemopoietic stem cells, and most immediately from common lymphoid precursors (i.e. capable of giving rise to all types of lymphocytes) that are present after birth in the bone marrow and undergo primary differentiation (ontogeny) into mature B and T cells (in the bone marrow and thymus, respectively) capable of responding to antigen via their antigen receptors. Of critical importance is the minimization of reactions against antigens present in normal tissues, a process which results in the negative selection (i.e. elimination) of large numbers of differentiating lymphocytes that could otherwise cause severe damage to normal cells and tissues (see Chapters 10 and 11). Although both B and T cells can be induced to proliferate in response to nonspecific signals (e.g. delivered by plant mitogens and some microorganisms), the process of generating a highly specific immune response requires effective antigen presentation – particularly, but not exclusively, by dendritic reticulum cells. Specific B cell responses may be T cell *independent*, e.g. through cross-linking of antigen receptors by bacterial polysaccharide antigens, or T cell *dependent*, when signals from T cells are also required for proliferation. Whereas B cells are capable of responding to intact (unprocessed) antigen, T cells respond to processed antigen, i.e. a small antigenic peptide (epitope) derived from a larger protein which is presented by the antigen-presenting cell in the context of MHC proteins.

In the case of B cells, the process of developing a specific immune response involves several elements. Naïve B cells initially encounter antigen in primary follicles of lymphoid tissue, usually presented by the rich complex of follicular dendritic cells in such follicles. Cells able to bind antigen to a sufficient degree proliferate, forming, in the process, a germinal center and converting the primary to a secondary lymphoid follicle. The formation of a germinal center requires the expression of a number of genes, a critical member of which is BCL6. The B cell antigen receptor is modified in the germinal center by a process known as affinity maturation, in which the 'fit' between antigen receptor and antigen is refined through mutation of the hypervariable (antigen binding) region of the antigen receptor and positive selection of cells able to bind more tightly to the antigen.

Lymphocytes that compete ineffectively for antigen do not receive the necessary survival signals and undergo programmed cell death, or apoptosis (see Chapters 12 and 17). Cells that compete effectively receive appropriate stimulation by both antigen and T cells able to interact with the same antigen. Such cells may undergo class switching – i.e. associating the antigen binding site to a different 'constant' region, which governs many aspects of antibodies' role in immune responses (for example, blood stream versus mucosal surface protection) and differentiate on the one hand into plasma cells – specialized antibody-producing cell (see Chapter 14) – and on the other into long-lived resting memory B cells which, by virtue of their high affinity receptor, retain memory of the antigen such that a rapid yet highly specific reaction can occur at the time of a future encounter.

The majority of T cells have antigen receptors consisting of $\alpha\beta$ chains and are primarily concerned with the regulation of immune responses (CD4+ cells) or the destruction of cells containing foreign antigens, fragments of which are expressed on their surface in the context of MHC proteins (CD8+ cells) (see Chapter 9). CD4 cells comprise the bulk of T cells, and, correspondingly, T cell neoplasms more often derive from CD4+ cells than from CD8+ cells. A much smaller class of T cells (5 percent of all T cells), those whose antigen receptors consist of $\gamma\delta$ chains have a more limited ability to recognize antigens than $\alpha\beta$ T cells, are not MHC restricted in their reactivity, generally do not express either CD4 or CD8 and are primarily found in the spleen and epithelial sites, where lymphomas expressing $\gamma\delta$ antigen receptors also generally occur. NK cells do not express antigen receptor molecules themselves, but do express other proteins that comprise a part of the entire antigen receptor complex, e.g. CD3.

This elementary understanding of the immune system provides the foundation for understanding lymphoid neoplasia, for lymphoid neoplasms can, for the most part, be clearly identified as the neoplastic counterparts of cells at various stages of differentiation (see below). In the B cell lineage, for example, there are precursor B cell neoplasms (generally presenting as ALL/lymphoblastic lymphoma), mature but naïve B cell neoplasms (mantle cell lymphoma), a number of neoplasms that relate to the germinal center (follicular lymphoma, diffuse large B cell lymphoma, Burkitt lymphoma and Hodgkin disease), and tumors that are considered to be post-germinal center neoplasms, such as chronic lymphocytic leukemia/small lymphocytic lymphoma, and neoplasms with variable degrees of plasmacytic differentiation. T cell tumors are less easy to classify beyond precursor T cell neoplasms (ALL/lymphoblastic lymphoma) and mature T cell neoplasms. The latter fall into various groups, largely related to the tissue of origin (skin, nasal sinuses, intestine, etc).

Lymphoid neoplasms resemble their normal cell counterparts

The use of reagents developed in the context of understanding the immune system soon led to the recognition that lymphoid neoplasms could be frequently seen to closely resemble specific normal cell types within each of the major lineages and at various stages of differentiation. While the normal counterpart cells of some lymphoid neoplasms have still to be identified, the principle that lymphoid neoplasms arise from defects in the regulation of the proliferation, differentiation and viability of normal lymphoid cells is well established. This principle also leads to a general understanding of the clinical behavior of lymphoid neoplasms, including their patterns of organ involvement and proliferative rates; for in order to accomplish the critically important task of maintaining surveillance of the blood stream and tissues for foreign antigens, lymphoid cells must circulate throughout the body, in blood, lymph and most tissues, and be able to home to appropriate locations in lymphoid structures where the microenvironment supports the development or reactivation of specific immune responses.

The diverse needs of an effective surveillance system are met by different lymphocyte populations with phenotypes and surface receptors relevant to their roles. MALT lymphocytes, for example, must be able to home to and accumulate in lymphoid structures in mucosal surfaces (such as the Peyer's patches), and to interact with specialized cells that comprise the epithelial barriers separating the internal milieu from the external world. These requirements dictate the need for lymphocytes to be able to traverse the basement membranes of appropriate blood and lymphatic vessels at sites they are able to recognize through receptors that bind to cognate ligands on specialized endothelial cells, e.g. the endothelial cells associated with high endothelial venules of secondary lymphoid organs, except spleen (see Chapter 16). In addition to homing to existing lymphoid structures, lymphocytes, in conjunction with dendritic cells and macrophages, also form functional lymphoid structures ('tertiary' lymphoid aggregates) in tissues that normally lack organized lymphoid tissue (see Chapters 12 and 13). Finally, lymphoid cells must also accumulate at sites of inflammation, especially chronic inflammation, interacting with, attracting and activating other cells essential to the immune response via the secretion of cytokines and chemokines (see Chapter 15). The need for normal lymphocytes to undertake broad surveillance of the tissues of the body accounts for the fact that even indolent lymphomas may be widespread when first detected, while differences in migration and homing patterns of different lymphocyte populations are relevant to the differences in the clinical sites of disease in different lymphoid neoplasms – at least, to the extent that lymphoid neoplasms retain the behavioral characteristics of their normal cell counterparts. These may be modified, sometimes drastically, by molecular genetic lesions, particularly those associated with neoplastic progression.

Abrogation of normal apoptotic pathways

Apoptosis is inherent to the processes of lymphocyte ontogeny, and the regulation of the immune response. Unwanted (e.g. self-reactive) or genetically damaged cells, cells infected by microorganisms, cells that fail to generate a functional antigen receptor and cells that have served their purpose in the context of an immune response, must all be destroyed. The various differentiation 'checkpoints' which ensure that only functionally competent lymphocytes survive, as well as the regulation of proliferation in the course of an immune response, create significant barriers to lymphomagenesis. Thus, the induction of neoplasia entails the inhibition of apoptosis – whether at a specific differentiation checkpoint, or in the context of immune regulations. In general, only some of the pathways leading to apoptosis are inactivated during lymphogenesis; in fact neoplastic cells are often finely balanced between cell death and cell survival and alteration of the balance in favor of apoptosis is one of the mechanisms whereby chemotherapy and radiation are able to destroy neoplastic lymphoid cells.

The immune system itself must also be subject to immunosurveillance for infections – many viruses are lymphotropic, and infected cells must be prevented from undergoing inappropriate proliferation, or destroyed. Interestingly, defects in the immune system, whether genetic or acquired, more commonly result in lymphoid neoplasia than in solid tumors (Kaposi sarcoma and conjunctival carcinoma in acquired immune deficiency syndrome [AIDS] are exceptions). In part, this is a consequence of the failure of mechanisms that normally limit the numbers of virus-infected cells.

CLONAL NATURE OF LYMPHOID NEOPLASIA

The vast majority of lymphoid neoplasms (those arising in the context of immunodeficiency may be an exception) are clonal, i.e. derive from a single cell. This is because molecular genetic lesions are the ultimate cause of lymphoid neoplasia (see Chapter 25) and the occurrence of an appropriate combination of genetic lesions in the same cell is extremely unlikely to occur. However, some genetic lesions, such as those associated with the integrity of the genome, may increase the likelihood that other genetic lesions will arise, increasing both the risk and the rate of development of neoplasia in the cell that first developed a genetic lesion. Infection of many cells by a virus that can contribute to neoplasia also increases the likelihood of the conjunction of the required set of molecular abnormalities (viral proteins can provide the equivalent of genetic lesions) in a single cell.

Malignant clones are not always frozen at a particular stage of differentiation, although for almost all lymphoid neoplasms, differentiation beyond a specific point is prevented, at least for the bulk of the population of neoplastic cells. In the case of myeloma there is evidence that the molecular genetic abnormalities are also present in less differentiated cells (see Chapter 14). Some neoplasms are generally manifested at more than one stage of differentiation, such as follicular lymphomas, which contain varying numbers of centrocytes and centroblasts. Malignant, or premalignant clones, may also evolve as cells differentiate, perhaps because some lymphogenetic molecular lesions are more likely to occur at particular stages of differentiation. Translocations involving antigen receptor genes, for example, would seem more likely to occur in immature cells, in which antigen-receptor gene rearrangements occur, but if differentiation is not inhibited, the partly transformed clone could develop additional lymphogenetic lesions at a later stage of differentiation. This seems to occur in follicular lymphoma (see Chapter 23) in which the characteristic 14;18 translocations, which involve the heavy chain immunoglobulin locus, bear the hallmarks of errors in the normal process of immunoglobulin gene rearrangement, even though the lymphoid cells are clearly the neoplastic counterparts of germinal center cells (see Chapters 11 and 24). One possible explanation is that translocated cells may acquire the additional genetic lesions required for neoplastic transformation in the germinal follicle. Failure to develop additional lesions may result in persistence of partially transformed clones (the equivalent, perhaps of carcinoma *in situ*). This notion is supported by the ease of finding 14;18 translocations in normal individuals in lymphocytes which otherwise appear normal – although their lifespan may be greatly prolonged.

The *transformation* of indolent to aggressive lymphomas probably result. from further abrogation of differentiation in a malignant clone, such that the neoplasm is manifested as a more immature neoplasm. If the more immature elements of a malignant clone are sufficiently immature, they may retain pluripotential properties such that additional molecular lesions could result in a lineage switch – the blastic forms of chronic myeloid leukemia, for example, include both acute myeloid leukemia and acute lymphoblastic leukemia (ALL).

Even if the cell of origin (i.e. the cell in which the neoplasia-inducing molecular genetic lesions occur) is relatively mature, it remains possible that the potential of the neoplastic cells to give rise to progeny cells varies – as is believed to be the case in other neoplasms. In some tumors it has been demonstrated that only a fraction of the neoplastic cells have the capacity to grow in immunodeficient mice, suggesting that, whether or not related to the normal

process of lymphocyte differentiation, the cells which continuously replenish lymphoid neoplasms *in vivo*, i.e. the tumor stem cells, are present in a minority. How these differ from the remainder of the neoplastic cells remains unknown, although their self-renewal potential appears to be handed on to only a small fraction of their progeny cells and in some cases they may be morphologically distinguishable. It is debatable as to whether the small fraction of prolymphocytes in chronic lymphocytic leukemia, which appear to be the replicating cells (see Chapter 27), should be considered as tumor stem cells.

EPIDEMIOLOGY OF LYMPHOID NEOPLASIA – THE MACROENVIRONMENT

Lymphoid neoplasms, like all neoplasms, arise as a consequence of interactions between the environment (in its broadest sense) and genetic factors (see Part 2). Since lymphoid leukemias and lymphomas are neoplasms of the system responsible for protecting the individual against potentially fatal invasion by pathogenic microorganisms, the cells of the immune system are exposed to a broad range of environmental agents. Bacteria, viruses, drugs and environmental chemicals have all been associated with the development of lymphoid neoplasia (see Part 2). In this respect, a parallel might be drawn with epithelial surfaces, which provide a barrier of a different kind, although close cooperation between epithelial cells and the immune system is very much in evidence (see Chapter 13) and some microorganisms have been implicated in both lymphoid and epithelial tumors (e.g. *Helicobacter pylori* and EBV). Incidence rates of individual diseases, and therefore groups of diseases (such as non-Hodgkin lymphoma) vary with country and populations (see Chapter 2 and Fig. 1.1), and although, overall, incidence rates increase with age, peak age-specific incidence rates also vary with individual diseases – and even with the 'same' disease in different countries (Figs 1.2 and 1.3). In Europe and the USA, the incidence rates of non-Hodgkin lymphoma peak between ages 55 and 80 years.

For present purposes, four main pathogenetic pathways through which environmental agents act can be considered, each of which operates via its ability to induce hyperplasia of specific cell populations, increasing, thereby, the risk of the development of a pathogenetically relevant molecular genetic abnormality – an absolute requirement for neoplasia.

- Chronic stimulation of the antigen receptor (a major driver of proliferation), frequently in conjunction with other lymphocyte growth-promoting receptors (e.g. CD40, via CD40 ligand on T cells).
- Alterations in the balance or regulation of lymphocyte subtypes through prior infection, which may move the immune system towards either a Th1 or Th2 response (see Chapter 15), or result in the impairment of the actions of regulatory cells (e.g. in acquired immunodeficiencies – see Chapter 25).

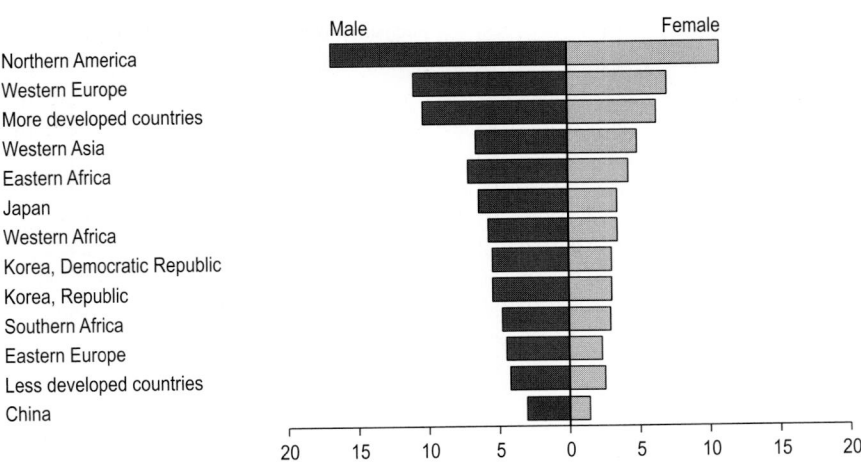

Figure 1.1 Incidence rates (age-standardized to a world population) per 100 000, all ages, of non-Hodgkin lymphoma in selected regions and countries. (Source: GLOBOCAN 2002.)

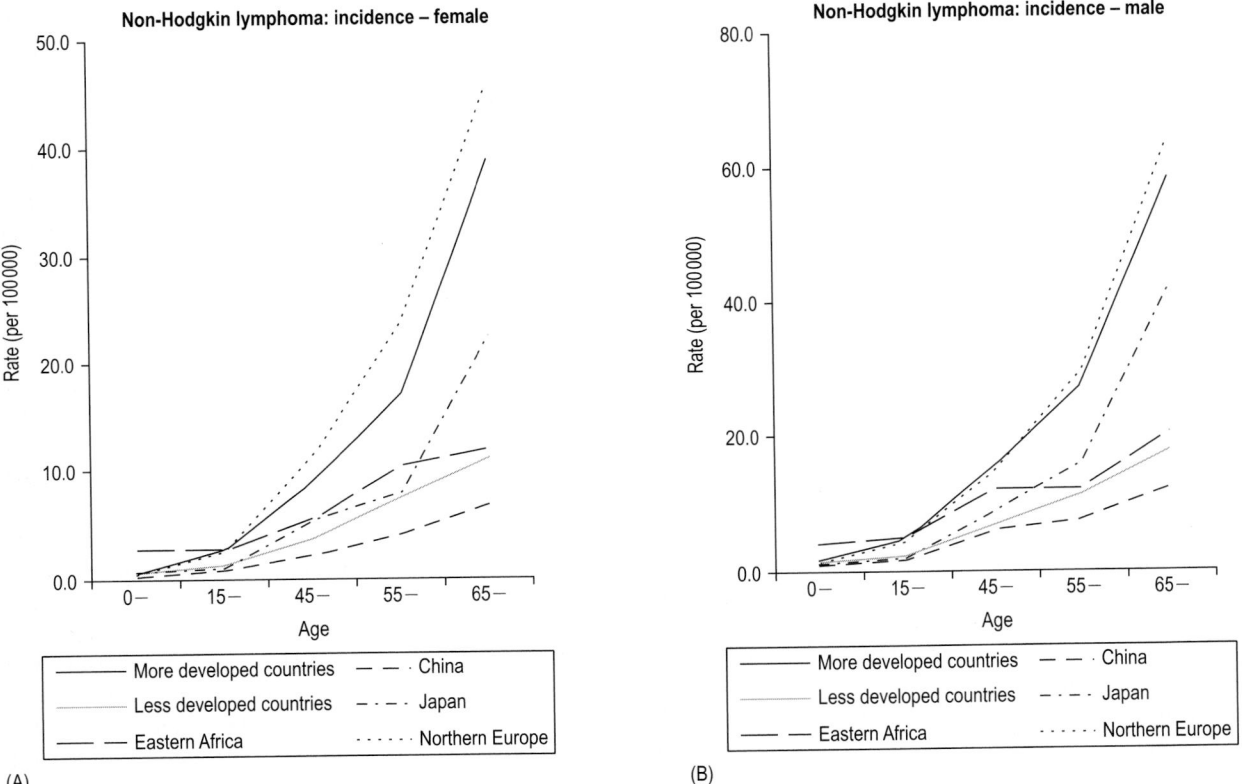

(A)

(B)

Figure 1.2 (A) Age-specific incidence rates of non-Hodgkin lymphoma in females for more and less developed countries and in selected regions. (B) Age-specific incidence rates of non-Hodgkin lymphoma in males for more and less developed countries and in selected regions. (Source: GLOBOCAN 2002.)

- Direct damage to cell DNA through, for example, the generation of free radicals through exposure to various chemicals, or prolonged exposure to ultraviolet light (in skin) and potentially other forms of ionizing radiation. Such damage, if not rapidly repaired, or sufficient to induce apoptosis may create, or increase the risk of development of molecular genetic lesions directly relevant to lymphogenesis.

- Direct action on a relevant molecular pathway of one or more foreign genes (derived from a virus present in the lymphoid cell).

Included in all four items, and unique to lymphoid cells, is the occurrence of pathogenetically relevant molecular genetic abnormalities resulting from errors in recombinational events relating to antigen receptor generation, from

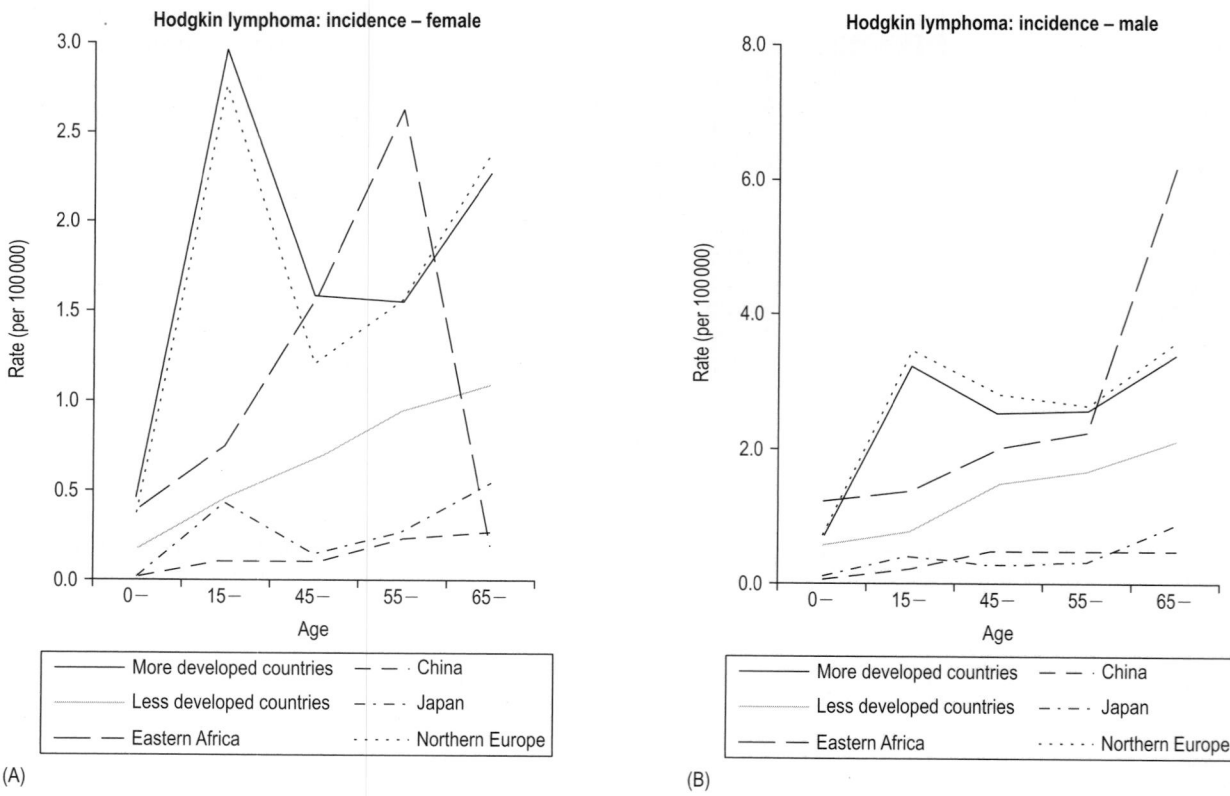

Figure 1.3 (A) Age-specific incidence rates of Hodgkin lymphoma in females for more and less developed countries and in selected regions. (B) Age-specific incidence rates of Hodgkin lymphoma in males for more and less developed countries and in selected regions. (Source: GLOBOCAN 2002.)

immunoglobulin class switching or from the somatic hypermutational mechanisms. These processes may, themselves, be influenced by the environment, e.g. as a consequence of infection-related lymphoid hyperplasia, but they may also be influenced by genetic factors – and often, both. Chronic inflammation, whether a consequence of chronic infections, e.g. with bacteria such as *Helicobacter pylori* and *Borrelia burgdorferi* associated with gastric MALT lymphomas and primary cutaneous lymphomas, respectively (see Chapter 8), or autoimmune disease, such as Sjögren syndrome and rheumatoid arthritis, may predispose to lymphoid neoplasia in several ways, including the induction of lymphoid hyperplasia as well as exposure to DNA-damaging radicals produced in the inflammatory process. Because of the need for multiple genetic abnormalities, the risk of developing a lymphoid neoplasm, even in the presence of one of the above-listed factors is not high, although in the presence of immunodeficiency, cells that would not normally contain sufficient molecular genetic abnormalities to induce neoplasia may behave as neoplastic cells.

Genetic predisposition to lymphoid neoplasia operates through greatly increasing the likelihood of occurrence of genetic abnormalities – in many cases, via the same mechanisms relevant to environmental agents (hence the possibility of synergy). Underlying inherited immunodeficiency syndromes, for example, cause impaired regulation of subpopulations of lymphoid cells. Some inherited immunodeficiency syndromes also influence the risk of the development of a molecular genetic lesion because they negatively influence DNA repair, as in ataxia-telangiectasia and Bloom syndrome, which are associated with chromosomal breakage syndromes and consequently an increased risk of translocations. In addition, genetic factors may influence apoptotic pathways. The autoimmune lymphoproliferative syndrome (ALPS) and the Li–Fraumeni syndrome, for example, are both associated with defects in apoptotic pathways and both predispose to lymphoid neoplasia. Inherited diseases generally result from mutations in single genes, e.g. the *ATM* gene in ataxia telangiectasia, the *BLM* gene in Bloom syndrome, the *FAS* (CD95) receptor (apoptosis inducing) in autoimmune lymphoproliferative syndrome (ALPS) and *TP53* in the Li–Fraumeni syndrome. Other families with predisposition to lymphoid neoplasms without identification of the genetic defect have been described. Many people, however, may be genetically predisposed to lymphoid neoplasia as a result of multiple single nucleotide polymorphisms that individually may have a small or negligible effect, but together create a significantly increased risk of developing lymphoid neoplasia.

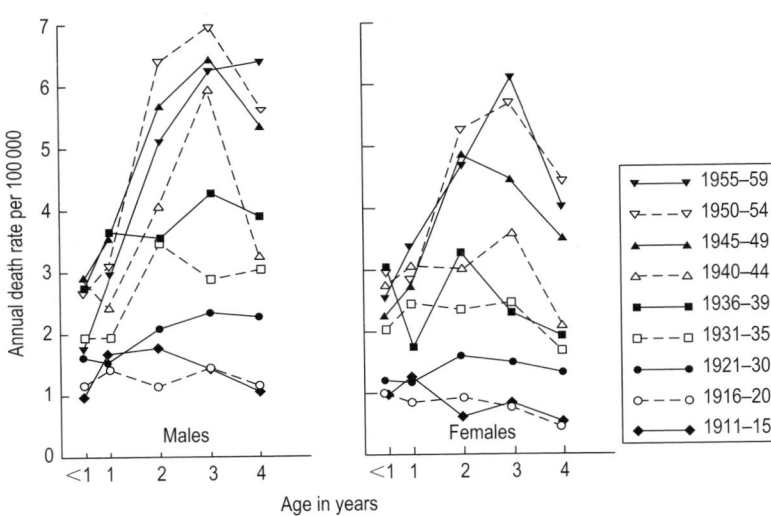

Figure 1.4 Mortality from leukemia in childhood in England and Wales 1911–59 (Registrar General's Statistics). In this era mortality and incidence were essentially synonymous. Although both myeloid and lymphoid leukemia are included, the development of the early age peak characteristic of acute lymphoblastic leukemia is unmistakable. (Reprinted with permission from Court-Brown WM, Doll R. *Br Med J* 1956.)

Such polymorphisms may also influence the outcome of treatment for lymphoid neoplasia.

Geographic and temporal differences

A number of observations are consistent with the probability that environmental factors that predispose to lymphoid neoplasia may do so either at the level of a broad range of neoplasms, e.g. of B cell neoplasms in general, or at the level of individual neoplasms. These possibilities, of course, are not mutually exclusive and may also be a function of age. Although there is a paucity of information, existing evidence suggests that lymphomas in general have a lower incidence in low- and middle-income countries than in high-income countries (Fig. 1.1). There is also evidence that in South-East Asia in particular, the proportion of B cell lymphomas, particularly those of germinal center origin, is lower than in, for example, the USA, where, as in other high-income countries, B cell lymphomas account for 80–85 percent of non-Hodgkin lymphomas. Moreover, the ratio between follicular lymphoma and diffuse large B cell lymphoma appears to be significantly lower in developing countries and in South-East Asia.[2–5] This, coupled to the lower incidence of lymphoma in developing countries suggests that the decreased incidence is mainly due to a paucity of B cell lymphomas, and particularly follicular lymphoma. This is consistent with the lower frequency of follicular lymphomas in several series reported in the USA (see Chapter 2) in the early to mid twentieth century, and also the failure to identify follicular lymphoma until the twentieth century, in spite of its highly characteristic histologic appearance and the increasing use of the microscope – suggesting that its incidence was previously very low. Follicular lymphoma, then, appears to be associated with some (unknown) aspect(s) of lifestyle or environment in high-income countries – with the exception of Japan. The possibility that transformation of follicular lymphoma to diffuse large B cell lymphoma occurs sooner, potentially

while the disease remains subclinical, in low-income countries or Japan, could partly account for these findings, but cannot explain the apparent lower overall incidence of B cell lymphomas in these countries.

Other striking geographic differences in the occurrence of lymphoid neoplasms are well described. One neoplasm of germinal center phenotype, for example, EBV-associated Burkitt lymphoma, has, in contrast to follicular lymphoma, its highest incidence in equatorial Africa, probably because of infection in infancy with both malaria and EBV (see Chapter 33). The age of infection with EBV may also account for the high frequency of EBV-associated Hodgkin disease in children in developing countries (see Chapter 7) but a different explanation must be found to account for the high frequency of NK/T cell nasal lymphoma in adults in Peru and parts of South-East Asia, in which approximately 80 percent are associated with EBV (see Chapter 39). Another virus, human T cell leukemia/lymphoma virus (HTLV1), accounts for the geographic distribution of adult T cell leukemia/lymphoma in parts of Japan and the Caribbean (see Chapter 6).

The existence of geographic or 'horizontal' differences in the incidence of lymphoid neoplasms suggests that temporal or 'vertical' differences may also be observed within the same country or region as the environment or lifestyle changes (as suggested above in the case in follicular lymphoma). Acute lymphoblastic leukemia, which is predominantly of precursor B cell type in high-income settings, is uncommon in equatorial Africa, accounting for only a small proportion of childhood malignancy, whereas in most other world regions ALL has a higher incidence and generally accounts for some 30 percent of childhood cancer.[6] This finding is also consistent with a historical observation; common ALL (the predominant form of precursor B cell ALL in high-income countries), based on its characteristic age peak in 2–5-year-olds, increased in incidence throughout the twentieth century, appearing in different populations, initially, that of England and Wales (Fig. 1.4), as the century progressed. In countries (and in particular

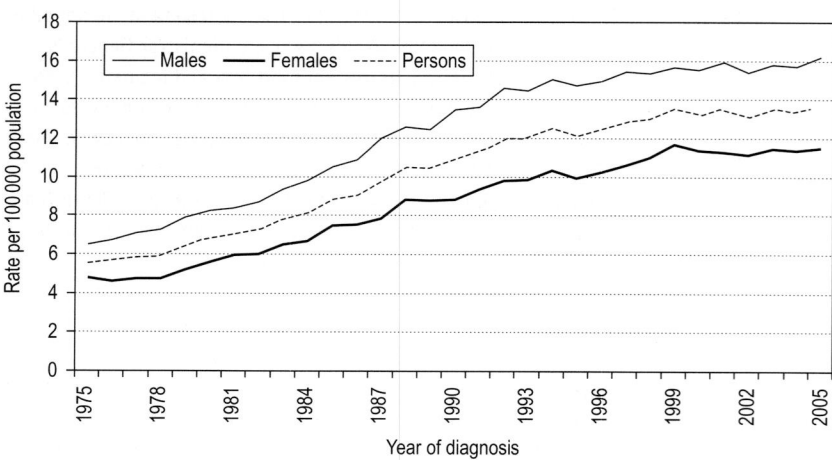

Figure 1.5   Age-standardized (European) incidence rates for non-Hodgkin lymphoma by sex, Great Britain, 1975–2005. Reprinted from Cancer Research UK, http://info. cancerresearchuk.org/cancerstats/types/nhl/ incidence/ with permission. Last accessed May 2009. Based on data from Court Brown WM, Doll R. Leukemia in childhood and young adult life. Trends in mortality in relation to aetiology. *Br Med J* 1961; 26: 982–92.

time periods) where this early age peak is not detectable, a much higher fraction of ALL in children is of T cell type.[7] These findings are consistent with common ALL being a disease of higher socioeconomic status, although the reasons for this remain largely hypothetical.

One additional piece of information consistent with the hypothesis that the incidence of many lymphoid neoplasms, with some notable exceptions, is in some way associated with socioeconomic or technological development is the recent trend towards a higher incidence of non-Hodgkin lymphoma in high-income countries. Between 1973 and 1995 the incidence rate increased by 2 percent per annum in the USA, although the rate of increase has leveled off sharply in recent years (see Chapter 3 and Fig. 1.5).

ANATOMIC LOCATIONS OF LYMPHOID NEOPLASIA – THE MICROENVIRONMENT

Just as lymphoid neoplasia is more or less likely to occur in different macroenvironmental contexts, there is considerable evidence that an appropriate microenvironment is also required. In many circumstances, macro- and microenvironments are closely linked, e.g. in the case of chronic infectious diseases that influence the relative proportions of lymphocyte subpopulations in the immune system, or even create appropriate microenvironments in tissues or organs, such as the tertiary lymphoid structures mentioned above. The patterns of involvement of different tissues or organs in particular lymphoid neoplasms also speaks to the importance of the microenvironment in supporting the growth of lymphoid neoplasms. Examples include the high frequency of involvement of the thymus in lymphoblastic lymphoma of T cell origin and mediastinal B cell lymphoma, and the high degree of tissue specificity of various peripheral (mature) T cell lymphomas – skin, nasal sinuses, spleen and intestine (the latter sometimes, but not always, in the context of a preceding gluten enteropathy). At a microscopic level, some lymphoid neoplasms can often be seen, at least in their earlier stages, to involve particular

microanatomic regions of lymphoid structures. Follicular lymphomas develop in germinal centers, and mantle cell and marginal cell lymphomas can be seen, at least, prior to massive invasion, to selectively involve the corresponding regions of lymphoid tissue. Sometimes extranodal regions may give rise to favored, or possibly, in the context of the malignant clones involved, exclusive, sites of involvement. Jaw tumors in African Burkitt lymphoma, for example, arise in and around the developing molar teeth in young children (even in Africa, jaw tumors are uncommon in teenagers and adults) while, characteristically, involvement of the breasts occurs in pubertal girls or lactating women (see Chapter 13). Involvement of peripheral lymph nodes in Burkitt lymphoma, which typically involves MALT tissues, is uncommon.

Role of normal cells in maintaining lymphoid neoplasms

A different, but related set of observations supporting an important role for the microenvironment in the development and maintenance of lymphoid neoplasia is derived from the presence of normal cells in lymphoid neoplasms. Dendritic reticulum cells, for example, are always present in follicular lymphoma and appear to be essential to the maintenance of the follicular architecture – and, along with other normal cells, the neoplastic state itself (see Chapter 32). The presence of infiltrating normal cells, particularly CD4+ T cells, in Hodgkin disease is likely to be important both for prevention of an immune response directed against the Sternberg–Reed cells, particularly when associated with EBV, as well as for the growth of the neoplasm (see Chapter 35).

It is quite probable that in many lymphoid neoplasms, the tumor cells are maintained as a consequence of interactions, sometimes via cell to cell contact and sometimes through the secretion of cytokines, between the neoplastic cells and the normal cells that comprise the microenvironment. Some lymphomas are infiltrated by particular normal cell populations (e.g. epithelial cells, macrophages, fibroblasts) that are attracted to the location by chemokines secreted by the neoplastic cells, e.g. the lymphohistoepithelial subtype of anaplastic large cell lymphoma, Hodgkin disease and NK/T cell lymphoma. Whether this represents an epiphenomenon, relating to the aberrant secretion of cyto/chemokines by the neoplastic cells, or whether such cells participate in maintaining the growth and viability of the neoplastic cells is, for the most part, unknown. Lymphoid neoplasms also, of course, require a blood supply, and as with other tumors, developing blood vessels and the microenvironment represent potential alternative targets for treatment.

THE SPECTRUM OF LYMPHOID NEOPLASMS AND THEIR CLASSIFICATION

Approaches to the classification of lymphoid neoplasms have evolved at an increasingly rapid rate. The clinical and gross morphologic characteristics of the early nineteenth century were supplemented progressively by microscopy, which, through improved instrumentation, the development of special stains, and more recently through the use of antibodies, now almost exclusively monoclonal antibodies, to interrogate cells for the expression of specific proteins, has allowed a continuous improvement in diagnostic accuracy, as well as the identification of new pathologic entities. Microscopy has also been essential to the development of cytogenetics and the use of molecular probes has permitted a range of additional tests to emerge, including techniques such as fluorescence in situ hybridization and spectral karyotyping that have enhanced the ability to detect structural chromosomal changes. These developments, stimulated by the recognition that lymphoid neoplasms, like all cancers, are caused by molecular genetic abnormalities, have been associated with new assays for the detection of molecular genetic abnormalities, including gross structural changes in specific genes, point mutations, and altered gene expression patterns (increased or decreased in comparison to various control cells). Modern classification is based on a combination of histopathology, immunophenotyping, cytogenetics and molecular characterization. Clinical features, such as the rate of progression and the pattern of organ and tissue involvement, although sometimes characteristic of particular pathological entities, is always subordinate to pathology in determining the diagnosis. Today, the World Health Organization (WHO) classification system of lymphoid neoplasms is the most widely used scheme (see Chapter 20) and is likely to remain so for the foreseeable future, although periodic revisions will continue to be undertaken as new or improved techniques permit resolution of the 'grey' areas of classification and concepts of what constitutes a disease entity evolve. Most lymphoid neoplasms can be related to specific normal cell types, particularly those in the B cell lineage, in which the phenotypes of neoplasms conform quite well to specific differentiation stages (see Chapters 9 and 20).

Precursor and mature cell neoplasms

All lymphoid neoplasms are derived from either NK/T cells, or B or T cell lymphocyte lineages, the relative proportions of each of the three major subtypes varying in different world regions, as described above, although at a global level the majority of lymphoid neoplasms are of B cell origin. The WHO classification subdivides lymphoid neoplasms into immature (lymphoblastic) neoplasms that arise in primary lymphoid tissues (where lymphocytes develop) and mature lymphoid neoplasms that arise in secondary lymphoid tissues (sites involved in the generation of immune responses). Since immature B lymphocytes develop in the bone marrow, the majority of immature B lymphoid neoplasms present as ALL, while immature T lymphocytes which migrate from the bone marrow to the thymus, where they undergo further differentiation, present either as leukemias or as lymphoblastic lymphomas – in either case, frequently with an enlarged thymus. Approximately 85–90 percent of lymphoblastic lymphomas (in high-income countries, at least) have a precursor T cell phenotype and the remainder a precursor B cell phenotype – almost the mirror image of the distribution in neoplasms that present as ALL. Lymphoblastic lymphomas can be readily distinguished from all other types of lymphoma by their expression of the enzyme terminal deoxyribonucleotide transferase (TdT), which has a role in the construction of a functional antigen receptor.

Mature B cell neoplasms

The subdivision of 'mature' B cell lymphomas into different categories is largely based on the relationship of the lymphoma to normal cells present in lymphoid follicles. The neoplastic counterparts of pregerminal center cells (e.g. mantle cell lymphoma) lack somatic hypervariable mutations in their immunoglobulin heavy chains while such mutations are readily detected in the neoplastic counterparts of germinal center cells (e.g. follicular lymphoma, Burkitt lymphoma and diffuse large B cell lymphoma) and postgerminal center lymphoid malignancies (immunoblastic lymphoma, chronic lymphocytic leukemia and plasma cell neoplasms). B cell neoplasms tend to have characteristic immunophenotypes and non-random chromosomal translocations, although the same translocation may be found in more than one type of neoplasm and several seemingly different translocations may occur in the same disease (see below).

Mature T cell neoplasms

T cell neoplasms cannot be subdivided in an analogous way, for no equivalent structure to the germinal center exists in the T cell lineage. However, T cell neoplasms are generally recognizable on the basis of immunophenotype as being derived, at least, in the majority of cases, from either CD8+ or CD4+ lineages. Most, therefore express $\alpha\beta$ T cell receptors. Examples of predominantly CD4+ neoplasms include mycosis fungoides/Sézary syndrome, primary cutaneous CD30 positive lymphoproliferative disorders, adult T cell leukemia/lymphoma and peripheral T cell lymphoma, unspecified. Examples of predominantly CD8+ neoplasms include subcutaneous panniculitis-like T cell lymphoma and enteropathy-type T cell lymphoma (especially the small- to medium-cell subtype). T cell prolymphocytic leukemia is 60 percent CD4+, 15 percent CD8+ and 25 percent CD4+, CD8+. Hepatosplenic T cell lymphoma, which is negative for both CD4 and CD8, is nearly always derived from $\gamma\delta$ T cells. Extranodal NK/T cell lymphoma of nasal type is also generally negative for CD4 and CD8, as well as surface CD3, although cytotoxic-granule-associated proteins are usually easily detectable.

Mature T cell lymphomas and NK cell neoplasms are also less readily divided into more and less indolent lymphomas than B cell neoplasms. Their classification, with the exception of the T cell leukemias, is, to a large extent, based on the sites or tissues of involvement and the tissue trophism they exhibit presumably derives from the role of their normal counterpart cells in tissue immunosurveillance – particular subsets being associated with particular tissues. A frequently used approach to classification is to divide mature T cell lymphoid neoplasms into leukemias, extranodal lymphomas and nodal lymphomas. The T cell leukemias include prolymphocytic leukemia, large granulocytic leukemia, aggressive NK cell leukemia and adult T cell lymphoma leukemia. Extranodal lymphomas include NK/T cell nasal lymphoma, enteropathy-type T cell lymphoma and hepatosplenic T cell lymphoma, cutaneous T cell lymphomas, including mycosis fungoides/Sézary syndrome and cutaneous anaplastic large cell lymphoma (which lack the *ALK* deregulating translocations present in a high proportion of other types of anaplastic large cell lymphomas). Nodal lymphomas include angioimmunoblastic T cell lymphoma and anaplastic large cell lymphoma. Although many genetic abnormalities have been described in T cell neoplasms, with some exceptions, such as anaplastic large cell lymphoma and the immature T cell neoplasms, rather few characteristic chromosomal translocations have been described.

MOLECULAR PATHOGENESIS OF LYMPHOID NEOPLASMS

All lymphoid neoplasms result from the presence of genetic abnormalities, including gross changes (e.g. chromosomal deletions, amplifications or translocations) or point mutations that disrupt the normal regulatory mechanisms that control cell growth, differentiation and viability. Chromosomal translocations, for the most part specific for particular diseases, are particularly characteristic of lymphoid neoplasia. The complex molecular pathways involved in lymphoid neoplasia include a large number of genes, many of which are common to fundamental pathways present in a broad range of cells (e.g. genes involved in the cell cycle and its regulation, or in the induction or inhibition of apoptosis) while other frequently involved genes reside on pathways that link important lymphocyte receptors (whether in the context of lymphocyte ontogeny or an immune response) to the pathways that control cell proliferation, differentiation and viability. Some molecular lesions – especially those that affect genes relevant to fundamental pathways – may occur in several lymphoid neoplasms (e.g. abnormalities in the inhibitors of cell cycle progression from G1 to S, such as p16 [INK4a] and p27 [KIP1]), while others, which relate more specifically to lymphoid cell biology, are characteristic of particular lymphoid neoplasms. Genetic specificity is likely to arise in part because expressed genes are much more vulnerable to damage, and in part because the pathways that must be modified in order to induce neoplasia differ in different subsets of lymphocytes. Genes involved in ontogeny, for example, are frequently deregulated, or their function modified by mutation or translocation in immature lymphoid neoplasms, while abnormal expression of BCL6 is frequent in tumors arising in germinal center cells (BCL6 is critically important to the process of affinity maturation of B cells in normal germinal centers, in which it prevents apoptosis and cell cycle arrest in cells undergoing somatic hypervariable region mutation by inhibiting TP53 and p21).

Although, for the most part, specific translocations are characteristic of a particular disease, on occasion, identical or very similar translocations may be found in different lymphoma subtypes. This is easily understood if each genetic lesion is considered in terms of the functional abnormality it confers – it would be surprising if there were not overlap in the functional requirements for lymphomagenesis among different, although generally, quite closely related neoplasms (e.g. t[8;14] in Burkitt lymphoma and diffuse large B cell lymphoma and 14;18 in follicular lymphoma and diffuse large B cell lymphoma). Sometimes, the constitutive expression of a gene is aberrant, as is the case for ALK-kinase, a gene that can be deregulated by several different translocations in anaplastic large cell lymphoma, and which is not expressed in normal lymphoid cells. This may be the consequence of a selective process, whereby a particular gene is especially suited to lymphomagenesis in a particular cellular milieu. Finally, different tumors of the same type may bear genetic lesions that involve closely related genes, or which may be present in the same molecular pathway, such that they give rise to closely similar functional end results (as occurs in MALT lymphomas, mantle cell lymphomas and anaplastic large cell lymphomas – see relevant chapters in Part 5).

Major types of translocation

In lymphoid neoplasms, chromosomal translocations fall into two main classes. In the first type, juxtaposition of antigen receptor gene sequences to another gene causes its overexpression through the influence of antigen receptor gene regulatory elements. A classical example of this is constitutive expression of MYC (a transcription factor that influences many aspects of cell physiology, including proliferation, differentiation, apoptosis and metabolism) resulting from the juxtaposition of *MYC* to heavy or light chain immunoglobulin genes (via t[8;14], t[8;22] or t[2;8] translocations) in Burkitt lymphoma. Similarly, BCL2 (an antiapoptotic protein) is constitutively expressed when *BCL2* is juxtaposed to immunoglobulin heavy chain sequences in follicular lymphoma.

The second major type of translocation results in the production of a fusion gene, i.e. a part of one gene is fused to a part of a second. When the component of the first gene includes its promoter sequence, which must be efficiently expressed in the normal counterpart of the neoplastic cell, it will induce abnormal expression of the gene to which it is fused. This occurs in diffuse large B cell lymphoma in which many different gene promoters can be fused to *BCL6*, resulting in its overexpression. In other circumstances, the fusion protein may have enhanced functional activity (e.g. BCR-ABL in some ALLs), or qualitatively different functional activity not shared by either of the component genes.

Occurrence of pathogenetic lesions in normal individuals

Considerable evidence exists that some of the apparently central molecular lesions of lymphoid neoplasms, such as t(14;18), which leads to the overexpression of *BCL2*, and the *TEL-AML1* fusion gene, which is associated with approximately 25 percent of precursor B cell ALLs, are present in normal individuals and at a much higher incidence than would be consistent with the incidence of the diseases associated with these translocations. This is consistent with the requirement for multiple genetic lesions for full neoplastic transformation and suggests that many people who never develop lymphoid neoplasia have some cells that contain potentially lymphomagenic lesions – not dissimilar from carcinoma *in situ* or other forms of premalignant epithelial lesions. Some of the translocations associated with childhood leukemias have been shown to be present *in utero*, strongly suggesting that maternal exposure to leukemogenic agents must have occurred. Such findings could represent the first steps toward prevention.

Genetic lesions in immature lymphoid neoplasms

In immature lymphoid neoplasms, genetic lesions that result in the disruption of the process of ontogeny are of particular importance, but can be illustrated here by only one or two examples. In precursor T cell ALL, approximately 50 percent of cases have mutations in the *NOTCH1*

gene (see Chapter 27), a member of a family of transmembrane receptors that is highly conserved, being first identified in *Drosophila*. In lymphoid cells, *NOTCH1* regulates the commitment and early development of T lymphocytes when its cytoplasmic portion is cleaved after ligand binding (a process that requires contact with ligand-bearing cells), and translocated to the nucleus, where it initiates a cascade of signaling events that modify the pattern of gene expression, including upregulation of the pre-T cell receptor protein that is required for $\alpha\beta$ T cell development (see Chapter 10).

Commitment to B cell differentiation requires the expression of two transcription factors, E12 and E14, derived by differential splicing from the *E2A* gene. They regulate the expression of multiple components of the B cell antigen receptor, including the heavy and light chain immunoglobulins themselves (see Chapter 11). In precursor B cell ALL, two translocations, t(1;19) and t(17;19) involving the *E2A* gene have been identified (see Chapter 27). In the 1;19 translocation, the fusion protein, E2A-PBX induces expression of another gene, *WNT16*, which is essential for cell viability and growth of the leukemic cells – its inhibition results in apoptosis.

Genetic lesions in mature lymphoid neoplasms

In mature lymphoid neoplasms, most molecular genetic abnormalities identified are in molecular pathways relevant to growth or apoptosis in a variety of cell types. In lymphoid cells, antigen receptor genes represent an important growth factor receptor and can induce proliferation when activated by their highly specific growth factors (antigens) and any required cellular cofactors. Hyperplasia of one or a number of clones can be caused by chronic antigenic stimulation, but there are relatively few examples where this mechanism is unequivocally fundamental to lymphomagenesis. Lymphomas associated with infections, such as MALT lymphomas are obvious candidates, particularly since eradication of the infection, e.g. *Helicobacter pylori* in the case of gastric MALT lymphomas, can be curative (see Chapter 67). However, it appears that the specificity for bacterial antigens is via T cells, which appear to provide the necessary cofactors for B cell replication. Such B cells bear molecular genetic lesions in the B cell antigen receptor pathway, obviating the need for B cell antigen receptor stimulation.

Although the identification of specific antigens of pathogenetic significance in lymphoid neoplasms not known to be associated with infections has been difficult, chronic antigenic stimulation of B cell receptors has been suggested in some neoplasms by the presence, in the antigen receptors of different tumors, of the same variable region segments as well, in some cases, as the same pattern of somatic hypervariable region mutation. These findings suggest that the antigen receptors bind the same antigen.

This has been demonstrated in both MALT lymphomas involving various tissues as well as chronic lymphocytic leukemia (see Chapters 25 and 27). Similarity of variable regions has not been described in other B cell neoplasms, but the possibility that different antigens may be involved in chronic antigenic stimulation, even in the same pathological entity, cannot be excluded. In some cases, the relevant antigens may be autoantigens – whether in the context of overt autoimmune disease or subclinical self-reactivity. Chronicity of antigenic stimulation would certainly be guaranteed in such cases. Chronic antigenic stimulation may help to induce neoplasia by increasing the risk of downstream genetic lesions in the antigen receptor pathway, e.g. in proteins that regulate nuclear factor (NF)-κB, a central transcription factor activated by antigenic stimulation in both B and T cells. As mentioned, MALT lymphomas provide a good example of this (see Chapters 25 and 33).

As a broad generalization, mature lymphoid neoplasms can be divided into those in which abnormal proliferation is the primary lesion, Burkitt lymphoma being, perhaps, the quintessential neoplasm in this regard, and those in which inhibition of apoptosis permits abnormal accumulation of a particular cell type(s), as, for example, occurs in chronic lymphocytic leukemia and follicular lymphoma. Highly proliferative tumors are clinically aggressive and consist of medium to large cells; in contrast, tumors in which there is over accumulation of a specific cell type (or closely related types) are frequently indolent and generally consist of small to medium cells. More indolent lymphomas can transform, through the acquisition of additional molecular genetic lesions, into neoplasms that proliferate rapidly. Even when proliferation appears to be the primary pathogenetic derangement, however, genes that would cause inappropriately proliferating cells (i.e. cells driven by virtue of a molecular lesion) to undergo apoptosis must be inhibited and differentiation must also be prevented for neoplasia to arise. Similarly, in indolent tumors, some degree of proliferation, in some cases at an earlier stage of differentiation in the neoplastic clone, is necessary to maintain tumor cell numbers.

Individual genes cannot always be designated as being exclusively involved in either proliferation or apoptosis. In fact, given the importance of achieving harmony among these pathways they must be linked, sometimes via the same gene, whose function may depend on the cellular context – i.e. the presence or absence of other proteins capable of specifically binding to it, with functional consequences. MYC, for example, can induce cell proliferation or apoptosis in different contexts, such that in proliferating cells driven by MYC, such as Burkitt lymphoma, its apoptosis-inducing effect must be inhibited. In some cases, mutually incompatible functions may be differentially influenced by the same gene. The tyrosine kinase gene, ALK, for example, which is ectopically expressed in anaplastic large cell lymphomas by several translocations, is, like other tyrosine kinases, involved in signaling pathways (see Chapter 40).

ALK activates phosphatidylinositol 3-kinase (PI3K), which in turn, via its downstream targets, activates an antiapoptotic pathway. ALK probably also activates cell proliferation, at least in part, through downregulation of p27KIP, an inhibitor of cell cycle progression at the G1/S interface.

Different genetic lesions may lead to similar pathobiologic consequences

There are many examples of different molecular lesions being present in the same category of lymphoid neoplasm. Frequently, these can be shown to lead to a similar or identical functional end result, such as the several translocations that result in different fusion genes involving ALK. Several different translocations can result in the activation of NF-κB in MALT lymphomas, or in the overexpression of BCL6 in diffuse large B cell lymphomas. In mantle cell lymphomas, different translocations result in the overexpression of either cyclin-D1, cyclin-D2 or cyclin-D3. Mutations in different regulatory genes of critical cellular pathways (e.g. cell cycle inhibitors or antiapoptotic genes) may also give rise to similar or identical functional end results. Together, these observations strongly suggest that particular lymphoid neoplasms result from the same set of functional abnormalities, although such functional abnormalities may be caused by different genetic abnormalities – frequently in the same molecular pathways. In addition, not only structural genetic lesions, but also epigenetic changes, or altered expression of regulatory microRNAs may be involved in the creation of the pathophysiologic changes required to induce lymphoid neoplasia.

Genesis of molecular lesions

The fundamental need to generate diversity of antigen receptors, in order for them to react efficiently with a wide range of antigens, is also relevant to the genesis of chromosomal abnormalities. This makes sense from the mechanistic perspective, since antigen receptors must be created by genetic recombination, such that their surrounding chromatin is open to the actions of recombinases and ligases. The importance of antigen receptor loci to chromosomal translocations in lymphoid neoplasia is supported by the high fraction of chromosomal translocations that involve antigen receptor genes in both B and T cells. In some cases, e.g. precursor B and T cell neoplasms and mantle cell lymphomas (see Chapter 24), the translocations appear to be mediated by the recombinases (RAG1 and RAG2) that mediate antigen receptor gene recombination, since the signal sequences that these enzymes recognize in cutting the DNA strands can be found in close proximity to the chromosomal breakpoint on the antigen receptor gene side of the translocation – and often cryptic RAG1/2 recognition sequences on the other. In follicular lymphoma at least some of the enzymes involved in normal VDJ recombination, possibly including RAG1/2 in some cases, are thought to be involved in mediating the translocation, consistent with the probability that the malignant clone extends back to the precursor cell level. In B cell neoplasms, the somatic hypervariable region mutational mechanism has also been implicated in the genesis of chromosomal translocation, e.g. in multiple myeloma. Other translocations appear to be mediated by the enzymatic machinery that mediates another recombinational event, namely, immunoglobulin class switching. Both class switching and somatic hypervariable region mutation take place in germinal centers and involve an enzyme known as activation induced deaminase (AID). This enzyme has been implicated in the genesis of many of the molecular abnormalities in B cell neoplasms whose normal counterpart cells are germinal center or postgerminal center cells (identifiable by the presence of somatic hypervariable mutations in their immunoglobulin genes). In general, translocations in more immature neoplasms tend to be mediated by enzymes involved in V(D)J joining, while translocations in more mature B cell neoplasms are more likely to be mediated by AID. Many DNA repair enzymes, some of which participate in the recombination processes described above, are likely to be also involved in the translocations observed in other tumors in which antigen receptor genes are not involved, e.g. T/NK cell neoplasms, but the evidence for this remains limited.

The somatic hypervariable region mutational mechanism is almost certainly involved in the generation of mutations in genes other than immunoglobulin molecules. In normal B cells, BCL6 and CD95/FAS, for example, are subject to mutation via this mechanism (see Chapter 25). In malignant B cell neoplasms a number of additional genes have been shown to carry mutations which have the molecular hallmarks of the hypervariable region mutational mechanism, including PIM1, MYC and PAX5. Such mutations, by altering interactions among these genes and other proteins to which they bind, make important contributions to lymphomagenesis.

MOLECULAR PROFILING

Ultimately, all of the characteristics of a neoplasm – from morphology to immunophenotype and cytokine expression – are consequences of the gene expression profile. This may be thought of as comprising two elements: first, the pattern of gene expression that derives from the normal counterpart lymphoid cell (the 'normal expression pattern') and second, deviations from this pattern relating to the neoplastic state, whether changes in the level of expression of the genes comprising the normal expression pattern (including absence of expression), the expression of additional genes brought about by the genetic abnormalities that create the neoplastic state and other differences resulting from genetic lesions that do not contribute to the neoplastic state. The recently acquired ability, using microarrays or other techniques, to study total or partial gene expression patterns of cell populations at RNA (including microRNAs and interfering RNAs, both of which are involved in the regulation of gene expression patterns) or protein levels is likely, therefore, to provide additional insights into pathogenesis, classification, neoplastic behavior and response to therapy.

The identification of sets of *signature genes*, i.e. genes that are almost identically expressed in all lymphoid neoplasms of a particular category can be of major help in both defining particular lymphoid neoplasms, and differentiating tumors that are difficult to separate using standard pathologic techniques (see Chapter 24). However, intermediate patterns of gene expression (i.e. that lie between the clearcut signatures of particular entities) may be observed. At some level, of course, every tumor is unique. These molecular 'gray areas' do not necessarily correspond to histopathological gray areas – some morphologically typical diffuse large B cell lymphomas, for example, have a typical Burkitt lymphoma molecular profile,[8] and it may be necessary to begin to overcome the longstanding assumption that the 'gold standard' of diagnosis is the histopathologic appearance (e.g. the separation between immunophenotypically similar tumors such as Burkitt lymphoma and diffuse large B cell lymphoma) – particularly since this includes a significant subjective element. Even immunophenotyping has reproducibility problems – not only do techniques vary, but definitions of positivity often vary from one laboratory to another. Ultimately, the molecular profile, which has the advantage of simultaneously examining many genes, is likely to usurp the present dominant position of histopathology, although agreement may need to be reached on the genes to be used in standardized diagnostic profiles, as well as on test procedures and analysis. It will also be important to decide whether purified tumor cells should be used to determine molecular profiles, or whether simultaneous study of the tumor cells in the context of their microenvironment is important – studying both may be valuable in some circumstances, depending on whether the profile is for purely diagnostic reasons or also to determine prognosis or the optimal treatment approach.

Molecular profiling has already been shown to be able to accurately distinguish benign processes from malignant neoplasms (e.g. inflammatory dermatoses from anaplastic large cell lymphoma), and can identify otherwise difficult to distinguish subgroups within tumor categories, such as germinal center and activated B cell subtypes of diffuse large B cell lymphoma (see Chapter 24). Molecular profiling also shows promise of identifying additional prognostic factors in the context of specific treatment regimens, and is likely to lead to additional information about pathogenetic pathways (see Chapter 85).

CLINICAL FEATURES

Malignant lymphoid neoplasms have a broad spectrum of presentation with considerable clinical overlap, since many quite different lymphoid neoplasms involve lymph nodes, spleen, bone marrow and often liver (see Chapter 41). Immature neoplasms are highly likely to involve the sites of differentiation of immature cells, namely the bone marrow and thymus. However, involvement of the thymus may also occur in mature 'mediastinal' B cell lymphomas, Hodgkin lymphoma, thymoma and many other benign and malignant diseases and both immature T and B cell neoplasms frequently involve peripheral lymph nodes, liver and spleen as well as the bone marrow. In mature lymphoid neoplasms, involvement of peripheral lymph nodes is the most frequent site of disease, but in some diseases lymph node involvement is much less prominent and, in some patients, may not occur at all, e.g., in myeloma, African Burkitt lymphoma, cutaneous T cell lymphomas, NK/T cell nasal lymphomas, enteropathy-associated T cell lymphomas and MALT lymphomas (see relevant chapters). While there is logic in the division of lymphomas into nodal and extranodal diseases, both are often present in the same patient. The clinical patterns of spread are, of course, determined by the molecular profile, which governs surface protein expression patterns, and thereby the tissues in which the malignant lymphoid cells can survive and proliferate.

In the presence of underlying predisposing conditions, lymphomas may be strongly suspected on clinical grounds in the presence of enlarging lymph nodes or suggestive symptomatology (e.g., relating to the gastrointestinal tract in enteropathy-related T cell lymphoma, pneumothorax in pyothorax-associated lymphoma). Rarely, lymphomas may involve only the eye or central nervous system (brain, extradural space or cranial nerves), which may present important diagnostic difficulties, especially in the absence of an underlying predisposing syndrome (such as HIV infection in the case of brain lymphoma). In AIDS patients, the pattern of lymphoma has been changed by the advent of antiretroviral therapy, and since major immunosuppression can be avoided for many years, the risk of lymphomas overall is much less, although the impact on Burkitt lymphoma, which occurs prior to major immunosuppression has been more difficult to document. Lymphomas with marked plasmacytoid differentiation, EBV-associated Hodgkin disease and also MALT lymphomas occur at higher frequency in AIDS patients than in the non-immunosuppressed population. Such patients are also more likely to develop HHV-8-associated primary effusion lymphoma.

Associated conditions not due to mass lesions

Patients sometimes present with symptoms and signs resulting from associated hematologic or metabolic abnormalities, such as hemolytic anemia, thrombocytopenia, infection, hypercalcemia, bone or joint pain, renal failure or hypoglycemia (see Chapter 44). Systemic symptoms, such as fever and weight loss, often labelled as 'B' symptoms, are a consequence of cytokine production by the neoplastic cells, or by normal infiltrating lymphocytes and macrophages. In patients with Hodgkin disease confined to the abdomen, such symptoms may be the presenting features, such that a high index of suspicion is important. A syndrome of high fever, liver failure and hemophagocytosis, usually virus associated, is associated with some T and NK cell neoplasms, particularly in South-East Asia. This syndrome sometimes occurs before and sometimes after the emergence of the neoplasm.

Age

Age is an important determinant of the type of lymphoid neoplasm. In children, ALL is generally (i.e. at a global level) the most frequent childhood malignancy, which, in the absence of significant bone marrow infiltration (arbitrarily set at 25 percent or more) is diagnosed as lymphoblastic lymphoma (which may rapidly progress to involve the bone marrow if untreated). Burkitt lymphoma accounts for perhaps 50 percent of childhood cancer in some equatorial African countries, although it has been displaced from its number one rank in others by the high incidence of AIDS-related Kaposi sarcoma. In the childhood age group, peripheral T cell lymphoma other than anaplastic large cell lymphoma, by far the commonest peripheral T cell lymphoma in children, accounts for only a small proportion of childhood lymphomas, and small cell lymphoma, marginal cell lymphoma, mantle cell lymphoma and follicular lymphoma are extremely rare. Mediastinal large cell lymphoma is more common in young adults, particularly women, whereas hepatosplenic lymphoma of T cells tends to occur in young men. Small lymphocytic lymphomas, follicular lymphomas, diffuse large B cell lymphomas, and many T cell lymphomas occur more often in the last two or three decades of life. Sometimes, the clinical pattern of a disease differs in different age groups – jaw tumors in African Burkitt lymphoma, for example, occur particularly in young children, and breast involvement in pubertal girls – although, interestingly, ovarian involvement can occur at any age. Other factors, discussed earlier, may also influence the site of disease, such as the genesis of an appropriate microenvironment at a specific body location – e.g., by an infectious process, which itself may be influenced by age. Underlying predisposing conditions, whether genetic or acquired, may also influence the age at which lymphoma occurs – in this case usually resulting in a shift towards a younger age.

The rate of progression of the disease may also be influenced by age or preexisting disease. Perhaps the most rapidly progressive is Burkitt lymphoma, where newly palpable masses may occur in the space of days and the rapid initiation of treatment is imperative. At the other extreme, some patients with follicular lymphoma or chronic lymphocytic leukemia may have stable disease, causing no significant symptoms, for many years. Even within individual diseases, the rate of progression may vary markedly from one patient to another.

Diagnosis

The diagnosis of lymphoid neoplasia with very rare exceptions can be made only by an examination of the cells that comprise the neoplasm. This entails biopsy of suspicious lesions within a time frame ranging from immediate (e.g. as part of an emergency situation, where, for example, the lymphoma has induced perforation of a viscus or intussusception, or is causing cord compression) to within a matter of a few weeks with slowly progressive lesions in which alternative diagnoses are possible and can be eliminated by appropriate tests. Histopathologic examination, including special studies, particularly immunophenotyping, remain the primary diagnostic procedure (see Chapters 44–46). The most definitive diagnoses are made when a combination of techniques is used, and, accordingly, cytogenetics, fluorescence in situ hybridization and/or examination of tumor tissue for the presence of specific molecular genetic lesions is increasingly undertaken as part of the routine diagnostic workup. The role of gene expression profiling in diagnostics is likely to increase with time, although small arrays of highly selected genes and alternative techniques such as quantitative polymerase chain reaction or immunophenotyping algorithms using a small number of antibodies selected on the basis of larger molecular profiles are likely to be introduced first, since such analyses are more widely accessible and less expensive. However, the decreasing cost of large microarrays and the introduction of improved analytic tools may lead sooner than expected to the routine use of arrays or other genomic studies not only for diagnostic purposes, but, perhaps, along with the detection of single nucleotide polymorphisms, to aid treatment decisions (see Chapter 85).

In some circumstances, particularly in low-resource settings, a needle aspirate of a node, mass, effusion, or the bone marrow may provide sufficient material for the establishment of a diagnosis, e.g. of African Burkitt lymphoma and ALL. However, whilst permitting good cytology, immunophenotyping and even cytogenetic and molecular studies, needle aspirates do not permit study of the characteristic changes of the normal architecture in lymphoid tissue, which is an important component of histologic diagnosis in many lymphoid neoplasms. In addition, needle aspiration provides relatively small quantities of material, reducing the number of special studies that can be performed and hence the diagnostic precision.

It is probable that telepathology will begin to play an increasing role in obtaining expert opinions, especially as diagnoses are best made by specialized hematopathologists. In smaller institutions or in low-resource settings, where hematopathologists are unavailable, electronic transmission of images, assuming sufficient quality of both the histologic and/or cytologic material and the image itself, can permit consultation both with respect to the samples available, and to advise special studies that may be indicated. In addition to consultation, telepathology may be used as a teaching tool. Conversely, however, the further development of simplified molecular techniques and automated analysis may, some day, render diagnosis a technical exercise such that the need for highly experienced, specialized pathologists will be reduced.

MANAGEMENT

Patients with lymphoma must sometimes undergo emergency treatment, particularly when lymphomas are rapidly progressive. Common emergencies arising from mass lesions include compression of vital structures (vena cavae, trachea, esophagus, spinal cord, bowel) or, occasionally, perforation of a viscus. Metabolic complications, particularly hyperuricemic renal failure, hypercalcemia, extreme anemia or thrombocytopenia and local or general infections may also require emergency treatment at the time of diagnosis. In such circumstances, lifesaving measures take precedence over diagnosis, but the introduction of specific therapy as early as possible is necessary to avoid worsening of the problem or further complications.

The extent of the disease (usually expressed as clinical or pathologic stage – see Chapter 47) is determined through clinical examination, bone marrow and often cerebrospinal fluid examination, and imaging studies, such as standard radiological examinations, ultrasound, computed tomography, magnetic resonance imaging, and occasionally positron emission tomography, a functional study which can also be valuable in determining whether a residual mass contains viable tumor (see Chapters 45 and 46). In low-resource settings, clinical examination supplemented by simple radiological and hematological tests may be all that is available or affordable (see Chapter 49). Computerized superimposition of anatomic and functional studies is now possible and may provide additional information in some cases, although high technology does not always lead to a better treatment outcome – indeed, in situations where treatment is delayed as a consequence, it can be deleterious. Theoretically, imaging could eventually provide diagnostic and prognostic information simultaneously, e.g. through the use of radiolabeled antibodies that identify specific tumor markers or patterns of gene expression. Even imaging of disease-specific fusion proteins may eventually be possible, but such techniques are unlikely to be realistic in the foreseeable future.

In addition to a precise diagnosis, the extent of disease, or 'stage', is important in deciding optimal therapy and in providing an indication of prognosis. In this regard, the application of staging schemes, some of which are designed for individual diseases (e.g. chronic lymphocytic leukemia) are not always sufficient to enable the oncologist to decide on optimal therapy, which may, particularly in indolent lymphomas, depend on other features, including the patient's clinical course or overall wellbeing. The International Prognostic Index, which includes age, performance status, a measure of tumor burden (clinical stage and lactate dehydrogenase concentration) and the number of extranodal sites (see Chapter 47), has been widely used in adults to determine prognosis (usually retrospectively), although less as a determinant of optimal therapy. In children, clinical stage and lactate dehydrogenase are often used together to determine the appropriate intensity of therapy.

Choice of therapy

The range of therapeutic options in lymphoid neoplasia is broad. In some indolent leukemias and lymphomas such as chronic lymphocytic leukemia and follicular lymphoma, which are producing minimal symptoms and progressing very slowly, if at all, a policy of 'watch and wait' may be adopted, with locoregional or simple chemotherapy being used as necessary to control symptoms. In the case of MALT lymphomas, a fraction respond well to antibiotic therapy or local surgery or radiation (see Chapter 71), while cutaneous T cell lymphomas may be controlled by locally applied chemotherapeutic drugs, skin irradiation or psoralen plus ultraviolet light. In nearly all other circumstances, systemic chemotherapy is the major element of treatment, but this too may vary in intensity, from single agents to intensive multidrug therapies sometimes requiring stem cell transplantation or mini-transplants. Although studied in first remission in both rapidly progressive lymphomas and advanced follicular lymphoma, intensive programs requiring stem cell rescue are rarely used in the context of primary therapy and are usually reserved for patients who relapse (see Chapter 60).

Although a small fraction of non-Hodgkin lymphomas appear to be localized, the use of exclusively local therapy (surgery or radiotherapy) is rarely successful (with the above-noted exceptions), and most diseases should be considered to be disseminated from the outset, such that except when the primary purpose is symptom control, single modality radiation therapy is rarely used (see Chapter 52). Radiation–chemotherapy combinations are more often used when disease is localized. Patients with primary CNS lymphoma have traditionally been treated with radiation, but recently, very good results have been achieved with regimens including high-dose methotrexate, suggesting that the presence of parenchymal brain lymphoma may no longer be an absolute indication for radiation therapy.

One of the more valuable approaches to therapy introduced in recent years is anti-CD20 (rituximab) therapy, which has been shown to be active as a single agent in indolent lymphomas, such as follicular lymphoma, and to improve survival rates when combined with chemotherapy in other B cell lymphomas such as diffuse large B cell lymphoma (see Chapters 76 and 91). Rituximab also appears to improve survival rates when used in addition to chemotherapy in the treatment of follicular lymphoma and mantle cell lymphoma and has a role in the management of B cell lymphomas associated with organ and bone marrow transplantation or with immunodeficiency diseases. Radioimmunoconjugates of anti-CD20 have also been shown to be active in B cell NHL, and although their use to date has largely been in the context of refractory or relapsed lymphoma, their role in primary therapy is currently under investigation.

Newer therapies, or therapies that have been under investigation for many years include vaccine therapies designed to raise responses against the immunoglobulin receptor idiotype antisense therapy, various monoclonal antibodies and a number of new drugs (see Part 9). The identification of specific targets in neoplastic cells followed by the development of drugs, particularly small molecules, directed against such targets, appears at the present time to have the greatest potential for the development of relatively nontoxic, curative therapy. Such a potential revolution in therapy more than justifies the intensification of efforts to develop detailed molecular profiles of lymphoid neoplasms of every category.

Prognosis

Lymphomas of immature lymphoid cells tend to have the best prognosis when treated with appropriate chemotherapy regimens and optimal supportive care (see Part 8). Children with ALL enjoy an overall cure rate, when treatment is optimal, of perhaps 80 percent, and those with B cell lymphomas or T cell lymphoblastic lymphoma even higher cure rates, although patients with central nervous system disease have a somewhat worse prognosis. Standard combination chemotherapy alone is presently able to cure approximately half of patients with diffuse large B cell lymphomas and more when rituximab is used (see Chapter 76), but patients with mantle cell lymphoma and peripheral T cell lymphomas other than anaplastic large cell lymphomas have a somewhat lower survival rate and many diseases are still considered incurable, particularly the more indolent lymphomas such as follicular lymphoma and chronic lymphocytic leukemia, although some of these patients may live for many years essentially symptom free.

One area that is likely to be further developed in the coming years is the significance of the expression of various markers to treatment outcome. The expression of various proteins, including BCL2, ZAP70, TP53 and many others, as well as single nucleotide polymorphisms, has been associated with prognosis in particular diseases. However, examination of the prognostic influence of the expression of single markers can be misleading, particularly in retrospective studies where treatment had not been standardized or was assumed to be sufficiently similar (e.g. 'doxorubicin-containing regimens') and prospective studies are essential. It is likely, however, that the use of multiple markers or 'signatures' may not only improve prognosis, but permit much greater individualization of therapy. Nonetheless, host factors (e.g. pharmacogenetics, comorbidities) as well as tumor factors, and the quality of care all influence outcome and will need to be included in any future algorithms designed to optimize therapy in individual patients.

KEY POINTS

- Lymphoid neoplasms are derived from lymphocytes, their precursors and their progeny.
- Prior to an understanding of the ontogeny of lymphocytes and their role in immune responses, the understanding and classification of lymphoid neoplasms was limited to relatively crude descriptions of clinical features, gross pathological appearances and morphology (primarily histology).
- Since lymphoid neoplasms are derived from cells which migrate throughout the body in the course of their normal function, standard concepts of staging used in solid cancers arising in specific organs have only limited application in lymphoid neoplasms, while the concepts of 'leukemia' and 'lymphoma' do not, in practice, separate discrete types of neoplasm. Even widespread lymphoid neoplasms can be effectively controlled and even cured.
- While lymphoid neoplasms phenotypically resemble their normal counterpart cells, the neoplastic clone may extend beyond the one or a small number of cell types that comprise the clinical neoplasm and more indolent lymphoid neoplasms may undergo 'transformation' into a more aggressive phenotype.
- Apoptosis is critical to normal lymphocyte ontogeny and to the regulation of immune responses, and it is probably true that all lymphoid neoplasms are able to bypass one or more 'checkpoints' that divert unwanted cells into apoptotic pathways. They remain susceptible, however, to apoptosis induced via other pathways.
- Lymphoid neoplasms, with the possible exception of those arising in immunodeficiency states are clonal; such clones may include cells at different stages of differentiation, some of which may be tumor stem cells.
- Lymphoid neoplasia arises primarily as a consequence of environmental factors, particularly certain chronic infections or exposure to chemicals, although some individuals, particularly those with underlying immunodeficiency (inherited or acquired), autoimmune diseases, or other genetic factors are at higher risk.
- Lymphoid neoplasms, require a microenvironment conducive to their survival, which may be a consequence of an external agent, or be present at certain ages or in particular physiological circumstances. Interactions between normal and neoplastic cells are probably essential to the maintenance of the neoplastic state.
- Classification (the most widely used system being that of the World Health Organization) is now largely based on the origin of cells from their normal counterparts, whose characteristics are retained at least in part, and utilizes a broad range of approaches to cell characterization as well as the identification of the molecular genetic abnormalities present.
- In effect, neoplasia generally recapitulates ontogeny and elements of immune responses in which normal regulatory mechanisms have been abrogated and/or replaced by aberrant regulatory elements.
- Genetic lesions are the proximate cause of lymphoid neoplasms; chromosomal translocations are particularly prominent and, to a large extent, tumor specific. However, other changes at chromosomal and DNA sequence levels involving relevant genes are essential to lymphomagenesis. Some tumor-specific chromosomal translocations can be detected in normal individuals who remain healthy.
- Viral genomes present in tumor cells may contribute to the neoplastic state.
- The genetic abnormalities are frequently mediated by enzymes responsible for genetic change during normal differentiation or immune reactions.
- Examination of broad gene expression patterns (molecular profiling) is playing an increasing role in defining diseases and is likely to play an increasing role in dictating therapy.
- Targeting specific cellular characteristics or genetic lesions is becoming increasingly important in the evolution of highly specific therapy.
- Treatment outcome depends upon the disease, its extent, host factors (age, comorbidities, underlying diseases, genetic factors), and the treatment itself.

REFERENCES

- ● = Key primary paper
- ◆ = Major review article

●1. Hodgkin T. On some morbid appearances of the absorbent glands and spleen. *Trans Med Chir Soc Lond* 1832; **xvii**: 68–114.
2. Lee SS, Cho KJ, Kim CW, Kang YK. Clinicopathological analysis of 501 non-Hodgkin's lymphomas in Korea according to the revised European-American classification of lymphoid neoplasms. *Histopathology* 1999; **35**: 345–54.

3. Chang KC, Huang GC, Jones D *et al.* Distribution and prognosis of WHO lymphoma subtypes in Taiwan reveals a low incidence of germinal-center derived tumors. *Leuk Lymphoma* 2004; **45**: 1375–84.

4. Aoki R, Karube K, Sugita Y *et al.* Distribution of malignant lymphoma in Japan: analysis of 2260 cases, 2001–2006. *Pathol Int* 2008; **58**: 174–82.

●5. Anderson JR, Armitage JO, Weisenburger DD. Epidemiology of the non-Hodgkin's lymphomas: distributions of the major subtypes differ by geographic locations. Non-Hodgkin's lymphoma classification project. *Ann Oncol* 1998; **9**: 717–20.

●6. Stiller CA, Parkin DM. International variations in the incidence of childhood lymphomas. *Paediatr Perinat Epidemiol* 1990; **4**: 303–24.

●7. Ramot B, Magrath I. Hypothesis: the environment is a major determinant of the immunological sub-type of lymphoma and acute lymphoblastic leukaemia in children. *Br J Haematol* 1982; **50**: 183–9.

●8. Hummel M, Bentink S, Berger H *et al.* Molecular mechanisms in malignant lymphomas network project of the deutsche krebshilfe. A biologic definition of Burkitt's lymphoma from transcriptional and genomic profiling. *N Engl J Med* 2006; **354**: 2419–30.

2

Historical perspective: the evolution of modern concepts of lymphoid neoplasia

IAN T MAGRATH

ORIGINS OF MODERN CONCEPTS OF LYMPHOID NEOPLASIA

Modern pathology has its foundations in the understanding of the structure of the human body that emerged in the Renaissance era, along with many other scientific and artistic advances. Vesalius' great book, *De Humani Corporis Fabrica*, published in seven volumes in 1543 and beautifully illustrated by a student of the Venetian painter, Titian, established the importance of dissection of the human body to an understanding of human anatomy. Over 100 years later, Thomas Bartholin (1616–80) and Olaus Rudbeck (1630–1702) almost simultaneously discovered the lymphatic system – or rather, the connection, via the thoracic duct, between lymph vessels draining the intestine and the bloodstream. The role of the lymphatic system in immunity, however, was to remain unknown for centuries. Similarly, there could be no understanding of human disease until the emergence of modern pathology in the course of the eighteenth and nineteenth centuries, when it became evident that diseases could be understood through an examination of their effects on the body – a remarkably novel idea in a world that had subscribed, since

the time of Hippocrates, to the theory that disease results from an imbalance in 'vital forces' or *humors*.

Giovanni Battista Morgagni (1682–1771) is credited with initiating the science of morbid anatomy (anatomic pathology). His revolutionary notion that disease is caused by malfunction of one or more organs was based on 500 case histories and autopsies conducted at the University of Padua, as well as his earlier experiences in Bologna and the observations of some of his teachers, among them, Valsalva. In 1761, in his eightieth year, Morgagni published his renowned treatise *De Sedibus et Causis Morborum per Anatomen Indagatis* [The Seats and Causes of Disease Investigated by Anatomy] in which he linked the symptoms of disease in life with the anatomic findings after death. Marie-Francois-Xavier Bichat (1771–1802), also a prodigious morbid anatomist (he is reputed to have performed 600 necropsies in a single winter, during which he lived in the autopsy room), was the first to introduce the concept of distinct *tissues*, which, he believed, provided the primary matrix for disease processes, thus going beyond Morgagni's organ theory. Bichat's work was carried out, however, without the aid of a microscope, even though Leeuwenhoek (1632–1723), using single, highly curved lenses, and Robert Hook (1635–1703), using a compound microscope of novel design, had made extensive microscopic observations over a century earlier. Indeed, it was Hook, in his famous book, *Micrographia*, published in 1665, who first used the term 'cell', in the context of the honeycomb-like spaces he observed in cork, which reminded him of the monks' cells in monasteries. Once again, the significance of this observation did not become apparent until much later.

Bichat's observations made it possible to correlate the symptoms of disease with the tissue affected (e.g. chest pain with involvement of the pleura), which led inexorably to the next major advance – the concept of pathophysiology. Johannes Müller (1801–58), unlike Bichat, used the microscope extensively and was able, through his broad erudition (he was a physiologist and ichthyologist as well as a comparative anatomist), to synthesize information from diverse sources. He made numerous important contributions to human physiology and anatomy, including observations on the chemistry of lymph, chyle and blood. He attempted to classify tumors on the basis of their histology as well as their physiologic and chemical characteristics – an approach similar in concept to that of the present era, but greatly handicapped by the vastly inferior tools then available. One of Müller's students, Theodor Schwann, was responsible, with Matthias Schleiden, for the *cell theory*, which was jointly published in 1839 and expressed the idea that cells are the basic building blocks of plants and animals and even give rise to nails, feathers and teeth. Müller himself recognized that cancers are also composed of cells, which, he suggested (wrongly), 'budded' out of intercellular elements in normal tissue – the so-called 'blastema theory'.

It was another of Müller's students, Rudolph Virchow (1821–1905), who provided the final element of the cell theory with his proposal that all cells, including cancer cells, arise from other cells. The cell theory, along with Darwin's theory of evolution and Pasteur's experimental studies, provided strong evidence against the prevailing notion of the times (dating back at least to Aristotle), that living organisms (even mice and crocodiles) could arise by spontaneous generation (*abiogenesis*) from fluids or decaying organic matter. Virchow's concept of cellular pathology, expounded in his treatise, *Cellularpathologie*, was first published in 1858. Like several of his illustrious forebears, he espoused careful observation and experiment as the fundamental tools of pathology and eschewed the still prevalent tendency to formulate speculative hypotheses. He made important observations on the anatomy and functions of the spleen and lymphoid tissues, and originated the terms *leukemia*, *lymphoma* and *lymphosarcoma*. His Berlin lecture series on malignant tumors, given during the winter of 1862, was published as *Die Krankhaften Geschwülste*, a work that launched the present era of neoplastic pathology.[1] Virchow's most distinguished student, Julius Cohnheim (1839–84), extended Virchow's observations and gave renewed emphasis to the importance of pathophysiology in understanding disease. Cohnheim was

the first to freeze pathological material for later examination and recognized that pus originated from white blood corpuscles. He also made important contributions to the emerging concepts of leukemia and lymphoma.

Hodgkin disease, leukemia and pseudoleukemia

In the middle of the past century, international communication was remarkably poor by modern standards and it is, therefore, not surprising that our modern concepts of what we now refer to as lymphoid neoplasia had multiple origins in the medical centers of Europe, and later, the USA. In the nineteenth century clinical medicine and pathology were not separate disciplines – in part because the tools available to classify and understand disease were remarkably limited and specialization was hardly warranted. Our modern understanding of lymphoid neoplasia began with sporadic descriptions of generalized lymph node swelling of unknown cause, often associated with splenic enlargement, published in the late eighteenth and nineteenth centuries. Among them were reports by Cruickshank, Craigie, Hodgkin, Wunderlich, Wilkes and Trousseau.[2–7] Hodgkin, in his classical paper of 1832, surmised that the lymph node enlargement he described was a primary process and not secondary to inflammation in adjacent tissue. Wilkes, although he had independently described primary lymphadenopathy,[5] became aware of Hodgkin's earlier contribution and was the first to use the term *Hodgkin's disease*,[8] which became the preferred term for lymphadenopathy of unknown origin in England, although in France, the same, ill-defined condition was referred to as *l'adenie*.[7] In 1844 and 1845, patients with idiopathic lymphadenopathy and hepatosplenomegaly associated with a white appearance of the blood at autopsy (antemortem examination of the blood at the time was possible, but rarely performed) were described in France (Alfred Donné), Germany (Rudolph Virchow) and Great Britain (David Craigie and John Bennet). Virchow referred to this condition as *Weisses Blut*[9] and subsequently renamed it *Leukämie*. Donné recognized the appearance of the blood to be due to an abnormal number of white cells, and Craigie and Bennett described patients with splenic or hepatosplenic 'tumors' who died from what they took to be suppuration of the blood.[10,11] This interpretation was not favored by Virchow, who, in his first publication on the topic[9] as well as in *Cellularpathologie*, remarked that leukemia was more often associated with splenomegaly than with lymphadenopathy, although both were often present. He also referred to 'splenic' and 'lymphatic' subdivisions, of leukemia, in part, based on the clinical features, and also on his ability to recognize microscopic differences in the types of white blood cells present in the bloodstream in each of these clinical variants. Although the cells associated with the splenic variety are poorly described by Virchow, 'comparatively large and perfectly developed with one or more nuclei … and in many cases bearing a strong resemblance to the cells of the spleen', the cells he observed in the lymphatic variant 'small, the nuclei large in proportion and single … while the cell wall is frequently in apposition to them such that an interval can scarcely be demonstrated' were surely small lymphocytes. We can be quite confident that Virchow was describing chronic myeloid and chronic lymphoid leukemias. It was not until 1889 that Wilhelm Ebstein (whose name is associated with Pel–Ebstein fever) introduced the term *acute leukemia* to differentiate more rapidly progressive leukemias from the chronic forms described many years before.

In 1862, Cohnheim used the term *Pseudoleukämie*,[12] to emphasize the absence of a high white blood cell count in a patient whose illness was otherwise indistinguishable from Virchow's *Leukämie*. The term *Pseudoleukämie* continued to be used in Germany to describe cases of idiopathic lymphadenopathy with or without hepatosplenomegaly. Thus, the relationship between leukemia and lymphoma was central to the first attempts to classify hematologic malignancies – a debate that has continued until the present day.

It is important to recognize that each of the designations *Hodgkin's disease*, *l'adenie* and *Pseudoleukämie* encompassed the whole range of malignant lymphomas (i.e. both Hodgkin and non-Hodgkin lymphomas) and quite probably acute leukemias with low white blood cell counts, as well as various non-neoplastic lymphadenopathies without a recognizable local cause. Wunderlich, for example, in his work on *Pseudoleukämie*, describes a 21-year-old with an acute febrile illness associated with marked malaise, generalized lymphadenopathy, hepatosplenomegaly and tonsillitis who recovered after some 4–5 weeks – perhaps a case of infectious mononucleosis.[13] And some of Hodgkin's original cases were shown, more than a century later, to be tuberculosis. In Osler's textbook of medicine,[14] published in 1892, all lymphomas are included under the general term *Hodgkin's disease*, which was stated to be synonymous with *Pseudoleukämie*, *general lymphadenoma* and *l'adénie*. Osler pointed out that a large majority of cases arise without any recognizable cause and that recovery is very rare. Both he and Dreschfeld[15] drew attention to the extremely variable clinical course, and referred to acute and chronic cases of Hodgkin's disease. In addition to the rate of progression, patients also appeared to fall into two main groups – those with localized disease and those with generalized lymph node swellings. This became an important consideration in early attempts to classify the non-leukemic cases of idiopathic lymphadenopathy, although clinical features, then, as now, were sufficiently overlapping as to provide a poor basis for classification – particularly since they evolve over time when untreated!

Lymphosarcoma versus hyperplasia

At the pathologic level, a frequent debate was whether diseases affecting the lymph nodes were malignant or hyperplastic – terms that were, at the time, ill defined. In *Die krankhaften Geschwülste*, Virchow wrote: 'insofar that true sarcomas of the usual kind also occur in lymph nodes, I propose to refer to such swellings as lymphosarcoma'. The word 'sarcoma' had been used as early as the second century CE by Galen (a Greek physician who cared for many leading citizens of the Roman Empire, including Marcus Aurelius), to refer to any fleshy, superficial tumor, but its use by Virchow clearly indicates an assumption of malignancy, which he attempted to differentiate on histologic grounds from 'simple hyperplasia' in which the appearance of the enlarged lymph nodes, at least with the primitive microscopes of the mid-nineteenth century, was indistinguishable from that of normal lymph nodes. This division was to continue into the twentieth century. Virchow recognized that patients with lymphosarcoma often had swelling in multiple lymph node areas, particularly the neck and axillae, which, as was also the case in leukemia, were characterized by progressive growth refractory to all available therapy. Kundrat, writing some 30 years after the introduction of the terms lymphosarcoma and pseudoleukemia, enlarged on Virchow's views and attempted to demonstrate that these diseases were separate entities. He considered, like Virchow, that *Lymphosarkom* was closely related to other sarcomata, i.e. cellular growths arising in connective tissue, and proposed that *Pseudoleukämie* was a form of 'lymphatic growth' more closely related to lymphoid hyperplasia.[16] In Kundrat's view, *Lymphosarkom* was confined to lymph nodes or lymphatic tissue in mucous membranes, although it tended to invade neighboring tissues and could spread directly from its local origin to other lymph node groups (in contrast to the presumed bloodstream spread of *Pseudoleukämie*). Involvement of the liver and spleen, if present, generally took the form of scattered nodules or masses, and involvement of the bone marrow was said to be rare. He referred to the progressive form of *Lymphosarkom* as *Lymphosarkomatosis*, which he still considered, on clinical grounds (i.e. the evolution of the disease from a single site, and the lack of diffuse involvement of liver, spleen and bone marrow), to be distinct from *Pseudoleukämia*, although more closely related to it than to other sarcomas (Cohnheim's index case of *Pseudoleukämia* had presented with a large splenic mass, general malaise and nose bleeds). Kundrat's clinicopathologic categories clearly do not correspond to modern disease categories – each must have encompassed many different entities, which, doubtless, also crossed Kundrat's dividing lines. Nevertheless, his work was widely known and he is sometimes (wrongly) credited with introducing the term 'lymphosarcoma' (referred to by some as 'Kundrat disease') and distinguishing lymphosarcoma from Hodgkin's disease and leukemia. Even though he could not, with the tools available to him, have accomplished such a separation, his ideas may well have influenced subsequent nomenclature while his separation of lymphosarcoma into localized versus generalized forms could be considered to herald our present division of lymphomas into clinical stages.

Ironically, Kundrat's classical paper of 1893,[16] in which he described *Lymphosarkomatosis* as a condition characterized by progressive anatomic involvement of adjacent lymph node areas, is more reminiscent of what we recognize today as Hodgkin lymphoma rather than non-Hodgkin lymphoma, although for much of the twentieth century *lymphosarcoma* was used as a generic term for lymphomas *other* than Hodgkin disease. Kundrat had paid only cursory attention to histology, which remained an ancillary investigation rather than a basis for distinguishing one disease from another, although this was soon to change. In the absence of more effective diagnostic tools, hypothetical classification schemes could not be tested, and many different ideas could therefore coexist. Dreschfeld, for example, writing in 1882,[15] considered *malignant lymphoma, lymphosarcoma, lymphosarcomatosis, l'adénie, lymphadénie, lymphadenoma, lymphadenosis and pseudoleukemia* (which he referred to as *pseudoleucocythemia*) to be synonyms for Hodgkin's disease – a view that was perhaps closest to the truth, since even the term Hodgkin's disease (used largely in England, where Dreschfeld was working at the time) still had no more specific sense than 'idiopathic lymphadenopathy'. In effect, each of these terms was the equivalent to the modern term *lymphoma* (more specifically, malignant lymphoma), a term that Virchow had introduced as a generic term for lymphatic tumors, formerly classified as 'lymphatic dyscrasias').

The significance of the differences in clinical characteristics, including the degree of spread and the rapidity of progression, remained a matter for speculation. Dreschfeld might today be referred to as a 'lumper' (and Kundrat a 'splitter'), but his ideas illustrate the difficulties faced in attempting to classify lymphoid neoplasia in the nineteenth century. He thought that *Hodgkin's disease*, or malignant lymphoma, was 'a specific inflammatory growth (a specific granuloma, if you like)' caused by an as yet unidentified infectious agent, which could present with either local involvement that became generalized (like Kundrat's *Lymphosarkomatosis*) or which could be generalized from the outset (like Cohnheim's *Pseudoleukämia*). He alluded to differences in the predominant location of the disease (superficial, thoracic or abdominal lymph nodes), but did not believe that there were fundamental 'structural differences' (i.e. histological differences) between 'benign' and 'malignant' lymphomas (referred to as *lymphadenoma* and *lymphosarcoma*, respectively, by others), only that the mixed cellular appearance (which included giant cells!) indicated an infectious etiology.

Dreschfeld did, however, believe, like Virchow and Kundrat, that there was a distinction between sarcomatous diseases of lymph nodes and 'hyperplastic' diseases of the blood forming organs and suggested, apparently on these grounds, that *acute Hodgkin's disease* might better be called *acute lymphosarcomatosis*. In agreement with Stevens,[17] Dreschfeld suggested that chronic Hodgkin's disease (generalized *ab initio*) was closely related to leukemia in that it resulted from hyperplasia of the blood-forming organs

(then thought to be the bone marrow, the spleen and the lymphatic glands). He suggested that such cases might 'more aptly be termed *chronic pseudoleukemia*' and, that, like leukemia, could be divided into lymphatic, splenic and myelogenic types, although the separate nature of the latter two, referring to primary involvement of the spleen and medulla (marrow) of the bones, respectively, remained in question.

These remarks serve largely to highlight the confusion that reigned in the late nineteenth century, and the marked variability in the use of terms originating in several countries that had, by now, been exported and made widely available to enterprising taxonomists across Europe. One might think of the second half of the nineteenth century as an era in which descriptions of lymphoid neoplasms, largely based on clinical features, but often supplemented by comments on histology were accumulated in the medical literature. Many of the terms associated with these descriptions remained in use well into the twentieth century, but meant different things to different people. Improvements in microscopes and histological techniques led gradually towards the identification of clinicopathological entities, but for the time being, clinical and gross pathological appearances remained the primary classification tools. Perhaps the clearest division was that between leukemia(s) and all other 'idiopathic' diseases of lymph nodes and spleen (pseudoleukemias and/or lymphosarcomas), a distinction that persisted into the twentieth and even twenty-first century. Ironically, we now recognize that the terms 'leukemia' and 'lymphoma' do not define discrete groups of diseases but, like the attempts to define diseases on the basis of clinical and gross pathologic appearances, are more relevant to modern staging systems than to pathologic classification.

EMERGENCE OF HISTOLOGIC CLASSIFICATION

Although Bichat is often considered to be the father of histology, it is curious that he made little or no use of the microscope, particularly since numerous microscopic observations had been made much earlier. It is probable that the failure to exploit the extraordinary potential of the microscope prior to the nineteenth century for the purposes of pathology was a consequence of the persistence of classical ideas of the nature of disease rather than simply the lack of availability of equipment or experience in microscopy. Even as ancient concepts were gradually superseded by the new science of pathologic anatomy, there was little attempt to move beyond gross description, even in major institutions. In future years, the slow introduction of new technology into clinical use would occur repeatedly as immunophenotyping and cytogenetics were developed and shown to be a valuable aid to classification. New tools, of course, require not only evaluation with respect to their utility, but also training in both the technology and the interpretation of results, both of which ensure that delay in their becoming routine is inevitable. Molecular techniques will doubtless face similar, if not greater delays because of the greater complexity and technological requirements, to say nothing of cost. Even so, it is somewhat surprising that as late as 1842, Rokitansky's great *Handbuch der pathologischen Anatomie* made no use of histology, although the microscopic study of tissues, aided by the discovery of the achromatic lens in the nineteenth century was, by now, well advanced. Histopathology owes much to Jacob Henle (1809–85), another of Müller's protégés, who wrote the first text on microscopic histology, *Allgemeine Anatomie*, published in 1841. By this time, greatly improved techniques in the hardening, sectioning and staining of tissues had been developed. Eventually, the concept of cells as the ultimate pathologic unit set the stage for rapid progress. Virchow devoted a third of *Cellularpathologie*, to normal (microscopic) histology and Cohnheim's text, *Vorlesungen über Allgemeine Pathologie*, written between 1877 and 1880, provided a solid foundation for modern pathology.

Dating from the latter part of the nineteenth century, there was continual improvement in the development of differential staining of cells in histologic preparations. Major contributions to staining techniques had been made by Paul Ehrlich (1854–1915). Encouraged by his cousin, the pathologist Carl Weigert, who had developed staining techniques for bacteria, and profiting from the recent synthesis of aniline dyes, Ehrlich enthusiastically set about the improved identification of cell types through the use of special stains. He was an expert chemist as well as a histologist (and later, a pioneer immunologist) who had been taught by several major figures in the field of pathology, including Cohnheim and Waldeyer. His doctoral thesis of 1878 was entitled 'Contributions to the theory and practice of histological staining' and Ehrlich developed staining methods for the tubercle bacillus as well as blood films; methods that provided the foundation on which many modern stains have been developed. He was able to distinguish, using a mixture of acid, basic and neutral dyes, three types of granulated white blood cell, 'acidophils', 'neutrophils' and 'basophils'), as well as megaloblasts and normoblasts. His aniline dyes enabled him to differentiate among a number of hematologic diseases and his work in this regard was summarized in an important book published with Adolf Lazarus in 1892 – *Histologie des Blutes*. The new staining techniques proved to be of great value in separating myeloid from lymphoid leukemias but in the absence of pathophysiologic understanding could make only limited contributions to lymphoma classification.

Histologic perspectives on Hodgkin disease and lymphosarcoma

Increasingly, in the latter years of the nineteenth century, histologic descriptions were provided in the lengthy case reports which comprised most of the medical publications of the era, such that inevitably, clinicopathologic correlations began to be made. In the second half of the nineteenth century, evidence for the value of histopathologic examination accumulated. Virchow, for example, had provided the morphologic basis for the classification of chronic leukemias, and Wunderlich reported the presence of binucleate and large multinucleate cells in the enlarged lymph nodes of a patient with *Pseudoleukämia* as early as 1858.[6] Precisely 40 years later, Sternberg described the histology (including the giant cells named after him, but previously recognized by Wunderlich) of what he considered to be 'a peculiar type of tuberculosis masquerading as *Pseudoleukämie*'.[18] Reflecting the growing importance of histology, Sternberg suggested that a diagnosis of *Pseudoleukämie* should only be entertained after histologic examination – or after the inoculation of involved tissue into animals failed to induce tuberculosis. In fact because of the ultimate development of tuberculosis in a high fraction of patients, Sternberg wondered whether, after separating 'clear-cut' cases of *Lymphosarkom* (i.e. neoplastic conditions), most of the remaining cases of *Pseudoleukämia* were not simply a manifestation of tuberculosis. In those days, tuberculosis was rampant and had always – as is the case today in many developing countries – to be included in the differential diagnosis of lymphadenopathy, particularly of the neck. An infectious etiology also seemed entirely consistent with Pel and Ebstein's descriptions of what, on the basis of the presence of a characteristic chronic relapsing fever and diffuse lymphadenopathy, they believed could be a different form of *Pseudoleukämia*.[19,20]

Debate over the question of whether Hodgkin disease is an infectious process or a malignant disease persisted for decades. Dorothy Reed,[21] however, writing a few years after Sternberg's publication, refuted his contention that the tubercle bacillus was causally involved (although she favored an infectious origin over the notion that it was a malignant disease). She emphasized the association of particular clinical features with a specific histologic appearance and, like Sternberg, described giant cells with one or multiple nuclei and prominent nucleoli dispersed among a mixture of cell types closely resembling a granuloma. Clinically, the cases she described nearly always began with cervical lymphadenopathy that rapidly spread to other nodal regions, the nodes being more mobile and discrete than is the case with sarcoma or tuberculosis. Of course, both Reed's and Sternberg's conceptions, like those of Hodgkin, must be interpreted in the context of the knowledge and ideas of the times in which their observations were made. Sternberg had referred to an unusual form of tuberculosis resembling *Pseudoleukämia*, and as pointed out by Coley in 1907,[22] Reed's clinical description was also sometimes seen in cases that had a histologic appearance of 'round cell sarcoma'.

Thus, the terminological disputes were by no means resolved by the histologic division that now became possible; Coley, who prefaced his remarks with the comment that 'Both pathologists and clinicians are widely at variance as to what constitutes Hodgkin's disease' was of the opinion, like many before him, that 'Hodgkin's disease' was a type of sarcoma (i.e. malignant) and there could 'hardly be a better name for the disease than *lymphosarcoma* (a view entirely consistent with our modern perspective – see Chapter 1). He also suggested that sarcomas might, in any event, be caused by a microorganism. Attempts to classify lymphoid neoplasms continued to suffer from the limited characterization then possible, although the description of Sternberg–Reed cells and the granuloma-like appearance of some idiopathic lymphomas (using the latter term in Virchow's original sense) created a precedent for histologic examination as an important component of diagnosis and permitted the recognition of a specific type of non-leukemic lymphoma, whatever its nature. Paltauf and his student, Sternberg, gave the disease a name consistent with its histologic appearance – *lymphogranulomatosis*,[23,24] whereas Reed used the generic term more widely used in English-speaking countries, but variably interpreted – Hodgkin's disease. Virchow, many years before, had described the cells present in 'lymphosarcoma' as small round cells, although he had also recognized the existence of lymphosarcoma in which the cells were of much larger size than a normal lymphocyte – a finding which others confirmed. The separation of non-leukemic lymphoid tumors into lymphogranulomatosis and lymphosarcoma (which persists today in the distinction, now somewhat artificial, between Hodgkin disease and non-Hodgkin lymphoma), the latter being further subdivided according to cell size, emerged rather than being formally proposed and might legitimately be considered the first histologic classification, although, as with all classifications prior to the modern era, it was not accepted by all.

By 1916, Ghon and Roman had begun to relate the cytology of lymphosarcomas to that of the cells of normal lymph nodes, and referred to *lymphocytic* and *lymphoblastic* forms.[25] This was the same year that Sternberg described mediastinal *leukosarcomatose*,[26] which, although not a homogeneous group, probably included cases of what is now known as lymphoblastic lymphoma. Ghon and Roman were aware of significant differences in the appearance of the nuclei of lymphosarcoma cells compared to normal lymphoid cells, and also recognized that many tumors consisted of mixtures of cell types – not only large and small lymphoid cells (that others had considered a mark of the degree of maturity of the cells), but also macrophage-like cells, sometimes multinucleate cells, and plasma cells. They likened the macrophage-like cells to reticulum cells (see below) and commented on their presence in normal lymphoid tissue. Ghon and Roman were clearly aware that some authors might diagnose cases as lymphogranuloma that would previously have been called lymphosarcoma. They also expressed uncertainty as to whether lymphosarcomatosis could be clearly separated from, on the one hand, leukemia/pseudoleukemia, which they considered, like others before them, to be of 'hyperplastic origin' and on the

other from sarcomas appearing in non-lymphoid locations. A close relationship between pseudoleukemia and leukemia was suggested by the observation that the former could evolve into the latter, and Ghon and Roman believed that these diseases involved the entire lymph node and probably all lymphatic tissue, while in lymphosarcoma a clear boundary between normal and abnormal lymphoid tissue could frequently be seen and normal and abnormal lymph nodes observed in the same patient. Ghon and Roman also made other important observations on the histology of lymphoid neoplasms that might be seen as the first glimmerings of concepts that remain important today. They reported that the number of cells in mitosis varied greatly from one tumor to another, and described 'dwarf cells' with a very dense, round nucleus – cells that would today surely be recognized as cells undergoing apoptosis. Presciently, they wondered whether this appearance was a consequence of cell damage.

Entities new and old

As if the confusion in terminology was not already sufficient,[27] new terms were introduced in the first half of the twentieth century. These arose in part as a result of the recognition of what appeared to be new disease entities with quite distinctive histologic appearances, and also because of the notion of a *reticuloendothelial system* that provided protection against diseases caused by microorganisms. Although this proved, in the end, to be a blind alley from the perspective of the classification of lymphoid neoplasm, it had a critically important role in the development of modern concepts, and particularly, the notion of lymphoid neoplasms as tumors of the immune system. It also led to wide acceptance of the idea, already apparent in Virchow's writings, that neoplasms could be understood not only in terms of the normal cells they derived from, but also in terms of cellular differentiation pathways (although the latter remained speculative for many decades). This led to a plethora of new terms for supposed disease entities defined on the basis of histologic appearances. Few of these terms remain in use today, in part because limitations in technical resources made both description and communication difficult (for example, only black and white drawings were used to illustrate histologic appearances), and hence consensus, even in individual countries, was largely impossible. Prior to the emergence of histology as a diagnostic tool, only pathologic entities with highly characteristic clinical features (e.g. mycosis fungoides [Box 2.1] and multiple myeloma [Box 2.2]) could be reproducibly diagnosed. Even with improved histologic techniques, the lack of clinical correlation (e.g. in the case of lymphogranuloma) led to more confusion than clarification. The recognition, however, of follicular lymphoma (Box 2.3) permitted, for perhaps the first time, the correlation of histology with clinical course and gave considerable impetus to the use of histology as a diagnostic tool.

BOX 2.1: Mycosis fungoides

Mycosis fungoides was recognized at about the same time as Hodgkin was describing primary disease of the 'absorbent glands and spleen'.[4] Alibert (1760–1837), a physician for skin diseases in Paris, first used the term for what was formerly referred to as 'framboesia', a fungating skin condition that had been recognized in West Africa (as pian) and the West Indies (as yaws).[28] As recorded by Kaposi (1837–1902),[29] Alibert believed the mushroom-like growth (hence his choice of nomenclature) on the face of a patient he described was related to syphilis. Kaposi, however, was confused by the observation that the disease may remain confined to the skin for long periods, but could involve underlying structures and even, uncommonly, the viscera. He suggested that it was one of the 'sarcoid tumors' in which he included sarcomatosis but thought the more invasive forms might well be related, following Paltauf's suggestion, to pseudoleukemia or lymphosarcoma.

BOX 2.2: Multiple myeloma

Multiple myeloma was described in the mid-nineteenth century. Bence Jones protein was discovered in the urine of a patient with severe bone pain in 1845 by William McKyntire, and quantitated, in the same patient by Henry Bence Jones who remarked on the association of this finding in other patients with 'softening of the bones', which was also found at autopsy in McKyntire's patient. The surgeon, John Dalyrimple, who performed the autopsy, described the presence of cells that, from his description, were almost certainly plasma cells. Von Rustizky first used the term 'multiple myeloma' in 1873 for the disease he encountered in another patient with multiple tumors in the bone marrow, which he therefore referred to, descriptively, as multiple myeloma. Carl Kahler reported a patient with bone pain in whom he recognized albuminuria and the same type of urinary protein described by Bence Jones. Autopsy, performed in 1887, also showed tumors in the ribs and vertebrae that contained large round cells. The term 'plasma cell' was first used in 1875 by Waldever, and although the function of such cells remained unknown, they were accurately described by Cajal in 1890. It was not until 1900 that they were recognized by Wright – who also developed the stain for blood cells that bears his name – as being the cells present in multiple myeloma. In Wright's patient, X-rays, only recently possible, revealed the characteristic lesions in ribs.

BOX 2.3: Giant follicular lymphoma

The occurrence of lymphomas with a follicular or nodular architecture had been recognized at least as early as 1902,[30] as reported by Ghon and Roman,[25] but received only sporadic mention in the literature until the independent descriptions by Brill *et al.* (1925) and Symmers (1927) of patients with lymphadenopathy and splenomegaly in which histologic studies revealed enlarged lymphoid follicles.[31,32] This histologically diagnosed disease had a generally protracted clinical course, and therefore generated considerable controversy as to whether it was simply a chronic, but benign hyperplastic state, as originally believed to be the case by Brill *et al.* and Symmers, or a truly neoplastic condition. That it could evolve into a rapidly progressive malignant lymphoma was, however, accepted by all.

Varying descriptions of the histology and clinical course of follicular lymphomas appear to reflect the range of diseases that originally fell under this rubric. Its relative rarity was such that it was difficult for any one individual to acquire a large experience. In fact, reports of series collected in the first half of this century suggest that follicular lymphoma comprised a much lower proportion of all lymphomas than is the case today. In two large series collected in the USA over many years and reported in 1954 and 1961, follicular lymphomas comprised just 4 percent and 13 percent of patients with non-Hodgkin lymphoma, respectively.[33,34] Although not population based, these data suggest that the incidence of follicular lymphoma was much lower in the early part of the twentieth century and before, which is consistent with the low frequency of follicular lymphomas in developing countries today. In both cases, the possibility of underdiagnosis because of the slow progression of the disease, at least before conversion to a diffuse lymphoma, or misdiagnosis as reactive hyperplasia, cannot be excluded, but neither would seem sufficient explanations of the low frequencies observed once the histologic descriptions had been published.

Gall *et al.*[35] described four main histologic forms of follicular lymphoma, which correspond to categories that are still recognized. Types 1, 2 and 3 were composed of follicles containing small cells, mixed small and large cells, and large cells, respectively. Type 4 referred to a variety in which there was a degree of confluence or 'rupture of follicles' such that a diagnosis of follicular lymphoma was sometimes difficult. Such cases were probably undergoing transformation to an aggressive diffuse B cell lymphoma.

The reticuloendothelial system

The concept of a protective reticuloendothelial system based on phagocytosis was stimulated by the developing concepts of the pathophysiology of inflammation and immunity that had begun to emerge in the last decades of the nineteenth century. The germ theory of the cause of disease had been well established by the work of Louis Pasteur (1822–95), who showed that microorganisms are present in the environment and not derived from spontaneous generation. When Jacob Henle's student, Robert Koch (1843–1910), discovered the tubercle bacillus in 1882, the discipline of microbiology was born. Antibodies were discovered by Emil Adolph von Behring (1854–1917), who demonstrated the existence of diphtheria antitoxins and won the first Nobel Prize for physiology and medicine for his development of a serum therapy for diphtheria and tetanus (published in *Die Blutserumtherapie* in 1892). The starting point for the understanding of the physiological mechanisms employed in protection against diseases caused by microorganisms, however, came from Elie Metchnikoff's (1845–1916) extensive studies on phagocytosis, including the phagocytosis of bacteria.[36] He was able to show this phenomenon in cells of the splenic pulp, lymph nodes, liver (Küppfer cells) and mononuclear cells circulating in the blood. Metchnikoff's work was instrumental to the development of Aschoff's notion of a phagocytic *reticuloendothelial* system.[37] Aschoff proposed that a number of widely distributed cell types that were already known, including the large *reticulum cells* in lymph nodes, certain *endothelial cells* (littoral cells) lining the lymph sinuses of lymph nodes and the venous sinuses of the spleen, bone marrow and liver, tissue histiocytes and some of the mononuclear cells of the blood, were all part of the same system. These large cells, known to be capable of taking up dyes introduced into the bloodstream, as well as engulfing colloidal suspensions of various materials, were seen to be the same cells that Metchnikoff had recognized as capable of engulfing bacteria. Such cells were also believed to synthesize fibres found in connective tissue that could be stained with silver (by reduction of silver oxide). These phagocytic cells appeared, thus, to comprise a network (hence the word 'reticulum') that was dispersed throughout the mesenchymal matrix of organs and tissues as well as in the endothelial cells lining blood and lymphatic sinuses (hence, *reticuloendothelial* system).

A NEW BASIS FOR CLASSIFICATION

The reticuloendothelial system was believed to be the component of lymph nodes, liver, spleen and bone marrow that was responsible for the production of both red and white blood cells. Further, its cellular constituents were believed to be identical to both the widely distributed phagocytic cells in normal tissues, as well as those present in the lesions of tuberculosis, typhoid fever, leprosy and various other infections – cells that had often been observed to contain bacteria and cellular debris in their cytoplasm, providing further evidence of their role in protecting against infection. Experiments in which the injection of particular material in animals influenced the formation of various antibodies provided evidence of the relationship

of the cells of the reticuloendothelial system to immunity against infection, and led to the reticuloendothelial system being considered as loosely synonymous with the 'immune system' particularly in the context of what we now refer to as lymphoid neoplasms, although the importance of lymphoid cells to immunity was not recognized until the last decades of the twentieth century. Although the term reticuloendothelial system remains in use, there is an increasing tendency to replace it by *mononuclear phagocytic system* to refer to the widely dispersed phagocytic cells involved in inflammatory responses and immunity. Some of these cells, or closely related cells, are critically important to the functions of lymphocytes – dendritic macrophages or reticular cells, for example, have a major role in antigen presentation to lymphocytes.

The discovery of the widely dispersed phagocytic system had a profound influence on early classification schemes of the lymphomas and leukemias, which were believed, largely erroneously, to derive directly from its cellular constituents. Although limited largely to the use of morphology to determine cellular origin, which gave rise to considerable license in interpreting the histogenetic origins of lymphoid neoplasms, and as a result, a number of erroneous conclusions (such as the notion of reticulum cell sarcoma), the concept provided, at last, a firm rationale for future classification schemes.

Reticulum cell sarcoma

Although the heterogenous histology of primary lymph node diseases had been known for decades, and the description of lymphogranuloma had created a major histological divide, Ewing was able to remark, in 1939, that beyond the existence of small cell and large cell lymphosarcomas, as reported originally by Virchow, there was no uniformity of opinion.[38] But by now the histological appearance of normal lymph nodes – important elements of the reticuloendothelial system – had been well studied (Fig. 2.1), and the structures and cells they contained provided the foundation on which to build classification schemes in terms of the cellular origins of various categories of lymph node neoplasms. Any of the cell types present in lymph nodes, including lymphoid cells (believed by many to arise from the germinal follicles), the endothelial cells lining the lymph node sinuses and reticulum cells interspersed among the lymphoid cells, were potential candidates for the origin of neoplasms. Both reticulum cells and endothelial cells were believed by many pathologists, e.g. Maximov,[40] to be derived from a single precursor cell of mesenchymal origin (that also gave rise to lymphocytes). Some believed they could recognize this mesenchymal precursor cell in lymph node sections; others thought the reticulum cell itself to be the 'mother cell'.[41,42]

Meanwhile, many pathologists (including Ewing), had begun to use the term *endothelial sarcoma* or *endothelioma of lymph nodes* to denote a tumor of large cell type that they

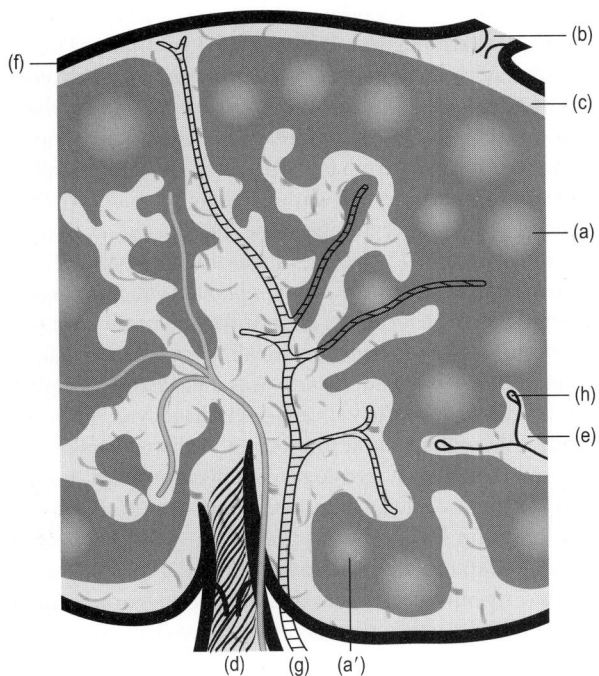

Figure 2.1 Normal lymph node (after Heudorfer K, *Z Anat u Entwickl* 1921; **365**: LXI). (a) Lymph follicle, (a') pseudofollicle, (b) afferent lymphatic, (c) cortical sinus, (d) efferent lymphatic, (e) medullary sinus, (f) capsule, (g) hilum vessels, (h) trabeculae. (Modified from Robb-Smith.[39])

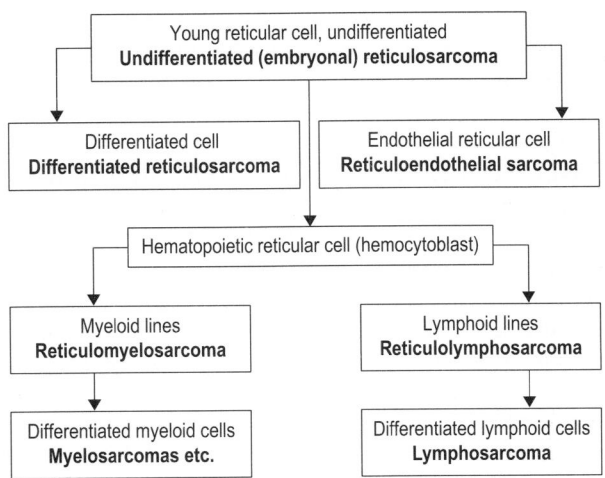

Figure 2.2 Oberling's perspective on sarcomatous tumors of the reticuloendothelial system.

believed arose from the endothelial lining cells of the lymph node sinuses,[43,44] although the concept of endothelioma of lymph nodes was not universally accepted.[45] Oberling, in France, subsequently introduced the terms *reticulosarcoma* and *reticuloendotheliosarcoma* in the context of a subset of bone tumors that he believed arose from reticuloendothelial tissue of the bone marrow and that were not, therefore, true bone tumors.[46] He thought they were very similar, if not identical, to the endotheliomas of lymph nodes and bone, that had been described by Ewing (who referred to the bone tumors he described as *diffuse endothelioma of bone* and *endothelial myeloma*).[44,47] Oberling described what he took to be undifferentiated or embryonic reticulosarcomas composed of syncytial masses arising from the primitive 'mesenchymal syncytium' of bone marrow. His conceptual scheme included more differentiated reticulosarcomas, among them a hematopoietic reticular cell (or hemocytoblast) whose still more differentiated forms were *reticulomyelosarcomas* and *reticulolymphosarcomas*, and most differentiated, *myélosarcome* and *lymphosarcome*, respectively (Fig. 2.2). At the time myelosarcomas were believed to be derived from *myeloblasts* or *myelocytes* – terms which referred to ill-defined bone marrow cells rather than the more precise sense in which they are used today (similarly, *myeloma* has nothing to do with modern myeloid cells). Finally, Oberling divided lymphosarcoma

into less (lymphoblastic) and more (lymphocytic) differentiated variants. His classification cannot be reconciled with modern classifications and probably encompassed true bone tumors. It is, however, important as one of the early classifications schemes based on the concept of a set of neoplasms derived from the reticuloendothelial system – whether in lymph nodes or the bone marrow – which can be subdivided according to their stage of differentiation.[48]

Not everyone agreed with Oberling's terminology. Roulet, discussing the tumors of lymph nodes,[49] preferred to delete the references to endothelial cells in the context of reticulum cell sarcoma, which he referred to as *Retothelsarkom*, as had his mentor, Rössle, since, he claimed, such tumors did not arise from the endothelial cells of lymph nodes sinuses but from the cells associated with the fibrous scaffolding (the *Reticulothelium* or *Retikulum*) of lymph nodes. Roulet accepted that both reticulum and endothelial cells had phagocytic properties and these, as well as the lymphoid cells, originated in undifferentiated mesenchymal cells. He also subscribed to the occurrence of undifferentiated and differentiated subtypes of reticulum cell sarcoma (based on production of argentophilic fibers in the latter), with intermediate forms possible. He considered *Retothelsarkom* to be the 'third' type of lymphosarcoma of lymph nodes, the first two being lymphocytic and lymphoblastic types. Roulet's classification had eliminated endothelial cells from consideration, but still subscribed to the idea that some lymphomas are derived from reticulum cells with phagocytic properties (or, as subsequently proposed in the USA, from histocytes). This erroneous idea was to persist for decades. Meanwhile, the concept that reticulum cell sarcoma was a disease arising either in lymph nodes or bone prompted numerous additional publications.[50,51] In Europe, particularly, the notion that lymphomas arise from the reticuloendothelial system led to the widespread use of the terms *reticuloendothelioses*, or *reticuloses* to refer to a broad range of diseases of the reticuloendothelial system. Consequently, reticulum cell sarcoma was preferred by some to lymphosarcoma as a generic term for what we refer to today as lymphoid neoplasms, only adding to the existing confusion.

EVOLUTION OF HISTOLOGIC CLASSIFICATION SCHEMES

Histologic classification was slow to evolve because of the limited understanding of the origins and functions of the cells that comprise lymphoid tissue. In the absence of experimental information, cellular differentiation pathways were largely speculative. The origins of neoplastic diseases were equally speculative, and existing terms continued to be used, often in different ways, while new terms were invented or older terms modified according to favored theories of histogenesis. In addition, the limited communication among pathologists meant that opportunities for developing consensus views were similarly limited. Communication across the Atlantic Ocean was particularly poor, such that American and European schools of pathology tended to evolve separately, although even by the beginning of the latter half of the twentieth century, it seemed to many that in spite of the multiple attempts at classification, little progress had been made. In a large review of lymphoid neoplasms from New York, published in 1958, earlier views were echoed in the statement that 'pathologists and clinicians have largely come to realize that the histological appearance does not define with much degree of certainty the clinical course, extent of involvement and prognosis of these diseases'.[52]

In the USA, however, a pivotal classification scheme had been published by Gall and Mallory in 1942.[53] This subsequently evolved into the widely used Rappaport classification,[54] which lurks behind the later Working Formulation for Clinical Usage published in 1982.[55] Gall and Mallory's classification, of course, did not emerge *de novo*, but superseded

that provided by Callender in his review of the American College of Pathologists' Registry of Lymphatic Tumors. Callender's classification was based on a mixture of cytologic, gross anatomic and clinical characteristics,[56] and, like that of Robb-Smith (see below), included leukemias, lymphomas and non-neoplastic lymphadenopathies (Table 2.1). Gall and Mallory proposed a much simpler scheme – essentially an inventory – based on cytology alone. They listed seven major types of lymphoma (Table 2.2), including two types of reticulum cell sarcoma – *stem cell lymphoma*, which, following Maximov, was believed to arise from an undifferentiated mesodermal cell able to give rise to all types of blood cell, and *clasmatocytic lymphoma*, which was believed to originate from differentiated cells with marked phagocytic properties, namely, macrophages and monocytes. Gall and Mallory had proposed their purely cytologic classification with 'no little hesitation' but avoided using anatomic distribution as a diagnostic criterion since they felt that nothing in the histologic character of an individual lesion permitted a reliable forecast as to its distribution in other parts of the body, or whether or not the blood picture would prove to be 'leukemic'. They even noted that while diffuse marrow involvement was found in the majority of leukemic patients, in some patients

Table 2.2 Gall and Mallory's classification of malignant lymphoma and number of cases in each category in their series from the Massachusetts General Hospital

1. Stem cell lymphoma	56	} 'Reticulum cell
2. Clasmatocytic lymphoma	71	sarcoma'
3. Lymphoblastic lymphoma	85	
4. Lymphocytic lymphoma	135	
5. Hodgkin's lymphoma	193	
6. Hodgkin's sarcoma	36	
7. Follicular lymphoma	42	

Table 2.1 Callender's classification of tumors and tumor-like conditions arising from lymphocyte stem cells, and monocyte or reticuloendothelial stem cells

| | | Reticulum cell | |
Adult cell type	Lymphocyte	Reticulocyte monocyte	Hodgkin's disease
I. Reactions	'Lymphoma'	Gaucher disease Lymphocytosis	Localized (sclerosing) Niemann–Pick disease
II. Neoplastic proliferations	Leukemic lymphocytoma 1. Chronic 2. Acute	Leukemic reticulocytoma (*synonym* monocytic leukemia)	
III. Neoplastic proliferations	Aleukemic lymphocytoma 1. Diffuse 2. Nodular	Aleukemic reticulocytoma	Generalized (cellular)
IV. Malignant tumors	Lymphosarcoma 1. Aleukemic 2. Leukemic (*synonym* lymphatic leukosarcoma)	Reticulum cell sarcoma	Sarcomatous

the bone marrow was normal, and in others, there was variability over time with respect to bone marrow involvement.

In Europe, Robb-Smith developed the idea expressed by Pullinger (incorporating Maximov's concept of an undifferentiated mesenchymal cell) that 'a group of diseases of the reticulum exists in which proliferation is possible into one or several of the possible cell progeny'. Robb-Smith proposed a rather complex histologic classification (Box 2.4) of 'reticuloses' [a] and 'reticulosarcoma' [b] of lymph nodes, these designations being used to indicate less (hyperplastic or *blastomatoid)* and more malignant (true *blastomata,* or neoplasms) subsets of diseases of the reticuloendothelial system.[39] His classification (Box 2.4), which was revised in 1947 and again in 1964, was the most widely used classification scheme in Europe until replaced by the German 'Kiel' classification, devised by Lennert and colleagues. The Kiel classification retained the concept of less and more malignant neoplasms, although now referring to them as low and high grade categories, and built on the Robb-Smith classification's central theme – that neoplasms were derived from different structures (and therefore, cell types) within lymph nodes.

Robb-Smith considered that only three structures within the lymph node were important from a histologic and consequently a pathologic standpoint. These were the lymphoid follicles of the cortex, the sinuses which surrounded the more peripheral *cortex* of the node and ramified throughout the central medulla, and the remainder of the nodal tissue in the cortex and medulla which, in his classification, referred to as 'medulla'. He noted that reticulin fibers were not present in the lymphoid follicles, but were apparent throughout the rest of the node. He also underlined the fact that pathological proliferations in lymph nodes were often associated with similar proliferations in the spleen, periportal hepatic tissue and bone marrow, supporting the notion that these were tumors of the reticuloendothelial system. His classification, in which pathologic processes derived from the lymphoid follicles, sinuses or medulla (categories A, B and C under section [a], Box 2.4) were further subdivided according to the differentiation of the proliferating cells into various cytologic subtypes, represented the most comprehensive effort to date to relate lymphoid neoplasms to their normal counterpart cells. While at first sight daunting, it included several quite familiar elements, although many diseases, in retrospect, were not individual pathologic entities and cannot, therefore, be related to individual modern diagnostic categories (e.g. histiocytic medullary reticulosis).

Follicular reticuloses encompassed follicular lymphoma and benign follicular processes. Sinus reticuloses, or endothelioses comprised tumors supposedly derived from undifferentiated mesenchymal cells and littoral cells of lymph sinuses (here, Maximov's contribution is evident) and occasionally, histiocytes. Medullary reticuloses included a broad range of pathologic processes of lymphoid, myeloid and reticulum cells as well as malignant histiocytoses (Letterer–Siwe disease) and storage diseases (e.g. Gaucher disease and Niemann–Pick disease). Robb-Smith

---

BOX 2.4: Robb-Smith's classification of the primary lymphadenopathies: reticulosis (benign) and reticulosarcoma (malignant)

(a)

A. Follicular reticuloses
   i. Lymphoid (follicular lymphoblastoma)
   ii. Myeloid
   iii. Lymphoid and histiocytic (Flemming's centers: reactive hyperplasia)
   iv. Giant cell and fibrillary

B. Sinus reticuloses (endothelioses)
   i. Histiocytic
   ii. Giant-cell histiocytic (Stengel–Wolbach sclerosis)
   iii. (?) Histiosyncytial

C. Medullary reticuloses
   i. Lymphoid (lymphoid leukosis)
   ii. Myeloid (myeloid leukosis and myeloid transformations)
   iii. Monocytic (monocytic leukosis)
   iv. Reticulum celled
   v. Storage reticulum celled (lipoidosis)
   vi. Histiocytic
   vii. Pro-histiocytic-fibrillary
   viii. Fibromyeloid (Hodgkin's disease)

In any of these conditions, free cellular elements may appear in the circulating blood.

(b)

A. Undifferentiated sarcoma
   1. Diffuse
   2. Trabecular

B. Differentiation to histioid cells
   1. Dicytosyncytial (fibrosyncytial) reticulosarcoma
   2. Dicytocytic (fibrillary) reticulosarcoma

C. Differentiation to hemic cells
   1. Lymphocytoma
      i. Lymphoblastic sarcoma
         a. Medullary
         b. Follicular
      ii. Lymphosarcoma
   2. 'Plasmacytoma'
   3. (Monocytoma)
   4. Myeloblastoma
   5. Erythroblastoma

D. Mixed type (polymorphic reticulosarcoma)

E. Differentiation of sinus lining cells
   1. Undifferentiated cell type (reticuloendotheliosarcoma)
   2. Differentiated cell type (histiocytoma)

D Corresponds to Hodgkin's sarcoma or malignant Hodgkin's disease.

felt it likely that myeloid cells, too, were derived from undifferentiated mesenchymal cells, consistent with the persisting idea that the cellular elements of the blood were derived from lymph nodes, or perhaps, from the reticuloendothelial system in general. The greater proportion of Hodgkin lymphoma, probably equivalent to what Jackson and Parker subsequently referred to as Hodgkin's granuloma (see below) was included as fibromyeloid medullary reticulosis (the importance of histologic appearances in defining categories is very much in evidence here). Lymphocyte-depleted Hodgkin disease, or 'Hodgkin's sarcoma' was included as a mixed type of reticulosarcoma (polymorphic). Among the malignant processes [b] Robb-Smith described what he believed to be less and more differentiated diseases derived, respectively, from reticulum cells, or their progeny, lymphoid and other blood cells. He did not believe that reticuloendothelial sarcomas occurred in lymph nodes, only in bone marrow, and suggested that cells filling lymph node sinuses were probably secondary deposits of anaplastic carcinomas. Interestingly, he used the term *leukosis*, rather than lymphoma or leukemia for many conditions, since identical abnormal cells to those identified in lymph nodes could often be found circulating in the blood. Thus, in contrast with the earlier distinction between leukemia and pseudoleukemia, and in line with modern thinking, Robb-Smith did not consider involvement of the peripheral blood to be indicative of a different disease.

Not surprisingly, classifications based on purely morphologic schemata, with minimal assistance from special stains and no real understanding of the immune system were less than satisfactory, as indicated by the proliferation of alternative classification schemes throughout the twentieth century. As pointed out by Stout in 1947,[57] even when the same term was used by different pathologists, they frequently used it in quite different ways. For example, Sugarbaker and Craver (1940) diagnosed 94 percent of their series of lymphomas as reticulosarcoma,[58] whereas Warren and Picena had included only 3.6 percent of their 1941 series in this category.[51]

Clinicopathologic correlations

Some histologic categories, at least, were by mid-century sufficiently defined that some clinicopathologic correlations could be made. Stout, for example, in analyzing the clinical course of 170 patients, 119 of whom had been treated with radiation and/or surgery, confirmed that while most lymphosarcomas (a term he used to indicate non-Hodgkin lymphomas) 'generally run a rapid and fatal course, there are a few of them that are slow and deliberate in their progress', an observation that had also been made by others. He recognized that patients with giant follicular lymphoma survived considerably longer than most other patients (36.8 percent of untreated, and 43.8 percent of treated patients survived for 5 years as compared with 23 percent of treated patients with either lymphocytic

lymphomas [a term he used for lymphomas consisting of smaller cells] or reticulum cell sarcomas [used for lymphomas consisting of larger cells]), although he could discern no clear difference in survival between patients with lymphocytic versus reticulum cell lymphosarcoma – 20 percent and 15 percent, respectively, survived 5 years, although less than 10 percent were alive at 10 years. Stout, like others before and since, noted that among patients with follicular lymphomas, those with a mixed follicular and diffuse pattern had a worse prognosis – survival was half that of patients with 'fully differentiated' follicular lymphosarcoma. He also recognized that extranodal lymphomas tended to have a better prognosis, in that 26 percent of 35 such patients were alive 10 years after treatment versus 7 percent of his 83 treated patients with nodal lymphomas. Most of these long-surviving extranodal lymphomas had primaries in the oral cavity, tonsil, nasopharynx, salivary glands and gastrointestinal tract, and probably included what subsequently became known as pseudolymphomas' and, more recently, lymphomas of mucosa-associated lymphoid tissue (MALT). Patients with extranodal lymphomas also more often had localized disease. In contrast, Stout reported that childhood lymphomas and lymphomas complicated by leukemia had a rapid and almost invariably fatal course.

Blind alleys

For years it had been assumed (correctly, as it turned out) that follicular lymphomas arose from the lymphoid follicles present in normal lymph nodes, although the true functional significance of these structures remained unknown. This more readily permitted the perpetuation of the speculation that reticulum cell sarcomas (a term increasingly used in the context of large cell lymphomas in the USA) were of quite different origin, and to easy acceptance of the theory that they were derived from phagocytic cells. Gall brought attention to some of the enigmas brought about by the lack of knowledge of the functional significance of lymph nodes structures[59] and Rappaport and colleagues published a paper in which they questioned whether the follicles seen in follicular lymphoma were truly the neoplastic counterparts of lymphoid follicles.[60] Gall and Rappaport,[61] in a departure from the earlier Gall and Mallory classification, proposed that follicular lymphomas be designated 'nodular', a term that had been used by Callender in his classification of lymphohematopoietic neoplasms in 1934.[56] Further, they suggested that all lymphomas could be either 'nodular' or 'diffuse', and that nodularity did not imply an origin from lymphoid follicles. Rappaport's classification, published in monograph form a decade later was almost identical, and represented the final version of a series of classification schemes evolved in the USA (Table 2.3).[54] It rapidly became the most widely used classification in the USA, perhaps in part because of its simplicity compared, for example, to the Robb-Smith

Table 2.3 Evolution of histologic classification systems of non-Hodgkin lymphomas in the USA

Custer and Bernhard	Gall and Mallory	Gall and Rappaport[a]	Rappaport[a]
Lymphosarcoma	Lymphocytic	Lymphocytic, WD	Lymphocytic, WD
	Lymphoblastic	Lymphocytic, PD	Lymphocytic, PD
		Histiocytic/lymphocytic	Histiocytic/ lymphocytic, mixed
Reticulum cell sarcoma	Stem cell	Stem cell ⎫ RCS	Histiocytic
	Clasmatocytic	Histiocytic ⎭	
Follicular	Follicular	Nodular (divided into all of the above subtypes)	Nodular (divided into all of the above subtypes)

[a]In these classification schemes, each cytological type of lymphoma is divided into diffuse and nodular forms (see text).
RSC, reticulum cell sarcoma; WD, well differentiated; PD, poorly differentiated.

classification, although, as was soon to become apparent, its simplicity did not reflect the reality of the gamut of lymphoid neoplasms.

Each of the two broad classes in the Rappaport system, nodular and diffuse, was divided into three categories: lymphomas consisting predominantly of small cells, lymphomas consisting predominantly of large cells and lymphomas in which there was a roughly equal mixture of small and large cells. Small cell lymphomas were referred to as 'well differentiated', intermediate as 'poorly differentiated' and large cell lymphomas as 'histiocytic' (instead of 'clasmatocytic,' indicating a phagocytic cell), the term used by Gall and Mallory. This system was subsequently modified to take into account the recently described lymphomas occurring in children, namely Burkitt lymphoma and lymphoblastic lymphoma.[62]

Repeated efforts to improve histologic and cytologic classification extended into the 1970s[63–65] but in the absence of a framework based on knowledge of cellular origins and differentiation pathways, such classifications relied largely upon descriptive morphology with, inevitably, a large subjective element. The absence of objective markers of specific diseases allowed the development of classification schemes to continue, in association with a constantly expanding nomenclature, which frequently hindered, rather than helped communication.

The importance of follicular lymphoma

The discovery of follicular lymphomas can be seen, in retrospect, as a major influence on lymphoma classification. Robb-Smith believed it important to distinguish proliferations in follicles from those in the rest of the lymphoid tissue, and germinal center cells were of great importance to Lennert's later work on lymphoma classification in Europe. Even before a functional understanding had been obtained, Lennert and his colleagues had performed a careful analysis of the cells present in normal germinal centers and recognized that these same cells were present in follicular lymphomas.[66–68] Lennert referred to the smaller lymphoid cells as 'germinocytes' (later, centrocytes) and

the larger ones as 'germinoblasts' (later centroblasts). He also recognized the presence of immunoblasts and the desmosome-bearing dendritic reticulum cell, a cell that had been described some years earlier[69] and which appeared to be found only in germinal centers. The dendritic reticulum cell had already been demonstrated to be associated, in some way, with antigen, and Lennert concluded that germinocytes and germinoblasts were transformed lymphocytes (Nowell had demonstrated the conversion of small lymphocytes into large 'blast' cells in 1960).[70] This seminal idea, based on meticulous cytological observations, was supported by the independent work of Lukes and Collins,[71] and Kojima and collaborators[72] and subsequently confirmed and elaborated upon when newer tools permitted the more detailed elucidation of the immunologic functions of the germinal center, which in turn provided the basis for our modern understanding of the origins of mature B cell neoplasms.

Hodgkin's disease

Since the linkage of a granulomatous appearance to the term 'Hodgkin's disease' subclassification, based on morphology alone, has continued. The understanding of the origin of the characteristic large cells of this disease, or set of diseases has only recently been determined. Clinical differences in the rate of progression of Hodgkin's disease had for long been observed, and Rosenthal, in 1936,[73] and Robb-Smith, some two years later,[39] attempted to relate histologic features to the clinical course of the disease. Rosenthal's proposal for histologic classification was not widely accepted, but provided the basis of Jackson and Parker's classification of 1944,[74] which had prognostic significance and became the standard classification for the next 20 years. Jackson and Parker proposed three histologic categories – the most frequently observed form of the disease, Hodgkin's granuloma (a term akin to lymphogranuloma), a less aggressive form, referred to as Hodgkin's paragranuloma, and an aggressive form that they called Hodgkin's sarcoma. The main drawback of this classification was that 80 percent of the cases fell into the granuloma category. Nevertheless, this classification sufficed for many years. Indeed, as techniques of radiation therapy improved, Peters, who was a pioneer in the development of modern treatment approaches, eventually demonstrated that the stage of disease at presentation was a better predictor of prognosis than histology.[75] Eventually, Lukes and Butler proposed a new classification based on an extensive study of servicemen with Hodgkin's disease, in which they described six categories based on the ratio of Sternberg–Reed cells to lymphocytes and the pattern of fibrosis.[76] In a subsequent meeting in Rye, New York,[77] a group of distinguished experts adopted a classification which included four categories (nodular sclerosing, mixed cellularity, lymphocyte predominant and lymphocyte depleted), which has served as the basis for classification ever since, although these categories are now referred to as 'classical' Hodgkin lymphoma to differentiate them from a more recently described subtype with variant Sternberg–Reed cells known as *nodular lymphocyte predominant* Hodgkin lymphoma (see Chapter 34).

Leukemia

Just a year after Virchow's subdivision of leukemia into splenic (myeloid) and lymphatic subtypes in 1856, Friedreich reported an acute form of the disease.[78] The ability to reproducibly differentiate between myeloid and lymphatic leukemia became possible much later, and only after advances in histology and cytology, particularly the use of the staining techniques developed by Ehrlich.[79] Türk is generally credited with the first modern description of chronic lymphocytic leukemia in 1903[80] and Ward noted the high frequency of acute lymphocytic leukemia in young children.[81] Like the lymphomas, the nature of diseases presenting as leukemia was vigorously debated. Most considered them to be neoplastic rather than of infectious origin, and in some leukemias the possibility that an infectious agent may be a predisposing factor remains a topic of research. The division into acute and chronic leukemia has persisted to the present day, although new entities, such as prolymphocytic leukemia and hairy cell leukemia have been described. It is also now well accepted that the terms 'leukemia' and 'lymphoma' relate to the clinical features of the disease rather than delineating pathologic subdivisions.

THE IMMUNOBIOLOGIC REVOLUTION

In the nineteenth century, immunology was an embryonic discipline. Immunity to some diseases after recovery (in those fortunate enough to recover) had been recognized, as well as the principle of vaccination, but the basis for this remained entirely unknown until the demonstration by von Behring of the presence of highly specific 'antitoxins' in the serum of patients who had recovered from diphtheria or tetanus, and the development of serum therapy for

these diseases. In 1904, Almoth Wright suggested that antibodies may coat bacteria and 'mark' them for phagocytosis – a process Wright referred to as opsoninization,[82] and one which would help link the later concept of a reticulo-endothelial system to the broader concept of an immune system. Michael Heidelberger was a major figure in the emergence of the field of immunochemistry. With his collaborators he showed that type-specific pneumococcal polysaccharide antigens could be precipitated by the relevant antibody[83] and, subsequently, that antibody could also cause agglutination of suspensions of antigen-bearing particles, including bacteria. He and his colleagues, Forrest Kendell and Elvin Kabat, were able to purify antibody and demonstrate that they were proteins – in fact, globulins.[84] This work was greatly expanded by Kabat, and Tai Te Wu, who not only demonstrated that antibodies are γ-globulins, but went on to identify the hypervariable, or complementarity-determining region and showed these regions to be the antigen-binding sites.[85] When techniques for amino-acid sequencing become available, Kabat and his collaborators produced an invaluable resource, *Sequences of proteins of immunological interest*, which includes sequence data for immunoglobulins, T cell antigen receptors and major histocompatibility complex proteins.[86]

The advances in the understanding of the nature of antibody were important to an understanding of the origins of lymphoid neoplasms, from both conceptual and practical perspectives. The critical observation was the recognition that antibodies are produced by lymphoid cells. As early as 1948, Fagreus had concluded that antibodies were produced by plasma cells,[87] a finding that was conformed within a few years by more sophisticated techniques. Then, in 1960, Nowell's discovery that exposure of small lymphocytes to phytohemagglutinin resulted in transformation to a large proliferating cell dispensed with the longstanding notion that the small lymphocyte is an end-stage cell.[70] After some years of uncertainty, the use of another plant extract, pokeweed mitogen, led to the recognition that suitably stimulated lymphocytes can synthesize immunoglobulin.[88] The stage was set for not only understanding the physiologic basis of immunity at both cellular and molecular levels, but also for the understanding of lymphoid neoplasms as malignant proliferations of cells of the immune system. In the 1970s it became clear that lymphocytes can be divided into two populations – B cells, which mediate humoral immunity and which bear surface immunoglobulin, and T cells, initially differentiated from B cells by their lack of surface immunoglobulin. T cells were subsequently shown to mediate cell-mediated immunity and also to regulate the proliferation of both B and T cells (see Chapter 9). The tools and methods required to make these observations, such as the fluorescent labeling techniques pioneered by Coons,[89] were also used to develop an understanding of the functional importance of the structural features of lymph nodes – knowledge that would prove to be essential to the understanding of lymphoid neoplasms and the confirmation of the earlier studies

Table 2.4 The first classification schemes based on immunologic concepts (although histologically defined)

Lennert *et al.* (1975)[91]	Lukes and Collins (1974)[92]
Low-grade malignant lymphomas	
Lymphocytoma	
B cell types	B cell
CLL, hairy cell leukemia	Small lymphocytic (CLL)
T cell types	T cell
Sézary syndrome (and	Sézary syndrome (and
mycosis fungoides?)	mycosis fungoides)
Others	
Immunocytoma	
(lymphoplasmacytoid)	
Lymphoplasmacytic	B cell
Lymphoplasmacytoid	Plasmacytoid lymphocyte
Polymorphic	
Germinocytoma (diffuse)	B cell
	Small cleaved FCC
	Large cleaved FCC
Germinoblastoma	
Follicular	Follicular
Follicular and diffuse	Follicular and diffuse
Nonsclerotic; sclerotic	Diffuse, with or without
(Bennett's type)	sclerosis
High-grade malignant lymphomas	
Germinoblastic sarcoma	
	B cell
	Large noncleaved FCC
Lymphoblastic sarcoma	
(including ALL)	
B cell types	B cell
Burkitt's tumor	Small noncleaved FCC
Non-Burkitt's tumor	Burkitt type
T cell type	T cell
Convoluted type of Lukes	Convoluted lymphocyte
Undefined	U cell (undefined)
Unclassifiable	Unclassifiable
Immunoblastic sarcoma	
	B cell
	Immunoblastic sarcoma
	T cell
	Immunoblastic sarcoma

CLL, chronic lymphocytic leukemia; FCC, follicular center cell.

performed by Lennert in Germany and Lukes and Collins in the USA – studies that had relied heavily on histologic and cytologic similarities between neoplastic cells and normal cells present in different microanatomic structures in lymphoid tissue (Table 2.4).[90–92] In the mid-1970s, monoclonal antibodies able to bind with exquisite specificity to epitopes on cellular proteins (sometimes carbohydrates) and therefore of immense value to the study of cell lineage markers in addition to many other wide-ranging applications were developed.[93]

Lymphocyte differentiation pathways and lymphoid neoplasia

Virchow's recognition that all cells arise from cells had implied that cellular differentiation must occur, but cytology alone had proved insufficient to elucidate differentiation pathways or to identify, with any degree of precision, the normal cells from which lymphoid neoplasms arise. Detailed characterization of the protein constituents of lymphoid cells, including lymphoid precursors, and of the cellular interactions that take place in the course of the immune response, permitted the gradual elucidation of the differentiation pathways of lymphoid cells, and the recognition of the importance of the bone marrow and thymus in lymphocyte ontogeny. It became clear that some neoplasms have the phenotype of lymphocyte precursors, namely acute lymphoblastic leukemia and lymphoblastic lymphoma and others the phenotype of mature lymphoid cells. Moreover, a number of lymphoid neoplasms were found to express T lymphocyte characteristics[94–96] and others were of the B lymphocyte lineage.[94,97,98] The goals of pioneer histopathologists, who had sought an understanding of lymphoid neoplasms in terms of normal histogenesis, but lacked the tools that would permit them to reproducibly differentiate normal cell types from each other and to relate them to particular lymphoid neoplasms, could finally be realized. Normal cells in the germinal centers and subsequently their adjacent structures, the mantle and marginal zones, could now be definitively shown to be the counterparts of the majority of the 'mature' lymphomas of B cell origin. Germinal centers, a term introduced by Flemming in 1885,[99] had for long been thought to be the site of lymphocyte production – a belief that proved to be partly true. Hellman had proposed, as early as 1921, a role for germinal centers in reactions against inflammatory or toxic insults (hence his term *Reaktionzentren*),[100] but their importance to the production of antibodies was not demonstrated until the early 1970s.[101]

The realization that germinal centers are the anatomic location in which primary humoral immune responses occur gave a new dimension to an understanding of the cellular origins of mature B cell lymphomas that account for the majority of all lymphomas. The new immunologic perspective clearly demonstrated that such neoplasms, as well as T lineage lymphomas with predominantly large cells, could not be derived from the phagocytic elements of lymph nodes, and that terms such as reticulum cell sarcoma, clasmatocytic lymphoma or histiocytic lymphoma were inappropriate.[102–105] However, non-neoplastic antigen-presenting follicular dendritic cells, which have a major role in creating the germinal centers of lymph nodes, are present in some more indolent lymphomas and were eventually recognized to be important to their follicular architecture, while in rare neoplasms, normal macrophages and epithelial cells can also be prominent due to the production of cytokines by the neoplastic cells (see Chapter 15).

The last purely histologic classification and the beginning of international consensus

It was many years before immunophenotyping was to become a routine part of pathologic diagnosis – this required familiarity with new technology as well as investments in sometimes expensive reagents, training in interpretation and more time to examine samples. Clinicians, at first, were largely unconvinced of the value of the new understanding of lymphoid malignancies to therapeutic decisions – in part because they continued to lump together several different categories for treatment purposes such that prognostic differences associated with immunophenotype were difficult to discern. Further, the problem that had dogged lymphoma pathologists for so long – the use of different terms for the same, or at least, overlapping entities, remained to be overcome. In the early 1980s there were six major classifications schemes in use. The difficulties this created in an age of air travel and greatly improved international communication through meetings and a plethora of journals led to a new era of collaboration whereby hematologic pathologists from many countries joined forces in an attempt to develop a consensus rather than each developing his or her own classification. In 1982, under the auspices of the US National Cancer Institute (NCI), a historic collaborative attempt to test the reproducibility and clinical relevance of the six major classification systems was undertaken by 12 pathologists. Because consensus building was a new idea in pathology, with the possible exception of the classification of Hodgkin disease, the collaboration was presented as an attempt to create a 'translation' system or 'formulation', i.e. to 'facilitate clinical comparisons of case reports and therapeutic trials' rather than to create yet another classification'.[55] In this study, the histologic slides and clinical records of 1175 cases of non-Hodgkin lymphoma were examined by the participating hematopathologists (six of whom had been instrumental in the development of one of the major classification scheme) and the diagnoses made were correlated with clinical information, primarily the outcome of therapy (patients had been treated with similar but not identical regimens). Although each of the extant classification schemes was shown to be able to identify different prognostic groups, an attempt was made to reach a consensus with respect to nomenclature. The resultant 'Working Formulation for Clinical Usage' separated lymphomas into 10 major categories on the basis of morphology alone (Table 2.5), each with a different survival expectancy. Survival curves for each of the 10 subtypes were rather evenly spread between 29 percent and 70 percent at 5 years, and this information was used to create three major prognostic groups which were referred to as low, intermediate

and high grade, perhaps in deference to the Kiel classification. Although terms from the Lukes and Collins scheme were used, the Working Formulation was, in effect, a descendent of the modified Rappaport classification. It quickly became used as a classification in its own right and largely replaced the Rappaport scheme in North America, although the Kiel classification, in successive versions, continued to predominate in Europe.

Even before the creation of the Working Formulation, immunologic techniques had been used to identify or improve the definition of a number of entities (most had been previously described with more or less precision on the basis of clinical and/or morphological characteristics) that were often referred to in different classification schemes by different names. These included lymphoblastic lymphoma,[95,96] centrocytic/mantle cell lymphoma, centrocytic/centroblastic/follicular lymphoma,[105–107] marginal cell lymphoma,[108,109] centroblastic, immunoblastic or diffuse large B cell lymphoma[105,110] and intestinal T cell lymphoma.[111] Moreover, classification systems with more of an immunobiologic basis, even if dependent exclusively on morphology, had been published – and had been included among those examined in the development of the Working Formulation (Table 2.5). It could, thus, be argued that the Working Formulation was outdated before it was published. But immunologic techniques did not become routine for many more years, during which time the Formulation continued to be used, although the existence of entities not included in the Formulation led to increasing difficulties in its application. It also became clear that even the combination of morphology and immunophenotyping provided insufficient precision to be sure that all of the recently defined categories were, in fact, discrete pathologic entities. Moreover, although more objective than morphology, variability in reagents and techniques used for immunophenotyping led, and continue to lead, to problems of reproducibility and interpretation among pathology laboratories. However, new technologies that were to prove to be of considerable importance to both the understanding of lymphoid neoplasia and its classification were simultaneously emerging.

BEYOND THE CELL: CYTOGENETICS AND MOLECULAR GENETICS

At the same time as the immunobiologic revolution was occurring, improvements in cytogenetic techniques led to the recognition by Rowley, in 1973, that the abnormally small G-group chromosome consistently present in chronic myeloid leukemia is caused by a translocation.[112] In 1982, Zech et al.[113] showed that the 14q+ abnormality discovered by Manolov and Manolova[114] in Burkitt lymphoma is also caused by a chromosomal translocation and, in the same year, Yunis et al. recognized characteristic chromosomal abnormalities in follicular lymphomas and some large cell lymphomas.[115] Thus it was demonstrated that specific

Table 2.5 The Working Formulation for Clinical Usage

Low grade	Intermediate grade	High grade
A. Small lymphocytic	D. Follicular large cell	H. Large cell immunoblastic
B. Follicular small-cleaved cell	E. Diffuse small cleaved cell	I. Lymphoblastic
C. Follicular mixed small-cleaved and large cell	F. Diffuse mixed small and large cell	J. Small non-cleaved cell (Burkitt's and non-Burkitt's type)
	G. Diffuse large cell	

Note: the Working Formulation was based on the following classification schemes: Rappaport,[54] Dorfman,[64] Lukes and Collins,[92] Kiel[106] and the British Lymphoma system.

genetic abnormalities are associated with particular neoplasms (although the story is, unfortunately, not quite so simple – see Chapter 22) and a potential new diagnostic tool, inconceivable in the first half of the twentieth century, had emerged. This advance was to prove as important as the new immunologic concepts in understanding the origins of lymphoid neoplasia, since the discovery of chromosomal translocations led naturally to questions concerning their functional significance. It was Burkitt lymphoma, a tumor first recognized as a clinicopathologic entity in Uganda in the late 1950s and early 1960s[116,117] that provided the critical insight which pointed the way to the answer to this question. Several investigators[118,119] demonstrated that in Burkitt lymphoma the characteristic chromosomal translocations result in the juxtaposition of immunoglobulin genes to a human gene bearing close similarity to the oncogene (MYC) of an avian retrovirus (myelocytomatosis virus, MC29) capable of inducing tumors in birds and of transforming human fibroblasts.[120] Although many years and a great deal of experimental work were required, this finding eventually led to a general understanding of the mechanism of deregulation of the human homolog of MYC and its role in the pathogenesis of Burkitt lymphoma (although even now, many details remain to be elucidated). The *MYC*–immunoglobulin translocations provided a model for understanding other, subsequently identified chromosomal translocations involving antigen receptor genes (i.e. immunoglobulin or T cell receptor), and led to the discovery of numerous other genes whose overexpression, or perhaps better stated, inappropriate expression, brought about by chromosomal translocation, is an important element in the genesis of lymphoid neoplasms (see Chapters 22 and 25).[121,122] Determining the function of these genes led to the elucidation of important mechanisms of neoplastic transformation, including the role of transcription factors, such as MYC and nuclear factor κB and the inhibition of apoptosis, e.g. by creating an imbalance between genes that promote apoptosis, such as *BAX*, and those that inhibit apoptosis, such as *BCL2* (see Chapter 17).

Cytogenetics and molecular genetic observations have refined our concepts of the nature of a pathologic entity, but new questions have arisen because of the frequent lack of congruity of cytogenetic or molecular genetic findings with histology or immunophenotype. In some cases, the same type of translocation is present in diseases which are histologically and/or phenotypically different, whereas in other circumstances, what appears to be the same disease on histologic, immunophenotypic and clinical grounds can be associated with several different chromosomal abnormalities.[123] This should not be surprising, since it is apparent that there are several molecular pathways to the same (or essentially the same) functional end result, such that there may be, on the one hand, a range, more or less narrow, of histologic and immunophenotypic characteristics for each molecularly defined entity and on the other hand, somewhat 'fuzzy' boundaries between different entities. In some cases a different line would be drawn when using histology versus immunophenotype or cyto- or molecular genetic abnormalities. Indeed, some categories such as diffuse large B cell lymphoma consist of several 'diseases' whichever of these criteria are used, with potentially different etiologies and differences in response to therapy. This has become even more apparent through molecular profiling, e.g. of aggressive B cell lymphomas.[124–126] Although molecular profiling (see Chapter 24) does appear able to provide a precise definition of each neoplastic entity, even molecular profiles may be intermediate between two well-defined neoplasms.[125] This is consistent with the concept that neoplastic behavior arises as a consequence of a set of molecular abnormalities occurring in lymphoid cells at specific stages of differentiation. Some neoplasms may be locked into an intermediate state, while in other cases, just as one cell type differentiates into another, so one neoplastic disease may also give rise to another – a process known as 'transformation' in which a relatively indolent neoplasm evolves (or at least, a clone of cells present in the neoplasm evolves) into a more aggressive neoplasm. Whereas the diagnosis itself provides significant ability to predict response to any given treatment regimen, cytogenetic or molecular characteristics, including single nucleotide polymorphisms (SNPs), that are not consistently present in a particular pathologic entity, may be associated with different clinical behavior, including response to treatment (see Chapter 85).[127–129]

Molecular techniques have also proved valuable in other ways. Clonal rearrangements of antigen receptor genes can be used to determine lineage in cases where histopathology is inconclusive,[111,130] or to provide evidence of value in determining whether a pathologic process is inflammatory or neoplastic (e.g. in angioimmunoblastic lymphadeno-pathy).[131] In all, there is little doubt that a combination of cytology, histology, immunophenotyping and molecular techniques has already led, and will continue to lead, to a more profound understanding of the nature of lymphoid neoplasia, which in turn, will have important implications for the development of optimal therapy, including therapy specifically targeted at molecular lesions. Molecular analysis also shows promise of eventually leading to an elucidation of the mechanisms whereby environmental factors, such as viruses and chemicals, predispose to the development of lymphoid neoplasms (see Part 2 of the book).[132,133]

PRESENT AND FUTURE

The Working Formulation for Clinical Usage was the last purely histologic classification of lymphomas. For this reason, it could not be effective as a 'translation system' since each of its morphologic categories were subsequently shown by immunohistochemical and cytogenetic analysis to include multiple types of lymphoid neoplasm. Thus, in retrospect, perhaps the most valuable outcome of the attempt to develop a classification that could be universally used lay not in the Formulation itself, but in the initiation of a new era of international collaboration among leading hematologic pathologists. Further collaborative efforts on the part of European and American pathologists were prompted by the discoveries made possible by the newer techniques and soon led to the development of a new classification scheme, the Revised European–American classification of Lymphoid Neoplasms (REAL).[134] This classification, which included immunophenotypic and cytogenetic information in the definitions, quite rapidly evolved into the World Health Organization (WHO) classification,[135] which is now widely considered to be the global diagnostic standard. The WHO classification will undergo periodic revision as new techniques are developed or existing techniques are refined and used for diagnostic purposes, but, importantly, modifications will be based on consensus reached by experts, thus avoiding the multiple interpretations of terms that has plagued the classification of lymphoid neoplasms since the early nineteenth century (see Chapter 18 for latest version).

It seems inevitable that molecular profiling, whether at RNA, micro-RNA or protein levels, will become of increasing diagnostic importance, since the gene expression profiles, in conjunction with mutations and polymorphisms (which may have functional consequences), reflect on the one hand the normal counterpart cell and on the other hand, the consequences of pathogenetic abnormalities, such that they must ultimately determine all of the biologic characteristics of tumor cells – including their cytology and histology, as well as their response to treatment (although this is likely to be modified by host factors, both genetic

and environmental). The new molecular tools will also lead to a much deeper understanding of lymphomagenesis, which will, in turn, give rise to improved classification and therefore permit a better understanding of treatment results and an improved ability to determine the value of specific treatment approaches in more precisely defined entities, although there is much research, including large clinical trials, that must be done before the full benefits of the molecular era can be realized. These recently developed technologies are still only available at major centers, so for some years, rather than replacing standard pathological techniques, molecular profiling, along with newer cytogenetic tests, such as fluorescent *in situ* hybridization, comparative genomic hybridization and whole genome scanning for polymorphisms, are likely to be used to improve the interpretation of histopathology and immunophenotyping, leading perhaps to specific immunophenotypic algorithms, such as that recently proposed by Hans *et al.* for diffuse large B cell lymphomas.[136] A number of technical or interpretive problems also need to be addressed, such as the variable presence of nonmalignant cells in the tumor (which may itself be of diagnostic and of potentially prognostic importance), and familiarity of pathologists and clinicians with these new tools and the interpretation of results. Although morphology is likely to remain an important element of the diagnostic armamentarium for the foreseeable future, it will surely ultimately be replaced by purely molecular techniques; although Virchow's recognition of the importance of the cell to the definition of neoplastic diseases remains as true today as it was one and a half centuries ago, it is the molecular milieu which ultimately defines the cell, and hence the neoplasm.

KEY POINTS

- Lymphoid neoplasms were first recognized as lymph node swellings (often accompanied by splenomegaly) that developed and progressed in the absence of any of the known explanations at the time (e.g. acute illness, local infection).
- Leukemia was observed initially at post mortem by the white color of the blood, usually also in patients with enlarged spleens and frequently with swollen lymph nodes.
- Virchow's view of 'cellular pathology' represented a major advance over previous concepts of disease, and led to the recognition that microscopic examination of tissue could be used as a basis for the classification of neoplasms. It has remained so until the present time, although its value has been enormously enhanced by the use of antibodies and molecular probes capable of identifying specific proteins, chromosomal translocations and molecular genetic lesions.

- In the absence of a firm conceptual foundation for classification, the first classification schemes were largely speculative.
- The identification of the reticuloendothelial system, antibodies and lymphocyte transformation led eventually to our present understanding of the immune system, which has finally provided the much needed conceptual basis for classification.
- New techniques at the level of the whole, or a part of the genome or proteome are likely to add greatly to our understanding of pathogenesis, classification, diagnosis and prognosis – with consequent benefits to treatment.

REFERENCES

- = Key primary paper
- = Major review article

- 1. Virchow R. *Die krankhaften Geschwülste.* Dreissig Vorlesungen gehalten wahrend des Winter-semesters 1862–1863 an der Universität zu Berlin. Berlin: Hirschwald, 1864–1865: 564–620.
- 2. Cruickshank W. *The anatomy of the absorbing vessels of the human body.* London: Nicol, 1786.
3. Craigie D. *Elements of general pathological anatomy.* Edinburgh: Black, 1828: 250.
- 4. Hodgkin T. On some morbid appearances of the absorbent glands and spleen. *Trans Med Chir Soc Lond* 1832; **xvii**: 68–114.
5. Wilks S. Cases of lardaceous disease and some allied affections, with remarks. *Guys Hosp Rep* 1856; **17**(Ser. II, vol. 2): 102–32.
6. Wunderlich CA. Zwei Fälle von progressiven muliplen Lymphdrüsenhypertrophien. *Arch Physiol Heilk* 1858; **12**: 122–31.
7. Trousseau A. De l'adénie. *Clin Méd l'Hotel-Dieu Paris* 1865; **3**: 555–81.
8. Wilks S. Cases of enlargement of the lymphatic glands and spleen (or, Hodgkin's disease), with remarks. *Guys Hosp Gaz* 1865; **23**: 528–32.
- 9. Virchow R. *Weisses Blut.* Neue Notizen aus dem Gebiet der Natur und Heilkunde (Froriep's Neue Notizen) 1845; **36**: 1–6.
- 10. Craigie D. Case of disease of the spleen in which death took place in consequence of purulent matter in the blood. *Edinburgh Med J* 1845; **64**: 400–13.
- 11. Bennett JH. Case of hypertrophy of the spleen and liver, in which death took place from suppuration of the blood. *Edinburgh Med J* 1845; **64**: 413–23.
12. Cohnheim J. Ein Fall von Pseudoleukämia. *Virchows Arch* 1862; **33**: 451–4.
13. Wunderlich CA. Pseudoleukämie, Hodgin'sche Krankheit oder multiple Lymphadenome ohne Leukämie. *Arch d Heilkunde* 1866: 531–52.
14. Osler W. *The principles and practice of medicine.* New York: Appleton and Company, 1892: 704–8.
15. Dreschfeld J. Clinical lecture on acute Hodgkin's (or pseudoleucocythemia). *Br Med J* 1882; **i**: 893–6.
- 16. Kundrat H. Über Lymphosarkomatosis. *Wien Klin Wochenschr* 1893; **6**: 211–13, 234–9.
17. Stevens. *Glasgow Med J* 1891.
18. Sternberg C. Über ein eigenartige unter dem Bilde der Pseudoleukämie verlaufende Tuberculose des Lymphatischen Apparates. *Z Heilk* 1898; **xix**: 21–90.
19. Pel PK. Pseudoleukämie oder chronisches Rückfallsfieber. *Berlin Klin Wochenschr* 1885; **24**: 644–6.
20. Ebstein W von. Das chronische Rückfallsfieber. *Berl kl Wochenschr* 1887; **24**: 565–8.
- 21. Reed DM. The pathological changes of Hodgkin's disease with special reference to its relation to tuberculosis. *Johns Hopkins Med J* 1902; **x**: 133–96.
22. Coley WB. Hodgkin's disease, a type of sarcoma. *N Y State J Med* 1907; **lxxxv**: 577–83.
23. Paltauf R. Lymphosarkom (lymphosarkomatose, pseudoleukämia, myelom, chlorom). *Ergeb Allg Pathol Pathol Anat* 1896; **3**: 652–91.
- 24. Sternberg C. Primärerkrankungen des lymphatischen und hämatopoetischen Apparates etc. *Ergeb Allg Pathol Pathol Anat* 1903; 9.
- 25. Ghon A, Roman B. Über Lymphosarkom. *Frankf Z Pathol* 1916; **xix**: 1.
26. Sternberg C. Leukosarkomatose and myeloblastenleukaamie. *Beitr Pathol* 1916; **61**: 75.
27. Ginsburg S. Lymphosarcoma and Hodgkin's disease: biologic characteristics. *Ann Intern Med* 1934; 14–36.
- 28. Alibert JLM. *Description des maladies de la peau, observé á l'hôpital Saint-Louis, et expositions des meilliers méthodes suivies pour le traitement.* Paris: Barrois L'Aine et Fils, 1806–1827.
- 29. Kaposi M. Mycosis fungoides (framboesia). In: *Pathology and treatment of diseases of the skin for practitioners and students.* New York: Willian Wood and Co, 1895: 593–8.
30. Borst M. *Die Lehre von den Geschwülsten.* Wiesbaden, 1902.
- 31. Brill NE, Baehr G, Rosenthal N. Generalized giant lymph follicle hyperplasia of the lymph nodes and spleen. *JAMA* 1925; **84**: 668–71.
- 32. Symmers D. Follicular lymphadenopathy with splenomegaly. A newly recognized disease of the lymphatic system. *Arch Pathol Lab Med* 1927; **3**: 816–20.
33. Evans TS, Doan CA. Giant follicle hyperplasia: a study of its incidence, histopathologic variability, and the frequency of sarcoma and secondary hypersplenic complications. *Ann Intern Med* 1954; **40**: 851–80.
34. Rosenberg SA, Diamond HD, Jaslowitz B, Craver LF. Lymphosarcoma: a review of 1269 cases. *Medicine* 1961; **40**: 31–84.

●35. Gall EA, Morrison HR, Scott AT. The follicular type of malignant lymphoma: a survey of 63 cases. *Ann Intern Med* 1941; **14**: 2073–90.

36. Metchnikoff E. Untersuchungen über die intracelluläre Verdauung bei wirbellosen Thieren. *Arb zool Inst Univ Wien* 1883; **5**: 141–68.

●37. Aschoff L. *Das retikuloendotheliale System. Vorträge über Pathologie.* Jena, 1905.

38. Ewing J. General pathology of lymphosarcoma. *Bull N Y Acad Med* 1939; **15**: 92–103.

●39. Robb-Smith AHT. Reticulosis and reticulosarcoma: histological classification. *J Pathol Bacteriol* 1938; **47**: 457–80.

40. Maximov AA. Relation of blood cells to connective tissues and endothelium. *Annu Rev Physiol* 1924; **iv**: 431.

41. Klemperer P. Relationship of the reticulum to diseases of the hematopoietic system. In: *Libman Anniversary Volumes*, Vol. 2. New York: The International Press, 1932: 665.

42. Medlar EM. An interpretation of the nature of Hodgkin's disease. *Am J Pathol* 1931; **7**: 499–513.

43. Oliver J. The relation of Hodgkin's disease to lymphosarcoma and endothelioma. *J Med Res* 1913; **xxix**: 191–207.

44. Ewing JJ. Endothelioma of lymph nodes. *J Med Res* 1913; **28**: 1.

●45. Willis RA. *The spread of tumors in the human body.* London: J and A Churchill Ltd, 1934.

46. Oberling C. Les réticulosarcomes et les réticuloendotheliosarcomes de la moelle osseuse (sarcomes d'Ewing). *Bull Assoc Fr Etud Cancer* 1928; **17**: 250–6.

47. Ewing JJ. Diffuse endothelioma of bone. *Proc N York Pathol Soc* 1921; **21**: 17–24.

●48. Rhoads CP. The reticulo-endothelial system. A general review. *N Engl J Med* 1928; **198**: 76–8.

49. Roulet F. Das Primäre Retothelesarkom der Lymph-knoten. *Virchows Arch Pathol Anat Physiol Klin Med* 1930; **277**: 15–47.

50. Parker F Jr, Jackson H Jr. Primary reticulum cell sarcoma of bone. *Surg Gynecol Obstet* 1939; **68**: 45–53.

51. Warren S, Picena JP. Reticulum cell sarcoma of lymph nodes. *Am J Pathol* 1941; **17**: 385–93.

●52. Rosenberg SA, Diamond HD, Dargeon HW, Craver LF. Lymphosarcoma in childhood. *N Engl J Med* 1958; **259**: 505–12.

●53. Gall EA, Mallory TB. Malignant lymphoma. A clinico-pathological survey of 618 cases. *Am J Pathol* 1942; **18**: 381–429.

●54. Rappaport H. Tumors of the hematopoietic system. In: *Atlas of tumor pathology, section iii, fascicle 8.* Washington, DC: Armed Forces Institute of Pathology, 1966: 97–161.

55. National Cancer Institute Sponsored Study of Classifications of Non-Hodgkin's Lymphomas. Summary and description of a working formulation for clinical usage. *Cancer* 1982; **49**: 2112–35.

●56. Callender GR. Tumors and tumor like conditions of the lymphocyte, the myelocyte, the erythrocyte and the reticulum cell. *Am J Pathol* 1934; **10**: 443–65.

57. Stout AP. The results of treatment of lymphosarcoma. *N Y State J Med* 1947; **47**: 158–64.

58. Sugarbaker ED, Craver LF. Lymphosarcoma: a study of 196 cases with biopsy. *JAMA* 1940; **115**: 17–23, 112–17.

59. Gall EA. Enigmas in lymphoma, reticulum cell sarcoma and mycosis fungoides. *Minn Med* 1955; **38**: 674–81.

60. Rappaport H, Winter WJ, Hicks EB. Follicular lymphoma. A re-evaluation of its position in the scheme of malignant lymphoma, based on a survey of 253 cases. *Cancer* 1956; **9**: 792–821.

61. Gall EA, Rappaport H. Seminar on diseases of lymph nodes and spleen. In: *Proceedings of the 23rd Annual Seminar of the American Society of Clinical Pathologists, October, 1957.* American Society of Clinical Pathologists, 1958.

62. Rappaport H, Braylan RC. In: Rebuck JW, Berard CW, Abell MR (eds). *The reticuloendothelial system.* International Academy of Pathology Monograph, no. 16. Baltimore: Williams and Wilkins, 1975: 1–19.

63. Bennett MH, Farrer-Brown G, Henry K *et al.* Classification of non-Hodgkin's lymphomas. *Lancet* 1974; **ii**: 405–6.

64. Dorfman RF. The non-Hodgkin's lymphomas. In: Rebuck JW, Berard CW, Abell MR (eds). *The reticuloendothelial system.* International Academy of Pathology Monograph, no. 16. Baltimore: Williams and Wilkins, 1975: 262–81.

65. Mathé G, Rappaport H, O'Conor GT *et al.* Histological and cytological typing of neoplastic diseases of hematopoietic and lymphoid tissues. *WHO international classification of diseases*, no. 14. Geneva: World Health Organization, 1976.

●66. Lennert K. Über die Erkennung von Keimzentrumszellen. In: Lymphknotenausstrich. *Klin Wochenschr* 1957; **35**: 1130–2.

67. Lennert K. *Pathologie der halslymphknoten.* Berlin: Springer Verlag, 1964.

●68. Lennert K. Follicular lymphoma. A tumor of germinal centers. *Gann Monograph Cancer Res* 1973; **15**: 217–23.

69. Maruyama K, Masuda T. Electron microscopic observation on the germinal center of the lymph node in guinea pigs sensitized with sheep erythrocytes. *Ann Rep Inst Virus Res Kyoto Univ* 1964; **7**: 149–52.

●70. Nowell PC. Phytohemagglutinin: an initiator of mitosis in cultures of normal human leukocytes. *Cancer Res* 1960; **20**: 462–6.

71. Lukes F, Collins RD. New observations on follicular lymphoma. *Gann Monograph Cancer Res* 1973; **15**: 209–15.

72. Kojima M, Imai Y, Mori N. A concept of follicular lymphoma. A proposal for the existence of a neoplasm originating from the germinal center. *Gann Monograph Cancer Res* 1973; **15**: 195–208.

73. Rosenthal SR. Significance of tissue lymphocytes in prognosis of lymphogranulomatosis. *Arch Pathol* 1936; **26**: 628–46.

●74. Jackson H Jr, Parker F. Hodgkin's disease, II, Pathology. *N Engl J Med* 1944; **231**: 35–44.

75. Peters MVA. Study of survivals in Hodgkin's disease treated radiologically. *AJR Am J Roentgenol* 1950; **63**: 299–311.

●76. Lukes RJ, Butler JJ. The pathology and nomenclature of Hodgkin's disease. *Cancer Res* 1966; **26**: 1063–81.

77. Lukes RJ, Craver LF, Hall TC *et al.* Report of the nomenclature committee in symposium: obstacles to the control of Hodgkin's disease. *Cancer Res* 1966; **26** (Part 1): 1311.

78. Friedreich N. Ein neuer fall von leukämie. *Arch Anat Pathol (Paris)* 1857; **12**: 37.

79. Ehrlich P. Farbenanolytische untersuchungen zur histologic and klinik des blutes. Berlin: Hirschwald, 1891.

80. Türk W. Ein system der lymphomatosen. *Wien Klin Wochenschr* 1903; **16**: 1073.

81. Ward G. Infective theory of acute leukaemia. *Br J Child Dis* 1917; **14**: 10–20.

82. Wright AE. On the need for abandoning much in immunology that has been regarded as assured. *Proc R Soc Med* 1942; **35**: 161–86.

83. Heidelberger M, Kendall FE. A quantitative study of the precipitin reaction between type III pneumococcus polysaccharide and purified homologous antibody. *J Exp Med* 1929; **50**: 809–23.

84. Heidelberger M. A 'pure' organic chemist's downward path: chapter 2. *Annu Rev Biochem* 1979; **48**: 1–21.

85. Wu TT, Kabat EA. An analysis of the sequences of the variable regions of Bence Jones proteins and myeloma light chains and their implications for antibody complementarity. *J Exp Med* 1970; **132**: 211–50.

86. Johnson G, Wu TT. Kabat data base and its implications: 30 years after the first variability plot. *Nucleic Acids Res* 2000; **28**: 214–18.

87. Fagreus A. Antibody production in relation to the development of plasma cells. *Acta Med Scand* 1948; **204**(Suppl).

88. Greaves MF, Flad HD. Effect of lymphocyte stimulants on specific antibody synthesis *in vitro*. *Nature* 1968; **219**: 975–8.

●89. Coons AH. The beginnings of immunofluorescence. *J Immunol* 1961; **87**: 499–503.

●90. Seligmann M, Grouet JC, Preud'Homme JL. The immunological diagnosis of human leukemias and lymphomas. An overview. In: Thierfelder S, Rodt H, Thiel E (eds). *Immunological diagnosis of leukemias and lymphomas*. Berlin: Springer Verlag, 1977: 1–16.

●91. Lennert K, Mohri N, Stein H *et al.* The histopathology of malignant lymphoma. *Br J Haematol* 1975; **31** (Suppl. II): 193–203.

92. Lukes RJ, Collins RD. Immunologic characterization of human malignant lymphomas. *Cancer* 1974; **34**: 1488–503.

●93. Köhler G, Milstein C. Continuous culture of fused cells secreting antibody of predefined specificity. *Nature* 1975; **256**: 495–7.

94. Magrath IT. Lymphocyte differentiation pathways – an essential basis for the comprehension of lymphoid neoplasia. *J Natl Cancer Inst* 1981; **67**: 501–14.

95. Stein H, Petersen N, Gaedicke G *et al.* Lymphoblastic lymphoma of convoluted or acid phosphatase type – a tumor of T precursor cells. *Int J Cancer* 1976; **17**: 292–5.

96. Smith JL, Clein GP, Barker CR *et al.* Characterisation of malignant mediastinal lymphoid neoplasm (Sternberg sarcoma) as thymic in origin. *Lancet* 1973; **i**: 74–7.

●97. Seligmann M, Preud'Homme JL, Brouet JC. B and T cell markers in human proliferative blood diseases and primary immunodeficiencies, with special reference to membrane bound immunoglobulins. *Transplant Rev* 1973; **16**: 85–113.

98. Brown G, Greaves MF, Lister TA *et al.* Expression of human T and B lymphocyte cell-surface markers on leukaemic cells. *Lancet* 1974; **2**: 753–5.

99. Flemming W. Studien über Regeneration der Gewebe. *Arch Mikrobiol Anat* 1885; **24**: 50.

100. Hellman T. Studien über das lymphoide Gewebe. Die Deutung der Sekundärfollikel. *Beitr Pathol Anat* 1921; **68**: 333.

101. Kojima M, Imai Y. Genesis and function of germinal center. *Gann Monograph Cancer Res* 1973; **15**: 1–24.

●102. Jaffe ES, Shevach EM, Frank MM *et al.* Nodular lymphoma – evidence for origin from follicular B lymphocytes. *N Engl J Med* 1974; **290**: 813–19.

103. Stein H, Gerdes J, Mason D. The normal and malignant germinal center. *Clin Adv Hematol Oncol* 1982; **11**: 531–59.

●104. Stein H, Lennert K, Feller AC *et al.* Immunohistological analysis of human lymphoma: correlation of histological and immunological categories. *Adv Cancer Res* 1984; **42**: 67–147.

●105. Harris NL, Nadler LM, Bhan AK. Immunohistologic characterization of two malignant lymphomas of germinal center type (centroblastic/centrocytic and centrocytic) with monoclonal antibodies: follicular and diffuse lymphomas of small cleaved cell types are related but distinct entities. *Am J Pathol* 1984; **117**: 262–72.

106. Takeshita M, Masuda Y, Sumiyoshi Y, Ohshima K *et al.* Clinicopathologic, enzyme and histochemical studies of centrocytic (mantle cell) lymphoma: comparison with other types of low-grade B cell lymphoma based on the updated Kiel classification. *Acta Pathol Jpn* 1993; **43**: 244–52.

●107. Zukerberg LR, Medeiros LJ, Ferry JA, Harris NL. Diffuse low-grade B-cell lymphomas. Four clinically distinct subtypes defined by a combination of morphologic and immunophenotypic features. *Am J Clin Pathol* 1993; **100**: 373–85.

●108. Isaacson P, Wright DH. Malignant lymphoma of mucosa-associated lymphoid tissue. A distinctive type of B-cell lymphoma. *Cancer* 1984; **52**: 1410–16.

109. Nizze H, Cogliatti SB, von Schilling C *et al.* Monocytoid B-cell lymphoma: morphological variants and relationship to low-grade B-cell lymphoma of the mucosa-associated lymphoid tissue. *Histopathology* 1991; **18**: 403–14.

110. Horning SJ, Doggett RS, Warnke RA *et al.* Clinical relevance of immunologic phenotype in diffuse large cell lymphoma. *Blood* 1984; **63**: 1209–15.

●111. Isaacson PG, O'Connor NT, Spencer J *et al.* Malignant histiocytosis of the intestine: a T-cell lymphoma. *Lancet* 1985; **2**: 688–91.

●112. Rowley JD. A new consistent chromosomal abnormality in chronic myelogenous leukemia identified by quinacrine fluorescence and Giemsa staining. *Nature* 1973; **243**: 290–1.

●113. Zech L, Hagland U, Nilsson K *et al.* Characteristic chromosomal abnormalities in biopsies and lymphoid-cell lines from patients with Burkitt's and non-Burkitt's lymphomas. *Int J Cancer* 1982; **17**: 47–56.

114. Manolov G, Manolova Y. Marker band in one chromosome 14 from Burkitt lymphomas. *Nature* 1972; **237**: 33–4.

115. Yunis JJ, Oken MM, Kaplan ME *et al.* Distinctive chromosomal abnormalities in histological subtypes of non-Hodgkin's lymphomas. *N Engl J Med* 1982; **307**: 1231–6.

●116. Burkitt D. A sarcoma involving the jaws in African children. *Br J Surg* 1958; **46**: 218–23.

●117. O'Conor G. Malignant lymphoma in African children. Cancer. II. A pathological entity. *Cancer* 1961; **14**: 270–83.

●118. Taub R, Kirsch I, Morton C *et al.* Translocation of the c-myc gene into the immunoglobulin heavy chain locus in human Burkitt lymphoma and murine plasmacytoma cells. *Proc Natl Acad Sci U S A* 1982; **79**: 7837.

●119. Dalla-Favera R, Bregni M, Erikson J *et al.* Human c-myc onc gene is located on the region of chromosome 8 that is translocated in Burkitt lymphoma cells. *Proc Natl Acad Sci U S A* 1982; **79**: 7824.

120. Lautenberger JA, Schulz RA, Garon CF *et al.* Molecular cloning of avian myelocytomatosis virus (MC29) transforming sequences. *Proc Natl Acad Sci U S A* 1981; **78**: 1518–22.

121. Bernicot I, Douet-Guilbert N, Le Bris MJ *et al.* Molecular cytogenetics of IGH rearrangements in non-Hodgkin B-cell lymphoma. *Cytogenet Genome Res* 2007; **118**: 345–52.

122. O'Neil J, Look AT. Mechanisms of transcription factor deregulation in lymphoid cell transformation. *Oncogene* 2007; **26**: 6838–49.

123. Herens C, Lambert F, Quintanilla-Martinez L *et al.* Cyclin D1-negative mantle cell lymphoma with cryptic t(12;14)(p13;q32) and cyclin D2 overexpression. *Blood* 2008; **111**: 1745–6.

●124. Alizadeh AA, Eisen MB, Davis RE *et al.* Distinct types of diffuse large B-cell lymphoma identified by gene expression profiling. *Nature* 2000; **403**: 503–11.

●125. Hummel M, Bentink S, Berger H *et al.* A biologic definition of Burkitt's lymphoma from transcriptional and genomic profiling. *N Engl J Med* 2006; **354**: 2419–30.

●126. Dave SS, Fu K, Wright GW *et al.* Lymphoma/leukemia molecular profiling project: molecular diagnosis of Burkitt's lymphoma. *N Engl J Med* 2006; **354**: 2431–42.

●127. Rosenwald A, Wright G, Chan WC *et al.* Lymphoma/leukemia molecular profiling project: the use of molecular profiling to predict survival after chemotherapy for diffuse large-B-cell lymphoma. *N Engl J Med* 2002; **346**: 1937–47.

128. Hohaus S, Mansueto G, Massini G. Glutathione-S-transferase genotypes influence prognosis in follicular non-Hodgkin's lymphoma. *Leuk Lymphoma* 2007; **48**: 564–9.

129. Lee JJ, Kim DH, Lee NY *et al.* Interleukin-10 gene polymorphism influences the prognosis of T-cell non-Hodgkin lymphomas. *Br J Haematol* 2007; **137**: 329–36.

130. Svachova M, Tichy M. PCR analysis of immunoglobulin heavy chain and TCR gene rearrangements in diagnosis of lymphoproliferative disorders on formalin-fixed, paraffin-embedded tissues. *Neoplasma* 2008; **55**: 36–41.

131. Feller A, Griesser H, Schilling C *et al.* Clonal gene rearrangement patterns correlate with immunophenotype and clinical parameters in patients with angio-immunoblastic lymphoadenopathy. *Am J Pathol* 1988; **133**: 549–56.

132. Franchini G. Molecular mechanisms of human T-cell leukemia/lymphotropic virus type I infection. *Blood* 1995; **86**: 3619–39.

133. Kirsch IR, Lipkowitz S. A measure of genomic instability and its relevance to lymphomagenesis. *Cancer Res* 1992; **52**(Suppl): s5545–46.

●134. Harris N, Jaffe ES, Stein H *et al.* A revised European–American classification of lymphoid neoplasms: a proposal from the international lymphoma study group. *Blood* 1994; **84**: 1361–92.

●135. Jaffe ES, Harris NL, Stein H, Vardiman JW (eds). *World Health Organization classification of tumors: pathology and genetics of tumors of haematopoietic and lymphoid tissues.* France: Lyon, IARC Press, 2001.

136. Hans CP, Weisenburger DD, Greiner TC *et al.* Confirmation of the molecular classification of diffuse large B-cell lymphoma by immunohistochemistry using a tissue microarray. *Blood* 2004; **103**: 275–82.

PART 2

EPIDEMIOLOGY

3

Descriptive epidemiology

CATHY BURTON, ANDREW JACK, PETER ADAMSON AND EVE ROMAN

INTRODUCTION

Classic descriptive epidemiology is concerned with the occurrence of disease in human populations in terms of the characteristics of person, place and time.[1] Of particular concern here are differences with age and between the sexes, as well as variations in the geographic distribution and trends over extended periods of time.

The descriptive epidemiology of hematologic malignancies has traditionally considered four broad disease groups – leukemia, multiple myeloma (MM), Hodgkin lymphoma (HL) and non-Hodgkin lymphoma (NHL). This classification, which predates the development of effective therapy, stems from the recognition of entities in the early part of the twentieth century. This was long before there was any real understanding of the relation between hematologic malignancies, the normal bone marrow and the immune system, and before anything was known about the cellular and genetic basis of malignant transformation.

Taxonomic concepts and models have considerable impact on descriptive epidemiologic observations, patterns and trends. Within oncology, this is particularly true for the lymphoid neoplasms. Accordingly, this chapter both begins and ends by considering some of the most important epidemiologic features.

SYSTEMS OF CLASSIFICATION

Classification has changed over the past few decades as innovative diagnostic methods and techniques have been developed and a new consensus reached on the definition of lymphoid neoplasms. The Working Formulation, which was developed as a method of translating between the many competing classifications in the early 1980s, rapidly became the standard in North America and many epidemiologic studies conducted there were based on this system. During the same time period a majority of European centers used the Kiel classification, making effective comparison of results between North America and Europe almost impossible. In 1994 the Revised European–American Lymphoma (REAL) classification was published and this rapidly became the standard in all countries of the world. For the first time, the REAL classification was based on the definition of clinicopathologic entities – a major departure from previous practice. Disease entities are characterized based on morphologic, phenotypic, genotypic and clinical data.[2] The principles defined in the REAL classification formed the basis for the development of the third edition of the World Health Organization (WHO) classification of hematologic malignancies. This 'International Classification of Diseases for Oncology' third edition (ICD-O-3) was published by the WHO in 2001. ICD-O-3 is now the internationally recognized standard classification for all hematologic malignancies.[3,4]

A key feature of ICD-O-3 is the recognition that lymphoid leukemia and lymphoma describe patterns of disease spread, rather than individual disease entities. In the past, the terms leukemia and lymphoma were often used somewhat arbitrarily, reflecting the patient's mode of presentation and/or initial investigation rather than the underlying disease. This is particularly important for the interpretation of epidemiologic data where leukemia and lymphoma are generally regarded as fundamentally different disease entities. A second key feature of the ICD-O-3 classification is the delineation of precursor from mature lymphoid neoplasms, which again is of considerable significance for the interpretation of epidemiologic data. Importantly, mature lymphoproliferative disorders are very diverse in terms of their cellular pathology, clinical features, prognosis and treatment. Of particular note is the recognition that Hodgkin lymphoma, although highly distinctive in many respects, is part of the spectrum of B cell malignancies. A fundamental manifestation of this relationship is the appreciation that composite lymphomas, where HL occurs alongside another B cell lymphoma, are now known to be relatively common.

The structure of ICD-O-3 has been shown to be highly effective as a tool in clinical practice, and its introduction has demonstrated the clinical and biologic diversity of many of the lymphoma subtypes that had been previously grouped together into the broad categories of high and low grade. Entities such as mantle cell lymphoma, extranodal marginal zone lymphoma and follicular lymphoma, for example, appear to have little in common, raising questions about the usefulness of epidemiologic studies that do not distinguish between these disease categories. By contrast, it is also important to recognize that clinically distinct subgroups, including the relatively common germinal center types of diffuse large B cell lymphoma and follicular lymphoma, may, in fact, be closely related at a cellular level.

CHANGES IN DIAGNOSTIC TECHNOLOGIES

The taxonomic progress of the past 20 years has only been possible because of marked advances in diagnostic techniques. The Working Formulation system was morphologically based and, as such, was highly subjective. By contrast the more objective WHO ICD-O-3 classification now defines disease entities in terms of immunophenotype, genetic abnormalities and clinical features. At the present time, the availability of effective methods for immunophenotyping and detection of genetic abnormalities mean that it is now possible to develop diagnostic strategies that ensure high levels of accuracy through extensive cross-validation of individual investigative results. The momentum created by the development of these new diagnostic technologies continues and, in this regard, the recent introduction of techniques for assessing global gene expression and more accurate and sensitive flow cytometry are particularly noteworthy. Importantly, modern imaging and endoscopic techniques are also impacting on the diagnostic accuracy of key clinical features including the pattern of tumor spread.

The introduction of new diagnostic technologies presents several challenges for the interpretation of epidemiologic data. Although ICD-O-3 is now widely used, the extent to which the diagnosis of individual patients is supported by modern diagnostic methods varies both within and between countries. In addition, the ever-increasing use of sensitive flow cytometric methods to examine peripheral blood samples (especially for chronic lymphocytic leukemia [CLL] and multiple myeloma) and endoscopic biopsies of the gastrointestinal tract mean that many more indolent lymphoproliferative disorders are coming to clinical attention now than would have done so in previous years. Surveillance of individuals, either known or suspected to be, at high risk of developing a lymphoproliferative disorder is also becoming common practice in many countries. The impact that changes such as these have had on the descriptive epidemiology of lymphoproliferative disorders is poorly understood.

Finally, the introduction of new diagnostic techniques is changing basic concepts of disease, and these developments will probably continue to accelerate as the biologic heterogeneity of lymphoproliferative disorders becomes even more apparent. It seems unlikely, however, that these new technologies and concepts will be adopted uniformly across all centers and countries, and it is possible that in the future an even greater variety of reporting practices, terminology and diagnostic accuracy will ensue. Paradoxically, such diversity could result in a recapitulation of the situation that existed prior to the introduction of ICD-O-3.

CANCER REGISTRATION

With a view to elucidating potential causes of disease, descriptive epidemiologic studies are routinely concerned with measures of disease incidence, prevalence, mortality and survival in specific well-defined populations and/or subgroups. The occurrence of cancer, unlike most other human diseases, is often monitored by national, or specialist, cancer registries. These registration data, which in their simplest form can be summarized as basic frequencies, are often related to 'population at risk' estimates generated from national, or local, censuses. The accuracy of the resulting incidence rate estimates are predicated on the underlying quality of both numerator and denominator data, and only when the ascertainment of both is complete, or the levels of completeness are known, can the true incidence of disease within the target population be estimated.

Several factors can affect the quality of the rates estimated from cancer registries and census data, and these need to be considered when interpreting patterns and trends. With respect to denominator data, official population censuses do not always guarantee accurate capture of important demographic characteristics. Furthermore, censuses are not carried out in all areas of the world, and in countries where they are the interval between them is usually 10 or 20 years. With respect to numerator data, cancer registration typically involves complex information gathering processes that utilize multiple data sources (e.g. death certificates, pathology reports and systems, hospital admission/discharge summaries), data formats (e.g. paper and computerized records) and methods of data abstraction (e.g. clerical and electronic). Furthermore, in contrast with vital registration and certain infectious disease notification systems, in countries where it occurs, cancer registration is often a voluntary (e.g. the UK) as opposed to a statutory (e.g. Norway) exercise.

For meaningful descriptive studies, it is essential to ensure that the initial diagnosis is accurate, particularly with respect to subtype, and that the coding system applied preserves as much diagnostic precision as possible – as it does in ICD-O-3, for example. Another important, but less frequently discussed, consideration is the certainty and accuracy of diagnosis. Interrater agreement is imperative, but in some instances only one observer assigns the diagnosis. One of the main problems for lymphoproliferative disorders concerns the reproducibility/interrater agreement for NHL diagnoses and their subsequent coding, particularly with the classification systems used before ICD-O-3 became the international standard. The study of trends over time requires the use of comparable data – particularly with respect to the coding of diagnoses. Disparities in coding have been highlighted in many studies. Using the Surveillance Epidemiology and End Results (SEER) program registry data, for example, 57–63 percent agreement was achieved using the Working Formulation classification systems[5] and 77 percent agreement among cases assigned to the ICD-O-2 codes. Other studies have demonstrated similar results.[6,7]

The impact that changes in data quality have on estimates of incidence and mortality, in addition to any real trends in risk and random variation, is difficult to estimate.[8] Analyses of spatial and temporal cancer incidence patterns can present particular difficulties, as observed trends may reflect factors which influence the number of cancer registrations that are made – as opposed to reflecting changes in underlying disease levels. With all disease surveillance systems, it is important to consider the impact that changes in the criteria for data collection may have. For example, shifting definitions of what amounts to a malignant condition, variations and refinements in diagnostic classifications, improvements in the effectiveness of cancer registration, as well as changes in the type and numbers of interventions performed – which may themselves result in detection and diagnosis of cancer. Although the existence of this myriad of potential problems is well known, their impact on data about lymphoid neoplasms has not been systematically assessed.

Even with the above caveats, routinely collected population-based cancer registry data are of unquestionable value in studying the descriptive epidemiology of hematologic and other malignancies. These data generally provide the most reliable information about cancer levels within the populations from which they are derived, and etiologic hypotheses that do not harmonize with descriptive trends often turn out to be wrong. It is also important to keep in mind that good quality descriptive data not only provide potential insights into the determinants of disease, but are also required for sensible health service provision and planning.

INTERNATIONAL VARIATION

Although cancer registration has a long history in many parts of the world, particularly in the more affluent countries of Europe and North America, most of the world's population still live in areas that are not covered by such systems. International variations in incidence, prevalence and mortality can be described, however, using data estimates provided by the Descriptive Epidemiology Group (www-dep.iarc.fr) of the International Agency for Research in Cancer (IARC). Data on cancer are always collected and complied after diagnosis, so in this sense the most recent statistics are always 'late'. The GLOBOCAN 2002 database contains the latest international estimates based on the most recent incidence, mortality and survival data available.[9] For Northern Europe, Australia, New Zealand, Israel, Central Europe and Canada estimates either come from entire national populations, or representative samples; for most of Russia and southern Europe, Japan and Korea, the USA and South America the estimates are derived from a mixture of data modeled on national mortality and regional cancer registries; and for the remaining areas, including much of Africa and large parts of Asia, less reliable estimates are based on locally collected data, frequency data and averages based on neighboring countries.[9]

Globally, it is estimated that around 449 000 people were newly diagnosed with a lymphoid malignancy in the year 2002, and that the number of people living with a lymphoid malignancy up to 5 years after diagnosis was in excess of 1.1 million.[10] Although ICD-O-3 is now the recognized standard for the classification of hematologic malignancies, many cancer registries still rely heavily on topographic coding systems, the most recent version being the International Classification of Diseases (ICD)-10.[10,11] Hence, the global estimates presented in Figure 3.1 are for HL (ICD-10 code C81), NHL (ICD-10 code C82-C85, C96) and multiple myeloma (ICD-10 codes C88, C90) combined, and represent estimated incidence rates for 2002. Data for chronic lymphoblastic lymphoma/leukemia (CLL) have been traditionally grouped with the leukemias, and are not included in Figure 3.1.

The geographic incidence patterns are dominated by the high rates in developed countries, where around 52 percent of the world's total lymphomas are diagnosed.[12] The patterns seen for each of the contributing malignancies (NHL, HL and multiple myeloma) are broadly similar to those shown in Figure 33.1, with rates being higher in men than women and markedly lower incidence rates being reported for less developed regions of the world. Globally, NHL accounts for around half of all lymphoproliferative disorders, and there is considerable variation in the estimated crude incidence rates across countries,

Incidence of all lymphoproliferative per 100 000 population – males

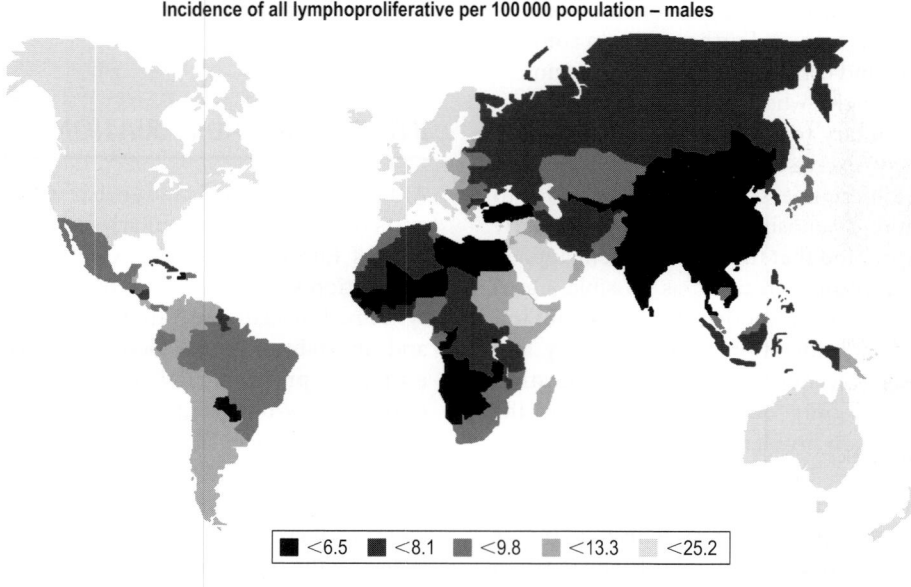

| ■ <6.5 | ■ <8.1 | ■ <9.8 | ▨ <13.3 | ▨ <25.2 |

Incidence of all lymphoproliferative per 100 000 population – females

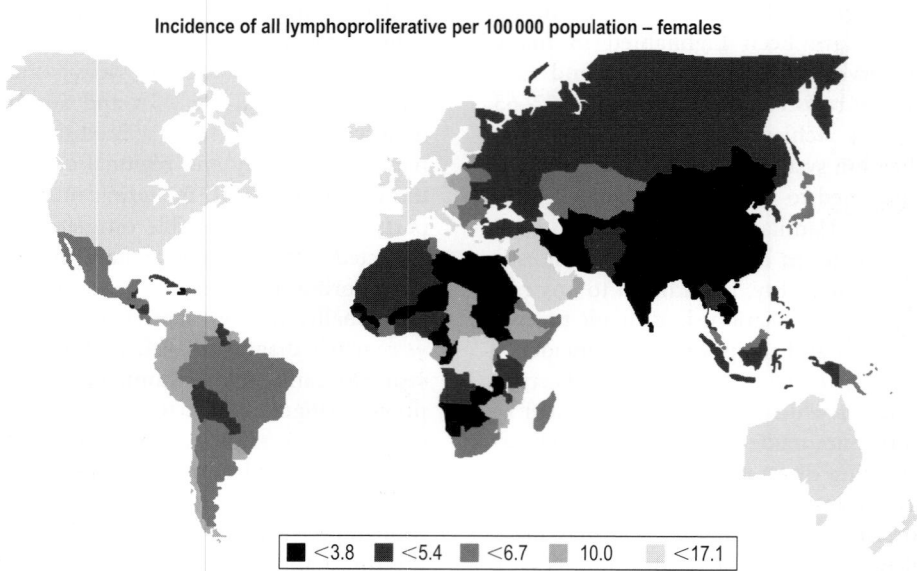

| ■ <3.8 | ■ <5.4 | ■ <6.7 | ▨ 10.0 | ▨ <17.1 |

Figure 3.1   Age-standardized (world) rates for non-Hodgkin lymphoma, Hodgkin lymphoma and multiple myeloma (Source: GLOBOCAN 2002.)

ranging from 1.6 to 17.1 cases per 100 000 persons per year (women) and 2.7 to 21.8 cases per 100 000 persons per year (men).

For both males and females, the incidence is highest in northern Europe and northern America, relatively high in other areas of Europe and Australia, and lowest in East and South East Asia. Western Asia is unusual in that there is a relatively high rate of lymphoma in this region (4.2 per 100 000 persons per year [women], 5.1 per 100 000 persons per year [men] for NHL and 1.7 per 100 000 persons per year [women], 2.4 per 100 000 persons per year [men] for HL). Hodgkin lymphoma accounts for a sixth of all lymphomas, with annual incidence rates worldwide ranging from 0.3 to 3.5 and 0.1 to 2.6 per 100 000 for men and

women, respectively. For both males and females, incidence is again highest in northern Europe and northern America, relatively high in other areas of Europe and Australia, and lowest in East and South East Asia. Multiple myeloma incidence rates are higher in men with age-standardized rates (world) around 1.7 per 100 000 per year (men) and 1.2 (women). Rates are highest in Australia/New Zealand, Europe and North America and lowest again in Africa and South Eastern Asia.

When evaluating global comparisons such as those shown in Figure 3.1, it is important to recall that data for large parts of the world are not necessarily reliable. Information gathering in Africa, for example, is particularly poor, although findings from the USA also suggest

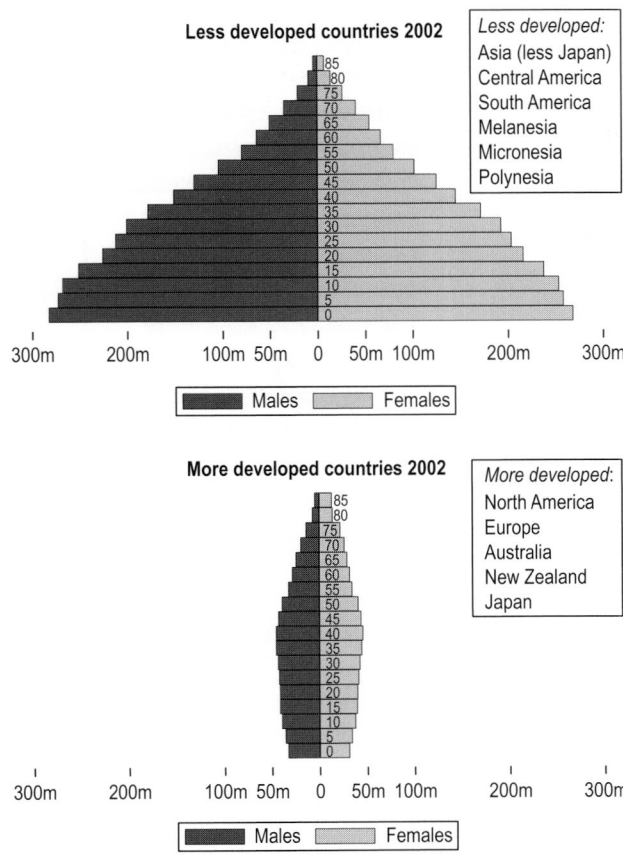

Figure 3.2 Population pyramids for less developed compared to more developed countries. Numbers (millions) in each 5-year age group. (Source: GLOBOCAN 2002.)

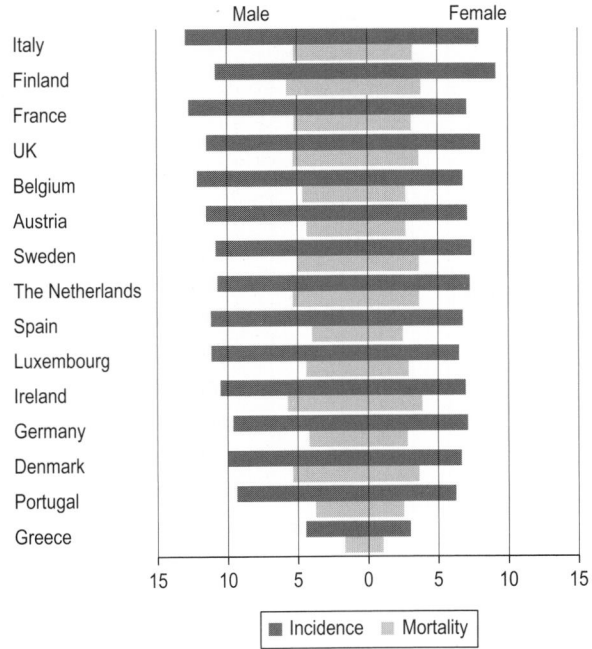

Figure 3.3 Non-Hodgkin lymphoma ranked incidence/mortality. Age-standardized rate (world) per 100 100 (all ages). (Source: GLOBOCAN 2002.)

that in both men and women the incidence of NHL, HL and multiple myeloma is greater among white people than among black people.[9,12,13] Nonetheless, given the complexities of the cancer registration process as well as the range of methods used for both data and subsequent parameter estimation (www-dep.iarc.fr), it is, perhaps, not surprising that the majority of non-hematologic cancers also show similar global patterns to those shown in Figure 3.1 in that there appears to be an increased incidence in developed countries.

A further interesting, but less frequently commented on feature of global estimates, such as those shown in Figure 3.1, is that the bulk of the world's population resides in areas of the world classified by most international agencies as 'less developed'. This is illustrated in Figure 3.2 which shows population pyramids for countries defined by GLOBOCAN either as more or as less developed. Population numbers are based on estimates from the United Nations. As can be seen, the differences in terms of both the absolute numbers of people and the age distributions are striking. Indeed, while the figures are particularly arresting at younger ages, even at older ages (65+ years) at which lymphoid malignancies are most common, the absolute numbers of people are still greater in countries classified as less

developed – around 263 million compared with around 175 million in developed countries.[9]

Data for the main neoplasm groups NHL, HL and multiple myeloma collated by IARC for the 15 member states of the European Union (EU) are shown in Figures 3.3, 3.4 and 3.5, respectively. These estimates were extracted from the GLOBOCAN 2002 Cancer Incidence, Mortality and Prevalence Worldwide,[9] and include both incidence and mortality for males and females positioned side by side, ranked in terms of decreasing overall incidence.

Overall, in the EU approximately 152 900 people were estimated to have been diagnosed with NHL in the 5 years up to 1995. In addition, over 28 630 people were estimated to have been diagnosed with HL – giving a total for the lymphomas of just over 181 000 and a figure in excess of 238 000 for all lymphoid neoplasms combined.

For NHL, incidence rates were reported to be highest in Italy and lowest in Greece, with the UK, Netherlands, France, Finland, Ireland and Italy all having rates above the EU average. Broadly speaking the variation between countries seen for incidence is mirrored by that seen for mortality. With respect to survival, estimates taken from the EUCAN database,[10] for 1-, 3- and 5-year survival, are similar for European registries covering the largest populations (Denmark, Finland, Italy, and UK) – typically 1-, 3- and 5-year survivals around 65–68 percent, 51–53 percent and over 45 percent, respectively, for both sexes. Importantly, there have been considerable improvements in survival since the 1970s, and many people who would have died then are now cured.[14]

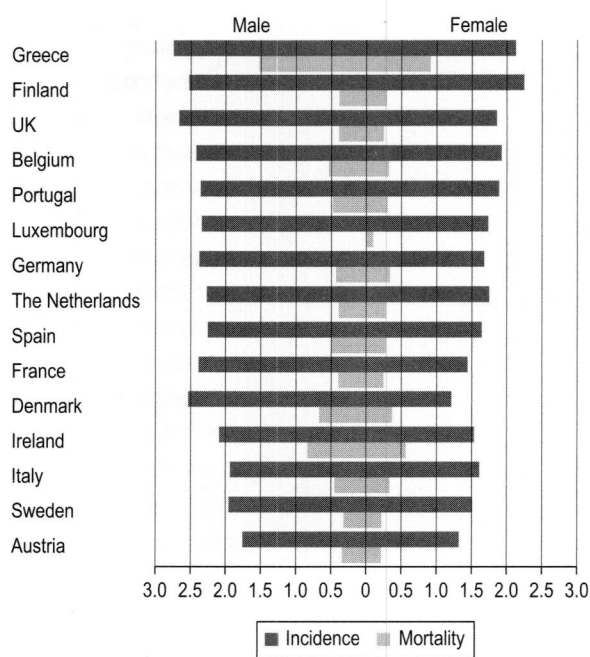

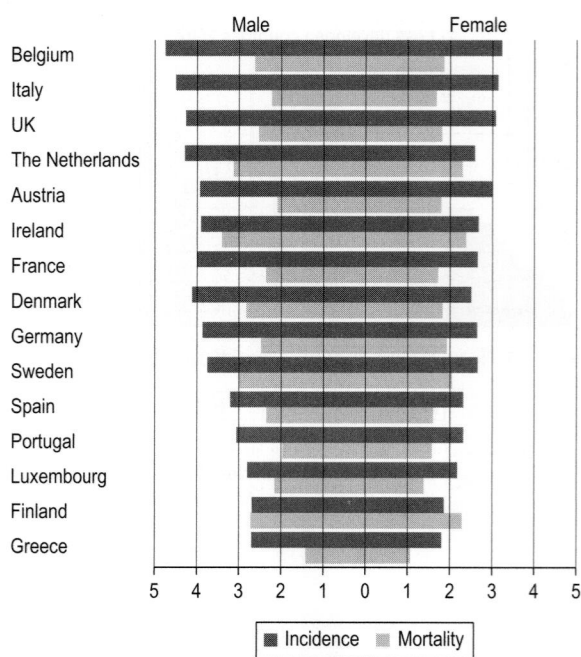

Figure 3.4 Hodgkin lymphoma ranked incidence/mortality. Age-standardized rate (world). Age-standardized rate (world) per 100 000 (all ages). (Source: GLOBOCAN 2002.)

Figure 3.5 Multiple myeloma ranked incidence/mortality. Age-standardized rate (world) per 100 000 (all ages). (Source: GLOBOCAN 2002.)

By contrast, HL is notable for quite large differences in incidence and mortality between EU countries. Finland and Greece appear to have the highest incidence with Greece also having the highest mortality. The lowest incidence and mortality rates appear to be in Sweden and Austria. In all countries in the EU there appears to be a male excess for both NHL and HL, the difference for HL being particularly marked in Austria and Greece, where the male-to-female incidence ratio appears to be approximately 1.4:1. Survival estimates for HL are much better than for NHL. Typically rates for 1-, 3- and 5-year survival are around 89 percent, 80 percent and 75 percent, respectively, for registries covering large populations. There is, however, a fair amount of variation, and a few of the smaller registries appear to have 1-year survival rates considerably higher than the EU average would predict. Similarly to NHL, improvements in treatment have resulted in sharp falls in HL mortality across the developed world.[14]

As with NHL and HL, incidence and mortality rates for multiple myeloma are higher in males than in females. Multiple myeloma is, however, associated with a higher case-fatality than either NHL or HL (there is no cure), and there is generally less variation in incidence and mortality across countries in the EU (Fig. 3.5). Although 1-year relative survival estimates usually lie within the range 60–86 percent, 5-year survival is very poor, typically in the range of 20–40 percent across the EU for both sexes. Unfortunately, in contrast to many other lymphoproliferative disorders, there has been little improvement in long-term survival for myeloma, although improvements have been made in median survival.[14]

The basic patterns described above are broadly similar to those seen in other parts of the developed world. The SEER program of the National Cancer Institute (NCI), for example, is a valuable source of information on cancer incidence and survival in the USA. It currently collects and publishes cancer incidence and survival estimates from population-based cancer registries covering approximately 26 percent of the US population.[15] SEER data for the years 1998–2002 suggest that incidence and mortality rates for NHL, HL and multiple myeloma in the USA are generally similar, if not a little higher, to EU averages; and that survival following diagnosis is broadly the same.

VARIATIONS WITH AGE AND SEX

Figures 3.6–3.9 show the number of new cases and age-specific incidence rates by age and sex in the UK for NHL, multiple myeloma and HL, respectively.[16] The UK patterns are similar to those reported for other developed countries with good-quality cancer registration data.

As is the case for most cancers, NHL and multiple myeloma are both principally diseases of the elderly, the incidence of both malignancies increasing as age increases (Figs 3.6 and 3.7). In agreement with the overall summary rates presented in Figures 3.3 and 3.5, the age-specific rates of both NHL and multiple myeloma are consistently higher in males than females. At older ages (80+ years), however, although the rate difference remains, the increased longevity of women means that in absolute terms more women than men are diagnosed.

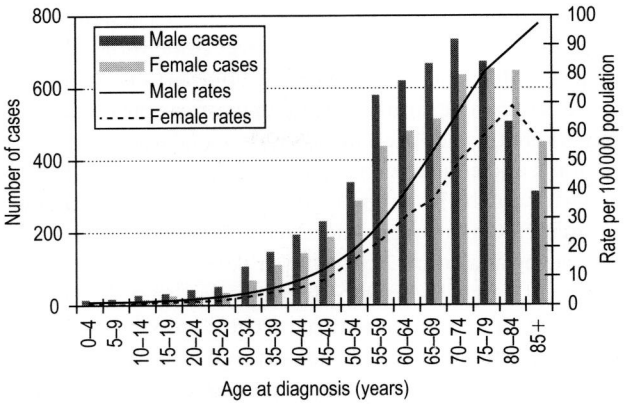

Figure 3.6   Age-specific incidence of non-Hodgkin lymphoma (UK 2004). (Source: Cancer Research UK [http:// info.cancerresearchuk.org/cancerstats/].)

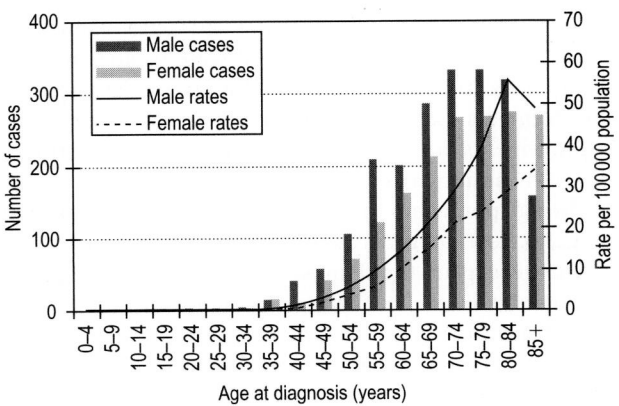

Figure 3.7   Age-specific incidence of multiple myeloma (UK 2004). (Source: Cancer Research UK [http:// info.cancerresearchuk.org/cancerstats/].)

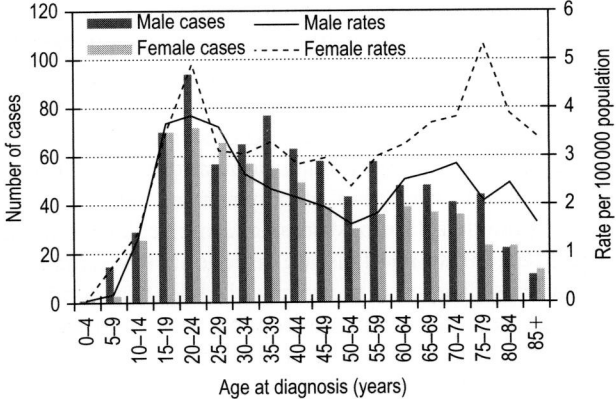

Figure 3.8   Age-specific incidence of Hodgkin lymphoma (2004 UK). (Source: Cancer Research UK [http://info.cancerresearchuk. org/cancerstats/].)

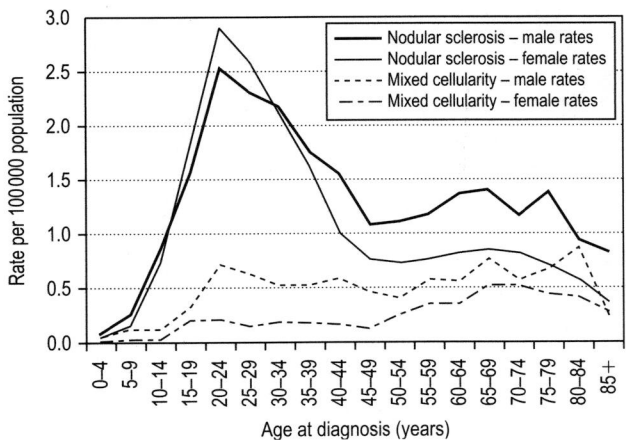

Figure 3.9   Age-specific incidence for Hodgkin lymphoma subtypes England 1995–2001. (Source: Cancer Research UK [http:// info.cancerresearchuk.org/cancerstats/].)

HL has unique epidemiologic features. The cause(s) of HL are largely unknown although certain infections and immune system factors have been implicated.[17] In marked contrast to NHL and myeloma, the HL incidence distribution has two peaks – one in young adults and one in the elderly (Fig. 3.8). Furthermore, the pattern seen in males and females varies with age – the male and female rates being more similar at younger ages than at older ages. These differences reflect differences in the sub-types of HL that typically occur within the different age strata (Fig. 3.9). Nodular sclerosis, with its pronounced peak in the late teenage and early twenties age ranges in both males and females, predominates in younger people. Furthermore, in contrast with other lymphoid malignancies, between the ages of 10 and 30 years this subtype of HL is more common in women than in men. The age and sex patterns seen for the mixed cellularity form of HL is similar to that of other lymphoproliferative disorders – the rates being consistently higher in males and increasing with age.

Interestingly, the estimated rates from GLOBOCAN 2002 for countries defined either as more or less developed,[9] show marked similarities with the patterns seen for the two main HL subtypes – nodular sclerosis (ICD10 C81.1) and mixed cellularity (ICD10 C81.2) (Fig. 3.9). The shape of the age distributions (0–651 years) for men and women in more developed countries (Fig. 3.10) are similar to those of nodular sclerosis (Fig. 3.9), the main differences being that the male rate remains consistently higher than the female rate and the distributions peak earlier in Figure 3.10 (around 15 years) than in Figure 3.9 (around 20 years). In the same way, the curves for the mixed cellularity form of HL are not dissimilar to those estimated for HL as a whole in less developed countries (Fig. 3.10).

The reasons underpinning the similarities between Figures 3.9 and 3.10 are probably complex, involving both

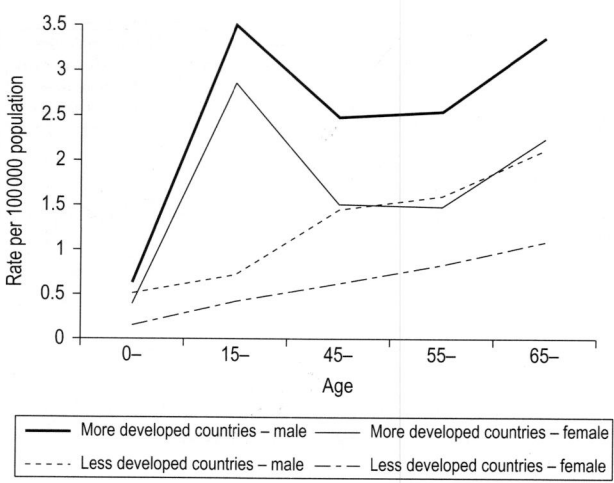

Figure 3.10 Incidence of Hodgkin lymphoma in more and less developed countries by age and sex. (Source: GLOBOCAN 2002.)

differences between countries with respect to their diagnostic and registration practices and differences in disease determinants. Etiologic issues relating to the determinants of HL, NHL and multiple myeloma that may impact on patterns such as these shown in Figures 3.8–3.10 are discussed in Chapter 35.

CURRENT ISSUES IN THE DESCRIPTIVE EPIDEMIOLOGY OF LYMPHOID NEOPLASMS

Descriptive epidemiologic observations often generate hypotheses that in turn form the basis of more detailed research, with theories that do not fit descriptive patterns being difficult to reconcile. The three topical areas we have chosen to highlight below are particularly germane to the descriptive epidemiology of lymphoid malignancies. We begin by considering issues relating to temporal trends, followed by geographic differences and end, as we began the chapter, with diagnostics.

TEMPORAL TRENDS: IS NON–HODGKIN LYMPHOMA INCREASING?

As cancer registration data are continuously improving in terms of both quality and completeness, estimates within countries and regions are often not truly comparable over time. This is particularly true for hematologic malignancies where diagnostics have, perhaps, altered more rapidly than for any other cancer. This means that it is especially difficult to evaluate present day incidence estimates against those generated in the past. For this reason IARC cautions that it is often the case that observed differences reflect changes in methodology, and temporal variations should not necessarily be interpreted as real time trend effects (www-dep.iarc.fr).

That having been said, monitoring disease trends over time is fundamental to descriptive epidemiology, such analyses often yielding important etiologic clues. Indeed, there are many examples in the field of cancer epidemiology where this has been the case – particularly in the occupational and environmental fields.[18] The temporal changes reported for NHL in recent decades are, unquestionably, dramatic. On average, rates have been reported to be increasing at around 2 percent per year over the last 30–40 years, although the rate of increase has now slowed and there are reports that it may have leveled off.[19,20] Naturally, these reported increases have captured both scientific and public attention – since any increase, if real, impacts greatly on public health.

Despite the caveats relating to changing diagnostic practices, the increasing numbers of cancer registrations seen for NHL have been interpreted by many as evidence for a genuine increase in the underlying level of disease.[21–23] Indeed, several investigators have concluded that the observed increases in the number of lymphoma registrations made over recent decades, and hence changes in incidence, reflect real changes in disease occurrence that are unlikely to be explained by changes in classification, advancements in diagnostic practice or generalized improvements in the completeness of cancer registration.[24] However, although recent studies have attempted to use modeling approaches to look at the possible contributions of age, period and generational (cohort) effects that could potentially explain the claimed rise in incidence, modeling the potential impact of changes in diagnostic practice is far from straightforward.[25–27]

There has been considerable speculation about the possible exposures and/or lifestyle changes that could have caused such a rapid rise in NHL incidence, and the potential etiologic role of many biologic, chemical and physical candidates is discussed in Chapter 4. If the increase is (or was) real, it has serious implications as the magnitude of the change suggests that one or more modern environmental causes may have driven the rate upwards. Clearly, if this is the case then knowing the cause – which could be one or more potentially modifiable risk factor(s) – would be of enormous public health importance. Nonetheless, as discussed earlier in this chapter, the role of artifact is difficult to evaluate since the introduction of more reliable and sensitive diagnostic techniques, for example, the ability of flow cytometry to detect small populations of abnormal cells and the introduction of polymerase chain reaction, allowing the detection of disease at a molecular level, has lowered the threshold of disease detection. Hence, many of the patients diagnosed today have indolent or asymptomatic disease, and it remains possible that the increasing numbers of registrations may be due, at least in part, to the recognition of new group(s) of patients that in previous decades would either not have been diagnosed at all, or would have been diagnosed at later ages. A recent study, part of the WHO Comprehensive Cancer Monitoring Project, summarized trends in incidence from HL and

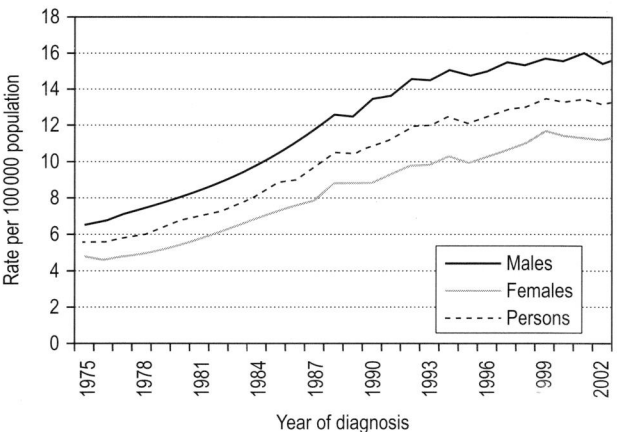

Figure 3.11 Age-standardized (European) incidence rates, non-Hodgkin lymphoma, by sex, Great Britain, 1975–2004. (Source: Cancer Research UK [http://info.cancerresearchuk.org/cancerstats/].)

Table 3.1 Comparison of non-Hodgkin lymphoma and Hodgkin lymphoma incidence per 100 000 population per year in Japan, Taiwan and India compared with Europe and North America

Country	Non-Hodgkin lymphoma		Hodgkin lymphoma	
	Male	Female	Male	Female
Japan	10.9	7.0	0.4	0.3
Taiwan	3.0	1.7	0.3	0.1
India	2.6	1.5	0.9	0.4
Europe	15.6	12.9	2.7	2.0
North America	22.0	17.2	3.5	2.6

Source: GLOBOCAN, 2002.[9]

NHL in 13 European countries where data were considered reliable and for which data were available for a sufficiently extended time period. Overall, there was a consistent increase in the number of registrations of NHL in both sexes in all countries studied, alongside decreases in HL in previous decades. More recently, however, there appears to be a leveling off of this trend. One could speculate that this plateau indicates stability in detection, diagnosis and registration and that this is the totality of disease in a population. Continued monitoring of contemporary data will reveal the extent to which this may be true.[19]

Two US studies using recent data reported a decline in the rate of increase.[20,28,29] Australian incidence data for New South Wales (NSW) for the period 1973–2003 show marked increases in NHL in both sexes up to the end of 1993. Data for the period 1994–2003, however, show a marked decline in the rate of increase – a leveling off.[30] A recently published study into time trends in incidence for NHL details findings for Sweden, Denmark and Finland over the period (1960–2003). This study concludes that the 'epidemic' increase of NHL has largely subsided.[31] Figure 3.11 shows data for Great Britain for the period 1975–2004 which also indicate a leveling off in the incidence for NHL in both sexes.

GEOGRAPHIC VARIATION: B CELL VERSUS T CELL LYMPHOMA

Analyses of data by histologic subtype are strongly suggestive of there being different causal mechanisms in operation for the different lymphoid subtypes, which could influence the large geographic variations seen for descriptive data such as those shown in Table 3.1.

These variations support the view that both future descriptive and etiologic epidemiologic studies of lymphomas should use ICD-O-3 or its successor, and that analyses should be performed separately for each subtype.[32] It is important, therefore, to pursue analyses that respect this heterogeneity. One fundamental issue deserving attention relates to the different underlying frequencies of B cell and T cell disease. Although descriptive epidemiology cannot be used to answer questions pertaining to the reasons for this variation in lineage occurrence, it is possible that examination of different patterns in different geographic locations may shed light on underlying etiologic mechanisms.

Data from Japan probably provides the most substantial evidence for geographic variation in lymphoma subtypes, particularly for T cell lymphoma which seem to be higher in Asian populations than in Europe and the USA. A recent pathologic review in Japan studied 3194 patients with malignant lymphoma. There were 3025 cases of NHL (comprising 2189 cases of B cell lymphoma, 796 cases of T cell lymphoma and 40 cases of unassignable lineage), 141 cases of HL, 10 cases of histiocytic/dendritic neoplasms and 18 cases who were unclassifiable.[33] Overall around 70 percent of the lymphomas were of B cell origin (33.3 percent diffuse large B cell lymphoma, 8.5 percent extranodal marginal zone lymphoma, 8.1 percent myeloma, 6.7 percent follicular lymphoma, 2.8 percent mantle cell lymphoma, 2.4 percent precursor B cell lymphoblastic leukemia/lymphoma, 1.3 percent small lymphocytic lymphoma, 1.1 percent plasmacytoma, 1 percent nodal marginal zone lymphoma and 1 percent Burkitt lymphoma) and 25 percent were of T cell origin (7.5 percent adult T cell leukemia/lymphoma, 6.7 percent peripheral T cell lymphoma of unspecified type, 2.6 percent extranodal nasal type natural killer/T cell lymphoma, 2.4 percent angioimmunoblastic T cell lymphoma, 1.7 percent precursor T lymphoblastic leukemia/lymphoma, 1.5 percent anaplastic large cell lymphoma and 1.2 percent mycosis fungoides/Sézary syndrome). The frequency of other B and T subtypes was less than 1 percent. It should be noted that the incidence of adult T cell leukaemia/lymphoma was influenced by an endemic area of human T cell leukemia virus type 1. The nodular sclerosis and mixed cellularity

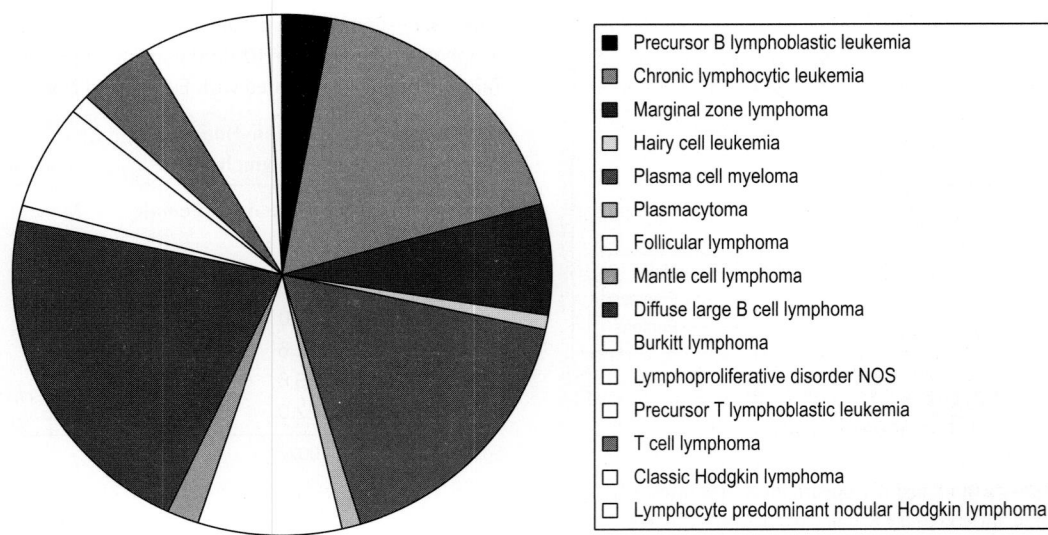

Figure 3.12 The distribution of lymphoid neoplasms. NOS, not otherwise specified. (Source: Haematological Malignancy Research Network [HMRN] September 2004–September 2007 [www.hmrn.org].)

types of HL occupied 1.8 percent and 1.6 percent, respectively. These data are clearly distinct from those described for Western countries, where T cell disease usually accounts for around 15 percent, at most.

Data from Taiwan show similar geographic patterns, supporting the suggestion of variation in incidence of subtypes.[34] A review of 200 consecutive cases in Mumbai, India, by a panel of five expert hematopathologists from the NHL Classification Project reported that 80 percent of NHLs were of B cell type (33.3 percent diffuse large B cell, 15.3 percent follicular lymphoma, 5.1 percent mantle cell lymphoma, 5.1 percent small lymphocytic lymphoma, 4.1 percent Burkitt lymphoma, 2.6 percent extranodal marginal zone lymphoma, 2.6 percent precursor B cell lymphoblastic leukemia/lymphoma, 1.5 percent plasmacytoma, 1.5 percent nodal marginal zone lymphoma and 1.5 percent mediastinal large cell lymphoma) and 18 percent were of T cell type (7.2 percent precursor T lymphoblastic leukemia/lymphoma, 4.1 percent anaplastic large cell lymphoma, 3.1 percent peripheral T cell lymphoma of unspecified type and 1.5 percent angioimmunoblastic T cell lymphoma). The immunophenotype could not be determined for the remaining 2 percent of patients.[35] Overall precursor T lymphoblastic leukemia/lymphoma was estimated to be commoner in India (7 percent) than the rest of the world (1–4 percent), and indolent B cell NHLs (30 percent) were less common than in the West. As compared with China and Japan, peripheral T cell lymphoma, extranodal nasal type natural killer/T cell lymphoma, and extranodal marginal zone B cell lymphoma of mucosa-associated lymphoid tissue (MALT lymphoma) were less common, but follicular lymphoma and small lymphocytic lymphoma were more common. These findings suggest that the distribution of B cell and T cell lymphomas in the Indian population, except for lymphoblastic lymphoma,

may fall somewhere between the Western and Oriental worlds. It is, however, important to recall that data ascertainment is an issue in India, and that these observations require replication and further research.

CHANGING DIAGNOSTICS

Hitherto, most descriptive epidemiologic investigations using cancer registration data have mainly concentrated on the broad disease groupings of NHL, HL and multiple myeloma as defined topographically by ICD-10, with information on CLL being grouped with leukemia (as opposed to lymphoma) as a whole. For this reason, thus far, descriptive data on CLL have not been presented in this chapter. As discussed at the beginning, however, the introduction of new diagnostic techniques is changing basic concepts of disease, and this process will possibly accelerate. As a consequence, in the future, descriptive information on CLL, as well as other hematologic groupings and subtypes recognized in ICD-O-3, should be more widely available. An example of the real spectrum of lymphoid malignancy is presented in Figure 3.12. This figure shows the proportion of each diagnosis that was collected during the first three years (2004–7) of the newly established population-based Haematological Malignancy Research Network (HMRN) in the UK. This specialist population-based register, serving the Yorkshire and Humberside regions of England (population approximately 3.7 million) collects the full spectrum of lymphoproliferative and other hematologic malignancies coded with expert review to ICD-O-3 (www.hmrn.org). Although the HMRN has not accrued enough patients to allow analyses of trends over time, it does provide an accurate representation of the distribution of lymphoid neoplasms in a well-defined population.

KEY POINTS

- Greater understanding of cellular pathology and the requirement to bring together disparate classifications, coupled with emerging techniques of immunophenotyping, cytogenetics and clinical imaging have led to the synthesis of the WHO ICD-O-3 classification of hematologic malignancies based on a description of clinical syndromes and molecular biology.
- Improvements in diagnostic technology and change in classification have led to the redefinition of lymphoid leukemia and lymphoma.
- Historical cancer registry data cannot be reliably converted from earlier classifications to more informative ones without loss of precision. Therefore comparisons between datasets are difficult to make and secular trends in incidence may be unreliable. Furthermore, increased detection of occult disease has impacted on the reported incidence, making global assessments of temporal changes in incidence virtually impossible.
- In the future, continuing change can be expected with the introduction of molecular classification techniques, some of which highlight similarities between disease entities previously regarded as unrelated, for example HL and mediastinal B cell lymphoma and germinal center diffuse large B cell lymphoma and follicular lymphoma. Currently, there are sparse data on comparative epidemiology between these disease entities.
- Lymphoma comprises numerous histologic subtypes and trends in incidence require surveillance and etiologic study of these subtypes. More research should be done to understand and implement reliable means of subtype classification – improvements in the molecular characterization of lymphoid neoplasms will lead to improved classification schemes which may further enlighten etiology.
- Descriptive epidemiology has an important role in contributing to the understanding of the pathogenesis of lymphoid neoplasms as it is clear geographic location, age, racial and gender variation occurs, without clear, identifiable reasons.
- Changes in diagnostic technology and classification highlight the need for a new approach to descriptive epidemiology, closely integrated with laboratory and clinical findings, designed to identify etiologic factors and clues to the pathogenesis of lymphoid neoplasms.

REFERENCES

● = Key primary paper
◆ = Major review article

●1. John M (ed) *A dictionary of epidemiology.* Oxford: Oxford Medical Publications, 1983.
●2. Cogliatti SB, Schmid U. Who is WHO and what was REAL? *Swiss Med Wkly* 2002; **132**: 607–17.
●3. Swerdlow SH, Campo E, Harris NL *et al. Tumours of the haemopoietic and lymphoid tissues.* IARC, 4th edition. 2008.
●4. Fritz A, Percy C, Jack A *et al. International classification of diseases for oncology,* 3rd edition. Geneva: World Health Organization, 2000.
●5. Dick FR, Van Lier S, Banks P *et al.* Comparison of methods of recording subclasses of non-Hodgkin's lymphoma for use in epidemiologic studies. *Am J Epidemiol* 1985; **122**: 542.
●6. Dick FR, Vanlier SF, Mckeen K *et al.* Nonconcurrence in abstracted diagnoses of non-Hodgkin's lymphoma. *J Natl Cancer Inst* 1987; **78**: 675–8.
●7. Neiman RS, Cain K, Ben Arieh Y *et al.* A comparison between the Rappaport Classification and Working Formulation in cooperative group trials: the ECOG experience. *Hematol Pathol* 1992; **6**: 61–70.
●8. Esteve J, Benhamou E, Raymond L. *Statistical methods in cancer research,* volume IV. IARC scientific publications no. 128. Lyon, 1994.
●9. Ferlay J, Bray F, Pisani P *et al. GLOBOCAN 2002 Cancer incidence, mortality and prevalence worldwide.* IARC Cancer Base No. 5, version 2.0. Lyon: IARC Press, 2004.
●10. Ferlay J, Bray F, Sankila R *et al. EUCAN: cancer incidence, mortality and prevalence in the European Union 1998.* IARC cancer base No. 4, version 5.0. Lyon: IARC Press, 1999.
●11. World Health Organization. *International statistical classification of diseases and health related problems, tenth revision.* Geneva: World Health Organization, 1994, 2008.
●12. Boyle P, Levin B. (eds) *World cancer report 2008.* Lyon: IARC, 2008.
◆13. Willett E, Roman E. Epidemiology. In: Marcus R (ed) *Lymphoma: diagnosis, pathology and treatment.* London: Cambridge University Press, 2008.
◆14. Quinn M, Wood H, Cooper N *et al.* (eds) *Cancer atlas of the United Kingdom and Ireland 1991–2000.* Studies on medical and population subjects 68, 2005.
●15. SEER: Surveillance Epidemiology and End Results, 2008. Available at: http://seer.cancer.gov/.
●16. Cancer stats. Cancer Research UK, 2008. Available at: http://info.cancerresearchuk.org/cancerstats/.
●17. Newton R, Crouch S, Ansell P *et al.* Hodgkin's lymphoma and infection: findings from a UK case–control study. *Br J Cancer* 2007; **97**: 1310–14.
●18. Schottenfeld D, Fraumeni J (eds) *Cancer epidemiology and prevention.* Oxford: Oxford University Press, 1996.
●19. Adamson P, Bray F, Costantini AS *et al.* Time trends in the registration of Hodgkin and non-Hodgkin lymphomas in Europe. *Eur J Cancer* 2007; **43**: 391–401.

●20. Clarke CA, Glaser SL. Changing incidence of non-Hodgkin lymphomas in the United States. *Cancer* 2002; **94**: 2015–23.

●21. Devesa SS, Fears T. Non-Hodgkin's lymphoma time trends: United States and international data. *Cancer Res* 1992; 52: s5432–40.

●22. Obrams GI, O'Conor G. The emerging epidemic of non-Hodgkin's lymphoma: current knowledge regarding etiological factors. Time trends and pathological classification: a summary. *Cancer Res* 1992; **52**: s5570.

●23. Carli PM, Boutron MC, Maynadie M *et al.* Increase in the incidence of non-Hodgkin's lymphomas: evidence for a recent sharp increase in France independent of AIDS. *Br J Cancer* 1994; **70**: 713–15.

●24. Liu S, Semenciw R, Mao Y. Increasing incidence of non-Hodgkin's lymphoma in Canada, 1970–1996: age-period-cohort analysis. *Hematol Oncol* 2003; **21**: 57–66.

●25. Holford TR, Zheng T, Mayne ST *et al.* Time trends of non-Hodgkin's lymphoma: are they real? What do they mean? *Cancer Res* 1992; **52**: s5443–6.

●26. Pollan M, Lopez-Abente G, Moreno C *et al.* Rising incidence of non-Hodgkin's lymphoma in Spain: analysis of period of diagnosis and cohort effects. *Cancer Epidemiol Biomarkers Prev* 1998; **7**: 621–5.

●27. Nordstrom M. Increasing incidence of non-Hodgkin's lymphomas in Sweden 1958–1992. *Oncol Rep* 1996; **3**: 645–9.

●28. Eltom MA, Jemal A, Mbulaiteye SM *et al.* Trends in Kaposi's sarcoma and non-Hodgkin's lymphoma incidence in the United States from 1973 through 1998. *J Natl Cancer Inst* 2002; **94**: 1204–10.

●29. Howe HL, Wingo PA, Thun MJ *et al.* Annual report to the nation on the status of cancer (1973 through 1998), featuring cancers with recent increasing trends. *J Natl Cancer Inst* 2001; **93**: 824–42.

●30. Tracey EA Roder, D, Bishop J *et al. Cancer in New South Wales. Incidence and mortality 2003, NSW Central Cancer Registry, Cancer Institute NSW 2005.*

●31. Sandin S, Hjalgrim H, Glimelius B *et al.* Incidence of non-Hodgkin's lymphoma in Sweden, Denmark, and Finland from 1960 through 2003: an epidemic that was. *Cancer Epidemiol Biomarkers Prev* 2006; **15**: 1295–300.

●32. Morton LM, Wang SS, Devesa SS *et al.* Lymphoma incidence patterns by WHO subtype in the United States, 1992–2001. *Blood* 2006; **107**: 265–76.

●33. The World Health Organization classification of malignant lymphomas in Japan: incidence of recently recognized entities. Lymphoma Study Group of Japanese Pathologists. *Pathol Int* 2000; **50**: 696–702.

●34. Chang KC, Huang GC, Jones D *et al.* Distribution and prognosis of WHO lymphoma subtypes in Taiwan reveals a low incidence of germinal-center derived tumors. *Leuk Lymphoma* 2004; **45**: 1375–84.

●35. Naresh KN, Agarwal B, Nathwani BN *et al.* Use of the World Health Organization (WHO) classification of non-Hodgkin's lymphoma in Mumbai, India: a review of 200 consecutive cases by a panel of five expert hematopathologists. *Leuk Lymphoma* 2004; **45**: 1569–77.

4

Causes and prevention of lymphoma

OLGA L VAN DER HEL AND PAOLO BOFFETTA

NON-HODGKIN LYMPHOMA

Non-Hodgkin lymphoma (NHL) represents a heterogeneous group of lymphocytic disorders ranging in aggressiveness from indolent cellular proliferation to highly aggressive and rapidly proliferative processes. As discussed in detail elsewhere in this volume, the incidence of NHL has risen steadily worldwide during the past two decades.[1] The causes of this upward trend are largely unknown, and in general the current understanding of the etiology of NHL is incomplete. More than 300 000 new cases of NHL are estimated to occur annually worldwide.[2]

Risk factors that have been suggested include familiar history of lymphoma, immunodeficiency (whether acquired, congenital or iatrogenic), infection with Epstein–Barr and other viruses, exposure to ultraviolet (UV) radiation, exposure to pesticides, solvents and hair dyes, as well as nutritional factors. Several of the observed associations suggest that altered immunologic function, either immunostimulation or immunosuppression, is a common mechanism in lymphomagenesis. Whereas the role of biologic agents and immunologic conditions is discussed in other parts of the volume, this chapter reviews risk factors related to lifestyle and those occurring in the general environment, including the workplace.

Occupational exposures

Many epidemiologic studies have investigated potential occupational risk factors for NHL,[3] with methods ranging from analyzing occupation (longest held occupation or full occupational history) to more specific approaches for exposure assessment such as self-reported exposure, job-exposure matrices, or expert assessment based on a detailed task description of the study subjects.

AGRICULTURE AND EXPOSURE TO PESTICIDES

The occupation that is most often found to be associated with an elevated risk of NHL is farming and agricultural work. Several studies have found an increased risk of NHL among farmers,[4–12] although some did not confirm this association.[13–18] A meta-analysis including 36 studies published up to 1997 resulted in an overall relative risk of NHL equal to 1.10 (95 percent confidence interval [CI] 1.03 to 1.19).[19] The factors responsible for the increased risk of NHL in farmers are not well understood, but most studies have focused on pesticides. However, farmers are also exposed to other agricultural chemicals, zoonotic viruses and UV light. All these factors are potentially carcinogenic and can lead to chronic antigen stimulation.

Pesticide exposure is one of the hypotheses proposed to explain an increased NHL risk in farmers. They can increase the risk of NHL through various mechanisms. Some pesticides are known to be genotoxic or tumor promoters, whereas others possess hormonal immunotoxic or hematotoxic properties.[20–22] A higher frequency of chromosomal aberrations, sister chromatide exchanges and micronuclei have been observed in peripheral blood lymphocytes of pesticide applicators and certain groups of farmers.[23] A recent case–control study showed that farming and exposure to selected pesticides were strongly related to t(14;18)-positive NHL but not to t(14;18)-negative NHL.[24] In a study of workers exposed to pentachlorophenol-containing pesticides, an increased blood level of pentachlorophenol was associated with severe T lymphocyte dysfunction.[25]

A number of studies aimed to investigate the effect of specific groups of pesticides. Phenoxy herbicides, which can be contaminated by dioxins, have been associated with an increased risk for NHL,[3,26–29] but positive associations have also been observed for insecticides based on organochlorines,[3,4,8,27,29,30] carbamate[29] and organophosphates,[29] as well as fungicides[29,31–33] and chlorophenols.[28] In general, however, results of studies looking at specific pesticides have not been consistent, precluding the possibility of a final evaluation of the etiologic role of these chemicals.

SOLVENTS

Occupations entailing exposure to solvents that have been associated with an increased NHL risk include dry-cleaning and laundry[34,35] metal working,[11,14,34,35] welding,[5,10,11,18,36] printing[34] and painting.[18] A recent review has been published.[37] Exposure to organic solvents including benzene, 1,3-butadiene, trichloroethylene, perchloroethylene, lead arsenate and paint thinners has repeatedly been associated with an increased risk of NHL,[3,17,18,28,38–40] although some studies did not observe an association.[31] Two studies indicate that associations are mainly specific to diffuse-type lymphomas, and not for follicular lymphomas.[34,41] Results for specific solvents have been largely inconsistent, as it can be illustrated by results on benzene exposure:[42] this agent was associated with an increased risk for NHL in one study,[10] but several other studies did not confirm the association.[17,41,43,44] Trichloroethylene (TCE) has been an industrial chemical for many years and its main use is for degreasing, as a generalized solvent and as a dry-cleaning agent. Also, ground water contamination is common. Therefore humans can be exposed to TCE occupationally as well as via the environment. The impact on NHL risk following TCE exposure were reviewed by Wartenberg and Siegel.[45] These authors identified an increased risk of NHL associated with TCE exposure of 1.9 (95 percent CI 1.3 to 2.8). Tetrachloroethylene is also used for degreasing and for dry-cleaning. There is some evidence for an increased risk of NHL. In a cohort in Finland (workers exposed to halogenated hydrocarbons) and two cohorts in USA (dry cleaners and workers at an aircraft maintenance facility) there was an elevated risk of NHL among workers who were mainly exposed to TCE.[46–48]

Solvents may exert immunotoxic effects, induce impairment or suppression of cell-mediated immunity and therefore have been associated with increased risk for NHL.[25,49–52] In particular, one study reported that workers with long-term exposure to solvents experienced a decrease in T lymphocyte (but not B lymphocyte) count.[50]

OCCUPATIONS ENTAILING EXPOSURE TO BIOLOGIC AGENTS

Associations found between NHL and several occupations with possible exposures to viruses and other biologic agents have supported the hypothesis that delayed infection may be a risk factor for NHL. Several studies have found statistically significant increased NHL risk for teachers,[11,53–56] suggesting that immunologic response to late exposure to human viruses carried by children may be a risk factor for NHL. An increased risk of NHL has also been observed for medical occupations,[5,14,34,35,54,55] although in medical professions a variety of other exposures may occur such as to ionizing radiation, anesthetics and antineoplastic drugs. Furthermore, an increased risk of NHL has been observed for meat workers exposed to a variety of animal products,[42,57–59] although a study of butchers did not confirm this result.[60] Occupational exposure to live cattle has been associated with NHL in several[14,61,62] but not all studies.[12,18,34] In a recent German study, the association between cattle and NHL was stronger and reached statistical significance for older age of first exposure,[62] suggesting that delayed viral exposure may explain the elevated NHL risk.

POLYCHLORINATED BIPHENYLS

Before being banned in the late 1970s, polychlorinated biphenyls (PCBs) were widely used in various industrial applications. Their compounds are characterized by long-term persistence and diffusion in the environment, and by bioaccumulation through the food chain. Food is the main route of exposure to the general population, but the highest exposures have occurred in occupational cohorts through inhalation or skin absorption in work environments.[63] A review of epidemiologic studies on workers occupationally exposed to PCB showed no excess risk for cancers of the lymphatic and hematopoietic system.[64] In contrast, one study found an increased risk for NHL for subjects when comparing PCB serum level in healthy individuals who eventually developed NHL and controls.[65]

ORGANIC DUSTS

Besides farmers, several other occupations exposed to organic dusts have been reported as having an increased NHL risk, such as grain millers[66] (exposed not only to grain and flour dust but also to pesticides), textile workers and knitters[41,55,67] (who can be exposed to textile dusts and dyes), and carpenters and cabinet makers,[26,53,68] (who are exposed to wood dust and solvents from glues). Wood dust exposure has been associated with a statistically significant increased NHL risk,[39,43] but not consistently.[18] Organic dust may exert an effect on lymphomagenesis through stimulation of the immune system; although a study looking at occupational exposure to immunologically active agents, acting predominantly through an immunoglobulin E-dependent hypersensitivity mechanism did not reveal an increased risk of NHL.[69]

OTHER OCCUPATIONAL EXPOSURES

A variety of other occupations and agents have been associated with an increased NHL risk. These include cutting, lubricating and mineral oils,[43,70,71] employment in motor-vehicle related industries,[11,18] and employment as motor-vehicle operator,[53,72] aircraft mechanic,[54] and hairdresser.[26,34,36,55,73] Three studies have found a statistically significant increased risk for NHL in fire fighters,[54,74,75] who can be exposed to wide variety of toxic gases and aerosols, including benzene. Finally, an increased risk of NHL has been reported for a variety of white collar occupations,[35,53,54] including, in particular, laboratory workers and chemists.[54,76–80]

Ethylene oxide is widely used as a chemical intermediate in the manufacture of products such as ethylene glycol antifreeze and non-ionic detergents. It is also used as a fumigant and in the sterilization of hospital equipment and cosmetics.[81] In a cohort of 18 235 workers exposed to ethylene oxide, a positive exposure–response trend was observed for NHL with a standardized mortality ratio (SMR) of 2.37 (95 percent CI 1.02 to 4.67) for the workers at highest exposure.[82] However, in another cohort of 2876 workers who were exposed to ethylene oxide there was no excess risk of NHL.[83]

Exposure to styrene has been high in the reinforced plastic industry. It is used to make products such as rubber, plastic, insulation, fibreglass, pipes, automobile parts, food containers and carpet banking. Results of studies of NHL in styrene-exposed workers vary, and the findings are not robust.[81] A recent update of an US cohort of workers exposed to styrene in the reinforced plastic industry did not find an excess in mortality related to NHL.[84]

Polychlorinated dibenzo-para-dioxins are formed as inadvertent byproducts during the production of chlorophenols and chlorophenoxy herbicides. Exposure to the conger 2,3,7,8,tetrachlorodibenzo-para-dioxins has been studied in several industrial cohorts and in the Seveso accident cohort. An increased risk for NHL was observed, although the relative risks were mostly nonsignificant and below 2.[63,85–88] However in the Seveso accident cohort, after a follow-up of 20 years, significant increase in mortality (relative risk [RR] 1.7, 95 percent CI 1.2 to 2.5) and morbidity (RR 1.8, 95 percent CI 1.2 to 2.6) of NHL was observed, consistent in both sexes.[89] Aside from the studies involving heavy exposure in industrial settings, exposure to dioxin is also possible from municipal solid waste incinerators. A cluster of patients with NHL was detected around a French municipal solid waste incinerator with high dioxin emissions. A case–control study in that area observed an increased risk of NHL of 2.3 (95 percent CI 1.4 to 3.8) among individuals living in the area with the highest dioxin concentration.[90]

Environmental factors

Although the separation between occupational and environmental factors is somewhat artificial, since agents occur in both settings, exposure to some agents occurs mainly in the general environment.

ULTRAVIOLET RADIATION

The epidemiologic evidence linking NHL risk to UV exposure is largely indirect. Ecological studies have observed parallel geographic patterns and temporal trends in NHL and skin melanoma,[91] and individuals with preexisting skin cancer have also been found to be at greater risk for NHL.[92–94] As discussed above, occupational studies have shown increased risk for NHL in farmers, who are exposed to solar radiation, and welders, who are exposed to artificial UV radiation. Both occupational groups are, however, exposed to other suspected risk factors for NHL as well, such as pesticides and solvents. Three studies looking at occupational UV exposure in outdoor occupations did not find an association[95,96] and studies looking at nonoccupational exposure to sunlight and NHL have been inconclusive.[97] A recent study from Australia reported results of a large case–control study providing weak support for the possibility that sun sensitivity increases risk of NHL,[92] while there was some suggestion that sun exposure itself was protective against NHL.[96] Another case–control study in Scandinavia found that a history of high UV exposure was associated with reduced risk of NHL.[93] UV radiation is known to induce immune suppression and induce the production of suppressor T lymphocytes in the skin as well as in locations remote to the site of exposure.[98] An additional mechanism to explain a role on UV radiation on lymphomagenesis is via $1,25(OH)_2D_3$, the active metabolite of vitamin D_3, which has been shown to decrease the proliferation of NHL cell lines,[99] to inhibit the cell cycle process, and downregulate T helper cell activity.[100]

IONIZING AND NONIONIZING RADIATION

Epidemiologic studies of populations exposed to ionizing radiation have found little evidence for an association with NHL. In a large study on X-ray workers, no excess of lymphoma was seen in over 27 000 radiologists in China.[101] Studies of atomic energy workers also find no evidence of a link between radiation and NHL.[102,103] A significant increase in the risk of mortality from lymphoma was observed in US radiologists who began to work between 1920 and 1939.[104] For nuclear workers, an increased risk of NHL was not found.[103,105–111] Three case–control studies evaluating the association between occupational radiation exposure and NHL did not find an increased risk of NHL among subjects that reported exposure to radiation.[18,43,112] Conflicting results have been reported on the association between NHL and electromagnetic fields. Studies from Canada[39] and Sweden[18] have reported an increased risk, whereas no association was observed in a study from Norway.[113] A study in Canadian electric utility workers showed no associations between indices of exposure to magnetic fields and NHL, but there was a suggestion of an association with exposure above electric field threshold cutoff points 10 and 40 V/m.[114] In two other studies among electric utility workers in USA and France no association with NHL was observed.[115,116]

DRINKING WATER CONTAMINANTS

Exposure to nitrates in drinking water has been suggested as a possible risk factor for NHL, but the available evidence is limited. In a case–control study of men from Minnesota, USA, no association was found with long-term exposure to nitrates.[117] In contrast, in Nebraska, long-term consumption of community water with high nitrate level was positively associated with NHL.[118] In another study from Sardinia, no association between nitrate concentration in community water supplies and NHL was observed.[119]

Lifestyle factors

BODY MASS INDEX

A threefold increased risk of NHL was reported for subjects with body mass index (BMI) equal or greater than 30 kg/m^2 in a case–control study from the USA.[120] A smaller, but still increased risk of NHL for subjects with a BMI of 35 kg/m^2 or greater was observed in a US cohort.[121] An association between BMI and NHL for women has been reported in a cohort from Sweden.[122] In contrast, a cohort study from the USA and a case–control study from Denmark and Sweden found no association between BMI or other anthropometric characteristics and NHL risk.[123,124] The evidence in favor of an association between high BMI and NHL is thus still limited and controversial.[125]

DIETARY FACTORS

There is limited evidence supporting diet or dietary components as risk factors for NHL.[125] Experimental evidence from animal studies suggests that greater fat and protein intake can alter immune function and increase risk of NHL.[126] High intake of fruit and vegetables, particularly cruciferous vegetables and fibers, has been suggested to be associated with a lower risk, whereas intake of specific carotenoids, vitamins A, C, E, or folate does not seem to be associated with NHL risk.[127,128]

High intake of meat, and of red meat in particular, was associated with a higher risk of NHL in several studies,[129–132] although this association was not confirmed in an Italian case–control study.[133] Conversely, fish intake was suggested to be protective against NHL development in several studies,[130,133–135] although one study reported no association.[127] Increased milk consumption has been associated with elevated NHL risk in two case–control studies and in one cohort study.[133,136,137] In contrast, two other studies could not confirm this association.[129,130] These results could be explained by the observation that a decrease in total fat intake may improve the immune status and long-term intake of large amounts of dietary protein

may increase immune tolerance.[129] The only study that has explored the association between dietary factors and specific NHL subtypes, has not provided evidence of heterogeneity of effects.[132]

There is no consistent evidence of an effect of use of supplements of vitamins A, C and E, and of multivitamins, on NHL risk.[138]

TOBACCO SMOKING

Most of the numerous epidemiologic studies investigating the role of smoking in the development of NHL did not report an increased risk of NHL overall.[139] Recently, a slight association between tobacco smoking and NHL was observed in a pooled analysis of 6594 cases and 8892 controls.[140] For subjects who ever smoked the increased risk of NHL was 1.07 (95 percent CI 1.00 to 1.15) and for current smokers the estimate was 1.10 (95 percent CI 1.00 to 1.20).[140] A large population-based case–control study conducted in the USA, which was not included in the pooled analysis[141] and two case–control studies that were included in the pooled analysis,[142,143] found that women, but not men, who had ever smoked were at increased risk to develop NHL. This sex difference could be explained by immunosuppression due to nicotine, which is influenced by genetic factors and sex.[144]

ALCOHOL DRINKING

There is limited literature on the effects of alcohol on the risk of NHL. Most of the available studies have not reported an association, but in one cohort[145] and three case–controls studies an inverse association has been observed.[120,146,147] A recent pooled analysis of nine case–control studies reported that people who drank alcohol were at lower risk of NHL (odds ratio [OR] 0.83; 95 percent CI 0.76 to 0.89), but no decreasing trend in risk was observed with increasing alcohol consumption. The protective effect of alcohol was particularly strong for Burkitt's lymphoma.[148]

HAIR DYE USE

Hair dyes contain chemicals that are carcinogenic and mutagenic in animals. The epidemiologic data on this topic are inconsistent. Several large studies have not detected an increased risk of NHL,[55,149–155] whereas others have reported a positive association, although mostly of small magnitude.[156–158] Studies that differentiate between products have suggested that the effect might be restricted to women using black hair products for more than 20 years, in particular with use of hair-coloring products before 1980.[151–153]

HORMONAL AND REPRODUCTIVE FACTORS

The incidence of NHL is approximately 50 percent higher in men than in women, but the reason for this gender difference is unknown. A hypothesis is that sex hormones partly have a role, since estrogen is known to influence immunocompetence.[159] However, a cohort study in Iowa did not find an association between menstrual or reproductive factors and NHL risk.[160]

Since pregnancy causes immunologic changes, it has been suggested that it could alter the incidence of NHL, but there is no clear evidence of an association of NHL with parity or age at first birth.[161]

PHYSICAL ACTIVITY

Laboratory evidence suggests an effect of physical activity on immune status, but few studies have addressed that issue in humans. A pooled analysis of occupational data from three case–control studies found no association between NHL and occupational physical activity measured by energy expenditure or sitting time.[162]

Medical conditions and medications

A history of immunologic disease has been linked to an increased risk of NHL, and this is reviewed in detail in Chapter 5. Other medical conditions have also been suspected to modify the risk of NHL, although the underlying mechanisms are not well understood. They are briefly reviewed in the following sections.

BLOOD TRANSFUSION

There is little evidence to support the hypothesis of an association between blood transfusion and NHL. In 1993, a cohort study reported a twofold elevated risk of NHL after blood transfusion.[163] Two other cohort studies also reported an increased risk of similar magnitude.[164,165] However, subsequent case–control studies have reported conflicting results.[166–172] The updated results of the initial cohort study continued to support the modestly increased risk, after adjustment for potentially confounding factors.[173] Blood transfusions have been shown to have a suppressive effect on the immune system; in addition they can cause engraftment of allogenic lymphoma cells from a donor with subclinical disease, and can transfer oncogenic viruses and chemical carcinogens.[167] The leukocyte and plasma fractions of blood transfusions are believed to mediate these immune-suppressive effects. Persons who receive transfusions are more susceptible to infections caused by blood–borne organisms. Yet, results are difficult to interpret because of differences and changes in blood transfusion practice in different countries and over time.[163]

USE OF MEDICATIONS

Many studies investigated the role of medication in the NHL etiology. In the USA, a case–control study used data from a medical care program to evaluate the risk of NHL after use of 14 common medications. Using a minimum of 5-year exposure lag between first notation and malignancy diagnosis, the risk of NHL was higher among subjects who were prescribed amphetamines (OR 2.2, 95 percent CI 1.1 to 4.8), lidocaine (OR 2.6, 95 percent CI 1.2 to 5.5) and meprobamate (OR 2.1, 95 percent CI 1.03 to 4.3).[174] Amphetamines were used primarily for weight control or for treatment of fatigue, depression or anxiety. Lidocaine was prescribed for tendonitis or bursitis, musculoskeletal or joint pain and local anesthesia for lacerations or other surgical procedures. Meprobamate was most often prescribed for anxiety and was also given for musculoskeletal pain and headaches.[174]

A few studies have examined the association between use of nonsteroidal anti-inflammatory drugs (NSAIDs), in particular aspirin, and risk of NHL. In 1992, a US case–control study found that women, but not men, with continuous use of aspirin or other pain relievers experienced an increased risk of NHL.[175] Similar results were observed in another US case–control study among women.[176] In contrast, a decreased risk of NHL was reported in a US study among men and women who ever used NSAIDs,[120] and no association between NSAID use and NHL was observed in a Dutch case–control study.[177] A US cohort reported a positive association between nonaspirin NSAID use and risk of NHL, but no dose–response was detected with frequency of use.[178] Recently, a case–control study revealed a decreased risk of NHL among men, but not among women. In contrast, regular use of acetaminophen was associated with elevated NHL risk among women, but not among men.[179]

Estrogen replacement therapy has been inconsistently linked to NHL risk. The Iowa women's cohort study in the USA did not find an association;[180] however, an update of that cohort revealed an weak positive association for NHL and a strong positive association for follicular NHL.[181] A Dutch study showed no statistically significant risk increase of NHL for women who used estrogens (hormone replacement therapy).[177] In contrast, a case–control in Connecticut, USA, found a decreased risk of NHL among women who used estrogen replacement therapy.[182]

In a case–control study in Yorkshire, UK, an increased risk for NHL was observed among subjects who took oral diabetic drugs (OR 2.4, $P = 0.02$) or used steroids (RR 1.7, $P = 0.006$).[183]

Subjects who had used medication such as aspirin, HMG-CoA reductase inhibitors, β-adrenergic blocking agents, and noninsulin-dependent diabetic medication had a decreased risk of NHL in a case–control study in Connecticut women.[182] In a US cohort of older women there was no association between NHL and nonestrogen steroid use or use of thyroid medications.[180] In a case–control study in USA, a reduced risk for NHL was associated with use of diazepam among men (OR 0.54, 95 percent CI 0.33 to 0.90), but no risk for NHL was associated with use of antibiotics, acetaminophen, medications for hypertension, steroids, or barbiturates; phenytoin sodium, allopurinol, insulin, or other drugs to control diabetes; or drugs to control weight for either men or women.[120] In the same study there was an increased risk of NHL with the use of cimetidine and other histamine H_2-receptor antagonists to treat ulcers.[120] In a cohort of glucocorticoids users, an elevated risk was found for NHL among those with 10–14 prescriptions (standardized incidence ratio [SIR] 2.68, 95 percent CI 1.16 to 5.29).[184]

DIAGNOSTIC X–RAY AND RADIATION THERAPY

Three studies reported no association between NHL and exposure to low level diagnostic X-ray procedures,[185] while a case–control study in Sweden observed an decreased risk of NHL among subjects having radiographic examinations (OR 0.6, 95 percent CI 0.3 to 0.9).[17] In a case–control study conducted in Yorkshire there was a decreased risk for NHL among subjects who received past diagnostic X-rays.[183] However in a US case–control study a history of diagnostic radiographic examinations was not associated with risk for NHL.[120] A pooled analysis of two studies in Sweden neither observed an association between radiographic examinations and NHL nor between radiation treatment and NHL.[17] A case–control study in Sweden revealed a significant association between NHL and radiation therapy, which was preserved even when radiation therapy within 10 years of NHL diagnosis was excluded (OR 2.07, 95 percent CI 1.24 to 3.44).[18]

HISTORY OF NONIMMUNOLOGIC DISEASES

Numerous studies have investigated the association between diabetes mellitus and NHL, but the results are inconclusive. A case–control study in Yorkshire found an OR of 2.0 (95 percent CI 1.1 to 3.7).[183] A prospective cohort study showed that women with a self-reported history of adult-onset diabetes have an increased risk of developing NHL.[180] Another study found that the prevalence of diabetes was high in patients with extranodal lymphoma, especially lymphoma in the head, nose and sinuses, central nervous system and orbit.[186] A cohort study in Denmark showed an increased risk for NHL with diabetes at older age as well, however the numbers were small.[187] Other studies did not find an association.[120,188–192]

Scarlet fever is caused by group A streptococcus. Epidemiologic studies have reported an increased risk of NHL (OR 3.2, 95 percent CI 1.4 to 7.2),[183] no association[192] or a reduced risk.[182] A history of duodenal ulceration was association with a decreased risk for NHL in a case–control study conducted in Yorkshire (OR 0.5, 95 percent CI 0.3 to 0.95), while history of malignancy (OR 2.1, 95 percent CI 1.2 to 3.7), kidney stones (OR 3.4, 95 percent 1.2 to 9.3), pneumonia (OR 2.6, 95 percent CI 1.1 to 6.6), and herpes zoster (OR 1.9, 95 percent CI 1.1 to 3.5) were associated with an increased risk of NHL.[183] In a case–control study in Los Angeles, USA, prior history of solid cancer was associated with significantly increased risk

of NHL.[175] However these diagnoses are self-reported and have not been independently validated. Similarly, in a US cohort of older women, those women who reported a previous cancer (excluding hematopoietic and lymphatic cancers) were at an increased risk of NHL (RR 1.66, 95 percent CI 1.02 to 2.69). There was limited power to detect site-specific associations.[180] Several epidemiologic studies have suggested an association between cutaneous melanoma and NHL. A pooled analysis of seven cohort studies revealed an increased risk of NHL (SIR 2.01, 95 percent CI 1.26 to 1.58) among cutaneous melanoma survivors.[94]

In an US cohort of older women no association was found between NHL and history of chronic colitis.[180] In a large case–control study from the USA, there was no evidence for NHL risk associated with heart diseases.[120] Among women, a reduced risk for NHL was associated with a history of rubella, whooping cough, cold sores and fever sores, canker sores, and tooth abscess.[120] An increased risk was found among women with nonthyroid-related endocrine gland disorders and among men who had a history of polio and gonorrhea.[120] In an Italian case–control study, the risk for NHL was not associated with asthma or ulcerative colitis.[192]

Conclusions and perspectives for prevention

The preceding paragraphs illustrate that studies investigating occupational, environmental and lifestyle-related risk factors of NHL have been valuable for generating hypotheses into the etiology of this malignancy. However, even for the most consistent findings (e.g. farming), the evidence is conflicting. For none of the agents and exposures reviewed here can one conclude that a causal association has been definitely established. This could be due to differences in circumstance of exposure between populations, differences in study design and exposure assessment methods, and lack of statistical power in individual studies because of small study size and low exposure prevalence. Furthermore, the available evidence might suffer from publication bias, as positive and statistically significant associations can be preferentially reported compared with null results. An additional limitation in the existing knowledge is the limited amount of results on specific NHL subtypes. Because of their limited study size, most epidemiologic studies looked at all NHL combined, but it is plausible that the risk factors are heterogeneous among NHL types, as suggested by the few studies that reported subtype-specific results.[39,42,140,148]

Large and international studies are needed to investigate the consistency in findings among populations and address the possible causes of inconsistencies. A promising approach in this direction is the establishment of InterLymph, an international consortium of NHL studies with comparable design, as tools to conduct large-scale, pooled analyses of environmental risk factors.[193]

Two large-scale pooled analyses of tobacco smoking and alcohol drinking, described above, have been recently published as part of the InterLymph collaboration.[140,148] Given the uncertainties in the etiology of this disease, the possibilities of primary prevention of NHL remain meager. One aspect worth noting is that most of the suspected risk factors discussed above have low prevalence of exposure in the general population, and even if a causal association were established, the removal of exposure (which in many instances would be difficult or impossible to achieve) would prevent only a small proportion of cases. A risk factor responsible for a relative risk of 1.5 with prevalence of exposure of 1 percent (e.g. solvents used for dry cleaning) would be responsible for only 0.3 percent of cases in the overall population, while a risk factor responsible for a relative risk of 1.2 with 30 percent exposure prevalence (e.g. tobacco smoking, high meat intake) would be responsible for 5 percent of all cases. Suspected risk factors with high prevalence of exposure therefore offer a better perspective for prevention.

HODGKIN LYMPHOMA

Hodgkin lymphoma (HL) is a malignancy that usually occurs in the lymph nodes. Its first description was in 1832 by Thomas Hodgkin (1798–1866). The incidence varies around the world and some remarkable geographic patterns are observed – this is discussed in detail elsewhere in this volume.

A subset of HL has been linked to the Epstein–Barr virus (EBV).[1] There is also evidence for a link between HL and infectious diseases, immune deficits and genetic susceptibility, which is discussed in other parts of this volume. This chapter reviews risk factors related to lifestyle and those occurring in the general environment, including the workplace.

Occupational exposures

OCCUPATIONS ENTAILING EXPOSURE TO BIOLOGIC AGENTS

Given the strong evidence for an etiologic role of infections in HL, an increased risk of HL among workers who may be in close contact with other people has been suggested. Examples include teachers[194,195] and physicians.[196] However, a survey in Boston, USA in the years 1960–70 found no increased risk of HL in teachers,[197] and other studies did not find an increased risk of HL in physicians and nurses.[197–199]

WOOD DUST AND WOOD-RELATED OCCUPATIONS

The first description of an increased risk of HL among men employed in woodworking or wood-related industries dates from 1967.[200] Since then, several studies have been conducted on workers in wood and related industries with inconsistent results. In five of 12 studies addressing the link between HL and working in the wood industry there was a statistically significant association as reviewed by McCunney.[201] The risk of HL associated with exposure to wood dust is analyzed in a pooled analysis of data from five cohort studies. There was no association between wood dust and HL.[202]

ORGANIC CHEMICALS, INCLUDING PESTICIDES

An extensive literature review on studies conducted to address the HL risk among occupational groups with exposure to organic chemicals concluded that those studies yielded inconsistent results.[201] An association between HL and benzene exposure was first reported in 1979 from a study based on death certificates,[203] but no risk was observed in a subsequent study of occupations involving benzene exposure.[204] In the rubber and refinery industries workers may be exposed to benzene either as a component or as the direct substance. Eighteen studies addressed the potential role of chemical exposure as a factor in the development of HL, but no consistent results were found.[201]

A meta-analysis of 30 studies of HL among farmers revealed a significant increased risk for farmers to develop HL (RR 1.25, 95 percent CI 1.11 to 1.42). No specific etiologic exposure was identified, but exposure commonly experienced by farmers (infectious microorganisms and insecticides) may contribute to the occurrence of the disease.[205] Studies of occupational exposure to phenoxy acids, chlorophenols and dioxins, including use of herbicides and pesticides, have been conflicting, increasing risk in some studies[206–210] and not in others.[26,85,211–214]

Lifestyle factors

NUTRITIONAL FACTORS

Concerning diet, a hospital-based case–control study was conducted in northern Italy. They found no association between wholegrain food, vegetables, fruit, fish or red meat intake and risk of HL,[135,215–217] whereas high consumption of ham and liver was associated with a significantly increased risk of HL.[133] There is no consistent evidence of an association between HL and specific dietary products.

A review of nine case–control studies on the association between infant breastfeeding and childhood cancer suggested that children who were never breastfed or breastfed for a short term have a higher risk of developing HL than those who were breastfed more than 6 months.[218]

TOBACCO SMOKING

The effect of tobacco consumption on HL has been investigated in several epidemiologic studies and two reported a significant increased risk of HL among smokers.[219,220]

The cohort study recruited 248 046 US veterans followed for 26 years. A 50 percent increased risk of developing HL was observed for current smokers.[219] In a case–control study current smokers had a significant 80 percent increased risk of HL, and there was a linear dose–response relationship with increasing packs per day, years and pack-years of smoking.[220] Several cohorts and case–control studies reported an increased but insignificant risk of HL ranging from 1.1 to 1.8 for smokers.[142,221–225] Additional case–control studies reported a decreased risk of HL, with OR between 0.8 and 0.9,[55,226,227] whereas another case–control study conducted in UK reported a significant protective effect of ever tobacco smoking on development of HL (OR 0.7, 95 percent CI 0.5 to 0.9).[228]

ALCOHOL DRINKING

Only two studies reported about a potential link between alcohol drinking and risk of HL. One study carried out in Yorkshire during the period 1979–84 included 248 cases of HL and reported significant inverse association for wine drinkers as well as for spirits drinkers.[228] The second study was a hospital-based case–control study conducted in Northern Italy and reported no association between alcohol intake and risk of HL.[133]

HORMONAL AND REPRODUCTIVE FACTORS

The incidence of HL is higher in men than in women. This difference may be explained at least in part by an influence of hormones or reproductive factors. A population-based study of women in Israel comparing HL cases diagnosed between 1960 and 1972 with matched controls reported that women with HL tended to have a lower parity than their controls.[229] A Norwegian cohort study investigating the effect of childbearing found that women with increasing parity had a lower risk of HL.[230] In contrast, a Slovakian study could not confirm previous reports of a protective effect of pregnancy for the HL risk.[231] A Swedish study of 917 women with HL and concomitant fertility information found a small and nonsignificantly reduced risk in parous versus nulliparous women.[232] A hospital-based Swedish study found that having children before the age of 30 compared with after 30 years of age showed a protective effect.[233]

Medical conditions and medications

TONSILLECTOMY

Several epidemiologic studies have addressed the question whether tonsillectomy is a risk factor for HL. This relates to the question of the role of biologic agents in HL etiology. Case–control studies have generated inconsistent results. A large population-based study found no association

between HL and tonsillectomy overall, but there was an increased risk in children with tonsillectomy before age 12.[234] In contrast, in a study from Italy it was found that young age at operation had a protective effect.[235] Two companion case–control studies in USA observed among older persons an increased HL risk, but the data are sparse.[236] The lack of a uniform association suggests either that tonsillectomy is not a causal factor, or when it is, its effect is complex and modified by factors related to family size.[237] Some positive findings have been explained by the confounding effect of social economic status and underlying disease.[235,236]

MEDICATION USE

In a population-based case–control study, regular aspirin use was associated with a 40 percent reduced risk of HL. Aspirin specifically inactivates nuclear factor (NF)-κB and NF-κB is constitutively active in HL cells. Inhibition of active NF-κB decreases proliferation and causes spontaneous apoptosis of Hodgkin cells.[238–240]

Family size and birth order

Family size may be a proxy for the overall probability of acquiring infections, i.e. the larger the family, the higher the probability that one member will bring home an infection. Birth order may be of importance for the age at exposure to common infections assuming that children of later birth order are more likely to be exposed to an infectious agent at an earlier age via their older siblings.[241] In a US study, the risk of developing HL among people with five or more siblings was half that among those with one or none. Furthermore, the risk was reduced among people of late birth order.[242] A case–control study in Yorkshire during 1979–84 supported small family size being a risk factor for HL.[228] In an Italian hospital-based study, a decrease in risk of HL was observed among subjects with large sibship size,[235] while a further Italian study did not observe an association between sibship and HL.[243] A register-based case–control study in Sweden investigated the effect of having older and younger siblings on HL risk. They found that number of older siblings was associated with a decreased risk of HL in young adults. This corroborates with previous reports indicating that individuals with more siblings and later birth order have a lower risk of HL in early adulthood.[244] In a case–control study in USA the analyses were stratified by age; among young adults and middle-aged persons, the risk of HL was associated with small family size, which was not the case among older people.[245] A study in Denmark among children and young adults reported that among children the risk of HL increase with increasing sibship size and among young adults the HL risk tended to decrease with increasing sibship size.[241]

Socioeconomic factors

Common infections are suspected to have a role in the development of HL. Such infections generally occur earlier in life under more crowded and less hygienic conditions, and it is hypothesized that low socioeconomic status (SES) can reflect an increased opportunity for exposure to those infections.[237] Therefore, the role of SES may differ in the development of HL in children, young adults and older adults. [245] Cohen and colleagues conducted the first study in 1964 among white male soldiers during World War II. Patients with HL were better educated, were of higher social economic class, and were more often unmarried at induction than army men in general.[246] In an Italian hospital-based study, a decrease in risk of HL was observed among subjects with low educational level,[235] and another study in Italy observed an association between HL and high educational level.[243] In a US case–control study the analyses were stratified by age; among young adults and middle-aged persons risk of HL was associated with single-family housing, and relative high maternal education. Among middle-aged persons, a similar pattern of social class risk factors was present. However, among older persons, risk was not associated with social class.[245] With growing enrollment of young children in nursery school, early exposure to other children now seems to be mediated more regularly through classmates at daycare and nursery school rather than siblings at home. A study in the USA found an inverse association between HL in young children and preschool attendance. This may implicate that HL is not associated with childhood SES itself, but rather with factors that influence age at exposure to infections during childhood.[247] However, among older adults aged 59–79 years, HL was associated with lower childhood SES but not with preschool attendance.

Conclusions and perspectives for prevention

In summary, epidemiologic studies indicate that environmental factors have a limited role in HL etiology. Some environmental factors that could be important in determining HL risk, such as number of siblings, birth order and SES, are likely to act as determinants of infection. There is evidence that risk of HL in children is associated with large family size and for young adults it is the opposite. These characteristics had also been observed in the epidemiology of polio-virus infection and suggested that young adults may develop HL as a rare consequence of late infection with a common infectious agent.[248] The role of infection with Epstein–Barr virus in causing HL is reviewed elsewhere in this volume; it is plausible that other infectious agents are also involved in HL etiology. Identification and control of biologic agents causally associated with HL remain the most promising approach for the prevention of this disease.

KEY POINTS

- Occupational, environmental and lifestyle-related risk factors have been valuable to generate hypotheses into the etiology of NHL and HL, but no causal association has been established.
- Farming has been often associated with increased NHL and HL risk.
- Occupational, environmental and lifestyle-related risk factors are likely to be heterogeneous among different NHL types.
- Large and international studies are needed to properly test etiologic hypotheses.
- Most suspected risk factors for NHL and HL have a low prevalence of exposure in the general population and their removal would probably prevent only a small proportion of cases.

REFERENCES

● = Key primary paper
◆ = Major review article

●1. Baris D, Zahm SH. Epidemiology of lymphomas. *Curr Opin Oncol* 2000; **12**: 383–94.
2. Ferlay J, Bray F, Pisani P, Parkin DM. *GLOBOCAN 2002 cancer incidence, mortality and prevalence worldwide*. IARC Cancer Base No. 5, version 2.0. Lyon: IARC Press, 2004.
◆3. Boffetta P, de Vocht F. Occupation and the risk of non-Hodgkin lymphoma. *Cancer Epidemiol Biomarkers Prev* 2007; **16**: 369–72.
4. Cantor KP, Blair A, Everett G *et al*. Pesticides and other agricultural risk factors for non-Hodgkin's lymphoma among men in Iowa and Minnesota. *Cancer Res* 1992; **52**: 2447–55.
5. Persson B, Fredriksson M, Olsen K *et al*. Some occupational exposures as risk factors for malignant lymphomas. *Cancer* 1993; **72**: 1773–8.
6. Amadori D, Nanni O, Falcini F *et al*. Chronic lymphocytic leukaemias and non-Hodgkin's lymphomas by histological type in farming-animal breeding workers: a population case–control study based on job titles. *Occup Environ Med* 1995; **52**: 374–9.
7. Kelleher C, Newell J, MacDonagh-White C *et al*. Incidence and occupational pattern of leukaemias, lymphomas, and testicular tumours in western Ireland over an 11 year period. *J Epidemiol Community Health* 1998; **52**: 651–6.
8. Blair A, Cantor KP, Zahm SH. Non-Hodgkin's lymphoma and agricultural use of the insecticide lindane. *Am J Ind Med* 1998; **33**: 82–7.
9. Simpson J, Roman E, Law G, Pannett B. Women's occupation and cancer: preliminary analysis of cancer registrations in England and Wales, 1971–1990. *Am J Ind Med* 1999; **36**: 172–85.

10. Fabbro-Peray P, Daures JP, Rossi JF. Environmental risk factors for non-Hodgkin's lymphoma: a population-based case–control study in Languedoc-Roussillon, France. *Cancer Causes Control* 2001; **12**: 201–12.

11. Zheng T, Blair A, Zhang Y *et al.* Occupation and risk of non-Hodgkin's lymphoma and chronic lymphocytic leukemia. *J Occup Environ Med* 2002; **44**: 469–74.

12. McDuffie HH, Pahwa P, Spinelli JJ *et al.* Canadian male farm residents, pesticide safety handling practices, exposure to animals and non-Hodgkin's lymphoma (NHL). *Am J Ind Med* 2002; **Suppl 2**: 54–61.

13. Franceschi S, Serraino D, Bidoli E *et al.* The epidemiology of non-Hodgkin's lymphoma in the north-east of Italy: a hospital-based case–control study. *Leuk Res* 1989; **13**: 465–72.

14. Skov T, Lynge E. Non-Hodgkin's lymphoma and occupation in Denmark. *Scand J Soc Med* 1991; **19**: 162–9.

15. Hanrahan LP, Anderson HA, Haskins LK *et al.* Wisconsin farmer cancer mortality, 1981 to 1990: selected malignancies. *J Rural Health* 1996; **12**: 273–7.

16. Cerhan JR, Cantor KP, Williamson K *et al.* Cancer mortality among Iowa farmers: recent results, time trends, and lifestyle factors (United States). *Cancer Causes Control* 1998; **9**: 311–19.

17. Persson B, Fredrikson M. Some risk factors for non-Hodgkin's lymphoma. *Int J Occup Med Environ Health* 1999; **12**: 135–42.

●18. Dryver E, Brandt L, Kauppinen T, Olsson H. Occupational exposures and non-Hodgkin's lymphoma in Southern Sweden. *Int J Occup Environ Health* 2004; **10**: 13–21.

◆19. Khuder SA, Schaub EA, Keller-Byrne JE. Meta-analyses of non-Hodgkin's lymphoma and farming. *Scand J Work Environ Health* 1998; **24**: 255–61.

20. Zahm SH, Blair A. Pesticides and non-Hodgkin's lymphoma. *Cancer Res* 1992; **52**: s5485–8.

21. Figgs LW, Holland NT, Rothmann N *et al.* Increased lymphocyte replicative index following 2,4-dichlorophenoxyacetic acid herbicide exposure. *Cancer Causes Control* 2000; **11**: 373–80.

22. Acquavella J, Doe J, Tomenson J *et al.* Epidemiologic studies of occupational pesticide exposure and cancer: regulatory risk assessments and biologic plausibility. *Ann Epidemiol* 2003; **13**: 1–7.

23. Bolognesi C. Genotoxicity of pesticides: a review of human biomonitoring studies. *Mutat Res* 2003; **543**: 251–72.

24. Schroeder JC, Olshan AF, Baric R *et al.* Agricultural risk factors for t(14;18) subtypes of non-Hodgkin's lymphoma. *Epidemiology* 2001; **12**: 701–9.

25. Tonn T, Esser C, Schneider EM *et al.* Persistence of decreased T-helper cell function in industrial workers 20 years after exposure to 2,3,7,8-tetrachlorodibenzo-p-dioxin. *Environ Health Perspect* 1996; **104**: 422–6.

26. Persson B, Dahlander AM, Fredriksson M *et al.* Malignant lymphomas and occupational exposures. *Br J Ind Med* 1989; **46**: 516–20.

27. Zahm SH, Weisenburger DD, Babbitt PA *et al.* A case–control study of non-Hodgkin's lymphoma and the herbicide 2,4-dichlorophenoxyacetic acid (2,4-D) in eastern Nebraska. *Epidemiology* 1990; **1**: 349–56.

28. Hardell L, Eriksson M, Degerman A. Exposure to phenoxyacetic acids, chlorophenols, or organic solvents in relation to histopathology, stage, and anatomical localization of non-Hodgkin's lymphoma. *Cancer Res* 1994; **54**: 2386–9.

29. McDuffie HH, Pahwa P, McLaughlin JR *et al.* Non-Hodgkin's lymphoma and specific pesticide exposures in men: cross-Canada study of pesticides and health. *Cancer Epidemiol Biomarkers Prev* 2001; **10**: 1155–63.

30. Quintana PJ, Delfino RJ, Korrick S *et al.* Adipose tissue levels of organochlorine pesticides and polychlorinated biphenyls and risk of non-Hodgkin's lymphoma. *Environ Health Perspect* 2004; **112**: 854–61.

31. Hardell L, Eriksson M. A case–control study of non-Hodgkin lymphoma and exposure to pesticides. *Cancer* 1999; **85**: 1353–60.

32. Miligi L, Costantini AS, Bolejack V *et al.* Non-Hodgkin's lymphoma, leukemia, and exposures in agriculture: results from the Italian multicenter case–control study. *Am J Ind Med* 2003; **44**: 627–36.

33. Hardell L, Eriksson M, Nordstrom M. Exposure to pesticides as risk factor for non-Hodgkin's lymphoma and hairy cell leukemia: pooled analysis of two Swedish case–control studies. *Leuk Lymphoma* 2002; **43**: 1043–9.

34. Blair A, Linos A, Stewart PA *et al.* Evaluation of risks for non-Hodgkin's lymphoma by occupation and industry exposures from a case–control study. *Am J Ind Med* 1993; **23**: 301–12.

35. Cano MI, Pollan M. Non-Hodgkin's lymphomas and occupation in Sweden. *Int Arch Occup Environ Health* 2001; **74**: 443–9.

36. Costantini AS, Miligi L, Vineis P. An Italian multicenter case–control study on malignant neoplasms of the hematolymphopoietic system. Hypothesis and preliminary results on work-related risks. WILL (Working Group on Hematolymphopoietic Malignancies in Italy). *Med Lav* 1998; **89**: 164–76.

◆37. Vineis P, Milizi L, Seniori Costentini A *et al.* Exposure to solvents and risk of non-Hodgkin lymphoma: clues on putative mechanisms. *Cancer Epidemiol Biomarkers Prev* 2007; **16**: 381–4.

38. Rego MA, Sousa CS, Kato M *et al.* Non-Hodgkin's lymphomas and organic solvents. *J Occup Environ Med* 2002; **44**: 874–81.

●39. Band PR, Le ND, Fang R, Gallagher R. Identification of occupational cancer risks in British Columbia: a population-based case–control study of 769 cases of non-Hodgkin's lymphoma analyzed by histopathology subtypes. *J Occup Environ Med* 2004; **46**: 479–89.

40. Olsson H, Brandt L. Risk of non-Hodgkin's lymphoma among men occupationally exposed to organic solvents. *Scand J Work Environ Health* 1988; **14**: 246–51.

41. Tatham L, Tolbert P, Kjeldsberg C. Occupational risk factors for subgroups of non-Hodgkin's lymphoma. *Epidemiology* 1997; **8**: 551–8.

◆42. Smith MT, Jones RM, Smith AH. Benzene exposure and risk of non-Hodgkin lymphoma. *Cancer Epidemiol Biomarkers Prev* 2007; **16**: 325–91.

43. Mao Y, Hu J, Ugnat AM, White K. Non-Hodgkin's lymphoma and occupational exposure to chemicals in Canada. Canadian Cancer Registries Epidemiology Research Group. *Ann Oncol* 2000; **11**(Suppl 1): 69–73.

44. Rinsky RA, Hornung RW, Silver SR, Tseng CY. Benzene exposure and hematopoietic mortality: a long-term epidemiologic risk assessment. *Am J Ind Med* 2002; **42**: 474–80.

◆45. Wartenberg D, Siegel SC. Carcinogenicity of trichloroethylene. *Environ Health Perspect* 2002; **110**: A13–14.

46. Anttila A, Pukkala E, Sallmen M *et al.* Cancer incidence among Finnish workers exposed to halogenated hydrocarbons. *J Occup Environ Med* 1995; **37**: 797–806.

47. Blair A, Stewart PA, Tolbert PE *et al.* Cancer and other causes of death among a cohort of dry cleaners. *Br J Ind Med* 1990; **47**: 162–8.

48. Spirtas R, Stewart PA, Lee JS *et al.* Retrospective cohort mortality study of workers at an aircraft maintenance facility, I. Epidemiological results. *Br J Ind Med* 1991; **48**: 515–30.

49. Daniel V, Huber W, Bauer K, Opelz G. Impaired in-vitro lymphocyte responses in patients with elevated pentachlorophenol (PCP) blood levels. *Arch Environ Health* 1995; **50**: 287–92.

50. Moszczynski P. Organic solvents and T lymphocytes. *Lancet* 1981; **i**: 438.

51. Ng HL, Araki S, Tanigawa T, Sakurai S. Selective decrease of the suppressor-inducer (CD4+CD45RA+) lymphocytes in workers exposed to benzidine and beta-naphthylamine. *Arch Environ Health* 1995; **50**: 196–9.

52. Hardell L, Axelson O. Environmental and occupational aspects on the etiology of non-Hodgkin's lymphoma. *Oncol Res* 1998; **10**: 1–5.

53. Linet MS, Malker HS, McLaughlin JK *et al.* Non-Hodgkin's lymphoma and occupation in Sweden: a registry based analysis. *Br J Ind Med* 1993; **50**: 79–84.

54. Figgs LW, Dosemeci M, Blair A. United States non-Hodgkin's lymphoma surveillance by occupation 1984–1989: a twenty-four state death certificate study. *Am J Ind Med* 1995; **27**: 817–35.

●55. Miligi L, Seniori CA, Crosignani P *et al.* Occupational, environmental, and life-style factors associated with the risk of hematolymphopoietic malignances in women. *Am J Ind Med* 1999; **36**: 60–9.

56. Bernstein L, Allen M, Anton-Culver H *et al.* High breast cancer incidence rates among California teachers: results from the California Teachers Study (United States). *Cancer Causes Control* 2002; **13**: 625–35.

57. Pearce NE, Sheppard RA, Smith AH, Teague CA. Non-Hodgkin's lymphoma and farming: an expanded case–control study. *Int J Cancer* 1987; **39**: 155–61.

58. Metayer C, Johnson ES, Rice JC. Nested case–control study of tumors of the hemopoietic and lymphatic systems among workers in the meat industry. *Am J Epidemiol* 1998; **147**: 727–38.

59. McLean D, Cheng S, 't Mannetje A *et al.* Mortality and cancer incidence in New Zealand meat workers. *Occup Environ Med* 2004; **61**: 541–7.

60. Boffetta P, Gridley G, Gustavsson P *et al.* Employment as butcher and cancer risk in a record-linkage study from Sweden. *Cancer Causes Control* 2000; **11**: 627–33.

61. Fritschi L, Johnson KC, Kliewer EV, Fry R. Animal-related occupations and the risk of leukemia, myeloma, and non-Hodgkin's lymphoma in Canada. *Cancer Causes Control* 2002; **13**: 563–71.

62. Becker N, Deeg E, Nieters A. Population-based study of lymphoma in Germany: rationale, study design and first results. *Leuk Res* 2004; **28**: 713–24.

63. Kogevinas M, Becher H, Benn T *et al.* Cancer mortality in workers exposed to phenoxy herbicides, chlorophenols, and dioxins. An expanded and updated international cohort study. *Am J Epidemiol* 1997; **145**: 1061–75.

◆64. Engel LS, Lan Q, Rothman N. Polychlorinated biphenyls and non-Hodgkin lymphoma. *Cancer Epidemiol Biomarkers Prev* 2007; **26**: 373–6.

●65. Rothman N, Cantor KP, Blair A *et al.* A nested case–control study of non-Hodgkin lymphoma and serum organochlorine residues. *Lancet* 1997; **350**: 240–4.

66. Alavanja MC, Blair A, Masters MN. Cancer mortality in the US flour industry. *J Natl Cancer Inst* 1990; **82**: 840–8.

67. Delzell E, Grufferman S. Cancer and other causes of death among female textile workers, 1976–78. *J Natl Cancer Inst* 1983; **71**: 735–40.

68. Eriksson M, Hardell L, Malker H, Weiner J. Malignant lymphoproliferative diseases in occupations with potential exposure to phenoxyacetic acids or dioxins: a register-based study. *Am J Ind Med* 1992; **22**: 305–12.

69. Kogevinas M, Zock JP, Alvaro T *et al.* Occupational exposure to immunologically active agents and risk for lymphoma. *Cancer Epidemiol Biomarkers Prev* 2004; **13**: 1814–18.

70. Pasqualetti P, Casale R, Colantonio D, Collacciani A. Occupational risk for hematological malignancies. *Am J Hematol* 1991; **38**: 147–9.

71. Hours M, Fevotte J, Ayzac L *et al.* Occupational exposure and malignant hemopathies: a case–control study in Lyon (France). *Rev Epidemiol Sante Publique* 1995; **43**: 231–41.

72. Holly EA, Lele C, Bracci P. Non-Hodgkin's lymphoma in homosexual men in the San Francisco Bay Area: occupational, chemical, and environmental exposures. *J Acquir Immune Defic Syndr Hum Retrovirol* 1997; **15**: 223–31.

73. Boffetta P, Andersen A, Lynge E *et al.* Employment as hairdresser and risk of ovarian cancer and non-Hodgkin's lymphomas among women. *J Occup Med* 1994; **36**: 61–5.

74. Sama SR, Martin TR, Davis LK, Kriebel D. Cancer incidence among Massachusetts firefighters, 1982–1986. *Am J Ind Med* 1990; **18**: 47–54.

75. Ma F, Lee DJ, Fleming LE, Dosemeci M. Race-specific cancer mortality in US firefighters: 1984–1993. *J Occup Environ Med* 1998; **40**: 1134–8.

76. Li FP, Fraumeni JF Jr, Mantel N, Miller RW. Cancer mortality among chemists. *J Natl Cancer Inst* 1969; **43**: 1159–64.

77. Olin GR, Ahlbom A. The cancer mortality among Swedish chemists graduated during three decades. A comparison with the general population and with a cohort of architects. *Environ Res* 1980; **22**: 154–61.

78. Carpenter L, Beral V, Roman E *et al.* Cancer in laboratory workers. *Lancet* 1991; **338**: 1080–81.

79. Belli S, Comba P, De Santis M *et al.* Mortality study of workers employed by the Italian National Institute of Health, 1960–1989. *Scand J Work Environ Health* 1992; **18**: 64–7.

80. Dosemeci M, Alavanja M, Vetter R *et al.* Mortality among laboratory workers employed at the U.S. Department of Agriculture. *Epidemiology* 1992; **3**: 258–62.

81. IARC Monographs on the evaluation of carcinogenic risks to humans, volume 60, Ethylene oxide. Lyons, France: IARC, 1994: 73–159.

82. Steenland K, Stayner L, Deddens J. Mortality analyses in a cohort of 18 235 ethylene oxide exposed workers: follow up extended from 1987 to 1998. *Occup Environ Med* 2004; **61**: 2–7.

83. Coggon D, Harris EC, Poole J, Palmer KT. Mortality of workers exposed to ethylene oxide: extended follow up of a British cohort. *Occup Environ Med* 2004; **61**: 358–62.

84. Ruder AM, Ward EM, Dong M *et al.* Mortality patterns among workers exposed to styrene in the reinforced plastic boatbuilding industry: an update. *Am J Ind Med* 2004; **45**: 165–76.

85. Fingerhut MA, Halperin WE, Marlow DA *et al.* Cancer mortality in workers exposed to 2,3,7,8-tetrachlorodibenzo-p-dioxin. *N Engl J Med* 1991; **324**: 212–18.

86. Kogevinas M, Kauppinen T, Winkelmann R *et al.* Soft tissue sarcoma and non-Hodgkin's lymphoma in workers exposed to phenoxy herbicides, chlorophenols, and dioxins: two nested case–control studies. *Epidemiology* 1995; **6**: 396–402.

87. Bertazzi A, Pesatori AC, Consonni D *et al.* Cancer incidence in a population accidentally exposed to 2,3,7,8-tetrachlorodibenzo-para-dioxin. *Epidemiology* 1993; **4**: 398–406.

88. Hooiveld M, Heederik DJ, Kogevinas M *et al.* Second follow-up of a Dutch cohort occupationally exposed to phenoxy herbicides, chlorophenols, and contaminants. *Am J Epidemiol* 1998; **147**: 891–901.

89. Pesatori AC, Consonni D, Bachetti S *et al.* Short- and long-term morbidity and mortality in the population exposed to dioxin after the 'Seveso accident'. *Ind Health* 2003; **41**: 127–38.

90. Floret N, Mauny F, Challier B *et al.* Dioxin emissions from a solid waste incinerator and risk of non-Hodgkin lymphoma. *Epidemiology* 2003; **14**: 392–8.

●91. Cartwright R, McNally R, Staines A. The increasing incidence of non-Hodgkin's lymphoma (NHL): the possible role of sunlight. *Leuk Lymphoma* 1994; **14**: 387–94.

92. Hughes AM, Armstrong BK, Vajdic CM *et al.* Pigmentary characteristics, sun sensitivity and non-Hodgkin lymphoma. *Int J Cancer* 2004; **110**: 429–34.

93. Smedby KE, Hjalgrim H, Melbye M *et al.* Ultraviolet radiation exposure and risk of malignant lymphomas. *J Natl Cancer Inst* 2005; **97**: 199–209.

◆94. Lens MB, Newton-Bishop JA. An association between cutaneous melanoma and non-Hodgkin's lymphoma: pooled analysis of published data with a review. *Ann Oncol* 2005; **16**: 460–5.

95. Freedman DM, Zahm SH, Dosemeci M. Residential and occupational exposure to sunlight and mortality from non-Hodgkin's lymphoma: composite (threefold) case–control study. *BMJ* 1997; **314**: 1451–5.

96. Hughes AM, Armstrong BK, Vajdic CM *et al.* Sun exposure may protect against non-Hodgkin lymphoma: a case–control study. *Int J Cancer* 2004; **112**: 865–71.

◆97. Armstrong BA, Kricker A. Sun exposure and non-Hodgkin lymphoma. *Cancer Epidemiol Biomarkers Prev* 2007; **16**: 396–400.

98. Cooper KD, Oberhelman L, Hamilton TA *et al.* UV exposure reduces immunization rates and promotes tolerance to epicutaneous antigens in humans: relationship to dose, CD1a-DR+ epidermal macrophage induction, and Langerhans cell depletion. *Proc Natl Acad Sci U S A* 1992; **89**: 8497–501.

99. Hickish T, Cunningham D, Colston K *et al.* The effect of 1,25-dihydroxyvitamin D3 on lymphoma cell lines and expression of vitamin D receptor in lymphoma. *Br J Cancer* 1993; **68**: 668–72.

100. Lemire JM. Immunomodulatory role of 1,25-dihydroxyvitamin D3. *J Cell Biochem* 1992; **49**: 26–31.

101. Wang JX, Inskip PD, Boice JD Jr *et al.* Cancer incidence among medical diagnostic X-ray workers in China, 1950 to 1985. *Int J Cancer* 1990; **45**: 889–95.

102. Gilbert ES, Fry SA, Wiggs LD *et al.* Analyses of combined mortality data on workers at the Hanford Site, Oak Ridge National Laboratory, and Rocky Flats Nuclear Weapons Plant. *Radiat Res* 1989; **120**: 19–35.

103. Kendall GM, Muirhead CR, MacGibbon BH *et al.* Mortality and occupational exposure to radiation: first analysis of the National Registry for Radiation Workers. *BMJ* 1992; **304**: 220–5.

104. Matanoski GM, Sartwell P, Elliott E *et al.* Cancer risks in radiologists and radiation workers. In: Boice JD, Fraumeni JF (eds) *Radiation carcinogenesis: epidemiology and biological significance.* New York: Raven Press, 1984.

105. Beral V, Inskip H, Fraser P *et al.* Mortality of employees of the United Kingdom Atomic Energy Authority, 1946–1979. *Br Med J (Clin Res Ed)* 1985; **291**: 440–7.

106. Gilbert ES, Omohundro E, Buchanan JA, Holter NA. Mortality of workers at the Hanford site: 1945–1986. *Health Phys* 1993; **64**: 577–90.

107. Wiggs LD, Cox-DeVore CA, Voelz GL. Mortality among a cohort of workers monitored for 210Po exposure: 1944–1972. *Health Phys* 1991; **61**: 71–6.

108. Liu Z, Lee TS, Kotek TJ. Mortality among workers in a thorium-processing plant – a second follow-up. *Scand J Work Environ Health* 1992; **18**: 162–8.

109. Darby SC, Kendall GM, Fell TP *et al*. Further follow up of mortality and incidence of cancer in men from the United Kingdom who participated in the United Kingdom's atmospheric nuclear weapon tests and experimental programmes. *BMJ* 1993; **307**: 1530–5.

110. Carpenter L, Higgins C, Douglas A *et al*. Combined analysis of mortality in three United Kingdom nuclear industry workforces, 1946–1988. *Radiat Res* 1994; **138**: 224–38.

111. Cardis E, Gilbert ES, Carpenter L *et al*. Effects of low doses and low dose rates of external ionizing radiation: cancer mortality among nuclear industry workers in three countries. *Radiat Res* 1995; **142**: 117–32.

112. Eheman CR, Tolbert PE, Coates RJ *et al*. Case-control assessment of the association between non-Hodgkin's lymphoma and occupational radiation with doses assessed using a job exposure matrix. *Am J Ind Med* 2000; **38**: 19–27.

113. Tynes T, Haldorsen T. Residential and occupational exposure to 50 Hz magnetic fields and hematological cancers in Norway. *Cancer Causes Control* 2003; **14**: 715–20.

114. Villeneuve PJ, Agnew DA, Miller AB, Corey PN. Non-Hodgkin's lymphoma among electric utility workers in Ontario: the evaluation of alternate indices of exposure to 60 Hz electric and magnetic fields. *Occup Environ Med* 2000; **57**: 249–57.

115. Sahl JD, Kelsh MA, Greenland S. Cohort and nested case–control studies of hematopoietic cancers and brain cancer among electric utility workers. *Epidemiology* 1993; **4**: 104–14.

116. Theriault G, Goldberg M, Miller AB *et al*. Cancer risks associated with occupational exposure to magnetic fields among electric utility workers in Ontario and Quebec, Canada, and France: 1970–1989. *Am J Epidemiol* 1994; **139**: 550–72.

117. Freedman DM, Cantor KP, Ward MH, Helzlsouer KJ. A case–control study of nitrate in drinking water and non-Hodgkin's lymphoma in Minnesota. *Arch Environ Health* 2000; **55**: 326–9.

118. Ward MH, Mark SD, Cantor KP *et al*. Drinking water nitrate and the risk of non-Hodgkin's lymphoma. *Epidemiology* 1996; **7**: 465–71.

119. Cocco P, Broccia G, Aru G *et al*. Nitrate in community water supplies and incidence of non-Hodgkin's lymphoma in Sardinia, Italy. *J Epidemiol Community Health* 2003; **57**: 510–11.

●120. Holly EA, Lele C, Bracci PM, McGrath MS. Case–control study of non-Hodgkin's lymphoma among women and heterosexual men in the San Francisco Bay Area, California. *Am J Epidemiol* 1999; **150**: 375–89.

121. Calle EE, Rodriguez C, Walker-Thurmond K, Thun MJ. Overweight, obesity, and mortality from cancer in a prospectively studied cohort of U.S. adults. *N Engl J Med* 2003; **348**: 1625–38.

122. Wolk A, Gridley G, Svensson M *et al*. A prospective study of obesity and cancer risk (Sweden). *Cancer Causes Control* 2001; **12**: 13–21.

123. Cerhan JR, Janney CA, Vachon CM *et al*. Anthropometric characteristics, physical activity, and risk of non-Hodgkin's lymphoma subtypes and B-cell chronic lymphocytic leukemia: a prospective study. *Am J Epidemiol* 2002; **156**: 527–35.

124. Chang ET, Hjalgrim H, Smedby KE *et al*. Body mass index and risk of malignant lymphoma in Scandinavian men and women. *J Natl Cancer Inst* 2005; **97**: 210–18.

◆125. Skibola CF. Obesity, diet and risk of non-Hodgkin lymphoma. *Cancer Epidemiol Biomarkers Prev* 2007; **16**: 392–3.

126. Cameron RG, Armstrong D, Clandinin MT, Cinader B. Changes in lymphoma development in female SJL/J mice as a function of the ratio in low polyunsaturated/high polyunsaturated fat diet. *Cancer Lett* 1986; **30**: 175–80.

127. Ward MH, Zahm SH, Weisenburger DD *et al*. Dietary factors and non-Hodgkin's lymphoma in Nebraska (United States). *Cancer Causes Control* 1994; **5**: 422–32.

128. Zhang SM, Hunter DJ, Rosner BA *et al*. Intakes of fruits, vegetables, and related nutrients and the risk of non-Hodgkin's lymphoma among women. *Cancer Epidemiol Biomarkers Prev* 2000; **9**: 477–85.

129. Zhang S, Hunter DJ, Rosner BA *et al*. Dietary fat and protein in relation to risk of non-Hodgkin's lymphoma among women. *J Natl Cancer Inst* 1999; **91**: 1751–8.

130. Chiu BC, Cerhan JR, Folsom AR *et al*. Diet and risk of non-Hodgkin lymphoma in older women. *JAMA* 1996; **275**: 1315–21.

131. De Stefani E, Fierro L, Barrios E, Ronco A. Tobacco, alcohol, diet and risk of non-Hodgkin's lymphoma: a case–control study in Uruguay. *Leuk Res* 1998; **22**: 445–52.

●132. Purdue MP, Bassani DG, Klar NS *et al*. Dietary factors and risk of non-Hodgkin lymphoma by histologic subtype: a case–control analysis. *Cancer Epidemiol Biomarkers Prev* 2004; **13**: 1665–76.

133. Tavani A, Pregnolato A, Negri E *et al*. Diet and risk of lymphoid neoplasms and soft tissue sarcomas. *Nutr Cancer* 1997; **27**: 256–60.

134. Fritschi L, Ambrosini GL, Kliewer EV *et al*. Dietary fish intake and risk of leukaemia, multiple myeloma, and non-Hodgkin lymphoma. *Cancer Epidemiol Biomarkers Prev* 2004; **13**: 532–7.

135. Fernandez E, Chatenoud L, La Vecchia C *et al*. Fish consumption and cancer risk. *Am J Clin Nutr* 1999; **70**: 85–90.

136. Franceschi S, Serraino D, Carbone A *et al*. Dietary factors and non-Hodgkin's lymphoma: a case–control study in the northeastern part of Italy. *Nutr Cancer* 1989; **12**: 333–41.

137. Ursin G, Bjelke E, Heuch I, Vollset SE. Milk consumption and cancer incidence: a Norwegian prospective study. *Br J Cancer* 1990; **61**: 456–9.

138. Zhang SM, Giovannucci EL, Hunter DJ *et al*. Vitamin supplement use and the risk of non-Hodgkin's lymphoma

among women and men. *Am J Epidemiol* 2001; **153**: 1056–63.

139. Kuper H, Boffetta P, Adami HO. Tobacco use and cancer causation: association by tumour type. *J Intern Med* 2002; **252**: 206–24.

◆140. Morton LM, Hartge P, Holford TR *et al.* Cigarette smoking and risk of non-Hodgkin lymphoma: a pooled analysis from the international lymphoma epidemiology consortium (InterLymph). *Cancer Epidemiol Biomarkers Prev* 2005; **14**: 925–33.

141. Zahm SH, Weisenburger DD, Holmes FF *et al.* Tobacco and non-Hodgkin's lymphoma: combined analysis of three case–control studies (United States). *Cancer Causes Control* 1997; **8**: 159–66.

142. Stagnaro E, Ramazzotti V, Crosignani P *et al.* Smoking and hematolymphopoietic malignancies. *Cancer Causes Control* 2001; **12**: 325–34.

143. Morton LM, Holford TR, Leaderer B *et al.* Cigarette smoking and risk of non-Hodgkin lymphoma subtypes among women. *Br J Cancer* 2003; **89**: 2087–92.

144. McAllister-Sistilli CG, Caggiula AR, Knopf S *et al.* The effects of nicotine on the immune system. *Psychoneuroendocrinology* 1998; **23**: 175–87.

145. Chiu BC, Cerhan JR, Gapstur SM *et al.* Alcohol consumption and non-Hodgkin lymphoma in a cohort of older women. *Br J Cancer* 1999; **80**: 1476–82.

146. Matsuo K, Hamajima N, Hirose K *et al.* Alcohol, smoking, and dietary status and susceptibility to malignant lymphoma in Japan: results of a hospital-based case–control study at Aichi Cancer Center. *Jpn J Cancer Res* 2001; **92**: 1011–17.

147. Kim JH, Bang YJ, Park BJ *et al.* Hepatitis B virus infection and B-cell non-Hodgkin's lymphoma in a hepatitis B endemic area: a case–control study. *Jpn J Cancer Res* 2002; **93**: 471–7.

◆148. Morton LM, Zheng T, Holford TR *et al.* Alcohol consumption and risk of non-Hodgkin lymphoma: a pooled analysis. *Lancet Oncol* 2005; **6**: 469–76.

149. Hennekens CH, Speizer FE, Rosner B *et al.* Use of permanent hair dyes and cancer among registered nurses. *Lancet* 1979; **1**: 1390–3.

150. Grodstein F, Hennekens CH, Colditz GA *et al.* A prospective study of permanent hair dye use and hematopoietic cancer. *J Natl Cancer Inst* 1994; **86**: 1466–70.

151. Thun MJ, Altekruse SF, Namboodiri MM *et al.* Hair dye use and risk of fatal cancers in U.S. women. *J Natl Cancer Inst* 1994; **86**: 210–15.

152. Holly EA, Lele C, Bracci PM. Hair-color products and risk for non-Hodgkin's lymphoma: a population-based study in the San Francisco bay area. *Am J Public Health* 1998; **88**: 1767–73.

153. Zhang Y, Holford TR, Leaderer B *et al.* Hair-coloring product use and risk of non-Hodgkin's lymphoma: a population-based case–control study in Connecticut. *Am J Epidemiol* 2004; **159**: 148–54.

154. Tavani A, Negri E, Franceschi S *et al.* Hair dye use and risk of lymphoid neoplasms and soft tissue sarcomas. *Int J Cancer* 2005; **113**: 629–31.

155. Benavente Y, Garcia N, Domingo-Domenech E *et al.* Regular use of hair dyes and risk of lymphoma in Spain. *Int J Epidemiol* 2005; **34**: 1118–22.

156. Cantor KP, Blair A, Everett G *et al.* Hair dye use and risk of leukemia and lymphoma. *Am J Public Health* 1988; **78**: 570–1.

157. Zahm SH, Weisenburger DD, Babbitt PA *et al.* Use of hair coloring products and the risk of lymphoma, multiple myeloma, and chronic lymphocytic leukemia. *Am J Public Health* 1992; **82**: 990–7.

◆158. Correa A, Jackson L, Mohan A *et al.* Use of hair dyes, hematopoietic neoplasms, and lymphomas: a literature review. II. Lymphomas and multiple myeloma. *Cancer Invest* 2000; **18**: 467–79.

159. Olsen NJ, Kovacs WJ. Gonadal steroids and immunity. *Endocr Rev* 1996; **17**: 369–84.

160. Cerhan JR, Habermann TM, Vachon CM *et al.* Menstrual and reproductive factors and risk of non-Hodgkin lymphoma: the Iowa women's health study (United States). *Cancer Causes Control* 2002; **13**: 131–6.

161. Adami HO, Tsaih S, Lambe M *et al.* Pregnancy and risk of non-Hodgkin's lymphoma: a prospective study. *Int J Cancer* 1997; **70**: 155–8.

162. Zahm SH, Hoffman-Goetz L, Dosemeci M *et al.* Occupational physical activity and non-Hodgkin's lymphoma. *Med Sci Sports Exerc* 1999; **31**: 566–71.

163. Cerhan JR, Wallace RB, Folsom AR *et al.* Transfusion history and cancer risk in older women. *Ann Intern Med* 1993; **119**: 8–15.

164. Blomberg J, Moller T, Olsson H *et al.* Cancer morbidity in blood recipients – results of a cohort study. *Eur J Cancer* 1993; **29A**: 2101–5.

165. Memon A, Doll R. A search for unknown blood-borne oncogenic viruses. *Int J Cancer* 1994; **58**: 366–8.

166. Adami J, Nyren O, Bergstrom R *et al.* Blood transfusion and non-Hodgkin lymphoma: lack of association. *Ann Intern Med* 1997; **127**: 365–71.

167. Zhang Y, Holford TR, Leaderer B *et al.* Blood transfusion and risk of non-Hodgkin's lymphoma in Connecticut women. *Am J Epidemiol* 2004; **160**: 325–30.

168. Anderson H, Brandt L, Ericson A *et al.* Blood transfusion at delivery and risk of subsequent malignant lymphoma in the mother. *Vox Sang* 1998; **75**: 145–8.

169. Nelson RA, Levine AM, Bernstein L. Blood transfusions and the risk of intermediate- or high-grade non-Hodgkin's lymphoma. *J Natl Cancer Inst* 1998; **90**: 1742–3.

170. Maguire-Boston EK, Suman V, Jacobsen SJ *et al.* Blood transfusion and risk of non-Hodgkin's lymphoma. *Am J Epidemiol* 1999; **149**: 1113–18.

171. Tavani A, Soler M, La Vecchia C, Franceschi S. Re: Blood transfusions and the risk of intermediate- or high-grade non-Hodgkin's lymphoma. *J Natl Cancer Inst* 1999; **91**: 1332–3.

172. Chow EJ, Holly EA. Blood transfusions as a risk factor for non-Hodgkin's lymphoma in the San Francisco Bay Area: a population-based study. *Am J Epidemiol* 2002; **155**: 725–31.

173. Cerhan JR, Wallace RB, Dick F *et al*. Blood transfusions and risk of non-Hodgkin's lymphoma subtypes and chronic lymphocytic leukemia. *Cancer Epidemiol Biomarkers Prev* 2001; **10**: 361–8.

174. Doody MM, Linet MS, Glass AG *et al*. Risks of non-Hodgkin's lymphoma, multiple myeloma, and leukemia associated with common medications. *Epidemiology* 1996; **7**: 131–9.

175. Bernstein L, Ross RK. Prior medication use and health history as risk factors for non-Hodgkin's lymphoma: preliminary results from a case–control study in Los Angeles County. *Cancer Res* 1992; **52**: s5510–15.

176. Kato I, Koenig KL, Shore RE *et al*. Use of anti-inflammatory and non-narcotic analgesic drugs and risk of non-Hodgkin's lymphoma (NHL) (United States). *Cancer Causes Control* 2002; **13**: 965–74.

177. Beiderbeck AB, Holly EA, Sturkenboom MC *et al*. No increased risk of non-Hodgkin's lymphoma with steroids, estrogens and psychotropics (Netherlands). *Cancer Causes Control* 2003; **14**: 639–44.

178. Cerhan JR, Anderson KE, Janney CA *et al*. Association of aspirin and other non-steroidal anti-inflammatory drug use with incidence of non-Hodgkin lymphoma. *Int J Cancer* 2003; **106**: 784–8.

179. Baker JA, Weiss JR, Czuczman MS *et al*. Regular use of aspirin or acetaminophen and risk of non-Hodgkin lymphoma. *Cancer Causes Control* 2005; **16**: 301–8.

180. Cerhan JR, Wallace RB, Folsom AR *et al*. Medical history risk factors for non-Hodgkin's lymphoma in older women. *J Natl Cancer Inst* 1997; **89**: 314–18.

181. Cerhan JR, Vachon CM, Habermann TM *et al*. Hormone replacement therapy and risk of non-Hodgkin lymphoma and chronic lymphocytic leukemia. *Cancer Epidemiol Biomarkers Prev* 2002; **11**: 1466–71.

182. Zhang Y, Holford TR, Leaderer B *et al*. Prior medical conditions and medication use and risk of non-Hodgkin lymphoma in Connecticut United States women. *Cancer Causes Control* 2004; **15**: 419–28.

●183. Cartwright RA, McKinney PA, O'Brien C *et al*. Non-Hodgkin's lymphoma: case–control epidemiological study in Yorkshire. *Leuk Res* 1988; **12**: 81–8.

184. Sorensen HT, Mellemkjaer L, Nielsen GL *et al*. Skin cancers and non-Hodgkin lymphoma among users of systemic glucocorticoids: a population-based cohort study. *J Natl Cancer Inst* 2004; **96**: 709–11.

●185. Boice JD, Jr. Radiation and non-Hodgkin's lymphoma. *Cancer Res* 1992; **52**: s5489–91.

186. Natazuka T, Manabe Y, Kono M, *et al*. Association between non-insulin dependent diabetes mellitus and non-Hodgkin's lymphoma. *BMJ* 1994; **309**: 1269.

187. Hjalgrim H, Frisch M, Ekbom A *et al*. Cancer and diabetes – a follow-up study of two population-based cohorts of diabetic patients. *J Intern Med* 1997; **241**: 471–5.

188. O'Mara BA, Byers T, Schoenfeld E. Diabetes mellitus and cancer risk: a multisite case–control study. *J Chronic Dis* 1985; **38**: 435–41.

189. Adami HO, McLaughlin J, Ekbom A *et al*. Cancer risk in patients with diabetes mellitus. *Cancer Causes Control* 1991; **2**: 307–14.

190. Wideroff L, Gridley G, Mellemkjaer L *et al*. Cancer incidence in a population-based cohort of patients hospitalized with diabetes mellitus in Denmark. *J Natl Cancer Inst* 1997; **89**: 1360–5.

191. Vineis P, Crosignani P, Sacerdote C *et al*. Haematopoietic cancer and medical history: a multicentre case–control study. *J Epidemiol Community Health* 2000; **54**: 431–6.

192. Tavani A, La Vecchia C, Franceschi S *et al*. Medical history and risk of Hodgkin's and non-Hodgkin's lymphomas. *Eur J Cancer Prev* 2000; **9**: 59–64.

●193. Boffetta P, Armstrong BK, Linet MS *et al*. Consortia in cancer epidemiology: lessons from InterLymph. *Cancer Epidemiol Biomarkers Prev* 2007; **16**: 197–9.

194. Milham S Jr. Letter: Hodgkin's disease as an occupational disease of schoolteachers. *N Engl J Med* 1974; **290**: 1329.

195. Fonte R, Grigis L, Grigis P, Franco G. Chemicals and Hodgkin's disease. *Lancet* 1982; **2**: 50.

196. Vianna NJ, Polan AK, Keogh MD, Greenwald P. Hodgkin's disease mortality among physicians. *Lancet* 1974; **2**: 131–3.

197. Grufferman S, Duong T, Cole P. Occupation and Hodgkin's disease. *J Natl Cancer Inst* 1976; **57**: 1193–5.

198. Matanoski GM, Sartwell PE, Elliott EA. Hodgkin's disease mortality among physicians [letter]. *Lancet* 1975; **i**: 926–7.

199. Smith PG, Kinlen LJ, Doll R. Letter: Hodgkin's disease mortality among physicians. *Lancet* 1974; **ii**: 525.

200. Milham S Jr, Hesser JE. Hodgkin's disease in woodworkers. *Lancet* 1967; **ii**: 136–7.

◆201. McCunney RJ. Hodgkin's disease, work, and the environment. A review. *J Occup Environ Med* 1999; **41**: 36–46.

◆202. Demers PA, Boffetta P, Kogevinas M *et al*. Pooled reanalysis of cancer mortality among five cohorts of workers in wood-related industries. *Scand J Work Environ Health* 1995; **21**: 179–90.

203. Vianna NJ, Polan A. Lymphomas and occupational benzene exposure. *Lancet* 1979; **1**: 1394–5.

204. Smith PR, Lickiss JN. Benzene and lymphomas. *Lancet* 1980; **i**: 719.

◆205. Khuder SA, Mutgi AB, Schaub EA, Tano BD. Meta-analysis of Hodgkin's disease among farmers. *Scand J Work Environ Health* 1999; **25**: 436–41.

206. Eriksson M, Hardell L, Berg NO *et al*. Soft-tissue sarcomas and exposure to chemical substances: a case-referent study. *Br J Ind Med* 1981; **38**: 27–33.

207. Hardell L, Eriksson M, Lenner P, Lundgren E. Malignant lymphoma and exposure to chemicals, especially organic solvents, chlorophenols and phenoxy acids: a case–control study. *Br J Cancer* 1981; **43**: 169–76.

208. Hardell L, Bengtsson NO. Epidemiological study of socioeconomic factors and clinical findings in Hodgkin's disease, and reanalysis of previous data regarding chemical exposure. *Br J Cancer* 1983; **48**: 217–25.

209. Wiklund K, Lindefors BM, Holm LE. Risk of malignant lymphoma in Swedish agricultural and forestry workers. *Br J Ind Med* 1988; **45**: 19–24.

210. Franceschi S, Bidoli E, La Vecchia C. Pregnancy and Hodgkin's disease. *Int J Cancer* 1994; **58**: 465–6.

211. Lynge E. A follow-up study of cancer incidence among workers in manufacture of phenoxy herbicides in Denmark. *Br J Cancer* 1985; **52**: 259–70.

212. Milham S Jr. Herbicides, occupation, and cancer. *Lancet* 1982; **i**: 1464–5.

213. Hoar SK, Blair A, Holmes FF *et al.* Agricultural herbicide use and risk of lymphoma and soft-tissue sarcoma. *JAMA* 1986; **256**: 1141–7.

214. Saracci R, Kogevinas M, Bertazzi PA *et al.* Cancer mortality in workers exposed to chlorophenoxy herbicides and chlorophenols. *Lancet* 1991; **338**: 1027–32.

215. Negri E, La Vecchia C, Franceschi S *et al.* Vegetable and fruit consumption and cancer risk. *Int J Cancer* 1991; **48**: 350–54.

216. Tavani A, La Vecchia C, Gallus S *et al.* Red meat intake and cancer risk: a study in Italy. *Int J Cancer* 2000; **86**: 425–8.

217. Chatenoud L, Tavani A, La Vecchia C *et al.* Whole grain food intake and cancer risk. *Int J Cancer* 1998; **77**: 24–8.

218. Davis MK. Review of the evidence for an association between infant feeding and childhood cancer. *Int J Cancer* 1998; **11**(Suppl): 29–33.

219. McLaughlin JK, Hrubec Z, Blot WJ, Fraumeni JF Jr. Smoking and cancer mortality among U.S. veterans: a 26-year follow-up. *Int J Cancer* 1995; **60**: 190–3.

220. Briggs NC, Hall HI, Brann EA *et al.* Cigarette smoking and risk of Hodgkin's disease: a population-based case–control study. *Am J Epidemiol* 2002; **156**: 1011–20.

221. Paffenbarger RS Jr., Wing AL, Hyde RT. Characteristics in youth indicative of adult-onset Hodgkin's disease. *J Natl Cancer Inst* 1977; **58**: 1489–91.

222. Matthews ML, Dougan LE, Thomas DC, Armstrong BK. Interpersonal linkage among Hodgkin's disease patients and controls in Western Australia. *Cancer* 1984; **54**: 2571–9.

223. Glaser SL, Keegan TH, Clarke CA *et al.* Smoking and Hodgkin lymphoma risk in women United States. *Cancer Causes Control* 2004; **15**: 387–97.

224. Adami J, Nyren O, Bergstrom R *et al.* Smoking and the risk of leukemia, lymphoma, and multiple myeloma (Sweden). *Cancer Causes Control* 1998; **9**: 49–56.

225. Siemiatycki J, Krewski D, Franco E, Kaiserman M. Associations between cigarette smoking and each of 21 types of cancer: a multi-site case–control study. *Int J Epidemiol* 1995; **24**: 504–14.

226. Gallus S, Giordano L, Altieri A *et al.* Cigarette smoking and risk of Hodgkin's disease. *Eur J Cancer Prev* 2004; **13**: 143–4.

227. Newell GR, Rawlings W, Kinnear BK *et al.* Case-control study of Hodgkin's disease. I. Results of the interview questionnaire. *J Natl Cancer Inst* 1973; **51**: 1437–41.

228. Bernard SM, Cartwright RA, Darwin CM *et al.* Hodgkin's disease: case-control epidemiological study in Yorkshire. *Br J Cancer* 1987; **55**: 85–90.

229. Abramson JH, Pridan H, Sacks MI *et al.* A case–control study of Hodgkin's disease in Israel. *J Natl Cancer Inst* 1978; **61**: 307–14.

●230. Kravdal O, Hansen S. Hodgkin's disease: the protective effect of childbearing. *Int J Cancer* 1993; **55**: 909–14.

231. Zwitter M, Zakelj MP, Kosmelj K. A case–control study of Hodgkin's disease and pregnancy. *Br J Cancer* 1996; **73**: 246–51.

232. Lambe M, Hsieh CC, Tsaih SW *et al.* Childbearing and the risk of Hodgkin's disease. *Cancer Epidemiol Biomarkers Prev* 1998; **7**: 831–4.

233. Olsson H, Olsson ML, Ranstam J. Late age at first full-term pregnancy as a risk factor for women with malignant lymphoma. *Neoplasma* 1990; **37**: 185–90.

234. Liaw KL, Adami J, Gridley G *et al.* Risk of Hodgkin's disease subsequent to tonsillectomy: a population-based cohort study in Sweden. *Int J Cancer* 1997; **72**: 711–13.

235. Bonelli L, Vitale V, Bistolfi F *et al.* Hodgkin's disease in adults: association with social factors and age at tonsillectomy. A case–control study. *Int J Cancer* 1990; **45**: 423–7.

236. Mueller N, Swanson GM, Hsieh CC, Cole P. Tonsillectomy and Hodgkin's disease: results from companion population-based studies. *J Natl Cancer Inst* 1987; **78**: 1–5.

237. Mueller NE. Hodgkin's disease. In: Schottenfeld D, Fraumeni JF (eds) *Cancer epidemiology and prevention*. New York: Oxford University Press, 1996: 893–919.

238. Bargou RC, Emmerich F, Krappmann D *et al.* Constitutive nuclear factor-kappaB-RelA activation is required for proliferation and survival of Hodgkin's disease tumor cells. *J Clin Invest* 1997; **100**: 2961–9.

◆239. Izban KF, Ergin M, Huang Q *et al.* Characterization of NF-kappaB expression in Hodgkin's disease: inhibition of constitutively expressed NF-kappaB results in spontaneous caspase-independent apoptosis in Hodgkin and Reed-Sternberg cells. *Mod Pathol* 2001; **14**: 297–310.

240. Hinz M, Loser P, Mathas S *et al.* Constitutive NF-kappaB maintains high expression of a characteristic gene network, including CD40, CD86, and a set of antiapoptotic genes in Hodgkin/Reed-Sternberg cells. *Blood* 2001; **97**: 2798–807.

241. Westergaard T, Melbye M, Pedersen JB *et al.* Birth order, sibship size and risk of Hodgkin's disease in children and young adults: a population-based study of 31 million person-years. *Int J Cancer* 1997; **72**: 977–81.

242. Gutensohn N, Cole P. Childhood social environment and Hodgkin's disease. *N Engl J Med* 1981; **304**: 135–40.

243. Serraino D, Franceschi S, Talamini R *et al.* Socio-economic indicators, infectious diseases and Hodgkin's disease. *Int J Cancer* 1991; **47**: 352–7.

244. Chang ET, Montgomery SM, Richiardi L *et al.* Number of siblings and risk of Hodgkin's lymphoma. *Cancer Epidemiol Biomarkers Prev* 2004; **13**: 1236–43.

245. Gutensohn NM. Social class and age at diagnosis of Hodgkin's disease: new epidemiologic evidence for the 'two-disease hypothesis'. *Cancer Treat Rep* 1982; **66**: 689–95.

246. Cohen BM, Smetana HF, Miller RW. Hodgkin's disease: long survival in a study of 388 World War II army cases. *Cancer* 1964; **17**: 856–66.

247. Chang ET, Zheng T, Weir EG *et al.* Childhood social environment and Hodgkin's lymphoma: new findings from a population-based case–control study. *Cancer Epidemiol Biomarkers Prev* 2004; **13**: 1361–70.

248. Gutensohn N, Cole P. Epidemiology of Hodgkin's disease in the young. *Int J Cancer* 1977; **19**: 595–604.

5

Immunologic and genetic predisposition

ALEXANDRA NIETERS AND CHRISTINE F SKIBOLA

INTRODUCTION

Most human cancers arise as a result of genetically influenced host responses to environmental causative factors. In some cases such as with familial cancer syndromes, the influence of an inherited genetic defect is great enough to predispose to the disease. The study of these cancer syndromes can provide mechanistic clues and identify molecular lesions that may give rise to malignancy. Though the risk of disease from these mutations may be great, their frequency in the population is low. Of perhaps greater significance on the population level are common genetic polymorphisms that may pose small increases in individual risk, but affect more people than cancer syndromes caused by inherited defects in major cancer genes. Moreover, gene–gene and gene–environment interactions are likely to result in a genetic predisposition to a 'high-risk' phenotype. These considerations may be particularly relevant to the study of lymphoid neoplasms. The inherent heterogeneity of lymphoma and the relatively subtle effects of common genetic polymorphisms make complex diseases such as lymphoma difficult to study. Surprisingly, candidate gene association studies have provided some valuable clues to date as to what genes and related pathways may be of relevance in lymphomagenesis. Some of these susceptibility alleles may be useful markers in the search for environmental causative agents. Furthermore, rapid technologic advances in high-throughput genotyping and bioinformatics have paved the way for an agnostic exploration of the entire genome to identify lymphoma risk alleles. This unbiased approach is likely to yield major benefits to lymphoma genetic research in the years to come.

Here we will concentrate on the genetics underlying leukemia, lymphoma and multiple myeloma including familial aggregations, associations with specific genetic syndromes, and common genetic polymorphisms with particular attention, where possible, to risk estimates.

FAMILY HISTORY OF HEMATOLOGIC MALIGNANCIES/LYMPHOMA

Familial aggregations for lymphoproliferative malignancies have been previously documented,[1–3] particularly for lymphomas and leukemias. Several large-scale studies have explored associations between family history of hematopoietic malignancy and lymphoma risk.[4–9] On the basis of a large Swedish family-cancer database, significant familial aggregation has been described for chronic lymphocytic leukemia/lymphoma (CLL).[4] In addition to a 7.5-fold elevated risk of CLL (relative risk [RR] 7.52, 95 percent CI 3.63 to 15.56), first-degree relatives of cases exhibited higher risks for non-Hodgkin lymphoma (NHL) (RR 1.45, 95 percent CI 0.98 to 2.16) and Hodgkin lymphoma (HL) (RR 2.35, 95 percent CI 1.08 to 5.08). Evaluation of 26 089 NHL cases and 58 960 matched controls of the combined Swedish family-cancer database and the Danish cancer registry reported that relatives of NHL cases exhibited an increased risk for NHL (RR 1.73, 95 percent CI 1.39 to 2.15), HL (RR 1.41, 95 percent CI 1.0–1.97), and CLL (RR 1.31, 95 percent CI 0.93 to 1.85), but not for multiple myeloma.[6] Risk of NHL was particularly evident for relatives of cases with an aggressive NHL subtype (RR 3.56, 95 percent CI 1.80 to 7.02). Further, a number of studies have reported an estimated doubling of NHL risk in first-degree relatives of affected cases.[2,8–12] An approximate twofold risk elevation has been reported in the largest pooled analysis of 10 211 NHL cases and 11 905 controls from the InterLymph consortium.[13] NHL risk was increased for individuals who reported first-degree relatives with NHL (odds ratio [OR] 1.5, 95 percent CI 1.2 to 1.9), HL (OR 1.6, 1.1 to 2.3) and leukemia (OR 1.4, 95 percent CI 1.2 to 2.7). Though the pattern of NHL heritability appeared to be uniform across NHL subtypes, noteworthy risk patterns differed by sex and type of hematopoietic neoplasm. Consistently for all subtypes, risk was highest among individuals who reported a brother with NHL. Other patterns were seen when first-degree relatives had HL or small lymphocytic leukemia/lymphoma (SLL)/CLL. If a first-degree relative had HL, NHL risk was highest if the relative was a parent (OR 1.7, 1.0 to 2.9). If a first-degree relative had leukemia, NHL risk was highest for women who reported a sister with leukemia (OR 3.0, 1.6 to 5.5).[13]

A large body of evidence supports an important familial component for HL.[2,5,14,15] A Scandinavian study of nearly 7500 HL cases and 10 500 controls found a threefold increased risk of HL (RR 3.11, 95 percent CI 1.82 to 5.29) in relatives of patients with HL.[5] Relative risks were higher in men than in women, a finding that is consistent with data from that of other studies. Individuals with familial HL had an earlier than average age at diagnosis,[5] which also has been reported by others.[14] The important role of genetic predisposition as an underlying cause of HL in young adulthood is further supported by data from a large twin study where monozygotic twins of patients with HL had an unusually high disease risk (standardized incidence ratio 99, 95 percent CI 48 to 182), while dizygotic twins of patients with HL had no increase in risk.[15]

In conclusion, the association of lymphoma risk with family history of hematopoietic malignancy suggests that genetic factors play an important etiologic role. Risks do not appear to vary considerably between histopathologic subtypes, suggesting common genetic pathways may be involved. Importantly, even though the risk to relatives of cases with lymphoproliferative tumors is significantly increased compared with risks in relatives of controls, the absolute excess risk of hematopoietic cancers is modest. For instance, the lifetime risk of lymphoproliferative malignancy in first-degree relatives of NHL cases was estimated to be 5 percent, about twice the absolute lifetime risk derived from the Surveillance Epidemiology and End Results data.[4–6]

INHERITED SYNDROMES

Many familial diseases involve rare inherited syndromes and germline mutations in tumor suppressor genes, proto-oncogenes or key genes involved in the regulation of DNA repair, apoptosis and immune response. However, due to their rare occurrence in the general population, and that affected individuals often die before reproductive age, these syndromes contribute only marginally to overall lymphoma risk. Since inherited immunodeficiency will be addressed in more detail in Chapter 24, only a brief overview of this topic will be presented here and is summarized in Table 5.1.

X-LINKED LYMPHOPROLIFERATIVE SYNDROME

X-linked lymphoproliferative syndrome (XLP) is a rare immune cell defect characterized by abnormal antiviral, antitumor and long-term humoral immune responses.[26] XLP is caused by germline mutations in the *SH2D1A* gene which encodes the adapter protein, signaling lymphocytic activation molecule-(SLAM) associated protein (SAP).[27] The clinical phenotypes of XLP include lymphoma (typically extranodal B cell NHL, usually of the Burkitt type), fulminant infectious mononucleosis and hypogammaglobulinemia. This protein and other factors of the SLAM family receptors regulate important aspects of lymphocyte function. A broad spectrum of abnormal immunologic features such as deregulated T helper (TH)1 and TH2 cytokine production, diminished cellular cytotoxicity, altered B cell differentiation, and disrupted natural killer T cell development are the consequence of SAP-deficiency.[27] One study on unrelated XLP families found a deletion of *SH2D1A* exon 1 and a splice site mutation in three boys with early-onset NHL.[28] None of these showed signs of prior Epstein–Barr virus (EBV) infection. Analyses of gene alterations in *SH2D1A* did not reveal any mutations in HL cases, non-endemic Burkitt lymphoma and Burkitt-type leukemia.[29] Further studies of SAP and the SLAM family receptors may provide insights into XLP and help elucidate underlying mechanisms involved in lymphomagenesis.

WISKOTT–ALDRICH SYNDROME

The Wiskott–Aldrich syndrome (WAS) is an X-linked recessive immunodeficiency characterized by thrombocytopenia, eczema, recurrent infections[27] and an increased risk of malignancy, most notably for NHL.[18] In the USA, incidence is approximately four per million live male births.[30] This syndrome is caused by as many as several hundred different mutations in the WAS protein (*WASP*) gene, that encodes a 502-amino acid protein involved in linking cellular signaling to regulation of cytoskeletal rearrangements in activated cells. Generally, missense mutations affecting the *WASP* – terminus result in X-linked thrombocytopenia, whereas C-terminal mutations and other extreme mutations result in WAS.[31] Clinical and laboratory information on 154 WAS patients revealed associated malignancies in 13 percent of patients mainly of the lymphoreticular system.[16] Furthermore, a particularly high risk of lymphomas (44 percent) has been seen in patients with specific splice site mutations in intron 6.[18]

Table 5.1 Inherited syndromes predisposing to lymphomas. Rare inherited syndromes and germline mutations in proto-oncogenes, tumor suppressor genes or key genes involved in the regulation of DNA repair or immune response constitute a small fraction of familial diseases. Although these syndromes account for a small number of lymphomas overall, they can provide clues to elucidate mechanisms underlying lymphomagenesis

Syndrome	Inheritance	Locus	OMIM	Gene, protein/Function	Lymphoma risk (reference)
Wiskott–Aldrich (WAS)	X-linked recessive	Xp11.23-p11.22	301000	WASP, WAS protein/key regulator of actin polymerization in hematopoietic cells	9–12% of WAS patients developed lymphoma.[14–17] Specific splice site mutations in intron 6 conferred a particularly high risk of lymphomas (44%)[18]
Ataxia telangiectasia (AT)	Autosomal recessive	11q22.3	208900	ATM, ATM protein/DNA damage detection	10–17% of AT patients will present with lymphoid malignancies in childhood or early adulthood[17,19]
Nijmegen breakage (NBS)	Autosomal recessive	8q21	251260	NBS1, nibrin/DS–DNA break repair	29% of 55 NBS patients developed lymphoma[20]
Bloom (BS)	Autosomal recessive	15q26.1	210900	BML, BML protein/DNA damage repair	13% of 168 individuals with BS developed lymphoma[21]
X-linked lymphoproliferative (XLP)	X-linked recessive	Xq25	308240	SH2D1A, SAP[a]/regulator of signaling pathways of various immune cells	30% of 272 XLP patients developed lymphoma[22]
Common variable immunodeficiency (CVID)	Variable	Several loci including 17p11.2	240500	Several, including TNFRSF13B, TACI[b]/class switch recombination	12–30-fold increased risk for lymphoma[17,23,24]
Li-Fraumeni (LFS)	Autosomal dominant	17p13.1, 9p21	151623	TP53, p53/DNA damage checkpoint	6.8% increased risk of lymphoma in 83 LFS families with and 16 LFS families without inherited TP53 mutations[25]

[a]Signaling lymphocytic activation molecule–associated protein.
[b]Transmembrane activator and calcium–modulator and cyclophilin ligand interactor.

ATAXIA TELANGIECTASIA

Ataxia telangiectasia (AT) is a rare autosomal recessive disorder characterized by telangiectasia, progressive ataxia, radiosensitivity, premature aging, immunologic deficiency and an elevated cancer risk. Genetic instability, abnormal sensitivity to ionizing radiation, altered DNA repair and disruptions of cell cycle checkpoints are the features of the AT phenotype at the cellular level. Individuals with AT show increased genomic instability associated with a 100-fold cancer excess, with the majority of cancers being of B and T cell origin, involving NHL, HL and several forms of leukemia.[32] Ten percent to 15 percent of AT patients will present with lymphoid malignancy in childhood or early adulthood.[19]

AT is caused by mutations of both alleles of the ataxia-telangiectasia mutated (ATM) gene located on chromosome 11q22–23. The biallelic germline mutations of the ATM gene result in a truncated protein in most AT patients. ATM encodes a 350-kDa protein kinase with homology to the catalytic domain of phosphoinositol-3-kinase and is an upstream mediator of a kinase cascade that links the detection of DNA damage to cell cycle progression, genetic recombination, and apoptosis.[33,34] ATM is implicated in the maintenance of genome integrity by activation of multiple cellular functions that prevent DNA damage from causing genetic instability.

Heterozygosity for ATM occurs with an estimated frequency of 0.2–1 percent in the general population. These carriers appear to be clinically normal, but have an increased risk for cancer, particularly of the breast.[35,36] A potential role of the ATM gene in lymphomagenesis has been suggested on the basis of studies on mutations in different lymphoma subtypes. Alterations of ATM are frequently detected in lymphoid malignancies and often consist of missense mutations.[37] These can be either acquired, as found in sporadic T cell prolymphocytic leukemia (T-PLL) and some other lymphoma subtypes, or they can be of germline origin as described in B-CLL, mantle cell lymphoma (MCL), and childhood acute lymphocytic leukemia (ALL). Germline mutations do occur in B-CLL patients;[38,39] however, they apparently do not account for familial clustering of B-CLL.[40] MCL is often characterized by deletion of one copy of the ATM gene[41] and missense mutations of germline and somatic origin have repeatedly been reported.[42,43] Loss of heterozygosity appears to be a rare event in HL.[44]

Several studies have explored single nucleotide polymorphisms (SNPs) in ATM in relation to lymphoma and leukemia risk. In a Japanese study, SNPs in the ATM gene have been associated with pediatric HL.[45] For three of these variants, functional relevance in ATM-mediated processes could be shown, supporting the notion that SNPs in the ATM gene may contribute to pediatric HL. Missense variants in ATM were found in two out of 23 pediatric HL cases from Israel.[46] Multiple rare ATM variants were observed more frequently in HL cases than controls in a US study.[47] Some recent studies have identified a role of ATM germline alterations in the risk of childhood B- and T-ALL.[48–50] In a study involving 103 pediatric T-ALL patients, five polymorphisms in the coding region of ATM were 2.6-fold more frequent in T-ALL patients compared to controls ($p = 0.06$) and associated with unfavorable outcome.[48] Three missense ATM variants were in fivefold excess (OR 4.9, 95 percent CI 1.2 to 18.2) in a group of 39 pediatric T-ALL patients compared to healthy controls.[49] Genomic missense alterations also have been detected in childhood B-precursor ALL. Two of 26 B-precursor ALL cases but none of the controls carried germline ATM alterations.[50] In a Danish study of 120 cases of lymphoid malignancy, a variant associated with aberrant splicing involving exon 9 (735C>T) was 5.6 times more frequent in diffuse large B cell lymphoma (DLBCL) patients compared to controls ($p = 0.026$).[51] In addition, several missense variants were overrepresented among cases. In a systematic evaluation of ATM germline variants common ATM alleles did not contribute to the risk of NHL, though rare putatively deleterious variants were overrepresented among mantle cell and marginal zone lymphomas.[52]

NIJMEGEN BREAKAGE SYNDROME

Nijmegen breakage syndrome (NBS) is an autosomal recessive disorder characterized by microcephaly, growth and mental retardation, immunodeficiency, hypersensitivity to ionizing radiation, chromosome instability and a high risk of malignancies, primarily of lymphoid origin. Of 55 patients with NBS, 40 percent developed cancer before age 21; more than 70 percent of these were B cell lymphomas.[20] The gene mutated in NBS, NBS1, is mapped to chromosome 8q21 encoding nibrin. In a complex with two other proteins, Mre11 and Rad50, nibrin participates in the repair of DNA double strand breaks.[53] In NBS patients, mutated nibrin cannot partake in repair of chromosomal breaks crucial for immunoglobulin and T cell receptor gene recombination. The common clinical and biologic features of AT can be explained by a partial overlap in the functional pathway of the ATM and nibrin proteins. Furthermore, nibrin is a substrate for phosphorylation by ATM. A deletion of five nucleotides in exon 6 of NBS1 (657del5) results in a truncated protein and has been found in approximately 90 percent of patients with NBS.[54] The majority of NBS patients are of Slavic origin and share the 657del5 founder mutation. Several sporadic NBS truncating mutations also have been detected in other ethnic groups.[55] In 25 individuals with mutations in both alleles, 22 developed lymphomas, most of them before age 15.[56]

Inconclusive data have been presented regarding the role of heterozygosity for the mutated NBS1 gene and cancer predisposition. Three studies did not find a major role of mutations in NBS1 in sporadic NHL;[57–59] however, in two of these, the low prevalence of the mutation in the respective populations will probably require larger sample sizes to establish whether an association exists. Among 68 Russian children with lymphoid tissue malignancies, Resnick et al.[55]

found two carriers of the 657del5 mutation, one case with pre-B cell ALL and one with Burkitt lymphoma. Further, a recent Polish study presented some evidence for a role of *NBS1* heterozygosity in predisposition to NHL and melanoma of the skin.[60] In another Polish study, the *NBS1* 657del5 mutation was more frequent in pediatric patients with ALL (OR 1.85, 95 percent CI 1.42 to 2.65) and NHL (OR 1.57, 95 percent CI 1.21 to 2.25) compared to controls.[61]

LI–FRAUMENI SYNDROME

Li–Fraumeni syndrome (LFS) is a rare autosomal disorder frequently associated with germline mutations in the *TP53* tumor suppressor gene. This syndrome is characterized by a high excess risk for all cancers, including B-CLL, ALL, HL, and Burkitt lymphoma. The prevalence of germline *TP53* mutations is approximately 0.01 percent in the general population, 0.1–1 percent among various cancer patients, and 5–10 percent among young patients with multiple cancers.[62] Analysis of data from 83 LFS families with and 16 LFS families without inherited *TP53* mutations revealed an occurrence of ALL and lymphoma at a frequency of 5.3 percent and 6.8 percent, respectively.[25]

In addition to the aforementioned diseases, several other rare inherited or congenital conditions, such as Bloom syndrome, common variable immunodeficiency syndrome, IgA deficiency, severe combined immunodeficiency (SCID), Duncan disease, autoimmune lymphoproliferative syndrome, and Down syndrome are all associated with a high risk of NHL and/or leukemia in children.[63]

CANDIDATE GENES

A number of association studies have examined polymorphisms in candidate genes and pathways that may be relevant

to the risk of lymphoid neoplasms. These include genetic variants affecting DNA methylation, synthesis and repair, those involved in immunoregulation, obesity and hormone production, and genes relevant to xenobiotic metabolism and oxidative stress. To date, most of these studies have been limited by size, further restricting the potential investigation of gene–gene and gene–environment interactions. Nonetheless, several genetic variants have been identified as potential susceptibility loci and have been replicated in more than one study, suggesting their relevance as true risk alleles (Tables 5.2–5.4). Larger studies involving dense mapping in these regions and more exploratory studies involving whole genome scans will help to further elucidate disease mechanisms and identify relevant pathways.

One-carbon metabolism

Folate is an essential micronutrient in humans and a carrier of single carbon units for methylation processes and nucleotide, protein and polyamine synthesis[64] (Fig. 5.1). Disruption of homeostasis in the one-carbon pool has been associated with altered risks of heart disease, neural tube defects, and cancer. Folic acid, vitamin B_6 and B_{12} deficiencies can influence DNA methylation patterns and hinder DNA synthesis and repair. Furthermore, functional variants in key folate genes are likely to alter the flux of one-carbon donors in these pathways, and have been repeatedly associated with disease susceptibility including lympho-hematopoietic malignancies.

5,10-METHYLENETETRAHYDROFOLATE REDUCTASE

5,10-Methylenetetrahydrofolate reductase (*MTHFR*), a key enzyme in the folate metabolic pathway, catalyzes the irreversible reduction of 5,10-methylenetetrahydrofolate

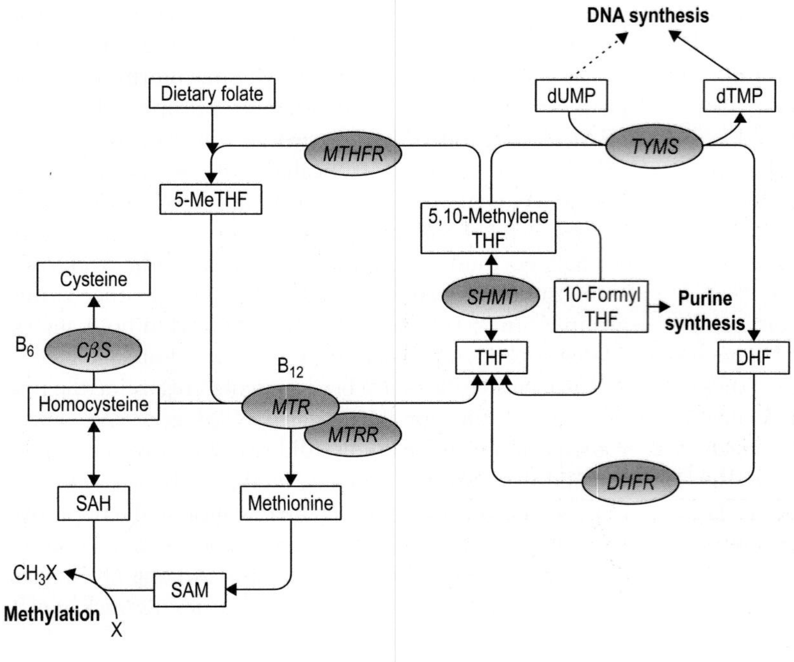

Figure 5.1 Simplified overview of the human folate metabolic pathway adapted from Skibola *et al.*[64] Metabolites: 5-MeTHF, 5-methyltetrahydrofolate; 5,10-methyleneTHF, 5,10-methylenetetrahydrofolate; 10-formylTHF, 10-formyltetrahydrofolate; SAM, S-adenosylmethionine; SAH, S-adenosylhomocysteine; DHF, dihydrofolate; THF, tetrahydrofolate; dTMP, deoxythymidine monophosphate; dUMP, deoxyuridine monophosphate. Enzymes: MTR, methionine synthase; MTRR, methionine synthase reductase; SHMT, serine hydroxymethyltransferase; MTHFR, 5,10-methylenetetrahydrofolate reductase; TYMS, thymidylate synthase; DHFR, dihydrofolate reductase; CβS cystathionine-β-synthase.

(methyleneTHF) to 5-methyltetrahydrofolate, the main circulatory form of folate and one-carbon donor for the remethylation of homocysteine to methionine (Fig. 5.1). Two frequent *MTHFR* polymorphisms (677C>T, Ala222Val; 1298A>C, Glu429Ala) have been described and their frequency varies substantially among Black, Caucasian and Asian populations.[65–67] These variants are in strong linkage disequilibrium (LD) and both appear to have functional effects. *MTHFR* 677C>T is located in the binding site for the enzyme cofactor flavin adenine dinucleotide that results in thermolability and reduced enzyme activity;[68,69] *MTHFR* 1298A>C lies within the S-adenosylmethionine-regulatory domain of the enzyme. Reduced MTHFR activity provides greater flux of folate for nucleotide synthesis, whereas DNA methylation may be hindered. These polymorphisms have been associated with pediatric and adult ALL[70–74] and lymphoma[64,73,75–77] (Table 5.2). Several studies report associations between NHL and the *MTHFR* 677C>T and 1298A>C alleles, though findings have been inconsistent.[64,73,77–82] In one large

US-based study of 1141 NHL cases and 949 controls, Lim *et al.* found no direct effect of variants in *MTHFR* (1298A>C) and NHL risk, however, they identified interaction between *MTHFR* 1298A>C and one-carbon nutrients, particularly methionine, in relation to NHL risk.[83] The Lim *et al.* study and others suggest important interactions between *MTHFR* SNPs and one-carbon donors and B vitamins, which may explain some of the inconsistencies observed in these studies.

METHIONINE SYNTHASE

Methionine synthase (*MTR*) encodes a vitamin B_{12}-dependent enzyme that catalyzes the remethylation of homocysteine to methionine; thus it plays a critical role in maintaining adequate intracellular methionine concentrations. The variant allele for an *MTR* SNP (2756A>G, Asp919Gly) has been inversely associated with follicular lymphoma (FL),[82] ALL,[73] and primary central nervous system lymphoma,[84] whereas an approximate twofold increased risk for lymphoma was

Table 5.2 Gene variants associated with non-Hodgkin lymphoma (NHL) risk – C1 metabolism and DNA repair

	Variant	Association
C1–metabolism		
MTHFR	Ala222Val, 677C>T, rs1801133	NHL (1.5 [0.97 to 2.2]);[64] NHL (0.58 [0.41 to 0.83]);[78] NHL (0.61 [0.45 to 0.82])[79] NS for NHL[73,77,80–82,91]
	1298A>C, rs1801131	NHL (1.7 [1.07 to 2.8]);[79] NS for NHL in[64,78,83] NHL with high vs. low methionine intake for 1298CC: (0.13 [0.04 to 0.39])[83]
MTR	Asp919Gly, rs1805087	NHL (2.0 [1.05 to 3.80]);[78] FL (0.41 [0.19 to 0.88]);[82] FL (0.49 [0.29 to 0.81];[91] NS in[64,77,83]
MTRR	66A>G, rs161870	Low-grade NHL (0.50 [0.25 to 0.99]);[73] DLBCL [1.56(1.03 to 2.38]);[79] NHL with high vs. low methionine intake (0.67 [0.47 to 0.97])[83]
SHMT1	1420C>T	NHL (0.75 [0.51 to 1.09]);[77] NHL (0.46 [0.23 to 0.93])[86]
TYMS	6bp del 3'UTR, rs16430	6bp-/- (and 3 linked SNPs): NHL (0.57 [0.34 to 0.94]), DLBCL (0.29 [0.10 to 0.82])[64] 6bp-/-: DLBCL (1.61 [0.99 to 2.60])[77]
	28-bp 2R>3R, rs699517	Multiple positive associations with NHL and 2R v 3R 28-bp repeat[77,79,86] 1 inverse association with FL[91] and 1 NS[64]
DNA repair		
LIG4	Thr9Ile, rs1805388	NHL (0.5 [0.3 to 0.9]);[92] NS in[93,94]
RAG1	Lys820Arg, rs2227973	NHL (2.7 [1.4 to 5.0]);[92] NS in[93,94]
WRN	rs4987236	NHL (0.7 [0.6 to 1.0]);[92] NS in[93]
	rs1346044	NHL (0.71 [0.56 to 0.91]);[93] NS[92,94]
BRCA2	rs766173	T cell NHL (3.97 [1.6 to 9.9]);[93] NS in[92,94]
	rs144848	T cell NHL (2.0 [1.2 to 3.3]);[92] NS in[93]
XRCC3	Thr241Met, rs861539	FL (1.62 [1.03 to 2.56]); MZL (2.60 [1.04 to 6.51]);[93] NS in[92,94,95]
	5'UTRC>T, rs3212024	FL (1.8 [1.1 to 2.8])[95]
H2AFX	–417G>A, rs2509049	NHL (0.54 [0.37 to 0.79]), FL, MCL[96]
MGMT	Val143Ile, rs2308321	FL [1.4 [1.0 to 2.0]);[93] NHL (2.6 [0.98 to 6.6])[95]

MTHFR, 5,10-methylenetetrahydrofolate reductase; *MTR*, 5-methyltetrahydrofolate-homocysteine methyltransferase; *MTRR*, 5-methyltetrahydrofolate-homocysteine methyltransferase reductase; *SHMT1*, serine hydroxymethyltransferase 1; *TYMS*, thymidylate synthetase; *LIG4*, ligase-4; *RAG1*, recombination activating gene 1; *WRN*, Werner–Syndrome helicase; *BRCA2*, breast cancer 2; *XCRR3*, X-ray repair complementing defective repair in Chinese hamster cells 3; *H2AFX*, H2A histone family member X; *MGMT*, O-6-methylguanine-DNA methyltransferase; NHL, non-Hodgkin lymphoma; FL, follicular lymphoma; DLBCL, diffuse large B cell lymphoma; NS, not significant.

seen in 919GlyGly homozygotes among Asians[78] (Table 5.2). However, no association was found for risk of DLBCL, multiple myeloma[82] and adult ALL.[85] In the latter study, some evidence for statistical interaction between *MTR* 2756A>G and a polymorphism in the serine hydroxymethyltransferase (*SHMT1* 1420C>T) gene was suggested. This gene encodes a vitamin B_6-dependent enzyme that catalyzes the reversible conversion of serine and tetrahydrofolate (THF) to glycine and methyleneTHF. Skibola *et al.* also found that carriers of the 1420T allele were at reduced risk for adult ALL compared to CC homozygotes.[85] Further, for NHL, the 1420T allele was associated with reduced risk in both a UK[77] and a Japanese study[86] (Table 5.2).

THYMIDYLATE SYNTHASE (TYMS)

The flux of deoxynucleotides for DNA synthesis is directly controlled by thymidylate synthase (TYMS) (Fig. 5.1). *TYMS* has a polymorphic 6-bp deletion (1494del6) in the 3'-untranslated region (UTR) that may influence RNA levels, and a tandem repeat sequence within the 5'-UTR containing a double or triple 28–bp repeat. Presence of the triple 28-bp repeat leads to enhanced gene expression that may increase conversion of deoxyuridine monophosphate (dUMP) to deoxythymidine monophosphate (dTMP), reducing the level of uracil that might otherwise be incorporated into DNA. Theoretically, this could limit DNA damage in rapidly dividing tissues that have the greatest requirement for DNA such as those involved in hematopoiesis. Skibola *et al.* found that those carrying one or two 28-bp triple-repeat alleles exhibited a significant 64 percent and 75 percent decrease in adult ALL risk, respectively.[85] Three case–control studies have investigated the role of *TYMS* polymorphisms in the risk of NHL, though results have been somewhat inconsistent. In an Asian study, those who harbored at least one double 28-bp repeat allele exhibited an increased risk for lymphoma,[86] NHL and T cell lymphoma,[79] whereas a British study found that the *TYMS* triple 28-bp repeat allele was associated with an increased risk of NHL[77] (Table 5.2). Furthermore, a US-based study found no association between the 28-bp repeat alleles and NHL risk; however, they did report a statistically significant inverse association of NHL risk with additional *TYMS* variants and constructed haplotypes.[64] Specifically, individuals who carried two copies of the 6-bp deletion in the 3'-UTR had a >40 percent reduced NHL risk estimate compared with non-deletion homozygotes, an effect which was more pronounced for DLCL. Interestingly, the British study found this same 6-bp deletion was positively associated with NHL risk[77] (Table 5.2). Two additional studies found no associations with *TYMS* gene variants.[79, 83]

OTHER ONE–CARBON METABOLISM ENZYMES

Transport of 5-methylTHF from the circulation to peripheral cells is facilitated by the reduced folate carrier (*RFC*). A non-synonymous SNP (*RFC* 80 G>A) associated with

higher plasma folate levels did not appear to alter NHL risk in a US and UK study.[64,77] Homocysteine can be remethylated to methionine by MTR or trans-sulfurated to cystathionine by cystathionine-β-synthase (CBS). A splice variant of *CBS* (844ins68) conferred an increased risk of primary central nervous system lymphoma (OR 2.43, 95 percent CI 0.90 to 6.61).[84] Methionine synthase reductase (MTRR) is an enzyme that maintains cellular levels of the co-factorial form of the MTR enzyme. Homozygous variants of a common *MTRR* polymorphism (66A>G) that was associated with neural tube defect risk under vitamin B_{12} deficiency exhibited a twofold risk reduction (OR 0.50, 95 percent CI 0.25 to 0.99) for low-grade NHL.[73] In an investigation of 30 variants in 18 genes among 1141 NHL cases and 949 controls, Lim *et al.* identified other NHL risk alleles in *CBS* and in four other genes involved in one-carbon metabolism: betaine-homocysteine methyltransferase (*BHMT*), folylpolyglutamate synthase (*FPGS*), 10-formyltetrahydrofolate dehydrogenase (*FTHFD*) and 5,10-methyltetrahydrofolate synthetase (*MTHFS*).[83] Interestingly, the last three of these showed an interaction with nutritional status, which highlights the need to integrate dietary data in risk assessment.

PROPOSED MECHANISMS OF FOLATE DEFICIENCY AND GENETIC VARIATION IN DISEASE RISK

Several mechanisms likely influence the risk of lymphohematopoietic malignancies associated with one-carbon metabolism. Disruptions in DNA methylation, either through hypomethylation of the promoter regions of proto-oncogenes, or hypermethylation of these regions in tumor suppressor genes, could result in selective growth, genomic instability, and induction of malignancy.[87] Furthermore, an increased rate of uracil misincorporation into DNA followed by extensive repair by uracil DNA glycosylase increases the likelihood of DNA double strand breaks due to erroneous excision repair processes. As a consequence, chromosomal instability, translocations, and other preneoplastic alterations may be induced potentially influencing malignant transformation, clonal expansion and pathogenesis. In an experimental model of folate deficiency, a 1000-fold increase in the rate of uracil misincorporation in DNA was observed resulting in a 50-fold increase in double strand breaks.[68] Particularly in fast replicating cells of the hematopoietic system, a sufficient supply of deoxynucleotides is essential for the maintenance of DNA integrity.

A number of studies have reported that the thermolabile *MTHFR677* T variant is a low-risk allele for ALL[70,71,73,88] and several mechanisms have been proposed. Reduced MTHFR enzyme activity provides a greater provision of one-carbon units available for purine and DNA synthesis, and enhances DNA repair mechanisms by reducing levels of uracil that might otherwise be incorporated in DNA (Fig. 5.1). However, reduced MTHFR enzyme activity also lowers the availability of *S*-adenosyl methionine (SAM) required for methylation processes resulting in hypomethylation of DNA, the effects of which are exacerbated under conditions of low folate status.[89,90] Thus, interactions between folate status and genetic variants in folate metabolism such as the *MTHFR* 677C>T or the *TYMS* 3′- or 5′-UTR polymorphisms are likely to explain some of the discrepancies in disease risk estimates being reported in various case-control studies. For example, the effects of some gene variants may seem less apparent in situations of adequate folate status. A point in hand is the inverse association between the *MTHFR* 677TT genotype and risk of childhood ALL among children in Canada born before but not after January 1996,[74] the approximate time Health Canada began recommending folic acid supplementation in pregnancy. Hence, additional studies, preferably with a prospective design and biomarkers, are needed that consider the complex interrelationship between genetics, folate, vitamin B_6 and B_{12} intakes, and other factors that may affect vitamin B status such as alcohol consumption. Furthermore, the integration of research on methylation status of lymphoma relevant candidate genes may help to shed light on epigenetic mechanisms linking genetic variability in one-carbon metabolism and lymphoma risk.

DNA REPAIR

Cellular DNA is damaged by alkylating and other chemical agents, oxidative stress, UV light and ionizing radiation. Mammalian cells have evolved numerous defence mechanisms to counterbalance these threats and to ensure genomic integrity.[97,98] Genetic factors that influence the elimination of damaged or deregulated cells through apoptosis and DNA repair processes are likely to play key roles in lympho-hematopoietic malignancies. The high risk of lymphoproliferative disorders in individuals that carry germline mutations in *ATM* and *NBS1*, two syndromes associated with aberrant repair of DNA double strand breaks, underscores the relevance of this pathway in lymphomagenesis. Double strand breaks occur physiologically during V(D)J recombination, the process responsible for the diversity of Ig and T cell receptors. Repair of these breaks is carried out by enzymes of the non-homologous end joining (NHEJ) pathway. For example, the *WRN* gene plays a crucial role in DNA double strand break repair (DSBR) and in other repair pathways. Mutations in this gene are associated with the autosomal recessive disorder, Werner syndrome, characterized by premature aging. However, more common *WRN* genetic variants have not been consistently associated with NHL[92,93] (Table 5.2). Polymorphisms in five other non-homologous end joining/DNA DSBR genes (*LIG4, RAG1, BRCA1, BRCA2, XRCC3*) and in the DNA DSBR checkpoint gene, *TP53*, also have not been consistently associated with NHL across studies.[92,94] An interesting finding was presented by Novik *et al.* where variation in a key histone gene involved in the detection of DNA DSBR, namely *H2AFX*, was associated with NHL.[96] Homozygosity for the A-allele upstream of

the translational start site of *H2AFX* (rs2509049) conferred a reduced risk for NHL. This finding will need to be tested in independent populations.

Variability in a DNA repair gene, O6-methyl-guanine-DNA-methyltransfersase (*MGMT*), was shown to modulate lymphoma risk.[92,94] The MGMT enzyme removes alkyl-DNA adducts and has an additional role in maintaining genomic stability. Hill *et al.* reported a positive but non-significant association of Ile143Val (rs2308321) and NHL and a statistically significant 1.4-fold increase in FL risk.[92] A meta-analysis including two further studies and a total of 573 FL cases and 1959 controls, presented a 30 percent increase in FL risk for carriers of the Val allele (95 percent CI 1.03 to 1.64), though DLBCL risk was not affected.[94] The Val allele of this polymorphism was shown to correlate with higher levels of nitrosamine-induced chromosome aberrations.[99]

In general, data on DNA-repair variants in relation to lymphomagenesis have so far been inconsistent (Table 5.2). There is little evidence yet to point to common DNA repair polymorphisms in disease risk.

Immunoregulatory genes

Genetic factors that influence immunoregulatory actions are likely to play a crucial role in the etiology of lympho-hematopoietic malignancies. Several candidate genes encoding proteins of critical relevance for the regulation of inflammatory processes, apoptosis, TH1/TH2 balance and host response to microorganisms have already been explored (Table 5.3). Several of these, such as tumor necrosis factor-alpha (*TNF*), are known as important autocrine growth regulators in lymphoid tumors and appear to have prognostic relevance.

TUMOR NECROSIS FACTOR (TNF)

TNF-α is a pro-inflammatory immunoregulatory cytokine that is a key mediator of T and B cell responses, natural killer cell activity, and dendritic cell maturation. Several polymorphisms at the *TNF* locus have been identified, including a functionally relevant −308G>A (rs1800629) SNP that has been associated with increased susceptibility for cerebral malaria, rheumatoid arthritis and Sjögren syndrome.[100,101] Functional studies revealed higher constitutional and inducible expression of TNF in whole blood of those carrying the −308A allele.[102,103] The *TNF* −308G>A and lymphotoxin-α (*LTA*) 252A>G (rs909253) polymorphisms are in strong LD. LTA is a related inflammatory cytokine that participates in similar signaling cascades as TNF.[104] Higher TNF expression associated with the −308A allele may augment antiapoptotic behavior in B cells and up-regulate pro-inflammatory effectors via the NF-κB pathway. TNF-mediated NF-κB activation induces several antiapoptotic factors including members of the BCL2 family, cellular inhibitors of apoptosis, and cell cycle regulators.[105] Thus, elevated TNF levels can promote chronic

Table 5.3   Gene variants associated with non–Hodgkin lymphoma (NHL) risk – immune regulation, obesity and energy regulation

Immune regulation

TNF	–308G>A, rs1800629	NHL (1.19 [1.05 to 1.33], DLBCL (1.29 [1.10 to 1.51]) AG vs GG, DLBCL (1.65 [1.16 to 2.34]) AA vs GG[106]
	–857C>T, rs1799724	NHL (0.59 [0.42 to 0.84]); FL (0.40 [0.23 to 0.68])[107]
LTA	252 A>G, rs909253	DLBCL (1.47 [1.18 to 1.84])[106]
TNFRSF5	–1C>T, rs1883832	FL (1.6 [1.1 to 2.4]),[108] (3 pooled studies, 1776 cases/2482 controls)
IL-4	–1098T>G	NHL (1.5 [1.1 to 2.1]);[109] T-NHL (3.8 [1.8 to 8.2]);[110] DLBCL (1.6 [1.1 to 2.4])[107]
IL-6	–174G>C, rs1800795	C allele: HL (0.29 [0.1 to 0.87]);[111] T-NHL (0.46 [0.23 to 0.92]);[110] NS for NHL, DLBCL, FL[106,107,109]
IL-10	–1082 A>G, rs1800896	–1082GG: DLBCL (1.23 [1.0 to 1.52]) 3575AA: DLBCL (1.11 [1.04 to 1.57]); TNF-308A/IL10_3575A: DLBCL (2.13 [1.37 to 3.32])[106]
	3575T>A, rs1800890	3575AA: DLBCL (2.1 [1.5 to 3.1])[107]
TLR4	Asp299Gly, rs4986790	MALT (2.76 [1.12 to 6.81]) and HL (1.80 [0.99 to 3.26]);[112] DLBCL (0.67 [0.45 to 0.99])[113]
TLR6	Ala427Val, rs5743815	NHL (5.20 [1.77, 15.3]) and subtypes[114]
CARD15	rs1715364	NHL (3.1 [1.1 to 8.8]);[113] DLBCL (10 [0.83 to 542])[106]

Obesity, energy regulation

CYP17A	rs743572	NHL (1.4 [0.95 to 2.1]), DLBCL (2.0 [1.1 to 3.5])[115]
		NHL (1.4 [1.02 to 2.03]), DLBCL (1.8 [1.1 to 2.7])[115]
CYP19A1	rs1870049	FL (3.0 [1.2 to 7.5])
	rs4774587	SLL (1.8 [1.1 to 3.0])[116]
ESR1	rs3020314	US study: FL (0.42 [0.23 to 0.77]); validated in German study (0.24 [0.06 to 0.94])[116]
COMT	Val108/158Met, (GA) rs4680	Bay Area NHL1: FL in women (2.0 [0.84 to 4.9])[117]
	+ others	Bay Area NHL2: DLBCL (1.8 [1.2 to 2.7])
LEP	–2548G>A, rs7799039	LEP –2548AA: NHL (1.4 [1.0 to 1.9]), FL (1.6 [1.1 to 2.3])[118]
	19 A>G, rs2167270	19G: NHL (1.6 [1.1 to 2.3]), FL (1.9 [1.0 to 3.6]);[119]
		19GG: NHL (1.4 [1.0 to 2.0]), FL (2.0 [1.3 to 3.3])[118]
LEPR	Gln223Arg, rs1137101	223ArgArg: FL among women (1.9 [1.0 to 3.6])[118]
		LEPR 223ArgArg/LEP–2548AA:NHL (2.3 [1.1 to 4.6, p = 0.02])[119]

TNF, tumor necrosis factor; *LTA*, lymphotoxin alpha; *TNFRSF5*, CD40 molecule, *TNF*, receptor superfamily member 5; *IL-4*, interleukin-4; *TLR4*, toll-like receptor 4; *CARD15*, recruitment domain family, member 15; *CYP17A*, cytochrome P450, family 17; *ESR1*, estrogen receptor 1; *COMT*, catechol-O-methyltransferase; *LEP*, leptin; *LEPR*, leptin receptor; NHL, non-Hodgkin lymphoma; DLBCL, diffuse large B cell lymphoma; FL, follicular lymphoma; HL, Hodgkin lymphoma; MALT, mucosa-associated lymphoid tissue lymphoma; SLL, small lymphocytic leukemia/lymphoma; NS, not significant.

inflammatory processes and enhance B cell survival, factors that may provide a milieu that favors lymphomagenesis.

Several studies have investigated the role of *TNF* polymorphisms in lymphomagenesis and/or prognosis. In the largest published study to date, pooled analyses of *TNF* and *LTA* genotyping data from eight European and North American case-control studies of the InterLymph Consortium[106] found that the *TNF –308G>A* SNP was associated with a 1.18 and 1.25-fold increased risk for the GA and AA genotypes, respectively among 2718 cases and 3118 controls (*p*-trend = 0.005). When restricted to cases with DLBCL (*n* = 1081 cases), there was a stronger gene-dosage effect of 1.29 and 1.65 for GA and AA genotypes, respectively. In contrast, no associations were found for FL (Table 5.3). In an updated pooled InterLymph analysis of more than 7000 NHL cases and 7000 controls this promoter variant was also associated with risk of marginal zone lymphomas (OR 2.7, *p*-trend=0.004) and mycosis fungoides (OR 2.1, *p*-trend=0.03), two further subtypes

with pro-inflammatory pathogenesis. *TNF –308A-LTA* 252G haplotypes have been associated with a negative prognosis for DLBCL[120] and multiple myeloma.[121] Other small studies reported null results between *TNF* polymorphisms and the risk of HL, CLL,[122] and multiple myeloma.[123] Additional SNPs in *TNF* (–857C>T, rs1799724 and –863C>A, rs1800630) have been associated with risk for NHL and FL,[107,124] gastric mucosa-associated lymphoid tissue lymphoma (MALT)[125,126] and adult T cell leukemia/lymphoma among human T-lymphotropic virus type I (HTLV-I) carriers.[127]

The *TNF* gene is located on chromosome 6p21 in the human leukocyte antigen (HLA) class III region in close proximity to other immunoregulatory factors such as leukocyte-specific transcript and allograft inflammatory factor. Interestingly, a variant in HLA-B associated transcript 2 (*BAT2*) (Val1883Leu, rs3132453) was significantly associated with NHL risk in a study of genetic variation in 1253 immune and inflammation genes explored among

458 NHL cases and 1253 controls.[114] To further clarify the role of this locus in lymphomagenesis, future studies should focus on fine mapping of the HLA region and functional characterization of variants in other genes in the proximity of the *TNF/LTA* locus.

TUMOR NECROSIS FACTOR SUPER FAMILY, MEMBER 5 (TNFRSF5)

CD40 and its ligand, *CD154*, are major co-stimulatory molecules whose interactions are important in humoral and cellular immunity. CD40-CD154 ligation is crucial for the maturation and activation of B cells, dendritic cells and other APCs. The C allele of a −1 C>T promoter SNP located in the Kozak sequence of the *TNFRSF5* gene (rs1883832) has been associated with enhanced CD40 translational efficiency and protein expression on B cells.[128,129] A pooled analyses of three case–control studies (total $n = 1776$ NHL cases, $n = 2482$ controls) revealed an increased risk of FL associated with the *TNFRSF5*–1TT genotype[108] (Table 5.3). Skibola *et al.* also found that healthy individuals with the −1T allele had reduced CD40 expression on dendritic cells and lower circulating CD40 levels.[108] These findings were recently further validated in EpiLymph in 1878 cases and 1904 controls where investigators found that the *TNFRSF5*–1TT genotype was associated with an increased risk of FL and DLBCL (Nieters *et al.* submitted for publication). Interestingly, in all study centers the *TNFRSF5*–1TT genotype was associated with an elevated risk of at least one of the two major NHL subtypes, DLBCL and FL, neoplasms that derive mainly in the germinal center (GC). CD40-CD154 ligation plays a pivotal role in centrocyte differentiation in the GC by up-regulating the NF-κB canonical pathway resulting in down-regulation of BCL6.[130] Low BCL6 activity permits differentiation of centrocytes into plasma cells and memory cells, allowing B cells to exit the GC. This process may be attenuated by the *TNFRSF5*–1TT genotype where low CD40 expression could hinder B and T cell interactions, allowing B cells to linger in GCs, undergoing further somatic hypermutation and proliferation. This may promote B cells with preneoplastic lesions to undergo malignancy.

CASPASES

Caspases (CASP) may also influence B cell apoptotic behavior and lymphoid tumor development as they are cysteine proteases that function in the cell death pathway. Inactivating mutations of the *CASP10* gene have been found in NHL[131] and preliminary studies suggest that genetic variants in caspase genes may influence NHL susceptibility.[132] In a population-based study of US women, variants in *CASP3* rs1049216 and *9* rs1052576 conferred reduced risks of NHL and FL. Also risk of marginal zone lymphoma and CLL were inversely affected by *CASP* gene

variants. If these preliminary findings are validated in larger studies, *CASP* genes may also be promising targets for treatment of lymphoid neoplasms.

INTERLEUKIN-4 AND -6

Interleukin (IL)-4 is the hallmark cytokine of TH2 cell immune response and signaling through its receptor, IL4R, crucial for B and T cell proliferation. Several polymorphisms in *IL-4* and *IL-4R* appear to be of functional importance and have been associated with various atopic and inflammatory conditions, outcomes of viral infections, and more recently, with lymphoma risk[107,109,110] (Table 5.3). The G-allele of a promoter polymorphism in *IL-4* (-1098T>G) was positively associated with NHL, T-NHL[110] and DLBCL.[107] These studies also reported an over-representation of a SNP (rs2107356) that alters gene expression of IL-4R among patients with DLBCL[109] and T-NHL.[110]

Elevated IL-6 levels have been detected in patients with lymphoid malignancies such as HL and multiple myeloma. IL-6 may influence lymphomagenesis through its effect on TH1/TH2 response, stimulation of T cell proliferation, or its function as a growth factor in lymphoid cells. A frequently studied *IL-6* promoter polymorphism (−174G>C, rs1800795) may modulate intracellular and plasma IL-6 levels, though results are conflicting.[109] A few studies have investigated this variant in relation to lympho-hematopoietic cancer risk. The −174C allele was inversely associated with risk of young adult HL[111] (Table 5.3), young adult nodular lymphocyte predominant HL,[133] and T-NHL,[110] but not NHL,[106,107,109] and CLL.[123,134]

INTERLEUKIN-10

IL-10 is a hallmark cytokine of regulatory T cells with an important function in modulating TH1 and TH2 immune responses.[135] Through feedback inhibition, IL-10 down-regulates proinflammatory cytokine production, notably TNF-α, and enhances survival and proliferation of B cells.[136] Furthermore, elevated IL-10 levels were indicators of poor prognosis and shorter survival for NHL[137] and CLL patients.[138] Several polymorphisms in the *IL-10* distal and proximal promoter elements may have functional relevance. The *IL-10* −1082A and −1082G alleles have been correlated with low and high IL-10 production, respectively. Pooled analyses of the 3575A>T (rs1800890) and −1082A>G (rs1800896) variants from the InterLymph Consortium[106] revealed that both *IL-10* SNPs were associated with DLBCL risk though not with FL (Table 5.3). An updated InterLymph analysis of more than 7000 NHL cases and more than 7000 controls revealed a 20 percent increased risk for DLBCL (*p*-trend = 0.016) and a 90 percent increased risk for extranodal marginal zone lymphoma among those homozygous for the 3575AA genotype (*p*-trend = 0.08). The GG genotype of IL-10 −1082 conferred a 70 percent elevation in risk for mantle cell lymphoma (p-trend = 0.04). An early study reported an elevated multiple myeloma risk in association with a high-producer IL-10 microsatellite genotype (136/136),[139] though IL-10 promoter SNPs (−592A>C, −819C>T and −1082A>G) did not affect risk.[139,140] In another study, elevated serum IL-10 and the −592CC genotype were associated with AIDS-related NHL (OR 1.6, 95 percent CI 1.1 to 2.3 for the 592CC genotype).[141]

Other immune regulatory variants

B CELL LYMPHOMA 6

B cell lymphoma 6 (BCL6) is a transcriptional repressor for a variety of target genes implicated in T and B cell maturation, apoptosis and cell cycle regulation. BCL6 is expressed early in GC formation and its down-regulation is critical for post-GC B cell maturation.[142] Frequent genetic alterations including translocations, deletions, and somatic mutations have been identified in DLBCL and FL subtypes. Evidence for a role of BCL6 SNPs in lymphomagenesis was reported by Lossos et al.[143] that found an intronic variant allele (397G>C) more frequent in FL cases than in controls (p = 0.01). This was not supported by a recent study,[144] though the 397G>C genotype correlated to a higher-grade transformation risk. In a population-based NHL case–control study of women in the USA, a common BCL6 variant (−195C>T, rs1056932) that alters a potential binding site for an exonic splicing enhancer was associated with a doubling of NHL risk (OR 2.2, 95 percent CI 1.5 to 3.3).[145] In a subtype analysis, compared with −195TT, the −195CC genotype was associated with an elevated risk for B cell lymphoma (OR 2.0, 95 percent CI 1.3 to 3.1), particularly CLL/SLL (OR 3.5, 95 percent CI 1.6 to 7.8), and T cell lymphoma (OR 5.2, 95 percent CI 2.0 to 13.3).

NOD2/CARD15 AND TLR

NOD2/CARD15 and TLR-4 are proinflammatory mediators that are integral in the first line of defense against viral and bacterial infection, providing non-specific protection against numerous pathogens. NOD2 exerts antimicrobial activity through a NF-κB-mediated pathway of inflammation and apoptosis.[146] A NOD2 C insertion at nucleotide 1007 (rs2066847) has been linked to autoimmune disorders such as Crohn disease and psoriasis.[147] Further, studies by the InterLymph consortium found that the NOD2 C insertion was associated with an elevated, but imprecise, elevated risk estimate for NHL and DLBCL in particular[106] (Table 5.3). This was supported in a pooled analysis of two population-based case–control studies of NHL from the San Francisco Bay Area and UK (CC vs. — OR = 3.1, 95 percent CI 1.1 to 8.8).[113] Due to its relative rarity in Caucasian populations, this polymorphism will need to be further investigated in larger future studies involving the InterLymph consortium

to determine its impact on lymphoma risk. The TLR4 gene facilitates proinflammatory cytokine release by human cells in response to lipopolysaccharide (LPS), mediates tolerance and multiple stages of B cell activation. A TLR4 polymorphism (Asp299Gly, rs4986790) in the extracellular domain attenuates receptor signaling, reduces IL-12 and interferon (IFN)-γ levels, and promotes an allergy-driven TH2 response. Recently, the TLR4 299Gly allele was inversely associated with the risk of gastric marginal zone lymphoma (GMZL)[148] and DLCL[113] (Table 5.3). The same variant was associated with increased risk of MALT lymphoma and HL in a population-based German study.[112] Nieters et al. also reported an elevated risk of FL associated with a TLR2 polymorphism (−16933T>A) that has been implicated in atopy and asthma.[149] TLR2 is another important pattern recognition receptor involved in the resolution of inflammation. The implication of TLR in lymphomagenesis is also supported by a recent study of genetic variation in 1253 immune and inflammatory genes and NHL risk among 458 patients with NHL and 484 controls.[114] One of the strongest findings was a rare variant in TLR6 (Val427Ala, rs5743815), which increased the risk of NHL and the main subtypes (CLL/SLL, FL, DLBCL) (Table 5.3). TLR6 forms heterodimers with TLR2 and upon activation promotes the secretion of proinflammatory cytokines. In that large-scale investigation, polymorphisms in several other genes of importance for the inflammatory and innate immune response have been associated with NHL risk including TRAF, RIPK3 and BAT2. This further supports the crucial role of variation in components of TNF and TLR signaling as risk alleles for lymphoid neoplasms.

HUMAN LEUKOCYTE ANTIGEN REGION

The human leukocyte antigen (HLA) region located on chromosome 6 (6p21.3) has now been entirely sequenced and approximately 220 genes have been defined. Many of these genes encode proteins that are likely to be involved in immune and inflammatory responses such as TNF, LTA, heat shock protein (HSP) 70 and prolactin.[150] Few studies have explored the association of HLA genes with lymphoid malignancies; existing reports are mainly for HL. Recently, genotyping was performed for >30 markers spanning the HLA region in EBV-positive and -negative HL cases (n = 200) and controls (n = 348).[151] Two consecutive markers, D6S265 and D6S510, located in the HLA class I region were associated with EBV-positive HL. Homozygotes for these alleles had odds ratios for EBV-positive HL of 8.3 (95 percent CI 2.5 to 27.4) and 7.1 (95 percent CI 1.9 to 26.3), respectively. These results suggest a role for inter-individual differences in the antigenic presentation of EBV antigens to cytotoxic T lymphocytes in the etiology of EBV-positive HL. Further, some studies have identified HL-associated HLA class II susceptibility alleles.[152–154] What has emerged from these studies is that HLA-DPB1*0301 appears to confer susceptibility, and DPB1*0201 resistance to HL. The former appears to be associated specifically with EBV-positive young adult HL.[154] Two studies provided evidence that HLA class II DRB1*1501 and DQB1*0602 alleles, or linked loci, may confer increased risk for sporadic and familial HL.[152,155] So far, only few studies have explored the association of HLA polymorphisms with NHL risk with inconclusive results.[156,157] The application of multiple genetic markers in the HLA region will help to elucidate the significance of variability in this region for all lymphoma histologies.

Obesity and energy regulation genes

Obesity can induce a state of chronic inflammation, leptin and insulin resistance and immune dysregulation.[158] An association between obesity and hematopoietic and lymphoreticular diseases has become evident, with increased risks reported for NHL, leukemia and multiple myeloma.[118,119,159–162] The potential relevance of obesity as a modulator of NHL susceptibility is underscored by recent genetic findings that report associations between NHL and polymorphisms in the leptin (LEP), leptin receptor (LEPR), ghrelin (GHRL) and neuropeptide Y (NPY) genes[118,119,163] (Table 5.3), which are key factors involved in body weight regulation. These same factors also exert major influences on humoral and cellular immune functions.

NPY, LEPTIN AND GHRELIN

Two SNPs in the LEP gene (−2548G>A, rs7799039 and 19A>G, rs2167270) that influence leptin levels;[164–166] and are associated with an obese phenotype[165,167–169] have been identified as susceptibility loci for NHL in two case–control studies based in the USA[119] and UK.[118] The US study found that relative to the LEP 19AA genotype, the LEP 19G allele was associated with up to a twofold increased risk of NHL, particularly FL (OR 1.9, 95 percent CI 1.0 to 3.6). Similar associations were observed in the UK study. Willett et al. also reported an increased risk of NHL, particularly FL, associated with the LEP −2548GA and −2548AA genotypes and a nonsynonomous variant in the leptin receptor gene (LEPR).[118]

In the US study population, three NPY variants (−485T>C, rs16147; 1258G>A, rs11557492 and 5671C>T, rs5574) and a rare functional polymorphism in NPY (1128 T>C, rs16139), all in close LD, were associated with up to a twofold increased risk for NHL, and particularly for FL.[163] NPY 1128T>C is a functional SNP that has been associated with elevated NPY levels, enhanced angiogenesis, and lymphocyte proliferation.[170] Further, Skibola et al. found that polymorphisms in the GHRL gene (−4427G>A, rs1629816, 5179A>G, rs35684) conferred a 20–70 percent reduced risk for NHL, especially for DLCL.[163] Thus, there is increasing evidence both from epidemiologic and genetic data to suggest that obesity may be a causal factor in the pathogenesis of NHL through its adverse action on immune system functions.

VITAMIN C RECEPTORS

A recent study identified NHL risk alleles in the vitamin C receptor genes, SLC23A1 and 2[116] that may provide indirect evidence to support epidemiologic data showing inverse associations between NHL and intakes of fruits and vegetables, which are primary sources of dietary vitamin C.[171,172] Skibola et al. found that homozygous variant genotypes for two closely linked intronic SLC23A1 SNPs, rs6596473 and rs11950646, were positively associated with FL in a US study and SLL/CLL in a second validation case–control study based in Germany (Table 5.4).[116] Furthermore, the homozygous genotype for SLC23A2 rs1715364 increased SLL/CLL risk in both the US and German studies (Table 5.4). SLC23A1 and 2 encode two vitamin C transport proteins, SVCT1 and 2, respectively. SVCT-1 is expressed in kidney, intestinal, hepatic and placental tissues and is critical for vitamin C absorption and reabsorption, whereas SVCT2 is expressed in most tissues and is essential for vitamin C bioaccumulation.[173] Thus, the influence of SLC23A1 and SLC23A2 genetic variation on NHL risk suggests that both vitamin C uptake and storage may be important factors that influence lymphomagenesis. Vitamin C is an essential enzyme cofactor in reactions catalyzed by several metal-dependent oxygenases. It also functions as a scavenger of reactive oxygen species and, thus, may play an important role in preventing oxidative stress induced DNA damage by quenching free radical formation.

Hormones

Extensive crosstalk exists between the endocrine and immune systems where hormones and their respective receptors influence immune and neuroendocrine functions. Expression of prolactin and estrogen receptors in lymphocytes, bone marrow, and in leukemia and lymphoma cell lines suggests that hormonal modulation may influence hematopoietic disease risk. Estrogen exerts multiple effects on lymphopoietic cells including the modulation of lymphocyte growth, antigen presentation, and production of antibodies.[174] Prolactin modulates cytokine production and promotes proliferation and survival of B cells, factors that could potentially influence disease risk. Elevated prolactin levels have been associated with progression of hematologic diseases such as multiple myeloma, AML and NHL.[175,176] However, there is less certainty regarding associations between exogenous estrogens (using postmenopausal hormones or oral contraceptives as a proxy of estimated exposure) and lymphoma/leukemia risk.

ESTROGEN SYNTHESIS, METABOLISM AND SIGNALING

Two studies based in the USA and the UK investigated the association of NHL with SNPs in the cytochrome P450 17A1 (CYP17A1) gene that encodes an enzyme involved in

Table 5.4 Gene variants associated with non-Hodgkin lymphoma (NHL) risk – oxidative stress and xenobiotic metabolism

Oxidative stress

Gene	Variant	Association
NOS2A	rs2297518	NHL (2.2 [1.1 to 4.4]), DLBCL (3.4 [1.5 to 7.8]), FL (2.6 [1.0 to 6.8])[179]
MPO	rs2333227	NHL (1.3 [1.1 to 1.5]), DLBCL[179]
PPARG	rs3856806	FL (3.0 [1.2 to 7.2]), SLL (0.5 [0.3 to 0.9])[179]
SOD2	Val16Ala rs4880	B cell lymphoma (1.3 [1.0 to 1.6])[179] MZL (0.45 [0.60 to 1.1])[180]
AKR1A1	rs2088102	NHL in women (1.7 [1.2 to 2.4]);[178] NS in[179]
CYBA	rs1049255	NHL (1.6 [1.1 to 2.4]), T cell lymphoma in women (3.5 [1.3 to 9.6]);[178] NS in[136,179]
GPX1	rs1050450	NHL (1.31 [1.06 to 1.62]), DLBCL, FL;[180] NS in[179]
SLC23A1	rs6596473, rs11950646	US study: (both SNPs) FL (1.8 [1.2 to 2.9]), German study: CLL/SLL (3.4 [0.91 to 13]); (2.6 [0.85 to 7.9]), DLBCL (0.4 [0.13 to 1.1])[116]
SLC23A2	rs1715364	US study: SLL/CLL (1.9 [1.2 to 3.1]), German study (1.8 [0.8 to 4.1])[116]

Xenobiotic metabolism

Gene	Variant	Association
GSTT1	Null	NHL (2.4 [1.94 to 3.22]);[182] GMZL (9.51 [4.57 to 19.81]);[183] MALT (1.8 [1.1 to 3.0]);[184] DLBCL [11 (7.9 to 18)][185]
GSTP1	1578A>G (Ile105Val) rs947894	DLBCL (0.2 [0.1 to 0.96]);[186] DLBCL (0.37 [0.17 to 0.81],[185] NS in[187]
	2293 C>T (Ala114Val) rs1799811	DLBCL (3.42 [1.26 to 9.38];[185] NS in[187]
NAT1	Slow acetylator	NHL in women (1.4 [0.9 to 2.3])[186]
	*10/*10 v *10-	NHL (1.60; 1.04 to 2.46)[188]; FL (2.06 [1.12 to 3.79])[188]
NAT2	Intermediate/rapid vs. slow-acetylators	FL (1.50 [1.11 to 2.02]), MZL (1.56 [0.98 to 2.49)[188] (interaction with smoking and hair dye use)[188,189]
PON1	Gln192Arg, rs662	NHL (2.55 [1.37 to 4.55]);[182] NS in[187]
	Leu55Met, rs854560	Met/Met: NHL (1.44 [1.00 to 2.08]), FL [2.12, (1.27 to 3.52]), T-NHL (2.93 [1.21 to 7.08])[187]
CYP2E1	−1054C>T, rs2031920	CT/TT: NHL (0.59 [0.37 to 0.93]);[187] NS in[192]

NOS2A, nitric oxide synthase 2A; *MPO*, myeloperoxidase; *PPARG*, peroxisome proliferator activated receptor gamma; *SOD2*, superoxide dismutase 2; *AKR1A1*, aldo-keto reductase family 1, member A1; *CYBA* ,cytochrome b-245, alpha polypeptide; *GPX1*, glutathione peroxidase 1; *SLC23A1*, sodium-dependent vitamin C transporter-1; *SLC23A2*, sodium-dependent vitamin C transporter-2; *GSTT1*, glutathione S transferase T1; *GSTP1*, glutathione S transferase P1; *NAT1*, N-acetyl transferase 1; *NAT2*, N-acetyltransferase 2; *PON1*, paraoxonase 1; *CYP2E1*, cytochrome P450, family 2, subfamily E, polypeptide 1; NHL, non-Hodgkin lymphoma; DLBCL, diffuse large B cell lymphoma; FL, follicular lymphoma; SLL, small lymphocytic leukemia/lymphoma; MZL, marginal zone lymphoma; CLL, chronic lymphocytic leukemia/lymphoma; GMZL, gastric marginal zone lymphoma; MALT, mucosa-associated lymphoid tissue lymphoma; NS, not significant.

estrogen and testosterone biosynthesis.[115,117] Both studies genotyped a −34T>C SNP (rs743572) in the 5′UTR of the *CYP17A1* gene where the −34C variant has been associated with elevated serum dehydroepiandrosterone sulfate and estradiol levels in pre-menopausal women.[177] The *CYP17A1* −34T>C variant was positively associated with NHL risk, particularly for DLCL (Table 5.3). The US study also investigated SNPs in the catechol-O-methyltransferase (*COMT*) gene including a functional 108/158Val>Met (rs4680) SNP that influences enzyme thermolability. COMT expresses an intracellular enzyme involved in estrogen metabolism that can alter circulating estrogen concentrations including catechol estrogens. The researchers found a marginally elevated risk of FL in women homozygous for the 108/158Met allele, while another SNP investigated (*COMT* 701A>G) was associated with a significant reduction in FL risk among women.[117] In the same study, Skibola *et al.* investigated a functional SNP in prolactin (*PRL* −1149G>T) associated with reduced lymphocyte prolactin levels. ORs for NHL and FL were reduced for *PRL* −1149TT carriers.[117] In a more recent report from the same investigators, which included a

validation study from Germany, they found an inverse association with an intronic estrogen receptor 1 (*ESR1*) 5029T>C variant (rs3020314) and risk of FL (Table 5.3).[116] Furthermore, SNPs in the *CYP19A1* gene (rs1870049, rs4774587) were also associated with FL and SLL/CLL risk in the US study. These results suggest that although lymphoma is not considered a classic endocrinologic tumor, interactions involving aberrant cross-talk between the neuroendocrine-immune networks may be involved in the pathogenesis of NHL.

OXIDATIVE STRESS

Reactive oxygen species (ROS) such as oxygen ions, hydrogen peroxides and other free radicals can oxidize various macromolecules including DNA, proteins and lipids. Increased production or elimination of ROS leads to oxidative stress and causes cellular damage which is implicated in a number of pathologic conditions including cancer. Antioxidant enzymes such as superoxide dismutase, catalase, and glutathione peroxidase protect cells from harmful effects of ROS. Several gene variants implicated in oxidative stress response pathways have been explored in NHL risk (Table 5.4), but few findings have been replicated.[178–180] An overall evaluation of 13 SNPs in 10 relevant genes revealed a significant association of the stress response pathway with DLBCL risk in a large US study.[179] Specifically, a variant (Ser608Leu, 2297518) in nitric oxide synthase 2A (NOS2A) that confers higher enzymatic activity and results in elevated nitric oxide levels[181] was over-represented among NHL cases (Table 5.4). A genetic variant (Pro197Leu, rs1050450) in the antioxidant enzyme glutathione peroxidase (GPX1) was associated with increased NHL risk in pooled UK and US studies[180] (OR 1.3, 95 percent CI 1.1 to 1.6). SNPs in nicotinamide adenine dinucleotide phosphate (NADPH) oxidation related genes such as member A1 of the aldo-keto reductase family 1 (AKR1A1) and cytochrome b-245 α polypeptide (CYBA), encoding a factor important in ROS production, affected NHL risk in a study among women in Connecticut.[178] The Tyr/Tyr genotype of a non-synonomous variant in CYBA (His72Tyr, rs1049255) was over-represented among NHL and T-NHL cases (Table 5.4). An increased risk between this SNP and NHL also was found in another independent study.[179]

Overall, there is no conclusive evidence to date that genetic variants that impair antioxidant capacity and promote oxidative stress have a significant role in lymphomageneses.

Xenobiotic metabolism genes

Environmental chemicals such as pesticides and solvents are suspected etiologic agents for lymphoma and are considered contributing factors to the increasing incidence of NHL during the last 30–40 years. Higher organisms have evolved two main classes of xenobiotic-metabolizing enzyme systems that constitute one of the first lines of defense against environmental chemicals. CYP450 enzymes are responsible for the metabolic activation of procarcinogens to genotoxic electrophilic intermediates. Phase II enzymes such as glutathione S-transferase (GST), N-acetyltransferases (NAT), and paraoxonase (PON) most often create more water-soluble and readily excretable conjugates. Genes that produce these enzymes are polymorphic and contribute to inter-individual differences in carcinogen metabolism. Furthermore, the identification of susceptibility alleles in these pathways can provide clues to particular classes of environmental lymphomagens.

CYP1A1, CYP1B1 AND CYP2E1

CYP1A1 is induced by and catalyzes oxidation of polycyclic aromatic hydrocarbons (PAHs). Several polymorphisms have been identified in the CYP1A1 gene. A polymorphism (CYP1A1*2, 3801C>T) and a closely linked non-synonymous SNP (CYP1A1*3, Ile462Val) result in increased enzyme activity and/or inducibility. The CYP1A1*2 polymorphism was associated with risk of childhood ALL,[190,191] but not NHL.[182,187,192] A non-synonomous variant in CYP1B1 (Val432Leu) was associated with a slightly elevated NHL risk (OR 1.3; 95 percent CI 1.0 to 1.7) in a large US-based study.[187] Compared to the Leu allele, the Val allele presented a higher enzymatic activity and increased oxidation of benzo(a)pyrene and formation of toxic intermediates.[193]

CYP2E1 is a crucial factor in the metabolic activation of several carcinogens, including nitrosamines, ethanol, benzene, and halogenated solvents. Functional polymorphisms that impair enzymatic activity have been identified in CYP2E1, though few studies have investigated CYP2E1 variants in hematologic malignancies. Associations have been reported between CYP2E1 polymorphisms and childhood ALL,[194] some with regard to prenatal exposure and child DNA variants.[195,196] One study found an inverse association of a promoter variant (−1054C>T, rs2031920) and NHL risk[187] (Table 5.4).

GSTM1, GSTT1 AND GSTP1

One of the important functions of GSTs is the detoxification of a wide range of environmental and non-environmental carcinogens, including benzene, organochlorine compounds, organophosphate pesticides, tobacco smoke, chemotherapeutic agents and reactive oxygen species.[197] Furthermore, these enzymes exhibit antioxidant activity. Three of the GST genes (GSTM1, GSTT1, GSTP1) have been studied in relation to risk of leukemia and lymphoma. Deletion polymorphisms have been identified in GSTM1 (GSTM1*0) and GSTT1 (GSTT1*0) that result in a loss of enzymatic activity.

No association was found between the GSTM1 null genotype and NHL.[182,186,192] However, several studies reported an elevated risk for NHL in GSTT1 null homozygotes[182–185] (Table 5.4). In a study of GMZL, a ninefold increased risk associated with the GSTT1 genotype was described.[183] Further, deletions of the GSTT1 gene were more frequent in patients with HL, especially in women below age 45 (OR 6.1, 95 percent CI 1.6–23).[198] The GSTP1 polymorphism did not modulate NHL risk in two studies;[186,192] however, in subtype-specific analysis, homozygotes of GSTP1 Val had a slightly elevated risk for marginal zone lymphoma and lower risk of DLBCL[185,186] (Table 5.4).

NAT1 AND NAT2

NAT enzymes are involved in the metabolism and detoxification of cytotoxic and carcinogenic compounds and ROS. They catalyze N-acetylation of aromatic and heterocyclic amines that generally result in detoxification of monocyclic aromatic amines. Furthermore, through O-acetylation of compounds, these enzymes contribute to carcinogenesis by forming acetoxy-ester intermediates which have the potential to generate DNA adducts.[199] The NAT locus comprises two functional genes (NAT1 and

NAT2) through which slow and fast acetylator genotypes are largely determined. Thus far, few studies have explored the role of these variants in lymphomagenesis.[182,186,188,189,200] In a large population-based US study of 1136 cases and 922 controls, individuals with the *NAT1**10/*10 genotype were at increased risk of NHL[188] (Table 5.4). Overall, the low *NAT2* acetylator genotype was not associated with NHL,[182,186,200] though one study reported a modestly elevated risk associated with the *NAT2* intermediate- and rapid acetylators[188] (Table 5.4). The first joint evaluation of these variants with environmental exposures found that risk differences for hair dye use were dependent upon *NAT1* and *NAT2* genotypes.[189] Women who used permanent, intense tone products before 1980 were at increased NHL risk if they carried the rapid/intermediate NAT2 phenotype (OR 3.3, 95 percent CI 1.3 to 8.6), but not if they were slow NAT2 acetylators (OR 1.5; 95 percent CI 0.6 to 3.6).

PON1

PON1 plays a major role in detoxification of organophosphates, suspected etiologic agents for NHL. A glutamine to arginine change in the *PON1* gene at codon 192 (Gln192Arg, rs662) determines substrate-dependent differences in the catalytic efficiency of hydrolysis of specific organophosphates.[201] A study by Kerridge *et al.* found that the 192Arg/Arg genotype was associated with a 2.6-fold increased risk for NHL[182] (Table 5.4). Interestingly, the 192Arg allele also has been associated with organophosphate toxicity in sheep farmers who dip their animals in the organophosphate pesticide, diazinon.[202,203] Lower rates of diazoxon hydrolysis were associated with the 192Arg allele, suggesting the 192Arg variant reduces the ability to detoxify organophosphates. A further study found no association with the Gln192Arg variant, but reported an increased risk for FL and T-NHL with another *PON-1* polymorphism (Leu55Met)[187] (Table 5.4). These findings may warrant the study of this and other functionally relevant variants in paraoxonase enzymes in lymphoma risk in farmers and other occupationally exposed subjects.

These studies suggest that genetic variability in a number of pathways involved in the activation and detoxification of xenobiotics may play a role in the etiology of leukemias and lymphomas. However, a more in-depth analysis of gene variants in conjunction with occupational and other environmental exposures will help to clarify whether specific genotype-exposure combinations exist, that confer particularly high individual risks of lymphoproliferative malignancies.

CONCLUSIONS

Genetic factors can contribute to lymphomagenesis either through inheritance of rare mutations associated with various cancer syndromes or, of more relevance on a population level, through inheritance of moderate susceptibility loci that interact with other gene variants and/or environmental exposures. Genetic studies of familial cancer syndromes that predispose to lymphoid malignancy and genetic association studies of disease susceptibility may provide valuable insights to clarify disease mechanisms and identify potentially relevant pathways in lymphomagenesis. Association studies may be more powerful than linkage studies in identifying genes that contribute to variation in complex traits where the joint distribution of phenotypes and genotypes in population samples can be examined. However, the subtle phenotypic effects of common alleles will require replication in multiple studies or within consortia such as InterLymph. Thus far, a limited number of SNPs have been validated in multiple case-control studies of lymphoid neoplasms using a candidate gene approach. Nonetheless, this is considered a huge success given the unlikely chances of nominating and validating SNP associations across studies. NHL SNP associations in *TNF*, *LTA*, *IL10* and *CARD15* have been validated in 14 studies within InterLymph in over 7000 cases and 7000 controls, and the functionally relevant *TNFRSF5* −1C>T SNP was associated with NHL in eight studies in over 3500 cases and 3500 controls. These studies suggest an important role for SNPs that influence innate and humoral immune responses as susceptibility factors for lymphoid neoplasms.

Another model that emerges from combined genetic and immunologic data emphasizes the importance of persistent inflammation in B cell lymphomagenesis (see Fig. 5.2).[204] Chronic inflammation leads to increased cellular turnover, and provides selective pressure that results in the emergence of cells that are at high risk for malignant transformation. The consistent associations found between B cell NHL with genetic variants that influence production of proinflammatory factors such as TNF-α and leptin, as well as the association of viral, bacterial, and other exogenous agents leading to persistent inflammation, suggest that this may be one relevant mechanism underlying lymphomagenesis. The association of genetic polymorphisms in *MTHFR*, *TYMS*, *MTR* and *SHMT* in NHL and/or ALL disease risk suggests that folate, which provides vital one-carbon donors for normal DNA synthesis, repair and methylation processes, may be a relevant pathway in lymphoma leukemogenesis. Deviations in the flux of folate due to genetic variation could result in selective growth and genomic instability and affect susceptibility to various cancers including lymphoma and leukemia. To date, findings among studies have been somewhat inconsistent, which may reflect differences in circulating folate levels between study populations. Further investigations are warranted that include dietary information to determine the influence of genetics and folic acid status on lympho-hematopoietic disease risk. Recent evidence from multiple-SNP genotyping projects suggests a role of variants in factors implicated in tumor invasion and metastasis also in the etiology of lymphomas, such as integrins (*ITGB2* and *ITGB3*) and members of the matrix metalloproteinase family (*MMP3*, *MMP9*).[114,116] Replication of these and other

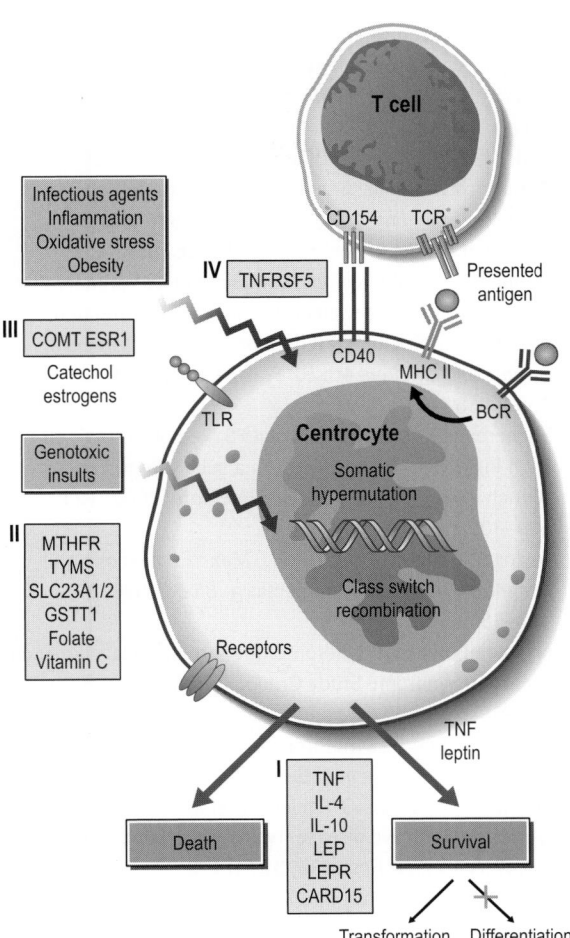

Figure 5.2 Overview of pathways and genetic variability implicated in lymphomagenesis. I. Factors that promote antigenic stimulation which include infectious agents such as Epstein–Barr virus, *Helicobacter pylori* and others, chronic inflammatory conditions such as obesity where there is an increase in production of proinflammatory cytokines such as leptin and tumor necrosis factor (TNF)-α and others from adipose tissue can promote enhanced B-cell survival and proliferation. The *TNF* and *LEP/LEPR* SNPs may mimic an obese state. The *CARD15* mutation may chronically activate alternative recognition receptors such as the TLRs that can lead to T-cell induced NF-κB activation, proinflammatory cytokine release and pro-survival signals. II. Sufficient dietary folate will minimize DNA double strand break repair (DSBR) and the level of chromosomal translocations. SNPs in one-carbon metabolizing genes (i.e. *MTHFR*, *TYMS*) may impact these processes. Variants in xenobiotic metabolizing genes (i.e. *GSTT1*) and oxidative stress response (i.e. *SLC23A1* and *SLC23A2)* may modulate levels of damage due to genotoxic agents. Sufficient vitamin C can play an anti-tumorigenic role by minimizing oxidative stress and supporting proper collagen formation and matrix stabilization. III. Polymorphisms in genes influencing synthesis of estrogens and catechol estrogens (i.e. *COMT* and *ESR1*) may be involved in the pathogenesis of NHL via aberrant crosstalk between the neuroendocrine-immune networks and genotoxic mechanisms, respectively. IV. SNPs in *TNFRSF5* may hinder B and T cell interactions and B cell differentiation resulting in increased rates of somatic hypermutation and proliferation in germinal centers that may support lymphomagenesis.

findings such as associations found with variants involving genes of lymphocyte trafficking and migration (*SELPLG* and *LSP1*), and vitamin C uptake and bioaccumulation (*SLC23A1*, *SLC23A2*), are urgently needed to elucidate the complex patho-mechanisms of lymphoid neoplasms.

Whole genome scan studies will soon provide more detailed information on the role of genetic host factors in the etiology of lymphoproliferative diseases. A thorough exposure assessment, if possible, using biomarkers and the WHO-defined classification of lymphoma subtypes also will be needed for assessment of gene–environment interactions and the identification of entity-specific gene variants. Overall, these studies will broaden our current understanding of important mechanistic pathways involved in lymphomagenesis and identify unfavorable allelic combinations that put individuals at particularly high risk of disease. Moreover, these studies will provide clues about environmental agents and lifestyle exposures that contribute to disease risk that may be translated to NHL screening, prevention or treatment regimens. Finally, these data will provide a framework for further investigation within the NHL consortium, InterLymph, where results from individual studies can be validated by other InterLymph case-control studies in pooled analyses and rarer NHL subtypes can be explored.

KEY POINTS

- A family history of hematologic malignancies is associated with a moderately increased risk of lymphoma and leukemia in first-degree relatives.
- Rare inherited syndromes, such as ataxia telangiectasia or Nijmegen breakage syndrome confer a highly elevated risk for lymphoid malignancy in childhood or early adulthood.
- Results from association studies suggest that genetic variants in one-carbon metabolism, such as *MTHFR*, and in immune response factors such as CD40 (*TNFRSF5*) or in inflammatory pathways, such as *TNF* and *LEP/LEPR*, appear to modulate the risk of lympho-hematopoietic malignancies.
- Most association studies to date are hampered by small sample sizes, which prohibit the investigation of gene–environment interactions.
- The large lymphoma consortium, InterLymph, will provide the means to replicate positive findings from individual studies and provide the power to investigate rare subtypes and interracial differences in disease susceptibility.

REFERENCES

● = Key primary paper
◆ = Major review article

◆1. Segel GB, Lichtman MA. Familial (inherited) leukemia, lymphoma, and myeloma: an overview. *Blood Cells Mol Dis* 2004; **32**: 246–61.

2. Linet MS, Pottern LM. Familial aggregation of hematopoietic malignancies and risk of non-Hodgkin's lymphoma. *Cancer Res* 1992; **52**(19 Suppl): s5468–73.

3. Houlston RS, Catovsky D, Yuille MR. Genetic susceptibility to chronic lymphocytic leukemia. *Leukemia* 2002; **16**: 1008–14.

●4. Goldin LR, Pfeiffer RM, Li X, Hemminki K. Familial risk of lymphoproliferative tumors in families of patients with chronic lymphocytic leukemia: results from the Swedish family-cancer database. *Blood* 2004; **104**: 1850–4.

●5. Goldin LR, Pfeiffer RM, Gridley G *et al.* Familial aggregation of Hodgkin lymphoma and related tumors. *Cancer* 2004; **100**: 1902–8.

6. Goldin LR, Landgren O, McMaster ML *et al.* Familial aggregation and heterogeneity of non-Hodgkin lymphoma in population-based samples. *Cancer Epidemiol Biomarkers Prev* 2005; **14**: 2402–6.

7. Daugherty SE, Pfeiffer RM, Mellemkjaer L *et al.* No evidence for anticipation in lymphoproliferative tumors in population-based samples. *Cancer Epidemiol Biomarkers Prev* 2005; **14**: 1245–50.

●8. Chang ET, Smedby KE, Hjalgrim H *et al.* Family history of hematopoietic malignancy and risk of lymphoma. *J Natl Cancer Inst* 2005; **97**: 1466–74.

●9. Altieri A, Bermejo JL, Hemminki K. Familial risk for non-Hodgkin lymphoma and other lymphoproliferative malignancies by histopathologic subtype: the Swedish Family-Cancer Database. *Blood* 2005; **106**: 668–72.

10. Pottern LM, Linet M, Blair A *et al.* Familial cancers associated with subtypes of leukemia and non-Hodgkin's lymphoma. *Leuk Res* 1991; **15**: 305–14.

11. Paltiel O, Schmit T, Adler B *et al.* The incidence of lymphoma in first-degree relatives of patients with Hodgkin disease and non-Hodgkin lymphoma: results and limitations of a registry-linked study. *Cancer* 2000; **88**: 2357–66.

12. Chatterjee N, Hartge P, Cerhan JR *et al.* Risk of non-Hodgkin's lymphoma and family history of lymphatic, hematologic, and other cancers. *Cancer Epidemiol Biomarkers Prev* 2004; **13**: 1415–21.

●13. Wang SS, Slager SL, Brennan P *et al.* Family history of hematopoietic malignancies and risk of non-Hodgkin lymphoma (NHL): a pooled analysis of 10 211 cases and 11 905 controls from the International Lymphoma Epidemiology Consortium (InterLymph). *Blood* 2007; **109**: 3479–88.

14. Ferraris AM, Racchi O, Rapezzi D *et al.* Familial Hodgkin's disease: a disease of young adulthood? *Ann Hematol* 1997; **74**: 131–4.

●15. Mack TM, Cozen W, Shibata DK *et al.* Concordance for Hodgkin's disease in identical twins suggesting genetic susceptibility to the young-adult form of the disease. *N Engl J Med* 1995; **332**: 413–18.

16. Sullivan KE, Mullen CA, Blaese RM, Winkelstein JA. A multiinstitutional survey of the Wiskott-Aldrich syndrome. *J Pediatr* 1994; **125**(6 Pt 1): 876–85.

17. Filipovich AH, Jyonouchi H, Gross TG, Shapiro RS. Hematologic and oncologic complications of primary and secondary immunodeficiencies, including EBV related disorders. In: Stiehm ER (ed.) *Immunologic disorders of infants and children,* 4th ed. Philadelphia, PA: Saunders, 1996: 855–88.

18. Shcherbina A, Candotti F, Rosen FS, Remold-O'Donnell E. High incidence of lymphomas in a subgroup of Wiskott-Aldrich syndrome patients. *Br J Haematol* 2003; **121**: 529–30.

19. Taylor AM, Metcalfe JA, Thick J, Mak YF. Leukemia and lymphoma in ataxia telangiectasia. *Blood* 1996; **87**: 423–38.

20. Nijmegen breakage syndrome. The International Nijmegen Breakage Syndrome Study Group. *Arch Dis Child* 2000; **82**: 400–6.

21. German J. Bloom's syndrome, XX. The first 100 cancers. *Cancer Genet Cytogenet* 1997; **93**: 100–6.

22. Seemayer TA, Gross TG, Egeler RM *et al.* X-linked lymphoproliferative disease: twenty-five years after the discovery. *Pediatr Res* 1995; **38**: 471–8.

23. Kinlen LJ, Webster AD, Bird AG *et al.* Prospective study of cancer in patients with hypogammaglobulinaemia. *Lancet* 1985; **1**: 263–6.

24. Mellemkjaer L, Hammarstrom L, Andersen V *et al.* Cancer risk among patients with IgA deficiency or common variable immunodeficiency and their relatives: a combined Danish and Swedish study. *Clin Exp Immunol* 2002; **130**: 495–500.

25. Olivier M, Goldgar DE, Sodha N *et al.* Li–Fraumeni and related syndromes: correlation between tumor type, family structure, and TP53 genotype. *Cancer Res* 2003; **63**: 6643–50.

26. Nichols KE, Ma CS, Cannons JL *et al.* Molecular and cellular pathogenesis of X-linked lymphoproliferative disease. *Immunol Rev* 2005; **203**: 180–99.

27. Burns S, Cory GO, Vainchenker W, Thrasher AJ. Mechanisms of WASp-mediated hematologic and immunologic disease. *Blood* 2004; **104**: 3454–62.

28. Brandau O, Schuster V, Weiss M *et al.* Epstein-Barr virus-negative boys with non-Hodgkin lymphoma are mutated in the SH2D1A gene, as are patients with X-linked lymphoproliferative disease (XLP). *Hum Mol Genet* 1999; **8**: 2407–13.

29. Parolini O, Kagerbauer B, Simonitsch-Klupp I, Ambros P, Jaeger U, Mann G *et al.* Analysis of SH2D1A mutations in patients with severe Epstein-Barr virus infections, Burkitt's lymphoma, and Hodgkin's lymphoma. *Ann Hematol* 2002; **81**: 441–7.

30. Perry GS III, Spector BD, Schuman LM *et al.* The Wiskott-Aldrich syndrome in the United States and Canada (1892–1979). *J Pediatr* 1980; **97**: 72–8.

31. Imai K, Nonoyama S, Ochs HD. WASP (Wiskott-Aldrich syndrome protein) gene mutations and phenotype. *Curr Opin Allergy Clin Immunol* 2003; **3**: 427–36.

32. Hecht F, Hecht BK. Cancer in ataxia-telangiectasia patients. *Cancer Genet Cytogenet* 1990; **46**: 9–19.

33. Khanna KK. Cancer risk and the ATM gene: a continuing debate. *J Natl Cancer Inst* 2000; **92**: 795–802.

34. Shiloh Y. ATM and related protein kinases: safeguarding genome integrity. *Nat Rev Cancer* 2003; **3**: 155–68.

●35. Olsen JH, Hahnemann JM, Borresen-Dale AL *et al.* Cancer in patients with ataxia-telangiectasia and in their relatives in the nordic countries. *J Natl Cancer Inst* 2001; **93**: 121–7.

●36. Thompson D, Duedal S, Kirner J *et al.* Cancer risks and mortality in heterozygous ATM mutation carriers. *J Natl Cancer Inst* 2005; **97**: 813–22.

37. Gumy-Pause F, Wacker P, Sappino AP. ATM gene and lymphoid malignancies. *Leukemia* 2004; **18**: 238–42.

38. Bullrich F, Rasio D, Kitada S *et al.* ATM mutations in B-cell chronic lymphocytic leukemia. *Cancer Res* 1999; **59**: 24–7.

●39. Stankovic T, Weber P, Stewart G *et al.* Inactivation of ataxia telangiectasia mutated gene in B-cell chronic lymphocytic leukaemia. *Lancet* 1999; **353**: 26–9.

40. Yuille MR, Condie A, Hudson CD *et al.* ATM mutations are rare in familial chronic lymphocytic leukemia. *Blood* 2002; **100**: 603–9.

41. Stilgenbauer S, Winkler D, Ott G *et al.* Molecular characterization of 11q deletions points to a pathogenic role of the ATM gene in mantle cell lymphoma. *Blood* 1999; **94**: 3262–4.

42. Schaffner C, Idler I, Stilgenbauer S *et al.* Mantle cell lymphoma is characterized by inactivation of the ATM gene. *Proc Natl Acad Sci U S A* 2000; **97**: 2773–8.

43. Camacho E, Hernandez L, Hernandez S *et al.* ATM gene inactivation in mantle cell lymphoma mainly occurs by truncating mutations and missense mutations involving the phosphatidylinositol-3 kinase domain and is associated with increasing numbers of chromosomal imbalances. *Blood* 2002; **99**: 238–44.

44. Lespinet V, Terraz F, Recher C *et al.* Single-cell analysis of loss of heterozygosity at the ATM gene locus in Hodgkin and Reed-Sternberg cells of Hodgkin's lymphoma: ATM loss of heterozygosity is a rare event. *Int J Cancer* 2005; **114**: 909–16.

45. Takagi M, Tsuchida R, Oguchi K *et al.* Identification and characterization of polymorphic variations of the ataxia telangiectasia mutated (ATM) gene in childhood Hodgkin disease. *Blood* 2004; **103**: 283–90.

46. Liberzon E, Avigad S, Yaniv I *et al.* Molecular variants of the ATM gene in Hodgkin's disease in children. *Br J Cancer* 2004; **90**: 522–5.

47. Offit K, Gilad S, Paglin S *et al.* Rare variants of ATM and risk for Hodgkin's disease and radiation-associated breast cancers. *Clin Cancer Res* 2002; **8**: 3813–19.

48. Meier M, den Boer ML, Hall AG *et al.* Relation between genetic variants of the ataxia telangiectasia-mutated (ATM) gene, drug resistance, clinical outcome and predisposition to childhood T-lineage acute lymphoblastic leukaemia. *Leukemia* 2005; **19**: 1887–95.

49. Liberzon E, Avigad S, Stark B *et al.* Germ-line ATM gene alterations are associated with susceptibility to sporadic T-cell acute lymphoblastic leukemia in children. *Genes Chromosomes Cancer* 2004; **39**: 161–6.

50. Gumy PF, Wacker P, Maillet P *et al.* ATM gene alterations in childhood acute lymphoblastic leukemias. *Hum Mutat* 2003; **21**: 554.

51. Gronbaek K, Worm J, Ralfkiaer E *et al.* ATM mutations are associated with inactivation of the ARF-TP53 tumor suppressor pathway in diffuse large B-cell lymphoma. *Blood* 2002; **100**: 1430–7.

52. Sipahimalani P, Spinelli JJ, MacArthur AC *et al.* A systematic evaluation of the ataxia telangiectasia mutated gene does not show an association with non-Hodgkin lymphoma. *Int J Cancer* 2007; **121**: 1967–75.

53. Carney JP, Maser RS, Olivares H *et al.* The hMre11/hRad50 protein complex and Nijmegen breakage syndrome: linkage of double-strand break repair to the cellular DNA damage response. *Cell* 1998; **93**: 477–86.

54. Varon R, Vissinga C, Platzer M *et al.* Nibrin, a novel DNA double-strand break repair protein, is mutated in Nijmegen breakage syndrome. *Cell* 1998; **93**: 467–76.

55. Resnick IB, Kondratenko I, Pashanov E *et al.* 657del5 mutation in the gene for Nijmegen breakage syndrome (NBS1) in a cohort of Russian children with lymphoid tissue malignancies and controls. *Am J Med Genet A* 2003; **120**: 174–9.

56. Wegner RD, Chrzanowsk KH, Sperling K, Stumm M. Ataxia-telangiectasia variants (Nijmegen breakage syndrome). In: Ochs HD, Smith CIE, Puck JM (eds). Primary immunodeficiency diseases, a molecular and genetic approach. Oxford University Press, 1999: 324–34.

57. Cerosaletti KM, Morrison VA, Sabath DE *et al.* Mutations and molecular variants of the NBS1 gene in non-Hodgkin lymphoma. *Genes Chromosomes Cancer* 2002; **35**: 282–6.

58. Stanulla M, Stumm M, Dieckvoss BO *et al.* No evidence for a major role of heterozygous deletion 657del5 within the NBS1 gene in the pathogenesis of non-Hodgkin's lymphoma of childhood and adolescence. *Br J Haematol* 2000; **109**: 117–20.

59. Rischewski J, Bismarck P, Kabisch H *et al.* The common deletion 657del5 in the Nibrin gene is not a major risk factor for B or T cell non-Hodgkin lymphoma in a pediatric population. *Leukemia* 2000; **14**: 1528–9.

60. Steffen J, Varon R, Mosor M *et al.* Increased cancer risk of heterozygotes with NBS1 germline mutations in Poland. *Int J Cancer* 2004; **111**: 67–71.

61. Chrzanowska KH, Piekutowska-Abramczuk D, Popowska E *et al.* Carrier frequency of mutation 657del5 in the NBS1 gene in a population of Polish pediatric patients with sporadic lymphoid malignancies. *Int J Cancer* 2006; **118**: 1269–74.

62. Imamura J, Miyoshi I, Koeffler HP. p53 in hematologic malignancies. *Blood* 1994; **84**: 2412–21.

◆63. Stiller CA. Epidemiology and genetics of childhood cancer. *Oncogene* 2004; **23**: 6429–44.

●64. Skibola CF, Forrest MS, Coppede F *et al.* Polymorphisms and haplotypes in folate-metabolizing genes and risk of non-Hodgkin lymphoma. *Blood* 2004; **104**: 2155–62.

65. Rosenberg N, Murata M, Ikeda Y *et al.* The frequent 5, 10-methylenetetrahydrofolate reductase C677T polymorphism is associated with a common haplotype in whites, Japanese, and Africans. *Am J Hum Genet* 2002; **70**: 758–62.

66. Botto LD, Yang Q. 5,10-Methylenetetrahydrofolate reductase gene variants and congenital anomalies: a HuGE review. *Am J Epidemiol* 2000; **151**: 862–77.

◆67. Robien K, Ulrich CM. 5,10-Methylenetetrahydrofolate reductase polymorphisms and leukemia risk: a HuGE minireview. *Am J Epidemiol* 2003; **157**: 571–82.

68. van der Put NM, Gabreels F, Stevens EM *et al.* A second common mutation in the methylenetetrahydrofolate reductase gene: an additional risk factor for neural-tube defects? *Am J Hum Genet* 1998; **62**: 1044–51.

69. Frosst P, Blom HJ, Milos R *et al.* A candidate genetic risk factor for vascular disease: a common mutation in methylenetetrahydrofolate reductase. *Nat Genet* 1995; **10**: 111–13.

●70. Skibola CF, Smith MT, Kane E *et al.* Polymorphisms in the methylenetetrahydrofolate reductase gene are associated with susceptibility to acute leukemia in adults. *Proc Natl Acad Sci U S A* 1999; **96**: 12810–15.

71. Wiemels JL, Smith RN, Taylor GM *et al.* Methylenetetrahydrofolate reductase (MTHFR) polymorphisms and risk of molecularly defined subtypes of childhood acute leukemia. *Proc Natl Acad Sci U S A* 2001; **98**: 4004–9.

72. Franco RF, Simoes BP, Tone LG *et al.* The methylenetetrahydrofolate reductase C677T gene polymorphism decreases the risk of childhood acute lymphocytic leukaemia. *Br J Haematol* 2001; **115**: 616–18.

73. Gemmati D, Ongaro A, Scapoli GL *et al.* Common gene polymorphisms in the metabolic folate and methylation pathway and the risk of acute lymphoblastic leukemia and non-Hodgkin's lymphoma in adults. *Cancer Epidemiol Biomarkers Prev* 2004; **13**: 787–94.

74. Krajinovic M, Lamothe S, Labuda D *et al.* Role of MTHFR genetic polymorphisms in the susceptibility to childhood acute lymphoblastic leukemia. *Blood* 2004; **103**: 252–7.

75. Gonzalez Ordonez AJ, Fernandez Carreira JM, Fernandez Alvarez CR *et al.* Normal frequencies of the C677T genotypes on the methylenetetrahydrofolate reductase (MTHFR) gene among lymphoproliferative disorders but not in multiple myeloma. *Leuk Lymphoma* 2000; **39**: 607–12.

76. Matsuo K, Suzuki R, Hamajima N *et al.* Association between polymorphisms of folate- and methionine-metabolizing enzymes and susceptibility to malignant lymphoma. *Blood* 2001; **97**: 3205–9.

77. Lightfoot TJ, Skibola CF, Willett EV *et al.* Risk of non-Hodgkin lymphoma associated with polymorphisms in folate-metabolizing genes. *Cancer Epidemiol Biomarkers Prev* 2005; **14**: 2999–3003.

78. Matsuo K, Hamajima N, Suzuki R *et al.* Methylenetetrahydrofolate reductase gene (MTHFR) polymorphisms and reduced risk of malignant lymphoma. *Am J Hematol* 2004b; **77**: 351–7.

79. Kim HN, Lee IK, Kim YK *et al.* Association between folate-metabolizing pathway polymorphism and non-Hodgkin lymphoma. *Br J Haematol* 2008; **140**: 287–94.

80. Toffoli G, Rossi D, Gaidano G *et al.* Methylenetetrahydrofolate reductase genotype in diffuse large B-cell lymphomas with and without hypermethylation of the DNA repair gene O6-methylguanine DNA methyltransferase. *Int J Biol Markers* 2003; **18**: 218–21.

81. Rudd MF, Sellick GS, Allinson R *et al.* MTHFR polymorphisms and risk of chronic lymphocytic leukemia. *Cancer Epidemiol Biomarkers Prev* 2004; **13**: 2268–70.

82. Lincz LF, Scorgie FE, Kerridge I *et al.* Methionine synthase genetic polymorphism MS A2756G alters susceptibility to follicular but not diffuse large B-cell non-Hodgkin's lymphoma or multiple myeloma. *Br J Haematol* 2003; **120**: 1051–4.

●83. Lim U, Wang SS, Hartge P *et al.* Gene-nutrient interactions among determinants of folate and one-carbon metabolism on the risk of non-Hodgkin lymphoma: NCI-SEER case-control study. *Blood* 2007; **109**: 3050–9.

84. Linnebank M, Schmidt S, Kolsch H *et al.* The methionine synthase polymorphism D919G alters susceptibility to primary central nervous system lymphoma. *Br J Cancer* 2004; **90**: 1969–71.

85. Skibola CF, Smith MT, Hubbard A *et al.* Polymorphisms in the thymidylate synthase and serine hydroxymethyltransferase genes and risk of adult acute lymphocytic leukemia. *Blood* 2002; **99**: 3786–91.

86. Hishida A, Matsuo K, Hamajima N *et al.* Associations between polymorphisms in the thymidylate synthase and serine hydroxymethyltransferase genes and susceptibility to malignant lymphoma. *Haematologica* 2003a; **88**: 159–66.

87. Bird AP. CpG-rich islands and the function of DNA methylation. *Nature* 1986; **321**: 209–13.

88. Oliveira E, Alves S, Quental S *et al.* The MTHFR C677T and A1298C polymorphisms and susceptibility to childhood acute lymphoblastic leukemia in Portugal. *J Pediatr Hematol Oncol* 2005; **27**: 425–9.

◆89. Friso S, Choi SW. Gene-nutrient interactions in one-carbon metabolism. *Curr Drug Metab* 2005; **6**: 37–46.

90. Friso S, Choi SW, Girelli D *et al.* A common mutation in the 5,10-methylenetetrahydrofolate reductase gene affects genomic DNA methylation through an interaction with folate status. *Proc Natl Acad Sci U S A* 2002; **99**: 5606–11.

91. Niclot S, Pruvot Q, Besson C et al. Implication of the folate-methionine metabolism pathways in susceptibility to follicular lymphomas. Blood 2006; **108**: 278–85.

92. Hill DA, Wang SS, Cerhan JR et al. Risk of Non-Hodgkin lymphoma (NHL) in relation to germline variation in DNA repair and related genes. Blood 2006; **108**: 3161–7.

93. Shen M, Zheng T, Lan Q et al. Polymorphisms in DNA repair genes and risk of non-Hodgkin lymphoma among women in Connecticut. Hum Genet 2006; **119**: 659–68.

94. Shen M, Purdue MP, Kricker A et al. Polymorphisms in DNA repair genes and risk of non-Hodgkin's lymphoma in New South Wales, Australia. Haematologica 2007; **92**: 1180–5.

95. Smedby KE, Lindgren CM, Hjalgrim H et al. Variation in DNA repair genes ERCC2, XRCC1, and XRCC3 and risk of follicular lymphoma. Cancer Epidemiol Biomarkers Prev 2006; **15**: 258–65.

96. Novik KL, Spinelli JJ, MacArthur AC et al. Genetic variation in H2AFX contributes to risk of non-Hodgkin lymphoma. Cancer Epidemiol Biomarkers Prev 2007; **16**: 1098–106.

97. Goode EL, Ulrich CM, Potter JD. Polymorphisms in DNA repair genes and associations with cancer risk. Cancer Epidemiol Biomarkers Prev 2002; **11**: 1513–30.

98. Madhusudan S, Middleton MR. The emerging role of DNA repair proteins as predictive, prognostic and therapeutic targets in cancer. Cancer Treat Rev 2005; **31**: 603–17.

99. Hill CE, Wickliffe JK, Wolfe KJ et al. The L84F and the I143V polymorphisms in the O6-methylguanine-DNA-methyltransferase (MGMT) gene increase human sensitivity to the genotoxic effects of the tobacco-specific nitrosamine carcinogen NNK. Pharmacogenet Genomics 2005; **15**: 571–8.

100. Hajeer AH, Hutchinson IV. TNF-alpha gene polymorphism: clinical and biological implications. Microsc Res Tech 2000; **50**: 216–28.

101. Bayley JP, Ottenhoff TH, Verweij CL. Is there a future for TNF promoter polymorphisms? Genes Immun 2004; **5**: 315–29.

102. Allen RD. Polymorphism of the human TNF-alpha promoter—random variation or functional diversity? Mol Immunol 1999; **36**: 1017–27.

103. Heesen M, Kunz D, Bachmann-Mennenga B et al. Linkage disequilibrium between tumor necrosis factor (TNF)-alpha-308 G/A promoter and TNF-beta NcoI polymorphisms: Association with TNF-alpha response of granulocytes to endotoxin stimulation. Crit Care Med 2003; **31**: 211–14.

104. Gommerman JL, Browning JL. Lymphotoxin/light, lymphoid microenvironments and autoimmune disease. Nat Rev Immunol 2003; **3**: 642–55.

◆105. Karin M, Greten FR. NF-kappaB: linking inflammation and immunity to cancer development and progression. Nat Rev Immunol 2005; **5**: 749–59.

●106. Rothman N, Skibola CF, Wang SS et al. Genetic variation in TNF and IL10 and risk of non-Hodgkin lymphoma: a report from the InterLymph Consortium. Lancet Oncol 2006; **7**: 27–38.

107. Purdue MP, Lan Q, Kricker A et al. Polymorphisms in immune function genes and risk of non-Hodgkin lymphoma: findings from the New South Wales non-Hodgkin Lymphoma Study. Carcinogenesis 2007; **28**: 704–12.

108. Skibola CF, Nieters A, Bracci PM et al. A functional TNFRSF5 gene variant is associated with risk of lymphoma. Blood 2008; **111**: 4348–54.

109. Wang SS, Cerhan JR, Hartge P et al. Common genetic variants in proinflammatory and other immunoregulatory genes and risk for non-Hodgkin lymphoma. Cancer Res 2006; **66**: 9771–80.

110. Lan Q, Zheng T, Rothman N et al. Cytokine polymorphisms in the Th1/Th2 pathway and susceptibility to non-Hodgkin lymphoma. Blood 2006; **107**: 4101–8.

111. Cozen W, Gill PS, Ingles SA et al. IL-6 levels and genotype are associated with risk of young adult Hodgkin lymphoma. Blood 2004; **103**: 3216–21.

112. Nieters A, Deeg E, Beckmann L, Becker N. Gene polymorphisms in Toll-like receptors-1,-2,-4,-5,-9, interleukin-10, and interleukin-10 receptor alpha and lymphoma risk. Genes Immun 2006; **7**: 615–24.

113. Forrest MS, Skibola CF, Lightfoot TJ et al. Polymorphisms in innate immunity genes and risk of non-Hodgkin lymphoma. Br J Haematol 2006; **134**: 180–3.

114. Cerhan JR, Ansell SM, Fredericksen ZS et al. Genetic variation in 1253 immune and inflammation genes and risk of non-Hodgkin lymphoma. Blood 2007; **110**: 4455–63.

115. Skibola CF, Lightfoot T, Agana L et al. Polymorphisms in cytochrome P450 17A1 and risk of non-Hodgkin lymphoma. Br J Haematol 2005; **129**: 618–21.

●116. Skibola CF, Bracci PM, Halperin E et al. Polymorphisms in the estrogen receptor 1 and vitamin C and matrix metalloproteinase gene families are associated with susceptibility to lymphoma. PLoS ONE 2008; **3**: e2816.

117. Skibola CF, Bracci PM, Paynter RA et al. Polymorphisms and haplotypes in the cytochrome P450 17A1, prolactin, and catechol-O-methyltransferase genes and non-Hodgkin lymphoma risk. Cancer Epidemiol Biomarkers Prev 2005; **14**: 2391–401.

118. Willett EV, Skibola CF, Adamson P et al. Non-Hodgkin's lymphoma, obesity and energy homeostasis polymorphisms. Br J Cancer 2005; **93**: 811–16.

●119. Skibola CF, Holly EA, Forrest MS et al. Body mass index, leptin and leptin receptor polymorphisms, and non-hodgkin lymphoma. Cancer Epidemiol Biomarkers Prev 2004; **13**: 779–86.

120. Warzocha K, Ribeiro P, Bienvenu J et al. Genetic polymorphisms in the tumor necrosis factor locus influence non-Hodgkin's lymphoma outcome. Blood 1998; **91**: 3574–81.

121. Davies FE, Rollinson SJ, Rawstron AC et al. High-producer haplotypes of tumor necrosis factor alpha and lymphotoxin alpha are associated with an increased risk

of myeloma and have an improved progression-free survival after treatment. *J Clin Oncol* 2000; **18**: 2843–51.

122. Wihlborg C, Sjoberg J, Intaglietta M *et al.* Tumour necrosis factor-alpha cytokine promoter gene polymorphism in Hodgkin's disease and chronic lymphocytic leukaemia. *Br J Haematol* 1999; **104**: 346–9.

123. Zheng C, Huang DR, Bergenbrant S *et al.* Interleukin 6, tumour necrosis factor alpha, interleukin 1beta and interleukin 1 receptor antagonist promoter or coding gene polymorphisms in multiple myeloma. *Br J Haematol* 2000; **109**: 39–45.

●124. Spink CF, Keen LJ, Mensah FK *et al.* Association between non-Hodgkin lymphoma and haplotypes in the TNF region. *Br J Haematol* 2006; **133**: 293–300.

125. Wu MS, Chen LT, Shun CT *et al.* Promoter polymorphisms of tumor necrosis factor-alpha are associated with risk of gastric mucosa-associated lymphoid tissue lymphoma. *Int J Cancer* 2004; **110**: 695–700.

126. Hellmig S, Fischbach W, Goebeler-Kolve ME *et al.* A functional promotor polymorphism of TNF-alpha is associated with primary gastric B-Cell lymphoma. *Am J Gastroenterol* 2005; **100**: 2644–9.

127. Tsukasaki K, Miller CW, Kubota T *et al.* Tumor necrosis factor alpha polymorphism associated with increased susceptibility to development of adult T-cell leukemia/lymphoma in human T-lymphotropic virus type 1 carriers. *Cancer Res* 2001; **61**: 3770–4.

128. Jacobson EM, Concepcion E, Oashi T, Tomer Y. A Graves' disease-associated Kozak sequence single-nucleotide polymorphism enhances the efficiency of CD40 gene translation: a case for translational pathophysiology. *Endocrinology* 2005; **146**: 2684–91.

129. Park JH, Chang HS, Park CS *et al.* Association analysis of CD40 polymorphisms with asthma and the level of serum total IgE. *Am J Respir Crit Care Med* 2007; **175**: 775–82.

130. Saito M, Gao J, Basso K *et al.* A signaling pathway mediating downregulation of BCL6 in germinal center B cells is blocked by BCL6 gene alterations in B cell lymphoma. *Cancer Cell* 2007; **12**: 280–92.

131. Shin MS, Kim HS, Kang CS *et al.* Inactivating mutations of CASP10 gene in non-Hodgkin lymphomas. *Blood* 2002; **99**: 4094–9.

132. Lan Q, Zheng T, Chanock S *et al.* Genetic variants in caspase genes and susceptibility to non-Hodgkin lymphoma. *Carcinogenesis* 2007; **28**: 823–7.

133. Cordano P, Lake A, Shield L *et al.* Effect of IL-6 promoter polymorphism on incidence and outcome in Hodgkin's lymphoma. *Br J Haematol* 2005; **128**: 493–5.

134. Hulkkonen J, Vilpo J, Vilpo L *et al.* Interleukin-1 beta, interleukin-1 receptor antagonist and interleukin-6 plasma levels and cytokine gene polymorphisms in chronic lymphocytic leukemia: correlation with prognostic parameters. *Haematologica* 2000; **85**: 600–6.

135. O'Garra A, Vieira P. Regulatory T cells and mechanisms of immune system control. *Nat Med* 2004; **10**: 801–5.

136. Khatri VP, Caligiuri MA. A review of the association between interleukin-10 and human B-cell malignancies. *Cancer Immunol Immunother* 1998; **46**: 239–44.

137. Blay JY, Burdin N, Rousset F *et al.* Serum interleukin-10 in non-Hodgkin's lymphoma: a prognostic factor. *Blood* 1993; **82**: 2169–74.

●138. Fayad L, Keating MJ, Reuben JM *et al.* Interleukin-6 and interleukin-10 levels in chronic lymphocytic leukemia: correlation with phenotypic characteristics and outcome. *Blood* 2001; **97**: 256–63.

●139. Zheng C, Huang D, Liu L *et al.* Interleukin-10 gene promoter polymorphisms in multiple myeloma. *Int J Cancer* 2001; **95**: 184–8.

140. Mazur G, Bogunia-Kubik K, Wrobel T *et al.* IL-6 and IL-10 promoter gene polymorphisms do not associate with the susceptibility for multiple myeloma. *Immunol Lett* 2005; **96**: 241–6.

141. Breen EC, Boscardin WJ, Detels R *et al.* Non-Hodgkin's B cell lymphoma in persons with acquired immunodeficiency syndrome is associated with increased serum levels of IL10, or the IL10 promoter – 592 C/C genotype. *Clin Immunol* 2003; **109**: 119–29.

142. Jardin F, Sahota SS. Targeted somatic mutation of the BCL6 proto-oncogene and its impact on lymphomagenesis. *Hematology* 2005; **10**: 115–29.

143. Lossos IS, Jones CD, Zehnder JL, Levy R. A polymorphism in the BCL-6 gene is associated with follicle center lymphoma. *Leuk Lymphoma* 2001; **42**: 1343–50.

144. Jardin F, Ruminy P, Parmentier F *et al.* Clinical and biological relevance of single-nucleotide polymorphisms and acquired somatic mutations of the BCL6 first intron in follicular lymphoma. *Leukemia* 2005; **19**: 1824–30.

145. Zhang Y, Lan Q, Rothman N *et al.* A putative exonic splicing polymorphism in the BCL6 gene and the risk of non-Hodgkin lymphoma. *J Natl Cancer Inst* 2005; **97**: 1616–18.

146. Chamaillard M, Philpott D, Girardin SE *et al.* Gene-environment interaction modulated by allelic heterogeneity in inflammatory diseases. *Proc Natl Acad Sci U S A* 2003; **100**: 3455–60.

147. Yamada R, Ymamoto K. Recent findings on genes associated with inflammatory disease. *Mutat Res* 2005; **573**: 136–51.

148. Hellmig S, Fischbach W, Goebeler-Kolve ME *et al.* Association study of a functional Toll-like receptor 4 polymorphism with susceptibility to gastric mucosa-associated lymphoid tissue lymphoma. *Leuk Lymphoma* 2005; **46**: 869–72.

149. Eder W, Klimecki W, Yu L *et al.* Toll-like receptor 2 as a major gene for asthma in children of European farmers. *J Allergy Clin Immunol* 2004; **113**: 482–8.

150. Complete sequence and gene map of a human major histocompatibility complex. The MHC Sequencing Consortium. *Nature* 1999; **401**: 921–3.

151. Diepstra A, Niens M, Vellenga E *et al.* Association with HLA class I in Epstein-Barr-virus-positive and with HLA

class III in Epstein-Barr-virus-negative Hodgkin's lymphoma. *Lancet* 2005; **365**: 2216–24.

152. Klitz W, Aldrich CL, Fildes N *et al*. Localization of predisposition to Hodgkin disease in the HLA class II region. *Am J Hum Genet* 1994; **54**: 497–505.

153. Taylor GM, Gokhale DA, Crowther D *et al*. Further investigation of the role of HLA-DPB1 in adult Hodgkin's disease (HD) suggests an influence on susceptibility to different HD subtypes. *Br J Cancer* 1999; **80**: 1405–11.

154. Alexander FE, Jarrett RF, Cartwright RA *et al*. Epstein-Barr Virus and HLA-DPB1-*0301 in young adult Hodgkin's disease: evidence for inherited susceptibility to Epstein-Barr Virus in cases that are EBV(+ve). *Cancer Epidemiol Biomarkers Prev* 2001; **10**: 705–9.

155. Harty LC, Lin AY, Goldstein AM *et al*. HLA-DR, HLA-DQ, and TAP genes in familial Hodgkin disease. *Blood* 2002; **99**: 690–3.

156. Nathalang O, Tatsumi N, Hino M *et al*. HLA class II polymorphism in Thai patients with non-Hodgkin's lymphoma. *Eur J Immunogenet* 1999; **26**: 389–92.

157. Al Tonbary Y, Abdel-Razek N, Zaghloul H *et al*. HLA class II polymorphism in Egyptian children with lymphomas. *Hematology* 2004; **9**: 139–45.

158. Marti A, Marcos A, Martinez JA. Obesity and immune function relationships. *Obes Rev* 2001; **2**: 131–40.

159. Pan SY, Johnson KC, Ugnat AM *et al*. Association of obesity and cancer risk in Canada. *Am J Epidemiol* 2004; **159**: 259–68.

●160. Calle EE, Rodriguez C, Walker-Thurmond K, Thun MJ. Overweight, obesity, and mortality from cancer in a prospectively studied cohort of U.S. adults. *N Engl J Med* 2003; **348**: 1625–38.

161. Cerhan JR, Bernstein L, Severson RK *et al*. Anthropometrics, physical activity, related medical conditions, and the risk of non-hodgkin lymphoma. *Cancer Causes Control* 2005; **16**: 1203–14.

●162. Willett EV, Morton LM, Hartge P *et al*. Interlymph Consortium. Non-Hodgkin lymphoma and obesity: a pooled analysis from the InterLymph Consortium. *Int J Cancer* 2008; **122**: 2062–70.

●163. Skibola DR, Smith MT, Bracci PM *et al*. Polymorphisms in ghrelin and neuropeptide Y genes are associated with non-Hodgkin lymphoma. *Cancer Epidemiol Biomarkers Prev* 2005; **14**: 1251–6.

164. Mammes O, Betoulle D, Aubert R *et al*. Novel polymorphisms in the 5′region of the LEP gene: association with leptin levels and response to low-calorie diet in human obesity. *Diabetes* 1998; **47**: 487–9.

165. Mammes O, Betoulle D, Aubert R *et al*. Association of the G-2548A polymorphism in the 5′region of the LEP gene with overweight. *Ann Hum Genet* 2000; **64**: 391–4.

166. Hager J, Clement K, Francke S *et al*. A polymorphism in the 5′untranslated region of the human ob gene is associated with low leptin levels. *Int J Obes Relat Metab Disord* 1998; **22**: 200–5.

167. Li WD, Reed DR, Lee JH *et al*. Sequence variants in the 5′flanking region of the leptin gene are associated with obesity in women. *Ann Hum Genet* 1999; **63**: 227–34.

168. Nieters A, Becker N, Linseisen J. Polymorphisms in candidate obesity genes and their interaction with dietary intake of n-6 polyunsaturated fatty acids affect obesity risk in a sub-sample of the EPIC-Heidelberg cohort. *Eur J Nutr* 2002; **41**: 210–21.

169. Jiang Y, Wilk JB, Borecki I *et al*. Common variants in the 5′region of the leptin gene are associated with body mass index in men from the National Heart, Lung, and Blood Institute Family Heart Study. *Am J Hum Genet* 2004; **75**: 220–30.

170. Ding B. Distribution of the NPY 1128C allele frequency in different populations. *J Neural Transm* 2003; **110**: 1199–204.

171. Chang ET, Smedby KE, Zhang SM *et al*. Dietary factors and risk of non-hodgkin lymphoma in men and women. *Cancer Epidemiol Biomarkers Prev* 2005; **14**: 512–20.

172. Talamini R, Polesel J, Montella M *et al*. Food groups and risk of non-Hodgkin lymphoma: a multicenter, case-control study in Italy. *Int J Cancer* 2006; **118**: 2871–6.

173. Kuo SM, MacLean ME, McCormick K, Wilson JX. Gender and sodium-ascorbate transporter isoforms determine ascorbate concentrations in mice. *J Nutr* 2004; **134**: 2216–21.

174. Olsen NJ, Kovacs WJ. Gonadal steroids and immunity. *Endocr Rev* 1996; **17**: 369–84.

175. Gado K, Rimanoczi E, Hasitz A *et al*. Elevated levels of serum prolactin in patients with advanced multiple myeloma. *Neuroimmunomodulation* 2001; **9**: 231–6.

176. Hooghe R, Merchav S, Gaidano G *et al*. A role for growth hormone and prolactin in leukaemia and lymphoma? *Cell Mol Life Sci* 1998; **54**: 1095–101.

177. Sharp L, Cardy AH, Cotton SC, Little J. CYP17 gene polymorphisms: prevalence and associations with hormone levels and related factors. a HuGE review. *Am J Epidemiol* 2004; **160**: 729–40.

178. Lan Q, Zheng T, Shen M *et al*. Genetic polymorphisms in the oxidative stress pathway and susceptibility to non-Hodgkin lymphoma. *Hum Genet* 2007; **121**: 161–8.

179. Wang SS, Davis S, Cerhan JR *et al*. Polymorphisms in oxidative stress genes and risk for non-Hodgkin lymphoma. *Carcinogenesis* 2006; **27**: 1828–34.

180. Lightfoot TJ, Skibola CF, Smith AG *et al*. Polymorphisms in the oxidative stress genes, superoxide dismutase, glutathione peroxidase and catalase and risk of non-Hodgkin's lymphoma. *Haematologica* 2006; **91**: 1222–7.

181. Shen J, Wang RT, Wang LW *et al*. A novel genetic polymorphism of inducible nitric oxide synthase is associated with an increased risk of gastric cancer. *World J Gastroenterol* 2004; **10**: 3278–83.

182. Kerridge I, Lincz L, Scorgie F *et al*. Association between xenobiotic gene polymorphisms and non-Hodgkin's lymphoma risk. *Br J Haematol* 2002; **118**: 477–81.

183. Rollinson S, Levene AP, Mensah FK *et al.* Gastric marginal zone lymphoma is associated with polymorphisms in genes involved in inflammatory response and antioxidative capacity. *Blood* 2003; **102**: 1007–11.
184. Wu MS, Shun CT, Huang SP *et al.* Effect of interleukin-1beta and glutathione S-transferase genotypes on the development of gastric mucosa-associated lymphoid tissue lymphoma. *Haematologica* 2004; **89**: 1015–17.
185. Al-Dayel F, Al-Rasheed M, Ibrahim M *et al.* Polymorphisms of drug-metabolizing enzymes CYP1A1, GSTT and GSTP contribute to the development of diffuse large B-cell lymphoma risk in the Saudi Arabian population. *Leuk Lymphoma* 2008; **49**: 122–9.
186. Chiu BC, Kolar C, Gapstur SM *et al.* Association of NAT and GST polymorphisms with non-Hodgkin's lymphoma: a population-based case-control study. *Br J Haematol* 2005; **128**: 610–15.
187. De Roos AJ, Gold LS, Wang S *et al.* Metabolic gene variants and risk of non-Hodgkin's lymphoma. *Cancer Epidemiol Biomarkers Prev* 2006; **15**: 1647–53.
188. Morton LM, Schenk M, Hein DW *et al.* Genetic variation in N-acetyltransferase 1 (NAT1) and 2 (NAT2) and risk of non-Hodgkin lymphoma. *Pharmacogenet Genomics* 2006; **16**: 537–45.
●189. Morton LM, Bernstein L, Wang SS *et al.* Hair dye use, genetic variation in N-acetyltransferase 1 (NAT1) and 2 (NAT2), and risk of non-Hodgkin lymphoma. *Carcinogenesis* 2007; **28**: 1759–64.
190. Krajinovic M, Labuda D, Richer C *et al.* Susceptibility to childhood acute lymphoblastic leukemia: influence of CYP1A1, CYP2D6, GSTM1, and GSTT1 genetic polymorphisms. *Blood* 1999; **93**: 1496–501.
191. Canalle R, Burim RV, Tone LG, Takahashi CS. Genetic polymorphisms and susceptibility to childhood acute lymphoblastic leukemia. *Environ Mol Mutagen* 2004; **43**: 100–9.
192. Sarmanova J, Benesova K, Gut I *et al.* Genetic polymorphisms of biotransformation enzymes in patients with Hodgkin's and non-Hodgkin's lymphomas. *Hum Mol Genet* 2001; **10**: 1265–73.
193. Shimada T, Watanabe J, Inoue K *et al.* Specificity of 17beta-oestradiol and benzo[a]pyrene oxidation by polymorphic human cytochrome P4501B1 variants substituted at residues 48, 119 and 432. *Xenobiotica* 2001; **31**: 163–76.
194. Krajinovic M, Sinnett H, Richer C *et al.* Role of NQO1, MPO and CYP2E1 genetic polymorphisms in the susceptibility to childhood acute lymphoblastic leukemia. *Int J Cancer* 2002; **97**: 230–6.
195. Infante-Rivard C, Krajinovic M, Labuda D, Sinnett D. Childhood acute lymphoblastic leukemia associated with parental alcohol consumption and polymorphisms of carcinogen-metabolizing genes. *Epidemiology* 2002; **13**: 277–81.
196. Infante-Rivard C, Amre D, Sinnett D. GSTT1 and CYP2E1 polymorphisms and trihalomethanes in drinking water: effect on childhood leukemia. *Environ Health Perspect* 2002; **110**: 591–3.
197. Kelada SN, Eaton DL, Wang SS *et al.* The role of genetic polymorphisms in environmental health. *Environ Health Perspect* 2003; **111**: 1055–64.
198. Hohaus S, Massini G, D'Alo' F *et al.* Association between glutathione S-transferase genotypes and Hodgkin's lymphoma risk and prognosis. *Clin Cancer Res* 2003; **9**: 3435–40.
199. Hein DW. Molecular genetics and function of NAT1 and NAT2: role in aromatic amine metabolism and carcinogenesis. *Mutat Res* 2002; **506–507**: 65–77.
200. Lemos MC, Cabrita FJ, Silva HA *et al.* Genetic polymorphism of CYP2D6, GSTM1 and NAT2 and susceptibility to haematological neoplasias. *Carcinogenesis* 1999; **20**: 1225–9.
201. Costa LG, Cole TB, Jarvik GP, Furlong CE. Functional genomic of the paraoxonase (PON1) polymorphisms: effects on pesticide sensitivity, cardiovascular disease, and drug metabolism. *Annu Rev Med* 2003; **54**: 371–92.
202. Mackness B, Durrington P, Povey A *et al.* Paraoxonase and susceptibility to organophosphorus poisoning in farmers dipping sheep. *Pharmacogenetics* 2003; **13**: 81–8.
203. Cherry N, Mackness M, Durrington P *et al.* Paraoxonase (PON1) polymorphisms in farmers attributing ill health to sheep dip. *Lancet* 2002; **359**: 763–4.
◆204. Gzulich AE, Vajdic CM, Coten W. Altered immunity as a risk factor for non-Hodgkin lymphoma. *Cancer Epidemiol Biomarkers Prev* 2007; **16**: 405–8.

6

Epidemiology of exogenous human retroviruses associated with hematologic malignancies

ROBERT NEWTON

EXOGENOUS HUMAN RETROVIRUSES

Exogenous retroviruses are distinguished by a RNA genome which replicates through the action of the enzyme reverse transcriptase, via a DNA intermediate that integrates into the host chromosomal DNA. They are among the first known viruses, although until the late 1970s and early 1980s, they had only been found in animals, usually in association with neoplastic disease. In 1908, Ellerman and Bang first demonstrated the transmission of leukemia among chickens by 'an agent that passed through a filter'. However, leukemia was not recognized as a malignant disease until the 1930s. It was Peyton Rous in 1911 who first demonstrated the acellular transmission of a solid tumor (sarcoma) between chickens (the term virus had not yet been coined). Although both conditions are now known to be caused by retroviruses, the research community was not receptive to the notion that a chronic disease may have an infectious cause and it was to be 55 years before Rous received the Nobel Prize for his seminal discovery. In 1936, Bittner demonstrated that predisposition to breast cancer in C3H mice was transmitted in breast milk; the cause was subsequently found to be the retrovirus mouse mammary tumor virus. In 1951 Gross discovered the first murine leukemia virus. Many other retroviruses have since been identified including the avian leukosis and bovine leukemia viruses. The first human retrovirus (human T cell leukemia virus [HTLV-1]) was identified by Gallo and colleagues in 1979 and the findings were published in 1980.[1] Three other retroviruses were subsequently identified – HTLV-2, and the human immunodeficiency viruses types 1 and 2. Although HTLV-2 was identified in a person with hairy cell leukemia, it has not been firmly linked with any human disease, while HTLV-1 and human immunodeficiency virus (HIV)-1 and 2 are important causes of morbidity and mortality. In addition to other malignant and nonmalignant diseases, in the year 2002, together these three viruses have been estimated to account for up to 40 000 cases of hematologic malignancy – more than any other known cause (Table 6.1).[2,3] The human retroviruses target cells of the immune system, particularly mature CD4+ T cells, impair their function and cause them either to grow abnormally (HTLV-1), or to die (HIV-1 and HIV-2). Infection, therefore, manifests with a range of diseases,

Table 6.1 Global burden (as measured by the number of newly diagnosed cases) of hematologic malignancies associated with infection by HTLV-1 and HIV in 2002[a]

Infection	Number of new cases of hematologic malignancy		
	Men	Women	Total
HTLV-1	2 160	1 180	3 340
HIV	25 700	10 300	36 100
Total	27 860	11 480	39 340

Note: In the same year, the Epstein–Barr virus is estimated to have caused about 35 000 cases of hematologic malignancy (80 percent of which were classified as Hodgkin lymphoma).
[a]Adapted from Parkin.[2]
HTLV, human T cell leukemia virus; HIV, human immunodeficiency virus.

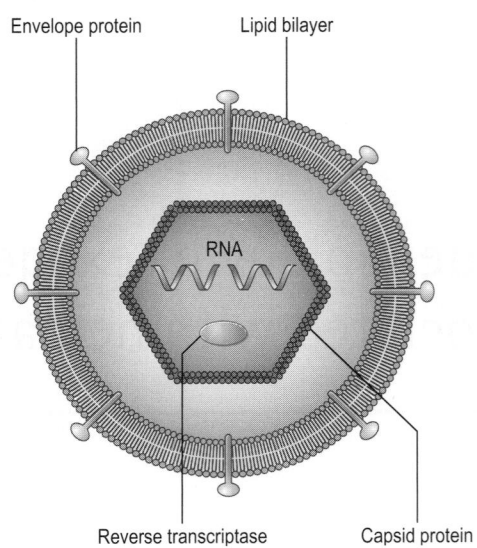

Figure 6.1 Schematic representation of a retrovirus.

including neurologic disorders, leukemia/lymphoma and the many conditions associated with HIV-AIDS (acquired immune deficiency syndrome).

Although there is considerable diversity between the various types of retrovirus, certain features are universal (Fig. 6.1). They are enveloped viruses, somewhat variable in size and shape, but usually about 100 nm in diameter. The outer envelope (a lipid bilayer derived from the plasma membrane of the host cell) carries virus-encoded glycoproteins and surrounds the viral capsid. The protein capsid encompasses the core which contains two molecules of RNA varying in size from about 8 kb to 11 kb, together with several molecules of RNA-dependent DNA polymerase (reverse transcriptase) – this enzyme converts the RNA genome into DNA, which then integrates into the host chromosome to form a provirus. Each retroviral genome contains at least three genes: *gag* (which encodes the internal core proteins), *pol* (encodes reverse transcriptase) and *env* (encodes the external envelope glycoproteins), which are bounded at either end by a regulatory sequence – the long terminal repeat (LTR) – which facilitates integration into the host chromosome and controls gene expression. The order of these genes within the genome does not vary:

LTR – gag – pol – env – LTR

Most retroviruses contain one or more additional genes that may be involved in the pathogenesis of associated diseases. Some of these represent RNA copies of genes that were inherited from eukaryotic hosts during evolution.

At infection, viral glycoproteins bind to specific receptors on the surface of the host cell, initiating fusion of the envelope with the cell membrane and inclusion into the cytoplasm of the viral core. This reaction is highly cell-specific and does much to determine the pathogenesis of different retroviruses. After the virion enters the cell, reverse transcriptase converts viral RNA into DNA which integrates randomly into the host cell genome. The integrated provirus may remain inactive or be transcribed into progeny viral RNA and into messenger RNA, which is translated to produce the viral structure and regulatory proteins. Progeny virions are assembled at the cell surface and acquire an envelope through the process of budding from the cell surface. When the genome of a retrovirus integrates into the germ line, it is passed on to following generations. Such 'endogenous' retrovirus sequences are thought to make up between 2 percent and 10 percent of the human genome and although most insertions have no known function, some have a role in host biology and others are thought to contribute to certain human diseases.[4]

HUMAN T CELL LEUKEMIA VIRUS-1

Epidemiology and transmission

Human T cell leukemia virus-1, the cause of adult T cell leukemia/lymphoma (ATLL), is an enveloped retrovirus, of the family *oncornavirinae*, containing two covalently bound genomic RNA strands, which are combined with several viral enzymes, including reverse transcriptase.[5,6] It is considered to be an ancient infection of humans and related retroviruses are common among Old World primates. The prevalence of infection with HTLV-1 varies widely, with high levels in diverse geographic areas (Fig. 6.2; reviewed by Proietti *et al.*[7]). The exact number of infected individuals worldwide is not known, but has been estimated to be between about 15–20 million people.[8,9] Antibodies against HTLV-1 are found in 5–15 percent of indigenous adult populations in southern Japan, the Caribbean, South America, central Africa, Papua New Guinea and the Solomon Islands. However, within endemic areas, clusters of especially high prevalence can occur; for example, in selected populations in southwestern

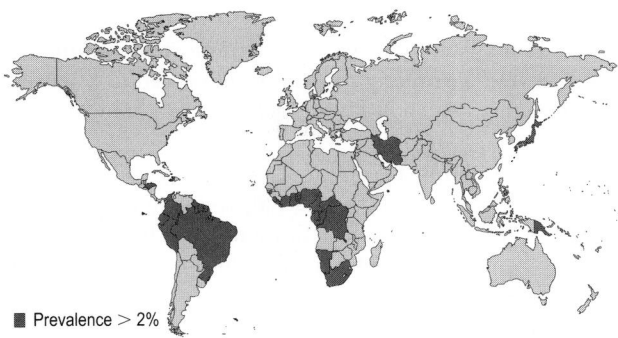

■ Prevalence > 2%

Figure 6.2 Map showing the distribution of endemic human T cell leukemia virus-1 infection. (Adapted from Proietti *et al.*[7] by Cancer Research UK.)

Table 6.2 Seroprevalence of antibodies against human T cell leukemia virus-1 in some endemic populations

Country	Ethnic group	Percentage seropositive (number positive/total)
Asia		
Japan	Japanese (Kyushu)	8 (241/3026)
Philippines	Aeta (south)	2 (17/746)
Iran	Mashadi Jew (north)	12 (24/208)
Africa		
Gabon	Black	8 (144/1874)
Zaire	Pygmy	6 (8/132)
Cameroon	Pygmy	20 (8/41)
Oceania		
Australia	Aborigine	6 (7/120)
Papua New Guinea	Melanesian	3 (26/972)
Americas		
Trinidad	Black	7 (56/797)
Panama	Amerindian	8 (27/337)
Columbia	Black	8 (17/226)
	Amerindian	4 (13/329)
	Amerindian (Orinoco)	32 (29/92)
Chile	Amerindian (north)	4 (9/214)
	Amerindian (south)	22 (10/45)

Adapted from Tajima and Takezaki.[12]

Japan and in Columbia, prevalence rates of more than 30 percent have been reported.[10,11] However, among these highly endemic populations, substantial variation in prevalence has been noted even between neighboring villages.[12] Carriers can be found elsewhere in the world, but are mostly individuals who moved from endemic areas, their offspring and sexual contacts and, among sex workers and intravenous drug users. Seroprevalence of HTLV-1 is generally less than 0.03 percent in blood donors from North America and Europe.[7,9]

It is important to note that most of the data on the prevalence of antibodies against HTLV-1 have come from studies of blood donors or other selected subpopulations, such as pregnant women, intravenous drug users or specific native groups, which are not necessarily representative of the general population. In addition, estimates from many studies are based on relatively small numbers of tested individuals (Table 6.2; reviewed by Tajima and Takezaki[12]).

In most, but not in all endemic areas, the seroprevalence of HTLV-1 increases with increasing age and is higher among females than among males.[11–15] The higher prevalence with age probably reflects not only the accumulation of seroconversions throughout the lifetime of those tested, but also an age-cohort effect due to declining seroprevalence over the past two decades. The higher prevalence among women may, in part, reflect more efficient sexual transmission from males to females than from females to males, although it has also been suggested that hormonal factors may affect susceptibility to infection.[16,17] In addition, several studies both in endemic and in nonendemic areas have reported that infection with HTLV-1 is more prevalent among people of lower socioeconomic status, suggesting that factors associated with poverty may influence the likelihood of transmission (reviewed by Proietti *et al.*[7]).

Three modes of transmission of HTLV-1 have been identified: from mother to child, via sex and by transfusion of infected cellular blood (for example, in blood products or through intravenous drug use). Infection occurs principally by passage of cells containing HTLV-1 proviral DNA,

rather than from infectious virions, perhaps explaining the relatively poor transmissibility of the virus. Mother-to-child transmission is the most frequent explanation for infection and occurs in about 20 percent of children of infected mothers.[18] Postnatal infection by breastfeeding is the primary route, while intrauterine and peripartum transmissions are very much less important.[19–21] The risk of transmission via infected lymphocytes in breast milk is related to maternal proviral load, high antibody titers and prolonged breastfeeding,[20,22] the risk being particularly high beyond about 6 months (Table 6.3; see Takahashi *et al.*[23] and Oki *et al.*[24]).

Sexual transmission is also an important method of spread of HTLV-1. As with other sexually transmitted infections (STIs), HTLV-1 seropositivity is associated with markers of sexual behavior such as number of lifetime sexual partners, unprotected sex, work in the sex industry and presence of other STIs.[25] Some studies have suggested that the likelihood of transmission is greater from male to female rather than from female to male, and HTLV-1 has certainly been found in the semen of infected men.[19,26]

The most efficient mode of transmission of HTLV-1 is via intravenous contact with infected blood or blood products. The risk of seroconversion following a transfusion of infected blood is between 40 percent and 60 percent, but is lower following cold storage of the blood product (presumably because the infected lymphocytes

Table 6.3 Prevalence of human T cell leukemia virus-1 (HTLV-1) among children of infected mothers in Japan, according to the method of infant feeding.

Method of infant feeding	Percentage of children infected with HTLV-1 (number infected/total)	
	Takahashi et al. (1991)[23]	Oki et al. (1992)[24]
Breastfed for less than 7 months	4 (4/90)	4 (1/26)
Breastfed for 7 or more months	14 (20/139)	25 (1/4)
Bottle-fed from birth	6 (9/158)	6 (10/177)

Data from Takahashi et al.[23] and Oki et al.[24]

die). In the past, such exposure was more frequent because blood donors were not screened for HTLV-1 – more recently, routine screening has been implemented in a number of places including Japan, the USA, Canada, Brazil and several European countries.[7,12,27,28] Sharing of contaminated needles by intravenous drug users is another important mode of parenteral transmission of HTLV-1 and infection has become endemic among drug users in several countries.[29–31]

Adult T cell leukemia/lymphoma

Human T cell leukemia virus type 1 is the main causal agent of ATLL, a disease characterized by malignant proliferation of CD4+ T lymphocytes. Clinical features include hypercalcemia, lymphadenopathy, skin lesions due to leukemic cell infiltration, involvement of the spleen and liver and immunodeficiency. The disease was first described as a distinct entity in Japan in the 1970s,[5,6] then among Caribbean immigrants living in the UK[32] and in other endemic areas (reviewed by Proietti,[7] IARC,[9] Tajima et al.[12] and Blattner et al.[33]). It represents a spectrum of clinical conditions and has subsequently been classified into four clinicopathologic subtypes: acute type (about 60 percent of all cases), lymphoma type (25 percent), chronic type (10 percent) and smoldering type (5 percent).[5–7] The prognosis of patients with acute ATLL is generally poor and few survive more than a matter of months following diagnosis.

ATLL occurs almost exclusively in areas where HTLV-1 is endemic, such as Japan, the Caribbean and west Africa, and cases described elsewhere have generally been in immigrants from those endemic regions, or their offspring. Early studies showed that infection with HTLV-1 is so closely associated with adult T cell leukemia, that it is now part of the diagnostic criteria used for defining the disease.[9] All antibody positive cases of adult T cell leukemia have monoclonally integrated HTLV-1 provirus in the malignant cells,

suggesting that the tumor is an outgrowth of an individual T cell clone. The virus is able to immortalize human T lymphocytes, a property that has been related to a specific viral gene *tax*, which has been identified as a transforming factor.[34]

ATLL develops in about 2–5 percent of HTLV-1-infected individuals and is especially frequent among those infected early in life (such as those infected by mother-to-child transmission).[35] Onset of disease occurs mostly in adult life, usually in the fourth or fifth decade and at least 20–30 years after infection with HTLV-1. In addition it is slightly more common among men than women, even though the underlying causal infection is more frequent among women. High anti-HTLV-1 antibodies and low anti-*tax* reactivity have been related to increased risk of ATLL, but the determinants of these are unclear.[36] Other factors associated with progression of infection to malignancy are suspected but not well described, including viral and host genetics, and environmental factors such as infecting dose.

Other human T cell leukemia virus–1–associated diseases

Decades before the discovery of HTLV-1, series of patients were reported from Martinique and Jamaica, with slowly progressive spastic paraparesis associated with sphincter disturbance and abnormalities of sensory perception and proprioception.[37,38] The condition has been reported to have occurred in people who were also diagnosed with ATLL and subsequent investigations demonstrated a high prevalence of HTLV-1 among cases.[7,39–41] It was later designated by a working group of the World Health Organization (WHO) as 'HTLV-1-associated myelopathy', or 'tropical spastic paraparesis' (HAM/TSP),[42] and is the second most common disease caused by infection with HTLV-1. Pathologically, it is characterized by progressive myelopathy and demyelination of the spinal cord motor neurons. Primary symptoms include limp (caused by stiffness of the lower limbs), bladder dysfunction, paresthesia, low back pain and impotence (in men). The principal immunologic features are the presence of high anti-HTLV-1 antibody titers in serum and cerebrospinal fluid, a high proviral load in peripheral blood cells and the presence of cytotoxic T cells, which recognize HTLV-1 *tax* gene products.[43] Up to 4 percent of HTLV-1 infected people can develop HAM/TSP, which more frequently affects women than men and can occur at younger ages than is seen for adult T cell leukemia.[44] Epidemiologic evidence suggests that it develops primarily among people who are infected with HTLV-1 via sexual transmission,[45,46] although it has been reported following blood transfusion.[47] Use of corticosteroids may confer some transient benefit, but the clinical course is progressive. Some of the features of HAM/TSP are described in Table 6.4, together with those of ATLL.

Table 6.4 Characteristics of adult T-cell leukemia/lymphoma (ATLL) and of human T cell leukemia virus-1 (HTLV-1) associated myelopathy/tropical spastic paraparesis (HAM)

	ATLL	HAM
Clinical features	Leukemia/lymphoma with cutaneous lesions and hypercalcemia	Spastic gait, dysuria and sensory disturbance
Age distribution	Mainly in adults 45 years and older	Can occur among young people, but usual age of onset 34–45 years
Sex distribution	More common among men	More common among women
Source of HTLV-1	Mainly vertical transmission	Mainly horizontal transmission
Latency	Usually more than 20 years	Can occur within months of infection
Cumulative risk	2–5%	1–4%

Adapted from Tajima and Takezaki.[12]

Uveitis is another common manifestation of infection with HTLV-1 and is characterized by relatively rapid onset of blurred vision, but with no change in visual acuity.[48] Again, the clinical course is progressive, although corticosteroids can induce remission that might last for several years. Inflammatory cells infected with HTLV-1 infiltrate ocular tissues, but the precise pathogenesis remains unclear. A variety of other conditions such as arthritis, polymyositis, alveolitis and immunosuppression have also been reported in relation to infection with HTLV-1[1,7, 9, 12] sometimes concurrent with ATLL or HAM/TSP.

Prevention

The prognosis of ATLL and HAM/TSP is poor and, despite the fact that passive and active immunization is effective in animal models, no preventive vaccine is yet available for humans.[9] Therefore, control and prevention of HTLV-1-associated diseases depends on limiting transmission of the virus by all three of the major routes. Prevention of mother-to-child transmission is likely to have the biggest impact. Perinatal transmission has been greatly reduced in Japan by advising infected women to use alternatives to breastfeeding. In some parts of the world, such as in Africa, the cessation of breastfeeding is not an option because it deprives the child of the protection conferred by maternal antibodies against various infections. However, short-term breastfeeding carries little risk of transmission and would be advisable. Unfortunately, such measures are dependent on a mother knowing her HTLV-1 status, which is rarely the case in the developing world. Several countries have introduced universal screening of blood donors and needle

exchange programs have been shown to be effective in limiting the spread of a number of infections, including HTLV-1 and HIV. Recommendations to prevent sexual transmission, such as condom use, are being emphasized in high-risk settings.

HUMAN IMMUNODEFICIENCY VIRUS TYPES 1 AND 2

Epidemiology and transmission

Human immunodeficiency viruses 1 and 2 are distinguished from HTLV-1 in that there is little evidence that either virus has a direct oncogenic effect in relation to the development of hematologic cancer or other malignancies. Instead, they appear to facilitate the development, via effects on the immune system, of a number of cancers, which are either known, or thought, to be caused by other underlying infectious agents or immune factors. For the purposes of this chapter where the abbreviation 'HIV' is used, it refers specifically to infection with HIV-1; reports on the association of cancers with HIV-2 are relatively infrequent and where they are discussed, the term 'HIV-2' will be used.

In the summer of 1981 in the USA, several cases of *Pneumocystis carinii* pneumonia and Kaposi sarcoma in young men were reported to the Centers for Disease Control and Prevention. It was subsequently recognized that the affected individuals were both homosexual and immunosuppressed and the condition was given the name of acquired immune deficiency syndrome, although its cause and modes of transmission were not immediately obvious. The HIV type 1 was discovered in 1983 by Barré-Sinoussi and colleagues[49] and firmly associated with AIDS in 1984.[50] In 1986, a second related type of HIV – the HIV-2 – was isolated from AIDS patients in western Africa, where it may have been present for decades.

Both HIV-1 and HIV-2 infect components of the human immune system, notably CD4+ T lymphocytes, macrophages and dendritic cells, ultimately killing the infected cell. Primary infection is associated with rapid viral replication (Fig. 6.3) and a range of symptoms including fever, generalized lymphadenopathy, rash, myalgia and joint pain. Within weeks, the immune system can recognize and destroy HIV-infected cells and antibodies against HIV are detectable (seroconversion), leading to a decline in viral load. There follows a period of clinical latency (measured in years), which inevitably ends as viral load rises again and the number of CD4+ immune cells declines. When the immune system is sufficiently damaged, the symptoms of AIDS become apparent – many of these conditions do not normally develop in people with an intact immune system and are usually associated with infections (bacterial, viral, fungal and parasitic). General symptoms such as fever, lymphadenopathy and weight loss are also common (for further details of AIDS-related

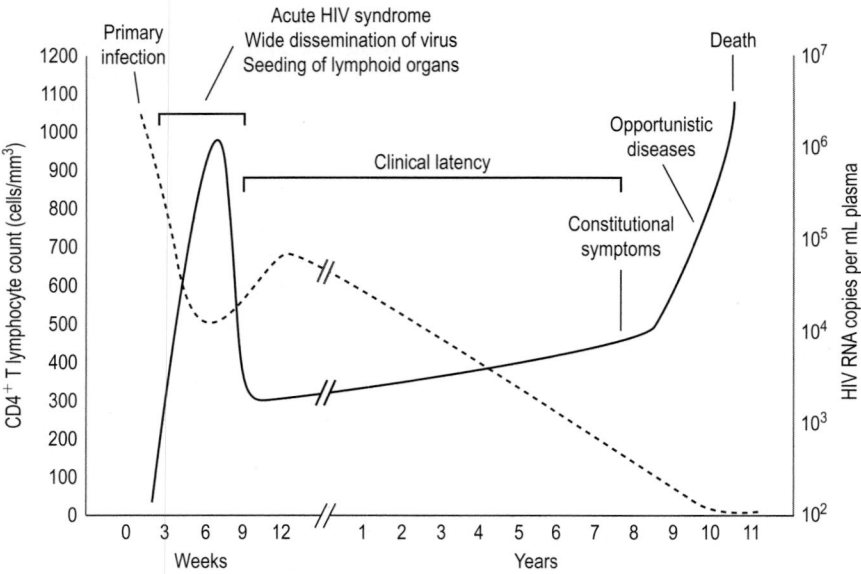

Figure 6.3   A graphical representation of changes in HIV viral load and CD4+ lymphocyte counts over time in an HIV-infected person.

diseases and symptom profiles, see www.cdc.gov/hiv). The rate of disease progression varies from person to person, but untreated HIV disease is inevitably fatal. Time from seroconversion to death among HIV-infected people is broadly similar among untreated individuals from developed and developing countries (about 10 years), although the rate of progression does vary markedly depending on the age at which someone is infected.[51,52] In general, greater age at infection is associated with a shorter time until death from AIDS, although mortality is also high among infants (Table 6.5).

Both HIV-1 and HIV-2 have the same modes of transmission and are associated with similar opportunistic infections and malignancies. However, in people infected with HIV-2, immunodeficiency generally develops more slowly and is less severe than among people infected with HIV-1. Similarly the virus is less infectious and has not spread as rapidly or as widely as HIV-1.

It is now generally accepted that HIV is descended from simian immunodeficiency viruses because of the striking similarities with certain strains of virus found in monkeys; HIV-2 corresponds to a virus found in sooty mangabeys (green monkeys), which are indigenous in western Africa and probably passed into humans on several occasions over the past century.[53,54] The likely source of HIV-1 infection is the chimpanzee species *Pan troglodytes troglodytes*, indigenous to southern Cameroon.[55,56] The evidence suggests that wild chimpanzees were infected simultaneously with two different strains of simian virus (one from a red-capped mangabey and the other from a greater spot-nosed monkey), that recombined to form a third virus that could be passed between chimpanzees and to people (probably via the consumption of bush meat). Hybridization of the two simian viruses is thought to have taken place when

Table 6.5   Percent of human immunodeficiency virus (HIV)-1-infected hemophiliac patients in the UK surviving 10 years following seroconversion

Age at seroconversion to HIV	Percent who survived 10 years
<15 years	86
15–34 years	72
35–54 years	45
55+ years	12

Data from Darby *et al.*[51]

a chimpanzee became infected with both strains of SIV having hunted and killed two species of monkey. The first human infection probably took place sometime in the first half of the past century.

Although the first cases of HIV disease were reported as recently as 1981, in 2005 there were estimated to be nearly 40 million people living with HIV, more than four million new infections and nearly three million deaths from AIDS (for the most up-to-date estimates see www.unaids.org). Of those infected, more than 17 million are women, nearly 2.5 million are children and almost 25 million live in sub-Saharan Africa (Fig. 6.4 and Table 6.6) – the majority of those infected (up to 90 percent) will not yet know it. The epidemic is also growing rapidly in eastern Europe and Central Asia, although declines in prevalence have been noted in Kenya, Zimbabwe, parts of Haiti and Burkina Faso and in several Indian states. Infections with HIV-2 are predominantly limited to west African nations including Cape Verde, Côte d'Ivoire, Gambia, Guinea-Bissau, Mali, Mauritania, Nigeria and Sierra Leone.

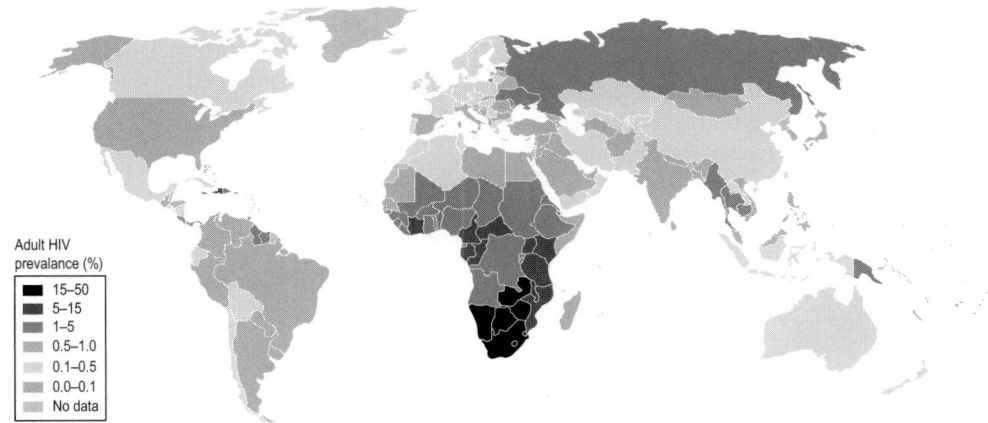

Figure 6.4   Global prevalence of HIV infection among adults in 2005. (Based on data from UNAIDS [www.unaids.org].)

Table 6.6   HIV infection – regional statistics for 2005

Region	People living with HIV	New infections in 2005	AIDS deaths in 2005	Adult prevalence (%)
Sub-Saharan Africa	24.5 million	2.7 million	2 million	6.1
Asia	8.3 million	930 000	600 000	0.4
Latin America	1.6 million	140 000	59 000	0.5
North America, Western and Central Europe	2 million	65 000	30 000	0.5
Eastern Europe and Central Asia	1.5 million	220 000	53 000	0.8
Middle East and North Africa	440 000	64 000	37 000	0.2
Caribbean	330 000	37 000	27 000	1.6
Oceania	78 000	7200	3400	0.3
TOTAL	**38.6 million**	**4.1 million**	**2.8 million**	**1**

Data from UNAIDS (www.unaids.org).

The three primary routes of transmission – sexual intercourse, blood contact and from mother to infant – were proposed on the basis of the epidemiology of AIDS, even before the identification of HIV. Of those, heterosexual transmission accounts for over 80 percent of new infections worldwide, while the importance of contact with infected blood products is declining in developed countries since the introduction of routine screening procedures in blood banks. In fact, the HIV is not as infectious as many other viruses (Table 6.7, references 57–64), but the spread of the epidemic is facilitated by the long period of infectiousness before an individual becomes ill or is even aware that they are infected (see Fig. 6.3).

Immunosuppression and non–Hodgkin lymphoma

It has long been thought that the immune system plays a vital role in the etiology of cancer. In 1965 the Nobel Laureate Sir McFarlane Burnet argued that immunosurveillance was a central mechanism by which tumor development was kept in check and predicted that individuals who were immunosuppressed would be at an increased risk of cancer.[65] It was already known that children with rare congenital defects of their immune system, such as X-linked gammaglobulinemia or ataxia telangiectasia, were at increased risk of non-Hodgkin lymphoma (including Burkitt-type tumors), but the number of children with such defects was exceedingly small and so it was not possible to classify more thoroughly the subtypes of non-Hodgkin lymphoma, or to tell whether they were also at an increased risk of other types of cancer.[66,67] Only since the 1970s, with the increasing use of immunosuppressive drugs in relation to tissue transplantation, has it been possible to investigate Burnet's hypothesis in detail. Studies of individuals on long-term immunosuppressive drug therapy showed that such people were at a greatly increased risk of certain, but not of all, types of cancer. The most marked increases were for non-Hodgkin lymphoma (the most commonly reported tumor in most studies of immunosuppressed transplant recipients), Kaposi sarcoma and squamous cell carcinoma of the skin.[68,69] Some studies, but not others, also reported an increase for Hodgkin lymphoma.[69]

Table 6.7 Estimated per act risk for acquisition of HIV by exposure route

Exposure route	Estimated infections per 10 000 exposures to an infected source
Blood transfusion	9000
Childbirth	2500
Needle sharing injection drug use	67
Unprotected receptive anal intercourse	50
Needle stick injury	30
Unprotected receptive penile-vaginal intercourse	10
Insertive anal intercourse	7
Unprotected insertive penile-vaginal intercourse	5
Receptive oral intercourse on a man	1
Insertive oral intercourse on a man	0.5

Based on references 57–64.

The findings in transplant recipients suggested that immunosuppression leads to the selective development of cancers that are caused by infectious or immune factors. The first specific infectious agent implicated as causing cancer in transplant recipients was the Epstein–Barr virus (EBV), which has been consistently identified in transplant-related lymphomas.[70] Indeed, most post-transplant lymphomas appear to arise as a result of an EBV driven lymphoproliferation and the Burkitt-type lymphomas are relatively less frequent.[9,71] The related gamma herpesvirus – human herpesvirus 8 (or Kaposi sarcoma-associated herpesvirus) – is the established cause of Kaposi sarcoma and of a rare form of non-Hodgkin lymphoma – primary effusion lymphoma – that also occurs among immunodeficient people albeit rarely.[71] The clinical course of the cancers that occur in immunosuppressed transplant recipients tend to be more aggressive than in the general population and it has also been noted that the cessation of immunosuppressive therapy can halt or even reverse tumor growth.[72]

Thus by the late 1970s, before the AIDS epidemic, it was widely believed that immunosuppression leads to the selective development of cancers that are caused by infectious agents or immune factors. However, because the immunodeficient tended to be ill for other reasons, it was not always clear whether the cancers that occurred among them were due to the immunodeficiency itself or to the underlying medical condition or related exposures or even to the immunosuppressive drugs.

Human immunodeficiency virus–associated non-Hodgkin lymphoma

Following a report published in 1984 of a series of 90 cases of non-Hodgkin lymphoma occurring in homosexual men with AIDS, three types – immunoblastic, Burkitt and central nervous system non-Hodgkin lymphomas – were categorized as being AIDS defining.[73,74] In developed countries, before effective treatment for HIV disease became available in the form of highly active antiretroviral therapy (HAART), people diagnosed with AIDS were about 60 times more likely than the general population to have non-Hodgkin lymphoma (and up to 1000 times more likely to have Burkitt lymphoma or central nervous system lymphomas).[75] Non-Hodgkin lymphoma was the AIDS-defining condition in about 3 percent of cases in developed countries (less in children with AIDS), although as many as 10–15 percent of those with HIV infection contracted the disease at some stage in their illness;[75–77] the prevalence of non-Hodgkin lymphoma in autopsy studies of HIV-infected individuals was as high as 20 percent.[78] This increased risk is of a similar order of magnitude to that in immunosuppressed transplant recipients and, for most, but not all, types of non-Hodgkin lymphoma, increases with increasing level of immunosuppression.[79,80] Consistent failure to detect HIV sequences within the tumor clone indicates that the virus does not directly cause transformation of B lymphocytes. All these factors suggest that the role of HIV in lymphomagenesis is indirect and related to its effects on immunoregulation. Interestingly, however, HIV-associated non-Hodgkin lymphomas differ in some respects from those lymphomas occurring in immunosuppressed transplant recipients, perhaps because the nature of the immunosuppression is different.

Non-Hodgkin lymphomas associated with HIV, although histologically heterogeneous, are characterized by an aggressive clinical course. High-grade disease is common and extranodal sites are often involved, with lesions in the central nervous system being rare except in the immunosuppressed. Three broad categories of HIV-associated non-Hodgkin lymphoma were initially described and can be distinguished by their clinical, histologic and epidemiologic features.[71,75] The most common type is a B cell immunoblastic tumor, the risk of which increases steadily with age. About a fifth of lymphomas in AIDS patients in the West are primary brain lymphomas and another fifth are Burkitt lymphomas. The risk of cerebral lymphomas in HIV-infected individuals does not change with age and that of Burkitt lymphomas peaks between 10 and 19 years of age, mirroring the epidemiologic pattern of sporadic Burkitt lymphoma in the USA. For all types, the risk is twice as high in men as it is in women, and in white people as it is in black people.[75]

More recently, this simplistic classification of AIDS-related lymphomas has been reviewed by the WHO, in an effort to better characterize disease entities and to standardize the increasingly complex nomenclature (Box 6.1, derived from reference 81).[81] Tumors are divided into 1) those that occur specifically in HIV infected people, 2) those that occur in other immunosuppressed groups as well and 3) those that also arise in immunocompetent people. The majority are diffuse large B-cell lymphomas, which are further subdivided into centroblastic and immunoblastic types. The immunoblastic tumors are characteristic of HIV disease and are strongly associated with EBV infection (malignant cells usually express EBV-encoded LMP-1).[82–86] In addition, they tend to lack *bcl-6* expression (a proto-oncogene which is selectively expressed in B cells located within germinal centres), but do express CD138 (normally expressed by B cells in the later stages of development), strongly suggesting the tumor arises from post-germinal centre lymphocytes. Conversely, the centroblastic subtype displays features similar to tumors found in the general population, is less clearly associated with EBV (malignant cells rarely express LMP-1), but does usually express *bcl-6*, suggesting a germinal centre origin.[86] Primary central nervous system lymphomas are generally of the immunoblastic diffuse large B-cell type and are almost always associated with EBV infection. LMP-1 is expressed on tumor cells and EBV-DNA is present in cerebrospinal fluid of affected individuals.[87]

Burkitt lymphoma, which accounts for between 20 percent and 30 percent of AIDS-related lymphomas, is associated with EBV infection in only about 30 percent of cases and is less clearly linked with immunodeficiency than other AIDS-related lymphomas.[88] Whereas central nervous system lymphomas occur in people with profound levels of immunosuppression (median CD4 counts of around 10–20 cells/mL) and other B cell tumors also occurring in late-stage HIV disease (median CD4 counts of about 70 cells/mL; similar to Kaposi sarcoma), Burkitt lymphoma can occur among people with relatively high CD4 counts.[89] Furthermore, the widespread introduction of antiretroviral therapy for HIV disease has seen a decline in the incidence of most non-Hodgkin lymphomas, with the exception of Burkitt lymphoma.[90] The increased B cell activation accompanying HIV infection may increase the likelihood of such mutational events. Burkitt lymphoma tumor cells are of germinal center origin and contain classic c-*myc* translocations. However, c-*myc*/immunoglobulin gene translocations can be found in circulating B cells in the peripheral blood of otherwise healthy HIV-seropositive individuals and their presence, in one study, did not correlate with the subsequent development of lymphoma, suggesting that further oncogenic steps may be required.[91]

As well as EBV, the related gamma herpesvirus, human herpesvirus 8 (HHV-8; or Kaposi sarcoma-associated herpesvirus) is known to cause a rare AIDS-related lymphoma – primary effusion lymphoma (PEL) – which classically presents with malignant effusions in the absence of an underlying tumor mass.[92] Immunoglobulin gene rearrangements indicate that the neoplastic cells are of B cell lineage, but do not express any B cell antigens on their surface. In addition to infections, several nonspecific host factors have also been suggested as playing a role in lymphomagenesis in HIV-infected individuals, such as disrupted immunosurveillance, chronic antigenic stimulation and cytokine dysregulation, all of which might be responsible for expanding the B cell population from which a lymphoma subsequently develops.

Antiviral therapy and lymphoma

Highly active antiretroviral therapy became widely available in North America, western Europe and Australia in 1996–7; since then, mortality rates from AIDS have fallen dramatically in developed countries.[93–97] In particular, the frequency of opportunistic infections has declined by 50–80 percent in the USA and Europe.[94,96] Therefore, despite also showing a decline in incidence since the introduction of HAART, there has been a relative increase in AIDS-related lymphomas as a percentage of first AIDS-defining illnesses. In one study from western Europe, the proportion of all AIDS-defining illnesses comprising non-Hodgkin lymphoma increased from 3.6 percent in 1994 to 4.9 percent in 1997,[98] and in another study, it increased from 4 percent in 1994, to almost 16 percent in 1998.[99] Similar results have been found in studies from North America and Australia.[100,101] However, in general, the incidence of the two major AIDS-related cancers, Kaposi sarcoma and non-Hodgkin lymphoma, has declined since

CANCER TYPE	Adjusted[a] incidence rate per 1000 per year (number)		Rate ratio[a] (RR) in 1997–99 versus 1992–96	
	1992–96	1997–99	RR	RR (95% CI)
Kaposi sarcoma	15.3 (1489)	4.9 (190)	0.32	
Non-Hodgkin lymphoma	6.2 (621)	3.6 (134)	0.58	
Hodgkin disease	0.5 (38)	0.4 (12)	0.77	
Cancer of the uterine cervix	1.1 (19)	2.1 (17)	1.88	
Other cancers[a]	1.8 (126)	1.7 (54)	0.96	

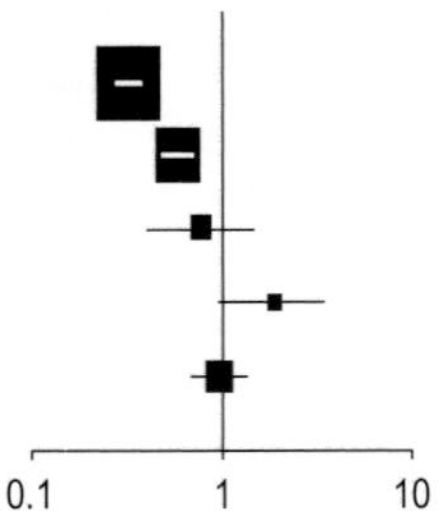

0.1   1   10

[a] Adjusted for study, age, sex and HIV risk group.

Figure 6.5 Changes in cancer incidence since the introduction of highly active antiretroviral therapy. RR, relative risk. (Derived from International Collaboration on HIV and Cancer.[90])

CANCER TYPE	Adjusted[a] incidence rate per 1000 per year (number)		Rate ratio[a] (RR) in 1997–99 versus 1992–96	
	1992–96	1997–99	RR (SE)	RR (99% CI)
Cerebral lymphoma	1.7 (138)	0.7 (24)	0.42 (0.09)	
Burkitt lymphoma	0.3 (26)	0.4 (13)	1.18 (0.41)	
Immunoblastic lymphoma	3.0 (246)	1.7 (54)	0.57 (0.09)	

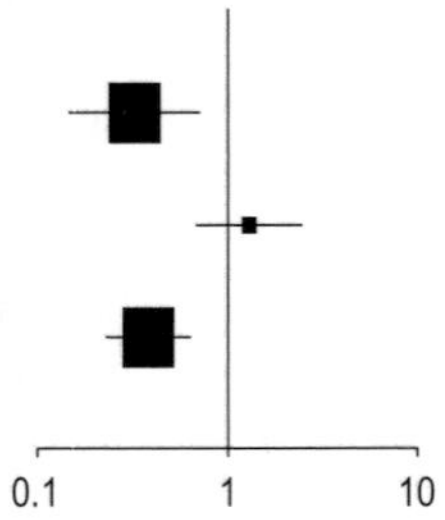

0.1   1   10

[a]Adjusted for study, age, sex and HIV risk group.

Figure 6.6 Changes in non-Hodgkin lymphoma incidence since the introduction of highly active antiretroviral therapy. RR, relative risk. (Derived from International Collaboration on HIV and Cancer.[90])

the introduction of HAART, by about 70 percent and 40 percent, respectively (Fig. 6.5; International Collaboration on HIV and Cancer[90]).

In a combined reanalysis of much of the worldwide data on this issue, the International Collaboration on HIV and Cancer[90] reported that, in relation to specific subtypes of AIDS-related lymphoma, the greatest declines were seen for cerebral lymphoma (58 percent decline), followed by immunoblastic lymphoma (43 percent decline); there was no evidence of a decline for Burkitt lymphoma (or Hodgkin lymphoma) since 1996 (Fig. 6.6). The greatest declines, therefore, have been seen for the tumors that tend to occur in people with the lowest CD4 counts.[89]

Human immunodeficiency virus–associated non-Hodgkin lymphoma in Africa

The majority of people with HIV disease live in the developing world and, in particular, in Africa. Despite this, relatively little is known about HIV-associated non-Hodgkin lymphomas occurring in Africa or other resource poor settings. Several studies have considered the risk of non-Hodgkin lymphoma in HIV-seropositive compared with HIV-seronegative individuals and in each, the relative risk in the HIV seropositives was considerably less than would be expected in the West – between about fivefold and 13-fold excess risks compared with HIV-uninfected

people.[102–105] The interpretation of this finding is complex. In those with HIV, the risk of non-Hodgkin lymphoma increases with increasing level of immunosuppression, by which time many Africans may have already died of something else, such as tuberculosis.[106,107] Also, the accurate diagnosis of a lymphoma requires relatively sophisticated technology, unavailable in many African countries, so it seems likely that some cases will be missed. However, even careful autopsy studies of HIV-infected individuals have identified fewer cases of non-Hodgkin lymphoma than have been found in similar studies in the West[78,108] and there have been only small increases in the incidence of non-Hodgkin lymphoma identified in cancer registry data from countries with a high prevalence of HIV, which contrasts with the explosion in the incidence of Kaposi's sarcoma.[109–113] Furthermore, HIV-infected people in the USA, who were born in Africa or the Caribbean, are at a lower risk of non-Hodgkin lymphoma than other HIV transmission groups.[75] This suggests that HIV-infected black Africans may indeed be at a lower risk of developing non-Hodgkin lymphoma than HIV-infected people in the West. These differences in the risk of non-Hodgkin lymphoma by race are not great, but may point to the importance of genetic factors, or more likely, environmental factors in the etiology of the disease.

Little is known about the histologic subtypes of lymphoma that occur in HIV-infected people from African or other developing countries. As in the West, the predominant type would appear to be immunoblastic tumors and cerebral lymphomas have been identified at autopsy.[108] Interestingly, however, the evidence concerning classical Burkitt lymphoma, which is endemic in parts of sub-Saharan Africa, in relation to HIV infection is mixed, although data are sparse.[105,108,114–118] Some studies have found associations between HIV infection and Burkitt lymphoma among adults,[117] whilst others have not.[118] Similarly, for children, the endemic form of Burkitt lymphoma was associated with HIV in one study,[105] but not in others.[114,115] Furthermore, in parts of Africa with a high prevalence of HIV infection, there is little evidence of an increase in the incidence of Burkitt lymphoma in those age groups most affected by HIV.[109–112]

Hematologic cancers and human immunodeficiency virus infection among children

Relative to adults, there are few published data from analytic studies on the risk of non-Hodgkin lymphoma and other cancers in HIV-infected children, primarily because both cancer and HIV infection are less common in children than in adults. It is notable that the spectrum of cancers affecting children in the general population is different from that in adults. Furthermore, unlike adults, the great majority of HIV-infected children acquire the virus in the first months of life, while the immune system is developing and prior to exposure to many other immunologic challenges.

A study from the USA showed that, subsequent to a diagnosis of AIDS, children were at an increased risk of non-Hodgkin lymphoma (based on 42 cases; including 'sporadic' Burkitt lymphoma, immunoblastic lymphoma and primary lymphoma of the brain), Kaposi sarcoma (based on four cases) and leiomyosarcoma (based on three cases).[119] Each of these cancers has been linked to infection with specific human herpesviruses.[116] Several other cohort studies from the USA and Europe have information on cancer incidence in HIV-infected children, but these data have not yet been published. However, even in combination, the numbers of cases of certain cancer sites or types is likely to be small.

Despite the fact that HIV infection is more prevalent in parts of sub-Saharan Africa than elsewhere, there is only one published study from Africa that investigated the scale of the excess risk of cancer in HIV-infected as compared with uninfected children (and none from elsewhere in the developing world).[105] The results from a small case–control study of childhood cancer in Uganda showed that HIV infection increased the risk both of Kaposi sarcoma and of the African endemic form of Burkitt lymphoma. Case series of HIV-infected children in Africa with cancer have suggested associations with non-Burkitt, non-Hodgkin lymphoma, but the risk has not been adequately quantified.[115]

Human immunodeficiency virus 2 and non–Hodgkin lymphoma

Reports on the impact of HIV-2 on the risk of non-Hodgkin lymphoma and other cancers are few, in part because of the limited geographic distribution of infection (predominantly in west Africa). In general for a given level of immunosuppression, those with HIV-2 appear to develop the same spectrum of diseases as those with HIV-1, including Kaposi sarcoma and non-Hodgkin lymphoma.[106,120–122] However, no formal observational studies of AIDS-related cancers among HIV-2 infected people have yet been published.

Hodgkin disease and HIV infection

There is some evidence that immunosuppressed transplant recipients are at a higher risk of Hodgkin lymphoma than the general population, but the relative risks are much smaller than for non-Hodgkin lymphoma.[69] Since the mid-1980s, there have also been a large number of case reports and case series of Hodgkin lymphoma occurring in HIV-seropositive individuals.[9] In this context, the disease is clinically unusual, generally presenting at a late stage, often with extranodal dissemination. The predominant histologic subtypes are mixed cellularity and lymphocyte depleted, which are relatively rare in the HIV-uninfected population. But, until recently, there was little evidence as to whether HIV infection actually increased the risk of Hodgkin lymphoma, although it clearly affected the way in which the tumor was manifest.

Several recent reports have identified excesses of Hodgkin disease in association with HIV infection, in cohort studies, or through linkage of AIDS and cancer registries.[123–131] The excess risk in HIV-infected individuals, compared with the uninfected, is usually between fivefold and 10-fold – much less than for non-Hodgkin lymphoma. This probably explains why excesses have not been consistently identified. In case–control studies from Africa (Rwanda, South Africa and Uganda, respectively) no excess risk of Hodgkin lymphoma has yet been identified in HIV-infected individuals, although the number of cases is relatively small.[102–105]

Little is known about risk factors for the etiology of Hodgkin lymphoma in HIV-infected individuals, but EBV DNA has been identified in tumor tissue from AIDS patients in some studies.[71,132,133] Although results are not completely consistent, this is also true of Hodgkin lymphoma in the HIV-uninfected population, in whom high antibody titers to EBV prior to disease onset have been found to be predictive of the subsequent development of the tumor.[134]

Other human immunodeficiency virus-associated malignancies

Although many cancers have been reported to be increased in people with HIV infection, for only a few is the evidence sufficiently strong and consistent that it is possible to conclude there is a definite increase in risk. It is well recognized that infection with HIV is causally associated with Kaposi sarcoma and non-Hodgkin lymphoma and, in light of data emerging from sub-Saharan Africa, with squamous cell carcinoma of the conjunctiva.[9,116,135–138] Recent evidence for some other cancers – anal cancer, cancer of the cervix, Hodgkin lymphoma and leiomyosarcoma in children – also suggests a definite increase in risk associated with HIV infection.[9,135]

The relative risks for HIV-seropositive compared with HIV-seronegative people for the cancers listed above tend to be very large – generally 10-fold or greater. There may be other cancers whose incidence is increased with HIV infection but, if so, they are probably rare, or the associated relative risks are not likely to be large. Increases in oral, testicular, skin, brain, lung, breast, thyroid and plasma cell cancers have been suggested,[9] but have yet to be confirmed.

Prevention of human immunodeficiency virus–associated lymphoma

Two issues must be addressed in relation to the control and prevention of HIV-associated cancers: first, adequate control of HIV infection itself and, second, control of the infections such as EBV and HHV-8 that are known to cause some HIV-associated cancers. Control and prevention of the relevant underlying causal viruses of several of the cancers described here is beyond the scope of this chapter, but preventive vaccines do not yet exist for these infections. Control of the impact of HIV infection can also be divided into two areas. The first involves limiting the onset of immunosuppression in infected individuals (with antiretroviral drugs) and has been discussed above. The second involves limiting the transmission of HIV itself.

In the absence of an effective vaccine, behavioral change is still the most important method of controlling the spread of HIV. Transmission of the virus in blood and blood products has been largely halted in developed countries, with the introduction of screening and education in combination with needle exchange programmes, which have been shown to be effective in reducing the spread of HIV among intravenous drug users. The bulk of transmission of HIV is sexual, however, and preventive activities include: reducing the number of sexual partners, modifying the types of sexual contact, and use of condoms. Several behavioral interventions in high-risk populations have been tried, with variable results, but continued education remains a high priority.

Recent interest has focused on other areas that may be important in reducing sexual transmission of HIV. There is some evidence suggesting that effective syndromic treatment of other STIs can reduce the transmission rate of HIV. There is also considerable interest in developing vaginal virucides to protect against HIV, particularly as they can be used unobtrusively by women, in situations where condom use is unacceptable. In addition, clinical trials of male circumcision to reduce infection are ongoing.

Perinatal transmission of HIV is the most common route of infection among children and is the source of almost all pediatric AIDS cases; almost 2.5 million children are currently living with HIV. In the absence of medical intervention around 25–30 percent of children born to infected mothers will themselves be infected with HIV. The use of antiretroviral therapies in pregnancy, labor and delivery and then to the newborn, together with elective cesarean section for women with high viral loads, can reduce transmission to less that 2 percent. Postnatal transmission of HIV from an infected mother to her child can occur through breastfeeding[139,140] and avoidance of breastfeeding by HIV-infected women is recommended if safe and affordable alternatives can be used.[141,142] However, throughout much of the developing world, such alternatives are not available. A key component in the success of any protocol to reduce mother-to-child transmission of HIV is that the mother must know her HIV status prior to delivery of the child. For this reason, voluntary testing of pregnant women is now actively encouraged in many countries. If properly applied, such approaches can almost eliminate mother-to-child transmission of HIV infection.

KEY POINTS

- Human T cell leukemia virus is the cause of adult T cell leukemia/lymphoma and several other conditions.
- HTLV-1 is most prevalent in parts of Japan, the Caribbean, South America, central America, Papua New Guinea and the Solomon Islands; elsewhere, it is rare except in certain high risk groups such as intravenous drug users.
- Three modes of transmission of HTLV-1 have been identified: from mother to child (via breast milk), via sex and by transfusion of infected cellular blood.
- In many parts of the world, prevalence of HTLV-1 is declining following changes to breast feeding behavior.
- HIV-1 and HIV-2 increase the risk of non-Hodgkin lymphoma (and many other conditions).
- HIV is one of the most significant global killers.
- Latest prevalence estimates for HIV are available at www.UNAIDS.com.
- Transmission is from mother to child, via sex and in infected blood products.
- The incidence of NHL has declined among people with HIV secondary to the widespread use of antiretroviral drugs.
- No vaccines are yet available for HTLV-1 or HIV.

REFERENCES

● = Key primary paper
◆ = Major review article

●1. Poiesz BJ, Ruscetti FW, Gazdar AF *et al.* Detection and isolation of type C retrovirus particles from fresh and cultured lymphocytes of a patient with cutaneous T-cell lymphoma. *Proc Natl Acad Sci U S A* 1980; **77**: 6134–8.

2. Parkin DM. The global health burden of infection-associated cancers in the year 2002. *Int J Cancer* 2006; 118: 3030–44.

3. Newton R, Hjalgrim H, Law G, Roman E. A review of the epidemiology of non-Hodgkin's lymphoma. In: Cunningham D, Morgan G, Miles A (eds) *Key advances in the effective management of non-Hodgkin's lymphoma.* London: Aesculapius Medical Press, 2004, 3–23.

4. de Parseval N, Heidmann T. Human endogenous retroviruses: from infectious elements to human genes. *Cytogenet Genome Res* 2005; **110**: 318–32.

●5. Uchiyama T, Yodoi J, Sagawa K *et al.* Adult T-cell leukemia: clinical and features of 16 cases. *Blood* 1977; **50**: 481–92.

6. Shimoyama M, Members of the Lymphoma Study Group. Diagnostic criteria and classification of clinical subtypes of adult T-cell leukaemia lymphoma. *Br J Haematol* 1991; **79**: 428–37.

◆7. Proietti FA, Carneiro-Proietti ABF, Catalan-Soares BC, Murphy EL. Global epidemiology of HTLV-1 infection and associated diseases. *Oncogene* 2005; **24**: 6058–68.

8. de Thé G, Kazanji M. An HTLV-I/II vaccine: from animal models to clinical trials. *J Acq Immun Def Synd Hum Retrovirol* 1996; **13**(Suppl 1): s191–8.

◆9. IARC monograph on the evaluation of carcinogenic risks to humans, Volume 67. Human immunodeficiency viruses and human T-cell lymphotropic viruses. France: Lyon, IARC, 1996, 4–140.

10. Yamaguchi K. Human T-lymphotropic virus type 1 in Japan. *Lancet* 1994; **343**: 213–16.

11. Mueller N, Okayama A, Stuver S, Tachibana N. Findings from the Miyazaki Cohort Study. *J Acq Immun Def Synd Hum Retrovirol* 1996; **13**(Suppl 1): s2–7.

12. Tajima K, Takezaki T. Human T-cell leukaemia virus type 1. In: Newton R, Beral V, Weiss R (eds) *Cancer surveys volume 33, infections and human cancer.* Cold Spring Harbor Laboratory Press, 1999, 191–211.

13. Kajiyama W, Kashiwaga S, Ikematsu H *et al.* Intrafamilial transmission on adult T-cell leukaemia virus. *J Infect Dis* 1986; **154**: 851–7.

14. Murphy EL, Figueroa JP, Gibbs WN *et al.* Human T-lymphotropic virus type 1 (HTLV-1) seroprevalence in Jamaica. I. Demographic determinants. *Am J Epidemiol* 1991; **133**: 1114–24.

15. Mueller N. The epidemiology of HTLV-1 infection. *Cancer Causes Control* 1991; **2**: 37–52.

16. Chavance M, Frery N, Valette I *et al.* Sex ratio of human T-lymphotropic virus type 1 infection and blood transfusion. *Am J Epidemiol* 1990; **131**: 395–9.

17. Nakashima K, Kashiwagi S, Kajiyama W *et al.* Sexual transmission of human T-lymphotropic virus type 1 among female prostitutes and among patients with sexually transmitted diseases in Fukuoka, Kyushu, Japan. *Am J Epidemiol* 1995; **141**: 305–11.

18. Tajima K, Hinuma Y. Epidemiology of HTLV-I/II in Japan and the world. *Gann Monograph on Cancer Research* 1992; **39**: 129–49.

19. Tajima K, Tominaga S, Suchi T *et al.* Epidemiological analysis of the distribution of antibody to adult T-cell leukaemia virus-associated antigen: possible horizontal transmission of adult T-cell leukaemia virus. *Jpn J Cancer Res* 1982; **73**: 893–901.

20. Kinoshita K, Hino S, Amagaski T *et al.* Demonstration of adult T-cell leukaemia virus antigen in milk from three seropositive mothers. *Jpn J Cancer Res* 1984; **75**: 103–5.

21. Fujino T, Nagata Y. HTLV-1 transmission from mother to child. *J Reprod Immunol* 2000; **47**: 197–206.

22. Ureta-Vidal A, Angelin-Duclos C, Tortevoye P *et al.* Mother-to-child transmission of human T-cell leukaemia/lymphoma virus type 1: implication of high antiviral antibody titer and high proviral load in carrier mothers. *Int J Cancer* 1999; **82**: 832–6.

23. Takahashi K, Takezaki T, Oki T *et al.* Inhibitory effect of maternal antibody on mother-to-child transmission of human T-lymphotropic virus type 1. *Int J Cancer* 1991; **49**: 673–7.

24. Oki T, Yoshinaga M, Otsuka H *et al.* A sero-epidemiological study on mother-to-child transmission of HTLV-1 in southern Kyushu, Japan. *Asia Oceania J Obstet Gynaecol* 1992; **18**: 371–7.

25. Belza MJ. For the Spanish group for the unlinked anonymous survey of HIV seroprevalence in STD patients. Prevalence of HIV, HTLV-1 and HTLV-2 among female sex workers in Spain, 2000–2001. *Eur J Epidemiol* 2004; **19**: 279–82.

26. Nakano S, Ando Y, Ichijo M *et al.* Search for possible routes of vertical and horizontal transmission of adult T-cell leukaemia virus. *Jpn J Cancer Res* 1984; **75**: 1044–5.

27. Taylor GP. The epidemiology of HTLV-1 in Europe. *J Acquir Immune Defic Syndr Hum Retrovirol* 1996; **13**(Suppl 1): s8–14.

28. Okochi K, Sato H, Hinuma Y. A retrospective study on transmission of adult T-cell leukaemia virus by blood transfusion: seroconversion in recipients. *Vox Sang* 1984; **46**: 245–53.

29. Feigal E, Murphy E, Vranizan K *et al.* Human T-cell lymphotropic virus types 1 and 2 in intravenous drug users in San Francisco: risk factors associated with seropositivity. *J Infect Dis* 1991; **164**: 36–42.

30. Etzel A, Shibata GY, Rozman M *et al.* HTLV-1 and HTLV-2 infections in HIV-infected individuals from Santos,

Brazil: seroprevalence and risk factors. *J Acquir Immune Defic Syndr Hum Retrovirol* 2001; **26**: 185–90.

31. Ehrlich GD, Poiesz BJ. Clinical and molecular parameters of HTLV-1 infection. *Clin Lab Med* 1988; **8**: 65–84.

32. Catovsky D, Greaves MF, Rose M *et al.* Adult T-cell lymphoma-leukaemia in blacks from the West Indies. *Lancet* 1982; **1**: 639–43.

33. Blattner WA, Saxinger C, Riedel D *et al.* A study of HTLV-1 and its associated risk factors in Trinidad and Tobago. *J Acquir Immune Defic Syndr* 1990; **3**: 1102–8.

34. Gallo RC. Human retroviruses after 20 years: a perspective from the past and prospects for their future control. *Immunol Rev* 2002; **185**: 236–65.

35. Murphy EL, Hanchard B, Figueroa JP *et al.* Modelling the risk of adult T-cell leukaemia/lymphoma in persons infected with human T-lymphotropic virus type 1. *Int J Cancer* 1989; **43**: 250–3.

36. Hisada M, Okayama A, Shioiri S *et al.* Risk factors for adult T-cell leukaemia among carriers of human T-lymphotropic virus type 1. *Blood* 1998; **92**: 2557–61.

37. Cruickshank EK. A neuropathic syndrome of uncertain origin; review of 100 cases. *West Indian Med J* 1956; **5**: 147–58.

38. Rodgers PE. The clinical features and aetiology of the neuropathic syndrome in Jamaica. *West Indian Med J* 1965; **14**: 36–47.

39. Gessain A, Barin F, Vernant JC *et al.* Antibodies to human T-lymphotropic virus type 1 in patients with tropical spastic paraparesis. *Lancet* 1985; **ii**: 407–10.

40. Kawai H, Nishida Y, Takagi M *et al.* HTLV-1 associated myelopathy (HAM) with adult T-cell leukaemia (ATL). *Rinsho Shinkeigaku* 1989; **29**: 588–92.

41. Kasahata N, Kawamura M, Shiota J *et al.* A case of acute type adult T-cell leukaemia and human T-lymphotropic virus type 1 associated myelopathy who presented meningitis and polyradiculoneuropathy and improved with steroid treatment. *No To Shinkei* 2000; **52**: 1003–6.

42. World Health Organization. Diagnostic guidelines of HAM/TSP. Virus diseases. Human lymphotropic virus type 1, HTLV-1. *Wkly Epidemiol Rec* 1989; **49**: 382–3.

43. Jacobson S, Shida H, McFarlin DE *et al.* Circulating CD8+ cytotoxic T lymphocytes specific for HTLV-1 pX in patients with HTLV-1 associated neurological disease. *Nature* 1990; **348**: 245–8.

44. Orland JR, Engstrom J, Fridey J *et al.* Prevalence and clinical features of HTLV neurologic disease in the HTLV outcomes study. *Neurology* 2003; **61**: 1588–94.

45. Kramer A, Maloney EM, Morgan OS *et al.* Risk factors and cofactors for human T-cell lymphotropic virus type 1 (HTLV-1) associated myelopathy/tropical spastic paraparesis (HAM/TSP) in Jamaica. *Am J Epidemiol* 1995; **142**: 1212–20.

46. Maloney EM, Cleghorn FR, Morgan OS *et al.* Incidence of HTLV-1 associated myelopathy/tropical spastic paraparesis (HAM/TSP) in Jamaica and Trinidad. *J Acquir Immune Defic Syndr Hum Retrovirol* 1998; **17**: 167–70.

47. Osame M, Izumo S, Igata A *et al.* Blood transfusion and HTLV-1 associated myelopathy. *Lancet* 1986; **2**: 104–5.

48. Mochizuki M, Tajima K, Watanabe T, Yamaguchi K. Human T lymphotropic virus type 1 uveitis. *Br J Ophthalmol* 1994; **78**: 149–54.

●49. Barré-Sinoussi F, Chermann JC, Rey F *et al.* Isolation of a T-lymphotropic retrovirus from a patient at risk for acquired immunodeficiency syndrome (AIDS). *Science* 1983; **220**: 868–71.

●50. Gallo RC, Salahuddin SZ, Popovic M *et al.* Frequent detection and isolation of cytopathic retrovirus (HTLV-III) from patients with AIDS and at risk for AIDS. *Science* 1984; **224**: 500–3.

51. Darby SC, Ewart DW, Giangrande PL *et al.* Importance of age at infection and HIV-1 for survival and development of AIDS in UK haemophilia population. UK Haemophilia Centre Director's Organization. *Lancet* 1996; **347**: 1573–9.

52. Morgan D, Mahe C, Mayanja B, Whitworth JA. Progression to symptomatic disease in people infected with HIV-1 in rural Uganda: prospective cohort study. *BMJ* 2002; **324**: 193–6.

53. Sharp PM, Bailes E, Chaudhuri RR *et al.* The origins of AIDS viruses: where and when? *Philos Trans R Soc Lond B Biol Sci* 2001; **356**: 867–76.

54. Santiago ML, Range F, Keele BF *et al.* Simian immunodeficiency virus infection in free-ranging sooty mangabeys (*Cercocebus atys atys*) from the Tai Forest, Cote d'Ivoire: implications for the origin of epidemic human immunodeficiency virus type 2. *J Virol* 2005; **79**: 1215–27.

55. Bailes E, Gao F, Bibollet-Ruche F *et al.* Hybrid origin of SIV in chimpanzees. *Science* 2003; **300**: 1713.

56. Keele BF, Van Heuverswyn F, Li Y *et al.* Chimpanzee reservoirs of pandemic and nonpandemic HIV-1. *Science* 2006; **313**: 523–6.

57. Donegan E, Stuart M, Niland JC *et al.* Infection with human immunodeficiency virus type 1 (HIV-1) among recipients of antibody-positive blood donations. *Ann Intern Med* 1990; **113**: 733–9.

58. European Study Group. Heterosexual transmission of HIV. Comparison of female to male and male to female transmission of HIV in 563 stable couples. *BMJ* 1992; **304**: 809–13.

59. Kaplan EH, Heimer R. HIV incidence among New Haven needle exchange participants: updated estimates from syringe tracking and testing data. *J Aquir Immune Defic Syndr Hum Retrovirol* 1995; **10**: 175–6.

60. Leynaert B, Downs AM, de Vincenzi I. Heterosexual transmission of human immunodeficiency virus: variability of infectivity throughout the course of infection. European Study Group on heterosexual transmission of HIV. *Am J Epidemiol* 1998; **148**: 88–96.

61. Bell DM. Occupational risk of human immunodeficiency virus infection in healthcare workers: an overview. *Am J Med* 1997; **102**: 9–15.

62. Varghese B, Maher JE, Peterman TA *et al.* Reducing the risk of sexual HIV transmission: quantifying the per-act risk for HIV on the basis of choice of partner, sex act and condom use. *Sex Transm Dis* 2002; **29**: 38–43.

63. Coovadia H. Antiretroviral agents – how best to protect infants from HIV and save their mothers from AIDS. *N Engl J Med* 2004; **351**: 289–92.

64. Smith DK, Grohskopf LA, Black RJ *et al.* Antiretroviral post-exposure prophylaxis after sexual, injection drug use or other non-occupational exposure to HIV in the United States. *MMWR* 2005; **54**: 1–20.

65. Burnet M. Somatic mutation and chronic disease. *Br Med J* 1965; **i**: 338–42.

66. Mueller BU, Pizzo PA. Cancer in children with primary or secondary immuno-deficiencies. *J Pediatr* 1995; **126**: 1–10.

67. Filipovich AH, Mathur A, Kamat D *et al.* Lymphoproliferative disorders and other tumours complicating immunodeficiencies. *Immunodeficiency* 1994; **5**: 91–112.

68. Kinlen LJ, Sheil AGR, Peto J, Doll R. Collaborative United Kingdom-Australasian study of cancer in patients treated with immunosuppressive drugs. *Br Med J* 1979; **ii**: 1461–6.

69. Birkeland SA, Storm HH, Lamm LU *et al.* Cancer risk after renal transplantation in the Nordic countries, 1964–1986. *Int J Cancer* 1995; **60**: 183–9.

70. Thomas JA, Crawford DH. EBV associated B-cell lymphoma in AIDS and after organ transplantation. *Lancet* 1989; **1**: 1075–6.

71. IARC monograph on the evaluation of carcinogenic risks to humans, volume 70. Epstein Barr virus and Kaposi's sarcoma virus/human herpesvirus 8. France: Lyon, IARC, 1997.

72. Starzl TE, Nalesnik MA, Porter KA *et al.* Reversibility of lymphomas and lymphoproliferative lesions developing under cyclosporin-steroid therapy. *Lancet* 1984; **i**: 583–7.

73. Ziegler JL, Beckstead JA, Volberding PA *et al.* Non-Hodgkin's lymphoma in 90 homosexual men. Relation to generalized lymphadenopathy and the acquired immunodeficiency syndrome. *N Engl J Med* 1984; **311**: 565–70.

74. Centers for Disease Control and Prevention. Revision of the case definition of acquired immunodeficiency syndrome for national reporting – United States. *MMWR* 1985; **34**: 373–5.

75. Beral V, Peterman TA, Berkelman R, Jaffe H. AIDS-associated non-Hodgkin lymphoma. *Lancet* 1991; **337**: 805–9.

76. Serraino D, Salamina G, Franceschi S *et al.* The epidemiology of non-Hodgkin's lymphoma in the World Health Organization European Region. *Br J Cancer* 1992; **66**: 912–16.

77. Lyter D, Besley D, Thackeray R *et al.* Incidence of malignancies in the Multicenter AIDS Cohort Study (MACS). *Proc ASCO* 1994; **13**: 50(A2).

78. Wilkes MS, Felix JC, Fortwin AH *et al.* Value of necropsy in acquired immunodeficiency syndrome. *Lancet* 1988; **ii**: 85–8.

79. Kinlen LJ. Immunologic factors, including AIDS. In: Schottenfeld D, Fraumeni JF (eds) *Cancer epidemiology and prevention*, 2nd ed. New York: Oxford University Press, 1996: 532–45.

80. Pluda JM, Venzon DJ, Tosato G *et al.* Parameters affecting the development of non-Hodgkin's lymphoma in patients with severe human immunodeficiency virus infection receiving anti-retroviral therapy. *Am J Clin Oncol* 1993; **11**: 1099–107.

81. Jaffe ES, Harris NL, Stein H, Vardinan JW (eds) *World Health Organization classification of tumours. Pathology and genetics of tumours of haematopoietic and lymphoid tissues.* France: Lyon, IARC Press, 2001: 260–3.

82. Ambinder RF. Epstein-Barr virus associated lymphoproliferations in the AIDS setting. *Eur J Cancer* 2001; **10**: 1209–16.

83. Hamilton-Dutoit SJ, Rea D, Raphael M *et al.* Epstein-Barr virus-latent gene expression and tumour cell phenotype in acquired immunodeficiency syndrome-related non-Hodgkin's lymphoma. Correlation of lymphoma phenotype with three distinct patterns of viral latency. *Am J Pathol* 1993; **143**: 1072–85.

84. Carbone A, Tirelli U, Gloghini A *et al.* Human immunodeficiency virus-associated systemic lymphomas may be subdivided into two main groups according to Epstein-Barr viral latent gene expression. *J Clin Oncol* 1993; **11**: 1674–81.

85. Carbone A, Gaidano G, Gloghini A *et al.* BCL-6 protein expression in AIDS-related non-Hodgkin's lymphomas: inverse relationship with Epstein-Barr virus-encoded latent membrane protein-1 expression. *Am J Pathol* 1997; **150**: 155–65.

86. Carbone A, Gloghini A, Larocca LM *et al.* Expression profile of MUM1/IRF4, BCL-6 and CD138/syndecan-1 defines novel histogenetic subsets of human immunodeficiency virus-related lymphomas. *Blood* 2001; **97**: 744–51.

87. Cingolani A, De Luca A, Larocca LM *et al.* Minimally invasive diagnosis of acquired immunodeficiency syndrome-related primary central nervous system lymphoma. *J Natl Cancer Inst* 1998; **90**: 364–9.

88. Herndier BG, Kaplan LD, McGrath MS. Pathogenesis of AIDS lymphomas. *AIDS* 1994; **8**: 1025–49.

89. Jones JL, Hanson DL, Dworkin MS *et al.* Effect of antiretroviral therapy on recent trends in selected cancers among HIV-infected persons. *J Acquir Immune Defic Synd* 1999; **21**: s11–17.

90. International Collaboration on HIV and Cancer. The impact of highly active anti-retroviral therapy on the incidence of cancer in people infected with the human immunodeficiency virus. *J Natl Cancer Inst* 2000; **92**: 1823–30.

91. Muller JR, Janz S, Goedert JJ *et al.* Persistence of immunoglobulin heavy chain /c-myc recombination-positive lymphocytes clones in the blood of human immunodeficiency virus-infected homosexual men. *Proc Natl Acad Sci U S A* 1995; **92**: 6577–81.

92. Cesarman E, Chang Y, Moore PS *et al*. Kaposi's sarcoma-associated herpesvirus-like DNA sequences in AIDS-related body-cavity-based lymphomas. *N Engl J Med* 1995; **332**: 1186–91.

93. Hogg RS, Heath KV, Yip B *et al*. Improved survival among HIV-infected individuals following initiation of antiviral therapy. *JAMA* 1998; **279**: 450–4.

94. Mocroft A, Vella S, Benfield TL *et al*. Changing patterns of mortality across Europe in patients infected with HIV-1. EuroSIDA Study Group. *Lancet* 1998; **352**: 1725–30.

95. Egger M, Hirschel B, Francioli P *et al*. Impact of new antiretroviral combination therapies in HIV infected patients in Switzerland: prospective multicentre study. Swiss HIV cohort study. *BMJ* 1997; **315**: 1194–9.

96. Palella FJ Jr, Delaney KM, Moorman AC *et al*. Declining morbidity and mortality among patients with advanced human immunodeficiency virus infection. HIV outpatient study investigators. *N Engl J Med* 1998; **338**: 853–60.

97. Detels R, Munoz A, McFarlane G *et al*. Effectiveness of potent antiretroviral therapy on time to AIDS and death in men with known HIV infection duration. Multicenter AIDS cohort study investigators. *JAMA* 1998; **280**: 1497–503.

98. Franceschi S, Dal Maso L, La Vecchia C. Advances in the epidemiology of HIV-associated non-Hodgkin's lymphoma and other lymphoid neoplasms. *Int J Cancer* 1999; **83**: 481–5.

99. Mocroft A, Katlama C, Johnson AM *et al*. AIDS across Europe, 1994–98: the EuroSIDA study. *Lancet* 2000; **356**: 291–6.

100. Rabkin CS, Testa MA, Huang J, Von Roenn JH. Kaposi's sarcoma and non-Hodgkin's lymphoma incidence trends in AIDS clinical trial group study participants. *J Acquir Immune Defic Syndr* 1999; **21**(Suppl): s31–3.

101. Dore GJ, Li Y, McDonald A *et al*. National HIV Surveillance Committee. Impact of highly active antiretroviral therapy on individual AIDS-defining illness incidence and survival in Australia. *J Acquir Immune Defic Syndr* 2002; **29**: 388–95.

102. Newton R, Grulich A, Beral V *et al*. Cancer and HIV infection in Rwanda. *Lancet* 1995; **345**: 1378–9.

103. Sitas F, Bezwoda WR, Levin V *et al*. Association between human immunodeficiency virus type 1 infection and cancer in the black population of Johannesburg and Soweto, South Africa. *Br J Cancer* 1997; **75**: 1704–7.

104. Sitas F, Pacell-Norman R, Carrara H *et al*. The spectrum of HIV-1 related cancers in South Africa. *Int J Cancer* 2000; **88**: 489–92.

105. Newton R, Ziegler J, Beral V *et al*. A case-control study of human immunodeficiency virus infection and cancer in adults and children residing in Kampala, Uganda. *Int J Cancer* 2001; **92**: 622–7.

106. Grant AD, Djomand G, De Cock KM. Natural history and spectrum of disease in adults with HIV/AIDS in Africa. *AIDS* 1997; **11**(Suppl B): s43–54.

107. Morgan D, Mahe C, Mayanja B *et al*. HIV-1 infection in rural Africa: is there a difference in median time to AIDS and survival compared with that in industrialized countries? *AIDS* 2002; **16**: 597–603.

108. Lucas SB, Diomande M, Hounnou A *et al*. HIV-associated lymphoma in Africa: an autopsy study on Côte D'Ivoire. *Int J Cancer* 1994; **59**: 20–4.

109. Wabinga HR, Parkin DM, Wabwire-Mangen F, Mugerwa JW. Cancer in Kampala, Uganda, in 1989–91: changes in incidence in the era of AIDS. *Int J Cancer* 1993; **54**: 26–36.

110. Parkin DM, Wabinga H, Nambooze S, Wabwire-Mangen F. AIDS-related cancers in Africa: maturation of the epidemic in Uganda. *AIDS* 1999; **13**: 2563–70.

111. Wabinga HR, Parkin DM, Wabwire-Mangen F, Nambooze S. Trends in cancer incidence in Kyadondo County, Uganda, 1960–1997. *Br J Cancer* 2000; **82**: 1585–92.

112. Bassett MT, Chokunonga E, Mauchaza B *et al*. Cancer in the African population of Harare, Zimbabwe in 1990–92. *Int J Cancer* 1995; **63**: 29–36.

113. Dedicoat M, Sitas F, Newton R. Cancer in rural KwaZulu/Natal. *S Afr Med J* 2003; **93**: 846–7.

114. Mbidde EK, Banura C, Kazura J *et al*. Non-Hodgkin's lymphoma (NHL) and HIV infection in Uganda. 5th International Conference in Africa, on AIDS, 1990; FPB: 1.

115. Sinfield RL, Molyneux EM, Banda K *et al*. The spectrum and presentation of paediatric malignancies in the HIV era: experience from Blantyre, Malawi, 1998–2003. *Paedr Blood Cancer* 2007; **48**: 515–20.

116. Newton R, Beral V, Weiss R. Human immunodeficiency virus infection and cancer. In: Newton R, Beral V, Weiss R (eds) *Cancer surveys volume 33, infections and human cancer*. USA: Cold Spring Harbor Laboratory Press, 1999.

117. Otieno MW, Remick SC, Whalen C. Adult Burkitt's lymphoma in patients with and without human immunodeficiency virus infection in Kenya. *Int J Cancer* 2001; **92**: 687–91.

118. Lazzi S, Ferrari F, Nyongo A *et al*. HIV-associated malignant lymphomas in Kenya (Equatorial Africa). *Hum Pathol* 1998; **29**: 1285–9.

119. Biggar RJ, Frisch M, Goedert JJ. Risk of cancer in children with AIDS. AIDS-Cancer match registry study group. *JAMA* 2000; **284**: 205–9.

120. Ariyoshi K, Schim van der Loeff M, Cook P *et al*. Kaposi's sarcoma in the Gambia, West Africa is less frequent in human immunodeficiency virus type 1 infection despite a high prevalence of human herpesvirus 8. *J Hum Virol* 1998; **1**: 185–6.

121. Colebunders R, De Vuyst H, Verstraeten T *et al*. A non-Hodgkin's lymphoma in a patient with HIV-2 infection. *Genitourin Med* 1995; **71**: 129.

122. Kempf W, Margolin DH, Dezube BJ *et al*. Clinicopathological characterization of an HIV-2-infected individual with two clonally unrelated primary lymphomas. *Am J Hematol* 2000; **65**: 302–6.

123. Hessol NA, Katz MH, Liu JY *et al*. Increased incidence of Hodgkin's disease in homosexual men with HIV infection. *Ann Intern Med* 1992; **117**: 309–11.

124. Reynolds P, Saunders LD, Layefsky ME, Lemp GF. The spectrum of acquired immunodeficiency syndrome (AIDS)-associated malignancies in San Francisco, 1980–1987. *Am J Epidemiol* 1993; **137**: 19–30.

125. Grulich A, Wan X, Law M *et al.* Rates of non-AIDS defining cancers in people with AIDS. *J Aquir Immune Defic Syndr Hum Retrovirol* 1997; **14**: a18.

126. Grulich AE, Wan X, Law MG *et al.* Risk of cancer in people with AIDS. *AIDS* 1999; **13**: 839–43.

127. Weiss SH, Karcnik T, Patel S *et al.* The ten-year cancer and HIV experience of the UMDNJ-University Hospital (UH) cancer registry: excess proportions of Hodgkin's lymphoma and lung cancer. *J Aquir Immune Defic Syndr Hum Retrovirol* 1997; **18**: a9.

128. Lyter DW, Bryant J, Thackeray R *et al.* Non-AIDS defining malignancies in the multicenter AIDS cohort study (MACS), 1984–1996. *J Acquir Immune Defic Syndr Hum Retrovirol* 1998; **17**.

129. Cooksley CD, Hwang L-Y, Waller DK, Ford CE. HIV-related malignancies: a community based study using a linkage of cancer registry and HIV registry data. *J Aquir Immune Defic Syndr Hum Retrovirol* 1998; **14**: a11.

130. Goedert JJ, Coté TR, Virgo P *et al.* Spectrum of AIDS-associated malignant disorders. *Lancet* 1998; **351**: 1833–9.

131. Franceschi S, Dal Maso L, Arniani S *et al.* Risk of cancer other than Kaposi's sacroma and non-Hodgkin's lymphoma in persons with AIDS in Italy. Cancer and AIDS registry linkage study. *Br J Cancer* 1998; **78**: 966–70.

132. Moran CA, Tuur S, Angritt P *et al.* Epstein-Barr virus in Hodgkin's disease from patients with human immunodeficiency virus infection. *Mod Pathol* 1992; **5**: 85–8.

133. Tirelli U, Errante D, Dolcetti R *et al.* Hodgkin's disease and human immunodeficiency virus infection: clinicopathologic and virologic features of 114 patients from the Italian cooperative group on AIDS and tumors. *J Clin Oncol* 1995; **13**: 1758–67.

134. Mueller N, Evans A, Harris NL *et al.* Hodgkin's disease and Epstein-Barr virus: altered antibody pattern before diagnosis. *N Engl J Med* 1989; **320**: 689–95.

135. Beral V, Newton R. Overview of the epidemiology of immunodeficiency associated cancers. *Natl Cancer Inst Monogr* 1998, **23**: 1–6.

136. Newton R. A review of the aetiology of squamous cell carcinoma of the conjunctiva. *Br J Cancer* 1996; **74**: 1511–13.

137. Waddell K, Downing R, Lucas S, Newton R. Corneo-conjunctival carcinoma associated with human immunodeficiency virus type-1 (HIV-1) in Uganda. *Eye* 2006; **20**: 893–9.

138. Waddell KM, Newton R. The aetiology and associations of conjunctival intraepithelial neoplasia – further evidence. *Br J Ophthalmol* 2007; **91**: 120–1.

139. Dunn DT, Newell ML, Ades AE, Peckham CS. Risk of human immunodeficiency virus type 1 transmission though breastfeeding. *Lancet* 1992; **340**: 585–8.

140. Miotti PG, Taha TET, Kumwenda MI *et al.* HIV transmission though breast-feeding: a study in Malawi. *JAMA* 1999; **282**: 744–9.

141. World Health Organization. *HIV and infant feeding guidelines for decision makers.* Geneva: World Health Organization, WHO/FRH/NUT/CHD 98.1.

142. World Health Organization. *The optimal duration of exclusive breast feeding: report of an expert consultation.* Switzerland: Geneva, 28–30 March 2001. Document ref WHO/NHD/01.09 Geneva: WHO, 2002.

7

Herpesviruses and lymphoma

RICHARD F AMBINDER

INTRODUCTION

Two herpesviruses (HHV) are associated with lymphoma and lymphoproliferative disease in man: Epstein–Barr virus (EBV) and Kaposi sarcoma-associated herpesvirus (KSHV, also referred to as HHV-8).[1] Both were first identified in tumors, both establish latency in B cell reservoirs that are maintained for life, and both are present in saliva.[2,3] Primary infection is commonly asymptomatic and most hosts do not develop tumors.[4] Immunocompromise appears to be important for the pathogenesis of some but not all of the virus-associated tumors. These similarities notwithstanding, the viruses and their associated lymphoproliferative diseases are quite different: EBV is ubiquitous whereas KSHV shows striking variation in its prevalence among populations; and EBV is associated with many different lymphomas and lymphoproliferative diseases whereas KSHV is associated with only a few. This chapter begins with an overview of the viruses and their associations with malignancies and then focuses on consideration of their associations with lymphoma.

Serologic evidence of EBV infection is consistently reported in greater than 90 percent of adults in every adult population that has been studied.[5] In contrast with ubiquitous EBV infection, serologic surveys show that KSHV is most prevalent in sub-Saharan Africa and certain populations in the Mediterranean. KSHV is rare in most other populations.[6–8] In areas of Africa, seropositivity is greater than 60 percent, in Italy and the Mediterranean area (10–15 percent); in northern Europe, Asia and the USA the seropositivity rates in the general population range from just 1 percent to 3 percent. Both viruses are detected in saliva.[9] In infancy premastication of food by mothers and use of shared eating utensils is likely to explain early EBV infection, whereas kissing and perhaps other sexual activities are associated with EBV transmission in adolescence and adulthood;[3] KSHV is also transmitted within families during childhood presumably by a salivary route. In men who have sex with men particular sexual behaviors (e.g. receptive anal intercourse, oral genital contact, oral anal contact) and numbers of sexual partners have been identified as risk factors.[10–14]

Primary infection with either virus may be asymptomatic or associated with febrile illness. The syndrome of infectious mononucleosis characterized by fever, pharyngitis, fatigue lymphadenopathy, splenomegaly and lymphocytosis often accompanies EBV seroconversion especially in adolescence or adulthood.[15] Symptoms generally resolve over days to weeks although fatigue may last for months. Primary infection with KSHV may also be accompanied by rash, and in at least some situations, lymphadenopathy and splenomegaly.[16–18]

EPSTEIN–BARR VIRUS BIOLOGY

Following EBV infection of resting B lymphocytes, the linear genome circularizes and viral gene expression leads to immortalization.[19–21] The resultant EBV 'lymphoblastoid' cell lines harbor episomes (typically 5–50 copies) and express at least 10 viral genes. Six viral proteins are required for transformation (Table 7.1).[22] Epstein–Bar nuclear antigen 1 (EBNA1) activates the viral latency replication and tethers viral episomes to chromosomes.[23] It is essential for

Table 7.1 Epstein–Barr virus genes

Gene	Function	Latent state	Lytic state
EBNA1	Binds to viral origin of latency replication, tethers viral episome to chromatin, transcriptional transactivator, required for immortalization	Yes	Yes
EBNA2	Mimics activated NOTCH (interacts with a cellular transcriptional repressor to activate transcription of target viral and cellular genes), required for immortalization	Yes	No
EBNA3A	Modulates NOTCH pathway, required for immortalization	Yes	No
EBNA3B	Modulates NOTCH pathway, required for immortalization	Yes	No
EBNA3C	Modulates NOTCH pathway, required for immortalization	Yes	No
LMP1	Constitutively active TNF receptor family molecule, activates nuclear factor κB and other signaling pathways, required for immortalization	Yes	Yes
LMP2	Interacts with signaling tyrosine kinases to mimic immunoglobulin signaling	Yes	No

latency in any host cell that is dividing. EBNA2 is a transcriptional transactivator that mimics activated NOTCH.[24] The viral protein activates viral latency promoters and cellular NOTCH pathway genes turning on cellular genes not normally expressed at this stage in B cell development. EBNA3 family members (EBNA3A, 3B, 3C) modulate this same signaling pathway. Latency membrane protein 1 (LMP1) is required for immortalization and resembles a constitutively activated CD40 molecule.[25,26] Its expression leads to activation of nuclear factor κB (NF-κB) and signaling through JNK/MAPK, p38/MAPK and STAT pathways; LMP-1 is associated with transformation in model systems.

Several viral transcripts are expressed in immortalized lymphocytes that are not required for immortalization. LMP-2A, an intrinsic membrane protein that includes an immunoreceptor tyrosine based activation motif (ITAM), is expressed.[27] This protein provides a tonic signal that mimics the signal associated with Ig receptor engagement.[28] This signal allows the survival of cells of B lineage that lack Ig expression (in a transgenic murine models and in human lymphocytes *in vitro*).[27,29,30] Two polymerase III transcripts, EBER1 and EBER2 do not code for protein but are abundant in latently infected cells. Their functions are unknown but a role in the modulation of pathways important in interferon response has been suggested.[31,32] Their abundant expression has made them practical tools for research and the clinical detection of virus in tumor by *in situ* hybridization (Fig. 7.1). Transcripts from the BamHI-A region of the genome encode open reading frames that are predicted to code for proteins but that have not been unambiguously demonstrated in natural infection or in tumors.[33–35] Micro-RNAs have also been identified in this region.[35]

Although immortalized lymphocytes have served as a valuable system for investigation of viral gene expression and its regulation, the patterns of viral gene regulation *in vivo* are more complex, and different patterns of viral gene expression are recognized in infected lymphocytes *in vivo* and in tumor tissue. These are illustrated in Figure 7.2. Latently infected B cells *in vivo* show very limited expression

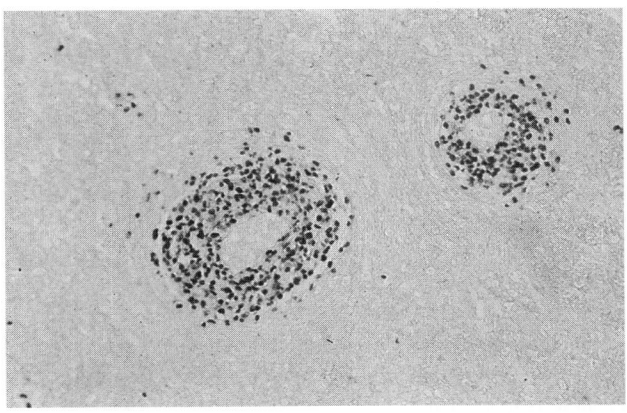

Figure 7.1 *In situ* hybridization showing EBER expression in primary central nervous system lymphoma arising in a patient with acquired immune deficiency syndrome. patient. The malignant B cells surround a blood vessel in brain.

of viral genes and are resting rather than cycling.[36–39] Reverse-transcriptase polymerase chain reaction (PCR) detects EBER RNA in blood mononuclear cells, and sometimes LMP2A and EBNA1 transcripts. However, analysis of cells at limiting dilution raises questions as to whether viral genes other than the EBERs are expressed in most infected cells. B cells that harbor virus generally carry hypermutated immunoglobulin genes.[21,39] The genesis of these virus-infected B cells expressing few viral genes is poorly understood. Some have suggested that a germinal center or germinal center-like reaction in which viral membrane proteins LMP1 and LMP2 have an important role.

Although immortalization of B lymphocytes serves as an attractive model for lymphomagenesis, the pattern of gene expression in immortalized lymphocytes is so different from that associated with most of the virus-associated tumors that a great deal of uncertainty exists as to the role that the viral genes actually play in tumors. For example, in Burkitt lymphoma EBNA1 and the EBERs are expressed. Although EBNA1 has been reported to have effects in a

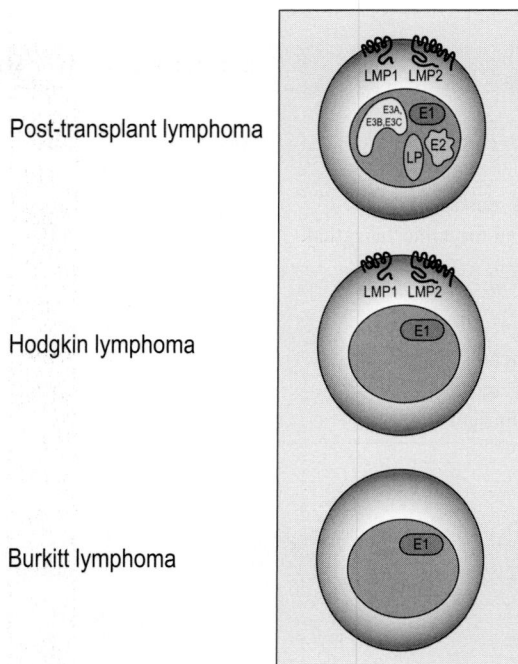

Post-transplant lymphoma

Hodgkin lymphoma

Burkitt lymphoma

Figure 7.2   Different patterns of Epstein–Barr virus (EBV) gene expression are associated with different lymphomas: EBV-associated Burkitt lymphoma expresses only a single nuclear protein (EBNA1; E1 on figure), whereas Hodgkin's lymphoma expresses EBNA1, LMP1 and LMP2A, and some post-transplant lymphomas express all of these proteins as well as EBNA2 (E2 on figure), EBNA3A (E3A on figure), EBNA3B (E3B on figure) and EBNA3C (E3C on figure).

murine transgenic model, others have disputed these conclusions and the role of the protein in the malignancy is uncertain.[40–42] Similarly the EBERs have been suggested by some but not others to have a critical role in maintaining the malignant phenotype.[31]

ASPECTS OF KAPOSI SARCOMA–ASSOCIATED HERPESVIRUS BIOLOGY

Kaposi sarcoma-associated herpesvirus also infects lymphocytes but infection does not result in immortalization. Most studies of viral gene expression *in vitro* have focused on primary effusion lymphoma cell lines. In these cell lines four latency genes are expressed. LANA1 is important in KSHV episomal maintenance. It also sequesters glycogen synthase kinase 3 (GSK3) in the nucleus, elevating levels of β catenin and promoting cell proliferation and interacts with p53 and pRb tumor suppressor proteins and induces lymphomas in a transgenic model.[43,44] LANA2 (also known as vIRF-3) is expressed only in B cells. It inhibits the apoptotic activity of p53.[45–47] vCYC functions as a B cell cdk6 regulator also promoting cell cycle.[48,49] vFLIP functions to block FAS-mediated apoptosis and upregulates NF-κB activity.[50–52]

Table 7.2   Kaposi sarcoma-associated herpesvirus genes

Gene	Function	Latent state	Lytic state
LANA1	Binds to origin of latency replication, interacts with GSK, p53, RB	Yes	No
vCYC	B cell cdk6 regulator	Yes	No
LANA2	Only expressed in B cells	Yes	No
vFLIP	Anti-apoptotic	Yes	No
vIL6	Mimics cellular cytokine	No	Yes
K1	Membrane signaling molecule, transforming in a variety of assays	No	Yes
vGCR	Membrane signaling molecule, transforming in a variety of assays		

Latent gene expression may not be sufficient for initiation or maintenance of lymphoid malignancy. Among the lytic genes of interest in this regard are K1, a transmembrane protein with a functional immunoreceptor tyrosine-based activation motif (ITAM) that can bind several signaling kinases. The gene substitutes for a herpesvirus samirii-transforming gene in a marmoset lymphoma model and leads to tumorigenesis in transgenic mice.[53] However, there is no evidence that it is actually expressed in lymphoma, so any contribution to transformation remains highly speculative. An interleukin 6 homolog, vIL-6, is encoded by the virus.[54] A recognized lymphocyte growth factor, a paracrine role seems likely.

KSHV-encoded genes that may be important in lymphomagenesis are listed in Table 7.2. These include latent and lytic genes and there is considerable debate as to whether latent gene expression is sufficient for neoplastic transformation and maintenance of the transformed state, or whether partial or abortive lytic cycle functions and the paracrine effects of these proteins may have required roles in pathogenesis.

STRAIN VARIATION

Strain variation is recognized in both viruses. Two strains of EBV are recognized that differ mainly in the *EBNA2* gene. Type 1 (or A) is more efficient at lymphocyte transformation *in vitro* and in tumorigenesis in a murine model than is Type 2 virus (or B).[55] Type A predominates in most EBV-associated malignancies including nasopharyngeal carcinoma, Hodgkin lymphoma, and post-transplant lymphoma.[56] However, type 2 (or B) infection is detected in African Burkitt lymphoma and tumors arising in men who have sex with men and are infected with the human immunodeficiency virus (HIV).[57,58] Strain variation has also been characterized in other viral genes. Variation in the sequences of *EBNA1*, *LMP1*, *LMP2* and *BZLF1* have all been suggested to be important in determining tumor

Table 7.3 Lymphoma and gammaherpesviruses

Lymphoma	Cell type	Comments
Diffuse large B cell lymphoma	B cell	In immunocompromised patients sometimes associated with EBV, rarely in immunocompetent patients
Primary central nervous system lymphoma	B cell	In AIDS, organ transplant recipients, congenital immunodeficiency associated with EBV; not associated in immunocompetent patients
Burkitt	B cell	Associated with EBV in malarial Africa but only variably in other parts of the world
Pyothorax	B cell	Always associated with EBV, arise in the setting of chronic inflammation
Post-transplant	B cell (usually)	Usually EBV associated, especially when arising within 2 years of transplantation
Hodgkin	B cell	In HIV, organ transplant and congenital immunodeficiency patients associated with EBV; also in at least 30% of patients without history of immunocompromise
Nasal lymphoma	T/NK cell	Virtually always associated with EBV
Angiocentric lymphoma	T cell	Very commonly associated with EBV
Primary effusion lymphoma	B cell	Associated with KSHV and usually with EBV

EBV, Epstein–Barr virus; KSHV, Kaposi sarcoma-associated herpesvirus; AIDS, acquired immune deficiency syndrome; HIV, human immunodeficiency virus.

association, although no clear consensus in this regard has emerged.[59–64] Strain variation in KSHV has also been intensively investigated.[65] Clear geographic/ethnic strain differences have been documented, but again there is no clear disease association.

GAMMAHERPESVIRUSES-ASSOCIATED NON-LYMPHOID MALIGNANCIES

Epstein–Barr virus is consistently associated with undifferentiated nasopharyngeal carcinoma in all populations and smooth cell mesenchymal tumors in the immunocompromised.[66,67] It is also associated with a minority of gastric cancers.[68,69] Geographic, ethnic or genetic differences play different roles in each of these tumors. Nasopharyngeal carcinoma is most common in particular southern Chinese, Indonesian, north African and Eskimo populations. Gastric cancers are most common in regions of Asia and Africa but at a first approximation the percentage of gastric cancers associated with EBV is invariant around the globe (approximately 10 percent). KSHV is associated with Kaposi sarcoma in all of its varieties including 'classical KS' in elderly men, particular of Mediterranean or Semitic extraction, 'endemic KS' in regions of Africa, 'post-transplant KS' in organ transplant recipients and acquired immune deficiency syndrome (AIDS) KS in HIV-infected patients.[70]

EPSTEIN–BARR VIRUS-ASSOCIATED LYMPHOMA

Lymphoid tumors of B, T and natural killer (NK) cell types may be EBV associated (Table 7.3). Three broad patterns

of latency viral gene expression are recognized.[71,72] Burkitt lymphoma shows the most restricted pattern. Only a single viral antigen is expressed in most tumor cells. Hodgkin lymphoma, some of the diffuse large B cell lymphomas in immunodeficient patients and extranodal NK/T cell lymphomas also express the latency membrane antigens (LMP1 and 2).[73,74] Some post-transplant lymphomas and EBV-associated AIDS lymphomas express all of the latency antigens including EBNA2, 3A, 3B and 3C.[75,76]

Burkitt lymphoma in malarial Africa shows a nearly 100 percent association with EBV. Viral gene expression is highly restricted with EBNA1 being the only viral protein consistently expressed (Fig. 7.2). However, heterogeneity of gene expression has been recognized in tumors.[77,78] In tissue culture, many Burkitt lymphoma cell lines have drifted to less restricted patterns of latency.[71] Burkitt lymphoma is rare in northern Europe, the USA and Canada and is rarely associated with EBV. In areas of Latin America and Asia there is an intermediate incidence of the tumor and an intermediate association with virus.[79]

Lymphoproliferative disorders in patients with congenital immunodeficiencies, with iatrogenically induced immunodeficiencies (such as lymphoproliferative disorders following transplantation), and HIV infection are associated with EBV. Many congenital immunodeficiencies including all varieties of severe combined immunodeficiency are associated with EBV B cell lymphoma.

In organ transplant recipients, EBV-associated lymphoproliferative disease develops as a function of the organ transplanted, the immunosuppressive regimen, the occurrence of graft rejection and patient characteristics (age, whether the recipient is EBV-seronegative).[80] Benign hyperplasia, polymorphic proliferations, and large cell lymphoma are all recognized.[81] The EBV-infected cells often show broad expression of viral latency antigens although there is considerable inter- and intra-tumor variation in patterns of expression.[75]

Approximately half of AIDS-associated lymphomas are EBV-associated.[82] The association is higher in central nervous system and immunoblastic lymphomas.[83] Both of these are lymphomas that tend to occur in persons with longstanding AIDS who have extremely low T cell counts; the association is lower in small noncleaved or large cell lymphomas, which tend to occur in nodal sites in persons with earlier-stage AIDS.[76] Burkitt lymphomas arising in AIDS patients are less likely to be EBV associated than other B cell lymphomas.[84,85] With the advent of effective antiretroviral therapy, the incidence of many HIV-associated lymphomas has decreased.[86–88]

Boys with X-linked lymphoproliferative disease frequently die during the acute phase of primary EBV infection;[89] EBV lymphoma occurs in many of the survivors. The genetic lesion has been mapped.[90–92] A short adaptor molecule normally expressed in activated T and NK cells is mutated or deleted. This is the signaling lymphocytic activation molecule (SLAM)-associated protein (SAP). The clinical features of X-linked lymphoproliferative disease may reflect a dysregulated cellular immune response as a consequence of the absence of functional SAP. Treatment with anti-CD20 (rituximab) at the time of primary EBV infection has led to rapid resolution of clinical symptoms and no progression of disease in preliminary reports.[93]

Lymphomatoid granulomatosis is a B cell tumor associated with EBV. It characteristically involves skin, lung, kidneys, and brain. Histologically it that shows regions of necrosis. In anecdotal reports that pattern of viral gene expression is similar to that of post-transplant lymphoma.[94,95]

Hodgkin's lymphoma originates from B lineage cells as demonstrated by the presence of characteristic immunoglobulin gene rearrangements. Epstein–Barr virus is detected in the Reed–Sternberg cells in approximately 30 percent of cases in north America and Europe but in a higher fraction of cases in Latin America, Africa and Asia.[96] The virus is also consistently detected in Hodgkin lymphoma arising in immunocompromised patients including HIV patients.[87] The pattern of viral gene expression is restricted but LMP2 and LMP1 are expressed at high levels. Hodgkin tumor cells never express immunoglobulin and in some instances show destructive mutations in the immunoglobulin coding regions that preclude expression. These tumors seem to almost invariably harbor virus and it has been suggested that expression of LMP2A may protect against apoptosis that normally ensures the death of B cells that do not express immunoglobulin.[97,98]

Pyothorax-associated lymphoma has been described principally in Japan.[99,100] It is of special interest because its existence underscores the importance of inflammatory cofactors in EBV-lymphomagenesis. These patients have a B cell malignancy arising in the pleural space and presenting as a solid mass (in contrast to primary effusion lymphoma that may present in the pleural space as a malignant effusion). In the preantibiotic era, treatment for tuberculosis involved therapeutic pneumothorax. In Japan, a common procedure for maintaining pneumothorax involved placement of ping pong balls in the pleural space. Chronic infection leading to pyothorax was the result. Tumors arose in the pleural space with a latency more than 20 years from the time of the pneumothorax.

Extranodal NK/T cell tumors are often EBV-associated. Nasal tumors in particular are almost always associated with EBV.[101,102] The virus is also present in most cases of NK cell leukemia and the presence of virus is one of the features that distinguishes it from a more indolent NK cell lymphoproliferative disorder.[103]

Other peripheral T cell lymphomas including angiocentric lymphoma and lymphoma arising in the setting of EBV-associated hemophagocytic syndrome are commonly EBV-associated. In all of these tumors, LMP1 and LMP2 are expressed but not EBNA2, 3A, 3B or 3C.[104]

LYMPHOMA ASSOCIATED WITH KAPOSI SARCOMA-ASSOCIATED HERPESVIRUS

Castleman disease refers to a polyclonal, non-neoplastic lymphoproliferative disorder.[105] Two different histologies are classically recognized: the hyaline vascular type and the less common plasma cell type. However, transitional and composite histologies are common. Disease may be multicentric or localized. Recurrent fevers, lymphadenopathy, hepatosplenomegaly and autoimmune phenomena are common in multicentric Castleman disease. Multicentric Castleman disease, particularly that with a plasma cell histology is commonly associated with KSHV infection.[106–108] Germinal centers are composed of small and large lymphocytes and the mantle zone is surrounded by sheets of mature-appearing plasma cells. KSHV-associated disease may be morphologically distinct with larger cells in the mantle zones containing prominent nucleoli. These plasmablasts express IgM.[109] A variety of immunohistochemical and in situ hybridization techniques show the presence of lytic and latency viral antigens in the plasmablasts located in the mantle zones of lymph nodes of patients with MCD. These cells are polyclonal B cells expressing IgMλ.[110–113] Castleman disease therapy remains ill-defined; however, evidence of lytic viral expression has led some to advocate ganciclovir or other antiviral therapy.[114]

Primary effusion lymphomas preferentially involve body cavities often in the absence of a tumor mass. For example they may present as malignant ascites or pleural effusions. Other extranodal and nodal sites may also be involved. These tumors carry KSHV and are often coinfected by EBV.[115,116] Surface marker expression is characteristic with activation-associated antigens often in the setting of low or absent B cell-associated antigens and immunoglobulin expression. Clonal immunoglobulin gene rearrangements and somatic hypermutation indicate a post-germinal cell stage of differentiation. Immunohistochemistry shows the presence LANA and other KSHV proteins in a variable proportion of neoplastic cells, in particular vIL-6. In addition, the majority of primary effusion lymphomas are coinfected with EBV, which can be detected by *in situ* hybridization to EBERs.[117,118]

KEY POINTS

- Both EBV and KSHV are associated with a heterogeneous group of tumors. Neither virus is associated with malignancy in any more than a tiny fraction of infected hosts except in circumstances of immunocompromise or specific (and rare) genetic lesions.
- Strain variation is well recognized but etiologic significance has yet to be defined.
- Both viruses are episomal in tumor tissue relying predominantly on host functions to replicate viral genomes.
- EBV is associated with B cell, T cell and NK cell tumors. KSHV is only known to be associated with B cell tumors.
- Primary effusion lymphoma always involves KSHV and usually involves EBV. The viral interactions remain poorly understood. Immunocompromise is a common feature of many of these lymphomas (post-transplant, AIDS-associated, congenital) but in others there is no clear association with immunocompromise (nasal lymphoma, angiocentric lymphoma).
- In pyothorax lymphoma, it seems clear that chronic inflammation plays a key role in pathogenesis.

REFERENCES

● = Key primary paper
◆ = Major review article

◆1. Engels EA. Infectious agents as cause of non-Hodgkin lymphoma. *Cancer Epidemiol Biomarkers Prev* 2007; **16**: 401–4.

●2. Chang Y, Cesarman E, Pessin MS *et al.* Identification of herpesvirus-like DNA sequences in AIDS-associated Kaposi's sarcoma. *Science* 1994; **266**: 1865–9.

3. Epstein MA. Reflections on Epstein-Barr virus: some recently resolved old uncertainties. *J Infect* 2001; **43**: 111–15.

◆4. Williams H, Crawford DH. Epstein-Barr virus: the impact of scientific advances on clinical practice. *Blood* 2006; **107**: 862–9.

5. Henle W, Henle G, Lennette ET. The Epstein-Barr virus. *Sci Am* 1979; **241**: 48–59.

6. Chatlynne LG, Lapps W, Handy M *et al.* Detection and titration of human herpesvirus-8-specific antibodies in sera from blood donors, acquired immunodeficiency syndrome patients, and Kaposi's sarcoma patients using a whole virus enzyme-linked immunosorbent assay. *Blood* 1998; **92**: 53–8.

7. Gao SJ, Kingsley L, Li M *et al.* KSHV antibodies among Americans, Italians and Ugandans with and without Kaposi's sarcoma. *Nat Med* 1996; **2**: 925–8.

8. Kedes DH, Operskalski E, Busch M *et al.* The seroepidemiology of human herpesvirus 8 (Kaposi's sarcoma-associated herpesvirus): distribution of infection in KS risk groups and evidence for sexual transmission. *Nat Med* 1996; **2**: 918–24.

9. Koelle DM, Huang ML, Chandran B *et al.* Frequent detection of Kaposi's sarcoma-associated herpesvirus (human herpesvirus 8) DNA in saliva of human immunodeficiency virus-infected men: clinical and immunologic correlates. *J Infect Dis* 1997; **176**: 94–102.

●10. Martin JN, Ganem DE, Osmond DH *et al.* Sexual transmission and the natural history of human herpesvirus 8 infection. *N Engl J Med* 1998; **338**: 948–54.

11. Smith NA, Sabin CA, Gopal R *et al.* Serologic evidence of human herpesvirus 8 transmission by homosexual but not heterosexual sex. *J Infect Dis* 1999; **180**: 600–6.

12. Dukers NH, Renwick N, Prins M *et al.* Risk factors for human herpesvirus 8 seropositivity and seroconversion in a cohort of homosexual men. *Am J Epidemiol* 2000; **151**: 213–24.

13. Grulich AE, Olsen SJ, Luo K *et al.* Kaposi's sarcoma-associated herpesvirus: a sexually transmissible infection? *J Acquir Immune Defic Syndr Hum Retrovirol* 1999; **20**: 387–93.

14. Pellett PE, Spira TJ, Bagasra O *et al.* Multicenter comparison of PCR assays for detection of human herpesvirus 8 DNA in semen. *J Clin Microbiol* 1999; **37**: 1298–301.

◆15. Cohen JI. Epstein-Barr virus infection. *N Engl J Med* 2000; **343**: 481–92.

16. Andreoni M, Sarmati L, Nicastri E *et al.* Primary human herpesvirus 8 infection in immunocompetent children. *JAMA* 2002; **287**: 1295–300.

17. Casper C, Wald A, Pauk J *et al.* Correlates of prevalent and incident Kaposi's sarcoma-associated herpesvirus infection in men who have sex with men. *J Infect Dis* 2002; **185**: 990–3.

18. Luppi M, Barozzi P, Guaraldi G *et al.* Human herpesvirus 8-associated diseases in solid-organ transplantation: importance of viral transmission from the donor. *Clin Infect Dis* 2003; **37**: 606–7. Author reply 607.

19. Diehl V, Henle G, Henle W, Kohn G. Demonstration of a herpes group virus in cultures of peripheral leukocytes from patients with infectious mononucleosis. *J Virol* 1968; **2**: 663–9.

20. Moss DJ, Pope JH. Assay of the infectivity of Epstein-Barr virus by transformation of human leucocytes *in vitro*. *J Gen Virol* 1972; **17**: 233–6.

21. Thorley-Lawson DA. Epstein-Barr virus: exploiting the immune system. *Nat Rev Immunol* 2001; **1**: 75–82.

22. Kieff E, Rickinson AB. Epstein-Barr virus and its replication. In: Fields BN, Knipe DM, Howley PM, Griffin DE (eds) *Fields virology*, 4th ed. Philadelphia: Lippincott Williams & Wilkins, 2001: 2511–73.

23. Hung SC, Kang MS, Kieff E. Maintenance of Epstein-Barr virus (EBV) oriP-based episomes requires EBV-encoded nuclear antigen-1 chromosome-binding domains, which can be replaced by high-mobility group-I or histone H1. *Proc Natl Acad Sci U S A* 2001; **98**: 1865–70.

24. Hayward SD. Viral interactions with the Notch pathway. *Semin Cancer Biol* 2004; **14**: 387–96.

25. Wu S, Xie P, Welsh K *et al.* LMP1 protein from the Epstein-Barr virus is a structural CD40 decoy in B lymphocytes for binding to TRAF3. *J Biol Chem* 2005; **280**: 33620–6.

26. Young LS, Rickinson AB. Epstein-Barr virus: 40 years on. *Nat Rev Cancer* 2004; **4**: 757–68.

27. Merchant M, Caldwell RG, Longnecker R. The LMP2A ITAM is essential for providing B cells with development and survival signals *in vivo*. *J Virol* 2000; **74**: 9115–24.

28. Portis T, Longnecker R. Epstein-Barr virus (EBV) LMP2A alters normal transcriptional regulation following B-cell receptor activation. *Virology* 2004; **318**: 524–33.

29. Chaganti S, Bell AI, Pastor NB *et al.* Epstein-Barr virus infection *in vitro* can rescue germinal center B cells with inactivated immunoglobulin genes. *Blood* 2005; **106**: 4249–52.

30. Mancao C, Altmann M, Jungnickel B, Hammerschmidt W. Rescue of 'crippled' germinal center B cells from apoptosis by Epstein-Barr virus. *Blood* 2005; **106**: 4339–44.

31. Ruf IK, Lackey KA, Warudkar S, Sample JT. Protection from interferon-induced apoptosis by Epstein-Barr virus small RNAs is not mediated by inhibition of PKR. *J Virol* 2005; **79**: 14562–9.

32. Wong HL, Wang X, Chang RC *et al.* Stable expression of EBERs in immortalized nasopharyngeal epithelial cells confers resistance to apoptotic stress. *Mol Carcinog* 2005; **44**: 92–101.

33. Chen H, Smith P, Ambinder RF, Hayward SD. Expression of Epstein-Barr virus BamHI-A rightward transcripts in latently infected B cells from peripheral blood. *Blood* 1999; **93**: 3026–32.

34. Thornburg NJ, Kusano S, Raab-Traub N. Identification of Epstein-Barr virus RK-BARF0-interacting proteins and characterization of expression pattern. *J Virol* 2004; **78**: 12848–56.

35. Pfeffer S, Sewer A, Lagos-Quintana M *et al.* Identification of microRNAs of the herpesvirus family. *Nat Methods* 2005; **2**: 269–76.

●36. Miyashita EM, Yang B, Babcock GJ, Thorley-Lawson DA. Identification of the site of Epstein-Barr virus persistence *in vivo* as a resting B cell. *J Virol* 1997; **71**: 4882–91.

37. Miyashita EM, Yang B, Lam KM *et al.* A novel form of Epstein-Barr virus latency in normal B cells *in vivo*. *Cell* 1995; **80**: 593–601.

38. Hochberg D, Middeldorp JM, Catalina M *et al.* Demonstration of the Burkitt's lymphoma Epstein-Barr virus phenotype in dividing latently infected memory cells *in vivo*. *Proc Natl Acad Sci U S A* 2004; **101**: 239–44.

39. Souza TA, Stollar BD, Sullivan JL *et al.* Peripheral B cells latently infected with Epstein-Barr virus display molecular hallmarks of classical antigen-selected memory B cells. *Proc Natl Acad Sci U S A* 2005; **102**: 18093–8.

●40. Wilson JB, Bell JL, Levine AJ. Expression of Epstein-Barr virus nuclear antigen-1 induces B cell neoplasia in transgenic mice. *EMBO J* 1996; **15**: 3117–26.

●41. Kang MS, Lu H, Yasui T *et al.* Epstein-Barr virus nuclear antigen 1 does not induce lymphoma in transgenic FVB mice. *Proc Natl Acad Sci U S A* 2005; **102**: 820–5.

42. Takada K. Role of Epstein-Barr virus in Burkitt's lymphoma. *Curr Top Microbiol Immunol* 2001; **258**: 141–51.

●43. Fujimuro M, Wu FY, ApRhys C *et al.* A novel viral mechanism for dysregulation of beta-catenin in Kaposi's sarcoma-associated herpesvirus latency. *Nat Med* 2003; **9**: 300–6.

44. Fakhari FD, Jeong JH, Kanan Y, Dittmer DP. The latency-associated nuclear antigen of Kaposi sarcoma-associated herpesvirus induces B cell hyperplasia and lymphoma. *J Clin Invest* 2006; **116**: 735–42.

45. Lubyova B, Kellum MJ, Frisancho AJ, Pitha PM. Kaposi's sarcoma-associated herpesvirus-encoded vIRF-3 stimulates the transcriptional activity of cellular IRF-3 and IRF-7. *J Biol Chem* 2004; **279**: 7643–54.

46. Burysek L, Pitha PM. Latently expressed human herpesvirus 8-encoded interferon regulatory factor 2 inhibits double-stranded RNA-activated protein kinase. *J Virol* 2001; **75**: 2345–52.

47. Rivas C, Thlick AE, Parravicini C *et al.* Kaposi's sarcoma-associated herpesvirus LANA2 is a B-cell-specific latent viral protein that inhibits p53. *J Virol* 2001; **75**: 429–38.

48. Chiou CJ, Poole LJ, Kim PS *et al.* Patterns of gene expression and a transactivation function exhibited by the vGCR (ORF74) chemokine receptor protein of Kaposi's sarcoma-associated herpesvirus. *J Virol* 2002; **76**: 3421–39.

49. Sturzl M, Hohenadl C, Zietz C *et al.* Expression of K13/v-FLIP gene of human herpesvirus 8 and apoptosis in Kaposi's sarcoma spindle cells. *J Natl Cancer Inst* 1999; **91**: 1725–33.

50. Chugh P, Matta H, Schamus S *et al.* Constitutive NF-kappaB activation, normal Fas-induced apoptosis, and increased incidence of lymphoma in human herpes virus 8 K13 transgenic mice. *Proc Natl Acad Sci U S A* 2005; **102**: 12885–90.

51. Grossmann C, Podgrabinska S, Skobe M, Ganem D. Activation of NF-kappaB by the latent vFLIP gene of Kaposi's sarcoma-associated herpesvirus is required for the spindle shape of virus-infected endothelial cells and contributes to their proinflammatory phenotype. *J Virol* 2006; **80**: 7179–85.

52. Guasparri I, Keller SA, Cesarman E. KSHV vFLIP is essential for the survival of infected lymphoma cells. *J Exp Med* 2004; **199**: 993–1003.

53. Lee H, Veazey R, Williams K *et al*. Deregulation of cell growth by the K1 gene of Kaposi's sarcoma-associated herpesvirus. *Nat Med* 1998; **4**: 435–40.

●54. Nicholas J, Ruvolo VR, Burns WH *et al*. Kaposi's sarcoma-associated human herpesvirus-8 encodes homologues of macrophage inflammatory protein-1 and interleukin-6. *Nat Med* 1997; **3**: 287–92.

55. Cohen JI, Wang F, Mannick J, Kieff E. Epstein-Barr virus nuclear protein 2 is a key determinant of lymphocyte transformation. *Proc Natl Acad Sci U S A* 1989; **86**: 9558–62.

56. Tao Q, Robertson KD, Manns A *et al*. Epstein-Barr virus (EBV) in endemic Burkitt's lymphoma: molecular analysis of primary tumor tissue. *Blood* 1998; **91**: 1373–81.

57. Yao QY, Croom-Carter DS, Tierney RJ *et al*. Epidemiology of infection with Epstein-Barr virus types 1 and 2: lessons from the study of a T-cell-immunocompromised hemophilic cohort. *J Virol* 1998; **72**: 4352–63.

58. Sculley TB, Apolloni A, Hurren L *et al*. Coinfection with A- and B-type Epstein-Barr virus in human immunodeficiency virus-positive subjects. *J Infect Dis* 1990; **162**: 643–8.

59. Bhatia K, Raj A, Guitierrez MI *et al*. Variation in the sequence of Epstein Barr virus nuclear antigen 1 in normal peripheral blood lymphocytes and in Burkitt's lymphomas. *Oncogene* 1996; **13**: 177–81.

60. Fassone L, Cingolani A, Martini M *et al*. Characterization of Epstein-Barr virus genotype in AIDS-related non-Hodgkin's lymphoma. *AIDS Res Hum Retroviruses* 2002; **18**: 19–26.

61. Schafer H, Berger C, Aepinus C *et al*. Molecular pathogenesis of Epstein-Barr virus associated posttransplant lymphomas: new insights through latent membrane protein 1 fingerprinting. *Transplantation* 2001; **72**: 492–6.

62. Gutierrez MI, Kingma DW, Sorbara L *et al*. Association of EBV strains, defined by multiple loci analyses, in non-Hodgkin lymphomas and reactive tissues from HIV positive and HIV negative patients. *Leuk Lymphoma* 2000; **37**: 425–9.

63. Edwards RH, Sitki-Green D, Moore DT, Raab-Traub N. Potential selection of LMP1 variants in nasopharyngeal carcinoma. *J Virol* 2004; **78**: 868–81.

64. Miller WE, Edwards RH, Walling DM, Raab-Traub N. Sequence variation in the Epstein-Barr virus latent membrane protein 1. *J Gen Virol* 1994; **75**: 2729–40.

65. Zong J, Ciufo DM, Viscidi R *et al*. Genotypic analysis at multiple loci across Kaposi's sarcoma herpesvirus (KSHV) DNA molecules: clustering patterns, novel variants and chimerism. *J Clin Virol* 2002; **23**: 119–48.

66. Lee ES, Locker J, Nalesnik M *et al*. The association of Epstein-Barr virus with smooth-muscle tumors occurring after organ transplantation. *N Engl J Med* 1995; **332**: 19–25.

67. Iezzoni JC, Gaffey MJ, Weiss LM. The role of Epstein-Barr virus in lymphoepithelioma-like carcinomas. *Am J Clin Pathol* 1995; **103**: 308–15.

68. Shibata D, Tokunaga M, Uemura Y *et al*. Association of Epstein-Barr virus with undifferentiated gastric carcinomas with intense lymphoid infiltration. Lymphoepithelioma-like carcinoma. *Am J Pathol* 1991; **139**: 469–74.

69. Shibata D, Weiss LM. Epstein-Barr virus-associated gastric adenocarcinoma. *Am J Pathol* 1992; **140**: 769–74.

70. Moore PS. The emergence of Kaposi's sarcoma-associated herpesvirus (human herpesvirus 8). *N Engl J Med* 2000; **343**: 1411–13.

71. Rowe M, Rowe DT, Gregory CD *et al*. Differences in B cell growth phenotype reflect novel patterns of Epstein-Barr virus latent gene expression in Burkitt's lymphoma cells. *EMBO J* 1987; **6**: 2743–51.

72. Thorley-Lawson DA, Gross A. Persistence of the Epstein-Barr virus and the origins of associated lymphomas. *N Engl J Med* 2004; **350**: 1328–37.

73. Murray PG, Constandinou CM, Crocker J *et al*. Analysis of major histocompatibility complex class I, TAP expression, and LMP2 epitope sequence in Epstein-Barr virus-positive Hodgkin's disease. *Blood* 1998; **92**: 2477–83.

74. Jaffe ES, Krenacs L, Kumar S *et al*. Extranodal peripheral T-cell and NK-cell neoplasms. *Am J Clin Pathol* 1999; **111**: s46–55.

75. Murray PG, Swinnen LJ, Constandinou CM *et al*. BCL-2 but not its Epstein-Barr virus-encoded homologue, BHRF1, is commonly expressed in posttransplantation lymphoproliferative disorders. *Blood* 1996; **87**: 706–11.

76. Hamilton-Dutoit SJ, Pallesen G, Franzmann MB *et al*. AIDS-related lymphoma. Histopathology, immunophenotype, and association with Epstein-Barr virus as demonstrated by *in situ* nucleic acid hybridization. *Am J Pathol* 1991; **138**: 149–63.

77. Niedobitek G, Agathanggelou A, Rowe M *et al*. Heterogeneous expression of Epstein-Barr virus latent proteins in endemic Burkitt's lymphoma. *Blood* 1995; **86**: 659–65.

78. Bacchi MM, Bacchi CE, Alvarenga M *et al*. Burkitt's lymphoma in Brazil: strong association with Epstein-Barr virus. *Mod Pathol* 1996; **9**: 63–7.

79. Gutierrez MI, Bhatia K, Barriga F *et al*. Molecular epidemiology of Burkitt's lymphoma from South America: differences in breakpoint location and Epstein-Barr virus association from tumors in other world regions. *Blood* 1992; **79**: 3261–6.

80. Swinnen LJ. Organ transplant-related lymphoma. *Curr Treat Options Oncol* 2001; **2**: 301–8.

81. Knowles DM. Immunodeficiency-associated lymphoproliferative disorders. *Mod Pathol* 1999; **12**: 200–17.

82. Carbone A. Emerging pathways in the development of AIDS-related lymphomas. *Lancet Oncol* 2003; **4**: 22–9.

●83. MacMahon EM, Glass JD, Hayward SD *et al*. Epstein-Barr virus in AIDS-related primary central nervous system lymphoma. *Lancet* 1991; **338**: 969–73.

●84. Subar M, Neri A, Inghirami G *et al*. Frequent c-myc oncogene activation and infrequent presence of

Epstein-Barr virus genome in AIDS-associated lymphoma. *Blood* 1988; **72**: 667–71.

85. Davi F, Delecluse HJ, Guiet P *et al.* Burkitt-like lymphomas in AIDS patients: characterization within a series of 103 human immunodeficiency virus-associated non-Hodgkin's lymphomas. Burkitt's lymphoma study group. *J Clin Oncol* 1998; **16**: 3788–95.

86. Frisch M, Smith E, Grulich A, Johansen C. Cancer in a population-based cohort of men and women in registered homosexual partnerships. *Am J Epidemiol* 2003; **157**: 966–72.

●87. Glaser SL, Clarke CA, Gulley ML *et al.* Population-based patterns of human immunodeficiency virus-related Hodgkin lymphoma in the Greater San Francisco Bay Area, 1988–1998. *Cancer* 2003; **98**: 300–9.

88. Jones JL, Hanson DL, Dworkin MS *et al.* Effect of antiretroviral therapy on recent trends in selected cancers among HIV-infected persons. Adult/adolescent spectrum of HIV disease project group. *J Acquir Immune Defic Syndr* 1999; **21**(Suppl 1): s11–17.

89. Morra M, Howie D, Grande MS *et al.* X-linked lymphoproliferative disease: a progressive immunodeficiency. *Annu Rev Immunol* 2001; **19**: 657–82.

90. Coffey AJ, Brooksbank RA, Brandau O *et al.* Host response to EBV infection in X-linked lymphoproliferative disease results from mutations in an SH2-domain encoding gene. *Nat Genet* 1998; **20**: 129–35.

91. Nichols KE, Harkin DP, Levitz S *et al.* Inactivating mutations in an SH2 domain-encoding gene in X-linked lymphoproliferative syndrome. *Proc Natl Acad Sci U S A* 1998; **95**: 13765–70.

92. Sayos J, Wu C, Morra M *et al.* The X-linked lymphoproliferative-disease gene product SAP regulates signals induced through the co-receptor SLAM. *Nature* 1998; **395**: 462–9.

93. Milone MC, Tsai DE, Hodinka RL *et al.* Treatment of primary Epstein-Barr virus infection in patients with X-linked lymphoproliferative disease using B-cell-directed therapy. *Blood* 2005; **105**: 994–6.

94. Beaty MW, Toro J, Sorbara L *et al.* Cutaneous lymphomatoid granulomatosis: correlation of clinical and biologic features. *Am J Surg Pathol* 2001; **25**: 1111–20.

95. Wilson WH, Kingma DW, Raffeld M *et al.* Association of lymphomatoid granulomatosis with Epstein-Barr viral infection of B lymphocytes and response to interferon-alpha 2b. *Blood* 1996; **87**: 4531–7.

●96. Glaser SL, Lin RJ, Stewart SL *et al.* Epstein-Barr virus-associated Hodgkin's disease: epidemiologic characteristics in international data. *Int J Cancer* 1997; **70**: 375–82.

◆97. Re D, Kuppers R, Diehl V. Molecular pathogenesis of Hodgkin's lymphoma. *J Clin Oncol* 2005; **23**: 6379–86.

98. Bechtel D, Kurth J, Unkel C, Kuppers R. Transformation of BCR-deficient germinal-center B cells by EBV supports a major role of the virus in the pathogenesis of Hodgkin and posttransplantation lymphomas. *Blood* 2005; **106**: 4345–50.

99. Copie-Bergman C, Niedobitek G, Mangham DC *et al.* Epstein-Barr virus in B-cell lymphomas associated with chronic suppurative inflammation. *J Pathol* 1997; **183**: 287–92.

100. Aozasa K, Takakuwa T, Nakatsuka S. Pyothorax-associated lymphoma: a lymphoma developing in chronic inflammation. *Adv Anat Pathol* 2005; **12**: 324–31.

101. Chiang AK, Tao Q, Srivastava G, Ho FC. Nasal NK- and T-cell lymphomas share the same type of Epstein-Barr virus latency as nasopharyngeal carcinoma and Hodgkin's disease. *Int J Cancer* 1996; **68**: 285–90.

102. Cheung MM, Chan JK, Wong KF. Natural killer cell neoplasms: a distinctive group of highly aggressive lymphomas/leukemias. *Semin Hematol* 2003; **40**: 221–32.

103. Hart DN, Baker BW, Inglis MJ *et al.* Epstein-Barr viral DNA in acute large granular lymphocyte (natural killer) leukemic cells. *Blood* 1992; **79**: 2116–23.

104. Weiss LM, Jaffe ES, Liu XF *et al.* Detection and localization of Epstein-Barr viral genomes in angioimmunoblastic lymphadenopathy and angioimmunoblastic lymphadenopathy-like lymphoma. *Blood* 1992; **79**: 1789–95.

105. Hall PA, Donaghy M, Cotter FE *et al.* An immunohistological and genotypic study of the plasma cell form of Castleman's disease. *Histopathology* 1989; **14**: 333–46. Discussion 429–332.

106. Soulier J, Grollet L, Oksenhendler E *et al.* Kaposi's sarcoma-associated herpesvirus-like DNA sequences in multicentric Castleman's disease. *Blood* 1995; **86**: 1276–80.

107. Larroche C, Cacoub P, Soulier J *et al.* Castleman's disease and lymphoma: report of eight cases in HIV-negative patients and literature review. *Am J Hematol* 2002; **69**: 119–26.

108. Suda T, Katano H, Delsol G *et al.* HHV-8 infection status of AIDS-unrelated and AIDS-associated multicentric Castleman's disease. *Pathol Int* 2001; **51**: 671–9.

109. Dupin N, Diss TL, Kellam P *et al.* HHV-8 is associated with a plasmablastic variant of Castleman disease that is linked to HHV-8-positive plasmablastic lymphoma. *Blood* 2000; **95**: 1406–12.

110. Du MQ, Liu H, Diss TC *et al.* Kaposi sarcoma-associated herpesvirus infects monotypic (IgM lambda) but polyclonal naive B cells in Castleman disease and associated lymphoproliferative disorders. *Blood* 2001; **97**: 2130–6.

111. Cannon JS, Nicholas J, Orenstein JM *et al.* Heterogeneity of viral IL-6 expression in HHV-8-associated diseases. *J Infect Dis* 1999; **180**: 824–8.

112. Parravinci C, Corbellino M, Paulli M *et al.* Expression of a virus-derived cytokine, KSHV vIL-6, in HIV-seronegative Castleman's disease. *Am J Pathol* 1997; **151**: 1517–22.

113. Staskus KA, Zhong W, Gebhard K *et al.* Kaposi's sarcoma-associated herpesvirus gene expression in endothelial (spindle) tumor cells. *J Virol* 1997; **71**: 715–19.

114. Casper C, Nichols WG, Huang ML *et al.* Remission of HHV-8 and HIV-associated multicentric Castleman disease with ganciclovir treatment. *Blood* 2004; **103**: 1632–4.

115. Nador RG, Cesarman E, Chadburn A *et al.* Primary effusion lymphoma: a distinct clinicopathologic entity associated with the Kaposi's sarcoma-associated herpes virus. *Blood* 1996; **88**: 645–56.

116. Cesarman E, Chang Y, Moore PS *et al.* Kaposi's sarcoma-associated herpesvirus-like DNA sequences in AIDS-related body-cavity-based lymphomas. *N Engl J Med* 1995; **332**: 1186–91.

117. Chadburn A, Hyjek E, Mathew S *et al.* KSHV-positive solid lymphomas represent an extra-cavitary variant of primary effusion lymphoma. *Am J Surg Pathol* 2004; **28**: 1401–16.

118. Engels EA, Pittaluga S, Whitby D *et al.* Immunoblastic lymphoma in persons with AIDS-associated Kaposi's sarcoma: a role for Kaposi's sarcoma-associated herpesvirus. *Mod Pathol* 2003; **16**: 424–9.

8

Other microorganisms associated with lymphoid neoplasms

SILVIA FRANCESCHI AND LUIGINO DAL MASO

INTRODUCTION

Lymphoid neoplasms are malignant diseases that arise from the lymphoid tissues.[1] As they are heterogeneous, in terms of histologic characteristics and anatomic site(s) of involvement, and have relatively low incidence rates (Chapter 3), the identification of the causes of lymphomas has turned out to be difficult. Several possible causative factors have been reported, including immunodeficiency, and, possibly, exposure to pesticides and radiation, smoking habits and several aspects of diet (Chapter 4).[2,3] An association between certain infectious agents, e.g. Epstein–Barr virus, human T cell leukemia virus, human immunodeficiency virus (HIV), and lymphoid neoplasms, is well established and has important implications from a prevention point of view (Chapters 6 and 7).[4]

This chapter will systematically review studies on the association between lymphoid neoplasms and selected microorganisms. In particular, the focus will be on the relationship between non-Hodgkin lymphoma (NHL) and other hemolymphopoietic neoplasms, with a few infections

relatively recently assessed as possible causes of lymphoma, i.e. hepatitis C virus (HCV), hepatitis B virus (HBV), Helicobacter pylori, Borrelia burgdorferi (Lyme disease) and Chlamydiae.

HEPATITIS C AND B VIRUS INFECTION

Hepatitis C virus is an RNA virus belonging to the family of flaviviruses. Approximately 170 million people are infected with HCV worldwide, making HCV a major public health problem.[5] HCV is hepatotrophic and causes hepatitis, liver cirrhosis and hepatocellular carcinoma.[6] HCV is also lymphotrophic and is involved in the etiology of essential mixed cryoglobulinemia, a lymphoproliferative disease that can evolve into B cell NHL (B NHL).[7]

Several studies found a high prevalence of HCV infection in patients with B cell lymphoproliferative disorders, particularly B NHL, including cases in which essential mixed cryoglobulinemia was absent.[8] The association between HCV and B NHL appears to have a strong regional connotation. Studies from Italy, Japan and California, USA, where the number of HCV carriers in the general population is relatively high (1–5 percent), showed the highest percentages (10–20 percent) of HCV carriers in patients with B NHL, whereas studies from central and northern Europe found none or very few HCV carriers among B NHL patients.[8]

Hepatitis B virus is a DNA virus, and causes, like HCV, hepatitis, liver cirrhosis and hepatocellular carcinoma. Infection with HBV is very common, with more than 400 million people chronically infected, mainly in Asia and Africa.[9] Since the 1980s, a very effective vaccine against HBV has been available, and its use is also spreading to developing countries.

Search strategy for identification of studies

Searches of MEDLINE and EMBASE for articles on hepatitis and lymphomas were conducted in order to identify the relevant literature. Additional articles were retrieved up to February 2008 in the reference lists of the identified papers and of large recent reviews.[2,3,10–12]

Inclusion criteria

The aim was the identification of all papers presenting the prevalence of HCV infection in NHL patients and in a control group. The definition of these control groups varied greatly between studies. They included patients with defined diseases such as lymphoproliferative diseases other than NHL, solid cancers, patients undergoing a given hospital procedure, such as a biopsy or a colonoscopy, blood donors, or population-based samples. Most recent studies have been designed as formal case–control or cohort studies, with clearly defined inclusion criteria for the control group, and estimates of odds ratios (ORs) or relative risks (RRs) adjusted for age, sex, and other potential confounding factors. The RR will also be used in tables for case–control studies, instead of OR. Patients with other lymphoproliferative diseases were never used as a control group in the present review, since these conditions may also be associated with HCV infection. Moreover, since the prevalence of HCV infection varied widely according to age and sex, these factors had to be taken into account. Therefore, only studies that fulfilled at least one of the following conditions were considered eligible:

1. sex- and age-adjusted RRs were presented
2. matching of cases and controls by age and sex was reported
3. some measure of age (mean or median or distribution) and sex ratio in cases and controls, and evidence of good comparability of the two groups, were provided.

Only in instances 2 and 3 did we compute crude RRs with 95 percent confidence intervals (CIs) computed according to the Wald method,[13] if not provided in the original publication.

To avoid multiple inclusions of the same data, whenever the same author appeared in more than one article, a check of the place and time of recruitment was conducted, and, in case of overlapping material, only the most recent publication was included. Only series with 100 or more cases were included for the overall analyses on NHL and hepatitis viruses. Findings for specific NHL subtypes and other lymphoid neoplasms were shown only when 20 or more cases were collected. All prospective studies (or case–control studies nested in a cohort) were included regardless of the number of lymphomas reported.

The main characteristics of studies with data on hepatitis viruses and lymphoid neoplasms included in the present review are summarized in Table 8.1.

Assessment of study quality

Several problems of comparability emerged among the retrieved studies. The definition of lymphoma adopted by the various authors differed. For example, some authors included chronic lymphocytic leukemia (CLL) among NHL cases, whereas others did not. Since CLL is similar to small lymphocytic lymphoma (SLL),[1] this histological type was included among NHL. The definition of NHL given by the author was used whenever possible. Patients with HIV infection were explicitly excluded in most studies, and studies including only HIV patients were not reviewed.[34] A record linkage study of subjects with HBV/HCV infections from Australia[35] and the cohort study of US veterans with and without HCV[36] were not included.

The method of testing HCV infection also differed between studies. Some studies relied only on enzyme-linked immunosorbent assay (ELISA) while others used also recombinant immunoblot assay (RIBA) confirmation and/or looked for HCV RNA. First generation ELISAs had unsatisfactory sensitivity and specificity, so our review considered only studies where second or third generation ELISAs were used. The presence of HCV RNA is the best marker for risk of hepatocellular carcinoma, but whether detection of HCV RNA, in addition to anti-HCV antibodies, is a requirement in the association between HCV and NHL is still unclear.

In respect to NHL classification, most studies used, or can be recoded into, the World Health Organization/Revised European–American classification of Lymphoid neoplasms (WHO/REAL)[1] classification. To reduce problems of misclassification between subcategories of NHL, since they were presented in different degrees of detail, only major NHL subtypes (e.g. diffuse large B cell (DLBC), follicular B cell (FBC), marginal zone (MZ), T cell and CLL/SLL) are discussed here. The separation of nodal or extranodal NHL, or NHL with or without liver or spleen involvement was possible only in a few studies.

Table 8.1 Relative risk (RR)[a] and 95 percent confidence interval (CI) of non-Hodgkin lymphoma (NHL) according to hepatitis C virus (HCV) infection status in case–control and cohort studies

First author	Year	Country	Comparison groups	NHL subtype (REAL/WHO)	NHL Men (%)	NHL Mean/median age (range)	NHL HCV+/HCV−	Controls HCV+/HCV−	RR (95% CI)
Case–control studies									
Zuckerman[14]	1997	USA	Hospital patients	Yes, WF[c]	53	52 (23–84)	26/94	6/108	5.0 (2.0 to 12.6)
Vallisa[15]	1999	Italy	Hospital patients[b]	Yes[c]	50	63	65/110	32/318	5.9 (3.6 to 9.4)
Mizorogi[16]	2000	Japan	Hospital patients[b]	Yes, WF	64	63 (24–87)	17/117	34/482	2.1 (1.1 to 3.8)
Pioltelli[17]	2000	Italy	Hospital patients[b]	Yes, WF[c]	63	63 (17–92)	48/252	66/781	2.3 (1.5 to 3.4)
Montella[18]	2001	Italy	Hospital patients	Yes, WF	56	59 (13–85)	28/83	17/209	3.7 (1.9 to 7.4)
Imai[19]	2002	Japan	Blood donors	Yes	54	63 (46–79)	23/164	9.6[d]	2.4 (1.4 to 3.4)[e]
Kim[20]	2002	South Korea	Hospital patients[b]	Yes, WF	60	52 (14–85)	7/207	19/846	1.5 (0.6 to 3.6)
Mele/Bianco[21,22]	2003	Italy	Hospital patients	Yes	64	– (≥15)	83/447	22/374	3.2 (1.9 to 5.2)
Cowgill[23]	2004	Egypt	Hospital patients	No[c]	60	48 (≥18)	94/126	52/170	2.7 (1.8 to 4.1)
Engels[24]	2004	USA	Population patients	Yes	54	57 (20–74)	32/781	14/670	1.9 (1.0 to 4.0)
Morton[25]	2004	USA	Population patients	Yes	0	64 (21–84)	8/456	5/529	1.9 (0.6 to 5.7)
Seve[26]	2004	France	Hospital patients	Yes[c]	58	60 (21–90)	6/206	20/954	1.3 (0.5 to 3.4)
Talamini[27]	2004	Italy	Hospital patients	Yes	53	59 (18–84)	44/181	45/459	2.6 (1.6 to 4.3)
Nieters[28]	2006	Europe	Population and hospital patients	Yes	55	59	25/351	22/577	1.9 (1.0 to 3.4)
Vajdic[29]	2006	Australia	Population patients	Yes	56	50	43/1304	41/1749	1.4 (0.9 to 2.2)
Spinelli[30]	2008	Canada	Population patients	Yes	54	– (20–79)	19/776	5/692	2.6 (0.9 to 7.4)
Cohort studies									
Ohsawa[31]	1999	Japan	Cohort of HCV patients	–[c]	100	63 (40–69)	4	1.9[d]	2.1 (0.6 to 5.4)
Rabkin[32]	2002	USA	Cancer free subjects	No[c,f]		53 (19–76)	0/57	0/95	
Duberg[33]	2005	Sweden	Cohort of HCV patients	No[c]	75	44 (31–82)	24	12.1[d]	2.0 (1.3 to 3.1)
Pooled									2.4 (2.0 to 3.0)

[a]Relative risks (RRs) adjusted at least by age and sex are in italics; elsewhere crude RRs (Wald 95 percent confidence intervals) were calculated.

[b]Includes non-hemolymphopoietic cancer cases.

[c]Includes only B cell NHL.

[d]NHL expected.

[g]OR adjusted for sex, age and birthplace.

[e]Observed/expected number of HCV+ from birth cohort and sex-matched blood donors.

[f]Nested case–control study.

WHO, World Health Organization; REAL, Revised European–American classification of lymphoid neoplasms; WF, Working Formulation.

To investigate the specificity of the association of HCV with NHL, the prevalence of HCV in patients with Hodgkin lymphoma (HL) and multiple myeloma, is also presented. Few studies presented results for leukemia other than CLL/SLL,[37] or other premalignant hemo-lymphoproliferative diseases, and therefore these neoplasms will not be considered in detail in this chapter.

Statistical methods

To provide a quantitative estimate of the risk of lymphoid neoplasms among HCV-positive individuals from all studies combined, the RRs and the corresponding 95 percent CIs were abstracted from published articles. Whenever available, we used the estimates adjusted for relevant confounding factors included in the original studies. When RRs were not given, they were computed from tabular data using Wald estimates.[13] We then calculated the summary RR and corresponding 95 percent CI using random effects models of DerSimonian and Laird.[38]

It should be kept in mind that the overall associations estimated by random effect models should be interpreted as the average of the RRs across studies[38] and the main sources of heterogeneity of RR estimates between available studies must be considered before drawing final conclusions on the real strength of the association between HCV and lymphomas.

Hepatitis C virus infection and non-Hodgkin lymphoma

Table 8.1 summarizes the main results of studies on NHL. The highest prevalence of HCV in a control group (over 20 percent) was reported in Egypt.[23] High prevalence (5–10 percent) was also found in Italy[15,17,18,21,22,27,39] and in Japan.[16,19] Conversely, relatively low HCV prevalence (less than 5 percent) was found in South Korea,[20] northern Europe,[26,28,33] the USA,[14,24,25,32] Australia[29] and Canada.[30]

The pooled RR from the 19 studies on HCV and NHL risk was 2.4 (95 percent CI 2.0 to 3.0), and significantly elevated RRs were found in most of them (12/19) (Table 8.1). The corresponding RR from 16 case–control studies was 2.5 (95 percent CI 2.0 to 3.1), based on 6444 cases (546 exposed), and the pooled RR from cohort studies was 2.0 (95 percent CI 1.3 to 3.1). Heterogeneity was found between individual case–control studies ($P < 0.01$) but not between case–control and cohort studies. The greatest source of heterogeneity seemed to be HCV prevalence in the NHL-free study population. Studies conducted in areas where HCV prevalence was above 5 percent showed more elevated RR (3.0; 95 percent CI 2.4 to 3.7) than studies conducted in lower-prevalence areas (1.7; 95 percent CI 1.3 to 2.2).[12,28,30] Heterogeneity emerged also between type of controls (RR of 2.8 for hospital-based and 1.6 for population-based case–control studies),[12,28,30] whereas no significant heterogeneity emerged by study periods (RR was 2.9 for studies published up to 2003 compared to 2.2 for studies published thereafter).

Sites of involvement and histologic subtype of non-Hodgkin lymphoma and hepatitis C virus infection

Some early studies found that HCV infection was more strongly related to extranodal NHL,[14,18] or to specific NHL sites of involvement (e.g. liver),[40] than to nodal NHL. However, two larger case–control studies[24,27] did not confirm these results and showed a similar strength of association between HCV infection and nodal and extranodal NHL (Table 8.2). Pooled RRs were 2.5 (95 percent CI 1.8 to 3.5) for nodal NHL, based on five studies and 887 cases, and 3.7 (95 percent CI 2.2 to 6.3) for extranodal NHL, based on 471 cases. The exclusion of the study by Zuckerman et al.,[14] which showed the highest RRs, notably for extranodal NHL, made the RR for nodal and extranodal NHL very similar (RR 2.4; 95 percent CI 1.7 to 3.7 and 3.1; 95 percent CI 2.1 to 4.6, respectively).

Table 8.2 Relative risk (RR)[a] and 95 percent confidence interval (CI) of nodal and extranodal non-Hodgkin lymphoma (NHL) according to hepatitis C virus (HCV) infection status in case–control studies

First author	Year	Country	Controls HCV+/HCV−	Primary nodal NHL HCV+/HCV−	RR (95% CI)	Extranodal NHL HCV+/HCV−	RR (95% CI)
Case–control studies							
Zuckerman[14]	1997	USA	6/108	16/79	3.6 (1.4 to 9.7)	10/15	12.0 (3.8 to 38)
Mizorogi[16]	2000	Japan	34/482	7/43	2.3 (1.0 to 5.5)	9/40	3.2 (1.4 to 7.1)
Montella[18]	2001	Italy	17/209	9/38	2.4 (0.9 to 5.9)	16/38	5.0 (2.3 to 10.8)
Engels[24]	2004	USA	14/670	22/518	2.0 (1.1 to 4.3)	10/263	1.8 (0.7 to 4.2)
Talamini[27]	2004	Italy	45/459	30/125	2.7 (1.5 to 4.6)	14/56	2.6 (1.3 to 5.3)
Pooled			116/1928	84/803	2.5 (1.8 to 3.5)	59/412	3.7 (2.2 to 6.3)

[a]Relative risks (RRs) adjusted at least by age and sex are in italics; elsewhere crude RR (Wald 95 percent confidence intervals) were calculated.

Some reports also suggested that the relationship between HCV and NHL may be confined to certain histologic subtypes of NHL, in particular lymphoplasmocytoid/immunocytoma or splenic lymphoma.[41]

Ten studies described in Table 8.1 were reevaluated to elucidate the association between HCV and specific NHL subtypes (Table 8.3).[1] Studies including at least 20 cases of specific subtypes are shown in Table 8.3. Only the most frequent and reproducible NHL subtypes, namely DLBC, FBC, MZ and T cell NHL, were presented and discussed. CLL/SLL are described in the following section. By and large, positive associations with HCV positivity were seen for different NHL histologic types. In particular, in the studies for which a RR could be computed (not equal 0), the RRs were 2.9 (95 percent CI 2.1 to 4.1) for DLBC (1544 cases), 2.4 (95 percent CI 1.4 to 4.1) for follicular NHL (925 cases), 3.4 (95 percent CI 2.1 to 5.2) for MZ (378 cases), and 1.4 (95 percent CI 0.8 to 2.5) for T cell NHL (347 cases). It is however, worth noticing that HCV positivities largely differ in series of follicular (3.8 percent) or T cell NHL (3.3 percent) compared to DLBC (10.1 or MZ NHL (8.0). In conclusion, even if an association between HCV and major B NHL subtypes emerged, the issue of whether the role of HCV varies by histologic type must be considered still an open one.

There seems to be only a weak association between HCV infection and T cell NHL, or at least epidemiologic evidence suggests that an RR greater than two can be excluded.

Hepatitis C virus infection and other hemolymphopoietic neoplasms

Table 8.4 shows the association of HCV with CLL/SLL, multiple myeloma (plasma cell myeloma according to the WHO classification)[1] and HL. The RRs for CLL/SLL in five studies ranged between 1.1 and 2.5, but in no study was the association with HCV infection statistically significant. However, the pooled RR was 1.5 (95 percent CI 1.0 to 2.3).

In respect to multiple myeloma, two studies, one case–control in Italy[18] and one cohort in Sweden[33] showed a significant association with HCV infection, with RRs of 4.5 (95 percent CI 1.9 to 10.7) and 2.4 (95 percent CI 1.0 to 5.0), respectively. However, two multicenter case–control studies, one from Italy[22] and one from Europe,[28] showed no increased risk in patients with multiple myeloma (Table 8.4).

Findings for HL suggested lack of association with HCV-positivity with a pooled estimate of the RR of 1.3 (Table 8.4). Notably, no significantly increased risk emerged in the largest study, based on 239 patients (OR 1.0, 95 percent CI 0.3 to 3.5).[28]

In respect to HCV infection and leukemia risk, Bianco et al.[22] reported on 49 cases of chronic myeloid leukemia (CML) (RR 2.3, 95 percent CI 0.8 to 6.4), 140 cases of acute myeloid leukemia (AML) (RR 1.3, 95 percent CI 0.6 to 2.9), and 54 cases of acute lymphocytic leukemia (ALL) (OR 2.4, 95 percent CI 0.8 to 7.1).

Gentile et al.[37] in a study on leukemia and HCV infection, found no association for ALL (67 cases; RR 1.3, 95 percent CI 0.5 to 3.5), for AML (172 cases; RR 1.5, 95 percent CI 0.8 to 2.9) or CML (125 cases; RR 0.3, 95 percent CI 0.1 to 1.1).

In conclusion, findings for CLL/SLL are compatible with those for the NHL types, but the evidence for an association with HCV infection is weak and less consistent for HL, multiple myeloma and T cell NHL. No conclusions can be drawn for leukemia, which has been studied very little in relation to HCV.

Hepatitis B virus infection and lymphomas

The possible association between HBV infection and NHL has been evaluated by much fewer studies than is the case for HCV infection (Table 8.5). In addition, the limited number of HBV markers that have been evaluated complicates the comparison of findings from different studies.

The presence of HBsAg indicates that the person is a chronic carrier of HBV whereas the presence of anti-HBsAg is generally interpreted as evidence of clearance of HBV infection. Anti-HBsAg is also found in people who were successfully vaccinated against HBV.

The only study specifically designed to evaluate the association between HBV and lymphomas was conducted in South Korea, where HBV was endemic before the introduction of the vaccine against HBV.[20] An association emerged between NHL and HBsAg-positivity (13 percent positivity among cases vs 9 percent among controls) with an RR of 3.9 (95 percent CI 1.9 to 7.9), but not with anti-HBsAg-positivity (58 percent positivity among cases vs 64 percent among controls; RR 0.8, 95 percent CI 0.6 to 1.2). Two studies conducted in Italy on HCV showed RRs of 4.9[17] and 4.1,[27] respectively, among HBV carriers. Ohsawa et al. in Japan,[31] detected HBsAg in the serum of 39 (2 percent) patients; HCV prevalence in Osaka blood donors was estimated to be 2.2 percent. The RR of all NHL among HBsAg-positive people was 4.4 (95 percent CI 2.8 to 6.9) and no heterogeneity was found between studies.

Hepatitis B virus infection is a serious global health problem with high worldwide prevalence,[42] the excess risk of NHL in patients with acute or chronic hepatitis may contribute non-negligibly to NHL, at least in HBV endemic countries. Therefore, additional studies on NHL and HBV are necessary, especially in low-resource countries.

Mechanisms of hepatitis viruses: pathogenic effect on lymphomas

The natural targets of HCV are hepatocytes and, possibly, B lymphocytes.[6] Presently, the mechanisms underlying the contribution of HCV to lymphomagenesis are not completely understood.

Table 8.3 Relative risk (RR)[a] estimates and corresponding 95 percent confidence intervals (CIs) of non-Hodgkin lymphoma according to hepatitis C virus (HCV) infection status by major histologic types

First author	Year	Country	Controls HCV+/HCV−	Diffuse large B cell HCV+/HCV−	Diffuse large B cell RR (95% CI)	Follicular B cell HCV+/HCV−	Follicular B cell RR (95% CI)	Marginal zone[b] HCV+/HCV−	Marginal zone[b] RR (95% CI)	T cell HCV+/HCV−	T cell RR (95% CI)
Vallisa[15]	1999	Italy	32/318	32/55	5.8 (3.3 to 10.2)	6/19	3.1 (1.2 to 8.2)	6/17	3.5 (1.3 to 9.5)	–	–
Mizorogi[16]	2000	Japan	34/482	9/43	3.4 (1.8 to 6.7)	–	–	–	–	0/23	0.0 (0.0 to 3.1)
Imai[19]	2002	Japan	1.6[c]	–	–	–	–	–	–	2/29	1.3 (0.0 to 3.1)
Mele/Bianco[21,22]	2003	Italy	22/374	39/176	3.8 (2.2 to 6.5)	11/68	2.8 (1.3 to 5.9)	7/33	3.6 (1.4 to 9.1)	4/26	2.2 (0.6 to 7.6)
Engels[24]	2004	USA	14/670	6/224	1.3 (0.5 to 3.8)	11/214	2.5 (1.1 to 5.5)	4/71	2.8 (0.9 to 8.4)	2/48	2.0 (0.4 to 6.5)
Morton[25]	2004	USA	5/529	2/133	1.6 (0.3 to 8.3)	4/103	4.1 (1.1 to 15.6)	–	–	0/34	0.0 (0.0 to 12.3)
Seve[26]	2004	France	20/954	2/107		0/31	0.0 (0.0 to 1.1)	4/29	6.6 (2.1 to 20.4)	–	–
Talamini[27]	2004	Italy	45/459	22/90	2.5 (1.4 to 4.4)	0/36		–	–	–	–
Nieters[28]	2006	Europe	41/1747	18/374	2.2 (1.2 to 3.9)	2/208	0.5 (0.1 to 2.1)	4/108	1.6 (0.6 to 4.5)	2/99	0.9 (0.2 to 3.7)
Spinelli[30]	2008	Canada	5/692	12/200	7.3 (2.1 to 25.0)	0/212	0.0 (0.0 to 3.6)	3/92	6.1 (1.1 to 33.9)	1/77	0.4 (0.0 to 6.1)
Pooled[d]			218/6225	142/1402	2.9 (2.1 to 4.1)	34/891	2.4 (1.4 to 4.1)	28/350	3.4 (8.1 to 5.2)	11/336	1.4 (0.8 to 2.5)

[a] Relative risks (RRs) adjusted at least by age and sex are *in italics*, otherwise crude RR (Wald 95 percent confidence intervals) were calculated.
[b] All types (mucosa-associated lymphoid tissue, splenic and nodal) included.
[c] NHL expected.
[d] Studies for which RR = 0 (variance could not be computed) were excluded.

Table 8.4 Relative risk (RR)[a] estimates and corresponding 95 percent confidence intervals (CI) of chronic lymphocytic leukemia/small lymphocytic lymphoma (CLL/SLL), multiple myeloma (MM), and Hodgkin lymphoma (HL) according to hepatitis C virus (HCV) infection status in case–control and cohort studies

First author	Year	Country	Controls HCV+/HCV–	CLL/SLL		MM		HL	
				HCV+/HCV–	RR (95% CI)	HCV+/HCV–	RR(95% CI)	HCV+/HCV–	RR (95% CI)
Case–control studies									
Montella[18]	2001	Italy	17/209	–	–	13/28	4.5 (1.9 to 11)	5/58	1.9 (0.6 to 6.3)
Bianco[22]	2004	Italy	22/374	11/107	1.8 (0.8 to 3.7)	5/102	0.6 (0.2 to 1.8)	5/152	1.2 (0.6 to 3.3)
Engels[24]	2004	USA	14/670	2/89	1.1 (0.3 to 3.5)	–	–	–	–
Morton[25]	2004	USA	5/529	1/43	2.5 (0.3 to 23)	–	–	–	–
Dal Maso[39]	2004	Italy	45/459	–	–	–	–	1/61	0.9 (0.1 to 7.2)
Nieters[28]	2006	Europe	41/1747	10/332	1.2 (0.6 to 2.4)	7/214	1.4 (0.6 to 3.2)	3/236	1.0 (0.3 to 3.5)
Cohort studies									
Rabkin[32]	2002	USA	0/95	–	–	0/24	–	–	–
Duberg[33]	2005	Sweden	–	4[b]	1.9 (0.5 to 5.0)	7[b]	2.4 (1.0 to 5.0)	–	–
Pooled[c]					1.5 (1.0 to 2.3)		1.7 (0.8 to 3.7)		1.3 (0.7 to 2.4)

[a]Relative risks (RRs) adjusted at least by age and sex are in italics; otherwise crude RR (Wald 95 percent confidence intervals) were calculated.
[b]Observed cases.
[c]Studies for which RR=0 (variance could not be computed) were excluded.

Table 8.5   Relative risk (RR)[a] estimates and corresponding 95 percent confidence intervals (CIs) of non-Hodgkin lymphoma according to markers of hepatitis B virus (HBV) infection

| First author | Year | Country | HBV marker | Positive/negative | | RR (95% CI) |
				Cases	Controls	
Pioltelli[17]	2000	Italy	HBsAg	23/277	14/833	4.9 (2.5 to 9.7)
Kim[20]	2002	South Korea	HBsAg	28/194	21/423	*3.9* (1.9 to 7.9)
			Anti-HBsAg	131/91	282/162	0.8 (0.6 to 1.2)
Talamini[27]	2004	Italy	HBsAg	8/157	4/341	*4.1*[b] (1.2 to 14.4)
			Anti-HBsAg	45/157	118/341	*0.8*[b] (0.6 to 1.3)
Pooled			HBsAg	59/628	42/1597	4.4 (2.8 to 6.9)

[a]Relative risks (RRs) adjusted at least by age and sex are *in italics*; elsewhere crude RR (Wald 95 percent confidence intervals) were calculated.
[b]Compared to anti-HbsAg negative.
HBsAg = HBV surface antigen.

A direct oncogenic role of HCV through B cell infection and deregulation has been hypothesized as the virus is lymphotropic.[43] However, only a small subset of the neoplastic cells in HCV-associated NHL harbor the viral genome or viral proteins, whereas these are frequently found in the stromal cells that surround the neoplastic ones.[44] It is therefore more likely that neoplastic transformation is causally linked to the chronic antigen stimulation (indirect effect) of B cells by HCV.[7] Immunoglobulin variable region genes expressed by B NHL cells from HCV-positive patients have been shown to exhibit somatic mutations indicative of an antigen-selection process.[45] Moreover, the histologic type of the majority of B NHL cells from HCV-positive patients is typical of germinal center and post germinal center B NHLs, again suggesting that lymphomagenesis occurs when B cells proliferate in response to a virus-associated antigen.[21,44] Notably, the sequences of B cell receptors in HCV-associated lymphoproliferations show a certain similarity with anti-HCV antibodies.[45]

Six distinct but related HCV genotypes and multiple subtypes have been identified.[6] In the USA and western Europe genotypes 1a and 1b are the most common, followed by genotypes 2 and 3. Other genotypes are rare in the USA and western Europe, but common in other areas, such as Egypt (genotype 4), South Africa (genotype 5), and southeast Asia (genotype 6). Knowledge of the genotype is important because it has been shown to have a predictive value in terms of the response to antiviral therapy in HCV-positive patients with chronic hepatitis.[6] However, no consistent difference in excess risk for NHL emerged between different genotypes in most of the studies.[14,19,21,27,28]

Summary of results on hepatitis virus infection and non-Hodgkin lymphoma

In summary, high prevalence was found in southern and eastern Europe and Japan, whereas very few HCV-positive individuals were found in Central and northern Europe.[8]

The highest prevalence so far (over 20 percent) has been reported in some areas of Egypt, probably related to mass use of intramuscular treatment of schistosomiasis.[8] Substantial variation in the prevalence of HCV positivity was also reported in case series of NHL in certain countries and world regions, e.g. Turkey, Asian countries other than Japan and North America.[8] Furthermore, despite the limitations of the information on the incidence and prevalence of HCV in different parts of the world, data on the incidence of hepatocellular carcinoma in different birth cohorts suggested that the spread of HCV might have occurred earlier in southern Europe and Japan than in the USA.

The prevalence of HCV infection among cancer-free subjects in the studies included in the present review (Table 8.1) reflects, therefore, the wide variations in HCV prevalence worldwide.

In HCV-endemic areas, high prevalence of infection among NHL patients may be found, even if no real association exists, and the choice of an appropriate control group is essential to providing an unbiased RR. Conversely, in countries where the prevalence of HCV is very low, or has only increased very recently, a moderate association between HCV and NHL can be undetectable in relatively small studies. Indeed, the association between HCV infection and NHL is not a strong one. The likeliest estimate of the RR of NHL among HCV-positive subjects, compared to HCV-negative ones, is between two and three. The strict inclusion criteria that we adopted in our present review may explain why our present estimates of the association between NHL and HCV tended to be lower than in previous reviews,[10,11] where, for instance, adjustment for age was not always required.[11]

In terms of attributable risks,[46] assuming an RR of 2, the fraction of NHL attributable to HCV infection would be more than 10 percent in a country such as Italy, where approximately 20 percent of NHL cases were found to be HCV positive.[27] In a country where the prevalence of HCV infection in the general population is 1 percent, the proportion of NHL attributable to HCV infection would be less than 1 percent; thus, it could have easily been missed in studies including a few hundred NHL cases.

Bias could have somewhat affected our present findings. Publication bias may have inflated the prevalence of HCV positivity in the NHL case series, and the RR estimates in early case–control studies.[8] The reactivation of HCV infection due to lymphoma-related immune suppression may account, at least in part, for the high HCV positivity found among lymphoma patients. However, reactivation of HCV infection has been reported after cytotoxic treatment,[20,27] but not in untreated HIV-negative NHL patients, who were included in some recent case–control studies.[21,27] Another potential problem is confounding. Several viruses are known to be involved in the etiopathogenesis of lymphomas[47] and others, not yet identified, may also be implicated. It is, therefore, conceivable that HCV may be a marker of some other unknown virus that uses the same transmission route as HCV and may constitute the real cause of NHL, regardless of HCV status. Finally, the definition for HCV infection is not totally consistent across studies. Some studies defined positivity as positivity for HCV antibodies only,[20] others as positivity for both HCV antibodies and HCV RNA,[23] while the majority classified as positive all individuals who were positive for either marker.[19,24,25,27,28]

Independent support to the role of HCV infection in a fraction of B NHL comes from the observation that regression of splenic lymphoma with villous lymphocytes could be achieved by treating HCV infection with interferon α and ribavirina.[48] The treatment of HCV with interferon α also resulted in remission of the lymphoma in one patient with immunocytoma[49] and of monoclonal B cell expansion in patients with mixed cryoglobulin.[50] In conclusion, HCV infection may be associated with an approximately two-fold increase in risk of B NHL, and the etiologic fraction of the disease attributable to HCV may be 10–15 percent in areas where HCV prevalence is high, and it is much smaller than in other areas. As only three case–control studies are available on the topic, no conclusion can be drawn on the involvement of HBV in lymphomagenesis.

HELICOBACTER PYLORI

H. pylori is a bacterium that infects the human gastric mucosa. The prevalence of H. pylori is strongly correlated to socioeconomic conditions, and is higher than 80 percent in middle-aged adults in many developing countries, compared with 20 percent in developed countries.[51] H. pylori infection in adults is usually chronic and does not heal without specific antimicrobial treatment.[51] H. pylori causes continuous gastric inflammation in virtually all infected individuals and induces a vigorous humoral and cellular immune response that contributes to tissue damage. Duodenal ulcer, gastric carcinoma and lymphoma (mucosa-associated lymphoid tissue, MALT NHL)

are among the possible long-term outcomes of H. pylori infection.

Here we summarize the epidemiological evidence of the association between H. pylori and lymphomas, in particular those originating from the stomach.

Association between *Helicobacter pylori* and lymphomas

The first large study to address the evaluation of H. pylori as a risk factor for gastric NHL was a case–control study nested in two large cohort studies[52] (Table 8.6). Between 1964 and 1991, approximately 300 000 people participating in various health screening programs were enrolled in the USA and Norway. Cancer cases diagnosed through 1991 were identified by record linkage to the respective cancer registries.

A total of 33 histologically confirmed gastric NHL and 31 non-gastric NHL (for comparative purposes) were identified and corresponding blood samples were tested for anti-H. pylori antibodies. For gastric NHL, approximately four controls were matched by date of birth, sex, date, and blood collection site. Control patients from the USA were matched to cases also by racial or ethnic group. For non-gastric NHL, approximately two controls were selected using the same matching criteria as for gastric NHL. H. pylori prevalence, tested by ELISA, was 85 percent and 65 percent in gastric and non-gastric NHL, respectively, compared to 55 percent and 59 percent in the two control groups. Thus, strong evidence emerged from this study of an association between H. pylori and gastric NHL (OR 6.3, 95 percent CI 2.0 to 19.9), but not for other NHLs (OR 1.2). The fraction of gastric NHL attributable to H. pylori in this population was 66 percent.

These findings were consistently reproduced by other studies. A case–control study conducted in Finland (see later in the chapter) to investigate the association between chlamydia infections and malignant lymphomas[53] confirmed that H. pylori-positivity is not associated (OR 0.8) with NHL or HL, of which gastric lymphoma would have constituted a very small fraction.

Xue et al.[54] conducted a meta-analysis of Chinese studies on the association between H. pylori, NHL and gastric cancer. Three case–control studies included totally 83 lymphomas of the stomach and 143 controls. The overall H. pylori prevalence was 88 percent among cases and 56 percent among controls (OR 5.7, 95 percent CI 2.7 to 12.0).

The large multicenter case–control study conducted in Spain evaluated the association between H. pylori and a large spectrum of lymphoma subtypes,[55] including 439 B NHL, 39 T cell NHL and 58 HL. Anti-H. pylori antibodies were found in 69 percent of all cases and 71 percent of controls and were not associated with an increased lymphoma risk. RRs were similar for B NHL, T cell NHL and HL (0.9, 0.7, and 0.8, respectively), and for nodal and extranodal lymphomas (OR 0.9 and 0.7, respectively). However, all four MALT lymphomas of the stomach, and

Table 8.6 Relative risk (RR)[a] estimates and corresponding 95% confidence intervals (CIs) of non-Hodgkin Lymphoma (NHL) according to *Helicobacter pylori* infection status

First author	Year	Country	Type of control	Type of case	H. pylori+ (%)/H. pylori– Cases	Controls	RR (95% CI)
Cohort studies							
Parsonnet[52]	1994	USA	Matched	Gastric NHL	28(85)/5	74/60	6.3 (2.0 to 19.9)
				Other NHL	20(65)/11	36/25	1.2 (0.5 to 3.0)
Case–control studies							
Anttila[53]	1998	Finland	Matched (blood donors)	All NHL	25(53)/28	27/26	0.8 (0.4 to 1.9)
				HL	4(21)/15	5/14	0.8 (0.2 to 3.4)
Xue[54]	2001	China	Not specified	Gastric NHL	73(88)/10	80/63	5.7 (2.7 to 12.0)
de Sanjosé[55]	2004	Spain	Hospital controls	B cell NHL	307(70)/122	430/173	*0.9* (0.7 to 1.1)
				T cell NHL	307(67)/122	430/173	*0.7* (0.4 to 1.5)
				HL	34(59)/24	430/173	*0.8* (0.5 to 1.5)

[a]Relative risks (RRs) adjusted at least by age and sex are in italics; elsewhere crude RR (Wald 95 percent confidence intervals) were calculated.
[b]Meta analyses of three case–control studies.
HL, Hodgkin lymphoma.

all 10 lymphomas of the stomach of other histological types, were *H. pylori* positive.

In conclusion, the association between *H. pylori* infection and gastric NHL is well established and entails an approximately sixfold increased risk. Contrary to HCV infection, which is associated with a broad spectrum of lymphomas, the association with *H. pylori* is restricted to gastric NHL, particularly gastric MALT, while *H. pylori* does not appear to be associated to any other hemolymphopoietic neoplasms.

Pathogenesis of gastric MALT lymphoma and effect of *H. pylori* eradication on MALT lymphoma

The role of *H. pylori* infection in the development of gastric MALT lymphoma is relatively well understood.[56] Bacterial colonization of the gastric mucosa by *H. pylori* triggers lymphoid infiltration and the formation of MALT. The bacterial infection induces and sustains an actively proliferating B cell population through direct (autoantigen) and indirect (intratumoral T cells specific for *H. pylori*) immunologic stimulation. Moreover, the bacterial infection provokes a neutrophilic response, which causes the release of oxygen free radicals. These reactive species may promote the acquisition of genetic abnormalities and malignant transformation of reactive B lymphocytes. A transformed clone carrying the translocation t(11;18)(q21;q21) can give origin to MALT lymphoma.[56]

Malignant clones without t(11;18)(q21;q21), but with other genetic abnormalities, such as trisomy 3 or microsatellite instability, depend critically on immune stimulation mediated by *H. pylori* for their expansion. In its early stages, the tumor can be successfully treated by eradication of the bacterium, whereas at later stages the tumor may escape its

H. pylori dependency through acquisition of additional genetic abnormalities. Finally, further genetic abnormalities, such as inactivation of the tumor suppressor genes *TP53* and *TP16*, can lead to high-grade transformation.[56]

The observations that gastric MALT lymphoma is strongly associated with *H. pylori* infection and that tumor-cell growth can be actively stimulated *in vitro* by the bacterium via T cells has led to many clinical investigations examining the effect of *H. pylori* eradication on tumor control.[57]

Over 70 percent of patients with gastric MALT lymphoma can achieve complete remission after *H. pylori* eradication.[56] In 50 percent of patients, the tumor clone can be detected by PCR clonality analysis on material obtained from post-remission biopsy samples, even though no histologic tumor lesion is detectable. The monoclonal tumor cell population decreases during long-term follow-up. Relapse after complete remission occurs in less than 10 percent of cases, and it is unclear whether this is caused by *H. pylori* reinfection. In cases of *H. pylori* reinfection, the tumor can again be cured by the eradication of the organism. In the absence of *H. pylori*, relapse is frequently a transient self-limiting event.[56,58]

Conversely, the role of *H. pylori* eradication in the treatment of *de novo* DLBC gastric lymphomas, or DLBC that evolved from MALT lymphoma, is less clear than for MALT. Most studies reported a complete remission of more than half DLBC after *H. pylori* eradication. However, as very few patients (<20) were included in each study and the follow-up was less than 3 years, the value of *H. pylori* eradication as a treatment modality in these cases remains to be definitively established.[57]

In conclusion, *H. pylori* eradication alone was demonstrated as an effective therapy for gastric MALT lymphoma and, possibly, for other gastric lymphomas associated with *H. pylori*.[56,57] The success of *H. pylori* eradication in the

Table 8.7　Prevalence of *Borrelia burgdorferi* and relative risk (RR)[a] estimates with corresponding 95 percent confidence intervals (CIs) of non-Hodgkin lymphoma (NHL)

First author	Year	Country	Type of cases	Type of controls	Positive (%)/negative Cases	Controls	Crude RR (95% CI)
Case series							
Cerroni[63]	1997	Austria	Cutaneous B NHL	–	9(18)/41	–	–
Wood[64]	2001	USA	Cutaneous B NHL	–	0(0)/38	–	–
Li[65]	2003	Taiwan	Cutaneous marginal zone B NHL	–	0(0)/24	–	–
Case–control studies							
Jelic[62]	1999	Yugoslavia	Cutaneous B NHL	Blood donors	12(55)/10	2/58	34.8 (6.7 to 179)
			Cutaneous T NHL	Blood donors	0(0)/10	2/58	0.0 (0.0 to 12.3)
			Other B NHL	Blood donors	4(5)/71	2/58	1.6 (0.3 to 9.2)
Goodlad[61]	2000	Scotland	Cutaneous B NHL	Melanoma patients[b]	7(35)/13	1(5)/19 }	21.0 (2.4 to 187)
				Dermatosis		0(0)/20 }	

[a] Wald 95 percent CIs were calculated.
[b] Controls matched to cases by age and sex.
B NHL, B cell NHL; T NHL, T cell NHL.

treatment of gastric MALT has created great hopes that the knowledge on the association between infectious agents and lymphomas may be exploited not only for prevention, but also for the treatment of lymphomas.

BORRELIA BURGDORFERI AND CUTANEOUS LYMPHOMAS

Lyme borreliosis is a multiorgan infection caused by tick-borne spirochetes of the *Borrelia burgdorferi* sensu lato. Using phylogenetic studies, *B. burgdorferi* can be subdivided into multiple genospecies (i.e. *B. burgdorferi* sensu stricto, *B. garinii* and *B. afzelii*) with different distribution worldwide.[59]

Common skin manifestations of Lyme borreliosis include erythema migrans, acrodermatitis chronica atrophicans, and lymphocytoma, a benign B cell lymphoproliferative process.[59] A few reports have suggested a positive association between *B. burgdorferi* and primary cutaneous B NHL (PCB NHL).[60]

Results on prevalence of *B. burgdorferi* in PCB NHL or other NHL subtypes in studies reporting at least 20 cases are presented in Table 8.7. In two studies[61,62] a comparison group was included. In a series of 50 PCB NHL, Cerroni *et al.*[63] identified DNA sequences for *B. burgdorferi* in 18 percent of cases, compared with a reported prevalence of 15 percent in the *B. burgdorferi*-endemic region in Austria, where the study had been carried out.

In two additional PCB NHL case series from different areas of the USA (38 cases)[64] and from Taiwan (24 cases),[65] no *B. burgdorferi*-specific DNA was detected in any PCB NHL cases. Jelic and colleagues[62] collected the largest series of PCB NHL in former Yugoslavia. They reported a high

proportion (55 percent) of antibody positivity for *B. burgdorferi* among PCB NHL cases (12/22), while the prevalence was 0 percent (10 cases) for T NHL, and 5 percent (4/75) for other B NHL. The excess risk of *B. burgdorferi*-positive PCB NHL was 35-fold using, as a control group, 30 breast cancer patients and 60 blood donors, whose *B. burgdorferi*-prevalence was 4 percent.

Goodlad *et al.*[61] conducted their case–control study in Scotland between 1978 and 1998. It included 20 PCB NHL and a control group of 40 age- and sex-matched patients, 20 with melanoma and 20 with inflammatory dermatosis. *B. burgdorferi* DNA, detected by nested PCR assay, was present in seven (35 percent) of PCB NHL compared to one (2.5 percent) control. The corresponding RR was 21.0 (95 percent CI 2.4 to 187).

Some caveats are needed in the interpretation of the findings on *B. burgdorferi* and PCB NHL. First, no clear ecological association has been found between incidence of Lyme disease and that of PCB NHL in the USA.[66] In addition, the distinction between PCB NHL and B cell lymphocytoma, that is clearly related to *B. burgdorferi* infections, is difficult[67] and may produce histologic misclassification between benign and malignant lymphoid neoplasms.

In conclusion, an association between *B. burgdorferi* and PCB NHL may exist in areas with high prevalence of Lyme borreliosis. However, the fraction of PCB NHL attributable to *B. burgdorferi* seems to be negligible.

CHLAMYDIA INFECTIONS AND LYMPHOMAS

Chlamydiae are obligate intracellular bacteria and are responsible for a wide spectrum of human diseases including respiratory, genital and ocular diseases.[49] They have a tendency to cause persistent infections. Some studies have suggested that *Chlamydia trachomatis* may contribute with human papillomavirus to the development of cervical cancer[68] and *C. pneumoniae* to lung cancer.[69] *C. psittaci* is the cause of psittacosis, a human lung infection caused by exposure to infected birds.

The first study that suggested an association between *C. trachomatis* infection and malignant lymphomas was a case–control study conducted in Finland.[53] Cases were subjects aged between 19 and 74 years (mean 53) with HL (19 cases) or NHL (53 cases). Controls were 72 healthy blood donors matched by age ($\pm$1 year), sex, residence, and time of sample collection.

Sera were screened for specific IgG antibodies against *C. pneumoniae* and *C. trachomatis* by micro-immunofluorescence (MIF) and ELISA. Immune complexes, markers of chronic infection, were also analyzed by MIF and ELISA.

Two-thirds of lymphoma cases and three-quarters of controls had IgG antibodies against *C. pneumoniae*, as determined by MIF. The ELISA test provided comparable results for *C. pneumoniae* but not for *C. trachomatis*. Antibodies against *C. trachomatis* were found in 10 percent and 42 percent of cases, and 6 percent and 22 percent of controls, respectively using MIF or ELISA.

C. pneumoniae-specific immune complexes were demonstrated in 63 percent of cases and 21 percent of controls, and corresponding *C. trachomatis* immune complexes in 20 percent of cases and in 2 percent of controls, using ELISA. The corresponding risk increase for lymphomas was 10-fold for both types of chlamydia-positive patients. The risk was nonsignificantly higher in men than women, and for HL compared to NHL.

Another study explored the association between chlamydia infections and the rare lymphoma of the ocular adnexa in Italy.[70] The presence of DNA of *C. pneumoniae*, *C. trachomatis* and *C. psittaci* was investigated among 40 histologically proven NHL of the ocular adnexa. Polymerase chain reaction assay was performed in tissue and peripheral blood mononuclear cell samples. None of the samples were positive for *C. pneumoniae* or *C. trachomatis*, while 32 (80 percent) of the 40 cases were positive for *C. psittaci*. Of 46 control subjects (20 with non-neoplastic conjunctival/orbital diseases and 26 with reactive lymphoadenopathies), only three (7 percent) were *C. psittaci* DNA-positive, leading to an unadjusted 50-fold increased risk. The study also showed evidence of lymphoma regression after *C. psittaci* eradication with doxycycline treatment. Ferreri *et al.*[70] therefore suggest yet another link between a chronic infection and a specific type of lymphoma at the same site (i.e. the ocular adnexa).

In conclusion, the involvement of some species of Chlamydiae in the development of at least some types of lymphomas probably exists. Thus, a very small proportion of lymphomas (<1 percent) may be attributable to chlamydial bacteria.

Shortly before the publication of the present chapter, the International Agency for Research on Cancer Monograph Working Group reported that sufficient evidence is available to conclude that chronic infection with HCV can cause non-Hodgkin lymphoma, especially B cell lymphoma.[71]

KEY POINTS

- HCV infection is associated with approximately a twofold to threefold increase in risk of B NHL and the etiologic fraction of the disease attributable to HCV may be 10–15 percent in areas where HCV infection is frequent, although much smaller in areas where HCV infection is rare. An association between all NHL and HbsAg positivity (i.e. chronic HBV-infection) has also been suggested by a few studies.
- No significant heterogeneity emerged in the association between HCV and major B NHL subtypes or by primary site (nodal/extranodal).
- It is unclear whether HCV infection is also associated with T cell NHL, multiple myeloma and CLL/SLL. No significant associations emerged for HL.
- The risk of gastric MALT lymphomas is approximately sixfold higher in individuals seropositive for *H. pylori* and pathogenetic studies demonstrated the role of *H. pylori* infection in the development of chronic gastritis and gastric MALT lymphoma. However, *H. pylori* does not appear to be associated with haemolymphopoietic neoplasms outside the stomach.
- *H. pylori* eradication is an effective therapy for gastric MALT lymphoma and, possibly, for other gastric lymphomas.
- The majority of PCB NHL arise through a pathway unrelated to *B. burgdorferi*. However, some PCB NHL responded to antibiotic therapy designed to treat *B. burgdorferi* infection.
- An association between *C. psittaci* and ocular adnexal lymphomas (able to regress after chlamydia eradication) has been recently suggested.
- A close relationship between certain infections and NHL types is proved and may have important implications for the prevention and treatment of a fraction of lymphomas.

ACKNOWLEDGMENTS

Financial support: Grant 20 G.3 from the Istituto Superiore di Sanità, Rome, Italy and grant from AIRC (Italian Association for Cancer Research). Grant from Oncosuisse (ICP OCS–01355–03–2003). The authors wish to thank Dr M Libra for useful comments and Mrs L Mei and T Perdrix-Thoma for editorial assistance.

REFERENCES

● = Key primary paper
◆ = Major review article

◆1. Jaffe ES, Harris NL, Stein H, Vardiman J. (eds) *World Health Organization classification of tumours: pathology and genetics of tumours of haematopoietic and lymphoid tissues.* Lyon: IARC Press, 2001.

◆2. Fisher SG, Fisher RI. The epidemiology of non-Hodgkin's lymphoma. *Oncogene* 2004; **23**: 6524–34.

3. Muller AM, Ihorst G, Mertelsmann R, Engelhardt M. Epidemiology of non-Hodgkin's lymphoma (NHL): trends, geographic distribution, and etiology. *Ann Hematol* 2005; **84**: 1–12.

◆4. Engels EA. Infections agents as causes of non-Hodgkin lymphoma. *Cancer Epidemiol Biomarkers Prev* 2007; **16**: 401–4.

5. Poynard T, Yuen MF, Ratziu V, Lai CL. Viral hepatitis C. *Lancet* 2003; **362**: 2095–100.

6. Lauer GM, Walker BD. Hepatitis C virus infection. *N Engl J Med* 2001; **345**: 41–52.

◆7. Gasparotto D, De Re V, Boiocchi M. Hepatitis C virus, B-cell proliferation and lymphomas. *Leuk Lymphoma* 2002; **43**: 747–51.

◆8. Negri E, Little D, Boiocchi M *et al.* B-cell non-Hodgkin's lymphoma and hepatitis C virus infection: a systematic review. *Int J Cancer* 2004; **111**: 1–8.

9. Lai CL, Ratziu V, Yuen MF, Poynard T. Viral hepatitis B. *Lancet* 2003; **362**: 2089–94.

10. Gisbert JP, Garcia-Buey L, Pajares JM, Moreno-Otero R. Prevalence of hepatitis C virus infection in B-cell non-Hodgkin's lymphoma: systematic review and meta-analysis. *Gastroenterology* 2003; **125**: 1723–32.

11. Matsuo K, Kusano A, Sugumar A *et al.* Effect of hepatitis C virus infection on the risk of non-Hodgkin's lymphoma: a meta-analysis of epidemiological studies. *Cancer Sci* 2004; **95**: 745–52.

◆12. Dal Maso L, Franceschi S. Hepatitis C virus and risk of lymphoma and other lymphoid neoplasms: a meta-analysis of epidemiologic studies. *Cancer Epidemiol Biomarkers Prev* 2006; **15**: 2078–85.

13. Breslow NE, Day NE. Statistical methods in cancer research, volume 1. The analysis of case–control studies. IARC scientific publication no 32. Lyon: International Agency for Research on Cancer, 1980.

14. Zuckerman E, Zuckerman T, Levine AM *et al.* Hepatitis C virus infection in patients with B-cell non-Hodgkin lymphoma. *Ann Intern Med* 1997; **127**: 423–8.

15. Vallisa D, Berté R, Rocca A *et al.* Association between hepatitis C virus and non-Hodgkin's lymphoma, and effects of viral infection on histologic subtype and clinical course. *Am J Med* 1999; **106**: 556–60.

16. Mizorogi F, Hiramoto J, Nozato A *et al.* Hepatitis C virus infection in patients with B-cell non-Hodgkin's lymphoma. *Intern Med* 2000; **39**: 112–17.

17. Pioltelli P, Gargantini L, Cassi E *et al.* Hepatitis C virus in non-Hodgkin's lymphoma. A reappraisal after a prospective case–control study of 300 patients. Lombart study group of HCV-lymphoma. *Am J Hematol* 2000; **64**: 95–100.

18. Montella M, Crispo A, Frigeri F *et al.* HCV and tumors correlated with immune system: a case–control study in an area of hyperendemicity. *Leuk Res* 2001; **25**: 775–81.

19. Imai Y, Ohsawa M, Tanaka H *et al.* High prevalence of HCV infection in patients with B-cell non-Hodgkin's lymphoma: comparison with birth cohort- and sex-matched blood donors in a Japanese population. *Hepatology* 2002; **35**: 974–6.

20. Kim JH, Bang YJ, Park BJ *et al.* Hepatitis B virus infection and B-cell non-Hodgkin's lymphoma in a hepatitis B endemic area: a case–control study. *Jpn J Cancer Res* 2002; **93**: 471–7.

21. Mele A, Pulsoni A, Bianco E *et al.* Hepatitis C virus and B-cell non-Hodgkin lymphomas: an Italian multicenter case–control study. *Blood* 2003; **102**: 996–9.

22. Bianco E, Marcucci F, Mele A *et al.* Prevalence of hepatitis C virus infection in lymphoproliferative diseases other than B-cell non-Hodgkin's lymphoma, and in myeloproliferative diseases: an Italian multi-center case–control study. *Haematologica* 2004; **89**: 70–6.

23. Cowgill KD, Loffredo CA, Eissa SA *et al.* Case–control study of non-Hodgkin's lymphoma and hepatitis C virus infection in Egypt. *Int J Epidemiol* 2004; **33**: 1034–9.

24. Engels EA, Chatterjee N, Cerhan JR *et al.* Hepatitis C virus infection and non-Hodgkin lymphoma: results of the NCI-SEER multi-center case–control study. *Int J Cancer* 2004; **111**: 76–80.

25. Morton L, Engels EA, Holford TR *et al.* Hepatitis C virus and risk of non-Hodgkin lymphoma: a population-based case–control study among Connecticut women. *Cancer Epidemiol Biomarkers Prev* 2004; **13**: 425–30.

26. Seve P, Renaudier P, Sasco AJ *et al.* Hepatitis C virus infection and B-cell non-Hodgkin's lymphoma: a cross-sectional study in Lyon, France. *Eur J Gastroenterol Hepatol* 2004; **16**: 1361–5.

27. Talamini R, Montella M, Crovatto M *et al.* Non-Hodgkin's lymphoma and hepatitis C virus: a case–control study from northern and southern Italy. *Int J Cancer* 2004; **110**: 380–5.

28. Nieters A, Kallinowski B, Brennan P *et al.* Hepatitis C and risk of lymphoma: results of the European multicenter case–control study EPILYMPH. *Gastroenterology* 2006; **131**: 1879–86.

29. Vajdic CM, Grulich AE, Caldor JM *et al.* Specific infections, infection-related behavior, and risk of non-Hodgkin lymphoma in adults. *Cancer Epidemiol Biomarkers Prev* 2006; **15**: 1102–8.

30. Spinelli JJ, Lai AS, Krajden M *et al.* Hepatitis C virus and risk of non-Hodgkin lymphoma in British Columbia, Canada. *Int J Cancer* 2008; **122**: 630–3.

31. Ohsawa M, Shingu N, Miwa H *et al.* Risk of non-Hodgkin's lymphoma in patients with hepatitis C virus infection. *Int J Cancer* 1999; **80**: 237–9.

32. Rabkin CS, Tess BH, Christianson RE *et al.* Prospective study of hepatitis C viral infection as a risk factor for subsequent B-cell neoplasia. *Blood* 2002; **99**: 4240–2.

33. Duberg AS, Nordstrom M, Torner A *et al.* Non-Hodgkin's lymphoma and other nonhepatic malignancies in Swedish patients with hepatitis C virus infection. *Hepatology* 2005; **41**: 652–9.

34. Franceschi S, Polesel J, Rickenbach M *et al.* Hepatitis C virus and non-Hodgkin's lymphoma: findings from the Swiss HIV Cohort Study. *Br J Cancer* 2006; **95**: 1598–602.

35. Amin J, Dore GJ, O'Connell DL *et al.* Cancer incidence in people with hepatitis B or C infection: a large community-based linkage study. *J Hepatol* 2006; **45**: 197–203.

36. Giordano TP, Henderson L, Landgren O *et al.* Risk of non-Hodgkin lymphoma and lymphoproliferative precursor diseases in US veterans with hepatitis C virus. *JAMA* 2007; **297**: 2010–17.

37. Gentile G, Mele A, Monarco B *et al.* Hepatitis B and C viruses, human T-cell lymphotropic virus types I and II, and leukemias: a case–control study. The Italian leukemia study group. *Cancer Epidemiol Biomarkers Prev* 1996; **5**: 227–30.

38. Normand SL. Meta-analysis: formulating, evaluating, combining, and reporting. *Stat Med* 1999; **18**: 321–59.

39. Dal Maso L, Talamini R, Montella M *et al.* Hepatitis B and C viruses and Hodgkin lymphoma: a case–control study from northern and southern Italy. *Haematologica* 2004; **89**: ELT17.

40. De Vita S, Zagonel V, Russo A *et al.* Hepatitis C virus, non-Hodgkin's lymphomas and hepatocellular carcinoma. *Br J Cancer* 1998; **77**: 2032–5.

41. Izumi T, Sasaki R, Miura Y, Okamoto H. Primary hepatosplenic lymphoma: association with hepatitis C virus infection. *Blood* 1996; **87**: 5380–1.

42. Lavanchy D. Hepatitis B virus epidemiology, disease burden, treatment, and current and emerging prevention and control measures. *J Viral Hepat* 2004; **11**: 97–107.

43. Sung VM, Shimodaira S, Doughty AL *et al.* Establishment of B-cell lymphoma cell lines persistently infected with hepatitis C virus *in vivo* and *in vitro*: the apoptotic effects of virus infection. *J Virol* 2003; **77**: 2134–46.

44. Sansonno D, De Vita S, Cornacchiulo V *et al.* Detection and distribution of hepatitis C virus-related proteins in lymph nodes of patients with type II mixed cryoglobulinemia and neoplastic or non-neoplastic lymphoproliferation. *Blood* 1996; **88**: 4638–45.

45. De Re V, De Vita S, Marzotto A *et al.* Pre-malignant and malignant lymphoproliferations in an HCV-infected type II mixed cryoglobulinemic patient are sequential phases of an antigen-driven pathological process. *Int J Cancer* 2000; **87**: 211–16.

46. Bruzzi P, Green SB, Byar DP *et al.* Estimating the population attributable risk for multiple risk factors using case–control data. *Am J Epidemiol* 1985; **122**: 904–14.

47. Pagano JS. Viruses and lymphomas. *N Engl J Med* 2002; **347**: 78–9.

48. Hermine O, Lefrere F, Bronowicki JP *et al.* Regression of splenic lymphoma with villous lymphocytes after treatment of hepatitis C virus infection. *N Engl J Med* 2002; **347**: 89–94.

49. Patriarca F, Silvestri F, Fanin R *et al.* Long-lasting complete remission of hepatitis C virus (HCV) infection and HCV-associated immunocytoma with alpha-interferon treatment. *Br J Haematol* 2001; **112**: 370–2.

50. Mazzaro C, Franzin F, Tulissi P *et al.* Regression of monoclonal B-cell expansion in patients affected by mixed cryoglobulinemia responsive to alpha-interferon therapy. *Cancer* 1996; **77**: 2604–13.

51. Suerbaum S, Michetti P. *Helicobacter pylori* infection. *N Engl J Med* 2002; **347**: 1175–86.

●52. Parsonnet J, Hansen S, Rodriguez L *et al.* *Helicobacter pylori* infection and gastric lymphoma. *N Engl J Med* 1994; **330**: 1267–71.

53. Anttila TI, Lehtinen T, Leinonen M *et al.* Serological evidence of an association between chlamydial infections and malignant lymphomas. *Br J Haematol* 1998; **103**: 150–6.

54. Xue FB, Xu YY, Wan Y *et al.* Association of *H. pylori* infection with gastric carcinoma: a meta analysis. *World J Gastroenterol* 2001; **7**: 801–4.

55. de Sanjosé S, Dickie A, Alvaro T *et al.* Helicobacter pylori and malignant lymphoma in Spain. *Cancer Epidemiol Biomarkers Prev* 2004; **13**: 944–8.

◆56. Du MQ, Isaccson PG. Gastric MALT lymphoma: from aetiology to treatment. *Lancet Oncol* 2002; **3**: 97–104.

◆57. Wündisch T, Kim TD, Thiede C *et al.* Etiology and therapy of helicobacter pylori-associated gastric lymphomas. *Ann Hematol* 2003; **82**: 535–45.

58. Stolte M, Bayerdorffer E, Morgner A *et al.* Helicobacter and gastric MALT lymphoma. *Gut* 2002; **50** (Suppl 3): III19–24.

59. Hengge UR, Tannapfel A, Tyring SK *et al.* Lyme borreliosis. *Lancet Infect Dis* 2003; **3**: 489–500.

60. Slater DN. *Borrelia burgdorferi*-associated primary cutaneous B-cell lymphoma. *Histopathology* 2001; **38**: 73–7.

61. Goodlad JR, Davidson MM, Hollowood K *et al.* Primary cutaneous B-cell lymphoma and *Borrelia burgdorferi* infection in patients from the Highlands of Scotland. *Am J Surg Pathol* 2000; **24**: 1279–85.

62. Jelic S, Filipovic-Ljeskovic I. Positive serology for Lyme disease borrelias in primary cutaneous B-cell lymphoma: a study in 22 patients; is it a fortuitous finding? *Hematol Oncol* 1999; **17**: 107–16.

63. Cerroni L, Zochling N, Putz B, Kerl H. Infection by *Borrelia burgdorferi* and cutaneous B-cell lymphoma. *J Cutan Pathol* 1997; **24**: 457–61.

64. Wood GS, Kamath NV, Guitart J *et al.* Absence of *Borrelia burgdorferi* DNA in cutaneous B-cell lymphomas from the United States. *J Cutan Pathol* 2001; **28**: 502–7.

65. Li C, Inagaki H, Kuo TT *et al.* Primary cutaneous marginal zone B-cell lymphoma: a molecular and clinicopathologic study of 24 Asian cases. *Am J Surg Pathol* 2003; **27**: 1061–9.

66. Munksgaard L, Frisch M, Melbye M, Hjalgrim H. Incidence patterns of Lyme disease and cutaneous B-cell non-Hodgkin's lymphoma in the United States. *Dermatology* 2000; **201**: 351–2.

67. Grange F, Wechsler J, Guillaume JC *et al.* Borrelia burgdorferi-associated lymphocytoma cutis simulating a primary cutaneous large B-cell lymphoma. *J Am Acad Dermatol* 2002; **47**: 530–4.

68. Smith JS, Bosetti C, Muñoz N *et al.* Chlamydia trachomatis and invasive cervical cancer: a pooled analysis of the IARC multicentric case–control study. *Int J Cancer* 2004; **111**: 431–9.

69. Littman AJ, Jackson LA, Vaughan TL. *Chlamydia pneumoniae* and lung cancer: epidemiologic evidence. *Cancer Epidemiol Biomarkers Prev* 2005; **14**: 773–8.

●70. Ferreri AJ, Guidoboni M, Ponzoni M *et al.* Evidence for an association between chlamydia psittaci and ocular adnexal lymphomas. *J Natl Cancer Inst* 2004; **96**: 586–94.

◆71. Bouvard V, Baan R, Stralf K *et al.* on behalf of the WHO International Agency for Research on Cancer Monograph Working Group. A review of human carcinogens – Part B: biological agents. *Lancet Oncol* 2009; **10**: 321–2.

IMMUNOBIOLOGY

PART 3

IMMUNOBIOLOGY

9

Overview of the immune system

RALF KÜPPERS

INTRODUCTION

The human body is constantly under threat to be colonized by infectious agents, in particular viruses, bacteria, and parasitic protozoans. While some of these are rather harmless, others can cause life-threatening diseases. During evolution, animals developed numerous specific defense mechanisms to be able to combat infectious agents. The simplest mechanisms involve physical barriers that prevent entry of pathogens into the body. These are the outer and inner epithelial layers of the body. A further layer of defense is provided by the production of substances that have toxic effects on infectious particles, such as the acidic condition in the stomach or bactericidal enzymes secreted into the saliva. However, these simple defense mechanisms are not sufficient to prevent life-threatening infections. A much more sophisticated defense system has evolved in vertebrates, the immune system. This system is most highly developed in mammals and involves numerous organs and cell types. Different arms and functions of the immune system can be distinguished for particular types of immune responses. Innate immune responses use a restricted set of receptors for pathogen recognition, whereas adaptive immune responses rely on antigen recognition by highly diverse antigen receptors on B and T lymphocytes. There are two types of adaptive immune responses. Cellular immune responses involve killing of pathogen-infected cells by cytotoxic T cells, whereas humoral immune responses are mediated through antibodies produced by B lymphocytes.

As lymphomas derive from B or T lymphocytes, this chapter is intended to give a brief introduction to the cells of the immune system, the organs involved, and the cellular interactions that play a role in immune responses. A more detailed description of lymphocytes and their functions and activities is provided in the following chapters of this book.

CELLS OF THE IMMUNE SYSTEM

All cells of the immune system derive from a common precursor, the hematopoietic stem cell, which itself is of mesenchymal origin. The hematopoietic stem cells give rise not only to the cells of the immune system, the leukocytes, but also to two other types of cells – the megakaryocytes and the erythrocytes. The main function of the megakaryocytes is the production of platelets, which are needed for blood clotting; erythrocytes are essential for the transport of oxygen from the lungs to all tissues of the body. The leukocytes, the white blood cells, can be distinguished into six main cell types: granulocytes, monocytes, dendritic cells, natural killer (NK) cells, B lymphocytes and T lymphocytes (Fig. 9.1). Granulocytes are further subdivided into

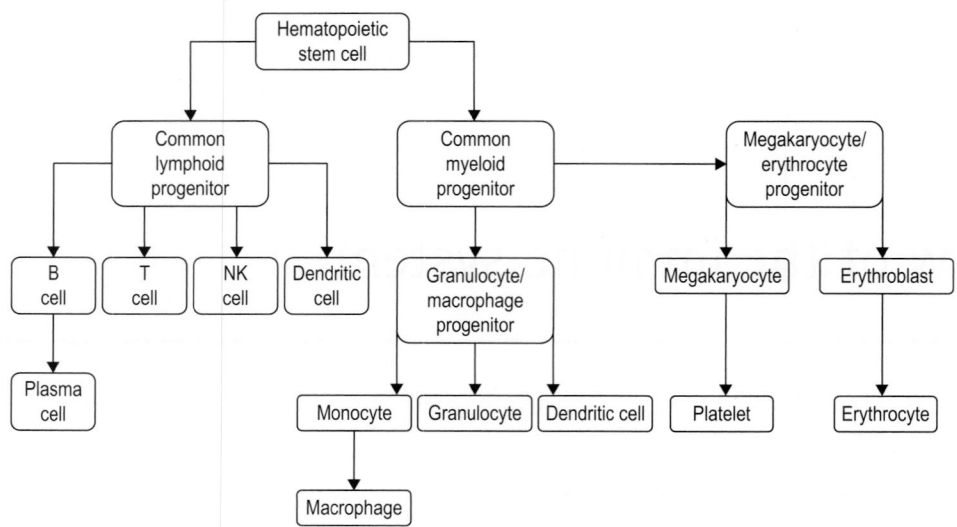

Figure 9.1   The hematopoietic system. Hematopoietic stem cells give rise to common lymphoid and common myeloid progenitors. B lymphocytes, T lymphocytes and natural killer (NK) cells develop from common lymphoid progenitors. Upon activation, B cells can further differentiate into antibody-secreting plasma cells. Common myeloid progenitors further differentiate into granulocyte/macrophage progenitors and megakaryocyte/erythrocyte progenitors. The former is the precursor of granulocytes and monocytes. Three types of granulocytes can be distinguished (not shown): neutrophils, eosinophils and basophils. In tissues, monocytes differentiate into macrophages. Dendritic cells can develop from lymphoid and myeloid precursors. The megakaryocyte/erythrocyte progenitor gives rise to megakaryocytes, from which platelets are produced, and erythroblasts, which differentiate further into erythrocytes.

neutrophils, basophils and eosinophils. These cells play an important role as a first line of defense, as we shall see later. Monocytes circulate through the blood and differentiate into macrophages when they enter tissues. The macrophages are phagocytic cells, as their name already indicates. They also function as antigen-presenting cells. Antigen presentation is also the main function of dendritic cells. Natural killer cells have the capacity to kill virus-infected cells and to some extent also cancer cells. B and T lymphocytes (also called B and T cells) express specific surface antigen receptors, which are somatically generated and highly diverse. Equipped with these antigen receptors, they can perform the most specific recognition and elimination of foreign antigens, and play an essential role for the generation of immunologic memory. If mature B cells are involved in immune responses, they can further differentiate either into long-lived memory B cells or they give rise to plasma cells, which are specialized in the production and secretion of large amounts of antibodies, a secreted form of the B cell antigen receptor, which is also called immunoglobulin (Ig). Also, T cells are subdivided into functionally diverse cell types. T helper (TH) cells are mainly involved in supporting and regulating immune responses involving B cells; cytotoxic T cells can directly kill target cells, such as virus-infected cells; and regulatory T cells play an important role in negatively regulating immune responses and preventing autoimmune diseases. The development of these various forms of leukocytes from hematopoietic stem cells occurs in a multistep differentiation process, involving intermediate precursor cells (Fig. 9.1). A myeloid precursor gives rise to monocytes, granulocytes and dendritic cells. A lymphoid precursor gives rise to NK cells, B cells, T cells and also dendritic cells.

ORGANS OF THE IMMUNE SYSTEM

The generation and function of cells of the immune system are linked to specific organs and histologic structures. The hematopoietic stem cells first reside in the liver during fetal development, but from around birth onward, these cells are found in the bone marrow, which is the main primary lymphoid organ. Most leukocytes differentiate into maturity in the bone marrow, the exception being T cells. T cell precursors migrate from the bone marrow into the thymus and undergo the final developmental processes of T cell differentiation in this organ, which hence also represents a primary lymphoid organ. Mature leukocytes leave the bone marrow (or thymus) and migrate through the body via the peripheral blood and the lymph. Some parts of immune responses take place directly at the site of entry of an infectious agent into the body, when leukocytes extravasate from the blood and enter tissues, as we will discuss below. Other arms of immune responses, in particular adaptive immune responses involving B and T cells, take place in specific organs of the immune system, the secondary lymphoid organs. These include lymph nodes, the spleen, the Peyer's patches of mucosal-associated lymphoid tissues (MALT), and the tonsils. The lymph nodes are histologically structured into areas rich in T cells (the

T cell zone) and B cell-rich areas (the B cell follicles). Cells can enter the lymph nodes through the blood or through afferent lymphatics. The spleen also harbors T cell areas, here called periarteriolar lymphoid sheaths (PALS), and B cell follicles. In addition, a B cell-rich marginal zone is found at sinus structures surrounding the B cell follicles, where the cells are in direct contact with the peripheral blood. A marginal zone stucture is also found in Peyer's patches. The lymphoid structures in the spleen together define the white pulp region, whereas in the large red pulp many erythrocytes are found, as in this region the turnover of erythrocytes takes place.

Organized lymphoid structures are usually confined to the primary and secondary lymphoid organs. However, in particular situations, such structures can also develop in extranodal sites. One of the best known examples is the induced lymphoid tissue in the submucosal area of the stomach as a consequence of persistent infection by *Helicobacter pylori*.[1] In addition, extranodal lymphoid infiltrates can develop in the course of certain autoimmune diseases. In rheumatoid arthritis, for example, follicular structures containing B cells, T cells, and dendritic cells can be found in the synovial tissue.[2]

INNATE IMMUNE RESPONSES

When infectious agents pass epithelial surfaces and enter the tissue, they usually first encounter macrophages, which are present in most tissues. Macrophages recognize conserved patterns of many viruses and bacteria by a limited set of pattern-recognition receptors. An important family of such receptors is the Toll-like receptors (TLR), of which eleven have been identified so far.[3] TLR4, for example, recognizes lipopolysaccharides (LPS), which are cell-wall components of many encapsulated bacteria. TLR9 recognizes unmethylated CpG dinucleotides, which are found in viral and bacterial DNA, whereas CpG dinucleotides are mostly methylated in human genomic DNA. Upon recognition of infectious agents, macrophages secrete a number of substances to attract other innate immune cells to the site of infection. Important factors secreted by macrophages are cytokines and chemokines. Cytokines often activate other immune cells when binding to specific receptors, whereas chemokines mediate the migration of cells toward the source of the chemokine. The cytokines and chemokines secreted from macrophages then initiate an inflammatory response: dilation of small blood vessels at the site of infection facilitates movement of neutrophils and monocytes out of the blood and into the tissue. The blood vessels also become more penetratable for blood plasma proteins, some of which have bactericidal functions. Monocytes entering the inflamed tissue differentiate into macrophages, thereby increasing the number of these phagocytic cells. Neutrophils are the other major phagocytic cell population in inflammation. Upon phagocytosis, macrophages and neutrophils produce toxic substances, including nitric oxide and other reactive oxygen species such as hydrogen peroxide, to kill the ingested infectious particles.

Natural killer cells are another important component of the innate immune system. These cells are activated by interferons and macrophage-derived cytokines, and are mainly involved in the response to intracellular pathogens. Natural killer cell killing is mediated by the release of cytotoxic granules that are bound to the surface of the target cells and subsequently induce the death of those cells. Thus, NK cell activity causes the death of the target cell, for example virus-infected human cells. This leads to the loss of the infected cells, but is usually beneficial for the immune response, as it prevents spreading of the virus. The effector functions of NK cells are controlled by distinct invariant groups of activating and inhibitory receptors.[4] The inhibitory receptors recognize MHC (major histocompatibility complex) class I molecules, which are expressed on nearly all somatic cells in the body. Some intracellular pathogens cause the downregulation of MHC class I molecules – likely as a means to evade the recognition of infected cells by cytotoxic T cells, which will be discussed further below – and hence become a target for NK cells. If the inhibitory receptors no longer inhibit NK cell activity, the activating receptors become dominant and induce NK cell killing of the target cells.

Besides the cell-based innate defense mechanisms, a sophisticated system of plasma proteins – the complement system – plays a key role in innate immune responses. One function of the complement system is to bind to pathogens and thereby mark them for recognition by complement receptor-expressing phagocytic cells a process called opsonization. Complement receptors are found on macrophages, granulocytes, dendritic cells and B cells. However, complement factors can also directly kill pathogens by building a membrane attack complex that introduces holes into the cell wall of certain bacteria, causing their lysis.

The innate immune response is a fast response, becoming effective within minutes and hours after encounter of invading pathogens. Often, this response is sufficient to eliminate the pathogens, so that no disease develops. However, there are many instances where pathogens have developed strategies to evade an efficient attack by the innate immune response. In these situations, the adaptive immune response that relies on B and T cells comes into effect and plays a crucial role for the immune response. As we will see, innate and adaptive immune responses are not strictly separated, and the adaptive immune response is often dependent on stimulation through innate immune cells. For example, macrophages not only function by phagocytosis of infectious agents but also by presenting pathogen-derived peptides to T cells for their activation. It has also become clear that TLR play an important role as costimulatory receptors in humoral immune responses.[5] Moreover, innate immune cells also play a role in adaptive immune responses as effector cells, for example when pathogens marked by antibodies are recognized and eliminated by macrophages expressing receptors for the antibodies (Fc receptors).

GENERATION OF B AND T CELLS

Generation of B cells

The main functions of B cells are mediated through their antibodies, which are composed of two identical heavy and light chains. These antibodies are built together with several coreceptor molecules to form the B cell antigen receptor (BCR) complex. In the antibody heavy and light chain, N-terminal variable regions and C-terminal constant regions can be distinguished. The variable (V) regions are the sites on the antibody that mediate antigen binding, whereas the constant regions are important for the three-dimensional structure of the molecule and, in the case of the heavy chain constant regions, also for the effector functions. To generate a highly diverse repertoire of antibodies for the recognition of a myriad of different foreign antigens, the variable regions of antibody heavy and light chains are generated by somatic recombination processes from separate gene segments. As a consequence, each

newly generated B cell will be equipped with a unique BCR. The enzymatic machinery that mediates the V gene recombination process is largely known and includes the lymphocyte-specific recombination activating (*RAG*) genes 1 and 2 and components of the nonhomologous DNA repair complex.[6] The RAG proteins generate DNA double-strand breaks at particular recombination signal sequences that flank the rearranging gene segments, and the intervening DNA between two rearranging gene segments is usually deleted from the chromosome.[6]

The ordered recombination processes and the subsequent selection processes define the multiple stages of B cell development (Fig. 9.2). B cell development starts from common lymphoid precursors, which are themselves generated from hematopoietic stem cells. First, recombination of diversity (D) and joining (J) gene segments for the variable region of the Ig heavy chain (D_H and J_H, respectively) occurs in pro-B cells. In the human, there are 27 D_H and 6 J_H gene segments available for this recombination process.[7,8] Often, D_H to J_H joining takes place on both IgH alleles, located on chromosome 14. In the next step, one of about 40 functional V gene segments (the exact number depends on the haplotype) is rearranged to a $D_H J_H$ joint.[9] During both recombination processes, additional diversity is generated at the joining sites by removal of a variable

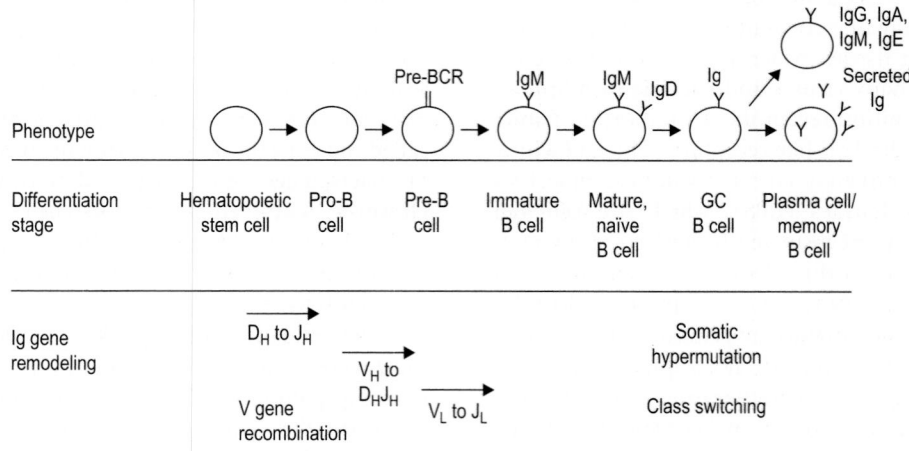

Figure 9.2 B cell development. B cell development is a multistage process, beginning with lymphoid precursors, which are themselves generated from hematopoietic stem cells. Lymphoid precursors in the bone marrow initiate B cell development when particular B cell transcription factors are expressed (e.g. early B cell factor and E2A) and heavy chain V gene rearrangements take place. First, D_H to J_H rearrangements are performed, and the cells carrying $D_H J_H$ joints are called pro-B cells. Next, V_H to $D_H J_H$ rearrangements occur. Such rearrangements can be productive or nonproductive. Only if a heavy chain can be expressed and assembled with a surrogate light chain will further development take place. B cell precursors harboring productive heavy chain rearrangements are termed pre-B cells. Light-chain gene rearrangements begin on the Igκ locus by V_κ to J_κ rearrangements. If the cells fail to generate a functional $V_\kappa J_\kappa$ rearrangement on either of the two alleles that can pair with the heavy chain, rearrangements will be performed on the Igλ locus. Cells that express a functional B cell receptor (BCR) on their surface have reached the immature B cell stage. At this stage, the BCR is expressed as an immunoglobulin (Ig) M molecule on the cell surface. The immature B cells are selected against expression of a strong autoreactive BCR, and if they survive this selection process, they differentiate into mature, naïve B cells that coexpress IgM and IgD through differential splicing and leave the bone marrow. In T-dependent immune responses, antigen-activated B cells differentiate into germinal center (GC) B cells, which undergo somatic hypermutation of the V-region genes and often also class switch recombination. Germinal center B cells can differentiate either into memory B cells or antibody-secreting plasma cells.

number of nucleotides from the ends of the rearranging gene segments and the addition of a few non-germ-line-encoded (N) nucleotides by a lymphocyte-specific enzyme, the terminal deoxynucleotidyl transferase. The $V_H D_H J_H$ rearrangements can be either in-frame or out-of-frame, as the reading frame that is defined by the translational start site in the V gene segment can be lost if the number of nucleotides between the last complete codon of the V_H gene segment and the first complete codon of the J_H gene segment is not a multiple of three, because then the constant parts of the Ig heavy chain, which follow downstream of the J_H gene segment, would not be read in the correct reading frame. Some rearrangements may also be nonfunctional because of the generation of a non-sense codon in the recombination process. If the first attempt to generate an in-frame $V_H D_H J_H$ fails, the pro-B cells can make a second attempt on the second IgH allele. If a B cell precursor can express a functional heavy chain together with a surrogate light chain as a pre-BCR, the pre-B cell stage of B cell development is reached. These pre-B cells undergo several rounds of division before they initiate Ig light-chain gene rearrangements.[10] There are two types of light chains, κ and λ, which are encoded by genes on chromosomes 2 and 22 in humans. The light chains are also composed of a variable and a constant region. However, the V regions of the light chain genes are only composed of two gene segments, V and J. In humans, there are about 30 V_κ and 5 J_κ gene segments available for the generation of V_κ region genes, and 40 V_λ and 4 J_λ genes for V_λ region genes.[11–15] Like during heavy chain rearrangements, loss of nucleotides and addition of N nucleotides at the V-J joining sites increases the diversity of the rearrangements. Initially, light chain rearrangements take place at the Igκ loci.[16] If a first V_κ-J_κ rearrangement is nonfunctional, there is not only the possibility to use the second allele for a new attempt, but it is usually also possible that further attempts are made on the originally rearranging allele, because V_κ segments located upstream of the rearranged one can rearrange to J_κ genes downstream of the one originally used. If all of these attempts do not lead to a productive light chain gene rearrangement that can pair with the heavy chain, the pre-B cell can undergo rearrangements at the Igλ loci. If a productive light chain gene rearrangement is finally generated, and if the heavy and light chains can pair and be expressed on the surface of the cell, the immature B cell stage is reached and further rearrangements are stopped. The BCR, which is expressed as an IgM molecule at this stage, is now tested for autoreactivity. Autoantigen binding can either reinduce further light chain gene rearrangements, a process called receptor editing, or the B cell can be eliminated by apoptosis.[17] If the immature B cell survives the negative selection against autoreactivity, it further differentiates into a mature, naïve (i.e. antigen-unexperienced) B cell that expresses its BCR in two isotypes, as IgM and IgD molecules. These isotypes of the BCR are composed of the same light chains and the same heavy chain V regions spliced to two different heavy chain constant region genes, the $C\mu$ gene for IgM and the $C\delta$ gene for IgD.

B cells are not only stringently selected for expression of an appropriate BCR during their development (first a pre-BCR at the pre-B cell stage and then a functional but nonautoreactive BCR at the immature B cell stage), but constantly throughout their life. Thus, even resting, mature B cells circulating through the body depend on tonic survival signals supplied by their BCR.[18,19] Additional selection processes for expression of a functional BCR will occur later in B cell differentiation, when B cells are engaged in T-dependent immune responses, as will be discussed later.

Generation of T cells

The antigen receptor of T cells is called the T cell receptor (TCR) and exists in two forms, as $\alpha\beta$ and $\gamma\delta$ TCR. The basic structure of the TCR chains is similar to that of the BCR chains. All chains have an N-terminal variable domain and a C-terminal constant domain. The variable domains of the β and δ chains are generated by somatic recombination of three gene segments (V, D, and J), whereas the variable domains of the α and γ chains are each composed of two gene segments (V and J).[20,21] Different to the BCR, the TCR consists of only two chains, either an α and β or a γ and δ chain. In addition, the TCR complex encompasses several proteins of the CD3 complex, which are essential for signaling. The somatic rearrangement processes that generate the TCR occur in a similar manner to the corresponding processes for the generation of the BCR, using the same enzymatic machinery. Most T cells in the periphery express an $\alpha\beta$ TCR. Importantly, the $\alpha\beta$ TCR recognizes antigen only in the context of MHC molecules, which present processed antigenic peptides to the TCR. There are two main types of MHC molecules, MHC class I and II, and distinct T cell subsets recognize antigen presented by them. MHC class I is recognized by the TCR in association with the CD8 coreceptor, whereas MHC class II is recognized by the TCR in association with the CD4 coreceptor.

The particular features of antigen recognition by the TCR have a major impact on T cell development, as it affords that T cells are selected to recognize either MHC class I molecules and express CD8, or to recognize MHC class II and express CD4. The T cells are generated from common lymphoid precursors that migrate from the fetal liver or bone marrow to the thymus, where they undergo the rearrangement processes to produce a TCR. First, rearrangements of TCRβ gene segments occur, and if these give rise to a productive TCRβ chain, V_α-J_α rearrangements occur at the TCRα locus. The differentiation steps of $\alpha\beta$ T cells are conventionally subdivided, based on expression of the CD4 and CD8 molecules, into a double negative, a double positive, and a CD4 or CD8 single positive stage. TCRβ gene rearrangements occur at the double negative stage of T cell development, followed by TCRα gene rearrangements in double positive T cell precursors. At the double positive stage, which represents the largest T cell lineage population in the thymus, a positive selection occurs that selects T cell precursors with a TCR that can recognize peptide/self-MHC complexes with appropriate affinity. If the precursor can interact with peptide/MHC class I molecules, it will become a CD8-positive cytotoxic T cell, whereas T cell precursors recognizing peptide/MHC class II complexes will become CD4-positive helper or regulatory T cells. T cell precursors that are not able to bind to one of the MHC complexes will die by neglect. A further selection process, negative selection, ensures that T cells with strong autoreactivity are counterselected and eliminated. Finally, the T cells will leave the thymus as mature CD4 or CD8 single positive T cells and circulate through the body.

The γδT cells are also generated in the thymus, and there are common precursors for γδ and αβT cells. Antigen recognition by the γδTCR is different from that of the αβTCR. MHC class I or II restriction is not involved in antigen recognition by γδ T cells and there is indication that the γδTCR can bind free antigen and/or antigen bound to unconventional MHC molecules. Some subsets of γδT cells, such as intraepithelial γδT cells, have a very limited TCR repertoire and in this regard resemble more the innate immune cells than typical lymphocytes of the adaptive immune system. A further subset of T cells generated in the thymus are NK T cells, which express an αβTCR of limited diversity that recognizes CD1 molecules instead of MHC class I or II.

CELLULAR IMMUNE RESPONSES

Cellular immune responses are essential for the elimination of intracellular pathogens (e.g. viruses and some bacteria) and are also involved in the activation of macrophages. Two types of T cells play a central role in these immune responses. CD8$^+$ cytotoxic T cells recognize pathogen-infected cells in the body and eliminate these cells to prevent further spread of the pathogens. Type 1 helper (TH1-type) CD4$^+$ T cells interact with macrophages and can activate these cells for improved function. The first critical step in cellular immune responses is the activation of the naive T cells. Binding of the TCR to peptide-loaded MHC molecules is not sufficient to activate naïve T cells, and costimulatory factors are needed. These are provided by professional antigen-presenting cells; that is, dendritic cells, macrophages and B cells. The most efficient of these are the dendritic cells. When dendritic cells in tissues take up antigen or are themselves infected by viruses, they migrate to the draining lymph nodes and here further differentiate into mature dendritic cells that upregulate costimulatory molecules for the activation of cytotoxic T cells, and present antigenic peptides on MHC class I complexes. Key costimulatory molecules are CD80 and CD86,

which can activate T cells by binding to the ligand CD28, which is expressed by T cells.[22] Upon initial activation of a T cell, further costimulatory molecules are expressed, such as CD40 ligand (CD40L).[23] Only if the same antigen-presenting cell provides the specific antigenic stimulation and the costimulatory signals will a naïve T cell be appropriately activated. This is an important safeguard against the unwanted activation of autoreactive cytotoxic T cells, as autoreactive T cells will normally not see autoantigen in the context of activated antigen-presenting cells. In some cytotoxic T cell responses, additional help is needed from T helper cells. For example, weakly stimulating antigen-presenting cells, like macrophages, can be activated by CD4$^+$ T helper cells, increasing their stimulatory function on cytotoxic T cells.

There are different effector functions of cytotoxic T cells to kill pathogen-infected target cells. First, they can secrete cytotoxic granules, the main component of which are perforin, granzymes and granulysin. Perforin is inserted into the target cell membrane and thereby produces pores through which granzyme and granulysin molecules can enter the cell. These molecules then induce apoptosis in the target cell. A second mechanism for cytotoxic T cell killing functions through the Fas ligand. This member of the tumor necrosis factor (TNF) family binds to the Fas receptor (also called CD95), which is expressed by many cells, and can induce apoptosis via activation of a caspase-dependent apoptosis pathway.[24] Caspases are a family of proteases that, following activation, can cleave many cellular proteins and are the main executioners of apoptosis.

Another arm of cellular immune responses are mediated by TH1-type CD4$^+$ T cells. When naïve CD4$^+$ T helper cells are activated by antigen-presenting cells, they will either differentiate into TH1- or TH2-type T helper cells. The factors that determine whether a naïve TH cell will become a TH1- or TH2-type T cell are not fully understood, but cytokines and other costimulatory factors are involved. The function of TH2 cells will be discussed later. Helper T cells recognize, with their TCR, cognate antigen presented to them on MHC class II molecules by the antigen-presenting cells. The activated TH1 cells will then activate macrophages presenting the antigenic peptide to them. The activation of the macrophages involves both cytokines, in particular interferon γ, and costimulatory surface receptors, such as the CD40-CD40 ligand pair.

T–INDEPENDENT IMMUNE RESPONSES

Certain antigens can induce B cell proliferation and antibody production largely independent of help by T cells. As such responses have initially been identified in athymic animals, they are called thymus independent or T-independent (TI) immune responses. Two types of TI responses are distinguished. In TI-1 reactions, B cell activators bind to specific receptors on B cells and induce their proliferation. A well-known example of such activators is bacterial LPS, which binds to LPS binding protein and activates the B cells through TLR4 signaling. As the recognition of LPS is mediated through receptors expressed on most B cells and not through the BCR, it causes a polyclonal B cell proliferation and differentiation.

T-independent type 2 (TI-2) responses are induced by strongly BCR-crosslinking antigens, in particular repetitive surface epitopes on bacteria. These are often polysaccharides, as they are found as cell wall components of encapsulated bacteria. As such bacteria are relatively resistant to elimination by phagocytic cells, TI-2 responses play an important role in controlling infections by encapsulated bacteria. The antibodies secreted during TI-2 responses are mostly of the IgM type, but class switching to particular IgG classes (see below for an introduction into class switching) is also observed.[25] While TI-2 responses are largely T cell independent, there is indication that such responses can be modulated in the presence of T cells. T-independent type 2 responses produce antibodies with relatively low affinity and do not undergo affinity maturation (see below) or produce long-lived memory B cells. There is indication that specific subsets of B cells are specialized in responding to TI-2 responses, in particular marginal zone B cells and perhaps B1 cells, a B cell subpopulation characterized by expression of the CD5 surface molecule.[25,26]

T-DEPENDENT IMMUNE RESPONSES

Extrafollicular reaction

T cell-dependent immune reactions are initiated when antigen-presenting dendritic cells that took up antigen in tissues move into the T cell areas of secondary lymphoid organs and present their antigen to TH cells in this microenvironment.[27] Antigen-specific T cells are activated and under appropriate conditions differentiate into activated TH2 cells, which are essential for humoral T dependent immune responses. B cells on their way through the secondary lymphoid organs also move through the T zone and, if they encounter activated TH2 cells recognizing the same antigen (but perhaps a different epitope), they will be trapped at the T zone–B zone border and be activated by stimulation through the TH2 cells.[28] For the antigen-specific interaction between B and T cells, the B cells internalize antigen bound to their BCR, process it and present peptide fragments of the antigens on their MHC class II molecules. These are recognized by the TCR/CD4 complex on the antigen-specific TH cells. Costimulatory interactions are essential for the full activation of the B cells, in particular interactions between CD80/CD86 on B cells and CD28 expressed by T cells, and CD40 on B cells and CD40L on T cells. Stimulation of the B cells induces a strong proliferation, causing the generation of foci of B cells at the T zone–B zone border.[27,28] Some B cells will quickly differentiate into plasma cells that produce a first wave of antigen-specific antibody. These plasma cells are short lived and produce antibody of usually low affinity. Other activated B cells of the primary foci will move into primary B cell follicles and initiate the next step of the T dependent humoral immune response – the germinal center (GC) reaction.[29] The extrafollicular reaction usually starts one or two days after infection and lasts for a few days.[28]

Germinal center reaction

The GC reaction takes place in B cell follicles after antigen-activated B cells migrate from the primary foci into these structures. B cell follicles composed mainly of B cells and a network of follicular dendritic cells (FDC) are called primary B cell follicles, whereas they are termed secondary follicles when they harbor the GC.[27] Follicular dendritic cells are a specific type of antigen-presenting cell as they present unprocessed antigen on their surface in the form of antigen–antibody complexes. Another essential component of the GC are antigen-specific TH cells, which also migrate into the B cell follicles. In the GC, the activated B cells start to vigorously proliferate and grow to large clones (Fig. 9.3). These proliferating GC B cells are called centroblasts. As a result, the resting B cells originally occupying the primary follicle are pushed aside and build a mantle zone around the GC. The proliferation of the centroblasts is accompanied by the activation of somatic hypermutation, a process by which single point mutations and also some small deletions or insertions are introduced at a very high rate specifically into the V-region genes of the antibody heavy and light chains.[30–32] The enzymatic machinery that mediates somatic hypermutation is not completely known, but the enzyme activation-induced cytidine deaminase (AID) is an essential compoment.[33] Somatic hypermutation is initiated when AID deaminates cytidine residues in the V-region DNA, giving rise to uracil, which is not a normal component of DNA, and these lesions can be further processed by various pathways involving components of DNA repair pathways and error-prone DNA polymerases.[34] The hypermutation process appears to be associated with DNA strand breaks, which might partly explain the occcasional occurrence of deletions or insertions.[30] Most of the somatic mutations will be disadvantageous, for example if they introduce stop codons or replacement mutations that prevent proper folding of the antibody polypeptide chains or lead to loss of antigen binding. Germinal center B cells with such unfavorable mutations will be very efficiently eliminated and undergo apoptosis.[35] The apoptotic cells will be taken up and digested by macrophages present in the GC. A few GC B cells that acquire affinity-increasing mutations will be positively selected by interaction with the FDC and the TH cells (Fig. 9.3). This selection largely takes place when centroblasts differentiate into resting GC B cells, termed centrocytes. Centroblasts are mainly located in a region of the GC that is called the dark zone, whereas FDC, TH cells and

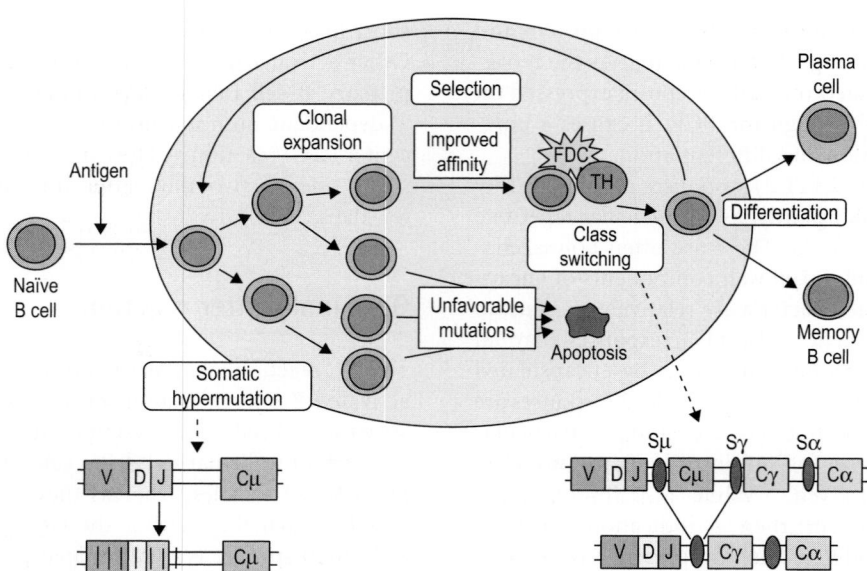

Figure 9.3 B cell differentiation in the germinal center. Mature B cells that are activated by antigen binding to their B cell receptor (BCR) and that receive help from antigen-specific T helper cells migrate into primary B cell follicles and initiate a vigorous proliferation. The proliferating B cells thereby generate a germinal center (GC). In the course of the proliferation the process of somatic hypermutation is initiated, which introduces mutations at a high rate into the immunoglobulin (Ig) V-region genes. Mutations that reduce the affinity of the antibody to the activating antigen or cause destruction of the BCR will lead to death of the GC B cells by apoptosis. Germinal center B cells acquiring affinity-increasing mutations will be positively selected by interaction with GC T helper (TH) cells and follicular dendritic cells (FDC). Usually, one can discriminate a dark zone of the GC enriched in proliferating GC B cells and a light zone enriched in nonproliferating GC B cells, T helper cells, and follicular dendritic cells (not shown). Germinal center B cells migrate back and forth between the dark and light zones and undergo multiple rounds of proliferation, mutation, and selection. Positively selected GC B cells can either differentiate into memory B cells or plasma cells and leave the GC.

centrocytes are concentrated in the light zone.[27] There is, however, also some proliferation of GC B cells in the light zone, and selection presumably also takes place in the dark zone.[36] It is likely that reiterative cycles of proliferation, mutation and selection occur, enabling an efficient stepwise improvement of affinity. Indeed, recent live-imaging studies confirmed that there is an extensive migration of GC B cells within the GC.[37–39] As a consequence of the stepwise selection for GC B cells with increased affinity for the immunizing antigen, an affinity maturation of the immune response occurs.

A large fraction of the GC B cells will switch their antibody isotype in a class switch recombination process. In this process, DNA strand breaks are introduced in particular switch regions located upstream of the IgH constant region genes, and the intervening DNA between the originally expressed Cμ gene and the downstream C$_H$ gene that is targeted for recombination is deleted from the chromosomes.[40] In the human, there are four Cγ genes, two Cα genes, and one Cε gene available for class switching. Each of these classes has particular effector functions. Notably, AID is not only essential for hypermutation but also for class switch recombination.[33,41]

Positively selected GC B cells will finally differentiate further and leave the GC. They can differentiate into

memory B cells or plasma cells.[27] The decision of whether a GC B cell will become a memory B cell or a plasma cell is regulated by the GC TH cells and perhaps also the FDC and involves both direct cellular interactions and cytokines.[42] The GC reaction usually becomes visible four to six days after immunization or infection and lasts for two to three weeks.

Memory B cells and plasma cells

Memory B cells are resting, long-lived cells that are generated in GC reactions.[43] Consequently, they are characterized by somatically mutated Ig V genes. Many of them also express class-switched BCR, and this has intially been the key phenotypic feature for their isolation. However, in particular in humans, there are also distinct subsets of IgM$^+$ B cells with somatically mutated V genes, and it has been proposed that these represent GC-derived memory B cells too.[44–46] Indeed, the mutated IgM$^+$ B cells share many functional and phenotypic features with class-switched memory B cells.[46] Most mutated IgM$^+$ B cells coexpress IgD and CD27 (a member of the TNF receptor [TNFR] family), but a small subset is characterized by low to absent IgD expression (IgM-only B cells).[44,47] As the vast majority of class-switched, IgM-only and mutated IgM$^+$IgD$^+$ B cells express

CD27, this marker may represent the first general marker for peripheral memory B cells.[47] CD27 is also expressed by most GC B cells and at high levels by plasma cells.[48,49] Moreover, CD27-negative class-switched B cells have also recently been identified in humans, indicating that some memory B cells lack CD27 expression.[50] There is currently controversial discussion on whether the mutated IgM-expressing B cells are indeed GC-derived memory B cells, or whether they originate from T-independent responses or from another developmental pathway with hypermutation active during primary antibody diversification.[51,52] These scenarios are based mainly on the finding that mutated IgM$^+$IgD$^+$CD27$^+$ B cells can be found in patients affected by X-linked hyper-IgM syndrome who apparently lack GC, and from the observation that many mutated IgM-positive B cells are found in the marginal zone of the spleen, which is thought to be mainly involved in T-independent immune responses.[51,52]

Memory B cells play an important role in immunity against pathogens, as they produce highly specific antibodies, are present in large numbers, and are quickly activated upon reencounter with the cognate antigen. Upon activation, a large fraction of antigen-specific memory B cells will differentiate into plasma cells.[53] To what extent reactivated memory B cells in recall responses undergo further GC reactions is unclear.

The plasma cells that are generated in GC reactions mainly home to the red pulp of the spleen, the lamina propria of the intestinal tissue, or the bone marrow. In the bone marrow, plasma cells seed specific niches in which they are supplied with survival signals.[54] It is still debated whether GC-derived plasma cells are intrinsically long lived, or whether the microenvironmental interactions in their bone marrow niches are the main regulators of plasma cell longevity.[54] Mature plasma cells no longer proliferate, but they can secrete antibodies for a long time.

RELATIONSHIP BETWEEN NORMAL LYMPHOCYTES AND LYMPHOMAS

When B cells undergo malignant transformation they usually retain many key features of their specific differentiation stage.[55,56] For example, in follicular lymphoma, the lymphoma cells grow in a follicular pattern in association with FDC and GC-type TH cells, they morphologically resemble centroblasts and centrocytes, they express many typical markers of GC B cells, and they show ongoing hypermutation activity of their rearranged Ig V genes.[57] Hence, there is little doubt that follicular lymphoma cells represent transformed GC B cells. The evaluation of genetic and phenotypic features in other lymphomas revealed that a surprisingly large number of them are related to the GC or post-GC stage of B cell differentiation.[55] Such GC B cell–associated lymphomas include – besides follicular lymphoma – Burkitt lymphoma, a subset of diffuse large B cell lymphomas, post-transplant lymphomas, and classical and lymphocyte-predominant Hodgkin lymphoma.[55] Also, it may well be that other lymphomas that show a post-GC phenotype underwent critical transformation steps in the GC, and that the cells either differentiated to a post-GC stage before final transformation, or that features of GC B cells were lost due to specific transforming events in GC B cell precursors of the lymphoma clones. For example, when a transforming event occurring in a GC B cell interferes with the somatic hypermutation process, the lymphoma would lack intraclonal V gene diversity and would hence appear in this regard as a post-GC – that is, memory – B cell. The retention of typical differentiation stage–associated phenotypic and gene expression patterns may well be of pathogenic relevance, as will be discussed below. An exception to the concept of retained differentiation-associated features in B cell lymphomas is represented by classical Hodgkin lymphoma, as the tumor cells in this malignancy (the Hodgkin and Reed-Sternberg cells) have lost or at least downregulated expression of the vast majority of typical B cell genes.[58,59] Perhaps, this dramatic reprogramming is associated with the presumed origin of these lymphoma cells from pre-apoptotic GC B cells (see Chapter 34 by Küppers, Hartmann and Hansmann).

Several factors can account for the high frequency of GC B cell-derived lymphomas. First, GC B cells physiologically undergo very strong and sustained proliferation, and it is presumably easier to sustain proliferation in already proliferating cells than inducing proliferation in a resting cell. Moreover, the high proliferation rate of GC B cells, which is also associated with the inhibition of particular cellular safeguard mechanisms,[60] may also increase the risk of acquiring DNA mutations during DNA replication. Second, GC B cells undergo Ig gene remodeling processes – somatic hypermutation and class switch recombination – that bear an inherent risk for genetic lesions.[30,61] This includes both the generation of chromosomal translocations and the acquisition of somatic mutations by mistargeted somatic hypermutation (see below). Thus, the GC, which is of key importance for efficient humoral adaptive immune responses, bears an inherent risk for the development of B cell lymphomas.

Attempts are also made to type human T cell lymphomas in a similar way to B cell lymphomas, to their specific cellular origin. In angioimmunoblastic lymphadenopathy with dysproteinema (AILD), a mature T cell lymphoma, the lymphoma cells show phenotypic features of GC TH cells and the cells are embedded in a network of FDC, indicating that this malignancy is derived from GC TH cells.[62] However, for most other T cell lymphomas, a specific assignment to distinct differentiation stages (besides the assigment to a CD4$^+$ or CD8$^+$ T cell origin) is more difficult. This is partly due to the fact that genetic traits of a particular differentiation stage, comparable to somatic Ig V gene mutations and class switching as a molecular trait for a (post) GC derivation of B cell lymphomas, does not exist for T cells.

MECHANISMS OF LYMPHOMA PATHOGENESIS

Genetic lesions

A hallmark of many B cell lymphomas are chromosomal translocations involving the Ig loci.[61,63] The breakpoints of these translocations in the Ig loci are at those positions in which DNA strand breaks are introduced during the physiological processes of V(D)J recombination, somatic hypermutation, and class switch recombination.[61,63] This indicates that the translocations happen as mistakes during these Ig gene remodeling processes. The causes for the breaks in the partner loci are less well understood, but may in some instances also involve DNA breaks introduced by the RAG enzymes or by targeting of somatic hypermutation to non-Ig loci.[64,65] The translocation partners are protooncogenes that upon translocation come under transcriptional control of the active Ig regulatory elements, in particular the Ig enhancers, causing their deregulated constitutive expression. Prototypic examples of such translocations involve the *BCL1*/IgH translocation in mantle cell lymphoma, the *BCL2*/IgH translocation in follicular lymphoma, and the *MYC*/IgH or *MYC*/IgL translocations in Burkitt lymphoma.[63] Similar translocations are also found in T cell lymphomas and leukemias; however, as class switching and somatic hypermutation does not occur in T cells, they are here associated with mistakes during TCR V gene rearrangements.[66] Other types of translocations in lymphomas, such as the *NPM*/*ALK* translocation in anaplastic large cell lymphoma or the *API2*/*MALT1* translocation in MALT lymphomas, do not involve TCR or BCR genes, but generate fusion proteins of two distinct genes.

Further genetic lesions found in lymphomas involve tumor suppressor genes, for example ATM in mantle cell lymphoma and B chronic lymphocytic leukemia, CD95 in diffuse large B cell lymphomas, TP53 in chronic lymphocytic leukemia and diffuse large B cell lymphomas, and IKBA in classical Hodgkin lymphoma.[67]

Microenvironmental factors

Genetic lesions to activate oncogenes or inactivate tumor suppressor genes are essential for lymphoma development. However, it has become increasingly clear that many lymphomas do not grow autonomously, but still depend on microenvironmental interactions and stimulation through their BCR for their growth.[67] Indeed, most B cell lymphomas still express a BCR, including subtypes with ongoing somatic hypermutation, where BCR-destructive mutations are apparently counterselected. In addition, chromosomal translocations targeting and thereby disrupting Ig loci are usually targeted to the nonexpressed Ig alleles. Thus, it appears that there is a selection for retained BCR expression in B cell lymphomas, and that the tonic BCR signaling that is critical for the survival of normal B cells also plays a role in many B cell lymphomas.[67,68] Moreover, several B cell lymphomas show evidence for triggering of their BCR by antigen. Often, the antigens appear to be autoantigens, which are constantly available for sustained signaling.[69] Also, viruses may in some instances provide an antigenic stimulus for B cell lymphomas, as is indicated from B cell lymphomas associated with chronic hepatitis C virus infection.[70]

The dependence of many B cell lymphomas on microenvironmental cellular interactions is well exemplified by follicular lymphoma. The follicular lymphoma cells grow in the typical GC microenvironment in close association with FDC and GC T helper cells. Follicular lymphoma cells do not grow in culture and quickly undergo apoptosis *in vitro*. However, when the lymphoma cells are cultured together with CD4$^+$ T cells, or with stromal cells and are stimulated with an antibody against CD40 (mimicking a main signal normally supplied by T cells), they survive for longer periods and undergo proliferation *in vitro*.[71,72] These observations support a critical role for stromal cells and CD4$^+$ T cells in follicular lymphoma growth. Another striking example for the role of extrinsic factors for lymphoma growth is provided by gastric MALT lymphomas, which are associated with infection by *Helicobacter pylori*. *H. pylori* establishes a chronic gastric infection and can activate T helper cells, which then stimulate MALT lymphoma B cells (which themselves frequently express autoreactive antibodies).[69,73,74] If the bacterial infection is cleared by antibiotic treatment, the lymphoma often completely regresses, demonstrating the dependence of the lymphoma cells on the stimulation provided indirectly by *H. pylori*.[74]

The role of viruses

Viruses are involved in the pathogenesis of several lymphomas. Epstein–Barr virus (EBV), a member of the herpesvirus family, is found in nearly all cases of endemic Burkitt lymphoma, in most post-transplant lymphomas, and in about 40 percent of Hodgkin lymphomas.[75] Epstein–Barr virus infects most humans and persists usually as a harmless passenger in B cells (at a frequency of about 1–10 infected cells per 10^6 B cells), but its transforming capacity is indicated from the fact that it can growth-transform B cells *in vitro*. In Hodgkin lymphoma and post-transplant lymphomas, among the latent EBV-encoded genes expressed in the lymphoma cells are two latent membrane proteins, LMP1 and LMP2a, that mimic key survival signals for B cells (i.e. CD40 signaling by LMP1, and BCR signaling by LMP2a).[76,77] Another member of the herpesvirus family, human herpes virus 8 (HHV-8), is found in all cases of the rare primary effusion lymphomas that mostly occur in acquired immune deficiency syndrome (AIDS) patients.[78] These lymphomas frequently show coinfection by EBV.[78] Viruses also play a role in the development of some T cell malignancies, such as human T cell lymphotrophic virus 1 (HTLV-1) in adult T cell leukemias in Asian countries.[79]

CONCLUSIONS

Humans are equipped with a multilayered immune system that is essential to combat a myriad of infectious agents and that is hence crucial for their survival. Many infections are quickly cleared by neutrophils, macrophages and NK cells in the innate immune response that uses conserved pathogen patterns for the recognition and elimination of the pathogens. However, when these mechanisms are unsuccessful, the adaptive immune response comes into play. The adaptive immune responses involve both cellular and humoral reactions, which are specialized for the elimination of intracellular and extracellular pathogens, respectively. B and T cells are the central players in adaptive immunity, but they interact with numerous other hematopoietic cell types, and a close interaction of lymphocytes with innate immune cells has become evident. The possibility to generate a practically limitless diversity of antigen receptors on T and B cells is a main factor for the power of the adaptive immune response. This diversification and adaptation of the immune response is most elaborated in B cells, where somatic hypermutation and class switching further diversifies and improves the immune response. However, it appears that the vigorous proliferation of antigen-activated B cells and their Ig gene remodeling processes also leads to an increased risk for the development of B cell lymphomas in rare instances. In the development of such lymphomas, key determinants for the survival of normal B cells – such as expression and stimulation through the BCR and microenvironmental interactions – play essential roles also in the survival and growth of the malignant cells.

KEY POINTS

- All cells of the immune system derive from a common precursor, the hematopoietic stem cell.
- The innate immune response is fast and uses conserved pathogen patterns for the recognition and elimination of the pathogens.
- The possibility to generate a practically limitless diversity of antigen receptors on T and B cells by gene rearrangement processes is a main factor for the power of the adaptive immune response.
- B and T cells are the key players of adaptive immune responses, but they also interact with cells of the innate immune system.
- Affinity maturation of humoral immune responses and immunologic memory are specific features of adaptive immune responses.
- The vigorously proliferating germinal center B cells undergoing immunoglobulin gene modifying processes are at particular risk to undergo malignant transformation.

- Key determinants for the survival of normal B cells also play essential roles in the survival and growth of B cell lymphomas.

REFERENCES

● = Key primary paper
◆ = Major review article

1. Wilson KT, Crabtree JE. Immunology of *Helicobacter pylori*: insights into the failure of the immune response and perspectives on vaccine studies. *Gastroenterology* 2007; **133**: 288–308.
2. Randen I, Mellbye OJ, Forre O, Natvig JB. The identification of germinal centres and follicular dendritic cell networks in rheumatoid synovial tissue. *Scand J Immunol* 1995; **41**: 481–6.
3. Takeda K, Akira S. Toll-like receptors in innate immunity. *Int Immunol* 2005; **17**: 1–14.
4. Moretta L, Moretta A. Killer immunoglobulin-like receptors. *Curr Opin Immunol* 2004; **16**: 626–33.
◆5. Lanzavecchia A, Sallusto F. Toll-like receptors and innate immunity in B-cell activation and antibody responses. *Curr Opin Immunol* 2007; **19**: 268–74.
●6. McBlane JF, van Gent DC, Ramsden DA *et al*. Cleavage at a V(D)J recombination signal requires only RAG1 and RAG2 proteins and occurs in two steps. *Cell* 1995; **83**: 387–95.
7. Corbett SJ, Tomlinson IM, Sonnhammer EL *et al*. Sequence of the human immunoglobulin diversity (D) segment locus: a systematic analysis provides no evidence for the use of DIR segments, inverted D segments, "minor" D segments or D-D recombination. *J Mol Biol* 1997; **270**: 587–97.
8. Ravetch JV, Siebenlist U, Korsmeyer S *et al*. Structure of the human immunoglobulin mu locus: characterization of embryonic and rearranged J and D genes. *Cell* 1981; **27**: 583–91.
9. Cook GP, Tomlinson IM. The human immunoglobulin VH repertoire. *Immunol Today* 1995; **16**: 237–42.
10. Melchers F, ten Boekel E, Seidl T *et al*. Repertoire selection by pre-B-cell receptors and B-cell receptors, and genetic control of B-cell development from immature to mature B cells. *Immunol Rev* 2000; **175**: 33–46.
11. Hieter PA, Maizel JV Jr, Leder P. Evolution of human immunoglobulin kappa J region genes. *J Biol Chem* 1982; **257**: 1516–22.
12. Kawasaki K, Minoshima S, Nakato E *et al*. One-megabase sequence analysis of the human immunoglobulin lambda gene locus. *Genome Res* 1997; **7**: 250–61.
13. Schäble KF, Zachau HG. The variable genes of the human immunoglobulin kappa locus. *Biol Chem Hoppe Seyler* 1993; **374**: 1001–22.
14. Vasicek TJ, Leder P. Structure and expression of the human immunoglobulin lambda genes. *J Exp Med* 1990; **172**: 609–20.

15. Williams SC, Frippiat JP, Tomlinson IM *et al.* Sequence and evolution of the human germline V lambda repertoire. *J Mol Biol* 1996; **264**: 220–32.

16. Bräuninger A, Goossens T, Rajewsky K, Küppers R. Regulation of immunoglobulin light chain gene rearrangements during early B cell development in the human. *Eur J Immunol* 2001; **31**: 3631–7.

17. Nemazee D. Receptor editing in lymphocyte development and central tolerance. *Nat Rev Immunol* 2006; **6**: 728–40.

18. Kraus M, Alimzhanov MB, Rajewsky N, Rajewsky K. Survival of resting mature B lymphocytes depends on BCR signaling via the Igalpha/beta heterodimer. *Cell* 2004; **117**: 787–800.

●19. Lam KP, Kühn R, Rajewsky K. In vivo ablation of surface immunoglobulin on mature B cells by inducible gene targeting results in rapid cell death. *Cell* 1997; **90**: 1073–83.

20. Arden B, Clark SP, Kabelitz D, Mak TW. Human T-cell receptor variable gene segment families. *Immunogenetics* 1995; **42**: 455–500.

21. Rowen L, Koop BF, Hood L. The complete 685-kilobase DNA sequence of the human beta T cell receptor locus. *Science* 1996; **272**: 1755–62.

22. Alegre ML, Frauwirth KA, Thompson CB. T-cell regulation by CD28 and CTLA-4. *Nat Rev Immunol* 2001; **1**: 220–8.

23. Grewal IS, Flavell RA. The role of CD40 ligand in costimulation and T-cell activation. *Immunol Rev* 1996; **153**: 85–106.

24. Peter ME, Krammer PH. Mechanisms of CD95 (APO-1/Fas)-mediated apoptosis. *Curr Opin Immunol* 1998; **10**: 545–51.

25. Zandvoort A, Timens W. The dual function of the splenic marginal zone: essential for initiation of anti-TI-2 responses but also vital in the general first-line defense against blood-borne antigens. *Clin Exp Immunol* 2002; **130**: 4–11.

26. Berland R, Wortis HH. Origins and functions of B-1 cells with notes on the role of CD5. *Annu Rev Immunol* 2002; **20**: 253–300.

◆27. MacLennan IC. Germinal centers. *Annu Rev Immunol* 1994; **12**: 117–39.

28. Jacob J, Kassir R, Kelsoe G. In situ studies of the primary immune response to (4-hydroxy-3-nitrophenyl)acetyl. I. The architecture and dynamics of responding cell populations. *J Exp Med* 1991; **173**: 1165–75.

29. Jacob J, Kelsoe G. In situ studies of the primary immune response to (4-hydroxy-3-nitrophenyl)acetyl. II. A common clonal origin for periarteriolar lymphoid sheath-associated foci and germinal centers. *J Exp Med* 1992; **176**: 679–87.

30. Goossens T, Klein U, Küppers R. Frequent occurrence of deletions and duplications during somatic hypermutation: Implications for oncogene translocations and heavy chain disease. *Proc Natl Acad Sci USA* 1998; **95**: 2463–8.

●31. Küppers R, Zhao M, Hansmann ML, Rajewsky K. Tracing B cell development in human germinal centres by molecular analysis of single cells picked from histological sections. *EMBO J* 1993; **12**: 4955–67.

32. Jacob J, Kelsoe G, Rajewsky K, Weiss U. Intraclonal generation of antibody mutants in germinal centres. *Nature* 1991; **354**: 389–92.

●33. Muramatsu M, Kinoshita K, Fagarasan S *et al.* Class switch recombination and hypermutation require activation-induced cytidine deaminase (AID), a potential RNA editing enzyme. *Cell* 2000; **102**: 553–63.

◆34. Di Noia JM, Neuberger MS. Molecular mechanisms of antibody somatic hypermutation. *Annu Rev Biochem* 2007; **76**: 1–22.

35. Liu YJ, Joshua DE, Williams GT *et al.* Mechanism of antigen-driven selection in germinal centres. *Nature* 1989; **342**: 929–31.

◆36. Allen CD, Okada T, Cyster JG. Germinal-center organization and cellular dynamics. *Immunity* 2007; **27**: 190–202.

37. Allen CD, Okada T, Tang HL, Cyster JG. Imaging of germinal center selection events during affinity maturation. *Science* 2007; **315**: 528–31.

38. Hauser AE, Junt T, Mempel TR *et al.* Definition of germinal-center B cell migration in vivo reveals predominant intrazonal circulation patterns. *Immunity* 2007; **26**: 655–67.

39. Schwickert TA, Lindquist RL, Shakhar G *et al.* In vivo imaging of germinal centres reveals a dynamic open structure. *Nature* 2007; **446**: 83–7.

40. Chaudhuri J, Alt FW. Class-switch recombination: interplay of transcription, DNA deamination and DNA repair. *Nat Rev Immunol* 2004; **4**: 541–52.

41. Revy P, Muto T, Levy Y *et al.* Activation-induced cytidine deaminase (AID) deficiency causes the autosomal recessive form of the Hyper-IgM syndrome (HIGM2). *Cell* 2000; **102**: 565–75.

42. Liu YJ, Arpin C. Germinal center development. *Immunol Rev* 1997; **156**: 111–26.

◆43. Rajewsky K. Clonal selection and learning in the antibody system. *Nature* 1996; **381**: 751–8.

44. Klein U, Küppers R, Rajewsky K. Evidence for a large compartment of IgM-expressing memory B cells in humans. *Blood* 1997; **89**: 1288–98.

●45. Klein U, Rajewsky K, Küppers R. Human immunoglobulin (Ig)M+IgD+ peripheral blood B cells expressing the CD27 cell surface antigen carry somatically mutated variable region genes: CD27 as a general marker for somatically mutated (memory) B cells. *J Exp Med* 1998; **188**: 1679–89.

46. Tangye SG, Good KL. Human IgM+CD27+ B cells: memory B cells or "memory" B cells? *J Immunol* 2007; **179**: 13–9.

47. Klein U, Küppers R, Rajewsky K. Human IgM+IgD+ B cells, the major B cell subset in the peripheral blood, express V kappa genes with no or little somatic mutation throughout life. *Eur J Immunol* 1993; **23**: 3272–7.

48. Jung J, Choe J, Li L, Choi YS. Regulation of CD27 expression in the course of germinal center B cell differentiation: the pivotal role of IL-10. *Eur J Immunol* 2000; **30**: 2437–43.

49. Odendahl M, Jacobi A, Hansen A *et al.* Disturbed peripheral B lymphocyte homeostasis in systemic lupus erythematosus. *J Immunol* 2000; **165**: 5970–9.

50. Fecteau JF, Cote G, Neron S. A new memory CD27-IgG+ B cell population in peripheral blood expressing VH genes with low frequency of somatic mutation. *J Immunol* 2006; **177**: 3728–36.

51. Kruetzmann S, Rosado MM, Weber H *et al.* Human immunoglobulin M memory B cells controlling Streptococcus pneumoniae infections are generated in the spleen. *J Exp Med* 2003; **197**: 939–45.

●52. Weller S, Faili A, Garcia C *et al.* CD40-CD40L independent Ig gene hypermutation suggests a second B cell diversification pathway in humans. *Proc Natl Acad Sci USA* 2001; **98**: 1166–70.

53. Arpin C, Banchereau J, Liu YJ. Memory B cells are biased towards terminal differentiation: a strategy that may prevent repertoire freezing. *J Exp Med* 1997; **186**: 931–40.

◆54. Radbruch A, Muehlinghaus G, Luger EO *et al.* Competence and competition: the challenge of becoming a long-lived plasma cell. *Nat Rev Immunol* 2006; **6**: 741–50.

◆55. Küppers R, Klein U, Hansmann M-L, Rajewsky K. Cellular origin of human B-cell lymphomas. *N Engl J Med* 1999; **341**: 1520–9.

56. Stevenson FK, Sahota SS, Ottensmeier CH *et al.* The occurrence and significance of V gene mutations in B cell-derived human malignancy. *Adv Cancer Res* 2001; **83**: 81–116.

57. Bende RJ, Smit LA, van Noesel CJ. Molecular pathways in follicular lymphoma. *Leukemia* 2007; **21**: 18–29.

58. Schwering I, Bräuninger A, Klein U *et al.* Loss of the B-lineage-specific gene expression program in Hodgkin and Reed-Sternberg cells of Hodgkin lymphoma. *Blood* 2003; **101**: 1505–12.

59. Stein H, Marafioti T, Foss HD *et al.* Down-regulation of BOB.1/OBF.1 and Oct2 in classical Hodgkin disease but not in lymphocyte predominant Hodgkin disease correlates with immunoglobulin transcription. *Blood* 2001; **97**: 496–501.

60. Phan RT, Dalla-Favera R. The BCL6 proto-oncogene suppresses p53 expression in germinal-centre B cells. *Nature* 2004; **432**: 635–9.

61. Küppers R, Dalla-Favera R. Mechanisms of chromosomal translocations in B cell lymphomas. *Oncogene* 2001; **20**: 5580–94.

62. Dunleavy K, Wilson WH, Jaffe ES. Angioimmunoblastic T cell lymphoma: pathobiological insights and clinical implications. *Curr Opin Hematol* 2007; **14**: 348–53.

63. Willis TG, Dyer MJ. The role of immunoglobulin translocations in the pathogenesis of B-cell malignancies. *Blood* 2000; **96**: 808–22.

64. Pasqualucci L, Neumeister P, Goossens T *et al.* Hypermutation of multiple proto-oncogenes in B-cell diffuse large-cell lymphomas. *Nature* 2001; **412**: 341–6.

65. Raghavan SC, Swanson PC, Ma Y, Lieber MR. Double-strand break formation by the RAG complex at the bcl-2 major breakpoint region and at other non-B DNA structures in vitro. *Mol Cell Biol* 2005; **25**: 5904–19.

66. Tycko B, Sklar J. Chromosomal translocations in lymphoid neoplasia: a reappraisal of the recombinase model. *Cancer Cells* 1990; **2**: 1–8.

◆67. Küppers R. Mechanisms of B-cell lymphoma pathogenesis. *Nat Rev Cancer* 2005; **5**: 251–62.

68. Gururajan M, Jennings CD, Bondada S. Constitutive B cell receptor signaling is critical for basal growth of B lymphoma. *J Immunol* 2006; **176**: 5715–9.

69. Bende RJ, Aarts WM, Riedl RG *et al.* Among B cell non-Hodgkin's lymphomas, MALT lymphomas express a unique antibody repertoire with frequent rheumatoid factor reactivity. *J Exp Med* 2005; **201**: 1229–41.

70. Quinn ER, Chan CH, Hadlock KG *et al.* The B-cell receptor of a hepatitis C virus (HCV)-associated non-Hodgkin lymphoma binds the viral E2 envelope protein, implicating HCV in lymphomagenesis. *Blood* 2001; **98**: 3745–9.

71. Johnson PW, Watt SM, Betts DR *et al.* Isolated follicular lymphoma cells are resistant to apoptosis and can be grown in vitro in the CD40/stromal cell system. *Blood* 1993; **82**: 1848–57.

72. Umetsu DT, Esserman L, Donlon TA *et al.* Induction of proliferation of human follicular (B type) lymphoma cells by cognate interaction with CD4+ T cell clones. *J Immunol* 1990; **144**: 2550–7.

73. Hussel T, Isaacson PG, Crabtree JE, Spencer J. *Helicobacter pylori*-specific tumour-infiltrating T cells provide contact dependent help for the growth of malignant B cells in low-grade gastric lymphoma of mucosa-associated lymphoid tissue. *J Pathol* 1996; **178**: 122–7.

●74. Wotherspoon AC, Doglioni C, Diss TC *et al.* Regression of primary low-grade B-cell gastric lymphoma of mucosa-associated lymphoid tissue after eradication of *Helicobacter pylori*. *Lancet* 1993; **342**: 575–7.

75. Young LS, Rickinson AB. Epstein-Barr virus: 40 years on. *Nat Rev Cancer* 2004; **4**: 757–68.

76. Küppers R. B cells under influence: transformation of B cells by Epstein-Barr virus. *Nat Rev Immunol* 2003; **3**: 801–12.

77. Mancao C, Hammerschmidt W. Epstein-Barr virus latent membrane protein 2A is a B-cell receptor mimic and essential for B-cell survival. *Blood* 2007; **110**: 3715–21.

78. Swaminathan S. Molecular biology of Epstein-Barr virus and Kaposi's sarcoma-associated herpesvirus. *Semin Hematol* 2003; **40**: 107–15.

79. Matsuoka M, Jeang KT. Human T-cell leukaemia virus type 1 (HTLV-1) infectivity and cellular transformation. *Nat Rev Cancer* 2007; **7**: 270–80.

10

Ontogeny of T and natural killer cells

YU-WAYE CHU AND RONALD GRESS

INTRODUCTION

T cell development is a complex process that encompasses fundamental concepts in immunology and developmental biology. The inherent complexity in T cell development relates in large part to the strict requirements of T cells in the elicitation of diverse yet specific immune responses that protect the host organism while at the same time avoiding indiscriminate attack against itself in the form of autoimmunity. As such, T cell development is replete with decisions regarding cell differentiation, survival, and death. T cell development is a critical area of research not only because of the insights into immunology, developmental biology, and cell biology, but also because of the clinical implications of T cell biology in the context of T cell neoplasms, immune homeostasis, and immune reconstitution in the setting of immunodeficient states including human immunodeficiency virus (HIV) infection, cancer, and immunodepleting therapies including chemotherapy and hematopoietic stem cell transplantation (HSCT). In addition to T cells, natural killer (NK) and NK-T cells (whose development is not discussed in this chapter) have emerged as important contributors in immune responses to pathogens and tumors for which insights into developmental programs are currently being characterized.

The purpose of this chapter is to describe salient phenotypic, anatomic, and functional events in T cell and NK cell ontogeny. The first part describes key phenotypic changes that occur as early T cell progenitors proceed through the program of T cell development. The second part of the chapter focuses on the thymus, the major organ of T cell development, and the anatomic microenvironments within the thymus that facilitate specific stages of thymocyte development. The third part of the chapter highlights critical checkpoints pertaining to T cell lineage commitment. The final part of the chapter focuses on NK cell development.

OVERVIEW OF T CELL DEVELOPMENT

Major phenotypic markers of T cell development

The program of T cell development is illustrated in Figure 10.1. In mammals, most of T cell development occurs in the thymus, and developing T cells within the thymus are referred to as thymocytes. T cells differ from other hematopoietically derived immune cells in that bone marrow-derived progenitor cells are required to migrate out of the bone marrow to an extramedullary site to undergo further development. The thymus itself lacks a pool of self-renewing progenitor cells and therefore requires continuous replenishment from bone marrow progenitors to maintain mature T cell production. Precursor cells enter the

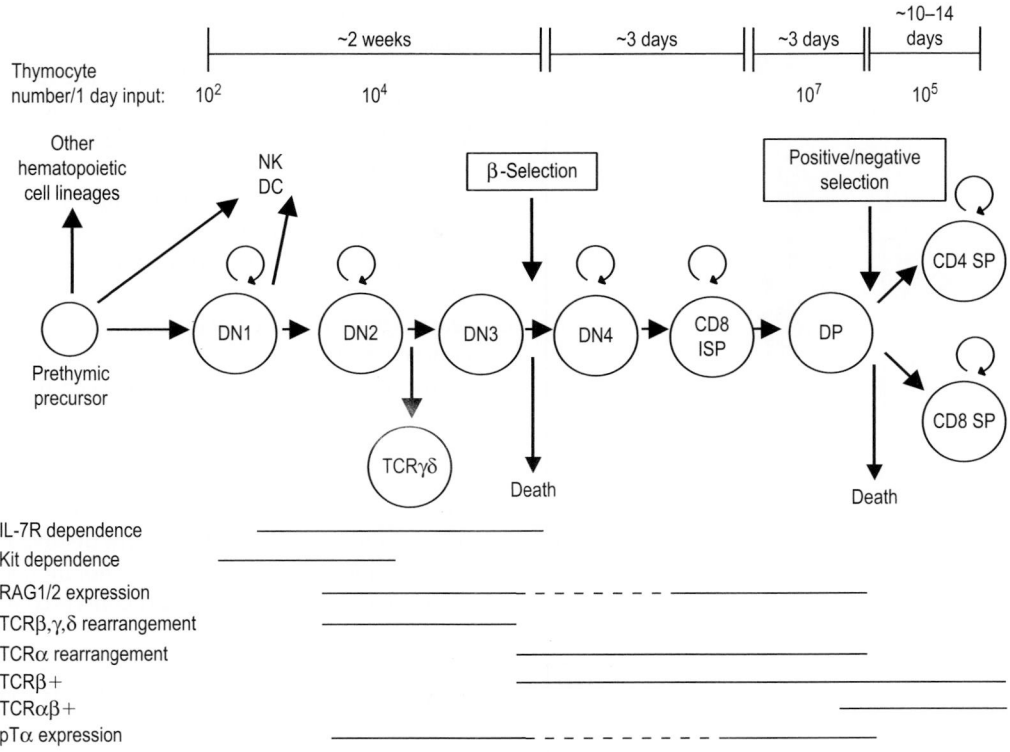

Figure 10.1   Program of T cell development. Shown is the course of T cell development in mice, indicating the phenotypic changes and functional events that occur from the entry of prethymic precursors through terminal maturation of T cells just prior to export. The number of thymocytes that are generated at each developmental stage from the import of a single day's worth of precursor cells is shown. Circular arrows indicate the stages in thymocyte development during which cell proliferation occurs. The red arrows indicate the major developmental checkpoints of β-selection and positive/negative selection, which are discussed in detail in the chapter text. Also shown are the patterns of IL-7 and Kit dependence, as both of these cytokines have been shown to have critical roles in early thymocyte development. Finally, patterns of RAG expression, TCR gene rearrangements, and expression of TCR components on the cell surface are indicated. Dotted lines indicate transient decreases in expression. DN, double negative; SP, single positive; TCR, T cell receptor; NK, natural killer cell; DC, dendritic cell.

thymus and begin a series of sequential maturational steps, beginning with commitment of the precursor cells to a T-lineage developmental program, followed by rearrangements in the T cell receptor (TCR) loci. T cell receptor rearrangements result in the production of a large population of cells with broad clonal recognition properties known as repertoire diversity. Subsequent to the formation of functional TCR, developing T cells undergo a complex selection process whereby cells with either nonfunctional or self-reactive TCR are eliminated. Cells that proceed through this selection process undergo additional maturational changes before being exported into the periphery as recent thymic emigrants (RTE). It is believed that the time course from entry of precursor cells to export of RTE is approximately four to five weeks, during which the daily influx of approximately 100 precursors leads to a 10^5-fold expansion in cell number, providing a sufficiently large pool of cells to ensure diversity in responses to foreign antigens.

In all mammals, T cell development in the thymus can be tracked by changes in the phenotype of developing thymocytes, as the thymus contains cells in multiple stages

of T cell development. Major phenotypic markers that are used to identify these populations include surface TCR$\alpha\beta$, TCR$\gamma\delta$, and the T cell coreceptors CD4 and CD8. Based on CD4 and CD8 coexpression, four major subsets of thymocytes can be identified by flow cytometry (Fig. 10.2). The most immature thymocytes are termed 'double negative' (DN) thymocytes. Because these cells lack TCR expression as well, they are often referred to as TCR$\alpha\beta^-$ CD4$^-$ CD8$^-$ 'triple negative' (TN) thymocytes. In mice, but not humans, developmental stages within the DN population can be further defined, based on coexpression patterns of the interleukin (IL)-2 receptor α-chain CD25 and the adhesion molecule CD44, into four progressive stages termed DN1 (CD44$^+$ CD25$^-$), DN2 (CD44$^+$ CD25$^+$), DN3 (CD44$^-$ CD25$^+$), and DN4 (CD44$^-$ CD25$^-$). As will be discussed, these phenotypic stages are associated with important functional events in T cell development.

Among the cells in the thymus that are in the latter part of intrathymic development, the largest population of thymocytes (accounting for approximately 80 percent of total thymocytes) express both CD4 and CD8 and are

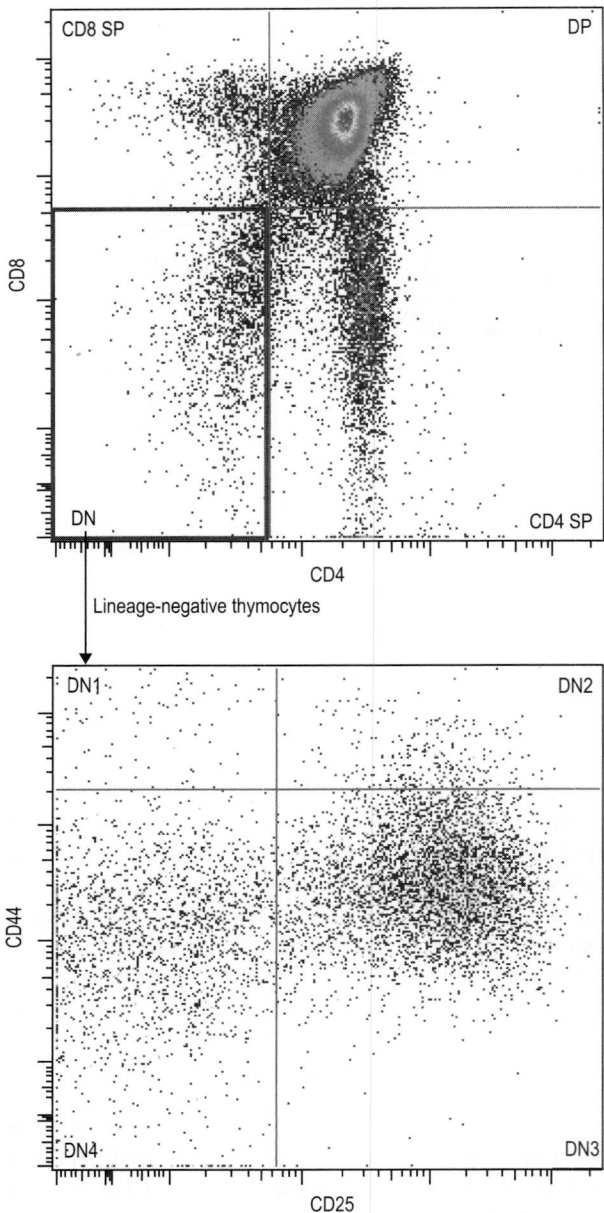

Figure 10.2   Flow cytometric profiles of thymus T cell subsets in mice. At the top are the four major thymocyte populations defined by expression patterns of the CD4 and CD8 coreceptor molecules. Double negative (DN) thymocytes are defined by the absence of CD4 and CD8 expression, double positive (DP) thymocytes are defined by the dual expression of CD4 and CD8, and single positive (SP) thymocytes are defined by the monoexpression of CD4 or CD8. At the bottom is an example of a flow cytometric profile of the DN1 through DN4 subsets, which are defined by the expression patterns of CD44 and CD25 on thymocytes lacking all known hematopoietic lineage markers, including erythrocytes, granulocytes, monocytes, macrophages, dendritic cells, B cells, and NK cells.

termed 'double positive' (DP) thymocytes. It is this population that undergoes the important processes of positive and negative selection that result in the programmed cell death of the vast majority of these cells based on the

appropriateness of TCR specificities. 'Single positive' (SP) CD4$^+$ CD8$^-$ and CD4$^-$ CD8$^+$ thymocytes, both of which also express high levels of TCR$\alpha\beta$, account for 10–15 percent of total thymocytes, constitute those cells that have survived positive and negative selection, and represent the most mature cells.

It is instructive to note that while most information on T cell development has been based on studies in murine models, it is apparent that most of these events, including immigration of multipotent progenitor cells, TCR gene rearrangement, and positive and negative selection, are conserved in humans as well as other mammals. Nevertheless, differences exist between mouse and human thymocytes based on cell-surface molecule expression.[1–3] These differences are listed in Table 10.1. Thus, while the phenotypic markers mentioned in the subsequent text are based on murine thymocyte cell markers, the important cellular and molecular mechanisms involved in T cell development, including cytokines, chemokines, and cell-surface molecules, are for the most part conserved in humans.

T cell receptor gene rearrangements

Complementing the phenotypic markers that define the major thymocyte subsets, TCR gene rearrangement is a well-defined molecular marker in T cell ontogeny. Successful progression to the more mature stages of T cell development is critically dependent on successful TCR gene rearrangement, which gives rise to receptor complexes important for intracellular signaling during positive and negative selection as well as mature T cell activation upon encounter with foreign antigen in the context of self-MHC (major histocompatibility complex) expression. In humans, there are four TCR loci corresponding to the TCR α, β, γ, and δ chains. In an organization that is similar to that of the immunoglobulin gene loci, each TCR loci is composed of variable (V) region and joining (J) region segments as well as a single constant (C) region exon. TCR β and δ loci additionally contain diversity (D) region genes. Rearrangements mediated by the RAG1 and RAG2 protein complex that result in the juxtaposition of V-J or V-D-J gene segments define the binding specificity of the TCR. Rearrangements in TCR β, γ, and δ chains occur first, during the DN2 stage of development, and are the primary determinants in both $\alpha\beta/\gamma\delta$ lineage commitment and β-selection. Rearrangements in the TCRα locus occur during the DN4 stage of T cell development just prior to the transition to the DP thymocyte stage and the initiation of positive and negative selection. Interestingly, in humans, TCR rearrangements, in addition to creating a broad repertoire of antigen receptors, have also been postulated to play a contributory role in the lineage commitment of a developing T cell to a TCR$\alpha\beta$ or TCR$\gamma\delta$ lineage.[4] In support of this, it is noted that the TCRδ locus resides within the TCRα locus in such a way that rearrangement of the latter necessarily results in the deletion of the former.

Table 10.1 Phenotypic markers of developing T cells in mice and humans[1–3]

Developmental stage	Mouse phenotype	Human phenotype
Earliest thymocyte precursor (Pre-T/B/NK)	Lin$^-$ CD44$^+$ CD25$^-$ Kit$^+$ NK1.1$^-$	CD34$^+$ CD38$^-$ CD7$^-$
Pro-T thymocyte	Lin$^-$ CD44$^+$ CD25$^-$ Kit$^+$ NK1.1$^-$ (DN1)	CD34$^+$ CD38$^+$ pTα^- CD1a$^-$
Pre/pro-T thymocyte	Lin$^-$ CD44$^+$ CD25$^+$ Kit$^+$ NK1.1$^-$ (DN2)	CD34$^+$ CD38$^+$ CD1a$^{+/-}$ pT$\alpha^{+/-}$
Pre-T thymocyte	Lin$^-$ CD44$^-$ Kit$^-$ CD25$^+$ HSA$^+$ (DN3)	CD34$^-$ CD38$^+$ pTα^+ CD1a$^+$ CD3ε^+
β-Selection	Lin$^-$ CD44$^-$ CD25$^+ \rightarrow$ CD25$^-$ (DN3: $\rightarrow$ DN4)	CD4$^{+/-}$ CD8$^-$ CD3$^{+/-}$ pTα^+ CD1a$^+$
TCRα rearrangement (ISP)	CD4$^-$ CD8$^+$ CD3$^{+/-}$ pTα^+	CD4$^+$ CD8$^-$ CD3$^{+/-}$ pTα^+ CD1a$^+$
DP thymocyte	CD4$^+$ CD8$^+$ CD3$^+$ pTα^-	CD4$^+$ CD8$^+$ CD3$^+$ pTα^- CD1a$^{+/-}$
SP thymocytes	CD3$^+$ CD4$^+$ (CD4SP)	CD1a$^-$ CD3$^+$ CD4$^+$ (CD4SP)
	or	*or*
	CD3$^+$ CD8$^+$ (CD8SP)	CD1a$^-$ CD3$^+$ CD8$^+$ (CD8SP)

Lin$^-$, lineage negative (lacking all hematopoietic surface markers); DN, double negative; DP, double positive; SP, single positive; HAS, heat-stable antigen (CD24); pTα, pre-T cell alpha receptor chain.

Overview of functional events in intrathymic T cell development

Figure 10.1 illustrates details in intrathymic T cell development with regard to phenotypic and functional changes in addition to showing the major thymocyte populations described above. Each of these processes is discussed in greater detail later in the chapter. These phenotypic changes occur as part of a regulated, coordinated program of gene regulation and expression that determines to a large extent the susceptibility of cells to survival and death signals.

Bone marrow–derived precursor cells enter the thymus and develop into early T lineage progenitors (ETPs), the phenotype of which is defined as the absence of lineage-specific markers, i.e., lineage-negative (lin$^-$), CD25$^-$, CD44^{hi}, Kit$^+$, and CD24 (heat stable antigen [HSA])^{lo}. These cells have been identified as the earliest intrathymic T cell precursors in mice.[5] Early T lineage progenitors give rise to the DN1 population and continue to maintain pluripotency,[6] with an ability to give rise to intrathymic NK and dendritic cells (DC). With the progression to the DN2 stage of thymocyte development, however, cells begin to adopt T-lineage specificity while losing the ability to differentiate into other cell types.[7] For example, it is also at the DN2 stage that lineage choices leading to TCR$\alpha\beta$ and TCR$\gamma\delta$ T cell differentiation are initiated. Additionally, DN2 thymocytes undergo six to ten rounds of cell division. Expression of RAG-1 and RAG-2 recombinases, which lead to the initiation of TCR γ, δ, and β rearrangement and the assembly of TCR complexes, is induced during the DN2 stage as well.

The DN3 stage is functionally associated with the first of three major developmental checkpoints that are TCR-dependent, known as β-selection, whereby cells are selected to proceed with T cell development on the basis of a productive TCRβ gene rearrangement. Following β-selection, surviving cells undergo a rapid proliferative burst of six to eight rounds of cell division,[8] cease to undergo additional TCRβ, TCRγ, and TCRδ rearrangements, begin TCRα rearrangements, and initiate CD4 and CD8 expression. Consequently, the time course of transition from DN3 through DN4 to the DP stage is very rapid.

The DP stage of T cell development is functionally highlighted by three selection events that are dependent on the assembly and binding characteristics of the TCR. The first involves rearrangements of the TCRα gene locus and the selection of those cells that are able to generate functional TCR$\alpha\beta$ complexes. Thymocytes that manage to produce TCR$\alpha\beta$ on their cell surfaces are subsequently subjected to *positive and negative selection*, which constitute the second major TCR-dependent developmental checkpoint. The efficiency and stringency of positive and negative selection is highlighted by the fact that numerically, DP cells represent the largest population of developing T cells in the thymus (see Fig. 10.2), yet approximately 95 percent of these cells are destined to die in the three days following their entry into the DP compartment.

Lineage commitment to a CD4 SP versus a CD8 SP thymocyte is the third major TCR-dependent developmental checkpoint. In addition to determining the fate of the cell, the nature of TCR-MHC interactions also determines the final differentiation fate of DP into CD4 SP or CD8 SP thymocytes. Ultimately, DP thymocytes with TCR that recognize MHC class II molecules develop into CD4$^+$ CD8$^-$ T cells while those that recognize MHC class I molecules develop into CD4$^-$ CD8$^+$ T cells. CD4 SP and CD8 SP thymocytes, once formed, remain in the thymus for an additional ten to fourteen days, during which they acquire additional maturational markers and undergo additional cell proliferation[9] before they are released into the periphery as mature naïve T cells.

ANATOMIC CORRELATES OF T CELL DEVELOPMENT

Thymus structure and ontogeny

As the thymus represents the major site of T cell development, a discussion on its anatomic and functional

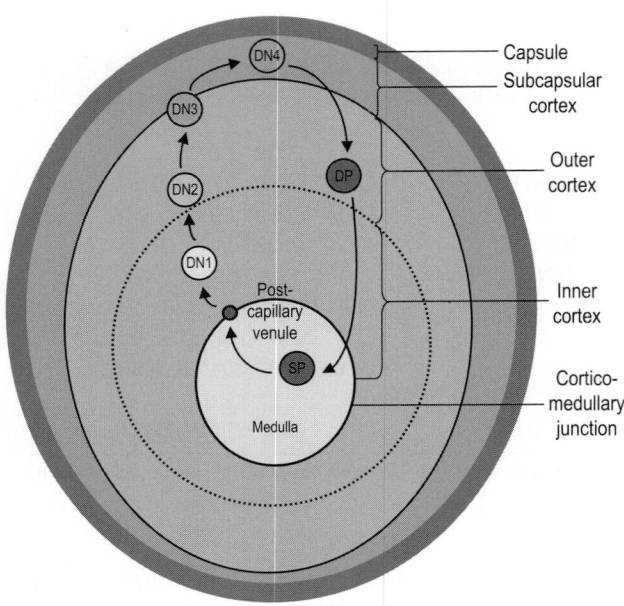

Figure 10.3 Scheme of thymus structure and thymocyte migration. The thymus is divided anatomically and functionally into three major areas: the subcapsular cortex, the cortex, and the medulla. Each of these three areas is defined by the composition of developing thymocytes, thymic epithelial cells, and other non-hematopoietic cell types (see text for details). The migration pattern of a developing thymocyte is shown. Precursor cells initially enter the thymus by way of post-capillary venules at the cortico-medullary junction. As part of their maturational program, these cells migrate outward toward the subcapsular cortex such that most double negative (DN) cells at the DN4 stage of development are concentrated at the subcapsular cortex. During positive selection, thymocytes reverse course and migrate back toward the medulla, at which time they enter the medulla as single positive (SP) thymocytes and ultimately exit the thymus.

organization is warranted. The thymus is composed of lobes that are delineated into discrete zones observable by light microscopy. The larger outer domain is termed the cortex, which is densely packed with thymocytes comprising the DN and DP lineages. The cortex surrounds the medulla, where most of the CD4$^+$ and CD8$^+$ SP thymocytes are found. Two additional regions of the thymus are important in the context of T cell development: the cortico-medullary junction and the subcapsular cortex (Fig. 10.3). Each of the aforementioned areas of the thymus is composed of specific mixtures of developing thymocytes, specialized stromal cells termed thymic epithelial cells, macrophages, and dendritic cells. The composition of these cell types contributes to the formation of developmental microenvironments, or niches, that are important to the orderly sequence of T cell development.

The thymus is a dynamic organ in that its size and degree of function are sensitive to age, fluctuations in its responses to neuroendocrine hormones and other non-immune specific growth factors, pharmacologic agents

such as corticosteroids and immunosuppressive drugs, and radiation. In healthy individuals, the thymus attains its greatest relative size and cellularity in the late fetal and early neonatal period, after which it undergoes progressive age-dependent loss of function.[10] Changes in the size of the thymus with age parallel changes in its function as measured by enumeration of phenotypically naïve peripheral T cells[11] and RTE.[12] While the factors contributing to the age-related decline in thymic function are numerous, many are related to changes in the developmental niches that are composed of developing thymocytes and the thymic epithelial cells described in the next section.

Thymic epithelial cells

Key to the development of thymic developmental niches is the formation of specialized thymic epithelial cells (TEC). Based on observations in mice, these cells are derived from the interaction of ectodermal and endodermal cells of the third pharyngeal pouch and neural crest-derived mesenchyme. Together, these cells generate a thymic epithelial primordium into which hematopoietic stem cells enter and serve as precursors to dendritic cells and macrophages, as well as developing lymphocytes.[13] In the mature thymus, several phenotypic and functional TEC subsets exist. These subsets are distinguished from one another based on cytokeratin expression patterns,[14,15] expression of unique combinations of cell-surface molecules, and secretion of cytokines, chemokines, and other factors.[16–18] These cell subsets are critical in the formation of developmental niches regulating T cell development. Importantly, evidence in mice exists that TEC subsets are derived from a TEC precursor pool concentrated at the cortico-medullary junction and that differentiation into mature cortical and medullary TEC populations is dependent on concomitant thymocyte development.[14,15,19,20] Thus, developmental niches in the thymus are defined by *both* developing thymocytes and TEC in a highly coordinated fashion.

Thymic epithelial cells serve three important functions. First, they serve as directors of thymocyte trafficking, directing developing T cells to the appropriate areas in the thymus in which to continue their developmental program. As shown in Figure 10.3, developing thymocytes proceed along a well-defined pathway, beginning with the recruitment of precursor cells into the thymus through the post-capillary venules in the cortico-medullary junction. During the DN1 through DN2 stage, thymocytes migrate from the cortico-medullary junction outward toward the subcapsular cortex. During this time, thymocytes undergo developmental and proliferative changes as previously described. The arrival in the subcapsular cortex corresponds to the phenotypic transition from DN2 to DN3. It is during this stage in the subcapsular cortex that thymocytes undergo β-selection, followed by additional rounds of cell proliferation in cells that survive this process (see Fig. 10.1).

Table 10.2   Selected chemokines/chemokine receptors in thymocyte development[7,19,21,23,30]

Chemokine receptor	Receptor expression pattern	Ligands	Ligand expression pattern	Functional roles
CCR4	CD69$^+$ DP CD69$^+$ CD62L^{lo} CD4SP	CCL17 (TARC) CCL22 (MDC)	Medullary DC Hassall's corpuscles; mTEC (hu)	Possible role in negative selection
CCR7	SP thymocytes TCR-stimulated DP DN1 and DN2 thymocytes	CCL19 (ELC, MIP-3β) CCL21 (SLC)	mTEC; medullary venule endothelium; CMJ mTEC; CMJ	(1) Migration of positively selected thymocytes in medulla (2) Thymic emigration (3) Migration of DN thymocytes to outer cortex (4) Recruitment of progenitors into fetal thymus
CCR9	Thymic precursors DP thymocytes SP thymocytes	CCL25 (TECK)	cTEC and mTEC	(1) Importation of T precursors into the thymus (2) Migration of DN2 and/or DN3 to outer cortex
CXCR4	DN1:DN4 thymocytes DP thymocytes SP thymocytes	CXCL12 (SDF-1α)	cTEC; medulla; CMJ Fibroblasts Hassall's corpuscles (hu)	(1) Migration of DN thymocytes to outer cortex (2) DN thymocyte development (3) Thymic emigration

DP, double positive; SP, single positive; DN, double negative; DC, dendritic cells; mTEC, medullary thymic epithelial cells; cTEC, cortical thymic epithelial cells; CMJ, cortico-medullary junction; (hu), data from human studies.

Subsequently, cells transitioning into the DP stage of development reverse their course and travel inward from the subcapsular cortex toward the medulla. During this time, thymocytes are positively and negatively selected based on TCR-MHC peptide interactions. Those cells that survive ultimately enter the medulla as SP thymocytes, where they complete their maturation prior to export into the periphery. Studies with adoptively transferred bone marrow-derived progenitor cells show that the time intervals where thymocytes reside in specific areas of the thymus correspond to the time course of their development.[21] The transit time from entry at the cortico-medullary junction to the subcapsular cortex is approximately fourteen days, corresponding to the DN1 to DN3 transition. β-Selection in the subcapsular cortex lasts for three days, and the transit time for DP thymocytes from the subcapsular cortex to the medulla, corresponding to positive and negative selection, lasts for three to seven days.[22]

Thymic epithelial cell-directed migration of developing thymocytes is carried out in part through the secretion of chemokines, expression of cell-surface adhesion molecules that interact with specific receptors on the developing thymocytes, and secretion of extracellular matrix (ECM) proteins.[23] Chemokines are small polypeptides that stimulate migration of responding cells through interaction with specific receptors containing a common pertussis toxin-sensitive, G1α protein-coupled seven-transmembrane motif.[24] Consistent with the temporal spatial distribution of developing thymocyte populations within the thymus (Fig. 10.3), TEC and thymocyte subsets are programmed

to express specific combinations of chemokine and chemokine receptors (Table 10.2). Consequently, developmental niches are in part defined by the pattern of chemokine secretion.[18] Among the chemokines and their receptors that have been implicated in T cell development,[24,25] two are mentioned here as examples to highlight the importance of chemokines as critical regulators of thymocyte migration. First, the chemokine receptor CCR7, which is expressed on DN1 and DN2 thymocytes and is the specific ligand for the chemokine CCL21, is required for the trafficking of these cells through the inner cortex toward the subcapsular cortex. The absence of CCR7 in mice results in the failure of thymocytes to develop past the DN2 stage and the accumulation of DN2 cells at the cortico-medullary junction.[26] Another chemokine that has been shown to play a critical role in T cell development involves the dependence of migration of DN3 thymocytes into the subcapsular cortex on TEC secretion of the chemokine CXCL12 (SDF-1α/β) and the expression of its receptor CXCR4 on thymocytes. Murine thymocytes lacking CXCR4, similar to those lacking CCR7, fail to migrate out of the cortico-medullary junction and demonstrate developmental arrest.[27] Moreover, CCL21-CCR7 and CXCL12-CXCR4 interactions, which are essential for the *outward* trafficking of DN thymocytes, are also important in the *inward* trafficking of DP thymocytes toward the medulla.[27–30]

In addition to chemokine receptors, thymocytes at various stages of development express different patterns of cell-adhesion molecules called integrins, which are linked to the actin cytoskeleton of the cell, and thus play a direct role in cell migration. Integrins interact with both cell-surface expressed ligands, including vascular cell-adhesion molecule-1 (VCAM1) and mucosal vascular addressin molecule-1 (MADCAM1), and ECM proteins including fibronectin, laminin-1 and laminin-5, and type IV collagen.[31] The specificity of integrin binding to its ligand is dependent on the combinatorial heterodimerization of component α and β chain subtypes. In mice, it has been shown that the developmental stage of thymocytes is associated with distinct patterns of integrin expression.[32] Moreover, the patterns of ECM proteins appear to be distinct within the thymus.[31] The net effect of the polarized expression of chemokines, surface molecules, ECM proteins by non-lymphocyte cells in the thymus, and their corresponding receptors on thymocytes is the directed trafficking of thymocytes in a regulated manner that is coincident with their development.

The second major function of TEC is their secretion of cytokines that confer survival, proliferative and/or pro-apoptotic signals to thymocytes. Recall that during the progression from the DN1 through DP developmental stage, thymocytes undergo regulated bursts of cell proliferation (see Fig. 10.1). The significance of these proliferative events in conjunction with productive TCR gene rearrangement is the establishment of a large pool of cells with functional TCR that are primed for positive and negative selection. Numerous cytokines and their receptors have been shown to be expressed by both TEC and thymocytes.[17] Two cytokines in particular, stem cell factor (SCF) and interleukin-7 (IL-7), and their respective receptors, KIT and the IL-7R, have been shown to be particularly important in promoting the survival and expansion of early DN thymocytes. As stated above, ETPs entering the thymus express KIT and expression is maintained through the DN2 developmental stage after which it is downregulated.[33] In mouse knockout models, absence of KIT results in profound loss of thymocyte number due to the absence of cell proliferation. Loss of KIT, on the other hand, does not abrogate the full spectrum of T cell development.[34] Loss of IL-7R, which is expressed in DN3 and DN4 thymocytes, also shows evidence of causing impaired thymocyte development.[34,35] IL-7R is a member of the cytokine receptors, including those for IL-2, IL-4, IL-9, and IL-15, which share the common γ chain (γc). This subunit is critical for intracellular signaling upon binding of the cytokine to the receptor. In mouse knockout models of IL-7, IL-7R, γc, or the intracellular signaling molecules JAK1 and JAK3 that are recruited by γc signaling, thymic cellularity is dramatically reduced, supporting the concept that IL-7 has a nonredundant role in thymocyte development.[36,37] In addition to its effect on early thymocyte survival and proliferation, IL-7 may also have effects on thymocyte differentiation into $\gamma\delta$ T cells from DN2 thymocytes,[38] control of TCR gene rearrangements,[39,40] as well as playing an important role during lineage commitment following positive selection.[41]

The third major function of TEC is the expression of surface molecules that provide critical signals that dictate lineage decisions and decisions that determine whether the developing T cell is destined to survive or die. Lineage commitment from pluripotent precursor cells into T cell-specific lineages following entry into the thymus is mediated by Notch-1 signaling. The Delta-like 1 ligand for Notch-1 is located on TEC. Interactions of MHC molecules on TEC and TCR on thymocytes determine cell fate during β-selection, positive and negative selection, and lineage commitment from DP to SP thymocytes.

KEY EVENTS IN INTRATHYMIC T CELL DEVELOPMENT

From the preceding discussion, it is clear that thymic T cell development is characterized by the formation of spatially defined developmental niches comprising developing thymocytes and TEC. The purpose of these niches is to provide an anatomic and functional framework in which developing thymocytes make decisions of lineage commitment and cell fate, i.e., survival versus death. These decision points are critical in generating a repertoire of peripheral T cells that is broad enough to generate specific immune responses against foreign antigens, yet restricted enough to prevent autoimmunity through attack on host cells. In addition to TCR$\alpha\beta^+$ T cells that form the majority of cells derived from DN precursors, NK cells, dendritic cells, and TCR$\gamma\delta^+$ T cells are also generated as a result of lineage choices along the T development pathway (see Fig. 10.1). The purpose of this section is to highlight the cellular and molecular changes that influence these decisions, from most immature to most mature: (1) commitment from immigrant pluripotent progenitor cells to T cells; (2) lineage commitment to TCR$\gamma\delta$ Tcells; (3) β-selection; (4) positive and negative selection; and (5) commitment from DP to CD4$^+$ versus CD8$^+$ SP thymocytes. It is instructive to again emphasize that these events require complex interactions between thymocytes and TEC, involving both direct cell-to-cell contacts and the secretion of cytokines, chemokines, and other growth factors.

Lineage commitment in early thymocyte precursors

The first decision point in the thymus concerns the lineage decision of an entering precursor cell to become a T cell. As was stated earlier, precursor cells destined to migrate to the thymus are derived from bone marrow hematopoietic cells. Early T-lineage precursors (lineage$^-$ CD44$^+$ CD25$^-$ Kit$^+$ cells in mice, CD34$^+$ CD38$^-$ cells in humans; see Table 10.1) define the earliest intrathymic T cell precursors. Even so, based on adoptive transfer studies in mice, cells contained in this population that immediately enter the thymus continue to have the capacity to differentiate into T cells, B cells, NK cells, and dendritic cells (Fig. 10.1).[7] While it remains unclear which specific pluripotent cell populations from the bone marrow give eventual rise to

Table 10.3 Selected transcription factors in T cell lineage commitment[3,60]

Transcription factor	Class	Effect of gene mutant on T cell development
RUNX1–CBFβ	Runt	Loss of pan-lineage hematopoiesis during embryonic development in Runx1 knockout; disruption in DN development during adult T cell development
MYB	Myb	Multilineage fetal hematopoiesis defect
PU.1	ETS	Loss of embryonic, but not postnatal, T cell development
IKAROS	Zn finger	Dominant negative: absent lymphoid development
		Null: loss of fetal, but not postnatal, T cell development; decreased CD8 SPs; TCRγδ development affected; possible effects on β-selection
GFI1	Zn finger	Block in DN2 generation
GATA3	Zn finger	*RAG−/−* chimeras: block in T cell development at or before DN1 stage
CREB	Basic/leucine ZIP	Null: block in fetal T cell development
		Dominant negative: normal T cell development; inhibited activation responses; increased apoptosis due to G1 cell cycle arrest
TCF1	HMG	Block in DN to DP transition; block in DN1 to DN2 transition
E2A	bHLH (class I)	Decreased thymocyte numbers, especially in DP population, due to partial block at DN1
HEB	bHLH (class I)	Partial block at DN to DP transition
ID3	bHLH (class V)	Transgenic: inhibition of TCRαβ cells; enhanced NK cell development; disruption of positive/negative selection
HES1	bHLH (class VI)	Block at DN3 stage; defect in DN1 and DN2 proliferative expansion
NFATc	NFAT	Decreased thymocyte cellularity due to partial block in ISP-DP transition

DN, double negative; DP, double positive; SP, single positive; ETS, E26-transformation specific; bHLH, basic helix-loop-helix; HMG, high mobility group; CBF, core binding factor; TCR, T cell receptor.

developing T cells in the thymus, or whether the beginnings of T-lineage commitment occur even prior to entry of cells into the bone marrow[42] or prior to their entry into the thymus,[43] it is clear that the thymic microenvironment plays an important role in the decision to promote commitment among the entering precursors to the T cell lineage.

Interactions of the cell-surface receptor Notch and its ligands exemplify the influence of extracellular signals in both mice and humans to promote lineage fate decisions in a wide variety of cell types.[44] In T cell development, binding of NOTCH1 on hematopoietic cell precursors to its Delta-like 1 ligand has been shown to be instrumental in promoting T cell specific development, specifically with respect to the T versus B cell lineage fate.[45–49] Delta-like 1 is expressed in cortical TEC[47] and interacts with NOTCH1 expressed on ETP in the thymus to initiate a cascade of intracellular events leading to alterations in DNA transcription.[50,51] Cells that do not receive sufficient signals through NOTCH1 are redirected toward B cell development.[52] In addition to directing precursor cells toward a T-lineage fate, NOTCH1 signaling appears to be important for lineage commitment at stages beyond the T/B lineage-commitment step. For example, *in vitro* studies in which DN2 thymocytes are cultured in the presence or absence of Delta-like 1-expressing stromal cells suggest that recurrent signaling through NOTCH1 is required for continuing T cell development, whereas the absence of such signaling leads to NK cell development.[47]

In addition to the NOTCH1 signaling pathway, signals of other molecules through hematopoietic cells are important

in supporting the maintenance of the T cell precursor pool, including the WNT signaling pathway[53,54] and hedgehog family of proteins.[55–57] The WNT pathway, for example, encompasses a class of secreted glycoproteins that mediate cell-to-cell communication during development. Binding of WNT to the Frizzled class of receptors leads to the accumulation of the protein β-catenin and its interaction with transcription factors of the T cell factor/lymphoid enhancer factor (TCF/LEF) family, of which TCF1 is specific to T cells and LEF1 is specific to T and B cells. Mouse knock-out models of TCF1 and β-catenin, which lead to a loss of DN4 thymocytes, demonstrate the importance of WNT signaling in the maintenance of these cell populations.[54,58] While these signaling pathways may involve unique sets of molecules involved in intracellular signaling events, it is probable that a substantial degree of interaction exists among them. In support of this, it has recently been shown that WNT signaling affects the transcriptional targets of NOTCH signaling and that this signal is required for the WNT-mediated maintenance of hematopoietic stem cells.[59]

Transcription factor expression resulting from external signals is instrumental in turning on genes that dictate the T cell lineage decision.[3,60] A list of selected transcription factors that are associated with early lineage commitment is shown in Table 10.3. The biological effects of genes controlled by these transcription factors include those that mediate cell survival and proliferation, as is the case for the JAK-STAT activation resulting from IL-7R signaling,[61] which, among its gene targets, leads to expression of the anti-apoptotic gene *BCL2*.[62,63] Transcriptional targets of

Notch-1 signaling, which include Hes-1 and Deltex,[64] are evidently important in mediating T- versus B-lineage decisions.[65] Nevertheless, the pattern of genes that are expressed as a result of these signaling pathways is complex[66] and may confer overlapping functions. Moreover, gene expression patterns in and of themselves may not necessarily determine T-lineage commitment, based on the observations of T-specific genes being expressed in hematopoietic stem cells in the bone marrow, prior to their immigration into the thymus.[63,67] Thus, the commitment of a bone marrow-derived progenitor cell to develop into a T cell involves a complex interplay of gene expression patterns, presumably leading to a genetic profile that favors T cell development while disfavoring development into other cell lineages.

$\alpha\beta/\gamma\delta$ T-lineage commitment

While most of the discussion about T cell development in the thymus focuses on the TCR$\alpha\beta$ development, TCR$\gamma\delta$ T cells also arise from the thymus. The roles of TCR$\gamma\delta$ T cells in the immune system, while not yet fully characterized, appear to be distinct from those of TCR$\alpha\beta$ T cells. TCR$\gamma\delta$ T cells, representing approximately 1–5 percent of circulating T cells in both humans and mice, have been shown to be involved in primary immune responses against infectious pathogens, immune regulation, and in wound repair.[68,69] Moreover, TCR$\gamma\delta$ T cells differ functionally at the cellular level from their TCR$\alpha\beta$ counterparts in that their activation is initiated in a non-MHC restricted fashion, and that the TCR$\gamma\delta$ T cells in specific anatomic sites such as the skin and gut have very restricted TCR repertoires.

TCR$\gamma\delta$ T cell development differs from TCR$\alpha\beta$ T cell development in several ways. First, TCR$\gamma\delta$ T cells do not proceed through the DP stage of development (see Fig. 10.1), leading to the supposition that the generation of TCR$\gamma\delta$ T cells represents an evolutionary precursor pathway to T cell development. Second, in both humans and mice, TCR$\gamma\delta$ T cells appear to develop in 'waves' that are based on specific rearrangements in TCRγ, which define anatomically specific populations of TCR$\gamma\delta$ T cells. Third, in addition to cells that develop in the thymus, a significant proportion of TCR$\gamma\delta$ T cells has been shown to develop in extrathymic sites.[70,71] For the remainder of this discussion, TCR$\gamma\delta$ development in the thymus will be discussed.

Many facets of thymic TCR$\gamma\delta$ T cell development remain incompletely understood. For example, while rearrangements in TCR γ and δ chain genes are initially detected during the DN2 stage of development,[72] concurrent with rearrangements in the TCRβ genes, the precise point at which TCR$\gamma\delta$ development diverges from TCR$\alpha\beta$ development and the signals that initiate TCR$\gamma\delta$ differentiation are incompletely understood. Central to this question is the relative importance of TCR gene rearrangement events in dictating TCR$\alpha\beta$ versus $\gamma\delta$ lineage choice. In this context, two models have been commonly used to describe the divergence of TCR$\alpha\beta$ and TCR$\gamma\delta$ T differentiation.

The first is a stochastic/selection model, whereby the decision to commit to either population is made prior to and independently of TCR gene rearrangements. Subsequent $\gamma\delta$TCR or pre-TCR signaling is required for further progression along the predetermined developmental pathway. Evidence in support of this model is based on the role of IL-7R signaling, in that a subset of DN2 thymocytes that express IL-7R, when injected intrathymically, had a higher potential to develop TCR$\gamma\delta$ T cells while the IL-7R-negative counterparts had a higher potential to develop into TCR$\alpha\beta$ T cells.[73] This is further supported by the finding that IL-7R signaling promotes rearrangements in TCRγ chain genes.[39,40] Another TCR-independent signal that has been implicated in TCR$\gamma\delta$ commitment is Notch. Several studies suggest that reduced Notch signaling favors the TCR$\gamma\delta$ fate over the TCR$\alpha\beta$ fate,[74] yet other studies appear to suggest the opposite.[75–77] Nevertheless, in all of these experimental models examining the role of Notch in TCR$\gamma\delta$ development, the skewing is not absolute in that TCR$\alpha\beta$ T cells continue to be produced. Other signaling events in addition to those induced by NOTCH and IL-7R are therefore likely to be involved in dictating TCR$\gamma\delta$ development.

The second model of TCR$\gamma\delta$ T cell development is an instructive model whereby expression of, and signaling through, either the TCR$\gamma\delta$ or the pre-TCR complex in itself dictates lineage fate. Evidence supporting this model includes the observation that TCR$\alpha\beta$ T cells are depleted of in-frame TCR γ and δ gene rearrangements,[78] while thymocytes expressing TCR$\gamma\delta$ in mice deficient in pTα, a component required for assembly of the pre-TCR complex (see below), are enriched for in-frame TCRβ rearrangements compared to wild-type mice.[79] Furthermore, in pTα-deficient mice, the thymus is characterized by drastic reductions in TCR$\alpha\beta$ T cells while the number of TCR$\gamma\delta$ T cells is increased.[80] Functionally, the $\gamma\delta$TCR complex differs from the pre-TCR complex with respect to interactions with CD3[81] and in utilization of intracellular signaling cascades[82,83] such that differential transcription factor expression ultimately plays a critical role in influencing TCR$\gamma\delta$ versus TCR$\alpha\beta$ development.[84] More recent data have extended the instructive model to incorporate TCR signal strength as an important parameter to determine TCR$\gamma\delta$ versus TCR$\alpha\beta$ lineage fate.[81,85] For example, presence or absence of signaling through a transgenic TCR$\gamma\delta$ through binding with its cognate ligand appears to determine TCR$\gamma\delta$ and TCR$\alpha\beta$ lineage fates, respectively, and attenuation of TCR$\gamma\delta$ signaling results in commitment to TCR$\alpha\beta$ lineage.[79] Furthermore, TCR$\gamma\delta$ versus TCR$\alpha\beta$ T cell lineage fate was shown to be influenced by the relative signal strengths conveyed by the TCR$\gamma\delta$ and pre-TCR complex, in that strong signals transduced by the TCR$\gamma\delta$ receptor promoted TCR$\gamma\delta$ T cell development, whereas weak signals transduced by the pre-TCR complex conferred commitment to TCR$\alpha\beta$ lineage.[86]

Despite the incomplete understanding of the precise mechanisms that dictate lineage decisions toward TCR$\alpha\beta$ or TCR$\gamma\delta$ lineages, it is clear that the process involves secreted molecules such as cytokines as well as contact-mediated interactions involving the TCRγδ and the pre-TCR complex. It is quite possible that the divergence of precursors to either population may not occur at a discrete stage of thymocyte development, but rather through a spectrum of lineage commitment potential within the DN2–DN4 stages that is defined in part anatomically by developmental niches in the thymus, as detailed earlier. These niches may be defined not only by the thymic epithelium, which constitutes the source of cytokines (IL-7) and cell-surface molecules (Notch and γδTCR-specific ligands), but also TCRαβ thymocytes, which have been shown to promote TCRγδ T cell development through a lymphotoxin-mediated pathway.[87,88]

β-Selection

β-Selection refers to the stage in T cell development where the developing T cell's fate is determined by its ability to successfully rearrange its TCRβ-chain genes. With β-selection, thymocytes become exclusively committed to T-lineage development. It also marks the first stage in intrathymic T cell development where the generation of functional TCR and its interactions with the microenvironment are the primary determinants of cell-fate decisions. In contrast to the recruitment of progenitor cells described in the previous section, where many signals (for example through the IL-7 receptor) activate genes that promote cell survival and proliferation, cells arising from β-selection have relatively little intrinsic survival potential. This is due in part to the loss of Bcl-2 expression from IL-7R signaling,[89] in contrast to cells committed to the TCRγδ lineage (see above), and induced expression of the pro-apoptotic surface receptor Fas.[90,91] Instead, cell survival in the absence of cytokines is almost entirely dependent on interactions involving expression of TCR-encoded genes, beginning with β-selection.

β-Selection is initiated upon the synthesis of the TCRβ chain protein following successful TCRβ gene rearrangement. Rearrangement of the TCRβ chain gene locus begins during the DN3 stage. Initially, Dβ gene segments rearrange with Jβ gene segments to form Dβ-Jβ rearrangements, followed by rearrangements with Vβ and the Cβ gene segments (see previous section on TCR gene rearrangements). Productive rearrangements lead to expression of the TCRβ chain, which associates with the invariant partner pTα chain to form a functional pre-TCR complex on the cell surface. That successful rearrangement of TCRβ chain genes is necessary or even sufficient for continued T cell development is illustrated by the finding that mice expressing a functionally rearranged TCRβ transgene can restore T cell development in RAG knockout mice.[92,93]

Once the pre-TCR complex is synthesized, a series of maturational events among the developing thymocytes is initiated. First, allelic exclusion is enforced, in that further TCRβ gene rearrangements, as well as TCRγ gene rearrangements, are halted as a result of the transient

phosphorylation and subsequent degradation of the RAG-2 protein[94,95] (RAG protein expression is reinduced for TCRα gene rearrangements following β-selection). Second, those cells that have a functional pre-TCR complex are programmed to undergo additional rounds of proliferation (approximately 100-fold) at the DN4 stage, prior to their entrance into the DP stage of development, in order to generate a sufficiently large number of precursors for positive selection.[96,97] As such, β-selection marks the beginning of the last significant round of proliferation prior to T cell export from the thymus. Third, cells undergo CD4, CD8, and TCRα transcriptional activation. Finally, in the absence of Bcl-2 expression, the expression of other anti-apoptotic molecules is induced, including BCL-X$_L$ and nuclear factor κB (NF-κB), which promote the survival of β-selected thymocytes. All of the signals that govern these processes originate from the pre-TCR complex, thus emphasizing the importance of successful assembly of the complex in subsequent T cell development. Interestingly, evidence strongly suggests that signaling through the pre-TCR complex is contingent on its assembly in the absence of any specific ligand, in contrast to the highly specific interactions with TCR during positive and negative selection, in that mutant forms of TCRβ and pTα lacking the extracellular domains can still proceed with β-selection.[98,99]

The pre-TCR is a complex of proteins consisting of the TCRβ chain, pTα chain, and the CD3 complex. The CD3 complex itself is composed of component chains termed γ, δ, ε, and ζ2. Most of the components of the pre-TCR play an important role in subsequent T cell development, as each contains elements involved in the recruitment and activation of intracellular signaling cascades that ultimately lead to induction of gene transcription (Fig. 10.4). An interesting characteristic of the pre-TCR complex is the absence of any identifiable ligand responsible for initiation of pre-TCR complex signaling. Instead, it appears that self-assembly of the pre-TCR complex is sufficient.[100] Following assembly, molecules that are directly recruited to and activated by the pre-TCR include the src kinase p56LCK, the tyrosine kinases ZAP70 and SYK, and the adapter proteins SLP-76 and LAT. All are critical components of the signaling cascade, as demonstrated by the absence of full T cell development in mouse models in which the genes encoding these proteins are deleted.[101–104] Following activation of SLP-76 and LAT, multiple signaling cascades are activated, including the induction of the RAS-dependent mitogen-activated protein (MAP) kinases MEK, ERK1/2, and p38 pathways, as well as calcium-mediated signaling pathways that are mediated by phospholipase Cγ (PLCγ).[105,106] These in turn activate transcription factors that result in the developmental stage-specific gene expression contributing to the phenotypic and functional series of events described above. Among the transcription factor families that have been shown to be important in β-selection are NF-κB, AP-1, NFAT, the HMG box transcription factors TCF-1 and LEF, the Egr family of transcription factors and the basic helix-loop-helix (bHLH) transcription factors.[107–114] More recent evidence has

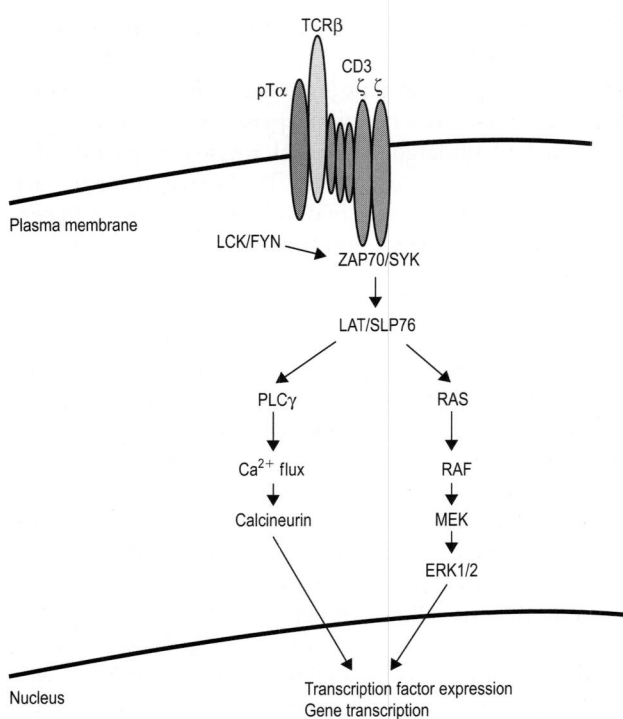

Figure 10.4 β-Selection. Shown are the components of the pre-T cell receptor (TCR) and selected intracellular signaling cascades initiated by pre-TCR assembly/signaling. See the text for details.

demonstrated the requirement of NOTCH signaling in β-selection that is independent of pTα signaling.[115] While many of the genes with expression are induced by these transcription factors, and their interactions with other products of gene transcription remain incompletely defined, it is clear that such integrations do exist and play an important role in the progression through β-selection.

Positive and negative selection

Once developing T cells have completed rearrangement of their TCRβ genes and have undergone β-selection, they exit from the DN stage of development and acquire phenotypic and functional characteristics of CD4$^+$ CD8$^+$ DP thymocytes (see Fig. 10.1). It is at this point that DP thymocytes undergo the processes of positive and negative selection, the purpose of which is to select a population of T cells that are (a) restricted to self-MHC (positive selection), and (b) tolerant to self-antigens (negative selection). Unlike β-selection, during which the assembly of the pre-TCR complex constitutes the critical checkpoint that determines the fate of the cell independently of its binding properties, in positive and negative selection both the successful gene rearrangements in TCRα chain genes and TCR$\alpha\beta$ (hereafter referred to as TCR) assembly and the nature of its interactions with MHC-peptide complexes presented by antigen-presenting cells (APC) are critical determinants in cell fate. In the context of positive and negative selection,

the peptides that are assembled with MHC represent those with structural homology to self-antigens, which confer different TCR-triggering thresholds than MHC-peptide complexes containing the identical MHC but with a foreign peptide that are encountered by mature T cells in the peripheral immune system. The life span of DP thymocytes is on average only three to four days,[116] which is relatively brief compared with the two weeks that elapse between the entry of bone marrow-derived precursors and the completion of β-selection. However, in this short period, the vast majority of cells (about 95 percent) die, while the few that survive (about 5 percent) undergo further lineage development into CD4$^+$ and CD8$^+$ SP thymocytes.

T cell development up to the DP stage, in addition to controlling lineage fates, generates a sufficiently large pool of precursor cells that, after positive and negative selection, yields a pool of mature T cells containing a broad repertoire of TCR specificities. In contributing to this diversity, TCRα gene rearrangements in DP thymocytes undergoing positive selection are not targeted for allelic exclusion, in contrast to TCRβ gene rearrangements during β-selection. In fact, up to one-third of mature T cells carry two productive TCRα rearrangements.[117] Cessation of TCRα gene rearrangements occurs only with engagement of the TCR, which leads to downregulation of RAG-1 recombinase expression.[118,119] The implication for this concept of *receptor editing*, whereby ongoing TCRα gene rearrangement leads to replacement of one TCR specificity by another, is evident in that it provides an additional layer of diversity independent of the size of the DP cell pool fated to undergo positive and negative selection.

Studies in murine models utilizing transgenes encoding TCRα and TCRβ chains of known specificity and affinity have led to the concept of thresholds in binding of both TCR as the prime determinants of positive and negative selection. TCR that establish *low*-affinity interactions with MHC-peptide complexes are *positively* selected for further development. In the absence of any interaction between TCR and MHC-peptide complexes, the thymocyte dies by neglect. Double positive thymocytes possess a number of biologic features that optimize their potential for positive selection; namely, the extreme dose–response sensitivity of the TCR to interact with MHC–peptide complexes compared with that of mature T cells,[120] and enhanced binding avidity of the CD4 and CD8 coreceptors to the MHC–peptide complex due to alterations in their glycosylation states.[121,122] Moreover, DP thymocytes themselves do not express class I or class II MHC, thus ensuring that interactions involving TCR on these cells are restricted primarily to MHC–peptide complexes expressed by TEC. That stimulation of DP thymocytes through the TCR occurs with a sensitivity threshold that is substantially lower than that of mature T cells helps to ensure that once out in the periphery, the now mature T cell will not be activated by the same low-affinity MHC–self-peptide interaction, but will instead be activated by high-affinity MHC–foreign peptide interactions in which the foreign peptides are generally structurally similar to the self-peptides that are involved in selection. Furthermore, the low-affinity interaction between TCR and MHC–peptide complexes permits selection of thymocytes with different TCR specificities selected by a single MHC–peptide complex.[123,124]

On the other hand, TCR that establish *high*-affinity interactions with MHC–self-peptide complexes are *negatively* selected and subsequently die. In further contrast to positive selection, negative selection also requires a second signal in addition to those induced by binding of TCR to MHC–peptide.[125,126] These signals are similar to signals required for mature T cell activation in the peripheral immune system.[127] The result of negative selection is a population of mature T cells that are not indiscriminately activated by high-affinity interactions with self-MHC or self-peptide. Consequently, the potential for autoimmunity is minimized. The importance of negative selection in the prevention of autoimmunity is highlighted by studies in the AIRE (autoimmune regulator) gene. AIRE is expressed in medullary TEC and functions as an inducer of transcription of a broad set of tissue-specific proteins and regulates their expression on medullary TEC.[128,129] Mutations in the Aire gene in both mice and humans results in systemic autoimmunity; this mutation defines the polyendocrine autoimmune disease APECED (autoimmune polyendocrinopathy-candidiasis-ectodermal dystrophy) or APS-1 (autoimmune polyglandular syndrome type 1) in humans.[130]

A corollary to the principle that positive and negative selection is dictated by TCR–MHC-peptide binding affinity is that these processes significantly differ with respect to the microenvironments in which they occur. Consistent with their absolute dependence on TCR interactions for survival, DP thymocytes have little intrinsic functionality and survivability outside of the thymic microenvironment. The dependence on TCR signaling for DP thymocyte survival underscores the importance of the role of cortical TEC, as these cells play a major role in presentation of MHC–peptide as well as of other surface molecules that may complement TCR–MHC-peptide interactions in promoting thymocyte development through positive selection.[131–133] On the other hand, medullary TEC appear to be the prime mediators of negative selection, as they are involved in Aire-induced presentation of self-tissue-specific antigens.[134,135] Additionally, cells other than TEC can also serve as APC for positive and negative selection. For example, negative selection involves signaling through accessory molecules, the ligands of which are found on hematopoietically derived dendritic cells in the medulla, leading to the notion that negative selection events, at least to class II MHC-restricted T cells, occur to a large degree in the medulla. Recent studies have in fact demonstrated that tissue-specific antigens expressed by medullary TEC are acquired by bone marrow-derived dendritic cells, which in turn mediate deletion of autoreactive thymocytes.[136] Finally, with respect to thymocyte migration, during positive selection DP thymocytes reverse their course within the thymus. After fourteen days from initial

seeding by multipotent precursor cells and migration from the cortico-medullary junction to the subcapsular cortex to complete T-lineage commitment and β-selection, DP thymocytes reverse course and in the three to four days during which they undergo positive selection, migrate back toward the medulla (see Fig. 10.3). While the precise molecules that are responsible for this reversed migration are not completely known, it is likely that the process involves interactions between chemokines secreted by TEC in the cortex and medulla and their respective receptors on DP thymocytes, the expression of which is likely regulated by TCR-mediated signaling.[28,137,138]

In addition to controlling the generation of conventional T cells whose TCR binding specificities are shaped by positive and negative selection, the thymus is also important in the generation of regulatory T cells (Tregs), defined phenotypically as $CD4^+ CD25^{hi} IL-7R\alpha^{lo}$.[139] Tregs play a critical role in regulating immune responses, including the prevention of autoimmunity,[140] inhibition of antitumor immunity,[141] and in the prevention of allograft rejection.[142] The hallmark of Treg cells is their expression of Foxp3 (forkhead box P3), anomalies of which result in the severe autoimmune disorder IPEX syndrome (immune dysregulation, polyendocrinopathy, X-linked) in humans. Induction of Foxp3 is critical for the effector functions of Tregs.[143] Medullary TEC and bone marrow-derived dendritic cells appear to play important roles in the generation of Tregs.[144,145] Despite the fact that the mechanism of Treg induction and the requirements for their selection in the thymus remain unknown, the critical role of medullary TEC in both negative selection of conventional T cells and the generation of Tregs establishes a potential link between the expression of tissue-specific antigens under the control of Aire expression and the modulation of peripheral T cell responses that preserve self-tolerance and minimize autoimmunity.[146]

Since positive and negative selection is largely dependent on interactions between TCR and MHC–peptide complexes, what are the differential mechanisms that drive a thymocyte to continued development versus death? Similar to β-selection, binding of MHC–peptide to the TCR initiates a cascade of intracellular signaling events mediated by the LCK-ZAP70-LAT pathway. However, in contrast to β-selection, where assembly of the pre-TCR complex itself initiates a linear sequence of signaling events, the signaling pathways in positive and negative selection diverge depending on the strength and duration of the interaction between the TCR and the MHC–peptide complex. This interaction appears to dictate the phosphorylation patterns in the signaling domains of the TCR, which in turn regulate the recruitment of signaling and adapter proteins to the TCR and subsequently the activation of intracellular signaling cascades. In support of this, mutations in specific TCR complex components have been shown to disrupt positive but not negative selection.[147,148] Differential activation of MAP kinase pathways by TCR signaling is an example of the divergent intracellular signaling pathways with positive and negative selection

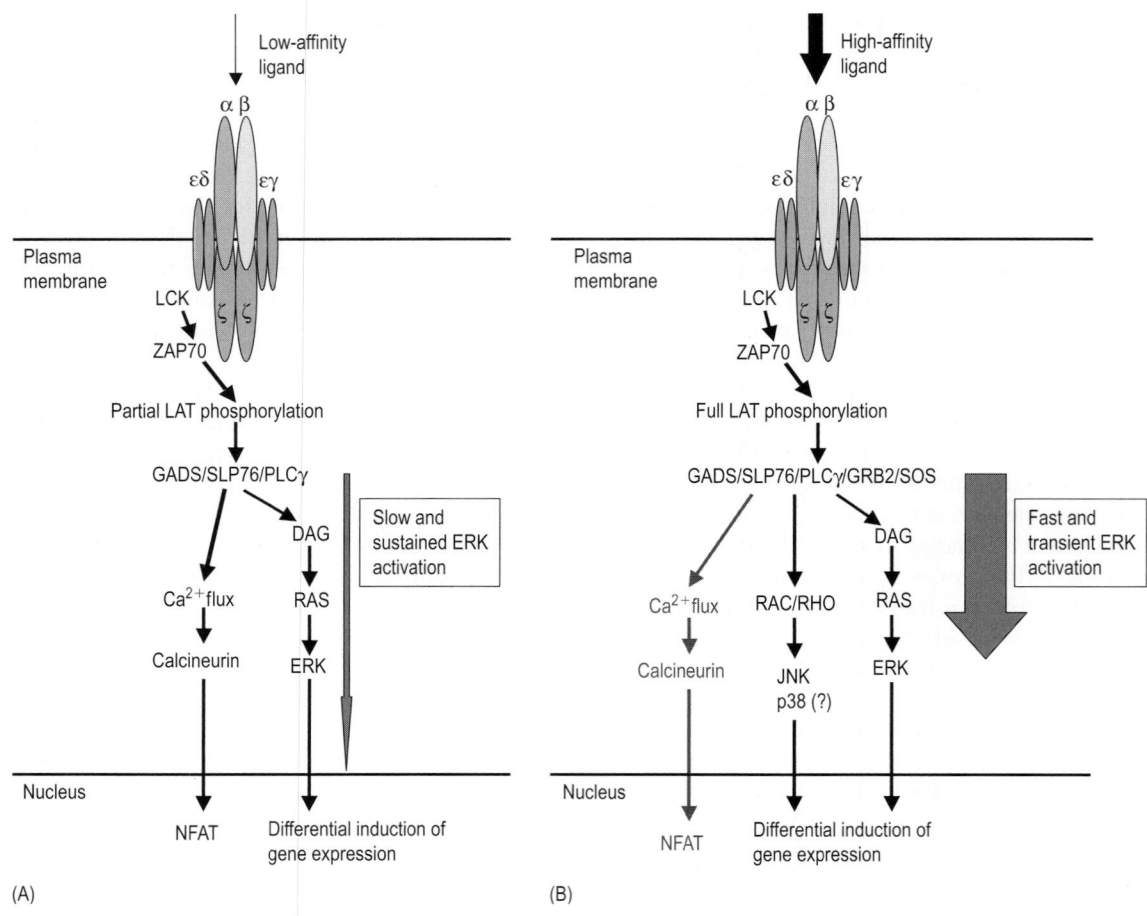

Figure 10.5 Positive and negative selection is dependent on differential signaling pathways that are dictated by T cell receptor (TCR) to major histocompatibility complex (MHC)–peptide interactions. (A) In positive selection, low-affinity interactions between the TCR and MHC–peptide complexes leads to a pattern of molecular signaling within the TCR complex that results in the partial phosphorylation of the LAT protein, which in turn leads to recruitment of GADS, SLP76, and phospholipase Cγ (PLCγ). This results in a cascade of intracellular signaling involving the slow and sustained activation of the mitogen-activated protein (MAP) kinase ERK, which then leads to differential induction of transcription factor activity and gene expression. Nuclear factor of activated T cells (NFAT) is also induced by intracellular signaling as a result of low-affinity TCR–MHC-peptide interactions through the calcineurin pathway and plays a role in positive selection. (B) In contrast, during negative selection, high-affinity interactions between the TCR and MHC–peptide complex results in a different pattern of intra-TCR complex signaling that results in the full phosphorylation of LAT. Consequently, GRB2 and SOS are additionally recruited to the GADS/SLP76/PLCγ complex. The composition and kinetics of the recruitment of these second messenger molecules result in the fast and transient induction of ERK, and lead to a pattern of gene expression distinct from that induced by positive selection. In addition, activation of NFAT does not appear to feature prominently in negative selection (light gray shading), whereas the induction of the MAP kinases JNK and possibly p38, both of which are activated through the RAC/RHO pathway, does.

(Fig. 10.5). MAP kinases have been implicated in many physiological processes including cell proliferation, differentiation, and death,[106] and have a role in β-selection (see earlier section). The three major groups of MAP kinases involved in T cell development – the extracellular signal-regulated protein kinases (ERK), the p38 MAP kinases, and the JUN N-terminal kinases (JNK) – are distinct with respect to the molecules that induce their expression and their downstream transcription factor targets. From studies utilizing mouse knockout models of MAP kinase signaling components, positive and negative selection result in qualitative and quantitative differences in the induction of MAP kinase signaling pathways, in that

positive selection is associated with a low sustained level of ERK activation, whereas negative selection occurs in response to a large burst of ERK activation and concomitant activation of JNK and p38.[149] The identity of the specific components of the TCR signaling complex that mediate this remains incompletely characterized, and may involve differential immunoreceptor tyrosine-based activation motifs (ITAM) phosphorylation patterns of the CD3 molecule[148,150,151] and/or in the α-connecting peptide motif (α-CPM) that links the CD3 δ chain to the TCRα chain.[147,152] Other signaling pathways are also involved in discriminating positive and negative selection, and, as is the case with negative selection, require signals in addition to TCR that include costimulatory molecules that are involved in peripheral T cell activation.[146] Differential signaling from the MAP kinase and other complementary signaling pathways, in turn, leads to activation of distinct sets of transcription factors that result in the expression of genes that dictate the ultimate outcome of cell fate. The full spectrum of the genes involved, their contributions to the effect on the positively and negatively selected thymocyte, and their interactions continue to be investigated.

CD4/CD8 lineage commitment

The final major lineage commitment made by developing thymocytes prior to their emigration as mature T cells is the decision to become a CD4+ T cell or a CD8+ T cell. This step is critical as each of these two populations, with respect to phenotype, immune responses, and responses to growth factors and cell interactions, are distinct. Key to these differences is the corecognition of MHC class II and MHC class I molecules by the CD4 and CD8, respectively, and the TCR. The two classes of MHC molecules convey different functions. MHC class I molecules alert the immune system to intracellular infection and target infected cells for destruction, whereas MHC class II molecules play a role in recruiting multiple immune populations to target extracellular infections. Thus, CD4 or CD8 coreceptor expression defines function in that CD4+ T cells, upon binding to MHC class II–foreign peptide complexes, are programmed to carry out helper and regulatory functions, while CD8+ T cells, upon binding to MHC class I–foreign peptide complexes, are programmed to have predominantly cytotoxic function. The critical nature of coreceptor–MHC interactions is underscored by the finding that mice lacking MHC class I were devoid of CD8 SP thymocytes while mice lacking MHC class II were devoid of CD4 SP thymocytes. The process by which a thymocyte that has survived positive and negative selection is chosen to either a CD4+ or CD8+ T cell fate is significant in the immune system as a whole because maintaining the proper proportion of CD4+ and CD8+ T cells is important in maintaining optimal defense against foreign pathogens as well as providing antitumor immunity.

The precursor pool for CD4+ and CD8+ T cells are the DP thymocytes. Differentiation into CD4+ and CD8+ SP thymocytes, therefore, requires a cessation in expression of the other coreceptor. How this is carried out has been the subject of intensive investigation, and the exact mechanisms remain incompletely elucidated. Studies to date have attempted to define the mechanisms that help determine CD4/CD8 lineage fates as illustrated in Figure 10.6. Similar to the models of development of TCRγδ cells described earlier, these models center on an instructional versus a stochastic/selection mechanism. The *instructional model* (Fig. 10.6A) postulates that TCR-coreceptor signals direct termination of the other coreceptor: T cell receptor–CD4 binding to MHC class II–peptide directs termination of CD8 expression, while TCR-CD8 binding to MHC class I–peptide directs termination of CD4 expression. The

stochastic/selection model (Fig. 10.6B), in contrast, postulates that the lineage choice to become a CD4+ or CD8+ T cell is made independently of TCR-coreceptor and that the latter serves to promote the survival of those preprogrammed cells upon appropriate binding to MHC–peptide during positive and negative selection. Evidence supporting either model has depended in large part on the experimental system used, and in fact suggests that, given the inherently broad range of overlapping affinities between TCR and coreceptors and their ligands, elements of both models may play a role in CD4 versus CD8 lineage commitment.[153] This has been further complicated by the fact that the transition from the DP to the SP thymocyte stage does not result from the direct termination of coreceptor transcription and expression, but from the transition of DP through a number of intermediate stages involving variable expression of CD4 and CD8 before establishment of the terminal phenotype.[153] These observations have led to the formulation of a third model of CD4/CD8 lineage commitment, the *kinetic signaling model* (Fig. 10.6C).[154,155] In this model, DP thymocytes that receive TCR signals during positive selection are automatically programmed to downregulate CD8 expression to form an intermediate population of CD4+ CD8lo thymocytes. Lineage commitment to CD4 SP or CD8 SP thymocytes is dependent on the persistence of signal generated by TCR and the coreceptor. In the situation where the signal persists, e.g., by co-engagement of MHC class II–specific TCR and the CD4 coreceptor or by persistence of TCR signaling in the absence of coreceptor signaling, CD4+ CD8lo intermediate thymocytes differentiate into CD4 SP thymocytes. If TCR-coreceptor signaling is terminated, e.g., by interaction of a MHC class I-specific TCR with the CD4 coreceptor or by very low-affinity interactions with MHC class I-specific TCR, then CD8 expression is reinduced and CD4 expression is terminated, thus leading to the development of CD8 SP thymocytes.[156]

Key to the mechanisms that define CD4/CD8 lineage commitment by each of the aforementioned models is the nature of the signal that is transmitted by the combination of TCR and coreceptor signaling. In contrast to positive and negative selection, where the binding affinity of the TCR to the MHC–peptide complex is the primary determinant of cell survival and cell death, both signal *strength* and *duration,* as determined by cooperative binding by TCR and coreceptor to MHC, appear to be the primary determinant of CD4 versus CD8 lineage commitment (Fig. 10.7). This 'strength of signal' model is based on a number of observations. The concept of signal strength contributing to CD4/CD8 lineage commitment is based in part on the finding that the cytoplasmic tails of CD4 and CD8 differ with respect to their ability to recruit p56LCK, in that CD4 is associated with almost 20-fold more p56LCK than the CD8α.[157–159] That the duration of signaling influences the CD4/CD8 lineage decision is based on the observation that duration of TCR signaling determines the CD4 versus CD8 T cell fate *in vitro.* Longer co-culture times of DP thymocytes from transgenic TCR mice with antigen-pulsed APC resulted in subsequent differentiation to CD4 SP thymo-cytes, while shorter co-culture times under otherwise identical conditions yielded CD8 SP thymocytes.[160]

Similar to positive and negative selection, the intracellular cascades involving LCK and the MAP kinase ERK appear to be directly involved in differential CD4 versus CD8 signaling. While both cascades are critical for both CD4 and CD8 T cell development, increased signaling through the LCK cascade appears to favor CD4 over CD8 SP thymocyte development, consistent with its increased recruitment to CD4, while increases in ERK activity similarly favor CD4 SP thymocyte development.[161–167] Other signaling molecules have also been implicated in CD4/CD8 lineage commitment, including integrins,[168] IL-7R signals,[154] and Notch,[169] although definitive evidence for their roles is inconclusive and, in the case of Notch, contradictory.[160,170] Not surprisingly, differential patterns in intracellular signaling lead to differential transcription factor activation that influences CD4 versus CD8 lineage decisions.[171–174] Moreover, the identification of transcription factors in normal CD4/CD8 lineage development has implications in the potential of these cells to undergo neoplastic transformation into lymphomas.[171,172] It is likely that multiple pathways confer overlapping effects on DP

thymocytes to directly promote CD4/CD8 lineage commitment and/or promote supportive functions, e.g., enhancing cell survival among thymocytes that have already committed to the CD4 or CD8 SP lineage.

While much investigation involving CD4/CD8 lineage commitment has focused on the effects on DP thymocytes themselves, the thymic microenvironment not surprisingly also plays a role. Given the large number of DP thymocytes in the thymic cortex, competition for developmental 'niches,' e.g., available TEC for MHC–peptide presentation, serves to influence the efficiency of positive selection.[116] Moreover, as discussed previously, that positive selection takes place predominantly in the cortex and negative selection takes place in the medulla further supports the importance of the thymic microenvironment for these processes. Within the context of CD4/CD8 lineage commitment, similar influences may hold in terms of competition for available MHC–peptide complexes to serve as ligands for TCR and coreceptor binding. Indeed, studies in chimeric mice with different mixtures of TCR selectable and nonselectable precursors have shown that CD4/CD8 lineage commitment in the selectable precursor population was dependent on their content relative to the nonselectable population, and that SP thymocyte development of these populations

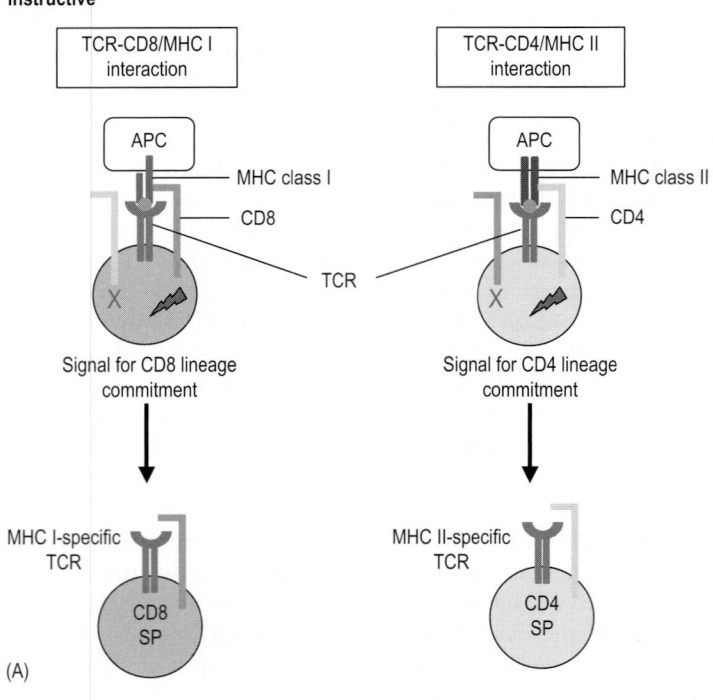

Figure 10.6   Models of CD4/CD8 lineage commitment. (A) The instructive model posits that commitment to the CD4 or CD8 lineage is dependent on unique signals that are transmitted through the T cell receptor (TCR)–coreceptor complex during interaction by double positive (DP) thymocytes with major histocompatibility complex (MHC)–peptide, such that the complex formed among TCR–MHC class I/peptide-CD8 yields a signal directing CD8 lineage commitment while TCR–MHC class II/peptide-CD4 yields a signal directing CD4 lineage commitment. (B) The stochastic/selection model proposes that precursor DP thymocytes are preprogrammed to downregulate CD4 or CD8 independent of TCR specificity. A cell that is programmed to express the wrong coreceptor ('Wrong') will die upon interaction between the TCR and its specific MHC–peptide complex because of the inability to transmit an appropriate survival signal through the coreceptor. In contrast, cells that are programmed to express the correct coreceptor ('Right') will successfully undergo lineage commitment because of

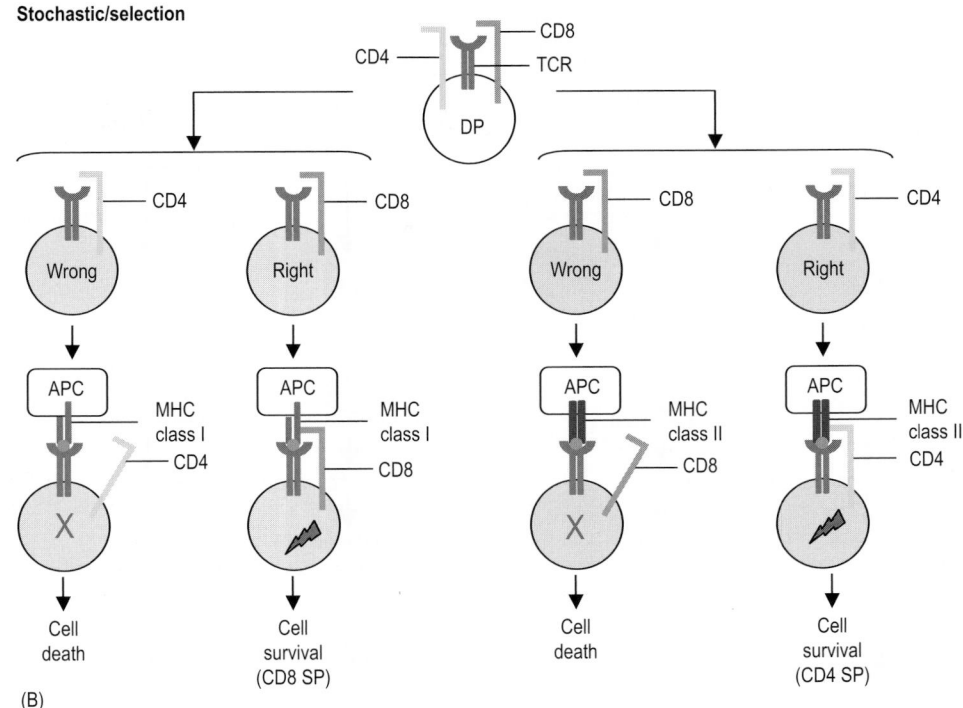

(B)

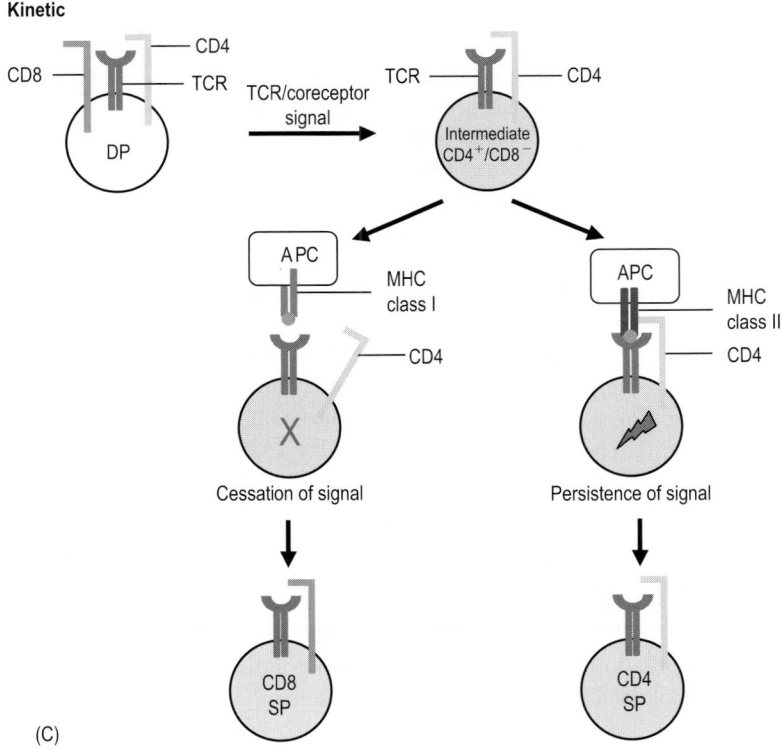

(C)

the transmission of survival signals through the coreceptor. (C) The kinetic signaling model stipulates that DP thymocytes, upon TCR-coreceptor signaling, terminate CD8 expression to form an intermediate CD4⁺/CD8⁻ population. Commitment to CD4 or CD8 single positive (SP) thymocytes is dependent on the duration of TCR-coreceptor signaling. In the case where cells express a MHC class I-specific TCR, the inability to transmit signals through CD8 upon interactions with MHC class I-peptide complexes leads to a cessation of signaling through the TCR, the termination of CD4 expression, reinduction of CD8 expression, and the development of CD8 SP thymocytes. In contrast, thymocytes containing MHC class II-specific TCR continue to receive signals through the CD4 coreceptor upon binding to MHC class II-peptide complexes and subsequently develop into CD4 SP thymocytes.

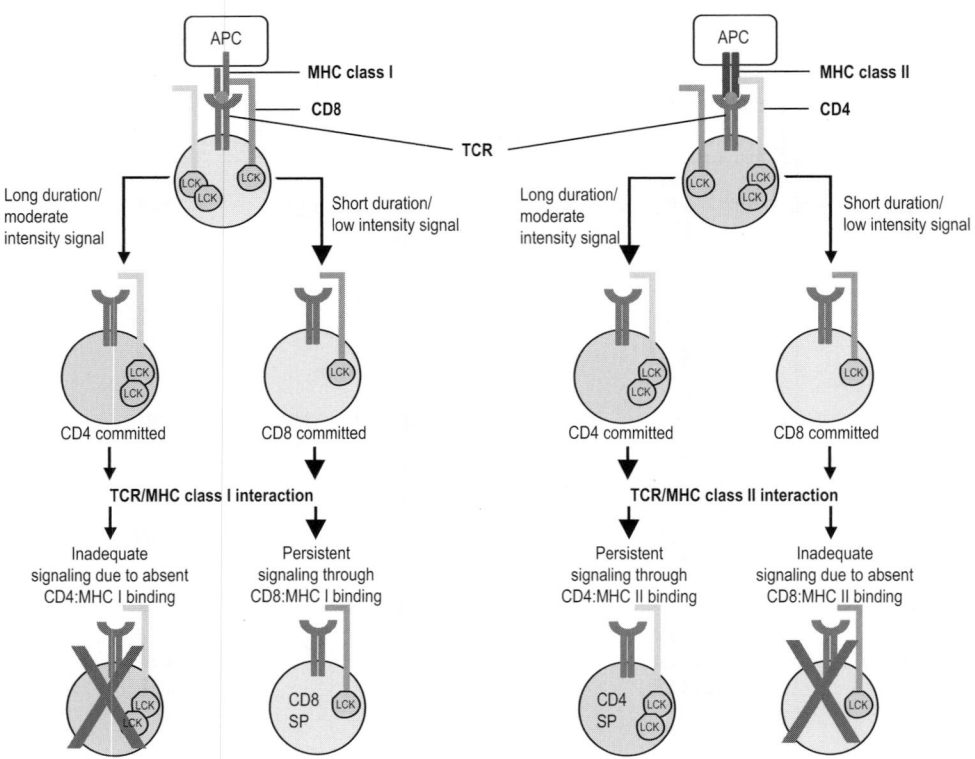

Figure 10.7   Strength of signal model. This model highlights the importance of signal intensity and duration through the CD4 and CD8 coreceptor as a determinant in CD4/CD8 lineage commitment. Based on the finding that CD4 associates with substantially higher numbers of LCK molecules than CD8, CD4-committed thymocytes are generated upon binding with an appropriate major histocompatibility complex (MHC) class II–peptide complex as a result of long duration/moderate intensity signals whereas CD8-committed cells are generated upon binding with an appropriate MHC class I–peptide complex as a result of short duration/low intensity signals. In the rarer instances of inappropriate lineage commitment (indicated by the thin arrows), where strong TCR binding to MHC class I–peptide results in long duration/moderate intensity signals leading to CD4 commitment or weak T cell receptor (TCR) binding to MHC class II–peptide results in short duration/low intensity signals leading to CD8 commitment, these cells will die because of the absence of the necessary survival signals transmitted through the inappropriately expressed coreceptor. APC, antigen-presenting cell; SP, single positive.

occurred in distinct areas of the medulla.[175] Observations such as these again confirm that the thymic microenvironment plays an important role in lineage commitment through the availability of TCR and coreceptor ligands as well as through additional contact-mediated and secreted factors to influence all stages of T cell development.

NATURAL KILLER CELL DEVELOPMENT

Natural killer cells comprise a population that is part of the innate immune system. Morphologically, NK cells are granular lymphocytes distinct from T cells and B cells, comprising about 15 percent of peripheral blood lymphocytes. The surface phenotype of NK cells is distinct from that of T cells and B cells in that they lack B and T cell antigen receptors; like T cells, the surface phenotype differs between mice and humans (Fig. 10.8). Natural killer cells utilize their own unique set of receptors that are configured such that recognition of host MHC molecules determines the nature of the effector response.[176] Natural killer

cells are found, in addition to the circulation, in peripheral tissues including the liver, peritoneum, and placenta. Consistent with their role in innate immunity, NK cells, unlike T cells, require no prior stimulus to initiate effector functions. Natural killer cells have been shown to play a role in early defense against microorganisms and tumor cells. In fact, the initial characterization of NK cells thirty years ago was based on their antitumor effects,[177,178] and they have been shown in mice and humans to contribute to improved outcome for individuals undergoing hematopoietic stem cell transplant for the treatment of leukemia.[179,180] Natural killer cell function is mediated through a number of pathways, including cell-mediated cytolysis,[181] antibody-dependent cellular cytotoxicity through the Fc-receptor complex (CD16) that enables NK cells to participate in the destruction of antibody-targeted cells, and the secretion of cytokines (including IFNγ, tumor necrosis factor (TNF), lymphotoxin β (LTβ), granulocyte macrophage colony-stimulating factor (GM-CSF), IL-10, and IL-13) that can recruit other immune cells to sites of immunologic insult and qualitatively influence the

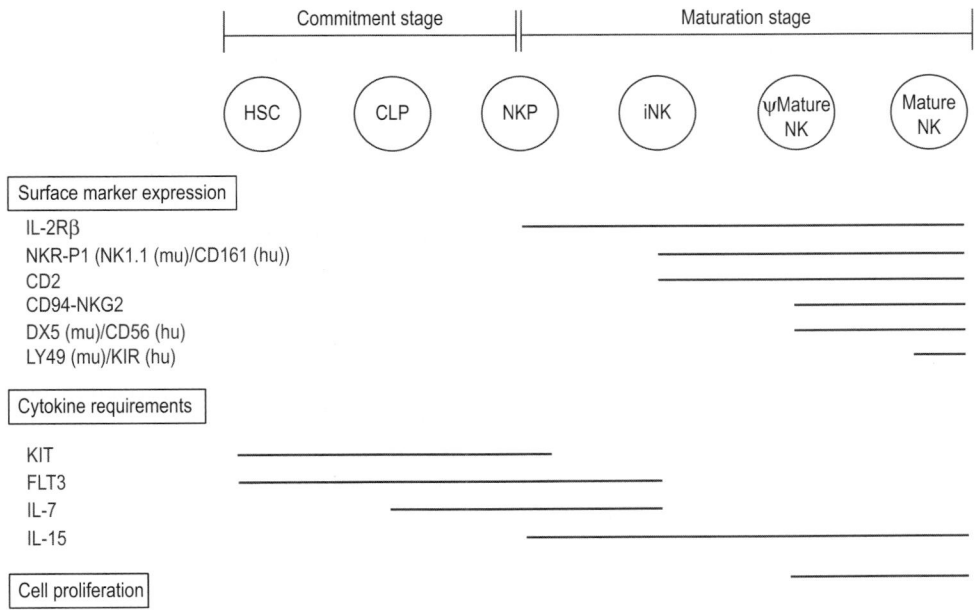

Figure 10.8   Natural killer (NK) cell development. In contrast to T cell development, which requires the migration of precursor cells from the bone marrow to the thymus, virtually all NK cell development is thought to occur in the bone marrow. In this two-stage model, the first stage is the commitment stage whereby NK precursors (NKP) develop from hematopoietic stem cells (HSC). The acquisition of the interleukin-2 (IL-2) receptor β chain (IL-2Rβ) is the culmination of the commitment stage. During the maturation stage, developing NK cells accumulate NK-specific markers such as the C-type lectin NK-cell receptor protein 1 (NKR-P1) and DX5 (mouse)/CD56 (human), as well as the CD94-NKG2 (mouse and human) and Ly49 (mouse)/KIR (human) receptors that dictate the target-cell specificity of NK cell function based on major histocompatibility complex (MHC) class I expression. Cytokine requirements for each of the developmental stages are also illustrated, highlighting the importance of KIT and FLT3 on NK cell development during the commitment stage and IL-15 during the maturation stage. Cell proliferation occurs after the acquisition of CD94-NKG2 and LY49/KIR. Not shown in the figure are the two populations of NK cells, cytolytic and cytokine-producing, that are seen in the peripheral immune system of humans (see text for details). These distinct NK cell populations are not found in mice. CLP, common lymphoid progenitor.

nature of the immune response.[182,183] Thus, despite the fact that NK cells are evolutionarily older than the cells involved in adaptive immunity, they remain critical components in the immune system, as evidenced by rare reported cases of NK cell deficiency in humans that demonstrate increased susceptibility to life-threatening viral infections and tumors.[184–186]

Despite the different phenotypic markers that define NK cells in humans and mice, NK cell development is similar in the two species. The developmental stages in NK cell development are fundamentally different from those of T cells. The first major difference is that NK cell development occurs predominantly in the bone marrow. The thymus plays a minor role in NK cell development; mice and humans (such as those individuals with DiGeorge syndrome) that lack a functional thymus have normal NK cell numbers.[187–189] Peripheral lymph nodes also are a potential site for extramedullary NK cell development,[190] as is the liver,[191] as both organs contain populations of immature NK cells. A second major difference that distinguishes NK cell development from T cell development is that NK cell development does not require events that are dependent on antigen receptor gene rearrangement. Natural killer

cells express a panel of non-rearranging activating and inhibitory receptors where relative signaling contributions from these receptors determine whether or not the NK cell is activated. However, this is not to suggest that NK cells are not subject to some alternate form of positive and negative selection. For example, in mice, NK receptor repertoire in mature NK cells appears to be influenced by MHC class I expression,[192,193] and is dependent on interactions with self-MHC class I ligands from surrounding cells.[194,195] Additional mechanisms that may play a role in the selection of the NK repertoire involve the asynchronous expression of NK receptors and their ligands during embryonic development.[193] The result of this selection process is the development of NK cells expressing inhibitory receptors recognizing self-MHC class I molecules. According to the 'missing-self' hypothesis, NK cells recognizing self-MHC class I would not result in activation because of the expression of these inhibitory receptors, whereas cells that lack or express low self-MHC class I molecules, such as a tumor cell or a virally infected cell, would result in NK cell activation and subsequent target-cell cytolysis.

Current models of NK cell development divide the process into two stages (Fig. 10.8). The first stage involves the generation of NK cell progenitors from hematopoietic stem cells (HSC). In the bone marrow, the earliest CD34[+] HSC give rise to cells termed common lymphoid progenitors (CLPs), which are the precursors for NK, T, and B cell populations. Natural killer cell precursors are generally identified by the expression of the IL-2 receptor β-chain (IL-2Rβ) in the absence of other hematopoietic cell markers in mice[196,197] and the ability to differentiate to mature NK cells in response to IL-2 or IL-15 in humans.[198,199] Development of NK precursors from CLPs requires the secretion of cytokines from bone marrow stromal cells, including KIT, FLT3, and IL-7.[200–202] While cytokine secretion alone appears to be sufficient for the generation of NK precursors,[201] contact between NK precursors and bone marrow stromal cells is required for subsequent differentiation of NK precursors into immature NK cells and ultimately mature NK cells, which constitutes the second stage of NK cell development. During this stage, NK cells express surface molecules that are characteristic of mature NK cells including the killer-cell immunoglobulin-like receptor (KIR) and its murine analogue Ly49, and the lectin-like receptor CD94-NKG2 in both species, that connote their effector functions through their acquisition of lytic and cytokine-production capabilities. Another molecule that is expressed in humans but not mice is CD56, which is commonly used as a marker for mature NK cells. Cell proliferation is also a hallmark of this developmental stage. Among the molecules that are important for continued NK cell development is lymphotoxin α (LTα). Lymphotoxin α-deficient mice lack NK cells.[203] Lymphotoxin α-mediated signals appear to play an important role in the production of IL-15, which is the central cytokine driving development of NK cells from NK precursors.[198,203–205] Interleukin-15, in turn, appears to function primarily as a cell proliferation and survival factor. For example, the anti-apoptotic molecule BCL2 is a candidate downstream target of IL-15 signaling in that NK cells containing the BCL2 transgene that are adoptively transferred into IL-15-deficient mice are able to survive.[206,207] Other cytokines, like IL-15, whose receptors transmit intracellular signals through the common γc chain, do not appear to have a critical role in NK cell development. Both IL-2 and IL-7 deficiencies do not appear to affect NK cell development,[36,197,208,209] although IL-2 deficiency does impair effector responses of mature NK cells.[208,210] The combination of cytokine and cell contact-mediated signaling results in the activation of transcription factors, of which Ikaros, Id2, ETS-1, MEF, and interferon regulatory factor 1 (IRF1) have been demonstrated to affect NK cell development.[211]

Once NK cell development in the bone marrow is complete, the cells are exported into the periphery where they are found in the blood, the lymphoid organs, and other organs such as the liver and the lung. In mice, NK cells labeled with fluorescent tracking dyes can be detected in the circulation for at least five weeks.[206] In humans there exists two peripheral populations of NK cells that are distinct with respect to their cytotoxic activity and their cytokine secretion patterns.[212] Cytolytic NK cells express high concentrations of KIR on their surfaces, contain abundant cytolytic granules, and are CD56[lo]. These cells function through several mechanisms, including the secretion of perforin and granzymes,[213] expression of surface molecules that are involved in contact-mediated cell death (including FAS ligand and tumor necrosis factor–related apoptosis-inducing ligand [TRAIL]),[213] and mediation of antibody-dependent cellular toxicity (ADCC) through expression of the Fc receptor (CD16) on opsonized target cells. Recent evidence suggests that CD16 expression is regulated by IL-21,[212,214] indicating that this cytokine plays a role in the latter stages of NK cell development.

In contrast, NK cells for which the primary role is cytokine secretion differ phenotypically from cytolytic NK cells in that they express lower KIR levels, contain few cytolytic granules, and are CD56[hi]. As was mentioned earlier, cytokines that are produced by these cells include IFNγ, TNF, LTβ, GM-CSF, IL-10, and IL-13. How these cytokines influence NK-mediated immune responses and how they play a role in interactions between NK cells and other cells involved in adaptive immunity remains to be characterized. Moreover, the developmental relationships between cytolytic and cytokine-producing NK cells, and the anatomic sites where they undergo terminal differentiation, are not completely known. Interestingly, the vast majority of circulating NK cells are CD56[lo], while the vast majority of NK cells residing in lymph nodes are CD56[hi].[215] Recent evidence suggests that CD56[lo] cytolytic NK cells are derived from the CD56[hi] cytokine-producing NK cell population, and that this conversion occurs in the lymph nodes under the influence of IL-2.[216]

CONCLUSION

Much insight has been gained in the understanding of T cell and NK cell development. Such understanding is important for several reasons. First, it provides extremely useful basic biologic models for delineating the molecules and pathways that are critical determinants in the progression from the most immature pluripotent stem cell to the terminally differentiated cell. Second, defining these pathways will have profound implications in understanding the molecular events that initiate and promote aberrant development of normal developing cells into tumor cells, and may lead to the identification of molecules that could serve as effective candidates for targeted antitumor therapy. Finally, understanding the forces that shape T cell and NK cell development can lead to therapeutic approaches for manipulating the immune system to selectively target and eliminate tumor cells without causing damage to normal cells, approaches clearly needed in current modes of immunotherapy such as allogeneic hematopoietic stem cell transplantation and donor lymphocyte infusions, where graft versus host disease is a major complication.

KEY POINTS

- T cell development takes place in the thymus, and requires a constant influx of bone marrow-derived progenitors to maintain adequate T cell production.
- The thymus is structurally and functionally divided into developmental niches that are defined by developing thymocytes and supporting stromal cells including thymic epithelial cells. Thymic epithelial cells play an important role in T cell development by directing thymocyte migration through the secretion of chemokines and extracellular matrix proteins, by supporting cell survival and proliferation through the secretion of cytokines, and by participating in the lineage commitment of developing thymocytes through the expression of cell surface molecules such as NOTCH1 ligands and MHC–peptide complexes.
- The role of early thymocyte development is to generate a large pool of thymocytes (10^5 cells/thymic progenitor cell) with a diverse TCR repertoire that ensures continued diversity following positive and negative selection, during which about 95 percent of cells die.
- The T cell receptor (TCR) plays a critical role in determining the fate of T cells at multiple stages of development, including β-selection, positive and negative selection, and CD4 versus CD8 lineage commitment.
- Natural killer (NK) cells play an important role in both innate and adaptive immunity. Unlike T cells, NK cell development occurs predominantly in the bone marrow. Interleukin-15 (IL-15) is a critical mediator in NK cell development.
- Understanding the mechanisms by which T cells and NK cells develop may provide insight into the cellular and molecular events that lead to the development of tumor cells. This may also provide insights into the treatment of these tumors as well as approaches to manipulate the immune system to enhance its ability to eliminate tumor cells.

REFERENCES

● = Key primary paper
◆ = Major review article

1. Blom B, Res PC, Spits H. T cell precursors in man and mice. *Crit Rev Immunol* 1998; **18**: 371–88.
2. Plum J, De Smedt M, Verhasselt B *et al.* Human T lymphopoiesis. In vitro and in vivo study models. *Ann N Y Acad Sci* 2000; **917**: 724–31.
3. Staal FJ, Weerkamp F, Langerak AW *et al.* Transcriptional control of T lymphocyte differentiation. *Stem Cells* 2001; **19**: 165–79.
4. Verschuren MC, Wolvers-Tettero IL, Breit TM *et al.* Preferential rearrangements of the T cell receptor-delta-deleting elements in human T cells. *J Immunol* 1997; **158**: 1208–16.
5. Allman D, Sambandam A, Kim S *et al.* Thymopoiesis independent of common lymphoid progenitors. *Nat Immunol* 2003; **4**: 168–74.
6. Porritt HE, Rumfelt LL, Tabrizifard S *et al.* Heterogeneity among DN1 prothymocytes reveals multiple progenitors with different capacities to generate T cell and non-T cell lineages. *Immunity* 2004; **20**: 735–45.
◆7. Bhandoola A, von Boehmer H, Petrie HT, Zuniga-Pfhucker JC. Commitment and developmental potential of extrathymic and intrathymic T cell precursors: plenty to choose from. *Immunity* 2007; **26**: 678–89.
8. Penit C, Lucas B, Vasseur F. Cell expansion and growth arrest phases during the transition from precursor (CD4-8-) to immature (CD4+8+) thymocytes in normal and genetically modified mice. *J Immunol* 1995; **154**: 5103–13.
9. Le Campion A, Lucas B, Dautigny N *et al.* Quantitative and qualitative adjustment of thymic T cell production by clonal expansion of premigrant thymocytes. *J Immunol* 2002; **168**: 1664–71.
10. Taub DD, Longo DL. Insights into thymic aging and regeneration. *Immunol Rev* 2005; **205**: 72–93.
11. Haynes BF, Markert ML, Sempowski GD *et al.* The role of the thymus in immune reconstitution in aging, bone marrow transplantation, and HIV-1 infection. *Annu Rev Immunol* 2000; **18**: 529–60.
●12. Douek DC, McFarland RD, Keiser PH *et al.* Changes in thymic function with age and during the treatment of HIV infection. *Nature* 1998; **396**: 690–5.
◆13. Anderson G, Moore NC, Owen JJ, Jenkinson EJ. Cellular interactions in thymocyte development. *Annu Rev Immunol* 1996; **14**: 73–99.
14. Klug DB, Carter C, Crouch E *et al.* Interdependence of cortical thymic epithelial cell differentiation and T-lineage commitment. *Proc Natl Acad Sci U S A* 1998; **95**: 11822–7.
15. Klug DB, Crouch E, Carter C *et al.* Transgenic expression of cyclin D1 in thymic epithelial precursors promotes epithelial and T cell development. *J Immunol* 2000; **164**: 1881–8.
16. Gray DH, Ueno T, Chidgey AP *et al.* Controlling the thymic microenvironment. *Curr Opin Immunol* 2005; **17**: 137–43.
17. Yarilin AA, Belyakov IM. Cytokines in the thymus: production and biological effects. *Curr Med Chem* 2004; **11**: 447–64.
18. Bleul CC, Boehm T. Chemokines define distinct microenvironments in the developing thymus. *Eur J Immunol* 2000; **30**: 3371–9.
19. van Ewijk W, Hollander G, Terhorst C *et al.* Stepwise development of thymic microenvironments in vivo is regulated by thymocyte subsets. *Development* 2000; **127**: 1583–91.

●20. Rossi SW, Jenkinson WE, Anderson G, Jenkinson EJ. Clonal analysis reveals a common progenitor for thymic cortical and medullary epithelium. *Nature* 2006; **441**: 988–91.

◆21. Petrie HT. Cell migration and the control of post-natal T-cell lymphopoiesis in the thymus. *Nat Rev Immunol* 2003; **3**: 859–66.

22. Shortman K, Egerton M, Spangrude GJ, Scollay R. The generation and fate of thymocytes. *Semin Immunol* 1990; **2**: 3–12.

23. Takahama Y. Journey through the thymus: stromal guides for T-cell development and selection. *Nat Rev Immunol* 2006; **6**: 127–35.

24. Norment AM, Bevan MJ. Role of chemokines in thymocyte development. *Semin Immunol* 2000; **12**: 445–55.

25. Takahama Y. Journey through the thymus: stromal guides for T-cell development and selection. *Nat Rev Immunol* 2006; **6**: 127–35.

●26. Misslitz A, Pabst O, Hintzen G *et al.* Thymic T cell development and progenitor localization depend on CCR7. *J Exp Med* 2004; **200**: 481–91.

27. Plotkin J, Prockop SE, Lepique A, Petrie HT. Critical role for CXCR4 signaling in progenitor localization and T cell differentiation in the postnatal thymus. *J Immunol* 2003; **171**: 4521–7.

28. Kwan J, Killeen N. CCR7 directs the migration of thymocytes into the thymic medulla. *J Immunol* 2004; **172**: 3999–4007.

29. Ueno T, Saito F, Gray DH *et al.* CCR7 signals are essential for cortex-medulla migration of developing thymocytes. *J Exp Med* 2004; **200**: 493–505.

30. Poznansky MC, Olszak IT, Evans RH *et al.* Thymocyte emigration is mediated by active movement away from stroma-derived factors. *J Clin Invest* 2002; **109**: 1101–10.

31. Savino W, Mendes-da-Cruz DA, Silva JS *et al.* Intrathymic T-cell migration: a combinatorial interplay of extracellular matrix and chemokines? *Trends Immunol* 2002; **23**: 305–13.

32. Prockop SE, Palencia S, Ryan CM *et al.* Stromal cells provide the matrix for migration of early lymphoid progenitors through the thymic cortex. *J Immunol* 2002; **169**: 4354–61.

33. Godfrey DI, Zlotnik A, Suda T. Phenotypic and functional characterization of c-kit expression during intrathymic T cell development. *J Immunol* 1992; **149**: 2281–5.

34. Rodewald HR, Kretzschmar K, Swat W, Takeda S. Intrathymically expressed c-kit ligand (stem cell factor) is a major factor driving expansion of very immature thymocytes in vivo. *Immunity* 1995; **3**: 313–19.

35. Peschon JJ, Morrissey PJ, Grabstein KH *et al.* Early lymphocyte expansion is severely impaired in interleukin 7 receptor-deficient mice. *J Exp Med* 1994; **180**: 1955–60.

36. von Freeden-Jeffry U, Vieira P, Lucian LA *et al.* Lymphopenia in interleukin (IL)-7 gene-deleted mice identifies IL-7 as a nonredundant cytokine. *J Exp Med* 1995; **181**: 1519–26.

37. Haks MC, Oosterwegel MA, Blom B *et al.* Cell-fate decisions in early T cell development: regulation by cytokine receptors and the pre-TCR. *Semin Immunol* 1999; **11**: 23–37.

38. El Kassar N, Lucas PJ, Klug DB *et al.* A dose effect of IL-7 on thymocyte development. *Blood* 2004; **104**: 1419–27.

39. Schlissel MS, Durum SD, Muegge K. The interleukin 7 receptor is required for T cell receptor gamma locus accessibility to the V(D)J recombinase. *J Exp Med* 2000; **191**: 1045–50.

40. Huang J, Durum SK, Muegge K. Cutting edge: histone acetylation and recombination at the TCR gamma locus follows IL-7 induction. *J Immunol* 2001; **167**: 6073–7.

41. Yu Q, Erman B, Bhandoola A *et al.* In vitro evidence that cytokine receptor signals are required for differentiation of double positive thymocytes into functionally mature CD8+ T cells. *J Exp Med* 2003; **197**: 475–87.

42. Petrie HT, Kincade PW. Many roads, one destination for T cell progenitors. *J Exp Med* 2005; **202**: 11–13.

43. Maillard I, Schwarz BA, Sambandam A *et al.* Notch-dependent T-lineage commitment occurs at extrathymic sites following bone marrow transplantation. *Blood* 2006; **107**: 3511–19.

44. Artavanis-Tsakonas S, Rand MD, Lake RJ *et al.* Notch signaling: cell fate control and signal integration in development. *Science* 1999; **284**: 770–6.

45. De Smedt M, Hoebeke I, Plum J *et al.* Human bone marrow CD34+ progenitor cells mature to T cells on OP9-DL1 stromal cell line without thymus microenvironment. *Blood Cells Mol Dis* 2004; **33**: 227–32.

46. La Motte-Mohs RN, Herer E, Zuniga-Pflucker JC. Induction of T-cell development from human cord blood hematopoietic stem cells by Delta-like 1 in vitro. *Blood* 2005; **105**: 1431–9.

47. Schmitt TM, Ciofani M, Petrie HT, Zuniga-Pflucker JC. Maintenance of T cell specification and differentiation requires recurrent notch receptor-ligand interactions. *J Exp Med* 2004; **200**: 469–79.

48. Schmitt TM, de Pooter RF, Gronski MA *et al.* Induction of T cell development and establishment of T cell competence from embryonic stem cells differentiated in vitro. *Nat Immunol* 2004; **5**: 410–17.

●49. Schmitt TM, Zuniga-Pflucker JC. Induction of T cell development from hematopoietic progenitor cells by delta-like-1 in vitro. *Immunity* 2002; **17**: 749–56.

50. Sambandam A, Maillard I, Zediak VP *et al.* Notch signaling controls the generation and differentiation of early T lineage progenitors. *Nat Immunol* 2005; **6**: 663–70.

◆51. von Boehmer H. Notch in lymphopoiesis and T cell polarization. *Nat Immunol* 2005; **6**: 641–2.

52. Pui JC, Allman D, Xu L *et al.* Notch1 expression in early lymphopoiesis influences B versus T lineage determination. *Immunity* 1999; **11**: 299–308.

53. van de Wetering M, de Lau W, Clevers H. WNT signaling and lymphocyte development. *Cell* 2002; **109(Suppl)**: S13–19.

54. Xu Y, Banerjee D, Huelsken J *et al.* Deletion of beta-catenin impairs T cell development. *Nat Immunol* 2003; **4**: 1177–82.

55. Gutierrez-Frias C, Sacedon R, Hernandez-Lopez C et al. Sonic hedgehog regulates early human thymocyte differentiation by counteracting the IL-7-induced development of CD34+ precursor cells. J Immunol 2004; **173**: 5046–53.

56. Outram SV, Varas A, Pepicelli CV, Crompton J. Hedgehog signaling regulates differentiation from double-negative to double-positive thymocyte. Immunity 2000; **13**: 187–97.

57. Shah DK, Hager-Theodorides AL, Outram SV et al. Reduced thymocyte development in sonic hedgehog knockout embryos. J Immunol 2004; **172**: 2296–306.

58. Schilham MW, Wilson A, Moerer P et al. Critical involvement of Tcf-1 in expansion of thymocytes. J Immunol 1998; **161**: 3984–91.

59. Duncan AW, Rattis FM, DiMascio LN et al. Integration of Notch and Wnt signaling in hematopoietic stem cell maintenance. Nat Immunol 2005; **6**: 314–22.

◆60. Rothenberg EV, Moore JE, Yui MA et al. Launching the T-cell-lineage developmental programme. Nat Rev Immunol 2008; **8**: 9–21.

61. Ihle JN, Thierfelder W, Teglund S et al. Signaling by the cytokine receptor superfamily. Ann N Y Acad Sci 1998; **865**: 1–9.

●62. Akashi K, Kondo M, von Freeden-Jeffry U et al. Bcl-2 rescues T lymphopoiesis in interleukin-7 receptor-deficient mice. Cell 1997; **89**: 1033–41.

63. Kondo M, Akashi K, Domen J et al. Bcl-2 rescues T lymphopoiesis, but not B or NK cell development, in common gamma chain-deficient mice. Immunity 1997; **7**: 155–62.

64. Choi JW, Pampeno C, Vukmanovic S, Meruelo D. Characterization of the transcriptional expression of Notch-1 signaling pathway members, Deltex and HES-1, in developing mouse thymocytes. Dev Comp Immunol 2002; **26**: 575–88.

65. Osborne B, Miele L. Notch and the immune system. Immunity 1999; **11**: 653–63.

66. Tydell CC, David-Fung ES, Moore JE et al. Molecular dissection of prethymic progenitor entry into the T lymphocyte developmental pathway. J Immunol 2007; **179**: 421–38.

67. Igarashi H, Gregory SC, Yokota T et al. Transcription from the RAG1 locus marks the earliest lymphocyte progenitors in bone marrow. Immunity 2002; **17**: 117–30.

68. Kaufmann SH. gamma/delta and other unconventional T lymphocytes: what do they see and what do they do? Proc Natl Acad Sci U S A 1996; **93**: 2272–9.

69. Jameson J, Ugarte K, Chen N et al. A role for skin gammadelta T cells in wound repair. Science 2002; **296**: 747–9.

70. McVay LD, Carding SR. Generation of human gammadelta T-cell repertoires. Crit Rev Immunol 1999; **19**: 431–60.

71. McVay LD, Jaswal SS, Kennedy C et al. The generation of human gammadelta T cell repertoires during fetal development. J Immunol 1998; **160**: 5851–60.

72. Capone M, Hockett RD Jr, Zlotnik A. Kinetics of T cell receptor beta, gamma, and delta rearrangements during adult thymic development: T cell receptor rearrangements are present in CD44(+)CD25(+) Pro-T thymocytes. Proc Natl Acad Sci U S A 1998; **95**: 12522–7.

73. Kang J, Volkmann A, Raulet DH. Evidence that gammadelta versus alphabeta T cell fate determination is initiated independently of T cell receptor signaling. J Exp Med 2001; **193**: 689–98.

●74. Washburn T, Schweighoffer E, Gridley T et al. Notch activity influences the alphabeta versus gammadelta T cell lineage decision. Cell 1997; **88**: 833–43.

75. Jiang R, Lan Y, Chapman HD et al. Defects in limb, craniofacial, and thymic development in Jagged2 mutant mice. Genes Dev 1998; **12**: 1046–57.

76. De Smedt M, Reynvoet K, Kerre T et al. Active form of Notch imposes T cell fate in human progenitor cells. J Immunol 2002; **169**: 3021–9.

77. Garcia-Peydro M, de Yebenes VG, Toribio ML. Sustained Notch1 signaling instructs the earliest human intrathymic precursors to adopt a gammadelta T-cell fate in fetal thymus organ culture. Blood 2003; **102**: 2444–51.

78. Dudley EC, Girardi M, Owen MJ, Hayday AC. Alpha beta and gamma delta T cells can share a late common precursor. Curr Biol 1995; **5**: 659–69.

79. Aifantis I, Azogui O, Feinberg J et al. On the role of the pre-T cell receptor in alphabeta versus gammadelta T lineage commitment. Immunity 1998; **9**: 649–55.

●80. Fehling HJ, Krotkova A, Saint-Ruf C, von Boehmer H. Crucial role of the pre-T-cell receptor alpha gene in development of alpha beta but not gamma delta T cells. Nature 1995; **375**: 795–8.

81. Hayes SM, Shores EW, Love PE. An architectural perspective on signaling by the pre-, alphabeta and gammadelta T cell receptors. Immunol Rev 2003; **191**: 28–37.

82. Mulroy T, Sen J. p38 MAP kinase activity modulates alpha beta T cell development. Eur J Immunol 2001; **31**: 3056–63.

83. Nunez-Cruz S, Aguado E, Richelme S et al. LAT regulates gammadelta T cell homeostasis and differentiation. Nat Immunol 2003; **4**: 999–1008.

84. Blom B, Heemskerk MH, Verschuren MC et al. Disruption of alpha beta but not of gamma delta T cell development by overexpression of the helix-loop-helix protein Id3 in committed T cell progenitors. Embo J 1999; **18**: 2793–802.

85. Pennington DJ, Silva-Santos B, Hayday AC et al. Gammadelta T cell development—having the strength to get there. Curr Opin Immunol 2005; **17**: 108–15.

●86. Hayes SM, Li L, Love PE. TCR signal strength influences alphabeta/gammadelta lineage fate. Immunity 2005; **22**: 583–93.

87. Pennington DJ, Silva-Santos B, Shires J et al. The inter-relatedness and interdependence of mouse T cell receptor gammadelta+ and alphabeta+ cells. Nat Immunol 2003; **4**: 991–8.

88. Silva-Santos B, Pennington DJ, Hayday AC. Lymphotoxin-mediated regulation of gammadelta cell differentiation by alphabeta T cell progenitors. Science 2005; **307**: 925–8.

89. Gratiot-Deans J, Merino R, Nunez G, Turka LA. Bcl-2 expression during T-cell development: early loss and late return occur at specific stages of commitment to differentiation and survival. *Proc Natl Acad Sci U S A* 1994; **91**: 10685–9.

90. Andjelic S, Drappa J, Lacy E *et al.* The onset of Fas expression parallels the acquisition of CD8 and CD4 in fetal and adult alpha beta thymocytes. *Int Immunol* 1994; **6**: 73–9.

91. Yokoyama T, Tanahashi M, Kobayashi Y *et al.* The expression of Bcl-2 family proteins (Bcl-2, Bcl-x, Bax, Bak and Bim) in human lymphocytes. *Immunol Lett* 2002; **81**: 107–13.

●92. Shinkai Y, Koyasu S, Nakayama K *et al.* Restoration of T cell development in RAG-2-deficient mice by functional TCR transgenes. *Science* 1993; **259**: 822–5.

◆93. von Boehmer H, Fehling HJ. Structure and function of the pre-T cell receptor. *Annu Rev Immunol* 1997; **15**: 433–52.

94. Levelt CN, Wang B, Ehrfeld A *et al.* Regulation of T cell receptor (TCR)-beta locus allelic exclusion and initiation of TCR-alpha locus rearrangement in immature thymocytes by signaling through the CD3 complex. *Eur J Immunol* 1995; **25**: 1257–61.

95. Senoo M, Shinkai Y. Regulation of Vbeta germline transcription in RAG-deficient mice by the CD3epsilon-mediated signals: implication of Vbeta transcriptional regulation in TCR beta allelic exclusion. *Int Immunol* 1998; **10**: 553–60.

96. Dudley EC, Petrie HT, Shah LM *et al.* T cell receptor beta chain gene rearrangement and selection during thymocyte development in adult mice. *Immunity* 1994; **1**: 83–93.

●97. Mallick CA, Dudley EC, Viney JL *et al.* Rearrangement and diversity of T cell receptor beta chain genes in thymocytes: a critical role for the beta chain in development. *Cell* 1993; **73**: 513–19.

98. Gibbons D, Douglas NC, Barber DF *et al.* The biological activity of natural and mutant pTalpha alleles. *J Exp Med* 2001; **194**: 695–703.

99. Irving BA, Alt FW, Killeen N. Thymocyte development in the absence of pre-T cell receptor extracellular immunoglobulin domains. *Science* 1998; **280**: 905–8.

100. Panigada M, Porcellini S, Barbier E *et al.* Constitutive endocytosis and degradation of the pre-T cell receptor. *J Exp Med* 2002; **195**: 1585–97.

101. Anderson SJ, Levin SD, Perlmutter RM. Protein tyrosine kinase p56lck controls allelic exclusion of T-cell receptor beta-chain genes. *Nature* 1993; **365**: 552–4.

102. Zhang W, Sommers CL, Burshtyn DN *et al.* Essential role of LAT in T cell development. *Immunity* 1999; **10**: 323–32.

103. Cheng AM, Negishi I, Anderson SJ *et al.* The Syk and ZAP-70 SH2-containing tyrosine kinases are implicated in pre-T cell receptor signaling. *Proc Natl Acad Sci U S A* 1997; **94**: 9797–801.

●104. Pivniouk V, Tsitsikov E, Swinton P *et al.* Impaired viability and profound block in thymocyte development in mice lacking the adaptor protein SLP-76. *Cell* 1998; **94**: 229–38.

105. Sen J. Signal transduction in thymus development. *Cell Mol Biol (Noisy-le-grand)* 2001; **47**: 197–215.

106. Rincon M, Flavell RA, Davis RJ. Signal transduction by MAP kinases in T lymphocytes. *Oncogene* 2001; **20**: 2490–7.

107. Sen J, Shinkai Y, Alt FW *et al.* Nuclear factors that mediate intrathymic signals are developmentally regulated. *J Exp Med* 1994; **180**: 2321–7.

108. Sen J, Venkataraman L, Shinkai Y *et al.* Expression and induction of nuclear factor-kappa B-related proteins in thymocytes. *J Immunol* 1995; **154**: 3213–21.

109. Zuniga-Pflucker JC, Schwartz HL, Lenardo MJ. Gene transcription in differentiating immature T cell receptor(neg) thymocytes resembles antigen-activated mature T cells. *J Exp Med* 1993; **178**: 1139–49.

110. Rincon M, Flavell RA. Regulation of AP-1 and NFAT transcription factors during thymic selection of T cells. *Mol Cell Biol* 1996; **16**: 1074–84.

111. Okamura RM, Sigvardsson M, Galceran J *et al.* Redundant regulation of T cell differentiation and TCRalpha gene expression by the transcription factors LEF-1 and TCF-1. *Immunity* 1998; **8**: 11–20.

112. Miyazaki T. Two distinct steps during thymocyte maturation from CD4-CD8- to CD4+CD8+ distinguished in the early growth response (Egr)-1 transgenic mice with a recombinase-activating gene-deficient background. *J Exp Med* 1997; **186**: 877–85.

113. Greenbaum S, Zhuang Y. Regulation of early lymphocyte development by E2A family proteins. *Semin Immunol* 2002; **14**: 405–14.

114. Engel I, Johns C, Bain G *et al.* Early thymocyte development is regulated by modulation of E2A protein activity. *J Exp Med* 2001; **194**: 733–45.

115. Maillard I, Tu L, Sambandam A *et al.* The requirement for Notch signaling at the beta-selection checkpoint in vivo is absolute and independent of the pre-T cell receptor. *J Exp Med* 2006; **203**: 2239–45.

●116. Huesmann M, Scott B, Kisielow P, von Boehmer H. Kinetics and efficacy of positive selection in the thymus of normal and T cell receptor transgenic mice. *Cell* 1991; **66**: 533–40.

117. Casanova JL, Romero P, Widmann C *et al.* T cell receptor genes in a series of class I major histocompatibility complex-restricted cytotoxic T lymphocyte clones specific for a Plasmodium berghei nonapeptide: implications for T cell allelic exclusion and antigen-specific repertoire. *J Exp Med* 1991; **174**: 1371–83.

118. Brandle D, Muller C, Rulicke T *et al.* Engagement of the T-cell receptor during positive selection in the thymus down-regulates RAG-1 expression. *Proc Natl Acad Sci U S A* 1992; **89**: 9529–33.

119. Borgulya P, Kishi H, Uematsu Y, von Boehmar H. Exclusion and inclusion of alpha and beta T cell receptor alleles. *Cell* 1992; **69**: 529–37.

120. Davey GM, Schober SL, Endrizzi BT *et al.* Preselection thymocytes are more sensitive to T cell receptor stimulation than mature T cells. *J Exp Med* 1998; **188**: 1867–74.

121. Daniels MA, Devine L, Miller JD et al. CD8 binding to MHC class I molecules is influenced by T cell maturation and glycosylation. Immunity 2001; 15: 1051–61.

122. Moody AM, Chui D, Reche PA et al. Developmentally regulated glycosylation of the CD8alphabeta coreceptor stalk modulates ligand binding. Cell 2001; 107: 501–12.

123. Chmielowski B, Muranski P, Ignatowicz L. In the normal repertoire of CD4+ T cells, a single class II MHC/peptide complex positively selects TCRs with various antigen specificities. J Immunol 1999; 162: 95–105.

●124. Ignatowicz L, Kappler J, Marrack P. The repertoire of T cells shaped by a single MHC/peptide ligand. Cell 1996; 84: 521–9.

125. Page DM, Kane LP, Allison JP, Hedrick SM. Two signals are required for negative selection of CD4+CD8+ thymocytes. J Immunol 1993; 151: 1868–80.

126. Aiba Y, Mazda O, Davis MM et al. Requirement of a second signal from antigen presenting cells in the clonal deletion of immature T cells. Int Immunol 1994; 6: 1475–83.

127. Li R, Page DM. Requirement for a complex array of costimulators in the negative selection of autoreactive thymocytes in vivo. J Immunol 2001; 166: 6050–6.

●128. Anderson MS, Venanzi ES, Chen Z et al. The cellular mechanism of Aire control of T cell tolerance. Immunity 2005; 23: 227–39.

129. Anderson MS, Venanzi ES, Klein L et al. Projection of an immunological self shadow within the thymus by the aire protein. Science 2002; 298: 1395–401.

130. Mathis D, Benoist C. Back to central tolerance. Immunity 2004; 20: 509–16.

131. Groves T, Parsons M, Miyamoto NG, Guidos CJ. TCR engagement of CD4+CD8+ thymocytes in vitro induces early aspects of positive selection, but not apoptosis. J Immunol 1997; 158: 65–75.

132. Cibotti R, Punt JA, Dash KS et al. Surface molecules that drive T cell development in vitro in the absence of thymic epithelium and in the absence of lineage-specific signals. Immunity 1997; 6: 245–55.

133. Laufer TM, Glimcher LH, Lo D. Using thymus anatomy to dissect T cell repertoire selection. Semin Immunol 1999; 11: 65–70.

134. Derbinski J, Schulte A, Kyewski B, Klein L. Promiscuous gene expression in medullary thymic epithelial cells mirrors the peripheral self. Nat Immunol 2001; 2: 1032–9.

◆135. Kyewski B, Derbinski J. Self-representation in the thymus: an extended view. Nat Rev Immunol 2004; 4: 688–98.

●136. Gallegos AM, Bevan MJ. Central tolerance to tissue-specific antigens mediated by direct and indirect antigen presentation. J Exp Med 2004; 200: 1039–49.

137. Campbell JJ, Pan J, Butcher EC et al. Cutting edge: developmental switches in chemokine responses during T cell maturation. J Immunol 1999; 163: 2353–7.

138. Witt CM, Raychaudhuri S, Schaefer B et al. Directed migration of positively selected thymocytes visualized in real time. PLoS Biol 2005; 3: e160.

139. Liu W, Putnam AL, Xu-Yu Z et al. CD127 expression inversely correlates with FoxP3 and suppressive function of human CD4+ T reg cells. J Exp Med 2006; 203: 1701–11.

140. Sakaguchi S, Setoguchi R, Yagi H, Nomura T. Naturally arising Foxp3-expressing CD25+CD4+ regulatory T cells in self-tolerance and autoimmune disease. Curr Top Microbiol Immunol 2006; 305: 51–66.

141. Beyer M, Schultze JL. Regulatory T cells in cancer. Blood 2006; 108: 804–11.

142. Joffre O, Santolaria T, Calise D et al. Prevention of acute and chronic allograft rejection with CD4+CD25+Foxp3+ regulatory T lymphocytes. Nat Med 2008; 14: 88–92.

143. Lin W, Haribhai D, Relland LM et al. Regulatory T cell development in the absence of functional Foxp3. Nat Immunol 2007; 8: 359–68.

144. Gavin MA, Rasmussen JP, Fontenot JD et al. Foxp3-dependent programme of regulatory T-cell differentiation. Nature 2007; 445: 771–5.

●145. Watanabe N, Wang YH, Lee HK et al. Hassall's corpuscles instruct dendritic cells to induce CD4+CD25+ regulatory T cells in human thymus. Nature 2005; 436: 1181–5.

146. Nomura T, Sakaguchi S. Foxp3 and Aire in thymus-generated Treg cells: a link in self-tolerance. Nat Immunol 2007; 8: 333–4.

147. Werlen G, Hausmann B, Palmer E. A motif in the alphabeta T-cell receptor controls positive selection by modulating ERK activity. Nature 2000; 406: 422–6.

148. Delgado P, Fernandez E, Dave V et al. CD3delta couples T-cell receptor signalling to ERK activation and thymocyte positive selection. Nature 2000; 406: 426–30.

◆149. Starr TK, Jameson SC, Hogquist KA. Positive and negative selection of T cells. Annu Rev Immunol 2003; 21: 139–76.

150. Madrenas J, Wange RL, Wang JL et al. Zeta phosphorylation without ZAP-70 activation induced by TCR antagonists or partial agonists. Science 1995; 267: 515–18.

151. Haks MC, Pepin E, van den Brakel JH et al. Contributions of the T cell receptor-associated CD3gamma-ITAM to thymocyte selection. J Exp Med 2002; 196: 1–13.

152. Backstrom BT, Muller U, Hausmann B, Palmer E. Positive selection through a motif in the alphabeta T cell receptor. Science 1998; 281: 835–8.

◆153. Germain RN. T-cell development and the CD4-CD8 lineage decision. Nat Rev Immunol 2002; 2: 309–22.

●154. Brugnera E, Bhandoola A, Cibotti R et al. Coreceptor reversal in the thymus: signaled CD4+8+ thymocytes initially terminate CD8 transcription even when differentiating into CD8+ T cells. Immunity 2000; 13: 59–71.

155. Bosselut R, Guinter TI, Sharrow SO, Singer A. Unraveling a revealing paradox: Why major histocompatibility complex I-signaled thymocytes 'paradoxically' appear as CD4+8lo transitional cells during positive selection of CD8+ T cells. J Exp Med 2003; 197: 1709–19.

156. Singer A. New perspectives on a developmental dilemma: the kinetic signaling model and the importance of signal duration for the CD4/CD8 lineage decision. Curr Opin Immunol 2002; 14: 207–15.

157. Itano A, Cado D, Chan FK, Robey E. A role for the cytoplasmic tail of the beta chain of CD8 in thymic selection. *Immunity* 1994; **1**: 287–90.

158. Seong RH, Chamberlain JW, Parnes JR *et al*. Signal for T-cell differentiation to a CD4 cell lineage is delivered by CD4 transmembrane region and/or cytoplasmic tail. *Nature* 1992; **356**: 718–20.

159. Campbell KS, Buder A, Deuschle U. Interactions between the amino-terminal domain of p56lck and cytoplasmic domains of CD4 and CD8 alpha in yeast. *Eur J Immunol* 1995; **25**: 2408–12.

● 160. Yasutomo K, Doyle C, Miele L *et al*. The duration of antigen receptor signalling determines CD4+ versus CD8+ T-cell lineage fate. *Nature* 2000; **404**: 506–10.

● 161. Hernandez-Hoyos G, Sohn SJ, Rothenberg EV, Alberola-Ila J. Lck activity controls CD4/CD8 T cell lineage commitment. *Immunity* 2000; **12**: 313–22.

162. Legname G, Seddon B, Lovatt M *et al*. Inducible expression of a p56Lck transgene reveals a central role for Lck in the differentiation of CD4 SP thymocytes. *Immunity* 2000; **12**: 537–46.

163. Pages G, Guerin S, Grall D *et al*. Defective thymocyte maturation in p44 MAP kinase (Erk 1) knockout mice. *Science* 1999; **286**: 1374–7.

164. Shao H, Wilkinson B, Lee B *et al*. Slow accumulation of active mitogen-activated protein kinase during thymocyte differentiation regulates the temporal pattern of transcription factor gene expression. *J Immunol* 1999; **163**: 603–10.

165. Sharp LL, Hedrick SM. Commitment to the CD4 lineage mediated by extracellular signal-related kinase mitogen-activated protein kinase and lck signaling. *J Immunol* 1999; **163**: 6598–605.

166. Sharp LL, Schwarz DA, Bott CM *et al*. The influence of the MAPK pathway on T cell lineage commitment. *Immunity* 1997; **7**: 609–18.

167. Wilkinson B, Kaye J. Requirement for sustained MAPK signaling in both CD4 and CD8 lineage commitment: a threshold model. *Cell Immunol* 2001; **211**: 86–95.

168. Schmeissner PJ, Xie H, Smilenov LB *et al*. Integrin functions play a key role in the differentiation of thymocytes in vivo. *J Immunol* 2001; **167**: 3715–24.

169. Robey E, Chang D, Itano A *et al*. An activated form of Notch influences the choice between CD4 and CD8 T cell lineages. *Cell* 1996; **87**: 483–92.

170. Wolfer A, Bakker T, Wilson A *et al*. Inactivation of Notch 1 in immature thymocytes does not perturb CD4 or CD8 T cell development. *Nat Immunol* 2001; **2**: 235–41.

171. Nawijn MC, Ferreira R, Dingjan GM *et al*. Enforced expression of GATA-3 during T cell development inhibits maturation of CD8 single-positive cells and induces thymic lymphoma in transgenic mice. *J Immunol* 2001; **167**: 715–23.

172. Fujii M, Hayashi K, Niki M *et al*. Overexpression of AML1 renders a T hybridoma resistant to T cell receptor-mediated apoptosis. *Oncogene* 1998; **17**: 1813–10.

173. Hayashi K, Abe N, Watanabe T *et al*. Overexpression of AML1 transcription factor drives thymocytes into the CD8 single-positive lineage. *J Immunol* 2001; **167**: 4957–65.

174. Telfer JC, Hedblom EE, Anderson MK *et al*. Localization of the domains in Runx transcription factors required for the repression of CD4 in thymocytes. *J Immunol* 2004; **172**: 4359–70.

175. Canelles M, Park ML, Schwartz OM. Fowlkes BJ. The influence of the thymic environment on the CD4-versus-CD8 T lineage decision. *Nat Immunol* 2003; **4**: 756–64.

◆ 176. Parham P. MHC class I molecules and KIRs in human history, health and survival. *Nat Rev Immunol* 2005; **5**: 201–14.

177. Herberman RB, Nunn ME, Lavrin DH. Natural cytotoxic reactivity of mouse lymphoid cells against syngeneic acid allogeneic tumors. I. Distribution of reactivity and specificity. *Int J Cancer* 1975; **16**: 216–29.

178. Pross HF, Jondal M. Cytotoxic lymphocytes from normal donors. A functional marker of human non-T lymphocytes. *Clin Exp Immunol* 1975; **21**: 226–35.

179. Hsu KC, Keever-Taylor CA, Wilton A *et al*. Improved outcome in HLA-identical sibling hematopoietic stem-cell transplantation for acute myelogenous leukemia predicted by KIR and HLA genotypes. *Blood* 2005; **105**: 4878–84.

● 180. Ruggeri L, Capanni M, Urbani E *et al*. Effectiveness of donor natural killer cell alloreactivity in mismatched hematopoietic transplants. *Science* 2002; **295**: 2097–100.

181. Smyth MJ, Hayakawa Y, Takeda K, Yagita H. New aspects of natural-killer-cell surveillance and therapy of cancer. *Nat Rev Cancer* 2002; **2**: 850–61.

182. Cooper MA, Fehniger TA, Turner SC *et al*. Human natural killer cells: a unique innate immunoregulatory role for the CD56(bright) subset. *Blood* 2001; **97**: 3146–51.

183. Lauwerys BR, Garot N, Renauld JC, Houssiau FA. Cytokine production and killer activity of NK/T-NK cells derived with IL-2, IL-15, or the combination of IL-12 and IL-18. *J Immunol* 2000; **165**: 1847–53.

184. Ballas ZK, Turner JM, Turner DA *et al*. A patient with simultaneous absence of 'classical' natural killer cells (CD3-, CD16+, and NKH1+) and expansion of CD3+, CD4-, CD8-, NKH1+ subset. *J Allergy Clin Immunol* 1990; **85**: 453–9.

185. Biron CA, Byron KS, Sullivan JL. Severe herpesvirus infections in an adolescent without natural killer cells. *N Engl J Med* 1989; **320**: 1731–5.

186. Joncas J, Monczak Y, Ghibu F *et al*. Brief report: killer cell defect and persistent immunological abnormalities in two patients with chronic active Epstein-Barr virus infection. *J Med Virol* 1989; **28**: 110–17.

187. Sirianni MC, Businco L, Seminara R, Aiuti F. Severe combined immunodeficiencies, primary T-cell defects and DiGeorge syndrome in humans: characterization by monoclonal antibodies and natural killer cell activity. *Clin Immunol Immunopathol* 1983; **28**: 361–70.

188. Sihvola M, Hurme M. The development of NK cell activity in thymectomized bone marrow chimaeras. *Immunology* 1984; **53**: 17–22.

189. Ramos SB, Garcia AB, Viana SR et al. Phenotypic and functional evaluation of natural killer cells in thymectomized children. Clin Immunol Immunopathol 1996; 81: 277–81.

190. Freud AG, Becknell B, Roychowdhury S et al. A human CD34(+) subset resides in lymph nodes and differentiates into CD56bright natural killer cells. Immunity 2005; 22: 295–304.

191. Kim S, Iizuka K, Kang HS et al. In vivo developmental stages in murine natural killer cell maturation. Nat Immunol 2002; 3: 523–8.

192. Raulet DH, Held W, Correa I et al. Specificity, tolerance and developmental regulation of natural killer cells defined by expression of class I-specific Ly49 receptors. Immunol Rev 1997; 155: 41–52.

◆193. Raulet DH, Vance RE, McMahon CW. Regulation of the natural killer cell receptor repertoire. Annu Rev Immunol 2001; 19: 291–330.

194. Johansson MH, Bieberich C, Jay G et al. Natural killer cell tolerance in mice with mosaic expression of major histocompatibility complex class I transgene. J Exp Med 1997; 186: 353–64.

195. Sykes M, Harty MW, Karlhofer FM et al. Hematopoietic cells and radioresistant host elements influence natural killer cell differentiation. J Exp Med 1993; 178: 223–9.

196. Ikawa T, Kawamoto H, Fujimoto S et al. Commitment of common T/Natural killer (NK) progenitors to unipotent T and NK progenitors in the murine fetal thymus revealed by a single progenitor assay. J Exp Med 1999; 190: 1617–26.

197. Rosmaraki EE, Douagi I, Roth C et al. Identification of committed NK cell progenitors in adult murine bone marrow. Eur J Immunol 2001; 31: 1900–9.

198. Yu H, Fehniger TA, Fuchshuber P et al. Flt3 ligand promotes the generation of a distinct CD34(+) human natural killer cell progenitor that responds to interleukin-15. Blood 1998; 92: 3647–57.

199. Shibuya A, Kojima H, Shibuya K et al. Enrichment of interleukin-2-responsive natural killer progenitors in human bone marrow. Blood 1993; 81: 1819–26.

200. Mrozek E, Anderson P, Caligiuri MA. Role of interleukin-15 in the development of human CD56+ natural killer cells from CD34+ hematopoietic progenitor cells. Blood 1996; 87: 2632–40.

201. Williams NS, Moore TA, Schatzle JD et al. Generation of lytic natural killer 1.1+, Ly-49- cells from multipotential murine bone marrow progenitors in a stroma-free culture: definition of cytokine requirements and developmental intermediates. J Exp Med 1997; 186: 1609–14.

202. Williams NS, Klem J, Puzanov IJ et al. Differentiation of NK1.1+, Ly49+ NK cells from flt3+ multipotent marrow progenitor cells. J Immunol 1999; 163: 2648–56.

203. Iizuka K, Chaplin DD, Wang Y et al. Requirement for membrane lymphotoxin in natural killer cell development. Proc Natl Acad Sci U S A 1999; 96: 6336–40.

204. Lodolce JP, Boone DL, Chai S et al. IL-15 receptor maintains lymphoid homeostasis by supporting lymphocyte homing and proliferation. Immunity 1998; 9: 669–76.

205. Kennedy MK, Glaccum M, Brown SN et al. Reversible defects in natural killer and memory CD8 T cell lineages in interleukin 15-deficient mice. J Exp Med 2000; 191: 771–80.

●206. Ranson T, Vosshenrich CA, Corcuff E et al. IL-15 is an essential mediator of peripheral NK-cell homeostasis. Blood 2003; 101: 4887–93.

207. Cooper MA, Bush JE, Fehniger TA et al. In vivo evidence for a dependence on interleukin 15 for survival of natural killer cells. Blood 2002; 100: 3633–38.

208. Kundig TM, Schorle H, Bachmann MF et al. Immune responses in interleukin-2-deficient mice. Science 1993; 262: 1059–61.

209. Puel A, Ziegler SF, Buckley RH et al. Defective IL7R expression in T(-)B(+)NK(+) severe combined immunodeficiency. Nat Genet 1998; 20: 394–7.

210. Sharfe N, Dadi HK, Shahar M, Roifman CM. Human immune disorder arising from mutation of the alpha chain of the interleukin-2 receptor. Proc Natl Acad Sci U S A 1997; 94: 3168–71.

211. Shibuya A. Development and functions of natural killer cells. Int J Hematol 2003; 78: 1–6.

◆212. Colucci F, Caligiuri MA, Di Santo JP et al. What does it take to make a natural killer? Nat Rev Immunol 2003; 3: 413–25.

213. Smyth MJ, Cretney E, Kelly JM et al. Activation of NK cell cytotoxicity. Mol Immunol 2005; 42: 501–10.

214. Parrish-Novak J, Foster DC, Holly RD, Clagg CH. Interleukin-21 and the IL-21 receptor: novel effectors of NK and T cell responses. J Leukoc Biol 2002; 72: 856–63.

215. Cooper MA, Fehniger TA, Caligiuri MA. The biology of human natural killer-cell subsets. Trends Immunol 2001; 22: 633–40.

216. Ferlazzo G, Thomas D, Lin SL et al. The abundant NK cells in human secondary lymphoid tissues require activation to express killer cell Ig-like receptors and become cytolytic. J Immunol 2004; 172: 1455–62.

11

Ontogeny of B cells

FRITZ MELCHERS

INTRODUCTION

A single pluripotent hematopoietic stem cell (pHSC) is capable of generating all the erythocytes, megakaryocytes, and blood platelets; all the cells of the myeloid cell lineages, such as monocytes, macrophages, dendritic cells, granulocytes (i.e., neutrophils, basophils, eosinophils, and mast cells), and osteoclasts; all the natural killer (NK) cells; the T lymphocytes – and the B lymphocytes. This chapter describes the major known molecular steps and cellular stages, and the interactions with the endogenous environment of cooperating cells, as well as with the exogenous environment of antigens and polyclonal activators, that begins with the generation of a pluripotent hematopoietic stem cell and finally leads to the deposition and use of mature B cells in different compartments of the immune system.

The major hallmark and specific feature of B cells is their capacity to produce immunoglobulins (Ig), to deposit them as antigen-specific receptors (B cell receptors, BCR) on their surface, and to respond to the recognition of specific antigen, or of polyclonal activators, by the generation of memory B cells and of plasma cells. Plasma cells secrete the Ig as antigen-specific Ig, also called antibodies

(as polyclonal Ig are respectively sometimes called 'natural antibodies'), into extracellular spaces such as the blood or – after transport through epithelial layers – the gut.

As mature B cells displaying Ig on their surface, they can also attract 'their' specific protein antigen with high avidity, take it up, process it, and present it as peptides complexed with major histocompatibility complex (MHC) class II molecules to helper T cells, i.e., act as antigen-specific antigen-presenting cells.

PLURIPOTENT HEMATOPOIETIC STEM CELLS

B lymphocytes, like all other cell lineages of blood, are generated – in mouse and man, throughout life – from pluripotent hematopoietic stem cells. These pHSCs derive from embryonal mesoderm, which also generates the environments of the hematopoietic system. These environments are the vascular endothelial cells that form blood and lymph vessels through which the blood cells travel and the microenvironmental niches, especially the bone and its mesenchyme-derived stromal cells, which interact with the pHSC and the progenitors of the different blood cell lineages (Fig. 11.1).[1]

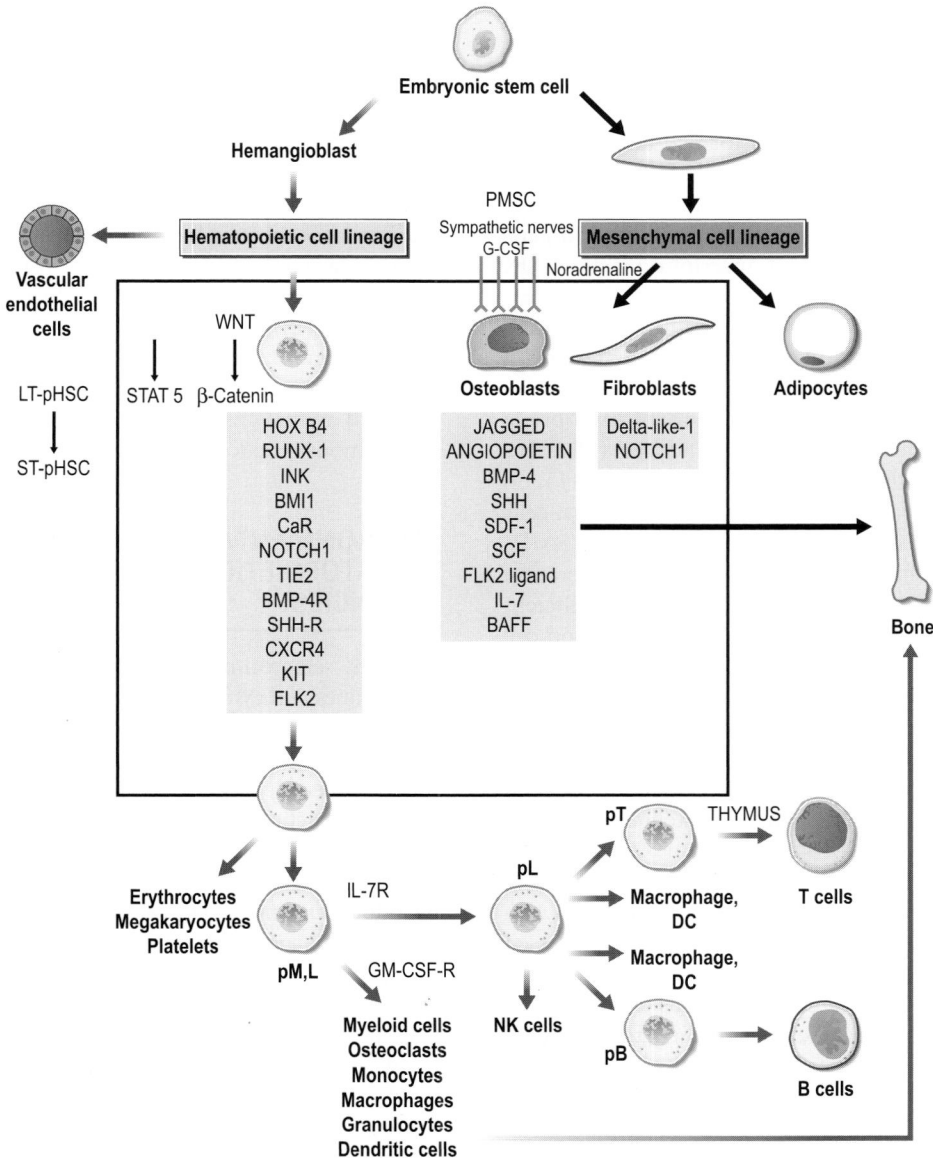

Figure 11.1   The 'niche' of pluripotent hematopoietic stem cells. Pluripotent hematopoietic stem cells (pHSC), especially those of long-term reconstitution potential (LT-pHSC), developed from common progenitors of vascular endothelium and hematopoietic cells express receptors – CaR, NOTCH1, TIE2, BMP-4R, SHH-R, CXCR4, KIT, and FLK2 – that signal via the WNT pathway including β-catenin and also via STAT5 to balance proliferation; that is, self-renewal and differentiation, i.e., pluripotency. The ligands for these receptors are provided by mesenchymal stem cell–derived osteoblasts and fibroblasts which, themselves, balance their differentiation to either osteoblasts, fibroblasts, or adipocytes. The ligands are JAGGED-1 and Delta-like-1 for NOTCH1, Angiopoietin for TIE2, BMP-4 for BMP-4R, SHH for SHH-R, SDF-1 (CXCL12) for CXCR4, SCF for KIT, and FLK2 ligand for FLK2. These so-called stromal cells also provide cytokines (e.g., interleukin-7 [IL-7]) for the later lymphoid progenitors. Since these stromal cells also provide the 'niche' for memory B cells and long-lived plasma cells, they may provide BAFF, for example, for long-term survival of such cells. The mesenchymal cell–derived stroma is innervated by sympathetic nerves that control apoptosis of the stroma with noradrenaline. For details see the text. pMSC, pluripotent mesenchymal stem cell; G-CSF, granulocyte colony-stimulating factor; GM-CSF, granulocyte macrophage colony-stimulating factor; ST-pHSC, Pluripotent hematopoietic stem cells of short-term reconstitution potential; DC, dendritic cell; NK, natural killer.

Five properties characterize a pHSC: the capacity to renew itself upon cell division; the pluripotency to develop into the various differentiation lineages of blood cells; the chemotaxis to home back to the bone marrow upon transplantation; the long-term reconstituting ability to, again, serve as a stem cell when used from the transplanted host in secondary transplantations; and the potency to protect a transplanted host from death as the consequence of lethal irradiation.[2–7]

Self-renewal

Pluripotent hematopoietic stem cells have the capacity to renew themselves upon cell division. Self-renewal can be symmetric, so that two pHSCs are formed after cell division, leading to an expansion of the pool of pHSCs. Several factors have been identified that control the self-renewing proliferation of pHSCs, most notably the Polycomb gene family member BMI1[8,9] and the transcription factor HOX B4;[10-16] gene expression of both is controlled by the nuclear factor NF-Ya.[17] The WNT signaling pathway, including β-catenin,[18-20] has been found to be involved in the control of pHSC proliferation. Hence, pHSCs can now be expanded and cloned in tissue cultures in the presence of appropriate cytokines, e.g., interleukin (IL)-3, IL-6, and stem cell factor (SCF; the ligand for the receptor tyrosine kinase, KIT), on a supportive layer of mesenchymally derived stromal cells (see Fig. 11.1). Thus, transgenic expression of NF-Ya, BMI1, HOX B4, or β-catenin favor long-term proliferation of pHSC, while at the same time may inhibit efficient hematopoietic differentiation into the different blood cell lineages.[21]

Mesenchyme-derived stromal cells provide molecules for several pHSC-cooperative, stimulatory interactions, among them SCF (interacting with KIT on pHSC),[22] angiopoietin (interacting with TIE2 on pHSC),[23,24] and bone morphogenic protein 4 (BMP-4; interacting with its receptor on pHSC).[25-27] Also, these stromal cells chemotactically attract pHSC through the production of CXCLI2 (SDF-1), interacting with its receptor CXCR4 on pHSC,[28-33] and Ca-2, the Ca^{2+}-receptor protein expressed on pHSC, probably sensing bone Ca^{2+} near the marrow of the bones.[34] Activation of these stromal cells (especially the osteoblasts among them), thereby forming the so-called 'hematopoietic cell niche,'[35] therefore results in subsequent activation or inhibition of pHSC activities. Furthermore, noradrenaline produced by sympathetic nerves in collaboration with as yet undefined actions of the stem cell-mobilizing cytokine, granulocyte colony-stimulating factor (G-CSF), induces apoptosis of stromal cells, thereby mobilizing pHSC to leave the bone marrow and enter blood circulation.[36-40] This offers molecular and cellular explanations for the links to stress of pHSC production and activation (Fig. 11.1).

Since the hematopoietic cell niches in bone marrow can be expected to have a constant, finite size, and since pHSCs – except for unusual, acute overactivations – are confined to the bone marrow of an adult, most pHSC cell proliferation should be asymmetric, leading to one pHSC and one further differentiated progenitor after division, hence maintaining pHSC pool sizes. Early progenitors of B lymphocyte development in mouse and man have been shown to decrease in absolute numbers in bone marrow during life.[41] Hence, it is reasonable to expect that absolute numbers of pHSC also decrease with age; however, they never disappear completely.

Pluripotency

A single pHSC can repopulate all cell lineages of blood and fill their respective compartments in the body with normal numbers of cells.[2-7] pHSC give rise to erythrocytes, megakaryocytes, and platelets, and also cells of the innate immune system, i.e., myeloid cells (such as monocytes, macrophages, various forms of dendritic cells, granulocytes such as basophils, neutrophils and eosinophils, and osteoclasts) as well as lymphoid cells (i.e., the various forms of natural killer cells) and, of the cells of the adaptive immune system, T and B lymphocytes. Pluripotency is controlled by the environment of cell contacts, chemokines, and cytokines provided by stromal cells, as well as by pHSC through autonomous genetic programs.

ENVIRONMENTAL INFLUENCES ON HEMATOPOIETIC DIFFERENTIATION POTENCIES

Different environmental influences (such as different chemokines and cytokines produced from, and cell contacts provided by, stromal cells) can induce the differentiation of a pHSC along different cell lineages of blood. Experimentally this has been documented most convincingly with cloned lines of genetically marked (i.e., D_HJ_H/D_HJ_H-rearranged) progenitor B cells of PAX5-deficient,[42-48] and later also of E2A-deficient, mice.[49] The PAX5-deficient progenitors can be induced in vitro to (D_HJ_H/D_HJ_H-rearranged) macrophages by macrophage colony-stimulating factor (M-CSF), to (D_HJ_H/D_HJ_H-rearranged) dendritic cells by granulocyte macrophage colony-stimulating factor (GM-CSF) and M-CSF, to (D_HJ_H/D_HJ_H-rearranged) granulocytes by GM-CSF and G-CSF, to (D_HJ_H/D_HJ_H-rearranged) natural killer cells by IL-2, to (D_HJ_H/D_HJ_H-rearranged) osteoclasts by tumor necrosis factor (TNF)-related activation-induced cytokine (TRANCE) expressed on mesenchyme-derived stromal cells, and to (D_HJ_H/D_HJ_H-rearranged) thymocytes by Notch-ligand Delta1, again expressed on stromal cells (Fig. 11.2).[48,50,51] Alternatively, these PAX-5-deficient progenitor cells can also be transgenetically marked by retroviral transfection with a marker gene, for example that encoding green fluorescent protein (GFP).[46]

The cooperating stromal cells appear to all belong to mesenchymal stem cell-derived epithelial cells, of which osteoblasts have been found to be stimulatory for some early hematopoietic progenitor functions, while differentiated adipocytes are either no longer stimulatory, or even inhibitory (author's unpublished observations). In part, this may be due to the spectrum of cytokines produced by these different stages of mesenchymal cell differentiation. Thus, in contrast to a series of stromal cell lines derived from wild-type mouse bone marrow, the OP9 stromal cell line derived from M-CSF-deficient mouse bone marrow stroma[52] cooperates in early hematopoiesis, even from

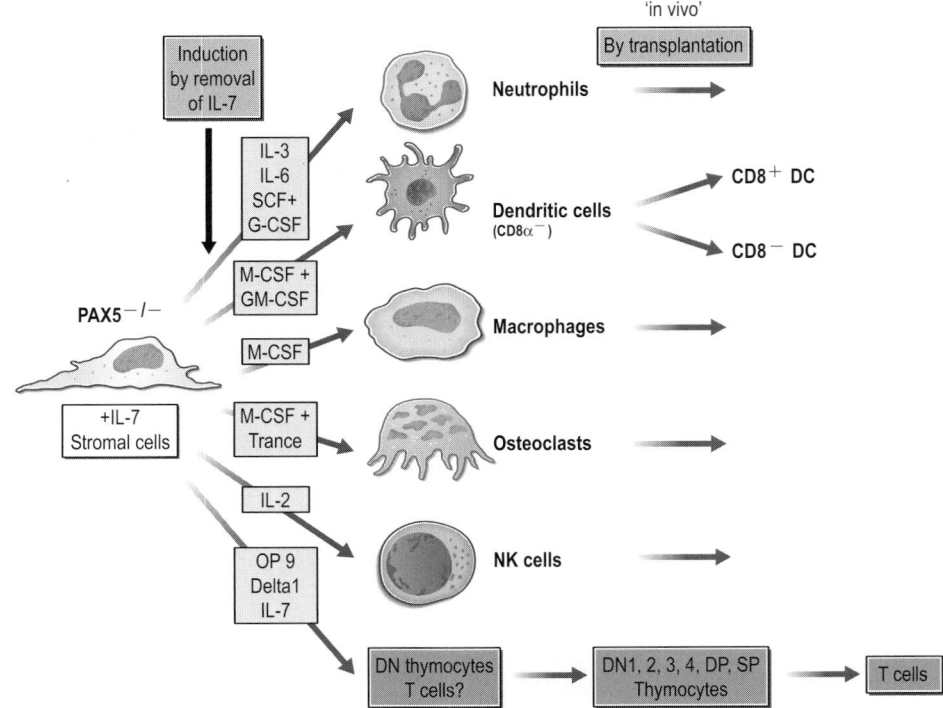

Figure 11.2 Pluripotency of pluripotent hematopoietic stem cells (pHSCs) *in vitro* and *in vivo*. Differentiation of pHSC is induced by different environmental conditions of the 'niche' described in Figure 11.1 and subsequent 'niches' providing the cytokines and cell contacts shown here. For details see the text. GM-CSF, granulocyte macrophage colony-stimulating factor; M-CSF, macrophage colony-stimulating factor; IL, interleukin; SCF, stem cell factor; DN, double negative; DP, double positive; SP, single positive; NK, natural killer.

embryonic stem cells, and, with transgenically expressed Notch-ligand Delta1, in the differentiation and proliferation of thymocytes *in vitro*,[53] and with transgenically expressed TRANCE,[44] in osteoclast development.

We do not know which microenvironmental influences positively stimulate the development of surface IgM (sIgM)[+] immature B cells from B-lineage-committed progenitors and precursors, in contrast to the other lineages in bone marrow described above. B-progenitors of wild-type mice differentiate spontaneously – without addition of cytokines or exposure to stromal cells – to sIgM[+] B lymphocytes.[54] Contrary to the lineage-inducing capacities of other cytokines, IL-7 locks D_HJ_H-rearranged preBI cells into their early stage of B-lineage differentiation. In the added presence of stromal cells (which provide, for example, SCF for interaction with the receptor tyrosine kinase KIT), these preBI cells proliferate but, again, do not differentiate to later stages of B cell development.[55]

HEMATOPOIETIC CELL-AUTONOMOUS INFLUENCES ON DIFFERENTIATION POTENCIES

The potencies of hematopoietic progenitors, stimulated by different microenvironmental influences, are controlled by sets of differentially expressed transcription factors (Fig. 11.3).

Hence, GATA1 controls erythroid development,[56,57] high levels of PU.I control myeloid cell development,[58–61] and low levels of PU.I and IKAROS control lymphoid development.[62–64] Expression of NOTCH1 accompanies development to the T lineage.[50] Ectopic expression of 'active' NOTCH1 allows early thymocyte development in the absence of a thymus and, at the same time, inhibits B cell development.[65] Ectopic expression of ID2 induces differentiation to the NK cell lineage[66–68] and, again, inhibits B cell development, possibly by forming heterodimeric complexes with E2A.[68] 'Inactive' NOTCH1, on the other hand, inhibits T cell development at the earliest, double negative (DN)1 stage of T cell development, but promotes B cell development even in the thymus.[69,70] NOTCH1 can also be inactivated by Lunatic Fringe[71] and by Deltex.[72] Such activations, again, lead to arrest of T cell development and stimulation of B cell development.

EXCLUSIVE B- VERSUS T-LYMPHOID LINEAGE DECISIONS

With the expression of low levels of PU.I and IKAROS, the major decision is made to become lymphoid-committed rather than myeloid-committed. At least a part of the CD19-negative, CD4[−]/CD8[−] DN, IL-7 receptor-expressing, receptor tyrosine kinases KIT and FLK2 double positive (DP) progenitor cell population has yet to make the decision

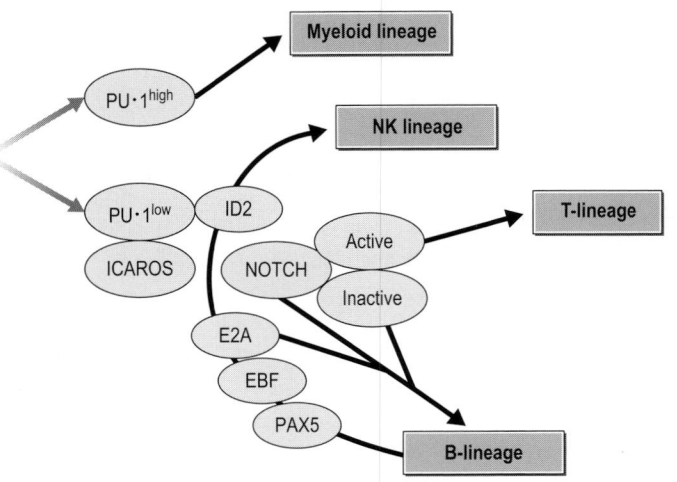

Figure 11.3 Transcription factors involved in decision of hematopoietic cell differentiation. Different levels of transcription factors (e.g., high versus low levels of PU.1) drive progenitors of myeloid/lymphoid differentiation either to myeloid or to lymphoid cells in complexes with, for example, homo- or heterodimeric forms of E2A to B-lineage, or E2A/Id2 to Nκ-lineage differentiation, in active or inactive forms of NOTCH1 to T- or to B-lineage, or in sequences of E2A/EBF and PAX5 to B-lineage differentiation. For details see the text. NK, natural killer.

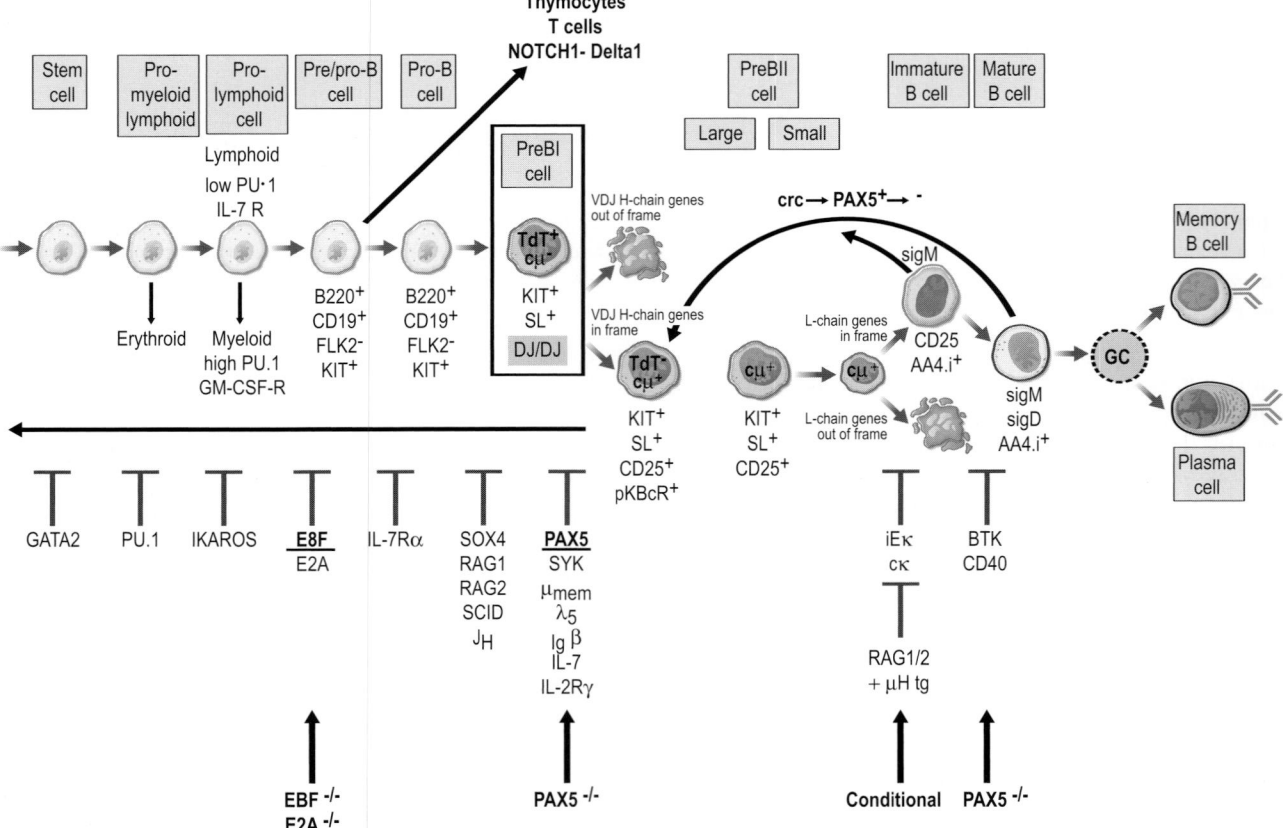

Figure 11.4 Stages of cellular differentiation of B lymphocytes from pluripotent hematopoietic stem cells and steps of de-/redifferentiation induced by deletion of PAX5 in preBI or mature B cells. Red arrows indicate the de-/redifferentiation, and the intensity of the arrows their rates. The figure also indicates the points of differentiation arrest induced by given mutations (for a review see [1]). The characterization of the different cellular stages is given by their expressions of surface-located as well as intracellular markers.

to enter either the T- or B-lymphoid lineage pathway of differentiation. These early lymphoid progenitors in the bone marrow express both the T-lymphoid lineage-specific preTα gene as well as the surrogate L chain-encoding V_{preB} and $\lambda 5$ genes (Fig. 11.4). In parallel, cellular functions control the proliferative expansion of DN2 to DN3 and DN4

and large DP (CD4$^+$ CD8$^+$) thymocytes once the precursors have migrated to the thymus, and surrogate light (SL) chain controls proliferative expansion of preBI to large preBII cells in the bone marrow. Hence, while these common lymphoid progenitors already express both surrogate chains as well as the rearrangement machinery (i.e., RAG1,

RAG-2, and terminal deoxynucleotidyl transferase [TdT]), they still have to commit themselves to the expression of only one of the two surrogate chains, and they have to open either T cell receptor TCR loci – TCRγ for exclusive VJ-rearrangement, TCRδ and β for exclusive DJ-rearrangements – and they have to express the genes encoding antigen receptor–anchoring proteins: for T cells the CD3 complex, for B cells Igα and Igβ. The net result of these decisions, described below for the B-lymphoid cell lineage, is that B-lineage cells do not express preTα, do not express CD3, and, most exclusively, do not enter D-J rearrangements at the TCRβ and δ loci.

MODES OF COMMITMENT TO THE B LYMPHOCYTE LINEAGE OF DIFFERENTIATION

In a cell that has made the decision to enter the lymphoid lineage of differentiation, Ikaros as well as low levels of PU.I contribute to the control of expression of the IL-7 receptor and the rearrangement machinery (i.e., RAG-1 and RAG-2), as well as to the expression of parts of the pre-lymphocyte receptor complexes, i.e., preTα and components of the CD3 complex, and VpreB/λ5 and the Igβ of the Igα/β complex. Thereafter, additional transcription factors contribute to the decisions to enter into further differentiation along the different lymphoid lineages (see Fig. 11.3).

E2A[73,74] and EBF[75–77] favor B cell development, and E2A- or EBF-deficient mice are arrested in B cell development, just as PAX5-deficient mice are.[78,79] However, E2A-deficient progenitor B cells carry no D_HJ_H rearrangements.[49] By contrast, PAX5 deficiency still allows D_H to J_H rearrangements on the Ig H chain loci to the same extent (i.e., on both alleles) as PAX5-proficient, wild-type progenitor B cells.[46] Transgenic expression of E2A[62] (but not of EBF or PAX5), or of important lineage-specific genes controlled by these early regulators (e.g., the IL-7 receptor[80]), induces autonomous, environment-independent, B-lineage-specific differentiation. Transfection and subsequent transgenic expression of the E47 component of E2A in nonlymphoid fibroblasts activates the TdT gene and the Ig H chain locus.[80] When, in addition, transgenic expression of the rearrangement machinery (i.e., RAG1 and RAG2) is provided in an embryonic kidney cell line, D_H to J_H rearrangements are induced at the endogenous Ig H chain loci.[81] Endogenous rearrangements at the L chain loci in the same nonlymphoid cells require more selective actions of transcription factors: in the RAG1/RAG2-transgenic cells E2A allows for endogenous V_K to J_K rearrangements, and EBF for V_α to J_β rearrangements.[81] Finally, myeloid cell differentiation can be autonomously induced by the transgenic expression of high levels of PU.I, or of the gene encoding the receptor for GM-CSF,[60] as lymphoid differentiation can be directed by the transgenic expression of the receptor for IL-7.[62] We expect that the different microenvironmental stimuli (cytokines, cell contacts) induce the different transcription factor-activating cell programs.

Both E2A-deficient as well as PAX5-deficient progenitor B cells can be grown – like wild-type preBI cells – for long periods and cloned on stromal cells in the presence of IL-7. In the case of PAX5-deficient pre-B cells, they are cell clones that are genetically identifiable by individual sets of D_HJ_H rearrangements at both Ig H chain alleles – just as wild-type, D_HJ_H-D_HJ_H-rearranged preBI cells are.[45,54] The same is true for RAG-deficient as well as SL chain-deficient CD19$^+$ pro/pre-B cells, the former without any D_HJ_H-rearranged Ig H chain loci, the latter with normally D_HJ_H/D_HJ_H-rearranged loci. Hence, the cellular differentiation program of the expression of the tyrosine kinases FLK2 and KIT and of CD19, accompanied by reactivity to IL-7 and to stromal cell interactions (which provide the ligands for FLK2 and KIT, and the cytokine IL-7), can become disconnected from the D_H to J_H rearrangement program in progenitor B cells (Fig. 11.4).

REVERSIBLE DECISIONS OF EXCLUSIVE B CELL DIFFERENTIATION – THE FLEXIBILITY OF PLURIPOTENT CELLS

The hierarchical structure of hematopoietic cell differentiation, shown in one of the two currently prevailing models in Figure 11.4, proposes that commitment to a given cell lineage, with concomitant loss of the respective pluripotency, or multipotency, is achieved in steps. In normal hematopoietic differentiation it is expected that these steps of differentiation are 'one-way streets,' in that they follow a precursor–product relationship. When PAX5-deficient,[79] and later E2A-deficient mice,[49] were analyzed for their hematopoietic potentials, this concept of hematopoietic cell differentiation became untenable.

Surprisingly, PAX5-deficient pro/pre-B cells, blocked in further B cell development, differentiate to all the possible hematopoietic cell lineages, i.e., erythroid, myeloid, NK, and T lymphoid cells. However, they do so at rates that are too slow to allow protection of the transplanted host from irradiation-induced death. PAX5-deficient cells home back to their original sites in bone marrow, retaining the original phenotype of KIT$^+$FLK2$^+$ CD19$^-$ IL-7Ra$^+$ SCA1$^+$ cells.[45,46] The same multipotency has also been seen with E2A-deficient pro-B cells.[49] By contrast, wild-type preBI cells do not home back to the bone marrow and, upon transplantation, give rise to a single wave of B cell development, mainly to B-1 type.[54] B-2-type B cells are developed when CD4$^+$ helper T cells, together with CD4$^+$CD25$^+$ regulatory T cells, are cotransplanted. Hence, neither wild-type preBI cells nor the PAX5-deficient progenitors are fully functional, pluripotent, long-term-reconstituting stem cells since they do not differentiate to all the hematopoietic cell lineages at appropriate rates to allow protection of the host from death by lethal irradiation.

The expression of PAX5 can be seen as the final, decisive step to commit hematopoietic progenitors to the B-lineage pathway of development. The importance of PAX5 in this commitment process is further documented by experiments in which LOX-flanked PAX5 has been 'knocked into' the PAX5 locus, rendering the locus conditionally inactivatable. When preBI cells of such conditionally PAX5-deficient preBI cells are treated with CRE recombinase, thus deleting the PAX5 locus, these wild-type preBI cells revert back to the PAX5-deficient pro/pre-B cell phenotype. They become inducible to enter erythroid, myeloid, NK, and T lymphoid development (Fig. 11.4).[82] T lymphoid cells in the thymus derived from the PAX5-inactivated, transplanted preBI B cells retain the $D_H J_H/D_H J_H$ rearrangements of the original pre-B cells.

When mature, $sIgM^+$ B cells of conditionally PAX5-deficient mice are rendered PAX5 deficient by treatment with CRE recombinase the cells revert back to a pre-B-like stage.[83] Reverted cells *in vitro* regain their IL-7 receptor expression and regain the capacity to respond to IL-7 by proliferation. Since these cells have already expressed a set of productively $V_H D_H J_H/V_L J_L$ rearranged Ig H/IgL chain loci (i.e., sIgMs with μH- and κL or δL chains), and since PAX5 deficiency leads to lack of SLP65 expression,[84] the resulting pre-B cells express a polyclonal spectrum of V_H domains on μH chains and reexpress SL chain (i.e., reexpress pre-BCRs), but cannot signal downregulation of SL chain expression. Hence they continue to proliferate, stimulated by IL-7. Interestingly, the induced PAX5 deficiency turns off the expression of the productively $V_L J_L$-rearranged L chain loci, i.e., of L chains, suggesting a tight regulation of L chain expression by PAX5. Transplantation *in vivo* of the CRE-induced, PAX5-deficient pre-B cells leads to repopulation by polyclonal μH chain-expressing thymocytes in the thymus, again without expression of the $V_L J_L$-rearranged L chain loci. It remains to be determined whether the CRE-induced PAX5 inactivation dedifferentiates these cells to a large preBII-cell-like, or to a pro/preBI-like stage of B cell differentiation.

EMBRYONIC DEVELOPMENT OF B LYMPHOCYTES

Three waves of hematopoietic cell developments colonize the mouse embryo.[84–86] The first begins in extra-embryonic tissue (i.e., in the yolk sac) at day 7 to 7.5 of development. This so-called 'primitive' hematopoiesis (which shows similarities to haematopoiesis in lower vertebrates) generates 'primitive' erythrocytes (synthesizing 'fetal' hemoglobin with globin γ and β H chains), megakaryocytes (with lower ploidy) and platelets, and myeloid cells (such as macrophages, with a special set of enzymes).[87] Lymphocytes are not generated. Mutations that affect 'primitive' hematopoiesis, leading to death of cells between days 8 and 11 of development, encode the transcription factors TAL1,[88–91] RBTN1 and RBTN2,[92–95] LMO2,[96]

GATA1,[97,98] and GATA2,[99] as well as the receptor tyrosine kinase Flk1 (Fig. 11.1).[100]

Although these 'primitive' blood cell lineages are developed at extra-embryonic, ventral sides of the embryo, they migrate to the embryonic dorsal sites as soon as blood circulation is established at day 8 to 9 of development by the development of vascular endothelium. At day 8.5 to 9 of mouse embryonic development the second wave of hematopoiesis is started within the intra-embryonic, anterior portion of the aorta-gonad-mesonephros (AGM) region.[101,102] Undifferentiated, apparently pluripotent stem cells[103] then migrate through the blood and colonize the rudiments of thymus and fetal liver. At these sites, the second so-called 'definitive' wave of hematopoiesis is initiated. It now generates erythrocytes producing adult-type hemoglobin (with α and β major globin), 'definitive' megakaryocytes and platelets, and adult-type myeloid cells. In thymus, several waves of thymopoiesis are initiated.

In fetal liver a first, apparently synchronous wave of B lymphocytes is generated.[104] Two other sites of embryonic B cell development, generating B cells with properties similar to those of fetal liver, are the embryonic sites of the placenta and the omentum.[105–110] Since these B cells do not express the enzyme TdT, they rearrange V(D)J segments of the Ig H and L chain loci without N-region diversity. The early waves of embryonic B cells preferentially home to the gut-associated lymphoid tissues (GALT), belong in large part to the B-1 types of B cells, and form a first line of defense and cohabitation, against and with, the developing intestinal bacterial flora.

The third wave of hematopoiesis (the second of 'definitive' hematopoiesis) starts in bone marrow between days 17 and 19 of development, i.e., at around birth of a mouse. It initiates a continuous process of hematopoietic cell generation throughout life. Bone marrow-derived B cells differ from fetal liver-derived ones as they express TdT and, hence, generate V(D)J-rearranged Ig H loci with N-region insertions. They generate not only B-1 cells but also conventional B cells, which populate the gut-associated lymphoid tissues and also the follicular regions of spleen and lymph nodes (see below).[111]

Mutations that selectively affect 'definitive' hematopoiesis include the transcription factors AML1[112] and CBF-β.[113] Since the waves of hematopoiesis involve cell migrations through the embryo, mutations in genes controlling this migration, e.g., α_1 and β_4 integrins[114–119] and the chemokine SDF-1 and its receptor CXCR4,[120–125] affect embryonic hematopoiesis (Fig. 11.1).

B LYMPHOCYTE COMPARTMENTS OF THE IMMUNE SYSTEM OF MICE AND HUMANS

The repertoires of B lymphocytes expressing immunoglobulin, i.e., antigen-specific BCR, are generated by stepwise rearrangements of the Ig H and Ig L chain gene segments, first by D_H to J_H, then by V_H to $D_H J_H$, and, finally, by V_L to

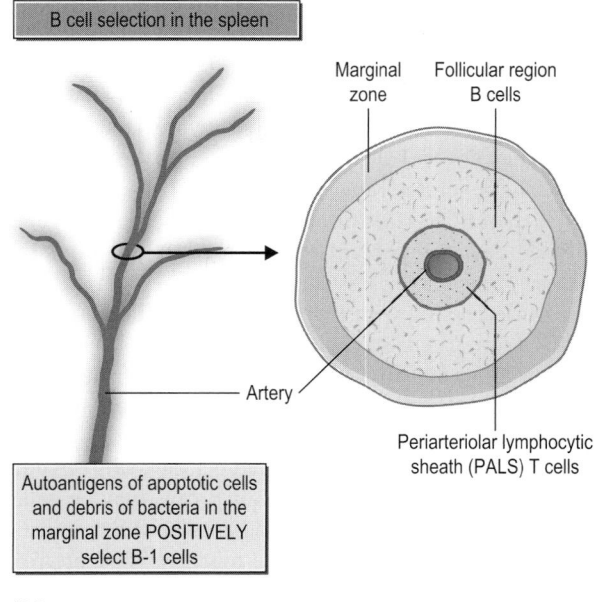

B cell selection in the spleen

Marginal zone

Follicular region B cells

Artery

Periarteriolar lymphocytic sheath (PALS) T cells

Autoantigens of apoptotic cells and debris of bacteria in the marginal zone POSITIVELY select B-1 cells

(A1)

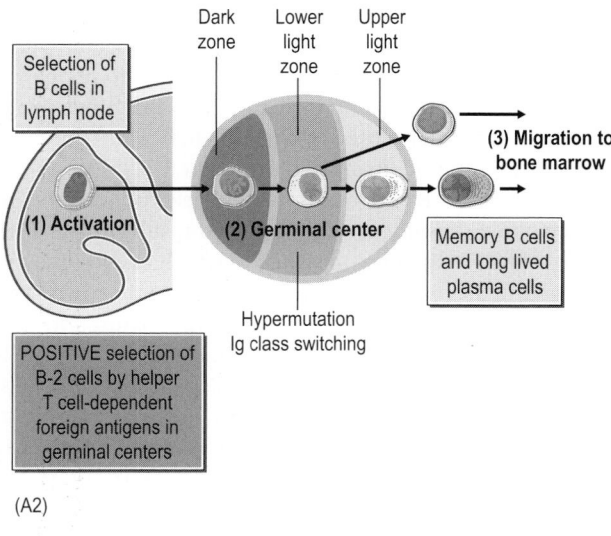

Selection of B cells in lymph node

Dark zone

Lower light zone

Upper light zone

(1) Activation

(2) Germinal center

(3) Migration to bone marrow

Memory B cells and long lived plasma cells

Hypermutation Ig class switching

POSITIVE selection of B-2 cells by helper T cell-dependent foreign antigens in germinal centers

(A2)

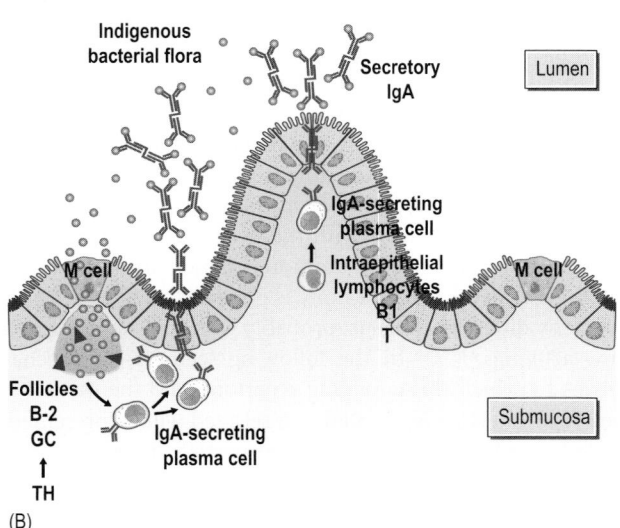

Indigenous bacterial flora

Secretory IgA

Lumen

IgA-secreting plasma cell

Intraepithelial lymphocytes

M cell

M cell

Follicles B-2 GC ↑ TH

IgA-secreting plasma cell

B1 T

Submucosa

(B)

Figure 11.5 Peripheral compartments of B lymphocytes within the immune system. (A) B lymphocytes generated in the bone marrow enter the spleen via the central artery. While T lymphocytes produced in the thymus, entering through the same route, become localized around and near this central artery as periarteriolar lymphocytic sheaths (PALS), the B cells become located in the follicular regions, in which germinal centers (GC) form when T cell-dependent antigens stimulate an immune response of these B cells. In the marginal zone, B cells meet the antigens that enter the spleen. (B) B lymphocytes generated in the bone marrow, and during embryonic development in fetal liver, become localized in follicular structures of the gut-associated lymphoid tissues (GALT) underneath flat epithelial M cells of the gut mucosa, as well as in the epithelium and the submucosa of the lamina propria in the form of single resting B cells as well as single, mostly IgA-secreting, plasma cells. The IgA is transported across the epithelium as secretory IgA and can bind to bacteria of the indigenous flora of the gut. In follicular structures below the M cells helper T cells (TH) can cooperate in a T cell–dependent immune response. For further details see the text.

J_L rearrangements. The rearrangements on the Ig H chain locus can be followed by replacement of the V_H segment in a $V_HD_HJ_H$-rearranged locus, as well as by secondary V_L to J_L rearrangements on an already V_LJ_L-rearranged L chain locus. If these rearrangements are made in-frame (i.e., if they are capable of generating Ig H and L chains by translation of the transcribed rearranged genes) and if the Ig H and L chains are capable of pairing (i.e., of forming Ig H/L chain heterodimers), then the BCRs can be expressed on the surface of, first, an immature B cell population, then a virgin mature B cell population, and, finally, after a response to antigen, a memory B cell population (for review, see [126–129]).

At least two major subcompartments of mature, BCR-expressing B lymphocytes are generated (Fig. 11.5). Approximately one-half of them are found in the follicular regions of spleen and lymph nodes and in the recirculating blood and lymph. They are often called conventional, or B-2-type, B cells. The other half is mainly found in the

GALT: for example, in Peyer's patches, either in follicular structures near the flat M-cell regions of the gut epithelia; or, often as single intraepithelial lymphocytes, in the lamina propria of the gut. A majority of these B cells appear to belong to the so-called B-1 subpopulation. In addition, B cells in the spleen are found in the marginal zone (MZ) surrounding the T cell-rich periarteriolar regions (periarteriolar lymphocytic sheaths; PALS) and the B cell-rich follicular regions.

While conventional, B-2-type B cells appear truly resting (i.e., in the G0 phase of the cell cycle), ignorant of autoantigens in their environment, and not (yet) recognized by foreign antigens, B-1 cells appear slightly activated – 'tickled' – by autoantigens as well as by foreign antigens present in the gut. Thus, food antigens as well as antigens of the indigenous bacterial flora of the gut might be recognized because they can access the lymphoid follicles in the epithelia lining gut by penetration through epithelial M cells.[130–132]

Conventional B-2-type B cells are most often triggered into responses by helper T cell-dependent antigens. These foreign antigens also stimulate helper T cells to cooperate with the follicular B cells in a response that takes place mainly in germinal centers within the follicular regions of secondary lymphoid organs. This induces B cells in a CD40-CD40 ligand (on B and T cells, respectively) cell-dependent and cytokine-dependent (e.g., IL-4 or transforming growth factor β [TGFβ]) fashion to switch to IgG, IgE, and IgA, and to hypermutate preferentially the V regions of the rearranged Ig H and L chain genes, leading to affinity maturation of B cells. The switched, hypermutated BCR-expressing B cells have the choice either to mature to Ig-secreting plasma cells, or to BCR-expressing memory cells. Both of them gain longevity in such a T cell-dependent response with half-life changed from a few days to weeks and months of survival in the immune system. The memory B cells and the long-lived plasma cells appear to leave the germinal centers to lodge in special niches in the bone marrow until they are recalled by a secondary challenge of the same antigen.

B-2 cells can also respond to T cell-independent antigens, i.e., in the absence of an activation of helper T cells and their cooperative actions on the B cells. In this situation the Ig-secreting cells that are generated produce mainly IgM, remain short-lived, and do not generate memory B cells.

By contrast to follicular B cells, gut-associated (maybe B-1 type) B cells often respond to antigen even in the absence of helper T cells, with Ig class switching mainly to IgA production. Hence, IgA-secreting plasma cells are abundant in the lamina propria. The IgA can transmigrate into the lumen of the gut, and may bind to food-derived antigens and to bacterial antigens of the indigenous flora. As much as one-third of the IgA levels found in the serum may be derived from T cell-independent stimulation of such gut-associated B cells.

Gut-associated B cells can also respond in a T cell-dependent fashion to form germinal centers, and generate long-lived, Ig class switched plasma cells and memory B cells. In such cases they are, or become, conventional B-2-type B cells. Germinal-center-like lymphoid aggregations form near the flat epithelium M cells.

In mice and humans the generation of B cell repertoires is continuous throughout life, fed from the pools of pluripotent hematopoietic progenitor cells, lymphoid and B-lineage-committed progenitors and precursors, and – maybe especially strongly in the B-1 compartment – from BCR-expressing (i.e., fully Ig gene-rearranged) B cells.

During life, the B-lineage-committed progenitor and precursor compartments appear to decrease by at least 100-fold, but never cease completely to generate B cells.[41] Therefore, the establishment of an unresponsive state to autoantigens should be achieved by mechanisms that remain operative throughout life. Continuous generation of B cells also implies that most peripheral B cells remain short lived and are replaced. Hence, chronic B cell stimulation with the danger of genetic transformations to premalignant and malignant states may be limited in time, unless these B cells become long lived.

V(D)J rearrangements of the Ig H and L chain loci generate a diversity of antigen-binding BCRs – during embryonic development in omentum and fetal liver without N-region diversity, and in adult bone marrow with N-region diversity introduced by the enzyme TdT at the V_H to D_H, and D_H to J_H, but not (in mouse) at the V_L to J_L joints. The generated repertoire of IgH/IgL chain combinations (i.e., of BCRs) is limited by the number of cells generated per day: 0.1 percent of the total B cell pool in a newborn, and maybe less than 0.001 percent in an adult, possibly decreasing with increasing age, as the frequencies of IL-7/stromal cell-clonable precursors have been seen to decrease 20- to 100-fold within a few months from birth in mice and from birth to 10 years of age in humans.[133,134] This means that in newborn mice with around 5×10^7 B cells, 5×10^4 cells may be generated per day, while in adult mice, with 5×10^8 B cells, 5×10^3 B cells may be generated. Humans, who show striking similarities to mice in the generation of B cells in bone marrow, have approximately 1000-fold higher numbers of B cells and should, therefore, also generate each day 1000-fold more B cells with newly formed BCRs.

It has been estimated that a large part – maybe more than 60 to 80 percent – of the newly generated repertoires of B cells, both of mice and humans, can bind autoantigens.[135] Many of them bind DNA, maybe because many of the V regions generated from the inherited gene segments encode positively charged arginine residues, which can interact in polar, noncovalent ways with the negatively charged phosphate groups of DNA. In addition, a large part of the originally generated B cell repertoire is polyreactive; that is, binds to many different antigens, probably with varying and often low activities.[135–141] In the following sections the mechanisms by which this emerging repertoire and the mature B cell repertoires are generated and selected will be presented. Cellular and molecular modes that participate in a positive response to foreign antigens and which contribute to the apparent unresponsiveness of the selected mature, resting B cell repertoires toward immunogenic stimulation by autoantigens will be discussed. Breaking of this unresponsiveness could lead to chronic pathological B cell responses, resulting in autoimmune diseases and B cell malignancies.

THE ROLE OF PRE–B CELL RECEPTORS IN REPERTOIRE SELECTIONS OF DEVELOPING B CELLS

After pluripotent hematopoietic stem cells have entered B lymphocyte development – that is, have expressed E2A, EBF, and PAX5, and have expressed the rearrangement machinery (i.e., the RAG1 and RAG2 genes) as well as the IL-7 receptor that controls much of the cytokine responsiveness of early B-lineage progenitors and precursors[129] – SL chain is expressed in the early lymphoid progenitors. Then D_H to J_H rearrangements begin in B220$^+$ but CD19$^-$ cells, which then change to express CD19, a B-lineage-specific

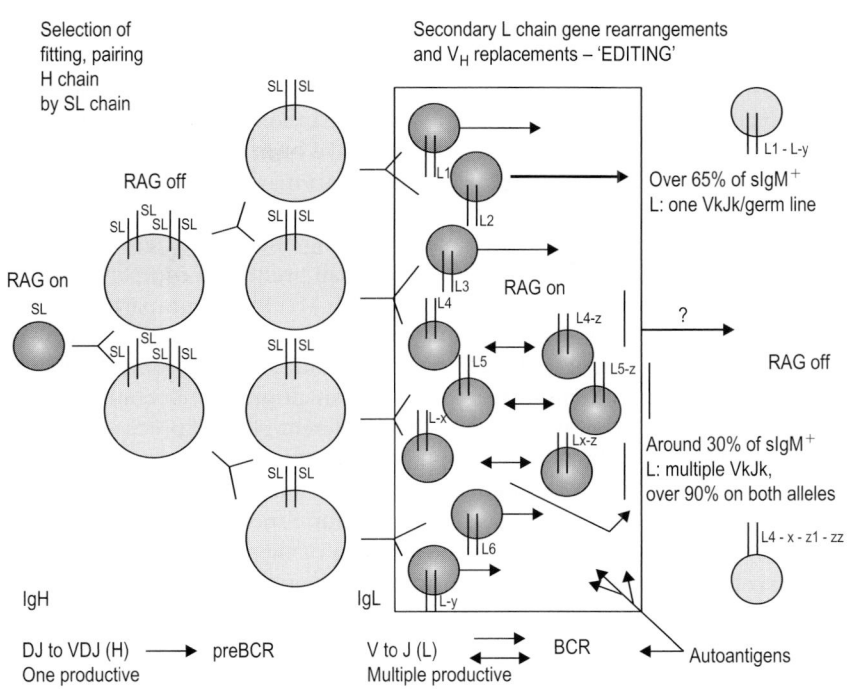

Figure 11.6 Cellularity of stages of B lymphocyte development, pre-B cell receptor-induced proliferative expansion of preBCR-expressing pre-B cells, and development of small preBII and immature B cells. In the latter two cellular stages, secondary rearrangements of L chain genes and secondary replacements of V_H-segments in $V_H D_H J_H$-rearranged H chain genes allow forth-and-back differentiation and result in 'editing' of antigen-specific BCR. Autoantigens are implicated in this process in the primary lymphoid organs, e.g., the bone marrow. For further details see the text.

surface membrane protein with regulatory functions for mature B cells. PreBI cells finally develop in which both Ig H chain alleles are $D_H J_H$ rearranged. In the mouse these $CD19^+$ $D_H J_H/D_H J_H$-rearranged preBI cells show capacities for extended profliferation *in vitro* on stromal cells in the presence of IL-7, so that such cells, isolated and cloned from fetal liver, can divide for more than 300 cell divisions without a loss of their stage of differentiation or their capacity to differentiate further down the lines of B cell developments.[129]

Further development is marked by V_H to $D_H J_H$ rearrangements that are initiated at the transition from preBI to large preBII cells (Fig. 11.6). It is not yet clear whether both $D_H J_H$-rearranged alleles of a pre-B cell are equally accessible for V_H to $D_H J_H$ rearrangements, or whether they differ in their methylation/demethylation status as the L chains loci do.[142] PreBI cells *in vitro* will enter V_H to $D_H J_H$ rearrangements as well as V_L to J_L rearrangements when IL-7 is removed from tissue cultures.[55] Whenever these rearrangements occur in-frame, and whenever the μH chains produced from such a productively rearranged IgH chain allele can pair with an SL chain, pre-B cell receptors (preBCR) are deposited at the cell surface. This signals the cell to turn off the rearrangement machinery, RAG1 and RAG2. If the rearrangement at the first $D_H J_H$ allele is productive, rearrangement at the second allele is turned off, possibly because the locus is rendered inaccessible for the rearrangement machinery, securing allelic exclusion at the Ig H chain locus so that one B cell produces only one type of H chain. Membrane-bound Ig μH chains signal the cell to turn off the rearrangement machinery and make the second, $D_H J_H$-rearranged Ig H chain allele inaccessible for further rearrangements.

The classical preBCR with SL chain appears not to be involved in this allelic exclusion.[143–145]

On the other hand, the preBCR signals proliferation so that the preBII cells are in cell cycle (i.e., large). At the same time the preBCR signals the preBII cell to turn off SL chain expression, thereby limiting the amount of SL chain available for preBCR formation. Hence, proliferative expansion of large preBII cells is limited, as SL chains are diluted out by cell division (Fig. 11.6). An individual V_H domain of a μH chain appears to be probed for pairing by the V_{preB} subunit of the SL chain, and this interaction may display different avidities depending on the structure of the V_H domain. Thus, different individual Ig μH chains may be expanded in large preBII cells to different extents, i.e., for different number of divisions. Mutations that abolish the proper structure of the preBCR (i.e., B-lineage progenitors deficient in V_{preBI} and V_{preBII} or $\lambda5$, or V_{preBI}, V_{preBII}, and $\lambda5$) or which interfere with preBCR signaling[145,146] abolish the proliferative expansion of large preBII cells.

It appears that the non-Ig portion of the $\lambda5$-subunit of SL chain is mandatory for the capacity of preBCRs to stimulate preBII cell proliferation.[147] This proliferation appears to be cell-autonomous, in that preBCRs on the surface of preBII cells could be either 'self-crosslinked,' or could be crosslinked by a linker molecule made by the preBII cells, inducing crosslinking of preBCRs via the non-Ig portions of the $\lambda5$ subunit of SL chain. In other experiments galectin-1[148] and heparan sulfate[149] have been seen to positively influence preBCR signaling. These negatively charged macromolecules may well interact with the seven positively charged arginine residues in the non-Ig portion of the $\lambda5$ protein and, hence, help to crosslink preBCRs.

Deletion of the gene encoding the adaptor protein Slp65 directly by targeted mutagenesis[150,151] or indirectly by targeted inactivation of PAX5 controlling Slp65 expression,[84] abolishes the capacity of large preBII cells to downregulate surrogate L chain expression. This leads to continued preBCR formation in dividing large preBII cells so that, in fact, Slp65-defective mice have a hyperplastic large preBII cell compartment. This chronic preBII cell proliferation is a breeding ground for secondary mutation so that, in a period of weeks, pre-B cell lymphomas (lymphocytic leukemias) develop in these mice.

In this view of B cell development, the preBCR does not use the complementarity-determining regions (CDRs) of the V_H domain of its μH chain to bind ligands that could induce proliferation. Therefore, the newly generated V_H-domain repertoire is not screened for antigen – i.e., autoantigen binding – but merely for fitness to pair, to be prepared for the eventual combination with conventional L chains. Thus, 'unfit' H chains are excluded that may have other unwanted properties such as the formation of self-aggregating immune complexes that might bear the danger of glomerulonephritis and vasculitis.[145]

In conclusion, the Ig H chain repertoire emerging from preBII cell expansion and entering L chain gene rearrangements should be fully autoreactive. This conclusion is also warranted by the observation that administration *in vivo* or *in vitro* of either autoantigens or Ig μH chain-specific and SL chain-specific monoclonal antibodies do not disturb – positively or negatively – the development of pre-B cells to the stage of an immature, $sIgM^+$ B cell.[152]

GENERATION OF IMMATURE, $sIgM^+$ B CELL REPERTOIRES

As SL chains become limiting in the proliferative expansion, because the preBCR turns off further SL chain synthesis, preBCR formation ceases and preBII cells exit the cell cycle. Hence, they fall into a resting state, the small preBII cell stage (Fig. 11.6).

These small preBII cells begin to reexpress the rearrangement machinery, i.e., RAG1 and RAG2. In human development, but not in mouse, they also reexpress TdT. Hence the emerging L chain repertoire can be expected to contain N-region sequences; that is, be more diverse than that of mice. The cells open the L chain gene loci, first detectable by the production of sterile transcripts. However, the D_HJ_H-rearranged H chain alleles remain inaccessible for the rearrangement machinery throughout further B cell development and mature B cell responses. This secures continued allelic exclusion of the H chain locus.

Hence, when large preBII cells finally exit the cell cycle and become small, V_L to J_L rearrangement becomes detectable.[153] Single-cell polymerase chain reaction (PCR) analyses have shown that a part of the small preBII compartment contains cells that have rearranged the L chain gene loci but do not express L chain proteins, hence do not express IgM on their surface. Another part of them appear to be nonproductively rearranged, and yet another part express L chains in their cytoplasm, but not (yet) on the surface. This may be because in some of them the preexisting μH chain may not have been able to pair with the L chain – and yet another part may already have expressed L chains on their surface but may have been exposed to autoantigens, downregulating the surface expression of IgM (see below). In the small preBII cell compartment, as well as in the immature, $sIgM^+$ B cell compartment, the rearrangement machinery remains expressed, i.e., active. Single-cell PCR analyses and analyses of intracellular L chain expression of this small preBII cell compartment indicate that all of these different types of precursor B cells may be present in this compartment.

In the mouse nearly one hundred functional $V\kappa$ segments can rearrange to four functional $J\kappa$ segments by either deletion or inversion of the intervening sequences, and multiple rearrangements on one allele are possible as long as J elements remain unrearranged. In a large proportion of the small preBII cells, multiple L chain gene rearrangements have been and still are taking place – and more frequently so than in the immature IgM^+ B cell compartment. Furthermore, productive rearrangements are often seen to be followed by nonproductive rearrangements suggesting that the L chains produced from the productive rearrangements were either incapable of pairing or led to the expression of sIgM on an immature B cell with specificity for an autoantigen present in the environment of the primary lymphoid organ. The reactions of the autoreactive sIgM on immature B cells stimulates a sustained expression of the rearrangement machinery and thereby allows 'editing' of the autoreactive IgM by a second L chain, with the chance to change its specificity away from autoreactivity. As a consequence, some small preBII cells are not only the precursors, but often also the products of immature $sIgM^+$ B cells (Fig. 11.6).[153–156]

Because of the reactivated expression of the rearrangement machinery in small preBII and immature B cells these two cellular compartments are also the most likely sites for any V_H replacements in the $V_HD_HJ_H$ rearranged alleles of the H chain locus.[157] Again, autoreactivity of a BCR could stimulate the replacement of the autoreactive V_H by a hopefully nonautoreactive V_H, rescuing such BCR-expressing immature B cells from apoptosis. If the second allele is D_HJ_H rearranged, that allele will remain VDJ nonrearranged. However, if the second allele happens to be nonproductively $V_HD_HJ_H$ rearranged – as is the case in approximately half of all developing and mature B cells – then the V_H of this second allele could also be replaced by a new V_H. In principle, it is even conceivable that a cell with two nonproductively $V_HD_HJ_H$-rearranged alleles could participate in V_H replacements, if the cells carrying these two nonproductive H chain alleles have not yet died. However, since the replacement reaction uses a fixed heptamer sequence upstream of the V to D joints, it should in most cases not alter the status of nonproductivity of rearrangements of this allele.

However, if the replacement reaction changes the status of nonproductivity or productivity, the developing B cell might begin to use that allele for H chain production. In a productively/nonproductively $V_HD_HJ_H$-rearranged cell this may even result in a double μH chain–producing cell, abolishing allelic exclusion. However, the ratio of $V_HD_HJ_H/D_HJ_H$ to $V_HD_HJ_H/V_HD_HJ_H$-rearranged cells does not change during B cell development from large preBII to mature B cells, suggesting that these replacement reactions cannot be of high impact for the total mature B cell repertoires.

Initially only one of the two IgκL alleles appears to be accessible for V_L to J_L rearrangements. This may be the consequence of a differential chromatin methylation and acetylation state of the two alleles.[142,158] For nearly two-thirds of all emerging B cells this initial status of the κL chain alleles is sufficient to generate a sIgM$^+$ B cell for the peripheral, mature pools of cells. Hence, for two-thirds of the developing and mature B cell repertoires allelic exclusion at the L chain loci is achieved by a single V_L to J_L rearrangement followed immediately by an apparent positive selection of an apparently acceptable μH chain–L chain combination of a BCR. This terminates the expression of the rearrangement machinery. These cells in the repertoires have only one V_L to J_L rearrangement, usually to the most proximal J_L segment on one allele, while the second allele remains in germ-line configuration. It is not yet clear how sIgM signals the termination of secondary rearrangements in these cells and whether occupancy by antigen is required for it, but it is reasonable to expect that surface deposition of the IgM is an essential part of this signal.[159,160]

Two-thirds of the potentially functional $V\kappa$ segments of the mouse κL chain locus are oriented in an opposite direction to the $J\kappa$ segments.[161–163] Hence, these two-thirds rearrange $V\kappa$ to $J\kappa$ by inversion of the intervening sequences on the chromosome, while the other one-third is in the same orientation – i.e., rearranges by deletion of the intervening sequences. Half of all $V\kappa$-$J\kappa$ joints sequenced from developing B cells are generated from only 10 percent of all available, potentially functional $V\kappa$ segments, and inversions and deletions occur at random; that is, in the 2:1 ratio expected from their existence in the genome.

The κL chain gene locus may open before the κL chain loci do[164] but rearrangements at the κ and λ loci are independent of each other. Thus, in $C\kappa$-deficient and $JC\kappa$-deficient mice, small preBII cells develop in normal numbers in the bone marrow, but only 15 to 25 percent of them carry a V_α-J_β–rearranged L chain locus. All others have all L chain loci in germ-line configuration.[165] Hence, the rate of V_L to J_L rearrangement appears five to ten times higher at the κL than at the λL locus, providing an explanation for the κL to λL ratio of 10:1 in mouse Ig molecules. This is also one of several cases where a given cellular state of B cell differentiation, in this case the small preBII cell stage, can be reached without concomitant Ig gene rearrangements and expressions.

The role of sIgM on immature B cells appears to be quite different whenever that sIgM$^+$ B cell encounters an autoantigen in the primary lymphoid organ. The rearrangement machinery is kept active, and the cell appears to open the second L chain allele for rearrangements. Hence, the single-cell PCR analyses of wild-type B-lineage cells with two rearrangement-competent κL chain alleles have shown that only a minority (around 5 percent) of all preBII cells containing secondary rearrangements retain this second allele in germ-line configuration. This suggests the possibility, and danger, that a B cell could produce two L chains from two productively rearranged L chain alleles.

NEGATIVE AND POSITIVE SELECTION – AND IGNORANCE OF THE REPERTOIRE OF DEVELOPING IMMATURE B CELLS

It has been estimated that more than half of all originally generated immature B cells display some level of autoreactivity to antigens of the environment of the B cell generating organ. These large numbers of immature sIgM$^+$ B cells with autoreactivity for autoantigens are first screened in the primary lymphoid organs and later at the second checkpoints in spleen (where immature B cells are also found).[166] While the strength of the signal through the BCR, a consequence of the avidity of the autoantigen toward the corresponding sIgM-expressing B cell, is thought to be the controlling influence on this repertoire selection process, the environment and the form of the antigen also appear to contribute to the fate of a B cell at these earliest repertoire checkpoints.[167–169] Such 'cooperating' influences on B cell repertoire selection are contributed by direct or indirect interactions with the constant regions of the BCR, for example its Fc portions.

Genetic deficiencies in complement components such as C1q, C4, serum amyloid protein, and complement receptor 2 (CR2), as well as secreted 'natural' serum IgM, lead to systemic autoimmune disease (systemic lupus erythematosus; SLE) with a preponderance of autoantibodies against single- and double-stranded DNA and a variety of other nuclear antigens. Such high-avidity autoantibodies are not found in normal, nondiseased individuals. These observations have suggested two models for the selection of the emerging B cell repertoires.[168] In one model, the maturing B cells are 'protected' from the stimulatory influence of autoantigens released as 'blebs' from apoptosing cells in the primary lymphoid organ because macrophages expressing complement receptors (C1qR for C1q, CRI for C4) efficiently take up and thereby remove apoptosing cells bound by 'natural' serum IgM and complexed with CIq and C4b. This model implicitly assumes that all developing B cells that make it to the mature stage are positively selected. It does not explain how the developing repertoire of immature B cells is purged of autoreactive cells, and does not take into account that immature B cells are sensitive to be induced to apoptosis rather than to proliferation as the mature B cells do, which not only proliferate but also mature to Ig-secreting plasma cells and memory B cells under the influence of the same stimuli.

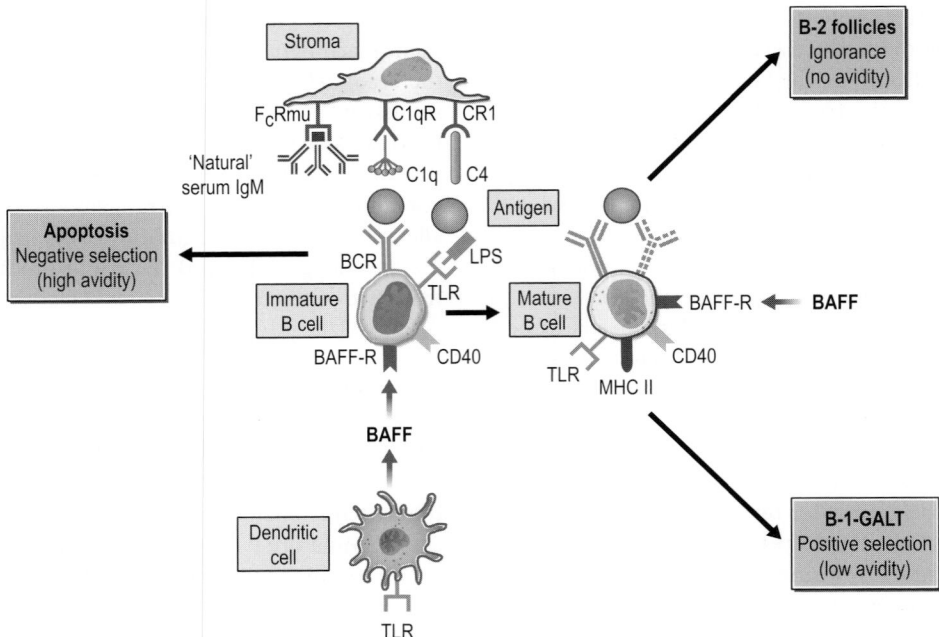

Figure 11.7   A proposed scenario for the selection of B cell repertoires in the primary lymphoid organs (e.g., in bone marrow) to either apoptosis (high avidity), positive selection (intermediate to low avidity) mostly into B-1 compartments mainly in gut-associated lymphoid tissues, or by no selection into follicles of spleen, mainly as B-2 conventional B cells (ignorance). Stromal cells with Fcμ-receptors, C1q-receptors, and CRI bind 'natural' serum IgM, C1q, and C4 in complex with antigen (usually autoantigens) that they present to BCRs on developing immature, surface IgM⁺ (B cell receptor [BCR]⁺) B cells, which can also bind such antigens by other receptors, such as Toll-like receptors (TLRs) if they contain TLR ligands. Dendritic cells provide BAFF, which can induce maturation of immature to mature B cells. While immature B cells are induced to apoptosis by antigen occupying BCRs, mature B cells are stimulated to proliferation and Ig secretion. For further details, see the text. MHC, major histocompatibility complex; LPS, lipopolysaccharide; GALT, gut-associated lymphoid tissues.

Negative selection and 'editing'

By contrast, the second model proposes that autoantigens from dying cells are 'presented' to the emerging repertoire of B cells by stromal cells in the primary lymphoid organs (Fig. 11.7).[168,170] These 'autoantigen-presenting cells' are suggested to be provided by microenvironmental stromal cells. They are expected to express C1q receptor and CRI, to bind C1q and C4, respectively, which in turn bind to surface IgM occupied by autoantigens on autoreactive B cells.[159] Depending on the strength of the interaction of the BCRs with autoantigens, and maybe also on the nature of the presenting cell (in bone marrow or spleen), this autoantigen-induced signaling can have different outcomes. It can lead to apoptosis of the B cell, if the avidity of autoantigen-BCR binding is high, hence leading to negative selection of the B cell repertoire. Such negative selection has been documented in a variety of experimental settings.[171–175] If BCR downregulation and reexpression of a secondary BCR due to 'editing' of a new L chain leading to a new, nonautoreative BCR occurs fast enough, this apoptosis may be avoided.

As an extension of this model, and to accommodate the apparent role of serum IgM in the B cell repertoire selection process, one could propose that the stromal cells also express receptors for 'natural' serum IgM (Fcμ receptors) to include serum IgM in these processes. In this way the serum IgM could also bind to autoantigens and then be able to fix C1q, creating a multiple bridge between the C1qR, CRI, and Fcμ receptor on stromal cells and the autoreactive BCR on the immature B cell, brought together by C1q, C4, serum IgM, and autoantigens.

Approximately 90 percent of the 2×10^7 sIgM⁺ immature B cells that are made each day in the bone marrow of a mouse never arrive at the immature sIgM⁺ B cell pool of the spleen, suggesting that a large portion of the initially generated B cell repertoires are negatively selected, and that most of the negative selection of the B cell repertoires occurs at the transit from bone marrow to spleen.[176,177] On the other hand, the vast majority (more than 90 percent) of all immature B cells in spleen make it into the mature B cell pool, suggesting that there remains only a very small portion of the immature B cell repertoire to be negatively selected in the spleen.

Ignorance

Emerging B cells with no apparent autoreactivity pass the two checkpoints in bone marrow and spleen as long as they express a surface membrane-deposited BCR. A variety of

Ig-transgenic mouse models support this view.[178] The ignored B cells enter the spleen via the terminal branches of the central arterioles and populate the follicular regions as conventional, B-2-type B cells. Initially they are short lived, with half-lives of 2 to 4 days. They then mature to longer-lived B cells, with half-lives longer than 6 weeks. The BCR complex with Igα and Igβ is mandatory for transition to the peripheral sIgM$^+$ B cell pools – no sIgM$^-$ B cells survive normally. The transition from short lived to long lived, from AA4.1$^+$ to AA4.1$^-$, and CD21$^-$/CD23$^-$ to CD21$^+$/CD23$^+$ cells is controlled by a series of genes, including *OBF*, *BTK*, and CD40. Thus, BTK$^-$/CD40$^-$ or BTK$^-$/OBF$^-$ double deficient mice have a strong defect at the transition from the immature, 'transitional' T1- and T2-type B cells to mature B cells (Fig. 11.7).[176] In addition, crosslinking of surface IgM by anti-IgM antibodies (possibly a polyclonal example of a crosslinking autoantigen) induces immature B cells of bone marrow as well as spleen (T1- and T2-type) to apoptosis. This apoptosis can be prevented by the transgenic expression of the antiapoptotic transgene *BCL2*, and is circumvented by polyclonal activation with lipopolysaccharide and with CD40-specific antibodies or CD40 ligand.

Deficiency in the expression of the TNF-family member BAFF (also called B-lys), or its receptor, BAFF-R, blocks the maturation of immature B cells into conventional, B-2-type B cells, but not to B-1-type B cells.[179–184] *In vitro*, BAFF induces polyclonal maturation of immature B cells from bone marrow and from spleen (type 1 and type 2) without proliferation. BAFF has been found in the sera of some SLE patients, as well as in the sera of NZB × NZW SLE autoimmune disease-prone mice. In these mice, administration of BAFF-specific antibodies prevents, or at least delays, the development of SLE disease. Therefore, excessive production of BAFF, administered at the sites of negative selection of immature B cells, could 'rescue' autoreactive B cells from deletion, leading to autoimmune reactivities in the peripheral mature conventional B cell repertoires. One major site of BAFF production has been found to be dendritic cells. Hence, in order to interfere with the deletion of autoreactive immature B cells, such dendritic cells would have to be localized near the sites of B cell deletion in bone marrow or spleen, and would have to be strongly activated to BAFF production to effect rapid maturation of autoreactive immature B cells before they are subjected to negative selection (Fig. 11.7). Such a scenario still needs to be investigated, and the observed partial rescue of B cell tolerance by T cell-independent antigens may be one experimental way to probe the molecular and cellular requirements for such competition with clonal deletion.

Positive selection

Autoreactive, in fact often polyreactive B cells,[185] can be positively selected and appear to accumulate in the B-1 compartments of the GALT, i.e., in the follicles below the M cells of the flat epithelium of the gut. Some are also found as single intraepithelial cells (Fig. 11.5). B cells within the marginal zone of the spleen also appear to be positively selected. However, it remains to be seen whether this major traffic intersection is, in fact, a selection site for newly generated (as well as possibly of recirculating) B cells. Potentially, these B cells could be in contact with cellular debris of dying blood cells and of killed bacteria, which are found at the same sites and which are about to be removed from the circulation. Many of the B cells have a B-1 phenotype.[186,187] B-1 B cells are often found to crossreact with a variety of autoantigens and bacterial antigens at low avidities. They appear mildly activated, or 'tickled,' and do not proliferate in their GALT, but appear to be long lived. Transplantation of B-1 cells into secondary hosts, in contrast to the transplantation of conventional B cells, is easy and repeatable in subsequent hosts. Even low numbers of B-1 cells will fully replenish the gut-associated lymphoid sites. This suggests that the low-avidity autoreactivity, combined with a polyreactivity to several antigens, could be the stimulatory influence for B-1 cells to replenish their lymphoid sites after transplantation and to attain longevity.[188,189]

Many positively selected B cells appear to be B-1 cells, and many are accumulated in the gut. B cells in the GALT, including the lamina propria, produce IgM and predominantly switch to IgA.[188] Secreted IgA traverses the epithelia associated with the secretory piece, which it acquires during the migration through the epithelial layer. On the luminal side it binds with low affinity and high crossreactivity to bacteria of the indigenous flora and to food antigens. Hence, the positive selection via low avidity of these (eventually IgA-producing and secreting) B-1 cells appears to possibly be useful for 'neutralizing' interactions of the secreted antibodies with potentially infectious bacteria of the gut flora.

At least in part this IgA production appears to be quite distinct from the Ig production elicited in a helper T cell-dependent inflammatory response of B cells in germinal centers of peripheral lymph nodes and the spleen. First, while the follicular B cell response beneath the M cells may be helper T cell-dependent (hence, germinal center-derived), the submucosal, intraepithelial response in the lamina propria can be helper T cell-independent. One-third of the IgA might derive from such T cell-independent B cell responses.[41] The expression of the Ig class switch-inducing AID gene (activation-induced cytidine deaminase)[190–192] is normally induced by a CD40 ligand–CD40 interaction. However, the cooperating cell providing the CD40 ligand in the GALT, especially in the intraepithelial spaces, is not known, and must not be a helper T cell. Furthermore, these B cell responses could be costimulated by other cell–cell contacts and cytokines that might not be typical for a T cell-dependent, germinal center response of B cells. Hypermutation of the V regions of the IgM, and later IgA, expressed and secreted by the lamina propria of the intestine B-1 cells could well occur in the AID-expressing, IgA class switching cells. However, the lack of the selection of better-fitting V-region mutants by bacterial antigens and the lack of germinal center formation, i.e., exclusive B cell proliferation, may decrease the probability to generate and select better-fitting antibacterial antibodies – as much as that also should decrease the probability of generating high-affinity autoreactive antibodies.

Conventional, follicular B-2-type B cells appear to need a response to a T cell-dependent antigen in a germinal center reaction – i.e., the cooperation with helper T cells in an interaction of CD40 ligand on the T cells with CD40 on the B cells – to acquire longevity. Since this interaction also induces AID, it induces class switch recombination and somatic hypermutation. Hence, the resulting long-lived memory B cells most often express somatically hypermutated Ig of classes other than IgM with specificities for the stimulating, selecting foreign antigen.

While B-1 B cells are apparently unable to be stimulated to longevity by BAFF, a member of the TNF family of cytokines, conventional B cells express BAFF-receptor (BAFF-R; a member of the TNF-receptor family), and respond to BAFF by polyclonal maturation to long-lived B cells (Figs 11.6 and 11.7).[193]

The TNF family ligands BAFF and APRIL, and their receptors BCMA, TACI, and BAFF-R, control the selection of short-lived immature B cells with no apparent positively (or negatively) selecting specificities for autoantigens to long-lived mature B cells. Experiments studying the *in vivo* administration of soluble BAFF-R ligands and of soluble decoy receptors, and the analysis of BAFF-transgenic, BAFF-deficient, and BAFF-R-deficient mice, as well as the *in vitro* responses of immature and mature B cells of BAFF (all reviewed elsewhere[193]), have shown that immature B cells from bone marrow and spleen (initially immature as well as 'transitional' B cells) and mature B cells respond to BAFF by polyclonal maturation to long-lived B cells without proliferation. BAFF and BAFF-R deficiencies arrest B cell development at the transition from immature to transitional B cells (Fig. 11.7). Although the action of BAFF *in vitro* is polyclonal and independent of BCR occupancy, it remains to be seen whether ligand selection through BCR occupancy plays a role in this selection of the conventional 'virgin' antigen-reactive mature B cells.

PERIPHERAL B CELLS WITHOUT IMMUNOGLOBULIN

In normal B cell development, B-lineage cells that cannot express Ig molecules on their surface are restricted to the primary lymphoid organs and will die there, usually with half-lives of 2 to 4 days. Experimentally induced ablation of surface Ig expression in peripheral mature B cells induces their rapid death.[194] Therefore, neither immature, nor mature, nor memory B cells, nor plasma cells without Ig expression can ever be detected in the peripheral lymphoid organs, and even most B cell tumors appear to be selected to express Ig. However, several observations, most of them

made *in vitro*, suggest that B-lineage cells from as early as the B-lineage-committed progenitor B cells and preBI cells can differentiate all the way to memory-phenotype-like and plasma-cell-like stages without ever expressing Ig. For example, L chain gene rearrangements can be induced by the removal of IL-7 in cells differentiating *in vitro* from preBI cells that have never expressed a μH chain, i.e., a preBCR. Cells with an immature B-cell-like phenotype develop.[195] Furthermore, transgenic expression of constitutively active forms of RAS[196] or RAF[197,198] induce RAG-deficient precursor cells to develop to cells with preBII immature B-like phenotypes. Immunoglobulin H chain rearrangement-deficient cells progress under such signaling to L chain gene rearrangements in preBII-like cells. In κ L chain rearrangement-deficient bone marrow, over 90 percent of the small preBII cells have the proper phenotype, but no L chain rearrangements, since rearrangements at the λL chain loci are so slow that they can only be detected in the remaining 10 percent of the small preBII cells.[165] Most striking is the development of RAG-deficient preBI cells (hence with Ig H and L chain loci in non-rearranged, germ-line configurations) *in vitro* in the stimulatory presence of CD40-specific monoclonal antibody and IL-4 to $S\mu$-$S\gamma$-switched cells with a mature phenotype (Fig. 11.6).[199] Hence, the differentiation of B-lineage cells is a stepwise process driven by cell–cell contacts and cytokines that can occur without the synthesis or surface deposition of Ig. The roles of the preBCR and BCR (Ig) also become apparent from these experiments: they control, positively and negatively, proliferation, anergy, and apoptosis of B-lineage cells and, thereby, ascertain the production of appropriate numbers of cells with selected specificities.

Viral infection of B cells by Epstein–Barr virus (EBV) may be another way by which the requirement of surface Ig deposition on B cells for their survival and use in the peripheral lymphoid organs may be circumvented. The EBV line encodes latent membrane proteins (LMP) of which LMP2A, a multispanning transmembrane protein, when expressed in B lymphocytes, can associate with Igα and Igβ and share with these two anchor proteins an immunoreceptor tyrosine-based activation motif (ITAM motif).[200–202] In fact, the phosphorylated form of the ITAM motif of LMP2A recruits tyrosine kinases and adapter proteins, which are also used by the BCR complex for signaling. In this way, LMP2A acts as a BCR analogue, supporting the selection into the peripheral mature B cell compartments of B cells lacking BCRs. High-level transgenic expression of LMP2A selectively recruits cells into the B-1 compartments (e.g., into the gut and intestine), while low-level expression promotes development of conventional, B-2-type and marginal zone B cells.[167]

Neither the high level or low level LMP2A-expressing BCR-negative B cell populations can be stimulated by T cell-dependent antigens to develop germinal centers in peripheral lymphoid organs, indicating that BCRs on the surface of B cells are needed for peripheral germinal center responses. By contrast, the low level, but not the high level

LMP2A expression (i.e., the conventional B-2 but not the B-1 cell-directed LMP2A) allows germinal centers to be formed in the gut. Hence, the role of BCRs in germinal center formation in the gut might be replaced by an antigen-unspecific mechanism of antigen uptake, which allows processing and presentation by MHC class II molecules to helper T cells. Alternatively these gut-associated BCR-deficient B cells might be stimulated by bystander helper T cells activated with bacteria of the gut, or by bacteria-derived polyclonal activators, such as lipopolysaccharide, lipoprotein, and so on (in the latter case via Toll-like receptor 2 [TLR2], TLR4, and other receptors[203]), or by other T-lineage cells or NK cells not restricted by the recognition of MHC class I and II/peptide complexes. In summary, T cell (or NK cell)-dependent, BCR-independent (maybe MHC class II-independent) activation of B cells in germinal centers can lead to germinal center responses, in which the activated B cells (as well as T or NK cells) can be expected to secrete proinflammatory cytokines such as interferon gamma (IFNγ), IL-1, IL-4, IL-5, IL-6, and TNFα as essential mediators of immune responses. Furthermore it has been observed in preBI cell-transplanted RAG-deficient mice, containing only preBI cell-derived B-1 cells, but no T cells, that one-third of the normal levels of IgA can be produced, apparently T cell-independently, mainly by cells in the intestinal lamina propria, without the formation of germinal centers. It is likely that these cells are also present in BCR-deficient, high level LMP2A-expressing lamina propria B-1 cells. Obviously they cannot produce IgA, but they can be expected, again, to respond to bacteria by the secretion of cytokines that might be of pro- or anti-inflammatory types.

In conclusion, the GALT-associated B cell compartments can develop even when the B cells do not express BCRs (and maybe also not MHC class II); that is, they can function in cellular responses of proliferation and differentiation to effector functions in an antigen-independent, maybe bacteria-dependent way, leading to proinflammatory (and maybe also antiinflammatory) responses. From all these results it becomes evident that peripheral mature B cells have important functions beyond their capacity to produce, secrete, class switch, and hypermutate antibodies in the regulation of immune reactions.

KEY POINTS

Key issues covered in this chapter:

- Embryonic and adult B cell development
- Immunoglobulin gene segment rearrangement
- B cell repertoires
- Structure and functions of gene B cell receptor
- B cell tolerance by negative repertoire selection

REFERENCES

● = Key primary paper
◆ = Major review article

1. Melchers F, Rolink A. B lymphocyte development and biology. In: Paul WE. (ed.) *Fundamental Immunology*, 4th edn. Philadelphia, PA: Lippincott-Raven, 1999; 183–224.

2. Jordan CT, Lemischka IR. Clonal and systemic analysis of long-term hematopoiesis in the mouse. *Genes Dev* 1990; **4**: 220–32.

3. Spangrude GJ, Smith L, Uchida N *et al.* Mouse hematopoietic stem cells. *Blood* 1991; **78**: 1395–402. Review.

4. Smith LG, Weissman IL, Heimfeld S. Clonal analysis of hematopoietic stem-cell differentiation in vivo. *Proc Natl Acad Sci U S A* 1991; **88**: 2788–92.

5. Morrison SJ, Uchida N, Weissman IL. The biology of hematopoietic stem cells. *Annu Rev Cell Dev Biol* 1995; **11**: 35–71. Review.

6. Osawa M, Hanada K, Hamada H, Nakauchi H. Long-term lymphohematopoietic reconstitution by a single CD34-low/negative hematopoietic stem cell. *Science* 1996; **273**: 242–5.

7. Osawa M, Nakamura K, Nishi N *et al.* In vivo self-renewal of c-Kit+ Sca-1+ Lin(low/-) hemopoietic stem cells. *J Immunol* 1996; **156**: 3207–14.

8. Iwama A, Oguro H, Negishi M *et al.* Enhanced self-renewal of hematopoietic stem cells mediated by the polycomb gene product Bmi-1. *Immunity* 2004; **21**: 843–51.

9. Park IK, Qian D, Kiel M *et al.* Bmi-1 is required for maintenance of adult self-renewing haematopoietic stem cells. *Nature* 2003; **423**: 302–5. Epub 2003 Apr 20.

10. Sauvageau G, Thorsteinsdottir U, Eaves CJ *et al.* Overexpression of HOXB4 in hematopoietic cells causes the selective expansion of more primitive populations in vitro and in vivo. *Genes Dev* 1995; **9**: 1753–65.

11. Helgason CD, Sauvageau G, Lawrence HJ *et al.* Overexpression of HOXB4 enhances the hematopoietic potential of embryonic stem cells differentiated in vitro. *Blood* 1996; **87**: 2740–9.

12. Thorsteinsdottir U, Sauvageau G, Humphries RK. Enhanced in vivo regenerative potential of HOXB4-transduced hematopoietic stem cells with regulation of their pool size. *Blood* 1999; **94**: 2605–12.

13. Kyba M, Perlingeiro RC, Daley GQ. HoxB4 confers definitive lymphoid-myeloid engraftment potential on embryonic stem cell and yolk sac hematopoietic progenitors. *Cell* 2002; **109**: 29–37.

14. Antonchuk J, Sauvageau G, Humphries RK. HOXB4-induced expansion of adult hematopoietic stem cells ex vivo. *Cell* 2002; **109**: 39–45.

15. Buske C, Feuring-Buske M, Abramovich C *et al.* Deregulated expression of HOXB4 enhances the primitive growth activity of human hematopoietic cells. *Blood* 2002; **100**: 862–8.

16. Krosl J, Austin P, Beslu N *et al.* In vitro expansion of hematopoietic stem cells by recombinant TAT-HOXB4 protein. *Nat Med* 2003; **9**: 1428–32. Epub 2003 Oct 26.

17. Zhu J, Giannola DM, Zhang Y et al. NF-Y cooperates with USF1/2 to induce the hematopoietic expression of HOXB4. *Blood* 2003; **102**: 2420–7. Epub 2003 Jun 5.

18. Baba Y, Garrett KP, Kincade PW. Constitutively active beta-catenin confers multilineage differentiation potential on lymphoid and myeloid progenitors. *Immunity* 2005; **23**: 599–609.

19. Duncan AW, Rattis FM, DiMascio LN et al. Integration of Notch and Wnt signaling in hematopoietic stem cell maintenance. *Nat Immunol* 2005; **6**: 314–22. Epub 2005 Jan 23.

20. Reya T, Duncan AW, Ailles L et al. A role for Wnt signalling in self-renewal of haematopoietic stem cells. *Nature* 2003; **423**: 409–14. Epub 2003 Apr 27.

21. Schiedlmeier B, Klump H, Will E et al. High-level ectopic HOXB4 expression confers a profound in vivo competitive growth advantage on human cord blood CD34+ cells, but impairs lymphomyeloid differentiation. *Blood* 2003; **101**: 1759–68. Epub 2002 Oct 24.

22. Gilliland DG, Griffin JD. The roles of FLT3 in hematopoiesis and leukemia. *Blood* 2002; **100**: 1532–42. Review.

23. Arai F, Hirao A, Ohmura M et al. Tie2/angiopoietin-1 signaling regulates hematopoietic stem cell quiescence in the bone marrow niche. *Cell* 2004; **118**: 149–61.

24. Zhang CC, Kaba M, Ge G et al. Angiopoietin-like proteins stimulate ex vivo expansion of hematopoietic stem cells. *Nat Med* 2006; **12**: 240–5. Epub 2006 Jan 22.

25. Maeno M, Mead PE, Kelley C et al. The role of BMP-4 and GATA-2 in the induction and differentiation of hematopoietic mesoderm in Xenopus laevis. *Blood* 1996; **88**: 1965–72.

26. Graff JM. Embryonic patterning: to BMP or not to BMP, that is the question. *Cell* 1997; **89**: 171–4. Review.

27. Hogan BL. Bone morphogenetic proteins in development. *Curr Opin Genet Dev* 1996; **6**: 432–8. Review.

28. Nagasawa T, Nakajima T, Tachibana K et al. Molecular cloning and characterization of a murine pre-B-cell growth-stimulating factor/stromal cell-derived factor 1 receptor, a murine homolog of the human immunodeficiency virus 1 entry coreceptor fusin. *Proc Natl Acad Sci U S A* 1996; **93**: 14726–9.

29. Egawa T, Kawabata K, Kawamoto H et al. The earliest stages of B cell development require a chemokine stromal cell-derived factor/pre-B cell growth-stimulating factor. *Immunity* 2001; **15**: 323–34.

30. Ma Q, Jones D, Springer TA. The chemokine receptor CXCR4 is required for the retention of B lineage and granulocytic precursors within the bone marrow microenvironment. *Immunity* 1999; **10**: 463–71.

31. Ma Q, Jones D, Borghesani PR et al. Impaired B-lymphopoiesis, myelopoiesis, and derailed cerebellar neuron migration in CXCR4- and SDF-1-deficient mice. *Proc Natl Acad Sci U S A* 1998; **95**: 9448–53.

32. Kawabata K, Ujikawa M, Egawa T et al. A cell-autonomous requirement for CXCR4 in long-term lymphoid and myeloid reconstitution. *Proc Natl Acad Sci U S A* 1999; **96**: 5663–7.

33. Melchers F, Rolink AG, Schaniel C. The role of chemokines in regulating cell migration during humoral immune responses. *Cell* 1999; **99**: 351–4. Review.

34. Adams GB, Chabner KT, Alley IR et al. Stem cell engraftment at the endosteal niche is specified by the calcium-sensing receptor. *Nature* 2006; **439**: 599–603. Epub 2005 Dec 28.

35. Wilson A, Trumpp A. Bone-marrow haematopoietic-stem-cell niches. *Nat Rev Immunol* 2006; **6**: 93–106. Review.

36. Osmond DG, Fulop GM, Opstelten D, Pretrangeli C. In vivo regulation of B lymphocyte production in the bone marrow: effects and mechanism of action of exogenous stimuli on pre-B cell proliferation and lymphocyte turnover. *Adv Exp Med Biol* 1985; **186**: 35–46.

37. Rico-Vargas SA, Potter M, Osmond DG. Perturbation of B cell genesis in the bone marrow of pristane-treated mice. Implications for plasmacytoma induction. *J Immunol* 1995; **154**: 2082–91.

38. Medina KL, Smithson G, Kincade PW. Suppression of B lymphopoiesis during normal pregnancy. *J Exp Med* 1993; **178**: 1507–15.

39. Medina KL, Garrett KP, Thompson LF et al. Identification of very early lymphoid precursors in bone marrow and their regulation by estrogen. *Nat Immunol* 2001; **2**: 718–24.

40. Katayama Y, Battista M, Kao WM et al. Signals from the sympathetic nervous system regulate hematopoietic stem cell egress from bone marrow. *Cell* 2006; **124**: 407–21.

41. Rolink A, Haasner D, Nishikawa S, Melchers F. Changes in frequencies of clonable pre B cells during life in different lymphoid organs of mice. *Blood* 1993; **81**: 2290–300.

42. Urbanek P, Wang ZQ, Fetka I et al. Complete block of early B cell differentiation and altered patterning of the posterior midbrain in mice lacking Pax5/BSAP. *Cell* 1994; **79**: 901–12.

43. Busslinger M, Urbanek P. The role of BSAP (Pax-5) in B-cell development. *Curr Opin Genet Dev* 1995 Oct; **5**: 595–601. Review.

44. Nutt SL, Heavey B, Rolink AG, Busslinger M. Commitment to the B-lymphoid lineage depends on the transcription factor Pax5. *Nature* 1999; **401**: 556–62.

45. Schaniel C, Bruno L, Melchers F, Rolink AG. Multiple hematopoietic cell lineages develop in vivo from transplanted Pax5-deficient pre-B I-cell clones. *Blood* 2002; **99**: 472–8.

46. Rolink AG, Nutt SL, Melchers F, Busslinger M. et al. Long-term in vivo reconstitution of T-cell development by Pax5-deficient B-cell progenitors. *Nature* 1999; **401**: 603–6.

47. Schebesta M, Heavey B, Busslinger M. Transcriptional control of B-cell development. *Curr Opin Immunol* 2002: **14**: 216–23. Review.

48. Rolink AG, Schaniel C, Melchers F. Stability and plasticity of wild-type and Pax5-deficient precursor B cells. *Immunol Rev* 2002; **187**: 87–95. Review.

49. Ikawa T, Kawamoto H, Wright LY, Murre C. Long-term cultured E2A-deficient hematopoietic progenitor cells are pluripotent. *Immunity* 2004; **20**: 349–60.

50. Radtke F, Wilson A, Mancini SJ, MacDonald HR. Notch regulation of lymphocyte development and function. *Nat Immunol* 2004; **5**: 247–53.

51. Hoflinger S, Kesavan K, Fuxa M *et al*. Analysis of Notch1 function by in vitro T cell differentiation of Pax5 mutant lymphoid progenitors. *J Immunol* 2004; **173**: 3935–44.

52. Nakano T, Kodama H, Honjo T. Generation of lymphohematopoietic cells from embryonic stem cells in culture. *Science* 1994; **265**: 1098–101.

53. Schmitt TM, de Pooter RF, Gronski MA *et al*. Induction of T cell development and establishment of T cell competence from embryonic stem cells differentiated in vitro. Nat Immunol 2004; **5**: 410–7. Epub 2004 Mar 21.

54. Rolink A, Kudo A, Karasuyama H *et al*. Long-term proliferating early pre B cell lines and clones with the potential to develop to surface Ig-positive, mitogen reactive B cells in vitro and in vivo. *EMBO J* 1991; **10**: 327–36.

55. Rolink A, Ghia P, Grawunder U *et al*. In-vitro analyses of mechanisms of B-cell development. *Semin Immunol* 1995; **7**: 155–67. Review.

56. Olsen AL, Stachura DL, Weiss MJ. Designer blood: creating hematopoietic lineages from embryonic stem cells. *Blood* 2006; **107**: 1265–75. Epub 2005 Oct 27.

57. Pan X, Ohneda O, Ohneda K *et al*. Graded levels of GATA-1 expression modulate survival, proliferation, and differentiation of erythroid progenitors. *J Biol Chem* 2005; **280**: 22385–94. Epub 2005 Apr 6.

58. Klemsz MJ, McKercher SR, Celada A *et al*. The macrophage and B cell-specific transcription factor PU.1 is related to the ets oncogene. *Cell* 1990; **61**: 113–24.

59. Hromas R, Orazi A, Neiman RS *et al*. Hematopoietic lineage- and stage-restricted expression of the ETS oncogene family member PU.1. *Blood* 1993; **82**: 2998–3004.

60. Singh H. Gene targeting reveals a hierarchy of transcription factors regulating specification of lymphoid cell fates. *Curr Opin Immunol* 1996; **8**: 160–5. Review.

61. Singh H, Medina KL, Pongubala JM. Contingent gene regulatory networks and B cell fate specification. *Proc Natl Acad Sci U S A* 2005; **102**: 4949–53. Epub 2005 Mar 23. Review.

62. Singh H, Pongubala JM. Gene regulatory networks and the determination of lymphoid cell fates. *Curr Opin Immunol* 2006; **18**: 116–20. Epub 2006 Feb 10.

63. Dakic A, Metcalf D, Di Rago L *et al*. PU.1 regulates the commitment of adult hematopoietic progenitors and restricts granulopoiesis. *J Exp Med* 2005; **201**: 1487–502.

64. Nutt SL, Metcalf D, D'Amico A *et al*. Dynamic regulation of PU.1 expression in multipotent hematopoietic progenitors. *J Exp Med* 2005; **201**: 221–31.

65. Pui JC, Allman D, Xu L *et al*. Notch1 expression in early lymphopoiesis influences B versus T lineage determination. *Immunity* 1999; **11**: 299–308.

66. Yokota Y, Mansouri A, Mori S *et al*. Development of peripheral lymphoid organs and natural killer cells depends on the helix-loop-helix inhibitor Id2. *Nature* 1999; **397**: 702–6.

67. Ikawa T, Fujimoto S, Kawamoto H *et al*. Commitment to natural killer cells requires the helix-loop-helix inhibitor Id2. *Proc Natl Acad Sci U S A* 2001; **98**: 5164–9. Epub 2001 Apr 10.

68. Engel I, Murre C. The function of E- and Id proteins in lymphocyte development. *Nat Rev Immunol* 2001; **1**: 193–9. Review.

69. Radtke F, Wilson A, Stark G *et al*. Deficient T cell fate specification in mice with an induced inactivation of Notch1. *Immunity* 1999; **10**: 547–58.

70. Wilson A, MacDonald HR, Radtke F. Notch 1-deficient common lymphoid precursors adopt a B cell fate in the thymus. *J Exp Med* 2001; **194**: 1003–12.

71. Koch U, Lacombe TA, Holland D *et al*. Subversion of the T/B lineage decision in the thymus by lunatic fringe-mediated inhibition of Notch-1. *Immunity* 2001; **15**: 225–36.

72. Izon DJ, Aster JC, He Y *et al*. Deltex1 redirects lymphoid progenitors to the B cell lineage by antagonizing Notch1. *Immunity* 2002; **16**: 231–43.

73. Bain G, Maandag EC, Izon DJ *et al*. E2A proteins are required for proper B cell development and initiation of immunoglobulin gene rearrangements. *Cell* 1994; **79**: 885–92.

74. Zhuang Y, Soriano P, Weintraub H. The helix-loop-helix gene E2A is required for B cell formation. *Cell* 1994; **79**: 875–84.

75. Lin H, Grosschedl R. Failure of B-cell differentiation in mice lacking the transcription factor EBF. *Nature* 1995; **376**: 263–7.

76. Sigvardsson M, O'Riordan M, Grosschedl R. EBF and E47 collaborate to induce expression of the endogenous immunoglobulin surrogate light chain genes. *Immunity* 1997; **7**: 25–36.

77. Kee BL, Murre C. Induction of early B cell factor (EBF) and multiple B lineage genes by the basic helix-loop-helix transcription factor E12. *J Exp Med* 1998; **188**: 699–713.

78. Roessler S, Grosschedl R. Role of transcription factors in commitment and differentiation of early B lymphoid cells. *Semin Immunol* 2006; **18**: 12–9. Epub 2006 Jan 23.

79. Busslinger M. Transcriptional control of early B cell development. *Annu Rev Immunol* 2004; **22**: 55–79. Review.

80. Choi JK, Shen CP, Radomska HS *et al*. E47 activates the Ig-heavy chain and TdT loci in non-B cells. *EMBO J* 1996; **15**: 5014–21.

81. Romanow WJ, Langerak AW, Goebel P *et al*. E2A and EBF act in synergy with the V(D)J recombinase to generate a diverse immunoglobulin repertoire in nonlymphoid cells. *Mol Cell* 2000; **5**: 343–53.

82. Mikkola I, Heavey B, Horcher M, Busslinger M. Reversion of B cell commitment upon loss of Pax5 expression. *Science* 2002; **297**: 110–3.

83. Schebesta M, Pfeffer PL, Busslinger M. Control of pre-BCR signaling by Pax5-dependent activation of the BLNK gene. *Immunity* 2002; **17**: 473–85.

84. Schebesta A, McManus S, Salvagiotto G et al. Transcription factor Pax5 activates the chromatin of key genes involved in B cell signaling, adhesion, migration, and immune function. *Immunity* 2007; **27**: 49–63.

85. Ling KW, Dzierzak E. Ontogeny and genetics of the hemato/lymphopoietic system. *Curr Opin Immunol* 2002; **14**: 186–91. Review.

86. Godin I, Cumano A. The hare and the tortoise: an embryonic haematopoietic race. *Nat Rev Immunol* 2002; **2**: 593–604. Review.

87. Cumano A, Ferraz JC, Klaine M et al. Intraembryonic, but not yolk sac hematopoietic precursors, isolated before circulation, provide long-term multilineage reconstitution. *Immunity* 2001; **15**: 477–85.

88. Shivdasani RA, Mayer EL, Orkin SH. Absence of blood formation in mice lacking the T-cell leukaemia oncoprotein tal-1/SCL. *Nature* 1995; **373**: 432–4.

89. Robb L, Elwood NJ, Elefanty AG et al. The scl gene product is required for the generation of all hematopoietic lineages in the adult mouse. *EMBO J* 1996; **15**: 4123–9.

90. Robb L, Lyons I, Li R et al. Absence of yolk sac hematopoiesis from mice with a targeted disruption of the scl gene. *Proc Natl Acad Sci U S A* 1995; **92**: 7075–9.

91. Porcher C, Swat W, Rockwell K et al. The T cell leukemia oncoprotein SCL/tal-1 is essential for development of all hematopoietic lineages. *Cell* 1996; **86**: 47–57.

92. Foroni L, Boehm T, White L et al. The rhombotin gene family encode related LIM-domain proteins whose differing expression suggests multiple roles in mouse development. *J Mol Biol* 1992; **226**: 747–61.

93. Valge-Archer VE, Osada H, Warren AJ et al. The LIM protein RBTN2 and the basic helix-loop-helix protein TAL1 are present in a complex in erythroid cells. *Proc Natl Acad Sci U S A* 1994; **91**: 8617–21.

94. Ono Y, Fukuhara N, Yoshie O. Transcriptional activity of TAL1 in T cell acute lymphoblastic leukemia (T-ALL) requires RBTN1 or -2 and induces TALLA1, a highly specific tumor marker of T-ALL. *J Biol Chem* 1997; **272**: 4576–81.

95. Warren AJ, Colledge WH, Carlton MB et al. The oncogenic cysteine-rich LIM domain protein rbtn2 is essential for erythroid development. *Cell* 1994; **78**: 45–57.

96. Yamada Y, Warren AJ, Dobson C et al. The T cell leukemia LIM protein Lmo2 is necessary for adult mouse hematopoiesis. *Proc Natl Acad Sci U S A* 1998; **95**: 3890–5.

97. Pevny L, Lin CS, D'Agati V et al. Development of hematopoietic cells lacking transcription factor GATA-1. *Development* 1995; **121**: 163–72.

98. Pevny L, Simon MC, Robertson E et al. Erythroid differentiation in chimaeric mice blocked by a targeted mutation in the gene for transcription factor GATA-1. *Nature* 1991; **349**: 257–60.

99. Tsai FY, Keller G, Kuo FC et al. An early haematopoietic defect in mice lacking the transcription factor GATA-2. *Nature* 1994; **371**: 221–6.

100. Shalaby F, Rossant J, Yamaguchi TP et al. Failure of blood-island formation and vasculogenesis in Flk-1-deficient mice. *Nature* 1995; **376**: 62–6.

101. Medvinsky A, Dzierzak E. Definitive hematopoiesis is autonomously initiated by the AGM region. *Cell* 1996; **86**: 897–906.

102. Cumano A, Dieterlen-Lievre F, Godin I. Lymphoid potential, probed before circulation in mouse, is restricted to caudal intraembryonic splanchnopleura. *Cell* 1996; **86**: 907–16.

103. Ohmura K, Kawamoto H, Lu M et al. Immature multipotent hemopoietic progenitors lacking long-term bone marrow-reconstituting activity in the aorta-gonad-mesonephros region of murine day 10 fetuses. *J Immunol* 2001; **166**: 3290–6.

104. Strasser A, Rolink A, Melchers F. One synchronous wave of B cell development in mouse fetal liver changes at day 16 of gestation from dependence to independence of a stromal cell environment. *J Exp Med* 1989; **170**: 1973–86.

105. Kincade PW. Formation of B lymphocytes in fetal and adult life. *Adv Immunol* 1981; **31**: 177–245. Review.

106. Owen JJ, Raff MC, Cooper MD. Studies on the generation of B lymphocytes in the mouse embryo. *Eur J Immunol* 1976; **5**: 468–73.

107. Melchers F. Murine embryonic B lymphocyte development in the placenta. *Nature* 1979; **277**: 219–21.

108. Gekas C, Dieterlen-Lievre F, Orkin SH, Mikkola HK. The placenta is a niche for hematopoietic stem cells. *Dev Cell* 2005; **8**: 365–75.

109. Ottersbach K, Dzierzak E. The murine placenta contains hematopoietic stem cells within the vascular labyrinth region. *Dev Cell* 2005; **8**: 377–87.

110. Solvason N, Kearney JF. The human fetal omentum: a site of B cell generation. *J Exp Med* 1992; **175**: 397–404.

111. Kincade PW, Igarashi H, Medina KL et al. Lymphoid lineage cells in adult murine bone marrow diverge from those of other blood cells at an early, hormone-sensitive stage. *Semin Immunol* 2002; **14**: 385–94. Review.

112. Okuda T, van Deursen J, Hiebert SW et al. AML1, the target of multiple chromosomal translocations in human leukemia, is essential for normal fetal liver hematopoiesis. *Cell* 1996; **84**: 321–30.

113. Sasaki K, Yagi H, Bronson RT et al. Absence of fetal liver hematopoiesis in mice deficient in transcriptional coactivator core binding factor beta. *Proc Natl Acad Sci U S A* 1996; **93**: 12359–63.

114. Nuez B, Michalovich D, Bygrave A et al. Defective haematopoiesis in fetal liver resulting from inactivation of the EKLF gene. *Nature* 1995; **375**: 316–8.

115. Hirsch E, Iglesias A, Potocnik AJ et al. Impaired migration but not differentiation of haematopoietic stem cells in the absence of beta1 integrins. *Nature* 1996; **380**: 171–5.

116. Potocnik AJ, Brakebusch C, Fassler R. Fetal and adult hematopoietic stem cells require beta1 integrin function for colonizing fetal liver, spleen, and bone marrow. *Immunity* 2000; **12**: 653–63.

117. Yang JT, Rayburn H, Hynes RO. Cell adhesion events mediated by alpha 4 integrins are essential in placental and cardiac development. *Development* 1995; **121**: 549–60.

118. Arroyo AG, Yang JT, Rayburn H, Hynes RO. Differential requirements for alpha4 integrins during fetal and adult hematopoiesis. *Cell* 1996; **85**: 997–1008.

119. Arroyo AG, Yang JT, Rayburn H, Hynes RO. Alpha4 integrins regulate the proliferation/differentiation balance of multilineage hematopoietic progenitors in vivo. *Immunity* 1999; **11**: 555–66.

120. Nagasawa T, Hirota S, Tachibana K *et al.* Defects of B-cell lymphopoiesis and bone-marrow myelopoiesis in mice lacking the CXC chemokine PBSF/SDF-1. *Nature* 1996; **382**: 635–8.

121. Egawa T, Kawabata K, Kawamoto H *et al.* The earliest stages of B cell development require a chemokine stromal cell-derived factor/pre-B cell growth-stimulating factor. *Immunity* 2001; **15**: 323–34.

122. Ma Q, Jones D, Borghesani PR *et al.* Impaired B-lymphopoiesis, myelopoiesis, and derailed cerebellar neuron migration in CXCR4- and SDF-1-deficient mice. *Proc Natl Acad Sci U S A* 1998; **95**: 9448–53.

123. Ma Q, Jones D, Springer TA. The chemokine receptor CXCR4 is required for the retention of B lineage and granulocytic precursors within the bone marrow microenvironment. *Immunity* 1999; **10**: 463–71.

124. Kawabata K, Ujikawa M, Egawa T *et al.* A cell-autonomous requirement for CXCR4 in long-term lymphoid and myeloid reconstitution. *Proc Natl Acad Sci U S A* 1999; **96**: 5663–7.

125. Melchers F, Rolink AG, Schaniel C. The role of chemokines in regulating cell migration during humoral immune responses. *Cell* 1999; **99**: 351–4. Review.

126. Rajewsky K. Clonal selection and learning in the antibody system. *Nature* 1996; **381**: 751–8. Review.

127. Schlissel MS. Regulating antigen-receptor gene assembly. *Nat Rev Immunol* 2003; **3**: 890–9. Review.

128. Nemazee D, Weigert M. Revising B cell receptors. *J Exp Med* 2000; **191**: 1813–7.

129. Melchers F, Kincade P. Early B cell development to a mature, antigen-sensitive cell. In: Honjo T, Alt FW. (eds) *Molecular Biology of B cells.* USA: Elsevier Science, 2004: 101–26.

130. Backhed F, Ley RE, Sonnenburg JL *et al.* Host-bacterial mutualism in the human intestine. *Science* 2005; **307**: 1915–20. Review.

131. Fagarasan S, Honjo T. Intestinal IgA synthesis: regulation of front-line body defences. *Nat Rev Immunol* 2003: 63–72. Review.

132. Hooper LV, Gordon JI. Commensal host-bacterial relationships in the gut. *Science* 2001; **292**: 1115–8. Review.

133. Ghia P, ten Boekel E, Rolink AG, Melchers F. B-cell development: a comparison between mouse and man. *Immunol Today* 1998; **19**: 480–5. Review.

134. Ghia P, Melchers F, Rolink AG. Age-dependent changes in B lymphocyte development in man and mouse. *Exp Gerontol* 2000; **35**: 159–65. Review.

135. Ait-Azzouzene D, Skog P, Retter M *et al.* Tolerance-induced receptor selection: scope, sensitivity, locus specificity, and relationship to lymphocyte-positive selection. *Immunol Rev* 2004; **197**: 219–30. Review. Erratum in: *Immunol Rev* 2004; **200**: 272.

136. Kearney JF. CD5+ B-cell networks. *Curr Opin Immunol* 1993; **5**: 223–6.

137. Chen X, Martin F, Forbush KA *et al.* Evidence for selection of a population of multi-reactive B cells into the splenic marginal zone. *Int Immunol* 1997; **9**: 27–41.

138. Martin F, Kearney JF. B-cell subsets and the mature preimmune repertoire. Marginal zone and B1 B cells as part of a 'natural immune memory'. *Immunol Rev* 2000; **175**: 70–9. Review.

139. Cancro MP, Kearney JF. B cell positive selection: road map to the primary repertoire? *J Immunol* 2004; **173**: 15–9. Review.

140. Notkins AL. Polyreactivity of antibody molecules. *Trends Immunol* 2004; **25**: 174–9. Review.

141. Wardemann H, Yurasov S, Schaefer A *et al.* Predominant autoantibody production by early human B cell precursors. *Science* 2003; **301**: 1374–7. Epub 2003 Aug 14.

142. Mostoslavsky R, Singh N, Kirillov A *et al.* Kappa chain monoallelic demethylation and the establishment of allelic exclusion. *Genes Dev* 1998; **12**: 1801–11.

143. Shimizu T, Mundt C, Licence S *et al.* VpreB1/VpreB2/lambda 5 triple-deficient mice show impaired B cell development but functional allelic exclusion of the IgH locus. *J Immunol* 2002; **168**: 6286–93.

144. Melchers F. The death of a dogma? *Nat Immunol* 2004; **5**: 1199–201.

145. Melchers F. The pre-B-cell receptor: selector of fitting immunoglobulin heavy chains for the B-cell repertoire. *Nat Rev Immunol* 2005; **5**: 578–84. Review.

146. Melchers F, ten Boekel E, Seidl T *et al.* Repertoire selection by pre-B-cell receptors and B-cell receptors, and genetic control of B-cell development from immature to mature B cells. *Immunol Rev* 2000; **175**: 33–46. Review.

147. Ohnishi K, Melchers F. The nonimmunoglobulin portion of lambda5 mediates cell-autonomous pre-B cell receptor signaling. *Nat Immunol* 2003; **4**: 849–56. Epub 2003 Aug 3.

148. Gauthier L, Rossi B, Roux F *et al.* Galectin-1 is a stromal cell ligand of the pre-B cell receptor (BCR) implicated in synapse formation between pre-B and stromal cells and in pre-BCR triggering. *Proc Natl Acad Sci U S A* 2002; **99**: 13014–9. Epub 2002 Sep 23.

149. Bradl H, Jack HM. Surrogate light chain-mediated interaction of a soluble pre-B cell receptor with adherent cell lines. *J Immunol* 2001; **167**: 6403–11.

150. Flemming A, Brummer T, Reth M, Jumaa H. The adaptor protein SLP-65 acts as a tumor suppressor that limits pre-B cell expansion. *Nat Immunol* 2003; **4**: 38–43. Epub 2002 Nov 18.

151. Jumaa H, Bossaller L, Portugal K *et al.* Deficiency of the adaptor SLP-65 in pre-B-cell acute lymphoblastic leukaemia. *Nature* 2003; **423**: 452–6.

152. Ceredig R, Rolink AG, Melchers F, Andersson J. The B cell receptor, but not the pre-B cell receptor, mediates arrest of B cell differentiation. *Eur J Immunol* 2000; **30**: 759–67.

153. Yamagami T, ten Boekel E, Andersson J et al. Frequencies of multiple IgL chain gene rearrangements in single normal or kappaL chain-deficient B lineage cells. Immunity 1999; 11: 317–27.

154. Gay D, Saunders T, Camper S, Weigert M. Receptor editing: an approach by autoreactive B cells to escape tolerance. J Exp Med 1993; 177: 999–1008.

155. Rolink A, Grawunder U, Haasner D et al. Immature surface Ig+ B cells can continue to rearrange kappa and lambda L chain gene loci. J Exp Med 1993; 178: 1263–70.

156. Tiegs SL, Russell DM, Nemazee D. Receptor editing in self-reactive bone marrow B cells. J Exp Med 1993; 177: 1009–20.

157. Nemazee D, Weigert M. Revising B cell receptors. J Exp Med 2000; 191: 1813–7.

158. Mostoslavsky R, Alt FW, Bassing CH. Chromatin dynamics and locus accessibility in the immune system. Nat Immunol 2003; 4: 603–6. Review.

159. Monroe JG. B-cell positive selection and peripheral homeostasis. Immunol Rev 2004; 197: 5–9. Review.

160. Dal Porto JM, Gauld SB, Merrell KT et al. B cell antigen receptor signaling 101. Mol Immunol 2004; 41: 599–613. Review.

161. Roschenthaler F, Kirschbaum T, Heim V et al. The 5′ part of the mouse immunoglobulin kappa locus. Eur J Immunol 1999; 29: 2065–71.

162. Kirschbaum T, Roschenthaler F, Bensch A et al. The central part of the mouse immunoglobulin kappa locus. Eur J Immunol 1999; 29: 2057–64.

163. Kirschbaum T, Pourrajabi S, Zocher I et al. The 3′ part of the immunoglobulin kappa locus of the mouse. Eur J Immunol 1998; 28: 1458–66.

164. Engel H, Rolink A, Weiss S et al. B cells are programmed to activate kappa and lambda for rearrangement at consecutive developmental stages. Eur J Immunol 1999; 29: 2167–76.

165. Yamagami T, ten Boekel E, Schaniel C et al. Four of five RAG-expressing JCkappa-/- small pre-BII cells have no L chain gene rearrangements: detection by high-efficiency single cell PCR. Immunity 1999; 11: 309–16.

166. Wardemann H, Boehm T, Dear N, Carsetti R. B-1a B cells that link the innate and adaptive immune responses are lacking in the absence of the spleen. J Exp Med 2002; 195: 771–80.

167. Casola S, Otipoby KL, Alimzhanov M et al. B cell receptor signal strength determines B cell fate. Nat Immunol 2004; 5: 317–27. Epub 2004 Feb 1.

168. Carroll MC. A protective role for innate immunity in systemic lupus erythematosus. Nat Rev Immunol 2004; 4: 825–31. Review.

169. Carroll MC. The complement system in regulation of adaptive immunity. Nat Immunol 2004; 5: 981–6. Review.

170. Melchers F, Rolink AR. B cell tolerance – how to make it and how to break it. Curr Top Microbiol Immunol (in press).

171. Nossal GJ, Pike BL. Clonal anergy: persistence in tolerant mice of antigen-binding B lymphocytes incapable of responding to antigen or mitogen. Proc Natl Acad Sci U S A 1980; 77: 1602–6.

172. Nemazee DA, Burki K. Clonal deletion of B lymphocytes in a transgenic mouse bearing anti-MHC class I antibody genes. Nature 1989; 337: 562–6.

173. Nemazee DA, Burki K. Clonal deletion of autoreactive B lymphocytes in bone marrow chimeras. Proc Natl Acad Sci U S A 1989; 86: 8039.

174. Nossal GJ. Cellular and molecular mechanisms of B lymphocyte tolerance. Adv Immunol 1992; 52: 283–331. Review.

175. Goodnow CC, Crosbie J, Adelstein S et al. Altered immunoglobulin expression and functional silencing of self-reactive B lymphocytes in transgenic mice. Nature 1988; 334: 676–82.

176. Rolink AG, Brocker T, Bluethmann H et al. Mutations affecting either generation or survival of cells influence the pool size of mature B cells. Immunity 1999; 10: 619–28.

177. Rolink AG, Schaniel C, Andersson J, Melchers F. Selection events operating at various stages in B cell development. Curr Opin Immunol 2001; 13: 202–7. Review.

178. Fields ML, Erikson J. The regulation of lupus-associated autoantibodies: immunoglobulin transgenic models. Curr Opin Immunol 2003; 15: 709–17. Review.

179. Rolink AG, Tschopp J, Schneider P, Melchers F. BAFF is a survival and maturation factor for mouse B cells. Eur J Immunol 2002; 32: 2004–10.

180. Rolink AG, Melchers F. BAFFled B cells survive and thrive: roles of BAFF in B-cell development. Curr Opin Immunol 2002; 14: 266–75.

181. Ng LG, Mackay CR, Mackay F. The BAFF/APRIL system: life beyond B lymphocytes. Mol Immunol 2005; 42: 763–72. Epub 2004 Dec 8. Review.

182. Moore PA, Belvedere O, Orr A et al. BLyS: member of the tumor necrosis factor family and B lymphocyte stimulator. Science 1999; 285: 260–3.

183. Schiemann B, Gommerman JL, Vora K et al. An essential role for BAFF in the normal development of B cells through a BCMA-independent pathway. Science 2001; 293: 2111–4. Epub 2001 Aug 16.

184. Gross JA, Dillon SR, Mudri S et al. TACI-Ig neutralizes molecules critical for B cell development and autoimmune disease. Impaired B cell maturation in mice lacking BLyS. Immunity 2001; 15: 289–302.

185. Leslie D, Lipsky P, Notkins AL. Autoantibodies as predictors of disease. J Clin Invest 2001; 108: 1417–22.

186. Hayakawa K, Asano M, Shinton SA et al. Positive selection of natural autoreactive B cells. Science 1999; 285: 113–6.

187. Stall AM, Adams S, Herzenberg LA, Kantor AB. Characteristics and development of the murine B-1b (Ly-1 B sister) cell population. Ann N Y Acad Sci 1992; 651: 33–43. Review.

188. Craig SW, Cebra JJ. Peyer's patches: an enriched source of precursors for IgA-producing immunocytes in the rabbit. J Exp Med 1971; 134: 188–200.

189. Forster I, Rajewsky K. The bulk of the peripheral B-cell pool in mice is stable and not rapidly renewed from the bone marrow. Proc Natl Acad Sci U S A 1990; 87: 4781–4.

190. Muramatsu M, Kinoshita K, Fagarasan S *et al.* Class switch recombination and hypermutation require activation-induced cytidine deaminase (AID), a potential RNA editing enzyme. *Cell* 2000; **102**: 553–63.

191. Revy P, Muto T, Levy Y *et al.* Activation-induced cytidine deaminase (AID) deficiency causes the autosomal recessive form of the Hyper-IgM syndrome (HIGM2). *Cell* 2000; **102**: 565–75.

192. Shinkura R, Ito S, Begum NA *et al.* Separate domains of AID are required for somatic hypermutation and class-switch recombination. *Nat Immunol* 2004; **5**: 707–12. Epub 2004 Jun 13.

193. Rolink AG, Melchers F. BAFFled B cells survive and thrive: roles of BAFF in B-cell development. *Curr Opin Immunol* 2002; **14**: 266–75.

194. Lam KP, Kuhn R, Rajewsky K. In vivo ablation of surface immunoglobulin on mature B cells by inducible gene targeting results in rapid cell death. *Cell* 1997; **90**: 1073–83.

195. Grawunder U, Haasner D, Melchers F, Rolink A. Rearrangement and expression of kappa light chain genes can occur without mu heavy chain expression during differentiation of pre-B cells. *Int Immunol* 1993; **5**: 1609–18.

196. Shaw AC, Swat W, Ferrini R *et al.* Activated Ras signals developmental progression of recombinase-activating gene (RAG)-deficient pro-B lymphocytes. *J Exp Med* 1999; **189**: 123–9.

197. Iritani BM, Forbush KA, Farrar MA, Perlmutter RM. Control of B cell development by Ras-mediated activation of Raf. *EMBO J* 1997; **16**: 7019–31.

198. Nagaoka H, Takahashi Y, Hayashi R *et al.* Ras mediates effector pathways responsible for pre-B cell survival, which is essential for the developmental progression to the late pre-B cell stage. *J Exp Med* 2000; **192**: 171–82.

199. Rolink A, Melchers F, Andersson J. The SCID but not the RAG-2 gene product is required for S mu-S epsilon heavy chain class switching. *Immunity* 1996; **5**: 319–30.

200. Gross AJ, Hochberg D, Rand WM, Thorley-Lawson DA. EBV and systemic lupus erythematosus: a new perspective. *J Immunol* 2005; **174**: 6599–607.

201. Fruehling S, Longnecker R. The immunoreceptor tyrosine-based activation motif of Epstein-Barr virus LMP2A is essential for blocking BCR-mediated signal transduction. *Virology* 1997; **235**: 241–51.

202. Caldwell RG, Wilson JB, Anderson SJ, Longnecker R. Epstein-Barr virus LMP2A drives B cell development and survival in the absence of normal B cell receptor signals. *Immunity* 1998; **9**: 405–11.

203. Akira S, Takeda K. Toll-like receptor signalling. *Nat Rev Immunol* 2004; **4**: 499–511. Review.

12

Cellular immunobiology of lymph nodes and spleen

IAN CM MACLENNAN, KARINE SERRE AND ELODIE MOHR

INTRODUCTION

Lymphocytes respond specifically to infection by proliferating and differentiating into immunological effectors, such as helper T cells, plasma cells, and cytotoxic lymphocytes. The proliferation of lymphocytes during immune responses can be very rapid and constraints on this growth are critical. Further, control of the specificity of the lymphocytes that are induced to become effectors affords protection from infection, while minimizing the chance of inducing autoimmunity or allergy.

The secondary lymphoid organs, including the spleen and lymph nodes (LN), play an essential role in achieving this balance between protection and self-damage. This chapter will not consider the other secondary lymphoid organs – the palatine tonsils and adenoids, Peyer's patches, and the appendix – or the small aggregates of lymphoid tissue found along the length of the gut and in the respiratory passages, which share some of the functions of the larger secondary lymphoid organs. This is covered in Chapter 13.

LYMPHOCYTE RECIRCULATION AND LYMPH NODE STRUCTURE

A high proportion of lymphocytes – the recirculating T and B cells – migrate constantly between the different secondary lymphoid organs (Box 12.1).[1] This migration is independent of antigen, but entry into the lymphoid tissues is critical for antigen engagement by lymphocytes and their recruitment into immune responses. The way in which this occurs will be described in relation to LN, which share common features with the other secondary lymphoid organs.

The dome-shaped cortex of LN is covered by the subcapsular lymphatic sinus. The sinus is fed by afferent lymphatic vessels that drain adjacent tissues and carry free antigen to the node as well as antigen-transporting cells. Drainage from the sinus is into intranodal lymphatic channels, which penetrate the cortex at intervals. These intranodal lymphatics are often convoluted and they meet in the medulla, where they form the efferent lymphatic

---

BOX 12.1: Passage of recirculating T and B cells through lymph nodes

Recirculating B and T cells both enter lymph nodes from the blood via high endothelial venules (HEV) (Plate 1).

There is no obvious interaction between the T and B cells at this stage and they follow different paths from the HEV.

The recirculating B cells traffic along the walls of intranodal lymphatics to the follicles.

Recirculating T cells enter the central T zone where they screen the surface of dendritic cells.

In the absence of interaction with antigen both cell types leave the node after some hours by entering the efferent lymph and so return to the blood.

BOX 12.2: CD4 T cell priming and differentiation

Naïve recirculating CD4 T cells are primed by making cognate interaction with dendritic cells in the T zones of secondary lymphoid organs.

The start of priming is associated with an initial period of adjustment followed by very rapid proliferation within the T zone.

As early as the third day some of the responding CD4 T cells start to leave the T zone; four categories of differentiated CD4 T cell are recognized:

- CD4 T cells that provide help to antigen-activated B cells in the T zone (Box 12.3);
- Effector CD4 T cells that leave the node and enter the blood from which they can pass to sites of inflammation;
- Follicular CD4 T cells that are involved in selection of GC B cells;
- Recirculating memory CD4 T cells.

(Plate 1, see plate section). The efferent lymphatic may be afferent to downstream LN, but the lymph eventually drains via a major lymphatic vessel, such as the thoracic duct, into the venous system. The perilymphatic tissues that surround the intranodal lymphatics are an important microenvironment for cellular and molecular interactions within LN.[2]

Four main lymph node tissue compartments

The cortical tissue is occupied mainly by follicles, which are visited by recirculating B cells (Plate 1).[3] Follicles make up the compartment where germinal centers (GCs) form.[4] The follicles lie adjacent to each other except where intranodal lymphatics are present. Beneath the cortex is a compartment known as the T zone. This is filled with dendritic cells (DC) and recirculating T lymphocytes.[5] A third LN compartment, the outer T zone, surrounds the intranodal lymphatics and extends beneath the follicles. Here B cells that have taken up antigen accumulate and make cognate interaction with primed T cells (Box 12.2).[6] Naïve recirculating B cells migrating to follicles traffic through the outer T zone.[1,7] In the base of the lymph node – the medulla – the perilymphatic tissues become the fourth LN compartment: the medullary cords. This compartment is associated with plasmablast growth and differentiation to plasma cells.[8]

Migration of recirculating lymphocytes into and within lymph nodes

Recirculating T and B lymphocytes enter LN through post-capillary venules, which are typically located in the outer T zone (Box 12.1).[9] These venules have specialized cuboidal endothelial cells; hence their common name – high endothelial venules (HEV). Expression of L-selectin (CD62L) is a hallmark of recirculating lymphocytes and enables them to bind reversibly to vascular addressins

expressed by HEV. The addressins in peripheral LN HEV are collectively termed peripheral node addressin (Plate 1B).[10] This molecular interaction slows movement of recirculating lymphocytes in the blood within HEV and enables them to bind more firmly to the vessel walls through integrins.[9] They then cross the endothelium under the guidance of the chemokines CCL21 (SLC) and CCL19 (ELC).[11] Both SLC and ELC bind to the lymphocyte surface counterstructure, CCR7. T and B cells, after crossing the wall of HEV, follow different paths, again guided by chemokine control. This divergent migration reflects the different ways in which T and B cells encounter and recognize antigen. T cell receptors of naïve recirculating T cells recognize processed antigenic peptides presented by major histocompatibility complex (MHC) molecules on the surface of T zone DC. By contrast, the B cell receptor for antigen (BCR) recognizes intact antigen. In response to SLC produced by DC, recirculating T cells associate with and migrate over the surface of T zone DC.[12] They move from one dendritic cell to another[5] and, if they do not encounter processed antigen they recognize, leave the node after 18 to 24 hours by entering the efferent lymphatic system.[13] B cells are guided, at least in part, by the chemokine BLC (CXCL13) through their cognate receptor CXCR5. They move from HEV to the walls of the intranodal lymphatics and migrate along these toward the follicles.[14] Their perilymphatic location may enable them to bind antigen in the lymph. In addition, certain dendritic-shaped cells are able to transport intact antigen via the afferent lymph and pass this to B cells.[15] The onward passage of B cells into follicles brings them in contact with another cell type that can hold intact antigen that is available to B cells. These are the follicular dendritic cells (FDC). Recirculating B cells in a LN that are not recruited into an antibody response leave the node by entering efferent lymph. This happens a little over 24 hours after they entered the node.[13] Once in the lymph the lymphocytes return to the blood and repeat the cycle by entering another secondary lymphoid organ.

High endothelial venules are found in all secondary lymphoid organs other than the spleen. In rodents, recirculating B and T cells leave the blood in the spleen by adhering to the wall of the marginal sinus and cross this to enter the outer T zone. Naïve recirculating T and B cells show little selectivity for entry to different secondary lymphoid tissues.[16] Conversely, recirculating memory T cells tend to recognize the vascular endothelium of the group of secondary lymphoid organs where their progenitors were recruited into an immune response.[17]

T AND B CELL RECRUITMENT INTO IMMUNE RESPONSES IN LYMPH NODES

CD4 T cell priming, differentiation, and dispersal

As mentioned above, recirculating CD4 T cells spend their time in secondary lymphoid tissues inspecting processed antigen on the surface of T zone DC (Box 12.2).[5] If cognate interaction between the CD4 T cells and the DC occurs with appropriate costimulation, mainly through engagement of the B7 family molecules (CD80, CD86), the T cell starts to respond to antigen. For the first 24 hours or so, the T cell and dendritic cell remain together. The responding CD4 T cells upregulate CD69 and CD25 and cease to express L-selectin or interleukin-7 (IL-7) receptor. During the second day after immunization they start to divide rapidly[18] and by 48 hours are found throughout the T zone. On the third day T cells start to leave the T zone. Some enter follicles where they may be involved in the selection of B cells in the follicular response.[19,20] Others leave the node, either as effector cells that enter sites of inflammation,[21] or memory CD4 T cells that recirculate through secondary lymphoid tissues. A fourth population of differentiated CD4 T cells that interacts with B cells that have taken up antigen, remains in the outer T zone (Box 12.3).[22]

B cell interaction with antigen and primed T cells

When limiting amounts of antigen are injected in one foot pad the response tends to be confined to the nodes of the same leg and does not spread to contralateral nodes. Thus in this situation B cells encounter the antigen within the LN. Large doses of antigen injected in the foot can produce responses in the nodes of all limbs. This is likely to be due to antigen disseminating to other nodes. B cells and DC

BOX 12.3: Cognate T cell interaction with B cells at the start of T-dependent antibody responses

A proportion of primed T cells become highly efficient at seeking out, interacting with, and providing help to B cells that have engaged antigen.

B cells that bind, take up, process, and present antigen become highly efficient at seeking out and interacting with the primed helper T cells.

Cognate interaction between these antigen-activated T and B cells occurs in the outer T zone.

If there is mutual recognition the B cells may start to proliferate and give rise to cells that enter follicular or extrafollicular antibody responses (Box 12.4).

---

that pick up antigen in the blood typically migrate into the outer T zones of the spleen.[22] Whether some enter LN is not clear.

There is a strong mutual attraction between B cells that have been activated by taking up antigen through their BCR and T cells that have been primed following interaction with processed antigen presented by DC.[22,23] The affinity between these cells does not exist before encounter with antigen; naïve T and B cells appear to pass each other, as ships in the night, during passage through secondary lymphoid tissue. At the bottom of a test tube, antigen-activated B cells can interact with naïve T cells.[24] The extent to which these interactions occur *in vivo* is less clear.

The two types of T-dependent antibody response

Recirculating B cells, by making cognate interaction with a primed T cell, can be induced to proliferate and differentiate in either follicular or extrafollicular antibody responses (Box 12.4). T-dependent extrafollicular responses provide early antibody, which can be critical for halting the spread of viral infection.[25] The antigen-binding structure of the antibody produced in extrafollicular responses is the same as that of the BCR of the B cells recruited into the response.[26] Typically, memory B cells are not produced. By contrast, in follicular antibody responses GCs are formed, there is memory B cell production,[27,28] and affinity maturation of the BCR of the responding B cells occurs.[29] Affinity maturation first involves hypermutation of the rearranged immunoglobulin (Ig) variable-region genes followed by selection of those B cells with high affinity for the antigen that induced the response.[4,30] The onset of antibody production is later than that occurring in extrafollicular responses, but the response is long-term and the high-affinity antibody production curtails reinfection and protects against exotoxins.

BOX 12.4: Follicular and extrafollicular antibody response induction

These antibody responses may be induced by specific inter-action of B cells with antigen, normally with T cell help or innate immune signals, or both of these.

B cells become B blasts, which start to proliferate in the outer T zone.

During the third day after recruitment into the response the B cells acquire characteristics that are associated with their differentiation in one of two ways:

- Some migrate to follicles and participate in the formation of germinal centers where they will proliferate, mutate their immunoglobulin variable-region genes, and are then subjected to an antigen and T-dependent selection process;
- Others become plasmablasts that proliferate and differentiate to plasma cells in extrafollicular foci.

BOX 12.5: Germinal center formation and function

Germinal centers (GC) are formed from a small number (around 3) of founding B cells.

B cells that have taken up antigen move to the outer T zone where they make cognate interaction with primed T cells. The B cells become B blasts in this site and, after 1 or 2 days, the blasts migrate into the follicular dentritic cell network. Here they start to coexpress BCL6 and AID and continue proliferating, forming a visible germinal cen-ter by around 3 days from the time of cognate T cell B cell interaction.

By this stage B cells in the GC have activated immuno-globulin variable-region hypermutation mechanisms.

On the fourth day some B cells start to leave the GC either to become plasma cells or memory B cells.

Cells leaving the GC appear to have been selected; they tend to have higher affinity than the cells that founded the GC. In addition, a substantial proportion of B-lineage cells within the GC undergo apoptosis, many as a consequence of failed selection.

CD4 T cells are found particularly at the junction of the GC and follicular mantle. The involvement of these in selec-tion is suggested by the finding that GC can form without T cells, but memory cells and plasma cells are not produced by such GC.

It is postulated that B cells receive positive selection sig-nals if they bind antigen, process this, and present it to GC T cells, and that B cells failing to do this die.

Extrafollicular antibody responses

T-dependent extrafollicular responses start with antigen uptake and presentation by DC leading to T cell priming as well as specific uptake of antigen by B cells through their BCR. This is followed by cognate interaction between the activated T and B cells.[22,31] B cells then go through a pre-proliferative phase of about one day. During this they may start to produce germ-line transcripts of one or more of the Ig heavy chain constant-region genes and the associated switch regions.[22] The production and processing of these transcripts is a necessary prelude to Ig class switching.[32] During the second day after the start of the response the B cells begin to proliferate and many of them accumulate Ig in their cytoplasm. Although, at this stage, a majority of the cells express low levels of syndecan-1 (CD138) – a plasma cell-associated molecule[25] – they do not yet express BLIMP1, a transcriptional regulator associated with plasma cell differentiation.[33] Ambiguity in differentiation is reflected by many cells coexpressing, with the CD138, BCL6, a molecule associated with GC B cells. At this stage the cells express activation-induced cytidine deaminase (AID), which is required both for Ig class switching and hypermutation of Ig variable-region genes. Some of the B cells undergo Ig class switch recombination.[34] During the third day after T-dependent B cell activation a proportion of the B blasts differentiate into plasmablasts as deduced from their expression of BLIMP1. Their expression of CXCR4 is associated with their movement down the peri-lymphatic zone to the medullary cords. The plasmablasts progressively reduce expression of PAX5, resulting in lowered expression of the BCR and associated molecules. At the same time the cells start to secrete Ig. When plas-mablasts reach the medullary cords AID expression is minimal, consequently Ig class switching ceases. Thus switching, with its associated danger of translocation, in extrafollicular responses occurs in the outer T zone. During the fifth day after T-dependent B cell activation plasmablasts come out of cell cycle and differentiate into plasma cells. Many of these are short lived.[35,36] This description of an extrafollicular response applies to T cell-dependent antibody responses in which either recirculat-ing or marginal zone (MZ) B cells are recruited in the response. Extrafollicular responses associated with B1 cells have some important differences and will be described later in this chapter.

Germinal center formation

The striking structures of GCs, illustrated in (Plate 2A, see plate section), result from expansion of a small number of B cell clones within a primary follicle (Box 12.5).[37,38] Primary follicles lack GCs. They contain a network of FDC and the spaces between the FDC are filled with small recirculating B cells. Additional stromal elements in the cortex produce the chemokine BLC (CXCL13),[39] which first attracts B cells to follicles. Tumor necrosis factor α (TNFα) and lymphotoxin produced by follicular B cells induce FDC to differentiate from progenitors.[40,41] The nature of FDC progenitors is still controversial. Mature FDC also produce BLC and this production increases during follicular responses.[42]

Follicular dendritic cells have the ability to take up and hold intact antigen for extended periods.[43,44] This antigen is acquired by active cellular transport, which is different in LN and the spleen. In LN the transporting cell is radiation resistant and has not been characterized. Conversely, in the spleen, radiation-sensitive MZ B cells transport the antigen.[45,46] The transport is not antigen specific, but is FcγR and C3R dependent.[47] Heterogeneity in FDC phenotype has been used to identify different compartments in human tonsil GCs.[48] There is some variation in the distribution of FDC of different phenotype in human LN and tonsils.[49]

The earliest stages of B cell recruitment into T-dependent follicular antibody responses are poorly characterized. During the third day after cognate B cell interaction with T cells, proliferating B cells can be identified in follicle centers.[7,38] These cells, unlike those entering an extrafollicular response, sustain PAX5 expression. BCL6, which represses the expression of BLIMP1, is strongly expressed.[50] These follicular B blasts grow exponentially within the FDC network.[38] During the fourth day the center of the follicle is filled with blasts and the small recirculating B cells now form a mantle round the GC. Studies in rat spleens indicate that on average GCs contain only three B cell clones and that each grows to become some 4000 cells within 96 hours.[38] When the clones reach this size, the GC divides into a dark and light zone (Plate 2A).

The dark zone of a GC consists of a collection of B blasts, which lie outside the dense FDC network and next to the outer T zone. The blasts in the dark zone have a cell cycle rate in the order of 6 to 7 hours and are termed centroblasts.[4] In the dark zone any FDC processes that are present are threadlike and widely spaced.[48] Typically the centroblasts are mixed with prominent macrophages that contain condensed chromatin granules (tingible bodies) derived from apoptotic centroblasts.

The light zone of a GC lies within the dense FDC network. The B cells in this zone are a mixture of blasts, particularly around the outer rim of the light zone, together with centrocytes, which are cells that are not actively dividing.[48] The ratio of blasts to centrocytes in the light zone of mouse GCs generally is higher than that seen in human GCs. Centrocytes typically have an irregularly shaped nucleus, sometimes with a deep cleft. The centroblasts in the GC and the centrocytes within a single GC appear to belong to the same clones, as assessed by analysis of the sequence of the CDR3 of Ig variable region genes.[51] Pulse-chase labeling experiments using tritiated thymidine[52] or 5-bromo-2′-deoxyuridine[38] indicate that centrocytes are derived from cells that have recently been in cell cycle. These two factors suggest that centrocytes are the progeny of centroblasts. Further, there is evidence that

following centrocyte selection a proportion of centrocytes become centroblasts.[53] The light zone of GC also contains a substantial number of CD4 T cells.[54] These T cells are not present in primary follicles and enter follicles from the third day after T cell priming. In primary antibody responses significant proliferation occurs among follicular T cells, but later in the response and during secondary responses this is very limited.[19] Typically, T cells in reactive human GCs are not in cell cycle as assessed by Ki-67 expression. In addition to the T cells, B cells, and FDC in the light zone there are macrophages. Like dark zone tingible body macrophages these contain debris from apoptotic cells.[48]

A working hypothesis for germinal center function

Germinal centers are sites of oligoclonal B cell growth and the output from GCs is memory B cells and plasma cells (Box 12.5).[36,55] Within the GC, Ig variable region-directed hypermutation is activated and this alters the structure of the antigen-binding sites on the BCR.[29] It appears that cells which retain affinity for the antigen that induced the response are positively selected, while those that lose the ability to bind this antigen die by apoptosis.[56] This can be deduced from the increase in affinity of antibody produced that occurs with time from immunization and the association of variable-region mutations with GC-derived plasma cells that produce high-affinity antibody.[57,58] The low levels of the anti-apoptotic proteins such as BCL2 in GC B cells reflects their vulnerability to apoptosis.[59] If GC B cells are taken from their microenvironment they spontaneously enter apoptosis.[56] This may serve two purposes in vivo. First, if centroblasts require signals from within the GC, growth beyond the confines of the GC would be prevented. Second, B cells that have lost affinity for foreign antigen through hypermutation will die because they fail to get positive selection signals that prevent apoptosis. Follicular dendritic cells may promote B cell survival within GC, for FDC have been shown to prevent apoptosis of B cells in culture.[60] Additional factors must be involved, as ectopic, albeit abortive, GC can develop in mice that lack FDC.[41] The role of FDC in sustaining centroblast survival is questionable, for there are only sparse FDC processes in the dark zone.[48]

Current evidence favors a two-stage process for centrocyte selection. First the cells engage antigen through their BCR. In vitro, strong crosslinking of the BCR can delay, but not prevent, apoptosis among GC B cells.[56] The second phase of centrocyte selection seems to involve cognate interaction with GC T cells. Evidence for this comes from studies showing that GC cells are prevented from entering apoptosis by signaling through B cell surface CD40.[56] This can be achieved by CD40 ligand (CD40L) expression by T cells induced during cognate interaction with B cells[53] or by treating B cells with agonistic antibodies against CD40[56] or recombinant CD40L.[61] Conjugates made between GC T cells and autologous centrocytes *in vitro* can inhibit apoptosis and induce the rapid formation of memory B cells and centroblasts; CD40 ligation is necessary but not sufficient to produce these effects.[53] The additional signals required are not clear. Various culture conditions have been described that will induce plasma cell differentiation from centrocytes *in vitro*, but the way in which centrocytes are induced to differentiate into plasma cells *in vivo* requires further study. T cells in human GC are uniformly CD4$^+$ CD45RO$^+$, but vary in their expression of the costimulatory molecules CD40L and CTLA-4. These molecules are present as preformed ligand within a proportion of GC T cells. The CD40L is rapidly brought to the cell surface on T cell receptor ligation,[54] but is also quickly downregulated when this binds to B cell-expressed CD40.[62] Immunoglobulin class switching can be triggered during centrocyte selection by cognate interaction with T cells,[63] but some memory B cells leaving GCs are nonswitched.[64] Some GC T cells, particularly in the middle of the light zone, express CD57; CD57$^-$ T cells are mainly located next to the follicular mantle.[48] CTLA-4 moderates the size of established GCs.[65]

OTHER FEATURES OF LYMPH NODES

Dendritic cells of the T zone are key regulators of T cell responses and T-dependent antibody responses; they also control the fine balance between the induction of adaptive immunity and the maintenance of self-tolerance.[66–68] Dendritic cells are heterogeneous bone marrow-derived cells. They have the common feature of presenting processed antigen to recirculating naïve and memory T cells.[69–71] T zone DC precursors reside outside secondary lymphoid tissues at sites where they can encounter antigen. These include the walls of the gut and respiratory tract and the skin. Dendritic cells are also found in the internal organs, blood, and lymph. Dendritic cells can be activated to take up antigen via a wide range of innate immune recognition receptors that are triggered directly or indirectly by components associated with microorganisms and viruses and products of tissue injury.[72] This induces antigen processing, phenotypic change in the DC, and migration to secondary lymphoid organs associated with the sites where the DC were activated. Thus DC activated in the skin migrate in afferent lymph to draining peripheral LN.[73] Similarly, mesenteric nodes receive DC activated in the wall of the gut, and the cervical nodes DC from the ear, nose, mouth, and throat. The migration of activated DC from internal organs, blood, and peritoneal cavities is mainly to the spleen.[66,74] This pathway also applies to foreign DC introduced in renal or cardiac allografts.[74] Some DC activated in internal organs also pass to secondary lymphoid organs other than the spleen, for allograft rejection proceeds in splenectomized individuals. Finally, some DC within the T zones of secondary lymphoid organs can take up, process, and present antigen.[75]

Marginal zones in lymph nodes

Marginal zones are normally associated with the spleen. Cells with a similar phenotype are also found in LN,[76] located along the inner wall of the subcapsular sinus. In peripheral LN these usually are small patches of cells,[77] but in mesenteric nodes in humans they can form a substantial layer of cells along the entire inner surface of the subcapsular sinus.[76] Marginal zone-like B cells in LN have a similar privileged access to antigen enjoyed by equivalent cells in the spleen,[78] Peyer's patches,[79] and tonsils.[80] Marginal zone B cells will be considered in more detail in relation to the spleen.

CD8 T cell responses in lymph nodes

CD8 T cells contribute to the clearance of viral and certain bacterial infections. After encounter with antigen, CD8 T cells differentiate into cytotoxic T lymphocytes (CTL), which form an essential arm of the adaptive immune response through the action of cytokines and cell-mediated cytotoxicity. While CD4 T cells recognize peptides derived from antigens and presented by major MHC class II molecules, CD8 T cells respond to peptides displayed on MHC class I molecules. Most of these peptides originate from proteins produced within the cell, although transfer of peptides derived from external proteins taken into the endosomal compartment has been reported.[81] As demonstrated for CD4 T cells,[82] naïve CD8 T cell activation depends almost exclusively on DC[83] that have processed and are presenting external antigens on MHC class I molecules.[84] This mechanism allows 'cross-presentation' of pathogen-infected cells and the priming of CTL responses against intracellular microbial infections.

CD8 T cell responses depend, at least partially, on CD4 T cells. This CD4 T cell influence can act at more than one level during CD8 T cell development in primary and secondary responses.[85,86] Mechanisms implicated include direct CD4 T cell–DC interaction (involving CD40-CD154) that increases the efficiency of DC in stimulating CD8 T cells.[87] CD40L expressed by CD4 cells may also directly interact with CD40 expressed by CD8 T cells.[88]

Elegant studies using two-photon microscopy have characterized the rapid formation of CD8 T cell clusters around DC.[5] A phase of relatively stable CD8 T cell interaction with DC occurring between 8 and 20 hours after injection of antigen is consistent with the formation of an immune synapse. This interaction leads to the upregulation of CD69, CD25, and CD44. Within a few hours CD8 T cells disengage from the DC and start to proliferate rapidly. Although both CD4 and CD8 T cells are activated in the T zone of LN it is still uncertain if they interact at the same time with the same DC.[89] While there are many similarities between CD4 and CD8 T cell stimulation they appear to have different programs of activation. For CD8 T cells, a relatively short engagement of the T cell receptor seems to be sufficient to initiate a program driving clonal expansion and differentiation.[90,91] Conversely, with CD4 T cells the initial antigen encounter is not sufficient to direct the whole process of proliferation and diversification. Rather there seems to be sequential cognate interactions and the end result can vary if the amount of antigen and its persistence differs during a response.[92,93]

LYMPH NODE DEVELOPMENT

There has been considerable recent advance in the understanding of the cellular and molecular events associated with LN development. A chain of signaling initiated by LN inducer cells seems critical. These cells, of hemopoietic origin, express CD4, but not CD3.[94] Their action seems to be through surface expression of lymphotoxin $\alpha 1\beta 2$ that interacts with lymphotoxin $\beta 1$ receptor expressed by stromal organizer cells. This interaction induces the expression of a series of adhesion molecules and chemokines, including the adhesion molecules ICAM-1 and VCAM-1 (respectively binding integrins LFA-1 and VLA-4), addressins such as MAdCAM-1, and chemokines CXCL13, CCL19, and CCL21.[95] The first elements in LN formation are outgrowths from lymph sacs and the interaction of lymphatic endothelium with mesenchymal elements. Different LN arise at different stages in ontogeny and have different requirements for development. Progress has been made in understanding how these processes can lead to the development of ectopic secondary lymphoid tissue in inflammatory disease, where lymphoid tissue inducers operate that are analogous to those involved in the formation of physiological secondary lymphoid tissue. The importance of these regulators of secondary lymphoid tissue development in supporting the spread of lymphoid neoplasms deserves further investigation.

STRUCTURE AND FUNCTIONS OF THE SPLEEN

The spleen is a multifunctional organ. Most of these functions are duplicated elsewhere in the body, explaining why the spleen is not essential for life, but this redundancy provided by duplication reflects the importance of these functions of the spleen.

Anatomically, the white pulp of the spleen is composed of islands of secondary lymphoid tissue that float in a sea of blood – the red pulp. The term white pulp describes its macroscopic appearance and reflects the perfusion of its tissues by capillaries. By contrast, the red appearance of the rest of the spleen results from its sinusoidal blood supply. The sinusoids are open blood channels with fenestrated endothelium, allowing direct contact of nonendothelial cells, including the red pulp macrophages, with blood. The red pulp blood sinuses pass over arrays of macrophages suspended on fibrous stroma – the cords of Billroth

(Plate 2C). In mouse spleen the red pulp physiologically contains active hemopoietic tissue,[96,97] while spleen from healthy humans generally does not.[98] Plasma cells are found along collagen bands in the red pulp of the spleen (Plate 2E). The collagen bands link suspended elements including the white pulp to the capsule, providing stability to the suspended elements and limiting splenic enlargement. It follows that splenomegally occurring in disease is likely to require remodeling of this scaffold of fibrous bands rather than simple inflation.

Blood enters the spleen through the splenic artery, which flows from the celiac axis. The splenic vein drains into the portal vein with the blood consequently being processed through the liver. The splenic artery forms several branches, which pass within the suspensory collagen bands described above, while terminal arterioles form the core of the secondary lymphoid tissue.

The white pulp structure

The white pulp structure is depicted in Plate 2A, B, E, and F. Arterioles in the center of each block of white pulp are surrounded by a T zone, which contains DC and recirculating T cells. These T zones are sometimes referred to as the periarteriolar lymphocytic sheaths (PALS). At intervals the T zone is surrounded by B cell follicles, which contain recirculating B cells and FDC; GC develop in these follicles. In addition to IgD[high], IgM[variable] recirculating B cells which dominate LN follicles,[3] splenic primary follicles and follicular mantles contain a substantial minority of IgM[high], IgD[low/−] B cells. Recent evidence indicates some of these IgM[high], IgD[low/−] cells are cells that migrate back and forth between the marginal zone and follicles;[99] others may be transitional B2 cells and yet others are B1 cells.[100]

The splenic T zones, unlike those in LN, lack high endothelial venules. The equivalent endothelial surface in rat and mouse spleen is provided by specialized vascular endothelium, termed the marginal sinus. This expresses the addressin MAdCAM-1 and surrounds the follicles and part of those sections of T zone not covered by follicles.[101] Recirculating T and B cells adhere to and pass across the marginal sinus into the white pulp. As in LN, recirculating T cells then pass to the DC-rich central T zone,[1] while the B cells migrate along the outer T zone to follicles.[1,102] In rats and mice the marginal sinus represents the border between the white and red pulp; all the tissues outside this are perfused by blood sinusoids. One lymphocyte compartment, the MZ, lies outside the marginal sinus in rats and mice. Human spleen also has a well-developed MZ,[78,101] but in this case the inner border of the blood sinusoidal system is located in the outer part of the MZ (Plate 2B).[103] Consequently the inner part is perfused by capillaries and belongs to the white pulp. Fine vessels branch off the central arterioles and feed into the MZ and red pulp blood sinusoids as well as the white pulp capillaries. Much of the white pulp is surrounded by MZ, but there are gaps in the MZ where the T zone links directly with the red pulp. These have been termed bridging channels and through these recirculating B and T cells return from the white pulp to the blood.[104] This area, particularly in mouse spleen, is associated with plasmablast growth during extrafollicular antibody responses (Plate 2E, F).[8,31] Recirculating T and B cells, leaving the white pulp, pass along the outside of these extrafollicular foci of plasmablasts.[19]

The red pulp structure

Outside the MZ blood passes through a filtering system provided by the macrophages attached to the cords of Billroth (Plate 2C). Blood passes over this macrophage bed before entering the open mouths of the venous sinuses that drain into the splenic vein. These macrophages of the cords of Billroth are highly efficient at removing opsonized particles, apoptotic cells, and effete red cells from the circulation. This efficiency can be seen in the spleens of patients with autoimmune cytopenias where opsonized blood cells are removed by these macrophages. Histologically, the spleens from these patients show those macrophages nearest the MZ engorged with blood cells while those nearest venous sinuses are empty. Thus this filter system works like an affinity column where the solution or suspension passes through increasingly less saturated absorbent.

In addition to the macrophages on the cords of Billroth the lymphocyte content of the red pulp is greater than one would expect from the lymphocyte content of the blood in the red pulp sinusoids. Many of these lymphocytes are IgD$^+$ B cells, but there is a prominent CD8$^+$ T cell population, which expresses little or no CD5. Within the spleen, hairy cell leukemia shows a striking predilection to accumulate in the splenic red pulp blood sinusoids without involving the white pulp. A physiological counterpart to this neoplasm has not been identified.

Immune responses in the spleen

Classically the spleen mounts antibody responses against antigens that gain access to the blood. Antigens given intravenously are clearly in the blood, but antigens given intraperitoneally also enter the blood rapidly. B cells passing through the blood should be able to bind antigen via their BCR. In addition, those B cells in the MZ and bone marrow B cells that are perfused by blood sinuses will also have access to blood-borne antigen. Although MZ B cells may engage antigen directly from the blood, it has been shown that immature DC have the capacity to transport intact bacterial antigens to MZ B cells.[105] B cells that have engaged antigen cross the marginal sinus and enter the outer T zone; there they are exquisitely efficient at interacting with primed T cells. For example, B cells taking up antigen from the blood have been shown to move to the outer

T zone of the spleen and make cognate interaction with primed T cells within 8 hours of intravenous immunization.[22] Marginal zone B cells responding to T-independent antigens show the same rapid translocation from the MZ to the outer T zone.[106] The kinetics of extrafollicular and follicular responses in the spleen are similar to those that have already been described for the LN. The main difference is that the spleen contains more MZ B cells and B1 cells. In addition, B1 cells that bind antigen in the peritoneal cavity can migrate to the spleen and mount an antibody response.[107] Extrafollicular responses by B1 cells can be very persistent and are associated with protracted proliferation of plasmablasts in extrafollicular foci. Recent studies suggest that there is also antigen-driven clonal expansion of B1 cells in response to certain T-independent antigens and that B cell clones expanded in this way can sustain extrafollicular antibody responses for months, without the need for replenishment by primary B lymphopoiesis.[100]

A proportion of plasma cells from GCs or extrafollicular foci that pass into the red pulp of the spleen find niches, which can sustain their long-term survival.[108,109] Analysis of the origin of these long-lived splenic plasma cells indicates that follicular and extrafollicular plasma cells compete with each other on an equal footing for these niches and there is no preference between switched and non-switched plasma cells.[35] More work is required to determine the nature of the signals that sustain plasma cell survival in these niches.

Immature B cell selection in the spleen

B cells are produced throughout life in the bone marrow of rodents and primates. The number produced[110] normally greatly exceeds the number required to sustain losses from the recirculating and MZ B cell pools.[111] Nevertheless, if there is selective depletion of peripheral B cells, the rate of repopulation from newly produced virgin B cells suggests that in this non-steady-state situation a high proportion of B cells can be selected to become mature recirculating or MZ B cells.[112] It appears that in steady-state conditions there is competition between newly produced naïve B cells for selection into the peripheral B cell pools. Studies using transgenic B cell receptors suggest that the affinity of immature B cells for ambient antigen influences positive selection into the recirculating or follicular B cells or B1 pools.[113–118] On the other hand, there is a likelihood of cells with strong affinity for soluble antigen failing to be selected,[119] while B cells binding cell-surface antigens are deleted if they are unable to lose autoreactivity by receptor editing.[120] Most cells other than those in the last category migrate to the spleen about 2 days after first expressing a BCR.[111] They enter the T zone but, unlike mature cells, fail to progress to follicles or the MZ unless they receive positive selection signals. The way in which immature B cells are selected to become MZ or recirculating B cells is still not well understood, but it seems likely that the process proceeds in the spleen. This does not seem to happen in LN, but there must be other sites of immature B cell selection as recirculating B cells are present in neonatally splenectomized rodents.

CONCLUDING REMARKS

The efficient working of the immune system depends on selective induction of lymphocyte proliferation and differentiation. Cell-cycle times of responding small lymphocytes can be as fast as 4 hours. In this situation it is critical that there is a constraint on growth. Examples of the way this happens are seen when the number of antigen-specific cells is artificially raised by the introduction in mice of transgenic antigen-specific receptors or the use of superantigens.[25,35] In both situations early excessive proliferation is followed by mass apoptosis, with the final number of effector and memory cells being similar to that in wild-type mice. Much of the control appears to be exercised by the cells and stroma of secondary lymphoid tissue. Genetic change resulting in at least partial independence from this control is key to lymphoma formation and progression.

KEY POINTS

- The lymph nodes and spleen together with other secondary lymphoid tissues provide sites where lymphocytes can encounter antigen and undergo regulated growth and differentiation.
- Regulation occurs through a requirement for naïve T cells to encounter antigen presented by dendritic cells in the T zone for them to be induced to proliferate and differentiate into one of a variety of effector cells or memory cells.
- Secondary lymphoid tissue provides sites where antigen-primed CD4 T cells can interact with B cells that have taken antigen through their surface immunoglobulin.
- B cells recruited into antibody responses either grow as plasmablasts in extrafollicular foci or form germinal centers.
- In germinal centers B cells mutate their immunoglobulin variable-region genes and then the cells with high affinity for antigen are positively selected and differentiate either into plasma cells or memory cells.
- Differences between CD4 and CD8 T cell responses are considered and the responses of recirculating, marginal zone B cells are compared with those of B1 cells.
- Mechanisms regulating lymphocyte proliferation, differentiation, and survival within secondary lymphoid tissues are considered in each section of the chapter.

REFERENCES

● = Key primary paper
◆ = Major review article

●1. Nieuwenhuis P, Ford WL. Comparative migration of B- and T-Lymphocytes in the rat spleen and LN. *Cell Immunol* 1976; **23**: 254–67.

●2. Katakai T, Hara T, Sugai M *et al.* LN fibroblastic reticular cells construct the stromal reticulum via contact with lymphocytes. *J Exp Med* 2004; **200**: 783–95.

●3. Gray D, MacLennan IC, Bazin H, Khan M. Migrant mu+ delta+ and static mu+ delta- B lymphocyte subsets. *Eur J Immunol* 1982; **12**: 564–9.

◆4. MacLennan IC. Germinal centers. *Annu Rev Immunol* 1994; **12**: 117–39.

●5. Mempel TR, Henrickson SE, Von Andrian UH. T-cell priming by DC in LN occurs in three distinct phases. *Nature* 2004; **427**: 154–9.

●6. MacLennan IC, Gulbranson-Judge A, Toellner KM *et al.* The changing preference of T and B cells for partners as T-dependent antibody responses develop. *Immunol Rev* 1997; **156**: 53–66.

●7. MacLennan IC, Liu YJ, Oldfield S *et al.* The evolution of B-cell clones. *Curr Top Microbiol Immunol* 1990; **159**: 37–63.

◆8. MacLennan IC, Toellner KM, Cunningham AF *et al.* Extrafollicular antibody responses. *Immunol Rev* 2003; **194**: 8–18.

●9. Warnock RA, Askari S, Butcher EC, von Andrian UH. Molecular mechanisms of lymphocyte homing to peripheral LN. *J Exp Med* 1998; **187**: 205–16.

●10. Berg EL, Mullowney AT, Andrew DP *et al.* Complexity and differential expression of carbohydrate epitopes associated with L-selectin recognition of high endothelial venules. *Am J Pathol* 1998; **152**: 469–77.

◆11. Miyasaka M, Tanaka T. Lymphocyte trafficking across high endothelial venules: dogmas and enigmas. *Nat Rev Immunol* 2004; **4**: 360–70.

◆12. Ebert LM, Schaerli P, Moser B. Chemokine-mediated control of T cell traffic in lymphoid and peripheral tissues. *Mol Immunol* 2005; **42**: 799–809.

●13. Howard JC. The life-span and recirculation of marrow-derived small lymphocytes from the rat thoracic duct. *J Exp Med* 1972; **135**: 185–99.

●14. Breitfeld D, Ohl L, Kremmer E *et al.* Follicular B helper T cells express CXC chemokine receptor 5, localize to B cell follicles, and support Ig production. *J Exp Med* 2000; **192**: 1545–52.

●15. Wykes M, Pombo A, Jenkins C, MacPherson GG. DC interact directly with naive B lymphocytes to transfer antigen and initiate class switching in a primary T-dependent response. *J Immunol* 1998; **161**: 1313–19.

●16. Williams MB, Butcher EC. Homing of naive and memory T lymphocyte subsets to Peyer's patches, LN, and spleen. *J Immunol* 1997; **159**: 1746–52.

17. Campbell DJ, Butcher EC. Rapid acquisition of tissue-specific homing phenotypes by CD4(+) T cells activated in cutaneous or mucosal lymphoid tissues. *J Exp Med* 2002; **195**: 135–41.

18. McSorley SJ, Asch S, Costalonga M *et al.* Tracking salmonella-specific CD4 T cells in vivo reveals a local mucosal response to a disseminated infection. *Immunity* 2002; **16**: 365–77.

19. Gulbranson-Judge A, MacLennan I. Sequential antigen-specific growth of T cells in the T zones and follicles in response to pigeon cytochrome c. *Eur J Immunol* 1996; **26**: 1830–7.

20. Garside P, Ingulli E, Merica RR *et al.* Visualization of specific B and T lymphocyte interactions in the LN. *Science* 1998; **281**: 96–9.

21. Campbell DJ, Kim CH, Butcher EC. Separable effector T cell populations specialized for B cell help or tissue inflammation. *Nat Immunol* 2001; **2**: 876–81.

22. Toellner KM, Gulbranson-Judge A, Taylor DR *et al.* Ig switch transcript production in vivo related to the site and time of antigen-specific B cell activation. *J Exp Med* 1996; **183**: 2303–12.

23. Casamayor-Palleja M, Mondiere P, Verschelde C *et al.* BCR ligation reprograms B cells for migration to the T zone and B-cell follicle sequentially. *Blood* 2002; **99**: 1913–21.

24. Croft M, Duncan DD, Swain SL. Response of naive antigen-specific CD4+ T cells in vitro: characteristics and antigen-presenting cell requirements. *J Exp Med* 1992; **176**: 1431–7.

25. Luther SA, Gulbranson-Judge A, Acha-Orbea H, MacLennan IC. Viral superantigen drives extrafollicular and follicular B cell differentiation leading to virus-specific antibody production. *J Exp Med* 1997; **185**: 551–62.

26. Jacob J, Kelsoe G. In situ studies of the primary immune response to (4-hydroxy-3-nitrophenyl)acetyl. II. A common clonal origin for periarteriolar lymphoid sheath-associated foci and GC. *J Exp Med* 1992; **176**: 679–87.

27. Coico RF, Bhogal BS, Thorbecke GJ. Relationship of GC in lymphoid tissue to immunologic memory. VI. Transfer of B cell memory with LN cells fractionated according to their receptors for peanut agglutinin. *J Immunol* 1983; **131**: 2254–7.

28. Klaus GG, Humphrey JH. The generation of memory cells. I. The role of C3 in the generation of B memory cells. *Immunology* 1977; **33**: 31–40.

29. Jacob J, Kelsoe G, Rajewsky K, Weisses U. Intraclonal generation of antibody mutants in germinal centres. *Nature* 1991; **354**: 389–92.

30. MacLennan IC, Gray D. Antigen-driven selection of virgin and memory B cells. *Immunol Rev* 1986; **91**: 61–85.

31. Jacob J, Kassir R, Kelsoe G. In situ studies of the primary immune response to (4-hydroxy-3-nitrophenyl)acetyl. I. The architecture and dynamics of responding cell populations. *J Exp Med* 1991; **173**: 1165–75.

32. Jung S, Rajewsky K, Radbruch A. Shutdown of class switch recombination by deletion of a switch region control element. *Science* 1993; **259**: 984–7.

33. Shaffer AL, Lin KI, Kuo TC *et al.* Blimp-1 orchestrates plasma cell differentiation by extinguishing the mature B cell gene expression program. *Immunity* 2002; **17**: 51–62.

34. Muramatsu M, Kinoshita K, Fagarasan S *et al.* Class switch recombination and hypermutation require activation-induced cytidine deaminase (AID), a potential RNA editing enzyme. *Cell* 2000; **102**: 553–63.

35. Sze DM, Toellner KM, Garcia de Vinuesa C *et al.* Intrinsic constraint on plasmablast growth and extrinsic limits of plasma cell survival. *J Exp Med* 2000; **192**: 813–21.

36. Smith KG, Hewitson TD, Nossal GJ, Tarlinton DM. The phenotype and fate of the antibody-forming cells of the splenic foci. *Eur J Immunol* 1996; **26**: 444–8.

37. Kroese FG, Wubbena AS, Seijen HG, Nieuwenhuis P. GC develop oligoclonally. *Eur J Immunol* 1987; **17**: 1069–72.

38. Liu YJ, Zhang J, Lane PJ *et al.* Sites of specific B cell activation in primary and secondary responses to T cell-dependent and T cell-independent antigens. *Eur J Immunol* 1991; **21**: 2951–62.

39. Carragher D, Johal R, Button A *et al.* A stroma-derived defect in NF-kappaB2-/- mice causes impaired LN development and lymphocyte recruitment. *J Immunol* 2004; **173**: 2271–9.

40. Futterer A, Mink K, Luz A *et al.* The lymphotoxin beta receptor controls organogenesis and affinity maturation in peripheral lymphoid tissues. *Immunity* 1998; **9**: 59–70.

41. Endres R, Alimzhanov MB, Plitz T *et al.* Mature follicular DC networks depend on expression of lymphotoxin beta receptor by radioresistant stromal cells and of lymphotoxin beta and tumor necrosis factor by B cells. *J Exp Med* 1999; **189**: 159–68.

42. Ansel KM, Ngo VN, Hyman PL *et al.* A chemokine-driven positive feedback loop organizes lymphoid follicles. *Nature* 2000; **406**: 309–14.

43. Mandel TE, Phipps RP, Abbot A, Tew JG. The follicular DC: long term antigen retention during immunity. *Immunol Rev* 1980; **53**: 29–59.

44. Tew JG, Mandel TE, Phipps RP, Szakal AK. Tissue localization and retention of antigen in relation to the immune response. *Am J Anat* 1984; **170**: 407–20.

45. Brown JC, De Jesus DG, Holborow EJ, Harris G. Lymphocyte-mediated transport of aggregated human gamma-globulin into germinal centre areas of normal mouse spleen. *Nature* 1970; **228**: 367–9.

46. Gray D, Kumararatne DS, Lortan J *et al.* Relation of intra-splenic migration of MZ B cells to antigen localization on follicular DC. *Immunology* 1984; **52**: 659–69.

47. Carroll MC. The role of complement and complement receptors in induction and regulation of immunity. *Annu Rev Immunol* 1998; **16**: 545–68.

●48. Hardie DL, Johnson GD, Khan M, MacLennan IC. Quantitative analysis of molecules which distinguish functional compartments within GC. *Eur J Immunol* 1993; **23**: 997–1004.

●49. Brachtel EF, Washiyama M, Johnson GD *et al.* Differences in the germinal centres of palatine tonsils and LN. *Scand J Immunol* 1996; **43**: 239–47.

●50. Reljic R, Wagner SD, Peakman LJ, Fearon DT. Suppression of signal transducer and activator of transcription 3-dependent B lymphocyte terminal differentiation by BCL-6. *J Exp Med* 2000; **192**: 1841–8.

●51. Kuppers R, Zhao M, Hansmann ML, Rajewsky K. Tracing B cell development in human germinal centres by molecular analysis of single cells picked from histological sections. *EMBO J* 1993; **12**: 4955–67.

●52. Hanna MG. An autoradiographic study of the germinal center in spleen white pulp during early intervals of the immune response. *Lab Invest* 1964; **13**: 95–104.

●53. Casamayor-Palleja M, Feuillard J, Ball J *et al.* Centrocytes rapidly adopt a memory B cell phenotype on co-culture with autologous germinal centre T cell-enriched preparations. *Int Immunol* 1996; **8**: 737–44.

●54. Casamayor-Palleja M, Khan M, MacLennan IC. A subset of CD4+ memory T cells contains preformed CD40 ligand that is rapidly but transiently expressed on their surface after activation through the T cell receptor complex. *J Exp Med* 1995; **181**: 1293–301.

●55. Dilosa RM, Maeda K, Masuda A *et al.* GC B cells and antibody production in the bone marrow. *J Immunol* 1991; **146**: 4071–7.

●56. Liu YJ, Joshua DE, Williams GT *et al.* Mechanism of antigen-driven selection in germinal centres. *Nature* 1989; **342**: 929–31.

●57. Berek C, Griffiths GM, Milstein C. Molecular events during maturation of the immune response to oxazolone. *Nature* 1985; **316**: 412–18.

●58. Griffiths GM, Berek C, Kaartinen M, Milstein C. Somatic mutation and the maturation of immune response to 2-phenyl oxazolone. *Nature* 1984; **312**: 271–5.

●59. Liu YJ, Mason DY, Johnson GD *et al.* GC cells express bcl-2 protein after activation by signals which prevent their entry into apoptosis. *Eur J Immunol* 1991; **21**: 1905–10.

●60. Petrasch SG, Kosco MH, Perez-Alvarez CJ *et al.* Proliferation of GC B lymphocytes in vitro by direct membrane contact with follicular DC. *Immunobiology* 1991; **183**: 451–62.

●61. Arpin C, Dechanet J, Van Kooten C *et al.* Generation of memory B cells and plasma cells in vitro. *Science* 1995; **268**: 720–2.

●62. Yellin MJ, Sippel K, Inghirami G *et al.* CD40 molecules induce down-modulation and endocytosis of T cell surface T cell-B cell activating molecule/CD40-L. Potential role in regulating helper effector function. *J Immunol* 1994; **152**: 598–608.

●63. Liu YJ, Malisan F, de Bouteiller O *et al.* Within GC, isotype switching of Ig genes occurs after the onset of somatic mutation. *Immunity* 1996; **4**: 241–50.

●64. Pascual V, Liu YJ, Magalski A *et al.* Analysis of somatic mutation in five B cell subsets of human tonsil. *J Exp Med* 1994; **180**: 329–39.

●65. Walker LS, Wiggett HE, Gaspal FM *et al.* Established T cell-driven GC B cell proliferation is independent of CD28 signaling but is tightly regulated through CTLA-4. *J Immunol* 2003; **170**: 91–8.

●66. Kamath AT, Henri S, Battye F *et al.* Developmental kinetics and lifespan of DC in mouse lymphoid organs. *Blood* 2002; **100**: 1734–41.

◆67. Shortman K, Heath WR. Immunity or tolerance? That is the question for DC. *Nat Immunol* 2001; **2**: 988–9.

◆68. Steinman RM, Hawiger D, Nussenzweig MC, *et al.* Tolerogenic dendritic cells. *Annu Rev Immunol* 2003; **21**: 685–711.

◆69. Ardavin C, Martinez del Hoyo G, Martin P *et al.* Origin and differentiation of DC. *Trends Immunol* 2001; **22**: 691–700.

◆70. Shortman K, Liu YJ. Mouse and human DC subtypes. *Nat Rev Immunol* 2002; **2**: 151–61.

◆71. Wilson NS, Villadangos JA. Lymphoid organ DC: beyond the Langerhans cells paradigm. *Immunol Cell Biol* 2004; **82**: 91–8.

◆72. Pulendran B. Immune activation: death, danger and DC. *Curr Biol* 2004; **14**: R30–2.

●73. Henri S, Vremec D, Kamath A *et al.* The DC populations of mouse LN. *J Immunol* 2001; **167**: 741–8.

◆74. Larsen CP, Morris PJ, Austyn JM. Migration of dendritic leukocytes from cardiac allografts into host spleens. A novel pathway for initiation of rejection. *J Exp Med* 1990; **171**: 307–14.

●75. Itano AA, McSorley SJ, Reinhardt RL *et al.* Distinct DC populations sequentially present antigen to CD4 T cells and stimulate different aspects of cell-mediated immunity. *Immunity* 2003; **19**: 47–57.

●76. Stein H, Bonk A, Tolksdorf G *et al.* Immunohistologic analysis of the organization of normal lymphoid tissue and non-Hodgkin's lymphomas. *J Histochem Cytochem* 1980; **28**: 746–60.

●77. Liu YJ, Oldfield S, MacLennan IC. Thymus-independent type 2 responses in lymph nodes. *Adv Exp Med Biol* 1988; **237**: 113–17.

◆78. MacLennan IC, Liu YJ. Marginal zone B cells respond both to polysaccharide antigens and protein antigens. *Res Immunol* 1991; **142**: 346–51.

●79. Spencer J, Finn T, Pulford KA *et al.* The human gut contains a novel population of B lymphocytes which resemble marginal zone cells. *Clin Exp Immunol* 1985; **62**: 607–12.

●80. Liu YJ, Barthelemy C, de Bouteiller O *et al.* Memory B cells from human tonsils colonize mucosal epithelium and directly present antigen to T cells by rapid up-regulation of B7-1 and B7-2.PG. *Immunity* 1995; **2**: 239–48.

◆81. Watts C. Capture and processing of exogenous antigens for presentation on MHC molecules. *Annu Rev Immunol* 1997; **15**: 821–50.

●82. Miller MJ, Safrina O, Parker I, Cahalan MD. Imaging the single cell dynamics of CD4+ T cell activation by dendritic cells in lymph nodes. *J Exp Med* 2004; **200**: 847–56.

●83. Jung S, Unutmaz D, Wong P *et al*. In vivo depletion of CD11c(+) dendritic cells abrogates priming of CD8(+) T cells by exogenous cell-associated antigens. *Immunity* 2002; **17**: 211–20.

●84. Ackerman AL, Kyritsis C, Tampe R, Cresswell P. Access of soluble antigens to the endoplasmic reticulum can explain cross-presentation by dendritic cells. *Nat Immunol* 2005; **6**: 107–13.

●85. Schoenberger SP, Toes RE, van der Voort EI *et al*. T-cell help for cytotoxic T lymphocytes is mediated by CD40-CD40L interactions. *Nature* 1998; **393**: 480–3.

●86. Ridge JP, Di Rosa F, Matzinger P. A conditioned dendritic cell can be a temporal bridge between a CD4+ T-helper and a T-killer cell. *Nature* 1998; **393**: 474–8.

◆87. Lanzavecchia A. Immunology. Licence to kill. *Nature* 1998; **393**: 413–14.

●88. Bourgeois C, Rocha B, Tanchot C. A role for CD40 expression on CD8+ T cells in the generation of CD8+ T cell memory. *Science* 2002; **297**: 2060–3.

●89. Smith CM, Wilson NS, Waithman J *et al*. Cognate CD4(+) T cell licensing of dendritic cells in CD8(+) T cell immunity. *Nat Immunol* 2004; **5**: 1143–8.

●90. Kaech SM, Ahmed R. Memory CD8+ T cell differentiation: initial antigen encounter triggers a developmental program in naive cells. *Nat Immunol* 2001; **2**: 415–22.

●91. van Stipdonk MJ, Lemmens EE, Schoenberger SP. Naive CTLs require a single brief period of antigenic stimulation for clonal expansion and differentiation. *Nat Immunol* 2001; **2**: 423–9.

●92. Obst R, van Santen HM, Mathis D, Benoist C. Antigen persistence is required throughout the expansion phase of a CD4(+) T cell response. *J Exp Med* 2005; **201**: 1555–65.

●93. Bajenoff M, Wurtz O, Guerder S. Repeated antigen exposure is necessary for the differentiation, but not the initial proliferation, of naive CD4(+) T cells. *J Immunol* 2002; **168**: 1723–9.

●94. Mebius RE, Rennert P, Weissman IL. Developing LN collect CD4+CD3- LTbeta+ cells that can differentiate to APC, NK cells, and follicular cells but not T or B cells. *Immunity* 1997; **7**: 493–504.

●95. Cupedo T, Mebius RE. Cellular interactions in lymph node development. *J Immunol* 2005; **174**: 21–5.

●96. Fukushima N, Nishina H, Koishihara Y, Ohkawa H. Enhanced hematopoiesis in vivo and in vitro by splenic stromal cells derived from the mouse with recombinant granulocyte colony-stimulating factor. *Blood* 1992; **80**: 1914–22.

●97. Yanai N, Satoh T, Obinata M. Endothelial cells create a hematopoietic inductive microenvironment preferential to erythropoiesis in the mouse spleen. *Cell Struct Funct* 1991; **16**: 87–93.

●98. Wilkins BS, Green A, Wild AE, Jones DB. Extramedullary haemopoiesis in fetal and adult human spleen: a quantitative immunohistological study. *Histopathology* 1994; **24**: 241–7.

●99. Cinamon G, Zachariah MA, Lam OM *et al*. Follicular shuttling of marginal zone B cells facilitates antigen transport. *Nat Immunol* 2008; **9**: 54–62.

●100. Hsu MC, Toellner KM, Vinuesa CG, MacLennan IC. B cell clones that sustain long-term plasmablast growth in T-independent extrafollicular antibody responses. *Proc Natl Acad Sci U S A* 2006; **103**: 5905–10.

●101. Kraal G, Schornagel K, Streeter PR *et al*. Expression of the mucosal vascular addressin, MAdCAM-1, on sinus-lining cells in the spleen. *Am J Pathol* 1995; **147**: 763–71.

●102. Lortan JE, Oldfield S, Roobottom CA, MacLennan IC. Migration of newly-produced virgin B cells from bone marrow to secondary lymphoid organs. *Adv Exp Med Biol* 1988; **237**: 87–92.

●103. Steiniger B, Barth P, Hellinger A. The perifollicular and marginal zone of the human splenic white pulp: do fibroblasts guide lymphocyte immigration? *Am J Pathol* 2001; **159**: 501–12.

●104. Mitchell J. Lymphocyte circulation in the spleen. Marginal zone bridging channels and their possible role in cell traffic. *Immunology* 1973; **24**: 93–107.

●105. Balazs M, Martin F, Zhou T, Kearney JF. Blood dendritic cells interact with splenic marginal zone B cells to initiate T-independent immune responses. *Immunity* 2002; **17**: 341–52.

●106. Vinuesa CG, Sunners Y, Pongracz J *et al*. Tracking the response of Xid B cells in vivo: TI-2 antigen induces migration and proliferation but Btk is essential for terminal differentiation. *Eur J Immunol* 2001; **31**: 1340–50.

●107. Watanabe N, Ikuta K, Fagarasan S *et al*. Migration and differentiation of autoreactive B-1 cells induced by activated gamma/delta T cells in antierythrocyte Ig transgenic mice. *J Exp Med* 2000; **192**: 1577–86.

●108. Manz RA, Lohning M, Cassese G *et al*. Survival of long-lived plasma cells is independent of antigen. *Int Immunol* 1998; **10**: 1703–11.

●109. Slifka MK, Antia R, Whitmire JK, Ahmed R. Humoral immunity due to long-lived plasma cells. *Immunity* 1998; **8**: 363–72.

●110. Osmond DG, Nossal GJ. Differentiation of lymphocytes in mouse bone marrow. II. Kinetics of maturation and renewal of antiglobulin-binding cells studied by double labeling. *Cell Immunol* 1974; **13**: 132–45.

●111. Chan EY, MacLennan IC. Only a small proportion of splenic B cells in adults are short-lived virgin cells. *Eur J Immunol* 1993; **23**: 357–63.

●112. Bazin H, Platteau B, MacLennan IC *et al*. B cell production in adult rats. *Adv Exp Med Biol* 1985; **186**: 65–71.

●113. Kretschmer K, Jungebloud A, Stopkowicz J *et al*. The selection of marginal zone B cells differs from that of B-1a cells. *J Immunol* 2003; **171**: 6495–501.

●114. Dammers PM, Kroese FG. Recruitment and selection of marginal zone B cells is independent of exogenous antigens. *Eur J Immunol* 2005; **35**: 2089–99.

◆115. Pillai S, Cariappa A, Moran ST. Positive selection and lineage commitment during peripheral B-lymphocyte development. *Immunol Rev* 2004; **197**: 206–18.

●116. Schneider P, Takatsuka H, Wilson A *et al.* Maturation of marginal zone and follicular B cells requires B cell activating factor of the tumor necrosis factor family and is independent of B cell maturation antigen. *J Exp Med* 2001; **194**: 1691–7.

●117. Baker N, Ehrenstein MR. Cutting edge: selection of B lymphocyte subsets is regulated by natural IgM. *J Immunol* 2002; **169**: 6686–90.

◆118. Allman D, Srivastava B, Lindsley RC. Alternative routes to maturity: branch points and pathways for generating follicular and marginal zone B cells. *Immunol Rev* 2004; **197**: 147–60.

●119. Cyster JG, Hartley SB, Goodnow CC. Competition for follicular niches excludes self-reactive cells from the recirculating B-cell repertoire. *Nature* 1994; **371**: 389–95.

●120. Hartley SB, Crosbie J, Brink R *et al.* Elimination from peripheral lymphoid tissues of self-reactive B lymphocytes recognizing membrane-bound antigens. *Nature* 1991; **353**: 765–9.

●121. Banerji S, Ni J, Wang SX *et al.* LYVE-1, a new homologue of the CD44 glycoprotein, is a lymph-specific receptor for hyaluronan. *J Cell Biol* 1999; **144**: 789–801.

13

Cellular immunobiology of extranodal lymphoid tissue

NADINE CERF–BENSUSSAN AND VALÉRIE GABORIAU-ROUTHIAU

INTRODUCTION

Immunologic homeostasis along the vast expanse of the mucosal epithelial surface is maintained by the mucosal immune system. This complex system, built up during the millions of years of coevolution with environmental antigens, promotes mutualistic interactions with commensal bacteria and tolerance to dietary or inhaled antigens and simultaneously functions as a potent first line of defense against invading pathogens.

The mucosal immune system can be schematically divided into inductive sites – where antigens sampled from mucosal surface stimulate cognate naïve T and B lymphocytes – and effector sites, where the effector cells, after extravasation and differentiation, can exert mature immune functions including production of antibodies and cytokines or cytotoxicity. Inductive sites comprise organized mucosal-associated lymphoid tissues and local/regional mucosa draining lymph nodes. The effector sites consist of different histologic compartments including lamina propria (LP) of various mucosae, the stroma of exocrine glands, and surface epithelia. The concept of Mucosal-Associated Lymphoid Tissues (MALT) originated from adoptive transfer experiments in mice suggesting that B cells derived from mesenteric and, to a lesser degree, from mediastinal or bronchial lymph nodes gave rise to immunoglobulin A

(IgA)-secreting cells that distributed into different mucosae.[1] MALT was therefore largely used as a synonym for 'common' mucosal immune system. The demonstration that mucosal immune responses are more compartmentalized than initially thought led to the revision of this concept and it was recently recommended that the term MALT be restricted to the organized lymphoid follicles and aggregates that are the origin of lymphocytes trafficking to mucosal effector sites and have in common the lack of afferent lymphatics and the ability to sample exogenous antigens directly from mucosal surfaces through a characteristic follicle-associated epithelium.[2,3] The most typical MALT structure is represented by Peyer's patches (PPs) in the mammalian small intestine. A large number of related structures are, however, described and subdivided according to anatomic regions. Their distribution and composition vary considerably with species. Their development is profoundly influenced by antigenic stimuli but also varies depending on the considered structures. Thus, PPs in humans and rodents, and tonsils in humans, initiate their development prenatally while other structures develop only after birth. This chapter will primarily focus on gut-associated lymphoid tissues (GALT), the best-studied part of the MALT, and then more briefly describe related structures associated with the oral cavity and the nasopharynx (represented by the Waldeyer's ring in humans) and with the bronchi (bronchi-associated lymphoid tissue; BALT). We will also summarize current views on the mechanisms that drive lymphocyte homing from inductive to mucosal effector sites and control the preferential differentiation of IgA-secreting cells in mucosal sites, and discuss how IgA and effector T cells may contribute to the protection of mucosae.

GUT–ASSOCIATED LYMPHOID TISSUE

Gut-associated lymphoid tissue comprises the PPs, the appendix, and isolated lymphoid follicles (ILFs), which are considered inductive sites for mucosal B and T cells. Lymphocyte-filled villi are rare T cell-dominated structures of unknown function described in the small intestine of rats and humans.[4] Cryptopatches have been described exclusively in mice and were initially thought to be the origin of a subset of intraepithelial lymphocytes. They more likely represent the precursors of murine ILFs. We will therefore focus our description on PPs and ILFs.

Peyer's patches

Peyer's patches, first described by Peyer in the seventeenth century, consist of a variable number of aggregated lymphoid follicles (from 5 to over 200) located at regular intervals on the antimesenteric border of the small intestine. In humans, they predominate in the ileum. Their central role in the induction of intestinal immune responses was demonstrated by the seminal experiments of Craig and Cebra who showed that isolated PPs lymphocytes from irradiated rabbits were able to repopulate the LP in IgA plasma cells.[5]

ONTOGENY OF PEYER'S PATCHES

The human PP precursor, composed of CD4$^+$ dendritic cells, can be seen at 11 weeks of gestation, and discrete T and B cell areas are visible between 16 and 19 weeks. Before birth, only primary follicles containing CD19$^+$ CD20$^+$ lymphocytes with a naïve phenotype (surface IgD$^+$/IgM$^+$) can be found and, except in cases of antenatal infections, no secondary follicles with germinal centers can be detected, emphasizing their dependency on antigenic stimulation. In humans, the number of macroscopically visible PPs increases from 50 at the beginning of the last trimester of pregnancy to 100 at birth. Their number is maximal (~250) in the mid-teens and decreases to ~100 after 70 years (for review, see [2]).

The multiple factors and successive steps involved in the antenatal development of PPs (Fig. 13.1) have been determined using mutant mice with defective lymphoid organogenesis. These studies indicate that the formation of PPs depends on the colonization of the gut wall during embryogenesis by hematopoietic lymphoid tissue inducers

(LTi) cells, which, following their interactions with resident stromal lymphoid tissue organizer (LTo) cells, aggregate on embryonic day 16.5 to generate PP precursors at sites where lymphatics have developed by budding and sprouting from venous endothelium, a step occurring between days 10.5 and 15.5 (for review, see [6,7]). Lymphoid tissue inducer cells express CD44, CD45, Thy-1, interleukin-7 receptor α (IL7-Rα), and KIT, but no other lineage markers except CD4, which is present on 50 to 75 percent of them. They are also characterized by the expression of the retinoic acid receptor-related orphan receptor γt (RORγt), a receptor indispensable for the appearance of LTi and the subsequent development of lymph nodes and PPs.[8] Lymphoid tissue inducer cells are detected at mouse embryonic day 12.5 in the proximal part of the intestine and are found in the whole intestinal wall by day 15.5 where they remain scattered. A recent study suggests that their aggregation is triggered by a subset of LTi cells, first detected on day 15.5, that lacks CD4 but expresses the dendritic marker CD11c and the receptor kinase Ret. This study further shows that signaling via Ret, initially known for its key role in the development of the mammalian enteric system, is also mandatory to initiate the aggregation of LTi cells and the formation of PPs' anlagen. Notably, one Ret ligand, ARTN, was detected in resident stromal LTo cells, suggesting that its release may induce the aggregation of LTi cells in predefined sites containing LTo cells.[9] Clustering of LTi cells may also be favored by the interactions of the integrin $\alpha_4\beta_1$ and the chemokine receptor CXCR5 on LTi cells with their respective ligands VCAM-1 and the CXCL13 chemokine produced by LTo cells.[7] The activation of PP LTi cells leads to the production of IL-7. This cytokine can be released by adjacent epithelial cells and may upregulate the production of the membrane lymphotoxin (LT) $\alpha1\beta2$ by LTi cells.[7] Via this cytokine, crucial for the subsequent steps of PPs development, LTi cells activate the LTβ receptor expressed on stromal LTo, initiating a signaling cascade leading to nuclear factor κB (NF-κB) activation through two pathways, one of which involves the kinase NIK, mandatory for the development of PPs and lymph nodes. Studies in mutant mice also point to the complementary role in NF-κB activation of the tumor necrosis factor (TNF) receptor p55 interacting either with TNFα, or with LTα3.[7] Nuclear factor κB activation then promotes the induction of VCAM-1 on LTo cells and induces their expression of several chemokines central in the anatomical and functional organization of the PPs and lymph nodes, including CXCL12 (SDF1), CXCL13, CCL19 (ELC), and CCL21 (SLC).[7,10] Activation of LTo cells thus results in positive feedback leading to further recruitment of LTi cells and later, between mouse embryonic days 17.5 and 18.5, of B and T cells (some of which also express LTα1β2) and of dendritic cells. The growing PPs partition subsequently into B cell follicles and T cell areas and develop high endothelial venules (HEVs) for the retention of circulating naïve lymphocytes.[6] Nevertheless PPs remain very small and unstimulated until

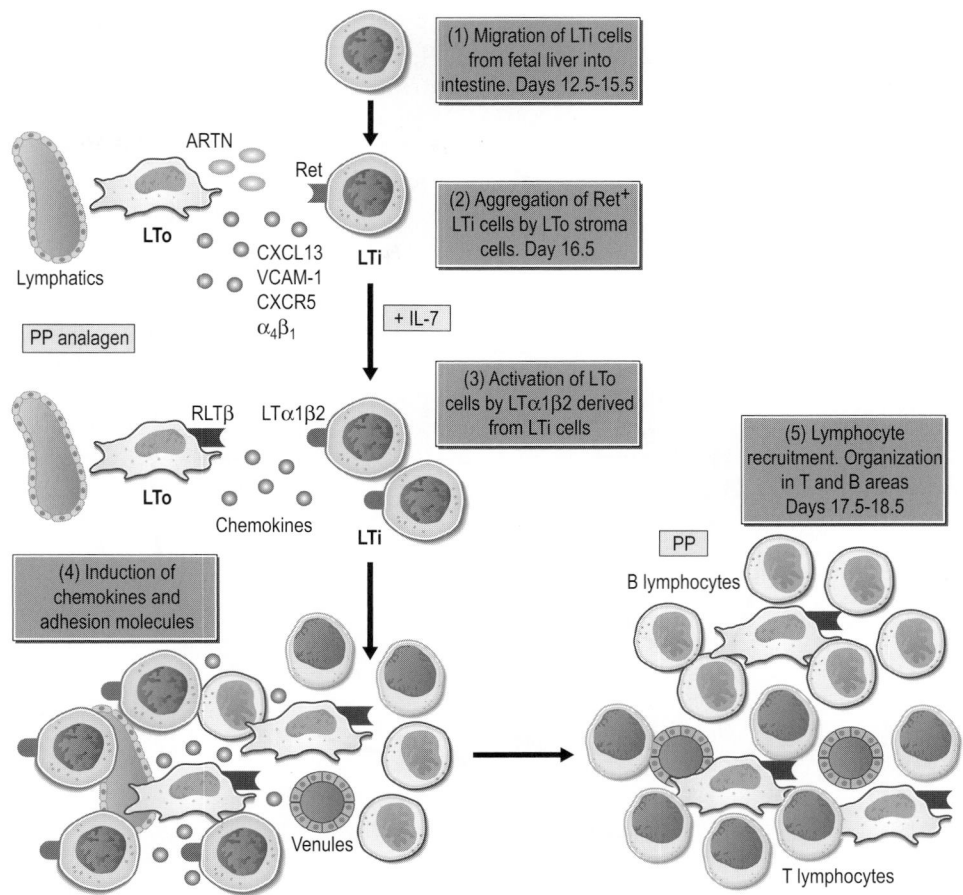

Figure 13.1   Main steps in the antenatal development of Peyer's patches (PPs) in mice. Between days 12.5 and 15.5 of gestation, lymphoid tissue inducer cells (LTi) of hematopoietic origin colonize the intestine from its proximal to distal parts. On day 16.5, LTi cells aggregate at sites where lymphatics have developed and which contain stromal lymphoid tissue organizer (LTo) cells. Aggregation is favored by signaling via Ret, expressed by a subset of LTi cells, and its ligand ARTN produced by LTo cells. Aggregation of LTi cells may also be promoted by CCL13, a chemokine produced by LTo cells and the integrin $\alpha_4\beta_1$ interacting with VCAM-1 on LTo cells. Subsequently, the NF-κB signaling cascade is triggered in LTo cells by LTi-derived lymphotoxin (LT) $\alpha1\beta2$, stimulating their expression of VCAM-1 and their production of several chemokines that promote lymphocyte recruitment and lymph node organogenesis. Differentiation of the epithelium overlaying the nascent follicle is initiated antenatally by unknown signals, probably derived from B cells. PPs remain small until birth when commensal bacteria stimulate the formation of germinal centers and the expansion of T cell areas.

birth. They develop further upon exposure to intraluminal bacteria that drive the proliferation of B and T blasts and result in the appearance of germinal centers and expansion of T areas.[11]

Parallel to the antenatal development of lymphoid follicles, differentiation of the overlying epithelium and of M cells (specialized epithelial cells – see below) probably occurs. *In vivo* studies in SCID mice and *in vitro* studies with human cells indeed indicate that PPs lymphocytes can induce the conversion of regular small intestinal epithelium into follicle-associated epithelium (FAE),[12] and M cells are observed before birth over PPs.[13] The nature of the inducing signals provided by the lymphocytes remains unknown although there is evidence of a prominent role of B cells.[14] As for the lymphoid tissue, antigenic stimulation can modulate the differentiation of the FAE: thus the number

of M cells in the FAE of rabbit PPs increased within 30 minutes after microbial challenge parallel to the recruitment of B cells in the FAE.[15]

FUNCTIONAL ANATOMY OF MATURE PEYER'S PATCHES

The organization of mature PPs, only partially overlapping with that of peripheral lymph nodes, serves their function in the induction of mucosal immune responses. In contrast to lymph nodes, they have no capsule, medulla, or afferent lymphatics. Made of a variable number of B follicles (5 to 200) separated by interfollicular T cell areas, they possess one specific area, the dome located over the B follicles (Fig. 13.2). This region deprived of villi directly bulges into the lumen and is overlaid by the FAE specialized in the sampling of intraluminal antigens.

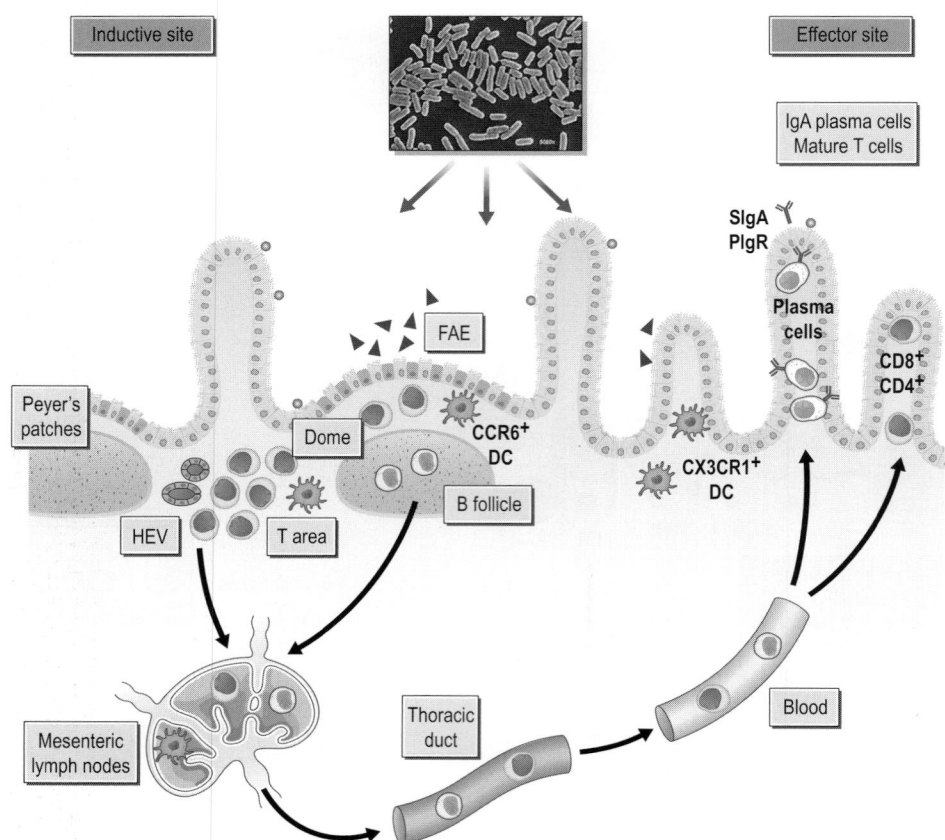

Figure 13.2   Functional organization of the intestinal immune system. Intraluminal antigens enter the mucosa, preferentially via the follicle-associated epithelium (FAE) covering the Peyers' patches (PPs) but also at a distance from PPs, either (in the case of soluble antigens) by epithelial endocytosis or (in the case of bacteria) via CX3CR1$^+$ dendritic cells (DC) that can emit dendrites between ileal epithelial cells. In PPs, intraluminal antigens are transported across M cells and delivered into the subepithelial area of the dome where they are captured by immature CCR6$^+$ DCs. The latter cells migrate toward the interfollicular T areas where they initiate T and B cell responses from naïve blood-derived lymphocytes recently migrated across high endothelial venules (HEV). B cells then migrate toward the B follicle where they undergo immunoglobulin class switch from IgM to IgA and somatic hypermutations. Activated T cells proliferate in the T areas. T and B cells leave PPs by the lymphatic network toward the mesenteric lymph nodes (MLNs). DCs loaded with antigens in lamina propria (LP) and PPs can migrate toward MLNs, where they can also initiate the activation of naïve B and T cells. After a short stay in MLNs, lymphocytes reenter lymphatics and join the thoracic duct that delivers them into the superior vena cava. Small lymphocytes are then distributed, via the bloodstream, to all lymphoid organs, while B and T blasts activated in PPs and MLNs preferentially home back into the intestinal mucosa due to their expression of gut-homing receptors acquired during their activation (see Fig. 13.3). Upon migration into LP, B blasts mature into plasma cells that preferentially secrete dimeric IgA. Polymeric IgA is transcytosed across epithelial cells by the polymeric immunoglobulin receptor (PIgR) and secreted into the lumen as secretory IgA (SIgA) associated with the external part of this receptor. After migration in the mucosa, CD4$^+$ T cells remain in the LP and differentiate into cytokine-producing cells. CD8$^+$ T cells migrate predominantly into the epithelium and can secrete cytokines or exert cytotoxic functions. For simplicity, isolated lymphoid follicles are not represented in this scheme; their role is discussed in the text.

ENTRANCE AND DISTRIBUTION OF LYMPHOCYTES INTO THE PEYER'S PATCHES

As in peripheral lymph nodes, PPs B and T lymphocytes are constantly renewed from the pool of circulating small lymphocytes. They enter the PPs in the interfollicular area through HEVs via the classical multistep process involving rolling, chemokine-mediated activation, and firm adherence, followed by transendothelial migration (Fig. 13.3). In PPs, these interactions involve the mucosal addressin MAdCAM-1 on the endothelium, and L-selectin (CD62L)

and the integrins $\alpha_4\beta_7$ and, to a lesser degree, LFA-1 on lymphocytes. Rolling is due to the interactions of MAdCAM-1 with $\alpha_4\beta_7$ weakly expressed on naïve lymphocytes and with CD62L able to interact with the glycosylated residues that decorate MAdCAM-1 in PPs. The second step of firm adhesion is mediated by $\alpha_4\beta_7$ and LFA-1 upon activation of their avidity conformation by $G_{\alpha i}$-induced signaling provided via the CCR7 receptor (for review, see[16,17]). CCR7 is expressed by naïve lymphocytes and a subset of memory T cells and is activated locally by its ligands, the

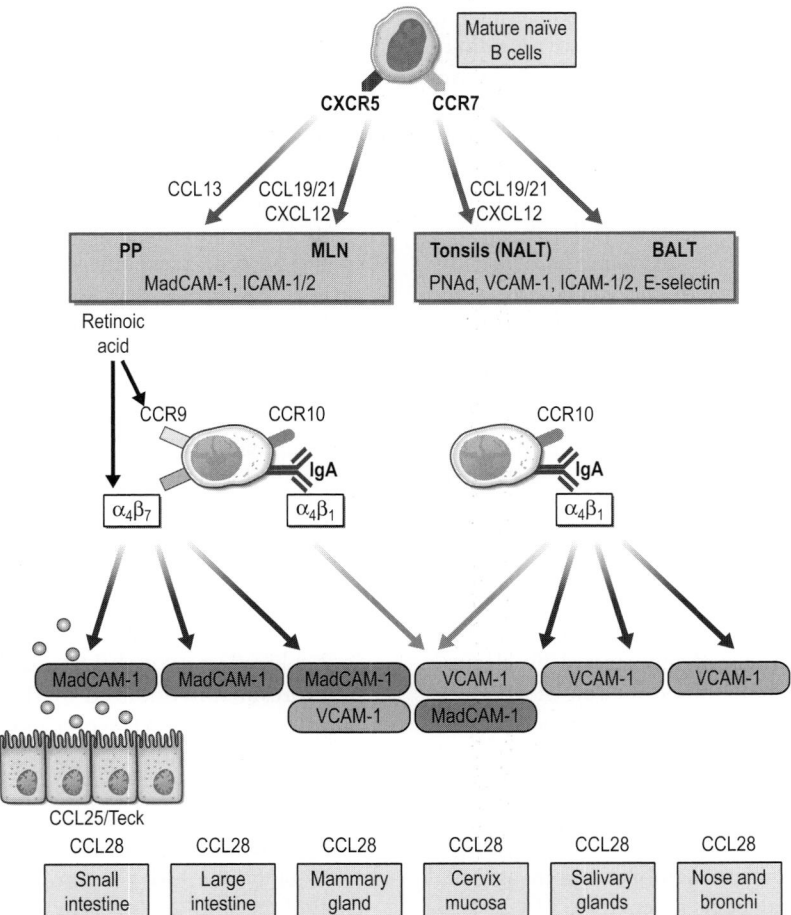

Figure 13.3 Schematical distribution of homing receptors and compartmentalization of mucosal B cell immune responses. Migration of naïve B (and T) lymphocytes circulating in permanence in the blood into mucosal-associated lymphoid tissues (MALT) and mesenteric lymph nodes (MLNs) is promoted by chemokines expressed at the surface of endothelium (in particular CCL19 and CCL21 interact with the CCR7 receptor on lymphocytes) and by adhesion molecules. In Peyer's patches (PPs) and MLNs, high endothelial venules (HEV) express MadCAM-1, which is able to interact with L-selectin and the $\alpha_4\beta_7$ integrin on naïve lymphocytes. In nasopharynx-associated lymphoid tissue (NALT) and bronchi-associated lymphoid tissue (BALT), HEVs express PNAd, VCAM-1, and ICAM-1/2 and therefore retain lymphocytes bearing L-selectin and the $\alpha_4\beta_1$ and LFA-1 integrins. In PPs and MLNs, adhesion may also be promoted by the interaction of LFA-1 on lymphocytes with ICAM-1/2 on HEVs. Other chemokines produced in lymph nodes such as CCL13 interacting with CXCR5, and CCL12 interacting with CXCR4, can promote the migration of lymphocytes into MALT and MLNs. During antigen priming of lymphocytes in PPs and MLNs, retinoic acid produced by mucosal dendritic cells drives the expression of CCR9, the ligand of the chemokine CCL25 produced by small intestinal epithelial cells, and upregulates $\alpha_4\beta_7$, the ligand of MAdCAM-1, on intestinal postcapillary venules. B cells (and T cells) primed in PPs and MLNs (which have lost L-selectin during activation) thus home back preferentially to the gut mucosa and the lactating mammary gland. By contrast, B (and T) blasts primed in NALT and BALT upregulate CCR28 and $\alpha_4\beta_1$, respective ligands for CCL10 and VCAM-1 expressed in non-intestinal effector mucosal sites. Differential expression of homing receptors results in compartmentalization of mucosal responses and should be taken into account in immunization protocols.

chemokines CCL21 (SLC) and CCL19. CCL21 is expressed by HEVs while CCL19 is produced by the perivascular stroma and translocated at the surface of endothelial cells.[18] After extravasation, T cells are retained in the interfollicular area by CCL19. The interfollicular area is thus characterized by the presence of T cells, of mature dendritic cells and macrophages, and the paucity of B cells. Approximately 70 percent of T cells are T cell receptor (TCR)$\alpha\beta$ CD4$^+$. Some of them express CD25, consistent with the role of the interfollicular area in the initiation of

the immune responses in PPs. TCR$\alpha\beta^+$CD8$^+$ cells are localized in a narrow band in the central portion of this region. In contrast, most extravasated B cells, which express the CXCR5 receptor, are attracted into the follicle by the chemokine CXCL13 synthesized by follicular reticular dendritic cells and other stromal cells in the follicle. A small number of CD4$^+$ T cells acquire CCR5 upon activation in the interfollicular area and migrate into the follicle where they exert a helper function in the induction of the germinal center and humoral response.[19] Peyer's patches'

B cell follicles thus consist of a mantle zone filled of predominantly surface IgM$^+$/IgD$^+$ B cells, surrounding a basally located germinal center containing B cell centroblasts, and centrocytes, associated with a network of follicular reticular dendritic cells, scattered CD4$^+$ T cells, dendritic cells, and tingible body macrophages. Consistent with the role of PPs as a major inductive site for IgA production, PP germinal centers are markedly enriched in B cells expressing surface IgA. A very precise description of the distribution of B cell surface markers in the mantle zone and germinal center of human PPs is reviewed elsewhere.[20]

ENTRANCE OF ANTIGENS INTO THE PEYER'S PATCHES

Peyer's patches lack afferent lymphatics and antigens are directly sampled from the lumen across the specialized epithelium that covers the dome (Fig. 13.4). This subepithelial region, located above the B follicle, is rich in T and B cells, macrophages, and immature dendritic cells and is overlaid by the specialized follicle-associated epithelium (for review, see [21]). Elective entrance of intraluminal antigens across the FAE has been demonstrated by electron microscopic studies, which identified the role of M cells in this transepithelial transport. The main characteristic of the FAE is indeed the presence of 5–10 percent M cells interspersed between enterocytes. M cells are polarized epithelial cells that form tight junctions with adjacent enterocytes but possess several distinctive features. Their basal domain, deprived of basement membrane, is invaginated into a large intraepithelial pocket penetrated by B cells, CD4$^+$ T lymphocytes, and macrophages from the subepithelial dome. Their apical membrane lacks a brush border and instead forms microfolds (hence the name M cells). The lack of hydrolytic brush-border enzymes and the very

thin glycocalyx promote the adherence of luminal macromolecules and microorganisms that can then be translocated due to the high endocytic activity of M cells. M cells can actively mediate clathrin-mediated endocytosis of ligand-coated particles, adherent macromolecules, and viruses. They can also conduct fluid-phase pinocytosis, actin-dependent phagocytosis, and macropinocytic engulfment. Perhaps due to the proximity of the basolateral pocket to the M cell apical surface, most endocytosed material escapes lysosomal degradation and is delivered within 10 to 15 minutes into the pocket in the immediate vicinity of dome macrophages and dendritic cells. Some viruses (reovirus) and bacteria (Yersinia) electively bind M cells but putative receptors have not yet been clearly identified. The oligosaccharides presented at the M cell apical membrane, distinct from those expressed by regular enterocytes, may be exploited by some microorganisms but this remains to be proven. Besides the presence of M cells, the FAE presents a biochemical face to the lumen that is distinct from that of the surrounding villous epithelium and further promotes antigen sampling. These particularities probably reflect the global transdifferentiation of the epithelium presumably induced by the close contact with lymphoid cells. Thus, FAE expresses low levels of brush-border hydrolases, contains few or no goblet or enteroendocrine cells, and does not secrete polymeric IgA. Moreover Paneth cells, specialized in the production of microbicidal products, are rare in follicle-associated crypts.[21]

Notably, the FAE predominantly expresses the CCL20 chemokine and can thereby attract or retain subsets of dendritic and lymphoid cells expressing its CCR6 ligand (Fig. 13.2).[22,23] Thus, CCR6−/− mice lack the dense subset of CD11c$^+$ CD11b$^+$ dendritic cells (DCs) normally present in the subepithelial area that is thought to capture

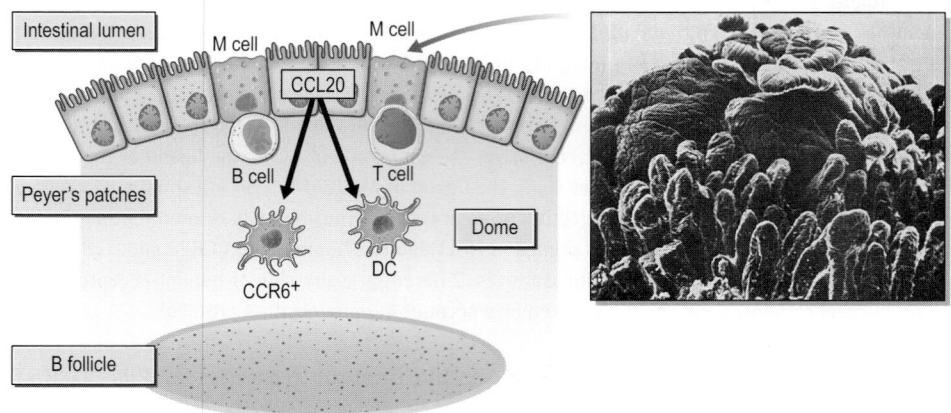

Figure 13.4 The follicle-associated epithelium. The scanning electron microscopic picture in the insert shows the flattened follicle-associated epithelium of the dome of a Peyer's patch (PP) bulging into the small intestinal lumen between adjacent villi. A schematic view of the follicle-associated epithelium is provided with M cells interspersed between regular columnar cells. M cells are deprived of basement membrane and immune cells present in the dome can push themselves into the folds of the cytoplasm of the M cells, thus coming close to the bowel lumen. M cells lack a brush border and have strong endocytic activities. They transport intact antigens from the lumen into the PPs where they can be captured by the numerous immature CCR6$^+$ dendritic cells (DC) attracted toward the dome epithelium by the CCL20 chemokine.

antigens transcytosing across M cells. This defect was suggested to explain the defective mucosal IgA responses of CCR6−/− mice.[22] Yet these mice also have a reduced number of PPs B cells and a profound defect in ILF formation.[23] A recent study showed that CCR6+ CD11c+ DCs are rapidly recruited into the dome of PPs upon FAE invasion by *Salmonella typhimurium* and are required for the activation of anti-*Salmonella* specific T cells and to limit bacterial dissemination.[24] Since CCL20 is constitutively expressed by the FAE, some other chemokine(s) probably promote(s) the *de novo* recruitment of CCR6+ DCs. Their production might be induced via the Toll-like receptors expressed by the FAE, since their stimulation by bacteria provokes the transient recruitment of DCs.[25]

INITIATION OF THE MUCOSAL IMMUNE RESPONSES IN PEYER'S PATCHES

Antigens sampled in the subepithelial dome are thought to be rapidly transported to the interfollicular area, the site of initiation of the immune responses. Thus, in mice fed intragastrically with fluorescent bacteria, bacteria were rapidly found in the CD11c+ immature dendritic cells of the PP dome.[26] Combined *in vitro* and *in vivo* experiments suggest that dome CD11c+ DCs stimulated by bacteria mature into antigen-presenting cells (APCs) and rapidly migrate toward the interfollicular areas, likely due to reciprocal CCR6 downmodulation and CCR7 upregulation.[27,28] In the interfollicular areas they can encounter recently extravasated naïve T and B cells and present the sampled antigens to those bearing a cognitive antigen receptor. Specific T cells proliferate in the interfollicular area, while a subset of activated helper T (TH) cells and activated surface IgM+ B cells enter the B follicle, a homing process largely driven by the interaction of CXCR5 on the latter cells and the CXCL13 chemokine produced by follicular reticular dendritic cells. In the follicle, B cells can undergo proliferation, class switch recombination (CSR), and somatic hypermutation (SHM).[29]

Isolated lymphoid follicles and cryptopatches

Besides PPs, the small intestine, particularly in its distal part, and the colon contain hundreds of ILFs. Their architecture resembles the single follicle of a PP, suggesting that both types of structures serve similar purposes. In contrast to PPs, however, ILFs do not form during ontogeny but are induced after birth.[6,30–32] Recent evidence indicates that ILFs are highly dynamic structures that develop in mice from the so-called cryptopatches under the influence of intraluminal stimuli.[32,33]

Crytopatches, described in mice, appear within the first two weeks after birth at the base of intestinal crypts as small clusters of mostly lineage-negative cells expressing the stem cell factor receptor KIT (CD117), the IL-7Rα chain, and RORγt,[31] a phenotype strikingly similar to that of fetal LTi cells necessary for the induction of secondary lymphoid organs. Cryptopatch formation requires, as for PPs and ILFs, the LTβ receptor, LTα, and RORγt.[6,30,31] Cryptopatches were initially thought to be the site of differentiation of the subset of nonconventional mouse CD8αα intraepithelial T lymphocytes (IEL; see below)[34] but several recent studies have cast doubt on this function. Thus, evidence has been provided of the thymic origin of mouse CD8αα IEL[35–37] and the latter cells were detected in large numbers in LTβ−/− mice lacking cryptopatches.[33] A more accepted current view is that cryptopatches develop into ILFs by the recruitment of lymphocytes, mainly B cells, in a process reminiscent of the fetal development of LNs and PPs but dependent on intraluminal stimuli. This proposal is supported by an extensive survey of lymphoid aggregates in the murine small intestine, which suggests a continuous spectrum from a few typical cryptopatches to mature ILFs containing a growing number of mature lymphocytes, mainly B cells but also T cells.[32,33] The size and numbers of ILFs is highly dependent on the microflora. Thus, ILFs undergo a considerable expansion in size and numbers in mice lacking the enzyme activation-induced cytidine deaminase (AID) that are unable to produce IgA and high-avidity immunoglobulins. These mice develop abnormally elevated intraluminal levels of anaerobic bacteria that likely drive ILF expansion since ILFs recover their normal size after antibiotic therapy.[38] The recruitment of B cells in the ILFs requires their expression of CCR6, but the CCR6 ligand and the signals provided by the flora to initiate this recruitment are not clearly delineated. These signals seem independent of any specific antigen recognition as well as of T cells,[39] pointing to the possible role of innate receptors. That cryptopatches develop into ILFs may explain why these structures have not been detected in the human, rat, and porcine intestine which, on the contrary, contain numerous ILFs.[33]

According to Newberry and Lorenz,[31] a mature mouse ILF contains approximately 70 percent B cells, a smaller population of TCRαβ+ CD4+ (~10 percent) and CD8+ (~3 percent) T cells, 8–10 percent CD11c+ DCs, and 10–15 percent IL-7Rα+ KIT+ cells. The B follicle contains a germinal center and occupies the central part of an enlarged and flattened villus with follicle-associated epithelium containing M cells. This central B cell area is surrounded by a layer of cells expressing KIT and IL-7R and by very numerous CD11c+ DCs. T cells do not form a discrete area and are rather scattered within the ILF. As in PPs, murine ILFs contain a large population of surface IgM+ B cells (mainly IgM^low IgD^high) but also a significant population of surface IgA+ B cells.[31,32] This finding, together with the observation that ILFs contain mRNA encoding activation-induced cytidine deaminase and Iμ-Cα transcripts,[40] suggests that ILFs are inductive sites for the initiation of IgA-committed immune responses in the intestine. However, their exact participation in the induction of mucosal responses is not clearly delineated. Thus, recent data indicate that they may contribute to intestinal secretory immunoglobulin A (SIgA) production but are, in contrast to PPs, unable to generate a specific SIgA against an epitope of tetanus toxoid carried by an attenuated strain of *S. typhimurium*.[41,42]

The role of mesenteric lymph nodes in the induction of intestinal immune responses

While mesenteric lymph nodes (MLNs) are excluded *stricto sensu* from the MALT,[2,3] they participate in the induction of mucosal immune responses following the migration of DCs loaded with lumen-derived antigens in PPs[26] (Fig. 13.2) and also in the LP. Notably, antigen-loaded DCs can be detected within a few hours in the murine LP following feeding with dietary soluble antigens which penetrate by endocytosis across the villus epithelium.[43] Dendritic cells present in the murine ileal LP can also sample intraluminal bacteria independently of PPs.[44,45] Thus, in response to the chemokine fractalkine (CX3CR1L) expressed by ileal murine enterocytes, CX3CR1$^+$ DCs (that are numerous in the LP) emit dendrites that are transiently thrust in-between epithelial cells into the lumen where they can capture intestinal bacteria before retracting into the LP and migrating toward MLNs.[44,46] Migration of DCs from the LP toward MLNs via intestinal lymphatics is observed in steady-state conditions but is drastically enhanced in inflammatory conditions.[47] The entrance of DCs into lymphatics stimulates the expression of the chemokine receptor CCR7,[48] which interacts with the chemokine CCL21 present on the lymphatic endolumen.[49] CCR7 may also promote the recruitment of DCs immigrating into the MLNs via the subcaspular sinus toward the interfollicular T cell areas which produce CCL19, the other ligand of CCR7. Indeed, as in PPs, interfollicular areas contain HEVs and are the site of initial encounter between antigen-loaded DCs and naïve T and B lymphocytes bearing the cognitive antigen receptor that have just entered MLNs.

A growing number of studies indicate that LP-derived DCs that migrate into MLNs are conditioned in the intestinal microenvironment by epithelial- and stromal-derived factors (for review, see [50]). These DCs, identified in mice by their expression of the CD103 (αEβ_7) integrin, serve several important functions discussed below, including imprinting intestinal homing specificity, driving IgA production, and promoting elective expansion and activation of regulatory T cells (reviewed elsewhere[17]). How the functions of the LP-derived DCs overlap with those of PP DCs is, however, not yet clear. Thus, the traffic of antigen-loaded DCs into MLNs seems mandatory for the induction of oral tolerance to soluble antigens while PPs are not absolutely necessary.[51] By contrast, a recent *in vivo* study in mice[52] raises questions about the role of MLNs in the induction of a specific IgA response against a pathogenic bacterium. In the latter study, the authors analyzed the humoral responses to an invasive strain of *S. typhimurium* that can cross the M cells and to a noninvasive strain that can only penetrate the LP (likely due to its capture by CX3CR1$^+$ DCs). Only the invasive strain of bacteria was found in PPs and could induce a specific intestinal SIgA response protective against a novel challenge. Both the invasive and noninvasive strains could, however, reach the MLNs and stimulate a systemic IgG response.[52]

Distribution of intestinal immune responses initiated in the GALT and MLNs to the mucosal effector sites across the hemolymphatic cycle

Lymphocyte recirculation studies performed in the 1970s demonstrated that IgA and T blasts sensitized to intraluminal stimuli in GALT migrate back into the intestinal mucosa via a hemolymphatic cycle that redistributes sensitized cells along the intestinal wall where they transform into mature plasma cells and effector T cells.[11,53,54] The steps that control this lymphocyte migration have been largely elucidated.

As in peripheral lymph nodes, lymphocyte and DC emigration from PPs occurs via the lymphatic network, which is very dense in the subserosal area below the follicle. Emigration from lymph nodes, initially thought to be a passive process, is in fact tightly regulated by a mechanism that is not entirely understood but involves interactions between the local gradient of phospholipid sphingosine 1-phosphate (S1P) and its S1P$_1$ receptor on lymphocytes and can be blocked by FTY720, an agonist of S1P$_1$.[55] Peyer's patch-derived lymphocytes and antigen-loaded DCs migrate via the mesenteric lymphatics – first into MLNs, where they stay transiently, allowing PP-derived blasts to initiate their maturation (attested to in the case of B cells by the appearance of intracytoplasmic IgA).[11] As discussed above, immigrating DCs loaded with antigen in PPs or the LP may also promote the sensitization of additional naïve lymphocytes recruited in MLNs via the blood. Lymphocytes leave MLNs via intestinal lymphatics and join the thoracic duct that delivers them into the superior vena cava and hence into the bloodstream.

Transfer experiments have demonstrated that small lymphocytes redistribute equally via the blood between all secondary lymphoid organs while blasts sensitized in GALT and present in MLNs redistribute mainly into the intestinal mucosa.[11,54] This homing of GALT-derived blasts was shown to result from the interactions of the $\alpha_4\beta_7$ integrin strongly expressed by these cells and of MAdCAM-1 expressed on post-capillary venules in the small intestinal and colonic LP.[17] The role of $\alpha_4\beta_7$ integrin in intestinal T cell lymphocyte homing is not absolute and may be compensated or completed by other integrins, particularly LFA-1 (αLβ_2) in inflamed intestine. Thus β_7-deficient and β_7-sufficient CD8$^+$ T cells were equally able to resolve enteric rotavirus infection[56] and LFA-1 plays a more important role than $\alpha_4\beta_7$ in the migration of alloreactive T cells into small intestinal grafts.[57]

Interestingly $\alpha_4\beta_7$ can mediate both the initial phase of rolling (as PP- and MLN-derived blasts lack L-selectin, which is lost during activation) and the second phase of arrest after activation of its high-avidity conformation by chemokines. In the small intestine, this activation signal is mainly provided by the chemokine CCL25, which is constitutively produced by the epithelium and translocated onto the luminal side of LP venules. CCL25 promotes integrin activation and lymphocyte adhesion by interacting with its receptor CCR9 strongly expressed by PP- and MLN-derived T and IgA blasts. In addition, CCL25 promotes the migration of CD8$^+$ effector cells from the LP into the epithelium. In the colon, the epithelium does not produce CCL25 but, like several other mucosal-associated epithelia, produces another chemokine CCL28 that attracts IgA plasma blasts bearing its CCR10 receptor. The chemokine driving the migration of T cells into the colon is not yet identified (for review, see [17,58,59]).

Expression of $\alpha_4\beta_7$ and CCR10 on GALT- and MLN-derived IgA blasts probably explains the capacity of the latter cells to migrate toward the lactating mammary gland, which contains MAdCAM-1$^+$ venules, and produce CCL28 (Fig. 13.3).[60] Accordingly, SIgA directed against maternal intestinal commensals or oral vaccines administered to the mother are detected in the colostrum and milk.[61] Newborns thus benefit from efficient passive immunization that helps them to cope with intestinal colonization, initiated during delivery, by bacteria derived from the maternal intestinal tract.[62] On the contrary, homing receptors acquired during sensitization in GALT do not drive the entrance of primed cells in other mucosae such as salivary glands and upper airways. In these sites, MAdCAM-1 is not expressed on vessels and is instead replaced by VCAM-1, a vascular adhesion molecule that interacts with the $\alpha_4\beta_1$ integrin that is not strongly expressed by blasts sensitized in GALT.[20]

The mechanisms that imprint gut-homing specificity into the small intestine have recently been elucidated. It was shown that gut-homing specificity is imparted to IgA and T cell blasts during their sensitization in PPs and MLNs by a subset of CD103$^+$ intestinal DCs that produce retinoic acid (Fig. 13.3). Thus, intestinal DCs (isolated either from PPs, MLNs, or the LP) but not splenic DCs can upregulate $\alpha_4\beta_7$ and CCR9 on T cells[17,63] and B cells[64] upon antigen activation. The effect of intestinal DCs is blocked by an antagonist of the retinoic acid receptor and, consistent with this finding, is reproduced by retinoic acid alone.[64] Notably, retinoic acid has no effect on CCR10 expression but can concomitantly reduce the expression of ligands for E- and P-selectin and, at lesser degree, of L-selectin, thus preventing imprinted cells from migrating outside mucosal sites.[64] The mechanisms underlying the elective production of retinoic acid by intestinal but not peripheral DCs remain, however, unclear (for discussion, see [17]). A contribution by enterocytes, also able to metabolize vitamin A in retinoic acid, is likely.[63] As described below, retinoic acid–producing DCs have been recently ascribed a major role in shaping the local immune responses. Besides their capacity to imprint gut-homing specificity, they drive the IgA humoral response[64] and promote in mice the generation of regulatory T cells at the expense of pro-inflammatory IL-17-producing T lymphocytes.[63,65]

The humoral response in the intestine

The humoral response in the intestine can be divided into four stages: predominant IgA induction in mucosal B cells; recirculation of IgA plasma blasts and homing into the intestinal mucosa; terminal B cell differentiation to plasma cells with local IgA production; and export of IgA through the intestinal epithelial layer.

The humoral response initiated in the PPs is indeed characterized by the predominance of IgA-specific CSR that allows substitution of the $C_H\mu$ by the $C_H\alpha$ constant region of immunoglobulins to produce IgA. Mice possess only one $C_H\alpha$ gene but humans have two genes, $C_H\alpha1$ and $C_H\alpha2$, located at the end of the constant immunoglobulin heavy-chain locus, and CSR leads to the production of either IgA1 or IgA2. The latter isotype is more resistant to proteases and is enriched in the lower part of the intestine. IgA-specific CSR is accomplished both by T cell-dependent and T cell-independent mechanisms (for review, see [20,66]).

T cell-dependent IgA CSR takes place in the germinal centers of PPs and may be necessary to generate high-avidity IgA mucosal responses (Fig. 13.5). It requires transforming growth factor β (TGFβ)[67] and CD40-CD40L interactions.[68] TGFβ promotes the first step of CSR – the germline transcription of the intronic Iα promoter 5' of the α locus – while signals via CD40 induce AID in germinal center B cells, the enzyme necessary both for CSR and SHM.[20,66] While IgA CSR can take place in ILFs and likely also in MLNs, the contribution of these lymphoid formations to the production of specific SIgA responses, presumably T cell-dependent, remain unclear, as discussed above.

Intestinal IgA production was found to be partially independent of T cells[69] and of CD40-CD40L engagement.[68] These findings led to the identification of other costimulatory signals for IgA-specific CSR. Two DC-derived cytokines, BAFF (B cell activating factor) and APRIL (aproliferation-inducing ligand), were found to stimulate T cell-independent IgA-specific CSR via their interactions with TACI (transmembrane activator and CAML interactor), one of their receptors on B cells that induces AID.[66] Expression of APRIL and BAFF has been detected in a subset of murine PP DCs.[70] The importance of this second pathway in the generation of IgA-producing cells in PPs is, however, unclear since IgA-specific CSR is severely impaired in PPs of CD40−/− mice.[68] This second pathway may rather serve a function outside PPs, in particular in the LP. Indeed, after many controversies, recent studies in humans[71] and mice[72] have provided strong evidence that IgA CSR can take place in the LP. Notably, it was shown that human colonocytes stimulated by bacteria via Toll receptors could release APRIL that triggered IgM-to-IgA2 or IgA1-to-IgA2 CSR in LP B cells. In addition, epithelial cells stimulated the production of APRIL and BAFF by LP

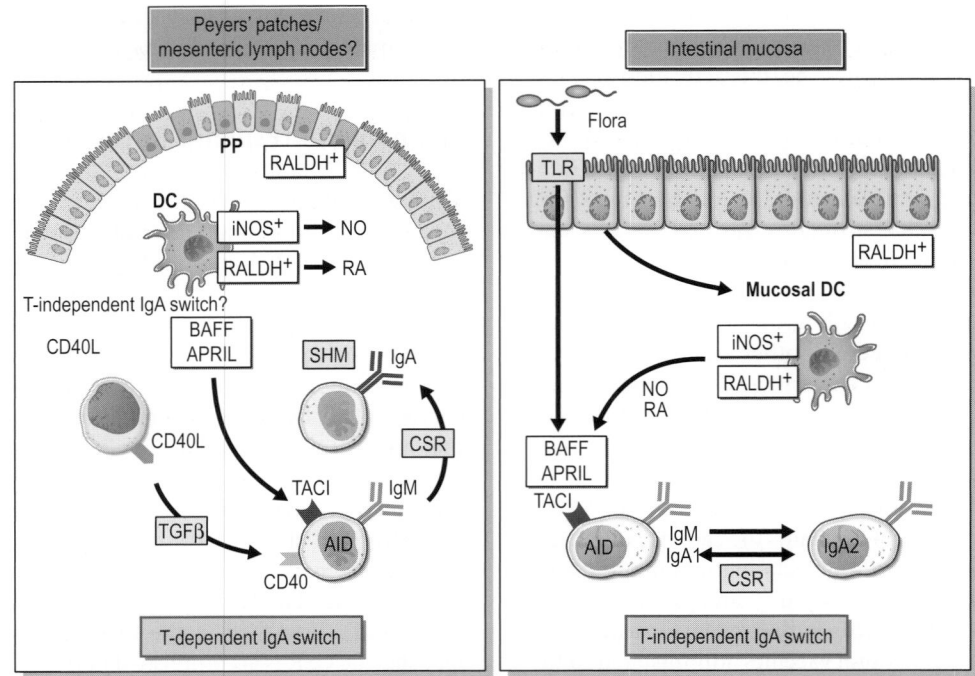

Figure 13.5   Intestinal sites of IgA class switch recombination. Class switch recombination (CSR) in mucosae, and particularly in the intestinal mucosa, predominantly leads to the production of immunoglobulin (Ig) A. T cell-dependent IgA CSR requires the interaction of CD40L on T cells and CD40 on B cells to induce the activation-induced cytidine deaminase (AID) enzyme, and of transforming growth factor β (TGFβ) to open the chromatin of the IgA locus. IgA avidity is increased by somatic hypermutation (SHM) in B follicle germinal centers. These events take place in Peyers' patches (PPs) and probably in mesenteric lymph nodes (MLNs), although the role of MLNs in the production of specific IgA has been questioned in a recent publication (see text). Mounting evidence indicates that the production of IgA of low avidity can occur independently of T cell help (T cell-independent CSR) in the intestinal mucosa. Thus, Toll-like receptor (TLR)-activated epithelial cells and mucosal dendritic cells produce BAFF and APRIL, two cytokines that induce AID and promote IgA CSR upon binding to their receptor, TACI, on B cells. Subsets of mucosal dendritic cells (that may overlap) express inducible NO synthase (iNOS) and/or retinal dehydrogenases (RALDH) and can produce nitric oxide (NO) and retinoic acid (RA), respectively. Both are able to enhance IgA switching independently of T cell help (see text). Enterocytes also express RALDH and may produce retinoic acid from dietary vitamin A and deliver it to dendritic cells (DCs). Recent evidence indicates that T cell-independent CSR takes place in the human colonic lamina propria and promotes CSR from IgM to IgA1 or from IgA1 to IgA2. The importance of the T cell-independent pathway in PPs and MLNs is unclear.

DCs that might thus relay and amplify the effect of enterocytes.[71] This extrafollicular pathway is currently thought to promote T cell-independent production of low-affinity IgA against commensal bacteria and, in humans, the production of IgA2 that is more resistant to proteases than IgA1 (discussed elsewhere[66]). These low-affinity SIgA seem indeed sufficient to reduce the translocation of commensal bacteria.[62]

Other mechanisms that participate in skewing CSR toward IgA in PPs and more generally in the intestine have been recently delineated and underscore the role of DCs conditioned in the intestinal microenvironment. One study demonstrates the role of the subset of intestinal DCs that constitutively produce retinoic acid. Thus, DCs isolated from PPs stimulated the *in vitro* production of IgA from murine naïve B cells activated by an anti-IgM antibody. This effect, independent of the presence of T cells, was blocked by an antagonist of the retinoic receptor and could be reproduced with DCs from peripheral lymph nodes (PLNs) in the presence of retinoic acid if added with

IL-6 and IL-5. Comparable results were obtained with human B cells and DCs derived from MLNs.[64] Confirming the *in vivo* role of retinoic acid, intestinal IgA production is profoundly impaired in mice or individuals with vitamin A deficiency and can be restored by vitamin A supplementation.[64] How retinoic acid can affect CSR remains, however, to be elucidated. A second mechanism recently described in mice may involve the production of nitric oxide (NO) by intestinal DCs stimulated by bacterial products via their Toll-like receptors.[70] Thus, TNF-producing and inducible NO synthase (iNOS)-producing DCs detected in PPs, MLNs, and LP but not in spleen were shown to be necessary for both T cell-dependent and T cell-independent IgA CSR. It was suggested that NO promotes expression of TGFβ receptor type II on B cells and of APRIL and BAFF in DCs.[70] The latter data are consistent with the central role of the commensal flora in the induction of intestinal IgA. It is not excluded that these TNF/iNOS-producing DCs are overlapping with the subset of DCs that produce retinoic acid.

Due to the preferential CSR toward IgA in GALT and in the mucosa, the intestinal LP contains a striking predominance (70–90 percent) of IgA plasma cells that form a considerable mass of antibody-secreting cells (estimated at 10^{10} per meter).[20] Thus, most large cells isolated from the human LP have the phenotype of terminally differentiated B cells (CD38$^+$ CD27$^+$ CD19$^+$/$^-$ CD20$^-$) with surface and/or intracellular IgA.[73] Studies in normal intestinal tissue sections indicate that 80 to 90 percent of plasma cells synthesize IgA, while 10 to 20 percent make IgM, and less than 5 percent make IgG. The proportion of IgA1 plasma cells, approximately 70 percent in the human duodenojejunum, decreases progressively toward the colon where the proportion of IgA2 increases to 65 percent (reviewed elsewhere[20,66]). One characteristic of plasma cells in mucosae, including the intestinal LP, is their synthesis of a J chain that allows the production of IgA dimers or polymers, collectively termed polymeric IgA (pIgA). The J chain also allows the assembly of pentameric IgM. Incorporation of the J chain in pIgA and in IgM is mandatory for their selective export into the intestinal lumen as it allows their binding to the receptor (pIgR) at the basal pole of enterocytes. Covalent linking stabilizes the interaction of pIgA (but not IgM) with the pIgR.[20] The polymeric Ig receptor carries its ligands across the epithelial cells by clathrin-mediated transcytosis.[74] After fusion of the apical endosome with the surface membrane and cleavage of the pIgR, the polymeric Ig is delivered into the intestinal lumen as secretory Ig bound to the extracellular part of the pIgR, also called secretory component (SC) (Fig. 13.2). The covalent coupling of pIgA to SC increases its stability in the intestinal lumen and gives rise to mucophilic properties.[75] Owing to the lack of covalent stabilization by SC, SIgM is less resistant to luminal degradation but SIgM provides compensatory mucosal defence in early infancy and selective IgA deficiency, explaining the variable susceptibility of IgA-deficient patients to mucosal infections.[66]

In cooperation with innate mucosal defence mechanisms,[76] the massive production of SIgA in the intestine (estimated at 40 mg/kg/day) has a major role in the exclusion of exogenous antigens present in the lumen. This function is important to maintaining the mutually beneficial relationship with the 10^{14} commensal bacteria comprising the intestinal microbiota. The microflora is the main physiologic inducer of SIgA. Thus levels of SIgA and LP plasma cells remain very low in germ-free mice but are induced within a few weeks following bacterial colonization.[69,77] Conversely, mice deficient in the AID enzyme develop microbial overgrowth and lymphoid hyperplasia.[38] This observation is reminiscent of cases of common variable immunodeficiency in humans and points not only to the role of SIgA in the intraluminal control of the microflora but also in an anti-inflammatory function able to prevent exaggerated stimulation of the immune system by intestinal commensals. A recent study further confirms the role of SIgA in maintaining intestinal homeostasis: production of a monoclonal IgA specific for the commensal bacterium *Bacteroides thetaiotaomicron* by a hybridoma implanted on the back of Rag$-$/$-$ mice prevented the innate immune response and the production of oxidative metabolites induced by this commensal in the ileum of the mice (that lack both B and T cells).[78] Interestingly, in this study the intestinal production of IgA, mainly directed against a capsular polysaccharide of *B. thetaiotaomicron*, induced mutations associated with the loss of this sugar and impaired growth, which may in turn limit local expansion of the bacterium.[78] While this study shows the role of specific IgA in containing commensal bacteria and maintaining intestinal homeostasis, it must be stressed that SIgA induced by the flora shows usually little specificity and low affinity[79] as well as a limited diversity (reviewed elsewhere[80]). It has therefore been proposed that induction of IgA by the flora is rather a primitive system (largely T-independent) in which the production of large amounts of antibody against bacterial surface molecules with relatively low affinity yet broad specificity is useful to limit colonization or penetration through the epithelial layer.[81] Secretory IgA may also serve important functions in the defence against a number of pathogens, particularly Gram-negative bacteria (e.g., *Salmonella*, *Shigella*), Giardia, and enteroviruses (rotavirus, echovirus, and poliovirus), as indicated by experimental studies in mice but also by the consequences of severe global B cell immunodeficiencies in humans (for review, see [66,82]). Unlike SIgA protection against the flora, efficient protection against pathogens requires T cell help and germinal centers, presumably to raise high-affinity antibodies.[66] Thus, while 'innate' SIgA induced by the flora could offer some early protection to naïve mice and decrease shedding of a virulent strain of *S. typhimurium*,[83] efficient protection against a challenge by a lethal dose of this pathogen requires a specific IgA response generated in PPs.[52]

In contrast to the well-established function in the exclusion of intraluminal antigens, SIgA was recently shown to behave as a Trojan horse, able to promote antigen entry into the mucosa. Secretory IgA was first shown to promote the translocation of bacteria such as Shigella across M cells in PPs and their capture by underlying DCs. It was postulated that SIgA may thereby help maintain an adaptive protective immune response.[84] In this study, the receptor that mediates reverse translocation of SIgA complexes was not identified. In a second recent publication on celiac disease, it was shown that SIgA complexed in the duodenal lumen to undigested gliadin peptides could be retrotranscytosed into the LP, a mechanism that may, in this pathological case, sustain the abnormal T cell response to gliadin and intestinal inflammation. Retrotransport of SIgA complexes was mediated by transferrin receptors, which were abnormally upregulated and expressed at the apical surface of enterocytes.[85] Identification of the receptor that mediates the retrotransport of SIgA complexes in PPs may help define whether the pathological retrotransport observed in celiac disease is a perversion in the villous epithelium of a physiological mechanism normally restricted to PPs.

Table 13.1 T cell subsets in the effector intestinal compartments

	CD4+ TCRαβ	CD8+ TCRαβ		TCRγδ		
		CD8 αβ	CD8 αα	CD8 αα	CD4− CD8−	TCR−
Mouse IEL	5–10%	20–40%	15–20%	30–50%	~0%	5–10%
Human IEL	5–15%	65–85%	<5%	2–5%	5–15%	2–15%
Lamina propria T cells	55–80%	30–40%	<2%	<1%	2–7%	
Antigen recognition[a]	MHC class II-restricted antigen recognition of exogenous antigens	MHC class I-restricted antigen recognition of	Self-antigens?	Putative antigens induced / Induced by stress on enterocytes?		
Putative functions[a]	Cytokine production	Cytokine production / Cytotoxicity	Regulation?	Cytokine production / Cytotoxicity	Regulation	??[b]

[a] Based on *in vitro* or *in vivo* studies in mice and *in vitro* studies in humans.
[b] Initially thought to be local precursors for T cell differentiation of intraepithelial T lymphocytes (IEL), their exact nature remains unclear; as T IEL, they can express NK receptors.

Intestinal T cell responses

T CELL SUBSETS IN THE EFFECTOR INTESTINAL COMPARTMENTS

Studies in mice have demonstrated that the majority of intestinal T cells are antigen-experienced T cells that first encountered their cognitive antigen in PPs (or perhaps in MLNs), and have migrated into the mucosa via the hemolymphatic pathway. Their appearance in the intestinal mucosa is thus strongly dependent on exposure to the microflora. These conventional T cells express TCRαβ and are distributed in the LP, where the majority (60–70 percent) are CD4+, and in epithelium, where they are mainly CD8+, expressing a regular heterodimeric CD8αβ molecule (Table 13.1).[86,87] In both compartments, and in humans as in mice, these conventional T cells have a skewed repertoire ascribed to the massive expansion of clones randomly selected by antigens (for review, see [88]). A second population of so-called nonconventional T cells has been described in the murine epithelium. These IEL are characterized by the expression of a homodimeric CD8αα molecule and contain both TCRαβ+ and TCRγδ+ cells, the latter cells being markedly enriched in the gut epithelium compared to the LP and other lymphoid compartments. CD8αα+ IEL show little dependence on the flora; they predominate in young mice and decrease in proportion over time as a consequence of the continuous influx and expansion of conventional T cells.[89,90] Their origin has been the subject of many controversies over the years. Recent data have led to a revision of the hypothesis that they differentiate locally in the gut wall and provide compelling evidence of the thymic origin of TCRαβ+CD8αα+ IEL, at least in thymus-competent mice.[35–37] Why they express a CD8αα homodimer has not been completely elucidated. Expression of CD8α and CD8β is regulated through the methylation and modulation of their promoters by a variety of factors, which have different effects in lymphocytes at different stages of maturation and/or activation. TCRγδ+ cells are usually CD4−CD8− in the periphery but a small subset can express CD8αα and this expression is apparently favored in the gut epithelium. Recent data suggest that CD8αα TCRαβ+ IELs derive from a subset of self-reactive double negative thymocytes and/or from effector memory CD8αβ T cells. The CD8αβ heterodimer is indeed a potent coreceptor of the T cell receptor, and can be lost during CD8 T cell activation. On the contrary, CD8αα can function as a negative regulator of the T cell receptor. Reinduction of CD8αα on these antigen-experienced cells when they enter the gut epithelium might be part of the mucosal immune regulation that mediates immune quiescence in the antigen-rich environment of the gut (for review, see [89]). Notably, CD8αα binds with a strong avidity to TL, a murine MHC class Ib molecule expressed on the laterobasal membrane of enterocytes. The consequences of this interaction on the functions of IEL remain, however, unclear.[91,92]

In humans, the LP contains, as in mice, a majority of TCRαβ+ CD4+ cells (60–70 percent versus 30–40 percent CD8αβ+) that bear the memory marker CD45R0. The epithelium is enriched in TCRγδ+ cells (approximately 15 percent in adults) and in CD8+ cells (65–85 percent). A CD8αα homodimer is found on a fraction of TCRγδ+ IEL (30 percent) but the vast majority of human CD8+ TCRαβ+ IEL bear, as their peripheral counterpart, the regular CD8αβ heterodimer (authors' unpublished data and [93]). The distinct expression of CD8 in mouse and human IEL may perhaps reflect the different regulation of CD8 in these species. In addition there is no human homolog of TL. In humans, fine-tuning of IEL activation may instead be modulated via NK receptors. Thus, human IELs express both activating and inhibitory NK receptors, the expression of which can be modulated in the intestinal microenvironment.[94] In the normal situation, expression of inhibitory receptors can increase the threshold of IEL activation via their TCR. By contrast, in celiac disease, activation of IELs and their cytotoxicity against epithelium is associated with downmodulation of inhibitory NK receptors and upregulation of activating NK receptors that promote an autoimmune attack of the epithelium.[94–97]

INTESTINAL T CELL RESPONSES

The outcome of intestinal T cell responses depends on the nature and form of the antigen. Administration of protein-soluble antigens such as ovalbumin results in antigen-specific tolerance both locally and systemically (for review, see[98]). Intestinal colonization by commensal bacteria is associated with the massive immigration of CD4 and CD8 T cells without evidence of mucosal damage,[69,87] probably due to the simultaneous recruitment of effector cells and regulatory T cells, the latter counterbalancing the proin-flammatory functions of the effector cells. This notion is supported by T cell transfer experiments in severe combined immune deficiency (SCID) and *Rag −/−* mice. The transfer of naïve CD4$^+$ T cells into these immunodeficient mice results in severe colitis due to their priming by commensal bacteria into effector cells producing interferon gamma and/or IL-17.[99,100] Colitis is prevented by the cotransfer of a reciprocal subset of CD4$^+$ cells containing regulatory T cells that act directly or via the induction of the anti-inflammatory cytokines IL-10 and TGFβ (for review, see[101,102]). Severe intestinal inflammation is, however, observed during invasion by pathogens, including invasive bacteria such as Shigella or Salmonella, viruses, and parasites. This inflammatory response is generally considered necessary for the elimination of pathogens but can be highly detrimental to the host, and even promote intestinal colonization by pathogenic bacteria through the eradication of the normal flora.[103]

PUTATIVE ROLES OF INTESTINAL T CELL SUBSETS IN MUCOSAL DEFENCE

CD4$^+$ T cells may serve several functions in the LP. Via IL-5 and IL-6, they can promote maturation of plasma cells and the production of SIgA that ensures that commensal bacteria or pathogens are contained within the intestinal lumen.[64] Via interferon gamma, they can stimulate phagocytosis by LP macrophages and the elimination of intracellular bacteria.[104] Via IL-17, they can recruit polymorphonuclear leucocytes, stimulate the production of microbicidal peptides, and thus enhance the barrier function of epithelial cells, thereby protecting against extracellular bacteria. In addition, IL-17 seems important for the defense against intracellular bacteria and fungal pathogens (for review, see[105]). At steady state, effector LP T cells may thus continuously provide help to eliminate commensals that have escaped exclusion by SIgA and epithelium-derived microbicidal substances. The importance of this function is illustrated by the onset of severe intestinal infections by opportunistic mycobacteria or Candida in patients with profound T cell immuno-deficiencies or with defective production of interferon gamma. The production of interferon gamma also seems essential to combating infection by virulent strains of Salmonella.[106]

Specific CD8αβ$^+$ TCRαβ T cells are elicited in the intestine in response to viruses such as reovirus and rotavirus and are thought to promote the rapid elimination of infected epithelial cells.[98] Their contribution to the defense against bacteria is not well delineated but is suggested by their increase during colonization by the flora and illustrated by the role of mouse CD8 T cells in the elimination of Listeria via the stimulation of innate immunity.[107]

The functions of nonconventional IELs are not well understood inasmuch as their ligands have not been identified. Intestinal TCRγδ IELs preferentially use Vγ7 in mice and Vδ1 in humans but, in marked contrast with murine skin TCRγδ IELs, which have an invariant TCR, they possess a diversified repertoire that differs in different individuals, arguing against the hypothesis of a unique epithelial ligand.[108,109] Intraepithelial T lymphocytes are thought to function as epithelial sentinels, activated in response to epithelial stress, but the consequences of their activation on epithelial homeostasis remain unclear. Depending on the models, they have been suggested to promote tissue repair, to be regulatory, or, on the contrary, to be cytotoxic, in particular *in vitro* against epithelial tumor lines (for review, see[109,110]). Murine CD8αα TCRαβ IELs are thought to be autoreactive T cells.[89] Rather surprisingly, they have been shown to downregulate the proinflammatory effects of conventional intestinal T cells in a mouse model of colitis.[111]

REGULATION OF INTESTINAL T CELL RESPONSES

How the intensity and nature of intestinal immune T cell responses are adjusted is under scrutiny. Recent data underscore the interplay between DCs and their local microenvironment, particularly the epithelium. At steady state, epithelial- or stromal-derived factors can shape LP and PP DCs into anti-inflammatory DCs. Thus, thymic stromal lymphopoietin, an IL-7-related cytokine produced by enterocytes, could condition DCs to induce non-inflammatory TH2 responses by inhibiting their production of IL-12, a TH1-skewing cytokine.[50,112] TGFβ produced by many cells in the intestine, including epithelial cells, down-modulates the proinflammatory functions of macrophages without altering their phagocytic functions and promotes the anti-inflammatory functions of DCs.[50,113] Finally retinoic acid-producing DCs not only promote the production of IgA and the acquisition of intestinal homing receptors (see above) but also stimulate the expansion/ activation of regulatory T cells in MLNs while they inhibit the differentiation of proinflammatory T cells producing IL-17.[65,114,115] Thus at steady state, the immune balance in the gut is tipped toward tolerance. Upon invasion by a pathogen, the profile of cytokines and chemokines synthesized by epithelial cells changes, due to the strong induction of the NF-κB and MAP-kinase pathways by signals provided by the pathogens through innate receptors of the Toll-like or NOD families. The release of chemokines such as CCL20 can attract CCR6$^+$ blood-derived monocytes that have not been conditioned in the intestinal microenvironment. These monocytes are thought to rapidly differentiate into proinflammatory DCs that promote the differentiation/activation of interferon gamma and/or IL-17-producing proinflammatory T cells.[50] In response to Toll-like receptors and via the production of cytokines such as IL-6, they may also inhibit regulatory T cells, thus reverting local immunoregulation toward inflammation.[116] If inflammation succeeds in eradicating the pathogen, factors produced in the microenvironment and regulatory T cells help restore quiescence. The severity of mucosal damage in patients with inflammatory bowel diseases and celiac disease (respectively associated with dysregulated local responses to the microflora or to the dietary antigen gluten) attests to the importance of these homeostatic mechanisms in the maintenance of quiescence at the steady state.

The complex function of GALT in preserving homeostasis in the intestinal mucosa is replicated in other mucosae by related lymphoid tissue; the nasopharynx-associated lymphoid tissue (NALT) in the nasopharynx and BALT in the bronchi. Their exact contribution to the mucosal immune responses has recently attracted much more attention but remains less well understood.

THE NASOPHARYNX–ASSOCIATED LYMPHOID TISSUE

In humans, NALT is represented by Waldeyer's ring, which includes the nasopharyngeal tonsil or adenoid attached to the roof of the pharynx, the paired tubal tonsils situated at the pharyngeal opening of the Eustachian tubes, the paired palatine tonsils positioned in the oropharynx, and the lingual tonsil on the posterior third of the tongue. Smaller subepithelial collections of lymphoid tissue in the pharyngeal mucosa complete the ring.[117] In addition, lymphoid tissue disseminated in the nasal mucosae reminiscent of the distribution of NALT in rodents (see below) has been described at autopsy in a subset of children who died during the first two years of life.[118]

Tonsils comprise a subepithelial compartment formed by numerous secondary lymphoid follicles (B cell areas) separated by interfollicular regions (T cell areas). They lack a capsule and are covered by an epithelium divided into two distinct parts. The surface epithelium lines the external face of the tonsils and protects it from antigen entry; it is made of squamous epithelium in the palatine and lingual tonsils, and of respiratory epithelium in pharyngeal and tubal tonsils. In contrast, the crypt epithelium serves as an active site for antigen sampling. It forms fissure-like invaginations, either as monocryptic units in lingual tonsils, or as polycryptic sometimes branching crypts in palatine and nasal tonsils. These crypts insinuate between follicles and considerably increase the surface exposed to intraluminal antigens. The crypt epithelium has a reticular morphology with strands of epithelial cells containing numerous lymphocytes and delineating a vast continuum of intercellular spaces infiltrated with T and B lymphocytes, macrophages, and DCs and containing numerous

capillary loops, some of which form HEVs at the border with B follicles. Several studies suggest that the crypt epithelium contains specialized epithelial cells with the functional properties and, to some extent, ultrastructural features of M cells. While the presence of true M cells is still debated, the uptake of tracers has been observed in the reticular crypt epithelium but not in the regular surface epithelium. The crypt epithelium is thus considered to be a very active site of antigen uptake.[117]

The role of NALT as a site at which mucosal responses are generated has been demonstrated in mice. Direct comparison with the situation in humans is, however, difficult, as NALT differs with respect to its distribution as well as its ontogeny. Thus, in mice, NALT is limited to bell-shaped paired structures located dorsally in the floor of the nasal cavity and is developed only after birth via mechanisms partly distinct from those involved in the formation of PPs (in particular, they are independent of RORγ, LTα and LTβ, and of IL-7).[119] By contrast, the development of human tonsils is antenatal and starts at the fourteenth week of gestation. Primary follicles are visible at 16 weeks and primitive crypts surrounded by richly vascularized capillaries and HEVs by 20 weeks.[117]

Nevertheless NALT in mice and humans probably share the ability to generate immune reactions. In both species, NALT HEVs express carbohydrates collectively named peripheral-node addressin (PNAd) and can thus recruit naïve lymphocytes bearing L-selectin.[117,119] In humans, these carbohydrates are presented by the CD34 molecule and recognized by the MECA-79 antibody. Human tonsil HEVs also express E-selectin, VCAM-1, and ICAM-1. The two last molecules are ligands for the integrins $\alpha_4\beta_1$ and LFA-1, respectively, and probably promote the second step of firm adhesion.[20,117] As in PPs, surface IgM$^+$ B cells can undergo CSR in the B follicle germinal center but they give rise to a higher proportion of IgG (55–72 percent) than IgA (18–30 percent) immunocytes as well as to IgD and IgM immunocytes. In the germinal centers of normal palatine tonsils and adenoids from children, these immunocytes often synthesize J chain (13–80 percent). The vast majority of IgA (95 percent) is IgA1.[120] Interestingly, a recent study in human palatine tonsils demonstrated that IgA CSR can also take place outside the B follicle in B cells scattered in the reticular crypt epithelium that respond to the AID-inducing factor, BAFF, secreted in large amounts by the crypt epithelium, probably in response to stimulation via Toll-like receptors.[121] In humans, patches of crypt epithelium in adenoids express the polymeric Ig receptor and may thus excrete SIgA, but this is not the case in palatine tonsils and it is thought that most immunocytes produced in NALT home to regional secretory effector sites.[120]

In mice, post-switch IgA-committed B cells generated in response to nasal immunization have been shown to express high levels of the integrin $\alpha_4\beta_1$ and of the chemokine receptor CCR10. These receptors can promote the migration of such B cells into nearby salivary glands but also into the respiratory and genitourinary tracts, which express the corresponding ligands CCL28 and VCAM-1.[2,119] Accordingly, in mice, nasal immunization has been shown to stimulate antigen-specific responses at these sites. Not only IgA responses, but also TH1 and TH2 cell-mediated responses have been observed.[119] In humans, Brandtzaeg and coworkers have provided evidence that a fraction of NALT-derived B cells are surface IgD^+/IgM^- $CD38^+$ B cells and can be used to track the pattern of migration of NALT-derived blasts. Consistent with data in mice, these authors observed that the latter cells are found in the cervical lymph nodes and in the upper aerodigestive tract (upper airways, lachrymal glands, and salivary glands) but not in the small intestine.[122] Investigations to identify homing markers on surface IgD^+/IgM^- $CD38^+$ B cells circulating in the blood revealed the presence of CCR10 and $\alpha_4\beta_1$ as well as of CCR7 and CD62L, while CCR9 and $\alpha_4\beta_7$ required for migration in the small intestine were low or absent. Brandtzaeg et al. suggested that the expression of CCR10 and $\alpha_4\beta_1$ explains why nasal immunization in humans elicits SIgA antibody defense preferentially in the upper airways and endocervix, while expression of CD62L and CCR7 may drive B cells to migrate to peripheral lymph nodes and thereby promote systemic antibody immune responses. They emphasized the fact that, given the pattern of homing receptors acquired during sensitization in NALT, nasal immunization is not an appropriate route to efficiently prime gut immune responses.[122] Finally, it is interesting to observe that combined tonsillectomy and adenoidectomy may reduce local IgA responses in children. However, this effect seems transient and less obvious in young adults (for review, see [120]).

BRONCHI-ASSOCIATED LYMPHOID TISSUE

Bronchi-associated lymphoid tissue has been described as clusters of B follicles surrounded by parafollicular areas of T cells included within the bronchial epithelium. The latter differentiates into a follicle-like epithelium lacking cilia and goblet cells and containing M cells with embedded lymphocytes.[123] Lymphocytes enter BALT in the parafollicular area via HEVs which, in marked contrast with HEVs in GALT, express PNAd and (very strongly) VCAM-1 but not MAdCAM-1. Homing into BALT was shown to depend on LFA-1 (probably interacting with ICAM-1 or ICAM-2) and on the interactions of PNAd with L-selectin on naïve lymphocytes and of VCAM-1 with $\alpha_4\beta_1$ on memory cells.[124] Large BALT aggregates are mainly observed in the upper airways at bifurcations of the bronchial tree. In addition, isolated lymphoid follicles covered by FAE and M cells and mainly comprised of B cells have been observed scattered in the bronchial epithelium. Studies in rats and rabbits, where BALT seems to be constantly present, indicate that the majority of the B cells in BALT express SIgA or SIgM (for review, see [123]).

The occurrence of BALT indeed differs considerably between species and it remains controversial whether BALT is exclusively inducible by inflammation and should, therefore, be considered as a secondary or rather a tertiary lymphoid organ. In humans, lympho-epithelium has been observed at 20 weeks of gestation in a small subset of noninfected fetuses, suggesting that BALT may occur at selected areas.[125] However, BALT is currently considered to be absent at birth in humans.[126] It can arise in a subset of children and adolescents, particularly in response to antigen stimulation.[126] In human adults, BALT has not been found in healthy individuals but it has been observed in cigarette smokers and in various pathological conditions, including diffuse panbronchiolitis and hypersensitivity pneumonitis.[127] Inducible BALT, consisting of numerous B cell follicles containing germinal centers and follicular dendritic cells surrounded by a loosely defined T cell area with HEVs, has been observed in peribronchial, perivascular, and interstitial areas in patients with pulmonary complications of Sjögren syndrome and rheumatoid arthritis.[128] Immunohistochemistry revealed the presence of the lymphoid-organizing chemokines CCL21 and CCL13, and of factors involved in CSR (BAFF, ICOS ligand).[128]

Inducible BALT has also been described after infection with influenza virus in mice genetically lacking both spleen and lymph nodes. The delayed but efficient and protective development of T and B cell responses against the virus in such mice pointed to the role of BALT in the induction of these responses.[129] It is, however, currently believed that the generation of primary immune responses to inhaled antigen in lungs and airways mainly takes place in mediastinal lymph nodes following the migration of DCs loaded with antigens into the airway mucosa, where they reside in large numbers. This is reminiscent of the role of intestinal DCs and MLNs in the generation of gut immune responses.[130,131] The circumstances in which a primary response was demonstrated in mouse inducible BALT are very artificial as the mice lacked a spleen and lymph nodes. The exact role of BALT in the generation of local immune responses is, therefore, debated. In the normal situation, where lymph nodes are present, the role of BALT in priming pulmonary immune responses may thus be minor. Instead, BALT may represent a site for expansion of memory B cells (discussed elsewhere[123]). Interestingly, a recent article suggests that regulatory T cells may have an important role in regulating the development of inducible BALT in mice.[132]

INDUCIBLE MALT-LIKE LYMPHOID ORGANS

The inducible development of BALT in response to exogenous antigens or autoantigens is reminiscent of the development of MALT-like structures in the salivary glands in Sjögren syndrome, in the thyroid gland in Hashimoto thyroiditis, and in the stomach of patients infected by Helicobacter pylori – all patients at high risk to develop MALT lymphomas. It is now clear that chronic inflammation can promote lymphoid neogenesis and the development of so-called tertiary lymphoid organs at a variety of locations through mechanisms that partially recapitulate normal lymphomagenesis. These tertiary lymphoid organs are highly plastic. They can be turned on by many different stimuli, including infectious and autoimmune diseases and graft rejection. Conversely they can be turned off by removing the antigenic stimulus. Their beneficial or, more likely, harmful roles have not yet been fully elucidated. They may promote autoimmunity by favoring local production of antibodies or T cell epitope spreading (for review, see [133,134]). Furthermore, there are many examples in which tertiary lymphoid organs, due to continuous antigenic stimulation, can be associated with oligo and subsequently clonal B cell proliferations, ultimately resulting in MALT B cell lymphomas. The sequence from neolymphogenesis toward MALT lymphomas has been particularly well demonstrated in *H. pylori*-induced gastritis where the growth of the lymphoma B cells can be stimulated by intra-tumoral *H. pylori*-specific T cells, while eradication of *H. pylori* with antibiotics leads to long-term regression of the lymphoma in a high proportion of patients (for review, see[135]).

CONCLUSION

Lymph nodes have appeared in mammals and evolved into highly sophisticated structures able to optimize the onset of immune responses. Gut-associated lymphoid tissues and mucosal-associated lymphoid tissues have developed specialized features adapted to their localization at the epithelial surfaces. Their strong interconnection with epithelial cells has resulted in the differentiation of a specialized epithelium able to sample antigens directly within these lymphoid organs, while epithelium-derived factors can modulate the function of immune cells, shape the properties of antigen-presenting cells, and adjust the nature of the humoral and cellular responses depending on the nature of antigens present at the mucosal surface. Thus, at the steady state, immune responses initiated in mucosal-associated lymphoid tissues are tuned to maintain local homeostasis despite continuous exposure of mucosae to commensal bacteria, while inflammatory signals triggered upon invasion by pathogens can result in strong proinflammatory responses that help eliminate pathogens. Interestingly, signals involved in the normal development of mucosal-associated lymphoid tissues can be reactivated by inflammatory signals provided either by chronic exposure to bacteria or during autoimmune reactions and result in the appearance of inducible MALT, a privileged site for the emergence of MALT-derived lymphomas. A better knowledge of the mechanisms that control the development of normal versus inducible MALT may help design new therapeutic strategies to prevent inducible MALT from evolving into lymphoma.

KEY POINTS

- The mucosal immune system is divided into inductive sites – where antigens sampled from the mucosal surface stimulate cognate naïve T and B lymphocytes – and effector sites – where effector cells after extravasation and differentiation exert mature immune functions.
- Peyer's patches, a major inductive site in the mammalian small intestine, represent the most typical MALT structure. Many related structures have been described but their distribution, composition, development, and functions vary considerably with species. Peyer's patches in humans and rodents and tonsils in humans initiate their development prenatally but other structures develop only after birth.
- Imprinting of homing receptors on lymphocytes during their sensitization in inductive sites directs their redistribution into mucosal effector compartments.
- The intestinal humoral response leads to a massive production of secretory IgA, necessary to confine exogenous antigens in the lumen. This function is important to maintain mutualistic relationships with the intestinal microbiota and protect the host against pathogenic bacteria and enteroviruses.
- The outcome of intestinal T cell responses depends on the nature of the antigen. Administration of soluble proteins results in antigen-specific tolerance both locally and systemically. In contrast, pathogenic bacteria and viruses elicit potent proinflammatory responses.
- The functions of NALT as an inductive site for mucosal responses have been demonstrated in mice. Direct comparison with the situation in humans is difficult as NALT differs by its distribution and ontogeny. In humans, nasal immunization in humans may elicit secretory IgA antibodies in the upper airways and endocervix and promote systemic IgG responses.
- The occurrence of BALT differs considerably between species and it remains controversial whether BALT is exclusively inducible or not.
- Chronic inflammation can promote the development of so-called tertiary lymphoid organs through mechanisms that partially recapitulate normal lymphomagenesis. Continuous antigenic stimulation in the latter organs can be associated with clonal B cell proliferations resulting in MALT B cell lymphomas.

ACKNOWLEDGMENTS

The authors thank Gérard Eberl for helpful discussions. INSERM U793 is supported by grants from INSERM, ANR, FRM, Fondation François Aupetit, Institut Danone, and Fondation Princesse Grace de Monaco.

REFERENCES

● = Key primary paper
◆ = Major review article

1. McDermott MR, Bienenstock J. Evidence for a common mucosal immunologic system. I. Migration of B immunoblasts into intestinal, respiratory, and genital tissues. *J Immunol* 1979; **122**: 1892–98.

2. Brandtzaeg P, Kiyono H, Pabst R, Russell M. Terminology: nomenclature of mucosa-associated lymphoid tissue. *Mucosal Immunology* 2008; **1**: 31–7.

3. Brandtzaeg P, Pabst R. Let's go mucosal: communication on slippery ground. *Trends Immunol* 2004; **25**: 570–7.

4. Moghaddami M, Cummins A, Mayrhofer G. Lymphocyte-filled villi: Comparison with other lymphoid aggregations in the mucosa of the human small intestine. *Gastroenterology* 1998; **115**: 1414–25.

5. Craig SW, Cebra JJ. Peyer's patches, an enriched source of precursors for IgA-producing lymphocytes in the rabbit. *J Exp Med* 1971; **134**: 188–200.

6. Eberl G. From induced to programmed lymphoid tissues: the long road to preempt pathogens. *Trends Immunol* 2007; **28**: 423–8.

◆7. Mebius RE. Organogenesis of lymphoid tissues. *Nat Rev Immunol* **3**: 2003; 292–303.

●8. Eberl G, Marmon S, Sunshine MJ *et al.* An essential function for the nuclear receptor RORγ(t) in the generation of fetal lymphoid tissue inducer cells. *Nat Immunol* 2004; **5**: 64–73.

9. Veiga-Fernandes H, Coles MC, Foster KE *et al.* Tyrosine kinase receptor RET is a key regulator of Peyer's patch organogenesis. *Nature* 2007; **446**: 547–51.

10. Ohl L, Bernhardt G, Pabst O, Forster R. Chemokines as organizers of primary and secondary lymphoid organs. *Semin Immunol* 2003; **15**: 249–55.

●11. Guy-Grand D, Griscelli C, Vassalli P. The gut-associated-lymphoid system: nature and properties of the large dividing cells. *Eur J Immunol* 1974; **4**: 435–43.

12. Kerneis S, Bogdanova A, Krahenbuhl J-P, Pringault E. Conversion by Peyer's patch lymphocytes of human enterocytes into M cells that transport bacteria. *Science* 1997; **277**: 949–52.

13. Moxey PC, Trier JS. Development of villus absorptive cells in the human fetal small intestine: a morphological and morphometric study. *Anat Rec* 1979; **195**: 463–82.

14. Golovkina TV, Shlomchik M, Hannum L, Chervonsky A. Organogenic role of B lymphocytes in mucosal immunity. *Science* 1999; **286**: 1965–8.

15. Borghesi C, Taussig MJ, Nicoletti C. Rapid appearance of M cells after microbial challenge is restricted at the periphery of the follicle-associated epithelium of Peyer's patch. *Lab Invest* 1999; **79**: 1393–1401.

16. Ebert LM, Schaerli P, Moser B. Chemokine-mediated control of T cell traffic in lymphoid and peripheral tissues. *Mol Immunol* 2005; **42**: 799–809.

◆17. Johansson-Lindbom B, Agace WW. Generation of gut-homing T cells and their localization to the small intestinal mucosa. *Immunol Rev* 2007; **215**: 226–42.

18. Baekkevold ES, Yamanaka T, Palframan RT *et al.* The CCR7 ligand ELC (CCL19) is transcytosed in high endothelial venules and mediates T cell recruitment. *J Exp Med* 2001; **193**: 1105–12.

19. Moser B, Schaerli P, Loetscher P *et al.* CXCR5(+) T cells: follicular homing takes center stage in T-helper-cell responses. *Trends Immunol* 2002; **23**: 250–4.

◆20. Brandtzaeg P, Johansen FE. Mucosal B cells: phenotypic characteristics, transcriptional regulation, and homing properties. *Immunol Rev* 2005; **206**: 32–63.

◆21. Neutra MR, Mantis NJ, Kraehenbuhl JP. Collaboration of epithelial cells with organized mucosal lymphoid tissues. *Nat Immunol* 2001; **2**: 1004–9.

22. Cook DN, Prosser DM, Forster R *et al.* CCR6 mediates dendritic cell localization, lymphocyte homeostasis, and immune responses in mucosal tissue. *Immunity* 2000; **12**: 495–503.

23. McDonald KG, McDonough JS, Wang C *et al.* CC chemokine receptor 6 expression by B lymphocytes is essential for the development of isolated lymphoid follicles. *Am J Pathol* 2007; **170**: 1229–40.

24. Salazar-Gonzalez RM, Niess JH, Zammit DJ *et al.* CCR6-mediated dendritic cell activation of pathogen-specific T cells in Peyer's patches. *Immunity* 2006; **24**: 623–32.

25. Chabot S, Wagner JS, Farrant S, Neutra MR. TLRs regulate the gatekeeping functions of the intestinal follicle-associated epithelium. *J Immunol* 2006; **176**: 4275–83.

●26. Macpherson AJ, Uhr T. Induction of protective IgA by intestinal dendritic cells carrying commensal bacteria. *Science* 2004; **303**: 1662–5.

27. Iwasaki A, Kelsall B. Localization of distinct Peyer's patch dendritic cell subsets and their recruitment by chemokines macrophage inflammatory protein (MIP)-3alpha, MIP-3beta, and secondary lymphoid organ chemokine. *J Exp Med* 2000; **191**: 1381–94.

28. Ruedl C, Hubele S. Maturation of Peyer's patch dendritic cells in vitro upon stimulation via cytokines or CD40 triggering. *Eur J Immunol* 1997; **27**: 1325–30.

29. Allen CD, Okada T, Cyster JG. Germinal-center organization and cellular dynamics. *Immunity* 2007; **27**: 190–202.

30. Lorenz RG, Chaplin DD, McDonald KG et al. Isolated lymphoid follicle formation is inducible and dependent upon lymphotoxin-sufficient B lymphocytes, lymphotoxin beta receptor, and TNF receptor I function. J Immunol 2003; **170**: 5475–82.

31. Newberry RD, Lorenz RG. Organizing a mucosal defense. Immunol Rev 2005; **206**: 6–21.

32. Pabst O, Herbrand H, Friedrichsen M et al. Adaptation of solitary intestinal lymphoid tissue in response to microbiota and chemokine receptor CCR7 signaling. J Immunol 2006; **177**: 6824–32.

●33. Pabst O, Herbrand H, Worbs T et al. Cryptopatches and isolated lymphoid follicles: dynamic lymphoid tissues dispensable for the generation of intraepithelial lymphocytes. Eur J Immunol 2005; **35**: 98–107.

34. Saito H, Kanamori Y, Takemori T et al. Generation of intestinal T cells from progenitors residing in gut cryptopatches. Science 1998; **280**: 275–8.

●35. Eberl G, Littman DR. Thymic origin of intestinal alphabeta T cells revealed by fate mapping of RORgammat+ cells. Science 2004; **305**: 248–51.

36. Gangadharan D, Lambolez F, Attinger A et al. Identification of pre- and postselection TCRalphabeta+ intraepithelial lymphocyte precursors in the thymus. Immunity 2006; **25**: 631–41.

●37. Guy-Grand D, Azogui O, Celli S et al. Extrathymic T cell lymphopoiesis: ontogeny and contribution to gut intraepithelial lymphocytes in athymic and euthymic mice. J Exp Med 2003; **197**: 333–41.

●38. Fagarasan S, Muramatsu M, Suzuki K et al. Critical roles of activation-induced cytidine deaminase in the homeostasis of gut flora. Science 2002; **298**: 1424–7.

39. McDonald KG, McDonough JS, Newberry RD. Adaptive immune responses are dispensable for isolated lymphoid follicle formation: antigen-naive, lymphotoxin-sufficient B lymphocytes drive the formation of mature isolated lymphoid follicles. J Immunol 2005; **174**: 5720–8.

40. Shikina T, Hiroi T, Iwatani K et al. IgA class switch occurs in the organized nasopharynx- and gut-associated lymphoid tissue, but not in the diffuse lamina propria of airways and gut. J Immunol 2004; **172**: 6259–64.

41. Hashizume T, Momoi F, Kurita-Ochiai T et al. Isolated lymphoid follicles are not IgA inductive sites for recombinant Salmonella. Biochem Biophys Res Commun 2007; **360**: 388–93.

42. Hashizume T, Togawa A, Nochi T et al. Peyer's patches are required for intestinal immunoglobulin a responses to Salmonella spp. Infect Immun 2008; **76**: 927–34.

43. Chirdo FG, Millington OR, Beacock-Sharp H, Mowat AM. Immunomodulatory dendritic cells in intestinal lamina propria. Eur J Immunol 2005; **35**: 1831–40.

●44. Niess JH, Brand S, Gu X et al. CX3CR1-mediated dendritic cell access to the intestinal lumen and bacterial clearance. Science 2005; **307**: 254–8.

●45. Rescigno M, Urbano M, Valzasina B et al. Dendritic cells express tight junction proteins and penetrate gut epithelial monolayers to sample bacteria. Nat Immunol 2004; **4**: 361–7.

46. Chieppa M, Rescigno M, Huang AY, Germain RN. Dynamic imaging of dendritic cell extension into the small bowel lumen in response to epithelial cell TLR engagement. J Exp Med 2006; **203**: 2841–52.

47. MacPherson GG, Jenkins CD, Stein MJ, Edwards C. Endotoxin-mediated dendritic cell release from the intestine. Characterization of released dendritic cells and TNF dependence. J Immunol 1995; **154**: 1317–22.

48. Jang MH, Sougawa N, Tanaka T et al. CCR7 is critically important for migration of dendritic cells in intestinal lamina propria to mesenteric lymph nodes. J Immunol 2006; **176**: 803–10.

49. Ohl L, Mohaupt M, Czeloth N et al. CCR7 governs skin dendritic cell migration under inflammatory and steady-state conditions. Immunity 2004; **21**: 279–88.

◆50. Iliev ID, Matteoli G, Rescigno M. The yin and yang of intestinal epithelial cells in controlling dendritic cell function. J Exp Med 2007; **204**: 2253–7.

51. Kraus TA, Brimnes J, Muong C et al. Induction of mucosal tolerance in Peyer's patch-deficient, ligated small bowel loops. J Clin Invest 2005; **115**: 2234–43.

52. Martinoli C, Chiavelli A, Rescigno M et al. Entry route of Salmonella typhimurium directs the type of induced immune response. Immunity 2007; **27**: 975–84.

53. Gowans JL, Knight EJ. The route of recirculation of lymphocytes in the rat. Proc R Soc London B 1964; **159**: 257–82.

●54. Husband A, Gowans J. The origin and antigen-dependent distribution of IgA-containing cells in the intestine. J Exp Med 1978; **148**: 1146–60.

55. Rosen H, Goetzl EJ. Sphingosine 1-phosphate and its receptors: an autocrine and paracrine network. Nat Rev Immunol 2005; **5**: 560–70.

56. Kuklin NA, Rott L, Darling J et al. $\alpha 4\beta 7$ independent pathway for CD8(+) T cell-mediated intestinal immunity to rotavirus. J Clin Invest 2000; **106**: 1541–52.

57. Sarnacki S, Auber F, Cretolle C et al. Blockade of the integrin alphaLbeta2 but not of integrins alpha4 and/or beta7 significantly prolongs intestinal allograft survival in mice. Gut 2000; **47**: 97–104.

58. Kunkel EJ, Butcher EC. Plasma-cell homing. Nat Rev Immunol 2003; **3**: 822–9.

59. Kunkel EJ, Campbell DJ, Butcher EC. Chemokines in lymphocyte trafficking and intestinal immunity. Microcirculation 2003; **10**: 313–23.

60. Bowman EP, Kuklin NA, Youngman KR et al. The intestinal chemokine thymus-expressed chemokine (CCL25) attracts IgA antibody-secreting cells. J Exp Med 2002; **195**: 269–75.

61. Van de Perre P. Transfer of antibody via mother's milk. Vaccine 2003; **21**: 3374–6.

62. Harris NL, Spoerri I, Schopfer JF et al. Mechanisms of neonatal mucosal antibody protection. J Immunol 2006; **177**: 6256–62.

63. Iwata M, Hirakiyama A, Eshima Y *et al.* Retinoic acid imprints gut-homing specificity on T cells. *Immunity* 2004; **21**: 527–38.

●64. Mora JR, Iwata M, Eksteen B *et al.* Generation of gut-homing IgA-secreting B cells by intestinal dendritic cells. *Science* 2006; **314**: 1157–60.

●65. Mucida D, Park Y, Kim G *et al.* Reciprocal TH17 and regulatory T cell differentiation mediated by retinoic acid. *Science* 2007; **317**: 256–60.

◆66. MacPherson AJ, McCoy KD, Johansen FE *et al.* The immune geography of IgA induction and function. *Mucosal Immunology* 2008; **1**: 11–22.

67. Klein J, Ju W, Heyer B *et al.* B cell-specific deficiency for Smad2 in vivo leads to defects in TGF-beta-directed IgA switching and changes in B cell fate. *J Immunol* 2006; **176**: 2389–96.

68. Bergqvist P, Gardby E, Stensson A *et al.* Gut IgA class switch recombination in the absence of CD40 does not occur in the lamina propria and is independent of germinal centers. *J Immunol* 2006; **177**: 7772–83.

69. Macpherson A, Hunziker L, McCoy K, Lamarre A. IgA responses in the intestinal mucosa against pathogenic and non-pathogenic microorganisms. *Microbes Infect* 2001; **3**: 1021–35.

70. Tezuka H, Abe Y, Iwata M *et al.* Regulation of IgA production by naturally occurring TNF/iNOS-producing dendritic cells. *Nature* 2007; **448**: 929–33.

●71. He B, Xu W, Santini PA *et al.* Intestinal bacteria trigger T cell-independent immunoglobulin A(2) class switching by inducing epithelial-cell secretion of the cytokine APRIL. *Immunity* 2007; **26**: 812–26.

72. Crouch EE, Li Z, Takizawa M *et al.* Regulation of AID expression in the immune response. *J Exp Med* 2007; **204**: 1145–56.

73. Farstad IN, Carlsen H, Morton HC *et al.* Immunoglobulin A cell distribution in the human small intestine: phenotypic and functional characteristics. *Immunology* 2000; **101**: 354–63.

74. Mostov K, Su T, ter Beest M. Polarized epithelial membrane traffic: conservation and plasticity. *Nat Cell Biol* 2003; **5**: 287–93.

75. Phalipon A, Cardona A, Kraehenbuhl JP *et al.* Secretory component: a new role in secretory IgA-mediated immune exclusion in vivo. *Immunity* 2002; **17**: 107–15.

76. Muller CA, Autenrieth IB, Peschel A. Innate defenses of the intestinal epithelial barrier. *Cell Mol Life Sci* 2005; **62**: 1297–307.

77. Moreau MC, Ducluzeau R, Guy-Grand D, Muller MC. Increase in the population of duodenal immunoglobulin A plasmocytes in axenic mice associated with different living or dead bacterial strains of intestinal origin. *Infect Immun* 1978; **21**: 532–9.

●78. Peterson DA, McNulty NP, Guruge JL, Gordon JI. IgA response to symbiotic bacteria as a mediator of gut homeostasis. *Cell Host Microbe* 2007; **2**: 328–39.

79. Jiang HQ, Thurnheer MC, Zuercher AW *et al.* Interactions of commensal gut microbes with subsets of B- and T-cells in the murine host. *Vaccine* 2004; **22**: 805–11.

◆80. Macpherson AJ. IgA adaptation to the presence of commensal bacteria in the intestine. *Curr Top Microbiol Immunol* 2006; **308**: 117–36.

81. Macpherson AJ, Geuking MB, McCoy KD. Immune responses that adapt the intestinal mucosa to commensal intestinal bacteria. *Immunology* 2005; **115**: 153–62.

82. Brandtzaeg P. Induction of secretory immunity and memory at mucosal surfaces. *Vaccine* 2007; **25**: 5467–84.

83. Wijburg OL, Uren TK, Simpfendorfer K *et al.* Innate secretory antibodies protect against natural Salmonella typhimurium infection. *J Exp Med* 2006; **203**: 21–6.

84. Kadaoui KA, Corthesy B. Secretory IgA mediates bacterial translocation to dendritic cells in mouse Peyer's patches with restriction to mucosal compartment. *J Immunol* 2007; **179**: 7751–7.

85. Matysiak-Budnik T, Moura IC, Arcos-Fajardo M *et al.* Secretory IgA mediates retrotranscytosis of intact gliadin peptides via the transferrin receptor in celiac disease. *J Exp Med* 2008; **205**: 143–54.

86. Arstila T, Arstila TP, Calbo S *et al.* Identical T cell clones are located within the mouse gut epithelium and lamina propia and circulate in the thoracic duct lymph. *J Exp Med* 2000; **191**: 823–34.

87. Guy-Grand D, Griscelli C, Vassalli P. The mouse gut T lymphocyte, a novel type of T cell. *J Exp Med* 1978; **148**: 1661–77.

88. Probert CS, Saubermann LJ, Balk S, Blumberg RS. Repertoire of the alpha beta T-cell receptor in the intestine. *Immunol Rev* 2007; **215**: 215–25.

89. Cheroutre H, Lambolez F. Doubting the TCR coreceptor function of CD8alphaalpha. *Immunity* 2008; **28**: 149–59.

90. Lambolez F, Kronenberg M, Cheroutre H. Thymic differentiation of TCR alpha beta(+) CD8 alpha alpha(+) IELs. *Immunol Rev* 2007; **215**: 178–88.

91. Leishman AJ, Naidenko OV, Attinger A *et al.* T cell responses modulated through interaction between CD8alphaalpha and the nonclassical MHC class I molecule, TL. *Science* 2001; **294**: 1936–9.

92. Pardigon N, Darche S, Kelsall B *et al.* The TL MHC class Ib molecule has only marginal effects on the activation, survival and trafficking of mouse small intestinal intraepithelial lymphocytes. *Int Immunol* 2004; **16**: 1305–13.

93. Jarry A, Cerf-Bensussan N, Brousse N *et al.* Subsets of CD3+(TCR$\alpha\beta$ or TCR$\gamma\alpha$) and CD3- lymphocytes isolated from normal human gut epithelium differ from their PBL counterparts. *Eur J Immunol* 1990; **20**: 1097–103.

94. Jabri B, Patey de Serre N, Cellier C *et al.* Selective expansion of intraepithelial lymphocytes expressing the HLA-E-specific natural killer receptor CD94 in celiac disease. *Gastroenterology* 2000; **118**: 867–79.

95. Hue S, Mention JJ, Monteiro RC *et al.* A direct role for NKG2D/MICA interaction in villous atrophy during celiac disease. *Immunity* 2004; **21**: 367–77.

96. Meresse B, Chen Z, Ciszewski C et al. Coordinated induction by IL15 of a TCR-independent NKG2D signaling pathway converts CTL into lymphokine-activated killer cells in celiac disease. *Immunity* 2004; **21**: 357–66.

97. Meresse B, Curran SA, Ciszewski C et al. Reprogramming of CTLs into natural killer-like cells in celiac disease. *J Exp Med* 2006; **203**: 1343–55.

98. Lefrancois L, Puddington L. Intestinal and pulmonary mucosal T cells: local heroes fight to maintain the status quo. *Annu Rev Immunol* 2006; **24**: 681–704.

99. Asseman C, Mauze S, Leach MW et al. An essential role for interleukin 10 in the function of regulatory T cells that inhibit intestinal inflammation. *J Exp Med* 1999; **190**: 995–1004.

100. Kullberg MC, Jankovic D, Feng CG et al. IL-23 plays a key role in Helicobacter hepaticus-induced T cell-dependent colitis. *J Exp Med* 2006; **203**: 2485–94.

♦101. Izcue A, Coombes JL, Powrie F. Regulatory T cells suppress systemic and mucosal immune activation to control intestinal inflammation. *Immunol Rev* 2006; **212**: 256–71.

102. Izcue A, Powrie F. Special regulatory T-cell review: Regulatory T cells and the intestinal tract–patrolling the frontier. *Immunology* 2008; **123**: 6–10.

●103. Stecher B, Robbiani R, Walker AW et al. Salmonella enterica serovar typhimurium exploits inflammation to compete with the intestinal microbiota. *PLoS Biol* 2007; **5**: 2177–89.

104. Deretic V, Singh S, Master S et al. Mycobacterium tuberculosis inhibition of phagolysosome biogenesis and autophagy as a host defence mechanism. *Cell Microbiol* 2006; **8**: 719–27.

105. Matsuzaki G, Umemura M. Interleukin-17 as an effector molecule of innate and acquired immunity against infections. *Microbiol Immunol* 2007; **51**: 1139–47.

106. Ravindran R, Foley J, Stoklasek T et al. Expression of T-bet by CD4 T cells is essential for resistance to Salmonella infection. *J Immunol* 2005; **175**: 4603–10.

107. Narni-Mancinelli E, Campisi L, Bassand D et al. Memory CD8+ T cells mediate antibacterial immunity via CCL3 activation of TNF/ROI+ phagocytes. *J Exp Med* 2007; **204**: 2075–87.

108. Holtmeier W, Chowers Y, Lumeng A et al. The δ T cell receptor repertoire in human colon and peripheral blood is oligoclonal irrespective of V region usage. *J Clin Invest* 1995; **96**: 1109–17.

109. O'Brien RL, Roark CL, Jin N et al. gammadelta T-cell receptors: functional correlations. *Immunol Rev* 2007; **215**: 77–88.

110. Nanno M, Shiohara T, Yamamoto H et al. gammadelta T cells: firefighters or fire boosters in the front lines of inflammatory responses. *Immunol Rev* 2007; **215**: 103–13.

111. Poussier P, Ning T, Banerjee D, Julius M. A unique subset of self-specific intraintestinal T cells maintains gut integrity. *J Exp Med* 2002; **195**: 1491–7.

●112. Rimoldi M, Chieppa M, Salucci V et al. Intestinal immune homeostasis is regulated by the crosstalk between epithelial cells and dendritic cells. *Nat Immunol* 2005; **6**: 507–14.

113. Smythies LE, Sellers M, Clements RH et al. Human intestinal macrophages display profound inflammatory anergy despite avid phagocytic and bacteriocidal activity. *J Clin Invest* 2005; **115**: 66–75.

●114. Coombes JL, Siddiqui KR, Arancibia-Carcamo CV et al. A functionally specialized population of mucosal CD103+ DCs induces Foxp3+ regulatory T cells via a TGF-beta and retinoic acid-dependent mechanism. *J Exp Med* 2007; **204**: 1757–64.

●115. Sun CM, Hall JA, Blank RB et al. Small intestine lamina propria dendritic cells promote de novo generation of Foxp3 T reg cells via retinoic acid. *J Exp Med* 2007; **204**: 1775–85.

116. Pasare C, Medzhitov R. Toll pathway-dependent blockade of CD4+CD25+ T cell-mediated suppression by dendritic cells. *Science* 2003; **299**: 1033–6.

♦117. Perry M, Whyte A. Immunology of the tonsils. *Immunol Today* 1998; **19**: 414–21.

118. Debertin AS, Tschernig T, Tonjes H et al. Nasal-associated lymphoid tissue (NALT): frequency and localization in young children. *Clin Exp Immunol* 2003; **134**: 503–7.

♦119. Kiyono H, Fukuyama S. NALT- versus Peyer's-patch-mediated mucosal immunity. *Nat Rev Immunol* 2004; **4**: 699–710.

120. Brandtzaeg P. Immunology of tonsils and adenoids: everything the ENT surgeon needs to know. *Int J Pediatr Otorhinolaryngol* 2003; **67** (Suppl 1): S69–76.

121. Xu W, He B, Chiu A et al. Epithelial cells trigger frontline immunoglobulin class switching through a pathway regulated by the inhibitor SLPI. *Nat Immunol* 2007; **8**: 294–303.

122. Johansen FE, Baekkevold ES, Carlsen HS et al. Regional induction of adhesion molecules and chemokine receptors explains disparate homing of human B cells to systemic and mucosal effector sites: dispersion from tonsils. *Blood* 2005; **106**: 593–600.

123. Bienenstock J, McDermott MR. Bronchus- and nasal-associated lymphoid tissues. *Immunol Rev* 2005; **206**: 22–31.

124. Xu B, Wagner N, Pham LN et al. Lymphocyte homing to bronchus-associated lymphoid tissue (BALT) is mediated by L-selectin/PNAd, alpha4beta1 integrin/VCAM-1, and LFA-1 adhesion pathways. *J Exp Med* 2003; **197**: 1255–67.

125. Gould SJ, Isaacson PG. Bronchus-associated lymphoid tissue (BALT) in human fetal and infant lung. *J Pathol* 1993; **169**: 229–34.

126. Debertin AS, Tschernig T, Schurmann A et al. Coincidence of different structures of mucosa-associated lymphoid tissue (MALT) in the respiratory tract of children: no indications for enhanced mucosal immunostimulation in sudden infant death syndrome (SIDS). *Clin Exp Immunol* 2006; **146**: 54–9.

127. Tschernig T, Pabst R. Bronchus-associated lymphoid tissue (BALT) is not present in the normal adult lung but in different diseases. *Pathobiology* 2000; **68**: 1–8.

●128. Rangel-Moreno J, Hartson L, Navarro C *et al.* Inducible bronchus-associated lymphoid tissue (iBALT) in patients with pulmonary complications of rheumatoid arthritis. *J Clin Invest* 2006; **116**: 3183–94.

●129. Moyron-Quiroz JE, Rangel-Moreno J, Kusser K *et al.* Role of inducible bronchus associated lymphoid tissue (iBALT) in respiratory immunity. *Nat Med* 2004; **10**: 927–34.

130. Cook DN, Bottomly K. Innate immune control of pulmonary dendritic cell trafficking. *Proc Am Thorac Soc* 2007; **4**: 234–9.

131. Langlois RA, Legge KL. Respiratory dendritic cells: mediators of tolerance and immunity. *Immunol Res* 2007; **39**: 128–45.

132. Kocks JR, Davalos-Misslitz AC, Hintzen G *et al.* Regulatory T cells interfere with the development of bronchus-associated lymphoid tissue. *J Exp Med* 2007; **204**: 723–34.

◆133. Drayton DL, Liao S, Mounzer RH, Ruddle NH. Lymphoid organ development: from ontogeny to neogenesis. *Nat Immunol* 2006; **7**: 344–53.

134. Eberl G. Inducible lymphoid tissues in the adult gut: recapitulation of a fetal developmental pathway? *Nat Rev Immunol* 2005; **5**: 413–20.

135. Du, MQ. MALT lymphoma: recent advances in aetiology and molecular genetics. *J Clin Exp Hematop* 2007; **47**: 31–42.

14

Biology of plasma cells

MICHAEL POTTER

GENERAL

The B lymphocyte/plasma cell lineage

The B lymphocyte/plasma cell lineage has three general developmental stages. In mammals the first takes place in the bone marrow. Here, closely linked but separate immunglobulin (Ig) structural genes that code for heavy (H) and light (L) chains are assembled and joined on the chromosome to form a template for transcription. For the H chain, four genes are rearranged from their germ-line configuration and brought together in two steps: first, one of 17–19 D_H genes is joined to one of the 5 J_H genes that are linked to $C\mu$; second, one of $\sim$100 functional V_H genes is joined to the 5'-selected D_H gene now joined to J_H and $C\mu$. For the L chain, where there is no D element, rearranged Ig DNA is formed by the joining of one of $\sim$50–100 V_L genes to one of 5 J_L genes. The newly synthesized H and L chains are folded, assembled, glycosylated, and then joined together to form the antigen-binding receptor, also called the B cell receptor (BCR). The complex steps in this process are described in Chapter 9. The second developmental stage takes place after the B lymphocyte, with its individual or idiotypic BCR, is released into the peripheral B cell pool where it circulates in and out of lymphoid tissues and inflammatory sites in search of a complementary antigenic structure. Appropriate binding to antigen by a T cell:B cell cognate interaction or by the BCR binding to intact antigenic macromolecules cause the B cell to proliferate and undergo clonal expansion. This process is described in Chapter 11. In the third and final developmental stage, the BCR-positive cell transforms into a professional Ig-secreting plasma cell, the subject of the present chapter. Very simplistically, the substeps in this process are the activated B lymphocyte becomes a plasmablast (with proliferative potential), then the plasmablast matures to intermediate plasma cell and finally to post-mitotic plasma cell. Some of the latter go on to become over-ripe: Mott cells. The anatomical sites where plasma cells develop are listed in Table 14.1.

The material discussed in this chapter deals with several issues of plasma cell biology, current knowledge of which is derived from studies in both humans and mice. Although the focus is on humans, the mouse provides a major source of experimental information, largely because it is possible to alter the genes that control B cell activation and differentiation to the plasma cell stage. Aside from the obvious differences in evolutionary history (greater than 20 Myr) – such as longevity, body structure, and societal lifestyles of the two species – there are well-known species differences in the detailed organization of the two immune systems; there are also many similarities. The differences need to be qualified when extrapolating principles from mouse to man. The differences in the composition of the peripheral B cell population, such as memory B cells, B1, B2 B cells, and splenic marginal zone cells, are discussed below. Nonetheless, the striking general similarities in the structure, function, and regulation of special genes make studies in the mouse of great potential value to understanding the generation of plasma cells in humans.

Activation of B lymphocytes to become plasma cells

The basic function of the plasma cell is the synthesis and massive export of Ig molecules into surrounding tissue spaces and plasma. When a B lymphocyte undergoes the transition to become a plasma cell, large groups of genes (the plasma cell program) are activated by transcription factors, such as BLIMP1, XBP1, and IRF4 (Fig. 14.1).[1] The organelle of protein secretion is the endoplasmic reticulum (ER). In plasma cells a structural permutation of the ER is a 'rough ER' (RER) that is studded with ribosomes. Here proteins are translated and liberated into cisternal spaces or lumens between the RER membranes, where they begin moving along the secretory pathway.[2] Proteins are folded and assembled into multichain structures in the RER, then transported to the Golgi and exported via the plasma membrane by

expulsion of packaged vescicles.[3] Here also, critical post-translational steps of N-glycosylation and some interchain disulfide bond formation take place.

Active protein synthesis for purposes of secreting large amounts of Ig (and other proteins in various other cell types) is regulated to cope with various kinds of stress that interfere with the synthesis, assembly, and folding of proteins in the ER. The coordinated activity of sensor proteins in the ER membranes, e.g., IRE1, PERK, and ATF6, trigger the unfolded protein response (UPR) by activating the transcription factor XBP1. When unfolded proteins accumulate in the cisternae of the ER, they can trigger the UPR response to downregulate protein synthesis, arrest growth, and even trigger apoptosis.[4,5]

In vitro differentiation of B cells to become plasma cells

It has been known for some time that murine B cells stimulated by bacterial lipopolysaccharide (LPS) can be activated *in vitro* and driven to the plasma cell stage.[6]

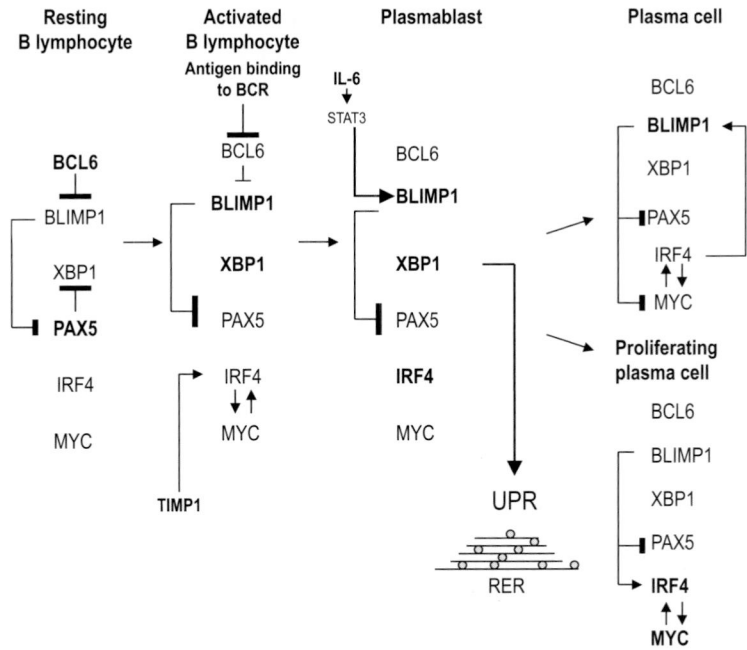

Figure 14.1   General scheme of lymphocyte to plasma cell transition based on reviews from several laboratories (see these articles for details).[37,111-116] While many of the studies were based on post-germinal center B cell differentiation in humans, the basic plan may be generally applicable to other modes of plasma cell origin. Future research will define significant details. Essentially, the basic changes in this process involve the upregulation and downregulation of six transcription factors: BCL6, XBP1, BLIMP1, PAX5, IRF4, and MYC. BLIMP1 (dominant factors are shown in bold), XBP1, and IRF4 direct the plasma cell program involved in immunoglobulin (Ig) secretion and rough endoplasmic reticulum (RER) elaboration. In resting B cells this program is suppressed by BCL6 and PAX5. Exogenous agents (e.g., antigen binding to the BCR) downregulate BCL6 and start the change to the plasma cell program. Proliferation of plasma cells is usually controlled and limited with IRF4 and MYC playing important roles. The formation of the extensive RER is determined chiefly by XBP1, which also activates the unfolded protein response (UPR). In neoplastic development and other conditions including multicentric Castleman disease, proliferation continues concomitantly with Ig secretion. An alteration in the interplay of IRF4 and MYC appears to be a critical regulatory step in this process.

An extensive literature exists on this subject. The relatively recent interest in innate immunity has greatly extended our understanding of the mechanism involved. A basic concept in innate immunity is that the mammalian host defenses can recognize pathogen-associated molecular patterns (PAMPS) via a set of 10–15 receptor molecules, the Toll-like receptors (TLR).[7] The Toll receptor for LPS on B cells is now recognized to be the Toll-like receptor TLR4, which is expressed constitutively in naïve murine B cells. Purified human naïve B cells isolated from the peripheral blood can also be activated *in vitro* to become Ig-secreting cells.[8] These cells were induced to proliferate and differentiate by BCR aggregation (with anti-IgM) or by the addition of irradiated T cells and TLR9 (receptor for CpG-DNA) and CpG oligodeoxynucleotide 2006, indicating the requirement for three activation signals. These investigators found that B cells triggered by anti-IgM upregulated TLR9 itself. They detected Ig secretion using the enzyme-linked immunosorbent spot (ELISPOT) assay. B cell activation that initiates proliferation and proceeds to the plasma cell stage is discussed in several reviews.[8–11]

A murine model system is available for studying ER biogenesis and Ig synthesis in the B cell line CH12, which can be induced by LPS to differentiate and become plasma cells.[12] In more recent studies with this cell line, a sharp upregulation of Ig H and L chain synthesis occurred 24 hours after addition of LPS. The activation of the UPR components preceded this elevation of Ig level.[4]

In this chapter the focus will be on the *in vivo* B lymphocyte activations that lead to the plasma cell transition, with emphasis given to the tissue microenvironments and factors that control this transition.

MAJOR *IN VIVO* SITES OF PLASMA CELL FORMATION

Following differentiation of the BCR the naïve B lymphocytes are released into the circulation to selectively enter tissue sites (spleen, lymph nodes [LN], Peyer's patches [PP], isolated lymphoid follicles [ILF]) where they have greatly increased opportunities to encounter a complementary antigenic structure. There are five major tissue sites where plasma cells develop from activated B lymphocytes, and these are summarized in Table 14.1. Not listed are memory B lymphocytes that are activated by antigen to the plasma cell stage, which may take place in any one of the sites listed, except possibly the bone marrow. An unresolved question concerns the role of antigen in the bone marrow site.

Rapid humoral responses

EXTRAFOLLICULAR REACTIONS

Several days are required to generate plasma cells that produce high-affinity antibodies to an antigen, and in this time an advancing microbial infection could overwhelm the organism. Most mammals, however, can rapidly respond to infection with a new agent by rapidly producing natural antibodies and antibodies from memory cells to deal with the immediate infection. Major tissue sites where rapid responses begin are, first, the T cell or extrafollicular zones in lymph nodes and spleen, and the marginal zones of the spleen. Early cognate responses in the extrafollicular spaces of lymphoid tissues are described in Chapter 12 (see also [22]).

Many of these early response antibodies are derived from antigen-inexperienced B cells and are polyreactive,

Table 14.1 Tissues in which plasma cells develop from B lymphocytes

Tissue site where B lymphocyte–plasmablast–plasma cell takes place	Characteristics	References
Extrafollicular T cell zone (TCZ) of lymph nodes, spleen	Antigen-activated B lymphocytes accumulate at the boundary of the follicles and the TCZ, become plasmablasts (PB), proliferate, and become short-lived plasma cells (PC)	13,14,15,16
Medullary cord lymph node, red pulp spleen	Activated B cells of three origins migrate to medullary cords and become PCs, B cells that have experienced germinal center reactions, B cells that have directly entered the cortex (via afferent lymphatics), or B cells that have been activated in the TCZ	17
Lamina propria (gastrointestinal tract, tonsils)	Activated B cells (blasts) or plasmablasts migrate into subepithelial lamina propria (LP) at the base of intestinal villi and then into the villus LP to become plasma cells	18,19
Bone marrow	Plasmablasts home to niches provided by stromal cells and mature to become long-lived plasma cells	20
Extralymphoid (ectopic) chronic inflammatory sites, inflammation-associated lymphoid neogenesis	Circulating B, T, and DC migrate to inflammatory and autoimmune sites of tissue destruction and chronic infections, where they assemble to form lymphoid tissues (lymphoid neogenesis) with varying degrees of complexity that can generate plasma cells; these tissues are antigen rich	21

i.e., they bind to multiple structurally unrelated epitopes.[23] Most have relatively low affinities for their antigenic targets or epitopes. Further, the structure of their binding sites may have specificities for epitopes that are widely distributed in nature, e.g., certain polysaccharides, CpG-rich DNA, and certain autoantigens. These antibodies are usually encoded by germ-line V_L, J_L, D_H, J_H, and V_H genes with minimal changes at the junction sites. These antibodies usually do not require somatic mutations to be functional and useful,[24] nor do they need cognate T cell help.

Thymus independent (TI-2) responses for the most part are initiated by antigenic macromolecules that have multiple repeating epitopes (for an excellent review, see[25]). Common natural antigens with repeating epitopes are polysaccharides on the surfaces of various microorganisms or viral capsid glycoproteins. The multivalent antigen can crosslink the BCRs on the surface and activate the B cell. This step may be sufficient to activate BCR signal transduction pathways (STP) and cause the cell to proliferate, clonally expand in numbers, and begin secreting antibody (Ab). The STP includes the Bruton tyrosine kinase (BTK) component that plays a singular role in TI-2 responses.[25] BTK deficiency is X linked and causes agammaglobulinemia in humans. The engagement and crosslinking alone of the BCRs, however, often is insufficient to drive the B cell to become a plasma cell. Mond and colleagues propose second signals are necessary that are supplied by engagement of PAMPS on microbial surfaces with TLRs on the B cells.[25] These signals first require the upregulation of TLR on the B cell surface, a step that is triggered by BCR engagement, and then the interaction of TLR with the PAMP drives the activated B cells to become Ig-secreting cells.[7,25] Other agents, including, hypothetically, T cells and their products, can supply these second signals as well.

MARGINAL ZONE B CELLS OF THE SPLEEN

A substantial portion of B cells capable of reacting rapidly with foreign antigens in humans and mice become concentrated and sequestered in the marginal zone (MZ) of the spleen, a special structure where blood is constantly filtered and antigens can be trapped by an abundance of macrophages.[26,27] Marginal zone B cells are thought to be preactivated and readily become plasmablasts and begin secreting IgM antibody when confronted with particulate antigens that have entered the circulation and become trapped in the MZ of the spleen. A major difference in human and mouse MZ B cell relates to their distribution in the lymphoid system. Marginal zone B cells in the mouse are usually sessile and splenic, while in humans they are circulating and found not only in the spleen but also in lymph nodes.[28] The phenotype of circulating and MZ B cells in humans is IgM^{hi} IgD^{lo}, $CD27^+$ $CD21^+$ $CD23^-$ $CDC1c^{hi}$. A high percentage (10–30 percent) of recirculating B lymphocytes possess the human MZ phenotype. In both humans and mice a fraction of the MZ humoral responses contains highly mutated V regions, further

supporting their association with antigen-experienced memory B cell clones.

B1 B CELLS AND CD5⁺ B CELLS

The B1/B2 subdivision of peripheral B cells is deeply entrenched in the literature, and there are major differences between humans and mice. B1 cells in both humans and mice are the predominant B lymphocyte in the fetus and neonate,[29] and this is the basis for interspecies homology. In both species B1 cells produce germ-line encoded antibodies with rare evidence of somatic hypermutations. The major differences in B1 cells are in adults. In adult mice, in contrast to humans, only a few B1 cells persist in the circulation and most are located in the peritoneal and pleural cavities. These possess the property of self-renewal. B1 cells in the mouse peritoneum have upregulated integrin genes that cause them to tightly bind to peritoneal surfaces where they are somewhat sessile. They can, however, be flushed out. Recently, it has been shown that peritoneal cavity (PerC) B1 cells can be mobilized into the circulation and then to the gut mucosa by downregulating these integrins.[30] CD5 is the characteristic marker of most but not all B1 cells in the mouse. However, in humans 10–25 percent of the B cells express CD5.[31] The commonality, however, between the species may reside in their relationship to fetal and neonatal B cell populations. In the mouse and humans, B1 cells are thought to be the source of serum IgM and natural antibodies.[31] Peritoneal cavity B1 cells in the mouse are the progenitors of 50 percent of the IgA-secreting plasma cells in the lamina propria (LP) of the gastrointestinal (GI) tract.[32,33] Following immunization with particulate bacterial antigens, B1 cells were found to be activated in the T cell zone/follicular border of the spleen to become Ig-secreting cells. A candidate homolog for the mouse B1 cell in humans is the $CD5^+$ IgM^+ IgD^+ cell in the peripheral blood.[31]

Germinal center–related immune responses

THE MEDULLARY CORD AND SPLENIC RED PULP PLASMA CELL

Common sites for plasma cell formation are the medullary cords in lymph nodes or the red pulp in spleen. Medullary cord plasma cell accumulations are seen in reactive plasmacytosis in humans.[35] The origin of the medullary cord plasma cell is not definitively established. Three sources of precursors are: (1) cells exiting from germinal center reactions in follicles; (2) B cells activated in the T cell zone, paracortex, or extrafollicular zone that migrate toward the hilus; or (3) B cells entering directly from the circulation through high endothelial venules (HEVs) or afferent lymphocytes. An excellent experimental model of medullary cord plasma cell development, though greatly exaggerated, is seen in the interleukin-6 (IL-6) transgenic mouse.

The late steps in the germinal center reaction are poorly defined. The step from centrocyte to small lymphocyte in the mantle zone, for example, is not clearly visualized as yet. Presumably the centrocytes enter the mantle zone as small lymphocytes and then go to the parenchyma of the lymphoid tissue on route to the circulation, initially by entering into the paracortex or T cell zone, then migrating toward the hilus of the node and efferent lymphatics to ultimately join the circulation and various homing sites, e.g., the bone marrow. Once the post-germinal center lymphocytes leave the germinal centers (GCs), they may become relieved of the suppressive actions of BCL6 and PAX5. The transcription factors B lymphocyte maturation factor (BLIMP1) and X-box binding protein-1 (XBP1) would now become upregulated to orchestrate the plasma cell program.[1] Some of these post-GC B cells transit through the paracortex or T cell zone and are activated to become plasmablasts in medullary cords.

The mechanism for selective plasmablast activation has not yet been elucidated but possibly involves cognate T:B interaction, T cell cytokine stimulation, or some other process. Specific cytokines such as IL-6 may be important intermediaries in this process and stimulate plasmablast activation and even plasmablast proliferation.[36] The plasmablasts in the medullary cords complete their maturation to the plasma cell stage, and the plasma cells presumably remain in this location. The decline of BCL6 expression also results in the upregulation of the IRF4 transcription factor, which appears to be required for post-GC lymphocytes and memory cells to become plasma cells. IRF4-deficient mice lack plasma cells derived from these precursors.[37]

THE LONG–LIVED BONE MARROW PLASMA CELL AND MEMORY B CELLS

In a recent and important review on long-lived plasma cells[20] extensive evidence has been provided supporting the concept that bone marrow plasma cells can maintain humoral memory for extensive periods of time, bordering in some extreme examples for a lifetime. This is based on the premise that activated B cells from different regions, but predominantly post-GC circulating plasmablasts, home to a limited number of protected niches in the bone marrow. Here the plasmablast matures under the protective influence of the stromal cells to become a long-lived (nondividing) plasma cell. It is thought that antigen does not activate the long-lived plasma cell through its BCR, as these receptors are greatly if not completely downregulated in plasma cells.

Memory B cells are difficult to define on the basis of specific cell-surface markers; the CD27 marker in humans is an exception. Many studies have, therefore, defined memory cells based on functional characteristics, such as isotype switches, somatic hypermutations in Ig genes, persistence of antibody long after initial exposure to antigen, and reactivation with reintroduction of antigen. Another problem in defining memory cells stems from the heterogeneity of the B cell population that is derived from different immunizations, both natural and induced.[38] Antigenic persistence, such as the stored immune complexes on follicular dendritic cells, certain unusual persisting antigens, or a

chronic (latent) viral infection,[39,40] may play a role in continued plasma cell formation.

The memory B cell population in humans is more clearly defined and consists of two general subdivisions: the classical memory pathways of post-GC class switched and somatically hypermutated B cells; and, second, a large fraction (~40 percent of the B cell pool) of $CD27^+ IgM^+ IgD^+$ cells that are not switched but have hypermutated BCRs.[41]

Gastrointestinal lamina propria plasma cells

The gastrointestinal-associated lymphoid tissues consist of PPs, ILFs,[42] mesenteric lymph nodes (MLNs), and the LP that contains T cells, B cells, dendritic cells, and a very large population of plasma cells. This gut- or mucosal-associated lymphoid system (GALT or MALT) in many ways is a distinct component of the immune system, both in its strategic location and way of handling antigens but also, as pathologists have noted, with its own unique pathology,[43] e.g., the MALT lymphomas.

The largest population of plasma cells in humans, mice, and other well-studied mammals resides in the subepithelial spaces (lamina propria) of the GI tract. They are positioned to secrete Ab for export into the lumen of the GI tract. An extensive series of investigations established that these LP plasma cells are a special population of plasma cells characterized by the predominant secretion of IgA. Antigens, including those in foods, bacteria, viruses, protozoa, and fungi, are taken up by dendritic cells. These antigen-presenting cells are critical in determining whether the antigen activates an immune response or leads to tolerance.[44] Recent studies have emphasized the importance of MLNs in determining whether the response to antigen results in tolerance or an active immune response.[45]

In mice, circulating $B220^+$ surface IgM $(sIgM)^+$ B cells enter through HEVs into the interfollicular regions of PP to begin their differentiation into IgA-secreting LP plasma cells. Antigens with PAMPs or entire microorganisms that have translocated across the mucosal epithelial barrier are taken up by dendritic cells. These interact with and activate B cells that can now gain access to the GCs of PP (and probably ILFs as well), where they respond to local stromal cells and cytokines to switch from $S\mu$ to $S\alpha$ to become $sIgA^+$ B cells This process upregulates $\alpha_4\beta_7$ and $\alpha_4\beta_1$ adhesion molecules and chemokine receptor CCR9. The $sIgA^+$ B cells enter the circulation or migrate directly through efferent lymphatics to the MLNs. The expression of the $\alpha_4\beta_7$ adhesion molecule endows the cell with the capacity to bind to the target adhesion molecule MAdCAM-1 that is expressed on gut-associated endothelial cells (for an excellent review, see [46]).

There is evidence that knockout mice that lack the lymphotoxin β receptor (LTβR$-/-$) that lack PP (but still form MLNs) can, nonetheless, develop mucosal IgA-secreting plasma cells.[47] Fagarasan and Honjo have provided experimental evidence that switching to IgA can take place in the gut LP without cells passing through germinal centers.[48] In the *aly/aly* (alymphoplasia) spontaneously mutant mice that lack PP and germinal centers it has been found that some naïve sIgM$^+$ B220$^+$ B cells can directly migrate to the intestinal LP where they can putatively activate the activation-induced cytidine deaminase (AID) enzyme and undergo class switch recombination to IgA production. It is not yet agreed upon that this process takes place in wild-type mice.[49,50]

The IgA molecules secreted by the intestinal LP plasma cells are dimers joined by J chains. These bind to the secretory component (SC) expressed on the surface of the columnar epithelial cells. The SC-IgA complex is endocytosed, the vesicle is transported across the epithelial cell, and the IgA molecule's contents are released into the lumen of the gut. It is here the IgA molecules exert their effector functions that impede the invasion of the body by bacteria, protozoa, and viruses. Another important function may be protection from toxins that can affect the viability of epithelial cells or the body in general. Immunoglobulin A can protect intestinal epithelial cells from the lethal action of ricin.[51] Other potential effector actions of these IgA molecules await further clarification. There are indications that IgA influences the ecology of the commensal anaerobic bacterial population in the GI tract.[52] Mice deficient for the AID enzyme and the ability to undergo somatic hypermutation develop dramatic changes in their gut flora. In these mice the colonic populations of bacteria are similar to normal but the upper regions of the small intestine become heavily populated with anaerobes.

PLASMA CELL ACCUMULATIONS

Lymphoid neogenesis and chronic inflammation

A remarkable feature of the lymphoid tissues is their ability to form new lymphoid structures by lymphoid neogenesis. In this process B and T lymphocytes, dendritic cells, and stromal cells (e.g., fibroblasts) aggregate and assemble into organized lymphoid neogenic structures. They may be even supplied by HEVs. These new lymphoid organoid structures are called tertiary lymphoid organs (TLOs). Tertiary lymphoid organs are heterogeneous and include ectopic germinal centers,[53] cryptopatches, and ILFs, and possibly other kinds of lymphoid aggregates that can vary in size and complexity.[54] In the larger lymphoid aggregates, the separation of T and B cell zones has been described. Plasma cells can be developed at TLO sites.

Tertiary lymphoid organ formation has been found in a variety of chronic inflammations: the synovial pannus in rheumatoid arthritis, myasthenia gravis, multiple sclerosis, Sjögren syndrome, Hashimoto thyroiditis, Graves disease, ulcerative colitis, chronic hepatitis C, Lyme disease, and many chronic infections.[55] Although many of these entities have different pathogenic origins, they do have in common an association with excessive antigen production.

There has been considerable recent interest in lymphoid neogenesis as a site of plasma cell formation.[21,56] In these

sites antigens are produced in abundance, e.g., chronic infections (Helicobacter, old Lyme disease, chronic hepatitis C, syphilitic lesions, some forms of tuberculosis) and in tissues undergoing autoimmune destruction (the joints in rheumatoid arthritis, the thyroid in Hashimoto thyroiditis, the salivary glands in Sjögren syndrome, and others). These tissues become infiltrated with macrophages, T cells, dendritic cells, fibroblasts, and B cells. This leads to a self-organization, in effect, of the lymphoid elements into follicle-like structures with peanut agglutinin PNA$^+$ germinal centers. Further, many of these structures contain plasma cells. Of special importance is that the plasma cells in these sites locally produce antibodies to the antigens or autoantigens generated at the sites.

Plasma cell accumulations are found in certain kinds of inflammation and with disorders of cytokine production. The best examples are associated with the overproduction of IL-6 and transforming growth factor β (TGFβ) of their signal transduction pathways. Extrafollicular B cell proliferation (in the apparent absence of follicles) has been described in humans.[57]

Castleman disease, IL-6 transgenic mice

Excessive plasma cell accumulations that are strongly suspected to result from overexpression of IL-6 occur in Castleman disease (CD).[58] Castleman disease (also known as angiofollicular lymph node hyperplasia, or giant lymph node hyperplasia) was first described in 1954 by Castleman as a lymphoproliferative disorder of unknown etiology.[59,60] The first patients were found to have greatly enlarged mediastinal lymph nodes. Pathologically, these nodes contained numerous enlarged follicles, about half of which contained plasma cells or plasmablasts that were arranged concentrically around the follicular mantle. Since this time, there has unfolded a growing understanding of this rare pathology that is still not defined fully. (See Casper[61] for a brief history of the first 50 years of CD.) A first pathogenetic milestone was the finding that CD could also involve multiple LNs, where it was associated with systemic clinical manifestations including fever, splenomegaly, and hyperimmunoglobulinemia. Life expectancy was reduced to around 24 months or less, and some patients developed secondary lymphomas. This form of CD was called multicentric CD (MCD). A second milestone was that there was an increased incidence of MCD in human immunodeficiency virus (HIV)–acquired immune deficiency syndrome (AIDS) patients,[62] and this led to the discovery that 14 of 14 HIV–AIDS patients with MCD carried a $\gamma 2$ or rhadino herpes virus (HHV-8), also known as Kaposi sarcoma herpes virus (KSHV).[63] The third milestone was the finding that HHV-8 encodes four highly relevant cytokine and chemokine genes: vIL-6, vCCL-2, vCCL-3, and vCCL-1.[64,65]

The presence of the vIL-6 gene is significant because Yoshizaki et al.[58] found that supernatants from cultured lymph nodes from four patients with MDC contained increased quantities of IL-6 and there was immunohis-tochemical evidence of IL-6 in the germinal centers. Interleukin-6 had been previously identified as a growth factor for mouse plasmacytomas *in vitro* and was implicated in the pathogenesis of pristane induction of plasma cell tumors in mice.[66] The Kishimoto laboratory developed strains of mice carrying the H-2L^D-hu-IL-6 IL-6 transgene.[67,68] It has been suggested that enforced overproduction of IL-6 by an IL-6 transgene in mice is a murine model of MCD.[69] Mice carrying the H-2L^D-hu-IL-6 transgene engineered by Suematsu et al.[68] develop generalized lymphadenopathy and splenomegaly beginning around six months of age. There is an extensive and progressive accumulation of plasma cells in the medullary cords of all lymph nodes, culminating in the virtual replacement of the node by plasma cells. The mantle zone ring-like arrangement of plasma cells has not been seen in the lymph nodes of mice carrying IL-6 transgenes. These mice also developed transplantable plasma cell tumors.

Excessive plasma cell accumulations have also been found in mice lacking the transcription factor C/EBP-β.[70] These mice develop lesions in mucosal tissues, suggesting increased susceptibility to infections. However, like the IL-6 transgenic mice, they develop lymphadenopathies associated with excessive accumulations of plasma cells involving the cervical and mesenteric lymph nodes, leading to the claim that C/EBP-β-deficient mice were another potential model of CD. Increased serum levels of IL-6 were also found. The observation that IL-6−/− C/EBP-β−/− mice did not develop lymphadenopathy, high levels of IL-6, or plasma cell accumulations further implicated IL-6 as the critical factor.[71] The mechanism proposed by Screpanti et al. is that C/EBP-β deficiency led to highly deregulated myeloid and B cell activities that increased IL-6 production.[70]

The viral IL-6 gene in HHV-8 shares many functional properties with human IL-6 but also has several differences relating to its mode of action and expression.[65,72] First, viral IL-6 was able to bypass the IL-6 receptor subunit gp80 and cause dimerization of the gp130 signal-transducing subunit, with resultant signaling through STAT1, STAT3, and C/EBP-β (transcription factors that regulate the acute phase response proteins). Second, there were many amino acid differences in the signal-transduction sequence, which showed only 28 percent homology, while the coding sequence has 62.2 percent homology with its human counterpart.[73]

The general implication of the available information is that the overproduction of IL-6 can lead to a dramatic accumulation of plasma cells in lymphoid tissues, creating generalized lymphadenopathy, and that in humans this can be associated with the subsequent development of Hodgkin disease or non-Hodgkin lymphomas. In contrast, the IL-6 transgenic mice develop plasma cell tumors at high incidence with varying grades of maturation.

Gastrointestinal plasma cell accumulations

Plasma cell accumulations in the LP of the GI tract are found in several diseases, such as familial juvenile polyposis (FJP), immunoproliferative small intestinal

disease (IPSID), and IL-10 deficiency created experimentally in mice, and have a complex pathogenesis. The character of the plasma cell infiltrates varies with the disease. The most dramatic of these disorders is IPSID, also known as alpha heavy chain disease or Mediterranean lymphoma. The LP is heavily infiltrated with lymphocytes and plasma cells.[74] Pathogenetic mechanisms in IPSID are discussed in Chapter 84 of this book.

Familial juvenile polyposis has an hereditary basis with defects in the *SMAD4* gene located on chr18q21.1 occurring in a high percentage of cases.[75] Pathogenetic mechanisms are becoming better defined as the predominant molecular lesions appear to be in the TGFβ signaling pathway.

Transforming growth factor β is produced by many cell types. The signaling pathway begins with the binding of TGFβ to the specific transmembrane receptor TGFβ RII. This triggers the phosphorylation of SMAD proteins that are nonenzymatic mediators of the pathway.[76,77] SMAD proteins form different heterodimeric complexes that can translocate to the nucleus where they govern several hundred gene targets by transcriptional activation or repression.[78,79] SMAD4 is the universal partner with regulatory SMADS 1, 2, and 3 and inhibitory SMADS (SMADS 6 and 7).

Transforming growth factor β is thought to be a negative regulator of immune responses by suppressing proliferation of both T and B lymphocytes. Blocking TGFβ signaling *in vivo* by various genetic manipulations (such as in the TGFβ and TGFβ RII knockout mice, the dominant negative TGFβ RII transgenic mouse, the inhibitory Smad7 transgenic mouse, the targeted inaction of Smad4 in T cells) leads to several biologic abnormalities notably plasma cell infiltrations in the LP of the GI tract, colitis, and benign and malignant neoplasia of the mucosal epithelium.[80]

Transforming growth factor β has several important actions in T cells including the differentiation of T cells and the effector functions of T cells. These alterations in T cell function can lead to inflammation in the LP and epithelial proliferation. Study of peripheral T cell development has focused for the last decade primarily on CD4$^+$ T helper type 1 (TH1) and TH2 differentiation and regulation. New components of the CD4 T cell subsets are CD4 TH17/IL-17 T cells[81,82] and the rediscovered T suppressor cell of Gershon, now called CD4$^+$ CD25$^+$ regulatory T cells.[83,84]

Familial juvenile polyposis in humans is characterized by hamartomatous polyps of the colon and rectum that contain intestinal epithelium and stroma, including the LP, that are infiltrated with lymphocytes and plasma cells.[85] An homologous model has been developed in mice in which the *Smad4* gene has been conditionally inactivated in T cells.[86] These mice develop hamartomatous polyps in the colon, rectum, duodenum, stomach, and oral cavity, some of which progress to become carcinomas.

Reactive plasmacytosis

Reactive plasmacytosis is rarely encountered clinically. It is manifested by a striking polyclonal expansion of circulating plasma cells and an increase in the bone marrow plasma cell population. It appears sporadically in a great variety of chronic autoimmune (e.g., rheumatoid arthritis), neoplastic, and infectious diseases.[35,87] Plasmacytosis appears also as an occasional and unusual manifestation in certain viral infections, e.g., hepatitis A,[88] Dengue,[89] and Epstein–Barr virus.[35] Bone marrow plasmacytosis has also been observed in idiopathic lymphadenopathy with polyclonal hyperimmunoglobulinemia (IPL).[90] The plasma cell accumulations in these processes though reaching great proportions are usually transient. The cells in the peripheral blood are both plasmablasts and mature plasmacytes, CD19[+], CD38[+], CD138[+], CD45[+], and CD11a[+].[35,91]

PROLIFERATION DISORDERS OF PLASMA CELLS

The terminal event in B cell development is the transformation of a B lymphocyte into an Ig-secreting plasma cell, which usually proceeds to a point where cell cycling ceases. There are intermediary cellular stages where both cell cycling and copious Ig secretion coexist in the same cell. We are beginning to appreciate the complexity of this process and its various manifestations. In the 1960s Guy Sainte-Marie, in a study of plasma cell accumulations in the medullary cords in mediastinal lymph nodes of normal laboratory rats, described stages of maturation in plasma cell development that were associated with an ordered number of cell divisions, a process he labeled 'plasmacytopoiesis.'[92,93] A progressive decrease in the nuclear diameter occurred during maturation. Plasmablasts with large nuclear diameters matured to an intermediary stage while undergoing active cell division, ultimately giving rise to a population of mature plasma cells associated with a decrease in mitotic activity. These striking but benign accumulations of plasma cells were the result of an undetermined antigenic stimulus. Similar plasma cell accumulations are found experimentally in IL-6 transgenic mice and in mice deficient for C/EBP-β[71] as well as clinically in Castleman disease, where there is an overproduction of IL-6.

Monoclonal gammopathy of undetermined significance

Monoclonal gammopathy of undetermined significance (MGUS) is characterized and distinguished clinically from multiple myeloma (MM) by serum monoclonal Ig level ranges from 0.5 to 3.0 g/L, the presence of less than 10 percent plasma cells in bone marrow analysis, and the absence of osteolytic bone lesions (for reviews, see [94,95]). It has been estimated that 3 percent of surveyed humans over the age of 50 years and 5 percent over the age of 70 can be shown to have a monoclonal Ig spike in their serum by zone electrophoresis or immunofixation. MGUS may remain asymptomatic indefinitely, which is the usual course, but about 1 percent of cases per year progress to become malignant

MM, Waldenstrom macroglobulinemia, or other serious lymphoproliferative disorder. This has been shown both prospectively[95] and retrospectively.[96] Defining the causes and nature of MGUS and the reasons for the transition to MM present important clinical and biological problems; monoclonal proliferations of plasma cells in MGUS occur with increasing frequency during aging in both humans and mice.[95,97–99]

GENOMIC INSTABILITY

An intriguing finding in MM is the high frequency of 14q32+-related chromosomal translocations (CTs) and many of these same CTs have also been found in MGUS plasma cells.[100,101] The recurring target genes to which the 14q32+ is joined are 11q13 (cyclin D1) – 15–18 percent in MM and 15–26 percent in MGUS and SMM (smoldering myeloma); 4p16 (FGFR3 and MMSET) – 10–18 percent in MM and 2–9 percent in MGS/SMM; 6p21 (cyclin D3) – 3–4 percent in MM; and 16q23 (Maf) – 2–9 percent in MM and 1–5 percent in MGUS/SHM.[101] Chromosomal rearrangements and t8;14(q24/q32) that affect the *MYC* locus are found infrequently in MM and less so in MGUS.[101–103] In general it has been concluded that CTs affecting a *MYC* locus are infrequent in the human disease and that when encountered they represent a later, progression event. It is of interest that many other rearrangements affecting the *MYC* locus in MM are not the t(8;14) but other more subtle changes, including translocations of *MYC* to non-Ig loci. The recurring CTs in MGUS suggest that these CTs activate genes that affect survival and proliferation of plasma cells. These may have arisen in post-GC B lymphocytes before the cells have matured to plasma cells.

RACE, AGE

It has been known for some time that the incidence of MM in Americans of African origin is higher than that in white subjects. This relationship also holds for MGUS. Landgren *et al.* have found a twofold higher incidence of MGUS in African Americans than in white subjects.[104] Also, a recent survey of men in Ghana has shown age-unrelated prevalence differences in MGUS as compared to United States (Olmsted County) white males. The prevalence in the 50–54/70–74-year-old men was 1.83/5.12 percent for Olmsted County Men, while for the Ghana men it was 5.33/5.38 percent (see [105]). The prevalence was much higher in the 50–54-year-old group. In other populations, mostly from Western countries and Japan,[106] the prevalence of MGUS is lower. In mice, inbred strain differences have been described.[99] These findings suggest that genetic factors may play a role in MGUS development; further environmental factors, such as prevalent infections as suggested by the Ghanian study, also may play a role.

CLONAL ORIGIN

The biology of MGUS is poorly understood, and the major question concerns the origin of the abnormal clone. Does

MGUS originate from the long-lived plasma cell population in the bone marrow or does the abnormal clone arise from a circulating B lymphocyte, a long-lived memory B cell precursor that expands over time and continuously gives rise to cells that home to bone marrow sites? Although there may be several explanations, one possibility is that the 14q32+/IgH switch region disorder develops in a germinal center B cell, because switching occurs in the germinal follicle. The mutant B lymphocyte and its progeny may recirculate or go through dormant phases. Some progeny possess an enhanced ability to compete with other memory cells for niches in the bone marrow cavities that are usually occupied by long-lived plasma cells. These cells, because of the mutations they carry (some in the form of a CT), may simply acquire a strategy for survival and limited proliferation in the bone marrow. Evidence supporting a B lymphocyte origin of MM is the finding that the myeloma protein idiotype can also be found on circulating B lymphocytes.[107–110] This suggests the MM plasma cells may be derived from a clone of B lymphocytes that persist along with the plasma cell clone.

Multiple myeloma

The pathogenesis of multiple myeloma and related neoplasms is discussed in Chapter 38.

KEY POINTS

- B lymphocyte to plasma cell transition can occur in different tissue sites.
- The transition of a B lymphocyte to become an Ig-secreting plasma cell is regulated by changes in transcription factors.
- Disorders in IL-6 production can lead to excessive plasma cell accumulations.
- Transition to the plasma cell is usually associated with cessation in cell cycling; however, in plasma cell neoplasia, the plasma cells retain proliferative potential.

REFERENCES

● = Key primary paper
◆ = Major review article

◆1. Calame KL, K-I Lin, Tunyaplin C. Regulatory mechanisms that determine the development and function of plasma cells. *Ann Rev Immunol* 2003; **21**: 205–30.

◆2. Lippincott-Schwartz J, Roberts TH, Hirschberg K. Secretory protein trafficking and organelle dynamics in living cells. *Annu Rev Cell Dev Biol* 2000; **16**: 557–89.

3. Hirschberg K, Miller CM, Ellenberg J *et al.* Kinetic analysis of secretory protein traffic and characterization of golgi to plasma membrane transport intermediates in living cells. *Cell Biol* 1998; **143**: 1485–503.

4. Gass JN, Gifford NM, Brewer JW. Activation of an unfolded protein response during differentiation of antibody-secreting B cells. *J Biol Chem* 2002; **277**: 49047–54.

5. Iwakoshi NN, Lee AH, Vallabhajosyula P *et al.* Plasma cell differentiation and the unfolded protein response intersect at the transcription factor XBP-1. *Nat Immunol* 2003; **4**: 321–9.

6. Melchers F, Andersson J. The kinetics of proliferation and maturation of mitogen-activated bone marrow-derived lymphocytes. *Eur J Immunol* 1974; **4**: 687–91.

7. Iwasaki A, Medzhitov R. Toll-like receptor control of the adaptive immune responses. *Nat Immunol* 2004; **5**: 987–95.

8. Ruprecht CR, Lanzavecchia A. Toll-like receptor stimulation as a third signal required for activation of human naive B cells. *Eur J Immunol* 2006; **36**: 810–16.

9. Peng SL, Signaling in B cells via Toll-like receptors. *Curr Opin Immunol* 2005; **17**: 230–6.

10. Fillatreau S, Manz RA. Tolls for B cells. *Eur J Immunol* 2006; **36**: 798–801.

11. Bernasconi NL, Onai N, Lanzavecchia A. A role for Toll-like receptors in acquired immunity: up-regulation of TLR9 by BCR triggering in naive B cells and constitutive expression in memory B cells. *Blood* 2003; **101**: 4500–4.

12. Wiest DL, Burkhardt JK, Hester S *et al.* Membrane biogenesis during B cell differentiation: most endoplasmic reticulum proteins are expressed coordinately. *J Cell Biol* 1990; **110**: 1501–11.

13. Garcia de Vinuesa, C, O'Leary P, Sze D *et al.* T-independent type 2 antigens induce B cell proliferation in multiple splenic sites, but exponential growth is confined to extrafollicular foci. *Eur J Immunol* 1999; **29**: 1314–23.

◆14. Cyster JG. Homing of antibody secreting cells. *Immunol Rev* 2003; **194**: 48–60.

◆15. Okada T, Cyster JG. B cell migration and interactions in the early phase of antibody responses. *Curr Opin Immunol* 2006; **18**: 278–85.

16. Jacob J, Kelsoe G. In situ studies of the primary immune response to (4-hydroxy-3-nitrophenyl) acetyl. II. A common clonal origin for periarteriolar lymphoid sheath-associated foci and germinal centers. *J Exp Med* 1992; **176**: 679–87.

17. Wehrli N, Legler DF, Finke D *et al.* Changing responsiveness to chemokines allows medullary plasmablasts to leave lymph nodes. *Eur J Immunol* 2001; **31**: 609–16.

18. Spahn TW, Kucharzik T. Modulating the intestinal immune system: the role of lymphotoxin and GALT organs. *Gut* 2004; **53**: 456–65.

19. Husband AJ, Gowans JL. The origin and antigen-dependent distribution of IgA-containing cells in the intestine. *J Exp Med* 1978; **148**: 1146–60.

◆20. Radbruch A, Muehlinghaus G, Luger EO *et al.* Competence and competition: the challenge of becoming a long-lived plasma cell. *Nat Rev Immunol* 2006; **6**: 741–50.

21. Aloisi F, Pujol-Borrell R. Lymphoid neogenesis in chronic inflammatory diseases. *Nat Rev Immunol* 2006; **6**: 205–17.

22. MacLennan IC, Toellner KM, Cunningham AF *et al*. Extrafollicular antibody responses. *Immunol Rev* 2003; **194**: 8–18.

23. Notkins AL. Polyreactivity of antibody molecules. *Trends Immunol* 2004; **25**: 174–9.

24. Casali P, Schettino EW, Structure and function of natural antibodies. *Curr Top Microbiol Immunol* 1996; **210**: 167–79.

25. Vos Q, Lees A, Wu ZQ *et al*. B-cell activation by T-cell-independent type 2 antigens as an integral part of the humoral immune response to pathogenic microorganisms. *Immunol Rev* 2000; **176**: 154–70.

26. Lopes-Carvalho T, Kearney JF. Marginal zone B cell physiology and disease. *Curr Dir Autoimmun* 2005; **8**: 91–123.

27. Mebius RE, Kraal G. Structure and function of the spleen. *Nat Rev Immunol* 2005; **5**: 606–16.

28. Weller S, Reynaud CA, Weill JC. Splenic marginal zone B cells in humans: where do they mutate their Ig receptor? *Eur J Immunol* 2005; **35**: 2789–92.

29. Hardy RR. B-1 B cell development. *J Immunol* 2006; **177**: 2749–54.

30. Ha SA, Tsuji M, Suzuki K *et al*. Regulation of B1 cell migration by signals through Toll-like receptors. *J Exp Med* 2006; **203**: 2541–50.

31. Dono M, Cerruti G, Zupo S. The CD5+ B-cell. *Int J Biochem Cell Biol* 2004; **36**: 2105–11.

32. Kroese FG, Butcher EC, Stall AM *et al*. Many of the IgA producing plasma cells in murine gut are derived from self-replenishing precursors in the peritoneal cavity. *Int Immunol* 1989; **1**: 75–84.

33. Rothstein TL. Cutting edge commentary: two B-1 or not to be one. *J Immunol* 2002; **168**: 4257–61.

34. Martin F, Oliver AM, Kearney JF. Marginal zone and B1 B cells unite in the early response against T-independent blood-borne particulate antigens. *Immunity* 2001; **14**: 617–29.

35. Jego G, Robillard N, Puthier D *et al*. Reactive plasmacytoses are expansions of plasmablasts retaining the capacity to differentiate into plasma cells. *Blood* 1999; **94**: 701–12.

36. Jego G, Bataille R, Pellat-Deceunynck C. Interleukin-6 is a growth factor for nonmalignant human plasmablasts. *Blood* 2001; **97**: 1817–22.

37. Klein U, Casola S, Cattoretti G *et al*. Transcription factor IRF4 controls plasma cell differentiation and class-switch recombination. *Nat Immunol* 2006; **7**: 773–82.

38. Anderson SM, Tomayko MM, Shlomchik MJ. Intrinsic properties of human and murine memory B cells. *Immunol Rev* 2006; **211**: 280–94.

39. Zinkernagel RM. On differences between immunity and immunological memory. *Curr Opin Immunol* 2002; **14**: 523–36.

40. Gray D, A role for antigen in the maintenance of immunological memory. *Nat Rev Immunol* 2002; **2**: 60–5.

41. Weller S, Braun MC, Tan BK *et al*. Human blood IgM 'memory' B cells are circulating splenic marginal zone B cells harboring a prediversified immunoglobulin repertoire. *Blood* 2004; **104**: 3647–54.

42. Hamada H, Hiroi T, Nishiyama Y *et al*. Identification of multiple isolated lymphoid follicles on the antimesenteric wall of the mouse small intestine. *J Immunol* 2002; **168**: 57–64.

43. Isaacson PG, Du MQ. Gastrointestinal lymphoma: where morphology meets molecular biology. *J Pathol* 2005; **205**: 255–74.

44. Macpherson AJ, Smith K. Mesenteric lymph nodes at the center of immune anatomy. *J Exp Med* 2006; **203**: 497–500.

45. Worbs T, Bode U, Yan S *et al*. Oral tolerance originates in the intestinal immune system and relies on antigen carriage by dendritic cells. *J Exp Med* 2006; **203**: 519–27.

46. Kunkel EJ, Butcher EC. Plasma-cell homing. *Nat Rev Immunol* 2003; **3**: 822–9.

47. Yamamoto M, Rennert P, McGhee JR *et al*. Alternate mucosal immune system: organized Peyer's patches are not required for IgA responses in the gastrointestinal tract. *J Immunol* 2000; **164**: 5184–91.

48. Suzuki K, Ha SA, Tsuji M, Fagarasan S. Intestinal IgA synthesis: a primitive form of adaptive immunity that regulates microbial communities in the gut. *Semin Immunol* 2007; **19**: 127–35.

49. Suzuki K, Meek B, Doi Y *et al*. Two distinctive pathways for recruitment of naive and primed IgM+ B cells to the gut lamina propria. *Proc Natl Acad Sci U S A* 2005; **102**: 2482–6.

50. Shikina T, Hiroi T, Iwatani K *et al*. IgA class switch occurs in the organized nasopharynx- and gut-associated lymphoid tissue, but not in the diffuse lamina propria of airways and gut. *J Immunol* 2004; **172**: 6259–64.

51. Mantis NJ, McGuinness CR, Sonoyi O *et al*. Immunoglobulin A antibodies against ricin A and B subunits protect epithelial cells from ricin intoxication. *Infect Immun* 2006; **74**: 3455–62.

52. Fagarasan S, Muramatsu M, Suzuki K *et al*. Critical roles of activation-induced cytidine deaminase in the homeostasis of gut flora. *Science* 2002; **298**: 1424–7.

53. Magalhaes R, Stiehl P, Morawietz L *et al*. Morphological and molecular pathology of the B cell response in synovitis of rheumatoid arthritis. *Virchows Arch* 2002; **441**: 415–27.

54. Newberry RD, Lorenz RG. Organizing a mucosal defense. *Immunol Rev* 2005; **206**: 6–21.

55. Drayton DL, Liao S, Mounzer RH, Ruddle NH. Lymphoid organ development: from ontogeny to neogenesis. *Nat Immunol* 2006; **7**: 344–53.

56. Thaunat O, Kerjaschki D, Nicoletti A. Is defective lymphatic drainage a trigger for lymphoid neogenesis? *Trends Immunol* 2006; **27**: 441–5.

57. Brighenti A, Andrulis M, Geissinger E *et al*. Extrafollicular proliferation of B cells in the absence of follicular hyperplasia: a distinct reaction pattern in lymph nodes

correlated with primary or recall type responses. *Histopathology* 2005; **47**: 90–100.

58. Yoshizaki K, Matsuda T, Nishimoto N *et al.* Pathogenic significance of interleukin-6 (IL-6/BSF-2) in Castleman's disease. *Blood* 1989; **74**: 1360–7.

59. Castleman B, Towne VW. Case records of the Massachusetts General Hospital: Case No. 40231. *N Engl J Med* 1954; **250**: 1001–5.

60. Castleman B, Iverson L, Menendez VP. Localized mediastinal lymphnode hyperplasia resembling thymoma. *Cancer* 1956; **9**: 822–30.

61. Casper C. The aetiology and management of Castleman disease at 50 years: translating pathophysiology to patient care. *Br J Haematol* 2005; **129**: 3–17.

62. Du MQ, Liu H, Diss TC *et al.* Kaposi sarcoma-associated herpesvirus infects monotypic (IgM lambda) but polyclonal naive B cells in Castleman disease and associated lymphoproliferative disorders. *Blood* 2001; **97**: 2130–6.

63. Soulier J, Grollet L, Oksenhendler E *et al.* Kaposi's sarcoma-associated herpesvirus-like DNA sequences in multicentric Castleman's disease. *Blood* 1995; **86**: 1276–80.

64. Jenner RG, Boshoff C. The molecular pathology of Kaposi's sarcoma-associated herpesvirus. *Biochim Biophys Acta* 2002; **1602**: 1–22.

65. Nicholas J. Human gammaherpesvirus cytokines and chemokine receptors. *J Interferon Cytokine Res* 2005; **25**: 373–83.

66. Nordan RP, Potter M. A macrophage-derived factor required by plasmacytomas for survival and proliferation in vitro. *Science* 1986; **233**: 566–9.

67. Suematsu S, Matsuda T, Aozasa K *et al.* IgG1 plasmacytosis in interleukin 6 transgenic mice. *Proc Natl Acad Sci USA* 1989; **86**: 7547–51.

68. Suematsu S, Matsusaka T, Matsuda T *et al.* Generation of plasmacytomas with the chromosomal translocation t(12;15) in interleukin 6 transgenic mice. *Proc Natl Acad Sci USA* 1992; **89**: 232–5.

69. Brandt SJ, Bodine DM, Dunbar CE, Neinhuis AW. Dysregulated interleukin 6 expression produces a syndrome resembling Castleman's disease in mice. *J Clin Invest* 1990; **86**: 592–9.

70. Screpanti I, Romani L, Musiani P *et al.* Lymphoproliferative disorder and imbalanced T-helper response in C/EBP beta-deficient mice. *EMBO J* 1995; **14**: 1932–41.

71. Screpanti I, Musiani P, Bellavia D *et al.* Inactivation of the IL-6 gene prevents development of multicentric Castleman's disease in C/EBP beta-deficient mice. *J Exp Med* 1996; **184**: 1561–6.

72. Meads MB, Medveczky PG. Kaposi's sarcoma-associated herpesvirus-encoded viral interleukin-6 is secreted and modified differently than human interleukin-6: evidence for a unique autocrine signaling mechanism. *J Biol Chem* 2004; **279**: 51793–803.

73. Moore PS, Boshoff C, Weiss RA, Chang Y. Molecular mimicry of human cytokine and cytokine response pathway genes by KSHV. *Science* 1996; **274**: 1739–44.

74. Al-Saleem T, Al-Mondhiry H. Immunoproliferative small intestinal disease (IPSID): a model for mature B-cell neoplasms. *Blood* 2005; **105**: 2274–80.

75. Merg A, Howe JR. Genetic conditions associated with intestinal juvenile polyps. *Am J Med Genet C Semin Med Genet* 2004; **129**: 44–55.

76. Derynck R, Zhang YE. Smad-dependent and Smad-independent pathways in TGF-beta family signalling. *Nature* 2003; **425**: 577–84.

77. Dennler, S, Goumans MJ, ten Dijke P. Transforming growth factor beta signal transduction. *J Leukoc Biol* 2002; **71**: 731–40.

78. ten Dijke, Hill CS. New insights into TGF-beta-Smad signalling. *Trends Biochem Sci* 2004; **29**: 265–73.

79. Massague J, Gomis RR. The logic of TGFbeta signaling. *FEBS Lett* 2006; **580**: 2811–20.

80. Letterio JJ. TGF-beta signaling in T cells: roles in lymphoid and epithelial neoplasia. *Oncogene* 2005; **24**: 5701–12.

81. Weaver CT, Harrington LE, Mangan PR *et al.* Th17: an effector CD4 T cell lineage with regulatory T cell ties. *Immunity* 2006; **24**: 677–88.

82. Iwakura Y, Ishigame H. The IL-23/IL-17 axis in inflammation. *J Clin Invest* 2006; **116**: 1218–22.

83. Jonuleit H, Schmitt E. The regulatory T cell family: distinct subsets and their interrelations. *J Immunol* 2003; **171**: 6323–7.

84. Becker C, Fantini MC, Neurath MF. TGF-beta as a T cell regulator in colitis and colon cancer. *Cytokine Growth Factor Rev* 2006; **17**: 97–106.

85. Schreibman IR, Baker M, Amos C, McGarruty TS. The hamartomatous polyposis syndromes: a clinical and molecular review. *Am J Gastroenterol* 2005; **100**: 476–90.

86. Kim BG, Li C, Qiao W *et al.* Smad4 signalling in T cells is required for suppression of gastrointestinal cancer. *Nature* 2006; **441**: 1015–9.

87. Gavarotti P, Boccadoro M, Redoglia V *et al.* Reactive plasmacytosis. Case report and review of the literature. *Acta Haematol* 1985; **73**: 108–10.

88. Wada T, Maeba H, Ikawa Y *et al.* Reactive peripheral blood plasmacytosis in a patient with acute hepatitis A. *Int J Hematol* 2007; **85**: 191–4.

89. Gawoski JM, Ooi WW. Dengue fever mimicking plasma cell leukemia. *Arch Pathol Lab Med* 2003; **127**: 1026–7.

90. Kojima M, Murayama K, Igarashi T *et al.* Bone marrow plasmacytosis in idiopathic plasmacytic lymphadenopathy with polyclonal hyperimmunoglobulinemia: a report of four cases. *Pathol Res Pract* 2007; **203**: 789–94.

91. Adams DO, Hamilton TA. The cell biology of macrophage activation. *Annu Rev Immunol* 1984; **2**: 283–318.

92. Sainte-Marie G. Study on plasmocytopoieses. I. Description of plasmocytes and of their mitoses in the mediastinal lymph nodes of ten-week-old rats. *Am J Anat* 1964; **114**: 207–33.

◆93. Sainte-Marie G. Cytokinetics of antibody formation. *J Cell Physiol* 1966; **67**(Suppl 1):109–28.

◆94. Kyle RA, Rajkumar SV. Monoclonal gammopathies of undetermined significance: a review. *Immunol Rev* 2003; **194**: 112–39.

95. Kyle RA, Rajkumar SV. Monoclonal gammopathy of undetermined significance and smoldering multiple myeloma. *Hematol Oncol Clin North Am* 2007; **21**: 1093–113, ix.

96. Steingrimsdottir H, Haraldsdottir V, Olafsson I *et al.* Monoclonal gammopathy: natural history studied with a retrospective approach. *Haematologica* 2007; **92**: 1131–4.

97. Radl J. Idiopathic paraproteinemia – a consequence of an age-related deficiency in the T immune system. *Clin Immunol Immunopathol* 1979; **14**: 251–5.

98. Radl J. Animal model of human disease. Benign monoclonal gammopathy (idiopathic paraproteinemia). *Am J Pathol* 1981; **105**: 91–3.

99. Radl J. Age-related monoclonal gammapathies: clinical lessons from the aging C57BL mouse. *Immunol Today* 1990; **11**: 234–6.

100. Fonseca R, Bailey RJ, Ahmann GJ *et al.* Genomic abnormalities in monoclonal gammopathy of undetermined significance. *Blood* 2002; **100**: 1417–24.

101. Bergsagel PL, Kuehl WM. Critical roles for immunoglobulin translocations and cyclin D dysregulation in multiple myeloma. *Immunol Rev* 2003; **194**: 96–104.

102. Shou Y, Martelli ML, Gabrea A *et al.* Diverse karyotypic abnormalities of the c-myc locus associated with c-myc dysregulation and tumor progression in multiple myeloma. *Proc Natl Acad Sci U S A* 2000; **97**: 228–33.

103. Avet-Loiseau H, Gerson F, Magrangeas F *et al.* Rearrangements of the c-myc oncogene are present in 15% of primary human multiple myeloma tumors. *Blood* 2001; **98**: 3082–6.

104. Landgren O, Katzmann JA, Hsing AW *et al.* Prevalence of monoclonal gammopathy of undetermined significance among men in Ghana. *Mayo Clin Proc* 2007; **82**: 1468–73.

105. Munshi NC. Monoclonal gammopathy of undetermined significance: genetic vs environmental etiologies. *Mayo Clin Proc* 2007; **82**: 1457–9.

106. Iwanaga M, Tagawa M, Tsukasaki K *et al.* Prevalence of monoclonal gammopathy of undetermined significance: study of 52,802 persons in Nagasaki City, Japan. *Mayo Clin Proc* 2007; **82**: 1474–9.

107. Mellstedt H, Hammarstrom S, Holm G. Monoclonal lymphocyte population in human plasma cell myeloma. *Clin Exp Immunol* 1974; **17**: 371–84.

108. Pilarski LM, Jensen GS. Monoclonal circulating B cells in multiple myeloma. A continuously differentiating, possibly invasive, population as defined by expression of CD45 isoforms and adhesion molecules. *Hematol Oncol Clin North Am* 1992; **6**: 297–322.

109. Kay NE, Leong T, Kyle RA *et al.* Circulating blood B cells in multiple myeloma: analysis and relationship to circulating clonal cells and clinical parameters in a cohort of patients entered on the Eastern Cooperative Oncology Group phase III E9486 clinical trial. *Blood* 1997; **90**: 340–5.

110. Billadeau D, Van Ness B, Kimlinger T *et al.* Clonal circulating cells are common in plasma cell proliferative disorders: a comparison of monoclonal gammopathy of undetermined significance, smoldering multiple myeloma, and active myeloma. *Blood* 1996; **88**: 289–96.

111. Shaffer AL, Emre NC, Lamy L *et al.* IRF4 addiction in multiple myeloma. *Nature* 2008; **454**: 226–31.

112. Kallies A, Hasbold J, Fairfax K *et al.* Initiation of plasma-cell differentiation is independent of the transcription factor Blimp-1. *Immunity* 2007; **26**: 555–66.

113. Guedez L, Martinez A, Zhao S *et al.* Tissue inhibitor of metalloproteinase 1 (TIMP-1) promotes plasmablastic differentiation of a Burkitt lymphoma cell line: implications in the pathogenesis of plasmacytic/plasmablastic tumors. *Blood* 2005; **105**: 1660–8.

114. Fairfax KA, Kallies A, Nutt SL, Tarlinton DM. Plasma cell development: from B-cell subsets to long-term survival niches. *Semin Immunol* 2008; **20**: 49–58.

◆115. Tarlinton D, Radbruch A, Hiepe F, Dömer T. Plasma cell differentiation and survival. *Curr Opin Immunol* 2008; **20**: 162–9.

116. van Anken E, Braakman I. Endoplasmic reticulum stress and the making of a professional secretory cell. *Crit Rev Biochem Mol Biol* 2005; **40**: 269–83.

15

Interleukins and lymphoid neoplasia

BRIAN F SKINNIDER AND TAK W MAK

INTRODUCTION

Cytokines are low-molecular-weight proteins that play a crucial role in the regulation of the immune response. They are produced by and act upon several different cell types, but lymphocytes are the main cell population that produces cytokines, and they in turn depend on them for their differentiation, proliferation, survival, and biologic activity. Since cytokines play such an important role in normal lymphocyte biology, it is not surprising that cytokines play a role in the biology of their malignant counterparts, the lymphoid neoplasms. As with normal lymphocytes, lymphoma cells are capable of producing and responding to cytokines, which can act as growth factors for lymphoma cells, and also contribute to an altered immune response that promotes the development and maintenance of lymphomas.

The activity of cytokines in lymphoid neoplasms is most evident in those tumors with a prominent non-neoplastic reactive infiltrate. The prime example of this phenomenon is Hodgkin lymphoma, but certain non-Hodgkin lymphomas may also demonstrate this feature. In these lymphoid neoplasms, the reactive infiltrate is thought to be recruited by cytokines produced by the malignant cells, and the reactive infiltrate in turn may be contributing to the growth of the malignant cell population, may be altering the immune response, or may simply be an innocuous epiphenomenon. The role of cytokines in lymphoid neoplasms has been most widely studied in Hodgkin lymphoma, and so the greater part of this chapter will deal with this particular disease. Although cytokine activity is most evident in lymphoid neoplasms with a prominent reactive component, many other types of lymphoid neoplasms without such a reactive infiltrate are influenced by cytokines.

The expression and activity of cytokines in lymphoid neoplasms can be studied by several methods, using both cell lines and primary tissue samples. Each approach has its limitations, such that a combination of strategies provides the most comprehensive information on the activity of a specific cytokine. Examination of cell lines allows for the study of the biologic activity of cytokines on proliferation, survival, and gene expression. However, many lymphoma cell lines are derived from treatment-resistant end-stage disease, and as such may not be representative of the disease as it presents in the typical patient. Examination of cytokine activity in tissues involved by lymphoid neoplasms is limited to the study of expression of cytokines, cytokine receptors, and downstream signaling molecules. Because cytokines act at very low concentrations, methods to determine cytokine expression in lymphoid neoplasms must be very sensitive. The most common methods include *in situ* hybridization to demonstrate mRNA expression, and immunohistochemistry to detect protein expression.

The activity of cytokines is complex. Many cytokines have multiple effects on different cells in the immune system. In the normal immune reaction, cytokines act in combination with other cytokines that may be antagonistic or synergistic in their activities. Cytokines act to recruit other cells that will produce other cytokines, resulting in a complex cytokine cascade reaction. This makes it difficult to understand the implication of the expression of a single cytokine in lymphoid neoplasms without knowledge of other cytokines. Therefore, the greatest understanding of cytokine activity in certain lymphoid neoplasms will be gained by the study of multiple cytokines in both cell culture and in a large group of primary cases using multiple techniques. Conversely, it is difficult to conclude the role of cytokines in lymphoid neoplasms in which only one or a small number of cytokines have been studied in a small number of cases.

A general understanding of normal cytokine production and effects is needed to understand their activities in lymphoid neoplasms. Many of the cytokines that play an important role in lymphomas are produced in the normal immune system by CD4$^+$ helper T cells, which can be divided into different cell types based on their cytokine production and subsequent roles in the regulation of immune responses. The biologic activity of the cytokines produced by different subsets of CD4$^+$ T cells will be discussed in the following section. In addition, the normal activity of chemokines and tumor necrosis factor (TNF) family members, as well as cytokine signaling, will also be discussed.

CYTOKINE BIOLOGY

TH1 and TH2 cytokines

The human adaptive immune response can be divided into two distinct branches: the humoral immune response, which targets extracellular pathogens by stimulating B cells to produce antibodies, and the cell-mediated immune response, which targets intracellular pathogens by activating CD8$^+$ cytotoxic T cells and macrophages. CD4$^+$ T cells are a main source of cytokine production in the normal immune system and play pivotal roles in the regulation of humoral and cell-mediated immune responses. CD4$^+$ T cells can be divided into two mutually exclusive subsets based on the pattern of cytokine production: T helper type 1 (TH1) and T helper type 2 (TH2) cells.[1]

T helper type 1 cells require interleukin-12 (IL-12) for their differentiation, and are characterized by the production of IL-2 and interferon gamma (IFNγ). These cytokines promote a cell-mediated immune response by inducing inflammatory reactions, stimulating T cell growth, activating microbicidal functions of macrophages, and assisting B cells to produce complement-fixing and opsonizing antibodies.

T helper type 2 cells require IL-4 for their differentiation, and are characterized by the production of IL-4, IL-5, IL-6, IL-9, IL-10, and IL-13. These cytokines act in concert to promote the production by B cells of non-complement-fixing antibodies of the immunoglobulin (Ig) G4 and IgE classes. Interleukin-4 and IL-13 share several biologic activities and play central roles in the humoral immune response. Interleukin-4 stimulates the proliferation and survival of B cells and stimulates Ig class switching. Interleukin-13 has similar biologic functions as IL-4, although it does not act as a TH2 cell differentiation factor. Interleukin-6 contributes to the humoral immune response by inducing differentiation of B cells into plasma cells. Interleukin-5 is a vital cytokine in the growth and differentiation of eosinophils, which are important effector cells in clearing extracellular pathogens. Interleukin-9 is a growth factor for T cells and mast cells and also potentiates IL-4-induced Ig class switching. Interleukin-10 acts to inhibit TH1 cell-mediated immune responses and also downregulates proinflammatory cytokine production.

Certain cytokines such as IL-3 and granulocyte and macrophage colony-stimulating factor (GM-CSF) can be produced by both TH1 and TH2 cells.

TH1 and TH2 cells are able to crossregulate each other, such that only one type of immune response will predominate. Therefore, IL-12 and IFNγ will suppress the differentiation of TH2 cells so that a cell-mediated immune response will predominate. Similarly, IL-4 and IL-10 will suppress TH1 cell differentiation such that a humoral immune response will predominate.

An imbalance of TH1 and TH2 response can be correlated with several human diseases.[2] Those diseases associated with a delayed-type hypersensitivity form of granulomatous immune response (such as mycobacterial infections) are associated with production of TH1-type cytokines. Those diseases typified by eosinophilia, increased IgE production, hypergammaglobulinemia, and autoantibody production (such as atopic asthma) are associated with an overproduction of TH2-type cytokines.

Regulatory T cells

While the majority of CD4$^+$ T cells belong to either the TH1 or TH2 subsets, other groups of CD4$^+$ T cells, called regulatory T (Treg) cells, have been identified that have a separate role in suppressing cell-mediated immune responses.[3,4] Multiple types of Treg cells have been characterized, including a naturally occurring population and those induced during an immune response. Naturally occurring Treg cells arise during T cell development in the thymus and are characterized by the expression of the IL-2 receptor α chain (CD25). They are also characterized by the expression of the transcription factor FOXP3, which appears to regulate the development of these naturally occurring Treg cells. These CD4$^+$ CD25$^+$ Treg cells comprise approximately 5–10 percent of all peripheral CD4$^+$ T cells. They express the $\alpha\beta$ T cell receptor and are activated in an antigen-specific fashion. Once activated they suppress the proliferation of both CD4$^+$ and CD8$^+$ CD25$^-$ T cells *in vitro* through a cell contact-dependent mechanism by inhibiting IL-2 expression in the responding cells. *In vivo* studies have also shown that IL-10 and transforming growth factor β (TGFβ) also play a role in suppression of immune responses by CD4$^+$ CD25$^+$ Treg cells, suggesting that there may be involvement of another cell type, such as an antigen-presenting cell or CD4$^+$ CD25$^-$ T cells. These naturally occurring Treg cells are thought to play an important role in maintenance of tolerance to self-antigens.

A second population of Treg cells is induced during normal immune responses in order to control and terminate the response when the inciting antigen is eliminated. Two populations of induced Treg cells have been characterized, known as T regulatory 1 (Tr1) cells and T helper type 3 (TH3) cells.[5] These do not express CD25 and are abundant in the intestines where their main function appears to be to prevent systemic immune responses to foreign antigens in foodstuffs. Tr1 and TH3 cells are generated in response to IL-10 and produce high levels of TGFβ (TH3 cells) or TGFβ and IL-10 (Tr1 cells). These two cytokines have potent anti-inflammatory properties and suppress the proliferation of CD4$^+$ T cells, the antigen-presenting capacity of antigen-presenting cells, and the production of immunoglobulin by B cells. It is not clear whether FOXP3 plays a role in the development of Tr1 or TH3 cells.

Chemokines

Chemokines are chemoattractant cytokines that regulate the selective migration of leukocytes through binding to specific chemokine receptors that are differentially expressed on various leukocyte populations.[6] Many of the chemokine receptors important in lymphoid neoplasms are differentially expressed on TH1 and TH2 cells, as well as the associated effector cells (such as macrophages in a TH1 response and eosinophils in a TH2 response). Therefore, many of these chemokines will amplify either a cell-mediated immune response (by attracting TH1 cells and monocytes, which will differentiate into activated macrophages) or a humoral immune response (by attracting TH2 cells and eosinophils).

TH1 cells differentially express chemokine receptor CCR5, while TH2 cells differentially express chemokine receptors CCR3 and CCR4. Therefore, ligands for CCR5, such as macrophage inflammatory protein (MIP)-1α and MIP-1β, selectively recruit TH1 cells. They also recruit monocytes (which express CCR5), important effector cells in the cell-mediated immune response. Similarly, ligands

for CCR3, such as eotaxin, selectively recruit TH2 cells. They also recruit eosinophils (which express CCR3), important effector cells in the humoral immune response.

The study of expression patterns of chemokines in lymphomas characterized by a prominent non-neoplastic reactive infiltrate can be correlated with the cellular constituents of the infiltrate. As well, in the study of T cell lymphoid neoplasms in which data on cytokine expression are limited, the expression patterns of chemokine receptors can be used as surrogate markers to indicate a TH1 or TH2 phenotype, as discussed below.

Tumor necrosis factor receptor and ligand families

Members of the TNF family of receptors and ligands play an important role in the regulation of the immune response, and have also been shown to play a role in the pathogenesis of different types of lymphoid neoplasms.[7,8] Tumor necrosis factor α (TNFα) is a cytokine that plays an important role in inflammation, tissue remodeling, and wound healing. Other members of the TNF family act as membrane-bound molecules, and as such may not be considered to be cytokines, but they share some important biologic activities and signaling mechanisms with TNFα such that they are included in this discussion. Two of these molecules, CD30 and CD40, have been shown to play a role in the pathogenesis of different lymphoid neoplasms.[8] The precise role of CD30 in regulation of the normal immune system is not well understood, but CD30 activation can have pleiotropic effects on different lymphoma cell lines, inducing apoptosis in certain cell lines, and stimulating proliferation in others. Activation of CD40 on B cells by T cells expressing CD40 ligand (CD40L) is required for the generation of T cell-dependent humoral immune responses. CD40 activation stimulates B cell proliferation and Ig class switching in conjunction with IL-4 and IL-13.

Epstein–Barr virus (EBV) is associated with the development of several types of lymphoid neoplasms. Epstein–Barr virus latent membrane protein 1 (LMP1) is a membrane-bound protein expressed in cells latently infected by EBV. LMP1 activates CD40 signaling pathways in a constitutive ligand-independent manner.[9]

Cytokine signaling

The activity of cytokines and their contribution to proliferation and survival of lymphoma cells can be studied by examining their signaling pathways. Two important pathways are the JANUS kinase (JAK)/signal transducer and activator of transcription (STAT) signaling pathway used by interleukins and other cytokines,[10] and the nuclear factor κB (NF-κB) signaling pathway utilized by TNF family members.[11]

Binding of cytokines with their cell-surface receptors results in multiple biologic activities through the activation of several intracellular signaling pathways. Most cytokine receptors utilize the JAK/STAT family of signaling proteins. Upon receptor activation by cytokine binding, one of three JAK family members (JAK1, JAK2, or JAK3) is activated, which then in turn activates a member of the STAT family (STAT1, STAT2, STAT3, STAT4, STAT5a, STAT5b, or STAT6) for the transduction of cytokine signals. STATs are latent transcription factors that reside in the cytoplasm and become activated by tyrosine phosphorylation by JAKs. Tyrosine phosphorylation allows for dimerization and localization into the nucleus, leading to transcriptional activation of multiple genes. Each JAK and STAT family member is activated by a distinct set of cytokines. STAT3, STAT5, and STAT6 have been identified in playing potential roles in oncogenesis. STAT3 is activated by IL-2, IL-6, IL-9, IL-10, and IL-15. STAT5a and STAT5b are activated by IL-2, IL-3, IL-5, IL-9, IL-15, and GM-CSF. STAT6 activation by cytokines is limited to IL-4 and IL-13.

Constitutive STAT activation has been shown to contribute to oncogenesis in a variety of neoplastic conditions.[12] Multiple solid tumors, including carcinomas of the breast, prostate, head and neck, and ovary, have demonstrable constitutive activation of STAT proteins, particularly STAT3.

Activation of TNF receptor family members can lead to cell survival through activation of NF-κB. The NF-κB family of transcription factors consists of RELA (p65), REL-B, c-REL, p50, and p52.[11] A functional NF-κB molecule is a heterodimer composed of these members, the major form being the RELA/p50 complex. These molecules are constitutively expressed in many cells, but are maintained in an inactive form in the cytoplasm by the inhibitor IκB (the most common form being IκBα), which prevents nuclear localization and transcriptional activity of NF-κB. Nuclear factor κB activation by TNF family members is mediated through TRAF molecules, which act as adapter proteins that bind to the cytoplasmic portion of the receptor and recruit other proteins to form a signaling complex that leads to the activation of the IκB kinase complex (IKK). IKK phosphorylates IκB, which allows for its degradation and subsequent release of NF-κB, allowing it to translocate to the nucleus where it activates the transcription of multiple genes involved in the inflammatory response as well as cell proliferation and survival.

Constitutive NF-κB activation has been implicated in development of a variety of neoplastic diseases.[13] Amplification of genes encoding NF-κB family members has been identified in a wide variety of hematolymphoid and solid tumors. Constitutive activation of NF-κB has been identified in several lymphoid neoplasms, including classical Hodgkin lymphoma (HL), activated B cell-like diffuse large B cell lymphomas, and acute lymphoblastoid leukemias, as well as in a wide variety of carcinomas. In several instances, constitutive NF-κB activation has been shown to contribute to proliferation and survival of the neoplastic cells.

CYTOKINES IN HODGKIN LYMPHOMA

Of all the lymphoid neoplasms, the role of cytokines has been studied in most depth in Hodgkin lymphoma. Histologically, HL is characterized by a minor component of malignant cells, the Reed–Sternberg (RS) cells, in a background of non-neoplastic reactive leukocytes that make up the majority of the clinically detected tumor. Hodgkin lymphoma comprises two distinct diseases: classical HL and nodular lymphocyte predominant HL. The vast majority of cases belong to the classical HL group, which will be the subject of this discussion. The most common subtype of classical HL is the nodular sclerosis variant, characterized by sclerotic fibrous bands dividing the lymphoma into nodules. The second-most-common subtype is the mixed cellularity variant, characterized by a mixed reactive background and lack of sclerotic bands. Hodgkin lymphoma is a highly curable lymphoma, with over 80 percent of patients achieving long-term cure with current therapeutic regimens.

The RS cell of classical HL has been shown to express multiple cytokines that play a role in RS cell proliferation and survival as well as recruitment of the reactive leukocyte component and also alteration of the immune response. The expression and activity of cytokines in Hodgkin lymphoma is summarized in Table 15.1, and a more detailed review can be found elsewhere.[14]

Cytokine expression in Reed–Sternberg cells

TH1 AND TH2 CYTOKINES

Reed–Sternberg cells demonstrate an overexpression of TH2 cytokines. Interleukin-13 is expressed in four of five RS cell lines and its expression has been demonstrated in primary RS cells in 93 percent of classical HL cases by *in situ* hybridization and immunohistochemistry.[15,16] Furthermore, the IL-13 receptor α1 chain is commonly expressed by RS cell lines and primary RS cells, and IL-13 has been shown to be a growth factor for two RS cell lines[17,18] (see discussion on RS cell growth below). Although IL-4 expression has been shown in some RS cell lines, it is not expressed by primary RS cells.[18–21]

Interleukin-5 is expressed by two of six RS cell lines, and has been demonstrated in primary RS cells in tumors characterized by tissue eosinophilia.[22] However, there is no evidence that IL-5 is an autocrine growth factor for RS cells. Interleukin-6 is expressed in five of seven RS cell lines and in 75 percent of primary RS cells.[20,23–26] Although IL-6 receptor components are also expressed by RS cells, there is no evidence that IL-6 acts as an autocrine growth factor. Interleukin-9 has been detected in primary RS cells by *in situ* hybridization in more than 50 percent of cases,[27] and exogenous IL-9 demonstrated a stimulatory growth effect on one RS cell line,[28] suggesting a role in RS cell proliferation. Interleukin-10 expression by primary RS cells

Table 15.1 Cytokines in Hodgkin lymphoma

Cytokine/ chemokine	Biologic activity	Expression in primary HL tissue	Predominant source of expression	Role as RS cell growth factor
TH2 cytokines/chemokines				
IL-4	TH2 cell differentiation; B cell proliferation and Ig switching	−		
IL-13	B cell proliferation and Ig switching	+++	RS cell	+
IL-5	Eosinophil growth and differentiation	+++	RS cell	
IL-6	Plasma cell differentiation	+++	RS cell	
IL-9	T cell/mast cell growth factor	++	RS cell	+
IL-10	Anti-inflammatory cytokine	+	RS cell	
TARC	TH2 cell recruitment	+++	RS cell	
MDC	TH2 cell recruitment	+++	RS cell	
Eotaxin	Eosinophil recruitment	++	RS cell; fibroblasts	
TH1 cytokines/chemokines				
IL-12	TH1 cell differentiation	+++	Lymphocytes	
IL-2	T cell growth factor; NK cell activation	+	RS cells; lymphocytes	
IFNγ	Macrophage activation	+	RS cells; lymphocytes	
IP-10	TH1 cell recruitment	+++	RS cells; reactive cells	
Mig	TH1 cell recruitment	+++	RS cells; reactive cells	
MIP-1α	TH1 cell, monocyte recruitment	+++	RS cells; reactive cells	
Other cytokines				
IL-3	Hematopoietic growth factor	+++	Lymphocytes	+
TNF family members and related molecules				
CD40L	B cell proliferation through CD 40 activation	+++	TH2 cells	+
CD30L	T cell stimulation through CD30 activation	+++	Eosinophils; mast cells	+
EBV LMP1	Ligand-independent growth stimulation	+	RS cells	+

+++, expressed in ≥75% of cases; ++, expressed in 50–74% of cases; +, expressed in 5–49% of cases; −, expressed in <5% of cases.
IL, interleukin; TARC, thymus- and activation-regulated chemokine; MDC, macrophage-derived chemokine; IFN, interferon; IP, inducible protein; Mig, monokine induced by interferonγ; MIP, macrophage inflammatory protein; EBV, Epstein–Barr virus; LMP, latent membrane protein; RS, Reed-Sternberg; HL, Hodgkin lymphoma; Ig, immunoglobulin; NK, natural killer.

has been demonstrated in a minority of cases, in which it is more commonly associated with EBV[+] cases compared to EBV[−] cases.[21] There is no evidence that it acts as a growth factor for RS cells.

TH1 cytokines are expressed at lower levels in Hodgkin lymphoma compared to TH2 cytokines. Interleukin-12 is not expressed by primary RS cells, but a variable number of IL-12[+] cells can be demonstrated in the majority of HL cases, and are present in higher numbers in EBV[+] cases.[29] Data on IL-2 expression in HL have been variable, but studies suggest that IL-2 is not produced by RS cells, but is expressed in a variable proportion of cells within the reactive infiltrate.[24,30,31] Although RS cells express components of the IL-2 receptor, there is no evidence to indicate a role as an autocrine growth factor for RS cells. Immunohistochemical studies show variable IFNγ expression in primary HL tissue, with higher levels seen in mixed cellularity cases compared with nodular sclerosis cases.[31,32]

Other cytokines that do not fit well into the TH1/TH2 paradigm are also expressed in HL. Interleukin-3 plays a role in the proliferation and differentiation of hematopoietic stem cells, and can be expressed by both TH1 and TH2 cells. Immunohistochemical studies on tissues involved by HL have identified IL-3Rα protein expression in RS cells in more than 90 percent of cases.[33] Exogenous IL-3 has been shown to stimulate the growth of several RS cell lines. Interleukin-3 does not appear to be expressed by RS cells, and therefore does not act as an autocrine growth factor, although increased IL-3 mRNA has been detected in HL tissues, most likely produced by T cells within the reactive infiltrate. Therefore, IL-3 is probably acting as a paracrine growth factor for RS cells.[33] TGFβ is a cytokine with potent anti-inflammatory properties, and is characteristically expressed in cases of nodular sclerosis HL. There are conflicting data on the exact cellular source of TGFβ, with some investigators identifying RS cells as the main producers,[34] while others suggest that eosinophils are the primary source.[35]

CHEMOKINES

The expression of chemokines and chemokine receptors has been recently studied in Hodgkin lymphoma and provides an explanation for the prominent non-neoplastic reactive infiltrate typical of this lymphoma. Most of the chemokines studied in HL play a role in either the humoral or cell-mediated immune response, with a predominant expression of chemokines associated with a TH2-mediated humoral immune response.

TH2-related chemokines include thymus- and activation-regulated chemokine (TARC), macrophage-derived chemokine (MDC), and eotaxin.[6] TARC and MDC attract cells that express chemokine receptor CCR4, expressed by normal TH2 cells. Eotaxin attracts cells that express CCR3, expressed by normal TH2 cells and eosinophils. TARC expression in RS cells was first discovered using serial gene expression analysis of RS cell lines.[36] Further studies using in situ hybridization and immunohistochemistry demonstrated TARC expression in RS cells in greater than 85 percent of primary classical HL cases.[36,37] Cases of nodular sclerosis HL demonstrated stronger expression of TARC compared to mixed cellularity cases. Although the expression of MDC in classical HL was not significantly different from normal lymphoid tissue, MDC expression was higher in nodular sclerosis HL compared to mixed cellularity cases.[32]

Eotaxin is also overexpressed in classical HL, with higher levels seen in nodular sclerosis cases.[32] Eotaxin expression correlated with the number of eosinophils, consistent with its biologic role in eosinophil recruitment. There are conflicting data as to the source of the eotaxin in classical HL tissue. One study showed eotaxin expression by RS cells,[32] while another study suggested that the major source of eotaxin in nodular sclerosis HL tissue was the fibroblasts.[38] These latter investigators demonstrated that eotaxin expression by cultured fibroblasts could be stimulated by TNFα produced by an RS cell line.

Several TH1-associated chemokines have been identified in classical HL, including inducible protein 10 (IP-10), monokine induced by IFNγ (Mig), MIP-1α, and MIP-1β.[32,39] These are expressed at higher levels in classical HL tissue compared to normal lymphoid tissue. As opposed to the TH2-associated chemokines, levels of IP-10, Mig-1, and MIP-1α were higher in mixed cellularity cases and those that were positive for EBV.

TNF FAMILY MEMBERS

Several TNF receptor and ligand family members are expressed in classical HL. CD40 and CD30 are expressed in RS cells in virtually all cases of classical HL,[28,40,41] and their role in RS cell proliferation and survival is discussed below.

The role of cytokines in Reed–Sternberg cell proliferation and survival

Several cytokines have been shown to have a role in RS cell proliferation and survival, including TNF ligand family members, IL-13, IL-3, and IL-9. The roles of TNF ligand family members and IL-13 have been more extensively studied, and will be the focus of this section.

The expression of CD40 and CD30 on RS cells and expression of CD40L and CD30L on surrounding cells in the reactive infiltrate allow for their contribution to RS cell proliferation and survival. CD40L is expressed on benign T cells in the reactive infiltrate.[40,42] These CD40L$^+$ T cells are increased in HL tissue compared to normal lymphoid tissue and are typically in close proximity to the RS cells. Activation of CD40 on RS cell lines increases survival in vitro.[28] CD30L is also expressed by cells in the reactive infiltrate, including eosinophils and mast cells.[43,44] Although activation of CD30 induces different biologic responses in various CD30$^+$ lymphoma cell lines, ranging from cell death to proliferation, activation of CD30 on RS cell lines has been shown to either increase proliferation or to have no effect.[45,46] The expression of EBV LMP1 in the cases of EBV$^+$ HL also allows for the activation of CD40 signaling pathways in a ligand-independent and constitutive manner.

CD30, CD40, and EBV LMP1 all activate NF-κB, and constitutive NF-κB has been identified in several HL cell lines.[47–49] The role of NF-κB in the biology of RS cells has been studied by overexpressing a dominant negative form of IκB, which binds to NF-κB but is not able to release it. These studies demonstrate the role of NK-κB in cell proliferation and protection from apoptosis.[50] NF-κB contributes to proliferation and survival in RS cell lines in part by upregulation of antiapoptotic proteins (including BCLX$_L$ and IAP2) and cell-cycle regulator cyclin D2.[51] NF-κB has also been shown to contribute to STAT5 overexpression and activation in RS cell lines.[52]

In addition to activation by TNF receptor family members and EBV LMP1, NF-κB can also be constitutively activated in RS cell lines by mutations of the IKBA gene. Mutations can lead to C-terminal truncated IκB-α proteins, which are ineffective in maintaining NF-κB in an inactive form in the cytoplasm.[53,54] However, these mutations have only been demonstrated in a minority of RS cell lines and primary HL tissues, and may not be a common mechanism for NF-κB activation in HL.

Interleukin-13 has also been identified as an autocrine growth factor for RS cell lines. Antibody-mediated neutralization of IL-13 in two RS cell lines (HDLM-2 and L-1236) led to a dose-dependent reduction in cell proliferation.[17,18] In L-1236 cells, IL-13 neutralization also led to the induction of apoptosis. Reed–Sternberg cell lines demonstrate constitutive STAT6 activation, and in the two IL-13-responsive RS cell lines, STAT6 activation was shown to be IL-13-dependent.[18] Nuclear localization of phosphorylated STAT6 was shown to be a common feature of RS cells in HL tissue and was more commonly seen in nodular sclerosis cases compared to mixed cellularity cases. The common expression of IL-13 and IL-13Rα1 and STAT6 activation in RS cells in HL tissue indicates that IL-13 signaling is functional in vivo. Using an animal model of HL, in which tumors are derived from the IL-13-responsive RS cell line HDLM-2, treatment with a soluble IL-13 decoy receptor via adenoviral-mediated gene transfer delayed tumor onset and led to regression or stabilization of established tumors.[55]

A role for IL-3 and IL-9 in growth of RS cells has also been demonstrated, but further study is needed. Exogenous IL-3 stimulates *in vitro* growth of RS cell lines, as well as decreasing apoptosis induced by serum starvation.[33] The primary source of IL-3 in HL tissues is most likely reactive T cells. Exogenous IL-9 had a moderate stimulatory effect on one RS cell line (KMH2).[28]

The role of cytokines in the reactive infiltrate in Hodgkin lymphoma

It is becoming increasingly clear that the non-neoplastic reactive infiltrate that is characteristic of Hodgkin lymphoma is not just a passive bystander in the pathogenesis of this lymphoid neoplasm. On the contrary, the reactive infiltrate probably contributes to the proliferation and survival of RS cells by directly stimulating the cells through membrane-bound receptors, and also maintains the lymphoma by preventing an effective antitumor immune response.

The composition of the reactive infiltrate can vary between cases of HL, but may include T cells, B cells, eosinophils, neutrophils, macrophages, plasma cells, and fibroblasts. The variation of the infiltrate components most likely depends on the chemokine expression pattern of each individual case.

Reactive T cells are a component of the reactive infiltrate in virtually all cases of HL. In immunocompetent patients, the overwhelming majority of these T cells are CD4$^+$. There are some conflicting data on the exact nature of these T cells, with different studies suggesting that these are predominantly TH2 cells or Treg cells. Poppema and van den Berg demonstrated that when CD4$^+$ T cells immediately surrounding the RS cells were isolated and stimulated, they produced both IL-4 and IFNγ, but not IL-2, a pattern more consistent with TH2 cells rather than TH1 or Treg cells.[56] However, a recent study by Marshall *et al.* demonstrated that the CD4$^+$ T cells from HL tissues did not produce a TH1 or TH2 cytokine response upon stimulation.[57] Rather, these tumor-infiltrating T cells contained large numbers of both CD4$^+$ CD25$^+$ Treg cells and Tr1 cells that secreted IL-10. The abundance of regulatory T cells would explain the local immunosuppression evident in HL tissues (discussed below). The authors suggested several mechanisms by which these regulatory T cells exert their immunosuppressive functions, including production of IL-10 and through cell-to-cell contact.

These data suggest that the T cells in HL do not exhibit TH1 characteristics, but consist of regulatory T cells or TH2 cells, or both. Both TH2 cells and CD4$^+$ CD25$^+$ Treg cells express chemokine receptor CCR4,[58,59] and are thus recruited to tissues involved by HL through the activity of chemokines TARC, MDC, and eotaxin that are produced by RS cells or other cells in the reactive infiltrate. CD4$^+$ T cells

are typically in close contact with the RS cells. The expression of CD40L on the T cell surface allows for activation of CD40 expressed by the RS cells,[42] promoting proliferation and survival of the RS cells through NF-κB signaling.

CD8$^+$ T cells are not a prominent component of the reactive infiltrate of HL and are not in close contact with RS cells as the CD4$^+$ cells are.[60] However, CD8$^+$ T cells are seen in higher numbers in EBV$^+$ cases of HL compared to EBV$^-$ cases.[61,62] This correlates with increased production of chemokines that support a TH1 immune response, such as IP-10, MIP-1α, and MIP-1β. However, these CD8$^+$ cells do not appear to be cytotoxic for EBV$^+$ RS cells. Although EBV-specific cytotoxic T cells can be detected in these patients' peripheral blood, no such EBV-specific CD8$^+$ cells can be detected within the tumors.[63] This defect of failure to penetrate the tumor or to function properly within the tumor environment is most likely due to the immunosuppressive effects of the Treg cells and/or TH2 cells that prevent an effective cell-mediated immune response against the tumor.

Eosinophils are another common component in the reactive infiltrate in tissues involved by HL. They are recruited by cytokines and chemokines produced by RS cells and other cells in the reactive infiltrate, and have the potential to contribute to RS cell proliferation and survival. Interleukin-3, IL-5, and GM-CSF are important cytokines regulating the differentiation and survival of eosinophils. Interleukin-5 is expressed by RS cells and correlates with the degree of tissue eosinophilia.[22] Eotaxin is a chemokine that recruits cells that express chemokine receptor CCR3, which is expressed by eosinophils. Eotaxin is expressed by tissue fibroblasts in tissues involved by HL and also correlates with the degree of eosinophilia.[32,38] Eotaxin expression is known to be upregulated by IL-13 and TNFα, which are commonly expressed by RS cells. CD30L expressed on eosinophils has the potential to stimulate RS cells through surface CD30 (expressed on RS cells in virtually all cases of classical HL), which can lead to proliferation and survival through activation of NF-κB.[43] CD30L is expressed at higher levels in circulating eosinophils from HL patients compared to healthy donors. Mast cells within the reactive infiltrate also express CD30L.[44]

Fibrosis is a characteristic feature of the nodular sclerosis subtype of HL. Cytokines play a role in the formation of these fibrotic bands, and the fibroblasts produce chemokines that amplify the recruitment of other components of the reactive infiltrate.[64] Multiple cytokines, including TGFβ, IL-13, and basic fibroblast growth factor (b-FGF), are produced by RS cells and are known to stimulate fibroblast proliferation and collagen production. In addition to potent anti-inflammatory properties, TGFβ has stimulatory effects on fibroblasts, and is characteristically produced by tissues involved by nodular sclerosis HL compared to other subtypes. The exact source of the TGFβ is unclear; both eosinophils and RS cells have been identified as potential sources. An imbalance of TH2 cytokines over TH1 cytokines has also been implicated in various disease processes characterized by fibrosis, including pulmonary and hepatic fibrosis.[65] In particular, IL-13 is able to stimulate collagen synthesis and also activate TGFβ production. The production of b-FGF has also been identified within RS cells and cells of the reactive infiltrate, where it is associated with the nodular sclerosis variant compared to other HL subtypes. Fibroblasts within the fibrous bands of nodular sclerosis HL have been shown to produce eotaxin, which attracts eosinophils and TH2 cells to the reactive infiltrate.

Cytokines and impaired cellular immunity in Hodgkin lymphoma

Patients with HL often demonstrate systemic defects in cell-mediated immunity, as demonstrated by increased sensitivity to bacterial, fungal, and viral infections, and delayed hypersensitivity to new and recall antigens.[66] In contrast, humoral immunity is often overactive, manifested by increased serum IgE levels.

Tissues involved by HL also demonstrate local defects in cell-mediated immunity. In patients with EBV$^+$ HL, EBV-specific cytotoxic T lymphocytes (CTLs) cannot be detected within tumor tissue, although circulating EBV-specific CTLs can be detected in the peripheral blood.[63] These data suggest a localized cell-mediated immune defect within the tumor microenvironment. This is most

likely due to the increased numbers of Treg cells within HL tissues as well as increased production of the potent anti-inflammatory cytokines TGFβ (predominantly in nodular sclerosis cases) and IL-10 (predominantly in EBV$^+$ cases) by RS cells or other cells in the reactive infiltrate. Additionally, the unbalanced production of TH2 cytokines in most cases of HL may also prevent an effective TH1-driven cell-mediated immune response.

Cytokines and Hodgkin lymphoma: summary

A close relationship exists between the RS cell and the non-neoplastic reactive infiltrate in the pathogenesis of HL. Cytokines and chemokines produced by RS cells recruit the reactive infiltrate, which, in turn, contributes to RS cell proliferation and survival as well as prevention of an effective antitumor immune response (Fig. 15.1).

Most cases of HL are characterized by the overproduction of TH2-type cytokines and chemokines, and constitutive activation of NF-κB. The production of TH2-type cytokines contributes to RS cell proliferation (particularly IL-13) and also leads to the characteristic reactive infiltrate that is often rich in eosinophils, TH2 cells, and Treg cells, as well as fibrosis in nodular sclerosis cases. Constitutive NF-κB activation is a characteristic feature of RS cells, contributing to their proliferation and survival as well as their

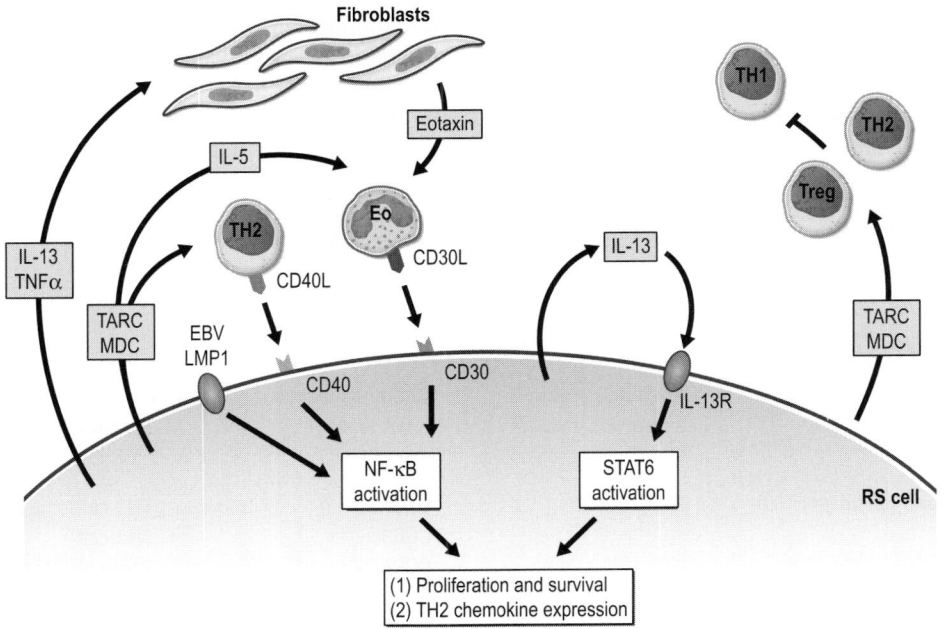

Figure 15.1 The role of cytokines and chemokines in Hodgkin lymphoma. Reed–Sternberg (RS) cells produce several T helper type 2 (TH2) cytokines and chemokines, including interleukin (IL)-13, IL-5, thymus- and activation-regulated chemokine (TARC), and macrophage-derived chemokine (MDC). Interleukin-13 acts as an autocrine growth factor. Interleukin-5, TARC, and MDC recruit the prominent reactive infiltrate including TH2 cells, eosinophils, and fibroblasts. The reactive infiltrate contributes to Reed–Sternberg cell proliferation through CD40 activation by TH2 cells and CD30 activation by eosinophils. The presence of TH2 cells and regulatory T (Treg) cells also acts to inhibit an effective TH1 cell–mediated immune response. EBV, Epstein–Barr virus; LMP1, latent membrane protein 1; NF-κB, nuclear factor κB; TNF, tumor necrosis factor.

overexpression of cytokines and chemokines. NF-κB activation of HL can occur through various mechanisms, including activation of CD30 and CD40 on the RS cell surface by their respective ligands on the surface of cells within the reactive infiltrate. Additionally, the expression of EBV LMP1 in those cases of HL associated with EBV infection also results in NF-κB activation. Finally, in a small subset of HL cases, mutations of the *IKBA* gene also result in constitutive NF-κB activation.

The systemic and local defects in cell-mediated immunity typically seen in patients with HL also contribute to tumor survival and are due to the various cytokines and chemokines produced by the tumor. The production of chemokines such as TARC and MDC by RS cells leads to the influx of Treg and TH2 cells, which both prevent an effective antitumor cell-mediated immune response. In addition to the suppressive activities of Treg cells, anti-inflammatory cytokines TGFβ and IL-10 are produced by other tumor constituents in cases of nodular sclerosis HL and EBV$^+$ HL, respectively.

Cytokines probably play an important role in the clinical progression of HL. Reed–Sternberg cells in almost all cases of HL are thought to arise from germinal center B cells that have lost the ability to express functional Ig molecules, a situation that would normally lead to apoptosis. Epstein–Barr virus infection is thought to play an important role in the survival of these cells, but EBV infection is not present in every case of HL. Cytokines such as IL-13 and TNF family members may contribute to the survival of these RS cell precursors, allowing for other transforming events to occur. The essential role of cytokines in the maintenance of HL is also supported by clinical and laboratory features of the disease. Hodgkin lymphoma characteristically starts at a single site (almost always a lymph node) and has an orderly and predictable pattern of progression, spreading in an orderly fashion to contiguous lymph nodes. This suggests that RS cells do not have the intrinsic ability to grow at any site, but require an appropriate microenvironment. Given the prominent production of cytokines in HL, it is postulated that the cytokines elaborated by RS cells in one lymph node group will spread to adjacent lymph nodes to produce the appropriate cellular background to support the continued growth of RS cells. This dependence of RS cells on the appropriate microenvironment for their survival and growth is also supported by the fact that the development of cell lines from RS cells in the laboratory is exceedingly difficult.

An understanding of the role of cytokines in the pathogenesis of HL may help to identify new therapeutic targets. New therapies may target cytokines and signaling pathways involved in the proliferation and survival of RS cells, as well as acting to reverse the local immunosuppression that assists in the tumor growth. Potential therapeutic molecules include antibody targeting TNF family members (CD30, CD40), IL-13, as well as multiple strategies to inhibit NF-κB signaling (including selective IKK inhibitors and targeting proteosomal degradation). Such potential biologically based strategies for HL are the subject of a recent review.[67]

CYTOKINES AND T CELL LYMPHOID NEOPLASMS

Normal T cells are the primary source of cytokine production within the immune system, and their growth and differentiation depends on the activity of several cytokines. Therefore, it would be expected that neoplasms arising from these cells have the potential to produce and respond to cytokines. Histologically, T cell lymphomas often have a polymorphous inflammatory background, which may correlate with cytokine activity. The relationship of cytokines and various T cell lymphomas is summarized in Table 15.2.

Table 15.2 Cytokines in T cell lymphomas

T cell lymphoma subtype	Possible cytokines as growth factors	Chemokine receptor expression	Possible lineage differentiation
Peripheral T cell lymphoma, unspecified	IL-2, IL-4	CXCR3 CCR3 CCR4	TH1 cell TH2 cell ?Treg cell (FOXP3$^+$) ?TH2 cell
Anaplastic large cell lymphoma	IL-6, IL-9	CCR3, CCR4	TH2 cell
Angioimmunoblastic T cell lymphoma	?	CXCR3	TH1 cell ?TH2 cell (IL-4, IL-6 expression)
Lennert lymphoma	IL-2, IL-6	CXCR3	TH1 cell
Mycosis fungoides	?	?	TH1 cell
Sézary syndrome	IL-7, IL-15	?	TH2 cell ?Treg cell (FOXP3$^+$)
Adult T cell leukemia/lymphoma	IL-2, IL-4	CCR4	Treg cell (FOXP3$^+$)

Peripheral T cell lymphoma, unspecified

These tumors are the most common subtype of T cell lymphomas seen in Western countries, and comprise cases of peripheral T cell lymphomas that do not have the characteristics of recognized subtypes of T cell lymphoid neoplasms. It is recognized that this is most probably a heterogeneous group of lymphomas that cannot be further subdivided based on current data. As a group, these are aggressive lymphomas and patients often have a poor response to therapy; only a small minority of patients achieve long-term cure. Most cases of peripheral T cell lymphoma, unspecified, are CD4$^+$ CD8$^-$, suggesting origin from helper T cells, and therefore the study of cytokine expression in these tumors has focused on cytokines produced by normal TH1 and TH2 cells.

Available data, although limited, suggest a direct role for cytokines as autocrine growth factors in peripheral T cell lymphomas. A cell line derived from a high-grade T cell non-Hodgkin lymphoma was shown to produce IL-2 and constitutively express high-affinity surface IL-2 receptors. Monoclonal antibodies against IL-2 and IL-2 receptors inhibited cell growth, indicating that IL-2 is acting as an autocrine growth factor for this cell line.[68] In another study from Saudi Arabia, freshly purified tumor cells from CD4$^+$ and CD8$^+$ peripheral T cell lymphomas secreted high levels of IL-4 after stimulation with anti-CD3, and IL-4 induced *in vitro* proliferation of the malignant cells.[69] These studies identify a possible role of both TH1 and TH2 cytokines as autocrine growth factors in peripheral T cell lymphomas, although study of a larger number of cases is needed.

Cytokine mRNA expression has been studied in primary peripheral T cell lymphoma samples. Using RNase protection assays and reverse transcription polymerase chain reaction (RT-PCR), Ho *et al.* found that peripheral T cell lymphomas from cases in Hong Kong produced a predominance of TH1 cytokines (IFNγ), with low or absent production of TH2 cytokines.[70] These investigators also found expression of immunosuppressive cytokines TGFβ and IL-10 at high frequencies. A German study examining cytokine expression by Northern analysis and *in situ* hybridization found variable cytokine expression.[19] There are significant geographic differences in the incidence of T cell lymphomas which may reflect different biologic factors in their pathogenesis. A deeper understanding of the expression and role of cytokines in peripheral T cell lymphomas will require more extensive study.

Several recent studies have examined the expression patterns of chemokine receptors in an attempt to identify different subtypes of peripheral T cell lymphomas.[71–74] Although cytokine expression was not directly studied, chemokine receptor expression can be used as a surrogate marker for identifying TH1 and TH2 subtypes. Tumors could be divided into prognostically distinct groups based on their expression of chemokine receptors. Those cases that expressed chemokine receptor CCR3, which is

expressed by normal TH2 cells, had a relatively good prognosis, while those that expressed the receptor CCR4, which is expressed by normal TH2 and Treg cells, had a poor prognosis. Those cases that expressed receptor CXCR3, which is expressed by normal TH1 cells, had an intermediate prognosis. One group found that CCR4 expression correlated with the expression of FOXP3, a transcription factor specific to Treg cells, and also correlated with a relatively poor prognosis.[74]

It is likely that this differential expression of chemokine receptors in peripheral T cell lymphomas correlates with different cytokine expression patterns. These various cytokines may contribute to proliferation and survival of the neoplastic clone and/or alter the antitumor immune response, leading to clinical and prognostic differences. For example, expression of CCR4 and FOXP3 in a subset of these lymphomas suggests a Treg phenotype. These neoplastic cells may have the same immunosuppressive activity as their benign counterpart Treg cells, possibly through the production of TGFβ and IL-10, which inhibits an effective antitumor immune response and may lead to the poor prognosis. If the role of cytokines in the biologic behavior of peripheral T cell lymphomas is confirmed by further study, then targeted therapies designed to alter the cytokine balance may provide additional benefit for these aggressive lymphomas.

Anaplastic large cell lymphoma

Anaplastic large cell lymphoma (ALCL) is a T cell lymphoma characterized by large pleomorphic cells and overexpression of CD30. A majority of cases are characterized by the expression of anaplastic lymphoma kinase (ALK) due to balanced chromosomal translocations involving the ALK gene on chromosome 2p23. Anaplastic large cell lymphoma typically demonstrates diffuse sheets of tumor cells without a significant inflammatory background, but a minority of cases can have a prominent background of histiocytes or, less commonly, neutrophils. Clinically, the expression of ALK is an important prognostic indicator, with ALK$^+$ ALCL having a five-year survival of approximately 80 percent, and ALK$^-$ cases a significantly worse prognosis.

The majority of ALCL cases are positive for CD4, suggesting a helper T cell phenotype. Cytokine expression has not been well studied in ALCL, but the expression of TH2 cytokines IL-9 and IL-6 has been identified. Merz *et al.* found IL-9 mRNA expression in two of six cases of ALCL and in one ALCL cell line.[27] However, IL-9 was not identified as an autocrine growth factor. Freshly isolated ALCL tumor cells in another study were found to be dependent on IL-6 for their growth.[75] Anaplastic large cell lymphoma does not express TH2 cytokine IL-13.[15] Studies examining chemokine receptor expression also support a TH2 phenotype in ALCL, with common expression of chemokine receptors CCR3 and CCR4 which are typically expressed by TH2 cells.[71,72] The role of cytokines in those cases of ALCL with a prominent reactive component has not been specifically studied.

Angioimmunoblastic T cell lymphoma

Angioimmunoblastic T cell lymphoma (AITL) is a peripheral T cell lymphoma typically associated with generalized lymphadenopathy, systemic symptoms, polyclonal hypergammaglobulinemia, and a frequent pruritic skin rash. It is an aggressive lymphoma with a median survival of less than three years. Patients often show evidence of immunodeficiency and often have expanded EBV$^+$ B cell clones within their lymph nodes, and are susceptible to infectious complications. Lymph node biopsies typically show tumor cells admixed with a reactive infiltrate of small lymphocytes, eosinophils, plasma cells, and histiocytes, and a vascular proliferation. These clinical and pathologic features indicate a potential role for cytokines in this disease.

Ohshima et al. demonstrated overexpression of both TH1 cytokines (IL-2 and IFNγ) and TH2 cytokines (IL-4, IL-5, IL-6, IL-13) in AITL compared to other T cell lymphomas.[76] Increased expression of pro-inflammatory cytokines (lymphotoxin [LT] and TNFα) has also been identified, particularly in those cases with a mixed cellular background.[77] Interleukin-4 was expressed more frequently in AITL compared to other T cell lymphomas, and correlated with the presence of hypergammaglobulinemia.[78] Interleukin-6 overexpression has also been associated with hypergammaglobulinemia and plasma cell infiltrates in the lymphoma.[79] However, studies of chemokine receptor analysis have shown CXCR3 expression, suggesting a TH1 phenotype to the lymphoma cells.[71,73]

These studies have shown a combination of TH1 and TH2 cytokine expression, but the role of cytokines in lymphoma proliferation and survival is unknown. Those cases associated with hypergammaglobulinemia appear to be associated with TH2 cytokines IL-4 and IL-6, which are involved in B cell and plasma cell proliferation and differentiation.

Lennert lymphoma

Lennert lymphoma (also known as lymphoepithelioid cell variant of peripheral T cell lymphoma) is characterized by a prominent reactive component of epithelioid histiocytes admixed with the malignant T cell population.

A CD4$^+$ T cell lymphoma cell line derived from a patient with Lennert lymphoma spontaneously produced IFNγ and proliferated in response to the addition of macrophages, macrophage-derived factor, or IL-2 to the culture.[80] This macrophage-derived factor was later identified as IL-6.[81] These in vitro data suggest a positive feedback loop operating in this lymphoma, in which IFNγ produced by the tumor cells promotes an exuberant

cell-mediated immune response characterized by a prominent macrophage infiltration. The macrophages, in turn, secrete cytokines, including IL-2 and IL-6, to promote the proliferation of the tumor cells. Immunohistochemical and in situ hybridization studies on tissues involved by Lennert lymphoma show an overexpression of chemokine receptor CXCR3,[71] consistent with a predominant TH1 cytokine phenotype, and confirm IFNγ overexpression.[78]

Cutaneous T cell lymphoma

Mycosis fungoides (MF) is the most common type of primary cutaneous T cell lymphoma, and is characterized by an epidermal and dermal infiltrate of atypical T cells, which are most often CD4$^+$. Sézary syndrome (SS) is a leukemic variant of MF, characterized by erythroderma, lymphadenopathy, and neoplastic T cells with cerebriform nuclei present in the peripheral blood (Sézary cells).

Skin involved by MF has been shown to express a TH1 cytokine profile, which shifts toward a TH2 cytokine profile in SS.[82-84] RT-PCR performed on epidermal tissue involved by MF demonstrated expression of IL-2 and IFNγ, but not IL-4, IL-5, or IL-10. In contrast, skin and peripheral blood samples from patients with SS showed a predominance of IL-4, IL-5, and IL-10 expression. Other investigators have also confirmed the TH2 cytokine profile in SS, also demonstrating expression of TH2 cytokines IL-6 and IL-13. The expression of IL-5 and IL-13 in cutaneous T cell lymphoma cell lines was shown to be dependent on STAT3 activation.[84]

Several cytokines have been identified as growth factors for cutaneous T cell lymphomas, including IL-7 and IL-15.[85] Interleukin-7 is a lymphoid progenitor stimulatory cytokine, while IL-15 has similar biologic properties to IL-2. Interleukin-7 and IL-15 have been shown to activate STAT proteins in cutaneous T cell lymphoma cell lines, including STAT2, STAT3, STAT5, and STAT6, and also lead to BCL2 overexpression.[85,86] Interleukin-15 is produced by Sézary cells, as well as by basal keratinocytes, suggesting both autocrine and paracrine stimulation.[87,88] Interleukin-7, on the other hand, does not appear to be produced by Sézary cells but is produced by keratinocytes, providing paracrine stimulation to the neoplastic lymphocytes in the epidermis and dermis. The TH2 cytokines IL-4, IL-9, and IL-13 have not been shown to be growth factors for cutaneous T cell lymphoma.

Cutaneous T cell lymphoma cell lines have also been shown to have a Treg phenotype, with overexpression of TGFβ and IL-10. An IL-7-dependent cell line from a patient with SS produced high levels of TGFβ. Freshly isolated CD4$^+$ cutaneous T cell lymphoma cells upregulated CD25 and FOXP3, and expressed high levels of IL-10 and TGFβ after encountering activated dendritic cells, a phenotype typical of Treg cells.[89] This may help to create an immunosuppressive anergic environment that allows for the survival of the malignant cells. Cytokine-based treatments to enhance a cell-mediated immune response (using IFNα, IFNγ, IL-12, or IL-2) may be of use in these patients.[90]

Adult T cell leukemia/lymphoma

Adult T cell leukemia/lymphoma (ATLL) is a T lymphoid neoplasm caused by the human T cell lymphotrophic virus 1 (HTLV-1). Patients typically have disseminated disease, with widespread involvement of lymph nodes and peripheral blood, and often have cutaneous involvement. The malignant cells are highly pleomorphic and are typically CD4$^+$ CD25$^+$ T cells. Adult T cell leukemia/lymphoma is typically an aggressive disease with a poor prognosis.

Human T cell lymphotrophic virus 1 is known to activate the expression of NF-κB, as well as various cytokines, including IL-2, IL-4, IL-10, and IL-13, and the receptors for IL-2 and IL-4.[91–95] The expression of IL-2 and IL-2 receptor allows for the potential autocrine activity of IL-2 in ATLL. Studies have shown that IL-2 and IL-4 stimulate proliferation of ATLL cells,[96,97] with IL-4 providing a stronger response. Interleukin-4 production by ATLL cells has not been demonstrated, and therefore may be acting as a paracrine factor secreted by surrounding reactive lymphocytes.

While the expression pattern of cytokines has not been well studied in ATLL, chemokine receptor studies have provided some information on the potential cell of origin. Adult T cell leukemia/lymphoma cells have been found to express chemokine receptor CCR4 and the transcription factor FOXP3,[72,98–100] indicating differentiation toward Treg cells. In keeping with the Treg phenotype, studies have shown that freshly isolated leukemic cells from patients with ATLL express IL-10, mediated through NF-κB activation.[91] The production of this immunosuppressive cytokine would prevent an effective antitumor immune response and allow for the survival and proliferation of the malignant cells. CCR4 expression (which correlates with FOXP3 expression) is associated with a poor prognosis and cutaneous involvement, and has been identified as a potentially useful therapeutic target for this aggressive disease.[98]

CYTOKINES AND B CELL LYMPHOID NEOPLASMS

B cells are not a major source of cytokines in the normal immune system, but rely upon them for many aspects of their biologic activity. Similarly, lymphoid neoplasms of B lineage do not commonly produce cytokines, but several subtypes rely on cytokine activity for proliferation and survival.

Diffuse large B cell lymphoma

Interleukin-6 is a potential growth and differentiation factor for diffuse large B cell lymphomas (DLBCL). One cell line derived from a DLBCL was shown to produce IL-6, and antibody-mediated neutralization inhibited proliferation.[101] In tissues involved by DLBCL, IL-6 is expressed in a minority of cases.[102–104] Its expression has been correlated with immunoblastic morphology of DLBCL.

T cell-rich B cell lymphoma (TCRBCL) is an uncommon variant of diffuse large B cell lymphoma in which the majority of cells within the tumor are non-neoplastic reactive T cells. Histiocytes can also be a component of the reactive infiltrate, and some authors use the term 'T cell/histiocyte-rich large B cell lymphoma' for these tumors. The neoplastic component – the large B cells – make up less than 10 percent of the tumor. The presence of a prominent reactive component to this lymphoma is very similar to HL, a diagnosis that often enters into the differential diagnosis. Unlike HL, TCRBCL is an aggressive lymphoma that typically presents with widespread disease, including bone marrow and liver involvement.

Because of the relative rarity of TCRBCL, it has not been well studied. In addition, somewhat different diagnostic criteria have been used in existing studies, a factor that has contributed to inconsistent results. A single study examined cytokine expression in TCRBCL, demonstrating expression of IL-4 by the large B cells and histiocytes by immunohistochemical methods in 16 of 18 cases.[105] In contrast, only one of 15 cases of conventional diffuse large B cell lymphoma showed strong IL-4 expression in histiocytes within the tumor. Interleukin-4 may be contributing to the T cell infiltration seen in this lymphoma, but further study is needed to confirm its role.

Multiple myeloma

Multiple myeloma is a neoplasm of the terminally differentiated B cell (the plasma cell), which is characterized by lytic bone lesions and a serum monoclonal protein. The primary site of involvement is the bone marrow, where bone marrow stromal cells produce cytokines involved in myeloma cell growth. Interleukin-6, a growth and differentiation factor for benign plasma cells, has been identified as a major paracrine growth factor for myeloma cells.[106,107] Although cells from some cases of myeloma can secrete IL-6, the major source is the bone marrow stromal cell. Myeloma cells can stimulate IL-6 production by these stromal cells through direct cell-to-cell contact as well as through the production of TNF-α, TGFβ, and vascular endothelial growth factor (VEGF), which leads to further production of IL-6.

Myeloma cells commonly express IL-6 receptors, and IL-6 binding contributes to growth, survival, and drug resistance in these cells. Multiple signaling pathways are activated, including the JAK/STAT pathway and phosphatidylinositol 3-kinase (PI3K)/AKT (protein kinase B; PKB) pathway.[106,107] Activation of STAT3 promotes myeloma cell survival through activation of antiapoptotic proteins of the BCL2 family, including BCLX$_L$ and MCL1.

Activation of the PI3K/Akt pathway contributes to resistance to dexamethasone, a drug that is often used in the treatment of this disease.

Other B cell lymphoid neoplasms

Multiple cytokines are produced by freshly isolated cells from low-grade B cell lymphomas including follicular lymphoma and marginal zone lymphoma, as well as mantle cell lymphoma.[108] These include TH1 cytokines (IL-2, IL-12, IFNγ), TH2 cytokines (IL-6, IL-10), and proinflammatory cytokines (IL-1, TNF-α, LTα). TH2 cytokines IL-4, IL-5, and IL-13 were not detected in unstimulated lymphoma cells, but they were produced in several of the lymphomas after stimulation with CD40 monoclonal antibody and IL-4.

The direct activity of cytokines in low-grade B cell lymphomas has been demonstrated in a limited number of studies. Freshly isolated cells from extranodal marginal B cell lymphomas of mucosal-associated lymphoid tissue (MALT lymphomas) required the activation of CD40 and IL-4 for their *in vitro* proliferation, and were induced to differentiate into immunoglobulin-secreting cells by IL-10.[109] The most likely source of these signals *in vivo* is the reactive T cells admixed with the tumor cells, providing evidence for the importance of the tumor microenvironment for this low-grade lymphoma.

Conflicting results have been reported for IL-3 as a growth factor for follicular lymphoma. One group found that addition of IL-3 to freshly isolated follicular lymphoma cells and a follicular lymphoma cell line stimulated proliferation, which could be abrogated by neutralizing antibodies to IL-3.[110] Follicular lymphoma cells have been shown to express IL-3 receptor, but not IL-3. The most likely source of IL-3 *in vivo* was thought to be the surrounding reactive T cells. However, in another study the investigators were not able to demonstrate that IL-3 was a growth stimulator for follicular lymphoma cells,[111] and therefore the role of IL-3 in follicular lymphoma requires further study.

CYTOKINES IN LYMPHOID NEOPLASMS: SUMMARY

Cytokines can contribute to the development and maintenance of lymphoid neoplasia in several ways. First, cytokines can be produced by lymphoma cells and contribute to their proliferation and survival as autocrine growth factors (particularly in classical HL). Second, cytokines and chemokines contribute to provide a suitable microenvironment for the survival of the neoplastic cells. While this is most apparent in tumors with a prominent non-neoplastic reactive infiltrate, such as HL, other neoplasms such as myeloma and low-grade B cell lymphomas, which have less prominent infiltrates, may still rely upon cytokines and other survival signals from surrounding non-neoplastic cells for their continued viability and possibly proliferation. Finally, cytokines play a role in sustaining the growth of several lymphoid neoplasms by altering the local immune response and preventing an effective antitumor reaction. In this area, increasing awareness of the role of Treg cells and the TH1/TH2 balance in lymphoid neoplasms is providing new information in the pathogenesis of not only lymphoid neoplasms, but other malignancies as well.

A better understanding of the role of cytokines and chemokines in the pathogenesis of lymphoid neoplasms will hopefully provide new strategies in the treatment of patients with these diseases. Targeting autocrine growth factors as well as manipulating the immune response in order to rectify cell-mediated immune defects that impair an effective antitumor response may prove to be of added benefit to these patients.

KEY POINTS

- Cytokines play a crucial role in the regulation of the immune system.
- Lymphocytes are the main producers of cytokines, and rely on them for their biologic activity.
- Malignant lymphocytes in lymphomas often retain the ability to produce and respond to cytokines.
- Hodgkin lymphoma is the quintessential example of cytokine activity in lymphoma, in which a prominent reactive immune infiltrate is thought to be recruited by cytokines, and likely contributes to growth and survival of the malignant cells.
- Many other lymphomas without a reactive inflammatory component have evidence of cytokine activity.
- Cytokines may be playing a role as growth factors in several lymphomas.
- Cytokines and their signaling pathways represent possible therapeutic targets in the treatment of patients with lymphoma.

REFERENCES

● = Key primary paper

◆ = Major review article

◆1. Mosmann TR, Coffman RL. TH1 and TH2 cells: different patterns of lymphokine secretion lead to different functional properties. *Annu Rev Immunol* 1989; **7**: 145–73.

2. Lucey DR, Clerici M, Shearer GM. Type 1 and type 2 cytokine dysregulation in human infectious, neoplastic, and inflammatory diseases. *Clin Microbiol Rev* 1996; **9**: 532–62.

3. Holm TL, Nielsen J, Claesson MH. CD4+CD25+ regulatory T cells: I. Phenotype and physiology. *APMIS* 2004; **112**: 629–41.

4. Nielsen J, Holm TL, Claesson MH. CD4+CD25+ regulatory T cells: II. Origin, disease models and clinical aspects. *APMIS* 2004; **112**: 642–50.

5. Mills KH, McGuirk P. Antigen-specific regulatory T cells – their induction and role in infection. *Semin Immunol* 2004; **16**: 107–17.

◆6. Zlotnik A, Yoshie O. Chemokines: a new classification system and their role in immunity. *Immunity* 2000; **12**: 121–7.

◆7. Locksley RM, Killeen N, Lenardo MJ. The TNF and TNF receptor superfamilies: integrating mammalian biology. *Cell* 2001; **104**: 487–501.

8. Younes A, Aggarwall BB. Clinical implications of the tumor necrosis factor family in benign and malignant hematologic disorders. *Cancer* 2003; **98**: 458–67.

9. Uchida J, Yasui T, Takaoka-Shichijo Y *et al.* Mimicry of CD40 signals by Epstein-Barr virus LMP1 in B lymphocyte responses. *Science* 1999; **286**: 300–3.

◆10. Leonard WJ, O'Shea JJ. Jaks and STATs: biological implications. *Annu Rev Immunol* 1998; **16**: 293–322.

◆11. Ghosh S, May MJ, Kopp EB. NF-kappa B and Rel proteins: evolutionarily conserved mediators of immune responses. *Annu Rev Immunol* 1998; **16**: 225–60.

12. Bowman T, Garcia R, Turkson J, Jove R. STATs in oncogenesis. *Oncogene* 2000; **19**: 2474–88.

13. Rayet B, Gelinas C. Aberrant rel/nfkb genes and activity in human cancer. *Oncogene* 1999; **18**: 6938–47.

◆14. Skinnider BF, Mak TW. The role of cytokines in classical Hodgkin lymphoma. *Blood* 2002; **99**: 4283–97.

15. Skinnider BF, Elia AJ, Gascoyne RD *et al.* Interleukin 13 and interleukin 13 receptor are frequently expressed by Hodgkin and Reed-Sternberg cells of Hodgkin lymphoma. *Blood* 2001; **97**: 250–5.

16. Ohshima K, Akaiwa M, Umeshita R *et al.* Interleukin-13 and interleukin-13 receptor in Hodgkin's disease: possible autocrine mechanism and involvement in fibrosis. *Histopathology* 2001; **38**: 368–75.

●17. Kapp U, Yeh WC, Patterson B *et al.* Interleukin 13 is secreted by and stimulates the growth of Hodgkin and Reed-Sternberg cells. *J Exp Med* 1999; **189**: 1939–46.

18. Skinnider BF, Elia AJ, Gascoyne RD *et al.* Signal transducer and activator of transcription 6 is frequently activated in Hodgkin and Reed-Sternberg cells of Hodgkin lymphoma. *Blood* 2002; **99**: 618–26.

19. Merz H, Fliedner A, Orscheschek K *et al.* Cytokine expression in T-cell lymphomas and Hodgkin's disease. Its possible implication in autocrine or paracrine production as a potential basis for neoplastic growth. *Am J Pathol* 1991; **139**: 1173–80.

20. Hsu SM, Xie SS, Hsu PL, Waldron JA Jr. Interleukin-6, but not interleukin-4, is expressed by Reed-Sternberg cells in Hodgkin's disease with or without histologic features of Castleman's disease. *Am J Pathol* 1992; **141**: 129–38.

21. Herbst H, Foss HD, Samol J *et al.* Frequent expression of interleukin-10 by Epstein-Barr virus-harboring tumor cells of Hodgkin's disease. *Blood* 1996; **87**: 2918–29.

22. Samoszuk M, Nansen L. Detection of interleukin-5 messenger RNA in Reed-Sternberg cells of Hodgkin's disease with eosinophilia. *Blood* 1990; **75**: 13–6.

23. Jucker M, Abts H, Li W *et al.* Expression of interleukin-6 and interleukin-6 receptor in Hodgkin's disease. *Blood* 1991; **77**: 2413–8.

24. Klein S, Jucker M, Diehl V, Tesch H. Production of multiple cytokines by Hodgkin's disease derived cell lines. *Hematol Oncol* 1992; **10**: 319–29.

25. Foss HD, Herbst H, Oelmann E *et al.* Lymphotoxin, tumour necrosis factor and interleukin-6 gene transcripts are present in Hodgkin and Reed-Sternberg cells of most Hodgkin's disease cases. *Br J Haematol* 1993; **84**: 627–35.

26. Herbst H, Samol J, Foss HD *et al.* Modulation of interleukin-6 expression in Hodgkin and Reed-Sternberg cells by Epstein-Barr virus. *J Pathol* 1997; **182**: 299–306.

27. Merz H, Houssiau FA, Orscheschek K *et al.* Interleukin-9 expression in human malignant lymphomas: unique association with Hodgkin's disease and large cell anaplastic lymphoma. *Blood* 1991; **78**: 1311–7.

28. Carbone A, Gloghini A, Gattei V *et al.* Expression of functional CD40 antigen on Reed-Sternberg cells and Hodgkin's disease cell lines. *Blood* 1995; **85**: 780–9.

29. Schwaller J, Tobler A, Niklaus G *et al.* Interleukin-12 expression in human lymphomas and nonneoplastic lymphoid disorders. *Blood* 1995; **85**: 2182–8.

30. Hsu SM, Tseng CK, Hsu PL. Expression of p55 (Tac) interleukin-2 receptor (IL-2R), but not p75 IL-2R, in cultured H-RS cells and H-RS cells in tissues. *Am J Pathol* 1990; **136**: 735–44.

31. Dukers DF, Jaspars LH, Vos W *et al.* Quantitative immunohistochemical analysis of cytokine profiles in Epstein-Barr virus-positive and -negative cases of Hodgkin's disease. *J Pathol* 2000; **190**: 143–9.

●32. Teruya-Feldstein J, Jaffe ES, Burd PR *et al.* Differential chemokine expression in tissues involved by Hodgkin's disease: direct correlation of eotaxin expression and tissue eosinophilia. *Blood* 1999; **93**: 2463–70.

33. Aldinucci D, Olivo K, Lorenzon D *et al.* The role of interleukin-3 in classical Hodgkin's disease. *Leuk Lymphoma* 2005; **46**: 303–11.

34. Kadin ME, Agnarsson BA, Ellingsworth LR, Newcom SR. Immunohistochemical evidence of a role for transforming growth factor beta in the pathogenesis of nodular sclerosing Hodgkin's disease. *Am J Pathol* 1990; **136**: 1209–14.

35. Kadin M, Butmarc J, Elovic A, Wong D. Eosinophils are the major source of transforming growth factor-beta 1 in nodular sclerosing Hodgkin's disease. *Am J Pathol* 1993; **142**: 11–16.

●36. van den Berg A, Visser L, Poppema S. High expression of the CC chemokine TARC in Reed-Sternberg cells. A possible explanation for the characteristic T-cell infiltrate in Hodgkin's lymphoma. *Am J Pathol* 1999; **154**: 1685–91.

37. Peh SC, Kim LH, Poppema S. TARC, a CC chemokine, is frequently expressed in classic Hodgkin's lymphoma but not in NLP Hodgkin's lymphoma, T-cell-rich B-cell lymphoma, and most cases of anaplastic large cell lymphoma. *Am J Surg Pathol* 2001; **25**: 925–9.

38. Jundt F, Anagnostopoulos I, Bommert K *et al.* Hodgkin/Reed-Sternberg cells induce fibroblasts to secrete eotaxin, a potent chemoattractant for T cells and eosinophils. *Blood* 1999; **94**: 2065–71.

39. Buri C, Korner M, Scharli P *et al.* CC chemokines and the receptors CCR3 and CCR5 are differentially expressed in the nonneoplastic leukocytic infiltrates of Hodgkin disease. *Blood* 2001; **97**: 1543–8.

40. Gruss HJ, Hirschstein D, Wright B *et al.* Expression and function of CD40 on Hodgkin and Reed-Sternberg cells and the possible relevance for Hodgkin's disease. *Blood* 1994; **84**: 2305–14.

41. Falini B, Pileri S, Pizzolo G *et al.* CD30 (Ki-1) molecule: a new cytokine receptor of the tumor necrosis factor receptor superfamily as a tool for diagnosis and immunotherapy. *Blood* 1995; **85**: 1–14.

42. Carbone A, Gloghini A, Gruss HJ, Pinto A. CD40 ligand is constitutively expressed in a subset of T cell lymphomas and on the microenvironmental reactive T cells of follicular lymphomas and Hodgkin's disease. *Am J Pathol* 1995; **147**: 912–22.

43. Pinto A, Aldinucci D, Gloghini A *et al.* Human eosinophils express functional CD30 ligand and stimulate proliferation of a Hodgkin's disease cell line. *Blood* 1996; **88**: 3299–305.

44. Molin D, Fischer M, Xiang Z *et al.* Mast cells express functional CD30 ligand and are the predominant CD30L-positive cells in Hodgkin's disease. *Br J Haematol* 2001; **114**: 616–23.

45. Smith CA, Gruss HJ, Davis T *et al.* CD30 antigen, a marker for Hodgkin's lymphoma, is a receptor whose ligand defines an emerging family of cytokines with homology to TNF. *Cell* 1993; **73**: 1349–60.

46. Hsu PL, Hsu SM. Autocrine growth regulation of CD30 ligand in CD30-expressing Reed-Sternberg cells: distinction between Hodgkin's disease and anaplastic large cell lymphoma. *Lab Invest* 2000; **80**: 1111–19.

47. Bargou RC, Leng C, Krappmann D *et al.* High-level nuclear NF-kappa B and Oct-2 is a common feature of cultured Hodgkin/Reed-Sternberg cells. *Blood* 1996; **87**: 4340–7.

●48. Wood KM, Roff M, Hay RT. Defective IkappaBalpha in Hodgkin cell lines with constitutively active NF-kappaB. *Oncogene* 1998; **16**: 2131–9.

49. Krappmann D, Emmerich F, Kordes U *et al.* Molecular mechanisms of constitutive NF-kappaB/Rel activation in Hodgkin/Reed-Sternberg cells. *Oncogene* 1999; **18**: 943–53.

●50. Bargou RC, Emmerich F, Krappmann D *et al.* Constitutive nuclear factor-kappaB-RelA activation is required for proliferation and survival of Hodgkin's disease tumor cells. *J Clin Invest* 1997; **100**: 2961–9.

51. Hinz M, Loser P, Mathas S *et al.* Constitutive NF-kappaB maintains high expression of a characteristic gene network, including CD40, CD86, and a set of antiapoptotic genes in Hodgkin/Reed-Sternberg cells. *Blood* 2001; **97**: 2798–807.

52. Hinz M, Lemke P, Anagnostopoulos I *et al.* Nuclear factor kappaB-dependent gene expression profiling of Hodgkin's disease tumor cells, pathogenetic significance, and link to constitutive signal transducer and activator of transcription 5a activity. *J Exp Med* 2002; **196**: 605–17.

53. Cabannes E, Khan G, Aillet F *et al.* Mutations in the IkBa gene in Hodgkin's disease suggest a tumour suppressor role for IkappaBalpha. *Oncogene* 1999; **18**: 3063–70.

54. Emmerich F, Meiser M, Hummel M *et al.* Overexpression of I kappa B alpha without inhibition of NF-kappaB activity and mutations in the I kappa B alpha gene in Reed-Sternberg cells. *Blood* 1999; **94**: 3129–34.

55. Trieu Y, Wen XY, Skinnider BF *et al.* Soluble interleukin-13Ralpha2 decoy receptor inhibits Hodgkin's lymphoma growth in vitro and in vivo. *Cancer Res* 2004; **64**: 3271–5.

56. Poppema S, van den Berg A. Interaction between host T cells and Reed-Sternberg cells in Hodgkin lymphomas. *Semin Cancer Biol* 2000; **10**: 345–50.

57. Marshall NA, Christie LE, Munro LR *et al.* Immunosuppressive regulatory T cells are abundant in the reactive lymphocytes of Hodgkin lymphoma. *Blood* 2004; **103**: 1755–62.

58. Sallusto F, Lanzavecchia A, Mackay CR. Chemokines and chemokine receptors in T-cell priming and Th1/Th2-mediated responses. *Immunol Today* 1998; **19**: 568–74.

59. Iellem A, Mariani M, Lang R *et al.* Unique chemotactic response profile and specific expression of chemokine receptors CCR4 and CCR8 by CD4(+)CD25(+) regulatory T cells. *J Exp Med* 2001; **194**: 847–53.

60. Poppema S, Bhan AK, Reinherz EL *et al.* In situ immunologic characterization of cellular constituents in lymph nodes and spleens involved by Hodgkin's disease. *Blood* 1982; **59**: 226–32.

61. Oudejans JJ, Jiwa NM, Kummer JA *et al.* Analysis of major histocompatibility complex class I expression on Reed-Sternberg cells in relation to the cytotoxic T-cell response in Epstein-Barr virus-positive and -negative Hodgkin's disease. *Blood* 1996; **87**: 3844–51.

62. Kandil A, Bazarbashi S, Mourad WA. The correlation of Epstein-Barr virus expression and lymphocyte subsets with the clinical presentation of nodular sclerosing Hodgkin disease. *Cancer* 2001; **91**: 1957–63.

63. Chapman AL, Rickinson AB, Thomas WA *et al.* Epstein-Barr virus-specific cytotoxic T lymphocyte responses in the blood and tumor site of Hodgkin's disease patients: implications for a T-cell-based therapy. *Cancer Res* 2001; **61**: 6219–26.

64. Aldinucci D, Lorenzon D, Olivo K *et al.* Interactions between tissue fibroblasts in lymph nodes and Hodgkin/Reed-Sternberg cells. *Leuk Lymphoma* 2004; **45**: 1731–9.

65. Sime PJ, O'Reilly KM. Fibrosis of the lung and other tissues: new concepts in pathogenesis and treatment. *Clin Immunol* 2001; **99**: 308–19.

♦66. Slivnick DJ, Ellis TM, Nawrocki JF, Fisher RI. The impact of Hodgkin's disease on the immune system. *Semin Oncol* 1990; **17**: 673–82.

♦67. Re D, Thomas RK, Behringer K, Diehl, V. From Hodgkin disease to Hodgkin lymphoma: biologic insights and therapeutic potential. *Blood* 2005; **105**: 4553–60.

68. Duprez V, Lenoir G, Dautry-Varsat A. Autocrine growth stimulation of a human T-cell lymphoma line by interleukin 2. *Proc Natl Acad Sci U S A* 1985; **82**: 6932–6.

69. Raziuddin S, Sheikha A, Abu-Eshy S, Al-Janadi M. Regulation of interleukin-4 production and cytokine-induced growth potential in peripheral T-cell non-Hodgkin's lymphomas. *Br J Haematol* 1998; **100**: 310–16.

70. Ho JW, Liang RH, Srivastava G. Preferential type 1-1 cytokine gene expressions in peripheral T-cell lymphomas. *Hematol Oncol* 1999; **17**: 117–29.

71. Jones D, O'Hara C, Kraus MD *et al.* Expression pattern of T-cell-associated chemokine receptors and their chemokines correlates with specific subtypes of T-cell non-Hodgkin lymphoma. *Blood* 2000; **96**: 685–90.

72. Ohshima K, Karube K, Kawano R *et al.* Classification of distinct subtypes of peripheral T-cell lymphoma unspecified, identified by chemokine and chemokine receptor expression: Analysis of prognosis. *Int J Oncol* 2004; **25**: 605–13.

73. Tsuchiya T, Ohshima K, Karube K *et al.* Th1, Th2, and activated T-cell marker and clinical prognosis in peripheral T-cell lymphoma, unspecified: comparison with AILD, ALCL, lymphoblastic lymphoma, and ATLL. *Blood* 2004; **103**: 236–41.

74. Ishida T, Inagaki H, Utsunomiya A *et al.* CXC chemokine receptor 3 and CC chemokine receptor 4 expression in T-cell and NK-cell lymphomas with special reference to clinicopathological significance for peripheral T-cell lymphoma, unspecified. *Clin Cancer Res* 2004; **10**: 5494–500.

75. Kubonishi I, Bandobashi K, Murata N *et al.* High serum levels of CA125 and interleukin-6 in a patient with Ki-1 lymphoma. *Br J Haematol* 1997; **98**: 450–2.

76. Ohshima KS, Suzumiya J, Kawasaki C *et al.* Cytoplasmic cytokines in lymphoproliferative disorders: multiple cytokine production in angioimmunoblastic lymphadenopathy with dysproteinemia. *Leuk Lymphoma* 2000; **38**: 541–5.

77. Foss HD, Anagnostopoulos I, Herbst H *et al.* Patterns of cytokine gene expression in peripheral T-cell lymphoma of angioimmunoblastic lymphadenopathy type. *Blood* 1995; **85**: 2862–9.

78. Ohnishi K, Ichikawa A, Kagami Y *et al.* Interleukin 4 and gamma-interferon may play a role in the histopathogenesis of peripheral T-cell lymphoma. *Cancer Res* 1990; **50**: 8028–33.

79. Hsu SM, Waldron JA Jr, Fink L *et al.* Pathogenic significance of interleukin-6 in angioimmunoblastic lymphadenopathy-type T-cell lymphoma. *Hum Pathol* 1993; **24**: 126–31.

80. Shimizu S, Takiguchi T, Sugai S *et al.* An established CD4+ T lymphoma cell line derived from a patient with so-called Lennert's lymphoma: possible roles of cytokines in histopathogenesis. *Blood* 1988; **71**: 196–203.

81. Shimizu S, Hirano T, Yoshioka R *et al.* Interleukin-6 (B-cell stimulatory factor 2)-dependent growth of a Lennert's lymphoma-derived T-cell line (KT-3). *Blood* 1988; **72**: 1826–8.

82. Saed G, Fivenson DP, Naidu Y, Nickoloff BJ. Mycosis fungoides exhibits a Th1-type cell-mediated cytokine profile whereas Sezary syndrome expresses a Th2-type profile. *J Invest Dermatol* 1994; **103**: 29–33.

83. Dummer R, Heald PW, Nestle FO *et al.* Sezary syndrome T-cell clones display T-helper 2 cytokines and express the accessory factor-1 (interferon-gamma receptor beta-chain). *Blood* 1996; **88**: 1383–9.

84. Nielsen M, Nissen MH, Gerwien J *et al.* Spontaneous interleukin-5 production in cutaneous T-cell lymphoma lines is mediated by constitutively activated Stat3. *Blood* 2002; **99**: 973–7.

85. Qin JZ, Zhang CL, Kamarashev J *et al.* Interleukin-7 and interleukin-15 regulate the expression of the bcl-2 and c-myb genes in cutaneous T-cell lymphoma cells. *Blood* 2001; **98**: 2778–83.

86. Qin JZ, Kamarashev J, Zhang CL *et al.* Constitutive and interleukin-7- and interleukin-15-stimulated DNA binding of STAT and novel factors in cutaneous T cell lymphoma cells. *J Invest Dermatol* 2001; **117**: 583–9.

87. Dobbeling U, Dummer R, Laine E *et al.* Interleukin-15 is an autocrine/paracrine viability factor for cutaneous T-cell lymphoma cells. *Blood* 1998; **92**: 252–8.

88. Leroy S, Dubois S, Tenaud I *et al.* Interleukin-15 expression in cutaneous T-cell lymphoma (mycosis fungoides and Sezary syndrome). *Br J Dermatol* 2001; **144**: 1016–23.

89. Berger CL, Tigelaar R, Cohen J *et al.* Cutaneous T-cell lymphoma: malignant proliferation of T-regulatory cells. *Blood* 2005; **105**: 1640–7.

90. Rook AH, Kuzel TM, Olsen EA. Cytokine therapy of cutaneous T-cell lymphoma: interferons, interleukin-12, and interleukin-2. *Hematol Oncol Clin North Am* 2003; **17**: 1435–48, ix.

91. Mori N, Gill PS, Mougdil T *et al.* Interleukin-10 gene expression in adult T-cell leukemia. *Blood* 1996; **88**: 1035–45.

92. Mori N, Shirakawa F, Murakami S *et al.* Characterization and regulation of interleukin-4 receptor in adult T-cell leukemia cells. *Eur J Haematol* 1996; **56**: 241–7.

93. Portis T, Harding JC, Ratner L. The contribution of NF-kappa B activity to spontaneous proliferation and resistance to apoptosis in human T-cell leukemia virus type 1 Tax-induced tumors. *Blood* 2001; **98**: 1200–8.

94. Ding W, Kim SJ, Nair AM *et al.* Human T-cell lymphotropic virus type 1 p12I enhances interleukin-2 production during T-cell activation. *J Virol* 2003; **77**: 11027–39.

95. Waldele K, Schneider G, Ruckes T, Grassmann R. Interleukin-13 overexpression by tax transactivation: a potential autocrine stimulus in human T-cell leukemia virus-infected lymphocytes. *J Virol* 2004; **78**: 6081–90.

96. Mori N, Yamashita U, Tanaka Y *et al.* Interleukin-4 induces proliferation of adult T-cell leukemia cells. *Eur J Haematol* 1993; **50**: 133–40.

97. Uchiyama T, Kamio M, Kodaka T *et al.* Leukemic cells from some adult T-cell leukemia patients proliferate in response to interleukin-4. *Blood* 1988; **72**: 1182–6.

98. Ishida T, Utsunomiya A, Iida S *et al.* Clinical significance of CCR4 expression in adult T-cell leukemia/lymphoma: its close association with skin involvement and unfavorable outcome. *Clin Cancer Res* 2003; **9**: 3625–34.

99. Ishida T, Iida S, Akatsuka Y *et al.* The CC chemokine receptor 4 as a novel specific molecular target for immunotherapy in adult T-cell leukemia/lymphoma. *Clin Cancer Res* 2004; **10**: 7529–39.

100. Karube K, Ohshima K, Tsuchiya T *et al.* Expression of FoxP3, a key molecule in CD4CD25 regulatory T cells, in adult T-cell leukaemia/lymphoma cells. *Br J Haematol* 2004; **126**: 81–4.

101. Yee C, Biondi A, Wang XH *et al.* A possible autocrine role for interleukin-6 in two lymphoma cell lines. *Blood* 1989; **74**: 798–804.

102. Freeman GJ, Freedman AS, Rabinowe SN *et al.* Interleukin 6 gene expression in normal and neoplastic B cells. *J Clin Invest* 1989; **83**: 1512–8.

103. Merz H, Fliedner A, Lehrnbecher T *et al.* Cytokine expression in B-cell non-Hodgkin lymphomas. *Hematol Oncol* 1990; **8**: 355–61.

104. Hsu SM, Xie SS, Waldron JA Jr. Functional heterogeneity and pathogenic significance of interleukin-6 in B-cell lymphomas. *Am J Pathol* 1992; **141**: 915–23.

105. Macon WR, Cousar JB, Waldron JA Jr, Hsu SM. Interleukin-4 may contribute to the abundant T-cell reaction and paucity of neoplastic B cells in T-cell-rich B-cell lymphomas. *Am J Pathol* 1992; **141**: 1031–6.

106. Potter M. Neoplastic development in plasma cells. *Immunol Rev* 2003; **194**: 177–95.

107. Hideshima T, Bergsagel PL, Kuehl WM, Anderson KC. Advances in biology of multiple myeloma: clinical applications. *Blood* 2004; **104**: 607–18.

108. Airoldi I, Guglielmino R, Ghiotto F *et al.* Cytokine gene expression in neoplastic B cells from human mantle cell, follicular, and marginal zone lymphomas and in their postulated normal counterparts. *Cancer Res* 2001; **61**: 1285–90.

109. Greiner A, Knorr C, Qin Y *et al.* Low-grade B cell lymphomas of mucosa-associated lymphoid tissue (MALT-type) require CD40-mediated signaling and Th2-type cytokines for in vitro growth and differentiation. *Am J Pathol* 1997; **150**: 1583–93.

110. Clayberger C, Luna-Fineman S, Lee JE *et al.* Interleukin 3 is a growth factor for human follicular B cell lymphoma. *J Exp Med* 1992; **175**: 371–6.

111. Shade RJ, Younes A. In vitro and in vivo biologic effects of interleukin-3 (IL-3) in follicular low-grade lymphoma. *Leuk Lymphoma* 1997; **26**: 17–25.

16

Lymphocyte homing and the dissemination of lymphoid malignancies

STEVEN T PALS AND DAVID JJ DE GORTER

INTRODUCTION

Specific recognition of foreign antigens and effective surveillance are the two mainstays of the body's defense against microbial invasion. Evolution has created great antigen-receptor diversity and has equipped lymphocytes with exquisite motility and migratory properties to accomplish these tasks. As discovered more than four decades ago by Gowans and Knight, mature lymphocytes recirculate, moving continuously from blood to tissue and back to the bloodstream again.[1] This recirculation is not random, but is guided by mechanisms allowing lymphocyte diapedesis at the correct site and directing their migration to the proper place in the tissues (for reviews, see [2–5]). Within the tissues, lymphocytes display a characteristic 'amoeboid' form of cell migration,[6] which represents a physically optimized migration mode that allows easy cell traffic toward and between different tissue compartments. This movement is directed by chemokines and stromal cell networks in the lymphoid microenvironments.[7,8] Lymphocyte-endothelial recognition plays a central role in controlling the access of specialized lymphocyte subsets to particular tissues, thus influencing the nature of local immune and inflammatory responses. At the molecular level, this 'homing' process is regulated by adhesion molecules in concert with chemokines (chemoattractant cytokines): lymphocyte subsets as well as endothelial cells specifically program their expression of adhesion molecules and chemokines/chemokine receptors, allowing lymphocytes to move selectively to specific functional compartments of the immune system, such as the mucosal-associated lymphoid tissue (MALT) and the skin.[2–5]

This chapter describes the basic principles of lymphocyte trafficking and discusses emerging evidence indicating that the molecular cues regulating this process also play a critical role in lymphoma dissemination. In cases of malignant transformation, the fact that lymphocytes are 'licensed to move' forms a serious threat to the organism, since it allows rapid tumor dissemination irrespective of the conventional anatomic boundaries limiting tumor spread in most solid tumors. The strikingly tissue-specific dissemination of, for example, malignant lymphomas of the mucosal-associated lymphoid tissues, cutaneous lymphomas, and multiple myeloma reflect basic rules of lymphocyte homing. A better understanding of the molecular mechanisms underlying this behavior may provide novel targets for treatment of lymphoma patients. For the convenience of the reader, an overview of the most important adhesion molecules and chemokine receptors involved in homing, their distribution on various lymphocyte subsets and non-Hodgkin lymphoma (NHL) subtypes, and their ligands, sites of interaction, and predominant role(s) in homing are given in Table 16.1.

LYMPHOCYTE RECIRCULATION AND HOMING

Lymphocytes: licensed to move

Cell migration is a universal process; most cell types in the body are capable of migrating at one or more distinct steps

Table 16.1 Adhesion molecules, chemokine receptors, and chemokines involved in lymphocyte homing and lymphoma dissemination

Receptor	Expression on lymphocytes	Expression on lymphomas	Ligands	Predominant sites of homing
Adhesion molecules			*Adhesion molecules*	
L-Selectin	Naïve T and B cells, central memory T cells	B-CLL, MCL, MZBL, nodal FL, DLBCL, nodal PTCL	PNAd (MAdCAM-1)	PLN
CLA	Skin-homing T cells	CTCL	E-Selectin	Skin
$\alpha_4\beta_7$	Naïve T and B cells (low), gut-homing T cells (high), IgA plasmablasts	GI-tract MCL (MLP), GI-tract MZBCL (maltoma), GI-tract FL, GI-tract PTCL (EA-TCL)	MAdCAM-1 (VCAM-1)	Gut
$\alpha E\beta_7$	Intraepithelial T cells	GI-tract PTCL, GI-tract MZBCLs	E-cadherin	Epithelium
$\alpha L\beta_2$ (LFA-1)	Broad expression on T and B cells	Broad expression on T and B cell lymphomas and MM	ICAM-1 ICAM-2	Multiple sites
$\alpha_4\beta_1$ (VLA-4)	Broad expression on T and B cells	Broad expression on T and B cell lymphomas and MM	VCAM-1	Inflammatory sites and bone marrow
Chemokine receptors			*Chemokines*	
CCR4	Skin-homing T cells	CTCL	CCL17 (TARC)	Skin
CCR7	Naïve T cells, central memory T cells	CTCL, MCL	CCL21 (SLC)	PLN
CCR9	Gut-homing T cells, intra-epithelial T cells, IgA plasmablasts	Unknown	CCL25 (TECK)	Intestinal mucosa and crypt epithelium
CCR10	Skin-homing T cells IgA plasma blasts	CTCL Unknown	CCL27 (CTAK) CCL28 (MEC)	Skin Intestine
CXCR4	Pre-B cells, B cells, plasma cells	Broad expression on T and B cell lymphomas and MM	CXCL12 (SDF-1)	Secondary lymphoid tissues and BM, migration to GCs
CXCR5	Mature B cells	Broad expression on T and B cell lymphomas	CXCL13 (BLC/BCA-1)	Migration to GCs in PLN and Peyer's patches

Only adhesion molecules, chemokines, and their receptors with major functions in tissue-specific lymphocyte homing are listed. The $\alpha\beta$ heterodimers belong to the integrin family.

CLA, cutaneous lymphocyte antigen; ICAM, intercellular adhesion molecule; LFA, lymphocyte function-associated; MAdCAM, mucosal addressin cell adhesion molecule; PNAd, peripheral lymph node addressin; VCAM, vascular cell adhesion molecule; VLA, very late antigens; B-CLL, B cell chronic lymphocytic leukemia; BM, bone marrow; MCL, mantle cell lymphoma; MLP, malignant lymphomatous polyposis; MZBL, marginal zone B cell lymphoma; FL, follicular lymphoma; DLBCL, diffuse large B cell lymphoma; PLN, peripheral lymph node; PTCL, peripheral T cell lymphoma; EA-TCL, enteropathy-associated T cell lymphoma; MM, multiple myeloma; CTCL, cutaneous T cell lymphomas; GC, germinal center; GI, gastrointestinal.

during their development and differentiation. This migration is essential for tissue morphogenesis and leukocyte trafficking, as well as for epithelial turnover and regeneration processes, such as wound healing. Furthermore, deregulated cell migration can take place in cancer, resulting in tumor invasion and metastasis. Given the highly diverse biological contexts of cell migration, it is not surprising that distinct cell migration strategies have emerged. These cell type-specific patterns of migration are acquired during differentiation and can be subdivided into at least three main migration modes, i.e., 'mesenchymal' and 'amoeboid' single cell migration, and 'collective' cell migration (Fig. 16.1).[6] The essential molecules that control and specify these different types of migration include adhesion molecules of the $\beta1$ and $\beta3$ integrin families that mediate interaction with the extracellular matrix (ECM); matrix

metalloproteinases (MMPs) and serine proteinases, such as uPA/uPAR, responsible for ECM degradation; cadherins and associated molecules that mediate stable intercellular adhesions; and signaling molecules that control the actin cytoskeleton, specifically the small GTPases RHOA, RAC, and CDC42 and their downstream effectors. In mesenchymal migration, which represents the archetype of cell migration, cells complete a migration sequence consisting of: (1) cell polarization driven by localized actin polymerization causing formation of a leading pseudopod; (2) attachment of this pseudopod to ECM ligands via $\beta1$ and $\beta3$ integrin clusters called focal adhesions, interaction sites which recruit cytoplasmic adapter, signaling, and cytoskeletal proteins as well as cell-surface proteases such as MMPs and the uPA/uPAR complex; (3) local proteolysis of the ECM, widening the space for forward movement of the

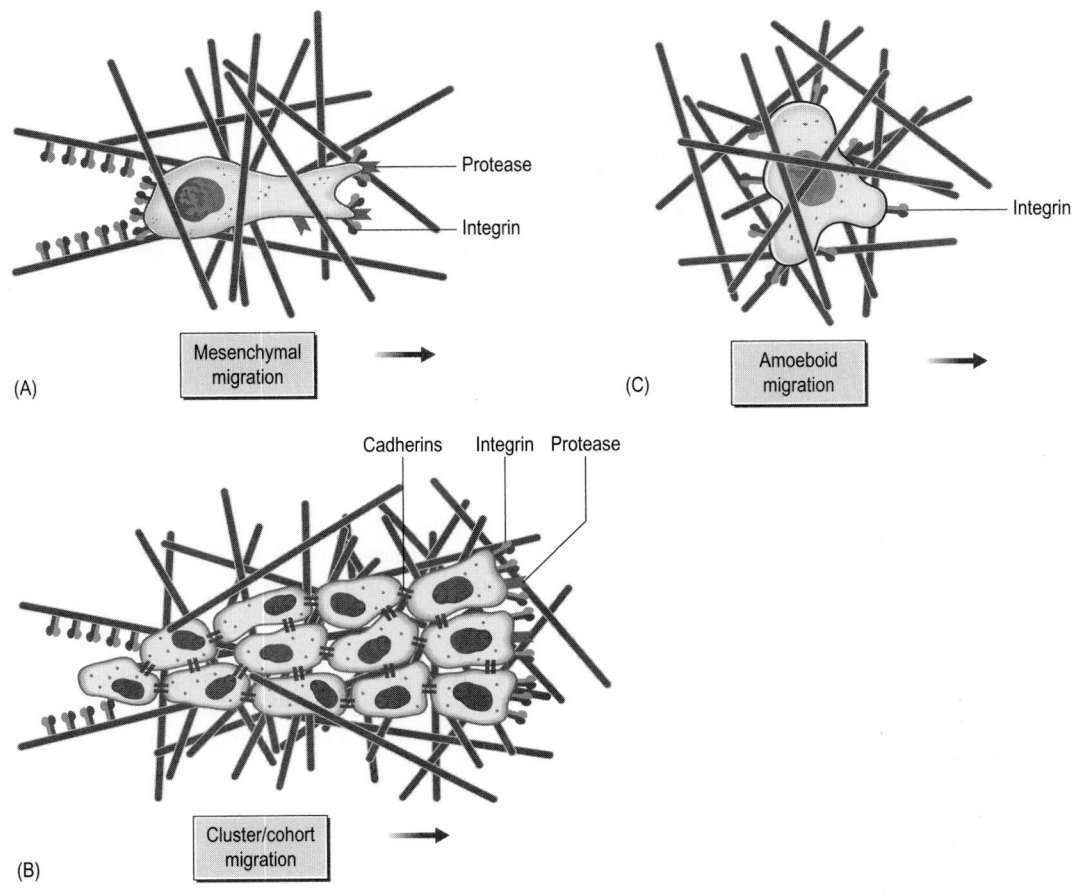

Figure 16.1   Diversity in cell migration strategies. In the tissue microenvironment different cell types exhibit distinct migration strategies. (A) Mesenchymal migration. Mesenchymal cells display an adhesive phenotype and develop a spindle shape. The elongated morphology is dependent on integrin-mediated adhesion and the presence of traction forces on both cell poles. Simultaneous with integrin and actin concentration at focal contacts, the cells recruit surface proteases to these substrate contact sites to digest and remodel the extracellular matrix, thus generating matrix defects that allow cell migration. Other cells may follow along the generated matrix defect creating a moving cell chain. (B) Cluster/cohort migration. Migrating cancer cell collectives utilize an integrin- and protease-dependent migration mode similar to mesenchymal migration but the migrating cells within the cohorts are interconnected by cadherins and gap-junctional communication. (C) Amoeboid migration. Lymphoid cells display a characteristic 'amoeboid' type of migration, in which integrin-mediated adhesion is dispensable and cell movement is driven by short-lived, relatively weak interactions with the substrate. The lack of focal contacts and high deformability of lymphocytes allows movement at high velocity, while the fast deformability of lymphocytes allows them to overcome matrix barriers by physical mechanisms, independent of proteolytic matrix degradation.[37]

cell; (4) activation of contractile proteins, like myosin II, and consequent shortening of membrane-anchored actin filaments; and (5) contraction of the cell, leading to retraction of its rear end and consequent forward movement (Fig. 16.1). This five-step migration program is typical for single cell migration of fibroblasts and keratinocytes as well as for single epithelial (cancer) cells that have undergone epithelial to mesenchymal transition (EMT), and represents a relatively slow process with migration velocities of 0.1–2 μm/min. Collective cell migration, as seen during wound healing and during the invasion of epithelial cancer cell collectives, uses the same integrin- and protease-dependent migration cycle, but in this migration type the cell junctions within the invasive collectives are stabilized

by cadherins and gap-junctional cell–cell communication (Fig. 16.1). Interestingly, recent studies indicate that lymphocytes do not conform to the classic five-step paradigm of cell migration. Instead they display a characteristic form of cell migration, which has been termed 'amoeboid' migration, since it mimics that of the amoeba *Dictyostelium discoideum*.[6] In this migration type, integrin-mediated adhesion is partially or completely dispensable and stable focal contacts are not formed, but cell movement is driven by short-lived, relatively weak interactions with the substrate. The lack of focal contacts and high deformability of lymphocytes allows movement at high velocity (2–30 μm/min). Moreover, the fast deformability of lymphocytes allows them to overcome matrix barriers by physical

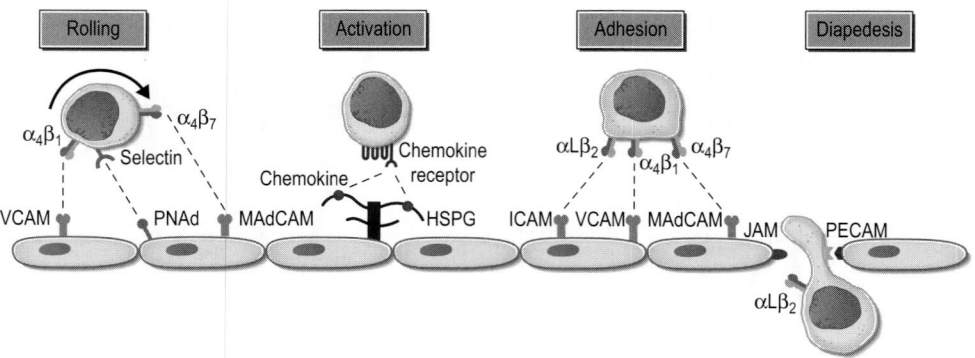

Figure 16.2 Lymphocyte interaction with endothelium. In the post-capillary venules, selectin–sialomucin interactions (or interactions mediated by integrin $\alpha_4\beta_1$ or $\alpha_4\beta_7$) mediate 'rolling' of lymphocytes on the endothelium. Chemokines, presented by heparan sulfate proteoglycans expressed on the endothelium, bind to chemokine receptors, which are G-protein-coupled receptors, leading to increased affinity/avidity integrins on the surface of lymphocytes. Interaction of these integrins with their ligands results in stable adhesion of lymphocytes to endothelium and in diapedesis, involving engagement with junction adhesion molecules (JAMs) and PECAM-1 (CD31). ICAM, intercellular adhesion molecule; MAdCAM, mucosal addressin cell adhesion molecule; PNAd, peripheral lymph node addressin; VCAM, vascular cell adhesion molecule; VLA, very late antigens; HSPG, heparan sulfate proteoglycan.

mechanisms, i.e, adaptation of shape to preformed matrix structures (contact guidance), extension of lateral footholds (elbowing), and squeezing through narrow spaces (contraction rings). Thus, lymphocyte migration is shape-change driven and lymphocytes use protease-independent physical mechanisms that allow easy cell traffic toward and between structurally different tissue compartments. Among higher eukaryotes, this migration type is only found in lymphocytes and other leukocytes, hematopoietic stem cells, and certain tumor cells.[6]

Lymphocyte–endothelial interaction, a multistep process

Lymphocyte exit from the bloodstream occurs via a series of interactions with vascular endothelium in specialized post-capillary venules, termed high endothelial venules (HEVs), in lymph nodes and Peyer's patches.[2] The initial step consists of a loose 'tethering' engagement, leading to a rolling movement of the lymphocyte over the vascular endothelium (Fig. 16.2). Generally, lymphocyte rolling is mediated by molecules of the selectin family, which are strategically localized on the tips of the cell membrane's microvilli,[9,10] allowing effective interaction with their sialomucin ligands. Under certain conditions, the integrins $\alpha_4\beta_1$ and $\alpha_4\beta_7$, and CD44 can also mediate rolling.[9,11–13] Lymphocyte rolling is transient and reversible, unless followed by a chemokine signal leading to integrin activation. Heparan sulfate proteoglycans (HSPGs) expressed on endothelium or extracellular matrix contribute to integrin activation and promote diapedesis by concentrating and presenting chemokines to their receptors. Heparan sulfate chain modifications can affect cytokine binding specificity and may add an additional level of complexity to the lymphocyte–endothelial cell interaction cascade. By interacting with their

G protein–coupled receptors and activating various signaling molecules including phosphatidylinositol 3-kinase (PI3K), Tec/Btk-family kinases, phospholipase C, and Ras-family GTPases,[14,15] chemokines like CXCL12 (SDF-1), CXCL13 (BCA/BLC), CCL21 (SLC), CXCL10 (IP10), and CCL17 (TARC) trigger affinity and avidity of lymphocyte integrins, resulting in rapid (milliseconds) lymphocyte arrest under flow conditions.[16–18] These integrins, specifically lymphocyte function-associated antigen (LFA)-1 ($\alpha L\beta_2$), $\alpha_4\beta_1$, and $\alpha_4\beta_7$, mediate stable adhesion and promote migration of lymphocytes across the vessel wall (Fig. 16.2). This transmigration is further promoted by interaction with junctional adhesion molecules (JAMs) and PECAM-1 (CD31).[19,20] Once in the tissue, the lymphocytes engage chemoattractant gradients, directing their migration to the correct microenvironment. The 'exit decision' of a given lymphocyte in the multistep lymphocyte–endothelial cell interaction model (Fig. 16.2) is determined by the unique combination of adhesion molecules and chemokine receptors on its cell surface. This 'homing signature' enables the cell to recognize and leave the blood at specialized endothelial 'address' sites expressing the relevant ligands, thus allowing tissue-specific homing.[2–5,18,21,22]

Tissue-specific lymphocyte homing

The homing signature of a lymphocyte is dependent on differentiation stage and antigenic experience. Mature naïve lymphocytes display a remarkable tropism for the various secondary lymphoid organs, and are generally excluded from nonlymphoid sites.[23] During the late stages of their ontogeny in the thymus and bone marrow, T cell and B cell precursors upregulate L-selectin as well as the chemokine receptor CCR7.[22] The ligands for these receptors, the peripheral lymph node addressin (PNAd) and the

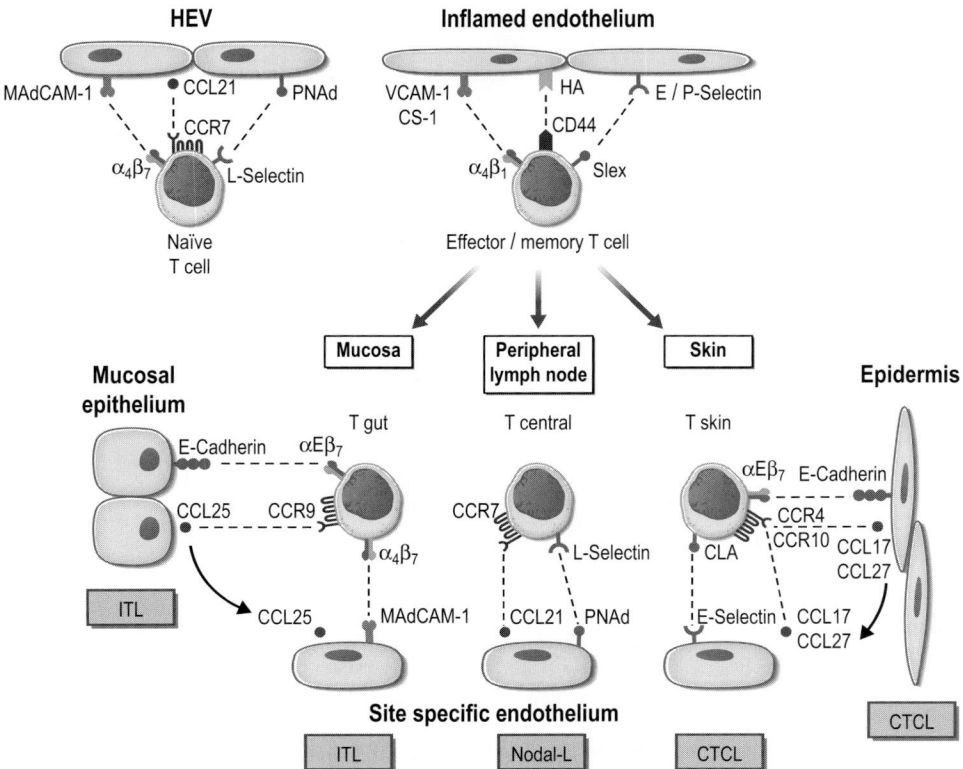

Figure 16.3 Lymphocyte trafficking and the tissue-specific dissemination of T cell lymphomas. Lymphocyte migration is strictly regulated by adhesion molecules and chemokine receptors on lymphocytes and their ligands expressed by the endothelium. Naïve T lymphocytes can home and recirculate via all secondary lymphoid tissues since they express both $\alpha_4\beta_7$ (for mucosal homing) and L-selectin (for homing to peripheral lymph nodes). Migration of activated T lymphocytes to sites of inflammation involves several receptor–ligand pairs, including selectin–sialomucin, $\alpha_4\beta_1$–VCAM-1, $\alpha_4\beta_1$–CS-1, and CD44–hyaluronate (HA) interactions. Upon antigen priming by dendritic cells, T lymphocytes become memory cells and acquire a 'homing signature,' i.e., a specific adhesion molecule and chemokine receptor make-up, which enables them to selectively home to specific tissue environments, thereby increasing the efficacy of immunosurveillance. The T cell non-Hodgkin lymphomas related to lymphocyte populations with tissue-specific homing properties are shown in the white boxes. These tumors usually display tissue-specific dissemination patterns and express homing receptors corresponding to the tissue of origin. ITL, intestinal T cell lymphoma; Nodal-L, nodal T cell lymphoma; CTCL, cutaneous T cell lymphoma.

chemokine CCL21, are expressed on the luminal surface of HEV (Fig. 16.3).[21,22] Naïve lymphocytes also express the integrin $\alpha_4\beta_7$, an important mediator of lymphocyte rolling and adhesion in the gut-associated lymphoid tissues. The combined expression of L-selectin, $\alpha_4\beta_7$, LFA-1, and CCR7 allows naïve lymphocytes access to both the peripheral and gut-associated lymphoid tissues, resulting in efficient surveillance of these crossroads of the immune system (Fig. 16.3).

In the absence of antigen stimulation, a naïve lymphocyte will exit the secondary lymphoid tissues via the efferent lymphatics and return to the recirculating lymphocyte pool.[1] Antigen engagement blocks this exit and results in clonal expansion of the antigen-specific lymphocyte and its differentiation into a functionally specialized effector or memory cell. As an integral part of this differentiation process, the homing signature of the lymphocyte is revised to a unique combination of adhesion molecules and chemokine receptors, allowing preferential exit from the

blood in the type of lymphoid tissue where the initial activation took place.[2,5,18,21–23] In addition, the newly acquired homing profile enables the lymphocyte to leave the blood in the nonlymphoid tissue draining to this lymph node. The molecular mechanisms controlling the reprogramming of the homing signature of lymphocytes are still incompletely understood. Recent studies indicate that interaction with dendritic cells (DCs) plays a crucial role. For example, it was demonstrated that priming of lymphocytes by mucosal DCs increases the expression of $\alpha_4\beta_7$ and CCR9, molecules that promote specific homing to the gut.[24–28] By contrast, activation by skin-derived DCs decreases $\alpha_4\beta_7$ and CCR9 expression but enhances expression of the skin-homing receptor cutaneous lymphocyte antigen (CLA).[29]

Currently, the best-characterized pathways of lymphocyte homing are those mediating homing to the gut-associated lymphoid tissue and skin (Fig. 16.3). Both intestine and skin represent barrier tissues exposed to high antigenic load and it is conceivable that these specialized

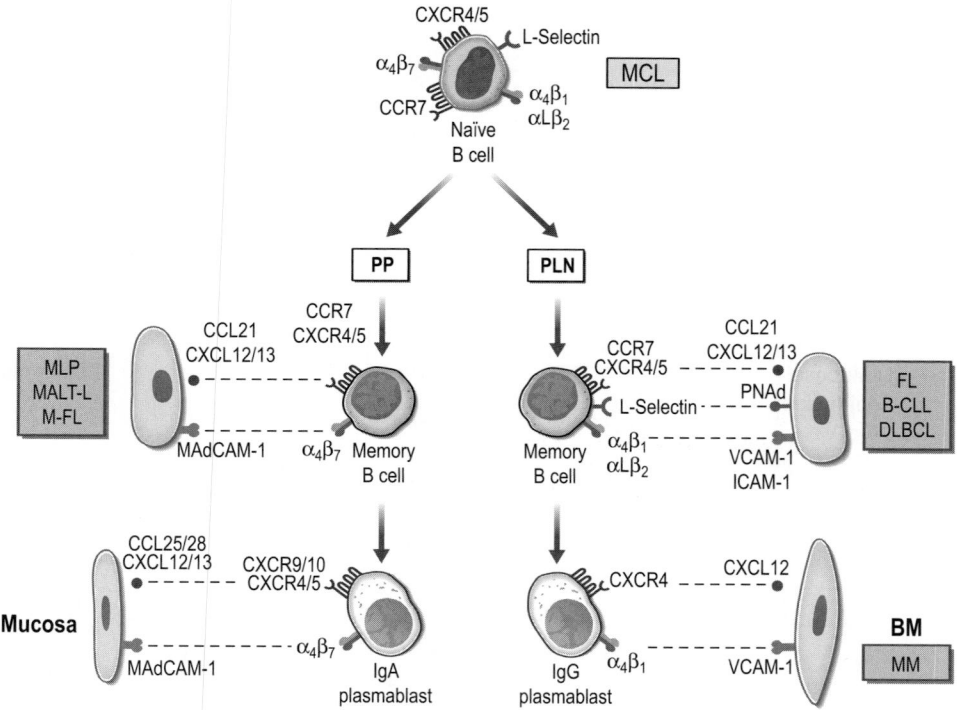

Figure 16.4   Adhesion molecule and chemokine receptor expression profiles of B lymphocyte subsets and related lymphoid malignancies. Naïve B lymphocytes coexpress L-selectin and $\alpha_4\beta_7$ enabling them to migrate to the mucosa as well as to peripheral lymph nodes (PLN). Germinal center reactions in Peyer's patches (PP) lead to generation of $\alpha_4\beta_7$-expressing memory B lymphocytes, which subsequently can differentiate into IgA-secreting plasma cells. Most memory B cells arising in lymph nodes, on the other hand, differentiate into IgG-secreting plasma cells. These cells express CXCR4 and the integrins $\alpha_4\beta_1$ and LFA-1, which can mediate homing to the bone marrow (BM), where these cells become long-lived plasma cells. The B cell malignancies related to lymphocyte populations with tissue-specific homing properties are shown in the white boxes. MCL, mantle cell lymphoma; MLP, malignant lymphomatous polyposis; MALT-L, MALT lymphoma; FL, follicular lymphoma; M-FL, mucosal follicular lymphoma; B-CLL, B cell chronic lymphocytic leukemia; DLBCL, diffuse large B cell lymphoma; MM, multiple myeloma.

pathways have evolved to segregate intestinal and cutaneous immunity, securing robust secondary immune responses to tissue-tropic pathogens. Effector/memory T cells with homing specificity for intestine and skin can be readily identified in the blood of normal individuals by their mutually exclusive expression of $\alpha_4\beta_7$ and CLA.[30] These molecules mediate rolling through interaction with their endothelial counter-receptors MAdCAM-1 and E-selectin, respectively (Fig. 16.3). After chemokine-triggered activation, $\alpha_4\beta_7$ also causes the arrest of intestinal lymphocytes on the endothelium. In addition to mediating T cell homing to the intestine, $\alpha_4\beta_7$ plays a crucial role in the migration of B cells and plasmablasts to Peyer's patches and the intestinal lamina propria (Fig. 16.4).[5,31] Unlike the gut- and skin-homing effector memory cell populations, the so-called central memory cells retain their expression of L-selectin (and CCR7) and continue to recirculate through peripheral lymph nodes.[3,32]

In addition to tissue-specific expression of adhesion molecules, site-specific production of chemokines plays a crucial role in the homing of cutaneous and intestinal T cells (Fig. 16.3). CLA$^+$ T cells selectively express CCR4 and

CCR10, whose ligands CCL17 (TARC) and CCL27 (CTAK) are presented on the luminal surface of post-capillary venules in the skin.[4] Blocking of these chemokine receptors impairs migration of CD4$^+$ lymphocytes to the skin.[33,34] CCR9 and its ligand CCL25 (TECK) play an analogous role in T cell recruitment to the intestine. CCR9 is expressed on a subset of T cells with strong $\alpha_4\beta_7$ expression, as well as by the T cells in the epithelium and lamina propria of the small intestine,[35] while CCL25 is produced by the epithelium of the small intestinal crypts and presented on the luminal surface of endothelial cells in intestinal post-capillary venules.[36] Blocking of CCL25 inhibits the accumulation of antigen-specific effector T cells in the intestinal mucosa.[37] B cell recruitment into lymph nodes requires combined expression of CCR7 and CXCR4 on the B cell. Entry into Peyer's patches, in addition, requires expression of CXCR5. In accordance with these receptor requirements, CCL21 and CXCL12 are displayed broadly on HEVs, while CXCL13 is found selectively on Peyer's patch HEVs.[38]

Apart from mediating T cell homing, CCL25/CCR9 interaction contributes to the migration of immunoglobulin A (IgA) plasmablasts to the small intestine. Plasmablast recruitment furthermore involves the epithelial chemokine CCL28 (MEC), which interacts with CCR10 on the plasmablasts (Fig. 16.4).[39] CCL28 is also expressed at other mucosal sites belonging to the common mucosal immune system.[31] Once they leave the bloodstream, lymphocytes will be recruited to specific tissue microenvironments by chemokine gradients and through interaction with stromal cell networks formed by fibroblastic reticular cells (FRC) and follicular dendritic cells (FDC).[7,8] For example, CCL25 recruits CCR9-expressing $CD8^+$ T cells from the intestinal lamina propria into the epithelium and enhances $\alpha E\beta_7$ integrin-mediated adhesion to epithelial E-cadherin.[35,37] CXCL12 and CXCL13 recruit B cells into distinct B cell compartments by interacting with CXCR4 and CXCR5, respectively. CXCL13 is specifically expressed by FDC in B cell follicles, and disruption of its function leads to a disturbed development of primary follicles and germinal centers in the spleen and Peyer's patches.[40–42] Within the germinal center, $\alpha_4\beta_1$ in concert with LFA-1 mediates interaction of B cells with FDC.[43] These B cell receptor-controlled integrin-mediated interactions inhibit apoptosis of germinal B cells and may be crucial for affinity maturation.[44–47]

THE MOLECULAR BASIS OF LYMPHOMA DISSEMINATION

A number of clinical observations suggest that conserved homing programs mediate the dissemination of non-Hodgkin lymphomas (NHLs).[48,49] For example, NHLs related to small recirculating lymphocytes, such as small lymphocytic lymphoma/chronic lymphocytic leukemia (SLL/CLL) and mantle cell lymphoma (MCL), usually show systemic dissemination at presentation, whereas NHLs related to lymphocytes undergoing active proliferation and differentiation, such as Burkitt lymphoma (BL) and diffuse large B cell lymphomas (DLBCL), often are initially localized. Furthermore, tumor dissemination to sites of trauma and inflammation is regularly observed in lymphoma patients, implying specific recruitment of tumor cells by locally produced chemokines and activated endothelium. Most strikingly, extranodal lymphomas arising in the gut-associated lymphoid tissues or the skin show a strong preference to disseminate to mucosal sites and skin, respectively.[48,49] Although they may eventually disseminate to (regional) lymph nodes, intestinal lymphomas will rarely disseminate to the skin and, vice versa, cutaneous lymphomas will seldom involve the intestine. In the following paragraphs, the molecular basis underlying the dissemination patterns of a number of distinct lymphoma subtypes will be discussed.

The dissemination of T-lineage lymphomas

Virtually all mature T-lineage lymphomas are derived from memory ($CD45RO^+$) T cells and collectively are designated 'peripheral' T cell lymphomas as opposed to 'central' (thymocyte-derived) precursor T cell neoplasms. Notwithstanding this shared derivation from antigen-experienced T cells, peripheral T cell lymphomas represent a heterogeneous group of tumors comprising several well-defined entities with distinctive molecular, pathological, and clinical characteristics.[48] For some decades, the tissue of primary presentation and dissemination pattern have been recognized as important criteria for the classification of these tumors into distinctive clinicopathological entities.[48] As will be discussed, this empirical practice can now be grounded on molecular data (Fig. 16.3).

Cutaneous T cell lymphoma (CTCL) represents a striking example of a lymphoma type displaying tissue-specific dissemination. Cutaneous T cell lymphomas usually express the cutaneous lymphocyte homing receptor CLA[50,51] as well as the chemokine receptor CCR4, often in combination with CCR10 and/or CXCR3.[52–56] The expression of these receptors, not only on tumor cells residing in the skin but also on circulating cells, permits these cells to home effectively to the skin. Interestingly, the tumor cells of mycosis fungoides (MF) and Sézary syndrome, two closely related CTCL subtypes, show markedly different homing signatures, which correspond to the distinctive dissemination patterns encountered in these diseases. Mycosis fungoides typically shows no or very little lymph node involvement during most of the disease course. In keeping with this finding, the tumor cells express low levels of the peripheral lymph node (PLN)-homing receptor L-selectin and CCR7. During MF progression, the development of lymph node involvement is accompanied by a loss of skin-specific chemokine receptors and upregulation of CCR7.[57] Sézary syndrome, by contrast, is characterized by extensive systemic involvement. Accordingly, the tumor cells in this disease coexpress the 'cutaneous' and 'PLN' homing signatures, i.e., they express L-selectin and CCR7 as well as CLA and CCR4.[56] In line with the strict physiological dichotomy between the skin- and gut-homing memory T cell populations, both CTCLs do not express the gut-homing receptor $\alpha_4\beta_7$. Notably, in adult T cell leukemia/lymphoma (ATLL), a systemic lymphoma, CCR4 expression was reported to be linked to skin dissemination.[58]

From the perspective of dissemination, intestinal T cell lymphomas (ITLs) represent the mirror-image of CTCLs. These ITLs, which are most often enteropathy-associated, express the mucosal-homing receptor $\alpha_4\beta_7$,[59] allowing them to interact with MAdCAM-1 on mucosal post-capillary venules, but lack CLA and L-selectin (Table 16.1).[60] Moreover, they generally express the integrin $\alpha E\beta_7$, which allows interaction with E-cadherin on the epithelial cells of the intestinal mucosa.[61] At present, no comprehensive studies of chemokine receptor expression in ITLs are available. A recent case report suggests that enteropathy-associated T cell lymphomas do not express the chemokine receptor CCR7,[62] which is consistent with the absence of PLN dissemination in these tumors.

Nodal T cell lymphomas represent a heterogeneous group of tumors, which can be subclassified into distinct entities based on molecular, pathological, and clinical criteria.[48] At least part of these lymphomas presumably is related to the central memory T cell subset.[32] Consistent with this notion, the vast majority of nodal T cell lymphomas express L-selectin, but lack the skin-homing receptor CLA as well as the mucosal-homing receptor $\alpha_4\beta_7$ (Table 16.1).[60] Anaplastic large cell lymphomas, however, are L-selectin negative, which may be related to their activated phenotype.[60] The expression pattern of chemokine receptors in nodal T cells has thus far been incompletely analyzed, but the available data suggest differential expression on specific lymphoma subtypes.[63,64] CCR4, the skin-homing chemokine receptor, is expressed on a minor subset of nodal T cell lymphomas, but approximately half of these tumors express the T helper type 1 (TH1) chemokine receptors CXCR3 and/or CCR5.[63,64] Expression of these receptors in peripheral T cell lymphoma, unspecified (PTCL-U) has been reported to be related to a favorable prognosis.[65]

The dissemination of B-lineage lymphomas

The trafficking pathways of T and B lymphocytes are markedly different, reflecting the distinctive functions of T and B cells in the immune system. Effective immunosurveillance against virally infected cells requires effector T cells to have physical access to nonlymphoid tissues. B cell effector function, by contrast, depends primarily on antibodies produced by plasma cells. These antibodies are solubilized in body fluids and hence can act at a distance, obviating the need for B cells to migrate to peripheral sites of antigenic insult, like the skin. Indeed, B cells are virtually undetectable in the normal skin.[66] B cell migration to the skin and other extralymphoid sites presumably occurs almost exclusively in the context of chronic inflammation driven by locally persistent antigen, including infectious agents, like *Borrelia burgdorferi* in the skin and *Helicobacter pylori* in the stomach, or autoantigens in, for example, Sjögren disease. This persistent antigenic stimulation can lead to neoformation of lymphoid tissue,[67,68] with local expression of vascular addressins and chemokines that are normally expressed in organized lymphoid tissues. These molecules are unrelated to the cues that recruit typical 'skin-homing T cells' and their malignant counterparts. At these sites of chronic antigenic stimulation, in the skin or at other extralymphoid sites like the stomach mucosa or the orbit, B cell lymphomas, in particular marginal zone and follicular lymphomas, can eventually arise.[69–71]

Naïve B cells need to recirculate freely through peripheral and mucosal lymphoid tissues to optimize their chances of meeting their cognate antigen, whereas B memory cells and plasmablasts have to migrate to specific lymphoid environments dedicated to their recall and effector functions. Like T cells, B cells consequently must adapt

their homing signature to their specific maturational stage (Fig. 16.4). These maturation-dependent profiles are largely conserved in B cell lymphomas and control their dissemination. For example, naïve B cells coexpress the PLN-homing receptor L-selectin and the intestinal-homing receptor $\alpha_4\beta_7$.[59] Combined expression of these molecules has also been reported on a subset of MCLs,[72] tumors which generally lack somatic hypermutations in their immunoglobulin variable genes (IgA), and are therefore presumably derived from naïve B cells.[73] Interestingly, $\alpha_4\beta_7$ expression in MCL is associated with a clinical presentation known as malignant lymphomatous polyposis (MLP) (Fig. 16.4), characterized by multifocal involvement of the gastrointestinal tract as well as widespread lymph node involvement.[72,74] It is noteworthy that MCLs with a primary nodal presentation are often $\alpha_4\beta_7$ negative but that $\alpha_4\beta_7$, when present, predicts multifocal digestive tract involvement.[74] In addition to the adhesion molecule profile of MCLs, the chemokine receptor profile of these tumors, which includes expression of CCR7 and CXCR4, also allows wide dissemination to both PLNs and mucosal sites.[75,76]

The intestinal-homing receptor $\alpha_4\beta_7$ (Fig. 16.4) is of key importance for the homing of normal memory B cells and IgA plasmablasts to the marginal zones of Peyer's patches and the intestinal lamina propria, respectively.[77] In striking parallel, the malignant counterparts of gut-homing memory cells, i.e., the low-grade marginal zone B cell lymphomas of the MALT, express $\alpha_4\beta_7$.[59] These tumors are believed to arise as a result of chronic antigenic stimulation, often associated with *Helicobacter pylori* infection. Although they coexpress L-selectin, intestinal MALT lymphomas remain localized or disseminate to other mucosal sites, but only rarely to PLNs.[48,59] Absence of antigenic stimulation within the peripheral lymph node microenvironment may explain the low incidence of MALT-type lymphoma growth at these sites.

Similar to intestinal MALT lymphomas, primary follicular lymphomas (FLs) of the gastrointestinal (GI) tract also express $\alpha_4\beta_7$ (Fig. 16.4).[78] These rare lymphomas resemble nodal FLs with respect to morphology and expression of typical germinal center markers such as CD10, CD38, and Bcl-6, and the presence of a Bcl-2 translocation.[78] However, in contrast to their nodal counterparts, they are often IgA positive, express $\alpha_4\beta_7$, and remain localized to the GI tract, suggesting that they represent a distinct entity that, like low-grade intestinal MALT lymphoma, originates from local antigen-responsive B cells.[78] Unlike these small cell B cell lymphomas, however, DLBCLs and Burkitt lymphomas with a primary intestinal localization do not express $\alpha_4\beta_7$.[59] In summary, $\alpha_4\beta_7$ expression is a hallmark of a number of typical GI tract B cell lymphomas and presumably plays an important role in the characteristic mucosal dissemination of these tumors.

As already pointed out, the major chemoattractants for B cells are CXCL12 and CXCL13, and these chemokines play a role at more than one trafficking checkpoint.[3–5,40–42] CXCL12 and CXCL13 are present on HEVs of lymph nodes and Peyer's patches[38] and are also present on HEV-like vessels at sites of lymphoid neogenesis, e.g., the salivary glands in Sjögren syndrome.[79] Furthermore, both CXCL12 and CXCL13 are important in the organization of germinal centers.[40–42] CXCL12 guides CXCR4-positive lymphocytes to the germinal center dark zones, whereas CXCL13 is produced by FDCs and attracts CXCR5-positive B cells into the light zones.[42] In line with their prominent function in the biology of B cell homing, the chemokine receptors CXCR4 and CXCR5 are widely expressed in B cell neoplasms including B cell chronic lymphocytic leukemia (B-CLL), hairy cell leukemia (HCL), MCL, MALT lymphomas, FL, and DLBCL, and can drive migration of lymphoma cells.[76,80–82] Ectopic chemokine expression at sites of chronic inflammation with lymphoid neogenesis presumably is a key factor in the selective homing of malignant B cells to these sites. In addition, autocrine expression of CXCL13 has been reported in FL[80] and primary central nervous system lymphomas.[83] Apart from chemokines, other cytokines, including hepatocyte growth factor (HGF), can also control integrin-mediated adhesion of malignant lymphocytes.[84] These autocrine and paracrine interactions may contribute to lymphoma organization and promote tumor growth.

Homing of normal plasma cells and myeloma cells

Differentiation of a B cell to a plasma cell is accompanied by a coordinated change in chemokine receptor expression.[85] Whereas CXCR5 and CCR7 are downregulated, resulting in loss of responsiveness to the B- and T-zone chemokines CXCL13, CCL19, and CCL21,[31,85] CXCR4, the receptor for CXCL12 (SDF-1), is upregulated (Fig. 16.4). The latter chemokine is constitutively expressed by bone marrow (BM) stromal cells[85–87] and, indeed, CXCL12/CXCR4 interaction is required for plasma cells homing to the BM, the major site of antibody production in adult life.[85,88] Within the BM microenvironment, cytokines like interleukin-6 (IL-6), produced by stromal cells, control the maturation and survival of plasma cells.[89,90] In addition, $\alpha_4\beta_1$-mediated interactions with fibronectin and VCAM-1 are also critical for plasma cell survival and longevity.[91,92]

As in normal plasma cell homing, CXCL12/CXCR4 interaction is also essential in the recruitment to and retention of multiple myeloma (MM) plasma cells in the BM. CXCL12 promotes transendothelial migration and induces $\alpha_4\beta_1$-mediated adhesion to VCAM-1 and fibronectin.[93] It should be noted that both normal and MM plasma cells also express other chemokine receptors besides CXCR4, like CXCR6, CCR6, CCR10, and CCR3.[87] Consequently, they have the potential to migrate in response to a variety of chemoattractants. Interestingly, the chemokine receptor CCR5 is expressed by MM cells but not by normal plasma cells,[94] while the BM of MM patients contains high levels of the CCR5 ligand CCL3 (MIP-1α).[95] CCL3, which was found to be secreted by the majority of MM cell lines as well as primary MMs,[96] does not only function as a chemoattractant for MM cells[94] but also possesses osteoclast stimulatory activity and may thus contribute to osteolytic bone disease.[96] On top of this, CCL3 may act as an autocrine growth and survival factor for MM.[94] Besides controlling proliferation and survival, several cytokines including insulin-like growth factor (IGF)-1, vascular endothelial growth factor (VEGF), and hepatocyte growth factor (HGF), can induce migration of MM cells.[97,98] Hence, multiple factors in the BM microenvironment may modulate homing of MM cells.

Blocking antibodies that prevent interaction of $\alpha_4\beta_1$ with its ligands fibronectin and VCAM-1, expressed by BM stromal cells, not only disturb chemoattractant-induced adhesion and migration of MM cells,[97,98] but also inhibit growth in a murine MM model.[99] This growth inhibition may be the consequence of defective MM cell homing. However, blocking of integrin-mediated interactions between MM cells and BM stromal cells may also disturb the niche required for MM cell expansion. Indeed, adhesion of human MM cells to BM stromal cells stimulates secretion of IL-6, which has potent proliferative and anti-apoptotic effects.[100] Also, the *Maf* oncogene, besides promoting expression of cyclin D2, also promotes expression of $\beta7$ integrins, thereby enhancing MM cell adhesion to BM stromal cells and increasing VEGF production,[101] which in turn stimulates MM cell growth and survival as well as angiogenesis. Although both long-lived plasma cells and MM cells are protected from apoptosis by integrin-mediated interactions with the BM stroma, the ability to proliferate in this environment is a unique property of MM cells. Cytokines including IL-6, HGF, and WNTs produced by BM stromal cells provide MM cells with proliferative and survival signals required for their expansion.[102–105] Of interest, $\alpha_4\beta_1$- and $\alpha_5\beta_1$-mediated adhesion to fibronectin can protect MM cells from drug-induced apoptosis, a phenomenon called cell adhesion-mediated drug resistance (CAM-DR).[106] Since various chemokines and growth factors produced in the BM stimulate integrin-mediated adhesion,[98,107,108] these cytokines can contribute to resistance of MM cells to treatment. Hence, integrins and their regulation by chemokines play a crucial role in the homing of MM cells to the BM and, moreover, contribute to the expansion of MM cells in the BM niche by mediating interaction with the BM stroma, which via 'outside-in signaling' generates growth and survival signals for the malignant plasma cells.

CONCLUSION

Although most cells in the body are capable of migrating at one or more distinct steps during their development and differentiation, the trafficking propensity of lymphocytes is unrivaled by that of any other somatic cell. The unique motility program and migratory properties endowed upon lymphocytes bears witness of the great evolutionary importance of effective immunosurveillance for the survival of higher vertebrates. Lymphocytes display a physically optimized amoeboid migration mode that allows flexible trafficking toward and between different tissue compartments, and utilize sophisticated recognition mechanisms to home to particular tissues, thus influencing the nature of local immune and inflammatory responses. At the molecular level, this homing process is regulated by adhesion molecules in concert with chemokines. Lymphomas represent the malignant counterparts of lymphocytes arrested at a specific stage of maturation. The studies discussed in this chapter clearly demonstrate that the selective and often strikingly tissue-specific dissemination of malignant lymphomas and MM is controlled by the same molecular mechanisms that also guide the homing of their normal lymphocyte counterparts. This implies that lymphoma dissemination, unlike the metastatic spread of other types of cancer, generally is not a reflection of tumor progression but rather of conserved physiological behavior. Targeting of the receptors that constitute the homing signature of malignant lymphocytes by, for example, blocking monoclonal antibodies or small molecule drugs, may present a novel means of therapeutic intervention in lymphoma patients: preventing the homing of circulating tumor cells to their natural environment may deprive the cells of essential growth and survival signals, causing cell death by anoikis (apoptosis resulting from a deprivation of signals from the extracellular matrix).

KEY POINTS

- The immune response is critically dependent on lymphocyte migration and recirculation; lymphocytes are 'licensed to move.'
- Adhesion molecules and chemokines/chemokine receptors direct lymphocyte 'homing' to specific tissues.
- Lymphoma dissemination often refects basic rules of lymphocyte homing.
- Unlike the metastatic spread of other cancers, lymphoma dissemination generally is not a reflection of tumor progression but of conserved physiological behaviour.
- Anoikis induction by targeting of homing receptors may present a novel means of therapeutic intervention in lymphoma.

REFERENCES

● = Key primary paper

◆ = Major review article

●1. Gowans JL, Knight EJ. The route of re-circulation of lymphocytes in the rat. *Proc R Soc Lond B Biol Sci* 1964; **159**: 257–82.

2. Butcher EC, Picker LJ. Lymphocyte homing and homeostasis. *Science* 1996; **272**: 60–6.

◆3. von Andrian UH, Mempel TR. Homing and cellular traffic in lymph nodes. *Nat Rev Immunol* 2003; **3**: 867–78.

4. Kunkel EJ, Butcher EC. Chemokines and the tissue-specific migration of lymphocytes. *Immunity* 2002; **16**: 1–4.

◆5. Salmi M, Jalkanen S. Lymphocyte homing to the gut: attraction, adhesion, and commitment. *Immunol Rev* 2005; **206**: 100–13.

◆6. Friedl P. Prespecification and plasticity: shifting mechanisms of cell migration. *Curr Opin Cell Biol* 2004; **16**: 14–23.

●7. Bajenoff M, Egen JG, Koo LY *et al.* Stromal cell networks regulate lymphocyte entry, migration, and territoriality in lymph nodes. *Immunity* 2006; **25**: 989–1001.

8. Mempel TR, Junt T, von Andrian UH. Rulers over randomness: stroma cells guide lymphocyte migration in lymph nodes. *Immunity* 2006; **25**: 867–9.

9. Bargatze RF, Jutila MA, Butcher EC. Distinct roles of L-selectin and integrins alpha 4 beta 7 and LFA-1 in lymphocyte homing to Peyer's patch-HEV in situ: the multistep model confirmed and refined. *Immunity* 1995; **3**: 99–108.

10. von Andrian UH, Hasslen SR, Nelson RD *et al.* A central role for microvillous receptor presentation in leukocyte adhesion under flow. *Cell* 1995; **82**: 989–99.

11. DeGrendele HC, Estess P, Picker LJ, Siegelman MH. CD44 and its ligand hyaluronate mediate rolling under physiologic flow: a novel lymphocyte-endothelial cell primary adhesion pathway. *J Exp Med* 1996; **183**: 1119–30.

12. Alon R, Kassner PD, Carr MW *et al.* The integrin VLA-4 supports tethering and rolling in flow on VCAM-1. *J Cell Biol* 1995; **128**: 1243–53.

13. Berlin C, Bargatze RF, Campbell JJ *et al.* Alpha 4 integrins mediate lymphocyte attachment and rolling under physiologic flow. *Cell* 1995; **80**: 413–22.

●14. de Gorter DJ, Beuling EA, Kersseboom R *et al.* Bruton's tyrosine kinase and phospholipase Cgamma2 mediate chemokine-controlled B cell migration and homing. *Immunity* 2007; **26**: 93–104.

◆15. Kinashi T. Intracellular signalling controlling integrin activation in lymphocytes. *Nat Rev Immunol* 2005; **5**: 546–59.

16. Lloyd AR, Oppenheim JJ, Kelvin DJ, Taub DD. Chemokines regulate T cell adherence to recombinant adhesion molecules and extracellular matrix proteins. *J Immunol* 1996; **156**: 932–8.

●17. Campbell JJ, Hedrick J, Zlotnik A *et al.* Chemokines and the arrest of lymphocytes rolling under flow conditions. *Science* 1998; **279**: 381–4.

●18. Campbell JJ, Haraldsen G, Pan J *et al.* The chemokine receptor CCR4 in vascular recognition by cutaneous but not intestinal memory T cells. *Nature* 1999; **400**: 776–80.

19. Johnson-Leger CA, Aurrand-Lions M, Beltraminelli N *et al.* Junctional adhesion molecule-2 (JAM-2) promotes lymphocyte transendothelial migration. *Blood* 2002; **100**: 2479–86.

20. Ebnet K, Suzuki A, Ohno S, Vestweber D. Junctional adhesion molecules (JAMs): more molecules with dual functions? *J Cell Sci* 2004; **117**: 19–29.

●21. Gunn MD, Tangemann K, Tam C *et al.* A chemokine expressed in lymphoid high endothelial venules promotes the adhesion and chemotaxis of naive T lymphocytes. *Proc Natl Acad Sci U S A* 1998; **95**: 258–63.

22. Warnock RA, Askari S, Butcher EC, von Andrian UH. Molecular mechanisms of lymphocyte homing to peripheral lymph nodes. *J Exp Med* 1998; **187**: 205–16.

◆23. Mackay CR. T-cell memory: the connection between function, phenotype and migration pathways. *Immunol Today* 1991; **12**: 189–92.

24. Johansson-Lindbom B, Svensson M, Pabst O *et al.* Functional specialization of gut CD103+ dendritic cells in the regulation of tissue-selective T cell homing. *J Exp Med* 2005; **202**: 1063–73.

●25. Mora JR, Bono MR, Manjunath N *et al.* Selective imprinting of gut-homing T cells by Peyer's patch dendritic cells. *Nature* 2003; **424**: 88–93.

26. Stagg AJ, Kamm MA, Knight SC. Intestinal dendritic cells increase T cell expression of alpha4beta7 integrin. *Eur J Immunol* 2002; **32**: 1445–54.

●27. Mora JR, Iwata M, Eksteen B *et al.* Generation of gut-homing IgA-secreting B cells by intestinal dendritic cells. *Science* 2006; **314**: 1157–60.

28. Johansen FE, Baekkevold ES, Carlsen HS *et al.* Regional induction of adhesion molecules and chemokine receptors explains disparate homing of human B cells to systemic and mucosal effector sites: dispersion from tonsils. *Blood* 2005; **106**: 593–600.

29. Mora JR, Cheng G, Picarella D *et al.* Reciprocal and dynamic control of CD8 T cell homing by dendritic cells from skin- and gut-associated lymphoid tissues. *J Exp Med* 2005; **201**: 303–16.

●30. Schweighoffer T, Tanaka Y, Tidswell M *et al.* Selective expression of integrin alpha 4 beta 7 on a subset of human CD4+ memory T cells with Hallmarks of gut-trophism.
J Immunol 1993; **151**: 717–29.

◆31. Kunkel EJ, Butcher EC. Plasma-cell homing. *Nat Rev Immunol* 2003; **3**: 822–9.

●32. Sallusto F, Lenig D, Forster R *et al.* Two subsets of memory T lymphocytes with distinct homing potentials and effector functions. *Nature* 1999; **401**: 708–12.

33. Reiss Y, Proudfoot AE, Power CA *et al.* CC chemokine receptor (CCR)4 and the CCR10 ligand cutaneous T cell-attracting chemokine (CTACK) in lymphocyte trafficking to inflamed skin. *J Exp Med* 2001; **194**: 1541–7.

●34. Homey B, Alenius H, Muller A *et al.* CCL27-CCR10 interactions regulate T cell-mediated skin inflammation. *Nat Med* 2002; **8**: 157–65.

35. Zabel BA, Agace WW, Campbell JJ *et al.* Human G protein-coupled receptor GPR-9-6/CC chemokine receptor 9 is selectively expressed on intestinal homing T lymphocytes, mucosal lymphocytes, and thymocytes and is required for thymus-expressed chemokine-mediated chemotaxis. *J Exp Med* 1999; **190**: 1241–56.

●36. Kunkel EJ, Campbell JJ, Haraldsen G *et al.* Lymphocyte CC chemokine receptor 9 and epithelial thymus-expressed chemokine (TECK) expression distinguish the small intestinal immune compartment: Epithelial expression of tissue-specific chemokines as an organizing principle in regional immunity. *J Exp Med* 2000; **192**: 761–8.

37. Svensson M, Marsal J, Ericsson A *et al.* CCL25 mediates the localization of recently activated CD8alphabeta(+) lymphocytes to the small-intestinal mucosa. *J Clin Invest* 2002; **110**: 1113–21.

38. Okada T, Ngo VN, Ekland EH *et al.* Chemokine requirements for B cell entry to lymph nodes and Peyer's patches. *J Exp Med* 2002; **196**: 65–75.

39. Kunkel EJ, Kim CH, Lazarus NH *et al.* CCR10 expression is a common feature of circulating and mucosal epithelial tissue IgA Ab-secreting cells. *J Clin Invest* 2003; **111**: 1001–10.

●40. Gunn MD, Ngo VN, Ansel KM *et al.* A B-cell-homing chemokine made in lymphoid follicles activates Burkitt's lymphoma receptor-1. *Nature* 1998; **391**: 799–803.

41. Forster R, Mattis AE, Kremmer E *et al.* A putative chemokine receptor, BLR1, directs B cell migration to defined lymphoid organs and specific anatomic compartments of the spleen. *Cell* 1996; **87**: 1037–47.

●42. Allen CD, Ansel KM, Low C *et al.* Germinal center dark and light zone organization is mediated by CXCR4 and CXCR5. *Nat Immunol* 2004; **5**: 943–52.

●43. Koopman G, Parmentier HK, Schuurman HJ *et al.* Adhesion of human B cells to follicular dendritic cells involves both the lymphocyte function-associated antigen 1/intercellular adhesion molecule 1 and very late antigen 4/vascular cell adhesion molecule 1 pathways. *J Exp Med* 1991; **173**: 1297–1304.

●44. Koopman G, Keehnen RM, Lindhout E *et al.* Adhesion through the LFA-1 (CD11a/CD18)-ICAM-1 (CD54) and the VLA-4 (CD49d)-VCAM-1 (CD106) pathways prevents apoptosis of germinal center B cells. *J Immunol* 1994; **152**: 3760–7.

45. Spaargaren M, Beuling EA, Rurup ML *et al.* The B cell antigen receptor controls integrin activity through Btk and PLCgamma2. *J Exp Med* 2003; **198**: 1539–50.

46. Carrasco YR, Fleire SJ, Cameron T *et al.* LFA-1/ICAM-1 interaction lowers the threshold of B cell activation by facilitating B cell adhesion and synapse formation. *Immunity* 2004; **20**: 589–99.

47. Carrasco YR, Batista FD. B-cell activation by membrane-bound antigens is facilitated by the interaction of VLA-4 with VCAM-1. *EMBO J* 2006; **25**: 889–99.

48. Jaffe E, Harris NL, Stein H, Vardiman JW. *Pathology and genetics of tumours of haematopoietics and lymphoid tissues.* Lyon: IARC Press 2001.

◆49. Pals ST, de Gorter DJJ, Spaargaren M. Lymphoma dissemination: the other face of lymphocyte homing. *Blood* 2007; **110**: 3102–11.

50. Meijer CJLM, Beljaards F, Horst E *et al.* Differences in antigen expression between primary cutaneous- and node-based T-cell lymphomas. *J Invest Dermatol* 1989; **92**: 479.

●51. Picker LJ, Michie SA, Rott LS, Butcher EC. A unique phenotype of skin-associated lymphocytes in humans. Preferential expression of the HECA-452 epitope by benign and malignant T cells at cutaneous sites. *Am J Pathol* 1990; **136**: 1053–68.

52. Ferenczi K, Fuhlbrigge RC, Pinkus J *et al.* Increased CCR4 expression in cutaneous T cell lymphoma. *J Invest Dermatol* 2002; **119**: 1405–10.

53. Kallinich T, Muche JM, Qin S *et al.* Chemokine receptor expression on neoplastic and reactive T cells in the skin at different stages of mycosis fungoides. *J Invest Dermatol* 2003; **121**: 1045–52.

54. Wenzel J, Gutgemann I, Distelmaier M *et al.* The role of cytotoxic skin-homing CD8+ lymphocytes in cutaneous cytotoxic T-cell lymphoma and pityriasis lichenoides. *J Am Acad Dermatol* 2005; **53**: 422–7.

55. Notohamiprodjo M, Segerer S, Huss R *et al.* CCR10 is expressed in cutaneous T-cell lymphoma. *Int J Cancer* 2005; **115**: 641–7.

●56. Sokolowska-Wojdylo M, Wenzel J, Gaffal E *et al.* Circulating clonal CLA(+) and CD4(+) T cells in Sezary syndrome express the skin-homing chemokine receptors CCR4 and CCR10 as well as the lymph node-homing chemokine receptor CCR7. *Br J Dermatol* 2005; **152**: 258–64.

●57. Kallinich T, Muche JM, Qin S *et al.* Chemokine receptor expression on neoplastic and reactive T cells in the skin at different stages of mycosis fungoides. *J Invest Dermatol* 2003; **121**: 1045–52.

58. Ishida T, Utsunomiya A, Iida S *et al.* Clinical significance of CCR4 expression in adult T-cell leukemia/lymphoma: its close association with skin involvement and unfavorable outcome. *Clin Cancer Res* 2003; **9**: 3625–34.

●59. Drillenburg P, van der Voort R, Koopman G *et al.* Preferential expression of the mucosal homing receptor integrin alpha 4 beta 7 in gastrointestinal non-Hodgkin's lymphomas. *Am J Pathol* 1997; **150**: 919–27.

60. Pals ST, Meijer CJ, Radaszkiewicz T *et al.* Expression of the human peripheral lymph node homing receptor (LECAM-1) in nodal and gastrointestinal non-Hodgkin's lymphomas. *Leukemia* 1991; **5**: 628–31.

61. Chott A, Dragosics B, Radaszkiewicz T. Peripheral T-cell lymphomas of the intestine. *Am J Pathol* 1992; **141**: 1361–71.

62. Shiratsuchi M, Suehiro Y, Yoshikawa Y *et al.* Extranodal multiple involvement of enteropathy-type T-cell lymphoma without expression of CC chemokine receptor 7. *Int J Hematol* 2004; **79**: 44–7.

●63. Jones D, O'Hara C, Kraus MD *et al.* Expression pattern of T-cell-associated chemokine receptors and their chemokines correlates with specific subtypes of T-cell non-Hodgkin lymphoma. *Blood* 2000; **96**: 685–90.

64. Ishida T, Inagaki H, Utsunomiya A *et al.* CXC chemokine receptor 3 and CC chemokine receptor 4 expression in T-cell and NK-cell lymphomas with special reference to clinicopathological significance for peripheral T-cell lymphoma, unspecified. *Clin Cancer Res* 2004; **10**: 5494–500.

65. Tsuchiya T, Ohshima K, Karube K *et al.* Th1, Th2, and activated T-cell marker and clinical prognosis in peripheral T-cell lymphoma, unspecified: comparison with AILD, ALCL, lymphoblastic lymphoma, and ATLL. *Blood* 2004; **103**: 236–41.

●66. Bos JD, de Boer OJ, Tibosch E *et al.* Skin-homing T lymphocytes: detection of cutaneous lymphocyte-associated antigen (CLA) by HECA-452 in normal human skin. *Arch Dermatol Res* 1993; **285**: 179–83.

67. Pals ST, Horst E, Scheper RJ, Meijer CJ. Mechanisms of human lymphocyte migration and their role in the pathogenesis of disease. *Immunol Rev* 1989; **108**: 111–33.

●68. Aloisi F, Pujol-Borrell R. Lymphoid neogenesis in chronic inflammatory diseases. *Nat Rev Immunol* 2006; **6**: 205–17.

69. Mori M, Manuelli C, Pimpinelli N *et al.* BCA-1, A B-cell chemoattractant signal, is constantly expressed in cutaneous lymphoproliferative B-cell disorders. *Eur J Cancer* 2003; **39**: 1625–31.

70. Chan CC, Shen D, Hackett JJ *et al.* Expression of chemokine receptors, CXCR4 and CXCR5, and chemokines, BLC and SDF-1, in the eyes of patients with primary intraocular lymphoma. *Ophthalmology* 2003; **110**: 421–6.

71. Mazzucchelli L, Blaser A, Kappeler A *et al.* BCA-1 is highly expressed in Helicobacter pylori-induced mucosa-associated lymphoid tissue and gastric lymphoma. *J Clin Invest* 1999; **104**: R49–54.

●72. Pals ST, Drillenburg P, Dragosics B *et al.* Expression of the mucosal homing receptor alpha 4 beta 7 in malignant lymphomatous polyposis of the intestine. *Gastroenterology* 1994; **107**: 1519–23.

◆73. Kuppers R. Mechanisms of B-cell lymphoma pathogenesis. *Nat Rev Cancer* 2005; **5**: 251–62.

●74. Geissmann F, Ruskone-Fourmestraux A, Hermine O *et al.* Homing receptor alpha4beta7 integrin expression predicts digestive tract involvement in mantle cell lymphoma. *Am J Pathol* 1998; **153**: 1701–5.

75. Corcione A, Arduino N, Ferretti E *et al.* CCL19 and CXCL12 trigger in vitro chemotaxis of human mantle cell lymphoma B cells. *Clin Cancer Res* 2004; **10**: 964–71.

76. Lopez-Giral S, Quintana NE, Cabrerizo M *et al.* Chemokine receptors that mediate B cell homing to secondary lymphoid tissues are highly expressed in B cell chronic lymphocytic leukemia and non-Hodgkin lymphomas with widespread nodular dissemination. *J Leukoc Biol* 2004; **76**: 462–71.

77. Youngman KR, Franco MA, Kuklin NA et al. Correlation of tissue distribution, developmental phenotype, and intestinal homing receptor expression of antigen-specific B cells during the murine anti-rotavirus immune response. J Immunol 2002; **168**: 2173–81.

78. Bende RJ, Smit LA, Bossenbroek JG et al. Primary follicular lymphoma of the small intestine: alpha4beta7 expression and immunoglobulin configuration suggest an origin from local antigen-experienced B cells. Am J Pathol 2003; **162**: 105–13.

79. Amft N, Curnow SJ, Scheel-Toellner D et al. Ectopic expression of the B cell-attracting chemokine BCA-1 (CXCL13) on endothelial cells and within lymphoid follicles contributes to the establishment of germinal center-like structures in Sjogren's syndrome. Arthritis Rheum 2001; **44**: 2633–41.

80. Husson H, Freedman AS, Cardoso AA et al. CXCL13 (BCA-1) is produced by follicular lymphoma cells: role in the accumulation of malignant B cells. Br J Haematol 2002; **119**: 492–5.

81. Burger JA, Kipps TJ. Chemokine receptors and stromal cells in the homing and homeostasis of chronic lymphocytic leukemia B cells. Leuk Lymphoma 2002; **43**: 461–6.

◆82. Trentin L, Cabrelle A, Facco M et al. Homeostatic chemokines drive migration of malignant B cells in patients with non-Hodgkin lymphomas. Blood 2004; **104**: 502–8.

83. Smith JR, Braziel RM, Paoletti S et al. Expression of B-cell-attracting chemokine 1 (CXCL13) by malignant lymphocytes and vascular endothelium in primary central nervous system lymphoma. Blood 2003; **101**: 815–21.

84. Tjin EP, Groen RW, Vogelzang I et al. Functional analysis of HGF/MET signaling and aberrant HGF-activator expression in diffuse large B-cell lymphoma. Blood 2006; **107**: 760–8.

●85. Hargreaves DC, Hyman PL, Lu TT et al. A coordinated change in chemokine responsiveness guides plasma cell movements. J Exp Med 2001; **194**: 45–56.

86. Hauser AE, Debes GF, Arce S et al. Chemotactic responsiveness toward ligands for CXCR3 and CXCR4 is regulated on plasma blasts during the time course of a memory immune response. J Immunol 2002; **169**: 1277–82.

87. Nakayama T, Hieshima K, Izawa D et al. Cutting edge: profile of chemokine receptor expression on human plasma cells accounts for their efficient recruitment to target tissues. J Immunol 2003; **170**: 1136–40.

●88. Ma Q, Jones D, Springer TA. The chemokine receptor CXCR4 is required for the retention of B lineage and granulocytic precursors within the bone marrow microenvironment. Immunity 1999; **10**: 463–71.

89. Roldan E, Rodriguez C, Navas G et al. Cytokine network regulating terminal maturation of human bone marrow B cells capable of spontaneous and high rate Ig secretion in vitro. J Immunol 1992; **149**: 2367–71.

90. Kawano MM, Mihara K, Huang N et al. Differentiation of early plasma cells on bone marrow stromal cells requires interleukin-6 for escaping from apoptosis. Blood 1995; **85**: 487–94.

●91. Roldan E, Garcia-Pardo A, Brieva JA et al. VLA-4-fibronectin interaction is required for the terminal differentiation of human bone marrow cells capable of spontaneous and high rate immunoglobulin secretion. J Exp Med 1992; **175**: 1739–47.

●92. Cassese G, Arce S, Hauser AE et al. Plasma cell survival is mediated by synergistic effects of cytokines and adhesion-dependent signals. J Immunol 2003; **171**: 1684–90.

93. Sanz-Rodriguez F, Hidalgo A, Teixido J et al. Chemokine stromal cell-derived factor-1alpha modulates VLA-4 integrin-mediated multiple myeloma cell adhesion to CS-1/fibronectin and VCAM-1. Blood 2001; **97**: 346–51.

94. Lentzsch S, Gries M, Janz M et al. Macrophage inflammatory protein 1-alpha (MIP-1 alpha) triggers migration and signaling cascades mediating survival and proliferation in multiple myeloma (MM) cells. Blood 2003; **101**: 3568–73.

95. Choi SJ, Cruz JC, Craig F et al. Macrophage inflammatory protein 1-alpha is a potential osteoclast stimulatory factor in multiple myeloma. Blood 2000; **96**: 671–5.

96. Abe M, Hiura K, Wilde J et al. Role for macrophage inflammatory protein (MIP)-1alpha and MIP-1beta in the development of osteolytic lesions in multiple myeloma. Blood 2002; **100**: 2195–202.

97. Tai YT, Podar K, Catley L et al. Insulin-like growth factor-1 induces adhesion and migration in human multiple myeloma cells via activation of beta1-integrin and phosphatidylinositol 3'-kinase/AKT signaling. Cancer Res 2003; **63**: 5850–8.

98. Podar K, Tai YT, Lin BK et al. Vascular endothelial growth factor-induced migration of multiple myeloma cells is associated with beta 1 integrin- and phosphatidylinositol 3-kinase-dependent PKC alpha activation. J Biol Chem 2002; **277**: 7875–81.

●99. Mori Y, Shimizu N, Dallas M et al. Anti-alpha4 integrin antibody suppresses the development of multiple myeloma and associated osteoclastic osteolysis. Blood 2004; **104**: 2149–54.

100. Uchiyama H, Barut BA, Mohrbacher AF et al. Adhesion of human myeloma-derived cell lines to bone marrow stromal cells stimulates interleukin-6 secretion. Blood 1993; **82**: 3712–20.

●101. Hurt EM, Wiestner A, Rosenwald A et al. Overexpression of c-maf is a frequent oncogenic event in multiple myeloma that promotes proliferation and pathological interactions with bone marrow stroma. Cancer Cell 2004; **5**: 191–9.

102. Kuehl WM, Bergsagel PL. Multiple myeloma: evolving genetic events and host interactions. Nat Rev Cancer 2002; **2**: 175–87.

103. Klein B, Zhang XG, Lu ZY, Bataille R. Interleukin-6 in human multiple myeloma. *Blood* 1995; **85**: 863–72.

104. Derksen PW, De Gorter DJ, Meijer HP *et al.* The hepatocyte growth factor/Met pathway controls proliferation and apoptosis in multiple myeloma. *Leukemia* 2003; **17**: 764–74.

●105. Derksen PW, Tjin E, Meijer HP *et al.* Illegitimate WNT signaling promotes proliferation of multiple myeloma cells. *Proc Natl Acad Sci U S A* 2004; **101**: 6122–7.

●106. Damiano JS, Cress AE, Hazlehurst LA *et al.* Cell adhesion mediated drug resistance (CAM-DR): role of integrins and resistance to apoptosis in human myeloma cell lines. *Blood* 1999; **93**: 1658–67.

107. Sanz-Rodriguez F, Hidalgo A, Teixido J. Chemokine stromal cell-derived factor-1alpha modulates VLA-4 integrin-mediated multiple myeloma cell adhesion to CS-1/fibronectin and VCAM-1. *Blood* 2001; **97**: 346–51.

108. Holt RU, Baykov V, Ro TB *et al.* Human myeloma cells adhere to fibronectin in response to hepatocyte growth factor. *Haematologica* 2005; **90**: 479–88.

17

Mouse models of human B lymphoid neoplasms

HERBERT C MORSE III, JERROLD M WARD AND MICHAEL A TEITELL

INTRODUCTION

The identification of T cells and B cells as subsets of lympho-cytes readily distinguished by phenotype and function her-alded a new era for the field of immunology. This milestone also marked the end of an epoch in which hematologic malignancies were categorized primarily on the basis of their cytology, histology, and clinical presentation. Classification schemes founded on recognition of microscopic features were gradually replaced by those emphasizing cell lineage and state of differentiation as defined by immunophenotyp-ing. Identification of distinctive chromosomal abnormali-ties in metaphase spreads foresaw the wealth of molecular genetic approaches that now belong to the armamentarium of a modern department of human hematopathology. The sum of approaches to diagnosis provided by clinical fea-tures, morphology, immunophenotype, and genetic charac-teristics was brought to bear in the 2001 World Health

Table 17.1   Relationships between classification of mouse and human B cell-lineage lymphomas

Human B cell neoplasm	Mouse B cell neoplasm
Precursor B cell neoplasm	Precursor B cell neoplasm
Precursor B lymphoblastic leukemia/lymphoma	Precursor B lymphoblastic leukemia/lymphoma
Mature B cell neoplasms	Mature B cell neoplasms
Chronic lymphocytic leukemia/small lymphocytic lymphoma	Small B cell lymphoma/leukemia
B cell prolymphocytic leukemia	
Lymphoplasmacytic lymphoma	
Splenic marginal zone lymphoma	Splenic marginal zone lymphoma
Hairy cell leukemia	
Plasma cell myeloma	
Solitary plasmacytoma of bone	
Extraosseus plasmacytoma	Extraosseus plasmacytoma
Extranodal marginal zone B cell lymphoma of mucosal-associated lymphoid tissue	
Nodal marginal zone lymphoma	
Follicular lymphoma	Follicular B cell lymphoma
Mantle cell lymphoma	
Diffuse large B cell lymphoma	Diffuse large B cell lymphoma
Morphologic variants:	Morphologic variants:
Centroblastic	Centroblastic
Immunoblastic	Immunoblastic
T cell/histiocyte-rich	Histiocyte associated
Subtypes:	Subtypes:
Mediastinal (thymic) large B cell lymphoma	Mediastinal (thymic) large B cell lymphoma
Intravascular large B cell lymphoma	
Primary effusion lymphoma	
Burkitt lymphoma/leukemia	
	Diffuse high-grade B cell blastic lymphoma/leukemia

Organization (WHO) classification of human hematopoietic neoplasms,[1] which has recently been updated.

An appreciation of the diversity and pathogenesis of mouse hematopoietic neoplasms has historically lagged far behind that of seemingly similar human malignancies. The spur to changing the *status quo* came from the remarkable progress made in manipulating the mouse genome. The use of transgenic (TG), knockout, knockin, and mutagenized mice to model human diseases has yielded a wealth of new strains, many of which unexpectedly develop hematologic malignancies. In addition, the rate at which the scientific community is generating mouse models of human cancer that require validation has grown almost exponentially. To optimize the utility of mouse models of human lymphoma and leukemia, community standards were developed for classifying both lymphoid and nonlymphoid neoplasms using systems that parallel the WHO schemes for human diseases.[2] These 'Bethesda proposals' were recognized to have inherent limitations due to lack of information on specific disorders and were designed to be open to revision with the development of new data.

This chapter will focus exclusively on B cell-lineage lymphomas, except for plasma cell-related neoplasms,

which are covered in Chapter 14. The classification scheme to be used here differs from that published in the Bethesda proposals, with changes suggested by information garnered from the literature and the experiences of our laboratories. The classification defines individual disease entities based on morphology, immunophenotype, genetic features, and state of differentiation in relation to a presumed cell of origin.

Table 17.1 lists the mouse lymphoma types distinguished by these characteristics and their closest human counterpart. This comparison shows that many disease entities recognized in humans do not have parallels in the mouse for either spontaneous diseases or those appearing in genetically engineered mice. Several factors are likely to have contributed to this discrepancy. First, much of our detailed knowledge about mouse B cell lymphomas comes from studies of a limited number of strains. The best-studied strains are NFS.V[+] congenic mice[3] and the AKXD recombinant inbred (RI) strains.[4–6] The NFS congenics and most of the RI strains express ecotropic murine leukemia viruses (MuLV) from endogenous germ-line loci at high levels from early in life. When MuLV infect somatic cells, their insertion into genomic DNA is inherently mutagenic.

Some of these mutagenic insertions result in the unprogrammed activation of cellular genes, some of which are protooncogenes that can participate in the process of transformation.[7] These contributions to disease pathogenesis in the mouse have no direct parallels in human B lymphomas that instead feature activation of protooncogenes induced by balanced chromosomal translocations. Translocations resulting in protooncogene activation do occur in the mouse, being found in almost all pristane-induced plasmacytomas of BALB/c mice[8] and rarely in diffuse large B cell lymphomas,[9] but they are certainly not the rule.

Second, there are significant differences between mouse and human immune systems in their development, structure, phenotype, and function.[10,11] For example, expression of CD23 and CD5 is mutually exclusive on mouse but not on human B cell subsets, and CD38 is downregulated on mouse germinal center (GC) B cells but upregulated in humans.[12] More important, perhaps, is that the spleen is the major secondary lymphoid organ of the mouse, whereas lymph nodes fill that niche in humans. In addition, the mouse spleen is responsible for extramedullary hematopoiesis throughout the animal's lifespan, while hematopoiesis in humans is confined to the bone marrow.

Finally, the genetic and epigenetic alterations required for neoplastic transformation sometimes differ for mouse and human.[13] As one example, programmed telomere shortening is viewed as a tumor-suppressor pathway in humans, with activation of telomerase being a requirement for averting replicative senescence. In contrast, telomerase is not repressed in murine somatic cells, and the cellular response to telomere damage differs for mice and humans.[14] A second example comes from studies of mice with targeted mutations of tumor-suppressor genes in which the phenotypes of mutant mice are sometimes highly discordant with the effects of the mutation in humans.[15] Species-specific differences in the immune system and the molecular circuitry required for transformation could thus make it difficult to model some human diseases in mice.

This difficulty is exemplified by efforts to develop a mouse model of Burkitt lymphoma by generating 'simple' MYC transgenics,[16–19] yeast artificial chromosome (YAC) transgenics with MYC inserted into the IgH locus[20,21] and, most recently, a knockin mouse with MYC inserted into the IgH locus in an orientation characteristic of most translocations in endemic Burkitt lymphoma and mouse plasmacytomas.[22] All these mice developed lymphomas with varying latency. Analyses of immunoglobulin (Ig) gene rearrangements and phenotypic analyses showed that the Eμ-MYC lymphomas included pre-B as well as IgM+ IgD- lymphomas, a phenotype consistent with immature or transitional B cells. The λ-MYC lymphomas were also found to have features of immature or transitional B cells and had non-mutated Ig genes. Approximately 25 percent of the MYC knockin lymphomas were lymphoblastic with a starry-sky appearance and expression of BCL6, a phenotype very much like human Burkitt lymphoma;[22] however, the Ig genes of these lymphomas did not contain somatic hypervariable region mutations,[23] whereas all human Burkitt lymphoma Ig genes contain such mutations to varying extents. Could some mouse B cells passage the GC without being mutated? Can Ig gene mutation occur outside the GC? The answer to the latter question has recently been shown to be 'yes.'[24] Answers to questions such as this will be critical for fully assessing the validity of a mouse model for a human disease.

These concerns are important to those involved in basic research efforts to understand the pathogenesis of mouse lymphomas or to develop mouse models of human cancers. Other scientific communities need only determine whether mice presented to them have a neoplasm and, if so, how to classify that tumor. In the former circumstance, many approaches can be applied to make diagnoses that contribute to understanding B cell pathogenesis. In the latter, histologic analysis of fixed sections stained with hematoxylin and eosin will sometimes be the only material available for diagnosis. The classification system described below for each lymphoma class is intended to be useful for both the basic research and applied science communities.

PRECURSOR B CELL LYMPHOBLASTIC LYMPHOMA/LEUKEMIA

Definition

Precursor B cell lymphoblastic lymphoma/leukemia (pre-B LBL) is a high-grade neoplasm of small to medium-sized, round, uniform precursor B cells arising in the bone marrow. A leukemic phase and spread to peripheral lymphoid and nonlymphoid tissues is frequently present.

Synonyms

Lymphoblastic lymphoma; lymphoblastic leukemia

Epidemiology of spontaneous disease

SL/Kh is a recombinant congenic mouse strain, derived from proto-SL and AKR strains, that develops pre-B LBL.[25,26] Tumors arise from a combination of host genetic factors and reintegration of endogenous MuLV provirus into several loci that include Stat5a, Stat5b, Evi3, c-MYC, and n-MYC.

Crosses between AKR and DBA/2 mice created 24 distinct AKXD RI strains with distinct MuLV proviral integration sites, most of which develop lymphoma.[4–6] Tumors classified as pre-B LBL on the basis of lymphoblastic cytology and the presence of clonal IgH rearrangements without detectable IgL clonality morphology arise in at least ten different AKXD RI strains, although analysis of additional phenotypic features of pre-B LBL have not yet been performed.[6]

Epidemiology of disease in genetically engineered mice

BCR-ABL^{p210} retrovirus-transduced bone marrow cells:[27–29] Infection of bone marrow (BM) cells from mice treated with 5-fluorouracil with a BCR-ABL^{p210}-expressing retrovirus followed by injection of lethally irradiated hosts yielded pre-B LBL in DBA/2 recipients, T cell acute lymphocytic leukemia (T-ALL) in C57BL/6 recipients, and other hematopoietic tumors in BALB/c recipients.

Metallothionein-1 promoter-BCR-ABL^{p190} TG:[30,31] Transgenic mice developed either chronic myeloid leukemia (CML) in blast crisis or pre-B LBL.

IgV$_H$-promoter-Eμ or retroviral LTR-BCR/v-ABL TG:[32] Transgenic mice expressing a synthetic BCR-ABL gene created by fusing *BCR* with *v-ABL* sequences developed either pre-B LBL or probably pre-T LBL.

BCR-ABL^{p190} knockin:[33] BCR-ABL inserted in-frame into exon 1 of the endogenous *BCR* locus by homologous recombination mimics half of the reciprocal translocation seen in Philadelphia (Ph)-positive cases. These *BCR-ABL^{p190}* 'knockin' mice developed pre-B LBL.

Eμ-MYC TG:[16] These mice developed pre-B LBL together with more mature lymphomas. Most tumors lacked IgL gene rearrangements and were surface immunoglobulin (sIg)$^-$. Crossing Eμ-*MYC* TG with Eμ-*PIM1* TG mice, which develop low-frequency pre-T LBL, resulted in congenital pre-B LBLs that were B220$^+$ and sIg$^-$.[34]

Eμ-BLK TG:[35] BLK is a Src family tyrosine kinase that associates with and signals from the pre-BCR and BCR.[36] Mice with a constitutively active *BLK* (Y495F) flanked by a H-2K promoter and Eμ developed pro-B and pre-B LBL along with intermediate single positive-stage thymic pre-T LBL. B cell-lineage tumors occurred in 45 percent of mice by 6 months. Activating lesions for the *Blk* homolog in human B and T cell tumors have not yet been described.

LTR-TEL/AML1 retrovirus-transduced BM cells:[37–39] A t(12;21)(p13;q22) occurs in 25 percent of pediatric and 3 percent of adult B-ALL cases, resulting in a *TEL/AML1* oncogene. TEL/AML1 retains the amino portion of the TEL protein fused to the AML1 DNA binding domain. TEL/AML1 may cause B-ALL by direct repression of AML1 target genes or by TEL inhibition of other ETS family proteins via binding through its pointed domain.[40–42] Transduction of wild-type or *p16^{Ink4a}*/p19^{Arf} null BM retrovirus was followed by adoptive transfer into lethally irradiated C57BL/6 mice. A low frequency of pre-B-ALL and T-ALL from the transduced wild-type donor cells and a higher frequency of an undetermined leukemia type was seen with the *p16^{Ink4a}*/p19^{Arf}-deficient cells.

Aiolos knockout:[43] Aiolos is a member of a kruppel-like zinc finger transcription factor family that binds DNA and regulates lymphocyte development and function. A knockout of Aiolos causes hyperproliferation and constitutive B cell activation followed by lymphadenopathy and evolution into probable B-LBL in 20 percent of mice. Alternatively, spliced Aiolos isoforms lacking a full complement of DNA binding domains in normal and leukemic human B cells have been reported, but their role in B cell transformation is not resolved.[44,45]

p16^{INK4a}/p19(p14)^{ARF} knockouts:[46] The *p16^{INK4a}/p19(p14)^{ARF}* genes overlap in the genome and encode tumor suppressor proteins that inhibit cancer formation.[47] Mice deficient in *p16^{Ink4a}/p19^{Arf}* developed mainly soft tissue sarcomas or B220$^+$ B cell lymphomas with prominent nucleoli that effaced lymph nodes. Although not further characterized, these features suggest a pre-B LBL phenotype. Deletion of *p16^{INK4a}/p14^{ARF}* occurs in 20 percent of B-ALL and 60 percent of T-ALL arising during childhood.[48] Also, DNA methylation of the *p16^{INK4a}* (but not of the *p14^{ARF}*) locus occurs in multiple types of non-Hodgkin lymphoma (NHL) and acute myeloid leukemia (AML), accompanied by loss of *p16^{INK4a}* expression.[49]

IL-7 TG:[50–53] Interleukin-7 (IL-7) and the IL-7/γcR regulate lymphopoiesis. Four distinct transgenic strains were generated to aberrantly express IL-7. A major histocompatibility complex (MHC)-II E$_α$ promoter-IL-7 transgene causes λ5 and EBF-expressing pre/pro-B/pro-B LBL with germ-line Ig genes.[53] Clonality is difficult to establish, and femurs are packed with lymphoid blast cells. There is accompanying lymphadenopathy. The tumor incidence varies by strain, with almost 100 percent of BALB/c and 25 percent of C57BL/6 mice developing morbid disease. Human lymphoid malignancies from IL-7 dysregulation have not been reported.

Histologic features

Pre-B LBL forms sheets of small to medium-sized blast cells in the bone marrow or infiltrated organs. The nuclei appear round to oval with condensed chromatin and a central, prominent nucleolus. There is a high nuclear:cytoplasmic ratio, with scant eosinophilic cytoplasm. A high mitotic index and abundant apoptosis can provide a 'starry-sky' appearance from macrophages stuffed with apoptotic debris (tingible body macrophages) that is histologically indistinguishable from that seen with pre-T LBL or more mature sIg$^+$ diffuse high-grade blastic B cell lymphoblastic lymphomas (DBLL), previously referred to as Burkitt-like.[2] Distinction is made from pre-T LBL, which are CD3$^+$ and B220$^-$, and DBLL, which are sIg$^+$ and contain rearranged IgL. Gross presentation may include lymphadenopathy without splenomegaly, a relatively unique occurrence for B cell lineage mouse tumors.

Immunologic features

Precursor B cells that by flow cytometry (fluorescence-activated cell sorting; FACS) are sIg$^-$, B220$^+$, CD19$^+$,

$CD43^{+/-}$, LY6d (ThB)$^+$, and by immunohistochemistry (IHC) are TdT$^+$.

Molecular features

Clonal population of precursor B cells with IgH gene rearrangement, typically of one allele and germ-line configuration of κ and λ IgL.

Postulated cell of origin

Bone marrow precursor B cell lymphoblast.

Comments

Mice containing BCR-ABL-infected BM or mice expressing either form of BCR-ABL (or bcr-v-abl) using transgenic, tetracycline-inducible or knockin technologies develop pre-B LBL with variable penetrance and strain dependence.[54] The p210 isoform of BCR-ABL generally does not result in B-ALL in humans. The human counterpart malignancies are pro-B and pre-B acute lymphoblastic leukemia (B-ALL) or B lymphoblastic lymphoma (B-LBL). Pre-B LBL shows similar histologic, cytologic, phenotypic, and molecular features in mice and humans.

SMALL B CELL LYMPHOMA/LEUKEMIA

Definition

A neoplasm of small, round, monomorphic B cells in the spleen and lymph nodes, sometimes admixed with prolymphocytes and paraimmunoblasts in pseudofollicles. Cases without leukemia (i.e., lymphoma) are more common than cases with leukemia.

Synonyms

Lymphocytic lymphoma; small lymphocytic lymphoma; chronic lymphocytic leukemia; well-differentiated lymphocytic lymphoma.

Epidemiology of spontaneous disease

Frequency was ~1 percent in AKXD RI strains and ~12 percent of all B cell lineage lymphomas in NFS.V$^+$.[55] The average age at diagnosis was ~400 days in NFS.V$^+$ mice. Uncommon in most commonly used mouse strains and stocks.

Epidemiology of disease in genetically engineered mice

$E\mu$-TCL1 TG:[56] Mice exhibited involvement of bone marrow at 2 months, spleen at 5 months, and leukemia

at 5 months with CD5$^+$CD11b$^+$Bcl-6$^-$ clonal B cells. Spleens often exhibited marked expansion of the marginal zone.

TRAF2DN/BCL-2 TG:[57] Transgenic mice exhibited splenic involvement at 10–16 months often associated with leukemia, ascites, and pleural effusion with CD5$^{+/-}$CD11b$^+$BCL6$^-$ B cells. Splenic marginal zone expansion was often present.

IL-5 TG:[58] Forty percent of mice presented with clonal CD5$^+$ B cell leukemia by 22 months of age.

Histologic features

Enlarged splenic white pulp filled with small lymphocytes and some larger prolymphocytes, with few mitotic or apoptotic figures (Plate 3, see plate section). Isolated accumulations of cells with features of immunoblasts can form proliferation centers similar to those seen in human chronic lymphocytic leukemia (CLL). A readily evident blood phase with predominantly small lymphocytes is seen in about 25 percent of cases. Extensive, diffuse infiltration of lymph nodes, lung, liver, and kidney can occur in the presence or absence of leukemia. Progression to immunoblastic lymphoma is rare, with immunoblasts and small lymphocytes cohabiting isolated areas, a possible parallel to Richter's transformation in human CLL.

Immunologic features

NFS.V$^+$ lymphomas were usually IgM$^+$B220^d CD5^d CD11b$^{+/-}$ by FACS and PAX5$^+$BCL6$^-$ by IHC.

Molecular features

Clonal IgH rearrangements. No major structural rearrangements of protooncogenes or tumor suppressor genes were identified in mice with spontaneous disease.

Postulated cell of origin

Not known. Immunoglobulin V-region sequencing required to determine whether pre- or post-GC.

Comments

Strains NZB and NZW, and genetically engineered strains including those listed above under induced diseases, regularly exhibit age-related expansions of populations of CD5$^+$ B cells in the peritoneum, spleen, and blood, sometimes sequentially. Expression of CD5 on mouse B cells is usually confined to a substantial proportion of B cells in the peritoneum and ~2 percent of B cells in the spleen.

SPLENIC MARGINAL ZONE B CELL LYMPHOMA

Definition

A neoplasm of cells from the splenic marginal zone presenting as low-, intermediate-, or high-grade disease that arises in the spleen and is almost always restricted to the spleen.

Synonyms

Splenic marginal zone lymphoma.

Epidemiology of spontaneous disease

The frequency of marginal zone lymphoma (MZL) was ~7 percent in NZB mice.[59] Marginal zone lymphoma accounted for ~35 percent of all neoplasms in NFS.V[+] and ~18 percent in AKXD strains.[55] The mean latency in NZB mice was ~450 days. In NFS.V[+] mice, the average age at diagnosis for low-, intermediate-, or high-grade disease was ~400 days.[60] In AKXD RI strains, the mean latency of predominantly low-grade disease was ~500 days.[6] A significant number of one-year-old TAN mice, a strain derived from a cross between NZB and NZW, also had MZL. Frequency is less than 1 percent in most commonly used mouse strains and stocks.

Epidemiology of disease in genetically engineered mice

In p53 knockouts,[61] MZL was diagnosed in ~35 percent of ex-breeder mice.

Histologic features

Three levels of progression have been described: MZL, MZL+, and MZL++ (Plate 4–6, see plate section). Marginal zone lymphoma is characterized by a substantially widened marginal zone comprising cells with normal cytology yielding a halo-like appearance around the follicles. Early lesions include hyperplastic marginal zone B cells with abundant eosinophilic cytoplasm and uniformly shaped nuclei. At this stage, mitoses are rare. With progression to MZL+, there is a merging of the marginal zones and the cells have taken on centroblastic features. Infiltration of the red pulp is often extensive, but follicles are usually intact. By the MZL++ stage, the spleen can be almost completely taken over by cells with centroblastic or, more rarely, immunoblastic morphology. The white pulp is usually rudimentary, consisting only of a periarteriolar lymphoid sheath (PALS). Mitoses are common. The lymphoma occasionally extends to the splenic node and rarely disseminates to the liver or other tissues. A leukemic phase is extremely rare.

Immunologic features

By FACS analysis, MZL – regardless of grade – expressed IgM at varying levels and little to no IgD.[60] Almost all cells expressed CD5 and CD45R(B200) at low levels and CD38 at high levels but were CD23[−]. Nearly half of cases expressed CD11B at low levels. By IHC, cases were consistently IgM[+]CD45R(B220)[dull]IgD[−]CD5[−].

Molecular features

Clonal for Ig gene rearrangements, with oligoclonality being more common among MZL than MZL+ or MZL++.[60,61] Rearrangements of cellular loci identified in MZL of AKXD RI strains included Nmyc1, Pim1, and Evi1 in ~16 percent of cases.[6] Marginal zone lymphoma of NFS.V[+] mice studied for common proviral integration sites identified three or more integrations at Stk10, Abcc5, Sox4, Mela, and Edh2.[62] Gfi1 was also identified as a common integration site (CIS) and was expressed at elevated levels in all grades of MZL.[62]

Postulated cell of origin

Splenic marginal zone B cell.

Comments

Non-splenic MZL in humans is associated with autoimmune diseases including, most prominently, Sjögren syndrome and Hashimoto thyroiditis.[63] Marginal zone lymphoma also occurs in association with infections caused by Helicobacter pylori, Chlamydia psittaci, and other agents. The observation that MZL occurs in autoimmune NZB mice and in the TAN strain, derived from a cross between NZB and NZW, suggests a possible etiologic link with human MZL. Shared low-affinity reactivity with autoantigens or repetitive bacterial antigens could be that tie. Autoimmune disease is generally not associated with these lymphomas in mice.

FOLLICULAR B CELL LYMPHOMA

Definition

Follicular B cell lymphoma (FBL) is a neoplasm comprising a mixture of B-lineage cells with cytologic features of centrocytes and centroblasts in varying proportions (Plates 7 and 8, see plate section).

Synonyms

Follicular lymphoma; centroblastic/centrocytic lymphoma; follicular center cell lymphoma, mixed; reticulum cell sarcoma, type B; lymphoma-pleiomorphic.

Epidemiology of spontaneous disease

This is the most common neoplasm in aging mice of many inbred strains. It accounts for 6 percent of cases in NFS.V$^+$ mice, 35 percent of cases in CFW strains, and 8 percent of cases in AKXD RI strains.[55] The average age at diagnosis is ~435 days for NFS.V$^+$ and ~400 days for the AKXD RI strains but ranges from 18 to 24 months in most other strains and stocks.

Epidemiology of disease in genetically engineered mice

Eμ-BCL2 TG:[64,65] Both TG lines of mice were reported to develop follicular hyperplasia that progressed to overt lymphoma. No increase in lymphoma incidence was found in later studies of the same strains.

MCL1 TG:[66] About 65 percent of mice presented with lymphoma by two years of age, most presenting with splenomegaly and lymphadenopathy. Around 20 percent of cases were FBL.

VAVP-BCL2 TG:[67] Approximately 60 percent of mice not dying previously with autoimmune disease succumbed to lymphoma between 10 and 18 months of age. Lymphoma development was preceded by increases in the number and size of GC and class-switched B cells with mutated Ig genes. The expanded GC phenotype was totally dependent on the presence of CD4$^+$ T cells.

Histologic features

Animals present most commonly with gross lesions of splenomegaly and varying degrees of enlargement of the mesenteric lymph node and Peyer's patches. In the spleen, the white pulp is expanded, appearing as white nodules that coalesce as the disease progresses. Occasionally, there is only a solitary large white nodule in the spleen. The smaller nodules are enlarged, sometimes with fused follicles with centrocytes and centroblasts as the chief cellular constituents. Normal small follicular B cells are pushed to the periphery, and the T cell zone is reduced or eliminated. In some mouse strains, tumors may arise within the PALS or inactive white pulp with no apparent relation to the GC. The proportions of centrocytes and centroblasts vary from case to case. The proportion of blasts should be less than 50 percent to differentiate the condition from diffuse large B cell lymphoma (DLBCL).

Immunologic features

By FACS, both the centrocytes and centroblasts in spontaneous cases were most often IgM$^+$IgD$^-$CD5^{dull}CD45R (B220)$^{dull\ to\ normal}$. By IHC, both populations were IgM$^+$ B220$^+$(Plates 9 and 10, see plate section).[68]

Molecular features

All cases examined in NFS.V$^+$ and AKXD mice were mono- or oligoclonal for Ig gene rearrangements.[3,6] No rearrangements in BCL2 were seen in large panels of FBL from NFS.V$^+$ mice or other inbred strains.[2] Genomic rearrangements of oncogenes or tumor suppressor genes were seen only for *Evi1* in AKXD mice.[6]

Postulated cell of origin

Germinal center centrocytes and centroblasts.

DIFFUSE LARGE B CELL LYMPHOMA

Definition

Diffuse large B cell lymphoma is a B cell neoplasm characterized by a diffuse proliferation of cells with large nuclei and distinctive cytologic features characteristic of each of the variants seen in spontaneous disease: centroblastic (CBL), immunoblastic (IBL), and histiocyte associated (HA) DLBCL.

DLBCL – centroblastic

SYNONYMS

Large cleaved follicular center lymphoma; centroblastic lymphoma.

EPIDEMIOLOGY OF SPONTANEOUS DISEASE

Centroblastic DLBCL accounted for ≈12 percent of cases in NFS.V$^+$ mice and 17 percent in CFW mice but were not observed among AKXD RI strain lymphomas.[55] The average age at diagnosis was ≈400 days in NFS.V$^+$ mice. The disease is uncommon in most commonly used strains and stocks of inbred mice.

HISTOLOGIC FEATURES

The white pulp is greatly expanded, with a population of cells with round nuclei, often with two nucleoli attached to the nuclear membrane, and a moderate amount of basophilic cytoplasm (Plate 11, see plate section). These are admixed to varying extents with smaller cells with characteristics of centrocytes. The diagnosis is readily made when over 70 percent of the cells are blasts. When the proportions of centrocytes and blasts range from 40 percent to 70 percent and the ratio varies in different fields, a distinction between FBL and DLBCL is difficult. In the classification system of Fredrickson and Harris,[68] CBL is subdivided into follicular, marginal zone, and diffuse to identify distinct regional origins for the first two and CBL of uncertain origin for the last. The lymphoma frequently infiltrates the lung, liver, and kidney and, less frequently, the bone marrow.

IMMUNOLOGIC FEATURES

By FACS, the tumors are IgM$^+$ or IgG$^+$, CD19$^+$, and B220$^+$ and often express CD5 at low levels. The tumors are almost uniformly BCL6$^+$ PAX5$^+$IRF8$^+$PU.1$^+$ by IHC, but CD138$^-$XBP1$^-$IRF4$^-$BLIMP$^-$.

MOLECULAR FEATURES

The tumors are clonal for Ig gene rearrangements, and rare cases have structural changes in BCL6.[9] Oligonucleotide microarray analyses have shown no clear distinctions between CBL subclassified as follicular or diffuse, suggesting similar origins from follicular B cells for both. By this methodology, both are readily distinguished from the centroblastic form of MZL, MZL++.

POSTULATED CELL OF ORIGIN

Germinal center dark zone centroblasts.

DLBCL – immunoblastic

SYNONYMS

Immunoblastic lymphoma.

EPIDEMIOLOGY OF SPONTANEOUS DISEASE

Immunoblastic lymphoma comprised ~8 percent of cases in NFS.V$^+$ mice and 4 percent in CFW mice, but was not observed among AKXD strain lymphomas.[55] The average age at diagnosis in NFS.V$^+$ mice was ~400 days.

HISTOLOGIC FEATURES

These are highly aggressive tumors populated by cells with large nuclei having dispersed chromatin and large, frequently bar-shaped nucleoli (Plate 12, see plate section). The cells are frequently admixed with centroblasts and centrocytes reflecting their probable origin in FBL or from a post-GC immunoblast.

IMMUNOLOGIC FEATURES

By FACS, surface Ig levels are very low and they are B220^{dull}. By IHC, almost all cases are BCL6$^+$ and PAX5$^+$ but IRF8$^-$XBP1$^-$IRF4$^-$PU.1$^-$BLIMP$^-$.

MOLECULAR FEATURES

Clonal for Ig gene organization.

PRESUMED CELL OF ORIGIN

Post-GC immunoblast.

DLBCL – histiocyte associated

SYNONYMS

Diffuse large cell lymphoma, histiocyte associated (DLCL[HS]).

EPIDEMIOLOGY OF SPONTANEOUS DISEASE

In AKXD RI strains, ~20 percent of lymphomas were HA, while only ~1 percent of NFS.V$^+$ lymphomas were diagnosed as such.[55] The average age at diagnosis for the AKXD RI strains was ~500 days. The disease is uncommon in commonly used strains and stocks of mice.

HISTOLOGIC FEATURES

All mice present with splenomegaly associated with a marked expansion of macrophages (histiocytes) with frothy eosinophilic cytoplasm and, usually, quite limited numbers of lymphocytes. The histiocytes often occupy the entire white pulp, obliterating the PALS and normal follicular structure, leaving patches of B cells pushed to the periphery. Most often, the lymphocytes have features characteristic of FBL or CBL although rare cases with features of MZL, small B cell lymphoma (SBL), or IBL have been observed. Lymphadenopathy was seen in about half of the cases and was associated with diffuse histiocytic infiltration.

IMMUNOLOGIC FEATURES

The histiocyte population is frequently positive for EMR1 (F4/80) and LGALS3 (Mac-2) by IHC, with the B cell populations clearly delineated by exclusive expression of PAX5.

MOLECULAR FEATURES

Frequently, the diagnosis can be made only after evaluating Ig gene organization and IHC staining. The presence of clonal Ig gene rearrangements and PAX5$^+$ populations of cells associated with a histologic picture dominated by histiocytes is diagnostic. The differential diagnosis is true histiocytic sarcoma. In some cases, clonal rearrangements of T cell receptor (TCR)β have also been observed.

PRESUMED CELL OF ORIGIN

Germinal center B cells for the B cell component, in most cases; tissue macrophages for the histiocytic component.

DLBCL in genetically engineered mice

T and B cell-lineage lymphomas and autoimmunity are among the most common unexpected features of transgenic and knockout mice.[69] The B cell neoplasms appearing in individual lines of such mice may span several histologic types, ranging from FBL to CBL and IBL and histiocyte-associated DLBCL (Plate 13, see plate section). They may resemble the spontaneous lymphomas of older mice of commonly used strains while developing in younger animals than in wild-type mice and having a more aggressive phenotype. It is important to distinguish induced from spontaneous tumors in genetically engineered mice. The genetic manipulation may simply accelerate the development of a disease seen in wild-type mice or may induce novel diseases not seen in conventional strains and stocks.

FEATURES OF GENETICALLY ENGINEERED MICE WITH DLBCL

Riz1 knockout:[70] About 37 percent of −/− and 19 percent of +/− mice killed between 18 and 22 months of age had clonal B cell lymphomas with histologic and cytologic features of centroblastic DLBCL.

H2-L^d-Il6 TG:[71] Between 6 and 19 months of age, many TG mice developed FBL or CBL that sometimes coexisted with plasmacytomas. The lymphomas were IgM$^+$CD19$^+$ CD45R(B220)$^+$. Several of the lymphomas had t(12;15) IgH/Myc translocations detectable by polymerase chain reaction (PCR) and/or Southern blotting.

Eμ-TCL1 TG:[72] Transgenic mice averaging ~12 months of age presented with splenomegaly and often with lymphadenopathy due to lymphomas. The tumors were classified as FBL, DLBCL(HA), CBL, and DBLL. The neoplasms were clonal, had mutated Ig genes, and were Bcl-6$^+$.

Bad knockouts:[73] About 20 percent of mice homozygous for a null allele developed clonal B cell lymphomas between 18 and 24 months of age. The lymphomas were surface IgM$^+$ or IgG$^+$ and were BCL6$^+$.

IμBCL6 knockins:[74] Mice with *BCL6* knocked into the IgH locus developed DLBCL and FBL beginning at 13 months of age. The lymphomas were clonal with mutated IgG genes and variably expressed some late GC markers such as IRF4. Trisomy 15 was common.

EμMYC knockins:[22,23] Mice with *MYC* knocked into the IgH locus 5′ of Eμ developed DLBCL between 6 and 21 months of age. Other B cell-lineage neoplasms included FBL, plasmacytomas, and DBLL. The DLBCL were clonal and Bcl-6$^+$IgM$^+$CD45R(B220)$^+$CD19$^+$.

PRESUMED CELL OF ORIGIN

Germinal center B cells.

DIFFUSE HIGH–GRADE BLASTIC B CELL LYMPHOMA/LEUKEMIA

Definition

Diffuse high-grade lymphoblastic lymphoma/leukemia is a highly aggressive neoplasm characterized by a uniform population of medium-size B cells usually associated with a high mitotic rate and extensive apoptosis, sometimes with a leukemic phase.

Synonyms

Lymphoblastic lymphoma; Burkitt and Burkitt-like lymphoma; DLBCL of lymphoblastic lymphoma subtype (DLBCL[LL]).

Epidemiology of spontaneous disease

Diffuse high-grade lymphoblastic lymphoma/leukemia accounted for ~20 percent of cases in NFS.V$^+$ mice and ~30 percent in AKXD RI strains and CFW mice.[55] The average age at diagnosis for NFS.V$^+$ mice was ~280 days and for AXKD RI strains was ~350 days. This disease is not frequent among commonly used inbred strains and stocks.

Epidemiology of disease in genetically engineered mice

Eμ-MYC TG: All TG mice with a particular construct[16] died with clonal lymphoma by 84 weeks of age, with a median time to diagnosis of ~90 days, while mice with a different construct[18] died with clonal lymphoma, with a mean time to diagnosis of ~115 days.

IgH/MYC YAC and EΔIgH/MYC YAC TG:[20,21] All mice died with clonal lymphoma before 20 weeks of age.

λ-MYC TG3:[19] All mice died with clonal lymphoma with an average age at diagnosis of ~125 days.

Histologic features

Cases present with lymphadenopathy and variable involvement of the spleen. Affected tissues are infiltrated with lymphoblasts: uniform cells of medium size with little cytoplasm, moderately dispersed chromatin, and indistinct nucleoli. These are associated with many mitotic figures and often with large numbers of tingible body macrophages ingesting apoptotic cells and leading to a starry-sky appearance (Plate 14, see plate section). In lymph nodes, early infiltration of the deep cortex progresses to total replacement of normal cells, with growth outside the capsule and into the fat. The spleen, when involved, exhibits diffuse infiltration of the red and white pulp. Perivascular and peribronchial infiltrates of the lungs and periportal live infiltrates are common.

Immunologic features

Diffuse high-grade lymphoblastic lymphoma/leukemia has a spectrum of surface phenotypes ranging from patterns similar to those of normal immature or transitional B cells – IgM$^+$IgD$^-$C1QR1(AA4.1)$^+$ – to that of cells that are Ig class switched and mutated for Ig V-region sequences. The less mature phenotype is characteristic of most lymphomas of Eμ-MYC, IgH/MYC YAC, EΔIgH/MYC YAC, and λ-MYC transgenic mice. More mature phenotypes are characteristic of many spontaneous DBLL of NFS.V$^+$ mice and some lymphomas of Eμ-TCL1 TG and EμMYC knockin mice along with many other genetically engineered mice.

Molecular features

The lymphomas are clonal for IgH and IgL rearrangements. Structural rearrangements of cellular genes, most due to proviral insertions, were found in pooled studies of NFS.V^{+}[3] and AKXD RI[6] lymphomas for *Zfp521* (*Evi3*) (11.9 percent), *Pim1* (5.6 percent), *Evi1* (4.8 percent), and *MYC* (0.8 percent). Lymphomas of λ-MYC were characterized by chromosomal instability and frequent biallelic deletions of *Cdkn2a* (p16).[19] Lymphomas of Eμ-MYC mice had frequent changes in the p19^{ARF}-MDM2-p53 tumor suppressor axis.[22]

Presumed cell of origin

Immature or transitional B cells for Eμ-MYC, IgH/MYC YAC, EΔIgH/MYC YAC, and λ-MYC transgenic mice. Probable GC or early post-GC cells for those with features similar to the DBLL of Eμ-TCL1 transgenic mice.

Comments

B cell-lineage lymphomas with lymphoblastic cytology but distinct from precursor B lymphoblastic neoplasms are seen at low to high frequency in many strains of genetically engineered mice and a number of conventional inbred strains. The lymphomas of λ-MYC transgenic mice were previously designated Burkitt lymphoma,[2] but the findings that Ig genes are not mutated and that they have a surface phenotype of transitional or immature B cells indicate that they differ from most human Burkitt lymphoma cases, suggesting that another designation is warranted. Mouse cases with similar histology and cytology occurring in mice other than the λ-MYC transgenic mice were previously designated Burkitt-like.[2] The findings that they rarely have structural alterations in *MYC* and do not overexpress *MYC* distinguish them from human Burkitt-like lymphomas.[1]

KEY POINTS

- Mouse B cell-lineage lymphomas comprise a spectrum of tumor types that can be distinguished through studies of their histologic, immunophenotypic, and molecular features and their relationship to a presumed cell of origin.

- Most detailed information on these lymphomas has come from studies of a limited number of mouse strains that express murine leukemia viruses at high levels, with the viruses acting as insertional mutagens.
- Some mouse lymphoma classes identified in high-virus mice exhibit many similarities to distinct lymphoma types in humans, whereas others appear to be species specific. There are many human B cell-lineage neoplasms that have no known counterpart in mice.
- Efforts to model human lymphomas in the mouse through genetic engineering have generally failed to produce accurate replicas but have generated invaluable information on the functions of oncogenes and tumor suppressor genes in normal B cell biology and their contributions to the transformed state in mice.
- The true utility of any mouse model will only be known when it has been rigorously dissected using the combined powers of histologic, immunophenotypic, genetic, and epigenetic analyses.

ACKNOWLEDGMENTS

This work was supported in part by the Intramural Research Program of the NIH, National Institute of Allergy and Infectious Diseases.

REFERENCES

● = Key primary paper
◆ = Major review article

◆1. Jaffe ES, Harris NL, Stein H, Vardiman JW. World Health Organization classification of tumors. Pathology and genetics. Tumors of haematopoietic and lymphoid tissues. Lyon: IARC Press, 2001.

◆2. Morse HC, Anver MR, Fredrickson TN *et al.* Bethesda proposals for classification of lymphoid neoplasms in mice. *Blood* 2002; **100**: 246–58.

●3. Hartley JW, Chattopadhyay SK, Lander MR *et al.* Accelerated appearance of multiple B cell lymphoma types in NFS/N mice congenic for ecotropic murine leukemia viruses. *Lab Invest* 2000; **80**: 159–69.

4. Mucenski ML, Taylor BA, Jenkins NA. AKXD recombinant inbred strains: models for studying the molecular genetic basis of murine lymphomas. *Mol Cell Biol* 1986; **6**: 4236–43.

5. Gilbert DJ, Neuman PE, Taylor BA, *et al.* Susceptibility of AKXD recombinant inbred mouse strains to lymphomas. *J Virol* 1993; **67**: 2083–90.

●6. Morse HC, Qi CF, Chattopadhyay SK *et al.* Combined histiologic and molecular features reveal previously unappreciated subsets of lymphoma in AKXD recombinant inbred mice. *Leuk Res* 2001; **25**: 719–33.

●7. Suzuki T, Shen HF, Akagi K *et al.* New genes involved in cancer identified by retroviral tagging. *Nat Genet* 2002; **32**: 166–74.

8. Potter M, Wiener F. Plasmacytomagenesis in mice – model of neoplastic development dependent upon chromosomal translocations. *Carcinogenesis* 1992; **13**: 1681–97.

9. Qi CF, Hori M, Coleman AE *et al.* Genomic organisation and expression of BCL6 in murine B-cell lymphomas. *Leuk Res* 2000; **24**: 719–32.

10. Gordon CJ, Grafton G, Wood PM *et al.* Modelling the human immune response: can mice be trusted? *Curr Opin Pharmacol* 2001; **1**: 431–8.

◆11. Mestas J, Hughes CCW. Of mice and not mend. Differences between mouse and human immunology. *J Immunol* 2004; **172**: 2731–8.

12. Oliver AM, Martin F, Kearney JF. Mouse Cd38 is down-regulated on germinal center B cells and mature plasma cells. *J Immunol* 1997; **158**: 1108–15.

◆13. Hahn WC, Weinberg RA. Modelling the molecular circuitry of cancer. *Nat Rev Cancer* 2002; **2**: 331–40.

14. Smogorzewska A, deLange T. Different telomere damage signaling pathways in human and mouse cells. *EMBO J* 2002; **21**: 4338–48.

15. Hooper ML. Tumor suppressor gene mutations in humans and mice: parallels and contrasts. *EMBO J* 1998; **17**: 6783–9.

●16. Adams JM, Harris AW, Pinkert CA *et al.* The c-*myc* oncogene driven by immunoglobulin enhancers induces lymphoid malignancy in transgenic mice. *Nature* 1985; **318**: 533–8.

17. Yukawa K, Kikutani H, Inomoto T *et al.* Strain dependency of B and T lymphoma development in immunoglobulin heavy chain enhancer (Eμ)-*myc* transgenic mice. *J Exp Med* 1989; **170**: 711–26.

18. Schmidt EV, Pattengale PK, Weir Leder P. Transgenic mice bearing the human c-myc gene activated by an immunoglobulin enhancer: a pre-B-cell lymphoma model. *Proc Natl Acad Sci U S A* 1988; **85**: 6047–51.

19. Kovalchuk AL, Qi CF, Torrey TA *et al.* Burkitt lymphoma in the mouse. *J Exp Med* 2000; **192**: 1183–90.

20. Butzler C, Zou X, Popov AV, Bruggemann M. Rapid induction of B-cell lymphomas in mice carrying a human IgH/c-*myc* YAC. *Oncogene* 1997; **14**: 1383–8.

21. Palomo C, Zou X, Nicholson IC *et al.* B-cell tumorigenesis in mice carrying a yeast artificial chromosome-based immunoglobulin heavy/c-*myc* translocus is independent of the heavy chain intron enhancer (Eμ). *Cancer Res* 1999; **59**: 5625–8.

22. Park SS, Kim JS, Han SS *et al.* Insertion of Myc into IgH induces B-cell lymphomas and plasmacytomas in mice. *Cancer Res* 2005; **65**: 1306–15.

23. Zhu D, Qi CF, Morse HC *et al.* Deregulated expression of the Myc cellular oncogene drives development of mouse

'Burkitt-like' lymphomas from naive B cells. *Blood* 2005; **105**: 2135–7.

24. William J, Euler C, Christensen S, Shlomchik MJ. Evolution of autoantibody responses via somatic hypermutation outside of germinal centers. *Science* 2002; **297**: 2066–70.

25. Yamada Y, Matsushiro H, Ogawa MS *et al.* Genetic predisposition to pre-B lymphomas in Sl Kh strain mice. *Cancer Res* 1994; **54**: 403–7.

26. Hiai H, Tsuruyama T, Yamada Y. Pre-B lymphomas in Sl/Kh mice: a multifactorial disease model. *Cancer Sci* 2003; **94**: 847–50.

27. Elefanty AG, Hariharan IK, Cory S. BCR-ABL, the hallmark of chronic myeloid-leukemia in man, induces multiple hematopoietic neoplasms in mice. *EMBO J* 1990; **9**: 1069–78.

28. Daley GQ, Vanetten RA, Baltimore D. Induction of chronic myelogenous leukemia in mice by the p210bcr/ABL gene of the Philadelphia chromosome. *Science* 1990; **247**: 824–30.

29. Kelliher MA, McLaughlin J, Witte ON, Rosenbergn N. Induction of a chronic myelogenous leukemia-like syndrome in mice with V-ABL and BCR/ABL. *Proc Natl Acad Sci U S A* 1990; **87**: 6649–53.

●30. Heisterkamp N, Jenster G, Tenhoeve J *et al.* Acute leukemia in BCR/ABL transgenic mice. *Nature* 1990; **344**: 251–3.

31. Voncken JW, Kaartinen V, Pattengale PK *et al.* BCR/ABL p210 and p190 cause distinct leukemia in transgenic mice. *Blood* 1995; **86**: 4603–11.

32. Hariharan IK, Harris AW, Crawford M *et al.* A BCR-V-ABL oncogene induces lymphomas in transgenic mice. *Mol Cell Biol* 1989; **9**: 2798–805.

33. Castellanos A, Pintado B, Weruaga E *et al.* A BCR-ABL^{p190} fusion gene made by homologous recombination causes B-cell acute lymphoblastic leukemias in chimeric mice with independence of the endogenous BCR product. *Blood* 1997; **90**: 2168–74.

34. Verbeek S, Vanlohuizen M, Vandervalk M *et al.* Mice bearing the E-μ-Myc and E-μ-Pim-1 transgenes develop pre-B-cell leukemia prenatally. *Mol Cell Biol* 1991; **11**: 1176–9.

35. Malek SN, Dordai DI, Reim J *et al.* Malignant transformation of early lymphoid progenitors in mice expressing an activated Blk tyrosine kinase. *Proc Natl Acad Sci U S A* 1998; **95**: 7351–6.

36. Lowell CA, Soriano P. Knockouts of Src-family kinases: stiff bones, wimpy T cells, and bad memories. *Genes Dev* 1996; **10**: 1845–57.

37. Golub TR, Barker GF, Bohlander SK *et al.* Fusion of the Tel gene on 12p13 to the AML1 gene on 21q22 in acute lymphoblastic leukemia. *Proc Natl Acad Sci U S A* 1995; **92**: 4917–21.

38. Romana SP, Poirel H, Leconiat M *et al.* High-frequency of t(12-21) in childhood B-lineage acute lymphoblastic leukemia. *Blood* 1995; **86**: 4263–9.

39. Romana SP, Mauchauffe M, Leconiat M *et al.* The t(12-21) of acute lymphoblastic leukemia results in a TEL-AML1 gene fusion. *Blood* 1995; **85**: 3662–70.

40. Hiebert SW, Sun WH, Davis JN *et al.* The t(12;21) translocation converts AML-1B from an activator to a

repressor of transcription. *Mol Cell Biol* 1996; **16**: 1349–55.

41. Fears S, Gavin M, Zhang DE *et al.* Functional characterization of ETV6 and ETV6/CBFA2 in the regulation of the MCSFR proximal promoter. *Proc Natl Acad Sci U S A* 1997; **94**: 1949–54.

42. Bernardin F, Yang YD, Cleaves R *et al.* TEL-AML1, expressed from t(12;21) in human acute lymphocytic leukemia, induces acute leukemia in mice. *Cancer Res* 2002; **62**: 3904–8.

43. Wang JH, Avitahl N, Cariappa A *et al.* Aiolos regulates B cell activation and maturation to effector state. *Immunity* 1998; **9**: 543–53.

44. Liippo J, Nera KP, Veistinen E *et al.* Both normal and leukemic B lymphocytes express multiple isoforms of the human *Aiolos* gene. *Eur J Immunol* 2001; **31**: 3469–74.

45. Schmitt C, Tonnelle C, Dalloul A *et al.* Aiolos and Ikaros: regulators of lymphocyte development, homeostasis and lymphoproliferation. *Apoptosis* 2002; **7**: 277–84.

46. Serrano M, Lee HW, Chin L *et al.* Role of the INK4a locus in tumor suppression and cell mortality. *Cell* 1996; **85**: 27–37.

47. Lowe SW, Sherr CJ. Tumor suppression by INK4a-ARF: progress and puzzles. *Curr Opin Genet Devel* 2003; **13**: 77–83.

48. Takeuchi S, Bartram CR, Seriu T *et al.* Analysis of a family of cyclin-dependent kinase inhibitors – p15/MTS2/INK4b, p16/MTS1/INK4a, and p18 genes in acute lymphoblastic leukemia of childhood. *Blood* 1995; **86**: 755–60.

♦49. French SW, Dawson DW, Miner MD *et al.* DNA methylation profiling: a new tool for evaluating hematologic malignancies. *Clin Immunol* 2002; **103**: 217–30.

50. Samaridis J, Casorati G, Traunecker A *et al.* Development of lymphocytes in interleukin 7-transgenic mice. *Eur J Immunol* 1991; **21**: 453–60.

51. Uehira M, Matsuda H, Hikita I *et al.* The development of dermatitis infiltrated by $\gamma\Delta$ T-cells in IL-7 transgenic mice. *Int Immunol* 1993; **5**: 1619–27.

52. Rich BE, Campos Torres J, Tepper RI *et al.* Cutaneous lymphoproliferation and lymphomas in interleukin-7 transgenic mice. *J Exp Med* 1993; **177**: 305–16.

53. Fisher AG, Burdet C, Bunce C *et al.* Lymphoproliferative disorders in IL-7 transgenic mice – expansion of immature B cells which retain macrophage potential. *Int Immunol* 1995; **7**: 415–23.

54. Wong S, Witte ON. Modeling Philadelphia chromosome positive leukemias. *Oncogene* 2001; **20**: 5644–59.

♦55. Morse HC III, McCarty T, Qi CF *et al.* B lymphoid neoplasms of mice: characteristics of naturally occurring and engineered diseases and relationships to human disorders. *Adv Immunol* 2004; **81**: 97–121.

56. Bichi R, Shinton SA, Martin ES *et al.* Human chronic lymphocytic leukemia modeled in mouse by targeted TCL1 expression. *Proc Natl Acad Sci U S A* 2002; **99**: 6955–60.

57. Zapata JM, Krajewska M, Morse HC *et al.* TNF receptor-associated factor (TRAF) domain and BCL-2 cooperate to induce small B cell lymphoma/chronic lymphocytic

leukemia in transgenic mice. *Proc Natl Acad Sci U S A* 2004; **101**: 16600–5.

58. Wen XS, Zhang DQ, Kikuchi Y *et al.* Transgene-mediated hyper-expression of IL-5 inhibits autoimmune disease but increases the risk of B cell chronic lymphocytic leukemia in a model of murine lupus. *Eur J Immunol* 2004; **34**: 2740–9.

59. Yumoto T, Yoshida Y, Yoshida H *et al.* Prelymphomatous and lymphomatous changes in splenomegaly of New Zealand black mice. *Acta Pathol Jpn* 1980; **30**: 171–86.

60. Fredrickson TN, Lennert K, Chattopadhyay SK *et al.* Splenic marginal zone lymphomas of mice. *Am J Pathol* 1999; **154**: 805–12.

61. Ward JM, Tadesse-Heath L, Perkins SN *et al.* Splenic marginal zone B-cell and thymic T-cell lymphomas in p53-deficient mice. *Lab Invest* 1999; **79**: 3–14.

62. Shin MS, Fredrickson TN, Hartley JW *et al.* High-throughput retroviral tagging for identification of genes involved in initiation and progression of mouse splenic marginal zone lymphomas. *Cancer Res* 2004; **64**: 4419–27.

63. Morse HC III, Kearney JF, Isaacson PG *et al.* Cells of the marginal zone – origins, function and neoplasia. *Leuk Res* 2001; **25**: 169–78.

64. McDonnell TJ, Korsmeyer SJ. Progression from lymphoid hyperplasia to high-grade malignant lymphoma in mice transgenic for the t(14,18). *Nature* 1991; **349**: 254–6.

65. Strasser A, Harris AW, Cory S. Eμ-BCL-2 transgene facilitates spontaneous transformation of early pre-B and immunoglobulin-secreting cells but not T cells. *Oncogene* 1993; **8**: 1–9.

66. Zhou P, Levy NB, Xie HY *et al.* MCL1 transgenic mice exhibit a high incidence of B-cell lymphoma manifested as a spectrum of histologic subtypes. *Blood* 2001; **97**: 3902–9.

67. Egle A, Harris AW, Bath ML *et al.* VavP-Bcl2 transgenic mice develop follicular lymphoma preceded by germinal center hyperplasia. *Blood* 2004; **103**: 2276–83.

68. Fredrickson TN, Harris AW. Atlas of mouse hematopathology. Amsterdam: Harwood Academic, 2000.

69. Taddesse-Heath L, Morse HC III. Lymphoma in genetically engineered mice. In: *Pathology of genetically engineered mice*. Ames: Iowa State University Press, 2000: 365–81.

70. Steele-Perkins G, Fang W, Yang XH *et al.* Tumor formation and inactivation of *Riz1*, an Rb-binding member of a nuclear protein-methyltransferase superfamily. *Genes Dev* 2001: **15**: 2250–62.

71. Kovalchuk AL, Kim JS, Park SS *et al.* IL-6 transgenic mouse model for extraosseous plasmacytoma. *Proc Natl Acad Sci U S A* 2002; **99**: 1509–14.

●72. Hoyer KK, French SW, Turner DE *et al.* Dysregulated TCL1 promotes multiple classes of mature B cell lymphoma. *Proc Natl Acad Sci U S A* 2002; **99**: 14392–7.

73. Ranger AM, Zha JP, Harada H *et al.* Bad-deficient mice develop diffuse large B cell lymphoma. *Proc Natl Acad Sci U S A* 2003; **100**: 9324–9.

●74. Cattoretti G, Pasqualucci L, Ballon G *et al.* Deregulated Bcl6 expression recapitulates the pathogenesis of human diffuse large B cell lymphomas in mice. *Cancer Cell* 2005; **7**: 445–55.

PART **4**

CLASSIFICATION AND PATHOGENESIS

18

Classification of lymphoid neoplasms

HK MÜLLER-HERMELINK AND E HARALAMBIEVA

INTRODUCTION

Classification of tumors is a major task of diagnostic pathology. Rudolf Virchow, 110 years ago, wrote in a conceptual speech on the anatomic understanding of disease and the tasks of pathologic research:[1] 'The research on the origin of diseases (the Latin "sedes morbi," quoting the famous book of Morgagni: De sedibus et causibus morborum[2]) has progressed from organs to tissues and from tissues to cells.' If we were to continue this reasoning today, we would complete the phrase: 'from cells to molecules and pathways.' This basic and functional understanding of biologic processes should govern the ideas of modern tumor classification – it still remains an idealistic goal, not reached in all tumor subtypes and hard to achieve in the individual diagnostic process.

Neoplastic tumors can be identified and typified by their morphologic features with high specificity and sensitivity. This is the great advantage of the histopathological approach to tumor categorization. Due to the development of new biopsy and imaging techniques, all tumors can be identified and classified by this easy and generally applicable method that has now been in use for over a century. However, the functional understanding of the biologic

processes underlying the morphologic appearances in the case of malignant lymphomas only reached a significant level when the complicated physiological behavior and the cellular interactions of the normal immune system became unveiled stepwise – a knowledge that is still incomplete.

Therefore, it is, in retrospect, not surprising that the interpretation of morphologic features of lymphomas, alone, resulted in different historical classification proposals that had several characteristics in common: (1) over-simplification and generalization; (2) lack of reproducibility by high inter- and even intraobserver variability; and (3) lack of second-line methods to prove or reject the descriptive interpretation. The modern biological approach was established in the Kiel classification[3,4] by correlating the morphologically defined subsets of malignant lymphomas to the cellular composition and reactive changes of the normal lymphoid tissue. However, it still reflected the incompleteness of immunological and genetic knowledge and the inability to integrate new and evolving knowledge in its purely cytomorphologic terminology.

Certain tumors of the lymphoid tissue have been recognized originally by their syndromatic clinical presentation regarding age, primary localization, and a characteristic morphology and/or ethnic prevalence. Often they were classified by eponyms acknowledging their first descriptors. The most prominent example is, of course, Hodgkin lymphoma (HL),[5] stratifying all lymphoid tumors into HL and non-Hodgkin lymphoma (NHL). Well-known NHL eponyms are Burkitt lymphoma,[6] Sternberg lymphosarcoma,[7] and giant follicular lymphosarcoma of Brill-Symmers[8] describing the characteristic presentation of endemic Burkitt lymphoma, mediastinal T lymphoblastic lymphoma, and follicular lymphoma, respectively. Some eponyms are still in use but now with a different significance, being aware that the original description may have overrated the characteristic presentation of a tumor that is now known to also occur under different clinical conditions. Therefore clinical presentation in the case of malignant lymphomas is neither sensitive nor specific enough to allow a classification system based on clinical features alone. However, the cited examples and the extranodal lymphomas discussed later show how important clinical features are and that histomorphology alone is also incomplete as a unique approach to lymphoma classification.

A different clinical approach as a classification system for lymphomas, in particular the NHLs, has been the outcome-oriented classification system of the so-called Working Formulation.[9] Based on the review of a large historical collection of cases serving as a reference, the cases were stratified according to survival probabilities and correlated to morphologic and clinical features. With the evolution of new treatment strategies and the impossibility to include new biological knowledge or to compare different patient groups, this approach proved to be unsatisfactory.

Classic cytogenetic studies and the interphase cytogenetic studies showed that many subtypes of malignant lymphoma are characterized by the occurrence of specific balanced translocations and their functional sequelae (discussed in Chapters 22–24).[10,11] Even if the classical translocation could not be demonstrated, as, for instance, in some t(14;18)-negative follicular lymphomas, various genetic[12] and/or epigenetic events resulted in functionally similar phenotypic effects on apoptosis resistance as in the translocation-positive cases. Different patterns of genomic gains and losses are associated with the different lymphoma entities and suggest a further stratification of diffuse large B cell lymphoma (DLBCL).[13] Therefore, many lymphomas are characterized by well-defined genetic alterations. They are the biological backbone of recent classifications of malignant lymphomas but, in practical terms, these are still applied more in research projects and less in routine diagnostic issues.

The majority of lymphoma classification in the last decade profited from the ever-increasing availability of specific monoclonal antibodies and improvement of immune histochemical techniques to detect the specific phenotypes of tumor cells in tissue sections. Hereby, the comparison of tumor cells to the corresponding normal cells of the immune system was established, as well as their characteristic topographical distribution and infiltration pattern. The demonstration of characteristic tumor-specific phenotypic alterations as a result of altered protein expression by genetic effects became a diagnostic tool.

For some lymphomas, infectious agents play a role as etiopathogenetic factors.[14–18] Epstein–Barr virus (EBV), human herpes virus 8 (HHV-8), and *Helicobacter pylori* are associated with different lymphoma subtypes. However, an identical infectious agent, e.g., EBV, may be causative for such different lymphomas as HL, nasal natural killer (NK)/T cell lymphoma, and endemic Burkitt lymphoma (and other nonlymphoid tumors). Furthermore, no major differences between EBV-positive and EBV-negative lymphomas of the same type have been identified. Therefore, the presence of these infectious agents does not establish a classification principle. They are considered to be preneoplastic conditions or risk factors that together with endogenous factors and conditions, e.g., genetic or acquired immune deficiency, in combination or alone, may initiate the neoplastic transformation process.

Starting with descriptive terms of the poorly defined lymphoid cell populations and their application to neoplastic cell populations, the classification of lymphoid neoplasms has now reached a high standard of evidence-based definition of tumor entities. New concepts, new entities, and elucidation of molecular pathways are constantly arising and have to be implemented in the classification system. In this respect, a classification has to be a living evolutionary process. The principles established in the Revised European–American Lymphoma (REAL) classification[19] and updated in the World Health Organization (WHO) classification[10,20] will also govern a new edition of the WHO classification (2008) and form the basis of this chapter.

CONCEPTUAL BASIS OF CLASSIFICATION

In the daily application of any classification by pathologists and clinicians we may paraphrase: 'Making a diagnosis is the act of assigning a name to a disease.'[21] In the past, much effort was focused on the creation of **names**, usually by one professional discipline, and their arrangement by principles formed the core of a classification system. As much as this approach was helpful to the teaching and learning of a classification, difficulties and inconsistencies arose by the fact that never could one principle alone account for and define all elements included in the system; as a rule, multiple factors were important and contributed differently to the definition of the diseases. Furthermore, practical issues complicated the diagnostic process, e.g., availability of the methods or clinical requirements of a therapeutic stratification, and the classification lost its value with respect to diagnostic specificity and accuracy. The new approach at making a diagnosis consists of the complex definition of the **disease**, using the information of many disciplines, which is then called an **entity**, as being one element in a list of diseases that constitute the actual sum of our knowledge in the field.[10,19] With new knowledge, diseases may split up to form new diseases, multiplying the number of names in the list, or they may be deleted and grouped with other names if convincing evidence becomes available to do so.

This list of names of entities, if internationally accepted, is named a classification and in reality establishes the creation of a **language** enabling communication, recognition of epidemiologic and ethnic prevalences, comparison of treatment protocols, and even international multicenter prospective trials. These important goals are the driving force for the **agreement** of specialists on the names in a given group of tumors, e.g., lymphomas, which has also to serve as a method to establish accuracy of the system, at least as long as it is based mainly on empirical evidence or common experience. Objective tests that are becoming available now to define the entities of a classification may be used to prove, complete, or even substitute in future the empirical knowledge. Agreement of specialists overrules the individual diagnosis and is also used in the **diagnostic panels** of multicenter studies to establish diagnostic accuracy and specificity by measuring the interobserver and intraobserver variability. Furthermore, it helps to define the use and value of ancillary tests and specific requirements for the definition of each entity.

BASIC UNITS OF CLASSIFICATION

Malignant lymphoid tumors are split up into the major categories of T cell, B cell, and HL.[10,11] In each major category, **entities** are listed that either constitute real diseases or groups of diseases listed together because subgrouping appears not to be meaningful. Within the entities, **variants** are defined by specific morphologic, immunohistochemical, or genetic features, often with variant clinical presentation or prognosis. **Prognostic factors** are defined within each entity separately, either by clinical features, e.g., grading or staging, or specific molecular, immunophenotypic, or morphologic features.

Entity

Each entity is defined by specific morphologic, immunohistological, (molecular) genetic, and clinical features. Each method contributes differently to the final diagnosis in different entities. Even if not all techniques are applied in an individual diagnostic approach, the definition of the entity is based on a characteristic and invariable combination of features that would be demonstrable and is tacitly presumed if the *de facto* demonstration is not performed or not available. The logistic approach to reach the complete information needed for a diagnosis may vary, but the results gained by all important methods must be available to the pathologist. By this integrated approach, specialized methodology and functional knowledge can be combined in the diagnostic process.[10,11]

The category of **provisional entity** has been introduced, if the evidence to define a certain type of tumor as an entity is still insufficient, in order to recognize these lymphomas separately in the classification. The decision whether they are accepted as a new entity can be taken later, on the basis of new data.

Entities listed in the classification of lymphoid neoplasms are, in the majority, real separate diseases differing from each other by all major criteria, e.g., mantle cell lymphoma (MCL) presenting with typical clinical, morphologic, genetic, and immunohistochemical findings. Interestingly, DLBCL and peripheral T cell lymphoma (PTCL) not otherwise specified (NOS) are considered to be heterogeneous, containing separate variants or entities that at present cannot be unanimously defined and which for clinical studies are grouped together. As expected, in view of additional data, some subentities have already or will split out from this pool and be defined as 'new' entities, e.g., primary mediastinal large B cell lymphoma[22] or some of the organ-based DLBCL, e.g., central nervous system (CNS) large B cell lymphoma. New entities not present in previous classifications may also be defined on the basis of new biological findings, e.g., the recognition of the hematodermic neoplasia of dendritic cell precursor cells[23,24] replacing blastoid NK cell lymphoma of the previous WHO classification.

Prognostic factor

Although the disease entities are the primary elements of the classification, there is considerable heterogeneity within most entities in respect to the probability of overall and disease-free survival, even after optimal treatment. In follicular lymphoma (as well as in other lymphoma entities), for example, some patients die within the first year after diagnosis from progressive untreatable disease whereas others survive for more than 25 years and do not show significant difference to the survival of age-matched controls. Thus, risk assessment is an important issue.

Clinically, the general risk assessment is performed according to the International Prognostic Index (IPI),[25] which provides important information concerning disease status and general patient characteristics. For many lymphoma types, the IPI clearly allows stratification in four quartiles, where grades I and II are low and low intermediate and grades III and IV are intermediate high and high risk classes. According to certain typical clinical features, the IPI has been modified for certain tumor entities, e.g., the Follicular Lymphoma International Prognostic Index (FLIPI)[26] for follicular lymphoma, achieving even more accurate predictive classes in the respective lymphoma entities.

All other prognostic factors are specific for and defined within each entity. As a consequence, the diagnosis of the correct entity is also the most important prognostic factor,[27,28] since treatment approaches and results vary considerably between the lymphoma entities and also the additional risk factors are dependent on the type of lymphoma.

Prognostic factors may be defined by morphology (blastoid versus classical MCL), immunohistochemistry (TP53 expression, Ki-67 in MCL[29,30]), genetic or molecular genetic features (del 13q or immunoglobulin heavy chain gene [IGH] somatic mutation pattern in chronic lymphocytic leukemia [CLL][31,32]), or clinical features (e.g., anemia in HL). Recently, gene expression profiling signatures have provided promising data in the definition of tumor-related or host-related risk profiles in the various lymphoma types.[30,33–37]

The value of prognostic factors to predict outcome-related events may vary considerably over time and especially in relation to new or different treatment protocols. The morphologic subclassification of classical HL as defined in the Rye classification originally correlated well to different outcome and survival characteristics, but now all subtypes of HL, irrespective of stage, show a similar high cure rate by new chemotherapy protocols. The benefit of R-CHOP (rituximab, cyclophosphamide, vincristine, doxorubicin, and prednisone) treatment in DLBCL in comparison to the traditional CHOP regimen in some clinical trials was attributable to the much better response rate of activated B cell (ABC)-like large B cell lymphoma, whereas germinal center B cell (GCB)-like DLBCL showed a less marked but still beneficial response after the addition of the anti-CD20 treatment.[38,39]

Although prognostic factors stratify a given lymphoma entity into subgroups, e.g., responders versus nonresponders, they do not define different entities. There may be, however, a certain terminological gray zone in cases where prognostic factors identify well-defined biological variants (see below) that respond to a different, more specific treatment (thus establishing the criteria of an entity by specific morphologic, immunohistochemical, genetic, and clinical features).

Variant

Variants are defined within the entities very often for clinical or morphologic reasons in order to validate a special clinical presentation or course, or a morphologic finding which might be of diagnostic or prognostic relevance. Accordingly, the definition of a variant may also be a prognostic factor.

The recognition and characterization of variants are correlated to the heterogeneity of each entity. For instance: (1) primary follicular lymphoma of the duodenum is considered to be a localized disease with little or almost no tendency to disseminate, despite the fact that morphology, immunophenotype, and presence of the t(14;18) translocation are similar to the nodal follicular lymphoma; (2) the diffuse variant of follicular lymphoma grade one is important to recognize in order to establish the diagnosis and also to correlate it with certain clinical (localized disease) and genetic (*BCL2*-negative, del 1q) features.

The recognition of variants may be considered as a first step in the hierarchical definition of new entities (variant → subentity, provisional entity → entity).

FUNCTIONAL ASPECTS OF CLASSIFICATION

Normal counterpart/differentiation arrest

Much of our knowledge of the different lymphoma entities originates from the continuous scientific progress in the fields of immunology and molecular genetics of normal

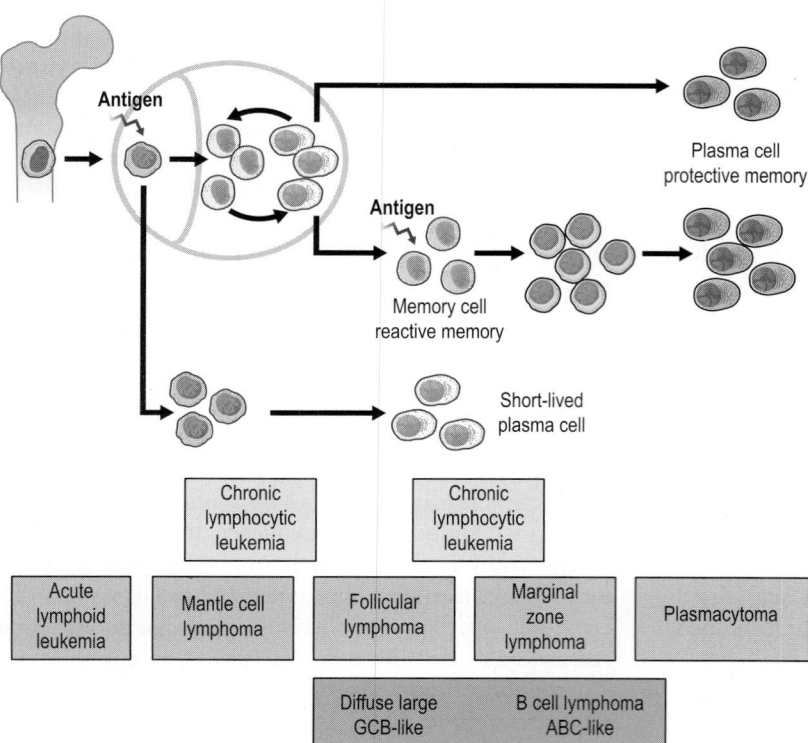

Figure 18.1 Correlation of major subtypes of B cell non-Hodgkin lymphoma to normal B cell development and differentiation. GCB, germinal center B cell; ABC, activated B cell.

B and T cells, as well as the recognition of specific onco-genic pathways in the different lymphomas.

The traditional approach of histopathological classification to define tumors according to their highest degree of differentiation in comparison to a hypothetical cell of origin has been applied for malignant lymphomas primarily in the Kiel classification. It postulated that the B cell NHLs represent frozen states in the successive phases of B cell development and antigen-driven differentiation. This concept originally had its strongest plausibility linking the cyto-morphologic features of neoplastic cells to the normal cells of the germinal center reaction. Meanwhile, it was verified for the vast majority of B cell NHL and strongly supported by immunohistochemical, phenotypic, and genetic data. Indeed, most B cell NHLs have a putative normal counterpart related to development and functional differentiation of B cells in adaptive and innate immune responses.

This close resemblance of the tumor cells in NHL to normal reactive B cell subpopulations – not only in respect to cytomorphology, but also in respect to the topography within the organized lymphoid tissue, to interactions with a normal microenvironment, differentiation capacity, and immunophenotype – was often taken as evidence suggesting the derivation of tumors from these corresponding normal counterparts. However, the histogenetic approach in lymphoma classification does not necessarily imply a direct transformation of a given normal cell type to its corresponding tumor cell. It rather characterizes the tumor according to an endpoint of differentiation, reached after oncogenic events in their precursor cells. Furthermore, the differentiation arrest may keep the tumor cells in a state of proliferation when physiological regulatory events would limit the population size, therefore representing itself as a major oncogenic event. For instance, in a subgroup of ABC-like DLBCL, inactivating mutations of *BLIMP1* were found, interfering with the terminal differentiation to plasma cells.[40]

In Figure 18.1 a simplified scheme of normal B cell development is provided and correlated with the major subtypes of B cell NHL. The resemblance extends not only to cytologic characteristics but also to early involvement and tumor growth pattern that often parallels the tissue distribution of the normal counterpart (Plate 15, see plate section). Unusual immunophenotypic variants in tumors may even reflect the presence of minor subpopulations in the reactive lymphoid tissue that remained unrecognized (e.g., CD10-negative, MUM1-positive follicular lymphoma probably corresponds to a follicular exit population also present in the normal germinal center response).

However, not for all lymphoid neoplasms has the putative normal counterpart been established. The initial transformation event in HL is linked to a germinal center B cell,[41,42] but the tumor-specific morphogenetic and immunophenotypic alterations are not found in reactive conditions. Similarly, anaplastic large cell lymphoma (ALCL) is probably derived from activated cytotoxic T cells but is morphologically and phenotypically different from all reactive counterparts. Hairy cell leukemia shows a highly

specific phenotype and clinical presentation, but so far the corresponding normal counterpart has not been defined.

In contrast to the B cells' differentiation pathways, the functional subpopulations of peripheral T and NK cells cannot be recognized morphologically. Tissue distribution patterns, cell-to-cell interactions, and activation stages are morphologically similar or identical in different T and NK cell subpopulations. Many specific subpopulations of peripheral T and NK cells have been recognized only recently (Fig. 18.2). Therefore, various subtypes of PTCL are still insufficiently correlated to their normal counterpart. Furthermore, the functional redundancy of cytotoxic effector cell populations is also mirrored by the fact that extranodal cytotoxic T/NK cell lymphomas are derived from different cytotoxic effector cells. Nevertheless, growing knowledge on T and NK cell maturation and differentiation models results in increasing recognition of the functional subpopulations corresponding to defined T cell lymphoma subtypes[43–45] and allows classification of nodal PTCL correctly with respect to immunophenotype of T cell subpopulation and differentiation/maturation stage of putative normal counterparts (Figs 18.2 and 18.3).[46]

Stem cell concept

The concept of normal counterparts has to be considered as the relevant backbone of the classification of lymphoid neoplasms; however, it is not directly correlated to the initial (primary) oncogenic events of tumor stem cells. As a rule, these primary oncogenic events consist of genetic alterations which occur in earlier steps of cellular differentiation than those represented by the respective normal counterpart of established lymphomas. The oncogenic translocations t(14;18) in follicular lymphoma and t(11;14) in MCL are related to the V(D)J rearrangement in the bone marrow pre-B cell[47] (and not in corresponding germinal center or mantle zone B cells). Many translocations are related to somatic hypermutation and to the activity of activation-induced cytidine deaminase (AID) in the germinal center reaction; others, identified in post-germinal center B cell neoplasia, e.g., DLBCL subtypes and plasmacytoma/multiple myeloma, occur during immunoglobulin class switch recombination (discussed in detail in Chapters 22 and 23).[47] Similarly, in HL, the primary transformation event takes place during the late germinal center reaction;[42] however, the tumor cells in classical HL show more similarities to post-germinal center B cells.

These examples may be interpreted, on the one hand, as evidence for the fact that the primary translocation is not enough and has to be followed by additional mutagenic events establishing the full neoplastic phenotype: increasingly these translocations, e.g., the t(14;18), are found in circulating B cells of the normal population[48,49] and it is even not proven that this finding is a predisposing factor for the later occurrence of a follicular lymphoma. On the other hand, the tumor stem cell or founder cell may develop and differentiate to a later stage of differentiation where the majority of offspring has a different phenotype. This behavior would be similar to the differentiation and amplification steps of other hematopoietic cells in the bone marrow.

It may also be interesting to consider clonal amplification and differentiation of B cells under the aspect of modern stem cell biology. B lymphocytes can activate telomerase and thus have the capacity of unlimited proliferation. Furthermore, the principal requirements of pluripotent stem cells, namely differentiation, clonal amplification, and self-renewal of stem cell candidates, are fulfilled at different steps of the B cell maturation and differentiation pathway (Fig. 18.4).

Lymphoid stem cells are derived from the pluripotent hemopoietic stem cells and give rise to B, T, and NK cells. By immunoglobulin (Ig) rearrangements, the idiotypic B cell receptor is generated. In a first selection, amplification, and differentiation process, the repertoire of naïve B cells is generated, a process that generates **heterogeneity (diversity)**. Under the influence of appropriate antigen stimulation, naïve B cells undergo a second selection, amplification,

and differentiation process in the germinal centers, giving rise either to plasma cells as terminal differentiation of effector cells or memory B cells with eventually class-switched, highly specialized, mutated Ig receptors. This process generates **specificity**. A third amplification and differentiation process takes place when memory B cells are restimulated by the same antigen in extrafollicular activation, which leads to the increased formation of long-lived plasma cells, a process generating specialized **effector cells**. These cells (or their precursors) are translocated back to the bone marrow where they constitute a '**defense organ**' producing more than 90 percent of circulating immunoglobulins of the serum. Whether this 'organ' of terminally differentiated effector cells is capable of regeneration in the bone marrow or is constantly replenished by circulating precursors is not completely clear. At least three steps in the normal B cell maturation and differentiation fulfill the prerequisites of stem cells: self-renewal of the precursors and differentiation leading to (temporary) end cells with different biological characteristics. In that process, phases of highly regulated proliferation, as well as different

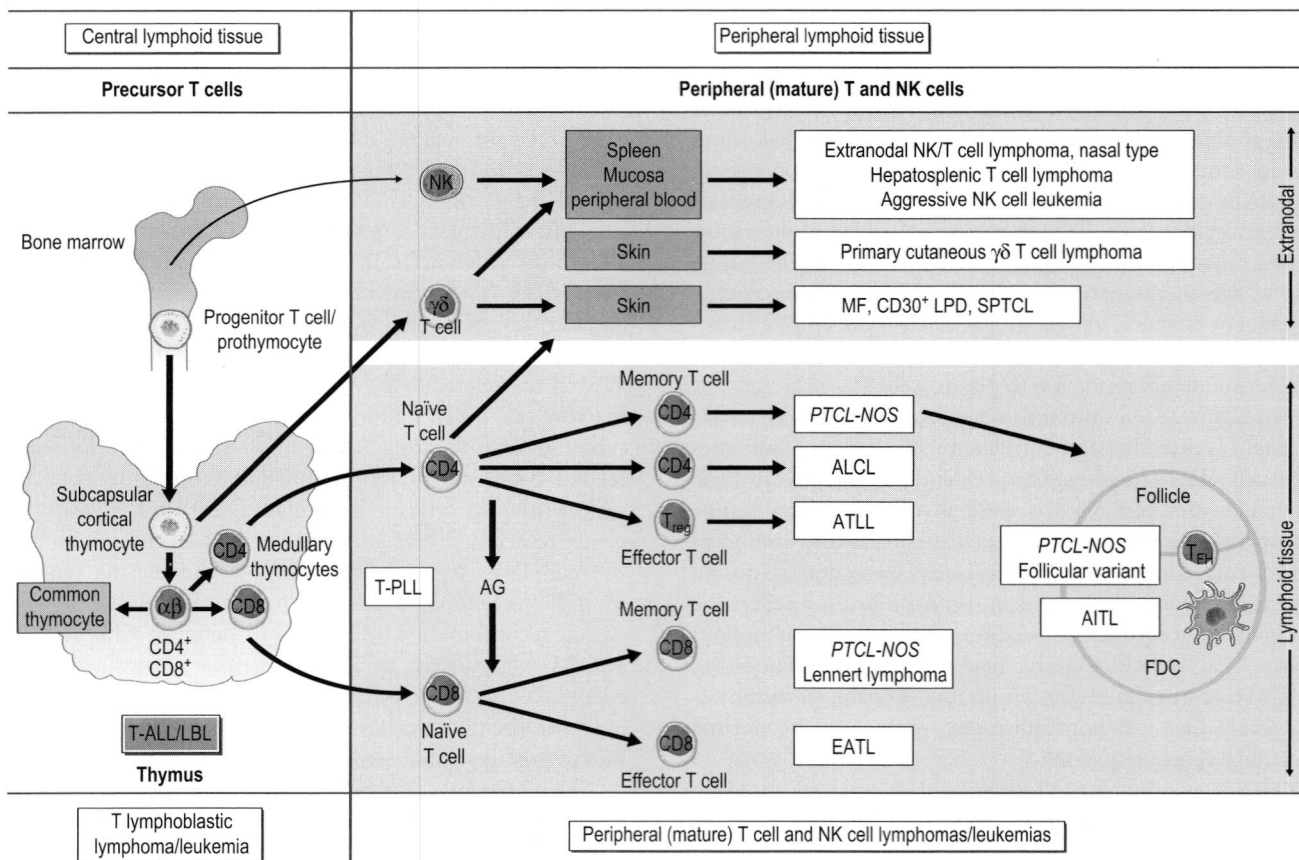

Figure 18.2 Correlation of peripheral T/natural killer (NK) cell lymphomas to different subpopulations of normal T and NK cells. T-ALL, T cell acute lymphoblastic leukemia; LBL, lymphoblastic lymphoma; T-PLL, T cell prolymphocytic leukemia; PTCL-NOS, peripheral T cell lymphoma, not otherwise specified; ALCL, anaplastic large cell lymphoma; ATLL, adult T cell leukemia/lymphoma; EATL, enteropathy-associated T cell lymphoma; AITL, angioimmunoblastic T cell lymphoma; MF, mycosis fungoides; LPD, lymphoproliferative disorder; SPTCL, subcutaneous panniculitis-like T cell lymphoma; T_FH, follicular helper T cells.

directly mutagenic events – i.e., V(D)J rearrangement, somatic hypermutation of Ig receptors, and Ig-switch recombination – take place and increase the risk of oncogenic events. Increasingly it becomes clear that different patterns of genetic alterations, translocations and chromosomal gains and losses, are related to these different phases of B cell development. It still remains an open question whether in the lymphoid neoplasms the respective neoplastic stem or precursor cells are present and play a role within the tumor tissue, in treatment responses, or in resistance, spread, or tumor heterogeneity and plasticity as discussed in the case of cancer stem cells.

Clonal evolution

The consecutive acquisition of genetic alterations in the tumor cell resulting in clonal heterogeneity and selection of subclones is referred to as clonal evolution. It is generally accepted that overt malignancy is a result of a multistep carcinogenesis process, although little is known on the transforming potential of the different early events in malignant lymphoma and, for example, how many genetic events are required and/or sufficient to cause malignancy.

In clinically overt lymphoma, the clonal evolution reflects the process of tumor progression and/or transformation. Different lymphoma subtypes are characterized by a different frequency and pathway of tumor progression, accompanied or not by major changes in the lymphoma phenotype.[50,51] Morphologic progression or transformation of lymphoma results in a tumor of different morphologic subtype, e.g., DLBCL or HL in indolent NHL. The distinction from a second, *de novo* lymphoma is based on the molecular comparison of both (primary and secondary) tumors and can not be accomplished by morphology alone. Clonal evolution can also occur without major phenotypic changes and result in increased chromosomal heterogeneity, leading to genomic instability and therapeutic resistance. The different pathways and time course of clonal evolution account, at least to some extent, for the varying clinical behavior and survival of patients with indolent NHL.

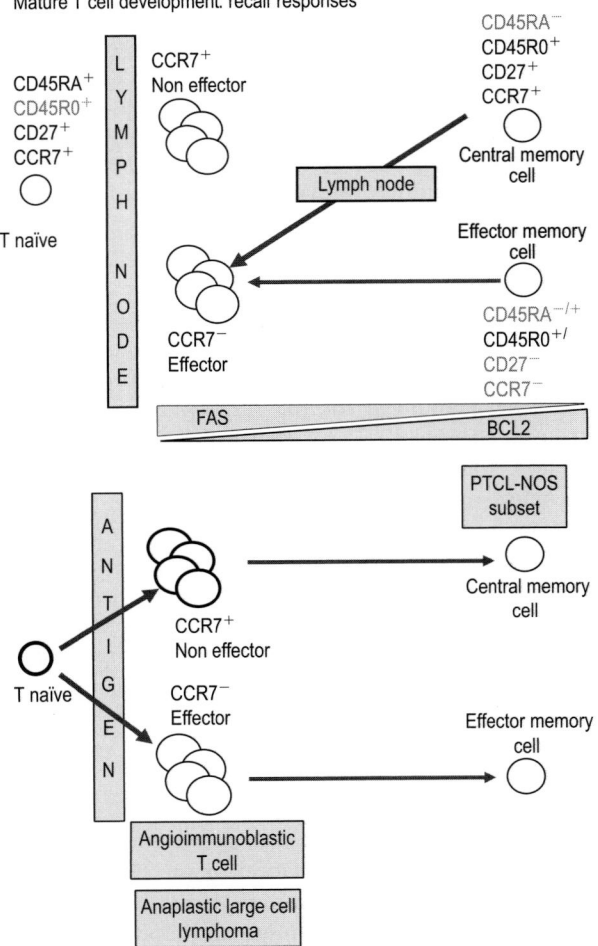

Figure 18.3 Correlation of nodal peripheral T cell lymphomas to functional differentiation after antigenic stimulation (independent of T cell subpopulation in adaptive immune responses).[46] PTCL-NOS, peripheral T cell lymphoma, not otherwise specified.

Etiology and pathogenesis

Current data indicate that infectious agents are linked to a significant number of lymphoid neoplasias.[17] Important

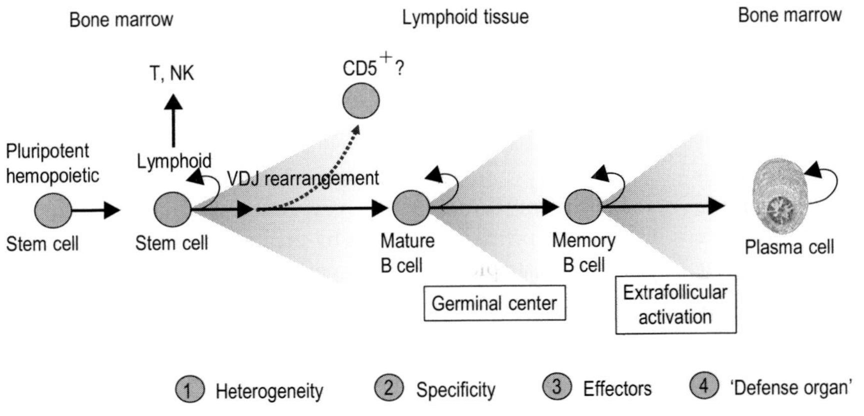

Figure 18.4 Successive stem cell and differentiation phases in normal B cell development. NK, natural killer.

examples represent the association of EBV with a variety of malignant lymphoma,[16] human T cell lymphotrophic virus type 1 (HTLV-1) with T cell leukemia/lymphoma, HHV-8 with primary effusion lymphoma, and *Helicobacter pylori* with gastric marginal zone B cell lymphoma of mucosal-associated lymphoid tissue (MALT) type.[15,18] Further infectious agents possibly contributing to the genesis of the marginal zone lymphoma at different extranodal sites are *Campylobacter jejuni* in immunoproliferative small intestinal disease (IPSID), *Borrelia burgdorferi* in primary cutaneous marginal zone B cell lymphoma (MZBL), *Chlamydia psittaci* in MZBL of ocular adnexae, and hepatitis C virus (HCV) in a subset of splenic marginal zone B cell lymphoma (SMZBL). The mechanisms by which these microorganisms are involved in lymphomagenesis are poorly understood and are discussed in Chapters 25 and 26.

The presence of infectious agents, however, does not influence considerably the classification of malignant lymphomas, due to the fact that a single etiologic agent may be linked to various malignancies/subtypes, e.g., EBV with classical HL, nasal type T/NK cell lymphoma, Burkitt lymphoma, DLBCL subtypes, and nasopharyngeal carcinoma. In addition, no significant variation in clinical presentation and outcome is seen depending on the presence or absence of an infectious agent in many lymphomas. For instance, EBV-positive and EBV-negative Burkitt lymphoma patients have similar clinical features and survival. In other instances, however, the identification of the respective associated infection has important clinical implications;[18] for example, gastric marginal zone lymphoma of MALT type may show complete regression upon *Helicobacter pylori* eradication therapy.

Genetic predisposition and ethnic prevalences are well documented for many lymphoma subtypes. Again, these factors do not reflect the lymphoma classification, since cases occurring out of the context of genetic or ethnic predisposition show no consistent biological or clinical difference.

PRINCIPLES AND METHODS OF CLASSIFICATION

The lymphoma diagnosis requires the histopathological and cytologic investigation of **formalin-fixed, paraffin-embedded** (FFPE) tissue, enabling a detailed immunophenotypic characterization of tumor cells and microenvironment and also some molecular and genetic studies. The novel, still experimental diagnostic tools of gene expression profiling and high resolution analysis of chromosomal imbalances, by single nucleotide polymorphism (SNP) array analysis, are only applicable if sufficient **fresh-frozen tumor tissue** (FFTT) is available. Classical cytogenetics requires a fresh tissue sample or vital tumor cells and its success rate varies highly depending on the number and quality of the acquired metaphases. Circulating lymphoma cells can be analyzed morphologically in blood smears and immunophenotyped by fluorescence-activated cell sorting (FACS) analysis. Primary cytologic diagnosis and classification of a

malignant lymphoma is in general discouraged or reserved for special clinical situations since the classification specificity and sensitivity are limited and identification of specific risk factors remains problematic. In remote topographical areas, e.g., mediastinum and retroperitoneum, computed tomography (CT)-guided histological core biopsies are frequently adequate and allow a definite diagnosis without major surgical intervention. In peripheral localizations a surgical biopsy is favored.

The routine workup at the centers and institutions involved in lymphoma diagnosis and treatment is based on their standard operation procedures (SOPs) approved by local ethics committees and documenting the logistics and availability of techniques in handling and storage of lymph node specimens for all the above mentioned needs. The sampling of FFPE tissue has a priority because of its importance for diagnostic purposes. Fresh-frozen tumor tissue is collected in cases of availability of sufficient material. The appropriate time frame in handling of the surgical biopsy should be guaranteed for the respective supplementary tests, e.g., adequate RNA for gene expression studies, vital cells for cytogenetics, or storage etc. The logistic coordination between different institutions involved in processing and testing of the material is essential. An optimal panel of investigations required for the correct diagnosis and clinical management of the patients in prospective trials should be set up in advance. By informed consent the patient may control and contribute to the adequate handling of his/her tumor biopsy material.

Morphology/histopathology

The histomorphologic approach allows the recognition and morphologic characterization of the tumor cells as well as of the cellular composition of the non-neoplastic microenvironment. The potentials and limitations of this approach are best illustrated by the Kiel classification of malignant lymphoma, where the concept of the normal counterparts for lymphoma categorization has been introduced. With few exceptions, the sensitivity of the histomorphology for lymphoma diagnosis and its distinction from reactive lesions is very high. Importantly, the correct morphologic orientation directs the consequent immunohistochemical and molecular genetic testing required for differential diagnosis or support of the morphologic conclusion.

The histopathological approach is to some extent limited by the empirical competence of the investigator, which may vary considerably, since lymphomas are relatively infrequent tumors and very heterogeneous. Therefore, after the primary diagnosis by the local pathologists, a centralized sample review is performed in many countries where experienced hematopathologists can apply the pertinent techniques for lymphoma diagnosis.

The highest levels of specificity using the morphologic approach to distinguish definitive lymphoma entities are reached in HL and certain B cell lymphomas. In classical HL the 'diagnostic' morphology of Reed–Sternberg (RS) cells and mononuclear Hodgkin cells and their variants in an 'appropriate' background of reactive cells and tissue alterations allows the diagnosis. Also, in nodular lymphocyte-predominant HL (NLPHL), the cytology of tumor cells and the characteristic lymphocytic and histiocytic (L&H) cells (now called LP – lymphocyte predominance), surrounded by collars or rosettes of activated lymphoid cells within enlarged, poorly defined nodular structures, is very typical. But even in such cases, a basic immunohistochemical workup for the phenotypic classification of tumor cells is recommended in order to exclude or confirm the diagnosis and to identify rare cases, e.g., morphologically classical HL with a cytotoxic T cell phenotype,[52] or diagnose lymphocyte-rich classical HL or gray zone variants with transition to T cell-rich B cell lymphoma (TCRBCL) in the case of NLPHL.[53,54]

In mature B cell lymphomas, chronic lymphocytic leukemia/small lymphocytic lymphoma (CLL/SLL), MCL, follicular lymphoma (FL), and marginal zone lymphomas (MZL) can be diagnosed by morphology in typical cases.[10,11,19,20,27] However, since these entities may show overlapping histological features and mimics – e.g., marginal zone distribution of CLL mimicking MZL, or MCL and CLL with (pseudo) follicular pattern mimicking FL or a mantle cell distribution, and MCL in situ mimicking reactive hyperplasia[55] (Plate 16, see plate section) – the establishment of the diagnostic immunohistochemical phenotype for each entity is a basic diagnostic prerequisite.

The role of the morphologic approach is less specific in DLBCL, in all peripheral T cell lymphomas, and all precursor neoplasms. Here immunohistochemistry, molecular techniques ranging from B and T cell clonality assays, in situ hybridization (fluorescence in situ hybridization [FISH] and/or EBV-encoded small RNA [EBER]) for cytogenetic alterations, and clinical data are frequently essential for the establishment of a proper diagnosis.

Immunohistochemistry

As mentioned before, immunohistochemistry analysis is a basic requirement for the establishment of lymphoma diagnosis. There are no standard approaches that are internationally agreed with respect to the recommended methods, antibodies, or detection systems. Although the reagents are now widely used all over the world, there are still considerable differences in sensitivity among different laboratories (even among specialized centers, as recently established in the Lunenburg Consortium[56]). Of note, the variation may depend on antibody clone selection, antigen retrieval methods, the detection, amplification, and developing systems using peroxidase or alkaline phosphatase, and the presence or absence of automatization. Nevertheless, as described in a large interlaboratory trial in Germany, despite great differences of staining intensity, the techniques

used for detection did only marginally influence the diagnostic result, which was mainly dependent on the selection of the 'proper' antibodies for a specific diagnostic problem.

Relevant controls are important for the correct evaluation of immunohistochemistry. The staining pattern of the relevant normal cells within all sections represents a sufficient internal control for the vast majority of the antibodies. External controls are indispensable when the relevant molecule is not present in the normal tissue, e.g., ALK1[57,58] or antibodies detecting infectious agents, or latent nuclear antigen (LNA) of HHV-8 or latent membrane protein 1 (LMP1) of EBV. 'False-negative' results in these conditions cannot be controlled directly as they may be due to tissue processing artifacts and can only be avoided when supplementary tests with higher sensitivity, e.g., EBER-hybridization for the detection of EBV, are available.

An economic use of antibodies in diagnostic immunohistochemistry is an important factor in any pathological laboratory. Costs cannot be requested for reactions that are not necessary or not essentially indicated for the diagnostic conclusion. The detailed immunophenotype of the different lymphoma entities is described in the relevant chapters of this book. There is no general agreement on a common primary panel of antibodies. However, certain antibodies (e.g., CD20, CD5, CD30, CD23, CD30, and Ki-67) in our experience are useful to define therapeutically relevant decisions in the majority of cases and allow an economically adequate decision on further diagnostic tests.

In a first approach, the distribution of T and B cells is documented by the detection of **CD20** and **CD5**. Abnormal distribution and infiltration of lymphoid tissue is easily detected. In the case of B cell lymphomas, CD20 recognizes a therapeutically relevant target antigen and CD5 allows the judgement on tumor-related coexpression of CD20 and CD5 in CLL/SLL and MCL. **CD23** detects the meshwork of normal or abnormal distributed follicular dendritic cells. In small B cell lymphomas, it accomplishes the phenotype of CLL/SLL, and negativity in a CD5/CD20-coexpressing tumor speaks in favor of MCL. CD23 may also be expressed in a minority of MZL that are CD5 negative. A very important antibody used in almost all of our cases is **Ki-67**. The detection of proliferating cells helps to distinguish tumor cells and reactive cells and detects tumor cells in a reactive background, e.g., in lymphohistiocytic ALCL. Also the lack of proliferation in follicles that are highly proliferating in reactive conditions is a hallmark of follicular lymphoma. Finally, **CD30** is essential for the detection and definition of Hodgkin cells and RS cells and the tumor cells of ALCL. In normal reactive changes of lymphoid tissue, CD30 is found in some extrafollicular B blasts considered to be plasmablasts.

In a second step, the tumor-specific phenotype can be completed, e.g., by staining cyclin D1 in a suspected MCL; CD10, BCL6, and BCL2 in a suspected Burkitt lymphoma or FL; or CD15 and LMP1 and PAX5 in HL. Secretory differentiation of any B cell lymphoma can be proven by kappa and lambda light chain staining. If the coexpression of CD5 and CD20 is difficult to evaluate due to a high T cell background, a CD3 stain as comparison to the distribution of CD5 is helpful. CD79a is usually negative in HL but positive in EBV-driven lymphoproliferative diseases and TCRBCL. CD79a is also longer expressed during secretory plasmacytic differentiation when CD20 physiologically is downregulated or when it is lost after anti-CD20 treatment. The diagnosis and subclassification of peripheral T cell lymphomas is more difficult (see below); cytotoxic markers (TIA1, granzyme B, and perforin), T cell differentiation antigens, CD56, beta F1, and EBER hybridization are important and should be done in specialized laboratories.[59] The most sensitive and specific demonstration of EBV in lymphoid neoplasms, by EBER *in situ* hybridization, is positive in all latency types of the virus; LMP1 can be shown by immunohistochemistry in latency type II and to a lesser extent in latency type III.

Genetic features

The contemporary molecular genetic studies of different cellular compartments of the immune system, as well as of lymphoid neoplasia, promoted significantly our ability to understand, identify, and therefore classify and treat different lymphoma entities. Consequently, certain genetic characteristics are incorporated in the current classification scheme. Many of these represent solitary aberrations, such as chromosomal translocations, deletions, amplifications, and mutations; others designate comprehensive genetic signatures of the tumor, provided by genome-wide SNP and comparative genomic hybridization (CGH) microarray platforms or gene expression and microRNA profiling studies. The latter are currently not applicable in routine practice. However, they have provided important surrogate markers for potential diagnostic and/or prognostic usage.

A detailed overview of lymphoma-associated genetic aberrations and their role in lymphomagenesis and disease progression is provided in Chapters 22–24. The important question to be addressed here is how these genetic abnormalities can be incorporated in the contemporary lymphoma diagnosis and classification.

Methodologically, many of the well-established molecular techniques are laborious and time consuming, and essentially are dependent on the availability of sufficient fresh/frozen biopsy material and therefore are not applicable in routine settings. Both practical and biological considerations favored the use of polymerase chain reaction (PCR), reverse transcription PCR (RT-PCR), and interphase FISH for regular detection of the listed genetic lesions on FFPE tissue.[60–62] These methods are restricted to a targeted detection of an already known abnormality and the presence of each particular lesion has to be approached individually. In these settings the pathologist is confronted with new responsibilities including the selection and setting up of the appropriate molecular diagnostic assay and interpretation of the results that, indeed, require a broad knowledge in the field of molecular genetics. Tissue sampling and histomorphologic composition of the material also affect the individual assay performance. For instance, in paraffin sections, interphase FISH generates various signal patterns[61] depending on the thickness of tissue sections, the size of the cells and nuclei, as well as the design of the FISH assay (segregation versus colocalization). In addition, a focal tissue infiltration pattern and high numbers of the admixed reactive cells decrease the sensitivity of the molecular test and eventually give rise to false-negative results.

It is generally believed that the presence of a clonal (molecular) genetic aberration is indicative for malignancy. However, it was shown that with sensitive molecular tests several lymphoma- and leukemia-specific genetic aberrations[48,49,63] (e.g., *BCL2/IGH*, *CCND1/IGH*) are detectable in peripheral blood and tissue samples of healthy individuals. The biological and clinical implications of this observation are not clear and are discussed in Chapter 22. It may limit the use of such markers, especially in follow-up of minimal residual disease.

Individual (molecular) genetic markers are highly characteristic for certain disease entities but they are not entirely specific[10] and restricted to one single entity. On the other hand, all lymphoma subtypes that are associated with characteristic genetic lesions also include cases lacking them (e.g., BCL2-negative FL, rare cyclin D1-negative MCL, etc.). One possible explanation is that the gene of interest may be deregulated by different genetic mechanisms (e.g., mutation of essential regulatory sites instead of translocation) or epigenetic factors (demethylation or histone acetylation), or even by alterations of different genes that may result in a similar functional effect. Therefore, although certain genetic lesions are strongly associated with a specific lymphoma subtype, in our view they are not an absolute defining criteria but give important information that should be interpreted in context of the other data available (histomorphology, immunophenotype, and clinical presentation).

Antigen receptor molecule (immunoglobulin and T cell receptor) rearrangements are widely used to document the cell lineage and clonality of lymphoid proliferation. In addition, the rearranged immunoglobulin genes, particularly, provide important information on the development stage of the cell of origin, influence of antigen, and tumor progression. **Southern blot** analysis represents a valuable method for the accurate characterization of immunoglobulin and T cell receptor (TCR) gene configuration; however, it requires sufficient fresh or frozen material and is time consuming. For routine purposes it is therefore widely abandoned in favor of PCR,[60,64–66] which is a powerful alternative that provides a rapid and massive amplification and therefore is used preferably. Usually IGH, TCRγ and TCRβ genes are analyzed and less commonly IGκ. The detection of a clonal rearrangement strongly correlates with the diagnosis of malignant lymphoma but is not an absolute proof. **False-positive results** overall are rare and may be due to technical reasons (contamination, poor DNA quality, or a small amount of template) or specified biological conditions.

Dominant B cell or T cell clones can be detected in patients with a compromised immune system, autoimmune disorders, non-neoplastic conditions such as *Helicobacter pylori* gastritis, inflammatory cutaneous disorders, etc. **False-negative results** are a frequent problem because of inadequate DNA template. However, they also result from altered binding of the primers to tumor sequences, related to somatic hypermutation or deletion of the region, usage of gene segments not targeted by the primers, or translocation or inversion, causing loss of or incorrect orientation of target sequences. For instance, in B cell lymphoma with a high degree of somatic hypermutation, as in FL and marginal zone B cell lymphoma (MZBCL) of MALT type, monoclonality is not detectable by PCR in up to 20 percent of the cases. Acute leukemias may show false-negative results due to incomplete V(D)J rearrangements.

Immunoglobulin and TCR rearrangements are usually lineage specific; however, **lineage infidelity** (or lineage promiscuity) may occur in precursor B and T cell neoplasia. In addition, secondary, usually EBV-associated, B cell proliferation arises in some T cell lymphoma (e.g., angioimmunoblastic T cell lymphoma). Furthermore, some B cell lymphomas may show clonally restricted tumor-infiltrating T cells. Therefore in these instances, a simultaneous *IGH* and *TCR* clonal rearrangement may be detected.

Nucleotide sequence analysis of variable regions of rearranged Ig genes[67] provides information on the development stage of the cell of origin, in cases of tumor transformation and relapse, and on the influence of antigen-dependent microheterogeneity (so-called ongoing mutations). Although not routinely tested, IGV gene mutational status can be used as important information to classify B cell lymphoma. Follicular lymphoma, as an example, shows high levels of somatic mutation with ongoing mutation, as their normal counterparts the germinal center B cells. Marginal zone B cell lymphomas show the mutation pattern of the post-germinal center cells, e.g., somatically hypermutated with no evidence of ongoing mutation. Interestingly, B-CLL splits with respect to the mutational status into two separate, clinically relevant subtypes: patients with mutated IgV genes and favorable prognosis, and patients with unmutated IgV genes and poor clinical outcome.[32]

Gene expression profiling (GEP) using high-throughput microarray technologies represents a powerful new approach to the molecular diagnosis of lymphoma.[37,44,68–71] The current diagnostic categories of NHL are associated with characteristic gene expression signatures. In addition, GEP identifies molecularly distinct subgroups of acute leukemias that are indistinguishable with current diagnostic methods. Furthermore, significant novel prognostic factors and recurrent oncogenic events as potential therapeutic targets have been recognized, as discussed in Chapter 24. Although GEP is still not used in routine settings, several initiatives are ongoing to objectively define lymphoproliferative diseases by this approach

Some of the results of GEP may be used as surrogate markers to demonstrate characteristic signatures or prognostic factors in different NHL. For instance, Hans and colleagues,[72] and independently other groups, approached DLBCL subclassification into GCB and non-GCB groups using a set of immunohistochemical markers. The important role of microenvironment factors, detected by GEP, as predictors of survival in FL patients was also consequently addressed by immunohistochemistry. Of note, gene expression at the RNA level does not always correlate with protein expression and, in addition, single markers as well as combinations of markers have a lower performance than GEP, which therefore cannot be simply substituted.

Clinical presentation

The specific clinical presentation with a predominant pattern of anatomical distribution influences to a large extent the correct lymphoma classification. For some entities it represents an essential diagnostic criterion, indicated in the disease nomenclature, e.g., primary mediastinal (thymic) large B cell lymphoma, hepatosplenic T cell lymphoma, T/NK cell lymphoma of nasal type, primary effusion lymphoma, or splenic marginal zone lymphoma.[10] Specific localization in other entities bears important clinical implications, e.g., follicular lymphoma of the duodenum infrequently disseminates; primary cutaneous follicle center lymphoma also has an indolent clinical course.[73] In other lymphoid neoplasms the diagnosis and classification is independent of the primary tumor localization. However, especially in different extranodal organ- or tissue-based lymphomas, the distribution of subtypes of lymphoma entities, such as germinal center type or activated B cell type of DLBCL, may vary considerably with its clinical implications. Therefore, in the WHO classification (2008) these organ-based lymphomas are treated as separate entities or provisional entities and localization of primary lymphoma manifestation has been recognized as a distinctive element of classification. Genetic variants of extranodal marginal zone B cell lymphomas of MALT types are distributed at typical and sometimes almost exclusive primary localizations.

Several disease entities may show alternating clinical presentation as leukemia or solid tumor (lymphoma) although they biologically represent a sole entity. In addition, lymphoma patients occasionally harbor in peripheral blood a variable number of circulating lymphoma cells that are detected only by sensitive molecular techniques or FACS. Therefore the term leukemia is used to characterize a predominant clinical presentation but not to designate a separate disease entity.

CLASSIFICATION OF MAJOR ENTITIES OF LYMPHOPROLIFERATIVE DISORDERS

Table 18.1 compares the three recent classifications of the lymphoid neoplasia. These three classification schemes show very few differences, reflecting the contemporary knowledge in the field. Unlike the previous classifications,

Table 18.1 Comparison of the three recent classifications of the lymphoid neoplasia

The revised European–American classification of lymphoid neoplasms (REAL) (1994)	World Health Organization (WHO) classification of lymphoid neoplasms (2001)	World Health Organization (WHO) classification of lymphoid neoplasms (2008)
B cell neoplasms	**B cell neoplasms**	**B cell neoplasms**
Precursor B cell neoplasm	*Precursor B cell neoplasm*	*Precursor B cell neoplasm*
Precursor B-lymphoblastic leukemia/lymphoma	Precursor B-lymphoblastic leukemia/lymphoma	Precursor B-lymphoblastic leukemia/lymphoma
Peripheral B cell neoplasms	*Mature B cell neoplasms*	*Mature B cell neoplasms*
Chronic lymphocytic leukemia/prolymphocytic leukemia/ lymphocytic lymphoma	Chronic lymphocytic leukemia/lymphocytic lymphoma	Chronic lymphocytic leukemia/lymphocytic lymphoma
	B cell prolymphocytic leukemia	B cell prolymphocytic leukemia
Lymphoplasmacytic lymphoma/immunocytoma	Lymphoplasmacytic lymphoma/Waldenström macroglobulinemia	Lymphoplasmacytic lymphoma
Provisional entity: splenic marginal zone lymphoma (± villous lymphocytes)	Splenic marginal zone lymphoma	Splenic marginal zone lymphoma
Hairy cell leukemia	Hairy cell leukemia	Hairy cell leukemia
		Alpha heavy chain disease
		Gamma heavy chain disease
		Mu heavy chain disease
Plasmacytoma/plasma cell myeloma	Plasma cell myeloma	Plasma cell myeloma
		Heavy and light chain deposition disease
	Solitary plasmacytoma of bone	Solitary plasmacytoma of bone
	Extraosseous plasmacytoma	Extraosseous plasmacytoma
Marginal zone B cell lymphoma, extranodal mucosal-associated lymphoid tissue type (± monocytoid B cells)	Extranodal marginal zone lymphoma of mucosal-associated lymphoid tissue (MALT lymphoma)	Extranodal marginal zone lymphoma of mucosal-associated lymphoid tissue (MALT lymphoma)
Provisional subtype: nodal marginal zone B cell lymphoma (± monocytoid B cells)	Nodal marginal zone B cell lymphoma	Nodal marginal zone B cell lymphoma
		Pediatric marginal zone lymphoma
Follicular center lymphoma, follicular	Follicular lymphoma	Follicular lymphoma
		Pediatric follicular lymphoma
		Primary cutaneous follicle center lymphoma
Provisional cytologic grades I (small cell), II (small and large cell), III (large cell)		
Provisional subtype: diffuse, predominantly small cell type		
Mantle cell lymphoma	Mantle cell lymphoma	Mantle cell lymphoma
Diffuse large B cell lymphoma	Diffuse large B cell lymphoma	Diffuse large B cell lymphoma, unspecified
		Variants :
		Morphologic: centroblastic, immunoblastic, plasmablastic, anaplastic

Molecular subtypes: GCB-like, ABC-like
Immunohistochemical: GCB-like, non-GCB-like, CD5-positive
Primary mediastinal (thymic) large B cell lymphoma
T cell/histiocyte-rich large B cell lymphoma
Intravascular large B cell lymphoma
Primary diffuse large B cell lymphoma of the CNS
Primary cutaneous diffuse large B cell lymphoma, leg type
ALK-positive diffuse large B cell lymphoma
Plasmablastic lymphoma, oral cavity type
Diffuse large B cell lymphoma associated with chronic inflammation
Primary effusion lymphoma
Lymphoma associated with HHV-8-associated multicentric Castleman disease
Burkitt lymphoma/leukemia
B cell lymphoma, with features intermediate between DLBCL and BL
B cell lymphoma, with features intermediate between DLBCL and CHL

B cell proliferations of variable malignant potential
Lymphomatoid granulomatosis
B cell post-transplant lymphoproliferative disorders
Other/non-transplant-associated iatrogenic immunodeficiency-associated B cell LPD
Age-related EBV+ DLBCL

T cell and NK cell neoplasm

Precursor T cell neoplasms
T cell lymphoblastic leukemia/lymphoma
NK cell lymphoblastic leukemia/lymphoma

Mature T cell and NK cell neoplasms
T cell prolymphocytic leukemia

T cell large granular lymphocytic leukemia

Indolent large granular NK cell lymphoproliferative disorder
Aggressive NK cell leukemia
Fulminant EBV+ T cell LPD of childhood
Adult T cell leukemia/lymphoma
Extranodal NK/T cell lymphoma

(Continued)

Subtype: primary mediastinal (thymic) B cell lymphoma
Mediastinal (thymic) large B cell lymphoma

Intravascular large B cell lymphoma

Primary effusion lymphoma

Burkitt lymphoma/leukemia

Burkitt lymphoma
Provisional entity: high-grade B cell lymphoma, Burkitt like

B cell proliferations of uncertain malignant potential
Lymphomatoid granulomatosis
Post-transplant lymphoproliferative disorder, polymorphic

T cell and putative NK cell neoplasm

Precursor T cell neoplasms
Precursor T lymphoblastic leukemia/lymphoma
Blastic NK cell lymphoma

Peripheral T cell and NK cell neoplasms
T cell chronic lymphocytic leukemia/prolymphocytic leukemia
Large granular lymphocyte leukemia: T cell type, NK cell type

Aggressive NK cell leukemia

Adult T cell leukemia/lymphoma
Angiocentric lymphoma

Table 18.1 Continued

The revised European-American classification of lymphoid neoplasms (REAL) (1994)	World Health Organization (WHO) classification of lymphoid neoplasms (2001)	World Health Organization (WHO) classification of lymphoid neoplasms (2008)
Intestinal T cell lymphoma (± enteropathy-associated)	Enteropathy-type T cell lymphoma	Enteropathy-associated T cell lymphoma
Provisional subtypes: hepatosplenic γδ T cell lymphoma	Hepatosplenic T cell lymphoma	Hepatosplenic T cell lymphoma
Provisional subtypes: subcutaneous panniculitis-like T cell lymphoma	Subcutaneous panniculitis-like T cell lymphoma	Subcutaneous panniculitis-like T cell lymphoma
Mycosis fungoides/Sézary syndrome	Mycosis fungoides	Mycosis fungoides
	Sézary syndrome	Sézary syndrome
	Primary cutaneous anaplastic large cell lymphoma	Primary cutaneous aggressive epidermotropic CD8-positive cytotoxic T cell lymphoma
		Cutaneous gamma–delta T cell lymphoma
		Primary cutaneous small/medium CD4-positive T cell lymphoma (provisional)
Peripheral T cell lymphoma, unspecified	Peripheral T cell lymphoma, unspecified	Peripheral T cell lymphoma, unspecified
Provisional cytologic categories: medium sized cell, mixed medium sized and large cell, large cell, lymphoepithelioid cell		Variants: follicular T cell lymphoma, lymphoepithelioid PTCL (Lennert)
Angioimmunoblastic T cell lymphoma	Angioimmunoblastic T cell lymphoma	Angioimmunoblastic T cell lymphoma
Anaplastic large cell lymphoma, CD30+, T and null cell type	Anaplastic large cell lymphoma	Anaplastic large cell lymphoma (ALCL), ALK positive
Provisional entity: anaplastic large cell lymphoma, Hodgkin like		Anaplastic large cell lymphoma (ALCL), ALK negative
T cell proliferation of uncertain malignant potential	**T cell proliferation of uncertain malignant potential**	**T cell proliferation of variable malignant potential**
		Cutaneous CD30+ LPD
Lymphomatoid papulosis	Lymphomatoid papulosis	Lymphomatoid papulosis
		Primary cutaneous anaplastic large cell lymphoma
		T cell PTLD
Hodgkin disease	**Hodgkin lymphoma**	**Hodgkin lymphoma**
Lymphocyte predominance	Nodular lymphocyte-predominant Hodgkin lymphoma	Nodular lymphocyte-predominant Hodgkin lymphoma
Classical Hodgkin disease	*Classical Hodgkin lymphoma*	*Classical Hodgkin lymphoma*
Nodular sclerosis	Nodular sclerosis classical Hodgkin lymphoma	Nodular sclerosis classical Hodgkin lymphoma
Provisional entity: lymphocyte-rich classical Hodgkin disease	Lymphocyte-rich classical Hodgkin lymphoma	Lymphocyte-rich classical Hodgkin lymphoma
Mixed cellularity	Mixed cellularity classical Hodgkin lymphoma	Mixed cellularity classical Hodgkin lymphoma
Lymphocyte depletion	Lymphocyte-depleted classical Hodgkin lymphoma	Lymphocyte-depleted classical Hodgkin lymphoma

The table compares the three recent classifications of the lymphoid neoplasia. These three classification schemes show very few differences, reflecting the contemporary knowledge in the field. In contrast to the previous classifications, they include all lymphoid neoplasms: Hodgkin disease, non-Hodgkin lymphomas, lymphoid leukemias, and plasma cell tumors.

GCB, germinal center B cell; ABC, activated B cell; ALK, anaplastic lymphoma kinase; HHV-8, human herpes virus 8; DLBCL, diffuse large B cell lymphoma; BL, Burkitt lymphoma; CHL, classical Hodgkin lymphoma; LPD, lymphoproliferative disorder; EBV, Epstein–Barr virus; NK, natural killer; PTCL, peripheral T cell lymphoma; PTLD, post-transplant lymphoproliferative disorder.

they include all lymphoid neoplasms: Hodgkin disease, non-Hodgkin lymphomas, lymphoid leukemias, and plasma cell tumors.

Precursor neoplasms

The classification of hematopoietic neoplasias reached consensus on the issue that precursor lymphoblastic leukemia and lymphoma biologically represent one disease entity and both terms can be used arbitrarily reflecting the predominant clinical presentation.[10] Depending on the early lineage commitment of the tumor cells, B-lymphoblastic leukemia/lymphoma (B-ALL), T-lymphoblastic leukemia/lymphoma (T-ALL), and NK-lymphoblastic leukemia/lymphoma are recognized. T-lymphoblastic neoplasms clinically present more frequently as a tumor mass, which commonly involves the anterior mediastinum and the thymus, and morphologically is composed from small to medium-sized cells with irregular, convoluted nuclei. Immunophenotype is needed to identify cell of origin and for differential diagnosis from other tumors. The tumor cells express CD10 and terminal deoxynucleotidyl transferase (TdT); B cell tumors express CD79a, PAX-5, and CD20 in a varying proportion of the cases. The T cell precursor phenotype is defined by cytoplasmic expression of CD3, frequent positivity for CD7, and coexpression of CD4 and CD8 and CD1a. Antigen receptor rearrangement studies are not reliable for lineage determination, due to the marked lineage infidelity of these neoplasms. Both T- and B-lymphoblastic leukemia/lymphoma are associated with various recurrent genetic lesions that should be identified when possible since they define different prognostic groups and facilitate stratification of the therapy.[74] B-ALL associated with particular genetic alterations – e.g., t(9;22), t(v;11q23), t(12;21), hyperdiploidy, hypodiploidy, t(5;14), and t(1;19) – are defined in the WHO classification (2008) as separate entities based partially on a specific clinical presentation and outcome and partially on gene profiling studies. Further genetic aberrations, for instance t(17;19) and *AML1* gene amplification, have important prognostic implication. Similarly, in T-ALL various genetic alterations, most frequently affecting TCR loci but also transcriptional factors such as HOX11 and HOX11L2, are recurrently identified. Activating mutations of *NOTCH1* gene are detected in approximately 50 percent of T-ALL patients, suggesting a possible therapeutic implication of *NOTCH1* pathway inhibitors. T-ALL-associated genetic alterations target key factors involved in early T cell development and leukemogenesis and bear prognostic implication; however, to date there are insufficient data to separate them into separate entities, in contrast to the situation with B-ALL.

Mature B cell lymphoma

Mature B cell lymphoma represents a heterogeneous group of common lymphoid neoplasias, with nodal and extranodal presentation, deriving from mature, naïve (pre-germinal center), germinal center, and post-germinal center B cells. Morphologically, two major subtypes are recognized: (1) lymphoma composed predominantly of large, blastic cells with high content of mitotic nuclei, frequent apoptosis, and necrosis; and (2) those characterized by tumor cells with small to medium-large mature nuclei and a relatively low proliferation rate. The latter group includes some neoplasias that in general can be easily recognized based on cytomorphology and architecture, for instance follicular lymphoma or chronic lymphocytic leukemia with characteristic pseudo-follicular growth pattern.

Among the low-proliferative, small to medium-sized tumor cells, an appropriate immunohistochemical panel of antibodies (pan-B cell marker [CD20], CD5, germinal center marker [CD10, BCL6], and BCL2) defines the CD10/BCL6-positive *follicular lymphoma*, the CD20/CD5-coexpressing neoplasms (which are further distinguished based on morphology and CD23 or cyclin D1 expression as *chronic lymphocytic leukemia* or *mantle cell lymphoma*), and the group of CD5/CD10-negative cases that are represented mainly by the different *marginal zone B cell lymphoma*. Some lymphoma cases can be difficult to distinguish from reactive lesions and in such instances aberrant immunophenotype (e.g., CD20/CD5 or CD10/BCL2 coexpression or light chain restriction) and/or detection of clonal immunoglobulin rearrangement would favor the diagnosis of lymphoma. The accurate diagnosis of different marginal zone B cell lymphoma subtypes (extranodal marginal zone B cell lymphoma, MALT type at a different localization, splenic marginal zone B cell lymphoma, and nodal marginal zone B cell lymphoma) is to a large extent dependent on the availability of appropriate clinical and laboratory data. Of note, these lymphomas frequently harbor a significant clonal plasma cell component that may cause a diagnostic bias between MZBL and lymphoplasmacytic lymphoma. *Waldenström macroglobulinemia* represents more a clinical syndrome characterized by serum IgM paraprotein and consequent hyperviscosity symptoms than a separate disease entity. In the WHO classification (2008), lymphoplasmacytic lymphoma with primary bone marrow involvement without significant nodal or spleen involvement may be recognized as a major representative of Waldenström macroglobulinemia. In addition, 10–15 percent of *multiple myeloma/plasmacytoma* express the pan-B cell-specific marker CD20 and present as a diagnostic pitfall mimicking B cell neoplasia with plasmacytoid differentiation. These tumors characteristically show small mature plasma cell morphology and are frequently associated with a translocation, t(11;14)(q13;q32), resulting in cyclin D1 overexpression.

Diffuse large B cell lymphoma is the prevalent category in the group of morphologically aggressive mature B cell lymphoma and accounts for at least 30 percent of all adult lymphomas. It represents a rather heterogeneous disease with a number of morphologic, immunophenotypic, and molecular variants and diverse clinical presentation and outcome that are discussed in detail in Chapter 35. Briefly, the diagnosis is based on the proliferation of large blastic cells, which harbor a B cell phenotype and display a relatively high proliferation rate. Primary mediastinal (thymic) large B cell lymphoma (PMBCL), intravascular large B cell lymphoma, and primary effusion lymphoma demonstrate specific clinical, morphologic, immunophenotypic, and molecular (genetic) features and are therefore recognized as distinct entities. For instance, PMBCL presents as a large anterior mediastinal tumor, predominantly in female patients in the third or fourth decade, morphologically composed of cohesive cells with abundant pale cytoplasm and distinct immunophenotype (CD45$^+$, CD20$^+$, CD5$^-$, CD10$^-$, CD23$^+$, CD30$^+$ variable), genetic features (amplification 2p23-p25/*REL*, +9p, +X), and specific transcriptional profile. Several former DLBCL variants are listed in the WHO (2008) classification scheme separately (see Table 18.1), which reflects the current diagnostic standard in specialized centers. Unfortunately, and regardless of all current diagnostic technologies, a 'gray zone' of lymphomas that encompasses a spectrum of histomorphologies and genetic features between *Burkitt lymphoma* and DLBCL, and between DLBCL and classical HL, still persists (these lymphomas are specifically discussed in Chapter 21). Since Burkitt lymphoma, DLBCL, and HL patients benefit from different therapeutic regimens, the diagnostic dilemma in this field may have important clinical implications and further studies in this field are therefore urgently needed.

Mature T/natural killer cell lymphoma

Mature T/NK cell lymphoma (Table 18.1) represent a group of clinically aggressive neoplasms, in which the consistent diagnosis and classification is more problematic in comparison to the mature B cell lymphoma due to the complex histomorphology, probably diverse subtypes, and relative low incidence in Western Europe and the United States.[10,11,59] The *morphology is nonspecific* since there is a significant overlap between different lymphoma subtypes and variation within an individual entity. The cellular composition ranges from small to medium-sized, sometimes 'clear' cells with minimal atypia to large anaplastic, occasionally Reed–Sternberg-like, multinucleated giant cells in an inflammatory background of small or activated reactive lymphocytes, including T cell subpopulations, eosinophils and neutrophils, epitheloid histiocytes, plasma cells, and high endothelial venules. Some PTCL show a characteristic proliferation of follicular dendritic cells. The morphologic features are in some cases suggestive of a T cell derivation. However, the cell lineage needs to be confirmed by immunophenotyping and/or TCR gene rearrangement studies. Pan-T cell markers (CD2, CD3, CD5, and CD7) are variably expressed and the aberrant immunophenotype with loss of one or more T cell antigens is in favor of malignancy. Most tumors harbor $\alpha\beta$ TCR, less than 10 percent $\gamma\delta$ TCR, and some, for instance like ALCL, lack the proteins of the

TCR complex, although the TCR is genetically rearranged and can be detected by PCR-based clonality analysis. Natural killer cell lymphomas also lack TCR and harbor only the ε chain of CD3, which can be identified in the cytoplasm with polyclonal anti-CD3 antibodies, in addition to inherent CD56/CD16 expression. A comprehensive immunophenotypic profile is compulsory for appropriate T/NK cell lymphoma subclassification; however, most of the markers show relative low specificity for the different subtypes of PTCL. Of particular value are data on clinical presentation, in respect to which there are four major T/NK cell lymphoma categories: (1) leukemic or disseminated; (2) extranodal; (3) cutaneous; and (4) nodal. With the major exception of the NPM/ALK chromosomal translocation (t(2;5)(p23;q35)) in ALK1-positive ALCL, there are few *recurrent genetic aberrations*. Of interest, recent studies indicated that intestinal (enteropathy-type) T cell lymphoma is associated with recurrent genomic gain in the 9q chromosome and identified two morphologically and genetically distinct subtypes.[75,76]

Hodgkin lymphoma

The current bulk of clinical, morphologic, immunophenotypic, and genetic data enable division of HL into two major groups: classical HL (CHL) comprising around 90–95 percent of all HL cases, and NLPHL in the remaining cases. Although many cardinal differences occur between these two groups, there are also more than expected shared features: for example, B cell-derived origin, loss of B cell identity, and constitutive nuclear factor κB (NF-κB) activation.[41,42,77,78] Moreover, it has become more and more evident that HL and NHL do share interfaces as individual diseases (primary mediastinal B cell lymphomas and CHL) as well as in the cases of composite lymphomas (CHL and CLL, CHL and DLBCL, and NLPHL and TCRBCL),[53,54,79] as discussed in Chapter 21. Of note, the subclassification of CHL into five morphologic subtypes – nodular sclerosis, mixed cellularity, lymphocyte rich, lymphocyte depleted, and unclassifiable – is important for clinical and morphologic recognition, but in the modern therapy era, the prognostic relevance of subclassification is minimized when patients at the same disease stage, and even in comparing all stages, are evaluated. Infrequent cases of CHL show T cell derivation, e.g., expression of cytotoxic molecules and clonally rearranged TCR.[52] The clinical implication of this observation is unclear; however, in some instances their differential diagnosis with ALCL with morphologic HL-like features is equivocal.

Plasmacytoma/multiple myeloma

Plasmacytoma/multiple myeloma (MM) represent neoplasias derived from terminally differentiated plasma cells, most frequently manifested as a multifocal bone marrow tumor, but also as a solitary bone or extramedullary lesion (Table 18.1). The diagnosis is based on the presence of a monotypic plasma cell proliferation, usually in combination with a serum monoclonal paraprotein and organ damage symptoms. The distinction between monoclonal gammopathy of undetermined significance (MGUS) and smoldering plasmacytoma is based more on clinical and laboratory values than histomorphologic criteria. Plasmacytoma/MM may be subclassified in different genetic variants and genetic risk factors. Importantly, most common plasmacytoma/ MM-associated genetic aberrations are identified with similar frequencies in MGUS patients. Extramedullary infiltration may occur in disease progression or as a primary disease with differing clinical implication. On the other hand, the differential diagnosis between (extramedullary) plasmacytoma and mature B cell lymphoma with extreme plasmacytic/secretory differentiation is complex and is based on a characterization of the proliferating cell component.

Lymphoproliferative disorders in immunocompromised patients

Lymphoproliferative disorders arising in immunodeficiency comprise a broad spectrum of pathological and clinical manifestations that are further discussed in Chapters 25 and 26. Various immunodeficiency conditions are associated with higher risk for development of lymphoproliferative disorders, including congenital immunodeficiencies, human immunodeficiency virus (HIV) infection–linked immunodeficiency, or post-transplant or methotrexate-related immunosuppression. Recently, similar disorders were reported in elderly patients without overt immunodeficiency and in a setting of malnutrition.[80] The distinction of separate entities is problematic since these encompass malignant lymphomas (most often of B cell phenotype) and polymorphic polyclonal and monoclonal lymphoproliferative and hyperplastic lesions frequently due to and associated with reactivation of or de novo EBV infection. Clinical manifestations are rather broad with common involvement of the extranodal sites and possibly rapid fatal outcome, progression to overt malignancy, or regression either spontaneously or upon discontinuation or reduction of the immunosuppressive therapy.[81,82]

The diagnosis is based on the availability of adequate clinical information with respect to the type of organ transplantion, type of immunosuppression, timing of the clinical onset, etc., as well as morphology (monomorphic versus polymorphic lesion), immunophenotype, demonstration of EBV infection (EBER in situ hybridization), molecular biological clonality analysis, and molecular genetic data.

Early stages/precursor lesions

The modern diagnostic approaches allow the identification of a number of malignant lymphomas at very early stages of their development and result in the definition of the so-called early stages and 'in situ' lesions[55,83] (Plate 15) in the WHO classification (2008). Good examples include 'in situ' follicular lymphoma with focal involvement of hyperplastic lymphoid follicles of architecturally preserved, reactive lymphoid tissue that can be recognized only by aberrant BCL2 protein expression. In most cases, follow-up data do not show progression to overt follicular lymphoma. It is suspected that in these cases the hyperplasia of t(14;18)-positive cells is equivalent to their occurrence in normal individuals.

On the other hand, 'in situ' mantle cell lymphoma presents with discrete infiltrates in the mantle zones of the reactive lymphoid follicles of morphologically non-neoplastic lymphoid tissue. The clinical and biological significance of this phenomenon is unclear. In some instances it may possibly represent a colonization of the respective normal lymphoid structures by circulating tumor cells from overt malignancy located elsewhere, or it manifests as a real, early lymphoma with high probability of progression to overt MCL. Therefore these possibilities should be indicated in the pathology report.

Other hematopoietic neoplasms, e.g., CLL and MM, are associated with defined **precursor conditions**: monoclonal B cell lymphocytosis (MBL) and MGUS,[84] respectively. These precursor conditions present in 3–5 percent of the general adult population 50 years of age or older, the vast majority of which never develop clinically overt malignancy. Long-term follow-up data from the Mayo Clinic indicate an average risk of progression to MM of approximately 1 percent per year in MGUS patients, depending on the size and the type of monoclonal protein and serum free light chain ratio. For instance, MGUS patients with monoclonal protein >15 g/L of non-IgG isotype and abnormal serum free kappa/lambda ratio had an up to 60 percent risk of developing MM in a 20-year period. In contrast, the risk of MM progression in the 20-year period is approximately 5 percent in MGUS patients with <15 g/L monoclonal protein, an IgG isotype, and lack of abnormal serum light chain ratio. While it is generally accepted that MBL confers increased probability of development of CLL, the precise degree of risk and the risk factors are unknown.

KEY POINTS

- Classification of the malignant lymphoma represents a list of disease entities, recognized by a panel of internationally accepted criteria.
- The relative impact of the defining criteria (e.g. morphology, immunophenotype, genetic, clinical presentation and course) varies significantly between different disease entities.
- Classification of the malignant lymphoma, in particular the definition of different disease entities, reflects the current knowledge in the field, and therefore represents a dynamic process.

REFERENCES

● = Key primary paper
◆ = Major review article

1. Virchow R. Morgagni und der anatomische Gedanke. *Berl Klin Wochenschr* 1894; **31**: 345–50.

2. Morgangni GB. *De sedibus et causibus morborum.* Venice, 1761.

3. Lennert K. *Malignant lymphoma others than Hodgkin's disease.* New York: Springer-Verlag, 1978.

4. Stansfeld AG, Diebold J, Noel H *et al.* Updated Kiel classification for lymphomas. *Lancet* 1988; **1**: 292–3.

5. Hodgkin T. On some morbid appearances of the absorbent glands and spleen. *Medico-Chirurgical Transactions* 1832; **17**: 68–114.

6. Burkitt D. A sarcoma involving the jaws in African children. *Br J Surg* 1958; **46**: 218–23.

7. Sternberg C. Über eine eigenartige unter dem Bilde der Pseudoleukämie verlaufende Tuberculose des lymphatischen Apparates. *Zeitschr Heilk* 1898; **19**: 21–90.

8. Brill NE, Baehr G, Rosenthal N. Generalized giant lymph follicle hyperplasia of lymph nodes and spleen; a hitherto undescribed type. *JAMA* 1925; **84**: 668–71.

9. National Cancer Institute sponsored study of classifications of non-Hodgkin's lymphomas: summary and description of a working formulation for clinical usage. The Non-Hodgkin's Lymphoma Pathologic Classification Project. *Cancer* 1982; **49**: 2112–35.

10. Jaffe ES, Harris NL, Stein H, Vardiman JW. *Pathology and genetics of tumours of haematopoietic and lymphoid tissues.* Lyon, France: IARC Press, 2001.

11. Knowles DM. *Neoplastic hematopathology*, 2nd Edn. Philadelphia, PA: Lippincott Williams & Wilkins, 2001.

12. Weinberg OK, Ai WZ, Mariappan MR *et al.* 'Minor' BCL2 breakpoints in follicular lymphoma: frequency and correlation with grade and disease presentation in 236 cases. *J Mol Diagn* 2007; **9**: 530–7.

13. Bea S, Zettl A, Wright G *et al.* Diffuse large B-cell lymphoma subgroups have distinct genetic profiles that influence tumor biology and improve gene-expression-based survival prediction. *Blood* 2005; **106**: 3183–90.

14. Du MQ, Bacon CM, Isaacson PG. Kaposi sarcoma-associated herpesvirus/human herpesvirus 8 and lymphoproliferative disorders. *J Clin Pathol* 2007; **60**: 1350–7.

15. Farinha P, Gascoyne RD. Molecular pathogenesis of mucosa-associated lymphoid tissue lymphoma. *J Clin Oncol* 2005; **23**: 6370–8.

16. Kutok JL, Wang F. Spectrum of Epstein-Barr virus-associated diseases. *Annu Rev Pathol* 2006; **1**: 375–404.

17. Pagano JS, Blaser M, Buendia MA *et al.* Infectious agents and cancer: criteria for a causal relation. *Semin Cancer Biol* 2004; **14**: 453–71.

18. Sagaert X, De Wolf-Peeters C, Noels H, Beans M. The pathogenesis of MALT lymphomas: where do we stand? *Leukemia* 2007; **21**: 389–96.

19. Harris NL, Jaffe ES, Stein H *et al.* A revised European-American classification of lymphoid neoplasms: a proposal from the International Lymphoma Study Group. *Blood* 1994; **84**: 1361–92.

20. Harris NL, Jaffe ES, Diebold J *et al.* World Health Organization classification of neoplastic diseases of the hematopoietic and lymphoid tissues: report of the Clinical Advisory Committee meeting-Airlie House, Virginia, November 1997. *J Clin Oncol* 1999; **17**: 3835–49.

21. Bohrod MG. What is a pathologic diagnosis? A prelude to computer diagnosis. *Pathol Annu* 1971; **6**: 197–208.

22. Rosenwald A, Wright G, Leroy K *et al.* Molecular diagnosis of primary mediastinal B cell lymphoma identifies a clinically favorable subgroup of diffuse large B cell lymphoma related to Hodgkin lymphoma. *J Exp Med* 2003; **198**: 851–62.

23. Petrella T, Comeau MR, Maynadie M *et al.* 'Agranular CD4+ CD56+ hematodermic neoplasm' (blastic NK-cell lymphoma) originates from a population of CD56+ precursor cells related to plasmacytoid monocytes. *Am J Surg Pathol* 2002; **26**: 852–62.

24. Herling M, Jones D. CD4+/CD56+ hematodermic tumor: the features of an evolving entity and its relationship to dendritic cells. *Am J Clin Pathol* 2007; **127**: 687–700.

25. A predictive model for aggressive non-Hodgkin's lymphoma. The International Non-Hodgkin's Lymphoma Prognostic Factors Project. *N Engl J Med* 1993; **329**: 987–94.

26. Solal-Celigny P, Roy P, Colombat P *et al.* Follicular lymphoma international prognostic index. *Blood* 2004; **104**: 1258–65.

27. A clinical evaluation of the International Lymphoma Study Group classification of non-Hodgkin's lymphoma. The Non-Hodgkin's Lymphoma Classification Project. *Blood* 1997; **89**: 3909–18.

28. Armitage JO, Weisenburger DD. New approach to classifying non-Hodgkin's lymphomas: clinical features of the major histologic subtypes. Non-Hodgkin's Lymphoma Classification Project. *J Clin Oncol* 1998; **16**: 2780–95.

29. Katzenberger T, Petzoldt C, Holler S *et al.* The Ki67 proliferation index is a quantitative indicator of clinical risk in mantle cell lymphoma. *Blood* 2006; **107**: 3407.

30. Rosenwald A, Wright G, Wiestner A *et al.* The proliferation gene expression signature is a quantitative integrator of oncogenic events that predicts survival in mantle cell lymphoma. *Cancer Cell* 2003; **3**: 185–97.

31. Dohner H, Stilgenbauer S, Dohner K *et al.* Chromosome aberrations in B-cell chronic lymphocytic leukemia: reassessment based on molecular cytogenetic analysis. *J Mol Med* 1999; **77**: 266–81.

32. Hamblin TJ, Davis Z, Gardiner A *et al.* Unmutated Ig V(H) genes are associated with a more aggressive form of chronic lymphocytic leukemia. *Blood* 1999; **94**: 1848–54.

33. Alizadeh AA, Eisen MB, Davis RE *et al.* Distinct types of diffuse large B-cell lymphoma identified by gene expression profiling. *Nature* 2000; **403**: 503–11.

34. Dave SS, Wright G, Tan B *et al.* Prediction of survival in follicular lymphoma based on molecular features of tumor-infiltrating immune cells. *N Engl J Med* 2004; **351**: 2159–69.

35. Lossos IS, Czerwinski DK, Alizadeh AA *et al.* Prediction of survival in diffuse large-B-cell lymphoma based on the expression of six genes. *N Engl J Med* 2004; **350**: 1828–37.

36. Rosenwald A, Wright G, Chan WC *et al.* The use of molecular profiling to predict survival after chemotherapy for diffuse large-B-cell lymphoma. *N Engl J Med* 2002; **346**: 1937–47.

37. Wright G, Tan B, Rosenwald A *et al.* A gene expression-based method to diagnose clinically distinct subgroups of diffuse large B cell lymphoma. *Proc Natl Acad Sci U S A* 2003; **100**: 9991–6.

38. Nyman H, Adde M, Karjalainen-Lindsberg ML *et al.* Prognostic impact of immunohistochemically defined germinal center phenotype in diffuse large B-cell lymphoma patients treated with immunochemotherapy. *Blood* 2007; **109**: 4930–5.

39. Wilson WH, Dunleavy K, Pittaluga S *et al.* Phase II study of dose-adjusted EPOCH and rituximab in untreated diffuse large B-cell lymphoma with analysis of germinal center and post-germinal center biomarkers. *J Clin Oncol* 2008; **26**: 2717–24.

40. Pasqualucci L, Compagno M, Houldsworth J *et al.* Inactivation of the PRDM1/BLIMP1 gene in diffuse large B cell lymphoma. *J Exp Med* 2006; **203**: 311–17.

41. Kuppers R, Rajewsky K, Zhao M *et al.* Hodgkin disease: Hodgkin and Reed-Sternberg cells picked from histological sections show clonal immunoglobulin gene rearrangements and appear to be derived from B cells at various stages of development. *Proc Natl Acad Sci U S A* 1994; **91**: 10962–6.

42. Kuppers R. Molecular biology of Hodgkin's lymphoma. *Adv Cancer Res* 2002; **84**: 277–312.

43. Grogg KL, Attygalle AD, Macon WR *et al.* Angioimmunoblastic T-cell lymphoma: a neoplasm of germinal-center T-helper cells? *Blood* 2005; **106**: 1501–2.

44. de Leval L, Rickman DS, Thielen C *et al.* The gene expression profile of nodal peripheral T-cell lymphoma demonstrates a molecular link between angioimmunoblastic T-cell lymphoma (AITL) and follicular helper T (TFH) cells. *Blood* 2007; **109**: 4952–63.

45. Rudiger T, Geissinger E, Muller-Hermelink HK *et al.* 'Normal counterparts' of nodal peripheral T-cell lymphoma. *Hematol Oncol* 2006; **24**: 175–80.

46. Geissinger E, Bonzheim I, Krenacs L *et al.* Nodal peripheral T-cell lymphomas correspond to distinct mature T-cell populations. *J Pathol* 2006; **210**: 172–80.

47. Kuppers R, Dalla-Favera R. Mechanisms of chromosomal translocations in B cell lymphomas. *Oncogene* 2001; **20**: 5580–94.

48. Limpens J, de Jong D, van Krieken JH *et al.* Bcl-2/JH rearrangements in benign lymphoid tissues with follicular hyperplasia. *Oncogene* 1991; **6**: 2271–6.

49. Janz S, Potter M, Rabkin CS *et al.* Lymphoma- and leukemia-associated chromosomal translocations in healthy individuals. *Genes Chromosomes Cancer* 2003; **36**: 211–23.

50. Hoglund M, Sehn L, Connors JM *et al.* Identification of cytogenetic subgroups and karyotypic pathways of clonal evolution in follicular lymphomas. *Genes Chromosomes Cancer* 2004; **39**: 195–204.

51. Johansson B, Mertens F, Mitelman F. Cytogenetic evolution patterns in non-Hodgkin's lymphoma. *Blood* 1995; **86**: 3905–14.

52. Muschen M, Rajewsky K, Brauninger A *et al.* Rare occurrence of classical Hodgkin's disease as a T cell lymphoma. *J Exp Med* 2000; **191**: 387–94.

53. Rudiger T, Ott G, Ott MM *et al.* Differential diagnosis between classic Hodgkin's lymphoma, T-cell-rich B-cell lymphoma, and paragranuloma by paraffin immunohistochemistry. *Am J Surg Pathol* 1998; **22**: 1184–91.

54. Rudiger T, Jaffe ES, Delsol G *et al.* Workshop report on Hodgkin's disease and related diseases ('grey zone' lymphoma). *Ann Oncol* 1998; **9**: S31–8.

55. Richard P, Vassallo J, Valmary S *et al.* 'In situ-like' mantle cell lymphoma: a report of two cases. *J Clin Pathol* 2006; **59**: 995–6.

56. de Jong D, Rosenwald A, Chhanabhai M *et al.* Immunohistochemical prognostic markers in diffuse large B-cell lymphoma: validation of tissue microarray as a prerequisite for broad clinical applications – a study from the Lunenburg Lymphoma Biomarker Consortium. *J Clin Oncol* 2007; **25**: 805–12.

57. Mason DY, Pulford KA, Bischof D *et al.* Nucleolar localization of the nucleophosmin-anaplastic lymphoma kinase is not required for malignant transformation. *Cancer Res* 1998; **58**: 1057–62.

58. Pulford K, Lamant L, Morris SW *et al.* Detection of anaplastic lymphoma kinase (ALK) and nucleolar protein nucleophosmin (NPM)-ALK proteins in normal and neoplastic cells with the monoclonal antibody ALK1. *Blood* 1997; **89**: 1394–404.

59. Chan JK. Peripheral T-cell and NK-cell neoplasms: an integrated approach to diagnosis. *Mod Pathol* 1999; **12**: 177–99.

60. van Krieken JH, Langerak AW, Macintyre EA *et al.* Improved reliability of lymphoma diagnostics via PCR-based clonality testing: report of the BIOMED-2 Concerted Action BHM4-CT98-3936. *Leukemia* 2007; **21**: 201–6.

61. Haralambieva E, Kleiverda K, Mason DY *et al.* Detection of three common translocation breakpoints in non-Hodgkin's lymphomas by fluorescence in situ hybridization on routine paraffin-embedded tissue sections. *J Pathol* 2002; **198**: 163–70.

62. Belaud-Rotureau MA, Parrens M, Dubus P *et al.* A comparative analysis of FISH, RT-PCR, PCR, and immunohistochemistry for the diagnosis of mantle cell lymphomas. *Mod Pathol* 2002; **15**: 517–25.

63. Hirt C, Schuler F, Dolken L *et al.* Low prevalence of circulating t(11;14)(q13;q32)-positive cells in the peripheral blood of healthy individuals as detected by real-time quantitative PCR. *Blood* 2004; **104**: 904–5.

64. Bruggemann M, White H, Gaulard P *et al.* Powerful strategy for polymerase chain reaction-based clonality assessment in T-cell malignancies Report of the BIOMED-2 Concerted Action BHM4 CT98-3936. *Leukemia* 2007; **21**: 215–21.

65. Evans PA, Pott C, Groenen PJ et al. Significantly improved PCR-based clonality testing in B-cell malignancies by use of multiple immunoglobulin gene targets. Report of the BIOMED-2 Concerted Action BHM4-CT98-3936. Leukemia 2007; 21: 207–14.

66. Muller-Hermelink HK, Greiner A. Molecular analysis of human immunoglobulin heavy chain variable genes (IgVH) in normal and malignant B cells. Am J Pathol 1998; 153: 1341–6.

67. Goossens T, Klein U, Kuppers R. Frequent occurrence of deletions and duplications during somatic hypermutation: implications for oncogene translocations and heavy chain disease. Proc Natl Acad Sci U S A 1998; 95: 2463–8.

68. Dave SS, Fu K, Wright GW et al. Molecular diagnosis of Burkitt's lymphoma. N Engl J Med 2006; 354: 2431–42.

69. Hummel M, Bentink S, Berger H et al. A biologic definition of Burkitt's lymphoma from transcriptional and genomic profiling. N Engl J Med 2006; 354: 2419–30.

70. Piccaluga PP, Agostinelli C, Califano A et al. Gene expression analysis of peripheral T cell lymphoma, unspecified, reveals distinct profiles and new potential therapeutic targets. J Clin Invest 2007; 117: 823–34.

71. Thompson MA, Stumph J, Henrickson SE et al. Differential gene expression in anaplastic lymphoma kinase-positive and anaplastic lymphoma kinase-negative anaplastic large cell lymphomas. Hum Pathol 2005; 36: 494–504.

72. Hans CP, Weisenburger DD, Greiner TC et al. Confirmation of the molecular classification of diffuse large B-cell lymphoma by immunohistochemistry using a tissue microarray. Blood 2004; 103: 275–82.

73. Burg G, Kempf W, Cozzio A et al. WHO/EORTC classification of cutaneous lymphomas 2005: histological and molecular aspects. J Cutan Pathol 2005; 32: 647–74.

74. Armstrong SA, Look AT. Molecular genetics of acute lymphoblastic leukemia. J Clin Oncol 2005; 23: 6306–15.

75. Deleeuw RJ, Zettl A, Klinker E et al. Whole-genome analysis and HLA genotyping of enteropathy-type T-cell lymphoma reveals 2 distinct lymphoma subtypes. Gastroenterology 2007; 132: 1902–11.

76. Zettl A, deLeeuw R, Haralambieva E, Mueller-Hermelink HK. et al. Enteropathy-type T-cell lymphoma. Am J Clin Pathol 2007; 127: 701–6.

77. Marafioti T, Hummel M, Anagnostopoulos I et al. Origin of nodular lymphocyte-predominant Hodgkin's disease from a clonal expansion of highly mutated germinal-center B cells. N Engl J Med 1997; 337: 453–8.

78. Mason DY, Banks PM, Chan J et al. Nodular lymphocyte predominance Hodgkin's disease. A distinct clinicopathological entity. Am J Surg Pathol 1994; 18: 526–30.

79. Boudova L, Torlakovic E, Delabie J et al. Nodular lymphocyte-predominant Hodgkin lymphoma with nodules resembling T-cell/histiocyte-rich B-cell lymphoma: differential diagnosis between nodular lymphocyte-predominant Hodgkin lymphoma and T-cell/histiocyte-rich B-cell lymphoma. Blood 2003; 102: 3753–8.

80. Shimoyama Y, Yamamoto K, Asano N et al. Age-related Epstein-Barr virus-associated B-cell lymphoproliferative disorders: special references to lymphomas surrounding this newly recognized clinicopathologic disease. Cancer Sci 2008; 99: 1085–91.

81. Knowles DM, Cesarman E, Chadburn A et al. Correlative morphologic and molecular genetic analysis demonstrates three distinct categories of posttransplantation lymphoproliferative disorders. Blood 1995; 85: 552–65.

82. Knowles DM. Immunodeficiency-associated lymphoproliferative disorders. Mod Pathol 1999; 12: 200–17.

83. Cong P, Raffeld M, Teruya-Feldstein J et al. In situ localization of follicular lymphoma: description and analysis by laser capture microdissection. Blood 2002; 99: 3376–82.

84. Landgren O, Kyle RA. Multiple myeloma, chronic lymphocytic leukaemia and associated precursor diseases. Br J Haematol 2007; 139: 717–23.

19

Borderlands between pathological entities: composite lymphomas

ELAINE S JAFFE AND WYNDHAM H WILSON

INTRODUCTION

Considerable progress has been made regarding the origin of the neoplastic cell in the lymphomas, both classical Hodgkin lymphoma (CHL) and the non-Hodgkin lymphomas (NHL). Regarding the Reed–Sternberg cell (RS) and mononuclear Hodgkin (H) cells, the neoplastic cells of CHL, recent evidence has indicated a B cell derivation in all or nearly all cases. If CHL is derived from an altered B lymphocyte, it is not surprising that areas of overlap with B cell NHL should occur both biologically and clinically (Fig. 19.1).[1] The HRS cell is a crippled B cell, incapable of immunoglobulin secretion.[2] Many other aspects of the B cell program are also suppressed in HRS cells.[3–5] The biological and molecular events leading to this state are complex, and not fully resolved.[6,7] These events may occur in the context of a relatively normal immune system as seen in most patients with CHL, or in the setting of immunodeficiency.[8–12] In addition, cells resembling RS cells and variants may be observed disease states not meeting all diagnostic criteria for CHL, and may represent early steps in the transformation to CHL.[11,13] The study of lymphomas at the interface of CHL and NHL may provide insight into the pathogenesis of *de novo* CHL, and the molecular and cellular events distinguishing it from NHL.

The term **gray zone lymphoma** has been used to describe a process at the histological, and also biological, interface between various types of lymphoma. It has been used in the context of CHL and NHL, and also nodular lymphocyte-predominant Hodgkin lymphoma (NLPHL) and B cell lymphomas, most commonly T cell/histiocyte-rich large B cell lymphoma (TCHRLBCL). Similarly, **synchronous lymphomas** of discordant histologies can involve a combination of Hodgkin lymphoma (HL) and NHL. Some of the first **metachronous lymphomas** described involved the late presentation of NHL following CHL (Table 19.1). However, the opposite sequence also occurs. Hodgkin lymphoma and NHL have long been regarded as distinct disease entities based on differences in pathology, immunophenotype, clinical features, and response to therapy. However, recent observations suggest that these disorders may be more closely related than previously thought,

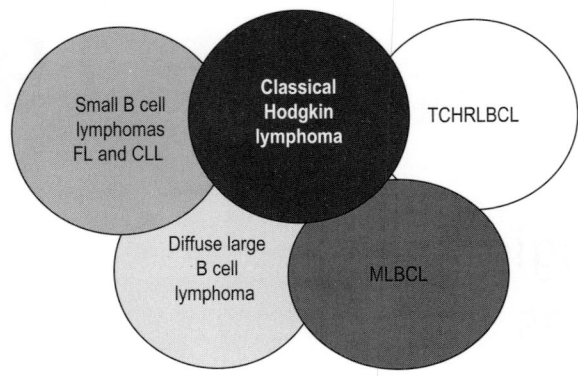

Figure 19.1   Classical Hodgkin lymphoma and other B cell lymphomas: composite lymphomas. Hodgkin lymphoma is derived from an altered B lymphocyte. The precise molecular events that result in the Reed–Sternberg cell are not fully elucidated. However, it is likely that these events can occur *de novo*, in a normal B cell; or secondarily, in a neoplastic B cell. Instances of composite lymphoma have been identified with classical Hodgkin lymphoma and a variety of B cell lymphomas, as indicated above. FL, follicular lymphoma; CLL, chronic lymphocytic leukemia; TCHRLBCL, T cell/histiocyte-rich large B cell lymphoma; MLBCL, mediastinal (thymic) large B cell lymphoma.

Table 19.1   Interrelationship between classical Hodgkin lymphoma and non-Hodgkin lymphomas

	NHL subtypes (%)	Association with EBV
NHL following CHL	Diffuse large B cell (45%)	14% of all B cell subtypes
	Burkitt/high-grade B, NOS (45%)	(Mainly in high grade subtypes)
	Other B cell (10%)	
Composite CHL/NHL	Follicular (45%)	No
	Large B cell (45%)	50% (in both CHL and NHL)
	Other B cell (10%)	No
CHL following NHL*	CLL	90% (in CHL)
	Follicular lymphoma	No
	Large B cell	No
	Mycosis fungoides	Often
	Other PTCL (rare)	Yes

(%) Approximate distribution of associated lymphomas and lymphocytic leukemias based on published data.
*Accurate relative incidence figures for CHL following NHL are not available; only most common associations are shown.
NHL, non-Hodgkin lymphoma; CHL, classical Hodgkin lymphoma; CLL, chronic lymphocytic leukemia; NOS, not otherwise specified; EBV, Epstein–Barr virus; ND, not determined, PTCL, peripheral T cell lymphomas.

and provide insight into the biology of gray zone and synchronous/metachronous lymphomas.

We limit the use of the term gray zone lymphoma to those cases in which there are morphologic, biological, and

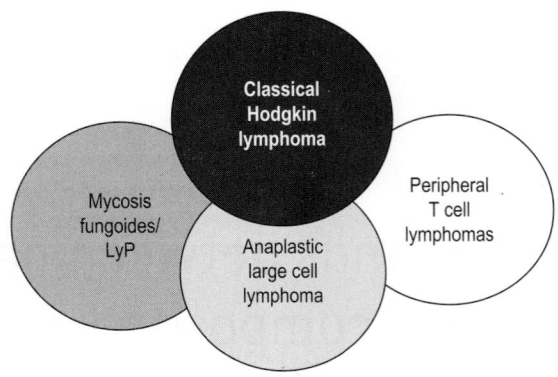

Figure 19.2   Classical Hodgkin lymphoma and non-Hodgkin lymphomas: morphologic gray zones. In contrast to true biological interfaces, morphologic interfaces occur between classical Hodgkin lymphoma and other non-Hodgkin lymphomas. These morphologic interfaces may provide problems in differential diagnosis, but do not reflect an underlying biological relationship. LyP, lymphomatoid papulosis.

clinical features suggesting overlap between HL and NHL.[14,15] For example, there are instances of gray zone lymphoma between both CHL and NLPHL and TCHRL-BCL. A similar but unrelated diagnostic issue involves those cases in which there may be diagnostic uncertainty, but not true biological overlap. The interface between anaplastic large cell lymphoma (ALCL) and CHL may be ambiguous histologically and immunophenotypically, but does not represent a biological gray zone (Fig. 19.2). Other benign and malignant conditions contain Reed–Sternberg-like cells that may mimic CHL. These conditions are best discussed in the context of differential diagnosis, and for the most part will not be covered here, as they do not represent a true biological borderland.

Historically, the term **composite lymphoma** has been used to describe two distinct cytological and architectural patterns of a lymphoma in the same biopsy site or mass.[16] This phenomenon is most often encountered in instances of histological progression, such as transformation of follicular lymphoma to a more aggressive diffuse large B cell lymphoma (DLBCL).[17] A collision of two clonally distinct forms of lymphoma is extremely rare, although well-documented cases have been described.[18] Prior to immunophenotypic and molecular studies identifying the cells of origin of NHL and their clonal relationships, the possibility that composite lymphomas might represent two distinct variants of lymphoma was more often entertained. However, early on, most instances of composite lymphoma were shown to be histological transformation of a low-grade lymphoma to a more high-grade process. This phenomenon is encountered in both B cell and T cell lymphomas. Chronic lymphocytic leukemia (CLL) may be associated with both DLBCL and CHL, both of which are considered forms of Richter syndrome.[19–22] Among the T cell malignancies, mycosis fungoides (MF) may undergo transformation to a large T cell lymphoma.[23]

Table 19.2 Summary of antigen expression in classical Hodgkin lymphoma, T cell histiocyte-rich large B cell lymphoma, and mediastinal large B cell lymphoma

	CD30	CD20	CD79a	CD15	EBV	Bcl-6	MAL
Classical HL	+	−/+	−	+	+/−	−	−/+
TCHRLBCL	−	+	+	−	−/+	+/−	−
MLBCL	−/+	+	−/+	−	−	+/−	+

HL, Hodgkin lymphoma; TCHRLBCL, T cell histiocyte-rich large B cell lymphoma; MLBCL, mediastinal large B cell lymphoma; EBV, Epstein–Barr virus.

Finally, the last type of discordance in morphology and immunophenotype occurs in lymphomas in which the neoplastic cell is capable of differentiating, either to a cell with a closely related lineage, or a cell with a quite distinct cell lineage. Chronic myelogenous leukemia is the classical example of this occurrence, in which a stem cell carrying the *BCR/ABL* translocation can differentiate along several lineages, resulting in the coexistence of neoplastic myeloid and B-lymphoid cells.[24] Among the B cell malignancies, marginal zone B cell lymphomas may show striking plasmacytoid differentiation.[25] A clonal relationship between T cell acute lymphocytic leukemia/lymphoblastic lymphoma and Langerhans cell histiocytosis has been more recently recognized.[26]

PATHOBIOLOGY AND DIAGNOSIS

INTERFACE BETWEEN CLASSICAL HODGKIN LYMPHOMA AND LARGE B CELL LYMPHOMAS

Hodgkin lymphoma and mediastinal large B cell lymphoma

One of the more common gray zone lymphomas, which also may present as a composite lymphoma, involves mediastinal (thymic) large B cell lymphoma (MLBCL) and nodular sclerosis (NS) CHL.[27] Nodular sclerosis CHL and MLBCL share a number of common clinical features. They both show a female predominance, present in young adults – albeit at a slightly older age in MLBCL – and involve the anterior mediastinum, thymus gland, and supraclavicular lymph nodes.[28–30] This form of lymphoma is included in the 2008 World Health Organization (WHO) classification as 'B cell lymphoma, unclassifiable, with features intermediate between diffuse large B cell lymphoma and classical Hodgkin lymphoma.'[31]

In gray zone lymphoma cases the histological and immunophenotypic features are transitional between NSCHL and MLBCL (Table 19.2).[27,32] Clusters of cells akin to lacunar cells or even classical RS cells may be seen in a background resembling MLBCL. In some cases the histology is composite, with some areas resembling NSCHL and other areas showing sheets of large B cells characteristic of MLBCL. The inflammatory background and pattern of sclerosis usually corresponds to the appearance of the neoplastic cells, resembling either NSCHL or MLBCL, respectively. Immunophenotypically, the features also are intermediate. Scattered RS-like cells will be CD30 positive, but CD15 positivity is more inconsistent. Interestingly, the CD30 antigen is often expressed in MLBCL.[33] The majority of the infiltrating cells are usually CD20 positive, sometimes with variable staining intensity. Both NSCHL and MLBCL are negative for immunoglobulin expression, so studies of immunoglobulin are noninformative.[34,35]

Mediastinal large B cell lymphoma has been reported following CHL, but in contrast to most NHLs that typically present ten years or longer after the diagnosis of HL, MLBCL presents early, frequently within one year.[36] This close association suggests a different pathogenesis for secondary MLBCL, compared to the late-occurring NHLs, and raises the likely possibility that these cases are clonally related to the CHL.[37] In two cases analyzed by polymerase chain reaction (PCR) of the immunoglobulin heavy chain (IGH) genes a clonal relationship was shown.[27] Nodular sclerosis CHL and MLBCL also share a number of molecular characteristics, such as *REL* amplification and gains on chromosome 9, suggesting molecular overlap as well.[38,39,40] Immunohistochemical studies of CHL and MLBCL also have shown similarities in the staining patterns for Rel and TRAF1, which differs from those seen in most other DLBCLs, and implicate activation of the nuclear factor κB (NF-κB) pathway in both neoplasms.[41] Recent studies have identified the *MAL* gene as aberrantly expressed in MLBCL, and *MAL* can be expressed in a proportion of mediastinal NSCHL, as well as mediastinal gray zone lymphomas.[27,42] Finally, recent studies from two groups have demonstrated similarities in the gene expression profile between MLBCL and CHL.[43,44]

The immunohistochemical phenotype of gray zone lymphomas is also 'transitional.' CD30 and CD15 are often positive, but in addition both CD20 and CD79a may be expressed in the neoplastic cells. The transcription factors OCT-2 and BOB.1, frequently suppressed in CHL, are usually positive in gray zone lymphomas.[27,32] Nearly all cases are negative for Epstein–Barr virus (EBV), arguing against a role for EBV in the process.

The clinical course in these patients is generally aggressive and many relapse following conventional treatment for CHL.

In addition, relapse often occurred at distant sites, such as kidneys or central nervous system, that are common for MLBCL. An unexpected finding is that most of these cases are seen in males. This fact is surprising since both NSCHL and MLBCL are more common in females than males.

Hodgkin lymphoma and T cell/histiocyte–rich large B cell lymphoma

In recent years, several groups have reported cases that histologically resemble CHL but have an immunophenotype of TCHRLBCL.[45–48] The neoplastic cells are strongly CD20 positive, but negative for CD30 and CD15. These cases may resemble either CHL or more often NLPHL.[48] Epithelial membrane antigen (EMA) is typically expressed in those TCHRLBCL resembling NLPHL, but is negative in many other cases.[48,50]

In a sense current understanding indicates that 'CHL' is in fact a form of TCHRLBCL.[51] In both diseases, the malignant cell is a B lymphocyte, and both have an inflammatory background comprised mostly of T cells.[52] However, they usually have qualitative differences. Classical HL, for example, shows significant variation among the HRS cells in B cell antigen expression and in morphologically borderline cases, in which all neoplastic cells are strongly CD20 positive, the diagnosis of TCHRLBCL is favored.[53,54] Clinically, TCHRLBCL has a more aggressive course than CHL and frequently does not adequately respond to conventional therapy for CHL.[47,49] Interestingly, the expression of B cell antigens by greater than 20 percent of malignant cells in HL was found to be an adverse prognostic factor by the German Hodgkin Study Group, and in more recent studies as well.[55,56] Other immunophenotypic markers may be of value in this differential diagnosis. Positivity for Bcl-6, CD79a, and leukocyte common antigen (LCA) favors TCHRLBCL, while staining for CD30, CD15, or latent membrane protein 1 (LMP-1) favors CHL. A common clonal origin has been identified in rare cases of CHL and TCHRLBCL occurring in the same patient, further suggesting that the distinction between CHL and TCHRLBCL is a biological gray zone.[57,58]

Hodgkin lymphoma and EBV–positive lymphoproliferative disorders

Patients with rheumatologic disorders on long-term methotrexate immunosuppression are at increased risk of developing EBV-positive lymphoproliferative disorders (LPD) that may resemble CHL and NHL.[11,59,60] The etiology is mostly likely from chronic immunosuppression, rather than direct oncogenic effects, since the atypical lymphoproliferations may regress when immunosuppression is withdrawn.[11,59] Similar EBV-positive LPD may be seen in the elderly.[61,62] These cases may present as a spectrum of EBV-positive B cell proliferations ranging from polymorphic B cell lymphomas, as seen in solid organ transplantation, to lymphomas resembling both CHL and DLBCL.[63] The cases of LPD that resemble CHL often occur in soft tissue or other non-nodal sites, whereas cases with more typical CHL features tend to present in lymph nodes. Immunohistochemical studies may help to distinguish typical CHL from LPD; the atypical cells in LPD are usually negative for CD15, although like CHL, CD30 may be positive, with antigenic expression induced by EBV.[64–66] Classical HL can occur rarely following solid organ transplantation, usually after many years, whereas Hodgkin-like LPD occurs earlier in the post-transplantation period.[67] An increased risk of CHL following allogeneic bone marrow transplantation also has been observed and virtually all cases are EBV positive.[68,69]

INTERFACE BETWEEN CLASSICAL HODGKIN LYMPHOMA AND ANAPLASTIC LARGE CELL LYMPHOMA

Classical HL and ALCL share some immunophenotypic features, such as CD30 antigen expression, which led to early speculation that they were related.[70,71] However, subsequent studies showed them to be distinct diseases without true biological or clinical overlap.[72] The neoplastic cells of ALCL usually express one or more T cell-associated antigens and have a cytotoxic phenotype, whereas the malignant cells of HL usually lack cytotoxic antigens such as TIA-1, granzyme B, and perforin.[73,74] One early report suggested that the t(2;5)(p23;q35), characteristic of ALCL, could be detected by a sensitive reverse transcription PCR (RT-PCR) method in some cases of CHL,[75] but this finding could not be confirmed by subsequent genetic or immunophenotypic studies.[76–80]

Hodgkin-related ALCL was initially described as a form of ALCL closely resembling HL.[81,82] The patients were often young males with mediastinal masses who responded poorly to conventional therapy for HL, but appeared to respond to third-generation NHL chemotherapy regimens. It is now apparent that most of these cases are aggressive forms of CHL, probably within the spectrum of grade II NSCHL, or mediastinal gray zone lymphomas.[27,63,77,83–85] The sheeting out of large numbers of CD30-positive cells, often without CD15 positivity, led investigators to favor ALCL. The poor prognosis associated with these cases may be related to the known poorer prognosis of massive mediastinal HL and grade II NSCHL.[86,87]

By contrast, some cases of ALCL histologically resemble NSCHL, having a vaguely nodular growth pattern and areas of fibrosis.[88] However, ALCL usually lacks a prominent inflammatory background of eosinophils, neutrophils, and plasma cells, although histiocytes may be abundant. Moreover, careful immunophenotypic evaluation usually reveals an absence of CD15, expression of EMA, and some T cell-associated antigens. Positivity for the anaplastic lymphoma kinase (ALK) tyrosine kinase may further confirm the diagnosis of ALCL.[80,83] Finally, mediastinal involvement is rare in ALCL, in contrast to its prevalence in NSCHL.

SYNCHRONOUS LYMPHOMAS

Synchronous lymphomas may be defined as the simultaneous occurrence of two lymphoma subtypes within a single patient. These may be further distinguished by presentations within the same anatomic site, termed *composite lymphoma*, and presentations in different sites, termed *discordant lymphoma*. Although the definition of composite lymphoma historically has been broadly applied to the presence of two variants of NHL, in most cases, phenotypic and genotypic studies have indicated that the two histologies are clonally related. For example, DLBCL that occur with follicular lymphomas are considered evidence of histologic progression within the same B cell clone.[17] As such, in recent years, the term composite lymphoma has been more narrowly defined to situations in which the clonal relationship of the two neoplasms is more ambiguous. As with the B cell NHL, an analysis of composite HL and NHL may shed light on the nature of molecular events associated with both malignancies.

Hodgkin and B cell non-Hodgkin lymphomas

Composite lymphoma may be more narrowly defined as the simultaneous occurrence of HL and NHL in the same anatomic site or biopsy specimen.[16,89] Composite HL and NHL most often represents a B cell NHL in association with CHL, usually of the nodular sclerosis or mixed cellularity subtype. The type of B cell NHL involved reflects the incidence of B cell lymphoma subtypes in the population, such that most composite lymphomas involve HL with follicular lymphoma or DLBCL.[57,58,90–92] Uncommonly, other types of B cell lymphoma may be seen in association with CHL, including marginal zone B cell lymphoma and mantle cell lymphoma.[93] The association of CLL with CHL has some distinctive features and will be discussed separately.

Biopsy specimens usually show a segregation of the two histologic patterns within the lymph node. However, in some instances the CHL and NHL may be more intertwined, such as some cases involving follicular lymphoma where the CHL may be found in the interfollicular paracortical regions. Immunohistochemical studies are usually required for the diagnosis of a composite lymphoma. The neoplastic cells of the CHL component should retain the classical phenotype of CHL: CD30 positive, CD15 positive, and negative for LCA and both B cell-associated and T cell-associated antigens. A minority of the RS cells in a composite lymphoma also may be CD20 positive, as seen in other cases of CHL.[53] Studies to show a clonal relationship are difficult to perform, as it is difficult to isolate the RS cells. However, in rare cases employing single-cell microdissection, a clonal relationship has been demonstrated.[57,94]

Epstein–Barr virus has been implicated in the pathogenesis of many cases of CHL, and is most often associated with the mixed cellularity and lymphocyte-depleted subtypes. Epstein–Barr virus also has been investigated in composite lymphomas, and in most cases studied, was concordantly expressed or not in both components.[95] Overall, approximately 33 percent of composite lymphomas are positive for EBV sequences in the neoplastic cells. In all EBV-positive cases, the NHL component was an aggressive B cell lymphoma, either DLBCL or Burkitt-like, whereas all composite follicular lymphoma and CHL cases were EBV negative. Only limited molecular studies have been applied to composite lymphomas. With the advent of techniques permitting the microdissection of individual tumor cells, it is likely that future studies will shed more light on the interrelationship of CHL and NHL in composite lymphomas.

The coexistence of CHL with NLPHL also has been rarely observed. In recent years NLPHL has been considered a distinct entity, separable from CHL in virtually all cases on morphologic, immunophenotypic, and clinical grounds.[96,97] Nodular lymphocyte-predominant HL has a mature B cell phenotype, and contains functional rather than crippled immunoglobulin genes.[98,99] Just as CHL may occur in the setting of a NHL of B cell phenotype, CHL has also been reported in association with rare cases of NLPHL.[100–102] The significance of this association is not fully explored. Rare cases of NLPHL may show expression of either CD15 or CD30 in the neoplastic lymphocytic and histiocytic (L&H) cells, raising the possibility that the published reports represent aberrant phenotypes in NLPHL.

Clinically, composite lymphomas present in an older age group with a median age of 63 years in one study.[90] This clinical presentation is more typical of the underlying NHL, and coincides with the second 'peak' seen in epidemiological studies of HL, in which a bimodal age distribution is seen. The prognosis for patients with composite HL and NHL is most dependent on the histologic subtype of the NHL identified.

A situation closely related to composite lymphoma is discordant lymphomas in which HL and NHL simultaneously present in different anatomic sites.[1] Only a small number of cases have been identified, perhaps because few patients undergo multiple simultaneous diagnostic biopsies at different sites. While the true frequency of discordant HL and NHL is difficult to assess, it nevertheless appears to be a rare phenomenon. The distribution of the NHL subtypes encountered is similar to that of composite lymphoma, with follicular lymphomas and DLBCL being the most frequent.

METACHRONOUS LYMPHOMAS

Patients with a history of lymphoma are at increased risk of developing a second clonally unrelated lymphoma. Although the risk is low over all lymphoma subtypes, it is mostly confined to specific lymphoma subtypes, such as NHL following HL and EBV-positive DLBCL following angioimmunoblastic T cell lymphoma, where the risk is not insignificant.

Non-Hodgkin lymphoma following Hodgkin lymphoma

Krikorian et al. were the first to report an increased incidence of NHL in patients successfully treated for HL with an actuarial risk of 4.4 percent.[103] Generally these are late-occurring events, typically at least 5 years after HL diagnosis, with a reported range of 1–26 years. Their etiology has been postulated to be related to the underlying defects in cell-mediated immunity that persist following treatment of HL, and interestingly their risk appears higher in patients with evidence of underlying immunodeficiency or immune suppression, such as low peripheral blood lymphocyte counts, advanced clinical stage, or systemic symptoms.[36,104,105] Histologically, DLBCL or high-grade B cell lymphomas such as Burkitt-like are most commonly seen, although low-grade lymphomas can also rarely occur, and the histology does not appear to be related to HL subtype or treatment.[36,105,106] Virtually all cases are of B cell phenotype, and most patients present with intraabdominal disease with pathologic and clinical features similar to aggressive B cell lymphomas seen in other immunodeficiency states, such as acquired immune deficiency syndrome (AIDS). Based on these findings, one might expect these secondary lymphomas to be EBV positive, but this is an uncommon finding; EBV encoded small RNA (EBER1) mRNA was only found in 2 of 14 (14 percent) NHL cases by in situ hybridization and two cases of simultaneous HL and DLBCL were also EBV negative.[95] The absence of EBV, however, does not preclude the etiologic role of immune deficiency. Parallels may be drawn with AIDS-related lymphomas where EBV-negative Burkitt lymphomas with MYC oncogene rearrangements are observed.[107] Indeed, a similar pathogenesis may be operative in secondary NHL where Burkitt-like lymphomas are also observed, along with evidence of polyclonal B cell hyperplasia and plasmacytosis, similar to human immunodeficiency virus (HIV)-positive patients. While these findings are of interest, they do not shed light on the clonal relationship between the CHL and secondary NHL. One case study, however, has provided evidence for two distinct B cell clones in the tumors using a single-cell microdissection assay and PCR amplification.[108]

Mediastinal large B cell lymphoma also has been reported following NSCHL, and in contrast to the late-occurring high-grade B cell lymphomas, occurs within a shorter time span following the initial diagnosis of CHL.[36,109] In one recent report, clonal identity by PCR of immunoglobulin heavy chain genes was identified.[27]

Hodgkin lymphoma following non-Hodgkin lymphoma

Compared to the risk of NHL following CHL, the risk of CHL following NHL is rare. Carrato et al. reported five cases occurring 5 to 23 years after a primary diagnosis of NHL.[110] Travis et al. reviewed the experience of the national Surveillance, Epidemiology, and End Results (SEER) Cancer Registry and found CHL to be the most common cancer following NHL, with an observed to expected risk ratio of 4.16:1, even more common than treatment-related leukemias.[111] In a recent study expanding on CHL following NHL, all cases involved a B cell NHL, mostly follicular lymphoma or DLBCL, with presentation at a median patient age of 54 years.[36] The median interval between NHL and CHL was five years, and most patients had received chemotherapy, either alone or in combination with radiation therapy. Nodular sclerosis CHL was the most common histologic subtype in this study, with lymph node presentation in all cases, and most patients responded to treatment. Classical HL has also been reported in association with T cell malignancies, most commonly MF and CLL.

As expected, the immunologic phenotypes of the CHL and NHL were discordant. In one study of Bcl-2 rearrangements investigated by PCR in 32 unselected cases of CHL, only two showed Bcl-2 rearrangements and both occurred in patients with a prior follicular lymphoma.[112] In one case, identical chromosomal breakpoints were identified in the CHL and the follicular lymphoma, suggesting a clonal relationship between the two tumors. However, given the sensitivity of PCR, it is difficult to rule out the presence of small numbers of contaminating follicular lymphoma B cells in the lymph node. In one reported case of CHL following MLBCL, a common IGH gene rearrangement was seen in both tumors.[27] In a separate study that investigated EBV in CHL following NHL, no EBV was found in the RS cells, a somewhat unexpected finding given the role of EBV in CHL following CLL.[95]

Hodgkin lymphoma and chronic lymphocytic leukemia

The development of lymphomas resembling CHL in patients with CLL is well recognized and had been considered a form of Richter transformation.[113,114] It was often assumed that these cases represented pleomorphic NHL resembling CHL rather than true CHL.[20,115,116] More recently, however, several groups have histologically and immunophenotypically documented the association of CHL and CLL.[21,22] Two histologic patterns are observed.[19,117] In one, the CHL is histologically segregated from the CLL, either involving a different lymph node or anatomic site or within a single lymph node.[117,118] In these cases, RS cells and variants are found in the usual cellular milieu of CHL with numerous T lymphocytes, plasma cells, eosinophils, and other inflammatory cells. The RS cells display a typical phenotype for classical HL and are usually EBV positive by in situ hybridization and CD20 is often expressed by some RS cells.

The second pattern, which is more frequently encountered, shows RS cells and variants in a background of otherwise typical CLL without the cellular background of CHL.[22,91] Although the RS cells are surrounded by small lymphocytes, closer inspection using immunohistochemistry shows they are rosetted by T cells, as is typical of CHL, with the surrounding B cells showing a classical CLL phenotype and monoclonality.[22] This process is considered a form of composite lymphoma, since both diseases are present in the same anatomic site. Immunohistochemical studies show a usual phenotype in the RS cells with CD30 and CD15 expression, and variable expression of some B cell antigens. Epstein–Barr virus appears to play a major role in the development of HL in this setting, with over 90 percent of cases studied showing EBV by *in situ* hybridization or staining for LMP-1.[119] While most of the background CLL cells are negative for EBV, a small number of EBV-positive cells are often found. In one study, EBV was identified in a small population of lymphocytes in the underlying CLL several years prior to the development of HL, suggesting EBV infection of CLL B lymphocytes may be an initial step in lymphomagenesis.[19] Rare cases of EBV-negative CHL have been described, indicating other mechanisms of lymphomagenesis.[120]

A recent study examined the clonal relationship between CLL and CHL using microdissection techniques and PCR amplification of *IGH* genes in two cases, and found identical IGH CDRIII sequences in the RS and CLL cells.[121] However, other studies have provided evidence for two distinct clones in the two components.[122,123] In a recent study we have found that the mutational status of the underlying CLL predicts for clonal identity between the two components. All cases of CHL arising in ZAP70-positive (unmutated) CLL were clonally unrelated, whereas CHL arising in ZAP70-negative (mutated) CLL shared clonal identity by PCR (unpublished data).

Clinically, the development of CHL in a patient with CLL usually portends an aggressive clinical course that is associated with advanced and poorly responsive disease.[117,119] The median survival is under two years following the diagnosis of CHL. It is interesting to speculate on the role of immune deficiency in the development of CHL following CLL. Patients with CLL typically display defects in both cellular and humoral immunity and have an increased risk of viral infections. In this regard, it has been suggested that treatment with fludarabine, which leads to profound lymphopenia, may increase the risk of secondary CHL.[124]

Hodgkin lymphoma and T cell lymphomas

Peripheral T cell lymphomas (PTCL) are much less often reported in association with CHL compared to B cell lymphomas.[125] On one hand, the relative risk of secondary CHL may be equivalent in both B and T cell lymphomas but PTCL are much less common, or the biology of PTCL may not predispose to secondary CHL. Alternatively, the difficulty in distinguishing CHL from PTCL may lead to

underreporting. Peripheral T cell lymphoma is associated with a prominent inflammatory background and may contain pleomorphic cells resembling RS cells that might incorrectly be considered a manifestation of the T cell malignancy instead of CHL. However, if the association of CHL with NHL is an indication of the clonal relationship of these disorders, as a B cell origin is likely for most cases of CHL, it is not surprising that CHL is rarely found with T cell lymphomas. In one well-documented case, cytogenetic studies were performed on both the CHL and the associated PTCL and two distinct clones were found.[126]

The most common association is that of CHL and MF with over 20 well-documented reports since 1979.[127–132] In cases of MF and CHL, the diagnosis of MF usually precedes CHL by months to years, supporting the view that some of these cases might represent pleomorphic T cell lymphomas simulating CHL. In other cases, however, the diagnosis of CHL may precede MF or the two disorders may present simultaneously.[127,133–135] Moreover, some reports employing molecular techniques found distinct clonal origins for CHL and MF,[131] showing in one instance a B cell origin for the malignant cells of CHL, and a T cell origin for MF.[132] A true association of MF and CHL is further supported by the diagnosis of CHL in the relatives of patients with MF.[136] In a large epidemiological study of 526 patients with MF or Sézary syndrome, 21 had first-degree relatives with lymphoma or leukemia, of which one-third were CHL. Such observations suggest these disorders may share genetically influenced pathways of oncogenesis.

Cells resembling RS cells both morphologically and immunophenotypically have been reported in a number of T cell lymphoproliferative disorders including MF, lymphomatoid papulosis (LyP), adult T cell leukemia/lymphoma (ATL), and PTCL unspecified.[137–142] Studies of an association between MF, LyP, and CHL are complicated by the existence of common morphologic and immunophenotypic characteristics, such as CD15 and CD30, making it difficult to distinguish CHL from Hodgkin-like lymphoproliferations.[137,143–146] In one case studied with molecular techniques, a common clonal T cell gene rearrangement was found in tissues involved by LyP, MF, and CHL, suggesting that these were all different manifestations of a single neoplastic clone.[147]

A relationship between CHL and MF, LyP, and primary cutaneous ALCL is further complicated by controversy as to whether a T cell form of CHL exists.[143,148] Although it is generally agreed that the vast majority of cases of CHL are of B cell origin, cases of CHL with a T cell immunophenotype and more rarely genotype have been described.[149–151] A T cell form of CHL raises certain conceptual issues, since lineage is generally considered one of the defining features of a disease entity. Do CHL and 'T cell CHL' share common pathogenetic mechanisms, or are the shared similarities more superficial in nature? The existence of a true T cell form of CHL is complicated by the recent description of PTCLs expressing both CD30 and CD15.[152] Two different histologic patterns were observed. In some of the cases there was a sheet-like growth of monomorphic large cells readily distinguished from CHL on morphological grounds. However, in a second subset of the cases the morphology more closely resembled that of CHL. Whether CHL of true T cell derivation truly exists remains to be determined.

Reed–Sternberg-like cells have also been observed in angioimmunoblastic T cell lymphoma and ATL.[139,140] A CHL histologic pattern appears to precede the development of acute ATL in the few published cases, with one report suggesting the RS-like cells were EBV-positive transformed B cells and not part of the neoplastic T cell process. In contrast to the neoplastic T cells, the RS-like cells lacked human T cell lymphotrophic virus 1 (HTLV-I)-associated sequences. A similar basis appears to underlie the RS-like cells in angioimmunoblastic T cell lymphomas.[139] In these cases, the RS-like cells contained EBV sequences and expressed CD20 and did not express T cell antigens. Notably, both ATL and angioimmunoblastic T cell lymphoma are malignancies associated with immune suppression and an increased risk of opportunistic infections, and the presence of EBV-transformed B cell blasts may be secondary to the underlying immunodeficiency. Epstein–Barr virus-positive B cell immunoblastic lymphomas also are seen in this setting.[153]

NODULAR LYMPHOCYTE–PREDOMINANT HODGKIN LYMPHOMA AND DIFFUSE LARGE B CELL LYMPHOMA

An association between NLPHL and DLBCL has been recognized for many years. Miettinen *et al.* first described diffuse DLBCL occurring 4 to 11 years after primary diagnosis of NLPHL in 5 of 51 patients.[102] A lower incidence of this phenomenon was encountered by Hansmann *et al.* in their series of NLPHL.[101] In recent years NLPHL has come to be accepted as distinct from other forms of CHL, and the malignant cells consistently have a B cell phenotype.[97,98,154] Thus, an association with aggressive B cell lymphomas was not unexpected. The long-term risk of DLBCL in a patient with NLPHL is in the range of 2–5 percent.

A close relationship between NLPHL and DLBCL was further suggested by the identification of cases in which both diagnoses were present in the same anatomic site – so-called composite lymphomas.[91,155] Immunophenotypic and genotypic studies have indicated a clonal relationship in all cases studied, whether composite or sequential.[156,157] The clinical significance of this association is ambiguous. In some series the occurrence of a more aggressive component has not necessarily led to a more aggressive clinical course.[125,155] However, other reports have suggested that DLBCL arising in the context of NLPHL behaves in a manner similar to *de novo* DLBCL.[158] Interestingly, the majority of these cases occurs in axillary lymph nodes. The axillary masses can be of large size, indicating that careful sectioning is necessary for accurate diagnosis.

NODULAR LYMPHOCYTE–PREDOMINANT HODGKIN LYMPHOMA AND T CELL/HISTIOCYTE-RICH LARGE B CELL LYMPHOMA

Although NLPHL and TCHRLBCL are considered distinct clinicopathologic entities, these diseases share a number of morphologic and immunophenotypic features, with cells resembling L&H-type cells seen in both conditions.[45,46,48] The neoplastic B cells in both disorders share a common immunophenotype: CD20$^+$, CD79a$^+$, EMA$^{+/-}$, CD15$^-$, CD30$^-$. Diffuse areas can be seen in NLPHL that can be very difficult to distinguish from *de novo* TCHRLBCL, and in particular it is often problematic to distinguish advanced stage NLPHL from TCHRLBCL. Clinically, when disseminated, both diseases have a very similar clinical behavior, and both have a male predominance.[49] Reports of both diseases occurring in the same patient and the existence of cases showing features of both entities have led to the hypothesis that NLPHL and TCHRLBCL may be related biologically.[15] Fan *et al.* reported three patients who developed NLPHL subsequent to DLBCL, one of whom initially presented with TCHRLBCL which recurred 5 years later in the same site as NLPHL.[159] Clonal identity of TCHRLBCL and NLPHL occurring in the same patient also has been reported.[160] In addition, a familial association of NLPHL and TCHRLBCL has been noted both in patients with the autoimmune lymphoproliferative syndrome, and sporadically.[15,161] However, studies comparing NLPHL and TCHRLBCL using comparative genomic hybridization (CGH) have questioned the association between these two entities.[162,163] Franke *et al.* used CGH to show that NLPHL demonstrates characteristic genomic imbalances, but comparison with CGH findings in TCHRLBCL demonstrated fewer genomic imbalances than in NLPHL, challenging the hypothesis that TCHRLBCL represents a progression from NLPHL.[162,163] Although some of the genomic imbalances differed in the two diseases, others were similar (e.g., gains of material in 4q and losses in 19/19p), raising the possibility that both NLPHL and TCHRLBCL might originate from a common precursor cell.

CLINICAL MANAGEMENT

Proper histological classification is fundamental to the selection of appropriate clinical treatment for lymphomas.[164] In some circumstances, however, the histology may bridge two lymphoma diagnoses that would otherwise indicate different treatment approaches. Gray zone lymphomas contain immunophenotypic and histologic features that are either shared or intermediate between two different lymphoma subtypes.[14] For clinical considerations, gray zone lymphomas should be differentiated from composite lymphomas, in which two distinct histological subtypes of lymphoma are seen. Divergent histologies can also simultaneously present in different lymph nodes, known as discordant lymphomas, and may or may not be clonally related. The metachronous occurrence of different lymphoma subtypes raises different biological and clinical issues from gray zone and synchronous lymphomas.[103] These usually arise in patients with known risk factors for a second lymphoma, such as NHL following CHL or CHL in patients with CLL. They may be temporally separated by months to years and treatment decisions are generally directed toward the most recent histology.

Virtually any combination of lymphomas can occur synchronously, and the subtypes will have a variable impact on treatment decisions. Foremost is the need to identify the treatment options for each lymphoma subtype and its stage, and to determine its curative potential and effect on survival. Treatment decisions should generally be guided by maximizing curative potential and the optimal treatment of the more aggressive subtype.

GRAY ZONE LYMPHOMAS

Morphologic gray zone lymphomas, i.e., cases with an indeterminate diagnosis due to ambiguous histologic or immunophenotypic features, do not present a clinical dilemma if the diagnosis can ultimately be resolved. These diagnostic problems can result from an inadequate or small biopsy specimen, or lack of available diagnostic techniques. Such cases, while presenting a diagnostic challenge, do not represent a true biological gray zone. They can, however, present a serious clinical problem if incorrectly diagnosed, such as can occur when distinguishing CHL from ALCL, where treatments are very different. The inclusion of immunophenotype and genetics into modern lymphoma classification systems such as the Revised European–American Lymphoma classification,[165] and its descendent, the World Health Organization system,[63] has reduced classification errors.[28] Nevertheless, some cases continue to present a diagnostic challenge and a diagnosis may be changed following disease evolution and/or larger tissue biopsies.

The impact of misdiagnosis of morphologic gray zone lymphoma was addressed by a study from the Groupe d'Etude des Lymphomes de l'Adulte (GELA) through a retrospective pathology review of 2855 cases entered on the LNH85 lymphoma protocol between 1987 and 1993.[85] Employing contemporary pathological definitions and immunohistochemistry, 77 (2.7 percent) of the cases were reclassified as CHL, with the most common previous diagnosis of ALCL (primarily CHL-like) (38 cases) or PTCL unspecified (25 cases). The reclassification of the ALCL CHL-like cases (30) to CHL reflects the current consensus that these cases represent grade 2 NSCHL.[166] The interface between some cases of CHL and ALCL or PTCL, however, can still present a diagnostic dilemma and requires the appropriate use of immunophenotype and genetic analyses. Clinically, the 5-year event-free survival of these misdiagnosed CHL cases was inferior to that reported by the International Database of Hodgkin Disease, and might suggest the inferior efficacy of NHL regimens over those developed for CHL. This conclusion is far from certain, given the retrospective nature of the study, and could equally likely reflect the poorer prognosis of grade 2 NSCHL.[86]

Biological gray zone lymphomas present a different clinical problem because they do not fit into a known histological subgroup and their rarity has precluded clinical studies.[14] Many of these cases contain biological and histological features intermediate between NSCHL and MLBCL. Treatment recommendations for gray zone lymphomas must be derived from an understanding of their biology and natural history, due to the lack of prospective clinical trials. Clinically, many of these cases present in mediastinal nodes, and as such, the clinical presentation is not particularly helpful in the differential diagnosis of NSCHL and MLBCL.[109,167] A superior vena caval syndrome is more common in MLBCL.

Both the morphology and immunophenotype of these cases may be ambiguous, with extensive sclerosis, scattered lacunar-type and RS-like cells, and focal CD30 positivity. However, the majority of the cells are generally CD20 positive. Clinically, these lymphomas often reach large size in the mediastinum before spreading outside the anatomical region, similar to both NSCHL and MLBCL. They have an aggressive clinical behavior.

Based on these findings, we favor doxorubicin-based regimens developed for aggressive DLBCL, but with the inclusion of rituximab.[168] We have recently had successful experience with the dose-adjusted EPOCH-rituximab regimen (infusional etoposide, vincristine, and doxorubicin with bolus cyclophosphamide, oral prednisone, and pharmacodynamic dose-adjustment plus rituximab) without radiation in mediastinal gray zone lymphoma and MLBCL.[169,170] Among 11 newly diagnosed patients with gray zone lymphoma treated with dose-adjusted-EPOCH-rituximab, ten (91%) achieved complete remission and one partial remission. At a median follow-up time of 4 years, overall survival and progression-free survival are 86 percent and 57 percent, respectively.[171] MACOP-B (methotrexate with leucovorin, doxorubicin, cyclophosphamide, vincristine, prednisone, and bleomycin) is an alternative chemotherapy regimen with activity in MLBCL.[172] However, Zinzani *et al.* reported that 70 percent of cases treated with MACOP-B in their study were persistently gallium avid at the end of chemotherapy and before receiving radiation therapy, compared to only one of eleven (9 percent) patients treated with dose-adjusted EPOCH alone.[169,172] These results suggest that radiation may not be necessary with the dose-adjusted EPOCH-rituximab regimen, although it is unknown if radiation can be avoided with MACOP-B and rituximab. Nonetheless, we have encountered occasional cases of gray zone lymphoma that have weak or variable expression of CD20, and believe such cases would likely benefit from radiation consolidation. Clearly, radiation consolidation should be used in all cases with localized disease in which there is an inadequate response to chemotherapy, as judged by computed tomography and positron emission tomography scans.

The mediastinal gray zone lymphomas serve as a good clinical model from which to base treatment recommendations for other types of gray zone lymphomas. In our experience, the anatomical distribution of other gray zone lymphomas, like those in the mediastinum, reflects the distribution of the associated histological subtypes.[14] Hence, gray zone lymphomas intermediate between CHL and TCHRLBCL tend to occur in peripheral lymph nodes. Similar to the mediastinal gray zone lymphomas, we recommend doxorubicin-based regimens designed for aggressive lymphomas, with the addition of rituximab. The role of radiation consolidation is more uncertain in these lymphomas, and suggests its use be restricted to patients with early stage disease and an inadequate response.

The clinical management of gray zone lymphomas in the setting of chronic immunosuppression presents a different set of complex issues. Clearly, in cases that resemble EBV-positive LPD in the post-transplant setting, the immunosuppression should be withdrawn and the patient observed for spontaneous regression. A similar approach might be followed in patients with lymph node involvement resembling more typical HL or even NHL, since some cases will spontaneously regress. However, if the lesions persist, conventional therapy is recommended and should be guided by the histological diagnosis.

SYNCHRONOUS LYMPHOMAS

Composite or discordant lymphomas raise different biological issues, compared to gray zone lymphomas, but are clinically more straightforward. Transformation of low-grade lymphoma to an aggressive large B cell lymphoma, best illustrated by follicular lymphomas, comprises the majority of composite or discordant lymphomas and reflects the natural history of these diseases.[173,174] In such circumstances, treatment is directed toward controlling the most aggressive lymphoma subtype, and frequently calls for a doxorubicin-based regimen.[175] Less common is the synchronous presentation of lymphoma subtypes that do not appear to share a common histologic root, although many of these cases are clonally related. The principle of treatment is similar to transformed lymphomas but the atypical histologic presentations suggest these tumors are biologically unique. Of course, histologically and clonally unrelated lymphomas do synchronously occur, some of which reflect risk factors associated with the underlying disease process, while others are simply sporadic. An example of the former includes the occurrence of EBV large B cell lymphoma in patients with angioimmunoblastic T cell lymphoma, whereas the latter cases can include virtually any combination of lymphoma subtypes.[153,176,177]

METACHRONOUS LYMPHOMAS

It is well recognized that lymphoma patients are at increased risk of developing a second lymphoma subtype, usually many years after the first presentation.[103] Most common is the late development of NHL following the curative treatment of HL, although the converse occurs as

well.[110,111,178] Clinically, treatment is directed toward the most recent lymphoma, and should entail standard treatment regimens. Anecdotally, however, the clinical outcome of these late lymphomas appears worse than similar histologies that present *de novo*, and raises the question of whether more aggressive treatment should be employed, such as stem cell transplant consolidation. In the absence of controlled trials, clinical decisions must be individualized and based on established clinical and biological precepts.

CONCLUSION

Clearly, the cases of CHL occurring in association with NHL, either as composite lymphomas or as secondary CHL, differ clinically from typical CHL. The patients are elderly, and the clinical behavior of the CHL is usually aggressive, especially in the context of CLL. The question may be posed: Are such cases truly CHL or do they represent a CHL-like transformation induced by EBV or other unknown causes? Until the molecular events that cause CHL are fully elucidated this question cannot be addressed. However, it is important for both the pathologist and clinician to be aware of these transformations, as they do impact on the clinical management of the patient. The study of such cases also may yield clues to the pathogenesis of usual CHL.

Metachronous lymphomas tend to have a worse outcome and a more aggressive clinical course compared to *de novo* presentations. Their biology, however, appears to be distinct from their *de novo* counterparts in many cases and likely accounts for much of the difference in clinical outcome, above and beyond the effects of prior treatment exposure. Biological gray zone lymphomas appear to have a particularly aggressive clinical course and represent a unique biological entity among lymphomas.

KEY POINTS

- Classical HL and NHL occur together with greater frequency than would be expected by chance alone.
- The association of CHL and NHL supports a lymphoid origin for the malignant cell of HL and, given the predominance of B cell NHL, would be consistent with a B cell origin in the majority of cases.
- A clonal relationship may exist between certain forms of CHL and NHL, most commonly follicular lymphoma and DLBCL and CLL.
- The data support the concept that CHL is a B cell malignancy, with the B cell program markedly suppressed, possibly by a virus such as EBV and/or other candidates yet to be identified.
- The late-occurring NHL in patients in remission for CHL are rarely EBV positive and may have a similar pathogenesis to the Burkitt-like lymphomas seen in association with HIV infection.

REFERENCES

● = Key primary paper
◆ = Major review article

1. Jaffe ES, Zarate-Osorno A, Medeiros LJ. The interrelationship of Hodgkin's disease and non-Hodgkin's lymphomas – lessons learned from composite and sequential malignancies. *Semin Diagn Pathol* 1992; **9**: 297–303.

◆2. Kuppers R, Schwering I, Brauninger A *et al.* Biology of Hodgkin's lymphoma. *Ann Oncol* 2002; **13**(Supply 1): 11–8.

●3. Schwering I, Brauninger A, Klein U *et al.* Loss of the B-lineage-specific gene expression program in Hodgkin and Reed-Sternberg cells of Hodgkin lymphoma. *Blood* 2003; **101**: 1505–12.

4. Mathas S, Janz M, Hummel F *et al.* Intrinsic inhibition of transcription factor E2A by HLH proteins ABF-1 and Id2 mediates reprogramming of neoplastic B cells in Hodgkin lymphoma. *Nat Immunol* 2006; **7**: 207–15.

●5. Renne C, Martin-Subero JI, Eickernjager M *et al.* Aberrant expression of ID2, a suppressor of B-cell-specific gene expression, in Hodgkin's lymphoma. *Am J Pathol* 2006; **169**: 655–64.

●6. Kanzler H, Kuppers R, Hansmann ML, Rajewsky K. Hodgkin and Reed-Sternberg cells in Hodgkin's disease represent the outgrowth of a dominant tumor clone derived from (crippled) germinal center B cells. *J Exp Med* 1996; **184**: 1495–505.

●7. Stein H, Marafioti T, Foss HD *et al.* Down-regulation of BOB.1/OBF.1 and Oct2 in classical Hodgkin disease but not in lymphocyte predominant Hodgkin disease correlates with immunoglobulin transcription. *Blood* 2001; **97**: 496–501.

8. Andrieu JM, Roithmann S, Tourani JM *et al.* Hodgkin's disease during HIV1 infection: the French registry experience. French Registry of HIV-associated tumors. *Ann Oncol* 1993; **4**: 635–41.

9. Levine AM. Hodgkin's disease in the setting of human immunodeficiency virus infection. *J Natl Cancer Inst Monogr* 1998; 37–42.

10. Bellas C, Santon A, Manzanal A *et al.* Pathological, immunological, and molecular features of Hodgkin's disease associated with HIV infection. Comparison with ordinary Hodgkin's disease. *Am J Surg Pathol* 1996; **20**: 1520–24.

●11. Kamel OW, Weiss LM, van de Rijn M *et al.* Hodgkin's disease and lymphoproliferations resembling Hodgkin's disease in patients receiving long-term low-dose methotrexate therapy. *Am J Surg Pathol* 1996; **20**: 1279–87.

12. Kumar S, Fend F, Quintanilla-Martinez L *et al.* Epstein-Barr virus-positive primary gastrointestinal Hodgkin's disease: association with inflammatory bowel disease and immunosuppression. *Am J Surg Pathol* 2000; **24**: 66–73.

●13. Poppema S, van Imhoff G, Torensma R, Smith J. Lymphadenopathy morphologically consistent with Hodgkin's disease associated with Epstein-Barr virus infection. *Am J Clin Pathol* 1985; **84**: 385–90.

◆14. Rudiger T, Jaffe ES, Delsol G *et al.* Workshop report on Hodgkin's disease and related diseases ('grey zone' lymphoma). *Ann Oncol* 1998; **9(Suppl 5)**: S31–8.

◆15. Rudiger T, Gascoyne RD, Jaffe ES *et al.* Workshop on the relationship between nodular lymphocyte predominant Hodgkin's lymphoma and T cell/histiocyte-rich B cell lymphoma. *Ann Oncol* 2002; **13**: 44–51.

16. Kim H, Hendrickson R, Dorfman R. Composite lymphoma. *Cancer* 1977; **40**: 959–76.

●17. Sander CA, Yano T, Clark HM *et al.* p53 mutation is associated with progression in follicular lymphomas. *Blood* 1993; **82**: 1994–2004.

●18. Fend F, Quintanilla-Martinez L, Kumar S *et al.* Composite low grade B-cell lymphomas with two immunophenotypically distinct cell populations are true biclonal lymphomas. A molecular analysis using laser capture microdissection. *Am J Pathol* 1999; **154**: 1857–66.

19. Rubin D, Hudnall SD, Aisenberg A *et al.* Richter's transformation of chronic lymphocytic leukemia with Hodgkin's-like cells is associated with Epstein-Barr virus intection. *Mod Pathol* 1994; **7**: 91–8.

20. Foucar K, Rydell RE. Richter's syndrome in chronic lymphocytic leukemia. *Cancer* 1980; **46**: 118–34.

21. Brecher M, Banks P. Hodgkin's disease variant of Richter's syndrome: report of eight cases. *Am J Clin Pathol* 1990; **93**: 333–9.

●22. Williams J, Schned A, Cotelingam JD, Jaffe ES. Chronic lymphocytic leukemia with coexistent Hodgkin's disease: Implications for the origin of the Reed-Sternberg cell. *Am J Surg Pathol* 1991; **15**: 33–42.

●23. Vergier B, de Muret A, Beylot-Barry M *et al.* Transformation of mycosis fungoides: clinicopathological and prognostic features of 45 cases. French Study Group of Cutaneous Lymphomas. *Blood* 2000; **95**: 2212–8.

24. Calabretta B, Perrotti D. The biology of CML blast crisis. *Blood* 2004; **103**: 4010–22.

25. Dogan A, Du M, Koulis A *et al.* Expression of lymphocyte homing receptors and vascular addressins in low-grade gastric B-cell lymphomas of mucosa-associated lymphoid tissue. *Am J Pathol* 1997; **151**: 1361–9.

●26. Feldman AL, Berthold F, Arceci R *et al.* Clonal relationship between precursor T-lymphoblastic leukaemia/lymphoma and Langerhans-cell histiocytosis. *Lancet Oncol* 2005; **6**: 435–7.

●27. Traverse-Glehen A, Pittaluga S, Gaulard P *et al.* Mediastinal gray zone lymphoma: the missing link between classic Hodgkin's lymphoma and mediastinal large B-cell lymphoma. *Am J Surg Pathol* 2005; **29**: 1411–21.

28. The Non-Hodgkin's Lymphoma Classification Project: A clinical evaluation of the International Lymphoma Study Group classification of non-Hodgkin's lymphoma. *Blood* 1997; **89**: 3909–18.

29. Lamarre L, Jacobson J, Aisenberg A, Harris N. Primary large cell lymphoma of the mediastinum. *Am J Surg Pathol* 1989; **13**: 730–39.

30. Moller P, Moldenhauer G, Momburg F *et al.* Mediastinal lymphoma of clear cell type is a tumor corresponding to terminal steps of B cell differentiation. *Blood* 1987; **69**: 1087–95.

31. Swerdlow SH, Campo E, Harris NL *et al. WHO classification of tumours of haematopoietic and lymphoid tissues*, 4th Edn. Lyon, France: International Agency for Research on Cancer; 2008.

32. Garcia JF, Mollejo M, Fraga M *et al.* Large B-cell lymphoma with Hodgkin's features. *Histopathology* 2005; **47**: 101–10.

33. Higgins JP, Warnke RA. CD30 expression is common in mediastinal large B-cell lymphoma. *Am J Clin Pathol* 1999; **112**: 241–7.

34. Kanavaros P, Gaulard P, Charlotte F *et al.* Discordant expression of immunoglobulin and its associated molecule mb-1/CD79a is frequently found in mediastinal large B-cell lymphomas. *Am J Pathol* 1995; **146**: 735–41.

35. Pileri SA, Gaidano G, Zinzani PL *et al.* Primary mediastinal B-cell lymphoma: high frequency of BCL-6 mutations and consistent expression of the transcription factors OCT-2, BOB.1, and PU.1 in the absence of immunoglobulins. *Am J Pathol* 2003; **162**: 243–53.

●36. Zarate OA, Medeiros LJ, Longo DL, Jaffe ES. Non-Hodgkin's lymphomas arising in patients successfully treated for Hodgkin's disease. A clinical, histologic, and immunophenotypic study of 14 cases. *Am J Surg Pathol* 1992; **16**: 885–95.

●37. Addis B, Isaacson P. Large cell lymphoma of the mediastinum: a B-cell tumor of probable thymic origin. *Histopathology* 1986; **10**: 379–90.

◆38. Barth TF, Leithauser F, Moller P. Mediastinal B-cell lymphoma, a lymphoma type with several characteristics unique among diffuse large B-cell lymphomas. *Ann Hematol* 2001; **80**: B49–53.

39. Joos S, Menz CK, Wrobel G *et al.* Classical Hodgkin lymphoma is characterized by recurrent copy number gains of the short arm of chromosome 2. *Blood* 2002; **99**: 1381–7.

40. Schmitz R, Hansmann ML, Bohle V *et al.* TNFAIP3 (A20) is a tumor suppressor gene in Hodgkin lymphoma and primary mediastinal B cell lymphoma. *J Exp Med* 2009; **206**: 981–90.

●41. Rodig SJ, Savage KJ, Nguyen V *et al.* TRAF1 expression and c-Rel activation are useful adjuncts in distinguishing classical Hodgkin lymphoma from a subset of morphologically or immunophenotypically similar lymphomas. *Am J Surg Pathol* 2005; **29**: 196–203.

●42. Copie-Bergman C, Gaulard P, Maouche-Chretien L *et al.* The MAL gene is expressed in primary mediastinal large B-cell lymphoma. *Blood* 1999; **94**: 3567–75.

●43. Rosenwald A, Wright G, Leroy K *et al.* Molecular diagnosis of primary mediastinal B cell lymphoma identifies a clinically favorable subgroup of diffuse large B cell lymphoma related to Hodgkin lymphoma. *J Exp Med* 2003; **198**: 851–62.

●44. Savage KJ, Monti S, Kutok JL *et al.* The molecular signature of mediastinal large B-cell lymphoma differs from that of other diffuse large B-cell lymphomas and shares features with classical Hodgkin lymphoma. *Blood* 2003; **102**: 3871–9.

●45. Chittal S, Brousset P, Voigt J, Delsol G. Large B-cell lymphoma rich in T-cells and simulating Hodgkin's disease. *Histopathology* 1991; **19**: 211–20.

●46. Delabie J, Vandenberghe E, Kennes C *et al.* Histiocyte-rich B-cell lymphoma. A distinct clinicopathologic entity possibly related to lymphocyte predominant Hodgkin's disease, paragranuloma subtype. *Am J Surg Pathol* 1992; **16**: 37–48.

47. McBride JA, Rodriguez J, Luthra R *et al.* T-cell rich B large-cell lymphoma simulating lymphocyte rich Hodgkin's disease. *Am J Surg Pathol* 1996; **20**: 193–201.

●48. Lim MS, Beaty M, Sorbara L *et al.* T-cell/histiocyte-rich large B-cell lymphoma: a heterogeneous entity with derivation from germinal center B cells. *Am J Surg Pathol* 2002; **26**: 1458–66.

●49. Achten R, Verhoef G, Vanuytsel L, De Wolf-Peeters C. T-cell/histiocyte–rich large B-cell lymphoma: a distinct clinicopathologic entity. *J Clin Oncol* 2002; **20**: 1269–77.

●50. Achten R, Verhoef G, Vanuytsel L, De Wolf-Peeters C. Histiocyte-rich, T-cell-rich B-cell lymphoma: a distinct diffuse large B-cell lymphoma subtype showing characteristic morphologic and immunophenotypic features. *Histopathology* 2002; **40**: 31–45.

51. Schwartz RS. Hodgkin's disease–time for a change. *N Engl J Med* 1997; **337**: 495–6.

52. Gruss HJ, Pinto A, Duyster J *et al.* Hodgkin's disease: a tumor with disturbed immunological pathways. *Immunol Today* 1997; **18**: 156–63.

●53. Schmid C, Pan L, Diss T, Tsaacson PG. Expression of B-cell antigens by Hodgkin's and Reed-Sternberg cells. *Am J Pathol* 1991; **139**: 701–7.

54. Zukerberg L, Collins A, Ferry J, Harris, N. Coexpression of CD15 and CD20 by Reed-Sternberg cells in Hodgkin's disease. *Am J Pathol* 1991; **139**: 475–83.

●55. von Wasielewski R, Mengel M, Fischer R *et al.* Classical Hodgkin's disease. Clinical impact of the immunophenotype. *Am J Pathol* 1997; **151**: 1123–30.

56. Portlock CS, Donnelly GB, Qin J *et al.* Adverse prognostic significance of CD20 positive Reed-Sternberg cells in classical Hodgkin's disease. *Br J Haematol* 2004; **125**: 701–8.

57. Brauninger A, Hansmann ML, Strickler JG *et al.* Identification of common germinal-center B-cell precursors in two patients with both Hodgkin's disease and non-Hodgkin's lymphoma. *N Engl J Med* 1999; **340**: 1239–47.

58. Bellan C, Lazzi S, Zazzi M *et al.* Immunoglobulin gene rearrangement analysis in composite Hodgkin disease and large B-cell lymphoma: evidence for receptor revision of immunoglobulin heavy chain variable region genes in

Hodgkin-Reed-Sternberg cells? *Diagn Mol Pathol* 2002; **11**: 2–8.

59. Georgescu L, Quinn GC, Schwartzman S, Paget SA. Lymphoma in patients with rheumatoid arthritis: association with the disease state or methotrexate treatment. *Semin Arthritis Rheum* 1997; **26**: 794–804.

60. Kamel OW, van de Rijn M, Weiss LM *et al.* Brief report: reversible lymphomas associated with Epstein-Barr virus occurring during methotrexate therapy for rheumatoid arthritis and dermatomyositis. *N Engl J Med* 1993; **328**: 1317–21.

61. Oyama T, Yamamoto K, Asano N *et al.* Age-related EBV-associated B-cell lymphoproliferative disorders constitute a distinct clinicopathologic group: a study of 96 patients. *Clin Cancer Res* 2007; **13**: 5124–32.

62. Schrager J, Pittaluga S, Raffeld M, Jaffe ES. EBV reactivation syndromes in adults without known immunodeficiency. *Mod Pathol* 2009; **22**(Suppl 1): 285A.

◆63. Jaffe ES, Harris NL, Stein H, Vardiman J. *Pathology and genetics of tumours of haematopoietic and lymphoid tissues.* Lyon, France: IARC Press, 2001.

64. Andreesen R, Osterholz J, Lohr GW, Bross KJ. A Hodgkin cell-specific antigen is expressed on a subset of auto- and alloactivated T (helper) lymphoblasts. *Blood* 1984; **63**: 1299–302.

65. Ansieau S, Scheffrahn I, Mosialos G *et al.* Tumor necrosis factor receptor-associated factor (TRAF)-1, TRAF-2, and TRAF-3 interact in vivo with the CD30 cytoplasmic domain; TRAF-2 mediates CD30-induced nuclear factor kappa B activation. *Proc Natl Acad Sci U S A* 1996; **93**: 14053–8.

66. Kanavaros P, Jiwa NM, de Bruin PC *et al.* High incidence of EBV genome in CD30-positive non-Hodgkin's lymphomas. *J Pathol* 1992; **168**: 307–15.

67. Schlieper G, Kurschat C, Donner A *et al.* Hodgkin disease-like posttransplantation lymphoproliferative disorder of donor origin in a renal allograft recipient. *Am J Kidney Dis* 2006; **47**: e37–41.

●68. Rowlings PA, Curtis RE, Passweg JR *et al.* Increased incidence of Hodgkin's disease after allogeneic bone marrow transplantation. *J Clin Oncol* 1999; **17**: 3122–7.

69. Zambelli A, Lilleri D, Baldanti F *et al.* Hodgkin's disease as unusual presentation of post-transplant lymphoproliferative disorder after autologous hematopoietic cell transplantation for malignant glioma. *BMC Cancer* 2005; **5**: 109.

70. Leoncini L, Del Vecchio M, Kraft R *et al.* Hodgkin's disease and CD30-positive anaplastic large cell lymphomas – a continuous spectrum of malignant disorders. *Am J Pathol* 1990; **137**: 1047–57.

●71. Stein H, Mason D, Gerdes J *et al.* The expression of the Hodgkin's disease associated antigen Ki-1 in reactive and neoplastic lymphoid tissue: evidence that Reed-Sternberg cells and histiocytic malignancies are derived from activated lymphoid cells. *Blood* 1985; **66**: 848–58.

◆72. Jaffe ES. Anaplastic large cell lymphoma: the shifting sands of diagnostic hematopathology. *Mod Pathol* 2001; **14**: 219–28.

73. Foss HD, Anagnostopoulos I, Araujo I *et al.* Anaplastic large-cell lymphomas of T-cell and null-cell phenotype express cytotoxic molecules. *Blood* 1996; **88**: 4005–11.

74. Krenacs L, Wellmann A, Sorbara L *et al.* Cytotoxic cell antigen expression in anaplastic large cell lymphomas of T- and null-cell type and Hodgkin's disease: evidence for distinct cellular origin. *Blood* 1997; **89**: 980–89.

75. Orscheschek K, Merz H, Hell J *et al.* Large-cell anaplastic lymphoma-specific translocation (t[2;5] [p23;q35]) in Hodgkin's disease: indication of a common pathogenesis? *Lancet* 1995; **345**: 87–90.

76. Wellman A, Otsuki T, Vogelbruch M *et al.* Analysis of the t(2;5) (p23;q35) translocation by reverse trasnscription-polymerase chain reaction in CD 30+ anaplastic large-cell lymphomas, in other non-Hodgkin's of T-cell phenotype, and in Hodgkin's disease. *Blood* 1995; **86**: 2321–8.

77. Nakamura S, Shiota M, Nakagawa A *et al.* Anaplastic large cell lymphoma: a distinct molecular pathologic entity: a reappraisal with special reference to p80(NPM/ALK) expression. *Am J Surg Pathol* 1997; **21**: 1420–32.

78. Chittal SM, Delsol G. The interface of Hodgkin's disease and anaplastic large cell lymphoma. *Cancer Surv* 1997; **30**: 87–105.

79. Weber-Matthiesen K, Deerberg-Wittram J, Rosenwald A *et al.* Translocation t(2;5) is not a primary event in Hodgkin's disease. Simultaneous immunophenotyping and interphase cytogenetics. *Am J Pathol* 1996; **149**: 463–8.

80. Pittaluga S, Wiodarska I, Pulford K *et al.* The monoclonal antibody ALK1 identifies a distinct morphological subtype of anaplastic large cell lymphoma associated with 2p23/ALK rearrangements. *Am J Pathol* 1997; **151**: 343–51.

81. Pileri S, Bocchia M, Baroni C *et al.* Anaplastic large cell lymphoma (CD30+/Ki-1+): results of a prospective clinicopathologic study of 69 cases. *Br J Haematol* 1994; **86**: 513–23.

82. Zinzani PL, Bendandi M, Martelli M *et al.* Anaplastic large-cell lymphoma: clinical and prognostic evaluation of 90 adult patients. *J Clin Oncol* 1996; **14**: 955–62.

●83. Benharroch D, Meguerian-Bedoyan Z, Lamant L *et al.* ALK-positive lymphoma: a single disease with a broad spectrum of morphology. *Blood* 1998; **91**: 2076–84.

84. MacLennan K, Bennett M, Tu A *et al.* Relationship of histopathologic features to survival and relapse in nodular sclerosing Hodgkin's disease. *Cancer* 1989; **64**: 1686–93.

85. Cazals-Hatem D, Andre M, Mounier N *et al.* Pathologic and clinical features of 77 Hodgkin's lymphoma patients treated in a lymphoma protocol (LNH87): a GELA study. *Am J Surg Pathol* 2001; **25**: 297–306.

86. Bennett MH, MacLennan KA, Easterling MJ *et al.* The prognostic significance of cellular subtypes in nodular sclerosing Hodgkin's disease: an analysis of 271 non-laparotomised cases (BNLI report no. 22). *Clin Radiol* 1983; **34**: 497–501.

87. DeVita VT Jr, Simon RM, Hubbard SM et al. Curability of advanced Hodgkin's disease with chemotherapy. Long-term follow-up of MOPP-treated patients at the National Cancer Institute. Ann Intern Med 1980; 92: 587–95.

88. Vassallo J, Lamant L, Brugieres L et al. ALK-positive anaplastic large cell lymphoma mimicking nodular sclerosis Hodgkin's lymphoma: report of 10 cases. Am J Surg Pathol 2006; 30: 223–9.

89. Custer R, Bernard W. The interrelationship of Hodgkin's disease and other lymphatic tumors. Am J Med Sci 1948; 216: 625–42.

●90. Gonzalez CL, Medeiros LJ, Jaffe ES. Composite lymphoma. A clinicopathologic analysis of nine patients with Hodgkin's disease and B-cell non-Hodgkin's lymphoma. Am J Clin Pathol 1991; 96: 81–9.

●91. Hansmann ML, Fellbaum C, Hui PK, Lennert K. Morphological and immunohistochemical investigation of non-Hodgkin's lymphoma combined with Hodgkin's disease. Histopathology 1989; 15: 35–48.

92. Paulli M, Rosso R, Kindl S et al. Nodular sclerosing Hodgkin's disease and large cell lymphoma. Immunophenotypic characterization of a composite case. Virchows Arch A Pathol Anat Histopathol 1992; 421: 271–5.

93. Aguilera NS, Howard LN, Brissette MD, Abbondanzo SL. Hodgkin's disease and an extranodal marginal zone B-cell lymphoma in the small intestine: an unusual composite lymphoma. Mod Pathol 1996; 9: 1020–6.

94. Kuppers R, Sousa AB, Baur AS et al. Common germinal-center B-cell origin of the malignant cells in two composite lymphomas, involving classical Hodgkin's disease and either follicular lymphoma or B-CLL. Mol Med 2001; 7: 285–92.

95. Kingma DW, Medeiros LJ, Barletta J et al. Epstein-Barr virus is infrequently identified in non-Hodgkin's lymphomas associated with Hodgkin's disease. Am J Surg Pathol 1994; 18: 48–61.

●96. Pinkus G, Said J. Hodgkin's disease, lymphocyte predominance type, nodular – further evidence for a B cell derivation: L&H variants of Reed-Sternberg cells express L26, a pan B cell marker. Am J Pathol 1988; 133: 211–7.

◆97. Mason D, Banks P, Chan J et al. Nodular lymphocyte predominance Hodgkin's disease: a distinct clinico-pathological entity. Am J Surg Pathol 1994; 18: 528–30.

●98. Marafioti T, Hummel M, Anagnostopoulos I et al. Origin of nodular lymphocyte-predominant Hodgkin's disease from a clonal expansion of highly mutated germinal-center B cells. N Engl J Med 1997; 337: 453–8.

99. Ohno T, Stribley JA, Wu G et al. Clonality in nodular lymphocyte-predominant Hodgkin's disease. N Engl J Med 1997; 337: 459–65.

100. Gelb AB, Dorfman RF, Warnke RA. Coexistence of nodular lymphocyte predominance Hodgkin's disease and Hodgkin's disease of the usual type. Am J Surg Pathol 1993; 17: 364–74.

●101. Hansmann M, Stein H, Fellbaum C et al. Nodular paragranuloma can transform into high-grade malignant lymphoma of B type. Hum Pathol 1989; 20: 1169–75.

102. Miettinen M, Franssila KO, Saxen E. Hodgkin's disease, lymphocytic predominance nodular. Increased risk for subsequent non-Hodgkin's lymphomas. Cancer 1983; 51: 2293–300.

103. Krikorian JG, Burke JS, Rosenberg SA, Kalpan HS. Occurrence of non-Hodgkin's lymphoma after therapy for Hodgkin's disease. N Engl J Med 1979; 300: 452–8.

104. Levy R, Kaplan HS. Impaired lymphocyte function in untreated Hodgkin's disease. N Engl J Med 1974; 290: 181–6.

105. Bennett M, MacLennan K, Hudson G, Hudson B. Non-Hodgkin's lymphoma arising in patients treated for Hodgkin's disease in the BNLI: a 20-year experience. Ann Oncol 1991; 2: 83–92.

106. Shimizu K, Hara K, Kunii A. Non-Hodgkin's lymphoma following Hodgkin's disease. A case report and immunohistochemical corroboration. Am J Clin Pathol 1986; 86: 370–4.

107. Gaidano G, Carbone A, Dalla-Favera R. Pathogenesis of AIDS-related lymphomas: molecular and histogenetic heterogeneity. Am J Pathol 1998; 152: 623–30.

108. Ohno T, Trenn G, Wu G et al. The clonal relationship between nodular sclerosis Hodgkin's disease with a clonal Reed-Sternberg cell population and a subsequent B-cell small non-cleaved cell lymphoma. Mod Pathol 1998; 11: 485–90.

109. Perrone T, Frizzera G, Rosai J. Mediastinal diffuse large-cell lymphoma with sclerosis. A clinicopathologic study of 60 cases. Am J Surg Pathol 1986; 10: 176–91.

110. Carrato A, Filippa D, Koziner B. Hodgkin's disease after treatment of non-Hodgkin's lymphoma. Cancer 1987; 60: 887–96.

111. Travis LB, Gonzalez CL, Hankey BF, Jaffe ES. Hodgkin's disease following non-Hodgkin's lymphoma. Cancer 1992; 69: 2337–42.

112. LeBrun DP, Ngan BY, Weiss LM et al. The bcl-2 oncogene in Hodgkin's disease arising in the setting of follicular non-Hodgkin's lymphoma. Blood 1994; 83: 223–30.

●113. Richter M. Generalized reticular cell sarcoma of lymph nodes associated with lymphocytic leukemia. Am J Pathol 1928; 4: 285–92.

114. Choi H, Keller RH. Coexistence of chronic lymphocytic leukemia and Hodgkin's disease. Cancer 1981; 48: 48–57.

115. Dick F, Maca R. The lymph node in chronic lymphocytic leukemia. Cancer 1978; 41: 283–92.

116. Caveriviere P, Mallem O, Al Saati T, Delsol G. Reed-Sternberg-like cells in Richter's syndrome express granulocytic-associated-antigen (Leu-M1). Am J Clin Pathol 1986; 85: 755–7.

117. Fayad L, Robertson LE, O'Brien S et al. Hodgkin's disease variant of Richter's syndrome: experience at a single institution. Leuk Lymphoma 1996; 23: 333–7.

118. Weisenberg E, Anastasi J, Adeyanju M *et al*. Hodgkin's disease associated with chronic lymphocytic leukemia. Eight additional cases, including two of the nodular lymphocyte predominant type. *Am J Clin Pathol* 1995; **103**: 479–84.

●119. Momose H, Jaffe ES, Shin SS *et al*. Chronic lymphocytic leukemia/small lymphocytic lymphoma with Reed-Sternberg-like cells and possible transformation to Hodgkin's disease. Mediation by Epstein-Barr virus. *Am J Surg Pathol* 1992; **16**: 859–67.

120. Cha I, Herndier BG, Glassberg AB, Hamill TR. A case of composite Hodgkin's disease and chronic lymphocytic leukemia in bone marrow. Lack of Epstein-Barr virus. *Arch Pathol Lab Med* 1996; **120**: 386–9.

●121. Ohno T, Smir BN, Weisenburger DD *et al*. Origin of the Hodgkin/Reed-Sternberg cells in chronic lymphocytic leukemia with 'Hodgkin's transformation'. *Blood* 1998; **91**: 1757–61.

●122. de Leval L, Vivario M, De Prijck B *et al*. Distinct clonal origin in two cases of Hodgkin's lymphoma variant of Richter's syndrome associated with EBV infection. *Am J Surg Pathol* 2004; **28**: 679–86.

123. Mao Z, Quintanilla-Martinez L, Raffeld M *et al*. IgVH mutational status and clonality analysis of Richter's transformation: diffuse large B-cell lymphoma and Hodgkin lymphoma in association with B-cell chronic lymphocytic leukemia (B-CLL) represent two different pathways of disease evolution. *Am J Surg Pathol* 2007; **31**: 1605–14.

◆124. Giles FJ, O'Brien SM, Keating MJ. Chronic lymphocytic leukemia in (Richter's) transformation. *Semin Oncol* 1998; **25**: 117–25.

◆125. Jaffe ES, Zarate-Osorno A, Kingma DW *et al*. The interrelationship between Hodgkin's disease and non-Hodgkin's lymphomas. *Ann Oncol* 1994; **5**: 7–11.

126. Wlodarska I, Delabie J, De Wolf-Peeters C *et al*. T-cell lymphoma developing in Hodgkin's disease: evidence for two clones. *J Pathol* 1993; **170**: 239–48.

127. Simrell CR, Boccia RV, Longo DL, Jaffe ES. Coexisting Hodgkin's disease and mycosis fungoides. Immunohistochemical proof of its existence. *Arch Pathol Lab Med* 1986; **110**: 1029–34.

128. Hawkins KA, Schinella R, Schwartz M *et al*. Simultaneous occurrence of mycosis fungoides and Hodgkin disease: clinical and histologic correlations in three cases with ultrastructural studies in two. *Am J Hematol* 1983; **14**: 355–62.

129. Clement M, Bhakri H, Monk B *et al*. Mycosis fungoides and Hodgkin's disease. *J R Soc Med* 1984; **77**: 1037–9.

130. Kaufman D, Gordon LI, Variakojis D *et al*. Successfully treated Hodgkin's disease followed by mycosis fungoides: case report and review of the literature. *Cutis* 1987; **39**: 291–6.

131. Brousset P, Lamant L, Viraben R *et al*. Hodgkin's disease following mycosis fungoides: phenotypic and molecular evidence for different tumour cell clones. *J Clin Pathol* 1996; **49**: 504–7.

132. Kremer M, Sandherr M, Geist B *et al*. Epstein-Barr virus-negative Hodgkin's lymphoma after mycosis fungoides: molecular evidence for distinct clonal origin. *Mod Pathol* 2001; **14**: 91–7.

133. Caya JG, Choi H, Tieu TM *et al*. Hodgkin's disease followed by mycosis fungoides in the same patient. Case report and literature review. *Cancer* 1984; **53**: 463–7.

134. Park CS, Chung HC, Lim HY *et al*. Coexisting mycosis fungoides and Hodgkin's disease as a composite lymphoma: a case report. *Yonsei Med J* 1991; **32**: 362–9.

135. Lipa M, Kunynetz R, Pawlowski D *et al*. The occurrence of mycosis fungoides in two patients with preexisting Hodgkin's disease. *Arch Dermatol* 1982; **118**: 563–7.

136. Greene MH, Pinto HA, Kant JA *et al*. Lymphomas and leukemias in the relatives of patients with mycosis fungoides. *Cancer* 1982; **49**: 737–41.

137. van der Putte SC, Toonstra J, Go DM, Van Unnik JA. Mycosis fungoides. Demonstration of a variant simulating Hodgkin's disease. A report of a case with a cytomorphological analysis. *Virchows Arch B Cell Pathol Incl Mol Pathol* 1982; **40**: 231–47.

138. Picard F, Dreyfus F, Le Guern M *et al*. Acute T-cell leukemia/lymphoma mimicking Hodgkin's disease with secondary HTLV I seroconversion. *Cancer* 1990; **66**: 1524–8.

139. Ohshima K, Kikuchi M, Yoshida T *et al*. Lymph nodes in incipient adult T-cell leukemia-lymphoma with Hodgkin's disease-like histologic features. *Cancer* 1991; **67**: 1622–8.

●140. Quintanilla-Martinez L, Fend F, Moguel LR *et al*. Peripheral T-cell lymphoma with Reed-Sternberg-like cells of B-cell phenotype and genotype associated with Epstein-Barr virus infection. *Am J Surg Pathol* 1999; **23**: 1233–40.

141. Paulli M, Berti E, Rosso R *et al*. CD30/Ki-1-positive lymphoproliferative disorders of the skin-clinicopathologic correlation and statistical analysis of 86 cases: a multicentric study from the European Organization for Research and Treatment of Cancer Cutaneous Lymphoma Project Group. *J Clin Oncol* 1995; **13**: 1343–54.

142. Kaudewitz P, Stein H, Plewig G *et al*. Hodgkin's disease followed by lymphomatoid papulosis. Immunophenotypic evidence for a close relationship between lymphomatoid papulosis and Hodgkin's disease. *J Am Acad Dermatol* 1990; **22**: 999–1006.

●143. Kadin ME, Drews R, Samel A *et al*. Hodgkin's lymphoma of T-cell type: clonal association with a CD30+ cutaneous lymphoma. *Hum Pathol* 2001; **32**: 1269–72.

144. Ralfkiaer E, Bosq J, Gatter KC *et al*. Expression of a Hodgkin and Reed-Sternberg cell associated antigen (Ki-1) in cutaneous lymphoid infiltrates. *Arch Dermatol Res* 1987; **279**: 285–92.

145. Wieczorek R, Suhrland M, Ramsay D *et al*. Leu-M1 antigen expression in advanced (tumor) stage mycosis fungoides. *Am J Clin Pathol* 1986; **86**: 25–32.

146. Scheen SR, Banks PM, Winkelmann RK. Morphologic heterogeneity of malignant lymphomas developing in mycosis fungoides. *Mayo Clin Proc* 1984; **59**: 95–106.

147. Davis T, Morton C, Miller-Cassman R *et al.* Hodgkin's disease, lymphomatoid papulosis, and cutaneous T-cell lymphoma derived from a common T-cell clone. *N Engl J Med* 1992; **326**: 1115–22.

148. Willenbrock K, Ichinohasama R, Kadin ME *et al.* T-cell variant of classical Hodgkin's lymphoma with nodal and cutaneous manifestations demonstrated by single-cell polymerase chain reaction. *Lab Invest* 2002; **82**: 1103–9.

149. Kadin ME, Muramoto L, Said J. Expression of T-cell antigens on Reed-Sternberg cells in a subset of patients with nodular sclerosing and mixed cellularity Hodgkin's disease. *Am J Pathol* 1988; **130**: 345–53.

150. Seitz V, Hummel M, Marafioti T *et al.* Detection of clonal T-cell receptor gamma-chain gene rearrangements in Reed-Sternberg cells of classic Hodgkin disease. *Blood* 2000; **95**: 3020–24.

151. Muschen M, Rajewsky K, Brauninger A *et al.* Rare occurrence of classical Hodgkin's disease as a T cell lymphoma. *J Exp Med* 2000; **191**: 387–94.

●152. Barry TS, Jaffe ES, Sorbara L *et al.* Peripheral T-cell lymphomas expressing CD30 and CD15. *Am J Surg Pathol* 2003; **27**: 1513–22.

153. Abruzzo LV, Schmidt K, Weiss LM *et al.* B-cell lymphoma after angioimmunoblastic lymphadenopathy: a case with oligoclonal gene rearrangements associated with Epstein-Barr virus. *Blood* 1993; **82**: 241–6.

●154. Timmens W, Visser L, Poppema S. Nodular lymphocyte predominance type of Hodgkin's disease is a germinal center lymphoma. *Lab Invest* 1986; **54**: 457–61.

●155. Sundeen JT, Cossman J, Jaffe ES *et al.* Lymphocyte predominant Hodgkin's disease, nodular subtype with coexistent "large cell lymphoma." Histological progression or composite malignancy? *Am J Surg Pathol* 1988; **12**: 599–606.

156. Greiner TC, Gascoyne RD, Anderson ME *et al.* Nodular lymphocyte-predominant Hodgkin's disease associated with large-cell lymphoma: analysis of Ig gene rearrangements by V-J polymerase chain reaction. *Blood* 1996; **88**: 657–66.

157. Wickert RS, Weisenburger DD, Tierens A *et al.* Clonal relationship between lymphocytic predominance Hodgkin's disease and concurrent or subsequent large-cell lymphoma of B lineage. *Blood* 1995; **86**: 2312–20.

158. Huang JZ, Weisenburger DD, Vose JM *et al.* Diffuse large B-cell lymphoma arising in nodular lymphocyte predominant Hodgkin lymphoma: a report of 21 cases from the Nebraska Lymphoma Study Group. *Leuk Lymphoma* 2004; **45**: 1551–7.

159. Fan Z, Natkunam Y, Bair E *et al.* Characterization of variant patterns of nodular lymphocyte predominant Hodgkin lymphoma with immunohistologic and clinical correlation. *Am J Surg Pathol* 2003; **27**: 1346–56.

160. Shimodaira S, Hidaka E, Katsuyama T. Clonal identity of nodular lymphocyte-predominant Hodgkin's disease and T-cell-rich B-cell lymphoma. *N Engl J Med* 2000; **343**: 1124–5.

●161. Straus SE, Jaffe ES, Puck JM *et al.* The development of lymphomas in families with autoimmune lymphoproliferative syndrome with germline Fas mutations and defective lymphocyte apoptosis. *Blood* 2001; **98**: 194–200.

162. Franke S, Wlodarska I, Maes B *et al.* Lymphocyte predominance Hodgkin disease is characterized by recurrent genomic imbalances. *Blood* 2001; **97**: 1845–53.

●163. Franke S, Wlodarska I, Maes B *et al.* Comparative genomic hybridization pattern distinguishes T-cell/histiocyte-rich B-cell lymphoma from nodular lymphocyte predominance Hodgkin's lymphoma. *Am J Pathol* 2002; **161**: 1861–7.

164. Jaffe ES, Harris NL, Diebold J, Muller-Hermelink HK. World Health Organization classification of neoplastic diseases of the hematopoietic and lymphoid tissues. A progress report. *Am J Clin Pathol* 1999; **111**: S8–12.

165. Harris NL, Jaffe ES, Stein H *et al.* A revised European-American classification of lymphoid neoplasms: a proposal from the International Lymphoma Study Group. *Blood* 1994; **84**: 1361–92.

166. Harris NL, Jaffe ES, Diebold J *et al.* World Health Organization classification of neoplastic diseases of the hematopoietic and lymphoid tissues: report of the Clinical Advisory Committee meeting-Airlie house, Virginia, November 1997. *J Clin Oncol* 1999; **17**: 3835–49.

167. Yonetani N, Kurata M, Nishikori M *et al.* Primary mediastinal large B-cell lymphoma: a comparative study with nodular sclerosis-type Hodgkin's disease. *Int J Hematol* 2001; **74**: 178–85.

168. Coiffier B, Lepage E, Briere J *et al.* CHOP chemotherapy plus rituximab compared with CHOP alone in elderly patients with diffuse large-B-cell lymphoma. *N Engl J Med* 2002; **346**: 235–42.

169. Wilson WH, Grossbard ML, Pittaluga S *et al.* Dose-adjusted EPOCH chemotherapy for untreated large B-cell lymphomas: a pharmacodynamic approach with high efficacy. *Blood* 2002; **99**: 2685–93.

170. Wilson WH, Gutierrez M, O'Connor P *et al.* The role of rituximab and chemotherapy in aggressive B-cell lymphoma: a preliminary report of dose-adjusted EPOCH-R. *Semin Oncol* 2002; **29**(1 Suppl 2): 41–7.

171. Dunleavy D, Pittaluga S, Grant N *et al.* Gray zone lymphomas: clinical and histological characteristics and treatment with dose-adjusted EPOCH-R. *Blood* 2008; **112**: 1228.

172. Zinzani PL, Martelli M, Magagnoli M *et al.* Treatment and clinical management of primary mediastinal large B-cell lymphoma with sclerosis: MACOP-B regimen and mediastinal radiotherapy monitored by (67)Gallium scan in 50 patients. *Blood* 1999; **94**: 3289–93.

173. Zelenetz AD, Chen TT, Levy R. Histologic transformation of follicular lymphoma to diffuse lymphoma represents

tumor progression by a single malignant B cell. *J Exp Med* 1991; **173**: 197–207.

174. Oviatt DL, Cousar JB, Collins RD *et al*. Malignant lymphomas of follicular center cell origin in humans. V. Incidence, clinical features, and prognostic implications of transformation of small cleaved cell nodular lymphoma. *Cancer* 1984; **53**: 1109–14.

175. Gutierrez M, Chabner BA, Pearson D *et al*. Role of a doxorubicin-containing regimen in relapsed and resistant lymphomas: an 8-year follow-up study of EPOCH. *J Clin Oncol* 2000; **18**: 3633–42.

176. Matsue K, Itoh M, Tsukuda K *et al*. Development of Epstein-Barr virus-associated B cell lymphoma after intensive treatment of patients with angioimmunoblastic lymphadenopathy with dysproteinemia. *Int J Hematol* 1998; **67**: 319–29.

177. Abruzzo LV, Rosales CM, Medeiros LJ *et al*. Epstein-Barr virus-positive B-cell lymphoproliferative disorders arising in immunodeficient patients previously treated with fludarabine for low-grade B-cell neoplasms. *Am J Surg Pathol* 2002; **26**: 630–36.

●178. Zarate OA, Medeiros LJ, Kingma DW *et al*. Hodgkin's disease following non-Hodgkin's lymphoma. A clinicopathologic and immunophenotypic study of nine cases. *Am J Surg Pathol* 1993; **17**: 123–32.

20

Chromosomal and molecular alterations in lymphoid malignancies: basic principles and detection methods

MARTIN JS DYER AND REINER SIEBERT

INTRODUCTION

Cancer is a genetic disease. All forms of malignancy are characterized by the presence of genetic abnormalities. Over and above point mutations at the level of DNA, gross changes at the chromosomal level can be detected in the vast majority of malignancies. By definition, these genetic aberrations are somatic in origin, and are thus not transmitted through the germ line. Many of these lesions are recurrent and are therefore considered to be pivotal to the pathogenesis of disease; in many instances, it is possible to confirm this hypothesis by recapitulating disease using mouse transgenic models that 'knock in' constructs that resemble human chromosomal translocations.[1]

This chapter is concerned with the description of the structural chromosomal lesions in lymphoid malignancies and their detection in routine clinical practice. These lesions have not only diagnostic but also prognostic and therapeutic applications and thus play an increasingly important role in patient management. The molecular origins and consequences of these lesions in terms of neoplastic transformation of normal B cells will be discussed elsewhere in this volume.

Our knowledge of the importance of genetic changes in tumorigenesis has evolved from observations spanning the last century. Historically, interest in the number and form of human chromosomes has paralleled developments in cytological techniques; early studies have been reviewed by

Hungerford.[2] Perhaps the most famous early observations are those of Boveri, who from his studies of the number of chromosomes in various tissues was the first to suggest a chromosomal cause of malignancy, through variation in the number of chromosomes. Confirmation of these speculations was some time in coming. It is perhaps surprising to recall that the precise number of human chromosomes was only determined unequivocally in 1956.[3]

Following the introduction of better methods for obtaining metaphases, the first recurrent chromosomal aberration in cancer, the derivative chromosome 22 from t(9;22)(q34;q11), the so-called 'Philadelphia chromosome' of chronic myeloid leukemia, was observed as a 'minute' chromosome in both Edinburgh and Philadelphia in 1959.[4] However, it was the development of banding techniques by Zech and colleagues in the late 1960s that led to significant progress in deciphering these abnormalities more objectively.[5]

Modern fluorescence *in situ* hybridization (FISH) and, more recently, array-based technologies now allow us to probe the cancer genome with unprecedented sensitivity, and discussion of these techniques and their application to routine clinical material forms the basis of much of this chapter.

HISTORICAL BACKGROUND: CHROMOSOMAL ABERRATIONS IN LYMPHOID NEOPLASMS

Before describing the astonishing recent progress in the field of chromosomal changes in lymphoid malignancies, it is as well to recall how things began. In 1972, Manolov and Manolova, in a seminal paper, described a 14q+ marker chromosome in Burkitt lymphoma (BL).[6] This was subsequently shown by Zech and colleagues to represent reciprocal transfer of material from chromosome 8, the recognition of the t(8;14)(q24;q32). Using radioactivity-based *in situ* hybridization methods, the 14q+ marker chromosome was shown to involve the immunoglobulin heavy chain (*IGH*) locus on chromosome 14q32. Other BL cases showed similar breaks on chromosome 8, but interchange with material on chromosomes 2 and 22, variant translocations that we now know involve the immunoglobulin kappa and lambda light chains, respectively. The history of how the direct involvement of the immunoglobulin loci with the *MYC* locus on chromosome 8 was discovered has been recounted in a wonderfully lively manner by George Klein.[7] *MYC-IG* translocations are also found in mice, particularly in pristine-induced plasmacytomas.

It has subsequently become apparent that *IG* translocations are a cytogenetic characteristic of many but not all forms of B cell malignancy; similarly, the T cell receptor (*TCR*) loci, with the exception of the *TCRG* locus on chromosome 7, are involved in recurrent chromosomal translocations in T cell malignancies (summarized in Table 20.1). Progress in defining cytogenetic abnormalities in human lymphoproliferative subgroups other than Burkitt

lymphoma was slow: in part this was due to a lack of histological consensus on the different subtypes of disease and in part due to the difficulties in obtaining metaphases from lymph nodal preparations, especially from indolent malignancies. For example, the t(11;14)(q13;q32) was originally described as being found in chronic lymphocytic leukemia (CLL); it is now clear that this translocation predominately occurs in mantle cell lymphoma (MCL) in leukemic phase, although a small subset of true t(11;14)(q13;q32)-positive CLL might possibly exist. The t(14;18)(q32;q21) was detected in cases of follicular lymphoma by Dr Shirou Fukuhara working in Janet Rowley's laboratory.[8,9] As with BL, the 14q32 breakpoints involved the *IGH* locus.

On his return to Kyoto, Japan, Fukuhara expanded this work in a remarkable way, defining many different 14q32 translocations in different subtypes of disease, leading to the suggestion that different subgroups of lymphoid malignancy might be defined by their specific *IG* translocations, a hypothesis borne out by subsequent molecular cloning experiments.[10] Detection of *IG* translocations in B cell malignancies is thus of central diagnostic importance in several clinical conditions, including detection of *MYC* translocations in Burkitt lymphoma and *CCND1* translocations in mantle cell lymphoma. Detection of these translocations may significantly alter therapy.

A MULTISTEP MODEL OF LYMPHOID TUMORIGENESIS

These fundamental cytogenetic studies and subsequent molecular genetic investigations have led to the concept that the neoplastic process in lymphoid malignancies follows a multistep model similar to that proposed for colorectal cancer and other tumors (Fig. 20.1). Like all cancers, lymphoid malignancies are clonal diseases; that is, all cells of an individual tumor are assumed to derive from one single, tumor-initiating cell. Whether the tumor-initiating cells for lymphoma and other mature B cell malignancies are stem cells *strictu sensu* (with capacity to differentiate down multiple lineages) and derive from B cell precursors or from more committed B cells remains to be determined. Recent remarkable experiments on the plasticity of mature B cells have shown that loss of *PAX-5* expression can result in dedifferentiation into T cells via uncommitted progenitors.[11] Similarly, expression of *CEBPA* in mature B cells can result in some of these cells becoming macrophages.[12] Thus mature B cells appear to maintain extraordinary lineage plasticity. The role of such lineage switches in human lymphoid malignancies remains unknown; for example, it is not known if B cell precursor acute lymphoblastic leukemia (BCP-ALL) derives from dedifferentiation of more mature B cells.

It is widely assumed that the first genetic events initiating tumorigenesis target this precursor cell population. All other cells of the tumor cell clone inherit this genetic change, which is therefore termed the '**primary**' genetic alteration. As shown in mouse transgenic models, the

Table 20.1 Examples of the most common recurrent cytogenetic markers associated with the diagnosis of lymphoid malignancies

Hematologic malignancy	Chromosomal aberration(s)	Gene(s) involved
B cell neoplasms		
B cell precursor acute lymphoblastic leukemia (BCP-ALL)	t(1;19)(q23;p13)	PBX1/TCF3
	t(12;21)(p13;q22)	TEL(ETV6)/AML1
	t(9;22)(q34;q11)	ABL/BCR
	t(4;11)(q21;q23)	AF4/MLL
	IGH translocations	All CEBP family members, ID4, BCL9, IL3 etc.
B cell chronic lymphocytic leukemia (CLL)	del(13q14), +12/+12q	DLEU2/miR15 and miR16
	del(11q22–23)	ATM (others?)
	del(17p13)	TP53 (others?)
Follicular lymphoma (FL)	t(14;18)(q32;q21) and variants	IGH/BCL2
	t(2;18) and t(18;22)	IGK/BCL2 and BCL2/IGL
Diffuse large B cell lymphoma (DLBCL)	t(14q32)	IGH
	t(3q27)	BCL6
		Both loci involved with many different partner genes
Mantle cell lymphoma (MCL)	t(11;14)(q13;q32)	CCND1/IGH
MALT lymphoma (MALT)	t(11;18)(q21;q21)	API2/MALT1
	t(14;18)(q32;q21)	IGH/MALT1
	t(1;14)(p22;q32)	BCL10/IGH
	t(3;14)(p21;q32)	FOXP1/IGH
Burkitt lymphoma/leukemia (BL)	t(8;14)(q24;q32) and variants	MYC/IGH
	t(2;8) and t(8;22)	IGK/MYC and MYC/IGL
Plasma cell myeloma (PCM)	t(11;14)(q13;q32)	CCND1/IGH
	t(4;14)(p16;q32)	FGFR3/IGH
	t(14;16)(q32;q23)	IGH/MAF
	t(8;14)(q24;q32)	MYC/IGH
	del(13q14)	unknown
Classical Hodgkin lymphomas (CHL)	Amplifications in 2p13-16	REL
	Amplifications in 9p24	JAK2 and others
	t(14q32)	IGH
T cell neoplasms		
Precursor T lymphoblastic leukemia (T-ALL)	Rearrangements in 14q11	TCRA-D
	Rearrangements in 7q35	TCRB
T cell prolymphocytic leukemia (T-PLL)	inv(14)(q11q32) and t(14;14) Also variant translocation	TCRA-D/TCL1
	t(X;14)(q28;q11)	MTCP1
Anaplastic large cell lymphoma (ALCL)	Rearrangements of 2p23, commonly t(2;5)(p23;q35)	ALK ALK/NPM

primary genetic alteration is frequently not sufficient to drive cancerogenesis.[13,14] Additional genetic changes are required for the full neoplastic phenotype of malignancy to emerge. These aberrations are usually called 'secondary' genetic changes. An important paradigm is that the 'primary' and 'secondary' events target synergistic combinations of genes, resulting in malignant transformation. Practically, this results in recurrent patterns of chromosomal changes within tumor types; specific chromosomal translocations are therefore often found in combination with other specific chromosomal changes, as discussed below. So-called 'tertiary' genetic events may occur in some malignancies and are associated with the transformation of an indolent malignancy to more aggressive forms. In the case of follicular lymphoma, there is a steady rate of approximately 3 percent of cases per annum of transformation to diffuse large B cell lymphoma (DLBCL) or on rare occasions to BCP-ALL. Various genetic changes have been associated with this event. What predisposes to such transformation events remains unknown.

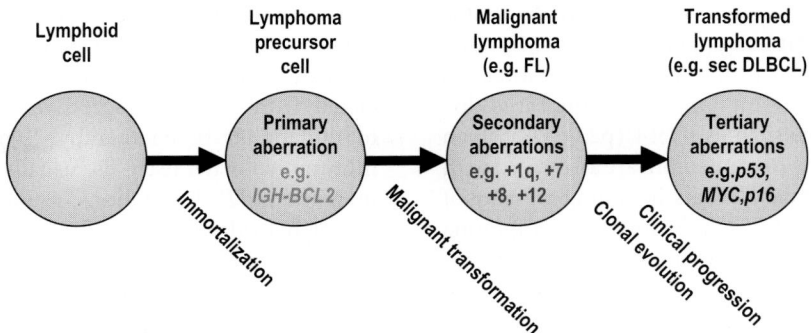

Figure 20.1   Simplified model of multistep lymphomagenesis using t(14;18)(q32;q21)-positive lymphoma as an example. The nature of the initial, 'primary' events that predispose to the generation of t(14;18)(q32;q21) and the precise nature of the cells in which these primary events occur are unknown. The rate of acquisition of 'secondary' events is presumably also very variable given the very variable nature of clinical progression of follicular lymphoma (FL). Different pathways involving different genetic lesions have been proposed for transformation of follicular lymphoma.[22] Various 'tertiary' genetic events including *MYC* translocations (to both *IG* and non-*IG* loci), *TP53* mutation (often as a consequence of complex unbalanced chromosomal translocations), and *p16/CDKN2A* deletion on chromosome 9p21 may lead to transformation to diffuse large B cell lymphoma (DLBCL), or more rarely to B cell precursor acute lymphoblastic leukemia. Again, at the current time, it is not possible to predict at diagnosis which patients are likely to progress on the basis of presenting genetic lesions. In most countries, and certainly in the United Kingdom, cytogenetic analysis is not routinely performed on follicular lymphoma nodal samples.

In lymphoid malignancies 'primary' and 'secondary' genetic aberrations show different features. 'Primary' genetic abnormalities are usually present in the stem line of a tumor, i.e., detectable in all tumor cells. In some instances, they occur as the sole detectable alteration in a tumor. In hematopoietic tumors, the known 'primary' aberrations are mostly thought to be chromosomal translocations (Table 20.1). Such translocations are highly conserved, i.e., they are present in the vast majority of tumors of a given subtype. This makes primary genetic alterations valuable diagnostic markers. However, it should be noted that some primary alterations might also constitute secondary changes in other subtypes of disease. *BCL2* chromosomal translocations for example, which underlie the pathogenesis of follicular lymphoma as primary events, may occur as secondary events in CLL (Plate 17, see plate section)[15] and *IG-MYC* fusions, the hallmark of Burkitt lymphoma, may occur as secondary events during disease progression in various subtypes of lymphoid malignancies like follicular, mantle cell, or diffuse large B cell lymphoma.

Several of the primary genetic alterations can also be detected in healthy individuals, sometimes at surprisingly high levels, again indicating that chromosomal translocations alone are not sufficient to induce lymphomagenesis.[16,17] Polymerase chain reaction (PCR) studies of *IGH* translocations involving the *BCL2* major breakpoint region or MBR (this being the site of about 50 percent of breakpoints in follicular lymphoma) have shown that in Western populations, some 60 percent of normal individuals will have detectable *IGH–BCL2* clones. This frequency increases with age. In some instances these clones may be large, comprising about one cell per five thousand. Moreover, they appear to be stable over several years.

Given that many aging individuals in Western societies have also been shown, using sensitive flow cytometry, to harbor clonal lymphocytes in the peripheral blood, and given that the incidence of monoclonal gammopathy increases dramatically with age, it is therefore likely that pre-malignant B cell populations are the norm in the elderly population, at least in the West. Similarly, high levels of several *IGH* translocations/fusion may be detected in individuals with polyclonal B cell lymphocytosis. This is a rare but benign condition found in middle-aged female tobacco smokers, associated with the appearance of bizarre, multinucleated B cells in the peripheral blood.[18] In neither instance does the presence of *IGH–BCL2* MBR fusion obviously lead to malignancy. These data raise many questions. How do these fusions not lead to malignancy? Do they genuinely represent translocations or might they be more localized insertions? In what type of B cells do these events occur? Is the *BCL2* gene deregulated as a consequence? What about other *IGH* translocations – are they present in normal B cells at comparable frequency? It is also clear from the pioneering work of Mel Greaves on identical twins with acute lymphoblastic leukemia (ALL) that chromosomal translocations constituting primary genetic aberrations can occur *in utero* but only generate ALL many years later, with the accumulation of multiple secondary genetic changes.[19]

'**Secondary**' genetic aberrations might be present only in a subset of cells of a given tumor and different secondary aberrations might even be present in distinct subclones of a tumor. Tumors of the same subtype (and harboring the same primary event) might thus show variation in terms of secondary aberrations. Nevertheless, the pattern of secondary changes is not random, but depends on the nature of the primary event. Indeed, some primary genetic alterations are hardly ever associated with any cytogenetically detectable secondary aberrations. An example is t(11;18) (q21;q21), resulting in *API2-MALT1* fusion in mucosal-associated lymphoid tissue (MALT) lymphomas.[20] In the same disease, other translocations such as t(1;14)(p22;q32), which results in deregulated *BCL10* expression, are associated with a conserved set of secondary events including trisomy of chromosomes 3, 12, and 18. Similarly, follicular lymphoma with t(14;18)(q32;q21) show different, distinctive patterns of secondary changes suggesting different pathways of germinal center B cell transformation.[21,22] T cell prolymphocytic leukemia (T-PLL), a rare but very aggressive malignancy of post-thymic T-cells, is characterized by an extraordinary conservation of both primary and secondary genetic changes.[23]

Secondary chromosomal alterations in lymphoid malignancies predominantly lead to gain or loss of genetic material, whereas recurrent, balanced translocations – with the exception of translocations affecting the *MYC* locus in chromosome band 8q24 – are uncommon as secondary events. The number of secondary and tertiary genetic aberrations usually increases during disease progression. As a consequence, it is a general rule that within a given tumor subtype the prognosis is inversely related to the complexity of secondary changes. Moreover, some individual secondary and tertiary aberrations, the most prominent being loss of 17p13, associated with inactivation of the *TP53* tumor suppressor, usually through mutation of the remaining allele, can serve as markers of disease progression and therapy resistance. This is most evident clinically in CLL, where loss of 17p13, usually detected by interphase FISH, is associated with rapidly progressive disease that is resistant to fludarabine-based therapy.[24] In terms of lymphoma, immunohistochemistry is usually used as a surrogate marker for *TP53* mutations; mutated TP53 protein has a longer half-life than wild-type protein, resulting in more ready detection. However, it should be noted that malignant B cells can tolerate high-level expression of TP53 without undergoing apoptosis and only about 30 percent of cases with TP53 staining by immunohistochemistry will in fact harbor *TP53* mutations.[25] How malignant B cells sustain high-level expression of apparently wild-type TP53 expression without undergoing apoptosis is not clear.

TYPES OF CHROMOSOMAL ABERRATIONS IN LYMPHOID NEOPLASIA

From the cytogenetic point of view, chromosomal aberrations can be grossly divided into two groups: **balanced aberrations** and **unbalanced aberrations**. In contrast to balanced changes, unbalanced aberrations are characterized by gain or loss of genetic material (shown diagrammatically in Fig. 20.2).

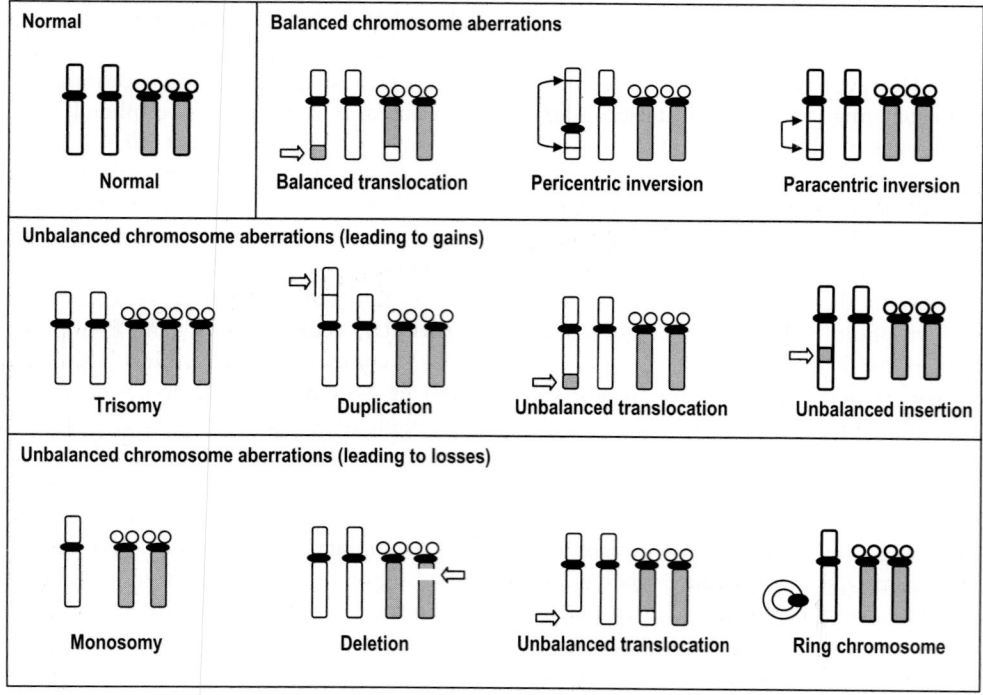

Figure 20.2 Chromosomal aberrations can be divided into two groups: balanced aberrations and unbalanced aberrations; unbalanced aberrations are characterized by gain or loss of genetic material.

Balanced chromosomal aberrations: translocations, inversions

Balanced chromosomal changes include translocations and inversions. Translocations are interchromosomal changes resulting from the exchange of genetic material between two chromosomes. In contrast, inversions constitute intrachromosomal aberrations derived from a 180° turn of part of a chromosome. Depending on whether the centromere is included in the inverted part or not, inversions are termed 'pericentric' or 'paracentric.' In neoplasms, both translocations and inversions predominately exert their transforming potential either through the creation of chimeric fusion genes resulting from in-frame fusion of genes normally found in separate chromosomal regions or, alternatively, deregulated and sometimes ectopic gene expression of a target gene.

In malignancy, translocations usually involve **dominant oncogenes**, whose expression results in either proliferation and/or blocked normal differentiation or suppressed apoptotic pathways. Examples of translocations or inversions in lymphoid malignancies leading to fusion genes are the t(2;5)(p23;q35) and inv(2)(p23q35) resulting in activation of the tyrosine kinase *ALK* through fusion to *NPM* and *ATIC*, respectively, in CD30-positive anaplastic large cell lymphoma (ALCL).[26] Examples for translocations and inversions driving lymphomagenesis through deregulation of expression are the t(14;18)(q32.3;q21) in follicular lymphoma and the inv(14)(q11q32.1) in T-PLL leading to activation of the *BCL2* and *TCL1* oncogenes via juxtaposition to the *IGH* and *TCRAD* loci, respectively. The majority of recurrent balanced chromosomal aberrations are supposed to be primary events in lymphoid neoplasms. It is noteworthy that within a disease subtype, different genetic alterations may nevertheless involve the same pathway, a good example being the involvement of both *BCL10* and *MALT1* genes in *IGH* translocation in MALT lymphoma.[27,28] These two proteins directly interact and are involved in signal transduction from the B cell receptor for antigen resulting in nuclear factor κB (NF-κB) activation.[29] Involvement of different members of one pathway within a given malignancy is a recurrent feature of many forms of malignancy.[30]

Unbalanced chromosomal aberrations associated with gains of chromosomal material: trisomies, duplications, unbalanced translocations, amplifications, and complicons

Gain of chromosomal material can derive from addition of single whole chromosomes described as trisomy (three chromosomes), tetrasomy (four chromosomes), etc. Typical examples are trisomy 12 in CLL as well as trisomies of chromosomes with odd and even numbers in hyperdiploid multiple myeloma and BCP-ALL, respectively. Trisomies can increase the modal chromosome number from normal 46 to more than 50 in the setting of hyperdiploidy. In

this regard it is important to distinguish gains of single chromosomes from alterations in ploidy, which derive from gains of a complete chromosome set (i.e., 23 chromosomes). Triploidy (69 chromosomes), tetraploidy (92 chromosomes), and higher ploidy, as well as variation of these (near-triploid, hypertriploid, etc.), can be a sign of tumor progression in many lymphoid malignancies, whereas particularly in classical Hodgkin lymphoma (CHL) it is a hallmark of the disease.[31,32]

In addition to whole chromosomes, partial chromosomes can also be gained, typically through intrachromosomal duplications or unbalanced translocations, in which one derivative chromosome is missing or added. The most extreme form of genomic gain is amplification, though it is a matter of debate where to set the border between genomic gains and amplifications. Cytogenetically, gene amplifications can be tightly clustered as a homogeneously staining region (HSR) on a single chromosome or appear as small double minutes (dmin) in metaphase spreads. Episomal amplification has also been described in rare instances.[33] Whilst cytogenetic evidence for high-level amplifications has been rare in lymphomas, recent array-based analyses have identified a number of recurrent sites of amplification, including *REL* in 2p13 or *MYC* in 8q24 in DLBCL.[34,35] Amplification of a very gene-poor region of 13q32 may also be found in some B cell lymphomas. For some time it was unclear what the target for this amplification might be; however, it now seems that this is a polycistronic microRNA (miRNA) gene cluster that synergizes with *MYC*.[36] These small non-coding RNA genes appear to play a role in several chromosomal abnormalities, including translocations and deletions as well as amplifications, in lymphoid malignancies as discussed below (please also see[37] for a review of their role in malignancy).

Amplifications are supposed to activate dominant oncogenes and might constitute a genetic mechanism comparable to chromosomal translocation; in some instances, for example *BCL11A*, the same gene locus may be involved in either event, indicating that different pathogenetic mechanisms may nevertheless have an identical outcome. In line with this assumption, overexpression of the activated oncogene can be mostly seen at the RNA or protein level in cases with high-level amplification. It has to be emphasized though that not all genes within a given amplicon need be transcriptionally activated. Rather, the amplicon might retain the chromatin structure of the region specific to a given cell type and might, thus, only increase expression of genes also normally expressed in this cellular context. Moreover, amplification of translocational junction segments resulting in fusion genes or transcriptional deregulation has been observed as a mechanism of lymphoma progression.[35,38] These so-called '**complicons**' might be indicators of a defect in DNA repair based on observations in mouse models.

In contrast to high-level amplification, the effect of low-level gains may be much less pronounced. Some studies have shown that gain of whole chromosomes (like trisomy

12 in CLL) or certain chromosome regions (like gain of 18q21 in DLBCL) is associated with increased expression of a set of genes located in the gained segments.[39] Nevertheless, the overall concordance between gene dosage and gene expression on a genome-wide level seems to be rather poor. There are a number of possible reasons for this including epigenetic mechanisms, transcription factor repertoires, and transchromosomal effects.

Unbalanced chromosomal aberrations associated with loss of chromosomal material: monosomies, deletions, and unbalanced translocations

Loss of chromosomal material can derive from deletion of a whole chromosome, described as monosomy, or of part of a chromosome due to a deletion or an unbalanced translocation. Complete loss of both alleles of a gene locus is described as homozygous deletion and, by definition, completely abrogates gene function. Although it has been shown that intrachromosomal deletion can lead to activation of oncogenes, e.g., via gene fusion,[40] the most prominent consequence of deletion is inactivation of tumor suppressor genes (TSGs). This is obvious in the case of homozygous deletions, which have been instrumental in identifying TSGs in lymphoid neoplasms. Many of these deletions are small, far beyond the detection limits of conventional cytogenetics; however, these can now be detected with unprecedented sensitivity using array-based methods as described below.[41] Table 20.2 lists a number of TSGs that have been shown to be inactivated in lymphoid neoplasms by homozygous loss.

Much more frequent than homozygous loss is deletion of only one allele. Mostly, this does not result in significantly reduced expression of genes normally expressed in the normal counterpart of the cancer cell, unless the second allele is silenced by epigenetic mechanisms such as DNA methylation or the presence of a mutation leading to nonsense-mediated RNA decay. An alternative mechanism of inactivation of a second allele of a TSG is a point or other mutation that influences function.[42] Such mutations may be dominant-negative over wild-type protein and

therefore may occur in the presence of wild-type protein; that is, without deletion of the other allele.

The most prominent examples of chromosomal deletions in lymphoid neoplasms are losses in the short arm of chromosome 17 or deletions in the long arm of chromosome 6q. For both regions, candidate TSGs have been TP53 and PRDM1/BLIMP1, respectively, which are inactivated by mutation in the remaining allele in a considerable number of cases; mutations of the latter occur particularly in the activated B cell subset of DLBCL.[43] Nevertheless, from cases lacking mutations of the second allele of these genes, as well as from cases showing different minimal regions of loss, derive evidence that additional TSGs are located in these chromosomal regions. In the case of chromosome 6, recent data point to A20/TNFAIP3 and PERP in 6q23.3 as additional TSGs.[44,45] In the case of 17p deletions, these usually arise in B cell malignancies as a consequence of unbalanced translocations resulting in loss of a large region of the short arm of chromosome 17. It has been suggested that other TSGs distal to TP53 may be implicated in the pathogenesis of B cell malignancies.[46]

Even with modern technologies, TSGs remain difficult to identify.[47] In contrast, molecular cloning of chromosomal translocations allows rapid identification of dominant oncogenes through their physical proximity to the translocation breakpoint.

Balanced chromosomal aberration with unbalanced effect: uniparental disomy

Biallelic inactivation of TSGs in a balanced setting can also derive from simultaneous loss of a wild-type allele and duplication of the mutated allele. Similar to a deletion, the effect of this event is loss of heterozygosity (LOH). For this kind of event, characterized by LOH without chromosomal deletion, the term 'partial uniparental disomy (pUPD)' has been introduced. The term 'pUPD' might not be the most appropriate as it could also include the possibility that both grandparental chromosomes from one parent are present. As this is not possible in a tumor deriving from a host with only one grandparental chromosome per parent, the term 'isodisomy' might probably be better. By studying mantle cell lymphoma cell lines, Nieländer et al. showed that pUPD is a recurrent event in lymphomas.[48] An increasing amount of data has shown that pUPD is a recurrent alteration in lymphoid and other hemopoietic neoplasms, which frequently affects regions that may harbor TSGs.[44,49,50] Overall, the contribution of this particular type of genetic change to neoplastic transformation remains to be determined.

BETWEEN CHROMOSOMES AND DNA: EPIGENETIC CHANGES IN LYMPHOID NEOPLASMS

The cytogenetic aberrations described above focus on the chromosome number and structure. In contrast, alterations

Table 20.2 Candidate tumor suppressor genes targeted by homozygous deletion in lymphoid malignancies (modified from[118])

Region of homozygous loss	Tumor suppressor gene
1p32.3	INK4C/P18
2q13	BIM
3p14.2	FHIT
9p21.3	INK4A/P16
11q14–q23	ATM
13q14.2	RB1
16p13.13	SOCS1
18q21.3	NOXA

at the molecular level described elsewhere in this volume focus on mutations detectable at the DNA. Nevertheless, this dichotomous view on cytogenetics and molecular genetics only poorly reflects the reality in a cell, where DNA and proteins are intimately linked within chromatin. Changes in chromatin composition, including both methylation of DNA or modification of histones, influence both chromosome stability and gene function. Chromatin modifications comprise part of the epigenome which denotes the entirety of hereditary information that affects gene activity without altering the DNA sequence itself. The best studied epigenetic change in cancer is DNA methylation at CpG sites. Globally, most lymphoid malignancies show reduced methylation levels. Such hypomethylation has been shown to confer chromosomal instability in a wide variety of malignancies.[51–53]

In contrast, CpG-rich promoter regions (called CpG islands) of TSGs recurrently show hypermethylation, which in addition to genomic deletion and mutation represents another mechanism resulting in TSG silencing. Table 20.3 gives an overview of some of the genes that have been described to undergo *de novo* methylation in lymphoid tumors. Methylated CpG sites can silence genes by impeding the binding of transcription factors directly, if they are located within the respective DNA recognition or binding sequences. Additionally, the presence of methylated sites recruits m^5CpG-binding proteins, which bind to the methylated DNA restricting access to other proteins. A transcriptional repressor machinery is recruited to the CpG island at the gene promoter, consisting of DNA methyltransferases (DNMTs), methyl-CpG-binding proteins (MBPs), histone

methyltransferases for lysine-9 of histone H3 (HMT K9H3), histone deacetylases (HDACs), and polycomb (PcGs) complexes. This molecular mechanism closely links changes in methylation patterns to histone modifications. Interestingly, recent reports suggest that histone marks established by PcG complexes at the stem cell stage predetermine which genes will suffer *de novo* methylation in cancer, which further supports the concept of a stem-cell origin of cancer. Transferring these observations from solid tumors to lymphomagenesis could lead to the hypothesis that the 'primary' chromosomal aberrations only arise or only have a transforming effect in progenitor cells which contain a polycomb signature resembling characteristics of stem cells. Arguing against this hypothesis are recent observations from mouse models showing that CpG-island methylation in lymphoma cells is driven by the 'primary' chromosomal change.[54] Further studies are required to shed light onto the intimate interaction between genetic and epigenetic changes in lymphomagenesis and to unravel whether DNA methylation is the prerequisite or the consequence of primary chromosomal aberrations to induce lymphomas. CpG hypermethylation is of potential therapeutic interest, since this process can be reversed pharmacologically using compounds such as 5′-azacytidine.

TECHNICAL APPROACHES TO DETECT CHROMOSOMAL ABERRATIONS

Current methods for the routine detection of chromosomal changes in lymphomas are based on conventional

Table 20.3   Summary of genes whose CpG islands have been reported to be hypermethylated in lymphoma (modified from [118,119])

Gene name	Function	Location	Malignancy
TP73	TP53 homologue	1p36.23	Burkitt lymphoma
IL12RB2	Interleukin 12 receptor, beta2 precursor	1p31.3	B cell malignancies
PROX1	Prospero related homobox 1	1q41	B cell malignancies
TWIST2	Basic helix–loop–helix protein	2q37	IGHV mutated CLL
RARB	Retinoic acid receptor β2 (thyroid steroid hormone receptor)	3p24.2	B cell malignancies
RASSF1A	ras effector homologue	3p21.31	Hodgkin lymphoma
CRBP1	Cellular retinol binding protein 1	3q23	B cell malignancies
CDKN2A (INK4A/p16)	Cyclin-dependent kinase inhibitor	9p21.3	Burkitt lymphoma
CDKN2B (INK4b/p15)	Cyclin-dependent kinase inhibitor 2B isoform 1	9p21.3	Burkitt lymphoma
DAPK1	Death-associated protein kinase	9q21.33	B cell lymphoma/CLL/Burkitt lymphoma
GSTP1	Glutathione S-transferase	10q13.2	PCNSL
MGMT	O6-methylguanine methyltransferase	10q26.3	DLBCL
p57 (KIP2, CDKN1C)	Cyclin-dependent kinase inhibitor 1C	11p15.4	B cell malignancies
CCND1	Cyclin D1	11q13.2	B cell malignancies
PTPN6 (SHP1)	Protein tyrosine phosphatase, non-receptor type	12p13.31	B-NHL
TSP1	Thrombospondin 1	15q14	PCNSL
TIMP2	Tissue inhibitor of metalloproteinase 2	17q25.3	PCNSL
TIMP3	Tissue inhibitor of metalloproteinase 3	22q12.3	PCNSL
AR	Androgen receptor	Xq12	Non-Hodgkin lymphoma

PCNSL, primary central nervous system lymphoma; CLL, chronic lymphocytic leukemia; DLBCL, diffuse large B cell lymphoma; NHL, non-Hodgkin lymphoma.

cytogenetic, molecular cytogenetic, and molecular genetic techniques.

Conventional cytogenetic methods

Conventional cytogenetic analysis is based on the study of metaphase chromosomes by staining techniques like Giemsa (G) or Reverse (R) banding. Viable tumor cells have to be obtained and cultured *in vitro* in order to obtain metaphases, rendering the availability of fresh material mandatory. Suitable mitogens can be applied to stimulate growth of tumor cells. Obtaining high-quality metaphases from mature lymphoproliferative disorders is often difficult, particularly from indolent malignancies. Another problem is the presence of residual normal cells. Nevertheless, in dedicated centers it is possible to obtain tumor metaphases in most cases, even in diseases such as CLL.[55] In principle, banding analysis is a genome-wide screening method that allows both numerical and structural abnormalities to be detected. However, the complete resolution of the karyotype can be hampered by chromosomal complexity or cryptic cytogenetic rearrangements, such as a reciprocal translocation involving subtelomeric regions or small imbalances.

Conventional cytogenetics must therefore be supplemented by a growing number of techniques to define objectively and comprehensively all other significant genetic lesions.

Fluorescence *in situ* hybridization–based methods

Molecular cytogenetics comprises a number of techniques based on FISH. Common to all these techniques is the principle that a fragment of labeled, single-stranded (ss) DNA or 'probe' is hybridized onto a ssDNA sample, where the probe will find its complementary sequence or 'target.' As the probe is labeled with a fluorescent dye, it will produce fluorescent signals at the place where the target is located within the nucleus. Molecular cytogenetic methods have evolved dramatically during recent years leading to the development of multiple variant techniques. Among these, single- and double-color FISH using satellite and locus-specific probes have special diagnostic applications. These probes can be applied to both metaphase and interphase cells and can detect the vast majority of numerical or structural chromosomal aberrations. For the detection of lymphoma-associated translocations by conventional interphase FISH, there are two main strategies. First, two differentially labeled probes spanning the respective breakpoints in both translocation partners (i.e., **double-color, double-fusion probes**) can be applied to detect a specific translocation with high sensitivity. On the other hand, two-color probes flanking the chromosomal breakpoints in one specific locus (i.e., **break-apart probes**) allow the detection of all the translocations affecting a 'promiscuous' gene partnering with several others (e.g.,

the *IGH, BCL6,* or *MYC* locus). Genomic imbalances can simply be detected by counting the number of signals of a locus-specific probe in comparison to that of a differentially labeled control probe hybridized simultaneously. As mentioned above, detection of *IGH* translocations is of particular importance in the diagnosis of B cell malignancies; commercial probe sets are now available that allow detection of all the common events.

An important advantage of interphase FISH is its suitability to study material embedded in paraffin. As many surgical biopsies (e.g., lymph nodes) reach the laboratory in an unfixed state only in few diagnostic centers, this is of increasing diagnostic relevance. Therefore, the application of FISH in paraffin-embedded material significantly widens the application range of this technique in the lymphoma diagnostic setting.[56]

Advanced fluorescence *in situ* hybridization–based methods

Most commercially available as well as other widely used conventional FISH assays are restricted to two, sometimes three, differently labeled probes. This limits the analyses to a maximum of three genetic loci or two chromosomal aberrations that can be targeted simultaneously. Multicolor interphase FISH approaches have been developed that allow the detection of multiple lymphoma-related rearrangements simultaneously.[57] Other FISH-based techniques such as multicolor karyotyping (M-FISH and SKY) allow visualization of each metaphase chromosome in a different color.[58,59] Although several studies using multicolor karyotyping have been published over the last decade, they are rarely used in the lymphoma diagnostic process today.[60] Its main application is the characterization of complex karyotypes in the research setting.

As the FISH technique does not destroy cell and tissue structure, FISH can be combined with assessment of morphology and, furthermore, also with fluorescence immunophenotyping. A technique combining these three features was developed in the early 1990s and was coined 'FICTION' (Fluorescence Immunophenotyping and Interphase Cytogenetics as a Tool for Investigation of Neoplasms).[61] This technique allows the detection of genetic aberrations in immunologically characterized cell populations, even if they present a minority in the tissue studied. Using this approach, the sensitivity of interphase FISH can be enhanced because only certain cell subpopulations are targeted. For example, this technique is especially suited to study CHL, in which the percentage of tumor cells in patient biopsies is certainly very low.[62,63]

Array-based methods

There are currently two main strategies to detect chromosomal changes with DNA microarrays: array-based comparative genomic hybridization (CGH) and single nucleotide polymorphism (SNP)-chips. The former has been developed from conventional 'chromosomal CGH,' which is based on the competitive hybridization of differentially labeled tumor and normal DNA onto metaphase spreads. Several seminal studies using conventional CGH have been performed in lymphomas, which resulted in a gross overview of chromosomal imbalance patterns in various subtypes of lymphoid neoplasms. These studies can be easily accessed via the Progenetix CGH database (www.progenetix.de). Nevertheless, most of these studies were limited by the resolution of the technique. Significant improvement came from CGH using microarrays containing spotted DNA fragments (frequently bacterial artificial chromosome [BAC] clones or now more frequently oligonucleotides), which allows a comprehensive high-resolution overview of chromosomal imbalances in a given sample. Single nucleotide polymorphism–chip analyses are usually based on a one-color microarray hybridization, and the fluorescence intensities are then compared to those obtained in normal controls with a dedicated software, so that an overview of chromosomal imbalances can be obtained. Furthermore, SNP-chips are also able to detect the so-called 'partial uniparental disomies,' e.g., loss of heterozygosity without loss of genetic material.

Several array-CGH studies have been published concerning lymphomas, which have led to a better characterization of chromosomal imbalances and the identification of novel lymphoma-related genes (www.progenetix.de and, for example, see [44,45,64,65]). An important point is that despite the great advantages of microarray-based genomic profiling in terms of resolution and genomic coverage, it cannot detect balanced chromosomal changes and the proportion of aberrant cells in the sample has to be over 30–50 percent to obtain reliable results.

Technical comparison

Among the methods described above, interphase FISH is one of the most advantageous for the routine diagnosis and follow-up of lymphoma patients with chromosomal translocations such as t(8;14)(q24;q32) and t(11;14) (q13;q32). The main virtues of the FISH technique are as follows:[66]

- It does not require tumor metaphases and therefore both archival and fresh material can be used;
- Nuclear morphology is maintained allowing techniques such as FICTION to be used;
- Depending on the probe design and type of alteration detected, the diagnostic cutoff can be less than 1 percent, allowing a great degree of sensitivity;
- It allows quantification of the tumor clone;
- It is not highly influenced by dispersal of chromosomal breakpoints – this is particularly important in certain chromosomal translocations such as those involving

MYC and CCND1 in lymphoma where the breakpoints can be scattered over many hundreds of kilobases;
- Due to the rapidity of the analysis; results can usually be obtained within 48 hours of receipt of samples;
- It requires a low labor intensity;
- It is suitable for automation.

The major disadvantage of FISH is that the rest of the genome, other than the regions being probed, remains uninvestigated. Therefore, wherever possible, it is important to include complementary screening techniques, especially conventional cytogenetics, which remains the 'gold standard' for obtaining an overview of chromosomal changes within a given population. Array-CGH can also be applied in the diagnostic setting to obtain a high-resolution picture of chromosomal imbalances but will not detect balanced events such as chromosomal translocations. Therefore, a combination of methods remains desirable if not essential for completeness of diagnosis. A current example is that of CLL. Recurrent deletions of chromosomes 11q22.3, 13q14, and 17p13 are seen in this disease; deletions of 11q22.3 and 17p13 are usually associated with progressive disease. However, disease progression may often be seen in the absence of any of these markers and, in some cases, regular conventional cytogenetics, which can be obtained in most cases of CLL, may often show complex abnormalities in cases of advanced disease.[55,67]

Molecular genetic methods

Molecular genetic methods for the detection of chromosomal changes in hematologic neoplasms are mainly based on PCR. These approaches are predominantly used for the detection of recurrent translocations leading to fusion genes and thus use RNA templates for detection (reverse transcription PCR [RT-PCR]). They find application principally in the diagnosis and monitoring of patients with acute leukemias, where such fusions are the norm. In the mature lymphoid malignancies, fusion transcripts are rare and the more common consequence is deregulated expression due to juxtaposition of the oncogene to transcriptional enhancers as discussed below. Such translocations therefore require genomic DNA for detection of the genomic fusion sequences. For regular PCR to be successful at detecting breaks in routine clinical material, both breakpoints must be clustered, since the limit of regular PCR is of the order of 2000 base pairs. This limitation can be overcome using long-distance (LD) PCR methods, which can amplify PCR products up to 30 000 base pairs; however, this technique is difficult to perform reliably and requires high-molecular-weight DNA that has been prepared from viable cells and not paraffin-fixed material. Long-distance PCR methods have been used for both BCL2 and MYC translocations.[68,69]

A variant of this technique is long-distance inverse or LDI-PCR. Its value is the ability to clone chromosomal translocation breakpoints with a single set of primers. This technique has been used for *IGH* translocations falling within both *IGHJ* and *IGHS* segments as well as many different *BCL6* translocations involving multiple different partner genes.[70–72] Again, LDI-PCR demands high-molecular-weight DNA, but here it is initially digested with restriction enzymes and then allowed to relegate overnight at low DNA concentrations, thus promoting circularization. DNA circles containing the known sequence can then be amplified using primers to these sequences to amplify around the resulting circle; resulting PCR products should therefore contain the translocation breakpoint. It is interesting to note that both the productive allele involved in normal *IGHV-D-J* recombination and the translocation breakpoint are usually coamplified in the same PCR reaction despite sometimes large differences in product size (see for example Figure 1 in reference 27, where the productive *VDJ* allele of 500 base pairs was coamplified with the translocated allele of 5500 base pairs). Although LDI-PCR from certain target sequences such as *IGHJ* and *BCL6* is a robust method, and continues to allow the definition of previously undescribed chromosomal translocations, the technique has not been used routinely. Interphase FISH allows much more rapid assessment of breaks at either locus, although the precise breakpoints cannot readily be defined precisely using these methods.

Future directions in diagnostic methods

It seems likely that the future of the detection of chromosomal changes in lymphoid malignancies will be twofold. On the one hand, it will be characterized by the application of current methods including conventional metaphase cytogenetics, FISH, array-CGH, and PCR and gene expression analysis in a more routine and comprehensive manner in all patients in order to establish a more complete picture of the genetic 'damage' within the neoplastic clone. In time, it is likely that these investigations will be supplemented by more advanced, upcoming techniques. For instance, the development of the next generation of DNA sequencers will allow the sequence of complete lymphoma genomes to be determined rapidly. This will certainly lead to the detection of novel recurrent genetic changes beyond the power of any of the current methods. On the other hand, the application of advanced screening methods will lead to the discovery of highly informative genetic markers that will be studied in the clinical setting with more accessible and cheaper techniques (e.g., FISH or PCR) for a better diagnosis, prediction of prognosis, and therapy stratification according to risk groups. The nature and number of specific tests to be used will depend not only on the disease subtype but also on the available therapies; an example of this is the development of mutations in the chimeric BCR-ABL kinase, which are associated with resistance to imatinib, but may nevertheless be sensitive to other tyrosine kinase inhibitors. The development and integration of such expensive tests (and expensive new therapies) into routine clinical practice will present major health economic problems.

RECURRENT CYTOGENETIC ABERRATIONS IN LYMPHOID MALIGNANCIES – COMMON THEMES

A detailed review of the primary and secondary genetic changes in distinct subtypes of lymphoid neoplasms will be detailed in the disease-specific chapters of this volume. Nevertheless, a compendium of the common recurrent cytogenetic abnormalities and, for the most part, cloned molecularly in lymphoid malignancies is given in Table 20.1.

In this final section, some themes common to cytogenetic aberrations across subtypes of lymphoid neoplasias will be discussed briefly. As mentioned previously, an important point is that synergistic interaction of dominant oncogenes and tumor suppressor genes is necessary for the full neoplastic phenotype to develop. Moreover, these events have to occur in an ordered, sequential manner; activation of an oncogene such as *MYC* may induce cell programmed cell death or apoptosis, if this pathway has not been previously blocked, for example either by prior activation of *BCL2* through chromosomal translocations (as occurs in transformed follicular lymphoma) or by p53 mutation (as occurs commonly in Burkitt lymphoma).[73–75] Another important point is that each subtype of B cell malignancy is characterized by a specific spectrum of molecular genetic abnormalities. Although some translocations do occur in multiple tumor types (such as *MYC* and *CCND1* and, to a lesser extent, *BCL2*), others (such as *MALT1* and *BCL10* translocations in MALT lymphoma) do not. Where cytogenetically identical translocations occur in more than one disease, molecular analysis may nevertheless show different breakpoints both within the translocated gene and with the *IGH* locus, implying different pathogenetic mechanisms. Detection of these chromosomal translocations has important clinical implications in terms of diagnosis, prognosis, and ultimately therapy, either directly by the development of targeted therapy, or in selection of more aggressive chemotherapeutic regimens. For example, MALT lymphomas with *BCL10* translocations follow a more aggressive clinical course. Interestingly, these translocations can be detected not only by high-level expression of Bcl-10 protein, but also by aberrant subcellular localization within the nucleus.[76] Similarly, *ALK* translocations in ALCL may be recognized through different patterns of ALK protein expression on immunohistochemistry.[77]

It is perhaps surprising that there is such considerable genetic heterogeneity among the B cell malignancies. Why are they not all B cells at all stages of differentiation, transformed by the same or similar mechanisms?

Chromosomal translocations in lymphoid malignancies

One of the many major successes of molecular biology in terms of oncological medicine has been the molecular dissection of chromosomal translocations either through a cytogenetic lead positional cloning approach or, more recently, through gene expression profiling. Cloning of translocation breakpoints leads directly to the involved gene(s) whose altered function(s) have dominant effects. As noted initially by Fukuhara, the *IG* loci, including both the *IGH* locus on 14q32 and both *IGK* and *IGL* light chain loci on chromosome 2p11 and 22q11, are recurrently involved in chromosomal translocations in B cell malignancies, especially B cell non-Hodgkin lymphoma and myeloma (Table 20.1). Diffuse large B cell lymphoma is characterized by the large number of partner genes involved. Chronic lymphocytic leukemia on the other hand is notable for its lack of *IG* translocations and, moreover, breaks at 14q32 in CLL may not always involve the *IGH* locus. Somewhat surprisingly, given that the enzymes necessary for generation of translocations are expressed at high level at this stage of B cell lymphopoiesis, most cases of BCP-ALL lack *IGH* translocations. However, use of interphase FISH for the *IGH* locus, which allows unequivocal detection of *IGH* translocations in a break-apart assay, has revealed a number of recurrent *IGH* chromosomal translocations in BCP-ALL.[78,79] Again, these translocations are specific for this BCP-ALL and are not found in more mature B cell malignancies.

IG translocations in malignant B cells may be multiple, involving both *IGH* and *IGL*. A common combination is that of an *IGH–BCL2* translocation in follicular lymphoma being associated with an *IGL-MYC* translocation occurring at transformation to DLBCL. Such cases are usually highly aggressive clinically and respond poorly to chemotherapy. *IGH* translocations may themselves be involved in secondary translocation events, resulting in marked cytogenetic complexity.[74,80]

Incidentally, gene deregulation may also occur as a consequence of insertion rather than translocation. Thus, both *BCL2* and *CCND1* have been observed to be inserted into the *IGH* locus in cases of follicular lymphoma and MCL, respectively; a similar event has been reported for the miRNA125b gene in BCP-ALL.[81,82] The frequency of insertional events in B cell malignancies is not known, again demanding metaphases cytogenetics to distinguish them from regular translocations. This is similar to the insertion of *PML* into the *RARA* locus in cases of acute promyelocytic leukemia that lack the characteristic t(15;17)(q21;q22) of the disease but nevertheless exhibit *PML-RARA* fusion. Although the biological consequences of the insertions would appear to be identical to regular translocations, their pathogenetic origins would appear to be very different, involving different DNA breaks.

Tumor suppressor genes in lymphoid malignancies

In contrast to translocations, efforts to identify TSGs have been much less successful. According to the Knudson hypothesis, which derived from studies on retinoblastoma,[42] TSGs would be loss-of-function mutations deriving from loss of one allele and mutation of the other. Thus, TSGs should be detected through first defining a minimally deleted region (nowadays done by either BAC or by SNP arrays) and then sequencing all the genes within; detection of coding mutations should then identify the culprit!

One of the major problems to this approach, however, has been the fact that deletions may be large (spanning several megabases of DNA), and may therefore contain many possible candidate genes. This problem may be overcome by the use of modern and cheaper high-throughput sequencing methods that allow sequencing of individual genomes. Detection of homozygous deletions is a strong indication of a TSG within the deleted region. Most of these deletions are well below the level of cytogenetic detection (some may only be a few kilobases in size). Thus far, the best described example of homozygous loss in lymphoid malignancies is the loss of the *CDKN1A* locus on chromosome 9p21. Homozygous loss is seen commonly in BCP-ALL. Deletion in more mature B cell malignancies is less common and associated with transformation to more aggressive forms of malignancy.

Using BAC arrays, homozygous deletions appear to be uncommon in B cell malignancies. Homozygous deletion of the *BIM* locus on chromosome 2q13 in MCL has been observed in a number of derived MCL cell lines.[83] BIM is a key pro-apoptotic BH3-only domain protein that binds directly to BCL2; its loss therefore should synergize with deregulated BCL2 expression. However, neither *BIM* deletions nor mutations have been observed in any primary cases. The reasons for the differences between primary clinical material and derived cell lines are not clear; if *BIM* deletion is an artifact of tissue culture, why is this only observed in MCL cell lines and not others? Other homozygous deletions in B cell malignancies have recently been described as noted in Table 20.2.

There are several problems with the detection of TSGs using positional approaches. Many deletions may not be associated with missense mutations within the coding regions of genes. In one study of mainly nonhematologic malignancies, homozygous deletions occurred in gene-poor regions.[84] From our own studies, sequencing of a 650 kilobase (kb) minimally deleted region of chromosome 8p21 typically seen in MCL in leukemic phase failed to identify any missense mutations within the remaining allele.[85] Therefore, this raises the question of whether these deletions are simply a reflection of increased 'genetic instability' associated with malignancy, or whether they really have some functional significance despite the lack of mutation demanded of the Knudson hypothesis. There are several possible explanations. First, loss of gene expression may not require mutation within the coding region of genes – loss of expression may follow deletions involving regulatory regions that may be many kilobases distant from the target gene. Second, epigenetic silencing of the remaining allele (or both alleles) may contribute significantly. Third, it appears that some deletions (like some amplifications described above) may in fact be very small and involve miRNAs; two of these small non-coding RNAs (miRNA-15 and miRNA-16) have been implicated in the deletion of chromosome 13q14 seen in at least 80 percent of CLL.[86,87] Although close homologs of these miRNA genes are found elsewhere in the genome, it has been postulated that loss of only one copy of a specific miRNA may have profound effects on translation of key target genes such as BCL2 (however, see[88]). The two miRNAs are located within another much larger non-coding RNA gene (DLEU2); the function of loss of this gene, which would accompany loss of the two miRNAs, and whose expression is either very low or undetectable in nearly all cases of CLL, has yet to be determined.[89] Interestingly, deletions of 13q14 are often associated with unbalanced chromosomal translocations in this locus; many different partner chromosomes are involved.[55] Whether these translocations have different consequences from interstitial deletions of 13q14 is not known.

Gains and amplifications in lymphoid malignancies

Genomic gains or amplifications are also common in B cell malignancies. Sometimes these may be detected by regular cytogenetics as, for example, trisomy of an entire chromosome. Trisomy 12, for example, is found not only in CLL but in many other subtypes of B cell malignancy. In CLL, trisomy 12 is associated with 'atypical' morphology of the malignant cells but in most instances is a secondary event, found only in a subclone and, moreover, progressive disease is not associated with an increase in the frequency of trisomy 12. These data raise doubts over the involvement of trisomy 12 in the pathogenesis of the disease, although gene expression data have shown high-level expression of genes on chromosome 12.[39]

Unlike other forms of malignancy, HSRs are uncommon in lymphoid malignancies. However, some regions may undergo high-level amplification. The best known of these is an amplicon on the short arm of chromosome 2, seen in primary mediastinal B cell lymphoma, CHL, and a subset of DLBCL.[62,90,91] This amplicon (which may be up to 256×) involves an ultraconserved region of DNA that contains two closely juxtaposed genes (separated by only 350 kb of DNA) of importance in normal B cell differentiation and transformation, REL and BCL11A. Determining which of these genes, or perhaps both (or perhaps even neither!), is the key target oncogene is not trivial. REL is an NF-κB family member and deregulated expression of this gene has been shown to have proliferative effects in a

chicken B cell system. Truncation of REL has also been seen in the RC-K8 mediastinal B cell lymphoma cell line as a consequence of chromosomal translocation. These and other data implicate REL as a key target of the amplification.[92] On the other hand, REL needs to be nuclear to exert its functions and one study in DLBCL failed to show correlation of nuclear REL in cases with the 2p16 amplicon.[34] BCL11A was cloned through its direct involvement in t(2;14)(p16;q32), which occurs in rare cases of CLL.[93] BCL11A is a DNA sequence-specific transcriptional repressor that binds directly to Bcl-6. BCL11A knockout mutant mice show a complete block in early B cell differentiation, but the ability of BCL11A to transform normal B cells has not yet been demonstrated.[94] BCL11A is a complex gene with multiple RNA isoforms, encoding proteins with very different properties. Interestingly, in mouse retroviral insertional models, overexpression of Bcl11a resulted in myeloid leukemias. It is likely that different subtypes of B cell malignancy with the 2p16 amplicon will utilize different genes. Resolution of the key targets will require detailed functional as well as molecular genetic analyses.

Other forms of genetic instability in lymphoid malignancies

Over and above the types of recurrent chromosomal abnormalities described above, two other forms of genetic damage commonly seen in B cell malignancies need to be mentioned. Somatic hypermutation (SHM) of the immunoglobulin V-region gene segments is needed in order to generate high-affinity antibodies during the germinal center reaction. This process, however, can also involve other genes resulting in loss of gene expression in some instances. A prime example of this process is loss in DLBCL of PRDM1/BLIMP1 expression of the activated B cell phenotype.[43]

On a much larger genetic scale, however, most B cell malignancies have acquired many apparently random and often surprisingly complex genetic events during their generation. This has been shown most clearly using multicolor M-FISH experiments in follicular lymphoma; careful dissection of these complex changes may allow recognition of different pathways of progression.[21] However, the contribution, if any, of these events to the pathogenesis of disease and whether any are of prognostic significance is uncertain. An important point though is that, as with chromosomal translocations, metaphase preparations are required to elucidate these events – they will not be detected using array-based methods.

Finally, it is interesting to note that metaphase studies in CLL have shown a large number of apparently random, and usually unbalanced, chromosomal translocations (see[55] and references therein). In this regard, CLL appears to differ from all other B cell malignancies; the error in DNA repair that underlies the disease remains unknown. Deletion of chromosome 13q is found in most cases although the consequences of this deletion remain unclear. Deletion of chromosome 17p, which is found often as a secondary event in aggressive and fludarabine-resistant cases, is usually associated with complex cytogenetic rearrangements of this chromosomal arm.[95] Mutation of *TP53* may occur in the absence of deletion of the other allele and may similarly be associated with poor prognosis disease, suggesting that *TP53* may, on occasion, function as a dominant oncogene as well as a TSG.

Inherited predispositions to B cell malignancies

Although most B cell malignancies appear to be sporadic, there is increasing evidence that several subtypes may have a significant genetic predisposition. First, in follicular lymphoma, there is unequivocal geographic variation, with a much lower incidence of this disease in China and Japan; this may be related to a much lower incidence of the t(14;18)(q32;q21), not only in B cell malignancies but also in normal individuals.[96] In Caucasian populations, about 60 percent of normal individuals will have PCR evidence for low levels of t(14;18)(q32;q21) but these are not found at the same incidence in either Japanese or Chinese individuals. The molecular basis for this variation remains unknown.

Second, a positive family history of lymphoproliferative disorders may be present in at least 5 percent of patients with CLL.[97] Chronic lymphocytic leukemia families are not comparable with *BRCA1* or *BRCA2* mutant families; there are usually only two or three family members affected in two or three generations. Genetic anticipation (that is, earlier onset in subsequent generations) appears to be a real phenomenon rather than an ascertainment bias: anticipation does not appear to reflect trinucleotide expansion as seen in neurological disorders. International collaborative linkage studies have been initiated and some preliminary results suggested that 11p11 may harbor a predisposing locus but this remains to be confirmed. Interested readers with suitable families are recommended to submit these families (www.icr.ac.uk/).

Very recently, it has been reported from studies of a family with an unusually large number of affected individuals, that a mutation in the 5′ regulatory region of the death-associated protein kinase 1 (*DAPK1*) gene, found on chromosome 9q22, may underlie the pathogenesis of some cases of familial CLL. Moreover, epigenetic silencing of this gene through aberrant promoter methylation was observed in a very high frequency of sporadic cases of CLL.[98] Inactivation of DAPK1 may result in loss of sensitivity to normal pro-apoptotic stimuli, allowing the persistence of cells otherwise destined to die by apoptosis. Thus, familial and sporadic cases may reflect the actions of different pathogenetic mechanisms converging on the one gene. However, these data need to be confirmed in other familial cases.

Familial predispositions for several other forms of B cell malignancy may also be found. The familial association for Hodgkin lymphoma (HL) is very high. According to data from the Swedish national cancer registry, the chance of a child of a parent with HL developing the disease is about eight times higher than for the population in general. Moreover, interestingly, there is a high degree of gender concordance; that is, the increased risk of HL within a given family will only be seen in one gender and not the other.[99] Similar gender concordance is seen for CLL as well. These and other data suggest linkage to the pseudo-autosomal region (PAR) of the sex chromosomes. Given the relatively small size of the PAR, this hypothesis is testable. Whether this region also contributes to the significant gender imbalances seen in other B cell malignancies such as MCL and hairy cell leukemia is not known.

The association of specific cytogenetic abnormalities with specific subtypes of lymphoid malignancy

The origin of the association of specific recurrent genetic abnormalities with specific subtypes of malignancy remains a fascinating problem.[100] Within the premalignant cell, two chromosomal breaks must occur at approximately the same time and then, in the case of a reciprocal translocation, the four ends juxtaposed. At first glance this seems impossible, given not only the size of the human genome, but also the structures associated with higher order chromatin. (An alternative view might be that such events are in fact common and nonspecific within the tumor stem cell compartment, but it is only the events that confer selective survival advantage that are 'seen' in the periphery.) However, it is now clear from both FISH and biochemical studies that the nucleus is highly organized, with genes being arranged in chromosomal 'territories' and with gene-specific intrachromosomal interactions. Such physical associations may predispose to chromosomal translocation.[101]

Nevertheless, the large number of *IGH* translocations in human B cell malignancies generates a number of problems. First, although physical proximity might explain how chromosomal translocations arise in general, it does not explain specificity. For example, why are *BCL10* and *MALT1* chromosomal translocations only seen in MALT lymphoma and not in other subtypes of disease? (Note that *MALT1* is located only five megabases centromeric of *BCL2* on chromosome 18q21.3.) Moreover, different breaks within both the *IG* loci and in the translocated oncogene may be seen in different subtypes of disease. *BCL2* breakpoints in follicular lymphoma are virtually always found in the 3′ untranslated region (UTR) of the gene, whereas *BCL2* breakpoints in CLL involving *IGK* or *IGL* involve the 5′ UTR about 250 kb telomeric. Rare cases of t(14;18) (q32;q21) involving *IGH* may also involve the 5′ region of *BCL2*; since the *IGH* breakpoints involve the *IGHJ* segments, from the organization of the *BCL2* gene, such translocations must also involve inversion of chromosome 18.[102] The precise molecular anatomy of these variants has yet to be determined. Similarly, as noted above, it is clear that in some instances, insertion rather than translocation may occur. Presumably such different events must have very different pathogenic mechanisms, although the end result – deregulated expression of *BCL2* – is identical.

Second, when do *IGH* translocations occur in the B cell differentiation pathway? It has been widely assumed, since the *IGH* breaks occur in regions of DNA that are involved in normal *VDJ* recombination, that these breaks occur as errors of *VDJ* recombination in B cell precursors within the bone marrow at a time when the recombination activating gene (RAG) enzymes are constitutively active. If correct, this observation would have significant therapeutic consequences, since it would imply that to cure diseases such as follicular lymphoma it would be necessary to deplete not only mature B cells but also the B cell precursors. However, it seems likely that this is in fact not the case and that most *IGH* translocations are in fact generated in mature B cells. For example, when both derivative chromosomes have been analyzed – in the case of the *IGH-BCL2* translocation of follicular lymphoma both the der(14) t(14;18) and the der(18)t(14;18) have been sequenced – in most instances, it is clear from the presence of *VDJ* sequences on the der(18) that *IGH-BCL2* translocation occurred after *VDJ* recombination.[103,104] Rare cases may involve *Sμ* sequences rather than the more usual *IGHJ* sequences, again suggesting that these breaks occur as errors in class switch recombination rather than *VDJ* recombination.[105] This leads to the suggestion that such translocations probably arise within the germinal center. Furthermore, in cases of CLL with t(14;18), cytogenetic/ FISH analysis has shown that these translocations may be found in only a fraction of cells, suggesting that they are secondary events arising in cells that have already undergone VDJ and perhaps class switch recombination (Fig. 20.2).

The enzymes considered important and the specific three-dimensional conformations of DNA that may predispose to chromosomal translocation have been discussed in another chapter (Chapter 21). It should also be noted, however, that many of the experimental data concerning the enzymes involved in *IG* chromosomal translocation genesis have been generated in mice, where the only common *IG* translocations involve *MYC*; the wide range of *IG* translocations seen in man do not appear to occur in mice.

CONCLUSIONS

In summary, progress in the molecular cytogenetic characterization of the lymphoid malignancies has been particularly rapid over the past fifty years. This is due mainly to the ready accessibility of tumor cells in the peripheral blood and the ability to culture lymphocytes and obtain good metaphase preparations from most subtypes of disease. Nevertheless, although all the common recurrent chromosomal translocations found in the lymphoid malignancies have been cloned, it is perhaps surprising that new ones continue to be identified in many different subgroups of hematological and other diseases and define novel pathways of transformation.[78,79,106] Similar abnormalities are also being discovered in other 'solid' malignancies as well; it is interesting to note that there is a commonality of genes involved in both types of malignancy.[107] Moreover, analysis of the cancer genome using newer whole-genome techniques and high-throughput genome-sequencing methods are beginning to reveal more completely the surprising complexity of the genetic damage underlying most cases of malignancy.[30,108]

In common with other forms of malignancy, B cell malignancies require the coordinated and sequential dysregulation of several dominant oncogenes and TSGs, arising through several different types of genetic event. How many different forms of molecular cytogenetic data are required at diagnosis to provide adequate information that will dictate therapy will vary with the different diseases. In BCP-ALL, the presence of a single chromosomal translocation may determine intensity of therapy. In the more indolent, 'evolutive' B cell malignancies, the situation is more complex. Some 85 percent of follicular lymphoma will exhibit t(14;18)(q32;q21) but within this group will be patients who remit spontaneously or enter durable complete remissions with single-agent chlorambucil, as well as patients who will fail to respond to combination chemotherapy. Genetic markers that indicate propensity to transformation to DLBCL are lacking. Similarly in CLL, with the exception of chromosome 17p deletions, which are associated with p53 mutations in most cases, there is a dearth of clinically useful prognostic markers that can be used rationally to tailor current therapies. In these malignancies it may be necessary to study the 'stem cell' or progenitor population rather than bulk tumors. On the other hand, if newer therapeutic approaches targeting, for example, Bcl-2 are as successful as they would appear to be *in vitro*, then the clinical necessity for such investigations might not be so pressing.[109,110] BH3 mimetics that interfere with the binding of apoptotic BH3-only proteins such as BIM to Bcl-2 result in rapid induction of apoptosis at very low concentrations, at least in cases of CLL.[111] These drugs, designed on the basis of the three-dimensional structure of the Bcl-2 family of proteins, are remarkable since they inhibit protein–protein interactions, something that has traditionally been difficult or impossible to achieve.

It should also be noted that the tumor microenvironment is now thought to play an important role in the pathogenesis of several forms of indolent B cell malignancy, including both follicular lymphoma and CLL. For the latter, specialized 'nurse cells' may maintain viability of the neoplastic clone.[112] The type, number, and degree of activation of various kinds of normal lymphocytes and lymphoma-associated macrophages and various subsets of T cells, as well as their localization within the neoplastic germinal center, may determine rates of progression of follicular lymphoma.[113,114]

In one study, it has been reported that the t(14;18)(q32;q21) may be found in the tumor neovasculature of patients with follicular lymphoma suggesting that malignant mature B cells may undergo lineage switch within the involved lymph node;[115] such lineage switches are reminiscent of those described experimentally for mature B cells with loss of PAX-5 expression or overexpression of CEBPA.[11,12] These data may have therapeutic implications if we are to use targeted therapy to cure these diseases – it may be necessary to deplete more than the one cell lineage for therapy to be ultimately successful and result in cure of the disease.

Delineating the pathways involved in the pathogenesis of malignancy has been a major aim of molecular and cellular biology over the last 30 years, with the aim of developing tumor-specific therapies. A successful example of this approach is the development of the tyrosine kinase inhibitor imatinib for the *BCR-ABL* fusion gene associated with chronic myeloid leukemia.[116] This is now the paradigm for other malignancies to emulate. Targeting TSGs remains more difficult since this requires some degree of restoration of normal gene function in all malignant cells. However, in the context of the TP53 pathway, it may be possible to restore some degree of normal function through small-molecule inhibitors that bind to the TP53 binding protein, MDM2.[117] To use these new and expensive drugs in an optimal manner, it is necessary to be able to detect the key molecular cytogenetic abnormalities in routine clinical samples.

KEY POINTS

- A specific spectrum of somatically-acquired genetic abnormalities underlies each subtype of lymphoid malignancy.
- Chromosomal translocations targeting the immunoglobulin loci are recurrent in B cell malignancies and result in deregulated expression of key oncogenes that drive the development of the disease.
- These cytogenetic changes can be detected by a combination of cytogenetic, molecular and immunohistochemical techniques.
- Some of these abnormalities may provide novel therapeutic targets, such as the high-level expression of the anti-apoptotic protein *BCL2* in follicular lymphoma.
- Detection of the key genetic events in lymphoid malignancy is therefore of paramount importance not only to allow precise diagnosis but also for selection of optimal therapy.

ACKNOWLEDGMENTS

We acknowledge with gratitude the help and collaboration of our many colleagues and patients in Leicester, London, and Kiel. We gratefully acknowledge funding from the UK Medical Research Council, Deutsche Krebshilfe, European Union, Lymphoma Research Foundation (NY), and Kinder-Krebsinitiative Buchholz/Holm-Seppensen.

REFERENCES

In view of space restraints, the number of references has been limited; we apologize to colleagues whose work is not cited here. Please contact the authors if additional information is required.

● = Key primary paper

◆ = Major review article

1. Forster A, Pannell R, Drynan L. Chromosomal translocation engineering to recapitulate primary events of human cancer. *Cold Spring Harb Symp Quant Biol* 2005; **70**: 275–82.

◆2. Hungerford DA. Some early studies on human chromosomes, 1879–1955. *Cytogenet Cell Genet* 1978; **20**: 1–11.

3. Tijo HJ, Levan A. The chromosome number of man. *Hereditas* 1956; **42**: 1–6.

4. Nowell P, Hungerford D. A minute chromosome in human granulocytic leukemia. *Science* 1960; **132**: 1497.

5. Caspersson T, Lomakka G, Zech L. The 24 fluorescence patterns of the human metaphase chromosomes – distinguishing characters and variability. *Hereditas* 1972; **67**: 89–102.

6. Manolov G, Manolova Y. Marker band in one chromosome 14 from Burkitt lymphomas. *Nature* 1972; **237**: 33–4.

◆7. Klein G. The road to the Ig/Myc translocation. In: Kirsch IR. (ed.) *The causes and consequences of chromosomal aberrations*. Boca Raton: CRC Press 1993: 481–503.

8. Fukuhara S, Rowley JD, Variakojis D, Golomb HM. Chromosome abnormalities in poorly differentiated lymphocytic lymphoma. *Cancer Res* 1979; **39**: 3119–28.

9. Fukuhara S, Nasu K, Kita K *et al.* Cytogenetic approaches to the clarification of pathogenesis in lymphoid malignancies: clinicopathologic characterization of 14q+ marker-positive non-T-cell malignancies. *Jpn J Clin Oncol* 1983; **13**: 461–75.

◆10. Willis TG, Dyer MJS. The role of immunoglobulin translocations in the pathogenesis of B-cell malignancies. *Blood* 2000; **96**: 808–22.

●11. Cobaleda C, Jochum W, Busslinger M. Conversion of mature B cells into T cells by dedifferentiation to uncommitted progenitors. *Nature* 2007; **449**: 473–7.

●12. Xie H, Ye M, Feng R, Graf T. Stepwise reprogramming of B cells into macrophages. *Cell* 2004; **117**: 663–76.

13. McDonnell TJ, Deane N, Platt FM *et al.* Bcl-2-immunoglobulin transgenic mice demonstrate extended B cell survival and follicular lymphoproliferation. *Cell* 1989; **57**: 79–88.

14. Bodrug SE, Warner BJ, Bath ML *et al.* Cyclin D1 transgene impedes lymphocyte maturation and collaborates in

lymphomagenesis with the myc gene. *EMBO J* 1994; **13**: 2124–30.

15. Leroux D, Hillion J, Monteil M *et al.* t(18;22)(q21;q11) with rearrangement of *BCL2* as a possible secondary change in a lymphocytic lymphoma. *Genes Chromosomes Cancer* 1991; **3**: 205–09.

16. Liu Y, Hernandez AM, Shibata D, Cortopassi GA. *BCL2* translocation frequency rises with age in humans. *Proc Natl Acad Sci U S A* 1994; **91**: 8910–14.

17. Roulland S, Navarro JM, Grenot P *et al.* Follicular lymphoma-like B cells in healthy individuals: a novel intermediate step in early lymphomagenesis. *J Exp Med* 2006; **203**: 2425–31.

18. Delage R, Roy J, Jacques L *et al.* Multiple bcl-2/Ig gene rearrangements in persistent polyclonal B-cell lymphocytosis. *Br J Haematol* 1997; **97**: 589–95.

◆19. Greaves MF, Wiemels J. Origins of chromosome translocations in childhood leukaemia. *Nat Rev Cancer* 2003; **3**: 639–49.

20. Starostik P, Patzner J, Greiner A *et al.* Gastric marginal zone B-cell lymphomas of MALT type develop along 2 distinct pathogenetic pathways. *Blood* 2002; **99**: 3–9.

21. Lestou VS, Gascoyne RD, Sehn L *et al.* Multicolour fluorescence in situ hybridization analysis of t(14;18)-positive follicular lymphoma and correlation with gene expression data and clinical outcome. *Br J Haematol* 2003; **122**: 745–59.

22. Höglund M, Sehn L, Connors JM *et al.* Identification of cytogenetic subgroups and karyotypic pathways of clonal evolution in follicular lymphomas. *Genes Chromosomes Cancer* 2004; **39**: 195–204.

23. Soulier J, Pierron G, Vecchione D *et al.* A complex pattern of recurrent chromosomal losses and gains in T-cell prolymphocytic leukemia. *Genes Chromosomes Cancer* 2001; **31**: 248–54.

24. Catovsky D, Richards S, Matutes E *et al.* Assessment of fludarabine plus cyclophosphamide for patients with chronic lymphocytic leukaemia (the LRF CLL4 Trial): a randomised controlled trial. *Lancet* 2007; **370**: 230–39.

25. Young KH, Weisenburger DD, Dave BJ *et al.* Mutations in the DNA-binding codons of TP53, which are associated with decreased expression of TRAILreceptor-2, predict for poor survival in diffuse large B-cell lymphoma. *Blood* 2007; **110**: 4396–405.

26. Amin HM, Lai R. Pathobiology of ALK+ anaplastic large-cell lymphoma. *Blood* 2007; **110**: 2259–67.

27. Willis TG, Jadayel DM, Du MQ *et al.* Bcl10 is involved in t(1;14)(p22;q32) of MALT B cell lymphoma and mutated in multiple tumor types. *Cell* 1999; **96**: 35–45.

28. Sanchez-Izquierdo D, Buchonnet G, Siebert R *et al.* MALT1 is deregulated by both chromosomal translocation and amplification in B-cell non-Hodgkin lymphoma. *Blood* 2003; **101**: 4539–46.

29. Thome M. CARMA1, BCL-10 and MALT1 in lymphocyte development and activation. *Nat Rev Immunol* 2004; **4**: 348–59.

30. Wood LD, Parsons DW, Jones S *et al.* The genomic landscapes of human breast and colorectal cancers. *Science* 2007; **318**: 1108–13.

31. Weber-Matthiesen K, Deerberg J, Poetsch M *et al.* Numerical chromosome aberrations are present within the CD30+ Hodgkin and Reed-Sternberg cells in 100 percent of analyzed cases of Hodgkin's disease. *Blood* 1995; **86**: 1464–8.

32. Ott G, Kalla J, Ott MM *et al.* Blastoid variants of mantle cell lymphoma: frequent bcl-1 rearrangements at the major translocation cluster region and tetraploid chromosome clones. *Blood* 1997; **89**: 1421–9.

33. Graux C, Cools J, Melotte C *et al.* Fusion of *NUP214* to *ABL1* on amplified episomes in T-cell acute lymphoblastic leukemia. *Nat Genet* 2004; **36**: 1084–9.

34. Houldsworth J, Olshen AB, Cattoretti G *et al.* Relationship between *REL* amplification, REL function, and clinical and biologic features in diffuse large B-cell lymphomas. *Blood* 2004; **103**: 1862–8.

35. Martín-Subero JI, Odero MD, Hernandez R *et al.* Amplification of *IGH/MYC* fusion in clinically aggressive *IGH/BCL2*-positive germinal center B-cell lymphomas. *Genes Chromosomes Cancer* 2005; **43**: 414–23.

36. He L, Thomson JM, Hemann MT *et al.* A microRNA polycistron as a potential human oncogene. *Nature* 2005; **435**: 828–33.

37. Calin GA, Croce CM. MicroRNA signatures in human cancers. *Nat Rev Cancer* 2006; **6**: 857–66.

38. Zhu C, Mills KD, Ferguson DO *et al.* Unrepaired DNA breaks in p53-deficient cells lead to oncogenic gene amplification subsequent to translocations. *Cell* 2002; **109**: 811–21.

39. Haslinger C, Schweifer N, Stilgenbauer S *et al.* Microarray gene expression profiling of B-cell chronic lymphocytic leukemia subgroups defined by genomic aberrations and VH mutation status. *J Clin Oncol* 2004; **22**: 3937–49.

40. Cools J, DeAngelo DJ, Gotlib J *et al.* A tyrosine kinase created by fusion of the *PDGFRA* and *FIP1L1* genes as a therapeutic target of imatinib in idiopathic hypereosinophilic syndrome. *N Engl J Med* 2003; **348**: 1201–14.

●41. Mestre-Escorihuela C, Rubio-Moscardo F, Richter JA *et al.* Homozygous deletions localize novel tumor suppressor genes in B-cell lymphomas. *Blood* 2007; **109**: 271–80.

42. Knudson AG. Two genetic hits (more or less) to cancer. *Nat Rev Cancer* 2001; **1**: 157–62.

43. Pasqualucci L, Compagno M, Houldsworth J *et al.* Inactivation of the *PRDM1/BLIMP1* gene in diffuse large B cell lymphoma. *J Exp Med* 2006; **203**: 311–17.

44. Ross CW, Ouillette PD, Saddler CM *et al.* Comprehensive analysis of copy number and allele status identifies multiple chromosome defects underlying follicular lymphoma pathogenesis. *Clin Cancer Res* 2007; **13**: 4777–85.

45. Honma K, Tsuzuki S, Nakagawa M *et al.* TNFAIP3 is the target gene of chromosome band 6q23.3-q24.1 loss in ocular adnexal marginal zone B cell lymphoma. *Genes Chromosomes Cancer* 2008; **47**: 1–7.

46. Stöcklein H, Smardova J, Macak J *et al.* Detailed mapping of chromosome 17p deletions reveals *HIC1* as a novel tumor suppressor gene candidate telomeric to *TP53* in diffuse large B-cell lymphoma. *Oncogene* 2008; **27**: 2613–25.

◆47. Devilee P, Cleton-Jansen AM, Cornelisse CJ. Ever since Knudson. *Trends Genet* 2001; **17**: 569–73.

48. Nielaender I, Martín-Subero JI, Wagner F *et al.* Partial uniparental disomy: a recurrent genetic mechanism alternative to chromosomal deletion in malignant lymphoma. *Leukemia* 2006; **20**: 904–5.

49. Fitzgibbon J, Iqbal S, Davies A *et al.* Genome-wide detection of recurring sites of uniparental disomy in follicular and transformed follicular lymphoma. *Leukemia* 2007; **21**: 1514–20.

50. Young BD, Debernardi S, Lillington DM *et al.* A role for mitotic recombination in leukemogenesis. *Adv Enzyme Regul* 2006; **46**: 90–7.

51. Eden A, Gaudet F, Waghmare A, Jaenisch R. Chromosomal instability and tumors promoted by DNA hypomethylation. *Science* 2003; **300**: 455.

52. Rodriguez J, Frigola J, Vendrell E *et al.* Chromosomal instability correlates with genome-wide DNA demethylation in human primary colorectal cancers. *Cancer Res* 2006; **66**: 8462–8.

53. Karpf AR, Matsui S. Genetic disruption of cytosine DNA methyltransferase enzymes induces chromosomal instability in human cancer cells. *Cancer Res* 2005; **65**: 8635–9.

54. Opavsky R, Wang SH, Trikha P *et al.* CpG island methylation in a mouse model of lymphoma is driven by the genetic configuration of tumor cells. *PLoS Genet* 2007; **3**: 1757–69.

55. Haferlach C, Dicker F, Schnittger S *et al.* Comprehensive genetic characterization of CLL: a study on 506 cases analysed with chromosome banding analysis, interphase FISH, IgV(H) status and immunophenotyping. *Leukemia* 2007; **21**: 2442–51.

◆56. Ventura RA, Martin-Subero JI, Jones M *et al.* FISH analysis for the detection of lymphoma-associated chromosomal abnormalities in routine paraffin-embedded tissue. *J Mol Diagn* 2006; **8**: 141–51.

57. Gesk S, Martín-Subero JI, Harder L *et al.* Molecular cytogenetic detection of chromosomal breakpoints in T-cell receptor gene loci. *Leukemia* 2003; **17**: 738–45.

58. Speicher MR, Gwyn Ballard S, Ward DC. Karyotyping human chromosomes by combinatorial multi-fluor FISH. *Nat Genet* 1996; **12**: 368–75.

59. Schröck E, du Manoir S, Veldman T *et al.* Multicolor spectral karyotyping of human chromosomes. *Science* 1996; **273**: 494–7.

60. Nanjangud G, Rao PH, Hegde A *et al.* Spectral karyotyping identifies new rearrangements, translocations, and clinical associations in diffuse large B-cell lymphoma. *Blood* 2002; **99**: 2554–61.

61. Martín-Subero JI, Chudoba I, Harder L *et al.* Multicolor-FICTION: expanding the possibilities of combined morphologic, immunophenotypic, and genetic single cell analyses. *Am J Pathol* 2002; **161**: 413–20.

62. Martín-Subero JI, Gesk S, Harder L *et al.* Recurrent involvement of the REL and BCL11A loci in classical Hodgkin lymphoma. *Blood* 2002; **99**: 1474–7.

63. Martín-Subero JI, Klapper W, Sotnikova A *et al.* Chromosomal breakpoints affecting immunoglobulin loci are recurrent in Hodgkin and Reed-Sternberg cells of classical Hodgkin lymphoma. *Cancer Res* 2006; **66**: 10332–8.

64. Wessendorf S, Schwaenen C, Kohlhammer H *et al.* Hidden gene amplifications in aggressive B-cell non-Hodgkin lymphomas detected by microarray-based comparative genomic hybridization. *Oncogene* 2003; **22**: 1425–9.

65. Rubio-Moscardo F, Climent J, Siebert R *et al.* Mantle-cell lymphoma genotypes identified with CGH to BAC microarrays define a leukemic subgroup of disease and predict patient outcome. *Blood* 2005; **105**: 4445–54.

66. Martín-Subero JI, Gesk S, Harder L *et al.* Interphase cytogenetics of hematological neoplasms under the perspective of the novel WHO classification. *Anticancer Res* 2003; **23**: 1139–48.

67. Dicker F, Schnittger S, Haferlach T *et al.* Immunostimulatory oligonucleotide-induced metaphase cytogenetics detect chromosomal aberrations in 80% of CLL patients: A study of 132 CLL cases with correlation to FISH, IgVH status, and CD38 expression. *Blood* 2006; **108**: 3152–60.

68. Akasaka T, Akasaka H, Yonetani N *et al.* Refinement of the *BCL2*/immunoglobulin heavy chain fusion gene in t(14;18)(q32;q21) by polymerase chain reaction amplification for long targets. *Genes Chromosomes Cancer* 1998; **21**: 17–29.

69. Karran EL, Sonoki T, Dyer MJS. Cloning of immunoglobulin chromosomal translocations by long-distance inverse polymerase chain reaction. *Methods Mol Med* 2005;**115**: 217–30.

●70. Willis TG, Jadayel DM, Coignet LJ *et al.* Rapid molecular cloning of rearrangements of the IGHJ locus using long-distance inverse polymerase chain reaction. *Blood* 1997; **90**: 2456–64.

71. Akasaka H, Akasaka T, Kurata M *et al.* Molecular anatomy of *BCL6* translocations revealed by long-distance polymerase chain reaction-based assays. *Cancer Res* 2000; **60**: 2335–41.

72. Sonoki T, Willis TG, Oscier DG *et al.* Rapid amplification of immunoglobulin heavy chain switch (IGHS) translocation breakpoints using long-distance inverse PCR. *Leukemia* 2004; **18**: 2026–31.

73. Fanidi A, Harrington EA, Evan GI. Cooperative interaction between *c-myc* and *bcl-2* proto-oncogenes. *Nature* 1992; **359**: 554–6.

74. Knezevich S, Ludkovski O, Salski C *et al.* Concurrent translocation of *BCL2* and *MYC* with a single immunoglobulin locus in high-grade B-cell lymphomas. *Leukemia* 2005; **19**: 659–63.

75. Farrell PJ, Allan GJ, Shanahan F *et al.* p53 is frequently mutated in Burkitt's lymphoma cell lines. *EMBO J* 1991; **10**: 2879–87.

76. Ye H, Dogan A, Karran L *et al.* BCL10 expression in normal and neoplastic lymphoid tissue. Nuclear localization in MALT lymphoma. *Am J Pathol* 2000; **157**: 1147–54.

77. Falini B, Pulford K, Pucciarini A *et al.* Lymphomas expressing ALK fusion protein(s) other than NPM-ALK. *Blood* 1999; **94**: 3509–15.

78. Akasaka T, Balasas T, Russell LJ *et al.* Five members of the *CEBP* transcription factor family are targeted by recurrent *IGH* translocations in B-cell precursor acute lymphoblastic leukemia (BCP-ALL). *Blood* 2007; **109**: 3451–61.

79. Russell LJ, Akasaka T, Majid A *et al.* t(6;14)(p22;q32): a new recurrent *IGH@* translocation involving ID4 in B-cell precursor acute lymphoblastic leukemia (BCP-ALL). *Blood* 2008; **111**: 387–91.

80. Dyer MJ, Lillington DM, Bastard C *et al.* Concurrent activation of MYC and BCL2 in B cell non-Hodgkin lymphoma cell lines by translocation of both oncogenes to the same immunoglobulin heavy chain locus. *Leukemia* 1996; **10**: 1198–208.

81. Vaandrager JW, Schuuring E, Philippo K, Kluin PM. V(D)J recombinase-mediated transposition of the *BCL2* gene to the *IGH* locus in follicular lymphoma. *Blood* 2000; **96**: 1947–52.

82. Sonoki T, Iwanaga E, Mitsuya H, Asou N. Insertion of microRNA-125b-1, a human homologue of lin-4, into a rearranged immunoglobulin heavy chain gene locus in a patient with precursor B-cell acute lymphoblastic leukemia. *Leukemia* 2005; **19**: 2009–10.

83. Tagawa H, Karnan S, Suzuki R *et al.* Genome-wide array-based CGH for mantle cell lymphoma: identification of homozygous deletions of the proapoptotic gene *BIM*. *Oncogene* 2005; **24**: 1348–58.

84. Cox C, Bignell G, Greenman C *et al.* A survey of homozygous deletions in human cancer genomes. *Proc Natl Acad Sci U S A* 2005; **102**: 4542–7.

85. Rubio-Moscardo F, Blesa D, Mestre C *et al.* Characterization of 8p21.3 chromosomal deletions in B-cell lymphoma: TRAIL-R1 and TRAIL-R2 as candidate dosage-dependent tumor suppressor genes. *Blood* 2005; **106**: 3214–22.

86. Cimmino A, Calin GA, Fabbri M *et al.* miR-15 and miR-16 induce apoptosis by targeting BCL2. *Proc Natl Acad Sci U S A* 2005; **102**: 13944–9.

87. Nicoloso MS, Kipps TJ, Croce CM, Calin GA. MicroRNAs in the pathogenesis of chronic lymphocytic leukaemia. *Br J Haematol* 2007; **139**: 709–16.

88. Fulci V, Chiaretti S, Goldoni M *et al.* Quantitative technologies establish a novel microRNA profile of chronic lymphocytic leukemia. *Blood* 2007; **109**: 4944–51.

89. Migliazza A, Bosch F, Komatsu H *et al.* Nucleotide sequence, transcription map, and mutation analysis of the 13q14 chromosomal region deleted in B-cell chronic lymphocytic leukemia. *Blood* 2001; **97**: 2098–104.

90. Joos S, Otaño-Joos MI, Ziegler S *et al.* Primary mediastinal (thymic) B-cell lymphoma is characterized by gains of chromosomal material including 9p and amplification of the *REL* gene. *Blood* 1996; **87**: 1571–8.

91. Beà S, Colomo L, López-Guillermo A *et al.* Clinicopathologic significance and prognostic value of chromosomal imbalances in diffuse large B-cell lymphomas. *J Clin Oncol* 2004; **22**: 3498–506.

92. Gilmore TD, Kalaitzidis D, Liang MC, Starczynowski DT. The c-Rel transcription factor and B-cell proliferation: a deal with the devil. *Oncogene* 2004; **23**: 2275–86.

93. Satterwhite E, Sonoki T, Willis TG *et al.* The *BCL11* gene family: involvement of *BCL11A* in lymphoid malignances. *Blood* 2001; **98**: 3413–20.

94. Liu P, Keller JR, Ortiz M *et al.* Bcl11a is essential for normal lymphoid development. *Nat Immunol* 2003; **4**: 525–32.

95. Fink SR, Smoley SA, Stockero KJ *et al.* Loss of TP53 is due to rearrangements involving chromosome region 17p10~p12 in chronic lymphocytic leukemia. *Cancer Genet Cytogenet* 2006; **167**: 177–81.

◆96. Biagi JJ, Seymour JF. Insights into the molecular pathogenesis of follicular lymphoma arising from analysis of geographic variation. *Blood* 2002; **99**: 4265–75.

97. Sellick GS, Catovsky D, Houlston RS. Familial chronic lymphocytic leukemia. *Semin Oncol* 2006; **33**: 195–201.

98. Raval A, Tanner SM, Byrd JC *et al.* Downregulation of death-associated protein kinase 1 (DAPK1) in chronic lymphocytic leukemia. *Cell* 2007; **129**: 879–90.

99. Altieri A, Hemminki K. The familial risk of Hodgkin's lymphoma ranks among the highest in the Swedish Family-Cancer Database. *Leukemia* 2006; **20**: 2062–3.

◆100. Barr FG. Translocations, cancer and the puzzle of specificity. *Nat Genet* 1998; **19**: 121–4.

101. Meaburn KJ, Misteli T. Cell biology: chromosome territories. *Nature* 2007; **445**: 379–81.

102. Dyer MJS, Oscier DG. The configuration of the immunoglobulin genes in B cell chronic lymphocytic leukemia. *Leukemia* 2002; **16**: 973–84.

103. Cotter F, Price C, Zucca E, Young BD. Direct sequence analysis of the 14q+ and 18q chromosome junctions in follicular lymphoma. *Blood* 1990; **76**: 131–5.

104. Stamatopoulos K, Kosmas C, Belessi C *et al.* t(14;18) chromosomal translocation in follicular lymphoma: an event occurring with almost equal frequency both at the D to J(H) and at later stages in the rearrangement process of the immunoglobulin heavy chain gene locus. *Br J Haematol* 1997; **99**: 866–72.

105. Fenton JA, Vaandrager JW, Aarts WM *et al.* Follicular lymphoma with a novel t(14;18) breakpoint involving the immunoglobulin heavy chain switch mu region indicates an origin from germinal center B cells. *Blood* 2002; **99**: 716–8.

106. Streubel B, Vinatzer U, Willheim M *et al.* Novel t(5;9)(q33;q22) fuses *ITK* to *SYK* in unspecified peripheral T-cell lymphoma. *Leukemia* 2006; **20**: 313–18.

107. Soda M, Choi YL, Enomoto M *et al*. Identification of the transforming *EML4-ALK* fusion gene in non-small-cell lung cancer. *Nature* 2007; **448**: 561–6.

●108. Mullighan CG, Goorha S, Radtke I *et al*. Genome-wide analysis of genetic alterations in acute lymphoblastic leukaemia. *Nature* 2007; **446**: 758–64.

109. Oltersdorf T, Elmore SW, Shoemaker AR *et al*. An inhibitor of Bcl-2 family proteins induces regression of solid tumours. *Nature* 2005; **435**: 677–81.

◆110. Fesik SW. Promoting apoptosis as a strategy for cancer drug discovery. *Nat Rev Cancer* 2005; **5**: 876–85.

111. Del Gaizo Moore V, Brown JR, Certo M *et al*. Chronic lymphocytic leukemia requires BCL2 to sequester prodeath BIM, explaining sensitivity to BCL2 antagonist ABT-737. *J Clin Invest* 2007; **117**: 112–21.

112. Burger JA, Tsukada N, Burger M *et al*. Blood-derived nurse-like cells protect chronic lymphocytic leukemia B cells from spontaneous apoptosis through stromal cell-derived factor-1. *Blood* 2000; **96**: 2655–63.

◆113. de Jong D. Molecular pathogenesis of follicular lymphoma: a cross talk of genetic and immunologic factors. *J Clin Oncol* 2005; **23**: 6358–63.

114. Glas AM, Knoops L, Delahaye L *et al*. Gene-expression and immunohistochemical study of specific T-cell subsets and accessory cell types in the transformation and prognosis of follicular lymphoma. *J Clin Oncol* 2007; **25**: 390–98.

115. Streubel B, Chott A, Huber D *et al*. Lymphoma-specific genetic aberrations in microvascular endothelial cells in B-cell lymphomas. *N Engl J Med* 2004; **351**: 250–59.

116. Sherbenou DW, Druker BJ. Applying the discovery of the Philadelphia chromosome. *J Clin Invest* 2007; **117**: 2067–74.

117. Kojima K, Konopleva M, McQueen T *et al*. Mdm2 inhibitor Nutlin-3a induces p53-mediated apoptosis by transcription-dependent and transcription-independent mechanisms and may overcome Atm-mediated resistance to fludarabine in chronic lymphocytic leukemia. *Blood* 2006; **108**: 993–1000.

118. Nieländer I, Bug S, Richter J *et al*. Combining array-based approaches for the identification of candidate tumor suppressor loci in mature lymphoid neoplasms. *APMIS* 2007; **115**: 1107–34.

119. Raval A, Lucas DM, Matkovic JJ *et al*. TWIST2 demonstrates differential methylation in immunoglobulin variable heavy chain mutated and unmutated chronic lymphocytic leukemia. *J Clin Oncol* 2005; **23**: 3877–85.

21

Molecular basis of chromosomal translocation

PHM KLUIN AND JEJ GUIKEMA

INTRODUCTION

Recurrent chromosomal translocations in lymphoid malignancies are found in a minority of precursor T cell acute lymphoblastic leukemia (T-ALL) and precursor B cell ALL (B-ALL) and in approximately 40 percent of all mature B cell lymphomas and multiple myeloma. In some B cell lymphomas such as mantle cell lymphoma, specific translocations are highly characteristic, and can be considered as a diagnostic criterion of the disease. In this chapter the most important mechanisms that are involved in chromosomal translocations will be described. Three different molecular configurations of chromosomal translocations with different oncogenic effects can be recognized.

- **Translocations with juxtaposition to foreign enhancers**. These are translocations with breakpoints outside the coding domain of the target gene and within the immunoglobulin (IG) or T cell receptor (TCR) genes, leading to juxtaposition of the target gene to foreign immunoglobulin (BCR) or TCR gene specific enhancers. In consequence, the target gene is deregulated/overexpressed. However, the target gene may keep its own promoter/enhancer region and, except for possible secondary alterations like mutations, the protein remains intact (no chimeric or fusion protein). An example is the t(11;14)(q13;q32) in mantle cell lymphoma where breakpoints may occur far upstream of the *CCND1*/cyclinD1 gene at 11q13, and juxtaposition of this gene to the IGH heavy chain intronic Eμ enhancer leads to a constitutive expression of cyclinD1, a gene that is not or very weakly expressed in normal B cells.

- **Translocations with promoter substitution**. These are translocations with breakpoints outside the coding domain of the target gene, but leading to the exchange of its promoter/enhancer region with another gene: promoter substitution. Dependent on the nature of the other gene, it may result in deregulation of the target gene; also in this situation, the overexpressed protein remains intact (except for possible secondary mutations). An example is formed by the various t(3;v)(q27;v) translocations where *BCL6* on 3q27 is the target gene, which is affected by juxtaposition to numerous different other genes. Approximately 5–10 percent of all follicular lymphomas and 30–40 percent of diffuse large B cell lymphomas (DLBCL) harbor these 3q27/*BCL6* translocations.

- **Translocations with the generation of fusion genes**. These are translocations with breakpoints within two genes (mostly intronic) leading to fusion of two genes and in consequence resulting in one or sometimes even two chimeric RNAs and proteins. An example is the t(11;18)(q21;q21) in mucosal-associated lymphoid tissue lymphomas of the stomach and lung, involving the *API2* and *MALT1* gene, leading to a chimeric *API2–MALT1* fusion transcript and protein. Another example is the t(2;5)(p23;q35) and its numerous variants in 40–60 percent of all anaplastic large cell lymphomas (ALCL), in which anaplastic large cell lymphoma kinase (*ALK*) is fused to nucleophosmin (*NPM*) or other genes.

Table 21.1   Translocations in lymphoid malignancies

Lymphoma	Translocation	Genes	Frequency	Probable origin	Mechanism at BCR/TCR locus	Mechanism non-TCR/Ig locus
Precursor T cell lymphoma/leukemia	Many	Variable	?	Pre-T	V(D)J-R	Partially RAG1/2-mediated
Anaplastic large cell lymphoma	t(2;5)(p23;q35) t(2;v)(p23;v)	ALK; variable[a]	40–60%	?	—	Unknown (fusion gene)
Precursor B cell lymphoma/leukemia	Many	Variable, only rarely IGH	Variable, age dependent	Pre-B	V(D)J-R	Unknown
Mantle cell lymphoma	t(11;14)(q13;q32)	CCND1; IGH	>95%	Pre-B	V(D)J-R	Unknown
Follicular lymphoma grade 1, 2, 3a	t(14;18)(q32;q21) t(3;v)(q27;v)	IGH; BCL2 BCL6; variable[b]	80%	Pre-B GC	V(D)J-R	Non-B configuration at MBR of BCL2; SHM at MBR[c] of BCL6?; other sites unknown
Follicular lymphoma grade 3b (+/− DLBCL component)	t(3;v)(q27;v) t(14;18)(q32;q21)	BCL6; variable[b] IGH; BCL2	30–50% 30%	GC? Pre-B?	SHM? V(D)J-R?	Unknown (breakpoints at ABR[c]); non-B configuration at MBR[c]
Burkitt lymphoma	t(8;14)(q24;q32), t(2;8)(p12;q24) t(8;22)(q24;q11)	IGH; MYC IGK; MYC MYC; IGL	80% <5% 10%	GC GC GC	SHM or CSR	Immediate 5' and intron I: SHM? AID mediated, H-DNA Other breakpoints unknown
Diffuse large B cell lymphoma	t(3;v)(q27;v) t(14;18)(q32;q21) t(8;14)(q24;q32),	BCL6; variable[b] IGH; BCL2 MYC; IGH	35–40% 15–20% 5–15%	GC Pre-B GC	— V(D)J-R SHM or CSR	SHM at MBR? Non-B configuration at MBR SHM?
Extranodal marginal zone lymphoma	t(11;18)(q21;q21) t(1;14)(p22;q32) t(14;18)(q32;q21) t(3;14)(p14;q32)	API2; MALT1 BCL10; IGH IGH; MALT1 FOXP1; IGH	Variable Variable Variable Variable	? GC? GC? GC?		Unknown/NHEJ (fusion gene) Unknown Unknown Unknown
Multiple myeloma	t(11;14)(q13;q32) t(4;32)(p16;q32)	CCND1; IGH FGFR3/MMSET; IGH	16% 15%	GC GC	CSR (SHM?) CSR	Unknown Unknown
	t(14;16)(q23;q32) t(6;14)(p21;q34) t(14;20)(q32;q11) t(8;v)(q24;v)	IGH; MAF CCND3; IGH IGH; MAFB MYC; variable	5% 3% 2% 15%	GC GC GC ?	CSR CSR CSR	Unknown Unknown Unknown Possibly not RAG1/2 or AID mediated

[a]Recurrent partners: 5q35 (nucleophosmin, NPM), 1q25 (tropomyosin TPM3), 3q35 (TRK fused gene, TFG), 2q35 (ATIC), 17q11-qter (clathrin), Xq11.2-q12 (moesin), 17q25 (ALO17), 22q11.2 (MYH9).

[b]Recurrent partners: 2p12 (IgK), 3;q29 (TFRC; transferrin receptor), 4p13 (RHOH; GTPase), 6p22 (H1F1 histone), 6p21.2 (PIM1); 7p12 (IKAROS), 8q24 (MYC?), 11q23 (OBF1, B cell transcriptional co-activator), 13q14 (L-plastin), 14q32.33 (IGH), 14q32.33 (HSP89alpha/HSP90), 15q22 (?), 16p13 (CIITA), 17q11 (?), 18p11.2 (EIF4A2), 22q11 (IgL) and others.

[c]Two breakpoint clusters (MBR [major translocation breakpoint cluster region] and ABR [alternative translocation breakpoint cluster region] at 3q27).

Pre-B, precursor B cells; Pre-T, precursor T cells; non-B config., non-B configuration of DNA (see text for details); DLBCL, diffuse large B cell lymphoma; GC, germinal center; SHM, somatic hypermutation; CSR, class switch recombination.

Chromosomal translocations can be reciprocal, i.e., without gross loss of DNA, or non-reciprocal, i.e., with loss or duplication of large DNA fragments. The occurrence and frequencies of these translocations in various types of lymphoproliferative disorders will be described in Chapters 22 and 24. A brief summary is given in Table 21.1.

To some extent, the mechanisms involved in the generation of chromosomal breakpoints mimic the physiological processes involved in V(D)J recombination in precursor B and T cells as well as the generation of somatic hypermutations (SHM) and class switch recombinations (CSR) that are specific for mature germinal center B cells.[1] These physiological processes, which are all mediated by

DNA double-strand breaks (DSBs), have been described in detail in Chapter 17. Table 21.2 shows the possible mechanisms and proteins that might be involved in the generation of chromosomal translocations.

During these physiological processes, only a few steps are really B cell or T cell specific, including the involvement of recombination activating genes 1 and 2 (RAG1/2) during the initiating step of normal V(D)J recombination in precursor B cells and precursor T cells and the involvement of activation-induced cytidine deaminase (AID) during SHM and CSR in mature germinal center B cells. All other steps are mediated by ubiquitous protein complexes that are also generally involved in DNA repair in non-B and non-T cells.

Table 21.2   Mechanisms and DNA structures that have been associated with normal rearrangements and chromosomal translocations in human lymphoproliferative disorders

	Normal V(D)J recombination	V(D)J-mediated translocation	Normal SHM	SHM-mediated translocation	Normal CSR	CSR-mediated translocation	Other translocations
Proteins							
RAG1/2, HMG1, HMG2	+	+	−	−	−	−	−
TdT	±	±	−	−	−	−	−
AID	−	−	+	+	+	+	?
UNG, APE1	−	−	+	?	+	+	?
TP53BP1/ATM/MDC1; NBS1/H2AX	+	?	?	?	+	+	?
Mismatch repair proteins	−	−	+	?	+	?	?
NHEJ: KU70/80, Artemis, DNA-PKcs, XRCC4, DNA ligase IV	+	+	+	+	+	+	?
Homologous recombination	−	−	−	−	−	−	?
Physical structure of DNA							
RSS	+	+	−	−	−	−	−
Cryptic RSS	−	±	−	−	−	−	−
Non-B DNA	−	+	−	+?	+?	+?	?
RGYW motif	−	−	+	+?	+	+	−
GC-rich regions	−	+	+	+	+	+	?−
CA repeats	−	?	−	−	−	−	?
Other repeats	−	−	−	−	−	−	?
SARs	−	±	−	−	−	−	?
DNAse-I hypersensitive sites	−	−?	−	−	−	−	?
Nuclear topology and transcriptional factories	+	+	+	+	+	+	+

RAG1/2, recombination activating genes 1/2; HMG1, HMG2, high mobility group protein 1 and 2; TdT, terminal deoxynucleotidyl transferase; AID, activation-induced cytidine deaminase; UNG, uracil DNA glycosylase; APE1, apurinic endonuclease 1; TP53BP1, tumor protein 53 binding protein 1; ATM, ataxia teleangiectasia mutated; MDC1, mediator of DNA damage checkpoint 1; NBS1, Nijmegen breakage syndrome 1; H2AX, H2A histone family, member X; NHEJ, nonhomologous end-joining; KU70/KU80, KU70/KU80 heterodimer; DNA-PKcs: protein kinase, DNA-activated, catalytic subunit; XRCC4, X-ray repair, complementing defective, in Chinese hamster, 4; RSS, recombination signal sequence; RGYW motif (R = A or G, Y = C or T, W = A or T); SAR, scaffold-associated region; MAR, matrix attachment region; SHM, somatic hypermutation; CSR, class switch recombination; GC, germinal center.

LYMPHOID-SPECIFIC EVENTS IN THE GENERATION OF CHROMOSOMAL TRANSLOCATIONS

As discussed in Chapters 9–14, TCR and BCR gene rearrangements are under control of the *RAG*1/2 genes and further modulated by dispensable proteins such as terminal deoxynucleotidyl transferase (TdT) and high mobility group proteins (HMG1 and HMG2). In normal T and B cells, RAG1/2 recognizes specific recognition sequences, the recombination signal sequences (RSS), that are present at both sides of the individual V, D, and J genes and consist of heptamer/nonamer sequences and a 12 or 23 base pair (bp) spacer.

The second mechanism is only seen in mature B cells, in particular germinal center B cells, and is associated with the generation of SHM and CSR. These processes are both associated with the activity of a large number of proteins, the most important and initiating protein being AID.

THE ROLE OF RAG1/2 IN CHROMOSOMAL BREAKPOINTS

In the last decade many authors investigated the mechanism by which RAG1/2 might be involved in the generation of chromosomal breaks involving non-TCR or non-BCR genes instead of physiological V(D)J recombinations. In almost all instances, one of the chromosomal partners is a TCR or BCR gene segment. The configuration of this part of the breakpoint, often with addition of so-called P-nucleotides and TdT-mediated N-nucleotides, strongly suggests that this part reflects a normal rearrangement as occurs in normal precursor T or B cells. This implies that we are almost certainly informed on the timing of the breakpoint as well: this should have occurred in precursor T or B cells at the moment of physiological V(D)J rearrangement.

What is the target of RAG1/2 in the non-TCR or non-BCR locus? Trying to understand this, one has to keep in mind the enormous diversity of these breakpoints. For instance the *BCL1*/11q13 breakpoints of the t(11;14)(q13;q32) in mantle cell lymphoma are dispersed over a very large region of more than 120 kilobases (kb), and only 40 percent of these breakpoints are clustered in an approximately 400 bp region called the major translocation cluster (MTC) of the region.[2] Similarly, many breakpoints at the *BCL2*/18q21 are scattered in the major breakpoint region (MBR) or minor cluster region (mcr) 3' of *BCL2*, whereas other breakpoints occur at the 5' end of the gene. In the past this randomness of targets has been explained by a model in which the non-BCR/TCR DNA is directly attacked by RAG1/RAG2, but these models have never been validated *in vivo*. Recently it has been suggested that RAG1/2-mediated breakpoints at non-IG sites may preferentially occur at CpG hotspots due to inadequate repair of cytosine deamination at hypermethylated sites.[3]

Few chromosomal translocations may be mediated by the evolutionarily conserved mechanism of transposition.[4,5] RAG1/2 might be an excellent enzyme to generate transposition since RAG1/2 is able to both cut at RSS sites and also to religate the same free ends ('open and shut'). Some exceptional cases of follicular lymphoma were described in which the *BCL2* locus might have been excised from the 18q21 region and inserted in the *IGH* locus and in which such a transposition might have functioned.[6]

Based on extensive studies, two different types of breakpoints might be distinguished:[7,8]

- Type A translocations show a normal RSS at the TCR or BCR and a cryptic RSS at the site of the non-BCR or non-TCR locus (Fig. 21.1A). Whereas the prototypic RSS contains a heptamer 5'-CACAGTG-3' and a nonamer 5'-ACAAAAACC-3' separated by a 12 or 23 ± 1 bp spacer, multiple sequences may actually function as a cryptic RSS. Even the 5'-CAC-3' of the heptamer is not always required for RAG1/2-mediated breakage. In fact some authors have suggested that cryptic RSS are present every 1–2 kb in the human genome, and that one-third of these sites might be cut by RAG1/2 in primary thymocyte DNA. How are we then protected against these ubiquitous and hazardous RAG1/2 attacks? Very likely most DNA is protected by chromatin structure and possibly RAG1/2 itself might be targeted to the TCR and BCR DNA by chromatin modalities. The ensuing breakpoints may be further modified by a resumed RAG1/2 activity. Examples of type A translocations are many breakpoints in T-ALL, for instance the recurrent t(11;14)(p13;q11) involving *LMO2* (Ttg-2/rhombotin-2) and *TCRdelta*, t(11;14)(p15;q11) involving *Ttg-1* and *TCRdelta*, t(10;14)(q24;q11) involving *HOX11* (Tcl-3) and *TCRdelta*, and t(7;9)(q34;q32) involving *TAL2* and *TCRB*.[9] Additionally a 100 kb interstitial deletion occurs at 1p32 in approximately 25 percent of all T-ALL and affects *SCL* (Tal-1) and *SIL* and is also mediated by recombination of cryptic RSS by

RAG1/2.[10] Interestingly, the breakpoint of the t(7;9)(q34;q32) is further modified by RAG1/2; however, the most simple unmodified form of the translocation already potentially leading to oncogene activation, can be found relatively frequently in thymocytes of normal children.[11] Detailed analysis of the breakpoint regions of the otherwise very common interstitial deletion of p16/CDKN2A on chromosome 9p21 in lymphomas also revealed cryptic RSS.[12]

- Type B translocations may be characterized by the invasion of blunt broken ends of DNA in a synaptic complex of the BCR or TCR, leading to a complex containing the two signal ends, the two coding ends, and the two blunt ends. Illegitimate repair using nonhomologous end-joining (NHEJ) mechanisms may then result in mixed joints leading to oncogene activation (Fig. 21.1B). In fact these breakpoints are mediated by the DNA repair mechanisms that are active during normal V(D)J recombination in precursor B or T cells. According to these authors, examples of these breakpoints should be the t(11;14)(q13;q32) in mantle cell lymphoma and t(14;18)(q21;q32) in follicular lymphoma as well as many breakpoints in T-ALL that do not contain any cryptic RSS.

Local factors might further contribute to the occurrence of breakpoints at certain sites in the genome. Generally, DNA is in a 'B configuration,' whereas local non-B configurations may exist of triplex DNA configurations (due to purine-pyrimidine tracts) or cruciform configurations (due to inverted repeats).[9,13–16] The MBR of *BCL2* is localized in the 3' untranslated region (UTR) of the gene at chromosome 18q21 and is involved in 70 percent of all t(14;18)(q21;q32) breakpoints. Within this region, the great majority of breakpoints occurs in a 150 bp region, and again within this region breakpoints are clustered at three sites, called peak I, II, and III. Non-B DNA configurations and possibly triplex configurations were identified at peak I and III, indicating that parts of the DNA are single stranded. The RAG complex indeed can efficiently nick this region of the MBR *in vitro* as well.[16,17] Previously, a so-called Z-DNA structure was described for the opposite 5' side of the *BCL2* gene that could mediate breakpoints in unusual t(2;18) or t(18;22) breakpoints.[18]

Specific structural features like the presence of Alu repeats, palindromes, DNA topoisomerase-II sites, scaffold-associated regions (SARs), and DNAse I hypersensitive sites all may contribute to the occurrence of DNA breaks.[13,19,20]

Furthermore, the higher-order spatial genome organization is a contributing factor in the formation of recurrent translocations. For instance, the inactive murine IGH locus has been demonstrated to be distributed at the periphery of the nucleus, possibly being associated with the nuclear lamina. In pro-B cells this interaction is disrupted, allowing this locus to undergo germ-line transcription.[21] In normal B cells *MYC*, *BCL2*, and the immunoglobulin loci,

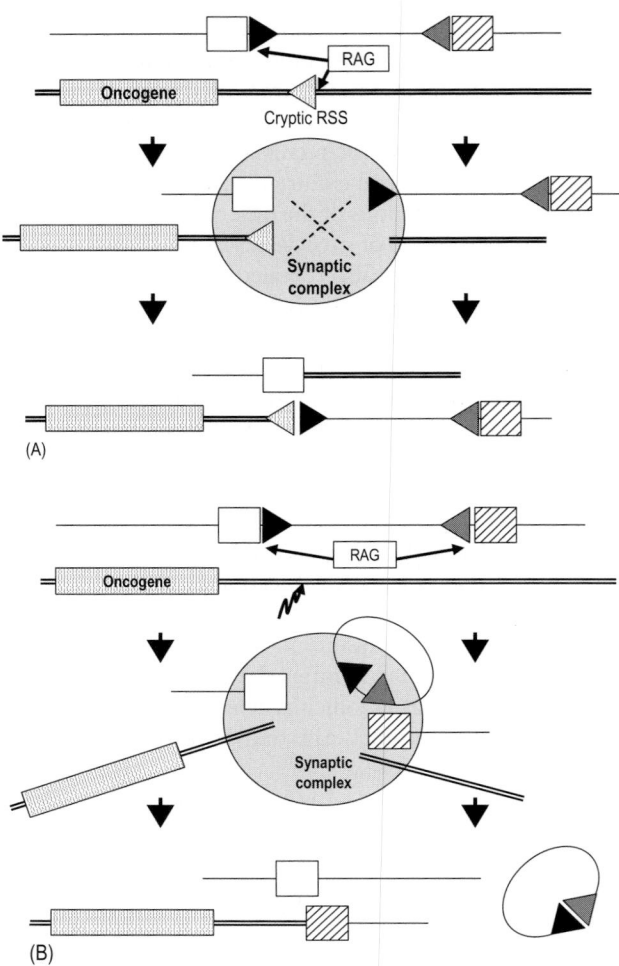

Figure 21.1 Two possible types of RAG1/2-mediated translocation. (A) According to this model, non-Ig and non-TCR loci involved in chromosomal translocations harbor cryptic recognition sites that can be attacked by RAG1/2. (B) According to model B, non-Ig and non-TCR loci involved in chromosomal translocations harbor no cryptic recognition sites but are broken by other mechanisms. For instance, an unusual non-B DNA configuration might be attacked by RAG1/2. RSS, recombination signal sequences.

which are recurrently translocated in various B cell lymphomas, are preferentially positioned in close spatial proximity relative to each other. This phenomenon has been found by quantitative measurement of fluorescence *in situ* hybridization (FISH) results in three-dimensional reconstructions of nuclei.[22–24] A recent study showed that the *IGH* and *MYC* loci are brought together in so-called nuclear 'transcription factories' that reflect dynamic nuclear domains containing active RNA polymerases.[25] This suggests that chromosomal regions involved in chromosomal translocations may be relatively nearby and therefore could be preferentially brought together in other structures upon breakage, such as a synaptic complex with the KU proteins (see later).

THE ROLE OF ACTIVATION–INDUCED CYTIDINE DEAMINASE IN CHROMOSOMAL BREAKPOINTS

Importantly, both CSR and the SHM process are instigated by AID activity, and both processes have been implicated in the generation of chromosomal translocations (see also Chapters 11 and 18; also reviewed by Dudley *et al.*[26]). This may be explained by the fact that during the generation of both CSR and SHM, DSBs are formed as an intermediate stage, making these processes vulnerable to illegitimate recombinations.[27] However, SHM mostly affects the VDJ region whereas CSR affects the more centromeric regions of the *IGH* locus. This specific targeting of different parts of the *IGH* locus is mediated by different domains of the AID protein: experiments with deletion mutants of the protein have shown that the carboxyl (COOH)-end mediates CSR whereas the amino (NH_2)-terminal end of AID mediates SHM.[28]

Many mature B cell lymphomas that originate from germinal center B cells harbor chromosomal breakpoints physically involving the *IGH* switch regions, suggesting that CSR is directly involved in the generation of these breakpoints. As a consequence, the expression of the involved oncogene is deregulated by juxtaposition to enhancers located in the *IGH* locus. Many recurrent translocation partners have been identified, of which the 8q24 locus harboring the *MYC* gene is the most prevalent and most extensively studied partner (see Table 21.1). Interestingly, spontaneous and pristane-induced mouse lymphomas almost invariably carry the t(12;15) chromosomal translocation with breakpoints in *MYC* (chromosome 15) and *IGH* (chromosome 12) loci.[5] This murine translocation is therefore considered as the prototype of the human variant translocation t(8;14)(q24;q34), which characterizes Burkitt lymphoma.[29]

The involvement of AID in these murine plasmacytomas has been thoroughly investigated[30–33] and most experimental data indeed suggest that AID is directly involved in the generation of chromosomal translocations between the *IGH* genes and the *MYC* locus in murine plasmacytomas.[30,31] Other work suggests that translocations between *IGH* S regions and *MYC* can also occur in an AID-independent fashion, but that the outgrowth of translocation-positive cells is dependent on AID.[33]

Activation-induced cytidine deaminase-mediated somatic mutations especially involve the first two kilobases immediately downstream of the V genes and are accompanied by the formation of small deletions or insertions, suggesting that this process of SHM might mediate chromosomal translocations as well. Indeed, chromosomal breakpoints in the VDJ region of Burkitt lymphomas that previously were interpreted as RAG1/2 mediated, now more likely appear to be a by-product of SHM and thus AID mediated.[1] This interpretation is supported by the fact that in contrast to the situation in mantle cell lymphoma and follicular lymphoma, the exact position of the breakpoint is often not at RSS sites but more 5′ in V genes themselves, i.e., more proximal to the VH promoter sites[34] (see Küppers and Dalla-Favera for review[1]). Further support for this hypothesis is derived from data obtained in interleukin-6 (IL-6) transgenic mice. These animals developed lymphoproliferative disorders with *MYC–IGH* breakpoints, a minor portion harboring *MYC–VDJ* breakpoints instead of *MYC–CH* breakpoints. In IL-6 transgenic AID$^{-/-}$ mice no translocations were formed. Furthermore, sequence analysis of the *IGH* locus immediately around the breakpoint revealed signs of NHEJ and a high load of somatic mutations, indicative of AID activity.[35]

Interestingly, SHM is shown to directly target non-Ig genes. This illegitimate SHM activity of non-Ig genes is largely restricted to normal germinal center B cells and mature B cell lymphomas, in particular DLBCL and to a lesser extent follicular lymphoma. In DLBCL the *MYC, PAX5, BCL6, PIM1, CD95,* and *RhoH/TTF* genes undergo somatic mutations that are biased to the AID hotspot RGYW sequence motif.[36,37] In consequence, these regions may be targets for the introduction of DSBs. This is illustrated for the *BCL6* gene in DLBCL. In DLBCL, SHM are found in 70 percent of the cases[38] and chromosomal translocations in 30–40 percent of the cases.[39] The positions of the mutations at the MBR of *BCL6* exactly match to the position of the chromosomal breakpoints in this region, which strongly suggests that many of these breakpoints have been generated by the SHM machinery itself.[40] Moreover, a part of these mutations affects hotspots that function as (negative) regulatory domains of the *BCL6* gene, and in consequence these specific mutations result in a higher expression of BCL6 protein.[41,42]

In parallel to the situation for the *BCL6* gene, a similar coincidence of the sites of mutations and chromosomal breakpoints in DLBCL have been found for *PIM1, MYC,* and *PAX5,* giving further evidence for the hypothesis that both events are mediated by AID.[1]

This vulnerability of non-BCR targets to AID is further substantiated for the *MYC* locus. The *MYC* gene has G-rich regions in the non-template strand, and transcribed plasmids carrying parts of the *MYC* locus bind AID protein *in vitro* as assessed by electron microscopy imaging.[43] Moreover, the promoter region of the *MYC* gene harbors regions of single-strand DNA, as shown by single-strand-specific S1 nuclease hypersensitivity and potassium-permanganate sensitivity mapping, identifying it as a potential AID substrate.[44] Finally, this region is also prone to DSB induction as it contains so-called mirror-repeat sequences that can adopt an H-DNA configuration.[45] Very recently it has been shown that the MYC promoter is essential in the formation of the MYC/IG translocation.[46]

DNA REPAIR AND THE GENERATION OF CHROMOSOMAL TRANSLOCATIONS

In normal B cells, and to a lesser extent T cells, a plethora of physiological protein complexes play multiple critical roles in the repair of DNA errors. These errors include base pair errors, nicks, and DNA DSBs. As previously described, RAG1/2 directly creates DNA DSBs and these breaks are generally resolved by components of NHEJ, either on the same allele leading to a normal recombination or on different chromosomes, leading to a translocation.

In contrast, the effects of AID are more subtle since in principle AID targets single cytidine residues only. These errors of single nucleotides can be repaired by base excision repair (BER); however, if there are multiple nearby errors, the risk of a DNA DSB increases. In more detail, AID alters DNA bases by deamination of deoxycytidine (dC) to produce deoxyuracil (dU). The BER component uracil DNA glycosylase (UNG) removes uracil from the DNA strand and the DNA sugar–phosphate backbone is subsequently nicked by apurinic endonucleases (APE).[47] This nick can now be resolved by filling in the gap by DNA polymerases and ligation by DNA ligases.

However, when multiple nearby nicks exist, as might occur in the GC-rich and repeat-rich *IGH* S-regions, this might lead to a DNA DSB. In consequence, the staggered DNA ends may be repaired by NHEJ. When such a NHEJ occurs within a switch region it may lead to a small internal deletion (as frequently seen for Sμ in mature B cells[48]), but when multiple switch regions are involved, it may lead to recombination between two different switch sites and in consequence to class switching.[49] Formation of S-S synapses may be further facilitated by a positional change of the intronic Eμ and 3′ Eα enhancers.[50]

Gene-targeting studies suggest the involvement of mismatch repair (MMR) in the conversion of single-stranded DNA nicks into DSB in CSR. According to this model, (U:G) mismatches remaining after incomplete action of UNG are recognized by the MSH2/MSH6 and MLH1/ PMS2 heterodimers, which recruit exonuclease I to the nearby nicks, which excises the mismatched DNA proceeding until the nearest nick on the opposite strand.[51] Similarly, biochemical experiments indicate that MSH2/ MSH6 is also involved in SHM mutation, by interacting with polymerase η.[52]

Apart from this role, mismatch repair proteins, in particular the heterodimer MUTSα (MSH2/MSH6), also seem to be involved in physiological CSR by promoting synapses between transcriptionally activated switch sites.[53] Moreover, MSH6 may play another role and function as a physical scaffold of the VH region of the *IGH* locus early in SHM.[53–56] Thus MSH6 might target AID to both the VH region and switch regions of this region.

Whereas there is ample evidence for a role in normal SHM and CSR, the role of mismatch repair in the generation of translocations is uncertain. Certainly, NHEJ is the primary repair mechanism involved in chromosomal translocations of B and T cell lymphomas, as the genes involved in the translocation obviously lack extensive homology needed for homologous recombination. Because of the lack of such a template, NHEJ often results in a final DNA sequence that differs from the original template. See elsewhere for a review of NHEJ in lymphomagenesis.[14,57,58]

In addition, it has recently been shown that a non-classical end-joining pathway that relies on microhomology can also mediate joining in S-S recombination as well as in chromosomal translocations involving IGH breaks.[59]

Components of NHEJ that are active in the repair of DSBs in lymphomas (both generated by RAG1/2 or AID) are KU70/KU80 (86 Da), DNA-PKcs, XRCC4/DNA ligase IV, Artemis, and XLF (also known as Cernunnos) and are illustrated in Figure 21.2. The KU70/KU80 heterodimer covers free DNA ends and recruits DNA-PKcs, which subsequently phosphorylate the KU proteins, XRCC4 and the Artemis nuclease.

DNA-PKcs autophosphorylation results in dissociation of DNA-PKcs from the free DNA termini. KU, DNA-PKcs, and XRCC4 all bring together the free DNA termini. In turn, XRCC4 forms a tight complex with DNA ligase IV. Several nucleases with different characteristics are active, one being Artemis that complexes with DNA-PKcs, but also Werner syndrome gene product (WRN) and MRE11, the latter being involved in the MRE11/RAD50/NBS1 complex. The result of this step is gap filling at the site of the free DNA termini. The whole repair process in which the termini are ligated is finished by a DNA polymerase X, in particular $POL\mu$.

Finally, DNA DSBs also result in activation of the 53BP1/ATM/MDC1Nbs1/H2AX proteins that rapidly accumulate at the site of the breakpoint. These proteins promote end joining of DNA ends and prevent DSBs from progressing into translocations by recruitment of DNA DSB repair proteins. DNA lesions that are unresolved may initiate a p53-mediated checkpoint, or may initiate a chromosomal translocation.[60,61] Absence of normal ATM and stabilization of DNA ends in repair complexes might therefore also explain the occurrence of abnormal translocations in patients with ataxia teleangiectasia.[62]

Certainly, DNA repair proteins play an important role in normal SHM and CSR, but only very little is known on their role in the generation of chromosomal translocations. In fact, apart from the role of several NHEJ proteins, it remains completely speculative whether and how the many other proteins are involved in these illegitimate events.

KEY POINTS

- RAG1/2 and AID play a key role in the generation of many chromosomal translocations in human B cell and T cell lymphomas as well as leukemias.
- RAG1/2 affects not only the recombination signal sequences of the BCR and TCR loci but likely also attacks other loci. Abnormal DNA structures such as a non-B configuration of the DNA at these loci may contribute to their vulnerability.
- AID is a key player in somatic hypermutation and class switch recombination of the BCR in normal B cells. There is ample evidence that AID affects several non-BCR loci as well, both by induction of somatic mutations but probably also by induction of DNA breakpoints, thereby causing chromosomal translocations.
- In contrast to these two highly lymphocyte-specific proteins, a plethora of DNA repair proteins contribute to normal V(D)J recombination, somatic hypermutation, and class switch recombination. However, their role in the generation of chromosomal translocations is less clear or at least uncertain.

REFERENCES

● = Key primary paper
◆ = Major review article

◆1. Küppers R, Dalla-Favera R. Mechanisms of chromosomal translocations in B cell lymphomas. *Oncogene* 2001; **20**: 5580–94.

●2. Vaandrager JW, Schuuring E, Zwikstra E *et al.* Direct visualization of dispersed 11q13 chromosomal translocations in mantle cell lymphoma by multi-color DNA fiber FISH. *Blood* 1996; **88**: 1177–82.

3. Tsai AG, Lu H, Raghavan SC *et al.* Human chromosomal translocations at CpG sites and a theoretical basis for their lineage and stage specificiy. *Cell* 2008; **135**: 1130–42.

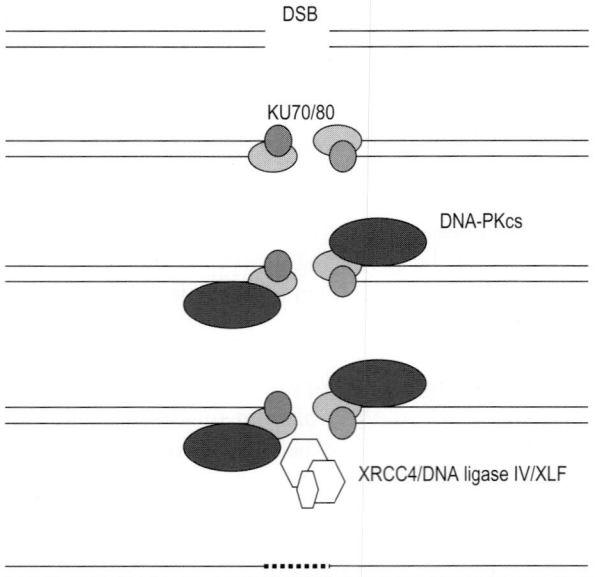

DSB

KU70/80

DNA-PKcs

XRCC4/DNA ligase IV/XLF

Figure 21.2   Schematic overview of nonhomologous end-joining (NHEJ). After initiation of the DNA double-strand break (DSB), free ends are recognized and bound by KU70/KU80 heterodimers, which recruit DNA-PKcs. Break ends are remodeled by nucleases such as Artemis, Mre11, and WRN. The XRCC4/DNA ligase IV complex interacts with the recently identified NHEJ factor XLF and religates DNA ends.

●4.   Hiom K, Melek M, Gellert M. DNA transposition by the RAG1 and RAG2 proteins: a possible source of oncogenic translocations. *Cell* 1998; **94**: 463–70.

●5.   Agrawal A, Eastman QM, Schatz DG. Transposition mediated by RAG1 and RAG2 and its implications for the evolution of the immune system. *Nature* 1998; **394**: 744–51.

●6.   Vaandrager JW, Schuuring E, Philippo K, Kluin PM. V(D)J recombinase-mediated transposition of the BCL2 gene to the IGH locus in follicular lymphoma. *Blood* 2000; **96**: 1947–52.

●7.   Marculescu R, Le T, Simon P *et al.* V(D)J-mediated translocations in lymphoid neoplasms: a functional assessment of genomic instability by cryptic sites. *J Exp Med* 2002; **195**: 85–98.

◆8.   Marculescu R, Vanura K, Montpellier B *et al.* Recombinase, chromosomal translocations and lymphoid neoplasia: targeting mistakes and repair failures. *DNA Repair (Amst)* 2006; **5**: 1246–58.

◆9.   Raghavan SC, Lieber MR. DNA structures at chromosomal translocation sites. *BioEssays* 2006; **28**: 480–94.

●10. Aplan PD, Lombardi DP, Ginsberg AM *et al.* Disruption of the human SCL locus by 'Illegitimate' V-(D)-J recombinase activity. *Science* 1990; **250**: 1426–9.

●11. Marculescu R, Vanura K, Le T *et al.* Distinct t(7;9)(q34;q32) breakpoints in healthy individuals and individuals with T-ALL. *Nat Genet* 2003; **33**: 342–4.

●12. Kitagawa Y, Inoue K, Sasaki S *et al.* Prevalent involvement of illegitimate V(D)J recombination in chromosome 9p21 deletions in lymphoid leukemia. *J Biol Chem* 2002; **277**: 46289–97.

●13. Kurahashi H, Inagaki H, Ohye T *et al.* Chromosomal translocations mediated by palindromic DNA. *Cell Cycle* 2006; **5**: 1297–303.

◆14. Aplan PD. Causes of oncogenic chromosomal translocation. *Trends Genet* 2006; **22**: 46–55.

●15. Raghavan SC, Chastain P, Lee JS *et al.* Evidence for a triplex DNA conformation at the bcl-2 major breakpoint region of the t(14;18) translocation. *J Biol Chem* 2005; **280**: 22749–60.

●16. Raghavan SC, Swanson PC, Wu X *et al.* A non-B-DNA structure at the Bcl-2 major breakpoint region is cleaved by the RAG complex. *Nature* 2004; **428**: 88–93.

●17. Raghavan SC, Swanson PC, Ma Y, Lieber MR. Double-strand break formation by the RAG complex at the bcl-2 major breakpoint region and at other non-B DNA structures in vitro. *Mol Cell Biol* 2005; **25**: 5904–19.

●18. Adachi M, Tsujimoto Y. Potential Z-DNA elements surround the breakpoints of chromosome translocation within the 5′ flanking region of bcl-2 gene. *Oncogene* 1990; **5**: 1653–7.

●19. Ramakrishnan M, Liu WM, DiCroce PA *et al.* Modulated binding of SATB1, a matrix attachment region protein, to the AT-rich sequence flanking the major breakpoint region of BCL2. *Mol Cell Biol* 2000; **20**: 868–77.

●20. Elliott B, Richardson C, Jasin M. Chromosomal translocation mechanisms at intronic alu elements in mammalian cells. *Mol Cell* 2005; **17**: 885–94.

●21. Kosak ST, Skok JA, Medina KL *et al.* Subnuclear compartmentalization of immunoglobulin loci during lymphocyte development. *Science* 2002; **296**: 158–62.

●22. Bartova E, Kozubek S, Jirsova P *et al.* Nuclear structure and gene activity in human differentiated cells. *J Struct Biol* 2002; **139**: 76–89.

●23. Kozubek S, Lukasova E, Ryznar L *et al.* Distribution of ABL and BCR genes in cell nuclei of normal and irradiated lymphocytes. *Blood* 1997; **89**: 4537–45.

●24. Roix JJ, McQueen PG, Munson PJ *et al.* Spatial proximity of translocation-prone gene loci in human lymphomas. *Nat Genet* 2003; **34**: 287–91.

●25. Osborne CS, Chakalova L, Mitchell JA *et al.* Myc dynamically and preferentially relocates to a transcription factory occupied by Igh. *PLoS Biol* 2007; **5**: 1763–72.

◆26. Dudley DD, Chaudhuri J, Bassing CH, Alt FW. Mechanism and control of V(D)J recombination versus class switch recombination: similarities and differences. *Adv Immunol* 2005; **86**: 43–112.

●27. Papavasiliou FN, Schatz DG. Cell-cycle-regulated DNA double-stranded breaks in somatic hypermutation of immunoglobulin genes. *Nature* 2000; **408**: 216–21.

●28. Shinkura R, Ito S, Begum NA *et al.* Separate domains of AID are required for somatic hypermutation and class-switch recombination. *Nat Immunol* 2004; **5**: 707–12.

◆29. Janz S. Myc translocations in B cell and plasma cell neoplasms. *DNA Repair (Amst)* 2006; **5**: 1213–24.

●30. Ramiro AR, Jankovic M, Callen E *et al.* Role of genomic instability and p53 in AID-induced c-myc-Igh translocations. *Nature* 2006; **440**: 105–9.

●31. Ramiro AR, Jankovic M, Eisenreich T *et al.* AID is required for c-myc/IgH chromosome translocations in vivo. *Cell* 2004; **118**: 431–8.

●32. Okazaki IM, Hiai H, Kakazu N *et al.* Constitutive expression of AID leads to tumorigenesis. *J Exp Med* 2003; **197**: 1173–81.

●33. Unniraman S, Zhou S, Schatz DG. Identification of an AID-independent pathway for chromosomal translocations between the Igh switch region and Myc. *Nat Immunol* 2004; **5**: 1117–23.

●34. Neri A, Barriga F, Knowles DM *et al.* Different regions of the immunoglobulin heavy-chain locus are involved in chromosomal translocations in distinct pathogenetic forms of Burkitt lymphomas. *Proc Natl Acad Sci U S A* 1988; **85**: 2748–52.

●35. Dorsett Y, Robbiani DF, Jankovic M *et al.* A role for AID in chromosome translocations between c-myc and the IgH variable region. *J Exp Med* 2007; **204**: 2225–32.

●36. Pasqualucci L, Migliazza A, Fracchiolla N *et al.* BCL-6 mutations in normal germinal center B cells: evidence of somatic hypermutation acting outside Ig loci. *Proc Natl Acad Sci U S A* 1998; **95**: 11816–21.

●37. Pasqualucci L, Neumeister P, Goossens T *et al.* Hypermutation of multiple proto-oncogenes in B-cell diffuse large-cell lymphomas. *Nature* 2001; **412**: 341–6.

●38. Migliazza A, Martinotti S, Chen W *et al.* Frequent somatic hypermutation of the 5' noncoding region of the BCL6 gene in B-cell lymphoma. *Proc Natl Acad Sci U S A* 1995; **92**: 12520–4.

●39. Ye BH, Chaganti S, Chang CC *et al.* Chromosomal translocations cause deregulated BCL6 expression by promoter substitution in B cell lymphoma. *EMBO J* 1995; **14**: 6209–17.

●40. Jardin F, Sahota SS. Targeted somatic mutation of the BCL6 proto-oncogene and its impact on lymphomagenesis. *Hematology* 2005; **10**: 115–29.

●41. Artiga MJ, Saez AI, Romero C *et al.* A short mutational hot spot in the first intron of BCL-6 is associated with increased BCL-6 expression and with longer overall survival in large B-cell lymphomas. *Am J Pathol* 2002; **160**: 1371–80.

●42. Wang X, Li Z, Naganuma A, Ye BH. Negative autoregulation of BCL-6 is bypassed by genetic alterations in diffuse large B cell lymphomas. *Proc Natl Acad Sci U S A* 2002; **99**: 15018–23.

●43. Duquette ML, Pham P, Goodman MF, Maizels N. AID binds to transcription-induced structures in c-MYC that map to regions associated with translocation and hypermutation. *Oncogene* 2005; **24**: 5791–8.

●44. Michelotti GA, Michelotti EF, Pullner A *et al.* Multiple single-stranded cis elements are associated with activated chromatin of the human c-myc gene in vivo. *Mol Cell Biol* 1996; **16**: 2656–69.

●45. Wang G, Vasquez KM. Naturally occurring H-DNA-forming sequences are mutagenic in mammalian cells. *Proc Natl Acad Sci U S A* 2004; **101**: 13448–53.

46. Robbiani DF, Bothmer A, Callen E *et al.* AID is required for the chromosomal breaks in c-myc that lead to c-myc/IgH translocations. *Cell* 2008; **135**: 1028–38.

●47. Guikema JE, Linehan EK, Tsuchimoto D *et al.* APE1- and APE2-dependent DNA breaks in immunoglobulin class switch recombination. *J Exp Med* 2007; **204**: 3017–26.

●48. Schrader CE, Linehan EK, Mochegova SN *et al.* Inducible DNA breaks in Ig S regions are dependent on AID and UNG. *J Exp Med* 2005; **202**: 561–8.

●49. Stavnezer J, Schrader CE. Mismatch repair converts AID-instigated nicks to double-strand breaks for antibody class-switch recombination. *Trends Genet* 2006; **22**: 23–8.

●50. Wuerffel R, Wang L, Grigera F *et al.* S-S synapsis during class switch recombination is promoted by distantly located transcriptional elements and activation-induced deaminase. *Immunity* 2007; **27**: 711–22.

●51. Schrader CE, Vardo J, Stavnezer J. Role for mismatch repair proteins Msh2, Mlh1, and Pms2 in immunoglobulin class switching shown by sequence analysis of recombination junctions. *J Exp Med* 2002; **195**: 367–73.

◆52. Goodman MF, Scharff MD. Identifying protein-protein interactions in somatic hypermutation. *J Exp Med* 2005; **201**: 493–6.

●53. Larson ED, Duquette ML, Cummings WJ *et al.* MutSalpha binds to and promotes synapsis of transcriptionally activated immunoglobulin switch regions. *Curr Biol* 2005; **15**: 470–4.

●54. Li Z, Zhao C, Iglesias-Ussel MD *et al.* The mismatch repair protein Msh6 influences the in vivo AID targeting to the Ig locus. *Immunity* 2006; **24**: 393–403.

●55. Bardwell PD, Woo CJ, Wei K *et al.* Altered somatic hypermutation and reduced class-switch recombination in exonuclease 1-mutant mice. *Nat Immunol* 2004; **5**: 224–9.

◆56. Min IM, Selsing E. Antibody class switch recombination: roles for switch sequences and mismatch repair proteins. *Adv Immunol* 2005; **87**: 297–328.

◆57. Lieber MR, Yu K, Raghavan SC. Roles of nonhomologous DNA end joining, V(D)J recombination, and class switch recombination in chromosomal translocations. *DNA Repair (Amst)* 2006; **5**: 1234–45.

●58. Ma Y, Lu H, Schwarz K, Lieber MR. Repair of double-strand DNA breaks by the human nonhomologous DNA end joining pathway: the iterative processing model. *Cell Cycle* 2005; **4**: 1193–200.

●59. Yan CT, Bobiola C, Souza EK *et al.* IgH class switching and translocations use a robust non-classical end-joining pathway. *Nature* 2007; **449**: 472–82.

●60. Pan-Hammarstrom Q, Lahdesmaki A, Zhao Y *et al.* Disparate roles of ATR and ATM in immunoglobulin class switch recombination and somatic hypermutation. *J Exp Med* 2006; **203**: 99–110.

●61. Franco S, Gostissa M, Zha S *et al.* H2AX prevents DNA breaks from progressing to chromosome breaks and translocations. *Mol Cell* 2006; **21**: 201–14.

●62. Bredemeyer AL, Sharma GG, Huang CY *et al.* ATM stabilizes DNA double-strand-break complexes during V(D)J recombination. *Nature* 2006; **442**: 466–70.

22

Genesis and consequences of genetic lesions in lymphoid neoplasms

DAVIDE ROSSI AND GIANLUCA GAIDANO

GENERAL CONCEPTS

Some general molecular features are shared by all lymphoid neoplasms: (1) molecular lesions predominantly affect genes regulating lymphoid maturation, cell cycle progression, and cell survival; (2) within a given clinico-pathological category, different genetic lesions in different patients may converge upon activation or disruption of the same molecular pathway; (3) many, though not all, genetic lesions are represented by recurrent and balanced chromosomal translocations; (4) the degree of generalized genomic instability is markedly lower than observed in solid cancers; and (5) a single genetic alteration is rarely, if ever, capable of driving the full development of a lymphoid neoplasm.

Some genetic alterations develop in precursor lymphoid cells, but are permissive for further maturation of the tumor clone, and display their oncogenic potential when the tumor cell population has reached a stage of differentiation consistent with mature lymphoid cells. Other genetic lesions, mainly involving transcription factors regulating early lymphoid maturation, do not allow the maturation of the tumor clone, and lead to precursor lymphoid neoplasia. In other instances, the genetic lesion is acquired by an already mature lymphoid cell, residing preferentially, but not exclusively, in mutagenic microenvironments, of which the germinal center (GC) is unequivocally the best example.

In addition to genetic lesions, other factors, provided by the host or derived from the tumor microenvironment, play a role in some lymphoid tumors of mature lymphoid cells. Because mature lymphoid cells express a fully competent antigen receptor, whereas precursor lymphoid cells do not, the role of antigen stimulation and selection in promoting tumor growth is restricted to mature lymphoid cell neoplasia. With the limits intrinsic to all generalizations, it appears that the pathogenesis of precursor lymphoid neoplasms may be predominantly ascribed to genetic lesions, whereas the development of mature lymphoid cell neoplasia, at least of some tumor types, is a multifactorial process characterized by the interplay between genetic lesions, antigen drive, microenvironmental stimuli, and host factors.

This chapter does not aim at providing an exhaustive coverage of the molecular lesions of lymphoid neoplasms, but rather aims at defining a general framework for understanding the molecular pathogenesis of lymphoid neoplasia. Emphasis will be placed on the basic mechanisms, rather than on single disease entities.

PRECURSOR LYMPHOID CELL NEOPLASMS

The pathogenesis of precursor lymphoid neoplasia is due to the somatic acquisition of recurrent genetic lesions that are represented mainly, though not exclusively, by chromosomal translocations.[1–3] Translocations of precursor lymphoid neoplasms (1) involve protooncogenes implicated in transcriptional regulation of lymphoid maturation, or, more rarely, in signal transduction; (2) identify leukemia subsets, which are characterized by specific gene expression profiles and, in some instances, may predict outcome; (3) tend to be mutually exclusive in a given patient; and (4) to a certain extent, share a common molecular genesis.[2–5] Attempts to model precursor lymphoid neoplasms in mice have indicated that most genetic lesions occurring in these neoplasms are by themselves insufficient to generate a full leukemic phenotype. Thus, cooperating oncogenic lesions are required.[5]

The genesis of many, but not all, genomic aberrations of precursor lymphoid cell neoplasms follows a unifying molecular mechanism involved in mediating translocations, insertions, and deletions in leukemogenic cells. This involves lymphocyte-specific genomic rearrangements mediated by the V(D)J recombinase enzyme complex (see also Chapter 23).[4] A partial summary of leukemogenic rearrangements proposed to be mediated by V(D)J recombinase is presented in Table 22.1. Overall, the high level of activity of the V(D)J recombinase system in lymphocytes during fetal and early childhood immunologic development presents a considerable risk to genomic stability.

Table 22.1 V(D)J-mediated chromosomal translocations

Translocation	Neoplasm	IG/TCR partner	Oncogene
t(1;7)(q34;q34)	T-ALL	TCRβ	LCK
t(1;14)(p34;q11)	T-ALL	TCRδ	TAL1
t(7;9)(q34;q32)	T-ALL	TCRβ	TAL2
t(7;11)(q34;p13)	T-ALL	TCRβ	LMO2
t(11;14)(p13;q11)	T-ALL	TCRδ	LMO2
t(11;14)(p15;q11)	T-ALL	TCRδ	LMO1
t(8;14)(q24;q11)	T-ALL	TCRα/δ	MYC
t(10;14)(q24;q11)	T-ALL	TCRα/δ	HOX11
t(14;21)(q11;q22)	T-ALL	TCRα	BHLHB1
inv(14)(q11;q32)	T-ALL	TCRδ	BCL11B
t(11;14)(q13;q32)	Mantle cell lymphoma	IGH	BCL1/ cyclin D1
t(14;18)(q32;q11)	Follicular lymphoma	IGH	BCL2

T-ALL, T cell acute lymphoblastic leukemia.

Surprisingly, V(D)J-mediated translocations appear to predominate in T cell acute lymphoblastic leukemia (T-ALL), whereas the genesis of chromosomal translocations in B cell lineage ALL is more heterogeneous.

THE UTERUS AS A SITE OF LEUKEMOGENESIS

A significant fraction of acute leukemias of infancy and childhood is believed to arise during intrauterine life.[6] Several lines of evidence are in support of this view, including (1) a common clonal origin of concordant leukemia in monozygotic twins;[6,7] (2) the presence of acquired identical genetic lesions in the leukemia clone and in archived neonatal blood spots (Guthrie cards) in children with leukemia;[8] and (3) the presence of functional leukemia fusion genes in cord blood samples.[9] The ALL types for which a uterine origin has been formally demonstrated include precursor B cell lineage ALL with TEL-AML1 chimeric transcripts or hyperdiploidy, infant pro-B lineage ALL with MLL-AF4 fusion, and T cell lineage ALL carrying NOTCH1 mutations.[6,7,10]

The twin and Guthrie card studies have provided important insights into the latency of ALL development.[6–8] Although most cases have a relatively brief postnatal latency (~6 months for infant ALL, 2–5 years for childhood ALL), latency is very variable and can occasionally be very protracted.[11] It is likely that average latency and cases of protracted latency reflect the time required for the accrual of secondary mutations that precipitate clinical leukemia. According to this model, a first (prenatal) hit would be followed by at least an additional (postnatal) hit.[6,7] This is also consistent with transgenic animal modeling: TEL-AML1 does contribute to leukemogenesis, but overt leukemia requires the presence of additional genetic changes.[12,13] Direct evidence for the presence of postnatal secondary genetic changes comes also from twin studies in which paired samples share the same initiating event, but have distinct secondary events, e.g., different TEL deletions or chromosome changes.[14] Also, ~1 percent of newborns have TEL-AML1-positive B-lineage clones, although the incidence of TEL-AML1-positive ALL is 100 times lower.[9] This observation indicates that leukemia initiation by chromosomal changes in utero is far more common than the rarity of the clinical disease would otherwise suggest. Because ALL biology is not different between twins and singletons, there is no basis for considering that leukemia might be uniquely initiated in utero only in the context of twinning. Therefore, the conclusion from the twin studies that leukemia can originate prenatally may apply more generally to pediatric patients.

HETEROTOPIC GENE EXPRESSION IN THE THYMUS

Key steps of thymocyte development are controlled by several transcriptional regulators, including the basic helix-loop-helix (bHLH) family of transcription factors and homeobox proteins.[15] In T-ALL, many of these proteins are misexpressed because of structural alterations, mainly chromosomal translocations, that cause deregulated

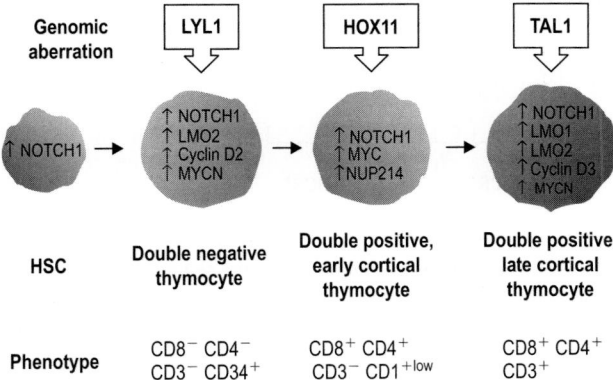

Figure 22.1 Different steps in thymocyte differentiation correlated with T cell acute lymphoblastic leukemia (T-ALL) molecular heterogeneity. Key steps of thymocyte development are controlled by several transcriptional regulators. Among these, the basic helix-loop-helix (bHLH) family of transcription factors and homeobox proteins are major players in T cell ontogeny. In T-ALL, many of these proteins are misexpressed because of structural alterations, mainly chromosomal translocations, that cause deregulated expression in thymocytes. LYL1$^+$ T-ALL shows an expression profile indicating maturation arrest at the earliest double negative stage of thymocyte differentiation. HOX11$^+$ cases develop to the early cortical double positive stage, whereas TAL1$^+$ cases are arrested at a late cortical double positive stage. The gene expression profiles that are characteristic of each stage of maturation arrest indicate multiple molecular pathways that can result in the transformation of T cell progenitors during development. HSC, hematopoietic stem cell.

expression in thymocytes (Fig. 22.1).[5] Chromosomal breakpoints in T-ALL often involve the TCRβ enhancer (7q34) or the TCRα/δ enhancer (14q11), both of which are highly active in committed T cell progenitors, resulting in the deregulated expression of transcription factor genes located at the breakpoint on the reciprocal chromosome (Table 22.2).[2,3,5,16]

Transcription factors belonging to the bHLH family share the bHLH motif allowing homo- or heterodimerization through the HLH domain, and DNA binding through the basic part of dimerized proteins.[17] In the normal thymus, the class A bHLH genes *E2A* and *HEB*, named the E proteins, are the bHLH transcription factors that are expressed physiologically. Conversely, the class B bHLH genes *LYL1*, *TAL1*, *TAL2*, and *bHLHB1* are not expressed in the normal thymus. These latter genes can be ectopically expressed in T-ALL, following juxtaposition to regulatory sequences (derived from TCR loci or other loci) that are highly active at the thymocyte stage.[5,16] Examples are: (1) *TAL1* activation due to t(1;14)(p32;q11) or due to submicroscopic interstitial deletions generating *SIL-TAL1* fusion genes;[18] (2) *LYL1* deregulation due to t(7;19)(q34;p13);[19] and (3) the rare chromosomal translocations t(7;9)(q34;q32) juxtaposing *TAL2* and TCRβ, and t(14;21)(q11;q22) juxtaposing *BHLH1* and TCRα.[20,21]

Homeobox (HOX) genes are key regulators of embryonic development and share a 61-amino-acid motif, the homeodomain, that serves as a DNA binding domain regulating transcription of target genes.[22] In addition to embryonal development, some *HOX* genes play a role in normal hematopoiesis, influencing stem cell renewal and lineage commitment. *HOXA* genes (A7, A9, A10, A11) are expressed during the early stages of human T cell development.[23] In knockout mice, the absence of specific *HOXA*

Table 22.2 Heterogeneity of chromosomal translocations causing heterotopic deregulation in T-ALL

Translocation	Oncogene	Partner	Functional consequence
Translocations (or other abnormalities) involving basic helix–loop–helix (bHLH) genes			
t(1;14)(p32;q11)	*TAL1*	TCRα/δ	Heterotopic deregulation
1p32 deletions (cryptic)	*TAL1*	SIL	Heterotopic deregulation
t(7;19)(q34;p13)	*LYL1*	TCRβ	Heterotopic deregulation
t(7;9)(q34;q32)	*TAL2*	TCRβ	Heterotopic deregulation
t(14;21)(q11;q22)	*BHLHB1*	TCRα/δ	Heterotopic deregulation
Translocations (or other abnormalities) involving homeobox (HOX) genes			
t(7;10)(q34;q24)	*TLX1*	TCRβ	Heterotopic deregulation
t(10;14)(q24;q11)	*TLX1*	TCRα/δ	Heterotopic deregulation
t(5;14)(q35;q11)	*TLX3*	TCRα/δ	Heterotopic deregulation
inv(7)(p15;q34)	*HOXA* cluster	TCRβ	Heterotopic deregulation
Translocations involving LIM-only domain (LMO) genes			
t(11;14)(p15;q11)	*LMO1*	TCRα/δ	Heterotopic deregulation
t(11;14)(p13;q11)	*LMO2*	TCRα/δ	Heterotopic deregulation
t(7;11)(q34;p13)	*LMO2*	TCRβ	Heterotopic deregulation

T-ALL, T cell acute lymphoblastic leukemia.

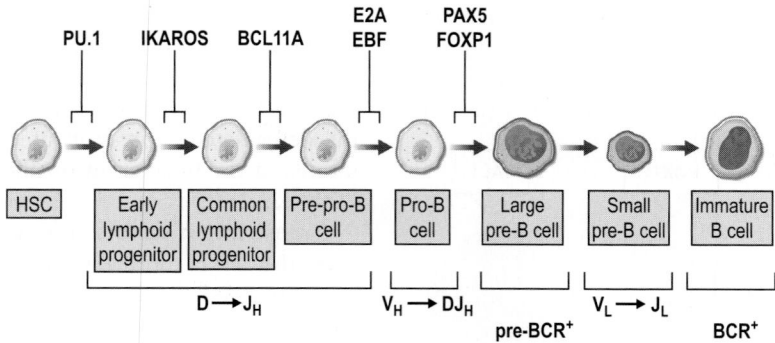

Figure 22.2 Early B cell differentiation in the bone marrow. Differentiation of lymphoid progenitors into mature B cells is a tightly regulated process coordinated by a hierarchical network of transcription factors. This process is accompanied by the sequential rearrangement of immunoglobulin receptor genes. At least seven transcription factors (PU.1, IKAROS, BCL11A, E2A, EBF, PAX5, and FOXP1) are involved in B cell progenitor differentiation (the predominant corresponding site of action is shown in the figure). D-J$_H$ rearrangements are initiated in early lymphocyte progenitors and are completed as the cell progresses to the common lymphocyte progenitor and pre-pro-B cell stage. V$_H$-DJ$_H$ recombination takes place in pro-B cells. Successful rearrangement is denoted by the expression of immunoglobulin (Ig)$_\mu$ protein in the pre-B cell receptor (BCR) of large pre-B cells. Subsequent rearrangement of the IG light chain locus in small pre-B cells results in the expression of the BCR in immature B cells. HSC, hematopoietic stem cell.

genes results in early block of thymocyte differentiation.[24] Conversely, overexpression of specific *HOXA* genes also results in defective T cell development.[25] In T-ALL, *HOXA* genes (especially *HOXA10* and *HOXA11*) can be upregulated as a consequence of an often cryptic inv(7) or t(7;7), which bring the TCRβ enhancer within the *HOXA* locus.[26]

Class II homeobox genes (also termed non-HOX genes or divergent homeobox genes) are dispersed throughout the genome and encode cofactors for HOX proteins that are not involved in homeotic transformation.[27] Their pattern of expression is restricted, being implicated in organogenesis and in differentiation of specific cell types. The *TLX1* and *TLX3* genes are involved in T-ALL. The *TLX1* homeobox gene has been identified as the gene located at the 10q24 breakpoint region of t(10;14)(q24;q11) and t(7;10)(q34;q24).[28] As a result of the juxtaposition with promoter elements of TCRα and TCRβ, respectively, the full-length protein is expressed at a high level. Deregulated expression of *TLX3* in T-ALL is in most cases caused by the cryptic translocation t(5;14)(q35;q32) juxtaposing *TLX3* to the distal region of *BCL11B*, a gene universally expressed during T cell differentiation.[29] *TLX3* is very similar to *TLX1*, and microarray studies indicate that *TLX1*[+] and *TLX3*[+] T-ALL cluster together, suggesting a common mechanism of action.[30,31]

In addition to bHLH transcription factors and homeobox genes, chromosomal translocations of T-ALL may also implicate LIM-only domain (LMO) genes, namely *LMO1* and *LMO2*. *LMO1* and *LMO2* encode proteins containing the LIM domains involved in protein–protein interactions and can be activated by translocation to the TCR enhancer loci or, in the case of *LMO2*, by deletion removing a negative regulator of *LMO2* expression.[32]

BLOCK OF DIFFERENTIATION IN PRECURSOR B CELL NEOPLASMS

Differentiation of lymphoid progenitors into mature B cells is a tightly regulated process coordinated by a hierarchical network of transcription factors and cytokines.[33] This process is accompanied by the sequential rearrangement of immunoglobulin receptor genes. At least seven transcription factors (PU.1, IKAROS, E2A, BCL11A, EBF, PAX5, and FOXP1) are involved in B cell progenitor differentiation. PU.1 and IKAROS are required for the development of early lymphoid precursors (Fig. 22.2).[33] The transcription factors E2A (TCF3), EBF, and BCL11A are crucial for the generation of early (pro-B) B cell precursors, and mice lacking E2A, EBF, or BCL11A show an arrest in B cell differentiation prior to the onset of IG gene rearrangement.[33] E2A and EBF also regulate expression of downstream transcription factors such as PAX5.[34] In turn, PAX5 is essential for B-lineage commitment and differentiation, and, together with FOXP1, promotes V(D)J recombination (Fig. 22.2).[34]

Several of the aforementioned transcription factors involved in B cell differentiation are implicated in precursor B cell neoplasia (Table 22.3 and Fig. 22.2).[5,33] The E2A transcription factor is involved in at least two types of chromosomal translocations, leading to fusion of the *E2A* gene with the homeobox gene *PBX1* or, alternatively, with *HLF*, a member of the PAR subfamily of bZIP transcription factors.[35–38] In both instances, the N-terminal transactivation domain of *E2A* is retained in the chimeric transcript and is fused to the DNA-binding domain of the partner gene.[35–38] Approximately 30 percent of B cell lineage ALL display structural alterations of *PAX5*, leading to loss of gene function.[39,40] Genetic lesions of *PAX5* include copy number alterations, focal deletions due to cryptic

Table 22.3 Chromosomal translocations in B cell lineage acute lymphoblastic leukemia

Translocation	Oncogene/fusion gene	Frequency in B cell lineage ALL	
		Children	Adult
t(12;21)(p12;q22)	TEL/AML1	25%	5%
t(1;19)(q23;p13)	E2A/PBX	5%	5%
t(17;19)(q22;p13)	E2A/HLF	Rare	Rare
der(11)(q23)	MLL	15%	10%
t(9;22)(q34;q11)	BCR/ABL	2–5%	20%

ALL, acute lymphoblastic leukemia.

translocations, and loss-of-function mutations that cluster in the DNA-binding paired domain and in the transactivation domain. Loss-of-function mutations or deletions lead to a reduction of the functional level of PAX5 and/or other key regulators of B cell differentiation. As a consequence, the altered leukemic progenitor is unable to normally differentiate beyond the pro-B cell stage of development.[39,40]

DEREGULATED SIGNAL TRANSDUCTION IN PRECURSOR LYMPHOID CELL NEOPLASIA

NOTCH1 encodes a regulatory transmembrane receptor that is expressed in hematopoietic stem cells and controls several steps in thymocyte specification and differentiation.[41] Upon interaction with ligands of the DLL and Jagged family, the intracellular domain of NOTCH translocates to the nucleus and activates the transcription of target genes.[41] Over 50 percent of T-ALL acquire activating mutations of NOTCH.[42] These mutations occur either in the heterodimerization domain, causing an unstable connection between the intracellular and the extracellular domains, or in the negative regulatory PEST domain.[42] Both types of NOTCH mutations lead to increased levels of NOTCH-dependent transcription, presumably by increasing nuclear NOTCH levels.

Aberrant signal transduction also plays a relevant role in B cell lineage ALL, as documented by the occurrence of t(9;22) translocations leading to BCR/ABL fusion genes in B cell lineage ALL of adulthood and of the elderly.[1–3]

MATURE LYMPHOID CELL NEOPLASMS

Neoplasms of mature lymphoid cells are far more heterogeneous than neoplasms of immature lymphoid cells in terms of: (1) histogenetic origin of the tumor cell population; (2) anatomical site of derivation; (3) characteristics of the tumor microenvironment (e.g., GC microenvironment versus bone marrow microenvironment); and (4) host immune function and infection status.[1] Because mature lymphoid cell neoplasms generally derive from lymphoid cells that have expressed functional antigen receptors at some timepoint of their history, endogenous and foreign antigens may also play a role in promoting tumor growth. The aforementioned factors interplay with the somatic acquisition of genetic lesions, which in many cases tend to associate specifically with a given disease entity.

THE TUMOR CELL

Tumor cells of mature lymphoid neoplasms experience several molecular events that may favor, directly or indirectly, neoplastic transformation. Examples of such molecular events include but are not restricted to: (1) signaling through antigen receptor; (2) acquisition of chromosomal translocations and somatic mutations due to genomic plasticity; (3) deregulation of the cell cycle machinery; (4) activation of the nuclear factor κB (NF-κB) master system; and (5) gain of foreign DNA material derived from oncogenic viruses.

The B cell receptor: antigen stimulation in mature B cell neoplasms

The heavy chain complementarity determining region 3 (HCDR3) of the B cell receptor (BCR) is created de novo by the VDJ recombination process (Fig. 22.3).[43] HCDR3 sequences are the principal determinant of specificity, at least in the primary B cell repertoire. Somatic hypermutation (SHM) of IG variable genes forms a second round of diversification after somatic recombination, which increases antibody diversity (Fig. 22.3).[43,44]

In recent years, chronic lymphocytic leukemia (CLL) has emerged as the prototype lymphoid disorder whose development, growth, and prognosis are affected by the molecular characteristics of the BCR expressed by leukemic cells.[45,46] Chronic lymphocytic leukemia that expresses unmutated IG variable genes tends to have an aggressive clinical course relative to patients expressing IG variable genes with somatic mutations.[47,48] The mutation status of IG variable genes has now entered the clinical practice of CLL, and is considered as one of the most powerful disease prognosticators. Despite the molecular difference in the mutation status of IG variable genes, gene expression profiling studies have shown that both CLL subsets resemble antigen-experienced and activated B cells, and that the profiles of mutated and unmutated CLL differ for only a few genes, which importantly include the ZAP70 protein tyrosine kinase.[45,46,49]

Several lines of experimental evidence indicate that CLL development might be influenced by antigen recognition and/or selection through the BCR. This evidence is based on: (1) skewed usage of IG genes; (2) stereotyped HCDR3 in the BCR; and (3) stereotyped mutations in the BCR. Chronic lymphocytic leukemia cells display a skewed usage

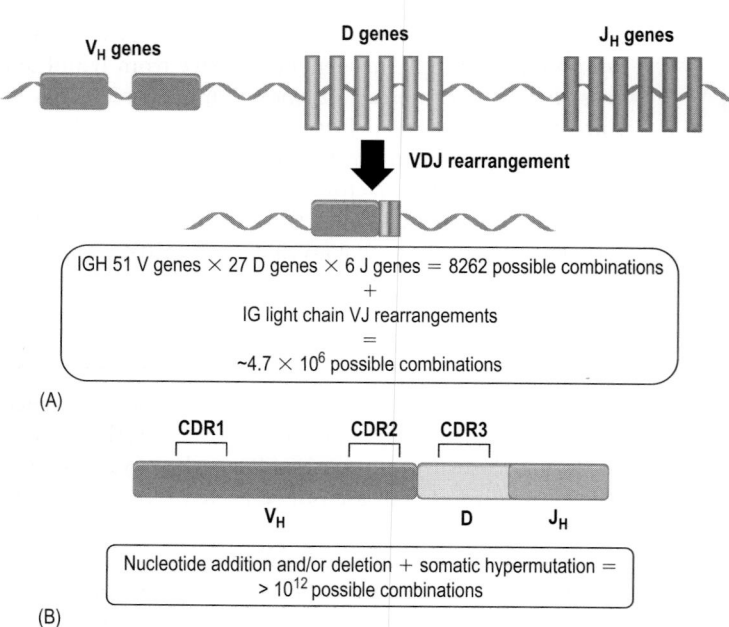

(A)

(B)

Figure 22.3   Molecular diversity of the B cell repertoire. Diversity of the B cell repertoire is ensured at multiple levels. (A) First, VDJ rearrangement in the heavy chain locus, coupled to rearrangements in the light chain loci, allows a combinatorial diversity exceeding 4×10^6 possible combinations. (B) Nucleotide additions/deletions and somatic hypermutation occurring in the germinal center further increases diversity of the B cell repertoire to greater than 10^{12} combinations.

of IG variable genes, with specific loci being utilized in CLL at a higher frequency than in the normal B cell repertoire.[50–55] Out of the more than fifty IG variable genes, usage of only ten accounts for more than 60 percent of CLL. Certain IG variable genes (e.g., IGHV1-69) are preferentially used in unmutated CLL, whereas others (e.g., IGHV3-7, IGHV3-23, IGHV4-34) are more frequent in mutated CLL.[50–55] Skewed usage of IG variable genes in CLL suggests that antigens or superantigens, or both, might be involved in leukemia development by stimulating proliferation of B cells that express surface immunoglobulin encoded by particular IG genes. From a clinical standpoint, usage of specific IG variable genes, e.g., IGHV3-21, may herald poor prognosis despite the presence of other favorable predictors in a given patient.[50–55]

A second piece of evidence corroborating the role of antigen stimulation in CLL comes from the observation that over 20 percent of CLL carry BCR whose HCDR3 sequences are closely homologous among mutated and unmutated cases.[54,55] These BCR have been named as 'stereotyped' BCR and have been grouped in clusters, whose number is constantly growing. The remarkable BCR similarity in unrelated and geographically distant cases implies the recognition of individual, discrete antigens or classes of structurally similar epitopes, likely operating a positive selection of the leukemic clone.[54,55] The nature of the involved antigens cannot be directly deduced from the IG gene sequences of the BCR expressed by CLL cells and is the subject of current investigations.

In addition to HCDR3 restriction, groups of CLL patients using certain IG variable genes carry shared, stereotyped mutations occurring across the entire IG variable sequence.[55] The presence of stereotyped mutations unequivocally documents that not only the HCDR3 but also other regions of the IG molecule could actively participate in antigen recognition,

and therefore be involved in the development and evolution of CLL clones.[55]

The BCR restriction observed in CLL is not a general phenomenon of B cell malignancies, but rather should be considered 'CLL biased,' since BCR restriction is very rare in other B cell lymphomas. The potential role of antigen stimulation through BCR activation in CLL is not limited to the chronic phase of the disease. In fact, recent evidence has documented that usage of an otherwise rarely used IG variable gene, namely *IGHV4-39*, is a powerful and independent predictor of CLL transformation to clonally related diffuse large B cell lymphoma, a poor prognosis event also known as Richter syndrome.[56]

The germinal center reaction as a site of chromosomal translocation and aberrant somatic hypermutation

After successfully rearranging V(D)J genes in the bone marrow, immunoglobulin M (IgM)-expressing B cells enter the periphery, where they come into contact with their cognate antigens in the presence of antigen-specific T cells. A fraction of B cells activated in this manner initiate the formation of oligoclonal GCs, in which they undergo two distinct IG diversification processes: (1) class switch recombination (CSR) and (2) SHM (Fig. 22.4).[57] Both CSR and SHM are involved in the genesis of several genetic lesions specific of mature B cell neoplasia (Fig. 22.5).[44,57,58]

CLASS SWITCH RECOMBINATION AND THE GENESIS OF CHROMOSOMAL TRANSLOCATIONS

During CSR, the membrane-expressed BCR, which is primarily encoded during development and maturation, is

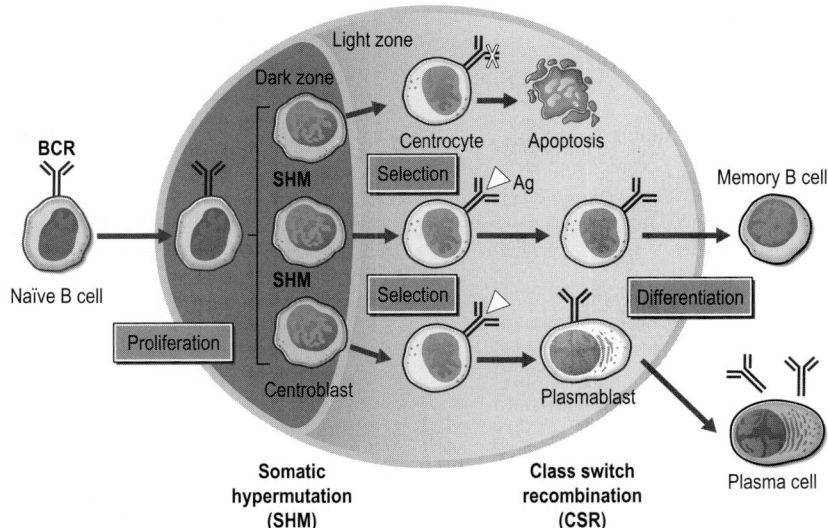

Figure 22.4 The germinal center reaction. Naïve B cells differentiate into centroblasts and undergo clonal expansion in the dark zone of the germinal center. During this process, somatic hypermutation (SHM) targets the IGV regions of the B cell receptor (BCR); some of these mutations may change the amino acid sequence and increase, or decrease, the BCR affinity for antigen (Ag). Centroblasts subsequently differentiate into centrocytes, which reside in the germinal center light zone. With help from T cells (not shown) and follicular dendritic cells (FDC), the mutated BCR is selected for antigen binding. Newly generated centrocytes whose mutations decreased BCR affinity for antigen undergo apoptosis and are removed. A subset of centrocytes undergoes class switch recombination. Antigen-selected centrocytes eventually differentiate into memory B cells or plasma cells.

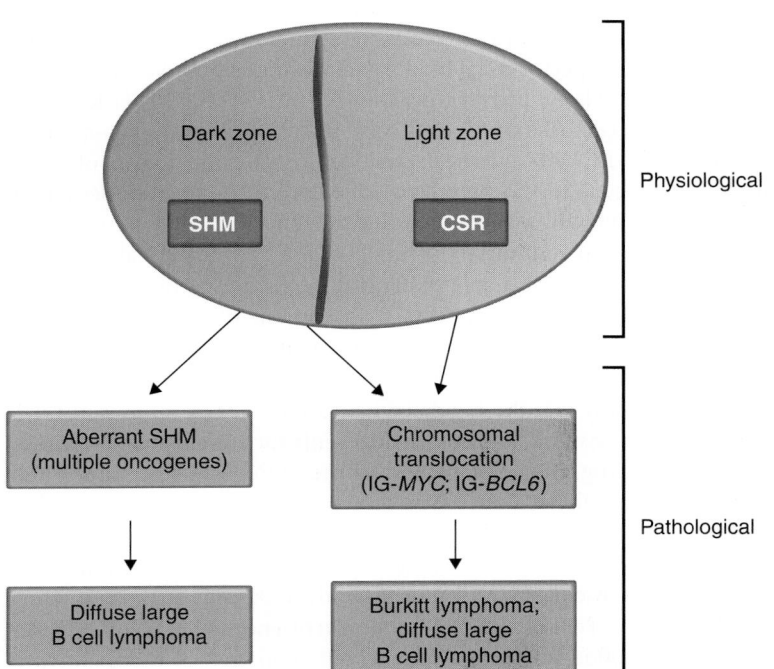

Figure 22.5 Genomic plasticity in the germinal center and pathological consequences in lymphomagenesis. Somatic hypermutation (SHM) and class switch recombination (CSR) are physiological events occurring in the germinal center dark zone and light zone, respectively. Errors in the processes of SHM or CSR at the IG loci or at non-IG loci result in the generation of free DNA ends that lead to chromosomal translocation (e.g., IG-*MYC* in Burkitt lymphoma and translocations involving *BCL6* and either IG or non-IG loci in diffuse large B cell lymphoma). Aberrant SHM affecting the 5′ regulatory or coding regions of multiple protooncogenes in diffuse large B cell lymphoma may cause deregulated expression or abnormal function of these genes.

replaced by a different BCR isotype. This genomic modification replaces the expressed μ constant region (Cμ) of the heavy chain locus with a downstream isotype Cγ, Cα, or Cε. Class switch recombination involves a recombination between two different repetitive switch (S) region sequences, located upstream of the constant region genes. Class switch recombination, as well as SHM, is initiated by the activity

of activation-induced cytidine deaminase (AID), an enzyme selectively expressed in GC B cells.[57–60]

A hallmark of mature B cell lymphomas is the presence of reciprocal chromosomal translocations that juxtapose loci encoding the IG genes to a protooncogene.[2,3] Some, though not all, chromosomal translocations of mature B cell lymphomas are due to the genomic plasticity caused

Table 22.4 Chromosomal translocations associated with class switch recombination

Translocation	Neoplasm	Oncogene	Partner gene
t(8;14)(q24;q32)	Burkitt lymphoma	MYC	IGH
t(14;19)(q32;q13)	Chronic lymphocytic leukemia	BCL3	IGH
t(3;14)(q26;q32)	Diffuse large B cell lymphoma	BCL6	IGH
t(9;14)(p13;q32)	Lymphoplasmacytic lymphoma	PAX5	IGH
t(4;14)(p16;q32)	Multiple myeloma	FGFR3; MMSET	IGH
t(14;16)(q32;q23)	Multiple myeloma	MAF	IGH
t(6;14)(p21;q32)	Multiple myeloma	Cyclin D3	IGH
t(14;20)(q32;q11)	Multiple myeloma	MAFB	IGH
t(11;14)(q13;q32)	Multiple myeloma	Cyclin D1	IGH

by CSR in the GC microenvironment (Table 22.4).[57–59] In the process of CSR, DNA double-strand break (DSB) intermediates generated in IG genes by this reaction are potent substrates for translocations by recombining with DSBs on a nonhomologous chromosome. Therefore, CSR, IG-associated breaks, and IG-involving translocations are initiated by a common mechanism involving DNA deamination. The formal proof that AID is required for GC-derived lymphomagenesis is based on the observation that AID deficiency prevents the formation of BCL6-dependent, GC-derived B cell non-Hodgkin lymphoma in lymphoma-prone animal models.[61]

Chromosomal translocations of B cell neoplasms that have the molecular clues of CSR-mediated translocations include (Table 22.4): (1) MYC translocations in Burkitt lymphoma and in a fraction of diffuse large B cell lymphoma; (2) BCL6 translocations in diffuse large B cell lymphoma; (3) PAX5 translocations in lymphoplasmacytic lymphoma; (4) the rare BCL3 translocation in CLL; and (5) an array of translocations involved in multiple myeloma.[58,59]

Chromosomal translocations involving the MYC proto-oncogene and antigen receptor loci have provided the first example of oncogene involvement in tumor-associated chromosomal abnormalities. The product of the MYC proto-oncogene is a ubiquitously expressed nuclear bHLH-LZIP phosphoprotein that functions as a transcriptional regulator controlling cell proliferation, differentiation, and apoptosis.[62] Via this mechanism, MYC regulates the expression of an unusually large number of target genes involved in the control of key cellular functions, including cell growth and cell cycle progression. Reverse engineering of networks linking coregulated genes from genome-wide expression profiles has led to the identification of MYC as a major hub in B cells, i.e., one of a few highly interconnected genes in a genome-wide network.[63] Consistent with its function as a hub, MYC controls a network comprising many genes, some of which are themselves provided with a hub function.[63] Expression of MYC is rapidly induced in quiescent cells upon mitogenic induction, suggesting that MYC plays a role in mediating the transition from quiescence to proliferation.[62] In addition to mediating cell proliferation, MYC is also implicated in blocking differentiation.[62] In the absence of a supportive

microenvironment providing adequate concentrations of growth stimuli, however, proliferation and/or block of differentiation are replaced by cellular apoptosis.[64]

In physiologic in vivo settings, MYC is mainly engaged in heterodimeric complexes with the related protein MAX, which stimulates transcription and cell proliferation.[62] In addition to MYC, MAX can also form homodimers and heterodimers with MAD and MXI1, two bHLH-LZIP proteins acting as negative regulators of transcription.[62] Since the levels of MAX tend to be stable throughout the cell cycle, the ratio of MYC/MAX heterodimers is controlled by the relative abundance of MYC, MAD, and MXI1.[62] As the ratio of MYC to MAD or MXI1 varies, the promoter activity of target genes is expected to be modulated in either a positive (when MYC levels are high) or negative (when MAD or MXI1 levels are high) fashion.[62] Therefore, in lymphoid tumors associated with MYC deregulation, constitutive expression of MYC leads to the prevalence of MYC/MAX heterodimers, thus inducing positive growth regulation.

In addition to its function as a transcriptional regulator, MYC is also able to control DNA replication via nontranscriptional pathways.[65] Initiation of DNA replication requires coordination between assembly of the prereplicative complex at replication origins during late mitosis and early G1, the regulated activation of these origins at G1/S transition, and epigenetic events such as chromatin remodeling. MYC interacts with the prereplicative complex and localizes to early sites of DNA synthesis.[65] Overexpression of MYC, as observed in lymphomas carrying MYC translocations, causes increased replication origin activity with subsequent DNA damage and checkpoint activation.[65]

The constitutive expression of a normal MYC protein can influence the growth and differentiation of B cells in vitro and in vivo, consistent with a role in B cell lymphomagenesis. In vitro, the expression of MYC oncogenes transfected into Epstein–Barr virus (EBV)-immortalized human B cells, a potential natural target for MYC activation in EBV-positive Burkitt lymphoma, leads to their malignant transformation.[66] Accordingly, antisense oligonucleotides directed against translocated MYC mRNA are able to revert tumorigenicity of Burkitt lymphoma.[67] In vivo, the targeted expression of MYC oncogenes in the B cell lineage of transgenic mice leads to the development of B cell malignancy at a relatively high frequency.[68]

Cytogenetic studies of non-Hodgkin lymphoma have demonstrated that chromosomal alterations affecting band 3q27 and several alternative partner chromosomes are a frequent recurrent abnormality in diffuse large B cell lymphoma.[2,3] The cloning of the 3q27 chromosomal breakpoints revealed the *BCL6* gene, a transcriptional repressor containing zinc fingers, a protein sequence motif able to mediate the protein binding to specific DNA sites.[69] The amino-terminal region of the BCL6 protein contains a domain, termed *POZ*, that is homologous to domains found also in several other zinc-finger transcription factors and acts as a protein–protein interface implicated in homo/heterodimerization processes. The pattern of BCL6 protein expression in human tissues is highly specific and high levels are specifically found in B cells.[70] In particular, *BCL6* expression is topographically restricted to the GC, where *BCL6* is expressed by both centroblasts and centrocytes, whereas expression of *BCL6* is absent in pre-GC B cells (naïve B cells) and post-GC B cells (memory B cells and plasma cells).[70] The observation that *BCL6* is expressed within the GC, but not before entrance into or after exit from the GC, led to the postulate that *BCL6* may be needed for GC development and sustainment, while its downregulation may be necessary for further differentiation of B cells. Consistent with this hypothesis, mice carrying the $Bcl6^{-/-}$ phenotype consistently fail to form the GC and display impairments in T cell-dependent antigen-specific IgG responses.[71]

BCL6 determines the ability of GC B cells to tolerate their extremely high proliferation rate while undergoing DNA remodeling by SHM and CSR. In fact, *BCL6* suppresses apoptotic and cell cycle arrest responses by directly suppressing *TP53* transcription and by suppressing the activation of the cell cycle arrest gene *p21*.[72,73] Therefore, *BCL6* may allow GC B cells to sustain the physiologic genotoxic stress associated with high proliferation, and sustain the DNA breaks that are induced by SHM and CSR without eliciting the *TP53*-dependent and *TP53*-independent growth arrest and apoptosis that would otherwise ensue.[72,73] In addition to responses to DNA damage, *BCL6* may also suppress the sensing of DNA damage itself by direct transcriptional suppression of ATR (ataxia-telangiectasia mutated and RAD3 related), one of the main sensors of DNA damage.[74] The activity of *BCL6* in controlling the cellular responses to genotoxic stress is, in turn, regulated by the levels of DNA damage by a signaling pathway promoting BCL6 degradation. Upon accumulation of DNA damage, ATM (ataxia-telangiectasia mutated) indirectly promotes ubiquitin-mediated proteasomal degradation of BCL6.[75]

Chromosomal translocations involving band 3q27 truncate *BCL6* within its 5′ flanking region within the first exon or within the first intron. *BCL6* rearrangements are detectable in 35 percent of cases of diffuse large B cell lymphoma and in a small fraction of follicular lymphoma.[69,76] Conversely, *BCL6* rearrangements are virtually absent in all other types of lymphoid neoplasms. The coding domain of the gene is left intact in all cases displaying *BCL6* rearrangements, whereas the 5′ regulatory sequences, which contain the *BCL6* promoter, are either truncated or, alternatively, completely removed. In all *BCL6* rearrangements, the entire coding sequence of *BCL6* is juxtaposed downstream to heterologous sequences which, based on cytogenetic data, may originate from different chromosomal sites in different patients. The common functional consequence of *BCL6* translocations is the juxtaposition of heterologous promoters to the *BCL6* coding domain, a mechanism called promoter substitution.[77] The substitution of the *BCL6* promoter by heterologous regulatory sequences causes deregulated *BCL6* expression in lymphomas carrying *BCL6* rearrangements. One feature shared by the heterologous promoters linked to rearranged *BCL6* alleles is that they are physiologically active in normal B cells and are not downregulated during the late stages of B cell differentiation.[77] Thus, *BCL6* rearrangements may prevent downregulation of *BCL6* and, in turn, block the differentiation of GC B cells toward the stage of plasma cells. In particular, *BCL6* translocations abrogate the NF-κB-mediated induction of the IRF4 transcription factor that, in normal B cells, represses *BCL6* expression.[78] Another way whereby *BCL6* contributes to lymphomagenesis is functional inactivation of *TP53*.[72] *BCL6* functions normally to suppress *TP53*-mediated apoptosis of GC B cells in response to DNA damage during the GC reaction. Constitutive expression of *BCL6* might decrease the *TP53*-mediated apoptotic response to DNA damage, promoting persistence of malignant clones.[72] *BCL6* transgenic mouse modeling provides further insights into the precise role of *BCL6* in lymphomagenesis.[79]

SOMATIC HYPERMUTATION: PHYSIOLOGICAL AND ABERRANT

The physiological function of SHM is to introduce non-templated point mutations in the variable region of rearranged IG genes.[44] Somatic hypermutation underlies the process of affinity maturation, which results in the preferential outgrowth of B cells expressing an immunoglobulin that has high affinity for its cognate antigen.[44,57] The mutations introduced by SHM are predominantly point mutations, although insertions and deletions are occasionally observed. Transitions are twice as frequent as transversions, and a high proportion of mutations target the hotspot motifs DGYW (where D denotes adenosine [A], guanosine [G], or thymidine [T]; Y denotes cytidine [C] or T; and W denotes A or T) and WRCH (where R denotes A or G; and H denotes T, C, or A), documenting that SHM is influenced by the primary DNA sequence.[44] The process of SHM is closely linked to transcription.[44] The mutation rate of an IG gene is proportional to the transcription rate of the locus, and mutations are confined to a 1–2 kilobase (kb) region downstream of the transcription start site.[44]

As for CSR, AID is required also for SHM.[44,57] Activation-induced cytidine deaminase acts directly on DNA, converting C to uridine (U) in IG variable and switch regions (Fig. 22.6). After AID initiates SHM by the deamination of C nucleotides, the resulting U·G mismatch may lead to mutations in several different ways. If the mismatch is not repaired before the onset of DNA replication, DNA polymerases will insert an A nucleotide opposite to U, thus creating a C→T and G→A transition. If, conversely, the U is removed by uracil DNA glycosylase (UNG), an abasic site is created, and its replication may give rise to either transitions or transversions. In addition to activating UNG-dependent base excision repair (BER), a U·G mismatch recruits the mismatch repair (MMR) machinery, which is thought to create mutations at A·T near the initiating U·G lesion, probably through an error-prone patch repair process. Remarkably, U nucleotides are frequently incorporated into the DNA of proliferating cells independently of AID activity. These U nucleotides are efficiently and accurately repaired by BER enzymes. During SHM, though, the U lesion is repaired in an error-prone manner, possibly because of saturation of the BER machinery. Thus, both AID-mediated deamination and error-prone DNA lesion repair are thought to be necessary for SHM.

Somatic hypermutation is not specific for IG genes, but in normal B cells it targets also other genes expressed in the GC, namely *BCL6* and *CD95/FAS*.[80–82] The molecular profile of SHM of *BCL6* and *CD95/FAS* reflects the features of mutations introduced in IG genes.[80–82] In some lymphomas deriving from GC B cells, mainly though not exclusively represented by diffuse large B cell lymphoma, SHM may misfire and target several protooncogenes, thus contributing to neoplastic transformation.[83–88] Malfunctioning of SHM in the context of lymphoma is termed aberrant SHM and the protooncogenes most frequently affected include *PIM1*, *MYC*, *RHOH* (*Ras* homologue gene-family member H), and *PAX5*.[83–88] Collectively, aberrant SHM of *PIM1*, *MYC*, *RHOH*, and *PAX5* occurs in ~70 percent of diffuse large B cell lymphoma, although the frequency of affected cases may be higher when considering that several genes other than *PIM1*, *MYC*, *RHOH*, and *PAX5* are involved, albeit more rarely.[83–88] The mutation frequency of non-IG genes is ~50–100-fold lower than that of IG variable genes, but the mutation profile (in terms of transition/transversion ratio or hotspot targeting) is similar in both physiological and aberrant SHM. Aberrant SHM can contribute to lymphomagenesis by mutating both regulatory and coding sequences in protooncogenes.[83–88] For example, mutations in *MYC* frequently target important functional domains and regulatory sequences, and mutations in the *BCL6* regulatory region have been shown to deregulate *BCL6* expression.[89–91] Also, SHM

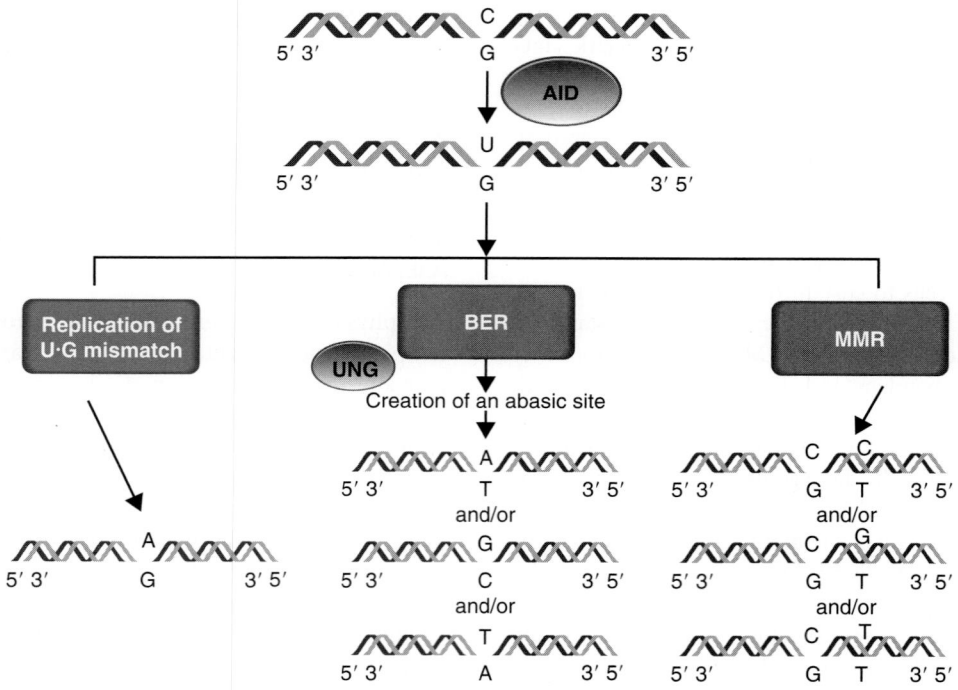

Figure 22.6   Generation of somatic hypermutation by activation-induced cytidine deaminase (AID). AID acts directly on DNA, converting C to U in IG variable and switch regions. After AID initiates somatic hypermutation (SHM) by the deamination of C nucleotides, the resulting U·G mismatch may lead to mutations in several different ways in an error-prone environment: (1) if the mismatch is not repaired before the onset of DNA replication, DNA polymerases will insert an A nucleotide opposite to U, thus creating a C>T and G>A transition; (2) if the U is removed by the uracil DNA glycosylase (UNG)-dependent base excision repair (BER), an abasic site is created, and its replication may give rise to either transitions or transversions; or (3) a U·G mismatch may also recruit the mismatch repair (MMR) machinery, which creates mutations at A·T near the initiating U·G lesion.

may promote chromosomal translocations of the targeted protooncogenes in the regions where SHM-derived mutations are located.

The origin of some mature lymphoid cell neoplasms may be traced to precursor B cells

The t(11;14)(q13;q32) translocation characterizes mantle cell lymphoma and juxtaposes the protooncogene *CCND1*, which encodes cyclin D1, at chromosome 11q13, to the IG heavy chain locus at 14q32.[92] This translocation occurs in the bone marrow in an early B cell at the pre-B stage of differentiation when the cell is initiating the IG gene rearrangement process with the recombination of the V(D)J segments (Table 22.1).[92] In contrast to other genetic lesions occurring at early B cell stages, such as those of precursor B cell neoplasms, the t(11;14) does not prevent further maturation of the tumor clone. Rather, the selective oncogenic advantage of this chromosomal translocation fully develops when these cells attain the differentiation stage of mature, though naïve, pre-GC B cells.

The *BCL2* gene was identified by molecular cloning of the t(14;18)(q32;q21) translocation, which occurs in virtually all cases of follicular lymphomas and in a proportion of diffuse large B cell lymphomas.[2,3] The translocation joins the *BCL2* gene at its 3' untranslated region to IGH sequences, resulting in deregulation of *BCL2* expression because of the nearby presence of IG transcriptional regulatory elements.[93] The consequence of the translocation is the presence within the cells of constitutively high levels of BCL2 protein, due to both increased transcription and more efficient processing of the *BCL2*/IG fusion allele. *BCL2* encodes a 26 kDa integral membrane protein localized to mitochondria, smooth endoplasmic reticulum, and perinuclear membrane.[93] BCL2 controls the cellular apoptotic threshold by preventing programmed cell death and is only one member of a family of apoptotic regulators. It is now clear that BCL2 exists as part of a high-molecular-weight complex generated through heterodimerization with BAX. The inherent ratio of BCL2 to BAX determines the functional activity of BCL2. When BAX is in excess, BAX homodimers dominate and cell death is accelerated; conversely, when BCL2 is in excess, as in lymphomas carrying *BCL2* rearrangements, BCL2/BAX heterodimers are the prevalent species and cell death is prevented.

BCL2 translocation is thought to occur early in ontogeny in a pre-B cell representing a precursor of follicular lymphoma (Table 22.1). In contrast to other genetic lesions occurring in pre-B cells and leading to B cell lineage ALL through a differentiative block of the target cells, *BCL2* rearrangements are permissive of B cell maturation to the stage of surface immunoglobulin M (sIgM)$^+$/sIgD$^+$ B cell. The pathogenicity of *BCL2* lesions in the context of follicular lymphoma is substantiated by the ability of *BCL2*-specific antisense oligonucleotides to inhibit the growth of human B cell lymphomas bearing *BCL2* translocations.[93]

In vivo, however, *BCL2* transgenes lead to a pattern of polyclonal hyperplasia of mature, long-lived B cells resting in G0, which, despite morphologic similarities, contrasts with the consistent monoclonality of follicular lymphoma. Hence the view that *BCL2* activation is not sufficient for follicular lymphoma development, and that other genetic lesions or host factors, including BCR stimulation by antigen, are required. With time, and analogous to the human disease, a fraction of *BCL2* transgenic mice progress to develop aggressive, clonal diffuse large cell lymphomas which have acquired additional genetic lesions.

Disordered cell cycle as a primary alteration in lymphomagenesis

Mantle cell lymphoma is the prototypic lymphoid neoplasm characterized by a primary genetic lesion, the t(11;14) translocation, that directly affects cell cycle regulators.[92] Mantle cell lymphoma derives from mature B cells that resemble naïve B cells and have not experienced the GC reaction. Consistent with its origin from pre-GC B cells, most cases of MCL have no or very few somatic mutations in IG variable genes. As a consequence of the t(11;14) translocation, cyclin D1, which is not expressed in normal B lymphocytes, becomes constitutively overexpressed.[92] The genetic alteration is thought to be the primary event in mantle cell lymphoma pathogenesis, facilitating the deregulation of cell cycle at G1-S phase transition. Cyclin D1 participates in the control of the G1 phase by binding to cyclin-dependent kinase 4 (CDK4) and CDK6. The hyperphosphorylation of RB1 by cyclin D1-CDK4 and cyclin D1-CDK6 causes the release of the E2F transcription factor and, consequently, progression of the cell into the S phase. Also, overexpression of cyclin D1 in mantle cell lymphoma cells titers the CDK inhibitor p27 into CDK4-cyclin D1 complexes rendering p27 incapable of inducing G1 arrest.

Additional genetic lesions of cell cycle regulators occur in highly proliferating mantle cell lymphoma variants (also known as blastoid variants), corroborating the notion that mantle cell lymphoma is in fact a disease characterized by disruption of cell cycle control.[92] The *CDKN2A* locus on chromosome 9p21 encodes the CDK4 inhibitor *INK4α* and the *P53* regulator *ARF*. Homozygous deletions of this locus have been detected in 20–30 percent of highly proliferative mantle cell lymphoma variants.[92] INK4α inhibits CDK4 and CDK6, and thus maintains the RB1 protein in its active, antiproliferative state. *INK4α* deletion and increased levels of cyclin D1 may therefore cooperate in promoting the G1-S phase transition in mantle cell lymphoma cells by increasing the intracellular amount of active cyclin D1-CDK complexes. Some mantle cell lymphomas with an intact *CDKN2A* locus display gene amplification and overexpression of *CDK4* or *BMI1*, a gene of the Polycomb group at 10p11 that participates in cell cycle control by acting as a transcriptional repressor of the *CDKN2A* locus.[92] This exemplifies how different genetic alterations in individual patients may converge upon disruption of the same pathogenetic pathway.

The master role of the nuclear factor κB system

The NF-κB signaling pathway is chronically active in a variety of tumor cell types. Such sustained activity of NF-κB leads to aberrant expression of NF-κB target genes, including loci involved in cell survival, cell proliferation, cell adhesion, and inflammation.[94] In lymphoid neoplasms, activation of the NF-κB system in tumor cells may be due to: (1) extracellular stimuli derived from the microenvironment, such as BAFF and APRIL, and acting on the tumor clone; and (2) molecular lesions intrinsic to the tumor clone and affecting genes belonging to or regulating the NF-κB system. Two sets of lymphoid neoplasms best exemplify the pathogenetic relevance of the NF-κB signaling pathway: multiple myeloma and marginal zone lymphoma.

Five subunits combine into hetero- and homodimers to create the NF-κB transcription factor family (p50, p52, Rel, p65/RelA, and RelB). Such dimers are inactive in the cytoplasm in most normal cells, due to the interaction of NF-κB dimers with IκB inhibitors (Fig. 22.7).[94] Activation of NF-κB signaling may follow two general pathways (Fig. 22.7). In the classical (or canonical) pathway IκB kinase complex (IKKβ) phosphorylates the inhibitory subunits IκBα, IκBβ, or IκBε, leading to their degradation in the proteasome. As a result, the NF-κB heterodimers p50/p65 and Rel/p65 accumulate in the nucleus. In the alternative (or non-canonical) pathway, IKKα homodimers phosphorylate p100/NFKB2, resulting in proteasomal removal of an inhibitory C-terminal domain and generating the NF-κB p52 subunit. As a consequence, p52/RelB heterodimers preferentially accumulate in the nucleus. These two pathways, however, show much interplay and overlap: many signals activate both NF-κB pathways, many of the same cytoplasmic effector proteins are used in both pathways, and many target genes are activated by both pathways.

Multiple myeloma, a tumor composed of plasma cells, is an eloquent example of how extrinsic stimuli activating NF-κB as well as genetic lesions causing constitutive NF-κB activation are both relevant for disease pathogenesis. Among B cell subsets, normal plasma cells have the highest expression of the NF-κB signature, which is induced by growth factors produced in the bone marrow microenvironment, including BAFF and APRIL. One step in multiple myeloma development is the progression from a microenvironment-dependent NF-κB activated state to an NF-κB activated state with reduced or abolished dependence on the microenvironment. In fact, constitutive nuclear activity of NF-κB is a very frequent feature of multiple myeloma cells, and represents the molecular target for small molecules interfering with NF-κB activity.

At least 20 percent of multiple myeloma cases carry mutations in genes encoding positive and negative regulators

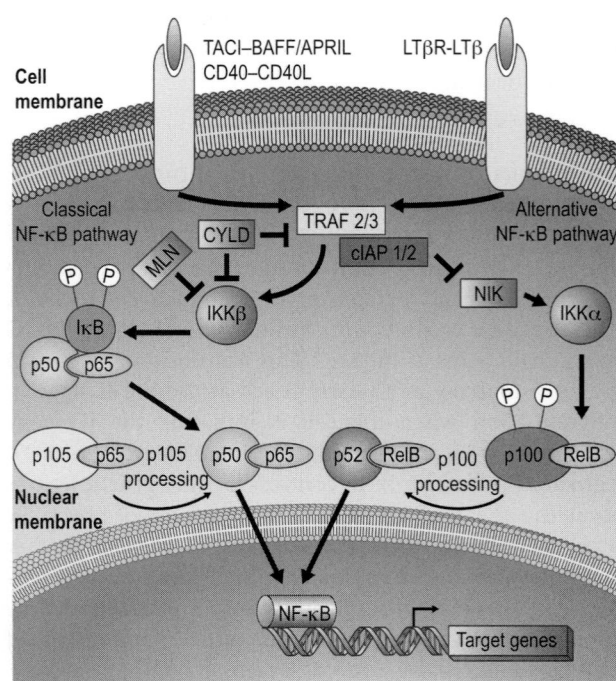

Figure 22.7 The nuclear factor κB (NF-κB) pathway and its involvement in multiple myeloma. Five subunits combine into hetero- and homodimers to create the NF-κB transcription factor family (p50, p52, Rel, p65/RelA, and RelB). Such dimers are inactive in the cytoplasm in most normal cells, due to the interaction of NF-κB dimers with IκB inhibitors. Activation of NF-κB signaling may follow two general pathways. In the classical (or canonical) pathway, IKKβ phosphorylates the inhibitory IκB molecule, leading to degradation (not shown) in the proteasome. As a result, the NF-κB heterodimers p50/p65 and Rel/p65 accumulate in the nucleus. In the alternative (or non-canonical) pathway, IKKα phosphorylates p100/NFKB2, resulting in proteasomal removal of an inhibitory C-terminal domain and generating the NF-κB p52 subunit. As a consequence, the p52/RelB heterodimers preferentially accumulate in the nucleus. Following translocation to the nucleus, p50/p65, Rel/p65, and p52/RelB activate transcription of target genes. In multiple myeloma, the NF-κB pathway is altered by several structural alterations. Inactivating mutations target the NF-κB negative regulators encoded by the *TRAF2*, *TRAF3*, *cIAP1/2*, and *CYLD* genes. Gain-of-function abnormalities affect the positive NF-κB regulators and effectors *LTBR*, *TACI*, *CD40*, *NIK*, and *NFKB2*.

of NF-κB signaling, and these mutations cause myeloma cells to have constitutive NF-κB activity (Fig. 22.7).[95,96] Genes in multiple myeloma that contain gain-of-function mutations (such as amplifications, translocations, or point mutations) for NF-κB signaling include receptors known to activate NF-κB (*CD40*, *LTβR*, and *TACI*), *NIK* (NF-κB-inducing kinase), NF-κB1 *P50/P105*, and NF-κB *P52/P100*. Overexpression of the *CD40*, *LTβR*, and *TACI* receptors may be sufficient to activate the NF-κB pathway, or might enhance the sensitivity of multiple myeloma cells to factors in the microenvironment. Overexpression of

NIK or NF-κB1 *P105* directly leads to constitutive activation of NF-κB. In the case of NF-κB2, a deletion of sequences in the *P100* IκB-like domain promotes processing of p100 to p52 and activation of the alternative NF-κB pathway.[95,96] Other mutations affect negative regulators of NF-κB and, by causing loss of function (through deletions, point mutations, or loss of heterozygosity) of NF-κB inhibitors, lead to NF-κB activation.[95,96] Negative regulators of NF-κB that are disrupted in multiple myeloma include the *TRAF2, TRAF3, cIAP1/2,* and *CYLD* genes. Overall, inactivation of *TRAF3* is the most frequent genetic alteration affecting NF-κB signaling in multiple myeloma.[95,96] Apart from underscoring the relevance of the NF-κB system in lymphoid neoplasms, the case of multiple myeloma documents how a plethora of different genetic abnormalities may converge upon a common result, i.e., NF-κB activation.

Mucosal-associated lymphoid tissue (MALT) lymphoma represent another setting in which the consequences of multiple distinct genetic lesions converge upon activation of NF-κB signaling.[97] Similar to multiple myeloma, in early stages of tumor development NF-κB activation is provided by extrinsic stimuli derived from the microenvironment.[97] With time, the tumor clone acquires and selects for genetic lesions that are capable of constitutively activating NF-κB signaling independent of extracellular stimuli.

In normal lymphoid tissues, signaling through the antigen receptor induces the interaction between the BCL10 and MALT1 proteins, which form a heterodimer and synergize to activate the downstream factor NF-κB. Expression of both BCL10 and MALT1 is restricted primarily to lymphoid tissues. In contrast to normal lymphoid tissues, MALT lymphomas display an array of chromosomal translocations that deregulate the expression of these two proteins.[2,3,97] Gastric MALT lymphoma has been investigated most extensively, and the role of NF-κB activation in this setting is known better than for MALT lymphomas arising at other sites.[97] In *Helicobacter pylori*-associated gastritis and during the early phases of MALT lymphoma development, antigens expressed by *H. pylori* in conjunction with specific T cells help stimulate the antigen receptor of polyclonal B cells and promote BCL10/MALT1 heterodimerization, thus activating NF-κB.[97] With time, a subclone with one of the characteristic MALT lymphoma translocations may emerge with an obvious growth advantage. Constitutive NF-κB activation ensues, eliminating the need for persistent infection and antigen stimulation.[97]

The t(1;14)(p22;q32) translocation of MALT lymphoma leads to *BCL10* overexpression, which, in turn, triggers MALT1 oligomerization and aberrant NF-κB activation.[97] In cases with t(14;18)(q32;q21), *MALT1* is overexpressed. Conceivably, MALT1 interacts with and stabilizes BCL10, causing its accumulation in the cytoplasm of tumor cells bearing the translocation. The t(11;18)(q21;q21) translocation causes the formation of a novel chimeric gene, *API2-MALT1*, and subsequent fusion protein. The chimeric protein is able to activate NF-κB directly, whereas neither wild-type *API2* nor *MALT1* alone have this activity.

Foreign DNA material in the tumor clone

An additional molecular mechanism implicated in development of mature lymphoid cell neoplasms, of both B and T cell lineage, is represented by the introduction of foreign DNA material into tumor cells via infection of the tumor clone by oncogenic viruses. Three oncogenic viruses are known to exert a direct pathogenetic effect in lymphomagenesis, including two herpesviruses, i.e., EBV and human herpes virus type 8 (HHV-8), and a retrovirus, i.e., human T cell lymphotrophic virus 1 (HTLV-1). The role of these viruses in lymphoid neoplasia is described in detail elsewhere in this book (see Chapters 6 and 7).

THE MICROENVIRONMENT

Since the early stages of cancer research, it has been thought that the microenvironment affects the growth of resident neoplastic cells by several mechanisms. As early as 1889, Stephen Paget advanced the 'seed and soil' hypothesis, whereby the establishment of tumor localizations in specific organs is influenced by interactions between cancer cells (the 'seed') and the microenvironment (the 'soil') of the involved organ. Among neoplasms of lymphoid cells, multiple myeloma best recapitulates the various strategies provided by the microenvironment, in this instance represented by the bone marrow milieu, and favoring tumor growth.

The behavior of multiple myeloma cells, at a biological and clinical level, appears not to be solely determined by their underlying genetic features. Instead, the pathophysiology of multiple myeloma appears to be significantly affected by a complex network of interactions between neoplastic plasma cells and the bone marrow milieu (Fig. 22.8).[98]

The main strategies whereby the bone marrow milieu supports multiple myeloma growth and survival are: (1) direct adhesion of plasma cells to bone marrow stromal cells; (2) paracrine or autocrine release of cytokines and growth factors; and (3) activation of signaling cascades in plasma cells.[98] Bone marrow stromal cells are able to support normal hematopoiesis *in vitro*, and their support of plasma cell growth recapitulates their physiological role in nurturing normal hematopoietic cells. Multiple myeloma plasma cells capitalize on the adhesive interaction with bone marrow stromal cells, which is mediated by several adhesion molecules including very late antigen 4 (VLA-4) and vascular cell adhesion molecule 1 (VCAM-1). In the bone, multiple myeloma cells cause the deregulated production of cytokines and growth factors involved in bone resorption and remodeling, of which some, namely interleukin-6 (IL-6), IL-1α, IL-1β, insulin-like growth factor 1 (IGF-1), hepatocyte growth factor (HGF), vascular endothelial growth factor (VEGF), tumor necrosis factor α (TNFα) and others, can also function to stimulate plasma cell growth and promote apoptotic resistance to conventional drugs, such as alkylating agents and dexamethasone.[98] As stated above, adhesion of multiple myeloma plasma

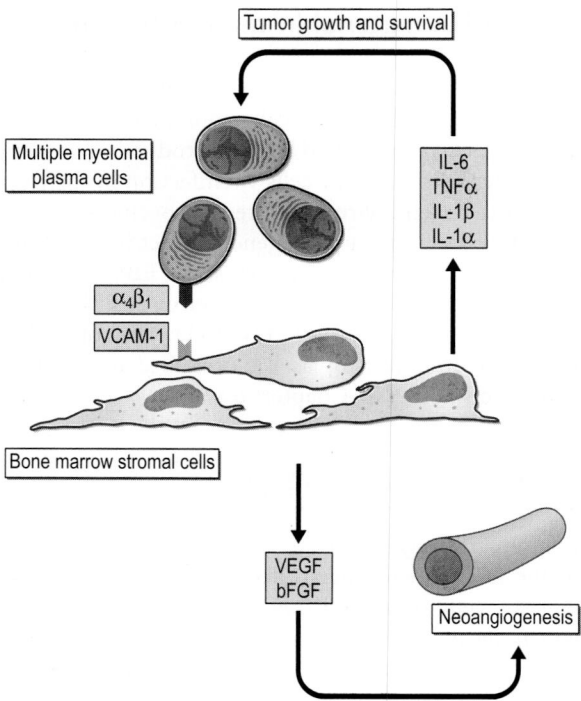

Figure 22.8 Interactions between multiple myeloma plasma cells and the bone marrow microenvironment. In the early phases of the disease, multiple myeloma is strictly dependent upon interactions with the surrounding microenvironment. Multiple myeloma plasma cells capitalize on the adhesive interaction with bone marrow stromal cells, which is mediated by several adhesion molecules including VLA-4 and VCAM-1. In the bone, multiple myeloma cells cause the deregulated production of cytokines and growth factors involved in bone resorption and remodeling, of which some, namely IL-6, IL-1α, IL-1β, IGF-1, HGF, VEGF, TNFα, and others, can also function to stimulate plasma cell growth and promote apoptotic resistance. Bone marrow stromal cells also release endothelial cell growth factors (VEGF, bFGF) that promote neoangiogenesis. VLA-4, very late antigen 4; VCAM-1, vascular cell adhesion molecule 1; IL, interleukin; IGF-1, insulin-like growth factor 1; HGF, hepatocyte growth factor; VEGF, vascular endothelial growth factor; TNFα, tumor necrosis factor α.

cells to bone marrow stromal cells is also capable of activating many growth- and survival-promoting cascades in the neoplastic clone. These pathways, which include the phosphatidylinositol 3-kinase (PI3K)/Akt/mTOR/p70S6K cascade, the IKKα/NF-κB pathway, as well as the Ras/Raf/MAPK and JAK/STAT3 signal transduction pathways, can be activated by upstream binding of cytokines to their receptors or by direct cell adhesion through adhesion-triggered kinase pathways.

The growth-promoting effect exerted by the microenvironment on multiple myeloma plasma cells is targeted by novel drugs, namely thalidomide, lenalidomide, and to a certain extent also bortezomib, which are highly active in this context. The realization that these novel drugs counteract or, in some cases, overcome the protective effects

exerted by the microenvironment on plasma cells provides indirect, but powerful, support to the importance of tumor–stromal interactions in multiple myeloma and has set a research model that is currently being explored in other lymphoid neoplasms. In advanced multiple myeloma, the accumulation of multiple genetic lesions in the multiple myeloma clone may render plasma cells totally independent of the bone marrow microenvironment, and hence favor the extramedullary localization and multiple drug resistance of neoplastic plasma cells, which may assume the features of plasma blasts.

THE HOST

The emergence and sustained growth of a lymphoid neoplasm may also be favored by factors provided by the host. These may be hereditary in a very minor fraction of cases, whereas most host factors involved in lymphoid tumorigenesis are of an acquired nature. The latter include the role of host infection by specific microorganisms and the host immune status.

The host genetic background

Familial aggregation is uncommon or virtually absent in both B cell and T cell lymphoid neoplasms, with the notable exception of a small fraction of CLL which has been reported to run in families in up to 10 percent of cases.[99] The evidence of high heritability has prompted investigators to conduct genome-wide searches for linkage in CLL families. A search of more than two hundred CLL families analyzed by a high-density genome-wide approach has identified possible loci of disease susceptibility mapping to 2q21, 6p22, and 18q21.[100] Such loci could be epistatic or act independently. Recently, one study has proposed downregulation of the death-associated protein kinase 1 (*DAPK1*) gene as a mechanism predisposing to CLL in a large family with multiple affected individuals.[101] *DAPK1* codes for a positive mediator of apoptosis and has been shown to be inactivated in multiple sporadic lymphoid neoplasms by promoter methylation.[102,103] Importantly, in CLL *DAPK1* appears not only to be a target in familial cases, but is also inactivated through epigenetic silencing in the majority of patients with the sporadic form of the disease.

Host infection with microorganisms associated with lymphomagenesis

Host infection by several microorganisms may contribute to mature B cell lymphomagenesis by providing foreign antigens that stimulate B cell growth and clonal expansion, or via other indirect mechanisms. The best example is represented by the association between *H. pylori* infection and gastric MALT lymphoma (see also Chapter 8). Other examples are infection by hepatitis C virus (HCV) and B cell lymphoma, and the emerging association between *Chlamydia psittaci* and marginal zone lymphoma of the ocular adnexa. In all instances, the association between infection and lymphoma has been initially documented based on epidemiological, rather than molecular, evidence. The pathogenetic link has been further strengthened empirically by achieving therapeutic response of the lymphoma through control or eradication of the infection.

For both *H. pylori* and HCV, and potentially also for *C. psittaci*, the general model holds that foreign antigens provided by the infectious microorganism perturb the microenvironment of lymphoid tissues, causing a driving force for B cell proliferation that may progress from poly- or oligoclonal expansion to monoclonal lymphoma. Additional mechanisms, including the microorganism-induced generation of toxic substances that may enhance B cell mutagenesis and DNA damage, have also been invoked.

Mature B cell lymphoma is the only category of lymphoid neoplasms for which microenvironmental stimuli provided by foreign antigens are known to play a role in tumor growth. The development of marginal zone lymphoma, particularly in its extranodal and splenic variants, appears particularly susceptible to the pathogenetic role of foreign antigens provided by infectious microorganisms.

HELICOBACTER PYLORI

Gastric MALT lymphoma is an eloquent example of the interplay between host infection, genesis of genetic lesions, and lymphomagenesis. *In vitro*, lymphoma growth is stimulated when lymphoma cells are exposed to the microorganism, through tumor-infiltrating T cells involving CD40 and CD40 ligand (CD40L) costimulatory molecules.[97] With disease progression, *H. pylori* may favor the accumulation of genetic lesions, partly owing to the release of reactive oxygen species (ROS) by neutrophils present in the area of chronic inflammation.[97] Interestingly, polymorphisms of the glutathione-S-transferase (GST) gene family may decrease enzyme activity and antioxidative capacity, thus favoring ROS accumulation.[104] The same polymorphisms predispose to MALT lymphoma development.[104] The potential relevance of ROS in the genesis of molecular lesions of MALT lymphoma is further supported by the frequent epigenetic inactivation of the *GSTP1* gene, a member of the GST family.[103] Because *GSTP1* plays an important role in scavenging ROS and their metabolites and protecting cells from DNA damage produced by these agents, its somatic inactivation in MALT lymphoma provides an additional mechanism favoring the accumulation of ROS and lymphomagenesis in the context of chronic gastric inflammation.[103]

Upon gain of genetic lesions, the growth of the MALT lymphoma clone may no longer require antigen stimulation, thus becoming independent of *H. pylori*.[97] Several genetic lesions specific for MALT lymphoma have been identified, including the chromosomal translocations t(1;14) (p22;q32), t(14;18)(q32;q21), t(11;18)(q21;q21), and t(3;14)

(p13;q32).[2,3,97] These chromosomal translocations occur with variable frequencies throughout the spectrum of MALT lymphomas.

OTHER BACTERIA

The list of bacterial species associated with marginal zone lymphoproliferations has grown longer with molecular investigations, and now includes *Campylobacter jejuni*, *Borrelia burgdorferi*, and *C. psittaci*, which have been associated with immunoproliferative small intestinal disease (also known as IPSID), cutaneous MALT lymphoma, and MALT lymphoma of the ocular adnexa, respectively.[105] In the instance of *C. psittaci* and MALT lymphoma of the ocular adnexa, the pathogenetic link is also suggested by response of the lymphoma to antibacterial therapy with tetracyclins.

HEPATITIS C VIRUS

The role of HCV in promoting lymphomagenesis is indirect and is mediated, at least in part, by the host immune response. Also, HCV has been suggested to favor mutations of IG genes and of protooncogenes by a 'hit and run' mechanism.[106] The high frequency of aberrant SHM of protooncogenes in HCV-related lymphoma may be due to the mutagenic pressure exerted by HCV.[85] Strong evidence for a pathogenetic role of HCV in at least some lymphoma types comes from the observation that targeting HCV itself, through the combination of alpha interferon and the antiviral agent ribavirin, is able to induce a therapeutic response in patients affected by splenic marginal zone lymphoma.[107]

The host immune system as a determinant of lymphomagenesis

Two major settings of immune system dysregulation are known to associate with lymphomagenesis: (1) immunodeficiency and (2) certain autoimmune conditions.

IMMUNODEFICIENCY

The interplay between immunodeficiency, viral infection, and genetic lesions in immunodeficiency-related lymphoma is covered elsewhere in this book (Chapter 24). Two general concepts should be kept in mind regarding immunodeficiency and lymphoid malignancies. First, the highest risk of lymphoid malignancies is carried by immunodeficiencies affecting primarily the T cell branch of the immune system. Second, all types of immunodeficiency predispose to neoplasms of mature lymphoid cells, which are of B cell origin in the overwhelming majority of cases. Precursor lymphoid cell neoplasms are not known to associate with immunodeficiency, and the association between immunodeficiency and T cell lymphoma is doubtful, with the exception of T cell prolymphocytic leukemia arising in ataxia telangiectasia patients.

AUTOIMMUNITY

Autoimmune disorders, both systemic and organ specific, may carry an increased risk of lymphoma development that is independent of immunosuppressive therapy (see also Chapter 28). The types of lymphoma vary upon the specific autoimmune setting, and most commonly include diffuse large B cell lymphoma (in rheumatoid arthritis and systemic lupus erythematosus), MALT lymphoma (in Sjögren syndrome and Hashimoto thyroiditis), and enteropathy-type T cell lymphoma (in celiac disease).[108] All autoimmunity-related lymphoid neoplasms are tumors of mature lymphoid cells, which have expressed antigen receptors at some timepoint of their history and, therefore, may have been stimulated by antigen. Notably, an association has been noted between severity of chronic inflammation and lymphoma risk in rheumatoid arthritis and in Sjögren syndrome, further reinforcing the notion that profound perturbation of the immune system is an important factor in lymphomagenesis.

KEY POINTS

- The pathogenesis of precursor lymphoid neoplasia is due to the somatic acquisition of recurrent genetic lesions, which are represented mainly, though not exclusively, by chromosomal translocations.
- The genesis of many, though not all, genomic aberrations of precursor lymphoid cell neoplasms follows a unifying molecular mechanism involving the V(D)J recombinase enzyme complex.
- The molecular characteristics of the B cell receptor expressed by tumor cells provide pathogenetic and prognostic information for some lymphoid neoplasms, namely chronic lymphocytic leukemia.
- Class switch recombination and/or somatic hypermutation are involved in the genesis of several genetic lesions specific of mature B cell neoplasia, including B cell non-Hodgkin lymphoma and multiple myeloma.
- The NF-κB system is targeted by molecular lesions intrinsic to the tumor clone of some types of mature lymphoid cell neoplasms.
- Introduction of foreign DNA material into tumor cells via infection of the tumor clone by oncogenic viruses is a mechanism of genetic lesion in some types of mature lymphoid cell neoplasms.
- Host factors, mainly represented by host infection by specific microorganisms and host immune status, may contribute to the development of mature lymphoid cell neoplasia.

ACKNOWLEDGMENTS

Work by the authors described in this chapter has been supported by Ricerca Sanitaria Finalizzata and Ricerca Scientifica Applicata, Regione Piemonte, Torino, Italy; PRIN 2006, Rome, Italy; Progetto Alfieri, Fondazione CRT, Torino, Italy; Novara-AIL Onlus, Associazione Franca Capurro per Novara Onlus, and Next Event, Novara, Italy.

REFERENCES

● = Key primary paper

◆ = Major review article

1. Jaffe ES, Harris NL, Stein H, Vardiman JW. *World Health Organization classification of tumours. Pathology and genetics of tumours of haematopoietic and lymphoid tissues*. Lyon, France: IARC Press 2001.
2. Mitelman F, Johansson B, Mertens F. (eds) Mitelman database of chromosome aberrations in cancer (2008). http://cgap.nci.nih.gov/Chromosomes/Mitelman
3. Atlas of genetics and cytogenetics in oncology and haematology. http://AtlasGeneticsOncology.org
◆4. Lieber MR, Yu K, Raghavan SC. Roles of nonhomologous DNA end joining, V(D)J recombination, and class switch recombination in chromosomal translocations. *DNA Repair* 2006; **5**: 1234–45.
◆5. O'Neil J, Look AT. Mechanisms of transcription factor deregulation in lymphoid cell transformation. *Oncogene* 2007; **26**: 6838–49.
◆6. Greaves MF, Maia AT, Wiemels JL, Ford AM. Leukemia in twins: lessons in natural history. *Blood* 2003; **102**: 2321–33.
◆7. Greaves M, Wiemels J. Origins of chromosome translocations in childhood leukaemia. *Nat Rev Cancer* 2003; **3**: 639–49.
8. Gale KB, Ford AM, Repp R *et al.* Backtracking leukemia to birth: identification of clonotypic gene fusion sequences in neonatal blood spots. *Proc Natl Acad Sci U S A* 1997; **94**: 13950–4.
9. Mori H, Colman SM, Xiao Z *et al.* Chromosome translocations and covert leukemic clones are generated during normal fetal development. *Proc Natl Acad Sci U S A* 2002; **99**: 8242–7.
10. Eguchi-Ishimae M, Eguchi M, Kempski H, Greaves M. *NOTCH*1 mutation can be an early, prenatal genetic event in T-ALL. *Blood* 2008; **111**: 376–8.
11. Maia AT, Koechling J, Corbett R *et al.* Protracted postnatal natural histories in childhood leukemia. *Genes Chromosomes Cancer* 2004; **39**: 335–40.
12. Bernardin F, Yang Y, Cleaves R *et al.* TEL-AML1, expressed from t(12;21) in human acute lymphocytic leukemia, induces acute leukemia in mice. *Cancer Res* 2002; **62**: 3904–8.
13. Hong D, Gupta R, Ancliff P *et al.* Initiating and cancer-propagating cells in TEL-AML1-associated childhood leukemia. *Science* 2008; **319**: 336–9.

14. Raynaud S, Cavé H, Baens M *et al.* The 12;21 translocation involving TEL and deletion of the other TEL allele: two frequently associated alterations found in childhood acute lymphoblastic leukemia. *Blood* 1996; **87**: 2891–9.

◆15. Rothenberg EV, Taghon T. Molecular genetics of T cell development. *Annu Rev Immunol* 2005; **23**: 601–49.

16. Graux C, Cools J, Michaux L *et al.* Cytogenetics and molecular genetics of T-cell acute lymphoblastic leukemia: from thymocyte to lymphoblast. *Leukemia* 2006; **20**: 1496–510.

17. Jones S. An overview of the basic helix-loop-helix proteins. *Genome Biol* 2004; **5**: 226.

18. Brown L, Cheng JT, Chen Q *et al.* Site-specific recombination of the tal-1 gene is a common occurrence in human T cell leukemia. *EMBO J* 1990; **9**: 3343–51.

19. Mellentin JD, Smith SD, Cleary ML. lyl-1, a novel gene altered by chromosomal translocation in T cell leukemia, codes for a protein with a helix-loop-helix DNA binding motif. *Cell* 1989; **58**: 77–83.

20. Xia Y, Brown L, Yang CY *et al.* TAL2, a helix-loop-helix gene activated by the t(7;9)(q34;q32) translocation in human T-cell leukemia. *Proc Natl Acad Sci U S A* 1991; **88**: 11416–20.

21. Wang J, Jani-Sait SN, Escalon EA *et al.* The t(14;21)(q11.2;q22) chromosomal translocation associated with T-cell acute lymphoblastic leukemia activates the BHLHB1 gene. *Proc Natl Acad Sci U S A* 2000; **97**: 3497–502.

22. Gehring WJ, Qian YQ, Billeter M *et al.* Homeodomain-DNA recognition. *Cell* 1994; **78**: 211–23.

23. Van Oostveen J, Bijl J, Raaphorst F *et al.* The role of homeobox genes in normal hematopoiesis and hematological malignancies. *Leukemia* 1999; **13**: 1675–90.

24. Izon DJ, Rozenfeld S, Fong ST *et al.* Loss of function of the homeobox gene Hoxa-9 perturbs early T-cell development and induces apoptosis in primitive thymocytes. *Blood* 1998; **92**: 383–93.

25. Kroon E, Krosl J, Thorsteinsdottir U *et al.* Hoxa9 transforms primary bone marrow cells through specific collaboration with Meis1a but not Pbx1b. *EMBO J* 1998; **17**: 3714–25.

26. Speleman F, Cauwelier B, Dastugue N *et al.* A new recurrent inversion, inv(7)(p15q34), leads to transcriptional activation of HOXA10 and HOXA11 in a subset of T-cell acute lymphoblastic leukemias. *Leukemia* 2005; **19**: 358–66.

27. Owens BM, Hawley RG. HOX and non-HOX homeobox genes in leukemic hematopoiesis. *Stem Cells* 2002; **20**: 364–79.

28. Hatano M, Roberts CW, Minden M *et al.* Deregulation of a homeobox gene, HOX11, by the t(10;14) in T cell leukemia. *Science* 1991; **253**: 79–82.

29. Bernard OA, Busson Le Coniat M, Ballerini P *et al.* A new recurrent and specific cryptic translocation, t(5;14)(q35;q32), is associated with expression of the Hox11 L2 gene in T acute lymphoblastic leukemia. *Leukemia* 2001; **15**: 1495–504.

●30. Ferrando AA, Neuberg DS, Staunton J *et al.* Gene expression signatures define novel oncogenic pathways in T cell acute lymphoblastic leukemia. *Cancer Cell* 2002; **1**: 75–87.

31. Soulier J, Clappier E, Cayuela JM *et al.* HOXA genes are included in genetic and biologic networks defining human acute T-cell leukemia (T-ALL). *Blood* 2005; **106**: 274–86.

32. Rabbits TH. LMO T-cell translocation oncogenes typify genes activated by chromosomal translocations that alter transcription and developmental processes. *Genes Dev* 1998; **12**: 2651–7.

33. Fuxa M, Skok JA. Transcriptional regulation in early B cell development. *Curr Opin Immunol* 2007; **19**: 129–36.

◆34. Cobaleda C, Schebesta A, Delogu A, Busslinger M. Pax5: the guardian of B cell identity and function. *Nat Immunol* 2007; **8**: 463–70.

35. Kamps MP, Murre C, Sun XH, Baltimore D. A new homeobox gene contributes the DNA binding domain of the t(1;19) translocation protein in pre-B ALL. *Cell* 1990; **60**: 547–55.

36. Nourse J, Mellentin JD, Galili N *et al.* Chromosomal translocation t(1;19) results in synthesis of a homeobox fusion mRNA that codes for a potential chimeric transcription factor. *Cell* 1990; **60**: 535–45.

37. Hunger SP, Ohyashiki K, Toyama K, Cleary ML. Hlf, a novel hepatic bZIP protein, shows altered DNA-binding properties following fusion to E2A in t(17;19) acute lymphoblastic leukemia. *Genes Dev* 1992; **6**: 1608–20.

38. Inaba T, Roberts WM, Shapiro LH *et al.* Fusion of the leucine zipper gene HLF to the E2A gene in human acute B-lineage leukemia. *Science* 1992; **257**: 531–4.

39. Kuiper RP, Schoenmakers EF, van Reijmersdal SV *et al.* High-resolution genomic profiling of childhood ALL reveals novel recurrent genetic lesions affecting pathways involved in lymphocyte differentiation and cell cycle progression. *Leukemia* 2007; **21**: 1258–66.

●40. Mullighan CG, Goorha S, Radtke I *et al.* Genome-wide analysis of genetic alterations in acute lymphoblastic leukemia. *Nature* 2007; **446**: 758–64.

◆41. Grabher C, von Boehmer H, Look AT. Notch1 activation in the molecular pathogenesis of T-cell acute lymphoblastic leukemia. *Nat Rev Cancer* 2006; **6**: 347–59.

●42. Weng AP, Ferrando AA, Lee W *et al.* Activating mutations of NOTCH1 in human T cell acute lymphoblastic leukemia. *Science* 2004; **306**: 269–71.

43. Maizels N. Immunoglobulin gene diversification. *Annu Rev Genet* 2005; **39**: 23–46.

44. Odegard VH, Schatz DG. Targeting of somatic hypermutation. *Nat Rev Immunol* 2006; **6**: 573–83.

◆45. Chiorazzi N, Rai KR, Ferrarini M. Chronic lymphocytic leukemia. *N Engl J Med* 2005; **352**: 804–15.

◆46. Montserrat E. New prognostic markers in CLL. *Hematology Am Soc Hematol Educ Program* 2006; 279–84.

●47. Damle RN, Wasil T, Fais F *et al.* Ig V gene mutation status and CD38 expression as novel prognostic indicators in chronic lymphocytic leukemia. *Blood* 1999; **94**: 1840–7.

●48. Hamblin TJ, Davis Z, Gardiner A *et al.* Unmutated Ig V(H) genes are associated with a more aggressive form of chronic lymphocytic leukemia. *Blood* 1999; **94**: 1848–54.

49. Crespo M, Bosch F, Villamor N *et al.* ZAP-70 expression as a surrogate for immunoglobulin-variable-region mutations in chronic lymphocytic leukemia. *N Engl J Med* 2003; **348**: 1764–75.

◆50. Chiorazzi N, Ferrarini M. B cell chronic lymphocytic leukemia: lessons learned from studies of the B cell antigen receptor. *Annu Rev Immunol* 2003; **21**: 841–94.

51. Capello D, Guarini A, Berra E *et al.* Evidence of biased immunoglobulin variable gene usage in highly stable B-cell chronic lymphocytic leukemia. *Leukemia* 2004; **18**: 1941–7.

52. Thorselius M, Krober A, Murray F *et al.* Strikingly homologous immunoglobulin gene rearrangements and poor outcome in VH3-21-using chronic lymphocytic leukemia patients independent of geographic origin and mutational status. *Blood* 2006; **107**: 2889–94.

53. Bomben R, Dal Bo M, Capello D *et al.* Comprehensive characterization of IGHV3-21-expressing B-cell chronic lymphocytic leukemia: an Italian multicenter study. *Blood* 2007; **109**: 2989–98.

54. Stamatopoulos K, Belessi C, Moreno C *et al.* Over 20% of patients with chronic lymphocytic leukemia carry stereotyped receptors: pathogenetic implications and clinical correlations. *Blood* 2007; **109**: 259–70.

55. Murray F, Darzentas N, Hadzidimitriou A *et al.* Stereotyped patterns of somatic hypermutation in subsets of patients with chronic lymphocytic leukemia: implications for the role of antigen selection in leukemogenesis. *Blood* 2008; **111**: 1524–33.

56. Rossi D, Cerri M, Capello D *et al.* Biological and clinical risk factors of chronic lymphocytic leukaemia transformation to Richter syndrome. *Br J Haematol* 2008; **142**: 202–15.

◆57. Klein U, Dalla-Favera R. Germinal centres: role in B-cell physiology and malignancy. *Nat Rev Immunol* 2008; **8**: 12–33.

58. Ramiro AR, Nussenzweig MC, Nussenzweig A. Switching on chromosomal translocations. *Cancer Res* 2006; **66**: 7837–9.

59. Edry E, Melamed D. Class switch recombination: a friend and a foe. *Clin Immunol* 2007; **123**: 244–51.

●60. Muramatsu M, Kinoshita K, Fagarasan S *et al.* Class switch recombination and hypermutation require activation-induced cytidine deaminase (AID), a potential RNA editing enzyme. *Cell* 2000; **102**: 553–63.

●61. Pasqualucci L, Bhagat G, Jankovic M *et al.* AID is required for germinal center-derived lymphomagenesis. *Nat Genetics* 2008; **40**: 108–12.

◆62. Grandori C, Cowley SM, James LP, Eisenman RN. The Myc/Max/Mad network and the transcriptional control of cell behavior. *Annu Rev Cell Dev Biol* 2000; **16**: 653–99.

63. Basso K, Margolin AA, Stolovitzky G *et al.* Reverse engineering of regulatory networks in human B cells. *Nat Genet* 2005; **4**: 382–90.

64. Evan GI, Wyllie AH, Gilbert CS *et al.* Induction of apoptosis in fibroblasts by c-myc protein. *Cell* 1992; **69**: 119–28.

65. Dominguez-Sola D, Ying CY, Grandori C *et al.* Non-transcriptional control of DNA replication by c-MYC. *Nature* 2007; **448**: 445–53.

●66. Lombardi L, Newcomb EW, Dalla-Favera R. Pathogenesis of Burkitt lymphoma: expression of an activated c-myc oncogene causes the tumorigenic conversion of EBV-infected human B lymphoblasts. *Cell* 1987; **49**: 161–70.

●67. McManaway ME, Neckers LM, Loke SL *et al.* Tumour-specific inhibition of lymphoma growth by an antisense oligodeoxynucleotide. *Lancet* 1990; **335**: 808–11.

●68. Adams JM, Harris AW, Pinkert CA *et al.* The c-myc oncogene driven by immunoglobulin enhancers induces lymphoid malignancy in transgenic mice. *Nature* 1985; **318**: 533–8.

●69. Ye BH, Lista F, Lo Coco F *et al.* Alterations of BCL-6, a novel zinc-finger gene, in diffuse large cell lymphoma. *Science* 1993; **262**: 747–50.

70. Cattoretti G, Chang C, Cechova K *et al.* BCL-6 protein is expressed in germinal-center B cells. *Blood* 1995; **86**: 45–53.

●71. Ye BH, Cattoretti G, Shen Q *et al.* The BCL-6 proto-oncogene controls germinal-centre formation and Th2-type inflammation. *Nat Genet* 1997; **16**: 161–70.

●72. Phan T, Dalla-Favera R. The BCL6 proto-oncogene suppresses p53 expression in germinal-centre B cells. *Nature* 2004; **432**: 635–9.

●73. Phan RT, Saito M, Basso K *et al.* BCL6 interacts with the transcription factor Miz-1 to suppress the cyclin-dependent kinase inhibitor p21 and cell cycle arrest in germinal center B cells. *Nat Immunol* 2005; **6**: 1054–60.

●74. Ranuncolo SM, Polo JM, Dierov J *et al.* Bcl-6 mediates the germinal center B cell phenotype and lymphomagenesis through transcriptional repression of the DNA-damage sensor ATR. *Nat Immunol* 2007; **8**: 705–14.

75. Phan RT, Saito M, Kitagawa Y *et al.* Genotoxic stress regulates expression of the proto-oncogene Bcl6 in germinal center B cells. *Nat Immunol* 2007; **8**: 1132–9.

76. Gaidano G, Lo Coco F, Ye BH *et al.* Rearrangements of the BCL-6 gene in acquired immunodeficiency syndrome-associated non-Hodgkin's lymphoma: association with diffuse large-cell subtype. *Blood* 1994; **84**: 397–402.

77. Ye BH, Chaganti S, Chang CC *et al.* Chromosomal translocations cause deregulated BCL6 expression by promoter substitution in B cell lymphoma. *EMBO J* 1995; **14**: 6209–17.

78. Saito M, Gao J, Basso K *et al.* A signaling pathway mediating downregulation of *BCL6* in germinal center B cells is blocked by *BCL6* gene alterations in B cell lymphoma. *Cancer Cell* 2007; **12**: 280–92.

●79. Cattoretti G, Pasqualucci L, Ballon G *et al.* Deregulated BCL6 expression recapitulates the pathogenesis of human diffuse large B cell lymphomas in mice. *Cancer Cell* 2005; **7**: 445–55.

80. Pasqualucci L, Migliazza A, Fracchiolla N *et al.* BCL-6 mutations in normal germinal center B cells: evidence of somatic hypermutation acting outside Ig loci. *Proc Natl Acad Sci U S A* 1998; **95**: 11816–21.

81. Capello D, Vitolo U, Pasqualucci L *et al.* Distribution and pattern of BCL-6 mutations throughout the spectrum of B-cell neoplasia. *Blood* 2000; **95**: 651–9.

82. Müschen M, Re D, Jungnickel B *et al.* Somatic mutation of the CD95 gene in human B cells as a side-effect of the germinal center reaction. *J Exp Med* 2000; **192**: 1833–40.

●83. Pasqualucci L, Neumeister P, Goossens T *et al.* Hypermutation of multiple proto-oncogenes in B-cell diffuse large-cell lymphomas. *Nature* 2001; **412**: 341–6.

84. Gaidano G, Pasqualucci L, Capello D *et al.* Aberrant somatic hypermutation in multiple subtypes of AIDS-associated non-Hodgkin lymphoma. *Blood* 2003; **102**: 1833–41.

85. Libra M, Capello D, Gloghini A *et al.* Analysis of aberrant somatic hypermutation (SHM) in non-Hodgkin lymphomas of patients with HCV infection. *J Pathol* 2005; **206**: 87–91.

86. Rossi D, Cerri M, Capello D *et al.* Aberrant somatic hypermutation in primary mediastinal large B-cell lymphoma. *Leukemia* 2005; **19**: 2363–6.

87. Liso A, Capello D, Marafioti T *et al.* Aberrant somatic hypermutation in tumor cells of nodular lymphocyte-predominant and classical Hodgkin's lymphoma. *Blood* 2006; **108**: 1013–20.

88. Rossi D, Berra E, Cerri M *et al.* Aberrant somatic hypermutation in transformation of follicular lymphoma and chronic lymphocytic leukemia to diffuse large B-cell lymphoma. *Haematologica* 2006; **91**: 1405–9.

●89. Bhatia K, Huppi K, Spangler G *et al.* Point mutations in the c-Myc transactivation domain are common in Burkitt's lymphoma and mouse plasmacytomas. *Nat Genet* 1993; **5**: 56–61.

90. Bhatia K, Spangler G, Gaidano G *et al.* Mutations in the coding region of c-myc occur frequently in acquired immunodeficiency syndrome-associated lymphomas. *Blood* 1994; **84**: 883–8.

91. Pasqualucci L, Migliazza A, Basso K *et al.* Mutations of the BCL6 proto-oncogene disrupt its negative autoregulation in diffuse large B-cell lymphoma. *Blood* 2003; **101**: 2914–23.

◆92. Jares P, Colomer D, Campo E. Genetic and molecular pathogenesis of mantle cell lymphoma: perspectives for new targeted therapies. *Nat Rev Cancer* 2007; **7**: 750–62.

93. Thomadaki H, Scorilas A. BCL2 family of apoptosis-related genes: functions and clinical implications in cancer. *Crit Rev Clin Lab Sci* 2006; **4**: 1–67.

94. Hoffmann A, Baltimore D. Circuitry of nuclear factor kappaB signaling. *Immunol Rev* 2006; **210**: 171–86.

●95. Annunziata CM, Davis RE, Demchenko Y *et al.* Frequent engagement of the classical and alternative NF-kappaB pathways by diverse genetic abnormalities in multiple myeloma. *Cancer Cell* 2007; **12**: 115–30.

●96. Keats JJ, Fonseca R, Chesi M *et al.* Promiscuous mutations activate the noncanonical NF-kappaB pathway in multiple myeloma. *Cancer Cell* 2007; **12**: 131–44.

◆97. Farinha P, Gascoyne RD. Molecular pathogenesis of mucosa-associated lymphoid tissue lymphoma. *J Clin Oncol* 2005; **23**: 6370–78.

98. Mitsiades C, Mitsiades NS, Richardson PG *et al.* Multiple myeloma: a prototypic disease model for the characterization and therapeutic targeting of interactions between tumor cells and their local microenvironment. *J Cell Biochem* 2007; **101**: 950–68.

99. Goldin LR, Caporaso NE. Family studies in chronic lymphocytic leukaemia and other lymphoproliferative tumours. *Br J Haematol* 2007; **139**: 774–9.

100. Sellick GS, Goldin LR, Wild RW *et al.* A high-density SNP genome-wide linkage search of 206 families identifies susceptibility loci for chronic lymphocytic leukemia. *Blood* 2007; **110**: 3326–33.

101. Raval A, Tanner SM, Byrd JC *et al.* Downregulation of death-associated protein kinase 1 (DAPK1) in chronic lymphocytic leukemia. *Cell* 2007; **129**: 879–90.

102. Rossi D, Gaidano G, Gloghini A *et al.* Frequent aberrant promoter hypermethylation of O6-methylguanine-DNA methyltransferase and death-associated protein kinase genes in immunodeficiency-related lymphomas. *Br J Haematol* 2003; **123**: 475–8.

103. Rossi D, Capello D, Gloghini A *et al.* Aberrant promoter methylation of multiple genes throughout the clinico-pathologic spectrum of B-cell neoplasia. *Haematologica* 2004; **89**: 154–64.

104. Rollinson S, Levene AP, Mensah FK *et al.* Gastric marginal zone lymphoma is associated with polymorphisms in genes involved in inflammatory response and antioxidative capacity. *Blood* 2003; **102**: 1007–11.

105. Parsonnet J, Isaacson PJ. Bacterial infection and MALT lymphoma. *N Engl J Med* 2004; **350**: 213–15.

106. Machida K, Cheng KT, Sung VM *et al.* Hepatitis C virus induces a mutator phenotype: enhanced mutations of immunoglobulin and protooncogenes. *Proc Natl Acad Sci U S A* 2004; **101**: 4262–7.

107. Hermine O, Lefrère F, Bronowicki JP *et al.* Regression of splenic lymphoma with villous lymphocytes after treatment of hepatitis C virus infection. *N Engl J Med* 2002; **347**: 89–94.

108. Ekström Smedby K, Baecklund E, Askling J. Malignant lymphomas in autoimmunity and inflammation: a review of risk, risk factors, and lymphoma characteristics. *Cancer Epidemiol Biomarkers Prev* 2006; **15**: 2069–77.

23

Gene expression patterns in lymphoma classification

ULF KLEIN

INTRODUCTION

Global gene expression profile (GEP) analysis, facilitated by the invention of DNA microarrays in the late 1990s that allowed the simultaneous screening of thousands of expressed genes, was poised from the beginning to have a major impact on the classification of the lymphoid neoplasms. While previously only relatively few cell-surface antigens or other markers, often in combination with morphological features, were used for the phenotypic characterization of lymphoid tumors, GEP analysis generates an enormous number of data points that become available for a more comprehensive comparative analysis of tumor entities. These methodological advances allow progress in a number of issues, including the identification of novel tumor subtypes, the cellular derivation of tumors, and the identification of tumor-associated gene expression patterns of potential therapeutic value.

DNA microarrays

The DNA microarrays, also referred to as gene chips, currently used in GEP analyses contain a large number of either polymerase chain reaction (PCR) products (cDNA

arrays) or shorter oligonucleotides (oligonucleotide arrays, e.g., from Affymetrix) representing distinct messenger RNA (mRNA) sequences that are spotted on glass slides.[1,2] RNA derived from the cells under study is first labeled using fluorescent molecules, followed by the hybridization to the microarrays. Finally, fluorescent signals which indicate hybridization between the labeled probe and the probe sets representing the genes on the microarray are measured by scanning of the gene chip. Hybridizations to cDNA arrays generally require two fluorochromes, while for the oligonucleotide system a single-color fluorochrome is sufficient. The output of such hybridizations is normalized gene expression data, which are then compared to each other using biostatistical methods in order to identify gene expression differences among the different cell types. The identification of cell type-specific microRNA signatures necessitated the development of specialized microarray platforms [3] or other detection mechanisms.[4]

Biostatistical analysis methods

The meaningful evaluation of the enormous number of data points generated in a GEP study required the development of biostatistical analysis methods that are able to

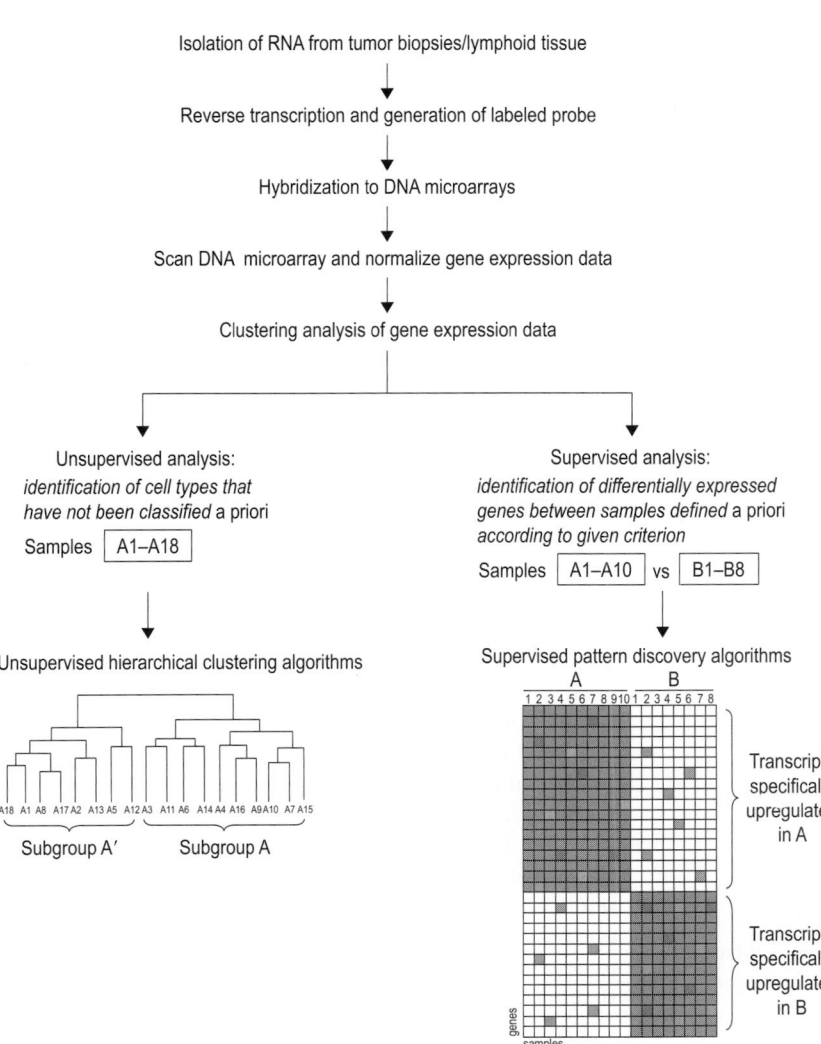

Isolation of RNA from tumor biopsies/lymphoid tissue

Reverse transcription and generation of labeled probe

Hybridization to DNA microarrays

Scan DNA microarray and normalize gene expression data

Clustering analysis of gene expression data

Unsupervised analysis:
*identification of cell types that
have not been classified* a priori

Samples   A1–A18

Unsupervised hierarchical clustering algorithms

Subgroup A′   Subgroup A

Supervised analysis:
*identification of differentially expressed
genes between samples defined* a priori
according to given criterion

Samples   A1–A10   vs   B1–B8

Supervised pattern discovery algorithms

A   B
1 2 3 4 5 6 7 8 9 10 1 2 3 4 5 6 7 8

Transcripts specifically upregulated in A

Transcripts specifically upregulated in B

genes
samples

Figure 23.1   Strategy for the identification of cell subtypes and differentially expressed genes between cell subtypes by gene expression profile analysis. Shown lower right, the matrix resulting from supervised learning of two subgroups (A1–A10 and B1–B8); gray and white identify upregulated and downregulated genes, respectively. Columns represent individual samples, rows correspond to genes. Shown lower left, the dendrogram resulting from unsupervised hierarchical clustering of samples from one group (A1–A18).

identify specific patterns of gene expression associated with the individual cell types. Generally, one distinguishes two approaches: unsupervised learning is applied in the identification of cell types which have not been classified *a priori*, whereas supervised learning allows the identification of differentially expressed genes between samples defined *a priori* according to a specific criterion, e.g., cell type, genotype, or clinical parameters (Fig. 23.1).[5,6]

Unsupervised learning, also referred to as unsupervised hierarchical cluster analysis, employs algorithms that seek out similarities among individual samples (e.g., tumor cases) of a larger panel, and branches the samples according to their relatedness to other samples. This type of analysis yields the characteristic *dendrogram*, where the length of the branches indicates the similarity between samples or genes, and higher-order branches identify related groups of samples or genes. Unsupervised hierarchical clustering may be extremely useful in the initial analysis of GEP data for two reasons: (1) a dendrogram immediately reveals the relationship of the tumor type under investigation to other tumor categories; and (2) unsupervised clustering may uncover gene expression differences that are due

to methodological variations, e.g., in sample collection, preparation, probe labeling, or hybridization. For example, a dendrogram generated from clustering purified and unpurified samples of a homogeneous tumor category typically shows two major branches that separate those groups, reflecting the presence of non-tumor tissue in the unpurified samples. Also, different cDNA synthesis protocols or labeling methods (one-step versus two-step labeling) can affect an unsupervised analysis, since the use of different reagents may influence the quality of full-length transcripts. Therefore, unsupervised hierarchical cluster analysis is unsuitable for the detection of biological gene expression differences between samples that were not processed in the same way.

Supervised learning, also referred to as supervised pattern discovery analysis, is the principal method for tumor class prediction and for the identification of genes specifically expressed in a tumor subtype. To this end, supervised learning employs an algorithm that identifies a set of genes that is able to reliably identify the respective tumor subtype in a classification analysis (Fig. 23.2). In a supervised analysis, a '*tester set*' that usually comprises a number of cases of

Generation of gene expression data from a set of biopsies
corresponding to different tumor subtypes

↓

Generation of a class predictor (classifier) based on the gene
expression data (learning panel)

↓

Applying the class predictor to an independent panel of cases

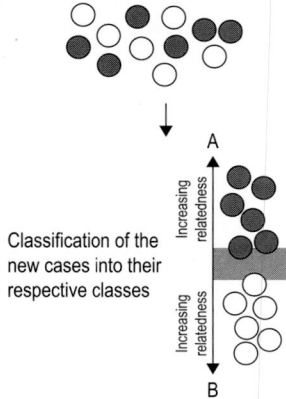

Classification of the
new cases into their
respective classes

Figure 23.2 Class predictors (classifiers): generation and testing of a class predictor by gene expression profile (GEP) analysis to identify tumor subtypes. A classifier is generated using GEP data from a set of biopsies corresponding to different tumor subtypes and applied to an unclassified (independent) panel. Tumor cases belonging to the two subgroups are identified by gray and white circles. The relatedness of the respective cases to either subtype is scored and quantified. The arrows in the diagram at the bottom denote increasing relatedness to either tumor subtype. The relatedness of cases inside the 'gray area' to either of the chronic lymphocytic leukemia subtypes does not reach statistical significance.

a well-defined class (e.g., phenotype) is compared to a 'control set' (which may include one or more phenotypically, genotypically, or otherwise defined traits) to extract gene expression differences. By applying stringent criteria to the algorithm, one is able to filter out genes whose expression differences relative to the control set do not achieve sufficient statistical significance, and/or to exclude genes which are not consistently upregulated across most or all samples of the tester set.

The validity of supervised learning was first demonstrated by the ability to distinguish acute lymphoblastic leukemia (ALL) from acute myeloid leukemia (AML) based only on their specific gene expression:[7] a class predictor (classifier) was generated on a tester panel that, without previous knowledge about the origin of tumor specimens of an independent panel, could classify those cases into either ALL or AML subgroups with 100 percent confidence level. Generally, classifiers can be tailored for the identification of various parameters, such as differences in the clinical prognosis among tumor cases. Although

numerous classification methods with different underlying algorithms have been reported, it is generally observed that if the gene expression differences between data sets are robust, independent classifiers yield virtually the same results. The ultimate proof for the value of a classifier is its ability to correctly separate an independent panel of tumor cases (i.e., excluding the cases on which the classifier was built) into the corresponding subtypes. The generation of a classifier by supervised learning does not require knowledge of the actual genes that build the classifier. However, supervised learning is also the tool of choice for the identification of tumor-associated genes with relevance for diagnosis, prognosis, and therapy.

Commonly used terms and definitions

The pattern of expressed genes identified by supervised or unsupervised learning that specifies a cell type or an otherwise defined 'class' is conventionally called a 'signature.' The output of unsupervised hierarchical clustering is the dendrogram that indicates the relatedness of the individual samples or genes to each other, often in combination with a colored matrix (sometimes also referred to as an 'Eisenplot') that depicts the transcript levels of each gene across the samples. Matrices are color coded, and the color scale identifies relative gene expression changes, typically as fold difference. It turned out to be extremely practical to represent GEP data by a matrix, since this enables the simultaneous portrayal of the expression changes of a large number of genes across a large number of samples, a circumstance that has the additional advantage of readily identifying outliers. Also, the results of supervised analyses are usually shown as colored matrices, often in combination with a statistical value which can be a P value or ζ-score. The latter corresponds to the average expression difference of a gene between the two groups of samples divided by the standard deviation of the gene across the samples, and can thus be significant even for a gene with a low fold-difference value if it is expressed at similar levels in all samples of the tester set.

Applications of gene expression profile analysis

Cell type-specific signatures and classifiers generated by GEP analyses can be extremely valuable for lymphoma classification and the identification of tumor-associated genes. First, the vast amount of data points ensuing from a GEP analysis may increase the chance of identifying novel tumor subtypes relative to single or multiple marker analyses. The availability of a large number of parameters may also lead to improvements in the diagnosis of morphologically similar but prognostically heterogeneous malignancies. Second, a comparative GEP analysis of a lymphoma versus 'healthy' lymphocytes may help to identify the normal cellular counterpart of the tumor, and may thus provide insights into the pathogenetic mechanisms underlying the tumor development. Third, GEP data from lymphomas may be specifically interrogated for the activity of a certain signaling pathway or a transcriptional response, and may thus provide clues about the activation, or distortion, of certain cellular signaling pathways.

Over the last several years, GEP data have been generated for most types of lymphoid malignancies as well as for the major subsets of normal B lymphocytes,[8–11] and the biostatistical analysis of those data could often shed new light on the classification and pathogenesis of lymphomas.[12,13] Evidently, the differences in the transcriptomes measured by GEP analyses represent only part of the biological changes in a cell, since translational and post-translational modifications remain undetectable. In the near future, GEP analyses will almost certainly be complemented by large-scale protein and tissue microarray analyses.[14,15]

This book chapter is aimed at introducing the use of large-scale GEP analysis in the study of lymphomas. Thus, with special emphasis on the methodological approaches, the following paragraphs address what we have learned so far about the classification of lymphoid malignancies, the relation of lymphoid malignancies to their normal cell of origin, and the pathogenetic mechanisms of lymphoma development.

CLASSIFICATION OF LYMPHOID MALIGNANCIES

Based on phenotype and morphological features, lymphoid malignancies have long been classified into major categories. Consistent with this notion, a GEP analysis using unsupervised hierarchical clustering separates a mixed panel of lymphoid tumors into the morphologically recognized subgroups (Fig. 23.3). In reality, however, certain categories of lymphoid malignancies show a marked clinical heterogeneity, thus hinting at the existence of biologically distinct subtypes within a lymphoma category that is presently recognized and treated as a single disease. A GEP analysis, which allows simultaneous monitoring of thousands of data points in a large panel of cases, represents an ideal tool for the identification of novel, biologically defined tumor subtypes. Experimentally, this goal can be approached in two ways: (1) by unsupervised clustering of cases of a single disease entity – a true class discovery experiment; or (2) by supervised analysis, if specific parameters are known that vary among individual tumor cases (Fig. 23.4). Those parameters may include differences in the clinical course, in specific phenotypic markers or mRNA transcripts, in genetic alterations such as chromosomal translocations or mutations in protooncogenes, or in the level of somatic hypermutation in immunoglobulin variable region (IGV) genes. The following paragraphs summarize what has been learned from GEP analyses in the attempts to decipher the heterogeneity of diffuse large

B cell lymphoma (DLBCL), B cell chronic lymphocytic leukemia (CLL), and pediatric ALL.

Diffuse large B cell lymphoma

Diffuse large B cell lymphoma is a malignancy of mature B cells that carry somatically mutated IGV genes. Diffuse large B cell lymphoma had long been recognized as a category of lymphoid malignancies with extensive clinical heterogeneity. The first GEP analysis of DLBCL cases made the groundbreaking discovery that this lymphoma entity can be separated into at least two distinct subtypes by virtue of their specific gene expression signatures.[16] One subtype was characterized by the expression of genes typical of germinal center (GC) B cells (GC-type DLBCL), the other by the expression of genes that are upregulated in in vitro-activated B cells (ABC-type DLBCL). In subsequent analyses on larger tumor panels, at least one additional DLBCL category could be identified by virtue of its distinct gene expression signature.[17,18] Of note, the discovery that DLBCL cases can be classified into biologically distinct subgroups has fueled a tremendous activity in the investigation of the pathogenic mechanisms of this disease.

There appears to be a correlation between particular DLBCL subtypes and patient survival, with the GC-type DLBCL showing a more benign clinical course.[16,17] While these findings led to the creation of a predictor that is able to classify DLBCL into clinically distinct subgroups with a high confidence, and independent of the particular DNA microarray platform used,[19] it remains to be seen whether the labor-intensive and costly GEP-based approaches will find their way into the clinical diagnosis of DLBCL. Ultimately, one would like to identify the minimal set of genes or gene products that can predict survival outcome. Toward this goal, a study reported that a combination of only six markers was sufficient to predict the clinical outcome of DLBCL in the panel analyzed.[20]

B cell chronic lymphocytic leukemia

Chronic lymphocytic leukemia is a malignancy of mature B cells. No common genetic lesion has as yet been identified in CLL. Although uniform in their morphology, CLL can be separated into cases that harbor somatic mutations in their IGV genes, or cases without somatic mutations.[21] These two subgroups also differ in their clinical prognosis; the IGV-mutated CLL show a more benign disease course than the IGV-unmutated CLL.[21] Today, the determination of the IGV gene mutational status of a CLL case represents a standard diagnostic procedure in many hospitals.

Gene expression profile analysis has been employed to identify the putative gene expression differences between the two genetically distinct CLL subgroups. Surprisingly, unsupervised analysis of a panel of CLL failed to cluster the IGV gene mutated and unmutated cases into separate

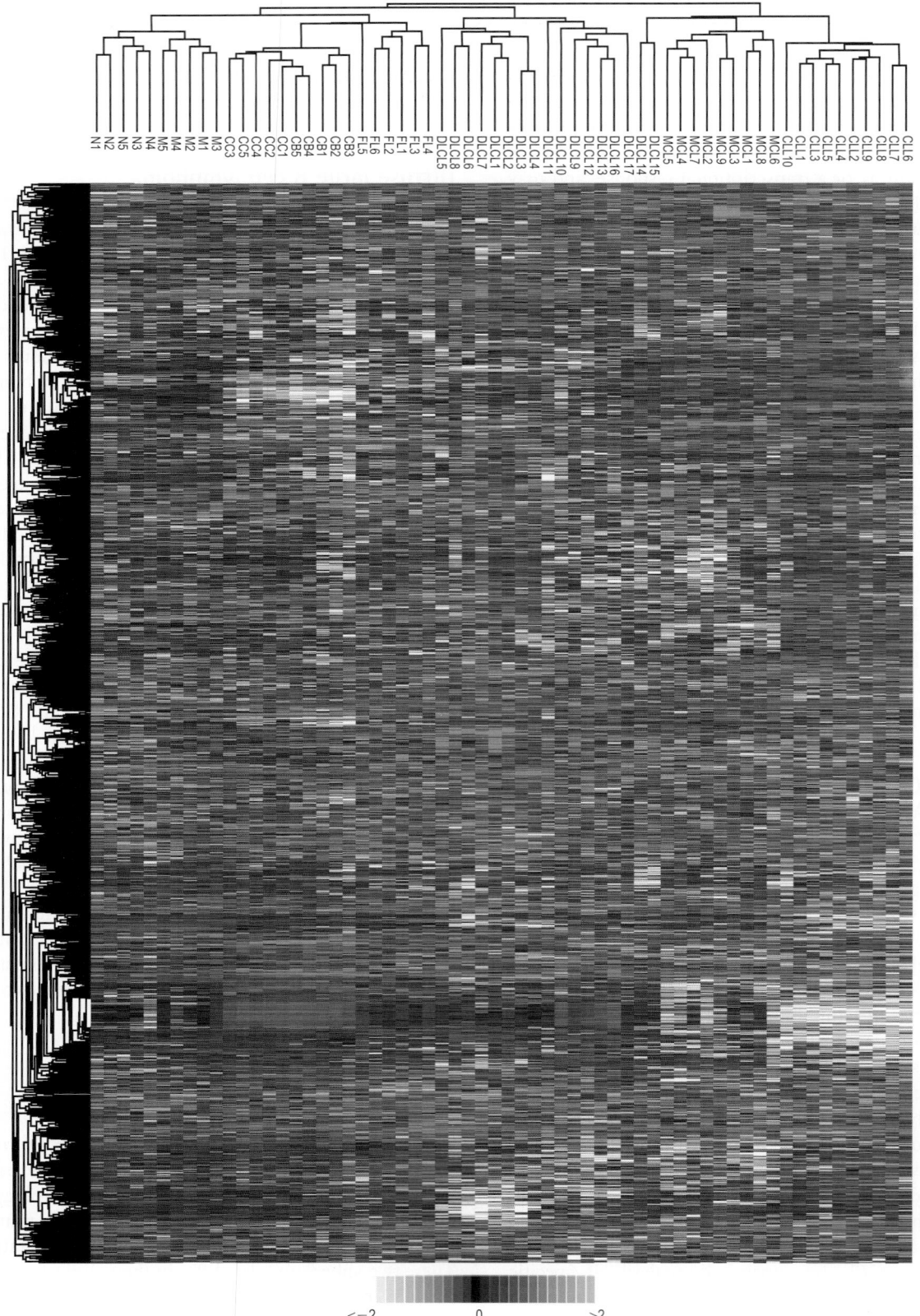

Figure 23.3 Unsupervised hierarchical clustering of normal B cell subpopulations and B cell-derived tumors. Unsupervised hierarchical clustering separates a mixed panel of lymphoid tumors into the morphologically recognized subgroups. Gene expression profile data from normal B cell subsets (N, naïve; M, memory; CB, GC centroblasts; CC, GC centrocytes) and various B cell tumors (DLCL, diffuse large B cell lymphoma; FL, follicular lymphoma; MCL, mantle cell lymphoma; CLL, B cell chronic lymphocytic leukemia) were clustered using the average linkage method. The dendrogram at the top shows the relatedness among the samples; the dendrogram at the left the relatedness among the genes. The matrix visualizes the relative expression of a given gene across the samples. Upregulated and downregulated genes are identified by different shades of gray, ranging from dark to light. Columns represent individual samples, rows correspond to genes.

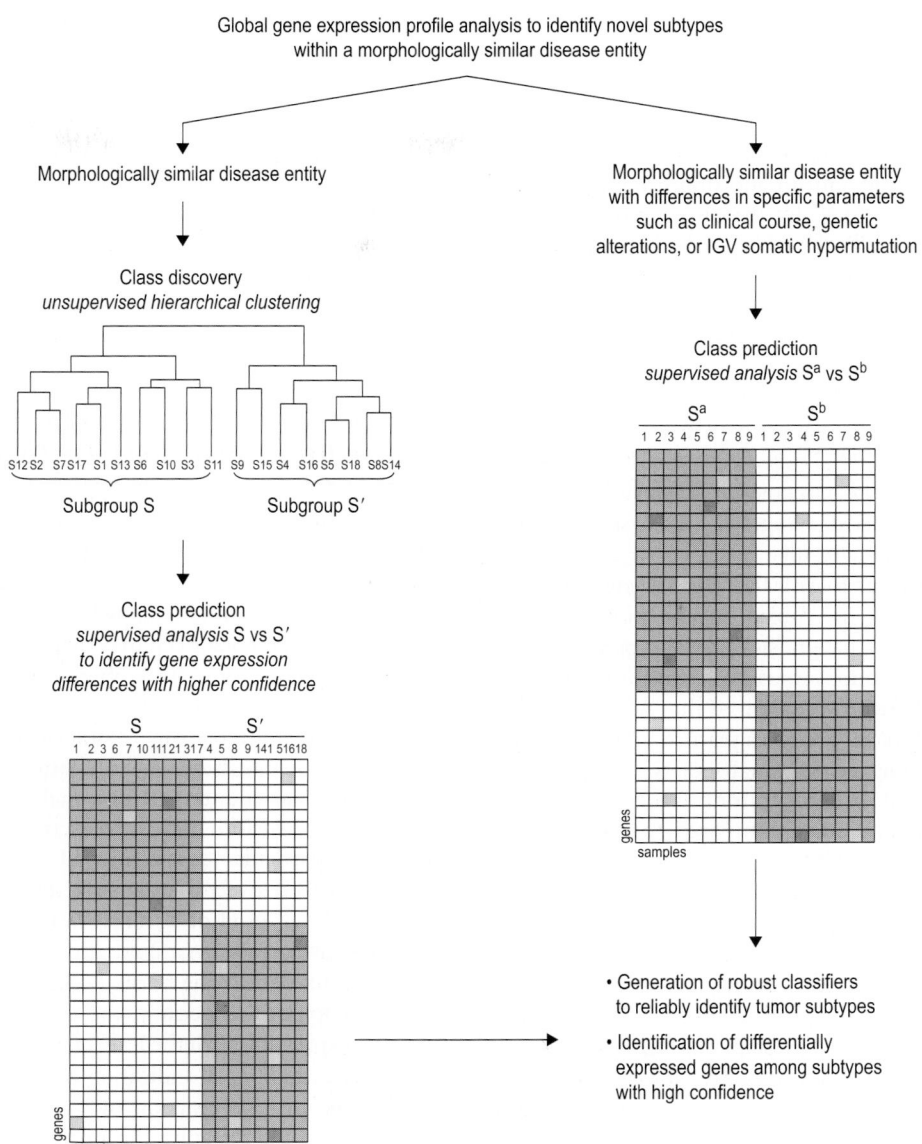

Figure 23.4 Identification of novel subtypes within a morphologically similar disease: the use of unsupervised (class discovery) and supervised (class prediction) analysis. Novel subtypes within a morphologically similar disease can be identified by unsupervised hierarchical clustering (left), and by supervised analysis (right). Unsupervised clustering can be employed for a true class discovery, in which novel subtypes are defined according to their gene expression signatures. This analysis may be followed by a class prediction step aiming at identifying gene expression differences with higher confidence. Supervised analysis is employed directly for class prediction in case other specific parameters, e.g., genomic alterations, differ among the individual cases of the disease entity. Gene expression profile data resulting from both approaches are then used to generate classifiers that allow the identification of tumor subtypes, and also to identify genes that are differentially expressed between the subtypes.

groups.[22,23] Rather, it turned out that all CLL show a homogeneous signature that is distinct from other tumor entities. Supervised analysis of the two CLL subgroups, however, could identify a pattern of genes (30–100 of more than 10 000 genes in two independent studies[22,23]) that in a classification analysis was able to correctly assign an independent panel of CLL cases into *IGV* gene mutated or unmutated subgroups. Among the genes whose expression was associated with an *IGV*-unmutated CLL genotype was

the tyrosine kinase ZAP70.[23] This discovery led to the development of a flow-cytometrical assay for Zap70 protein expression as a single marker for CLL diagnosis.[23,24] Of note, ZAP70 expression has been suggested to be more informative in the diagnosis of CLL subtypes than *IGV* gene analysis.[25] Several other gene products that were identified by supervised analysis of *IGV*-mutated versus unmutated CLL cases are currently being tested and evaluated for their potential value as diagnostic and prognostic markers.

Acute lymphoblastic leukemia

Pediatric acute B cell lymphoblastic leukemia (B-ALL) is characterized by the occurrence of specific genomic alterations. One study could separate the six known subtypes by unsupervised clustering, and in addition identified a further subtype that is defined by the absence of a specific cytogenetic abnormality.[26] The subtype-specific gene expression signatures may reflect changes in the normal transcriptional program of the tumor cell precursor inflicted by specific chromosomal translocations or other genomic alterations. Importantly, the corresponding signatures were strong enough to build classifiers that could identify the individual tumor classes at a high confidence level (i.e., more than 95 percent).[26,27] These studies are likely to have a profound impact on the diagnosis of pediatric leukemias, since the commonly used cytogenetic analysis does not always yield interpretable results.

A specific subtype of B-ALL that is characterized by a translocation involving the mixed-lineage leukemia gene (*MLL*) has a very poor prognosis. The comparative GEP analysis of this subgroup versus ALL without the MLL translocation, as well as AML, showed that ALL with MLL translocation displays a specific signature which exhibits features of a particular early hematopoietic progenitor.[28] The circumstance that this progenitor cell corresponds to a different developmental stage compared to those of the presumed normal cellular counterparts of AML and ALL without MLL translocation led to the suggestion that ALL with MLL translocation represents a separate disease.

A class discovery analysis performed on T cell-derived ALL revealed the existence of T-ALL subtypes that specifically overexpressed certain protooncogenes.[29] This overexpression, however, was not generally confined to cases that harbored a chromosomal abnormality (mostly a translocation) leading to the activation of the corresponding protooncogene, suggesting the existence of other mechanisms of deregulation. Thus, an unexpected and novel finding of this study turned out to be the identification of key markers that may be informative for the diagnosis of T-ALL cases without gross genomic alterations.

Other lymphoid malignancies

Gene expression profile analysis has now been successfully applied to the (sub)classification of several other lymphoma categories, including mantle cell lymphoma,[30] follicular lymphoma,[31] and Burkitt lymphoma.[32,33] A GEP analysis of a large panel of mantle cell lymphoma cases identified specific signatures that could predict the length of survival of the patients.[30] The same analysis also uncovered a quantitative correlation between a proliferation gene expression signature in mantle cell lymphoma and clinical prognosis. In the case of follicular lymphoma, gene expression patterns could be identified by supervised analysis that specifically correlated with either short or long survival.[31] The latter

study also exemplifies a characteristic feature of GEP analyses using whole biopsies as opposed to purified tumor cells: the gene expression signature of the survival predictor was actually derived from transcripts of nonmalignant immune cells that were present in the tumor at the time of diagnosis. In clinical diagnosis, Burkitt lymphoma and DLBCL, which require different treatment regimens, are sometimes difficult to distinguish based on their morphology alone. Gene expression profile analyses of large panels of Burkitt lymphoma and DLBCL cases revealed that Burkitt lymphoma can indeed be identified by a specific signature.[32,33]

RELATION OF LYMPHOID MALIGNANCIES TO THEIR NORMAL CELL OF ORIGIN

The identification of the normal cellular counterpart of a lymphoid neoplasia constitutes an important step toward the understanding of the pathogenetic mechanisms leading to lymphoma development. Knowing the differentiation stage of the tumor precursor cell may help to discern the disease-associated genes as well as aberrantly activated signaling pathways in the tumor cells, and may thus provide direct clues into the mechanism of transformation. It may not always be possible, however, to unambiguously identify the normal cellular counterpart of a malignancy. For example, one could envision that a transcriptional program that defines a particular developmental stage of a lymphocyte may be activated ectopically in a different developmental context as the result of a transforming event. Nevertheless, over the last decade, manifold attempts have been made in the quest to identify the normal cellular counterparts of the B cell neoplasms. Especially, the correlation of cell-surface marker expression with the level of *IGV* gene somatic hypermutation, which is an indication as to whether the cell has undergone the GC reaction of T cell-dependent immune responses, could separate the normal B lymphocytes into defined subpopulations. These subsets comprise (1) antigen-inexperienced naïve B cells; (2) GC B cells that undergo active somatic hypermutation (centroblasts) or are the precursors of post-GC cells (centroctyes); and (3) antigen-experienced memory B cells as well as plasma cells that carry somatically mutated *IGV* genes. These studies helped to lay down a B cell developmental 'scheme' that could assign several categories of B cell tumors to defined differentiation stages,[34-37] such as follicular lymphoma that is characterized by a follicular growth pattern with ongoing somatic hypermutation and may thus originate from a GC centroblast. In many cases, however, the normal cellular counterpart of a tumor entity remained enigmatic, as in the case of DLBCL and CLL. Therefore, the expectations were high that the mere quantity of data points resulting from a GEP analysis might help to uncover a developmental relationship between a malignant and a healthy cell.

One may assume that in an unsupervised hierarchical cluster analysis of gene expression data from normal and malignant B lymphocytes, the tumors cluster next to their most closely related normal subpopulation. However, in practice this is rarely observed, because usually the gene expression differences between transformed and normal cells are extremely large. As an additional complexity, the transcriptomes of developmentally distinct (normal) B cell subpopulations are often very similar.[8] Since a dendrogram is built from all gene expression values of all samples, large differences in the transcriptomes between groups of samples have a stronger influence on clustering than the small ones. These methodological restrictions of the unsupervised clustering can be overcome by first defining a B cell subset-specific gene expression pattern through supervised analysis, and then tracking this signature within the GEP data of the tumor (Plate 18, see plate section). This approach resembles the classification analysis described in the previous paragraph, although here the classifier is built on the differences in the transcriptomes of the various normal B cell subsets and then applied to the tumor samples.

Diffuse large B cell lymphoma

The first demonstration that GEP analyses may indeed yield insights into the relationships between lymphomas and distinct subsets of normal lymphocytes stems from the DLBCL profiling analysis by Louis Staudt and collaborators.[16] As a fact, virtually all DLBCL originate from the oncogenic transformation of cells that have diversified their *IGV* genes by somatic hypermutation. Diffuse large B cell lymphoma, however, comprises an extremely heterogeneous tumor category, and the morphological/histological presentation of the tumor cells did not immediately suggest a candidate normal cellular counterpart. Gene expression profile analyses made the intriguing finding that DLBCL cases can be separated into at least three biologically distinct subtypes.[16,17] In those studies, unsupervised analysis of a large panel of cases including DLBCL, various other tumor entities, and normal and *in vitro*-activated B lymphocytes revealed a correlation between the expression of specific genes and a particular cell type. Thus, the specific upregulation of a set of genes whose expression is associated with GC B cells and malignancies known to be derived from those cells led to the definition of a GC-specific signature. Likewise, an activated B cell-specific signature could be established. When DLBCL cases were clustered using the GC- and activated B cell-signature genes only, most of the DLBCL cases could be subdivided into either of the two groups.[16] It is now commonly assumed that the cell of origin of the GC type of DLBCL is a GC B cell, probably a centroblast. The normal cellular counterpart of ABC-type DLBCL is still enigmatic, since it is unclear which normal B cell corresponds to the *in vitro*-activated B cell.

B cell chronic lymphocytic leukemia

Chronic lymphocytic leukemia is unique among B cell malignancies in that the tumors can be subdivided into *IGV* gene somatically mutated and unmutated cases (see previous section). This observation initially led to the hypothesis that the *IGV* gene mutated subtype may originate from a cell that has acquired somatic mutations during GC transit, while the *IGV* gene unmutated subtype, despite showing evidence of antigenic selection, did not pass through the GC.[21] Since pre- and post-GC B cells differ in their transcriptomes,[8] this scenario would predict that the two CLL subgroups display distinct gene expression signatures. Surprisingly, however, GEP analysis demonstrated that both CLL subtypes show a homogeneous gene expression signature with only minor differences,[22,23] indicating that both CLL subtypes originate from the oncogenic transformation of a precursor cell of the same developmental stage. The observation that the cell-surface marker phenotype of CLL (CD5[+] CD23[+] CD27[+]) does not resemble that of any known normal B cell, and that an unsupervised cluster analysis of CLL cases and other malignant and normal B cells failed to reveal any relationships, called for a methodologically different approach in the attempt to elucidate the cellular derivation of CLL. First, the major human B cell subsets were purified from lymphoid tissue and GEP data were generated.[8] Then, supervised analysis was performed between the developmentally distinct subpopulations in a pairwise fashion in order to establish the individual B cell subset-specific signatures. Those signatures were then tracked in the GEP data of CLL, and a measure of statistical significance (*P* value) could be assigned to the relatedness between a CLL biopsy and the corresponding signatures. Following this approach, it was possible to uncover a relationship of both *IGV* gene mutated and unmutated CLL cases to antigen-experienced B cells,[22] which may include marginal zone and memory B cells. Furthermore, it has been reported that the *IGV* gene unmutated cases show evidence of activation by B cell receptor signaling.[23] Together, these findings may explain the puzzling observation that all CLLs show a common gene expression profile, but that *IGV* gene mutated and unmutated CLLs differ in the expression of a small set of genes.

Other lymphoid malignancies

The results of a comparative GEP analysis between hairy cell leukemia (HCL) and the normal B cell subsets suggested that the tumor cell precursor of HCL is phenotypically related to an antigen-experienced memory or marginal zone B cell,[38] as in the case of CLL (see above). Together, these findings point toward the existence of a category of tumors that may originate from the oncogenic transformation of antigen-experienced B cells that have passed the GC stage of B cell development, and that may include CLL and HCL.[39] Using a similar approach, the acquired immune deficiency syndrome (AIDS)-associated lymphoma subtype primary effusion lymphoma (PEL), whose tumor cells carry somatically mutated *IGV* genes and are characteristically infected by the Kaposi sarcoma-associated herpes virus (KSHV/human herpes virus 8

[HHV-8]), did not show any relatedness to the gene expression signatures of either GC B cells or memory B cells.[40] When PEL cases were then compared to the specific gene expression signature of Epstein–Barr virus (EBV)-transformed lymphoblastoid cell lines as well as cell lines derived from multiple myeloma, their transcriptomes displayed relatedness to both signatures,[40] suggesting that the precursor cell of PEL may represent a not fully differentiated plasma cell (plasmablast). Alternatively, the peculiar phenotype of PEL may, at least in part, be attributed to the activity of KSHV/HHV-8-encoded gene products.

Finally, cell lines derived from Hodgkin–Reed–Sternberg (H-RS) cells of classical Hodgkin lymphoma exhibited more relatedness in their GEP to the specific signature of EBV-transformed B cell lines than to those of any other B cell subset or plasma cells.[41] Interestingly, two independent GEP analyses of mediastinal large B cell lymphoma (MLBCL), a DLBCL subtype, uncovered a strong phenotypic relationship of MLBCL cases to classical Hodgkin lymphoma cell lines.[42,43] Together, these observations raise the possibility that a subset of B cell-derived malignancies, including classical Hodgkin lymphoma, MLBCL, and perhaps also the category of 'gray zone' lymphomas,[44,45] may originate from the oncogenic transformation of an as yet unidentified normal B cell, or that similar transforming mechanisms acting in the different tumor entities lead to the acquisition of a similar cell phenotype.

INSIGHTS INTO PATHOGENETIC MECHANISMS OF LYMPHOMA DEVELOPMENT

Gene expression profile analysis may be used as a tool to gain insights into the pathogenetic mechanisms of lymphoma development. The most straightforward way toward this goal is the generation of a tumor-specific gene expression pattern by a supervised analysis between a tumor entity and the respective control populations (Fig. 23.5). This pattern can then be analyzed for concerted changes in the expression of known downstream targets of signaling pathways or transcriptional activators/repressors with functions in survival or cell cycle regulation. The findings obtained from such approaches may help to inspire novel hypotheses on lymphoma pathogenesis, and, equally important, identify new markers or therapeutic targets. In the latter case, it is necessary to verify the expression of the transcript by other methods (PCR, Northern blot) and to further investigate the transcript structure, since the sequence of an mRNA is represented only partly on most types of DNA microarrays. In case the transcript encodes a polypeptide, the ultimate goal is to detect the gene product at the single-cell level by immunohistochemical analysis on tissue sections or by flow-cytometric analysis of lymphocyte populations.

Gene expression profile-based approaches may help to determine whether a specific gene product (e.g., a transcription factor) or a specific signaling pathway is functionally active in a tumor. In vitro systems can be devised

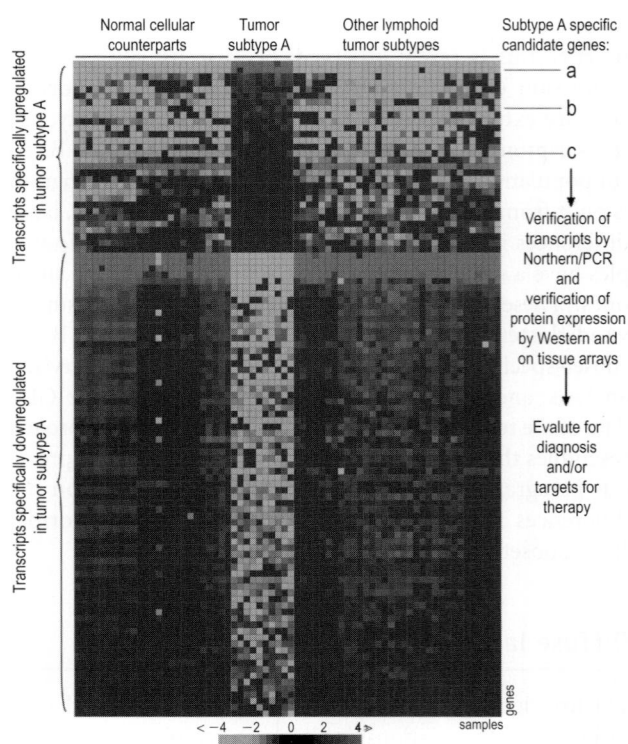

Figure 23.5 Identification of tumor-specific genes by supervised analysis. Genes specifically up- or downregulated in a tumor subtype relative to the various other lymphoid tumor categories and normal cellular counterparts are identified by supervised pattern discovery analysis. The expression of candidate genes of potential interest for diagnosis or therapy, e.g., cell-surface receptors or molecules involved in signaling, is verified by Northern blot or polymerase chain reaction (PCR) analysis and, at the protein level, by immunohistochemistry and Western blot analysis. Upregulated and downregulated genes are identified by different shades of gray, ranging from dark to light, respectively. Columns represent individual samples, rows correspond to genes.

that allow the deliberate activation of a specific signaling pathway or a transcriptional response, followed by the generation of GEP data. For example, cells can be activated *in vitro* through receptor–ligand interaction, or a transcription factor not normally active in a cell line can be introduced into the cells by transfection or viral transduction (Fig. 23.6). The transcriptional consequences of such single-parameter manipulations are identified by supervised analysis and then tracked in the GEP data of a tumor, potentially verifying the activity of the specific signaling pathway or transcriptional response in the tumor cells. Similarly, one can investigate the transcriptional consequences of a putative tumor suppressor following its reintroduction into a cell line with a homozygous deletion of the gene. The list of suitable experimental systems is much longer and includes RNA interference-mediated silencing of genes as well as the investigation of the effects of pharmacological compounds.

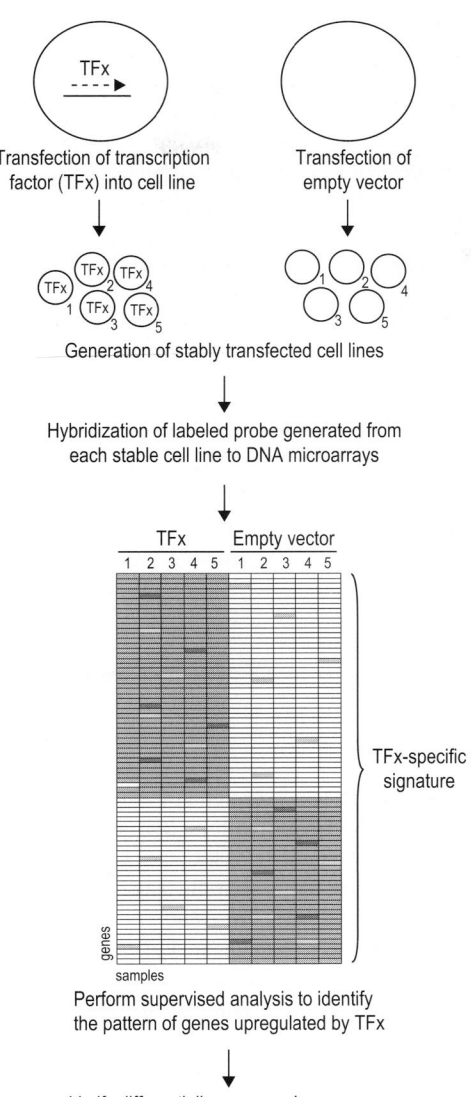

Figure 23.6 Tracking a transcriptional response in normal and malignant cells using a gene expression profile-based approach. A transcription factor-specific gene expression signature is generated *in vitro*, followed by tracking of the respective signature in normal or malignant cells. A cell line is transfected with a gene encoding a transcription factor (left) or empty vector as a control (right). Stably transfected cell lines are generated. Gene expression profile analysis is performed to identify a signature of genes whose expression is regulated directly or indirectly by the transcription factor. Following verification, the specific signature can then be tracked in tumors.

Identification of tumor-specific gene expression

Supervised analysis has been employed for the identification of genes that are specifically expressed in a tumor or tumor subtype. Several thus-identified gene products were further investigated and found to be useful for a more

refined diagnosis of CLL[24] or HCL,[24,46] or to represent candidate genes involved in the pathogenesis of Hodgkin lymphoma.[47,48]

A finding of the GEP analysis on MLL[28,49] (see above) may have direct implications for the mechanism of transformation of this tumor entity: among the genes of the MLL-specific signature, the subset of the HOX genes represents known target genes of the MLL fusion-gene product generated by the corresponding chromosomal translocation. One of the HOX genes, *HOXA9*, can induce leukemia in mice if overexpressed, suggesting that this gene product (or other family members) might be critically involved in MLL tumorigenesis. The case of MLL demonstrates that a gene product whose expression is the direct cause of a genomic alteration can establish a unique transcriptional program in the tumor cells. Gene expression profile analysis of MLL against ALL and AML cases also identified the FMS-like tyrosine kinase 3 (*FLT3*) gene whose expression was specifically upregulated in MLL, and which was subsequently shown to have activating mutations in MLL.[50] The therapeutic potential of FLT3 inhibitors was tested in a xenograft mouse model of this leukemia where the application of a pharmacological FLT3 inhibitor led to a substantial inhibition of leukemic progression,[50] suggesting that the targeted inhibition of this gene product in human leukemias may be developed into a promising therapeutic approach.

In an attempt to elucidate the transforming events of T cell-derived leukemias, a GEP analysis that compared different leukemic subgroups among each other and to normal T cell subpopulations was able to identify gene products with crucial roles in the T cell leukemogenic pathways, including the HOX11L2 transcription factor.[29] The same analysis also revealed that overexpression of the transcription factors that characterize the T-ALL subtypes was not generally associated with chromosomal translocations that were previously thought to be the underlying cause for their deregulated expression. In summary, the GEP analyses performed on the pediatric leukemias proved to be highly successful in the identification of key oncogenic factors and could thereby spur the development of new hypotheses on leukemogenesis.

Dissecting cellular pathways in normal and transformed cells

Whole transcriptome analyses can be extremely useful in the identification of the downstream effects of major gene expression regulators. This is particularly true for *in vitro* systems that measure the transcriptional consequences of the expression of an exogenous gene product by GEP analysis. The first analysis of this kind centered on the *MYC* protooncogene[51] that is constitutively expressed in Burkitt lymphoma and DLBCL subgroups as the result of a chromosomal translocation. This analysis could identify a large number of previously unknown *MYC* target genes with roles in cell growth and proliferation. Similarly, exogenous expression of the B cell lymphoma 6 (*BCL6*) protooncogene, a master regulator of GC B cell development, led to the identification of previously unknown relationships with other major transcriptional programs that are involved in the cellular differentiation of GC B cells.[52] Since lymphomas frequently show deregulated expression of *BCL6*, elucidating its function in normal B cells may help to understand the role of this transcriptional repressor in lymphoma development.

A hallmark of T cell-dependent antibody responses is the stimulation of B cells through the CD40 cell-surface receptor, a tumor necrosis factor (TNF) receptor family member, although the nature of the B cell subpopulation(s) that is subjected to CD40 stimulation remained elusive. Downstream effects of CD40 stimulation include the activation of the nuclear factor κB (NF-κB) signaling pathway. A GEP-based approach was employed in order to determine at which B cell developmental stage CD40 stimulation occurs. First, a CD40 activation-specific signature was established by supervised analysis of GEP data derived from CD40-stimulated versus unstimulated cells of a B cell line *in vitro*. Then, the expression of those 'signature genes' was tracked in the GEP data of the normal B cell subsets using biostatistical analysis methods.[53] Contrary to the widely accepted view, this analysis suggested that the majority of GC B cells is not subjected to CD40 stimulation and/or activation of the NF-κB pathway. Further evidence for the inactivity of the NF-κB pathway in the majority of GC B cells comes from an independent work.[10] The results of these studies are consistent with the hypothesis that in a T cell-dependent immune response, CD40 stimulation shows a biphasic pattern in that it is required at the B cell activation step, and then later at the completion of the GC reaction when the cell is instructed to differentiate into a post-GC B cell. Since the NF-κB pathway is activated in several lymphoma entities,[54] including DLBCL,[55] it will be important to find out whether NF-κB activation in those tumors is aberrant or whether it can be attributed to the normal physiology of the tumor precursor cell.

While the GEP-based identification of an active signaling pathway or transcriptional response in a cell can provide new insights into the physiology of this cell type, one should caution that the data interpretation might be obscured by the connectivity of cell signaling pathways *in vivo*. Computational biology is beginning to address this issue, and outgoing from the analysis of cellular networks of lower organisms,[56] it has now become possible to study the more complex network interactions of the higher eukaryotes. For example, the approach of reverse engineering of gene regulatory networks is aimed at reconstructing cellular networks using GEP data of cell types known to differ in the expression of a key gene product or signaling pathway.[57] In the near future, computational biology will undoubtedly have a major impact on the dissection of physiologic as well as pathologic networks in human lymphocytes.

KEY POINTS

Key issues covered in this chapter

- Classification of lymphoid malignancies.
- Relation of lymphoid malignancies to their normal cell of origin.
- Insights into the pathogenetic mechanisms of lymphoma development.

ACKNOWLEDGMENTS

I would like to thank Riccardo Dalla-Favera, Andrea Califano, Gustavo Stolovitzky, Yuhai Tu, Katia Basso, and Laura Pasqualucci for discussion and for their constant input in some of the GEP experiments described in this chapter.

REFERENCES

● = Key primary paper
◆ = Major review article

◆1. Brown PO, Botstein D. Exploring the new world of the genome with DNA microarrays. *Nat Genet* 1999; **21**: 33–7.

◆2. Lockhart DJ, Dong H, Byrne MC *et al*. Expression monitoring by hybridization to high-density oligonucleotide arrays. *Nat Biotechnol* 1996; **14**: 1675–1680.

●3. Calin GA, Ferracin M, Cimmino A *et al*. A microRNA signature associated with prognosis and progression in chronic lymphocytic leukemia. *N Engl J Med* 2005; **353**: 1793–801.

●4. Lu J, Getz G, Miska EA *et al*. MicroRNA expression profiles classify human cancers. *Nature* 2005; **435**: 834–8.

●5. Eisen MB, Spellman PT, Brown PO, Botstein D. Cluster analysis and display of genome-wide expression patterns. *Proc Natl Acad Sci U S A* 1998; **95**: 14863–8.

●6. Califano A, Stolovitzky G, Tu Y. Analysis of gene expression microarrays for phenotype classification. *Proc Int Conf Intell Syst Mol Biol* 2000; **8**: 75–85.

●7. Golub TR, Slonim DK, Tamayo P *et al*. Molecular classification of cancer: class discovery and class prediction by gene expression monitoring. *Science* 1999; **286**: 531–7.

●8. Klein U, Tu Y, Stolovitzky GA *et al*. Transcriptional analysis of the B-cell germinal center reaction. *Proc Natl Acad Sci U S A* 2003; **100**: 2639–44.

●9. Shen Y, Iqbal J, Xiao L *et al*. Distinct gene expression profiles in different B-cell compartments in human peripheral lymphoid organs. *BMC Immunol* 2004; **5**: 20.

◆10. Shaffer AL, Rosenwald A, Hurt EM *et al*. Signatures of the immune response. *Immunity* 2001; **15**: 375–85.

●11. Underhill GH, George D, Bremer EG, Kansas GS. Gene expression profiling reveals a highly specialized genetic program of plasma cells. *Blood* 2003; **101**: 4013–21.

◆12. Staudt LM. Gene expression profiling of lymphoid malignancies. *Annu Rev Med* 2002; **53**: 303–18.

◆13. Ebert BL, Golub TR. Genomic approaches to hematologic malignancies. *Blood* 2004; **104**: 923–32.

●14. Hedvat CV, Hegde A, Chaganti RS *et al.* Application of tissue microarray technology to the study of non-Hodgkin's and Hodgkin's lymphoma. *Hum Pathol* 2002; **33**: 968–74.

●15. Hans CP, Weisenburger DD, Greiner TC *et al.* Confirmation of the molecular classification of diffuse large B-cell lymphoma by immunohistochemistry using a tissue microarray. *Blood* 2004; **103**: 275–82.

●16. Alizadeh AA, Eisen MB, Davis RE *et al.* Distinct types of diffuse large B-cell lymphoma identified by gene expression profiling. *Nature* 2000; **403**: 503–11.

●17. Rosenwald A, Wright G, Chan WC *et al.* The use of molecular profiling to predict survival after chemotherapy for diffuse large-B-cell lymphoma. *N Engl J Med* 2002; **346**: 1937–47.

●18. Shipp MA, Ross KN, Tamayo P *et al.* Diffuse large B-cell lymphoma outcome prediction by gene-expression profiling and supervised machine learning. *Nat Med* 2002; **8**: 68–74.

●19. Wright G, Tan B, Rosenwald A *et al.* A gene expression-based method to diagnose clinically distinct subgroups of diffuse large B-cell lymphoma. *Proc Natl Acad Sci U S A* 2003; **100**: 9991–6.

●20. Lossos IS, Czerwinski DK, Alizadeh AA *et al.* Prediction of survival in diffuse large-B-cell lymphoma based on the expression of six genes. *N Engl J Med* 2004; **350**: 1828–37.

◆21. Chiorazzi N, Ferrarini M. B-cell chronic lymphocytic leukemia: lessons learned from studies of the B-cell antigen receptor. *Annu Rev Immunol* 2003; **21**: 841–94.

●22. Klein U, Tu Y, Stolovitzky GA *et al.* Gene expression profiling of B-cell chronic lymphocytic leukemia reveals a homogeneous phenotype related to memory B-cells. *J Exp Med* 2001; **194**: 1625–38.

●23. Rosenwald A, Alizadeh AA, Widhopf G *et al.* Relation of gene expression phenotype to immunoglobulin mutation genotype in B-cell chronic lymphocytic leukemia. *J Exp Med* 2001; **194**: 1639–47.

●24. Crespo M, Bosch F, Villamor N *et al.* ZAP-70 expression as a surrogate for immunoglobulin-variable-region mutations in chronic lymphocytic leukemia. *N Engl J Med* 2003; **348**: 1764–75.

●25. Rassenti LZ, Huynh L, Toy TL *et al.* ZAP-70 compared with immunoglobulin heavy-chain gene mutation status as a predictor of disease progression in chronic lymphocytic leukemia. *N Engl J Med* 2004; **351**: 893–901.

●26. Yeoh EJ, Ross ME, Shurtleff SA *et al.* Classification, subtype discovery, and prediction of outcome in pediatric acute lymphoblastic leukemia by gene expression profiling. *Cancer Cell* 2002; **1**: 133–43.

●27. Ross ME, Zhou X, Song G *et al.* Classification of pediatric acute lymphoblastic leukemia by gene expression profiling. *Blood* 2003; **102**: 2951–9.

●28. Armstrong SA, Staunton JE, Silverman LB *et al.* MLL translocations specify a distinct gene expression profile that distinguishes a unique leukemia. *Nat Genet* 2002; **30**: 41–7.

●29. Ferrando AA, Neuberg DS, Staunton J *et al.* Gene expression signatures define novel oncogenic pathways in T-cell acute lymphoblastic leukemia. *Cancer Cell* 2002; **1**: 75–87.

●30. Rosenwald A, Wright G, Wiestner A *et al.* The proliferation gene expression signature is a quantitative integrator of oncogenic events that predicts survival in mantle cell lymphoma. *Cancer Cell* 2003; **3**: 185–97.

●31. Dave SS, Wright G, Tan B *et al.* Prediction of survival in follicular lymphoma based on molecular features of tumor-infiltrating immune cells. *N Engl J Med* 2004; **351**: 2159–69.

●32. Dave SS, Fu K, Wright GW *et al.* Molecular diagnosis of Burkitt's lymphoma. *N Engl J Med* 2006; **354**: 2431–42.

●33. Hummel M, Bentink S, Berger H *et al.* A biologic definition of Burkitt's lymphoma from transcriptional and genomic profiling. *N Engl J Med* 2006; **354**: 2419–30.

◆34. Küppers R, Klein U, Hansmann ML, Rajewsky K. Cellular origin of human B-cell lymphomas. *N Engl J Med* 1999; **341**: 1520–29.

◆35. Stevenson F, Sahota S, Zhu D *et al.* Insight into the origin and clonal history of B-cell tumors as revealed by analysis of immunoglobulin variable region genes. *Immunol Rev* 1998; **162**: 247–59.

◆36. Klein U, Goossens T, Fischer M *et al.* Somatic hypermutation in normal and transformed human B-cells. *Immunol Rev* 1998; **162**: 261–80.

●37. Pascual V, Liu YJ, Magalski A *et al.* Analysis of somatic mutation in five B-cell subsets of human tonsil. *J Exp Med* 1994; **180**: 329–39.

●38. Basso K, Liso A, Tiacci E *et al.* Gene expression profiling of hairy cell leukemia reveals a phenotype related to memory B-cells with altered expression of chemokine and adhesion receptors. *J Exp Med* 2004; **199**: 59–68.

◆39. Klein U, Dalla-Favera R. New insights into the phenotype and cell derivation of B-cell chronic lymphocytic leukemia. *Curr Top Microbiol Immunol* 2005; **294**: 31–49.

●40. Klein U, Gloghini A, Gaidano G *et al.* Gene expression profile analysis of AIDS-related primary effusion lymphoma (PEL) suggests a plasmablastic derivation and identifies PEL-specific transcripts. *Blood* 2003; **101**: 4115–21.

●41. Küppers R, Klein U, Schwering I *et al.* Identification of Hodgkin and Reed-Sternberg cell-specific genes by gene expression profiling. *J Clin Invest* 2003; **111**: 529–37.

●42. Rosenwald A, Wright G, Leroy K *et al.* Molecular diagnosis of primary mediastinal B-cell lymphoma identifies a clinically favorable subgroup of diffuse large B-cell lymphoma related to Hodgkin lymphoma. *J Exp Med* 2003; **198**: 851–62.

●43. Savage KJ, Monti S, Kutok JL *et al.* The molecular signature of mediastinal large B-cell lymphoma differs from that of other diffuse large B-cell lymphomas and shares features with classical Hodgkin lymphoma. *Blood* 2003; **102**: 3871–9.

◆44. Poppema S, Kluiver JL, Atayar C *et al.* Report: workshop on mediastinal grey zone lymphoma. *Eur J Haematol Suppl* 2005; 45–52.

◆45. Stein H, Johrens K, Anagnostopoulos I. Non-mediastinal grey zone lymphomas and report from the workshop. *Eur J Haematol Suppl* 2005; 42–4.

●46. Falini B, Tiacci E, Liso A *et al.* Simple diagnostic assay for hairy cell leukaemia by immunocytochemical detection of annexin A1 (ANXA1). *Lancet* 2004; **363**: 1869–70.

●47. Hinz M, Lemke P, Anagnostopoulos I *et al.* Nuclear factor kappaB-dependent gene expression profiling of Hodgkin's disease tumor cells, pathogenetic significance, and link to constitutive signal transducer and activator of transcription 5a activity. *J Exp Med* 2002; **196**: 605–17.

●48. Janz M, Hummel M, Truss M *et al.* Classical Hodgkin lymphoma is characterized by high constitutive expression of activating transcription factor 3 (ATF3), which promotes viability of Hodgkin/Reed-Sternberg cells. *Blood* 2006; **107**: 2536–9.

●49. Ferrando AA, Armstrong SA, Neuberg DS *et al.* Gene expression signatures in MLL-rearranged T-lineage and B-precursor acute leukemias: dominance of HOX dysregulation. *Blood* 2003; **102**: 262–8.

●50. Armstrong SA, Kung AL, Mabon ME *et al.* Inhibition of FLT3 in MLL. Validation of a therapeutic target identified by gene expression based classification. *Cancer Cell* 2003; **3**: 173–83.

●51. Coller HA, Grandori C, Tamayo P *et al.* Expression analysis with oligonucleotide microarrays reveals that MYC regulates genes involved in growth, cell cycle, signaling, and adhesion. *Proc Natl Acad Sci U S A* 2000; **97**: 3260–65.

●52. Shaffer AL, Yu X, He Y *et al.* BCL6 represses genes that function in lymphocyte differentiation, inflammation, and cell cycle control. *Immunity* 2000; **13**: 199–212.

●53. Basso K, Klein U, Niu H *et al.* Tracking CD40 signaling during germinal center development. *Blood* 2004; **104**: 4088–96.

◆54. Jost PJ, Ruland J. Aberrant NF-kappaB signaling in lymphoma: mechanisms, consequences, and therapeutic implications. *Blood* 2007; **109**: 2700–7.

●55. Davis RE, Brown KD, Siebenlist U, Staudt LM. Constitutive nuclear factor kappaB activity is required for survival of activated B-cell-like diffuse large B-cell lymphoma cells. *J Exp Med* 2001; **194**: 1861–74.

●56. Jeong H, Tombor B, Albert R *et al.* The large-scale organization of metabolic networks. *Nature* 2000; **407**: 651–4.

●57. Basso K, Margolin AA, Stolovitzky G *et al.* Reverse engineering of regulatory networks in human B-cells. *Nat Genet* 2005; **37**: 382–90.

24

Immunodeficiency, inherited and acquired, and lymphomagenesis

DAVIDE ROSSI, DANIELA CAPELLO AND GIANLUCA GAIDANO

GENERAL CONCEPTS

The World Health Organization (WHO) classification of hematopoietic tumors recognizes four broad settings of immunodeficiency conditions associated with an increased incidence of lymphoma. These are (1) primary immunodeficiency; (2) infection with the human immunodeficiency virus (HIV); (3) iatrogenic immunosuppression in patients who have received solid organ or bone marrow transplantation; and (4) iatrogenic immunosuppression associated with methotrexate treatment for autoimmune diseases.[1]

The first evidence of a link between immunodeficiency and lymphoma stemmed from the increased incidence of lymphoproliferative diseases observed in individuals with inherited immunodeficiencies and other forms of primary immunodeficiency.[2] Among inherited immunodeficiencies, the highest incidence of lymphoma occurs in T cell defects, including severe combined immune deficiency (SCID), CD40 ligand deficiency, Wiskott–Aldrich syndrome, and ataxia telangiectasia, which display a 100-fold increased risk of lymphoma.[3] Epidemiological studies have shown that lymphoma ranks as the most frequent tumor associated with SCID, CD40 ligand deficiency, Wiskott–Aldrich syndrome, and ataxia telangiectasia, generally comprising 80 percent of cancers developing in these syndromes.[3] Among other primary immunodeficiencies, the highest incidence of lymphoma is found in common variable immunodeficiency (CVID) disease.[3] In this disease, lymphoma is the most frequently associated cancer, approximating 50 percent of tumors affecting CVID patients. In particular, CVID patients display a high relative risk of non-Hodgkin lymphoma (NHL), ranging from 30 to 400 in different series.[4–6]

Since the outburst of HIV infection in 1981, the incidence of HIV-related lymphomas has been rising steadily and in 1987 the Centers for Disease Control (CDC) in Atlanta recognized NHL as an acquired immunodeficiency syndrome (AIDS)-defining illness.[7] In the era preceding the introduction of highly active antiretroviral therapy (HAART), NHL represented the second most frequent cancer associated with HIV after Kaposi sarcoma.[8] Following the introduction of HAART, the frequency of systemic HIV-related lymphomas has remained substantially unmodified despite more effective antiretroviral therapy, whereas the frequency of Kaposi sarcoma has reduced strikingly. Therefore, HIV-related lymphomas are now the most frequent tumor type associated with HIV.[9–13]

Since the original report in 1969, it has been well established that there is an increased incidence of neoplasms, especially lymphoproliferative disorders, in transplant recipients of both solid organ and bone marrow.[14] The risk of developing a post-transplant lymphoproliferative disorder (PTLD) varies depending upon the type of transplanted organ, the host's age at transplantation, and the

Table 24.1　Relative risk for development of post-transplant lymphoproliferative disorders[15]

Transplanted organ	
Pancreas	0.6%
Liver	1–2%
Kidney	0.3–3%
Heart	1.8–9.8%
Lung	3.7–7.9%
Heart and lung	4.6–12.5%
Unmanipulated bone marrow	0–0.4%
T cell-depleted bone marrow	6–9%
Mismatched T cell-depleted bone marrow	16–24%
Immunosuppressive regimen	
PND + AZT	1–4.9%
CSA ± PND	0–1.5%
CSA + PND + AZT	3.8–8%
OKT3/ALG + CSA + PND + AZT	12.5%

PND, prednisone; AZT, azathioprine; CSA, cyclosporin A; OKT3/ALG, antilymphocyte globulin.

immunosuppressive regimen used (Table 24.1).[15] In the case of solid organ transplantation, the overall incidence of PTLD is approximately 1–2 percent. In bone marrow transplant recipients, the incidence of PTLD is 0.5 percent after HLA-matched noncomplicated transplants, and 25 percent after T cell-depleted highly immunosuppressed transplants (Table 24.1).[15]

Methotrexate treatment for autoimmune diseases may predispose to the development of lymphoma.[16–19] The frequency of methotrexate-associated lymphoma is not known. Notably, the vast majority of these lymphomas has been seen in patients with rheumatoid arthritis.[17–19] Since patients with rheumatoid arthritis are estimated to have a 2–20-fold increased risk of lymphoma in the absence of methotrexate, it remains controversial whether methotrexate *per se* increases the risk of lymphoma.[18]

Immunodeficiency-related lymphomas display several common features, irrespective of the underlying immunosuppressive condition.[1] These include a preferential representation by NHL, involvement of extranodal and unusual sites, high-grade histopathology, aggressive clinical behavior, B cell lineage derivation, and frequent association with Epstein–Barr virus (EBV) infection.[1] Despite these common features, immunodeficiency-related lymphomas display a high degree of clinico-pathologic, histogenetic, and molecular heterogeneity. At the clinico-pathologic level, primary immunodeficiency-related lymphomas are mostly represented by diffuse large B cell lymphoma (DLBCL).[1] Human immunodeficiency virus-related lymphomas may be classified according to the WHO classification into: (1) systemic NHL, including Burkitt/Burkitt-like lymphoma (BL/BLL) and DLBCL; (2) primary central nervous system lymphoma (PCNSL); (3) primary effusion lymphoma (PEL); (4) plasmablastic lymphoma of the oral cavity (PBL); and (5) Hodgkin lymphoma (HL).[1] Post-transplant

lymphoproliferative disorders may be classified according to the WHO classification into: (1) early lesions, generally represented by EBV-driven polyclonal lymphoproliferation; and (2) true monoclonal diseases, comprising polymorphic PTLD (P-PTLD) and monomorphic PTLD.[1] Monomorphic PTLD are further distinguished into BL/BLL, DLBCL, multiple myeloma, and HL.[1]

This chapter will focus on the histogenesis and molecular pathogenesis of immunodeficiency-related lymphoma, with special emphasis on HIV-related lymphomas and on PTLD, which are the most frequent types of lymphomas associated with immunodeficiency. Lymphomas arising in the context of primary immunodeficiencies and methotrexate-associated lymphoma will also be briefly reviewed.

MOLECULAR HISTOGENESIS OF IMMUNODEFICIENCY-RELATED LYMPHOMA

The histogenesis of immunodeficiency-related lymphoma has been elucidated by the application of a model exploiting genotypic and phenotypic markers and allowing the distinction of mature B cells into different compartments, namely virgin B cells, germinal center (GC) B cells, and post-GC B cells (Fig. 24.1).[20] The most informative genotypic marker is represented by somatic hypermutation (SHM) of immunoglobulin variable (*IGV*) genes, which takes place in the GC microenvironment. Positivity for *IGV* SHM indicates that a given B cell tumor derives from GC or post-GC B cells. The presence of ongoing *IGV* mutations, documented by intraclonal heterogeneity, indicates that the lymphoma clone reflects centroblasts experiencing the GC reaction, whereas absence of intraclonal heterogeneity suggests derivation from late centrocytes or post-GC B cells that have terminated the GC reaction (Fig. 24.1). Phenotypic markers of histogenesis include the BCL6, MUM1, and CD138 proteins and contribute to the distinction between GC and post-GC B cells. Expression of BCL6 clusters with the GC stage of differentiation, MUM1 positivity clusters with B cells exiting the GC and with post-GC B cells, and CD138 is a marker of pre-terminal B cell differentiation (Fig. 24.1).

Based on *IGV* gene analysis, virtually all HIV-NHL derive from GC-experienced B cells. A small fraction of HIV-BL and HIV-DLBCL, mainly of centroblastic morphology, carries ongoing *IGV* mutations, denoting an origin from centroblasts, whereas most cases of HIV-DLBCL, HIV-BL, HIV-PCNSL, and HIV-PEL carry stable *IGV* mutations, denoting a centrocyte or post-GC origin.[21] A fraction (60 percent) of HIV-PBL is devoid of *IGV* mutations and apparently originates from pre-GC B cells.[21,22]

Phenotypic analysis of HIV-lymphoma reveals that: (1) 100 percent of HIV-BL, 50 percent of HIV-DLBCL, and 30 percent of HIV-PCNSL are BCL6[+]/MUM1[−]/CD138[−], denoting a centroblast–centrocyte origin; (2) 20 percent of HIV-PCNSL and 20 percent of HIV-DLBCL are

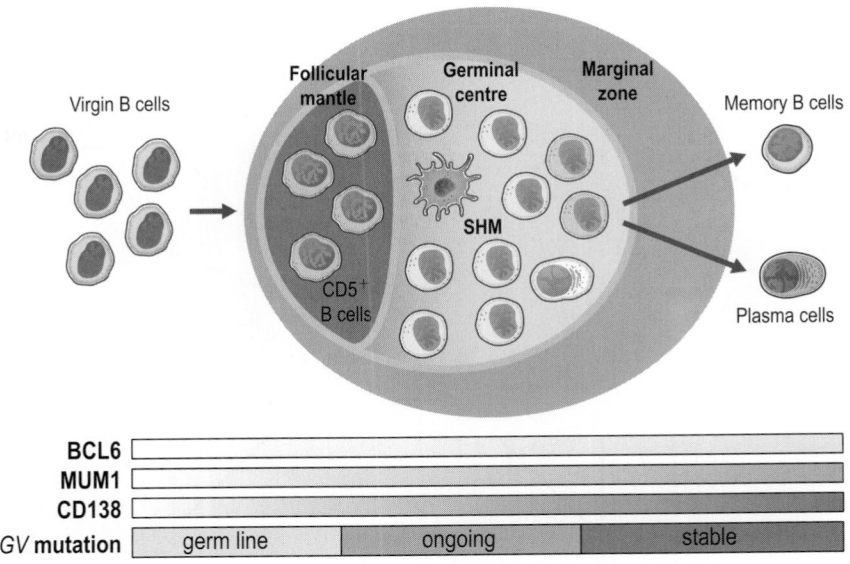

Figure 24.1   Genotypic markers of B cell histogenesis are mainly represented by somatic hypermutation (SHM) of immunoglobulin variable (*IGV*) genes, which takes place in the germinal center (GC) microenvironment. Positivity for *IGV* mutations indicates that a given lymphoma derives from GC or post-GC B cells. The presence of ongoing *IGV* mutations suggests that the lymphoma reflects centroblasts experiencing the GC reaction. The presence of stable *IGV* mutations is consistent with derivation from late centrocytes or post-GC B cells that have terminated the GC reaction. Phenotypic markers of B cell lymphoma histogenesis are represented by the BCL6, MUM1, and CD138 proteins. Expression of BCL6 clusters with the GC stage of differentiation, MUM1 positivity clusters with B cells exiting the GC and with post-GC B cells, and CD138 is a marker of pre-terminal B cell differentiation.

BCL6$^-$/MUM1$^+$/CD138$^-$, denoting a late centrocyte origin; (3) 30 percent of HIV-DLBCL, 50 percent of HIV-PCNSL, 100 percent of HIV-PEL, 100 percent of HIV-PBL, and 100 percent of HIV-HL are BCL6$^-$/MUM1$^+$/CD138$^+$, denoting a post-GC immunoblastic-plasmablastic origin.[22,23] Among EBV-infected HIV lymphoma, expression of latent membrane protein 1 (LMP1) is mutually exclusive with expression of BCL6 and clusters with the BCL6$^-$/CD138$^+$ phenotype, suggesting that the GC stage is not permissive for LMP1 expression and that post-GC maturation is an essential requirement for LMP1 expression in B cell tumors.[24] By combining genotypic and phenotypic data, the histogenetic model of HIV-NHL shows that, at variance with lymphoma of similar histology arising in the immunocompetent host, only a small fraction of HIV-BL and HIV-DLBCL displays centroblastic features, while the majority of HIV-NHL arises from late centrocytes or post-GC B cells (Fig. 24.2).

IGV analysis of monoclonal PTLD arising after solid organ transplantation reveals that: (1) 25 percent of P-PTLD and 10 percent of DLBCL carry unmutated *IGV* genes, denoting a pre-GC origin; (2) 100 percent of BL and 25 percent of DLBCL, mainly of centroblastic morphology, carry ongoing *IGV* mutations, denoting an origin from centroblasts; and (3) 75 percent of P-PTLD and 65 percent of DLBCL carry stable *IGV* mutations, denoting a centrocyte or post-GC origin.[25,26] The fact that *IGV* mutations occur in the overwhelming majority of PTLD documents that malignant

transformation targets GC B cells and their descendants both in EBV-positive and EBV-negative cases.[25,26]

Analysis of phenotypic markers of histogenesis identifies three predominant profiles of PTLD arising after solid organ transplantation (Fig. 24.3).[25,26] Post-transplant lymphoproliferative disorders belonging to the first histogenetic category express the BCL6$^+$/MUM1$^{+/-}$/CD138$^-$ profile and reflect B cells actively experiencing the GC reaction. These PTLD associate with ongoing SHM and are morphologically classified as DLBCL centroblastic or as BL/BLL. A second category of PTLD reflects the BCL6$^-$/MUM1$^+$/CD138$^-$ phenotype and comprises 65 percent of P-PTLD and 30 percent of DLBCL, mainly with immunoblastic features. This PTLD subset putatively derives from B cells that have concluded the GC reaction but have not yet undergone terminal differentiation. The BCL6$^-$/MUM1$^+$/CD138$^-$ profile is common among PTLD, but is rare among HIV-related lymphomas, underscoring biological differences between these two groups of immunodeficiency-related lymphomas.[22,23,25,26] A third group of PTLD is reminiscent of post-GC and pre-terminally differentiated B cells that show the BCL6$^-$/MUM1$^+$/CD138$^+$ phenotype and, if EBV-positive, express the LMP1 antigen. These PTLD are morphologically represented by either P-PTLD (35 percent of cases) or DLBCL immunoblastic. The BCL6$^-$/MUM1$^+$/CD138$^+$ histogenetic profile is shared also by many HIV-related lymphomas.[23] Analogous to PTLD after solid organ transplantation, phenotypic analysis of monoclonal

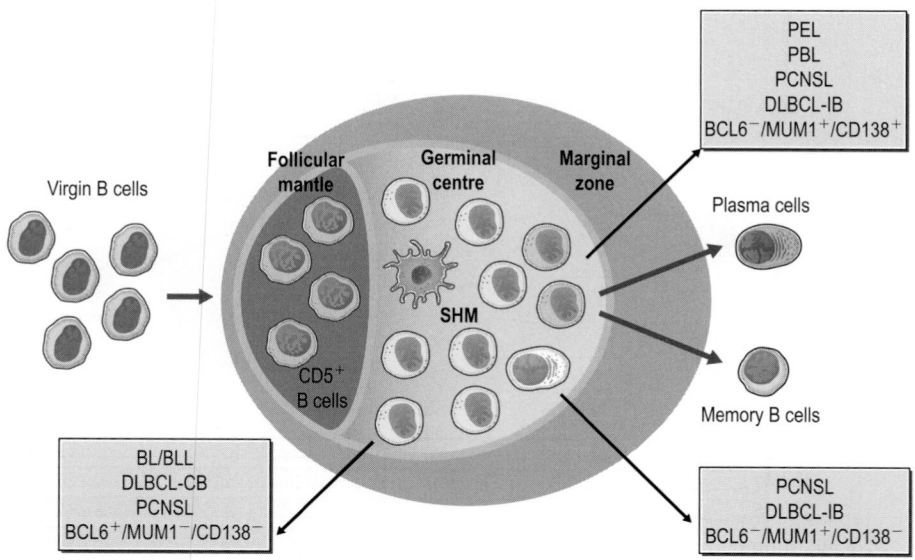

Figure 24.2   Model of human immunodeficiency virus (HIV) non-Hodgkin lymphoma (NHL) histogenesis based on the expression of the phenotypic markers BCL6, MUM1, and CD138. The majority of HIV-NHL, namely diffuse large B cell lymphoma showing immunoblastic morphology (DLBCL-IB), a fraction of primary central nervous system lymphoma (PCNSL), plasmablastic lymphoma (PBL), and primary effusion lymphoma (PEL), display the BCL6$^-$/MUM1$^+$/CD138$^+$ profile, denoting an immunoblastic–plasmablastic origin. A fraction of DLBCL-IB and PCNSL are BCL6$^-$/MUM1$^+$/CD138$^-$, denoting a late centrocyte origin. Burkitt/Burkitt-like lymphoma (BL/BLL), diffuse large B cell lymphoma with centroblastic morphology (DLBCL-CB), and a fraction of PCNSL are BCL6$^+$/MUM1$^-$/CD138$^-$, denoting a centroblast–centrocyte origin. SHM, somatic hypermutation.

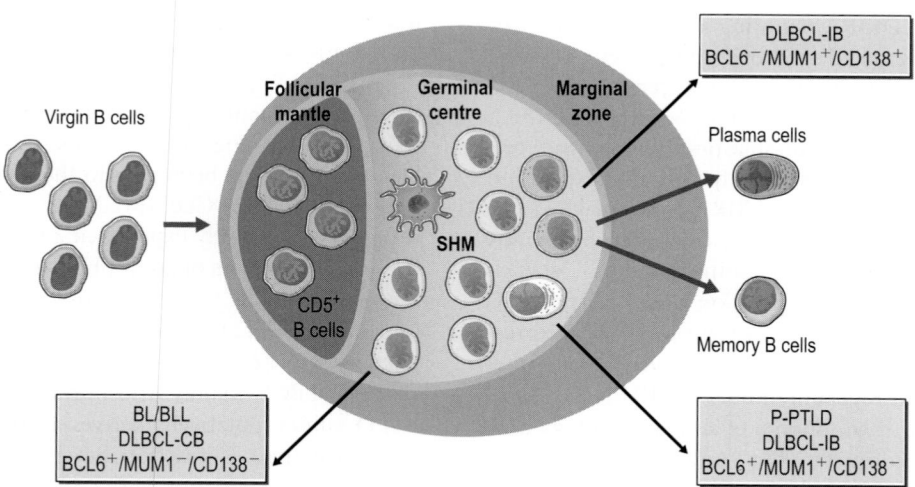

Figure 24.3   Model of post-transplant lymphoproliferative disorders (PTLD) histogenesis based on the expression of the phenotypic markers BCL6, MUM1, and CD138. The majority of PTLD, namely diffuse large B cell lymphoma showing immunoblastic morphology (DLBCL-IB) and polymorphic PTLD (P-PTLD), carry the BCL6$^-$/MUM1$^+$/CD138$^-$ profile, denoting a late centrocyte origin. A fraction of DLBCL-IB are BCL6$^-$/MUM1$^+$/CD138$^+$, denoting an immunoblastic–plasmablastic origin. Burkitt/Burkitt-like lymphoma (BL/BLL) and diffuse large B cell lymphoma with centroblastic morphology (DLBCL-CB) are BCL6$^+$/MUM1$^-$/CD138$^-$, denoting a centroblast–centrocyte origin.

PTLD after bone marrow transplantation indicates that 70 percent of PTLD show the BCL6$^-$/MUM1$^+$/CD138$^-$ signature, while the remaining 30 percent of cases are BCL6$^-$/MUM1$^+$/CD138$^+$.[27]

The histogenesis of primary immunodeficiency-associated lymphoma is relatively obscure, although molecular analysis suggests that CVID-NHL derive from centrocytes or post-GC B cells.[28]

MOLECULAR PATHOGENESIS OF IMMUNODEFICIENCY–RELATED LYMPHOMA

Genetic background of the host

The genetic background of the immunodeficient host may predispose to lymphoma development. Polymorphisms of several genes belonging to the chemokine-cytokine pathways are known to influence the risk of developing HIV-NHL. A first example is represented by the chemokine stromal cell-derived factor 1 (SDF1) gene, which encodes a potent mitogen, chemoattractant, and differentiating agent for B cells.[29] The SDF1 gene carries a genetic polymorphism termed SDF13'A, leading to the substitution of A for G at position 881 of the 3' untranslated region. Human immunodeficiency virus-infected patients harboring both the homozygous and heterozygous SDF1-3'A variant are at two- to fivefold increased risk for NHL development.[30] Increased levels of SDF1 in peripheral blood mononuclear cells have been observed in HIV-NHL patients.[31] Whether increased expression of SDF1 is a consequence of SDF1-3'A polymorphism is still unclear.[31]

CCR5 is a chemokine receptor expressed on lymphocytes and acts as a coreceptor for HIV. A 32 base pair (bp) deletion in the coding region of CCR5 (CCR5 Δ32) is a polymorphism that prevents the expression of the receptor on the cell surface, thus conferring T cell protection against HIV infection and leading to lower HIV viral load and delayed progression to AIDS.[32] CCR5Δ32 variant is also associated to a threefold reduction of the risk of HIV-NHL development.[30,33] Protection against HIV-NHL may be mediated through better-preserved immune surveillance and reduced chronic immune stimulation by HIV. In fact, since CCR5 is expressed on B cells and its stimulation enhances B cell proliferation, lack of CCR5 expression may be associated to a reduced response of B cells to chemokines.[34]

Interleukin (IL)-10 is a B cell stimulatory cytokine that is able to enhance the proliferation of lymphoma cells. Several experimental data suggest a role of IL-10 in HIV lymphomagenesis.[35,36] The IL-10 gene polymorphism at nucleotide 592 leads to the substitution of A to C in the promoter region of the gene causing increased expression of IL-10 and is associated to an increased risk of lymphoma in HIV-infected patients.[37]

Host genetic defects may *per se* favor lymphomagenesis also in the context of congenital primary immunodeficiency, as exemplified by germ-line mutations of the *ATM* (ataxia telangiectasia mutated) gene that are responsible for ataxia telangiectasia.[38] *ATM* encodes a nuclear protein kinase involved in the detection of DNA double-strand breaks, transmission of cell cycle arrest, and proapoptotic signals.[39,40] Most mutations in ATM result in truncation and destabilization of the protein. Disruption of the ATM protein in ataxia telangiectasia patients predisposes to genetic instability, accumulation of DNA damage, and transformation.[39,40] The pathogenetic role of ATM disruption is supported by the observation that knockout mice for the *ATM* gene frequently develop thymic lymphoma.[41] ATM is involved in the regulation of immunoglobulin (Ig) gene recombination, and aberrations of this process may contribute to genetic instability and lymphomagenesis in ATM-deficient lymphocytes.[42,43] This hypothesis is supported by the observation that the onset of thymic lymphoma is greatly suppressed in ATM and recombination activating gene 2 (RAG2) null mice, which are totally deficient in VDJ recombination because of abrogation of RAG2.[44]

Antigen stimulation

The persistent generalized lymphadenopathy (PGL) syndrome, a condition characterized by polyclonal B cell expansion, precedes the development of HIV-NHL in one-third of individuals and increases the risk of HIV-NHL by 800–900-fold.[45] Furthermore, 20 percent of PGL contain one or more discrete bands of immunoglobulin gene rearrangement but none of the genetic lesions typically associated with HIV-NHL. The presence of oligoclonal B cell expansions in the context of PGL may represent lymphoma precursors.[46] This notion is formally documented by an immunogenetic longitudinal study showing that the same *IGV* rearrangement detected in a case of HIV-NHL was already present in the patient's bone marrow together with other B cell clones three years before the diagnosis of lymphoma.[47] These epidemiological and molecular observations suggest that a pathogenetic relationship may exist between B cell hyperplasia, antigen stimulation, and HIV-NHL.

Insights into the pathogenetic role of antigen stimulation in HIV-NHL are provided by the detailed analysis of *IGV* genes. In general terms, HIV-NHL show the molecular clues of antigen stimulation, since 65 percent of cases select mutations in order to maintain intact the *IGV* framework region structure and 30 percent select mutations apt at increasing antigen binding affinity.[21] Remarkably, 30 percent of HIV-NHL rearrange the same *IgV* gene, namely the *VH4-34* gene, whose usage is biased in comparison to normal B cells.[21,48–53] The putative antigens involved in HIV-NHL pathogenesis have not been identified yet, but it is presumed that they are self-antigens rather than HIV antigens. Intriguingly, *VH4-34* is involved in autoimmunity since it is rearranged in *IGV* reacting against DNA and cardiolipin.[54] Moreover, several HIV-NHL have been formally demonstrated to produce antibodies directed against autoantigens such as actin, Ig, and cell-surface proteins.[55–57]

IGV mutations generated by the SHM mechanism may introduce new sites of link for oligosaccharides on the Ig protein. In the immunocompetent host, this phenomenon is specific for B-NHL derived from GC cells.[58] Immunoglobulin glycosylation may alter the biochemical properties of the Ig by enhancing or reducing the affinity for the antigen. Furthermore, it may activate the B cell receptor (BCR) in an antigen-independent fashion by mediating the interaction with lectins of the microenvironment.[59] The acquisition of novel sites of Ig glycosylation occurs in ~40 percent

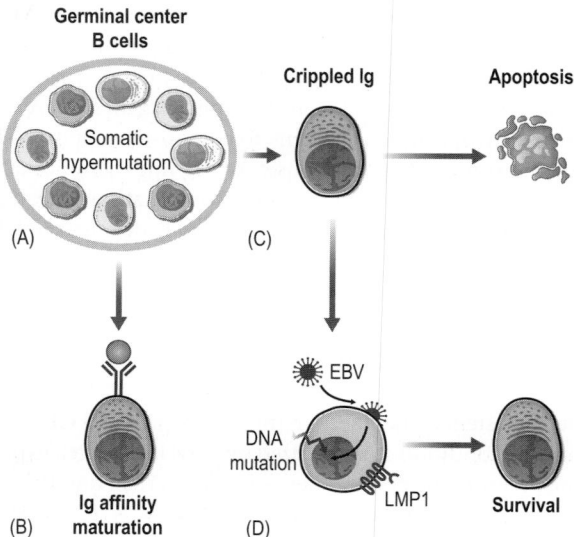

Figure 24.4 Pathogenetic model of post-transplant lymphoproliferative disorders (PTLD). (A) The somatic hypermutation (SHM) process affecting the immunoglobulin (Ig) variable region genes within the germinal center is aimed at increasing the affinity of the B cell receptor (BCR) for the antigen. (B) B cells that have successfully undergone affinity maturation for the antigen are positively selected and rescued from apoptosis. (C) On the contrary, B cells failing this process are induced to apoptosis. (D) A relevant fraction of PTLD fail to express the BCR, mainly due to crippling mutations of immunoglobulin genes introduced by the SHM process, and thus are predisposed to programmed cell death. The putative mechanisms that rescue PTLD from apoptosis are represented by latent membrane protein 1 (LMP1) expression and/or molecular lesions affecting genes regulating apoptosis. EBV, Epstein–Barr virus.

of HIV-NHL, further supporting the role of antigen stimulation and BCR activation in the pathogenesis of these lymphomas.[60]

The pathogenetic role of antigen stimulation in PTLD is less evident, since ~50 percent of PTLD derive from B cells that have lost the ability to express a functional BCR.[25,26,61,62] A frequent cause of BCR inactivation in PTLD is represented by crippling mutations of *IGV* genes, which are generated by the SHM process and introduce stop codons in originally in-frame rearrangements.[26,61,62] Since the expression of a functional BCR is crucial for B cell survival, PTLD lacking BCR are thought to acquire the ability to escape apoptotic death in the absence of antigen stimulation. Epstein–Barr virus infection has been proposed as a mechanism of apoptotic rescue in PTLD with nonfunctional BCR, although other mechanisms might also be involved (Fig. 24.4).[25,26,61,62]

Among the 50 percent of PTLD displaying a functional BCR, molecular signs of antigen stimulation are documented in a fraction of cases. In fact, approximately 60 percent of PTLD with functional BCR select mutations in order to maintain intact the *IGV* framework region structure, and

30 percent select mutations apt to increase antigen binding affinity.[25,26] Overusage of specific *IGV* genes known to be involved in autoimmune phenomena, as observed in HIV-NHL, does not appear to be a distinctive feature of PTLD.[25,26] Despite their origin from GC B cells, and at a variance with HIV-NHL, the acquisition of novel sites of *IGV* glycosylation is a rare event in PTLD.[60] This observation is consistent with the hypothesis that BCR stimulation does not play a major pathogenetic role in many PTLD.

The role of antigen stimulation in lymphomas associated with primary immunodeficiency is largely unknown. However, a role for chronic antigen stimulation is suggested by the marked lymphoid hyperplasia in the lung and gastrointestinal tract of many CVID patients. These lymphoid lesions of CVID patients display oligoclonal or monoclonal *IGV* rearrangements, which may predispose to the development of lymphoma.[63,64]

Viral infection

Infection by oncogenic viruses is a major mechanism in the pathogenesis of lymphoma arising in the context of immunodeficiency of the T cell compartment. Oncogenic viruses may act through direct and indirect mechanisms. Oncogenic viruses acting through a direct mechanism and involved in immunodeficiency-related lymphoma are EBV and human herpes virus 8 (HHV-8). These viruses are able to infect and transform B cells. The association between viral infection and tumor development can be understood in the context of viral strategies to ensure persistent infection, namely prevention of death of infected cells, enhancement of their proliferation to maintain the infected reservoir, and evasion of the immune system.

Viruses acting through indirect mechanisms and involved in immunodeficiency-related lymphoma include HIV and hepatitis C virus (HCV). These viruses predispose to lymphoma by modifying the microenvironment through the reduction of immune surveillance and/or enhancement of B cell proliferation.

EPSTEIN–BARR VIRUS

Epstein–Barr virus is a double-strand DNA virus belonging to the γ herpesvirus family. Epstein–Barr virus targets B lymphocytes and, after acute infection, the virus DNA forms a circle and persists as an episome in the nuclei of resting memory B cells establishing a latent infection.[65] In latently infected B cells, EBV encodes a series of viral proteins that interact with or exhibit homology to a variety of signal transducers, cytokines, and antiapoptotic human molecules. These proteins are EBV nuclear antigens (EBNA)1, EBNA2, EBNA3A, EBNA3B, EBNA3C, EBNALP, and LMP1, LMP2A, and LMP2B. Beside these proteins, EBV-encoded nontranslated RNAs (EBER) are transcribed in latently infected B cells.[65] Based on the pattern of expression of the latency genes, three types of latent infection have been described: (1) latency I, which is defined by the expression of EBER and EBNA1; (2) latency II, which is characterized by the expression of EBER, EBNA1, LMP1, and LMP2; and (3) latecy III, denoted by the expression of EBER, all EBNAs, LMP1, and LMP2.[65]

Several lines of evidence suggest that EBV infection has a major pathogenetic role in immunodeficiency-related lymphoma. First, EBV infects ~50 percent of HIV-NHL, ~60–80 percent of PTLD, 80–100 percent of HIV-HL and post-transplant HL, and the majority of congenital immunodeficiency-related NHL and methotrexate-associated NHL.[66] Second, in many cases, EBV infection is monoclonal, consistent with the hypothesis that the virus has been present in the tumor progenitor cell since the early phases of its clonal expansion.[67] Third, EBV-infected B cells are present in increased numbers in blood and tissues of patients who subsequently developed HIV-NHL.[68–73] Furthermore, decrease of EBV-specific cytotoxic T cells and increase in EBV viral load is strongly associated with both HIV-NHL and PLTD development.[74–76] Fourth, treatment of PTLD with autologous EBV-specific cytotoxic T cells results in viral load control and tumor size reduction.[77] Finally, the EBNA2 and LMP1 genes expressed during latent infection have true oncogenic activity and thus are presumed to be involved in lymphomagenesis.[78,79]

EBNA2 is a transcriptional coactivator that regulates both viral latency genes, for example *LMP1* and *LMP2*, and many cellular genes involved in proliferation and survival, including *MYC*.[78–80] EBNA2 does not bind directly to the DNA but interacts with other transcription factors, namely the viral transcription factor Cp1 and the cell transcription factor RBP-Jk involved in the NOTCH1 signaling pathway.[81] This pathway is well known to be involved in lymphomagenesis, since *NOTCH1* is a protooncogene frequently activated by mutation/translocation in T cell lymphoblastic lymphoma.[82]

Two main types (1 and 2) of EBV are distinguished on the basis of sequence variation in the EBNA2 protein. Despite type 2 EBV frequently infecting immunosuppressed individuals, no clear correlation has been identified between EBV strain and lymphoma development.[83–88]

LMP1 is an integral membrane protein expressed on the surface of infected B cells. LMP1 is a well-recognized oncogene, since its expression in transgenic mice leads to the development of B cell lymphoma.[65,66] LMP1 is involved in transformation by acting as constitutively active CD40, a receptor that physiologically provides a signal for proliferation and survival to B cells. LMP1 mimics CD40 by binding the same cytoplasmic signal transduction molecules, namely the tumor necrosis factor (TNF)-receptor-associated factors (TRAFs).[89] TRAFs, in turn, activate at least four signaling pathways represented by nuclear factor κB (NF-κB), Jun NH$_2$-terminal kinase, p38 mitogen-activated protein kinase, and Janus kinase. These molecules affect diverse signaling cascades that lead to enhanced expression of B cell adesion molecules, activation markers, MYC, and the antiapoptotic factors BCL2 and A20 (Fig. 24.5).[90–93]

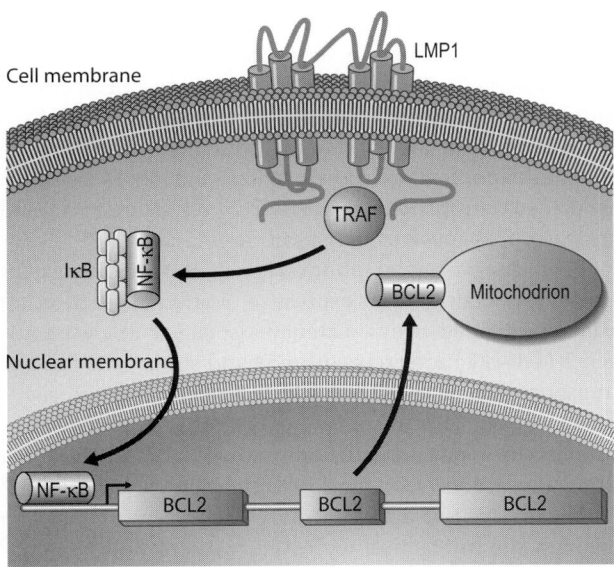

Figure 24.5   The role of Epstein–Barr virus (EBV) latent membrane protein 1 (LMP1) in promoting survival in human immunodeficiency virus (HIV) non-Hodgkin lymphoma and post-transplant lymphoproliferative disorders. LMP1 is the viral homologue of the family of the cellular tumor necrosis factor (TNF) receptors. LMP1 acts as a constitutively activated TNF receptor. LMP1 binds the TNF-receptor-associated factor (TRAF), which then activates the nuclear factor κB (NF-κB) transcription factor. NF-κB, after the degradation of the inhibitory protein IκB, reaches the nucleus where it promotes the expression of several genes, including the antiapoptotic gene *BCL2*.

Other EBV-encoded genes, though not strictly transforming, may also be involved in lymphomagenesis. LMP2A is an integral membrane protein that contains an immunoreceptor tyrosine-based activation motif. This motif is similar to that present in BCR coreceptors CD79a and CD79b and transmits activating signals after BCR stimulation.[78] LMP2A binds and thus sequesters tyrosine kinases from the BCR, resulting in inhibition of BCR signaling. This prevents unwanted antigen-triggered activation of infected B cells that would otherwise cause the entry into lytic cycle.[78] On the other hand, LMP2A is also able to stimulate the BCR-associated tyrosine kinases providing an important survival signal to B cells.[79] EBER1 and EBER2 are short-strand non-coding RNAs expressed in all forms of latent infection. EBERs seem to be involved in inducing autocrine IL-10 secretion by BL cells, which might stimulate growth of infected neoplastic B cells and suppress cytotoxic T cells.[66] In addition, EBERs might mediate resistance of BL cells to interferon α (IFNα).[78]

HUMAN HERPES VIRUS 8

Human herpes virus 8 is a double-strand DNA virus belonging to the γ herpesvirus family. Similar to EBV, HHV-8 establishes a lifelong latent infection in which the viral DNA persists as an episome in the nuclei of infected cells.[94–97] Human herpes virus 8 infects 100 percent of PEL arising in immunocompromised hosts.[98–102] A number of HHV-8 genes are homologous to human genes involved in proliferation, antiapoptosis, and angiogenesis and cytokines which are able to transform human cells *in vitro* and/or *in vivo*, and are potentially involved in lymphomagenesis.[94–97]

Primary effusion lymphomas are characterized by latent HHV-8 infection and express a restricted pattern of HHV-8-encoded genes. Latency-associated nuclear antigen 1 (LANA1) interacts with p53 and suppresses the p53 transcriptional activity and ability to induce apoptosis.[103] Furthermore, LANA1 binds to the retinoblastoma (Rb) protein, thus releasing the transcription factor E2F that upregulates genes involved in cell cycle progression.[104] Finally, LANA1 is able to induce the expression of IL-6 through the interaction with AP1 transcription factor.[105] v-Cyclin encodes a homologue of human cyclin D2.[94,97,106] Similar to cyclin D2, v-cyclin contributes to Rb phosphorylation by activating cyclin-dependent kinases. Phosphorylated Rb then releases the E2F transcription factor, thus cooperating with LANA1 in inducing cell cycle acceleration.[97] In contrast to human cyclin D2, v-cyclin is resistant to inhibition by p16, p21, and p27, a family of cyclin-dependent kinase inhibitors that physiologically block cell cycle progression.[106–108] Overall, v-cyclin permits circumvention of normal cell cycle checkpoints and leads to constitutive cell cycling. vIL-6 is homologous to human IL-6 and has anti-apoptotic and growth-promoting functions.[109]

HUMAN IMMUNODEFICIENCY VIRUS

Although HIV is able to transform B cells in experimental models, several lines of evidence have clearly demonstrated that HIV does not infect the HIV-NHL clone.[110–112] Rather, it is generally accepted that HIV acts through indirect mechanisms including immunosuppression, antigen stimulation, and cytokine deregulation.

In general, the development of many HIV-NHL is strictly related to the degree and duration of T cell immunodeficiency. In fact, based on pre-HAART data, the greater risk of HIV-NHL occurs when CD4$^+$ T cells are fewer than 50/μl and when this degree of immunosuppression persists for more than 24 months.[113–115] Moreover, fewer tumor-infiltrating T cells are present in HIV-NHL compared to immunocompetent NHL, suggesting a failure in local T cell response.[116] Beside the degree of immunosuppression, also the quality of T cell impairment represents a risk factor, since a decrease of EBV-specific cytotoxic T cells correlates with HIV-NHL development.[74,117] The correlation between severity of immune deficit and risk of lymphoma is also documented by primate models, in which malignant lymphomas develop 5 to 15 months after simian immunodeficiency virus infection and coincidentally with the onset of severe immunosuppression.[118] The relationship between degree of immune deficit and lymphoma has been corroborated by the observation of reduced risk of lymphoma development in the HAART era.[9–13,119–123] In particular, HAART has a major impact on the risk of lymphoma occurring at low CD4 levels, such as DLBCL immunoblastic and PCNSL. In contrast, the risk of BL and HL, which seem to occur in the context of a more preserved immune system, are not influenced by HAART (Table 24.2).[9] Despite the strong correlation between severity of T cell deficit and HIV-NHL development, at least one category of HIV-NHL, namely HIV-BL/BLL, may arise also in the context of a relatively well-preserved immune system.[123]

Some lines of evidence indicate that the role of HIV in lymphomagenesis is more complex than initially thought and is not merely recapitulated by immunodeficiency. Human immunodeficiency virus may contribute more directly to HIV-NHL development via infection of

Table 24.2   Incidence rates of human immunodeficiency virus-related lymphoma[9]

	Incidence rate per 1000 per year		Rate ratio (RR) for 1997–1999 vs 1992–1996
	1992–1996	1997–1999	
All non-Hodgkin lymphomas	6.2	3.6	0.58 (SE 0.06)*
Immunoblastic lymphoma	3.0	1.7	0.57 (SE 0.09)*
Burkitt lymphoma	0.3	0.4	1.18 (SE 0.41)
Primary central nervous system lymphoma	1.7	0.7	0.42 (SE 0.09)*
Hodgkin lymphoma	0.5	0.4	0.77 (SE 0.26)

Data shown are incidence rates of human immunodeficiency virus (HIV)-related lymphoma in 1992 through 1996 and in 1997 through 1999 and rate ratios (RRs) of incidence rates in 1992 through 1996 compared to 1997 through 1999, by study (International Collaboration on HIV and Cancer).[9]
Statistically significant change in the risk.
SE, standard error.

nonmalignant bystander cells that interact with lymphoma. Human immunodeficiency virus infection of microvascular endothelial cells stimulates surface expression of CD40 through the viral proteins Tat and Vpu. Ligation of CD40 on endothelial cells by CD40 ligand expressed on HIV-NHL increases lymphoma cell attachment via vascular cell-adhesion molecule-1 (VCAM-1).[124–126] Direct cell–cell contact, allowing proximity to cytokines produced by endothelial cells, may promote HIV-NHL proliferation and the outgrowth of malignant foci at extranodal sites. Moreover, HIV-infected cells secrete the Tat protein in the extracellular compartment, thus inducing HIV-NHL cell migration in the extravascular compartment in a paracrine fashion through the vascular endothelial growth factor (VEGF) pathway.[124–126]

In an animal model, Tat acts as an oncogene since Tat transgenic mice develop B cell lymphoma.[127] The oncogenic activity of Tat is presumed to be a consequence of cell cycle perturbation. In fact, Tat is able to bind and inactivate RB2/p130, resulting in accumulation of the transcription factor E2F4 as well as induction of cell cycle regulatory genes such as cyclin A, cyclin B, and p107. Furthermore, Tat directly binds and activates E2F4, bypassing the checkpoint of RB2/p130.[128–131] How Tat may contribute to HIV-NHL in humans is unclear, since HIV-NHL cells do not carry HIV infection.

HEPATITIS C VIRUS

Several epidemiological studies and metaanalysis have underlined the association between HCV infection and NHL in the immunocompetent host. In B cells infected *in vitro*, HCV induces a mutator phenotype characterized by enhanced somatic hypermutation of *IGV* and *BCL6* genes and introduction of mutations in the p53 and β-catenin genes.[132] However, because only a subset of NHL cells harbor the viral genome or proteins *in vivo*, the current pathogenetic hypothesis holds that HCV may act on B cells indirectly through chronic antigen stimulation, as suggested by the identification of molecular clues of antigen stimulation in HCV-related NHL and by the expression of HCV-specific *IGV* in a fraction of HCV-related NHL.[133,134]

Although coinfection with HCV is frequent in HIV-infected patients, studies from both the USA and Italy have documented that the risk of NHL is similar in HCV-negative/HIV-positive and HCV-positive/HIV-positive patients, suggesting that HCV does not contribute significantly to HIV-related lymphomagenesis.[135–137] Regarding PTLD, scanty epidemiological data suggest an association between HCV infection and the development of PTLD.[138–140]

SV40

Based on the paradigm of other lymphoma-related viruses, SV40 has several features predicting a pathogenetic role: it is lymphotropic, it is capable of transforming B cells *in vitro*, and induces B cell lymphomas in animals. SV40

exerts its transforming activity through the large T antigen viral gene. Although two reports described a high prevalence of SV40 in NHL, including HIV-NHL,[141,142] the association between SV40 and NHL or HIV-NHL has been subseqently denied by large molecular, immuno-histochemical, and serological studies.[143–148]

Molecular pathways

Infection by oncogenic viruses is a pathogenetic mechanism often necessary but not sufficient to develop immunodeficiency-related lymphoma. Progression to overt lymphoma requires the accumulation of genetic lesions leading to the activation of protooncogenes by chromosomal translocation or inactivation of tumor suppressor genes by mutation, deletion, and/or DNA methylation. At variance with lymphoma arising in the immunocompetent host, whose genome is relatively stable, a fraction of HIV-NHL and PTLD is characterized by microsatellite instability due to defects in the DNA mismatch repair machinery.[149] These cases are characterized by a mutator phenotype, thus predisposing the tumor cells to accumulate mutations in several genes, including the proapoptotic factors *BAX* and *CASPASE-5* and the DNA repair gene *RAD50*.[149] The explanation of why immunodeficiency-related lymphoma displays a mutator phenotype, which is otherwise exceptional in lymphomas of the immunocompetent host, is speculative. One hypothesis is that the mutator phenotype, by introducing missense mutations changing the amino acid sequence of proteins, may generate numerous neoantigens at the tumor-cell surface. In the immunocompetent host, the immune system is capable of recognizing and eliminating tumor cells carrying such neoantigens, thus promptly abrogating lymphoma subclones characterized by the mutator phenotype. On the other hand, in the context of immunodeficiency, the host immune system might be less prone to recognize and eliminate such highly immunogenic lymphoma cells.

To date, a fraction of protooncogenes and tumor suppressor genes has been recognized to be frequently involved in immunodeficiency-related lymphoma, including *MYC*, *BCL6*, *p53*, O[6]-methylguanine-DNA methyltransferase (*MGMT*), *death-associated protein kinase* (*DAPK*), *p73*, *PIM1*, *PAX5*, and *RHOH/TTF*.

MYC

Chromosomal breaks at 8q24 are found in 100 percent of HIV-BL and post-transplant BL.[150–153] All 8q24 breaks lead to a common final consequence: deregulated expression of the *MYC* protooncogene. Depending on the Ig locus involved, the *MYC* gene may participate in three distinct translocations.[154,155] In 80 percent of cases, the translocation involves Ig heavy chain genes, leading to t(8;14)(q24;q32). In the remaining 20 percent of cases, *MYC* juxtaposes either to Igκ, leading to t(2;8)(p11;q24) (15 percent of cases), or to Igλ, leading to t(8;22) (q24;q11) (5 percent of cases). In the case of t(8;14), the *MYC* breakpoint involves sequences on chromosome 8 within *MYC*, which is deprived of its exon 1, and sequences on chromosome 14 in proximity to the Igμ switch region.[155] Furthermore, *MYC* alleles involved by t(8;14) consistently harbor small mutations mapping within the exon 2 coding sequence, leading to amino acid substitution in the *MYC* protein.[156,157] The cDNA transcribed by translocated *MYC* alleles includes *MYC* exons 2 and 3 and gives rise to a normally sized *MYC* protein.

The common functional effect of t(8;14), t(2;8), and t(8;22) is that *MYC* translocated alleles undergo constitutive expression in tumor cells. Conversely, under physiologic conditions, MYC levels are tightly regulated during B cell proliferation and differentiation, and *MYC* is not expressed in normal GC cells, the presumed counterpart of BL. Chromosomal translocations cause *MYC* deregulation by at least two distinct mechanisms. First, translocated *MYC* alleles are juxtaposed to heterologous regulatory elements derived from Ig loci. Second, the 5′ regulatory regions of *MYC* are consistently affected by structural alterations that are supposed to modify their responsiveness to cellular factors regulating *MYC* expression. In HIV and post-transplant BL, a 400 bp region spanning the first exon/first intron junction, and containing several potentially relevant regulatory domains, is consistently mutated in translocated *MYC* alleles.

In addition to transcriptional deregulation, oncogenic conversion of *MYC* is also thought to stem from amino acid substitutions in *MYC* exon 2, which affect the amino-terminal transcriptional activation domain (TAD) of the gene and are found in 30–40 percent of HIV-NHL.[156,157] The high prevalence of these mutations suggests a biologic role for these alterations in lymphomagenesis. Although under normal conditions the activity of the MYC transactivation domain is suppressed by protein–protein interactions with the pRB-related protein p107, MYC proteins carrying exon 2 mutations can escape the p107-mediated modulation.[158] The mechanism of resistance of mutant *MYC* proteins to p107-mediated suppression is not known, although it is not caused by the disruption of the physical interactions between MYC and p107. Rather, *MYC* exon 2 mutations may confer resistance to p107-mediated phosphorylation, which is essential for the suppression effect of p107.[158]

Several lines of experimental evidence document that the deregulated expression of *MYC* can influence the growth of B cells *in vitro* and *in vivo*. *In vitro*, the expression of *MYC* oncogenes transfected into EBV-immortalized human B cells, a potential natural target for *MYC* activation in EBV-positive BL, leads to their malignant transformation.[159] In addition, antisense oligonucleotides directed against translocated *MYC* alleles are able to revert the tumorigenicity of BL.[160] *In vivo*, the targeted expression of *MYC* oncogenes in the B cell lineage of transgenic mice leads to the development of B cell malignancies at a high

rate.[161,162] Overexpression of *MYC* in primary cells results in cell cycle arrest and apoptosis mediated by the induction of p19 that sequesters MDM2, thus leading to the activation of p53. The ability of *MYC* to induce apoptosis explains why transgenic mice for *MYC* usually develop clonal B cell malignancies only after the accumulation of alterations in the *p53* pathway, which counteract *MYC*-induced apoptosis.[163]

The product of the *MYC* protooncogene is a ubiquitously expressed nuclear basic helix-loop-helix/leucine zipper (bHLH-LZ) phosphoprotein that functions as a transcriptional regulator.[164] In B cells, MYC is in the center of one of the major networks of pathways controlling proliferation, differentiation, and apoptosis. The pleiotropic activity of MYC is suggested by the functional heterogeneity of its numerous target genes.

Expression of *MYC* is rapidly induced in quiescent cells upon mitogenic induction, suggesting that *MYC* plays a role in mediating the transition from quiescence to proliferation. In addition to mediating cell proliferation, *MYC* is also implicated in blocking differentiation. In the absence of a supportive microenvironment providing adequate concentrations of growth stimuli, however, proliferation and/or block of differentiation are replaced by cellular apoptosis.[163] The biochemical mechanisms by which *MYC* achieves its various functions have been clarified to a certain extent.[164] In physiologic *in vivo* settings, MYC is mainly engaged in heterodimeric complexes with the related protein MAX, which stimulates transcription and cell proliferation. In addition to MYC, MAX can also form homodimers as well as heterodimers with MAD and MXI1, two bHLH-LZ proteins that act as negative regulators of transcription. Because the levels of MAX tend to be stable throughout the cell cycle, the ratio of MYC/MAX heterodimers is controlled by the relative abundance of MYC, MAD, and MXI1. As the ratio of MYC to MAD or MXI1 varies, the promoter activity of target genes is expected to be modulated in either a positive (when MYC levels are high) or negative (when MAD or MXI1 levels are high) fashion. Therefore, in lymphoid tumors associated with *MYC* deregulation, it is conceivable that constitutive expression of *MYC* leads to the predominance of MYC/MAX heterodimers, thus inducing positive growth regulation.[164]

MYC promotes proliferation through the induction of genes involved in cell cycle control such as *CDK4*, *ID2*, *CDC25A*, cyclin D1, cyclin D2, cyclin A, and cyclin E. Additionally *MYC* suppresses growth-arresting genes, including *P15*, *P21*, and *P27*.[165]

MYC has a direct role in induction of the activity of telomerase, which has the function of preserving chromosome integrity by maintaining telomere length during the life span of a cell. MYC activates telomerase by inducing expression of its catalytic subunit, telomerase reverse transcriptase (TERT), through interaction with the numerous MYC binding sites contained in the *TERT* promoter.[166] *MYC* and *TERT* are expressed in normal and transformed proliferating cells and downregulated in quiescent and terminally differentiated cells. *MYC* and *TERT* can induce immortalization when constitutively expressed, thus supporting the pathogenetic role of *MYC* and *TERT* interaction.[166]

MYC induces the activity of *protein kinase A* (*PKA*), a key effector of cyclic adenosine monophosphate (cAMP)-mediated signal transduction, by inducing the transcription of the gene encoding the PKA catalytic subunit.[167] The relevance of MYC-induced PKA activity is supported by the observation that expression of the PKA catalytic subunit induces transformation of transfected cells and that *MYC* transformation can be reverted by pharmacological inhibition of PKA.[167]

The *lactate dehydrogenase-A* gene (*LDH-A*), whose product participates in normal anaerobic glycolysis and is frequently increased in human cancers, is a target of MYC.[168] MYC-induced transformation requires *LDH-A* overexpression, as documented by the observation that lowering *LDH-A* levels with antisense oligonucleotides abrogates MYC-transformed cell growth, in particular under hypoxic conditions.[168] These observations suggest that increased *LDH-A* mediated by *MYC* deregulation is necessary for the growth of a cell mass that has an hypoxic internal microenvironment.[168]

BCL6

Chromosomal alterations affecting band 3q27 and involving the *BCL6* gene occur in ~60 percent of CVID-DLBCL and ~20 percent of HIV-DLBCL.[28,151,169] These alterations are predominantly represented by reciprocal translocations between the 3q27 region and several alternative partner chromosomes, including, although not restricted to, the sites of the Ig genes at 14q32 (Ig heavy chain), 2p11 (Igκ), and 22q11 (Igλ). The variability of the partner chromosomes juxtaposed to 3q27 suggests that these abnormalities belong to the group of 'promiscuous' translocations, which involve a fixed chromosome breakpoint on one side and, on the other side, different chromosomal partners in different cases.

The *BCL6* gene is a transcriptional repressor belonging to a family of transcription factors containing zinc fingers, a protein sequence motif that can mediate the protein binding to specific DNA sites.[170] The amino-terminal region of the BCL6 protein contains a domain, called POZ, that is homologous to domains that are also found in several other zinc-finger transcription factors. Apparently, the POZ domain acts as a protein–protein interface implicated in homo/heterodimerization processes. These structural features of the BCL6 protein are consistent with functional studies indicating that *BCL6* can indeed function as a transcriptional repressor that inhibits the expression of genes carrying its specific DNA-binding motif.[170]

The pattern of BCL6 protein expression in human tissues is highly restricted, and high levels are specifically found in B cells. In particular, BCL6 expression is topographically restricted to the GC, where BCL6 is expressed by both centroblasts and centrocytes, whereas expression of BCL6 is absent in pre-GC and post-GC B cells.[171] Clarification of the precise role of BCL6 in physiologic immune processes has been provided by knockout animal models carrying biallelically disrupted *BCL6* genes. Mice carrying the $Bcl6^{-/-}$ phenotype consistently fail to form GC.[172] Consistent with the lack of GC formation, $Bcl6^{-/-}$ mice also display impaired T cell–dependent, antigen-specific IgG responses.[172] Overall, these observations demonstrate that *BCL6* is needed for GC development and survival, whereas its downregulation may be necessary for further differentiation of B cells.

Chromosomal translocations involving band 3q27 truncate the *BCL6* gene within its 5' flanking region, within the first exon or within the first intron.[173] The coding domain of the *BCL6* gene is left intact in all cases, whereas the 5' regulatory sequences, which contain the *BCL6* promoter, are either truncated or, alternatively, completely removed.[173] In all *BCL6* rearrangements, the entire coding sequence of *BCL6* is juxtaposed downstream to heterologous sequences that, based on cytogenetic data, may originate from different chromosomal sites in different patients.[173] The common functional consequence of *BCL6* translocations is the juxtaposition of heterologous promoters to the *BCL6* coding domain, a mechanism called promoter substitution. The substitution of the *BCL6* promoter by heterologous regulatory sequences causes deregulated *BCL6* expression in DLBCL carrying *BCL6* rearrangements. One feature shared by the heterologous promoters linked to rearranged *BCL6* alleles is that they are physiologically active in normal B cells and are not downregulated during the late stages of B cell differentiation. Thus, *BCL6* rearrangements may prevent downregulation of *BCL6* and, in turn, block the differentiation of GC B cells toward plasma cells.

In addition to rearrangements, the *BCL6* gene may be altered by other mechanisms. In 100 percent of CVID-DLBCL, ~70 percent of HIV-NHL, and ~50 percent of PTLD the *BCL6* gene is affected by multiple, often biallelic, mutations introduced by the SHM mechanism, which selectively cluster within the 5' non-coding regions of the gene.[28,174,175] The DNA sequences most frequently affected by mutations lie near the *BCL6* promoter region and overlap with the major cluster of chromosomal breaks at 3q27, suggesting that mutations and rearrangements may be selected for their ability to alter the same region, which, conceivably, regulates the normal expression of *BCL6*. A specific subset of such mutations causes deregulated *BCL6* transcription. These mutations affect two adjacent BCL6 binding sites located in the first non-coding exon of the gene, and prevent BCL6 from binding its own promoter, thereby disrupting the negative autoregulatory circuit that normally controls its expression.[176]

The oncogenic role of *BCL6* rearrangements is supported by a transgenic model of mice carrying *BCL6* alleles rearranged with the Ig heavy chain Iμ promoter, thus mimicking chromosomal translocations found in human DLBCL.[177] These transgenic mice constitutively express

BCL6 and initially display increased GC formation and altered post-GC differentiation. Subsequently, mice develop a polyclonal–oligoglonal lymphoproliferative syndrome that culminates, upon the accumulation of additional genetic lesions, with the development of lymphomas displaying features typical of human DLBCL.[177]

The pathogenetic role of *BCL6* in lymphoma is supported by the biologic functions of BCL6. BCL6 represses a group of genes involved in B cell activation and terminal differentiation, namely *BLIMP1*, and cell cycle control, namely *Cyclin D2* and *P27*.[178] Therefore, the lack of GC formation in *BCL6* knockout mice could be partially a consequence of the absence of proliferative and differentiation signals that are dependent upon *BCL6*.

BCL6 interacts with the MYC pathway. BLIMP1 is a transcription repressor for *MYC* and inhibition of BCL6 induces BLIMP1, which in turn downregulates *MYC* causing cell cycle arrest. On the other hand, BCL6 overexpression could activate *MYC* through the repression of BLIMP1.[179]

The altered expression of *BCL6* may also repress genes involved in apoptosis. BCL6 directly suppresses *P53* expression by binding the *P53* promoter.[180] Moreover, BCL6 is able to indirectly suppress p53 through the interaction with the MDM2 pathway.[180] In experimental models, constitutive expression of BCL6 protects B cells from apoptosis induced by DNA damage, suggesting that an important function of BCL6 is to allow GC to tolerate the physiological DNA breaks required for Ig class switch recombination and SHM without inducing p53-dependent apoptosis.[180] This phenomenon may contribute to B cell lymphomagenesis by allowing the accumulation of aberrant genetic lesions caused by the misfire of the switch recombination and SHM mechanisms.

P53

Mutations of *P53* are detected in 60 percent of HIV-BL and in a fraction of post-transplant DLBCL.[111,151,152,181] Mutations of *P53* tend to be clustered in conserved regions spanning from the coding sequence of exon 5 through exon 9 and encoding the *P53* DNA binding domain. *P53* is a transcription factor that induces expression of genes involved in cell cycle arrest or apoptosis in response to a variety of toxic or oncogenic stimuli.[165] Negative regulation of cell cycle progression by *P53* is mediated by induction of *P21*, a cyclin kinase inhibitor that neutralizes the activity of cyclin E.[165] Missense mutations of *P53* usually result in the inability to transactivate its target genes, as reflected by the loss of *P21* expression in *P53* mutant lymphoma.[165]

DNA METHYLATION

Aberrant promoter hypermethylation is an epigenetic alteration that targets specific DNA sequences called 'CpG islands' located within the regulatory regions of human genes.[182] Consequently, aberrant hypermethylation of 'CpG islands' causes repression of gene transcription and represents a mechanism for tumor suppressor gene inactivation alternative to mutations/deletions of the locus.[182] Aberrant promoter hypermethylation has been documented as a relevant mechanism of lymphomagenesis in immunocompromised hosts, targeting multiple and functionally heterogeneous lymphoma-related genes.

The *MGMT* gene is frequently inactivated through aberrant promoter hypermethylation in NHL of the immunocompromised host. Hypermethylation of *MGMT* has been detected in 30 percent of HIV-NHL, 60 percent of PTLD, and 40 percent of CVID-NHL.[183] *MGMT* is a DNA repair gene whose product removes mutagenic and cytotoxic adducts introduced in the DNA from environmental and therapeutic alkylating agents.[184] The potential role of *MGMT* in lymphoma stems from the fact that *MGMT* inactivation favors lymphomagenesis in knockout mice.[185] Consistent with the protective function of *MGMT* against spontaneous and alkylator-induced G to A transitions in human DNA, *MGMT* inactivation may cause tumors by generating genetic instability and acquisition of *P53* and *RAS* point mutations.[186,187]

Another gene frequently targeted by aberrant promoter hypermethylation in NHL of the immunocompromised host is *DAPK*. Hypermethylation of *DAPK* occurs in 80 percent of HIV-NHL, 80 percent of PTLD, and 60 percent of CVID-NHL.[183] DAPK is a pro-apoptotic serine-threonine kinase involved in the extrinsic pathway of apoptosis initiated by IFNγ, TNF-α, and Fas ligand.[188] In addition, *DAPK* also participates to counteract *MYC*-induced transformation by activating the *P53* checkpoint and favoring *MYC*-induced apoptosis.[189] Consequently, inactivation of *DAPK* prevents apoptosis triggered by death receptors and weakens the apoptotic response secondary to *MYC* activation.

The *P73* gene is a candidate tumor suppressor gene sharing structural and functional similarities with *P53* and is involved in cell cycle control and apoptosis.[190] Hypermethylation of *P73* is restricted to 15 percent of HIV-NHL, 20 percent of PTLD, and 20 percent of CVID-NHL.[183]

ABERRANT SOMATIC HYPERMUTATION

In normal physiology, the SHM process introduces mainly single nucleotide substitutions into the *IGV* genes of GC B cells in order to produce antibodies with high affinity for the antigen. Somatic hypermutation is not physiologically restricted to *IGV* sequences, since at least two non-Ig genes, *BCL6* and *FAS/CD95*, accumulate mutations in normal GC B cells.[191] In over half of patients with DLBCL of the immunocompetent host, the SHM process appears to misfire and aberrantly target multiple loci, including well-known protooncogenes implicated in the pathogenesis of lymphoid malignancies (*PIM1*, *PAX5*, *RHOH/TTF*, and *MYC*).[192] *PIM1* encodes a serine-threonine kinase and is occasionally involved in DLBCL-associated chromosomal translocations.[193] *PAX5* encodes a B cell-specific transcription factor essential for B-lineage commitment and differentiation and is involved in translocations in about 50 percent of lymphoplasmacytic lymphoma.[194] *RHOH/ TTF* encodes a small GTP-binding protein belonging to the *RAS* superfamily and is involved in rare instances of lymphoma translocations.[195]

Mutations affecting *PIM1, PAX5, RHOH/TTF,* and *MYC* in lymphoma mimic the molecular features of the physiological SHM process, but they do not occur at a significant level in normal GC B cells or in other B cell malignancies suggesting a malfunction of SHM associated to NHL. On this basis, this phenomenon has been called aberrant SHM.[192]

Aberrant SHM is involved in the pathogenesis of NHL arising in the immunocompromised host. Overall, aberrant SHM has been observed in 50 percent of HIV-NHL, at a frequency of 10 percent in the case of *PIM1,* 20 percent in the case of *PAX5,* 20 percent in the case of *RHOH/TTF,* and 25 percent in the case of *MYC.*[196] Aberrant SHM has also been detected in 30 percent of PTLD. Overall, *PIM1* was mutated in 15 percent, *PAX5* in 15 percent, *RHOH/TTF* in 5 percent, and *MYC* in 10 percent of PTLD.[197]

Based on the distribution and type of mutations, aberrant SHM may alter the function of *PIM1, PAX5, RHOH/TTF,* and *MYC* with two modalities. First, because mutations cluster around the gene 5′ regulatory regions, mutations may deregulate gene transcription. Second, a subset of mutations of *MYC* and *PIM1* lead to amino acid substitutions and, consequently, may alter the biochemical and/or structural properties of the protein.

Moreover, the sequences of *PIM1, PAX5, RHOH/TTF,* and *MYC* targeted by aberrant SHM largely overlap with the breakpoint regions involved in chromosomal translocations affecting the same genes. On this basis, it has been speculated that aberrant SHM may represent a mechanism of genomic instability favoring the development of lymphoma-associated chromosomal translocation.

CLINICO–PATHOLOGIC ENTITIES

Human immunodeficiency virus–related lymphoma

HIV-BL/BLL

Viral infection of HIV-BL/BLL cells is mainly represented by EBV infection, which is restricted to approximately 30 percent of cases.[111] Epstein–Barr virus infection in HIV-BL/BLL, as well as in other HIV-related lymphomas, is generally monoclonal, consistent with the hypothesis that the virus had been present in the tumor progenitor cells since the early phases of clonal expansion and thus putatively contributed to lymphoma development.[198] The precise role of EBV in the pathogenesis of Burkitt lymphoma, however, remains controversial. Epstein–Barr virus-positive HIV-BL/BLL display a latency I type of EBV infection, thus they carry EBNA1 and EBERs, but fail to express

the EBV transforming antigens EBNA2 and LMP1, which are key inducers of the transformed phenotype in other B cell models.[78] Several findings indicate a possible role for EBV as a secondary event in the promotion of BL/BLL transformation after the acquisition of *MYC* translocation. First, EBERs can induce the expression of IL-10 and mediate resistance to interferon, which might support tumor growth and survival.[199] Second, expression of EBERs is positively regulated by *MYC.*[200] As the EBERs are thought to have antiapoptotic activity, sustained expression of EBERs might counteract the pro-apoptotic effect of *MYC* deregulation by chromosomal translocation. Third, the comparison of gene expression profiles between EBV-infected and EBV-negative BL cell lines allowed the identification of a number of genes putatively regulated by EBV infection.[201,202] By clustering gene expression based on the putative gene function, EBV infection in BL cell lines seems to upregulate antiapoptotic pathways, as well as STAT transcription factor pathways, which ultimately induce interferon response genes. Also, EBV infection may upregulate the TNF receptor pathways, which are able to activate NF-κB, and downregulate genes involved in the cell cycle. Finally, introduction of latency I genes in EBV-negative BL cell lines restores their tumorigenicity by increased resistance to apoptosis mediated by BCL-2 and decreased expression of MYC.[203]

An alternative hypothesis is that HIV-BL/BLL may derive from EBV-transformed B cells that in the course of malignant transformation have lost the expression of most EBV transforming genes.[204] This selection pressure could stem from the incompatibility of the EBNA2 and *MYC* programs or from a need to downregulate the expression of immunogenic EBV proteins. This notion is supported by the identification of BL cases that fail to perform a latency III program because a deletion of the *EBNA2* gene specifically abrogated the expression of EBNA2.[204]

The profile of molecular lesions of HIV-BL/BLL includes activation of *MYC* in 100 percent of cases, inactivation of *P53* in 60 percent of cases, and point mutations of *BCL6* in 70 percent of cases.[111,152,153,156,157,169,174] DNA methylation affects *MGMT* in 25 percent, *DAPK* in 90 percent, and *P73* in 20 percent of HIV-BL/BLL.[183] Aberrant SHM involves *PIM1* in 10 percent, *PAX5* in 30 percent, and *RHOH/TTF* in 20 percent of HIV-BL/BLL (Table 24.3).[196]

HIV-DLBCL

The molecular pathogenesis of HIV-DLBCL involves infection by EBV in 80 percent of cases.[111] However, only a proportion of infected cases, mainly those categorized as immunoblastic lymphoma, express the EBV-encoded LMP1 protein, which exerts a transforming role for B cells.[23] Apart from EBV infection, the only genetic alterations associated with HIV-DLBCL are represented by rearrangements of *BCL6,* which occur in 20 percent of cases, and *BCL6* mutations, observed in 70 percent of cases.[111,169,174] DNA methylation affects *MGMT* in 30 percent, *DAPK* in

Table 24.3 Genetic lesions associated with immunodeficiency-related lymphoma

	BCL6 R	BCL6 M	MYC R	P53	MYC M	PAX5	PIM1	RHOH/TTF	MGMT	DAPK	EBV	HHV-8
HIV-lymphoma												
Diffuse large B cell lymphoma	20%	70%	–	–	30%	20%	20%	20%	30%	80%	80%	–
Burkitt lymphoma	–	70%	100%	60%	40%	30%	10%	20%	25%	90%	30%	–
Primary central nervous system lymphoma	–	70%	–	–	25%	–	–	25%	–	25%	50%	–
Primary effusion lymphoma	–	70%	–	–	20%	20%	–	30%	65%	80%	90%	100%
Plasmablastic lymphoma	–	10%	–	–	na	na	na	na	na	na	60%	–
Hodgkin lymphoma	na	na	na	na	na	na	na	na	na	na	100%	–
Post-transplant lymphoproliferative disorders												
Polymorphic	–	40%	–	–	–	–	–	–	50%	75%	100%	–
Monomorphic	Rare	90%	Rare	Rare	15%	25%	–	5%	50%	85%	50–90%	Rare
Hodgkin lymphoma	na	na	na	na	na	na	na	na	na	na	100%	–
Methotrexate–associated lymphoma	na	na	na	na	na	na	na	na	na	na	100%	–
CVID–associated lymphoma	60%	100%	–	–	na	na	na	na	40%	50%	–	–

HIV, human immunodeficiency virus; CVID, common variable immunodeficiency; R, rearrangement; –, absent; na, not available; M, mutation.

80 percent, and *P73* in 10 percent of HIV-DLBCL.[183] Aberrant SHM involves *PIM1* in 20 percent, *PAX5* in 20 percent, *RHOH/TTF* in 20 percent, and *MYC* in 30 percent of HIV-DLBCL (Table 24.3).[196]

HIV–PCNSL

Human immunodeficiency virus–PCNSL is characterized by the consistent infection of the tumor clone by EBV.[111] Approximately 50 percent of cases express the EBV-encoded transforming protein LMP1, suggesting a direct role of the virus in the pathogenesis of these lymphomas.[24] At the molecular level, *BCL6* mutations are observed in 70 percent of cases.[174] DNA methylation affects *DAPK* in 25 percent of HIV-PCNSL.[183] Aberrant SHM involves *RHOH/TTF* in 25 percent and *MYC* in 25 percent of HIV-PCNSL (Table 24.3).[196]

HIV–PEL

Human herpes virus 8 infection occurs in 100 percent of HIV-PEL.[98,102] Epstein–Barr virus infection occurs in 90 percent of HIV-PEL but fails to express LMP1.[98,102] At the molecular level, HIV-PEL is characterized by a complex karyotype and recurrent chromosomal abnormalities such as trisomy 7, trisomy 12, and breaks at 1q21–q25.[205,206] Mutations of *BCL6* occur in 70 percent of cases while other HIV-NHL-associated lesions, namely *MYC* and *BCL6* rearrangements or *P53* mutations, are absent.[98,102] DNA methylation affects *MGMT* in 65 percent, *DAPK* in 80 percent, and *P73* in 10 percent of HIV-PEL.[183] Aberrant SHM involves *PAX5* in 20 percent, *RHOH/TTF* in 30 percent, and *MYC* in 20 percent of HIV-PEL (Table 24.3).[196]

Gene expression profiling studies have shown that PEL display a common profile that is clearly distinct from all NHL of immunocompetent hosts and HIV-NHL subtypes and, in contrast to those, is not related to GC or memory B cells. The gene expression profile of PEL is defined as plasmablastic because it shows features of both immunoblasts, identified by EBV-transformed lymphoblastoid cell lines and HIV immunoblastic lymphoma, and plasma cells, as defined by multiple myeloma cell lines. Also, gene expression profiling studies have identified a set of genes specifically expressed in PEL tumor cells. Their expression has been validated at the protein level, suggesting their potential pathogenetic and clinical significance.[207,208] Interestingly, a gene expression profile similar to that of PEL has also been identified in a subset of solid-based lymphomas carrying HHV-8 infection.[209] Because pathobiological features of HHV-8-positive solid lymphomas closely mimic those of PEL, it has been suggested that HHV-8-positive solid lymphomas should be considered as a tissue-based variant of classical PEL.[209]

HIV–PBL

The molecular pathophysiology of HIV-PBL is poorly understood. Infection by EBV occurs in approximately 60 percent of cases, although expression of LMP1 is restricted to a fraction of cases. *BCL6* mutations are restricted to 10 percent of HIV-PBL (Table 24.3).[22,210,211]

HIV–HL

To date, the only pathogenetic lesion asssociated to HIV-HL is EBV infection, which occurs in 80–100 percent of cases and is always associated with LMP1 expression (Table 24.3).[212]

Post-transplant lymphoproliferative disorders

POLYMORPHIC–PTLD

The molecular pathogenesis of P-PTLD involves infection by EBV in virtually all cases and expression of the transforming proteins EBNA2 and LMP1.[66] Apart from EBV infection, the only genetic alteration associated with P-PTLD is represented by *BCL6* mutations, which are observed in 40 percent of cases and correlate with improved outcome and response to immunosuppressive therapy withdrawal.[175,213] DNA methylation affects *MGMT* in 50 percent, *DAPK* in 75 percent, and *P73* in 50 percent of P-PTLD.[183] Aberrant SHM is not involved in P-PTLD (Table 24.3).[197]

MONOMORPHIC PTLD

Epstein–Barr virus infection has been detected in 50–90 percent of monomorphic PTLD.[15,66,151] The prevalence of EBV infection does not significantly differ among the single clinico-pathologic entities. The most relevant predictor of EBV status is the time of PTLD onset after transplantation. In fact, EBV-negative PTLD arise at a median time of 50–60 months post-transplant compared to 6–10 months in EBV-positive PTLD.[214,215] Moreover, nearly half of PTLD arising 20 months or later post-transplant fail to show evidence of EBV infection.[216] Human herpes virus 8 infection is restricted to the rare PEL arising in the post-transplant setting.[101,102] The most frequent genetic lesion of monomorphic PTLD is represented by *BCL6* mutations, occurring in 90 percent of cases. Other molecular lesions are generally restricted to a small fraction of cases and are represented by *MYC* rearrangement, mutations of *p53* and *N-RAS*, and 9p deletion.[151,217] DNA methylation affects *MGMT* in 50 percent, *DAPK* in 85 percent, and *P73* in 15 percent of monomorphic PTLD.[183] Aberrant SHM involves *PAX5* in 25 percent, *RHOH/TTF* in 5 percent, and *MYC* in 15 percent of monomorphic PTLD (Table 24.3).[197] The role of antigen stimulation and selection in PTLD appears to be limited when compared to HIV-NHL.[218]

Recent studies based on genome-wide technologies revealed recurrent lesions among PTLD.[219] Chromosomes 5p and 11p were commonly gained in PTLD-DLBCL, whereas chromosome 12p was the most frequent target of deletions.[219] Loss of heterozygosity (LOH) did not always match DNA loss and chromosome 10 seemed to be targeted by uniparental disomy in PTLD.[219] Small deletions and gains, involving both known (*BCL2* and *PAX5*) and unknown genes (*ZDHHC14*), were identified by genome-wide approaches.[219] These data suggest that PTLD share, at a lower frequency, common genetic aberrations with DLBCL from immunocompetent patients. The demonstration of 9p13 amplification emphasizes the importance of *PAX5* in PTLD. The combination of DNA copy number and LOH assessment leads to the hypothesis that uniparental disomy may be a potential mechanism in PTLD pathogenesis.[219]

POST-TRANSPLANT-HL

The molecular pathogenesis of post-transplant HL is largely unknown. Epstein–Barr virus infection occurs in 100 percent of cases and is always associated with LMP1 expression (Table 24.3).[15]

Non–Hodgkin lymphoma related to other immunodeficiency conditions

CVID-DLBCL

CVID-DLBCL lack EBV and HHV-8 infection, as well as other genetic lesions commonly associated with DLBCL of the immunocompetent host, including *BCL-2* and *MYC* rearrangement, *REL* amplification, and *P53* mutations.[28] All CVID-DLBCL carry *BCL6* mutations and two-thirds *BCL6* rearrangement.[28] DNA methylation affects *MGMT* in 40 percent, *DAPK* in 50 percent, and *p73* in 20 percent of CVID-DLBCL (Table 24.3).[183]

ATAXIA TELANGIECTASIA–ASSOCIATED T CELL PROLYMPHOCYTIC LEUKEMIA

Ataxia telangiectasia–associated T cell prolymphocytic leukemia is characterized by the chromosomal abnormalities inv(14), t(14;14), or t(X;14).[38] These rearrangements result in the juxtaposition of the T cell receptor (TCR) gene regulatory elements to the *TCL1* gene at chromosome 14 and its homologue, the *MTCP1* gene, at Xq28.[220] Transgenic animals overexpressing either the *TCL1* or *MTCP1* gene develop mature T cell leukemias, indicating that these genes are directly involved in leukemogenesis.[220] *TCL1* is an Akt kinase coactivator. Akt, the cellular homologue of the transforming viral oncogene v-Akt, is a serine-threonine kinase that plays a central role in the regulation of cell survival and proliferation. TCL1 binds to Akt and mediates the formation of oligomeric TCL1-Akt high-molecular-weight protein complexes. Within these protein complexes, Akt is preferentially phosphorylated and activated.[220]

METHOTREXATE-ASSOCIATED LYMPHOMA

The molecular pathogenesis of methotrexate-associated-lymphoma is poorly understood. Most cases display a

DLBCL histology and carry EBV infection. In line with the possible pathogenetic role of EBV in methotrexate-associated lymphoma, *in vitro* and *in vivo* experimental models suggest that methotrexate treatment may induce EBV reactivation (Table 24.3).[221]

KEY POINTS

- Immunodeficiency conditions associated with increased incidence of lymphoma include primary immunodeficiency, HIV infection, iatrogenic immunosuppression in transplant recipients and methotrexate treatment for autoimmune diseases.
- Immunodeficiency-related lymphomas display common features, irrespective of the underlying immunodeficiency condition.
- Common characteristics of immunodeficiency-related lymphomas include preferential representation of non-Hodgkin lymphoma, involvement of extranodal and unusual sites, aggressive pathology and clinical behavior, B cell lineage derivation, and frequent association with EBV infection.
- The molecular histogenesis of immunodeficiency-related lymphomas may be traced in most cases to germinal center or post-germinal center B cells.
- Factors involved in the molecular pathogenesis of immunodeficiency-related lymphoma comprise the genetic background of the host, chronic antigen stimulation, accumulation of genetic and epigenetic alterations in the tumor cell, and clonal infection by oncogenic viruses.

REFERENCES

● = Key primary paper

◆ = Major review article

1. Jaffe ES, Harris NL, Stein H, Vardiman JW. *World Health Organization classification of tumours, pathology and genetics of tumours of haematopoietic and lymphoid tissues.* Lyon, France: IARC Press, 2001.

●2. Immunodeficiency disease and malignancy. Various immunologic deficiencies of man and the role of immune processes in the control of malignant disease. *Ann Intern Med* 1972; **77**: 605–28.

◆3. Beral V, Newton R. Overview of the epidemiology of immunodeficiency-associated cancers. *J Natl Cancer Inst Monogr* 1998; **23**: 1–6.

4. Kinlen LJ, Webster AD, Bird AG *et al.* Prospective study of cancer in patients with hypogammaglobulinaemia. *Lancet* 1985; **1**: 263–6.

5. Cunningham-Rundles C, Siegal FP, Cunningham-Rundles S, Lieberman P. Incidence of cancer in 98 patients with common varied immunodeficiency. *J Clin Immunol* 1987; **7**: 294–9.

6. Mellemkjaer L, Hammarstrom L, Andersen V *et al*. Cancer risk among patients with IgA deficiency or common variable immunodeficiency and their relatives: a combined Danish and Swedish study. *Clin Exp Immunol* 2002; **130**: 495–500.

7. Centers for Disease Control. Revision of the CDC surveillance case definition for acquired immunodeficiency syndrome. *MMWR Morb Mortal Wkly Rep* 1987; **36(Suppl 1)**: 1S–15S.

◆8. Levine AM. AIDS-related malignancies: the emerging epidemic. *J Natl Cancer Inst* 1993; **85**: 1382–97.

●9. International Collaboration on HIV and Cancer. Highly active antiretroviral therapy and incidence of cancer in human immunodeficiency virus-infected adults. *J Natl Cancer Inst* 2000; **92**: 1823–30.

10. Eltom MA, Jemal A, Mbulaiteye SM *et al*. Trends in Kaposi's sarcoma and non-Hodgkin's lymphoma incidence in the United States from 1973 through 1998. *J Natl Cancer Inst* 2002; **94**: 1204–10.

11. Matthews GV, Bower M, Mandalia S *et al*. Changes in acquired immunodeficiency syndrome-related lymphoma since the introduction of highly active antiretroviral therapy. *Blood* 2000; **96**: 2730–34.

12. Besson C, Goubar A, Gabarre J *et al*. Changes in AIDS-related lymphoma since the era of highly active antiretroviral therapy. *Blood* 2001; **98**: 2339–44.

13. Kirk O, Pedersen C, Cozzi-Lepri A *et al*. Non-Hodgkin lymphoma in HIV-infected patients in the era of highly active antiretroviral therapy. *Blood* 2001; **98**: 3406–12.

14. McKhann CF. Primary malignancy in patients undergoing immunosuppression for renal transplantation. *Transplantation* 1969; **8**: 209–12.

15. Frizzera G. Atypical lymphoproliferative disorders. In: Knowles DM (ed.) *Neoplastic hemopathology*, 2nd Edn. Philadelphia, PA: Lippincott Williams and Wilkins, 2001: 569–622.

16. Salloum E, Cooper DL, Howe G *et al*. Spontaneous regression of lymphoproliferative disorders in patients treated with methotrexate for rheumatoid arthritis and other rheumatic diseases. *J Clin Oncol* 1996; **14**: 1943–9.

17. Dawson TM, Starkebaum G, Wod BL *et al*. Epstein-Barr virus, methotrexate and lymphoma in patients with rheumatoid arthritis and primary Sjogren's syndrome: case series. *J Rheumatol* 2001; **28**: 47–53.

18. Mariette X, Cazals-Hatem D, Warszawki J *et al*. Lymphomas in rheumatoid arthritis patients treated with methotrexate: a 3-year prospective study in France. *Blood* 2002; **99**: 3909–15.

19. Wolfe F, Michaud K. Lymphoma in rheumatoid arthritis: the effect of methotrexate and anti-tumor necrosis factor therapy in 18,572 patients. *Arthritis Rheum* 2004; **50**: 1740–51.

20. Gaidano G, Carbone A. MUM1: a step ahead toward the understanding of lymphoma histogenesis. *Leukemia* 2000; **14**: 563–6.

21. Capello D, Berra E, Cerri M *et al*. Molecular analysis of immunoglobulin variable genes in HIV-related non-Hodgkin lymphoma: implications for disease pathogenesis and histogenesis. *Blood* 2005; **106**: 330a.

22. Gaidano G, Cerri M, Capello D *et al*. Molecular histogenesis of plasmablastic lymphoma of the oral cavity. *Br J Haematol* 2002; **119**: 622–8.

●23. Carbone A, Gloghini A, Larocca LM *et al*. Expression profile of MUM1/IRF4, BCL-6, and CD138/syndecan-1 defines novel histogenetic subsets of human immunodeficiency virus-related lymphomas. *Blood* 2001; **97**: 744–51.

24. Carbone A, Gaidano G, Gloghini A *et al*. BCL-6 protein expression in AIDS-related non-Hodgkin's lymphomas: inverse relationship with Epstein-Barr virus-encoded latent membrane protein-1 expression. *Am J Pathol* 1997; **150**: 155–65.

●25. Capello D, Cerri M, Muti G *et al*. Molecular histogenesis of posttransplantation lymphoproliferative disorders. *Blood* 2003; **102**: 3775–85.

◆26. Capello D, Rossi D, Gaidano G. Post-transplant lymphoproliferative disorders: molecular basis of disease histogenesis and pathogenesis. *Hematol Oncol* 2005; **23**: 61–7.

27. Abed N, Casper JT, Camitta BM *et al*. Evaluation of histogenesis of B-lymphocytes in pediatric EBV-related post-transplant lymphoproliferative disorders. *Bone Marrow Transplant* 2004; **33**: 321–7.

28. Ariatti C, Vivenza D, Capello D *et al*. Common-variable immunodeficiency-related lymphomas associate with mutations and rearrangements of BCL-6: pathogenetic and histogenetic implications. *Hum Pathol* 2000; **31**: 871–3.

29. Cyster JG. Homing of antibody secreting cells. *Immunol Rev* 2003; **194**: 48–60.

30. Rabkin CS, Yang Q, Goedert JJ *et al*. Chemokine and chemokine receptor gene variants and risk of non-Hodgkin's lymphoma in human immunodeficiency virus-1-infected individuals. *Blood* 1999; **93**: 1838–42.

31. Sei S, O'Neill DP, Stewart SK *et al*. Increased level of stromal cell-derived factor-1 mRNA in peripheral blood mononuclear cells from children with AIDS-related lymphoma. *Cancer Res* 2001; **61**: 5028–37.

32. Hogan CM, Hammer SM. Host determinants in HIV infection and disease. Part 2: genetic factors and implications for antiretroviral therapeutics. *Ann Intern Med* 2001; **134**: 978–96.

33. Dean M, Jacobson LP, McFarlane G *et al*. Reduced risk of AIDS lymphoma in individuals heterozygous for the CCR5-delta32 mutation. *Cancer Res* 1999; **59**: 3561–4.

34. Ganju RK, Brubaker SA, Chernock RD *et al*. Beta-chemokine receptor CCR5 signals through SHP1, SHP2, and Syk. *J Biol Chem* 2000; **275**: 17263–8.

35. Benjamin D, Knobloch TJ, Dayton MA. Human B-cell interleukin-10: B-cell lines derived from patients with acquired immunodeficiency syndrome and Burkitt's lymphoma constitutively secrete large quantities of interleukin-10. *Blood* 1992; **80**: 1289–98.

36. Masood R, Zhang Y, Bond MW et al. Interleukin-10 is an autocrine growth factor for acquired immunodeficiency syndrome-related B-cell lymphoma. Blood 1995; 85: 3423–30.

37. Breen EC, Boscardin WJ, Detels R et al. Non-Hodgkin's B cell lymphoma in persons with acquired immunodeficiency syndrome is associated with increased serum levels of IL10, or the IL10 promoter -592 C/C genotype. Clin Immunol 2003; 109: 119–29.

38. Taylor AMR, Metcalfe JA, Thick J, Mak YF. Leukemia and lymphoma in ataxia telangiectasia. Blood 1996; 87: 423–38.

39. Gumy-Pause F, Wacker P, Sappino AP. ATM gene and lymphoid malignancies. Leukemia 2004; 18: 238–42.

40. Boultwood J. Ataxia telangiectasia gene mutations in leukaemia and lymphoma. J Clin Pathol 2001; 54: 512–16.

41. Barlow C, Hirotsune S, Paylor R et al. Atm-deficient mice: a paradigm of ataxia telangiectasia. Cell 1996; 86: 159–71.

42. Lumsden JM, McCarty T, Petiniot LK et al. Immunoglobulin class switch recombination is impaired in Atm-deficient mice. J Exp Med 2004; 200: 1111–21.

43. Reina-San-Martin B, Chen HT, Nussenzweig A, Nussenzweig MC. ATM is required for efficient recombination between immunoglobulin switch regions. J Exp Med 2004; 200: 1103–10.

44. Liao MJ, Van Dyke T. Critical role for Atm in suppressing V(D)J recombination-driven thymic lymphoma. Genes Dev 1999; 13: 1246–50.

●45. Ziegler JL, Beckstead JA, Volberding PA et al. Non-Hodgkin's lymphoma in 90 homosexual men. Relation to generalized lymphadenopathy and the acquired immunodeficiency syndrome. N Engl J Med 1984; 311: 565–70.

●46. Pelicci PG, Knowles DM 2nd, Arlin ZA et al. Multiple monoclonal B cell expansions and c-myc oncogene rearrangements in acquired immune deficiency syndrome-related lymphoproliferative disorders. Implications for lymphomagenesis. J Exp Med 1986; 164: 2049–60.

47. Przybylski GK, Goldman J, Ng VL et al. Evidence for early B-cell activation preceding the development of Epstein-Barr virus-negative acquired immunodeficiency syndrome-related lymphoma. Blood 1996; 88: 4620–9.

48. Bessudo A, Cherepakhin V, Johnson TA et al. Favored use of immunoglobulin V(H)4 genes in AIDS-associated B-cell lymphoma. Blood 1996; 88: 252–60.

49. Matolcsy A, Nador RG, Cesarman E, Knowles DM. Immunoglobulin VH gene mutational analysis suggests that primary effusion lymphomas derive from different stages of B-cell maturation. Am J Pathol 1998; 153: 1609–14.

50. Delecluse HJ, Hummel M, Marafioti T et al. Common and HIV-related diffuse large B-cell lymphomas differ in their immunoglobulin gene mutation pattern. J Pathol 1999; 188: 133–8.

51. Fais F, Gaidano G, Capello D et al. Immunoglobulin V region gene use and structure suggest antigen selection in AIDS-related primary effusion lymphomas. Leukemia 1999; 13: 1093–9.

52. Julien S, Radosavljevic M, Labouret N et al. AIDS primary central nervous system lymphoma: molecular analysis of the expressed VH genes and possible implications for lymphomagenesis. J Immunol 1999; 162: 1551–8.

53. Bellan C, Lazzi S, Hummel M et al. Immunoglobulin gene analysis reveals 2 distinct cells of origin for EBV-positive and EBV-negative Burkitt lymphomas. Blood 2005; 106: 1031–6.

54. Link JM, Schroeder HW Jr. Clues to the etiology of autoimmune diseases through analysis of immunoglobulin genes. Arthritis Res 2002; 4: 80–83.

55. Ng VL, Hurt MH, Fein CL et al. IgMs produced by two acquired immune deficiency syndrome lymphoma cell lines: Ig binding specificity and VH-gene putative somatic mutation analysis. Blood 1994; 83: 1067–78.

56. Riboldi P, Gaidano G, Schettino EW et al. Two acquired immunodeficiency syndrome-associated Burkitt's lymphomas produce specific anti-i IgM cold agglutinins using somatically mutated VH4-21 segments. Blood 1994; 83: 2952–61.

57. Cunto-Amesty G, Przybylski G, Honczarenko M et al. Evidence that immunoglobulin specificities of AIDS-related lymphoma are not directed to HIV-related antigens. Blood 2000; 95: 1393–9.

58. Zhu D, McCarthy H, Ottensmeier CH et al. Acquisition of potential N-glycosylation sites in the immunoglobulin variable region by the somatic mutation is a distinctive feature of follicular lymphoma. Blood 2002; 99: 2562–8.

59. Rudd PM, Elliott T, Cresswell P et al. Glycosylation and the immune system. Science 2001; 291: 2370–6.

60. Forconi F, Capello D, Berra E et al. Incidence of novel N-glycosylation sites in the B-cell receptor of lymphomas associated with immunodeficiency. Br J Haematol 2004; 124: 604–9.

●61. Bräuninger A, Spieker T, Mottok A et al. Epstein-Barr virus (EBV)-positive lymphoproliferations in post-transplant patients show immunoglobulin V gene mutation patterns suggesting interference of EBV with normal B cell differentiation processes. Eur J Immunol 2003; 33: 1593–602.

●62. Timms JM, Bell A, Flavell JR et al. Target cells of Epstein-Barr-virus (EBV)-positive post-transplant lymphoproliferative disease: similarities to EBV-positive Hodgkin's lymphoma. Lancet 2003; 361: 217–23.

63. Laszewski MJ, Kemp JD, Goeken JA et al. Clonal immunoglobulin gene rearrangement in nodular lymphoid hyperplasia of the gastrointestinal tract associated with common variable immunodeficiency. Am J Clin Pathol 1990; 94: 338–43.

64. Chiaramonte C, Glick SN. Nodular lymphoid hyperplasia of the small bowel complicated by jejunal lymphoma in a patient with common variable immune deficiency syndrome. Am J Roentgenol 1994; 163: 1118–9.

◆65. Cohen JI. Epstein-Barr virus infection. N Engl J Med 2000; 343: 481–92.

66. Cohen JI. Benign and malignant Epstein-Barr virus-associated B-cell lymphoproliferative diseases. Semin Hematol 2003; 40: 116–23.

67. Shibata D, Weiss LM, Nathwani BN et al. Epstein-Barr virus in benign lymph node biopsies from individuals infected with the human immunodeficiency virus is

associated with concurrent or subsequent development of non-Hodgkin's lymphoma. *Blood* 1991; **77**: 1527–33.

68. Lei KIK, Chan LYS, Chan WY *et al.* Quantitative analysis of circulating cell-free Epstein-Barr virus (EBV) DNA levels in patients with EBV-associated lymphoid malignancies. *Br J Haematol* 2000; **111**: 239–46.

69. Stevens SJC, Verschuuren EAM, Pronk I *et al.* Frequent monitoring of Epstein-Barr virus DNA load in unfractioned whole blood is essential for early detection of posttransplant lymphoproliferative disease in high risk patients. *Blood* 2001; **97**: 1165–71.

70. van Baarle D, Wolthers KC, Hovenkamp E *et al.* Absolute level of Epstein-Barr virus in human immunodeficiency virus type 1 infection is not predictive of AIDS-related non-Hodgkin lymphoma. *J Infect Dis* 2002; **186**: 405–9.

71. Muti G, Klersy C, Baldanti F *et al.* Epstein-Barr virus (EBV) load and interleukin-10 in EBV-positive and EBV-negative post-transplant lymphoproliferative disorders. *Br J Haematol* 2003; **122**: 927–33.

72. Piriou E, van Dort K, Nanlohy NM *et al.* Altered EBV viral load setpoint after HIV seroconversion is in accordance with lack of predictive value of EBV load for the occurrence of AIDS-related non-Hodgkin lymphoma. *J Immunol* 2004; **172**: 6931–7.

73. Fan H, Kim SC, Chima CO *et al.* Epstein-Barr viral load as a marker of lymphoma in AIDS patients. *J Med Virol* 2005; **75**: 59–69.

74. Kersten MJ, Klein MR, Holwerda AM *et al.* Epstein-Barr virus-specific cytotoxic T cell responses in HIV-1 infection: different kinetics in patients progressing to opportunistic infection or non-Hodgkin lymphoma. *J Clin Invest* 1997; **99**: 1525–33.

75. Baudouin V, Dehee A, Pedron-Grossetete B *et al.* Relationship between CD8+ T-cell phenotype and function, Epstein-Barr virus load and clinical outcome in pediatric renal transplant recipients: a prospective study. *Transplantation* 2004; **77**: 1706–13.

76. Davis JE, Sherritt MA, Bahradwaj M *et al.* Determining virological, serological and immunological parameters of EBV infection in the development of PTLD. *Int Immunol* 2004; **16**: 983–9.

77. Comoli P, Maccario R, Locateli F *et al.* Treatment of EBV-related post-renal transplant lymphoproliferative disease with a tailored regimen including EBV-specific T cells. *Am J Transplant* 2005; **5**: 1415–22.

♦78. Küppers R. B cells under influence: transformation of B cells by Epstein-Barr virus. *Nat Rev Immunol* 2003; **3**: 801–12.

♦79. Thompson MP, Kurzrock R. Epstein-Barr virus and cancer. *Clin Cancer Res* 2004; **10**: 803–21.

80. Kaiser C, Laux G, Eick D *et al.* The proto-oncogene c-myc is a direct target gene of Epstein-Barr virus nuclear antigen 2. *J Virol* 1999; **73**; 4481–4.

81. Hayward SD. Viral interactions with the Notch pathway. *Semin Cancer Biol* 2004; **14**: 387–96.

82. Armstrong SA, Look AT. Molecular genetics of acute lymphoblastic leukemia. *J Clin Oncol* 2005; **23**: 6306–15.

83. Boyle MJ, Sewell WA, Sculley TB *et al.* Subtypes of Epstein-Barr virus in human immunodeficiency virus-associated non-Hodgkin lymphoma. *Blood* 1991; **78**: 3004–11.

84. Goldschmidts WL, Bhatia K, Johnson JF *et al.* Epstein-Barr virus genotypes in AIDS-associated lymphomas are similar to those in endemic Burkitt's lymphomas. *Leukemia* 1992; **6**: 875–8.

85. Khanim F, Yao QY, Niedobitek G *et al.* Analysis of Epstein-Barr virus gene polymorphisms in normal donors and in virus-associated tumors from different geographic locations. *Blood* 1996; **88**: 3491–501.

86. van Baarle D, Hovenkamp E, Kersten MJ *et al.* Direct Epstein-Barr virus (EBV) typing on peripheral blood mononuclear cells: no association between EBV type 2 infection or superinfection and the development of acquired immunodeficiency syndrome-related non-Hodgkin's lymphoma. *Blood* 1999; **93**: 3949–55.

87. Fassone L, Bhatia K, Gutierrez M *et al.* Molecular profile of Epstein-Barr virus infection in HHV-8-positive primary effusion lymphoma. *Leukemia* 2000; **14**: 271–7.

88. Fassone L, Cingolani A, Martini M *et al.* Characterization of Epstein-Barr virus genotype in AIDS-related non-Hodgkin's lymphoma. *AIDS Res Hum Retroviruses* 2002; **18**: 19–26.

89. Liebowitz D. Epstein-Barr virus and a cellular signalling pathway in lymphomas from immunosuppressed patients. *N Engl J Med* 1998; **338**: 1413–21.

90. Huen DS, Henderson SA, Croom-Carter D, Rowe M. The Epstein-Barr virus latent membrane protein-1 (LMP1) mediates activation of NF-kappa B and cell surface phenotype via two effector regions in its carboxy-terminal cytoplasmic domain. *Oncogene* 1995; **10**: 549–60.

91. Eliopoulos AG, Young LS. Activation of the cJun N-terminal kinase (JNK) pathway by the Epstein-Barr virus-encoded latent membrane protein 1 (LMP1). *Oncogene* 1998; **16**: 1731–42.

92. Eliopoulos AG, Gallagher NJ, Blake SM *et al.* Activation of the p38 mitogen-activated protein kinase pathway by Epstein-Barr virus-encoded latent membrane protein 1 coregulates interleukin-6 and interleukin-8 production. *J Biol Chem* 1999; **274**: 16085–96.

93. Gires O, Kohlhuber F, Kilger E *et al.* Latent membrane protein 1 of Epstein-Barr virus interacts with JAK3 and activates STAT proteins. *EMBO J* 1999; **18**: 3064–73.

94. Cathomas G. Kaposi's sarcoma-associated herpesvirus (KSHV)/human herpesvirus 8 (HHV-8) as a tumour virus. *Herpes* 2003; **10**: 72–6.

95. Swaminathan S. Molecular biology of Epstein-Barr virus and Kaposi's sarcoma-associated virus. *Semin Hematol* 2003; **40**: 107–15.

96. Aoki Y, Tosato G. Pathogenesis and manifestations of human herpesvirus-8-associated disorders. *Semin Hematol* 2003; **40**: 143–53.

97. Verschuren E, Jones N, Evan GI. The cell cycle and how it is steered by Kaposi's sarcoma-associated herpesvirus cyclin. *J Gen Virol* 2004; **85**: 1347–61.

●98. Cesarman E, Chang Y, Moore PS *et al.* Kaposi's sarcoma-associated herpesvirus-like DNA sequences in AIDS-related body-cavity-based lymphomas. *N Engl J Med* 1995; **332**: 1186–91.

●99. Carbone A, Gloghini A, Vaccher E et al. Kaposi's sarcoma-associated herpesvirus DNA sequences in AIDS-related and AIDS-unrelated lymphomatous effusions. Br J Haematol 1996; 94: 533–43.

100. Nador RG, Cesarman E, Chadburn A et al. Primary effusion lymphoma: a distinct clinicopathologic entity associated with the Kaposi's sarcoma-associated herpes virus. Blood 1996; 88: 645–56.

101. Jones D, Ballestas ME, Kaye KM et al. Primary-effusion lymphoma and Kaposi's sarcoma in a cardiac-transplant recipient. N Engl J Med 1998; 339: 444–9.

◆102. Gaidano G, Carbone A. Primary effusion lymphoma: a liquid phase lymphoma of fluid-filled body cavities. Adv Cancer Res 2001; 80: 115–46.

103. Rivas C, Thlick AE, Parravicini C et al. Kaposi's sarcoma-associated herpesvirus LANA2 is a B-cell-specific latent viral protein that inhibits p53. J Virol 2001; 75: 429–38.

104. An FQ, Compitello N, Horwitz E et al. The latency-associated nuclear antigen of Kaposi's sarcoma-associated herpesvirus modulates cellular gene expression and protects lymphoid cells from p16 INK4A-induced cell cycle arrest. J Biol Chem 2005; 280: 3862–74.

105. An J, Lichtenstein AK, Brent G, Rettig MB. The Kaposi sarcoma-associated herpesvirus (KSHV) induces cellular interleukin 6 expression: role of the KSHV latency-associated nuclear antigen and the AP1 response element. Blood 2002; 99: 649–54.

106. Carbone A, Gloghini A, Bontempo D et al. Proliferation in HHV-8-positive primary effusion lymphomas is associated with expression of HHV-8 cyclin but independent of p27(kip1). Am J Pathol 2000; 156: 1209–15.

107. Jarviluoma A, Koopal S, Rasanen S et al. KSHV viral cyclin binds to p27KIP1 in primary effusion lymphomas. Blood 2004; 104: 3349–54.

108. Sarek G, Jarviluoma A, Ojala P. KSHV viral cyclin inactivates p27KIP1 through Ser10 and Thr187 phosphorylation in proliferating primary effusion lymphomas. Blood 2006; 107: 725–32.

109. Klouche M, Carruba G, Castagnetta L, Rose-John S. Virokines in the pathogenesis of cancer: focus on human herpesvirus 8. Ann N Y Acad Sci 2004; 1028: 329–39.

●110. Laurence J, Astrin SM. Human immunodeficiency virus induction of malignant transformation in human B lymphocytes. Proc Natl Acad Sci U S A 1991; 88: 7635–9.

111. Ballerini P, Gaidano G, Gong JZ et al. Multiple genetic lesions in acquired immunodeficiency syndrome-related non-Hodgkin's lymphoma. Blood 1993; 81: 166–76.

112. Gaidano G, Parsa NZ, Tassi V et al. In vitro establishment of AIDS-related lymphoma cell lines: phenotypic characterization, oncogene and tumor suppressor gene lesions, and heterogeneity in Epstein-Barr virus infection. Leukemia 1993; 7: 1621–9.

113. Pluda JM, Yarchoan R, Jaffe ES et al. Development of non-Hodgkin lymphoma in a cohort of patients with severe human immunodeficiency virus (HIV) infection on long-term antiretroviral therapy. Ann Intern Med 1990; 113: 276–82.

114. Yarchoan R, Venzon DJ, Pluda JM et al. CD4 count and the risk for death in patients infected with HIV receiving antiretroviral therapy. Ann Intern Med 1991; 115: 184–9.

115. Pluda JM, Venzon DJ, Tosato G et al. Parameters affecting the development of non-Hodgkin's lymphoma in patients with severe human immunodeficiency virus infection receiving antiretroviral therapy. J Clin Oncol 1993; 11: 1099–107.

116. List AF, Spier CM, Miller TP, Grogan TM. Deficient tumor-infiltrating T-lymphocyte response in malignant lymphoma: relationship to HLA expression and host immunocompetence. Leukemia 1993; 7: 398–403.

117. van Baarle D, Hovenkamp E, Callan MF et al. Dysfunctional Epstein-Barr virus (EBV)-specific CD8(+) T lymphocytes and increased EBV load in HIV-1 infected individuals progressing to AIDS-related non-Hodgkin lymphoma. Blood 2001; 98: 146–55.

118. Habis A, Baskin GB, Murphey-Corb M, Levy LS. Simian AIDS-associated lymphoma in rhesus and cynomolgus monkeys recapitulates the primary pathobiological features of AIDS-associated non-Hodgkin's lymphoma. AIDS Res Hum Retroviruses 1999; 15: 1389–98.

119. Ledergerber B, Egger M, Erard V et al. AIDS-related opportunistic illnesses occurring after initiation of potent antiretroviral therapy: the Swiss HIV Cohort Study. JAMA 1999; 282: 2220–6.

120. Mocroft A, Katlama C, Johnson AM et al. AIDS across Europe, 1994–98: the EuroSIDA study. Lancet 2000; 356: 291–6.

121. Frisch M, Biggar RJ, Engels EA, Goedert JJ. Association of cancer with AIDS-related immunosuppression in adults. JAMA 2001; 285: 1736–45.

122. Stebbing J, Gazzard B, Mandalia S et al. Antiretroviral treatment regimens and immune parameters in the prevention of systemic AIDS-related non-Hodgkin's lymphoma. J Clin Oncol 2004; 22: 2177–83.

123. Lim ST, Karim R, Nathwani BN et al. AIDS-related Burkitt's lymphoma versus diffuse large-cell lymphoma in the pre-highly active antiretroviral therapy (HAART) and HAART eras: significant differences in survival with standard chemotherapy. J Clin Oncol 2005; 23: 4430–8.

124. Moses AV, Williams SE, Strussenberg JG et al. HIV-1 induction of CD40 on endothelial cells promotes the outgrowth of AIDS-associated B-cell lymphomas. Nat Med 1997; 3: 1242–9.

125. Chirivi RG, Taraboletti G, Bani MR et al. Human immunodeficiency virus-1 (HIV-1)-Tat protein promotes migration of acquired immunodeficiency syndrome-related lymphoma cells and enhances their adhesion to endothelial cells. Blood 1999; 94: 1747–54.

126. Henderson WW, Ruhl R, Lewis P et al. Human immunodeficiency virus (HIV) type 1 Vpu induces the expression of CD40 in endothelial cells and regulates HIV-induced adhesion of B-lymphoma cells. J Virol 2004; 78: 4408–20.

127. Kundu RK, Sangiorgi F, Wu LY et al. Expression of the human immunodeficiency virus-Tat gene in lymphoid

tissues of transgenic mice is associated with B-cell lymphoma. *Blood* 1999; **94**: 275–82.

128. Ambrosino C, Palmieri C, Puca A *et al*. Physical and functional interaction of HIV-1 Tat with E2F-4, a transcriptional regulator of mammalian cell cycle. *J Biol Chem* 2002; **277**: 31448–58.

129. Lazzi S, Bellan C, De Falco G *et al*. Expression of RB2/p130 tumor-suppressor gene in AIDS-related non-Hodgkin's lymphomas: implications for disease pathogenesis. *Hum Pathol* 2002; **33**: 723–31.

130. De Falco G, Bellan C, Lazzi S *et al*. Interaction between HIV-1 Tat and pRb2/p130: a possible mechanism in the pathogenesis of AIDS-related neoplasms. *Oncogene* 2003; **22**: 6214–9.

131. Bellan C, Lazzi S, De Falco G *et al*. Burkitt's lymphoma: new insights into molecular pathogenesis. *J Clin Pathol* 2003; **56**: 188–92.

132. Machida K, Cheng KT, Sung VM *et al*. Hepatitis C virus induces a mutator phenotype: enhanced mutations of immunoglobulin and protooncogenes. *Proc Natl Acad Sci U S A* 2004; **101**: 4262–7.

133. Ivanovski M, Silvestri F, Pozzato G *et al*. Somatic hypermutation, clonal diversity, and preferential expression of the VH 51p1/VL kv325 immunoglobulin gene combination in hepatitis C virus-associated immunocytomas. *Blood* 1998; **91**: 2433–42.

134. Chan CH, Hadlock KG, Foung SK, Levy S. V(H)1-69 gene is preferentially used by hepatitis C virus-associated B cell lymphomas and by normal B cells responding to the E2 viral antigen. *Blood* 2001; **97**: 1023–6.

135. Gisbert JP, Garcia-Buey L, Pajares JM, Moreno-Otero R. Prevalence of hepatitis C virus infection in B-cell non-Hodgkin's lymphoma: systematic review and meta-analysis. *Gastroenterology* 2003; **125**: 1723–32.

136. Matsuo K, Kusano A, Sugumar A *et al*. Effect of hepatitis C virus infection on the risk of non-Hodgkin's lymphoma: a meta-analysis of epidemiological studies. *Cancer Sci* 2004; **95**: 745–52.

137. Negri E, Little D, Boiocchi M *et al*. B-cell non-Hodgkin's lymphoma and hepatitis C virus infection: a systematic review. *Int J Cancer* 2004; **111**: 1–8.

138. Hezode C, Duvoux C, Germanidis G *et al*. Role of hepatitis C virus in lymphoproliferative disorders after liver transplantation. *Hepatology* 1999; **30**: 775–8.

139. Buda A, Caforio A, Calabrese F *et al*. Lymphoproliferative disorders in heart transplant recipients: role of hepatitis C virus (HCV) and Epstein-Barr virus (EBV) infection. *Transpl Int* 2000; **13**: S402–5.

140. McLaughlin K, Wajstaub S, Marotta P *et al*. Increased risk for posttransplant lymphoproliferative disease in recipients of liver transplants with hepatitis C. *Liver Transpl* 2000; **6**: 570–4.

141. Shivapurkar N, Harada K, Reddy J *et al*. Presence of simian virus 40 DNA sequences in human lymphomas. *Lancet* 2002; **359**: 851–2.

142. Vilchez RA, Madden CR, Kozinetz CA *et al*. Association between simian virus 40 and non-Hodgkin lymphoma. *Lancet* 2002; **359**: 817–23.

143. Capello D, Rossi D, Gaudino G *et al*. Simian virus 40 infection in lymphoproliferative disorders. *Lancet* 2003; **36**: 88–9.

144. Engels EA, Katki HA, Nielsen NM *et al*. Cancer incidence in Denmark following exposure to poliovirus vaccine contaminated with simian virus 40. *J Natl Cancer Inst* 2003; **95**: 532–9.

145. MacKenzie J, Wilson KS, Perry J *et al*. Association between simian virus 40 DNA and lymphoma in the United kingdom. *J Natl Cancer Inst* 2003; **95**: 1001–3.

146. Engels EA, Viscidi RP, Galloway DA *et al*. Case-control study of simian virus 40 and non-Hodgkin lymphoma in the United States. *J Natl Cancer Inst* 2004; **96**: 1368–74.

147. Brousset P, de Araujo V, Gascoyne RD. Immunohistochemical investigation of SV40 large T antigen in Hodgkin and non-Hodgkin's lymphoma. *Int J Cancer* 2004; **112**: 533–5.

148. Engels EA, Chen J, Hartge P *et al*. Antibody responses to simian virus 40 T antigen: a case-control study of non-Hodgkin lymphoma. *Cancer Epidemiol Biomarkers Prev* 2005; **14**: 521–4.

●149. Duval A, Raphael M, Brennetot C *et al*. The mutator pathway is a feature if immunodeficiency-related lymphomas. *Proc Natl Acad Sci U S A* 2004; **101**: 5002–7.

◆150. Carbone A. Emerging pathways in the development of AIDS-related lymphomas. *Lancet Oncol* 2003; **4**: 22–9.

●151. Knowles DM, Cesarman E, Chadburn A *et al*. Correlative morphologic and molecular genetic analysis demonstrates three distinct categories of posttransplantation lymphoproliferative disorders. *Blood* 1995; **85**: 552–65.

152. Gaidano G, Pastore C, Gloghini A *et al*. Genetic heterogeneity of AIDS-related small non-cleaved cell lymphoma. *Br J Haematol* 1997; **98**: 726–32.

153. Davi F, Delecluse HJ, Guiet P *et al*. Burkitt-like lymphomas in AIDS patients: characterization within a series of 103 human immunodeficiency virus-associated non-Hodgkin's lymphomas. Burkitt's Lymphoma Study Group. *J Clin Oncol* 1998; **16**: 3788–95.

●154. Dalla-Favera R, Martinotti S, Gallo RC *et al*. Translocation and rearrangements of the c-myc oncogene locus in human undifferentiated B-cell lymphomas. *Science* 1983; **219**: 963–7.

155. Pelicci PG, Knowles DM 2nd, Magrath I, Dalla-Favera R. Chromosomal breakpoints and structural alterations of the c-myc locus differ in endemic and sporadic forms of Burkitt lymphoma. *Proc Natl Acad Sci U S A* 1986; **83**: 2984–8.

156. Clark HM, Yano T, Otsuki T *et al*. Mutations in the coding region of c-MYC in AIDS-associated and other aggressive lymphomas. *Cancer Res* 1994; **54**: 3383–6.

●157. Bhatia K, Spangler G, Gaidano G *et al*. Mutations in the coding region of c-myc occur frequently in acquired immunodeficiency syndrome-associated lymphomas. *Blood* 1994; **84**: 883–8.

158. Gu W, Bhatia K, Magrath IT *et al*. Binding and suppression of the Myc transcriptional activation domain by p107. *Science* 1994; **264**: 251–4.

159. Lombardi L, Newcomb EW, Dalla-Favera R. Pathogenesis of Burkitt lymphoma: expression of an activated c-myc oncogene causes the tumorigenic conversion of EBV-infected human B lymphoblasts. *Cell* 1987; **49**: 161–70.

160. McManaway ME, Neckers LM, Loke SL *et al.* Tumour-specific inhibition of lymphoma growth by an antisense oligodeoxynucleotide. *Lancet* 1990; **335**: 808–11.

161. Adams JM, Harris AW, Pinkert CA *et al.* The c-myc oncogene driven by immunoglobulin enhancers induces lymphoid malignancy in transgenic mice. *Nature* 1985; **318**: 533–8.

162. Zhu D, Qi CF, Morse HC 3rd *et al.* Deregulated expression of the MYC cellular oncogenes drives development of mouse 'Burkitt-like' lymphomas from naïve B cells. *Blood* 2005; **105**: 2135–7.

163. Eischen CM, Weber JD, Roussel MF *et al.* Disruption of the ARF-Mdm2-p53 tumor suppressor pathway in Myc-induced lymphomagenesis. *Genes Dev* 1999; **13**: 2658–69.

164. Adhikary S, Eilers M. Transcriptional regulation and transformation by Myc proteins. *Nat Rev Mol Cell Biol* 2005; **6**: 635–45.

165. Sanchez-Beato M, Sanchez-Aguilera A, Piris MA. Cell cycle deregulation in B-cell lymphomas. *Blood* 2003; **101**: 1220–35.

166. Wu KJ, Grandori C, Amacker M *et al.* Direct activation of TERT transcription by c-MYC. *Nat Genet* 1999; **21**: 220–4.

167. Wu KJ, Mattioli M, Morse HC 3rd, Dalla-Favera R. c-MYC activates protein kinase A (PKA) by direct transcriptional activation of the PKA catalytic subunit beta (PKA-Cbeta) gene. *Oncogene* 2002; **21**: 7872–82.

168. Shim H, Dolde C, Lewis BC *et al.* c-MYC transactivation of LDH-A: implications for tumor metabolism and growth. *Proc Natl Acad Sci U S A* 1997; **94**: 6658–63.

●169. Gaidano G, Lo Coco F, Ye BH *et al.* Rearrangements of the BCL-6 gene in acquired immunodeficiency syndrome-associated non-Hodgkin's lymphoma: association with diffuse large-cell subtype. *Blood* 1994; **84**: 397–402.

170. Pasqualucci L, Bereschenko O, Niu H *et al.* Molecular pathogenesis of non-Hodgkin's lymphoma: the role of Bcl-6. *Leuk Lymphoma* 2003; **44**: S5–S12.

171. Cattoretti G, Chang CC, Cechova K *et al.* BCL-6 protein is expressed in germinal-center B cells. *Blood* 1995; **86**: 45–53.

172. Ye BH, Cattoretti G, Shen Q *et al.* The BCL-6 proto-oncogene controls germinal-centre formation and Th2-type inflammation. *Nat Genet* 1997; **16**: 161–70.

173. Ye BH, Lista F, Lo Coco F *et al.* Alterations of a zinc finger-encoding gene, BCL-6, in diffuse large-cell lymphoma. *Science* 1993; **262**: 747–50.

●174. Gaidano G, Carbone A, Pastore C *et al.* Frequent mutation of the 5′ noncoding region of the BCL-6 gene in acquired immunodeficiency syndrome related non-Hodgkin's lymphomas. *Blood* 1997; **89**: 3755–62.

●175. Cesarman E, Chadburn A, Liu YF *et al.* BCL-6 gene mutations in posttransplantation lymphoproliferative disorders predict response to therapy and clinical outcome. *Blood* 1998; **92**: 2294–302.

176. Pasqualucci L, Migliazza A, Basso K *et al.* Mutations of the BCL6 proto-oncogene disrupt its negative autoregulation in diffuse large B-cell lymphoma. *Blood* 2003; **101**: 2914–23.

177. Cattoretti G, Pasqualucci L, Ballon G *et al.* Deregulated BCL6 expression recapitulates the pathogenesis of human diffuse large B cell lymphomas in mice. *Cancer Cell* 2005; **7**: 445–55.

178. Shaffer AL, Yu X, He Y *et al.* BCL-6 represses genes that function in lymphocyte differentiation, inflammation, and cell cycle control. *Immunity* 2000; **13**: 199–212.

179. Lin Y, Wong K, Calame K. Repression of c-myc transcription by Blimp-1, an inducer of terminal B cell differentiation. *Science* 1997; **276**: 596–9.

180. Phan RT, Dalla-Favera R. The BCL-6 proto-oncogene suppresses p53 expression in germinal-centre B cells. *Nature* 2004; **432**: 635–9.

181. Nakamura H, Said JW, Miller CW, Koeffler HP. Mutation and protein expression of p53 in acquired immunodeficiency syndrome-related lymphomas. *Blood* 1993; **82**: 920–6.

182. Das PM, Singal R. DNA methylation and cancer. *J Clin Oncol* 2004; **22**: 4632–42.

183. Rossi D, Gaidano G, Gloghini A *et al.* Frequent aberrant promoter hypermethylation of O6-methylguanine-DNA methyltransferase and death-associated protein kinase genes in immunodeficiency-related lymphomas. *Br J Haematol* 2003; **123**: 475–8.

184. Gerson SL. MGMT: its role in cancer aetiology and cancer therapeutics. *Nat Rev Cancer* 2004; **4**: 296–307.

185. Sakumi K, Shiraishi A, Shimizu S *et al.* Methylnitrosourea-induced tumorigenesis in MGMT gene knockout mice. *Cancer Res* 1997; **57**: 2415–18.

186. Esteller M, Toyota M, Sanchez-Cespedes M *et al.* Inactivation of the DNA repair gene O6-methylguanine-DNA methyltransferase by promoter hypermethylation is associated with G to A mutations in K-ras in colorectal tumorigenesis. *Cancer Res* 2000; **60**: 2368–71.

187. Esteller M, Risques RA, Toyota M *et al.* Promoter hypermethylation of the DNA repair gene O(6)-methylguanine-DNA methyltransferase is associated with the presence of G:C to A:T transition mutations in p53 in human colorectal tumorigenesis. *Cancer Res* 2001; **61**: 4689–92.

188. Ng MH. Death associated protein kinase: from regulation of apoptosis to tumor suppressive functions and B cell malignancies. *Apoptosis* 2002; **7**: 261–70.

189. Raveh T, Droguett G, Horwitz MS *et al.* DAP kinase activates a p19ARF/p53-mediated apoptotic checkpoint to suppress oncogenic transformation. *Nat Cell Biol* 2001; **3**: 1–7.

190. Moll UM, Slade N. p63 and p73: roles in development and tumor formation. *Mol Cancer Res* 2004; **2**: 371–86.

191. Küppers R. Somatic hypermutation and B cell receptor selection in normal and transformed human B cells. *Ann N Y Acad Sci* 2003; **987**: 173–9.

192. Pasqualucci L, Neumeister P, Goossens T *et al.* Hypermutation of multiple proto-oncogenes in B-cell diffuse large-cell lymphomas. *Nature* 2001; **412**: 341–6.

193. Bachmann M, Moroy T. The serine/threonine kinase Pim-1. *Int J Biochem Cell Biol* 2005; **37**: 726–30.

194. Singh H, Medina KL, Pongubala JM. Contingent gene regulatory networks and B cell fate specification. *Proc Natl Acad Sci U S A* 2005; **102**: 4949–53.

195. Preudhomme C, Roumier C, Hildebrand MP *et al*. Nonrandom 4p13 rearrangements of the RhoH/TTF gene, encoding a GTP-binding protein, in non-Hodgkin's lymphoma and multiple myeloma. *Oncogene* 2000; **19**: 2023–32.

●196. Gaidano G, Pasqualucci L, Capello D *et al*. Aberrant somatic hypermutation in multiple subtypes of AIDS-associated non-Hodgkin lymphoma. *Blood* 2003; **102**: 1833–41.

197. Cerri M, Capello D, Muti G *et al*. Aberrant somatic hypermutation in post-transplant lymphoproliferative disorders. *Br J Haematol* 2004; **127**: 362–4.

198. Neri A, Barriga F, Inghirami G *et al*. Epstein-Barr virus infection precedes clonal expansion in Burkitt's and acquired immunodeficiency syndrome-associated lymphoma. *Blood* 1991; **77**: 1092–5.

199. Takada K, Nanbo A. The role of EBERs in oncogenesis. *Semin Cancer Biol* 2001; **11**: 461–7.

200. Niller HH, Salamon D, Ilg K *et al*. The in vivo binding site for oncoprotein c-Myc in the promoter for Epstein-Barr virus (EBV) encoding RNA (EBER) 1 suggests a specific role for EBV in lymphomagenesis. *Med Sci Monit* 2003; **9**: 1–9.

201. Baran-Maeszak F, Fagard R, Girard B *et al*. Gene array identification of Epstein Barr virus-regulated cellular genes in EBV-converted Burkitt lymphoma cell lines. *Lab Invest* 2002; **82**: 1463–79.

202. Cerimele F, Battle T, Lynch R *et al*. Reactive oxygen signalling and MAPK activation distinguish Epstein-Barr virus (EBV)-positive versus EBV-negative Burkitt's lymphoma. *Proc Natl Acad Sci U S A* 2005; **102**: 175–9.

203. Ruf IK, Rhyne PW, Yang H *et al*. Epstein-Barr virus regulates c-MYC, apoptosis and tumorigenicity in Burkitt lymphoma. *Mol Cell Biol* 1999; **19**: 1651–60.

204. Kelly G, Bell A, Rickinson A. Epstein-Barr virus-associated Burkitt lymphomagenesis selects for downregulation of the nuclear antigen EBNA2. *Nat Med* 2002; **8**: 1098–104.

205. Gaidano G, Capello D, Cilia AM *et al*. Genetic characterization of HHV-8/KSHV-positive primary effusion lymphoma reveals frequent mutations of BCL6: implications for disease pathogenesis and histogenesis. *Genes Chromosomes Cancer* 1999; **24**: 16–23.

206. Wilson KS, McKenna RW, Kroft SH *et al*. Primary effusion lymphomas exhibit complex and recurrent cytogenetic abnormalities. *Br J Haematol* 2002; **116**: 113–21.

●207. Klein U, Gloghini A, Gaidano G *et al*. Gene expression profile analysis of AIDS-related primary effusion lymphoma (PEL) suggests a plasmablastic derivation and identifies PEL-specific transcripts. *Blood* 2003; **101**: 4115–21.

208. Fan W, Bubman D, Chadburn A *et al*. Distinct subsets of primary effusion lymphoma can be identified based on their cellular gene expression profile and viral association. *J Virol* 2005; **79**: 1244–51.

209. Carbone A, Gloghini A, Vaccher E *et al*. Kaposi's sarcoma-associated herpesvirus/human herpesvirus type 8-positive solid lymphomas: a tissue-based variant of primary effusion lymphoma. *J Mol Diagn* 2005; **7**:17–27.

●210. Delecluse HJ, Anagnostopoulos I, Dallenbach F *et al*. Plasmablastic lymphomas of the oral cavity: a new entity associated with the human immunodeficiency virus infection. *Blood* 1997; **89**: 1413–20.

211. Carbone A, Gaidano G, Gloghini A *et al*. AIDS-related plasmablastic lymphomas of the oral cavity and jaws: a diagnostic dilemma. *Ann Otol Rhinol Laryngol* 1999; **108**: 95–9.

●212. Carbone A, Gloghini A, Larocca LM *et al*. Human immunodeficiency virus-associated Hodgkin's disease derives from post-germinal center B cells. *Blood* 1999; **93**: 2319–26.

213. Lucioni M, Capello D, Riboni R *et al*. B-cell posttransplant lymphoproliferative disorders in heart and/or lung recipients: clinical and molecular-histogenetic study of 17 cases from a single institution. *Transplantation* 2006; **82**: 1013–23.

214. Leblond V, Davi F, Charlotte F *et al*. Posttransplant lymphoproliferative disorders not associated with Epstein-Barr virus: a distinct entity? *J Clin Oncol* 1998; **16**: 2052–9.

215. Nelson BP, Nalesnik MA, Bahler DW *et al*. Epstein-Barr virus-negative post-transplant lymphoproliferative disorders: a distinct entity? *Am J Surg Pathol* 2000; **24**: 375–85.

216. Dotti G, Fiocchi R, Motta T *et al*. Epstein-Barr virus-negative lymphoproliferate disorders in long-term survivors after heart, kidney, and liver transplant. *Transplantation* 2000; **69**: 827–33.

217. Wood A, Angus B, Kestevan P *et al*. Alpha interferon gene deletions in post-transplant lymphoma. *Br J Haematol* 1997; **98**: 1002–3.

218. Capello D, Cerri M, Muti G *et al*. Analysis of immunoglobulin heavy and light chain variable genes in post-transplant lymphoproliferative disorders. *Hematol Oncol* 2006; **24**: 212–19.

219. Rinaldi A, Kwee I, Poretti G *et al*. Comparative genome-wide profiling of post-transplant lymphoproliferative disorders and diffuse large B-cell lymphomas. *Br J Haematol* 2006; **134**: 27–36.

220. Pekarsky Y, Zanesi N, Aqeilan R, Croce CM. Tcl1 as a model for lymphomagenesis. *Hematol Oncol Clin North Am* 2004; **18**: 863–79.

221. Feng WH, Cohen JI, Fisher S *et al*. Reactivation of latent Epstein-Barr virus by methotrexate: a potential contributor to methotrexate-associated lymphomas. *J Natl Cancer Inst* 2004; **96**: 1691–702.

25

Chronic inflammation, including autoimmunity, and lymphomagenesis

SA PILERI, C AGOSTINELLI, C CAMPIDELLI, F BACCI, E SABATTINI, M GIUNTI, A PILERI,
M PICCIOLI, S RIGHI, M ROSSI, C FERRI AND PP PICCALUGA

Malignant lymphomas can develop within the context of a preexisting chronic inflammatory disorder that may or may not sustain autoimmune phenomena. Basically, the preexisting disorder causes long-lasting reactive lymphoid proliferation with possible emergence of clones carrying chromosomal or genetic aberrations that confer them an advantage over the others in terms of cell proliferation and/or resistance to apoptosis, but are insufficient to carry a tumoral growth. Such aberrations can be facilitated, for instance, by high oxidative levels that generate genomic instability. Defects of the immune surveillance and/or DNA repair mechanisms may further contribute to the survival of the aberrant cells. One of these clones may then develop further abnormalities leading to neoplastic transformation with disconnection from the microenvironment, progressive substitution of the inflammatory milieu, and possible spread through the body. This model of lymphomagenesis (reactive population → clonal selection → malignant transformation) was first demonstrated in human immunodeficiency virus (HIV)-positive patients developing aggressive B cell lymphomas.[1] During the last few decades, it has been extended to a series of lymphoid tumors/clonal lymphoid proliferations ensuing from a chronic inflammation more often sustained by an infective agent. In the following text, the main categories of clonal lymphoproliferations/malignant lymphomas developing within this setting will be discussed in the light of the terminology and concepts introduced first by the Revised European–American Lymphoma (REAL) classification[2] and more recently adopted by the World Health Organization (WHO).[3] They will be divided into three groups depending on their biological significance and correlation with infectious agents and/or an autoimmune background, although the latter two factors are often simultaneously at work. It should be noted that an autoimmune disease will be considered only when it actually represents a favoring condition, but not as a lymphoma-related manifestation. In addition, the term 'atypical lymphoproliferative disorder'[4–6] will be intentionally avoided as it often refers to conditions – like Kikuki lymphadenitis[7] – that can mimic the clinical presentation and/or morphologic features of malignant lymphomas, but do not actually represent lymphoid tumors.

MONOCLONAL PROLIFERATIONS OF UNCERTAIN SIGNIFICANCE

The term monoclonal lymphoproliferative disorder of undetermined significance (MLDUS) was coined to identify lymphoid infiltrates that are often encountered in hepatitis C virus (HCV)-positive patients with type II mixed cryoglobulinemia (MC) and show a prevalent B cell composition with monotonous appearance and immunoglobulin (Ig) monotypic restriction.[8–10] These infiltrates have also been regarded as 'early lymphomas,' since they are sustained by lymphoid components indistinguishable from those of B cell chronic lymphocytic leukemia (CLL) and lympho-plasmacytic lymphoma (LPL).[8–10] However, unlike frank malignant lymphomas, they tend to remain unmodified for years or even decades and are followed by overt lymphoid tumors in about 10 percent of cases.[11,12] These characteristics justify the proposed term of MLDUS.[8–10] Of interest, type II MC-related MLDUS has its highest incidence in the same geographic areas as where approximately 30 percent of 'idiopathic' B cell lymphoma (BCL) patients also display HCV positivity, and where an increased prevalence of HCV genotype 2a/c has been observed in both MC and BCL.[10,13]

In general, cryoglobulinemia is a condition characterized by the presence of one or more immunoglobulins in the serum, which reversibly precipitate at temperatures below 37°C.[14–16] Cryoglobulinemia type I, composed of single monoclonal Ig, represents a paraproteinemia generally associated to lymphoid tumors (LPL, multiple myeloma, etc.).[9,10] It is asymptomatic *per se*, with the exception of the hyperviscosity syndrome. Mixed cryoglobulinemia, type II (polyclonal IgG–monoclonal IgM) or type III (polyclonal IgG–polyclonal IgM), is an immune complex-mediated systemic vasculitis (leukocytoclastic vasculitis) involving small vessels. Mixed cryoglobulinemia may be secondary to various immunologic, hematologic, and infectious diseases, or can represent a distinct disorder, called in the past 'essential' MC.[8–10,17–19] Since the causative role of HCV has been definitely established, the term 'essential' now refers to only a small percentage of patients.[8–10,20] There are no diagnostic criteria for MC. Classification guidelines include: detection of mixed cryoglobulinemia; hypocomplementemia (low C4); leukocytoclastic vasculitis; the typical clinical triad of purpura, weakness, and arthralgias; and multiple organ involvement (liver, kidney, peripheral nerves, and skin).[10]

Type II MC-associated MLDUS presents two main pathological patterns: CLL-like and LPL-like.[8–10,17–21] In the authors' experience, the former is more frequent than the latter. It is characterized by CD79a$^+$/CD5$^+$/CD23$^+$ lymphoid infiltrates in the liver and bone marrow, which consist of small lymphocytes, prolymphocytes, and para-immunoblasts and show moderate Ig expression with monotypic restriction at immunohistochemistry. In serial biopsies, these infiltrates tend to remain unmodified in the bone marrow and may undergo spontaneous regression in the liver in case of cirrhotic evolution, as reported by Monteverde *et al.* in 14 patients with type II MC-related MLDUS.[19] Notably, regression of lymphoid infiltrates in the bone marrow has been observed following antiviral treatment with interferon alone or associated with ribavirin.[11] The high frequency of lymphoplasmacytic/immunocytic morphology reported by others likely reflects the different terminologies used through time (see next paragraph). In any case, the rare cases still classifiable as LPL-like MLDUS

are sustained by a CD79a$^+$/CD5$^-$/CD23$^{-/+}$ population, which consists of small lymphocytes, lymphoplasmacytoid elements, and plasma cells, and expresses cytoplasmic monotypic Ig at high levels.

Only a few studies have been performed at the molecular level. First, the analysis of the B cell component by microdissection immunoglobulin heavy chain gene (IGVH)-polymerase chain reaction (PCR) in 35 portal lymphoid infiltrates from 11 HCV-positive patients (seven with and four without MC type II) showed a single band in 21 infiltrates, two bands in 10, and three bands in 4 cases.[22] Comparison of the IGVH-PCR amplicates obtained from different lymphoid aggregates of the same biopsy revealed that they differed in size. These findings suggest that in the liver each aggregate derives from the proliferation of one or a few unrelated founder B cells. Thus, in spite of the monotypic pattern shown by immunohistochemistry, the lymphoproliferation might be sustained by more than one clone. This hypothesis is strengthened by the observation of De Vita *et al.* that the pattern of B cell expansion in 12/15 bone marrow biopsies from HCV-positive patients with type II MC-associated MLDUS was oligoclonal.[21] Such findings are not surprising if one considers that, in spite of its morphologic and immunohistochemical features, MLDUS does correspond to an Ig production that contains both a polyclonal (IgG) component and a monoclonal (IgM) paraprotein. Within the complex spectrum of HCV-associated lymphoid proliferations, MLDUS can be regarded as a potential but not compulsory step between immune reaction and overt lymphoma (see below on HCV infection and lymphoproliferation).

As a corollary of the above mentioned data, one should be reminded that HCV infection is seen in about 15 percent of patients with monoclonal gammopathy of undetermined significance (MGUS) without cryoglobulinemia.[23] Andreone *et al.* have studied 239 HCV-positive and 98 HCV-negative patients with chronic liver disease. In their series, a monoclonal band in the serum (most often IgG/λ) was detected in 11 percent of HCV-positive patients and 1 percent of HCV-negative individuals ($P = 0.004$). The prevalence of HCV genotype 2a/c was higher in patients with monoclonal gammopathies than in those without (50 percent vs 18 percent; $P = 0.009$). At clinico-pathological analysis, most cases were regarded as examples of MGUS. These cases were characterized by discrete interstitial infiltrates in the bone marrow by typical plasma cells, which not always showed a clear-cut monotypic nature at immunohistochemical analysis; this finding was likely due to the extent of the clone responsible for the M-spike in the serum, which was not sufficiently large to modify the ratio between κ- and λ-producing plasma cells (2–3:1 under physiological conditions). In a few cases, the monoclonal component was sustained by an overt myeloma (see below). These cases of MGUS in HCV-positive patients should be taken apart from the above mentioned MLDUS because of the histologic pattern, usual lack of cryoglobulinemia, and type of M-component in the serum.

MALIGNANT LYMPHOMAS DEVELOPING WITHIN THE CONTEXT OF A CHRONIC INFECTIVE INFLAMMATION

Hepatitis C virus chronic infection–related lymphomas

The prevalence of HCV infection varies significantly all over the world.[9,10] Interestingly, in the geographic areas with a higher incidence of the infection, HCV-positive patients seem to be significantly more at risk of developing a malignant lymphoma than HCV-negative individuals.[9,10,24–27] Although all subtypes of lymphoid tumor can occur in HCV-positive patients, including – in the authors' experience – peripheral T cell lymphoma (PTCL) and Hodgkin lymphoma, by no means is there a definite prevalence of peripheral B cell lymphomas. Only a small minority of these tumors develop in patients with a previous history of MLDUS;[8,9,18] this finding strengthens the concept that lymphomas in HCV-positive patients do not necessarily stem from a preexisting lymphoproliferation, but the virus *per se* might play a relevant role in the process of lymphomagenesis.[9,10,24–26,28,29] The following sections will focus on the more common histotypes of *de novo* malignant lymphoma recorded in HCV-positive patients.

CLL AND LPL

Both these types of lymphoma can be encountered in HCV-positive patients, although in the experience of the authors and other groups they do not represent the commonest histotypes.[29,30] Interestingly, Silvestri *et al.*[26,28,31] reported an impressive association between HCV infection and the 'lymphoplasmacytoid/lymphoplasmacytic immunocytoma' of the updated Kiel classification.[32] The definition of the latter is, however, broader than the one of lymphoplasmacytic lymphoma of the current REAL/WHO classification.[2,3] Thus, it is possible that some mix-up between CLL and LPL was made. In addition, it is unclear whether Silvestri *et al.*[26,28,31] also included in the HCV-positive group examples of MLDUS; this cannot be excluded, taking into account that 94 percent of their HCV-positive immunocytomas were associated with type II MC and all showed a lymphoid infiltrate in the bone marrow significantly lower than that recorded in HCV-unrelated immunocytomas.

MARGINAL ZONE LYMPHOMA

Marginal zone lymphoma (MZL) is rather commonly observed in HCV-positive patients. All the varieties of the tumor can be recorded: extranodal, nodal, and splenic. It has been suggested that in the cases occurring in the node or at extranodal sites other than the stomach, the virus might play the same pathogenetic role as *Helicobacter pylori* in the development of gastric MZL (see below).[11,29,33] The two agents, however, do not seem to be mutually exclusive,

as contemporary positivities for HCV and *H. pylori* have been registered in some instances. Special interest has recently been aroused by the regression of splenic MZL in HCV-positive patients following the clearance of the virus by interferon and ribavirin, a finding that strengthens the cause–effect relationship between HCV infection and lymphoma.[11,34] Within this context, one should be reminded that the usage of specific *IGVH* gene segments has been recorded in HCV-positive patients with both nodal and splenic MZL.[35] In particular, the preferential usage of the V_H 1–69 segment with similar complementarity-determining region 3 s (CDR3s) suggests the presence of a common antigen, probably an HCV antigen epitope, involved in B cell selection, a fact which can also explain possible tumor regression following HCV eradication.

FOLLICULAR LYMPHOMA

Follicular lymphoma represents one of the commonest variety of malignant lymphoma encountered in HCV-positive patients.[29] The possible role of HCV infection in favoring the development of the t(14;18) translocation will be discussed below in the section on HCV infection and lymphoproliferation.

DIFFUSE LARGE B CELL LYMPHOMA

Diffuse large B cell lymphoma (DLBCL) is the commonest form of lymphoid tumor among HCV-positive patients (40–50 percent of cases).[29,30,36] Recently, a new clinicopathologic variant of DLBCL has been described in Japan and the USA, which primarily presents in the liver and sometimes in the spleen and is associated in 71 percent of cases with HCV infection.[37] No study has so far addressed the question as to whether DLBCL in HCV-positive patients carries molecular characteristics (such as a specific gene expression profile) that differ from those reported in HCV-negative cases.

MULTIPLE MYELOMA

The tumor may be detected in HCV-positive individuals (see above) but is indeed rare. Attention should be paid to the so-called extramedullary plasma cell tumors; in fact, most often they correspond to MZL with marked plasma cell differentiation, as shown by immunohistochemistry that – besides monotypic plasma cells – reveals a small B cell component carrying CD27 and possibly the immunoglobulin superfamily receptor translocation-associated 1 (IRTA-1) molecule.[38]

Hepatitis C virus infection and lymphoproliferation

Given the well-known HCV lymphotropism,[39] a direct role of the virus in B cell expansion has been initially hypothesized on the basis of the high frequency of HCV RNA-positive lymphocytes in the peripheral blood and bone marrow of cryoglobulinemic patients, along with the significant percentage of individuals developing malignant lymphomas.[40] Moreover, in patients with chronic HCV infection and BCL, the presence of viral genomic sequences in pathological samples was demonstrated by reverse transcription PCR (RT-PCR), *in situ* hybridization, and immunohistochemical techniques.[41] However, HCV is an RNA virus without reverse transcriptase activity, a fact that prevents its integration in the host genome with possible deregulation of cell functions.

Thus, it is conceivable that HCV exerts an indirect oncogenic action. Special attention has been paid to the possible role of the core protein, although this does not significantly modify the main signaling and transduction pathways.[42] The potential effect of co-infection by HCV and other lymphotropic viruses has been ruled out by two different studies,[43,44] even though *in vitro* experiments have shown that Epstein–Barr virus (EBV) nuclear antigen 1 (EBNA-1) can enhance HCV replication.[45] Several reports have outlined that HCV infection can cause chronic stimulation of the lymphatic system through viral epitopes, autoantigen production, and/or molecular mimicry.[46] The latter has been suggested by the detection of anti-GOR antibodies, which crossreact with both the HCV core and GOR nuclear antigen. However, the pathogenetic role played by these antibodies is still unknown.

Another hypothesis has pointed to the association between HCV and very low density lipoprotein (VLDL) that would induce a T-independent primordial B cell population producing monoclonal Ig with WA idiotype.[47] The rheumatoid factor (RF) activity of WA clones would be a consequence of somatic mutations induced after the stimulation by HCV–VLDL complexes. In this context, the evolution to BCL might be due to the accumulation of stochastic genetic aberrations.[47] Laboratory investigations in HCV-positive type II MC suggest the relevance of B cell chronic stimulation by HCV epitopes that might support the emergence of B cell clones with favorable and/or dominant genetic characteristics. Such a hypothesis recalls the role of *H. pylori* in the development of MZL of the stomach, for which different steps are required: from a polyclonal immune response to oligo-monoclonal phases through the acquisition of genetic modifications. The observation that the HCV E2 protein binds *in vitro* to CD81 (a quite ubiquitous tetraspannin that is well represented on the surface of B cells) has suggested that such interaction might represent one of the causes of the strong and sustained polyclonal stimulation of the B cell compartment.[48] However, a role of the HCV E2/CD81 complex in the pathogenesis of MC and eventually BCL seems to be unlikely due to the lack of sequence homologies between monoclonal rheumatoid factor (mRF) WA, the main mRF in HCV-related type II MC, and anti-HCV E2 antibody.[49]

In the light of the supposed multistep progression of HCV-related lymphoid proliferations, special emphasis has been given to the frequent occurrence of t(14;18) translocation or *BCL2* gene rearrangements in HCV-positive subjects.[50] The consequence of these events is the overexpression of BCL2 protein that leads to inhibition of apoptosis and abnormal B cell survival. Interestingly, the significant prevalence of t(14;18) translocation recorded in individuals with HCV hepatitis (37–38 percent vs 1–2 percent of the normal population) becomes impressive in patients with HCV-related type II MC (85 percent).[50] Several studies – conducted in cohorts from different countries by utilizing similar or complementary techniques[51] – have confirmed that peripheral B cells of HCV-positive patients show frequent association among the above mentioned aberrations, antiapoptotic BCL2 protein overexpression, imbalance of the BCL2/BAX ratio, and clonal expansion. Some observations in patients undergoing antiviral treatment suggest that the maintenance of the expanded B cell clone(s) needs viral replication.[52]

In conclusion, one can hypothesize that during chronic HCV infection several factors, including the interaction between HCV E2 protein and CD81 molecule, the high viral variability, and the persistent infection of both hepatic and lymphoid cells, may favor a sustained and strong B cell activation. The latter may in turn favor the emergence of t(14;18) translocation or other mutagenic effects with BCL2 protein overexpression that is responsible for abnormally prolonged B cell survival. Some predisposing factors, such as a peculiar susceptibility of RF-producing B cells to undergo activation, as well as the presence of HCV epitopes that selectively activate these cells, may result in an elevated production of IgM RF. The prolonged survival of activated B cells favors the development of the MC syndrome and eventually MLDUS. Similarly, the abnormal B cell survival may represent a predisposing condition for further genetic aberrations (such as those involving the *MYC*, *P53*, *BCL6* genes, etc.) that might lead to frank B cell malignancy within the context of or independently of a preexisting type II MC-associated MLDUS. Such a multistep process has found some objective confirmation in the identification of three discrete stages of differentiation of V_H 1–69 B cells in HCV-positive patients with type II MC-associated MLDUS and BCL: naïve (small sized, IgM^{high}, IgD^{high}, CD38$^+$, CD27$^-$, CD21^{high}, CD95$^-$, CD5$^-$), 'early memory' (medium sized, IgM^{high}, IgD^{low}, CD38$^-$, CD27$^+$, CD21^{low}, CD95$^+$, CD5$^+$), and 'late memory' (large sized, IgM^{low}, IgD^{low}, CD38$^-$, CD27^{low}, CD21$^{low/-}$, CD95$^-$, CD5$^-$).[53]

Chronic bacterial infection and extranodal marginal zone lymphoma

In the REAL/WHO classification,[2,3] the term extranodal marginal zone lymphoma (EMZL) is by definition restricted to tumors consisting of slowly proliferating small elements provided with centrocyte-like or monocytoid morphology and associated or not with plasmacytoid differentiation, which are thought to stem from marginal zone (MZ) cells of the mucosal-associated lymphoid tissue (MALT) and share with them phenotypic and molecular characteristics, including IRTA-1 gene expression.[54] According to the original description, these neoplasms are also called MALT lymphomas.[2,3,55]

Mucosal-associated lymphoid tissue is physiologically present in the intestine, where it gives rise to the Peyer patches, and develops *de novo* in the stomach, thyroid, salivary glands, skin, lung, bronchi, etc., due to an inflammatory stimulus produced by an infective agent and/or an autoimmune phenomenon.[55] Following antigen stimulation, MALT elements migrate from the mucosa to the regional nodes, where they complete their functional orientation: 98 percent of these elements return to the original anatomic site, while the remaining ones move to other sites where the MALT system is also represented.[55] The traffic of migrating cells is controlled via a homing receptor ($\alpha_4\beta_7$ integrin) and an adhesion molecule, mucosal vascular addressin molecule-1 (MAdCAM1).[56]

Because of its high prevalence and clinical relevance, MZL of the stomach has been the subject of impressive research activity, which has allowed better understanding of its characteristics including lymphoepithelial lesion formation, multicentricity, pathogenetic relationships to *H. pylori* infection, and susceptibility to antibiotics.

In particular, the pathogenetic link between *H. pylori* chronic gastritis and gastric MZL was first postulated based on epidemiological data showing that the tumor had a higher incidence in geographic areas with endemic *H. pylori* infection.[12,57] The subsequent demonstration – both at the experimental and patient level – of the sensitivity of part of gastric MZL to the antibiotics used for *H. pylori* eradication gave further confirmation of such a link.[12,58–61] Recently, it has been shown that *H. heilmannii* can play the same role in Japanese patients.[62] On pathogenetic grounds, it seems that some *H. pylori* strains (such as the CagA) induce interleukin (IL)-8 production by epithelial elements with activation of neutrophils, increased oxidation, and high risk of genomic alterations.[55,63] This situation might facilitate the onset and survival of clones with the replication error repair phenotype that are incapable of DNA damage repair, especially in subjects with IL-1 RN 2/2 and glutathione-*S*-transferase GST T1 genotypes.[55,64] Within this context, some clones carrying specific chromosomal abnormalities might take advantage over the others, producing a MALT lymphoma whose growth may or may not need microenvironmental support (i.e., *H. pylori* stimulation and T cell cooperation). The latter point is of practical relevance since it affects the susceptibility or insensitivity to antibiotics. During the course of the disease, the cases sensitive to *H. pylori*-eradicating therapies can undergo further clonal progression due to additional genomic aberrations that make the growth independent of the microenvironment. Finally, point mutations or loss of homozygosity of the *P53* gene, *P16* deletion, and *MYC*

rearrangements may produce the switch of the growth from low-grade to high-grade histology.[65]

In the light of the above depicted scenario, it is not surprising that following preliminary reports which suggested that most gastric MZL could regress following *H. pylori* eradication, it is now clear that this event actually occurs in only 50–55 percent of cases.[55] Interestingly, besides the regression of a gastric tumor, antibiotic therapy may at times produce disappearance of a contemporary extranodal MZL at another anatomic site; in one of these cases, a clonal relationship between the two tumors was recently documented in the literature.[66] Ultrasound endoscopy has shown that regression is unlikely in cases with infiltration of the muscularis propria or entire gastric wall, as well as in patients with perigastric lymph node involvement.[67]

Cytogenetic and molecular studies have shown that gastric MZL is characterized by recurrent chromosomal aberrations, which influence its invasive potential and possible response to antibiotics.[68,69] In particular, three chromosomal aberrations have been detected – t(1;14), t(11;18), and t(14;18) – that are possibly involved in the process of lymphomagenesis and affect the course of the disease.[68,69] Translocation t(1;14)(p22;q32) is exceedingly rare and causes the transfer of the *BCL10* gene close to the Ig enhancer on chromosome 14, thus producing overexpression of the corresponding product, which accumulates at the nuclear level and may be provided with oncogenic activity.[70,71] Such a translocation can represent the original lymphoma-promoting event or can occur within a neoplastic population already carrying other chromosomal abnormalities, such as trisomy 3; in any case, it produces insensitivity to antibiotic therapy in the stomach.[71]

Translocation t(11;18)(q21;q21) is detected in 30–35 percent of gastric MZL and produces the formation of the fusion gene *API2-MALT1*.[72] Interestingly, this aberration, which can be reliably detected in routine material by appropriate PCR studies,[73] is also associated with BCL10 protein accumulation within the nucleus of neoplastic cells.[70,71] The explanation of how the same phenomenon can be pursued by seemingly unrelated translocations lies in the observation that under physiologic conditions *BCL10* and *MALT1* products form a strong and specific complex.[74] In particular, BCL10 mediates the oligomerization of the MALT1 caspase-like domain with subsequent activation of the IκB kinase (IKK) complex through an unknown mechanism, setting in motion a cascade of events leading to nuclear factor κB (NF-κB) induction.[75] Furthermore, the API2-MALT1 fusion protein itself seems to strongly activate NF-κB and to show dependence upon the same downstream signaling pathway.[76] Thus, both the BCL10–MALT1 complex and API2-MALT1 fusion protein might activate a common route that originates with the oligomerization-dependent activation of the MALT1 caspase-like domain and leads to resistance to antibiotic therapy.[73–77] Notably, besides antibiotic resistance, t(11;18) is characterized by a higher potential of local infiltration and at-distance spread,[73] as well as by the lack of other chromosomal abnormalities and progression to a more aggressive tumor.[73] Epidemiological studies have recently shown that the translocation is (1) even more frequent in the lung than in the stomach[78] and (2) found also in roughly a half of the rare examples of gastric *H. pylori*–negative MZL,[79] thus further supporting the concept that tumors carrying t(11;18) do not need *H. pylori* stimulation for their growth and maintenance.

The translocation t(14;18)(q32;q21) has been a matter of long debate in the literature. In fact, some authors thought that the translocation at times found in extranodal MZL could correspond to the one typically found in follicular lymphoma (FL) and involving the *BCL2* gene.[2,3] In reality, the t(14;18) of MZL does not affect *BCL2* but *MALT1*, by possibly following the same pathogenetic pathway as t(1;14) and t(11;18). According to the few data in the literature, the translocation involving the Ig enhancer and *MALT1* gene seems to be more frequent at anatomic sites other than the gastrointestinal tract and, like t(1;14), to occur either as the sole genetic abnormality or in conjunction with trisomy 3 and/or 18.[80,81] It should always be distinguished from the translocation involving the *BCL2* gene by fluorescence *in situ* hybridization (FISH) and/or PCR analysis, particularly in light of the fact that FL may at times show prominent MZ differentiation, thus blurring the morphologic borders between the two tumors.[82] Features of MZ differentiation may also occur in mantle cell lymphoma (MCL);[83] under these circumstances, the occurrence of t(11;14) and cyclin D1 overexpression, along with the lack of t(1;14), t(11;18), or t(14;18), does allow the firm distinction of this aggressive neoplasm from MZL. Finally, a novel translocation, t(3;14)(p14.1;q32), has recently been described in EMZL involving the *IGVH* and *FOXP1* genes.[84]

A particular issue relates to the occurrence of a large B cell lymphoma in the stomach as well as at any other MALT site. Several authors have named this tumor 'high-grade MZ/MALT lymphoma.' The latter term has found no room in the REAL/WHO classification[2,3] because of the following reasons: (1) the label 'MALT' lymphoma is by definition restricted to neoplasms showing small cell size and derivation from MALT MZ elements; (2) there is no evidence that a large B cell lymphoma occurring *de novo* at a MALT site is derived from MZ cells; and (3) the clonal relationship between a MZL and a large B cell neoplasm simultaneously detected in the same organ should be molecularly proven, as the latter can actually represent the blastic phase of the former, but might also develop as a second, unrelated neoplasm. In the few cases in which a clonal progression from indolent to aggressive lymphoma has been proven, a loss of expression of $\alpha_4\beta_7$ integrin and L-selectin has been recorded and supposed to take part in the transforming event.[56]

Another issue deals with the response to antibiotic therapy and follow-up of patients with gastric MZL and *H. pylori* infection. First, morphology represents the most effective tool to assess lymphoma regression, as PCR studies can show a monoclonal signal even years following therapy in the absence of any sign of disease relapse.[61] Second, the monitoring of these patients should be performed according to clear-cut guidelines, similar to the ones proposed by the International Extranodal Lymphoma Study Group (IELSG): the first biopsy should be performed one month after the end of the antibiotic treatment to assess *H. pylori* eradication; a second exam should be carried out three months later by taking multiple samples from the area where the diagnosis of lymphoma was originally made and at distant sites in order to evaluate the tumor response.[61] Each sample should be histologically analyzed at different levels to be sure that foci of the disease are not neglected. Recently, a new histological score has been proposed.[85] In principle, in the case of no response to *H. pylori* eradication, the bioptic material should be analyzed by molecular techniques in order to check the possible occurrence of chromosomal aberrations, which would prevent the successful application of antibiotics, thus leading to different treatment options (such as chemotherapy, surgery, radiation therapy, and/or immunotherapy). On the other hand, cases that do show a significant improvement after antibiotic therapy should be indefinitely periodically studied in order to evaluate the maintenance of disease remission or the possible relapse or progression.

The model of gastric *H. pylori*-associated lymphoma has played a role of pivotal value in the field of EMZL. In fact, a significant correlation between chronic infection by bacterial infections and other EMZL has recently been demonstrated. This holds true for *Borrelia burgdorferi*,[86] *Campylobacter jejuni*,[87] *Chlamydia psittaci*,[88,89] *Chlamydia pneumoniae*,[89] *Chlamydia trachomatis*,[89] and *Mycobacterium avium*[90] infections that may trigger the development of MZL in the skin, small intestine (so-called immunoproliferative small intestine disease [IPSID]), ocular adnexal tissues, and lung. Interestingly, all these tumors show, at least in part, sensitivity to specific antibiotics. In addition, IPSID can carry t(9;14) involving the *PAX5* gene.[91]

Epstein–Barr virus infection-related lymphomas

The borders of this section are not sharply defined. In fact, EBV is thought to be involved in the pathogenesis of numerous malignant lymphomas, at least as a cofactor.[92,93]

Primary infection by EBV evokes two main responses, depending on the age of the affected subject and/or maturity of the immune system. If the primary infection occurs in early childhood, the immune response and clinical picture is usually asymptomatic, but the majority of infected older children or adults develop infectious mononucleosis (IM).[93] Following primary infection, an individual maintains a lifelong latent virus infection in which the latency and the eventual virus-driven lymphoproliferation is kept in check by the host immune surveillance.[93] Low-level virus production does occur in the oropharyngeal region, which results in the constant circulation of a few infected B cells (1 in 10^6) in the peripheral blood. Epstein–Barr virus in episomal form is present in normal epithelial and lymphoid cells of the oropharynx by causing different types of latent infection that confer a strong protection against apoptosis and may directly exert a carcinogenic effect by inducing the production of transforming proteins, such as the latent membrane protein 1 (LMP1).[93,94] Such a situation may be altered by a depression of the immune system due to genetic predisposition, concurrent infections with other agents, or iatrogenic conditions. Under these circumstances, there is an increased risk of developing a malignant lymphoma due to the escape of a clone with a survival advantage as the consequence of the protection from apoptosis exerted by the virus and the occurrence of genetic aberrations induced by EBV itself or stochastic events.[95] Such an incident may occur abruptly without previous clinical manifestations – such as in a proportion of classical Hodgkin lymphoma (CHL) cases and natural killer (NK)/T cell lymphoma of the nasal type[2,3] – or develop in patients with a patent inflammatory process.[96] This section will mainly focus on EBV-related/driven lymphomas that develop within the context of a protracted reactive lymphoid proliferation.

BURKITT LYMPHOMA

The first example is endemic Burkitt lymphoma (BL).[2,3] This is characteristically detected in children/adolescents living in the malaria belt of Central Africa and has typical (1) morphology (cohesive growth of highly proliferating medium-sized cells with deeply basophilic, vacuolated cytoplasm and round nuclei with reticulated chromatin and multiple nucleoli, intermingled with starry-sky macrophages phagocytozing nuclear debris);[2,3] (2) phenotype (CD10$^+$, BCL6$^+$, CD38$^+$, BCL2$^-$, Ki-67 = almost 100 percent);[97] and (3) chromosomal aberrations involving the *MYC* gene [i.e., t(8;14)].[2,3,98] Recently, a proportion of endemic BL, however, has been found to differ from this prototypic description by showing plasmacytoid differentiation with CD138 expression, CD30 positivity, and lack of *MYC* rearrangement in 40 percent, 30 percent, and 15 percent of cases, respectively.[99] Neoplastic cells show regular EBV integration in their genome.[98] The virus, however, is not the only causative agent of the tumor. In fact, different conditions can contribute to its development, which represents a classical example of multistep lymphomagenesis. According to van den Bosch,[100] the patients display chronic stimulation of the B cell system due to malaria infection. Subsequent or simultaneous EBV integration induces protection of B cell clones from apoptosis. Further events may be represented by Arbovirus infection (transmitted by mosquitoes, and which boosts the immune reaction) and mutagenic effects of plants, such as *Euphorbia tirucalli*, which are used by children as curative drugs or toys. The latter factor might favor the occurrence of *MYC* rearrangement that definitely transforms an immortalized

selected clone into BL. Such a fascinating hypothesis fits quite well with the histogenesis of African BL, but cannot be applied to the isomorphic form sporadically occurring in Western countries.[2,3] In fact, the latter display EBV integration in a proportion of cases, reaching the 50 percent value in HIV-positive patients, and carry different translocations involving the *MYC* gene [t(2;8) or t(8;22)].[98,100] According to recently published results, it appears that EBV-positive (both endemic and sporadic) and EBV-negative BL (usually sporadic) may originate from two distinct subsets of B cells, pointing to a particular role for the germinal center reaction in the pathogenesis of these tumors.[101] The different types of *MYC* translocation reported in BL may also be related to the different stages of B cell maturation.

PYOTHORAX–ASSOCIATED LYMPHOMA/DLBCL ASSOCIATED WITH CHRONIC INFLAMMATION

Pyothorax-associated lymphoma (PAL) is a pivotal example of DLBCL emerging within the context of chronic inflammation.[102,103] The latter corresponds to pyothorax lasting some decades and resulting from artificial pneumothorax for the treatment of pulmonary tuberculosis or tuberculous pleuritis. Pyothorax-associated lymphoma was first described among Japanese patients,[103] but can actually also occur in Western countries.[104] The patients are predominantly males (male:female ratio = 12.3:1) in the seventh decade of life; the disease is aggressive with dismal prognosis (survival at 5 years about 20 percent). On morphologic grounds, PAL is generally sustained by a DLBCL with features of plasmablastic differentiation, although a T cell origin has exceptionally been recorded.[105] Immunophenotyping displays: (1) monotypic cytoplasmic Ig restriction (that parallels *IGVH* and *IGVL* gene clonal rearrangements); (2) common expression of CD45, B cell markers (CD20, CD79a, CD45RA), and BCL2 protein; (3) high Ki-67 marking; and (4) variable positivity for CD138, interferon regulatory factor 4 (IRF4), and CD30. Notably, most cases reveal EBV integration as shown by the detection of EBV encoded small RNA 1/2 (EBER1/2) at *in situ* hybridization and EBNA2 and LMP1 at immunohistochemistry.[104] Conversely to pleural effusion lymphoma (PEL), PAL does not seem related to human herpes virus 8 (HHV-8) infection. Recent molecular studies have evidenced alterations of the *ATM* and *ATR* genes that might play a role in the process of lymphomagenesis, along with a local immune defect.[106] In particular, the loss of function of such genes can boost the DNA damage produced by free radicals and oxidative stress occurring within the inflammatory lesion. In addition, gene expression profiling has evidenced a set of 348 genes differentially expressed in PAL and nodal DLBCL: these are involved in apoptosis, interferon response, and signal transduction.[107] Finally, it has been noted that tumors with the same characteristics as PAL can occur in the site of metallic implants,[108] pacemaker pockets,[109] or long-standing tuberculous infection.[110]

EPSTEIN–BARR VIRUS-POSITIVE DLBCL OF THE 'ELDERLY'

This is an EBV-positive clonal lymphoid proliferation that occurs in patients over the age of 50 years and without any known immunodeficiency or prior lymphoma.[111] Cases of lymphomatoid granulomatosis, IM, plasmablastic lymphoma, primary effusion lymphoma, and DLBCL associated with chronic inflammation are excluded by definition. The prevalence of EBV-positive DLBCL increases with increasing patient age, with the highest proportion (20–25 percent) seen in those over 90 years of age.[111] The tumor is believed to be related to immunological deterioration or senescence in immunity that is part of the aging process.[111] It presents more often with extranodal disease and behaves aggressively with a median survival of about two years. The neoplastic population may be polymorphic and consist of large cells only. Reed–Sternberg-like elements are commonly found, as well as areas of geographic necrosis.[111] CD20, CD79a, and IRF4 are usually expressed, while CD10 and BCL6 are negative. CD30 is variably present, but CD15 is absent. Epstein–Barr virus is shown by EBER *in situ* hybridization: LMP1 and EBNA2 are detected in 94 percent and 28 percent of cases, respectively.[111]

MALIGNANT LYMPHOMAS DEVELOPING IN IMMUNODEFICIENT PATIENTS

The vast majority of these tumors is indeed related to EBV infection. However, the immune suppression can correspond to different settings that actually sustain a chronic inflammation/reactive lymphoid proliferation.[112–115]

Within this context, one should first of all consider lymphoproliferations associated with *primary immune disorders*, such as ataxia telangiectasia (AT), Wiskott–Aldrich syndrome (WAS), common variable immunodeficiency (CVID), severe combined immune deficiency (SCID), X-linked lymphoproliferative syndrome (XLP), Nijmegen breakage syndrome (NBS), hyper-IgM syndrome, and autoimmune lymphoproliferative syndrome (ALPS).[3] Besides fatal IM (which although characterized by unrestricted polyclonal reaction to EBV infection can turn lethal because of multiorgan failure brought on by anomalous cytotoxic T and NK cell activities and possible hemophagocytic syndrome[92,116–118]), patients with the above mentioned conditions are at risk of developing DLBCL or, more rarely, CHL or PTCL.[3] The lymphomagenic event is frequently preceded by lymphoid hyperplasia or marked plasmacytosis, which can be polyclonal, oligoclonal, or even monoclonal (but self-limiting) and may occur both in the lymph node and at extranodal sites (such as the gastrointestinal tract, liver, gallbladder, and bone marrow). In ALPS, the hyperplastic changes are at times misinterpreted as malignant lymphoma because of the detection of florid germinal centers and prominent paracortical expansion.[119] They reflect the occurrence of *FAS* gene mutations with block of apoptosis, which itself represents a predisposing condition for the development of malignant lymphoma.[120]

A peculiar form of DLBCL is the one included within the spectrum of the so-called lymphomatoid granulomatosis.[121] The latter is an EBV-driven lymphoproliferative disorder[122] that occurs not only in patients with the congenital immunodeficiency, but also in individuals with acquired deficit of the immune response produced by HIV infection or immunosuppression following organ transplantation or with reduced immune function evidenced by clinical or laboratory analysis.[3] The process recognizes three morphologic grades: grade I, sustained by a polymorphic infiltrate lacking cytological atypia; grade II, characterized by the presence of some blasts within a polymorphic background; and grade III, corresponding to an overt DLBCL, often of the T cell-rich type. Interestingly, these three grades relate to the number of EBV-positive B cells and encompass different molecular situations that range from the polyclonality of grade I to clear-cut *IGVH* gene monoclonal rearrangement of grade III. The process shows typical angioinvasiveness and angiocentricity that lead to necrosis and possible vanishing of the lymphoid infiltrates that occurs in the forms of nodules in the lung, brain, kidney, liver, and skin. Lymphomatoid granulomatosis is usually an aggressive disease with a median survival of about two years, although grade III forms may respond to chemotherapy and those of grade I or II to interferon-alpha 2b.[3,123,124]

A more detailed description of immunodeficiency-related lymphoproliferations is found in Chapter 25.

Kaposi sarcoma herpes virus/human herpes virus 8-related lymphoproliferations

Kaposi sarcoma herpes virus/HHV-8 is quite typically associated with lymphoid proliferations.[3] Pleural effusion lymphoma is a prototypic example of such an event. Another interesting association is the one with Castleman disease (CD).[125] This entity – whose nature is still a matter of debate (chronic unspecific inflammation? hamartoma?) – displays three different morphologic varieties (hyaline-vascular, plasmacellular, and mixed) and two presentation modalities (isolated and multicentric). The hyaline-vascular (HV) form is characterized by follicles with a wide mantle zone with onion-skin appearance and a regressed germinal center transformed into a hyaline mass rich in follicular dendritic cells (FDCs) and perforated by vessels. The follicles are separated by an expanded paracortex that contains numerous high endothelial venules. The plasma cell (PC) variant shows normal follicles with florid germinal centers and an extremely abundant plasmacellular component between follicles. Finally, the mixed form displays a combination of the two previously described patterns. The latter finding favors the viewpoint that the different varieties of CD are not different entities, but belong to the morphologic spectrum of the same process. The three above mentioned variants can present as an isolated mass that – in spite of its size (up to 10 cm across) – may be asymptomatic and occur at different sites, the mediastinum being the most commonly affected site.[125] Notably, solitary PC-CD (fewer than 20 percent of cases) is observed in slightly younger individuals than the commoner HV variant (third decade vs fourth decade) and is frequently associated with anemia and elevated erythrocyte sedimentation rate (ESR).[125] In the case of multicentric presentation, the process contemporarily involves multiple lymph nodes. Multicentric CD occurs in the fifth to sixth decade and is often associated with systemic symptoms and abnormal laboratory findings (elevated ESR, anemia, thrombocytopenia, or elevated transaminase values).[125] Conversely to isolated CD that is usually cured by surgery, multicentric CD implies a rather severe prognosis, especially in cases of association with the POEMS (polyneuropathy, organomegaly, endocrinopathy, monoclonal proteins, and skin changes) syndrome.[125,126] Many different therapeutic options have been proposed (chemotherapy, radiation therapy, immune modulators, monoclonal antibodies, and antiviral therapy), but no consensus on a standard strategy has been reached yet. Finally, all variants of CD (both isolated and multicentric) can occur in HIV-positive and HIV-negative patients.[125] Four major problems merit attention in the field of CD: clonality, viral stimulation, pathogenesis, and possible association with malignant lymphomas. Molecular studies show that a proportion of multicentric CD cases, especially of the PC type, carry monoclonal *IGVH* gene rearrangements; these cases may undergo transformation into an overt malignant lymphoma, are frequently associated with POEMS syndrome, and behave more aggressively.[125,127] The relevance of a viral infection in the development of CD has been the subject of a long debate in the literature. As the state of the art, a significant correlation with KSHV/HHV-8 is largely accepted: in particular, evidence of infected lymphoid cells is recorded in about 40 percent of the HIV-negative cases and in most if not all the HIV-positive cases, irrespectively of the morphologic variant.[128] On pathogenetic grounds, the initial step of CD might be the production of IL-6 by mantle B cells, stimulated in the majority of cases by KSHV/HHV-8 (which induces production of a viral IL-6 analogue by infected cells) and in a minority by a not-yet identified endogenous or exogenous factor.[129] Local elaboration of IL-6 and, in turn, vascular endothelial growth factor (VEGF), produces the characteristic B cell proliferation and vascularization of CD. In patients with multicentric CD, systemic symptoms may result from the circulation of IL-6 or IL-6-producing B lymphocytes, the generation of excess antibodies, or disseminated HHV-8 infection.[130] Finally, association with malignant lymphoma has been repeatedly reported in the literature: although more commonly recorded in patients with multicentric CD, it can also occur in isolated CD cases. All types of lymphoma have been detected in conjunction with CD, from CLL to CHL,[125,131] although the incidence of plasmablastic lymphoma seems to be somewhat higher.[132] Within this context, one should be reminded that CD may be associated with FDC sarcoma: a pathogenetic link between the two

entities has been proposed, although it is still a matter of speculation.[133]

MALIGNANT LYMPHOMAS AND AUTOIMMUNE DISEASES

Although basically differing in their pathogenesis, diagnostics, and treatment, autoimmune diseases and malignant lymphomas share a series of factors. Deregulation of apoptosis occurs in both conditions: it may be sustained by an excess of B cell activating factor (BAFF), mutation of CD95/Fas ligand, or overexpression of the BCL-2 protein.[134] The latter two phenomena affect, for example, T cells of patients with Sjögren syndrome (SS) leading to persisting autoreactive B cell clones in the exocrine glands that have a lymphomatous potential.[135] The recent detection of Fas$^{+/-}$ mutations (so-called Canale-Smith syndrome) represents a further example of the close relationships between malignant lymphomas and autoimmune diseases.[136] Infections by bacteria (*H. pylori*) or viruses (EBV, HCV, HIV, and human T cell lymphotrophic virus 1) can be concomitant, thus blurring the borders between idiopathic autoimmune disease and the above mentioned bacteria- or virus-driven lymphoid proliferations. For instance, it is a matter of debate whether the diagnosis of SS – an autoimmune disease that mainly affects the exocrine glands and presents with dryness of the mouth and eyes – should be made in HCV-positive patients.[137] Exclusion criteria have been proposed,[138] however, that are applicable to only 15 percent of HCV-positive subjects with SS. In fact, the latter can also show anti-La/SS-B and anti-Ro/SS-A antibodies.[137] In general, HCV-associated SS reveals a predilection for older males and higher prevalence of cryoglobulinemia, RF, and hypocomplementemia, along with cutaneous vasculitis and peripheral neuropathy.[137] Expansion of CD5$^+$ cells can be detected in both autoimmune diseases and malignant lymphomas, although are polyclonal/oligoclonal in the former and monoclonal in the latter.[136] Changes in the cytokine network (e.g., IL-3, IL-4, surface IL-2 receptor, and interferon γ) have also been recorded.[136] Based on these elements, it is not surprising that patients with autoimmune diseases are at risk of developing malignant lymphomas. Marginal zone lymphomas are not infrequently observed in the course of Hashimoto thyroiditis, in the small bowel of patients with gluten-sensitive enteropathy, and in subjects with SS;[136] transition from reactive lymphoid proliferation to overt malignant lymphoma has been convincingly documented. On the other hand, the correlation between autoimmune diseases and malignant lymphomas is looser in other settings: although patients with lupus erythematosus and rheumatoid arthritis are also at risk of malignant lymphoma, it is unclear whether or not this is due to the disease itself or to the drugs used in therapy.[136]

Finally, peripheral T cell lymphoma of the enteropathy type (ETL) developing in patients with celiac disease represents another example of malignant lymphoma ensuing from a reactive lymphoid proliferation.[3,139] Genetic predisposition and gliadin exposure play a pivotal role in the development of celiac disease.[140] The diagnosis is made on the detection of malabsorption, anemia, and osteoporosis, as well as the presence of anti-endomysial and anti-gliadin antibodies.[140] Microscopic examination shows intestinal changes ranging from an increase of intraepithelial CD8 T lymphocytes (IEL) in a normal mucosa (40 per 100 enterocytes) to villous atrophy and crypt hyperplasia.[140] All these findings can regress following a gluten-free diet. Failure to the latter leads some of the patients to develop refractory sprue.[140,141] These patients may have normal IEL and benefit from immunosuppressive therapy or show abnormal IEL (lacking CD3ε, CD8, or T cell receptor and harboring T cell receptor clonal rearrangements).[141] Abnormal IEL are considered as a cryptic or *in situ* form of ETL.[142] Interestingly, ETL can also develop in patients with celiac disease without an atypical phase.[140] Recent studies have shown that celiac disease corresponds to a T helper 1 (TH1)-mediated inflammatory response with increase of IFNγ, IL-18, and transcription factor T-bet.[143,144] The latter is expressed by all CD8$^+$ and CD4$^+$ T cells in celiac disease, restricted to CD8$^+$ elements in cryptic ETL, and is variable in overt ETL (with total negativity of cases with anaplastic morphology).[3]

Within this context, one should quote the iatrogenic lymphoproliferative disorders (ILPDs) that arise in patients treated with immunosuppressive drugs for autoimmune diseases such as rheumatoid arthritis, inflammatory bowel disease, psoriasis, and psoriasic arthritis. These processes usually present with the morphologic and molecular features of frank malignant lymphomas that only in part carry EBV integration.[145] Methotrexate[146] was the first reported immunosuppressive drug to be associated with ILPDs, followed by other agents including the tumor necrosis factor α (TNFα) blockers infliximab and etanercept.[147,148] Interestingly, a striking association between hepatosplenic T cell lymphoma and the administration of infliximab in combination with azathioprin and/or 6-mercaptopurine has recently been reported.[149] Therapy withdrawal produces at least partial ILPD regression in about 60 percent of patients receiving methotrexate but not TNFα blockers.[149]

KEY POINTS

- Malignant lymphomas can develop within the context of chronic inflammation irrespective of the condition that sustains it.
- This is the result of prolonged lymphoid proliferation, possible high oxidative levels, impaired immune surveillance, and/or a defect of DNA repair, which cause the onset and selection of aberrant clones. Due to progressive accumulation of chromosomal or genetic alterations, the latter eventually undergo malignant transformation.
- The resulting model of lymphomagenesis can be summarized as follows: reactive population → clonal selection → malignant transformation.
- Such a model can be first applied to HCV-driven lymphoproliferative reactions that lead to monoclonal proliferations of uncertain significance and/or overt malignant lymphoma such as chronic lymphocytic leukemia, lymphoplasmacytic lymphoma, marginal zone lymphoma, follicular lymphoma, diffuse large B cell lymphoma, or multiple myeloma.
- Second, it attains chronic bacterial infections (due to *Helicobacter pylori*, *Borrelia burgdorferi*, *Campylobacter jejuni*, *Chlamydia psittaci*, *Chlamydia pneumoniae*, *Chlamydia trachomatis*, and *Mycobacterium avium*) and extranodal marginal zone lymphoma.
- Third, it corresponds to a series of EBV- or HHV-8–related lymphomas, as clearly outlined in the recently published *WHO Classification of Tumours of the Haematopoietic and Lymphoid Tissues*.

REFERENCES

● = Key primary paper

◆ = Major review article

●1. Pelicci PG, Knowles DM 2nd, Arlin ZA *et al.* Multiple monoclonal B cell expansions and c-myc oncogene rearrangements in acquired immune deficiency syndrome-related lymphoproliferative disorders. Implications for lymphomagenesis. *J Exp Med* 1986; **164**: 2049–60.

◆2. Harris NL, Jaffe ES, Stein H *et al.* A revised European-American classification of lymphoid neoplasms: a proposal from the International Lymphoma Study Group. *Blood* 1994; **84**: 1361–92.

◆3. Swerdlow SH, Campo E, Harris NL *et al.* (eds) *WHO classification of tumours of haematopoietic and lymphoid tissues*, 4th edn. Lyon: IARC Press, 2008.

●4. Attygalle AD, Liu H, Shirali S *et al.* Atypical marginal zone hyperplasia of mucosa-associated lymphoid tissue: a reactive condition of childhood showing immunoglobulin lambda light-chain restriction. *Blood* 2004; **104**: 3343–8.

5. Kojima M, Motoori T, Hosomura Y *et al.* Atypical lymphoplasmacytic and immunoblastic proliferation from rheumatoid arthritis: a case report. *Pathol Res Pract* 2006; **202**: 51–4.

6. Ma YC, Shyur SD, Ho TY *et al.* Wiskott-Aldrich syndrome complicated by an atypical lymphoproliferative

disorder: a case report. *J Microbiol Immunol Infect* 2005; **38**: 289–92.

7.   Pileri SA, Pileri A, Yasukawa K *et al.* The karma of Kikuchi's disease. *Clin Immunol* 2005; **114**: 27–9.

◆8. Monteverde A, Pileri S. Lymphoproliferative diseases of uncertain classification. *Ann Ital Med Int* 1991; **6**: 162–70.

9.   Ferri C, Pileri S, Zignego AL *et al.* Hepatitis C virus, B-cell disorders, and non-Hodgkin's lymphoma. In: Goedert JJ. (ed.) *Infectious causes of cancer. Targets for intervention.* Totowa, New Jersey: National Cancer Institute, The Humana Press Inc., 2000: 349–68.

10. Ferri C, Zignego AL, Pileri SA. Cryoglobulins. *J Clin Pathol* 2002; **55**: 4–13.

●11. Arcaini L, Paulli M, Boveri E *et al.* Marginal zone-related neoplasms of splenic and nodal origin. *Haematologica* 2003; **88**: 80–93.

12. Muller AM, Ihorst G, Mertelsmann R, Engelhardt M. Epidemiology of non-Hodgkin's lymphoma (NHL): trends, geographic distribution, and etiology. *Ann Hematol* 2005; **84**: 1–12.

13. Lenzi M, Johnson PJ, McFarlane IG *et al.* Antibodies to hepatitis C virus in autoimmune liver disease: evidence for geographical heterogeneity. *Lancet* 1991; **338**: 277–80.

14. Meltzer M, Franklin EC. Cryoglobulinemia – a study of twenty-nine patients. I. IgG and IgM cryoglobulins and factors affecting cryoprecipitability. *Am J Med* 1966; **40**: 828–36.

15. Meltzer M, Franklin EC, Elias K *et al.* Cryoglobulinemia – a clinical and laboratory study. II. Cryoglobulins with rheumatoid factor activity. *Am J Med* 1966; **40**: 837–56.

16. Brouet JC, Clauvel JP, Danon F *et al.* Biologic and clinical significance of cryoglobulins. A report of 86 cases. *Am J Med* 1974; **57**: 775–88.

●17. Monteverde A, Rivano MT, Allegra GC *et al.* Essential mixed cryoglobulinemia, type II: a manifestation of a low-grade malignant lymphoma? Clinical-morphological study of 12 cases with special reference to immunohistochemical findings in liver frozen sections. *Acta Haematol* 1988; **79**: 20–5.

18. Monteverde A, Ballare M, Bertoncelli MC *et al.* Lymphoproliferation in type II mixed cryoglobulinemia. *Clin Exp Rheumatol* 1995; **13**(Suppl 13): S141–7.

19. Monteverde A, Ballare M, Pileri S. *et al.* Hepatic lymphoid aggregates in chronic hepatitis C and mixed cryoglobulinemia. *Springer Semin Immunopathol* 1997; **19**: 99–110.

●20. Ferri C, Greco F, Longombardo G *et al.* Association between hepatitis C virus and mixed cryoglobulinemia. *Clin Exp Rheumatol* 1991; **9**: 621–4.

21. De Vita S, De Re V, Gasparotto D *et al.* Oligoclonal non-neoplastic B cell expansion is the key feature of type II mixed cryoglobulinemia: clinical and molecular findings do not support a bone marrow pathologic diagnosis of indolent B cell lymphoma. *Arthritis Rheum* 2000; **43**: 94–102.

22. Magalini AR, Facchetti F, Salvi L *et al.* Clonality of B-cells in portal lymphoid infiltrates of HCV-infected livers. *J Pathol* 1998; **185**: 86–90.

23. Andreone P, Zignego AL, Cursaro C *et al.* Prevalence of monoclonal gammopathies in patients with hepatitis C virus infection. *Ann Intern Med* 1998; **129**: 294–8.

24. Luppi M, Grazia Ferrari M, Bonaccorsi G *et al.* Hepatitis C virus infection in subsets of neoplastic lymphoproliferations not associated with cryoglobulinemia. *Leukemia* 1996; **10**: 351–5.

25. Pioltelli P, Zehender G, Monti G *et al.* HCV and non-Hodgkin lymphoma. *Lancet* 1996; **347**: 624–5.

26. Silvestri F, Pipan C, Barillari G *et al.* Prevalence of hepatitis C virus infection in patients with lymphoproliferative disorders. *Blood* 1996; **87**: 4296–301.

27. Gisbert JP, Garcia-Buey L, Arranz R *et al.* The prevalence of hepatitis C virus infection in patients with non-Hodgkin's lymphoma. *Eur J Gastroenterol Hepatol* 2004; **16**: 135–8.

28. Silvestri F, Baccarani M. Hepatitis C virus-related lymphomas. *Br J Haematol* 1997; **99**: 475–80.

29. Luppi M, Longo G, Ferrari MG *et al.* Clinico-pathological characterization of hepatitis C virus-related B-cell non-Hodgkin's lymphomas without symptomatic cryoglobulinemia. *Ann Oncol* 1998; **9**: 495–8.

30. Trepo C, Berthillon P, Vitvitski L. HCV and lymphoproliferative diseases. *Ann Oncol* 1998; **9**: 469–70.

31. Silvestri F, Sperotto A, Fanin R. Hepatitis C and lymphoma. *Curr Oncol Rep* 2000; **2**: 172–5.

32. Stansfeld AG, Diebold J, Noel H *et al.* Updated Kiel classification for lymphomas. *Lancet* 1988; **1**: 292–3.

33. De Vita S, Sansonno D, Dolcetti R *et al.* Hepatitis C virus within a malignant lymphoma lesion in the course of type II mixed cryoglobulinemia. *Blood* 1995; **86**: 1887–92.

●34. Hermine O, Lefrere F, Bronowicki JP *et al.* Regression of splenic lymphoma with villous lymphocytes after treatment of hepatitis C virus infection. *N Engl J Med* 2002; **347**: 89–94.

35. Marasca R, Vaccari P, Luppi M *et al.* Immunoglobulin gene mutations and frequent use of VH1-69 and VH4-34 segments in hepatitis C virus-positive and hepatitis C virus-negative nodal marginal zone B-cell lymphoma. *Am J Pathol* 2001; **159**: 253–61.

●36. Ramos-Casals M, Trejo O, Garcia-Carrasco M *et al.* Triple association between hepatitis C virus infection, systemic autoimmune diseases, and B cell lymphoma. *J Rheumatol* 2004; **31**: 495–9.

37. Izumi T, Sasaki R, Miura Y, Okamoto H. Primary hepatosplenic lymphoma: association with hepatitis C virus infection. *Blood* 1996; **87**: 5380–1.

38. Went P, Ascani S, Strom E *et al.* Nodal marginal-zone lymphoma associated with monoclonal light-chain and heavy-chain deposition disease. *Lancet Oncol* 2004; **5**: 381–3.

39. Zignego AL, Macchia D, Monti M *et al.* Infection of peripheral mononuclear blood cells by hepatitis C virus. *J Hepatol* 1992; **15**: 382–6.

40. Zignego AL, Ferri C, Monti M *et al.* Hepatitis C virus as a lymphotropic agent: evidence and pathogenetic implications. *Clin Exp Rheumatol* 1995; **13(Suppl 13)**: S33–7.

41. Sansonno D, Iacobelli AR, Cornacchiulo V *et al.* Detection of hepatitis C virus (HCV) proteins by immunofluorescence and HCV RNA genomic sequences by non-isotopic in situ hybridization in bone marrow and peripheral blood mononuclear cells of chronically HCV-infected patients. *Clin Exp Immunol* 1996; **103**: 414–21.

42. Giannini C, Caini P, Giannelli F *et al.* Hepatitis C virus core protein expression in human B-cell lines does not significantly modify main proliferative and apoptosis pathways. *J Gen Virol* 2002; **83**: 1665–71.

43. Ferri C, Lo Jacono F, Monti M *et al.* Lymphotropic virus infection of peripheral blood mononuclear cells in B-cell non-Hodgkin's lymphoma. *Acta Haematol* 1997; **98**: 89–94.

44. Bates I, Bedu-Addo G, Jarrett RF *et al.* B-lymphotropic viruses in a novel tropical splenic lymphoma. *Br J Haematol* 2001; **112**: 161–6.

45. Sugawara Y, Makuuchi M, Kato N *et al.* Enhancement of hepatitis C virus replication by Epstein-Barr virus-encoded nuclear antigen 1. *EMBO J* 1999; **18**: 5755–60.

●46. Ferri C, Longombardo G, La Civita L *et al.* Hepatitis C virus chronic infection as a common cause of mixed cryoglobulinaemia and autoimmune liver disease. *J Intern Med* 1994; **236**: 31–6.

◆47. Agnello V. Hepatitis C virus infection and type II cryoglobulinemia: an immunological perspective. *Hepatology* 1997; **26**: 1375–9.

48. Pileri P, Uematsu Y, Campagnoli S *et al.* Binding of hepatitis C virus to CD81. *Science* 1998; **282**: 938–41.

49. Knight G, Agnello V. WA monoclonal rheumatoid factors and non-Hodgkin lymphoma. *Blood* 2001; **97**: 3319–21.

●50. Zignego AL, Ferri C, Giannelli F *et al.* Prevalence of bcl-2 rearrangement in patients with hepatitis C virus-related mixed cryoglobulinemia with or without B-cell lymphomas. *Ann Intern Med* 2002; **137**: 571–80.

51. Zuckerman E, Zuckerman T, Sahar D *et al.* The effect of antiviral therapy on t(14;18) translocation and immunoglobulin gene rearrangement in patients with chronic hepatitis C virus infection. *Blood* 2001; **97**: 1555–9.

52. Carbonari M, Caprini E, Tedesco T *et al.* Hepatitis C virus drives the unconstrained monoclonal expansion of VH1-69-expressing memory B cells in type II cryoglobulinemia: a model of infection-driven lymphomagenesis. *J Immunol* 2005; **174**: 6532–9.

53. Giannelli F, Moscarella S, Giannini C *et al.* Effect of antiviral treatment in patients with chronic HCV infection and t(14;18) translocation. *Blood* 2003; **102**: 1196–201.

●54. Falini B, Tiacci E, Pucciarini A *et al.* Expression of the IRTA1 receptor identifies intraepithelial and subepithelial marginal zone B cells of the mucosa-associated lymphoid tissue (MALT). *Blood* 2003; **102**: 3684–92.

◆55. Isaacson PG. Gastric MALT lymphoma: from concept to cure. *Ann Oncol* 1999; **10**: 637–45.

56. Liu YX, Yoshino T, Ohara N *et al.* Loss of expression of alpha4beta7 integrin and L-selectin is associated with high-grade progression of low-grade MALT lymphoma. *Mod Pathol* 2001; **14**: 798–805.

57. Doglioni C, Wotherspoon AC, Moschini A *et al.* High incidence of primary gastric lymphoma in northeastern Italy. *Lancet* 1992; **339**: 834–5.

●58. Wotherspoon AC, Doglioni C, Diss TC *et al.* Regression of primary low-grade B-cell gastric lymphoma of mucosa-associated lymphoid tissue type after eradication of *Helicobacter pylori*. *Lancet* 1993; **342**: 575–7.

59. Wotherspoon AC, Doglioni C, de Boni M *et al.* Antibiotic treatment for low-grade gastric MALT lymphoma. *Lancet* 1994; **343**: 1503.

60. Neubauer A, Thiede C, Morgner A *et al.* Cure of *Helicobacter pylori* infection and duration of remission of low-grade gastric mucosa-associated lymphoid tissue lymphoma. *J Natl Cancer Inst* 1997; **89**: 1350–5.

61. Bertoni F, Conconi A, Capella C *et al.* Molecular follow-up in gastric mucosa-associated lymphoid tissue lymphomas: early analysis of the LY03 cooperative trial. *Blood* 2002; **99**: 2541–4.

62. Okiyama Y, Matsuzawa K, Hidaka E *et al.* *Helicobacter heilmannii* infection: clinical, endoscopic and histopathological features in Japanese patients. *Pathol Int* 2005; **55**: 398–404.

●63. Lenze D, Berg E, Volkmer-Engert R *et al.* Influence of antigen on the development of MALT lymphoma. *Blood* 2006; **107**: 1141–8.

64. Rollinson S, Levene AP, Mensah FK *et al.* Gastric marginal zone lymphoma is associated with polymorphisms in genes involved in inflammatory response and antioxidative capacity. *Blood* 2003; **102**: 1007–11.

65. Du MQ. Molecular biology of gastric MALT lymphoma: application in clinical management. *Hematology* 2002; **7**: 339–44.

66. Caletti G, Togliani T, Fusaroli P *et al.* Consecutive regression of concurrent laryngeal and gastric MALT lymphoma after anti-*Helicobacter pylori* therapy. *Gastroenterology* 2003; **124**: 537–43.

67. Caletti G, Zinzani PL, Fusaroli P *et al.* The importance of endoscopic ultrasonography in the management of low-grade gastric mucosa-associated lymphoid tissue lymphoma. *Aliment Pharmacol Ther* 2002; **16**: 1715–22.

◆68. Farinha P, Gascoyne RD. Molecular pathogenesis of mucosa-associated lymphoid tissue lymphoma. *J Clin Oncol* 2005; **23**: 6370–8.

69. Inagaki H, Nakamura T, Li C *et al.* Gastric MALT lymphomas are divided into three groups based on responsiveness to *Helicobacter Pylori* eradication and detection of API2-MALT1 fusion. *Am J Surg Pathol* 2004; **28**: 1560–7.

70. Maes B, Demunter A, Peeters B, De Wolf-Peeters C. BCL10 mutation does not represent an important pathogenic mechanism in gastric MALT-type lymphoma, and the presence of the API2-MLT fusion is associated

with aberrant nuclear BCL10 expression. *Blood* 2002; **99**: 1398–404.

71. Ye H, Gong L, Liu H *et al.* Strong BCL10 nuclear expression identifies gastric MALT lymphomas that do not respond to *H pylori* eradication. *Gut* 2006; **55**: 137–8.

72. Baens M, Maes B, Steyls A *et al.* The product of the t(11;18), an API2-MLT fusion, marks nearly half of gastric MALT type lymphomas without large cell proliferation. *Am J Pathol* 2000; **156**: 1433–9.

73. Liu H, Ye H, Ruskone-Fourmestraux A *et al.* T(11;18) is a marker for all stage gastric MALT lymphomas that will not respond to *H. pylori* eradication. *Gastroenterology* 2002; **122**: 1286–94.

74. Nakamura K, Senda T, Sato K *et al.* Accumulation of BCL10 at the perinuclear region is required for the BCL10-mediated nuclear factor-kappa B activation. *Pathobiology* 2005; **72**: 191–202.

●75. Lucas PC, Yonezumi M, Inohara N *et al.* Bcl10 and MALT1, independent targets of chromosomal translocation in malt lymphoma, cooperate in a novel NF-kappa B signaling pathway. *J Biol Chem* 2001; **276**: 19012–9.

●76. Ho L, Davis RE, Conne B *et al.* MALT1 and the API2-MALT1 fusion act between CD40 and IKK and confer NF-kappa B-dependent proliferative advantage and resistance against FAS-induced cell death in B cells. *Blood* 2005; **105**: 2891–9.

77. Yeh KH, Kuo SH, Chen LT *et al.* Nuclear expression of BCL10 or nuclear factor kappa B helps predict *Helicobacter pylori*-independent status of low-grade gastric mucosa-associated lymphoid tissue lymphomas with or without t(11;18)(q21;q21). *Blood* 2005; **106**: 1037–41.

●78. Okabe M, Inagaki H, Ohshima K *et al.* API2-MALT1 fusion defines a distinctive clinicopathologic subtype in pulmonary extranodal marginal zone B-cell lymphoma of mucosa-associated lymphoid tissue. *Am J Pathol* 2003; **162**: 1113–22.

79. Ye H, Liu H, Raderer M *et al.* High incidence of t(11;18)(q21;q21) in *Helicobacter pylori*-negative gastric MALT lymphoma. *Blood* 2003; **101**: 2547–50.

●80. Streubel B, Lamprecht A, Dierlamm J *et al.* T(14;18)(q32;q21) involving IGH and MALT1 is a frequent chromosomal aberration in MALT lymphoma. *Blood* 2003; **101**: 2335–9.

81. Ye H, Gong L, Liu H *et al.* MALT lymphoma with t(14;18)(q32;q21)/IGH-MALT1 is characterized by strong cytoplasmic MALT1 and BCL10 expression. *J Pathol* 2005; **205**: 293–301.

82. Yegappan S, Schnitzer B, Hsi ED. Follicular lymphoma with marginal zone differentiation: microdissection demonstrates the t(14;18) in both the follicular and marginal zone components. *Mod Pathol* 2001; **14**: 191–6.

83. Anagnostopoulos I, Foss HD, Hummel M *et al.* Extranodal mantle cell lymphoma mimicking marginal zone cell lymphoma. *Histopathology* 2001; **39**: 561–5.

●84. Streubel B, Vinatzer U, Lamprecht A *et al.* T(3;14)(p14.1;q32) involving IGH and FOXP1 is a novel recurrent chromosomal aberration in MALT lymphoma. *Leukemia* 2005; **19**: 652–8.

●85. Copie-Bergman C, Gaulard P, Lavergne-Slove A *et al.* Proposal for a new histological grading system for post-treatment evaluation of gastric MALT lymphoma. *Gut* 2003; **52**: 1656.

●86. Goodlad JR, Davidson MM, Hollowood K *et al.* Primary cutaneous B-cell lymphoma and *Borrelia burgdorferi* infection in patients from the Highlands of Scotland. *Am J Surg Pathol* 2000; **24**: 1279–85.

●87. Lecuit M, Abachin E, Martin A *et al.* Immunoproliferative small intestinal disease associated with *Campylobacter jejuni*. *N Engl J Med* 2004; **350**: 239–48.

●88. Ferreri AJ, Ponzoni M, Guidoboni M *et al.* Regression of ocular adnexal lymphoma after *Chlamydia psittaci*-eradicating antibiotic therapy. *J Clin Oncol* 2005; **23**: 5067–73.

●89. Chanudet E, Adam P, Nicholson AG *et al.* Chlamydiae and Mycoplasma infections in pulmonary MALT lymphoma. *Br J Cancer* 2007; **97**: 949–51.PMID: 17876330

●90. Gaur S, Trayner E, Aish L, Weinstein R. Bronchus-associated lymphoid tissue lymphoma arising in a patient with bronchiectasis and chronic *Mycobacterium avium* infection. *Am J Hematol* 2004; **77**: 22–5.

◆91. Al-Saleem T, Al-Mondhiry H. Immunoproliferative small intestinal disease (IPSID): a model for mature B-cell neoplasms. *Blood* 2005; **105**: 2274–80.

◆92. Cohen JI. Benign and malignant Epstein-Barr virus-associated B-cell lymphoproliferative diseases. *Semin Hematol* 2003; **40**: 116–23.

93. Greiner T. Atypical immune lymphoproliferations. In: Hoffman R, Benz EJ, Shattil SJ *et al.* (eds) *Hematology. Basic principles and practice.* Philadelphia, PA: Elsevier Churchill Livingstone, 2005: 1561–74.

94. Herbst H, Dallenbach F, Hummel M *et al.* Epstein-Barr virus latent membrane protein expression in Hodgkin and Reed-Sternberg cells. *Proc Natl Acad Sci U S A* 1991; **88**: 4766–70.

95. Okano M, Thiele GM, Davis JR *et al.* Epstein-Barr virus and human diseases: recent advances in diagnosis. *Clin Microbiol Rev* 1988; **1**: 300–12.

●96. Aozasa K, Takakuwa T, Nakatsuka S. Pyothorax-associated lymphoma: a lymphoma developing in chronic inflammation. *Adv Anat Pathol* 2005; **12**: 324–31.

97. Spina D, Leoncini L, Megha T *et al.* Cellular kinetic and phenotypic heterogeneity in and among Burkitt's and Burkitt-like lymphomas. *J Pathol* 1997; **182**: 145–50.

◆98. Bellan C, Lazzi S, De Falco G *et al.* Burkitt's lymphoma: new insights into molecular pathogenesis. *J Clin Pathol* 2003; **56**: 188–92.

●99. Tumwine LK, Campidelli C, Righi S *et al.* B-cell non-Hodgkin lymphomas in Uganda: an immunohistochemical appraisal on tissue microarray. *Hum Pathol* 2008; **39**: 817–23.

◆100. van den Bosch CA. Is endemic Burkitt's lymphoma an alliance between three infections and a tumour promoter? *Lancet Oncol* 2004; **5**: 738–46.

●101. Bellan C, Lazzi S, Hummel M *et al.* Immunoglobulin gene analysis reveals 2 distinct cells of origin for EBV-positive and EBV-negative Burkitt lymphomas. *Blood* 2005; **106**: 1031-6.

102. Fukayama M, Ibuka T, Hayashi Y *et al.* Epstein-Barr virus in pyothorax-associated pleural lymphoma. *Am J Pathol* 1993; **143**: 1044-9.

◆103. Nakatsuka S, Yao M, Hoshida Y *et al.* Pyothorax-associated lymphoma: a review of 106 cases. *J Clin Oncol* 2002; **20**: 4255-60.

104. Ascani S, Piccioli M, Poggi S *et al.* Pyothorax-associated lymphoma: description of the first two cases detected in Italy. *Ann Oncol* 1997; **8**: 1133-8.

105. Hashizume T, Aozasa K, Tomita Y, Matsushita K. Pyothorax-associated T-cell lymphoma: a case report. *Jpn J Clin Oncol* 2003; **33**: 145-7.

106. Liu A, Takakuwa T, Fujita S *et al.* Alterations of DNA damage-response genes ATM and ATR in pyothorax-associated lymphoma. *Lab Invest* 2005; **85**: 436-46.

107. Nishiu M, Tomita Y, Nakatsuka S *et al.* Distinct pattern of gene expression in pyothorax-associated lymphoma (PAL), a lymphoma developing in long-standing inflammation. *Cancer Sci* 2004; **95**: 828-34.

●108. Cheuk W, Chan AC, Chan JK *et al.* Metallic implant-associated lymphoma: a distinct subgroup of large B-cell lymphoma related to pyothorax-associated lymphoma? *Am J Surg Pathol* 2005; **29**: 832-6.

●109. Hojo N, Yakushijin Y, Narumi H *et al.* Non-Hodgkin's lymphoma developing in a pacemaker pocket. *Int J Hematol* 2003; **77**: 387-90.

●110. Molinie V, Pouchot J, Navratil E *et al.* Primary Epstein-Barr virus-related non-Hodgkin's lymphoma of the pleural cavity following long-standing tuberculous empyema. *Arch Pathol Lab Med* 1996; **120**: 288-91.

●111. Oyama T, Yamamoto K, Asano N *et al.* Age-related EBV-associated B-cell lymphoproliferative disorders constitute a distinct clinicopathologic group: a study of 96 patients. *Clin Cancer Res* 2007; **13**: 5124-32.

◆112. Gilmour KC, Gaspar HB. Pathogenesis and diagnosis of X-linked lymphoproliferative disease. *Expert Rev Mol Diagn* 2003; **3**: 549-61.

◆113. Knowles DM. Etiology and pathogenesis of AIDS-related non-Hodgkin's lymphoma. *Hematol Oncol Clin North Am* 2003; **17**: 785-820.

◆114. Bleesing JJ. Autoimmune lymphoproliferative syndrome (ALPS). *Curr Pharm Des* 2003; **9**: 265-78.

115. Smets F, Latinne D, Bazin H *et al.* Ratio between Epstein-Barr viral load and anti-Epstein-Barr virus specific T-cell response as a predictive marker of posttransplant lymphoproliferative disease. *Transplantation* 2002; **73**: 1603-10.

116. Quintanilla-Martinez L, Kumar S, Fend F *et al.* Fulminant EBV(+) T-cell lymphoproliferative disorder following acute/chronic EBV infection: a distinct clinicopathologic syndrome. *Blood* 2000; **96**: 443-51.

117. van Laar JA, Buysse CM, Vossen AC *et al.* Epstein-Barr viral load assessment in immunocompetent patients with fulminant infectious mononucleosis. *Arch Intern Med* 2002; **162**: 837-9.

118. Wick MJ, Woronzoff-Dashkoff KP, McGlennen RC. The molecular characterization of fatal infectious mononucleosis. *Am J Clin Pathol* 2002; **117**: 582-8.

119. Lim MS, Straus SE, Dale JK *et al.* Pathological findings in human autoimmune lymphoproliferative syndrome. *Am J Pathol* 1998; **153**: 1541-50.

120. Poppema S, Maggio E, van den Berg A. Development of lymphoma in Autoimmune Lymphoproliferative Syndrome (ALPS) and its relationship to Fas gene mutations. *Leuk Lymphoma* 2004; **45**: 423-31.

◆121. Percik R, Serr J, Segal G *et al.* Lymphomatoid granulomatosis: a diagnostic challenge. *Isr Med Assoc J* 2005; **7**: 198-9.

122. Katzenstein AL, Peiper SC. Detection of Epstein-Barr virus genomes in lymphomatoid granulomatosis: analysis of 29 cases by the polymerase chain reaction technique. *Mod Pathol* 1990; **3**: 435-41.

123. Hagberg H. Review of lymphomatoid granulomatosis treated with rituximab and chemotherapy. *Clin Adv Hematol Oncol* 2003; **1**: 660.

124. Rao R, Vugman G, Leslie WT *et al.* Lymphomatoid granulomatosis treated with rituximab and chemotherapy. *Clin Adv Hematol Oncol* 2003; **1**: 658-60.

◆125. Casper C. The aetiology and management of Castleman disease at 50 years: translating pathophysiology to patient care. *Br J Haematol* 2005; **129**: 3-17.

126. Dispenzieri A, Kyle RA, Lacy MQ *et al.* POEMS syndrome: definitions and long-term outcome. *Blood* 2003; **101**: 2496-506.

127. Hanson CA, Frizzera G, Patton DF *et al.* Clonal rearrangement for immunoglobulin and T-cell receptor genes in systemic Castleman's disease. Association with Epstein-Barr virus. *Am J Pathol* 1988; **131**: 84-91.

128. Soulier J, Grollet L, Oksenhendler E *et al.* Kaposi's sarcoma-associated herpesvirus-like DNA sequences in multicentric Castleman's disease. *Blood* 1995; **86**: 1276-80.

129. Aoki Y, Jaffe ES, Chang Y *et al.* Angiogenesis and hematopoiesis induced by Kaposi's sarcoma-associated herpesvirus-encoded interleukin-6. *Blood* 1999; **93**: 4034-43.

130. Nishi J, Arimura K, Utsunomiya A *et al.* Expression of vascular endothelial growth factor in sera and lymph nodes of the plasma cell type of Castleman's disease. *Br J Haematol* 1999; **104**: 482-5.

131. Zarate-Osorno A, Medeiros LJ, Danon AD, Neiman RS. Hodgkin's disease with coexistent Castleman-like histologic features. A report of three cases. *Arch Pathol Lab Med* 1994; **118**: 270-4.

132. Dupin N, Diss TL, Kellam P *et al.* HHV-8 is associated with a plasmablastic variant of Castleman disease that is linked to HHV-8-positive plasmablastic lymphoma. *Blood* 2000; **95**: 1406-12.

133. Pileri SA, Grogan TM, Harris NL *et al*. Tumours of histiocytes and accessory dendritic cells: an immunohistochemical approach to classification from the International Lymphoma Study Group based on 61 cases. *Histopathology* 2002; **41**: 1–29.

134. Greil R, Anether G, Johrer K, Tinhofer I. Tracking death dealing by Fas and TRAIL in lymphatic neoplastic disorders: pathways, targets, and therapeutic tools. *J Leukoc Biol* 2003; **74**: 311–30.

●135. Szodoray P, Jonsson R. The BAFF/APRIL system in systemic autoimmune diseases with a special emphasis on Sjogren's syndrome. *Scand J Immunol* 2005; **62**: 421–8.

136. Varoczy L, Gergely L, Zeher M *et al*. Malignant lymphoma-associated autoimmune diseases – a descriptive epidemiological study. *Rheumatol Int* 2002; **22**: 233–7.

◆137. Ramos-Casals M, De Vita S, Tzioufas AG. Hepatitis C virus, Sjogren's syndrome and B-cell lymphoma: linking infection, autoimmunity and cancer. *Autoimmun Rev* 2005; **4**: 8–15.

138. Vitali C, Bombardieri S, Jonsson R. Classification criteria for Sjogren's syndrome: a revised version of the European criteria proposed by the American-European Consensus Group. *Ann Rheum Dis* 2002; **61**: 554–8.

◆139. Brousse N, Meijer JW. Malignant complications of coeliac disease. *Best Pract Res Clin Gastroenterol* 2005; **19**: 401–12.

140. Johrens K, Anagnostopoulos I, Stein H. T-bet expression patterns in coeliac disease, cryptic and overt enteropathy-type T-cell lymphoma. *Histopathology* 2005; **47**: 368–74.

141. Culliford AN, Green PH. Refractory sprue. *Curr Gastroenterol Rep* 2003; **5**: 373–8.

142. Daum S, Hummel M, Weiss D *et al*. Refractory sprue syndrome with clonal intraepithelial lymphocytes evolving into overt enteropathy-type intestinal T-cell lymphoma. *Digestion* 2000; **62**: 60–5.

143. Monteleone I, Monteleone G, Del Vecchio Blanco G *et al*. Regulation of the T helper cell type 1 transcription factor T-bet in coeliac disease mucosa. *Gut* 2004; **53**: 1090–5.

144. Matsuoka K, Inoue N, Sato T *et al*. T-bet upregulation and subsequent interleukin 12 stimulation are essential for induction of Th1 mediated immunopathology in Crohn's disease. *Gut* 2004; **53**: 1303–8.

●145. Abruzzo LV, Rosales CM, Medeiros LJ *et al*. Epstein-Barr virus-positive B-cell lymphoproliferative disorders arising in immunodeficient patients previously treated with fludarabine for low-grade B-cell neoplasms. *Am J Surg Pathol* 2002; **26**: 630–6.

●146. Mariette X, Cazals-Hatem D, Warszawki J *et al*. Lymphomas in rheumatoid arthritis patients treated with methotrexate: a 3-year prospective study in France. *Blood* 2002; **99**: 3909–15.

◆147. Callen JP. Complications and adverse reactions in the use of newer biologic agents. *Semin Cutan Med Surg* 2007; **26**: 6–14.

148. Wolfe F, Michaud K. The effect of methotrexate and anti-tumor necrosis factor therapy on the risk of lymphoma in rheumatoid arthritis in 19,562 patients during 89,710 person-years of observation. *Arthritis Rheum* 2007; **56**: 1433–9.

149. Mackey AC, Green L, Liang LC *et al*. Hepatosplenic T cell lymphoma associated with infliximab use in young patients treated for inflammatory bowel disease. *J Pediatr Gastroenterol Nutr* 2007; **44**: 265–7.

PATHOLOGY AND PATHOGENESIS OF SPECIFIC LYMPHOMAS

26

Lymphoblastic lymphomas and leukemias

JENNIFER O'NEIL AND A THOMAS LOOK

INTRODUCTION

Normal lymphoid cell populations undergo diverse, clonal rearrangements of their IG or TCR genes, followed by highly regulated proliferation of the cells that successfully complete these genetic changes. This developmental process generates B and T cells with the specificities needed to support a fully competent immune system. When a lymphoid progenitor cell becomes genetically altered through somatic changes, the result can be dysregulated proliferation and clonal expansion, eventually leading to acute lymphoblastic leukemia (ALL). In most cases, the pathobiology of transformed lymphoid cells reflects the altered expression of genes whose products contribute to the normal phenotypes of B and T cell progenitors, but it may also involve the aberrant expression of otherwise quiescent genes.

Because leukemic blasts represent the clonal expansion of hematopoietic progenitors that are blocked in differentiation at discrete stages of development, they provide large uniform populations for molecular and functional analyses. Leukemic cells duplicate most of the features of normal lymphoid progenitors and provide models for elucidating the regulatory cascades disrupted by specific genetic changes. For instance, molecular studies of chromosomal breakpoint regions in ALL cells have identified genes whose protein products are transcription factors that often control the expression of developmentally important genes.[1–4] In fact, much of the recent progress in understanding ALL pathobiology has come from the study of rearranged or mutated genes and their associated proteins.

CLONAL ORIGIN OF LEUKEMIC LYMPHOID CELLS

Human ALL arises from a single progenitor cell that has undergone genetic damage leading to dysregulated growth and arrested differentiation. Evidence that each leukemic cell has descended from a single transformed progenitor comes from cytogenetic studies showing common numerical and structural chromosomal abnormalities within discrete leukemic cell populations. The clonal development of leukemic cell populations is further demonstrated by precise rearrangements of IG or TCR genes, as compared with the heterogeneous pattern of rearrangements observed in populations of normal T and B lymphocytes.[5,6]

LINEAGE-SPECIFIC FEATURES OF LEUKEMIC LYMPHOBLASTS

An important advance in the understanding and treatment of ALL was the realization that malignant lymphoblasts share many of the features of normal lymphoid progenitors.[7,8] Thus, ALL cells rearrange their IG and TCR genes and express components of antigen receptor molecules and other differentiation-linked cell surface glycoproteins in ways that correspond to features of developing normal B and T lymphocytes. In many cases, leukemic cells appear to represent the clonal expansion of a lymphoid progenitor that is blocked in an early stage of B or T cell differentiation.[9] However, with better understanding of the normal patterns of antigen-independent lymphoid cell development, it has become clear that leukemic lymphoblasts can show asynchronous gene expression with subtle variations in phenotype.[10] Hence, it should not be surprising that in some cases of ALL, the blast cell phenotypes differ from those of normal lymphocyte progenitors, presumably because of aberrant regulation of gene expression. In addition, recent advances in the identification of 'tumor stem cells' raise the possibility that subsets of ALL may arise from minor populations of immature hematopoetic stem cells. Still, the general concept that leukemic cells should be classified according to their 'normal' developmental stage remains an important one, providing a basis for the study of immunophenotype-specific genetic changes and for the assignment of patients to phenotype-directed therapy.

B cell lymphoblastic lymphoma and acute lymphoblastic leukemia

B lineage lymphoblastic lymphoma (LBL) and B cell leukemia are identified by classic cytomorphology and the detection of surface immunoglobulin on leukemic blasts. This rare phenotype accounts for only 2–3 percent of ALL cases, and the lymphoblasts generally have a distinct morphology, with deeply basophilic cytoplasm containing prominent vacuoles; this morphologic pattern is designated L3 in the French–American–British (FAB) system.[11–13] Prominent clinical features include concomitant extramedullary lymphomatous masses in the abdomen or head and neck, frequent involvement of the central nervous system and cranial nerves, and hyperuricemia with acute renal failure due to uric acid nephropathy. Most investigators believe that acute B cell leukemia is a disseminated form of B cell LBL or Burkitt lymphoma, as these conditions share common cytogenetic, molecular genetic, immunologic, cytologic and clinical features.[14]

Acute B cell leukemia does not respond well to chemotherapy traditionally used for childhood ALL. However, outstanding results, typified by event-free survival (EFS) rates of nearly 90 percent, have been obtained with treatments designed for B cell LBL, which utilize cyclophosphamide and a rapid rotation of antimetabolites in high dosages.[14–18] Thus, B cell leukemia is the first form of ALL to be recognized as a distinct clinical entity based on immunophenotypic and cytogenetic features, and the first to be treated by separate protocols designed specifically for the leukemia's unique features.

Pre-B and early pre-B acute lymphoblastic leukemia

Approximately 80 percent of ALL patients have lymphoblasts with phenotypes corresponding to those of B cell progenitors.[12,19] Although early B lineage, these leukemias are sIg–, differentiating them from B cell ALL. Almost all lymphoblastic lymphomas are either sIg+ or T cell lineage. These cases can be identified on the basis of cell surface expression of CD19 and at least one other recognized B lineage-associated antigen: CD20, CD24, CD22, CD21, or CD79;[12,19] 90–95 percent of B lineage ALL cases also express CD10 (CALLA [Common ALL Antigen]). The lymphoblasts may also express nuclear TdT, or CD34, a surface glycoprotein of unknown function whose normal expression in hematopoiesis is restricted to lymphoid and hematopoietic precursors. About one-fourth of B progenitor ALL cases express cytoplasmic Ig μ heavy-chain proteins and are designated pre-B cell ALL. Pre-B cases were originally shown to have a worse long-term response to therapy compared to early pre-B cases, an observation that was later attributed to the presence of a specific t(1;19) in about one-fourth of the pre-B cases.[20] The poor outcome of standard therapy in children and adults with the balanced t(1;19)(q23;p13) extended to the unbalanced der(19)t(1;19)(q23;p13) variants of this translocation.[21,22] However, with the introduction of more intensive treatment regimens, the prognosis for patients with t(1;19)+ ALL has improved significantly,[16,23] although this revised outlook appears restricted to the subgroup with an unbalanced der(19)t(1;19) (q23;p13).[24]

T cell acute lymphoblastic leukemia

Leukemias of T cell precursors are identified and classified according to the expression of T cell-associated surface antigens which are expressed during normal thymocyte differentiation.[25] In this tightly regulated process, the earliest T cell precursors are characterized by the lack of expression of CD4 and CD8 surface markers. These double-negative thymocytes express CD7, TdT and cytoplasmic CD3, and proceed through four different stages of development (DN1 to DN4) defined by the expression of CD44 and CD25, after which the TCRβ gene becomes rearranged, driving the production of intermediate single-positive cells (ISPs) with a surface phenotype of CD4+, CD8–, CD3– that differentiate into early double-positive (CD4+, CD8+) cells. Subsequently, these double-positive progenitors acquire surface CD1 and differentiate into late cortical thymocytes showing a loss of CD1 and a gain of surface CD3 expression. This T cell developmental process ends when mature CD4+ or CD8+ single-positive cells are produced.[26]

The clinical features most closely associated with T cell ALL are high blood leukocyte counts, a predominance in boys and men, central nervous system involvement, and radiographic evidence of a thymic mass in about half of cases at presentation. Historically, patients with T cell ALL have had an adverse prognosis by comparison to patients with B lineage ALL, but this gap has narrowed with wider use of intensive chemotherapy.[27,28] Some authors contend that expression of specific antigens, including CD1 and/or coexpression of CD4 and CD8, CD2, CD5, CD10, or the coexpression of six or more T cell markers may identify subgroups of T cell ALL patients with better responses to therapy,[27–31] but this argument remains controversial.

The human antigen-specific TCR molecule is a heterodimer composed of disulfide-linked α and β polypeptide subunits, each encoded by gene families containing variable, joining and constant sequence elements that rearrange at the DNA level to generate diversity, in a manner analogous to the IG genes. Hence, rearrangement of the TCRα/β genes can be used to establish clonality and lineage derivation within leukemias of T cell progenitors.

GENETIC BASIS OF LYMPHOID LEUKEMIA

Multiple somatically acquired genetic abnormalities are responsible for the malignant transformation and disordered cell growth and differentiation seen in ALL. These include microscopically evident chromosomal rearrangements as well as lesions detectable only by molecular analysis of lymphoblast DNA. The ability to identify these changes in a precise, consistent manner and to relate them to the clinical course of the disease has led to risk-specific therapy for ALL. It is worth noting that most children with leukemia have normal constitutional karyotypes, indicating that the genetic abnormalities in their leukemic cells are acquired somatically and are restricted to the malignant clone.

Central role of transcriptional control genes

Chromosomal translocations are found in 75 percent of ALL cases (Fig. 26.1).[13,32] Molecular studies of the breakpoints of specific chromosomal translocations of human leukemic cells have focused on transcription factor genes (Table 26.1), whose alteration leads to the differentiation arrest and aberrant growth of leukemic lymphoid progenitors.[1,3,4] Rabbitts has aptly described a key group of regulatory transcription factors as the products of 'master genes'.[33] In his model, the nuclear proteins encoded by these genes act positively to upregulate critical target genes or negatively to interfere with normal regulatory pathways. The net effect is disruption of gene regulatory cascades that control and coordinate the expression of large numbers of proteins required for the completion of lymphoid cell

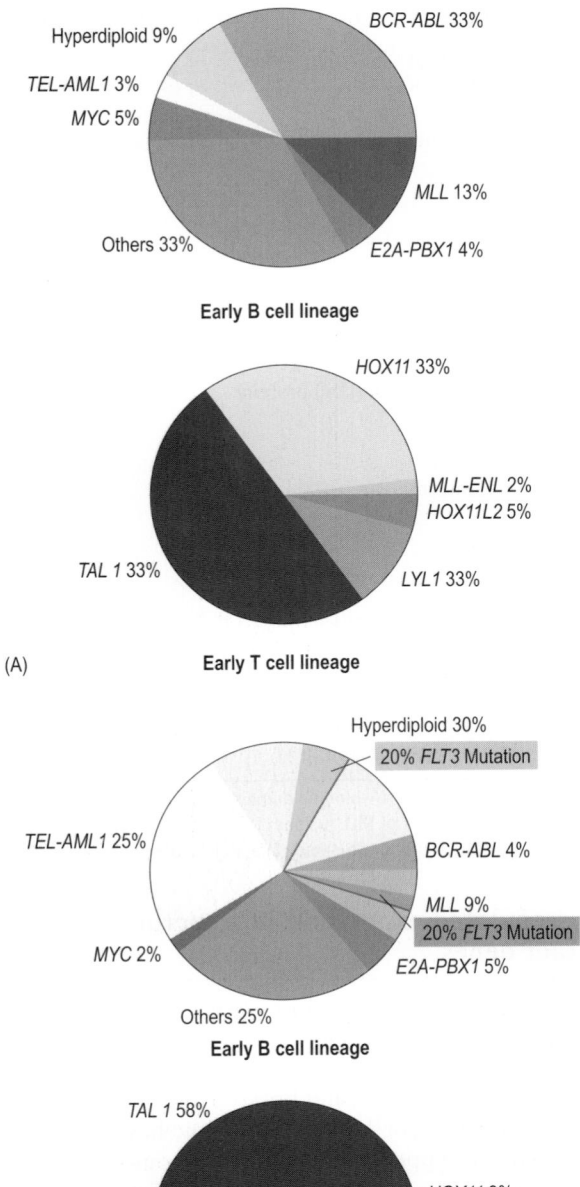

Figure 26.1 Chromosomal abnormalities in acute lymphoblastic leukemia. The relative frequencies of chromosomal aberrations found in lymphoblastic leukemias are shown for adult (A) and childhood (B) acute lymphoblastic leukemias.

differentiation programs. Disruption of transcription factors in leukemic blasts can occur by the dysregulated expression of intact genes, the creation of chimeric transcription factors or by mutation of the transcription factor.

Table 26.1   Transcription genes affected by chromosomal breakpoints in the acute lymphoblastic leukemias

Family[a]	Translocation	Affected gene	Disease
Basic helix-loop-helix (bHLH) proteins	t(8;14)(q24;q32)	MYC	Burkitt lymphoma
	t(2;8)(p12;q24)	MYC	and B cell ALL
	t(8;22)(q24;q11)	MYC	
	t(8;14)(q24;q11)	MYC	T cell ALL
	t(7;19)(q35;p13)	LYL1	T cell ALL
	t(1;14)(p32;q11)	TAL1	T cell ALL
	t(7;9)(q35;q34)	TAL2	T cell ALL
	t(14;21)(q11.2;q22)	BHLHB1	T cell ALL
Cysteine-rich (LIM) proteins	t(11;14)(p15;q11)	LMO1	T cell ALL
	t(11;14)(p13;q11)	LMO2	T cell ALL
	t(7;11)(q35;p13)	LMO2	T cell ALL
Homeodomain (HOX) proteins	t(10;14)(q24;q11)	HOX11	T cell ALL
	t(7;10)(q35;q24)	HOX11	T cell ALL
	t(5;14)(q35;q32.2)	HOX11L2	T cell ALL
	t(1;19)(q23;p13)	E2A-PBX1	Pre-B cell ALL
Basic-region/leucine-zipper (bZIP) proteins	t(17;19)(q22;p13)	E2A-HLF	EPB ALL
A-T hook minor groove binding proteins[b]	t(4;11)(q21;q23)	MLL-AF4	EPB ALL
	t(11;19)(q23;p13.3)	MLL-ENL	ALL or AML
ETS-like (TEL, ERG) proteins	t(12;21)(p13;q22)	TEL-AML1	ALL
Runt homology (AML1)	t(12;21)(p13;q22)	TEL-AML1	ALL

[a]Based on DNA-binding domain
[b]Partial list of MLL fusions
AML, acute myeloid leukemia; ALL, acute lymphoblastic leukemia; EPB, early pre-B.

Dysregulated expression of structurally intact genes

ACTIVATION OF MYC IN B CELL ACUTE LYMPHOBLASTIC LEUKEMIA

In B cell acute leukemia and Burkitt lymphoma, translocation of one allele of *MYC*, a prototypic basic helix-loop-helix/leucine zipper gene on chromosome 8, into the vicinity of an IG gene, either the heavy-chain gene on chromosome 14q32 or the κ or λ light-chain genes on chromosomes 2 and 22, leads to dysregulation of that allele.[34–42] In the predominant t(8;14) translocation, the involved *MYC* locus is translocated into the heavy-chain gene on chromosome 14, adjacent to the coding sequences of the IG constant region.[34–36] The coding sequences of the IG variable region generally are reciprocally translocated to the distal tip of chromosome 8. In variant translocations, the *MYC* gene remains on chromosome 8, and portions of the respective light-chain genes are translocated to that chromosome downstream of the *MYC* locus.[37–41]

MYC:MAX heterodimers bind to canonical hexameric E-box DNA sequences (5'-CACGTG-3') where they activate transcription.[43] MAX can also heterodimerize with other bHLHZip proteins, including MAD,[44] MXI-1 (MAD2)[45] and MNT.[46] Whereas transcriptional activation by MYC:MAX complexes promotes proliferation, binding by MAD:MAX and other MAX heterodimers

produces opposite effects; for example, MAD inhibits MYC function both by competing with MYC for binding to MAX and by directly inhibiting transcription.

Briefly, dysregulated expression of *MYC* due to the t(8;14) results in higher concentration of MYC:MAX complexes relative to MAX:MAD and hence to transcriptional cell proliferation. Among the genes activated by MYC, many encode proteins that probably have important roles in transformation, including those known to participate in cell division, growth, death, metabolism, adhesion and motility.[47] Others, however, are repressed by MYC through poorly understood mechanisms. It seems important that some of the effects of MYC on cell cycle regulation are mediated by repression of the cell cycle inhibitors p27 and p21, which synergize with the transcriptional activation of CDC25A, a protein phosphatase that activates the cyclin-associated kinases CDK2 and CDK4.[48–50] Finally MYC targets also include the *ARF* tumor suppressor,[51] the catalytic subunit of human telomerase,[52,53] and genes involved in nucleotide and protein biosynthesis pathways, any of which could contribute to ALL pathobiology.

BHLH, LIM AND HOX GENES IN T ACUTE LYMPHOBLASTIC LEUKEMIA

In leukemias with a T cell phenotype, chromosomal breakpoints consistently involve the TCR enhancer (7q34) or the TCRα/δ enhancer (14q11), both of which are highly active

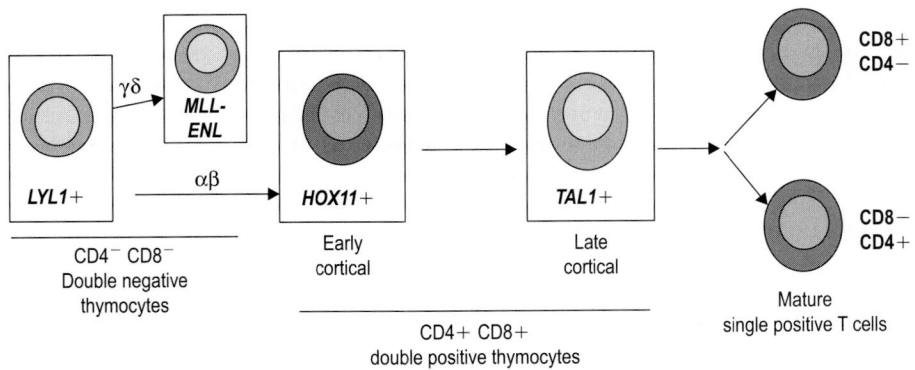

Figure 26.2 Thymocyte development is a tightly regulated process in which progenitor cells undergo sequential stages of differentiation, proliferation, lineage commitment and selection that result in the production of functionally competent mature T cells. Microarray gene expression profiling shows that T cell acute lymphoblastic leukemia (T-ALL) lymphoblasts expressing high levels of the *LYL1* transcription factor oncogene undergo an early arrest at the double-negative thymocyte (CD4−, CD8−) stage of development. In T-ALL cases with aberrant expression of *HOX11*, the leukemic cells show a developmental arrest at the double-positive (CD4+, CD8+) early cortical stage of thymocyte differentiation, whereas those with aberrant expression of *TAL1* are arrested at the double positive late cortical stage. T-ALL cells with expression of the *MLL-ENL* fusion gene are characterized by an early arrest of differentiation with a gene expression signature that indicates commitment to the gamma-delta lineage. (Reprinted from *Hematology*, 4th edition, Hoffman, Pathobiology of acute lymphoblastic leukemia, Chapter 63, 2004, with permission from Elsevier.)

in committed T cell progenitors and can cause dysregulated expression of transcription factor genes located at the breakpoint on the reciprocal chromosome involved in these phenotype-specific rearrangements.[54] The affected transcription factors include:

- genes encoding bHLH family members, such as *TAL1*,[55,56] *TAL2*,[57] *LYL1*,[58] *MYC*,[59–61] and *bHLHb1*[62]
- *LMO* genes, such as *LMO1* and *LMO2* [63–65]
- the orphan homeobox genes *HOX11* and *HOX11L2*.[66–72]

The observation that T-ALL oncogenes act as master transcriptional regulators during the embryonic development of specific organ systems suggests that their aberrant expression in T cell precursors may contribute to the onset of leukemia by disrupting the mechanisms that control cell proliferation, differentiation and survival during the discrete steps of normal T cell development.

The best characterized of these genes is *TAL1*, which is altered by the t(1;14) or by site-specific deletions in approximately a fourth of childhood T-ALL cases.[73–78] *TAL1* is aberrantly expressed in the leukemic cells of 60 percent of children and 45 percent of adults with T-ALL (Fig. 26.2). TAL1 acts as a master regulatory protein during early hematopoietic development and is required for the generation of all blood cell lineages,[79,80] however, it does not seem to be required for the generation and function of hemopoietic stem cells during adult hematopoiesis.[81] This class II bHLH transcription factor binds to DNA by forming heterodimers with class I bHLH factors such as E2A and HEB.[82] The observation that loss of E2A function induces T cell leukemias in mice,[83,84] and that the DNA-binding

domain of TAL1 is dispensable for transformation[85] in transgenic mouse models, supports the notion that TAL1 mediated inhibition of E2A plays a critical role in the pathogenesis of T-ALL. A recent study demonstrating accelerated leukemogenesis in TAL1 transgenic mice on a E2A or HEB heterozygous background shows that inhibition of HEB as well as E2A contributes to transformation by TAL1.[86]

The LIM-only domain genes, *LMO1/RBTN1/TTG1* and *LMO2/RBTN2/TTG2*,[63–65] encode proteins that contain cysteine-rich LIM domains involved in protein–protein interactions. LMO2 interacts with TAL1 in erythroid cells as part of a pentameric complex that also includes E47, GATA1 and LDB1.[87–89] Moreover, homozygous disruption of *LMO2* in mice causes the same phenotype as described above for *TAL1* knockout mice, indicating that the multiprotein complex involving LMO2 and TAL1 is required for normal hematopoietic development.[90,91] In addition, overexpression of *LMO1* or *LMO2* in thymocytes of transgenic mice leads to T cell lymphomas,[92–96] and accelerates the onset of leukemias in *TAL1* transgenic mice.[97,98] Activation of LMO2 is also implicated in gene therapy induced T-ALL that occurred in two patients in a recent gene therapy clinical trial for X-linked severe combined immunodeficiency.[99] In both patients, the retroviral vector inserted near the *LMO2* gene resulting in overexpression of LMO2.[100]

The homeodomain gene *HOX11* was originally isolated from the recurrent t(10;14)(q24;q11) in T-ALL[66,68,70,71] and is aberrantly expressed in 3–5 percent of pediatric and up to 30 percent of adult T-ALL cases (Fig. 26.1).[67,101,102] Like other *HOX* genes, *HOX11* plays an important role in embryonic development, and functions as a master transcriptional regulator necessary for the genesis of the spleen.[103,104] In the mouse embryo, *Hox11* expression can be detected in the branchial arches, restricted areas of the hindbrain and the splenic primordium,[105,106] where it is required for the survival of early splenic progenitors.[104] The proposed function of HOX11 as a transcriptional regulator, is supported by the presence of both a 61-amino acid, helix-turn-helix DNA-binding domain (or homeodomain) and by the localization of the HOX11 protein in the cell nucleus.[72] Recent data suggest that HOX11 may contribute to T cell transformation by blocking T cell differentiation and deregulating the cell cycle by blocking PP1/PP2A phosphatase activity.[107,108]

A second *HOX11* family member, *HOX11L2*, has been implicated in the pathogenesis of human T-ALL through characterization of the t(5;14)(q35;q32), a cryptic chromosomal rearrangement detectable only by fluorescence *in situ* hybridization (FISH) and by chromosome painting techniques.[69] This translocation leads to the etopic expression of *HOX11L2*, possibly by bringing it under the influence of regulatory elements in the *CTIP2/ BCL11B* gene, which is highly expressed during T cell differentiation. In contrast to the predominance of *HOX11* expression in adult T-ALL cases, both the t(5;14) and expression of *HOX11L2* can be detected in 20–25 percent of children but in only 5 percent of adults with T-ALL (Fig. 27.1).[67,102,109,110] The role of HOX11L2 as a master transcriptional regulator upstream of important pathways involved in cell fate determination is supported by its importance during embryonic development. In mice, *Hox11l2* expression is essential for normal development of the ventral medullary respiratory center. As a result *Hox11l2* deficient mice die soon after birth due to respiratory failure that resembles congenital central hypoventilation syndrome in humans.[111]

HOX11 and HOX11L2 are closely related in structure, and have a high degree of homology at the amino acid level, especially in the homeobox domain, where their sequences differ by only three amino acids. The high level of structural homology in their DNA-binding domains supports the hypothesis that HOX11 and HOX11L2 may induce T-ALL through regulation of the same transcriptional targets, however, activation of *HOX11* and *HOX11L2* seem to be associated with clinically relevant differences that may result, at least in part, from differences in their mechanisms of action. The expression of *HOX11* is associated with a favorable prognosis both in children and in adults,[2,54,101] while expression of *HOX11L2* has been associated with a high incidence of relapse in children with T-ALL.[2,109] A new recurrent translocation has been recognized that targets and dysregualtes expression from the whole HOXA cluster. Gene expression analysis demonstrates that this subgroup shares aspects of the gene expression signature characteristic of *HOX11-* and *HOX11L2*-overexpressing T-ALLs.[112]

Recently, the analysis of gene expression profiling using oligonucleotide microarrays has shown that the expression of different transcription factor oncogenes such as *TAL1*, *LYL1*, *HOX11* and *HOX11L2* is associated with distinct gene expression profiles. These unique signatures resemble those of thymocytes blocked at discrete stages of T cell development (Fig. 27.2) and suggest that transcription factor oncogenes contribute to the pathogenesis of T-ALL by interfering with critical regulatory networks that control cell proliferation, survival and differentiation during T cell development.[2] Although *TAL1*, *LMO2* and *HOX11* are all involved in translocations with the T cell receptor locus, all three of these genes have been shown to be over-expressed in cases in which no translocation in detected. A recent study has shown that these genes can be biallelically activated suggesting that in some leukemias there is a mutation in a pathway that normally downregulates these genes during T cell differentiation.[113]

NOTCH IN T ACUTE LYMPHOBLASTIC LEUKEMIA

The *TAN1* gene, which shares homology with the *Drosophila notch* gene, is involved in the t(7;9) translocation leading to its relocation to the TCRβ locus and dysregulated expression.[114] This translocation is very rare, occurring in less than 1 percent of T-ALLs. Bone marrow reconstitution experiments in the mouse have demonstrated that similar forms of activated NOTCH1 are potent inducers of T-ALL.[115] Although the mechanism through which NOTCH1 signaling promotes T-ALL is not known, NOTCH1 has been shown to play essential roles in normal T cell development, most notably at the level of T cell commitment.[116] NOTCH1 has also been shown to inhibit the transcription factor E47 that is essential for both B and T cell development.[117] Therefore, NOTCH1 may contribute to leukemogenesis by altering T development through inhibition of E47.

Recent studies have demonstrated a broader involvement of *NOTCH1* in T-ALL. Activating mutations in *NOTCH1* were detected in over 50 percent of T-ALL patient samples[118] (Fig. 26.3). The mutations were detected in all subtypes of T-ALL and were found in two regions of the NOTCH1 protein. Missense mutations in the heterodimerization domain activate NOTCH signaling by altering the interaction between the transmembrane subunit and the inhibitory extracellular subunit of NOTCH1. In addition, frameshift and point mutations that introduce premature stop codons are observed, which delete the C-terminal PEST destruction sequences and thereby increase ICN1 stability and signaling activity.[119]

The *NOTCH* genes encode single pass transmembrane receptors that regulate apoptosis, proliferation and cell fate determination in multicellular organisms. Pro-NOTCH1 is cleaved to produce a NOTCH1 heterodimer that is presented on the cell surface. Binding of NOTCH ligands, such as Delta and Serrate, initiates a series of additional proteolytic cleavages in NOTCH1. The last of these cleavages, which is catalyzed by γ-secretase, results in the release of the intracellular domain of NOTCH1 (ICN), permitting it to

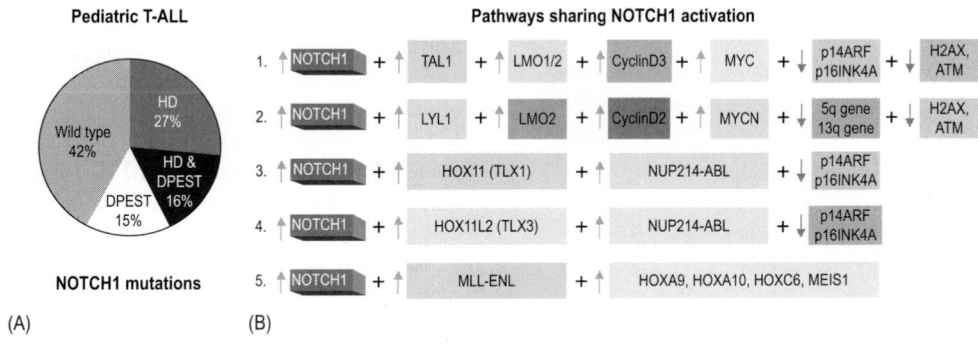

Figure 26.3 Frequency of *NOTCH1* mutations and the role of multistep molecular pathways in the pathogenesis of T cell acute lymphoblastic leukemia (T-ALL). (A) NOTCH1 missense mutations were identified within the heterodimerization domain (HD) in 27 percent of childhood T-ALL blasts, truncating mutations that deleted the PEST destruction box (DPEST) were identified in 15%, and both regions were simultaneously mutated in the same *NOTCH1* gene of 16 percent of cases, providing evidence for multi-hit mutagenesis affecting a single oncogene in primary T-ALL samples at diagnosis. Only 42 percent of cases had unmutated *NOTCH1* genes. (B) These mutations were shown to occur in each of the at least five multistep molecular pathways that can lead to the transformation of T cell progenitors during development, suggesting that some form of NOTCH pathway disruption may be required as a first step regardless of the additional genes that ultimately become mutated. *HOX11+*, *HOX11L2+* and *TAL1+* cases show high levels of *MYC* expression and share the loss of the tumor suppressor genes *p16/INK4A* and *p14/ARF* on chromosome 9p. *HOX11+* and *HOX11L2+* often have a novel *NUP214-ABL* episomal fusion gene, which may render these T-ALLs sensitive to imatinib. *LYL1+* cases show high levels of expression of *MYCN* and frequently have deletions affecting as yet unidentified loci on chromosomal arms 5q and 13q. Finally, *MLL-ENL+* cases have low levels of expression of *MYC* and other genes involved in cell growth and proliferation. This subset of T-ALL cases express high levels of HOXA9, HOXA10 and HOXC6, in concert with the *HOX* gene regulator *MEIS1*, which is different from other T-ALL cases, but similar to other cases. (Reprinted from *J Clin Oncol*, 10; 23(26), Armstrong SA and Look, AT, Molecular genetics of acute lymphoblastic leukemia, 6306–15, 2005, with permission from the American Society of Clinical Oncology.)

translocate to the nucleus and form part of a multiprotein complex that regulates gene transcription (Fig. 26.4). Treatment of T-ALL cell lines with mutations in *NOTCH1* with γ-secretase inhibitors led to G_0/G_1 arrest demonstrating that the cells are dependent on NOTCH signaling for growth and suggesting that activation of NOTCH may contribute to the pathogenesis of T-ALL by promoting cell cycle progression.[118] The γ-secretase enzyme also cleaves the amyloid precursor protein leading to the production of plaques in Alzheimer's patients. As a result, γ-secretase inhibitors have already been developed for use as drugs. Clinical trials are currently under way to determine if NOTCH pathway inhibitors will be efficacious in treating patients with T-ALL.

OTHER GENES ACTIVATED BY TRANSLOCATION

Transcription factors are not the only genes activated by translocation to the sites of the IG or TCR genes. In cases of B-precursor ALL carrying the t(5;14), for example, the *IL3* gene is activated by juxtaposition with the IG heavy-chain locus.[120,121] In T cell ALL, relocation to the TCRβ locus activates expression of the *LCK* tyrosine kinase genes in cases with the t(1;7).[122–124]

Recently, a unique fusion gene resulting in ABL kinase activation has been identified in T-ALL. This fusion results from a small deletion that removes an approximately 500 kb segment of chromosome 9 with breakpoints within one

of the introns of the *NUP214* gene and within the first intron of *ABL*. This deleted fragment is ligated as a circular episome that encodes a fusion gene between amino terminal sequences of NUP214 and the ABL kinase. It is maintained and amplified as an episomal structure lacking a centrosome, and is small enough that it does not appear as a double-minute chromatin body and can only be visualized cytogenetically by FISH analysis for the affected genes. The NUP214-ABL fusion occurs in the subset of cases with activated HOX11 or HOX11L2 homeobox transcription factors.[125]

Chimeric transcription factor genes

Formation of chimeric proteins whose functional domains come from two normally separate genes represents another mechanism of aberrant transcription factor activation. Chromosomal translocations produce a chimeric protein by fusing the DNA-binding, dimerization and transactivation regions of discrete genes.

E2A-PBX1 FUSION GENES IN PRE-B ACUTE LYMPHOBLASTIC LEUKEMIA

A well-known example of a chimeric transcription factor with oncogenic potential is the *E2A-PBX1* rearrangement, which results from the t(1;19)(q23;p13) chromosomal

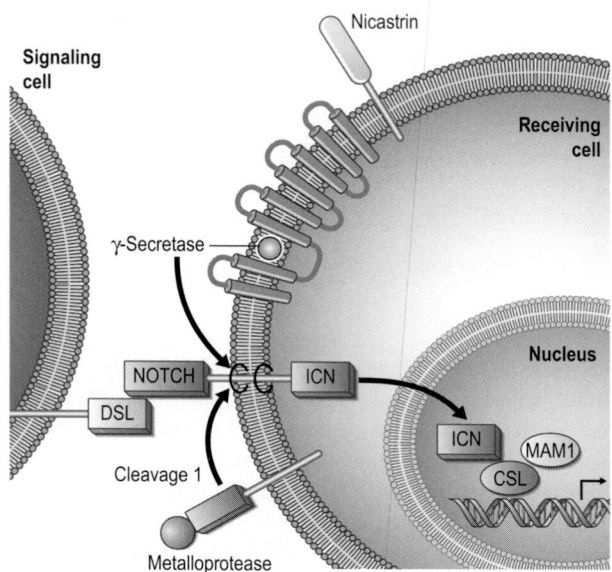

Figure 26.4 Activation of NOTCH signaling via extracellular and intracellular proteolytic cleavage and nuclear translocation of the intracellular NOTCH domain (ICN). Interaction with delta serrate ligand (DSL) stimulates NOTCH extracellular cleavage by metalloproteases and intracellular cleavage by gamma-secretase. After proteolytic cleavage, the ICN moves to the nucleus where it interacts with Mastermind-like proteins (MAM1) and the CSL DNA-binding component to regulate gene expression. (Reprinted from *J Clin Oncol*, 10;**23**(26), Armstrong SA and Look, AT, Molecular genetics of acute lymphoblastic leukemia, 6306–15, 2005, with permission from the American Society of Clinical Oncology.)

translocation present in 3–5 percent of all B lineage ALLs and in 25 percent of cases with a pre-B phenotype.[54] This translocation fuses the *E2A* gene on chromosome 19 to a homeobox gene (*PBX1*) on chromosome 1, leading to the expression of several forms of hybrid E2A-PBX1 oncoproteins. *PBX1* is related to the *Drosophila exd* gene, a homeotic gene that plays a role in segmental development through its ability to heterodimerize with and alter the downstream regulatory programs of the products of the *HOMC* major homeobox genes. The hybrid proteins resulting from the t(1;19) contain the amino-terminal trans-activation domains of E2A (AD1 and AD2)[126–128] and the DNA-binding domain of PBX1, enabling the fusion proteins to function as chimeric transcription factors.[129–131]

The transforming potential of *E2A-PBX1* was first demonstrated by the rapid induction of acute myeloid leukemia (AML) in lethally irradiated mice repopulated with bone marrow stem cells that had been infected with recombinant retroviruses containing *E2A-PBX1* genes.[132] The fusion has also been shown to transform NIH-3T3 fibroblasts and induce T cell lymphomas in transgenic mice.[133,134] Additional studies have shown that deletion of one of the E2A activation domains diminishes its

transforming activity, while deletion of the PBX1 homeodomain has no effect.[132,134] However, the homeodomain and flanking sequences are required for interactions with other HOX proteins and for optimal binding of E2A-PBX1 to specific DNA sequences.[135–139] It thus appears that complex interactions between E2A-PBX1 and other HOX proteins target the fusion protein to specific target genes whose activation is critical to lymphoid cell transformation.

Patients whose leukemic blasts express *E2A-PBX1* have a poor prognosis when treated with conventional antimetabolite-based therapy.[20] However, the poor prognosis of these patients can be overcome by the use of more intensive therapy,[140–142] demonstrating the importance of detecting *E2A-PBX1* fusion at diagnosis.

E2A–HLF FUSION GENES IN EARLY PRE-B ACUTE LYMPHOBLASTIC LEUKEMIA

The t(17;19) is a rare recurrent chromosomal translocation that fuses the amino-terminal transactivation domains of E2A to the C-terminal DNA binding and dimerization domains of HLF,[143,144] which belongs to the PAR subfamily of bZIP transcription factors. Although E2A-HLF can bind DNA either as a homodimer or as a heterodimer with HLF and related proteins, no other PAR proteins are expressed at detectable levels in leukemic cells, and the E2A-HLF fusion appears to bind DNA as a homodimer in cells harboring the t(17;19). Like E2A-PBX1, E2A-HLF can transform NIH-3T3 fibroblasts, a process that requires the HLF leucine zipper domain and the E2A transactivation domains.[145] E2A-HLF can also induce lymphoid tumors in transgenic mice.[146]

A major consequence of the activation of E2A-HLF in lymphoid precursors is dysregulation of the mechanisms that control programmed cell death in lymphoid progenitors. Expression of a dominant-negative form of E2A-HLF in t(17;19)-carrying cell lines blocks E2A-HLF function and results in apoptosis.[147] In normal pro-B lymphocytes, expression of E2A-HLF reversed interleukin (IL)-3-dependent and p53-induced apoptosis.

HLF is the mammalian homologue of the nematode protein CES-2, which regulates the death of specific nerve cells in *Caenorhabditis elegans*.[147–149] CES-2 is necessary for the death of the sister cells of a specific pair of serotoninergic neurons during worm development. CES-2 induces apoptosis by inhibiting the expression of *ces-1*, a pro-survival gene that normally inhibits programmed cell death by antagonizing the activity of the pro-apoptotic factor EGL1. This pathway which is highly evolutionarily conserved is disrupted by E2A-HLF fusion. Thus, in contrast to the proapoptotic role of CES-2 in the worm via repression of CES-1, E2A-HLF blocks apoptosis by inducing the expression of *SLUG*, a *ces-1* homologue normally responsible for protecting hematopoietic progenitors from DNA-damage-induced apoptosis[150–153] (Fig. 26.5).

The t(17;19) is very rare, ocurring in less than 1 percent of ALL cases, and is typically seen in adolescents and

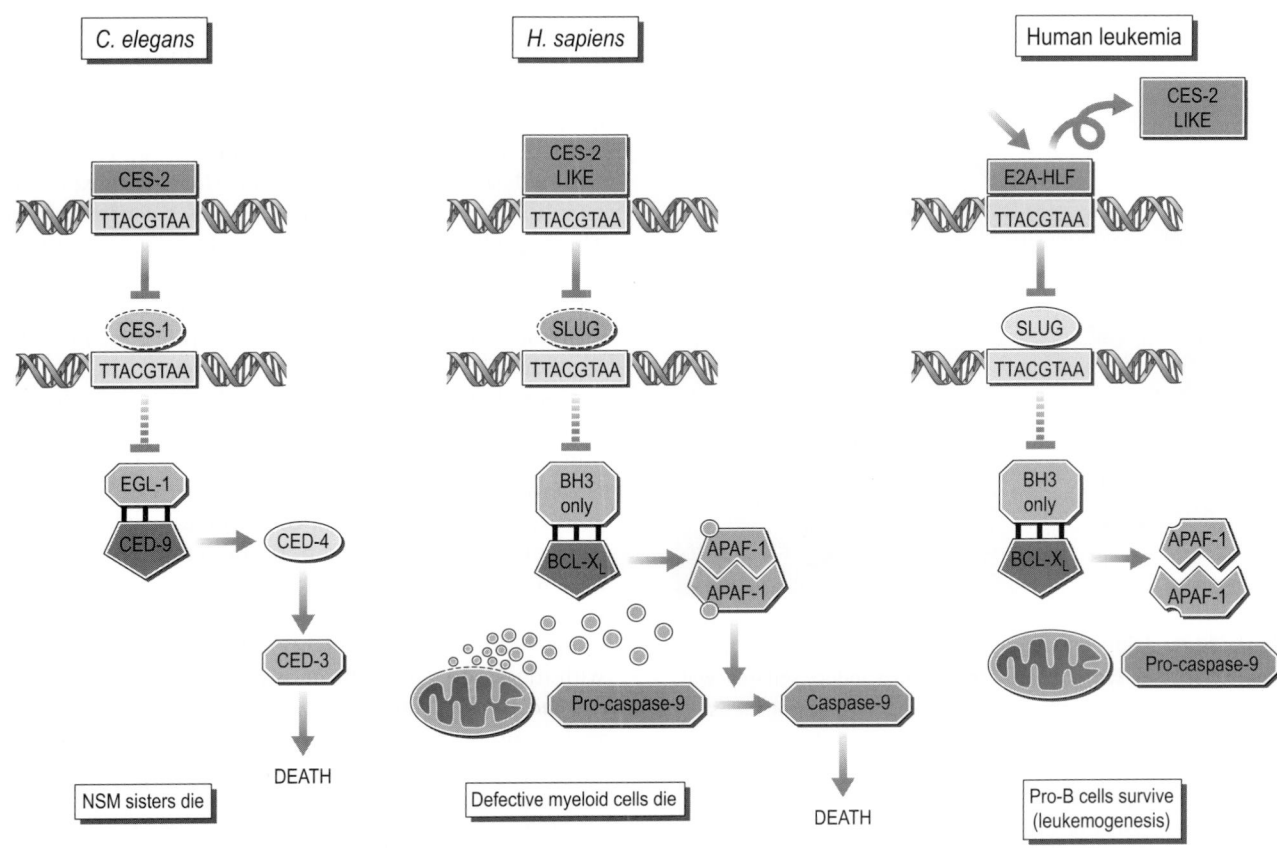

Figure 26.5 Models of conserved cell death specification pathways and the role of E2A-HLF in leukemogenesis. In the nematode *C. elegans* the CES-2 protein negatively regulates *ces-1* to induce the activation of a cell death pathway that results in the apoptosis of two serotononergic neurons (NSM sisters). This pathway presumably involves the transcriptional activation of *egl1*, whose product is a proapoptotic factor that binds to and inhibits CED-9, preventing it from inhibiting the CED-4 and CED-3 cell death effectors. In humans a similar cell death pathway regulates the survival of myeloid progenitors during hematopoiesis. In this system, a CES-2 homologue negatively controls the expression of *SLUG* (*ces-1* homologue), which presumably downregulates apoptosis by inhibiting a BH3-only family member (*egl1* homologue). In the absence of SLUG the upregulation of this BH3-only factor blocks the activity of antiapoptotic molecules such as BCL-2 and BCL-X$_L$, triggering the release of cytochrome C from the mitochondria and the activation of downstream apoptotic effector molecules (APAF-1, Caspase-9). Because E2A-HLF and CES-2 recognize the same DNA sequence, expression of this chimeric oncoprotein with its strong transactivation domains induces expression of *SLUG* which subsequently results in the inhibition of the expression of a BH3 only gene responsible for cell death activation in Pro-B cells. (Reprinted from *Hematology*, 4th edition, Hoffman, Pathobiology of acute lymphoblastic leukemia, Chapter 63, 2004, with permission from Elsevier.)

patients who present with associated intravascular coagulation and hypercalcemia at diagnosis. Although the clinical significance of the t(17;19) is unclear, each of seven patients whose blasts expressed *E2A-HLF* died of leukemia despite aggressive therapy.[54] It seems likely that resistance to chemotherapy in these cases is mediated by the role of E2A-HLF in inhibiting apoptosis.

MLL FUSION GENES

Translocations involving chromosome 11 band q23 occur in approximately 80 percent of infant ALL cases.[54] The gene bisected by 11q23 translocations is designated *MLL* and encodes a protein that shares significant sequence homology with trithorax, a *Drosophila* regulator of homeotic gene

function during fly embryogenesis.[154–157] Trithorax regulates homeotic genes in the *Antennapedia* and *Bithorax* complexes of the fly and is required for normal head, thorax, and abdomen development.[158] The MLL protein shares three regions of homology with trithorax, including two central zinc-finger domains and a 210-amino acid C-terminal SET domain. The *MLL* SET domain contains a histone H3/lysine 4 methyl transferase activity that plays a critical role in the regulation of *HOX* gene expression (Fig. 26.6).[159,160] Other structural features of *MLL* include three A-T hook domains near the N-terminus that are thought to bind the minor groove of DNA in AT-rich regions, and a 47-amino acid region of homology with the noncatalytic domains of human DNA methyltransferase.[161,162] *MLL* localization and stability depend on proteolytic post-translational processing by

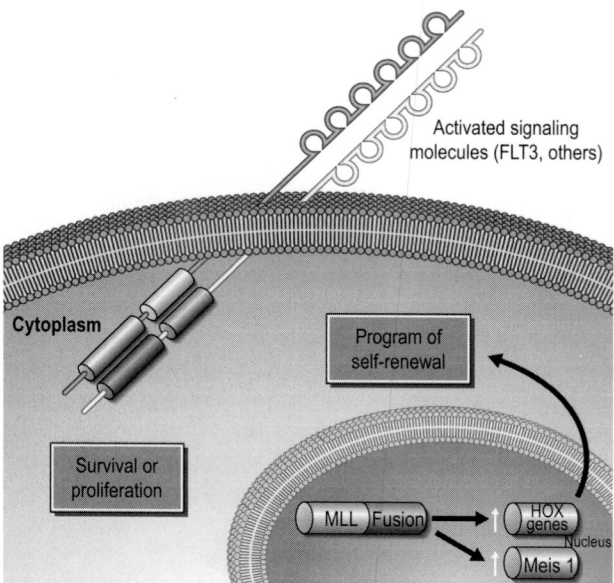

Figure 26.6 Multistep pathogenesis of *MLL*-rearranged lymphoblastic leukemias. *MLL* translocations induce self-renewal in hematopoietic progenitors as a first step in leukemogenesis. The presence of FLT3 mutations in *MLL*-rearranged ALLs support activation of FLT3 or other kinases as cooperating events in this disease. Clinical trials designed to assess the efficacy of FLT3 inhibitors in *MLL*-rearranged ALL are being developed. (Reprinted from *J Clin Oncol*, 10;23(26), Armstrong SA and Look, AT, Molecular genetics of acute lymphoblastic leukemia, 6306–15, 2005, with permission from the American Society of Clinical Oncology.)

taspase 1, a specialized protease that cleaves the *MLL* protein into N-terminal and C-terminal fragments that remain associated through intramolecular protein–protein interaction domains.[163,164]

Translocation breakpoints cluster in an 8.5 kb region of *MLL* between exons 5 and 11 and fuse the N-terminal region of *MLL*, containing the A-T hook and methyltransferase domains, to a variety of partner proteins. Although the role of each partner protein in leukemogenesis has not been fully determined, it appears that at least some of them may contribute functional domains to the fusion. For example, the t(4;11), t(9;11) and t(11;19)(q23;p13.3) fuse *MLL* to *AF4*, *AF9* and *ENL*, respectively. All three of these partners are small serine/proline-rich proteins with nuclear localization signals, suggesting that they may function as transcriptional transactivators. An unrelated gene, *ELL*, is fused to *MLL* by the t(11;19)(q23;p13.1).[165,166] *ELL* was also independently isolated as an RNA polymerase II elongation factor.[167] Still other partners seem to have no transcriptional activity but to contribute a dimerization domain to the fusion protein that results in homo-oligomerization of the N-terminal portion of MLL.[168,169]

Homologous recombination techniques have recently been used to create mice lacking one or both copies of *Mll*,

the murine homologue of *MLL*. *Mll* heterozygous mice demonstrated the effects of haploinsufficiency, including anemia, thrombocytopenia, and reduced numbers of B lymphocytes. The mice also showed homeotic transformations of the cervical, thoracic, and lumbar regions that reflected shifts in the pattern of *Hox* gene expression, establishing a crucial role for *Mll* in *Hox* gene regulation. These results are consistent with other data suggesting a role for *Hox* genes in normal hematopoiesis. Mice with homozygous loss of *Mll* died *in utero* and lacked *Hox* gene expression, further supporting a key role for *Mll* in *Hox* regulation.[170]

Formal proof that *MLL* fusions play a critical role in the development of leukemias has come from the generation of murine models of *MLL*-induced leukemias. Chimeric mice harboring a *MLL-AF9* fusion gene generated by homologous recombination developed leukemias with a latency of 4–12 months.[171] Retroviral transduction of *MLL-ENL*, MLL-ELL and MLL-CBP fusion genes in hemopoietic precursors induces transformation upon transplantation into recipient mice.[172–174] Similar results were recently obtained with models in which chromosomal translocations involving the *Mll* locus are induced by directed interchromosomal recombination in mice, a strategy that reproduces experimentally the initiating events in the pathogenesis of *MLL*-rearranged leukemias.[175–177]

Microarray gene expression analysis of *MLL*-rearranged B-lineage leukemias has shown that these tumors have a characteristic gene expression signature that includes the upregulation of several *HOX* genes and the expression of numerous myeloid markers.[178,179] Both early B- and T cell ALLs with *MLL* rearrangements showed a characteristic upregulation of specific *HOX* genes including *HOXA9*, *HOXA10*, *HOXC6* and the *HOX* gene regulator *MEIS1*.[178–180] These results, together with the demonstration that HOXA9 is required for the transformation of hemopoietic precursors by MLL fusion oncogenes in murine leukemia models,[181] emphasize the central role of *HOX* gene dysregulation in the pathogenesis of *MLL*-rearranged leukemias.

The receptor tyrosine kinase FLT3 was recently found to be highly expressed in *MLL*-rearranged ALL as compared to other acute leukemias.[178] Further study uncovered that 20 percent of *MLL*-rearranged ALL samples possess activating mutations in the activation loop region[182] (Fig. 26.6). These data support the idea that leukemogenic fusion proteins such as MLL-fusions cooperate with activated kinases to promote leukemogenesis.[183] Furthermore, FLT3 inhibitors appear to have activity against *MLL*-rearranged and hyperdiploid ALL, *in vitro* and in murine models.[184,185] Clinical trials to assess the efficacy of FLT3 inhibitors in *MLL*-rearranged ALL are in development.

CALM–AF10 FUSION GENE IN T ACUTE LYMPHOBLASTIC LEUKEMIA

The t(10;11)(p13;q14) detected in approximately 3–10 percent of T-ALL cases and in occasional AML cases results in the fusion of *CALM*, encoding a protein with high homology to the murine clathrin assembly protein AP3; with *AF10*, a gene identified as an MLL partner in the MLL-AF10 fusion resulting from the t(10;11)(p13;q23).[186] Although the mechanism of action of CALM-AF10 is still poorly understood, the expression of this fusion transcript has been associated with early arrest in T cell development and to differentiation into the γ-δ lineage in T-ALL.[187] Microarray expression analysis has revealed that CALM-AF10 cases overexpress *HOXA* genes and the oncogene *BMI1* that suppresses the p16 and p19 cell cycle inhibitors.[188]

TEL-AML-1(ETV6-RUNX1) FUSION GENE IN EARLY PRE-B ACUTE LYMPHOBLASTIC LEUKEMIA

The t(12;21) translocation which creates the *TEL-AML1* fusion gene is the most common genetic lesion in pediatric ALL, occurring in 20–25 percent of B lineage cases, but is much less common in adult ALL.[54] The chimeric protein contains the helix-loop-helix (HLH) domain of TEL fused to nearly all of AML1, including both the transactivation domain and the DNA- and protein-binding Runt homology domain. Both the *TEL* and *AML1* genes are found in other leukemia-associated translocations. *TEL* was first identified in a fusion with the platelet-derived growth factor receptor gene (*PDGFRB*) created by the t(5;12) in chronic myelomonocytic leukemia and is also fused to *ABL*, *MN1*, and *EVI1* in AML, and to *JAK2* in T-ALL. AML1 is the DNA-binding component of the AML1-CBFβ transcription factor complex disrupted by the t(8;21), t(3;21), and inv(16) in AML, making it the most common target of chromosomal translocations in leukemia. In addition, inactivating mutations of AML1 occur in AML and the amplifications of the AML locus occur in pediatric ALL.[189,190]

Lack of expression of genes normally upregulated by *AML1* probably has a role in *TEL-AML1*-induced transformation. Evidence in support of this model includes the interference of AML1-dependent transcriptional transactivation by TEL-AML1 *in vitro*,[191] and the interaction of TEL-AML1, but not normal AML1, with N-Cor, a component of the nuclear coreceptor complex with histone deacetylase activity. In fact, *TEL-AML1*-mediated gene repression can be reversed by treatment with HDAC inhibitors suggesting that these drugs may be useful therapeutic agents for *TEL-AML1* patients.[192] The observation that the nontranslocated copy of *TEL* is frequently deleted in *TEL-AML1* leukemias suggests that the leukemogenic effect of TEL-AML1 may be mediated, at least in part, by loss of function of the *TEL* gene.[193–196]

TEL-AML1 expression is associated with an excellent prognosis, with EFS rates of approximately 90 percent in a variety of studies.[54] However, a recent analysis found that age at diagnosis and leukocyte count were independent predictors of outcome suggesting that these factors should be taken into account when treating *TEL-AML1* patients.[197]

Tyrosine kinase genes: *BCR–ABL*

The 22q chromosomal marker, often called the Philadelphia (Ph) chromosome, which arises from the t(9;22)(q34;q11), was originally identified in patients with chronic myelogenous leukemia (CML), although it is also found in about 4 percent of childhood cases and 25 percent of adult cases of ALL.[54] The t(9;22) breakpoints on the distal tip of the long arm of chromosome 9 are scattered over a distance of nearly 200 kb within the first intron of the *ABL* protooncogene, upstream of the tyrosine kinase domain.[198–200] The t(9;22) generates a *BCR-ABL* fusion gene, consisting of 5′ (upstream) sequences from *BCR* and 3′ (downstream) sequences of *ABL*. The fusion transcript found in CML (M-*BCR* breakpoint) encodes a 210 kDa hybrid protein (p210), whereas fusions typically present in ALL (M-*BCR*) encode a 190 kDa protein (p190).[201–203] Both types of fusions generate chimeric oncoproteins that are activated as a tyrosine-specific protein kinase, similar to the V-ABL protein.[204–206]

The ABL tyrosine kinase is localized both in the nucleus and in the cytoplasm of proliferating cells. It is activated by DNA damage downstream of ATM and appears to promote p53-mediated growth arrest.[207–210] Mice deficient in ABL develop a wasting syndrome and die soon after birth.[211,212] In contrast to the nuclear and cytoplasmic distribution of ABL, the BCR-ABL fusion oncoprotein is cytoplasmic and shows increased tyrosine kinase activity.[213,214] When expressed in murine hematopoietic precursors, both p190 and p210 transform hematopoietic cells *in vitro* and induce a syndrome similar to chronic myeloid leukemia (CML) in mice.[215–218] Transformation by the BCR-ABL oncoprotein involves activation of the RAS/MAPK pathway, PI3 and JUN kinases, CBL and CRKL, Janus kinases (JAKS)-signal transducers and activators of transcription (STAT), nuclear factor (NF)-κB, SRC, and cyclin D1.[219–226] Among these targets, RAS, JUN kinase and PI3 kinase pathways are involved in the induction of cell proliferation.[227] The BCR-ABL oncoprotein affects multiple aspects of cell homeostasis, including apoptosis, differentiation and cell adhesion. An important cellular effect of BCR-ABL is the induction of cellular resistance to DNA damage agents such as cytostatic drugs and irradiation. After DNA damage, BCR-ABL extends the duration of the G2/M cell cycle checkpoint and facilitates DNA repair. It also upregulates the antiapoptotic $BCLX_L$ gene, contributing to the suppression of apoptotic cell death.[228]

BCR-ABL expression is associated with an extremely poor prognosis in ALL patients despite treatment on contemporary protocols for high-risk disease.[229–231] Until recently, it was believed that the only curative treatment for Ph chromosome-positive ALL was bone marrow transplantation in first remission; however, a subset of these patients, primarily those with low blood leukocyte counts at diagnosis, may be cured with the use of standard intensive chemotherapy.[232,233] Similarly, Ph-positive leukemia patients with a good initial response to steroid/intrathecal methrotexate therapy have a more favorable prognosis than patients without this feature.[233,234]

The development of imatinib mesylate (STI-571/Gleevac), a pharmacologic tyrosine kinase inhibitor targeting the BCR-ABL oncoprotein, has opened novel therapeutic opportunities for the management of Ph-positive ALL. Initial phase I clinical studies with this agent showed marked antileukemic activity in patients with CML[235] or BCR-ABL-positive ALL.[236] Although the effectiveness of imatinib mesylate against BCR-ABL-positive leukemias has been confirmed in phase II trials,[237–239] its utility single agent is limited by the rapid development of drug resistance[240,241] underscoring the need to integrate imatinib into combination chemotherapy regimens for BCR-ABL-positive leukemias[242,243] and to develop other novel tyrosine kinase inhibitors.[244,245]

Tumor suppressor genes

Loss of function of a tumor suppressor protein, occurring through deletion or mutational inactivation of both chromosomal loci of the gene that encodes it, leads to malignant transformation. Knudson first proposed that inactivation of both alleles of a single locus is needed to initiate the development of retinoblastoma, basing his ideas on the observed frequencies of hereditary and sporadic forms of this disease.[246] Allelic loss of defined regions of many different chromosomes has been linked to specific types of human tumors. By analogy with the findings in retinoblastoma, a reasonable hypothesis is that each of these regions harbors a tumor suppressor gene whose product is uniquely involved in the inhibition of cell cycle progression and promotion of terminal differentiation of the normal cells that give rise to these different types of tumors. Tumor suppressor genes that play an important role in ALL include *p53* and the *p16* locus.

p53, located on chromosome 17, band p13, is mutated or lost through chromosomal deletion in a wide variety of human tumors,[247] including colon cancer, lung cancer, breast cancer and osteosarcoma. Families with Li–Fraumeni syndrome, which predisposes to a variety of cancers including sarcomas, brain tumors, leukemias, adrenocortical carcinomas and premenopausal breast cancers, have germline mutations in the *p53* gene.[248–251] *p53* encodes a 53 kDa transcription factor that functions as a cell cycle and apoptosis checkpoint regulator.[247,252–256] The p53 protein is increased by DNA damage, blocks cell division at G_1 to allow DNA repair, and activates apoptosis in cells that have sustained DNA damage.[257–262] The mechanism of p53 activation is triggered by the loss of activity of MDM2 after DNA damage (via ATM) or oncogenic stress (via p14/ARF). As a negative regulator of p53, MDM-2 induces the ubiquitination of p53 and its degradation by the proteasome. Hence, when MDM2 activity is abolished, p53 accumulates and certain cell cycle regulatory genes such as *p21(WAF1/CIP1/SDI1/CAP20)* and proapoptotic factor

genes such as *BAX*, *PUMA* and *NOXA* are transcriptionally activated.

p53 is also inactivated in a variety of hematopoietic malignancies, including B cell ALL and Burkitt's lymphoma, but is mutated or deleted in less than 3 percent of pediatric B-precursor or T cell ALL cases at diagnosis.[263–265] It thus appears to play a limited role in the etiology of pediatric leukemia. However, *p53* mutations are seen in approximately 25 percent of relapsed T cell ALL cases, suggesting a role for *p53* inactivation in the development of resistant disease.[263,264] In addition, *p53* mutations were detected in three of 10 ALL patients who failed on induction therapy or suffered early relapse, further supporting a role for *p53* inactivation in disease progression.[266,267]

The cyclin-dependent kinase inhibitors (CDKIs), which include p15 (INK4B/MTS2), p16 (INK4A/MTS1/CDKN2), p18 (INK4C), p19 (INK4D), p21 (WAF1/CIP1/SDI1/CAP20), p27 (KIP1), and p57 (KIP2) constitute a family of tumor suppressors that negatively regulate the cell cycle by inhibiting cyclin-dependent kinase (CDK) phosphorylation of pRB.[268] The *INK4A* locus, located on the short arm of chromosome band 9q21, contains two different tumor suppressor genes, *p16INK4A* and *p14ARF* (*p19ARF* in mice),[269,270] each with a distinct promoter and first exon but common second and third exons. Despite this close relationship at the genomic level, p16 and p14 have totally unrelated amino acid sequences as they use different reading frames in their common second and third exons.[271] A third tumor suppressor gene, the cyclin-dependent kinase inhibitor *p15INK4B*, also resides in this region.[272,273] p16INK4A and p15INK4B directly inhibit cyclin D-CDK4/6 complexes and interfere with cell cycle progression. Cyclin D-CDK4/6 complexes promote entry into S phase through phosphorylation of the retinoblastoma protein, pRB, leading to the release of transcription factors, such as E2F, that promote entry into S phase. By contrast, p14ARF lacks a direct effect on the cell cycle machinery acting instead to stabilize and upregulate p53 through the inhibition of MDM2.[273–276] The role of the *INK4a* locus in tumorigenesis was confirmed by selective targeted deletion of *p16* and *p19* in mice. *p16*-deficient mice (with intact *p19*) as well as *p19*-deficient mice (with intact *p16*) develop tumors (primarily lymphomas and fibrosarcomas).[269,277,278]

The short arm of chromosome 9 is the most frequent target of chromosomal alterations in human cancer. In particular, human leukemias and lymphomas show a high frequency of 9p21 deletions involving both the *p16INK4A/p14ARF* and the *p15INK4B* loci. Epigenetic silencing of these tumor suppressor genes through hypermethylation of their promoter sequences represents an alternative mechanism of gene inactivation. While *p16INK4A/p14ARF* and *p15INK4B* are homozygously deleted in 20–30 percent of B-precursor ALL cases and in 70–80 percent of T cell ALL cases, epigenetic silencing of the *p15INK4B* promoter has been observed in 44 percent of primary B lineage ALLs.[279–291]

The clinical impact of *p15INK4B* and *p16INK4A/ p14ARF* deletions in ALL remains controversial. On the one hand, homozygous *p16* deletion is related to high-risk features at diagnosis and to an increased risk of relapse and death in childhood ALL,[290,292,293] while on the other, *p15INK4B* and *p16INK4A/p14ARF* deletions were not associated with clinical outcome in a study of adult ALL cases.[294] Interpretation of the clinical significance of the inactivation of these tumor suppressor genes must also take into account alternative mechanisms of gene inactivation, such as aberrant methylation of *p15INK4B* promoter sequences, which has been associated with epigenetic silencing of this locus and a worse outcome in adult ALL cases.[295]

Identification of recurring chromosomal deletion syndromes in human ALL indicates that other tumor suppressor loci may be involved in this disease. These syndromes, which affect the long arm of chromosome 6, the short arm of chromosome 9, or the short arm of chromosome 12, can each be found in leukemic cells from approximately 10 percent of patients with ALL by standard cytogenetic analysis, making them among the most frequent cytogenetic abnormalities in this disease. Functional deletion can result either from interstitial deletion of the involved chromosome arm or from derivative chromosomes that result from unbalanced chromosomal translocations. For each chromosome, the deleted regions overlap a single target region, which may contain key tumor suppressor genes, whose loss could be an important step in leukemic transformation.

Deletions of the long arm of chromosome 6 are consistently found in about 10 percent of cases of ALL.[296] Interstitial deletions affecting bands 6q15-q24 have been reported most frequently; translocations with breakpoints within this region are also common. Band q21 of chromosome 6 seems to be involved in each of the abnormalities, suggesting that the target gene(s) resides in this region. Deletions of chromosome 6q occur with equal frequency in pro-B, pre-B and T cell cases.

Deletions or translocations involving the short arm of chromosome 12 are also found in about 10 percent of ALL cases, with most clustered around band 12p13.[296] These cases generally have a B-precursor phenotype, and the blast cells usually express CD10 and HLA-DR on the cell surface. Abnormalities of the short arm of chromosome 12 are rarely found in T-ALL cases. Translocations involving chromosome 12p13 may be balanced or unbalanced and can involve multiple different donor chromosomes. Molecular studies, however, have revealed that the majority of translocations involving 12p13 are cryptic 12;21 translocations, resulting in the *TEL-AML1* fusion. In the cases with unbalanced translocations, DNA sequences distal to the breakpoint are lost from the affected homologue and subsequently from the leukemic cell genome, so the result is similar to that of interstitial deletion. The frequency of deletions involving the 12p13 region suggests that these lesions primarily inactivate one allele of a tumor

suppressor gene in this chromosomal region. Although the *TEL* and *p27KIP1* genes may be targets of deletion in these cases, neither locus is inactivated by point mutations in childhood ALL cases with loss of heterozygosity (LOH) in 12p, possibly implicating additional tumor suppressor genes in this region, although *TEL* or *p27KIP1* haploinsufficiency could also contribute to leukemic transformation.[193,297]

Mutated *RAS* genes

Protooncogenes of the *RAS* family – *HRAS*, *KRAS*, and *NRAS* – encode 21 kDa proteins that are associated with the inner surface of the cytoplasmic membrane. These proteins bind guanidine nucleotides and function as intermediates in signal transduction pathways that regulate the growth of cells. The *RAS* protooncogenes are activated to the status of transforming oncogenes by somatic mutations that alter the amino acids specified by codons 12, 13 or 61. Human tumor DNAs were initially found to contain activated homologues of either *HRAS* or *KRAS*,[298,299] protooncogenes that were identified on the basis of their homology with viral oncogenes. Mutated *RAS* genes also bind guanine nucleotides, but have diminished capacity to hydrolyze guanidine triphosphate (GTP) to GDP. Transforming properties of activated RAS proteins may result from their inability to hydrolyze GTP, which could play an important role in modulating signal transduction.

The transforming potential of human *RAS* genes activated by point mutation has been documented in experimental systems. The *RAS* oncogenes will transform NIH-3T3 murine fibroblasts *in vitro*, and will collaborate with other oncogenes to transform primary cultures of embryo fibroblasts.[300–303] In addition, their role in mammalian tumorigenesis has been documented in carcinogen-induced animal tumor model systems.[304–306]

Activated *NRAS* genes appear to be preferentially involved in hematopoietic malignances. They were detected in the myeloid cell lines HL-60, KG1, and Rc2A;[171,307] in fresh leukemic cell samples from patients with AML or CML;[308–310] and in lymphoblastic leukemias with a T cell immunophenotype.[311] In AML, *NRAS* gene mutations involving codon 13 or 61 were found in approximately 20 percent of cases, regardless of morphologic subtype.[312,313] Mutation of codon 12 of the *KRAS* gene was also observed in two of the 37 cases studied.[312] In a study of lymphoblasts from children with ALL, two of 19 patients showed mutated *NRAS* genes, both involving codon 12.[312] Mutated *RAS* genes have also been documented in patients with preleukemic syndromes, indicating the potential involvement.

Abnormalities of leukemia cell ploidy

Abnormalities of chromosome number, which generally occur in the absence of specific chromosomal translocations, have important prognostic implications in childhood ALL.[314–316] In an analysis of patients treated in St Jude Total Therapy Studies IX and X, chromosome number as determined by karyotyping was the strongest single predictor of outcome: patients with hyperdiploidy >50 chromosomes had the best response to therapy.[316] Hyperdiploid ALL patients can also be identified rapidly by flow cytometric measurement of the DNA of leukemic blast cells, in which nuclei stained with a DNA-specific dye are analyzed for the amount of DNA per cell.[317]

Found in 25–30 percent of childhood ALL cases, hyperdiploidy >50 chromosomes in the leukemic clone is one of the most powerful means of identifying patients with a very good prognosis.[54] Patients with this chromosomal feature typically present with favorable prognostic indicators, such as age between 2 and 10 years, a low white blood cell count, and an early pre-B immunophenotype, and can expect cure rates of 80–90 percent.[318–320] DNA index >1.16, determined by flow cytometry and corresponding to more than 52 chromosomes per leukemic cell, predicts a similar outstanding response to therapy.[318] Even so, one can find considerable heterogeneity within this favorable subgroup: for example, patients with 51–56 chromosomes per leukemic cell fare less well on standard chemotherapy than do those with 56–67 chromosomes.[319] Moreover, about two-thirds of hyperdiploid ALL cases show additional chromosomal abnormalities that confer a less favorable prognosis.[321] The mechanism accounting for the favorable outcome of patients with hyperdiploid ALL remains elusive, but may reflect an increased sensitivity to antimetabolite therapy[322] and diminished protection from bone marrow stroma-secreted factors against drug-induced cell death.[323]

Present in 8–15 percent of pediatric ALL cases,[54] hyperdiploidy of 47–50 chromosomes (DNA index greater >1.00 but <1.16)[318] identifies a subgroup with unfavorable prognostic features at diagnosis, such as older age, higher WBC count and higher serum LDH levels.[319,324] Originally considered to have an intermediate prognosis,[325] these patients have shown improved responses to contemporary chemotherapy regimens.[319]

Near haploidy (<30 chromosomes), a rare numeric chromosomal abnormality, carries a very poor prognosis.[54] In a recent cooperative group study,[326] children with hypodiploid ALL fared worse than those without this abnormality. Overall, adults with ALL have significantly fewer numeric chromosomal abnormalities than do children, and the prognostic impact of these changes has been limited.[294] In a large series of adult ALL cases,[23] hypodiploidy was the only numeric abnormality with prognostic value and was associated with a poor outcome.[23]

FUTURE DIRECTIONS

Gene expression analysis of ALL samples has demonstrated that different molecular subsets of the disease have different gene expression signatures demonstrating the heterogeneity of the disease. The success of imatinib for *BCR-ABL* positive leukemia has indicated the promise of molecularly targeted therapies for leukemia and cancer in general. The discovery of activation of the NOTCH pathway in T-ALL patients has led to the opening of clinical trials with γ-secretase inhibitors. Gene expression analysis has identified activation of the FLT3 pathway in MLL rearranged leukemia providing another rational target for drug therapy. Future leukemia research should focus on defining the molecular events that contribute to transformation in each subtype of lymphoid leukemia. Microarray expression analysis combined with emerging technologies such as RNAi and ChIP-on-chip analysis hold promise in reaching this goal. We imagine that in the future, molecular-targeted therapies will be available for all pathways activated in leukemia and that patients will be given compounds that target the pathways activated by the oncoproteins expressed in their leukemic blasts. Because these drugs will be more specific they should be less toxic and have fewer long-term side effects than current chemotherapeutics.

KEY POINTS

- Lymphoblastic leukemia and lymphoma are clonal diseases.
- Lymphoblastic leukemias are classified according to their developmental stage, i.e., pre-B ALL, B-ALL and T-ALL.
- Aberrant expression of transcription factor genes, either intact or chimeric as a result of a chromosomal translocation, is a common feature of the diseases.
- Understanding the transcription factors deregulated in lymphoblastic leukemias as well as the gene expression changes downstream of these factors enables the development of targeted therapeutics.

ACKNOWLEDGMENTS

We thank Eric Smith and Scott Armstrong for assistance with the figures. This work is supported in part by the National Cancer Institute, NIH (grants CA 68484 (ATL), CA 109901 (JO and ATL), and T32 HL007623 (JO).

REFERENCES

● = Key primary paper
◆ = Major review article

1. Cleary ML. Oncogenic conversion of transcription factors by chromosomal translocations. *Cell* 1991; **66**: 619–22.

2. Ferrando AA, Neuberg DS, Staunton J et al. Gene expression signatures define novel oncogenic pathways in T cell acute lymphoblastic leukemia. *Cancer Cell* 2002; **1**: 75–87.

3. Look AT. Oncogenic transcription factors in the human acute leukemias. *Science* 1997; **278**: 1059–64.

4. Rabbitts TH. Chromosomal translocations in human cancer. *Nature* 1994; **372**: 143–9.

5. Arnold A, Cossman J, Bakhshi A et al. Immunoglobulin-gene rearrangements as unique clonal markers in human lymphoid neoplasms. *N Engl J Med* 1983; **309**: 1593–9.

6. Waldmann TA, Davis MM, Bongiovanni KF, Korsmeyer SJ. Rearrangements of genes for the antigen receptor on T cells as markers of lineage and clonality in human lymphoid neoplasms. *N Engl J Med* 1985; **313**: 776–83.

7. Sen L, Borella L. Clinical importance of lymphoblasts with T markers in childhood acute leukemia. *N Engl J Med* 1975; **292**: 828–32.

8. Kersey J, Nesbit M, Hallgren H et al. Evidence for origin of certain childhood acute lymphoblastic leukemias and lymphomas in thymus-derived lymphocytes. *Cancer* 1975; **36**: 1348–52.

9. Greaves MF. Differentiation-linked leukemogenesis in lymphocytes. *Science* 1986; **234**: 697–704.

10. Hurwitz CA, Loken MR, Graham ML et al. Asynchronous antigen expression in B lineage acute lymphoblastic leukemia. *Blood* 1988; **72**: 299–307.

11. Bennett JM, Catovsky D, Daniel MT et al. The morphological classification of acute lymphoblastic leukaemia: concordance among observers and clinical correlations. *Br J Haematol* 1981; **47**: 553–61.

12. Pui CH. Childhood leukemias. *N Engl J Med* 1995; **332**: 1618–30.

13. Pui CH, Crist WM, Look AT. Biology and clinical significance of cytogenetic abnormalities in childhood acute lymphoblastic leukemia. *Blood* 1990; **76**: 1449–63.

14. Murphy SB, Bowman WP, Abromowitch M et al. Results of treatment of advanced-stage Burkitt's lymphoma and B cell (SIg+) acute lymphoblastic leukemia with high-dose fractionated cyclophosphamide and coordinated high-dose methotrexate and cytarabine. *J Clin Oncol* 1986; **4**: 1732–9.

15. Patte C, Philip T, Rodary C et al. Improved survival rate in children with stage III and IV B cell non-Hodgkin's lymphoma and leukemia using multi-agent chemotherapy: results of a study of 114 children from the French Pediatric Oncology Society. *J Clin Oncol* 1986; **4**: 1219–26.

16. Patte C, Philip T, Rodary C et al. High survival rate in advanced-stage B-cell lymphomas and leukemias without CNS involvement with a short intensive polychemotherapy: results from the French Pediatric Oncology Society of a randomized trial of 216 children. *J Clin Oncol* 1991; **9**: 123–32.

17. Schwenn MR, Blattner SR, Lynch E, Weinstein HJ. HiC-COM: a 2-month intensive chemotherapy regimen for children with stage III and IV Burkitt's lymphoma and B-cell acute lymphoblastic leukemia. *J Clin Oncol* 1991; **9**: 133–8.

18. Reiter A, Schrappe M, Ludwig WD et al. Favorable outcome of B-cell acute lymphoblastic leukemia in childhood: a report of three consecutive studies of the BFM group. *Blood* 1992; **80**: 2471–8.

19. Pui CH, Behm FG, Crist WM. Clinical and biologic relevance of immunologic marker studies in childhood acute lymphoblastic leukemia. *Blood* 1993; **82**: 343–62.

20. Crist WM, Carroll AJ, Shuster JJ et al. Poor prognosis of children with pre-B acute lymphoblastic leukemia is associated with the t(1;19)(q23;p13): a Pediatric Oncology Group study. *Blood* 1990; **76**: 117–22.

21. Cytogenetic abnormalities in adult acute lymphoblastic leukemia: correlations with hematologic findings outcome. A Collaborative Study of the Group Francais de Cytogenetique Hematologique. *Blood* 1996; **87**: 3135–42.

22. Secker-Walker LM, Berger R, Fenaux P et al. Prognostic significance of the balanced t(1;19) and unbalanced der(19)t(1;19) translocations in acute lymphoblastic leukemia. *Leukemia* 1992; **6**: 363–9.

23. Secker-Walker LM, Prentice HG, Durrant J et al. Cytogenetics adds independent prognostic information in adults with acute lymphoblastic leukaemia on MRC trial UKALL XA. MRC Adult Leukaemia Working Party. *Br J Haematol* 1997; **96**: 601–10.

24. Uckun FM, Sensel MG, Sather HN et al. Clinical significance of translocation t(1;19) in childhood acute lymphoblastic leukemia in the context of contemporary therapies: a report from the Children's Cancer Group. *J Clin Oncol* 1998; **16**: 527–35.

25. Reinherz EL, Schlossman SF. Current concepts in immunology: regulation of the immune response–inducer and suppressor T-lymphocyte subsets in human beings. *N Engl J Med* 1980; **303**: 370–3.

26. Staal FJ, Weerkamp F, Langerak AW et al. Transcriptional control of t lymphocyte differentiation. *Stem Cells* 2001; **19**: 165–79.

27. Uckun FM, Steinherz PG, Sather H et al. CD2 antigen expression on leukemic cells as a predictor of event-free survival after chemotherapy for T-lineage acute lymphoblastic leukemia: a Children's Cancer Group study. *Blood* 1996; **88**: 4288–95.

28. Czuczman MS, Dodge RK, Stewart CC et al. Value of immunophenotype in intensively treated adult acute lymphoblastic leukemia: cancer and leukemia Group B study 8364. *Blood* 1999; **93**: 3931–9.

29. Shuster JJ, Falletta JM, Pullen DJ et al. Prognostic factors in childhood T-cell acute lymphoblastic leukemia: a Pediatric Oncology Group study. *Blood* 1990; **75**: 166–73.

30. Pui CH, Behm FG, Singh B et al. Heterogeneity of presenting features and their relation to treatment outcome in 120 children with T-cell acute lymphoblastic leukemia. *Blood* 1990; **75**: 174–9.

31. Niehues T, Kapaun P, Harms DO et al. A classification based on T cell selection-related phenotypes identifies a subgroup of childhood T-ALL with favorable outcome in the COALL studies. *Leukemia* 1999; **13**: 614–17.

32. Williams DL, Look AT, Melvin SL *et al.* New chromosomal translocations correlate with specific immunophenotypes of childhood acute lymphoblastic leukemia. *Cell* 1984; **36**: 101–9.

33. Rabbitts TH. Translocations, master genes, and differences between the origins of acute and chronic leukemias. *Cell* 1991; **67**: 641–4.

34. Dalla-Favera R, Bregni M, Erikson J *et al.* Human c-myc onc gene is located on the region of chromosome 8 that is translocated in Burkitt lymphoma cells. *Proc Natl Acad Sci U S A* 1982; **79**: 7824–7.

35. Taub R, Kirsch I, Morton C *et al.* Translocation of the c-myc gene into the immunoglobulin heavy chain locus in human Burkitt lymphoma and murine plasmacytoma cells. *Proc Natl Acad Sci U S A* 1982; **79**: 7837–41.

36. Adams JM, Gerondakis S, Webb E *et al.* Cellular myc oncogene is altered by chromosome translocation to an immunoglobulin locus in murine plasmacytomas and is rearranged similarly in human Burkitt lymphomas. *Proc Natl Acad Sci U S A* 1983; **80**: 1982–6.

37. Erikson J, Nishikura K, ar-Rushdi A *et al.* Translocation of an immunoglobulin kappa locus to a region 3′ of an unrearranged c-myc oncogene enhances c-myc transcription. *Proc Natl Acad Sci U S A* 1983; **80**: 7581–5.

38. Croce CM, Thierfelder W, Erikson J *et al.* Transcriptional activation of an unrearranged and untranslocated c-myc oncogene by translocation of a C lambda locus in Burkitt. *Proc Natl Acad Sci U S A* 1983; **80**: 6922–6.

39. Emanuel BS, Selden JR, Chaganti RS *et al.* The 2p breakpoint of a 2;8 translocation in Burkitt lymphoma interrupts the V kappa locus. *Proc Natl Acad Sci U S A* 1984; **81**: 2444–6.

40. Hollis GF, Mitchell KF, Battey J *et al.* A variant translocation places the lambda immunoglobulin genes 3′ to the c-myc oncogene in Burkitt's lymphoma. *Nature* 1984; **307**: 752–5.

41. Rappold GA, Hameister H, Cremer T *et al.* c-myc and immunoglobulin kappa light chain constant genes are on the 8q+ chromosome of three Burkitt lymphoma lines with t(2;8) translocations. *EMBO J* 1984; **3**: 2951–5.

42. Taub R, Kelly K, Battey J *et al.* A novel alteration in the structure of an activated c-myc gene in a variant t(2;8) Burkitt lymphoma. *Cell* 1984; **37**: 511–20.

43. Grandori C, Mac J, Siebelt F *et al.* Myc-Max heterodimers activate a DEAD box gene and interact with multiple E box-related sites *in vivo*. *EMBO J* 1996; **15**: 4344–57.

44. Ayer DE, Kretzner L, Eisenman RN. Mad: a heterodimeric partner for Max that antagonizes Myc transcriptional activity. *Cell* 1993; **72**: 211–22.

45. Foley KP, Eisenman RN. Two MAD tails: what the recent knockouts of Mad1 and Mxi1 tell us about the MYC/MAX/MAD network. *Biochim Biophys Acta* 1999; **1423**: m37–47.

46. Hurlin PJ, Queva C, Eisenman RN. Mnt: a novel Max-interacting protein and Myc antagonist. *Curr Top Microbiol Immunol* 1997; **224**: 115–21.

47. Coller HA, Grandori C, Tamayo P *et al.* Expression analysis with oligonucleotide microarrays reveals that MYC regulates genes involved in growth, cell cycle, signaling, and adhesion. *Proc Natl Acad Sci U S A* 2000; **97**: 3260–5.

48. Mateyak MK, Obaya AJ, Sedivy JM. c-Myc regulates cyclin D-Cdk4 and -Cdk6 activity but affects cell cycle progression at multiple independent points. *Mol Cell Biol* 1999; **19**: 4672–83.

49. Muller D, Bouchard C, Rudolph B *et al.* Cdk2-dependent phosphorylation of p27 facilitates its Myc-induced release from cyclin E/cdk2 complexes. *Oncogene* 1997; **15**: 2561–76.

50. Galaktionov K, Chen X, Beach D. Cdc25 cell-cycle phosphatase as a target of c-myc. *Nature* 1996; **382**: 511–17.

51. Zindy F, Eischen CM, Randle DH *et al.* Myc signaling via the ARF tumor suppressor regulates p53-dependent apoptosis and immortalization. *Genes Dev* 1998; **12**: 2424–33.

52. Wang J, Xie LY, Allan S *et al.* Myc activates telomerase. *Genes Dev* 1998; **12**: 1769–74.

53. Wu KJ, Grandori C, Amacker M *et al.* Direct activation of TERT transcription by c-MYC. *Nat Genet* 1999; **21**: 220–4.

54. Ferrando AA, Look AT. Clinical implications of recurring chromosomal and associated molecular abnormalities in acute lymphoblastic leukemia. *Semin Hematol* 2000; **37**: 381–95.

55. Begley CG, Aplan PD, Davey MP *et al.* Chromosomal translocation in a human leukemic stem-cell line disrupts the T-cell antigen receptor delta-chain diversity region and results in a previously unreported fusion transcript. *Proc Natl Acad Sci U S A* 1989; **86**: 2031–5.

56. Chen Q, Cheng JT, Tasi LH *et al.* The tal gene undergoes chromosome translocation in T cell leukemia and potentially encodes a helix-loop-helix protein. *EMBO J* 1990; **9**: 415–24.

57. Xia Y, Brown L, Yang CY *et al.* TAL2, a helix-loop-helix gene activated by the (7;9)(q34;q32) translocation in human T-cell leukemia. *Proc Natl Acad Sci U S A* 1991; **88**: 11416–20.

58. Mellentin JD, Smith SD, Cleary ML. lyl-1, a novel gene altered by chromosomal translocation in T cell leukemia, codes for a protein with a helix-loop-helix DNA binding motif. *Cell* 1989; **58**: 77–83.

59. Finger LR, Harvey RC, Moore RC *et al.* A common mechanism of chromosomal translocation in T- and B-cell neoplasia. *Science* 1986; **234**: 982–5.

60. McKeithan TW, Shima EA, Le Beau MM *et al.* Molecular cloning of the breakpoint junction of a human chromosomal 8;14 translocation involving the T-cell receptor alpha-chain gene and sequences on the 3′ side of MYC. *Proc Natl Acad Sci U S A* 1986; **83**: 6636–40.

61. Shima EA, Le Beau MM, McKeithan TW *et al.* Gene encoding the alpha chain of the T-cell receptor is moved immediately downstream of c-myc in a chromosomal 8;14 translocation in a cell line from a human T-cell leukemia. *Proc Natl Acad Sci U S A* 1986; **83**: 3439–43.

62. Wang J, Jani-Sait SN, Escalon EA *et al*. The t(14;21) (q11.2;q22) chromosomal translocation associated with T-cell acute lymphoblastic leukemia activates the BHLHB1 gene. *Proc Natl Acad Sci U S A* 2000; **97**: 3497–502.

63. McGuire EA, Hockett RD, Pollock KM *et al*. The t(11;14)(p15;q11) in a T-cell acute lymphoblastic leukemia cell line activates multiple transcripts, including Ttg-1, a gene encoding a potential zinc finger protein. *Mol Cell Biol* 1989; **9**: 2124–32.

64. Boehm T, Foroni L, Kaneko Y *et al*. The rhombotin family of cysteine-rich LIM-domain oncogenes: distinct members are involved in T-cell translocations to human chromosomes 11p15 and 11p13. *Proc Natl Acad Sci U S A* 1991; **88**: 4367–71.

65. Royer-Pokora B, Loos U, Ludwig WD. TTG-2, a new gene encoding a cysteine-rich protein with the LIM motif, is overexpressed in acute T-cell leukaemia with the t(11;14)(p13;q11). *Oncogene* 1991; **6**: 1887–93.

66. Hatano M, Roberts CW, Minden M *et al*. Deregulation of a homeobox gene, HOX11, by the t(10;14) in T cell leukemia. *Science* 1991; **253**: 79–82.

67. Ferrando AA, Look AT. Gene expression profiling in T-cell acute lymphoblastic leukemia. *Semin Hematol* 2003; **40**: 274–80.

68. Kennedy MA, Gonzalez-Sarmiento R, Kees UR *et al*. HOX11, a homeobox-containing T-cell oncogene on human chromosome 10q24. *Proc Natl Acad Sci U S A* 1991; **88**: 8900–4.

69. Bernard OA, Busson-LeConiat M, Ballerini P *et al*. A new recurrent and specific cryptic translocation, t(5;14)(q35;q32), is associated with expression of the Hox11L2 gene in T acute lymphoblastic leukemia. *Leukemia* 2001; **15**: 1495–504.

70. Lu M, Gong ZY, Shen WF, Ho AD. The tcl-3 proto-oncogene altered by chromosomal translocation in T-cell leukemia codes for a homeobox protein. *EMBO J* 1991; **10**: 2905–10.

71. Dube ID, Kamel-Reid S, Yuan CC *et al*. A novel human homeobox gene lies at the chromosome 10 breakpoint in lymphoid neoplasias with chromosomal translocation t(10;14). *Blood* 1991; **78**: 2996–3003.

72. Dear TN, Sanchez-Garcia I, Rabbitts TH. The HOX11 gene encodes a DNA-binding nuclear transcription factor belonging to a distinct family of homeobox genes. *Proc Natl Acad Sci U S A* 1993; **90**: 4431–5.

73. Brown L, Cheng JT, Chen Q *et al*. Site-specific recombination of the tal-1 gene is a common occurrence in human T cell leukemia. *EMBO J* 1990; **9**: 3343–51.

74. Aplan PD, Lombardi DP, Kirsch IR. Structural characterization of SIL, a gene frequently disrupted in T-cell acute lymphoblastic leukemia. *Mol Cell Biol* 1991; **11**: 5462–9.

75. Bernard O, Lecointe N, Jonveaux P *et al*. Two site-specific deletions and t(1;14) translocation restricted to human T-cell acute leukemias disrupt the 5' part of the tal-1 gene. *Oncogene* 1991; **6**: 1477–88.

76. Aplan PD, Lombardi DP, Reaman GH *et al*. Involvement of the putative hematopoietic transcription factor SCL in

77. T-cell acute lymphoblastic leukemia. *Blood* 1992; **79**: 1327–33.

77. Breit TM, Mol EJ, Wolvers-Tettero IL *et al*. Site-specific deletions involving the tal-1 and sil genes are restricted to cells of the T cell receptor alpha/beta lineage: T cell receptor delta gene deletion mechanism affects multiple genes. *J Exp Med* 1993; **177**: 965–77.

78. Bash RO, Hall S, Timmons CF *et al*. Does activation of the TAL1 gene occur in a majority of patients with T-cell acute lymphoblastic leukemia? A pediatric oncology group study. *Blood* 1995; **86**: 666–76.

79. Shivdasani RA, Mayer EL, Orkin SH. Absence of blood formation in mice lacking the T-cell leukaemia oncoprotein tal-1/SCL. *Nature* 1995; **373**: 432–4.

80. Robb L, Lyons I, Li R *et al*. Absence of yolk sac hematopoiesis from mice with a targeted disruption of the scl gene. *Proc Natl Acad Sci U S A* 1995; **92**: 7075–9.

81. Mikkola HK, Klintman J, Yang H *et al*. Haematopoietic stem cells retain long-term repopulating activity and multipotency in the absence of stem-cell leukaemia SCL/tal-1 gene. *Nature* 2003; **421**: 547–51.

82. Baer R. TAL1, TAL2 and LYL1: a family of basic helix-loop-helix proteins implicated in T cell acute leukaemia. *Semin Cancer Biol* 1993; **4**: 341–7.

83. Bain G, Engel I, Robanus Maandag EC *et al*. E2A deficiency leads to abnormalities in alphabeta T-cell development and to rapid development of T-cell lymphomas. *Mol Cell Biol* 1997; **17**: 4782–91.

84. Yan W, Young AZ, Soares VC *et al*. High incidence of T-cell tumors in E2A-null mice and E2A/Id1 double-knockout mice. *Mol Cell Biol* 1997; **17**: 7317–27.

85. O'Neil J, Billa M, Oikemus S, Kelliher M. The DNA binding activity of TAL-1 is not required to induce leukemia/lymphoma in mice. *Oncogene* 2001; **20**: 3897–905.

86. O'Neil J, Shank J, Cusson N *et al*. TAL1/SCL induces leukemia by inhibiting the transcriptional activity of E47/HEB. *Cancer Cell* 2004; **5**: 587–96.

87. Wadman I, Li J, Bash RO *et al*. Specific *in vivo* association between the bHLH and LIM proteins implicated in human T cell leukemia. *EMBO J* 1994; **13**: 4831–9.

88. Valge-Archer VE, Osada H, Warren AJ *et al*. The LIM protein RBTN2 and the basic helix-loop-helix protein TAL1 are present in a complex in erythroid cells. *Proc Natl Acad Sci USA* 1994; **91**: 8617–21.

89. Osada H, Grutz GG, Axelson H *et al*. LIM-only protein Lmo2 forms a protein complex with erythroid transcription factor GATA-1. *Leukemia* 1997; **11(Suppl 3)**: 307–12.

90. Porcher C, Swat W, Rockwell K *et al*. The T cell leukemia oncoprotein SCL/tal-1 is essential for development of all hematopoietic lineages. *Cell* 1996; **86**: 47–57.

91. Warren AJ, Colledge WH, Carlton MB *et al*. The oncogenic cysteine-rich LIM domain protein rbtn2 is essential for erythroid development. *Cell* 1994; **78**: 45–57.

92. McGuire EA, Rintoul CE, Sclar GM, Korsmeyer SJ. Thymic overexpression of Ttg-1 in transgenic mice results in T-cell acute lymphoblastic leukemia/lymphoma. *Mol Cell Biol* 1992; **12**: 4186–96.

93. Fisch P, Boehm T, Lavenir I et al. T-cell acute lymphoblastic lymphoma induced in transgenic mice by the RBTN1 and RBTN2 LIM-domain genes. *Oncogene* 1992; **7**: 2389–97.

94. Larson RC, Fisch P, Larson TA et al. T cell tumours of disparate phenotype in mice transgenic for Rbtn-2. *Oncogene* 1994; **9**: 3675–81.

95. Larson RC, Osada H, Larson TA et al. The oncogenic LIM protein Rbtn2 causes thymic developmental aberrations that precede malignancy in transgenic mice. *Oncogene* 1995; **11**: 853–62.

96. Neale GA, Rehg JE, Goorha RM. Ectopic expression of rhombotin-2 causes selective expansion of CD4-CD8- lymphocytes in the thymus and T-cell tumors in transgenic mice. *Blood* 1995; **86**: 3060–71.

97. Chervinsky DS, Zhao XF, Lam DH et al. Disordered T-cell development and T-cell malignancies in SCL LMO1 double-transgenic mice: parallels with E2A-deficient mice. *Mol Cell Biol* 1999; **19**: 5025–35.

98. Larson RC, Lavenir I, Larson TA et al. Protein dimerization between Lmo2 (Rbtn2) and Tal1 alters thymocyte development and potentiates T cell tumorigenesis in transgenic mice. *EMBO J* 1996; **15**: 1021–7.

99. Hacein-Bey-Abina S, von Kalle C, Schmidt M et al. A serious adverse event after successful gene therapy for X-linked severe combined immunodeficiency. *N Engl J Med* 2003; **348**: 255–6.

100. Hacein-Bey-Abina S, Von Kalle C, Schmidt M et al. LMO2-associated clonal T cell proliferation in two patients after gene therapy for SCID-X1. *Science* 2003; **302**: 415–19.

101. Kees UR, Heerema NA, Kumar R et al. Expression of HOX11 in childhood T-lineage acute lymphoblastic leukaemia can occur in the absence of cytogenetic aberration at 10q24: a study from the Children's Cancer Group (CCG). *Leukemia* 2003; **17**: 887–93.

102. Berger R, Dastugue N, Busson M et al. t(5;14)/HOX11L2-positive T-cell acute lymphoblastic leukemia. A collaborative study of the Groupe Francais de Cytogenetique Hematologique (GFCH). *Leukemia* 2003; **17**: 1851–7.

103. Roberts CW, Shutter JR, Korsmeyer SJ. Hox11 controls the genesis of the spleen. *Nature* 1994; **368**: 747–9.

104. Dear TN, Colledge WH, Carlton MB et al. The Hox11 gene is essential for cell survival during spleen development. *Development* 1995; **121**: 2909–15.

105. Raju K, Tang S, Dube ID et al. Characterization and developmental expression of Tlx-1, the murine homolog of HOX11. *Mech Dev* 1993; **44**: 51–64.

106. Roberts CW, Sonder AM, Lumsden A, Korsmeyer SJ. Development expression of Hox11 and specification of splenic cell fate. *Am J Pathol* 1995; **146**: 1089–101.

107. Riz I, Hawley RG. G1/S transcriptional networks modulated by the HOX11/TLX1 oncogene of T-cell acute lymphoblastic leukemia. *Oncogene* 2005; **24**: 5561–75.

108. Owens BM, Hawley TS, Spain LM et al. TLX1/HOX11-mediated disruption of primary thymocyte differentiation prior to the CD4+CD8+ double-positive stage. *Br J Haematol* 2006; **132**: 216–29.

109. Ballerini P, Blaise A, Busson-Le Coniat M et al. HOX11L2 expression defines a clinical subtype of pediatric T-ALL associated with poor prognosis. *Blood* 2002; **100**: 991–7.

110. Mauvieux L, Leymarie V, Helias C et al. High incidence of Hox11L2 expression in children with T-ALL. *Leukemia* 2002; **16**: 2417–22.

111. Shirasawa S, Arata A, Onimaru H et al. Rnx deficiency results in congenital central hypoventilation. *Nat Genet* 2000; **24**: 287–90.

112. Soulier J, Clappier E, Cayuela JM et al. HOXA genes are included in genetic and biologic networks defining human acute T-cell leukemia (T-ALL). *Blood* 2005; **106**: 274–86.

113. Ferrando AA, Herblot S, Palomero T et al. Biallelic transcriptional activation of oncogenic transcription factors in T-cell acute lymphoblastic leukemia. *Blood* 2004; **103**: 1909–11.

114. Ellisen LW, Bird J, West DC et al. TAN-1, the human homolog of the Drosophila notch gene, is broken by chromosomal translocations in T lymphoblastic neoplasms. *Cell* 1991; **66**: 649–61.

115. Pear WS, Aster JC, Scott ML et al. Exclusive development of T cell neoplasms in mice transplanted with bone marrow expressing activated Notch alleles. *J Exp Med* 1996; **183**: 2283–91.

116. Pear WS, Radtke F. Notch signaling in lymphopoiesis. *Semin Immunol* 2003; **15**: 69–79.

117. Ordentlich P, Lin A, Shen CP et al. Notch inhibition of E47 supports the existence of a novel signaling pathway. *Mol Cell Biol* 1998; **18**: 2230–9.

118. Weng AP, Ferrando AA, Lee W et al. Activating mutations of NOTCH1 in human T cell acute lymphoblastic leukemia. *Science* 2004; **306**: 269–71.

119. Grabher C, von Boehmer H, Look AT. Notch 1 activation in the molecular pathogenesis of T-cell acute lymphoblastic leukaemia. *Nat Rev Cancer* 2006; **6**: 347–59.

120. Meeker TC, Hardy D, Willman C, et al. Activation of the interleukin-3 gene by chromosome translocation in acute lymphocytic leukemia with eosinophilia. *Blood* 1990; **76**: 285–9.

121. Grimaldi JC, Meeker TC. The t(5;14) chromosomal translocation in a case of acute lymphocytic leukemia joins the interleukin-3 gene to the immunoglobulin heavy chain gene. *Blood* 1989; **73**: 2081–5.

122. Tycko B, Smith SD, Sklar J. Chromosomal translocations joining LCK and TCRB loci in human T cell leukemia. *J Exp Med* 1991; **174**: 867–73.

123. Burnett RC, David JC, Harden AM et al. The LCK gene is involved in the t(1;7)(p34;q34) in the T-cell acute lymphoblastic leukemia derived cell line, HSB-2. *Genes Chromosomes Cancer* 1991; **3**: 461–7.

124. Wright DD, Sefton BM, Kamps MP. Oncogenic activation of the Lck protein accompanies translocation of the LCK gene in the human HSB2 T-cell leukemia. *Mol Cell Biol* 1994; **14**: 2429–37.

125. Graux C, Cools J, Melotte C et al. Fusion of NUP214 to ABL1 on amplified episomes in T-cell acute lymphoblastic leukemia. *Nat Genet* 2004; **36**: 1084–9.

126. Kamps MP, Murre C, Sun XH, Baltimore D. A new homeobox gene contributes the DNA binding domain of the t(1;19) translocation protein in pre-B ALL. *Cell* 1990; **60**: 547–55.

127. Nourse J, Mellentin JD, Galili N *et al.* Chromosomal translocation t(1;19) results in synthesis of a homeobox fusion mRNA that codes for a potential chimeric transcription factor. *Cell* 1990; **60**: 535–45.

128. Mellentin JD, Nourse J, Hunger SP *et al.* Molecular analysis of the t(1;19) breakpoint cluster region in pre-B cell acute lymphoblastic leukemias. *Genes Chromosomes Cancer* 1990; **2**: 239–47.

129. Van Dijk MA, Voorhoeve PM, Murre C. Pbx1 is converted into a transcriptional activator upon acquiring the N-terminal region of E2A in pre-B-cell acute lymphoblastoid leukemia. *Proc Natl Acad Sci U S A* 1993; **90**: 6061–5.

130. LeBrun DP, Cleary ML. Fusion with E2A alters the transcriptional properties of the homeodomain protein PBX1 in t(1;19) leukemias. *Oncogene* 1994; **9**: 1641–7.

131. Lu Q, Wright DD, Kamps MP. Fusion with E2A converts the Pbx1 homeodomain protein into a constitutive transcriptional activator in human leukemias carrying the t(1;19) translocation. *Mol Cell Biol* 1994; **14**: 3938–48.

132. Kamps MP, Baltimore D. E2A-Pbx1, the t(1;19) translocation protein of human pre-B-cell acute lymphocytic leukemia, causes acute myeloid leukemia in mice. *Mol Cell Biol* 1993; **13**: 351–7.

133. Dedera DA, Waller EK, LeBrun DP *et al.* Chimeric homeobox gene E2A-PBX1 induces proliferation, apoptosis, and malignant lymphomas in transgenic mice. *Cell* 1993; **74**: 833–43.

134. Monica K, LeBrun DP, Dedera DA *et al.* Transformation properties of the E2a-Pbx1 chimeric oncoprotein: fusion with E2a is essential, but the Pbx1 homeodomain is dispensable. *Mol Cell Biol* 1994; **14**: 8304–14.

135. Chang CP, Shen WF, Rozenfeld S *et al.* Pbx proteins display hexapeptide-dependent cooperative DNA binding with a subset of Hox proteins. *Genes Dev* 1995; **9**: 663–74.

136. van Dijk MA, Peltenburg LT, Murre C. Hox gene products modulate the DNA binding activity of Pbx1 and Pbx2. *Mech Dev* 1995; **52**: 99–108.

137. Lu Q, Knoepfler PS, Scheele J *et al.* Both Pbx1 and E2A-Pbx1 bind the DNA motif ATCAATCAA cooperatively with the products of multiple murine Hox genes, some of which are themselves oncogenes. *Mol Cell Biol* 1995; **15**: 3786–95.

138. Knoepfler PS, Kamps MP. The pentapeptide motif of Hox proteins is required for cooperative DNA binding with Pbx1, physically contacts Pbx1, and enhances DNA binding by Pbx1. *Mol Cell Biol* 1995; **15**: 5811–19.

139. Chang CP, de Vivo I, Cleary ML. The Hox cooperativity motif of the chimeric oncoprotein E2a-Pbx1 is necessary and sufficient for oncogenesis. *Mol Cell Biol* 1997; **17**: 81–8.

140. Raimondi SC, Behm FG, Roberson PK *et al.* Cytogenetics of pre-B-cell acute lymphoblastic leukemia with emphasis on prognostic implications of the t(1;19). *J Clin Oncol* 1990; **8**: 1380–8.

141. Pui CH, Crist WM. Cytogenetic abnormalities in childhood acute lymphoblastic leukemia correlates with clinical features and treatment outcome. *Leuk Lymphoma* 1992; **7**: 259–74.

142. Rivera GK, Raimondi SC, Hancock ML *et al.* Improved outcome in childhood acute lymphoblastic leukaemia with reinforced early treatment and rotational combination chemotherapy. *Lancet* 1991; **337**: 61–6.

143. Hunger SP, Ohyashiki K, Toyama K, Cleary ML. Hlf, a novel hepatic bZIP protein, shows altered DNA-binding properties following fusion to E2A in t(17;19) acute lymphoblastic leukemia. *Genes Dev* 1992; **6**: 1608–20.

144. Inaba T, Roberts WM, Shapiro LH *et al.* Fusion of the leucine zipper gene HLF to the E2A gene in human acute B-lineage leukemia. *Science* 1992; **257**: 531–4.

145. Yoshihara T, Inaba T, Shapiro LH *et al.* E2A-HLF-mediated cell transformation requires both the trans-activation domains of E2A and the leucine zipper dimerization domain of HLF. *Mol Cell Biol* 1995; **15**: 3247–55.

146. Hunger SP. Chromosomal translocations involving the E2A gene in acute lymphoblastic leukemia: clinical features and molecular pathogenesis. *Blood* 1996; **87**: 1211–24.

147. Inaba T, Inukai T, Yoshihara T *et al.* Reversal of apoptosis by the leukaemia-associated E2A-HLF chimaeric transcription factor. *Nature* 1996; **382**: 541–4.

148. Metzstein MM, Hengartner MO, Tsung N *et al.* Transcriptional regulator of programmed cell death encoded by *Caenorhabditis elegans* gene ces-2. *Nature* 1996; **382**: 545–7.

149. Thompson CB. Transcription. A fate worse than death. *Nature* 1996; **382**: 492–3.

150. Inukai T, Inoue A, Kurosawa H *et al.* SLUG, a ces-1-related zinc finger transcription factor gene with antiapoptotic activity, is a downstream target of the E2A-HLF oncoprotein. *Mol Cell* 1999; **4**: 343–52.

151. Metzstein MM, Horvitz HR. The C. elegans cell death specification gene ces-1 encodes a snail family zinc finger protein. *Mol Cell* 1999; **4**: 309–19.

152. Inoue A, Seidel MG, Wu W *et al.* Slug, a highly conserved zinc finger transcriptional repressor, protects hematopoietic progenitor cells from radiation-induced apoptosis *in vivo*. *Cancer Cell* 2002; **2**: 279–88.

153. Wu WS, Heinrichs S, Xu D *et al.* Slug antagonizes p53-mediated apoptosis of hematopoietic progenitors by repressing puma. *Cell* 2005; **123**: 641–53.

154. Ziemin-van der Poel S, McCabe NR, Gill HJ *et al.* Identification of a gene, MLL, that spans the breakpoint in 11q23 translocations associated with human leukemias. *Proc Natl Acad Sci U S A* 1991; **88**: 10735–9.

155. Tkachuk DC, Kohler S, Cleary ML. Involvement of a homolog of Drosophila trithorax by 11q23 chromosomal translocations in acute leukemias. *Cell* 1992; **71**: 691–700.

156. Gu Y, Nakamura T, Alder H *et al.* The t(4;11) chromosome translocation of human acute leukemias fuses the ALL-1 gene, related to *Drosophila trithorax*, to the AF-4 gene. *Cell* 1992; **71**: 701–8.

157. Djabali M, Selleri L, Parry P *et al.* A trithorax-like gene is interrupted by chromosome 11q23 translocations in acute leukaemias. *Nat Genet* 1992; **2**: 113–18.

158. Mazo AM, Huang DH, Mozer BA, Dawid IB. The trithorax gene, a trans-acting regulator of the bithorax complex in Drosophila, encodes a protein with zinc-binding domains. *Proc Natl Acad Sci U S A* 1990; **87**: 2112–16.

159. Milne TA, Briggs SD, Brock HW *et al.* MLL targets SET domain methyltransferase activity to Hox gene promoters. *Mol Cell* 2002; **10**: 1107–17.

160. Yokoyama A, Wang Z, Wysocka J *et al.* Leukemia proto-oncoprotein MLL forms a SET1-like histone methyltransferase complex with menin to regulate Hox gene expression. *Mol Cell Biol* 2004; **24**: 5639–49.

161. Reeves R, Nissen MS. The A.T-DNA-binding domain of mammalian high mobility group I chromosomal proteins. A novel peptide motif for recognizing DNA structure. *J Biol Chem* 1990; **265**: 8573–82.

162. Ma Q, Alder H, Nelson KK *et al.* Analysis of the murine All-1 gene reveals conserved domains with human ALL-1 and identifies a motif shared with DNA methyltransferases. *Proc Natl Acad Sci U S A* 1993; **90**: 6350–4.

163. Yokoyama A, Kitabayashi I, Ayton PM *et al.* Leukemia proto-oncoprotein MLL is proteolytically processed into 2 fragments with opposite transcriptional properties. *Blood* 2002; **100**: 3710–18.

164. Hsieh JJ, Ernst P, Erdjument-Bromage H *et al.* Proteolytic cleavage of MLL generates a complex of N- and C-terminal fragments that confers protein stability and subnuclear localization. *Mol Cell Biol* 2003; **23**: 186–94.

165. Thirman MJ, Levitan DA, Kobayashi H *et al.* Cloning of ELL, a gene that fuses to MLL in a t(11;19)(q23;p13.1) in acute myeloid leukemia. *Proc Natl Acad Sci U S A* 1994; **91**: 12110–14.

166. Mitani K, Kanda Y, Ogawa S *et al.* Cloning of several species of MLL/MEN chimeric cDNAs in myeloid leukemia with t(11;19)(q23;p13.1) translocation. *Blood* 1995; **85**: 2017–24.

167. Shilatifard A, Lane WS, Jackson KW *et al.* An RNA polymerase II elongation factor encoded by the human ELL gene. *Science* 1996; **271**: 1873–6.

168. So CW, Lin M, Ayton PM *et al.* Dimerization contributes to oncogenic activation of MLL chimeras in acute leukemias. *Cancer Cell* 2003; **4**: 99–110.

169. Hsu K, Look AT. Turning on a dimer: new insights into MLL chimeras. *Cancer Cell* 2003; **4**: 81–3.

170. Yu BD, Hanson RD, Hess JL *et al.* MLL, a mammalian trithorax-group gene, functions as a transcriptional maintenance factor in morphogenesis. *Proc Natl Acad Sci U S A* 1998; **95**: 10632–6.

171. Corral J, Lavenir I, Impey H *et al.* An Mll-AF9 fusion gene made by homologous recombination causes acute leukemia in chimeric mice: a method to create fusion oncogenes. *Cell* 1996; **85**: 853–61.

172. Zeisig BB, Garcia-Cuellar MP, Winkler TH, Slany RK. The oncoprotein MLL-ENL disturbs hematopoietic lineage determination and transforms a biphenotypic lymphoid/myeloid cell. *Oncogene* 2003; **22**: 1629–37.

173. Lavau C, Luo RT, Du C, Thirman MJ. Retrovirus-mediated gene transfer of MLL-ELL transforms primary myeloid progenitors and causes acute myeloid leukemias in mice. *Proc Natl Acad Sci U S A* 2000; **97**: 10984–9.

174. Lavau C, Du C, Thirman M, Zeleznik-Le N. Chromatin-related properties of CBP fused to MLL generate a myelodysplastic-like syndrome that evolves into myeloid leukemia. *EMBO J* 2000; **19**: 4655–64.

175. Forster A, Pannell R, Drynan LF *et al.* Engineering de novo reciprocal chromosomal translocations associated with Mll to replicate primary events of human cancer. *Cancer Cell* 2003; **3**: 449–58.

176. Drynan LF, Pannell R, Forster A *et al.* Mll fusions generated by Cre-loxP-mediated de novo translocations can induce lineage reassignment in tumorigenesis. *EMBO J* 2005; **24**: 3136–46.

177. Metzler M, Forster A, Pannell R *et al.* A conditional model of MLL-AF4 B-cell tumourigenesis using invertor technology. *Oncogene* 2006; **25**: 3093–103.

178. Armstrong SA, Staunton JE, Silverman LB *et al.* MLL translocations specify a distinct gene expression profile that distinguishes a unique leukemia. *Nat Genet* 2002; **30**: 41–7.

179. Yeoh EJ, Ross ME, Shurtleff SA *et al.* Classification, subtype discovery, and prediction of outcome in pediatric acute lymphoblastic leukemia by gene expression profiling. *Cancer Cell* 2002; **1**: 133–43.

180. Ferrando AA, Armstrong SA, Neuberg DS *et al.* Gene expression signatures in MLL-rearranged T-lineage and B-precursor acute leukemias: dominance of HOX dysregulation. *Blood* 2003; **102**: 262–68.

181. Ayton PM, Cleary ML. Transformation of myeloid progenitors by MLL oncoproteins is dependent on Hoxa7 and Hoxa9. *Genes Dev* 2003; **17**: 2298–307.

182. Armstrong SA, Kung AL, Mabon ME *et al.* Inhibition of FLT3 in MLL. Validation of a therapeutic target identified by gene expression based classification. *Cancer Cell* 2003; **3**: 173–83.

183. Gilliland DG. Molecular genetics of human leukemias: new insights into therapy. *Semin Hematol* 2002; **39**: 6–11.

184. Brown P, Levis M, Shurtleff S *et al.* FLT3 inhibition selectively kills childhood acute lymphoblastic leukemia cells with high levels of FLT3 expression. *Blood* 2005; **105**: 812–20.

185. Armstrong SA, Mabon ME, Silverman LB *et al.* FLT3 mutations in childhood acute lymphoblastic leukemia. *Blood* 2004; **103**: 3544–6.

186. Dreyling MH, Martinez-Climent JA, Zheng M *et al.* The t(10;11)(p13;q14) in the U937 cell line results in the fusion of the AF10 gene and CALM, encoding a new member of the AP-3 clathrin assembly protein family. *Proc Natl Acad Sci U S A* 1996; **93**: 4804–9.

187. Asnafi V, Radford-Weiss I, Dastugue N *et al.* CALM-AF10 is a common fusion transcript in T-ALL and is specific to the TCRgammadelta lineage. *Blood* 2003; **102**: 1000–6.

188. Dik WA, Brahim W, Braun C *et al.* CALM-AF10+ T-ALL expression profiles are characterized by overexpression of HOXA and BMI1 oncogenes. *Leukemia* 2005; **19**: 1948–57.

189. Song WJ, Sullivan MG, Legare RD *et al.* Haploinsufficiency of CBFA2 causes familial thrombocytopenia with

propensity to develop acute myelogenous leukaemia. *Nat Genet* 1999; **23**: 166–75.

190. Roumier C, Fenaux P, Lafage M *et al.* New mechanisms of AML1 gene alteration in hematological malignancies. *Leukemia* 2003; **17**: 9–16.

191. Hiebert SW, Sun W, Davis JN *et al.* The t(12;21) translocation converts AML-1B from an activator to a repressor of transcription. *Mol Cell Biol* 1996; **16**: 1349–55.

192. Fenrick R, Amann JM, Lutterbach B *et al.* Both TEL and AML-1 contribute repression domains to the t(12;21) fusion protein. *Mol Cell Biol* 1999; **19**: 6566–74.

193. Cave H, Cacheux V, Raynaud S *et al.* ETV6 is the target of chromosome 12p deletions in t(12;21) childhood acute lymphocytic leukemia. *Leukemia* 1997; **11**: 1459–64.

194. Jousset C, Carron C, Boureux A *et al.* A domain of TEL conserved in a subset of ETS proteins defines a specific oligomerization interface essential to the mitogenic properties of the TEL-PDGFR beta oncoprotein. *EMBO J* 1997; **16**: 69–82.

195. McLean TW, Ringold S, Neuberg D *et al.* TEL/AML-1 dimerizes and is associated with a favorable outcome in childhood acute lymphoblastic leukemia. *Blood* 1996; **88**: 4252–8.

196. Takeuchi S, Seriu T, Bartram CR *et al.* TEL is one of the targets for deletion on 12p in many cases of childhood B-lineage acute lymphoblastic leukemia. *Leukemia* 1997; **11**: 1220–3.

197. Loh ML, Goldwasser MA, Silverman LB *et al.* Prospective analysis of TEL/AML1 positive patients treated on Dana-Farber Cancer Institute Consortium Protocol 95–01. *Blood* 2006; **107**: 4508–13.

198. Heisterkamp N, Stephenson JR, Groffen J *et al.* Localization of the c-abl oncogene adjacent to a translocation break point in chronic myelocytic leukaemia. *Nature* 1983; **306**: 239–42.

199. Leibowitz D, Schaefer-Rego K, Popenoe DW *et al.* Variable breakpoints on the Philadelphia chromosome in chronic myelogenous leukemia. *Blood* 1985; **66**: 243–5.

200. Grosveld G, Verwoerd T, van Agthoven T *et al.* The chronic myelocytic cell line K562 contains a breakpoint in bcr and produces a chimeric bcr/c-abl transcript. *Mol Cell Biol* 1986; **6**: 607–16.

201. Chan LC, Karhi KK, Rayter SI *et al.* A novel abl protein expressed in Philadelphia chromosome positive acute lymphoblastic leukaemia. *Nature* 1987; **325**: 635–7.

202. Clark SS, McLaughlin J, Crist WM *et al.* Unique forms of the abl tyrosine kinase distinguish Ph1-positive CML from Ph1-positive ALL. *Science* 1987; **235**: 85–8.

203. Kurzrock R, Shtalrid M, Romero P *et al.* A novel c-abl protein product in Philadelphia-positive acute lymphoblastic leukaemia. *Nature* 1987; **325**: 631–5.

204. Konopka JB, Watanabe SM, Witte ON. An alteration of the human c-abl protein in K562 leukemia cells unmasks associated tyrosine kinase activity. *Cell* 1984; **37**: 1035–42.

205. Kloetzer W, Kurzrock R, Smith L *et al.* The human cellular abl gene product in the chronic myelogenous leukemia cell line K562 has an associated tyrosine protein kinase activity. *Virology* 1985; **140**: 230–8.

206. Naldini L, Stacchini A, Cirillo DM *et al.* Phosphotyrosine antibodies identify the p210c-abl tyrosine kinase and proteins phosphorylated on tyrosine in human chronic myelogenous leukemia cells. *Mol Cell Biol* 1986; **6**: 1803–11.

207. Kharbanda S, Ren R, Pandey P *et al.* Activation of the c-Abl tyrosine kinase in the stress response to DNA-damaging agents. *Nature* 1995; **376**: 785–8.

208. Sawyers CL, McLaughlin J, Goga A *et al.* The nuclear tyrosine kinase c-Abl negatively regulates cell growth. *Cell* 1994; **77**: 121–31.

209. Mattioni T, Jackson PK, Bchini-Hooft van Huijsduijnen O, Picard D. Cell cycle arrest by tyrosine kinase Abl involves altered early mitogenic response. *Oncogene* 1995; **10**: 1325–33.

210. Goga A, Liu X, Hambuch TM *et al.* p53 dependent growth suppression by the c-Abl nuclear tyrosine kinase. *Oncogene* 1995; **11**: 791–9.

211. Tybulewicz VL, Crawford CE, Jackson PK *et al.* Neonatal lethality and lymphopenia in mice with a homozygous disruption of the c-abl proto-oncogene. *Cell* 1991; **65**: 1153–63.

212. Schwartzberg PL, Stall AM, Hardin JD *et al.* Mice homozygous for the ablm1 mutation show poor viability and depletion of selected B and T cell populations. *Cell* 1991; **65**: 1165–75.

213. Van Etten RA, Jackson P, Baltimore D. The mouse type IV c-abl gene product is a nuclear protein, and activation of transforming ability is associated with cytoplasmic localization. *Cell* 1989; **58**: 669–78.

214. Lugo TG, Pendergast AM, Muller AJ, Witte ON. Tyrosine kinase activity and transformation potency of bcr-abl oncogene products. *Science* 1990; **247**: 1079–82.

215. Daley GQ, Baltimore D. Transformation of an interleukin 3-dependent hematopoietic cell line by the chronic myelogenous leukemia-specific P210bcr/abl protein. *Proc Natl Acad Sci U S A* 1988; **85**: 9312–6.

216. Elefanty AG, Hariharan IK, Cory S. bcr-abl, the hallmark of chronic myeloid leukaemia in man, induces multiple haemopoietic neoplasms in mice. *EMBO J* 1990; **9**: 1069–78.

217. Gishizky ML, Johnson-White J, Witte ON. Efficient transplantation of BCR-ABL-induced chronic myelogenous leukemia-like syndrome in mice. *Proc Natl Acad Sci U S A* 1993; **90**: 3755–9.

218. Kelliher M, Knott A, McLaughlin J *et al.* Differences in oncogenic potency but not target cell specificity distinguish the two forms of the BCR/ABL oncogene. *Mol Cell Biol* 1991; **11**: 4710–16.

219. Cortez D, Reuther G, Pendergast AM. The Bcr-Abl tyrosine kinase activates mitogenic signaling pathways and stimulates G1-to-S phase transition in hematopoietic cells. *Oncogene* 1997; **15**: 2333–42.

220. Varticovski L, Daley GQ, Jackson P *et al.* Activation of phosphatidylinositol 3-kinase in cells expressing abl oncogene variants. *Mol Cell Biol* 1991; **11**: 1107–13.

221. Reuther JY, Reuther GW, Cortez D *et al.* A requirement for NF-kappaB activation in Bcr-Abl-mediated transformation. *Genes Dev* 1998; **12**: 968–81.

222. Carlesso N, Frank DA, Griffin JD. Tyrosyl phosphorylation and DNA binding activity of signal transducers and activators of transcription (STAT) proteins in hematopoietic cell lines transformed by Bcr/Abl. *J Exp Med* 1996; **183**: 811–20.

223. Raitano AB, Halpern JR, Hambuch TM, Sawyers CL. The Bcr-Abl leukemia oncogene activates Jun kinase and requires Jun for transformation. *Proc Natl Acad Sci U S A* 1995; **92**: 11746–50.

224. Sawyers CL, McLaughlin J, Witte ON. Genetic requirement for Ras in the transformation of fibroblasts and hematopoietic cells by the Bcr-Abl oncogene. *J Exp Med* 1995; **181**: 307–13.

225. Skorski T, Kanakaraj P, Nieborowska-Skorska M *et al.* Phosphatidylinositol-3 kinase activity is regulated by BCR/ABL and is required for the growth of Philadelphia chromosome-positive cells. *Blood* 1995; **86**: 726–36.

226. Skorski T, Bellacosa A, Nieborowska-Skorska M, *et al.* Transformation of hematopoietic cells by BCR/ABL requires activation of a PI-3k/Akt-dependent pathway. *EMBO J* 1997; **16**: 6151–61.

227. Sattler M, Griffin JD. Molecular mechanisms of transformation by the BCR-ABL oncogene. *Semin Hematol* 2003; **40**: 4–10.

228. Skorski T. BCR/ABL regulates response to DNA damage: the role in resistance to genotoxic treatment and in genomic instability. *Oncogene* 2002; **21**: 8591–604.

229. Ribeiro RC, Abromowitch M, Raimondi SC *et al.* Clinical and biologic hallmarks of the Philadelphia chromosome in childhood acute lymphoblastic leukemia. *Blood* 1987; **70**: 948–53.

230. Crist W, Carroll A, Shuster J *et al.* Philadelphia chromosome positive childhood acute lymphoblastic leukemia: clinical and cytogenetic characteristics and treatment outcome. A pediatric oncology group study. *Blood* 1990; **76**: 489–94.

231. Fletcher JA, Lynch EA, Kimball VM *et al.* Translocation (9;22) is associated with extremely poor prognosis in intensively treated children with acute lymphoblastic leukemia. *Blood* 1991; **77**: 435–9.

232. Roberts WM, Rivera GK, Raimondi SC *et al.* Intensive chemotherapy for Philadelphia-chromosome-positive acute lymphoblastic leukaemia. *Lancet* 1994; **343**: 331–2.

233. Arico M, Valsecchi MG, Camitta B *et al.* Outcome of treatment in children with Philadelphia chromosome-positive acute lymphoblastic leukemia. *N Engl J Med* 2000; **342**: 998–1006.

234. Schrappe M, Arico M, Harbott J *et al.* Philadelphia chromosome-positive (Ph+) childhood acute lymphoblastic leukemia: good initial steroid response allows early prediction of a favorable treatment outcome. *Blood* 1998; **92**: 2730–41.

235. Druker BJ, Talpaz M, Resta DJ *et al.* Efficacy and safety of a specific inhibitor of the BCR-ABL tyrosine kinase in chronic myeloid leukemia. *N Engl J Med* 2001; **344**: 1031–7.

236. Druker BJ, Sawyers CL, Kantarjian H *et al.* Activity of a specific inhibitor of the BCR-ABL tyrosine kinase in the blast crisis of chronic myeloid leukemia and acute lymphoblastic leukemia with the Philadelphia chromosome. *N Engl J Med* 2001; **344**: 1038–42.

237. Kantarjian H, Sawyers C, Hochhaus A *et al.* Hematologic and cytogenetic responses to imatinib mesylate in chronic myelogenous leukemia. *N Engl J Med* 2002; **346**: 645–52.

238. Sawyers CL, Hochhaus A, Feldman E *et al.* Imatinib induces hematologic and cytogenetic responses in patients with chronic myelogenous leukemia in myeloid blast crisis: results of a phase II study. *Blood* 2002; **99**: 3530–9.

239. Talpaz M, Silver RT, Druker BJ *et al.* Imatinib induces durable hematologic and cytogenetic responses in patients with accelerated phase chronic myeloid leukemia: results of a phase 2 study. *Blood* 2002; **99**: 1928–37.

240. von Bubnoff N, Peschel C, Duyster J. Resistance of Philadelphia-chromosome positive leukemia towards the kinase inhibitor imatinib (STI571, Glivec): a targeted oncoprotein strikes back. *Leukemia* 2003; **17**: 829–38.

241. Gorre ME, Sawyers CL. Molecular mechanisms of resistance to STI571 in chronic myeloid leukemia. *Curr Opin Hematol* 2002; **9**: 303–7.

242. Guilhot F, Gardembas M, Rousselot P *et al.* Imatinib in combination with cytarabine for the treatment of Philadelphia-positive chronic myelogenous leukemia chronic-phase patients: rationale and design of phase I/II trials. *Semin Hematol* 2003; **40**: 92–7.

243. Thiesing JT, Ohno-Jones S, Kolibaba KS, Druker BJ. Efficacy of STI571, an abl tyrosine kinase inhibitor, in conjunction with other antileukemic agents against bcr-abl-positive cells. *Blood* 2000; **96**: 3195–9.

244. Huron DR, Gorre ME, Kraker AJ *et al.* A novel pyridopyrimidine inhibitor of abl kinase is a picomolar inhibitor of Bcr-abl-driven K562 cells and is effective against STI571-resistant Bcr-abl mutants. *Clin Cancer Res* 2003; **9**: 1267–73.

245. Wisniewski D, Lambek CL, Liu C *et al.* Characterization of potent inhibitors of the Bcr-Abl and the c-kit receptor tyrosine kinases. *Cancer Res* 2002; **62**: 4244–55.

246. Knudson AG Jr. Mutation and cancer: statistical study of retinoblastoma. *Proc Natl Acad Sci U S A* 1971; **68**: 820–3.

247. Nigro JM, Baker SJ, Preisinger AC *et al.* Mutations in the p53 gene occur in diverse human tumour types. *Nature* 1989; **342**: 705–8.

248. Li FP, Fraumeni JF, Jr., Mulvihill JJ *et al.* A cancer family syndrome in twenty-four kindreds. *Cancer Res* 1988; **48**: 5358–62.

249. Malkin D, Li FP, Strong LC *et al.* Germ line p53 mutations in a familial syndrome of breast cancer, sarcomas, and other neoplasms. *Science* 1990; **250**: 1233–8.

250. Srivastava S, Zou ZQ, Pirollo K *et al.* Germ-line transmission of a mutated p53 gene in a cancer-prone family with Li-Fraumeni syndrome. *Nature* 1990; **348**: 747–9.

251. Frebourg T, Friend SH. Cancer risks from germline p53 mutations. *J Clin Invest* 1992; **90**: 1637–41.

252. Levine AJ. p53, the cellular gatekeeper for growth and division. *Cell* 1997; **88**: 323–31.

253. Matlashewski G, Lamb P, Pim D *et al.* Isolation and characterization of a human p53 cDNA clone: expression of the human p53 gene. *EMBO J* 1984; **3**: 3257–62.

254. Zakut-Houri R, Bienz-Tadmor B, Givol D, Oren M. Human p53 cellular tumor antigen: cDNA sequence and expression in COS cells. *EMBO J* 1985; **4**: 1251–5.

255. Baker SJ, Fearon ER, Nigro JM *et al.* Chromosome 17 deletions and p53 gene mutations in colorectal carcinomas. *Science* 1989; **244**: 217–21.

256. Baker SJ, Markowitz S, Fearon ER *et al.* Suppression of human colorectal carcinoma cell growth by wild-type p53. *Science* 1990; **249**: 912–15.

257. Funk WD, Pak DT, Karas RH *et al.* A transcriptionally active DNA-binding site for human p53 protein complexes. *Mol Cell Biol* 1992; **12**: 2866–71.

258. el-Deiry WS, Kern SE, Pietenpol JA *et al.* Definition of a consensus binding site for p53. *Nat Genet* 1992; **1**: 45–9.

259. Farmer G, Bargonetti J, Zhu H *et al.* Wild-type p53 activates transcription *in vitro. Nature* 1992; **358**: 83–6.

260. Fields S, Jang SK. Presence of a potent transcription activating sequence in the p53 protein. *Science* 1990; **249**: 1046–9.

261. Kern SE, Kinzler KW, Bruskin A *et al.* Identification of p53 as a sequence-specific DNA-binding protein. *Science* 1991; **252**: 1708–11.

262. Kastan MB, Onyekwere O, Sidransky D *et al.* Participation of p53 protein in the cellular response to DNA damage. *Cancer Res* 1991; **51**: 6304–11.

263. Hsiao MH, Yu AL, Yeargin J *et al.* Nonhereditary p53 mutations in T-cell acute lymphoblastic leukemia are associated with the relapse phase. *Blood* 1994; **83**: 2922–30.

264. Diccianni MB, Yu J, Hsiao M *et al.* Clinical significance of p53 mutations in relapsed T-cell acute lymphoblastic leukemia. *Blood* 1994; **84**: 3105–12.

265. Wada M, Bartram CR, Nakamura H *et al.* Analysis of p53 mutations in a large series of lymphoid hematologic malignancies of childhood. *Blood* 1993; **82**: 3163–9.

266. Marks DI, Kurz BW, Link MP *et al.* High incidence of potential p53 inactivation in poor outcome childhood acute lymphoblastic leukemia at diagnosis. *Blood* 1996; **87**: 1155–61.

267. Marks DI, Kurz BW, Link MP *et al.* Altered expression of p53 and mdm-2 proteins at diagnosis is associated with early treatment failure in childhood acute lymphoblastic leukemia. *J Clin Oncol* 1997; **15**: 1158–62.

268. Sherr CJ, Roberts JM. Inhibitors of mammalian G1 cyclin-dependent kinases. *Genes Dev* 1995; **9**: 1149–63.

269. Kamijo T, Zindy F, Roussel MF *et al.* Tumor suppression at the mouse INK4a locus mediated by the alternative reading frame product p19ARF. *Cell* 1997; **91**: 649–59.

270. Quelle DE, Zindy F, Ashmun RA, Sherr CJ. Alternative reading frames of the INK4a tumor suppressor gene encode two unrelated proteins capable of inducing cell cycle arrest. *Cell* 1995; **83**: 993–1000.

271. Sidransky D. Two tracks but one race? Cancer genetics. *Curr Biol* 1996; **6**: 523–5.

272. Kamb A, Gruis NA, Weaver-Feldhaus J *et al.* A cell cycle regulator potentially involved in genesis of many tumor types. *Science* 1994; **264**: 436–40.

273. Nobori T, Miura K, Wu DJ *et al.* Deletions of the cyclin-dependent kinase-4 inhibitor gene in multiple human cancers. *Nature* 1994; **368**: 753–6.

274. Zhang Y, Xiong Y, Yarbrough WG. ARF promotes MDM2 degradation and stabilizes p53: ARF-INK4a locus deletion impairs both the Rb and p53 tumor suppression pathways. *Cell* 1998; **92**: 725–34.

275. Pomerantz J, Schreiber-Agus N, Liegeois NJ *et al.* The Ink4a tumor suppressor gene product, p19Arf, interacts with MDM2 and neutralizes MDM2's inhibition of p53. *Cell* 1998; **92**: 713–23.

276. Ashcroft M, Vousden KH. Regulation of p53 stability. *Oncogene* 1999; **18**: 7637–43.

277. Sharpless NE, Bardeesy N, Lee KH *et al.* Loss of p16Ink4a with retention of p19Arf predisposes mice to tumorigenesis. *Nature* 2001; **413**: 86–91.

278. Krimpenfort P, Quon KC, Mooi WJ *et al.* Loss of p16Ink4a confers susceptibility to metastatic melanoma in mice. *Nature* 2001; **413**: 83–6.

279. Hebert J, Cayuela JM, Berkeley J, Sigaux F. Candidate tumor-suppressor genes MTS1 (p16INK4A) and MTS2 (p15INK4B) display frequent homozygous deletions in primary cells from T- but not from B-cell lineage acute lymphoblastic leukemias. *Blood* 1994; **84**: 4038–44.

280. Quesnel B, Preudhomme C, Philippe N *et al.* p16 gene homozygous deletions in acute lymphoblastic leukemia. *Blood* 1995; **85**: 657–63.

281. Haidar MA, Cao XB, Manshouri T *et al.* p16INK4A and p15INK4B gene deletions in primary leukemias. *Blood* 1995; **86**: 311–15.

282. Fizzotti M, Cimino G, Pisegna S *et al.* Detection of homozygous deletions of the cyclin-dependent kinase 4 inhibitor (p16) gene in acute lymphoblastic leukemia and association with adverse prognostic features. *Blood* 1995; **85**: 2685–90.

283. Rasool O, Heyman M, Brandter LB *et al.* p15ink4B and p16ink4 gene inactivation in acute lymphocytic leukemia. *Blood* 1995; **85**: 3431–6.

284. Okuda T, Shurtleff SA, Valentine MB *et al.* Frequent deletion of p16INK4a/MTS1 and p15INK4b/MTS2 in pediatric acute lymphoblastic leukemia. *Blood* 1995; **85**: 2321–30.

285. Hirama T, Koeffler HP. Role of the cyclin-dependent kinase inhibitors in the development of cancer. *Blood* 1995; **86**: 841–54.

286. Iolascon A, Faienza MF, Coppola B *et al.* Homozygous deletions of cyclin-dependent kinase inhibitor genes, p16(INK4A) and p18, in childhood T cell lineage acute lymphoblastic leukemias. *Leukemia* 1996; **10**: 255–60.

287. Nakao M, Yokota S, Kaneko H *et al.* Alterations of CDKN2 gene structure in childhood acute lymphoblastic leukemia: mutations of CDKN2 are observed preferentially in T lineage. *Leukemia* 1996; **10**: 249–54.

288. Cayuela JM, Madani A, Sanhes L et al. Multiple tumor-suppressor gene 1 inactivation is the most frequent genetic alteration in T-cell acute lymphoblastic leukemia. Blood 1996; 87: 2180–6.

289. Takeuchi S, Bartram CR, Seriu T et al. Analysis of a family of cyclin-dependent kinase inhibitors: p15/MTS2/INK4B, p16/MTS1/INK4A, and p18 genes in acute lymphoblastic leukemia of childhood. Blood 1995; 86: 755–60.

290. Heyman M, Rasool O, Borgonovo Brandter L et al. Prognostic importance of p15INK4B and p16INK4 gene inactivation in childhood acute lymphocytic leukemia. J Clin Oncol 1996; 14: 1512–20.

291. Drexler HG. Review of alterations of the cyclin-dependent kinase inhibitor INK4 family genes p15, p16, p18 and p19 in human leukemia-lymphoma cells. Leukemia 1998; 12: 845–59.

292. Kees UR, Burton PR, Lu C, Baker DL. Homozygous deletion of the p16/MTS1 gene in pediatric acute lymphoblastic leukemia is associated with unfavorable clinical outcome. Blood 1997; 89: 4161–6.

293. Yamada Y, Hatta Y, Murata K et al. Deletions of p15 and/or p16 genes as a poor-prognosis factor in adult T-cell leukemia. J Clin Oncol 1997; 15: 1778–85.

294. Faderl S, Kantarjian HM, Manshouri T et al. The prognostic significance of p16INK4a/p14ARF and p15INK4b deletions in adult acute lymphoblastic leukemia. Clin Cancer Res 1999; 5: 1855–61.

295. Wong IH, Ng MH, Huang DP, Lee JC. Aberrant p15 promoter methylation in adult and childhood acute leukemias of nearly all morphologic subtypes: potential prognostic implications. Blood 2000; 95: 1942–9.

296. Raimondi SC. Current status of cytogenetic research in childhood acute lymphoblastic leukemia. Blood 1993; 81: 2237–51.

297. Stegmaier K, Takeuchi S, Golub TR et al. Mutational analysis of the candidate tumor suppressor genes TEL and KIP1 in childhood acute lymphoblastic leukemia. Cancer Res 1996; 56: 1413–17.

298. Der CJ, Krontiris TG, Cooper GM. Transforming genes of human bladder and lung carcinoma cell lines are homologous to the ras genes of Harvey and Kirsten sarcoma viruses. Proc Natl Acad Sci U S A 1982; 79: 3637–40.

299. Parada LF, Tabin CJ, Shih C, Weinberg RA. Human EJ bladder carcinoma oncogene is homologue of Harvey sarcoma virus ras gene. Nature 1982; 297: 474–8.

300. Land H, Parada LF, Weinberg RA. Cellular oncogenes and multistep carcinogenesis. Science 1983; 222: 771–8.

301. Land H, Parada LF, Weinberg RA. Tumorigenic conversion of primary embryo fibroblasts requires at least two cooperating oncogenes. Nature 1983; 304: 596–602.

302. Eliyahu D, Raz A, Gruss P et al. Participation of p53 cellular tumour antigen in transformation of normal embryonic cells. Nature 1984; 312: 646–9.

303. Parada LF, Land H, Weinberg RA et al. Cooperation between gene encoding p53 tumour antigen and ras in cellular transformation. Nature 1984; 312: 649–51.

304. Balmain A, Pragnell IB. Mouse skin carcinomas induced in vivo by chemical carcinogens have a transforming Harvey-ras oncogene. Nature 1983; 303: 72–4.

305. Sukumar S, Notario V, Martin-Zanca D, Barbacid M. Induction of mammary carcinomas in rats by nitroso-methylurea involves malignant activation of H-ras-1 locus by single point mutations. Nature 1983; 306: 658–61.

306. Guerrero I, Calzada P, Mayer A, Pellicer A. A molecular approach to leukemogenesis: mouse lymphomas contain an activated c-ras oncogene. Proc Natl Acad Sci U S A 1984; 81: 202–5.

307. Murray MJ, Cunningham JM, Parada LF et al. The HL-60 transforming sequence: a ras oncogene coexisting with altered myc genes in hematopoietic tumors. Cell 1983; 33: 749–57.

308. Bos JL, Toksoz D, Marshall CJ et al. Amino-acid substitutions at codon 13 of the N-ras oncogene in human acute myeloid leukaemia. Nature 1985; 315: 726–30.

309. Gambke C, Signer E, Moroni C. Activation of N-ras gene in bone marrow cells from a patient with acute myeloblastic leukaemia. Nature 1984; 307: 476–8.

310. Hirai H, Tanaka S, Azuma M et al. Transforming genes in human leukemia cells. Blood 1985; 66: 1371–8.

311. Souyri M, Fleissner E. Identification by transfection of transforming sequences in DNA of human T-cell leukemias. Proc Natl Acad Sci U S A 1983; 80: 6676–9.

312. Bos JL, Verlaan-de Vries M, van der Eb AJ et al. Mutations in N-ras predominate in acute myeloid leukemia. Blood 1987; 69: 1237–41.

313. Rodenhuis S, Bos JL, Slater RM et al. Absence of oncogene amplifications and occasional activation of N-ras in lymphoblastic leukemia of childhood. Blood 1986; 67: 1698–704.

314. Swansbury GJ, Secker-Walker LM, Lawler SD et al. Chromosomal findings in acute lymphoblastic leukaemia of childhood: an independent prognostic factor. Lancet 1981; 2: 249–50.

315. Secker-Walker LM, Swansbury GJ, Hardisty RM et al. Cytogenetics of acute lymphoblastic leukaemia in children as a factor in the prediction of long-term survival. Br J Haematol 1982; 52: 389–99.

316. Williams DL, Tsiatis A, Brodeur GM et al. Prognostic importance of chromosome number in 136 untreated children with acute lymphoblastic leukemia. Blood 1982; 60: 864–71.

317. Look AT, Roberson PK, Williams DL et al. Prognostic importance of blast cell DNA content in childhood acute lymphoblastic leukemia. Blood 1985; 65: 1079–86.

318. Trueworthy R, Shuster J, Look T et al. Ploidy of lymphoblasts is the strongest predictor of treatment outcome in B-progenitor cell acute lymphoblastic leukemia of childhood: a Pediatric Oncology Group study. J Clin Oncol 1992; 10: 606–13.

319. Raimondi SC, Pui CH, Hancock ML et al. Heterogeneity of hyperdiploid (51–67) childhood acute lymphoblastic leukemia. Leukemia 1996; 10: 213–24.

320. Martinez-Climent JA. Molecular cytogenetics of childhood hematological malignancies. *Leukemia* 1997; **11**: 1999–2021.

321. Pui CH, Raimondi SC, Dodge RK *et al.* Prognostic importance of structural chromosomal abnormalities in children with hyperdiploid (greater than 50 chromosomes) acute lymphoblastic leukemia. *Blood* 1989; **73**: 1963–7.

322. Belkov VM, Krynetski EY, Schuetz JD *et al.* Reduced folate carrier expression in acute lymphoblastic leukemia: a mechanism for ploidy but not lineage differences in methotrexate accumulation. *Blood* 1999; **93**: 1643–50.

323. Ito C, Kumagai M, Manabe A *et al.* Hyperdiploid acute lymphoblastic leukemia with 51 to 65 chromosomes: a distinct biological entity with a marked propensity to undergo apoptosis. *Blood* 1999; **93**: 315–20.

324. Raimondi SC, Roberson PK, Pui CH *et al.* Hyperdiploid (47–50) acute lymphoblastic leukemia in children. *Blood* 1992; **79**: 3245–52.

325. Cortes JE, Kantarjian HM. Acute lymphoblastic leukemia. A comprehensive review with emphasis on biology and therapy. *Cancer* 1995; **76**: 2393–417.

326. Heerema NA, Nachman JB, Sather HN *et al.* Hypodiploidy with less than 45 chromosomes confers adverse risk in childhood acute lymphoblastic leukemia: a report from the children's cancer group. *Blood* 1999; **94**: 4036–45.

Chronic lymphoid leukemias and μ heavy chain disease

ERIC D HSI

INTRODUCTION

This chapter will cover a subset of the mature lymphoid leukemias of small lymphocytes including chronic lymphocytic leukemia (CLL), B prolymphocytic leukemia (B-PLL), T cell large granular lymphocyte leukemia (T-LGL), and T prolymphocytic leukemia (T-PLL). We will also cover the rare μ heavy chain disease. Other B cell leukemias and lymphomas of small lymphocytes such as hairy cell leukemia, splenic lymphoma with villous lymphocytes, other marginal lymphomas, mantle cell lymphoma, lymphoplasmacytic lymphoma and follicular lymphoma are covered in other chapters.

CHRONIC LYMPHOCYTIC LEUKEMIA

Chronic lymphocytic leukemia is the most common leukemia in the Western world. The age-adjusted estimated annual incidence in the USA is approximately 3.4/100 000.[1] The median age at diagnosis is approximately 65 years with a 2:1 male to female ratio. Chronic lymphocytic leukemia is an indolent leukemia with a disease course that can often span more than 15 years. In fact, many patients may die with their disease rather than from it. Effective therapies do exist that can induce remissions, but relapses inevitably occur. Thus, CLL is currently considered incurable in the vast majority of cases and new therapies are needed.

Table 27.1 Staging systems for chronic lymphocytic leukemia

Staging system	Stage	Clinical features	Median survival (years)
Rai			
Low risk	0	Lymphocytosis	14.5
Intermediate risk	I	Lymphocytosis, lymphadenopathy	7.5
	II	Lymphocytosis, hepatomegaly and/or splenomegaly	
High risk	III	Lymphocytosis, anemia <110 g/L	2.5
	IV	Lymphocytosis, thrombocytopenia <100 × 10^9/L	
Binet	A	Normal hemoglobin, platelets, <3 node-bearing areas	14
	B	Normal hemoglobin, platelets, ≥3 node-bearing areas	5
	C	Anemia (<100 g/L) and/or thrombocytopenia (<1 × 10^9/L)	2.5

Clinical features

Patients present with lymphocytosis (greater than 5.0×10^9/L, by definition persistent for at least 3 months)[2] and are often asymptomatic. Others may have symptoms relating to organ involvement (splenomegaly, hepatomegaly) or lymphadenopathy. Anemia and other cytopenias are often present due to immune hemolysis related to the leukemia or simple bone marrow replacement by leukemic infiltrates. Chronic lymphocytic leukemia may progress with increasing numbers of prolymphocytes in the blood or patients may experience transformation to a large cell lymphoma (Richter syndrome), heralded by a sudden change in symptoms or rapid localized lymph node enlargement. Staging systems such as the Rai or Binet staging systems are used to predict prognosis in CLL patients (Table 27.1).[3,4] While these systems are useful in stratifying patients, predicting outcome in intermediate stage patients is still difficult. Much work has been devoted to identifying biologic predictors of disease outcome (to be discussed).

Morphologic features

The peripheral blood smear of patients with CLL is characterized by a variable lymphocytosis that may uncommonly reach over 500×10^9/L. The lymphocytes are typically small and round with condensed nuclear chromatin that is often mottled due to areas of extreme condensation alternating with lighter areas, imparting a 'soccer ball' or 'cracked' chromatin pattern (Plate 19, see plate section). The cytoplasm is usually scanty. On an individual cell basis, they may be indistinguishable from normal mature lymphocytes. Variation from this typical form is acceptable within the spectrum of CLL and some cases may have substantial numbers (>10 percent) of cells demonstrating nuclear irregularity and/or moderate amounts of pale blue cytoplasm (Plate 20, see plate section). Some studies have associated such variant morphology with worse outcome.[5,6] Prolymphocytes are present in varying proportions. These cells are approximately 1.5–2 times larger than the typical CLL cells with slightly open chromatin and a central nucleolus. Cases in which prolymphocytes comprise greater than 10 percent but less than 55 percent of the lymphocytes have been termed 'mixed cell' CLL or CLL/PL in the original French–American–British classification scheme[7] but this has been dropped in the revised World Health Organization (WHO) classification.[8] Increased numbers of prolymphocytes have been associated with a poor prognosis (greater than 5×10^9/L)[9] and certain genetic abnormalities such as TP53 abnormalities and trisomy 12.[9–11]

Four major patterns of bone marrow involvement are recognized: nodular, interstitial, mixed and diffuse. The nodular pattern is composed of non-paratrabecular lymphoid aggregates. The cells are similar in appearance to those in the lymph node – small and round with condensed chromatin. Proliferation centers can be seen. In the interstitial pattern the lymphocytes infiltrate around preserved fat spaces, admixed with varying amounts of residual hematopoietic elements. The diffuse pattern shows complete replacement of the marrow space by sheets of leukemia cells and has been associated with advanced disease and an unfavorable prognosis (Plate 21, see plate section).[12–14]

Transformation to prolymphocytic leukemia is defined by >55 percent prolymphocytes and is usually characterized by worsening symptoms, loss of response to therapy and poor prognosis.[15] Richter's syndrome (transformation to an aggressive NHL) occurs in approximately 3–4 percent of patients. The transformation usually takes the form of aggressive higher grade lymphomas such as diffuse large B cell lymphoma and survival is short.[16] Unusual transformations/second malignancies such as Hodgkin lymphoma, acute lymphoblastic leukemia and multiple myeloma have been reported.[17,18] Of note, Reed–Sternberg-like cells in some patients with Hodgkin-like transformation have been shown to be Epstein–Barr virus (EBV)-positive and clonally related to the CLL.[19–21]

IMMUNOPHENOTYPE

Multiparameter flow cytometric immunophenotyping is helpful in confirming the diagnosis of CLL and should be done in all cases. The typical immunophenotype has been well characterized. Cells in CLL express CD5, CD19, CD20, CD22, CD23 and restricted surface immunoglobulin light chain. The expression of CD20 and immunoglobulin is usually dim. Heavy chain expression is usually of the IgM and IgD type. FMC7 and CD79b are absent or only dimly expressed.[22,23] Deviation from this typical immunophenotype occurs, and scoring systems have been proposed to help quantify the likelihood that the diagnosis is CLL.[23]

One caveat to the presence of restricted light chain expression is the existence of rare cases of biclonal CLL in which a kappa CLL clone and a lambda CLL clone are seen. Cases might seem polytypic but have the other immunophenotypic features of CLL and, on molecular analysis, show biclonal rearrangement patterns.

Recently, two additional markers have been shown to be important in the prognosis of CLL. CD38 is a marker that, initially, was thought to correlate well with *IGH* variable region (*IGHV*) mutational status (see below).[24] The correlation has subsequently been proven to be imperfect but it has been shown in numerous studies that CD38 expression is a poor prognostic indicator in CLL.[25] Several studies have also shown it to be independent of other clinical parameters.[25–27] The most commonly used cutoff for defining positivity for CD38 is 30 percent CD38+ leukemic cells, but some studies have considered as little as 7 percent as the cutoff.[25,28] The intracellular nonreceptor tyrosine kinase ZAP70 has been recently shown to correlate fairly well with *IGHV* mutational status and can also be assessed by flow cytometry or immunohistochemistry. Expression in >20 percent of CLL cells is associated with germline *IGHV* genes and a poor prognosis.[29,30]

With sensitive flow cytometric approaches, it has recently been found that a small proportion of people have minute B cell clones with the phenotype of CLL. In addition, first-degree relatives of patients with clinical CLL have a higher incidence of these minute CLL clones in peripheral blood.[31,32] The significance of these 'incidental' findings is as yet unknown but raises questions about the biology of CLL and risk factors for its development. Currently, presence of a CLL-like clone at levels less than 5×10^9/L without cytopenias are considered in the spectrum of 'monoclonal B-cell lymphocytosis', with a risk of progression to CLL in the range of 1–2 percent per year.[2,33]

MOLECULAR GENETICS

Interphase fluorescence *in situ* hybridization studies have revealed many common genetic abnormalities that also have clinical importance (Table 27.2).[34] Deletion 13q is the most common abnormality and is associated with typical morphology and good prognosis. Trisomy 12 is associated

Table 27.2 Frequency of chromosomal abnormalities[a][34]

Aberration	Percentage of cases
13q deletion	55
11q deletion	18
Trisomy 12	16
17p deletion	7
6q deletion	6
Trisomy 8q	5
t(14q32)	4
Trisomy 3q	3
Normal	18

[a]Defined by fluorescence *in situ* hybridization; some cases may have more than one abnormality.

with atypical morphology and intermediate prognosis. Deletion of 17p involving TP53 is uncommon but associated with a very poor prognosis.

IGHV mutational status has been shown to be an independent predictor of outcome in CLL.[24,35] *IGHV* mutational status can be characterized as unmutated based on greater than or equal to 98 percent homology to the germline sequence. Patients whose CLL cells have unmutated *IGHV* generally have a poorer prognosis than patients whose CLL cells have mutated *IGHV* genes. It is currently debatable whether, as one would expect from the paradigm of normal B cell development, unmutated CLL corresponds to a naïve B cell stage and mutated CLL corresponds with memory B cell stage. However, gene expression profiling suggests the two subtypes of CLL are quite closely related and supports a memory B cell origin for both types.[36] Regardless, ZAP70 was identified through these studies as one molecule that was important in distinguishing mutated (ZAP70 negative) and nonmutated CLL (ZAP-positive) and was associated with shorter time to treatment from diagnosis.[36,37]

Pathogenesis

The pathogenesis of CLL is unknown. Three areas of recent investigation include following up of information gained from expression profiling studies (such as the consequences of ZAP70 expression), micro-RNAs, and microenvironmental factors. Despite low levels of surface expressed immunoglobulin, signaling through the B cell receptor is possible. ZAP70 expression has shown to augment signaling via IgM ligation in CLL cells as measured by phosphorylation of downstream mediators such as Syk, BLNK and PLC and calcium flux.[38] This increased signaling might lead to enhanced proliferation or survival of the leukemic cell.[39]

Most recently, micro-RNAs have been shown to be important in the biology of CLL; miR-15 and miR-16 (which share a common precursor) are located at the site

Table 27.3   Immunophenotype and molecular genetic features of B cell lymphoproliferative disorders

	CD5	CD10	CD20	CD23	CD79b	FMC7	CD103	CD123	sIg	t(14;18)	t(11;14)
CLL	+	−	+(dim)	+	−/+(dim)	−/+(dim)	−	−	+/−(dim)	−	−
MCL	+	−	+	−	+	+	−	−	+	−	+
MZL	−	−	+	−/+	+	+	−/+	−	+	−	−
HCL	−	−/+	+	−	+	+	+	+	+	−	−
FCL	−	+	+	−/+	+	+	−	−	+/−	+	−

of chromosome 13 deletion. These micro-RNAs, negative regulators of BCL2, are deleted or downregulated in over 65 percent of CLL cases examined.[40,41] Levels of these negative regulators are inversely proportional to BCL-2 expression in CLL. This suggests that micro-RNAs may be important in altering the balance of apoptosis. Other alterations in micro-RNA genes may affect other oncogenes important in CLL.[40–42] Expression profiling of micro-RNAs has shown prognostic relevance in CLL, with a 13 micro-RNA gene signature correlating with ZAP70 expression, *IGH* mutation status and disease progression. Furthermore, germline mutations in micro-RNAs in CLL patients, including miR-15/16 precursor, have been identified.

Interactions in the microenvironment are now being recognized as important in survival of CLL cells. Through contact with nurse-like stromal cells and bone marrow stromal cells, prosurvival effects are mediated through molecules such as stromal-derived factor 1 (SDF1) and its receptor CXCR4 on CLL cells. Paracrine loops involving tumor necrosis factor (TNF) family ligands such as BAFF and APRIL also appear to be important in regulating leukemic cell survival.[43–47] Such studies may lead to further elucidation of the pathogenesis of CLL, development of new biologic predictors of outcome, and new therapeutic strategies.[48]

Differential diagnosis

The differential diagnosis of CLL includes other B cell leukemias and peripheralized lymphoma, particularly mantle cell lymphoma (MCL), marginal zone lymphoma and follicular lymphoma (FL). Given the phenotypic and morphologic similarities, leukemic MCL is an important consideration. Morphologically, MCL cells may show slight nuclear irregularities and occasional intermediate-sized cells. Flow cytometry is extremely helpful. While both CLL and MCL express CD5, CD23 is expressed in most cases of CLL and is absent in MCL. Other useful features include bright CD20 and surface Ig expression in MCL. CD79b and FMC-7 are typically dim or absent in CLL but strongly expressed in MCL. The t(11;14)(q13;q32) involving *IGH* and *CCND-1* can confirm a diagnosis of leukemic MCL with the caveat that some cases of myeloma may also have this translocation. However, a plasma cell leukemia would not coexpress CD20 and CD5. Table 27.3 shows the phenotypic and

genetic features of the various B cell lymphoproliferative disorders. Peripheralized FL may also have individual cells that resemble CLL cells but always has at least occasional, and often many, deeply clefted cells. Expression of CD10 and lack of CD5 is the rule in FL. Presence of a t(14;18) (q32;q21) is strong evidence against CLL and favors FL. Splenic marginal zone lymphoma will typically have occasional cells that have abundant cytoplasm and/or cytoplasmic villous projections. The immunophenotype is that of an immunoglobulin light chain restricted, CD5-negative lymphoproliferative disorder. Rare cases of marginal zone lymphoma may express CD5.[49] Some cases of CLL do show atypical features such as irregular nuclei or mild deviation from the normal immunophenotype.[6] However, elimination of other serious considerations using combined morphology, flow cytometry and, when needed, molecular studies, allows a confident diagnosis in most cases.

Occasional cases of T-PLL can mimic CLL but careful attention to the morphologic features (small nucleoli) and flow cytometric immunophenotype make distinction straightforward. Likewise, some cells of acute lymphoblastic leukemia (ALL with a French–American–British L-1 morphologic subtype) might have small cells resembling CLL but close attention to morphologic details such as chromatin pattern and immunophenotyping permits distinction from CLL.

Persistent polyclonal B cell lymphocytosis might be mistaken for a B cell leukemia. This disorder presents most commonly in female smokers with a modest lymphocytosis composed of polyclonal B cells, which may coexpress CD5.[50] Deeply clefted lymphocytes are present which makes confusion with CLL less likely than other entities such as leukemic FL. In fact, *BCL2/IGH* translocations have been detected in these cases but are also polyclonal.[51] Immunophenotyping, as the name implies, shows polytypic B cells. As noted above, patients with fewer than 5×10^9/L circulating monoclonal B lymphocytes without lymphadenopathy or cytopenias due to marrow involvement by CLL cells may be considered as monoclonal B cell lymphocytosis, rather than CLL.[2]

Prognosis

As noted above, the prognosis varies depending on stage and biologic marker studies. Still, the disease course is measured in years to decades. A conservative approach to therapy is often taken (watch and wait), withholding treatment until the patient becomes symptomatic. Current approved therapies are generally aimed at symptomatic disease and are not curative. Recently, nucleoside analogues such as fludarabine have become prominent in first-line therapies. Combination with other agents such as cyclophosphamide or monoclonal antibodies are being studied.[52]

B PROLYMPHOCYTIC LEUKEMIA

Prolymphocytic leukemia is defined as a B cell leukemia that is composed of >55 percent prolymphocytes in the peripheral blood.[7,53] PLL can arise from preexisting CLL (prolymphocytic transformation of CLL), in which case this should be noted in the diagnosis. We consider the *de novo* form in this section. *De novo* PLL is a rare disorder. Our concept of PLL is evolving, since cases of leukemia with >55 percent prolymphocytes appears to be a heterogeneous group of diseases encompassing transformed CLL, nucleolated variants of MCL and *de novo* PLL.[54–56]

Clinical features

Patients are usually older (median age 70) with a male predominance, presenting with splenomegaly, high leukocyte count (often >100 × 10^9/L), and usually lack significant lympadenopathy.[8,57] Cytopenias are common, usually due to marrow replacement.

Morphologic features

The peripheral blood smear shows numerous (>55 percent) prolymphocytes, characterized by intermediate size, slightly dispersed chromatin, and a prominent central nucleolus. The cytoplasm is pale blue and moderate to abundant in amount. The nuclear contours are classically round but indentations can be seen. The bone marrow often shows extensive involvement with intermediate-sized cells containing small nucleoli. The spleen may show white pulp involvement with or without red pulp involvement. Again the cells are round, intermediate in size and show small central nucleoli in tissue section (Plate 22–24, see plate section). The presence of occasional cells with more clefted, enlarged cells with inconspicuous nucleoli may suggest a variant of MCL.

Immunophenotype

The reported immunophenotype of PLL is variable, likely because previous reports have included several entities (listed above). PLL expresses CD19, CD20 (bright), CD79b, FMC-7 and sIg. CD5 may be expressed in some cases; however, prior data concerning CD5 expression may be inaccurate due to differences in inclusion criteria. Recent series

that attempted to exclude MCL show expression of CD5 in only minority of cases (31 percent).[58] Strong expression of cyclin D1 strongly suggests a nucleolated variant of MCL and essentially excludes PLL.

Molecular genetics

Rearranged immunoglobulin genes are present. Given the confusion in the precise definition related to MCL, the molecular genetic features of PLL are not yet precisely defined. The t(11;l4)(q13;q32) resulting in an *IGH/CCND1* fusion is present in a minority (20 percent of some series) of previously reported PLL. However, these cases are best considered a variant of MCL.[54] Other nonspecific abnormalities reported in PLL include TP53 abnormalities (deletion or mutation in 75 percent of cases) and deletions of 13q14 (55 percent of cases) and 11q23 (39 percent of cases).[59,60]

Pathogenesis

Little is known regarding the pathogenesis of PLL, particularly when MCL is excluded. Genetic changes have been associated with CLL/PLL and PLL and include abnormalities in TP53 and acquisition of 11q22.3–23.1 (ATM) deletion.[61,62]

Differential diagnosis

The differential diagnosis of a leukemia composed of prolymphocytes includes transformed CLL, MCL variant, T-PLL and variant hairy cell leukemia (HCL). History of CLL allows one reasonably to diagnose a case of B cell leukemia with >55 percent prolymphocytes as prolymphocytic transformation of CLL. Presence of t(11;14) (q13;q32) or strong cyclin D1 expression allows one to confirm a diagnosis of MCL. T-PLL cells may resemble B cell PLL cells morphologically because of the presence of nucleoli, although the T-PLL cells tend to have more nuclear irregularities and the chromatin may be more condensed. Immunophenotyping easily identifies a T cell process in T-PLL. The hairy cell variant (HCLv) may have small nucleoli but still have some cytoplasmic features of HCL that are not seen in PLL. Presence of CD103 and generally lower white count are seen in HCLv. Once these are excluded, PLL is the most likely diagnosis.

Prognosis

Prolymphocytic leukemia is usually an aggressive disease although a subset of cases will not follow a rapidly progressive course that does not appear to be predictable. Older age, anemia and presence of TP53 abnormalities may indicate more aggressive disease.[63] Therapy has not been uniform for this uncommon disease and has varied from low-grade alkylator-based therapy to more aggressive anthracycline-containing regimens. More recently, nucleoside analogs such as cladribine and monoclonal antibody therapy with agents such as alemtuzumab have been successfully used.[63–66]

T CELL LARGE GRANULAR LYMPHOCYTIC LEUKEMIA

T cell large granular lymphocytic leukemia (T-LGL) is an indolent T cell leukemia that occurs most commonly in patients with a median age of 55 years. It was first recognized as a syndrome of increased large granular lymphocytes and chronic neutropenia.[67] Its neoplastic nature was confirmed by demonstrating clonal cytogenetic abnormalities and careful clinicopathologic characterization defined its morphologic and immunophenotypic features.[68,69] Some authors consider several variants. The most common is T cell LGL. Less common types are natural killer cell (NK)-LGL, chronic T cell lymphocytosis, and chronic NK cell lymphocytosis. The neoplastic nature of the latter two is the subject of debate. We will focus predominantly on the most common T cell LGL.

Diagnostic criteria traditionally have been clonal T-LGL lymphocytosis $>2 \times 10^9$/L for >6 months. However, some patients may have much lower lymphocyte levels and, in practice, some patients may require therapy prior to the requisite 6 months. Clinically autoimmune disorders such as rheumatoid arthritis are commonly present and T-LGL patients usually have associated cytopenias, which are often the major causes of morbidity for patients. Other recently described clinical associations include bone marrow failure syndromes such as paroxysmal nocturnal hemoglobinuria, aplastic anemia, myelodysplasia and red cell aplasia, suggesting an important role for immune dysregulation as part of the pathogenesis of this disease.[70] Patients vary widely in age but the median age at diagnosis is 60 years.[71] Approximately two-thirds of patients are symptomatic, usually due to cytopenias such as neutropenia. 'B' symptoms are seen in about one-third of patients. Organomegaly can be present in a minority of patients. As mentioned, patients usually have increased LGLs with most patients having LGL counts between 2 and 10 $\times$ 10^9/L.

Morphology and immunophenotype

In the peripheral blood, one sees large granular lymphocytes that may only be modestly increased in number and are cytologically normal (Plate 25, see plate section). Since the normal number of LGLs is low (less than 520/μL) this can be easily overlooked.[72] Thus, the diagnosis is often difficult to make due to the low level of circulating leukemia cells without special studies such as flow cytometry or T cell receptor gene rearrangement studies. The most common immunophenotype is a CD3+/CD8+ T cell that also expresses CD57 and cytotoxic proteins such as TIA1 and Granzyme B. Gene rearrangement studies should be done in all suspected cases and demonstrate T cell clonality, although such assays may reveal an oligoclonal pattern in the background of a dominant clone.[73] Polymerase chain reaction (PCR) assays are preferred since the sensitivity is generally slightly better than Southern blot studies.[74]

Bone marrow findings aided by immunohistochemistry in T-GLL have only recently been described.[75,76] As in the blood, bone marrow involvement can be subtle (Plate 26, see plate section). Bone marrow cellularity is usually increased although normocellularity or hypocellularity can be seen. A left shift in granulocytic cells is common, perhaps as a compensatory mechanism in patients with neutropenia, along with a relative increase in erythroid elements.[75,76] Megakaryocytes are normal. The lymphoid infiltrate is best seen by immunostaining and consists of an interstitial clustering of 8 or more CD8+ or TIA1+ T cells or 6 or more Granzyme B+ cells is characteristic of LGL and not seen in other reactive conditions. A subtle intravascular/intrasinusoidal pattern is also present, again seen best with the aid of immunostains (Plate 27, see plate section).[76]

With the availability of antibodies having specificity to many of the TCR-Vβ families, a new modality that is useful in the diagnosis of T-LGL is flow cytometry for specific Vβ families as a rapid and specific way to document skewed T cell repertoire and thus T cell clonality.[73,77] Lima and colleagues showed an 81 percent sensitivity and 100 percent specificity when 60 percent of the total CD4+ or CD8+[bright] cells used a single Vβ family.[77] Using a commercially available kit consisting of 24 Vβ family antibodies in a multicolor format to decrease the number of tubes used in the assay, we have demonstrated good performance in variety of T cell leukemias, which may obviate the need for molecular studies.[78] However, because of incomplete T cell repertoire coverage, a negative result must be further investigated with molecular studies. Such a flow cytometric assay also has the advantage of determining the particular Vβ family used by the leukemia for potential immunologic studies and may be a useful way to monitor therapy as has been done in Sézary syndrome.[79]

The uncommon indolent NK cell variant lacks CD3 but expresses CD16 and CD56.[69,72,80,81] Such patients may present without symptoms or may have difficulties due to cytopenias. Rare patients had vasculitis or nephrotic syndrome. This disease should be distinguished from aggressive NK cell leukemia, which although of a similar immunophenotype, presents in younger patients with organomegaly, B symptoms, and lacks an association with rheumatoid arthritis.[72,82] It is uncertain whether this indolent NK cell type of leukemia is truly neoplastic due to difficulty in demonstrating monoclonality in NK cells and whether this should be considered as a variant of T-LGL or as in indolent variant of aggressive NK cell leukemia. However, recent advances in our understanding of the biology of NK cells and their receptors may allow the determination of clonality in NK cells. A restricted pattern of CD158a and CD158b expression has been shown in NK leukemias, most often the CD158a-/CD158b- subset.[83]

Molecular genetics

T cell receptor gene rearrangement studies should demonstrate monoclonally rearranged antigen receptor genes. This has become a very important diagnostic tool to confirm the diagnosis and differentiate reactive conditions such as autoimmune disease or viral infection. In clinically borderline cases it should be noted that monoclonal T cell populations can be seen, particularly in elderly patients.[84] No specific chromosomal abnormalities have been identified.

Pathogenesis

Prior studies have pointed to abnormal apoptosis regulation as a mechanism both of the leukemic cell survival and as a cause for some of the cytopenias. Despite expression of both CD95 and CD95L,[85] the leukemic LGL cells are resistant to CD95 mediated death, perhaps due to abnormal STAT3 activation. Granular lymphocytic leukemia cells were found to contain activated STAT3 and inhibition of JAK3 with the tyrphostin AG-490 or direct inhibition with STAT3 antisense lead to apoptosis, perhaps through decreasing levels of the antiapoptotic protein MCL1.[86] In a separate line of investigation aimed at examining the role of background of autoimmunity in these patients, analysis of the complementary determining region (representing the antigen binding portion of the T cell receptor) revealed a common clonotype in two separate patients with T-LGL. There was also similarity in other immunodominant clonotypes between other patients. These data suggest antigen selection pressure may be involved in the pathogenesis of T-LGL.[87] Most recently, interactions with dendritic cells has been investigated. Dendritic cells derived from the bone marrow but not from the peripheral blood from T-LGL patients have been shown to support proliferation of LGL cells.[88] Furthermore, immunohistochemical studies in bone marrow from these patients suggest physical interaction between LGL cells and dendritic cells. This interaction was not seen in control marrows.[88] This suggests a role for dendritic cells and antigen stimulation in bone marrow in the development of LGL lymphoproliferative disorders.

Differential diagnosis

The differential diagnosis of T-LGL includes reactive nonclonal LGL expansions secondary to viral infection, skin disorders, and idiopathic thrombocytopenic purpura. These are often transient with relatively modest increases in LGLs. Clonality studies usually are negative. Features supporting the diagnosis of LGL rather than reactive processes are clinical features such as persistent cytopenias and persistence of a T cell clone over time.

Prognosis

The course of T-LGL is generally indolent. In a multicenter series of 151 patients followed for a mean time of 29 months, most patients had nonprogressive disease.[89] However, some patients experienced more aggressive disease and death within 4 years was seen in 19 patients.[89] Factors associated with poor outcome included fever at diagnosis and low percentage of LGLs in blood.[89] In another relatively large series, Dhodapkar et al. reported 31 percent of patients required no therapy.[90] Median survival was 161 months.[90] Indicators of poor outcome included low neutrophil count and 'B' symptoms/infection.[90] As more patients are studied and uniform diagnostic criteria are used, more reliable prognostic indicators will be defined. Treatment is often a combination of supportive for cytopenias cyclosporine or methotrexate with or without corticosteroids.[71]

T PROLYMPHOCYTIC LEUKEMIA

T-PLL is an uncommon T cell lymphoproliferative disorder of mature post-thymic T cells characterized by occurrence in older adults (median age 69 years), with a male predominance. It represents approximately 2 percent of small lymphoid leukemias in adults.[91] Some confusion regarding this disease has been present in the past due to inconsistent terminology such as T chronic lymphocytic leukemia (T-CLL). This may have led to confusion with B-CLL and T-GLL. The current WHO classification does not recognize 'T-CLL' as an entity and most cases of T-CLL (once other leukemic T cell processes such as Sézary syndrome, adult T cell leukemia lymphoma, and T-LGL) are examples of T-PLL.[92,93] Some confusion also exists because the name 'prolymphocytic leukemia' to some implies a morphologic identity with B-PLL; this is an erroneous implication as detailed below.

Clinical features

Patients present with hepatosplenomegaly, lymphadenopathy, skin lesions and marked leukocytosis (over 100×10^9/L in 75 percent of cases).[91] Cytopenias such as anemia and thrombocytopenia are common. The clinical course is generally aggressive; however, an indolent phase has been recognized.[94]

Morphology

The morphologic spectrum of T-PLL is variable.[95] The leukemic cells often are small to intermediate in size with slight to marked nuclear irregularities. The chromatin is condensed and nucleoli are present but usually not as prominent as seen in B-PLL. Nuclear contours are sound to irregular and the irregularities can be quite marked. The cytoplasm is usually lightly basophilic, agranular, and cytoplasmic blebs can be found in some cases (Plate 28, see plate section). A minority of cases (approximately 20 percent) can be composed of small cells that may mimic typical B-CLL (so-called small cell variant of T-PLL).

Bone marrow involvement is often extensive and present in an interstitial and diffuse pattern. Cutaneous involvement can be present in approximately 25–30 percent of patients and most commonly manifests as indurated erythema. Histologically the pattern of infiltration is usually perivascular and periadnexal. Epidermotropism is not a feature.[96] This pattern is not specific and knowledge of the complete clinical picture is required for one to make a diagnosis of cutaneous involvement by T-PLL rather than primary cutaneous T cell lymphoma. Splenic involvement is characterized by red and white pulp involvement while paracortical involvement may be seen in lymph node. Hepatic involvement is frequent and infiltration of sinusoids is seen (Plate 29, see plate section).

Immunophenotype

Flow cytometric immunophenotypic is required to confirm the T cell lineage of this leukemia. The common immunophenotype is CD2+, CD3+, CD4+, CD5+, CD7+, CD8−, CD19−, CD20−, CD26+, TdT− and CD1a−. While most cases (60 percent) are CD4+, a minority (25 percent) coexpress CD4 and CD8, and occasional cases are CD4−/CD8+ (15 percent).[91] TCL1 expression is present in over 70 percent of cases of T-PLL and, although expressed in other lymphoid malignancy such as B cell lymphoma and CLL, appears to be specific for this entity when considering other T cell leukemic processes that might enter the differential diagnosis including T-LGL and Sézary syndrome.[97]

Molecular genetics

Cytogenetic analysis of T-PLL has shown frequent abnormalities of 14q32.1. Inv14(q11;q32.1) or 1(14;14)(q11;q32.1) is found in the majority (70 percent) of cases.[98]

Pathogenesis

Recent work has identified *TCL1* as the oncogene at 14q32.1 of particular pathogenetic importance in T-PLL. Interestingly, the TCL1 homolog MTCP-1, located at Xq28, is also involved in translocation with the TCRα/β locus at 14q11. Transgenic mice overexpressing these genes develop T-PLL-like leukemias, thus demonstrating the importance of these gene products in leukemogenesis.[99,100]

The mechanism by which TCL1 overexpression promotes leukemia appears to relate to its function as a cofactor for AKT activation, resulting in nuclear localization of AKT and enhance cell proliferation and survival.[100–102]

Differential diagnosis

The differential diagnosis of T-PLL includes other B cell leukemias, acute lymphoblastic leukemia, T-LGL, adult T cell leukemia/lymphoma, and Sézary syndrome. B cell leukemias can be excluded by basic immunophenotyping that shows expression of pan B cell antigens and lack of T cell antigens. Acute lymphoblastic leukemias can also be excluded by morphologic examination demonstrating the fine chromatin of blasts that is not seen in T-PLL. Phenotyping would also differentiate precursor lymphoblastic processes since these express such early precursor markers as CD1a, TdT and the CD34. These markers would not be present in a post-thymic T-cell. ATLL can be excluded by typical clinical presentation, ethnic/geographic considerations, and presence of human T lymphotrophic virus (HTLV) 1 that is characteristic of ATLL. Sézary syndrome can be excluded by history of mycosis fungoides and clinical features such as erythroderma. Phenotypic differences such as expression of CD26 (absent in most cases of Sézary syndrome) and loss of CD7 (seen in most cases of Sézary syndrome) also may be of help. Finally, as mentioned, expression of TCL1 in the specific setting of a mature T cell leukemia appears to be fairly specific for T-PLL.[97]

Prognosis

The disease course is usually aggressive with short survival (<1 year).[91] Recently, an indolent presentation has been recognized; however, even these patients will convert to a more aggressive course typical of T-PLL with short survival.[94] A few reports of indolent T cell PLL are appearing with complex karyotypes.[104,105] Therapy with alemtuzumab has resulted in complete responses in a high proportion of cases and may improve the outlook for many patients.[106,107]

μ HEAVY CHAIN DISEASE

First reported in 1969, μ heavy chain disease (μHCD) is an extremely rare occurrence with less than 40 reported cases in the literature.[108–111] It is characterized by abnormal IgM heavy chain that is incapable of forming an intact immunoglobulin molecule. Light chain is synthesized and Bence Jones protein can be seen. It occupies a place between plasma cell dyscrasia and lymphoid leukemia with regard to clinical features and is covered here due to its potential similarity to CLL and Waldenstrom macroglobulinemia (lymphoplasmacytic lymphoma).

Clinical features

μ Heavy chain disease appears to have a slight male predominance and occurs with a median age of approximately 58 years (range 15–80).[110] Most patients appear to have a lymphoproliferative disorder such as CLL, Waldenstrom macroglobulinemia, myeloma or other lymphoma. Associated findings include hepatosplenomegaly, anemia and lymphoadenopathy.[111] Monoclonal protein by serum protein electrophoresis can show a spike in a minority of patients. Hypogammaglobulinemia is seen in approximately half of the patients.[111] By definition, μ heavy chain can be demonstrated by immunoelectrophoresis or immunofixation. Unlike γ or α HCD, over half of μHCD patients can have detectable Bence Jones proteinuria.[111] The median duration of survival from diagnosis is 24 months. Amyloidosis has been reported in rare patients and appears to portend a short survival.[112]

Morphology

The characteristic finding is in the bone marrow with increased plasma cells, lymphocytes, or lymphoplasmacytic cells. Plasmacytosis appears to be common (18/20 cases). In most cases (13/18), the plasma cells contain clear cytoplasmic vacuoles.[110] Although this feature can also be seen in plasma cell myeloma, it is rather uncommon.

Immunophenotype and molecular genetics

Given the rarity of this entity, there are few data on particular immunophenotypic or molecular genetic characteristics. Some work has been done in characterizing the heavy chain protein component in these patients. It appears that there are usually deletions of the V-region with normal constant regions resulting in a truncated heavy chain and inability to pair with light chains.[113,114] Detailed molecular investigations on one case revealed a single-base deletion resulting in a stop codon in the variable region and also a deletion/insertion that caused loss of the J4 donor splice site. This would result in an RNA splice between the leader region and first constant region and a shortened μ-chain RNA lacking variable region sequences.[115,116]

Pathogenesis

Again, given the rarity, little is known regarding pathogenesis of this disorder.

Differential diagnosis

The differential diagnosis includes lymphoproliferative disorders such as CLL and lymphoplasmacytic lymphoma and plasma cell myeloma. Distinction from lymphoproliferative disorders is based on detection of a monotypic B cell component typical of CLL or LPL. These entities will not have heavy chain only when examined for paraproteins. Plasma cell myeloma can be diagnosed by adhering to typical laboratory (high levels of serum paraprotein and/or Bence Jones protein), radiologic (lytic bone lesions), and pathologic findings (atypical plasmacytosis in bone marrow, usually greater than 10 percent with displacement of hematopoietic elements between fatty spaces.

Prognosis

Few data exist due to the rarity of disease. However, in a review of 23 patients, 16 patients received therapy.[117] Therapy was heterogeneous and individually tailored depending on the type of underlying lymphoproliferative disorder. The median survival was 7.4 years with most of the known causes of deaths being unrelated to the underlying disease.[116]

KEY POINTS

- CLL is a biologically and pathologically heterogeneous disease. Flow cytometric analysis is required in all patients to establish a diagnosis. Prognostic information is available from biologic markers such as CD38, ZAP-70, *IGH* mutational status, and FISH analysis for TP53 deletion.
- *De novo* B-PLL should be distinguished from nucleolated variants of MCL and progression of CLL.
- T-LGL is an indolent disorder. Patients often do not have a lymphocytosis and a high index of suspicious is needed to establish a diagnosis.
- Flow cytometry for T-LGL can now identify the specific TCR Vβ receptor family used in most cases. *TCR* gene rearrangement remains the best technique for documenting monoclonality.
- T-PLL must be distinguished from other forms of T cell leukemia such as adult T cell leukemia/lymphoma
- μ HCD is an extremely uncommon disorder and appears to be a clinicopathologic entity characterized by μ heavy chain only in serum or urine and marrow plasmacytosis/lymphocytosis.

REFERENCES

● = Key primary paper
◆ = Major review article

1. Redaelli A, Laskin BL, Stephens JM *et al.* The clinical and epidemiological burden of chronic lymphocytic

leukaemia. *Eur J Cancer Care (Engl)* 2004; **13**: 279–87.

2. Hallek M, Cheson BD, Catovsky D *et al.* Guidlines for the diagnosis and treatment of chronic lymphocytic leukemia: a report from the International Workshop on Chronic Lymphocytic Leukemia updating the National Cancer Institute Working Group 1996 Guidelines. Blood 2008; **111**: 5446–56.

3. Binet JL, Auquier A, Dighiero G *et al.* A new prognostic classification of chronic lymphocytic leukemia derived from a multivariate survival analysis. *Cancer* 1981; **48**: 198–206.

4. Rai KR, Han T. Prognostic factors and clinical staging in chronic lymphocytic leukemia. *Hematol Oncol Clin North Am* 1990; **4**: 447–56.

5. Oscier DG, Matutes E, Copplestone A *et al.* Atypical lymphocyte morphology: an adverse prognostic factor for disease progression in stage A CLL independent of trisomy 12. *Br J Haematol* 1997; **98**: 934–9.

6. Frater JL, McCarron KF, Hammel JP *et al.* Typical and atypical chronic lymphocytic leukaemia differ clinically and immunophenotypically. *Am J Clin Pathol* 2001; **116**: 655–64.

◆7. Bennett JM, Catovsky D, Daniel MT *et al.* Proposals for the classification of chronic (mature) B and T lymphoid leukaemias. French-American-British (FAB) Cooperative Group. *J Clin Pathol* 1989; **42**: 567–84.

◆8. Swerdlow SH, Campo E, Harris NL *et al. WHO classification of tumours of haematopoietic and lymphoid tissues.* Lyon: IARC Press, 2008.

9. Vallespi T, Montserrat E, Sanz MA. Chronic lymphocytic leukaemia: prognostic value of lymphocyte morphological subtypes. A multivariate survival analysis in 146 patients. *Br J Haematol* 1991; **77**: 478–85.

10. Lens D, Dyer MJ, Garcia-Marco JM *et al.* p53 abnormalities in CLL are associated with excess of prolymphocytes and poor prognosis. *Br J Haematol* 1997; **99**: 848–57.

11. Matutes E, Oscier D, Garcia-Marco J *et al.* Trisomy 12 defines a group of CLL with atypical morphology: correlation between cytogenetic, clinical and laboratory features in 544 patients. *Br J Haematol* 1996; **92**: 382–8.

12. Montserrat E, Villamor N, Reverter JC *et al.* Bone marrow assessment in B-cell chronic lymphocytic leukaemia: aspirate or biopsy? A comparative study in 258 patients. *Br J Haematol* 1996; **93**: 111–16.

13. Raphael M, Chastang C, Binet JL. Is bone marrow biopsy a prognostic parameter in B-CLL? *Nouv Rev Fr Hematol* 1988; **30**: 377–8.

14. Rozman C, Montserrat E, Rodriguez-Fernandez JM *et al.* Bone marrow histologic pattern – the best single prognostic parameter in chronic lymphocytic leukemia: a multivariate survival analysis of 329 cases. *Blood* 1984; **64**: 642–8.

15. Kjeldsberg CR, Marty J. Prolymphocytic transformation of chronic lymphocytic leukemia. *Cancer* 1981; **48**: 2447–57.

16. Foucar K, Rydell RE. Richter's syndrome in chronic lymphocytic leukemia. *Cancer* 1980; **46**: 118–34.

17. Foon KA, Gale RP. Clinical transformation of chronic lymphocytic leukemia. *Nouv Rev Fr Hematol* 1988; **30**: 385–8.

18. Fayad L, Robertson LE, O'Brien S *et al.* Hodgkin's disease variant of Richter's syndrome: experience at a single institution. *Leuk Lymphoma* 1996; **23**: 333–7.

19. Kanzler H, Kuppers R, Helmes S *et al.* Hodgkin and Reed-Sternberg-like cells in B-cell chronic lymphocytic leukemia represent the outgrowth of single germinal-center B-cell-derived clones: potential precursors of Hodgkin and Reed-Sternberg cells in Hodgkin's disease. *Blood* 2000; **95**: 1023–31.

20. Rubin D, Hudnall SD, Aisenberg A *et al.* Richter's transformation of chronic lymphocytic leukemia with Hodgkin's-like cells is associated with Epstein-Barr virus infection. *Mod Pathol* 1994; **7**: 91–8.

21. Ohno T, Smir BN, Weisenburger DD *et al.* Origin of the Hodgkin/Reed-Sternberg cells in chronic lymphocytic leukemia with 'Hodgkin's transformation'. *Blood* 1998; **91**: 1757–61.

22. McCarron KF, Hammel JP, Hsi ED. Usefulness of CD79b expression in the diagnosis of B-cell chronic lymphoproliferative disorders. *Am J Clin Pathol* 2000; **113**: 805–13.

●23. Matutes E, Owusu-Ankomah K, Morilla R *et al.* The immunological profile of B-cell disorders and proposal of a scoring system for the diagnosis of CLL. *Leukemia* 1994; **8**: 1640–5.

●24. Damle RN, Wasil T, Fais F *et al.* Ig V gene mutation status and CD38 expression As novel prognostic indicators in chronic lymphocytic leukemia. *Blood* 1999; **94**: 1840–7.

●25. Hamblin TJ, Orchard JA, Ibbotson RE *et al.* CD38 expression and immunoglobulin variable region mutations are independent prognostic variables in chronic lymphocytic leukemia, but CD38 expression may vary during the course of the disease. *Blood* 2002; **99**: 1023–9.

26. Del Poeta G, Maurillo L, Venditti A *et al.* Clinical significance of CD38 expression in chronic lymphocytic leukemia. *Blood* 2001; **98**: 2633–9.

27. Hsi ED, Kopecky KJ, Appelbaum FR *et al.* Prognostic significance of CD38 and CD20 expression as assessed by quantitative flow cytometry in chronic lymphocytic leukemia (CLL). *Br J Haematol* 2003; **120**: 1017–25.

28. Krober A, Seiler T, Benner A *et al.* V(H) mutation status, CD38 expression level, genomic aberrations, and survival in chronic lymphocytic leukemia. *Blood* 2002; **100**: 1410–16.

29. Orchard JA, Ibbotson RE, Davis Z *et al.* ZAP-70 expression and prognosis in chronic lymphocytic leukaemia. *Lancet* 2004; **363**: 105–11.

30. Rassenti LZ, Huynh L, Toy TL *et al.* ZAP-70 compared with immunoglobulin heavy-chain gene mutation status as a predictor of disease progression in chronic lymphocytic leukemia. *N Engl J Med* 2004; **351**: 893–901.

31. Rawstron AC, Yuille MR, Fuller J et al. Inherited predisposition to CLL is detectable as subclinical monoclonal B-lymphocyte expansion. Blood 2002; 100: 2289–90.

32. Rawstron AC, Green MJ, Kuzmicki A et al. Monoclonal B lymphocytes with the characteristics of 'indolent' chronic lymphocytic leukemia are present in 3.5% of adults with normal blood counts. Blood 2002; 100: 635–9.

33. Rawstron AC, Bennett FL, O'Connor SJ et al. Monoclonal B-Cell lymphocytosis and chronic lymphocytic leukemia. N Engl J Med 2008; 359: 575–83.

●34. Dohner H, Stilgenbauer S, Benner A et al. Genomic alterations and survival in chronic lymphocytic leukemia. N Engl J Med 2000; 343: 1910–16.

35. Hamblin TJ, Davis Z, Gardiner A et al. Unmutated Ig V(H) genes are associated with a more aggressive form of chronic lymphocytic leukemia. Blood 1999; 94: 1848–54.

●36. Rosenwald A, Alizadeh AA, Widhopf G et al. Relation of gene expression phenotype to immunoglobulin mutation genotype in B cell chronic lymphocytic leukemia. J Exp Med 2001; 194: 1639–47.

37. Wiestner A, Rosenwald A, Barry TS et al. ZAP-70 expression identifies a chronic lymphocytic leukemia subtype with unmutated immunoglobulin genes, inferior clinical outcome, and distinct gene expression profile. Blood 2003; 101: 4944–51.

38. Chen L, Apgar J, Huynh L et al. ZAP-70 directly enhances IgM signaling in chronic lymphocytic leukemia. Blood 2005; 105: 2036–41.

39. Bernal A, Pastore RD, Asgary Z et al. Survival of leukemic B cells promoted by engagement of the antigen receptor. Blood 2001; 98: 3050–7.

40. Cimmino A, Calin GA, Fabbri M et al. miR-15 and miR-16 induce apoptosis by targeting BCL2. Proc Natl Acad Sci U S A 2005; 102: 13944–9.

41. Calin GA, Dumitru CD, Shimizu M et al. Frequent deletions and down-regulation of micro-RNA genes miR15 and miR16 at 13q14 in chronic lymphocytic leukemia. Proc Natl Acad Sci U S A 2002; 99: 15524–9.

42. Calin GA, Liu CG, Sevignani C et al. MicroRNA profiling reveals distinct signatures in B cell chronic lymphocytic leukemias. Proc Natl Acad Sci U S A 2004; 101: 11755–60.

43. Nishio M, Endo T, Tsukada N et al. Nurselike cells express BAFF and APRIL, which can promote survival of chronic lymphocytic leukemia cells via a paracrine pathway distinct from that of SDF-1alpha. Blood 2005; 106: 1012–20.

44. Tsukada N, Burger JA, Zvaifler NJ et al. Distinctive features of 'nurselike' cells that differentiate in the context of chronic lymphocytic leukemia. Blood 2002; 99: 1030–7.

45. Burger JA, Tsukada N, Burger M et al. Blood-derived nurse-like cells protect chronic lymphocytic leukemia B cells from spontaneous apoptosis through stromal cell-derived factor-1. Blood 2000; 96: 2655–63.

46. Burger JA, Burger M, Kipps TJ. Chronic lymphocytic leukemia B cells express functional CXCR4 chemokine receptors that mediate spontaneous migration beneath bone marrow stromal cells. Blood 1999; 94: 3658–67.

47. Nishii K, Katayama N, Miwa H et al. Survival of human leukaemic B-cell precursors is supported by stromal cells and cytokines: association with the expression of bcl-2 protein. Br J Haematol 1999; 105: 701–10.

●48. Calin GA, Ferracin M, Cimmino A et al. A MicroRNA signature associated with prognosis and progression in chronic lymphocytic leukemia. N Engl J Med 2005; 353: 1793–801.

49. Matutes E, Morilla R, Owusu-Ankomah K et al. The immunophenotype of splenic lymphoma with villous lymphocytes and its relevance to the differential diagnosis with other B-cell disorders. Blood 1994; 83: 1558–62.

50. Lush CJ, Vora AJ, Campbell AC et al. Polyclonal CD5 + B-lymphocytosis resembling chronic lymphocytic leukaemia. Br J Haematol 1991; 79: 119–20.

51. Delage R, Roy J, Jacques L et al. All patients with persistent polyclonal B cell lymphocytosis present Bcl-2/Ig gene rearrangements. Leuk Lymphoma 1998; 31: 567–74.

◆52. Hallek M. Chronic lymphocytic leukemia (CLL): first-line treatment. Hematol Am Soc Hematol Educ Program 2005; 285–91.

53. Galton DA, Goldman JM, Wiltshaw E et al. Prolymphocytic leukemia. Br J Haematol 1974; 27: 7–23.

●54. Schlette E, Bueso-Ramos C, Giles F et al. Mature B-cell leukemias with more than 55 percent prolymphocytes. A heterogeneous group that includes an unusual variant of mantle cell lymphoma. Am J Clin Pathol 2001; 115: 571–81.

◆55. Hsi ED, Frater JL. Advances in the diagnosis and classification of chronic lymphoproliferative disorders. Cancer Treat Res 2004; 121: 145–65.

56. Wong KF, So CC, Chan JK. Nucleolated variant of mantle cell lymphoma with leukemic manifestations mimicking prolymphocytic leukemia. Am J Clin Pathol 2002; 117: 246–51.

57. Melo JV, Catovsky D, Galton DA. The relationship between chronic lymphocytic leukaemia and prolymphocytic leukaemia I. Clinical and laboratory features of 300 patients and characterization of an intermediate group. Br J Haematol 1986; 63: 377–87.

●58. Ruchlemer R, Parry-Jones N, Brito-Babapulle V et al. B-prolymphocytic leukaemia with t(11;14) revisited: a splenomegalic form of mantle cell lymphoma evolving with leukaemia. Br J Haematol 2004; 125: 330–6.

59. Lens D, Matutes E, Catovsky D et al. Frequent deletions at 11q23 and 13q14 in B cell prolymphocytic leukemia (B-PLL). Leukemia 2000; 14: 427–30.

60. Lens D, De Schouwer PJ, Hamoudi RA et al. p53 abnormalities in B-cell prolymphocytic leukemia. Blood 1997; 89: 2015–23.

61. Bacher U, Kern W, Schoch C et al. Discrimination of chronic lymphocytic leukemia (CLL) and CLL/PL by

cytomorphology can clearly be correlated to specific genetic markers as investigated by interphase fluorescence *in situ* hybridization (FISH). *Ann Hematol* 2004; **83**: 349–55.

62. Cuneo A, Bigoni R, Rigolin GM *et al.* Late appearance of the 11q22.3–23.1 deletion involving the ATM locus in B-cell chronic lymphocytic leukemia and related disorders. Clinico-biological significance. *Haematologica* 2002; **87**: 44–51.

63. Hercher C, Robain M, Davi F *et al.* A multicentric study of 41 cases of B-prolymphocytic leukemia: two evolutive forms. *Leuk Lymphoma* 2001; **42**: 981–7.

64. McCune SL, Gockerman JP, Moore JO *et al.* Alemtuzumab in relapsed or refractory chronic lymphocytic leukemia and prolymphocytic leukemia. *Leuk Lymphoma* 2002; **43**: 1007–11.

65. Saven A, Lee T, Schlutz M *et al.* Major activity of cladribine in patients with de novo B-cell prolymphocytic leukemia. *J Clin Oncol* 1997; **15**: 37–43.

66. Shvidel L, Shtalrid M, Bassous L *et al.* B-cell prolymphocytic leukemia: a survey of 35 patients emphasizing heterogeneity, prognostic factors and evidence for a group with an indolent course. *Leuk Lymphoma* 1999; **33**: 169–79.

67. McKenna RW, Parkin J, Kersey JH *et al.* Chronic lymphoproliferative disorder with unusual clinical, morphologic, ultrastructural and membrane surface marker characteristics. *Am J Med* 1977; **62**: 588–96.

68. Loughran TP Jr, Kadin ME, Starkebaum G *et al.* Leukemia of large granular lymphocytes: association with clonal chromosomal abnormalities and autoimmune neutropenia, thrombocytopenia, and hemolytic anemia. *Ann Intern Med* 1985; **102**: 169–75.

◆69. Loughran TP Jr. Clonal diseases of large granular lymphocytes. *Blood* 1993; **82**: 1–14.

70. Karadimitris A, Li K, Notaro R *et al.* Association of clonal T-cell large granular lymphocyte disease and paroxysmal nocturnal haemoglobinuria (PNH): further evidence for a pathogenetic link between T cells, aplastic anaemia and PNH. *Br J Haematol* 2001; **115**: 1010–14.

◆71. Lamy T, Loughran TP Jr. Clinical features of large granular lymphocyte leukemia. *Semin Hematol* 2003; **40**: 185–95.

72. Lamy T, Loughran TP Jr. Current concepts: large granular lymphocyte leukemia. *Blood Rev* 1999; **13**: 230–40.

73. Langerak AW, van Den BR, Wolvers-Tettero IL *et al.* Molecular and flow cytometric analysis of the Vbeta repertoire for clonality assessment in mature TCRalphabeta T-cell proliferations. *Blood* 2001; **98**: 165–73.

74. Alkan S, Cosar E, Ergin M *et al.* Detection of T-cell receptor-gamma gene rearrangement in lymphoproliferative disorders by temperature gradient gel electrophoresis. *Arch Pathol Lab Med* 2001; **125**: 202–7.

75. Evans HL, Burks E, Viswanatha D *et al.* Utility of immunohistochemistry in bone marrow evaluation of T-lineage large granular lymphocyte leukemia. *Hum Pathol* 2000; **31**: 1266–73.

76. Morice WG, Kurtin PJ, Tefferi A *et al.* Distinct bone marrow findings in T-cell granular lymphocytic leukemia revealed by paraffin section immunoperoxidase stains for CD8, TIA-1, and granzyme B. *Blood* 2002; **99**: 268–74.

77. Lima M, Almeida J, Santos AH *et al.* Immunophenotypic analysis of the TCR-Vbeta repertoire in 98 persistent expansions of CD3(+)/TCR-alphabeta(+) large granular lymphocytes: utility in assessing clonality and insights into the pathogenesis of the disease. *Am J Pathol* 2001; **159**: 1861–8.

●78. Beck RC, Stahl S, O'Keefe CL *et al.* Detection of mature T cell leukemias by flow cytometry using anti-T cell receptor Vb antibodies. *Am J Clin Pathol* 2003; **120**: 785–94.

79. Ingen-Housz-Oro S, Bussel A, Flageul B *et al.* A prospective study on the evolution of the T-cell repertoire in patients with Sezary syndrome treated by extracorporeal photopheresis. *Blood* 2002; **100**: 2168–74.

●80. Morice WG, Leibson PJ, Tefferi A. Natural killer cells and the syndrome of chronic natural killer cell lymphocytosis. *Leuk Lymphoma* 2001; **41**: 277–84.

81. Rabbani GR, Phyliky RL, Tefferi A. A long-term study of patients with chronic natural killer cell lymphocytosis. *Br J Haematol* 1999; **106**: 960–6.

82. Imamura N, Kusunoki Y, Kawa-Ha K *et al.* Aggressive natural killer cell leukaemia/lymphoma: report of four cases and review of the literature. Possible existence of a new clinical entity originating from the third lineage of lymphoid cells. *Br J Haematol* 1990; **75**: 49–59.

83. Zambello R, Trentin L, Ciccone E *et al.* Phenotypic diversity of natural killer (NK) populations in patients with NK-type lymphoproliferative disease of granular lymphocytes. *Blood* 1993; **81**: 2381–5.

84. Posnett DN, Sinha R, Kabak S *et al.* Clonal populations of T cells in normal elderly humans: the T cell equivalent to 'benign monoclonal gammapathy'. *J Exp Med* 1994; **179**: 609–18.

85. Lamy T, Liu JH, Landowski TH *et al.* Dysregulation of CD95/CD95 ligand-apoptotic pathway in CD3(+) large granular lymphocyte leukemia. *Blood* 1998; **92**: 4771–7.

86. Epling-Burnette PK, Liu JH, Catlett-Falcone R *et al.* Inhibition of STAT3 signaling leads to apoptosis of leukemic large granular lymphocytes and decreased Mcl-1 expression. *J Clin Invest* 2001; **107**: 351–62.

87. Wlodarski MW, O'Keefe C, Howe EC *et al.* Pathologic clonal cytotoxic T-cell responses: nonrandom nature of the T-cell-receptor restriction in large granular lymphocyte leukemia. *Blood* 2005; **106**: 2769–80.

88. Zambello R, Berno T, Cannas G *et al.* Phenotypic and functional analyses of dendritic cells in patients with lymphoproliferative disease of granular lymphocytes (LDGL). *Blood* 2005; **106**: 3926–31.

89. Pandolfi F, Loughran TP Jr, Starkebaum G *et al.* Clinical course and prognosis of the lymphoproliferative disease of granular lymphocytes. A multicenter study. *Cancer* 1990; **65**: 341–8.

90. Dhodapkar MV, Li CY, Lust JA *et al.* Clinical spectrum of clonal proliferations of T-large granular lymphocytes: a T-cell clonopathy of undetermined significance? *Blood* 1994; **84**: 1620–7.

●91. Matutes E, Brito-Babapulle V, Swansbury J *et al.* Clinical and laboratory features of 78 cases of T-prolymphocytic leukemia. *Blood* 1991; **78**: 3269–74.

92. Hoyer JD, Ross CW, Li CY *et al.* True T-cell chronic lymphocytic leukemia: a morphologic and immunophenotypic study of 25 cases. *Blood* 1995; **86**: 1163–9.

93. Matutes E, Catovsky D. Similarities between T-cell chronic lymphocytic leukemia and the small-cell variant of T-prolymphocytic leukemia. *Blood* 1996; **87**: 3520–1.

94. Garand R, Goasguen J, Brizard A *et al.* Indolent course as a relatively frequent presentation in T-prolymphocytic leukaemia. Groupe Francais d'Hematologie Cellulaire. *Br J Haematol* 1998; **103**: 488–94.

◆95. Matutes E, Garcia TJ, O'Brien M *et al.* The morphological spectrum of T-prolymphocytic leukemia. *Br J Haematol* 1986; **64**: 111–24.

96. Mallett RB, Matutes E, Catovsky D *et al.* Cutaneous infiltration in T-cell prolymphocytic leukaemia. *Br J Dermatol* 1995; **132**: 263–6.

●97. Herling M, Khoury JD, Washington LT *et al.* A systematic approach to diagnosis of mature T-cell leukemias reveals heterogeneity among WHO categories. *Blood* 2004; **104**: 328–35.

98. Maljaei SH, Brito-Babapulle V, Hiorns LR *et al.* Abnormalities of chromosomes 8, 11, 14, and X in T-prolymphocytic leukemia studied by fluorescence *in situ* hybridization. *Cancer Genet Cytogenet* 1998; **103**: 110–16.

●99. Virgilio L, Lazzeri C, Bichi R *et al.* Deregulated expression of TCL1 causes T cell leukemia in mice. *Proc Natl Acad Sci U S A* 1998; **95**: 3885–9.

100. Gritti C, Dastot H, Soulier J *et al.* Transgenic mice for MTCP1 develop T-cell prolymphocytic leukemia. *Blood* 1998; **92**: 368–73.

101. Laine J, Kunstle G, Obata T *et al.* The protooncogene TCL1 is an Akt kinase coactivator. *Mol Cell* 2000; **6**: 395–407.

102. Pekarsky Y, Zanesi N, Aqeilan R *et al.* Tcl1 as a model for lymphomagenesis. *Hematol Oncol Clin North Am* 2004; **18**: 863–79, ix.

103. Pekarsky Y, Koval A, Hallas C *et al.* Tcl1 enhances Akt kinase activity and mediates its nuclear translocation. *Proc Natl Acad Sci U S A* 2000; **97**: 3028–33.

104. Soma L, Cornfield DB, Prager D *et al.* Unusually indolent T-cell prolymphocytic leukemia associated with a complex karyotype: is this T-cell chronic lymphocytic leukemia? *Am J Hematol* 2002; **71**: 224–6.

105. Yokohama A, Karasawa M, Takada S *et al.* Prolonged survival in two cases of T-prolymphocytic leukemias with complex hypodiploid chromosomal abnormalities. *J Med* 2000; **31**: 183–94.

◆106. Cao TM, Coutre SE. T-cell prolymphocytic leukemia: update and focus on alemtuzumab (Campath-1H). *Hematology* 2003; **8**: 1–6.

107. Dearden CE, Matutes E, Cazin B *et al.* High remission rate in T-cell prolymphocytic leukemia with CAMPATH-1H. *Blood* 2001; **98**: 1721–6.

108. Forte FA, Prelli F, Yount WJ *et al.* Heavy chain disease of the m (gM) type: report of the first case. *Blood* 1970; **36**: 137–44.

109. Fermand JP, Brouet JC. Heavy-chain diseases. *Hematol Oncol Clin North Am* 1999; **13**: 1281–94.

◆110. Wahner-Roedler DL, Kyle RA. Heavy chain diseases. *Best Pract Res Clin Haematol* 2005; **18**: 729–46.

111. Wahner-Roedler DL, Kyle RA. Mu-heavy chain disease: presentation as a benign monoclonal gammopathy. *Am J Hematol* 1992; **40**: 56–60.

112. Kinoshita K, Yamagata T, Nozaki Y *et al.* Mu-heavy chain disease associated with systemic amyloidosis. *Hematology* 2004; **9**: 135–7.

113. Barnikol-Watanabe S, Mihaesco E, Mihaesco C *et al.* The primary structure of mu-chain-disease protein BOT. Peculiar amino-acid sequence of the N-terminal 42 positions. *Hoppe Seylers Z Physiol Chem* 1984; **365**: 105–18.

114. Franklin EC, Frangione B, Prelli F. The defect in mu heavy chain disease protein GLI. *J Immunol* 1976; **116**: 1194–5.

115. Bakhshi A, Guglielmi P, Siebenlist U *et al.* A DNA insertion/deletion necessitates an aberrant RNA splice accounting for a mu heavy chain disease protein. *Proc Natl Acad Sci U S A* 1986; **83**: 2689–93.

116. Bakhshi A, Guglielmi P, Coligan JE *et al.* A pre-translational defect in a case of human mu heavy chain disease. *Mol Immunol* 1986; **23**: 725–32.

◆117. Wahner-Roedler DL, Witzig TE, Loehrer LL *et al.* Gamma-heavy chain disease: review of 23 cases. *Medicine (Baltimore)* 2003; **82**: 236–50.

28

Hairy cell leukemia

BRUNANGELO FALINI AND ENRICO TIACCI

INTRODUCTION

Hairy cell leukemia (HCL) is an unusual B cell chronic lymphoproliferative disorder that was first described as *Leukämische reticuloendotheliose* by Ewald in 1923.[1] More than 30 years later, Bouroncle identified HCL as a distinct disease entity.[2] Although the biology, pathogenesis and etiology of HCL are still poorly understood, remarkable progress has been made over the past 50 years in diagnosis and therapy of this pathologic entity.

Typical features of HCL are pancytopenia, marked splenomegaly and bone marrow, spleen, and liver infiltration by leukemic cells with 'hairy' morphology, which circulate, usually in low numbers, in peripheral blood.[3–5] Although HCL is recognized as a clonal B cell malignancy, there is no agreement about which normal B cell developmental stage leukemic hairy cells should be assigned to. Many patients have an indolent course with no or few symptoms, and others have splenomegaly-related symptoms or life-threatening pancytopenia requiring treatment.[6] HCL provides an excellent model for understanding cytokine and growth factor deregulation in human neoplasms and for developing new drugs.[7] The introduction of purine analogs, 2-chlorodeoxyadenosine (2-CDA) and 2′-deoxycoformycin (2′-DCF) into clinical practice[6] has changed the natural history of the disease.[8–10] In fact, most patients who have achieved a complete remission with these agents might live as long as age-matched controls.

CLINICAL AND LABORATORY FINDINGS

Hairy cell leukemia accounts for about 2 percent of lymphoid leukemias.[5] Its incidence is similar in Europe and the USA, with about 3 cases per 1 million population per year. Typical HCL is very rare in Japan. Median age at diagnosis is approximately 50 years and there is a 4:1 male preponderance.[11] The incidence of HCL is greater in Caucasians than in black people.[11] The classic presentation of HCL is that of a white, middle-aged man with marked splenomegaly, pancytopenia and circulating leukemic cells that exhibit typical surface projections ('hairy appearance').[8] Patients may have anemia-related fatigue or weakness, infections due to marked neutropenia, and/or abdominal discomfort produced by splenomegaly. In about 25 percent of patients, HCL is diagnosed through incidentally finding splenomegaly or an abnormal peripheral blood cell count.

More than two-thirds of HCL patients show pancytopenia, which is usually caused by bone marrow failure secondary to leukemic infiltration combined with splenic sequestration; the others show diverse combinations of

Table 28.1 Clinicopathologic features of hairy cell leukemia (HCL) and HCL-like disorders

Findings	HCL	HCLv	SLVL
Morphology	1–2 times the size of lymphocyte; indistinct nucleoli; fine hair-like projections[a]	Morphologic intermediate between hairy cells and prolymphocytes[b]	Smaller than hairy cells; less abundant hairy projections, largely confined to cell poles
WBC count	Usually low	Usually high	Usually normal or slightly raised
Splenomegaly	Prominent	Prominent	Prominent
Lymphadenopathy	Absent	Absent	Variable
Ig spike	No	No	IgM (60%)
Response to IFN or PA	Excellent	Poor/no response	Scarce
TRAP	Present in most cases	Absent or weak	Present, but usually weak
CD20	+	+	+
CD103	+	−/+	−/+
CD25	+	−/+	−/+
Annexin A1[c]	+	−	−

[a]Resembling ruffles; [b]unlike typical HCL, leukemic cells show evident nucleoli; [c]identified in fixed tissues/cytospins.
+, positive; −/+, usually negative; −, negative.
HCLv, hairy cell leukemia variant; SLVL, splenic lymphoma with villous lymphocytes; WBC, white blood cell; Ig, immunoglobulin; IFN, interferon; PA, purine analogs; TRAP, tartrate-resistant acid phosphatase.

cytopenias. Severe thrombocytopenia or neutropenia affects 30–40 percent of patients.[12] Monocytopenia is a consistent feature of HCL but its cause remains unclear.[8–10] At presentation, splenomegaly is observed in approximately 80 percent of patients with the spleen being palpable 5 cm below the left ribcage in about 60 percent of cases. In one large study, the weight of the spleen at splenectomy ranged from 250 g to 4600 g (median 1300 g).[13] Splenic rupture is very rare. The liver is enlarged in approximately 30 percent of patients. Clinical lymphadenopathy is usually absent at diagnosis, but internal lymphadenopathy may occasionally develop after a prolonged course of disease.[14] Osteolytic lesions of the axial skeleton, most frequently of the upper femurs, are observed in less than 5 percent of HCL patients.[15] The main clinical and laboratory findings of HCL are summarized in Table 28.1.

SITES OF INVOLVEMENT AND MORPHOLOGIC FEATURES

Leukemic hairy cells circulate in peripheral blood and infiltrate the bone marrow, spleen and liver, sparing the lymph nodes. This characteristic HCL distribution pattern probably depends on tumour cell expression of several adhesion molecules and chemokine receptors.

Peripheral blood

Circulating leukemic hairy cells vary in number at diagnosis. Most patients present with pancytopenia but 10–20 percent have a 'leukemia-like' presentation, i.e. white blood cell count >10 × 10^9/L, with >50 percent hairy cells.[8–10]

Circulating hairy cells are small-to-medium sized lymphoid cells, 1.5 times to twice as large as a small lymphocyte (Plate 30A, see plate section). Bigger than B chronic lymphocytic leukemia (CLL) cells, hairy cells may have round, oval, kidney or dumb-bell shaped nuclei. The chromatin is homogeneous, spongy, ground-glass-like in appearance with less clumping than normal lymphocytes. Nucleoli are absent or indistinct. The abundant cytoplasm is pale blue-grey in color with irregular fine cytoplasmic projections at its periphery (Plate 30A,B). In about 40 percent of HCL cases, the cytoplasm contains vacuoles or rod-shaped inclusions which are the counterparts of the ribosomal–lamella complexes seen on electron microscopy.[3] A correct diagnosis of HCL can be made on the basis of the characteristic 'hairy' morphology, which may be hard to detect in patients with marked pancytopenia. In these cases, the tartrate-resistant acid phosphatase (TRAP) assay[16] and/or immunophenotyping (see below) are particularly helpful.

Bone marrow

In all patients with HCL, the bone marrow is infiltrated and is usually hard to aspirate ('punctio sicca') due to reticulin fibrosis and interdigitation of hairy cell projections.[3,17] Therefore, examination of bone marrow biopsy sections plays a critical role in diagnosis.

In HCL, normal hemopoietic cells are always fewer in number. Granulopoiesis and monocytopoiesis are usually markedly reduced, whereas erythroid precursors and megakaryocytes are relatively spared. Bone marrow infiltration varies from patchy (with no preference for paratrabecular location) to complete. The nodular pattern observed in other chronic lymphoproliferative disorders is not a feature of HCL.[3,17] Histologically, HCL is easily diagnosed, with its typical round, oval or bean-shaped nuclei that are widely separated from each other by the abundant pale, water-clear cytoplasm surrounding them ('fried-egg' appearance)[3,17] (Plate 30C). Mitotic figures are rare. Mast cells are often numerous. Extravasated red blood cells are frequently seen between the hairy cells; blood lakes resembling those observed in the spleen may also be present. Reticulin fibrosis, as visualized in silver-stained sections, is always increased, often very markedly (Plate 30D). Hairy cell involvement is quantified by the hairy cell index which is derived from bone marrow cellularity and the percentage of hairy cells (percent cellularity $\times$ percent hairy cells/10^4).[13]

Spleen and other tissues

The cut surface of the spleen is characteristically beefy red, because the HCL cells consistently involve the red pulp. Unlike other B cell lymphoproliferative disorders, the splenic white pulp is not expanded and is actually atrophic. Hairy cells diffusely infiltrate the red pulp cords and adhere to the endothelial lining of the sinuses, damaging the sinus wall[18] and forming typical blood-filled pseudo-sinuses ('angiomatous lakes') lined by hairy cells.[19] These pseudosinuses contribute to the splenic red cell pooling that is typical of HCL.

Hairy cells frequently infiltrate the liver sinusoids, lying free within the lumen or in close association with the endothelium and adjacent hepatocytes (Plate 31, see plate section).[20] Involvement of sinusoids is variable and does not correlate with the number of circulating HCL cells.[20] Sinusoids can be congested and dilated, sometimes mimicking peliosis hepatic.[20] Periportal spaces are also infiltrated. Portal infiltration may be associated with reticulin fibrosis but the general architecture of the liver remains intact and, therefore, cirrhosis is rare.[20] Angiomatous lesions may be present.[19] Lymph node infiltration is rare and, when present, is restricted to the paracortex and medulla, sparing the B cell follicles.[5]

DIAGNOSTIC TOOLS

Tartrate–resistant acid phosphatase activity

Acid phosphatase activity resistant to inhibition by L(+)tartaric acid phosphate (TRAP activity) has been traditionally used to confirm the diagnosis of HCL.[16] TRAP activity in leukemic hairy cells is due to isoenzyme 5, which is one of the seven acid phosphatase isoenzymes found in human leukocytes.[16] This cytochemical reaction is usually performed on blood smears, buffy coat preparations or cytospins. The percentage of TRAP-positive leukemic cells varies markedly from one HCL patient to another and TRAP activity may even occasionally be negative in HCL. Furthermore, a number of neoplasms derived from B and

even T cells may occasionally show TRAP activity. Another limitation of the TRAP reaction is that it cannot be carried out in fixed/decalcified bone marrow trephines, because of denaturation of enzymatic activity.[21] For all these reasons, when diagnosing HCL many hematology centers now prefer immunophenotyping to TRAP cytochemistry. For immunophenotyping, the panel of antibodies now includes also a reagent that detects the TRAP enzyme by immuno-histochemistry, even in routine paraffin sections.[22]

Immunophenotyping

Many different procedures are suitable for analysis of HCL immunophenotype. Flow cytometry is good diagnostic technique because, with their distinctive light scatter pattern and immunophenotype, hairy cells are easily identified even when constituting <1 percent of the peripheral blood or bone marrow cell population.[23] Alternatively, HCL can be detected by immunocytochemical staining of smears, buffy coats or cytocentrifuge preparations.[24] Some HCL markers such as CD20, CD79a, DBA44, CD68 and cyclin D1, can be identified in paraffin sections from routine bone marrow biopsies.[25–27] Although not specific for HCL, these markers are useful in confirming the clinical and morphologic diagnosis and assessing the extent of bone marrow infiltration at diagnosis.

At flow cytometry, strong CD45 expression on hairy cells is shown as a bright signal, with increased forward and side scatter, resembling that of large lymphocytes or monocytes. Hairy cells exhibit moderate to bright positivity for surface Ig and about 40 percent of HCL cases carry multiple Ig isotypes.[28] HCL cells show strong surface positivity for the mature B cell markers CD19, CD20, CD22 and CD79a (Plate 30B; Plate 31B). In addition to the conventional B cell antigens, the leukemic hairy cells express macrophage molecules such as CD68 and several activation antigens, including CD25, CD11c, FCM7[29] and CD103, an α subunit of the α/β integrin molecule found on mucosal T cells and HCL cells.[30,31] The as yet unknown antigen that is recognized by the monoclonal antibody DBA44[26] is variably expressed in HCL (Plate 30E). Cyclin-D1 is overexpressed in most HCL cases,[27] but the underlying mechanism is unknown since HCL cells lack the BCL1 rearrangements that are typical of mantle cell lymphoma and multiple myeloma.[32,33] Leukemic hairy cells are negative for CD5, CD23, the germinal center-associated marker BCL6[5] and the plasma cell-associated molecules MUM1/IRF4 and CD138 (Plate 30F). CD10 is usually absent in HCL (Plate 31C), but it is observed in about 10 percent of cases.[34,35] CD10+ HCL cases appear to be morphologically and clinically similar to the CD10-negative cases.[34]

DIFFERENTIAL DIAGNOSIS

Immunocytochemistry plays a crucial role in the diagnosis of HCL when leukopenia is marked and hairy cells are hard to find in the peripheral blood smear. Morphologic and immunocytochemical examination of a buffy coat or cytospins prepared from Ficoll-separated mononuclear blood cells may hold the clue to diagnosis.[24] Suitable markers are CD20, DBA-44, CD11c and CD103, and the results always need to be correlated with morphologic findings ('hairy appearance'). In some preparations, immunocytochemistry serves to highlight the 'hairy' features of leukemic cells, thus facilitating diagnosis. Flow cytometry panels should include reagent combinations such as CD19/CD11c and CD19/CD103 so that B cells may be evaluated for coexpression of these HCL-associated antigens.[36]

A minority of HCL patients present with a severely hypoplastic bone marrow and little hairy cell infiltration and when splenomegaly is absent (about 10 percent of cases)[8] these findings risk being misdiagnosed as aplastic anemia. In such difficult cases, immunohistochemistry serves to identify leukemic hairy cells.[5,26] In other patients, HCL with spindle appearance may occasionally resemble systemic mastocytosis, but clinical findings and phenotype, e.g. positivity for CD20 (absent in mastocytes) and negativity for tryptase (positive in mastocytes) confirm the diagnosis of HCL.

Differentiating between hairy cell leukemia and HCL–like disorders

More arduous is distinguishing HCL from HCL variant (HCLv) and splenic lymphoma with villous lymphocytes (SLVL), as all are associated with marked splenomegaly and circulating neoplastic cells with 'hairy' appearance. This is a crucial diagnostic step, since HCLv and SLVL show no or partial response to interferon (IFN) α and purine analogs,[8] and HCV-related splenic marginal zone lymphoma/SLVL may even require antiviral therapy.[37] The main clinical and laboratory features of SLVL and HCLv are summarized in Table 28.1.

SPLENIC LYMPHOMA WITH VILLOUS LYMPHOCYTES

Splenomegaly and varying combinations of lymphocytosis and cytopenias characterize the presentation of SLVL.[38] Lymphadenopathy is usually absent. Most patients show a modest increase in the white cell count. Circulating leukemic cells display 'hairy features' and are usually smaller than typical HCL cells. They have round nuclei with coarse chromatin and occasional nucleoli; the cytoplasm is generally scanty and basophilic. Not infrequently, the leukemic cells are elongated with a spindle-shape appearance. Villous surfaces are frequently polarized and plasmacytoid features are also present.[38] In the bone marrow biopsy, the infiltration pattern is frequently intrasinusoidal.[39] Cells are negative for CD5 and CD23; CD103 and CD25 are variably expressed. Cells are frequently TRAP negative. Annexin A1, a specific marker of HCL, is consistently negative in SLVL (Plate 32A–D, see plate section). Microscopic examination of the spleen reveals a picture of splenic marginal zone lymphoma.[40]

HAIRY CELL LEUKEMIA VARIANT

Hairy cell leukemia variant is a very rare pathologic condition in which the bone marrow and spleen histology resembles HCL.[41] Patients usually present with marked splenomegaly and a high peripheral WBC count. Unlike HCL, monocytopenia is absent. Leukemic cells in HCLv show an intermediate morphology, falling between typical hairy cells and prolymphocytes; the nucleus is round or oval with a prominent nucleolus and the villous cytoplasm is moderately basophilic.[41] The HCL variant responds poorly to IFNα and purine analogues.[41] In HCLv tumour cells usually lack CD25 and sometimes also CD103. They are often TRAP-negative. Annexin A1, a highly specific marker for typical HCL (Plate 32A,B), is negative in HCLv[42] suggesting that HCLv is a different type of B cell lymphoma rather than just a morphologic variant of HCL. Accordingly, in the new WHO-2008 classification of lymphoid neoplasms, HCLv is now included in the category of splenic B-cell lymphoma/leukemia, unclassifiable.[43]

Differentiating between HCL and HCL-like disorders relies mainly on immunohistochemistry. At immunostaining for CD20, SLVL shows a rather characteristic intrasinusoidal pattern of infiltration (Plate 32E,F)[39] which, unfortunately, is not specific, since HCL and HCLv also sometimes show this staining pattern.[44] Although several molecules, including CD11c, FCM7, CD103, HC2, CD25, CD123 (interleukin [IL]-3Rα) and DBA44, have been reported to differentiate between HCL and HCL-like neoplasms, none appears to be entirely specific for HCL.[5,45] In order to improve diagnostic accuracy, an HCL scoring system based on multiple phenotypic markers has been proposed. Despite this, diagnosis remains controversial in a certain percentage of cases.[46]

Identifying annexin A1 as specifically one of the most upregulated genes in HCL[47] (as compared with other B cell lymphomas) led to the development of a simple, inexpensive and specific diagnostic assay using an anti-annexin A1 monoclonal antibody.[42] Notably, immunohistochemistry on a large cohort of lymphoma patients has confirmed annexin A1 expression in HCL (Plate 32A,B) and lack of it in all other B cell neoplasms (100 percent specificity), including HCLv and SLVL (Plate 32C,D middle right panel).[42] As annexin A1 is physiologically expressed in some normal cell populations such as myeloid precursors, a subset of T cells and monocytes,[42] labeling for annexin A1 must always be run in parallel with a B cell antigen (e.g. CD20) (Plate 32F) so as to ensure immunostaining results are interpreted correctly. Why annexin A1 is so strongly expressed in leukemic hairy cells is unclear. It may be implicated in some HCL features such as homing and phagocytosis (see below), which suggests expression is due to neoplastic transformation rather than derivation from a subset of normal B cells expressing annexin A1 (apparently not detectable in normal tissues).

The coexistence of HCL and a diffuse large B cell lymphoma is extremely rare and the relationship between the two diseases has not been conclusively established. One report found no clonal relationship[48] while in another study, the diffuse large B cell lymphoma was claimed to be of HCL origin, because of the results of immunophenotyping and the TRAP reaction.[49]

Monitoring of minimal residual disease

Monitoring of HCL minimal residual disease after therapy with interferon or purine analogs is done by immunohistochemistry on tissue sections or by flow cytometry.[50] At immunohistochemistry, CD20 is a more suitable marker than DBA44, since the latter is variably expressed in HCL. As these markers are also expressed in normal B cells, identification of residual leukemic cells mostly relies on the presence of the typical 'hairy' morphology, a feature which is not always easily detectable in tissue sections. The anti-annexin A1 antibody is not suitable for detecting minimal infiltrates of HCL cells, since the reactivity of normal, adjacent cells, especially myeloid precursors, makes it difficult to interpret the immunohistologic results. Using immunohistochemical techniques, the incidence of minimal residual disease in HCL patients treated with 2-chloro-deoxyadenosine ranges from about 10 percent to 50 percent.[51,52] Persistence of minimal residual disease has been also confirmed by molecular studies (polymerase chain reaction [PCR] with clonospecific probes).[53] Because of the very low proliferative index of leukemic hairy cells, the clinical significance of detecting minimal residual disease remains uncertain.

BIOLOGIC FEATURES OF HAIRY CELL LEUKEMIA CELLS

Despite remarkable progress in the diagnosis and therapy of HCL, several of its unique biologic features remain obscure. We do not yet fully understand from which mature B cell subset is HCL derived. HCL differs from most mature B cell tumors because it usually lacks chromosomal translocations and lymphadenopathy. Additional peculiarities that are rarely seen in other B cell neoplasms, include hairy morphology, selective homing of leukemic cells to bone marrow, liver and spleen, bone marrow fibrosis, monocyte–macrophage features, and exquisite sensitivity to IFNα and purine analogs.[6,54]

Unlike other B cell malignancies, where gene expression profiling usually reveals unrecognized subsets of the disease,[55] the molecular signature of HCL appears to be uniform,[47] suggesting it is a single disease entity, which is consistent with its homogeneous morphology and clinical behavior. Gene expression profiling analysis of primary HCL cells and other studies have also shed light on the peculiar biologic features of HCL.

Cellular origin and pathogenesis of HCL

Hairy cell leukemia represents a clonal expansion of mature B cells[56] with activation features.[57] Morphologically or phenotypically HCL cells differ from all known peripheral B cell subpopulations, and their cell of origin has long been a matter of debate.[58–62]

HCL cells express switched Ig isotypes,[28] carry somatic Ig variable (V) gene mutations in >85 percent of cases,[63–67] and exhibit some intraclonal *IGV* gene diversification.[28,63,67] It has accordingly been suggested that HCL is histogenetically related to germinal center,[67] possibly deriving from a B cell population that has been arrested at a point of isotype switching before deletional recombination, i.e. before exiting the germinal center.[28,63]

A more appealing hypothesis is that HCL derives from a post-germinal center B cell. Gene expression profiling studies have recently shown HCL cells are more closely related to memory B cell than to other B cell populations such as naïve, germinal center, lymphoblastoid and plasma cells[47] (Plate 33, see plate section). However, it is not yet clear which lymphoid compartment the putative normal B cell counterpart of HCL belongs to. In fact, normal memory B cells are heterogeneous and are found in diverse peripheral lymphoid tissues.[68–70] As lymphadenopathy is clinically irrelevant in HCL, other organs, i.e. bone marrow and spleen, appear to be the most probable candidates as location sites for the normal HCL B cell counterpart. Difficulties in identifying the normal counterpart of HCL may also reflect the neoplastic transformation process. In fact, different expression patterns of several cytokines, chemokine receptors and adhesion molecules[47] in HCL as compared to normal memory B cells might account for the divergence in homing, morphology, and phenotype between HCL and its normal counterpart.

Adhesion and homing properties of hairy cell leukemia cells

A variety of adhesion molecules and homing receptors expressed on the surface of HCL cells probably play important roles in regulating the traffic of leukemic cells in circulation and determining their preferential homing to some lympho-hemopoietic compartments. An hypothetical scheme of how these molecules interact with each to another to dictate tumor dissemination in HCL is shown in Plate 34, see plate section. In particular, homing of leukemic hairy cells to sinusoid-rich tissues[71] may be linked to an interaction between the intrinsically activated $\alpha_4\beta_1$ integrin (VLA-4) in HCL cells[72] and its cellular ligand vascular cell adhesion molecule (VCAM)-1 in bone marrow, splenic and hepatic sinusoids (Plate 34). Similarly, HCL expression of $\alpha_v\beta_3$, the vitronectin receptor, has been associated with homing to, and motility in, the vitronectin-rich splenic red pulp.[73] HCL cells may eventually replace sinusoid lining cells, thus accounting for the splenic pseudosinuses and hepatic angiomatous lesions described in HCL.[19] The receptor for macrophage colony-stimulating factor (c-*fms*) is highly expressed in HCL cells[74] and could be involved in the movement of leukemic cells towards splenic red pulp through interaction with the macrophage-colony stimulating factor secreted by resident macrophages.[74]

Other genes that are specifically upregulated in HCL may contribute to the HCL propensity to remain confined to blood-related compartments. They include *TIMP1*, *TIMP4*, and *RECK*[47] (Plate 34), all of which counteract the activity of metalloproteinases (MMPs) that promote local invasion, metastases and angiogenesis.[75,76] Annexin A1, which is strongly upregulated in HCL,[47] may also hamper leukemic hairy cell extravasation by blocking the trans-endothelial migration of leukocytes[77] (Plate 34).

Lack of clinically noteworthy lymph node involvement in HCL patients may be explained by leukemic cell down-regulation of some chemokine receptors,[47] such as CXCR5[78] or CCR7[47] that are required for homing to B cell follicles and lymph nodes[79,80] (Plate 34).

Adhesion properties of leukemic hairy cells may also affect their response to certain drugs, such as IFN-α. Thus, in the absence of cell adhesion, IFN-α induces apoptosis by sensitizing HCL cells to killing by autocrine tumor necrosis factor (TNF).[81] This sensitization occurs at least in part through IFN-α-induced downregulation of inhibitors of apoptosis.[81]

Bone marrow fibrosis

Formation of bone marrow fibrosis, a characteristic feature of HCL,[3] appears closely linked to the adhesion properties of leukemic hairy cells and their ability to interact with the bone marrow microenvironment. Fibrosis is caused by the assembly of a fibronectin matrix[82] and by deposition of fine argyrophilic reticulin fibers,[3] e.g. individual or small bundles of mainly type III collagen fibrils, that are detectable by silver-nitrate-based stains (Plate 30D).[3] Fibronectin is synthesized by the leukemic hairy cells and the HCL cell's autocrine secretion of basic fibroblast growth factor (bFGF) plays a major role in promoting this process.[83] Production of bFGF is in turn triggered when the CD44H and CD44v3 isoforms of CD44[83,84] (which are both expressed in HCL cells) bind with hyaluronan.[84] Moreover, CD44v3 also acts as a coreceptor of bFGF and is essential for optimal bFGF stimulation of leukemic cells.[83] This explains why fibrosis in HCL is observed only in hyaluron-rich anatomic compartments, such as bone marrow stroma and hepatic portal tracts, but not in the spleen or in the hepatic sinusoids where the extracellular matrix does not contain hyaluran.[29]

In HCL, reticulin fiber formation is due, not to increased fibroblast proliferation, but rather to adjacent marrow fibroblasts synthesizing and depositing extracellular matrix proteins (mainly type III collagen).[85] Indeed, leukemic hairy cells produce and secrete large amounts of activated transforming growth factor beta 1 (TGFβ1)[86,87] which induces type-III collagen synthesis and deposition. Accordingly, the fine meshwork of reticulin fibrosis which is typical of HCL clearly differs from the thick type I collagen fibrosis observed in idiopathic myelofibrosis,[88] in which fibroblast proliferation is the prominent event.

Hairy morphology

Although recognized as the hallmark of HCL, the hairy appearance of leukemic cells still remains without a definitive explanation. It may result from the oncogenic event(s) underlying HCL or reflect the leukemic cell's derivation from a hypothetical subset of 'hairy' memory B cells.

Interaction of the cytoskeleton-binding protein pp52 (LSP1)[89] with F-actin-rich cytoskeleton arrays in the surface projections of HCL cells has been proposed as underlying the 'hairy' appearance.[90] Notably, IFNα reduces pp52 levels and blunts the hairy projections of HCL cells, which return to a more rounded shape.[90,91] Constitutively activated Rho GTPases are also thought to play a key role in the *in vitro* persistence of hairy features of the leukemic cells.[92,93]

Gene expression profiling analysis highlights a number of HCL-specific genes that could well be implicated in the biological features of HCL, including the 'hairy' phenotype (Table 28.2). *GAS7* and *EPB41L2* are good candidates.[47] Originally associated with neuronal cells where it is required for neurite outgrowth,[94,95] Gas-7 assembles actin filaments and cross-links them into bundles. When overexpressed in NIH3T3 cells, it induces formation of cell protrusions where it colocalizes with F-actin.[96] EPB41L2 (protein 4.1G) is a nonerythroid member of the 4.1-family of cytoskeletal proteins[97] that could also play a role in the development of the 'hairy' phenotype. Interestingly, protein 4.1G interacts with F-actin and might be involved in maintaining the shape and structural integrity of neuronal cell membranes.[98]

Monocyte–macrophagic properties of hairy cell leukemia cells

Peculiar to HCL cells is their capability to phagocytose latex particles, zymosan and bacteria,[99] which is closely related to their membrane's active state and cytoskeletal reorganization. A number of findings point to annexin A1 and actin as mediators of this activity. In macrophages, annexin A1 stimulates actin cytoskeleton reorganization and enhances phagocytic uptake of zymosan particles and apoptotic cells. Macrophages from annexin A1-null mice show a markedly attenuated phagocytic ability.[100,101] Moreover, human monocytes phagocytose *Brucella suis* by recruiting F-actin microfilaments and annexin A1-associated phagosomal structures locally at the cell surface.[102]

Common to HCL and the mononuclear phagocytic system are not only functional features but also various markers of phagocytosis that include TRAP activity,[16] M-CSF-R,[103] CD11c,[104] and the macrophage-restricted CD68 isoform.[25] Gene expression profiling analysis has expanded the list of HCL-associated monocyte/macrophage-associated molecules even further.[47] Newly discovered overexpressed genes include those encoding:

- the carboxypeptidase vitellogenic-like (CPVL), a putative lysosomal serine-carboxypeptidase[105]

Table 28.2   Genes putatively involved in biologic features of hairy cell leukemia (HCL)

Gene name	Gene symbol	Putative features
Burkitt lymphoma receptor 1	BLR1/CXCR5	Dissemination pattern
Growth arrest-specific 7	GAS7	Hairy morphology
Tissue inhibitor of metalloprotein	TIMP1	Dissemination pattern
Protein tyrosine phosphatase, receptor type M	PTPRM	Adhesion properties
Annexin-A1	ANXA1	Adhesion, dissemination pattern, phagocytosis
Carboxypeptidase, vitellogenic-like	CPVL	'Monocyte-macrophage' features
FMS-like tyrosine kinase 2	FGFR1/FLT2	Marrow fibrosis
Fms-related tyrosyne kinase 3	FLT3	HCL growth, marrow fibrosis
Syndecan 3 (N-syndecan)	SDC3	Adhesion properties
Interleukin 3 receptor alpha subunit	IL3Rα	HCL growth
CD63 antigen	CD63	'Monocyte-macrophage' features
Cyclin D1	CCND1	HCL growth
Erythrocyte membrane protein band 4 1-like2	EPB41L2	Hairy morphology
Tumor necrosis factor receptor superfamily member 1A	TNFRSF1A	Response to interferon
Fibroblast growth factor 2 (basic)	FGF2	HCL growth
Beta actin	Beta actin	Adhesion properties, hairy morphology
Tissue inhibitor of metalloproteinase 4	TIMP4	Dissemination pattern
Thrombospodin-1	Thrombospodin-1	Dissemination pattern

A complete list of the genes which are specifically downregulated or overexpressed in HCL cells as compared to normal B cells and other B cell neoplasms is available at: www.jem.org/cgi/content/full/jem.20031175/DC1

- CD63 (LAMP3), a tetraspanin component of endosomal/lysosomal membranes[106,107]
- CD85d (MIR10), an inhibitory immunoreceptor whose binding to its HLA-G ligand dramatically increases myelo-monocytic cell production of TGFβ1[108]
- c-Maf, a transcription factor[47] whose deregulated expression can induce macrophage differentiation.[109,110]

OPEN QUESTIONS AND FUTURE DIRECTIONS

In spite of the remarkable progress in the diagnosis and therapy of HCL, several aspects of this disease still remain to be elucidated. The HCL variant is a still poorly defined entity.[43,111] The biologic overlap between HCL and SLVL has not yet been fully explored[112–114] and, to achieve this goal, gene expression profiling studies should be designed to compare these entities.

Better understanding of the HCL cell of origin could be achieved through immunohistochemical studies using antibodies raised against molecules that are specifically upregulated in HCL.[47]

Even today, nothing is known about the genetic lesion(s) underlying HCL which are likely to be, at least partly, responsible for the highly activated phenotype of the leukemic cells. Cytogenetic studies in HCL are sparse[115] mainly because often there are not sufficient cells for analysis (due to severe pancytopenia or 'dry tap'). The difficulty in inducing hairy cells to proliferate and in obtaining hairy cells metaphases adds to the problem. The use of the anti-CD40 monoclonal antibody to stimulate HCL proliferation has been proposed.[116] Although some patients show clonal chromosomal abnormalities which are both structural (gains and losses) and numerical[117,118] in nature, none is specific for HCL. The hypothesis that HCL derives from the malignant transformation of a memory B cell suggests that, like B-CLL,[119] its molecular pathogenesis may be related to amplifications and deletions rather than to reciprocal chromosomal translocations. Future efforts should exploit progress in molecular biology to identify key players in the pathogenesis of HCL, recognition of which should, in turn, lead to establishing new specific therapeutic targets.

ACKNOWLEDGMENTS

E. Tiacci is supported by Grant 2008/14 from the European Hematology Association.

KEY POINTS

- Hairy cell leukemia (HCL) is are rare indolent B cell neoplasm.
- Clinically, HCL presents with pancytopenia (including monocytopenia), circulating leukemic hairy cells (usually in low numbers), and hepatosplenomegaly. Lymphadenopathy is usually absent.

- Pathologically, HCL cells show a distinctive dissemination pattern (bone marrow, peripheral blood, spleen and liver).
- Owing to 'dry tap', diagnosis is frequently made in bone marrow biopsy (a typical 'fried-egg' histological pattern).
- The leukemic hairy cells express B cell markers and other typical molecules, such as CD103 and annexin A1.
- Among B cell lymphomas, annexin A1 is specific for HCL and serves as a marker to distinguish it from SLVL and HCL variant (HCLv).
- In the WHO-2008, HCLv is now included in the category of splenic B cell lymphoma/leukemia unclassifiable.
- HCL shows a distinctive gene expression profile that explains many of the biological properties of leukemic hairy cells, including hairy morphology, adhesion properties, monocyte–macrophage features, dissemination pattern and bone marrow fibrosis.
- Genetic alteration(s) underlying HCL remain unknown.

REFERENCES

- = Key primary paper
- ◆ = Major review article

1. Ewald O. Die Leukämische reticuloendotheliose. *Dtsch Arch Klin Med* 1923; **142**: 222.
- 2. Bouroncle BA. Leukemic reticuloendotheliosis (hairy cell leukemia). *Blood* 1979; **53**: 412–36.
3. Brunning RB. *Tumors of the bone marrow* (AFIP Atlas of Tumor Pathology, Series 3, Vol. 9). Michigan: Armed Forces Institute of Pathology, 1994.
- ◆4. Harris NL, Jaffe ES, Stein H *et al.* A revised European-American classification of lymphoid neoplasms: a proposal from the International Lymphoma study group. *Blood* 1994; **84**: 1361–92.
- ◆5. Foucar K, Falini B, Catovsky D, Stein H. Hairy cell leukemia. In: Swerdlow SH, Campo E, Harris NL *et al.* (eds) *WHO classification of tumours of haematopoietic and lymphoid tissues.* Lyon: IARC Press, 2008: 188–90.
6. Mey U, Strehl J, Gorschluter M *et al.* Advances in the treatment of hairy-cell leukaemia. *Lancet Oncol* 2003; **4**: 86–94.
7. Carson DA, Leoni LM. Hairy-cell leukaemia as a model for drug development. *Best Pract Res Clin Haematol* 2003; **16**: 83–9.
- ◆8. Zakarija A, Peterson LC, Tallman M. Hairy cell leukemia. In: Hoffman R. (ed.) *Hematology: basic principles and practice.* Edinburgh: Elsevier, Churchill Livingstone, 2009: 1349–58.
9. Else M, Ruchlemer R, Osuji N *et al.* Long remissions in hairy cell leukemia with purine analogs: a report of 219 patients with a median follow-up of 12.5 years. *Cancer* 2005; **104**: 2442–8.
10. Chadha P, Rademaker AW, Mendiratta P *et al.* Treatment of hairy cell leukemia with 2-chlorodeoxyadenosine (2-CdA): long-term follow-up of the Northwestern University experience. *Blood* 2005; **106**: 241–6.
11. Morton LM, Wang SS, Devesa SS *et al.* Lymphoma incidence patterns by WHO subtype in the United States, 1992–2001. *Blood* 2006; **107**: 265–76.
12. Frassoldati A, Lamparelli T, Federico M *et al.* Hairy cell leukemia: a clinical review based on 725 cases of the Italian Cooperative Group (ICGHCL). Italian cooperative group for hairy cell leukemia. *Leuk Lymphoma* 1994; **13**: 307–16.
13. Golomb HM, Vardiman JW. Response to splenectomy in 65 patients with hairy cell leukemia: an evaluation of spleen weight and bone marrow involvement. *Blood* 1983; **61**: 349–52.
14. Hakimian D, Tallman MS, Hogan DK *et al.* Prospective evaluation of internal adenopathy in a cohort of 43 patients with hairy cell leukemia. *J Clin Oncol* 1994; **12**: 268–72.
15. Lembersky BC, Ratain MJ, Golomb HM. Skeletal complications in hairy cell leukemia: diagnosis and therapy. *J Clin Oncol* 1988; **6**: 1280–4.
- ◆16. Yam LT, Janckila AJ, Li CY, Lam WK. Cytochemistry of tartrate-resistant acid phosphatase: 15 years' experience. *Leukemia* 1987; **1**: 285–8.
- 17. Burke JS. The value of the bone-marrow biopsy in the diagnosis of hairy cell leukemia. *Am J Clin Pathol* 1978; **70**: 876–84.
18. Pilon VA, Davey FR, Gordon GB. Splenic alterations in hairy cell leukemia. *Arch Pathol Lab Med* 1981; **105**: 577–81.
19. Nanba K, Soban EJ, Bowling MC, Berard CW. Splenic pseudosinuses and hepatic angiomatous lesions. Distinctive features of hairy cell leukemia. *Am J Clin Pathol* 1977; **67**: 415–26.
20. Yam LT, Janckila AJ, Chan CH, Li CY. Hepatic involvement in hairy cell leukemia. *Cancer* 1983; **51**: 1497–504.
21. Beckstead JH, Halverson PS, Ries CA, Bainton DF. Enzyme histochemistry and immunohistochemistry on biopsy specimens of pathologic human bone marrow. *Blood* 1981; **57**: 1088–98.
22. Janckila AJ, Cardwell EM, Yam LT, Li CY. Hairy cell identification by immunohistochemistry of tartrate-resistant acid phosphatase. *Blood* 1995; **85**: 2839–44.
23. Cornfield DB, Mitchell Nelson DM, Rimsza LM *et al.* The diagnosis of hairy cell leukemia can be established by flow cytometric analysis of peripheral blood, even in patients with low levels of circulating malignant cells. *Am J Hematol* 2001; **67**: 223–6.
24. Falini B, Pulford K, Erber WN *et al.* Use of a panel of monoclonal antibodies for the diagnosis of hairy cell leukaemia. An immunocytochemical study of 36 cases. *Histopathology* 1986; **10**: 671–87.
25. Falini B, Flenghi L, Pileri S *et al.* PG-M1: a new monoclonal antibody directed against a fixative-resistant epitope on the macrophage-restricted form of the CD68 molecule. *Am J Pathol* 1993; **142**: 1359–72.

26. Hounieu H, Chittal SM, al Saati T *et al.* Hairy cell leukemia. Diagnosis of bone marrow involvement in paraffin-embedded sections with monoclonal antibody DBA.44. *Am J Clin Pathol* 1992; **98**: 26–33.

27. Miranda RN, Briggs RC, Kinney MC *et al.* Immunohistochemical detection of cyclin D1 using optimized conditions is highly specific for mantle cell lymphoma and hairy cell leukemia. *Mod Pathol* 2000; **13**: 1308–14.

●28. Forconi F, Sahota SS, Raspadori D *et al.* Tumor cells of hairy cell leukemia express multiple clonally related immunoglobulin isotypes via RNA splicing. *Blood* 2001; **98**: 1174–81.

29. Allsup DJ, Cawley JC. Diagnosis, biology and treatment of hairy-cell leukaemia. *Clin Exp Med* 2004; **4**: 132–8.

30. Flenghi L, Spinozzi F, Stein H *et al.* LF61: a new monoclonal antibody directed against a trimeric molecule (150 kDa, 125 kDa, 105 kDa) associated with hairy cell leukaemia. *Br J Haematol* 1990; **76**: 451–9.

31. Schwarting R, Dienemann D, Kruschwitz M *et al.* Specificities of monoclonal antibodies B-ly7 and HML-1 are identical. *Blood* 1990; **75**: 320–1.

32. Fernandez V, Hartmann E, Ott G *et al.* Pathogenesis of mantle-cell lymphoma: all oncogenic roads lead to dysregulation of cell cycle and DNA damage response pathways. *J Clin Oncol* 2005; **23**: 6364–9.

33. Bergsagel PL, Kuehl WM. Molecular pathogenesis and a consequent classification of multiple myeloma. *J Clin Oncol* 2005; **23**: 6333–8.

34. Jasionowski TM, Hartung L, Greenwood JH *et al.* Analysis of CD10+ hairy cell leukemia. *Am J Clin Pathol* 2003; **120**: 228–35.

35. Chen YH, Tallman MS, Goolsby C, Peterson L. Immunophenotypic variations in hairy cell leukemia. *Am J Clin Pathol* 2006; **125**: 1–9.

36. Robbins BA, Ellison DJ, Spinosa JC *et al.* Diagnostic application of two-color flow cytometry in 161 cases of hairy cell leukemia. *Blood* 1993; **82**: 1277–87.

37. Hermine O, Lefrere F, Bronowicki JP *et al.* Regression of splenic lymphoma with villous lymphocytes after treatment of hepatitis C virus infection. *N Engl J Med* 2002; **347**: 89–94.

◆38. Catovsky D, Matutes E. Splenic lymphoma with circulating villous lymphocytes/splenic marginal-zone lymphoma. *Semin Hematol* 1999; **36**: 148–54.

39. Labouyrie E, Marit G, Vial JP, *et al.* Intrasinusoidal bone marrow involvement by splenic lymphoma with villous lymphocytes: a helpful immunohistologic feature. *Mod Pathol* 1997; **10**: 1015–20.

40. Isaacson PG, Piris MA, Berger F *et al.* Splenic B-cell marginal zone lymphoma. In: Swerdlow SH, Campo E, Harris NL *et al.* (eds) *WHO classification of tumours of haematopoietic and lymphoid tissues.* Lyon: IARC Press, 2008: 185–7.

◆41. Matutes E, Wotherspoon A, Catovsky D. The variant form of hairy-cell leukaemia. *Best Pract Res Clin Haematol* 2003; **16**: 41–56.

●42. Falini B, Tiacci E, Liso A *et al.* Simple diagnostic assay for hairy cell leukaemia by immunocytochemical detection of annexin A1 (ANXA1). *Lancet* 2004; **363**: 1869–70.

43. Piris M, Foucar K, Nollejo M *et al.* Splenic B-cell lymphoma/leukemia, unclassifiable. In: Swerdlow SH, Campo E, Harris NL *et al.* (eds) *Who classification of tumours of haematopoietic and lymphoid tissues.* Lyon: IARC Press, 2008: 191–3.

44. Ya-In C, Brandwein J, Pantalony D, Chang H. Hairy cell leukemia variant with features of intrasinusoidal bone marrow involvement. *Arch Pathol Lab Med* 2005; **129**: 395–8.

45. Del Giudice I, Matutes E, Morilla R *et al.* The diagnostic value of CD123 in B-cell disorders with hairy or villous lymphocytes. *Haematologica* 2004; **89**: 303–8.

46. Matutes E, Morilla R, Owusu-Ankomah K *et al.* The immunophenotype of hairy cell leukemia (HCL). Proposal for a scoring system to distinguish HCL from B-cell disorders with hairy or villous lymphocytes. *Leuk Lymphoma* 1994; **14(Suppl 1)**: 57–61.

●47. Basso K, Liso A, Tiacci E *et al.* Gene expression profiling of hairy cell leukemia reveals a phenotype related to memory B cells with altered expression of chemokine and adhesion receptors. *J Exp Med* 2004; **199**: 59–68.

48. Downing JR, Grossi CE, Smedberg CT, Burrows PD. Diffuse large cell lymphoma in a patient with hairy cell leukemia: immunoglobulin gene analysis reveals separate clonal origins. *Blood* 1986; **67**: 739–44.

49. Sun T, Grupka N, Klein C. Transformation of hairy cell leukemia to high-grade lymphoma: a case report and review of the literature. *Hum Pathol* 2004; **35**: 1423–6.

50. Sausville JE, Salloum RG, Sorbara L *et al.* Minimal residual disease detection in hairy cell leukemia. Comparison of flow cytometric immunophenotyping with clonal analysis using consensus primer polymerase chain reaction for the heavy chain gene. *Am J Clin Pathol* 2003; **119**: 213–17.

51. Ellison DJ, Sharpe RW, Robbins BA *et al.* Immunomorphologic analysis of bone marrow biopsies after treatment with 2-chlorodeoxyadenosine for hairy cell leukemia. *Blood* 1994; **84**: 4310–15.

52. Wheaton S, Tallman MS, Hakimian D, Peterson L. Minimal residual disease may predict bone marrow relapse in patients with hairy cell leukemia treated with 2-chlorodeoxyadenosine. *Blood* 1996; **87**: 1556–60.

53. Filleul B, Delannoy A, Ferrant A *et al.* A single course of 2-chloro-deoxyadenosine does not eradicate leukemic cells in hairy cell leukemia patients in complete remission. *Leukemia* 1994; **8**: 1153–6.

54. Goodman GR, Bethel KJ, Saven A. Hairy cell leukemia: an update. *Curr Opin Hematol* 2003; **10**: 258–66.

◆55. Staudt LM. Molecular diagnosis of the hematologic cancers. *N Engl J Med* 2003; **348**: 1777–85.

●56. Korsmeyer SJ, Greene WC, Cossman J *et al.* Rearrangement and expression of immunoglobulin genes and expression of Tac antigen in hairy cell leukemia. *Proc Natl Acad Sci U S A* 1983; **80**: 4522–6.

57. Burthem J, Zuzel M, Cawley JC. What is the nature of the hairy cell and why should we be interested? *Br J Haematol* 1997; **97**: 511–14.

58. Anderson KC, Boyd AW, Fisher DC *et al*. Hairy cell leukemia: a tumor of pre-plasma cells. *Blood* 1985; **65**: 620–9.

59. van den Oord JJ, de Wolf-Peeters C, Desmet VJ. Hairy cell leukemia: a B-lymphocytic disorder derived from splenic marginal zone lymphocytes? *Blut* 1985; **50**: 191–4.

60. Burke JS, Sheibani K. Hairy cells and monocytoid B lymphocytes: are they related? *Leukemia* 1987; **1**: 298–300.

61. Posnett DN, Wang CY, Chiorazzi N *et al*. An antigen characteristic of hairy cell leukemia cells is expressed on certain activated B cells. *J Immunol* 1984; **133**: 1635–40.

62. Visser L, Shaw A, Slupsky J *et al*. Monoclonal antibodies reactive with hairy cell leukemia. *Blood* 1989; **74**: 320–5.

●63. Forconi F, Sahota SS, Raspadori D *et al*. Hairy cell leukemia: at the crossroad of somatic mutation and isotype switch. *Blood* 2004; **104**: 3312–17.

64. Maloum K, Magnac C, Azgui Z *et al*. VH gene expression in hairy cell leukaemia. *Br J Haematol* 1998; **101**: 171–8.

65. Miranda RN, Cousar JB, Hammer RD *et al*. Somatic mutation analysis of IgH variable regions reveals that tumor cells of most parafollicular (monocytoid) B-cell lymphoma, splenic marginal zone B-cell lymphoma, and some hairy cell leukemia are composed of memory B lymphocytes. *Hum Pathol* 1999; **30**: 306–12.

66. Vanhentenrijk V, Tierens A, Wlodarska I *et al*. V(H) gene analysis of hairy cell leukemia reveals a homogeneous mutation status and suggests its marginal zone B-cell origin. *Leukemia* 2004; **18**: 1729–32.

67. Thorselius M, Walsh SH, Thunberg U *et al*. Heterogeneous somatic hypermutation status confounds the cell of origin in hairy cell leukemia. *Leuk Res* 2005; **29**: 153–8.

◆68. MacLennan IC, Toellner KM, Cunningham AF *et al*. Extrafollicular antibody responses. *Immunol Rev* 2003; **194**: 8–18.

◆69. McHeyzer-Williams LJ, McHeyzer-Williams MG. Antigen-specific memory B cell development. *Annu Rev Immunol* 2005; **23**: 487–513.

◆70. Carsetti R, Rosado MM, Wardmann H. Peripheral development of B cells in mouse and man. *Immunol Rev* 2004; **197**: 179–91.

●71. Vincent AM, Burthem J, Brew R, Cawley JC. Endothelial interactions of hairy cells: the importance of alpha 4 beta 1 in the unusual tissue distribution of the disorder. *Blood* 1996; **88**: 3945–52.

72. Csanaky G, Matutes E, Vass JA *et al*. Adhesion receptors on peripheral blood leukemic B cells. A comparative study on B cell chronic lymphocytic leukemia and related lymphoma/leukemias. *Leukemia* 1997; **11**: 408–15.

●73. Burthem J, Baker PK, Hunt JA, Cawley JC. Hairy cell interactions with extracellular matrix: expression of specific integrin receptors and their role in the cell's response to specific adhesive proteins. *Blood* 1994; **84**: 873–82.

74. Burthem J, Baker PK, Hunt JA, Cawley JC. The function of c-fms in hairy-cell leukemia: macrophage colony-stimulating factor stimulates hairy-cell movement. *Blood* 1994; **83**: 1381–9.

75. Freije JM, Balbin M, Pendas AM *et al*. Matrix metalloproteinases and tumor progression. *Adv Exp Med Biol* 2003; **532**: 91–107.

◆76. Jiang Y, Goldberg ID, Shi YE. Complex roles of tissue inhibitors of metalloproteinases in cancer. *Oncogene* 2002; **21**: 2245–52.

77. Perretti M, Ingegnoli F, Wheller SK *et al*. Annexin 1 modulates monocyte-endothelial cell interaction *in vitro* and cell migration *in vivo* in the human SCID mouse transplantation model. *J Immunol* 2002; **169**: 2085–92.

78. Durig J, Schmucker U, Duhrsen U. Differential expression of chemokine receptors in B cell malignancies. *Leukemia* 2001; **15**: 752–6.

●79. Forster R, Mattis AE, Kremmer E *et al*. A putative chemokine receptor, BLR1, directs B cell migration to defined lymphoid organs and specific anatomic compartments of the spleen. *Cell* 1996; **87**: 1037–47.

●80. Forster R, Schubel A, Breitfeld D *et al*. CCR7 coordinates the primary immune response by establishing functional microenvironments in secondary lymphoid organs. *Cell* 1999; **99**: 23–33.

●81. Baker PK, Pettitt AR, Slupsky JR *et al*. Response of hairy cells to IFN-alpha involves induction of apoptosis through autocrine TNF-alpha and protection by adhesion. *Blood* 2002; **100**: 647–53.

●82. Burthem J, Cawley JC. The bone marrow fibrosis of hairy-cell leukemia is caused by the synthesis and assembly of a fibronectin matrix by the hairy cells. *Blood* 1994; **83**: 497–504.

●83. Aziz KA, Till KJ, Chen H *et al*. The role of autocrine FGF-2 in the distinctive bone marrow fibrosis of hairy-cell leukaemia (HCL). *Blood* 2003; **10**: 10.

●84. Aziz KA, Till KJ, Zuzel M, Cawley JC. Involvement of CD44-hyaluronan interaction in malignant cell homing and fibronectin synthesis in hairy cell leukemia. *Blood* 2000; **96**: 3161–7.

●85. Shehata M, Schwarzmeier JD, Hilgarth M *et al*. TGF-beta1 induces bone marrow reticulin fibrosis in hairy cell leukemia. *J Clin Invest* 2004; **113**: 676–85.

86. Kimura A, Katoh O, Hyodo H, Kuramoto A. Transforming growth factor-beta regulates growth as well as collagen and fibronectin synthesis of human marrow fibroblasts. *Br J Haematol* 1989; **72**: 486–91.

●87. Gruber G, Schwarzmeier JD, Shehata M *et al*. Basic fibroblast growth factor is expressed by CD19/CD11c-positive cells in hairy cell leukemia. *Blood* 1999; **94**: 1077–85.

88. Lisse I, Hasselbalch H, Junker P. Bone marrow stroma in idiopathic myelofibrosis and other haematological diseases. An immunohistochemical study. *APMIS* 1991; **99**: 171–8.

89. Jongstra-Bilen J, Janmey PA, Hartwig JH *et al*. The lymphocyte-specific protein LSP1 binds to F-actin and to the cytoskeleton through its COOH-terminal basic domain. *J Cell Biol* 1992; **118**: 1443–53.

●90. Miyoshi EK, Stewart PL, Kincade PW *et al.* Aberrant expression and localization of the cytoskeleton-binding pp52 (LSP1) protein in hairy cell leukemia. *Leuk Res* 2001; **25**: 57–67.

91. Harvey W, Srour EF, Turner R *et al.* Characterization of a new cell line (ESKOL) resembling hairy-cell leukemia: a model for oncogene regulation and late B-cell differentiation. *Leuk Res* 1991; **15**: 733–44.

92. Zhang X, Machii T, Matsumura I *et al.* Constitutively activated Rho guanosine triphosphatases regulate the growth and morphology of hairy cell leukemia cells. *Int J Hematol* 2003; **77**: 263–73.

●93. Chaigne-Delalande B, Deuve L, Reuzeau E *et al.* RhoGTPases and p53 are involved in the morphological appearance and interferon-α response of hairy cells. *Am J Pathol* 2006; **168**: 562–73.

94. Ju YT, Chang AC, She BR *et al.* gas7: a gene expressed preferentially in growth-arrested fibroblasts and terminally differentiated Purkinje neurons affects neurite formation. *Proc Natl Acad Sci U S A* 1998; **95**: 11423–8.

95. Chao CC, Su LJ, Sun NK *et al.* Involvement of Gas7 in nerve growth factor-independent and dependent cell processes in PC12 cells. *J Neurosci Res* 2003; **74**: 248–54.

●96. She BR, Liou GG, Lin-Chao S. Association of the growth-arrest-specific protein Gas7 with F-actin induces reorganization of microfilaments and promotes membrane outgrowth. *Exp Cell Res* 2002; **273**: 34–44.

97. Parra M, Gascard P, Walensky LD *et al.* Cloning and characterization of 4.1G (EPB41L2), a new member of the skeletal protein 4.1 (EPB41) gene family. *Genomics* 1998; **49**: 298–306.

98. Kontrogianni-Konstantopoulos A, Frye CS, Benz EJ Jr, Huang SC. The prototypical 4.1R-10-kDa domain and the 4.1g-10-kDa paralog mediate fodrin-actin complex formation. *J Biol Chem* 2001; **276**: 20679–87.

99. Rosner MC, Golomb HM. Phagocytic capacity of hairy cells from seventeen patients. *Virchows Arch B Cell Pathol Incl Mol Pathol* 1982; **40**: 327–37.

100. Yona S, Buckingham JC, Perretti M, Flower RJ. Stimulus-specific defect in the phagocytic pathways of annexin 1 null macrophages. *Br J Pharmacol* 2004; **142**: 890–8.

101. Fan X, Krahling S, Smith D *et al.* Macrophage surface expression of annexins I and II in the phagocytosis of apoptotic lymphocytes. *Mol Biol Cell* 2004; **15**: 2863–72.

102. Kusumawati A, Cazevieille C, Porte F *et al.* Early events and implication of F-actin and annexin I associated structures in the phagocytic uptake of Brucella suis by the J-774A.1 murine cell line and human monocytes. *Microb Pathog* 2000; **28**: 343–52.

103. Till KJ, Lopez A, Slupsky J, Cawley JC. C-fms protein expression by B-cells, with particular reference to the hairy cells of hairy-cell leukaemia. *Br J Haematol* 1993; **83**: 223–31.

104. Schwarting R, Stein H, Wang CY. The monoclonal antibodies alpha S-HCL 1 (alpha Leu-14) and alpha S-HCL 3 (alpha Leu-M5) allow the diagnosis of hairy cell leukemia. *Blood* 1985; **65**: 974–83.

105. Mahoney JA, Ntolosi B, DaSilva RP *et al.* Cloning and characterization of CPVL, a novel serine carboxypeptidase, from human macrophages. *Genomics* 2001; **72**: 243–51.

106. Koyama Y, Suzuki M, Yoshida T. CD63, a member of tetraspan transmembrane protein family, induces cellular spreading by reaction with monoclonal antibody on substrata. *Biochem Biophys Res Commun* 1998; **246**: 841–6.

107. Metzelaar MJ, Schuurman HJ, Heijnen HF *et al.* Biochemical and immunohistochemical characteristics of CD62 and CD63 monoclonal antibodies. Expression of GMP-140 and LIMP-CD63 (CD63 antigen) in human lymphoid tissues. *Virchows Arch B Cell Pathol Incl Mol Pathol* 1991; **61**: 269–77.

108. McIntire RH, Morales PJ, Petroff MG *et al.* Recombinant HLA-G5 and -G6 drive U937 myelomonocytic cell production of TGF-beta1. *J Leukoc Biol* 2004; **76**: 1220–8.

109. Cao S, Liu J, Song L, Ma X. The protooncogene c-Maf is an essential transcription factor for IL-10 gene expression in macrophages. *J Immunol* 2005; **174**: 3484–92.

110. Hegde SP, Zhao J, Ashmun RA, Shapiro LH. c-Maf induces monocytic differentiation and apoptosis in bipotent myeloid progenitors. *Blood* 1999; **94**: 1578–89.

111. Cessna MH, Hartung L, Tripp S *et al.* Hairy cell leukemia variant: fact or fiction. *Am J Clin Pathol* 2005; **123**: 132–8.

112. Troen G, Nygaard V, Jenssen TK *et al.* Constitutive expression of the AP-1 transcription factors c-jun, junD, junB, and c-fos and the marginal zone B-cell transcription factor Notch2 in splenic marginal zone lymphoma. *J Mol Diagn* 2004; **6**: 297–307.

113. Thieblemont C, Nasser V, Felman P *et al.* Small lymphocytic lymphoma, marginal zone B-cell lymphoma, and mantle cell lymphoma exhibit distinct gene-expression profiles allowing molecular diagnosis. *Blood* 2004; **103**: 2727–37.

114. Ruiz-Ballesteros E, Mollejo M, Rodriguez A *et al.* Splenic marginal zone lymphoma: proposal of new diagnostic and prognostic markers identified after tissue and cDNA microarray analysis. *Blood* 2005; **106**: 1831–8.

115. Campbell LJ. Cytogenetics of lymphomas. *Pathology* 2005; **37**: 493–507.

116. Kluin-Nelemans HC, Beverstock GC, Mollevanger P *et al.* Proliferation and cytogenetic analysis of hairy cell leukemia upon stimulation via the CD40 antigen. *Blood* 1994; **84**: 3134–41.

117. Sambani C, Trafalis DT, Mitsoulis-Mentzikoff C *et al.* Clonal chromosome rearrangements in hairy cell leukemia: personal experience and review of literature. *Cancer Genet Cytogenet* 2001; **129**: 138–44.

118. Andersen CL, Gruszka-Westwood A, Ostergaard M *et al.* A narrow deletion of 7q is common to HCL, and SMZL, but not CLL. *Eur J Haematol* 2004; **72**: 390–402.

◆119. Klein U, Dalla-Favera R. New insights into the phenotype and cell derivation of B cell chronic lymphocytic leukemia. *Curr Top Microbiol Immunol* 2005; **294**: 31–49.

29

Mantle cell lymphoma

ELIAS CAMPO AND OLGA BALAGUÉ

DEFINITION

Mantle cell lymphoma (MCL) is a lymphoid neoplasm characterized by a monomorphic proliferation of small- to medium-sized lymphoid cells with irregular nuclei of B cell phenotype commonly coexpressing CD5.[1] The genetic hallmark of this neoplasm is the t(11;14)(q13;q32) translocation that leads to a constitutive deregulation and overexpression of cyclin D1 and plays an important pathogenetic role in the development of the tumor. This entity includes different categories of lymphomas recognized in previous classifications such as the centrocytic lymphoma, lymphocytic lymphoma of intermediate differentiation, intermediate lymphocytic lymphoma and mantle zone lymphoma.[2,3] The clinical behavior is very aggressive and few patients may be considered cured or reach long survival with current therapeutic protocols. Better knowledge of this disease and emergence of a new generation of drugs are facilitating the design of new therapeutic strategies that may overcome the resistance of

this aggressive lymphoma to conventional treatments, thereby improving the life expectancy of the patients.

EPIDEMIOLOGY

Mantle cell lymphoma represents 3–10 percent of all non-Hodgkin lymphomas (NHLs) and occurs in elderly males (male to female ratio 1.6–6.8:1) with a median age of approximately 60 years (range 29–85). Occasional cases of MCL have been identified in families in which another member had developed a lymphoid neoplasm. The tumor in the second generation tends to appear at an earlier age than in the parent, a phenomenon known as anticipation that also occurs in chronic lymphocytic leukemia (CLL) families and suggest a genetic predisposition.[4] However, the genetic mechanisms underlying this familial association are unknown. Recent studies have identified certain single nucleotide polymorphisms of the TRAIL receptor

DR4 and *CD5* genes at higher frequency in MCL patients than in the normal control population.[5]

ONTOGENY

Mantle cell lymphoma is derived in most cases from a subset of naïve pregerminal center B cells expressing CD5. Human CD5-positive B cells are present in fetal lymphoid tissues and blood, and decrease with age. The distribution of tumor cells surrounding germinal centers and the expression of several genes normally expressed by naïve and normal follicular mantle zone B cells such as IgM/IgD and alkaline phosphatase have supported the relationship of this tumor to cells of the primary lymphoid follicle or the mantle cells of secondary follicles.[2] The identification of no or very little somatic mutations in immunoglobulin genes of most cases of MCL has confirmed its origin from pregerminal center cells. The analyses of the JH/*BCL1* breakpoints have suggested that this translocation is predominantly generated during a primary DH-JH rearrangement in early B cells in opposition to the JH/*BCL2* in the t(14;18) translocation, which seems to occur during secondary rearrangements at a later stage of B cell differentiation.[6] However, recent studies indicate that 20–30 percent of MCLs may show somatic hypermutations in the immunoglobulin genes although at lower level than in diffuse large B cell lymphomas. A biased use of the VH3-21, VH3-24 and VH4-34 genes has been detected in MCL, suggesting that these tumors may originate from specific subsets of B cells.[6–9] Contrary to CLL, tumors with VH3-21 genes mainly occur in unmutated MCL, show a tendency to have longer survival,[7,8] and seem to have less genomic imbalances.[10] The mutational status of the VH genes in MCL does not correlate with survival or ZAP70 expression.[8,11] Interestingly, MCL with a leukemic, non-nodal clinical presentation frequently has mutated VH genes and may be associated with a longer survival (see below).[9] A frequent use of the VH4-39 immunoglobulin family gene in the tumor cells has been observed in leukemic patients.[12]

Mantle cell lymphoma expresses activation-induced cytidine deaminase (AID) at variable levels, but usually higher than in normal naïve B cells, suggesting that it may be a tumor-associated phenomenon.[13,14] The AID expression in MCL is unrelated to the presence of somatic mutations in the *Ig* gene, but seems to correlate with the presence of ongoing class switch recombination of the *Ig* gene.[13] This pattern of AID expression in MCL differs from the pattern observed in other lymphomas where AID expression correlates with somatic hypermutations or a germinal center phenotype, and also from the pattern observed in CLL, where AID is highly expressed in unmutated ZAP70-positive CLL but not in mutated and ZAP70-negative tumors.[13,14]

MORPHOLOGIC CHARACTERISTICS

Architectural patterns

MCL usually effaces the lymph node architecture showing three growth patterns: mantle zone, nodular or diffuse (Plate 35, see plate section). The mantle zone pattern is characterized by an expansion of the follicle mantle area by tumor cells surrounding a reactive 'naked' germinal center.[15] This pattern may be associated with partial preservation of the nodal architecture and it may be difficult to distinguish from follicular or mantle cell hyperplasias.[16] Early involvement of lymph nodes by MCL occurs in the mantle zone area.[17,18] The nodular pattern is characterized by a solid tumor growth without evidence of residual germinal centers. This pattern may raise the differential diagnosis with follicular lymphoma (Table 29.1). Residual germinal centers may also be seen in tumors with a more diffuse pattern, although in these cases they may only be identified focally. Most of the cases show a combination of these patterns with predominance of the diffuse (80 percent) or nodular (15–20 percent). A pure mantle zone pattern is very uncommon (less than 5 percent of the cases) but it may be observed focally usually associated with a nodular pattern.[19]

Table 29.1   Differential diagnostic between mantle cell lymphoma (MCL) and other lymphomas

Entity	MCL lymphoma variant	Features suggestive of MCL	Useful markers
CLL	Typical or small-round cell	Absence of prolymphocytes or paraimmunoblasts and proliferation centers	CD23, cyclin D1, p27
FL	Nodular diffuse	Monotonous cell population; less nuclear irregularities; absence of centroblasts	CD10, BCL6, cyclin D1, p27
MZL	MZL-like	Absence of mantle cell cuff; monotonous cell population; no immunoblasts or plasma cells; finely dispersed chromatin	Cyclin D1, CD5, MUM1, p27
DLBCL	Pleomorphic	Irregular nuclei; finely dispersed chromatin; small nucleoli	Cyclin D1, BCL6, MUM1
Acute leukemia	Blastic	Immunophenotype	Cyclin D1
HCL	MCL with clear cell cytoplasm	Irregular nuclei	Annexin I

CLL, chronic lymphocytic leukemia; FL, follicular lymphoma; MZL, marginal zone lymphoma; DLBCL, diffuse large B cell lymphoma; HCL, hairy cell leukemia.

Cytologic variants

Two main cytologic variants of MCL have been recognized, classical and blastoid. Classical (common or typical) MCLs are characterized by a monotonous proliferation of small- to medium-sized lymphoid cells with scant cytoplasm, variably irregular nuclei, evenly distributed condensed chromatin and inconspicuous nucleoli (Plate 36, see plate section). Large cells with abundant cytoplasm or prominent nucleoli are rare or absent and, when present, they may correspond to reactive centroblasts of residual germinal centers overrun by lymphoma cells. Occasional cases may show a predominance of small lymphocytes with rounded nuclei (Plate 36). This variant may be difficult to distinguish from chronic lymphocytic leukemia/small lymphocytic lymphoma (CLL/SLL). However, proliferation centers (growth centers) or isolated prolymphocytes and paraimmunoblasts are characteristically absent in MCL (Table 29.1). Proliferative activity in typical and small cell MCL may vary from case to case but is usually lower than 1–2 mitoses per high power field (HPF). However, some tumors with a typical morphology may show a relatively high mitotic index similar to the blastoid variants, and the patients may have an aggressive clinical course.[20] Scattered epithelioid histiocytes with eosinophilic cytoplasm are relatively common, but well-formed microgranulomas are not usually seen (Plate 36, see plate section). These histiocytes do not generally contain phagocytosis of apoptotic bodies. Nuclei of follicular dendritic cells with the typical aspect of overlapping nuclei, delicate nuclear membrane, and 'empty' chromatin appearance are frequently identified. In some cases, hyalinized small vessels may be seen scattered throughout the tumor.

Blastoid MCL is a more aggressive variant whose morphology ranges from a monotonous population of cells resembling lymphoblasts to a more pleomorphic appearance with larger irregular cells (Plate 36). The term blastoid, proposed by the World Health Organization (WHO) classification, includes the two previously recognized blastic and pleomorphic variants that may represent the ends of a morphologic spectrum, since transitional areas between these subtypes may be observed in some cases.[1] Blastic MCL is characterized by a monotonous population of medium-sized lymphocytes with scant cytoplasm, rounded nuclei with finely dispersed chromatin and inconspicuous nucleoli. These cases may resemble lymphoblastic lymphoma or nodal involvement by acute myeloid leukemia. The mitotic index is very high with more than 2–3 mitoses per HPF. Histiocytes with tingible bodies and a 'starry sky' pattern may be seen (Plate 37). Mantle cell lymphomas with a more pleomorphic or large cell morphology were initially designated in the Kiel classification as 'anaplastic' centrocytic lymphomas or centroblastic lymphomas of the 'centrocytoid' subtype. These tumors are composed of a more heterogeneous population of large cells with ovoid or irregular cleaved nuclei, finely dispersed chromatin and small distinct nucleoli (Plate 36). The mitotic index is high but usually lower than in blastic cases.

In some of these cases, mitotic figures may show a striking hyperchromatic staining with an apparent high number of chromosomes. This finding is usually associated with the presence of tetraploid clones.[21] This pleomorphic variant may be difficult to distinguish from large cell lymphomas. However, the nuclear characteristics with cleaved contours, finely disperse chromatin, and the discordance between the large size of the nuclei and a relatively small nucleoli may suggest a mantle cell origin. Ancillary studies are mandatory in these cases to confirm the diagnosis (Table 29.1). Some leukemic MCL described as 'prolymphocytic variants' of MCL may in fact represent leukemic forms of the pleomorphic subtype of MCL.[22]

All these morphologic variants should be considered as a spectrum and some tumors may show overlapping cytologic features. Particularly, some cases may show transitional areas between classical and pleomorphic variants with cells that may be difficult to define whether they are classical or pleomorphic. In occasional cases areas of classical and pleomorphic morphology may be identified in different parts of the same lymph node.[19]

Some cases may have a variable number of cells with more abundant pale cytoplasm mimicking monocytoid B cells (Plate 38, see plate section).[23] The nucleus of these cells may have a blastoid or classical morphology but the peculiar cytoplasm may raise the differential diagnosis of marginal zone lymphomas or hairy cell leukemia. In some cases, these monocytoid-like cells may even expand to the marginal zone of lymphoid follicles outside an apparent preserved mantle zone. CD5 and cyclin D1 positivity are crucial in the diagnosis of this variant (Table 29.1).

Bone marrow and peripheral blood

Bone marrow infiltration, independently of an apparent peripheral blood involvement, occurs in 50–91 percent of the patients[24,25] and is detected more frequently in core biopsies than aspirates.[25] Mantle cell lymphoma usually infiltrates the bone marrow with a mixed pattern combining nodular and paratrabecular or nodular and interstitial features. Isolated paratrabecular aggregates or pure interstitial infiltrates are rare. In some cases, a diffuse infiltration of the marrow may be seen. The degree of infiltration does not seem to correlate with the histologic variants of MCL identified in lymph node biopsies, architectural patterns, or survival of the patients.[25]

The cytologic appearance of tumor cells in peripheral blood and bone marrow aspirates shows a similar spectrum as in tissue samples (Plate 39, see plate section). Circulating cells in most MCL usually show a mixture of small- to medium-sized cells with scant cytoplasm, prominent nuclear irregularities, and reticular chromatin. Some cells may have rounded nuclei but the chromatin does not have the clumped appearance seen in CLL. Leukemic blastic MCL may mimic acute leukemia with medium to large size, high nuclear–cytoplasmic ratio, fine disperse chromatin and relatively small or inconspicuous nucleoli. Some cases of leukemic MCL may show very large atypical cells with prominent nucleoli that probably correspond to the leukemic phase of the pleomorphic variant of MCL.[22] In fact, some of these cases have hyperdiploid karyotypes and have been associated with a pleomorphic variant of MCL in the lymph nodes. Most cases previously diagnosed as B prolymphocytic leukemia carrying the t(11,14) translocation and cyclin D1 overexpression probably correspond to leukemic MCL.[22]

Spleen

Macroscopically, splenic involvement by MCL shows a generalized micronodular pattern, which may occasionally be associated with perivascular infiltration (Plate 40, see plate section). Histologically, the differential diagnosis of MCL and other small cell lymphomas in the spleen may be difficult.[26] White pulp nodules are enlarged with a variable involvement of the red pulp. Residual 'naked' germinal centers are found in 50 percent of the cases. Tumor cells show the similar monotonous morphology as in other locations. Interestingly, some cases may show a 'marginal zone'-like area at the periphery of the nodules, comprising cells with more abundant pale cytoplasm.[26] Spontaneous splenic rupture has been reported in occasional MCL.

Gastrointestinal tract

A typical presentation of MCL in the gastrointestinal tract is the 'lymphomatoid polyposis', in which multiple lymphoid polyps are identified in the small and large bowel that may be associated with large tumoral masses, usually ileocecal, and regional lymphadenopathy (Plate 41, see plate section).[27] Although relatively characteristic of MCL, this clinical presentation may also be caused by other NHLs, particularly follicular lymphoma and marginal zone lymphoma of the mucosa-associated lymphoid tissue (MALT) type. Gastrointestinal involvement without the macroscopic appearance of polyposis may also occur. In these cases, superficial ulcers, large tumor masses or diffuse thickening of the mucosa are common macroscopic findings. Microscopic infiltration of gastrointestinal mucosa by MCL without apparent macroscopic lesions is very common although rarely changes the clinical management of the patients.[28] In some cases, glandular infiltration by tumor cells may mimic lymphoepithelial lesions, thus making the differential diagnosis with marginal zone lymphomas difficult. However, the scarcity of these lesions and the monotonous aspect of the lymphoid infiltrate should suggest a diagnosis of MCL. Interestingly, MCLs, as well as other NHLs involving gastrointestinal mucosa, express $\alpha 4\beta 7$ integrin, a homing receptor which binds to MadCAM-1 adhesion molecule selectively expressed in endothelial cells of mucosas.[29]

Histologic progression

Studies of sequential biopsies have shown that the histologic pattern of MCLs remains relatively stable during the evolution of the disease.[30] In some cases, obliteration of residual germinal centers and nodular progression to a more diffuse pattern may be observed in serial biopsies.[30] Interestingly, some cases may show an oscillating course with changing patterns during the evolution of the disease.[31] Increased numbers of larger blastic cells and mitotic figures may be seen in 20–25 percent of the patients. However, most blastic MCLs are detected at diagnosis, and cytologic progression from typical MCL to a pure blastic variant is relatively uncommon in sequential biopsies,[30] although it may be detected more frequently at autopsies.[31] A clonal relationship has been demonstrated in occasional cases of progression from typical to blastoid MCL.[32] In some cases, tumor progression is associated with development of an overt leukemic phase.[2]

Composite mantle cell lymphoma and other lymphoid neoplasms

Composite lymphomas including MCL and a second malignant lymphoma in the same site have been described in some patients. The second lymphomas detected in association with MCL have been follicular lymphoma,[33,34] CLL/SLL,[33] plasmacytoma,[35] multiple myeloma[36] and Hodgkin lymphoma.[37,38] Clonal analysis have indicated that the MCL and the associated lymphoma are of different origin in most of the cases. However, two cases showed a common clone specific IgH rearrangement in the MCL and the associated follicular or Hodgkin lymphoma, suggesting the unusual evolution of a malignant single clone resulting in two morphologic, phenotypic and molecular distinct lymphomas.[34,37]

IMMUNOPHENOTYPE

Mantle cell lymphoma has a characteristic phenotype expressing the B cell markers CD19, CD20, CD22, CD79a-b and FCM7 whereas CD23 and the germinal center associated antigens BCL6 and CD10 are usually negative (Plate 42, see plate section). In addition, similarly to CLL/SLL, MCL is commonly positive for the T cell associated antigens CD5 and CD43. Surface immunoglobulins are of moderate to strong intensity with frequent coexpression of IgM and IgD with λ light chain more frequently expressed than κ. Some MCL cases may show phenotypic variants that do not exclude the diagnosis. Thus, some tumors may be CD5 negative, particularly among blastoid variants, and dim CD23 may be detected by flow cytometry in a number of cases.[39] CD8 and CD7[40] positivity by flow cytometry has been reported in isolated cases of MCL. Occasional MCL may show BCL6 staining whereas CD10 positivity has been documented in some cases by flow cytometry.[41–43] Follicular dendritic cells (FDCs) are usually prominent in MCL and its nodular or diffuse growth pattern may account in part for the architectural pattern observed in the hematoxylin and eosin staining (Plate 42). In nodular cases, a dense and concentric meshwork of FDCs may represent colonization of preexisting follicular centers by tumor cells, whereas a loose and irregular pattern may correspond to expansion of primary follicles.[2]

Cyclin D1 and p27 expression

Cyclin D1 expression is a constant and highly specific phenomenon in MCL associated with the specific t(11;14) translocation of this lymphoma (see below).[44] Different antibodies allow the immunohistochemical detection of cyclin D1 in routinely processed tissues and it is a crucial criterion in the diagnosis of this tumor (Plate 43, see plate section).[45] However, this technique may be difficult and unsatisfactory results are frequently obtained in many laboratories. Optimized protocols, including the use of more than one antibody in some difficult cases, demonstrate the expression of cyclin D1 in virtually all tumors.[46] However, occasional MCL with a proven t(11;14) translocation may rend a negative immunohistochemical result. This technical problem has to be distinguished from the rare true cyclin D1-negative MCL that is related to the overexpression of cyclin D2 or D3 (see below). Cyclin D1 is always detected in the nucleus of the cells, although the intensity may vary from cell to cell and case to case (Plate 43). Cyclin D1 is also detected in the nucleus of histiocytes, endothelial cells and epithelial cells that may be used as internal positive control.

Cyclin D1 detection in bone marrow trephines may require particular attention. In the occasional cases in which immunohistochemistry is not successful or in leukemic cases with no tissue available quantitative reverse transcriptase polymerase chain reaction[47] may be useful. In addition to MCL, cyclin D1 expression may be detected in 25 percent of multiple myeloma carrying the t(11;14) translocation, amplification of the gene, or without apparent structural alterations of the gene.[48] Low levels of cyclin D1 are also detected in hairy cell leukemia and this expression is not related to BCL1 rearrangements.[49] All other lymphoid neoplasms are negative. The detection of cyclin D1 in occasional cases with an initial diagnosis of CLL, B prolymphocytic leukemia or splenic marginal zone lymphomas carrying the t(11;14) translocation is now controversial because most of these cases have been reinterpreted as MCL.[22,23,44] However, cyclin D1 expression may be detected in cases with clear morphology and phenotype of CLL, particularly in the proliferation growth centers, in the absence of the t(11;14) translocation.[50]

Immunohistochemical detection of the cyclin-dependent kinase inhibitor p27[Kip1] is also useful in the differential diagnosis of MCL. p27[Kip1] expression in NHL is usually inversely related to the proliferative activity of the cells. Thus, it is strongly expressed in CLL, follicular lymphomas, and marginal zone lymphomas, but it has negative or low expression in large cell lymphomas. Interestingly, p27 staining in MCL is independent of the proliferative rate and is usually negative in classical MCL and positive in blastoid variants.[51] Hairy cell leukemia (HCL) is also negative or very weakly positive.[52] The mechanisms involved in this peculiar p27[Kip1] staining pattern in MCL and HCL are not fully understood (see below), but this staining may be useful in the differential diagnosis of these tumors, particularly when cyclin D1 staining fails (Table 29.1).[52]

Cyclin D1-negative mantle cell lymphoma

A microarray study of MCL identified a small subset of small B cell lymphomas with morphology, phenotype and global expression profile undistinguishable from conventional MCL but negative for cyclin D1 expression both at protein and mRNA level.[53] These cases also had a similar clinical presentation and follow up and carried similar chromosomal imbalances as conventional MCL. Interestingly, these cases had a high expression of cyclin D2 or cyclin D3 suggesting that overexpression of these two G1 cyclins may be an alternative mechanism to cyclin D1 overexpression in the pathogenesis of MCL. Intriguingly, none of these cases had chromosomal abnormalities involving the gene locus of these two cyclins and therefore the oncogenic mechanism is not known.[54] This 'true' cyclin D1-negative MCL is rare and should be distinguished from other types of small B cell lymphomas mimicking MCL.[55] These differences may be difficult because some cases may even be CD5 positive and CD23 negative but the prognosis is significantly better than in true MCL with cyclin D1 overexpression, which indicates that they may correspond to different entities including atypical B-CLL, CD5 positive marginal zone lymphomas or lymphoplasmacytoid lymphomas.[55] These observations emphasize the need to confirm the diagnosis of MCL by genetic or molecular studies when cyclin D1 expression cannot be reliably demonstrated. Given the important clinical impact of the diagnosis of MCL, the identification of the true cyclin D1-negative MCL or other small B cell lymphomas mimicking MCL has to be made with great caution. Further studies are needed to better define this subset of tumors.

CYTOGENETIC FINDINGS

The characteristic cytogenetic alteration in MCL is the t(11;14)(q13;q32). This translocation is detected by conventional cytogenetics in up to 65 percent of MCLs. However, using different fluorescent in situ hybridization (FISH) techniques, it can be found in virtually all cases of MCL (Plate 44, see plate section).[56,57] FISH probes may identify atypical presentations of this translocation more frequently than initially recognized. These atypical presentations include cryptic insertions of the cyclin D1 gene into the 14q32 region on apparently normal chromosomes, duplication of the cyclin D1/IgH region, and complex rearrangements fusing other chromosome fragments with the cyclin D1/IgH rearranged region.[58] In addition, occasional cases of variant translocations fusing the cyclin D1 locus on 11q13 to the λ light chain on chromosome 22q11 or κ light chain on 2p11 have been described.[59]

The initial studies reporting the t(11;14) translocation in other lymphoproliferative disorders were in all likelihood misdiagnosed MCL.[60] However, t(11;14) translocations have been identified in occasional atypical CLL, 20–30 percent of prolymphocytic leukemias, occasional splenic marginal zone lymphomas (SMZLs) with villous lymphocytes[61] and 5 percent of multiple myelomas.[60] B prolymphocytic leukemia was defined before MCL was identified as a distinct entity and probably most of these cases correspond to pleomorphic MCL.[22] Molecular analysis of this translocation in MCL and multiple myeloma suggests that the mechanism in these tumors is different, with an error in the V-D-J recombination in MCL and in the switch recombination process in myeloma.[62] The presence of the t(11;14) translocation in CLL and SMZL is now questionable since this cases probably represent a variant of indolent MCL. Interestingly, all these cases seem to have relatively common clinical and genetic features since most of these patients present with a non-nodal leukemic expression, indolent clinical course, frequent splenomegaly and mutated immunoglobulin genes.[9] Interestingly, three cases with the variant translocation t(2;11)(p11;q13) and the IgK-cyclin D1 rearrangement had the features of non-nodal indolent leukemic, CD5 negative, small B cell lymphomas with splenomegaly and mutated Ig genes.[59]

Cytogenetic studies including conventional analysis,[63] FISH,[64] comparative genomic hybridization (CGH)[65,66] and array-based CGH[12,67–69] have revealed a high number of secondary chromosomal alterations in MCL. The most common secondary alterations are losses of chromosome 1p, 6q, 8p, 9p, 10p, 11q, 13 and 17p, and gains in 3q, 7p, 8q, 12q, 18q and Xq (Table 29.2). Losses of chromosome 8p have been associated with leukemic presentation in some studies[70] but not in others. Blastoid variants have more complex karyotypes, and high level DNA amplifications, than typical variants.[21,65] In addition, certain chromosomal imbalances such as gains of 3q, 7p and 12q and losses of 17p are significantly more frequent in blastoid than typical variants. Interestingly, tetraploidy is more frequent in pleomorphic (80 percent) and blastic variants (36 percent) than in typical MCLs (8 percent).[21] Chromosome 8q24 alterations, including the t(8;14)(q24;q32) and variants, have been identified in occasional blastoid MCL with very aggressive clinical course.[71,72]

Table 29.2 Copy number changes by comparative genomic hybridization (CGH) in mantle cell lymphoma

	Altered cases Percent (range)
CGH gains	
3q25–q29	48 (37–70)
7p15–p22	25 (4–27)
8q22–q24	25 (10–32)
12q13	23 (4–30)
18q21	21 (7–26)
CGH losses	
1p13–p32	25 (24–33)
6q14–q27	29 (13–37)
8p21–p23	41 (7–79)
9p21–p24	23 (7–30)
9q	18 (3–20)
11q21–q23	26 (19–36)
13q	45 (32–63)
17p13	22 (4–30)

MOLECULAR CHARACTERISTICS

t(11;14) translocation and cyclin D1 overexpression

The t(11;14) translocation juxtaposes the *Ig* heavy chain joining region in chromosome 14 to a region on 11q13 designated *BCL1* (B cell lymphoma/leukemia 1).[2,3] Most rearrangements (30–55 percent) occur in a region known as the major translocation cluster (MTC), whereas up to 10–20 percent of cases may have breakpoints in additional distal regions. The MTC breakpoints occur within a relatively small region of around 80 bp on chromosome 11 and in the 5′ area of one of the Ig JH regions on chromosome 14, making it possible to detect this translocation by polymerase chain reaction (PCR).[73]

Studies on a chromosome 11 inversion, inv(11)(p15;q13), in parathyroid adenomas led to the characterization of a new gene designated *PRAD1*, for parathyroid adenomatosis. This gene was located approximately 120 kb downstream of the original *BCL1* locus and was considered the candidate oncogene activated by the t(11;14) translocation.[2,3] The sequence of *PRAD1* showed a high homology with other cyclins and it was recognized as a novel member of the family, cyclin D1, involved in G1 regulation. The gene was then renamed *CCND1* or cyclin D1.[2,3]

Cyclin D1 is not normally expressed in lymphocytes or myeloid cells but it is constantly expressed in MCLs indicating an important role in the pathogenesis of this lymphoma.[44] mRNA studies have shown the expression of two major transcripts of 4.5 and 1.5 kb. Both transcripts contain the whole coding region of the gene and differ in the length of the 3′ untranslated region. Some MCLs express aberrant transcripts of altered size instead of the 4.5 kb message. Interestingly, tumors with aberrant transcripts show very high levels of expression[44] and higher proliferation.[53,74] Molecular analyses of these cases have shown the loss of AUUUA destabilizing sequences at the 3' region, which results in an increased half-life of cyclin D1 truncated transcripts. These anomalous truncated messages are due to rearrangements at the 3' region of the gene that usually coexist with a regular 5' breakpoint on the same allele.[75,76] These double rearrangements at the 5' and 3' region of the gene constitute a peculiar phenomenon in MCL. It has been suggested that they may favor the initial deregulation of the gene (5' rearrangement) and, in some cases, a subsequent stabilization of the mRNA transcripts (3' rearrangement).[75]

Cyclin D1 gene has a frequent polymorphism in the final codon of exon 4 that may modify the splice donor signal between exon and intron 4, thus generating a transcript variant, named transcript b, coding for a shorter protein missing the whole exon 5.[77] These alternative transcripts and proteins are expressed in several normal and neoplastic tissues including mantle cell lymphomas.[77,78] Although this polymorphism has been associated with differences in prognosis and clinical presentation in several solid tumors, it does not seem to have an impact on survival in MCL patients.[78,79]

Cyclin D1 oncogenic mechanisms

Cyclin D1 may function as an oncogene cooperating with other oncogenes, generally *MYC* and *RAS*. However, the oncogenic mechanisms of cyclin D1 are not well understood. Cyclin D1 participates in the control of the G1 phase by binding to the cyclin dependent kinases (CDK) 4 and 6.[2] The complexes phosphorylate retinoblastoma (Rb) leading to the inactivation of its suppressor effect on the cell cycle progression. Hyperphosphorylation of Rb releases important transcription factors, such as E2F, that participate in the regulation of other genes involved in cell cycle progression. Cyclin D1 also binds physically to Rb and may overcome the growth suppressing effect of Rb independently of its phosphorylation. In MCL, retinoblastoma seems to be normally expressed in all cases and no mutations in functional domains have been detected.[80] However, it is hyperphosphorylated, particularly in blastic variants with high proliferative activity.[81] These findings suggest than cyclin D1 may play a role in these tumors by overcoming the suppressive effect of Rb.

Mantle cell lymphoma may also have impaired control of late G1 phase and G1 to S phase transition. This step is regulated by the cyclin E/CDK2 complex and the cyclin kinase inhibitor p27^{Kip1}. In NHL other than MCL, p27^{Kip1} protein expression is inversely related to the proliferation activity of the tumors.[51] However, in MCL p27^{Kip1} immunohistochemical detection is lost in typical MCL but it is paradoxically positive in blastic variants. No structural alterations of the p27^{Kip1} gene have been found. The mechanisms

for this peculiar detection of p27^{Kip1} in MCL is not clear but may include both an increased p27 protein degradation by the proteasome pathway,[82] and sequestration by the overexpressed cyclin D1, rendering it inaccessible to antibody detection.[83] p27^{Kip1} inhibits the complexes between CDK2 and cyclin E at the end of G1 phase. Increased degradation and/or blocking p27^{Kip1} by cyclin D1 would release the activation of these complexes and allow the cell to progress to the following cell cycle phases.[51] All these observations indicate that cyclin D1 deregulation plays an important role in the development of MCL, probably overcoming the suppressive effect of Rb and p27^{Kip1}. In addition to these mechanisms, cyclin D1 may have also an important oncogenic potential independently of its catalytic function by acting as a transcriptional modulator of multiple genes.[84,85] However, whether this transcriptional function is present in MCL is not known.

Deregulation of cell cycle

In addition to the deregulation of cyclin D1, other elements of the cell cycle regulatory pathway are also disrupted in MCL. One of the major differences between typical and blastoid MCL variants is the proliferative activity of the tumors and several studies have demonstrated that proliferation is the most important biologic prognostic parameter in MCL.[53,86] These observations indicate that deregulation of cell cycle by different oncogenic events are important mechanisms in the development but also the progression of the disease. Highly proliferative and clinically aggressive MCL carry oncogenic alterations in elements of the two major regulatory pathways of the cell cycle and senescence which include the *P16INK4a/CDK4/ Rb* and the *ARF/MDM2/P53* genes (Fig. 29.1). Thus, some aggressive tumors have a simultaneous inactivation of both pathways by homozygous deletions of the whole *INK4/ARF* locus on chromosome 9p21. This locus encodes for two key regulatory elements of the two pathways, the CDK4 inhibitor p16INK4A and the p53 regulatory gene p14ARF. Homozygous deletions of this locus occurs in around 20–30 percent of blastoid or highly proliferative MCL but in less than 5 percent of cases with classical morphology.[20,87] p16INK4a acts as an inhibitor of CDK 4 and 6 and thus maintains the Rb protein in its active, antiproliferative state. p16INK4a deletion and increased levels of cyclin D1 may therefore cooperate in promoting G1/S phase transition in MCL cells by increasing the intracellular amount of active cyclin D1/CDK complexes. Interestingly, a few MCL cases with wild-type status of the INK4a/*ARF* locus show gene amplification and high expression of *BMI1*, a gene that participates in cell cycle control by acting as an oncogenic transcriptional repressor of the INK4a/*ARF* locus.[88] The INK4a/*ARF* locus is inactivated in other lymphomas by hypermethylation of the promoter region but this phenomenon seems uncommon and of uncertain significance in MCL.[89] Inactivation of other CDK inhibitors such as

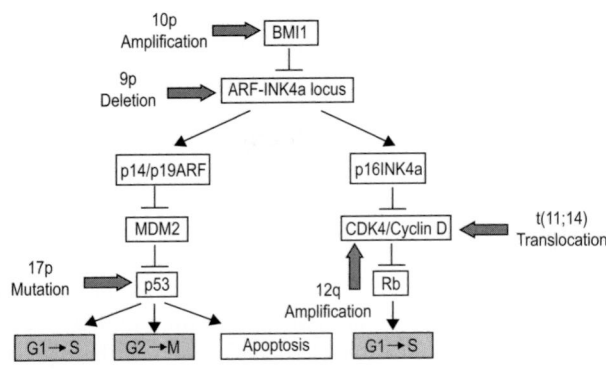

Figure 29.1 Cell cycle pathways deregulated in MCL. Clinically aggressive MCL carry oncogenic alterations in elements of the two major regulatory pathways of the cell cycle and senescence which include the *P16INK4a/CDK4/Rb* and the *ARF/MDM2/p53* genes. Both pathways are related at the INK4a–ARF locus, which encodes for p14ARF and p16INK4a. p16INK4a deletion and increased levels of cyclin D1 and CDK4 cooperate in promoting G1/S-phase transition in MCL cells. p14ARF stabilizes p53 preventing its MDM2-mediated degradation. In MCL, p14ARF deletions and *P53* mutations lead to inactivation of p53 protein.

p15INK4b, p18INK4c and p21Waf1 has been found in occasional blastic MCLs.[87,90]

The genomic locus of *P16INK4a* also encodes for a second transcript, *P14ARF*, whose expression is equally affected by homozygous deletions of the INK4a/*ARF* locus in MCL. p14ARF is encoded by the same exon 2 used by p16INK4a but an alternative exon 1 (exon 1β). The main function of p14ARF is to stabilize the p53 protein by preventing its MDM2-mediated degradation. Since in MCL as well as in other B cell lymphoma subtypes genomic deletions of the INK4a/*ARF* locus usually affect both the *P16INK4a* and the *P14ARF* genes, inactivation of this locus leads to simultaneous inhibition of the cell cycle regulatory and the p53 pathway (Fig. 29.1).

P53 is frequently targeted by genetic alterations in MCL patients. p53 is a key transcription factor that is upregulated in response to cellular stress such as DNA damage leading to cell cycle arrest or apoptosis. *P53* mutations are rarely observed in classical MCL with a low proliferative activity but they are found in approximately 30 percent of blastoid MCL cases, usually associated with 17p deletions, with a high proliferation rate and associated with a poor prognosis.[91] As an alternative mechanism to *P53* inactivation, high levels of MDM2 can be detected in a small subset of MCL cases.[92] However, the mechanism of upregulated MDM2 expression is not clear, since no correlations with DNA copy number changes have been found.

Very recently, genomic amplifications of *CDK4* leading to CDK4 mRNA and protein overexpression were described in a subset of highly aggressive blastoid MCL.[92] Interestingly, *CDK4* amplifications almost exclusively occurred in MCL cases with a wild-type status of the

INK4a/*ARF* locus suggesting that *CDK4* amplifications may represent yet another alternative pathogenetic mechanism of disrupting the G1/S phase cell cycle regulatory checkpoint in MCL. The fact that *CDK4* amplification occurs in association with *P53* mutations suggests that tumors obtain a selective advantage, inactivating the two *ARF/MDM2/P53* and *P16/CDK4/Rb* pathways (Fig. 29.1). The double inactivation of these pathways may occur by homozygous deletions of the *INKa/ARF* locus, *BMI1* amplification, or simultaneous mutations of *P53* and amplification or overexpression of CDK4. In fact the survival analysis of patients with these alterations indicate that patients with INK4a/*ARF* deletions or simultaneous aberrations of *P53* and *CDK4* have a significant shorter median survival than patients with isolated alterations of *P53* or *CDK4* and patients with no alterations in any of these genes.[92]

Deregulation of the DNA damage response pathway

The high number of chromosomal alterations and the common occurrence of tetraploid karyotypes in a subset of aggressive MCL cases suggest that alterations in the DNA damage response pathways and mitotic checkpoints may constitute another important pathogenetic mechanism in this lymphoma subtype. One of the most frequently observed secondary cytogenetic alterations in MCL are deletions in the chromosomal region 11q22-23 where the *ATM* gene is located.[93] *ATM* mutations have been detected in 40–75 percent of MCL and they mainly affect the PI3 kinase domain or lead to truncations of the ATM protein.[94] *ATM* encodes for a phosphoprotein kinase that belongs to the PI3 kinase-related superfamily and plays a central role in the cellular response to DNA damage. Importantly, ATM is required for the activation of p53 in response to DNA damage and during normal immunoglobulin V-D-J recombination and controls phosphorylation of effector genes such as *P53*, *MDM2*, *BRCA1*, *CHK2* and *NBS1*.[95]

ATM inactivation in MCL is associated with a high number of chromosomal alterations suggesting that it may, at least in part, be responsible for the chromosomal instability in these tumors.[94] The finding that *ATM* alterations occur in classical and blastoid MCL variants at similar frequencies and do not appear to be associated with tumor cell proliferation or the clinical behavior of the disease raises the possibility that ATM alterations represent a very early phenomenon or a predisposing event in these neoplasms. In line with this hypothesis, heterozygous germline *ATM* mutations have been described in occasional MCL patients in whom the tumor cells had subsequently lost the wild-type allele.[94]

Downstream targets of ATM in the DNA damage pathway may occasionally be altered in MCL as well (Fig. 29.2). CHK2 and CHK1 are two kinases that act downstream of ATM and prevent cell cycle progression in response to ATM and ATR activation after DNA damage is detected.[95]

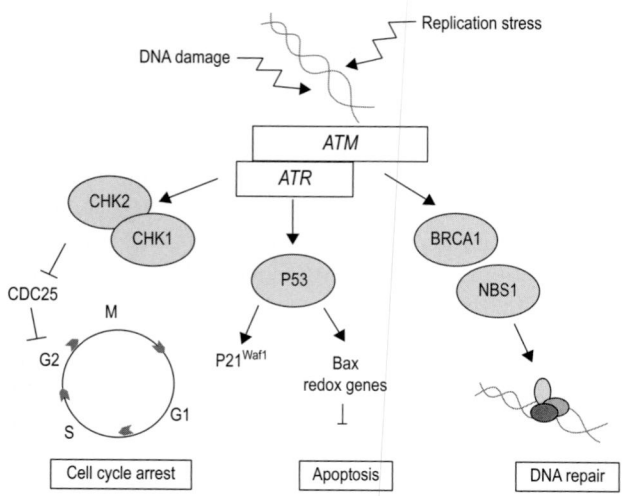

Figure 29.2 Deregulation of the DNA damage response pathway. ATM inactivation by mutation and deletions of 11q22 is frequently detected in mantle cell lymphoma (MCL). ATM plays a central role in DNA damage response and during normal immunoglobulin V-D-J recombination, activates p53 and controls phosphorylation of effector genes such as *P53*, *MDM2*, *BRCA1*, *CHK2* and *NBS1*. ATM inactivation may allow accumulation of additional chromosomal aberrations. ATM and germline *CHK2* gene mutations raise the possibility of these genetic alterations as a very early event in these neoplasms.

CHK2 stabilizes and activates p53 by phosphorylating the p53 binding site for MDM2 and blocks cell cycle progression at the G2/M phase by inhibiting Cdc25c. Although decreased protein levels and mutations of *CHK2* are rare events in B-NHL, these alterations have been described in a subset of MCL with a high number of chromosomal imbalances.[96] Importantly, germline *CHK2* mutations observed in some MCL patients raise the possibility that these mutations may predispose to the development of MCL analogous to germline *ATM* mutations.[96,97] Similarly, CHK1 protein is downregulated in occasional cases of MCL, but as yet no mutations of the gene have been found.[98]

Other oncogenic events

The high number of genetic alterations observed in MCL has promoted the search for additional potential targets of these chromosomal aberrations involved in the pathogenesis of these tumors. *MYC* is overexpressed in 38 percent of the tumors with a slightly higher frequency in blastoid than in typical variants and its overexpression levels are of prognostic significance.[99,100] Although occasional *MYC* gene amplification and rearrangements have been observed in blastoid MCL variants, these alterations are relatively uncommon and associated with an aggressive clinical course.[65,71,72,99] *BCL2* gene amplification and homozygous deletions of the proapoptotic *BIM* gene have been

observed in MCL cell lines but the presence of these alterations in primary tumors is not well kown.[69,101]

Mantle cell lymphoma gene expression profile

Several studies have analyzed the global expression profile of MCL, showing a specific expression pattern different from other B cell neoplasms.[53,61,102,103] Overexpression of cell cycle-related genes is a constant finding in these studies and the quantification of a small subset of these genes allows definition of groups of patients with markedly different survival.[53] MCL seems to have also a relatively high expression of genes related to multidrug resistance.[61] MCL with high levels of 3′ truncated cyclin D1 mRNA transcripts has a higher expression of proliferation-associated genes.[53,74]

MANTLE CELL LYMPHOMA CELL LINES AND ANIMAL MODELS

In the past years, several cell lines have been derived from MCL. Some other cell lines, obtained before this entity was well defined, have been reinterpreted as originating in these tumors (Table 29.3).[101] The characterization of these cell lines is irregular but provides a broad spectrum of the phenotypic, genetic and molecular characteristics of MCL. Cyclin D1 is expressed in all the lines examined although at different levels. Interestingly, JVM-2, derived from a B-prolymphocytic leukemia, now considered as a morphologic variant of MCL, also expressed cyclin D2. Several MCL cell lines are infected by the Epstein–Barr virus (EBV). The presence of the virus in the cell lines is a marked difference with primary tumors in which the virus has never been demonstrated. This may be a limitation to compare certain studies in cell lines and primary tumors. The genetic alterations observed in these cell lines reproduce the complex karyotypes of the primary tumors. Curiously, NCEB-1 carries five to eight stable murine chromosomes and expresses both human and murine BCL2 protein.[105] The functional significance of this finding is not known but it is curious that this cell line has been relatively resistant to different drug treatments in *in vitro* experiments.[106] Similarly to the findings in human tumors, most of the cell lines show an alternative inactivation of the *P53* and *P16INK4A* genes. In addition to cell lines, some authors have used animal models to study this disease experimentally. Unfortunately, transgenic animals overexpressing cyclin D1 generate lymphomas that are not similar to human MCL.[107] An alternative model is the use MCL cell lines as xenografts on immunodeficient mice. These grafts seem to retain the properties of human tumors with disseminated and leukemic disease, which may be used for experimental studies of new drugs and treatments.[108]

Table 29.3 Mantle cell lymphoma (MCL) cell lines carrying the t(11;14)(q13;q32) translocation (modified from Salaverria et al.[101] and Bea et al.[104])

	HBL2	JVM2	SP-49/-50B/-53	REC1	NCEB1	GRANTA-519	Mino	Z138	JEKO1	M1	UPN1	UPN2	MAVER-1
Age/gender	84/M	63/F	58/F	61/F	57/M	58/F	64/M	70/M	78/F	58/M	52/M	57/M	77/M
Original diagnosis	DLCL	PLL	ILL	MCL	DCb/CcL	MCL	MCL	Blastoid MCL	MCL	Blastoid MCL	Blastoid MCL	MCL	MCL
Sample	LN	PB	PB	LN	PB	PB	PB	BM	PB	PB	Pleural effusion	Pleural effusion	PB
Cyclin D1 overexpression	++	+	+	++	+	+	+	++	+		++	++	+
CD5	-	+	-		+	-	+	-	+	+	+	+	+
CD23	+	+	-		+	+	-	-	-	-	-	+	-
EBV	-	+	-/+/-	-	+	+	-	-	-	+	-	-	-
Ploidy	2N	2N	3N	2N-	4N-	2N-	3N+	2N+	3N-	2N+	2N-	3N+	2N
CC/M-FISH/SKY	Yes	Yes	Yes	Yes	Yes	Yes	Yes	Yes	Yes	Yes	Yes	Yes	Yes
mCGH/aCGH	Yes	Yes	Yes	Yes	Yes	Yes		Yes	Yes	Yes	Yes	Yes	Yes
P53 status	del/mut	wt/wt		wt/wt	del/mut	del/wt	uPD/mut	wt/[b]	del/mut		del/mut	del/mut	del/mut
ATM status		wt/wt		wt/[b]	del/[a,b]	del/mut[a]			ampl/[b]		c/polymorph	c/mut	del/[b]
P16INK4A status	hom del	wt/[c]		hom del	wt	hom del		hom del	del/[b]				hom del
P16ink4a exp WB	-	+	-		+		+	-	+				-
Other oncogenes	BCL2 amp					BCL2 amp	BCL2 amp	BCL2 amp	MYC amp		MYCR amp	MYCR	MYCR amp

[a]ATM protein expression negative; [b]mutational analysis not performed; [c]deletions not analyzed.

+, positive expression; ++ strong expression; -, negative/no detectable expression.

M, male; F, female; DLCL, diffuse large cell lymphoma; PLL, prolymphocytic leukemia; ILL, intermediate lymphocytic lymphoma; DCbCcL, diffuse centroblastic centrocytic lymphoma; CC, conventional cytogenetics; M-FISH, multicolor fluorescence in situ hybridization; SKY, multicolor spectral karyotyping; mCGH, metaphase comparative genomic hybridization; BM, bone marrow; EBV, Epstein–Barr virus; LN, lymph node; PB, peripheral blood; WB, Western blot; uPD, uniparental disomy detected by SNP array (100 K); aCGH, array comparative genomic hybridization; del, heterozygous deletion; mut, mutated; hom del, homozygous deletion; wt, wild type.

CLINICAL CHARACTERISTICS AND EVOLUTION

Most MCL patients present with stage IV disease with generalized lymphadenopathy and bone marrow involvement. Bulky disease and B symptoms are less common.[30,86,109] Hepatosplenomegaly is relatively frequent and massive splenomegaly is observed in 30–60 percent of the cases. Some patients have prominent splenomegaly with minimal or absent peripheral lymphadenopathy. This presentation is usually associated with peripheral blood involvement and the tumors seem to have a more indolent behavior than conventional MCL with nodal presentation.[9] Extranodal involvement is almost constant in MCL but not always clinically relevant. Tumor involvement in more than two extranodal sites is observed in 30–50 percent of the patients but an extranodal presentation without apparent nodal involvement occurs in only 4–15 percent of the cases. Asymptomatic involvement of the gastrointestinal tract with no macroscopic lesions is very common, but the detection of this microscopic infiltration rarely modifies the clinical management of the patients.[28] Clinical manifestations due to gastrointestinal involvement have been reported in 10–25 percent of the patients. Patients with 'lymphomatoid polyposis' may present with abdominal pain and melena. Central nervous system (CNS) involvement occurs in 10–20 percent of the patients. In contrast to other extranodal sites, CNS involvement usually appears as a late event in the evolution of the patients and is part of a resistant disease or generalized relapse with ominous significance.[110] Other extranodal sites commonly involved are the Waldeyer ring, lung and pleura (5–20 percent). Less common localizations are skin, breast, soft tissues, thyroid, salivary glands, peripheral nerves, conjunctiva and orbit.[30]

Peripheral blood involvement at diagnosis varies among studies depending in part on the definition of the disease. Conventional examination may detect leukemic involvement at diagnosis in 20–70 percent of the patients. Atypical lymphoid cells may be observed in the peripheral blood in the absence of lymphocytosis[24] and they may be detected by flow cytometry in virtually all the patients. Leukemic involvement may also appear during the evolution of the disease and may represent a manifestation of disease progression. Some patients may present with a very aggressive leukemic form mimicking acute leukemia. These cases have blastoid morphology, complex karyotypes, occasionally with 8q24 anomalies, and very rapid evolution with a median survival of only three months.[71,111]

Anemia and thrombocytopenia occur in 10–40 percent of the patients and high levels of lactate dehydrogenase (LDH) and β_2-microglobulin levels are detected in approximately 50 percent of the cases. A monoclonal serum component, usually at low levels, has been reported in 10–30 percent of the patients.[86] However, the immunoglobulin isotype is different in the serum and tumor cell surface in some cases. A second neoplasm detected before, concomitantly, or after the diagnosis of MCL, has been reported in 12–21 percent of the patients with a certain predominance of urinary tract tumors, suggesting that patients with MCL have an increased incidence of second malignancies.[30,112]

Clinical evolution in MCL patients is aggressive. The median overall survival in different series is around 3–4 years. Complete remission with conventional chemotherapy is only obtained in 6–35 percent of cases, although it has reached 50 percent in some series.[31,86,108] However, the disease-free survival period is short and very few patients achieve long-term remission. After relapse, patients may have a relatively slow course for several months with enlargement of lymph nodes and increased resistance to chemotherapy, which is followed by a more rapid and progressive evolution in a final accelerated phase. Although the initial clinical presentation of blastoid variants is relatively similar to typical MCL, the clinical evolution is much more aggressive.[86,113] Patients with blastoid MCL have a poor response to therapy and usually fail to achieve complete remissions. Absence of complete remission in these patients is associated with a rapid progressive course of the disease and death. In patients with complete remission, the duration of the response is usually short and virtually all patients relapse in less than one year.[113]

PROGNOSTIC PARAMETERS

Retrospective studies have analyzed the prognostic significance of different morphologic, genetic, molecular and clinical parameters in MCL.

Morphologic characteristics

The mantle zone pattern has been associated with more frequent localized disease and longer survival. However, the number of cases with this particular pattern is low in most series.[19,30,31,86] A predominant nodular growth pattern has been associated with better survival than a diffuse pattern in some studies[19] but not in others,[30,31] probably due to the frequent overlap and difficulty in defining the limits between them. Several studies have shown that blastoid morphology is associated with poor prognosis, with a median survival of approximately 14–18 months, significantly shorter than the 50 months of patients with classical morphology.[30,86,113] Blastoid morphology reflects several biologic factors related to poor prognosis such as high proliferation[86] complex karyotypes[65] and molecular alterations.[92] In multivariate analysis, both the architectural pattern and cytologic variant lose their predictive value in favor of the proliferative activity of the tumors.[19,30,86]

Proliferative activity

Early studies of centrocytic lymphoma had recognized that an increased mitotic index was an important prognostic parameter. The exact number of mitosis for which prognostic significance was shown varied, but a mitotic rate greater than 1.5–2.5 mitosis per HPF generally indicated a more aggressive course.[30,86] Concordantly, a high proliferative index recognized by Ki-67 is a good predictor of poor survival.[86] High proliferation is usually associated with a blastoid morphology but there are tumors with classical cytology that have high proliferative activity and are also associated with a rapid clinical course. The microarray analysis of the global expression profile in MCL has confirmed that the quantification of the proliferation signature is the best predictor factor of survival. Interestingly, the quantification of this signature is very discriminative allowing the identification of patients with median survival ranging from less than 1 year to more than 6 years.[53] New molecular proliferative markers recognized by immunohistochemistry such as topoisomerase II-α or MCM6 may be useful in routinely processed samples and may improve the predictive value of the Ki-67 detection.[114,115]

Genetic aberrations

FISH and CGH studies have shown a more aggressive clinical evolution in patients with complex karyotypes.[10,64,65] In particular, the number of chromosomal gains in chromosomes 3q, 12q and Xq, and losses in 9p and 17p are associated with shorter survival. An array CGH study has identified the loss of 9p21, 9q21-q22 and 17p13 as a predictor of poor survival whereas the loss of 1p21 was associated with better prognosis.[12]

Molecular alterations

Molecular studies have identified the inactivation of *P53* and *P16INK4a* as predictors of shortened survival. These alterations are closely related to the proliferative activity of the tumors and it has been suggested that this increased proliferation represents an integrator of different oncogenic events.[53,87,91] However, the presence of simultaneous oncogenic events in the two major cell cycle regulatory pathways *P16/CDK4* and *ARF/P53* in MCL has been shown to be associated with poor survival, which was independent of the Ki-67 proliferative index, suggesting that these oncogenic aberrations may have some influence on the behavior of the tumors independently of the proliferation.[92]

Clinical parameters

The main clinical parameters associated with poor prognosis are advanced age (>65–70 years), poor performance status, advanced stage, splenomegaly, elevated LDH, low albumin serum levels, bulky disease and anemia.[30,31,86,116] Multivariate analyses in some series have not confirmed the independent prognostic value of leukemic involvement at diagnosis.[113] The International Prognostic Index has been found to be of prognostic value in some series, but not in others,[30,86] probably because most of the patients fall into high-risk categories. Some patients with a very indolent clinical course have been identified. These patients may not require treatment for more than 5 years. Although they present with a non-nodal disease and leukemic expression, precise criteria to determine the management of these patients have not been defined.

TREATMENT OF MANTLE CELL LYMPHOMA

Treatment of patients with MCL remains a challenge. Conventional chemotherapeutic regimens, mainly based on the CHOP (cyclophosphamide, vincristine, doxorubicin and prednisolone) combination, have been extensively used in these patients. These regimens obtain a relatively high number of responses but the tumor relapses virtually in all patients, who eventually die of the disease. In the past few years, new strategies have appeared including therapies targeting crucial biologic cellular pathways, which may change the management and outcome in these patients.[117,118]

The combination of the anti-CD20 antibody rituximab to standard CHOP seems to increase the response rate and duration but does not increase the global outcome of the patients.[119] Intensive chemotherapy regimens such as hyperCVAD also obtain high number of complete remissions and the combination with rituximab may give similar results than the additional stem cell transplantation previously proposed in these patients.[120] This intensive regimen is not recommended for older patients (>65 years) due to higher toxicity and the shorter disease-free survival time. Purine nucleoside analogs have been proposed for relapsed patients or patients who are not candidates for stem cell transplantation. Particularly the combination of fludarabine, cyclophosphamide and mitoxantrone (FCM) with rituximab seems to improve the response rate and survival of relapsed patients. 2-Chlorodeoxyadenosine (2-CDA) has been used in combination with mitoxantrone.[118] These combinations may be useful for patients in advanced age or not tolerating anthracyclines. Several strategies based on stem cell transplantation have been proposed in MCL. If the patient is eligible for this therapy, an autologous stem cell transplant has been recommended after complete remission is achieved with an R-CHOP (rituximab, cyclophosphamide, vincristine, doxorubicin and prednisolone) regimen.[118]

A large number of new therapeutic agents targeting molecular pathways involved in the pathogenesis of this lymphoma are being proposed. The results of two separate phase II clinical trials conducted in relapsed or refractory MCL treated with the proteasome inhibitor bortezomib have shown promising results in relapsed patients intensively treated, with an overall response rate greater than 40 percent and a relatively long duration of the responses.[121,122] Although the inhibition of the proteasome may target several cell pathways including p53 and nuclear factor-κB, it seems that bortezomib induces cytotoxicity in MCL cells through the induction of the proapoptotic protein Noxa.[123]

mTOR (mammalian target of rapamycin) inhibitors have also been proposed as promising agents for cancer therapy.[118] Other new agents with attractive potential in MCL are mTOR inhibitors such as the rapamycin analog temsirolimus, flavopyridole, an inhibitor of CDKs, thalidomide or its analogs and histone deacetylase inhibitors.[117, 118] These compounds alone or in combination with standard chemotherapy may improve the outcome of MCL patients. Given the aggressive behavior of this tumor and the new therapeutic possibilities, patients should be advised to participate in quality clinical trials that may provide useful information in the coming years.[118]

KEY POINTS

- MCL is an aggressive neoplasm genetically characterized by the presence of the t(11;14) translocation leading to the overexpression of cyclin D1.
- Morphologically, MCL is characterized by the proliferation of a spectrum of atypical lymphoid cells, ranging from small cells with irregular nuclei to blastoid variants with pleomorphic or blastic nuclei.
- The phenotype of MCL is characterized by the expression of mature B cell antigens and CD5, but is negative for CD23 and CD10. Cyclin D1 is consistently expressed. A very small subset of cyclin D1 negative MCL have been recognized but this diagnosis has to be made with caution.
- Patients with MCL commonly present with disseminated disease, generalized lymphadenopathy and frequent extranodal and peripheral blood involvement. The clinical course is usually aggressive.
- The proliferative activity is the best prognostic parameter and may help discriminate between patients with a short median survival of less than 1 year and patients with median survival longer than 6 years.
- Current therapeutic strategies include a combination of CHOP-rituximab as well as intensive protocols. Studies of new therapeutic agents including the proteasome inhibitor bortezomib have provided promising results.

REFERENCES

● = Key primary paper
◆ = Major review article

1. Jaffe ES, Harris NL, Stein H, Vardiman JW. *World Health Organization classification of tumors. Pathology and genetics of tumours of haematopoietic and lymphoid tissues.* Lyon: IARC Press, 2001.
◆2. Campo E, Raffeld M, Jaffe ES. Mantle-cell lymphoma. *Semin Hematol* 1999; **36**: 115–27.
◆3. Swerdlow SH, Williams ME. From centrocytic to mantle cell lymphoma: a clinicopathologic and molecular review of 3 decades. *Hum Pathol* 2002; **33**: 7–20.
4. Tort F, Camacho E, Bosch F *et al.* Familial lymphoid neoplasms in patients with mantle cell lymphoma. *Haematologica* 2004; **89**: 314–19.
5. Fernandez V, Jares P, Bea S *et al.* Frequent polymorphic changes but not mutations of TRAIL receptors DR4 and DR5 in mantle cell lymphoma and other B-cell lymphoid neoplasms. *Haematologica* 2004; **89**: 1322–31.
6. Welzel N, Le T, Marculescu R *et al.* Templated nucleotide addition and immunoglobulin JH-gene utilization in t(11;14) junctions: implications for the mechanism of translocation and the origin of mantle cell lymphoma. *Cancer Res* 2001; **61**: 1629–36.
7. Camacho FI, Algara P, Rodriguez A *et al.* Molecular heterogeneity in MCL defined by the use of specific VH genes and the frequency of somatic mutations. *Blood* 2003; **101**: 4042–6.
8. Kienle D, Krober A, Katzenberger T *et al.* VH mutation status and VDJ rearrangement structure in mantle cell lymphoma: correlation with genomic aberrations, clinical characteristics, and outcome. *Blood* 2003; **102**: 3003–9.
●9. Orchard J, Garand R, Davis Z *et al.* A subset of t(11;14) lymphoma with mantle cell features displays mutated IgVH genes and includes patients with good prognosis, nonnodal disease. *Blood* 2003; **101**: 4975–81.
10. Thelander EF, Walsh SH, Thorselius M *et al.* Mantle cell lymphomas with clonal immunoglobulin V(H)3–21 gene rearrangements exhibit fewer genomic imbalances than mantle cell lymphomas utilizing other immunoglobulin V(H) genes. *Mod Pathol* 2005; **18**: 331–9.
11. Carreras J, Villamor N, Colomo L *et al.* Immunohistochemical analysis of ZAP-70 expression in B-cell lymphoid neoplasms. *J Pathol* 2005; **205**: 507–13.
12. Rubio-Moscardo F, Climent J, Siebert R *et al.* Mantle-cell lymphoma genotypes identified with CGH to BAC microarrays define a leukemic subgroup of disease and predict patient outcome. *Blood* 2005; **105**: 4445–54.
13. Babbage G, Garand R, Robillard N *et al.* Mantle cell lymphoma with t(11;14) and unmutated or mutated VH genes expresses AID and undergoes isotype switch events. *Blood* 2004; **103**: 2795–98.
14. Guikema JE, Rosati S, Akkermans K *et al.* Quantitative RT-PCR analysis of activation-induced cytidine deaminase expression in tissue samples from mantle cell lymphoma and B-cell chronic lymphocytic leukemia patients. *Blood* 2005; **105**: 2997–8.
15. Majlis A, Pugh WC, Rodriguez MA *et al.* Mantle cell lymphoma: correlation of clinical outcome and biologic features with three histologic variants. *J Clin Oncol* 1997; **15**: 1664–71.

16. Hunt JP, Chan JA, Samoszuk M et al. Hyperplasia of mantle/marginal zone B cells with clear cytoplasm in peripheral lymph nodes. A clinicopathologic study of 35 cases. Am J Clin Pathol 2001; **116**: 550–9.

17. Espinet B, Sole F, Pedro C et al. Clonal proliferation of cyclin D1-positive mantle lymphocytes in an asymptomatic patient: an early-stage event in the development or an indolent form of a mantle cell lymphoma? Hum Pathol 2005; **36**: 1232–7.

18. Nodit L, Bahler DW, Jacobs SA et al. Indolent mantle cell lymphoma with nodal involvement and mutated immunoglobulin heavy chain genes. Hum Pathol 2003; **34**: 1030–4.

●19. Tiemann M, Schrader C, Klapper W et al. Histopathology, cell proliferation indices and clinical outcome in 304 patients with mantle cell lymphoma (MCL): a clinicopathological study from the European MCL Network. Br J Haematol 2005; **131**: 29–38.

20. Dreyling MH, Bullinger L, Ott G et al. Alterations of the cyclin D1/p16-pRB pathway in mantle cell lymphoma. Cancer Res 1997; **57**: 4608–14.

●21. Ott G, Kalla J, Ott MM et al. Blastoid variants of mantle cell lymphoma: frequent bcl-1 rearrangements at the major translocation cluster region and tetraploid chromosome clones. Blood 1997; **89**: 1421–9.

22. Ruchlemer R, Parry-Jones N, Brito-Babapulle V et al. B-prolymphocytic leukaemia with t(11;14) revisited: a splenomegalic form of mantle cell lymphoma evolving with leukaemia. Br J Haematol 2004; **125**: 330–6.

23. Swerdlow SH, Zukerberg LR, Yang WI et al. The morphologic spectrum of non-Hodgkin's lymphomas with BCL1/cyclin D1 gene rearrangements. Am J Surg Pathol 1996; **20**: 627–40.

24. Pittaluga S, Verhoef G, Criel A et al. Prognostic significance of bone marrow trephine and peripheral blood smears in 55 patients with mantle cell lymphoma. Leuk Lymphoma 1996; **21**: 115–25.

25. Cohen PL, Kurtin PJ, Donovan KA, Hanson CA. Bone marrow and peripheral blood involvement in mantle cell lymphoma. Br J Haematol 1998; **101**: 302–10.

26. Piris MA, Mollejo M, Campo E et al. A marginal zone pattern may be found in different varieties of non-Hodgkin's lymphoma: the morphology and immunohistology of splenic involvement by B-cell lymphomas simulating splenic marginal zone lymphoma. Histopathology 1998; **33**: 230–9.

27. Isaacson PG, Maclennan KA, Subbuswamy SG. Multiple lymphomatous polyposis of the gastro-intestinal tract. Histopathology 1984; **8**: 641–56.

28. Romaguera JE, Medeiros LJ, Hagemeister FB et al. Frequency of gastrointestinal involvement and its clinical significance in mantle cell lymphoma. Cancer 2003; **97**: 586–91.

29. Drillenburg P, van der Voort R, Koopman G et al. Preferential expression of the mucosal homing receptor integrin alpha 4 beta 7 in gastrointestinal non-Hodgkin's lymphomas. Am J Pathol 1997; **150**: 919–27.

30. Argatoff LH, Connors JM, Klasa RJ et al. Mantle cell lymphoma: a clinicopathologic study of 80 cases. Blood 1997; **89**: 2067–78.

31. Norton AJ, Matthews J, Pappa V et al. Mantle cell lymphoma: Natural history defined in a serially biopsied population over a 20-year period. Ann Oncol 1995; **6**: 249–56.

32. Laszlo T, Matolcsy A. Blastic transformation of mantle cell lymphoma: genetic evidence for a clonal link between the two stages of the tumour. Histopathology 1999; **35**: 355–9.

33. Fend F, Quintanilla-Martinez L, Kumar S et al. Composite low grade B-cell lymphomas with two immunophenotypically distinct cell populations are true biclonal lymphomas. A molecular analysis using laser capture microdissection. Am J Pathol 1999; **154**: 1857–66.

34. Tsang P, Pan L, Cesarman E et al. A distinctive composite lymphoma consisting of clonally related mantle cell lymphoma and follicle center cell lymphoma. Hum Pathol 1999; **30**: 988–92.

35. Cachia AR, Diss TC, Isaacson PG. Composite mantle-cell lymphoma and plasmacytoma. Hum Pathol 1997; **28**: 1291–5.

36. Yamaguchi M, Ohno T, Miyata E et al. Analysis of clonal relationship using single-cell polymerase chain reaction in a patient with concomitant mantle cell lymphoma and multiple myeloma. Int J Hematol 2001; **73**: 383–5.

37. Tinguely M, Rosenquist R, Sundstrom C et al. Analysis of a clonally related mantle cell and Hodgkin lymphoma indicates Epstein-Barr virus infection of a Hodgkin/Reed-Sternberg cell precursor in a germinal center. Am J Surg Pathol 2003; **27**: 1483–8.

38. Caleo A, Sanchez-Aguilera A, Rodriguez S et al. Composite Hodgkin lymphoma and mantle cell lymphoma: two clonally unrelated tumors. Am J Surg Pathol 2003; **27**: 1577–80.

39. Gong JZ, Lagoo AS, Peters D et al. Value of CD23 determination by flow cytometry in differentiating mantle cell lymphoma from chronic lymphocytic leukemia/small lymphocytic lymphoma. Am J Clin Pathol 2001; **116**: 893–7.

40. Kaleem Z, White G, Zutter MM. Aberrant expression of T-cell-associated antigens on B-cell non-Hodgkin lymphomas. Am J Clin Pathol 2001; **115**: 396–403.

41. Camacho FI, Garcia JF, Cigudosa JC et al. Aberrant Bcl6 protein expression in mantle cell lymphoma. Am J Surg Pathol 2004; **28**: 1051–6.

42. Bangerter M, Hildebrand A, Griesshammer M. Immunophenotypic analysis of simultaneous specimens from different sites from the same patient with malignant lymphoma. Cytopathology 2001; **12**: 168–76.

43. Natkunam Y, Warnke RA, Montgomery K et al. Analysis of MUM1/IRF4 protein expression using tissue microarrays and immunohistochemistry. Mod Pathol 2001; **14**: 686–94.

●44.   Bosch F, Jares P, Campo E et al. PRAD-1/Cyclin D1 gene overexpression in chronic lymphoproliferative disorders: a highly specific marker of mantle cell lymphoma. Blood 1994; 84: 2726–32.

45.   Ott MM, Helbing A, Ott G et al. bcl-1 rearrangement and cyclin D1 protein expression in mantle cell lymphoma. J Pathol 1996; 179: 238–42.

46.   Torlakovic E, Nielsen S, Vyberg M. Antibody selection in immunohistochemical detection of cyclin D1 in mantle cell lymphoma. Am J Clin Pathol 2005; 124: 782–9.

47.   Suzuki R, Takemura K, Tsutsumi M et al. Detection of cyclin D1 overexpression by real-time reverse-transcriptase-mediated quantitative polymerase chain reaction for the diagnosis of mantle cell lymphoma. Am J Pathol 2001; 159: 425–9.

48.   Hoechtlen-Vollmar W, Menzel G, Bartl R et al. Amplification of cyclin D1 gene in multiple myeloma: clinical and prognostic relevance. Br J Haematol 2000; 109: 30–8.

49.   Bosch F, Campo E, Jares P et al. Increased expression of the PRAD-1/CCND1 gene in hairy cell leukaemia. Br J Haematol 1995; 91: 1025–30.

50.   O'Malley DP, Vance GH, Orazi A. Chronic lymphocytic leukemia/small lymphocytic lymphoma with trisomy 12 and focal cyclin d1 expression: a potential diagnostic pitfall. Arch Pathol Lab Med 2005; 129: 92–5.

51.   Quintanilla-Martinez L, Thieblemont C, Fend F et al. Mantle cell lymphomas lack expression of p27Kip1, a cyclin-dependent kinase inhibitor. Am J Pathol 1998; 153: 175–82.

52.   Kremer M, Dirnhofer S, Nickl A et al. p27(Kip1) immunostaining for the differential diagnosis of small b-cell neoplasms in trephine bone marrow biopsies. Mod Pathol 2001; 14: 1022–9.

●53.   Rosenwald A, Wright G, Wiestner A et al. The proliferation gene expression signature is a quantitative integrator of oncogenic events that predicts survival in mantle cell lymphoma. Cancer Cell 2003; 3: 185–97.

●54.   Fu K, Weisenburger DD, Greiner TC et al. Cyclin D1-negative mantle cell lymphoma: a clinicopathologic study based on gene expression profiling. Blood 2005; 106: 4315–21.

55.   Yatabe Y, Suzuki R, Tobinai K et al. Significance of cyclin D1 overexpression for the diagnosis of mantle cell lymphoma: a clinicopathologic comparison of cyclin D1-positive MCL and cyclin D1-negative MCL-like B-cell lymphoma. Blood 2000; 95: 2253–61.

56.   Bigoni R, Negrini M, Veronese ML et al. Characterization of t(11;14) translocation in mantle cell lymphoma by fluorescent in situ hybridization. Oncogene 1996; 13: 797–802.

●57.   Vaandrager JW, Schuuring E, Zwikstra E et al. Direct visualization of dispersed 11q13 chromosomal translocations in mantle cell lymphoma by multicolor DNA fiber fluorescence in situ hybridization. Blood 1996; 88: 1177–82.

58.   Gazzo S, Felman P, Berger F et al. Atypical cytogenetic presentation of t(11;14) in mantle cell lymphoma. Haematologica 2005; 90: 1708–9.

59.   Wlodarska I, Meeus P, Stul M et al. Variant t(2;11)(p11;q13) associated with the IgK-CCND1 rearrangement is a recurrent translocation in leukemic small-cell B-non-Hodgkin lymphoma. Leukemia 2004; 18: 1705–10.

◆60.   Raffeld M, Jaffe ES. bcl-1, t(11;14), and mantle cell-derived lymphomas. Blood 1991; 78: 259–63.

61.   Thieblemont C, Nasser V, Felman P et al. Small lymphocytic lymphoma, marginal zone B-cell lymphoma, and mantle cell lymphoma exhibit distinct gene-expression profiles allowing molecular diagnosis. Blood 2004; 103: 2727–37.

62.   Chesi M, Bergsagel PL, Brents LA et al. Dysregulation of cyclin D1 by translocation into an IgH gamma switch region in two multiple myeloma cell lines. Blood 1996; 88: 674–81.

63.   Wlodarska I, Pittaluga S, Hagemeijer A et al. Secondary chromosome changes in mantle cell lymphoma. Haematologica 1999; 84: 594–9.

64.   Cuneo A, Bigoni R, Rigolin GM et al. Cytogenetic profile of lymphoma of follicle mantle lineage: correlation with clinicobiologic features. Blood 1999; 93: 1372–80.

●65.   Bea S, Ribas M, Hernandez JM et al. Increased number of chromosomal imbalances and high-level DNA amplifications in mantle cell lymphoma are associated with blastoid variants. Blood 1999; 93: 4365–74.

66.   Bentz M, Plesch A, Bullinger L et al. t(11;14)-positive mantle cell lymphomas exhibit complex karyotypes and share similarities with B-cell chronic lymphocytic leukemia. Genes Chromosomes Cancer 2000; 27: 285–94.

67.   Kohlhammer H, Schwaenen C, Wessendorf S et al. Genomic DNA-chip hybridization in t(11;14)-positive mantle cell lymphomas shows a high frequency of aberrations and allows a refined characterization of consensus regions. Blood 2004; 104: 795–801.

68.   Schraders M, Pfundt R, Straatman HM et al. Novel chromosomal imbalances in mantle cell lymphoma detected by genome-wide array-based comparative genomic hybridization. Blood 2005; 105: 1686–93.

69.   Tagawa H, Karnan S, Suzuki R et al. Genome-wide array-based CGH for mantle cell lymphoma: identification of homozygous deletions of the proapoptotic gene BIM. Oncogene 2005; 24: 1348–58.

70.   Martinez-Climent JA, Vizcarra E, Sanchez D et al. Loss of a novel tumor suppressor gene locus at chromosome 8p is associated with leukemic mantle cell lymphoma. Blood 2001; 98: 3479–82.

71.   Vaishampayan UN, Mohamed AN, Dugan MC et al. Blastic mantle cell lymphoma associated with Burkitt-type translocation and hypodiploidy. Br J Haematol 2001; 115: 66–8.

72.   Au WY, Horsman DE, Viswanatha DS et al. 8q24 translocations in blastic transformation of mantle cell lymphoma. Haematologica 2000; 85: 1225–7.

73. van Dongen JJ, Langerak AW, Bruggemann M et al. Design and standardization of PCR primers and protocols for detection of clonal immunoglobulin and T-cell receptor gene recombinations in suspect lymphoproliferations: report of the BIOMED-2 Concerted Action BMH4-CT98-3936. *Leukemia* 2003; **17**: 2257–317.

74. Sander B, Flygare J, Porwit-MacDonald A et al. Mantle cell lymphomas with low levels of cyclin D1 long mRNA transcripts are highly proliferative and can be discriminated by elevated cyclin A2 and cyclin B1. *Int J Cancer* 2005; **117**: 418–30.

75. de Boer CJ, Vaandrager JW, van Krieken JH et al. Visualization of mono-allelic chromosomal aberrations 3' and 5' of the cyclin D1 gene in mantle cell lymphoma using DNA fiber fluorescence *in situ* hybridization. *Oncogene* 1997; **15**: 1599–603.

76. Rimokh R, Berger F, Delsol G et al. Detection of the chromosomal translocation t(11;14) by polymerase chain reaction in mantle cell lymphomas. *Blood* 1994; **83**: 1871–5.

77. Betticher DC, Thatcher N, Altermatt HJ et al. Alternate splicing produces a novel cyclin D1 transcript. *Oncogene* 1995; **11**: 1005–11.

78. Howe D, Lynas C. The cyclin D1 alternative transcripts [a] and [b] are expressed in normal and malignant lymphocytes and their relative levels are influenced by the polymorphism at codon 241. *Haematologica* 2001; **86**: 563–9.

79. Bala S, Peltomaki P. CYCLIN D1 as a genetic modifier in hereditary nonpolyposis colorectal cancer. *Cancer Res* 2001; **61**: 6042–5.

80. Zukerberg LR, Benedict WF, Arnold A et al. Expression of the retinoblastoma protein in low-grade B-cell lymphoma: relationship to cyclin D1. *Blood* 1996; **88**: 268–76.

81. Jares P, Campo E, Pinyol M et al. Expression of retinoblastoma gene product (pRb) in mantle cell lymphomas. Correlation with cyclin D1 (PRAD1/CCND1) mRNA levels and proliferative activity. *Am J Pathol* 1996; **148**: 1591–600.

82. Chiarle R, Budel LM, Skolnik J et al. Increased proteasome degradation of cyclin-dependent kinase inhibitor p27 is associated with a decreased overall survival in mantle cell lymphoma. *Blood* 2000; **95**: 619–26.

83. Quintanilla-Martinez L, Davies-Hill T, Fend F et al. Sequestration of p27Kip1 protein by cyclin D1 in typical and blastic variants of mantle cell lymphoma (MCL): implications for pathogenesis. *Blood* 2003; **101**: 3181–7.

84. Coqueret O. Linking cyclins to transcriptional control. *Gene* 2002; **299**: 35–55.

85. Lamb J, Ramaswamy S, Ford HL et al. A mechanism of cyclin D1 action encoded in the patterns of gene expression in human cancer. *Cell* 2003; **114**: 323–34.

86. Bosch F, Lopez-Guillermo A, Campo E et al. Mantle cell lymphoma: presenting features, response to therapy, and prognostic factors. *Cancer* 1998; **82**: 567–75.

87. Pinyol M, Hernandez L, Cazorla M et al. Deletions and loss of expression of p16INK4a and p21Waf1 genes are associated with aggressive variants of mantle cell lymphomas. *Blood* 1997; **89**: 272–80.

88. Bea S, Tort F, Pinyol M et al. BMI-1 gene amplification and overexpression in hematological malignancies occur mainly in mantle cell lymphomas. *Cancer Res* 2001; **61**: 2409–12.

89. Hutter G, Scheubner M, Zimmermann Y et al. Differential effect of epigenetic alterations and genomic deletions of CDK inhibitors [p16(INK4a), p15(INK4b), p14(ARF)] in mantle cell lymphoma. Genes chromosomes. *Cancer* 2006; **45**: 203–10.

90. Williams ME, Whitefield M, Swerdlow SH. Analysis of the cyclin-dependent kinase inhibitors p18 and p19 in mantle-cell lymphoma and chronic lymphocytic leukemia. *Ann Oncol* 1997;**8**(Suppl 2):71–3.

91. Hernandez L, Fest T, Cazorla M et al. p53 gene mutations and protein overexpression are associated with aggressive variants of mantle cell lymphomas. *Blood* 1996; **87**: 3351–9.

92. Hernandez L, Bea S, Pinyol M et al. CDK4 and MDM2 gene alterations mainly occur in highly proliferative and aggressive mantle cell lymphomas with wild-typeINK4a/ARF locus. *Cancer Res* 2005; **65**: 2199–206.

93. Stilgenbauer S, Winkler D, Ott G et al. Molecular characterization of 11q deletions points to a pathogenic role of the ATM gene in mantle cell lymphoma. *Blood* 1999; **94**: 3262–4.

94. Camacho E, Hernandez L, Hernandez S et al. ATM gene inactivation in mantle cell lymphoma mainly occurs by truncating mutations and missense mutations involving the phosphatidylinositol-3 kinase domain and is associated with increasing numbers of chromosomal imbalances. *Blood* 2002; **99**: 238–44.

95. Zhou BB, Elledge SJ. The DNA damage response: putting checkpoints in perspective. *Nature* 2000; **408**: 433–9.

96. Tort F, Hernandez S, Bea S et al. CHK2-decreased protein expression and infrequent genetic alterations mainly occur in aggressive types of non-Hodgkin lymphomas. *Blood* 2002; **100**: 4602–8.

97. Hangaishi A, Ogawa S, Qiao Y et al. Mutations of Chk2 in primary hematopoietic neoplasms. *Blood* 2002; **99**: 3075–7.

98. Tort F, Hernandez S, Bea S et al. Checkpoint kinase 1 (CHK1) protein and mRNA expression is downregulated in aggressive variants of human lymphoid neoplasms. *Leukemia* 2005; **19**: 112–17.

99. Hernandez L, Hernandez S, Bea S et al. c-myc mRNA expression and genomic alterations in mantle cell lymphomas and other nodal non-Hodgkin's lymphomas. *Leukemia* 1999; **13**: 2087–93.

100. Nagy B, Lundan T, Larramendy ML et al. Abnormal expression of apoptosis-related genes in haematological malignancies: overexpression of MYC is poor prognostic sign in mantle cell lymphoma. *Br J Haematol* 2003; **120**: 434–41.

101. Salaverria I, Perez-Galan P, Colomer D, Campo E. Mantle cell lymphoma: from pathology and molecular pathogenesis to new therapeutic perspectives. *Haematologica* 2006; **91**: 11–16.

102. Martinez N, Camacho FI, Algara P *et al.* The molecular signature of mantle cell lymphoma reveals multiple signals favoring cell survival. *Cancer Res* 2003; **63**: 8226–32.

103. Islam TC, Asplund AC, Lindvall JM *et al.* High level of cannabinoid receptor 1, absence of regulator of G protein signalling 13 and differential expression of cyclin D1 in mantle cell lymphoma. *Leukemia* 2003; **17**: 1880–90.

104. Bea S, Salaverria I, Armengol L *et al.* Uniparental disomies, homozygous deletions, amplifications, and target genes in mantle cell lymphoma revealed by integrative high-resolution whole-genome profiling. *Blood* 2009; **113**: 3059–69.

105. Camps J, Salaverria I, Garcia MJ *et al.* Genomic imbalances and patterns of karyotypic variability in mantle-cell lymphoma cell lines. *Leuk Res* 2006; **30**: 923–34.

106. Ferrer A, Marce S, Bellosillo B *et al.* Activation of mitochondrial apoptotic pathway in mantle cell lymphoma: high sensitivity to mitoxantrone in cases with functional DNA-damage response genes. *Oncogene* 2004; **23**: 8941–9.

107. Gladden AB, Woolery R, Aggarwal P *et al.* Expression of constitutively nuclear cyclin D1 in murine lymphocytes induces B-cell lymphoma. *Oncogene* 2006; **25**: 998–1007.

108. M'kacher R, Farace F, Bennaceur-Griscelli A *et al.* Blastoid mantle cell lymphoma: evidence for nonrandom cytogenetic abnormalities additional to t(11;14) and generation of a mouse model. *Cancer Genet Cytogenet* 2003; **143**: 32–8.

109. Teodorovic I, Pittaluga S, Kluin-Nelemans JC *et al.* Efficacy of four different regimens in 64 mantle-cell lymphoma cases: clinicopathologic comparison with 498 other non-Hodgkin's lymphoma subtypes. European Organization for the Research and Treatment of Cancer Lymphoma Cooperative Group. *J Clin Oncol* 1995; **13**: 2819–26.

110. Montserrat E, Bosch F, Lopez-Guillermo A *et al.* CNS involvement in mantle-cell lymphoma. *J Clin Oncol* 1996; **14**: 941–4.

111. Viswanatha DS, Foucar K, Berry BR *et al.* Blastic mantle cell leukemia: an unusual presentation of blastic mantle cell lymphoma. *Mod Pathol* 2000; **13**: 825–33.

112. Barista I, Cabanillas F, Romaguera JE *et al.* Is there an increased rate of additional malignancies in patients with mantle cell lymphoma? *Ann Oncol* 2002; **13**: 318–22.

113. Bernard M, Gressin R, Lefrere F *et al.* Blastic variant of mantle cell lymphoma: a rare but highly aggressive subtype. *Leukemia* 2001; **15**: 1785–91.

114. Schrader C, Meusers P, Brittinger G *et al.* Topoisomerase IIalpha expression in mantle cell lymphoma: a marker of cell proliferation and a prognostic factor for clinical outcome. *Leukemia* 2004; **18**: 1200–6.

115. Schrader C, Janssen D, Klapper W *et al.* Minichromosome maintenance protein 6, a proliferation marker superior to Ki-67 and independent predictor of survival in patients with mantle cell lymphoma. *Br J Cancer* 2005; **93**: 939–45.

116. Pittaluga S, Wlodarska I, Stul MS *et al.* Mantle cell lymphoma: A clinicopathologic study of 55 cases. *Histopathology* 1995; **26**: 17–24.

117. O'connor OA. Targeting histones and proteasomes: new strategies for the treatment of lymphoma. *J Clin Oncol* 2005; **23**: 6429–36.

◆118. Witzig TE. Current treatment approaches for mantle-cell lymphoma. *J Clin Oncol* 2005; **23**: 6409–14.

119. Lenz G, Dreyling M, Hoster E *et al.* Immunochemotherapy with rituximab and cyclophosphamide, doxorubicin, vincristine, and prednisone significantly improves response and time to treatment failure, but not long-term outcome in patients with previously untreated mantle cell lymphoma: results of a prospective randomized trial of the German Low Grade Lymphoma Study Group (GLSG). *J Clin Oncol* 2005; **23**: 1984–92.

120. Romaguera JE, Fayad L, Rodriguez MA *et al.* High rate of durable remissions after treatment of newly diagnosed aggressive mantle-cell lymphoma with rituximab plus hyper-CVAD alternating with rituximab plus high-dose methotrexate and cytarabine. *J Clin Oncol* 2005; **23**: 7013–23.

●121. Goy A, Younes A, McLaughlin P *et al.* Phase II study of proteasome inhibitor bortezomib in relapsed or refractory B-cell non-Hodgkin's lymphoma. *J Clin Oncol* 2005; **23**: 667–75.

●122. O'connor OA, Wright J, Moskowitz C *et al.* Phase II clinical experience with the novel proteasome inhibitor bortezomib in patients with indolent non-Hodgkin's lymphoma and mantle cell lymphoma. *J Clin Oncol* 2005; **23**: 676–84.

●123. Perez-Galan P, Roue G, Villamor N *et al.* The proteasome inhibitor bortezomib induces apoptosis in mantle cell lymphoma through generation of ROS species and Noxa activation independent of p53 status. *Blood* 2006; **107**: 257–64.

30

Marginal zone lymphomas

DENNIS WRIGHT

INTRODUCTION

This chapter discusses three different categories of lymphoma:

- extranodal marginal zone lymphoma (EMZL);
- nodal marginal zone lymphoma (NMZL);
- splenic marginal zone lymphoma (SMZL).

The three categories share several characteristics besides occupation of the marginal zone around reactive germinal follicles.

Cell morphology

The neoplastic cells may have elongated, twisted nuclei, resembling those of small centrocytes of follicle centers. These are often referred to as centrocytoid cells. The cells may also have oval nuclei and relatively abundant pale staining cytoplasm – so-called monocytoid cells – or they may appear as small lymphocytes with variable numbers of interspersed blast cells. These appearances are to some extent fixation dependent and intermediate cytology may be seen.

Plasma cell differentiation

Plasma cell differentiation may be seen in all three categories, but it is more common and more prominent in extranodal than is usual in nodal or SMZLs. Tumors showing plasma cell differentiation may be associated with a monoclonal serum protein.

Follicular colonization

It is a characteristic of all three categories of marginal zone lymphoma to colonize preexisting reactive germinal follicles. This leads to progressive dispersion of the follicle center cells. Sometimes the only evidence of a preexisting follicle is the demonstration by immunohistochemistry of follicular dendritic cells at the center of a tumor nodule.

Tumor progression

All three tumors may show progression to large B cell lymphoma. This progression is least common in SMZL.

Despite these similarities these tumors appear to arise from functionally different subsets of marginal zone B cells and their pathogenesis appears to proceed along different pathways. Generally they are clinically distinct, although in individual cases it might be difficult to determine whether NMZL is primary or secondary to one of the other subtypes. The cytogenetic characteristics of the three subgroups show differences, for example whereas the most frequent cytogenetic abnormality seen in SMZL is 7q deletion, this is not seen in EMZL which often exhibits characteristic chromosomal translocations and trisomies.

EXTRANODAL MARGINAL ZONE B CELL LYMPHOMA

History and definition

Extranodal marginal zone B cell lymphoma was first described by Isaacson and Wright,[1,2] who attempted to relate the morphology and behavior of these tumors to that of the physiologic mucosa-associated lymphoid tissue (MALT). Tumors at all sites have the characteristics of marginal zone B cell lymphoma showing, to varying degrees, clear cytoplasm, plasma cell differentiation, follicular colonization and lymphoepithelial lesions. In the past the reactive components of these tumors together with their indolent behavior led to the use of the term pseudolymphoma. Distinguishing EMZL from reactive/inflammatory processes may still present problems in some cases, however, developments in immunohistochemistry and molecular techniques to determine clonality have largely overcome this problem.

Morphology

The cytology of EMZL as described above may be centrocytoid, monocytoid or small lymphocytic with blast cells. In well-fixed preparations these cells are usually seen to have clear cytoplasm. In a biopsy the monomorphism of these cells in large groups or sheets will often be the first indication of a neoplastic rather than a reactive lymphoid process. Plasmacytoid/plasmacytic differentiation is common in EMZL and the monotypia of these cells with regard to light chain expression is strong evidence of a neoplastic process. The presence of large numbers of reactive plasma cells in a biopsy may be confusing or misleading. Interpretation is aided by the fact that reactive plasma cells are usually intermingled with other lymphoid cells whereas

neoplastic plasma cells often occur as zones of monomorphic cells. Immunoperoxidase staining for immunoglobulin also differs between reactive and neoplastic plasma cells; the former staining black and the latter usually having a paler brown color. Immunostaining for CD3 and CD5 will usually show large numbers of T cells in EMZL.

EMZL arise on an inflammatory background of acquired MALT. Reactive lymphoid follicles may be present within infiltrates of marginal zone B cells. Over time, however, follicular colonization by the neoplastic cells will gradually obliterate the follicles, sometimes giving the tumor an overall nodular appearance. In such cases staining with follicular dendritic cell markers (CD21, CD23, CD35) will usually reveal the dispersed remains of these cells. This is a valuable diagnostic aid, particularly in small biopsy specimens. Variable numbers of B cell blasts are seen in most EMZLs. These are not evidence of transformation, which should only be considered in the presence of large aggregates of blast cells.[3]

Lymphoepithelium is a characteristic feature of MALT in which large numbers of T and B cells singly infiltrate the overlying epithelium. Lymphoepithelial lesions are a characteristic feature of EMZL. These differ from non-neoplastic lymphoepithelium in that clusters of neoplastic marginal zone B cells infiltrate between epithelial cells, often resulting in the distortion and degeneration of epithelial structures. The appearance of lymphoepithelial lesions varies at different sites, presumably related to the structure and kinetics of the epithelium involved. In diagnostic biopsies lymphoepithelial lesions can often be highlighted with immunohistochemical stains for cytokeratins. Lymphoepithelial lesions have been reported in inflammatory gastritis but they are not as well defined or prominent as those seen in EMZL.[4]

STOMACH

Typical lymphoepithelial lesions occur at the base of gastric glands as intraepithelial clusters of marginal zone cells. Eventually the epithelial cells undergo degenerative changes and are seen as irregular clusters or single cells with eosinophilic cytoplasm.

SMALL INTESTINE

Immunoproliferative small intestinal disease (IPSID) shows characteristic lymphoepithelial lesions within crypt epithelium. This neoplasm shows marked plasma cell differentiation, but the plasma cells, as in all EMZLs, do not contribute to the lymphoepithelial lesions.

LUNG

Lymphoepithelial lesions may be seen in bronchial and bronchiolar epithelium. Staining for keratin often highlights a complex lacework of alveolar lining cells among the neoplastic cells.

SALIVARY GLAND

Lymphoepithelial lesions involve ductular epithelium, often showing large collections of marginal zone cells surrounded by attenuated ductal epithelium. Epimyoepithelial islands are a characteristic feature of Sjögren disease and are seen in many salivary EMZL. In themselves they are not diagnostic of EMZL. However, in EMZL they become infiltrated by marginal zone cells which eventually form a broad zone around them. At this stage they are a recognizable feature of EMZL.[5]

THYROID

In the thyroid gland, marginal zone lymphoma cells break into thyroid follicles. Rounded collections of marginal zone cells surrounded by attenuated thyroid epithelial cells, highlighted by stains for B cells or cytokeratins, are a characteristic diagnostic feature of this lymphoma.

OTHER EXTRANODAL MARGINAL ZONE LYMPHOMAS

Lymphoepithelial lesions have been described in EMZL at other sites, providing a valuable diagnostic feature. However, lymphoepithelial lesions are not found in all EMZLs and diagnosis is less dependent on this feature now that marginal zone lymphoma cells can be more reliably identified by their morphology and phenotype.

Epidemiology

EMZL accounts for 7–8 percent of all B cell lymphomas and over half of these are primary gastric lymphomas. Geographic variations in the prevalence of some EMZL presumably relates to the prevalence of underlying etiologic factors that may include genetic susceptibility.

Etiologic factors

The oropharyngeal tonsils and Peyer patches in the terminal ileum form prominent collections of MALT. However, EMZL is uncommon at these sites, more typically occurring at sites of acquired inflammatory or reactive lymphoid tissue.

STOMACH

The normal stomach is devoid of MALT. Infection with *Helicobacter pylori* leads to the acquisition of lymphoid tissue in the mucosa and submucosa with features of MALT. It is believed that this is the precursor lesion of gastric EMZL.[6] *H. pylori* can be demonstrated morphologically in gastric EMZL and approximately 70 percent of cases show tumor regression following eradication of the organism with antibiotic therapy. Isaacson and his coworkers showed that dispersed cells from gastric EMZL die within 5 days if cultured under standard conditions. If heat-killed *H. pylori* are, however, added to the culture, the tumor cells undergo proliferation and form clusters. This response was shown to be T cell dependent, interleukin 2 dependent and *H. pylori* substrain specific. Intratumoral T cells have been shown to be the source of this T cell specificity and presumably account for the localization of the tumor for long periods to the gastric mucosa.[7,8] In addition to the induction of MALT, *H. pylori* infection is associated with a brisk polymorph reaction. Free radicals associated with this inflammatory reaction may result in DNA damage, genetic abnormalities and the emergence of neoplastic B cells.[9,10]

SMALL INTESTINE

In its early stages, IPSID responds to tetracycline, ampicillin or metronidazole treatment, suggesting that it might have an infectious etiology. However, the search for a specific agent has been largely unsuccessful. Lecuit *et al.* demonstrated the presence of *Campylobacter jejuni*-specific sequences in intestinal tissue from a patient who showed a spectacular response to antimicrobial treatment. *In situ* hybridization and immunohistochemistry on this case and four of six archival cases identified *C. jejuni* antigens.[11] Larger studies are needed to clarify the possible role of *C. jejuni* in the pathogenesis of IPSID.

SALIVARY GLAND

Patients with Sjögren syndrome are at increased risk of developing EMZL of the salivary gland. An Italian study showed that of 33 patients with salivary gland EMZL, 15 had a history of Sjögren syndrome, 2 of other autoimmune diseases and 7 of hepatitis C virus (HCV) infection. No patient had both Sjögren syndrome and HCV infection.[12] The high incidence of HCV infection in patients with salivary EMZL reported from Italy is not seen in areas with a low prevalence of HCV infection in the wider community.

SKIN

The identification of marginal zone lymphoma of the skin has been greatly aided by advances in immunohistochemistry. In a review of 300 primary B cell lymphomas of the skin, Senff *et al.* found 71 patients with primary cutaneous marginal zone lymphoma.[13] Infection with *Borrelia burgdorferi*, the agent of Lyme disease, may be associated with lymphoid aggregates in the skin. Following a report of four cases of cutaneous EMZL associated with *B. burgdorferi* infection,[14] more studies from Europe reported polymerase chain reaction (PCR)-detected *B. burgdorferi* DNA in 7/20 primary cutaneous B cell lymphomas (5/12 EMZL, 1/5 follicle center cell lymphomas and 1/3 diffuse large B cell lymphomas) and in a later study 54/80 cutaneous EMZL.[15,16] Studies in the USA and Asia have, however, failed to detect an association between *B. burgdorferi* infection and cutaneous EMZL.[17,18] This may reflect the well-known genetic and phenotypic differences between strains of *B. burgdorferi* in Europe and the USA.

OCULAR ADNEXAL TISSUES

A study from Italy to determine whether chlamydial infection is associated with ocular adnexal lymphomas found that 32/40 (80 percent) biopsies contained *Chlamydia psittaci* DNA. Treatment with doxycycline resulted in complete tumor regression in two, partial regression in two and minimal regression in 3/7 patients studied.[19] In contrast, *C. psittaci* was not detected in ocular adnexal lymphomas from the USA.[20,21] Chanudet *et al.* have recently reported a study of 142 ocular adnexal EMZL, 53 non-marginal zone lymphomas and 51 ocular adnexal biopsies without lymphoproliferative disease from six geographic regions.[22] They used PCR to detect DNA from *C. psittaci*, *Chlamydia trachomatis*, *Chlamydia pneumoniae*, herpes virus simplex 1 and 2 and adenovirus 8 and 19. *C. psittaci* was found in 22 of the ocular adnexal EMZLs; considerably higher than the two control groups. A remarkable finding was the large variation in the prevalence of *C. psittaci* in different geographic regions (Germany 47 percent, the USA 35 percent, the Netherlands 29 percent, Italy 13 percent, the UK 12 percent and southern China 11 percent).[22] These figures suggest that if *C. psittaci* is etiologically related to ocular adnexal EMZL strain variants may be important or the molecular characteristics of the lymphomas may vary in different regions.

THYROID

Chronic thyroiditis and Hashimoto disease are precursor lesions of thyroid EMZL. No infectious agents have been implicated in this lymphoma and it may be that chronic antigenic drive by thyroid autoantigens is sufficient for oncogenic progression.

THYMUS

Thymic EMZL is rare. The largest series of 15 cases reported showed a female predominance (12F:3M) and a strong association with Sjögren syndrome. Plasma cell differentiation was present in all cases and 13/15 cases expressed IgA in contrast with the expression of IgM by most EMZL other than IPSID. The majority of patients reported with primary thymic EMZL have been Asian.[23]

Immunophenotype

Surface IgM is expressed on most EMZLs, with cytoplasmic staining of the cells showing plasma cell differentiation. Other heavy chains are much less frequently expressed except in thymic EMZL which usually expresses IgA[23] and IPSID in which α heavy chain without demonstrable light chains is synthesized.[24,25] Extranodal marginal zone lymphoma cells express CD20 and CD79a, the latter being

particularly useful since it highlights plasma cell differentiation. The tumor cells are negative for CD5, CD10 and CD23 in contrast with most other small B cell lymphomas. They stain weakly for CD21 and CD35 though these two markers are more useful in highlighting follicular dendritic cells and thus identifying colonized follicles. The majority of EMZLs contain large numbers of T cells identified by stains for CD3 and CD5. Staining for immunoglobulin light chains is useful in differentiating monotypic (neoplastic) from polytypic (reactive) plasma cells. In common with other small B cell lymphomas EMZL are BCL2 positive, this antibody may however be useful in identifying BCL2 negative residual reactive follicle centers in the tumor.

Many MALT lymphomas are characterized by chromosomal translocations involving the *BCL10* gene on chromosome 1 or the *MALT1* gene on chromosome 18 (see below). These translocations are associated with abnormal expression of the gene products. In normal lymphoid tissues BCL10 and MALT1 proteins are expressed mainly in the cytoplasm, most strongly in follicle center centroblasts and less strongly in centrocytes. They are expressed weakly in marginal zone cells and are usually absent or weakly expressed in mantle cells. Neoplasms arising from follicle center or mantle cells show a similar pattern of expression.

t(14;18)(q32;q21) positive MALT lymphoma cells show strong cytoplasmic, sometimes perinuclear, expression of MALT1 and BCL10. MALT lymphomas bearing the t(1;14)(q22;q32) show weak to negative cytoplasmic staining for MALT1 but strong nuclear expression of BCL10. t(11;18)(q21;q21) positive tumors show weak cytoplasmic staining for MALT1 and weak to moderate nuclear positivity for BCL10. However, up to 20 percent of translocation negative tumors show a similar staining pattern.[26]

Genetics

IMMUNOGLOBULIN GENES

The immunoglobulin genes are rearranged and show somatic mutations consistent with postgerminal center derivation and in keeping with the frequent plasma cell differentiation seen in these tumors.[27,28] Analysis of the immunoglobulin produced by gastric EMZL has shown reactivity against autoantigens but not against *H. pylori*.[29,30] In a recent comparison of *IGVH* complementary determining regions (CDR), from a large number of B cell lymphomas with CDR sequences in Gen Bank, 8 of 45 gastric EMZL and 13 of 32 salivary gland EMZL expressed B cell antigen receptors with strong CDR3 homology to rheumatoid factor (RF). Rheumatoid factor binding reactivity was confirmed in a selection of cases by *in vitro* binding studies. In this study RF-CDR3 homology and t(11;18) were mutually exclusive and RF-CDR3 homology was not found in any of 19 pulmonary EMZL.[31] In contrast to these findings Lenze *et al.* amplified and cloned immunoglobulin gene rearrangements from seven EMZLs and expressed these as single chain fragment variable antibodies.[32] These were tested on

Table 30.1   Chromosomal abnormalities detected in extranodal marginal zone lymphoma

	Ye *et al.* 2005[26]	Streubel *et al.* 2004[34]	Sagaert *et al.* 2006[33]
Number of cases	423	252	77
t(11;18)(q21;q21) *AP12/MALT1*	67 (15.8%)	34 (13.5%)	8 (10.3%)
t(1;14)(q22;q32) *BCL10/IGH*	12 (2.8%)	4 (1.6%)	1 (1.3%)
t(14;18)(q32;q21) *IGH/MALT1*	9 (2.1%)	27 (10.8%)	2 (2.6%)
Translocation negative	335 (79.1%)	187 (74.2%)	66 (85.7%)
Trisomy 3		78 (30.9%)	
Trisomy 18		28 (11.2%)	

human tissues using immunohistochemistry and on an expression library of 30 000 human proteins and on *H. pylori* lysates using western blotting. They found that the majority of tumor immunoglobulins showed no detectable reactivity against antigens. They concluded that tumor immunoglobulins do not have a significant role in the stimulation and proliferation of MALT lymphoma B cells and that tumor infiltrating T cells are more likely to stimulate the B cells by other receptors.[32]

CYTOGENETIC ABNORMALITIES AND ONCOGENES

A number of chromosomal abnormalities have been detected in EMZL including trisomies of chromosomes 3, 12 and 18, and a number of chromosomal translocations that appear to be specific for these tumors (Table 30.1).[26,33,34] These translocations are all mutually exclusive and show marked variation between MALT lymphomas at different sites.

- **t(11;18)(q21;q21):** This is the most common chromosomal translocation associated with EMZL, occurring in 25 percent of gastric lymphomas, 40 percent of pulmonary lymphomas and 5–15 percent of ocular adnexal lymphomas, but rarely at other sites.[10,34,35] This translocation fuses the *AP12* gene on chromosome 11 with the *MALT1* gene on chromosome 18. AP12 inhibits proteins involved in apoptosis. MALT1 activates nuclear factor (NF)-κB, a major transcriptional regulator. The AP12–MALT1 fusion protein protects cells from apoptosis dependent on its ability to activate NF-κB.[36] In gastric EMZL t(11;18) is more common in cases that show tumor spread. It is not associated with other chromosomal abnormalities and tumors bearing this translocation rarely undergo high-grade transformation. t(11;18)-positive gastric EMZL, unlike the majority of cases without this translocation, does not regress following *H. pylori* eradication.[37–39]
- **t(1;14)(q22;q32):** In common with translocation-negative EMZL, t(1;14)(q22;q32) is frequently associated with trisomies of chromosomes 3, 12 and 18. This translocation occurs in approximately

8 percent of pulmonary and 4 percent of gastric EMZL.[10,39] It is not seen in other lymphomas. Gastric cases are frequently of advanced stage and do not respond to *H. pylori* eradication. t(1;14)(q22;q32) brings the *BCL10* gene on chromosome 1 under the influence of the immunoglobulin heavy chain enhancer on chromosome 14 resulting in deregulation. Bcl10 overexpression leads to NF-κB activation. Tumors harboring t(11;14) show strong aberrant nuclear expression of *BCL10*.[6] t(1;2)(q22;p12) is a rare variant of an immunoglobulin BCL10 translocation involving the *BCL10* gene on chromosome 1 and the κ light chain enhancer on chromosome 2.[40]

- **t(14;18)(q32;q21):** This translocation has been found in lung, ocular adnexal, salivary gland, liver and skin EMZL but is uncommon in gastric EMZL.[34] t(14;18) characterizes follicle center cell lymphomas involving the immunoglobulin heavy chain locus and the *BCL2* gene, however, in EMZL the 18q breakpoint involves the *MALT1* gene. The translocation brings the *MALT1* gene under the influence of the enhancer region of the immunoglobulin heavy chain gene and results in its over expression. High levels of cytoplasmic MALT1 and BCL10 are seen in the tumor cells; together they lead to NF-κB activation.[6]
- **t(3;14)(p14.1;q32):** Cytogenetic analysis of a thyroid EMZL led to the identification of this translocation. The breakpoints were found to involve the immunoglobulin heavy chain locus and the *FOXP1* gene (forkhead protein transcription factor). Fluorescence *in situ* hybridization (FISH) screening of 91 marginal zone lymphomas showed the translocation in nine cases, comprising thyroid (3/6), ocular adnexal (4/20) and skin (2/20). Extranodal marginal zone lymphoma of the stomach, salivary gland and lung was negative as were splenic and NMZLs. Most of the cases showing t(3;14) harbored additional genetic abnormalities such as trisomy 3.[41] This translocation and the three classic EMZL translocations discussed above are mutually exclusive. Sagaert *et al.*[42] used immunohistochemistry to detect expression of FOXP1 and FISH to identify structural or numerical aberrations of the *FOXP1*, *BCL10* and *MALT1* genes

on 70 EMZLs. These were divided into 53 cases showing monomorphic histology and 17 that contained scattered activated B blasts and were categorized as polymorphic. Eight cases showed strong nuclear expression of FOXP1; only one of these had monomorphic histology. Five had transformed to diffuse large B cell lymphoma, one of which was t(3;14)(p14.1;q32) positive and four showed trisomy 3 + 18. They conclude that EMZL with polymorphic histology showing strong nuclear expression of FOXP1 and trisomy 3 and 18 are at risk of transforming to diffuse large B cell lymphoma. In a study of 275 B cell non-Hodgkin lymphoma (NHL) including 102 diffuse large B cell lymphomas and 122 EMZLs. Haralambieva et al.[43] found five with translocations involving the FOXP1 locus. These were all diffuse large B cell lymphomas (3 gastrointestinal, 1 thyroid, 1 lymph node); none of the EMZL showed FOXP1 translocations. The IgH gene was the translocation partner in only two cases. Other studies have shown that the nuclear expression of FOXP1 in diffuse large B cell lymphomas is associated with a poor prognosis.[44,45]

- **Trisomy/polysomy of chromosomes 3 and 18**: The incidence of trisomy 3 reported in low-grade EMZL varies from 20 percent to 60 percent.[46,47] Trisomy/polysomy 3 is rarely seen in tumors that have t(11;18)(q21;q21) or t(14;18)(q32;q21), but is seen in tumors bearing t(1;14)(q22;q32) or t(3;14)(p14.1;q32) as well as tumors that have no translocations. Trisomy/polysomy 3 alone may be associated with upregulation of the FOXP1 gene.[42] Similarly trisomy/polysomy 18 may result in MALT1 amplification. Saegert et al. found that 10 out of 18 cases with trisomy/polysomy 18 showed aberrant BCL10 expression; presumably resulting from the close association between the MALT1 and BCL10 proteins.[33] There is a higher incidence of trisomy/polysomy in high grade than low grade ENMZ involving chromosomes 12 and 18, although trisomy 3 is seen more frequently in low grade tumors.[48]

Prognosis and predictive factors

EMZL occur at many sites, appears to have differing etiologies at these sites, exhibits a range of cytogenetic abnormalities and presents at different clinical stages. All of these factors may influence progression and survival. Most tumors run an indolent course even when disseminated. Seventy percent or more of low-stage gastric lymphomas regress following eradication of H. pylori, entering into prolonged remission or cure. Low-stage tumors that have transformed into diffuse large B cell lymphomas may also regress following eradication of H. pylori.[49,50] Tumors carrying the AP12–MALT1 translocation do not usually respond in this way and require treatment with radiation therapy or chemotherapy. These tumors, however, do not develop secondary cytogenetic abnormalities and do not progress to large cell lymphoma.[37] In contrast EMZLs bearing the FOXP1–IGH translocation or showing nuclear expression of FOXP1 show transformation to large cell lymphoma and have a poor clinical outcome.[42] Similarly tumors with the BCL10–IGH translocation are typically of advanced stage and do not respond to H. pylori eradication. Independent of translocations, nuclear expression of BCL10 or NF-κB predicts H. pylori independent status in both small cell and large cell (diffuse large B cell lymphoma) gastric EMZL.[51,52]

Are diffuse large B cell lymphomas at extranodal sites high-grade marginal zone lymphomas?

The World Health Organization (WHO) classification[3] states that the term 'high-grade MALT lymphoma' should not be used, and the term 'MALT lymphoma' should not be applied to large B cell lymphoma, even if it has arisen in a MALT site. It has been known for many years that the low grade and high grade components of gastric MALT lymphomas show identical light chain restriction.[53] It was subsequently shown that both components share common clone specific immunoglobulin heavy chain rearrangements.[54] More recently it has been established that low-stage, high-grade gastric lymphomas respond to H. pylori eradication with long-term remissions.[49,50] Differences in the response of the low-grade and high-grade components of gastric EMZL have been shown to be related to clonal differences between these components as detected by IgH gene sequencing.[55] Barth et al. performed transcriptional profiling on a series of low-grade/high-grade gastrointestinal marginal zone lymphomas and diffuse large B cell lymphomas without evidence of low-grade tumor. The profound similarity of the blastic diffuse large B cell lymphomas to primary large B cell lymphomas strongly suggested that that these also were blastic marginal zone lymphomas.[56]

Progression to high-grade EMZL is associated with aneuploidy and rarely occurs in t(11;18)(q21;q21) positive tumors. This progression is however a feature of t(1;14)(q22;q32) positive tumors, those with FOXP1 abnormalities as well as many tumors bearing no recognizable translocations. It may be significant that four of the five diffuse large B cell lymphomas bearing FOXP1 translocations reported by Haralambiever et al.[43] were at extranodal sites. It should be noted that high-grade EMZL can express the follicle center phenotype (CD10+ BCL6+). However, if the Bcl6 staining was categorized as diffusely dense or sporadic, gastric diffuse large B cell lymphomas of germinal center phenotype fell into the former group, and high-grade MALT together with about a third of de novo diffuse large B cell lymphomas into the latter.[57] Lymphoepithelial lesions have been described in large B cell lymphomas at extranodal sites, but it is uncertain how reliable these are as a marker of marginal zone lymphoma origin.[58] It seems probable that many extranodal diffuse large B cell lymphomas are in fact high-grade EMZL.

NODAL MARGINAL ZONE B CELL LYMPHOMA

Definition

Nodal marginal zone B cell lymphoma (NMZL) is a primary nodal B cell neoplasm that morphologically resembles lymph nodes involved by marginal zone lymphomas of extranodal or splenic types, but without evidence of extranodal or splenic disease.

In patients with extranodal (MALT) lymphoma, Hashimoto thyroiditis or Sjogren syndrome, nodal involvement by marginal zone lymphoma should be considered secondary involvement by MALT lymphoma.[59]

NMZL was first designated as monocytoid B cell lymphoma, then as parafollicular B cell lymphoma until its relationship to marginal zone B cells was established by Piris et al.[60,61] It was clear from the outset that there was an overlap between NMZL and MALT lymphoma in many publications. Thus Campo et al. reported 36 cases of NMZL.[62] Six of these showed morphologic and phenotypic characteristics similar to those of SMZL and 30 were more like MALT-type lymphomas. Seven of 16 (44 percent) of patients with follow up showed evidence of extranodal lymphoma. The WHO definition (above) attempts to avoid this overlap by excluding cases with extranodal or splenic disease from this category. In our present state of knowledge of this disease this may be reasonable but it does not provide a watertight definition since extranodal disease may be occult or have a different immunoglobulin gene rearrangement. This problem is well illustrated by the report of 21 cases of NMZLs, selected using WHO criteria. On follow up two of these patients developed splenomegaly and one breast and skin involvement.[63] Assuming that the splenomegaly is due to involvement of the spleen by marginal zone lymphoma does this represent SMZLs presenting initially with lymphadenopathy or primary NMZL that has spread to the spleen? Similarly does the case with breast and skin involvement represent EMZL that presented with lymphadenopathy or NMZL that has spread to extranodal sites?

Sites of involvement

In the above report of 21 patients selected, using WHO criteria,[63] 15 had cervical and 10 paraaortic lymph node involvement. Eight patients had both abdominal and peripheral lymph node involvement. Infiltration of the bone marrow was present in 62 percent and circulating atypical cells or blood lymphocytosis was observed in 23 percent.

Clinical features

The median age in five reported series varied between 54 and 63 years and most series showed a female preponderance.[64–68] The majority of patients have disseminated disease with between 68 percent and 77 percent in stage III–IV. Despite this advanced stage the performance status of 81 percent was good. A third of patients had a monoclonal immunoglobulin band in the peripheral blood but none had cryoglobulinemia. As with SMZL, the incidence of hepatitis C positivity varies with geographic region. Arcaini et al.[64] (Italy) found HCV antibodies in the serum of 24 percent of their patients. Camacho et al.[65] (Spain) found antibodies to HCV in 2 of 10 patients studied.

Pediatric nodal marginal zone lymphoma

Taddesse-Heath et al.[69] described the clinicopathologic findings in 48 cases of NMZL in children and young adults (ages 2–29 years). Primary NMZL comprised the majority of cases and occurred most commonly in young males (median age 16 years, male/female ratio 5.4:1) presenting with localized lymphadenopathy, having a low rate of recurrence and an excellent prognosis. A commonly observed feature of these cases was the disruption of residual germinal centers either by mantle cells or marginal zone cells giving an appearance resembling progressive transformation of germinal centers (PTGC). The authors suggest that there may be a relationship between nodal marginal zone lymphoma and PTGC in the pediatric age group, noting that both have their highest prevalence in young males. The cases reported in this paper showed immunoglobulin light chain monotypia and CD43 expression, but not all were confirmed as being monoclonal by molecular examination. In a subsequent study of atypical marginal zone hyperplasia in childhood, Attygalle et al. reported six cases (4 tonsils, 2 appendixes) in which the marginal zone cells expressed CD43 and showed λ light chain restriction, but in which the sequencing of the immunoglobulin genes showed them to be polyclonal.[70] A similar finding has been reported in Kaposi sarcoma herpes virus-associated Castleman disease in which cells show λ light chain monotypia but are polyclonal on molecular analysis.[71] These studies illustrate the need to confirm monoclonality using molecular techniques and not to rely on light chain monotypia alone and possibly indicate that some of the cases reported by Taddesse-Heath et al. may have been reactive rather than neoplastic.

Morphology

The classic appearance of NMZL is of a node that has retained some of its normal architecture in which the follicles are surrounded by cells with clear cytoplasm. These cells may appear as small lymphocytes, centrocytoid cells or monocytoid cells. Variable numbers of scattered blast cells occur among these small cells; these do not, however, form sheets or large aggregates. Such a feature would indicate transformation to a diffuse large B cell lymphoma. Progressive follicular colonization eventually obscures the reactive follicles leading to a more diffuse appearance, though some degree of nodularity is usually retained. Plasmacytoid/plasmacytic differentiation is common in NMZL. The plasmacytoid/plasmacytic cells occur as aggregates or sheets rather than as scattered cells.

A feature seen mainly in some cervical nodes is the presence of sheets or clusters of epithelioid histiocytes. Characteristically variable sized aggregates of tumor cells may be surrounded by epithelioid histiocytes.[72] Lymph nodes with this appearance were previously categorized as immunocytomas with a high content of epithelioid cells.[73] In at least some cases this appearance is associated with spread of salivary gland MALT lymphoma in patients with Sjögren syndrome. As such it should not be included under the heading of nodal marginal zone lymphoma.

The ease of performance and associated lower morbidity of trephine biopsies has led to their increased use for lymph node biopsies. It is possible to obtain a reliable diagnosis of NMZL on such biopsies with the use of morphology and immunohistochemistry which can identify the phenotype of the tumor cells, the presence of residual follicular dendritic cells (CD21+, CD23+, CD35+) and plasmacytoid/plasmacytic differentiation with light chain restriction.

Immunohistochemistry

The tumor cells express the B cell markers CD20 and CD79a and half the cases coexpress CD43. BCL2 is positive in almost all cases; BCL6 is focally expressed in some cases, often in blast cells. Nuclear expression of BCL10 is not seen. The majority of tumors express IgM with κ light chain and almost half of these coexpress IgD.[63,66]

Differential diagnosis

The differential diagnosis of NMZL is with reactive lymphadenopathy and other small B cell lymphomas. Follicular lymphoma with marginal zone differentiation might be thought to mimic NMZL. However, morphology and immunohistochemistry should usually clearly distinguish between the neoplastic follicles of follicular lymphoma and the reactive follicles seen in NMZL. There has long been confusion between lymphoplasmacytic lymphoma and marginal zone lymphomas showing plasma cell differentiation. Although marginal zone lymphomas may show clonal immunoglobulin bands in the serum these do not usually reach the high levels seen in lymphoplasmacytic lymphoma. Lymphoplasmacytic lymphomas do not show the cytologic features and follicular colonization that characterizes marginal zone lymphomas.

Genetics

In the majority of NMZLs studied the immunoglobulin genes have been rearranged and mutated, indicating post-germinal center origin, with some tumors showing evidence of antigen-driven mutations. In a study of 14 NMZL, Traverse-Glehen et al.[74] found overusage of the VH4 family whereas Camacho et al. found VH3 gene usage in 4 of 5 cases.[65] In a study of 10 cases of NMZL from Italy 3/5 HCV-positive cases showed VH1 gene usage whereas 3/5 HCV-negative cases used the VH4 family of genes.[75]

The translocations that characterize many cases of EMZL and 7q deletions that are found in a proportion of SMZLs are not seen in NMZL. Trisomy 3, 7, 12 and 18 have been reported as well as del 6q and t(2;14)(q27;q32) in a minority of patients with NMZL. It is of interest that in a study of 131 primary nodal follicular lymphomas with t(14;18)(q32;q21) 35 were found to exhibit some degree of marginal zone differentiation. These cases showed a significant increase in secondary cytogenetic aberrations including trisomy 3.[76]

Prognosis and predictive factors

Nodal marginal zone lymphoma is considered to be an indolent lymphoma despite its usual presentation with advanced stage disease. Camacho et al. reported a 5 year overall survival probability of 79 percent with a failure free survival probability of only 22 percent due to persistence of disease.[65] Nathwani et al. found that the 5-year overall survival of patients with NMZL (56 percent) was less than that for EMZL (81 percent).[68]

SPLENIC MARGINAL ZONE LYMPHOMA

The WHO classification recognizes SMZL as a distinct but uncommon subtype of mature B cell lymphoma.[77] Previously described as splenic lymphoma with villous lymphocytes[78] the term SMZL was first applied by Schmid et al.[79] This tumor is said to represent less than 1 percent of lymphoid neoplasms. It is, however, likely to be a common lymphoma encountered in resected spleens, partly because splenic resection remains a therapeutic option for this disease.

Sites of involvement

The spleen, splenic hilar lymph nodes and bone marrow are involved and are the usual source of diagnostic material. Neoplastic cells are found in the blood in most cases especially if subjected to flow cytometric analysis as well as the examination of standard blood films. It is probable that the liver will show microscopic involvement in all cases. Peripheral lymph node involvement is not a feature of this neoplasm.

Clinical features

The median age of patients is 68 years with a male to female ratio of 1:1.8. Patients present with variable degrees of splenomegaly. Villous lymphocytes can usually be detected in blood films. These cells often have relatively abundant clear cytoplasm with short polar villous projections on some of the cells. Patients may have autoimmune thrombocytopenia and/or anaemia. A small monoclonal IgM band is found in the serum of some patients. Type II cryoglobulinemia associated with hepatitis C infection is seen in rare cases.[80]

Morphology

Recorded spleen weights are from 270 g to 5500 g with a median of 1750 g. In the majority of cases the cut surface of the spleen in SMZL shows multiple diffusely spread small white nodules (miliary nodules), characteristic of most small B cell lymphomas other than hairy cell leukemia. Histologic examination shows that these nodules are white pulp follicles that have undergone varying degrees of follicular colonization. In the early stages persistent reactive germinal centers and a defined mantle cell layer may be seen surrounded by marginal zone cells. In most cases, however, much of the reactive follicle is replaced by tumor cells with an outer layer of cells showing marginal zone morphology. This zone always contains a variable number of dispersed blast cells. Between the colonized primary follicles there are often smaller satellite nodules of tumor cells that frequently have small aggregates of epithelioid cells at their center. The red pulp (cords and sinusoids) contain a diffuse infiltrate of tumor cells which in some cases may obscure the nodular component.[81] The density of this infiltrate is highlighted in sections stained for CD20 or CD79a. In a review of 85 cases of SMZL, Mollejo et al.[82] identified four cases that showed a diffuse infiltration of the spleen without evidence of follicular colonization or residual reactive follicles. Bone marrow infiltration occurred in all four cases and peripheral blood involvement in two. All four cases showed p53 mutations or anomalous p53 staining. Two cases had skin involvement. The authors proposed this is a variant of SMZL. In a previous study of 59 patients with splenic lymphoma with villous lymphocytes (SLVL), 11 were found to have p53 abnormalities which were associated with a more aggressive disease course and poor prognosis.[83] Plasma cell differentiation can occur in SMZL and may be seen in residual germinal centers.

The splenic hilar lymph nodes usually show some preservation of the sinus structure. The lymphoid element has an overall nodular configuration. Reactive germinal centers and mantle zones are rarely clearly defined, the whole nodule being composed of small lymphocytes with interspersed blast cells. The outer marginal zone cells do not usually show the clear cytoplasm that characterizes the marginal zone cells in the spleen.

Splenic marginal zone cells in the bone marrow have a nodular distribution with a more diffuse background distribution. The nodules usually correspond to colonized follicles, follicular dendritic cells can usually be detected by immunohistochemistry but defined germinal centers are not usually seen. The diffuse infiltrate is often intrasinusoidal, a feature that is considered to be characteristic of SMZL and to differentiate it from most other small B cell lymphomas.[84,85]

Immunophenotype

The tumor cells of SMZL express surface IgM and IgD which has been recorded in between 33 and 46 percent of cases. Expression of IgD is weaker than that seen on residual reactive mantle cells. The tumor cells express CD20 and CD79a but, with the exception of a small number of cases, are negative for CD5, CD10, CD23 and CD43. This profile is useful in differentiating the tumor from B chronic lymphocytic leukemia/small lymphocytic lymphoma and mantle cell lymphoma, which are both usually CD5 positive. The absence of CD10 staining may be helpful in distinguishing SMZL from follicular lymphoma, any residual CD10 positive germinal center cells in SMZL will be BCL2 negative in contrast to BCL2 positive neoplastic follicular lymphoma cells. In well-fixed specimens immunoglobulin light chain restriction can usually be demonstrated in the blast cells within the marginal zone aiding the differentiation from reactive marginal zone proliferations. The demonstration of dendritic reticulum cells with CD21, CD23 or CD35 can be helpful in identifying the 'skeletal remains' of colonized follicles.

Genetics

ANTIGEN RECEPTOR GENES

Early studies reported that immunoglobulin heavy and light chain genes are rearranged and that most cases have somatic mutations. These studies, however, were based on small numbers of patients. Later larger studies have shown that between a third and half the tumors have unmutated immunoglobulin genes. These studies have also shown ongoing mutations, evidence of antigen selection and restricted VH gene usage; suggesting that the tumors may be driven by selective antigens. Tumors with unmutated genes are more likely to express IgD, to have 7q31 deletions and to be associated with a poorer overall survival.[81,86–89]

CYTOGENETIC ABNORMALITIES AND ONCOGENES

Studies by Oscier and colleagues showed that 26–31 percent of cases with a diagnosis of splenic lymphoma with villous lymphocytes showed abnormalities of chromosome 7 including del(7)(q22-32) and del(7)(q34-36).[90] Mateo et al.[91] studied 20 cases of splenic lymphoma with villous lymphocytes and 26 controls, using conventional cytogenetics and PCR, of 13 microsatellite loci spanning 7q21 to 7q36 to investigate tissue samples from 20 SMZLs and 26 control small B cell lymphomas. They detected allelic loss in 8/20 SMZLs and 2/26 controls and concluded that 7q31-32 may be used as a genetic marker of SMZL. There was an increased frequency of death due to tumor progression or large cell transformation among patients whose tumors showed 7q loss. The difference was, however, of only borderline significance. The authors suggest that the 7q31 region may contain a tumor suppressor gene.[91] Corcoran et al.[92] studied four SMZL patients with translocations involving 7q. They found the 7q breakpoints to be close to the transcription start of the cyclin dependent kinase (CDK) 6 gene, and in two patients there was overexpression of CDK6 protein in tumor cells. They suggest that dysregulation of the CDK6 gene may contribute to the genesis of SMZL.[92] The translocations that characterize many EMZLs have not been reported in SMZL.[35]

GENE EXPRESSION STUDIES

Ruiz-Ballesteros et al.[93] studied 44 SMZLs using cDNA microarray expression and tissue microarray. They found a largely homogeneous signature implying the existence of a single molecular entity. They observed deregulation of genes involved in B cell receptor signaling and downregulation of genes located in 7q31 in all cases. In a study of 24 cases of SMZL Troen et al. found upregulation of the AP1 transcription factors C-JUN, JUND, JUNB and C-FOS, together with upregulation of NOTCH2, a transcription factor that induces marginal zone B cell differentiation.[94]

Prognosis and predictive factors

Splenic marginal zone lymphoma is an indolent lymphoma and patients often show long-term survival following splenectomy alone. Shorter survival has been reported to be associated with CD38 expression, naïve IGVH genes and expression of NF-κB pathway genes. In common with other small B cell lymphomas, SMZL may undergo transformation to diffuse large B cell lymphoma. Camacho et al.[95] reported 12 such cases in which large cell lymphoma most frequently presented in peripheral lymph nodes. These 12 cases represented 13 percent of their cases of SMZL with adequate follow up, a lower incidence of transformation than seen in other small B cell lymphomas.

Splenic marginal zone lymphoma and hepatitis C virus infection

Restricted IGVH gene usage in SMZL suggests that this tumor may be antigen driven. Hepatitis C virus drives the unrestrained clonal expansion of VH1-69-expressing memory B cells in type II cryoglobulinemia, a model of infection-driven lymphomagenesis.[96,97] In a series of 17 HCV-associated NHLs (mostly diffuse large B cell lymphomas) the CDR3 sequences expressed by the tumor cells showed homology for antibody specific for the E2 protein of HCV. A number of studies have demonstrated potential oncogenic effects of HCV core protein and E2 protein.[98] The most convincing evidence of an etiologic role for HCV in SLVL comes from a report of nine patients with SLVL and HCV infection and six patients with SLVL who were HCV negative and were treated with interferon α with or without ribavirin. Eight patients in the first group had complete remission with loss of detectable HCV RNA, one patient showed partial remission and the HCV negative controls showed no response.[99] In a later publication the same group reported 18 patients with SLVL, type II cryoglobulinemia and HCV infection as a new entity. Fourteen patients responded to treatment with interferon α with or without ribavirin with a complete hematologic response after clearance of HCV RNA. Four patients showed complete or partial hematologic response with incomplete clearance of HCV RNA. Monoclonal immunoglobulin gene rearrangements persisted in the responders, indicating subclinical persistence of the neoplastic clones.[100] This syndrome appears to be uncommon outside areas with high HCV endemicity.

KEY POINTS

- Nodal, splenic and extranodal marginal zone lymphomas (MALT) represent very different and distinct entities all captured under the rubric of marginal zone lymphoma (MZL).
- The diagnosis of MZL in most cases requires an open biopsy or at least a biopsy of sufficient size to delineate architectural features.
- MZLs represent a group of lymphomas most convincingly associated with an infectious etiology.
- Some MALT lymphomas at different anatomic sites will regress with antibiotic therapy alone.
- Most of the translocations that characterize MALT lymphomas upregulate the NF-κB signaling pathway and the frequency of specific translocations will vary with anatomic site.

REFERENCES

● = Key primary paper

◆ = Major review article

1. Isaacson P, Wright DH. Malignant lymphoma of mucosa associated lymphoid tissue. A distinctive type of B-cell lymphoma. Cancer 1983; 52: 1410–16.

●2. Isaacson P, Wright DH. Extranodal malignant lymphoma arising from mucosa-associated lymphoid tissue. *Cancer* 1984; **53**: 2515–24.

◆3. Isaacson PG, Chott A, Nakamura S *et al.* Extranodal marginal zone lymphoma of mucosa-associated lymphoid tissue (MALT lymphoma). In: Swerdlow SH, Campo E, Harris NL *et al. WHO classification of tumours of haematopoietic and lymphoid tissues.* Lyon: IARC Press, 2008: 214–17.

◆4. Bacon CM, Du M-Q, Dogan A. Mucosa-associated lymphoid tissue (MALT) lymphoma: a practical guide for pathologists. *J Clin Pathol* 2007; **60**: 361–72.

5. Hyjek E, Smith WJ, Isaacson PG. Primary B-cell lymphoma of salivary glands and its relationship to myoepithelial sialadenitis. *Human Pathol* 1998; **19**: 766–76.

◆6. Isaacson PG, Du M-Q. MALT lymphoma: from morphology to molecules. *Nat Rev Cancer* 2004; **4**: 644–53.

7. Hussel T, Isaacson PG, Crabtree JE, Spencer J. The response of cells from low grade B-cell gastric lymphomas of mucosa-associated lymphoid tissue to *Helicobacter pylori*. *Lancet* 1993; **342**: 571–4.

8. Hussel T, Isaacson PG, Crabtree JE, Spencer J. *Helicobacter pylori*-specific tumour-infiltrating T cells provide contact dependent help for the growth of malignant B cells in low-grade gastric lymphoma of mucosa associated lymphoid tissue. *J Pathol* 1996; **178**: 111–12.

9. Rollinson S, Levene AP, Mensah FK *et al.* Gastric marginal zone lymphoma is associated with polymorphisms in genes involved in inflammatory response and antioxidative capacity. *Blood* 2003; **102**: 1007–11.

10. Ye H, Liu H, Attygalle A *et al.* Variable frequencies of t(11;18)(q21;q21) in MALT lymphomas of different sites: significant association with CagA strains of *H. pylori* in gastric MALT lymphoma. *Blood* 2003; **102**: 1012–18.

11. Lecuit M, Abachin E, Martin A *et al.* Immunoproliferative small intestinal disease associated with Campylobacter jejuni. *N Engl J Med* 2004; **350**: 239–48.

12. Ambrosetti A, Zanotti R, Pattaro C *et al.* Most cases of primary salivary mucosa-associated lymphoid tissue lymphoma are associated either with Sjögren syndrome or hepatitis C infection. *Br J Haematol* 2004; **126**: 43–9.

13. Senff NJ, Hoefnagel JJ, Jansen PM *et al.* Reclassification of 300 primary cutaneous B-cell lymphomas according to the new WHO-EORTC classification for cutaneous lymphomas: comparison with previous classifications and identification of prognostic markers. *J Clin Oncol* 2007; **25**: 1581–7.

14. Garbe C, Stein H, Dienemann D, Orfanos CE. *Borrelia burgdorferi*-associated cutaneous B-cell lymphoma: clinical and immunohistologic characterization of four cases. *J Am Acad Dermatol* 1991; **24**: 584–90.

15. Goodlad JR, Davidson MM, Hollowood K *et al.* Primary cutaneous B-cell lymphoma and *Borrelia burgdorferi* infection in patients from the highlands of Scotland. *Am J Surg Pathol* 2000; **24**: 1279–85.

16. Colli C, Leinweber B, Mulleger R *et al. Borrelia burgdorferi*-associated lymphocytoma cutis: clinicopathologic, immunophenotypic, and molecular study of 106 cases. *J Cutan Pathol* 2004; **31**: 232–40.

17. Wood GS, Kamath NV, Guitart J *et al.* Absence of *Borrelia burgdorferi* DNA in cutaneous B-cell lymphomas from the United States. *J Cutan Pathol* 2001; **28**: 502–7.

18. Li C, Inagaki H, Kuo TT *et al.* Primary cutaneous marginal zone B-cell lymphoma: a molecular and clinicopathologic study of 24 Asian cases. *Am J Surg Pathol* 2003; **27**: 1061–9.

19. Ferreri AJM, Guidoboni M, Ponzoni M *et al.* Evidence for an association between *Chlamydia psittaci* and ocular adnexal lymphomas. *J Natl Cancer Inst* 2004; **96**: 586–94.

20. Zhang GS, Winter JN, Variakojis D *et al.* Lack of an association between *Chlamydia psittaci* and ocular adnexal lymphomas. *Leuk Lymphoma* 2007; **48**: 577–83.

21. Ruiz A, Reischl U, Swerdlow SH *et al.* Extranodal marginal zone B-cell lymphomas of the ocular adnexal: multiparameter analysis of 34 cases including interphase molecular cytogenetics and PCR for *Chlamydia psittaci*. *Am J Surg Pathol* 2007; **31**: 792–802.

22. Chanudet E, Zhou Y, Bacon CM *et al. Chlamydia psittaci* is variably associated with ocular adnexal MALT lymphoma in different geographical regions. *J Pathol* 2006; **209**: 344–51.

●23. Inagaki H, Chan JKC, Ng JWM *et al.* Primary thymic extranodal marginal zone B-cell lymphoma of mucosa associated lymphoid tissue type exhibits distinctive clinicopathological and molecular features. *Am J Pathol* 2002; **160**: 1435–43.

24. Price SK. Immunoproliferative small intestinal disease: a study of 13 cases with alpha heavy chain disease. *Histopathology* 1990; **17**: 7–17.

25. Al-Saleem T, Al-Mondhiry H. Immunoproliferative small intestinal disease (IPSID): a model for mature B-cell neoplasms. *Blood* 2005; **105**: 2274–80.

26. Ye H, Gong L, Liu H *et al.* MALT lymphoma with t(14;18)(q32;q21)/IGH-MALT1 is characterized by strong cytoplasmic MALT1 and BCL10 expression. *J Pathol* 2005; **205**: 293–301.

27. Qin Y, Greiner A, Trunk M J *et al.* Somatic hypermutation in low grade mucosa-associated lymphoid tissue-type B-cell lymphoma. *Blood* 1995; **86**: 3528–34.

28. Qin Y, Greiner A, Hallas C *et al.* Intraclonal offspring expansion of gastric low-grade MALT-type lymphoma: evidence for the role of antigen-driven high-affinity mutation in lymphomagenesis. *Lab Invest* 1997; **76**: 477–85.

29. Hussell T, Isaacson PG, Crabtree JE. Immunoglobulin specificity of low grade B cell gastrointestinal lymphoma of mucosa-associated lymphoid tissue (MALT) type. *Am J Pathol* 1993; **142**: 285–92.

30. Du M, Diss T C, Xu C *et al.* Ongoing mutation in MALT lymphoma immunoglobulin gene suggests that antigen stimulation plays a role in the clonal expansion. *Leukemia* 1996; **10**: 1190–7.

31. Bende RJ, Aarts WM, Riedl RG *et al*. Among B-cell non-Hodgkin's lymphomas, MALT lymphomas express a unique antibody repertoire with frequent rheumatoid factor reactivity. *J Exp Med* 2005; **201**: 1229–41.

32. Lenze D, Berg E, Volkmer-Engert R *et al*. Influence of antigen on the development of MALT lymphoma. *Blood* 2006; **107**: 1141–8.

33. Sagaert X, Laurent M, Baens M *et al*. MALT1 and BCL10 aberrations in MALT lymphomas and their effect on the expression of BCL10 in the tumour cells. *Mod Pathol* 2006; **19**: 225–32.

34. Streubel B, Simonitsch-Klupp I, Mullauer L *et al*. Variable frequencies of MALT lymphoma-associated genetic aberrations in MALT lymphomas of different sites. *Leukemia* 2004; **18**: 1722–6.

35. Remstein ED, James CD, Kurtin PJ. Incidence and subtype specificity of AP12-MALT1 fusion translocations in extranodal, nodal, and splenic marginal zone lymphomas. *Am J Pathol* 2000; **156**: 1183–8.

36. Ho L, Davis E, Conne B *et al*. MALT1 and the AP12-MALT1 fusion act between CD40 and IKK and confer NF-kB-dependent proliferative advantage and resistance against FAS-induced cell death in B-cells. *Blood* 2005; **105**: 2891–9.

●37. Starostik P, Patzner J, Greiner A *et al*. Gastric marginal zone B-cell lymphomas of MALT type develop along 2 distinct pathogenetic pathways. *Blood* 2002; **99**: 3–9.

38. Liu H, Ye H, Ruskone-Fourmestraux A *et al*. T(11;18) is a marker for all stage gastric MALT lymphomas that will not respond to *H. pylori* eradication. *Gastroenterology* 2002; **122**: 1286–94.

39. Inagaki H, Nakamura T, Chunmei L *et al*. Gastric MALT lymphomas are divided into three groups based on responsiveness to *Helicobacter pylori* eradication and detection of AP12-MALT1 fusion. *Am J Surg Pathol* 2004; **28**: 1560–7.

40. Achuthan R, Bell SM, Leek JP *et al*. Novel translocation of the BCL10 gene in a case of mucosa associated lymphoid tissue lymphoma. *Genes Chromosomes Cancer* 2000; **29**: 347–9.

41. Streubel B, Vinatzer U, Lamprecht A *et al*. T(3;14)(p14.1;q32) involving IGH and FOXP1 is a novel recurrent chromosomal aberration in MALT lymphoma. *Leukemia* 2005; **19**: 652–8.

●42. Sagaert X, de Paepe P, Libbrecht L *et al*. Forkhead box protein P1 expression in mucosa-associated lymphoid tissue lymphomas predicts poor prognosis and transformation to diffuse large B-cell lymphoma. *J Clin Oncol* 2006; **24**: 2490–7.

43. Haralambieva E, Adam P, Ventura R *et al*. Genetic rearrangement of FOXP1 is predominantly detected in a subset of diffuse large B-cell lymphomas with extranodal presentation. *Leukemia* 2006; **20**: 1300–3.

44. Barrans SL, Fenton JA, Banham A *et al*. Strong expression of FOXP1 identifies a distinct subset of diffuse large B-cell lymphoma (DLBCL) patients with poor outcome. *Blood* 2004; **104**: 2933–5.

45. Banham AH, Connors JM, Brown PJ *et al*. Expression of the FOXP1 transcription factor is strongly associated with inferior survival in patients with diffuse large B-cell lymphoma. *Clin Cancer Res* 2005; **11**: 1065–72.

46. Wotherspoon AC, Finn TM, Isaacson PG. Trisomy 3 in low-grade B-cell lymphomas of mucosa-associated lymphoid tissue. *Blood* 1995; **85**: 2000–4.

47. Ott G, Kalla J, Steinhoff A *et al*. Trisomy 3 is not a common feature in malignant lymphomas of mucosa-associated lymphoid tissue type. *Am J Pathol* 1998; **153**: 689–94.

48. Hoeve MA, Gisbertz IA, Schouten HC *et al*. Gastric low-grade MALT lymphoma, high-grade MALT lymphoma and diffuse large B-cell lymphoma show frequent differences of trisomy. *Leukemia* 1999; **13**: 799–807.

49. Morgner A, Miehlke S, Fischbach W *et al*. Complete remission of primary high-grade B-cell gastric lymphoma after cure of *Helicobacter pylori* infection. *J Clin Oncol* 2001; **19**: 2041–8.

50. Chen LT, Lin JT, Tai JJ *et al*. Long-term results of anti-*Helicobacter pylori* therapy in early-stage gastric high-grade transformed MALT lymphoma. *J Natl Cancer Inst* 2005; **97**: 1345–53.

51. Kuo SH, Chen LT, Yeh KH *et al*. Nuclear expression of BCL10 or nuclear factor kappa B predicts *Helicobacter pylori*-independent status of early stage high grade gastric mucosa-associated lymphoid tissue lymphomas. *J Clin Oncol* 2004; **22**: 3491–7.

52. Yeh KH, Kuo SH, Chen LT *et al*. Nuclear expression of BCL10 or nuclear factor kappa B helps predict *Helicobacter pylori*-independent status of low-grade gastric mucosa associated lymphoid tissue lymphomas with or without t(11;18)(q21;q21). *Blood* 2005; **106**: 1037–41.

53. Chan JK, Ng CS, Isaacson PG *et al*. Relationship between high-grade lymphoma and low-grade B-cell mucosa-associated lymphoid tissue lymphoma (MALToma) of the stomach. *Am J Pathol* 1990; **136**: 1153–64.

54. Peng H, Du M, Diss TC *et al*. Genetic evidence for a clonal link between low and high-grade components in gastric MALT B-cell lymphoma. *Histopathology* 1997; **30**: 425–9.

55. Kuo SH, Chen LT, Wu MS *et al*. Differential response to *H. pylori* eradication therapy of co-existing diffuse large B-cell lymphoma and Malt lymphoma of stomach – significance of tumour cell clonality and BCL10 expression. *J Pathol* 2007; **211**: 296–304.

56. Barth TFE, Barth CA, Kestler HA *et al*. Transcriptional profiling suggests that secondary and primary large B-cell lymphomas of the gastrointestinal (GI) tract are blastic variants of GI marginal zone lymphoma. *J Pathol* 2007; **211**: 305–13.

57. Kwon MS, Go JH, Choi SC *et al*. Critical evaluation of Bcl-6 protein expression in diffuse large B-cell lymphoma of the stomach and small intestine. *Am J Surg Pathol* 2003; **27**: 790–8.

58. Bateman AC, Wright DH. Epitheliotropism in high-grade lymphomas of mucosal-associated lymphoid tissue. *Histopathology* 1993; **23**: 409–15.

◆59. Isaacson PG, Harris NL, Nathwani BN *et al.* Nodal marginal B-cell lymphoma. In: Jaffe ES, Harris NL, Stein H, Vardiman JW (eds) *World Health Organization Pathology and genetics of tumours of haematopoietic and lymphoid tissues.* Lyon: IARC Press, p. 161.

60. Cousar JB, McGinn DL, Glick AD *et al.* Report of an unusual lymphoma arising from parafollicular B-lymphocytes (PBLs) or so-called 'monocytoid' lymphocytes. *Am J Clin Pathol* 1987; **87**: 121–8.

61. Piris MA, Rivas C, Morente M *et al.* Monocytoid B-cell lymphoma, a tumour related to the marginal zone. *Histopathology* 1988; **48**: 383–92.

62. Campo E, Miquel R, Krenacs L *et al.* Primary nodal marginal zone lymphomas of splenic and MALT type. *Am J Surg Pathol* 1999; **23**: 59–68.

63. Traverse-Glehen A, Felman P, Callot-Bauchu E *et al.* A clinicopathological study of nodal marginal zone B-cell lymphoma. A report on 21 cases. *Histopathology* 2006; **48**: 162–73.

64. Arcaini L, Paulli M, Burcheri S *et al.* Primary nodal marginal zone B-cell lymphoma: clinical features and prognostic assessment of a rare disease. *Br J Haematology* 2006; **136**: 301–4.

65. Camacho FI, Algara P, Mollejo M *et al.* Nodal marginal zone lymphoma: a heterogeneous tumor. *Am J Surg Pathol* 2003; **27**: 762–71.

66. Berger F, Felman P, Thieblemont C *et al.* Non-MALT marginal zone B-cell lymphomas: a description of clinical presentation and outcome in 124 patients. *Blood* 2000; **95**: 1950–6.

67. Armitage JO, Weisenburger DD. New approach to classifying non-Hodgkin's lymphomas: clinical features of the major histologic subtypes. Non-Hodgkin's lymphoma classification project. *J Clin Oncol* 1988; **16**: 2780–95.

68. Nathwani BN, Anderson JR, Armitage JO *et al.* Marginal zone B-cell lymphoma: A clinical comparison of nodal and mucosa-associated lymphoid tissue types. Non-Hodgkin's lymphoma classification project. *J Clin Oncol* 1999; **17**: 2486–92.

69. Taddesse-Heath L, Pittaluga S, Sorbara L *et al.* Marginal zone B-cell lymphoma in children and young adults. *Am J Surg Pathol* 2003; **27**: 522–31.

70. Attygalle AD, Liu H, Shirali S *et al.* Atypical marginal zone hyperplasia of mucosa-associated lymphoid tissue: a reactive condition of childhood showing immunoglobulin lambda light-chain restriction. *Blood* 2004; **104**: 3343–8.

71. Du MQ, Liu H, Diss TC *et al.* Kaposi sarcoma-associated herpes virus infects monotypic (IgMλ) but polyclonal naive B cells in Castleman disease and associated lymphoproliferative disorders. *Blood* 2001; **97**: 2130–6.

72. Ortiz-Hidalgo C, Wright DH. The morphological spectrum of monocytoid B-cell lymphoma and its relationship to lymphomas of mucosa-associated lymphoid tissue. *Histopathology* 1992; **21**: 555–61.

73. Patsouris E, Noel H, Lennert K. Lymphoplasmacytic/lymphoplasmacytoid immunocytomas with a high content of epithelioid cells. Histologic and immunohistochemical findings. *Am J Surg Pathol* 1990; **14**: 660–70.

74. Traverse-Glehen A, Davi F, Ben SE *et al.* Analysis of VH genes in marginal zone lymphoma reveals marked heterogeneity between splenic and nodal tumors and suggests the existence of clonal selection. *Haematologica* 2005; **90**: 470–8.

75. Marasca R, Vaccari P, Luppi M *et al.* Immunoglobulin gene mutations and frequent use of VH1–69 and VH4–34 segments in hepatitis C virus-positive and hepatitis C virus-negative nodal marginal zone B-cell lymphoma. *Am J Pathol* 2001; **159**: 253–61.

76. Torlakovic EE, Aamot HV, Heim S. A marginal zone phenotype in follicular lymphoma with t(14;18) is associated with secondary cytogenetic aberrations typical of marginal zone lymphoma. *J Pathol* 2006; **209**: 258–64.

◆77. Isaacson PG, Berger F, Piris MA *et al.* Splenic marginal zone lymphoma. In: Jaffe ES, Harris NL, Stein H, Vardiman JW (eds) *World Health Organization Classification of Tumours. Pathology and genetics of tumours of haematopoietic and lymphoid tissues.* Lyon: IARC Press, 2001: 135–7.

78. Melo JV, Hegde U, Parreira A *et al.* Splenic B cell lymphoma with circulating villous lymphocytes: differential diagnosis of B-cell leukaemias with large spleens. *J Clin Pathol* 1987; **40**: 642–51.

79. Schmid C, Kirkham N, Diss TC, Isaacson PG. Splenic marginal zone cell lymphoma. *Am J Surg Pathol* 1992; **16**: 455–66.

80. Franco V, Florena AM, Iannitto E *et al.* Splenic marginal zone lymphoma. *Blood* 2003; **101**: 2464–72.

81. Papadaki T, Stamatopoulos K, Belessi C *et al.* Splenic marginal zone lymphoma: one or more entities? A histological, immunohistochemical and molecular study of 42 cases. *Am J Surg Pathol* 2007; **31**: 438–46.

82. Mollejo M, Algara P, Mateo MS *et al.* Splenic small B-cell lymphoma with predominant red pulp involvement: a diffuse variant of splenic marginal zone lymphoma. *Histopathology* 2002; **40**: 22–30.

83. Gruszka-Westwood AM, Hamoudi RA, Matutes E *et al.* p53 abnormalities in splenic lymphoma with villous lymphocytes. *Blood* 2001; **97**: 3552–8.

84. Franco V, Florena AM, Campasi G. Intrasinusoidal bone marrow infiltration: a possible hallmark of splenic lymphoma. *Histopathology* 1996; **29**: 571–5.

85. Labouyrie E, Marit G, Vial J *et al.* Intrasinusoidal bone marrow involvement by splenic lymphoma with villous lymphocytes: a helpful histologic feature. *Mod Pathol* 1997; **10**: 1015–20.

86. Zhu D, Oscier DG, Stevenson FK. Splenic lymphoma with villous lymphocytes involves B cells with extensively mutated Ig heavy chain variable region genes. *Blood* 1995; **85**: 1603–7.

87. Bahler DW, Pindzola JA, Swerdlow SH. Splenic marginal zone lymphomas appear to originate from different B cell types. *Am J Pathol* 2002; **161**: 81–8.

88. Algara P, Mateo MS, Sanches-Beato M *et al.* Analysis of the IgV$_H$ somatic mutations in splenic marginal zone

lymphoma defines a group of unmutated cases with frequent 7q deletion and adverse clinical course. *Blood* 2002; **99**: 1299–304.

89. Tierens A, Delabie J, Malecka A *et al.* Splenic marginal zone lymphoma with villous lymphocytes shows on-going immunoglobulin gene mutations. *Am J Pathol* 2003; **162**: 681–9.

90. Oscier DG, Gardiner A, Mould S. Structural abnormalities of chromosome 7q in chronic lymphoproliferative disorders. *Cancer Genet Cytogenet* 1996; **92**: 24–7.

91. Mateo M, Mollejo M, Villuendas R *et al.* 7q 31–32 allelic loss is a frequent finding in splenic marginal zone lymphoma. *Am J Pathol* 1999; **154**: 1583–9.

92. Corcoran MM, Mould SJ, Orchard JA *et al.* Dysregulation of cyclin dependent kinase 6 expression in splenic marginal zone lymphoma through chromosome 7q translocations. *Oncogene* 1999; **18**: 6271–7.

93. Ruiz-Ballesteros E, Mollejo M, Rodriguez A *et al.* Splenic marginal zone lymphoma: proposal of new diagnostic and prognostic markers identified after tissue and cDNA microarray analysis. *Blood* 2005; **106**: 1831–8.

94. Troen G, Nygaard V, Jenssen T-K *et al.* Constitutive expression of the AP-1 transcription factors C-jun, junD, junB and c-fos and the marginal zone B-cell transcription factor notch2 in splenic marginal zone lymphoma. *J Mol Diagn* 2004; **6**: 297–307.

95. Camacho F, Mollejo M, Mateo M-S *et al.* Progression to large B-cell lymphoma in splenic marginal zone lymphoma: a description of a series of 12 cases. *Am J Surg Pathol* 2001; **25**: 1268–76.

96. Carbonari M, Caprini E, Tedesco T *et al.* Hepatitis C virus drives the unconstrained monoclonal expansion of V_H 1–69 expressing memory B cells in type II cryoglobulinaemia: a model of infection-driven lymphomagenesis. *J Immunol* 2005; **174**: 6532–9.

97. DeRe V, DeVita S, Marzotto A *et al.* Sequence analysis of the immunoglobulin antigen receptor of hepatitis C virus-associated non-Hodgkin lymphomas suggests that the malignant cells are derived from the rheumatoid factor-producing cells that occur mainly in type II cryoglobulinemia. *Blood* 2000; **96**: 3578–84.

98. Machida K, Cheng KT-H, Pavio N *et al.* Hepatitis C virus E2-CD81 interaction induces hypermutation of the immunoglobulin gene in B cells. *J Virol* 2005; **79**: 8079–89.

99. Hermine O, Lefrere F, Bronowicki J-P *et al.* Regression of splenic lymphoma with villous lymphocytes after treatment of hepatitis C virus infection. *N Engl J Med* 2002; **347**: 89–94.

●100. Saadoun D, Suarez F, Lefrere F *et al.* Splenic lymphoma with villous lymphocytes associated with type II cryoglobulinemia and HCV infection: a new entity? *Blood* 2005; **105**: 74–6.

31

Follicular lymphoma

RANDY D GASCOYNE

INTRODUCTION

Follicular lymphoma (FL) represents the second most common subtype (22 percent) of non-Hodgkin lymphoma (NHL) after diffuse large B cell lymphoma (DLBCL), based on a large international NHL validation study.[1] In North America, FL represents the most common histologic subtype, accounting for 32 percent of all NHLs.[2] FL is imminently treatable, but most patients present with advanced stage disease and cannot be cured by conventional therapy. Follicular lymphoma is characterized by marked clinical heterogeneity, with median survivals in the range of 8–10 years, but with a wide range of outcomes. Some patients will survive in excess of 25 years, while 15–20 percent will die of transformed/aggressive FL within the first 3 years following diagnosis. Thus, the prevalence of FL is significant. The frequency of transformation is variably reported and generally portends a poor prognosis.[3–11] Several recent single institution studies suggest that transformation occurs at a steady-state of approximately 3 percent per year and may possibly plateau at 15–17 years, suggesting that only half of the patients are at risk.[11]

For several decades, asymptomatic FL patients with slow growing disease were followed under a policy of observation. This watch and wait approach provided an excellent opportunity to study the natural history of FL, particularly the opportunity to serially sample lymph node biopsy material over time in patients who may have never been exposed to treatment.[12] The luxury afforded by indolent clinical behavior in at least a subset of patients facilitated the in-depth study of molecular alterations that characterize disease progression over time. Much has already been learned by studying sequential biopsy material in FL, however, much more is now possible with the advent of genome-wide analysis platforms that should facilitate a detailed examination of these cancer genomes, somewhat similar to the analysis of multistep molecular progression in colon cancer.[13–16]

Several recent randomized clinical trials have confirmed a survival benefit for patients with FL treated with chemotherapy regimens to which the monoclonal anti-CD20 antibody, rituximab, has been added.[17–20] For the first time in several decades, newer therapies may be changing the clinical course of FL, leading to improvements in overall survival.[21–23] These steady improvements in treatment approaches combined with ever-shrinking biopsy size may make longitudinal correlative studies impossible in the future. Judicious use of existing bio-repositories of FL is thus of paramount importance. The treatment of FL is discussed in detail in Chapter 67.

DEFINITION

Follicular lymphoma is a lymphoid neoplasm of follicle center B cells that includes a variable mixture of small

Table 31.1 Clinicopathologic features distinguishing grade 3a and 3b follicular lymphoma (FL)

Features	Grade 3a FL	Grade 3b FL
Clinical		
Bone marrow involvement	67%	20%
Cell type in BM	Typically centrocytes	Concordant centroblasts more often present
Morphologic		
Diffuse areas	Uncommon	Common
Demarcation of follicles	Usually sharp	Often poorly defined, merging with areas resembling DLBCL
Immunophenotypic		
CD10	~100%	50%
BCL2	73%	69%
P53	9%	31%
Cytoplasmic immunoglobulin	0%	44%
Cytogenetic alterations		
t(14;18)	73%	13%
3q27 (BCL6) translocations	18%	44%
Mean number of karyotypic alterations	6.5	8.9

centrocytes and larger centroblasts and possesses at least a partial follicular architecture.[24] Most but not all cases harbor the genetic hallmark of this lymphoma, the t(14;18) (q32;q21.3), resulting in the deregulated expression of the BCL2 oncogene under control of the IGH enhancer element residing at chromosome 14q32.[25] This group of lymphomas has been identified in previous classifications as:[26–30]

- nodular, poorly differentiated lymphocytic lymphoma, mixed lymphocytic–histiocytic, histiocytic and undifferentiated (Rappaport);
- centroblastic/centrocytic follicular, follicular and diffuse, centroblastic, follicular (Kiel);
- small cleaved, large cleaved, small noncleaved or large noncleaved follicle center cell (follicular) (Lukes and Collins);
- follicular small cleaved, mixed, large or small noncleaved (Working Formulation);
- follicle center lymphoma, follicular (Revised European–American Lymphoma classification).

The current World Health Organization (WHO) classification recognizes three histologic grades of FL and two uncommon variants.[24] These are listed in Table 31.1. Grade 3a has >15 centroblasts per high power field (HPF) within the neoplastic follicles, but centrocytes are also present. Grade 3b has solid sheets of centroblasts only. Two variants are recognized, including diffuse follicle center cell lymphoma and cutaneous follicle center cell lymphoma. These will be discussed in detail later in this chapter.

EPIDEMIOLOGY

Follicular lymphoma comprises 22 percent of all lymphomas worldwide and approximately 70 percent of all indolent lymphomas.[1] In North America, FL is the most common histologic subtype of NHL. In contrast to North America, the incidence is lower in Europe, and even less common in Asia and in underdeveloped countries.[2] As the incidence of lymphoma is generally low in the same countries where FL is low, the incidence becomes very low. The annual incidence of FL in North America is 3.44 per 100 000 population in contrast with 0.15–0.38 per 100 000 in Asian countries.[31] Follicular lymphoma is predominantly a disease of middle-aged and elderly individuals, with a media age of 59 years at diagnosis.[1,32] There is a slight female predominance. Children are rarely affected, and the clinicopathologic and biologic features are different from those of adults, and will be discussed in more detail later in this chapter.[33–35] Familial cases of FL or those occurring in twins are extremely rare.[36,37] Little is known regarding the etiology of FL. Epidemiologic studies from the late 1980s suggested a possible link to environmental factors, including fertilizers and pesticides.[38] More recently, large-scale genetic epidemiologic studies have been possible due in part to the formation of consortia such as the InterLymph group.[39] A number of promising candidate genes and epidemiologic factors are beginning to emerge that convey either increased or decreased relative risk for the development of FL.[40–44] Candidate genes include many involved in cell signaling and immune response. Single nucleotide polymorphisms (SNPs) of genes such as caspase 3, caspase 9, tumor necrosis factor (TNF) and toll-like receptors have recently been implicated in affecting the risk for the development of FL.[40–42] More recently, an inverse relationship between sun exposure and FL development has been suggested, possibly mediated by a polymorphism of the vitamin D receptor gene.[45] As additional studies are performed more candidate susceptibility genes will be identified, many providing new insights into the biology of FL.

ONTOGENY

Follicular lymphoma is derived from germinal center B cells showing many features in common with normal follicle center cells. Most cases (85 percent) are characterized by a balanced translocation, the t(14;18)(q32;q21) that appears to be a pivotal disease-initiating event.[46,47] In humans, several distinct genes code for the immunoglobulin molecules. In normal B cells the gene segments (V [variable], D [diversity] and J [joining]) coding for a full length variable region of immunoglobulin are discontinuous, and thus must be recombined at the level of the DNA.[48] For the immunoglobulin heavy chain (IGH) locus there are 123 V region, 27 D region and 6 J region gene segments and recombination is random, thus significant diversity is possible simply based on the various VDJ combinations (so-called combinatorial diversity).[49] This occurs by a complicated system involving specific recombination recognition sequences (RRSs) in the primary DNA sequence, two RAG (recombinase activating genes, RAG1 and RAG2) genes and the nuclear enzyme terminal deoxynucleotidyl transferase (Tdt), capable of randomly adding base pairs to the end of a single strand of DNA in the absence of a template strand. Although DNA breakage and recombination are tightly controlled, a modicum of imprecision occurs, resulting in further sequence diversity.[48] All of these features contribute to the diversity of the immunoglobulin molecules by producing in-frame VDJ sequences of variable length and primary base pair sequence.

The molecular anatomy of the t(14;18) genetic alteration suggests that it occurs prior to antigen exposure in an immature B cell in the bone marrow that expresses nuclear Tdt and results from an error in primary VDJ gene recombination induced by the RAG complex.[50,51] The majority of the IGH breaks in BCL2 translocated cases involve the 5' end of a J region gene segment. This appears to be a RAG-induced alteration.[52] Initial studies of FL cases with t(14;18) suggested that the RAG complex in predisposed B cells recognizes RRSs on chromosome 18 within the BCL2 gene, leading to the abnormal fusion of chromosome 14 to chromosome 18 and the deregulated constitutive expression of the BCL2 gene. Overexpression of BCL2, an antiapoptotic molecule, would thus confer a survival advantage on B cells harboring this alteration. More recent studies could not confirm the presence of RRSs within the well-defined breakpoint regions of the BCL2 gene, suggesting that another mechanism may be responsible for the translocation. Proximity of the two chromosomes within the interphase nucleus has been proposed as a possible mechanism underlying the t(14;18) as well as other translocations, and more recently, the tendency for several of the BCL2 breakpoint regions to form areas of single-stranded DNA (so-called 'non-B DNA') that then fall under attack by the RAG complex, resulting in illegitimate recombination with the IGH locus on chromosome 14q32.[53] Alternative mechanisms have been proposed, including those involving templated nucleotide insertions.[54] This mechanism suggests that two separate steps occur: one involving VDJ recombination

and the other involving somatic hypermutation (SHM). Moreover, these data infer continued expression of RAG enzymes in late stages of B cell differentiation, raising the possibility that in some cases the t(14;18) may occur in the germinal center.

Regardless of the underlying mechanism, the random addition of N-nucleotides at the sites of DNA breakage suggests that the translocation occurs at an immature stage of differentiation when nuclear Tdt is actively expressed. This putative lymphoma precursor cell is then left with the capacity to differentiate. It exits the bone marrow and then seeds germinal centers in peripheral lymph node sites. Within germinal centers these cells rapidly divide and undergo rounds of DNA breakage characteristic of the germinal center milieu, in particular, SHM and class switch recombination (CSR).[55,56] These two molecular mechanisms are critical to the normal process of affinity maturation that helps fine-tune the diversity of the antibody response. Both induce double-strand DNA breakage and require the presence of activation-induced cytidine deaminase (AID). In some cases of FL the molecular anatomy of the translocated allele indicates that the t(14;18) occurs at a later stage of B cell differentiation, as the IGH breakpoints on chromosome 14q32 involve the switch region.[57] These unusual variants suggest that some translocations may occur in the germinal center, but in the majority of cases the BCL2 translocation arises in a cell within the bone marrow. Follicular lymphomas show all the hallmarks of germinal center B cells, including a high load of somatic mutations and in 80 percent of cases, class-switch recombination, the latter affecting both the translocated and the productive alleles. The translocated allele disrupts the IGV region and is often accompanied by deletion of the IgM-IgD region, however, on the productive allele this region is spared and so FLs commonly typically express surface IgM and IgD. This creates an allelic paradox whereby a cell that has undergone CSR continues to express IgM. Because these cells overexpress BCL2, they survive in the harsh environment of the germinal center and are prone to acquire further genetic changes. In contrast with VDJ recombination, during which double-strand DNA breaks are introduced by the RAG site-specific endonuclease, CSR and SHM are initiated by AID; AID is a single-stranded DNA deaminase that targets cytidine residues, thereby creating uracil-guanine mismatches in DNA, which are processed by a number of error-prone DNA repair enzymes, producing mutations and/or double-strand DNA breaks.

PATHOLOGY

Morphologic characteristics

ARCHITECTURAL FEATURES

Follicular lymphoma recapitulates the architecture, cytologic findings and phenotype of normal germinal centers and thus typically grows in a nodular pattern.[24] Polarity, defined as the presence of both light and dark zones within the germinal center, is a characteristic feature of benign follicles. This feature is virtually never seen in the neoplastic follicles of FL. In most lymph nodes involved by FL, the malignant follicles efface the normal architecture, obliterate the sinuses and frequently extend into the perinodal fat. The follicles are often closely packed and form a back-to-back pattern with effacement of normal mantle zones.[58] Some diffuse areas may be seen, but in most cases these are not prominent. The follicles may be poorly defined, making recognition difficult without the use of immunohistochemistry for follicular dendritic cells (FDCs). Similarly, an interfollicular component is variably present, but should not be confused with a true diffuse pattern. A purely diffuse variant of FL exists (a subset were previously recognized as diffuse small cleaved cell lymphoma) and typically shares immunophenotypic and genetic features with otherwise typical FL (see below). These cases are exceedingly rare. Much more frequent are cases of FL with poorly defined follicles that are mistaken for diffuse lymphomas. In 10–15 percent of cases of FL, areas of marginal zone differentiation are found.[59,60] This feature is recognized as a pale zone immediately surrounding the neoplastic follicles and is made up of cells resembling marginal zone or monocytoid B cells. This area of marginal zone differentiation is usually four to five cells thick and can be seen as a prominent halo surrounding the neoplastic follicles. This feature is not to be confused with the so-called 'inside-out' follicular architecture where larger centroblasts surround the small centrocytes of otherwise typical grade 1 FL.[61] Follicular lymphoma is often accompanied by sclerosis that may be within the follicles and/or in the interfollicular zones.[62] The clinical significance of sclerosis has recently been analyzed (see section on prognostic parameters).[63] A floral variant of FL exists that can morphologically mimic progressive transformation of germinal centers.[64] The clinical significance of this finding is uncertain.

CYTOLOGIC FEATURES

Most cases of FL are composed of two cell types that similarly make up the germinal center B cells of reactive lymphoid follicles. Centrocytes are small cells with angulated, twisted nuclei, inconspicuous nucleoli and scant amounts of pale cytoplasm. The second major cell type of FL is the centroblast. These are large cells with large nuclei, open chromatin, two to three peripheral nucleoli often adjacent to the nuclear membrane and a thin rim of amphophilic cytoplasm. The latter feature is more easily appreciated with Giemsa stains typically used in Europe that highlight the basophilic cytoplasm of centroblasts. Some cases of FL show a predominance of large centrocytes, but their presence does no alter the grading (see below).[24] A sizable minority of FL cases show ambiguous cytology characterized by large numbers of medium-sized cells resembling small centroblasts. Although recognition of such cases as FL is easy, precise grading is very difficult.[16] Caution may be required

when grading FL samples as some cases show significant increases in FDCs. These cells should not be confused with centroblasts, but rather are the antigen-presenting cells of both the benign and the malignant follicles.

Follicular lymphoma is graded by the proportion of centroblasts.[65] When non-doxorubicin-containing regimens are used for treatment, grading may be predictive of survival.[24] The reproducibility of grading remains controversial and thus its clinical significance is unresolved. Follicular lymphoma cases with 0–5 centroblasts per HPF within neoplastic follicles are grade 1 (Plate 45, see plate section). Grade 2 cases have 6–15 large centroblasts per HPF and grade 3a has >15 large centroblasts per HPF. Grade 3 FL is subdivided into 3a and 3b in which grade 3a still shows residual small centrocytes, whereas grade 3b FL shows a true follicular pattern with sheets of centroblasts within the follicles.[24] In many cases of FL there is variability in cytologic composition between follicles and between different anatomic sites.[66] This variability should be noted as should as the presence of true diffuse areas. The latter appears to represent early histologic transformation and is therefore probably a harbinger of more aggressive behavior.

A number of variant cytologic features may also be encountered in FL biopsies. As noted above, an increase in large centrocytes may be seen, but these do not alter the grading.[24] Only the number of large transformed cells within follicles, i.e. centroblasts contribute to the histologic grade. Rare cases of FL show intracytoplasmic immunoglobulin deposits, typically within centrocytes and are referred to as signet ring cell lymphoma.[67] Occasional cases of FL show plasma cell differentiation, both within the follicles and in the interfollicular zones that are clonally related to the tumor cells.[68] Uncommonly the presence of marginal zone differentiation may exist within the follicles as opposed to the usual architectural pattern of forming halos around the follicles.[60] Lastly, 'blastoid' morphologic features may be seen rarely in FL often accompanied by an increase in mitotic activity.[69] This finding makes grading extremely difficult.

Both benign and neoplastic follicles contain variable numbers of reactive cellular components other than B cells. This includes FDCs, reactive T cells, endothelial cells and macrophages. In FL samples with obvious clonal light chain restriction, some of the B cells will show expression of the other light chain and thus represent benign B cells.

Interfollicular involvement is variably present in FL and probably represents a special form of lymphoid trafficking.[70,71] The neoplastic cells within this zone tend to be smaller, have more clumped chromatin and display a more round nuclear contour in contrast to typical centrocytes. These cells are easily confused with reactive T cells. As discussed below, the interfollicular component also shows a significant alteration of their immunophenotype.[70]

Peripheral blood involvement

Circulating lymphoma cells may be seen in the peripheral blood of FL patients and may indicate an unfavorable prognosis independent of stage.[72–74] The reported frequency varies between 5 percent and 20 percent at diagnosis. The lymphoma cells range from scanty to abundant, but may not be accompanied by a lymphocytosis. The lymphoma cells show a very high nuclear/cytoplasmic ratio with virtually no visible cytoplasm, irregular nuclei often with a deep cleft (so-called buttock cells), an indistinct nucleolus and relatively clumped, mature chromatin.

Bone marrow involvement

The bone marrow shows involvement in FL in 25–50 percent of cases.[29,72,75] Typically the infiltrates are paratrabecular and composed of mostly small centrocytes. This is also the case for grades 2 and 3a FL, where the bone marrow is frequently a lesser cytologic grade.[76,77] However, in some cases admixed large centroblasts are also seen dependent on histologic grade. The endosteal surface of the bony trabeculae characteristically shows a thin rim of fibrosis and appears relatively hypocellular. Other patterns including diffuse, interstitial, nodular and follicular can also be seen.[76,78,79] Trephine biopsies often reveal evidence of FL involvement in comparison to bone marrow aspirates and clot sections. This finding in part explains the better yield using the bone marrow biopsy samples for staging purposes and the frequent lack of contribution from ancillary studies including flow cytometry and/or molecular genetic investigations.[80] Immunohistochemical studies are of value for recognizing the expression of CD20 and CD10, but must be interpreted with caution, as most infiltrates show a generous admixture of reactive cells (T cells, macrophages, etc.) mimicking the neoplastic follicles in lymph nodes. Moreover, the expression of CD10 is often weak or negative in comparison to the lymph node in the same patient. This is the only small B cell lymphoma that characteristically shows FDC meshworks underlying many of the BM infiltrates.[81]

Splenic involvement

Follicular lymphoma involves the spleen at a frequency of 25–55 percent based on studies from the staging laparotomy era.[66] The cut surface is typically studded with numerous nodules that occupy the white pulp. Spill over into the red pulp is frequent. The dominant cell type is centrocytes, dependent on histologic grade, and there may be marginal zone differentiation.

Grade 3 FL

Grades 3a versus 3b FL are distinguished by the presence of some residual centrocytes in 3a.[24] Grade 3b FL is composed of at least some follicular structures showing sheets of centroblasts, but characteristically is accompanied by diffuse areas (Plate 46, see plate section).[82] Grade 3b FL with a purely follicular architecture is extremely uncommon. Previous studies examining the clinical impact of grade 3 FL (follicular large cell lymphoma) did not distinguish between 3a and 3b and thus, must be interpreted with caution. A number of correlative sciences studies have examined the differences between grades 3a and 3b FL.[82–89]

Grade 1 through grade 3a FL represent opposite ends of a continuum defining a single biologic entity, which characteristically shows increasing numbers of centroblasts, increasing proliferation and thus, increasing pace of disease if not treated with anthracycline-containing chemotherapy regimens. All FLs within this spectrum show a similar immunophenotype that typically includes expression of CD10, BCL6 and BCL2. The vast majority of grades 1–3a FL harbor t(14;18), but show more cytogenetic complexity with increasing grade.[47] Thus, grade 1 through grade 3a FL are considered part of the spectrum of a single biologic entity.

Grade 3b FL on the other hand shows a number of features more reminiscent of de novo DLBCL.[82] In particular, areas of sheet-like growth of centroblasts are very common. Involvement of the staging BM is less frequent in comparison to grade 3a FL. CD10 is expressed in only 50 percent of FL 3b cases. Similarly, the expression of BCL2 is also slightly reduced in comparison and the frequency of cytoplasmic immunoglobulin and p53 expression is increased in 3b FL.[82] The t(14;18) is identified in only 13 percent of cases, while 3q27 (BCL6) translocations are found in 44 percent of grade 3b FL in comparison with 18 percent in grade 3a. Moreover, the t(14;18) and t(3;14)(q27;q32) or variants are mutually exclusive in grade 3b FL, but can coexist in grade 1 through grade 3a FL.[47,89,90] The implication from all of these data is that grade 3b FL is more akin to de novo DLBCL and thus should be treated in a similar manner.[91] However, the few studies that have examined this issue have not shown convincing data that a clinical difference exists between grades 3a and 3b FL.[88,92,93] In fact, it appears that the presence of diffuse areas accounting for >50 percent of the surface area of the biopsy was the only factor distinguishing patients with inferior overall and event-free survival. The proper interpretation of these results requires some context; as diffuse, sheet-like growth accounting for >50 percent of the biopsy is by definition a composite histology, including both FL and DLBCL. In summary, the clinical relevance of distinguishing between grade 3a vs 3b FL has not been universally accepted.[94] Contributing to the clinical uncertainty is the clear acknowledgement that reproducible morphologic distinction between these two subtypes is poor. See Table 31.1 for features distinguishing between FL grades 3a and 3b.

Follicular lymphoma variants

PRIMARY CUTANEOUS FOLLICLE CENTER CELL LYMPHOMA

Skin involvement can occur in otherwise typical systemic FL and would produce infiltrates that are morphologically, immunophenotypically and genetically similar to their nodal counterparts.[95] However, follicle center cell lymphomas (FCCLs) may arise primarily in the skin and only involve that extranodal site.[96–102] These cases may exhibit important differences from nodal FL. Cutaneous FCCL tend to occur on the head (particularly the scalp) and trunk producing single or grouped erythematous papules and nodules without accompanying nodal involvement. The infiltrates are composed of a mixture of centrocytes and centroblasts, but distinct follicle formation may be less well defined. They tend to be higher histologic grade in comparison to nodal FL. The malignant cells typically express CD10 and BCL6, but expression of BCL2 protein is much less common than nodal counterparts. Similarly, the presence of the t(14;18) is reported much less frequently, suggesting that many of these cases represent a distinct biology.[102] These cases are very amenable to local therapeutic maneuvers in contrast with systemic FL.

DIFFUSE VARIANT OF FL

A purely diffuse variant of FL is rare. In most cases it results from an inability to appreciate subtle follicle formation and/or failure to perform immunohistochemistry for FDCs. By definition, diffuse follicular lymphoma consists of a completely diffuse infiltrate of predominantly small centrocytes with scattered, admixed centroblasts. Dependent on the number of centroblasts, grades 1 (<5 large transformed cells per HPF) and 2 (5–15 large transformed cells per HPF) can be recognized.[24] Distinction from other diffuse small B cell lymphomas may be difficult. By definition, the tumor cells express both CD10 and BCL6 and are typically BCL2 positive. Molecular evidence of a t(14;18) should be present or investigated in suspected cases. This is most easily accomplished using fluorescence in situ hybridization or alternatively polymerase chain reaction (PCR) techniques. A diffuse component composed of large centroblasts should be separately designated, for example, 'diffuse follicular lymphoma, grade 2, with diffuse large B cell lymphoma'. This is a harbinger of early histologic transformation of FL (see below).

IN SITU FOLLICULAR LYMPHOMA

A rare form of FL is referred to as in situ FL.[103] It is almost certainly underreported as it is very difficult to appreciate based on routine histologic sections. As a result, BCL2 immunohistochemistry is not performed and cases go unnoticed. The typical findings are those of a slightly enlarged lymph node with mostly reactive lymphoid follicles. A small proportion of the follicles harbor large numbers of strongly BCL2 positive centrocytes, producing a striking pattern following immunostaining. Molecular studies have shown that these follicles are clonal and frequently also show BCL2 gene rearrangements. The surrounding reactive follicles are polyclonal. Laser-capture microdissection of adjacent neoplastic follicles in cases of in situ FL show identical rearrangements; suggesting homing to and early colonization of reactive follicles.[103] Studies suggest that in almost half of the cases the findings represent early FL. The remaining cases may represent the early

stages of FL or a preneoplastic event requiring additional genetic alterations before frank neoplasia can develop. In situ FL should be distinguished from 'early FL', in which lymph nodes harbor clear evidence of FL, but also show scattered reactive lymphoid follicles.[104] These typically do not show the characteristic BCL2 staining pattern associated with in situ FL, but have been shown to be associated with favorable clinical findings and improved survival.

PEDIATRIC FOLLICULAR LYMPHOMA

As noted previously in this chapter, the development of FL in preadolescent patients is quite rare.[35] In the pediatric age group, FL accounts for only 0.8–2.9 percent of all lymphomas.[105,106] In contrast with typical FL in adults, pediatric patients with FL appear to have distinct clinical, pathologic and biologic features. For example, pediatric cases typically present with limited stage disease, often confined to the head and neck, show mostly grades 2 and 3 histology and characteristically lack both BCL2 protein expression and evidence of t(14;18). This tumor appears to be highly curable with infrequent relapses.[33] Primary testicular lymphomas are extremely rare, but interestingly all published cases have shown grade 3 FL.[107] These cases also appear to represent a distinct biology, as cases are consistently BCL2 negative and do not show evidence of a BCL2 rearrangement. Reported cases express BCL6 and approximately half of the cases express CD10. In aggregate, these findings suggest that both pediatric FL and primary testicular FL in children derive from a completely different pathogenesis from FL in adults.[107,108]

PRIMARY DUODENAL FOLLICULAR LYMPHOMA

Extranodal FL is significantly less common than nodal disease. Primary FLs of the duodenum represent a very uncommon form of FL, but one with distinctive clinicopathologic features.[109–111] Virtually all cases present with localized disease (stages 1/2) in and around the ampulla of Vater, many not showing progression after long periods of simple observation. Most cases express BCL2, BCL6 and CD10.[112] A few cases with karyotypic data frequently show an isolated t(14;18) as the sole cytogenetic alteration. This intriguing finding suggests that primary duodenal FL may be cytogenetically stable, analogous to MALT lymphomas with t(11;18) (see Chapter 31).

COMPOSITE HISTOLOGIES

Biopsies showing FL together with another histologic diagnosis have been infrequently reported. The most common composite histology is typical FL with areas of DLBCL. As indicated earlier, any area of true DLBCL must be separately reported in cases of FL.[24] This finding is uncommon in grades 1 and 2 FL, is slightly more common in grade 3a FL and is almost an expected finding in grade 3b FL (see the section on transformation).

Follicular lymphomas occurring simultaneously with other B cell or T cell lymphomas may be difficult to recognize and thus are infrequently reported. The combination of FL with classical Hodgkin lymphoma is well recognized.[113–115] In most cases, molecular studies have shown a clonal relationship between isolated Reed–Sternberg cells and the FL B cells, suggesting a common clonal ancestry for both tumors.[114]

IMMUNOPHENOTYPE

The neoplastic cells of FL exhibit the typical immunophenotype of germinal center B cells and show monoclonal light chain expression in most cases. The tumor cells are usually surface immunoglobulin positive (IgM ± IgD, occasionally IgG, rarely IgA) and express either κ or λ light chains.[24] Pan-B cell antigens are also expressed including CD19, CD20, CD22, CD79a and PAX5. The neoplastic cells characteristically express CD10 and the nuclear antigen BCL6 (Plate 47, see plate section).[116,117] Occasional cases express CD43, particularly grade 3 FL. Most cases of FL express BCL2 protein, the result of deregulated expression of the BCL2 gene following the characteristic translocation t(14;18)(q32;q21). Rarely cases harbor a BCL2 rearrangement but fail to express the protein. A subset of these can be shown to express BCL2 protein if an alternative antibody is used, suggesting that some cases delete the epitope detected by the commonly used commercial antibody (Dako, clone 124).[118] Approximately 10–15 percent of cases of FL lack the t(14;18) and may show rearrangement of the BCL6 gene on chromosome 3q27 (see below).[87] Despite the absence of t(14;18), some of these cases express BCL2 protein, possibly resulting from copy number gain of the BCL2 gene (gains of chromosome 18q).[119] The remaining cases typically do not express BCL2, but may express other members of the BCL2 family of anti-apoptotic molecules, including $BCLX_L$, BAD and BAK.[120,121] More recently, a subset of FL cases has been recognized that lack expression of CD10. This group of CD10-negative FL cases tend to occur in older patients, typically show grade 3 morphology, fail to express BCL2 and characteristically express MUM1. These cases appear to be enriched for BCL6 translocations and may show more aggressive clinical behavior.[83,84]

In typical FL there is a variable, but well-recognized interfollicular component. It is estimated to be present in >90 percent of cases, but the presence of these interfollicular neoplastic B cells may be very subtle.[70] If these cells are plentiful, this particular feature can be used to help establish a diagnosis of FL and may represent a specialized form of cell trafficking characterized by cells that assume a different morphology and immunophenotype. These interfollicular FL cells tend to be smaller in size than typical centrocytes, show more rounded nuclear contours and more clumped chromatin. Expression of CD10 tends to be weaker and these cells are much less proliferative than neoplastic cells within the follicle centers. Cases of FL with prominent marginal zone differentiation characteristically show complete down-regulation of both CD10 and BCL6.

The nodules of FL typically show tight meshworks of FDCs that are easily identified using immunohistochemical stains for CD21, CD23, CD35 or CNA-42. Reactive T cells are present in varying numbers and can be demonstrated using antibodies to CD3. Variable subsets of these reactive T cells express CD4, CD8, CD57 and/or nuclear FOXP3. The distribution and absolute numbers of these cells appear to play a significant role in the biology and prognosis of FL.[122] Admixed reactive macrophages in variable numbers and distribution are also identified. The surrounding mantle zones contain polytypic reactive small B cells.

CYTOGENETIC FINDINGS

The genetic hallmark of FL present in 85 percent of cases in North America is the t(14;18)(q32;q21).[47,123] This translocation is seen in other lymphoma subtypes.[124–126] The frequency of t(14;18) in FL varies considerably from study to study; influenced by geography as well as variation in case selection and the methodology used to detect the translocation.[127] The frequency in North America (80–90 percent) is higher than European centers (70–80 percent), while the lowest frequency is reported in Asia (40–60 percent).[31,128–132] Rare cases show variant BCL2 translocations, including t(2;18)(p12;q21) and t(18;22)(q21;q11) involving the light chain genes κ and λ, respectively.[47,133] Translocations involving the BCL6 oncogene on chromosome 3q27 are seen in about 10–15 percent of cases.[82,90,134] Transgenic animal models placing the BCL2 oncogene under control of the Eμ IGH enhancer element demonstrated florid reactive follicular hyperplasia in the majority of the litter animals.[135] In time, approximately 50 percent of the mice develop an aggressive lymphoma, typically accompanied by additional cytogenetic alterations including acquired MYC translocations. These data suggest that a BCL2 translocation alone is insufficient to produce tumor formation. In human FL samples, patients with an isolated t(14;18) are uncommon, accounting for <5 percent of t(14;18)-positive cases and appears to be restricted to grade 1 histology (Plate 48, see plate section).[47] The implication from the animal studies is that other abnormalities are present in these t(14;18)-only cases, but are below the level of detection using standard G-banding karyotyping techniques.

In addition to balanced translocations, FL reveals a number of different alterations including genomic amplifications, deletions, inversions, insertions and infrequent ring chromosomes. The malignant cells show frequent secondary alterations in addition to the t(14;18), the total number of which varies with the histologic grade. Grade 1 FL reveals an average of 4.8 secondary changes, grade 2 FL 6.5 and grade 3 FL 19.0.[47] Combining all grades of FL, the most common alterations include +7, +X, +12, deletion 6q13–26, +18 or

+der(18) and isochromosome 17q.[90,136–139] Polyploidy and marker chromosomes are more common in grade 3 FL.[140] In particular, grade 3b FL shows a much lower frequency of t(14;18) (approximately 10–15 percent) and increased frequency of BCL6 translocations, mimicking the frequency identified in large series of DLBCL.[82,91] More refined karyotyping strategies such as multicolor FISH and spectral karyotyping (SKY) have shown additional alterations less apparent from G-banding, including alterations of 1p36, 3q27–29, 12q, 17q, +18/18q+ and +21.[137,141] Comparative genomic hybridization (CGH) studies have provided further resolution of the genomic changes in FL, particularly gains and losses.[136,138] Loss of chromosomal material at 6q25–27 has been associated with inferior survival. Genome-wide SNP chips are useful for assessing gains and losses in FL at a higher resolution than standard chromosomal CGH. These studies have provided evidence for acquired uniparental disomy (UPD), also known as copy-neutral loss of heterozygosity, on chromosomes 6p, 9p, 12q and 17p in FL progression.[142] More recently, Ross and colleagues analyzed flow-sorted, purified FL B cells from 58 cases and demonstrated a number of important observations.[143] First, deletion and/or UPD involving chromosome 1p36.3 is the second most common alteration in FL genomes, suggesting the presence of a tumor suppressor gene at this site. Second, they confirmed the complexity of 6q deletions in FL and implicated two possible genes, TNFAIP3 and PERP at chromosome 6q23.3–24.1. In 8 percent of cases this region showed homozygous deletion. Lastly, they confirmed a region of UPD involving chromosome 6p in 30 percent of FL patients. Elegant work by Höglund and colleagues using computational analyses has revealed distinct pathways of clonal evolution of karyotypes in FL.[139] Following a t(14;18), distinct pathways involving +7/+8, +18/18q+/der(18), +1q or 6q– can be recognized followed by a common set of deletions that characterize later changes of clonal evolution.[139]

MOLECULAR GENETICS FINDINGS

As noted above, the hallmark of FL is t(14;18) that leads to the constitutive expression of the BCL2 gene.[25] The translocation involves the 5′ end of a J region gene segment and thus abrogates a functional VDJ rearrangement from the translocated allele. Given that most FL cases express surface immunoglobulin, the normal chromosome 14 allele undergoes a functional rearrangement of the IGH locus (VDJ rearrangement) in order to generate an intact variable region gene. As FL shares molecular features of normal germinal center B cells, FL samples show frequent somatic hypermutation of the variable region of both heavy and light chain genes as well as evidence of on-going mutation, the latter showing a mutational pattern suggesting antigen-driven clonal selection.[144] Follicular lymphoma shows a lower frequency of clonality using consensus IGH PCR strategies that employ framework 3 region primers. This is

mainly due to the marked SHM that targets the CDR3 region of the IGH locus and leads to failed JH primer binding.[145,146] The breakpoints involving the BCL2 gene tend to cluster, a finding that has facilitated the development of PCR strategies to detect translocations.[147,148] The majority of breakpoints cluster in the 3′ noncoding region of the third exon known as the major breakpoint region (mbr). Other breakpoints include the minor cluster region (mcr), the intermediate cluster region (icr) and the variable cluster region (vcr).[127,149] Many previous molecular studies underestimated the frequency of BCL2 translocations in FL, choosing to study only mbr and mcr breakpoints. The involvement of the icr has recently been shown to be more frequent than the mcr, both in Europe and North America.[150,151] In the past PCR approaches suffered from a high false-negative rate due to the wide distribution of breakpoint regions, but more recent strategies using multiplex PCR techniques have shown improvements in detection rates.[148] FISH studies have proven to be the most robust method for detecting the t(14;18) (Plate 48) and perhaps more importantly, are easily adaptable to paraffin-embedded material. In particular, disaggregating the nuclei of formalin fixed material prior to analyses provides technically excellent results using FISH strategies.[152]

The second most frequent balanced translocation in FL (10–12 percent) involves juxtaposition of the BCL6 gene at chromosome 3q27 with one of the three immunoglobulin loci in form of t(3;14)(q27;q32), t(2;3)(p12;q27) or t(3;22) (q27;q11), or with a non-immunoglobulin locus.[153–155] BCL6 translocations may coexist with t(14;18) in grades 1 or 2 FL, but appear to be mutually exclusive in grade 3b FL.[47,89,90] In the latter FL subtype, the presence of BCL6 translocations tends to be associated with a lack of BCL2 protein expression, CD10-negativity and expression of MUM1.[82,84] Mutations of the 5′ noncoding region of the BCL6 oncogene occur in normal germinal center B cells as a result of targeting by the somatic hypermutation apparatus, but occur at a tenth of the frequency of IGH mutations. BCL6 mutations are found in 60 percent of FL cases and may play a role in histologic transformation (see below).[156]

GENE EXPRESSION PROFILING

Genome-wide transcription profiling has been successfully applied to samples of FL, providing important insight into the biology of the disease as well as molecular predictors of survival.[16,157–159] One of the original studies of expression profiling of FL analyzed flow-sorted purified neoplastic B cells and determined a list of differentially expressed genes in comparison to normal germinal center B cells.[157] Genes that were either up or downregulated were discovered with the former, showing a good correlation with copy number gains as determined by cytogenetics.[141] As a result of the approach of using purified neoplastic B cells, gene signatures derived from non-neoplastic cells in the tumor biopsies were not analyzable. A number of additional studies have now been published using whole frozen FL biopsy samples with somewhat differing results.[16,158] The latter may be the result of using different microarray platforms, variable methodology and bioinformatics tools for analysis in addition to differences in patient selection. Dave et al. studied 191 frozen FL biopsy samples to determine molecular predictors of overall survival.[158] Ten gene expression signatures predictive of outcome were found, five associated with favorable survival and five associated with inferior survival. However, two dominant signatures accounted for the most discriminate outcomes and appeared to be derived from non-neoplastic cells in the tumor microenvironment. One called immune response-1 was associated with favorable survival and contained many T cell genes and a few monocyte-derived genes. The other called immune response-2 was associated with inferior survival and was mostly a monocyte/antigen presenting cell (FDC) gene signature. Combining these two signatures into a molecular predictor score allowed the prediction of very disparate survivals for patients with newly diagnosed FL. Glas et al., using a non-commercial microarray platform, studied a cohort of FL patients grouped according to outcome and biopsy-proven histologic transformation.[16,159] These authors defined an 81-gene model capable of predicting immediate clinical behavior following biopsy, either diagnostic or at relapse, but were unable to determine any expression profiles associated with long-term survival or transformation risk. In a follow-up study of patients with early or late transformation, these same authors were unable to determine a consistent expression profile associated with early (<3 years from diagnosis) transformation, but did find that biopsies with increased intra-follicular CD4+ T cells determined using immunohistochemistry were more likely to transform early (see below).[159] The single consistent conclusion from these studies is that non-neoplastic cells in the microenvironment of FL are major contributors to the biology, transformation risk and clinical outcome of FL.

TRANSFORMATION

Histologic transformation is variably reported in FL, ranging from 4 percent to 68 percent.[3–7] This is in part due to a lack of strict criteria used to define transformation and the use of different classifications in the previous literature.[160] In the current era the diagnosis of transformation is further hampered because of a growing reliance on fine needle aspiration and needle core biopsy techniques used to assess clinically suspicious anatomic sites. Transformation when it occurs is a dominant clinical event.[11,161,162] It is often heralded by a change in the clinical course, such as a marked enlargement of a single nodal site of disease, the development of significant extranodal disease, a marked increase in serum lactate dehydrogenase (LDH) or hypercalcemia.[10]

Overall survival following transformation is significantly shortened, in part because patients are older and have frequently been exposed to a number of prior therapies for FL. It is important to note that some cases of FL demonstrate an aggressive clinical course in the absence of biopsy-proven histologic transformation. This probably reflects the profile of molecular and cytogenetic changes that characterize the malignant clone and/or a contribution by immune cells in the tumor microenvironment. When transformation is confirmed, the most frequent histologic type is DLBCL.[160] The usual scenario is a grade 1 FL at diagnosis, followed at a later date by a biopsy showing DLBCL with sheets of centroblasts. However, a number of other histologies can be seen, including Burkitt-like lymphoma, so-called blastoid or blastic transformation, Tdt-positive lymphoblastic lymphoma and classical Hodgkin lymphoma.[160,163–167] Cases described as Burkitt-like often show histologic findings intermediate between Burkitt lymphoma and DLBCL, so-called 'gray zone' lymphomas.[164] Moreover, biopsies showing histologic transformation of previous FL may be very difficult to classify using a classification scheme (WHO) largely based on primary diagnostic biopsies. In addition, the morphologic aspects of transformation specimens may be affected by prior therapy, further confounding reproducible classification.

The criteria for diagnosis of transformation are intended to be the same as those used for corresponding de novo biopsies, i.e. sheets of large lymphoid cells expressing at least one B lineage defining marker, lacking markers of other lymphoid lineages.[24] However, consensus criteria for defining early transformation in a background of FL are not agreed upon. Typically, if one identifies sheet-like areas of interfollicular large B cells with little intervening small lymphocytes, many pathologists would recognize this as a focus of early transformation. Unresolved, however, is the problem of the definition of a 'sheet' of large B cells. A small survey of eight expert hematopathologists was unable to reach consensus regarding the following issues (unpublished observations, 2007):

- the clinical relevance of sheet-like growth of interfollicular large B cells in a background of FL
- what was the definition of a 'sheet' of large B cells
- what features constitute early transformation.

Moreover, no agreement was possible regarding how such cases should be reported. Should these large B cell areas simply be included as a comment in a report or should they dictate a formal diagnosis of composite histology lymphoma, e.g. FL and a focus of DLBCL? These issues remain unresolved and thus are critical to recognizing the ambiguity surrounding diagnostic criteria for recognizing histologic transformation of FL. This uncertainty in diagnosis further confounds the interpretation of clinical outcome data following transformation.

With the exception of an associated increase in the proliferation rate (Ki-67), transformation is not defined using immunophenotypic criteria. Occasional cases show a phenotypic shift with loss of previously positive antigens such as BCL2, CD10 or BCL6, but typically the immunophenotypic features of the FL are preserved following transformation. Of potential diagnostic benefit might be the use of p53 (gain of expression) and p16 (loss of expression) immunohistochemistry, as alteration of the expression of either of these two proteins accompanied by morphologic evidence of large B cells would support a diagnosis of transformation.[13-15]

The majority of previous studies have confirmed a clonal relationship between the initial FL and the subsequent diffuse aggressive lymphoma, in keeping with a true transformation process.[168] However, some conflicting data exist. BCL2 rearrangements are stable clonal markers and most studies that have examined their presence in paired samples of FL with subsequent DLBCL show identical rearrangements in both biopsies. Alternatively, a review of published reports of cytogenetic profiles from paired samples shows somewhat discrepant findings.[133,169,170] Many cases show clonal karyotypes in paired samples with evidence of additional alterations in the transformed biopsy, while other cases show less clonal evolution in the DLBCL sample. This result suggests that the transformation sample represents outgrowth of a preexisting subclone of the FL.[171,172] Follicular lymphoma is a germinal center-derived neoplasm with evidence of ongoing somatic mutation of the B cell receptor. Previous studies have shown that the pattern of IGH mutations suggest initial antigen selection followed by clonal expansion.[144,173] Both histologic transformation and relapse of FL are thought to result from this process. Moreover, the initial studies using anti-idiotype therapy in FL clearly established a role for SHM and its contribution to the generation of antibody diversity in FL. Patients treated with passive administration of anti-idiotype antibodies rapidly became resistant to this treatment as their tumor cells mutated their B cell receptor, proving an important role for SHM acting under the selective pressure of treatment.[174] However, similar to the cytogenetic data described above, subclone selection rather than ongoing clonal evolution and B cell receptor editing may be responsible. Follicular lymphoma transformation is probably a heterogeneous process and several mechanisms are responsible.

Studies of paired specimens of FL and subsequent DLBCL have been instrumental for our understanding of the molecular events that underlie transformation. In summary, these data clearly show that histologic transformation is a molecularly diverse process. Several studies have defined a key role for the p53 tumor suppressor gene localized to chromosome 17p13.1.[13,14] An analysis of paired specimens showed both loss of heterozygosity (LOH) and/or the typical scenario of deletion followed by mutation of the remaining allele (classical Knudsen model) when comparing FL samples with their subsequent transformed biopsy. Evidence supporting an important role for p53 mutations was seen in 25–30 percent of cases. Similarly, loss of another tumor suppressor gene, p16 (chromosome 9p21) due to hypermethylation, mutation or deletion may account for an even greater number of cases of FL transformation. In a cohort of paired samples, p16 loss was found in 80 percent of the transformed biopsies but none of the preexisting FL specimens.[15]

Additional cytogenetic alterations that appear to contribute to histologic transformation include gain of chromosome 7, deletion of chromosome 6q and amplification of 12q13–14.[175-178] Mutations in the 5' non-coding region of the BCL6 gene, translocations involving the BCL6 oncogene, as well as mutations in the open reading frame of BCL2 have also been described as acquired genetic alterations contributing to transformation.[179-183]

One of the first candidates identified in the transformation process was the MYC oncogene.[163] In contrast to the classical scenario of loss of tumor suppressor genes (e.g. p53 or p16) as described above, MYC is a dominant oncogene and thus, translocations or other mechanisms that lead to deregulated overexpression of MYC are pivotal to the transformation process. Yano and colleagues described a comparison of FL and paired DLBCL samples whereby MYC alterations were infrequently, but almost exclusively found in the transformed biopsies.[163] The acquisition of a secondary MYC alteration on a background of a t(14;18) would be expected to be an unwanted event and has been shown to carry a grave prognosis.[164] As described previously, the associated morphologic spectrum that follows is diverse, resulting in typical DLBCLs, other cases resembling Burkitt-like cases and still others with the classical appearance of lymphoblastic lymphoma. So-called 'dual-translocation' or 'double-hit' lymphomas may arise de novo as initial manifestations of NHL.[164,184,185] In fact, half of the reported cases share this clinical evolution, suggesting that MYC deregulation followed closely on the heels of the t(14;18), abrogating a clinical history of antecedent FL. The cytogenetic correlates of these dual-translocation lymphomas are also varied, but distinct from de novo Burkitt lymphoma, as half of the MYC translocations involve light chain loci as opposed to the IGH locus on chromosome 14q32. This likely results from the fact that one of the chromosome 14 alleles is already involved in a translocation with BCL2, leaving the normal chromosome 14 allele to undergo a functional VDJ rearrangement.

Lastly, gene expression profiling studies addressing the molecular characteristics of FL transformation have begun to emerge.[16,159,161,186-188] Although most studies are small and difficult to compare, some unifying hypotheses emerge. First, FL transformation is a heterogeneous process and may indeed be a common morphologic consequence of a number of molecular alterations. Second, common themes include increasing the expression of genes involved in metabolic pathways, the mitotic apparatus, p38 MAP kinase and MYC targets identified in the transformed biopsies. Third, and not unexpected, the expression profile of the transformed biopsy is reminiscent of a germinal center B cell-like profile (so-called GCB type). More recently, a role for non-neoplastic cells in the transformation process has been suggested. FL biopsies with increased numbers of activated CD4+ T cells within the neoplastic follicles appear to be at increased risk of early transformation.[159] Other studies suggest a possible role for cytotoxic T cells, benign B cells and perhaps also T regulatory cells in the transformation process (unpublished observations, 2007). A dynamic interaction between the tumor cells and non-neoplastic cells in the microenvironment appears to be important in FL biology. It can be hypothesized that the clinical diversity identified in cohorts of FL results from the fact that some FL patients are dominated by molecular alterations intrinsic to the malignant cells, while others may be influenced more by cross-talk emanating from the reactive cells in the tumor microenvironment. More studies are required to fully understand the interplay and the underlying mechanisms involved.

PROGNOSTIC PARAMETERS

Clinical indices

A number of clinical and biologic prognostic factors have been implicated in FL.[189–192] With median survivals in the range of 8–10 years, FL shows marked heterogeneity in clinical outcomes. Some patients progress or transform early while others are alive without therapy after more than a decade. In most reported series, roughly 15–20 percent of newly diagnosed FL patients are dead within 3 years, contrasting with a similar frequency of patients surviving beyond 25 years. Understanding the clinical and biologic correlates that underlie this diverse spectrum of outcomes is the subject of much investigation.

A number of multi-parameter clinical indices have been developed to predict prognosis in FL.[189,193,194] The international prognostic index (IPI) was originally developed for aggressive lymphomas, and it also distinguishes distinct outcomes in FL patients. However, few patients are assigned to the high-risk (IPI 4/5) category making it of less practical value. In 2004 a new index was developed specifically for FL, known as the FLIPI (FL international prognostic index) index.[189] It consists of five adverse parameters including:

- age (>60 years)
- stage (Ann Arbor stages III–IV)
- serum LDH (elevated)
- number of nodal sites (>4 sites)
- hemoglobin (<120 g/L).

Patients can then be divided into three risk groups; low, intermediate and high, with 10-year overall survival rates of 71 percent, 51 percent and 36 percent, respectively. In contrast to the IPI, the FLIPI distributes patients into three roughly equal groups.

Biologic indices

A number of biologic factors have been identified as prognostic factors in FL. These are detailed in Table 31.2. Although reproducible grading is fraught with difficulty, increasing histologic grade in FL is associated with inferior survival in some but not all series.[195,196] The impact of grade is only apparent when patients are treated with non-anthracycline-containing chemotherapy regimens.[24] The addition of anthracycline to the therapy appears to abrogate the prognostic impact of grade 3 FL. As most of the cases of FL with a predominance of large centroblasts are presumably grade 3a, the implication from the WHO publication is that patients with grade 3a FL derive significant benefit from the use of curative anthracycline-containing regimens.[24] The proliferation rate in FL shows an imperfect relationship with grade, with proliferation increasing with advancing histologic grade.[196] A subset of FL cases show discordance, characterized by low-grade histology and an increased proliferative rate. These cases appear to show more aggressive clinical behavior.[197] Diffuse areas in FL are very common in grade 3b FL and decrease in frequency with diminishing grade. For grades 1 through 3a they probably represent areas of early transformation and thus not surprisingly are associated with inferior survival. In a recent study of grade 3 FL patients treated with anthracycline-containing regimens, histologic grade did not impact survival, but the presence of diffuse areas comprising >50 percent of the cross-section of the biopsy was associated with decreased survival.[88] In many centers these cases would be diagnosed as composite histology lymphomas, encompassing both FL grade 3 and DLBCL, and thus would be expected to show a more aggressive course. The impact of diffuse areas in grades 1 and 2 FL is less clear, in part due to a lack of agreement on criteria used to define their presence (described in detail in the transformation section). Intuitively, a diffuse growth pattern probably represents early transformation, but further study is required to determine the true clinical impact of this finding. The presence of marginal zone differentiation in FL had been associated with diminished survival, but this finding could not be confirmed in three other recent studies.[60,190] In contrast with DLBCL and non-lymphoid malignancies, increased small vessel density in FL has been associated with improved survival in FL.[198] A recent evaluation of prognostic indices in advanced stage FL revealed sclerosis in 14 percent of patients, which was shown to be prognostic for both overall survival and time to treatment failure and was independent of the FLIPI.[63]

A growing number of immunophenotypic markers have been shown to be of prognostic importance in FL, including proteins related to apoptotic signaling, stage of differentiation, cell cycle and immune response.[122,159,190,191,199–206] Follicular lymphoma cases lacking expression of BCL2 appear to demonstrate improved survival. Increased expression of BCLX$_L$ is also associated with poor prognosis.[120] High ratios of BCL2/BAK and BCL2/BAX have also been

Table 31.2   Biologic prognostic factors in follicular lymphoma (FL)

Biomarker	Impact on survival	Comments
Morphology		
Histological grade	Survival worsens with increasing grade	Dependent on therapy. Doxorubicin-containing regimens seem to abrogate the effect
Proliferative rate	Controversial	Some studies suggest that more proliferative tumors do worse
Architecture (diffuse areas)	Worse	Studies suggest that >50% diffuse areas portends an inferior survival. Such cases are in essence composite histologies of FL/DLBCL
Grade 3a vs 3b	Controversial	Most studies have not shown a survival difference despite clear biologic differences
Microenvironment		
CD4+ T cells	Controversial	IHC studies show variable results, whereas flow cytometry suggests little impact on survival
CD8+ T cells	Controversial	IHC studies show little impact, whereas flow studies suggest variable results
Regulatory T cells	Controversial	Some studies suggest that increased Treg cells are favorable, while others suggest the opposite
Macrophages	Worse	Studies show inferior survival associated with increased CD68+ cells
Microvessel density	Controversial	
Follicular dendritic cells	Worse	Studies show that an immature FDC phenotype or disruption of the FDC meshwork is an unfavorable prognostic feature
Immunophenotype		
BCL6 protein	Favorable	
CD10	Favorable	
BCL2/BCL2/BAX ratio/BAK	Worse	Studies show that high ratios favoring BCL2 are associated with diminished survival
MCL1	Worse	Increased expression of MCL1 associated with a worse outcome
BCLX$_L$	Worse	Antiapoptotic protein, increased expression associated with worse survival
MUM1	Worse	
Cyclin B1	Favorable	Increased expression associated with favorable response to CHOP chemotherapy
p53	Worse	Associated with transformation
MDM2	Worse	Associated with increased risk of transformation
PU.1	Favorable	
Cytogenetics		
MYC	Worse	Presence of translocation associated with transformation
P16	Worse	Loss of the p16 locus associated with transformation
P53	Worse	Associated with transformation
BCL6	Controversial	Some studies suggest that 3q27 translocations are associated with risk of transformation
Gene expression		
Microenvironment	Variable	Immune response (IR)-1 favorable/IR-2 unfavorable

IHC, immunohistochemistry; FDC, follicular dendritic cell; CHOP, cyclophosphamide, vincristine, doxorubicin and prednisolone.

shown to predict for early death in FL patients.[199] The majority of FL cases express both BCL6 and CD10. Increased levels of expression of BCL6 have been associated with improved survival.[206] More recently it has been suggested that a unique subgroup of FL exists characterized by a CD10-negative, MUM1-positive immunophenotype. This profile appears to identify a group of FL patients that tends to be older, has more frequent grade 3 morphology, has diffuse areas, a higher proliferative rate, characteristically lacks

the t(14;18) and may have more frequent *BCL6* translocations. These patients appear to show more aggressive behavior, but the significance of this finding requires confirmation from the study of additional patient cohorts.[83,84] PU.1 is an ETS-domain transcription factor critical for B cell development. It has recently been shown that cases of FL expressing PU.1 have improved survival, a finding that was independent of the FLIPI.[205] Cell cycle regulators have been studied in FL, with several shown to have prognostic importance. The expression of p53, which is imperfectly correlated with *P53* mutations, is associated with diminished survival in FL.[191] Key regulators of p53, such as p21 and MDM2, are also correlated with survival.[207] Loss of p16 expression is similarly associated with decreased survival.[15] It is important to recall that all of these molecular cell cycle alterations are also associated with histologic transformation as discussed earlier in this chapter. Lastly, in patients treated with CHOP chemotherapy, increased expression of cyclin B1 was associated with improved survival.[208] A small number of other proteins involving unrelated pathways have also been implicated as prognostic biomarkers in FL. Increased expression of SOCS3, a member of the JAK-STAT pathway, is reported to be an adverse prognostic marker in FL.[209] Similarly, overexpression of YY.1, a zinc-finger protein involved in regulating interleukin (IL) 4 expression has recently been linked with shortened survival in FL.[210]

A number of cytogenetic and molecular alterations have been shown to affect survival in patients with FL.[90] Cases with isolated t(14;18) as the sole cytogenetic abnormality have improved survival. Increasing chromosomal complexity may predict for inferior survival, but interestingly polyploidy alone was not a predictor.[140] Cytogenetic alterations associated with inferior survival include gains such as +7, +12q13-14, +X, +18q and +21.[136,138,141] Loss of chromosomal material including deletion 6q, −9p21 and −17p13 have also been associated with inferior survival.[90] Although the precise locus of chromosome 6q has not been defined, −9p21 and −17p13 correspond to *p16* and *p53* loss, respectively. Translocations involving the *BCL6* oncogene have been suggested to predict for early transformation.[180] *MYC* translocations are rare in *de novo* FL, but their presence is associated with decreased survival. Translocations of *MYC* as a secondary, acquired abnormality are clearly associated with transformation and a markedly poor survival.[164] Additional regions implicated in FL transformation include deletion of 1p36.3 and gain of 6p22.3.[211]

The precise role of the non-neoplastic cells in the tumor microenvironment in FL is as yet incompletely defined, but several cell types have been implicated as contributors to outcome in patients with FL. Studies from the late 1980s suggested that increased CD4+ T cells were associated with spontaneous remissions in FL.[212] More recently, both the absolute number and architectural distribution of CD4+ T cells have been studied, with somewhat conflicting results.[159,200,202,213] One study found that increased CD4+ T cells were linked with favorable clinical behavior, while other studies could not confirm a prognostic role for these cells.[202,204,213] In contrast, increased intra-follicular CD4+ T cells were recently associated with an increased risk of early transformation, a finding somewhat at odds with the numerical data.[159] Enumeration of CD4+ T cells using flow cytometry did not show any prognostic impact in FL.[200,213] The role of CD8+ T cells is similarly confounded by conflicting data in FL. Some studies have suggested an association with improved outcome, while others suggest the opposite finding.[122,204,213,214] The gene

expression profiling data discussed earlier in this chapter did implicate CD8+ T cells (immune response-1) as predictors of improved overall survival.[158,215] Clearly, additional studies are required to resolve the precise contribution of these non-neoplastic cells to survival in FL. Regulatory T cells (Treg) are a subset of cells expressing CD4, CD25 and a nuclear transcription factor FOXP3. These cells have a role in regulating effector T cell populations and their presence has been associated with inferior survival in epithelial malignancies as a result of creating an immunosuppressive microenvironment that allows tumor cells to escape the host immune response. In FL, the role and prognostic relevance of these cells is controversial, as some studies suggest an association with favorable outcome whereas other studies suggest the opposite.[204,216] It may well be that the role of different T cell populations in the microenvironment of FL is context dependent, affected significantly by the clinical features of the patients and the treatments given. Further studies are clearly required.

Increased CD68+ macrophages have been associated with inferior survival in some, but not all studies.[159,190,201] Similarly, the role of FDCs expressing CD21 is unclear. Some studies have suggested that an immature FDC immunophenotype correlates with early progression, while other studies could not confirm these findings.[217] Recently, disruption of the FDC meshwork has been implicated as a predictor of early histologic transformation in FL.[159,218]

Lastly, novel strategies to examine the microenvironment and constitutional genetics have begun to explore the role of the host in FL biology and outcome prediction. Single nucleotide polymorphisms, SNPs, are single base-pair changes in the germline DNA that occur in healthy individuals. They represent but one form of genetic variation among individuals. A SNP for the *FcγRIIIa* gene has been shown to predict survival in FL patients following therapy with single-agent rituximab, an anti-CD20 monoclonal antibody.[219–221] The implication is that immune effector cells such as macrophages and possibly natural killer cells that mediate their effects through antibody-dependent cellular cytotoxicity and complement-mediated cell lysis, differentially bind the Fc portion of rituximab, dependent on the particular variant of FcR coded for in the host genome. The affinity of binding therefore, appears to impact the efficacy of rituximab as a single therapeutic agent. It remains unclear whether FcR polymorphisms will hold their prognostic significance in FL patients treated in the era of immunochemotherapy (R-CHOP [rituximab, cyclophosphamide, vincristine, doxorubicin and prednisolone]).[222]

Cerhan and colleagues recently examined the role of additional immune response SNPs in FL and found that four genes, *IL8, IL2, IL12B* and *IL1RN*, together with clinical and demographic factors, could be used to construct an outcome predictor that identified three risk groups with 5-year overall survival estimates of 96 percent (low risk), 72 percent (intermediate risk) and 58 percent (high risk).[192] These patients were variably treated and importantly, were treated prior to the introduction of rituximab into routine clinical practice. These tantalizing new data require validation in additional patient cohorts of FL.

Additional adverse prognostic factors include any degree of bone marrow involvement, presence of a molecular clone in the peripheral blood or bone marrow, an increase in the absolute lymphocyte count, elevated β_2-microglobulin and low serum albumin.[73,78,189,193,222–224]

PATHOGENESIS

The etiology of FL is largely unknown. Rare familial cases have been described. Previous epidemiologic studies suggested a role for exposure to fertilizers and pesticides.[38] More recently, genetic predisposition linked to certain immune response and DNA repair[225] genes have begun to emerge.[41,44] Two major themes have evolved to explain the pathogenesis of FL:

- a primary genetic model based on accumulating genomic alterations and clonal selection of neoplastic B cells
- a model based on the composition and function of the microenvironment in which the non-neoplastic cells exert a dominant effect on the behavior of the tumor cells.

Both will be discussed and a unifying theme presented.

Genetic model

Central to the genetics and pathogenesis of FL is the t(14;18)(q32;q21) that leads to the constitutive expression of BCL2 protein. The majority of FL biopsies harbor this balanced translocation. Those cases lacking the t(14;18) may deregulate *BCL2* via other mechanisms (increased gene copy number for example) and thus still aberrantly express the BCL2 protein, or alternatively, overexpress other antiapoptotic family members such as PI3K/AKT/BAD, MCL1, survivin or BCLX$_L$.[121] The net effect remains the same; the neoplastic cells are protected from apoptotic cell death during B cell selection in nonmalignant germinal centers. Therefore, a key pathogenic event in the biology of FL is a switch away from the default program of normal germinal center B cells. The vast majority of germinal center B cells die via programmed cell death, while FL B cells are inappropriately rescued as long-lived, mitotically quiescent cells. Translocations involving the *BCL6* gene occur in a subset of FL cases and appear to be enriched in cases lacking expression of CD10, expressing MUM1 or cases with grade 3b histology.[84,91] Some FLs show mutations in the 5′ noncoding region of the *BCL6* gene and a proportion result in deregulated expression of BCL6. The molecular anatomy of both the *BCL6* translocated and *BCL6* mutated cases suggest that these molecular events occur in cells within the germinal center.[134,226,227] The resultant deregulated BCL6 expression likely keeps cells within the germinal center microenvironment and produces a block in terminal B cell differentiation

as an additional oncogenic mechanism in a subset of FL. This feature may be in common with a subset of DLBCL of the activated B cell type.[228–230]

As described in detail in the ontogeny section, the weight of evidence, with a few exceptions, favors that the disease-initiating t(14;18) translocation occurs within an immature pro-B cell in the bone marrow.[231] In part, this appears to be a RAG-mediated event, although alternative mechanisms have been proposed.[53,54,232] The net effect is that the *BCL2* gene is juxtaposed to the *IGH* gene, resulting in increased *BCL2* transcription and resistance to apoptosis. In normal cells *BCL2* transcription is initiated from the dominant P1 promoter, but cells with the translocation preferentially deregulate transcription from the normally minor P2 promoter. Recent data suggest that specific regions of the 3′ *IGH* enhancer region, notably the HS12 site, are critical to the promoter shift in cells harboring the t(14;18), that subsequently lead to deregulated expression of the BCL2 protein.[233] Importantly, these antigen-naïve B cells exit the bone marrow and seed peripheral lymphoid niches, and eventually enter germinal centers.

Germinal centers are the site of two important mechanisms that contribute to the generation of normal antibody diversity; namely SHM and CSR. FL cells show two hallmarks of germinal center B cells. First, FL cells show ongoing SHM, resulting in intraclonal heterogeneity.[56] The pattern of these mutations, as evidenced by contrasting the ratio of replacement to silent mutations between the framework regions (FR) and the complementary determining regions (CDR) of *IGH*, suggests a process of antigen-driven clonal selection. Moreover, the clonal expansion of FL is subsequent to antigen selection.[144] Within the germinal centers these t(14;18)-positive cells are antigenically selected and then clonally expanded, all the while in a milieu where double-stranded chromosomal breakage is encouraged. The variable region heavy chain genes in FL acquire sequence motifs by SHM that serve as sites for *N*-glycosylation.[234] This accumulation of motifs available for the addition of oligosaccharides is not seen in normal germinal center B cells. In FL, these alterations primarily involve the CDRs. Although this phenomenon occurs in other germinal center-derived tumors such as Burkitt lymphoma and DLBCL, it is most pronounced in FL. Retention of the B cell receptor (BCR) is found in the vast majority of FL cases, suggesting that stimulation through surface Ig may be important in the pathogenesis of FL. It is hypothesized that the introduction of *N*-glycosylation sites into the BCR may allow consistent interaction with some unknown lectin in the follicle and thus obviates the need for persistent antigen.[235] The lack of common V$_H$ gene use in FL and the heterogeneity of mutations make the likelihood of a common antigen remote. Thus, the t(14;18) is considered to be the first hit, but on its own is not completely tumorigenic. This is further supported by *BCL2* transgenic animal models showing that mice harboring the transgene develop florid lymphoid hyperplasia, but only a subset develop lymphoma following a long latency period.[135] The almost universal presence of

N-glycosylation might therefore represent the second hit in a multistep process of follicular lymphomagenesis.[235]

It has recently been demonstrated that as many as 50 percent of normal individuals may have infrequent cells harboring the t(14;18) in their peripheral blood and/or bone marrow.[231,236] These can be detected using sensitive PCR strategies. The use of cell enrichment techniques prior to PCR suggests that the presence of these cells may be even more common in specific B cell subsets.[237] Factors that appear to increase the frequency of *BCL2* rearrangements in healthy individuals include increasing age, male sex and smoking. However, the presence of these rare cells harboring the t(14;18) has not been associated with an increased risk of developing FL and thus it was previously hypothesized that these cells were probably naïve B cells and simply died prior to establishing a clinically evident tumor. More recently it was shown that these same t(14;18)-bearing cells have indeed undergone class-switch recombination and thus have transited the germinal center.[231,238] These cells appear to represent a unique subclass of IgM memory B cells that share immunophenotypic similarities with FL. The likelihood is that in most individuals these cells never develop additional alterations that confer a malignant phenotype. However, in at-risk individuals these cells may survive, allowing them to continue to traffic between the blood, bone marrow and lymph nodes. In some healthy individuals these t(14;18)-positive follicular-like B cells persist and even expand, supporting the concept that pre-malignant niches may exist that allow the maintenance and/or proliferation of these cells.[236] Perhaps as a result of their unique genetic features and the ability to stave-off apoptotic cell death, these t(14;18)-positive cells can reenter germinal centers and undergo further rounds of proliferation and SHM. Under the right conditions, possibly related to host genetics, microenvironmental factors, encounter with cognate antigen, *N*-glycosylation, some other cause of tonic BCR signaling or the acquisition of secondary genetic alterations, these cells may progress to clinically overt FL in a small number of so-called healthy individuals. Further study is required to resolve this hypothesis.

Cytogenetic data have in part provided support for a simple Darwinian model that favors selection and clonal evolution with accumulating genetic damage, resulting in a growth advantage for the neoplastic B cells in FL.[139,239] First, most FLs harbor additional cytogenetic alterations beyond the t(14;18). A number of publications have confirmed that secondary cytogenetic alterations increase with histologic grade, increasing from a median of 4.8, 6.5 and 19 for grades 1, 2 and 3 FL, respectively.[47] The few cases that show an isolated t(14;18) as the sole karyotypic alteration are characteristic of grade 1 histology. Moreover, rare cases of *in situ* FL with a clonal karyotype show the same finding, but in only a proportion of the metaphases (unpublished observations, 2005). Second, as detailed in the section on transformation, a number of cytogenetic alterations have been associated with transformation to DLBCL, as has karyotypic complexity in some series. Using statistical tools, Höglund and colleagues were able to map unique pathways of clonal evolution in FL samples, suggesting a temporal pattern of cytogenetic progression.[139] Specific alterations have also been associated with survival. Correlation of genetic change with gene expression also suggests a relationship, at least for upregulated genes and regions of chromosomal gain.[141] In aggregate, these data support a model of increasing genetic complexity associated with clonal evolution. However, several lines of evidence question an exclusively genetic model of FL pathogenesis. For example, analyses of paired specimens using laser-capture microdissection or classical cytogenetic techniques suggest that some cases of FL progression result from subclone selection rather than ongoing clonal evolution over time.[169,172] Karyotypes in a large percentage of transformed biopsies show overlapping, but fewer alterations than the original diagnostic FL sample.[171] Similarly, recent data from paired sample analyses using genome-wide SNP chips suggest that some cases of transformed FL arise by divergence from a common malignant ancestor cell rather than by clonal evolution from an antecedent FL.[142] These results are also supported by the single cell data arising from the analysis of composite histologies that include both FL and classical Hodgkin lymphoma, where the Reed–Sternberg cells and the FL B cells show a common ancestry.[114] These findings raise the possibility of FL stem cells, but it is difficult to imagine a precursor stem cell that antecedes the germinal center. The presence of SHM and CSR in most reported cases place this ancestral cell at the germinal center stage of development. It may well be that in some cases primary genetic alterations dominate the biology and clinical behavior of FL, while others show a preferentially greater influence by microenvironmental factors. The genetic model would favor that the accumulation of genetic alterations in the tumor cells dictates autonomous growth characteristics and risk of transformation, and controls the composition of the microenvironment of the lymph node. We will return to this point following a discussion of the role of the microenvironment in FL pathogenesis.

Immunologic model

The follicular growth pattern, the morphologic similarity to normal centrocytes and centroblasts, the immunophenotype and the molecular features of somatic mutation of *IGH* genes together with intraclonal sequence diversity establishes FL as a tumor of germinal center B cells. Evidence supports that the neoplastic B cells require the follicular microenvironment for their clonal expansion and survival.[240] Follicular lymphoma is one of several NHLs in which the microenvironment appears to play a pivotal role in the biology and perhaps the clinical outcome of patients.[158,159] A growing body of data implicates an important role for cross-talk between the tumor cells and various immune response, stromal and antigen-presenting cells in the tumor microenvironment.[241]

The neoplastic follicle, like the reactive follicle, is rich in a number of immune-related cells such as T cells, macrophages and FDCs. It is likely that clonal expansion and CSR require signals from these cells and involve costimulatory molecules including CD40, CD40L, CD28, ICOS and IL-4. FL cell lines do not exist, primarily because FL B cells fail to grow *in vitro* without recapitulating their microenvironment in the form of feeder layers, cytokines or the addition of non-neoplastic cells that mimic their germinal center niche.[240] These data suggest that early in the development of FL the malignant B cells require the close company of the constituents of the germinal center milieu. Recent gene expression studies and analyses of tissue microarrays lend themselves to similar conclusions.[158,159] The gene expression signatures of non-neoplastic cells in the tumor microenvironment appear to have a dominant impact on survival. Moreover, one molecular predictor was built using diagnostic biopsies of FL, a finding that is somewhat contrary to the concept of clonal evolution over time.[158] Another gene expression predictor of immediate clinical behavior following diagnosis or at relapse included several genes that point to mediators of a cellular immune response, including macrophages, follicular dendritic cells and various subsets of T cells.[16] These data suggest important cross-talk between the FL B cells and the non-neoplastic immune response cells in the tumoral microenvironment. Spontaneous remissions are well described in FL patients and suggest a role for an anti-tumor host immune response. The clinical efficacy of tumor vaccines and allogeneic bone marrow transplantation similarly rely on the concept of unique tumor antigens coupled with an active immune response to the tumor cells. Very recent data implicate a role for host genetics, as several immune response genes, including *IL2, IL8, IL12B,* and *IL1RN* were shown to predict overall survival in patients with FL.[192] These findings require validation in additional patient cohorts.

Factors that predict transformation risk also implicate the microenvironment, including the number of activated CD4+ T cells within the follicles, the dissolution of the FDC meshworks as well as their maturity and/or functional status.[159] Concomitant with histologic transformation, the FL B cells appear to gain autonomous growth characteristics and no longer require the growth-supporting niche offered by the follicular microenvironment. Thus, the resultant DLBCL loses its follicular growth pattern and is associated with dissolution of the FDC meshworks and loss of much of the accompanying T cells.[218] Therefore, a primary immunologic theory of pathogenesis would suggest that many of the genetic alterations in the tumor B cells are 'noise', and that the microenvironment controls the growth potential of the FL cells and determines the risk of histologic transformation.

Unifying model of pathogenesis

The shape of the overall survival curve in FL highlights the marked clinical heterogeneity characteristic of this lymphoma. It is unlikely that a simple genetic or immunologic model alone can be developed to easily explain the pathogenesis of FL. A more likely scenario is that FL is a balance between genetic and microenvironmental factors that may differentially influence the growth of the tumor cells and the clinical course of the patient. For example, those patients who transform early and pursue an aggressive clinical course may be more 'genetically driven', as their tumors may be less influenced by the non-neoplastic cells in the microenvironment and are more affected by acquired genetic alterations that confer enhanced growth potential and transformation risk. Genomic alterations known to dramatically influence the clinical course of FL include loss of *p53*, loss of *p16* and translocations of *MYC*. However, a purely genetic model in FL is confounded by the possibility that several different mechanisms may be contributing to the observed genomic alterations. Some DNA alterations may reflect true clonal selection while others are simply genetic 'noise' as a consequence of extended survival in the germinal center where double-strand DNA breakage is physiologic. In contrast to DLBCL where the SHM mechanism is aberrant and numerous other genes show evidence of mutations (e.g. *PIM1, MYC, RhoH/TTF,* and *PAX5*), in FL the affected genes appear only to include *IGH* variable region genes and *BCL6*.[242] Thus, the SHM machinery does not appear to be aberrantly functioning in FL, but if this process underlies many of the molecular alterations in FL genomes, these may be the result of defective downstream events including double-strand DNA repair or DNA-damage checkpoint function. Thus, the plethora of cytogenetic alterations in FL may simply reflect passive accumulation of rescued, long-lived B cells spending an extended period of time within the harsh germinal center microenvironment.

Some patients with FL experience very aggressive clinical behavior that is not a result of transformation. Macrophage content at diagnosis may represent a surrogate for such patients, suggesting that some microenvironmental factors can dictate early progressions.[190] In this scenario the microenvironment would be seen as nurturing, creating a trophic environment favoring tumor cell growth. Moreover, some features of the microenvironment may drive transformation, acting as a selection pressure for mutations that favor autonomous growth potential.

Alternatively, some patients with relapsing and remitting courses over many years may be primarily 'microenvironmentally driven', where tumor genomes are relatively stable and do not acquire deleterious genetic alterations that favor autonomous growth, but instead the neoplastic B cells are heavily influenced by non-neoplastic T cells and accessory cells in the biopsy samples. In such cases, genetic alterations may occur, but predominantly represent 'noise' as described above. In these patients, it can be hypothesized that the microenvironment tightly regulates the growth of the tumoral cells, suggesting an active immune response. Of great interest is the recent observation that certain genotypes for immune response genes heavily influence prognosis in FL, suggesting the possibility that host genetics determines both the composition and functionality of the tumor microenvironment.[192]

In summary, the diverse clinical spectrum of FL patients likely reflects a dynamic interaction between somewhat competing influences; functional intrinsic genomic alterations that provide the tumor cells with a growth advantage and immunologic factors within the tumoral microenvironment that either favor the neoplastic cells and/or drive transformation or alternatively, actively suppress growth of the FL B cells in favor of the host. The longitudinal analysis of large cohorts of FL patients followed for lengthy periods of time appear to identify two major clinical subgroups of patients. One group is at risk for transformation that occurs at a constant rate of 3 percent per year. The frequency and perhaps the rate of transformation may be affected by clinical features, biologic factors and treatment. However, a group of similar frequency exists that may never transform. These patients are not surprisingly enriched within the group of long-term FL survivors. In one study, transformations beyond 16 years were not seen.[11] The proposed clinical subgroups of FL and the hypothetical influence of pathogenic mechanisms are highlighted in (Plate 49, see plate section).

KEY POINTS

Clinical

- 22–32 percent of all NHLs.
- Median age ~65 years, slight female predominance.
- Most patients present with advanced stage.
- Spontaneous remissions can occur.
- Frequent bone marrow involvement, significant leukemic component uncommon.
- Survival improved with rituximab-containing regimens.

Morphology/immunophenotype

- True follicular growth pattern in most cases.
- Grading depends on number of centrocytes versus centroblasts.
- Grade 3b may be more akin to *de novo* DLBCL.
- A number of morphologic variants.
- Germinal center neoplasm expressing CD10 and BCL6.
- Deregulated BCL2 protein expression central to pathogenesis in most cases.

Cytogenetics/molecular genetics

- t(14;18) in 85 percent of cases.
- *IGH* shows somatic mutations and pattern of ongoing mutations.

- *BCL6* translocations occur ~10–15 percent, mutations of 5′ noncoding region of *BCL6*.

Pathogenesis

- FL best explained by a combined genetic and immunologic model.
- The balance of these two influences varies between cases, thus some patients are genetically driven and others are more influenced by immune-related cells in the microenvironment.

REFERENCES

● = Key primary paper

◆ = Major review article

●1. Anonymous. A clinical evaluation of the international lymphoma study group classification of non-Hodgkin's lymphoma. The non-Hodgkin's lymphoma classification project. *Blood* 1997; **89**: 3909–18.

2. Anderson JR, Armitage JO, Weisenburger DD. Epidemiology of the non-Hodgkin's lymphomas: distributions of the major subtypes differ by geographic locations. Non-Hodgkin's lymphoma classification project. *Ann Oncol* 1998; **9**: 717–20.

3. Garvin AJ, Simon RM, Osborne CK *et al.* An autopsy study of histologic progression in non-Hodgkin's lymphomas. 192 cases from the National Cancer Institute. *Cancer* 1983; **52**: 393–8.

4. Qazi R, Aisenberg AC, Long JC. The natural history of nodular lymphoma. *Cancer* 1976; **37**: 1923–7.

5. Cullen MH, Lister TA, Brearley RI *et al.* Histological transformation of non-Hodgkin's lymphoma: a prospective study. *Cancer* 1979; **44**: 645–51.

6. Hubbard SM, Chabner BA, DeVita VT Jr. *et al.* Histologic progression in non-Hodgkin's lymphoma. *Blood* 1982; **59**: 258–64.

7. Acker B, Hoppe RT, Colby TV *et al.* Histologic conversion in the non-Hodgkin's lymphomas. *J Clin Oncol* 1983; **1**: 11–16.

8. Oviatt DL, Cousar JB, Collins RD *et al.* Malignant lymphomas of follicular center cell origin in humans. V. Incidence, clinical features, and prognostic implications of transformation of small cleaved cell nodular lymphoma. *Cancer* 1984; **53**: 1109–14.

9. Ersboll J, Schultz HB, Pedersen-Bjergaard J, Nissen NI. Follicular low-grade non-Hodgkin's lymphoma: long-term outcome with or without tumor progression. *Eur J Haematol* 1989; **42**: 155–63.

10. Al-Tourah A, Chhanabhai M, Gill K *et al.* Incidence, predictive factors and outcome of transformed lymphoma: a population-based study from British Columbia. *Ann Oncol* 2005; **16**: 64.

●11. Montoto S, Davies AJ, Matthews J *et al.* Risk and clinical implications of transformation of follicular lymphoma to diffuse large B-cell lymphoma. *J Clin Oncol* 2007; **25**: 2426–33.

12. Horning SJ, Rosenberg SA. The natural history of initially untreated low-grade non-Hodgkin's lymphomas. *N Engl J Med* 1984; **311**: 1471–5.

13. Sander CA, Yano T, Clark HM *et al.* p53 mutation is associated with progression in follicular lymphomas. *Blood* 1993; **82**: 1994–2004.

14. Lo Coco F, Gaidano G, Louie DC *et al.* p53 mutations are associated with histologic transformation of follicular lymphoma. *Blood* 1993; **82**: 2289–95.

15. Elenitoba-Johnson KS, Gascoyne RD, Lim MS *et al.* Homozygous deletions at chromosome 9p21 involving p16 and p15 are associated with histologic progression in follicle center lymphoma. *Blood* 1998; **91**: 4677–85.

●16. Glas AM, Kersten MJ, Delahaye LJ *et al.* Gene expression profiling in follicular lymphoma to assess clinical aggressiveness and to guide the choice of treatment. *Blood* 2005; **105**: 301–7.

17. Marcus R, Imrie K, Belch A *et al.* CVP chemotherapy plus rituximab compared with CVP as first-line treatment for advanced follicular lymphoma. *Blood* 2005; **105**: 1417–23.

18. Hiddemann W, Kneba M, Dreyling M *et al.* Frontline therapy with rituximab added to the combination of cyclophosphamide, doxorubicin, vincristine, and prednisone (CHOP) significantly improves the outcome for patients with advanced-stage follicular lymphoma compared with therapy with CHOP alone: results of a prospective randomized study of the German low-grade lymphoma study group. *Blood* 2005; **106**: 3725–32.

19. Sacchi S, Pozzi S, Marcheselli L *et al.* Introduction of rituximab in front-line and salvage therapies has improved outcome of advanced-stage follicular lymphoma patients. *Cancer* 2007; **109**: 2077–82.

20. Herold M, Haas A, Srock S *et al.* Rituximab added to first-line mitoxantrone, chlorambucil, and prednisolone chemotherapy followed by interferon maintenance prolongs survival in patients with advanced follicular lymphoma: an East German study group hematology and oncology study. *J Clin Oncol* 2007; **25**: 1986–92.

21. Fisher RI, LeBlanc M, Press OW *et al.* New treatment options have changed the survival of patients with follicular lymphoma. *J Clin Oncol* 2005; **23**: 8447–52.

22. Liu Q, Fayad L, Cabanillas F *et al.* Improvement of overall and failure-free survival in stage IV follicular lymphoma: 25 years of treatment experience at The University of Texas M.D. Anderson Cancer Center. *J Clin Oncol* 2006; **24**: 1582–9.

23. Swenson WT, Wooldridge JE, Lynch CF *et al.* Improved survival of follicular lymphoma patients in the United States. *J Clin Oncol* 2005; **23**: 5019–26.

24. Jaffe ES, Harris NL, Stein H, Vardiman JW. *World Health Organization classification of tumours. pathology and genetics: tumours of haematopoietic and lymphoid tissues.* Lyon: IARC Press, 2001.

25. Tsujimoto Y, Finger LR, Yunis J *et al.* Cloning of the chromosome breakpoint of neoplastic B cells with the t(14;18) chromosome translocation. *Science* 1984; **226**: 1097–9.

26. Hicks EB, Rappaport H, Winter WJ. Follicular lymphoma; a re-evaluation of its position in the scheme of malignant lymphoma, based on a survey of 253 cases. *Cancer* 1956; **9**: 792–821.

27. Lukes RJ, Collins RD. Immunologic characterization of human malignant lymphomas. *Cancer* 1974; **34(Suppl)**:1488–503.

28. Lennert K. Morphology and classification of malignant lymphomas and so-called reticuloses. *Acta Neuropathol Suppl (Berl)* 1975; **Suppl 16**: 1–16.

29. Anonymous. National Cancer Institute sponsored study of classifications of non-Hodgkin's lymphomas: summary and description of a working formulation for clinical usage. The non-Hodgkin's lymphoma pathologic classification project. *Cancer* 1982; **49**: 2112–35.

30. Harris NL, Jaffe ES, Stein H *et al.* A revised European-American classification of lymphoid neoplasms: a proposal from the International Lymphoma Study Group. *Blood* 1994; **84**: 1361–92.

31. Biagi JJ, Seymour JF. Insights into the molecular pathogenesis of follicular lymphoma arising from analysis of geographic variation. *Blood* 2002; **99**: 4265–75.

32. Armitage JO, Weisenburger DD. New approach to classifying non-Hodgkin's lymphomas: clinical features of the major histologic subtypes. Non-Hodgkin's lymphoma classification project. *J Clin Oncol* 1998; **16**: 2780–95.

33. Atra A, Meller ST, Stevens RS *et al.* Conservative management of follicular non-Hodgkin's lymphoma in childhood. *Br J Haematol* 1998; **103**: 220–3.

34. Frizzera G, Murphy SB. Follicular (nodular) lymphoma in childhood: a rare clinical-pathological entity. Report of eight cases from four cancer centers. *Cancer* 1979; **44**: 2218–35.

35. Lorsbach RB, Shay-Seymore D, Moore J *et al.* Clinicopathologic analysis of follicular lymphoma occurring in children. *Blood* 2002; **99**: 1959–64.

36. Last KW, Goff LK, Summers KE *et al.* Familial follicular lymphoma: a case report with molecular analysis. *Br J Haematol* 2000; **110**: 744–5.

37. Marco F, Manjon R, Richard C *et al.* Simultaneous occurrence of follicular lymphoma in two monozygotic twins. *Br J Haematol* 1999; **107**: 461–2.

38. Harrington DS, Ye YL, Weisenburger DD *et al.* Malignant lymphoma in Nebraska and Guangzhou, China: a comparative study. *Hum Pathol* 1987; **18**: 924–8.

39. Rothman N, Skibola CF, Wang SS *et al.* Genetic variation in TNF and IL10 and risk of non-Hodgkin lymphoma: a report from the InterLymph Consortium. *Lancet Oncol* 2006; **7**: 27–38.

40. Nieters A, Beckmann L, Deeg E, Becker N. Gene polymorphisms in Toll-like receptors, interleukin-10, and

interleukin-10 receptor alpha and lymphoma risk. *Genes Immun* 2006; **7**: 615–24.

41. Purdue MP, Lan Q, Kricker A *et al.* Polymorphisms in immune function genes and risk of non-Hodgkin lymphoma: findings from the New South Wales non-Hodgkin lymphoma study. *Carcinogenesis* 2007; **28**: 704–12.

42. Lan Q, Zheng T, Chanock S *et al.* Genetic variants in caspase genes and susceptibility to non-Hodgkin lymphoma. *Carcinogenesis* 2007; **28**: 823–7.

43. Wang SS, Slager SL, Brennan P *et al.* Family history of hematopoietic malignancies and risk of non-Hodgkin lymphoma (NHL): a pooled analysis of 10,211 cases and 11,905 controls from the InterLymph Consortium. *Blood* 2007; **109**: 3479–88.

44. Novik KL, Spinelli JJ, MacArthur AC *et al.* Genetic variation in H2AFX contributes to risk of non-Hodgkin lymphoma. *Cancer Epidemiol Biomarkers Prev* 2007; **16**: 1098–106.

45. Purdue MP, Hartge P, Davis S *et al.* Sun exposure, vitamin D receptor gene polymorphisms and risk of non-Hodgkin lymphoma. *Cancer Causes Control* 2007; **18**: 989–99.

46. Horsman DE, Gascoyne RD, Coupland RW *et al.* Comparison of cytogenetic analysis, southern analysis, and polymerase chain reaction for the detection of t(14; 18) in follicular lymphoma. *Am J Clin Pathol* 1995; **103**: 472–8.

•47. Horsman DE, Connors JM, Pantzar T, Gascoyne RD. Analysis of secondary chromosomal alterations in 165 cases of follicular lymphoma with t(14;18). *Genes Chromosomes Cancer* 2001; **30**: 375–82.

48. Tonegawa S. Somatic generation of antibody diversity. *Nature* 1983; **302**: 575–81.

49. Gellert M. V(D)J recombination: RAG proteins, repair factors, and regulation. *Annu Rev Biochem* 2002; **71**: 101–32.

50. Bakhshi A, Jensen JP, Goldman P *et al.* Cloning the chromosomal breakpoint of t(14;18) human lymphomas: clustering around JH on chromosome 14 and near a transcriptional unit on 18. *Cell* 1985; **41**: 899–906.

51. Bakhshi A, Wright JJ, Graninger W *et al.* Mechanism of the t(14;18) chromosomal translocation: structural analysis of both derivative 14 and 18 reciprocal partners. *Proc Natl Acad Sci U S A* 1987; **84**: 2396–400.

52. Cotter F, Price C, Zucca E, Young BD. Direct sequence analysis of the 14q+ and 18q- chromosome junctions in follicular lymphoma. *Blood* 1990; **76**: 131–5.

53. Raghavan SC, Swanson PC, Wu X *et al.* A non-B-DNA structure at the Bcl-2 major breakpoint region is cleaved by the RAG complex. *Nature* 2004; **428**: 88–93.

54. Jager U, Bocskor S, Le T *et al.* Follicular lymphomas' BCL-2/IgH junctions contain templated nucleotide insertions: novel insights into the mechanism of t(14;18) translocation. *Blood* 2000; **95**: 3520–9.

55. Kuppers R, Dalla-Favera R. Mechanisms of chromosomal translocations in B cell lymphomas. *Oncogene* 2001; **20**: 5580–94.

◆56. Kuppers R. Mechanisms of B-cell lymphoma pathogenesis. *Nat Rev Cancer* 2005; **5**: 251–62.

57. Fenton JA, Vaandrager JW, Aarts WM *et al.* Follicular lymphoma with a novel t(14;18) breakpoint involving the immunoglobulin heavy chain switch mu region indicates an origin from germinal center B cells. *Blood* 2002; **99**: 716–18.

58. Nathwani BN, Winberg CD, Diamond LW *et al.* Morphologic criteria for the differentiation of follicular lymphoma from florid reactive follicular hyperplasia: a study of 80 cases. *Cancer* 1981; **48**: 1794–806.

59. Abou-Elella A, Shafer MT, Wan XY *et al.* Lymphomas with follicular and monocytoid B-cell components. Evidence for a common clonal origin from follicle center cells. *Am J Clin Pathol* 2000; **114**: 516–22.

60. Nathwani BN, Anderson JR, Armitage JO *et al.* Clinical significance of follicular lymphoma with monocytoid B cells. Non-Hodgkin's lymphoma classification project. *Hum Pathol* 1999; **30**: 263–8.

61. Cleary KR, Osborne BM, Butler JJ. Lymph node infarction foreshadowing malignant lymphoma. *Am J Surg Pathol* 1982; **6**: 435–42.

62. Waldron JA Jr, Newcomer LN, Katz ME, Cadman E. Sclerosing variants of follicular center cell lymphomas presenting in the retroperitoneum. *Cancer* 1983; **52**: 712–20.

63. Klapper W, Hoster E, Rolver L *et al.* Tumor sclerosis but not cell proliferation or malignancy grade is a prognostic marker in advanced-stage follicular lymphoma: the german low grade lymphoma study group. *J Clin Oncol* 2007; **25**: 3330–6.

64. Osborne BM, Butler JJ. Follicular lymphoma mimicking progressive transformation of germinal centers. *Am J Clin Pathol* 1987; **88**: 264–9.

65. Mann RB, Berard CW. Criteria for the cytologic subclassification of follicular lymphomas: a proposed alternative method. *Hematol Oncol* 1983; **1**: 187–92.

66. Kim H, Dorfman RF. Morphological studies of 84 untreated patients subjected to laparotomy for the staging of non-Hodgkin's lymphomas. *Cancer* 1974; **33**: 657–74.

67. Harris M, Eyden B, Read G. Signet ring cell lymphoma: a rare variant of follicular lymphoma. *J Clin Pathol* 1981; **34**: 884–91.

68. Keith TA, Cousar JB, Glick AD *et al.* Plasmacytic differentiation in follicular center cell (FCC) lymphomas. *Am J Clin Pathol* 1985; **84**: 283–90.

69. Natkunam Y, Warnke RA, Zehnder JL *et al.* Blastic/blastoid transformation of follicular lymphoma: immunohistologic and molecular analyses of five cases. *Am J Surg Pathol* 2000; **24**: 525–34.

70. Dogan A, Du MQ, Aiello A *et al.* Follicular lymphomas contain a clonally linked but phenotypically distinct neoplastic B-cell population in the interfollicular zone. *Blood* 1998; **91**: 4708–14.

71. Harris NL, Bhan AK. Distribution of T-cell subsets in follicular and diffuse lymphomas of B-cell type. *Am J Pathol* 1983; **113**: 172–80.

72. Criel A, Pittaluga S, Verhoef G et al. Small B cell NHL and their leukemic counterpart: differences in subtyping and assessment of leukemic spread. Leukemia 1996; 10: 848–53.

73. Siddiqui M, Ristow K, Markovic SN et al. Absolute lymphocyte count predicts overall survival in follicular lymphomas. Br J Haematol 2006; 134: 596–601.

74. Behl D, Ristow K, Markovic SN et al. Absolute lymphocyte count predicts therapeutic efficacy of rituximab therapy in follicular lymphomas. Br J Haematol 2007; 137: 409–15.

75. Foucar K. Bone marrow pathology, 2nd ed. Chicago: ASCP Press, 2001.

76. Arber DA, George TI. Bone marrow biopsy involvement by non-Hodgkin's lymphoma: frequency of lymphoma types, patterns, blood involvement, and discordance with other sites in 450 specimens. Am J Surg Pathol 2005; 29: 1549–57.

77. Bognar A, Csernus B, Bodor C et al. Clonal selection in the bone marrow involvement of follicular lymphoma. Leukemia 2005; 19: 1656–62.

78. Canioni D, Brice P, Lepage E et al. Bone marrow histological patterns can predict survival of patients with grade 1 or 2 follicular lymphoma: a study from the Groupe d'Etude des Lymphomes Folliculaires. Br J Haematol 2004; 126: 364–71.

79. Torlakovic E, Torlakovic G, Brunning RD. Follicular pattern of bone marrow involvement by follicular lymphoma. Am J Clin Pathol 2002; 118: 780–6.

80. Iancu D, Hao S, Lin P et al. Follicular lymphoma in staging bone marrow specimens: correlation of histologic findings with the results of flow cytometry immunophenotypic analysis. Arch Pathol Lab Med 2007; 131: 282–7.

81. Kremer M, Quintanilla-Martinez L, Nahrig J et al. Immunohistochemistry in bone marrow pathology: a useful adjunct for morphologic diagnosis. Virchows Arch 2005; 447: 920–37.

●82. Ott G, Katzenberger T, Lohr A et al. Cytomorphologic, immunohistochemical, and cytogenetic profiles of follicular lymphoma: 2 types of follicular lymphoma grade 3. Blood 2002; 99: 3806–12.

83. Naresh KN. MUM1 expression dichotomises follicular lymphoma into predominantly, MUM1-negative low-grade and MUM1-positive high-grade subtypes. Haematologica 2007; 92: 267–8.

84. Karube K, Guo Y, Suzumiya J et al. CD10-MUM1+ follicular lymphoma lacks BCL2 gene translocation and shows characteristic biologic and clinical features. Blood 2007; 109: 3076–9.

85. Karube K, Guo Y, Hiroyuki T et al. BCL6 gene amplification/3q27 gain is associated with unique clinicopathological characteristics among follicular lymphoma without BCL2 gene translocation. Mod Pathol [Epub 23 May 2008].

86. Bosga-Bouwer AG, van den Berg A, Haralambieva E et al. Molecular, cytogenetic, and immunophenotypic characterization of follicular lymphoma grade 3B; a

separate entity or part of the spectrum of diffuse large B-cell lymphoma or follicular lymphoma? Hum Pathol 2006; 37: 528–33.

87. Guo Y, Karube K, Kawano R et al. Low-grade follicular lymphoma with t(14;18) presents a homogeneous disease entity otherwise the rest comprises minor groups of heterogeneous disease entities with Bcl2 amplification, Bcl6 translocation or other gene aberrances. Leukemia 2005; 19: 1058–63.

88. Hans CP, Weisenburger DD, Vose JM et al. A significant diffuse component predicts for inferior survival in grade 3 follicular lymphoma, but cytologic subtypes do not predict survival. Blood 2003; 101: 2363–7.

89. Bosga-Bouwer AG, van Imhoff GW, Boonstra R et al. Follicular lymphoma grade 3B includes 3 cytogenetically defined subgroups with primary t(14;18), 3q27, or other translocations: t(14;18) and 3q27 are mutually exclusive. Blood 2003; 101: 1149–54.

90. Tilly H, Rossi A, Stamatoullas A et al. Prognostic value of chromosomal abnormalities in follicular lymphoma. Blood 1994; 84: 1043–9.

91. Katzenberger T, Ott G, Klein T et al. Cytogenetic alterations affecting BCL6 are predominantly found in follicular lymphomas grade 3B with a diffuse large B-cell component. Am J Pathol 2004; 165: 481–90.

92. Chau I, Jones R, Cunningham D et al. Outcome of follicular lymphoma grade 3: is anthracycline necessary as front-line therapy? Br J Cancer 2003; 89: 36–42.

93. Ganti AK, Weisenburger DD, Smith LM et al. Patients with grade 3 follicular lymphoma have prolonged relapse-free survival following anthracycline-based chemotherapy: the Nebraska lymphoma study group experience. Ann Oncol 2006; 17: 920–7.

94. Gascoyne RD. Hematopathology approaches to diagnosis and prognosis of indolent B-cell lymphomas. Hematology Am Soc Hematol Educ Program 2005: 299–306.

95. Jaffe ES, Sander CA, Flaig MJ. Cutaneous lymphomas: a proposal for a unified approach to classification using the R.E.A.L./WHO classification. Ann Oncol 2000; 11(Suppl 1): 17–21.

96. Cerroni L, Arzberger E, Putz B et al. Primary cutaneous follicle center cell lymphoma with follicular growth pattern. Blood 2000; 95: 3922–8.

97. Aguilera NS, Tomaszewski MM, Moad JC et al. Cutaneous follicle center lymphoma: a clinicopathologic study of 19 cases. Mod Pathol 2001; 14: 828–35.

98. de Leval L, Harris NL, Longtine J et al. Cutaneous b-cell lymphomas of follicular and marginal zone types: use of Bcl-6, CD10, Bcl-2, and CD21 in differential diagnosis and classification. Am J Surg Pathol 2001; 25: 732–41.

99. Franco R, Fernandez-Vazquez A, Rodriguez-Peralto JL et al. Cutaneous follicular B-cell lymphoma: description of a series of 18 cases. Am J Surg Pathol 2001; 25: 875–83.

100. Mirza I, Macpherson N, Paproski S et al. Primary cutaneous follicular lymphoma: an assessment of clinical,

histopathologic, immunophenotypic, and molecular features. *J Clin Oncol* 2002; **20**: 647–55.

101. Kim BK, Surti U, Pandya A *et al.* Clinicopathologic, immunophenotypic, and molecular cytogenetic fluorescence *in situ* hybridization analysis of primary and secondary cutaneous follicular lymphomas. *Am J Surg Pathol* 2005; **29**: 69–82.

102. Willemze R, Jaffe ES, Burg G *et al.* WHO–EORTC classification for cutaneous lymphomas. *Blood* 2005; **105**: 3768–85.

103. Cong P, Raffeld M, Teruya-Feldstein J *et al.* In situ localization of follicular lymphoma: description and analysis by laser capture microdissection. *Blood* 2002; **99**: 3376–82.

104. Adam P, Katzenberger T, Eifert M *et al.* Presence of preserved reactive germinal centers in follicular lymphoma is a strong histopathologic indicator of limited disease stage. *Am J Surg Pathol* 2005; **29**: 1661–4.

105. Murphy SB, Fairclough DL, Hutchison RE, Berard CW. Non-Hodgkin's lymphomas of childhood: an analysis of the histology, staging, and response to treatment of 338 cases at a single institution. *J Clin Oncol* 1989; **7**: 186–93.

106. Pinto A, Hutchison RE, Grant LH *et al.* Follicular lymphomas in pediatric patients. *Mod Pathol* 1990; **3**: 308–13.

107. Pileri SA, Sabattini E, Rosito P *et al.* Primary follicular lymphoma of the testis in childhood: an entity with peculiar clinical and molecular characteristics. *J Clin Pathol* 2002; **55**: 684–8.

108. Finn LS, Viswanatha DS, Belasco JB *et al.* Primary follicular lymphoma of the testis in childhood. *Cancer* 1999; **85**: 1626–35.

109. LeBrun DP, Kamel OW, Cleary ML *et al.* Follicular lymphomas of the gastrointestinal tract. Pathologic features in 31 cases and bcl-2 oncogenic protein expression. *Am J Pathol* 1992; **140**: 1327–35.

110. Yoshino T, Miyake K, Ichimura K *et al.* Increased incidence of follicular lymphoma in the duodenum. *Am J Surg Pathol* 2000; **24**: 688–93.

111. Born P, Vieth M, Stolte M. Follicular lymphoma of the duodenum. *Endoscopy* 2007; **39 (Suppl 1)**: E39.

112. Shia J, Teruya-Feldstein J, Pan D *et al.* Primary follicular lymphoma of the gastrointestinal tract: a clinical and pathologic study of 26 cases. *Am J Surg Pathol* 2002; **26**: 216–24.

113. Gonzalez CL, Medeiros LJ, Jaffe ES. Composite lymphoma. A clinicopathologic analysis of nine patients with Hodgkin's disease and B-cell non-Hodgkin's lymphoma. *Am J Clin Pathol* 1991; **96**: 81–9.

114. Brauninger A, Hansmann ML, Strickler JG *et al.* Identification of common germinal-center B-cell precursors in two patients with both Hodgkin's disease and non-Hodgkin's lymphoma. *N Engl J Med* 1999; **340**: 1239–47.

115. Schmitz R, Renne C, Rosenquist R *et al.* Insights into the multistep transformation process of lymphomas: IgH-associated translocations and tumor suppressor gene mutations in clonally related composite Hodgkin's and non-Hodgkin's lymphomas. *Leukemia* 2005; **19**: 1452–8.

116. Dogan A, Bagdi E, Munson P, Isaacson PG. CD10 and BCL-6 expression in paraffin sections of normal lymphoid tissue and B-cell lymphomas. *Am J Surg Pathol* 2000; **24**: 846–52.

117. Dunphy CH, Polski JM, Lance Evans H, Gardner LJ. Paraffin immunoreactivity of CD10, CDw75, and Bcl-6 in follicle center cell lymphoma. *Leuk Lymphoma* 2001; **41**: 585–92.

118. Schraders M, de Jong D, Kluin P *et al.* Lack of Bcl-2 expression in follicular lymphoma may be caused by mutations in the BCL2 gene or by absence of the t(14;18) translocation. *J Pathol* 2005; **205**: 329–35.

119. Horsman DE, Okamoto I, Ludkovski O *et al.* Follicular lymphoma lacking the t(14;18)(q32;q21): identification of two disease subtypes. *Br J Haematol* 2003; **120**: 424–33.

120. Zhao WL, Daneshpouy ME, Mounier N *et al.* Prognostic significance of bcl-xL gene expression and apoptotic cell counts in follicular lymphoma. *Blood* 2004; **103**: 695–7.

121. Zha H, Raffeld M, Charboneau L *et al.* Similarities of prosurvival signals in Bcl-2-positive and Bcl-2-negative follicular lymphomas identified by reverse phase protein microarray. *Lab Invest* 2004; **84**: 235–44.

122. Alvaro T, Lejeune M, Salvado M-T *et al.* Immunohistochemical patterns of reactive microenvironment are associated with clinicobiologic behavior in follicular lymphoma patients. *J Clin Oncol* 2006; **24**: 5350–7.

123. Fukuhara S, Rowley JD, Variakojis D, Golomb HM. Chromosome abnormalities in poorly differentiated lymphocytic lymphoma. *Cancer Res* 1979; **39**: 3119–28.

124. Armitage JO, Sanger WG, Weisenburger DD *et al.* Correlation of secondary cytogenetic abnormalities with histologic appearance in non-Hodgkin's lymphomas bearing t(14;18)(q32;q21). *J Natl Cancer Inst* 1988; **80**: 576–80.

125. Weiss LM, Warnke RA, Sklar J, Cleary ML. Molecular analysis of the t(14;18) chromosomal translocation in malignant lymphomas. *N Engl J Med* 1987; **317**: 1185–9.

126. Aisenberg AC, Wilkes BM, Jacobson JO. The bcl-2 gene is rearranged in many diffuse B-cell lymphomas. *Blood* 1988; **71**: 969–72.

127. Aster JC, Longtine JA. Detection of BCL2 rearrangements in follicular lymphoma. *Am J Pathol* 2002; **160**: 759–63.

128. Loke SL, Pittaluga S, Srivastava G *et al.* Translocation of bcl-2 gene in non-Hodgkin's lymphomas in Hong Kong Chinese. *Br J Haematol* 1990; **76**: 65–9.

129. Takechi M, Tanaka K, Hashimoto T *et al.* Cytogenetic, molecular biological and clinical study of B-cell lymphomas with 14;18 translocation in Japanese patients. *Leukemia* 1991; **5**: 1069–75.

130. Chen PM, Lin SH, Seto M *et al.* Rearrangement of bcl-2 genes in malignant lymphomas in Chinese patients. *Cancer* 1993; **72**: 3701–6.

131. Johnson A, Brun A, Dictor M *et al.* Incidence and prognostic significance of t(14;18) translocation in follicle center cell lymphoma of low and high grade.

A report from southern Sweden. *Ann Oncol* 1995; **6**: 789–94.

132. Segel MJ, Paltiel O, Zimran A *et al.* Geographic variance in the frequency of the t(14;18) translocation in follicular lymphoma: an Israeli series compared to the world. *Blood Cells Mol Dis* 1998; **24**: 62–72.

133. Knutsen T. Cytogenetic mechanisms in the pathogenesis and progression of follicular lymphoma. *Cancer Surv* 1997; **30**: 163–92.

134. Jardin F, Gaulard P, Buchonnet G *et al.* Follicular lymphoma without t(14;18) and with BCL-6 rearrangement: a lymphoma subtype with distinct pathological, molecular and clinical characteristics. *Leukemia* 2002; **16**: 2309–17.

135. McDonnell TJ, Korsmeyer SJ. Progression from lymphoid hyperplasia to high-grade malignant lymphoma in mice transgenic for the t(14;18). *Nature* 1991; **349**: 254–6.

136. Bentz M, Werner CA, Dohner H *et al.* High incidence of chromosomal imbalances and gene amplifications in the classical follicular variant of follicle center lymphoma. *Blood* 1996; **88**: 1437–44.

137. Fan YS, Rizkalla K. Comprehensive cytogenetic analysis including multicolor spectral karyotyping and interphase fluorescence *in situ* hybridization in lymphoma diagnosis. a summary of 154 cases. *Cancer Genet Cytogenet* 2003; **143**: 73–9.

138. Viardot A, Barth TF, Moller P *et al.* Cytogenetic evolution of follicular lymphoma. *Semin Cancer Biol* 2003; **13**: 183–90.

●139. Höglund M, Sehn L, Connors JM *et al.* Identification of cytogenetic subgroups and karyotypic pathways of clonal evolution in follicular lymphomas. *Genes Chromosomes Cancer* 2004; **39**: 195–204.

140. James GK, Horsman DE, Connors JM *et al.* Clinicopathological analysis of follicular lymphoma with a polyploid karyotype. *Leuk Lymphoma* 1998; **28**: 383–9.

141. Lestou VS, Gascoyne RD, Sehn L *et al.* Multicolour fluorescence *in situ* hybridization analysis of t(14;18)-positive follicular lymphoma and correlation with gene expression data and clinical outcome. *Br J Haematol* 2003; **122**: 745–59.

142. Fitzgibbon J, Iqbal S, Davies A *et al.* Genome-wide detection of recurring sites of uniparental disomy in follicular and transformed follicular lymphoma. *Leukemia* 2007; **21**: 1514–20.

●143. Ross CW, Ouillette PD, Saddler CM *et al.* Comprehensive analysis of copy number and allele status identifies multiple chromosome defects underlying follicular lymphoma pathogenesis. *Clin Cancer Res* 2007; **13**: 4777–85.

144. Zelenetz AD, Chen TT, Levy R. Clonal expansion in follicular lymphoma occurs subsequent to antigenic selection. *J Exp Med* 1992; **176**: 1137–48.

145. Bagg A, Braziel RM, Arber DA *et al.* Immunoglobulin heavy chain gene analysis in lymphomas: a multi-center study demonstrating the heterogeneity of performance of polymerase chain reaction assays. *J Mol Diagn* 2002; **4**: 81–9.

146. Diss TC, Peng H, Wotherspoon AC *et al.* Detection of monoclonality in low-grade B-cell lymphomas using the polymerase chain reaction is dependent on primer selection and lymphoma type. *J Pathol* 1993; **169**: 291–5.

147. van Dongen JJ, Langerak AW, Bruggemann M *et al.* Design and standardization of PCR primers and protocols for detection of clonal immunoglobulin and T-cell receptor gene recombinations in suspect lymphoproliferations: report of the BIOMED-2 Concerted Action BMH4-CT98-3936. *Leukemia* 2003; **17**: 2257–317.

148. Liu H, Bench AJ, Bacon CM *et al.* A practical strategy for the routine use of BIOMED-2 PCR assays for detection of B- and T-cell clonality in diagnostic haematopathology. *Br J Haematol* 2007; **138**: 31–43.

149. Albinger-Hegyi A, Hochreutener B, Abdou MT *et al.* High frequency of t(14;18)-translocation breakpoints outside of major breakpoint and minor cluster regions in follicular lymphomas: improved polymerase chain reaction protocols for their detection. *Am J Pathol* 2002; **160**: 823–32.

150. Batstone PJ, Goodlad JR. Efficacy of screening the intermediate cluster region of the bcl2 gene in follicular lymphomas by PCR. *J Clin Pathol* 2005; **58**: 81–2.

151. Weinberg OK, Ai WZ, Mariappan MR *et al.* Minor BCL2 breakpoints in follicular lymphoma. Frequency and correlation with grade and disease presentation in 236 cases. *J Mol Diagn* 2007; **9**: 530–7.

152. Paternoster SF, Brockman SR, McClure RF *et al.* A new method to extract nuclei from paraffin-embedded tissue to study lymphomas using interphase fluorescence *in situ* hybridization. *Am J Pathol* 2002; **160**: 1967–72.

153. Leroux D, Stul M, Sotto JJ *et al.* Translocation t(3;22)(q23;q11) in three patients with diffuse large B cell lymphoma. *Leukemia* 1990; **4**: 373–6.

154. Bastard C, Tilly H, Lenormand B *et al.* Translocations involving band 3q27 and Ig gene regions in non-Hodgkin's lymphoma. *Blood* 1992; **79**: 2527–31.

155. Deweindt C, Kerckaert JP, Tilly H *et al.* Cloning of a breakpoint cluster region at band 3q27 involved in human non-Hodgkin's lymphoma. *Genes Chromosomes Cancer* 1993; **8**: 149–54.

156. Migliazza A, Martinotti S, Chen W *et al.* Frequent somatic hypermutation of the 5′ noncoding region of the BCL6 gene in B-cell lymphoma. *Proc Natl Acad Sci U S A* 1995; **92**: 12520–4.

157. Husson H, Carideo EG, Neuberg D *et al.* Gene expression profiling of follicular lymphoma and normal germinal center B cells using cDNA arrays. *Blood* 2002; **99**: 282–9.

●158. Dave SS, Wright G, Tan B *et al.* Prediction of survival in follicular lymphoma based on molecular features of tumor-infiltrating immune cells. *N Engl J Med* 2004; **351**: 2159–69.

●159. Glas AM, Knoops L, Delahaye L *et al.* Gene-expression and immunohistochemical study of specific T-cell subsets and accessory cell types in the transformation and prognosis of follicular lymphoma. *J Clin Oncol* 2007; **25**: 390–8.

160. Muller-Hermelink HK, Zettl A, Pfeifer W, Ott G. Pathology of lymphoma progression. *Histopathology* 2001; **38**: 285–306.

161. Davies AJ, Rosenwald A, Wright G *et al.* Transformation of follicular lymphoma to diffuse large B-cell lymphoma proceeds by distinct oncogenic mechanisms. *Br J Haematol* 2007; **136**: 286–93.

162. Gine E, Lopez-Guillermo A, Montoto S *et al.* FLIPI and histological subtype are the most important predicting factors of histological transformation in follicular lymphoma. *Ann Oncol* 2005; **16**: 106.

163. Yano T, Jaffe ES, Longo DL, Raffeld M. MYC rearrangements in histologically progressed follicular lymphomas. *Blood* 1992; **80**: 758–67.

164. Macpherson N, Lesack D, Klasa R *et al.* Small noncleaved, non-Burkitt's (Burkitt-Like) lymphoma: cytogenetics predict outcome and reflect clinical presentation. *J Clin Oncol* 1999; **17**: 1558–67.

165. Mukhopadhyay S, Readling J, Cotter PD *et al.* Transformation of follicular lymphoma to Burkitt-like lymphoma within a single lymph node. *Hum Pathol* 2005; **36**: 571–5.

166. Agarwal AM, Agarwal N, Glenn MJ, Lim MS. Blastic transformation of low-grade follicular lymphoma. *J Clin Oncol* 2007; **25**: 2326–8.

167. de Jong D, Voetdijk BM, Beverstock GC *et al.* Activation of the c-myc oncogene in a precursor-B-cell blast crisis of follicular lymphoma, presenting as composite lymphoma. *N Engl J Med* 1988; **318**: 1373–8.

168. Boonstra R, Bosga-Bouwer A, Mastik M *et al.* Identification of chromosomal copy number changes associated with transformation of follicular lymphoma to diffuse large B-cell lymphoma. *Hum Pathol* 2003; **34**: 915–23.

169. Whang-Peng J, Knutsen T, Jaffe ES *et al.* Sequential analysis of 43 patients with non-Hodgkin's lymphoma: clinical correlations with cytogenetic, histologic, immunophenotyping, and molecular studies. *Blood* 1995; **85**: 203–16.

170. Johansson B, Mertens F, Mitelman F. Cytogenetic evolution patterns in non-Hodgkin's lymphoma. *Blood* 1995; **86**: 3905–14.

171. Johnson NA, Al-Tourah A, Horsman DE *et al.* Insights into disease evolution of transformed follicular lymphoma derived from cytogenetics. *Blood* 2005; **106**: a180.

172. Aarts WM, Bende RJ, Bossenbroek JG *et al.* Variable heavy-chain gene analysis of follicular lymphomas: subclone selection rather than clonal evolution over time. *Blood* 2001; **98**: 238–40.

173. Zelenetz AD, Chen TT, Levy R. Histologic transformation of follicular lymphoma to diffuse lymphoma represents tumor progression by a single malignant B cell. *J Exp Med* 1991; **173**: 197–207.

174. Meeker T, Lowder J, Cleary ML *et al.* Emergence of idiotype variants during treatment of B-cell lymphoma with anti-idiotype antibodies. *N Engl J Med* 1985; **312**: 1658–65.

175. Hough RE, Goepel JR, Alcock HE *et al.* Copy number gain at 12q12–14 may be important in the transformation from follicular lymphoma to diffuse large B cell lymphoma. *Br J Cancer* 2001; **84**: 499–503.

176. Martinez-Climent JA, Alizadeh AA, Segraves R *et al.* Transformation of follicular lymphoma to diffuse large cell lymphoma is associated with a heterogeneous set of DNA copy number and gene expression alterations. *Blood* 2003; **101**: 3109–17.

177. Bernell P, Jacobsson B, Liliemark J *et al.* Gain of chromosome 7 marks the progression from indolent to aggressive follicle centre lymphoma and is a common finding in patients with diffuse large B-cell lymphoma: a study by FISH. *Br J Haematol* 1998; **101**: 487–91.

178. Lossos IS. Higher-grade transformation of follicular lymphoma – a continuous enigma. *Leukemia* 2005; **19**: 1331–3.

179. Matolcsy A, Warnke RA, Knowles DM. Somatic mutations of the translocated bcl-2 gene are associated with morphologic transformation of follicular lymphoma to diffuse large-cell lymphoma. *Ann Oncol* 1997; **8**: 119–22.

180. Akasaka T, Lossos IS, Levy R. BCL6 gene translocation in follicular lymphoma: a harbinger of eventual transformation to diffuse aggressive lymphoma. *Blood* 2003; **102**: 1443–8.

181. Lossos IS, Levy R. Higher-grade transformation of follicle center lymphoma is associated with somatic mutation of the 5' noncoding regulatory region of the BCL-6 gene. *Blood* 2000; **96**: 635–9.

182. Lossos IS, Warnke R, Levy R. BCL-6 mRNA expression in higher grade transformation of follicle center lymphoma: correlation with somatic mutations in the 5' regulatory region of the BCL-6 gene. *Leukemia* 2002; **16**: 1857–62.

183. Szereday Z, Csernus B, Nagy M *et al.* Somatic mutation of the 5' noncoding region of the BCL-6 gene is associated with intraclonal diversity and clonal selection in histological transformation of follicular lymphoma. *Am J Pathol* 2000; **156**: 1017–24.

184. Lee JT, Innes DJ Jr, Williams ME. Sequential bcl-2 and c-myc oncogene rearrangements associated with the clinical transformation of non-Hodgkin's lymphoma. *J Clin Invest* 1989; **84**: 1454–9.

185. Brito-Babapulle V, Crawford A, Khokhar T *et al.* Translocations t(14;18) and t(8;14) with rearranged bcl-2 and c-myc in a case presenting as B-ALL (L3). *Leukemia* 1991; **5**: 83–7.

186. Lossos IS, Alizadeh AA, Diehn M *et al.* Transformation of follicular lymphoma to diffuse large-cell lymphoma: Alternative patterns with increased or decreased expression of c-myc and its regulated genes. *Proc Natl Acad Sci U S A* 2002; **99**: 8886–91.

187. de Vos S, Hofmann WK, Grogan TM *et al.* Gene expression profile of serial samples of transformed B-cell lymphomas. *Lab Invest* 2003; **83**: 271–85.

188. Elenitoba-Johnson KS, Jenson SD, Abbott RT et al. Involvement of multiple signaling pathways in follicular lymphoma transformation: p38-mitogen-activated protein kinase as a target for therapy. Proc Natl Acad Sci U S A 2003; 100: 7259–64.

●189. Solal-Celigny P, Roy P, Colombat P et al. Follicular lymphoma international prognostic index. Blood 2004; 104: 1258–65.

●190. Farinha P, Masoudi H, Skinnider BF et al. Analysis of multiple biomarkers shows that lymphoma-associated macrophage (LAM) content is an independent predictor of survival in follicular lymphoma (FL). Blood 2005; 106: 2169–74.

191. Davies AJ. Clinical and molecular prognostic factors in follicular lymphoma. Curr Oncol Rep 2006; 8: 359–67.

●192. Cerhan JR, Wang S, Maurer MJ et al. Prognostic significance of host immune gene polymorphisms in follicular lymphoma survival. Blood 2007; 109: 5439–46.

193. Federico M, Vitolo U, Zinzani PL et al. Prognosis of follicular lymphoma: a predictive model based on a retrospective analysis of 987 cases. Intergruppo Italiano Linfomi. Blood 2000; 95: 783–9.

194. Lopez-Guillermo A, Montserrat E, Bosch F et al. Applicability of the International Index for aggressive lymphomas to patients with low-grade lymphoma. J Clin Oncol 1994; 12: 1343–8.

195. Miller TP, LeBlanc M, Grogan TM, Fisher RI. Follicular lymphomas: do histologic subtypes predict outcome? Hematol Oncol Clin North Am 1997; 11: 893–900.

196. Martin AR, Weisenburger DD, Chan WC et al. Prognostic value of cellular proliferation and histologic grade in follicular lymphoma. Blood 1995; 85: 3671–8.

197. Wang SA, Wang L, Hochberg EP et al. Low histologic grade follicular lymphoma with high proliferation index: morphologic and clinical features. Am J Surg Pathol 2005; 29: 1490–6.

198. Koster A, van Krieken JH, Mackenzie MA et al. Increased vascularization predicts favorable outcome in follicular lymphoma. Clin Cancer Res 2005; 11: 154–61.

199. Gulmann C, Espina V, Petricoin E III et al. Proteomic analysis of apoptotic pathways reveals prognostic factors in follicular lymphoma. Clin Cancer Res 2005; 11: 5847–55.

200. Ai WYZ, Czerwinski DK, Horning S et al. Tumor-infiltrating T cells are not predictive of clinical outcome in follicular lymphoma. Blood 2006; 108: a824.

201. Canioni D, Salles G, Mounier N et al. The poor prognosis value of high intra-tumoral macrophage count in follicular lymphoma patients requires selection of appropriate cut-off and can be circumvented by rituximab therapy. J Clin Oncol 2008; 26: 440–6.

202. Lee AM, Clear AJ, Calaminici M et al. Number of CD4+ cells and location of forkhead box protein P3-positive cells in diagnostic follicular lymphoma tissue microarrays correlates with outcome. J Clin Oncol 2006; 24: 5052–9.

203. Alvaro T, Lejeune M, Camacho FI et al. The presence of STAT1-positive tumor-associated macrophages and their relation to outcome in patients with follicular lymphoma. Haematologica 2006; 91: 1605–12.

204. Carreras J, Lopez-Guillermo A, Fox BC et al. High numbers of tumor-infiltrating FOXP3-positive regulatory T cells are associated with improved overall survival in follicular lymphoma. Blood 2006; 108: 2957–64.

205. Torlakovic EE, Bilalovic N, Golouh R et al. Prognostic significance of PU.1 in follicular lymphoma. J Pathol 2006; 209: 352–9.

206. Bilalovic N, Blystad AK, Golouh R et al. Expression of bcl-6 and CD10 protein is associated with longer overall survival and time to treatment failure in follicular lymphoma. Am J Clin Pathol 2004; 121: 3 42.

207. Moller MB, Nielsen O, Pedersen NT. Frequent alteration of MDM2 and p53 in the molecular progression of recurring non-Hodgkin's lymphoma. Histopathology 2002; 41: 322–30.

208. Bjorck E, Ek S, Landgren O et al. High expression of cyclin B1 predicts a favorable outcome in patients with follicular lymphoma. Blood 2005; 105: 2908–15.

209. Krishnadasan R, Bifulco C, Kim J et al. Overexpression of SOCS3 is associated with decreased survival in a cohort of patients with de novo follicular lymphoma. Br J Haematol 2006; 135: 72–5.

210. Sakhinia E, Glennie C, Hoyland JA et al. Clinical quantitation of diagnostic and predictive gene expression levels in follicular and diffuse large B-cell lymphoma by RT-PCR gene expression profiling. Blood 2007; 109: 3922–8.

211. Cheung KJ, Shah SP, Steidl C et al. Genome-wide profiling of follicular lymphoma by array comparative genomic hybridization reveals prognostically significant DNA copy number imbalances. Blood 2009; 113: 137–48.

212. Strickler JG, Copenhaver CM, Rojas VA et al. Comparison of 'host cell infiltrates' in patients with follicular lymphoma with and without spontaneous regression. Am J Clin Pathol 1988; 90: 257–61.

213. Farinha P, Han J, Al-Tourah A et al. The tumor microenvironment measured by flow cytometry predicts overall survival and transformation risk in follicular lymphoma. Blood 2006; 108: a2406.

214. Wahlin BE, Sander B, Christensson B, Kimby E. CD8+ T-cell content in diagnostic lymph nodes measured by flow cytometry is a predictor of survival in follicular lymphoma. Clin Cancer Res 2007; 13: 388–97.

215. Dave S. Gene expression profiling and outcome prediction in non-Hodgkin lymphoma. Biol Blood Marrow Transplant 2006; 12: 50–2.

216. Farinha P, Campo E, Banham A et al. The architectural pattern of FOXP3+ T cells is an independent predictor of survival in patients with follicular lymphoma (FL). Mod Pathol 2006; 19: a1043.

217. Chang KC, Huang X, Medeiros LJ, Jones D. Germinal centre-like versus undifferentiated stromal immunophenotypes in follicular lymphoma. J Pathol 2003; 201: 404–12.

218. Shiozawa E, Yamochi-Onizuka T, Yamochi T et al. Disappearance of CD21-positive follicular dendritic cells

preceding the transformation of follicular lymphoma: immunohistological study of the transformation using CD21, p53, Ki-67, and P-glycoprotein. *Pathol Res Pract* 2003; **199**: 293–302.

219. Cartron G, Watier H, Golay J, Solal-Celigny P. From the bench to the bedside: ways to improve rituximab efficacy. *Blood* 2004; **104**: 2635–42.

220. Cartron G, Dacheux L, Salles G *et al.* Therapeutic activity of humanized anti-CD20 monoclonal antibody and polymorphism in IgG Fc receptor FcgammaRIIIa gene. *Blood* 2002; **99**: 754–8.

221. Weng WK, Levy R. Two immunoglobulin G fragment C receptor polymorphisms independently predict response to rituximab in patients with follicular lymphoma. *J Clin Oncol* 2003; **21**: 3940–7.

222. Carlotti E, Palumbo GA, Oldani E *et al.* FcgammaRIIIA and FcgammaRIIA polymorphisms do not predict clinical outcome of follicular non-Hodgkin's lymphoma patients treated with sequential CHOP and rituximab. *Haematologica* 2007; **92**: 1127–30.

223. Romaguera JE, McLaughlin P, North L *et al.* Multivariate analysis of prognostic factors in stage IV follicular low-grade lymphoma: a risk model. *J Clin Oncol* 1991; **9**: 762–9.

224. Seymour JF, Pro B, Fuller LM *et al.* Long-term follow-up of a prospective study of combined modality therapy for stage I-II indolent non-Hodgkin's lymphoma. *J Clin Oncol* 2003; **21**: 2115–22.

225. Wang SS, Cozen W, Cerhan JR *et al.* Immune mechanisms in non-Hodgkin lymphoma: joint effects of the TNF G308A and IL10 T3575A polymorphisms with non-Hodgkin lymphoma risk factors. *Cancer Res* 2007; **67**: 5042–54.

226. Ruminy P, Jardin F, Picquenot JM *et al.* Two patterns of chromosomal breakpoint locations on the immunoglobulin heavy-chain locus in B-cell lymphomas with t(3;14)(q27;q32): relevance to histology. *Oncogene* 2006; **25**: 4947–54.

227. Jardin F, Ruminy P, Parmentier F *et al.* Clinical and biological relevance of single-nucleotide polymorphisms and acquired somatic mutations of the BCL6 first intron in follicular lymphoma. *Leukemia* 2005; **19**: 1824–30.

228. Phan RT, Saito M, Basso K *et al.* BCL6 interacts with the transcription factor Miz-1 to suppress the cyclin-dependent kinase inhibitor p21 and cell cycle arrest in germinal center B cells. *Nat Immunol* 2005; **6**: 1054–60.

229. Cattoretti G, Pasqualucci L, Ballon G *et al.* Deregulated BCL6 expression recapitulates the pathogenesis of human diffuse large B cell lymphomas in mice. *Cancer Cell* 2005; **7**: 445–55.

230. Phan RT, Dalla-Favera R. The BCL6 proto-oncogene suppresses p53 expression in germinal-centre B cells. *Nature* 2004; **432**: 635–9.

●231. Roulland S, Navarro JM, Grenot P *et al.* Follicular lymphoma-like B cells in healthy individuals: a novel intermediate step in early lymphomagenesis. *J Exp Med* 2006; **203**: 2425–31.

232. Nadel B, Marculescu R, Le T *et al.* Novel insights into the mechanism of t(14;18)(q32;q21) translocation in follicular lymphoma. *Leuk Lymphoma* 2001; **42**: 1181–94.

233. Duan H, Heckman CA, Boxer LM. The immunoglobulin heavy-chain gene 3′ enhancers deregulate bcl-2 promoter usage in t(14;18) lymphoma cells. *Oncogene* 2007; **26**: 2635–41.

234. Zhu D, McCarthy H, Ottensmeier CH *et al.* Acquisition of potential N-glycosylation sites in the immunoglobulin variable region by somatic mutation is a distinctive feature of follicular lymphoma. *Blood* 2002; **99**: 2562–8.

235. McCann KJ, Johnson PW, Stevenson FK, Ottensmeier CH. Universal N-glycosylation sites introduced into the B-cell receptor of follicular lymphoma by somatic mutation: a second tumorigenic event? *Leukemia* 2006; **20**: 530–4.

236. Roulland S, Lebailly P, Lecluse Y *et al.* Long-term clonal persistence and evolution of t(14;18)-bearing B cells in healthy individuals. *Leukemia* 2006; **20**: 158–62.

237. Hirt C, Dolken G, Janz S, Rabkin CS. Distribution of t(14;18)-positive, putative lymphoma precursor cells among B-cell subsets in healthy individuals. *Br J Haematol* 2007; **138**: 349–53.

238. Staudt LM. A closer look at follicular lymphoma. *N Engl J Med* 2007; **356**: 741–2.

239. Yunis JJ, Oken MM, Kaplan ME *et al.* Distinctive chromosomal abnormalities in histologic subtypes of non-Hodgkin's lymphoma. *N Engl J Med* 1982; **307**: 1231–6.

240. Eray M, Postila V, Eeva J *et al.* Follicular lymphoma cell lines, an *in vitro* model for antigenic selection and cytokine-mediated growth regulation of germinal centre B cells. *Scand J Immunol* 2003; **57**: 545–55.

◆241. de Jong D. Molecular pathogenesis of follicular lymphoma: a cross talk of genetic and immunologic factors. *J Clin Oncol* 2005; **23**: 6358–63.

242. Pasqualucci L, Neumeister P, Goossens T *et al.* Hypermutation of multiple proto-oncogenes in B-cell diffuse large-cell lymphomas. *Nature* 2001; **412**: 341–6.

Burkitt lymphoma

IAN T MAGRATH

INTRODUCTION

Burkitt lymphoma (BL) was first recognized as a distinct clinicopathologic entity in Africa. The eponymous designation is probably well deserved, since Denis Burkitt, a surgeon working in Kampala, Uganda, can literally be said to have put the tumor 'on the map' even though others, primarily pathologists,[1–5] had recognized the high frequency of both jaw tumors and lymphomas in African children prior to the publication of Burkitt's classical paper in 1958.[6] Burkitt reported 38 Ugandan children with an unusual 'sarcoma' of the jaw that was by far the most frequent childhood cancer in the Kampala Cancer Registry. He described the characteristic clinical features of the jaw tumors and the unusual pattern of associated sites of involvement (in part based on autopsies) that included intra-abdominal organs, and salivary and endocrine glands, but rarely the spleen or lymph nodes. At about the same time, O'Conor and Davis, pathologists also working at Mulago Hospital, Kampala, who had been conducting a survey of the malignant tumors of children diagnosed in their department (the major reference center for Uganda), confirmed Davis's much earlier observation[2] that approximately half of all the childhood cancers in the Mulago series were tumors of the reticuloendothelial system.[7] O'Conor provided the first detailed histopathologic description of the cases described by Burkitt, which he recognized as lymphomas.[8]

In view of the unusual, but characteristic features of what became known as the 'African lymphoma', Burkitt and colleagues decided to examine its continental distribution. Using the simplest of methodologic approaches (questionnaires, illustrated leaflets and visits, by road and air, to more than 50 hospitals in East and Central Africa), Burkitt found that the clinical syndrome occurred at high frequency in a broad band across Africa, extending roughly 15° north and south of the Equator.[9] Within this region there were significant differences – the tumor was not seen in the highlands (above 1000 m) but was common in lowland areas such as river valleys, with a southern prolongation along the coastal plain of Mozambique. A similar distribution with respect to height above sea level was later shown in another high incidence area, Papua New Guinea.[10] This apparent altitude barrier, which did not apply to other types of lymphoma, strongly suggested that climate, and particularly temperature, was a critical determinant of the distribution of the tumor in Africa, and that, consequently, it could be caused by an insect-vectored virus. Haddow, who was then the Director of the Ugandan Virus Research Institute, showed that the distribution of BL matched the distribution of predetermined climate zones (based on temperature and rainfall) in equatorial Africa,[11] to within

5 percent. These climate zones had already been shown to correlate with the distribution of various mosquitoes.

After hearing a lecture given by Burkitt at the Middlesex Hospital in London, Epstein, a pathologist, obtained fresh BL tumor from Kampala to test the vectored-virus hypothesis by electron microscopic examination of tumor cells. Although Epstein could not detect virus particles in fresh biopsies, along with his colleague, Barr, he developed continuously growing cell lines from the tumor cells. In the first of these cell lines, designated EB1 (Epstein–Barr 1), Epstein and colleagues detected herpes-like virus particles, subsequently referred to as Epstein–Barr virus (EBV), in a small percentage of the cells.[12] Soon after, Gertrude and Werner Henle, working in Philadelphia, developed immunofluorescent techniques able to show the presence of antibodies in human sera that recognized viral antigens present in the cell lines, enabling them and others to conduct serologic studies of EBV infection in human populations.[13,14] Using such techniques, it has been estimated that EBV infects 90 percent of the world's population, although the age of primary infection varies with socioeconomic status. In low-income populations, antibodies are universally acquired in early childhood (in equatorial Africa, mostly prior to the lower age-limit of BL – 2 years) but in high-income populations, virus acquisition occurs primarily in adolescence and early adulthood,[15] when it is frequently associated with infectious mononucleosis.[16,17] Very few individuals in high socioeconomic groups are never infected. The age of acquisition of EBV, as first proposed by de Thé,[18] is likely to be important to the pathogenetic role of EBV in BL, since in poorer countries, the majority of BL cases are EBV associated (Fig. 32.1). In contrast, in high-income countries, rather few BL cases (10–20 percent) are EBV positive.[19] Even within countries (and doubtless, over time), the frequency of EBV-associated BL may vary in different populations, probably largely due to differences or changes in socioeconomic status and consequently, the age of acquisition of EBV.[20,21] Thus, although the geographic distribution of BL led to the discovery of EBV, this virus, which is not vectored by arthropods, cannot account for the climate-associated distribution of BL in Africa.

The discovery of the chromosomal translocations associated with BL[22] was a critical step in understanding its molecular pathogenesis. The first translocation discovered was a reciprocal chromosomal exchange between the locus of the *MYC* gene on chromosome 8 and the heavy chain immunoglobulin gene locus on chromosome 14.[23,24] Subsequently, less frequently observed reciprocal translocations involving the *MYC* locus and the light chain immunoglobulin gene loci on either chromosomes 2 (κ) or 22 (λ), often referred to as 'variant' translocations, were identified.[25] There are limited data on the relative frequency of the translocations associated with BL in different world regions although existing information suggests that the majority in all world regions are 8;14 translocations. Recognition of the consequences of the translocations coupled to an ever more complete understanding of the

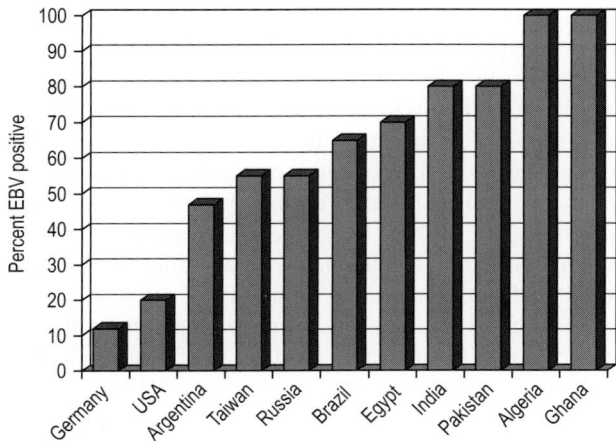

Figure 32.1   Fraction of Epstein–Barr virus (EBV)-positive cases among all cases of Burkitt lymphoma in published series from the countries indicated. These series have been collected over time, and may not be fully representative of the various populations in each country. They do serve to indicate that the majority of cases of Burkitt lymphoma in most countries are EBV positive. In high-income countries, most cases of Burkitt lymphoma are EBV negative.

mechanisms used by EBV to persist throughout the life of its host and to infect almost the entire human population, has provided insights into the pathogenesis of BL. In EBV-negative BL, specific molecular lesions presumably substitute functionally for the pathogenetic contributions of EBV. The incidence of this type of BL is presumably lower because EBV infects many cells, such that the chance that a *MYC*-immunoglobulin (*MYC*–Ig) translocation will occur in an EBV-infected cell (or vice versa) is much greater than the likelihood that the required set of molecular changes in the absence of EBV will occur in a single cell. This provides a possible explanation for the predominance of EBV-positive tumors and the generally higher incidence of BL in developing countries, where EBV infection occurs at an early age. In equatorial Africa (generally referred to simply as 'Africa' in this chapter), for example, the incidence rate is from 5 to 10 per 100 000 in children younger than 15 years – as much as 50 times the incidence in high-income countries. Hence the terms endemic and sporadic are frequently applied to these two main types of BL. BL is also increased in frequency in persons with human immunodeficiency virus (HIV) infection, although, interestingly, only about a third of HIV+ BLs are associated with EBV. BL in this context will be discussed in Chapter 81 and not dealt with here.

MALARIA AND AFRICAN BURKITT LYMPHOMA

In the same year that EBV was discovered, Dalldorf proposed that malaria, which is also transmitted by a mosquito vector and has a similar distribution to other mosquito vec-tored diseases, might predispose to BL.[26] The subsequent recognition that BL is of B cell origin[27] and that malaria is associated with polyclonal B cell hyperplasia[28] gave signifi-cant support to this hypothesis. Children in equatorial Africa have elevated serum levels of immunoglobulin (Ig) G, much of which is directed against malarial antigens, and splenomegaly, both a consequence of universal (holo-endemic) infection by malaria. Malaria-induced hyperplasia could predispose children to BL simply by virtue of increas-ing the number of target cells for neoplastic transformation, but because of the increased production of B cells, entailing molecular rearrangements of immunoglobulin genes, malaria could also predispose to the development of chro-mosomal translocations relevant to the pathogenesis of BL, i.e. those in which *MYC* is juxtaposed to an Ig gene (see below). However, it is clear that malaria-induced B cell hyperplasia does not predispose to B cell lymphoid neo-plasms in general. Acute precursor B cell leukemia, for example, is not increased in incidence in African children – indeed, the reverse appears to be the case,[29] as noted origi-nally by Burchenal.[30] Malaria does, however, increase the pool of EBV-carrying B cells as well as the production of virus in lymphoid tissue (potentially able to infect additional B cells), which results in an increase in the plasma level of viral DNA and the quantity of virus in saliva,[31] the primary route of transmission. By both increasing EBV transmission and the number of EBV-infected B cells as well as the prob-ability that a *MYC*–Ig translocation will occur (for which there is, as yet, no objective evidence), malaria could act at both population and individual levels in predisposing to BL.

In addition to the observations from Africa in the 1960s that the distribution of holoendemic malaria and BL coincide (rare islands of apparent discrepancy have been described), several other epidemiologic observations favor the hypothesis that the one predisposes to the other. BL for example, occurs at higher frequency in rural regions, where parasitemia rates are higher.[32] In highland regions, where malaria is much less prevalent, BL occurs at a later age. Such individuals appear to be at increased risk for BL if they migrate to regions of high malaria prevalence later in life.[33]

There are several reports of fluctuations in the incidence of BL corresponding to variations in malarial prevalence. In the 1960s, for example, a period of documented reduc-tion in BL in the Mengo districts of Uganda was associated with a reduction in infant mortality[33] believed to be related to improved malaria control. In early epidemiologic stud-ies carried out by Burkitt and colleagues, BL was essentially unknown in the islands of Zanzibar and Pemba, which, at the time, were also largely free of malaria due to an effec-tive eradication program based on DDT spraying. After the suspension of the eradication program, there has been a resurgence of malaria in Zanzibar, accompanied by a rise in the incidence of BL[34] Similarly, observations have been made in other tropical regions where malaria parasitemia rates, particularly with *Plasmodium falciparum*, are high,[35] although information is limited on the incidence of BL in

relationship to malaria prevalence or to the prevalence of various *Plasmodium* spp. in many relevant regions, such as equatorial Latin America.

In 1989, an attempt to directly study the relationship between BL and malaria was undertaken in the North Mara district of Tanzania. After some years of observation of the BL and malaria rates, malaria was suppressed with prophylactic chloroquine, which resulted in a marked drop in the incidence of BL and a return to prior levels after the cessation of prophylaxis.[36] Unfortunately, the results of this trial, although very suggestive, cannot be said to be definitive, since there was a slight dip in incidence prior to the introduction of chloroquine and an increase in inci-dence even before prophylaxis was stopped. This reflects the difficulties inherent in such studies, e.g. the problem of ensuring that prophylactic chloroquine is taken correctly throughout the study period by the test group and is not taken by the control group, and the necessity for very large populations to be studied, ideally over long time periods, to overcome the large natural fluctuations in BL incidence that will always occur in small populations.

Finally, animal models also support the hypothesis that malaria predisposes to BL – *Plasmodium yeolii*-infected mice, for example, are at increased risk to develop lymphoid neo-plasms, particularly when infected by a leukemia virus.[37] In all, although direct evidence remains elusive, a rather con-vincing case can be made for the possibility that malaria is the underlying reason for the particularly high incidence of BL in equatorial Africa and other tropical regions. It remains possi-ble, however, that other parasites or infections prevalent in Africa, by contributing to alterations in the cellular composi-tion of the immune system, may also influence the likelihood of the development of BL. In antigen stimulated athymic mice, for example, chronic nematode infestation (endemic in African children) predisposes to lymphomagenesis.[38] With the development of new approaches to the control of para-sitic diseases, such as a vaccine against malaria, new opportu-nities to study the associations between malaria and the incidence of BL will arise. This is not simply of scientific inter-est. Vaccination against malaria could prove to be an impor-tant means of preventing BL in holoendemic malarious areas.

EPSTEIN–BARR VIRUS ASSOCIATION WITH BURKITT LYMPHOMA

For some years after the discovery of EBV it was not clear why virus particles, and subsequently, viral proteins reac-tive with the sera of patients with BL, were detectable in only a few percent of the cells of continuously growing cell lines derived from fresh BL tumor cells. The discovery of virus-coded nuclear proteins, called EBV nuclear anti-gens, or EBNAs (in all, six such proteins were eventually identified – see Chapter 7) led to the demonstration that viral proteins, and therefore viral genomes, are present in all cells in EBV-positive BL cell lines. It has subsequently been shown that virus is generally present as multiple extrachromosomal DNA copies (there are rare exceptions), referred to as plasmids, in all EBV-containing cell lines, but virus production, triggered by the expression of the 'Zebra' or *Zba* gene and followed by cell lysis, occurs only in a small proportion of such cells (see Chapter 7). Progression to cell lysis in individual cells becomes an irreversible process early in the chain of molecular events, i.e. before virus particles are produced; once initiated, the inhibition of virus production by aciclovir does not prevent cell lysis.[39] This means that only latent viral genes, i.e. those that are critical to the persistence of EBV infection in a cell and its progeny, but not genes associated with virus production, can be expressed in tumor cells. Lytic cycle genes may be expressed in a small number of tumor cells, as is the case for cell lines, but such cells are destined to die.[40] Virus production, for example, has been demonstrated in tumor cells surrounding phagocytic macrophages (responsible for the classic 'starry sky' appearance) in EBV-positive tumors.[41] There is experimental confirmation that inducing the virus lytic cycle, e.g. by transfection with the Zebra gene regulated by an appropriate promoter, is incompatible with cell survival.[39] Thus, induction of the lytic cycle represents a novel approach to the treatment of EBV-associated tumors.[39–42]

Epstein–Barr virus latent and lytic virus cycles in normal and neoplastic cells

In 1968, Pope and colleagues demonstrated that EBV can transform B cells *in vitro*,[43] seemingly providing strong, if circumstantial evidence for a pathogenetic role for EBV in BL. Later it became clear that the viral latent genes responsible for the transformation of normal B cells *in vitro* (and not with virus production) are also responsible for what has been called the 'growth cycle' *in vivo*. This pattern of viral gene expression is orchestrated by EBNA2, which regulates the expression of the other growth cycle genes that comprise what has been called the latency III pattern – in which all six nuclear antigens and three membrane antigens are expressed. The induction of B cell proliferation presumably relates to augmentation of the number of virus-carrying cells shortly after primary infection, which may also be a necessary antecedent to the creation of a sufficient pool of memory cells in which EBV maintains permanent residence (see Chapter 7). While the EBV-infected population in the tonsils of normal EBV-positive individuals includes both naïve B cells (i.e. IgM+, IgD+ cells that have not been exposed to antigen and whose immunoglobulin genes do not contain somatically induced hypervariable region mutations) and memory B cells (IgD–), only IgD+ cells are found to express the latency III pattern. Such cells also express the activation antigen, CD80, not present on resting cells and can be found only when infectious virus is also present.[44] A reasonable explanation of these data is that naïve B cells, after infection in the mantle zone of the tonsil (at primary infection or subsequently, via

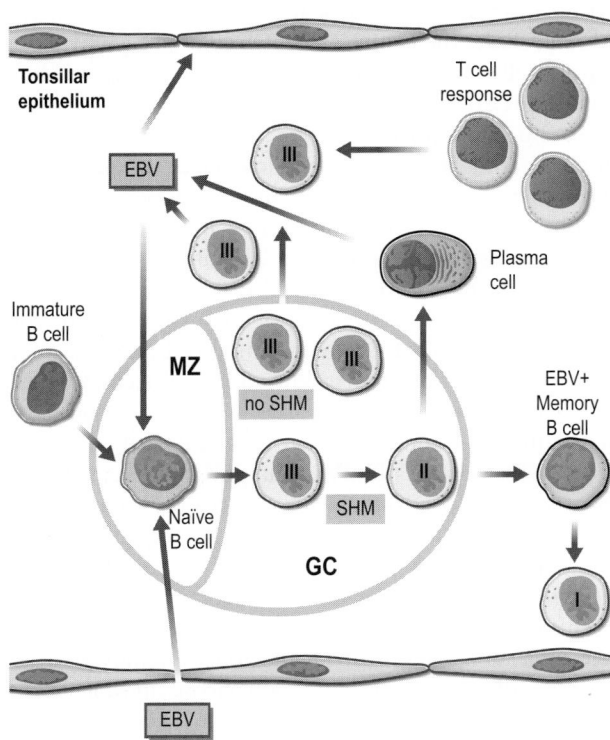

Figure 32.2 Diagram showing events in a germinal center in the Waldeyer ring following exposure to Epstein–Barr virus (EBV). In the acute event both germinal center (GC) cells and naïve B cells in the mantle zone (MZ) and potentially, also memory B cells may be infected and transformed via the EBV growth program (latency III pattern). The available evidence suggests that it is the infected naïve B cells, which undergo somatic hypervariable region mutation (SHM) that give rise to the EBV reservoir that persists after acute infection. Infected germinal center cells may be involved in amplifying the EBV copy number, but they do not undergo SHM and, once a T cell response develops, are largely destroyed by cytotoxic T cells. After acute infectious mononucleosis, such cells are difficult to find in normal tonsils although cells expressing the latency II pattern can be identified. The latency I phenotype – that of EBV+ BL – has been described only in dividing memory B cells, which may be the normal counterpart cell of EBV+ BL. EBV– BL may be the neoplastic counterpart of a particular type of germinal center cell.

virus producing cells – see below), passage into the germinal center and undergo immunoglobulin gene hypervariable region mutations and class switching just like uninfected, antigen-stimulated cells (see Chapter 12). Some of these EBV infected cells enter the peripheral blood as resting memory (IgD–) B cells (Fig. 32.2) – analysis of individual EBV-infected cells in peripheral blood has shown the invariable presence of the hallmarks of passage through the germinal center and the specific signature of antigen selection.[45] At first sight, this is surprising, since the EBV latent genes, *LMP1* and *LMP2a*, appear able to provide the necessary signals for B cells to survive the passage through a germinal center in the absence of antigen stimulation; LMP1 provides the equivalent of CD40 binding and T cell help, as well as the induction of activation induced cytidine deaminase (AID), a key element of both somatic hypermutation and immunoglobulin class switching, while LMP2a simulates antigen receptor signaling. Thus, antigen might appear to be unnecessary for cell survival. However, the lack of stop codons or aberrant mutations in circulating EBV-containing memory cells suggests that antigen selection has, indeed, occurred. LMP2a and LMP1, then, rather than overcoming the need for antigen, may simply favor the prolonged survival of EBV-containing cells; LMP2a may amplify growth stimulation by low-affinity antigens, whereas LMP-1 may ensure cell entry into the memory compartment rather than undergoing terminal differentiation into plasma cells. Carriage of EBV in true antigen-selected memory cells could be advantageous to virus persistence since periodic amplification of the cell clone – and persistence of its contained virus – would be induced by exposure to the relevant antigen stored by dendritic reticular cells.

This interpretation of available evidence appears to contrast with observations made in tonsils removed from patients with acute infectious mononucleosis, in which it has been shown that only occasional germinal center cells are positive for virus. Such cells express the growth program but do not undergo continued hypervariable region mutation of Ig genes (Fig. 32.2).[46] Recent evidence suggest that this results from EBNA2 inhibition of AID.[47] Such cells are found in tonsillar lymph nodes only in acute infectious mononucleosis, a time when the T cell immune response has not fully developed, and their major role may be amplification of viral genomes early in the infectious process. They appear to be derived from direct infection of memory B cells or germinal center cells rather than naïve B cells, and probably do not contribute to the pool of EBV-containing memory B cells in the peripheral blood (which is of the order of 1–10 per million B cells). After the acute infection, these cells, which may be unable to exit the growth phase, are probably largely eradicated in normal individuals, by cytotoxic T cells directed against latent antigens.[48] They can continue to proliferate, however, in the presence of various types of immunosuppression when they may be manifested as lymphoid hyperplasia ane even evolve into neoplasms (see Chapter 20).

In patients who have recovered from acute infectious mononucleosis, activated EBV-containing cells in tonsillar germinal centers manifest a latency II pattern, in which EBNA1 is transcribed from a different promoter (Q) from that used in latency III, and LMP1 and LMP2a are also expressed.[49] This pattern is also seen in nasopharyngeal carcinoma and Hodgkin disease, and may be a transient state observed in naïve cells in the process of shutting down the growth program (latency III); switching off EBNA2 may be necessary to allow somatic hypervariable region mutation. The latency II pattern could also occur in EBV-containing memory cells undergoing periodic amplification to ensure the persistence of EBV.[50] Interestingly, resting small lymphocytes in the peripheral blood that contain EBV appear to express no viral proteins (thus have no risk of elimination by T cells), although rare EBV containing (confirmed by the presence of the small RNA molecule, EBER) memory cells that divide while still in peripheral blood, express only a single viral protein, EBNA-1, transcribed from the Q promoter. This pattern, known as latency I, is found in EBV-positive BL.[51–53] Such cells appear to be the closest normal counterpart cell to EBV-positive BL,[51–54] although the tumor cell phenotype may be influenced by other molecular changes associated with the neoplastic state. EBNA1 is a DNA-binding protein involved in anchoring EBV genomes within the nucleus and ensuring their replication and equal subdivision into daughter cells. Hence, its presence is essential to the maintenance of viral genomes in dividing cells, whether malignant or not (see Chapter 7). In addition to EBNA1, EBV-positive BL cells also express small RNA EBER molecules and EBV microRNAs, whose gene regulatory functions may be important in maintaining the latency I state.[55]

Some EBV-infected cells in lymphoid tissue, particularly in tonsils, undergo terminal differentiation to plasma cells. They continue to produce virus which can infect other lymphocytes or epithelial cells in the nasopharynx (Fig. 32.2).[56] Virus production (and possibly, persistence) also takes place in epithelial cells overlying the tonsils, which are shed and undergo lysis.[57] Virus which enters the saliva in this way can be transmitted to other individuals. EBV clearly takes advantage of the normal pathways of B cell differentiation in order to persist indefinitely in a healthy host while continuously releasing infectious virus into saliva. This explains how it infects perhaps 90 percent of the adult population of the world. The patterns of EBV gene expression in its associated B cell neoplasms are consistent with patterns observed in normal B cells at different stages of differentiation, suggesting that each EBV-associated lymphoma (Hodgkin lymphoma, BL and B cell lymphomas in immunosuppressed individuals) arises in a different cellular context corresponding to a specific phase of the EBV life cycle (see Chapter 7). It is noteworthy that EBV predominantly takes up residence in B lymphocytes of mucosal-associated lymphoid tissue (MALT),[58] and, as might be expected, in order to maintain the virus–host balance in this circumstance, CD8+ T cells able to home to tonsillar sites have been shown to be enriched in individuals infected with EBV many years before.[59] This is consistent with the pattern of sites of involvement of neoplasms associated with EBV. In BL, peripheral lymph node involvement is uncommon but extranodal sites that are frequently involved in MALT lymphomas, such as the gastrointestinal tract, buccal and pharyngeal structures, salivary glands, orbit, endocrine glands and breast, are also frequently involved in BL.[60]

Avoiding immune surveillance

Of great importance, both to viral latency and to EBV's presumptive role in lymphomagenesis, at least in BL, is the observation that EBNA1 is not immunogenic – it contains a glycine–alanine repeat sequence which inhibits ubiquitin degradation and, consequently, major histocompatibility complex (MHC) class I-restricted presentation of EBNA-1 derived peptides.[61] Thus, although there are some conflicting findings in the literature, it would appear that EBNA1, unlike all other EBV latent genes, is poorly recognized by T cells, ensuring that neither the EBV reservoir in memory B cells, nor EBV-associated BL, excite an immune response. Other mechanisms permitting BL to escape immune surveillance include downregulation of human leukocyte antigen (HLA) class I antigens and cell adhesion molecules, a low level of expression of peptide transporters (TAP) involved in antigen loading of HLA class I complexes and deficiencies in EBNA1-specific T cell responses.[62,63] This pattern of gene expression is likely to be related to the differentiation stage of the normal counterpart cells of BL, since it can be at least partially reversed by crosslinking CD40 receptors.[64] However, a role for MYC overexpression in this process cannot be excluded since in at least one EBV-transformed B cell line, which, under normal circumstances has high levels of expression of adhesion molecules and HLA class I complexes, conditionally induced MYC expression has been shown to be associated with downregulation of these proteins, and reduced immunogenicity.[65]

Pathogenetic contribution of Epstein–Barr virus

Given the limited expression of EBV genes in BL, the candidates for maintenance of the neoplastic state are EBNA-1, and potentially the small RNA molecules known as EBERS, as well as microRNAs.[56] Although only achieved, to date, in a single laboratory, the predisposition of EBNA1 transgenic mice to develop B cell lymphomas with a similar phenotype to BL[66] and the demonstration of more rapid appearance of tumors when these mice are crossed with mice transgenic for an Ig-activated MYC gene[67] has provided support for a role for EBNA1. In contrast, there appears to be an antagonistic relationship with respect to surface phenotype and growth patterns between the latent genes expressed in the EBV growth cycle, particularly EBNA2, and MYC (see below).[68] These findings may be relevant to the sequence of pathogenetic events in BL[69] and their relationship to B cell differentiation. In the doubly transgenic mice referred to above, both the antiapoptic protein, BCLxL (BCL2-like X protein, long), and Ig-recombinase activating genes (RAG) are induced in EBNA1-expressing preneoplastic cells,[70] suggesting that EBNA1 may reduce the likelihood of apoptosis and possibly predispose to the development of chromosomal translocations involving Ig sequences. Indeed, both EBNA1 and EBERS have been shown to inhibit apoptosis.[71–75] MicroRNAs have the ability to inhibit the expression of many genes, but their role, if any, in pathogenesis remains to be elucidated. If EBV is to enter the memory cell compartment, it needs to reduce the risk of apoptosis at all stages of its lifecycle, and, not surprisingly, all three EBV latency programs of gene expression in B cells are associated with inhibition of apoptosis.[76] It remains possible, therefore, that some of the pathogenetic lesions relevant to lymphomagenesis develop in premalignant cells that express other EBNAs – not just EBNA1, e.g. cells passaging through germinal follicles. One important requirement for lymphomagenesis in BL is that apoptosis induced by a deregulated MYC gene is suppressed. Apoptosis can, of course, be inhibited by genetic lesions unrelated to virus infection but the likelihood of oncogenesis occurring in an EBV-infected cell is greatly increased because EBV is present in many cells. There is some evidence that EBNA1 and EBERs may also be involved in nonapoptotic mechanisms of lymphomagenesis,[77,78] but the relative importance of such alternative pathways remains unknown.

Apoptosis also occurs in B cells that fail to create, by genetic recombination, a functional B cell receptor (BCR) comprising heavy and light Ig chains, which is expressed by the vast majority of BLs. This may indicate that the cells in which a neoplasia-inducing transformation occurs have already passed beyond the stage of both heavy and light chain Ig gene rearrangement, or, alternatively, that a functional BCR is a requirement for lymphomagenesis. The likelihood that EBV persists in antigen-selected memory B cells and the observation that only dividing memory cells have the latency I pattern required in BL could account for the need for a functional BCR in EBV-positive BL, but passage through the germinal center, regardless of EBV association, may impose a similar requirement. BCL6, which is expressed in germinal center cells and in BL, protects cells undergoing hypervariable region mutation from apoptosis and may also help create an environment conducive to the persistence of genetic lesions (see Chapter 20).

Epstein–Barr virus strain differences

Since in some virus-associated neoplasms (those associated with human papilloma virus [HPV], for example) the vital genotype influences oncogenic potential, mutations or polymorphic variants of EBV genes could also be relevant to the ability of EBV to contribute to neoplasia. Multiple polymorphisms have been described in many EBV genes, including the latent genes and, although only EBNA1 is expressed in BL, it remains possible that polymorphisms in other genes are important to lymphomagenesis. Such polymorphisms could, for example, influence the size of the EBV-infected B cell pool. Major sequence differences in EBNA2, initially detected as antigenic differences,[79] as well as polymorphisms in other EBNAs[80,81] have led to the recognition of two major types of EBV, A and B (or 1 and 2). Intermediate types have also been identified.[82] Cells transformed by type A or B viruses have differing abilities to survive in vitro, although whether the same applies in vivo is unknown.[83] Type B virus has been shown to have a higher frequency in African BL than in BL in other world regions, but type B EBV also appears to be more prevalent in the normal African population.[84] A deletion in the carboxy terminal region of LMP1 has been reported to be more often present in EBV-associated neoplasms, including BL,[85] but this may also reflect differences in the geographic distribution of variant forms of LMP1 rather than being of pathogenetic importance.[86,87] Similarly, sequence differences in the Zebra gene promoter in various pathologic conditions[88] are of unknown significance. Geographic differences in viral gene polymorphisms could also arise from genetic differences in the infected human populations rather than simply from geographic separation over time. Type B EBV, for example, is more prevalent in both African BL- and HIV-associated EBV,[89] raising the possibility that differences in the immune system (in Africans, potentially associated with malaria) may influence the prevalence of different strains.[90] This leaves open the possibility that viral strain differences may influence the incidence of EBV-positive BL.

The EBV polymorphisms discussed so far relate to genes not expressed in BL. Potentially more important are polymorphisms in *EBNA1*. Such polymorphisms – sufficient to result in antigenic differences – have been described,[90–92] but once again, there appear to be geographic differences in the prevalence of such polymorphisms, although this does not necessarily rule out differences in oncogenic potential.[93] In nasopharyngeal carcinoma, in contrast, there is evidence that a particular EBNA1 subtype is more frequently associated with this disease and that this is not simply due to geographic variations in distribution.[94,95]

MOLECULAR ABNORMALITIES IN BURKITT LYMPHOMA

Although not unique to BL, chromosomal translocations (8;14,8;22 or 2;8) that result in the juxtaposition of the *MYC* gene, normally located on chromosome 8, and one of the heavy or light chain Ig gene loci, normally located on chromosomes 14, 2 or 22[23,24,57] are a characteristic feature of this disease. In the more frequent 8;14 translocations, the *MYC* gene, or at least its coding region, is moved to a location distal (i.e. telomeric) to or into the IgH locus. Since *MYC* is transcribed in a telomeric direction, breakpoints in this case are 5′ of the gene or in the 5′ part of the gene (i.e. first exon or intron). In the variant translocations the breakpoints are 3′ of *MYC*, which remains on chromosome 8 while light-chain sequences from chromosomes 22 or 2 are translocated to chromosome 8 telomeric to *MYC* (Fig. 32.3). The vast majority of breakpoints on chromosome 8 are located between some 200 kb 5′ and 50 kb 3′ of *MYC*.[96] A high fraction of BLs contain few or no additional cytogenetic abnormalities other than the *MYC*–Ig translocations, suggesting that genome stability is relatively intact compared with other lymphomas, such as diffuse large B cell lymphoma.[97] The most frequent additional cytogenetic changes are abnormalities on chromosome 1q[98,99] which have been associated with a worse prognosis, at least in sporadic BL.[100]

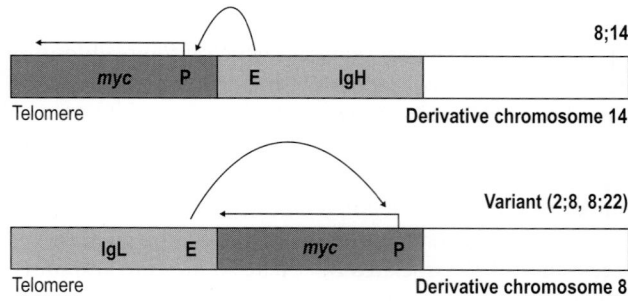

Figure 32.3 Diagrammatic depiction of the 8;14 and variant translocations in BL. In the former, *MYC* is translocated to chromosome 14 telomeric to or into the IgH locus. In the variant translocations, the *MYC* gene remains on chromosome 8 and light chain sequences (IgL) from either chromosome 22 (λ) or 2 (κ) are translocated telomeric to *MYC*. In both cases, enhancer elements associated with the immunoglobulin sequences, coupled to damage to the promoter regions of *MYC* (see Fig. 32.4) result in deregulation of *MYC*. Straight arrows indicate direction of transcription.

Translocations in relationship to B cell differentiation

It cannot be by chance that a B cell lymphoma carries translocations involving Ig genes. Being transcriptionally active early in the process of B cell differentiation, these genes are accessible to enzymes that mediate the molecular rearrangements required for the creation of functional Ig heavy and light chain genes and hence the BCR. Some of these enzymes could also mediate chromosomal translocation (see Chapter 28). Translocation could also occur, however, after antigen stimulation of a naïve B cell and passage through a germinal center, possibly related to somatic mutation of the hypervariable region and switch recombination (see Chapters 9 and 12). In follicular lymphomas there is strong evidence that the signal sequences involved in Ig heavy chain gene rearrangement (VDJ joining) are present at the chromosomal junctions in the associated 14;18 translocations, but site-specific recombination of this kind is not a characteristic feature of translocations in BL that involve the DJ regions of the Ig μ gene, although this has been reported,[101,102] as has site-specific translocation via the κ J region.[103] Translocations involving DJ heavy chain (rarely, V) regions appear to occur somewhat more frequently in BL in poorer countries – seemingly, for example, occurring in the majority of 8;14 translocations in African BL (Table 32.1).[104,105] Translocations involving Ig heavy chain switch regions are correspondingly less common in African Bl but account for the majority of translocations in, for example, European BL (see below).

Although the location of the chromosomal breakpoints on chromosome 14 could relate to the timing of the translocation in relationship to B cell differentiation, the observation that RAG1 and RAG2, which are necessary for VDJ joining

Table 32.1 Breakpoint locations as a percentage of total cases in each of the designated regions on chromosome 8 (*MYC* locus) and chromosome 14 in Burkitt lymphomas from various countries (see Fig. 32.4 for a map of *MYC* restriction enzyme sites)

Breakpoint location; *MYC* locus	Ghana	Brazil	Argentina/Chile	Algeria	USA
Outside HindIII	74	50	30	21	9
Immediately 5′	22	25	48	36	31
1st exon or 1st intron	4	25	22	43	60
Switch μ	22	20	38	7	31
Other Ig	78	80	62	93	69
Number of tumors[a]	23	24	27	14	32

[a]Including cell lines and biopsies (six cell lines from Ghana, 14 from Algeria and 12 from USA).

to occur, are expressed at high levels in EBV-bearing B cells[106] and, as mentioned above, in lymphoid cells in mice transgenic for EBNA1, indicates that this is not necessarily so. Since EBV, in some circumstances, activates the Ig hypervariable region mutation mechanism,[107] it remains possible that EBV infection of B cells could predispose to translocations involving both DJ and switch regions regardless of the stage of B cell differentiation. Circumstantial evidence that EBV may influence the likelihood of translocations involving the Ig heavy chain locus, and that translocations could, at least sometimes, occur in immature B cells, has been provided by the observation that Ig translocations occur frequently in pro-B cell lines derived by EBV-induced transformation (immortalization) of immature B cells present in fetal liver.[108] These cell lines, although immature, tended to have breakpoints in the switch immunoglobulin region, providing evidence that switch region recombination can, in some circumstances, be illegitimate and does not necessarily imply that the translocation occurred in a germinal center cell. Indeed, normal class switching involves the deletion of the μ and δ regions of the immunoglobulin locus, but this rarely occurs in BL translocations involving the Ig switch region,[109] suggesting that translocations are generally not 'mistakes' occurring during physiologic immunoglobulin gene recombinations, i.e. VDJ joining or class switching, but are simply more likely to occur in the same chromosomal locations which, by virtue of their accessibility to recombinases, constitute 'fragile sites' in B cells. However, this perspective may be an oversimplification: in experimental models, immature B cells expressing RAG (whose predominant location, after birth, is the bone marrow) may sometimes be found in peripheral lymphoid tissue, e.g. as a consequence of infection, including malaria,[110] while secondary VDJ recombination has been described in germinal center cells, and may be relevant to the generation or remodeling of translocations occurring in B cell neoplasms.[111,112] It would seem that the final molecular genetic arrangement may well be a consequence of more than one recombinational event, possibly occurring in more than one anatomic site and at different points in the course of B cell differentiation. Moreover, the translocational mechanism may differ from one tumor to another.

Molecular differences in Burkitt lymphoma from different geographic regions

Differences in chromosome 8 breakpoint locations in 8;14 translocations are strongly associated with geographic location (Fig. 32.4 and Table 32.1). In equatorial African BL breakpoint locations within the first exon or intron of *MYC* are uncommon (4 percent in one study), while in BL from the USA this is by far the most common breakpoint location (60 percent).[105] In Latin America, and North Africa, breakpoint locations appear to be intermediate between these two patterns, consistent with the possibility that differences may relate to socioeconomic status (compare Brazil with Argentina/Chile in Table 32.1). Differences in breakpoint locations in immunoglobulin regions also appear to be marked, with most African tumors having breakpoints in the VDJ region, and most European tumors in the switch region.[104,109] Differences in the frequency of immunoglobulin hypervariable region mutations in African BL versus non-African BL have also been reported (see below). A possible explanation of these findings is that they reflect differences in the normal counterpart cells of various BL subtypes. Since EBV is associated with most cases of BL outside the high-income countries, and differences in EBV association with specific breakpoint locations have not been identified,[105] it seems unlikely that the presence or absence of EBV accounts for these differences.[105]

Consequences of the *MYC*–Ig translocations

There is considerable evidence to support the conclusion that the functional consequence of the *MYC*–Ig translocations is the deregulation (inappropriate activation) of *MYC*. This gene is an important transcription factor belonging to the basic helix-loop-helix (b-HLH) family. It forms heterodimers with several partner b-HLH proteins which, through binding to a specific DNA sequence known as a core E-box element, regulate the expression of a large number of genes involved in cell cycle progression, ribosome biogenesis, protein synthesis, mitochondrial function, cell metabolism (including induction of lactate dehydrogenase-A, which is

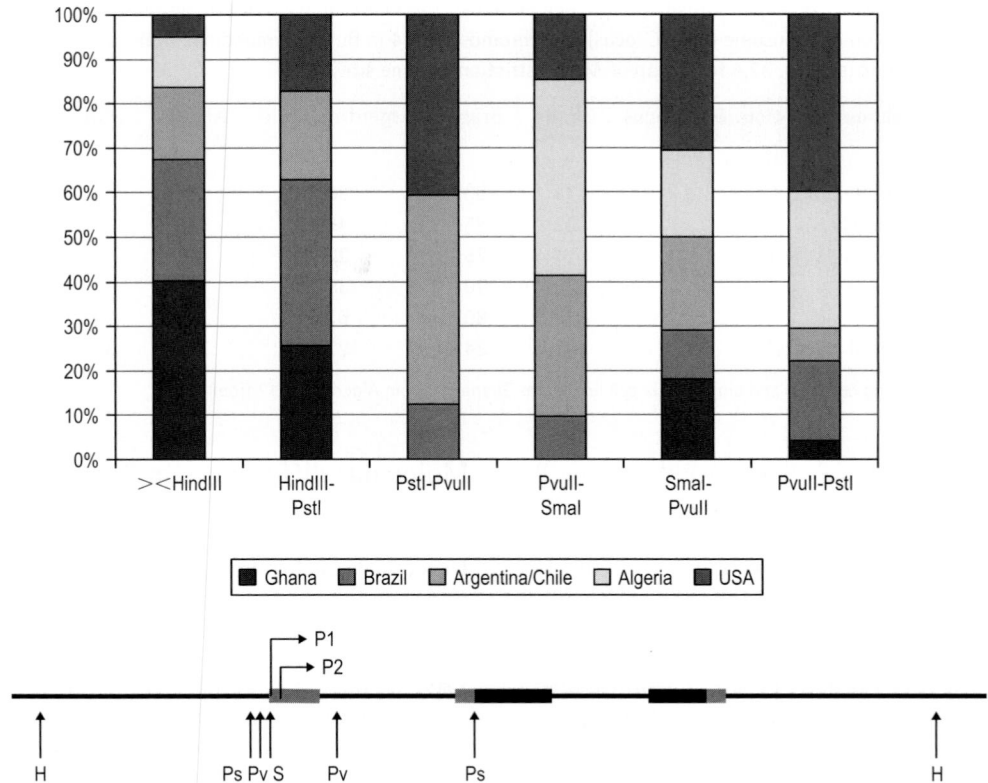

Figure 32.4   Proportions of breakpoint locations in a series of cell lines or tumour biopsies accounted for by countries in various world regions (Ghana, 23, 6 being cell lines, Brazil 24, all biopsies, Argentina and Chile, 27, all being biopsies, Algeria, 14, all cell lines, and USA, 32, 12 being cell lines). The breakpoints were classified according to the restriction fragments into which they fell (where multiple restriction enzyme sites for the same enzyme are present, the fragment reads from left to the first appropriate fragment). The percentages in each column were calculated by adding the percentages of each breakpoint location in each country provided in part in Table 32.1. A map of the relevant restriction enzyme sites is shown below the histogram. Note that in some regions breakpoints were not observed in some restriction fragments. H = HindIII, Ps = PstI, Pv = PvuII, S = SmaI. The country with the highest proportion of breakpoints outside HindIII is Ghana, with progressively smaller fractions in Brazil, Argentina/Chile, Algeria and the USA. No breakpoints between PstI and SmaI immediately upstream of P1 were observed in the Ghanaian samples and there were seemingly large differences in the precise locations of the immediately 5μ breakpoints in different countries, although some of these differences may be due to sample sizes.

elevated in BL), cell differentiation, cell adhesion, apoptosis and telomere maintenance (Fig. 32.5).[112–116] Recent studies have shown that in BL cells MYC predominantly forms heterodimers with MAX. MYC/MAX complexes are generally associated with activation of transcription and occupy approximately 15 percent of gene promoters tested.[117] Heterodimers not involving MYC, such as MAX/MAX, MAX/MAD and MAX/MXI1 compete with MYC/MAX in binding to DNA and repress transcription. A majority of the MYC target genes undergo changes in transcription in response to alterations in the cellular level of MYC (since MAX levels are relatively constant), although the C-terminal domain of MYC also binds other proteins involved in transcriptional regulation, e.g. YY1 transcription factor (YY1), and general transcription factor 2 (GTF2), such that the MYC level is not the sole determinant of MYC function. In an appropriate cellular and molecular context (e.g. when stimulated by growth factors), MYC protein induces cellular

proliferation. When the context is inappropriate, it induces apoptosis. In BL cells, it seems that either EBNA1, the small EBER RNAs, or lesions in genes that link MYC to apoptotic pathways, e.g., via the tumor suppressor protein, ARF (alternate reading frame), and BCL2-like 11 apoptosis facilitator (Bim), or lesions in genes in the apoptotic pathway itself, prevent apoptosis that would otherwise result from inappropriate activation of MYC.[118] This allows the proliferation of the genetically abnormal cell. Many observations related to the cooperation of genes involved in oncogenesis have been made in experimental models, particularly mice transgenic for *MYC* coupled to an immunoglobulin gene regulatory element. Such mice are prone to the development of B cell lymphoid neoplasms, some morphologically and biologically very similar to BL (see Chapter 17).[114,118–121] In addition, models of this kind allow the examination of the cell types which are present in the pre-malignant state in different genetic contexts.

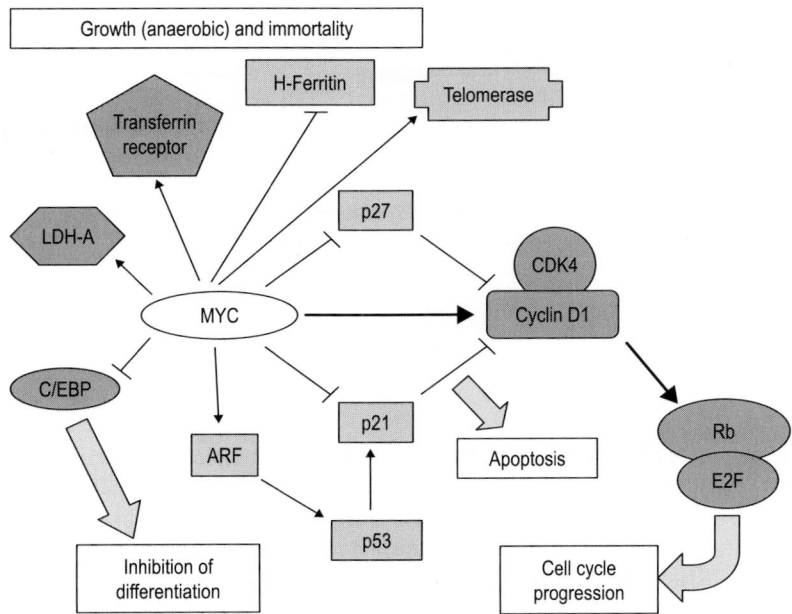

Figure 32.5 Schematic showing some of the important molecular pathways regulated by MYC. Some of these have very different outcomes, e.g. growth versus apoptosis. The pathway taken by a cell depends on its environment (particularly growth factors), the relative levels of MYC as well as those of the smaller basic helix-loop-helix (b-HLH) molecules, such as MAD and MXI1, which can bind to MAX and compete for the MYC/MAX binding sites in gene promoters, and the presence of other MYC-binding proteins. Burkitt lymphoma (BL) cells may be balanced precariously on this interface, which is one potential explanation of the high degree of chemosensitivity of BL (cells are readily tipped into apoptosis). Not all pathways or steps in each pathway are shown. Note that MYC stabilizes transferrin receptors, and influences iron metabolism, both necessary for cell growth, and also affects glycolysis. It is likely to be involved in both p53-dependent as well as p53-independent pathways (not shown). MYC may also be involved in protein and nucleotide synthesis (not shown). Inhibition of differentiation results in part from the drive to proliferation, but may also involve the regulation of genes in other molecular pathways.

Recently published evidence indicates that normal germinal center cells do not express MYC,[122] but instead use an alternative molecular pathway to drive cell proliferation. Since memory cells are normally in a resting state, they do not express MYC either. It is reasonable to conclude that MYC expression in BL is an exclusive effect of the chromosomal translocation, and hence, that this is a primary component of lymphomagenesis. In addition to transgenic mouse experiments, this conclusion is supported by the observations that inhibition of MYC expression by antisense molecules specific for *MYC* messenger RNA,[123,124] by anti-IgM, which downregulate both MYC and IgM,[125] or by a peptide nucleic acid complementary to a specific Eμ intronic sequence[126] causes cessation of proliferation in BL cell lines and frequently induces apoptosis, particularly in EBV-negative cell lines.

Antagonism between Myc and the Epstein–Barr virus growth program

There is substantial evidence that EBV does not drive proliferation in EBV-positive BL. Even though EBV is capable of transforming B cells, this is dependent on EBNA2, the key protein in the EBV growth program. However, EBNA2 is immunogenic and induces the expression of several other immunogenic EBV latent genes. This results in the self-limitation of the EBV transformation process and once a specific immune response has been generated, cells expressing the growth program are rapidly destroyed. MYC can also drive proliferation in EBV-transformed B cells, in which its conditional overexpression is able to compensate for the lack of expression of EBNA2 and LMP1.[127] Interestingly, EBNA2 downregulates IgM expression in EBV transformed cell lines as well as in cell lines containing *MYC*–Ig translocations in which it simultaneously also downregulates *MYC*, causing growth arrest.[128] This accounts for the invariable absence of EBNA2 expression in BL where its presence is not only not needed, but would be deleterious. In fact, although some of the target genes of these two transcription factors, MYC and EBNA2, are the same,[129] others, including cell surface proteins differ and when MYC replaces EBNA2 in EBV transformed B-cells, the cell morphology changes from lymphoblastoid to typical BL; CD10 is upregulated and cell surface activation markers known to be upregulated by EBNA2 are downregulated.[68] The ability to replace EBV transforming genes by MYC is consistent with the idea that EBV's role in the pathogenesis of BL is primarily to inhibit apoptosis, whereas Myc provides the proliferative drive. The change in phenotype associate with MYC expression, however, also provides a note of caution in equating neoplastic cells with a

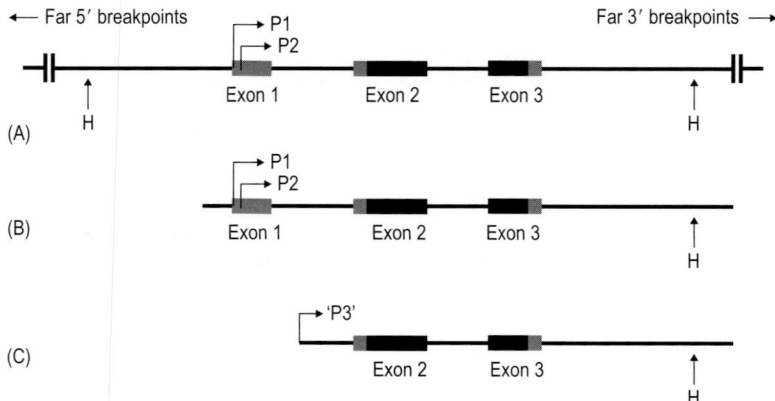

Figure 32.6   Structural consequences of the MYC-Ig chromosomal translocation. (A) Most endemic tumors with an 8;14 translocation and tumors with a variant translocation have a grossly intact *MYC* gene since breakpoints are far 5′ or 3′ of the gene, although there are point mutations in both regulatory and protein coding regions. (B) In approximately a third of Burkitt lymphomas (BLs) in the USA and North Africa, and almost a half in Argentina and Chile, but small fractions in endemic and Brazilian tumors, the breakpoint is in the 5′ regulatory region of the gene, i.e. between the 5′ HindIII site and SmaI site immediately adjacent to P1 (see Fig. 32.4). (C) In 60 percent of BLs from the USA, the breakpoint is downstream of P1, either in the first exon or first intron.

specific normal counterpart, since the phenotype may be partly or wholly a consequence of the abnormally high or low expression of specific genes rather than an indicator of the normal counterpart cells. Moreover, such changes in phenotype are likely to have functional consequences. For example, whereas crosslinking of surface immunoglobulin (normally by antigen) inhibits apoptosis in germinal center cells[130] crosslinking by anti-Ig in BL cell lines suppresses growth (probably since the translocations result in *MYC* being regulated by Ig sequences), induce EBV production[131] and may induce apoptosis.

Immunoglobulin hypervariable region mutations and Burkitt lymphoma subtype

Although a role for antigen in the pathogenesis of BL has not been defined, somatically induced hypervariable region mutations, that are essential to the adapation of antibody to specific antigens in normal germinal center cells, have been described by a number of investigators. Mutation frequencies are generally higher in African and acquired immune deficiency syndrome (AIDS)-related BL (approximately 5 percent vs 1 percent in sporadic BL)[132–134] and some have reported a lack evidence for antigen selection or continued accumulation of mutations in sporadic BL.[134] Even the highest hypervariable region mutation frequencies in BL are significantly lower (by a factor of 2) than the frequencies observed in follicular lymphomas (11–12 percent) in which there is clear evidence of antigen selection and continued accumulation of mutations.[135] This would be consistent with a differentiation block occurring at the early centroblast stage, prior to antigen selection, in sporadic, EBV-negative BL, and at the late germinal center or memory cell stage, post antigen selection, for African, EBV-positive BL.[134]

The differences in hypervariable region mutation rates parallel the differences in chromosomal breakpoint locations in BL in Africa versus, for example, Europe. Moreover, tumors with a breakpoint 5′ of *MYC* (predominantly African BL) have higher levels of MYC expression than those with breakpoints in the first exon or intron of *MYC* (predominantly non-African BL).[136] These findings are also consistent with the possibility that the translocations occur in cells at different stages of differentiation in BL occurring in different geographic locations and environmental circumstances.

Mechanism of activation of *MYC*

Since the breakpoint locations on chromosome 8, i.e. in relationship to *MYC*, vary quite markedly in 8;14 translocations – from several hundred kilobases upstream or downstream (in the variant translocations) of *MYC*, to within the first exon or intron of the gene itself,[137] there are large differences in the degree to which the genetic elements that regulate *MYC* remain intact (Fig. 32.6). As described, the three main patterns of gross structural change to *MYC* also vary in frequency in different geographic regions. Thus, the mechanism of activation of *MYC* must differ correspondingly. Regardless of the degree to which the regulatory elements of *MYC* are damaged by mutations or removed by the translocation, deregulation requires the influence of enhancer elements present in the immunoglobulin sequences juxtaposed to *MYC* by the translocation. In chromosome 8 breakpoints that are not within the gene itself, there is a shift in the pattern of promoter usage, such that the P1 promoter is more active than P2 (the reverse of normal). This change appears to be a hallmark of abnormal *MYC* activation when the chromosomal breakpoint is upstream of P1, and appears to require the preservation of regulatory elements (binding sites for regulatory proteins) adjacent to the coding region – either the preservation of positive elements, and/or the, inactivation of negative regulatory elements by deletion or mutation. Of particular importance appears to be the inactivation, by point mutations, of a transcriptional elongation inhibitory element located in exon 1 of MYC.[112,138–141] Although transcription-activating enhancer elements in the adjacent immunoglobulin locus may sometimes be distant from the MYC regulatory region, there is evidence that this is overcome through folding of the DNA strands, such that immunoglobulin and MYC regulatory elements are approximated.[142] In tumors in which the breakpoint is downstream of P1 and P2, transcription begins from a relatively ill-defined region within the first intron. This does not prevent the expression of the full length protein, since the predominant Myc protein, p64, is initiated in exon 2.

In addition to point mutations in the regulatory elements of MYC, mutations are also found in the protein coding region.[143,144] The genesis of these mutations is unclear, but the somatic hypervariable region mutational mechanism may, at least in some circumstances, be able to induce mutations in MYC genes juxtaposed by the translocations to immunoglobulin sequences.[145,146] Mutations that inhibit the binding of transcriptional repressors are probably of particular importance to the activation of MYC whereas those in critical locations in the Myc protein may have a variety of consequences including an altered ability of Myc to bind other proteins, such as proteins on apoptotic pathways,[147–150] or to be ubiquinated, thereby inhibiting proteosomal degradation of Myc and increasing its half-life.[151]

Other molecular abnormalities

A number of additional molecular abnormalities have been described in BL, particularly those involving apoptotic pathways. Mutations in p53, for example, are very frequent in both cell lines and fresh tumor cells,[152,153] and when absent are associated with other lesions that inactivate the ARF–MDM2–p53 apoptotic pathway.[154,155] Experimental data support the importance of this pathway that is initiated by DNA damage – inhibition of normal p53 increases the tumorigenicity of BL cell lines, while restoration of p53 function reduces tumorigenicity or may induce apoptosis.[152,156] Mutations or other abnormalities in pro-apoptotic proteins such as BAX (BCL2 associated X protein), BCLXs (BCL2-like X protein, short) and BAK (BCL2 antagonist/killer) inactivate other apoptotic pathways, including the CD95 (Fas)-receptor-mediated pathways,[156] and there may be variable expression of several inhibitors of apoptosis including cIAP-1 and cIAP-2.[157,158] Some of the observed genetic abnormalities result from epigenetic suppression of transcription, e.g. by DNA methylation.[159] This has been described for p73[160] and cell cycle inhibitors such as p16.[159,161] Occasional mutations in

cell cycle inhibitors have also been described,[162] and mutations in BCL6 are nearly always present.[146,163] These genetic and epigenetic changes, although broad in range can be seen to primarily affect pathways relating to progression through the cell cycle or the inhibition of apoptosis.

Alternative molecular mechanisms of lymphomagenesis

Recently, the absence of a MYC–Ig translocation in tumors with typical or atypical BL morphology has been described. In such cases, MYC deregulation is brought about by a different mechanism, either a translocation involving the MYC locus and a non-immunoglobulin locus,[98,164] or amplification of the MYC gene.[165] Even in cell lines bearing MYC–Ig translocations, MYC amplification may occur, sometimes as extrachromosomal copies.[166] These findings support the interpretation that the deregulation of MYC comprises one of the critical elements (another being the inhibition of apoptosis) in the pathogenesis of BL. It also raises the question, however, as to how BL should be defined, and the relationship between histopathological and molecular characteristics.

THE DEFINITION OF BURKITT LYMPHOMA

Burkitt's original description was of a clinical syndrome, not a pathologic entity. After O'Conor's detailed histopathological description[8] morphologically indistinguishable neoplasms were reported from the USA and the UK[166–168] and soon after, from other countries. Doubts continued, however, for some years as to whether a characteristic clinical syndrome (particularly jaw involvement) should be a requirement for diagnosis. In 1967 a consensus was reached on a formal pathologic definition by a group of 18 hematopathologists[169] who met in Washington, DC, under the auspices of the World Health Organization (WHO) and the International Agency for Research on Cancer. The majority view of the panel was that 'the eponym Burkitt's tumor is best applied to a malignant neoplasm of the haemopoietic system composed of a predominant and characteristic cell type' regardless of geographic origin. Whether or not involvement of the bone marrow, which occurs in less than 10 percent of African BLs, should exclude the diagnosis was for long debated,[170] in part because the research focus moved from Africa to the USA and Europe, where a higher proportion of cases present as leukemia (acute lymphocytic leukemia [ALL]). In 1980, an arbitrary cut-off of 25 percent blast cells in the bone marrow was proposed to distinguish between lymphomas and leukemias in children, and the term acute B cell leukaemia (i.e. the L3 type of acute lymphoblastic leukaemia in the French–American–British classification)[171] became widely used by pediatric oncologists. It remains in use today although it is clear that diffuse involvement of the bone marrow (localized involvement occurs in jaw and other sites of bone involvement) does not imply a different pathological entity. A second area of controversy has for long been the distinction between BL and diffuse large B cell lymphomas (DLBCLs), particularly in adults, in whom large B cell lymphomas have a much higher incidence than BL. At a histological level, cases intermediate between classic BL and classic DLBCL have long been recognized in the USA. Such tumors have many larger cells (BL cells are said to be of 'intermediate' size), or a more immunoblastic appearance, characterized particularly by the presence of a large single large nucleolus in a significant number of cells. The distinction among these categories has always included a large subjective element and reproducibility among pathologists has been poor. In earlier classification schemes the intermediate types were grouped with BL as 'undifferentiated lymphoma' or 'small noncleaved cell lymphoma', each category being divided into Burkitt and non-Burkitt types. These classification schemes did not take account of immunophenotype, such that these categories were rather heterogeneous. Burkitt lymphoma has for long been recognized as a tumor of B cell origin in view of the readily detectable expression of surface immunoglobulin, most often IgM (and either κ or λ light chains) and the constantly increasing repertoire of monoclonal antibodies led to the identification of an increasing array of B cell markers, including CD19, CD20, CD22, and CD79a and BCL6. CD10, which is present on both immature B cells and germinal center cells, is also essentially always expressed in BL, but by only a small fraction of DLBCLs. High levels of Ki67 are also invariably expressed, indicating that essentially all BL tumor cells are proliferating. CD5, CD23 and terminal deoxyribonucleotide transferase (TdT), which is expressed by neoplasms with immature immunophenotypes are not expressed and BCL2 is generally thought to be rarely expressed (but see below). Among these various markers, the expression of high levels of Ki67 and to a lesser extent of CD10 (which is expressed by some DLBCLs) in an 'aggressive' B cell lymphoma are particularly characteristic of BL.

In the Revised European–American Lymphoma (REAL) classification, published in 1994,[172] the middle ground between BL and DLBCL was occupied by Burkitt-like lymphoma (BLL), a provisional category, since it was unclear whether this was a truly separate disease, or simply histologically atypical BL or DLBCL. The morphological appearances of these three categories are shown in Plate 50, (see plate section) but morphological distinction has proved to be poorly reproducible. The authors of the REAL classification, for example, were able to agree on the distinction between BLL and DLBCL only 53 percent of the time.[173] The first WHO classification,[174] which was based on the REAL system, included BLL as a variant of BL in spite of the fact that most pathologists favored considering BLL to be a subtype of DLBCL. Clinicians felt that tumors diagnosed as BLL are more aggressive than the majority of DLBCL, having both a higher growth fraction and poorer response to therapies used for DLBCL.[173,175,176]

An additional category, atypical BL (aBL), in which there is evidence or strong 'presumption' of the presence of a chromosomal translocation typical of BL was also included in the WHO classification in which both BLL and aBL were defined as B cell tumors intermediate in appearance between BL and DLBCL with a very high growth fraction (close to 100 percent), as assessed by the level of reactivity with Ki67 or an equivalent monoclonal antibody. In the latest WHO (2008) classification (see Chapter 18) a category known as 'B-cell lymphoma, with features intermediate between DLBCL and BL' is still included. Morphology however, as well as immunophenotyping and all other clinicopathologic characteristics of any malignant tumor are ultimately determined by the gene expression profile and altered function of proteins resulting from the major structural changes and/or point mutations in genes that are responsible for the neoplastic state. It is difficult, therefore, to escape the conclusion that definitions must ultimately be made in molecular terms. Although, given the many molecular changes that occur in neoplastic cells, the precise description of the molecular characteristics of tumors may also fail to yield precise dividing lines, the objective nature, and potential to examine large numbers of genes by array techniques (whether at RNA, micro-RNA or protein levels), make microarray analysis a potentially more precise tool than morphology in providing a definition of a BL and identifying differences in the largely histologically defined BL, 'BLL' and DLBCL. Two recent publications in which the gene profile at an RNA level was examined in sporadic, almost exclusively EBV negative BL, and compared with that of tumors diagnosed as BLL/aBL and DLBCL, have provided considerable insight in this regard.[98,177]

A molecular definition

In both of these publications a molecular definition of BL was obtained by studying gene expression profiles of a reference set of typical BLs with respect to morphology, immunophenotype and the presence of MYC–Ig chromosomal translocations. In each case, a set of genes could be identified that demonstrated a high degree of similarity of expression in the reference set of BL. The expression profile of tumors possessing this BL signature, referred to here as 'molecular BL' (mBL) was then compared with that of additional tumors diagnosed as BL, BLL, aBL or DLBCL. In one of these studies,[97] 36 tumors had a very similar gene expression profile (more than 95 percent similarity) to the eight BLs in the reference set. These cases consistently expressed CD10 and BCL6; most (88 percent of the total of 44 mBLs) had a characteristic MYC–Ig translocation and 76 percent had minimal additional karyotypic abnormalities. No mBLs had a chromosomal abnormality involving BCL6, and only one had a 14;18 translocation involving BCL2, although 21 percent expressed BCL2. Remarkably, however, 11 of the additional 36 cases of mBL had morphology typical of DLBCL and four were unclassifiable B cell lymphomas. The remaining cases were classified as aBL based on BLL histology or a deviant immunophenotype (21) or were unclassified (4). Among 128 lymphomas in which expression profiles were less than 5 percent similar to the mBL signature (non-mBL), one was diagnosed as BL lymphoma-leukemia, 3 (2 percent) were diagnosed as aBL and 115 (90 percent) had typical DLBCL morphology (the remaining 9 cases were unclassified). CD10 was expressed in 21 percent of the 128 cases, only 4 percent had a typical *MYC*–Ig translocation, 11 percent carried a 14;18 translocation, 24 percent had a translocation involving *BCL-6* and 71 percent had a complex karyotype. In tumors with between 5 percent and 95 percent similarity to the mBL profile, i.e. neither mBL nor non-mBL, 81 percent had morphology typical of DLBCL, none had BL morphology and only 8 percent were diagnosed as aBL. More than half expressed CD10, 33 percent had *MYC*–Ig translocations and 21 percent translocations involving *MYC*, but not an Ig locus. Somewhat more (21 percent) had 14;18 translocations than non-mBL and rather fewer (15 percent), BCL6 translocations (Table 32.2). In the second reported study,[177] 48 percent of the 45 cases diagnosed morphologically as BL or aBL were children and all but one were also mBL – as were the 25 'morphologically verified' cases used as the control panel. However, nine cases originally diagnosed as BL or aBL but reclassified on review by a panel of experts as DLBCL or unclassified aggressive B cell lymphoma also had a molecular profile of mBL.

These findings indicate that most tumors diagnosed as BL or BLL (aBL) using WHO criteria have a similar molecular profile – that of classic BL – but a significant fraction *of* mBL cases (13 percent and 25 percent in the two studies) have the morphological features of DLBCL! The converse does not apply – typical BL morphology is essentially never associated with a DLBCL molecular profile (mDLBCL). DBLCL, at least in Europe and the USA has a much higher incidence than BL or BLL/aBL (or tumors intermediate

Table 32.2 Characteristics of molecularly defined diffuse B cell lymphomas (based on 220 cases)[a]

	Molecular BL (%)	Intermediate (%)	Nonmolecular BL (%)
Morphology			
BL	18	0	0
aBL	48	8	2
DLBCL	25	81	90
Other B-NHL	9	10	7
CD10 expression			
Negative	0	43	79
Positive	100	57	21
ABC/GCB signature[b]			
ABC	0	17	39
GCB	91	71	35
Unclassified	9	13	26
Myc translocation			
Myc-Ig	88	33	4
Myc-non-Ig	2	21	3
Myc-negative	9	46	93
BCL2–Ig translocation			
Negative	98	79	89
Positive	2	21	11
BCL6 translocation			
Negative	100	85	76
Positive	0	15	24
Complexity of karyotype			
Myc-simple	76	13	0
Myc-complex	13	40	7
Myc-negative	11	47	93

[a]Data from Hummel *et al.*[97] There were 44 cases of molecularly defined BL, including the reference set of eight 'core' cases. Similarity to the core group was measured as being between zero (no resemblance) and one (identical) on the basis of the gene expression profile. Molecularly defined BL had an index of expression similarity of >0.95. Those with an index of <0.05 (128 cases) were considered non-molecular BL. The remaining cases (48) were classified as 'intermediate'.
[b]Activated B cell (ABC) versus germinal center cell (GCB) profile.
BL, Burkitt lymphoma; aBl, atypical BL; DLBCL, diffuse large B cell lymphoma, B-NHL, B non-Hodgkin lymphoma.

between BL and DLBCL) and the majority of such cases – over 90 percent – will have a DLBCL molecular profile. Interestingly, in tumors defined by Hummel *et al.*,[97] as having a molecular profile intermediate between mBL and mDLBCL the majority of such cases were diagnosed morphologically as DLBCL, the remainder being equally divided between aBL and unclassified lymphomas. Over half (54 percent) of these tumors had a deregulated *MYC* gene, but in 21 percent of these the mechanism of deregulation was not via a *MYC–Ig* translocation. Moreover, lymphomas with an intermediate profile tended to have more complex karyotypic changes than either BL or DLBCL and a higher frequency of 14;18 translocations, suggesting that many of these lymphomas may have evolved from a subclinical B cell lymphoma of another category, particularly follicular lymphomas, a high fraction of which carry 14;18 translocations. This is consistent with the ability of BCL2 to cooperate with MYC in accelerating B cell tumor development in transgenic mice, with the well recognized evolution, both morphologically and karyotypically, of follicular lymphomas into a BL or BLL, and with the occasional presence of both *MYC–Ig* and *BCL2* translocations in the same lymphoma (a situation that generally results in the absence of surface Ig expression).[178–180] Deregulation of *MYC* associated with transformation into a more aggressive lymphoma has also been observed in small cell and mantle cell lymphomas.[181,182] Indeed, rare immature B cell neoplasms[183] and, at the other end of the spectrum, a significant fraction of plasma cell tumors, may also carry a deregulated *MYC* gene, resulting from either a *MYC–Ig* translocation, or a different mechanism.[184] Interestingly, DLBCLs with a *MYC–Ig* translocation were found by Dave *et al.* [177] to have a mDLBCL rather than mBL expression profile, although such tumors tend to have a much higher frequency of immunoglobulin gene hypervariable region mutations.[185] Whether these tumors might have fallen into the intermediate category of Hummel *et al.* is not known. However, it is clear that the majority of cases of BLL/aBL have a mBL profile, and appear to result from *de novo* lymphomagenesis supporting the clinical impression that these tumors are much closer to BL than to DLBCL – indeed, based on a molecular diagnosis, BLL would appear to represent a histological variant of BL – a variability that can extend to DLBCL. Whether the small fraction of morphological DLBCL with an mBL profile should be identified via, perhaps, a simpler set of molecular parameters, and treated as BL will need to be explored. In children this is not an issue since it is known that DLBCL in this age group, which is predominantly of germinal center phenotype,[186] has an excellent outcome when treated identically to BL. Moreover, since the more indolent lymphomas are very unusual in children and 14;18 translocations have not been identified in childhood DLBCL,[187] it is probable that the intermediate molecular profile will be correspondingly infrequent in this age group. It would be interesting, however, to determine the fraction of childhood DLBCLs that have a mBL profile.

Gene expression profiling has also provided additional evidence for the phenotypic resemblance of sporadic EBV-negative BL to germinal center cells. In lymphomas with characteristic DLBCL morphology there are several molecularly defined subtypes. In addition to mediastinal B cell lymphoma, the two major subdivisions have profiles resembling either germinal center cells or activated lymphocytes.[188,189] Both mBL and lymphomas with intermediate gene expression profiles express the signature genes of germinal center cells, whereas this is true of only approximately a third of molecularly defined DLBCL in adults.[97] However, clear differences in the pattern of expression of four subsets of signature genes in mBL versus mDLBCL of germinal center type have been identified by Dave *et al.*;[177] mBL expressed both MYC target genes and a subset of genes expressed in normal germinal centre cells at a higher level, while MHC class I genes and nuclear factor κB (NF-κB) target genes were expressed at lower levels. The higher expression of a subset of germinal center cell genes is consistent with the suggestion, based on the low frequency of somatic hypervariable region mutations, that sporadic BL is the neoplastic counterpart of an early germinal center cell, but could also relate to an origin from specific types of lymphoid tissue (e.g. MALT in the case of BL).

It remains to study the gene expression profiles of African BL and EBV-positive sporadic BL, as well as AIDS-related BL. It may also prove possible to identify sets of genes that are associated with the morphology of typical BL and DLBCL, respectively. Such a finding would provide further insights into the classification aggressive B cell lymphomas that phenotypically resemble germinal center cells, and could lead to a greater understanding of the immunobiology of the germinal center itself. It could also have implications for the role of morphology in diagnosis and treatment.

KEY POINTS

- Burkitt lymphoma (BL) was first recognized as a clinical syndrome and pathological entity some 50 years ago in Kampala, Uganda
- Its geographical distribution in Africa is similar to that of arthropods, giving rise to the hypothesis that BL is caused by a vectored virus. This led directly to the discover of Epstein–Barr virus (EBV), associated with more than 50 percent of BL cases worldwide, and several other diseases, but EBV is not insect vectored.
- Infection in infancy with both malaria and EBV appear to markedly predispose to BL, but the primary molecular lesion is one of several translocations (or even other molecular abnormalities) that lead to deregulation of the *MYC* gene, which controls many important

cellular pathways. Absence of malaria and early EBV infection is associated with a low incidence of BL, more often EBV negative.

- Although it is possible that some of the translocations occur in immature B lymphoid cells, passage through the lymphoid germinal center may be a requirement for the development of BL – and also for entry of EBV into the memory B cell population, where it persists for life. This may relate to the protection of germinal follicle cells from apoptosis during somatic hypervariable region mutation of immunoglobulins as antibodies refine their ability to bind to a specific antigen. This environment would be conducive to the persistence of cells bearing translocations and mutations, making oncogenesis more likely.
- The polyclonal activation of B cells by malaria, which increases the number of circulating EBV-containing cells may also predispose to the translocations (or their persistence) that are critical to the genesis of BL.
- The classical histopathological appearance of BL is distinctive; the medium sized cells have a high nuclear to cytoplasmic ratio, fenestrated nuclear reticulin, 2–5 prominent nucleoli and vacuolated basophilic cytoplasm.
- Although most cases of BL are histologically characteristic, an identical molecular profile can be seen in almost all BL-like/atypical BL with morphology intermediate between BL and diffuse large B cell lympoma (DLBCL) and a fraction of DLBCL, suggesting that true BL may occur throughout the morphological spectrum from BL through BL-like to DLBCL This may be important in determining optimal therapy.

REFERENCES

● = Key primary paper
◆ = Major review article

1. Smith EC, Elmes BGT. Malignant disease in natives of Nigeria. *Ann Trop Med Parasitol* 1934; **28**: 461–512.
2. Davies JNP. Reticuloendothelial tumours. *East Afr Med J* 1948; **25**: 117.
3. Edington GM. Malignant disease in the Gold Coast. *Br J Cancer* 1956; **10**: 41–54.
4. Thijs A. Considérations sur les tumeurs malignes des indigénes du Congo belge et du Ruanda-Urundi. A propos de 2,536 cas. *Ann Soc Belg Med Trop* 1957; **37**: 483–514.
5. De Smet MP. Observations cliniques de tumeurs malignes des tissus réticuloendothéliaux et des tissus hémolymphopoiétiques au Congo. *Ann Soc Belg Med Trop* 1956; **36**: 53–70.
●6. Burkitt D. A sarcoma involving the jaws in African children. *Br J Surg* 1958; **46**: 218–23.
7. O'Conor GT, Davies JNP. Malignant tumors in African children with special reference to malignant lymphomas. *J Pediatr* 1960; **56**: 526–35.
●8. O'Conor G. Malignant lymphoma in African children. Cancer II. A pathological entity. *Cancer* 1961; **14**: 270–83.
●9. Burkitt D. Determining the climatic limitations of a children's cancer common in Africa. *Br Med J* 1962; **ii**: 1019–26.
10. Booth K, Burkitt DP, Bassett DJ *et al*. Burkitt lymphoma in Papua, New Guinea. *Br J Cancer* 1967; **21**: 657–64.
11. Haddow AJ. An improved map for the study of Burkitt's lymphoma syndrome in Africa. *East Afr Med J* 1963; **40**: 429–32.
●12. Epstein MA, Achong BG, Barr YM. Viral particles in cultured lymphoblasts from Burkitt's lymphoma. *Lancet* 1964; **i**: 702–3.
●13. Henle G, Henle W. Immunofluorescence in cells derived from Burkitt's lymphoma. *J Bacteriol* 1966; **91**: 1248–56.
14. Henle G, Henle W, Clifford P *et al*. Antibodies to EB virus in Burkitt's lymphoma and control groups. *J Natl Cancer Inst* 1969; **43**: 1147–57.
●15. Sumaya CV, Henle W, Henle G *et al*. Seroepidemiologic study of Epstein–Barr virus infections in a rural community. *J Infect Dis* 1975; **131**: 403–8.
16. Diehl V, Henle G, Henle W, Kohn G. Demonstration of a herpes group virus in cultures of peripheral leukocytes from patients with infectious mononucleosis. *J Virol* 1968; **2**: 663–9.
17. Niederman JC, Miller G, Pearson HA *et al*. Infectious mononucleosis. Epstein-Barr-virus shedding in saliva and the oropharynx. *N Engl J Med* 1976; **294**: 1355–9.
18. de-Thé G. Epstein-Barr virus behavior in different populations and implications for control of Epstein-Barr virus-associated tumors. *Cancer Res* 1976; **36**: 692–5.
19. Karajannis MA, Hummel M, Oschlies I *et al*. A Epstein-Barr virus infection in Western European pediatric non-Hodgkin lymphomas. *Blood* 2003; **102**: 4244.
20. Klumb CE, Hassan R, De Oliveira DE *et al*. Geographic variation in Epstein-Barr virus-associated Burkitt's lymphoma in children from Brazil. *Int J Cancer* 2004; **108**: 66.
21. Figueira-Silva CM, Pereira FE. Prevalence of Epstein-Barr virus antibodies in healthy children and adolescents in Vitoria, State of Espirito Santo, Brazil. *Rev Soc Bras Med Trop* 2004; **37**: 409–12.
●22. Zech L, Haglund U, Nilsson K *et al*. Characteristic chromosomal abnormalities in biopsies and lymphoid-cell lines from patients with Burkitt and non-Burkitt lymphomas. *Int J Cancer* 1976; **17**: 47.

●23.   Taub R, Kirsch I, Morton C *et al.* Translocation of the c-myc gene into the immunoglobulin heavy chain locus in human Burkitt lymphoma and murine plasmacytoma cells. *Proc Natl Acad Sci U S A* 1982; **79**: 7837.

●24.   Dalla-Favera R, Bregni M, Erikson J *et al.* Human c-myc onc gene is located on the region of chromosome 8 that is translocated in Burkitt lymphoma cells. *Proc Natl Acad Sci U S A* 1982; **79**: 7824.

●25.   Bernheim A, Berger R, Lenoir G. Cytogenetic studies on African Burkitt's lymphoma cell lines; t(8;14), t(2;8) and t(8;22) translocations. *Cancer Genet Cytogenet* 1981; **3**: 307–15.

●26.   Dalldorf G, Linsell CA, Marnhart FE, Martyn R. An epidemiological approach to the lymphomas of African children and Burkitt's sarcoma of the jaws. *Perspect Biol Med* 1964; **7**: 435–49.

27.   Osunkoya BO, McFarlane H, Luzzatto L *et al.* Immunoglobin synthesis by fresh biopsy cells and established cell lines from Burkitt's lymphoma. *Immunology* 1968; **14**: 851–60.

28.   Daniel-Ribeiro C, de Oliveira-Ferreira J, Banic DM, Galvao-Castro B. Can malaria-associated polyclonal B-lymphocyte activation interfere with the development of anti-sporozoite specific immunity? *Trans R Soc Trop Med Hyg* 1989; **83**: 289–92.

29.   Childhood cancer. In: Parkin DM, Ferlay J, Hamdi-Cherif M *et al.* (eds) *Cancer in Africa. Epidemiology and prevention.* IARC Scientific Publications No. 153. France: Lyon, IARC Press, 2003: 381–96.

30.   Burchenal JH. Burkitt's tumor as a stalking horse for leukemia. *JAMA* 1972; **222**: 1165.

31.   Donati D, Espmark E, Kironde F *et al.* Clearance of circulating Epstein-Barr virus DNA in children with acute malaria after antimalaria treatment. *J Infect Dis* 2006; **193**: 971–7.

32.   Gardiner CN, Biggar RJ, Collins W, Nkrumah F. Malaria in urban and rural areas of southern Ghana: a survey of parasitaemia and of anti-malarial practice. *J Trop Pediatr* 1984; **30**: 296–9.

●33.   Morrow RJ, Kisuule A, Pike MC, Smith PG. Burkitt's lymphoma in the Mengo districts of Uganda: epidemiologic features and their relationship to malaria. *J Natl Cancer Inst* 1976; **56**: 479–83.

●34.   Matola YG, Mwita U, Masoud AE. Malaria in the islands of Zanzibar and Pemba 11 years after the suspension of a malaria eradication programme. *Cent Afr J Med* 1984; **30**: 91–2, 95–6.

35.   Morrow RH Jr. Epidemiological evidence for the role of falciparum malaria in the pathogenesis of Burkitt's lymphoma. *IARC Sci Publ* 1985; **60**: 177–86.

●36.   Geser A, Brubaker G, Draper CC. Effect of a malaria suppression program on the incidence of African Burkitt's lymphoma. *Am J Epidemiol* 1989; **129**: 740–52.

37.   Wedderburn N. Effect of concurrent malarial infection on development of virus-induced lymphoma in Balb-c mice. *Lancet* 1970; **ii**: 1114–6.

38.   Baird SM, Beattie GM, Lannom RA *et al.* Induction of lymphoma in antigenically stimulated athymic mice. *Cancer Res* 1982; **42**: 198–206.

39.   Gutierrez MI, Judde JG, Magrath IT, Bhatia KG. Switching viral latency to viral lysis: a novel therapeutic approach for Epstein-Barr virus-associated neoplasia. *Cancer Res* 1996; **56**: 969–72.

40.   Gutierrez MI, Bhatia K, Magrath I. Replicative viral DNA in Epstein-Barr virus associated Burkitt's lymphoma biopsies. *Leuk Res* 1993; **17**: 285–9.

41.   Fujita S, Buziba N, Kumatori A, Senba M *et al.* Early stage of Epstein-Barr virus lytic infection leading to the 'starry sky' pattern formation in endemic Burkitt lymphoma. *Arch Pathol Lab Med* 2004; **128**: 549–52.

42.   Feng WH, Hong G, Delecluse HJ, Kenney SC. Lytic induction therapy for Epstein-Barr virus-positive B-cell lymphomas. *J Virol* 2004; **78**: 1893–902.

●43.   Pope JH, Home MK, Scott W. Transformation of foetal human leukocytes *in vitro* by filtrates of a human leukemia cell line containing herpes-like virus. *Int J Cancer* 1968; **3**: 857–66.

●44.   Joseph AM, Babcock GJ, Thorley-Lawson DA. Cells expressing the Epstein-Barr virus growth program are present in and restricted to the naive B-cell subset of healthy tonsils. *J Virol* 2000; **74**: 9964–71.

●45.   Souza TA, Stollar BD, Sullivan JL *et al.* Peripheral B cells latently infected with Epstein-Barr virus display molecular hallmarks of classical antigen-selected memory B cells. *Proc Natl Acad Sci U S A* 2005; **102**: 18093–8.

●46.   Kurth J, Hansmann ML, Rajewsky K, Kuppers R. Epstein-Barr virus-infected B cells expanding in germinal centers of infectious mononucleosis patients do not participate in the germinal center reaction. *Proc Natl Acad Sci U S A* 2003; **100**: 4730–5.

●47.   Tobollik S, Meyer L, Buettner M *et al.* Epstein-Barr-virus nuclear antigen 2 inhibits AID expression during EBV-driven B cell growth. *Blood* 2006; **108**: 3859–64.

48.   Hislop AD, Annels NE, Gudgeon NH *et al.* Epitope-specific evolution of human CD8(+) T cell responses from primary to persistent phases of Epstein-Barr virus infection. *J Exp Med* 2002; **195**: 893–905.

●49.   Babcock GJ, Thorley-Lawson DA. Tonsillar memory B cells, latently infected with Epstein-Barr virus, express the restricted pattern of latent genes previously found only in Epstein-Barr virus-associated tumors. *Proc Natl Acad Sci U S A* 2000; **97**: 12250–5.

◆50.   Thorley-Lawson DA, Allday MJ. The curious case of the tumor virus: 50 years of Burkitt's lymphoma. *Nat Rev Microbiol* 2008; **12**: 913–24.

●51.   Hochberg D, Middeldorp JM, Catalina M *et al.* Demonstration of the Burkitt's lymphoma Epstein-Barr virus phenotype in dividing latently infected memory cells *in vivo. Proc Natl Acad Sci U S A* 2004; **101**: 239–44.

52. Tao Q, Robertson KD, Manns A *et al.* Epstein-Barr virus (EBV) in endemic Burkitt's lymphoma: molecular analysis of primary tumor tissue. *Blood* 1998; **91**:1373–81.

●53. Chen F, Zou JZ, di Renzo L *et al.* A subpopulation of normal B cells latently infected with Epstein-Barr virus resembles Burkitt lymphoma cells in expressing EBNA-1 but not EBNA-2 or LMP1. *J Virol* 1995; **69**: 3752–8.

◆54. Magrath IT. The pathogenesis of Burkitt's lymphoma. In: Klein G, Van de Woude G. (eds) *Adv Cancer Res* 1990; **55**: 133–270.

55. Cai X, Schafer A, Lu S *et al.* Epstein-Barr virus microRNAs are evolutionarily conserved and differentially expressed. *PLoS Pathog* 2006; **2**: 236–47.

56. Laichalk LL, Thorley-Lawson DA. Terminal differentiation into plasma cells initiates the replicative cycle of Epstein-Barr virus *in vivo. J Virol* 2005; **79**: 1296–307.

57. Pegtel DM, Middeldorp J, Thorley-Lawson DA. Epstein-Barr virus infection in ex vivo tonsil epithelial cell cultures of asymptomatic carriers. *J Virol* 2004; **78**: 12613–24.

58. Laichalk LL, Hochberg D, Babcock GJ *et al.* The dispersal of mucosal memory B cells: evidence from persistent EBV infection. *Immunity* 2002; **16**: 745–54.

●59. Hislop AD, Kuo M, Drake-Lee AB *et al.* Tonsillar homing of Epstein-Barr virus-specific CD8+ T cells and the virus-host balance. *J Clin Invest* 2005; **115**: 2546–55.

◆60. Magrath IT. African Burkitt's lymphoma. History, biology, clinical features, and treatment. *Am J Pediatr Hematol Oncol* 1991; **13**: 222–46.

61. Levitskaya J, Sharipo A, Leonchiks A *et al.* Inhibition of ubiquitin/proteasome-dependent protein degradation by the Gly-Ala repeat domain of the Epstein-Barr virus nuclear antigen 1. *Proc Natl Acad Sci U S A* 1997; **94**: 12616–21.

●62. Rowe M, Khanna R, Jacob CA *et al.* Restoration of endogenous antigen processing in Burkitt's lymphoma cells by Epstein-Barr virus latent membrane protein-1: coordinate up-regulation of peptide transporters and HLA-class I antigen expression. *Eur J Immunol* 1995; **25**: 1374–84.

●63. Moorman AM, Heller KN, Chelimo K *et al.* Children with endemic Burkitt lymphoma are deficient in EBNA1-specific IFN-gamma T cell responses. *Int J Cancer* 2003; **124**: 1721–6.

●64. Khanna R, Cooper L, Kienzle N *et al.* Engagement of CD40 antigen with soluble CD40 ligand up-regulates peptide transporter expression and restores endogenous processing function in Burkitt's lymphoma cells. *J Immunol* 1997; **159**: 5782–5.

●65. Staege MS, Lee SP, Frisan T *et al.* MYC overexpression imposes a nonimmunogenic phenotype on Epstein-Barr virus-infected B cells. *Proc Natl Acad Sci U S A* 2002; **99**: 4550–5.

●66. Wilson JB, Bell JL, Levine AJ. Expression of Epstein-Barr virus nuclear antigen-1 induces B cell neoplasia in transgenic mice. *EMBO J* 1996; **15**: 3117–26.

●67. Drotar ME, Silva S, Barone E *et al.* Epstein-Barr virus nuclear antigen-1 and Myc cooperate in lymphomagenesis. *Int J Cancer* 2003; **106**: 388–95.

●68. Pajic A, Staege MS, Dudziak D *et al.* Antagonistic effects of c-myc and Epstein-Barr virus latent genes on the phenotype of human B cells. *Int J Cancer* 2001; **93**: 810–16.

69. Gutierrez MI, Bhatia K, Cherney B *et al.* Intraclonal molecular heterogeneity suggests a hierarchy of pathogenetic events in Burkitt's lymphoma. *Ann Oncol* 1997; **8**: 987–94.

●70. Tsimbouri P, Drotar ME, Coy JL, Wilson JB. bcl-xL and RAG genes are induced and the response to IL-2 enhanced in EmuEBNA-1 transgenic mouse lymphocytes. *Oncogene* 2002; **21**: 5182–7.

71. Ruf IK, Rhyne PW, Yang H *et al.* Epstein-Barr virus regulates c-MYC, apoptosis, and tumorigenicity in Burkitt lymphoma. *Mol Cell Biol* 1999; **19**: 1651–60.

72. Kennedy G, Komano J, Sugden B. Epstein-Barr virus provides a survival factor to Burkitt's lymphomas. *Proc Natl Acad Sci U S A* 2003; **100**: 14269–74.

73. Hammerschmidt W, Sugden B. Epstein-Barr virus sustains Burkitt's lymphomas and Hodgkin's disease. *Trends Mol Med* 2004; **10**: 331–6.

●74. Hong M, Murai Y, Kutsuna T *et al.* Suppression of Epstein-Barr nuclear antigen 1 (EBNA1) by RNA interference inhibits proliferation of EBV-positive Burkitt's lymphoma cells. *J Cancer Res Clin Oncol* 2006; **132**: 1–8.

75. Nanbo A, Inoue K, Adachi-Takasawa K, Takada K. Epstein-Barr virus RNA confers resistance to interferon-alpha-induced apoptosis in Burkitt's lymphoma. *EMBO J* 2002; **21**: 954–65.

●76. Kelly GL, Milner AE, Baldwin GS *et al.* Three restricted forms of Epstein-Barr virus latency counteracting apoptosis in c-myc-expressing Burkitt lymphoma cells. *Proc Natl Acad Sci U S A* 2006; **103**: 14935–40.

●77. Nanbo A, Takada K. The role of Epstein-Barr virus-encoded small RNAs (EBERs) in oncogenesis. *Rev Med Virol* 2002; **12**: 321–6.

78. Ruf IK, Rhyne PW, Yang C *et al.* Epstein-Barr virus small RNAs potentiate tumorigenicity of Burkitt lymphoma cells independently of an effect on apoptosis. *J Virol* 2000; **74**: 10223–8.

79. Wallace LE, Young LS, Rowe M *et al.* Epstein-Barr virus-specific T-cell recognition of B-cell transformants expressing different EBNA 2 antigens. *Int J Cancer* 1987; **39**: 373–9.

80. Rowe M, Young LS, Cadwallader K *et al.* Distinction between Epstein-Barr virus type A (EBNA 2A) and type B (EBNA 2B) isolates extends to the EBNA 3

family of nuclear proteins. *J Virol* 1989; **63**: 1031–9.

81. Sample J, Young L, Martin B *et al.* Epstein-Barr virus types 1 and 2 differ in their EBNA-3A, EBNA-3B, and EBNA-3C genes. *J Virol* 1990; **64**: 4084–92.

82. Kim SM, Kang SH, Lee WK. Identification of two types of naturally-occurring intertypic recombinants of Epstein-Barr virus. *Mol Cells* 2006; **21**: 302–7.

●83. Rickinson AB, Young LS, Rowe M. Influence of the Epstein-Barr virus nuclear antigen EBNA 2 on the growth phenotype of virus-transformed B cells. *J Virol* 1987; **61**: 1310–17.

84. Young LS, Yao QY, Rooney CM *et al.* New type B isolates of Epstein-Barr virus from Burkitt's lymphoma and from normal individuals in endemic areas. *J Gen Virol* 1987; **68**: 2853–62.

85. Tacyildiz N, Cavdar AO, Ertem U *et al.* Unusually high frequency of a 69-bp deletion within the carboxy terminus of the LMP-1 oncogene of Epstein-Barr virus detected in Burkitt's lymphoma of Turkish children. *Leukemia* 1998; **12**: 1796–805.

86. Chen WG, Chen YY, Bacchi MM *et al.* Genotyping of Epstein-Barr virus in Brazilian Burkitt's lymphoma and reactive lymphoid tissue. Type A with a high prevalence of deletions within the latent membrane protein gene. *Am J Pathol* 1996; **148**: 17–23.

87. Mansoor A, Stevenson MS, Li RZ *et al.* Prevalence of Epstein-Barr viral sequences and EBV LMP1 oncogene deletions in Burkitt's lymphoma from Pakistan: epidemiological correlations. *Hum Pathol* 1997; **28**: 283–8.

88. Gutierrez MI, Ibrahim MM, Dale JK *et al.* Discrete alterations in the BZLF1 promoter in tumor and non-tumor-associated Epstein-Barr virus. *J Natl Cancer Inst* 2002; **94**: 1757–63.

89. Goldschmidts WL, Bhatia K, Johnson JF *et al.* Epstein-Barr virus genotypes in AIDS-associated lymphomas are similar to those in endemic Burkitt's lymphomas. *Leukemia* 1992; **6**: 875–8.

●90. Gutierrez MI, Raj A, Spangler G *et al.* Sequence variations in EBNA-1 may dictate restriction of tissue distribution of Epstein-Barr virus in normal and tumour cells. *J Gen Virol* 1997; **78**: 1663–70.

91. MacKenzie J, Gray D, Pinto-Paes R *et al.* Analysis of Epstein-Barr virus (EBV) nuclear antigen 1 subtypes in EBV-associated lymphomas from Brazil and the United Kingdom. *J Gen Virol* 1999; **80**: 2741–5.

92. Habeshaw G, Yao QY, Bell AI *et al.* Epstein-Barr virus nuclear antigen 1 sequences in endemic and sporadic Burkitt's lymphoma reflect virus strains prevalent in different geographic areas. *J Virol* 1999; **73**: 965–75.

●93. MacKenzie J, Gray D, Pinto-Paes R *et al.* Analysis of Epstein-Barr virus (EBV) nuclear antigen 1 subtypes in EBV-associated lymphomas from Brazil and the United Kingdom. *J Gen Virol* 1999; **80**: 2741–5.

94. Zhang XS, Wang HH, Hu LF *et al.* V-val subtype of Epstein-Barr virus nuclear antigen 1 preferentially exists

in biopsies of nasopharyngeal carcinoma. *Cancer Lett* 2004; **211**: 11–18.

95. Wang WY, Chien YC, Jan JS *et al.* Consistent sequence variation of Epstein-Barr virus nuclear antigen 1 in primary tumor and peripheral blood cells of patients with nasopharyngeal carcinoma. *Clin Cancer Res* 2002; **8**: 2586–90.

96. Haralambieva E, Schuuring E, Rosati S *et al.* Interphase fluorescence *in situ* hybridization for detection of 8q24/MYC breakpoints on routine histologic sections: validation in Burkitt lymphomas from three geographic regions. *Genes Chromosomes Cancer* 2004; **40**: 10–18.

●97. Hummel M, Bentink S, Berger H *et al.* Molecular mechanisms in malignant lymphomas network project of the Deutsche Krebshilfe. A biologic definition of Burkitt's lymphoma from transcriptional and genomic profiling. *N Engl J Med* 2006; **354**: 2419–30.

98. Zivkovic T, Chudoba I, Bokemeyer C, Dierlamm J. Multicolour banding provides a detailed characterisation of structural abnormalities of chromosome 1 in Burkitt lymphoma. *Br J Haematol* 2006; **132**: 2.

99. Polito P, Cilia AM, Gloghini A *et al.* High frequency of EBV association with non-random abnormalities of the chromosome region 1q21–25 in AIDS-related Burkitt's lymphoma-derived cell lines. *Int J Cancer* 1995; **61**: 370–4.

100. Garcia JL, Hernandez JM, Gutierrez NC *et al.* Abnormalities on 1q and 7q are associated with poor outcome in sporadic Burkitt's lymphoma. A cytogenetic and comparative genomic hybridization study. *Leukemia* 2003; **17**: 2016–24.

101. Haluska FG, Finver S, Tsujimoto Y, Croce CM. The t(8;14) chromosomal translocation occurring in B-cell malignancies results from mistakes in V-D-J joining. *Nature* 1986; **324**: 158–61.

102. Haluska FG, Tsujimoto Y, Croce CM. The t(8;14) chromosome translocation of the Burkitt lymphoma cell line Daudi occurred during immunoglobulin gene rearrangement and involved the heavy chain diversity region. *Proc Natl Acad Sci U S A* 1987; **84**: 6835–9.

103. Hartl P, Lipp M. Generation of a variant t(2;8) translocation of Burkitt's lymphoma by site-specific recombination via the kappa light-chain joining signals. *Mol Cell Biol* 1987; **7**: 2037–45.

●104. Neri A, Barriga F, Knowles DM *et al.* Different regions of the immunoglobulin heavy-chain locus are involved in chromosomal translocations in distinct pathogenetic forms of Burkitt lymphoma. *Proc Natl Acad Sci U S A* 1988; **85**: 2748–52.

●105. Gutierrez MI, Bhatia K, Barriga F *et al.* Molecular epidemiology of Burkitt's lymphoma from South America: differences in breakpoint location and Epstein-Barr virus association from tumors in other world regions. *Blood* 1992; **79**: 3261–6.

●106. Kuhn-Hallek I, Sage DR, Stein L *et al.* Expression of recombination activating genes (RAG-1 and RAG-2) in

Epstein-Barr virus-bearing B cells. *Blood* 1995; **85**: 1289–99.

●107. Epeldegui M, Hung YP, McQuay A *et al*. Infection of human B cells with Epstein-Barr virus results in the expression of somatic hypermutation-inducing molecules and in the accrual of oncogene mutations. *Mol Immunol* 2007; **44**: 934–42.

108. Altiok E, Klein G, Zech L *et al*. Epstein-Barr virus-transformed pro-B cells are prone to illegitimate recombination between the switch region of the mu chain gene and other chromosomes. *Proc Natl Acad Sci U S A* 1989; **86**: 6333–7.

●109. Guikema JE, de Boer C, Haralambieva E *et al*. IGH switch breakpoints in Burkitt lymphoma: exclusive involvement of noncanonical class switch recombination. *Genes Chromosomes Cancer* 2006; **45**: 808–19.

110. Nagaoka J H, Gonzalez-Aseguinolaza G *et al*. Immunization and infection change the number of recombination activating gene (RAG)-expressing B cells in the periphery by altering immature lymphocyte production. *Adv Exp Med Biol* 2000; **191**: 2113–20.

111. Davila M, Foster S, Kelsoe G, Yang K. A role for secondary V(D)J recombination in oncogenic chromosomal translocations? *Adv Cancer Res* 2001; **81**: 61–92.

◆112. Hecht JL, Aster JC. Molecular biology of Burkitt's lymphoma. *J Clin Oncol* 2000; **18**: 3707–21.

113. Boxer LM, Dang CV. Translocations involving c-myc and c-myc function. *Oncogene* 2001; **20**: 5595–610.

●114. Janz S. Myc translocations in B cell and plasma cell neoplasms. *DNA Repair (Amst)* 2006; **5**: 1213–24.

●115. Cowling VH, Cole MD. Mechanism of transcriptional activation by the Myc oncoproteins. *Semin Cancer Biol* 2006; **16**: 242–52.

◆116. Dang CV, O'Donnell KA, Zeller KI *et al*. The c-Myc target gene network. *Semin Cancer Biol* 2006; **16**: 253–64.

117. Li Z, Van Calcar S, Qu C *et al*. A global transcriptional regulatory role for c-Myc in Burkitt's lymphoma cells. *Proc Natl Acad Sci U S A* 2003; **100**: 8164–9.

●118. Egle A, Harris A, Bouillet P, Cory S. Bim is a suppressor of Myc-induced mouse B-cell leukemia. *PNAS* 2004; **101**: 6164–9.

119. Kovalchuk AL, Qi CF, Torrey TA *et al*. Burkitt lymphoma in the mouse. *J Exp Med* 2000; **192**: 1183–90.

120. Park SS, Kim JS, Tessarollo L *et al*. Insertion of c-Myc into Igh induces B-cell and plasma-cell neoplasms in mice. *Cancer Res* 2005; **65**: 1306–15.

◆121. Arvanitis C, Felsher DW. Conditional transgenic models define how MYC initiates and maintains tumorigenesis. *Semin Cancer Biol* 2006; **16**: 313–17.

122. Klein U, Dalla-Favera R. Germinal centres: role of B-cell physiology and malignancy. *Nat Rev Immunol* 2008; **8**: 22–33.

123. McManaway ME, Neckers LM, Loke SL *et al*. Tumour-specific inhibition of lymphoma growth by an antisense oligodeoxynucleotide. *Lancet* 1990; **335**: 808–11.

124. Williams SA, Gillan ER, Knoppel E *et al*. Effects of phosphodiester and phosphorothioate antisense oligodeoxynucleotides on cell lines which overexpress c-myc: implications for the treatment of Burkitt's lymphoma. *Ann Oncol* 1997; **8(Suppl 1)**: 25–30.

●125. Arasi VE, Lieberman R, Sandlund J *et al*. Antiimmunoglobulin inhibition of Burkitt's lymphoma cell proliferation and concurrent reduction of c-myc and mu heavy chain gene expression. *Cancer Res* 1989; **49**: 3235–41.

●126. Cutrona G, Carpaneto EM, Ponzanelli A *et al*. Inhibition of the translocated *c-myc* in Burkitt's lymphoma by a PNA complementary to the $E\mu$ enhancer. *Cancer Research* 2003; **63**: 6144–8.

●127. Polack A, Hortnagel K, Pajic A *et al*. c-myc activation renders proliferation of Epstein-Barr virus (EBV)-transformed cells independent of EBV nuclear antigen 2 and latent membrane protein 1. *Proc Natl Acad Sci U S A* 1996; **93**: 10411–16.

●128. Jochner N, Eick D, Zimber-Strobl U *et al*. Epstein-Barr virus nuclear antigen 2 is a transcriptional suppressor of the immunoglobulin mu gene: implications for the expression of the translocated c-myc gene in Burkitt's lymphoma cells. *EMBO J* 1996; **15**: 375–82.

129. Schlee M, Krug T, Gires O *et al*. Identification of Epstein-Barr virus (EBV) nuclear antigen 2 (EBNA-2) target proteins by proteome analysis: activation of EBNA-2 in conditionally immortalized B cells reflects early events after infection of primary B cells by EBV. *J Virol* 2004; **78**: 3941–52.

130. Knox KA, Finney M, Milner AE *et al*. Second-messenger pathways involved in the regulation of survival in germinal-centre B cells and in Burkitt lymphoma lines. *Int J Cancer* 1992; **52**: 959–66.

131. Takada K. Cross-linking of cell surface immunoglobulins induces Epstein-Barr virus in Burkitt lymphoma lines. *Int J Cancer* 1984; **33**: 27–32.

132. Chapman CJ, Wright D, Stevenson FK. Insight into Burkitt's lymphoma from immunoglobulin variable region gene analysis. *Leuk Lymphoma* 1998; **30(3–4)**: 257–67.

●133. Isobe K, Tamaru J, Nakamura S *et al*. VH gene analysis in sporadic Burkitt's lymphoma: somatic mutation and intraclonal diversity with special reference to the tumor cells involving germinal center. *Leuk Lymphoma* 2002; **43**: 159–64.

●134. Bellan C, Lazzi S, Hummel M *et al*. Immunoglobulin gene analysis reveals 2 distinct cells of origin for EBV-positive and EBV-negative Burkitt lymphomas. *Blood* 2005; **106**: 1031–6.

135. Tamaru J, Hummel M, Marafioti T *et al*. Burkitt's lymphomas express VH genes with a moderate number of antigen-selected somatic mutations. *Am J Pathol* 1995; **147**: 1398–407.

●136. Wilda M, Busch K, Klose I et al. Level of MYC overexpression in pediatric Burkitt's lymphoma is strongly dependent on genomic breakpoint location within the MYC locus. Genes Chromosomes Cancer 2004; 41: 178–82.

●137. Joos S, Falk MH, Lichter P et al. Variable breakpoints in Burkitt lymphoma cells with chromosomal t(8;14) translocation separate c-myc and the IgH locus up to several hundred kb. Hum Mol Genet 1992; 1: 625–32.

138. Jain VK, Judde JG, Max EE, Magrath IT. Variable IgH chain enhancer activity in Burkitt's lymphomas suggests an additional, direct mechanism of c-myc deregulation. J Immunol 1993; 150: 5418–28.

139. Raschke EE, Albert T, Eick D. Transcriptional regulation of the Ig kappa gene by promoter-proximal pausing of RNA polymerase II. J Immunol 1999; 163: 4375–82.

140. Wittekindt NE, Hortnagel K, Geltinger C, Polack A. Activation of c-myc promoter P1 by immunoglobulin kappa gene enhancers in Burkitt lymphoma: functional characterization of the intron enhancer motifs kappaB, E box 1 and E box 2, and of the 3' enhancer motif PU. Nucleic Acids Res 2000; 28: 800–8.

141. Hu HM, Arcinas M, Boxer LM. A Myc-associated zinc finger protein-related factor binding site is required for the deregulation of c-myc expression by the immunoglobulin heavy chain gene enhancers in Burkitt's lymphoma. J Biol Chem 2002; 277: 9819–24.

142. Ratsch A, Joos S, Kioschis P, Lichter P. Topological organization of the MYC/IGK locus in Burkitt's lymphoma cells assessed by nuclear halo preparations. Exp Cell Res 2002; 273: 12–20.

●143. Bhatia K, Huppi K, Spangler G et al. Point mutations in the c-Myc transactivation domain are common in Burkitt's lymphoma and mouse plasmacytomas. Nat Genet 1993; 5: 56–61.

●◆144. Bhatia K, Spangler G, Hamdy N, Magrath I. Mutations in the coding region of c-myc occur independently of mutations in the regulatory regions and are predominantly associated with myc/Ig translocation. Curr Top Microbiol Immunol 1995; 194: 389–98.

145. Bemark M, Neuberger MS. The c-MYC allele that is translocated into the IgH locus undergoes constitutive hypermutation in a Burkitt's lymphoma line. Oncogene 2000; 19: 3404–10.

146. Gaidano G, Pasqualucci L, Capello D et al. Aberrant somatic hypermutation in multiple subtypes of AIDS-associated non-Hodgkin lymphoma. Blood 2003; 102: 1833–41.

●147. Gu W, Bhatia K, Magrath IT et al. Binding and suppression of the Myc transcriptional activation domain by p107. Science 1994; 264: 251–4.

●148. Hemann MT, Bric A, Teruya-Feldstein J et al. Evasion of the p53 tumour surveillance network by tumour-derived MYC mutants. Nature 2005; 436: 807–11.

◆149. Dang CV, O'Donnell KA, Juopperi T. The great MYC escape in tumorigenesis. Cancer Cell 2005; 8: 177–8.

150. Eischen CM, Roussel MF, Korsmeyer SJ, Cleveland JL. Bax loss impairs Myc-induced apoptosis and circumvents the selection of p53 mutations during Myc-mediated lymphomagenesis. Mol Cell Biol 2001; 21: 7653–62.

●151. Gregory MA, Hann SR. c-Myc proteolysis by the ubiquitin-proteasome pathway: stabilization of c-Myc in Burkitt's lymphoma cells. Mol Cell Biol 2000; 20: 2423–35.

●152. Cherney BW, Bhatia KG, Sgadari C et al. Role of the p53 tumor suppressor gene in the tumorigenicity of Burkitt's lymphoma cells. Cancer Res 1997; 57: 2508–15.

153. Wiman KG, Magnusson KP, Ramqvist T, Klein G. Mutant p53 detected in a majority of Burkitt lymphoma cell lines by monoclonal antibody PAb240. Oncogene 1991; 6: 1633–9.

●154. Lindstrom MS, Klangby U, Wiman KG. p14ARF homozygous deletion or MDM2 overexpression in Burkitt lymphoma lines carrying wild type p53. Oncogene 2001; 20: 2171–7.

●155. Wilda M, Bruch J, Harder L et al. Inactivation of the ARF-MDM-2-p53 pathway in sporadic Burkitt's lymphoma in children. Leukemia 2004; 18: 584–8.

156. Ramqvist T, Magnusson KP, Wang Y et al. Wild-type p53 induces apoptosis in a Burkitt lymphoma (BL) line that carries mutant p53. Oncogene 1993; 8: 1495–500.

157. Gutierrez MI, Cherney B, Hussain A et al. Bax is frequently compromised in Burkitt's lymphomas with irreversible resistance to Fas-induced apoptosis. Cancer Res 1999; 59: 696–703.

158. Doucet JP, Hussain A, Al-Rasheed M et al. Differences in the expression of apoptotic proteins in Burkitt's lymphoma cell lines: potential models for screening apoptosis-inducing agents. Leuk Lymphoma 2004; 45: 357–62.

◆159. Lindstrom MS, Wiman KG. Role of genetic and epigenetic changes in Burkitt lymphoma. Semin Cancer Biol 2002; 12: 381–7.

160. Corn PG, Kuerbitz SJ, van Noesel MM et al. Transcriptional silencing of the p73 gene in acute lymphoblastic leukemia and Burkitt's lymphoma is associated with 5' CpG island methylation. Cancer Res 1999; 59: 3352–6.

161. Klangby U, Okan I, Magnusson KP et al. p16/INK4a and p15/INK4b gene methylation and absence of p16/INK4a mRNA and protein expression in Burkitt's lymphoma. Blood 1998; 91: 1680–7.

162. Bhatia K, Fan S, Spangler G et al. A mutant p21 cyclin-dependent kinase inhibitor isolated from a Burkitt's lymphoma. Cancer Res 1995; 55: 1431–5.

●163. Capello D, Carbone A, Pastore C et al. Point mutations of the BCL-6 gene in Burkitt's lymphoma. Br J Haematol 1997; 99: 168–70.

●164. Mossafa H, Damotte D, Jenabian A et al. Non-Hodgkin's lymphomas with Burkitt-like cells are associated with c-Myc amplification and poor prognosis. *Leuk Lymphoma* 2006; **47**: 1885–93.

●165. Khaira P, James CD, Leffak M. Amplification of the translocated c-myc genes in three Burkitt lymphoma cell lines. *Gene* 1998; **211**: 101–8.

166. O'Conor G, Rappaport H, Smith EB. Childhood lymphoma resembling Burkitt's tumor in the United States. *Cancer* 1965; **18**; 411–17.

167. Dorfman RF. Childhood lymphosarcoma in St Louis, Missouri, clinically and histologically resembling Burkitt's tumor. *Cancer* 1965; **18**: 418–30.

168. Wright DH. Burkitt's tumour in England. A comparison with childhood lymphosarcoma. *Int J Cancer* 1966; **1**: 503–14.

●169. Berard C, O'Conor GT, Thomas LB, Torloni H. Histopathological definition of Burkitt's tumour. *Bull World Health Organization* 1969; **40**: 601.

170. Magrath IT, Ziegler JL. Bone marrow involvement in Burkitt's lymphoma and its relationship to acute B-cell leukaemia. *Leuk Res* 1980; **4**: 33.

171. Murphy SB, Hustu O. A randomized trial of combined modality therapy of childhood non-Hodgkin's lymphoma. *Cancer* 1980; **45**: 630–7.

●172. Harris N, Jaffe E, Stein H *et al.* A revised European-American classification of lymphoid neoplasms: a proposal from the International Lymphoma Study Group. *Blood* 1994; **84**: 1361–92.

●173. The Non-Hodgkin's Lymphoma Classification Project. A clinical evaluation of the International Lymphoma Study Group classification of non-Hodgkin's lymphoma. *Blood* 1997; **89**: 3909–18.

●174. Jaffe ES, Harris NL, Stein H, Vardiman JW (eds) *World Health Organization classification of tumors: pathology and genetics of tumors of haematopoietic and lymphoid tissues.* Lyon: IARC Press, 2001.

●175. Harris NL, Jaffe ES, Diebold J *et al.* World Health Organization Classification of neoplastic diseases of the hematopoietic and lymphoid tissues: report of the clinical advisory committee meeting – Airlie House, Virginia, November 1997. *J Clin Oncol* 1999; **17**: 3835–49.

176. Braziel RM, Arber DA, Slovak ML. The Burkitt-like lymphomas: a Southwest Oncology Group study delineating phenotypic, genotypic, and clinical features. *Blood* 2001; **15**: 3713–20.

●177. Dave SS, Fu K, Wright GW *et al.* For the Lymphoma/ Leukemia Molecular Profiling Project: molecular diagnosis of Burkitt's lymphoma. *N Engl J Med* 2006; **354**: 2431–42.

178. Knezevich S, Ludkovski O, Salski C *et al.* Concurrent translocation of BCL2 and MYC with a single immunoglobulin locus in high-grade B-cell lymphomas. *Leukemia* 2005; **19**: 659–63.

●179. Tomita N, Nakamura N, Kanamori H *et al.* Atypical Burkitt lymphoma arising from follicular lymphoma: demonstration by polymerase chain reaction following laser capture microdissection and by fluorescence *in situ* hybridization on paraffin-embedded tissue sections. *Am J Surg Pathol* 2005; **29**: 121–4.

●180. Kanungo A, Medeiros LJ, Abruzzo LV, Lin P. Lymphoid neoplasms associated with concurrent t(14;18) and 8q24/c-MYC translocation generally have a poor prognosis. *Mod Pathol* 2006; **19**: 25–33.

181. Au WY, Horsman DE, Gascoyne RD *et al.* The spectrum of lymphoma with 8q24 aberrations: a clinical, pathological and cytogenetic study of 87 consecutive cases. *Leuk Lymphoma* 2004; **45**: 519–28.

182. Au WY, Horsman DE, Viswanatha DS *et al.* 8q24 Translocations in blastic transformation of mantle cell lymphoma. *Haematologica* 2000; **85**: 1225–7.

183. Loh ML, Samson Y, Motte E *et al.* Translocation (2;8)(p12;q24) associated with a cryptic t(12;21) (p13;q22) TEL/AML1 gene rearrangement in a child with acute lymphoblastic leukaemia. *Cancer Genet Cytogenet* 2000; **122**: 79–82.

184. Avet-Loiseau H, Gerson F, Magrangeas F *et al.* Intergroupe francophone du myelome. Rearrangements of the c-myc oncogene are present in 15 percent of primary human multiple myeloma tumors. *Blood* 2001; **98**: 3082–6.

●185. Nakamura N, Nakamine H, Tamaru J *et al.* The distinction between Burkitt lymphoma and diffuse large B-cell lymphoma with c-myc rearrangement. *Mod Pathol* 2002; **15**: 771–6.

186. Oschlies I, Klapper W, Zimmermann M *et al.* Diffuse large B-cell lymphoma in pediatric patients belongs predominantly to the germinal-center type B-cell lymphomas: a clinicopathologic analysis of cases included in the German BFM (Berlin-Frankfurt-Munster) multicenter trial. *Blood* 2006; **107**: 4047–52.

187. Dave BJ, Weisenburger DD, Higgins CM *et al.* Cytogenetics and fluorescence *in situ* hybridization studies of diffuse large B-cell lymphoma in children and young adults. *Cancer Genet Cytogenet* 2004; **153**: 115–21.

188. Alizadeh AA, Eisen MB, Davis RE *et al.* Distinct types of diffuse large B-cell lymphoma identified by gene expression profiling. *Nature* 2000; **403**: 503–11.

189. Rosenwald A, Wright G, Chan WC *et al.* The use of molecular profiling to predict survival after chemotherapy for diffuse large B-cell lymphoma. *N Engl J Med* 2002; **346**: 1937–57.

33

Diffuse large B cell lymphomas

LAURENCE DE LEVAL AND NANCY LEE HARRIS

INTRODUCTION

Diffuse large B cell lymphoma (DLBCL) is the most common adult non-Hodgkin lymphoma worldwide,[1] accounting for 30–40 percent of all cases. This group of tumors encompasses marked biologic heterogeneity and highly variable clinical course. Median age at presentation is in the seventh decade, but the disease also affects children or younger adults. DLBCL may occur *de novo*, or arise as a transformation from an underlying small B cell lymphoma. Patients present with variable combinations of nodal and/or extranodal involvement (Fig. 33.1), and present variable responses to therapy. Although most patients respond initially to chemotherapy, less than half are cured by currently available therapy.[2] Pathologically, the biologic heterogeneity of DLBCL is reflected in variable morphology, immunophenotype, cytogenetic alterations and molecular genetic features. Accordingly, in the World Health Organization (WHO) classification, in addition to the 'usual' form of DLBCL (DLBCL, not otherwise specified) which comprises the majority of the cases, several variants have been separated as distinct entities by virtue of distinctive immunophenotypic and/or clinical and pathologic features (Box 33.1).[3]

DIFFUSE LARGE B CELL LYMPHOMA OF THE USUAL TYPE

Morphology

DLBCL is defined as a diffuse proliferation of large neoplastic lymphoid cells with nuclear size equal or exceeding normal macrophage nuclei or more than twice the size of a normal lymphocyte.[3] Grossly, DLBCL appears as a mass-forming tissue with 'fish-flesh' white homogeneous appearance. Lymph nodes involved by DLBCL are typically enlarged, often with completely obliterated tissue architecture, although partial involvement may be seen. The centroblastic, immunoblastic and anaplastic variants of DLBCL represent the usual morphologic types, with centroblastic being the most common (about 75 percent of cases).[3] Centroblasts are large noncleaved lymphoid cells resembling the proliferating cells of the germinal center with oval to round vesicular nuclei, with fine chromatin and multiple membrane-bound nucleoli, and scanty amphophilic to basophilic cytoplasm. Immunoblasts have an oval or round nucleus with opened chromatin and a large central solitary nucleolus, and abundant deeply basophilic cytoplasm. Lymphomas comprising more than

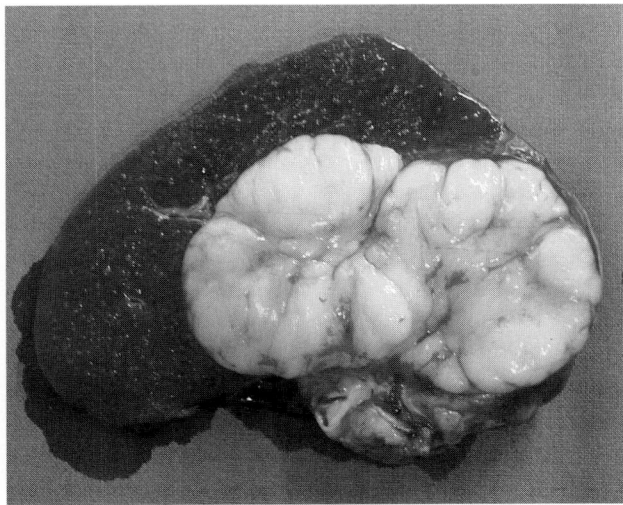

Figure 33.1 Diffuse large B-cell lymphoma of the spleen. The tumor manifests macroscopically as a bulging white fleshy mass.

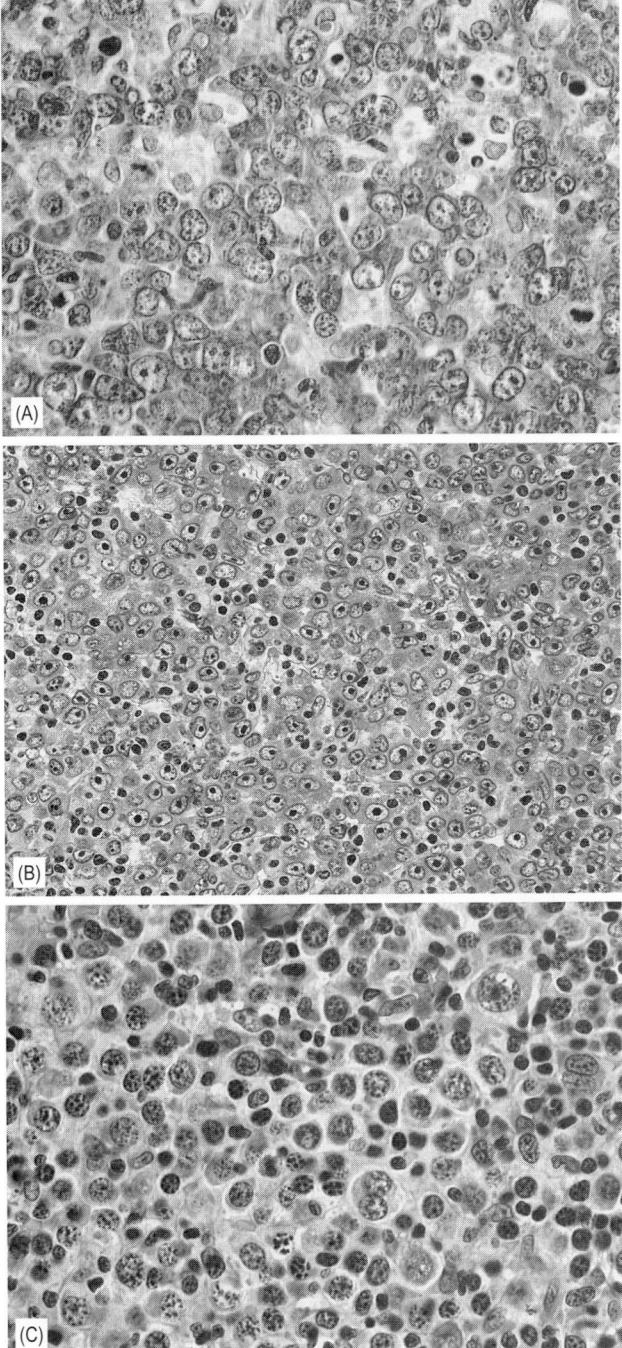

Figure 33.2 Centroblastic and immunoblastic variants of diffuse large B cell lymphoma. (A) Centroblastic lymphoma; (B) immunoblastic lymphoma; (C) immunoblastic lymphoma with plasmacytic differentiation (×400).

BOX 33.1: DIFFUSE LARGE B CELL LYMPHOMAS (DLBCL)

- Usual DLBCL (morphologic variants: centroblastic, immunoblastic, anaplastic)
- T cell/histiocyte-rich large B cell lymphoma (THRLBCL)
- Plasmablastic lymphoma
- Anaplastic lymphoma kinase-positive DLBCL
- Primary mediastinal (thymic) large B cell lymphoma (PMLBCL)
- Primary DLBCL of the central nervous system
- Primary cutaneous DLBCL, leg type
- Primary effusion lymphoma (PEL)
- DLBCL associated with chronic inflammation
- Intravascular large B cell lymphoma (IVLBCL)
- Epstein–Barr virus (EBV) DLBCL of the elderly
- Lymphomatoid granulomatosis

---

10 percent centroblasts fall into the category of centroblastic lymphoma, which includes the monomorphic and polymorphic variants (Fig. 33.2A). Centroblastic lymphomas may harbor multilobulated nuclei, a feature encountered frequently in primary osseous DLBCL.[4] Tumors comprising 90 percent immunoblasts or more are classified as immunoblastic (Fig. 33.2B). Immunoblastic tumors may show plasmacytic differentiation (Fig. 33.2C). The anaplastic variant of DLBCL (Plate 51, see plate section) is characterized by large pleomorphic cells, sometimes resembling Reed–Sternberg cells, forming cohesive sheets and showing a sinusoidal pattern of growth that may mimic carcinoma.

The intra- and interobserver reproducibility of cytologic subclassification has always been low.[5] Immunoblast-rich and anaplastic DLBCLs have been found to have a worse prognosis in several studies; however, there is no consensus on the usefulness of histologic subtyping of DLBCL.[6–11]

Bone marrow involvement in DLBCL, seen in about 15 percent of the cases, may appear either as a large cell infiltrate, or slightly more often as an infiltrate of small atypical B cells – so-called 'discordant' marrow involvement.[12] The latter is not associated with a worse prognosis than cases without marrow involvement;[13] however, these patients may be at risk for late relapses.[14]

Immunophenotype

Diffuse large B cell lymphomas usually express CD45 and pan-B cell antigens, such as CD19, CD20, CD45RA, CD79a, and the nuclear transcription factor PAX5, but may lack one or more of these.[15,16] Chimeric antibodies directed against CD20 (rituximab) are now commonly used in combination with standard therapies, for the treatment of DLBCLs.[17] Enrollment into trials with rituximab requires demonstration of expression of CD20 in tumor cells, and conversely therapy of B cell lymphoma with rituximab can result in the loss of CD20 antigen expression.[18] The majority of DLBCLs express monotypic surface immunoglobulin (sIg – usually IgM), which is detectable on frozen sections or by flow cytometry and only rarely on paraffin sections. Cytoplasmic Ig expression, a feature of secretory normal B cells, can be demonstrated in a minority of DLBCL cases, usually those with immunoblastic morphology. In DLBCL the cell cycle fraction is variable, ranging from 30 percent to 100 percent, but is typically high (median values around 65 percent).[19] Expression of CD30, which is characteristic of the anaplastic variant, may be seen occasionally in other morphologic types.

DLBCLs variably express antigens normally associated with specific stages of physiologic B cell differentiation (Fig. 33.3). BCL2 protein expression, normally downregulated in germinal center (GC) B cells,[20] is evidenced in 30 percent to 60 percent of DLBCLs.[21–23] BCL6, a zinc-finger nuclear factor normally expressed in GC B cells and acting as a transcriptional repressor[24] is expressed in the majority of DLBCLs, ranging from 60 percent to 90 percent in various series.[22,25–27] Typically, a variable fraction of tumor nuclei are stained, and a cutoff of 10 percent to 30 percent positive nuclei is usually used for considering a tumor as positive. The CD10 membrane metalloproteinase is another GC antigen[28] which is expressed in 20 to 40 percent of DLBCL cases.[26,29,30] The staining is usually homogeneous throughout the tumor. Cases that are positive for CD10 usually coexpress BCL6, but the reverse is not true. MUM1/IRF4 transcription factor is an 'early' post-germinal center antigen which denotes the final step of intra-GC B cell differentiation and subsequent steps of maturation towards plasma cells.[31] Unlike normal B cells where expression of MUM1 and BCL6 is mutually exclusive, in DLBCLs, MUM1 is detected in 50 percent to 75 percent of the cases, with or without BCL6 expression.[32] VS38c and CD138 are markers of later post-GC B cells and plasma cells. VS38c is a nonlineage-specific antibody that is reactive with a rough endoplasmic reticulum protein,[33] and CD138 (syndecan-1) a transmembrane glycoprotein receptor for several extracellular matrix proteins.[34] Whereas VS38c and CD138 react with neoplastic plasma cells and a

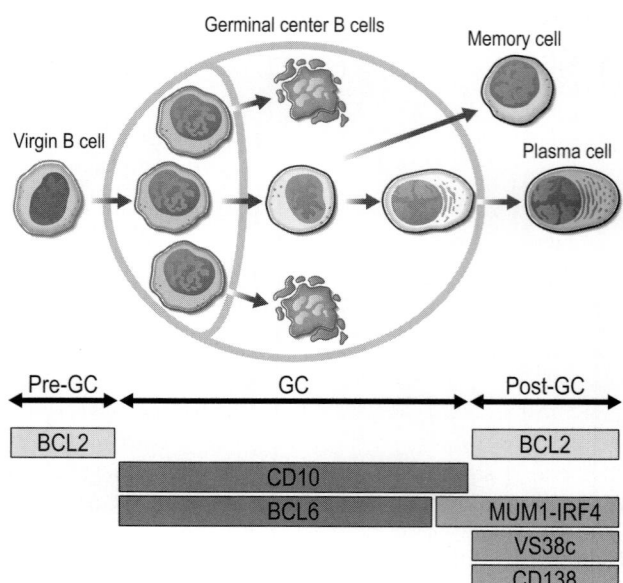

Figure 33.3 Expression of stage-specific differentiation antigens in relation to normal B cell differentiation, i.e. pre-germinal center (GC), GC and post-GC stages. Pre-GC B cells are virgin B cells. Cells comprising the GC consist of small blast cells, centroblasts, centrocytes and occasional plasma cells (from left to right). B cells exiting the GC differentiate either towards memory cells or immunoglobulin-secreting plasma cells. BCL2 is expressed at the pre-GC and post-GC stages of differentiation but is downregulated in GC B cells. Normal GC B cells express CD10 and BCL6. The latter antigen may be lost by late GC B cells, which in turn acquire MUM1 expression. MUM1, VS38c and CD138 are expressed by post-GC B cells. While MUM1 may be acquired late in the GC reaction, VS38c and CD138 expression is usually restricted to cells exhibiting plasmacytic differentiation and to plasma cells.

subset of small B cell lymphomas showing plasmacytic differentiation, usual DLBCLs are very infrequently reactive with these markers. In contrast they are often expressed in subsets of AIDS-associated lymphomas thought to arise from more terminally differentiated B cells, and lymphomas with plasmablastic features.

About 10 percent of *de novo* DLBCLs (i.e. excluding Richter's syndrome) express CD5. CD5+ DLBCLs are negative for cyclin D1 expression, distinguishing them from blastoid mantle cell lymphoma. Most CD5+ DLBCLs have a centroblastic morphology, are negative for CD10 and positive for BCL6 protein.[29,35]

Genetic features

At the genetic level most DLBCLs have been shown to harbor somatic mutations in the variable regions of their *IG* genes, and hence are thought to derive from antigen-exposed B cells that have migrated to or passed through the GC – either GC or post-GC B cells.[36,37]

Table 33.1 Recurrent genetic alterations in diffuse large B cell lymphoma

Gene	Location	Genetic alteration	Frequency (%)	Functional consequence
BCL6	3q27	Translocation t(3;)	25–40	Promotor substitution → BCL6 deregulation
		Somatic hypermutations	75	? BCL6 deregulation
BCL2	18q21	Translocation t(14;18)	15–20	BCL2 overexpression, antiapoptotic effect
		Gene amplification	25	BCL2 overexpression, antiapoptotic effect
MYC	8q24	Translocation t(8;14)	10	Myc overexpression, increased cell proliferation
FAS	10q24	Somatic hypermutations	20	Impaired apoptosis
P53	17p	Point mutations, deletions	20	Functional inactivation of p53

At variance with other B cell lymphoma entities, no single genetic aberration typifies DLBCL. Several mechanisms of genetic lesions are encountered: chromosomal translocations, aberrant somatic hypermutation and others common to all malignancies including point mutations, gene amplifications and deletions. Many cases exhibit complex karyotypes. Recurrent chromosomal translocations occur in about 50 percent of the cases[38] and genetic imbalances in as many as 67 percent.[39] The most frequently deregulated protooncogenes, BCL6, BCL2 and MYC, share a common mechanism whereby chromosomal translocation brings the target gene under inappropriate control of an immunoglobulin regulatory gene. Table 33.1 summarizes the most frequent recurrent genetic alterations in DLBCL.

CHROMOSOMAL TRANSLOCATIONS

- **BCL6**: Chromosomal translocations involving the BCL6 gene at the 3q27 locus represent the most common genetic abnormalities in DLBCL, occurring in 25 percent to 40 percent of the cases.[40,41] BCL6 translocations involve either the immunoglobulin IG (heavy or light chain) loci or other genes (variant translocation partners), and result in BCL6 deregulated expression as a consequence of promotor substitution. Furthermore, up to 75 percent of DLBCL cases display multiple somatic mutations clustering in the 5′ noncoding region of the gene, probably derived by the somatic hypermutation process and frequently occurring in the absence of translocations.[41,42] Although the functional consequences of most mutations remains largely unknown, some may cause BCL6 deregulation.[42] The BCL6 transcription factor plays a critical role in GC development[43] and represses genes involved in lymphocyte activation and differentiation, in cell cycle control and inflammation.[44] The down-regulation of BCL6 may be necessary for GC B cells to differentiate into memory cells and plasma cells. In DLBCL, dysregulated constitutive expression of BCL6 may lead to maturation arrest and confer a proliferative advantage. Recent studies have identified a mechanism whereby BCL6 may regulate GC reaction and lymphomagenesis via down-modulation and functional inactivation of

the p53 tumor suppressor gene, allowing GC B cells to tolerate genomic alterations and promoting the persistence of malignant clones.[45] Clinically, BCL6 rearrangements occur primarily in de novo DLBCL.[46] Attempts to evaluate the prognostic impact of BCL6 gene rearrangements have yielded divergent results.[47–53] The partner gene in BCL6 translocation (IG versus non-IG) may be prognostically relevant.[53,54]

- **BCL2**: Translocation of the BCL2 gene to the immunoglobulin heavy chain promotor, i.e. t(14;18) occurs in 15 percent to 20 percent of DLBCL cases.[55] The resulting overexpression of BCL2 antiapoptotic protein may confer a survival advantage and contribute to lymphomagenesis. Besides BCL2 translocation, BCL2 gene amplification represents another important mechanism for BCL2 protein overexpression in DLBCL.[56,57] In contrast with the adverse prognostic significance of BCL2 overexpression,[27,58] detection of the BCL2 translocation alone has no predictive value on the survival.[50,59,60] Because the t(14;18) is the hallmark of follicular lymphoma and transformed follicular lymphomas may be indistinguishable from de novo DLBCL, the reported frequencies of t(14;18) in DLBCL series may depend on how accurately tumors and patients were included.

- **MYC**: Deregulation of the MYC oncogene, the hallmark of Burkitt lymphoma, also occurs in approximately 10 percent of DLBCL cases.[50,61] MYC expression is strongly associated with cell proliferation and negatively correlated with cell differentiation, and MYC rearrangement in DLBCL has been found to carry a negative prognostic significance.[62] A subset of DLBCLs with MYC rearrangement also carry a t(14;18) (double hit lymphomas); these may show features partially overlapping those of Burkitt lymphoma and are extremely resistant to therapy.[63,64]

SOMATIC HYPERMUTATIONS

Somatic hypermutation in normal GC B cells targets IG as well as non-IG genes including BCL6 and FAS.[65] FAS mutations have been found in up to about 20 percent of DLBCLs,[66] likely acting in a dominant-negative manner by

Table 33.2   Characteristics of the diffuse large B cell lymphoma (DLBCL) molecular subgroups identified by gene expression profiling

	GCB DLBCL	ABC DLBCL
Overexpressed genes	CD10, BCL6, HGAL, LMO2	MUM1/IRF4, XBP1, CD44, FOXP1
Postulated cell of origin	Germinal center B cell	Postgerminal center B cell
Ongoing IG mutations	Yes	No
Genetic alterations and oncogenic mechanisms	t(14;18)(q32;q21): BCL2 translocation	t(3;)(q27;): BCL6 translocation
	REL amplification at 2p	PRDM1/BLIMP1 inactivation
	Gains at 12q12	Trisomy 3, trisomy 18
		Deletion 6q
		Constitutive NF-κB activation
Clinical outcome	Favorable	Unfavorable
	60% 5-year survival	35% 5-year survival

destabilizing trimeric Fas proapoptotic receptors physiologically involved in the initiation of caspase-induced apoptosis. In a large proportion of DLBCLs, an aberrant hypermutation activity may target multiple other proto-oncogenes, including *MYC*, *PIM1*, *PAX5* and *RhoH/TTF*.[67] Although a comprehensive functional characterization of these genetic alterations is lacking, they may represent a powerful mechanism of transformation, because they may have an effect on multiple genes. Furthermore, some of the hypermutable genes are susceptible to chromosomal translocations in the same region, consistent with a role for hypermutation in generating translocations by DNA double-strand breaks.[67]

OTHER GENETIC ALTERATIONS

Inactivation of the *p53* tumor suppressor gene by point mutations or gene deletion is found in about 20 percent of DLBCLs. Although occurring rarely as an isolated event in DLBCL, inactivation of *p53* has been associated with clinical drug resistance and poor outcome.[68,69]

The reported amplification of the 2p12–16 region in up to 14 percent of DLBCLs has focused attention on the *REL* gene mapped at this locus, because *REL* encodes a component of the nuclear factor (NF)-κB heterodimer, and several lines of evidence point at the possible role of constitutive of NF-κB activation in sustaining survival and growth of various tumors.[70] Recent data, however, indicate that 2p12–16 amplifications do not lead to abnormal *REL* activation, and are in fact more common in DLBCL subsets with no evidence of NF-κB activation, suggesting a different target at this locus.[71,72]

Numerous chromosomal imbalances have been observed in DLBCL, some of which may influence prognosis. Poor outcome has been associated with alterations of chromosomes 1q, 3p, 5, 7q, and 14.[73] Defects with no clear influence on prognosis include abnormalities on Xq, 7q, 12q and 6q. The role of these alterations in DLBCL pathogenesis is unclear.[74]

Molecular features – gene expression profiling

The landmark gene expression profiling study of DLBCL using a specialized cDNA microarray (Lymphochip), identified two distinct molecular DLBCL subgroups, namely the GC B cell-like DLBCL (GCB DLBCL) harboring a gene expression profile similar to that of GC B cells, and the activated B cell-like DLBCL (ABC DLBCL), with a gene expression profile similar to that of *in vitro* mitogenically activated peripheral blood cells.[75] In a subsequent study of a larger number of cases, an additional third subgroup was described, which did not express genes characteristic of either GC- or ABC-like signatures (type 3). Interestingly, the 'cell of origin' signature was prognostically meaningful, as patients with GC-like DLBCLs had significantly better outcomes than those with ABC-like and type 3 DLBCLs, with 5-years survivals of 60 percent, 35 percent and 39 percent, respectively (Plate 52, see plate section).[75,76]

The notion that the GCB and ABC subgroups represent pathogenetically distinct types of DLBCLs since then has been further supported by additional studies having demonstrated different genetic features and oncogenic mechanisms in the two subgroups (Table 33.2). The t(14;18)(q32;q21) translocation and chromosomal amplifications of the *REL* locus at 2p occur predominantly if not exclusively in the GCB group.[76–78] *BCL6* translocations are three times more common in ABC than in GCB DLBCLs.[41] Chromosomal deletion or mutational inactivation of the *PRDM1/BLIMP1* that functions as a mediator of plasmacytic differentiation is a mechanism of differentiation block in ABC tumors and is not found in the GCB subtype.[79,80] By comparative genomic hybridization, ABC tumors have frequent trisomy 3, gains of 3q and 18q21–q22, and losses of 6q21–q22, whereas GCB DLBCLs have frequent gains of 12q12.[81] Activation of the NF-κB signaling pathways is a feature of the ABC subgroup, and interference with this pathway selectively kills this type of DLBCL,[70,82] which might represent an interesting

Table 33.3 Prognostic biomarkers in diffuse large B cell lymphoma (DLBCL)

Molecular marker	Biological function	High expression correlation with outcome
HLA-II	Immune response	Favorable
Ki-67	Proliferation	Unfavorable
p53 mutation	Cell cycle control	Unfavorable
BCL2	Inhibition of apoptosis	Unfavorable[a]
Survivin	Inhibition of apoptosis	Unfavorable
sCD44, CD44v6	Adhesion molecules, lymphocyte homing and dissemination	Unfavorable
ICAM-1	Adhesion molecule, lymphocyte trafficking	Unfavorable
BCL6	Transcriptional repressor, GC marker	Favorable[a]
MUM1	Transcription factor, post-GC marker	Unfavorable
CD5	T cell lineage antigen	Unfavorable
GC-like immunophenotype	Reflective of GCB molecular subtype	Favorable[a]
Non-GC-like immunophenotype	Reflective of ABC molecular subtype	Unfavorable[a]
FOXP1	Transcription factor	Unfavorable
PKCβ	Enhances B cell proliferation and survival	Unfavorable
LMO2	GC marker	Favorable[b]

[a]Association not confirmed for DLBCL patients treated with immunochemotherapy.
[b]Association confirmed for DLBCL patients treated with immunochemotherapy.
HLA, human leukocyte antigen; ICAM, intercellular adhesion molecule; GC, germinal center

therapeutic option for ABC DLBCL patients. The activation of the NF-κB pathway in ABC tumors relies upon the CARD11/MALT1/BCL10 signaling complex which activates the central kinase of the NF-κB pathway.[83] A subset of ABC DLBCL has a high expression of STAT3 as well as interleukin-6 (IL-6) and/or IL-10, and such cell lines are selectively killed by STAT3 inhibitors.[84] All GCB DLBCL are characterized by ongoing somatic hypermutations in their IG genes, whereas the majority of ABC tumors are not.[85] GCB and ABC DLBCLs also present distinct activities of the IL-4 signaling pathway.[86]

Other expression profiling studies have identified alternative subgroups of DLBCL based on biologically meaningful gene expression signatures. In particular, in the study by Monti et al., three subgroups were identified:[87] the 'OxPhos' group, characterized by increased expression of genes associated with oxidative phosphorylation such as BCL2, the 'BCR/Proliferation' group, enriched in B cell receptor and cell-cycle regulatory genes, and the 'Host Response' group with increased expression of genes related to the inflammatory/immune response. Importantly, these subgroups did not differ in respect with survival.

Prognostic biomarkers

Although prognosis of individual patients is highly variable, the International Prognosis Index (IPI), based on five clinical parameters (age, performance status, stage, number of extranodal sites, serum lactate dehydrogenase), has proven to be very valuable to define prognostic subgroups in DLBCL.[88] This index is used to assess an individual patient's risk; however, these clinical variables probably represent surrogates for the intrinsic cellular and molecular heterogeneity within DLBCL. Moreover, patients with identical IPI still exhibit marked variability in survival, suggesting residual heterogeneity within each category. Several individual markers linked to different biologic aspects of the disease have been studied with respect to their correlation with distinct clinical features and/or outcome (for review see de Leval and Harris[89] and Lossos and Morgensztern[90]). More recently, novel biomarkers and signatures derived from DNA microarray analysis of DLBCL have also been identified. A summary is given in Table 33.3.

Importantly, the prognostic parameters are dependent on the management strategies of the patients. Since the introduction of rituximab in the therapeutic protocols of DLBCL the prognosis has improved significantly,[91] and the IPI seems to partly lose some of its robustness.[92] The predictive value of some biomarkers validated in the pre-rituximab era seem to be overcome by the new immunochemotherapy protocols,[93] and others need to be reevaluated.

INDIVIDUAL BIOMARKERS

- Immune response markers. Loss of human leukocyte antigens on neoplastic B cells, probably contributing to poor in vivo antitumor immune response, has been correlated with extranodal disease and poor survival.[94–96] Loss of expression of other membrane molecules important for T cell activation, such as CD54 and CD86, has been found to be associated with low numbers of tumor-infiltrating T lymphocytes, a feature predictive of shorter relapse-free survival.[97,98] Conversely, an increased number of activated CD4+ cells in DLBCLs has been correlated with a better prognosis.[99,100] Interestingly, these findings correlate with those derived from microarray-based analysis, as the major histocompatibility complex (MHC) class II gene-expression signature was found to be predictive of a good outcome in DLBCL.[76]

- Markers involved in the control of proliferation and apoptosis. The prognostic value of Ki-67 expression, a nuclear antigen reflecting actively cycling cells, has been the subject of several studies in the past, usually showing that a high proliferative index (>60 percent or >80 percent) is an adverse prognostic factor.[101] In the recent years, only a few studies have reassessed the prognostic significance of Ki-67 staining and while some confirmed an inverse correlation between proliferation and survival,[102] others failed to confirm these findings.[27,103] The p53 tumor suppressor gene encodes a protein that monitors DNA integrity by arresting cells at G1 or programming them to cell death when DNA replication is defective or when DNA is damaged. Functional inactivation of p53, reflected by p53-positive p21-negative immunophenotype,[104] has been associated with clinical drug resistance and poor outcome.[68,69] Multiple large-scale trials have established an association between BCL2 expression and decreased disease-free or overall survival in DLBCL, and an impact on overall survival independent of the IPI was demonstrated in two studies.[27,58,60,102,105] Strikingly, despite an overall concordance of the results of these studies, there was considerable variation in the cut-off used to classify BCL2-positive and -negative cases, and the significance of an intermediate or heterogeneous expression was ambiguous (Plate 53, see plate section). Importantly, the negative predictive value of BCL2 expression appears to be abrogated by the addition of rituximab to chemotherapy.[93] Survivin, a member of the inhibitor of apoptosis protein family normally undetectable in normal adult tissues, was expressed in 60 percent of DLBCL cases in one study and was an independent predictor of decreased survival.[106]

- Adhesion molecules. CD44, a family of cell surface adhesion glycoproteins acting as receptors for hyaluronate, is important for normal lymphocyte development, homing and activation.[107] In addition to the 'standard' CD44 isoform (CD44s) also expressed by normal lymphocytes, DLBCLs may express larger splice variants (CD44v) especially those containing exon v6/7 encoded sequences which confer metastatic behavior in carcinoma cell lines.[108,109] In DLBCL, expression of CD44s has been associated with advanced stage disease and shortened survival, and in one study was a powerful prognosticator of reduced survival in patients presenting with localized nodal

disease.[110–112] Expression of the CD44v6 isoform was found to correlate with disease stage[113] and in two studies to be an independent predictor of poor survival.[114,115] Intercellular adhesion molecule (ICAM)-1 is a cell-surface receptor belonging to the immunoglobulin superfamily. Low surface expression of ICAM-1 in patients with aggressive non-Hodgkin lymphoma has been correlated with advanced stage, extranodal involvement, bone marrow infiltration and poor outcome.[116]

- Differentiation antigens. Several investigators found a positive impact of high BCL6 expression (assessed at the mRNA or protein level) on the outcome of DLBCL patients treated with standard chemotherapy.[117,118] In patients treated with combined immunochemotherapy, the beneficial effect of BCL6 positivity seems to be abrogated.[119] The prognostic significance of CD10 expression in DLBCLs is controversial, since several studies using immunohistochemistry on paraffin sections found either no difference in outcome between patients with CD10+ and CD10– tumors[27,29,120] or an association between CD10 reactivity and a better outcome.[37,121] MUM1 expression by more than 30 percent lymphoma cells has been associated with a significantly worse outcome in DLBCL patients.[118] CD5+ DLBCLs are reported to occur in elderly women, with a predilection for extranodal involvement, especially bone marrow and spleen,[35,122] and to be associated with shorter survival in comparison with CD5-negative tumors.[29] Recent genetic and molecular studies suggest that the genomic imbalances and the gene expression signature of CD5-positive DLBCLs are similar to those of the ABC-like subgroup of DLBCLs.[123,124]

BIOMARKERS AND SIGNATURES DERIVED FROM DNA MICROARRAYS ANALYSIS

- Immunohistochemical panels. Based on gene expression profiling data and given the prognostic significance of the molecular subtypes of DLBCL, immunohistochemical algorithms have been developed as surrogates for the gene expression signatures, to classify the tumors as with a GC-like or non-GC-like immunophenotype and to predict survival in DLBCL patients. Different investigators have used various combinations of two markers or more, and a GC-like phenotype has been variably defined as coexpression of both BCL6 and CD10,[105,125] as expression of BCL6 and/or CD10 without expression of the post-germinal center markers MUM1 and CD138,[126] or as expression of CD10 or BCL6 in the absence of MUM1 expression in the Hans classifier.[118] The immunohistochemical classification based on Hans algorithm correlates with the cDNA classification and is the most widely used, but the concordance is imperfect.[118] In addition, immunohistochemistry allows semiquantitative measurements, and suffers from considerable problems in reproducibility as well as intra- and inter-observer variation.[127] Whereas several studies demonstrated the favorable predictive value of the GC-like immunophenotype,[105,118,125,126,128,129] others failed to show such correlation, even though similar classifiers were employed.[27,130] In the study by Colomo et al., BCL6+/CD10+ DLBCLs did not have a different outcome, but tended to be disseminated and showed a centroblastic morphology.[27] Another study also suggested that late relapses from DLBCL preferentially occur in patients whose primary tumors have GC-like features.[131] Recent reports suggest that the combination of rituximab to chemotherapy may eliminate the prognostic value of immunohistochemically defined GC and non-GC immunophenotypes.[132]

- Molecular predictors. Outcome predictors, based on the expression of a limited number of genes and potentially amenable to routine quantification by real time RT-PCR, have been developed.[76,133] For example, gene expression measurements of 17 genes is representative of four signatures, namely the GC-related expression profile, the lymph node signature, the proliferation signature and the MHC class II signature, have been combined into a model allowing risk classification.[76] Using another mathematical approach, Lossos et al. developed an outcome predictor based on the expression of six genes (LMO2, BCL6, FN1 associated with favorable prognosis, and CCND2, SCYA3 and BCL2, associated with unfavorable outcome).[134]
- Novel biomarkers. Other potentially interesting novel biomarkers have been identified by gene expression profiling studies. For example, high levels of expression of the forkhead box protein 1 (FOXP1) transcription factor, a gene clustering within the ABC-like signature, identify a group of patients with a particularly poor outcome.[135,136] The protein kinase C β gene, found to be overexpressed at the mRNA level in a group of DLBCLs refractory to chemotherapy, by comparison with curable tumors,[133] has been validated at the protein level as predictive of inferior survival.[137] Expression of the LMO2 protein associated with the GCB molecular subtype of DLBCL, has been shown to be a strong predictor of better outcome for patients treated by chemotherapy with or without rituximab.[138]

T CELL/HISTIOCYTE–RICH LARGE B CELL LYMPHOMA

In the T cell/histiocyte-rich variant of DLBCL (THRLBCL), there are few large neoplastic B cells scattered in a background of non-neoplastic T cells with or without histiocytes.

Small B cells are rare or absent. The growth pattern is diffuse or vaguely nodular, and may be associated with fine sclerosis (Plate 54A, see plate section). THRLBCL usually presents in middle-aged or older male adults, often with advanced-stage disease and frequent involvement of spleen (typically as a micronodular pattern involving the white pulp),[139] liver and bone marrow.

The disease is morphologically heterogeneous as the large cells may resemble lymphocytic and histiocytic cells, centroblasts or immunoblasts, or classic Reed–Sternberg cells (Plate 54B).[140] They are uniformly positive for CD45 and B cell-associated antigens (Plate 54C), may be positive for CD30 and EMA, but are negative for CD15, and in most cases are strongly positive for BCL6, while they are usually negative for CD10 and variably express BCL2.[140–142] There is no association with Epstein–Barr virus (EBV) infection. The reactive cells are mature T cells (Plate 54D) comprising variable proportions of CD4- and CD8-positive cells and few CD57-positive cells, in contrast to nodular lymphocyte predominant Hodgkin lymphoma (NLPHL).

Cytogenetic data for THRLBCL are scarcely available; in two cases a near-tetraploid karyotype was documented.[143,144] Many cases may in fact contain polyploid tumor cells, as suggested by fluorescence in situ hybridization (FISH) studies.[145] BCL2 and BCL6 gene rearrangements are found less frequently than in usual DLBCLs.[87,140] Microdissected neoplastic cells harbor somatic hypermutations with a pattern of mutations suggestive of antigen selection and intra-clonal diversity.[145] These features, together with strong BCL6 expression are interpreted as evidence for derivation from a precursor of GC origin. Due to the very few numbers of neoplastic B cells, PCR may fail to disclose the clonal immunoglobulin heavy-chain gene rearrangement.

The factors responsible for the reduced B cell numbers and increased reactive infiltrate in THRLBCL are not well understood. Production of cytokines may contribute to the abundant reactive infiltrate, and high levels of IL-4 have been demonstrated in some cases.[146] Tumor cell apoptosis, perhaps mediated by cytotoxic T cells and facilitated by low levels of BCL2 expression, may partly account for the decreased number of neoplastic B cells.[147] In a molecular profiling study of a large series of de novo DLBCLs, most THRLBCL cases fell into a discrete subset characterized by 'host inflammatory response' including increased expression of T/NK cell receptor and activation pathway components, complement cascade members, macrophage/dendritic cell markers and inflammatory mediators.[87]

A controversial issue concerns the possible relationship between THRLBCL and NLPHL. In both diseases, the neoplastic cells exhibit similar morphologic and immuno-phenotypic features, while the distinctive features are the architecture of the lymphoproliferation (THRLBCL, diffuse or vaguely nodular with no follicular dendritic cell meshworks versus NLPHL, at least partly nodular in association with follicular dendritic cells) and the nature of the associated background (T cell-rich with few CD57-positive cells in THRLBCL versus B cell-rich with many CD57-positive cells in NLPHL). The distinction is crucial as THRLBCL is an aggressive neoplasm while NLPHL usually pursues a relatively indolent clinical course. It has been suggested that the two diseases are also linked by a biologic continuum,[148] as there have been occasional reports of composite lesions in the same lymph node or in subsequent biopsies, and both diseases may evolve to usual DLBCL, so that with current diagnostic criteria there remains a 'gray zone' of cases of uncertain classification.[149] However, by comparative genomic hybridization the profiles of THRLBCL and NLPHL showed shared as well as distinctive features, especially in the number of genomic imbalances (lower in THRLBCL) and their distribution; these findings argue against the concept of a continuum between the two diseases but could be consistent with the hypothesis of a common precursor cell.[150] It is currently recommended that the diagnosis of THRLBCL should be restricted to *de novo* cases and not be applied in patients with a history of NLPHL.

Some studies have suggested that THRLBCL follows a more aggressive clinical course than 'usual' DLBCL;[151] however, other reports indicate that the outcome of THRLBCL patients is equivalent to that observed in patients with usual DLBCL.[152,153]

PLASMABLASTIC LYMPHOMA

Plasmablastic lymphoma designates a group of tumors that have a morphologic appearance suggestive of high-grade lymphoma, and an immunophenotypic profile of plasma cells. It was initially described as rare variant of DLBCL occurring in the oral cavity in HIV-infected patients.[154] Since the original description, its spectrum has expanded as similar lesions have been reported in immunocompetent patients and/or in other anatomic locations in HIV-infected individuals including other extranodal sites (anorectal region, nasopharynx, intestines) and lymph nodes.[155–160] These tumors are locally invasive, disseminate to extraoral sites and have a highly aggressive clinical behavior,[154] but improved survival outcomes have been reported more recently, since the advent of highly active anti-retroviral therapy (HAART).

Plasmablastic lymphoma encompasses a morphologic spectrum. It usually presents as a diffuse proliferation of medium to large immunoblastic cells harboring a central nucleolus, displaying a more or less cohesive appearance (Fig. 33.4A, B).[154,160] These tumors exhibit a high proliferation rate, many cases show frequent apoptotic cells or single cell necrosis, and a starry-sky pattern may be seen.[160] A subset of tumors show plasmacytic differentiation and contain a range of cells showing a morphologic continuum up to mature plasma cells.[158,160]

Plasmablastic lymphoma is characterized by absent or weak expression of CD45 and B cell-associated antigens (CD20–, CD45RA–, CD79a±), strong expression of plasma cell-associated antigens (MUM1, CD138, CD38, VS38c) (Fig. 33.4C). Monotypic expression of cytoplasmic immunoglobulins (usually of the IgG or IgA type) is detected in a variable proportion of the cases. Expression of BCL6 is usually lacking.

The Epstein–Barr virus is detected in the majority of the cases; the tumor cells are positive for EBV-encoded small RNAs (EBERs) by *in situ* hybridization, and lack EBV-associated proteins, such as EBNA2 and LMP1, consistent with a type I latency.[154,161,162] Although the potential implication of human herpes virus 8 (HHV8) in plasmablastic lymphoma remains a controversial matter,[163,164] virtually all cases are negative for HHV8-associated latent nuclear antigen 1 (LANA-1) by immunohistochemistry.[154,158,165,166]

Genetic alterations associated with plasmablastic lymphoma are not described. The tumors do not appear to carry *BCL2* gene rearrangements. A subset of cases carry hypermutations with a pattern suggestive of antigen selection in some cases and thus conceivably derive from post-GC B

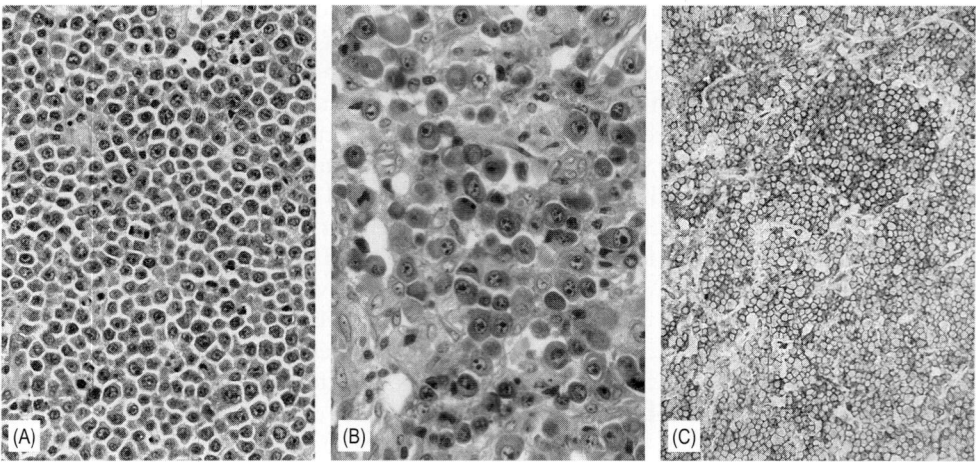

Figure 33.4 Plasmablastic lymphoma presenting as an oral mass in an HIV-positive man. The tumor consists of a (A) diffuse proliferation of large cells with abundant mitotic activity (×63) showing, (B) immunoblastic/plasmablastic features (×40), and (C) strong membranous positivity for CD138 (×200).

cells, whereas another fraction of these lymphomas carry unmutated immunoglobulin genes and appear to originate from naïve B cells that have undergone preterminal differentiation outside the GC.[167]

The differential diagnosis includes other neoplasms with plasmablastic features, with or without plasmacytic differentiation towards mature cells. These features indeed can also be identified in other aggressive large B cell lymphomas and plasma cell neoplasms, including some DLBCLs in immunocompromised and immunocompetent individuals, extramedullary dedifferentiated plasma cell myelomas and plasmacytomas,[165] HHV8-expressing solid lymphoid neoplasms,[168,169] and ALK-expressing DLBCL.[158,165] These latter two entities are discussed in more detail below.

ANAPLASTIC LYMPHOMA KINASE–POSITIVE LARGE B CELL LYMPHOMA

This very rare neoplasm initially described by Delsol et al.[170] is composed of large immunoblast-like cells with round pale nuclei, prominent central nucleoli and abundant cytoplasm with occasional morphologic evidence of plasmablastic differentiation suggested by a clear juxtanuclear area (Plate 55A, B, see plate section).

By immunohistochemistry, the tumor cells are weakly positive for CD45 and negative for expression of B cell antigens (CD20– and CD79a–) (Plate 55C, D), are positive for markers of plasma cell differentiation (VS38c+, CD138+), express cytoplasmic IgA. These tumors are also strongly positive for EMA but lack CD30 expression. A subset of cases may also express CD4 and CD57. In most cases ALK antibody produces a membranous and granular cytoplasmic pattern of staining (Plate 55E), as a consequence of t(2;17) translocation involving the clathrin gene (CTCL) at 17q23 and the ALK gene at 2p23.[171–173] A few cases of ALK-positive DLBCL express the NPM-ALK fusion as a consequence of a t(2;5) (p23;q35),[123,174] and these show a nuclear and diffuse cytoplasmic ALK staining.

Clinically, the disease shows a clear male predominance, affecting mostly adults, is often disseminated and is associated with a poor response to chemotherapy, commonly with fatal outcome.

PRIMARY MEDIASTINAL (THYMIC) LARGE B CELL LYMPHOMA

Primary mediastinal large B cell lymphoma (PMLBCL) comprises 7 percent of large B cell lymphomas and 2.4 percent of all non-Hodgkin lymphomas.[8,175] It tends to occur in young patients (median age about 35 years), and affects women more commonly than men. Patients present with an anterior mediastinal mass, and symptoms related to local invasion (superior vena cava syndrome [most frequently], airway obstruction, pleural and/or pericardial effusion).[176,177] The mass is often 'bulky' (>10 cm in diameter)

and locally invasive, infiltrating intrathoracic structures. Contiguous extension to the supraclavicular region is sometimes observed. Most patients have stage I or II disease at presentation. B symptoms may be present. Bone marrow involvement is extremely rare. Leukemia is never observed; however, hematogenous spread occurs during progression, as evidenced by dissemination to extranodal sites, including lung, liver, kidneys, adrenals, ovaries, brain, and the gastrointestinal tract.[177,178]

The tumor appears to arise in the thymus,[179] and residual thymic parenchyma is occasionally seen in the biopsies. The growth pattern is diffuse, and PMLBCL is morphologically heterogeneous; however, individual cases tend to be monomorphic. The presence of fine compartmentalizing sclerosis is a common feature (Plate 56A, see plate section).[179,180] The tumor is composed of medium to large-sized cells that resemble centroblasts, often with abundant clear or pale cytoplasm (Plate 56B). The nuclei are irregularly round or ovoid, sometimes multilobulated, usually with small nucleoli.[181] Rare cases may have larger cells with abundant cytoplasm and prominent nucleoli, resembling Reed– Sternberg cells and giving rise to a differential diagnosis with classic Hodgkin lymphoma.[182] Mitotic activity is high, similar to other large-cell lymphomas. The center of the lesion contains predominantly neoplastic cells. However, at the periphery of the mass, a variable number of reactive cells such as lymphocytes, macrophages and granulocytes may be present. The tumor cells express the B cell-associated antigens CD19, CD20, and CD79a, but 70 percent of the cases are negative for surface immunoglobulin, although immunoglobulin genes are rearranged and despite expression of the transcription factors BOB1, OCT2 and PU1.[183] The tumor cells also often have defective expression of human leukocyte antigen (HLA) class I and/or class II molecules.[184,185] Most cases express BCL6, often together with MUM1/IRF4; 25–30 percent are positive for CD10 expression; most cases express BCL2 and CD23 and a variable proportion of cases also express CD30, often weakly and on a subset of the tumor cells (Plate 56C).[183,186,187] Expression of the MAL gene, which is associated with T cell development, the IL-4-induced gene 1 (FIG1), and TNF-receptor-associated factor 1 (TRAF1) especially when combined with nuclear REL localization, have been shown to be characteristic of PMLBCL.[188–192]

The tumor cells carry isotype-switched IG genes with a high load of somatic mutations and no evidence of ongoing mutations.[193] More than half of the cases also carry BCL6 gene mutations.[183,194] Altogether these genetic features suggest an origin from an activated GC or post-GC B cell, which is consistent with the observed immunophenotype (non-GC-like in most cases).[183,186] So-called 'asteroid' B cells, present in the thymic medulla and having an immunophenotype similar to that of those found in PMLBCL, have been postulated as the cell of origin for PMLBCL.[187,195–197]

In contrast to DLBCL, PMLBCL rarely have either BCL2 rearrangements or translocations involving BCL6.[198] The

Table 33.4 Overlap in biologic and morphologic features between primary mediastinal large B cell lymphoma (PMLBCL) and classic Hodgkin lymphoma, nodular sclerosis type (NSHL)

Clinical presentation	Young adults
	Female predominance
	Mediastinal mass with involvement of thymus and supraclavicular nodes
	Localized disease (stages I–II)
Morphology	Fibrosis
	Cytologic overlap between Reed–Sternberg cells and tumor cells in PMLBCL
Immunophenotype	Absence or decreased expression of sIg and HLA
	CD30 expression
	MUM1 expression
Genetic features	Gain at 2p15: *REL* locus
	Gain at 9p24: *JAK2* locus
Molecular features	Decreased expression of the B cell receptor signaling pathway
	Constitutive NF-κB activation
	Activation of the cytokine-JAK-STAT pathway
	High expression of extracellular matrix elements
	Overexpression of the TNF family members
	Aberrant activation of tyrosine kinases and the PI3K/AKT pathway

Mediastinal gray zone lymphomas with features transitional between NSHL and PMLBCL
Composite and metachronous lymphomas in the same patient (clonal identity proven in some cases)

most frequent genetic abnormalities are gains in chromosomes 9p24 (in up to 75 percent of cases) and 2p (in about 50 percent of cases), including gains at the *JAK2* locus on 9p and *BCL11* and *REL* on 2p.[199–201] Other recurrent chromosomal gains are described at 2p, 6p, 7q, 9p, 12, and X. The 9p aberration is a chromosomal marker in PMLBCL, since it is very rare in other nodal and extranodal B cell lymphomas[200] but, interestingly, is detectable in about 25 percent of classic Hodgkin lymphoma.[202] In addition to chromosomal gains, recent array-comparative genomic hybridization (aGCH)-based studies have evidenced that recurrent genomic losses involving several chromosomes (1p, 3p, 4q, 6q, 7p, and 17p) also occur frequently in PMLBCL.[201,203]

Two studies have compared the gene-expression profiles of PMLBCL with those of DLBCL of other sites (Plate 57, see plate section).[191,204] Both groups found distinct gene expression patterns that were able to reliably diagnose PMLBCL and distinguish it from other DLBCLs. The PMLBCL signature included several genes previously reported to be expressed at high levels in this disease, including the cell-surface protein and lipid-raft component MAL, and the interleukin 4-induced gene. Interestingly, there were also striking similarities between the expression profile of PMLBCL and that of classic Hodgkin lymphoma, especially low levels of expression of multiple B cell signaling components and coreceptors and high expression of cytokine pathways components, tumor necrosis factor (TNF) family members, and extracellular matrix elements. These observations are of particular interest because both PMLBCL and the most common type of classic Hodgkin lymphoma, nodular sclerosis

Hodgkin lymphoma, have similar clinical presentations and overlapping morphologic, immunophenotypical and genetic features (Table 33.4). Evidence of activation of the NF-κB pathway, known to enhance the survival of Reed–Sternberg cells,[205] was also found in PMLBCL.[191] Moreover, NF-κB activation is also required for cell survival of a MLBL cell line,[72] suggesting that this may represent a shared survival pathway in PMLBCL and cHL. In classic Hodgkin lymphoma, several factors have been identified that may be involved causally in the activation of the NF-κB pathway, including amplifications of the *REL* locus at 2p, frequently present in Reed–Sternberg cells,[206–208] deleterious mutations in the IkBα gene in up to 30 percent of cases,[209,210] and expression of EBV-associated latent membrane protein 1 (LMP1).[211] Conversely, the mechanisms involved in activation of the NF-κB pathway in PMLBCL are poorly understood. It is unclear whether *REL* amplification is causally related, as there is imperfect correlation between nuclear REL accumulation, *REL* amplification and *REL* mRNA abundance.[72,192,212] Mutations of IkBα gene are not detected in PMLBCL.[213] Altered JAK/STAT signaling manifested by constitutive activation of STAT5 and STAT6, represents another alteration common to both PMLBCL and classic Hodgkin lymphoma,[214–217] frequently related to defective SOCS, as a consequence of gene deletion or deleterious mutations.[217,218] Aberrant tyrosine kinase activities (involving JAK2, RON and TIE tyrosine kinases not expressed in normal B cells) and activation of the PI3K/AKT pathway was recently identified as a further shared pathogenic mechanism in PMLBCL and classic Hodgkin lymphoma.[219]

The identification of a molecular link between PMLBCL and classic Hodgkin lymphoma also supports the hypothesis that there may be some pathogenic overlap between the two diseases. Mediastinal 'grey zone' lymphomas have been described, that represent a range of tumors having characteristics of both PMLBCL and HL.[182,220] Such cases may indicate that there is a spectrum of lymphomas along a continuum between PMLBCL and Hodgkin lymphoma.[221]

Clinically, PMLBCL is an aggressive lymphoma, and its relative responsiveness to treatment is controversial. Although PMLBCL was initially believed to carry a peculiar adverse prognostic,[222] other studies subsequently showed an overall survival rate similar to or higher than that of other DLBCLs.[176,223,224] Analyses of patients with PMLBCL treated before the advent of rituximab use suggest that the treatment has an overall failure rate of 40 percent.[225]

PRIMARY EFFUSION LYMPHOMA

Primary effusion lymphoma (PEL), originally identified in patients with acquired immune deficiency syndrome (AIDS) and described as 'body cavity-based lymphoma', is a neoplasm of large B cells usually presenting as effusions in serous cavities, generally with no formation of tumor masses. The majority of PELs occur exclusively as malignant effusions, but there are cases with concomitant or subsequent solid tissue involvement, that appear to be part of the same clinicopathologic spectrum. The tumor cells are characteristically infected by the Kaposi sarcoma-associated herpesvirus/HHV8 and most cases are coinfected with EBV.[226–228] The disease carries an adverse prognosis with a median survival of 6 months.[229]

Primary effusion lymphoma is composed of large pleomorphic cells with morphologic features bridging those of immunoblastic and anaplastic lymphoma (Fig. 33.5). The majority of PELs exhibit a distinctive immunophenotype: they express CD45 but lack expression of B cell antigens (CD19, CD20, CD79a, PAX5) and surface immunoglobulin and are positive for MUM1 and CD138 as well as for non-lineage-associated antigens (CD30, CD38, HLA-DR and EMA).[230,231]

Although the majority of PEL cases are coinfected by HHV8 and EBV, the studies on PEL pathogenesis highlight the role of HHV8.[232–234] The latency-associated nuclear antigen (LANA-1) is the only HHV8 gene consistently highly expressed, while lytic gene products are inconsistently expressed or absent. LANA1 plays a pivotal role in HHV8 episomal persistence in interacting with and influencing several cellular genes, thereby contributing to the growth of PEL cells, which require cytokines and factors from the host. In HIV-infected patients, in addition to systemic immunodeficiency a direct contribution to disease pathogenesis is exerted by the HIV protein Tat, which induces cellular and HHV8 genes that are pro-proliferative and proinflammatory. EBV infection does not appear to be determinant for PEL development, since expression of LMP1 and EBNA2,

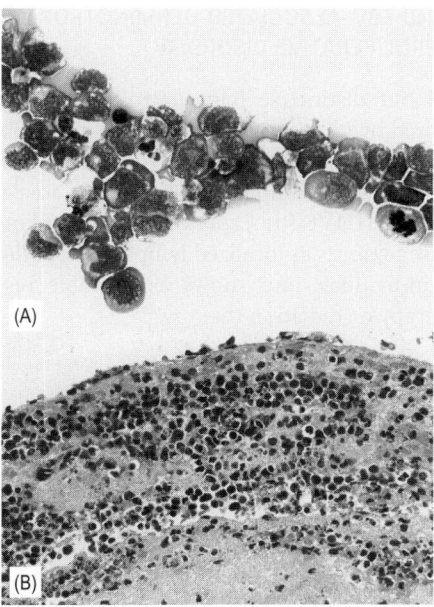

Figure 33.5   Primary effusion lymphoma. (A) Smear obtained from a pleural fluid showing large pleomorphic cells with abundant basophilic and sometimes vacuolated cytoplasm (×400). (B) Tissue section of a pleural biopsy (×200).

the major EBV growth transforming factors, is usually absent. Since EBV immortalizes B cells *in vitro* but HHV8 does not, EBV must play an important role as a cofactor in PEL development, but once these lymphomas develop, HHV8 appears to be the driving force.

PELs harbor clonally rearranged and mutated immunoglobulin genes whose sequences show evidence for antigen selection.[235] Gene expression profile studies have documented that PELs are more closely related to neoplastic plasma cells and EBV-positive immunoblasts than to other malignant B cells, suggesting a plasmablastic derivation.[236,237]

Other HHV8-positive lymphomas

LARGE B CELL LYMPHOMA ARISING IN HHV8-ASSOCIATED MULTICENTRIC CASTLEMAN DISEASE

This lymphoproliferation occurs in HIV-infected individuals with multicentric Castleman disease. It manifests in the mantle zones and interfollicular areas as clusters or sheets (microlymphomas) of large plasmablastic CD20+/– HHV8+ EBV– cells expressing cytoplasmic IgMλ and being either polyclonal or monoclonal.[238] These foci of microlymphoma may have a spontaneous smoldering evolution or progress toward an aggressive HHV8+ plasmablastic monoclonal lymphoma with massive nodal or splenic involvement or marked by a leukemic phase, and a short median survival.[239]

HHV8- AND EBV-ASSOCIATED GERMINOTROPIC LYMPHOPROLIFERATIVE DISORDER

This rare but distinctive lymphoproliferative disorder is characterized by oligoclonal or polyclonal plasmablasts that involve the germinal centers of the lymphoid follicles, forming confluent aggregates. These plasmablasts are positive for both EBV and HHV8 and express viral interleukin 6 (vIL6). The disease presents as localized lymphadenopathy in HIV-negative individuals and shows a favorable response to chemotherapy or radiation therapy.[240]

EXTRA–CAVITARY PELs

Recently there have been reports of HHV8-positive solid lymphomas presenting as extranodal masses with no associated effusions. Most cases occurred in HIV-positive individuals. These lymphomas exhibited a PEL-like morphology, and immunophenotypic and genotypic features similar to those of PELs, except for a slightly more frequent expression of B cell antigens and sIg (both positive in 25 percent of the cases). Thus, these HHV8-positive solid lymphomas are thought to belong to the spectrum of PEL and have been designated 'solid PELs' or 'extracavitary PELs'.[73,168]

DIFFUSE LARGE B CELL LYMPHOMA ASSOCIATED WITH CHRONIC INFLAMMATION

Pyothorax-associated lymphoma (PAL) is the prototypic form of a DLBCL occurring in the context of chronic inflammation and showing an association with EBV. PAL is a rare disease that develops in the pleural cavity of patients with a history of longstanding pyothorax. Most cases have been reported in Japan,[241–244] and only few cases in western countries.[245]

PAL affects elderly patients with a median age in the seventh decade and a strong male predominance (male/female ratio:12/1 in the largest Japanese series). The patients have a 30- to 40-year history of pyothorax or chronic pleuritis resulting from artificial pneumothorax for treatment of pulmonary tuberculosis or, less often, tuberculous pleuritis. Approximately two-thirds of patients have localized disease at diagnosis. The most common presenting symptoms are chest and/or back pain, fever and weight loss, while respiratory symptoms are less common. Imaging studies demonstrate a pleural-based tumor mass that often shows direct invasion to adjacent structures such as the chest wall and lung.

Histologically, PAL is similar to usual DLBCL, often of the immunoblastic type with frequent plasmacytoid or anaplastic features. Angiocentric or angioinvasive features with areas of necrosis are often observed (Plate 58A, B, see plate section).[245,246] The tumor cells are CD45+, variably express CD20 and are usually positive for CD79a (Plate 58C). They are negative for CD10 and BCL6, while they uniformly express MUM1 (Plate 58D) and variably express CD138, a phenotype suggestive of late GC/post-GC cells. Most cases are positive for BCL2. CD30 can be expressed. Aberrant coexpression of T cell-associated antigens (CD2, CD3 and/or CD4) has been reported in several cases. Some cases lack expression of lineage-specific antigens or express T cell-associated antigens only. Most cases contain a monoclonal form of the EBV DNA and display a type III latency phenotype, with expression of EBERs and EBNA2 and variable expression of LMP1 (Plate 58E).[247] In contrast with PEL, HHV8 has not been detected in most cases of PAL tested.[248,249] A comparison of the biologic and pathologic features of DLBCL associated with chronic inflammation and PEL is presented in Table 33.5.

Genetic alterations in PAL are not well characterized. PAL cell lines harbor complex karyotypes with numerical and multiple structural rearrangements.[250] *MYC* amplification appears to be frequent as it was found in 4/5 cases in a small study.[251] More than 70 percent of PAL cases have mutations in the *p53* gene. Molecular genetic studies usually demonstrate monoclonal *IGH* rearrangement and polyclonal T cell receptor gene rearrangement, even in cases with a dual B cell and T cell phenotype. PALs carry a high rate of somatic hypermutations without ongoing mutations of their *IG* genes, and in many cases the *IG* gene rearrangements appear to be nonproductive.[252,253] These findings indicate derivation from post-GC or crippled post-GC B cells which should be destined to death and might be rescued by EBV infection.[253] By gene expression profiling, the molecular signature of PAL differs from that of nodal DLBCL including differential expression of genes involved in apoptosis, interferon response and signal transduction.[254]

The disease mechanism of PAL has not yet been entirely clarified. The homogeneous clinicopathologic features of PAL suggest that chronic inflammation may promote the growth of the neoplastic B cells. The strong association with EBV and the viral gene expression pattern detected in most cases are features similar to those seen in post-transplant lymphoproliferative disorders, suggesting that a possibly localized immune defect may contribute to the development of PAL. Chronic inflammation may create a microenvironment that is less accessible to T cell immune surveillance, allowing the transformation of EBV-infected cells to proceed, and indeed the density of tumor-infiltrating T cells has been found to be significantly lower in PAL as compared to other nodal or extranodal DLBCL.[251] Chronic inflammation may also contribute to the development of PAL by providing local production of cytokines such as IL-6, that acts as a growth factor on PAL cell lines.[250] Conversely, the immunosuppressive cytokine IL-10 demonstrated produced *in vitro* by PAL cell lines may contribute to induce local immunosuppression.[255]

Occasional cases of EBV-positive lymphomas complicating long-standing chronic suppuration have been described in other extranodal sites (bone or joint lymphomas in the setting of chronic osteomyelitis or in association with metallic

Table 33.5 Comparison of body cavity lymphomas

	Primary effusion lymphoma	DLBCL associated with chronic inflammation
Clinical setting	AIDS patients	Chronic pyothorax/pleuritis
	Young to middle aged men	Elderly men
Presentation	Effusions in serous cavities, usually no tumor mass	Pleural-based tumor mass
Frequency	1–2% of AIDS NHLs	Overall rare: exceptional in Western countries, more frequent in Japan
Morphology	Large pleomorphic cells	DLBCL, immunoblastic
		Angiocentric features
		Abundant necrosis
HHV8	+	–
EBV	+	+
Immunophenotype		
CD45	+	+
B cell antigens	–	+/–
Ig expression	–	+/–
GC markers	–	–
Post-GC markers	+	+
T cell antigens	–	–/+ (CD2, CD3, CD4)
Non-lineage markers	CD30+ EMA+	CD30–
Genetic features	IGH rearrangement	IGH rearrangement
	IGH mutations	IGH mutations
		MYC amplification
Prognosis	Poor	Heterogeneous, 20–35% 5-year survival

AIDS, acquired immune deficiency syndrome; DLBCL, diffuse large B cell lymphoma; EBV, Epstein–Barr virus; GC, germinal center; HHV8, human herpes virus 8; NHL, non-Hodgkin lymphoma.

implants, and skin lymphoma in a patient with chronic venous ulcer), with clinical and pathologic features similar to those of PAL, and may be part of the same disease spectrum.[256,257]

The outcome of the disease is somewhat heterogeneous. The estimated 5-year survival rate ranges between 20 percent and 35 percent.[243,244] Adverse prognostic factors include advanced clinical stage, elevated lactate dehydrogenase (LDH) levels and the male sex.[244] Some patients may achieve durable remission with appropriate treatments.

INTRAVASCULAR LARGE B CELL LYMPHOMA

Intravascular large B cell lymphoma (IVLBCL) is a rare subtype of extranodal DLBCL characterized by a disseminated intravascular proliferation of lymphoma cells, involving small blood vessels, particularly capillaries, without an obvious extravascular tumor mass or leukemia.[258–260] This disease, first described in 1959 as angioendotheliomatosis proliferans and thought to be of endothelial origin,[261] has also been variously designated later as intravascular lymphomatosis and angiotropic lymphoma.[262] It is an aggressive and disseminated malignancy that affects elderly patients, without gender predominance. Patients present with a variety of symptoms related to organ dysfunction

secondary to vascular occlusion. B symptoms or fever constitute the dominant presenting feature in some patients. The skin and the brain are the most frequently involved organs, resulting in skin lesions (plaques or nodules) or variable neurologic symptoms according to the affected region of the brain (Fig. 33.6A). Lymph node involvement is rare. Bone marrow sinusoidal involvement is frequent, in association with hepatosplenic involvement and pancytopenia.[260] IVLBCL may also occur in association with solid tumors, for example carcinomas or hemangiomas.[263–265]

Cases of IVLBCL associated with an hemophagocytic syndrome (HPS) have been reported in Asian patients under the designation 'Asian variant of IVLBCL.' These cases are characterized by pancytopenia, hepatosplenomegaly and bone marrow involvement whereas they usually lack any neurologic or cutaneous abnormalities.[266–269]

Histologically (Fig. 33.6B, C), the neoplastic lymphoid cells are mainly lodged in the lumina of small vessels in many organs, and a limited perivascular infiltration is occasionally seen. Malignant cells are rarely seen in cerebrospinal fluid or blood. The tumor cells may resemble centroblasts or immunoblasts, and express B cell associated antigens CD19, CD20, CD79a and HLA-DR (Fig. 33.6D). In a subset of cases (30–40 percent) the B cells coexpress CD5.[269–271] Although many cases express BCL2, they usually lack the t(14;18) translocation.[271–274] Expression of BCL6 and CD10 is rather

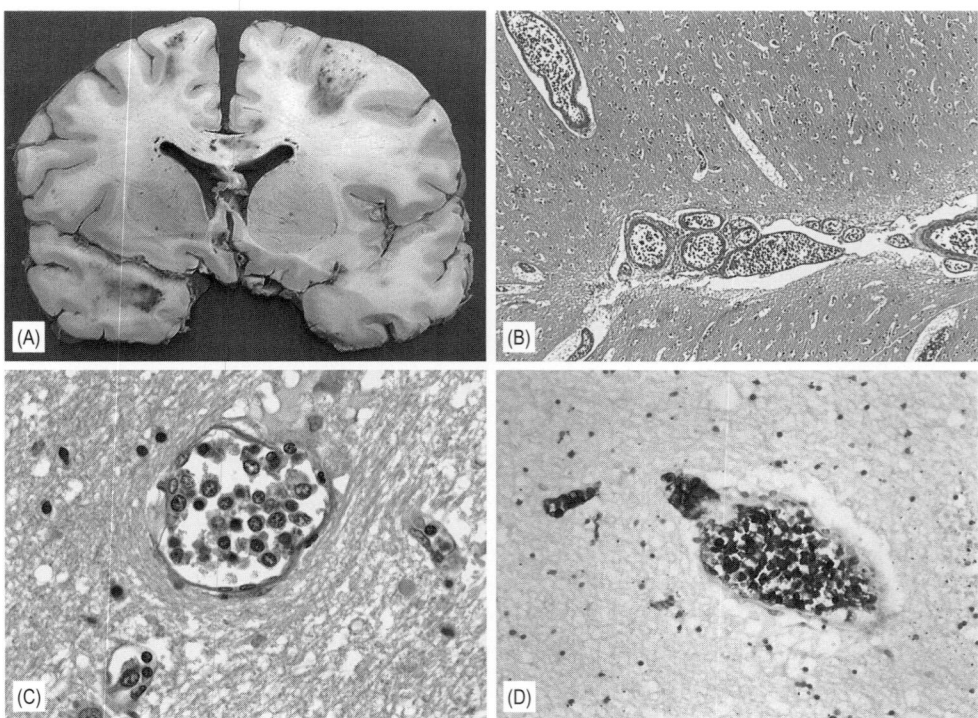

Figure 33.6 Intravascular large B cell lymphoma. (A) In this autopsy case, the brain displays numerous punctate hemorrhagic lesions in the cortex and the white matter. (B) The meningeal and cerebral vessels are filled with nucleated cells with no tissue extravasation (×50). (C) Large lymphoid cells occupy the vessel luminae (×400). (D) The intravascular cells stain for CD20 (immunoperoxidase, ×200).

infrequent whereas MUM1 expression is common.[272] Serum prostatic acid phosphatase (PAP) may be a tumor marker for IVLBCL, useful for the screening and assessment of disease activity and responses to treatment, the source of seric PAP likely being the intravascular lymphoma cells.[275] EBV appears to play no role in IVLBCL.

Karyotypic data have been reported in less than 20 cases, all of which harbored complex cytogenetic abnormalities.[269,273] Translocations involving common oncogenes implicated in B cell lymphoma (BCL1, BCL2, BCL6, MYC) have not been encountered. In one study 5/6 cases had hypermutated IG genes, suggesting an origin from post-GC cells.[276]

The mechanism responsible for the predilection of IVLBCL for blood vessels is not known. Defective expression of specific surface molecules, like CD29 and CD54, that are necessary for transvascular migration, has been incriminated in some cases.[277] It remains unclear whether there is any mechanistic relationship between CD5 expression, frequently reported in IVLBCL,[259,270,271] and the intravascular localization of the tumor cells.

Accurate and timely diagnosis of IVLBCL is still a problematic issue, and many cases are diagnosed at autopsy. If a timely diagnosis is made and chemotherapy instituted, complete or partial response is observed in more than half of the patients, and long-term survival appears to be possible, but overall survival is disappointing (around 33 percent at 3 years), with a relevant impact of diagnostic delay

and lethal complications.[260,278] Improved clinical outcomes are reported in patients treated by rituximab in addition to chemotherapy.[279] IVLBCL patients with disease limited to the skin at presentation ('cutaneous variant') have a much more favorable clinical behavior, especially in cases with a single lesion.[260]

EBV-POSITIVE DIFFUSE LARGE B CELL LYMPHOMAS

EBV infection is implicated in several lymphoid malignancies in both immunocompromised and immunocompetent individuals. EBV-positive lymphoproliferations composed of large B cells fall into several entities (Table 33.6). In addition to those already described earlier in this chapter, two additional EBV-associated DLBCL entities will be discussed: EBV-positive DLBCL occurring in elderly patients and lymphomatoid granulomatosis.

EBV-positive DLBCL of the elderly

Age-related EBV-positive DLBCL occurs in elderly patients (over 50 years, median eighth decade) without HIV infection or any known immune deficiency syndrome.[279–282] It is believed to be related to the deterioration of the immune function caused by immune senescence. The disease presents in lymph nodes or more commonly in

Table 33.6 Large B cell lymphoproliferations associated with Epstein–Barr virus (EBV) infection

In the setting of systemic immunodeficiency	
EBV+ diffuse large B cell lymphoma (DLBCL)	Congenital immunodeficiency syndromes
	Human immunodeficiency virus (HIV) infection
	Post-transplantation lymphoproliferative disorder
	Autoimmune disease ± methotrexate therapy
Plasmablastic lymphoma	HIV infection
Primary effusion lymphoma (PEL)	HIV infection
Extracavitary/solid PEL	HIV infection
Lymphomatoid granulomatosis	Congenital immunodeficiency syndromes, HIV infection
	post-transplantation
	Reduced immune function of uncertain cause
In the setting of presumably compromised immune function	
Pyothorax-associated lymphoma (PAL)	Chronic pyothorax, local immune compromise
EBV + DLBCL of the elderly	Elderly patients, immune senescence
In immunocompetent individuals	
HHV8 + EBV+ germinotropic lymphoproliferative disorder	

HHV8, human herpes virus 8.

various extranodal sites (skin, tonsil, stomach). The disease appears as a monomorphous large-cell lymphoproliferation or commonly as a polymorphous infiltrate including a variable inflammatory background. Reed–Sternberg-like cells are commonly seen and may be numerous. Angiocentricity and extensive necrosis are frequent. The tumor cells express CD20 and CD79a, are positive for EBERs, LMP1 and EBNA2, and variably express CD30 but are negative for CD15. The differential diagnosis with EBV+ classical Hodgkin lymphoma may be difficult. The clinical course is inferior to that of patients with EBV-negative DLBCLs. The presence of B symptoms and age older than 70 represent additional adverse prognostic factors.

Lymphomatoid granulomatosis

Lymphomatoid granulomatosis (LYG) was first described by Liebow *et al.* as a rare and unique angiocentric and angiodestructive lymphoproliferative process in the lungs,[283] represents an EBV-positive B cell proliferation associated with an exuberant T cell reaction.[284–287] Lymphomatoid granulomatosis encompasses a spectrum of histologic grades (1–3) and clinical aggressiveness related to the proportion of EBV-positive large B cells, with grade 3 lesions being assimilated to EBV-positive DLBCL.

Lymphomatoid granulomatosis affects patients of all ages, often between the fourth and sixth decades, with a slight male predominance.[288] Patients typically present with lung involvement and respiratory symptoms, mostly cough and dyspnea, and multiple bilateral nodular opacities predominating in the lower lobes on chest X-ray.[289] The central nervous system, kidneys, skin and subcutaneous tissue are also commonly involved.[290] Lymphoid organs are usually strikingly spared. Immunosuppression is a predisposing factor. The lesions may occur in the setting of

HIV, post-transplantation and in patients receiving iatrogenic immunosuppression for other disorders (steroids, methotrexate).[291]

Histologically, LYG consists of a polymorphous cellular infiltrate including lymphocytes, histiocytes, plasma cells and varying numbers of large atypical lymphoid cells, exhibiting an angioinvasive pattern (particularly affecting muscle veins and arterioles) with or without associated infarct-type necrosis (Fig. 33.7, A–C). The vascular tropism of the infiltrate; the cellular infiltrate is mainly parietal, raising the endothelium, but superimposed thrombosis is rare.[283] The large atypical cells are CD45+ CD20+ B cells expressing EBERs, LMP1 and EBNA2 (Fig. 33.7D).[284,287,292,293] Variable loss of CD20 expression may be seen, possibly as a consequence of EBV-induced downregulation.[294] Coexpression of CD43 by the B cells has been shown in some cases.[287] CD30 antigen expression is sometimes found.[295] The smaller lymphocytes consist mostly of CD3+ T cells, predominantly CD4-positive.[296,297] LYG is graded (1–3) according to the number of large B cells.[298] The average B cell proliferation index correlates with grade and in is similar to that of DLBCL in grade 3 lesions.[294] The ability to demonstrate monoclonal *IGH* gene rearrangement by PCR correlates closely with histologic grade and the proportion of EBV-positive cells, and analysis for T cell receptor γ-chain gene rearrangements is usually negative.[284,290] The nature of genetic alterations in LYG is unknown.

The pathologic and clinical features of LYG are somewhat related to those of post-transplant or HIV-associated EBV-positive lymphoproliferative disorders, and the pattern of viral protein expression in these diseases is similar. An important distinction lies in the abundant associated reactive T cell-rich background in LYG. The factor(s) driving the prominent T cell background in LYG are unknown, but the low proliferation index of reactive cells in LYG probably indicates recruitment from the circulation.[294]

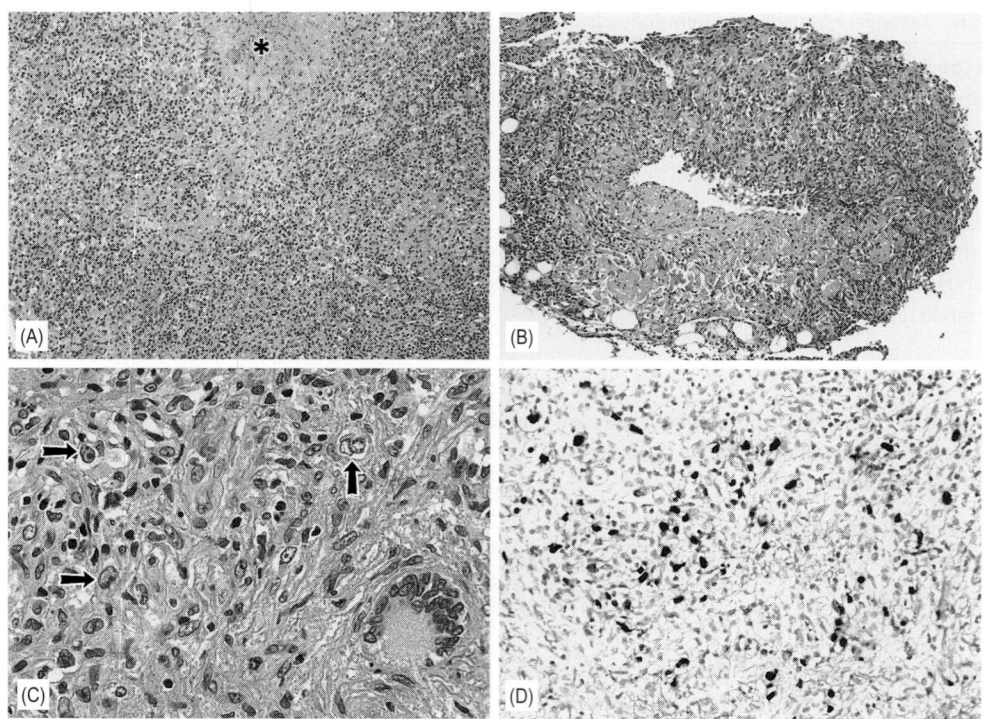

Figure 33.7 Lymphomatoid granulomatosis. (A) Lymphomatoid granulomatosis consists of a polymorphic lymphohistiocytic infiltrate with foci of necrosis (*) and a vaguely granulomatous appearance (×100). (B) There is destructive infiltration of the walls of arterial vessels without superimposed thrombosis (×100). (C) Scattered large atypical lymphoid cells (arrow) are dispersed among a reactive lymphohistiocytic infiltrate (×400). (D) The large lymphoid cells are positive for Epstein–Barr virus-encoded RNAs (EBERs) (*in situ* hybridization, ×200).

The chemokines interferon γ-inducible protein-10 (IP-10) and the monokine induced by interferon γ (Mig), which are induced by EBV, are overexpressed by reactive cells in LYG lesions and have been implicated in mediating the tissue necrosis and vascular damage in pulmonary LYG. These agents inhibit angiogenesis, promote T cell adhesion to endothelial cells and directly damage the endothelium. IP-10 is also increased in the serum of patients with LYG, suggesting that it could also act at distant sites.[299]

Grade 3 LYG cases fulfill the criteria for DLBCL in a T cell rich background, and may be clinically aggressive. The efficacy of rituximab for the treatment of LYG lesions has been reported recently in a few cases.[300,301]

somatic hypermutations targeting *BCL6*, *BCL2* and *cMYC* protooncogenes.
- Several molecular markers may aid at prognosticating outcome for individual patients.
- Primary mediastinal large B cell lymphoma displays clinical, pathologic and molecular features which are distinct from those of non-mediastinal diffuse large B cell and which bear a resemblance to Hodgkin lymphoma, nodular sclerosis type, another lymphoma frequently involving the mediastinum.

KEY POINTS

- DLBCL represents a heterogeneous group of neoplasms, including morphologic and phenotypic variants, molecular and immunophenotypic subgroups, subtypes and clinicopathologic entities.
- Most DLBCLs derive from antigen-experienced B cells, the most common genetic lesions identified are chromosomal translocations and

REFERENCES

● = Key primary paper
◆ = Major review article

1. Anderson JR, Armitage JO, Weisenburger DD. Epidemiology of the non-Hodgkin's lymphomas: distributions of the major subtypes differ by geographic locations. Non-Hodgkin's lymphoma classification project. *Ann Oncol* 1998; **9**: 717–20.
◆2. Coiffier B. State-of-the-art therapeutics: diffuse large B-cell lymphoma. *J Clin Oncol* 2005; **23**: 6387–93.

3. Swerdlow SH, Campo E, Harris NL. *et al. WHO classification of tumours of haematopoietic and lymphoid tissues.* Lyon: IARC Press, 2008.

4. Pettit CK, Zukerberg LR, Gray MH *et al.* Primary lymphoma of bone. A B-cell neoplasm with a high frequency of multilobated cells. *Am J Surg Pathol* 1990; **14**: 329–34.

5. Harris NL, Jaffe ES, Stein H *et al.* A revised European-American classification of lymphoid neoplasms: a proposal from the International Lymphoma Study Group. *Blood* 1994; **84**: 1361–92.

6. Engelhard M, Brittinger G, Huhn D *et al.* Subclassification of diffuse large B-cell lymphomas according to the Kiel classification: distinction of centroblastic and immunoblastic lymphomas is a significant prognostic risk factor. *Blood* 1997; **89**: 2291–7.

7. Fernandez de Sevilla S, Romagosa V, Domingo-Claros A *et al.* Diffuse large B-cell lymhpoma: is morphologic subdivision useful in clinical management? *Eur J Haematol* 1998; **60**: 202–08.

8. Armitage JO, Weisenburger DD. New approach to classifying non-Hodgkin's lymphomas: clinical features of the major histologic subtypes. Non-Hodgkin's lymphoma classification project. *J Clin Oncol* 1998; **16**: 2780–95.

9. Baars JW, de Jong D, Willemse EM *et al.* Diffuse large B-cell non-Hodgkin lymphomas: the clinical relevance of histological subclassification. *Br J Cancer* 1999; **79**: 1770–6.

10. Lai R, Medeiros LJ, Dabbagh L *et al.* Sinusoidal CD30-positive large B-cell lymphoma: a morphologic mimic of anaplastic large cell lymphoma. *Mod Pathol* 2000; **13**: 223–8.

11. Diebold J, Anderson JR, Armitage JO *et al.* Diffuse large B-cell lymphoma: a clinicopathologic analysis of 444 cases classified according to the updated Kiel classification. *Leuk Lymphoma* 2002; **43**: 97–104.

12. Kremer M, Spitzer M, Mandl-Weber S *et al.* Discordant bone marrow involvement in diffuse large B-cell lymphoma: comparative molecular analysis reveals a heterogeneous group of disorders. *Lab Invest* 2003; **83**: 107–14.

13. Fisher DE, Jacobson JO, Ault KA, Harris NL. Diffuse large cell lymphoma with discordant bone marrow histology. Clinical features and biological implications. *Cancer* 1989; **64**: 1879–87.

14. Cabanillas F, Velasquez WS, Hagemeister FB *et al.* Clinical, biologic, and histologic features of late relapses in diffuse large cell lymphoma. *Blood* 1992; **79**: 1024–8.

15. Knowles D. Immunophenotypic markers useful in the diagnosis and classification of hematopoietic neoplasms. In: Knowles D. (ed.) *Neoplastic hematopathology.* Philadelphia: Lippincott Williams & Wilkins, 2001: 93–226.

16. Torlakovic E, Torlakovic G, Nguyen P *et al.* The value of anti-Pax-5 immunostaining in routinely fixed and paraffin-embedded sections. A novel pan pre-B and B-cell marker. *Am J Surg Pathol* 2002; **26**: 1143–50.

17. Coiffier B. Rituximab in the treatment of diffuse large B-cell lymphomas. *Semin Oncol* 2002; **29**: 30–5.

18. Davis T, Czerwinski K, Levy R. Therapy of B-cell lymphoma with anti-CD20 antibodies can result in the loss of CD20 antigen expression. *Clin Cancer Res* 1999; **5**: 611–15.

19. Hall P, Richards M, Gregory W *et al.* The prognostic value of Ki67 immunostaining in non-Hodgkin's lymphoma. *J Pathol* 1988; **154**: 223–35.

20. Pezzella F, Tse AG, Cordell JL *et al.* Expression of the bcl-2 oncogene protein is not specific for the 14;18 chromosomal translocation. *Am J Pathol* 1990; **137**: 225–32.

21. Piris M, Pezella F, Martinez-Montero J *et al.* p53 and bcl-2 expression in high-grade B-cell lymphomas: correlation with survival time. *Br J Cancer* 1994; **69**: 337–41.

22. Skinnider BF, Horsman DE, Dupuis B, Gascoyne RD. Bcl-6 and Bcl-2 protein expression in diffuse large B-cell lymphoma and follicular lymphoma: correlation with 3q27 and 18q21 chromosomal abnormalities. *Hum Pathol* 1999; **30**: 803–8.

23. Rantanen S, Monni O, Joensuu H *et al.* Causes and consequences of bcl2 overexpression in diffuse large B-cell lymphoma. *Leuk Lymphoma* 2001; **42**: 1089–98.

24. Seyfert VL, Allman D, He Y, Staudt LM. Transcriptional repression by the proto-oncogene BCL-6. *Oncogene* 1996; **12**: 2331–42.

25. Onizuka T, Moriyama M, Yamochi T *et al.* BCL-6 gene product, a 92- to 98-kD nuclear phosphoprotein, is highly expressed in germinal center B cells and their neoplastic counterparts. *Blood* 1995; **86**: 28–37.

26. Dogan A, Bagdi E, Munson P, Isaacson P. CD10 and bcl-6 expression in paraffin sections of normal lymphoid tissue and B-cell lymphomas. *Am J Surg Pathol* 2000; **24**: 846–52.

27. Colomo L, Lopez-Guillermo A, Perales M *et al.* Clinical impact of the differentiation profile assessed by immunophenotyping in patients with diffuse large B-cell lymphoma. *Blood* 2003; **101**: 78–84.

28. McIntosh GG, Lodge AJ, Watson P *et al.* NCL-CD10-270: a new monoclonal antibody recognizing CD10 in paraffin-embedded tissue. *Am J Pathol* 1999; **154**: 77–82.

29. Harada S, Suzuki R, Uehira K *et al.* Molecular and immunological dissection of diffuse large B cell lymphoma: CD5+, and CD5− with CD10+ groups may constitute clinically relevant subtypes. *Leukemia* 1999; **13**: 1441–7.

30. King B, Chen C, Locker J *et al.* Immunophenotypic and genotypic markers of follicular center cell neoplasia in diffuse large B-cell lymphoma. *Mod Pathol* 2000; **13**: 1219–31.

31. Falini B, Fizzotti M, Pucciarini A *et al.* A monoclonal antibody (MUM1p) detects expression of the MUM1/IRF4 protein in a subset of germinal center B cells, plasma cells, and activated T cells. *Blood* 2000; **95**: 2084–92.

32. Natkunam Y, Warnke R, Montgomery K *et al.* Analysis of MUM1/IRF4 protein expression using tissue microarrays and immunohistochemistry. *Mod Pathol* 2001; **14**: 686–94.

33. Banham AH, Turley H, Pulford K *et al.* The plasma cell associated antigen detectable by antibody VS38 is the p63 rough endoplasmic reticulum protein. *J Clin Pathol* 1997; **50**: 485–9.

34. Sanderson RD, Lalor P, Bernfield M. B lymphocytes express and lose syndecan at specific stages of differentiation. *Cell Regul* 1989; **1**: 27–35.

35. Yamaguchi M, Seto M, Okamoto M *et al.* De novo CD5+ diffuse large B-cell lymphoma: a clinicopathologic study of 109 patients. *Blood* 2002; **99**: 815–21.

◆36. Kuppers R, Klein U, Hansmann ML, Rajewsky K. Cellular origin of human B-cell lymphomas. *N Engl J Med* 1999; **341**: 1520–9.

37. Ohshima K, Kawasaki C, Muta K *et al.* CD10 and Bcl10 expression in diffuse large B-cell lymphoma: CD10 is a marker of improved prognosis. *Histopathology* 2001; **39**: 156–62.

38. Chaganti RS, Nanjangud G, Schmidt H, Teruya-Feldstein J. Recurring chromosomal abnormalities in non-Hodgkin's lymphoma: biologic and clinical significance. *Semin Hematol* 2000; **37**: 396–411.

39. Bea S, Colomo L, Lopez-Guillermo A *et al.* Clinicopathologic significance and prognostic value of chromosomal imbalances in diffuse large B-cell lymphomas. *J Clin Oncol* 2004; **22**: 3498–506.

◆40. Pasqualucci L, Bereschenko O, Niu H *et al.* Molecular pathogenesis of non-Hodgkin's lymphoma: the role of Bcl-6. *Leuk Lymphoma* 2003; **44**(Suppl 3): s5–12.

●41. Iqbal J, Greiner TC, Patel K *et al.* Distinctive patterns of BCL6 molecular alterations and their functional consequences in different subgroups of diffuse large B-cell lymphoma. *Leukemia* 2007; **21**: 2332–43.

42. Pasqualucci L, Migliazza A, Basso K *et al.* Mutations of the BCL6 proto-oncogene disrupt its negative autoregulation in diffuse large B-cell lymphoma. *Blood* 2003; **101**: 2914–23.

43. Ye BH, Cattoretti G, Shen Q *et al.* The BCL-6 proto-oncogene controls germinal-centre formation and Th2- type inflammation. *Nat Genet* 1997; **16**: 161–70.

44. Dent A, Vasanwala F, Toney L. Regulation of gene expression by the proto-oncogene BCL-6. *Crit Rev Oncol Hematol* 2002; **41**: 1–9.

45. Phan RT, Dalla-Favera R. The BCL6 proto-oncogene suppresses p53 expression in germinal-centre B cells. *Nature* 2004; **432**: 635–9.

46. Ye BH, Lista F, Lo Coco F *et al.* Alterations of a zinc finger-encoding gene, BCL-6, in diffuse large-cell lymphoma. *Science* 1993; **262**: 747–50.

47. Lo Coco F, Ye BH, Lista F *et al.* Rearrangements of the BCL6 gene in diffuse large cell non-Hodgkin's lymphoma. *Blood* 1994; **83**: 1757–9.

48. Bastard C, Deweindt C, Kerckaert JP *et al.* LAZ3 rearrangements in non-Hodgkin's lymphoma: correlation with histology, immunophenotype, karyotype, and clinical outcome in 217 patients. *Blood* 1994; **83**: 2423–7.

49. Pescarmona E, De Sanctis V, Pistilli A *et al.* Pathogenetic and clinical implications of Bcl-6 and Bcl-2 gene configuration in nodal diffuse large B-cell lymphomas. *J Pathol* 1997; **183**: 281–6.

50. Kramer MH, Hermans J, Wijburg E *et al.* Clinical relevance of BCL2, BCL6, and MYC rearrangements in diffuse large B-cell lymphoma. *Blood* 1998; **92**: 3152–62.

51. Jerkeman M, Aman P, Cavallin-Stahl E *et al.* Prognostic implications of BCL6 rearrangement in uniformly treated patients with diffuse large B cell lymphoma – a Nordic Lymphoma Group study. *Int J Oncol* 2002; **20**: 161–5.

52. Barrans S, O'Connor S, Evans P *et al.* Rearrangement of the BCL6 locus at 3q27 is an independent poor prognostic factor in nodal diffuse large B-cell lymphoma. *Br J Haematol* 2002; **117**: 322–32.

53. Niitsu N, Okamoto M, Nakamura N *et al.* Prognostic impact of chromosomal alteration of 3q27 on nodal B-cell lymphoma: correlation with histology, immunophenotype, karyotype, and clinical outcome in 329 consecutive patients. *Leuk Res* 2007; **31**: 1191–7.

54. Ueda C, Akasaka T, Ohno H. Non-immunoglobulin/BCL6 gene fusion in diffuse large B-cell lymphoma: prognostic implications. *Leuk Lymphoma* 2002; **43**: 1375–81.

55. Jacobson J, Wilkes B, Kwaiatkowski D *et al.* Bcl-2 rearrangements in de novo diffuse large cell lymphoma. Association with distinctive clinical features. *Cancer* 1993; **72**: 231–6.

56. Rao PH, Houldsworth J, Dyomina K *et al.* Chromosomal and gene amplification in diffuse large B-cell lymphoma. *Blood* 1998; **92**: 234–40.

57. Monni O, Joensuu H, Franssila K *et al.* BCL2 overexpression associated with chromosomal amplification in diffuse large B-cell lymphoma. *Blood* 1997; **90**: 1168–74.

●58. Hermine O, Haioun C, Lepage E *et al.* Prognostic significance of bcl-2 protein expression in aggressive non-Hodgkin's lymphoma. Groupe d'Etude des Lymphomes de l'Adulte (GELA). *Blood* 1996; **87**: 265–72.

59. Hill ME, MacLennan KA, Cunningham DC *et al.* Prognostic significance of BCL-2 expression and bcl-2 major breakpoint region rearrangement in diffuse large cell non-Hodgkin's lymphoma: a British National Lymphoma Investigation Study. *Blood* 1996; **88**: 1046–51.

60. Gascoyne RD, Adomat SA, Krajewski S *et al.* Prognostic significance of Bcl-2 protein expression and Bcl-2 gene rearrangement in diffuse aggressive non-Hodgkin's lymphoma. *Blood* 1997; **90**: 244–51.

●61. Yunis JJ, Mayer MG, Arnesen MA *et al.* bcl-2 and other genomic alterations in the prognosis of large-cell lymphoma. *N Engl J Med* 1989; **320**: 1047–54.

62. Au WY, Horsman DE, Gascoyne RD *et al.* The spectrum of lymphoma with 8q24 aberrations: a clinical, pathological and cytogenetic study of 87 consecutive cases. *Leuk Lymphoma* 2004; **45**: 519–28.

●63. Hummel M, Bentink S, Berger H *et al.* A biologic definition of Burkitt's lymphoma from transcriptional and genomic profiling. *N Engl J Med* 2006; **354**: 2419–30.

64. Le Gouill S, Talmant P, Touzeau C *et al.* The clinical presentation and prognosis of diffuse large B-cell lymphoma with t(14;18) and 8q24/c-MYC rearrangement. *Haematologica* 2007; **92**: 1335–42.

65. Pasqualucci L, Migliazza A, Fracchiolla N *et al.* BCL-6 mutations in normal germinal center B cells: evidence of somatic hypermutation acting outside Ig loci. *Proc Natl Acad Sci U S A* 1998; **95**: 11816–21.

66. Muschen M, Rajewsky K, Kronke M, Kuppers R. The origin of CD95-gene mutations in B-cell lymphoma. *Trends Immunol* 2002; **23**: 75–80.

●67. Pasqualucci L, Neumeister P, Goossens T *et al.* Hypermutation of multiple proto-oncogenes in B-cell diffuse large-cell lymphomas. *Nature* 2001; **412**: 341–6.

68. Wilson W, Teruya-Feldstein J, Fest T *et al.* Relationship of p53, bcl-2, and tumor proliferation to clinical drug resistance in non-Hodgkin's lymphomas. *Blood* 1997; **89**: 601–9.

●69. Ichikawa A, Kinoshita T, Watanabe T *et al.* Mutations of the p53 gene as a prognostic factor in aggressive B-cell lymphoma. *N Engl J Med* 1997; **337**: 529–34.

●70. Davis RE, Brown KD, Siebenlist U, Staudt LM. Constitutive nuclear factor kappaB activity is required for survival of activated B cell-like diffuse large B cell lymphoma cells. *J Exp Med* 2001; **194**: 1861–74.

71. Houldsworth J, Olshen AB, Cattoretti G *et al.* Relationship between REL amplification, REL function, and clinical and biologic features in diffuse large B-cell lymphomas. *Blood* 2004; **103**: 1862–8.

●72. Feuerhake F, Kutok JL, Monti S *et al.* NFκB activity, function, and target-gene signatures in primary mediastinal large B-cell lymphoma and diffuse large B-cell lymphoma subtypes. *Blood* 2005; **106**: 1392–9.

73. Carbone A, Gloghini A, Vaccher E *et al.* Kaposi's sarcoma-associated herpesvirus/human herpesvirus type 8-positive solid lymphomas: a tissue-based variant of primary effusion lymphoma. *J Mol Diagn* 2005; **7**: 17–27.

◆74. Abramson JS, Shipp MA. Advances in the biology and therapy of diffuse large B-cell lymphoma: moving toward a molecularly targeted approach. *Blood* 2005; **106**: 1164–74.

●75. Alizadeh AA, Eisen MB, Davis RE *et al.* Distinct types of diffuse large B-cell lymphoma identified by gene expression profiling. *Nature* 2000; **403**: 503–11.

76. Rosenwald A, Wright G, Chan WC *et al.* The use of molecular profiling to predict survival after chemotherapy for diffuse large-B-cell lymphoma. *N Engl J Med* 2002; **346**: 1937–47.

77. Nanjangud G, Rao PH, Hegde A *et al.* Spectral karyotyping identifies new rearrangements, translocations, and clinical associations in diffuse large B-cell lymphoma. *Blood* 2002; **99**: 2554–61.

78. Huang JZ, Sanger WG, Greiner TC *et al.* The t(14;18) defines a unique subset of diffuse large B-cell lymphoma with a germinal center B-cell gene expression profile. *Blood* 2002; **99**: 2285–90.

79. Pasqualucci L, Compagno M, Houldsworth J *et al.* Inactivation of the PRDM1/BLIMP1 gene in diffuse large B cell lymphoma. *J Exp Med* 2006; **203**: 311–17.

80. Tam W, Gomez M, Chadburn A *et al.* Mutational analysis of PRDM1 indicates a tumor-suppressor role in diffuse large B-cell lymphomas. *Blood* 2006; **107**: 4090–100.

81. Bea S, Zettl A, Wright G *et al.* Diffuse large B-cell lymphoma subgroups have distinct genetic profiles that influence tumor biology and improve gene expression-based survival prediction. *Blood* 2005; **106**: 3183–90.

82. Lam LT, Davis RE, Pierce J *et al.* Small molecule inhibitors of IkappaB kinase are selectively toxic for subgroups of diffuse large B-cell lymphoma defined by gene expression profiling. *Clin Cancer Res* 2005; **11**: 28–40.

83. Ngo VN, Davis RE, Lamy L *et al.* A loss-of-function RNA interference screen for molecular targets in cancer. *Nature* 2006; **441**: 106–10.

84. Lam LT, Wright G, Davis RE *et al.* Cooperative signaling through the signal transducer and activator of transcription 3 and nuclear factor-κB pathways in subtypes of diffuse large B-cell lymphoma. *Blood* 2008; **111**: 3701–13.

85. Lossos IS, Alizadeh AA, Eisen MB *et al.* Ongoing immunoglobulin somatic mutation in germinal center B cell-like but not in activated B cell-like diffuse large cell lymphomas. *Proc Natl Acad Sci U S A* 2000; **97**: 10209–13.

86. Lu X, Nechushtan H, Ding F *et al.* Distinct IL-4-induced gene expression, proliferation, and intracellular signaling in germinal center B-cell-like and activated B-cell-like diffuse large-cell lymphomas. *Blood* 2005; **105**: 2924–32.

●87. Monti S, Savage KJ, Kutok JL *et al.* Molecular profiling of diffuse large B-cell lymphoma identifies robust subtypes including one characterized by host inflammatory response. *Blood* 2005; **105**: 1851–61.

●88. A predictive model for aggressive non-Hodgkin's lymphoma. The international non-Hodgkin's lymphoma prognostic factors project. *N Engl J Med* 1993; **329**: 987–94.

89. de Leval L, Harris NL. Variability in immunophenotype in diffuse large B-cell lymphoma and its clinical relevance. *Histopathology* 2003; **43**: 509–28.

◆90. Lossos IS, Morgensztern D. Prognostic biomarkers in diffuse large B-cell lymphoma. *J Clin Oncol* 2006; **24**: 995–1007.

91. Coiffier B. Rituximab therapy in malignant lymphoma. *Oncogene* 2007; **26**: 3603–13.

92. Sehn LH, Berry B, Chhanabhai M *et al.* The revised International Prognostic Index (R-IPI) is a better predictor of outcome than the standard IPI for patients with diffuse large B-cell lymphoma treated with R-CHOP. *Blood* 2007; **109**: 1857–61.

93. Mounier N, Briere J, Gisselbrecht C *et al.* Rituximab plus CHOP (R-CHOP) overcomes bcl-2–associated resistance to chemotherapy in elderly patients with diffuse large B-cell lymphoma (DLBCL). *Blood* 2003; **101**: 4279–84.

94. Miller T, Lippman S, Spier C *et al.* HLA-DR (Ia) immune phenotype predicts outcome for patients with diffuse large cell lymphoma. *J Clin Invest* 1988; **82**: 370–2.

95. Riemersma S, Jordanova E, Schop R *et al.* Extensive genetic alterations of the HLA region, including homozygous deletions of HLA class II genes in B-cell lymphomas arising in immune-privileged sites. *Blood* 2000; **96**: 3569–73.

96. Rimsza LM, Roberts RA, Miller TP *et al.* Loss of MHC class II gene and protein expression in diffuse large B-cell lymphoma is related to decreased tumor immunosurveillance and poor patient survival regardless of other prognostic factors: a follow-up study from the

Leukemia and Lymphoma Molecular Profiling Project. *Blood* 2004; **103**: 4251–8.

97. Lippman S, Spier C, Miller T *et al.* Tumor-infiltrating T-lymphocytes in B-cell diffuse large cell lymphoma related to disease course. *Mod Pathol* 1990; **3**: 361–7.

98. Stopeck A, Gessner A, Miller T *et al.* Loss of B7.2 (CD86) and intercellular adhesion molecule 1 (CD54) expression is associated with decreased tumor-infiltrating T lymphocytes in diffuse B-cell large-cell lymphoma. *Clin Cancer Res* 2000; **6**: 3904–9.

99. Ansell S, Stenson M, Habermann T *et al.* CD4+ T-cell immune response to large B-cell non-Hodgkin's lymphoma predicts patient outcome. *J Clin Oncol* 2001; **19**: 720–6.

100. Xu Y, Kroft S, McKenna R, Aquino D. Prognostic significance of tumour-infiltrating lymphocytes and T-cell subsets in de novo diffuse large B-cell lymhpoma: a multiparametric flow cytometry study. *Br J Haematol* 2000; **112**: 945–9.

101. Miller T, Grogan T, Dahlberg S *et al.* Prognostic significance of the KI-67-associated proliferative antigen in aggressive non-Hodgkin's lymphomas: a prospective Southwest Oncology Group trial. *Blood* 1994; **83**: 1460–6.

102. Sanchez E, Chacon I, Plaza MM *et al.* Clinical outcome in diffuse large B-cell lymphoma is dependent on the relationship between different cell-cycle regulator proteins. *J Clin Oncol* 1998; **16**: 1931–9.

103. Saez AI, Saez AJ, Artiga MJ *et al.* Building an outcome predictor model for diffuse large B-cell lymphoma. *Am J Pathol* 2004; **164**: 613–22.

104. Leroy K, Haioun C, Lepage E *et al.* p53 gene mutations are associated with poor survival in low and low-intermediate risk diffuse large B-cell lymphoma. *Ann Oncol* 2002; **13**: 1108–15.

105. Barrans SL, Carter I, Owen RG *et al.* Germinal center phenotype and bcl-2 expression combined with the International Prognostic Index improves patient risk stratification in diffuse large B-cell lymphoma. *Blood* 2002; **99**: 1136–43.

106. Adida C, Haioun C, Gaulard P *et al.* Prognostic significance of survivin expression in diffuse large B-cell lymphoma. *Blood* 2000; **96**: 1921–5.

107. Lesley J, Hyman R, Kincade PW. CD44 and its interaction with extracellular matrix. *Adv Immunol* 1993; **54**: 271–335.

108. Salles G, Zain M, Jiang WM *et al.* Alternatively spliced CD44 transcripts in diffuse large-cell lymphomas: characterization and comparison with normal activated B cells and epithelial malignancies. *Blood* 1993; **82**: 3539–47.

109. Drillenburg P, Pals S. Cell adhesion molecules in lymphoma dissemination. *Blood* 2000; **95**: 1900–10.

110. Pals ST, Horst E, Ossekoppele GJ *et al.* Expression of lymphocyte homing receptor as a mechanism of dissemination in non-Hodgkin's lymphoma. *Blood* 1989; **73**: 885–8.

111. Horst E, Meijer CJ, Radaskiewicz T *et al.* Expression of a human homing receptor (CD44) in lymphoid malignancies and related stages of lymphoid development. *Leukemia* 1990; **4**: 383–9.

112. Drillenburg P, Wielenga VJ, Kramer MH *et al.* CD44 expression predicts disease outcome in localized large B cell lymphoma. *Leukemia* 1999; **13**: 1448–55.

113. Tzankov A, Pehrs AC, Zimpfer A *et al.* Prognostic significance of CD44 expression in diffuse large B cell lymphoma of activated and germinal centre B cell-like types: a tissue microarray analysis of 90 cases. *J Clin Pathol* 2003; **56**: 747–52.

114. Stauder R, Eisterer W, Thaler J, Gunther U. CD44 variant isoforms in non-Hodgkin's lymphoma: a new independent prognostic factor. *Blood* 1995; **85**: 2885–99.

115. Inagaki H, Banno S, Wakita A *et al.* Prognostic significance of CD44v6 in diffuse large B-cell lymphoma. *Mod Pathol* 1999; **12**: 546–52.

116. Terol MJ, Lopez-Guillermo A, Bosch F *et al.* Expression of the adhesion molecule ICAM-1 in non-Hodgkin's lymphoma: relationship with tumor dissemination and prognostic importance. *J Clin Oncol* 1998; **16**: 35–40.

117. Lossos IS, Jones CD, Warnke R *et al.* Expression of a single gene, BCL-6, strongly predicts survival in patients with diffuse large B-cell lymphoma. *Blood* 2001; **98**: 945–51.

●118. Hans CP, Weisenburger DD, Greiner TC *et al.* Confirmation of the molecular classification of diffuse large B-cell lymphoma by immunohistochemistry using a tissue microarray. *Blood* 2004; **103**: 275–82.

119. Winter JN, Weller EA, Horning SJ *et al.* Prognostic significance of Bcl-6 protein expression in DLBCL treated with CHOP or R-CHOP: a prospective correlative study. *Blood* 2006; **107**: 4207–13.

120. Fabiani B, Delmer A, Lepage E *et al.* CD10 expression in diffuse large B-cell lymphomas does not influence survival. *Virchows Arch* 2004; **445**: 545–51.

121. Go J, Yang W, Ree H. CD10 expression in primary intestinal large B-cell lymphomas. *Arch Path Lab Med* 2002; **126**: 956–60.

122. Kroft SH, Howard MS, Picker LJ *et al.* De novo CD5+ diffuse large B-cell lymphomas. A heterogeneous group containing an unusual form of splenic lymphoma. *Am J Clin Pathol* 2000; **114**: 523–33.

123. Adam P, Katzenberger T, Seeberger H *et al.* A case of a diffuse large B-cell lymphoma of plasmablastic type associated with the t(2;5)(p23;q35) chromosome translocation. *Am J Surg Pathol* 2003; **27**: 1473–6.

124. Tagawa H, Suguro M, Tsuzuki S *et al.* Comparison of genome profiles for identification of distinct subgroups of diffuse large B-cell lymphoma. *Blood* 2005; **106**: 1770–7.

125. de Leval L, Braaten KM, Ancukiewicz M *et al.* Diffuse large B-cell lymphoma of bone: an analysis of differentiation-associated antigens with clinical correlation. *Am J Surg Pathol* 2003; **27**: 1269–77.

126. Chang CC, McClintock S, Cleveland RP *et al.* Immunohistochemical expression patterns of germinal center and activation B-cell markers correlate with prognosis in diffuse large B-cell lymphoma. *Am J Surg Pathol* 2004; **28**: 464–70.

●127. de Jong D, Rosenwald A, Chhanabhai M *et al.* Immunohistochemical prognostic markers in diffuse large

B-cell lymphoma: validation of tissue microarray as a prerequisite for broad clinical applications – a study from the Lunenburg Lymphoma Biomarker Consortium. *J Clin Oncol* 2007; **25**: 805–12.

128. Berglund M, Thunberg U, Amini RM *et al*. Evaluation of immunophenotype in diffuse large B-cell lymphoma and its impact on prognosis. *Mod Pathol* 2005; **18**: 1113–20.

129. Zinzani PL, Dirnhofer S, Sabattini E *et al*. Identification of outcome predictors in diffuse large B-cell lymphoma. Immunohistochemical profiling of homogeneously treated de novo tumors with nodal presentation on tissue micro-arrays. *Haematologica* 2005; **90**: 341–7.

130. De Paepe P, Achten R, Verhoef G *et al*. Large cleaved and immunoblastic lymphoma may represent two distinct clinicopathologic entities within the group of diffuse large B-cell lymphomas. *J Clin Oncol* 2005; **23**: 7060–8.

131. de Jong D, Glas AM, Boerrigter L *et al*. Very late relapse in diffuse large B-cell lymphoma represents clonally related disease and is marked by germinal center cell features. *Blood* 2003; **102**: 324–7.

132. Nyman H, Adde M, Karjalainen-Lindsberg ML *et al*. Prognostic impact of immunohistochemically defined germinal center phenotype in diffuse large B-cell lymphoma patients treated with immunochemotherapy. *Blood* 2007; **109**: 4930–5.

●133. Shipp MA, Ross KN, Tamayo P *et al*. Diffuse large B-cell lymphoma outcome prediction by gene-expression profiling and supervised machine learning. *Nat Med* 2002; **8**: 68–74.

●134. Lossos IS, Czerwinski DK, Alizadeh AA *et al*. Prediction of survival in diffuse large-B-cell lymphoma based on the expression of six genes. *N Engl J Med* 2004; **350**: 1828–37.

●135. Barrans SL, Fenton JA, Banham A *et al*. Strong expression of FOXP1 identifies a distinct subset of diffuse large B-cell lymphoma (DLBCL) patients with poor outcome. *Blood* 2004; **104**: 2933–5.

136. Banham AH, Connors JM, Brown PJ *et al*. Expression of the FOXP1 transcription factor is strongly associated with inferior survival in patients with diffuse large B-cell lymphoma. *Clin Cancer Res* 2005; **11**: 1065–72.

137. Hans CP, Weisenburger DD, Greiner TC *et al*. Expression of PKC-beta or cyclin D2 predicts for inferior survival in diffuse large B-cell lymphoma. *Mod Pathol* 2005; **18**: 1377–84.

138. Natkunam Y, Farinha P, Hsi ED *et al*. LMO2 protein expression predicts survival in patients with diffuse large B-cell lymphoma treated with anthracycline-based chemotherapy with and without rituximab. *J Clin Oncol* 2008; **26**: 447–54.

●139. Dogan A, Burke JS, Goteri G *et al*. Micronodular T-cell/histiocyte-rich large B-cell lymphoma of the spleen: histology, immunophenotype, and differential diagnosis. *Am J Surg Pathol* 2003; **27**: 903–11.

●140. Lim MS, Beaty M, Sorbara L *et al*. T-cell/histiocyte-rich large B-cell lymphoma: a heterogeneous entity with derivation from germinal center B cells. *Am J Surg Pathol* 2002; **26**: 1458–66.

●141. Achten R, Verhoef G, Vanuytsel L, De Wolf-Peeters C. Histiocyte-rich, T-cell-rich B-cell lymphoma: a distinct diffuse large B-cell lymphoma subtype showing characteristic morphologic and immunophenotypic features. *Histopathology* 2002; **40**: 31–45.

142. Fraga M, Sanchez-Verde L, Forteza J *et al*. T-cell/histiocyte-rich large B-cell lymphoma is a disseminated aggressive neoplasm: differential diagnosis from Hodgkin's lymphoma. *Histopathology* 2002; **41**: 216–29.

143. La Starza R, Aventin A, Falzetti D *et al*. 14q+ chromosome marker in a T-cell-rich B-cell lymphoma. *J Pathol* 1996; **178**: 227–31.

144. de Leval L, Harris NL, Lampertz S, Herens C. T-cell/histiocyte-rich large B-cell lymphoma associated with a near-tetraploid karyotype and complex genetic abnormalities. *APMIS* 2006; **114**: 474–8.

145. Brauninger A, Kuppers R, Spieker T *et al*. Molecular analysis of single B cells from T-cell-rich B-cell lymphoma shows the derivation of the tumor cells from mutating germinal center B cells and exemplifies means by which immunoglobulin genes are modified in germinal center B cells. *Blood* 1999; **93**: 2679–87.

146. Macon WR, Cousar JB, Waldron JA Jr, Hsu SM. Interleukin-4 may contribute to the abundant T-cell reaction and paucity of neoplastic B cells in T-cell-rich B-cell lymphomas. *Am J Pathol* 1992; **141**: 1031–6.

147. Felgar RE, Steward KR, Cousar JB, Macon WR. T-cell-rich large-B-cell lymphomas contain non-activated CD8+ cytolytic T cells, show increased tumor cell apoptosis, and have lower Bcl-2 expression than diffuse large-B-cell lymphomas. *Am J Pathol* 1998; 153: 1707–15.

148. Schmidt U, Metz KA, Leder LD. T-cell-rich B-cell lymphoma and lymphocyte-predominant Hodgkin's disease: two closely related entities? *Br J Haematol* 1995; **90**: 398–403.

149. Rudiger T, Gascoyne RD, Jaffe ES *et al*. Workshop on the relationship between nodular lymphocyte predominant Hodgkin's lymphoma and T cell/histiocyte-rich B cell lymphoma. *Ann Oncol* 2002; **13**(Suppl 1): 44–51.

150. Franke S, Wlodarska I, Maes B *et al*. Comparative genomic hybridization pattern distinguishes T-cell/histiocyte-rich B-cell lymphoma from nodular lymphocyte predominance Hodgkin's lymphoma. *Am J Pathol* 2002; **161**: 1861–7.

151. Maes B, Anastasopoulou A, Kluin-Nelemans JC *et al*. Among diffuse large B-cell lymphomas, T-cell-rich/histiocyte-rich BCL and CD30+ anaplastic B-cell subtypes exhibit distinct clinical features. *Ann Oncol* 2001; **12**: 853–8.

●152. Bouabdallah R, Mounier N, Guettier C *et al*. T-cell/histiocyte-rich large B-cell lymphomas and classical diffuse large B-cell lymphomas have similar outcome after chemotherapy: a matched-control analysis. *J Clin Oncol* 2003; **21**: 1271–7.

153. Aki H, Tuzuner N, Ongoren S *et al*. T-cell-rich B-cell lymphoma: a clinicopathologic study of 21 cases and comparison with 43 cases of diffuse large B-cell lymphoma. *Leuk Res* 2004; **28**: 229–36.

●154. Delecluse HJ, Anagnostopoulos I, Dallenbach F et al. Plasmablastic lymphomas of the oral cavity: a new entity associated with the human immunodeficiency virus infection. *Blood* 1997; **89**: 1413–20.

155. Chetty R, Hlatswayo N, Muc R et al. Plasmablastic lymphoma in HIV+ patients: an expanding spectrum. *Histopathology* 2003; **42**: 605–9.

156. Lin Y, Rodrigues GD, Turner JF, Vasef MA. Plasmablastic lymphoma of the lung: report of a unique case and review of the literature. *Arch Pathol Lab Med* 2001; **125**: 282–5.

157. Hausermann P, Khanna N, Buess M et al. Cutaneous plasmablastic lymphoma in an HIV-positive male: an unrecognized cutaneous manifestation. *Dermatology* 2004; **208**: 287–90.

●158. Colomo L, Loong F, Rives S et al. Diffuse large B-cell lymphomas with plasmablastic differentiation represent a heterogeneous group of disease entities. *Am J Surg Pathol* 2004; **28**: 736–47.

159. Schichman SA, McClure R, Schaefer RF, Mehta P. HIV and plasmablastic lymphoma manifesting in sinus, testicles, and bones: a further expansion of the disease spectrum. *Am J Hematol* 2004; **77**: 291–5.

●160. Dong HY, Scadden DT, de Leval L et al. Plasmablastic lymphoma in HIV-positive patients: an aggressive epstein-barr virus-associated extramedullary plasmacytic neoplasm. *Am J Surg Pathol* 2005; **29**: 1633–41.

161. Teruya-Feldstein J, Chiao E, Filippa DA et al. CD20-negative large-cell lymphoma with plasmablastic features: a clinically heterogenous spectrum in both HIV-positive and -negative patients. *Ann Oncol* 2004; **15**: 1673–9.

162. Carbone A, Gloghini A, Larocca LM et al. Expression profile of MUM1/IRF4, BCL-6, and CD138/syndecan-1 defines novel histogenetic subsets of human immunodeficiency virus-related lymphomas. *Blood* 2001; **97**: 744–51.

163. Cioc AM, Allen C, Kalmar JR et al. Oral plasmablastic lymphomas in AIDS patients are associated with human herpesvirus 8. *Am J Surg Pathol* 2004; **28**: 41–6.

164. Zanetto U, Martin CA, Sapia S et al. Re: Cioc AM, Allen C, Kalmar J et al. Oral plasmablastic lymphomas in AIDS patients are associated with human herpesvirus 8. *Am J Surg Pathol* 2004; **25**: 41–46. *Am J Surg Pathol* 2004; **28**: 1537–8 [author reply 8].

165. Vega F, Chang CC, Medeiros LJ et al. Plasmablastic lymphomas and plasmablastic plasma cell myelomas have nearly identical immunophenotypic profiles. *Mod Pathol* 2005; **18**: 806–15.

166. Goedhals J, Beukes CA, Hardie D. HHV8 in plasmablastic lymphoma. *Am J Surg Pathol* 2008; **32**: 172.

167. Gaidano G, Cerri M, Capello D et al. Molecular histogenesis of plasmablastic lymphoma of the oral cavity. *Br J Haematol* 2002; **119**: 622–8.

●168. Chadburn A, Hyjek E, Mathew S et al. KSHV-positive solid lymphomas represent an extra-cavitary variant of primary effusion lymphoma. *Am J Surg Pathol* 2004; **28**: 1401–16.

169. Deloose ST, Smit LA, Pals FT et al. High incidence of Kaposi sarcoma-associated herpesvirus infection in HIV-related solid immunoblastic/plasmablastic diffuse large B-cell lymphoma. *Leukemia* 2005; **19**: 851–5.

170. Delsol G, Lamant L, Mariame B et al. A new subtype of large B-cell lymphoma expressing the ALK kinase and lacking the 2; 5 translocation. *Blood* 1997; **89**: 1483–90.

171. Chikatsu N, Kojima H, Suzukawa K et al. ALK+, CD30-, CD20- large B-cell lymphoma containing anaplastic lymphoma kinase (ALK) fused to clathrin heavy chain gene (CLTC). *Mod Pathol* 2003; **16**: 828–32.

●172. Gascoyne RD, Lamant L, Martin-Subero JI et al. ALK-positive diffuse large B-cell lymphoma is associated with Clathrin-ALK rearrangements: report of 6 cases. *Blood* 2003; **102**: 2568–73.

173. De Paepe P, Baens M, van Krieken H et al. ALK activation by the CLTC-ALK fusion is a recurrent event in large B-cell lymphoma. *Blood* 2003; **102**: 2638–41.

●174. Onciu M, Behm FG, Downing JR et al. ALK-positive plasmablastic B-cell lymphoma with expression of the NPM-ALK fusion transcript: report of 2 cases. *Blood* 2003; **102**: 2642–4.

175. A clinical evaluation of the International Lymphoma Study Group classification of non-Hodgkin's lymphoma. The non-Hodgkin's lymphoma classification project. *Blood* 1997; **89**: 3909–18.

176. Jacobson J, Aisenberg A, Lamarre L et al. Mediastinal large cell lymphoma: an uncommon subset of adult lymphoma curable with combined modality therapy. *Cancer* 1988; **62**: 1893–8.

●177. Cazals-Hatem D, Lepage E, Brice P et al. Primary mediastinal large B-cell lymphoma. A clinicopathologic study of 141 cases compared with 916 nonmediastinal large B-cell lymphomas, a GELA ('Groupe d'Etude des Lymphomes de l'Adulte') study. *Am J Surg Pathol* 1996; **20**: 877–88.

178. Bishop PC, Wilson WH, Pearson D et al. CNS involvement in primary mediastinal large B-cell lymphoma. *J Clin Oncol* 1999; **17**: 2479–85.

179. Lamarre L, Jacobson JO, Aisenberg AC, Harris NL. Primary large cell lymphoma of the mediastinum. A histologic and immunophenotypic study of 29 cases. *Am J Surg Pathol* 1989; **13**: 730–9.

◆180. Barth TF, Leithauser F, Joos S et al. Mediastinal (thymic) large B-cell lymphoma: where do we stand? *Lancet Oncol* 2002; **3**: 229–34.

181. Moller P, Matthaei-Maurer DU, Hofmann WJ et al. Immunophenotypic similarities of mediastinal clear-cell lymphoma and sinusoidal (monocytoid) B cells. *Int J Cancer* 1989; **43**: 10–16.

182. Rudiger T, Jaffe ES, Delsol G et al. Workshop report on Hodgkin's disease and related diseases ('grey zone' lymphoma). *Ann Oncol* 1998; **9**(Suppl 5):s31–8.

183. Pileri SA, Gaidano G, Zinzani PL et al. Primary mediastinal B-cell lymphoma: high frequency of BCL-6 mutations and consistent expression of the transcription factors OCT-2, BOB.1, and PU.1 in the absence of immunoglobulins. *Am J Pathol* 2003; **162**: 243–53.

184. Moller P, Moldenhauer G, Momburg F et al. Mediastinal lymphoma of clear cell type is a tumor corresponding to

terminal steps of B cell differentiation. *Blood* 1987; **69**: 1087–95.

185. Momburg F, Herrmann B, Moldenhauer G, Möller P. B-cell lymphomas of high-grade malignancy frequently lack HLA-DR, -DP and -DQ antigens and associated invariant chain. *Int J Cancer* 1987; **40**: 598–603.

186. de Leval L, Ferry JA, Falini B *et al.* Expression of bcl-6 and CD10 in primary mediastinal large B-cell lymphoma: evidence for derivation from germinal center B cells? *Am J Surg Pathol* 2001; **25**: 1277–82.

187. Calaminici M, Piper K, Lee AM, Norton AJ. CD23 expression in mediastinal large B-cell lymphomas. *Histopathology* 2004; **45**: 619–24.

188. Copie-Bergman C, Gaulard P, Maouche-Chretien L *et al.* The MAL gene is expressed in primary mediastinal large B-cell lymphoma. *Blood* 1999; **94**: 3567–75.

●189. Copie-Bergman C, Plonquet A, Alonso MA *et al.* MAL expression in lymphoid cells: further evidence for MAL as a distinct molecular marker of primary mediastinal large B-cell lymphomas. *Mod Pathol* 2002; **15**: 1172–80.

190. Copie-Bergman C, Boulland ML, Dehoulle C *et al.* Interleukin 4-induced gene 1 is activated in primary mediastinal large B-cell lymphoma. *Blood* 2003; **101**: 2756–61.

●191. Savage KJ, Monti S, Kutok JL *et al.* The molecular signature of mediastinal large B-cell lymphoma differs from that of other diffuse large B-cell lymphomas and shares features with classical Hodgkin's lymphoma. *Blood* 2003; **102**: 3871–9.

192. Rodig SJ, Savage KJ, LaCasce AS *et al.* Expression of TRAF1 and nuclear c-Rel distinguishes primary mediastinal large cell lymphoma from other types of diffuse large B-cell lymphoma. *Am J Surg Pathol* 2007; **31**: 106–12.

193. Leithauser F, Bauerle M, Huynh MQ, Moller P. Isotype-switched immunoglobulin genes with a high load of somatic hypermutation and lack of ongoing mutational activity are prevalent in mediastinal B-cell lymphoma. *Blood* 2001; **98**: 2762–70.

194. Malpeli G, Barbi S, Moore PS *et al.* Primary mediastinal B-cell lymphoma: hypermutation of the BCL6 gene targets motifs different from those in diffuse large B-cell and follicular lymphomas. *Haematologica* 2004; **89**: 1091–9.

●195. Addis BJ, Isaacson PG. Large cell lymphoma of the mediastinum: a B-cell tumour of probable thymic origin. *Histopathology* 1986; **10**: 379–90.

196. Isaacson PG, Norton AJ, Addis BJ. The human thymus contains a novel population of B lymphocytes. *Lancet* 1987; **2**: 1488–91.

197. Hofmann WJ, Momburg F, Moller P, Otto HF. Intra- and extrathymic B cells in physiologic and pathologic conditions. Immunohistochemical study on normal thymus and lymphofollicular hyperplasia of the thymus. *Virchows Arch A Pathol Anat Histopathol* 1988; **412**: 431–42.

198. Tsang P, Cesarman E, Chadburn A *et al.* Molecular characterization of primary mediastinal B cell lymphoma. *Am J Pathol* 1996; **148**: 2017–25.

199. Joos S, Otano-Joos MI, Ziegler S *et al.* Primary mediastinal (thymic) B-cell lymphoma is characterized by gains of

chromosomal material including 9p and amplification of the REL gene. *Blood* 1996; **87**: 1571–8.

200. Bentz M, Barth TF, Bruderlein S *et al.* Gain of chromosome arm 9p is characteristic of primary mediastinal B-cell lymphoma (MBL): comprehensive molecular cytogenetic analysis and presentation of a novel MBL cell line. *Genes Chromosomes Cancer* 2001; **30**: 393–401.

201. Wessendorf S, Barth TF, Viardot A *et al.* Further delineation of chromosomal consensus regions in primary mediastinal B-cell lymphomas: an analysis of 37 tumor samples using high-resolution genomic profiling (array-CGH). *Leukemia* 2007; **21**: 2463–9.

202. Joos S, Granzow M, Holtgreve-Grez H *et al.* Hodgkin's lymphoma cell lines are characterized by frequent aberrations on chromosomes 2p and 9p including REL and JAK2. *Int J Cancer* 2003; **103**: 489–95.

203. Kimm LR, deLeeuw RJ, Savage KJ *et al.* Frequent occurrence of deletions in primary mediastinal B-cell lymphoma. *Genes Chromosomes Cancer* 2007; **46**: 1090–7.

●204. Rosenwald A, Wright G, Leroy K *et al.* Molecular diagnosis of primary mediastinal B cell lymphoma identifies a clinically favorable subgroup of diffuse large B cell lymphoma related to Hodgkin lymphoma. *J Exp Med* 2003; **198**: 851–62.

205. Kuppers R, Schwering I, Brauninger A *et al.* Biology of Hodgkin's lymphoma. *Ann Oncol* 2002; **13**(Suppl 1): 11–18.

206. Joos S, Kupper M, Ohl S *et al.* Genomic imbalances including amplification of the tyrosine kinase gene JAK2 in CD30+ Hodgkin cells. *Cancer Res* 2000; **60**: 549–52.

207. Joos S, Menz CK, Wrobel G *et al.* Classical Hodgkin lymphoma is characterized by recurrent copy number gains of the short arm of chromosome 2. *Blood* 2002; **99**: 1381–7.

208. Martin-Subero JI, Gesk S, Harder L *et al.* Recurrent involvement of the REL and BCL11A loci in classical Hodgkin lymphoma. *Blood* 2002; **99**: 1474–7.

209. Cabannes E, Khan G, Aillet F *et al.* Mutations in the IkBa gene in Hodgkin's disease suggest a tumour suppressor role for IkappaBalpha. *Oncogene* 1999; **18**: 3063–70.

210. Jungnickel B, Staratschek-Jox A, Brauninger A *et al.* Clonal deleterious mutations in the IkappaBalpha gene in the malignant cells in Hodgkin's lymphoma. *J Exp Med* 2000; **191**: 395–402.

211. Kuppers R. B cells under influence: transformation of B cells by Epstein-Barr virus. *Nat Rev Immunol* 2003; **3**: 801–12.

212. Weniger MA, Gesk S, Ehrlich S *et al.* Gains of REL in primary mediastinal B-cell lymphoma coincide with nuclear accumulation of REL protein. *Genes Chromosomes Cancer* 2007; **46**: 406–15.

213. Takahashi H, Feuerhake F, Monti S *et al.* Lack of IKBA coding region mutations in primary mediastinal large B-cell lymphoma and the host response subtype of diffuse large B-cell lymphoma. *Blood* 2006; **107**: 844–5.

214. Guiter C, Dusanter-Fourt I, Copie-Bergman C *et al.* Constitutive STAT6 activation in primary mediastinal large B-cell lymphoma. *Blood* 2004; **104**: 543–9.

215. Skinnider BF, Elia AJ, Gascoyne RD *et al*. Signal transducer and activator of transcription 6 is frequently activated in Hodgkin and Reed–Sternberg cells of Hodgkin lymphoma. *Blood* 2002; **99**: 618–26.

216. Hinz M, Lemke P, Anagnostopoulos I *et al*. Nuclear factor kappaB-dependent gene expression profiling of Hodgkin's disease tumor cells, pathogenetic significance, and link to constitutive signal transducer and activator of transcription 5a activity. *J Exp Med* 2002; **196**: 605–17.

●217. Melzner I, Bucur AJ, Bruderlein S *et al*. Biallelic mutation of SOCS-1 impairs JAK2 degradation and sustains phospho-JAK2 action in the MedB-1 mediastinal lymphoma line. *Blood* 2005; **105**: 2535–42.

218. Weniger MA, Melzner I, Menz CK *et al*. Mutations of the tumor suppressor gene SOCS-1 in classical Hodgkin lymphoma are frequent and associated with nuclear phospho-STAT5 accumulation. *Oncogene* 2006; **25**: 2679–84.

219. Renne C, Willenbrock K, Martin-Subero JI *et al*. High expression of several tyrosine kinases and activation of the PI3K/AKT pathway in mediastinal large B cell lymphoma reveals further similarities to Hodgkin lymphoma. *Leukemia* 2007; **21**: 780–7.

◆220. Calvo KR, Traverse-Glehen A, Pittaluga S, Jaffe ES. Molecular profiling provides evidence of primary mediastinal large B-cell lymphoma as a distinct entity related to classic Hodgkin lymphoma: implications for mediastinal gray zone lymphomas as an intermediate form of B-cell lymphoma. *Adv Anat Pathol* 2004; **11**: 227–38.

221. Traverse-Glehen A, Pittaluga S, Gaulard P *et al*. Mediastinal gray zone lymphoma: the missing link between classic Hodgkin's lymphoma and mediastinal large B-cell lymphoma. *Am J Surg Pathol* 2005; **29**: 1411–21.

222. Haioun C, Gaulard P, Roudot-Thoraval F *et al*. Mediastinal diffuse large-cell lymphoma with sclerosis: a condition with a poor prognosis. *Am J Clin Oncol* 1989; **12**: 425–9.

223. Lazzarino M, Orlandi E, Paulli M *et al*. Primary mediastinal B-cell lymphoma with sclerosis: an aggressive tumor with distinctive clinical and pathologic features [see comments]. *J Clin Oncol* 1993; **11**: 2306–13.

224. Abou-Elella AA, Weisenburger DD, Vose JM *et al*. Primary mediastinal large B-cell lymphoma: a clinicopathologic study of 43 patients from the Nebraska Lymphoma Study Group. *J Clin Oncol* 1999; **17**: 784–90.

225. van Besien K, Kelta M, Bahaguna P. Primary mediastinal B-cell lymphoma: a review of pathology and management. *J Clin Oncol* 2001; **19**: 1855–64.

●226. Cesarman E, Chang Y, Moore PS *et al*. Kaposi's sarcoma-associated herpesvirus-like DNA sequences in AIDS-related body-cavity-based lymphomas. *N Engl J Med* 1995; **332**: 1186–91.

227. Horenstein MG, Nador RG, Chadburn A *et al*. Epstein-Barr virus latent gene expression in primary effusion lymphomas containing Kaposi's sarcoma-associated herpesvirus/human herpesvirus-8. *Blood* 1997; **90**: 1186–91.

228. Cesarman E, Nador RG, Aozasa K *et al*. Kaposi's sarcoma-associated herpesvirus in non-AIDS related lymphomas occurring in body cavities. *Am J Pathol* 1996; **149**: 53–7.

229. Boulanger E, Gerard L, Gabarre J *et al*. Prognostic factors and outcome of human herpesvirus 8-associated primary effusion lymphoma in patients with AIDS. *J Clin Oncol* 2005; **23**: 4372–80.

230. Carbone A, Cilia AM, Gloghini A *et al*. Establishment and characterization of EBV-positive and EBV-negative primary effusion lymphoma cell lines harbouring human herpesvirus type-8. *Br J Haematol* 1998; **102**: 1081–9.

231. Gaidano G, Gloghini A, Gattei V *et al*. Association of Kaposi's sarcoma-associated herpesvirus-positive primary effusion lymphoma with expression of the CD138/syndecan-1 antigen. *Blood* 1997; **90**: 4894–900.

232. Cesarman E, Knowles DM. The role of Kaposi's sarcoma-associated herpesvirus (KSHV/HHV-8) in lymphoproliferative diseases. *Semin Cancer Biol* 1999; **9**: 165–74.

◆233. Ascoli V, Lo-Coco F. Body cavity lymphoma. *Curr Opin Pulm Med* 2002; **8**: 317–22.

234. Fan W, Bubman D, Chadburn A *et al*. Distinct subsets of primary effusion lymphoma can be identified based on their cellular gene expression profile and viral association. *J Virol* 2005; **79**: 1244–51.

235. Matolcsy A, Nador RG, Cesarman E, Knowles DM. Immunoglobulin VH gene mutational analysis suggests that primary effusion lymphomas derive from different stages of B cell maturation. *Am J Pathol* 1998; **153**: 1609–14.

236. Klein U, Gloghini A, Gaidano G *et al*. Gene expression profile analysis of AIDS-related primary effusion lymphoma (PEL) suggests a plasmablastic derivation and identifies PEL-specific transcripts. *Blood* 2003; **101**: 4115–21.

237. Jenner RG, Maillard K, Cattini N *et al*. Kaposi's sarcoma-associated herpesvirus-infected primary effusion lymphoma has a plasma cell gene expression profile. *Proc Natl Acad Sci U S A* 2003; **100**: 10399–404.

●238. Dupin N, Diss TL, Kellam P *et al*. HHV-8 is associated with a plasmablastic variant of Castleman disease that is linked to HHV-8-positive plasmablastic lymphoma. *Blood* 2000; **95**: 1406–12.

239. Oksenhendler E, Boulanger E, Galicier L *et al*. High incidence of Kaposi sarcoma-associated herpesvirus-related non-Hodgkin lymphoma in patients with HIV infection and multicentric Castleman disease. *Blood* 2002; **99**: 2331–6.

●240. Du MQ, Diss TC, Liu H *et al*. KSHV- and EBV-associated germinotropic lymphoproliferative disorder. *Blood* 2002; **100**: 3415–18.

241. Iuchi K, Ichimiya A, Akashi A *et al*. Non-Hodgkin's lymphoma of the pleural cavity developing from long-standing pyothorax. *Cancer* 1987; **60**: 1771–5.

242. Iuchi K, Aozasa K, Yamamoto S *et al*. Non-Hodgkin's lymphoma of the pleural cavity developing from long-standing pyothorax. Summary of clinical and pathological findings in thirty-seven cases. *Jpn J Clin Oncol* 1989; **19**: 249–57.

243. Nakatsuka S, Yao M, Hoshida Y *et al*. Pyothorax-associated lymphoma: a review of 106 cases. *J Clin Oncol* 2002; **20**: 4255–60.

◆244. Narimatsu H, Ota Y, Kami M *et al*. Clinicopathological features of pyothorax-associated lymphoma; a

245. Petitjean B, Jardin F, Joly B et al. Pyothorax-associated lymphoma: a peculiar clinicopathologic entity derived from B cells at late stage of differentiation and with occasional aberrant dual B- and T-cell phenotype. Am J Surg Pathol 2002; 26: 724–32.

246. Androulaki A, Drakos E, Hatzianastassiou D et al. Pyothorax-associated lymphoma (PAL): a western case with marked angiocentricity and review of the literature. Histopathology 2004; 44: 69–76.

247. Fukayama M, Ibuka T, Hayashi Y et al. Epstein-Barr virus in pyothorax-associated pleural lymphoma. Am J Pathol 1993; 143: 1044–9.

248. Ascani S, Piccioli M, Poggi S et al. Pyothorax-associated lymphoma: description of the first two cases detected in Italy. Ann Oncol 1997; 8: 1133–8.

249. O'Donovan M, Silva I, Uhlmann V et al. Expression profile of human herpesvirus 8 (HHV-8) in pyothorax associated lymphoma and in effusion lymphoma. Mol Pathol 2001; 54: 80–5.

250. Kanno H, Aozasa K. Mechanism for the development of pyothorax-associated lymphoma. Pathol Int 1998; 48: 653–64.

251. Yamato H, Ohshima K, Suzumiya J, Kikuchi M. Evidence for local immunosuppression and demonstration of c-myc amplification in pyothorax-associated lymphoma. Histopathology 2001; 39: 163–71.

252. Miwa H, Takakuwa T, Nakatsuka S et al. DNA sequences of the immunoglobulin heavy chain variable region gene in pyothorax-associated lymphoma. Oncology 2002; 62: 241–50.

253. Takakuwa T, Tresnasari K, Rahadiani N et al. Cell origin of pyothorax-associated lymphoma: a lymphoma strongly associated with Epstein-Barr virus infection. Leukemia 2008; 22: 620–7.

254. Nishiu M, Tomita Y, Nakatsuka S et al. Distinct pattern of gene expression in pyothorax-associated lymphoma (PAL), a lymphoma developing in long-standing inflammation. Cancer Sci 2004; 95: 828–34.

255. Kanno H, Naka N, Yasunaga Y, Aozasa K. Role of an immunosuppressive cytokine, interleukin-10, in the development of pyothorax-associated lymphoma. Leukemia 1997; 11(Suppl 3): 525–6.

256. Copie-Bergman C, Niedobitek G, Mangham DC et al. Epstein-Barr virus in B-cell lymphomas associated with chronic suppurative inflammation. J Pathol 1997; 183: 287–92.

257. Cheuk W, Chan AC, Chan JK et al. Metallic implant-associated lymphoma: a distinct subgroup of large B-cell lymphoma related to pyothorax-associated lymphoma? Am J Surg Pathol 2005; 29: 832–6.

258. Gatter K, Warnke R. Intravascular large B-cell lymphoma. In: Vardiman J (ed.). Pathology and genetics of tumours of haematopoietic and lymphoid tissues. Lyon: IARC Press, 2001:177–8.

259. Ferry JA, Harris NL, Picker LJ et al. Intravascular lymphomatosis (malignant angioendotheliomatosis). A B-cell neoplasm expressing surface homing receptors. Mod Pathol 1988; 1: 444–52.

260. Ferreri AJ, Campo E, Seymour JF et al. Intravascular lymphoma: clinical presentation, natural history, management and prognostic factors in a series of 38 cases, with special emphasis on the 'cutaneous variant'. Br J Haematol 2004; 127: 173–83.

261. Pfleger L, Tappeiner J. On the recognition of systematized endotheliomatosis of the cutaneous blood vessels (reticuloendotheliosis?). Hautarzt 1959; 10: 359–63.

262. Wick MR, Mills SE, Scheithauer BW et al. Reassessment of malignant 'angioendotheliomatosis'. Evidence in favor of its reclassification as 'intravascular lymphomatosis'. Am J Surg Pathol 1986; 10: 112–23.

263. Rubin MA, Cossman J, Freter CE, Azumi N. Intravascular large cell lymphoma coexisting within hemangiomas of the skin. Am J Surg Pathol 1997; 21: 860–4.

264. Wang BY, Strauchen JA, Rabinowitz D et al. Renal cell carcinoma with intravascular lymphomatosis: a case report of unusual collision tumors with review of the literature. Arch Pathol Lab Med 2001; 125: 1239–41.

265. Nixon BK, Kussick SJ, Carlon MJ, Rubin BP. Intravascular large B-cell lymphoma involving hemangiomas: an unusual presentation of a rare neoplasm. Mod Pathol 2005; 18: 1121–6.

266. Murase T, Nakamura S, Tashiro K et al. Malignant histiocytosis-like B-cell lymphoma, a distinct pathologic variant of intravascular lymphomatosis: a report of five cases and review of the literature. Br J Haematol 1997; 99: 656–64.

267. Murase T, Nakamura S. An Asian variant of intravascular lymphomatosis: an updated review of malignant histiocytosis-like B-cell lymphoma. Leuk Lymphoma 1999; 33: 459–73.

268. Murase T, Nakamura S, Kawauchi K et al. An Asian variant of intravascular large B-cell lymphoma: clinical, pathological and cytogenetic approaches to diffuse large B-cell lymphoma associated with haemophagocytic syndrome. Br J Haematol 2000; 111: 826–34.

269. Ferreri AJ, Dognini GP, Campo E et al. International Extranodal Lymphoma Study Group (IELSG). Variations in clinical presentation, frequency of hemophagocytosis and clinical behavior of intravascular lymphoma diagnosed in different geographical regions. Haematologica 2007; 92: 486–92.

270. Khalidi HS, Brynes RK, Browne P et al. Intravascular large B-cell lymphoma: the CD5 antigen is expressed by a subset of cases. Mod Pathol 1998; 11: 983–8.

271. Estalilla OC, Koo CH, Brynes RK, Medeiros LJ. Intravascular large B-cell lymphoma. A report of five cases initially diagnosed by bone marrow biopsy. Am J Clin Pathol 1999; 112: 248–55.

272. Yegappan S, Coupland R, Arber DA et al. Angiotropic lymphoma: an immunophenotypically and clinically heterogeneous lymphoma. Mod Pathol 2001; 14: 1147–56.

273. Khoury H, Dalal BI, Nantel SH. Intravascular lymphoma presenting with bone marrow involvement and leukemic phase. *Leuk Lymphoma* 2003; **44**: 1043–7.

274. Vieites B, Fraga M, Lopez-Presas E *et al.* Detection of t(14;18) translocation in a case of intravascular large B-cell lymphoma: a germinal centre cell origin in a subset of these lymphomas? *Histopathology* 2005; **46**: 466–8.

275. Seki K, Miyakoshi S, Lee GH *et al.* Prostatic acid phosphatase is a possible tumor marker for intravascular large B-cell lymphoma. *Am J Surg Pathol* 2004; **28**: 1384–8.

276. Kanda M, Suzumiya J, Ohshima K *et al.* Analysis of the immunoglobulin heavy chain gene variable region of intravascular large B-cell lymphoma. *Virchows Arch* 2001; **439**: 540–6.

277. Ponzoni M, Arrigoni G, Gould VE *et al.* Lack of CD 29 (beta1 integrin) and CD 54 (ICAM-1) adhesion molecules in intravascular lymphomatosis. *Hum Pathol* 2000; **31**: 220–6.

278. DiGiuseppe JA, Nelson WG, Seifter EJ *et al.* Intravascular lymphomatosis: a clinicopathologic study of 10 cases and assessment of response to chemotherapy. *J Clin Oncol* 1994; **12**: 2573–9.

279. Shimada K, Matsue K, Yamamoto K *et al.* Retrospective analysis of intravascular large B-cell lymphoma treated with rituximab-containing chemotherapy as reported by the IVL study group in Japan. *J Clin Oncol* 2008; **26**: 3189–95.

●280. Oyama T, Ichimura K, Suzuki R *et al.* Senile EBV+ B-cell lymphoproliferative disorders: a clinicopathologic study of 22 patients. *Am J Surg Pathol* 2003; **27**: 16–26.

◆281. Shimoyama Y, Oyama T, Asano N *et al.* Senile Epstein-Barr virus-associated B-cell lymphoproliferative disorders: a mini review. *J Clin Exp Hematop* 2006; **46**: 1–4.

282. Oyama T, Yamamoto K, Asano N *et al.* Age-related EBV-associated B-cell lymphoproliferative disorders constitute a distinct clinicopathologic group: a study of 96 patients. *Clin Cancer Res* 2007; **13**: 5124–32.

283. Liebow AA, Carrington CR, Friedman PJ. Lymphomatoid granulomatosis. *Hum Pathol* 1972; **3**: 457–558.

●284. Guinee D Jr., Jaffe E, Kingma D *et al.* Pulmonary lymphomatoid granulomatosis. Evidence for a proliferation of Epstein-Barr virus infected B-lymphocytes with a prominent T-cell component and vasculitis. *Am J Surg Pathol* 1994; **18**: 753–64.

285. Haque AK, Myers JL, Hudnall SD *et al.* Pulmonary lymphomatoid granulomatosis in acquired immunodeficiency syndrome: lesions with Epstein-Barr virus infection. *Mod Pathol* 1998; **11**: 347–56.

286. Katzenstein AL, Peiper SC. Detection of Epstein-Barr virus genomes in lymphomatoid granulomatosis: analysis of 29 cases by the polymerase chain reaction technique. *Mod Pathol* 1990; **3**: 435–41.

287. Myers JL, Kurtin PJ, Katzenstein AL *et al.* Lymphomatoid granulomatosis. Evidence of immunophenotypic diversity and relationship to Epstein-Barr virus infection. *Am J Surg Pathol* 1995; **19**: 1300–12.

288. Katzenstein A, Carrington C, Liebow A. Lymphomatoid granulomatosis: a clinicopathologic study of 152 cases. *Cancer* 1979; **43**: 360–73.

289. Cadranel J, Wislez M, Antoine M. Primary pulmonary lymphoma. *Eur Respir J* 2002; **20**: 750–62.

290. Beaty MW, Toro J, Sorbara L *et al.* Cutaneous lymphomatoid granulomatosis: correlation of clinical and biologic features. *Am J Surg Pathol* 2001; **25**: 1111–20.

291. Saxena A, Dyker KM, Angel S *et al.* Posttransplant diffuse large B-cell lymphoma of 'lymphomatoid granulomatosis' type. *Virchows Arch* 2002; **441**: 622–8.

292. Nicholson AG, Wotherspoon AC, Diss TC *et al.* Lymphomatoid granulomatosis: evidence that some cases represent Epstein-Barr virus-associated B-cell lymphoma. *Histopathology* 1996; **29**: 317–24.

293. Taniere P, Thivolet-Bejui F, Vitrey D *et al.* Lymphomatoid granulomatosis—a report on four cases: evidence for B phenotype of the tumoral cells. *Eur Respir J* 1998; **12**: 102–6.

294. Guinee DG Jr., Perkins SL, Travis WD *et al.* Proliferation and cellular phenotype in lymphomatoid granulomatosis: implications of a higher proliferation index in B cells. *Am J Surg Pathol* 1998; **22**: 1093–100.

295. Sabourin JC, Kanavaros P, Briere J *et al.* Epstein-Barr virus (EBV) genomes and EBV-encoded latent membrane protein (LMP) in pulmonary lymphomas occurring in nonimmunocompromised patients. *Am J Surg Pathol* 1993; **17**: 995–1002.

296. Gaulard P, Henni T, Marolleau JP *et al.* Lethal midline granuloma (polymorphic reticulosis) and lymphomatoid granulomatosis. Evidence for a monoclonal T-cell lymphoproliferative disorder. *Cancer* 1988; **62**: 705–10.

297. Medeiros L, Peiper S, Elwood L *et al.* Angiocentric immunoproliferative lesions: a molecular analysis of eight cases. *Hum Pathol* 1991; **22**: 1150–7.

298. Lipford E, Margolich J, Longo D *et al.* Angiocentric immunoproliferative lesions: a clinicopathologic spectrum of post-thymic T cell proliferations. *Blood* 1988; **5**: 1674–81.

299. Teruya-Feldstein J, Jaffe ES, Burd PR *et al.* The role of Mig, the monokine induced by interferon-gamma, and IP-10, the interferon-gamma-inducible protein-10, in tissue necrosis and vascular damage associated with Epstein-Barr virus-positive lymphoproliferative disease. *Blood* 1997; **90**: 4099–105.

300. Moudir-Thomas C, Foulet-Roge A, Plat M *et al.* Efficacy of rituximab in lymphomatoid granulomatosis. *Rev Mal Respir* 2004; **21**: 1157–61.

301. Jordan K, Grothey A, Grothe W *et al.* Successful treatment of mediastinal lymphomatoid granulomatosis with rituximab monotherapy. *Eur J Haematol* 2005; **74**: 263–6.

34

Hodgkin lymphoma

MARTIN-LEO HANSMANN, SYLVIA HARTMANN AND RALF KÜPPERS

INTRODUCTION

In non-Hodgkin lymphomas (NHL) the predominance of the tumor cell population is one of the leading features, whereas in Hodgkin lymphoma (HL) the tumor cells are a minor population. It seems that interaction of the rare malignant tumor cells in HL with reactive cells modulates the surrounding tissue, induces a specific morphologic and immunohistochemical picture and triggers lymphoma growth. The diagnosis of HL has to be established by a pathologist who examines histologic sections showing the typical morphologic and immunohistochemical features of this disease. These features are:

- The lymphoid tissue contains scattered large mononuclear and multinucleated tumor cells, so-called Hodgkin and Reed–Sternberg (HRS) cells, which represent a minority compared with the cells in the surrounding tissue.
- The architecture of the lymphoid tissue infiltrated by the neoplastic cells is destroyed. In most cases reactive T cells are the dominating cell population.
- HRS cells are often surrounded by rosetting T cells.

Hodgkin lymphomas usually arise in lymph nodes and can spread secondarily to other lymph nodes as well as other lymphoid and extranodal organs, such as liver and bone marrow. HRS cells are usually not found in the peripheral blood. Although histology is the gold standard for the diagnosis of this disease, a cytologic diagnosis may be useful in special cases. Several features of HL, such as the rarity of the tumor cells, fibrosis of the tissue and partial involvement of lymph nodes, may hamper the cytologic diagnosis of HL and make it difficult to distinguish it from a spectrum of differential diagnoses including Epstein–Barr virus (EBV) infection and NHLs.

In HL the morphologic features of HRS cells, their number, the lymphohistiocytic background, the amount of eosinophilic and neutrophilic granulocytes as well as dendritic cells and fibrosis may vary considerably. These histomorphologic variations of HL infiltrates reflect a biologic and clinical spectrum which has led to several attempts for subclassifications.

SUBCLASSIFICATION OF HODGKIN LYMPHOMA

The current opinion based on histomorphologic, biologic and clinical findings is that HL can be grouped in two disease entities: classical HL and nodular lymphocyte-predominant

HL (NLPHL). There are several reasons that speak in favor of this distinction:

- Clinically classical HL and NLPHL behave differently.
- The tumor cells of both entities show special and distinct cytologic features and immune profiles as well as biologic markers.
- The lymphohistiocytic background in classical HL is mainly dominated by T cells and in NLPHL by B cells.

CLASSICAL HODGKIN LYMPHOMA

Classical HL is defined by the typical HRS cells and the characteristic lymphohistiocytic background. Based on differences in the morphology of the HRS cells and the histologic picture and composition, classical HL is subdivided in the current World Health Organization (WHO) lymphoma classification into nodular sclerosis HL (NSHL), mixed cellularity HL (MCHL), lymphocyte-rich classical HL (LRCHL) and lymphocyte-depleted HL (LDHL) (Table 34.1).[1,2] Classical Hodgkin cells are mononuclear, and Reed–Sternberg cells are bi- or multinucleated cells which are 3–10 times larger in diameter than normal lymphocytes. Their nuclei are round or slightly lobulated and contain a large prominent nucleolus. The nuclear membrane is prominent. HRS cells have abundant, slightly to moderately, sometimes also strongly basophilic cytoplasm. Although there is usually a broad morphologic and cytologic spectrum of HRS cells, one has to find at least a few typical binucleated cells with classical features to establish the diagnosis of HL. From molecular biologic studies it is known that HRS cells derive from preapoptotic cells (see below), a fact that is reflected in HL cell variants known for a long time as 'mummified' cells. These tumor cells show features of apoptosis, such as condensed cytoplasm and pycnotic nuclei.

HRS cells alone are not sufficient to establish the diagnosis of HL. The environment too should show a characteristic composition. Small lymphocytes, mainly CD3- and CD4-positive T cells, are usually dominating. B cells (CD20+, CD19+) and small to moderate amounts of plasma cells can be found. Preexisting B cell areas such as lymph follicles and germinal centers (GC) seem to be replaced by the lymphohistiocytic infiltrate of HL. Eosinophilic granulocytes can be numerous and necrosis may occur. Characteristically, necrotic areas are surrounded by tumor cells and varying amounts of eosinophilic granulocytes.

IMMUNOHISTOCHEMICAL FEATURES OF HRS CELLS IN CLASSICAL HODGKIN LYMPHOMA

The immunophenotype of HRS cells can be extremely variable. A common diagnostic feature of the tumor cell population is their positivity for CD30 in all and CD15 in most of the cases as well as their negativity for CD45 (Table 34.1).[3] CD30 is usually strongly expressed on the outer cell membrane and in variable amounts in the cytoplasm, especially in the Golgi field. A similar distribution pattern of immunoreactivity is seen with CD15. Whereas CD30 is an activation marker which can be found also on other lymphoid cells under reactive (e.g. infectious mononucleosis) and neoplastic conditions (B and T cell lymphomas), CD15 is usually confined to the tumor cells of HL and not expressed in other B or T cell neoplasias.

Table 34.1 Subtypes of Hodgkin lymphoma (HL) and selected characteristic features

Type of HL	Percent of cases	Phenotype of tumor cells	EBV+ cases (percent)	B cells (environment)	T cells (environment)	Pattern	Specific features
Nodular sclerosis	70		20	a/b	c/b	Nodular	Lacunar HRS cells, >1 nodule surrounded by sclerotic bands, eosinophils
Mixed cellularity	15	CD30+, CD15+, CD45–, CD20–	50	a/b	c/b	Diffuse/ nodular	Epitheloid cells, remnants of B cell areas, eosinophils
Lymphocyte-rich classical	5		40	c/b	b/a	Nodular/ diffuse	Nodular B cell infiltrates, occasionally including germinal centers with broad mantle zones
Lymphocyte depleted	1		20	a	a	Diffuse	Strong fibrosis possible
Nodular lymphocyte predominant	5	CD30–, CD15–, CD45+, CD20+,?	0	c/b	a/b (CD57+)	Nodular	LP variant of HRS cells, B cell nodules, varying amounts of T cells (CD57+)

a, few; b, some; c, many.
LP, lymphocyte-predominant.

Positivity for CD15 can be seen in histiocytes and myeloid cells in different stages of development. Although in nearly all cases (with the exception of a few T cell-derived HL) HRS cells are derived from GC B cells, they usually lack B cell markers such as CD20 and CD79a (see below). However, in a minority of cases varying amounts of HRS cells may show a membrane-bound positivity for CD20 and/ or CD79a.[4–7] This feature can be a sign of worse prognosis.[8] Nearly all HRS cells are positive for the proliferation-associated nuclear antigen Ki-67.[9] They are usually negative for EMA (epithelial membrane antigen) and never express the anaplastic lymphoma kinase (ALK).[10] In about 20–40 percent of cases in western Europe, EBV can be detected in the tumor cells either by *in situ* hybridization for EBER transcripts or by immunohistochemistry visualizing LMP1.[11] Transcription factors such as OCT2, BOB1 and PU1 are mostly negative and MUM1 and PAX5 are usually positive, depending on the case and the sensitivity of the immunohistochemical detection system.[6,12–16] Interestingly, HRS cells can express T cell markers such as CD3, CD4 and cytotoxic markers such as granzyme B and TIA1 in rare cases.[17–20] However, this T cell or cytotoxic phenotype often does not reflect a T cell origin of HRS cells, as also in such cases HRS cells are mostly B cell derived (discussed below).

NODULAR SCLEROSIS HODGKIN LYMPHOMA

Typical for NSHL are nodular infiltrates that are surrounded by collagen bands (at least one nodule) and the occurrence of lacunar-type HRS cells (Plate 59, see plate section). NSHL is the HL subtype most often found (approximately 70 percent of classical HL). In approximately 80 percent of cases the mediastinum is involved. In addition, cervical, axillary and inguinal lymph nodes, spleen, lung or the bone marrow can be affected. Lacunar cells usually can be detected using low magnification. These cells show a pale broad cytoplasm which is retracted (due to an embedding artifact) so that they seem to be localized in a lacuna (Plate 59C). The nuclei are lobated and the nucleoli are usually smaller than those of classical HRS cells. However, as in other types of HL, a broad spectrum of tumor cells ranging from blast-like cells to classical HRS can occur.

Although a grading of NSHL is not required for routine diagnostic purposes, it may be applied in clinical studies. In grade 1 about 75 percent or more of the nodules show a few HRS or lacunar cells in a background of reactive lymphocytes and histiocytes. Grade 2 has increased numbers of tumor cells in at least 25 percent of the nodules and may partially show pictures of LDHL (British National Lymphoma Investigation [BNLI]).[21] The immunophenotype of lacunar cells is comparable with that of typical HRS cells (Plate 59D) with the speciality that CD15 can be negative in the lacunar cells in about half of the cases.

MIXED CELLULARITY HODGKIN LYMPHOMA

The typical features of the nodular sclerosis subtype are lacking in MCHL, such as sclerotic bands and large amounts of lacunar cells. The infiltrate consists of small lymphohistiocytic cells, eosinophiles and neutrophils (Plate 60, see plate section). Epitheloid histiocytes may sometimes occur and are found solitary or in clusters. Occasionally epitheloid cell granulomas are found. The lymph node architecture may be completely or partly effaced. The tumor cells are localized in nodular or diffuse or sometimes in interfollicular areas. About 15 percent of cases of HL are accounted for by MCHL, and it is often found in advanced stages (III and IV), involving peripheral lymph nodes, occasionally the spleen and bone marrow, liver and other organs, but usually not in the mediastinum.

LYMPHOCYTE-RICH CLASSICAL HODGKIN LYMPHOMA

Lymphocyte-rich classical Hodgkin lymphoma is a rare subtype comprising approximately 5 percent of all HL cases. It can grow in a nodular or in rare cases in a diffuse pattern (Plate 61A). The nodular parts may show a high content of small B cells. Sometimes one finds GC or remnants of GC surrounded by broad mantle zones, which can harbor HRS cells. Some of the HRS cells in LRCHL may exhibit features of the tumor cells in NLPHL, so that it may be difficult or even impossible in some cases to differentiate LRCHL from NLPHL on the basis of morphology alone.[22] Usually neutrophilic and eosinophilic granulocytes are absent or found in small numbers in vessels or in between the HL infiltrates. In those cases of LRCHL that show a diffuse infiltration pattern, the small lymphocyte is the predominant cell type (Plate 61B). In some cases many histiocytes and/or epitheloid histiocytes forming clusters may occur.

Although LRCHL and NLPHL may be morphologically very similar or even indistinguishable, the immunophenotype of the HRS cells allows a clear differentiation. In LRCHL the immunophenotype of the HRS cells is identical to other subtypes of classical HL. The tumor cells are positive for CD30 (Plate 61C), usually positive for CD15 and generally negative for CD20.[22,23] Only in rare cases a CD20 positivity of some HRS cells can be seen. The tumor cells are often found in so-called expanded IgM- and IgD-positive mantle zones. Sometimes remnants of GC include meshworks of CD21-positive follicular dendritic cells which may surround the tumor cells. Characteristically in the diffuse parts of this HL subtype small reactive CD3-positive T cells are the major cell population.

LYMPHOCYTE-DEPLETED HODGKIN LYMPHOMA

Lymphocyte-depleted Hodgkin lymphoma is a very rare subtype (<1 percent of all HL cases) which is characterized by a diffuse infiltration pattern of classical HL showing numerous HRS cells and/or depletion of reactive lymphohistiocytic cells (Plate 62, see plate section). The subtype of LDHL has been 'cleaned up' in the last years using immunohistochemistry to separate this entity from NHL such as ALK-positive and ALK-negative anaplastic or pleomorphic large cell lymphomas. LDHL has also to be differentiated from a tumor cell-rich variant of NSHL. There are many synonyms for this rare entity such as Hodgkin sarcoma (Jackson and Parker),[24] lymphocytic depletion, diffuse fibrosis and reticular type (Lukes and Buttler),[25] lymphocytic depletion (Rye)[26] and lymphocyte depletion (Revised European–American Lymphoma [REAL] classification).[27] Principally two different forms of LDHL occur, one with many HRS cells which can be more or less pleomorphic and a few reactive lymphocytes, and another form that is characterized by a diffuse fibrosis with few lymphocytes and few to moderate amounts of tumor cells. In any case, the amount of lymphocytes compared with other subtypes of HL is low. The immunohistochemical properties of HRS cells and reactive lymphocytes is identical to the other subtypes of classical HL.

NODULAR LYMPHOCYTE–PREDOMINANT HODGKIN LYMPHOMA

In NLPHL, as in classical HL, most often cervical lymph nodes are involved, followed by axillary and inguinal lymph nodes. These are usually larger than those seen in classical HL and typically show a size between 2 cm and 10 cm in diameter. The sections microscopically often reveal a nodular architecture and typically a small rim of uninvolved lymphoid tissue (Plate 63A,B). The histologic picture is reflected by the fact that NLPHL is a monoclonal B cell neoplasia growing in more or less nodular pattern. The tumor cells – the LP cells (lymphocyte-predominant Reed–Sternberg cell variant) – are surrounded by T cells and often large amounts of B cells in a meshwork of follicular dendritic cells (Plate 63D). A completely pure diffuse form of lymphocyte predominant HL may exist. However, in such rare cases T cell-rich large B cell lymphoma or LRCHL should be excluded.

The tumor cells of LP-type are found in a totally or partially nodular background of small lymphocytes (most of them CD20-positive), histiocytes, and epitheloid histocytes (Plate 64, see plate section). LP cells are large cells that have a large often lobulated nucleus with small- to medium-sized nucleoli and a thin nuclear membrane. The nucleoli are usually smaller than those in classical HRS cells. The cytoplasm is usually broad and slightly to moderately basophilic. It can be difficult to differentiate LP cells from centroblasts. However, centroblasts are usually smaller. B cell markers, especially CD20, are very useful to identify LP cells (Plate 64, see plate section). The tumor cells are often found in small clusters inside at the outer border or between the nodules. In addition to CD20 the tumor cells express CD79a, BCL6 and CD45 in nearly all cases (Plate 63C).[4,28,29] They are negative for CD30 and CD15.[30,31] Other markers can be helpful for identification of these cells, e.g. CD75, EMA, J-chain and transcription factors such as OCT2, BOB1, PU1 and MUM1.[13,16,32] Some of these markers are necessary for the immunoglobulin synthesis, which is intact in the LP cells in contrast to classical HRS cells (see below). Like classical HRS cells, LP cells are positive for Ki-67 and often show rosetting CD3-positive T cells (Plate 64A).[22] CD57-positive T cells, a subset of GC T helper cells, can be numerous and may also form rosettes.[30,33] Sometimes the LP cells have close contact to follicular dendritic cells and their processes.

DIFFERENTIAL DIAGNOSIS

Hodgkin lymphoma and its subtypes show a broad spectrum of tumor cell infiltration patterns, lymphohistiocytic backgrounds and marker constellations. For the correct diagnosis, a variety of differential diagnoses have to be considered. Nodular infiltration patterns are usually accompanied by B-zone-specific follicular dendritic cells in a background of small B lymphocytes and minor T cell populations. Diffuse infiltration areas are typically lacking follicular dendritic cells and are dominated by small T lymphocytes and varying amounts of epitheloid venules. Histiocytes can occur in both instances. Especially epitheloid histiocytes will be found in areas of diffuse infiltration and characteristically in NLPHL. The most common variant NSHL usually lacks epitheloid histiocytes or shows only few of them. Considering the different subtypes of HL, their infiltration patterns and the morphology of the tumor cells, the following differential diagnoses may be of importance. Classical HL as well as NLPHL have to be differentiated from:

- reactive lesions
- NHLs
- nonlymphoid tumors (in rare instances).

REACTIVE CONDITIONS THAT MAY SIMULATE HODGKIN LYMPHOMA

Typical HRS cells including their variants such as immunoblast-like cells can occur in viral infections especially caused by EBV. The HRS- or Hodgkin-like cells in infectious mononucleosis, the acute EBV infection, are typically found in a background of small lymphocytes of T and B cell-type. Especially tonsils infected by EBV can give similar pictures as infiltrates of HL. Often necrotic areas caused by the viral infection develop. Characteristically, these HRS cells are EBV-positive, Ki-67-positive, CD30-positive, but lack CD15 expression.[34] Only the complete histologic composition of the lesion and immunohistologic marker constellation helps in this important differential diagnosis. Another typical reactive condition mimicking HL is the so-called interfollicular Hodgkinoid lymphadenitis, which may be similar to a partial infiltration of lymph nodes by HL. Immunoblasts can resemble HRS cells but lack CD15 expression.[35]

Also necrotizing and granulomatous lymphadenitis can easily be confused with HL. Special attention should be paid to large cells surrounding the necrotic areas which are often epitheloid histiocytes with large nuclei and nucleoli mimicking Hodgkin cells. Finally, monocytoid reactions with blasts showing features of Hodgkin cells may occur. However, in these cases the typical background of HL is absent and the blast cells do not show the typical marker profile of classical HL with exception of CD30 expression.

The most important differential diagnosis of a reactive condition to NLPHL are progressively transformed GC. The latter are benign lesions that are enlarged GC composed of increased numbers of mantle zone B cells.[36,37] The progressively transformed GC are round, sometimes solitary or multiple and usually reactive lymphoid follicles are seen between them. Tumor cells such as LP cells are never found. In contrast, in NLPHL the nodules are closely packed and form tumors. An epitheloid cell reaction which is rare in progressively transformed GC is usually found in NLPHL. The diagnostic LP cells can be seen in routine sections and more easily by immunostainings using B cell markers (CD20, CD19).

DIFFERENTIAL DIAGNOSIS BETWEEN HODGKIN LYMPHOMA AND OTHER MALIGNANCIES

Several NHL can require a differential diagnosis to HL. These include large cell B cell lymphomas which can simulate NSHL. Especially small biopsies from the mediastinum can make this differential diagnosis extremely difficult, because HRS cells may express also partly B cell markers under certain conditions. T cell-rich B cell lymphoma can be very similar either to MCHL or diffuse or T cell-rich variant of NLPHL. Also follicular lymphomas grade 1 and 2 may show similar features as NLPHL. HL can be mimicked by angioimmunoblastic T cell lymphoma and peripheral T cell lymphoma of Lennert-type. However, these T cell lymphomas have no or very few HRS cells which may be CD30-positive but usually lack CD15.[38,39] The main differential diagnosis to LDHL are diffuse large B cell lymphomas and ALK lymphomas. Whereas ALK lymphomas are always ALK positive, HL is never positive for the ALK protein.[10]

Also nonlymphoid neoplasias can be a differential diagnosis of classical HL, such as carcinoma, malignant melanoma and different types of sarcomas.[40] Immunohistochemical stainings usually help in these special conditions.

RELATIONS AND POSSIBLE COMBINATIONS OF HODGKIN LYMPHOMA AND NON-HODGKIN LYMPHOMA

In rare cases, an HL and an NHL may occur in the same patient: in the same or in different localizations as well as simultaneously or subsequently. Such composite lymphomas often share a common clonal origin, but may also represent two independent malignancies (see also below). Most composite lymphomas represent combinations of a B cell NHL with classical HL.[41,42] The B cell lymphoma component is often a follicular lymphoma or a diffuse large B cell lymphoma. Much more seldom are marginal zone lymphomas and mantle cell lymphomas as well as B cell chronic lymphocytic leukaemia combined with HL. In rare cases of classical HL, combinations with T cell lymphomas occur.[43–45]

NLPHL has a relatively high incidence (3.5 percent of cases) of transformation to diffuse large B cell lymphoma.[46,47] Also transitions of NLPHL to T cell-rich B cell lymphoma may occur. The latter can be subclassified in at least two types according to the morphology of the tumor cells. They may be either of LP cell-type or resemble large blasts of large B cell lymphomas.

CELLULAR ORIGIN OF HRS AND LP CELLS

LP cells of NLPHL express multiple B cell markers (e.g. CD20, CD79, sIg, OCT2, PAX5) and lack expression of markers of other lineages, indicating that these cells derive from mature B cells (Plate 65, see plate section).[2,4,13,31] In addition, the detection of BCL6 in LP cells together with the follicular growth pattern and the association with typical constituents of GC, i.e. CD57+ T helper cells and follicular dendritic cells, pointed to a close relationship to GC B cells.[28,48] This was substantiated by single cell studies for rearranged immunoglobulin V genes with microdissected LP cells. The LP cells carried clonal IG gene rearrangements that in all cases were somatically mutated.[49–52] Thus, LP cells represent a monoclonal population of tumor cells in a patient. Moreover, as somatic hypermutation is specifically taking place in GC B cells,[53] these findings pointed to a derivation of the LP cells from GC or post GC B cells. Importantly, in a fraction of cases, intraclonal V gene diversification was observed, showing hypermutation activity during clonal expansion of the LP cells.[49–51] This argues for a GC derivation of the cells, as hypermutation activity is silenced in post GC B cells. LP cells indeed express AID, the main regulator of somatic hypermutation.[54]

The cellular origin of the HRS cells of classical HL has been debated much more and remained a mystery for a long time. This was mainly due to the unusual phenotype of HRS cells that did not resemble any normal hematopoietic cell (see above). Microdissected HRS cells were tested for a potential B cell origin by analyzing them for the presence of rearranged *IGV* genes.[50] The first study showed that HRS cells represent clonal populations of mature B cells in each of the cases analyzed.[50] These findings were initially questioned by other studies, which reported either lack of rearrangements or frequent polyclonal *IG* genes,[55–58] but later work confirmed the original studies.[59–65] HRS cells of nearly all cases analyzed carried somatically mutated V genes, indicating a derivation from cells that underwent a GC reaction. At variance to the LP cells, HRS cell clones did not show significant intraclonal V gene diversification, demonstrating that the hypermutation machinery was not active any more during clonal expansion of these lymphoma cells.[50,59–65] Surprisingly, in about 25 percent of cases analyzed, somatic mutations were identified that rendered originally functional V region genes nonfunctional.[50,59–65] Such obviously crippling mutations included small deletions that led to a loss of the correct reading-frame and nonsense mutations, generating stop codons. Destructive mutations can happen in GC B cells, but normally would cause their immediate elimination by apoptosis, as GC B cells are stringently selected for the expression of a (high-affinity) B cell receptor.[66] Therefore, the finding of HRS cell clones with destructive mutations indicates that these cells are derived from a population of preapoptotic GC B cells that were rescued by some mechanism from apoptosis. Whether also the remaining cases of classical HL are derived from preapoptotic GC B cells is less clear. However, most GC B cells undergo apoptosis not because of deletions or nonsense mutations, but because of replacement mutations that, for example, prevent proper folding of the *IG* heavy or light chain genes or reduce the affinity to the selecting antigen. Such mutations can not be easily identified as disadvantageous on V gene sequencing. Thus, if one assumes that HRS cells as a rule derive from the population of GC B cells induced to undergo apoptosis, one would indeed expect to find clearly crippling mutations only in a fraction of cases. It is consequently an attractive scenario that not only the 25 percent of cases with obviously crippling mutations but also the (majority of the) remaining cases originate from preapoptotic GC B cells.[67] There are a few cases of classical HL with unmutated V genes.[68,69] Such cases may derive from the transformation of naïve B cells. However, as GC founder cells start to proliferate and become prone to apoptosis even before the onset of somatic hypermutation,[70] it may well be that these cases reflect transformation of early GC B cells.

The cellular derivation of HRS cells from GC B cells is also supported by molecular analysis of composite lymphomas. In such lymphomas, an HL and an NHL are found in the same patient. In most composite lymphomas, a clonal relationship of the HRS and the NHL tumor cells was demonstrated by *IG* gene analysis.[59,69,71–76] In combination of HL with follicular lymphomas or diffuse large B cell lymphomas, the rearranged and mutated V genes showed a striking pattern of both shared as well as separate somatic mutations.[59,72–74] Therefore, the common

precursor of the lymphomas was a GC B cell which had already acquired some somatic mutations, and the two distinct lymphomas developed from separate daughter cells of that common precursor which are characterized by the distinct mutations.

As there are cases of HL in which the HRS cells express several typical T cell markers, such as CD4, granzyme B or perforin, and as two of the cell lines established from classical HL are of T lineage origin (see below), such cases were analysed for a potential T cell origin, by performing single cell PCR for rearranged *TCRβ* or *γ* genes. Clonal *TCR* gene rearrangements were identified in some of the cases with TCR marker expression.[45,77–79] Remarkably, most HRS clones with expression of multiple T cell markers nevertheless represented transformed B cells. Overall, it appears that perhaps 1–2 percent of cases of classical HL originate from transformed T cells.

THE LOST B CELL PHENOTYPE OF HRS CELLS

It was already known from early immunophenotypic studies (see above) that HRS cells of classical HL do not express a number of typical B cell molecules, such as CD20, CD79b, sIg, OCT2 and PU1.[5,6,12–14] When it became clear that HRS cells nevertheless derive from mature B cells, this motivated a genome-wide analysis for the B cell phenotype of HRS cells. A genechip analysis comparing the expression of typical B cell markers in HL cell lines with other B cell lymphomas and normal B cells revealed that there is a global loss of the B cell phenotype in HRS cells, including low or undetectable expression of many surface molecules (e.g. CD37, CD53), components of important signaling pathways in B cells (e.g. SYK, BLK, SLP65) and transcription factors (e.g. PUB, AMYB, SPIB).[80] Notably, this downregulation does not involve molecules that are involved in antigen presentation and interaction with T helper cells (CD80, CD86, major histocompatibility complex [MHC] class II).[80,81] Although also a few other lymphomas show a partial loss of expression of the typical B cell expression pattern, HRS cells are unique among all lymphomas in the extent to which they lost their B cell phenotype.[82]

Curiously, although many typical B cell genes are downregulated in HRS cells, PAX5, a master regulator for B cell lineage commitment and maintenance, and E2A, another transcription factor positively regulating many B cell genes, are still expressed in most cases of HL.[15,83] The reasons why these factors fail to induce the typical B cell gene expression programme are only partly understood. Factors likely contributing to the suppression of the B cell phenotype are ABF1 and ID2, which both inhibit the function of E2A and which show aberrant expression in HRS cells.[83–85] Moreover, HRS cells express activated NOTCH1, which normally supports T cell differentiation in lymphoid precursors by inhibiting B cell differentiation.[86] For at least a fraction of the B cell-specific genes their silencing in HRS cells is stabilized by epigenetic mechanisms, as for several genes (e.g. *CD19*, *CD79b*, *BOB1*) methylation of their promoter regions has been demonstrated.[87–89]

What could be the reason for this peculiar reprogramming of the HRS cells? One may speculate that this is related to the origin of HRS cells from crippled GC B cells.[80] B cells are normally under very strict selection to express a functional BCR, and in the GC in particular a high affinity receptor. Thus, when a GC B cell acquires disadvantageous mutations, there is a strong B cell intrinsic selection to induce apoptosis. By escaping from the B cell gene expression program, the cells may escape this selection pressure to undergo apoptosis. Consequently, there would be a selective advantage to downregulate the B cell-specific gene programme. Perhaps, it is the so far largely unknown transforming events involved in HRS cell pathogenesis target genes that cause this reprogramming.

CELL LINE MODELS

Numerous attempts have been made to establish *in vitro* growing cell lines from HL tissues. The vast majority of attempts failed, and only a few cell lines have been generated (Table 34.2). Importantly, all successful attempts were associated with heavily pretreated patients and the lines were not established from lymph node biopsies, but from peripheral blood, bone marrow or plural effusions.[93,101] This might indicate that HRS cells can grow in culture only if they have already become independent from the lymph node microenvironment for their survival in the patients. Perhaps, the cells had acquired additional transforming events in the patients treated with chemo- and/or radiation therapy. The fact that the cell lines originate from patients with advanced disease should be kept in mind

when using these lines to study the biology of HRS cells. Moreover, although the lines mostly used share many features with primary HRS cells, molecular proof that the lines derive from the HRS cells in the patients is available only for one of them, L1236.[62] One cell line originally regarded as a HL cell line, line CO, was recently shown to originate from a cell culture contamination by a T cell leukemia cell line.[98] Cell line HDMyz is most likely also not derived from HRS cells, as it phenotypically differs in key aspects from the HRS cells of the patient it was established from.[99] Moreover, HDMyz lacks *IG* and *TCR* gene rearrangements, and is suggested to be of myeloid origin, whereas all classical HL cases studied so far in detail could be assigned either to a B or T cell origin (see above). Cell lines L428, L540, L591, L1236, KMH-2 and HDLM-2 are currently available and considered as classical HL cell lines. Two of these lines, HDLM-2 and L540 are of T cell origin, so that T cell lines are overpresented, considering the low frequency of T cell-derived HL cases. On the other hand, only one of the lines is EBV-positive (L591), which is curious as about 40 percent of cases of classical HL harbor EBV-infected HRS cells (see below). When using this line to study the role of EBV in HRS cells, it needs to be considered that L591 does not show the typical expression pattern of EBV genes usually seen in HRS cells in the tissue.[100] One cell line, DEV, was originally reported as being also derived from a case of classical HL, but a reevaluation of the case led to a reassignment of this line to NLPHL.[102] Thus, this line is currently the only *in vitro* model for LP cells. Cell line HKB-1 was recently established from a pediatric case of HL, but little further studies with this line have so far been reported.[96]

Although the number of HL cell lines is low and they may not be representative of HRS cells in early stages of the disease, they have been very valuable in many aspects.

Table 34.2 Features of Hodgkin lymphoma (HL) cell lines[a]

Cell line	Subtype of HL	Cellular origin	B cell markers	T cell markers	EBV	Mutations in tumor suppressor genes or oncogenes	Reference
L428	Classical	B cell			–	IKBA, IKBE, SOCS1, TP53	90
L540	Classical	T cell			–		91,92
L591[b]	Classical	B cell	CD19, CD20	CD2	+		91
L1236	Classical	B cell			–	CD95, SOCS1, TP53	93
KMH-2	Classical	B cell			–	IKBA	94
HDLM-2	Classical	T cell		CD2	–	SOCS1, TP53	95
HKB-1	Classical	B cell	CD19, CD20		–		96
DEV	NLPHL	B cell	CD20, CD22		–		97

[a]Several additional cell lines have been published. However, for some of them, it is not known whether the lines are still existing (HD70, HO, ZO, SUP-HD1). Cell line CO has been identified as a cell culture contamination,[98] and HD-MyZ is of myeloid origin and differs phenotypically considerably from the HRS cells of the patient it was established from, suggesting that this line is not derived from HRS cells.[99]
[b]L591 shows an EBV gene expression pattern (latency III) untypical for EBV-positive HRS cells in biopsies.[100]
EBV, Epstein–Barr virus; NLPHL, nodular lymphocyte-predominant HL.

Many features of HRS cells were initially identified in HL cell lines and later confirmed in primary HRS cells in biopsies. Due to the rarity of primary HRS cells, the lines are also the only available tool to perform functional studies with HRS cells. In addition, as there is no mouse model existing for HL, transplantation of HL cell line cells into immunodeficient mice is still the only way to study the behavior of HRS cells in the context of a whole organism, for example to test novel treatment strategies.

CYTOGENETIC FEATURES OF HRS AND LP CELLS

Many attempts were made to elucidate the cytogenetic profile of HRS cells.[103] The low number of tumor cells, the rare occurrence of mitoses and the poor morphology of metaphase chromosomes has vastly hampered classical cytogenetic analysis of HRS and LP cells. Two-thirds of the HL cases analyzed by means of this method present with aneuploidy, most of them showing a triploid or tetraploid chromosome set, independently of histopathologic subtype. This was confirmed by fluorescence immunophenotyping and interphase cytogenetics as a tool for investigation of neoplasms (FICTION) where an even higher percentage of HRS cells displayed numerical chromosome aberrations, which occurred as clonal as well as subclonal events.[104] Furthermore, additional marker chromosomes were frequently found. Overall, HRS cells displayed more gains than losses of chromosomes. Additional copies of chromosomes 2, 5, 9, 12 and 19 were commonly found whereas chromosomes 13, 21 and Y presented in diminished copy numbers.[105–107]

Comparative genomic hybridization of microdissected HRS cells revealed a closer insight into these copy number aberrations.[108] Regions of gain could be confined to 2p (54 percent of cases), 12q (37 percent of cases), 17p (27 percent of cases), 9p (24 percent of cases) and 16p (24 percent of cases) and regions of loss to 13q (22 percent of cases), and X (12 percent of cases), mostly in agreement with classical cytogenetic data. Regions were considered to be gained if the fold change was at least 1.25, which represents five versus four copies in a tetraploid chromosome set. Occasional high copy number amplifications were observed in 17.5 percent of cases when a fold change above 2 was recorded. The most commonly gained region was related to chromosome 2p13-16, where the oncogenes REL, a member of the nuclear factor (NF)-κB transcription factor family, and BCL11A, a zinc-finger transcription factor, are located. Both genes were found to be frequently amplified in classical HL by fluorescence in situ hybridization (FISH) and FICTION.[109] As some cases featured solely a REL gain without a change of the BCL11A locus, the more important role was assigned to REL. Genomic gains of REL correlated with increased expression of the REL protein through a gene dosage effect.[110] Chromosome 9p24 is another chromosomal region which was amplified in three HL cell lines

and several primary cases.[108,111,112] Here, JAK2 is located, coding for a tyrosine kinase involved in the JAK/STAT pathway.

Concerning cytogenetic features of NLPHL, even fewer studies have been conducted so far. A cytogenetically aberrant clone in NLPHL was first described in 1986.[113] Several characteristic copy number changes in NLPHL were found by comparative genomic hybridization of microdissected LP cells.[114] Gains present in more than a third of investigated cases included 1p, 1q, 2q, 3p, 3q, 4q, 5q, 6p, 6q, 8q, 11q, 12q, Xp and Xq. Losses were located to 6p, 10p, 11q, 16p and 17.[115] A higher number of aberrations registered in NLPHL than in classical HL might be due to differences in the applied techniques.

Translocations in B cell lymphomas frequently include the IG loci, since these are exposed to somatic gene rearrangements and somatic hypermutation.[116] While recurring translocations to these loci have been described for most B cell NHL, a characteristic translocation for classical HL has not yet been identified. In a recent large-scale study the frequency of translocations involving the IG loci in classical HL was determined. Approximately 20 percent of the cases investigated showed translocations with involvement of the IGH locus, and a few cases had translocations affecting the Ig light chain loci.[116] A recurrent translocation partner could not be identified, still in single cases a juxtaposition of BCL6, MYC, BCL3 or REL to the IGH locus was detected.[116,117] Translocations of BCL2 and CCND1 to the IGH locus in HRS cells have been described in three rare cases of composite lymphomas, involving a classical HL and a clonally related follicular lymphoma or mantle cell lymphoma.[118] HRS cells showed the same translocations as the NHL parts of these lymphomas. Thus, the translocations happened in a common precursor of the two parts of the composite lymphomas as an early shared transforming event. Since Ig transcription and enhancer activity is downregulated in classical HL, the importance of translocations to IG loci remains unclear. Perhaps, the mechanism in these instances is not via IG enhancer driven deregulated oncogene expression, but through structural alterations of protooncogenes or inactivation of tumor suppressor genes.

The frequent detection of a specific translocation involving the NPM and ALK genes on chromosomes 5 and 2, respectively, in large cell anaplastic lymphoma, which shares several key features with classical HL, prompted several studies of this translocation in HL. Although initial investigations reported detection of such translocations, numerous large studies could not confirm the initial findings, indicating that HRS cells usually lack translocations involving NPM and ALK.[119,120]

A high number of other translocations concerning various breakpoints has been observed, implying so-called *jumping translocations*. These include translocations of one chromosomal breakpoint to different chromosomes in different tumor cells of the same tumor clone in the same patient.[121] The breakpoints involved in jumping translocations in classical HL are often located to ribosomal DNA regions.[122] Another interesting point is the occurrence of segmental chromosomal aberrations – multiple copies of a gene segment which are translocated and inserted into different parts of the genome resulting in an increased gene dosage, as was also found for *JAK2* in HL cell lines and one primary case.[111,123] These inserts often colocalize to amplified ribosomal DNA, which can also be inserted in various chromosomal regions.[122,123] These findings highlight chromosomal instability and intraclonal variability in classical HL.

Another mechanism being discussed as causing chromosomal instability are centrosome aberrations. Centrosomes play a major role in maintenance of a balanced chromosome segregation in mitosis and show defects in most solid tumors. A consequence of acquisition of multiple centrosomes may be the formation of giant cells. So far only few cases of classical HL have been investigated concerning centrosomes. HRS cells displaying multiple centrosomes were all multinucleated featuring the importance of centrosomes in cytokinesis.[123]

NLPHL showed in 48 percent of cases recurrent rearrangements of *BCL6*, an oncogene with transcription repressor function.[124] Different translocation partners of *BCL6* were identified. Translocations of *BCL6* to the *IGH* locus in 38 percent of NLPHL have been confirmed by an independent study.[125] Immunohistochemical expression of BCL6 protein in LP cells was found in all cases tested.[124]

ONCOGENES AND TUMOR SUPPRESSOR GENES

A number of oncogenes and tumor suppressor genes were analyzed for mutations in HRS cells. HRS cells and HL cell lines express the tumor suppressor gene *CD95* (*FAS*), and HL cell lines are resistant to apoptosis induction by CD95 triggering.[126] An analysis of HRS cells for mutations of *CD95* identified mutations in only 2/30 cases and one of three cell lines (Table 34.3).[132,133] It is, however, remarkable that patients affected by the autoimmune lymphoproliferative syndrome with germline mutations in the *CD95* gene show a 51-fold increased risk to develop HL.[144] The insensitivity of the HL cell lines against CD95 triggering motivated also a study for potential mutations in downstream CD95 signaling components, i.e. caspase 8, 10 and *FADD*, but no mutations were found in these genes.[134]

Isolated HRS were analyzed for mutations in the *TP53* gene in three studies. Mutations were identified in only 3/39 cases, indicating that *TP53* mutations do not play a major role in HL.[128–130] However, these studies were restricted to the analysis of exons 5–8 or 5–9, where normally *TP53* mutations cluster, and recent studies identified *TP53* mutations involving other exons of the gene in 3/6 HL cell lines.[131,145] Thus, HRS cells may potentially harbor *TP53* mutations more frequently than indicated from the earlier studies.

HRS cells show constitutive activity of the transcription factor NF-κB, and inactivation of this factor in HL cell

Table 34.3 Oncogene and tumor suppressor gene alterations in HRS and LP cells

Gene name	Type of alteration	Mutated cell lines/ cell lines analyzed	Mutated cases/ cases analyzed	Reference
NRAS	Somatic mutations	NA	0/12	127
TP53	Somatic mutations	3/6	3/39	128–131
CD95	Somatic mutations	1/3	2/30	132,133
Caspase 8	Somatic mutations	0/4	0/10	134
Caspase 10	Somatic mutations	0/4	0/10	134
FADD	Somatic mutations	0/4	0/10	134
SOCS1	Somatic mutations	3/5	8/19	135
JAK2	Somatic mutations	0/5	0/16	136
IKBA[a]	Somatic mutations	2/6	5/23	137–139
IKBE	Somatic mutations	1/6	1/6	140
ASHM[b]	Somatic mutations	NA	5/9 (classical HL) 8/10 (NLPHL)	141
JAK2	Chromosomal gains	3/4	3/11	111,112
REL	Chromosomal gains	3/4	33/70	109,111
BCL6	Translocations	1/1 (NLPHL)	0/40 (classical HL) 16/47 (NLPHL)	124,125
BCL2	Translocations		3/143	118,142,143

If not other specified, numbers refer to classical Hodgkin lymphoma (HL). When also LP cells of nodular lymphocyte-predominant HL (NLPHL) were studied, this is indicated.
[a]The true frequency of HL cases with mutations in the IKBA gene may be higher than indicated from the three studies, as in one of the studies, only part of the gene was amplified and sequenced, and another of the studies was restricted to the identification of cases with deletions or insertions.
[b]ASHM, aberrant somatic hypermutation; four genes affected by ASHM were analyzed (*PAX5, PIM5, MYC, RHO/TTF*), the numbers given in the table refer to cases having mutations in at least one of the four genes.
NA, not analyzed.

lines induces their death (see below).[146] It was shown that HRS cells harbor somatic inactivating mutation in the gene of the main inhibitor of NF-κB, i.e. *IKBA*, in about 20 percent of cases and two of six HL cell lines, suggesting that IKBA acts as a tumor suppressor gene in HL (Table 34.3).[137–139] Mutations were also found in the *IKBE* gene, coding for another inhibitor of NF-κB, in one cell line and one of six cases analyzed.[140]

HRS cells show constitutive activity of the JAK/STAT signaling pathway (see below), and this may partly be caused by genomic gains of the *JAK2* gene in a fraction of cases, as discussed above. Since the *JAK2* gene can also be activated by a particular missense mutation in exon 2, as it is frequently found in polycythemia vera and chronic myeloid leukemia, isolated HRS cells were also analyzed for this mutation, but none of the 16 HL and 4 HL cell lines showed a mutation.[136] Interestingly, however, mutations were frequently found (8/19 cases and 3/5 HL cell lines) in *SOCS1*, an inhibitor of STAT signaling (Table 34.3).[135] Most mutations resulted in premature termination of translation and hence shortened proteins lacking the functional critical SOCS box domain.

Aberrant somatic hypermutation of several proto-oncogenes, affecting *MYC*, *PAX5*, *RHO/TTF* and *PIM1*, has been identified as a pathogenetic mechanism in diffuse large B cell lymphomas.[147] These mutations probably happen as an aberrant activity of the somatic hypermutation machinery, as they show the typical mutation patterns of *IGV* gene mutations and are like V gene mutations restricted to a region about 1.5 kb downstream of the gene promoter. Aberrant somatic hypermutation was not found in normal GC B cells or various other GC-derived B cell NHLs.[147] A recent analysis of microdissected HRS and LP cells revealed that mutations were present in at least one of the four genes in 80 percent of NLPHL and 55 percent of classical HL.[141] The functional relevance of these mutations is difficult to discern, but some mutations in 5′ noncoding regions may influence gene expression and missense mutations in coding regions may alter protein function. The identification of frequent aberrant somatic hypermutation in NLPHL and classical HL indicates unexpected shared genetic lesions with diffuse large B cell lymphomas.

Tumor suppressor genes can not only be inactivated by somatic mutations, but also by epigenetic mechanisms, in particular through DNA hypermethylation of their promoters. For two candidate tumor suppressor genes, *p18(INK4c)* and *RASSF1A*, frequent epigenetic silencing has been reported in isolated HRS cells.[148,149]

Taken together, so far only a few recurrent genetic alterations have been found in HRS and LP cells, suggesting that key transforming events remain to be identified. The pathogenesis of classical HL appears to be quite diverse, as oncogene or tumor suppressor gene mutations were mostly found only in a fraction of cases. Notably, however, it appears that distinct genetic lesions can contribute to the deregulated activation of particular survival pathways, such as gains of *JAK2* or mutations of *SOCS1* activating STAT signaling.

EPSTEIN–BARR VIRUS AND OTHER VIRUSES IN HODGKIN LYMPHOMA PATHOGENESIS

Epstein–Barr virus is a γ herpes virus that was initially identified based on its association with endemic Burkitt lymphoma in Africa, where it is present in the lymphoma cells in more than 90 percent of cases. It is a DNA virus with a 172 kb large genome coding for more than 90 genes. The viral genome is present as a circular episome in infected cells. The virus can establish a latent infection in B cells in which up to nine viral proteins can be expressed. In 1989, EBV was detected by *in situ* hybridization in HRS cells of classical HL.[150,151] Southern blot studies indicated that the infection was a clonal event, i.e. occurring likely in the tumor clone precursor.[150,151] In Western countries about 30–40 percent of HL show EBV-positive HRS cells, while in childhood cases in Central and South America, the association can reach up to 90 percent.[11] EBV is not found in NLPHL, and among classical HL cases, it is predominantly present in mixed cellularity cases (Table 34.1).[11]

EBV is present in HRS cells in a latent state, and three protein-coding and two noncoding RNAs are expressed.[152] The EBER and BART RNAs do not code for proteins, and their function is largely unclear, although there is indication that EBER might induce expression of the immunosuppressive cytokine interleukin-10 (IL-10) and may play a role in regulating the interferon response in virally infected cells.[153] EBERs are expressed at very high level and can be detected by *in situ* hybridization, which is the most reliable method to detect EBV in tissue sections. The EBV nuclear antigen 1 (EBNA1) is expressed in all proliferating EBV-infected cells, as it is essential for the replication of the viral genome. Whether EBNA1 has an oncogenic potential is still controversially discussed. The other two proteins expressed in EBV-infected HRS cells are LMP1 and LMP2A. LMP1 bears a cytoplasmic motif that resembles the signalling motifs of the CD40 receptor, which is a main costimulatory molecule for T cell–B cell interaction and is critical for the survival of GC B cells, mainly by activating NF-κB.[154] LMP1 molecules associate in the cell membrane and transmit a constitutive signal without binding of any ligand. Hence, this viral protein probably acts as an oncogene, contributing to constitutive NF-κB activity in EBV-infected HRS cells. The oncogenic potential of LMP1 is directly demonstrated in fibroblast transformation assays and by the development of lymphoid malignancies in LMP1 transgenic mice.[155,156] LMP2A has a cytoplasmic motif called ITAM (immunoreceptor tyrosine-based activating motif) which is also found in the coreceptors CD79a and CD79b of the B cell receptor, and which mediate B cell receptor signaling to downstream tyrosine kinases.[157] LMP2A appears to be able to replace the tonic survival signal normally mediated by the B cell receptor.[158,159] This critical function of EBV in HL pathogenesis is strongly supported by the observation that practically all cases of classical HL in which the HRS cell clone carries destructive somatic *IGV* gene mutations that prevent B cell receptor expression (e.g. stop codons) are EBV-positive.[160] Thus, it appears that a GC B cell which acquired disadvantageous mutations impairing expression of surface Ig can survive and in rare instances develop into an HRS cell clone only if EBV is present in the cells. This striking association between EBV and HRS cells with crippled B cell receptor underscores the pathogenetic role of EBV in a subset of cases of HL.

As EBV is found only in a fraction of cases of classical HL, there has been an intensive search for other viruses involved in HL pathogenesis. Studies for a potential role of HHV-6, HHV-7, HHV-8, SV40, HTLV-1 and 2, adenoviruses and polyoma viruses all yielded negative results.[11,161] Recently, it was reported that measles virus can be found in about 50 percent of HL cases.[162] However, a detailed and highly sensitive reverse transcription polymerase chain reaction (RT-PCR) analysis of microdissected HRS cells (including cells from the cases originally reported as measles virus-positive) showed that measles virus was not present in the HRS cells of the cases investigated,[163] in line with another recent investigation.[164] There is, nevertheless, still interest in the search for novel viruses in HL, particularly since epidemiologic studies indicate an involvement of late exposure to an infectious agent in young adult HL patients in Western countries – and this patient group is mostly EBV negative.[11,165] Finally, it has also been discussed that initially all cases of HL were EBV positive, but that the virus is lost in a fraction of cases later in the course of the disease (hit-and-run scenario). While loss of the virus is difficult to disprove, attempts to identify remnants of the EBV genome integrated into the cellular genome in EBV-negative cases yielded only negative results.[166] Moreover, patients developing HL relatively shortly after an acute primary infection with EBV (infectious mononucleosis), are regularly EBV positive, indirectly also arguing against a hit-and-run scenario.[167,168]

ACTIVATION OF MULTIPLE SIGNALING PATHWAYS IN HRS CELLS

In normal B cells, activation of signaling pathways is transient and strictly regulated. In HRS cells, multiple signaling pathways and key transcription factors are constitutively activated. As inhibition of these pathways in HL cell lines shows significant effects on survival and/or proliferation, the activity of these signaling modules plays a major role in HL pathogenesis.

NF-κB is a family of dimeric transcription factors that have key roles in inflammatory and immunologic processes. It is usually retained in the cytoplasm by binding to inhibitors of NF-κB, the IκBs. When NF-κB signaling is initiated, an IκB kinase complex phosphorylates the IκBs, leading to their proteasomal degradation. This releases the

NF-κB factors which translocate into the nucleus and activate the transcription of multiple genes. HRS cells express the NF-κB factors P50, P52, P65 (RELA), RELB and CREL, and NF-κB is found in the cytoplasm and the nucleus, showing constitutive activity of these factors.[169–172] NF-κB is essential for HRS cell survival, as its inactivation in HL cell lines causes apoptosis of the cells.[146] A multitude of genes are activated by NF-κB in HRS cells, including antiapoptotic genes (*BCLXL*, *IAP2*), chemokines and cytokines (*IL13*, *CX3CL1*), and other transcription factors (*STAT5*, *SPIB*).[173,174] There is a remarkably long list of genetic and nongenetic factors that presumably contribute to NF-κB activation in HRS cells: genomic gains of the *REL* gene (see above), somatic mutations in the *IKBA* and *IKBE* genes (see above), activation of cell surface receptors CD30, CD40, RANK, TACI, BCMA and NOTCH1, and expression of the viral *LMP1* gene in EBV+ cases of HL.[86,154,175–179]

Aberrant tyrosine kinase activities are a frequent finding in several tumor types. Expression of seven receptor tyrosine kinases (RTK) has been observed in HRS cells in classical HL.[180,181] One of these RTKs, MET, is also expressed in normal GC B cells, but the other six (PDGFRA, DDR2, EPHB1, RON, TRKA and TRKB) are not normally expressed by B cells and hence show aberrant expression in HRS cells. These RTKs were each expressed in HRS cells of 30–70 percent of classicalal HL cases, with largely varying patterns.[180,181] The highest frequency of expression is found in EBV-negative NSHL, and the lowest in EBV-positive mixed cellularity HL.[182] Cases coexpressing several RTKs were largely EBV–, suggesting that strong RTK signaling could at least partially replace EBV in HRS cell pathogenesis.[182] Expression of multiple RTKs is unique for classical HL and primary mediastinal B cell lymphomas, as other lymphomas derived from mature B cells rarely express RTKs.[183] With antibodies specific for activated forms of three RTKs it was shown that the RTKs were activated in large fractions of cases, which is also supported by elevated phospho-tyrosine levels in HRS cells.[180] Detection of RTK ligands in HL tissues indicates that activation of the RTKs can be due to autocrine (PDGFRA and EPHB1) and paracrine (TRKA and DDR2) stimulation.[180] For one HRS cell line with coexpression of PDGFRA and the ligand PDGFA, the use of a PDGFRA-specific inhibitor demonstrated the importance of PDGFRA signaling for growth of the cell line.[180]

Signaling through cytokine receptors is mainly mediated through the JAK/STAT pathway. Upon activation of the cytokine receptors, JAK kinases are phosphorylated and subsequently phosphorylate STAT transcription factors which then translocate as dimers into the nucleus and activate transcription of target genes. Besides cytokine receptors, STATs can also be activated by RTKs and seven transmembrane receptors. In HRS cells, STAT3 and STAT6 are frequently activated, and STAT5 in a smaller fraction of cases.[184–186] Inhibition of cytokine signaling or STAT activity impairs proliferation and induces apoptosis of HL cell lines, supporting an important role for STAT signaling in HL.[184–187] Multiple factors presumably contribute to the constitutive STAT activity: genomic amplification of the *JAK2* gene and frequent deleterious mutations of *SOCS1* (see above), autocrine stimulation through expression of IL-13 and IL-13 receptor by HRS cells,[188] stimulation through other cytokines and activity of multiple RTKs, as discussed above.

Activation of the serine/threonine kinase AKT by phosphatidylinositol 3-kinase (PI3K) is another key signaling pathway for survival in lymphocytes. Most cases of classical HL express the active, phosphorylated form of AKT in the HRS cells, display phosphorylation of known downstream targets of AKT, and inhibition of this kinase in HL cell lines promotes cell cycle arrest and apoptosis.[189,190] Thus, the PI3K/AKT pathway is constitutively active in HRS cells and this pathway plays an essential role in HRS cell growth and survival. PI3K may be activated through CD40, CD30, RANK and RTK signaling, and in EBV-positive cases through the LMP1 and LMP2A proteins.[189,190]

Mitogen-activated protein kinases (MAPK) are serine/threonine kinases that can be activated by various extracellular stimuli and that regulate apoptosis, proliferation and differentiation. HRS cells express active forms of several members of this family, i.e. extracellular signal-related kinase (ERK) 1/2 and 5.[191,192] Inhibition of ERK activity shows antiproliferative activity in HL cell lines.[192] Similar to PI3K/AKT signaling, the MAPK/ERK pathway is activated in HRS cells by signaling through CD30, CD40, RANK, and perhaps RTKs.[192]

AP1 transcription factors are composed of homo- or heterodimers of members of the JUN, FOS and ATF families. In HRS cells, overexpression of CJUN and JUNB is found, and AP1 activity promotes proliferation and activates multiple target genes in HRS cells.[193] The expression of JUNB is regulated by NF-κB, whereas there is an autoregulatory mechanism promoting CJUN expression.[193] CD30 is among the targets of AP1 in HRS cells, and hence, AP1-induced CD30 expression may in a positive feedback loop through activation of NF-κB contribute to AP1 overexpression.[194]

ANTIAPOPTOTIC MECHANISMS IN HRS CELLS

As HRS cells are presumably derived from preapoptotic GC B cells, it is obvious that antiapoptotic mechanisms are essential for survival of the cells and establishment of the malignant clone. Several key factors for survival of HRS cells have already been discussed, such as constitutive NF-κB activity and PI3K/AKT signaling. Considering the two main apoptotic pathways, the extrinsic, death receptor-mediated pathway and the intrinsic, mitochondria-associated pathway, there is indication for specific inhibition of both pathways. HRS cells express the death receptor CD95, but are insensitive against CD95 stimulation and mostly lack mutations in the *CD95* gene or components of the death-inducing signaling complex (caspases

8 and 10, FADD) (see above). Importantly, HRS cells express high levels of the antiapoptotic cellular FLICE-inhibitory protein (CFLIP), and downregulation of CFLIP sensitizes HL cell lines for CD95-induced apoptosis, indicating that CFLIP plays an essential role in inhibiting death receptor mediated apoptosis of HRS cells.[195,196] HRS cells also show malfunctions of the intrinsic apoptosis pathway, which involves a cascade of caspases. Caspase activity is negatively regulated by a group of proteins designated as inhibitors of apoptosis (IAP). One member of this family, XIAP is strongly expressed by HRS cells.[197] Inhibition of XIAP in HL cell lines restored sensitivity of the cells to caspase-3-mediated apoptosis.[197]

HRS CELLS IN THEIR MICROENVIRONMENT

As discussed above, the microenvironment in HL is characterized by a mixed cellular infiltrate with HRS cells themselves usually accounting for less than 1 percent of the cellular infiltrate. The cellular infiltrate resembles an inflammatory response, as it is composed of T and B lymphocytes, neutrophils, eosinophils, mast cells, macrophages and plasma cells (Fig. 34.1). HRS cells produce a variety of cytokines and chemokines, suggesting that they actively regulate the nonmalignant infiltrate. For example, T helper 2 cells are attracted by secretion of the chemokine TARC, one of the most highly transcribed genes in HRS cells.[198] By secretion of CCL5, HRS cells recruit mast cells.[199] These cells express CD30 ligand and thereby may stimulate NF-κB activity in the CD30-positive HRS cells. Eosinophils are attracted into HL tissues by CCL11 (eotaxin) and CCL28 (MEC). CCL28 is secreted by the HRS cells, and there is indication that HRS cells induce fibroblasts to secrete CCL11.[200–202]

CD4+ T cells represent the largest cell population in the classical HL tissues. It was initially thought that these cells represent T helper cells of the TH2-type. For example, they secrete the TH2 cytokine IL-10, but not the TH1 cytokine interferon (IFN) γ. However, recent studies revealed that many HL-infiltrating CD4+ T cells have a phenotype resembling regulatory T cells (Tregs): expression of CD25, CTLA4, LAG3 and FOXP3, and secretion of IL-10 but not IL-4, as seen in HL-infiltrating CD4+ T cells, are hallmarks of Tregs.[203–205] It seems the Treg population is not homogenous, as many LAG3+ T cells do not coexpress FOXP3, and the T cells directly rosetting around the HRS cells are specifically enriched for CCR4+FOXP3+ Treg cells.[203–205]

The Treg cells probably contribute to the immunosuppressive microenvironment in classical HL and help to rescue the HRS cells from an attack by cytotoxic T cells. Indeed, suppressive effects of HL-infiltrating Tregs on cytotoxic T cells were shown *in vitro*.[203–205] This immunosuppression seems to be particularly important in EBV-positive cases of classical HL, as HRS cells express viral antigens that are principally targets for cytotoxic T cells. Another factor contributing to the immunosuppressive

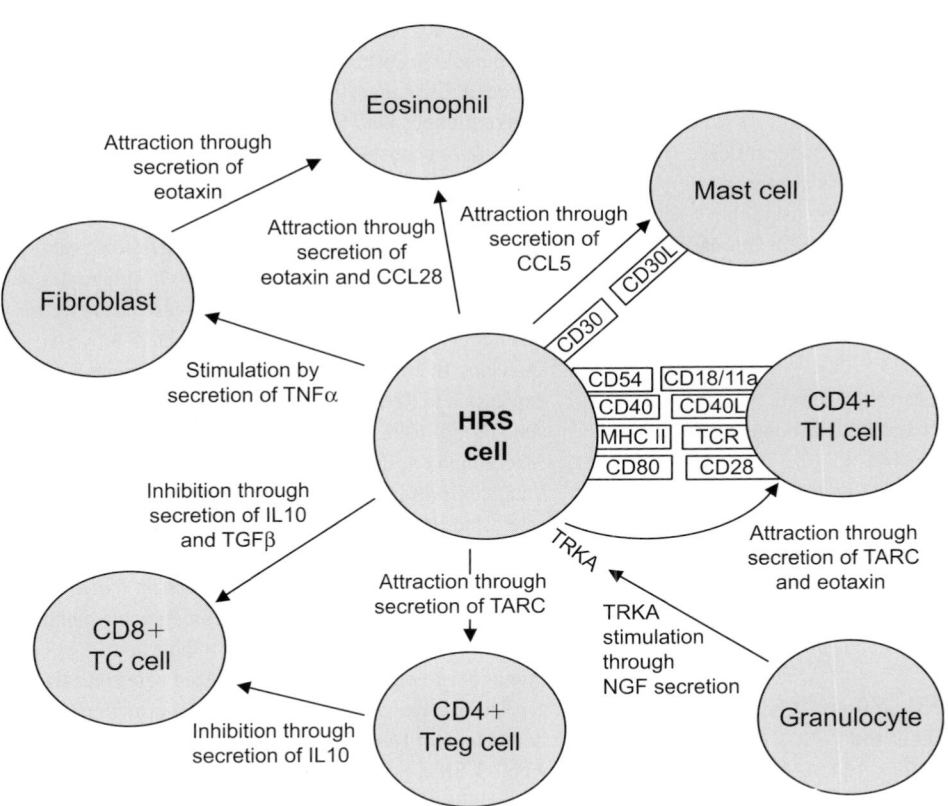

Figure 34.1 Cellular interactions in the classical Hodgkin lymphoma (HL) microenvironment. Shown are key interactions between HRS cells and other types of cells in the microenvironment of classical HL tissues. Direct cellular interactions and interactions mediated by secretion of cytokines or chemokines are depicted. TC cell, cytotoxic T cell; TH cell, T helper cell.

microenvironment is presumably represented by prostaglandin E_2, which is found at elevated levels in classical HL and which impairs CD4 helper functions.[206] However, the infiltrating CD4+ T cells do not only have suppressive functions on other infiltrating cells, but they (or a subset of them) also most likely have helper functions for the HRS cells. For example, HRS cells express CD40 and IL-13 receptor, whereas infiltrating T cells express CD40L and IL-13, and there is evidence that these interactions have stimulatory effects for HRS cells.[175,176,207] Notably, CD40L expression is particularly seen on the surface of T cells in direct contact with HRS cells.[176] The fact that HRS cells have lost expression of nearly all B cell-specific genes but have retained expression of genes important for antigen-presenting cell functions and interaction with T helper cells (MHC class II, CD40, CD80, CD86) further indicates an important role of the HRS cell/CD4+ T cell interaction for HRS cell pathogenesis.

- HL is unique among human hematologic malignancies in several aspects. The tumor cells are exceptionally rare in the tissue, and many indications support the view that the mixed cellular infiltrate in the lymphoma is essential for HRS cells' survival and growth.
- HRS cells in classical HL have undergone a dramatic reprogramming of their phenotype, which no longer resembles that of B cells.
- HRS cells have activated multiple signaling pathways that contribute to the survival of the cells.
- Relatively few recurrent genetic lesions have been identified, and it appears that various combinations of genetic events contribute to malignant transformation.

KEY POINTS

- Our understanding of the biology and pathogenesis of HL has made considerable progress in the past years, although much is still to be learnt.
- Both HRS and LP cells derive in most cases from GC B cells, in the case of classical HRS cells most likely from preapoptotic cells.

REFERENCES

- ● = Key primary paper
- ◆ = Major review article

1. Jaffe ES, Harris NL, Stein H, Vardiman JW. *WHO classification of tumors: pathology and genetics of tumors of haematopoietic and lymphoid tissues.* Lyon: IARC Press, 2001.

2. Chittal SM, Caveriviere P, Schwarting R *et al.* Monoclonal antibodies in the diagnosis of Hodgkin's disease. The search for a rational panel. *Am J Surg Pathol* 1988; **12**: 9–21.

3. Vasef MA, Alsabeh R, Medeiros LJ, Weiss LM. Immunophenotype of Reed–Sternberg and Hodgkin's cells in sequential biopsy specimens of Hodgkin's disease: a paraffin-section immunohistochemical study using the heat-induced epitope retrieval method. *Am J Clin Pathol* 1997; **108**: 54–9.

4. Korkolopoulou P, Cordell J, Jones M *et al.* The expression of the B-cell marker mb-1 (CD79a) in Hodgkin's disease. *Histopathology* 1994; **24**: 511–15.

5. Kuzu I, Delsol G, Jones M *et al.* Expression of the Ig-associated heterodimer (mb-1 and B29) in Hodgkin's disease. *Histopathology* 1993; **22**: 141–4.

6. Watanabe K, Yamashita Y, Nakayama A *et al.* Varied B-cell immunophenotypes of Hodgkin/Reed–Sternberg cells in classic Hodgkin's disease. *Histopathology* 2000; **36**: 353–61.

7. Drexler HG. Recent results on the biology of Hodgkin and Reed–Sternberg cells, I. Biopsy material. *Leuk Lymphoma* 1992; **8**: 283–313.

8. von Wasielewski R, Mengel M, Fischer R *et al.* Classical Hodgkin's disease. Clinical impact of the immunophenotype. *Am J Pathol* 1997; **151**: 1123–30.

9. Hell K, Lorenzen J, Hansmann ML *et al.* Expression of the proliferating cell nuclear antigen in the different types of Hodgkin's disease. *Am J Clin Pathol* 1993; **99**: 598–603.

10. Herbst H, Anagnostopoulos J, Heinze B *et al.* ALK gene products in anaplastic large cell lymphomas and Hodgkin's disease. *Blood* 1995; **86**: 1694–700.

11. Jarrett RF, MacKenzie J. Epstein-Barr virus and other candidate viruses in the pathogenesis of Hodgkin's disease. *Semin Hematol* 1999; **36**: 260–9.

12. Re D, Müschen M, Ahmadi T *et al.* Oct-2 and Bob-1 deficiency in Hodgkin and Reed Sternberg cells. *Cancer Res* 2001; **61**: 2080–4.

13. Stein H, Marafioti T, Foss HD *et al.* Down-regulation of BOB.1/OBF.1 and Oct2 in classical Hodgkin disease but not in lymphocyte predominant Hodgkin disease correlates with immunoglobulin transcription. *Blood* 2001; **97**: 496–501.

14. Torlakovic E, Tierens A, Dang HD, Delabie J. The transcription factor PU.1, necessary for B-cell development is expressed in lymphocyte predominance, but not classical Hodgkin's disease. *Am J Pathol* 2001; **159**: 1807–14.

15. Foss HD, Reusch R, Demel G *et al.* Frequent expression of the B-cell-specific activator protein in Reed–Sternberg cells of classical Hodgkin's disease provides further evidence for its B-cell origin. *Blood* 1999; **94**: 3108–13.

16. Falini B, Fizzotti M, Pucciarini A *et al.* A monoclonal antibody (MUM1p) detects expression of the MUM1/IRF4 protein in a subset of germinal center B cells, plasma cells, and activated T cells. *Blood* 2000; **95**: 2084–92.

17. Felgar RE, Macon WR, Kinney MC *et al.* TIA-1 expression in lymphoid neoplasms. Identification of subsets with cytotoxic T lymphocyte or natural killer cell differentiation. *Am J Pathol* 1997; **150**: 1893–900.

18. Foss HD, Anagnostopoulos I, Araujo I *et al.* Anaplastic large-cell lymphomas of T-cell and null-cell phenotype express cytotoxic molecules. *Blood* 1996; **88**: 4005–11.

19. Krenacs L, Wellmann A, Sorbara L *et al.* Cytotoxic cell antigen expression in anaplastic large cell lymphomas of T- and null-cell type and Hodgkin's disease: evidence for distinct cellular origin. *Blood* 1997; **89**: 980–9.

20. Oudejans JJ, Kummer JA, Jiwa M *et al.* Granzyme B expression in Reed–Sternberg cells of Hodgkin's disease. *Am J Pathol* 1996; **148**: 233–40.

21. MacLennan KA, Bennett MH, Vaughan Hudson B, Vaughan Hudson G. Diagnosis and grading of nodular sclerosing Hodgkin's disease: a study of 2190 patients. *Int Rev Exp Pathol* 1992; **33**: 27–51.

22. Anagnostopoulos I, Hansmann ML, Franssila K *et al.* European Task Force on Lymphoma project on lymphocyte predominance Hodgkin disease: histologic and immunohistologic analysis of submitted cases reveals 2 types of Hodgkin disease with a nodular growth pattern and abundant lymphocytes. *Blood* 2000; **96**: 1889–99.

23. Falini B, Stein H, Pileri S *et al.* Expression of lymphoid-associated antigens on Hodgkin's and Reed–Sternberg cells of Hodgkin's disease. An immunocytochemical study on lymph node cytospins using monoclonal antibodies. *Histopathology* 1987; **11**: 1229–42.

24. Jackson HJ, Parker FJ. *Hodgkin's disease and allied disorders.* New York: Oxford University Press, 1947.

25. Lukes RJ, Butler JJ. The pathology and nomenclature of Hodgkin's disease. *Cancer Res* 1966; **26**: 1063–83.

26. Lukes RJ, Butler JJ, Hicks EB. Natural history of Hodgkin's disease as related to its pathological picture. *Cancer* 1966; **19**: 317–44.

27. Harris NL, Jaffe ES, Stein H *et al.* A revised European-American classification of lymphoid neoplasms: a proposal from the International Lymphoma Study Group. *Blood* 1994; **84**: 1361–92.

28. Carbone A, Gloghini A, Gaidano G *et al.* Expression status of BCL-6 and syndecan-1 identifies distinct histogenetic subtypes of Hodgkin's disease. *Blood* 1998; **92**: 2220–8.

29. Pinkus GS, Said JW. Hodgkin's disease, lymphocyte predominance type, nodular – a distinct entity? Unique staining profile for L&H variants of Reed–Sternberg cells defined by monoclonal antibodies to leukocyte common antigen, granulocyte-specific antigen, and B-cell-specific antigen. *Am J Pathol* 1985; **118**: 1–6.

30. Hansmann ML, Fellbaum C, Hui PK, Zwingers T. Correlation of content of B cells and Leu7-positive cells with subtype and stage in lymphocyte predominance type Hodgkin's disease. *J Cancer Res Clin Oncol* 1988; **114**: 405–10.

31. Stein H, Hansmann ML, Lennert K *et al.* Reed–Sternberg and Hodgkin cells in lymphocyte-predominant Hodgkin's

disease of nodular subtype contain J chain. *Am J Clin Pathol* 1986; **86**: 292–7.

32. Marafioti T, Mancini C, Ascani S *et al.* Leukocyte-specific phosphoprotein-1 and PU.1: two useful markers for distinguishing T-cell-rich B-cell lymphoma from lymphocyte-predominant Hodgkin's disease. *Haematologica* 2004; **89**: 957–64.

33. Kamel OW, Gelb AB, Shibuya RB, Warnke RA. Leu 7 (CD57) reactivity distinguishes nodular lymphocyte predominance Hodgkin's disease from nodular sclerosing Hodgkin's disease, T-cell-rich B-cell lymphoma and follicular lymphoma. *Am J Pathol* 1993; **142**: 541–6.

34. Fellbaum C, Hansmann ML, Parwaresch MR, Lennert K. Monoclonal antibodies Ki-B3 and Leu-M1 discriminate giant cells of infectious mononucleosis and of Hodgkin's disease. *Hum Pathol* 1988; **19**: 1168–73.

35. Fellbaum C, Hansmann ML, Lennert K. Lymphadenitis mimicking Hodgkin's disease. *Histopathology* 1988; **12**: 253–62.

36. Hansmann ML, Fellbaum C, Hui PK, Moubayed P. Progressive transformation of germinal centers with and without association to Hodgkin's disease. *Am J Clin Pathol* 1990; **93**: 219–26.

37. Nguyen PL, Ferry JA, Harris NL. Progressive transformation of germinal centers and nodular lymphocyte predominance Hodgkin's disease: a comparative immunohistochemical study. *Am J Surg Pathol* 1999; **23**: 27–33.

38. Patsouris E, Noel H, Lennert K. Histological and immunohistological findings in lymphoepithelioid cell lymphoma (Lennert's lymphoma). *Am J Surg Pathol* 1988; **12**: 341–50.

39. Patsouris E, Noel H, Lennert K. Angioimmunoblastic lymphadenopathy – type of T-cell lymphoma with a high content of epithelioid cells. Histopathology and comparison with lymphoepithelioid cell lymphoma. *Am J Surg Pathol* 1989; **13**: 262–75.

40. Weiss LM, Warnke RA, Hansmann ML *et al.* Pathology of Hodgkin lymphoma. In: Hoppe RT, Mauch PM, Armitage JO *et al.* (eds) *Hodgkin lymphoma*, 2nd ed. Philadelphia: Lippincott Williams and Wilkins, 2007.

41. Hansmann ML, Fellbaum C, Hui PK, Lennert K. Morphological and immunohistochemical investigation of non-Hodgkin's lymphoma combined with Hodgkin's disease. *Histopathology* 1989; **15**: 35–48.

42. Jaffe ES, Zarate-Osorno A, Kingma DW *et al.* The interrelationship between Hodgkin's disease and non-Hodgkin's lymphomas. *Ann Oncol* 1994; **5**(Suppl 1): 7–11.

43. Bennett MH, MacLennan KA, Vaughan Hudson G, Vaughan Hudson B. Non-Hodgkin's lymphoma arising in patients treated for Hodgkin's disease in the BNLI: a 20-year experience. British National Lymphoma Investigation. *Ann Oncol* 1991; **2**(Suppl 2): 83–92.

44. Steinhoff M, Hummel M, Assaf C *et al.* Cutaneous T cell lymphoma and classic Hodgkin lymphoma of the B cell type within a single lymph node: composite lymphoma. *J Clin Pathol* 2004; **57**: 329–31.

45. Willenbrock K, Ichinohasama R, Kadin ME *et al.* T-cell variant of classical Hodgkin's lymphoma with nodal and cutaneous manifestations demonstrated by single-cell polymerase chain reaction. *Lab Invest* 2002; **82**: 1103–9.

46. Hansmann ML, Stein H, Fellbaum C *et al.* Nodular paragranuloma can transform into high-grade malignant lymphoma of B type. *Hum Pathol* 1989; **20**: 1169–75.

47. Miettinen M, Franssila KO, Saxen E. Hodgkin's disease, lymphocytic predominance nodular. Increased risk for subsequent non-Hodgkin's lymphomas. *Cancer* 1983; **51**: 2293–300.

48. Timens W, Visser L, Poppema S. Nodular lymphocyte predominance type of Hodgkin's disease is a germinal center lymphoma. *Lab Invest* 1986; **54**: 457–61.

●49. Braeuninger A, Küppers R, Strickler JG *et al.* Hodgkin and Reed–Sternberg cells in lymphocyte predominant Hodgkin disease represent clonal populations of germinal center-derived tumor B cells. *Proc Natl Acad Sci U S A* 1997; **94**: 9337–42.

●50. Küppers R, Rajewsky K, Zhao M *et al.* Hodgkin disease: Hodgkin and Reed–Sternberg cells picked from histological sections show clonal immunoglobulin gene rearrangements and appear to be derived from B cells at various stages of development. *Proc Natl Acad Sci U S A* 1994; **91**: 10962–6.

●51. Marafioti T, Hummel M, Anagnostopoulos I *et al.* Origin of nodular lymphocyte-predominant Hodgkin's disease from a clonal expansion of highly mutated germinal-center B cells. *N Engl J Med* 1997; **337**: 453–8.

●52. Ohno T, Stribley JA, Wu G *et al.* Clonality in nodular lymphocyte-predominant Hodgkin's disease. *N Engl J Med* 1997; **337**: 459–65.

53. Küppers R, Zhao M, Hansmann ML, Rajewsky K. Tracing B cell development in human germinal centres by molecular analysis of single cells picked from histological sections. *EMBO J* 1993; **12**: 4955–67.

54. Greiner A, Tobollik S, Buettner M *et al.* Differential expression of activation-induced cytidine deaminase (AID) in nodular lymphocyte-predominant and classical Hodgkin lymphoma. *J Pathol* 2005; **205**: 541–7.

55. Delabie J, Tierens A, Gavriil T *et al.* Phenotype, genotype and clonality of Reed–Sternberg cells in nodular sclerosis Hodgkin's disease: results of a single-cell study. *Br J Haematol* 1996; **94**: 198–205.

56. Delabie J, Tierens A, Wu G *et al.* Lymphocyte predominance Hodgkin's disease: lineage and clonality determination using a single-cell assay. *Blood* 1994; **84**: 3291–8.

57. Hummel M, Ziemann K, Lammert H *et al.* Hodgkin's disease with monoclonal and polyclonal populations of Reed–Sternberg cells. *N Engl J Med* 1995; **333**: 901–6.

58. Roth J, Daus H, Trümper L *et al.* Detection of immunoglobulin heavy-chain gene rearrangement at the single-cell level in malignant lymphomas: no rearrangement is found in Hodgkin and Reed–Sternberg cells. *Int J Cancer* 1994; **57**: 799–804.

●59. Bräuninger A, Hansmann ML, Strickler JG *et al.* Identification of common germinal-center B-cell precursors in two patients with both Hodgkin's disease and non-Hodgkin's lymphoma. *N Engl J Med* 1999; **340**: 1239–47.

60. Bräuninger A, Wacker HH, Rajewsky K *et al.* Typing the histogenetic origin of the tumor cells of lymphocyte-rich classical Hodgkin's lymphoma in relation to tumor cells of classical and lymphocyte-predominance Hodgkin's lymphoma. *Cancer Res* 2003; **63**: 1644–51.

61. Irsch J, Nitsch S, Hansmann ML *et al.* Isolation of viable Hodgkin and Reed–Sternberg cells from Hodgkin disease tissues. *Proc Natl Acad Sci U S A* 1998; **95**: 10117–22.

62. Kanzler H, Hansmann ML, Kapp U *et al.* Molecular single cell analysis demonstrates the derivation of a peripheral blood-derived cell line (L1236) from the Hodgkin/Reed–Sternberg cells of a Hodgkin's lymphoma patient. *Blood* 1996; **87**: 3429–36.

●63. Kanzler H, Küppers R, Hansmann ML, Rajewsky K. Hodgkin and Reed–Sternberg cells in Hodgkin's disease represent the outgrowth of a dominant tumor clone derived from (crippled) germinal center B cells. *J Exp Med* 1996; **184**: 1495–505.

64. Marafioti T, Hummel M, Foss H-D *et al.* Hodgkin and Reed–Sternberg cells represent an expansion of a single clone originating from a germinal center B-cell with functional immunoglobulin gene rearrangements but defective immunoglobulin transcription. *Blood* 2000; **95**: 1443–50.

65. Vockerodt M, Soares M, Kanzler H *et al.* Detection of clonal Hodgkin and Reed–Sternberg cells with identical somatically mutated and rearranged VH genes in different biopsies in relapsed Hodgkin's disease. *Blood* 1998; **92**: 2899–907.

◆66. Rajewsky K. Clonal selection and learning in the antibody system. *Nature* 1996; **381**: 751–8.

◆67. Küppers R, Rajewsky K. The origin of Hodgkin and Reed/Sternberg cells in Hodgkin's disease. *Annu Rev Immunol* 1998; **16**: 471–93.

68. Müschen M, Küppers R, Spieker T *et al.* Molecular single-cell analysis of Hodgkin- and Reed–Sternberg cells harboring unmutated immunoglobulin variable region genes. *Lab Invest* 2001; **81**: 289–95.

69. Rosenquist R, Roos G, Erlanson M *et al.* Clonally related splenic marginal zone lymphoma and Hodgkin lymphoma with unmutated V gene rearrangements and a 15-yr time gap between diagnoses. *Eur J Haematol* 2004; **73**: 210–14.

70. Lebecque S, de Bouteiller O, Arpin C *et al.* Germinal center founder cells display propensity for apoptosis before onset of somatic mutation. *J Exp Med* 1997; **185**: 563–71.

71. Bellan C, Lazzi S, Zazzi M *et al.* Immunoglobulin gene rearrangement analysis in composite Hodgkin disease and large B-cell lymphoma: evidence for receptor revision of immunoglobulin heavy chain variable region genes in Hodgkin-Reed–Sternberg cells? *Diagn Mol Pathol* 2002; **11**: 2–8.

72. Küppers R, Sousa AB, Baur AS *et al.* Common germinal-center B-cell origin of the malignant cells in two composite lymphomas, involving classical Hodgkin's disease and either follicular lymphoma or B-CLL. *Mol Med* 2001; **7**: 285–92.

73. Marafioti T, Hummel M, Anagnostopoulos I *et al.* Classical Hodgkin's disease and follicular lymphoma originating from the same germinal center B cell. *J Clin Oncol* 1999; **17**: 3804–9.

74. Rosenquist R, Menestrina F, Lestani M *et al.* Indications for peripheral light-chain revision and somatic hypermutation without a functional B-cell receptor in precursors of a composite diffuse large B-cell and Hodgkin's lymphoma. *Lab Invest* 2004; **84**: 253–62.

75. Tinguely M, Rosenquist R, Sundstrom C *et al.* Analysis of a clonally related mantle cell and Hodgkin lymphoma indicates Epstein-Barr virus infection of a Hodgkin/Reed–Sternberg cell precursor in a germinal center. *Am J Surg Pathol* 2003; **27**: 1483–8.

76. van den Berg A, Maggio E, Rust R *et al.* Clonal relation in a case of CLL, ALCL, and Hodgkin composite lymphoma. *Blood* 2002; **100**: 1425–9.

●77. Müschen M, Rajewsky K, Bräuninger A *et al.* Rare occurrence of classical Hodgkin's disease as a T cell lymphoma. *J Exp Med* 2000; **191**: 387–94.

●78. Seitz V, Hummel M, Marafioti T *et al.* Detection of clonal T-cell receptor gamma-chain gene rearrangements in Reed–Sternberg cells of classic Hodgkin disease. *Blood* 2000; **95**: 3020–4.

79. Tzankov A, Bourgau C, Kaiser A *et al.* Rare expression of T-cell markers in classical Hodgkin's lymphoma. *Mod Pathol* 2005; **18**: 1542–9.

●80. Schwering I, Bräuninger A, Klein U *et al.* Loss of the B-lineage-specific gene expression program in Hodgkin and Reed–Sternberg cells of Hodgkin lymphoma. *Blood* 2003; **101**: 1505–12.

81. Poppema S. Immunology of Hodgkin's disease. *Baillieres Clin Haematol* 1996; **9**: 447–57.

◆82. Küppers R. Mechanisms of B-cell lymphoma pathogenesis. *Nat Rev Cancer* 2005; **5**: 251–62.

●83. Mathas S, Janz M, Hummel F *et al.* Intrinsic inhibition of transcription factor E2A by HLH proteins ABF-1 and Id2 mediates reprogramming of neoplastic B cells in Hodgkin lymphoma. *Nat Immunol* 2006; **7**: 207–15.

84. Küppers R, Klein U, Schwering I *et al.* Identification of Hodgkin and Reed–Sternberg cell-specific genes by gene expression profiling. *J Clin Invest* 2003; **111**: 529–37.

85. Renné C, Martin-Subero JI, Eickernjager M *et al.* Aberrant expression of ID2, a suppressor of B-cell-specific gene expression, in Hodgkin's lymphoma. *Am J Pathol* 2006; **169**: 655–64.

●86. Jundt F, Anagnostopoulos I, Förster R *et al.* Activated Notch 1 signaling promotes tumor cell proliferation and survival in Hodgkin and anaplastic large cell lymphoma. *Blood* 2001; **99**: 3398–403.

87. Doerr JR, Malone CS, Fike FM *et al.* Patterned CpG methylation of silenced B cell gene promoters in classical Hodgkin lymphoma-derived and primary effusion lymphoma cell lines. *J Mol Biol* 2005; **350**: 631–40.

●88. Ushmorov A, Leithäuser F, Sakk O *et al.* Epigenetic processes play a major role in B-cell-specific gene silencing in classical Hodgkin lymphoma. *Blood* 2005; **107**: 2493–500.

89. Ushmorov A, Ritz O, Hummel M *et al.* Epigenetic silencing of the immunoglobulin heavy-chain gene in classical Hodgkin lymphoma-derived cell lines contributes to the loss of immunoglobulin expression. *Blood* 2004; **104**: 3326–34.

90. Schaadt M, Fonatsch C, Kirchner H, Diehl V. Establishment of a malignant, Epstein-Barr-virus (EBV)-negative cell-line from the pleura effusion of a patient with Hodgkin's disease. *Blut* 1979; **38**: 185–90.

91. Diehl V, Kirchner HH, Burrichter H *et al.* Characteristics of Hodgkin's disease-derived cell lines. *Cancer Treat Rep* 1982; **66**: 615–32.

92. Diehl V, Kirchner HH, Schaadt M *et al.* Hodgkin's disease: establishment and characterization of four *in vitro* cell lines. *J Cancer Res Clin Oncol* 1981; **101**: 111–24.

93. Wolf J, Kapp U, Bohlen H *et al.* Peripheral blood mononuclear cells of a patient with advanced Hodgkin's lymphoma give rise to permanently growing Hodgkin-Reed Sternberg cells. *Blood* 1996; **87**: 3418–28.

94. Kamesaki H, Fukuhara S, Tatsumi E *et al.* Cytochemical, immunologic, chromosomal, and molecular genetic analysis of a novel cell line derived from Hodgkin's disease. *Blood* 1986; **68**: 285–92.

95. Drexler HG, Gaedicke G, Lok MS *et al.* Hodgkin's disease derived cell lines HDLM-2 and L-428: comparison of morphology, immunological and isoenzyme profiles. *Leuk Res* 1986; **10**: 487–500.

96. Wagner HJ, Klintworth F, Jabs W *et al.* Characterization of the novel, pediatric Hodgkin disease-derived cell line HKB-1. *Med Pediatr Oncol* 1998; **31**: 138–43.

97. Poppema S, De Jong B, Atmosoerodjo J *et al.* Morphologic, immunologic, enzyme histochemical and chromosomal analysis of a cell line derived from Hodgkin's disease. Evidence for a B-cell origin of Sternberg-Reed cells. *Cancer* 1985; **55**: 683–90.

98. Drexler HG, Dirks WG, MacLeod RA. False human hematopoietic cell lines: cross-contaminations and misinterpretations. *Leukemia* 1999; **13**: 1601–7.

99. Stein H, Diehl V, Marafioti T *et al.* The nature of Reed–Sternberg cells, lymphocytic and histiocytic cells and their molecular biology in Hodgkin' disease. In: Armitage JO, Diehl V, Hoppe RT, Weiss I. (eds) *Hodgkin's disease.* Philadelphia: Lippincott Williams and Wilkins, 1999: 121–37.

100. Vockerodt M, Belge G, Kube D *et al.* An unbalanced translocation involving chromosome 14 is the probable cause for loss of potentially functional rearranged immunoglobulin heavy chain genes in the Epstein-Barr

virus-positive Hodgkin's lymphoma-derived cell line L591. *Br J Haematol* 2002; **119**: 640–6.

101. Drexler HG. Recent results on the biology of Hodgkin and Reed–Sternberg cells, II. Continuous cell lines. *Leuk Lymphoma* 1993; **9**: 1–25.

102. van den Berg A, Kroesen BJ, Kooistra K *et al.* High expression of B-cell receptor inducible gene BIC in all subtypes of Hodgkin lymphoma. *Genes Chromosomes Cancer* 2003; **37**: 20–8.

103. Atkin NB. Cytogenetics of Hodgkin's disease. *Cytogenet Cell Genet* 1998; **80**: 23–7.

●104. Weber-Matthiesen K, Deerberg J, Poetsch M *et al.* Numerical chromosome aberrations are present within the CD30+ Hodgkin and Reed–Sternberg cells in 100% of analyzed cases of Hodgkin's disease. *Blood* 1995; **86**: 1464–8.

105. Dohner H, Bloomfield CD, Frizzera G *et al.* Recurring chromosome abnormalities in Hodgkin's disease. *Genes Chromosomes Cancer* 1992; **5**: 392–8.

106. Schouten HC, Sanger WG, Duggan M *et al.* Chromosomal abnormalities in Hodgkin's disease. *Blood* 1989; **73**: 2149–54.

107. Tilly H, Bastard C, Delastre T *et al.* Cytogenetic studies in untreated Hodgkin's disease. *Blood* 1991; **77**: 1298–304.

●108. Joos S, Menz CK, Wrobel G *et al.* Classical Hodgkin lymphoma is characterized by recurrent copy number gains of the short arm of chromosome 2. *Blood* 2002; **99**: 1381–7.

●109. Martin-Subero JI, Gesk S, Harder L *et al.* Recurrent involvement of the REL and BCL11A loci in classical Hodgkin lymphoma. *Blood* 2002; **99**: 1474–7.

110. Barth TF, Martin-Subero JI, Joos S *et al.* Gains of 2p involving the REL locus correlate with nuclear c-Rel protein accumulation in neoplastic cells of classical Hodgkin lymphoma. *Blood* 2003; **101**: 3681–6.

111. Joos S, Granzow M, Holtgreve-Grez H *et al.* Hodgkin's lymphoma cell lines are characterized by frequent aberrations on chromosomes 2p and 9p including REL and JAK2. *Int J Cancer* 2003; **103**: 489–95.

112. Joos S, Küpper M, Ohl S *et al.* Genomic imbalances including amplification of the tyrosine kinase gene JAK2 in CD30+ Hodgkin cells. *Cancer Res* 2000; **60**: 549–52.

113. Hansmann ML, Godde-Salz E, Hui PK *et al.* Cytogenetic findings in nodular paragranuloma (Hodgkin's disease with lymphocytic predominance; nodular) and in progressively transformed germinal centers. *Cancer Genet Cytogenet* 1986; **21**: 319–25.

114. Franke S, Wlodarska I, Maes B *et al.* Lymphocyte predominance Hodgkin disease is characterized by recurrent genomic imbalances. *Blood* 2001; **97**: 1845–53.

◆115. Küppers R, Klein U, Hansmann M-L, Rajewsky K. Cellular origin of human B-cell lymphomas. *N Engl J Med* 1999; **341**: 1520–9.

116. Martin-Subero JI, Klapper W, Sotnikova A *et al.* Chromosomal breakpoints affecting immunoglobulin loci are recurrent in Hodgkin and Reed–Sternberg cells

of classical Hodgkin lymphoma. *Cancer Res* 2006; **66**: 10332–8.

117. Martin-Subero JI, Wlodarska I, Bastard C *et al.* Chromosomal rearrangements involving the BCL3 locus are recurrent in classical Hodgkin and peripheral T-cell lymphoma. *Blood* 2006; **108**: 401–2.

●118. Schmitz R, Renné C, Rosenquist R *et al.* Insight into the multistep transformation process of lymphomas: IgH-associated translocations and tumor suppressor gene mutations in clonally related composite Hodgkin's and non-Hodgkin's lymphomas. *Leukemia* 2005; **19**: 1452–8.

119. Weber-Matthiesen K, Deerberg-Wittram J, Rosenwald A *et al.* Translocation t(2;5) is not a primary event in Hodgkin's disease. Simultaneous immunophenotyping and interphase cytogenetics. *Am J Pathol* 1996; **149**: 463–8.

120. Weiss LM, Lopategui JR, Sun LH *et al.* Absence of the t(2;5) in Hodgkin's disease. *Blood* 1995; **85**: 2845–7.

121. Falzetti D, Crescenzi B, Matteuci C *et al.* Genomic instability and recurrent breakpoints are main cytogenetic findings in Hodgkin's disease. *Haematologica* 1999; **84**: 298–305.

122. MacLeod RA, Spitzer D, Bar-Am I *et al.* Karyotypic dissection of Hodgkin's disease cell lines reveals ectopic subtelomeres and ribosomal DNA at sites of multiple jumping translocations and genomic amplification. *Leukemia* 2000; **14**: 1803–14.

123. Martin-Subero JI, Knippschild U, Harder L *et al.* Segmental chromosomal aberrations and centrosome amplifications: pathogenetic mechanisms in Hodgkin and Reed–Sternberg cells of classical Hodgkin's lymphoma? *Leukemia* 2003; **17**: 2214–19.

●124. Wlodarska I, Nooyen P, Maes B *et al.* Frequent occurrence of BCL6 rearrangements in nodular lymphocyte predominance Hodgkin lymphoma but not in classical Hodgkin lymphoma. *Blood* 2003; **101**: 706–10.

125. Renné C, Martin-Subero JI, Hansmann ML, Siebert R. Molecular cytogenetic analyses of immunoglobulin loci in nodular lymphocyte predominant Hodgkin's lymphoma reveal a recurrent IGH-BCL6 juxtaposition. *J Mol Diagn* 2005; **7**: 352–6.

126. Re D, Hofmann A, Wolf J *et al.* Cultivated H-RS cells are resistant to CD95L-mediated apoptosis despite expression of wild-type CD95. *Exp Hematol* 2000; **28**: 31–5.

127. Trümper L, Pfreundschuh M, Jacobs G *et al.* N-ras genes are not mutated in Hodgkin and Reed–Sternberg cells: results from single cell polymerase chain-reaction examinations. *Leukemia* 1996; **10**: 727–30.

128. Küpper M, Joos S, Von Bonin F *et al.* MDM2 gene amplification and lack of p53 point mutations in Hodgkin and Reed–Sternberg cells: results from single-cell polymerase chain reaction and molecular cytogenetic studies. *Br J Haematol* 2001; **112**: 768–75.

129. Maggio EM, Stekelenburg E, Van den Berg A, Poppema S. TP53 gene mutations in Hodgkin lymphoma are infrequent and not associated with absence of Epstein-Barr virus. *Int J Cancer* 2001; **94**: 60–6.

130. Montesinos-Rongen M, Roers A, Küppers R *et al.* Mutation of the p53 gene is not a typical feature of Hodgkin and Reed–Sternberg cells in Hodgkin's disease. *Blood* 1999; **94**: 1755–60.

131. Feuerborn A, Moritz C, Von Bonin F *et al.* Dysfunctional p53 deletion mutants in cell lines derived from Hodgkin's lymphoma. *Leuk Lymphoma* 2006; **47**: 1932–40.

132. Maggio EM, van den Berg A, de Jong D *et al.* Low frequency of FAS mutations in Reed–Sternberg cells of Hodgkin's lymphoma. *Am J Pathol* 2003; **162**: 29–35.

133. Müschen M, Re D, Bräuninger A *et al.* Somatic mutations of the CD95 gene in Hodgkin and Reed–Sternberg cells. *Cancer Res* 2000; **60**: 5640–3.

134. Thomas RK, Schmitz R, Harttrampf AC *et al.* Apoptosis-resistant phenotype of classical Hodgkin's lymphoma is not mediated by somatic mutations within genes encoding members of the death-inducing signaling complex (DISC). *Leukemia* 2005; **19**: 1079–82.

●135. Weniger MA, Melzner I, Menz CK *et al.* Mutations of the tumor suppressor gene SOCS-1 in classical Hodgkin lymphoma are frequent and associated with nuclear phospho-STAT5 accumulation. *Oncogene* 2006; **25**: 2679–84.

136. Melzner I, Weniger MA, Menz CK, Möller P. Absence of the JAK2 V617F activating mutation in classical Hodgkin lymphoma and primary mediastinal B-cell lymphoma. *Leukemia* 2006; **20**: 157–8.

●137. Cabannes E, Khan G, Aillet F *et al.* Mutations in the IκBα gene in Hodgkin's disease suggest a tumour suppressor role for IκBα. *Oncogene* 1999; **18**: 3063–70.

●138. Emmerich F, Meiser M, Hummel M *et al.* Overexpression of I kappa B alpha without inhibition of NF-kappaB activity and mutations in the I kappa B alpha gene in Reed–Sternberg cells. *Blood* 1999; **94**: 3129–34.

●139. Jungnickel B, Staratschek-Jox A, Bräuninger A *et al.* Clonal deleterious mutations in the IκBα gene in the malignant cells in Hodgkin's disease. *J Exp Med* 2000; **191**: 395–401.

140. Emmerich F, Theurich S, Hummel M *et al.* Inactivating I kappa B epsilon mutations in Hodgkin/Reed–Sternberg cells. *J Pathol* 2003; **201**: 413–20.

141. Liso A, Capello D, Marafioti T *et al.* Aberrant somatic hypermutation in tumor cells of nodular-lymphocyte-predominant and classic Hodgkin lymphoma. *Blood* 2006; **108**: 1013–20.

142. Gravel S, Delsol G, Al Saati T. Single-cell analysis of the t(14;18)(q32;p21) chromosomal translocation in Hodgkin's disease demonstrates the absence of this transformation in neoplastic Hodgkin and Reed–Sternberg cells. *Blood* 1998; **91**: 2866–74.

143. Poppema S, Kaleta J, Hepperle B. Chromosomal abnormalities in patients with Hodgkin's disease: evidence for frequent involvement of the 14q chromosomal region but infrequent bcl-2 gene rearrangement in Reed–Sternberg cells. *J Natl Cancer Inst* 1992; **84**: 1789–93.

144. Straus SE, Jaffe ES, Puck JM *et al.* The development of lymphomas in families with autoimmune lymphoproliferative syndrome with germline Fas mutations and defective lymphocyte apoptosis. *Blood* 2001; **98**: 194–200.

145. Janz M, Stuhmer T, Vassilev LT, Bargou RC. Pharmacologic activation of p53-dependent and p53-independent apoptotic pathways in Hodgkin/Reed-Sternberg cells. *Leukemia* 2007; **21**: 772–9.

●146. Bargou RC, Emmerich F, Krappmann D *et al.* Constitutive nuclear factor-kappaB-RelA activation is required for proliferation and survival of Hodgkin's disease tumor cells. *J Clin Invest* 1997; **100**: 2961–9.

147. Pasqualucci L, Neumeister P, Goossens T *et al.* Hypermutation of multiple proto-oncogenes in B-cell diffuse large-cell lymphomas. *Nature* 2001; **412**: 341–6.

148. Murray PG, Qiu GH, Fu L *et al.* Frequent epigenetic inactivation of the RASSF1A tumor suppressor gene in Hodgkin's lymphoma. *Oncogene* 2004; **23**: 1326–31.

149. Sanchez-Aguilera A, Delgado J, Camacho FI *et al.* Silencing of the p18INK4c gene by promoter hypermethylation in Reed-Sternberg cells in Hodgkin lymphomas. *Blood* 2004; **103**: 2351–7.

150. Anagnostopoulos I, Herbst H, Niedobitek G, Stein H. Demonstration of monoclonal EBV genomes in Hodgkin's disease and Ki1-positive anaplastic large cell lymphoma by combined Southern blot and *in situ* hybridization. *Blood* 1989; **74**: 810–16.

151. Weiss LM, Movahed LA, Warnke RA, Sklar J. Detection of Epstein-Barr viral genomes in Reed-Sternberg cells of Hodgkin's disease. *N Engl J Med* 1989; **320**: 502–6.

152. Young LS, Dawson CW, Eliopoulos AG. The expression and function of Epstein-Barr virus encoded latent genes. *Mol Pathol* 2000; **53**: 238–47.

153. Kitagawa N, Goto M, Kurozumi K *et al.* Epstein-Barr virus-encoded poly(A)(-) RNA supports Burkitt's lymphoma growth through interleukin-10 induction. *EMBO J* 2000; **19**: 6742–50.

154. Kilger E, Kieser A, Baumann M, Hammerschmidt W. Epstein-Barr virus-mediated B-cell proliferation is dependent upon latent membrane protein 1, which simulates an activated CD40 receptor. *EMBO J* 1998; **17**: 1700–9.

155. Kaye KM, Izumi KM, Kieff E. Epstein-Barr virus latent membrane protein 1 is essential for B-lymphocyte growth transformation. *Proc Natl Acad Sci U S A* 1993; **90**: 9150–4.

156. Kulwichit W, Edwards RH, Davenport EM *et al.* Expression of the Epstein-Barr virus latent membrane protein 1 induces B cell lymphoma in transgenic mice. *Proc Natl Acad Sci U S A* 1998; **95**: 11963–8.

157. Alber G, Kim KM, Weiser P *et al.* Molecular mimicry of the antigen receptor signalling motif by transmembrane proteins of the Epstein-Barr virus and the bovine leukemia virus. *Curr Biol* 1993; **3**: 333–9.

158. Caldwell RG, Wilson JB, Anderson SJ, Longnecker R. Epstein-Barr virus LMP2A drives B cell development and survival in the absence of normal B cell receptor signals. *Immunity* 1998; **9**: 405–11.

159. Casola S, Otipoby KL, Alimzhanov M *et al.* B cell receptor signal strength determines B cell fate. *Nat Immunol* 2004; **5**: 317–27.

160. Bräuninger A, Schmitz R, Bechtel D *et al.* Molecular biology of Hodgkin and Reed/Sternberg cells in Hodgkin's lymphoma. *Int J Cancer* 2006; **118**: 1853–61.

161. Wilson KS, Gallagher A, Freeland JM *et al.* Viruses and Hodgkin lymphoma: no evidence of polyomavirus genomes in tumor biopsies. *Leuk Lymphoma* 2006; **47**: 1315–21.

162. Benharroch D, Shemer-Avni Y, Myint YY *et al.* Measles virus: evidence of an association with Hodgkin's disease. *Br J Cancer* 2004; **91**: 572–9.

163. Maggio E, Benharroch D, Gopas J *et al.* Absence of measles virus genome and transcripts in Hodgkin-Reed/Sternberg cells of a cohort of Hodgkin lymphoma patients. *Int J Cancer* 2007; **121**: 448–53.

164. Wilson KS, Freeland JM, Gallagher A *et al.* Measles virus and classical Hodgkin lymphoma: No evidence for a direct association. *Int J Cancer* 2007; **121**: 442–7.

165. Gutensohn N, Cole P. Epidemiology of Hodgkin's disease. *Semin Oncol* 1980; **7**: 92–102.

166. Staratschek-Jox A, Kotkowski S, Belge G *et al.* Detection of Epstein-Barr virus in Hodgkin-Reed-Sternberg cells. No evidence for the persistence of integrated viral fragments in latent membrane protein-1 (LMP-1)-negative classical Hodgkin's disease. *Am J Pathol* 2000; **156**: 209–16.

167. Hjalgrim H, Askling J, Sorensen P *et al.* Risk of Hodgkin's disease and other cancers after infectious mononucleosis. *J Natl Cancer Inst* 2000; **92**: 1522–8.

168. Hjalgrim H, Smedby KE, Rostgaard K *et al.* Infectious mononucleosis, childhood social environment, and risk of Hodgkin lymphoma. *Cancer Res* 2007; **67**: 2382–8.

169. Bargou RC, Leng C, Krappmann D *et al.* High-level nuclear NF-kappa B and Oct-2 is a common feature of cultured Hodgkin/Reed-Sternberg cells. *Blood* 1996; **87**: 4340–7.

170. Izban KF, Ergin M, Huang Q *et al.* Characterization of NF-κB expression in Hodgkin's disease: inhibition of constitutively expressed NF-κB results in spontaneous caspase-independent apoptosis in Hodgkin and Reed-Sternberg cells. *Mod Pathol* 2001; **14**: 297–310.

171. Nonaka M, Horie R, Itoh K *et al.* Aberrant NF-kappaB2/p52 expression in Hodgkin/Reed-Sternberg cells and CD30-transformed rat fibroblasts. *Oncogene* 2005; **24**: 3976–86.

172. Rodig SJ, Savage KJ, Nguyen V *et al.* TRAF1 expression and c-Rel activation are useful adjuncts in distinguishing classical Hodgkin lymphoma from a subset of morphologically or immunophenotypically similar lymphomas. *Am J Surg Pathol* 2005; **29**: 196–203.

173. Hinz M, Lemke P, Anagnostopoulos I *et al.* Nuclear factor kappaB-dependent gene expression profiling of Hodgkin's disease tumor cells, pathogenetic significance, and link to constitutive signal transducer and activator of transcription 5a activity. *J Exp Med* 2002; **196**: 605–17.

174. Hinz M, Loser P, Mathas S *et al.* Constitutive NF-kappaB maintains high expression of a characteristic gene network, including CD40, CD86, and a set of antiapoptotic genes in Hodgkin/Reed-Sternberg cells. *Blood* 2001; **97**: 2798–807.

175. Carbone A, Gloghini A, Gattei V *et al.* Expression of functional CD40 antigen on Reed-Sternberg cells and Hodgkin's disease cell lines. *Blood* 1995; **85**: 780–9.

176. Carbone A, Gloghini A, Gruss HJ, Pinto A. CD40 ligand is constitutively expressed in a subset of T cell lymphomas and on the microenvironmental reactive T cells of follicular lymphomas and Hodgkin's disease. *Am J Pathol* 1995; **147**: 912–22.

177. Chiu A, Xu W, He B *et al.* Hodgkin lymphoma cells express TACI and BCMA receptors and generate survival and proliferation signals in response to BAFF and APRIL. *Blood* 2007; **109**: 729–39.

178. Fiumara P, Snell V, Li Y *et al.* Functional expression of receptor activator of nuclear factor kappaB in Hodgkin disease cell lines. *Blood* 2001; **98**: 2784–90.

179. Horie R, Watanabe T, Morishita Y *et al.* Ligand-independent signaling by overexpressed CD30 drives NF-kappaB activation in Hodgkin-Reed–Sternberg cells. *Oncogene* 2002; **21**: 2493–503.

●180. Renné C, Willenbrock K, Küppers R *et al.* Autocrine and paracrine activated receptor tyrosine kinases in classical Hodgkin lymphoma. *Blood* 2005; **105**: 4051–9.

181. Teofili L, Di Febo AL, Pierconti F *et al.* Expression of the c-met proto-oncogene and its ligand, hepatocyte growth factor, in Hodgkin disease. *Blood* 2001; **97**: 1063–9.

182. Renné C, Hinsch N, Willenbrock K *et al.* The aberrant coexpression of several receptor tyrosine kinases is largely restricted to EBV-negative cases of classical Hodgkin's lymphoma. *Int J Cancer* 2007; **120**: 2504–9.

183. Renné C, Willenbrock K, Martin-Subero JI *et al.* High expression of several tyrosine kinases and activation of the PI3K/AKT pathway in mediastinal large B cell lymphoma reveals further similarities to Hodgkin lymphoma. *Leukemia* 2007; **21**: 780–7.

184. Baus D, Pfitzner E. Specific function of STAT3, SOCS1, and SOCS3 in the regulation of proliferation and survival of classical Hodgkin lymphoma cells. *Int J Cancer* 2006; **118**: 1404–13.

185. Kube D, Holtick U, Vockerodt M *et al.* STAT3 is constitutively activated in Hodgkin cell lines. *Blood* 2001; **98**: 762–70.

●186. Skinnider BF, Elia AJ, Gascoyne RD *et al.* Signal transducer and activator of transcription 6 is frequently activated in Hodgkin and Reed–Sternberg cells of Hodgkin lymphoma. *Blood* 2002; **99**: 618–26.

187. Holtick U, Vockerodt M, Pinkert D *et al.* STAT3 is essential for Hodgkin lymphoma cell proliferation and is a target of tyrphostin AG17 which confers sensitization for apoptosis. *Leukemia* 2005; **19**: 936–44.

188. Skinnider BF, Elia AJ, Gascoyne RD *et al.* Interleukin 13 and interleukin 13 receptor are frequently expressed by Hodgkin and Reed–Sternberg cells of Hodgkin lymphoma. *Blood* 2001; **97**: 250–5.

189. Dutton A, Reynolds GM, Dawson CW *et al.* Constitutive activation of phosphatidyl-inositide 3 kinase contributes to the survival of Hodgkin's lymphoma cells through a mechanism involving Akt kinase and mTOR. *J Pathol* 2005; **205**: 498–506.

190. Georgakis GV, Li Y, Rassidakis GZ *et al.* Inhibition of the phosphatidylinositol-3 kinase/Akt promotes G1 cell cycle arrest and apoptosis in Hodgkin lymphoma. *Br J Haematol* 2006; **132**: 503–11.

191. Nagel S, Burek C, Venturini L *et al.* Comprehensive analysis of homeobox genes in Hodgkin lymphoma cell lines identifies dysregulated expression of HOXB9 mediated via ERK5 signaling and BMI1. *Blood* 2007; **109**: 3015–23.

192. Zheng B, Fiumara P, Li YV *et al.* MEK/ERK pathway is aberrantly active in Hodgkin disease: a signaling pathway shared by CD30, CD40, and RANK that regulates cell proliferation and survival. *Blood* 2003; **102**: 1019–27.

●193. Mathas S, Hinz M, Anagnostopoulos I *et al.* Aberrantly expressed c-Jun and JunB are a hallmark of Hodgkin lymphoma cells, stimulate proliferation and synergize with NF-kappa B. *EMBO J* 2002; **21**: 4104–13.

194. Watanabe M, Sasaki M, Itoh K *et al.* JunB induced by constitutive CD30-extracellular signal-regulated kinase 1/2 mitogen-activated protein kinase signaling activates the CD30 promoter in anaplastic large cell lymphoma and Reed–Sternberg cells of Hodgkin lymphoma. *Cancer Res* 2005; **65**: 7628–34.

●195. Dutton A, O'Neil JD, Milner AE *et al.* Expression of the cellular FLICE-inhibitory protein (c-FLIP) protects Hodgkin's lymphoma cells from autonomous Fas-mediated death. *Proc Natl Acad Sci U S A* 2004; **101**: 6611–16.

●196. Mathas S, Lietz A, Anagnostopoulos I *et al.* c-FLIP mediates resistance of Hodgkin/Reed–Sternberg cells to death receptor-induced apoptosis. *J Exp Med* 2004; **199**: 1041–52.

●197. Kashkar H, Haefs C, Shin H *et al.* XIAP-mediated caspase inhibition in Hodgkin's lymphoma-derived B cells. *J Exp Med* 2003; **198**: 341–7.

●198. van den Berg A, Visser L, Poppema S. High expression of the CC chemokine TARC in Reed–Sternberg cells. A possible explanation for the characteristic T-cell infiltration Hodgkin's lymphoma. *Am J Pathol* 1999; **154**: 1685–91.

199. Fischer M, Juremalm M, Olsson N *et al.* Expression of CCL5/RANTES by Hodgkin and Reed–Sternberg cells and its possible role in the recruitment of mast cells into lymphomatous tissue. *Int J Cancer* 2003; **107**: 197–201.

200. Hanamoto H, Nakayama T, Miyazato H *et al.* Expression of CCL28 by Reed–Sternberg cells defines a major subtype of classical Hodgkin's disease with frequent infiltration of eosinophils and/or plasma cells. *Am J Pathol* 2004; **164**: 997–1006.

201. Jundt F, Anagnostopoulos I, Bommert K *et al.* Hodgkin/Reed–Sternberg cells induce fibroblasts to secrete eotaxin, a potent chemoattractant for T cells and eosinophils. *Blood* 1999; **94**: 2065–71.

202. Teruya-Feldstein J, Jaffe E, Burd PR *et al.* Differential chemokine expression in tissues involved by Hodgkin's disease: direct correlation of eotaxin expression and tissue eosinophilia. *Blood* 1999; **93**: 2463–70.

203. Gandhi MK, Lambley E, Duraiswamy J *et al.* Expression of LAG-3 by tumor-infiltrating lymphocytes is coincident

with the suppression of latent membrane antigen-specific CD8+ T-cell function in Hodgkin lymphoma patients. *Blood* 2006; **108**: 2280-9.

204. Ishida T, Ishii T, Inagaki A *et al.* Specific recruitment of CC chemokine receptor 4-positive regulatory T cells in Hodgkin lymphoma fosters immune privilege. *Cancer Res* 2006; **66**: 5716-22.

●205. Marshall NA, Christie LE, Munro LR *et al.* Immunosuppressive regulatory T cells are abundant in the reactive lymphocytes of Hodgkin lymphoma. *Blood* 2004; **103**: 1755-62.

206. Chemnitz JM, Driesen J, Classen S *et al.* Prostaglandin E2 impairs CD4+ T cell activation by inhibition of lck: implications in Hodgkin's lymphoma. *Cancer Res* 2006; **66**: 1114-22.

207. Atayar C, Poppema S, Visser L, van den Berg A. Cytokine gene expression profile distinguishes CD4+/CD57+ T cells of the nodular lymphocyte predominance type of Hodgkin's lymphoma from their tonsillar counterparts. *J Pathol* 2006; **208**: 423-30.

35

Plasma cell neoplasms

MW JENNER AND GJ MORGAN

INTRODUCTION

This chapter will cover the pathologic features and pathogenesis of plasma cell neoplasms, including the premalignant condition monoclonal gammopathy of uncertain significance (MGUS), multiple myeloma, plasma cell leukemia and monoclonal immunoglobulin deposition diseases.

The plasma cell neoplasms result from the proliferation of a single clone of terminally differentiated immunoglobulin-secreting B cells known as plasma cells. These disorders are characterized by the presence of a monoclonal immunoglobulin product (M band) in the urine or serum. The clinical and pathologic sequelae result from a combination of the consequences of deposition of this monoclonal protein and the direct effects of plasma cell infiltration in the bone marrow and other tissues.

NORMAL PLASMA CELL DEVELOPMENT

Plasma cells are mature B cells derived from a common lymphoid progenitor that has the capacity to develop in to T, B or natural killer (NK) cells.[1] Plasma cell differentiation requires passage of B cells through both the bone marrow and peripheral lymph nodes and relies on three key processes to modify immunoglobulin heavy chain (IgH) genes: VDJ recombination, somatic hypermutation and IgH switch recombination (Fig. 35.1). This results in the ability to generate diverse, high affinity, antibodies able to

recognize the vast range of antigens necessary for an effective secondary immune response.[2]

Immunoglobulin heavy chain rearrangement occurs in the bone marrow

Presence of the transcription factors E2A,[3] EBF[4] and Pax-5[5] allow passage of the common lymphoid progenitor through pro-B and pre-B cell stages of maturation within the bone marrow. The pro-B cell acquires CD19 expression, undergoes IgH VDJ gene rearrangement then develops cytoplasmic μ immunoglobulin expression, characteristic of a pre-B cell. Expression of a B cell receptor completes the precursor stage of B cell development and the release of a virgin B cell into the circulation. This stage of B cell development occurs in the bone marrow and is described in detail below.

A normal immunoglobulin molecule is made up from two heavy chains and two light chains. The heavy chain gene complexes are located on chromosome region 14q32, the κ light chain gene complex is at 2p12 and the λ light chain gene complex at 22q11. Heavy chain genes are rearranged prior to light chain genes.[6] IgH variable region genes are made up of three groups of gene segment: variable (V), diversity (D) and joining (J). The V gene segments encode for two out of three of the complementarity-determining regions (CDR 1 and 2) that determine the antigen specificity within the heavy chain V region. The third hypervariable region (CDR-3) is encoded by the joining of

Bone marrow

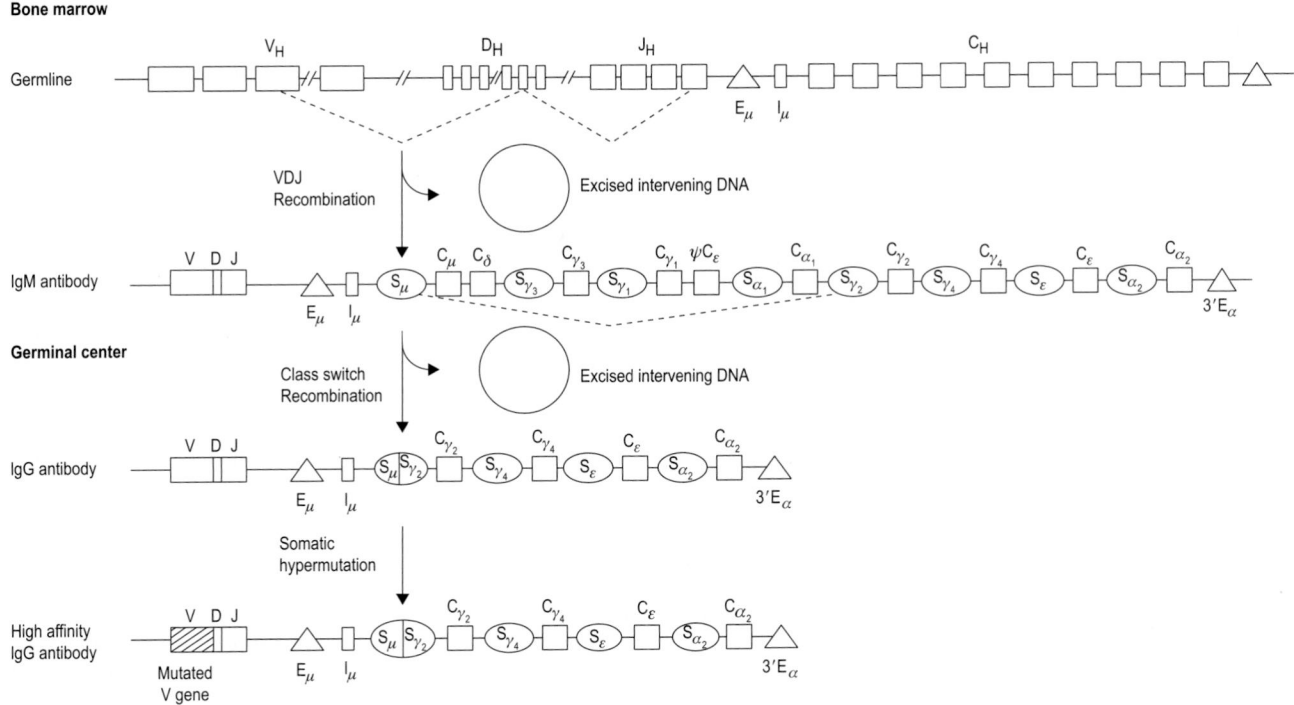

Figure 35.1   Reorganization of the immunoglobulin heavy chain locus to generate high affinity IgG or IgA antibody. In the germline configuration (line 1), the immunoglobulin heavy chain (IgH) gene variable region consists of clusters of gene segments encoding variable (V_H), diversity (D_H) and joining (J_H) exons upstream of the E_μ and I_μ enhancers and constant region (C_H) exons. VDJ recombination occurs in the bone marrow (lines 1 and 2) resulting in the formation of a VDJ rearranged gene unit capable of generating IgM antibody. Intervening DNA is excised as DNA circles. Class switch recombination occurs in the germinal center of the lymph node (lines 2 and 3). A repetitive switch region is located upstream of each IgH constant region. A breakpoint and recombination process occurs between switch regions with deletion of intervening DNA resulting in the association of the VDJ unit to another constant region exon. In this example, recombination occurs between the S_μ and S_{γ_2} regions resulting in a sequence from which an IgG_2 antibody can be generated. Somatic hypermutation of the V gene (line 4) occurs simultaneously with class switch recombination to generate a unique DNA sequence capable of producing high affinity antibody.

one D segment and one J segment with the downstream end of one of the V segments. This VDJ rearrangement requires recombination activating genes 1 and 2 (*RAG1* and *RAG2*) to introduce double stranded DNA breaks in regions flanking the genes to be rearranged,[7] then 'looping out' and deletion of intervening D and J gene segments and rejoining by the nonhomologous end-joining (NHEJ) pathway to form a DJ pair. This is followed by further looping out and deletion of intervening V gene segments to form a uniquely rearranged VDJ sequence. This process results in further variability in antigen specificity because the joining of the D to J and V to DJ segments is inexact and extra nucleotides may be added or subtracted, thus forming additional diversity in the CDR-3.[8] Subsequent rearrangement of the V and J segments of the light chain (IgL) gene allows the cell to fully express an IgH–IgL protein complex on the cell surface, to escape apoptosis and become an IgM-expressing virgin B cell. These cells then develop the ability to express IgD along with IgM and leave the bone marrow to circulate in the blood as naïve or virgin B cells. These cells have the capability to differentiate

into plasma cells and memory B cells, having encountered their cognate antigen.

Somatic hypermutation and class switch recombination occur in the lymph node

Further differentiation of virgin B cells requires T cell interaction, which occurs in the extrafollicular T zones of lymph nodes. Here the B cells are exposed to antigen and they either differentiate into mature short-lived IgM-secreting plasma cells that form the primary immune response or undergo blast transformation and migrate to the germinal center. Germinal center blast cells, known as centroblasts, are exposed to antigen and costimulatory responses on dendritic cells to develop a secondary response. Somatic hypermutation (SHM) occurs when B cells are exposed to antigen and introduces point mutations in to the V regions of the rearranged heavy and light chain genes, resulting in mutant immunoglobulin molecules on the cell surface, some of which will bind antigen more strongly than the original immunoglobulin. These are preferentially selected, protected from apoptosis by binding to follicular dendritic cells and give rise to affinity maturation.[9] The centroblasts then undergo class switch recombination (CSR) which allows the maturing B cell to produce different immunoglobulin isotypes with the same antigen affinity and specificity but different physiologic functions. This is of particular importance in multiple myeloma as the vast majority of chromosomal translocations that occur in the malignant plasma cell occur at the switch translocation 14q32 IgH locus. Both SHM and CSR occur only in antigen-stimulated B cells and require the activated B cell-specific enzyme activation-induced cytidine deaminase (AID).[10]

The IgH locus is arranged as a series of constant genes encoding a heavy chain isotype class, each one preceded by a switch region, except for $C\delta$. These switch regions consist of a repeat sequence. IgM, which is expressed on the immature B cell, is produced following mRNA transcription from the rearranged IgH variable region to the $C\mu$ gene. In order for the cell to express other isotypes, the switch regions of the locus recombine and the intervening DNA is 'looped out' and deleted. For example, excision of $C\mu$ to $C\alpha_1$ leads to production of an IgG_2 immunoglobulin (see Fig. 36.1). These IgG or IgA secreting cells either differentiate into memory B cells or plasmablasts, which migrate to the bone marrow and mature in to plasma cells.

Normal plasma cell development and the relationship with multiple myeloma

The above physiologic processes result in myeloma plasma cells being heavily mutated with no intraclonal variation in their mutational pattern and carrying isotype switched genes. More than 80 percent of the samples are IgG or IgA and only approximately 5 percent are IgM, IgD or IgE, with the remainder not secreting heavy chain.[11] Class switch recombination is disrupted in 40–50 percent of myeloma cases when recombination occurs at the switch regions within the IgH locus, not with other constant regions of the same chromosome but with other partner chromosomes, juxtaposing oncogenes in to the proximity of powerful IgH enhancers, which then drive aberrant expression of the juxtaposed oncogenes, a process known as aberrant class switch recombination.[12] This is discussed in more detail below.

PATHOGENESIS AND PATHOLOGY OF PLASMA CELL NEOPLASMS

Multiple myeloma is the most common of the plasma cell disorders and consists of a multifocal bone marrow centered proliferation of neoplastic plasma cells, characterized by the production of a monoclonal protein (the paraprotein), bone marrow failure, skeletal destruction and hypercalcemia.

The disorder is frequently preceded by MGUS, followed by asymptomatic and smoldering myeloma progressing to symptomatic myeloma, extramedullary myeloma and plasma cell leukemia. The progression through these stages of the disease is discussed in the following sections.

Multiple myeloma

MULTIPLE MYELOMA EPIDEMIOLOGY

Myeloma comprises around 10–15 percent of all hematologic malignancies, 1 percent of all cancers and has an incidence of 7.0 per 100 000 males and 5.9 per 100 000 females in England in 2005[13] and 6.7 per 100 000 males and 4.3 per 100 000 females in the USA (age adjusted to the 2000 US standard population) in 2004. The incidence rises with age. There is considerable racial variation with incidence in black males and females of 14.1/100 000 and 9.3/100 000, respectively, in the USA in 2004.[14] There is an apparently low incidence in the Chinese population. These racial variations appear to be retained after migration to new countries suggesting an inherited explanation for the racial differences rather than an environmental one.

MULTIPLE MYELOMA ETIOLOGY

Epidemiologic studies have been carried out extensively to identify risk factors associated with multiple myeloma. An association with radiation exposure, as seen in survivors of the World War II atomic bombs, was initially proposed[15] although subsequent studies have not clearly established a link,[16] nor with groups occupationally or therapeutically exposed to radiation. There is also a suggestion of an association with farming, paper producers, wood workers and exposure to a variety of chemicals including petroleum and materials associated with plastic and rubber manufacture.[17] There are families reported to have several cases of myeloma. Whether this is due to shared environmental factors or hereditary factors is unknown but under investigation.[18–20] Genetic studies have focused on single nucleotide polymorphisms (SNPs) involved in the inflammatory response (interleukin [IL]-6, IL-10 and tumor necrosis factor [TNF]-α), signaling (IKB) and DNA repair.[21–24]

MULTIPLE MYELOMA BIOLOGY

The cell of origin

The main phenotypic features of myeloma plasma cells include abnormal localization within the bone marrow with the replacement of normal bone elements and dysregulation of immunoglobulin secretion. There is much debate and controversy, however, regarding the exact site of origin and nature of the proliferating cell. Normal bone marrow plasma cells are derived from cells that have passed through a germinal center in a lymph node or other organ. Within the germinal center, cells undergo somatic hypermutation, class switch recombination and selection by antigen binding affinity, with only cells with high binding affinity surviving to become plasma cells. In myeloma the immunoglobulin genes from individual myeloma plasma cells show the same pattern of hypermutation, consistent with the clonal expansion of a single postgerminal center B cell.[25] This contrasts with the situation in MGUS where there is intraclonal variation in the pattern of mutation, suggesting that MGUS is the result of transformation of a virgin or memory B cell, the progeny of which continue to pass through the normal process of germinal center selection before becoming plasma cells.[26] Some studies have detected clonal VDJ sequences linked to the μ heavy chain suggesting the presence of a pre-switched cell as part of the myeloma clone or the presence of a marginal zone memory B cell.[27,28] However, these findings are controversial.

Primary genetic events in the pathogenesis of myeloma

- *Recurrent genetic abnormalities characterize myeloma*: Multiple myeloma is a heterogeneous disease with no single unifying pathogenic event. Conventional cytogenetic studies show that the karyotypes in myeloma are normal in 60–70 percent of cases due to the frequently low plasma cell yields in unselected bone marrow samples and the low proliferative index of plasma cells.[29–31] This contrasts with interphase fluorescent *in situ* hybridization (FISH) studies performed on selected plasma cells that have abnormalities in approximately 80 percent of cases. Interphase FISH has revealed the presence of recurrent genetic abnormalities.[32,33] The genetic abnormalities in myeloma are both structural, most commonly translocations involving IgH at 14q32, and numerical, consisting of recurrent gains or losses of whole chromosomes or smaller regions. These numerical abnormalities have been used to classify myeloma into two genetic subtypes: hyperdiploid and non-hyperdiploid. Hyperdiploidy (48–74 chromosomes) is present in almost 50 percent of cases in which there is an identifiable karyotypic abnormality and is characterized by gain particularly of chromosomes 3, 5, 7, 9, 11, 15 and 19, with a low

incidence of chromosome 13 deletions and IgH translocations.[34–36] The non-hyperdiploid cases (fewer than 48 or greater than 74 chromosomes) most frequently have deletions of all or part of chromosome 13 and/or rearrangements of IgH at 14q32. Advances in array-based technology in recent years have shed greater insight into additional genetic events associated with these primary abnormalities.

- *Illegitimate class switch recombination events involving IgH at 14q32*: Illegitimate immunoglobulin class switch recombination results in the translocation of regions of DNA, carrying oncogenes, into the strong enhancers of the IgH region and consequently oncogene dysregulation. Almost 100 percent of human myeloma cell lines have been found to have translocations involving the gene encoding the immunoglobulin heavy chain at 14q32. Most of these occur at the switch regions corresponding to the site of class switch recombination in the development of the normal plasma cell. Over half of myeloma cases have illegitimate IgH translocations.[12] The frequency of these is constant at diagnosis and relapse suggesting that these are primary rather than secondary genetic events. In addition, IgH translocations are present in up to 50 percent of MGUS cases, adding further support to this theory.[37] There are five common recurrently occurring translocation partners (Table 35.1): 11q13, 4p16, 6p21, 16q23 and 20q11.[38–42] Although the translocation t(8;14) does occur in multiple myeloma, the translocations involving *MYC* on chromosome 8 are often complex and are more common in advanced disease suggesting that this is a secondary event[43] (see below).

- *Translocations involving 11q13*: The t(11;14)(q13;q32) occurs in 15–20 percent of myeloma patients and leads to overexpression of cyclin D1 (*CCND1*).[41,44] The majority of the IgH breakpoints occur in the IgH switch region and on chromosome 11 in a region 100–330 kb centromeric to *CCND1*.[45] Cyclin D1 is a cell cycle regulator that is not normally expressed in normal proliferating lymphoid cells. Cyclin D1, D2 and D3 are expressed in overlapping patterns in

Table 35.1 Partner chromosomes most frequently involved in primary IgH translocations in multiple myeloma

Chromosomal partner	Candidate oncogene	Localization	Frequency (percent)	Function	Prognosis
11q13	Cyclin D1	der(14)	15–20	Cell cycle regulator	? Favorable
4p16	FGFR3; MMSET	der (14); der (4)	10–15	Receptor tyrosine kinase; epigenetic regulation of gene expression	Unfavorable
16q23	MAF	der (14)	5–12	Transcription factor	Unfavorable
6p21	Cyclin D3	der (14)	4–6	Cell cycle regulator	Unknown
20q11	MAFB	der (14)	2	Transcription factor	? Unfavorable

different cell types. In response to growth factors, cyclin D expression is up regulated. This results in phosphorylation of retinoblastoma protein via the cyclin-dependent kinases CDK-4 or CDK-6, leading to the transition of the cell through the G1 to S phase of the cell cycle. The role of *CCND1* overexpression in myeloma oncogenesis is unclear. Conventional cytogenetic data suggested an adverse prognosis associated with this translocation,[46] however, more recent FISH data suggest a favorable or neutral effect on prognosis.[47–49]

- *Translocations involving 4p16*: The t(4;14)(p16;q32) is present in 2–10 percent of MGUS[37,50,51] and 10–15 percent of multiple myeloma cases using FISH.[40,44] It cannot be detected by conventional cytogenetics due to the telomeric location of the breakpoint on chromosome 4. This translocation leads to dysregulated expression of two potential oncogenes: fibroblast growth factor receptor 3 (*FGFR3*) due to the juxtaposition of this gene within the switch region of the IgH gene on the derivative chromosome 14 and Wolf–Hirschhorn syndrome candidate 1 (*WHSC1*), also known as multiple myeloma SET domain (*MMSET*) which is dysregulated on the reciprocal chromosome 4.[40,52,53] *FGFR3* is a receptor tyrosine kinase. It is not usually expressed in plasma cells and its oncogenic potential is controversial. Overexpression of *FGFR3* in myeloma cell lines promotes proliferation and prevents apoptosis.[54] Mice transplanted with bone marrow with ectopic *FGFR3* expression developed B cell malignancies.[55] Inhibition of *FGFR3* in human myeloma cell lines and a mouse model induces plasma cell differentiation and apoptosis.[56] Preclinical studies of a small molecule inhibitor of *FGFR3* and an anti-*FGFR3* antibody have shown a cytotoxic effect in *FGFR3* overexpressing cell lines and primary myeloma cells and an antitumor effect in a xenograft mouse model.[57,58] However, *FGFR3* overexpression in isolation does not directly lead to myeloma given its existence in MGUS. In addition, *FGFR3* is only expressed in 75 percent of t(4;14) positive myeloma cases yet the translocation is associated with an adverse clinical prognosis irrespective of *FGFR3* expression. In most cases the lack of *FGFR3* expression has been associated with loss of the der(14) chromosome although cases with der(14) still present have been reported.[59,60] The der(4) IgH-MMSET transcript is detectable in all t(4;14) positive patients at diagnosis and relapse and results in overexpression of *MMSET* transcripts in all cases with the t(4;14) suggesting that *MMSET* may be the key gene dysregulated by the translocation.[61] *MMSET* is a complex gene with 9 splice variants and results in at least three protein isoforms. The exact functional activity of *MMSET* is unknown but a recent study suggests that at least one isoform has a transcriptional repressor role.[62] The t(4;14) is found in 10–15 percent of all myeloma cases

but 30 percent of IgA myeloma. It is associated with an adverse clinical outcome with shorter progression free survival and overall survival and resistance to alkylating agents at relapse.[47,63] There is a strong association with deletion 13 which is also associated with adverse outcome.[64]

- *Translocations involving 6p21*: A rarely occurring IgH translocation t(6;14)(p21;q32) is present in one of 30 myeloma cell lines and 4 percent of primary myeloma samples.[42] The translocation juxtaposes the γ4 switch region to a 6p21 sequence approximately 65 kb centromeric to the cyclin D3 gene (*CCND3*) and results in its overexpression. As with *CCND1* this leads to cellular proliferation.

- *Translocations involving 16q23*: The transcription factor *MAF* is overexpressed following translocation t(14;16)(q32;q23) in 5–12 percent of tumors.[39,65,66] The consequence of *MAF* overexpression is increased *CCND2* activity, stimulation of cell cycle progression and altered bone marrow stromal interactions.[67]

- *Translocations involving 20q11*: The t(14;20)(q32;q11) has been reported in myeloma cell lines and rarely in patient samples.[38] It results in overexpression of *MAFB*, another transcription factor that is not usually expressed in plasma cells. It has also been shown to transform chicken embryonic fibroblasts when overexpressed and also results in high *CCND2* expression. It may be associated with an adverse clinical outcome but there are inadequate data to support this at present.

- *Other translocation partners*: In up to half of myeloma cases with an IgH translocation demonstrated by FISH the partner chromosome is not one of the common partners identified above. There are numerous reports of other IgH translocations involving regions such as 12p13 (*CCND2*), 8q24 (*MAFA*) and nuclear factor-κB (NF-κB)-inducing kinase (NIK or *MAP3K14*),[68,69] although as yet there is insufficient evidence to determine whether these are primary or secondary events.

- *Deletion 13*: Monoallelic deletion of 13q (del(13q)) is one of the most frequent abnormalities in myeloma, detected by interphase FISH in approximately 20 percent of MGUS, 50 percent of untreated myeloma cases and 75 percent of plasma cell leukemia or human myeloma cell lines (HMCLs).[70–73] Typically there is deletion of one copy of the entire chromosome 13 or of 13q rather than an interstitial deletion.[74,75] A minimally deleted region has been mapped to band 13q14 the location of the retinoblastoma gene (*RB1*), a known tumor suppressor gene but there is increasing evidence that there is no consistently deleted region. However, studies on other tumor types have shown that both copies of *RB1* must be deleted or inactivated in order to eliminate its tumor suppressor function, a situation that rarely arises in multiple myeloma. It is therefore not clear whether this gene or another gene is the key tumor suppressor gene involved in the pathogenesis of myeloma. Deletion 13 is almost always present in cases with a t(4;14) or t(14;16) suggesting that it may have a role both early in the pathogenesis of the malignant clone as well as in progression of the disease.[70] Deletion of chromosome 13 is an adverse prognostic marker if detected by conventional cytogenetics and is also an independent prognostic marker when detected by interphase FISH although this effect is less strong.[76–80] Other studies suggest that given the high correlation between del(13q) with the high-risk translocations t(4;14) and t(14;16), it is actually these translocations that confer the poor risk associated with del(13q) rather than the deletion itself.[47]

- *Hyperdiploidy*: Hyperdiploidy is found in 40–60 percent of myeloma patients[31,34,81,82] and is also observed in MGUS suggesting that it is a primary genetic event.[83] The mechanism and primary genetic events leading to hyperdiploidy is unknown. The most frequently gained chromosomes are 3, 5, 7, 9, 11, 15 and 19. IgH translocations are rarely seen in this group and chromosome 13 deletions are less frequent which may explain the more favorable prognosis when hyperdiploidy is detected by conventional cytogenetics.[36] Use of gene expression profiling and array based comparative genomic hybridization (aCGH) techniques has led to attempts to subclassify hyperdiploid myeloma based on prognosis (see below).

Associated genetic and epigenetic events in myeloma pathogenesis and progression

- *Other recurrent gains and losses*: Use of aCGH techniques in which myeloma plasma cell DNA is hybridized to probes on a glass slide or commercial array has resulted in the identification of additional recurrent numerical abnormalities in addition to deletion 13 and the trisomies associated with hyperdiploid myeloma. Most commonly identified copy number changes are gains of 1q and deletions of 1p, 6q, 8p, 16q, 17p and X.[75,84] Using FISH or aCGH, gains of 1q have been identified in a third of tumors and have been associated both with adverse prognosis and with progression from MGUS to myeloma.[85–87] 1q21 gains are associated with t(4;14) and t(14;16) and more proliferative myeloma and there is debate as to whether 1q21 gain is an independent prognostic marker.[88] The target gene responsible for the poor prognosis of 1q gains has been proposed as being *CKS1B* at 1q21 but the region of gain is frequently the whole of 1q and in those cases with a minimal region of gain it spans several megabases.[75] However, overexpression of CKS-1B leads to cell proliferation and *CKS1B* inhibition with shRNA results in apoptosis suggesting that it remains a likely candidate.[89] Deletions of 1p occur in 20 percent of cases and are associated with an adverse prognosis although the key

region and genes are not determined.[90] Two studies have suggested a poor prognosis associated with deletions of 16q[84,91] with two potential candidate tumor suppressor genes being identified, *CYLD* at 16q12 and *WWOX* at 16q23, also the site of the breakpoint in t(14;16) myeloma.

- *Deletion of* TP53 *and other tumor suppressor genes*: Monoallelic deletion of 17p13, the location of the tumor suppressor gene *TP53* is identified in approximately 10 percent of intramedullary myelomas but up to 40 percent of advanced cases. *TP53* regulates genomic stability and is frequently mutated or deleted in other human cancers. It is associated with adverse clinical parameters, extramedullary myeloma and shorter survival.[92–96] Mutations of *TP53* are infrequent in myeloma cases even with deletion of 17p but in one study there was a strong association with poor prognosis although also with other unfavorable genetic factors such as t(4;14) and t(14;16).[97] It therefore remains uncertain as to whether *TP53* is the key gene on 17p. *PTEN*, the product of which promotes apoptosis, has also been reported to be potentially significant as a tumor suppressor gene in myeloma pathogenesis, again most likely associated with disease progression.[98] Using a combination of aCGH and expression arrays to investigate potential tumor suppressor genes, mutations resulting in activation of the NF-κB pathway have been identified in 17 percent of myeloma cases, the most frequent of which being inactivating abnormalities of the tumor suppressor gene *TRAF3*.[99] It has been proposed that patients with low *TRAF3* expression respond more favorably to the proteosome inhibitor bortezomib but this requires validation in additional studies. Other studies integrating gene expression with copy number have identified that *CDKN2C* (p18), a regulator of cell cycle progression, is homozygously deleted in both HMCLs and up to 10 percent of patient samples with an association with increased proliferation.[100,101] There is also paradoxical high expression of *CDKN2C* in a proportion of the most proliferative tumors by an as yet poorly understood mechanism.

- *MYC translocations*: Unlike the primary translocations that generally occur in the IgH switch regions, the translocations responsible for secondary events are more variable and complex. *MYC* is not expressed in resting germinal center cells or mature plasma cells but is expressed in myeloma cell lines. In Burkitt's lymphoma, *MYC* is reciprocally translocated with Ig gene loci as a universal primary genetic event. This t(8;14) is only rarely identified in myeloma patient samples. However, in 19/20 HMCLs and 15–40 percent of primary tumor samples, complex *MYC* structural abnormalities were detected by FISH.[102,103] The proportion of cases involved increases with advanced disease. The *MYC* abnormalities consist of complex translocations and insertions that are usually nonreciprocal and may involve three chromosomes. Associated deletions, inversions, duplications and amplifications are sometimes seen. The finding of the *MYC* karyotypic abnormalities in only a proportion of tumor cells is further evidence for these being a late event responsible for disease progression rather than primary events.

- *Mutational events*: Activating mutations of *RAS* oncogenes are found in 30–40 percent of myeloma tumor samples at the time of diagnosis and 45 percent HMCLs but only 5 percent of MGUS plasma cells, suggesting that the acquisition of *RAS* mutations is important for progression.[92] Mutations have been reported in *NRAS* and *KRAS* but not *HRAS*. Activating mutations of *RAS* enhance growth and lead to independence from growth factors such as IL-6 *in vitro* and are associated with a worse prognosis.[104] As well as being overexpressed as a result of t(4;14), *FGFR3* is also mutated in a small proportion of myeloma cases. This appears to be a secondary event that contributes to pathogenesis. It has been observed that mutations of *RAS* and *FGFR3* do not occur in the same myeloma cells. Both have an overlapping role in tumor progression acting via the MAP kinase pathway.[105]

- *Epigenetic phenomena: DNA methylation*. There is increasing evidence that carcinogenesis results not only from translocations, deletions and mutations affecting the DNA sequence but also epigenetic phenomena. Aberrant methylation of gene promoter regions is associated with loss of gene function. This is an alternative means to mutation by which tumor suppressor gene function is disrupted. One tumor suppressor gene implicated in myeloma pathogenesis is *CDKN2A* which encodes two transcripts: INK-4a (also known as p16) and ARF. p16 inhibits phosphorylation of Rb and hence progression of cells from the G1 to S phase of the cell cycle. ARF stabilizes p53. p16 is silenced by promoter hypermethylation (see below) in 15–35 percent of MGUS and primary myeloma plasma cells and most HMCLs.[106–108] The demethylating agent 5-deoxyazacytadine restored *CDKN2A* expression and induced G1 growth arrest in HMCL.[109] In one study, one of 11 potential tumor suppressor genes was hypermethylated in 80 percent of myeloma patient samples. In comparison with normal bone marrow samples, the genes most frequently methylated in myeloma patient samples were *SOCS1*, *CDKN2A*, *CDH1* (E-cadherin), *DAPK1* and *TP73*. There was a significantly higher methylation frequency of *CDKN2A*, *DAPK1* and *CDH01* in plasma cell leukemia in comparison with intramedullary myeloma supporting the hypothesis of an accumulation of both genetic and epigenetic events as myeloma progresses.[110] Several studies initially suggested that methylation of *CDKN2A* was associated with a poor prognosis,[107,108] however, more recent studies have called this into question with the conclusion that *CDKN2A* methylation is a marker for overall genetic

Table 35.2 TC expression groups identified in myeloma by RNA expression profiling. Groups 1–4 correspond to recurrent IgH translocations and groups 5–8 correspond to cases without a primary IgH translocation but with differential expression of one of the D cyclins

Group	Cyclin D	Ig translocation (gene)	Percent
1	3	t(6;14) (*CCND3*)	4
2	1	t(11;14) (*CCND1*)	17
3	2	t(14;16) and t(14;20) (*MAF* and *MAFB*)	9
4	2	t(4;14) (*FGFR3/MMSET*)	11
5	2	–	21
6	2 +1 (low)	–	6
7	1 (low)	–	32
8	none	–	1

change associated with progression without specific clinical consequences.[111,112] Hypermethylation of *SOCS1* has no impact on survival.[113] Hypermethylation is potentially reversible and demethylating drugs have been shown to have some effect in other hematologic malignancies.

- *Molecular classifications of myeloma*: The advent of array-based approaches has revolutionized the understanding of the chromosomal regions and genes involved in myeloma pathogenesis and prognosis. The initial studies of global gene expression in myeloma enabled the identification of genes characterizing the different stages of the myeloma transition from MGUS through to myeloma.[114,115] In addition, it has been possible to categorize cases by gene expression profiles typical for a given translocation group. This finding and the observation that most myeloma cases overexpress one or more of the cyclin D genes led to the development of the TC classification (translocation, cyclin D) (Table 35.2). This classifies myeloma in to one of eight subgroups based on translocations and cyclin genes differentially expressed. Four are based on oncogenes dysregulated by the five recurrent translocations and the other four by increased expression of cyclin D1 and/or D2 compared to normal bone marrow plasma cells.[116] While the TC classification is unable to firmly identify hyperdiploid myeloma, Zhan and colleagues performed an unsupervised clustering to identify seven tumor groups (Table 35.3) with much overlap with the TC system but also defining the hyperdiploid group and groups with specific clinical outcomes such as low bone disease and more proliferative disease.[117]

Both gene expression and mapping studies have attempted to subclassify hyperdiploid myeloma. In one recent analysis, four signatures could be defined in hyperdiploid cases with specific clinical outcomes such as the

Table 35.3 University of Arkansas for Medical Science (UAMS) molecular classification of myeloma

Subtype	Classification	Genetic group	Clinical associations	Percent
PR	Proliferation	Any	Abnormal cytogenetics, high β_2-microglobulin, high lactate dehydrogenase, low albumin	11
LB	Low bone disease	Any	Low incidence of MRI bone lesions	14
MS	MMSET	t(4;14)	High β_2-microglobulin, low albumin	16
HY	Hyperdiploid	Hyperdiploid		28
CD-1	CCND-1 and CCND-3	t(6;14) and t(11;14)		7
CD-2	CCND-1 and CCND-3	t(6;14) and t(11;14)		15
MF	MAF and MAFB	t(14;16) and t(14;20)	High β_2-microglobulin, low albumin	9

MRI, magnetic resonance imaging.

poor prognosis associated with expression of cancer testis antigens.[118] In a separate aCGH study, hyperdiploid cases with 1q gain, chromosome 13 deletion and trisomy 11 had an inferior progression free survival.[84] Gene expression signatures have also been generated to identify an MGUS-like myeloma signature[119] and a 70-gene high-risk signature with overexpressed genes predominantly mapping to 1q and underexpressed genes mapping to 1p. A 17-gene subset has been shown to predict outcome as well as the 70-gene model.[120] This high-risk signature has been validated in other datasets[121] but there is uncertainty at present as to how applicable the different classification systems are clinically and across a range of different datasets.

Multistep model of myeloma pathogenesis

A multistep model of the pathogenesis of myeloma has been proposed[122] where an immortalizing event occurs in the germinal center, most frequently a primary IgH translocation at the time of class switch recombination and somatic hypermutation. It is speculated that those tumors that do not have an IgH translocation either activate oncogenes or inactivate tumor suppressor genes as a result of spillover of IgH switch recombination or somatic hypermutation to non-Ig loci. The ectopic expression of an oncogene that results from an IgH translocation causes proliferation of the plasma cell. The role of a possible tumor suppressor gene on chromosome 13 and its role as an initiating or secondary event remains under debate. Activating mutations of *RAS* and *FGFR* may be factors heralding the progression from MGUS. Further mutations involving *TP53*, methylation of other tumor suppressor genes and secondary translocations that dysregulate *MYC* lead to further progression such as extramedullary disease. Additional deletions such as 1p or 16q are likely to be of importance as well as gains or 1q and mutations affecting the NF-κB pathway. These latter events are most likely related to disease progression but their timing is not yet clear. The multistep model is summarized in Figure 35.2.

Bone marrow microenvironment

The evolution of the malignant plasma cell clone in myeloma is not only determined by the genetic background of the clonal cells but also their two-way interaction with the bone marrow microenvironment. Myeloma cells disturb normal skeletal homeostasis resulting in lytic bone disease and the bone marrow environment produces growth stimulatory factors and provides relative protection from apoptosis.[123–125] The bone marrow microenvironment consists of the extracellular matrix along with five main types of stromal cells: 'fibroblastic' stromal cells, osteoblasts, osteoclasts, vascular endothelial cells and lymphocytes. There is a complex interaction between these cells and myeloma plasma cells mediated by a combination of cytokines, receptors and adhesion molecules. In order for intramedullary myeloma to develop, a series of events needs to take place:

- *Homing of plasma cells and adhesion molecules*: The normal plasma cell undergoes immunoglobulin heavy chain rearrangement and somatic hypermutation in the germinal center of the peripheral lymph nodes where longlived IgG or IgA secreting plasma cells are generated. These migrate to the bone marrow which is the major site for immunoglobulin production as part of the secondary immune response. The malignant plasma cell in all but the most advanced extramedullary cases such as plasma cell leukemia also has a preference for the bone marrow. Key chemoattractants involved in this process include stromal-derived factor 1α (SDF-1α)[126] and insulin-like growth factor 1 (IGF-1)[127] secreted by bone marrow endothelial and stromal cells. Plasma cells express numerous surface adhesion molecules including syndecan-1 (CD138) and very late antigen-4 (VLA-4, α4β1), responsible for binding to the extracellular matrix proteins type I collagen and fibronectin, respectively. Other adhesion molecules on myeloma plasma cells include VLA-5, intercellular adhesion molecule-1 (ICAM-1) and leukocyte function-associated antigen-1 (LFA-1, CD11a). Vascular cell adhesion molecule-1 (VCAM-1, CD106) is expressed on bone marrow stromal cells (BMSCs) and binding of plasma cells via VLA-4 is thought to be important in osteolytic bone disease.[128,129]
- *TNF-α, IL-6 and IGF-1*: TNF-α is an important cytokine that upregulates the expression of adhesion molecules LFA-1, VLA-1, ICAM-1 and VCAM-1. This

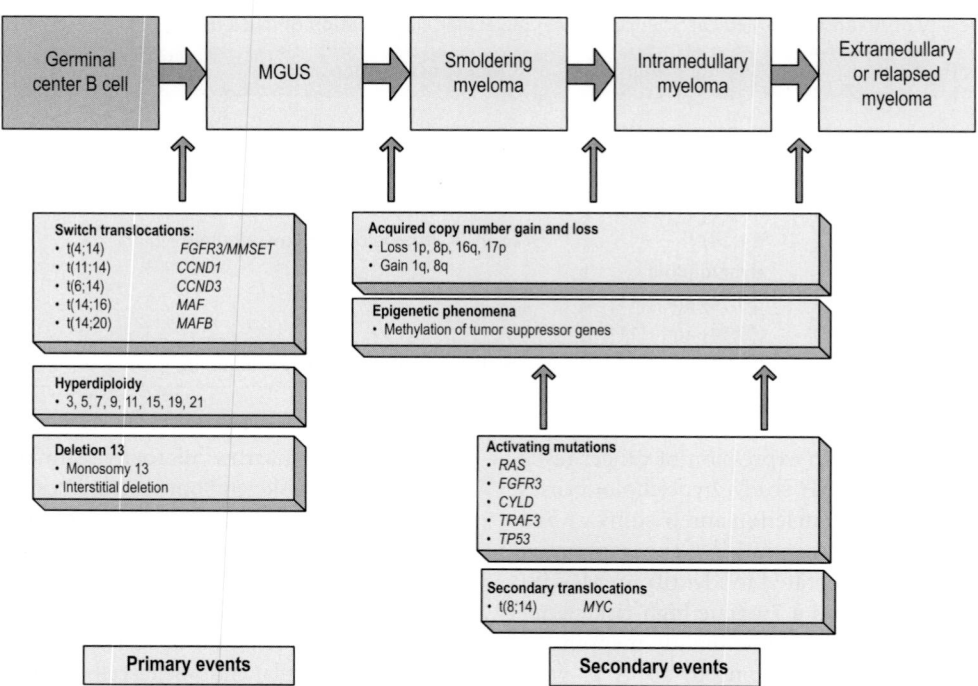

Figure 35.2 Multistep model of myeloma pathogenesis. Primary events responsible for the development of the malignant B cell clone include switch translocations, hyperdiploidy and deletion of all or part of chromosome 13. Secondary events responsible for progression from monoclonal gammopathy of uncertain significance (MGUS) to myeloma include recurrent amplifications and deletions and epigenetic phenomena such as methylation of tumor-suppressor genes. Late events include activating mutations and secondary translocations.

increases adhesion between myeloma cells and BMSCs. This adhesion triggers NF-κB-dependent transcription and secretion of IL-6, a key cytokine.[130,131] IL-6 is a key cytokine in the growth and survival of myeloma cells. It is predominantly produced by BMSCs in a paracrine fashion[132] but there is some autocrine production by myeloma cells. Its production is upregulated by adhesion and by cytokines TNF-α, VEGF and IL-1β.[130,133] IL-6 induces myeloma cell growth and survival via specific signal transduction pathways including the JAK2/STAT3, RAS/RAF/MAPK and MEK/ERK pathways.[134] STAT3 activation induces increased expression of the BCL2 family members BCLxL and myeloid cell factor-1 (MCL1). These are antiapoptotic proteins and key survival factors in myeloma cells. Apoptosis can be induced by blocking MCL1 directly or inhibiting JAK or STAT. MCL1 has therefore been shown to be essential for the survival of human myeloma cells *in vitro*[135,136] and is also overexpressed *in vivo* with high levels correlating with early relapse and shorter survival.[137] IL-6 also has a role in drug resistance by protecting the myeloma cells against dexamethasone-induced apoptosis via P13-K/Akt signaling and inactivation of caspase-9.[138] X-box binding protein-1 (XBP1), a transcription factor that induces the differentiation of B cells to plasma cells is also induced by IL-6.[139] Levels of serum IL-6 and IL-6 receptor (IL-6R) are of prognostic relevance as a reflection of tumor proliferation but clinical trials

of antibodies or small molecule antagonists of IL-6 or IL-6R have only shown transient responses.[140,141] IGF-1, produced by fibroblasts and osteoclasts, also induces proliferation and survival of myeloma cells via MEK/ERK and P13-K/Akt pathways. It also triggers phosphorylation of forkhead transcription factor (FKHR). Preclinical trials of IGF-1 receptor antagonists have shown antimyeloma activity.[142,143]

- *Angiogenic growth factors*: Angiogenesis is suggested to have a role in the pathogenesis of disease progression and plasma cell migration. Both basic fibroblast growth factor (bFGF) and vascular endothelial growth factor (VEGF) are involved in the induction of new vessel formation and have been suggested as paracrine growth factors for the multiple myeloma plasma cell.[133,144] Plasma cells secrete VEGF and so can influence stromal cells possessing VEGF receptors. VEGF promotes IL-6 production by BMSCs in a positive feedback fashion, thereby promoting myeloma cell growth and survival. This may be one mechanism for the observed upregulation of IL-6 secretion from stroma and increased tumor cell growth. Angiogenesis is correlated with disease activity, with a low level in MGUS and smoldering myeloma compared with active myeloma.[145] Low levels of microvessel density are associated with a more favorable prognosis[146] whereas higher levels are associated with advanced disease.[147] The degree of angiogenesis is also related to the plasma cell labeling index.[145] The role of the

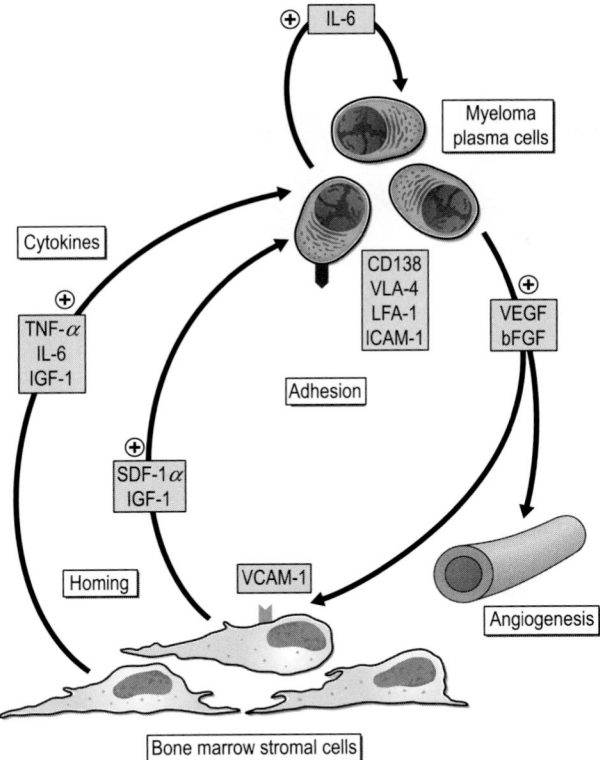

Figure 35.3 Plasma cell and bone marrow stromal cell (BMSC) interactions. Chemokines produced by BMSCs induce homing of plasma cells (PCs) to the bone marrow and adhesion via molecules on PCs and BMSCs. Adhesion triggers production of cytokines that promote growth and survival of the plasma cell. The plasma cells produce autocrine factors and angiogeneic growth factors that both stimulate new vessel formation and directly influence BMSCs in a positive feedback loop resulting in tumor proliferation. For full explanation of cytokines, adhesion molecules and angiogenic growth factors, see text.

bone marrow environment is key in the pathogenesis of multiple myeloma. The complex interaction between the cytokines, receptors and adhesion molecules is summarized in Figure 35.3.

Multiple myeloma bone disease

- *Myeloma bone disease and normal bone metabolism*: A major clinical feature of multiple myeloma is the development of lytic bone disease and generalized osteoporosis. Over 85 percent of myeloma patients have bone disease and thus it is a major cause of morbidity and mortality. The pathologic feature underlying the bone disease in multiple myeloma is an uncoupling of bone resorption by osteoclasts from bone formation by osteoblasts so that resorption predominates.[148] A critical factor in the bone remodeling process is the receptor activator of NF-κB ligand (RANKL), osteoprotegerin (OPG) system (Fig. 35.4A). RANKL is a cytokine primarily

produced by BMSCs, osteoblasts and by activated T cells.[149–151] Its presence has also been demonstrated on malignant plasma cells.[152,153] In the bone marrow, RANKL exists in both membrane bound and soluble forms. It can increase bone resorption by actions increasing both osteoclast formation and osteoclast activity. RANKL is unique, as *in vitro* it can produce these effects in the absence of supporting osteoblastic stromal cell lines, on which many other systems regulating bone turnover would depend.[154–156] It is a member of the TNF family and exerts its effects in the bone marrow via its receptor RANK. RANK is expressed on chondrocytes, mature osteoclasts and on their hemopoietic precursors. Engagement by its ligand RANKL is associated with precursor cell differentiation and maturation to osteoclasts.[157] In normal bone, homeostasis is achieved by a balance between the bone resorbing effects of the RANK/RANKL combination and soluble OPG, which is also a member of the TNF receptor family. OPG prevents bone resorption by acting as a decoy receptor, preventing the action of RANKL on its physiologic receptor RANK, thereby inhibiting the upregulation, proliferation and fusion of osteoclast precursors to produce mature osteoclasts.[157] Evidence for the intricate role of OPG in bone homeostasis and its effects when deregulated come from a number of sources. Overexpression of OPG in mice results in osteopetrosis, whereas knockout mice develop osteopenia.[158,159] The balance of bone resorption and formation is affected by other systemic and local factors that can act either directly or via other pathways to influence bone turnover. Those commonly recognized to have a significant role include glucocorticoids, 1,25-dihydroxyvitamin D3, parathyroid hormone (PTH), prostaglandins and cytokines (including IL-1, IL-3, IL-6, IL-7, IL-11 and TNF-α among others) (Fig. 35.4B).

- *Cytokines involved in myeloma bone disease*: The concept of a single 'osteoclast activating factor' (IL-1) mediating bone resorption has evolved to the description of a complex cocktail of cytokines including RANK/RANKL and OPG alongside other chemokines that are either produced by, or under the influence of, infiltrating multiple myeloma tumor cells. These cytokines (as outlined above) modify the marrow microenvironment, upregulating *RANKL* expression and secretion by both stroma and osteoblasts.[160] Destruction of bone matrix induced by multiple myeloma and its cellular interactions is accompanied by further cytokine release including IL-6, bFGF and IGFs. These help maintain expansion of the malignant clone in addition to inducing the plasma cells to release parathyroid hormone related protein (PTHrP). PTHrP from the malignant plasma cells further increases bone resorption, upregulating RANKL expression and perpetuating the cycle of bone destruction. It has also been suggested that syndecan-1

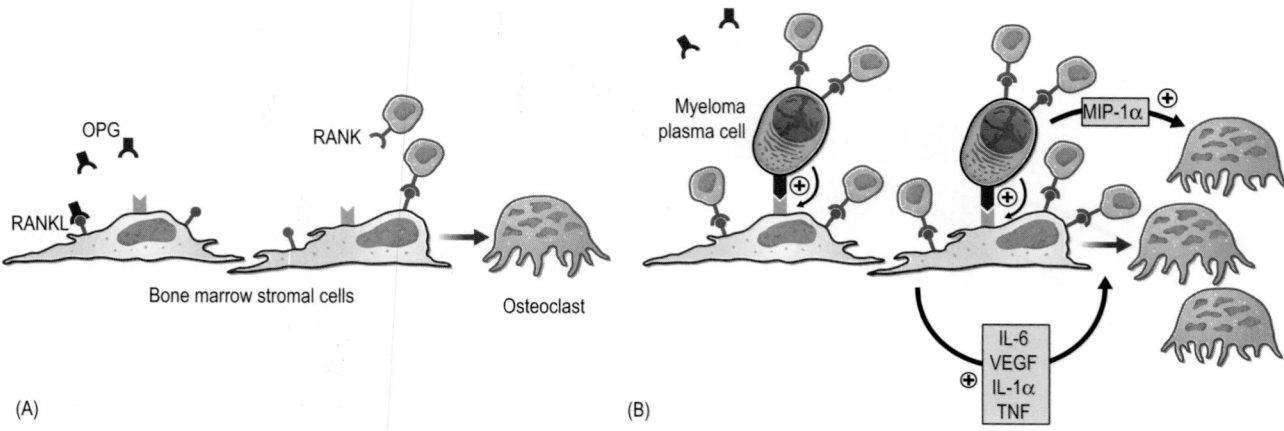

Figure 35.4 Dysregulation of bone homeostasis in multiple myeloma. (A) In the normal bone marrow, receptor activator of nuclear factor-κB ligand (RANKL) is expressed on bone marrow stromal cells (BMSCs). Interaction of RANKL with RANK on osteoclast precursors promotes their maturation in to osteoclasts. Osteoprotegerin (OPG) blocks the binding between RANK and RANKL thereby regulating osteoclast maturation and bone resorption. (B) In multiple myeloma, adhesion between myeloma plasma cells (PCs) and BMSCs results in overexpression of RANKL on BMSCs and PCs and downregulation of OPG. This results in increased production of macrophage inhibitory protein-1α (MIP-1α) by plasma cells and numerous other cytokines by BMSCs to induce osteoclast maturation and increased bone resorption, leading to lytic bone disease. For full explanation of cytokines, see text.

(CD138) expressed on the surface of and secreted from the myeloma cell can bind soluble OPG, thus preventing its inhibitory effects on RANKL function, further increasing osteoclast activity.[161] IL-3 is found at significantly greater levels in the bone marrow plasma of myeloma cases relative to normal controls. IL-3 can induce osteoclast formation and indirectly inhibit osteoblast formation.[162,163] IL-7 is also elevated in marrow plasma samples from myeloma patients and is a potent inhibitor of osteoblast differentiation by several mechanisms.[164,165] IL-11 exerts effects on bone through the RANK/RANKL/OPG system and is produced by both MM bone marrow stroma and osteoblasts.[166] IL-11 upregulates expression of RANKL on these cells inducing osteoclastogenesis and bone resorption as well as having inhibitory actions on new bone formation.[156] Further complexity is added to these interactions by the description of hepatocyte growth factor (HGF) being produced by the malignant plasma cell. HGF has the ability to upregulate IL-11 production from osteoblasts further contributing to bone damage.[167,168] Malignant plasma cells both produce and upregulate IL-6 production by the bone marrow stroma, osteoclasts and the osteoblasts. One consequence of upregulated IL-6 production is to increase the effects of hormones mediating bone resorption such as PTHrP;[169] IL-6 also acts as a growth factor for osteoclasts[170,171] and as a survival factor for the malignant plasma cells. These actions are potentiated by IL-1α, which is also a potent stimulator of bone resorption in its own right[172,173] alongside IL-1β, and the soluble IL-6 receptor (sIL-6). TNF-α and TNF-β (lymphotoxin-α) also have a major role.

They are both present in multiple myeloma marrow culture supernatant, are implicated in bone disease, in the hypercalcemia of malignancy, and can stimulate osteoclastogenesis.[174–177] They are known to activate RANK on osteoclast precursors and drive a transcription factor transduction cascade involving NF-κB, triggering osteoclast maturation and hence bone resorption. VEGF may also mimic the role of macrophage colony-stimulating factor (M-CSF) increasing early osteoclast development[178] alongside direct stimulation of resorptive activity[179] and hence mediate bone destruction by more than one route.

- *Chemokines and their receptors*: Chemokines are important in both the normal and pathologic behavior of lymphocytes. A member of this family of molecules, macrophage inhibitory protein-1α (MIP-1α), has been described as an osteoclast stimulatory factor. MIP-1α mRNA expression in bone marrow from patients at different stages of disease correlated with more advanced active disease.[180] MIP-1α induces osteoclast formation both independently of RANKL and via RANKL and IL-6.[181,182] Gene expression profiling has shown MIP-1α to be closely correlated with bone destruction in myeloma.[183] This all supports MIP-1α being an important osteoclast stimulator in patients with active multiple myeloma.

- *Wnt signaling pathway and DKK1*: The Wnt signaling pathway regulates plasma cell differentiation and also appears important in the development of myeloma bone disease.[184] Wnt signaling promotes proliferation and survival of osteoblasts. Several inhibitors have been identified including dickkopf (DKK1) and secreted frizzled-related protein (sFRP).[185] Mice lacking a single allele of DKK1 had increased bone mass[186] whereas transgenic overexpression of DKK1 results in osteopenia.[187] Elevated DKK1 levels appear to indirectly increase osteoclastogenesis by upregulating osteoblast expression of OPG and downregulating RANKL expression.[188,189] Using gene expression arrays, levels of DKK1 have been associated with the development of focal bone lesions in myeloma patients.[190] These studies indicate that DKK1 appears to be a key regulator of both normal bone physiology and myeloma pathophysiology.

The interaction between different cytokines and chemokines responsible for myeloma bone disease is summarized in Figure 35.4B. Improved understanding of the pathophysiology of myeloma bone disease will give further scope for the development of targeted therapy to treat and prevent this complication of myeloma. The major agents used at present are the bisphosphonates which directly inhibit osteoclast activity but also have direct antimyeloma effects by inhibiting IL-6 production from the bone marrow stroma. Both RANKL monoclonal antibodies and recombinant OPG are undergoing investigation as to their potential effects in myeloma bone disease.[148]

MULTIPLE MYELOMA PATHOLOGY

The diagnosis of multiple myeloma requires a combination of clinical, radiologic and pathologic features. Table 35.4 summarizes the classification of MGUS, smoldering (asymptomatic) myeloma, symptomatic myeloma, solitary plasmacytoma of bone and extramedullary myeloma, and Table 35.5 outlines myeloma-related organ or tissue impairment (ROTI) as defined by the International Myeloma Working Group.[191] The International Scoring System (ISS) (Table 35.6) has recently been devised and provides a simple and reliable way of staging and risk stratifying myeloma patients.[192] For further details of diagnosis and other staging systems see relevant chapters.

Ultimately, the diagnosis of myeloma or related plasma cell neoplasms requires the identification of clonal plasma cells within the bone marrow or other tissues. The classic pathologic features are discussed below, many of which have been alluded to previously in this chapter.

Morphology

Multiple myeloma is characterized by an excess of plasma cells in the bone marrow. They are rarely found in the peripheral blood except in cases of plasma cell leukemia (see below). In myeloma, plasma cells range from those with a mature morphology, indistinguishable from normal plasma cells, to those with an immature, pleiomorphic appearance.[193] Mature plasma cells are generally oval with abundant basophilic cytoplasm, an eccentric round nucleus with 'clock-face' chromatin and a perinuclear hof corresponding to the Golgi zone, the site of immunoglobulin

processing (Plate 66, see plate section). Immature 'plasmablasts' have dispersed nuclear chromatin, a high nuclear/cytoplasmic ratio and a prominent nucleolus. Plasmablastic features occur in approximately 10 percent of myeloma patients and rarely occur in reactive conditions therefore can be regarded as being neoplastic. Plasmablastic morphology is associated with a poor prognosis. No single morphologic feature is pathognomonic of malignancy as features such as binuclearity or trinuclearity are found in 1–5 percent of reactive plasma cells. However, bizarre multinuclearity is considered neoplastic. Other features more common in neoplastic plasma cells include Mott cells (multiple pale blue–grey intracytoplasmic grape-like inclusions), Russell bodies (cherry red inclusions), flame cells (vermilion-staining glycogen-rich IgA) and Dutcher bodies (intranuclear inclusions) all of which are occasionally found in reactive conditions such as chronic inflammatory disorders. These are all visual manifestations of condensed or crystallized immunoglobulin either in the cytoplasm or invaginated into the nucleus in the case of Dutcher bodies.

Immunophenotype

The typical immunophenotype of normal plasma cells is cIg+, CD19+, CD20−, CD27+, CD28−, CD38+, CD43+, CD45−, CD56− CD58−, CD81+, CD117−, CD126−, and CD138+. This contrasts with malignant plasma cells which are typically CD19− and CD56+.[194–197] CD19 loss in the malignant clone reflects altered expression of the *PAX5* gene.[198] CD56 and CD58 are adhesion molecules that are important in bone marrow localization. Positivity for CD20, CD117 and CD28 expression as well as loss of expression of CD27 also indicates the presence of malignant plasma cells in a proportion of cases.[197] Later in myeloma progression, CD56 expression is lost, which is one factor that may encourage progression from intramedullary to extramedullary disease including plasma cell leukemia.[199]

Histopathology and immunohistochemistry

On bone marrow trephine biopsy, myeloma is characterized by an excess of plasma cells. In reactive conditions the plasma cells are typically found in small clusters around arterioles. In myeloma, plasma cells are often present in large foci, nodules or sheets, sometimes replacing much of the normal hematopoietic tissue. Aside from this mass effect, the morphologic features discussed above can help distinguish a reactive from a malignant plasma cell infiltrate. Rarely is a reactive infiltrate greater than 30 percent.

Immunohistochemistry can help to confirm a typical myeloma phenotype with cytoplasmic expression of either κ or λ, negativity for CD19 and positivity for CD38, CD56 and CD138. These can help distinguish a clonal from a polyclonal reactive plasmacytosis. Proliferation antigens such as Ki-67 can also be studied. Ki-67 expression in plasma cells correlates with a plasmablastic morphology, advanced disease and a worse prognosis.[200] Cyclin D1 and

Table 35.4 Classification of monoclonal gammopathy of uncertain significance (MGUS), smoldering (asymptomatic) myeloma, symptomatic myeloma, solitary plasmacytoma of bone and extramedullary myeloma

	MGUS	Smoldering myeloma	Symptomatic myeloma	Solitary plasmacytoma of bone	Extramedullary myeloma	Multiple solitary plasmacytomas
Serum M-protein	<30 g/L	≥30 g/L and/or	Present (serum or urine)	Nil or small	Nil or small	Nil or small
Bone marrow clonal plasma cells (percent)	<10	≥10	Usually ≥10	Nil	Nil	Nil
Related organ or tissue impairment (see Table 36.5)	Nil	Nil	Present	Nil including normal skeletal survey/MRI except bone lesion	Nil including normal skeletal survey/MRI	Nil except bone lesion(s)
Skeletal survey and/or MRI spine and pelvis	Normal	Normal	Lytic lesions, osteoporosis or compression fractures usually present	Normal	Normal	Normal
Other	No evidence of other B cell proliferative disorders			Single area of bone destruction due to clonal plasma cells	Extramedullary tumor of clonal plasma cells	More than one localized area of bone destruction or extramedullary tumor of clonal plasma cells which may be recurrent

MRI, magnetic resonance imaging.

Table 35.5 Myeloma-related organ or tissue impairment (end organ damage) (ROTI) due to the plasma cell proliferative process

Organ/tissue	Abnormality
Calcium levels increased	Serum calcium >0.25 mmol/L above the upper limit of normal or >2.75 mmol/L
Renal insufficiency	Creatinine >173 μmol/L
Anemia	Hemoglobin 20 g/L below the lower limit of normal or hemoglobin <100 g/L
Bone lesions	Lytic lesions or osteoporosis with compression fractures (MRI or CT may clarify)
Other	Symptomatic hyperviscosity, amyloidosis, recurrent bacterial infections (>2 episodes in 12 months)

CT, computed tomography; MRI, magnetic resonance imaging.

Table 35.6 International Staging System for multiple myeloma

Stage	Criteria	Median survival (months)
I	Serum β_2-microglobulin <3.5 mg/L; serum albumin ≥3.5 g/dL	62
II	Not stage I or II	44
III	Serum β_2-microglobulin ≥5.5 mg/L	29

FGFR3 overexpression can also be assessed by immunohistochemistry as a surrogate marker for the t(11;14) and t(4;14), respectively. However, FGFR3 expression is not fully sensitive for all cases with t(4;14) as FGFR3 expression is lost in 25 percent of t(4;14) positive cases.[201] P53 overexpression by immunohistochemistry is associated with increased grade and stage.[202,203]

Cytogenetics

The typical primary immunoglobulin translocations, 13q deletions and activating mutations are discussed above.

Monoclonal gammopathy of undetermined significance

Monoclonal gammopathy of undetermined significance describes a low level of paraprotein in the absence of other clinical features of multiple myeloma, Waldenstrom macroglobulinemia or other B cell lymphoproliferative disorders. It is estimated that the clone must increase to approximately 5×10^9 cells before enough immunoglobulin is produced to be recognized as a monoclonal 'spike'

(M protein) in serum protein electrophoresis. The serum paraprotein level is usually less then 30 g/L with usually little or no urinary M protein and no abnormality in the total protein or globulin level. Clonal bone marrow plasmacytosis is less than 10 percent. There is no evidence of associated clinical symptoms and signs or pathologic features to suggest end organ damage.

MGUS EPIDEMIOLOGY AND ETIOLOGY

The prevalence increases with age with 1 percent of the population under the age of 60 years and 4–5 percent of the population above the age of 80 years being affected. The incidence is not fully determined but in one registry study was 16/100 000 per year in all age groups and 100/100 000 in those over the age of 70 years.[204] By definition the clone is stable and the M protein concentration usually remains static for years. However, it cannot be regarded as a benign condition. Prolonged follow-up of a large group has shown that 6–34 percent of patients progress to symptomatic myeloma, Waldenstrom macroglobulinemia, lymphoma, chronic lymphocytic leukemia or amyloidosis after 10 years, dependent on the level of the M band. Overall, the risk of progression is approximately 1 percent per year.[205] The etiology and cytogenetic and molecular findings in MGUS are described in the myeloma section above.

MGUS PATHOLOGY AND PROGRESSION

The peripheral blood picture is usually normal with no evidence of anemia. Clonal plasma cells are present within the bone marrow and represent 5–10 percent or less of the total nucleated cell number and have an interstitial distribution. Using flow cytometry it is possible to identify plasma cells with both a normal and 'myeloma' phenotype (CD38++, CD19+ and CD56− vs CD38+, CD19− and CD56+). Early data suggest that patients can have three patterns: phenotypically normal but genotypically abnormal plasma cells, a mixture of phenotypically normal and myeloma plasma cells and those with just a myeloma phenotype. Those with only a myeloma phenotype have a higher rate of progression to myeloma.[206,207] Following malignant transformation the paraprotein is always the same isotype as in the MGUS state although those with an IgA or IgM paraprotein are more likely to progress than those with IgG.[205]

Solitary plasmacytomas and extramedullary myeloma

Plasmacytomas are clonal proliferations of plasma cells that are cytologically and immunophenotypically identical to those of myeloma but confined to a local osseous (solitary plasmacytoma of bone) or extraosseous (extraosseous plasmacytoma) growth pattern.

Solitary plasmacytoma of bone (SBP) is a localized plasma cell tumor consisting of typical myeloma plasma cells which appears as a single radiographic lytic lesion. There are no other lytic lesions by radiography nor any evidence of bone marrow plasmacytosis or end organ damage (see Table 35.5). Approximately 50 percent of cases have a detectable paraprotein, usually of a low level. The genetic features of solitary plasmacytoma have not been well studied. Approximately 90 percent of patients are successfully treated with local radiation therapy although greater than 75 percent subsequently progress to myeloma, most likely as a result of occult asymptomatic myeloma not having been identified at the time of diagnosis of the plasmacytoma. Those who do progress appear to have a good response to chemotherapy and longer progression-free survival than *de novo* myeloma.[208]

Solitary extraosseous plasmacytomas (SEP) are less common than SBP but have a better prognosis as the majority can be cured by local radiation therapy. By definition there is no bone marrow plasmacytosis or other end organ damage. Almost 90 percent arise in the head and neck, especially the upper respiratory tract in mucosa-associated tissues. A monoclonal paraprotein occurs in 25 percent of cases with relapse risk of less than 30 percent. Approximately 15 percent progress to myeloma.[209]

In stark contrast to solitary plasmacytomas, secondary extramedullary myeloma is generally an aggressive form of myeloma with a very poor outlook. Extramedullary disease is not infrequent at relapse, particularly following high dose therapy. By anatomical location and morphology it is not always possible to distinguish solitary plasmacytoma from extramedullary myeloma but cyclin D1 and CD56 are virtually absent from SEP, yet usually present in extramedullary myeloma. The absence of CD56 in SEP may be due to failure to acquire this molecule rather than loss of this adhesion molecule as in the case of plasma cell leukemia.[202] Solitary plasmacytomas have a lower incidence of t(11;14), but a similar incidence of other IgH translocations, 13q deletions and hyperdiploidy, in comparison with myeloma cases.[210]

Plasma cell leukemia

Plasma cell leukemia (PCL) is defined as circulating peripheral blood plasma cells exceeding 2×10^9/l or 20 percent of peripheral white blood cells.[211] The spectrum of morphology is broad, ranging from mature plasma cells to blastic forms. It may be a presenting diagnosis (primary PCL) or evolve as a terminal feature of progressive myeloma (secondary PCL). PCL is more commonly seen in light-chain myeloma and less commonly in IgA myeloma. The clinical features are otherwise similar to intramedullary myeloma although bone disease is less frequent and lymphadenopathy and organomegaly are more frequent. The immunophenotype is similar to myeloma but there is lower expression of some adhesion molecules such as CD56, the loss of which may explain the escape of the plasma cells from the bone marrow. Primary IgH translocations occur with a similar frequency to intramedullary myeloma but hypodiploidy,

especially deletion 13q is significantly more common in PCL, whereas hyperdiploidy is rare. Methylation of known tumor suppressor genes is higher in PCL. Inactivation of *TP53* by mutation or deletion occurs in the majority of cases. These findings are consistent with the significantly worse prognosis found in plasma cell leukemia and support the hypothesis that an accumulation of genetic events is responsible for progressive, poor prognosis disease.[92,212]

Monoclonal immunoglobulin deposition diseases

AL AMYLOIDOSIS

AL amyloidosis is a protein conformation disorder associated with a clonal plasma cell dyscrasia. Deposition of extracellular monoclonal immunoglobulin light chain in an abnormal insoluble fibrillar form results in multiple organ damage. It produces a diagnostic apple green birefringence when viewed under polarized light following Congo red staining. This deposition most commonly occurs in the heart, kidneys, liver, bowel and nerves as well as the tongue and soft tissues. The clinical features result from progressive dysfunction of these organs. The natural history without therapy is of 80 percent mortality within 2 years.[213]

Epidemiology

The age-adjusted incidence of AL amyloidosis in the USA is between 5.1 and 12.8 per million person-years with a median age between 50 and 70 years.[214] The sex incidence is equal. In 80 percent a paraprotein is detected and 20 percent have overt myeloma. In contrast, 10–15 percent of myeloma patients have some degree of amyloidosis. There is also an association with MGUS, Waldenstrom macroglobulinemia and other lymphoid malignancies.

Pathophysiology

AL amyloidosis develops as a result of the production of monoclonal light chain from a clone of plasma cells. AL amyloid fibrils are derived from the N-terminal region of the light chain and consist of whole or part of the variable (VL) domain.[215] λ light chains predominate. Each fibril consists of filaments mainly composed of proteins arranged in a β-pleated sheet configuration. The exact mechanism for production of fibrils from filaments is unknown but particular clonal light chains or fragments have an inherited propensity to form amyloid by their ability to exist in partly unfolded states. Once the process has been initiated it may progress exponentially as further amyloid protein is deposited on the amyloid template. Amyloid fibrils are insoluble and relatively resistant to proteolytic degradation. However, deposition is not irreversible but reflects an imbalance between production of the precursor protein and resorption.[216]

The clonal amyloidogenic cells are typically present within the bone marrow although are occasionally located in the tissues and responsible for localized amyloidosis.[213] One study proposes that within the bone marrow this amyloidogenic clone consists not only of typical mature plasma cells but lymphoid and lymphoplasmacytoid cells, suggesting that the bone marrow infiltration may be greater than suggested by conventional morphology alone.[217] Clonal, post-switched B cells can also be identified in the peripheral blood and it is suggested that these may be the source of the bone marrow plasma cells.[218]

Bone marrow plasma cells in AL amyloid have a low proliferative index consistent with the overall clinical picture. Conventional cytogenetic analysis is therefore generally unsuccessful. FISH studies identify both numeric chromosomal abnormalities such as trisomies, gains of 1q and monosomies including deletion 13q at a similar frequency to MGUS.[219–221] Studies also identify the presence of the IgH translocations t(11;14) and t(4;14) confirming these to be early pathogenic events as in MGUS and myeloma.[219,221–223] Gene expression studies have identified a 12 gene signature of AL amyloidosis although this is yet to be evaluated in other studies.[224]

MONOCLONAL LIGHT AND HEAVY CHAIN DEPOSITION DISEASES

Monoclonal light and heavy chain deposition diseases are rare plasma cell neoplasms that secrete abnormal light or heavy chain or both. These do not form amyloid β-pleated sheets, bind Congo red or contain amyloid P-component but deposition in tissues causes organ dysfunction. All are very rare and usually occur in association with MGUS or myeloma. Deposition in light-chain deposition disease (LCDD) and heavy-chain deposition disease (HCDD) most commonly affects the kidneys, liver, heart, nerves and blood vessels.[225]

Light–chain deposition disease

The monoclonal immunoglobulin product is produced by neoplastic plasma cells and has undergone structural change due to deletion and mutational events. In LCDD the primary defect involves multiple mutations of the Ig light chain variable region. The consequence of this is immunoglobulin with altered properties or aberrant glycosylation which result in increased tissue deposition.[226] Histologically there are prominent monoclonal immunoglobulin deposits that are not amyloid in nature and do not stain with Congo red. They are frequently seen in the glomerular and tubular basement membranes. κ light chains predominate in LCDD and are apparent by immunohistochemistry. The classic feature is the presence of prominent, smooth, ribbon-like linear peritubular deposits of monotypic immunoglobulin along the outer edge of the tubular basement membrane. Usually there is no plasma cell infiltrate in the visceral organs but there is a bone marrow plasmacytosis found in approximately half of cases with confirmed myeloma in a total of 25 percent of cases in one report.[227]

Heavy chain deposition diseases

In HCDD there is deletion of the CH1 constant domain and usually the VH region resulting in production of a monoclonal immunoglobulin molecule with truncated heavy chain and no light chain. The variable regions also contain a high level of somatic mutation, deletions and insertions of sequences of unknown origin in the rearranged genes. These abnormal heavy chains are prone to tissue deposition with pathologic sequelae. These rare B cell neoplasms are morphologically, genetically and immunophenotypically heterogeneous but the unifying feature is the production of an abnormal serum immunoglobulin component. The pathologic immunoglobulin is either IgA (α HCD), IgG (γ HCD) or IgM (μ HCD). The heavy chain immunoglobulin is incomplete and incapable of full assembly thereby producing partial immunoglobulin molecules of varying size. There may or may not be a characteristic immunoglobulin spike by conventional electrophoresis and therefore immunoelectropheresis, immunoselection or immunofixation may be required.[225]

- α HCD: α HCD is a variant of extranodal marginal zone B cell lymphoma or mucosal-associated lymphoid tissue (MALT) in which defective α heavy chains are secreted. It typically involves the gastrointestinal tract, especially proximal, resulting in malabsorption. It is alternatively known as immunoproliferative small intestinal disease (IPSID). There is a peak in the second and third decades and it is most common around the Mediterranean with an association with low standards of living.[228] It is classified histologically into three stages, A–C. Stage A disease is characterized by a dense mucosal infiltrate of small lymphocytes and plasma cells of the small bowel mucosal lamina propria. In stage B atypical plasmacytic or lymphoplasmacytic cells are present, associated with subtotal or total villous atrophy. Aggregates and sheets of dystrophic plasmablasts and immunoblasts with submucosal invasion and ulceration typify progression to a higher grade large-cell lymphoplasmacytic and immunoblastic lymphoma (stage C).[229] The rate of progression from low- to high-grade lymphoma is not known. Serum protein electrophoresis may not identify a paraprotein but an abnormal α heavy chain can more reliably be identified by immunoelectrophoresis. Alternatively, abnormal α heavy chain in the absence of light chains can be identified by immunohistochemistry or immunofluoresence of small bowel biopsy specimens.[225]
- Unlike other variants of MALT lymphoma, IPSID does not tend to have the t(11;18) translocation. One reported translocation, t(9;14), involves the PAX5 gene, important in normal B cell development.[230,231] Although typical multiple myeloma aberrant class switch translocations are not found in IPSID, other translocations involving either the immunoglobulin heavy chain locus on chromosome 14 or the light chain

loci on chromosomes 2 and 22 encoding κ and λ light chains, respectively, have been reported.[232]

- *Campylobacter jejuni* infection of the gut has been reported to be associated with the development of IPSID, including a dramatic response to antibiotic therapy.[233] The mechanism for development of the disease is not clear but it is proposed that there may also be an association with impaired humoral and cellular immunity, either due to genetic predisposition or acquired factors such as the modulatory effects of *Vibrio cholerae* toxins. One theory is that as a result of chronic antigenic stimulation within the gut, a proliferation of IgA-producing plasma cells results. Somatic mutation within these cells results in an occasional mutated B cell with deletion of the variable heavy chain gene region and therefore a clone of abnormal plasma cells producing truncated α heavy chain is produced. The absence of variable region determinants may allow these cells to escape normal immune regulatory control and therefore gain a proliferative advantage.[234] The role of further initiating and disease progression events is unknown although Pax-5 warrants further study in this context.

- γ *HCD*: This is a lymphoplasmacytic neoplasm that appears to be a variant of lymphoplasmacytic lymphoma characterized by the production of a truncated γ chain that does not bind light chains and hence cannot form a complete immunoglobulin molecule. It is rare with a median age of 60 years. The tumor involves lymph nodes, spleen, bone marrow and blood. The lymphoplasmacytoid cells express pan-B cell markers and cytoplasmic γ heavy chain without light chain and are negative for CD5 and CD10.[234] General systemic symptoms predominate including lymphadenopathy but not bone pain as lytic bone disease is not a feature of this disease. Circulating plasma cells or lymphocytes in the blood may have the appearance of plasma cell leukemia or chronic lymphocytic leukemia. The immunophenotype is of a mature B cell neoplasm with monoclonal cytoplasmic gamma chain without light chain. No apparent proliferative disease is identified in 9–17 percent of patients but an underlying autoimmune disease is usually associated in these cases. The exact cell of origin and its genetics have not been well studied.[225]

- μ *HCD*: μ HCD is very rare and often resembles chronic lymphocytic leukemia (CLL) with a defective μ heavy chain lacking a variable region. The disease involves bone marrow, spleen, liver and peripheral blood. In the bone marrow there are characteristic vacuolated plasma cells and small, round lymphocytes more typical of CLL. It is a slowly progressive disease in which the genetics is not well characterized.[225]

KEY POINTS

- Plasma cell neoplasms result from the proliferation of a clone of terminally differentiated B cells that have undergone VDJ rearrangement, class switch recombination and somatic hypermutation.
- Plasma cell neoplasms form a spectrum from MGUS, through to multiple myeloma and plasma cell leukemia; MGUS progresses to multiple myeloma at approximately 1 percent per annum.
- MGUS and multiple myeloma can be broadly classified in to hyperdiploid and non-hyperdiploid based on chromosomal number with the hyperdiploid group having a better prognosis. Translocations involving the immunoglobulin heavy chain and deletions of all or part of chromosome 13 are associated with the non-hyperdiploid group.
- The acquisition of additional genetic and epigenetic events characterizes the transition from intramedullary to extramedullary myeloma.
- The interaction between BMSCs and plasma cells is essential in order for myeloma to develop and progress. The key cytokines produced by BMSCs include TNF-α, IL-6 and IGF-1.
- Multiple myeloma bone disease is driven by plasma cell and bone marrow stromal cell adhesion upregulating the RANK/RANKL system resulting in increased osteoclast activity and bone resorption.
- Monoclonal immunoglobulin deposition diseases in the form of AL amyloidosis, light and heavy chain diseases are the consequence of abnormal monoclonal light or heavy chain production and resultant pathologic tissue deposition.

REFERENCES

- • = Key primary paper
- ◆ = Major review article

1. Kondo M, Weissman IL, Akashi K. Identification of clonogenic common lymphoid progenitors in mouse bone marrow. *Cell* 1997; **91**: 661–72.
- •2. Tonegawa S. Somatic generation of antibody diversity. *Nature* 1983; **302**: 575–81.
3. Bain G, Maandag EC, Izon DJ *et al*. E2A proteins are required for proper B cell development and initiation of immunoglobulin gene rearrangements. *Cell* 1994; **79**: 885–92.

4. Lin H, Grosschedl R. Failure of B-cell differentiation in mice lacking the transcription factor EBF. *Nature* 1995; **376**: 263–7.

●5. Nutt SL, Heavey B, Rolink AG, Busslinger M. Commitment to the B-lymphoid lineage depends on the transcription factor Pax5. *Nature* 1999; **401**: 556–62.

6. Alt FW, Yancopoulos GD, Blackwell TK *et al*. Ordered rearrangement of immunoglobulin heavy chain variable region segments. *EMBO J* 1984; **3**: 1209–19.

7. Oettinger MA, Schatz DG, Gorka C, Baltimore D. RAG-1 and RAG-2, adjacent genes that synergistically activate V(D)J recombination. *Science* 1990; **248**: 1517–23.

8. Bassing CH, Swat W, Alt FW. The mechanism and regulation of chromosomal V(D)J recombination. *Cell* 2002; **109(Suppl)**: s45–55.

9. Papavasiliou FN, Schatz DG. Somatic hypermutation of immunoglobulin genes: merging mechanisms for genetic diversity. *Cell* 2002; **109(Suppl)**: s35–44.

◆10. Martin A, Scharff MD. AID and mismatch repair in antibody diversification. *Nat Rev Immunol* 2002; **2**: 605–14.

●11. Kyle RA. Multiple myeloma: review of 869 cases. *Mayo Clin Proc* 1975; **50**: 29–40.

●12. Bergsagel PL, Chesi M, Nardini E *et al*. Promiscuous translocations into immunoglobulin heavy chain switch regions in multiple myeloma. *Proc Natl Acad Sci U S A* 1996; **93**: 13931–6.

13. Office for National Statistics. *Cancer statistics – registrations, England, 2005*. Series MB1 no36. London: Office for National Statistics, 2008.

14. Ries LAG, Melbert D, Krapcho M *et al*. *SEER Cancer Statistics Review, 1975–2004*. Bethesda: National Cancer Institute, 2007.

15. Ichimaru M, Ishimaru T, Mikami M, Matsunaga M. Multiple myeloma among atomic bomb survivors in Hiroshima and Nagasaki, 1950–76: relationship to radiation dose absorbed by marrow. *J Natl Cancer Inst* 1982; **69**: 323–8.

16. Preston DL, Kusumi S, Tomonaga M *et al*. Cancer incidence in atomic bomb survivors. Part III. Leukemia, lymphoma and multiple myeloma, 1950–1987. *Radiat Res* 1994; **137**: s68–97.

◆17. Riedel DA, Pottern LM. The epidemiology of multiple myeloma. *Hematol Oncol Clin North Am* 1992; **6**: 225–47.

18. Grosbois B, Jego P, Attal M *et al*. Familial multiple myeloma: report of fifteen families. *Br J Haematol* 1999; **105**: 768–70.

19. Lynch H, Watson P, Tarantolo S *et al*. Phenotypic heterogeneity in multiple myeloma families. *J Clin Oncol* 2005; **23**: 685–93.

20. Lynch HT, Sanger WG, Pirruccello S *et al*. Familial multiple myeloma: a family study and review of the literature. *J Natl Cancer Inst* 2001; **93**: 1479–83.

21. Dring AM, Davies FE, Rollinson SJ *et al*. Interleukin 6, tumour necrosis factor alpha and lymphotoxin alpha polymorphisms in monoclonal gammopathy of uncertain significance and multiple myeloma. *Br J Haematol* 2001; **112**: 249–51.

22. Mazur G, Bogunia-Kubik K, Wrobel T *et al*. IL-6 and IL-10 promoter gene polymorphisms do not associate with the susceptibility for multiple myeloma. *Immunol Lett* 2005; **96**: 241–6.

23. Parker KM, Ma MH, Manyak S *et al*. Identification of polymorphisms of the IkappaBalpha gene associated with an increased risk of multiple myeloma. *Cancer Genet Cytogenet* 2002; **137**: 43–8.

24. Roddam PL, Rollinson S, O'Driscoll M *et al*. Genetic variants of NHEJ DNA ligase IV can affect the risk of developing multiple myeloma, a tumour characterised by aberrant class switch recombination. *J Med Genet* 2002; **39**: 900–5.

●25. Bakkus MH, Van Riet I, Van Camp B, Thielemans K. Evidence that the clonogenic cell in multiple myeloma originates from a pre-switched but somatically mutated B cell. *Br J Haematol* 1994; **87**: 68–74.

●26. Sahota SS, Leo R, Hamblin TJ, Stevenson FK. Ig VH gene mutational patterns indicate different tumor cell status in human myeloma and monoclonal gammopathy of undetermined significance. *Blood* 1996; **87**: 746–55.

27. Pilarski LM, Mant MJ, Ruether BA. Pre-B cells in peripheral blood of multiple myeloma patients. *Blood* 1985; **66**: 416–22.

28. Szczepek AJ, Seeberger K, Wizniak J *et al*. A high frequency of circulating B cells share clonotypic Ig heavy-chain VDJ rearrangements with autologous bone marrow plasma cells in multiple myeloma, as measured by single-cell and *in situ* reverse transcriptase-polymerase chain reaction. *Blood* 1998; **92**: 2844–55.

29. Calasanz MJ, Cigudosa JC, Odero MD *et al*. Cytogenetic analysis of 280 patients with multiple myeloma and related disorders: primary breakpoints and clinical correlations. *Genes Chromosomes Cancer* 1997; **18**: 84–93.

●30. Dewald GW, Kyle RA, Hicks GA, Greipp PR. The clinical significance of cytogenetic studies in 100 patients with multiple myeloma, plasma cell leukemia, or amyloidosis. *Blood* 1985; **66**: 380–90.

31. Sawyer JR, Waldron JA, Jagannath S, Barlogie B. Cytogenetic findings in 200 patients with multiple myeloma. *Cancer Genet Cytogenet* 1995; **82**: 41–9.

●32. Drach J, Schuster J, Nowotny H *et al*. Multiple myeloma: high incidence of chromosomal aneuploidy as detected by interphase fluorescence *in situ* hybridization. *Cancer Res* 1995; **55**: 3854–9.

◆33. Fonseca R, Barlogie B, Bataille R *et al*. Genetics and cytogenetics of multiple myeloma: a workshop report. *Cancer Res* 2004; **64**: 1546–58.

34. Debes-Marun CS, Dewald GW, Bryant S *et al*. Chromosome abnormalities clustering and its implications for pathogenesis and prognosis in myeloma. *Leukemia* 2003; **17**: 427–36.

●35. Fonseca R, Debes-Marun CS, Picken EB *et al*. The recurrent IgH translocations are highly associated with nonhyperdiploid variant multiple myeloma. *Blood* 2003; **102**: 2562–7.

36. Smadja N, Leroux D, Soulier J *et al.* Further cytogenetic characterization of multiple myeloma confirms that 14q32 translocations are a very rare event in hyperdiploid cases. *Genes Chromosomes Cancer* 2003; **38**: 234–9.

●37. Avet-Loiseau H, Facon T, Daviet A *et al.* 14q32 translocations and monosomy 13 observed in monoclonal gammopathy of undetermined significance delineate a multistep process for the oncogenesis of multiple myeloma. Intergroupe Francophone du Myelome. *Cancer Res* 1999; **59**: 4546–50.

38. Boersma-Vreugdenhil GR, Kuipers J, Van Stralen E *et al.* The recurrent translocation t(14;20)(q32;q12) in multiple myeloma results in aberrant expression of MAFB: a molecular and genetic analysis of the chromosomal breakpoint. *Br J Haematol* 2004; **126**: 355–63.

●39. Chesi M, Bergsagel PL, Shonukan OO *et al.* Frequent dysregulation of the c-maf proto-oncogene at 16q23 by translocation to an Ig locus in multiple myeloma. *Blood* 1998; **91**: 4457–63.

●40. Chesi M, Nardini E, Brents LA *et al.* Frequent translocation t(4;14)(p16.3;q32.3) in multiple myeloma is associated with increased expression and activating mutations of fibroblast growth factor receptor 3. *Nat Genet* 1997; **16**: 260–4.

41. Fonseca R, Witzig TE, Gertz MA *et al.* Multiple myeloma and the translocation t(11;14)(q13;q32): a report on 13 cases. *Br J Haematol* 1998; **101**: 296–301.

42. Shaughnessy JJ, Gabrea A, Qi Y *et al.* Cyclin D3 at 6p21 is dysregulated by recurrent chromosomal translocations to immunoglobulin loci in multiple myeloma. *Blood* 2001; **98**: 217–23.

43. Bergsagel PL, Nardini E, Brents L *et al.* IgH translocations in multiple myeloma: a nearly universal event that rarely involves c-myc. *Curr Top Microbiol Immunol* 1997; **224**: 283–7.

●44. Avet-Loiseau H, Li JY, Facon T *et al.* High incidence of translocations t(11;14)(q13;q32) and t(4;14)(p16;q32) in patients with plasma cell malignancies. *Cancer Res* 1998; **58**: 5640–5.

45. Ronchetti D, Finelli P, Richelda R *et al.* Molecular analysis of 11q13 breakpoints in multiple myeloma. *Blood* 1999; **93**: 1330–7.

46. Fonseca R, Hoyer JD, Aguayo P *et al.* Clinical significance of the translocation (11;14)(q13;q32) in multiple myeloma. *Leuk Lymphoma* 1999; **35**: 599–605.

●47. Avet-Loiseau H, Attal M, Moreau P *et al.* Genetic abnormalities and survival in multiple myeloma: the experience of the Intergroupe Francophone du Myélome. *Blood* 2007; **109**: 3489–95.

●48. Fonseca R, Blood EA, Oken MM *et al.* Myeloma and the t(11;14)(q13;q32); evidence for a biologically defined unique subset of patients. *Blood* 2002; **99**: 3735–41.

49. Gertz MA, Lacy MQ, Dispenzieri A *et al.* Clinical implications of t(11;14)(q13;q32), t(4;14)(p16.3;q32),

and –17p13 in myeloma patients treated with high-dose therapy. *Blood* 2005; **106**: 2837–40.

50. Fonseca R, Bailey RJ, Ahmann GJ *et al.* Genomic abnormalities in monoclonal gammopathy of undetermined significance. *Blood* 2002; **100**: 1417–24.

51. Kaufmann H, Ackermann J, Baldia C *et al.* Both IGH translocations and chromosome 13q deletions are early events in monoclonal gammopathy of undetermined significance and do not evolve during transition to multiple myeloma. *Leukemia* 2004; **18**: 1879–82.

●52. Chesi M, Nardini E, Lim RS *et al.* The t(4;14) translocation in myeloma dysregulates both FGFR3 and a novel gene, MMSET, resulting in IgH/MMSET hybrid transcripts. *Blood* 1998; **92**: 3025–34.

●53. Richelda R, Ronchetti D, Baldini L *et al.* A novel chromosomal translocation t(4; 14)(p16.3; q32) in multiple myeloma involves the fibroblast growth-factor receptor 3 gene. *Blood* 1997; **90**: 4062–70.

54. Plowright EE, Li Z, Bergsagel PL *et al.* Ectopic expression of fibroblast growth factor receptor 3 promotes myeloma cell proliferation and prevents apoptosis. *Blood* 2000; **95**: 992–8.

55. Li Z, Zhu YX, Plowright EE *et al.* The myeloma-associated oncogene fibroblast growth factor receptor 3 is transforming in hematopoietic cells. *Blood* 2001; **97**: 2413–19.

56. Trudel S, Ely S, Farooqi Y *et al.* Inhibition of fibroblast growth factor receptor 3 induces differentiation and apoptosis in t(4;14) myeloma. *Blood* 2004; **103**: 3521–8.

57. Trudel S, Li ZH, Wei E *et al.* CHIR-258, a novel, multitargeted tyrosine kinase inhibitor for the potential treatment of t(4;14) multiple myeloma. *Blood* 2005; **105**: 2941–8.

58. Trudel S, Stewart AK, Rom E *et al.* The inhibitory anti-FGFR3 antibody, PRO-001, is cytotoxic to t(4;14) multiple myeloma cells. *Blood* 2006; **107**: 4039–46.

●59. Keats JJ, Reiman T, Maxwell CA *et al.* In multiple myeloma, t(4;14)(p16;q32) is an adverse prognostic factor irrespective of FGFR3 expression. *Blood* 2003; **101**: 1520–9.

60. Santra M, Zhan F, Tian E *et al.* A subset of multiple myeloma harboring the t(4;14)(p16;q32) translocation lacks FGFR3 expression but maintains an IGH/MMSET fusion transcript. *Blood* 2003; **101**: 2374–6.

61. Keats JJ, Maxwell CA, Taylor BJ *et al.* Overexpression of transcripts originating from the MMSET locus characterizes all t(4;14)(p16;q32)-positive multiple myeloma patients. *Blood* 2005; **105**: 4060–9.

62. Todoerti K, Ronchetti D, Agnelli L *et al.* Transcription repression activity is associated with the type I isoform of the MMSET gene involved in t(4;14) in multiple myeloma. *Br J Haematol* 2005; **131**: 214–18.

63. Jaksic W, Trudel S, Chang H *et al.* Clinical outcomes in t(4;14) multiple myeloma: a chemotherapy-sensitive disease characterized by rapid relapse and alkylating agent resistance. *J Clin Oncol* 2005; **23**: 7069–73.

●64. Fonseca R, Oken MM, Greipp PR. The t(4;14)(p16.3;q32) is strongly associated with chromosome 13 abnormalities in both multiple myeloma and monoclonal gammopathy of undetermined significance. *Blood* 2001; **98**: 1271–2.

●65. Sawyer J, Lukacs J, Thomas E *et al.* Multicolour spectral karyotyping identifies new translocations and a recurring pathway for chromosome loss in multiple myeloma. *Br J Haematol* 2001; **112**: 167–74.

66. Sawyer JR, Lukacs JL, Munshi N *et al.* Identification of new nonrandom translocations in multiple myeloma with multicolor spectral karyotyping. *Blood* 1998; **92**: 4269–78.

67. Hurt EM, Wiestner A, Rosenwald A *et al.* Overexpression of c-maf is a frequent oncogenic event in multiple myeloma that promotes proliferation and pathological interactions with bone marrow stroma. *Cancer Cell* 2004; **5**: 191–9.

●68. Annunziata CM, Davis RE, Demchenko Y *et al.* Frequent engagement of the classical and alternative NF-kappaB pathways by diverse genetic abnormalities in multiple myeloma. *Cancer Cell* 2007; **12**: 115–30.

69. Hanamura I, Iida S, Ueda R *et al.* Identification of three novel chromosomal translocation partners involving the immunoglobulin loci in newly diagnosed myeloma and human myeloma cell lines. *ASH Annual Meeting Abstracts* 2005; **106**: 1552.

70. Avet-Loiseau H, Facon T, Grosbois B *et al.* Oncogenesis of multiple myeloma: 14q32 and 13q chromosomal abnormalities are not randomly distributed, but correlate with natural history, immunological features, and clinical presentation. *Blood* 2002; **99**: 2185–91.

71. Gutiérrez NC, Hernández JM, García JL *et al.* Differences in genetic changes between multiple myeloma and plasma cell leukemia demonstrated by comparative genomic hybridization. *Leukemia* 2001; **15**: 840–5.

72. Königsberg R, Ackermann J, Kaufmann H *et al.* Deletions of chromosome 13q in monoclonal gammopathy of undetermined significance. *Leukemia* 2000; **14**: 1975–9.

73. Rasillo A, Tabernero MD, Sánchez ML *et al.* Fluorescence *in situ* hybridization analysis of aneuploidization patterns in monoclonal gammopathy of undetermined significance versus multiple myeloma and plasma cell leukemia. *Cancer* 2003; **97**: 601–9.

74. Fonseca R, Oken MM, Harrington D *et al.* Deletions of chromosome 13 in multiple myeloma identified by interphase FISH usually denote large deletions of the q arm or monosomy. *Leukemia* 2001; **15**: 981–6.

●75. Walker BA, Leone PE, Jenner MW *et al.* Integration of global SNP-based mapping and expression arrays reveals key regions, mechanisms, and genes important in the pathogenesis of multiple myeloma. *Blood* 2006; **108**: 1733–43.

76. Chiecchio L, Protheroe RK, Ibrahim AH *et al.* Deletion of chromosome 13 detected by conventional cytogenetics is a critical prognostic factor in myeloma. *Leukemia* 2006; **20**: 1610–17.

77. Kaufmann H, Krömer E, Nösslinger T *et al.* Both chromosome 13 abnormalities by metaphase cytogenetics and deletion of 13q by interphase FISH only are prognostically relevant in multiple myeloma. *Eur J Haematol* 2003; **71**: 179–83.

78. Kröger N, Schilling G, Einsele H *et al.* Deletion of chromosome band 13q14 as detected by fluorescence *in situ* hybridization is a prognostic factor in patients with multiple myeloma who are receiving allogeneic dose-reduced stem cell transplantation. *Blood* 2004; **103**: 4056–61.

●79. Smadja NV, Bastard C, Brigaudeau C *et al.* Hypodiploidy is a major prognostic factor in multiple myeloma. *Blood* 2001; **98**: 2229–38.

●80. Zojer N, Königsberg R, Ackermann J *et al.* Deletion of 13q14 remains an independent adverse prognostic variable in multiple myeloma despite its frequent detection by interphase fluorescence *in situ* hybridization. *Blood* 2000; **95**: 1925–30.

81. Nilsson T, Höglund M, Lenhoff S *et al.* A pooled analysis of karyotypic patterns, breakpoints and imbalances in 783 cytogenetically abnormal multiple myelomas reveals frequently involved chromosome segments as well as significant age- and sex-related differences. *Br J Haematol* 2003; **120**: 960–9.

82. Smadja N, Fruchart C, Isnard F *et al.* Chromosomal analysis in multiple myeloma: cytogenetic evidence of two different diseases. *Leukemia* 1998; **12**: 960–9.

83. Chng WJ, Van Wier SA, Ahmann GJ *et al.* A validated FISH trisomy index demonstrates the hyperdiploid and nonhyperdiploid dichotomy in MGUS. *Blood* 2005; **106**: 2156–61.

●84. Carrasco DR, Tonon G, Huang Y *et al.* High-resolution genomic profiles define distinct clinico-pathogenetic subgroups of multiple myeloma patients. *Cancer Cell* 2006; **9**: 313–25.

●85. Hanamura I, Stewart JP, Huang Y *et al.* Frequent gain of chromosome band 1q21 in plasma-cell dyscrasias detected by fluorescence *in situ* hybridization: incidence increases from MGUS to relapsed myeloma and is related to prognosis and disease progression following tandem stem-cell transplantation. *Blood* 2006; **108**: 1724–32.

86. Chang H, Qi X, Trieu Y *et al.* Multiple myeloma patients with CKS1B gene amplification have a shorter progression-free survival post-autologous stem cell transplantation. *Br J Haematol* 2006; **135**: 486–91.

87. Chang H, Yeung J, Xu W *et al.* Significant increase of CKS1B amplification from monoclonal gammopathy of undetermined significance to multiple myeloma and plasma cell leukaemia as demonstrated by interphase fluorescence *in situ* hybridisation. *Br J Haematol* 2006; **134**: 613–15.

88. Fonseca R, Van Wier SA, Chng WJ *et al.* Prognostic value of chromosome 1q21 gain by fluorescent *in situ* hybridization and increase CKS1B expression in myeloma. *Leukemia* 2006; **20**: 2034–40.

89. Zhan F, Colla S, Wu X *et al.* CKS1B, overexpressed in aggressive disease, regulates multiple myeloma growth and survival through SKP2- and p27Kip1-dependent and -independent mechanisms. *Blood* 2007; **109**: 4995–5001.

90. Chang H, Ning Y, Qi X *et al.* Chromosome 1p21 deletion is a novel prognostic marker in patients with multiple myeloma. *Br J Haematol* 2007; **139**: 51–4.

91. Jenner MW, Leone PE, Walker BA *et al.* Gene mapping and expression analysis of 16q loss of heterozygosity identifies WWOX and CYLD as being important in determining clinical outcome in multiple myeloma. *Blood* 2007; **110**: 3291–300.

92. Tiedemann RE, Gonzalez-Paz N, Kyle RA *et al.* Genetic aberrations and survival in plasma cell leukemia. *Leukemia* 2008; **22**: 1044–52.

93. Chang H, Qi C, Yi QL *et al.* p53 gene deletion detected by fluorescence *in situ* hybridization is an adverse prognostic factor for patients with multiple myeloma following autologous stem cell transplantation. *Blood* 2005; **105**: 358–60.

94. Chang H, Sloan S, Li D, Stewart AK. Multiple myeloma involving central nervous system: high frequency of chromosome 17p13.1 (p53) deletions. *Br J Haematol* 2004; **127**: 280–4.

95. Königsberg R, Zojer N, Ackermann J *et al.* Predictive role of interphase cytogenetics for survival of patients with multiple myeloma. *J Clin Oncol* 2000; **18**: 804–12.

●96. Fonseca R, Blood E, Rue M *et al.* Clinical and biologic implications of recurrent genomic aberrations in myeloma. *Blood* 2003; **101**: 4569–75.

97. Chng WJ, Price-Troska T, Gonzalez-Paz N *et al.* Clinical significance of TP53 mutation in myeloma. *Leukemia* 2007; **21**: 582–4.

98. Chang H, Qi XY, Claudio J *et al.* Analysis of PTEN deletions and mutations in multiple myeloma. *Leuk Res* 2006; **30**: 262–5.

●99. Keats JJ, Fonseca R, Chesi M *et al.* Promiscuous mutations activate the noncanonical NF-kappaB pathway in multiple myeloma. *Cancer Cell* 2007; **12**: 131–44.

100. Dib A, Peterson TR, Raducha-Grace L *et al.* Paradoxical expression of INK4c in proliferative multiple myeloma tumors: bi-allelic deletion vs increased expression. *Cell Div* 2006; **1**: 23.

101. Leone PE, Walker BA, Jenner MW *et al.* Deletions of CDKN2C in multiple myeloma: biological and clinical implications. *Clin Cancer Res* 2008; **14**: 6033–41.

102. Avet-Loiseau H, Gerson F, Magrangeas F *et al.* Rearrangements of the c-myc oncogene are present in 15% of primary human multiple myeloma tumors. *Blood* 2001; **98**: 3082–6.

103. Fabris S, Storlazzi CT, Baldini L *et al.* Heterogeneous pattern of chromosomal breakpoints involving the MYC locus in multiple myeloma. *Genes Chromosomes Cancer* 2003; **37**: 261–9.

104. Liu P, Leong T, Quam L *et al.* Activating mutations of N- and K-ras in multiple myeloma show different clinical associations: analysis of the Eastern Cooperative Oncology Group Phase III Trial. *Blood* 1996; **88**: 2699–706.

105. Chesi M, Brents LA, Ely SA *et al.* Activated fibroblast growth factor receptor 3 is an oncogene that contributes to tumor progression in multiple myeloma. *Blood* 2001; **97**: 729–36.

106. González M, Mateos MV, García-Sanz R *et al.* De novo methylation of tumor suppressor gene p16/INK4a is a frequent finding in multiple myeloma patients at diagnosis. *Leukemia* 2000; **14**: 183–7.

107. Guillerm G, Depil S, Wolowiec D, Quesnel B. Different prognostic values of p15(INK4b) and p16(INK4a) gene methylations in multiple myeloma. *Haematologica* 2003; **88**: 476–8.

108. Mateos MV, García-Sanz R, López-Pérez R *et al.* Methylation is an inactivating mechanism of the p16 gene in multiple myeloma associated with high plasma cell proliferation and short survival. *Br J Haematol* 2002; **118**: 1034–40.

109. Lavelle D, DeSimone J, Hankewych M *et al.* Decitabine induces cell cycle arrest at the G1 phase via p21(WAF1) and the G2/M phase via the p38 MAP kinase pathway. *Leuk Res* 2003; **27**: 999–1007.

110. Galm O, Wilop S, Reichelt J *et al.* DNA methylation changes in multiple myeloma. *Leukemia* 2004; **18**: 1687–92.

111. Dib A, Barlogie B, Shaughnessy JDJ, Kuehl WM. Methylation and expression of the p16INK4A tumor suppressor gene in multiple myeloma. *Blood* 2007; **109**: 1337–8.

112. Gonzalez-Paz N, Chng WJ, McClure RF *et al.* Tumor suppressor p16 methylation in multiple myeloma: biological and clinical implications. *Blood* 2007; **109**: 1228–32.

113. Depil S, Saudemont A, Quesnel B. SOCS-1 gene methylation is frequent but does not appear to have prognostic value in patients with multiple myeloma. *Leukemia* 2003; **17**: 1678–9.

●114. Davies FE, Dring AM, Li C *et al.* Insights into the multistep transformation of MGUS to myeloma using microarray expression analysis. *Blood* 2003; **102**: 4504–11.

●115. Zhan F, Hardin J, Kordsmeier B *et al.* Global gene expression profiling of multiple myeloma, monoclonal gammopathy of undetermined significance, and normal bone marrow plasma cells. *Blood* 2002; **99**: 1745–57.

●116. Bergsagel PL, Kuehl WM, Zhan F *et al.* Cyclin D dysregulation: an early and unifying pathogenic event in multiple myeloma. *Blood* 2005; **106**: 296–303.

●117. Zhan F, Huang Y, Colla S *et al.* The molecular classification of multiple myeloma. *Blood* 2006; **108**: 2020–8.

118. Chng WJ, Kumar S, Vanwier S *et al.* Molecular dissection of hyperdiploid multiple myeloma by gene expression profiling. *Cancer Res* 2007; **67**: 2982–9.

119. Zhan F, Barlogie B, Arzoumanian V *et al.* Gene-expression signature of benign monoclonal gammopathy evident in multiple myeloma is linked to good prognosis. *Blood* 2007; **109**: 1692–700.

●120. Shaughnessy JDJ, Zhan F, Burington BE et al. A validated gene expression model of high-risk multiple myeloma is defined by deregulated expression of genes mapping to chromosome 1. Blood 2007; **109**: 2276–84.

121. Zhan F, Barlogie B, Mulligan G et al. High-risk myeloma: a gene expression based risk-stratification model for newly diagnosed multiple myeloma treated with high-dose therapy is predictive of outcome in relapsed disease treated with single-agent bortezomib or high-dose dexamethasone. Blood 2008; **111**: 968–9.

◆122. Kuehl WM, Bergsagel PL. Multiple myeloma: evolving genetic events and host interactions. Nat Rev Cancer 2002; **2**: 175–87.

123. Barillé S, Collette M, Bataille R, Amiot M. Myeloma cells upregulate interleukin-6 secretion in osteoblastic cells through cell-to-cell contact but downregulate osteocalcin. Blood 1995; **86**: 3151–9.

124. Caligaris-Cappio F, Gregoretti MG, Merico F et al. Bone marrow microenvironment and the progression of multiple myeloma. Leuk Lymphoma 1992; **8**: 15–22.

◆125. Cook G, Dumbar M, Franklin IM. The role of adhesion molecules in multiple myeloma. Acta Haematol 1997; **97**: 81–9.

126. Sanz-Rodríguez F, Hidalgo A, Teixidó J. Chemokine stromal cell-derived factor-1alpha modulates VLA-4 integrin-mediated multiple myeloma cell adhesion to CS-1/fibronectin and VCAM-1. Blood 2001; **97**: 346–51.

127. Asosingh K, Günthert U, Bakkus MH et al. In vivo induction of insulin-like growth factor-I receptor and CD44v6 confers homing and adhesion to murine multiple myeloma cells. Cancer Res 2000; **60**: 3096–104.

128. Michigami T, Shimizu N, Williams PJ et al. Cell-cell contact between marrow stromal cells and myeloma cells via VCAM-1 and alpha(4)beta(1)-integrin enhances production of osteoclast-stimulating activity. Blood 2000; **96**: 1953–60.

129. Vacca A, Di Loreto M, Ribatti D et al. Bone marrow of patients with active multiple myeloma: angiogenesis and plasma cell adhesion molecules LFA-1, VLA-4, LAM-1, and CD44. Am J Hematol 1995; **50**: 9–14.

130. Hideshima T, Chauhan D, Schlossman R et al. The role of tumor necrosis factor alpha in the pathophysiology of human multiple myeloma: therapeutic applications. Oncogene 2001; **20**: 4519–27.

131. Thomas X, Anglaret B, Magaud JP et al. Interdependence between cytokines and cell adhesion molecules to induce interleukin-6 production by stromal cells in myeloma. Leuk Lymphoma 1998; **32**: 107–19.

●132. Klein B, Zhang XG, Lu ZY, Bataille R. Interleukin-6 in human multiple myeloma. Blood 1995; **85**: 863–72.

133. Dankbar B, Padró T, Leo R et al. Vascular endothelial growth factor and interleukin-6 in paracrine tumor-stromal cell interactions in multiple myeloma. Blood 2000; **95**: 2630–6.

◆134. Hideshima T, Podar K, Chauhan D, Anderson KC. Cytokines and signal transduction. Best Pract Res Clin Haematol 2005; **18**: 509–24.

135. Derenne S, Monia B, Dean NM et al. Antisense strategy shows that Mcl-1 rather than Bcl-2 or Bcl-x(L) is an essential survival protein of human myeloma cells. Blood 2002; **100**: 194–9.

●136. Zhang B, Gojo I, Fenton RG. Myeloid cell factor-1 is a critical survival factor for multiple myeloma. Blood 2002; **99**: 1885–93.

137. Wuillème-Toumi S, Robillard N, Gomez P et al. Mcl-1 is overexpressed in multiple myeloma and associated with relapse and shorter survival. Leukemia 2005; **19**: 1248–52.

138. Hideshima T, Nakamura N, Chauhan D, Anderson KC. Biologic sequelae of interleukin-6 induced PI3-K/Akt signaling in multiple myeloma. Oncogene 2001; **20**: 5991–6000.

●139. Reimold AM, Iwakoshi NN, Manis J et al. Plasma cell differentiation requires the transcription factor XBP-1. Nature 2001; **412**: 300–7.

140. Bataille R, Barlogie B, Lu ZY et al. Biologic effects of anti-interleukin-6 murine monoclonal antibody in advanced multiple myeloma. Blood 1995; **86**: 685–91.

141. Moreau P, Harousseau JL, Wijdenes J et al. A combination of anti-interleukin 6 murine monoclonal antibody with dexamethasone and high-dose melphalan induces high complete response rates in advanced multiple myeloma. Br J Haematol 2000; **109**: 661–4.

◆142. Hideshima T, Bergsagel PL, Kuehl WM, Anderson KC. Advances in biology of multiple myeloma: clinical applications. Blood 2004; **104**: 607–18.

◆143. Hideshima T, Mitsiades C, Tonon G et al. Understanding multiple myeloma pathogenesis in the bone marrow to identify new therapeutic targets. Nat Rev Cancer 2007; **7**: 585–98.

144. Bisping G, Leo R, Wenning D et al. Paracrine interactions of basic fibroblast growth factor and interleukin-6 in multiple myeloma. Blood 2003; **101**: 2775–83.

145. Rajkumar S, Mesa R, Fonseca R et al. Bone marrow angiogenesis in 400 patients with monoclonal gammopathy of undetermined significance, multiple myeloma, and primary amyloidosis. Clin Cancer Res 2002; **8**: 2210–16.

146. Rajkumar SV, Fonseca R, Witzig TE et al. Bone marrow angiogenesis in patients achieving complete response after stem cell transplantation for multiple myeloma. Leukemia 1999; **13**: 469–72.

147. Ribatti D, Vacca A, Nico B et al. Bone marrow angiogenesis and mast cell density increase simultaneously with progression of human multiple myeloma. Br J Cancer 1999; **79**: 451–5.

148. Esteve FR, Roodman GD. Pathophysiology of myeloma bone disease. Best Pract Res Clin Haematol 2007; **20**: 613–24.

◆149. Marie P, Debiais F, Cohen-Solal M, de Vernejoul MC. New factors controlling bone remodeling. Joint Bone Spine 2000; **67**: 150–6.

150. Martin TJ, Ng KW. Mechanisms by which cells of the osteoblast lineage control osteoclast formation and activity. J Cell Biochem 1994; **56**: 357–66.

◆151. Suda T, Takahashi N, Martin TJ. Modulation of osteoclast differentiation. *Endocr Rev* 1992; **13**: 66–80.

152. Sezer O, Heider U, Jakob C *et al*. Immunocytochemistry reveals RANKL expression of myeloma cells. *Blood* 2002; **99**: 4646–7.

153. Sezer O, Heider U, Zavrski I *et al*. RANK ligand and osteoprotegerin in myeloma bone disease. *Blood* 2003; **101**: 2094–8.

154. Matsuzaki K, Udagawa N, Takahashi N *et al*. Osteoclast differentiation factor (ODF) induces osteoclast-like cell formation in human peripheral blood mononuclear cell cultures. *Biochem Biophys Res Commun* 1998; **246**: 199–204.

155. Quinn JM, Elliott J, Gillespie MT, Martin TJ. A combination of osteoclast differentiation factor and macrophage-colony stimulating factor is sufficient for both human and mouse osteoclast formation *in vitro*. *Endocrinology* 1998; **139**: 4424–7.

●156. Yasuda H, Shima N, Nakagawa N *et al*. Osteoclast differentiation factor is a ligand for osteoprotegerin/ osteoclastogenesis-inhibitory factor and is identical to TRANCE/RANKL. *Proc Natl Acad Sci U S A* 1998; **95**: 3597–602.

157. Lacey D, Timms E, Tan H *et al*. Osteoprotegerin ligand is a cytokine that regulates osteoclast differentiation and activation. *Cell* 1998; **93**: 165–76.

158. Mizuno A, Amizuka N, Irie K *et al*. Severe osteoporosis in mice lacking osteoclastogenesis inhibitory factor/osteoprotegerin. *Biochem Biophys Res Commun* 1998; **247**: 610–15.

●159. Simonet WS, Lacey DL, Dunstan CR *et al*. Osteoprotegerin: a novel secreted protein involved in the regulation of bone density. *Cell* 1997; **89**: 309–19.

160. Roux S, Meignin V, Quillard J *et al*. RANK (receptor activator of nuclear factor-kappaB) and RANKL expression in multiple myeloma. *Br J Haematol* 2002; **117**: 86–92.

◆161. Tricot G. New insights into role of microenvironment in multiple myeloma. *Lancet* 2000; **355**: 248–50.

162. Ehrlich LA, Chung HY, Ghobrial I *et al*. IL-3 is a potential inhibitor of osteoblast differentiation in multiple myeloma. *Blood* 2005; **106**: 1407–14.

163. Lee JW, Chung HY, Ehrlich LA *et al*. IL-3 expression by myeloma cells increases both osteoclast formation and growth of myeloma cells. *Blood* 2004; **103**: 2308–15.

164. Giuliani N, Colla S, Morandi F *et al*. Myeloma cells block RUNX2/CBFA1 activity in human bone marrow osteoblast progenitors and inhibit osteoblast formation and differentiation. *Blood* 2005; **106**: 2472–83.

165. Toraldo G, Roggia C, Qian WP *et al*. IL-7 induces bone loss *in vivo* by induction of receptor activator of nuclear factor kappa B ligand and tumor necrosis factor alpha from T cells. *Proc Natl Acad Sci U S A* 2003; **100**: 125–30.

166. Paul SR, Bennett F, Calvetti JA *et al*. Molecular cloning of a cDNA encoding interleukin 11, a stromal cell-derived lymphopoietic and hematopoietic cytokine. *Proc Natl Acad Sci U S A* 1990; **87**: 7512–16.

167. Borset M, Hjorth-Hansen H, Seidel C *et al*. Hepatocyte growth factor and its receptor c-met in multiple myeloma. *Blood* 1996; **88**: 3998–4004.

168. Hjertner O, Torgersen ML, Seidel C *et al*. Hepatocyte growth factor (HGF) induces interleukin-11 secretion from osteoblasts: a possible role for HGF in myeloma-associated osteolytic bone disease. *Blood* 1999; **94**: 3883–8.

169. de la Mata J, Uy HL, Guise TA *et al*. Interleukin-6 enhances hypercalcemia and bone resorption mediated by parathyroid hormone-related protein *in vivo*. *J Clin Invest* 1995; **95**: 2846–52.

170. Kurihara N, Bertolini D, Suda T *et al*. IL-6 stimulates osteoclast-like multinucleated cell formation in long term human marrow cultures by inducing IL-1 release. *J Immunol* 1990; **144**: 4226–30.

171. Löwik CW, van der Pluijm G, Bloys H *et al*. Parathyroid hormone (PTH) and PTH-like protein (PLP) stimulate interleukin-6 production by osteogenic cells: a possible role of interleukin-6 in osteoclastogenesis. *Biochem Biophys Res Commun* 1989; **162**: 1546–52.

172. Fried RM, Voelkel EF, Rice RH *et al*. Two squamous cell carcinomas not associated with humoral hypercalcemia produce a potent bone resorption-stimulating factor which is interleukin-1 alpha. *Endocrinology* 1989; **125**: 742–51.

173. Sato K, Fujii Y, Kasono K *et al*. Parathyroid hormone-related protein and interleukin-1 alpha synergistically stimulate bone resorption *in vitro* and increase the serum calcium concentration in mice *in vivo*. *Endocrinology* 1989; **124**: 2172–8.

174. Lichtenstein A, Berenson J, Norman D *et al*. Production of cytokines by bone marrow cells obtained from patients with multiple myeloma. *Blood* 1989; **74**: 1266–73.

●175. Mundy GR, Raisz LG, Cooper RA *et al*. Evidence for the secretion of an osteoclast stimulating factor in myeloma. *N Engl J Med* 1974; **291**: 1041–6.

176. Pfeilschifter J, Chenu C, Bird A *et al*. Interleukin-1 and tumor necrosis factor stimulate the formation of human osteoclastlike cells *in vitro*. *J Bone Miner Res* 1989; **4**: 113–18.

177. Yoneda T, Alsina MA, Chavez JB *et al*. Evidence that tumor necrosis factor plays a pathogenetic role in the paraneoplastic syndromes of cachexia, hypercalcemia, and leukocytosis in a human tumor in nude mice. *J Clin Invest* 1991; **87**: 977–85.

178. Niida S, Kaku M, Amano H *et al*. Vascular endothelial growth factor can substitute for macrophage colony-stimulating factor in the support of osteoclastic bone resorption. *J Exp Med* 1999; **190**: 293–8.

179. Nakagawa M, Kaneda T, Arakawa T *et al*. Vascular endothelial growth factor (VEGF) directly enhances osteoclastic bone resorption and survival of mature osteoclasts. *FEBS Lett* 2000; **473**: 161–4.

●180. Choi SJ, Cruz JC, Craig F *et al*. Macrophage inflammatory protein 1-alpha is a potential osteoclast stimulatory factor in multiple myeloma. *Blood* 2000; **96**: 671–5.

●181. Abe M, Hiura K, Wilde J *et al.* Role for macrophage inflammatory protein (MIP)-1alpha and MIP-1beta in the development of osteolytic lesions in multiple myeloma. *Blood* 2002; **100**: 2195–202.

182. Han JH, Choi SJ, Kurihara N *et al.* Macrophage inflammatory protein-1alpha is an osteoclastogenic factor in myeloma that is independent of receptor activator of nuclear factor kappaB ligand. *Blood* 2001; **97**: 3349–53.

183. Magrangeas F, Nasser V, Avet-Loiseau H *et al.* Gene expression profiling of multiple myeloma reveals molecular portraits in relation to the pathogenesis of the disease. *Blood* 2003; **101**: 4998–5006.

184. Qiang YW, Endo Y, Rubin JS, Rudikoff S. Wnt signaling in B-cell neoplasia. *Oncogene* 2003; **22**: 1536–45.

185. Westendorf JJ, Kahler RA, Schroeder TM. Wnt signaling in osteoblasts and bone diseases. *Gene* 2004; **341**: 19–39.

186. Morvan F, Boulukos K, Clement-Lacroix P *et al.* Deletion of a single allele of the Dkk1 gene leads to an increase in bone formation and bone mass. *J Bone Miner Res* 2006; **21**: 934–45.

187. Li J, Sarosi I, Cattley RC *et al.* Dkk1-mediated inhibition of Wnt signaling in bone results in osteopenia. *Bone* 2006; **39**: 754–66.

188. Glass DA 2nd, Bialek P, Ahn JD *et al.* Canonical Wnt signaling in differentiated osteoblasts controls osteoclast differentiation. *Dev Cell* 2005; **8**: 751–64.

189. Spencer GJ, Utting JC, Etheridge SL *et al.* Wnt signalling in osteoblasts regulates expression of the receptor activator of NFkappaB ligand and inhibits osteoclastogenesis *in vitro*. *J Cell Sci* 2006; **119**: 1283–96.

●190. Tian E, Zhan F, Walker R *et al.* The role of the Wnt-signaling antagonist DKK1 in the development of osteolytic lesions in multiple myeloma. *N Engl J Med* 2003; **349**: 2483–94.

●191. Criteria for the classification of monoclonal gammopathies, multiple myeloma and related disorders: a report of the International Myeloma Working Group. *Br J Haematol* 2003; **121**: 749–57.

●192. Greipp PR, San Miguel J, Durie BG *et al.* International staging system for multiple myeloma. *J Clin Oncol* 2005; **23**: 3412–20.

◆193. Grogan TM, Spier CM. The B cell immunoproliferative disorders including multiple myeloma and amyloidosis. In: Knowles DM (ed.) *Neoplastic hematopathology*, 2nd ed. Philadelphia: Lippincott Williams and Wilkins, 2001: 1235–66.

●194. Harada H, Kawano MM, Huang N *et al.* Phenotypic difference of normal plasma cells from mature myeloma cells. *Blood* 1993; **81**: 2658–63.

195. Rawstron AC, Fenton JA, Ashcroft J *et al.* The interleukin-6 receptor alpha-chain (CD126) is expressed by neoplastic but not normal plasma cells. *Blood* 2000; **96**: 3880–6.

196. San Miguel JF, Caballero MD, Gonzalez M *et al.* Immunological phenotype of neoplasms involving the B cell in the last step of differentiation. *Br J Haematol* 1986; **62**: 75–83.

197. Rawstron AC, Orfao A, Beksac M *et al.* Report of the European Myeloma Network on multiparametric flow cytometry in multiple myeloma and related disorders. *Haematologica* 2008; **93**: 431–8.

198. Mahmoud MS, Huang N, Nobuyoshi M *et al.* Altered expression of Pax-5 gene in human myeloma cells. *Blood* 1996; **87**: 4311–15.

199. Pellat-Deceunynck C, Barillé S, Jego G *et al.* The absence of CD56 (NCAM) on malignant plasma cells is a hallmark of plasma cell leukemia and of a special subset of multiple myeloma. *Leukemia* 1998; **12**: 1977–82.

200. Alexandrakis MG, Passam FH, Kyriakou DS *et al.* Ki-67 proliferation index: correlation with prognostic parameters and outcome in multiple myeloma. *Am J Clin Oncol* 2004; **27**: 8–13.

201. Chang H, Stewart AK, Qi XY *et al.* Immunohistochemistry accurately predicts FGFR3 aberrant expression and t(4;14) in multiple myeloma. *Blood* 2005; **106**: 353–5.

202. Kremer M, Ott G, Nathrath M *et al.* Primary extramedullary plasmacytoma and multiple myeloma: phenotypic differences revealed by immunohistochemical analysis. *J Pathol* 2005; **205**: 92–101.

203. Pruneri G, Carboni N, Baldini L *et al.* Cell cycle regulators in multiple myeloma: prognostic implications of p53 nuclear accumulation. *Hum Pathol* 2003; **34**: 41–7.

204. Ong F, Hermans J, Noordijk EM *et al.* A population-based registry on paraproteinaemia in The Netherlands. Comprehensive cancer centre West Leiden, The Netherlands. *Br J Haematol* 1997; **99**: 914–20.

●205. Kyle R, Therneau T, Rajkumar S *et al.* A long-term study of prognosis in monoclonal gammopathy of undetermined significance. *N Engl J Med* 2002; **346**: 564–9.

206. Pérez-Persona E, Vidriales MB, Mateo G *et al.* New criteria to identify risk of progression in monoclonal gammopathy of uncertain significance and smoldering multiple myeloma based on multiparameter flow cytometry analysis of bone marrow plasma cells. *Blood* 2007; **110**: 2586–92.

207. Rawstron AC, Fenton JAL, Gonzalez D *et al.* High-risk MGUS: identification by immunophenotype, karyotype, and clonal homogeneity. *ASH Annual Meeting Abstracts* 2003; **102**: 116.

◆208. Dimopoulos MA, Moulopoulos LA, Maniatis A, Alexanian R. Solitary plasmacytoma of bone and asymptomatic multiple myeloma. *Blood* 2000; **96**: 2037–44.

◆209. Dimopoulos MA, Kiamouris C, Moulopoulos LA. Solitary plasmacytoma of bone and extramedullary plasmacytoma. *Hematol Oncol Clin North Am* 1999; **13**: 1249–57.

210. Bink K, Haralambieva E, Kremer M *et al.* Primary extramedullary plasmacytoma: similarities with and differences from multiple myeloma revealed by interphase cytogenetics. *Haematologica* 2008; **93**: 623–6.

211. Kyle R, Maldonado J, Bayrd E. Plasma cell leukemia. Report on 17 cases. *Arch Intern Med* 1974; **133**: 813–18.

212. García-Sanz R, Orfão A, González M *et al.* Primary plasma cell leukemia: clinical, immunophenotypic, DNA ploidy, and cytogenetic characteristics. *Blood* 1999; **93**: 1032–7.

213. Kyle R, Gertz M. Primary systemic amyloidosis: clinical and laboratory features in 474 cases. *Semin Hematol* 1995; **32**: 45–59.

214. Kyle R, Linos A, Beard C *et al.* Incidence and natural history of primary systemic amyloidosis in Olmsted County, Minnesota, 1950 through 1989. *Blood* 1992; **79**: 1817–22.

●215. Glenner GG, Terry W, Harada M *et al.* Amyloid fibril proteins: proof of homology with immunoglobulin light chains by sequence analyses. *Science* 1971; **172**: 1150–1.

◆216. Falk RH, Comenzo RL, Skinner M. The systemic amyloidoses. *N Engl J Med* 1997; **337**: 898–909.

217. Perfetti V, Vignarelli MC, Casarini S *et al.* Biological features of the clone involved in primary amyloidosis (AL). *Leukemia* 2001; **15**: 195–202.

218. McElroy EAJ, Witzig TE, Gertz MA *et al.* Detection of monoclonal plasma cells in the peripheral blood of patients with primary amyloidosis. *Br J Haematol* 1998; **100**: 326–7.

219. Bochtler T, Hegenbart U, Cremer FW *et al.* Evaluation of the cytogenetic aberration pattern in amyloid light chain amyloidosis as compared to monoclonal gammopathy of undetermined significance reveals common pathways of karyotypic instability. *Blood* 2008; **111**: 4700–5.

220. Fonseca R, Ahmann GJ, Jalal SM *et al.* Chromosomal abnormalities in systemic amyloidosis. *Br J Haematol* 1998; **103**: 704–10.

221. Harrison CJ, Mazzullo H, Ross FM *et al.* Translocations of 14q32 and deletions of 13q14 are common chromosomal abnormalities in systemic amyloidosis. *Br J Haematol* 2002; **117**: 427–35.

222. Hayman SR, Bailey RJ, Jalal SM *et al.* Translocations involving the immunoglobulin heavy-chain locus are possible early genetic events in patients with primary systemic amyloidosis. *Blood* 2001; **98**: 2266–8.

223. Perfetti V, Coluccia AM, Intini D *et al.* Translocation T(4;14)(p16.3;q32) is a recurrent genetic lesion in primary amyloidosis. *Am J Pathol* 2001; **158**: 1599–603.

224. Abraham RS, Ballman KV, Dispenzieri A *et al.* Functional gene expression analysis of clonal plasma cells identifies a unique molecular profile for light chain amyloidosis. *Blood* 2005; **105**: 794–803.

◆225. Wahner-Roedler DL, Kyle RA. Heavy chain diseases. *Best Pract Res Clin Haematol* 2005; **18**: 729–46.

226. Cogné M, Silvain C, Khamlichi AA, Preud'homme JL. Structurally abnormal immunoglobulins in human immunoproliferative disorders. *Blood* 1992; **79**: 2181–95.

◆227. Buxbaum J, Gallo G. Nonamyloidotic monoclonal immunoglobulin deposition disease. Light-chain, heavy-chain, and light- and heavy-chain deposition diseases. *Hematol Oncol Clin North Am* 1999; **13**: 1235–48.

◆228. Fine KD, Stone MJ. Alpha-heavy chain disease, Mediterranean lymphoma, and immunoproliferative small intestinal disease: a review of clinicopathological features, pathogenesis, and differential diagnosis. *Am J Gastroenterol* 1999; **94**: 1139–52.

229. Galian A, Lecestre MJ, Scotto J *et al.* Pathological study of alpha-chain disease, with special emphasis on evolution. *Cancer* 1977; **39**: 2081–101.

230. Iida S, Rao PH, Nallasivam P *et al.* The t(9;14)(p13;q32) chromosomal translocation associated with lymphoplasmacytoid lymphoma involves the PAX-5 gene. *Blood* 1996; **88**: 4110–17.

231. Pellet P, Berger R, Bernheim A *et al.* Molecular analysis of a t(9;14)(p11;q32) translocation occurring in a case of human alpha heavy chain disease. *Oncogene* 1989; **4**: 653–7.

◆232. Al-Saleem T, Al-Mondhiry H. Immunoproliferative small intestinal disease (IPSID): a model for mature B-cell neoplasms. *Blood* 2005; **105**: 2274–80.

233. Lecuit M, Abachin E, Martin A *et al.* Immunoproliferative small intestinal disease associated with Campylobacter jejuni. *N Engl J Med* 2004; **350**: 239–48.

◆234. Grogan TM, Van Camp B, Kyle RA. Plasma cell neoplasms. In: Jaffe ES, Harris NL, Stein H, Vardiman JW. (eds) *Pathology and genetics of tumours of haematopoietic and lymphoid tissues.* Lyon: IARC Press, 2001: 142–56.

36

Natural killer (NK) cell neoplasms

WAH CHEUK AND JOHN KC CHAN

INTRODUCTION

Natural killer (NK) cells are lymphocytes with the morphology of large granular lymphocyte (LGL), immunophenotype of surface CD3−, CD56+ and germline configuration of T cell receptor (TCR) genes.[1,2] They are termed 'natural killer' because of their ability to lyse viral-infected cells and tumor cells in a major histocompatibility complex (MHC) unrestricted manner without prior sensitization. In contrast to B and T lymphocytes, they lack the ability to generate antigen-specific receptors by somatic gene rearrangements. Phenotypically, NK cells resemble activated cytotoxic CD8+ T cells with respect to cell surface receptors and effector molecules, but in contrast to the latter, the cytotoxic molecules and cytokines are already present and do not have to be synthesized upon antigenic stimulation, enabling the cells to provide early rapid response against pathogenic agents and thus represent an important arm of the innate immune system. On the other hand, the cytokines, e.g. interferon γ (IFN-γ), tumor necrosis factor α (TNF-α), and granulocyte macrophage colony-stimulating factor (GM-CSF) produced by NK cells can regulate the development of acquired specific immunity. Thus, NK cells can be conceived as the third lymphocyte lineage bridging the innate and adaptive immune systems.[3]

NK cells have two major mechanisms of activation: target recognition and cytokine stimulation.[4] There is a wide repertoire of invariant and constitutionally expressed receptors on NK cells. Each NK cell expresses its own repertoire of stimulatory and inhibitory NK receptors. Target recognition depends on integration and balance of the activation of the stimulatory receptors (such as killer cell immunoglobulin-like receptor [KIR] S family and CD94/NKG2C) and inhibitory receptors (such as KIR L family and CD94/NKG2A).[5] Activation of the stimulatory receptors can trigger perforin-dependent and Fas-Fas ligand (FasL) system killing as well as production of cytokines (such as IFN-γ, TNF-α and GM-CSF) and chemokines (Mig, MIP-1α), the two major effector mechanisms of NK cells.[6–9] Activation of the inhibitory receptors specific for MHC class I molecules on target cells, on the other hand, prevents NK cell activation and killing, providing the basis for the 'missing-self' hypothesis.[10] Alternatively, NK cells can be triggered by cytokines and chemokines (such as IFNα/β, interleukin [IL]-12, IL-15 and IL-18) produced by infected or activated dendritic cells and macrophages.[11]

Natural killer cell development

Natural killer cells have a unique development pathway distinct from B and T lymphocytes. They can develop normally in mice with severe combined immunodeficiency or athymic nude mice that lack T cells.[12–14] The development of NK cells occurs in the bone marrow. The earliest step shares a common pathway with other lymphocytes, involving the commitment of hematopoietic stem cell to the lymphoid lineage, giving rise to common lymphoid progenitors which are destined to form NK, T and B cells (Fig. 36.1).[15] This is followed by the differentiation to a bipotential T/NK progenitor, which can give rise to T cells and NK cells but not to other lineages.[16] The common ancestor for T and NK cells is consistent with the close resemblance of phenotype between mature NK cells and effector T cells. Development of bipotential T/NK progenitor to unipotent NK cell progenitor is characterized by the acquisition of IL-2/15Rβ subunit (CD122) in the cells, which renders

them responsive to IL-15, a critical cytokine that plays an essential role in subsequent development of NK cells.[16,17] In the late phase of development, NK precursors acquire cell surface receptors and undergo proliferation to become phenotypically and functionally mature NK cells.[18]

Mature peripheral NK cells that have exited the bone marrow are found primarily in the peripheral blood as LGLs (constituting around 4–15 percent of mononuclear cells), red pulp of the spleen (3–4 percent of lymphocytes), sinusoids of the liver, peritoneal cavity and the uterus.[3] They are very scanty in non-inflammatory lymph nodes, nasopharynx or tonsils, and are histologically indistinguishable from small B or T lymphocytes.[19] The half-life of mature NK cells in the periphery is about 7–10 days.[20] They undergo low level of proliferation to maintain homeostasis until they encounter a stimulus such as viral infection.[21] They then proliferate in an initial non-specific mode, followed by a selective proliferation of NK cells expressing the specific stimulatory receptors, in a manner reminiscent of T cell clonal expansion except that the NK cell antigen receptors are predetermined and unchangeable. This phase is followed by a resolution phase during which the number of NK cells rapidly returns to normal.

Immunophenotype and genotype of NK cells

NK cells bear a close developmental relationship with T cells as they share a common bipotential NK/T progenitor cell ancestor.[22,23] These two cell types also exhibit considerable immunophenotypic overlap. While NK cells variably

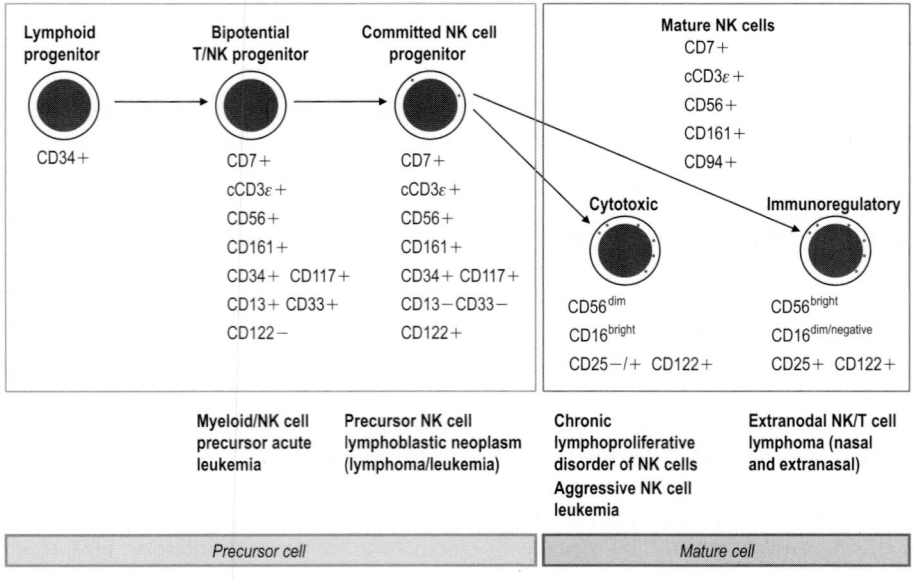

Figure 36.1   Schematic diagram to show the immunophenotypes of natural killer (NK) cells in different stages of development. The various NK cell neoplasms can be aligned to the corresponding stages of NK cell development.

express T-associated markers such as CD2, CD7 and CD8, subsets of cytotoxic T cells also express NK-associated markers such as CD16, CD56 and CD57.[1,7,24,25]

The fundamental feature that distinguishes NK cells from T cells is the germline configuration of the TCR genes, which results in failure to assemble the TCR molecule and complete CD3 complex on the cell membrane. CD3 is a TCR-associated protein, including two CD3ε chains, one CD3γ chain, one CD3δ chain and a ζ homodimer.[26] Natural killer cells only contain ε and ζ chains of CD3 in the cytoplasm. Currently, demonstration of the conformational epitope of the complete CD3 complex on the cell surface requires fresh or frozen tissue (using flow cytometry, frozen section immunohistochemistry or cytologic smear immunocytochemistry) and application of antibodies such as Leu-4, T3, OKT-3 and UCHT-1. This is often referred to as 'surface CD3' (sCD3),[27] a hallmark of T cells and characteristically absent in NK cells. Intracytoplasmic CD3ε chain in NK cells can be demonstrated in paraffin or frozen sections using anti-CD3ε antiserum, or CD3ε monoclonal antibodies such as PS-1 and LN-10; this is often referred to as 'cytoplasmic CD3ε' (cCD3ε) or 'cytoplasmic CD3' (cCD3). These CD3ε antibodies also stain the CD3ε component of the complete CD3 molecule in the cytoplasm or cell surface of T cells.[27–32] In summary, the working definition of NK cell includes a combination of surface TCR−, sCD3−, cCD3ε+, CD56+ and germline TCR genes.[33,34]

Currently CD56 is the most important and sensitive NK cell marker; it is an isoform of neural cell adhesion molecule (N-CAM) and shows homophilic binding to CD56 molecules on other cells.[26] Two functionally distinct subsets of NK cells can be recognized based on the density of surface CD56 expression.[2] Approximately 90 percent of NK cells express a low density of CD56 (CD56^{dim}) and the remaining 10 percent a high density of CD56 (CD56^{bright}). The former subset also expresses CD16+ CD25−/+ and mainly acts as a mediator of natural cytotoxicity and antibody-dependent cell cytotoxicity, whereas the latter is CD16− CD25+ and serves as an immunoregulator through production of cytokines.[2]

Natural killer cell neoplasms

Natural killer cell neoplasms are tumors of putative NK-cell lineage. These neoplasms are often designated 'NK/T cell' instead of simply 'NK cell' because while this category comprises predominantly genuine NK cell neoplasms, it also includes some lymphomas indeterminate between NK and T lineage as well as some cytotoxic T cell lymphomas showing similar clinicopathologic features.[35] The term 'NK/T cell' should not be confused with the recently described cell type known as natural killer T cell (NKT cell).[36] The latter represents a subset of T cells with innate-like lymphocyte and immunoregulatory properties that is characterized by conserved TCR (invariant

Vα14-Vα18 rearrangement) which recognizes glycolipids presented by the class I-like molecule CD1d.[36]

In the 2001 World Health Organization (WHO) classification, three neoplasms of putative NK cell lineage are recognized: extranodal NK/T cell lymphoma, aggressive NK-cell leukemia and blastic NK cell lymphoma.[35,37] The list has been modified and expanded with increased knowledge of NK cell neoplasms (Fig. 36.1).[38] Based on similarities in phenotype between the tumor cells and the normal NK cell counterparts in different stages of development,[39] the spectrum of NK cell neoplasms can be grouped as precursor NK cell neoplasms or mature NK cell neoplasms, similar to the classification schemes for B cell and T cell neoplasm (Fig. 36.1).

PRECURSOR NATURAL KILLER CELL NEOPLASMS

Precursor NK cell neoplasm is a group of rare diseases most frequently manifesting as leukemia, reflecting the habitat of normal NK cell precursors in the bone marrow. Because of the rarity and lack of consistent diagnostic criteria, the clinicopathologic features of this group of neoplasms are still poorly characterized.

Myeloid/NK cell precursor acute leukemia is a myeloid antigen-positive leukemia conceivably originating from bipotential T/NK progenitor cells.[40,41] It is characterized by myeloperoxidase-negative and Sudan Black B-negative blasts with the immunophenotype of CD7+, CD56+, cCD3−/+, sCD3−, myeloid antigens (CD13 or CD33) + and TdT−, and germline TCR and IgH genes. This tumor is currently included under acute myeloid leukemia M0, but with a distinctive CD7+, CD56+ immunophenotype, younger median age (median 46 years) and more frequent extramedullary (lymph node and mediastinal) involvement.[42] Although these cases are generally chemosensitive to myeloid leukemia regimens, relapse is frequent and the prognosis is poor.

Precursor NK cell acute lymphoblastic leukemia, conceptually derived from committed NK progenitor cells, is characterized by lymphoblasts with occasional azurophilic granules, immunophenotype of CD56+, cCD3−/+, sCD3−, B cell antigen negative and myeloid antigen negative, and germline configurations for TCR and IgH genes.[43]

Blastic NK cell lymphoma has been thought to represent the lymphomatous form of precursor NK cell acute lymphoblastic leukemia.[41] Recent findings, however, indicate that most cases represent neoplasms of precursor plasmacytoid dendritic cells, and very few cases represent genuine precursor NK cell lymphoblastic lymphoma.[41,44]

MATURE NATURAL KILLER CELL NEOPLASMS

Mature NK neoplasms, accounting for over 85 percent of NK cell neoplasms,[45] comprise **extranodal NK/T cell lymphoma** and **aggressive NK cell leukemia** (Table 36.1).

Table 36.1 Comparison between extranodal natural killer (NK)/T cell lymphoma, aggressive NK cell leukemia and so-called blastic NK cell lymphoma

	Nasal NK/T cell lymphoma	Extranasal NK/T cell lymphoma	Aggressive NK cell leukemia	Blastic plasmacytoid dendritic cell neoplasm (so-called blastic NK cell lymphoma)
Age (median)	53 years	50 years	39 years	65 years
Sex (M:F ratio)	3:1	3:1	1:1	2.4:1
Racial predilection	More common in Asians, Mexicans and South Americans			None
Clinical presentation	Ulcerative-destructive or mass lesion of upper aerodigestive tract; most have early stage disease (80% stage I/II)	Multiple extranodal lesions (skin, gastrointestinal tract, testis and soft tissue), without lymphadenopathy; most have high stage disease (stage III/IV)	Marked systemic symptoms, hepatosplenomegaly, cytopenia	Localized or disseminated skin nodules, plaques, and bruise-like lesions, lymphadenopathy, bone marrow involvement
Pathology	Mixed populations of small, medium-sized and large cells with variable degrees of atypia; geographic coagulative necrosis; angiocentric-angioinvasive growth		Circulating atypical large granular lymphocytes	Permeative growth of lymphoblast-like cells, without coagulative necrosis
Immunophenotype	cCD3ε+, sCD3−, CD56+, cytotoxic markers+, CD4−, CD123−; CD16+ in aggressive NK cell leukemia			cCD3−/+, sCD3− CD56+, cytotoxic markers−, CD4+, CD123+, CD16−
Epstein–Barr virus association (%)	~100	>90	~100	None
Postulated nature of neoplastic cells	Mature NK cells	Mature NK cells	Mature NK cells (CD56^{dim} CD16+ subset)	Precursor plasmacytoid dendritic cell
Clinical outcome	Aggressive, with long-term survival of 30–40%	Highly aggressive, with long-term survival of 10–20% only	Fulminant clinical course, usually unresponsive to therapy	Highly aggressive; almost invariably relapses after initial response

They occur almost exclusively in extranodal sites, and only very rare cases of primary nodal NK cell lymphoma have been reported.[46–48] Extranodal NK/T cell lymphoma shares many similarities with aggressive NK cell leukemia, such as the presence of azurophilic granules, immunophenotype (CD2+, sCD3−, CD56+), genotype (germline configuration of TCR genes), Epstein–Barr virus (EBV) association, and high prevalence in Asian populations. Therefore, it can be argued that they represent the lymphomatous and leukemic manifestations of the same disease. However, the significant differences in clinical presentation, age of disease onset, prognosis and genetic aberrations of these two entities suggest otherwise.

Chronic lymphoproliferative disorder of NK cells is a rare entity characterized by chronic expansion of mature-looking NK LGLs in the peripheral blood.[28,49–52] At least some cases represent clonal proliferations of NK cells.

EXTRANODAL NATURAL KILLER/T CELL LYMPHOMA

Definition

Extranodal NK/T cell lymphoma is a group of extranodal lymphomas characterized by frequent necrosis, angiocentric growth, cytotoxic phenotype and a strong association with EBV.[35] This designation replaces the less specific term 'angiocentric lymphoma' in the Revised European–American Lymphoma (REAL) classification,[53] and the once popular but non-specific term 'polymorphic reticulosis'.[54] The qualifier 'nasal-type' is often applied as the nasal cavity is the commonest site of involvement and the prototypic site in the initial characterization of the disease.[35,55]

The concept of 'angiocentric immunoproliferative lesions' was proposed in the 1980s for a family of extranodal lymphoid proliferations characterized by prominent angiocentric-angiodestructive growth, necrosis, and a polymorphic cellular infiltrate.[56] It was considered a T cell lymphoproliferative disorder encompassing benign lymphocytic vasculitis, polymorphic reticulosis, lymphomatoid granulomatosis and angiocentric lymphoma. More recent studies based on paraffin section immunohistochemistry (which permits much better cytomorphologic correlation) and molecular studies have shown that most examples of polymorphic reticulosis represent NK/T cell lymphoma, while lymphomatoid granulomatosis represents a peculiar form of T cell-rich large B cell lymphoproliferative disorder with a strong EBV association.[57–60]

Epidemiology

Extranodal NK/T cell lymphoma is an uncommon tumor with a predilection for Asians, Mexicans and South Americans, accounting for approximately 6 percent of all non-Hodgkin lymphomas in these populations in comparison to less than 1.5 percent in Western populations.[7,48,61,62] It is the commonest histologic type of primary nasal lymphoma in Asian populations.[63–65] Natural killer/T cell lymphoma arising in children or young adults can be preceded by various EBV-associated lymphoproliferative diseases such as hypersensitivity to mosquito bites, chronic active EBV infection, hemophagocytic syndrome and hydroa vacciniforme-like eruptions.[66]

Clinical manifestations

Extranodal NK/T cell lymphoma most commonly affects adults with a median age of 50–53 years and a male predominance (M:F = 3 to 1).[7,63,67]

Nasal NK/T cell lymphomas arise in the nasal cavity, nasopharynx or upper aerodigestive tract, causing progressive destructive and ulcerative lesions (so-called midfacial destructive disease) or mass lesions. Clinical manifestations are nasal obstruction, nasal bleeding, foul-smelling nasal discharge, facial swelling, proptosis and impairment of extraocular movement. The tumor frequently spreads to the adjacent anatomic structures such as the paranasal sinuses, orbit, palate, oral cavity and oropharynx, and is typically associated with bone erosion.[68]

Extranasal NK/T cell lymphoma most commonly involves the skin, gastrointestinal tract, salivary gland, testis and soft tissues, which are also the sites that nasal NK/T cell lymphoma tends to disseminate to during the course of the disease.[7,67,69–78] It has been postulated that these sites richly express CD56/N-CAM, favoring homing of the CD56+ lymphoma cells through homophilic binding.[79,80] Systemic symptoms such as fever, malaise and weight loss are common. The skin lesions take the form of multiple nodules or plaques, which commonly ulcerate with a necrotic center. Intestinal lesions often manifest as perforation, attributable

to the prominent tissue necrosis. Involvement of the testis or soft tissues usually manifests as mass lesions. Other extranodal sites can also be involved. Some unusual sites of involvement include the brain,[81] uterus,[82] lung[83] and adrenal gland.[84] A rare cutaneous form of intravascular NK-cell lymphoma has also been described.[85]

Clinical course and treatment

Nasal NK/T cell lymphoma usually presents as early stage disease (80 percent stage I and II).[63,86,87] Bone marrow involvement occurs in less than 10 percent of patients.[88] Some nasal NK/T cell lymphomas remain locally invasive even in terminal cases, but others show dissemination either early or late during the course of the disease, most commonly affecting skin, liver, lymph node, gastrointestinal tract and testis (Plate 67, see plate section).[63] Hemophagocytic syndrome may complicate the disease in some patients.[89] Radiation therapy, either alone or given upfront in combination with chemotherapy, is the single most important key to successful outcome in patients with nasal NK/T cell lymphoma.[39,90–92] The overall response rate ranges from 60 percent to 83 percent, and the reported 5-year survival rate is 40–78 percent. Despite high initial response rate, local and systemic relapses are frequent, varying from 17 percent to 77 percent,[93,94] with 50 percent being most commonly reported.[95,96] Chemotherapy is the treatment of choice for stage III/IV disease.[97] Anthracycline-based regimens such as CHOP (cyclophosphamide, vincristine, doxorubicin and prednisolone) have traditionally been used, but the results are disappointing, with the overall 5-year survival rate for advanced disease being only approximately 10 percent.[63,98] Recently, promising clinical outcome has been reported with chemotherapeutic regimens such as DeVIC (dexamethasone, etoposide, ifosfamide, and carboplatin) and L-asparaginase.[99,100] High-dose chemotherapy with autologous or allogeneic stem cell support is an alternative method of treatment, but the reported survival benefit requires further confirmation.[101–105]

In contrast to nasal NK/T cell lymphoma, patients with extranasal NK/T cell lymphoma often present at high stage (stage III or IV), with involvement of multiple anatomic sites. Systemic involvement occurs early in the clinical course.[67] Chemotherapy is the main stay of treatment, but unfortunately response is poor. The long-term remission rate of this highly aggressive lymphoma is less than 10 percent.[62,66,106] Nonetheless, rare cases of primary cutaneous NK/T cell lymphoma may pursue a protracted or waxing and waning clinical course; currently it is not possible to identify such cases from among those with an aggressive behavior.[7,107]

Prognostic factors

The most important prognostic factors are clinical stage and international prognostic index (IPI). Patients with stage I or II diseases demonstrate a better 2-year overall survival compared with stage III or IV patients. Patients with IPI ≤ 1 have a superior 20-year overall survival in comparison to those with IPI ≥ 2, irrespective of treatment.[62,108]

The commonly used Ann Arbor staging system is not ideal for nasal NK/T cell lymphoma because the extent of local involvement and tumor burden are not taken into consideration, and all cases would be classified as stage IE as long as there is only contiguous spread of the tumor. Hence, an integrative prognostic model incorporating the B symptoms, stage, lactate dehydrogenase level and regional lymph node status has been proposed, which shows better prognostic discrimination as compared with the IPI or Ann Arbor stage.[109] For Ann Arbor stage I/II disease, local invasion, defined as bony invasion or destruction or skin invasion, is a predictor for low probability of complete remission and reduced survival.[110] High levels of circulating EBV DNA at presentation and presence of EBV-positive cells in bone marrow biopsy also predict a poor survival.[111–113]

The prognostic value of histologic grading is controversial,[35,63,114] but a recent large series shows that >40 percent of large cells or a Ki-67 index of >50 percent predicts a worse overall survival for nasal NK/T cell lymphoma.[106] Lack of CD94 expression, expression of cyclooxygenase 2, absence of granzyme B-protease inhibitor 9 or low apoptosis index has been reported to correlate with a poor prognosis.[115–117]

Disease monitoring

NK cells lack a clonal marker, making molecular analysis for residual disease difficult. Circulating EBV DNA has been shown to be useful in disease monitoring, and a high titer is correlated with extensive disease, unfavorable response to treatment and poor survival.[111,112] Aberrant promoter methylation leading to gene silencing can be used as a surrogate tumor marker for NK/T cell neoplasms.[118] Commonly hypermethylated genes include *P73, retinoic acid receptor B,* and *death-associated protein kinase.* With methylation-specific PCR, aberrant methylation has been shown to be more sensitive than morphologic or immunophenotypic examination for detecting minimum residual lymphoma.[119] The level of metastases suppressor protein nm23-H1 is also found to be significantly increased in NK/T cell lymphomas, and high titer is correlated with a poor prognosis.[120]

Morphology

NASAL NATURAL KILLER/T CELL LYMPHOMA

The affected nasal mucosa is frequently ulcerated and necrotic (Plate 68, see plate section), and the adjacent surface epithelium can undergo squamous metaplasia with florid pseudoepitheliomatous hyperplasia (Plate 69, see plate section). The mucosal glands are often pushed apart or destroyed by the lymphoma cells, and some glandular

epithelial cells can exhibit cytoplasmic clearing, probably as a form of cytotoxic injury (Plate 70, see plate section).[7,35,34,121] The tumor cells, often intimately admixed with inflammatory cells and fibrinous exudates, are predominantly medium sized, but there can be variable numbers of small or large neoplastic cells which in some cases form the dominant populations (Plates 71, 72, see plate section).[7,36] They possess irregularly folded, angulated or serpentine-shaped nuclei with dense to granular chromatin, inconspicuous to small nucleoli and a variable amount of pale cytoplasm.[7,122,123] In Giemsa-stained touch preparations, azurophilic cytoplasmic granules are often detectable (Plate 73, see plate section). Mitotic figures are readily found, even in small cell-predominant lesions. Many apoptotic bodies are often scattered among the lymphoma cells. Angioinvasion and geographic necrosis comprising ghost shadows of necrotic cells, karyorrhectic debris and fibrinoid exudate are frequently found (Plate 74, see plate section).

EXTRANASAL NATURAL KILLER/T CELL LYMPHOMA

In the skin, there is a perivascular, periadnexal or diffuse infiltrate of lymphoma cells in the mid and deep dermis, with or without subcutaneous involvement (Plate 75, see plate section). Coagulative necrosis of the dermis and ulceration are common (Plate 76, see plate section). The lymphoma cells often exhibit epidermotropism (Plate 77, see plate section), and this may be mediated by expression of receptor for CXCR3, a chemoattractant cytokine that regulates leukocyte migration to specific tissue sites.[124] Invasion of the skin appendages is more frequently seen in metastatic than primary cutaneous NK/T cell lymphoma.[107,125] In the subcutaneous tissue, the lymphoma cells infiltrate among the adipocytes, producing a panniculitis-like picture with fat necrosis (Plate 78, see plate section),[67,126] simulating subcutaneous panniculitis-like T cell lymphoma.

In the intestine, there is usually transmural infiltration by lymphoma cells. Extensive coagulative necrosis, deep ulcers and perforation are common (Plates 79, 80, see plate section).[67,127] In the testis, there is infiltration of the interstitium by dense sheets of lymphoma cells, often accompanied by angiodestruction and necrosis (Plate 81, see plate section).[69] The seminiferous tubules are lost, atrophic or infiltrated by lymphoma cells. In the soft tissues, there is a permeative growth of tumor cells, prominent destruction of skeletal muscle fibers and invasion of the nerves. The muscle fibers may show flocculent necrosis or there can be drop-out of individual muscle cells leaving behind empty spaces (Plate 82, see plate section).[77]

Immunophenotype

The typical immunophenotype of extranodal NK/T cell lymphoma is: CD2+, sCD3−, cCD3ε+, CD5−, and

CD56+ (Plate 83, see plate section).[55,128–131] CD56 is the most consistently expressed NK marker, while CD16 and CD57 are usually negative (Plate 84A, see plate section). Cytotoxic molecules such as TIA1, granzyme B and perforin are almost always positive (Plate 84B),[7,132–134] and they probably mediate the tissue injury and cell death commonly observed in this lymphoma type.[135,136] CD43 and CD45RO are commonly positive, and CD7 is occasionally expressed. Other T cell-associated antigens such as CD4, CD5, CD8, TCRαβ, TCRγδ are usually negative.[7,24,25,67,129,137,138] Both Fas (CD95) and FasL (CD178) are frequently expressed,[139,140] and the Fas-FasL system has been postulated to play a role in tumor apoptosis and vascular injury. There can be variable expression of CD30, especially in cases rich in large cells. The proliferative fraction as demonstrated by Ki-67 immunostaining is usually high (>70 percent), even for small cell predominant lesions.[7]

Nasal lymphomas that are CD56− but demonstrate a cCD3ε+, cytotoxic molecule+, EBV+ phenotype are currently included within the category of nasal NK/T cell lymphoma.[35,141] Some of them are probably NK cell lymphomas lacking CD56 expression, while others are cytotoxic T cell lymphomas as evidenced by sCD3 expression. Some of the latter express αβ-TCR or γδ-TCR.[140,142,143] The clinical features and morphology of the CD56− group are indistinguishable from the CD56+ group. On the other hand, the nasal lymphomas that show a cCD3ε+, CD56−, cytotoxic molecule−, EBV-phenotype are classified as peripheral T cell lymphoma unspecified.

Most NK/T cell lymphomas express the NK cell receptor CD94/NKG2, but only some express KIRs.[24,25,137] However, NK cell receptors are not specific for NK neoplasms, but are also expressed by some cytotoxic T cell lymphomas and hepatosplenic T cell lymphomas. Nonetheless, demonstration of a skewed NK-cell repertoire by flow cytometry using antibodies against KIRs, CD94 and NKG2A may imply a monoclonal NK cell proliferation.[144]

Genetics features

The TCR and Ig genes are in germline configuration in the majority of cases; the rare cases with a cytotoxic T cell phenotype may show rearrangements of the TCR genes.[7,65,131,133,138,145–147] There is a very strong association with EBV, except for occasional extranasal cases, especially in Caucasians.[7,148] The EBV exists in a clonal episomal form in the tumor cells, and shows a type II latency pattern (EBNA1+, EBNA2–6–, LMP1+).[134,149,150] Despite expression of type II latency, immunostaining for EBV–LMP1 is not a reliable way to demonstrate EBV in NK/T cell lymphomas, because the expression is often very weak and focal. In situ hybridization for EBV-encoded early RNA (EBER) is the most reliable method to demonstrate EBV in this lymphoma type (Plate 85, see plate section). The EBV

is usually of subtype A, with a high frequency of 30-base pair deletion of the LMP1 gene.[134,149,150]

Partial deletion of the FAS gene at the death and transmembrane domains occurs in some cases, which disrupts the FasL/Fas signaling pathway, thereby protecting the lymphoma cells from apoptosis.[151] p53 protein overexpression occurs in 45–86 percent of NK/T cell lymphomas, while P53 gene mutation is found in 24–62 percent of cases, with some variation in frequencies reported from different populations.[152–154] P53 mutation has been found to correlate with large cell morphology and advanced stage at presentation.[155] Mutations of the βcatenin, KRAS and CKIT genes are detected in 22 percent, 14 percent and 6–26 percent respectively, but the significance is currently not clear.[154,156]

Demonstration of KIR repertoire restriction by RT-PCR can support the monoclonal nature of NK/T cell lymphoma. Taken together with germline TCR genes, this finding further confirms the true NK lineage of the lymphoma in most cases.[157] However, KIR repertoire restriction per se is not specific for NK cell lymphomas, and can also be observed in some T cell lymphomas with a cytotoxic phenotype.

Complex chromosomal abnormalities have been found in extranodal NK/T cell lymphomas.[122,158–161] On conventional cytogenetic and comparative genomic hybridization (CGH) studies, the commonest changes are 2q+, 6q−, 8p−, 11q−, 12q−, 13q−, 15q+, 17q+, and 22q+. Specific chromosomal translocations have not been identified, but translocations involving the 8p23 breakpoint are reported in a number of cases.[162–164]

Differential diagnosis

The main differential diagnoses are inflammatory or reactive lesions (such as fungal or mycobacterial infections and Wegener granulomatosis) and other lymphoid malignancies (such as lymphomatoid granulomatosis, diffuse large B cell lymphoma and T cell lymphoma). A correct diagnosis requires a high index of suspicion for any necrotic ulcerated lesions in patients of susceptible ethnic groups, liberal use of immunohistochemical stainings (such as CD56 and cytotoxic markers) and in situ hybridization for EBER.

Cases composed predominantly of small cells or a mixture of cell types can be difficult to distinguish from a reactive lesion (Plate 86, see plate section). Features favoring a diagnosis of NK/T cell lymphoma include prominent destructive growth (such as wide separation of mucosal glands and angioinvasion) and cytologic atypia (many unexplained medium-sized cells or clear cells). Demonstration of sheets of CD56+ or EBER+ cells would provide strong support for a diagnosis of lymphoma because there should be few positive cells in the normal mucosa or reactive lesions. One potential caveat is that herpes simplex infection may evoke striking proliferation of CD56+ T cells, but these cells are CD4+ and EBER−.[165]

In contrast to lymphomatoid granulomatosis in which the neoplastic cells express B lineage markers, NK/T cell lymphoma usually does not exhibit the histologic feature of large atypical cells scattered in a background of small lymphocytes, and furthermore characteristically expresses cCD3ε and CD56. Lymphomas of the upper aerodigestive tract with a cCD3ε+ CD56+ phenotype are almost certainly NK/T cell lymphomas, but lymphomas occurring in extranasal sites (such as skin and intestine) with a similar immunophenotype can represent other lymphoma types, such as cutaneous γδ-T cell lymphoma and enteropathy-associated T cell lymphoma. Demonstration of EBV will help to support a diagnosis of NK/T cell lymphoma because the lymphoma types in the differential diagnoses are often EBV negative.

Atypical proliferation of NK cells producing superficial erosions of the gastrointestinal tract has been reported in a patient with anti-gliadin antibodies but absence of full-blown celiac disease.[166] These lesions are relatively circumscribed and superficial, and the CD56-positive NK cells are negative for EBER. The benign nature of the disease is further confirmed by the non-progressive course and improvement with gluten-free diet.

Etiology and pathogenesis

Epstein–Barr virus appears to play a critical role in the etiology and pathogenesis of extranodal NK/T cell lymphomas. There is almost consistent association of nasal NK/T cell lymphomas with EBV (90–100 percent) irrespective of the ethnic origin of the patients.[61,67,133,134,145,167–173] NK/T cell lymphomas occurring in immunocompromised renal transplant recipients are also all associated with EBV.[174–177] Patients with EBV-associated lymphoproliferative disorders (such as chronic active EBV infection, EBV-associated hemophagocytic syndrome, hypersensitivity to mosquito bites, hydroa vacciniforme-like eruptions), a group of rare diseases endemic in Japan and Korea characterized by monoclonal or oligoclonal proliferation of EBV-infected T or NK cells, are more prone to develop frank NK/T cell lymphoma.[66,178,179] The EBV gene incorporated into the genome of tumor cells exists in a clonal episomal form, implying that EBV is etiologically important and not merely a bystander.[123] Furthermore, the disease activity correlates well with the quantity of EBV DNA in the serum, probably due to shedding of EBV from the proliferating tumor cells.[111,180]

The strong predilection of NK/T cell lymphoma in certain regions of the world suggests that ethnicity is an important predisposing factor. However, it is currently unclear whether ethnicity acts via genetic composition or pattern of EBV infection among these populations.[181]

EBV is also responsible for some of the characteristic morphological features and clinical manifestations of NK/T cell lymphomas. Angiocentric growth, reported in 25–100 percent of cases,[7,182] has been found to be associated with EBV-related upregulation of integrin subunits αM.[183] EBV-induced monokines and chemokines such as Mig and IP-10 have been suggested to play an important role in the fibrinoid necrosis and endothelial cell damage, features which are also frequently seen in other EBV-related lesions such as infectious mononucleosis and lymphomatoid granulomatosis.[184] Upregulation of EBV-related cytokines and chemokines has been postulated to play a role in the induction of hemophagocytic syndrome that sometimes complicates NK/T cell lymphoma.[185]

AGGRESSIVE NATURAL KILLER CELL LEUKEMIA

Definition

Aggressive NK cell leukemia, also known as aggressive NK cell leukemia/lymphoma, is a neoplasm of NK cells with primary involvement of peripheral blood and bone marrow and a fulminant clinical course.[186,187] Since bone marrow involvement is usually not extensive and peripheral lymphadenopathy is not uncommon, the term 'leukemia/lymphoma' may more accurately describe the entity.

Epidemiology and etiology

The disease occurs with a much higher frequency in Asians compared with Caucasians,[188] and thus ethnic factors may play a role in disease susceptibility similar to extranodal NK/T cell lymphoma. It is strongly associated with EBV.[28,67,189–196] Rare cases may evolve from chronic lymphoproliferative disorder of NK cells[197] or extranodal NK/T cell lymphoma.[198]

Clinical manifestations

The patients are typically adolescents or young adults with a median age in the third decade, but older patients can also be affected.[67,87,137,186,190,192,193,195,196,199–201] There is no sex predilection.

The typical presentations are fever, hepatosplenomegaly, lymphadenopathy and a leukemic blood picture.[67,87,137,186,190,192,193,195,196,199–201] The patients are often very ill, with malaise, significant weight loss, jaundice and sometimes disseminated intravascular coagulopathy or hemophagocytic syndrome.[195,202] Skin lesions are uncommon, but some patients may have nonspecific skin rash. Serum lactate dehydrogenase level is often markedly elevated, as is circulating FasL.[203, 204] It has been postulated that systemic shedding of large quantities of FasL from the lymphoma cells may contribute to the multiorgan failure commonly seen in patients with aggressive NK cell leukemia – binding of FasL to Fas, which is normally expressed in many different cell types (such as liver and kidney), results in apoptosis of the Fas-bearing cells and hence organ damage.

Treatment and clinical course

The disease is almost invariably fatal, with a median survival of less than 2 months.[195,196] It is frequently complicated by coagulopathy, bleeding and multiorgan failure. Response to chemotherapy is usually poor. Previously this has been attributed to frequent presence of P-glycoprotein, a multidrug resistance gene 1-encoded protein on the NK cell membrane that extrudes cytotoxic drugs such as vincristine and anthracyclin.[205] A recent report, however, indicates that the P-glycoprotein expressed by NK cells is 'dysfunctional' and unable to extrude anthracyclin.[206] These observations warrant reevaluation of the use of anthracycline-containing regimens.[195,196] Another promising chemotherapeutic agent is L-asparaginase.[101] There have been reports on success of bone marrow transplantation, but the disease usually relapses.[67,87,186,188,193,207,208] Presence of B symptoms, high IPI and poor therapeutic response are unfavorable prognostic factors.[207,208]

Morphology

Circulating leukemic cells range from scanty to abundant, accounting for less than 5 percent to over 80 percent of lymphocytes. They often exhibit a range of appearances in an individual case, from normal-looking LGLs to immature and atypical-looking LGLs. They have round nuclei with condensed chromatin, or larger nuclei with mild irregular foldings (Plate 87, see plate section). In some cases, there are conspicuous nucleoli, which when present strongly supports a diagnosis of aggressive NK cell leukemia over chronic lymphoproliferative disorder of NK cells (Plate 88, see plate section).[39] The cytoplasm is moderate to abundant in amount, and is lightly basophilic, with variable numbers of fine and occasionally coarse azurophilic granules. In the bone marrow, the involvement ranges from diffuse interstitial to subtle and patchy, with LGLs constituting 6–92 percent of all nucleated cells (Plates 89, 90, see plate section).[207]

In histologic sections of involved tissues, there is a diffuse, destructive and permeative infiltrate consisting of monomorphous cells with round or irregular nuclei, fairly condensed chromatin, and a thin to moderate rim of pale or amphophilic cytoplasm (Plate 91, see plate section). Interspersed apoptotic bodies and zonal cell death are common. Angioinvasive-angiodestructive growth is also frequently noted.[67,193]

Immunophenotype and molecular findings

The immunophenotype is similar to that of extranodal NK/T cell lymphoma, i.e. CD2+, sCD3−, cCD3ε+, CD56+, CD57−, cytotoxic markers+.[67,87,137,186,188,190,192,193,199–201,207,208] CD16 expression is seen in approximately 50–75 percent of cases.[205] Since CD16 is usually not expressed in other hematolymphoid malignancies including extranodal NK/T cell lymphoma, it has been suggested to be a marker for aggressive NK leukemia.[207] Based on frequent expression of CD16 and lack of CD25, aggressive NK leukemia has been hypothesized to be derived from the CD16+ CD56^dim subclass of NK cells.[207] The TCR genes are typically germline. Epstein–Barr virus is demonstrated in >90 percent of cases.[28,67,189–192,207,208]

Although previous comparative genomic hybridization (CGH) studies suggest similar genetic changes in aggressive NK leukemia and extranodal NK/T cell lymphoma, such as 3p+, 6q−, 11q−, 12q+,[123,158] a recent array-based CGH study reveals significant differences between the two diseases.[161] For instance, 7p− 17p− and 1q+ are frequent in aggressive NK leukemia, but not in extranodal NK/T cell lymphoma. The 6q− commonly found in the latter is not observed in cases of aggressive NK cell leukemia included in that series.

Differential diagnosis

Aggressive NK cell leukemia must be distinguished from the much more common **T cell LGL (T-LGL) leukemia**, which is EBV negative and frequently pursues an indolent clinical course.[49,201] Patients with T-LGL leukemia are generally older (mean 55–65 years), and commonly present with infection, hepatosplenomegaly, pure red cell aplasia or neutropenia, and may be associated with rheumatoid arthritis. While both T-LGL leukemia and aggressive NK cell leukemia are characterized by circulating lymphoid cells with azurophilic granules, the lymphoid cells in the former do not exhibit atypia or immature appearance as commonly observed in the latter. The T-LGL leukemia cells show a sCD3+, CD4−, CD8+ phenotype and rearranged TCR genes; CD56 is usually negative.

Chronic lymphoproliferative disorder of NK cells (see next section) differs from aggressive NK cell leukemia in the good clinical condition, lack of hepatosplenomegaly, indolent course, absence of atypia in the LGL, frequent expression of CD57, and lack of association with EBV (Table 36.2).[28,201]

In lymph nodes, aggressive NK cell leukemia may mimic **Kikuchi lymphadenitis** because the neoplastic cells can resemble plasmacytoid dendritic cells and there are many apoptotic bodies.[66,209] Features against a diagnosis of Kikuchi lymphadenitis include diffuse instead of discrete patchy nodal involvement, monotonous cellular infiltrate, extensive perinodal infiltrate and presence of many CD56+ cells.

Since the number of neoplastic cells in the peripheral blood and bone marrow may be low, the distinction of aggressive NK cell leukemia from **high-stage extranodal NK/T cell lymphoma** can be difficult in some cases, but this is more a matter of semantics.

Table 36.2 Comparison between aggressive natural killer (NK) cell leukemia and chronic lymphoproliferative disorder of NK cells

	Aggressive NK cell leukemia	Chronic lymphoproliferative disorder of NK cells
Age	Younger, with mean age of 39 years	Older, with mean age of 60.5 years
M:F ratio	1:1	7:1
Clinical presentation	Fever, systemic symptoms, hepatosplenomegaly, cytopenia	Usually asymptomatic, but some patients may have cytopenia, vasculitis or neuropathy; fever is uncommon
Hepatosplenomegaly	Common	Uncommon
Morphology of circulating large granular lymphocytes	Can be mature looking or immature looking	Always mature looking
Immunophenotype	sCD3– CD56+ CD16–/+	sCD3– CD56+ CD16+
Association with Epstein–Barr virus	~100%	No
Clinical behavior	Fulminant clinical course, usually unresponsive to therapy	Indolent and non-progressive course; very rare case may transform to an aggressive phase
Treatment	Acute lymphoblastic leukemia-type induction chemotherapy	Watch and wait, or immunosuppressive therapy

CHRONIC LYMPHOPROLIFERATIVE DISORDER OF NK CELLS

Definition

Chronic lymphoproliferative disorder of NK cells, also known as chronic NK lymphocytosis, chronic NK cell LGL leukemia or NK cell LGL lymphocytosis, is characterized by persistent expansion of mature-looking NK LGLs in the peripheral blood, and a nonprogressive clinical course.[28,49–52,210,211] The diagnostic criteria include the following:

- persistent increase in LGLs for more than 6 months
- LGL count over 2×10^9/L
- LGL showing an NK-cell immunophenotype of sCD3–, CD56–/+, CD16+
- absence of an obvious cause for the NK lymphocytosis.

Clinical manifestation and clinical course

The patients are usually over 40 years of age (mean 60.5 years). Most are asymptomatic and incidentally found to have persistent increase in circulating NK cells. There is no fever, lymphadenopathy, hepatosplenomegaly or neutropenia. Others are symptomatic, presenting with cytopenias (such as pure red cell aplasia or cyclical neutropenia), cutaneous vasculitis, peripheral neuropathy, nephrotic syndrome or splenomegaly.[49,212,213]

The clinical course is chronic and nonprogressive, and the disease may even remit spontaneously.[201,210,214] Treatment options include watchful waiting for asymptomatic patients,

and immunosuppressive therapy for clinically symptomatic patients.[215]

Rarely, abrupt transformation to an aggressive phase resembling aggressive NK cell leukemia can occur, but there is no association with EBV.[197,201,216] There is also a reported case of transformation to extranodal NK cell lymphoma, although the supervening neoplasm is also negative for EBV.[217]

Pathologic, immunophenotypic and molecular features

The circulating LGLs are mature looking, being indistinguishable from their normal counterparts (Plate 92, see plate section). They usually exhibit an NK cell immunophenotype of CD2+, sCD3–, CD56+, CD16+. CD57 is also commonly positive.[28] However, in some cases, CD56 expression is negative or dim.[218] While CD94 is commonly positive, KIR expression is usually restricted to one type.[219,220]

The TCR genes are in germline configuration, and there is no association with EBV.[28,49,210,221–223] Similar to patients with T cell LGL leukemia, antibodies to human T cell lymphotropic virus-I (HTLV-1) envelope protein are frequently detected (73 percent of patients), but there is no evidence of HTLV nuclei acid by polymerase chain reaction (PCR) analysis. The significance of this finding is currently unclear.[224]

Is this a neoplastic or reactive natural killer cell proliferation?

Since it is difficult to determine clonality of NK cells, it is unclear whether chronic lymphoproliferative disorder of

NK cells is a neoplastic (clonal) or reactive (polyclonal) condition. In one study on CD3− LGL proliferation, clonal molecular analysis using X-linked gene markers failed to provide evidence of clonality, suggesting that this is a reactive condition.[225] However, at least a proportion of cases exhibit clonal molecular markers based on X chromosome inactivation pattern or chromosomal aberrations, suggesting a neoplastic process.[211,218,222,223,226,227]

Differential diagnosis

It is most important to distinguish chronic lymphoproliferative disorder of NK cells from aggressive NK cell leukemia (Table 36.2). On the other hand, transient increase in circulating NK cells should not be diagnosed as chronic lymphoproliferative disorder of NK cells. The former can occur in patients with viral infection, autoimmune diseases, idiopathic thrombocytopenic purpura, malignancies or solid organ transplantation, and the LGL count is usually below 3–4×10^9/L.[228–231] The demonstration of a restricted pattern of KIR receptor expression is a helpful feature supporting a diagnosis of chronic lymphoproliferative disorder of NK cells.[219,220]

SO-CALLED BLASTIC NATURAL KILLER CELL LYMPHOMA

Definition

Blastic NK cell lymphoma is a neoplasm consisting of lymphoblast-like cells with a CD56+, cCD3−/+, sCD3−, CD4−/+ immunophenotype and germline TCR genes. This tumor was tentatively considered an NK cell neoplasm in the 2001 WHO classification because of CD56 expression, absence of sCD3 and germline T cell receptor.[232–234]

Heterogeneity of 'blastic natural killer cell lymphoma' and misnomer

The vast majority of so-called blastic NK cell lymphomas express CD4.[235–239] Recent studies suggest that this subgroup is a tumor of precursor plasmacytoid dendritic cells rather than NK cells, and has therefore been named **CD4+ CD56+ hematodermic neoplasm or blastic plasmacytoid dendritic cell neoplasm**.[240,241] Plasmacytoid dendritic cell (formerly known as plasmacytoid monocyte) is a newly identified subset of dendritic cells, characterized by plasma cell-like morphology and unique surface phenotype (CD4+, CD123+, BDCA+, HLA-DR+) in the absence of common lineage markers (CD3, CD11c, CD13, CD14, CD16, CD19, CD20 and CD34).[242,243] A small subset of plasmacytoid dendritic cells in the blood and activated plasmacytoid dendritic cells have been shown to express CD56.[240,244] The finding of CD123 (interleukin 3 receptor α) expression in practically all cases of CD4+ blastic NK cell lymphoma provides the first evidence that it may originate from plasmacytoid dendritic cells.[240,245] BDCA2, a cell surface protein selectively expressed on plasmacytoid dendritic cells,[246] has also been demonstrated in a high proportion of cases.[247,248] Functional studies of cultured tumor cells show production of IFN-α in response to viral challenge, which is a key functional property of plasmacytoid dendritic cells.[249]

On the other hand, the nature of the smaller numbers of CD4− blastic NK cell lymphoma remains uncertain. They probably include precursor NK cell lymphoblastic lymphoma/leukemia,[43,44,250,251] myeloid/NK cell precursor acute leukemia,[67,236,250,252,253] and possibly some 'genuine' NK-cell lymphomas.[254]

Epidemiology and etiology

So-called blastic NK cell lymphoma, be it CD4+ or CD4−, is a rare neoplasm with no obvious racial predilection.[253,255] The etiology is unknown, and there is no association with EBV.

Blastic plasmacytoid dendritic cell neoplasm (CD4+CD56+ hematodermic neoplasm)

CLINICAL MANIFESTATIONS

The peak age is in the sixth decade, but children can also be affected.[251,255,256] There is a male predilection of 2.4 to 1.[234,235,251,253,255,257,258] There is a propensity to involve the skin, followed by lymph node and bone marrow.[241,251,259] Most patients present with solitary or multiple cutaneous nodules or plaques with or without lymphadenopathy. The skin lesions are usually over 1 cm in size, often with a purple color (Plate 93, see plate section).[258] The bone marrow is involved at presentation in about half of the patients. Leukemia may be the initial presentation in a proportion of cases or appears during the course of the disease.[251] Patients with leukemic presentation often have hepatosplenomegaly.

TREATMENT AND CLINICAL COURSE

The tumor pursues an aggressive relentless course, with early systemic dissemination.[234,241,251,253,255,257,258,260] Radiation therapy and/or chemotherapy generally produces a good initial response in 70–75 percent of cases. Unfortunately, relapses occur in 90 percent of these cases, resulting in an average survival of only 14 months. In some patients, the disease may evolve to acute myeloid or myelomonocytic leukemia, attesting to the plasticity of the neoplastic cells.[234,235,258,261] L-Asparaginase has been used successfully in pediatric cases.[262] Rare long-term survivals have been reported following bone marrow transplantation.[251,258,263]

Favorable prognostic factors include young age, low leukocyte count, skin-confined disease, TdT expression and lack of BDCA2 expression.[247,251,260]

MORPHOLOGY

Blastic plasmacytoid dendritic cell neoplasm is characterized by a diffuse, dense, monotonous cellular infiltrate, usually showing remarkably uniform cell density throughout the involved tissues (Plate 94, see plate section). The medium-sized neoplastic cells possess round, oval, mildly convoluted or folded nuclei, fine chromatin, inconspicuous nucleoli, and a thin rim of pale cytoplasm (Plate 95, see plate section). Mitotic figures are readily found. Rarely, Homer–Wright-type rosettes are present.[252] There is insinuation of the collagen bundles by tumor cells, sometimes producing a single-file pattern (Plate 94B). Angioinvasive growth and coagulative necrosis are usually not seen.

In the skin, typically the entire dermis, and sometimes the subcutaneous tissue, is replaced by a diffuse permeative tumor infiltrate (Plate 94). The epidermis is spared. Rarely, there is periadnexal accentuation. In the lymph node, the normal architecture is totally effaced by diffuse sheets of tumor cells, or there is only partial involvement of the paracortex (Plate 96, see plate section).

Peripheral blood smears show blast cells with round or mildly irregular, eccentrically placed nuclei, and one to several nucleoli. There is a moderate amount of lightly basophilic cytoplasm, and azurophilic cytoplasmic granules are generally absent. Palisaded small vacuoles are sometimes seen at the periphery of the cell body. Pseudopodia-shaped cytoplasmic extensions are sometimes found.[258] The affected bone marrow is hypercellular, with large numbers of monotonous tumor cells. When myeloid tissue remains, dysplastic features can be seen, particularly in the megakaryocyte lineage.[241]

IMMUNOPHENOTYPE

Blastic plasmacytoid dendritic cell neoplasms are typically CD4+, CD56+, sCD3−, CD123+, and BDCA2+ (Plate 97, see plate section).[241,247,248] TCL1 (T cell leukemia 1) and CLA (cutaneous lymphocyte-associated antigen) are frequently positive, and the expression of the TCL1 can be useful in distinction from myelomonocytic leukemia cutis.[264,265] CD2 and CD7 expression are variable, and other T and B cell markers are generally negative except CD43 and CD45RO. Rare cases can express cCD3ε.[260] Cytotoxic markers are usually negative. The expression of TdT varies among different series and the average positivity rate is around 59 percent (Plate 98, see plate section);[235,251] its expression exhibits an inverse correlation with BDCA2, which is a marker for the more mature plasmacytoid dendritic cells.[247] Positivity for CD68 (up to 52 percent) has been reported in some series, with a characteristic dot-like pattern in the Golgi zone,[251,255,258,266] but other cytochemical (myeloperoxidase, Sudan Black B, esterases) and immunocytochemical markers of myeloid and monocytic cells (myeloperoxidase, CD11c, CD13, CD14, CD33, lysozyme) should be negative.

MOLECULAR FINDINGS

TCR genes are in germline configuration. With rare exceptions, EBV genome is absent.[267] Cytogenetic abnormalities are complex and varied, but recurrent events include 6q abnormalities and aberrations in chromosomes 1, 5q, 7, 9, 12p, 13 and 15.[234,251,253,257,258,268,269] Rare cases with del(5q), a relatively common cytogenetic finding in myelodysplastic syndromes, have been reported.[266]

DIFFERENTIAL DIAGNOSIS

Blastic plasmacytoid dendritic cell neoplasm morphologically resembles **T cell or B-cell precursor lymphoblastic lymphoma/leukemia**, but usually exhibits a slightly greater amount of cytoplasm such that the nuclei do not appear as crowded. The latter expresses multiple T lineage markers (such as CD7, CD2, CD3) or B lineage markers (such as CD79a, PAX5, CD19) in addition to TdT. Expression of CD56 in T cell or B-cell precursor lymphoblastic lymphoma/leukemia is extremely rare, and the TCR or Ig genes are rearranged.

Myeloid leukemia or myeloid sarcoma usually shows more distinct nucleoli, and the cytoplasm is usually eosinophilic, sometimes with identifiable granules. Some cases can express CD56, but most cases are immunoreactive for myeloperoxidase, CD117 and other myeloid markers (such as CD13, CD15 and CD33).

Blastoid mantle cell lymphoma uncommonly shows cutaneous involvement. It is a B cell lymphoma (CD20+ CD3−) with characteristic expression of cyclin D1. CD56 is negative.

Myeloid/NK cell acute leukemia or myeloid/NK cell precursor acute leukemia is an uncommon form of acute leukemia expressing markers of both myeloid cells (such as CD13, CD15, CD33, and variably CD34 and myeloperoxidase) and NK cells (CD56 and variably CD7).[40,270] It differs from CD4+ CD56+ hematodermic neoplasm in the predominantly leukemic manifestations, infrequent presentation as cutaneous lesions, and lack of expression of CD4.

Sometimes the neoplastic cells of blastic plasmacytoid dendritic cell neoplasm do not appear obviously blastic in small biopsies due to compression artifact, rendering distinction from **extranodal NK/T cell lymphoma** difficult. In contrast to the latter, CD4, CD123 and TdT are often positive, while cytotoxic markers and EBV are negative.

CD4–negative subset of blastic natural killer cell lymphoma

It is likely that most cases represent precursor NK-cell lymphoblastic neoplasms, which may show a predominantly leukemic or lymphomatous presentation. It is a rare disease with a median age of onset at 55 years. Lymphadenopathy, hepatosplenomegaly and mediastinal involvement are common, while skin involvement is rare.[44,251] In the leukemic cases, there is frequently severe thrombocytopenia.[251] The prognosis is poor.

The neoplastic cells usually show a CD2−/+, sCD3−, cCD3−/+, CD4−, CD7+, CD56+, CD123−, TdT+ immunophenotype.[44] CD16 and CD34 are frequently expressed.[251,254]

KEY POINTS

- NK cells are lymphocytes with the morphology of large granular lymphocytes, the immunophenotype of surface CD3−, cytoplasmic CD3ε+, CD56+ and the germline configuration of T cell receptor genes.
- NK cell neoplasms can be grouped as precursor and mature NK cell neoplasms.
- Precursor NK cell neoplasms include entities such as myeloid/NK cell precursor acute leukemia and NK cell lymphoblastic leukemia/lymphoma; these rare entities are difficult to define and have not been well characterized.
- Mature NK cell neoplasms include extranodal NK/T cell lymphoma and aggressive NK cell leukemia. They are highly aggressive tumors that occur almost exclusively in extranodal sites (the prototypic site being the nasal cavity). Pathologically, they are characterized by a neoplastic lymphoid cell infiltrate with frequent apoptosis, necrosis and angioinvasion. Like the normal NK cells, they show an immunophenotype of CD2+, surface CD3−, cytoplasmic CD3ε+, CD56+, and germline T cell receptor genes. There is a near constant association with EBV.
- Aggressive NK cell leukemia must be distinguished from chronic lymphoproliferative disorder of NK cells, which is characterized by persistent expansion of mature-looking NK large granular lymphocytes in the peripheral blood, and a nonprogressive clinical course. In contrast to the former, there is no fever, lymphadenopathy, hepatosplenomegaly or association with EBV.
- The entity previously known as blastic NK cell lymphoma mostly represents a tumor of precursor plasmacytoid dendritic cells.

REFERENCES

● = Key primary paper
◆ = Major review article

◆1. Robertson MJ, Ritz J. Biology and clinical relevance of human NK cells. *Blood* 1990; **76**: 2421–38.
2. Farag S, VanDeusen J, Fehniger T, Caligiuri M. Biology and clinical impact of human natural killer cells. *Int J Hematol* 2003; **78**: 7–17.
◆3. Trinchieri G. Biology of natural killer cells. *Adv Immunol* 1989; **47**: 187–376.
4. Yokoyama WM, Kim SC, French AR. The dynamic life of natural killer cells. *Annu Rev Immunol* 2004; **22**: 405–29.
◆5. Lanier LL. NK cell recognition. *Annu Rev Immunol* 2005; **23**: 225–74.
6. Andrews DM, Scalzo AA, Yokoyama WM *et al.* Functional interactions between dendritic cells and NK cells during viral infection. *Nat Immunol* 2003; **4**: 175–81.
◆7. Chan JK. Natural killer cell neoplasms. *Anat Pathol* 1998; **3**: 77–145.
8. Liu CC, Young LH, Young JD. Lymphocyte-mediated cytolysis and disease. *N Engl J Med* 1996; **335**: 1651–9.
9. Russell JH, Ley TJ. Lymphocyte-mediated cytotoxicity. *Annu Rev Immunol* 2002; **20**: 323–70.
10. Ljunggren HG, Karre K. In search of the 'missing self': MHC molecules and NK cell recognition. *Immuol Today* 1990; **11**: 237–44.
11. Zitvogel L. Dendritic and natural killer cells cooperate in the control/switch of innate immunity. *J Exp Med* 2002; **195**: f9–14.
12. Dorshkind K, Pollack SB, Bosma MJ, Phillips RA. Natural killer (NK) cells are present in mice with severe combined immunodeficiency (scid). *J Immunol* 1985; **134**: 3798–801.
13. Kiessling R, Klein E, Pross H, Wigzell H. Natural killer cells in the mouse, II. Cytotoxic cells with specificity for mouse Moloney leukemia cells. Characteristics of the killer cell. *Eur J Immunol* 1975; **5**: 117–21.
14. Herberman RB, Nunn ME, Lavrin DH. Natural cytotoxic reactivity of mouse lymphoid cells against syngeneic and allogeneic tumors, I. Distribution of reactivity and specificity. *Int J Cancer* 1975; **16**: 216.
15. Kondo M, Weissman IL, Akashi K. Identification of clonogenic common lymphoid progenitors in mouse bone marrow. *Cell* 1997; **91**: 661–72.
16. Douagi I, Colucci F, Di Santo J, Cumano A. Identification of the earliest prethymic bipotent T/NK progenitor in murine fetal liver. *Blood* 2002; **99**: 463–71.
17. Liu CC, Perussia B, Young JD. The emerging role of IL-15 in NK-cell development. *Immuol Today* 2000; **21**: 113–16.
18. Kim S, Iizuka K, Kang HS *et al.* In vivo developmental stages in murine natural killer cell maturation. *Nat Immunol* 2002; **3**: 523–8.
19. Tsang WY, Chan JK, Ng CS, Pau MY. Utility of a paraffin section-reactive CD56 antibody (123C3) for

characterization and diagnosis of lymphomas. *Am J Surg Pathol* 1996; **20**: 202–10.

20. Prlic M, Blazar BR, Farrar MA, Jameson SC. In vivo survival and homeostatic proliferation of natural killer cells. *J Exp Med* 2003; **197**: 967–76.

21. Dokun AO, Kims S, Smith HR *et al.* Specific and nonspecific NK cell activation during virus infection. *Nat Immunol* 2001; **2**: 951–6.

22. Spits H, Blom B, Jaleco AC *et al.* Early stages in the development of human T, natural killer and thymic dendritic cells. *Immunol Rev* 1998; **165**: 75–86.

◆23. Moretta L, Bottino C, Pende D *et al.* Human natural killer cells: their origin, receptors and function. *Eur J Immunol* 2002; **32**: 1205–11.

24. Haedicke W, Ho FC, Chott A *et al.* Expression of CD94/NKG2A and killer immunoglobulin-like receptors in NK cells and a subset of extranodal cytotoxic T-cell lymphomas. *Blood* 2000; **95**: 3628–30.

25. Dukers DF, Vermeer MH, Jaspars LH *et al.* Expression of killer cell inhibitory receptors is restricted to true NK cell lymphomas and a subset of intestinal enteropathy-type T cell lymphomas with a cytotoxic phenotype. *J Clin Pathol* 2001; **54**: 224–8.

26. Barclay AN, Brown MH, Law SKA *et al. The leukocyte antigen factsbook*, 2nd ed. San Diego: Academic Press, 1997.

27. Chan JK, Tsang WY, Pau MY. Discordant CD3 expression in lymphomas when studied on frozen and paraffin sections. *Hum Pathol* 1995; **26**: 1139–43.

◆28. Oshimi K. Lymphoproliferative disorders of natural killer cells. *Int J Hematol* 1996; **63**: 279–90.

29. Mason DY, Cordell J, Brown M *et al.* Detection of T cells in paraffin wax embedded tissue using antibodies against a peptide sequence from the CD3 antigen. *J Clin Pathol* 1989; **42**: 1194–200.

30. Steward M, Bishop R, Piggott NH *et al.* Production and characterization of a new monoclonal antibody effective in recognizing the CD3 T-cell associated antigen in formalin-fixed embedded tissue. *Histopathology* 1997; **30**: 16–22.

31. Lanier LL, Chang C, Spits H, Phillips JH. Expression of cytoplasmic CD3 epsilon proteins in activated human adult natural killer (NK) cells and CD3 gamma, delta, epsilon complexes in fetal NK cells. Implications for the relationship of NK and T lymphocytes. *J Immunol* 1992; **149**: 1876–80.

◆32. Spits H, Lanier LL, Phillips JH. Development of human T and natural killer cells. *Blood* 1995; **85**: 2654–70.

33. Lanier LL, Phillips JH, Hackett J Jr *et al.* Natural killer cells: definition of a cell type rather than a function. *J Immunol* 1986; **137**: 2735–9.

34. Moretta A, Bottino C, Mingari MC *et al.* What is a natural killer cell? *Nat Immunol* 2002; **3**: 6–8.

35. Chan JKC, Jaffe ES, Ralfkiaer E. Extranodal NK/T-cell lymphoma, nasal type. In: Jaffe ES, Harris NL, Stein H, Vardiman JW. (eds) *Pathology and genetics, tumours of haematopoietic and lymphoid tissues. World Health*

Organization classification of tumours. Lyon: IARC Press, 2001: 204–7.

36. Godfrey DI, MacDonald HR, Kronenberg M *et al.* NKT cells: What's in a name? *Nat Rev Immunol* 2004; **4**: 231–7.

37. Chan JKC, Jaffe ES, Ralfkiaer E. Blastic NK-cell lymphoma. In: Jaffe ES, Harris NL, Stein H, Vardiman JW. (eds) *Pathology and genetics, tumours of haematopoietic and lymphoid tissues. World Health Organization classification of tumours.* Lyon: IARC Press, 2001: 214–15.

38. Jaffe ES, Harris NL, Stein H *et al.* Introduction and overview of the classification of the lymphoid neoplasms. In: Swerdlow SH, Campo E, Harris NL *et al.* (eds) *WHO classification of tumours of haematopoietic and lymphoid tissues.* Lyon: IARC, 2008: 157–66.

◆39. Oshimi K. Leukemia and lymphoma of natural killer lineage cells. *Int J Hematol* 2003; **78**: 18–23.

●40. Suzuki R, Yamamoto K, Seto M *et al.* CD7+ and CD56+ myeloid/natural killer cell precursor acute leukemia: a distinct hematolymphoid disease entity. *Blood* 1997; **90**: 2417–28.

41. Suzuki R, Nakamura S. Malignancies of natural killer (NK) cell precursor: myeloid/NK cell precursor acute leukemia and blastic NK cell lymphoma/leukemia. *Leuk Res* 1999; **23**: 615–24.

42. Suzuki R, Murata M, Kami M *et al.* Prognostic significance of CD7+CD56+ phenotype and chromosome 5 abnormalities for acute myeloid leukemia M0. *Int J Hematol* 2003; **77**: 482–9.

43. Nakamura F, Tatsumi E, Kawano S *et al.* Acute lymphoblastic leukemia/lymphoblastic lymphoma of natural killer (NK) lineage: quest for another NK-lineage neoplasm [letter; comment]. *Blood* 1997; **89**: 4665–6.

44. Karube K, Ohshima K, Tsuchiya T *et al.* Non-B, non-T neoplasms with lymphoblast morphology. Further characterization and classification. *Am J Surg Pathol* 2003; **27**: 1366–74.

45. Oshimi K, Kawa K, Nakamura S *et al.* NK-cell neoplasms in Japan. *Hematology* 2005; **10**: 237–45.

46. Ohshima K, Suzumiya J, Sugihara M *et al.* Clinical, immunohistochemical and phenotypic features of aggressive nodal cytotoxic lymphomas, including alpha/beta, gamma/delta T-cell and natural killer cell types. *Virchows Arch* 1999; **435**: 92–100.

47. Kagami Y, Suzuki R, Taji H *et al.* Nodal cytotoxic lymphoma spectrum: a clinicopathologic study of 66 patients. *Am J Surg Pathol* 1999; **23**: 1184–200.

48. Au WY, Ma SK, Chim CS *et al.* Clinicopathologic features and treatment outcome of mature T-cell and natural killer-cell lymphomas diagnosed according to the World Health Organization classification scheme: a single center experience of 10 years. *Ann Oncol* 2005; **16**: 206–14.

49. Loughran TP Jr. Clonal diseases of large granular lymphocytes. *Blood* 1993; **82**: 1–14.

50. Rabbani GR, Phyliky RL, Tefferi A. A long-term study of patients with chronic natural killer cell lymphocytosis. *Br J Haematol* 1999; **106**: 960–6.

●51. Tefferi A, Li CY, Witzig TE *et al*. Chronic natural killer cell lymphocytosis: a descriptive clinical study. *Blood* 1994; **84**: 2721–5.

52. Tefferi A. Chronic natural killer cell lymphocytosis. *Leuk Lymphoma* 1996; **20**: 245–8.

53. Chan JK, Banks PM, Cleary ML *et al*. A proposal for classification of lymphoid neoplasms (by the International Lymphoma Study Group). *Histopathology* 1994; **25**: 517–36.

54. Eichel BS, Harrison EG Jr, Devine KD *et al*. Primary lymphoma of the nose including a relationship to lethal midline granuloma. *Am J Surg* 1966; **112**: 597–605.

●55. Ng CS, Chan JK, Lo ST. Expression of natural killer cell markers in non-Hodgkin's lymphomas. *Hum Pathol* 1987; **18**: 1257–62.

56. Jaffe ES. Pathologic and clinical spectrum of post-thymic T-cell malignancies. *Cancer Invest* 1984; **2**: 413–26.

57. Guinee D, Jaffe E, Kingma D. Pulmonary lymphomatoid granulomatosis: evidence of Epstein-Barr virus infected B-lymphocytes with a predominant T-cell component and vasculitis. *Am J Surg Pathol* 1994; **18**: 753–64.

58. Takahashi N, Miura I, Chubachi A *et al*. A clinicopathological study of 20 patients with T/natural killer (NK)-cell lymphoma-associated hemophagocytic syndrome with special reference to nasal and nasal-type NK/T-cell lymphoma. *Int J Hematol* 2001; **74**: 303–8.

●59. Myers JL, Kurtin PJ, Katzenstein AL *et al*. Lymphomatoid granulomatosis. Evidence of immunophenotypic diversity and relationship to Epstein-Barr virus infection. *Am J Surg Pathol* 1995; **19**: 1300–12.

60. Wilson WH, Kingma DW, Raffeld M *et al*. Association of lymphomatoid granulomatosis with Epstein-Barr viral infection of B lymphocytes and response to interferon-alpha 2b. *Blood* 1996; **87**: 4531–7.

61. Arber DA, Weiss LM, Albujar PF *et al*. Nasal lymphomas in Peru. High incidence of T-cell immunophenotype and Epstein-Barr virus infection [see comments]. *Am J Surg Pathol* 1993; **17**: 392–9.

62. Lymphoma Study Group of Japanese pathologists. The World Health Organization Classification of malignant lymphomas in Japan: incidence of recently recognized entities. *Pathol Int* 2000; **50**: 696–702.

●63. Cheung MM, Chan JK, Lau WH *et al*. Primary non-Hodgkin's lymphoma of the nose and nasopharynx: clinical features, tumor immunophenotype, and treatment outcome in 113 patients. *J Clin Oncol* 1998; **16**: 70–7.

64. Ko YH, Ree HJ, Kim WS *et al*. Clinicopathologic and genotypic study of extranodal nasal-type natural killer/T-cell lymphoma and natural killer precursor lymphoma among Koreans. *Cancer* 2000; **89**: 2106–16.

65. Nakamura S, Katoh E, Koshikawa T *et al*. Clinicopathologic study of nasal T/NK-cell lymphoma among the Japanese. *Pathol Int* 1997; **47**: 38–53.

66. Nitta Y, Iwatsuki K, Kimura H *et al*. Fatal natural killer cell lymphoma arising in a patient with a crop of Epstein-Barr

virus-associated disorders. *Eur J Dermatol* 2005; **15**: 503–6.

●67. Chan JK, Sin VC, Wong KF *et al*. Nonnasal lymphoma expressing the natural killer cell marker CD56: a clinicopathologic study of 49 cases of an uncommon aggressive neoplasm. *Blood* 1997; **89**: 4501–13.

68. Liang R. Nasal T/NK-cell lymphoma. In: Canellos GP, Lister TA, Young BD. (eds) *The lymphomas*, 2nd ed. Philadelphia: Saunders Elsevier, 2006: 451–5.

69. Chan JK, Tsang WY, Lau WH *et al*. Aggressive T/natural killer cell lymphoma presenting as testicular tumor. *Cancer* 1996; **77**: 1198–205.

70. Chan JK, Tsang WY, Hui PK *et al*. T- and T/natural killer-cell lymphomas of the salivary gland: a clinicopathologic, immunohistochemical and molecular study of six cases. *Hum Pathol* 1997; **28**: 238–45.

●71. Wong KF, Chan JK, Ng CS *et al*. CD56 (NKH1)-positive hematolymphoid malignancies: an aggressive neoplasm featuring frequent cutaneous/mucosal involvement, cytoplasmic azurophilic granules, and angiocentricity. *Hum Pathol* 1992; **23**: 798–804.

72. Wong KF, Chan JK, Ng CS. CD56 (NCAM)-positive malignant lymphoma. *Leuk Lymphoma* 1994; **14**: 29–36.

73. Takeshita M, Kimura N, Suzumiya J *et al*. Angiocentric lymphoma with granulomatous panniculitis in the skin expressing natural killer cell and large granular T-cell phenotypes. *Virchows Arch* 1994; **425**: 499–504.

74. Misago N, Ohshima K, Aiura S *et al*. Primary cutaneous T-cell lymphoma with an angiocentric growth pattern: association with Epstein-Barr virus. *Br J Dermatol* 1996; **135**: 638–43.

75. Katoh A, Ohshima K, Kanda M *et al*. Gastrointestinal T cell lymphoma: predominant cytotoxic phenotypes, including alpha/beta, gamma/delta T cell and natural killer cells. *Leuk Lymphoma* 2000; **39**: 97–111.

76. Abe Y, Muta K, Ohshima K *et al*. Subcutaneous panniculitis by Epstein-Barr virus-infected natural killer (NK) cell proliferation terminating in aggressive subcutaneous NK cell lymphoma. *Am J Hematol* 2000; **64**: 221–5.

77. Goodlad JR, Fletcher CDM, Chan JKC, Suster S. Primary soft tissue lymphoma: an analysis of 37 cases, (abstr). *J Pathol* 1996; **179**(Suppl): a42.

78. Miyamoto T, Yoshino T, Takehisa T *et al*. Cutaneous presentation of nasal/nasal type T/NK cell lymphoma: clinicopathological findings of four cases. *Br J Dermatol* 1998; **139**: 481–7.

79. Nakamura S, Suchi T, Koshikawa T *et al*. Clinicopathologic study of CD56 (NCAM)-positive angiocentric lymphoma occurring in sites other than the upper and lower respiratory tract. *Am J Surg Pathol* 1995; **19**: 284–96.

●80. Kern WF, Spier CM, Hanneman EH *et al*. Neural cell adhesion molecule-positive peripheral T-cell lymphoma: a rare variant with a propensity for unusual sites of involvement. *Blood* 1992; **79**: 2432–7.

81. Kaluza V, Rao DS, Said JW, de Vos S. Primary extranodal nasal-type natural killer/T-cell lymphoma of the brain: a case report. *Hum Pathol* 2006; **37**: 769–72.

82. Briese J, Noack F, Harland A, Horny HP. Primary extranodal NK/T cell lymphoma ('nasal type') of the endometrium: report of an unusual case diagnosed at autopsy. *Gynecol Obstet Invest* 2006; **61**: 164–6.

83. Laohaburanakit P, Hardin KA. NK/T cell lymphoma of the lung: a case report and review of literature. *Thorax* 2006; **61**: 267–70.

84. Thompson MA, Habra MA, Routbort MJ *et al.* Primary adrenal natural killer/T-cell nasal type lymphoma: first case report in adults. *Am J Hematol* 2007; **82**: 299–303.

85. Kuo TT, Chen MJ, Kuo MC. Cutaneous intravascular NK-cell lymphoma: report of a rare variant associated with Epstein-Barr virus. *Am J Surg Pathol* 2006; **30**: 1197–201.

86. Liang R, Todd D, Chan TK *et al.* Nasal lymphoma. A retrospective analysis of 60 cases. *Cancer* 1990; **66**: 2205–9.

●87. Kwong YL, Chan AC, Liang R *et al.* CD56+ NK lymphomas: clinicopathological features and prognosis. *Br J Haematol* 1997; **97**: 821–9.

88. Wong KF, Chan JK, Cheung MM, So JC. Bone marrow involvement by nasal NK cell lymphoma at diagnosis is uncommon. *Am J Clin Pathol* 2001; **115**: 266–70.

89. Ng CS, Chan JK, Cheng PN, Szeto SC. Nasal T-cell lymphoma associated with hemophagocytic syndrome. *Cancer* 1986; **58**: 67–71.

90. Kwong YL. Natural killer-cell malignancies: diagnosis and treatment. *Leukemia* 2005; **19**: 2186–94.

●91. Li YX, Yao B, Jin J *et al.* Radiotherapy as primary treatment for stage IE and IIE nasal natural killer/T-cell lymphoma. *J Clin Oncol* 2006; **24**: 181–9.

92. Ribrag V, Ell Hajj M, Janot F *et al.* Early locoregional high-dose radiotherapy is associated with long-term disease control in localized primary angiocentric lymphoma of the nose and nasopharynx. *Leukemia* 2001; **15**: 1123–6.

93. You JY, Chi KH, Yang MH *et al.* Radiation therapy versus chemotherapy as initial treatment for localized nasal natural killer (NK)/T-cell lymphoma: a single institute survey in Taiwan. *Ann Oncol* 2004; **15**: 618–25.

94. Koom WS, Chung EJ, Yang WI *et al.* Angiocentric T-cell and NK/T-cell lymphomas: radiotherapeutic viewpoints. *Int J Radiat Oncol Biol Phys* 2004; **59**: 1127–37.

95. Cheung MM, Chan JK, Lau WH *et al.* Early stage nasal NK/T-cell lymphoma: clinical outcome, prognostic factors, and the effect of treatment modality. *Int J Radiat Oncol Biol Phys* 2002; **54**: 182–90.

96. Kim GE, Cho JH, Yang WI *et al.* Angiocentric lymphoma of the head and neck: patterns of systemic failure after radiation treatment. *J Clin Oncol* 2000; **18**: 54–63.

97. Cheung MM, Chan JK, Wong KF. Natural killer cell neoplasms: a distinctive group of highly aggressive lymphomas/leukemias. *Semin Hematol* 2003; **40**: 221–32.

98. Liang R, Todd D, Chan TK *et al.* Treatment outcome and prognostic factors for primary nasal lymphoma. *J Clin Oncol* 1995; **13**: 666–70.

99. Yamaguchi M, Shoko O, Yoshihito N. Treatment outcome of nasal NK-cell lymphoma: a report of 12 consecutively diagnosed cases and a review of the literature. *J Clin Exp Hematopathol* 2001; **41**: 93–9.

100. Nagafuji K, Fujisaki T, Arima F, Ohshima K. L-Asparaginase induced durable remission of relapsed nasal NK/T-cell lymphoma after autologous peripheral blood stem cell transplantation. *Int J Hematol* 2001; **74**: 447–50.

101. Liang R, Chen F, Lee CK *et al.* Autologous bone marrow transplantation for primary nasal T/NK cell lymphoma. *Bone Marrow Transplant* 1997; **19**: 91–3.

102. Au WY, Lie AK, Liang R *et al.* Autologous stem cell transplantation for nasal NK/T-cell lymphoma: a progress report on its value. *Ann Oncol* 2003; **14**: 1673–6.

103. Murashige N, Kami M, Kishi Y *et al.* Allogeneic haematopoietic stem cell transplantation as a promising treatment for natural killer-cell neoplasms. *Br J Haematol* 2005; **130**: 561–7.

104. Kim HJ, Bang SM, Lee J *et al.* High-dose chemotherapy with autologous stem cell transplantation in extranodal NK/T-cell lymphoma: a retrospective comparison with non-transplantation cases. *Bone Marrow Transplant* 2006; **37**: 819–24.

105. Suzuki R, Suzumiya J, Nakamura S *et al.* Hematopoietic stem cell transplantation for natural killer-cell lineage neoplasms. *Bone Marrow Transplant* 2006; **37**: 425–31.

106. Au WY, Weisenburger DD, Intraqumtoruchai T *et al.* Clinical differences between nasal and extranasal natural killer/T-cell lymphoma: a study of 136 cases from the International Peripheral T-cell Lympoma Project. *Blood* 2009; **113**: 3931–7.

107. Chang SE, Yoon GS, Huh J *et al.* Comparison of primary and secondary cutaneous CD56+ NK/T cell lymphomas. *Appl Immunohistochem Mol Morphol* 2002; **10**: 163–70.

●108. Chim CS, Ma SY, Au WY *et al.* Primary nasal natural killer cell lymphoma: long-term treatment outcome and relationship with the International Prognostic Index. *Blood* 2004; **103**: 216–21.

109. Lee J, Suh C, Park YH *et al.* Extranodal natural killer T-cell lymphoma, nasal-type: a prognostic model from a retrospective multicenter study. *J Clin Oncol* 2006; **24**: 612–18.

●110. Kim TM, Park YH, Lee SY *et al.* Local tumor invasiveness is more predictive of survival than International Prognostic Index in stage I(E)/II(E) extranodal NK/T-cell lymphoma, nasal type. *Blood* 2005; **106**: 3785–90.

●111. Au WY, Pang A, Choy C *et al.* Quantification of circulating Epstein-Barr virus (EBV) DNA in the diagnosis and monitoring of natural killer cell and EBV-positive lymphomas in immunocompetent patients. *Blood* 2004; **104**: 243–9.

112. Lei KI, Chan LY, Chan WY *et al.* Diagnostic and prognostic implications of circulating cell-free Epstein-Barr virus DNA in natural killer/T-cell lymphoma. *Clin Cancer Res* 2002; **8**: 29–34.

113. Huang WT, Chang KC, Huang GC *et al.* Bone marrow that is positive for Epstein-Barr virus encoded RNA-1 by in situ hybridization is related with a poor prognosis in patients with extranodal natural killer/T-cell lymphoma, nasal type. *Haematologica* 2005; **90**: 1063–9.

114. Ho FC, Choy D, Loke SL *et al.* Polymorphic reticulosis and conventional lymphomas of the nose and upper aerodigestive tract: a clinicopathologic study of 70 cases, and immunophenotypic studies of 16 cases. *Hum Pathol* 1990; **21**: 1041–50.

115. Shim SJ, Yang WI, Shin E *et al.* Clinical significance of cyclooxygenase-2 expression in extranodal natural killer (NK)/T-cell lymphoma, nasal type. *Int J Radiat Oncol Biol Phys* 2007; **67**: 31–8.

116. Bossard C, Belhadj K, Reyes F *et al.* Expression of the granzyme B inhibitor PI9 predicts outcome in nasal NK/T-cell lymphoma: results of a Western series of 48 patients treated with first-line polychemotherapy within the Groupe d'Etude des Lymphomes de l'Adulte (GELA) trials. *Blood* 2007; **109**: 2183–9.

117. Lin CW, Chen YH, Chuang YC *et al.* CD94 transcripts imply a better prognosis in nasal-type extranodal NK/T-cell lymphoma. *Blood* 2003; **102**: 2623–31.

●118. Siu LL, Chan JK, Wong KF, Kwong YL. Specific patterns of gene methylation in natural killer cell lymphomas: p73 is consistently involved. *Am J Pathol* 2002; **160**: 59–66.

119. Siu LL, Chan JK, Wong KF *et al.* Aberrant promoter CpG methylation as a molecular marker for disease monitoring in natural killer cell lymphomas. *Br J Haematol* 2003; **122**: 70–7.

120. Niitsu N, Okamoto M, Honma Y *et al.* Serum levels of the nm23-H1 protein and their clinical implication in extranodal NK/T-cell lymphoma. *Leukemia* 2003; **17**: 987–90.

121. Krasne DL, Warnke RA, Weiss LM. Malignant lymphoma presenting as pseudoepitheliomatous hyperplasia. A report of two cases. *Am J Surg Pathol* 1988; **12**: 835–42.

122. Chinen K, Kaneko Y, Izumo T *et al.* Nasal natural killer cell/t-cell lymphoma showing cellular morphology mimicking normal lymphocytes. *Arch Pathol Lab Med* 2002; **126**: 602–5.

123. Siu LL, Chan JK, Kwong YL. Natural killer cell malignancies: clinicopathologic and molecular features. *Histol Histopathol* 2002; **17**: 539–54.

124. Yagi H, Seo N, Ohshima A *et al.* Chemokine receptor expression in cutaneous T cell and NK/T-cell lymphomas: immunohistochemical staining and *in vitro* chemotactic assay. *Am J Surg Pathol* 2006; **30**: 1111–19.

125. Chan JK, Sin VC, Ng CS, Lau WH. Cutaneous relapse of nasal T-cell lymphoma clinically mimicking erythema multiforme. *Pathology* 1989; **21**: 164–8.

126. Natkunam Y, Smoller BR, Zehnder JL *et al.* Aggressive cutaneous NK and NK-like T-cell lymphomas: clinicopathologic, immunohistochemical, and molecular analyses of 12 cases. *Am J Surg Pathol* 1999; **23**: 571–81.

127. Chim CS, Au WY, Shek TW *et al.* Primary CD56 positive lymphomas of the gastrointestinal tract. *Cancer* 2001; **91**: 525–33.

●128. Chan JK, Ng CS, Lau WH, Lo ST. Most nasal/nasopharyngeal lymphomas are peripheral T-cell neoplasms. *Am J Surg Pathol* 1987; **11**: 418–29.

129. Chan JKC, Ng CS, Tsang WY. Nasal/nasopharyngeal lymphomas: an immunohistochemical analysis of 57 cases on frozen tissues [abstract]. *Mod Pathol* 1993; **6**: a87.

130. Petrella T, Delfau-Larue MH, Caillot D *et al.* Nasopharyngeal lymphomas: further evidence for a natural killer cell origin. *Hum Pathol* 1996; **27**: 827–33.

131. Ohno T, Yamaguchi M, Oka K *et al.* Frequent expression of CD3 epsilon in CD3 (Leu 4)-negative nasal T-cell lymphomas. *Leukemia* 1995; **9**: 44–52.

132. Mori N, Yatabe Y, Oka K *et al.* Expression of perforin in nasal lymphoma. Additional evidence of its natural killer cell derivation. *Am J Pathol* 1996; **149**: 699–705.

133. Gaal K, Sun NC, Hernandez AM, Arber DA. Sinonasal NK/T-cell lymphomas in the United States. *Am J Surg Pathol* 2000; **24**: 1511–17.

134. Elenitoba-Johnson KS, Zarate-Osorno A, Meneses A *et al.* Cytotoxic granular protein expression, Epstein-Barr virus strain type, and latent membrane protein-1 oncogene deletions in nasal T- lymphocyte/natural killer cell lymphomas from Mexico. *Mod Pathol* 1998; **11**: 754–61.

135. Ng CS, Lo ST, Chan JK, Chan WC. CD56+ putative natural killer cell lymphomas: production of cytolytic effectors and related proteins mediating tumor cell apoptosis? *Hum Pathol* 1997; **28**: 1276–82.

136. Takeshita M, Yamamoto M, Kikuchi M *et al.* Angiodestruction and tissue necrosis of skin-involving CD56+ NK/T-cell lymphoma are influenced by expression of cell adhesion molecules and cytotoxic granule and apoptosis-related proteins. *Am J Clin Pathol* 2000; **113**: 201–11.

137. Mori KL, Egashira M, Oshimi K. Differentiation stage of natural killer cell-lineage lymphoproliferative disorders based on phenotypic analysis. *Br J Haematol* 2001; **115**: 225–8.

138. Emile JF, Boulland ML, Haioun C *et al.* CD5−CD56+ T-cell receptor silent peripheral T-cell lymphomas are natural killer cell lymphomas. *Blood* 1996; **87**: 1466–73.

139. Ng CS, Lo ST, Chan JK. Peripheral T and putative natural killer cell lymphomas commonly coexpress CD95 and CD95 ligand. *Hum Pathol* 1999; **30**: 48–53.

140. Ohshima K, Suzumiya J, Shimazaki K *et al.* Nasal T/NK cell lymphomas commonly express perforin and Fas ligand: important mediators of tissue damage. *Histopathology* 1997; **31**: 444–50.

141. Cuadra-Garcia I, Proulx GM, Wu CL *et al.* Sinonasal lymphoma: a clinicopathologic analysis of 58 cases from

the Massachusetts General Hospital. *Am J Surg Pathol* 1999; **23**: 1356–69.

142. Kanavaros P, Lescs MC, Briere J *et al.* Nasal T-cell lymphoma: a clinicopathologic entity associated with peculiar phenotype and with Epstein–Barr virus. *Blood* 1993; **81**: 2688–95.

143. Nagata H, Konno A, Kimura N *et al.* Characterization of novel natural killer (NK)-cell and gammadelta T-cell lines established from primary lesions of nasal T/NK-cell lymphomas associated with the Epstein–Barr virus. *Blood* 2001; **97**: 708–13.

144. Sawada A, Sato E, Koyama M *et al.* NK-cell repertoire is feasible for diagnosing Epstein-Barr virus-infected NK-cell lymphoproliferative disease and evaluating the treatment effect. *Am J Hematol* 2006; **81**: 576–81.

145. Ho FC, Srivastava G, Loke SL *et al.* Presence of Epstein–Barr virus DNA in nasal lymphomas of B and 'T' cell type. *Hematol Oncol* 1990; **8**: 271–81.

146. Suzumiya J, Takeshita M, Kimura N *et al.* Expression of adult and fetal natural killer cell markers in sinonasal lymphomas. *Blood* 1994; **83**: 2255–60.

147. Rodriguez J, Romaguera JE, Manning J *et al.* Nasal-type T/NK lymphomas: a clinicopathologic study of 13 cases. *Leuk Lymphoma* 2000; **39**: 139–44.

148. Martin AR, Chan WC, Perry DA *et al.* Aggressive natural killer cell lymphoma of the small intestine. *Mod Pathol* 1995; **8**: 467–72.

149. Chiang AK, Wong KY, Liang AC, Srivastava G. Comparative analysis of Epstein-Barr virus gene polymorphisms in nasal T/NK-cell lymphomas and normal nasal tissues: implications on virus strain selection in malignancy. *Int J Cancer* 1999; **80**: 356–64.

150. Suzumiya J, Ohshima K, Takeshita M *et al.* Nasal lymphomas in Japan: a high prevalence of Epstein-Barr virus type A and deletion within the latent membrane protein gene. *Leuk Lymphoma* 1999; **35**: 567–78.

151. Shen L, Liang AC, Lu L *et al.* Frequent deletion of Fas gene sequences encoding death and transmembrane domains in nasal natural killer/T-cell lymphomas. *Am J Pathol* 2002; **161**: 2123–31.

152. Li T, Hongyo T, Syaifudin M *et al.* Mutations of the p53 gene in nasal NK/T-cell lymphoma. *Lab Invest* 2000; **80**: 493–9.

153. Quintanilla-Martinez L, Franklin JL, Guerrero I *et al.* Histological and immunophenotypic profile of nasal NK/T cell lymphomas from Peru: high prevalence of p53 overexpression. *Hum Pathol* 1999; **30**: 849–55.

154. Hongyo T, Hoshida Y, Nakatsuka S *et al.* p53, K-ras, c-kit and beta-catenin gene mutations in sinonasal NK/T-cell lymphoma in Korea and Japan. *Oncol Rep* 2005; **13**: 265–71.

155. Quintanilla-Martinez L, Kremer M, Keller G *et al.* p53 mutations in nasal natural killer/T-cell lymphoma from Mexico: association with large cell morphology and advanced disease. *Am J Pathol* 2001; **159**: 2095–105.

156. Li T, Zhang B, Ye Y, Yin H. Immunohistochemical and genetic analysis of Chinese nasal natural killer/T-cell lymphomas. *Hum Pathol* 2006; **37**: 54–60.

157. Lin CW, Lee WH, Chang CL *et al.* Restricted killer cell immunoglobulin-like receptor repertoire without T-cell receptor gamma rearrangement supports a true natural killer-cell lineage in a subset of sinonasal lymphomas. *Am J Pathol* 2001; **159**: 1671–9.

158. Wong KF, Zhang YM, Chan JK. Cytogenetic abnormalities in natural killer cell lymphoma/leukaemia – is there a consistent pattern? *Leuk Lymphoma* 1999; **34**: 241–50.

159. Tien HF, Su IJ, Tang JL *et al.* Clonal chromosomal abnormalities as direct evidence for clonality in nasal T/natural killer cell lymphomas. *Br J Haematol* 1997; **97**: 621–5.

160. Ko YH, Choi KE, Han JH *et al.* Comparative genomic hybridization study of nasal-type NK/T-cell lymphoma. *Cytometry* 2001; **46**: 85–91.

161. Nakashima Y, Tagawa H, Suzuki R *et al.* Genome-wide array-based comparative genomic hybridization of natural killer cell lymphoma/leukemia: different genomic alteration patterns of aggressive NK-cell leukemia and extranodal Nk/T-cell lymphoma, nasal type. *Genes Chromosomes Cancer* 2005; **44**: 247–55.

162. Wong N, Wong KF, Chan JK, Johnson PJ. Chromosomal translocations are common in natural killer-cell lymphoma/leukemia as shown by spectral karyotyping. *Hum Pathol* 2000; **31**: 771–4.

163. MacLeod RAF, Nagel S, Kaufmann M *et al.* Multicolor-FISH analysis of a natural killer cell line (NK-92). *Leuk Res* 2002; **26**: 1027–33.

164. Cheung MM, Chan JK, Wong KH. Early stage nasal NK/T cell lymphoma: preliminary result of intensifying treatment with concurrent chemo-radiation and high dose chemotherapy [abstract]. *Ann Oncol* 2002; **12(s2)**: 82.

165. Taddesse-Heath L, Feldman JI, Fahle GA *et al.* Florid CD4+, CD56+ T-cell infiltrate associated with Herpes simplex infection simulating nasal NK-/T-cell lymphoma. *Mod Pathol* 2003; **16**: 166–72.

166. Vega F, Chang CC, Schwartz MR *et al.* Atypical NK-cell proliferation of the gastrointestinal tract in a patient with antigliadin antibodies but not celiac disease. *Am J Surg Pathol* 2006; **30**: 539–44.

167. Weiss LM, Chang KL. Association with the Epstein–Barr virus with hematolymphoid neoplasm. *Adv Anat Pathol* 1996; **3**: 1–15.

168. Jaffe ES. Nasal and nasal-type T/NK cell lymphoma: a unique form of lymphoma associated with the Epstein-Barr virus [comment]. *Histopathology* 1995; **27**: 581–3.

169. Chan JK, Yip TT, Tsang WY *et al.* Detection of Epstein-Barr viral RNA in malignant lymphomas of the upper aerodigestive tract. *Am J Surg Pathol* 1994; **18**: 938–46.

170. Kanavaros P, Briere J, Lescs MC, Gaulard P. Epstein-Barr virus in non-Hodgkin's lymphomas of the upper respiratory tract: association with sinonasal localization and expression of NK and/or T-cell antigens by tumour cells. *J Pathol* 1996; **178**: 297–302.

171. Tomita Y, Ohsawa M, Qiu K *et al.* Epstein-Barr virus in lymphoproliferative diseases in the sino-nasal

region: close association with CD56+ immunophenotype and polymorphic- reticulosis morphology. *Int J Cancer* 1997; **70**: 9–13.

172. Tsang WY, Chan JK, Yip TT *et al.* In situ localization of Epstein-Barr virus encoded RNA in non-nasal/ nasopharyngeal CD56-positive and CD56-negative T-cell lymphomas. *Hum Pathol* 1994; **25**: 758–65.

●173. van Gorp J, Weiping L, Jacobse K *et al.* Epstein–Barr virus in nasal T-cell lymphomas (polymorphic reticulosis/ midline malignant reticulosis) in western China. *J Pathol* 1994; **173**: 81–7.

174. Kwong YL, Lam CC, Chan TM. Post-transplantation lymphoproliferative disease of natural killer cell lineage: a clinicopathological and molecular analysis. *Br J Haematol* 2000; **110**: 197–202.

175. Stadlmann S, Fend F, Moser P *et al.* Epstein–Barr virus-associated extranodal NK/T-cell lymphoma, nasal type of the hypopharynx, in a renal allograft recipient: case report and review of literature. *Hum Pathol* 2001; **32**: 1264–8.

176. Hoshida Y, Li T, Dong Z *et al.* Lymphoproliferative disorders in renal transplant patients in Japan. *Int J Cancer* 2001; **91**: 869–75.

177. Hoshida Y, Hongyo T, Nakatsuka S *et al.* Gene mutations in lymphoproliferative disorders of T and NK/T cell phenotypes developing in renal transplant patients. *Lab Invest* 2002; **82**: 257–64.

178. Kimura H, Hoshino Y, Kanegane H *et al.* Clinical and virologic characteristics of chronic active Epstein-Barr virus infection. *Blood* 2001; **98**: 280–6.

179. Yachie A, Kanegane H, Kasahara Y. Epstein-Barr virus-associated T-/natural killer cell lymphoproliferative diseases. *Semin Hematol* 2003; **40**: 124–32.

180. Chan KC, Zhang J, Chan AT *et al.* Molecular characterization of circulating Epstein-Barr virus (EBV) DNA in the diagnosis and monitoring of natural killer cell and EBV-positive lymphomas in immunocompetent patients. *Cancer Res* 2003; **63**: 2028–32.

181. Peh SC, Quen QW. Nasal and nasal-type natural killer (NK)/T-cell lymphoma: immunophenotype and Epstein-Barr virus (EBV) association. *Med J Malaysia* 2003; **58**: 196–204.

●182. Jaffe ES, Chan JK, Su IJ *et al.* Report of the Workshop on nasal and related extranodal angiocentric T/natural killer cell lymphomas: definitions, differential diagnosis, and epidemiology. *Am J Surg Pathol* 1996; **20**: 103–11.

183. Liu A, Nakatsuka S, Yang WI *et al.* Expression of cell adhesion molecules and chemokine receptors: angioinvasiveness in nasal NK/T-cell lymphoma. *Oncol Rep* 2005; **13**: 613–20.

184. Teruya-Feldstein J, Jaffe ES, Burd PR *et al.* The role of Mig, the monokine induced by interferon-gamma, and IP-10, the interferon-gamma-inducible protein-10, in tissue necrosis and vascular damage associated with Epstein-Barr virus-positive lymphoproliferative disease. *Blood* 1997; **90**: 4099–105.

185. Teruya-Feldstein J, Setsuda J, Yao X *et al.* MIP-1alpha expression in tissues from patients with hemophagocytic syndrome. *Lab Invest* 1999; **79**: 1583–90.

●186. Imamura N, Kusunoki Y, Kawa-Ha K *et al.* Aggressive natural killer cell leukaemia/lymphoma: report of four cases and review of the literature. Possible existence of a new clinical entity originating from the third lineage of lymphoid cells. *Br J Haematol* 1990; **75**: 49–59.

187. Chan JKC, Wong KF, Jaffe ES, Ralfkiaer E. Aggressive NK-cell leukemia. In: Jaffe ES, Harris NL, Stein H, Vardiman JW. (eds) *Pathology and genetics, tumours of haematopoietic and lymphoid tissues. World Health Organization classification of tumours.* Lyon: IARC Press, 2001: 198–200.

188. Kwong YL, Wong KF, Chan LC *et al.* Large granular lymphocyte leukemia. A study of nine cases in a Chinese population. *Am J Clin Pathol* 1995; **103**: 76–81.

189. Gelb AB, van de Rijn M, Regula DP Jr *et al.* Epstein-Barr virus-associated natural killer-large granular lymphocyte leukemia. *Hum Pathol* 1994; **25**: 953–60.

190. Hart DN, Baker BW, Inglis MJ *et al.* Epstein-Barr viral DNA in acute large granular lymphocyte (natural killer) leukemic cells [see comments]. *Blood* 1992; **79**: 2116–23.

●191. Kawa-Ha K, Ishihara S, Ninomiya T *et al.* CD3−negative lymphoproliferative disease of granular lymphocytes containing Epstein-Barr viral DNA. *J Clin Invest* 1989; **84**: 51–5.

192. Shimodaira S, Ishida F, Kobayashi H *et al.* The detection of clonal proliferation in granular lymphocyte-proliferative disorders of natural killer cell lineage. *Br J Haematol* 1995; **90**: 578–84.

193. Mori N, Yamashita Y, Tsuzuki T *et al.* Lymphomatous features of aggressive NK cell leukaemia/lymphoma with massive necrosis, haemophagocytosis and EB virus infection. *Histopathology* 2000; **37**: 363–71.

194. Murdock J, Jaffe ES, Wilson WH *et al.* Aggressive natural killer cell leukaemia/lymphoma: case report, use of telesynergy and review of the literature. *Leuk Lymphoma* 2004; **45**: 1269–73.

195. Chang SE, Lee SY, Choi JH *et al.* Cutaneous dissemination of nasal NK/T-cell lymphoma with bone marrow, liver and lung involvement. *Clin Exp Dermatol* 2002; **27**: 120–2.

196. Suzuki K, Ohshima K, Karube K *et al.* Clinicopathological states of Epstein-Barr virus-associated T/NK-cell lymphoproliferative disorders (severe chronic active EBV infection) of children and young adults. *Int J Oncol* 2004; **24**: 1165–74.

197. Ohno Y, Amakawa R, Fukuhara S *et al.* Acute transformation of chronic large granular lymphocyte leukemia associated with additional chromosome abnormality. *Cancer* 1989; **64**: 63–7.

198. Soler J, Bordes R, Ortuno F *et al.* Aggressive natural killer cell leukaemia/lymphoma in two patients with lethal midline granuloma. *Br J Haematol* 1994; **86**: 659–62.

199. Chou WC, Chiang IP, Tang JL *et al.* Clonal disease of natural killer large granular lymphocytes in Taiwan. *Br J Haematol* 1998; **103**: 1124–8.

200. Engellenner W, Golightly M. Large granular lymphocyte leukemia. *Lab Med* 1991; **22**: 454–6.

201. Oshimi K, Yamada O, Kaneko T *et al.* Laboratory findings and clinical courses of 33 patients with granular lymphocyte-proliferative disorders. *Leukemia* 1993; **7**: 782–8.

202. Okuda T, Sakamoto S, Deguchi T *et al.* Hemophagocytic syndrome associated with aggressive natural killer cell leukemia. *Am J Hematol* 1991; **38**: 321–3.

203. Sato K, Kimura F, Nakamura Y *et al.* An aggressive nasal lymphoma accompanied by high levels of soluble Fas ligand. *Br J Haematol* 1996; **94**: 379–82.

204. Tanaka M, Suda T, Haze K *et al.* Fas ligand in human serum. *Nat Med* 1996; **2**: 317–22.

205. Egashira M, Kawamata N, Sugimoto K *et al.* P-glycoprotein expression on normal and abnormally expanded natural killer cells and inhibition of P-glycoprotein function by cyclosporin A and its analogue, PSC833. *Blood* 1999; **93**: 599–606.

206. Trambas C, Wang Z, Cianfriglia M, Woods G. Evidence that natural killer cells express mini P-glycoproteins but not classic 170 kDa P-glycoprotein. *Br J Haematol* 2001; **114**: 177–84.

207. Suzuki R, Suzumiya J, Nakamura S *et al.* Aggressive natural killer-cell leukemia revisited: large granular lymphocyte leukemia of cytotoxic NK cells. *Leukemia* 2004; **18**: 763–70.

208. Song SY, Kim WS, Ko YH *et al.* Aggressive natural killer cell leukemia: clinical features and treatment outcome. *Haematologica* 2002; **87**: 1343–5.

209. Tsang WY, Chan JK, Ng CS. Kikuchi's lymphadenitis. A morphologic analysis of 75 cases with special reference to unusual features. *Am J Surg Pathol* 1994; **18**: 219–31.

210. Chan WC, Link S, Mawle A *et al.* Heterogeneity of large granular lymphocyte proliferations: delineation of two major subtypes. *Blood* 1986; **68**: 1142–53.

211. Chan WC, Gu LB, Masih A *et al.* Large granular lymphocyte proliferation with the natural killer-cell phenotype. *Am J Clin Pathol* 1992; **97**: 353–8.

212. Bassan R, Rambaldi A, Abbate M *et al.* Association of NK-cell lymphoproliferative disease and nephrotic syndrome. *Am J Clin Pathol* 1990; **94**: 334–8.

213. Lamy T, Loughran TP Jr. Clinical features of large granular lymphocyte leukemia. *Semin Hematol* 2003; **40**: 185–95.

214. Kingreen D, Siegert W. Chronic lymphatic leukemias of T and NK cell type. *Leukemia* 1997; **11**(Suppl 2): s46–9.

215. Sokol L, Loughran TP Jr. Large granular lymphocyte leukemia. *Oncologist* 2006; **11**: 263–73.

216. Ohno T, Kanoh T, Arita Y *et al.* Fulminant clonal expansion of large granular lymphocytes. Characterization of their morphology, phenotype, genotype, and function. *Cancer* 1988; **62**: 1918–27.

217. Huang Q, Chang KL, Gaal KK, Weiss LM. An aggressive extranodal NK-cell lymphoma arising from indolent NK-cell lymphoproliferative disorder. *Am J Surg Pathol* 2005; **29**: 1540–3.

218. Lima M, Almeida J, Montero AG *et al.* Clinicobiological, immunophenotypic, and molecular characteristics of monoclonal CD56−/+dim chronic natural killer cell large granular lymphocytosis. *Am J Pathol* 2004; **165**: 1117–27.

219. Zambello R, Semenzato G. Natural killer receptors in patients with lymphoproliferative diseases of granular lymphocytes. *Semin Hematol* 2003; **40**: 201–12.

220. Epling-Burnette PK, Painter JS, Chaurasia P *et al.* Dysregulated NK receptor expression in patients with lymphoproliferative disease of granular lymphocytes. *Blood* 2004; **103**: 3431–9.

221. Hara J, Yumura-Yagi K, Tagawa S *et al.* Molecular analysis of T cell receptor and CD3 genes in CD3− large granular lymphocytes (LGLs): evidence for the existence of CD3− LGLs committed to the T cell lineage. *Leukemia* 1990; **4**: 580–3.

222. Cantoni C, de Totero D, Lauria F *et al.* Phenotypic, functional and molecular analysis of CD3-LGL expansions indicates a relationship to two different CD3− normal counterparts. *Br J Haematol* 1994; **86**: 740–5.

223. Kelly A, Richards SJ, Sivakumaran M *et al.* Clonality of CD3 negative large granular lymphocyte proliferations determined by PCR based X-inactivation studies. *J Clin Pathol* 1994; **47**: 399–404.

224. Loughran TP Jr, Hadlock KG, Yang Q *et al.* Seroreactivity to an envelope protein of human T-cell leukemia/lymphoma virus in patients with CD3− (natural killer) lymphoproliferative disease of granular lymphocytes. *Blood* 1997; **90**: 1977–81.

225. Nash R, McSweeney P, Zambello R *et al.* Clonal studies of CD3− lymphoproliferative disease of granular lymphocytes. *Blood* 1993; **81**: 2363–8.

226. Tefferi A, Greipp PR, Leibson PJ, Thibodeau SN. Demonstration of clonality, by X-linked DNA analysis, in chronic natural killer cell lymphocytosis and successful therapy with oral cyclophosphamide. *Leukemia* 1992; **6**: 477–80.

227. Taniwaki M, Tagawa S, Nishigaki H *et al.* Chromosomal abnormalities define clonal proliferation in CD3− large granular lymphocyte leukemia. *Am J Hematol* 1990; **33**: 32–8.

228. Gorochov G, Debre P, Leblond V *et al.* Oligoclonal expansion of CD8+ CD57+ T cells with restricted T-cell receptor beta chain variability after bone marrow transplantation. *Blood* 1994; **83**: 587–95.

229. Halwani F, Guttmann RD, Ste-Croix H, Prud'homme GJ. Identification of natural suppressor cells in long-term renal allograft recipients. *Transplantation* 1992; **54**: 973–7.

230. Schwab R, Szabo P, Manavalan JS *et al.* Expanded CD4+ and CD8+ T cell clones in elderly humans. *J Immunol* 1997; **158**: 4493–9.

231. Smith PR, Cavenagh JD, Milne T *et al.* Benign monoclonal expansion of CD8+ lymphocytes in HIV infection. *J Clin Pathol* 2000; **53**: 177–81.

232. Jaffe ES, Ralfkiaer E. Mature T-cell and NK-cell neoplasms: introduction. In: Jaffe ES, Harris NL, Stein H,

Vardiman J. (eds) *Pathology and genetics, tumours of haematopoietic and lymphoid tissues. World Health Organization classification of tumours.* Lyon: IARC Press, 2001: 191–4.

233. Plum J, De Smedt M, Verhasselt B *et al. In vitro* intrathymic differentiation kinetics of human fetal liver CD34+CD38- progenitors reveals a phenotypically defined dendritic/T-NK precursor split. *J Immunol* 1999; **162**: 60–8.

234. DiGiuseppe JA, Louie DC, Williams JE *et al.* Blastic natural killer cell leukemia/lymphoma: a clinicopathologic study. *Am J Surg Pathol* 1997; **21**: 1223–30.

235. Khoury JD, Medeiros LJ, Manning JT *et al.* CD56(+) TdT(+) blastic natural killer cell tumor of the skin: a primitive systemic malignancy related to myelomonocytic leukemia. *Cancer* 2002; **94**: 2401–8.

236. Kobashi Y, Nakamura S, Sasajima Y *et al.* Inconsistent association of Epstein-Barr virus with CD56 (NCAM)-positive angiocentric lymphoma occurring in sites other than the upper and lower respiratory tract. *Histopathology* 1996; **28**: 111–20.

237. Koita H, Suzumiya J, Ohshima K *et al.* Lymphoblastic lymphoma expressing natural killer cell phenotype with involvement of the mediastinum and nasal cavity. *Am J Surg Pathol* 1997; **21**: 242–8.

238. Nakamura S, Koshikawa T, Yatabe Y, Suchi T. Lymphoblastic lymphoma expressing CD56 and TdT [letter; comment]. *Am J Surg Pathol* 1998; **22**: 135–7.

239. Santucci M, Pimpinelli N, Massi D *et al.* Cytotoxic/natural killer cell cutaneous lymphomas. Report of EORTC cutaneous lymphoma task force workshop. *Cancer* 2003; **97**: 610–27.

240. Petrella T, Comeau MR, Maynadie M *et al.* 'Agranular CD4+ CD56+ hematodermic neoplasm' (blastic NK-cell lymphoma) originates from a population of CD56+ precursor cells related to plasmacytoid monocytes. *Am J Surg Pathol* 2002; **26**: 852–62.

●241. Petrella T, Bagot M, Willemze R *et al.* Blastic NK-cell lymphomas (agranular CD4+CD56+ hematodermic neoplasms): a review. *Am J Clin Pathol* 2005; **123**: 662–75.

242. Grouard G, Rissoan MC, Filgueira L *et al.* The enigmatic plasmacytoid T cells develop into dendritic cells with interleukin (IL)-3 and CD40-ligand. *J Exp Med* 1997; **185**: 1101–11.

♦243. Colonna M, Trinchieri G, Liu YJ. Plasmacytoid dendritic cells in immunity. *Nat Immunol* 2004; **5**: 1219–26.

244. MacDonald KP, Munster DJ, Clark GJ *et al.* Characterization of human blood dendritic cell subsets. *Blood* 2002; **100**: 4512–20.

245. Chaperot L, Bendriss N, Manches O *et al.* Identification of a leukemic counterpart of the plasmacytoid dendritic cells. *Blood* 2001; **97**: 3210–17.

246. Dzionek A, Fuchs A, Schmidt P *et al.* BDCA-2, BDCA-3, and BDCA-4: three markers for distinct subsets of dendritic cells in human peripheral blood. *J Immunol* 2000; **165**: 6037–46.

247. Jaye DL, Geigerman CM, Herling M *et al.* Expression of the plasmacytoid dendritic cell marker BDCA-2 supports a spectrum of maturation among CD4+ CD56+ hematodermic neoplasms. *Mod Pathol* 2006; **19**: 1555–62.

●248. Urosevic M, Conrad C, Kamarashev J *et al.* CD4+CD56+ hematodermic neoplasms bear a plasmacytoid dendritic cell phenotype. *Hum Pathol* 2005; **36**: 1020–4.

249. Maeda T, Murata K, Fukushima T *et al.* A novel plasmacytoid dendritic cell line, CAL-1, established from a patient with blastic natural killer cell lymphoma. *Int J Hematol* 2005; **81**: 148–54.

250. Ichinohasama R, Endoh K, Ishizawa K *et al.* Thymic lymphoblastic lymphoma of committed natural killer cell precursor origin: a case report. *Cancer* 1996; **77**: 2592–603.

251. Suzuki R, Nakamura S, Suzumiya J *et al.* Blastic natural killer cell lymphoma/leukemia (CD56-positive blastic tumor): prognostication and categorization according to anatomic sites of involvement. *Cancer* 2005; **104**: 1022–31.

252. Ko YH, Kim SH, Ree HJ. Blastic NK-cell lymphoma expressing terminal deoxynucleotidyl transferase with Homer-Wright type pseudorosettes formation. *Histopathology* 1998; **33**: 547–53.

253. Bayerl MG, Rakozy CK, Mohamed AN *et al.* Blastic natural killer cell lymphoma/leukemia: a report of seven cases. *Am J Clin Pathol* 2002; **117**: 41–50.

254. Argyrakos T, Rontogianni D, Karmiris T *et al.* Blastic natural killer (NK)-cell lymphoma: report of an unusual CD4 negative case and review of the CD4 negative neoplasms with blastic features in the literature. *Leuk Lymphoma* 2004; **45**: 2127–33.

255. Cong P, Raffeld M, Jaffe E. Blastic NK cell lymphoma/leukemia: a clinicopathological study of 23 cases [abstract]. *Mod Pathol* 2001; **14**: a160.

256. Natkunam Y, Cherry AM, Cornbleet PJ. Natural killer cell precursor acute lymphoma/leukemia presenting in an infant. *Arch Pathol Lab Med* 2001; **125**: 413–18.

257. Kameoka J, Ichinohasama R, Tanaka M *et al.* A cutaneous agranular CD2- CD4+ CD56+ 'lymphoma': report of two cases and review of the literature. *Am J Clin Pathol* 1998; **110**: 478–88.

258. Feuillard J, Jacob MC, Valensi F *et al.* Clinical and biologic features of CD4(+)CD56(+) malignancies. *Blood* 2002; **99**: 1556–63.

259. Jacob MC, Chaperot L, Mossuz P *et al.* CD4+ CD56+ lineage negative malignancies: a new entity developed from malignant early plasmacytoid dendritic cells. *Haematologica* 2003; **88**: 941–55.

260. Bekkenk MW, Jansen PM, Meijer CJ, Willemze R. CD56+ hematological neoplasms presenting in the skin: a retrospective analysis of 23 new cases and 130 cases from the literature. *Ann Oncol* 2004; **15**: 1097–108.

261. Alvarez-Larran A, Villamor N, Hernndez-Boluda JC *et al.* Blastic natural killer cell leukemia/lymphoma presenting as overt leukemia. *Clin Lymphoma* 2001; **2**: 178–82.

262. Hyakuna N, Toguchi S, Higa T *et al.* Childhood blastic NK cell leukemia successfully treated with L-asparaginase and allogeneic bone marrow transplantation. *Pediatr Blood Cancer* 2004; **42**: 631–4.

263. Knudsen H, Gronbaek K, thor Straten P *et al.* A case of lymphoblastoid natural killer (NK)-cell lymphoma: association with the NK-cell receptor complex CD94/NKG2 and TP53 intragenic deletion. *Br J Dermatol* 2002; **146**: 148–53.

264. Herling M, Teitell MA, Shen RR *et al.* TCL1 expression in plasmacytoid dendritic cells (DC2s) and the related CD4+ CD56+ blastic tumors of skin. *Blood* 2003; **101**: 5007–9.

265. Petrella T, Meijer CJ, Dalac S *et al.* TCL1 and CLA expression in agranular CD4/CD56 hematodermic neoplasms (blastic NK-cell lymphomas) and leukemia cutis. *Am J Clin Pathol* 2004; **122**: 307–13.

266. Petrella T, Dalac S, Maynadie M *et al.* CD4+ CD56+ cutaneous neoplasms: a distinct hematological entity? Groupe Francais d'Etude des Lymphomes Cutanes (GFELC). *Am J Surg Pathol* 1999; **23**: 137–46.

267. Ling TC, Harris M, Craven NM. Epstein-Barr virus-positive blastoid nasal T/natural killer-cell lymphoma in a Caucasian. *Br J Dermatol* 2002; **146**: 700–3.

268. Rakozy CK, Mohamed AN, Vo TD *et al.* CD56+/CD4+ lymphomas and leukemias are morphologically, immunophenotypically, cytogenetically, and clinically diverse. *Am J Clin Pathol* 2001; **116**: 168–76.

269. Leroux D, Mugneret F, Callanan M *et al.* CD4(+), CD56(+) DC2 acute leukemia is characterized by recurrent clonal chromosomal changes affecting 6 major targets: a study of 21 cases by the Groupe Francais de Cytogenetique Hematologique. *Blood* 2002; **99**: 4154–9.

270. Scott AA, Head DR, Kopecky KJ *et al.* HLA-DR-, CD33+, CD56+, CD16– myeloid/natural killer cell acute leukemia: a previously unrecognized form of acute leukemia potentially misdiagnosed as French-American-British acute myeloid leukemia-M3. *Blood* 1994; **84**: 244–55.

37

Anaplastic large cell lymphoma

GEORGES DELSOL, ESTELLE ESPINOS, SYLVIE GIURIATO, PIERRE BROUSSET,
LAURENCE LAMANT AND FABIENNE MEGGETTO

INTRODUCTION

In 1985, Stein and coworkers[1] recognized a subgroup of tumors with large-sized cells showing bizarre morphologic features, prominent sinusoidal invasion and expressing the Ki-1 antigen (now referred to as the CD30 molecule). These tumors were designated as 'Ki-1 lymphoma'.[1] Subsequently, a number of tumors were diagnosed as 'Ki-1 lymphoma', simply because they consisted of large cells, positive for the CD30 antigen, whatever their B, T or null cell phenotype. Later, the term 'Ki-1 lymphoma' was replaced by 'anaplastic large cell lymphoma' (ALCL). In the literature, cases described as ALCL are heterogeneous in terms of clinical, morphologic, phenotypic and cytogenetic features. In the World Health Organization (WHO) classification of hematopoietic neoplasms, only systemic ALCL of T or null phenotype is recognized as a distinct entity.[2] In 1994, Morris and coworkers showed that ALCL is associated with a t(2;5)(p23;q35) translocation which involves the anaplastic lymphoma kinase (ALK) gene at 2p23 that encodes a tyrosine kinase receptor, belonging to the insulin receptor superfamily and the NPM gene at 5q35 encoding nucleophosmin, a nucleolar-associated phosphoprotein.[3] The resultant NPM-ALK fusion protein is now detectable by immunohistochemistry using anti-Alk antibodies (ALK1).[4,5]

Primary systemic ALCL negative for the ALK protein is not reproducibly distinguishable on morphologic grounds from ALK-positive ALCL. This neoplasm, by definition, shows extensive staining for CD30 and lacks ALK protein and B cell markers. There is continuing controversy as to whether cases that lack ALK expression should: (i) continue to be grouped with ALK-positive ALCLs within a single category; (ii) be assigned to the broad category of 'peripheral T cell lymphoma, not otherwise specified'; or (iii) be considered an independent entity. It is of importance to resolve this uncertainty because of its clinical implications. Indeed, the clinical course of ALK-positive ALCLs compared to ALK-negative ones suggests that the latter represent a different (possibly heterogeneous) entity. Such a hypothesis has been reinforced by the results of gene profiling analysis (see below). In the 2008 WHO classification ALK-negative ALCL is considered as a provisional entity different from ALK-positive ALCL.[6]

Primary cutaneous ALCLs are included in the broad spectrum of 'Primary cutaneous CD30-positive T cell lymphoproliferative disorders' which have distinct clinical features.[7] Secondary systemic CD30-positive lymphomas with anaplastic morphology which may arise from mycosis fungoides or Hodgkin disease are also excluded from this entity. B cell lymphomas consisting of a predominant population of cells with anaplastic morphology and positive for CD30 are classified in the category of diffuse large B cell lymphoma.

CLINICAL FEATURES

Anaplastic large cell lymphomas account for 5 percent of all non-Hodgkin lymphoma and 10–30 percent of childhood lymphomas.[8] Anaplastic large cell lymphoma expressing X-ALK fusion protein is most frequent in the first three decades of life and shows a slight male predominance.[9,10] Occasional cases occur in human immunodeficiency virus (HIV)-positive patients or after solid-organ transplantation (personal observation, 2002). The majority of patients (70 percent) with systemic ALCL present with advanced stage III–IV disease with peripheral and/or abdominal lymphadenopathy, often associated with extranodal infiltrates and involvement of the bone marrow.[8,10] Patients often show B symptoms (75 percent), especially high fever.[8,10]

Primary systemic ALCLs positive for the ALK protein frequently involve both lymph nodes and extranodal sites. Extranodal sites commonly involved include skin (21 percent), bone (17 percent), soft tissues (17 percent), lung (11 percent) and liver (8 percent).[8,10,11] Retinal infiltration responsible for blindness and placental involvement have also been reported.[12] Involvement of the gut and central nervous system (CNS) is rare. However, occasional cases of primary gastric or central nervous system (CNS) ALCLs have been observed (unpublished observations). Mediastinal disease is less frequent than in Hodgkin disease. Bone marrow involvement is often subtle with only scattered malignant cells that are difficult to detect by routine bone marrow biopsies. However, positive bone marrow biopsies increase significantly (30–50 percent) when immunohistochemical stains for CD30, epithelial membrane antigen (EMA) and/or ALK are used.[13]

Most patients have circulating antibodies against NPM-ALK protein and these antibodies may persist in patients in apparent complete remission.[14]

No pathogenic factor has been demonstrated so far. However, in rare cases, an association with insect stings has been suggested (personal unpublished observation, 2008).

Primary systemic ALCL negative for the ALK protein involves both lymph nodes and extranodal tissues, although the latter sites are less commonly involved than in ALK-positive ALCL.[8] Unlike ALK-positive, the peak incidence of ALK-negative ALCL is in adults (40–65 years) although cases can occur at any age.[8,15] There is no clear male or female predominance.

MORPHOLOGIC FEATURES

Anaplastic large cell lymphomas that are Alk-positive show a broad spectrum of features, ranging from small cell neoplasms which many pathologists might have categorized as pleomorphic T-cell lymphomas, to cases at the opposite extreme in which very large cells predominate[5,9,16–20] (Plate 99A–D, F, see plate section). However, all cases share one common feature, notably the presence of a population of large cells with a highly characteristic morphology (Plate 99A, D, F). The nucleus lays eccentrically within these cells and is horseshoe or kidney shaped. These cells have been referred to as 'hallmark' cells (Plate 99A, D, F) because they

are present in all morphologic variants.[9] In most cases, cells with 'crown-like' or doughnut-shaped nuclei can also be seen. Nucleoli are less prominent than in Reed–Sternberg cells and often an eosinophilic region is seen near the nucleus, probably representing a prominent Golgi apparatus.[2,9] On lymph node imprints, lymphoma cells show vacuolated cytoplasm. Prominent inclusion-like nucleoli are relatively uncommon, aiding in the differential diagnosis with Hodgkin lymphoma.[21]

ALCLs are among the most polymorphic hematopoietic neoplasms. Five morphologic patterns are recognized in the 2008 WHO classification.[6]

- **Anaplastic large cell lymphoma, 'common pattern':** This accounts for 60 percent of cases and is predominantly composed of pleomorphic large cells with hallmark features as described above. Tumor cells with more monomorphic, rounded nuclei also occur (sometimes designated as monomorphic ALCL).[9,22] Characteristically, these tumors show a sinusoidal growth pattern which may mimic a metastatic tumor (Plate 99A–C).

- **Anaplastic large cell lymphoma, lymphohistiocytic pattern (5–10 percent):** This is characterized by tumor cells admixed with a large number of histiocytes[9,20,23] (Plate 99D). The histiocytes may mask the malignant cells which are often smaller than in the common type (Plate 99D, E). This morphologic variant may be extremely difficult to recognize without immunohistochemical study and is commonly misdiagnosed as histiocyte-rich lymphadenitis.

- **Anaplastic large cell lymphoma, small cell pattern (5–10 percent):** This shows a predominant population of small to medium-sized neoplastic cells with irregular nuclei (Plate 99F, G).[9,18,19] Hallmark cells are always present and are often concentrated around blood vessels (Plate 99H).[9] This morphologic variant of ALCL is often misdiagnosed as peripheral T-cell lymphoma 'not otherwise specified' (NOS) by conventional examination. When the blood is involved, atypical cells reminiscent of flower-like cells can be noted in smear preparations.[24,25] Small cell and lymphohistiocytic variants are probably closely related.[26,27]

- **Anaplastic large cell lymphoma, Hodgkin-like pattern (1–3 percent):** This tumor with ALK-positive neoplastic cells has been recently reported.[28] These tumors show features resembling Hodgkin lymphoma (HL) with a vaguely nodular fibrosis associated with capsular thickening and a significant number of tumor cells resembling classic Reed–Sternberg cells associated with hallmark cells.[28] In the past, tumors with these features have been referred to as 'Hodgkin's-like' ALCLs. However, most of them are negative for ALK and are more likely to be classic Hodgkin lymphoma rich in neoplastic cells. Since the description of ALCL, the existence of a 'Hodgkin-like' form has been the subject of controversy.[29,30] This controversy stems from the fact that before the availability of ALK1 antibody, there was no definite criteria to differentiate ALCL from HL. Thus, there were a number of reports dealing with 'Hodgkin-related'[31] or 'Hodgkin-like' ALCL.[32] The controversy was further amplified by the report by Orscheschek et al.,[33] who suggested that HL and ALCL were closely related, since they were able to demonstrate t(2;5)(p23;q35) in about 70–80 percent of HL. However, these results have not been confirmed by multiple studies using a variety of techniques.[34,35] It is now largely recognized that ALCL and HL are distinct entities and, despite the fact that there may be a morphologic overlap between ALCL and HL, there is no true biological borderline. It is possible that cases diagnosed as ALCL rich in neutrophils or eosinophils are also true HL.[36,37] Consequently, we think that lesions showing morphologic features of nodular sclerosing Hodgkin lymphoma (NSHL) with or without sinusoidal growth pattern, should not be diagnosed as Hodgkin-like ALCL unless they are positive for ALK. If they are negative for ALK protein, these lesions should be considered as HL and treated as such.[28]

- **Anaplastic large cell lymphoma with 'composite pattern' (15 percent)**: This is characterized by more than one pattern in a single lymph node biopsy. Furthermore, relapses may reveal morphologic features different from those seen initially.[6,9]
- **Other histological patterns**: These include tumors showing cells with monomorphic, rounded nuclei, either as the predominant population or mixed with more pleomorphic cells, cases rich in multinucleated neoplastic giant cells or displaying sarcomatoid features.[16] Tumors consisting of a predominant population of 'signet ring'-like cells[9] are rare and possibly related to the hypocellular morphologic variant.[38] Of note, in rare cases, malignant cells are exceedingly scarce, scattered in an otherwise reactive lymph node.

IMMUNOPHENOTYPE

Even if morphologic features of most ALCLs suggest the diagnosis, definitive diagnosis cannot be made without immunohistochemistry. The latter is critical in the diagnosis of some variants of ALCL. All ALCLs are positive for CD30. Neoplastic cells show a strong CD30 staining on the cell membrane and in the Golgi region (Plate 99B, C). In the small cell variant, the strongest immunostaining is seen in the large cells. Smaller tumor cells may be only weakly positive or even negative for CD30.[9] In the lymphohistiocytic and small cell variants, the neoplastic cells often cluster around blood vessels and can be highlighted by immunostaining using

antibodies to CD30, ALK and/or cytotoxic molecules (Plate 99H).[9] The majority of ALCLs are positive for EMA[9,39] but, in some cases, only a proportion of malignant cells is positive.

The majority of ALCLs express one or more T cell antigens and/or NK cell antigens.[1,8,9,40] However, due to loss of several pan T-cell antigens, some cases may have an apparent 'null cell phenotype'. CD3, the most widely used pan-T cell marker, is negative in more than 75 percent of cases.[9] CD5 and CD7 are often negative as well, whereas CD2 and CD4 are positive in a significant proportion of cases. CD43 is expressed by more than two-thirds of the cases, but this antigen lacks lineage specificity. Furthermore, most cases exhibit positivity for the cytotoxic associated antigens Tia-1, granzyme B, and/or perforin.[41,42] CD8 is usually negative, but rare CD8-positive cases exist. Occasional cases are positive for CD68/KP1 but not CD68/PGM1. Tumor cells are variably positive for CD45[39] but strongly positive for CD25 on frozen sections.[1,39] Blood group antigens H and Y (detected with monoclonal antibody BNH.9) have been reported in more than 50 percent of the cases.[43] CD15 expression is rarely observed and, when present, only a small proportion of the neoplastic cells are stained.[9] ALCLs are consistently negative for EBV[44] (i.e. EBER and LMP1). Most Alk-positive ALCLs are negative for BCL2.[45]

ALK expression is detectable in 60–85 percent of the cases. The ALK staining may be cytoplasmic and nuclear or it may be restricted either to the nucleus or to the cytoplasm (see below) (Plates 99G, 100, see plate section). ALK expression is virtually specific for ALCL since it is absent from all postnatal normal human tissues except rare cells in the brain.[4] ALK is expressed in rare human neoplasms other than ALCL (see Table 37.1).

GENETIC/MOLECULAR FINDINGS (PLATE 100, TABLE 37.1)

Approximately 90 percent of ALCLs show clonal rearrangement of the T cell receptor (TCR) genes irrespective of whether they express T cell antigens or not.[41] Recurrent chromosomal translocations play an important role in many human lymphoid tumors and are often responsible for the deregulation of genes involved in the control of normal cell proliferation. Anaplastic large cell lymphomas are associated with translocations which involve the *ALK* gene at 2p23 which is normally silent in lymphoid cells.[3,51,52] Originally, ALCL was considered to be strongly linked with the t(2;5)(p23;q35).[3,44,53] This translocation fuses the gene at 5q35 encoding nucleophosmin (*NPM*), a nucleolar-associated phosphoprotein, with the gene coding for the *ALK*, at 2p23.[3,44,53] The resultant hybrid gene encodes a chimeric 80 kD protein in which 40 percent of the N-terminal portion of NPM is fused to the complete intracytoplasmic portion of ALK. However, several studies have shown that about 30 percent of ALK-positive ALCLs are associated with other cytogenetic abnormalities in

Table 37.1   Tumors associated with Alk oncogenic protein

Tumors	ALK fusion proteins
Hematopoietic neoplasms	
Anaplastic large cell lymphoma	NPM-ALK; TPM3-ALK; ATIC-ALK; CLTC-ALK; TFG-ALK; MYH9-ALK; MSN-ALK; ALO17-ALK
Diffuse B cell lymphoma	CLTC-ALK (most cases); NPM-ALK (few cases)[c]
Histiocytic proliferations[a]	TPM3-ALK
Non-hematopoietic neoplasms	
Inflammatory myofibroblastic tumors	TPM3-ALK; TPM4-ALK; CLTC-ALK; RANBP2-ALK; CARS-ALK; SEC31L1-ALK
Neuroblastoma[b]	ALK full-length
Rhabdomyosarcoma[b]	ALK full-length
Nonsmall cell lung tumors	EML4- ALK; TFG-ALK

[a]J Chan.[65]

[b]The oncogenic role of ALK protein in these tumors is not yet elucidated (no prognostic significance).

[c]Some cases express both Cltc-Alk and the full-length Alk protein.

ALK, anaplastic lymphoma kinase; NPM, nucleophosmin; TPM3/4, non-muscular tropomyosin; ATIC, amino-terminus of 5-aminoimidazole-4-carboxamide ribonucleotide formyltransferase/IMP cyclohydrolase; CLTC, clathrin heavy polypeptide; TFG, TRK-fused gene, three different fusion proteins have been described (TFG-ALK$_{short}$, TFG-ALK$_{long}$ and TFG-ALK$_{Xlong}$); MYH9, myosin heavy chain 9; MSN, moesin; ALO17, ALK lymphoma oligomerization partner on chromosome 17; RANBP2, RAN binding protein 2, also known as NUP358; CARS, cysteinyl-tRNA synthetase enzyme; SEC31L1, SEC31-like 1; EML4, echinoderm microtubule-associated protein-like 4.

which *ALK* gene at 2p23 is known to be fused to *TPM3, TPM4, TFG, ATIC, CLTC, MSN, MYH9* and *ALO17* genes.[40,48–50,54–58] All of these translocations result in the expression of chimeric *ALK* transcripts which are translated into ALK fusion proteins with unrestrained tyrosine kinase activity and oncogenic properties. Antibodies recognizing the intracellular portion of ALK react with the full-length ALK protein and all X-ALK fusion proteins. However, the ALK staining pattern is dependent on the ALCL-associated translocations and their resultant ALK fusion proteins (Plate 100).[3,4,34] The classic t(2;5)(p23;q35) leads to positive staining for ALK in the nucleolus, nucleus and the cytoplasm (Plates 99H, xx).[46] In the variant translocations, Alk partners lack nuclear localization signal but they are known to have oligomerization domain located in their amino-terminal portion that could induce dimerization of the chimeric proteins and activation of ALK catalytic domain, i.e. the autophosphorylation of ALK protein.[54] In rare cases, *MSN* (moesin) gene at chromosome Xq11-12, is fused to *ALK* gene and these cases show a distinct ALK membrane restricted staining pattern, probably due to the binding properties of the N-terminal domain of moesin to cell-membrane associated proteins.[57] In these cases, the *ALK* breakpoint, as well as in the *MYH9-ALK* rearrangement,[55] is different from that described in all other translocations and occurs within the exonic sequence coding for the juxtamembrane portion of Alk.[55,57] Of note is that cases with variant translocations will be negative by standard RT-PCR using primers that are specific for the *ALK* and *NPM* genes. Therefore, immunohistochemistry is more reliable than molecular tests for the diagnosis of ALCL.

All X-ALK fusion proteins associated with ALCL are phosphorylated as demonstrated using antibodies detecting phosphorylated X-ALK protein.[59] The fact that oncogenic potential of NPM-ALK is dependent on its tyrosine phosphorylation level underlines the possible implication of tyrosine phosphatases in some down-regulation process. Interestingly, it has been recently demonstrated that SHP1 phosphatase acts as a negative regulator of NPM-ALK phosphorylation and ALCL cell proliferation.[60]

OTHER NEOPLASMS POSITIVE FOR ALK PROTEIN (TABLE 37.1)

- **Diffuse large B cell lymphoma with immunoblastic/plasmablastic morphology expressing ALK protein:**[61] This rare large cell lymphoma consists of monomorphic large plasmablast/immunoblast-like cells with large central nucleoli showing a tendency to invade lymphatic sinuses. At low magnification, these tumors resemble ALCL but they lack CD30. These lymphomas express EMA (as do ALCLs) but also contain intracytoplasmic Ig (usually IgA) of a single light chain type. They usually lack lineage-associated leukocyte antigens (CD3, CD20, CD79a), with the exception in some cases of CD4 and CD57. These tumors express weakly or may even be negative for the leukocyte common antigen CD45.[61,62] These tumors are strongly positive for ALK protein and characteristically show a restricted granular cytoplasmic staining highly indicative of the expression of CLTC-ALK protein and the t(2;17)(p23;q23).[62,63] Few cases may show a cytoplasmic, nuclear and nucleolar Alk staining pattern as seen in ALCL and are associated with NPM-ALK protein and the t(2;5)(p23;q35).[64] Alk-positive diffuse large B cell lymphomas typically follow an aggressive course. This type of lymphoma must be differentiated from other large B cell lymphomas showing a sinusoidal growth pattern, such as so-called 'microvillous lymphomas' which are negative for Alk.

This lymphoma is considered as a distinct entity in the 2008 WHO classification.[6]

- **A novel histiocytic proliferation expressing TPM3-ALK fusion protein**: Recently, J Chan and CW Chow have observed an undescribed histiocytic proliferation positive for Alk protein.[65] Such a proliferation occurs in newborns (3 weeks old) presenting with massive hepatosplenomegaly and a few petechia. Histology of the liver shows portal and sinusoidal infiltration by histiocytes. Rare cells show phagocytosis of red cells or lymphocytes. These cells are positive for CD68 and ALK. The latter staining is restricted to the cytoplasm with membrane reinforcement. Molecular analysis in one case showed *TPM3-ALK* mRNA in agreement with the Alk staining pattern usually observed in ALCL expressing Tpm3-Alk fusion protein.[65]

- **Some nonhematopoietic neoplasms**: These may be positive for ALK but are easily morphologically distinguished from ALCLs. As originally reported by Morris *et al.*,[3] occasional rhabdomyosarcoma can express the full-length ALK protein (200 kD).[5] Some inflammatory myofibroblastic tumors may also be associated with *ALK* gene rearrangement at 2p23.[66] Some neuroblastomas can also express full-length ALK protein but, in contrast to ALCL, the staining is weak.[67] Recently, ALK protein expression has been described in nonsmall cell lung tumors. In these tumors, which account for less than 5 percent of cases, ALK protein is fused to EML4, a microtubule-associated protein.[68,69]

GENE EXPRESSION PROFILING OF ANAPLASTIC LARGE CELL LYMPHOMAS

The recent development of DNA microarrays has provided new biological insights into lymphoproliferative disorders. This approach has mainly been used for B cell lymphomas, in particular diffuse large B cell lymphoma and follicular lymphoma.[70–74] In a recent study, a gene expression profiling analysis has been performed on a series of 32 systemic ALCLs (of which 25 are positive for the oncogenic ALK protein).[75] The supervised analysis by class comparison between ALK-positive and ALK-negative ALCLs provided distinct molecular signatures.

Among the 117 genes overexpressed in ALK-positive ALCLs, *BCL6, PTPN12, SERPIN A1* and *C/EBPβ* are the four top genes, being overexpressed with the most significant *P* value. This overexpression was also confirmed at the protein level, since a nuclear staining for C/EBPβ was detected in 97 percent of ALK-positive cases and in only 5 percent of ALK-negative cases. This finding is in agreement with the recently reported results, by Jundt and coworkers,[76] demonstrating in ALCL cell lines that the overexpression of C/EBPβ, via the AKT/mTOR (mammalian target of rapamycin) pathway activation, led to increased cell proliferation. A body of evidence suggests that C/EBPβ proteins play a central role in the balance between cell differentiation and proliferation, depending on the ratio between the main isoforms (i.e. LAP and LIP) transcribed from a single mRNA. Given that the expression of the LIP isoform of C/EBPβ, which promotes cell proliferation, is depending on the activation of the AKT/mTOR pathway, therapeutic drugs like rapamycin targeting this pathway could be used to treat ALK-positive ALCLs as suggested by Vega *et al.*[77] As already reported, the great majority of ALK-positive cases were positively stained by BCL6 antibody (80 percent). The expression of the tyrosine phosphatase PTPN12 (also named Ptp-PEST), described as a negative regulator of ABL kinase activity,[78] has never been reported in lymphoma. However, it was recently shown that SHP1, another protein tyrosine phosphatase, is expressed in ALK-positive ALCL and involved in NPM-ALK dephosphorylation.[60] A potentially interesting gene overexpressed in Alk-positive ALCLs is the *SERPIN A1* gene, which encodes a plasma serine proteinase inhibitor. In a recent study, Serpin A1 expression was correlated with the clinical status of patients and the *SERPIN A1* mRNA level was higher in patients presenting with extranodal dissemination. These data, together with the pattern of expression of Serpin A1 in ALK-positive tumors, suggest that Serpin A1 has an invasion-promoting effect in ALCL.[79]

The molecular signature of ALK-negative ALCLs consisted of 186 genes and included overexpression of four genes (*CCR7, CNTFR, IL22* and *IL21*) with the most significant *P* value. However, the functional categories of the genes overexpressed in ALK-negative ALCLs did not provide any obvious clues to the molecular mechanism(s) underlying this tumor subtype, since these genes tended to be associated with nonspecific biologic functions.

EXPERIMENTAL STUDIES, TRANSGENIC MOUSE MODELS AND ALK INHIBITORS

Experimental analysis of the transforming properties of X–ALK fusion proteins

The results observed both *in vitro* and *in vivo* with stably transfected NIH3T3 cells confirm the transforming properties of the X-ALK variants as well as the tumorigenicity of X-ALK-expressing cells in nude mice.[80] In the study by Armstrong and coworkers,[80] the NPM-ALK, TPM3-ALK, TFG-ALK, CLTC-ALK and ATIC-ALK fusion proteins were tyrosine phosphorylated and functional in NIH3T3 transfected cells as demonstrated by using *in vitro* kinase assay. In addition, NIH3T3 transfected cells showed the same subcellular distribution of the X-ALK proteins as seen in human ALCL. However, these effects, including growth properties and proliferation rates of NIH3T3 transfected cells were dependent on the level of X-ALK fusion proteins and on the ALK partners. Indeed, the analysis of NIH3T3 clones expressing increasing amount of NPM-ALK, TFG-ALK, CLTC-ALK, or ATIC-ALK showed a significant correlation between the level of fusion proteins and the proliferation rate (except for TPM3-ALK). However, cells expressing TPM3-ALK protein were found to be much more invasive *in vitro* than the other X-ALK expressing cells. The biologic behaviour of cells expressing TPM3-ALK protein, different from NIH3T3 cells expressing the other X-ALK variants, suggests that the partner of ALK may serve additional functions for oncogenesis other than promoting homo-oligomerization with resultant kinase activation.[80] Such a difference in the biologic behavior of TPM3-ALK versus the other X-ALK expressing cells has not yet been elucidated as well as its clinical relevance.

Transgenic models

The development of animal models for ALK oncogene-induced tumorigenesis is critical to understand the molecular mechanisms underlying tumor development and to evaluate, *in vivo*, the efficiency of ALK-specific tyrosine kinase inhibitors. To drive expression of NPM-ALK in the T cell lineage, three strategies have been used. *NPM-ALK* cDNA was cloned either downstream of murine *CD4*,[81] *Vav*[82] or *Lck* promoters.[83] Transgenic mice with enforced NPM-ALK expression under the regulation of the *CD4* promoter developed clonal lymphoproliferative diseases represented mainly by thymic lymphomas and plasma cells tumors, including multiple myeloma.[81] Using the hematopoietic cell specific *Vav* promoter, transgenic mice developed lymphomas that displayed B lineage features with aberrant coexpression of myeloid markers.[82] More recently, by using the *Lck* promoter, NPM-ALK expression was limited to early T cells[83] and mice died from lymphoma characterized by thymic and lymph node involvement as well as extranodal infiltration by large-sized tumor cells.

Of note, adoptive transfer of *NPM-ALK* retrovirally transduced bone marrow cells resulted in the generation of chimeric mouse models, developing B cell lymphomas, plasmacytomas and more rarely histiocyte-rich lymphoma depending on the low or high level of NPM-ALK expression.[84,85] Lange *et al.* reported that the transfer of *NPM-ALK* transduced bone marrow cells into lethally irradiated interleukin (IL)-9 transgenic mice led to the development of either T lymphoblastic lymphomas, plasmacytomas or diffuse large B cell lymphomas.[86] Overall, none of these models are strictly comparable with human ALCL and no conditional mouse models for NPM-ALK expression have been reported so far.

ALK tyrosine kinase inhibitors

ALK tyrosine kinase activity is essential for tumorigenesis, as demonstrated using either transformed cell lines or animal models. Therefore, the targeted inactivation of ALK offers a rational approach for the treatment of ALK-dependent tumors. Several strategies (reviewed by Pulford *et al.*[87]) have been developed to inhibit Alk signaling. They include gene therapy, *ALK* RNA targeted approaches and

immunotherapy. In addition, the development of ALK tyrosine kinase specific inhibitors has been motivated by the success of the STI-571 (Gleevec) compound which targets the ABL, KIT and PDGFR tyrosine kinases. Only a few ALK inhibitors, validated on high-throughput enzymatic assay and/or Alk-positive cell lines, have been reported so far. In general, their efficiency and selectivity should be improved and further *in vivo* studies are expected to determine their bioavailability and their toxicity.

ALK inhibition has been reported using herbimycin A[88] or 17-allylamino, 17-demethoxygeldanamycin molecules.[89] These compounds prevent NPM-ALK /Hsp90 stabilization, leading to premature proteosomal degradation of the oncogenic ALK protein. Fused pyrrolocarbazole (FP) derived small molecules (CEP-14083 and CEP-14513), by inhibiting NPM-ALK phosphorylation, induce proliferative arrest and apoptotic cell death.[90] 5-Aryl-pyridone-3-carboxamide derivates have been recently discovered as ALK ATP-competitive inhibitors.[91] In this context, a recent study describes computer modeling of ALK kinase domain that should help in the design of ALK ATP-competitive inhibitors.[92] Finally, STAT3 inhibitors (WHI-131 and WHI-154) directly inhibit Npm-Alk enzymatic activity and signaling.[93] Another Stat3 inhibitor, JSI-124 (cucurbitacin I), increases NPM-ALK proteosomal degradation.[94] Recently, two small molecules, NVP-TAE684 and PF-2341066, have been identified as potent inhibitors of ALK.[95,96] However, until now, none of these ALK inhibitors have been tested in clinical trials.

CLINICAL COURSE AND PROGNOSTIC FACTORS

The international prognostic index (IPI) appears to be of some value in predicting outcome, although less so than in other variants of lymphoma.[5,97] The most important prognostic indicator in ALCL is ALK positivity, which has been associated with a favorable prognosis in series from North America, Europe, and Japan.[5,97,98] No differences have been found between NPM-ALK-positive tumors and tumors showing variant translocations involving *ALK* and fusion partners other than *NPM*.[5,97] The overall 5-year survival rate in ALK-positive ALCLs is close to 80 percent, in contrast to only 40 percent in ALK-negative cases. Relapses are not uncommon (30 percent of cases), but often remain sensitive to chemotherapy.[99] In a recent study, using gene expression profiling of ALCLs, the pattern discovery based on an extensive cluster analysis using the most varying genes across a series of 32 samples showed a robust bi-partition of the ALCL tumor samples in two clusters. Cases of the first cluster were mostly ALCLs with common-type morphology, while the second cluster was enriched with cases diagnosed as morphologic variant ALCL (i.e. small cell variant and 'mixed ALCL'). In addition, patients in the first group were Ann Arbor stage I/II at diagnosis while those in the second group presented with advanced stage disease (i.e. Ann Arbor stage III/IV). Most importantly, a significant number of patients in the latter group developed early relapse (i.e. at most, 1 year after diagnosis). These results based on a limited number of cases may have clinical implications since they suggest that tumors in patients that relapse within one year after diagnosis express a set of genes which could be of clinical and therapeutic value.[75]

The available data indicate that the clinical outcome of ALK-negative ALCL with conventional therapy is clearly poorer than that of ALK-positive ALCL.[100]

KEY POINTS

Clinical

- 5 percent of all NHLs.
- Most frequent in the first three decades, slight male predominance.
- Most patients present with advanced stage.
- Frequent extranodal involvement (skin: 30 percent of cases).
- Frequent occult bone marrow involvement; some patients present with leukemic cells.
- 5 year overall survival: ALK+ = 70–80 percent; ALK−: 40–50 percent.

Morphology/immunophenotype

- ALK-positive ALCL is a distinct entity; ALK-negative ALCL is a provisional entity.
- Five morphological patterns of ALK+ ALCL (2008 WHO classification).
- All cases show characteristic cells designated as 'hallmark cells'.
- ALCL (both ALK+ and ALK−) are of T/null phenotype and strongly positive for CD30 and EMA.
- Other rare neoplasms may be positive for ALK

Cytogenetics/molecular genetics

- t(2;5)/*NPM-ALK* in 75 percent of cases; t(1;2)/*TPM3-ALK* in 15 percent of cases.
- Molecular signature of ALK+ ALCL: *BCL6+, SERPIN.A1+, CEBPB+, PTPN12+*.
- Molecular signature of ALK-ALCL: *CCR7+, CNTFR+, IL22+, IL21+*.

Pathogenesis

- Autophosphorylation of X-ALK protein is responsible for its oncogenic properties.
- Transgenic mice expressing ALK develop lymphoproliferative disorders (B>T).
- Some ALK tyrosine kinase inhibitors are in pre-clinical development.

REFERENCES

● = Key primary paper
◆ = Major review article

●1. Stein H, Mason DY, Gerdes J et al. The expression of the Hodgkin's disease associated antigen Ki-1 in reactive and neoplastic lymphoid tissue: evidence that Reed-Sternberg cells and histiocytic malignancies are derived from activated lymphoid cells. Blood 1985; 66: 848–58.

●2. Delsol G, Ralfkiaer E, Stein H et al. Anaplastic large cell lymphoma. Primary systemic (T/Null cell type). In: Jaffe ES, Harris NL, Stein H, Vardiman JW. (eds) World Health Organization (WHO) classification of tumours pathology and genetics of tumours of haematopoietic and lymphoid tissues. Lyon: IARC Press, 2001: 230–5.

●3. Morris SW, Kirstein MN, Valentine MB et al. Fusion of a kinase gene, ALK, to a nucleolar protein gene, NPM, in non-Hodgkin's lymphoma. Science 1994; 263: 1281–4.

4. Pulford K, Lamant L, Morris SW et al. Detection of anaplastic lymphoma kinase (ALK) and nucleolar protein nucleophosmin (NPM)-ALK proteins in normal and neoplastic cells with the monoclonal antibody ALK1. Blood 1997; 89: 1394–404.

5. Falini B, Bigerna B, Fizzotti M et al. ALK expression defines a distinct group of T/null lymphomas ('ALK lymphomas') with a wide morphological spectrum. Am J Pathol 1998; 153: 875–86.

●◆6. Swerdlow SH, Campo E, Harris NL et al. (eds) WHO classification of tumours of haematopoietic and lymphoid tissues. Lyon: IARC, 2008.

7. Ralfkiaer E, Delsol G, Willemze R, Jaffe ES. Primary cutaneous CD30-positive T-cell lymphoproliferative disorders. In: Jaffe ES, Harris NL, Stein H, Vardiman JW. (eds) World Health Organization (WHO) classification of tumours pathology and genetics of tumours of haematopoietic and lymphoid tissues. Lyon: IARC Press, 2001: 221–4.

8. Stein H, Foss HD, Durkop H et al. CD30(+) anaplastic large cell lymphoma: a review of its histopathologic, genetic, and clinical features. Blood 2000; 96: 3681–95.

9. Benharroch D, Meguerian-Bedoyan Z, Lamant L et al. ALK-positive lymphoma: a single disease with a broad spectrum of morphology. Blood 1998; 91: 2076–84.

10. Brugieres L, Deley MC, Pacquement H et al. CD30(+) anaplastic large-cell lymphoma in children: analysis of 82 patients enrolled in two consecutive studies of the French Society of Pediatric Oncology. Blood 1998; 92: 3591–8.

11. Bakshi NA, Ross CW, Finn WG et al. ALK-positive anaplastic large cell lymphoma with primary bone involvement in children. Am J Clin Pathol 2006; 125: 57–63.

12. Meguerian-Bedoyan Z, Lamant L, Hopfner C et al. Anaplastic large cell lymphoma of maternal origin involving the placenta: case report and literature survey. Am J Surg Pathol 1997; 21: 1236–41.

13. Fraga M, Brousset P, Schlaifer D *et al.* Bone marrow involvement in anaplastic large cell lymphoma. Immunohistochemical detection of minimal disease and its prognostic significance. *Am J Clin Pathol* 1995; **103**: 82–9.

14. Pulford K, Falini B, Banham AH *et al.* Immune response to the ALK oncogenic tyrosine kinase in patients with anaplastic large-cell lymphoma. *Blood* 2000; **96**: 1605–7.

15. Falini B. Anaplastic large cell lymphoma: pathological, molecular and clinical features. *Br J Haematol* 2001; **114**: 741–60.

16. Chan JK, Buchanan R, Fletcher CD. Sarcomatoid variant of anaplastic large-cell Ki-1 lymphoma. *Am J Surg Pathol* 1990; **14**: 983–8.

17. Falini B, Pileri S, Zinzani PL *et al.* ALK+ lymphoma: clinico-pathological findings and outcome. *Blood* 1999; **93**: 2697–706.

18. Jaffe ES. *Malignant histiocytosis and true histiocytic lymphomas.* Philadelphia: WB Sanders, 1995.

19. Kinney MC, Collins RD, Greer JP *et al.* A small-cell-predominant variant of primary Ki-1 (CD30)+ T-cell lymphoma. *Am J Surg Pathol* 1993; **17**: 859–68.

20. Pileri SA, Pulford K, Mori S *et al.* Frequent expression of the NPM-ALK chimeric fusion protein in anaplastic large-cell lymphoma, lympho-histiocytic type. *Am J Pathol* 1997; **150**: 1207–11.

21. Nakamura S, Shiota M, Nakagawa A *et al.* Anaplastic large cell lymphoma: a distinct molecular pathologic entity: a reappraisal with special reference to p80(NPM/ALK) expression. *Am J Surg Pathol* 1997; **21**: 1420–32.

22. Hodges KB, Collins RD, Greer JP *et al.* Transformation of the small cell variant Ki-1+ lymphoma to anaplastic large cell lymphoma: pathologic and clinical features. *Am J Surg Pathol* 1999; **23**: 49–58.

23. Pileri S, Falini B, Delsol G *et al.* Lymphohistiocytic T-cell lymphoma (anaplastic large cell lymphoma CD30+/Ki-1 + with a high content of reactive histiocytes). *Histopathology* 1990; **16**: 383–91.

24. Bayle C, Charpentier A, Duchayne E *et al.* Leukaemic presentation of small cell variant anaplastic large cell lymphoma: report of four cases. *Br J Haematol* 1999; **104**: 680–8.

25. Chhanabhai M, Britten C, Klasa R, Gascoyne RD. t(2;5) positive lymphoma with peripheral blood involvement. *Leuk Lymphoma* 1998; **28**: 415–22.

26. Jaffe ES. Anaplastic large cell lymphoma: the shifting sands of diagnostic hematopathology. *Mod Pathol* 2001; **14**: 219–28.

27. Jaffe ES, Harris NL, Stein H, Vardiman JW. *World Health Organization classification of tumours. Pathology and genetics: tumours of haematopoietic and lymphoid tissues.* Lyon: IARC Press, 2001.

28. Vassallo J, Lamant L, Brugieres L *et al.* ALK-positive anaplastic large cell lymphoma mimicking nodular sclerosis Hodgkin's lymphoma: report of 10 cases. *Am J Surg Pathol* 2006; **30**: 223–9.

29. Harris NL, Jaffe ES, Stein H *et al.* A revised European-American classification of lymphoid neoplasms: a proposal from the International Lymphoma Study Group. *Blood* 1994; **84**: 1361–92.

30. Stein H, Dallenbach F. Diffuse large cell lymphomas of B and T cell type. In: Knowles DM (ed.) *Neoplastic hematopathology.* Baltimore: Williams and Wilkins, 1992: 675–714.

31. Pileri S, Bocchia M, Baroni CD *et al.* Anaplastic large cell lymphoma (CD30 +/Ki-1+): results of a prospective clinico-pathological study of 69 cases. *Br J Haematol* 1994; **86**: 513–23.

32. Zinzani PL, Martelli M, Magagnoli M *et al.* Anaplastic large cell lymphoma Hodgkin's-like: a randomized trial of ABVD versus MACOP-B with and without radiation therapy. *Blood* 1998; **92**: 790–4.

33. Orscheschek K, Merz H, Hell J *et al.* Large-cell anaplastic lymphoma-specific translocation (t[2;5] [p23;q35]) in Hodgkin's disease: indication of a common pathogenesis. *Lancet* 1995; **345**: 87–90.

34. Lamant L, Meggetto F, al Saati T *et al.* High incidence of the t(2;5)(p23;q35) translocation in anaplastic large cell lymphoma and its lack of detection in Hodgkin's disease. Comparison of cytogenetic analysis, reverse transcriptase-polymerase chain reaction, and P-80 immunostaining. *Blood* 1996; **87**: 284–91.

35. Weiss LM, Lopategui JR, Sun LH *et al.* Absence of the t(2;5) in Hodgkin's disease. *Blood* 1995; **85**: 2845–7.

36. Mann KP, Hall B, Kamino H *et al.* Neutrophil-rich, Ki-1-positive anaplastic large-cell malignant lymphoma. *Am J Surg Pathol* 1995; **19**: 407–16.

37. McCluggage WG, Walsh MY, Bharucha H. Anaplastic large cell malignant lymphoma with extensive eosinophilic or neutrophilic infiltration. *Histopathology* 1998; **32**: 110–15.

38. Cheuk W, Hill RW, Bacchi C *et al.* Hypocellular anaplastic large cell lymphoma mimicking inflammatory lesions of lymph nodes. *Am J Surg Pathol* 2000; **24**: 1537–43.

●39. Delsol G, Al Saati T, Gatter KC *et al.* Coexpression of epithelial membrane antigen (EMA), Ki-1, and interleukin-2 receptor by anaplastic large cell lymphomas. Diagnostic value in so-called malignant histiocytosis. *Am J Pathol* 1988; **130**: 59–70.

40. Meech SJ, McGavran L, Odom LF *et al.* Unusual childhood extramedullary hematologic malignancy with natural killer cell properties that contains tropomyosin 4–anaplastic lymphoma kinase gene fusion. *Blood* 2001; **98**: 1209–16.

41. Foss HD, Anagnostopoulos I, Araujo I *et al.* Anaplastic large-cell lymphomas of T-cell and null-cell phenotype express cytotoxic molecules. *Blood* 1996; **88**: 4005–11.

42. Krenacs L, Wellmann A, Sorbara L *et al.* Cytotoxic cell antigen expression in anaplastic large cell lymphomas of T- and null-cell type and Hodgkin's disease: evidence for distinct cellular origin. *Blood* 1997; **89**: 980–9.

43. Delsol G, Blancher A, al Saati T *et al.* Antibody BNH9 detects red blood cell-related antigens on anaplastic large cell (CD30+) lymphomas. *Br J Cancer* 1991; **64**: 321–6.

44. Brousset P, Rochaix P, Chittal S *et al.* High incidence of Epstein-Barr virus detection in Hodgkin's disease and

absence of detection in anaplastic large-cell lymphoma in children. *Histopathology* 1993; **23**: 189–91.

45. Villalva C, Bougrine F, Delsol G, Brousset P. Bcl-2 expression in anaplastic large cell lymphoma. *Am J Pathol* 2001; **158**: 1889–90.

●46. Mason DY, Pulford KA, Bischof D *et al.* Nucleolar localization of the nucleophosmin-anaplastic lymphoma kinase is not required for malignant transformation. *Cancer Res* 1998; **58**: 1057–62.

47. Bischof D, Pulford K, Mason DY, Morris SW. Role of the nucleophosmin (NPM) portion of the non-Hodgkin's lymphoma-associated NPM-anaplastic lymphoma kinase fusion protein in oncogenesis. *Mol Cell Biol* 1997; **17**: 2312–25.

●48. Hernandez L, Pinyol M, Hernandez S *et al.* TRK-fused gene (TFG) is a new partner of ALK in anaplastic large cell lymphoma producing two structurally different TFG-ALK translocations. *Blood* 1999; **94**: 3265–8.

●49. Trinei M, Lanfrancone L, Campo E *et al.* A new variant anaplastic lymphoma kinase (ALK)-fusion protein (ATIC-ALK) in a case of ALK-positive anaplastic large cell lymphoma. *Cancer Res* 2000; **60**: 793–8.

●50. Touriol C, Greenland C, Lamant L *et al.* Further demonstration of the diversity of chromosomal changes involving 2p23 in ALK-positive lymphoma: 2 cases expressing ALK kinase fused to CLTCL (clathrin chain polypeptide-like). *Blood* 2000; **95**: 3204–7.

◆51. Amin HM, Lai R. Pathobiology of ALK+ anaplastic large-cell lymphoma. *Blood* 2007; **110**: 2259–67.

◆52. Chiarle R, Voena C, Ambrogio C *et al.* The anaplastic lymphoma kinase in the pathogenesis of cancer. *Nat Rev Cancer* 2008; **8**: 11–23.

◆53. Duyster J, Bai RY, Morris SW. Translocations involving anaplastic lymphoma kinase (ALK). *Oncogene* 2001; **20**: 5623–37.

●54. Lamant L, Dastugue N, Pulford K *et al.* A new fusion gene TPM3-ALK in anaplastic large cell lymphoma created by a (1;2)(q25;p23) translocation. *Blood* 1999; **93**: 3088–95.

●55. Lamant L, Gascoyne RD, Duplantier MM *et al.* Non-muscle myosin heavy chain (MYH9): a new partner fused to ALK in anaplastic large cell lymphoma. *Genes Chromosomes Cancer* 2003; **37**: 427–32.

●56. Rosenwald A, Ott G, Pulford K *et al.* t(1;2)(q21;p23) and t(2;3)(p23;q21): two novel variant translocations of the t(2;5)(p23;q35) in anaplastic large cell lymphoma. *Blood* 1999; **94**: 362–4.

●57. Tort F, Pinyol M, Pulford K *et al.* Molecular characterization of a new ALK translocation involving moesin (MSN-ALK) in anaplastic large cell lymphoma. *Lab Invest* 2001; **81**: 419–26.

●58. Wlodarska I, De Wolf-Peeters C, Falini B *et al.* The cryptic inv(2)(p23q35) defines a new molecular genetic subtype of ALK-positive anaplastic large-cell lymphoma. *Blood* 1998; **92**: 2688–95.

59. Pulford K, Delsol G, Roncador G *et al.* Immunohistochemical screening for oncogenic tyrosine kinase activation. *J Pathol* 1999; **187**: 588–93.

60. Honorat JF, Ragab A, Lamant L *et al.* SHP1 tyrosine phosphatase negatively regulates NPM-ALK tyrosine kinase signaling. *Blood* 2006; **107**: 4130–8.

61. Delsol G, Lamant L, Mariame B *et al.* A new subtype of large B-cell lymphoma expressing the ALK kinase and lacking the 2; 5 translocation. *Blood* 1997; **89**: 1483–90.

●62. Gascoyne RD, Lamant L, Martin-Subero JI *et al.* ALK-positive diffuse large B-cell lymphoma is associated with Clathrin-ALK rearrangements: report of 6 cases. *Blood* 2003; **102**: 2568–73.

63. De Paepe P, Baens M, van Krieken H *et al.* ALK activation by the CLTC-ALK fusion is a recurrent event in large B-cell lymphoma. *Blood* 2003; **102**: 2638–41.

64. Adam P, Katzenberger T, Seeberger H *et al.* A case of a diffuse large B-cell lymphoma of plasmablastic type associated with the t(2;5)(p23;q35) chromosome translocation. *Am J Surg Pathol* 2003; **27**: 1473–6.

●65. Chan JKC, Lamant L, Algar E *et al.* ALK+ histiocytosis: a novel type of systemic histiocytic proliferative disorder of infancy. *Blood* 2008; **112**: 2965–8.

●66. Griffin CA, Hawkins AL, Dvorak C *et al.* Recurrent involvement of 2p23 in inflammatory myofibroblastic tumors. *Cancer Res* 1999; **59**: 2776–80.

●67. Lamant L, Pulford K, Bischof D *et al.* Expression of the ALK tyrosine kinase gene in neuroblastoma. *Am J Pathol* 2000; **156**: 1711–21.

68. Rikova K, Guo A, Zeng Q *et al.* Global survey of phosphotyrosine signaling identifies oncogenic kinases in lung cancer. *Cell* 2007; **131**: 1190–203.

●69. Soda M, Choi YL, Enomoto M *et al.* Identification of the transforming EML4-ALK fusion gene in non-small-cell lung cancer. *Nature* 2007; **448**: 561–6.

70. Alizadeh AA, Eisen MB, Davis RE *et al.* Distinct types of diffuse large B-cell lymphoma identified by gene expression profiling. *Nature* 2000; **403**: 503–11.

71. Rosenwald A, Wright G, Chan WC *et al.* The use of molecular profiling to predict survival after chemotherapy for diffuse large-B-cell lymphoma. *N Engl J Med* 2002; **346**: 1937–47.

72. Shipp MA, Ross KN, Tamayo P *et al.* Diffuse large B-cell lymphoma outcome prediction by gene-expression profiling and supervised machine learning. *Nat Med* 2002; **8**: 68–74.

73. Wright G, Tan B, Rosenwald A *et al.* A gene expression-based method to diagnose clinically distinct subgroups of diffuse large B cell lymphoma. *Proc Natl Acad Sci U S A* 2003; **100**: 9991–6.

74. Dave SS, Wright G, Tan B *et al.* Prediction of survival in follicular lymphoma based on molecular features of tumor-infiltrating immune cells. *N Engl J Med* 2004; **351**: 2159–69.

●75. Lamant L, De Reynies A, Duplantier M *et al.* Gene expression profiling of systemic anaplastic large cell lymphoma reveals differences depending on ALK status and two distinct morphological ALK+ subtype. *Blood* 2007; **109**: 2156–64.

76. Jundt F, Raetzel N, Muller C *et al.* A rapamycin derivative (everolimus) controls proliferation through down-regulation

of truncated CCAAT enhancer binding protein {beta} and NF-{kappa}B activity in Hodgkin and anaplastic large cell lymphomas. *Blood* 2005; **106**: 1801–7.

77. Vega F, Medeiros LJ, Leventaki V *et al.* Activation of mammalian target of rapamycin signaling pathway contributes to tumor cell survival in anaplastic lymphoma kinase-positive anaplastic large cell lymphoma. *Cancer Res* 2006; **66**: 6589–97.

78. Cong F, Spencer S, Cote JF *et al.* Cytoskeletal protein PSTPIP1 directs the PEST-type protein tyrosine phosphatase to the c-Abl kinase to mediate Abl dephosphorylation. *Mol Cell* 2000; **6**: 1413–23.

79. Duplantier MM, Lamant L, Sabourdy F *et al.* Serpin A1 is overexpressed in ALK(+) anaplastic large cell lymphoma and its expression correlates with extranodal dissemination. *Leukemia* 2006; **20**: 1848–54.

80. Armstrong F, Duplantier MM, Trempat P *et al.* Differential effects of X-ALK fusion proteins on proliferation, transformation, and invasion properties of NIH3T3 cells. *Oncogene* 2004; **23**: 6071–82.

81. Chiarle R, Gong JZ, Guasparri I *et al.* NPM-ALK transgenic mice spontaneously develop T-cell lymphomas and plasma cell tumors. *Blood* 2003; **101**: 1919–27.

82. Turner SD, Tooze R, Maclennan K, Alexander DR. Vav-promoter regulated oncogenic fusion protein NPM-ALK in transgenic mice causes B-cell lymphomas with hyperactive Jun kinase. *Oncogene* 2003; **22**: 7750–61.

83. Jager R, Hahne J, Jacob A *et al.* Mice transgenic for NPM-ALK develop non-Hodgkin lymphomas. *Anticancer Res* 2005; **25**: 3191–6.

84. Kuefer MU, Look AT, Pulford K *et al.* Retrovirus-mediated gene transfer of NPM-ALK causes lymphoid malignancy in mice. *Blood* 1997; **90**: 2901–10.

85. Miething C, Grundler R, Fend F *et al.* The oncogenic fusion protein nucleophosmin-anaplastic lymphoma kinase (NPM-ALK) induces two distinct malignant phenotypes in a murine retroviral transplantation model. *Oncogene* 2003; **22**: 4642–7.

86. Lange K, Uckert W, Blankenstein T *et al.* Overexpression of NPM-ALK induces different types of malignant lymphomas in IL-9 transgenic mice. *Oncogene* 2003; **22**: 517–27.

♦87. Pulford K, Lamant L, Espinos E *et al.* The emerging normal and disease-related roles of anaplastic lymphoma kinase. *Cell Mol Life Sci* 2004; **61**: 2939–53.

88. Turturro F, Arnold MD, Frist AY, Pulford K. Model of inhibition of the NPM-ALK kinase activity by herbimycin A. *Clin Cancer Res* 2002; **8**: 240–5.

89. Bonvini P, Gastaldi T, Falini B, Rosolen A. Nucleophosmin-anaplastic lymphoma kinase (NPM-ALK), a novel Hsp90-client tyrosine kinase: down-regulation of NPM-ALK expression and tyrosine phosphorylation in

ALK(+) CD30(+) lymphoma cells by the Hsp90 antagonist 17-allylamino,17-demethoxygeldanamycin. *Cancer Res* 2002; **62**: 1559–66.

90. Wan W, Albom MS, Lu L *et al.* Anaplastic lymphoma kinase activity is essential for the proliferation and survival of anaplastic large-cell lymphoma cells. *Blood* 2006; **107**: 1617–23.

91. Li R, Xue L, Zhu T *et al.* Design and synthesis of 5-aryl-pyridone-carboxamides as inhibitors of anaplastic lymphoma kinase. *J Med Chem* 2006; **49**: 1006–15.

92. Gunby RH, Ahmed S, Sottocornola R *et al.* Structural insights into the ATP binding pocket of the anaplastic lymphoma kinase by site-directed mutagenesis, inhibitor binding analysis, and homology modeling. *J Med Chem* 2006; **49**: 5759–68.

93. Marzec M, Kasprzycka M, Ptasznik A *et al.* Inhibition of ALK enzymatic activity in T-cell lymphoma cells induces apoptosis and suppresses proliferation and STAT3 phosphorylation independently of Jak3. *Lab Invest* 2005; **85**: 1544–54.

94. Shi X, Franko B, Frantz C *et al.* JSI-124 (cucurbitacin I) inhibits Janus kinase-3/signal transducer and activator of transcription-3 signalling, downregulates nucleophosmin-anaplastic lymphoma kinase (ALK), and induces apoptosis in ALK-positive anaplastic large cell lymphoma cells. *Br J Haematol* 2006; **135**: 26–32.

95. Galkin AV, Melnick JS, Kim S *et al.* Identification of NVP-TAE684, a potent, selective, and efficacious inhibitor of NPM-ALK. *Proc Natl Acad Sci U S A* 2007;**104**:270–5.

96. Christensen JG, Zou HY, Arango ME *et al.* Cytoreductive antitumor activity of PF-2341066, a novel inhibitor of anaplastic lymphoma kinase and c-Met, in experimental models of anaplastic large-cell lymphoma. *Mol Cancer Ther* 2007;**6**:3314–22.

●97. Gascoyne RD, Aoun P, Wu D *et al.* Prognostic significance of anaplastic lymphoma kinase (ALK) protein expression in adults with anaplastic large cell lymphoma. *Blood* 1999; **93**: 3913–21.

98. Shiota M, Nakamura S, Ichinohasama R *et al.* Anaplastic large cell lymphomas expressing the novel chimeric protein p80NPM/ALK: a distinct clinicopathologic entity. *Blood* 1995; **86**: 1954–60.

●99. Brugieres L, Quartier P, Le Deley MC *et al.* Relapses of childhood anaplastic large-cell lymphoma: treatment results in a series of 41 children – a report from the French society of pediatric oncology. *Ann Oncol* 2000; **11**: 53–8.

100. ten Berge RL, de Bruin PC, Oudejans JJ *et al.* ALK-negative anaplastic large-cell lymphoma demonstrates similar poor prognosis to peripheral T-cell lymphoma, unspecified. *Histopathology* 2003; **43**: 462–9.

38

Mycosis fungoides and Sézary syndrome: pathophysiology and pathology

KAREN TARASZKA, EARL J GLUSAC, LYNN D WILSON AND MICHAEL GIRARDI

PATHOPHYSIOLOGY

Cutaneous T cell lymphoma (CTCL) encompasses a wide range of disorders with various manifestations, clinical courses and therapeutic considerations. Mycosis fungoides (MF) is the most common form of CTCL in which the skin may be variably affected by flat patches, thin plaques or tumors. Sézary syndrome (SS) is a more aggressive form of CTCL in which there is diffuse skin involvement (erythroderma) and substantial peripheral blood involvement. MF/SS is a malignancy of the skin-homing population of T lymphocytes. The fact that a proportion of patients with MF will eventually progress to SS, as well as the corollary observation that after treatment, a patient previously with SS may demonstrate lesions typical of MF, indicates that MF and SS are different manifestations of the same malignancy. Fundamental to their clinical manifestations, the clonal T cells in MF/SS utilize the same mechanisms as normal T lymphocytes to infiltrate/populate the skin. Especially relevant in more advanced disease, like normal recirculating T cells, MF/SS cells may also traffic to variably involve the lymph nodes and peripheral blood. MF/SS cells will express a particular T cell receptor (TCR) and demonstrate an activated, memory phenotype. Within the compartments of skin, lymph nodes, and blood, MF/SS cells are further characterized by their resistance to apoptosis, clonal expansion, and capacity to exert regulatory effects on the remaining T cell repertoire/populations. Hence, a detailed consideration of normal T cell physiology is fundamental to the understanding of the pathogenesis of CTCL.

Skin dependence

The molecular interactions involved in the ability of malignant T cells to migrate to and reside in the skin are part of the normal physiology of immunosurveillance of the skin (reviewed in Kupper and Fuhlbrigge,[1] summarized in Table 38.1). MF/SS may be considered a malignancy of skin-homing T cells which express the cell surface receptor called cutaneous lymphocyte-associated antigen (CLA).[2] CLA is produced by an inducible carbohydrate modification of a ubiquitously expressed T cell surface protein, PSGL1, through post-translational modification of PSGL1 by $\alpha(1,3)$-fucosyltransferase VII.[8] CLA facilitates homing of memory T cells to the skin by mediating tethering and rolling via E-selectin (CD62E) on dermal post-capillary endothelial cells. E-selectin expression is upregulated by proinflammatory cytokines such as interleukin (IL)-1 and tumor necrosis factor (TNF)-α. As T cells circulate through post-capillary venules, the first step in lymphocyte homing is rolling on endothelial selectins, followed by chemokine receptor activation, integrin-mediated firm adhesion between the lymphocyte and endothelial cells and, finally, tissue extravasation.

Table 38.1   Molecular interactions involved in T lymphocytes homing to and resident in the skin

T cell surface molecule	Ligand	Role	Identified in MF/SS (reference)
CLA	E-selectin	Mediates rolling and tethering on endothelial cells	2
CCR4	CCL17 (TARC) expressed by basal keratinocytes and present on dermal endothelial cells	Epidermotropism; triggers integrin activation	3,4
	CCL22 (MDC) expressed by Langerhans cells and dermal dendritic cells	Epidermotropism and interaction with dendritic cells	4
CCR7	CCL21 (SLC)	Homing to lymph nodes	5
Integrins			
$\alpha_4\beta_1$	VCAM-1 on endothelial cells	Firm adhesion	
$\alpha_L\beta_2$ (LFA1)	ICAM family on endothelial cells and Langerhans cells	Firm adhesion; retention in epidermis	
$\alpha_E\beta_7$	E-cadherin on keratinocytes and Langerhans cells	Retention in epidermis	6
CCR10	CCL27 (CTACK) expressed by basal keratinocytes and present on dermal endothelial cells	Epidermotropism; triggers integrin activation	5
CXCR3	CXCL9 (Mig), CXCL10 (IP-10), CXCL11 (IP-9) on basal keratinocytes	Epidermotropism	7

CLA, cutaneous lymphocyte-associated antigen; CCR, CC-chemokine receptor; TARC, thymus and activation-regulated chemokine; MDC, macrophage-derived chemokine; CCL, CC chemokine ligands; IP, interferon-γ-inducible protein; LFA, lymphocyte function-associated antigen; VCAM, vascular cell adhesion molecule; ICAM, intercellular adhesion molecule; Mig, monokine induced by interferon-γ.

Activation of G-protein–coupled chemokine receptors

Chemokines have two conserved internal disulfide loops and are named based on whether the two amino-terminal cysteine residues are adjacent [CC] or are separated by one amino acid [CXC]. Chemokine receptors are named numerically depending on whether they bind CC or CXC chemokines, e.g. CCR1, CCR2, CXCR1 and CXCR2. The chemokines are named numerically as CC or CXC ligands [L], e.g. CCL1, CCL2, CXCL1 and CXCL2. Migrating T cells trigger a conformational change in cell surface integrins allowing firm adhesion to the endothelial cell. CCR-4 and its ligands, thymus and activation-regulated chemokine (TARC, CCL17) and macrophage-derived chemokine (MDC, CCL22), are expressed in normal skin and in lesions of CTCL.[3,4] (TARC is found on dermal post-capillary venules and is capable of inducing integrin-dependent adhesion.) In addition, serum TARC levels are elevated in MF patients as compared with psoriasis patients and healthy controls.[3] Furthermore, in the peripheral blood of CTCL patients with peripheral blood involvement, there is a dramatically increased number of CLA+ CCR4+ T lymphocytes.[4] The interaction between CCR4 and TARC has been shown to be crucial in the homing of CLA+ memory T cells to the skin.[9] In addition, almost all malignant SS cells express the skin homing chemokine receptor CCR10 that binds CCL27 present on dermal

endothelial cells.[5] Firm adhesion and arrest of circulating T cells to the dermal post-capillary venule is mediated via integrins $\alpha_4\beta_1$ and $\alpha_L\beta_2$ (LFA1) on T cells interacting with VCAM-1 and the ICAM family expressed on endothelial cells, respectively.

After diapedesis (migration across the vascular wall), chemokines again play a chemoattractant role in T cell migration within the dermis and epidermis. In addition to expression on dermal endothelial cells, the CC-chemokine, TARC, is present on basal keratinocytes/epidermis and may contribute to epidermotropism.[4] Another CC-chemokine and CCR-4 ligand, MDC, is found on dendritic cells in the epidermis and dermis (Langerhans cells and dermal dendritic cells, respectively) suggesting a role in cell adhesion and signaling between dendritic cells and T lymphocytes.[4,10] Within the epidermis, CTCL cells congregate around Langerhans cells to form Pautrier microabscesses, the histologic *sine qua non* of CTCL. In addition, cutaneous T cell-attracting chemokine (CTACK, CCL27) is expressed preferentially by basal keratinocytes and selectively chemoattracts CLA+ memory T cells via CCR10.[11] Basal keratinocytes release CCL27 protein into the extracellular matrix, and CCL27 is displayed on dermal endothelial cells.[11] Basal keratinocytes also express IP9 (CXCL11), IP10 (CXCL10) and Mig (CXCL9), which are all chemoattractants for activated CXCR3+ T cells.[7] Furthermore, CTCL cells have been shown to express the integrin $\alpha_E\beta_7$,[6] which binds to E-cadherin[12] on keratinocytes and Langerhans cells and is responsible for retention of lymphocytes at epithelial sites.[13] Therefore, CTCL cells are equipped not only to migrate from the blood to the skin, but also to take residence in the epidermis.

As ICAM family members and VCAM-1 are expressed on endothelial cells throughout the body, the specificity of skin-homing is conferred by the combination of CLA and CCR4. While it is clear that early CTCL is a malignancy of CLA+CCR4+ 'cutaneous T cells', it is less clear where and when in disease progression the genetic and/or epigenetic events occur that confer the eventual loss of dependence on the skin environment. Once again, clues to CTCL behavior are found in the understanding of normal T cell physiology. A portion of benign and malignant CLA+CCR4+ cells will also express CD62L and CCR7.[5,14] Memory T cells retaining expression of L-selectin and CCR7 are referred to as central memory T cells.[15] L-selectin, which is predominantly found on naïve T lymphocytes, mediates rolling in peripheral lymph nodes via PNAd. CCR7 is activated by secondary lymphoid organ chemokine (SLC, CCL21) expressed in post-capillary venules and in T cell zones of the spleen and lymph nodes, and SLC is responsible for T cell and dendritic cell migration to the lymph nodes and spleen.[16] Thus, central memory T cells maintain the ability to circulate through lymph nodes, efficiently stimulate dendritic cells, and differentiate into CCR7-effector cells upon secondary stimulation. Therefore, it appears that CTCL progression, characterized in part by increasing involvement of the blood and lymph nodes, mimics features of normal T cell differentiation along the central memory pathway.[15]

The skin-homing characteristic of CTCL cells has several therapeutic implications. Since MF is a lymphoma that typically first declares itself in the skin as patches or plaques, it often presents early in its disease evolution, relative to other non-Hodgkin lymphomas. It is true that even patients with limited patch/plaque MF involvement can have a detectable clonal population in their blood and/or lymph nodes;[17,18] nevertheless, early MF cells behave as though they are dependent on stimulation within the epidermal environment, probably through interactions with Langerhans cells, keratinocytes, and/or other infiltrating cells. Thus, for limited patch/plaque MF, skin-directed therapies are often appropriate, potentially simultaneously targeting both the malignant T cells and the facilitating environment, e.g. stimulating Langerhans cells.

Emergence of a malignant clone

CLONAL EXPANSION

MF/SS arises from a clonal expansion of T lymphocytes and detection of a clonal population of T lymphocytes has been exploited for diagnostic purposes.[19] During T lymphocyte maturation, TCR variable (V), diversity (D) and joining (J) gene segments are rearranged, resulting in a unique genomic DNA configuration. Southern blot analysis has been replaced by the more sensitive, less time consuming and less expensive polymerase chain reaction (PCR) analysis to identify rearrangements of the γ chain of the TCR (TCRγ), even in early MF.[17,20] Clonal T cell populations can be identified in MF in more than 90 percent of cases. False negatives may occur because the tumor cell density is less than the detection threshold, failure of the PCR primers to detect all TCR gene rearrangements or deletion of gene rearrangements. Molecular identification of a clonal population of T lymphocytes often can facilitate the diagnosis of MF, especially in cases where typical clinical findings and histology are consistent with, but not classic for, MF and in erythrodermic MF, in which histology is often not diagnostic.[21] Care should be taken to correlate the clinical and histologic findings with the molecular studies, since clonal TCR rearrangements are sometimes found in lymphomatoid papulosis,[22] pityriasis lichenoides chronica,[22] pityriasis lichenoides et varioliformis acuta,[23] pseudolymphoma, lichen planus,[24] and lichen sclerosis et atrophicus.[25] In addition, if detection of the same clone is evident within more than one MF lesion, or in the same patient over time, there is a more significant risk of disease progression.[26] While PCR can detect the physiologic recirculation of malignant cells in the peripheral blood of patients with varying degrees of tumor burden, including limited patch/plaque disease, SS is characterized by dominance of the malignant clone with diminution of the normal T lymphocytes. One marker demonstrating the decrease in normal T lymphocytes is the reduction of the normal CD8+ lymphocyte population. As the disease progresses, CD8+ T lymphocytes are frequently decreased in skin lesions[27] and in the peripheral blood.[28]

MOLECULAR ABNORMALITIES

In several non-cutaneous T cell leukemias and lymphomas, clear associations with specific mutations and chromosomal abnormalities have been identified in which direct effects on the expression of oncogenes and/or inactivation of tumor suppressor genes would be expected to result in clonal expansion. Although the underlying molecular pathogenesis of MF and SS is still poorly understood, specific abnormalities are beginning to be identified and are summarized in Table 38.2 (reviewed by Smoller et al.[29]).

Comparative genomic hybridization (CGH) analysis, a wide-scale survey for chromosomal aberrations, has revealed chromosomal gains and losses in the advanced stages of MF and SS and, thus, provides a means to focus on the genes critical to the pathogenesis of MF and SS.[47,48] Chromosomal changes are not typically observed in limited patch/plaque stage. The advanced stages of MF and SS share a similar pattern of changes including loss on chromosomes 1p, 6q, 10q/10, 13q, 17p and 19 and gain on chromosomes 8q/8, 17q and 18, further evidence that these disorders share a common pathogenesis and represent a spectrum of disease. Furthermore, the number of chromosomal aberrations

Table 38.2 Summary of molecular abnormalities in MF and SS

Protein function	Gene	Molecular mechanism	Diseases involved	References
DNA repair	MLH1	Loss of function via methylation	MF	30
	MGMT	Loss of function via methylation	MF	31
Regulation of cell cycle	P53	Loss of function via mutation or deletion	MF ($\geq$IIB)/SS	32–34
	P15/P16	Loss of function via methylation, mutation or deletion	MF ($\geq$IIB)/SS	35,36
Apoptosis	FAS	Loss of function via mutation or dysfunctional splice variant	MF/SS	37–39
	BCL2	Decreased expression	MF/SS	40,41
Transcription factor	JUNB	Gain in function via chromosomal amplification	MF/SS	40,41
	NFκB2	Gain in function via mutation	MF/cell lines	42,43
	GATA3	Increased expression	SS	41
	STAT3	Constitutive expression	MF ($\geq$IIB)/SS/cell lines	44,45
	STAT5	Dysregulated expression of a truncated form	SS	46

correlates with clinical stage, and the chromosomal aberrations in malignant T cells coincide with clonal TCR rearrangements.[49] Moreover, microsatellite instability, a high propensity towards genetic instability that is characteristic of the hereditary non-polyposis colorectal cancer syndrome (HNPCC), has been detected in a portion of patients with MF.[30] Microsatellite instability is more prevalent in advanced forms of MF, suggesting that this phenomenon contributes to disease progression.

Molecular abnormalities in MF and SS have been identified in genes involved in DNA repair, regulation of the cell cycle, apoptosis and transcriptional regulation (Table 38.2). Hypermethylation of two DNA repair enzymes have been reported in MF. The promoter region of MLH1, a DNA mismatch repair enzyme, is hypermethylated in MF resulting in decreased MLH1 expression, whereas germline mutations in MLH1 have been identified in the HNPCC syndrome.[30] In addition, there is a report of hypermethylation of the O^6-methylguanine DNA methyl-transferase (MGMT) gene in patients with plaque and tumor-stage MF.[31] MGMT is a DNA repair enzyme that removes adducts from O^6 position of guanine, the preferred site of attack by many carcinogens and chemotherapeutic alkylating agents including carmustine (BCNU). Thus, loss of function of MGMT is anticipated to increase susceptibility to carcinogenesis and may suggest a good response to alkylating agents.

Gene alterations resulting in the loss of function of negative regulators of cell cycle progression including p53, p16 and p15 are observed in MF and SS. These genes block progression to S phase and allow time for DNA repair or eventual apoptosis. The p53 tumor suppressor gene, found on chromosome 17p, is the most commonly mutated gene in human malignancy. The loss of p53 function through mutation and deletion is restricted to tumor-stage MF and

SS, suggesting an association with disease progression.[32–34] Other negative regulators of cell cycle progression, the cyclin-dependent kinase inhibitors p16(INK4a)/CDKN2a and p15(INK4b), are also frequently inactivated in MF and SS via promoter hypermethylation, mutation or deletion.[35,36]

Cutaneous T cell lymphoma is a malignancy of activated T cells that appear to have a defect in apoptosis (i.e. programmed cell death), a process that would normally limit cell T cell proliferation and excessive activities after persistent TCR engagement and maintenance of T cell homeostasis. One insight into this phenomenon is the observation that SS express CD85j/immunoglobulin-like transcript 2, an inhibitory receptor analogous to killer cells immunoglobulin-like receptors (KIRs). CD85j+ SS are resistant to activation-induced cell death.[50] In addition, MF/SS cells have shown a decrease in Fas (CD95) expression with advancing disease, as well as a variety of mutated splice-variants[37–39] and thus they are resistant to Fas ligand (FASL) induction of apoptosis. Thus, MF/SS cells may avoid anti-tumor FasL+ CD8+ cytotoxic T cells that may have otherwise eliminated the malignant cells. On the other hand, MF/SS cells have been noted to have the capacity to express FasL which would endow them with the potential to eliminate anti-tumor cytotoxic T cells.[51,52] In contrast, the antiapoptotic gene BCL2 is underexpressed in the malignant cells in the skin and peripheral blood.[40,41] In summary, MF/SS cells resist apoptosis through loss of Fas and expression of inhibitory receptors that protect MF/SS from activation-induced cell death. These mechanisms may contribute to the accumulation of malignant T lymphocytes in the skin and peripheral blood.

In addition to demonstrating the skin-homing capabilities as previously discussed, T lymphocytes in MF/SS turn on the expression of cell surface receptors, signaling molecules and cytokines that execute specific effector functions.

Reactive T cells are typically present in the skin as a mixture of CD4 and CD8 subsets (normal CD4:CD8 ratio 1:1–1:6) and express mature T cell markers including CD2, CD3, CD5 and CD7. MF cells frequently have low expression of CD3, the TCR coreceptor involved in signaling, and lose expression of maturation markers including CD2, CD5, CD7, CD26, CD49 and CD60. CD158k is expressed by the majority of CD4+ peripheral blood lymphocytes in patients with SS,[53] compared to healthy individuals where CD158k is expressed on a small percentage of natural killer (NK) cells and CD3+CD8+ T cells. CD158k/KIR3DL2 is a member of the KIR family that inhibits natural killer cell cytotoxicity upon recognition of major histocompatibility complex (MHC) class I molecules. Moreover, circulating CD4+CD158k+ corresponds to the malignant cells bearing a clonal TCR rearrangement.[54] In addition, malignant cells in tumor stage MF express CD158k along with the cells of lymphomatoid papulosis, CD4+CD30+ and CD8+ large cell pleomorphic cutaneous T cell lymphoma, but not the infiltrating T cells in patch/plaque stage MF.[55]

Both by examination of clonal T lymphocytes in skin biopsy specimens and in the peripheral blood of leukemic patients, MF cells commonly express several activation markers including CD45RO, PCNA and CD25 (the α chain of the IL-2 receptor [IL-2R]). CD45RO is a marker of previously activated or memory T cells, and CD45RO is found on skin-infiltrating T cells in MF[56] and in the peripheral blood of patients with erythrodermic MF.[57] PCNA is a marker of G1 and G/S phases of the cell cycle and can be used to quantify proliferation. PCNA is observed in the nuclei of infiltrating cells in the skin biopsies of MF patients and positively correlates with advanced clinical stage.[58] Engagement of the high-affinity IL-2R triggers T cell growth. The IL-2R is composed of an α (CD25), β (CD122) and γ (CD132) chain. IL-2Rα (CD25) expression is restricted to activated T cells, which have recently encountered antigen. In healthy individuals, less than 5 percent of peripheral T cells express IL-2Rα. Aberrant expression of IL-2Rα has been described in MF.[56] The activated state of MF cells also make them a somewhat selective target for biologic therapy. For example, denileukin diftitox, a recombinant fusion protein of a portion of diphtheria toxin conjugated to IL-2, originally designed to target activated T lymphocytes in cutaneous inflammatory disease, allows for the disruption of cellular protein synthesis in cells expressing the IL-2 receptor[59] and is approved for treatment of mycosis fungoides.[60]

Following IL-2 and other cytokine receptor stimulation on activated T lymphocytes, several intracellular proteins in the JAK/STAT signaling pathway undergo phosphorylation. Malignant T cells in MF tumors have constitutive activation of STAT3 in vivo. In contrast, constitutive activation of STAT3 is not found in the T cells in patch/plaque lesions. STAT3 protects tumor cells from apoptosis in vitro.[44] Constitutively activated STAT3 has been shown to mediate the production of two T helper-2 (TH2) cytokines, IL-5 and IL-13, in MF cell lines.[61] MF/SS cell lines have constitutively active, tyrosine-phosphylated STAT3, which leads to constitutive expression of SOCS3. In normal T cells, SOCS3 serves as a negative regulator of JAK/STAT activation and down-regulates STAT3 activation. However, cell lines established from MF patients, SOCS3 does not diminish STAT3 activation. SOCS3 itself is not mutated in MF cell lines. SOCS3 overexpression in MF cell lines blocks interferon (IFN)-α mediated growth inhibition.[45] In the peripheral blood cells of SS patients, there is dysregulated expression of the carboxy-terminal truncated form of STAT5, and thus, loss of IL-2 inducible STAT5-dependent gene expression of BCL2, PIM1 and CISH by the full-length STAT5 isoform.[46]

In SS, the pathogenic cell type typically is a malignant CD4+ helper T cell that expresses a TH2 phenotype.[62] TH2 cells produce IL-4, IL-5, and IL-10, which stimulates class-switching to IgE, enhances the differentiation and activation of eosinophils, and suppresses TH1 differentiation, respectively. Diminished TH1 activity results in impaired cell-mediated immunity. Overexpression of GATA3 and JUNB likely play a role in the bias towards the TH2 phenotype. Gene expression analysis of peripheral blood leukocytes of leukemic MF/SS patients demonstrates hyperexpression of GATA3, a major transcription factor mediating TH2 differentiation, and JUNB, a major regulator of IL-4 expression.[41] Microarray, real-time PCR and immunophenotypic analyses have revealed chromosomal amplification and confirmed increased protein expression of JunB in some patients with MF and SS.[40] There is evidence for constitutive expression of another transcription factor NF-κB2 in MF.[42] The NF-κB family of transcription factors is critical for regulation of gene expression for cytokine production, cellular differentiation and apoptosis. Deletion in the regulatory binding site for NF-κB2 has been identified, suggesting a mechanism for constitutive activation.[42]

Treatments used in advanced MF and SS, including photopheresis and IFNα, have been shown to promote TH1 differentiation and suppress TH2 differentiation. Photopheresis induces apoptosis of the malignant cells with potential resultant loading of dendritic cells with apoptotic bodies and enhanced cell-mediated immune response versus the malignant cells. Treatment with photopheresis[63] or IFNα[64] restores production of TH1 cytokines. IL-12 is also a potent stimulator of IFNγ production and TH1 differentiation. Antigen-presenting cells (APCs) including dendritic cells and B cells, from patients with SS have impaired IL-12 production. On engagement of CD3/TCR, CD4+CD7– tumor cells have defective induction of CD40L compared to polyclonal CD4+CD7+ cells from the same patients and to healthy controls.[65] Deficient IL-12 production by APCs can be restored by treatment with recombinant soluble, hexameric CD40L that simulates engagement by a membrane-bound receptor.[65] Treatment of SS cells with IL-12 also suppresses the TH2 phenotype and promotes TH1 differentiation.[65] In addition, topical imiquimod is a potent stimulator of local production TH1 cytokines including IFNα, IFNγ and

IL-12. It also up upregulates expression of TNFα and enhances antigen presentation by Langerhans cells. These characteristics have led to its trial in the treatment of limited patch/plaque MF in case studies.[66] Bacterial DNA containing unmethylated nucleotides with the sequence motif CpG is recognized by APCs via toll-like receptor (TLR)-9. Activation of APCs via TLR9 leads to production of IFNα and TH1 differentiation. CpG alone or along with IL-15 restores IFNα production and activation of antitumor activity by natural killer cells and CD8+ cytotoxic T cells.[67]

Disease of T regulatory cells

Early observations in CTCL patients revealed that clonal expansion within the blood had suppressive effects on normal (nonmalignant) T cell counts, partially reflected in the CD4:CD8 ratio. More recently, complementary determining region 3 (CDR3) size spectratyping in which TCR diversity is evaluated using reverse transcriptase polymerase chain reaction (RT-PCR) with primers to the constant and variable regions of the TCRβ chain has been used to study the TCR diversity in stage I to stage IV disease. In healthy individuals, a Gaussian distribution of CDR3 length is observed in all TCRβ chains. As expected, the spectratype of the expanded malignant clone reveals a single peak, which is monoclonal by sequencing. In addition, clonal and oligoclonal populations as well as loss of normal T cells (deletion of other Vβ families) were identified, even in patients with early disease.[68] This finding suggests that MF/SS is not simply an expansion of a single malignant clone, but also that there may be profound abnormalities within the normal repertoire of peripheral T cells which may further contribute to the immunodeficient state in patients with this disease. The persistence of the malignant clone and its dominance over other nonmalignant T cells implies a disorder in the regulation of the normal population of T cells in MF/SS.

One mechanism by which the malignant MF/SS cells likely exert immunosuppressive effects is their capacity to function similar to T regulatory (Treg) cells. Treg cells are divided into two categories:

- natural (or constitutive) Treg, typically with a CD25+CD4+ phenotype, which develop in the thymus and enter the peripheral tissues to control immune responses
- inducible (or adaptive) Treg cells, which are generated in the periphery when naïve T cells encounter antigen presented by immature dendritic cells.

Natural Treg have intracellular expression of the transcriptional repressor FOXP3. Adaptive Treg cells mediate suppression through the secretion of inhibitory cytokines IL-10 and TGFβ. SS cells cultured with peripheral dendritic cells upregulate expression of CD25 and FOXP3 and secrete immunosuppressive cytokines IL-10 and TGFβ.[69]

This may represent an *in vitro* correlate of the Pautrier microabscess, where Langerhans cells may be stimulating the CTCL cells to manifest Treg activity with the net effect of local immunosuppression.

Furthermore, CTCL cells can produce extraordinary amounts of soluble IL-2 receptor, which may competitively bind IL-2 necessary for normal T cell activation.[70] Taken together these phenomena (Treg activity, TH2 cytokine production, soluble IL-2 receptor secretion) likely account for the increased risk of secondary malignancy and infections in CTCL patients.[71]

PATHOLOGY

Mycosis fungoides is among the most protean of diseases and poses great challenges to clinicians and pathologists alike. No other neoplasm is so closely mimicked by a wide variety disorders, most of which are non-neoplastic. Like most disorders, MF is readily diagnosed in its well-developed form. Establishing minimal histopathologic criteria necessary for a diagnosis of MF has proved challenging. Indeed, the accuracy of diagnosis of MF has sometimes been likened to a coin toss. One study on the histologic diagnosis of MF suggested that an accurate diagnosis can be rendered approximately half of the time.[72] Other studies have suggested better ability to diagnose MF but have drastically overdiagnosed control cases as MF.[73] These studies and others suggest that we have not yet established adequate criteria to diagnose or dismiss MF consistently.[74]

There are several important reasons why MF is so difficult to diagnose:

- *MF is a clinicopathologic diagnosis.*[75] The 'history' the pathologist often receives is 'rule out MF'. It is often unclear in such cases whether the clinician believes the patient likely has MF or, rather, an inflammatory disease, with MF at the bottom of the differential diagnosis. A variety of other conclusions are also possible.
- *Treatment alters the histopathologic features of MF.* At the time of biopsy, patients have often failed standard treatments for a presumed exanthem, including topical steroids. It should be noted that topical steroids appear to diminish or erase the epidermotropic features of MF.[76]
- *MF has a wide variety of clinical and histopathologic variants.*[77] While the diagnosis of standard patch stage MF is difficult enough, the existence of a variety of challenging variants complicates the matter.
- *Clinically, early MF often looks more like an exanthem than a neoplasm.*[78]
- *Mycosis fungoides very often looks like an exanthem histologically as well.* As such, a clinical misdiagnosis may be supported by a congruous if inaccurate histologic impression. This can readily occur, as the

cells of early MF often do not show significant morphologic differences from those of inflammatory conditions.[76,79]

- *Mycosis fungoides does not resemble merely a few different inflammatory processes under the microscope; it resembles many*. Shapiro and Pinto in an analysis of 222 MF biopsies, demonstrated that virtually every inflammatory pattern developed by Clark and Ackerman can be seen in MF.[80] The most common patterns encountered are **psoriasiform**, **lichenoid** and **psoriasiform/lichenoid**. Less common patterns include **superficial perivascular**, **superficial perivascular and interstitial**, **vacuolar**, **psoriasiform/spongiotic**, **spongiotic/psoriasiform/lichenoid**, **nodular**, **superficial** and **deep perivascular** and **interstitial**, **diffuse** and **folliculitic**. Rare patterns include **spongiotic**, **vasculitic**, **vesicular** and **panniculitic**. As such, in order to become skilled at the histopathologic diagnosis of MF, one must become expert at the diagnosis of inflammatory skin disorders. Often, one can only 'rule out MF' by making another diagnosis.
- *MF resembles inflammatory disorders not to a small degree but, frequently, to a large degree*. Lymphocytes typically infiltrate the basal layer in MF, interacting with Langerhans cells.[76,79,81] This feature is seen in a wide variety of other inflammatory conditions and is, in fact, typical of some of them, including lichen sclerosis et atrophicus.[82,83]

Ancillary studies

It is logical to ask whether, if histopathology is often inadequate to diagnose early MF, can ancillary studies identify this challenging condition? Immunophenotyping has been widely utilized for MF. Early hopes centered on increased CD4:CD8 ratio, but it has been subsequently demonstrated that most inflammatory disorders are CD4 predominant, and, of course, some examples of cutaneous T cell lymphoma are CD8 positive. Immunophenotyping is clearly helpful in plaque and tumor stage MF, where loss of the common T cell antigens CD2, CD3 and/or CD5 may be seen.[84,85] Such losses are not seen, however, in patch stage disease. Loss of CD7 is sometimes still touted as useful,[86] but loss of CD7 can be seen as frequently in inflammatory conditions as in early MF.[84,85,87] Additionally, it is important to bear in mind that immunohistochemical analysis of T cell infiltrates relies upon identifying antigen *loss*. It must be kept in mind that, even with adequate controls, it is more difficult to be certain about absence of staining than positive staining. At Yale University and at some other MF centers, immunohistochemistry is generally reserved until after a diagnosis of cutaneous T cell lymphoma has been established. It is then employed to identify aggressive subsets of cutaneous T cell lymphoma, such as γ/δ lymphoma or aggressive variants of CD8 positive lymphoma.

Less controversial is the use of T cell receptor gene rearrangements (TCR) via polymerase chain reaction (PCR). It is important to keep a variety of caveats in mind, however, in the interpretation of TCR results. It should be noted that up to half of patients with indubitable patch stage MF will not demonstrate a clone via PCR.[88–92] Furthermore, investigation of patients *without* indubitable MF is fraught with even greater difficulty. Patients described as having 'parapsoriasis',[93] 'pre-MF'[89] or as 'borderline'[89] can show clonality rates of significantly less than 50 percent. It is also important be aware that clones can be identified in disorders that we do not categorize as malignant. A few of these include cutaneous lymphoid hyperplasia,[20,93] pityriasis lichenoides et varioliformis acuta,[23,94,95] pigmented purpuric eruption,[96] lichen sclerosis,[25] and even lichen planus.[24]

As such, it is fair to say that there is no 'magic bullet'. It is also likely fair to say that the gold standard for the diagnosis of MF remains in the realm of clinical/histologic/molecular correlation. As such, histopathology remains a key factor.

Specific histopathologic features of mycosis fungoides

There have been many excellent descriptive studies regarding MF.[79,80,97,98] From such studies we know a great deal about histologic features of MF, but we know less regarding which criteria are most specific for this disorder. More recently, controlled and blinded studies of MF versus controls have been undertaken, and such studies have provided helpful information. As virtually any histopathologic feature of MF can be seen in a variety of other conditions, knowledge of criterion specificity is important.

The histopathologic features of MF can be divided into: epidermotropic pattern; cellular morphology; and ancillary histologic features. **Pattern of epidermotropism** can be thought of as a subset of pattern analysis, one uniquely important to MF. Recent studies have highlighted two important features of epidermotropic pattern: Pautrier microabscesses and the presence of lymphocytes within the epidermis which are larger than those within the dermis. These features are present in a minority of cases. They are important in that they are relatively specific for MF, a disorder with few specific histopathologic features. Lymphocytes within the epidermis, which are larger than those within the dermis are seen in approximately 20 percent of examples of patch stage MF and in few or no control cases[81] (and also Burg G *et al.* International society for cutaneous lymphoma – early mycosis fungoides study project [manuscript in preparation]; Plate 101, see plate section). This feature reflects the tendency of neoplastic cells of MF to home to the epidermis, while the dermis typically contains a significant admixture of non-neoplastic cells. In early MF, few neoplastic cells may be present in any given biopsy.[84,99] As a result, many of the histologic features assessed are not of tumor per se, but reaction pattern to tumor.

Pautrier microabscesses are better known as a specific feature of MF. Their incidence has varied widely among reports and has ranged from 4 percent to 37 percent (Burg G et al. International society for cutaneous lymphoma – early mycosis fungoides study project [manuscript in preparation]).[81,100] This variation is likely reflective of how 'early' the lesions are and how one defines a Pautrier microabscess. Strictly defined Pautrier microabscesses have been described as 'sharply marginated clusters of atypical lymphoid cells that are closely apposed to one another with uniform cytologic features, with no plasma or fibrin deposition or significant cytopathic changes in the surrounding keratinocytes' (Plate 102, see plate section). Defined in this strict manner, Pautrier microabscesses are uncommon in early MF. Studies of MF without regard to stage have demonstrated Pautrier microabscesses in approximately 20 percent of biopsies.[92,97,101]

Several histologic features of epidermotropism have been shown to be less specific for MF, but more sensitive, including epidermotropism associated with a paucity of spongiosis (disproportionate epidermotropism).[79] Disproportionate epidermotropism is difficult to reproducibly define, and the recent blinded studies have not attempted to rigorously delineate it. Disproportionate epidermotropism of at least 'moderate degree' is seen in approximately 58 percent of MF cases and approximately a quarter of controls.[81]

Like disproportionate epidermotropism, basilar epidermotropism is readily identified when it is florid. This feature has been likened to 'a string of pearls' or 'toy soldiers'. There is no accepted lower limit for this criterion, however. Moderate basilar epidermotropism (one to five basal lymphocytes per 20 × field) has been identified in more than two-thirds of MF cases and fewer than a quarter of controls.[81] If one defines basilar epidermotropism as the presence of any four contiguous lymphocytes within the basal, it becomes a more specific but less sensitive feature (93 percent specificity, 17 percent sensitivity for early MF).[98]

'Pagetoid spread' of intraepidermal lymphocytes (lymphocytes at all leads of the epidermis) has not been touted in the American literature as a common histopathologic feature in early MF biopsies. Blinded studies performed in Europe have found a pagetoid pattern of intraepidermal lymphocytes in 0–33 percent of early MF cases.[98,100] This feature highlights the suggestion that lymphocytes high in the epidermis may be more significant than basilar lymphocytes in some differentials.[79] Of note, Toro et al. found that atypical lymphocytes in the upper epidermis are useful in distinguishing purpuric MF from an increasingly confounding mimic, persistent pigmented purpuric eruption, many examples of which exhibit prominent basilar lymphocytes.[96]

Regarding **cellular morphology** in MF, much has been written on the topic, but cytologic features have proved difficult to quantify in routinely processed, paraffin embedded tissue. Convoluted nuclei appear to be present in more than two-thirds of examples of MF and fewer than a third of control cases.[81] Some studies have suggested that the presence of 'strikingly convoluted nuclei' in the epidermis or dermis is among the best discriminators of MF from controls (Burg G et al. International society for cutaneous lymphoma – early mycosis fungoides study project [manuscript in preparation]). Recently, 'medium-large cerebriform lymphocytes' in the epidermis (lymphocytes 7–9 μm in diameter, approximating the width of basal keratinocyte nuclei) has been touted as the most reliable indicator of early MF (Plate 103, see plate section).[100] These data are in contrast to other studies, which have suggested that atypical lymphocytes are not often present and are generally not as helpful as architectural features in early MF.[79,92,97]

While many clues to a diagnosis of MF can be gathered from **ancillary histologic features**, recent studies of MF versus controls have called into question the usefulness of some of the more characteristic ones. Many histopathologists carefully assess for papillary dermal fibrosis, frequently entrapping lymphocytes. Papillary dermal fibrosis alone, however, has not been found to be a statistically significant discriminator between MF and its mimics in controlled studies (Burg G et al. International society for cutaneous lymphoma – early mycosis fungoides study project [manuscript in preparation]).[81,100] This feature is typical of late patch and of plaque stage MF but appears more indicative of chronicity than etiology.

Another ancillary feature, 'haloed lymphocytes', has been shown to be more useful, however. Haloed lymphocytes show a vacuole around them, evident at even relative low magnification. The cause of this feature is unknown, but it is thought to result from artifactual contraction of the more abundant cytoplasm of neoplastic lymphocytes or their poor cohesion to keratinocytes.[79,81,97] Haloed lymphocytes are not typically identified in frozen sections.[81,97,98,101] Halos are a seemingly ubiquitous feature in routinely processed, paraffin embedded tissue, however, there is apparent variation in the degree of haloing among laboratories. In addition, haloed cells are best evaluated in the upper epidermis rather than within the basal layer, where they may be confused with melanocytes.[79] In one large American study, haloed lymphocytes were found in most MF biopsies and were the best single discriminator of MF from inflammatory stimulants.[81] A similar study from Europe found haloed lymphocytes to be a very specific but relatively insensitive feature of CTCL (100 percent specificity, 13 percent sensitivity) (Burg G et al. International society for cutaneous lymphoma – early mycosis fungoides study project [manuscript in preparation]). Other ancillary features that may support a diagnosis of MF but which have not been addressed in blinded studies, include the co-presence of eosinophils and plasma cells and regions of fine, dry parakeratosis, alternating with broader regions of orthokeratosis.[80]

Plaque stage MF is generally not so laden with difficulties as patch stage disease.[102] One sees, by definition, involvement of the reticular dermis in plaque stage MF (Plate 104, see plate section). This is usually accompanied by the aforementioned epidermal and papillary dermal changes typical of MF. In difficult examples of plaque stage disease, ancillary studies, including immunohistochemistry and gene rearrangement studies, are often helpful.[84,85,88] Additionally, histopathologists generally demonstrate a high degree of accuracy in the diagnosis of **tumor stage MF**. Clinically and histopathologically, the presence of a neoplasm is evident at this stage, and cytologic atypia is greater. MF tumors may retain their epidermotropic capacity or lose it, and they may be comprised of small- to medium-sized convoluted lymphocytes or large transformed ones.

Histopathology of Sézary syndrome

Regarding the leukemic variant of cutaneous T cell lymphoma, SS, it is fair to say that, compared to patch stage MF, histologic diagnosis goes from difficult to more difficult. Buechner and Winkelmann's classical treatise on this condition showed that only 15 percent of cases showed an epidermotropic pattern.[103] Other studies have demonstrated increased spongiosis,[80] diminished disproportionate exocytosis,[104] fewer basilar lymphocytes,[104] fewer convoluted lymphocytes,[104] increased acanthosis[105] and fewer Pautrier microabscesses[105] as compared to MF. One well-documented study of SS found that a third of patients showed only chronic spongiotic changes and no histologic evidence of lymphoma in original or repeat biopsies. Of note, this group showed no better survival than other patients within the study. In some patients with SS, the exanthem may represent a nonspecific chronic spongiotic response to a primarily leukemic process.[106]

It is important to bear in mind that the gold standard for the diagnosis of MF remains within the realm of clinical/histologic/molecular correlation. Histopathology plays a critical role in the diagnosis of MF, but the final determination rests upon somewhat of a gestalt synthesis of various clinical and laboratory findings. Familiarity with sensitivity and specificity of criteria for MF, in conjunction with extensive knowledge of disorders within the differential diagnosis of MF (inflammatory dermatopathology), is helpful in the diagnosis of this challenging condition.

KEY POINTS

- The molecular interactions involved in the ability of MF/SS cells to migrate to and reside in the skin are operative in the normal physiology of immunosurveillance of the skin. As a malignancy of 'cutaneous T cells', MF/SS cells often display a CLA+CCR-4+ phenotype.
- MF/SS is an immunosuppressive malignancy. Even at early stages, the normal T cell repertoire may be compromised. MF/SS cells may also function as T regulatory cells.

- There is accumulation of data on the specific defects that allow for the clonal expansion of MF/SS cells including resistance to apoptosis, genomic instability, and loss of cell cycle controls.
- Detection of clonality by TCR gene rearrangement analyses using PCR is a powerful tool and may help in the diagnosis of MF/SS. However, it is possible to obtain false positives in several inflammatory diseases that may have expanded T cells clones.
- MF/SS may be difficult to diagnose, and more than many other malignancies, requires a clinico-histologic correlation. Nevertheless, a detailed understanding of the spectrum of histologic features of MF/SS and the appropriate use of ancillary studies greatly aids in the diagnostic challenge.

REFERENCES

● = Key primary paper

◆ = Major review article

●1. Kupper TS, Fuhlbrigge RC. Immune surveillance in the skin: mechanisms and clinical consequences. *Nat Rev Immunol* 2004; **4**: 211–22.

2. Borowitz MJ, Weidner A, Olsen EA, Picker LJ. Abnormalities of circulating T-cell subpopulations in patients with cutaneous T-cell lymphoma: cutaneous lymphocyte-associated antigen expression on T cells correlates with extent of disease. *Leukemia* 1993; **7**: 859–63.

●3. Kakinuma T, Sugaya M, Nakamura K *et al.* Thymus and activation-regulated chemokine (TARC/CCL17) in mycosis fungoides: Serum TARC levels reflect the disease activity of mycosis fungoides. *J Am Acad Dermatol* 2003; **48**: 23–30.

4. Ferenczi K, Fuhlbrigge RC, Pinkus JL *et al.* Increased CCR4 expression in cutaneous T cell lymphoma. *J Invest Dermatol* 2002; **119**: 1405–10.

5. Sokolowska-Wojdylo M, Wenzel J, Gaffal E *et al.* Circulating clonal CLA+ and CD4+ T cells in Sezary syndrome express the skin-homing chemokine receptors CCR4 and CCR10 as well as the lymph node-homing chemokine receptor CCR7. *Brit J Dermatol* 2005; **152**: 258–64.

6. Schechner JS, Edelson RL, McNiff JM *et al.* Integrins alpha4beta7 and alphaEbeta7 are expressed on epidermotropic T cells in cutaneous T cell lymphoma and spongiotic dermatitis. *Lab Invest* 1999; **79**: 601–7.

7. Tensen CP, Flier J, Van Der Raaij-Helmer EM *et al.* Human IP-9: a keratinocyte-derived high affinity CXC-chemokine ligand for the IP-10/Mig receptor (CXCR3). *J Invest Dermatol* 1999; **112**: 716–22.

8. Fuhlbrigge RC, Kieffer JD, Armerding D, Kupper TS. Cutaneous lymphocyte antigen is a specialized form of PSGL-1 expressed on skin-homing T cells. *Science* 1997; **389**: 978–81.

9. Campbell JJ, Haraldsen G, Pan J *et al.* The chemokine receptor CCR4 in vascular recognition by cutaneous but not intestinal memory T cells. *Nature* 1999; **400**: 776–80.

10. Katuo F, Ohtani H, Nakayama T *et al.* Macrophage-derived chemokine (MDC/CCL22) and CCR4 are involved in the formation of T lymphocyte-dendritic cell clusters in human inflamed skin and secondary lymphoid tissue. *Am J Pathol* 2001; **158**: 1263–70.

11. Homey B, Alenius H, Mueller A *et al.* CCL27-CCR10 interactions regulate T cell-mediated skin inflammation. *Nat Med* 2002; **8**: 157–65.

12. Taraszka KS, Higgins JM, Tan K *et al.* Molecular basis for leukocyte integrin alpha(E)beta adhesion to epithelial (E)-cadherin. *J Exp Med* 2000; **191**: 1555–67.

13. Schon MP, Arya A, Murphy EA *et al.* Mucosal T lymphocyte numbers are selectively reduced in integrin alphaE (CD103)-deficient mice. *J Immunol* 1999; **162**: 6641–9.

14. Campbell JJ, Murphy KE, Kunkel EJ *et al.* CCR7 expression and memory T cell diversity in humans. *J Immunol* 2001; **166**: 877–84.

15. Sallusto F, Lenig D, Forster R *et al.* Two subsets of memory T lymphocytes with distinct homing potentials and effector functions. *Nature* 1999; **401**: 708–12.

16. Gunn MD, Kyuwa S, Tam C *et al.* Mice lacking expression of secondary lymphoid organ chemokine have defects in lymphocyte homing and dendritic cell localization. *J Exp Med* 1999; **189**: 451–60.

17. Benhattar J, Delacretaz F, Martin P *et al.* Improved polymerase chain reaction detection of clonal T-cell lymphoid neoplasms. *Diagn Mol Pathol* 1995; **4**: 108–12.

18. Slack DN, McCarthy KP, Wiedemann LM, Sloane JP. Evaluation of sensitivity, specificity, and reproducibility of an optimized method for detecting clonal rearrangements of immunoglobulin and T-cell receptor genes in formalin-fixed, paraffin-embedded sections. *Diagn Mol Pathol* 1993; **2**: 223–32.

19. Holm N, Flaig MJ, Yazdi AS, Sander CA. The value of molecular analysis by PCR in the diagnosis of cutaneous lymphocytic infiltrates. *J Cutan Pathol* 2002; **29**: 447–52.

●20. Wood GS, Tung RM, Haeffner AC *et al.* Detection of clonal T-cell receptor gamma gene rearrangements in early mycosis fungoides/Sezary syndrome by polymerase chain reaction and denaturing gradient gel electrophoresis (PCR/DGGE). *J Invest Dermatol* 1994; **103**: 34–41.

21. Cherny S, Mraz S, Su L *et al.* Heteroduplex analysis of T-cell receptor gamma gene rearrangement as an adjuvant diagnostic tool in skin biopsies for erythroderma. *J Cutan Pathol* 2001; **28**: 351–5.

22. Theodorou I, Delfau-Larue MH, Bigorgne C *et al.* Cutaneous T-cell infiltrates: analysis of T-cell receptor gamma gene rearrangement by polymerase chain reaction and denaturing gradient gel electrophoresis. *Blood* 1995; **86**: 305–10.

23. Weinberg JM, Kristal L, Chooback L *et al.* The clonal nature of pityriasis lichenoides. *Arch Dermatol* 2002; **138**: 1063–7.

24. Schiller PI, Flaig MJ, Puchta U *et al.* Detection of clonal T cells in lichen planus. *Arch Dermatol Res* 2000; **292**: 568–9.

25. Lukowsky A, Muche JM, Sterry W, Audring H. Detection of expanded T cell clones in skin biopsy samples of patients with lichen sclerosus et atrophicus by T cell receptor-gamma polymerase chain reaction assays. *J Invest Dermatol* 2000; **115**: 254–9.

26. Vega F, Luthra R, Medeiros LJ *et al.* Clonal heterogeneity in mycosis fungoides and its relationship to clinical course. *Blood* 2002; **100**: 3369–73.

●27. Hoppe RT, Medeiros LJ, Warnke RA, Wood GS. CD8-positive tumor-infiltrating lymphocytes influence the long-term survival of patients with mycosis fungoides. *J Am Acad Dermatol* 1995; **32**: 448–53.

●28. Heald P, Yan SL, Edelson R. Profound deficiency in normal circulating T cells in erythrodermic cutaneous T-cell lymphoma. *Arch Dermatol* 1994; **130**: 198–203.

29. Smoller BR, Santucci M, Wood GS, Whittaker SJ. Histopathology and genetics of cutaneous T-cell lymphoma. *Hematol Oncol Clin North Am* 2003; **17**: 1277–311.

30. Scarisbrick JJ, Mitchell TJ, Calonje E *et al.* Microsatellite instability is associated with hypermethylation of the hMLH1 gene and reduced gene expression in mycosis fungoides. *J Invest Dermatol* 2003; **121**: 894–901.

31. Gallardo F, Esteller M, Pugol RM *et al.* Methylation status of the p15, p16 and MGMT promoter genes in primary cutaneous T-cell lymphomas. *Haematologica* 2004; **89**: 1401–3.

32. McGregor JM, Crook T, Fraser-Andrews EA *et al.* Spectrum of p53 gene mutations suggests a possible role for ultraviolet radiation in the pathogenesis of advanced cutaneous lymphomas. *J Invest Dermatol* 1999; **112**: 317–21.

●33. Lauritzen AF, Vejlsgaard GL, Hou-Jensen K, Ralfkiaer E. p53 protein expression in cutaneous T-cell lymphomas. *Brit J Dermatol* 1995; **133**: 32–6.

34. Marrogi AJ, Khan MA, Vonderheid EC *et al.* p53 tumor suppressor gene mutations in transformed cutaneous T-cell lymphoma: a study of 12 cases. *J Cutan Pathol* 1999; **26**: 369–78.

35. Navas IC, Algara P, Mateo M *et al.* p16(INK4a) is selectively silenced in the tumoral progression of mycosis fungoides. *Lab Invest* 2002; **82**: 123–33.

36. Scarisbrick JJ, Woolford AJ, Calonje E *et al.* Frequent abnormalities of the p15 and p16 genes in mycosis fungoides and Sézary syndrome. *J Invest Dermatol* 2002; **118**: 493–9.

37. Dereure O, Levi E, Vonderheid EC, Kadin ME. Infrequent Fas mutations but no Bax or p53 mutations in early mycosis fungoides: a possible mechanism for the accumulation of malignant T lymphocytes in the skin. *J Invest Dermatol* 2002; **118**: 949–56.

38. Nagasawa T, Takakuwa T, Takayama H *et al.* Fas gene mutations in mycosis fungoides: analysis of laser

capture-microdissected specimens from cutaneous lesions. *Oncology* 2004; **67**: 130–4.

39. van Doorn R, Dijkman R, Vermeer MH *et al.* A novel splice variant of the Fas gene in patients with cutaneous T-cell lymphoma. *Cancer Res* 2002; **62**: 5389–92.

40. Mao X, Orchard G, Lillington DM *et al.* BCL2 and JUNB abnormalities in primary cutaneous lymphomas. *Br J Dermatol* 2004; **151**: 546–56.

41. Kari L, Loboda A, Nebozhyn M *et al.* Classification and prediction of survival in patients with the leukemic phase of cutaneous T cell lymphoma. *J Exp Med* 2003; **197**: 1477–88.

42. Izban KF, Ergin M, Qin JZ *et al.* Constitutive expression of NF-kappa B is a characteristic feature of mycosis fungoides: implications for apoptosis resistance and pathogenesis. *Hum Pathol* 2002; **31**: 1482–90.

●43. Migliazza A, Lombardi L, Rocchi M *et al.* Heterogeneous chromosomal aberrations generate 3′ truncations of the NFKB2/lyt-10 gene in lymphoid malignancies. *Blood* 1994; **84**: 3850.

44. Sommer VH, Clemmensen OJ, Nielsen O *et al.* In vivo activation of STAT3 in cutaneous T-cell lymphoma. Evidence for an apoptotic function of STAT3. *Leukemia* 2004; **18**: 1288–95.

45. Brender C, Lovato P, Sommer VH *et al.* Constitutive SOCS-3 expression protects T-cell lymphoma against growth inhibition by IFNalpha. *Leukemia* 2005; **19**: 209–13.

46. Mitchell TJ, Whittaker SJ, John S. Dysregulated expression of COOH-terminally truncated Stat5 and loss of IL2-inducible Stat5-dependent gene expression in Sezary syndrome. *Cancer Res* 2003; **63**: 9048–54.

●47. Fischer TC, Gellrich S, Muche JM *et al.* Genomic aberrations and survival in cutaneous T cell lymphomas. *J Invest Dermatol* 2004; **122**: 579–86.

48. Mao X, Lillington D, Scarisbrick JJ *et al.* Molecular cytogenetic analysis of cutaneous T-cell lymphomas: identification of common genetic alterations in Sezary syndrome and mycosis fungoides. *Br J Dermatol* 2002; **147**: 464–75.

49. Marcus Muche J, Karenko L, Gellrich S *et al.* Cellular coincidence of clonal T cell receptor rearrangements and complex clonal chromosomal aberrations – a hallmark of malignancy in cutaneous T cell lymphoma. *J Invest Dermatol* 2004; **122**: 574–8.

50. Nikolova M, Musette P, Bagot M *et al.* Engagement of ILT2/CD85j in Sezary syndrome cells inhibits their CD3/TCR signaling. *Blood* 2002; **100**: 1019–25.

51. Ni X, Hazarika P, Zhang C *et al.* Fas ligand expression by neoplastic T lymphocytes mediates elimination of CD8+ cytotoxic T lymphocytes in mycosis fungoides: a potential mechanism of tumor immune escape? *Clin Cancer Res* 2001; **7**: 2682–92.

●52. Zoi-Toli O, Vermeer MH, De Vries E *et al.* Expression of Fas and Fas-ligand in primary cutaneous T-cell lymphoma (CTCL): association between lack of Fas expression and aggressive types of CTCL. *Br J Dermatol* 2000; **143**: 313–19.

53. Bagot M, Moretta A, Sivori S *et al.* CD4(+) cutaneous T-cell lymphoma cells express the p140-killer cell immunoglobulin-like receptor. *Blood* 2001; **97**: 1388–91.

54. Poszepczynska-Guigne E, Schiavon V, D'Incan M *et al.* CD158k/KIR3DL2 is a new phenotypic marker of Sezary cells: relevance for the diagnosis and follow-up of Sezary syndrome. *J Invest Dermatol* 2004; **122**: 820–3.

●55. Wechsler J, Bagot M, Nikolova M *et al.* Killer cell immunoglobulin-like receptor expression delineates in situ Sezary syndrome lymphocytes. *J Pathol* 2003; **199**: 77–83.

●56. Nagatani T, Matsuzaki T, Iemoto G *et al.* Comparative study of cutaneous T-cell lymphoma and adult T-cell leukemia/lymphoma. Clinical, histopathologic, and immunohistochemical analyses. *Cancer* 1990; **66**: 2380–6.

57. Heald PW, Yan SL, Edelson RL *et al.* Skin-selective lymphocyte homing mechanisms in the pathogenesis of leukemic cutaneous T-cell lymphoma. *J Invest Dermatol* 1993; **101**: 222–6.

58. Neish C, Charlry M, Jegasothy B *et al.* Proliferation cell nuclear antigen and soluble interleukin 2 receptor levels in cutaneous T cell lymphoma: correlation with advanced clinical diseases. *J Dermatol Sci* 1994; **8**: 11–17.

59. Gottlieb SL, Gilleaudeau P, Johnson R *et al.* Response of psoriasis to a lymphocyte-selective toxin (DAB389IL-2) suggests a primary immune, but not keratinocyte, pathogenic basis. *Nat Med* 1995; **1**: 442–7.

60. Olsen E, Duvic M, Frankel A *et al.* Pivotal phase III trial of two dose levels of denileukin diftitox for the treatment of cutaneous T-cell lymphoma. *J Clin Oncol* 2001; **19**: 376–88.

61. Nielsen M, Nissen MH, Gerwien J *et al.* Spontaneous interleukin-5 production in cutaneous T-cell lymphoma lines is mediated by constitutively activated Stat3. *Blood* 2002; **99**: 973–7.

62. Vowels BR, Lessin SR, Cassin M *et al.* Th2 cytokine mRNA expression in skin in cutaneous T-cell lymphoma. *J Invest Dermatol* 1994; **103**: 669–73.

63. Di Renzo M, Rubegni P, De Aloe G *et al.* Extracorporeal photochemotherapy restores Th1/Th2 imbalance in patients with early stages of cutaneous T-cell lymphoma. *Immunology* 1997; **92**: 99–103.

64. Rook AH, Kubin M, Cassin M *et al.* IL-12 reverses cytokine and immune abnormalities in Sezary syndrome. *J Immunol* 1995; **154**: 1491–8.

65. French LE, Huard B, Wysocka M *et al.* Impaired CD40L signaling is a cause of defective IL-12 and TNF-alpha production in Sezary syndrome: circumvention by hexameric soluble CD40L. *Blood* 2005; **105**: 219–25.

66. Suchin KR, Junkins-Hopkins JM, Rook AH. Treatment of Stage IA cutaneous T-cell lymphoma with topical application of the immune response modifier imiquimod. *Arch Dermatol* 2002; **138**: 1137–9.

67. Wysocka M, Benoit BM, Newton S *et al.* Enhancement of the host immune responses in cutaneous T cell lymphoma by CpG oligodeoxynucleotides and IL-15. *Blood* 2004; **104**: 4142–29.

●68. Yawalkar N, Ferenczi K, Jones DA et al. Profound loss of T-cell receptor repertoire complexity in cutaneous T-cell lymphoma. Blood 2003; 102: 4059–66.

●69. Berger CL, Tigelaar R, Cohen J et al. Cutaneous T-cell lymphoma: malignant proliferation of T-regulatory cells. Blood 2005; 105: 1640–7.

70. Vonderheid EC, Zhang Q, Lessin SR et al. Use of serum soluble interleukin-2 receptor levels to monitor the progression of cutaneous T-cell lymphoma. J Am Acad Dermatol 1998; 38: 207–20.

71. Kantor AF, Curtis RE, Vonderheid EC et al. Risk of second malignancy after cutaneous T-cell lymphoma. Cancer 1989; 63: 1612–15.

72. Santucci M, Burg G, Feller AC. Interrater and intrarater reliability of histologic criteria in early cutaneous T-cell lymphoma. Dermatol Clin 1994; 12: 323–7.

●73. Olerud JE, Kulin PA, Chew DE, et al. Cutaneous T-cell lymphoma. Evaluation of pretreatment skin biopsy specimens by a panel of pathologists. Arch Dermatol 1992; 128: 501–7.

74. Burg G, Zwingers T, Staegemeir E, Santucci M. Interrater and intrarater variabilities in the evaluation of cutaneous lymphoproliferative T-cell infiltrates. Dermatol Clin 1994; 12: 311.

●75. Glusac EJ, Shapiro PE, McNiff JM. Cutaneous T-cell lymphoma. Refinement in the application of controversial histologic criteria. Dermatol Clin 1999; 17: 601–14.

76. Ming M, LeBoit PE. Can dermatopathologists reliably make the diagnosis of mycosis fungoides? If not, who can? Arch Dermatol 2000; 136: 543–6.

77. LeBoit PE. Variants of mycosis fungoides and related cutaneous T-cell lymphomas. Semin Diag Pathol 1991; 8: 773–81.

78. Zackheim HS, McCalmont TH. Mycosis fungoides: the great imitator. J Am Acad Dermatol 2002; 47: 914–18.

79. Sanchez JL, Ackerman AB. The patch stage of mycosis fungoides. Am J Dermatopathol 1979; 1: 5–26.

80. Shapiro PE, Pinto FJ. The histologic spectrum of mycosis fungoides/Sezary syndrome (cutaneous T-cell lymphoma). A review of 222 biopsies, including newly described patterns and the earliest pathologic changes. Am J Surg Pathol 1994; 18: 645–67.

●81. Smoller BR, Bishop K, Glusac EJ, et al. Reassessment of histologic parameters in the diagnosis of mycosis fungoides. Am J Surg Pathol 1995; 19: 1423–30.

82. Fung MA, LeBoit PE. Light microscopic criteria for the diagnosis of early vulvar lichen sclerosus. A comparison with lichen planus. Am J Surg Pathol 1998; 22: 473–8.

83. Citarella L, Massone C, Kerl H, Cerroni L. Lichen sclerosus with histopathologic features simulating early mycosis fungoides. Am J Dermatopathol 2003; 25: 463–5.

84. Ralfkiaer E. Immunohistological markers for the diagnosis of cutaneous lymphomas. Semin Diagn Pathol 1991; 8: 62–72.

85. Ralfkiaer E. Controversies and discussion on early diagnosis of cutaneous T-cell lymphoma. Phenotyping. Dermatol Clin 1994; 12: 329–34.

86. Ormsby A, Bergfeld WF, Tubbs RR, Hsi ED. Evaluation of a new paraffin-reactive CD7 T-cell deletion marker and a polymerase chain reaction-based T-cell receptor gene rearrangement assay: implications for diagnosis of mycosis fungoides in community clinical practice. J Am Acad Dermatol 2001; 45: 405–13.

87. Payne CM, Spier CM, Grogan TM et al. Nuclear contour irregularity correlates with Leu-9-, Leu-8- cells in benign lymphoid infiltrates of skin. An ultrastructural morphometric and quantitative immunophenotypic analysis suggesting the normal T-cell counterpart to the malignant mycosis fungoides/Sezary cell. Am J Dermatopathol 1988; 10: 377–89.

88. Bachelez H, Bioul L, Flageul B et al. Detection of clonal T-cell receptor gamma gene rearrangements with the use of the polymerase chain reaction in cutaneous lesions of mycosis fungoides and Sezary syndrome. Arch Dermatol 1995; 131: 1027–31.

89. Aston-Key M, Diss TC, Du MQ. The value of the polymerase chain reaction in the diagnosis of cutaneous T-cell infiltrates. Am J Surg Pathol 1997; 21: 743–47.

90. Tok J, Szabolcs J, Silvers DN et al. Detection of clonal T-cell receptor gamma chain gene rearrangements by polymerase chain reaction and denaturing gradient gel electrophoresis (PCR/DGGE) in archival specimens from patients with early cutaneous T-cell lymphoma: correlation of histologic findings with PCR/DGGE. J Am Acad Dermatol 1998; 38: 453–60.

91. Bergman R, Faclieru D, Sahar D et al. Immunophenotyping and T-cell receptor gamma gene rearrangement analysis as an adjunct to the histopathologic diagnosis of mycosis fungoides. J Am Acad Dermatol 1998; 39: 554–9.

●92. Massone C, Kodama K, Kerl H, Cerroni L. Histopathologic features of early (patch) lesions of mycosis fungoides: a morphologic study on 745 biopsy specimens from 427 patients. Am J Surg Pathol 2005; 29: 550–60.

93. Staib G, Sterry W. Use of polymerase chain reaction in the detection of clones in lymphoproliferative diseases of the skin. Recent Results Cancer Res 1995; 139: 239–47.

94. Weiss LM, Wood GS, Ellisen LW et al. Clonal T-cell populations in pityriasis lichenoides et varioliformis acuta (Mucha-Habermann disease). Am J Pathol 1987; 126: 417–21.

95. Dereure O, Levi E, Kadin ME. T-Cell clonality in pityriasis lichenoides et varioliformis acuta. Arch Dermatol 2000; 136: 1483–6.

96. Toro JR, Sander CA, LeBoit PE. Persistent pigmented purpuric dermatitis and mycosis fungoides: simulant, precursor, or both? A study by light microscopy and molecular methods. Am J Dermatopathol 1997; 19: 108–18.

97. Nickoloff BJ. Light-microscopic assessment of 100 patients with patch/plaque-stage mycosis fungoides. Am J Dermatopathol 1988; 10: 469–77.

98. Smith NP. Histologic criteria for early diagnosis of cutaneous T-cell lymphoma. Dermatol Clin 1994; 12: 315–22.

99. Bagot M, Wechsler J, Lescs MC *et al.* Intraepidermal localization of the clone in cutaneous T-cell lymphoma. *J Am Acad Dermatol* 1992; **27**: 589.

100. Santucci M, Biggeri A, Feller AC *et al.* Efficacy of histologic criteria for diagnosing early mycosis fungoides. An EORTC cutaneous lymphoma study group investigation. *Am J Surg Pathol* 2000; **24**: 40–50.

101. El Darouti M, Marzouk SA, Horn TD. Failure of detection of mucin in the clear halos around the epidermotropic lymphocytes in mycosis fungoides. *J Cutan Pathol* 2000; **27**: 183–5.

102. Lefeber WP, Robinson JK, Clendenning WE *et al.* Attempts to enhance light microscopic diagnosis of cutaneous T-cell lymphoma (mycosis fungoides). *Arch Dermatol* 1981; **117**: 408–11.

●103. Buechner SA, Winkelmann RK. Sezary syndrome: a clinicopathologic study of 39 cases. *Arch Dermatol* 1983; **119**: 979–86.

104. Kohler S, Kim YH, Smoller BR. Histologic criteria for the diagnosis of erythrodermic mycosis fungoides and Sezary syndrome: a critical reappraisal. *J Cutan Pathol* 1997; **24**: 292–7.

105. Kamarashev J, Burg G, Kempf M *et al.* Comparative analysis of histological and immunohistological features in mycosis fungoides and Sezary syndrome. *J Cutan Pathol* 1998; **25**: 407–12.

106. Trotter MJ, Whittaker SJ, Orchard GE, Smith NP. Cutaneous histopathology of Sezary syndrome: a study of 41 cases with a proven circulating T-cell clone. *J Cutan Pathol* 1997; **24**: 286–91.

39

Other peripheral T cell lymphomas: pathology and molecular pathogenesis

PHILIPPE GAULARD AND JEHAN DUPUIS

INTRODUCTION

T cell lymphomas are a heterogeneous group of neoplasms with variable clinical presentations, morphologic patterns, phenotypes and underlying genetic abnormalities. They are divided into precursor T cell (lymphoblastic) neoplasms of thymic origin, and mature (peripheral) post-thymic lymphomas. The latter are designated as peripheral T cell lymphomas (PTCLs), which account for about 10–15 percent of non-Hodgkin lymphomas in most Western countries, with a great geographic variation.[1,2] Indeed, they are more frequent in Asia and their frequency varies from 1.5 percent in Vancouver to around 20 percent in Hong Kong.[3] This may at least partly reflect the involvement of viruses in their pathogeny such as human T lymphotrophic virus type 1 (HTLV-1) and Epstein–Barr virus (EBV), whose presence is increased in some regions, especially in Asian countries.

Historically, the classification of malignant lymphomas was based on histology, which included cytologic features and growth patterns. The Kiel classification was the first to recognize some histopathologic entities among T cell neoplasms, with relatively well-defined characteristics (angioimmunoblastic, lymphoblastic, etc.). However, several studies have recognized the limitations of morphology as the defining criteria for these entities and the use of phenotypic and molecular tools has proved to be essential in the diagnostic work-up of T cell lymphomas. Despite significant progress made in recent years in understanding their pathogenesis, the primary genetic event has been recognized in only a few entities such as the translocations involving *ALK* (anaplastic lymphoma kinase) in anaplastic large cell lymphoma. These tumors may originate from different, sometimes tissue-specific, subsets of T cells (CD4, CD8, cytotoxic, $\alpha\beta$, $\gamma\delta$) or natural killer (NK) cells. However, as opposed to most B cell lymphomas, the precise normal cell counterpart of many PTCL subtypes remains largely unknown. Thus, the phenotype, the site of origin, the clinical presentation, and the relationship with certain antigens (such as EBV, gliadin) seem to be very important aspects in the definition of these entities.

As for B cell lymphomas, the concept of clinicopathologic entities has been introduced in the REAL classification[4] with a list of 'T cell and putative NK cell neoplasms', which has been slightly modified in the two successive editions of the WHO classification (Box 39.1).[5] Many of these entities are obviously organ-specific (i.e. mycosis fungoides, enteropathy-associated, hepatosplenic, nasal NK/T). Due to the phenotypic and functional properties shared by some cytotoxic T cells and NK cells, the list includes T and NK cell tumors, some entities showing some diversity in terms of cell lineage. Besides well-defined entities, this list comprises others which are just morphologic subtypes without clinical and biologic relevance, the prototype of which being the 'PTCL, not otherwise specified' (PTCL-NOS) category.

The clinical evolution of T cell lymphomas is usually aggressive and the present therapeutic strategies are limited. Therapies which have cured a significant proportion of

---

BOX 39.1: World Health Organization (WHO) classification for T cell neoplasms

Precursor T lymphoblastic lymphoma/leukemia

Mature T and NK cell neoplasms

- Leukemic/disseminated
  - T cell prolymphocytic leukemia
  - T cell large granular lymphocytic leukemia
  - Chronic lymphoproliferative disorders of NK cells
  - Aggressive NK cell leukemia
  - EBV-positive T cell lymphoproliferative disorders of childhood
  - Adult T cell leukemia/lymphoma (HTLV-1 +)
- Nodal
  - Peripheral T cell lymphoma, not otherwise specified
  - Angioimmunoblastic T cell lymphoma
  - Anaplastic large cell lymphoma, ALK positive
  - Anaplastic large cell lymphoma, ALK negative
- Extranodal
  - Extranodal NK/T cell lymphomas, nasal type
  - Enteropathy-associated T cell lymphoma
  - Hepatosplenic T cell lymphoma
  - Subcutaneous panniculitis-like T cell lymphoma
  - Primary cutaneous $\gamma\delta$ T cell lymphoma
  - Mycosis fungoides/Sézary syndrome
  - Primary cutaneous CD30-positive T cell lymphoproliferative disorders

---

other subtypes of aggressive lymphomas, such as diffuse large B cell lymphoma, have proved to be less efficient in most PTCL subtypes. The heterogeneity of these tumors and their relatively low incidence are important limiting factors for the establishment of more satisfactory therapies.

We will successively describe the morphologic, biologic and clinical aspects of the different entities. PTCLs can be divided into three groups according to their predominant leukemic, nodal or extranodal clinical presentation (Box 39.1). Most PTCLs present as nodal neoplasms. The latter comprise two distinct and relatively frequent entities with clinical and biologic significance: angioimmunoblastic T cell lymphoma (AITL) and primary systemic anaplastic large cell lymphoma (ALCL) whereas the PTCL, NOS groups the cases which cannot be classified in any other entity of T or NK cell lymphomas. Anaplastic large cell lymphoma is discussed in another section of this book (see Chapter 38). Among T and NK cell lymphomas with extranodal presentation, NK cell lymphomas and mycosis fungoides/Sézary syndrome are described in Chapters 34 and 36, respectively.

ADULT T CELL LEUKEMIA/LYMPHOMA (HTLV-1 RELATED)

Adult T cell leukemia/lymphoma (ATLL) is a peripheral T cell neoplasm that is caused by the human T cell leukemia virus type 1 (HTLV-1). Despite a heterogeneous clinical presentation, the disease is usually disseminated and follows an aggressive clinical course.

The disease occurs in adult patients originating from endemic areas for the HTLV-1 retrovirus (mostly Japan, the Caribbean islands and parts of Central Africa). It develops in 2 percent to 4 percent of carriers for HTLV-1. From the time of viral infection to the occurrence of the lymphoma, there is a long latency (20–40 years). The epidemiology of HTLV-1 infection and ATLL is covered in more detail in Chapter 6.

Clinical features

The clinical presentation of HTLV-1 related T cell lymphomas/leukemias is heterogeneous. The neoplastic cells are most often highly pleomorphic lymphoid cells which are often recognized on the blood film as so-called 'flower cells' because of their polylobated nuclei. At presentation, the most common sites of involvement are lymph nodes (72 percent), skin (53 percent), liver (47 percent), spleen (25 percent) and manifestations related to hypercalcemia due to lytic bone lesions are present in 25 percent of patients. Diagnostic criteria and separation into four distinct clinical subtypes have been proposed by the Japanese Lymphoma Study Group in 1991:[6]

- The smoldering type is defined by the presence of 5 percent or more abnormal T lymphocytes in the peripheral blood, without hyperlymphocytosis (i.e. less than 4×10^9 lymphocytes/L), no hypercalcemia, lactate deshydrogenase (LDH) value of up to 1.5 times the normal upper limit, no lymphadenopathy, no involvement of liver, spleen, central nervous system (CNS), bone and gastrointestinal tract, and neither ascites nor pleural effusion. Skin and pulmonary lesions may be present. In case of less than 5 percent abnormal T lymphocytes in the peripheral blood, at least one of histologically proven skin or pulmonary lesion should be present.

- In the chronic type, absolute lymphocytosis (4×10^9/L or more) is present with T lymphocytosis more than 3.5×10^9/L, LDH value up to twice the normal upper limit, no hypercalcemia, no involvement of CNS, bone and gastrointestinal tract, and neither ascites nor pleural effusion. Lymphadenopathy and involvement of the liver, spleen, skin, and lung may be present, and 5 percent or more abnormal T lymphocytes are seen in the peripheral blood in most cases.

- The lymphoma type is characterized by a mainly tumoral presentation, without significant leukemic (peripheral blood) involvement: no lymphocytosis, 1 percent or less abnormal T lymphocytes in the blood, and histologically proven lymphadenopathy with or without extranodal lesions.

- The acute type includes the remaining ATLL patients who usually have leukemic manifestations and tumor lesions, but are not classified as any of the three other types.

In the work cited above, a total of 818 ATLL patients with a mean age of 57 years, diagnosed from 1983 to 1987, were analyzed using these criteria. The median overall survival was 6.2 months for the acute type, 10.2 months for the lymphoma type, 24.3 months for the chronic type, and not yet reached for the smoldering type with a median follow-up period of 13 months after diagnosis for surviving patients. The chronic form can be further subdivided into unfavorable and favorable forms based on the following parameters: serum albumin, LDH level, blood urea nitrogen and expression of the Mib1/Ki67 antigen in tumor biopsies.[7]

The disease is resistant to conventional chemotherapy-based approaches. Different therapies have been proposed to overcome this poor prognosis (reviewed in[8]): intensive combination chemotherapy, high-dose therapy with autologous or allogeneic stem-cell transplant, and the introduction of newer agents such as monoclonal antibodies, antiretroviral therapy or arsenic trioxide.

Histopathology

Morphologic aspects also are heterogeneous. In the acute and lymphoma forms, the most characteristic feature is a pleomorphic tumor cell population composed of predominant medium-sized to large cells showing lobated nuclei with coarsely clumped chromatin and basophilic cytoplasm

(Plate 105, see plate section). Particularly striking is the pleomorphism with marked variation in the size of the nuclei which typically show multiple indentations (flower cells). A small proportion of large transformed cells expressing CD30, sometimes resembling Reed–Sternberg cells, may be present. In the skin, epidermal infiltration with Pautrier-like microabcesses are frequently found and these lesions may resemble those of mycosis fungoides. In the chronic and smoldering forms, the cells are usually small with less atypia. The skin is involved by a sparse dermal infiltrate with hyperkeratosis of the overlying dermis.

A Hodgkin-like variant characterized by an expansion of the paracortical areas of the lymph nodes by small to medium-sized lymphocytes with scattered CD30+, CD15+ Reed–Sternberg-like cells is reported. These cells are EBV-positive B lymphocytes which are thought to be secondary to the underlying immunodeficiency in patients with ATLL.[9] For diagnostic purposes, the presence of abnormal 'flower' cells within the peripheral blood is common and constitutes a good diagnostic criterion for ATLL. Due to the large spectrum of clinical presentation and the non-specific morphologic features, serologic tests for HTLV-1 and search for CD25 and/or FOXP3 expression should be considered in T cell lymphoma patients originating from endemic areas for HTLV-1.

Phenotype and genotype

The classical phenotype is that of helper T cells (CD3+, CD2+, CD4+) with frequent CD7 antigen loss. Very characteristic is the expression of CD25 (interleukin [IL]-2 receptor) antigen. Rare cases are CD8+ or CD4+/CD8+. The TCR genes are clonally rearranged and cytogenetic studies have not yet identified specific recurrent alterations. Southern blot analysis is useful to demonstrate the clonal integration of the virus into the DNA of the neoplastic cells.

Genetics and pathogenesis

The onset of ATLL is preceded by oligoclonal expansion of HTLV-1-infected T cells. These clonal populations result from the expression of the major viral transactivator protein TAX which activates a number of cellular genes (including IL-2, IL-15, etc. and their receptors) and plays an important role in HTLV-1 transformation and resistance to apoptosis, in part through the activation of the NF-κB pathway.[8]

HTLV-1 is transmitted mainly by cell-to-cell contact through a viral synapse, free virions having almost no efficiency in transmitting infection. HTLV-1 can infect multiple cell types (including synovial cells, B and T lymphocytes) and the cellular receptor of HTLV-1 has been identified as the glucose transporter type 1 (GLUT-1).[10] Recently, it has been shown that neuropilin-1 (NRP1), the receptor for semaphorin-3A and VEGF-A165 and a member of the immune synapse, is also a physical and functional partner of HTLV-1 envelope (Env) proteins. GLUT-1, NRP1, and

Env form ternary complexes in transfected cells, suggesting that the HTLV-1 receptor has a multicomponent nature.[11] After transmission, reverse transcription generates proviral DNA from the genomic viral RNA and the provirus is then integrated into the host genome by a viral integrase. Most infected cells have only one copy of the virus.

After infection, the viral copy number will increase both by infection of non-infected cells by cell-to-cell contact and by clonal proliferation of infected cells. As mentioned above, the TAX protein plays a major role in this last phenomenon by acting on many cellular pathways, resulting in enhanced proliferation and inhibition of apoptosis. These pathways include: activation of NF-κB, of cAMP responsive-element binding protein, upregulation of antiapoptotic proteins, repression of p53 (reviewed in Grassmann et al.,[12] Mortreux et al.[13] and Gatza et al.[14]). Therefore, *TAX* acts as a potent oncogene by promoting proliferation and invasiveness of HTLV-1-infected T cells in the early stages after infection. The role of the TAX protein in the latter stages of the disease is nevertheless controversial, because no expression of the protein is found in the tumor cells from patients with established ATLL.[15] TAX is a major target of cytotoxic lymphocytes, and TAX-expressing cells are continuously eliminated from the circulation by these cells.[16,17] One hypothesis is that tumor cells need to acquire supplemental genetic abnormalities in order to escape immune surveillance, thus allowing the expansion of transformed, non-TAX-expressing T cells. An alternative explanation might be that TAX expression could be limited to certain tumor sites outside the bloodstream.[8]

Complex karyotypes with multiple chromosomal breaks[13] and aneuploidy are more frequent in the acute and lymphoma forms. No specific genetic alteration has been identified in ATLL cells except for mutations of p53 and deletion of p16, which are associated with poor prognosis.[18] A DNA-chip analysis of the transcriptional profile of ATLL cells[19] revealed aberrantly transcribed genes such as tumor suppressor in lung cancer 1 *(TSLC1)*, a molecule associated with cell adhesion. Epigenetic changes might also be implicated in the acquisition of a TAX-independent transformed phenotype (reviewed by Taylor et al.[20]).

The tumor cells of ATLL patients have been shown to possess immunosuppressive activity *in vitro*, thus contributing to the profound immune deficiency with frequent infections seen in these patients. ATLL cells have been demonstrated to express the FOXP3 protein, a specific marker for regulatory/suppressive CD4+/CD25+ T cells,[21,22] as well as the chemokine receptor CCR4, which is also characteristic of this type of cell.[23] The physiologic counterpart of ATLL tumor cells is thus thought to correspond to HTLV-1 infected CD4+/CD25+ regulatory T cells.

In summary, ATLL represents a relatively rare complication of infection by the HTLV-1 retrovirus which results from the acquisition of a transformed phenotype by HTLV-1-infected regulatory T cells, through virus-mediated and virus-independent pathways. The multiplicity and complexity of the transformation process is reflected by the heterogeneous clinical and pathologic pictures, which are dominated by a poor prognosis. The development of innovative therapies is of paramount importance, as the results of conventional approaches have proven unsatisfying.

T CELL LYMPHOMAS WITH PREDOMINANTLY NODAL PRESENTATION (EXCLUDING ANAPLASTIC LARGE CELL LYMPHOMA)

ANGIOIMMUNOBLASTIC T CELL LYMPHOMA

Angioimmunoblastic T cell lymphoma is the second most frequent subtype of peripheral T cell lymphoma in the Western world, accounting for about 25–30 percent of PTCLs and up to 2–4 percent of all lymphomas.[1,3,24] The disease was first recognized in the mid-1970s by several groups, who gave it different names: 'immunoblastic lymphadenopathy',[25] 'lymphogranulomatosis X'[26] and 'angioimmunoblastic lymphadenopathy with dysproteinemia' (AILD).[27] For a while, the latter term has been the most commonly used. The disease was essentially felt to be an atypical reactive process or premalignant lesion with an increased risk of progression to lymphoma. In 1979, Shimoyama and colleagues described AILD as being a T cell lymphoma, and thus called it 'immunoblastic lymphadenopathy-like T cell lymphoma'.[28] At the end of the 1980s, cytogenetics and molecular studies for clonality documented that the vast majority if not all cases of so-called AILD were monoclonal T cell proliferations. Thus, this lesion was designated as a peripheral-node-based T cell lymphoma, which was included in the updated Kiel classification[29] and has been further recognized as a distinct clinicopathologic entity in the REAL and WHO classifications and is currently designated 'angioimmunoblastic T cell lymphoma (AITL)'.

Clinical features

Table 39.1 summarizes the main clinical characteristics of AITL according to the literature.[30–33] The disease most often arises in elderly patients, with a median age around 60 years. The clinical presentation plays a role in defining AITL as a 'real' clinico-pathologic entity. Indeed, besides its peculiar morphologic aspect, AITL discloses a distinct clinical presentation with systemic symptoms including fever and weight loss, generalized lymph node swelling, frequent skin rash and a common aggressive clinical behavior.[3,24,30–38] Splenomegaly is frequent, as well as bone marrow involvement, and polyarthritis may be seen. Eosinophilia, hypergammaglobulinemia and autoimmune biologic manifestations such as autoimmune hemolytic anemia with positive Coombs test are common, and are significantly more frequent within this entity than in other PTCL subtypes.[24] The clinical behavior is aggressive with a 10–40 percent

Table 39.1   Main clinical characteristics of angioimmunoblastic T cell lymphoma

First author	N	Stage III–IV	Eosinophilia	Hyper-γ globulinemia	B symptoms	Median age	Positive Coomb test	Skin rash	SMG
Frizzera[27]	24	24/24	7/24	12/22	7/24	68	8/14	9/24	17/23
Lukes[25]	32	21/29	4/12	13/14	13/22	57	3/7	8/20	11/16
Pautier[30]	33	31/33	13/33	16/33	28/33	62	14/33	11/33	24/33
Aozasa[31]	44	37/44	14/44	28/44	12/44	64	–	12/44	17/44
Lachenal[32]	77	71/77	25/75	37/73	59/77	64	38/66	35/77	39/77
Mourad[33]	157	126/156	12/38	73/146	112/155	62	30/92	46/154	86/155

SMG, splenomegaly.

5-year overall survival rate despite aggressive chemotherapy.[3,24,32,33,35–38] However, some patients may have a past history of fluctuating lymph node enlargement, and spontaneous remissions might occur during such episodes.

It has been reported that some patients have a history of drug use, including allergic manifestations to antibiotics (reviewed by Dogan et al.[39]). However, these manifestations more likely belong to the spectrum of clinical manifestations (skin rash) specific to the disease, and are not related to drugs prescribed for a systemic illness more or less mimicking an infectious condition.

Histopathology

Morphologically (Plate 106, see plate section), AITL – in its full picture – is characterized by: (1) an effacement of the normal lymph node architecture, usually with disappearance of follicles, frequent spreading throughout the lymph node capsule, but preservation of the peripheral cortical sinuses; (2) a proliferation of arborizing high endothelial venules frequently associated with PAS-positive material; (3) a polymorphic infiltrate comprising abundant reactive cells, i.e. small lymphocytes, eosinophils, plasmocytes, histiocytes or epithelioid cells, and scattered transformed large lymphoid B cells (sometimes showing a Reed–Sternberg-cell-like appearance); (4) an increase of follicular dentritic cells (FDC) realizing large irregular networks better recognized by specific stainings; and (5) a variable neoplastic cellular content made of slightly atypical small- to medium-sized T cells with abundant clear or pale cytoplasm. These atypical cells are distributed throughout the paracortex, either as scattered single cells or often as small aggregates with a tendency for perivascular distribution (Plate 106). Immunofluorescence staining with antibodies directed against T cell receptor Vβ-family-specific epitopes has shown that the neoplastic component is often less abundant than the reactive background and may even comprise only a minority of the T cell compartment.[40] This minimal neoplastic cell component is often difficult to recognize on morphology alone. CD3 and/or CD5 stainings are useful to highlight their subtle cytological atypia, as well as the more recently described characteristic markers CD10, CXCL13 and PD1 (see below). Demonstration of TCR clonality is often important along with the background of clinical and biologic features.

In the absence of accepted specific molecular markers, the morphologic spectrum of variation in AITL is not yet fully determined. Three architectural patterns have been recently reported.[41] The most common pattern, designated as pattern III according to Attygalle, shows a complete effacement of the normal architecture, without normal B cell follicles. Pattern I characterizes the relatively unfrequent cases of AITL with hyperplastic germinal centers with ill-defined borders without clearly developed mantle zone (also sometimes referred to as 'early phase')[42] (Plate 107A, see plate section) whereas pattern II shows occasional regressing or depleted follicles with concentrically arranged FDC. In both patterns I and II, the atypical polymorphic infiltrate extends beyond the follicles, thus predominating within the paracortical areas. According to the cell content, other morphologic variants have been recognized, including a form rich in epithelioid cell clusters (Plate 107B) which probably at least partly corresponds to cases previously reported as Lennert lymphoma,[43] and a variant with prominent clear cell clusters. In addition, up to 40 percent of cases disclose marked cytologic atypia with a high number of pleomorphic medium to large cells and may show a continuous spectrum with PTCL, NOS. This cytologic grading does not seem to have any clinical impact.[33,44] In a few cases, a transition from pattern I to a diffuse pattern has been noted as well as an increase in T cell immunoblasts over time.[5,39,41,42,45] Finally, numerous B blasts are found in 15–20 percent of cases,[44,46] some of which may even develop an EBV-associated diffuse large cell B cell lymphoma.[45,47] Many patients are found to have involvement of extranodal sites at the time of diagnosis, especially skin and bone marrow. The histopathologic features mimic the features observed in the lymph node, with vascular hyperplasia and polymorphic infiltrates.[48,49] However, due to the focal involvement in these organs, the identification of the neoplastic component is even more difficult, often requiring immunohistochemistry and molecular studies to be demonstrated.

Expertise might be required to distinguish AITL from other conditions which can mimic AITL, including dysimmune reactive processes, classical Hodgkin lymphoma of mixed cellularity subtype, T cell/histiocyte-rich diffuse large B cell lymphoma and EBV-senile lymphoproliferative disorders. These problematic diagnoses occur when the tumor component is minimal and difficult to recognize on morphology alone.

Genotype and phenotype

Southern blot analysis or polymerase chain reaction (PCR) strategies reveal a monoclonal or oligoclonal rearrangement of T cell receptor (TCR) genes in most cases and more variably, a clonal or oligoclonal expansion of B cells.[39] Published series underscore the presence of a monoclonal T cell population in 70–100 percent of cases. In the recent large BIOMED study,[50] PCR for γ and β genes failed to demonstrate clonal rearrangement in 8 percent and 11 percent of cases, respectively, and combined PCR analysis for β, γ and δ genes resulted in the demonstration of T cell clonality in 95 percent. In one study with sequential samples, multiple different clones appearing and disappearing over time have been found.[51] It is tempting to speculate that the failure to detect clonal populations in a small subset of patients is purely technical, due to minor neoplastic infiltrate below the level of detection by molecular techniques. Nevertheless, in a study performed on micromanipulated cells, TCRβ gene rearrangements were not detected, even at a single cell resolution, in those cases in which no clone was found by whole-tissue DNA analysis.[52] In this study, T cell clones from 4/10 cases showing oligoclonal TCR rearrangements were found to express similar TCRβ chains, indicating a potential role of antigen triggering the oligoclonal expansions observed in some cases of AITL.

A peculiar observation in AITL is the presence of a clonal or oligoclonal expansion of B cells in 20–40 percent of cases, as demonstrated by PCR techniques.[39,41,53,54] This observation appears to be a characteristic feature of AITL, with a 32 percent rate of immunoglobulin heavy and/or light chain genes rearrangement in AITL, compared with 9 percent in PTCL, NOS (and 0 percent in anaplastic large cell lymphoma in the BIOMED study).[50] It is thought to reflect the expansion of EBV-infected B immunoblasts with a restriction in their repertoire,[55] which, in some patients can give rise to a proliferation with features of an EBV-positive diffuse large B cell lymphoma.[45–47]

Phenotypic studies in AITL have shown that the neoplastic cells are mature $\alpha\beta$T cells with a CD3+ CD4+ phenotype that frequently show a CD7 T cell antigen loss and sometimes low or heterogeneous CD4 expression.[56] Immunohistochemistry typically shows a predominant infiltrate of CD3+ T cells with scattered large CD20+ B immunoblasts which may show Reed–Sternberg-cell-like features,[57] and are CD30+, sometimes CD15+, EBV-positive transformed cells. Immunohistochemistry is helpful to highlight the cytologic atypia within the T cell population and to demonstrate the proliferation of follicular dendritic cells (FDCs), which is regarded as one of the hallmarks of AITL.[58] It is recognized by stainings with CD21, CD23, CD35, or CNA-42 antibodies, with a better sensitivity for CD21 than CD23 and CNA-42.[59] However, it can be minimal or absent in early cases (pattern I) and can be lost in advanced cases with transformed features whereas it realizes disrupted networks inside the interfollicular areas surrounding arborizing venules in classical diffuse AITL (pattern III).[40,52] Neoplastic cells are admixed with an abundant population of CD4+ and CD8+ reactive T cells. The number of CD8+ cells can dominate the CD4+ cells in some cases and might even show mild atypia. Earlier studies describing CD8+ AITL cases have probably been misled by this appearance. These CD8+ cells are low-proliferating lymphocytes which most probably represent an exaggerated activated cytotoxic reaction.[60,61]

Recently, Attygalle and colleagues reported that CD10, an antigen normally expressed by immature lymphocytes, germinal center B cells and their derived-tumor cells, was also expressed by the neoplastic cells of most AITL cases, and could be used as an objective diagnostic marker.[41] CD10 expression by neoplastic cells of AITL has been reported in up to 90 percent of cases, but with a great variation in the number of positive cells from case to case. As demonstrated by flow cytometry (personal observations and references 62–65), CD10-positive T cells may account only for a fraction of the neoplastic cells. In cases with hyperplastic germinal centers, they are predominantly located at the rim of reactive germinal centers, sometimes within the follicle centers and, whatever the pattern, have a tendency to show an intimate association with the FDC meshwork.[39,41,56] CD10 positivity has been initially described as an aberrant expression, but might in fact reflect an origin from a peculiar subset of CD10 positive T cells as CD10 has been recently shown in a few benign T cells with a predominant follicular distribution.[56,66] Neoplastic cells in AITL have been shown to express BCL6[41,56,63,67] (in the absence of mutations in the 5' non-coding region of the gene), and CD57 has been scored as positive in rare cases.[44]

Recently, a population of T cells termed follicular B helper T cells (T_{FH}) specialized in B cell help and defined by a specific CD4+/CD45RO+/CXCR5+/CCR7−/CD57+ phenotype has been recognized.[68] These T_{FH} cells display a unique gene expression profile compared with other helper T cell populations and expression of CXCL13 and BCL6 were recognized as characteristic features of these cells, which are distributed in the light zone of the germinal centers.[69,70] Several arguments have provided convergent lines of evidence that AITL arises from this population of activated T cells which home to the follicles: some studies have shown that the neoplastic cells in AITL express markers such as CXCR3 and CD69 along with CD4 and BCL6, compatible with a T_{FH} origin.[71–73] Selective expression of the B cell attractant chemokine CXCL13 has been demonstrated in the atypical T cells of most AITL cases.[56,74,75] By double stainings, CXCL13 positive cells were demonstrated to correspond to CD10-positive T cells.[56] Interestingly,

CXCL13 was also found in CD10-negative AITL. Other follicular B helper T cell-associated antigens such as CXCR5, PD1 and SAP have also be shown to be expressed in AITL (see Plate 108, see plate section).[76–78] Finally, gene-expression profile studies have shown that AITL posseses a distinct expression profile reminiscent of T_{FH} cells[79,80] (Plate 108). The origin from T_{FH} cells might explain the frequent perifollicular or intrafollicular distribution of neoplastic cells in AITL,[41,81] as well as the features consistent with B cell stimulation, including follicular hyperplasia, hypergammaglobulinemia and large B blast expansion sometimes culminating in overt B cell lymphoma, which are seen in a proportion of AITL. The relationship between AITL and intrafollicular PTCLs as described by de Leval[82] (see above) remains to be established. Occasional cases of PTCL, NOS have been reported to express CD10 and/or CXCL13 or PD1, and/or to disclose overlapping molecular features with AITL.[56,75,79] At least some of these cases were reported to have borderline morphologic and phenotypic features with AITL and future studies with these markers will be helpful to delineate the morphologic spectrum of AITL.

Genetics and pathogenesis

According to the few existing cytogenetic studies, 70–90 percent of AITL patients have chromosomal alterations.[39] The most recurrent abnormalities are trisomy 3, trisomy 5 and gain of an X chromosome which are not specific of AITL, being also observed in other PTCL subtypes. A recurrent t(7;14)(q35;q11) translocation has been reported in three cases. According to two recent fluorescent in situ hybridization (FISH)-based studies, chromosomal breakpoints affecting the TCRα/δ (14q11) and TCRβ (7q35) gene loci appear to be rare events, being observed in only one out of 54 AITLs.[83,84] Besides the clonal alterations, Schlegelberger and coworkers showed the presence of unrelated clones in around half the patients, supporting a multistep process with the occurrence of chromosomal aberrations in different cells because of genetic instability.[85] It is not yet established whether the EBV-positive B blasts could have genetic alterations explaining the observed genetic heterogeneity.[39] Using a matrix-based comparative genomic hybridization (CGH) approach, complex genetic imbalances were found in AITL, with the more common recurrent changes being gains of 22q, 19 and 11q13 and losses of 13q.[86] In this last study, trisomies 3 and 5 were rare events.

Several infectious agents, especially lymphotropic viruses, have been reported to be associated with AITL. Polymerase chain reaction studies showed HHV-6B genome in almost half of the cases,[39,87] but HHV-6 was not found inside T cells by immunohistochemistry. The presence of HHV-8, which has been detected by PCR in occasionnal cases,[39] was also not confirmed by immunohistochemistry. Due to its virtually constant presence in AITL lymph nodes, the role of EBV has been postulated. Indeed, EBV has been detected by in situ hybridization with EBER probes in 80–95 percent of AITL. Double-labeling techniques as well as analysis obtained from microdissected cells have revealed that EBV-infected cells correspond to the scattered B immunoblasts.[55,87,88] Although the exact role of EBV in the pathogenesis of AITL remains unknown, it is highly suggested that EBV is reactivated within these B cells as a consequence of immunosuppression with reduced cytotoxic activity and secretion of growth factors favoring the expansion of EBV-infected B cells in a primary T cell disorder. It is admitted that AITL patients disclose immunologic deficiency. In keeping with the minor B cell clones found in a proportion of cases, the EBV genome is found to be clonal using Southern blot techniques.[89] These EBV-positive cells frequently have a type II latency with expression of LMP1.

The inflammatory background and the proliferation of FDCs, as well as the systemic and biologic manifestations seen in AITL patients, suggest the involvement of different cytokines and chemokines. In situ hybridization techniques and DNA array studies of cytokines and chemokines and their receptors have found increased expression of IFN-γ, lymphotoxin, TNFα, IL-2, IL-4, IL-6 and IL-13.[90,91] Vascular endothelial growth factor (VEGF), a major angiogenic cytokine that is expressed on different cell types including lymphoma cells, stromal cells and endothelial cells in AITL,[92,93] may explain the prominent vascularization observed in AITL. In addition, the expression of its receptor on endothelial cells surrounding the lymphoma component suggests the possibility of some paracrine and/or autocrine loop.[93] The molecular profile of AITL is characterized by a strong microenvironment imprint with overexpression of B cell- and follicular dendritic cell-related genes, chemokines and genes related to extracellular matrix and vascular biology,[79,94] with a specific deregulation of several genes including VEGF.[80] The possible implication of the NF-κB pathway in this disease does not seem to be confirmed by a recent study.[80] Considering genes known to be involved in B cell lymphomagenesis, p53 mutations are rarely found in AITL, and p53 expression seems often restricted to the scattered EBV-positive B blasts.[95] Very recently, a role for MAF, a (T_{H2}-specific) transcription factor that activates the expression of IL-4 and IL-10 and might also function as an oncogene in multiple myeloma, has been proposed in AITL: indeed, it was recently shown that transgenic mice for MAF developed T cell lymphoma[96] and expression of MAF has been observed in neoplastic T cells in most AITL cases by immunohistochemistry.[97]

PERIPHERAL T CELL LYMPHOMA, NOT OTHERWISE SPECIFIED

The term 'peripheral T cell lymphoma, unspecified (PTCL, NOS)' designates the vast group of predominantly nodal PTCLs which do not correspond to any recognizable ('specified') subtype of T cell lymphoma. Although the Kiel classification (which was the first to separate B and T cell lymphomas) defined multiple subtypes within this category (mainly pleomorphic small-, medium- and large-cell types),[29] these were not retained inside the REAL[4] and WHO[5] classifications, because of a perceived lack of evidence of diagnostic reproducibility and clinical significance. Studies focusing on diagnostic reproducibility of these categories found at best moderately good inter-observer consensus.[98] Hence, all cases are lumped together inside the – often described as a wastebasket – 'PTCL, not otherwise specified' category. Nevertheless, the WHO classification recognizes three rare morphologic variants designated lymphoepithelioid, follicular and T-zone PTCL, NOS. It is likely that individual clinicopathologic entities will be delineated in the future from this broad group of malignancies.

As a whole, PTCL, NOS represents the most frequent category among T cell neoplasms in Western countries, accounting for 29–68 percent of cases.[1,3,24,36,37,99–101] The reported lower relative frequency in case series from Asia might be due to the overrepresentation of nasal-type NK/T cell lymphoma in these populations.[102]

Clinical features

Despite their morphologic heterogeneity, clinical characteristics at diagnosis show a remarkable homogeneity between patient series (Table 39.2).[3,24,36–38,100–107] PTCL, NOS almost exclusively affects adult patients with a median age around 60 years. A male predominance is found in all studies (in the order of 60 percent), and the reasons for this remain to be understood. Most patients exhibit generalized lymphadenopathy, hepatosplenomegaly (advanced-stage disease is found in 70–80 percent of patients), and bone marrow involvement is found in a third of cases. Constitutional symptoms, including fever, weight loss and night sweats, are common (30 percent). Although most patients present with predominantly nodal disease, some patients with predominant or even exclusive extranodal disease might be classified as PTCL, NOS. These cases do not by definition show any of the characteristics of the extranodal disease entities of the WHO classification, such as hepatosplenic, etc.

The clinical course is aggressive, although complete remission is obtained with multiagent chemotherapy in around 50 percent of cases, a rate which is lower than the ones observed in diffuse large B cell lymphoma, the most frequent type of agressive lymphoma.[24] In most studies (Table 39.2), there is an elevated proportion of patients with unfavorable characteristics according to the International Prognostic Index (IPI) for aggressive lymphomas. However, these unfavorable characteristics alone do not explain the dismal prognosis associated with non-anaplastic PTCL in general, and PTCL, NOS in particular. As shown in Table 39.2, long-term survival does not exceed 30 percent in most series. In multivariate analysis, T cell phenotype retains a negative prognostic impact independently from other prognostic factors such as those of the IPI. A prognostic score differing slightly from the IPI has been proposed based on a retrospective multicentric Italian study: this score includes age, performance status, LDH level and the presence of bone marrow involvement, and separates patients in four risk groups with 5-year overall survival rates ranging from 18 percent to 62 percent according to risk stratification.[108]

Table 39.2 Main clinical characteristics of peripheral T cell lymphoma, not otherwise specified (PTCL, NOS)

First author, year	N	Median age	Percent Male	Percent B symptoms	Percent BM involvement	Percent Stage III–IV	Percent IPI >2	Percent CR	Percent 5-year OS	Median survival (months)
Zaja, 1997[103]	23	55	70	43	30	83	56	47	–	34
Ascani, 1997[36]	78	50	75	43	28	72	–	50	–	17
Gisselbrecht, 1998[24]	142	66% > 60	65	52	32	79	–	53	37	–
Lopez-Guillermo, 1998[37]	95	52% > 60	61	57	41	79	46	47	–	22
Armitage, 1998[104]	76	61	55	50	36	80	–	–	25	14
Pellatt, 2002[100]	35	57	68	51	20	54	–	40	40	16
Kim, 2002[102]	31	54	65	52	32	71	39	52	–	18
Rüdiger, 2002[3]	53	59	–	41	–	>60	60	–	26	–
Savage, 2004[38]	117	64	61	38	26	67	69	64	35	–
Kojima, 2004[105]	36	68	58	47	60	83	72	39	<25	–
Au, 2005[106]	24	54	79	–	–	58	–	42	–	12
Sonnen, 2005[101]	70	55	57	38	23	68	32	55	45	–
Dupuis, 2006[107]	110	60	68	–	36	84	44	50	30	–

BM, bone marrow; IPI, International Prognostic Index; CR, complete remission; OS, overall survival.

Histopathology

On histopathology, most PTCL, NOS are characterized by a heterogeneous cellular composition. There is usually a mixture of small, medium and large atypical lymphoid cells. In fact, cytologic appearance is very variable from case to case. They may show preferential involvement of the paracortical areas of lymph nodes. An inflammatory background can be seen, consisting of eosinophils, plasma cells, and histiocytes or epithelioid cells. The positive diagnosis of PTCL relies on both morphology and immunohistochemistry using a panel of antibodies comprising at least CD20 and CD3.

Most PTCL, NOS fall into the pleomorphic lymphoma category according to the Kiel classification, with a mixture of small, medium-sized and large atypical lymphoid cells showing nuclear pleomorphism, i.e. variations in the shape of the nuclei of the neoplastic cells. Most cases are composed of medium-sized and large cells and were referred to as 'pleomorphic medium-sized and large cell lymphoma' (Plate 109A, see plate section).[109] Occasional giant cells expressing CD30 which may ressemble Reed–Sternberg cells can be seen.[110] Some PTCL, NOS consisting of a uniform population of large cells expressing CD30 may be difficult to distinguish from ALK-negative anaplastic large cell lymphomas (ALCL) (Plate 109B, C). The latter do show a prognosis intermediate between that of PTCL, NOS and ALK-positive ALCL.[111–113] Thus, the border between CD30-positive PTCL, NOS and ALK-negative ALCL is ill-defined (and relies heavily on morphology alone), but this distinction may be clinically relevant. Very rarely, PTCL, NOS are composed of a relatively uniform population of large cells with a round nucleus and sometimes solitary nucleolus, referred to as 'immunoblastic T cell lymphoma' in the past. Cases composed of a relatively monotonous proliferation of pleomorphic small cells without a significant population of large cells – 'pleomorphic small-cell type' (Plate 109D) according to the Kiel classification – are rare and should be carefully distinguished from lymph node involvements by chronic ATLL (see above), T-PLL or mycosis fungoides/Sézary's syndrome.

Other cases might correspond to peculiar morphologic variants, some of which are recognized inside the WHO classification.

LYMPHOEPITHELIOID VARIANT (ALSO KNOWN AS LENNERT LYMPHOMA)

This variant is characterized by the presence of numerous small clusters of epithelioid histiocytes within a diffuse proliferation of small to medium-sized cells with slight nuclear irregularities (Plate 109D, E). The search for atypia within the T cell population, the effacement of the architecture and the absence of Reed–Sternberg cells are essential diagnostic criteria. This variant was first described to be of T helper origin, but there is now evidence for a derivation from CD8+ cytotoxic T cells expressing cytotoxic granule-associated proteins.[114,115] It is not clear whether these cases show specific clinical features compared with the rest of PTCL, NOS. Given the performance of immunohistochemistry on routinely fixed specimens, it appears that many of the cases reported in the past as lymphoepithelioid/ Lennert lymphoma based on morphology correspond to other lymphoma entities, especially AITL with a high content of epithelioid cells, and Hodgkin lymphoma, and that the diagnosis of this PTCL variant should be rarely considered.[116] Differential diagnosis might prove difficult between this entity and some cases of Hodgkin lymphoma, epithelioid-rich AITL, and some forms of B cell lymphoma with an important histiocytic component.[43]

T–ZONE VARIANT

In this very rare variant, the tumor cells develop between rare preserved or even hyperplastic follicles inside the interfollicular or T-zone. The tumor cells consist of small to medium-sized lymphocytes showing only moderate nuclear polymorphism. Scattered large cells (T immunoblasts) are often seen. The tumor cells show a helper CD4+/CD8−, nontoxic phenotype. The process may be mistaken for benign paracortical hyperplasia. The differential diagnosis with angioimmunoblastic T cell lymphoma with hyperplastic follicles might prove difficult and the search for clusters of clear cells is essential. The clinical context as well as the absence of interdigitated cells are also important to eliminate nodal involvement by mycosis fungoides/ Sézary syndrome.[109] It has been suggested that this variant may be associated with a more indolent course.[117]

Other variants, not included inside the WHO classification, have also been described.

FOLLICULAR VARIANT

In the past few years, several cases of PTCL, NOS in which the tumor cells showed a predominant follicular involvement with intrafollicular aggregates of medium-sized T cells with clear cytoplasm (mimicking follicular lymphoma), or small aggregates located within large B cell follicles – thus mimicking nodular lymphocyte-predominant Hodgkin lymphoma – or inside the expanded mantle zone of B cell follicles have been reported.[82,118–123] These cases show a CD4−positive helper T cell phenotype and may express the germinal-center associated proteins BCL6 and/or CD10, as well as CD57.[82,120–121] According to a recent study, this variant might be associated to a t(5;9) translocation (see below).[122] The link between this follicular variant and the subset of follicular helper T cells, which is recognized to be the cell of origin of angioimmunoblastic T cell lymphoma, is underlined by the fact that these cases consistently express follicular helper T cell associated molecules such as CXCL13 and PD1.[123] The possibility that this variant might represent a peculiar stage of AITL has been proposed.[118,123]

Phenotype and genotype

The vast majority of PTCL-U disclose expression of CD3 in neoplastic cells as shown by immunohistochemistry in paraffin-embedded tissue sections. The latter demonstrates the mature T cell phenotype (i.e. Tdt- and CD1a-negative) of the neoplastic cells. Deletion of one of the pan T cell antigens (CD3, CD5, CD2 or CD7) is seen in 75 percent of cases, with CD7 antigen being the most frequently lost.[3] Regarding the expression of the major subset antigens CD4 and CD8, a CD4+/CD8− phenotype is more frequent than a CD8+/CD4− phenotype, although a double negative CD4−/CD8− or double positive CD4+/CD8+ phenotype[124] has been reported in one series using a tissue microarray-based approach.[3,105,124] In fact, the precise immunophenotypical pattern of tumor cells is variable, reproducing that of the main T cell subsets corresponding to their supposed physiologic counterparts. As not all T cells contained inside a diagnostic specimen correspond to tumor cells, determination of which markers are specifically expressed by tumor versus reactive cells might prove challenging. Geissinger and coworkers[125] developed a polymerase chain reaction assay to define the clonally rearranged TCRVβ segment in order to specifically identify the neoplastic population in immunohistochemically stained slides, detecting the corresponding epitope with segment-specific antibodies. In nine of 14 cases, less than 50 percent of T cells expressed the clonally rearranged TCRVβ segment. Phenotypes defined in double stains differed from those obtained by conventional immunohistochemistry in many cases.

Expression of cytotoxic molecules is a hallmark of CD8-positive $\alpha\beta$ T cells, $\gamma\delta$ T cells, NK-like T cells and NK cells. Immunohistochemical detection of cytotoxic granule-associated proteins such as TIA1 and granzyme B help identify these subgroups.[124,126–129] The percentage of PTCL, NOS expressing cytotoxic proteins is variable according to published data.[61,124,129] In a recent study, Asano and coworkers[129] detected the expression of at least one of these proteins in 41 of 100 cases of PTCL, NOS. These patients had peculiar presenting characteristics, including frequent extranodal disease sites, younger age, less male predominance, and frequent adverse prognostic factors of the IPI. Expression of cytotoxic molecules was found by this group to be associated with an adverse prognosis in a multivariate analysis of survival. This was not confirmed by Went and colleagues,[124] who found expression of TIA1 and granzyme B in 27 percent and 2 percent of cases, respectively, without any association with survival. It is likely that these lymphomas represent the neoplastic counterparts of cytotoxic T cell subsets, with the disease showing a preference for extranodal MALT localizations,[127] albeit many are classified as PTCL, NOS according to WHO criteria.

Clonal rearrangements of the TCR genes are physiologically found in the vast majority of normal peripheral T cells. In PTCL, NOS, 90 percent to 100 percent of cases show a detectable rearrangement of the γ and β TCR genes.[50,130] In most cases, this leads to the expression of a TCR on the cell surface, mostly of the $\alpha\beta$ subtype.[124,131] In the largest study conducted to date,[124] expression of the βF1 antigen was found in 97 percent of 133 cases of PTCL, NOS. Some rare cases not corresponding to hepatosplenic $\gamma\delta$ entity do express a $\gamma\delta$ surface receptor; these cases show preferential extranodal involvement.[61,128,132,133]

Pathogenesis

TH1–TH2 PROFILE

Among effector helper T (Th) cells, two main functional subsets are identified according to their cytokine-production profile. Th1 cells produce interferonγ, TNFα and lymphotoxin and promote cell-mediated immunity, while Th2 cells secrete IL-4, -5, -10 and have an important role in antibody-mediated immune responses. Different authors have focused on the expression pattern of several chemokines and chemokine receptors associated with these subsets to identify different subclasses among PTCL: Jones et al.[72] studied the expression of the Th1-associated chemokine receptor CXCR3, whose expression was found in 17/39 patients with PTCL, NOS, whereas the Th2-associated receptor CCR4 was found in a mostly nonoverlapping subgroup of 4/15 PTCL, NOS. Ishida et al.[134] also found a heterogeneous expression of CXCR3 and CCR4 in PTCL, NOS, and associated CCR4 expression with a worse prognosis. Interestingly, they found an association between expression of CCR4 and the regulatory T cell associated protein FOXP3, suggesting an association with an immunocompromised state. Tsuchiya et al.[73] also separated PTCL, NOS cases according to their respective expression of Th1 or Th2 associated markers (such as CXCR3 and ST2(L) respectively). In this series, a worse prognosis was found among patients expressing neither Th1 or Th2 markers than among those expressing one or more of these markers. In a separate work including gene expression profiling studies focusing on chemokines and chemokine receptors,[135] the same group separated 134 cases of PTCL, NOS in three groups: CCR4 type ($n = 42$), CCR3 type ($n = 31$) and CXCR3 type ($n = 54$). Each group had significantly different survival times, with CCR4 type showing the worst prognosis.

A more recently described subset among helper T cells is the one termed follicular helper T cells. Expression of the chemokine CXCL13, which is associated with this subgroup was found in a small subgroup of PTCL, NOS showing borderline characteristics with angioimmunoblastic T cell lymphoma.[56,75] Gene expression profiling studies have shown traces of the TFH signature in CD30− PTCL, NOS suggesting that the AITL spectrum might be wider than suspected and might comprise borderline cases with PTCL, NOS.[79]

CYTOGENETICS

Classical cytogenetic studies in PTCL, NOS have not identified any specific recurrent genetic alterations, with the notable exception of t(5;9) (see below). Most reports are based on a low number of cases, but indicate abnormal findings in a majority of cases.[136–138] By comparative genomic hybridization, Zettl and coworkers[139] identified recurrent chromosomal losses on chromosomes 13q, 6q, 9p, 10q, 12q and 5q in PTCL, NOS and found recurrent gains in the 7q22-qter region. Interestingly, they also identified high-level amplification of the 12p13 region to be restricted to cytotoxic PTCL, NOS. Another group, using a matrix-based CGH approach, identified gains in 17q11-q25, 8 (including the MYC locus at 8q24) and 22q, and losses of 13q and 9p21-q33 as the most frequent imbalances in PTCL, NOS.[86] Such findings underline the complexity and multiplicity of pathogenic mechanisms associated with the diverse populations of tumor cells composing PTCL, NOS. More recently, a novel recurrent t(5;9) (q33;q22) chromosomal translocation has been reported in a subset of PTCL, NOS.[123] Among these cases, most presented with predominant involvement of follicles as described by de Leval *et al.*[82] Interestingly, this translocation fuses the IL-2-inducible T cell kinase (*ITK*) to the signal-transducing protein kinase (*SYK*). The development of FISH and RT-PCR strategies to detect such translocations would allow in the future the recognition of new clinicopathologic entities in this ill-defined group of PTCL, NOS based on specific genetic alterations with possible prognostic or therapeutic implications.

DNA ARRAY STUDIES

Several groups have reported results regarding gene-expression profile analysis in PTCL, NOS. Martinez-Delgado and colleagues analyzed 42 cases of T cell lymphomas (among which 19 cases of PTCL, NOS) using a specific cDNA microarray containing 6386 cancer-related genes.[140] Unsupervised clustering clearly separated PTCLs from T lymphoblastic lymphoma. An important fraction of the genes significantly overexpressed in PTCLs were found to be involved in immune response as well as in the NF-κB signaling pathway. On a separate analysis focusing on 109 NF-κB related genes, the same group reported[141] reduced expression of NF-κB related genes in a third of PTCLs, whereas the other two-thirds showed a high expression of these genes. This dichotomy was found inside each category of PTCL, except anaplastic large cell lymphoma. Reduced expression of NF-κB associated genes was associated with an adverse prognosis. Using the same array and also a custom oligonucleotide microarray comprising 2745 genes, the same group identified five gene clusters using unsupervised hierarchical clustering, among which two essentially contained proliferation-associated genes. The 14 most correlated genes formed a signature termed proliferation core signature, which was associated with decreased patient survival.[142]

By using a different cDNA microarray containing 7874 clones related to carcinogenesis to study 59 cases of T cell lymphoma – including 32 PTCL, NOS – Ballester and coworkers defined three distinct molecular subgroups among PTCL, NOS, termed U1 to U3.[94] The PTCL-U1 gene expression signature was characterized by the overexpression of genes known to be associated with poor outcome in various tumor types, such as overexpression of CCND2. The PTCL-U2 subtype disclosed high expression of genes involved in translation, signal transduction and apoptosis. Its signature included NF-κB-1 and BCL2. The PTCL-U3 signature was mainly characterized by genes related to the macrophage/histiocyte lineage. Most of these cases showed an abundant reactive histiocytic component and some had been classified as Lennert lymphomas.

Two groups performed gene expression profiling studies in PTCL, NOS using pangenomic Affymetrix microarrays: in the study by Piccaluga and colleagues, PTCL, NOS was shown to have an expression profile close to that of activated T cells, with two different subgroups being identified based on the similarity of their profile with that of normal helper CD4+ and cytotoxic CD8+ T cells, respectively. Surprisingly, this molecular subgrouping was poorly correlated with the expression of the CD4 and/or CD8 antigens on tissue sections. PTCL, NOSs differed from their normal counterparts by deregulation of genes classically related to proliferation, apoptosis, cell adhesion, and matrix remodeling.[143] In the study by de Leval and colleagues, genes overexpressed in PTCL, NOS in comparison with other PTCL subtypes were also reflective of nonspecific cellular functions, notably protein ubiquitination, regulation of transcription and metabolism.[79]

OTHER MOLECULAR FINDINGS

Overexpression of the p53 key regulator protein and mutations of the gene have been associated with an adverse prognosis in PTCL. p53-positive patients show a more frequent expression of the anti-apoptotic protein BCL2, and less frequent expression of p21.[95,144–146] Jung and colleagues[147] found an adverse prognosis only in the group of PTCL coexpressing BCL2 and p53.

Association of PTCL, NOS with EBV has been first described in the late 1980s.[148] The frequency of EBV detection varies with the technique used, and seems to approach 40 percent with the most sensitive technique, namely EBV-encoded small RNA-*in situ* hybridization (EBER-ISH).[107] D'Amore and colleagues[149] reported that the association with EBV (as detected by EBER-ISH) was associated with a worse outcome in a population of various T cell lymphomas. Nevertheless, the prognostic signification of the presence of EBV inside each PTCL category was not studied independently. In a homogeneous series of 110 patients with nodal PTCL, NOS, the presence of EBV was associated with a worse prognosis only in the elderly population.[107] The means by which EBV might play a role in oncogenesis in these types of tumor is not well understood, although recent studies have suggested a potential oncogenic role for EBERs through the induction of cytokine secretion.[150] EBV-associated PTCL has been associated with high levels of circulating TNFα,[151] a cytokine that plays a role in the pathogenesis of the hemophagocytic syndrome sometimes associated with this disease.[152]

In conclusion, PTCL, NOS appears as an heterogeneous category most likely grouping the neoplastic counterparts of many different normal T cell subsets, at different stages of differentiation. The frontiers between this category and better-defined entities of the WHO classification such as ALK-negative ALCL and AITL might be difficult to define, and some borderline cases do exist. The limited knowledge regarding underlying genetic abnormalities results in the absence of specific diagnostic markers for these malignancies.

T CELL LYMPHOMAS WITH PREDOMINANTLY EXTRANODAL PRESENTATION (EXCLUDING MYCOSIS FUNGOIDES, SÉZARY SYNDROME AND CUTANEOUS ANAPLASTIC LARGE CELL LYMPHOMA)

Extranodal T and NK cell lymphomas are relatively rare diseases, with the important exception of high frequency of nasal-type NK/T cell lymphomas in Asian populations. They comprise several clinicopathologic entities that were included in the REAL classification as distinct or provisional entities. Among them, angiocentric lymphoma was renamed 'nasal NK/T cell lymphoma' following a consensus workshop.[153] It appears that several entities are defined by their site of origin, their clinical features, their cellular origin and/or their possible association with specific antigens, whereas morphology is not specific.

ENTEROPATHY-ASSOCIATED T CELL LYMPHOMA

Enteropathy-associated T cell lymphoma (EATL) designates a rare T cell lymphoma entity which derives from intestinal intraepithelial lymphocytes, mainly arises in the small intestine, and appears to be a complication of celiac disease or gluten-sensitive enteropathy. It was first thought that the lymphoma was a cause of malabsorption, but several arguments have subsequently shown that the malabsorption was the consequence of celiac disease.[154] Based on the expression of histiocytic makers,[155] small intestinal lymphoma was first believed to originate from histiocytes and designated 'malignant histiocytosis of the intestine'. Demonstration of T cell antigens and of clonal rearrangements of TCR genes, proved the disease to be a unique entity of T cell lineage,[156] coined 'enteropathy-associated T cell lymphoma'. The term 'enteropathy-type T cell lymphoma' had been preferred in the previous WHO classification.

The disease is rare in most parts of the world, with a predilection for countries with a high prevalence of celiac disease such as western Europe and North America where approximately 0.5 percent of the populations suffer from the disease. Its prevalence also seems high in North Africa, and India, but the disease is rare in Black Africans and Japanese.[157] Like celiac disease, it shows a close linkage to specific HLA-DQ2/DQ8 alleles.

Large series of well-documented cases of EATL are rare and the diagnostic criteria are variable, mainly based on the initial presentation as an intestinal T cell lymphoma whereas the presence of a context of enteropathy and/or a CD103-positive phenotype are rarely documented, the latter antigen being only detectable on frozen samples. Therefore, several series may contain cases of other T cell lymphomas presenting in the gastrointestinal tract, especially the nasal-type NK/T cell lymphomas.

Clinical features

Enteropathy-associated T cell lymphoma presents in adults, with a median age of 50 years. In 30–60 percent of cases, patients have a prior history of celiac disease, sometimes with loss of response to gluten-free diet. In the remaining cases, patients have no peculiar clinical history and EATL is the first manifestation of latent celiac disease. Enteropathy-associated T cell lymphoma presents as multiple jejunal or ileal tumors or ulcers, frequently associated with mesenteric lymph node involvement, and EATL is commonly revealed by intestinal perforation or occlusion with many patients undergoing small bowel resection for acute abdominal emergencies. Other sites of involvement in the gastrointestinal tract (stomach, colon), and other mucosa (e.g. lung, breast, liver) or skin have been reported. Enteropathy-associated T cell lymphoma has been recognized to have a poor prognosis, with reported 5-year survival rate of 20 percent, probably related to a poor performance status in many patients,[158] even after high-dose polychemotherapy regimen.[159] During the course of the disease, dissemination to mesenteric lymph nodes, spleen, liver, bone marrow and other extranodal sites such as skin or lung, can occur.

It is admitted that refractory celiac disease and chronic ulcerative jejunitis, which are other recognized complications of celiac disease, are conditions closely related to EATL which may be regarded as a 'low-grade' intraepithelial T cell lymphoma.[160]

Histopathology

Enteropathy-associated T cell lymphoma exhibits a morphologic spectrum from small-cell variants to tumors composed of large immunoblastic or even anaplastic cells.[161,162] The most characteristic appearence is that of an ulcerated pleomorphic tumor composed of a variable proportion of medium and large malignant cells with more or less irregular nuclei, which invades the wall of the intestine (Plate 110, see plate section). In some instances, multilobated cells with prominent nucleoli, more or less resembling

Reed–Sternberg cells, are present. Histology is often complicated by the presence of necrosis and a large inflammatory component. Some cases are particularly rich in eosinophils. The demonstration of atypical T cells may require immunohistochemistry. The presence of intraepithelial tumor cells within the crypts is very characteristic, although it may be difficult to identify in the presence of prominent ulcerative lesions of the mucosa. Enteropathy-associated T cell lymphoma typically discloses features of enteropathy at a distance from the tumor with villous atrophy, crypt hyperplasia and an increase in intra-epithelial lymphocytes. However, these features may be lacking, especially when the patient is on a gluten-free diet or when the tumor occurs in the distal small intestine. A small cell variant composed of monomorphic small to medium-sized cells with a regular round nucleus and marked epitheliotropism has been reported which was believed to belong to the entity, in view of its cytotoxic profile.[163] Refractory celiac sprue and ulcerative jejunitis are characterized by an intraepithelial proliferation of lymphocytes without significant cytologic atypia. Based on the the finding of T cell clonality which parallels the loss of CD8 antigen, together with sCD3 and TCR,[164] and by the observation that patients with these lesions subsequently develop overt EATL, these lesions are now recognized as a cryptic form of EATL corresponding to a 'low-grade' intraepithelial EATL.[165]

Phenotype and genotype

Tumor cells express CD3, CD7 and CD2 but usually lack CD5. They are frequently CD4−/CD8−, more rarely CD8+ or even CD4+. They are derived from intraepithelial lymphocytes as supported by their CD103 (HML-1/αEβ7 integrin) phenotype (on frozen material). The ligand of CD103, E-cadherin, is expressed on epithelial cells. Tumor cells express TIA1, perforin and granzyme B granule associated molecules indicating their derivation from activated cytotoxic cells (Plate 110C). CD56 is only occasionally expressed and CD30 is variable. An abnormal phenotype with absence of CD5 and CD8 can be observed in the intraepithelial lymphocytes in the adjacent enteropathic mucosa. The great majority of the reported cases have an $\alpha\beta$ T cell origin, although rare $\gamma\delta$ cases have been reported[132] and reviewed,[166] as well as exceptional cases with a NK cell phenotype.[167] This apparent heterogeneous cell type might reflect the heterogeneity of IEL, which comprises in humans at least three cell subsets, e.g CD3+ TCR$\alpha\beta$+/CD8+ (70 percent), CD3+ TCR$\gamma\delta$+ (15 percent) (CD4−/CD8− or CD8$\alpha\alpha$), and CD3− CD7+ TCR$\alpha\beta$−/ TCR$\gamma\delta$− cells. Like normal intraepithelial lymphocytes, ETLs have been occasionally shown to express some CD94 and/or CD158a NK cell receptors.[168,169] Expression of a novel serine protease, granzyme M, is in agreement with derivation from lymphocytes involved in innate immunity.[170] The small cell variant has a distinct CD8+, CD56+ phenotype. Although it has been included as a variant of

EATL in the WHO classification, a context of celiac disease has not been reported in this group.[163]

TCRγ and/or β genes are clonally rearranged. The same clonal TCR rearrangement may be found in different sites at a distance from the intestine, including the colon and stomach, indicating the tendency of the disease to disseminate, even at the stage of refractory celiac sprue.[171]

Genetics and pathogeny

EATL is a model of T cell lymphomagenesis occurring in patients with a specific genetic background resulting in susceptibility to chronic antigen stimulation through gliadin. The role of gliadin hypersensitivity in the pathogenesis of the disease, especially the strong association with celiac disease and the in vivo demonstration of the increase and activation state of intraepithelial lymphocytes in celiac disease, is well established.[172] The genetic events associated with the multistep process involved in the accumulation of IEL in celiac disease and tumor development are largely unknown. In celiac disease, IL-15 secretion and increased susceptibility to genetic instability have been shown to promote the polyclonal expansion of intraepithelial lymphocytes.[173] In refractory sprue, which is regarded as a first step towards malignant transformation in which cell growth appears independent of gliadin, a recurrent structural chromosomal partial trisomy 1q22-q44 has been proposed as a frequent early event.[174] According to recent genetic studies using comparative genomic hybridization and FISH, the progression to overt lymphoma, i.e. transformation, invasion and dissemination, appears to be associated with additional oncogenic events. Amplifications at the 9q33–34 locus is the most frequent aberration found in 40–60 percent of cases.[175,176] This region contains two candidate genes, ABL1 and especially NOTCH1, which are preferentially amplified in EATL.[177] Aberrations at 9q33–34 appear, however, not completely specific, being also found in a small percentage (20 percent) of PTCL, NOS.[139] Loss of heterozygosity at chromosome 9p21, a region which harbors the tumor suppressor genes P16/INK4a, P15/INK4b and P14/ARF has been associated with progression being found in a proportion of EATL, especially in tumors with large cell morphology, not in ulcerative jejunitis,[178] whereas p53 seems frequently overexpressed despite the absence of detectable mutations of the gene.[178] Interestingly, based on genetic differences, it has been recently proposed that monomorphic small cell variant and pleomorphic EATLs could follow different oncogenic pathways, with fewer allelic imbalances and a lower frequency of microsatellite instability in the monomorphic EATLs.[176] In addition with its rare occurence in patients with celiac disease[163] and its peculiar phenotype, the relationship between the small cell variant and enteropathy will need further clarification. Despite some controversies, it appears that EATL is typically not associated with EBV, a feature which is of value for the differential diagnosis with nasal-type NK/T cell lymphoma. Its prevalence might, however, be higher in Mexican populations than among European cases.[163,179]

In summary, the classification of a T cell lymphoma within the EATL category may be difficult, even in the intestine. Indeed, no clinical evidence of enteropathy is found in a number of intestinal T cell lymphoma, since the disease frequently occurs in patients with asymptomatic villous atrophy (silent celiac disease), or in patients without history of gluten-sensitive enteropathy or malabsorption. In these cases, it is difficult to conclude to a definitive diagnosis of EATL. The search for villous atrophy, an increase of intraepithelial lymphocytes in adjacent mucosa, a specific CD103 phenotype on fresh tissue and the absence of EBV are important features for the diagnosis of EATL, as well as serology for IgA antiendomysial and IgG antigliadin antibodies. The demonstration of 9q gain observed in about 60 percent of cases could also be of value. On the contrary, the presence of an angiocentric pattern, EBV association and/or NK cell phenotype are strong arguments for a 'nasal-type' intestinal NK/T cell lymphoma.

HEPATOSPLENIC T CELL LYMPHOMA

Hepatosplenic T cell lymphoma (HSTL) is a rare aggressive subtype of extranodal lymphoma, which was first recognized in 1990 on the basis of its uniform clinicopathologic aspects and its $\gamma\delta$ phenotype.[131,180,181] The latter has been part of the definition of the entity, initially named *hepatosplenic $\gamma\delta$ T cell lymphoma* in the REAL classification.[4] Recently, similar cases with a $\alpha\beta$ phenotype have been described, and the term 'hepatosplenic T cell lymphoma' has been preferred in the current WHO classification.[5]

HSTL is rare, with approximately 100 cases reported.[166,182,183] Its incidence, however, might be underestimated as its features are not typical for lymphoma, and due to the difficulty in assessing the $\gamma\delta$ T cell origin on routine specimens. A number of cases have been reported in patients with immune manifestations or in patients receiving long-term immunosuppressive therapy for solid organ transplantation. In this context, HSTL is regarded as a late-onset post-transplantation lymphoproliferative disorder of host origin.[183,184] Cases occurring in patients followed for Crohn's disease, acute myeloid leukemia, EBV+ lymphoproliferative disorders, or falciparum malaria have been observed.[183,185–187] Recently, an association has been noted between the use of the antitumor necrosis factor agent infliximab along with concomitant purine analogs and the development of HSTL, in particular in younger patients with inflamatory bowel disease.[188]

Clinical features

The disease occurs mainly in young adults with a male predominance (median age around 35 years),[133,166,182,183] with few reports in children. Patients present with marked splenomegaly and often hepatomegaly, but without lymphadenopathy. Most patients have B symptoms.[166,182,183,189,190] Thrombocytopenia is a constant feature, associated with anemia and/or leucopenia in about half of the patients. Lymphocytosis is uncommon although, after careful examination of blood smears, a minor population of atypical lymphoid cells can be identified in some patients.[183,191] The association with a hemophagocytic syndrome has been occasionally mentioned.

The disease has a highly aggressive course. According to a recent series on 21 cases, median survival was 16 months and, despite consolidative or salvage high-dose therapy with stem cell transplantation in many of them, only two patients survived in complete response at 42 and 52 months.[183] Based on individual reports, the efficacy of platinum-cytarabine-based induction regimen and recently of 2'-deoxyconformcin[192,193] has been suggested, supported by the *in vitro* selective cytotoxic effect of 2'-deoxyconformcin on $\gamma\delta$ tumoral T cells.[192] Cytologic progression to large cell lymphoma with slight pleomorphism or with blastic appearance is frequently seen during the course of the disease. During progression, phenotypic changes may occur, such as loss of $\gamma\delta$ T cell receptor leading to a 'TCR-silent' phenotype (βF1−/TCRδ-1−).[194]

Histopathology

The neoplastic cells are usually monomorphic, small to medium-sized cells with a round/oval or slightly irregular nucleus with inconspicuous nucleoli. They show a common abundant pale cytoplasm. These cells are located preferentially in the sinusoids of the liver, the cords and sinuses of the splenic red pulp and the sinuses of the bone marrow.[194]

At splenectomy, the *spleen* is usually massively enlarged – commonly weighing 1000–3500 g – without any gross lesions identifiable, and without hilar lymph nodes enlargement. Histopathology shows marked reduction of the white pulp whereas the red pulp is diffusely invaded by a more or less dense neoplastic infiltration. The neoplastic cells are present within the cords of the red pulp and, at a variable extend from case to case, within more or less dilated sinuses (Plate 111A). Histiocytes are often numerous with, in rare cases, showing evidence of erythrophagocytosis. Hilar lymph nodes, although not significantly enlarged, commonly show some involvement confined to sinuses or perisinusal areas.[195]

Histologic involvement of the liver is quite constant. It is characterized by a sinusoidal pattern in all cases, which can realize pseudopeliotic lesions.[180] Additional mild portal and periportal lymphomatous infiltrate may be observed, but is not predominant.

Bone marrow involvement (Plate 111B, C) appears rather constant when trephine biopsies are carefully investigated by a combined histologic and immunohistochemical approach. It is distinguished by a characteristic sinusal pattern of infiltration. The initial bone marrow specimens are commonly hypercellular with trilineage hyperplasia, and may at first examination be confused with myelodysplastic or myeloproliferative syndrome. The marrow lymphoma infiltration is discrete, often subtle and difficult to recognize in routine H&E-stained sections: it consists of slightly atypical small to medium-sized lymphoid cells forming indian files or aggregates within more or less dilated sinuses, which are strongly highlighted by CD3 immunostaining.[189,191,196] Together with the peculiar sinusal distribution in the bone marrow, the demonstration of a CD3+, CD5−, TIA1+ phenotype appears characteristic, if not specific, of HSTL. Careful examination of aspirate smears may be helpful to identify the few atypical lymphoid cells which are sometimes described as blast-like cells and may in some instances contain fine cytoplasmic granules. Above all, it allows immunophenotyping on fresh cell suspension by flow cytometry, enabling the determination of the $\gamma\delta$ origin of the neoplastic cells in most cases.

Cytologic variants, i.e. large cells or those with blastic appearance, have been occasionally observed at diagnosis but frequently occur with progression during the course of the disease. In addition, at a late disease stage, the pattern of bone marrow involvement has a tendency to become more intense and diffuse, not only sinusal.

Phenotype and genotype

Tumor cells express CD3, CD2 and often CD7, but usually lack CD5. They are CD4−/CD8− or more rarely CD4−/CD8+. Most cases are CD56+, but CD57 is negative. They may express CD16. They have a nonactivated cytotoxic phenotype, i.e. TIA1+, without expression of granzyme B and perforin,[61,189] with the exception of rare cases with blastic appearance. Cytotoxic activity has been demonstrated in a few cases.[186] HSTL is negative for CD25 and CD30 activation antigens. Expression of killer immunoglobulin-like receptors (KIRs) and of CD94/NKG2A has been recently reported in several cases.[169,197] On frozen sections or flow cytometry, the majority of cases express the $\gamma\delta$ T cell receptor, as shown by the βF1-/TCRδ-1+ phenotype. Most HSTL of $\gamma\delta$ type, but not all, seem to be derived from the subset of $\gamma\delta$ T cells having rearranged the Vδ1 gene as revealed by molecular studies and the positive staining with the δTCS 1 antibody.[131,181,183,198,199] $\gamma\delta$ HSTL express the serine protease granzyme M, a finding consistent with a derivation from lymphocytes involved in innate immunity.[170] Recently, HSTL with an $\alpha\beta$ T cell receptor phenotype (βF1+/TCRδ-1−) have been reported.[200-202] On the basis of similar clinicopathologic and cytogenetic aspects, they are considered a variant of the more common $\gamma\delta$ form of the disease.[5]

It is noteworthy that determination of the $\alpha\beta$ or $\gamma\delta$ T cell origin may be difficult to establish in a number of cases due to the absence of a reliable marker for $\gamma\delta$ T cells in routinely fixed specimens (see above). In the absence of frozen samples, flow cytometric analysis on marrow aspirate smears is highly recommended.

Irrespective of their $\gamma\delta$ or $\alpha\beta$ phenotype, HSTL show a clonal rearrangement of the TCRγ gene, as demonstrated by PCR studies used in routine practice. Southern blot or PCR studies have demonstrated a rearrangement, usually biallelic, of the TCR δ chain,[181,183,199] in accordance with a genotype of $\gamma\delta$ T cells. Unproductive rearrangements of the β chain have been reported in some HSTL of $\gamma\delta$ T cell origin, following the same observation in normal $\gamma\delta$ T cells.[181,198] In addition to the clonal rearrangement of γ chain, $\alpha\beta$ cases disclose a clonal rearrangement of the TCRβ chain genes.[200,202]

Genetics and pathogeny

By conventional cytogenetics and FISH studies published in approximatively 40 cases,[203] most $\gamma\delta$ HSTL have been characterized by the presence of an isochromosome 7q (i[7][q10]).[203,204] The latter occasionally has appeared as the sole karyotypic abnormality, suggesting the primary role of this recurrent karyotypic abnormality in the pathogenesis of the disease. In addition to trisomy 8 and loss of chromosome Y, an increased number of 7q signals have been found in progressive cases indicating a tendency to multiply the i(7)(q10) chromosome during evolution of the disease.[203] Interestingly, i(7)(q10) has also been found in hepatosplenic cases with $\alpha\beta$-phenotype,[200-202] thus further supporting that both $\gamma\delta$ and $\alpha\beta$ cases may represent variants of the same entity. The biologic significance of i(7)(q10) is not established. Despite a strict correlation between i(7)(q10) and HSTL, this aberration is not associated exclusively with this type of lymphoma, since isochromosome 7q can be seen in other malignant disorders, such as acute myeloid leukemia, acute lymphoblastic leukemia, myelodysplastic syndrome and Wilms tumor.

So far, no viral association (HTLV-1 and -2, HIV, HHV-8, HCV) has been reported. One case has been reported in a patient positive for HHV-6. The vast majority of cases do not show EBV association as well, with the exception of rare cases with cytologic features of transformation, suggesting that EBV might be regarded as a secondary event.[166]

HSTL is supposed to be derived from a subset of immature nonactivated cytotoxic T cells, mostly $\gamma\delta$ showing predilection homing in the splenic red pulp.[205] It has been proposed that both $\alpha\beta$ and $\gamma\delta$ variants could originate from NK/T cells which comprise subsets of $\alpha\beta$ and $\gamma\delta$ cells with similar cytolytic properties and which participate with NK cells in the innate immune system. Several cases have been reported in patients with immune deficiency – mainly patients receiving long-term immunosuppressive therapy for solid organ transplantation – or auto-immune diseases. From these observations and in view of the functional properties of normal $\gamma\delta$ T cells, it is tempting to speculate that chronic antigen stimulation in the setting of immune defect could play a role in the pathogenesis of the disease. As an example, expansion of $\gamma\delta$ T cells is observed in peripheral blood in recipients of renal allografts as well as in autoimmune diseases and *in vitro* studies have shown that human $\gamma\delta$ T cells display an alloreactive response to various leukocyte antigen molecules.[183] Recently,[197] an aberrant dim or absent CD94 expression was found, along with a frequent expression of multiple KIR isoforms, an unexpected feature in memory T cells. As KIR expression is induced by chronic antigenic stimulation, the expression of multiple KIR isoforms could be indicative of this kind of process in HSTL. KIR expression could also be implicated in neoplastic transformation.[197]

In conclusion, the demonstration of a CD3+, CD5−, CD8−, TIA1+, granzyme B− phenotype of the sinusal infiltrate in routine bone marrow biopsy specimens provides a very strong indicator that a case represents HSTL and helps to distinguish HSTL from other lymphoma entities which commonly present with hepatosplenic disease and show an infiltration of the splenic red pulp. These are mainly T or NK cell neoplasms – i.e. aggressive NK cell lymphoma/leukemia, T cell large granular lymphocyte leukemia – and, among B cell neoplasms, hairy cell leukemia and splenic marginal zone lymphoma. Their main clinical, histopathologic, phenotypic and genetic features are summarized in Table 39.3.

SUBCUTANEOUS PANNICULITIS–LIKE T CELL LYMPHOMA

Subcutaneous panniculitis-like T cell lymphoma (SPLTCL) is defined as a cytotoxic T cell lymphoma with preferential involvement of subcutaneous tissue, often associated with tumor necrosis and karyorrhexis.[5] It is likely that SPLTCL was previously designated as histiocytic cytophagic panniculitis, a lesion initially thought to be a histiocytic malignancy. Since its first description in 1991[206] as a lymphoma characterized by the primary involvement of the subcutaneous fat tissue and the frequent association with a hemophagocytic syndrome (i.e. fever, pancytopenia, hepatosplenomegaly, elevated liver enzymes, hemophagocytosis in the bone marrow or other sites, etc.), SPLTCL is now recognized as a separate entity inside the extranodal T cell lymphoma group of the WHO classification.[5] More recent studies have pointed out that cases with an $\alpha\beta$ phenotype and those with a $\gamma\delta$ phenotype (around 25 percent of all cases) disclosed differences in histopathologic and immunologic features as well as in clinical outcomes. Therefore, in the WHO/EORTC classification of cutaneous lymphomas, published in 2005[207] as well as in the WHO classification of tumors of hematopoietic and lymphoid tissues updated in 2008,[5] the term SPLTCL is only proposed for cases with an $\alpha\beta$ phenotype, those expressing $\gamma\delta$ TCR being referred to as 'cutaneous $\gamma\delta$ T cell lymphoma' ($\gamma\delta$CTCL), a category which may belong to this group of $\gamma\delta$ T cell lymphomas with mucocutaneous presentation (see below). SPLTCL is one of the rarest PTCL subtypes, with approximately 200 cases reported in the world literature.[208] In the present chapter, we will indicate the clinical and pathologic differences observed among the $\alpha\beta$ type (referred to as SPLTCL) and the $\gamma\delta$ type (referred to as $\gamma\delta$ CTCL), which are summarized in Table 39.4.

Clinical features

The disease occurs in adults as well as in children. It shows a broad age range with, according to the largest retrospective literature analysis reported to date on 156 cases, a median age of 39 years (range 0.5–84 years). There were roughly equal numbers of male and female patients. Patients present with solitary or often multiple subcutaneous nodules, which can only occasionally present superficial ulcerations and/or necrosis. The most common localizations are on the extremities and the trunk. Dissemination outside the skin is rare, but a few cases with localization to the lung,[209] pleura[210] and peripheral blood[211] have been reported.

The hemophagocytic syndrome is present in a third of cases, and is associated with a worst prognosis. Cases of the $\gamma\delta$ genotype ($\gamma\delta$ CTCL) seem to be more often complicated by this phenomenon. Associations with myeloproliferative syndromes (one case each of polycythemia vera and myelofibrosis with myeloid metaplasia), multiple sclerosis and rheumatoid arthritis have been reported. Prognosis has been reported to be poor, with a median survival of 27 months. However, based on the few reports with appropriate investigations of TCR expression,[212,213] the 5-year median survival for $\alpha\beta$ SPLTCL patients may reach 80 percent whereas a median survival of 15 months has been reported for patients with a $\gamma\delta$ CTCL.[214] Proposed treatments include conventional anthracyclin-based chemotherapy, purine analogs and, for $\gamma\delta$ CTCL, intensive therapy followed by autologous or allogeneic stem-cell transplantation.

Histopathology

By definition, the neoplastic cellular infiltrate extends diffusely throughout the subcutaneous fat tissue simulating a panniculitis. The cytologic aspect is variable from case to case with forms composed of a predominance of slightly atypical small lymphoid cells to forms with a predominance of medium to large neoplastic cells. These cells often adopt a rimming configuration around adipocytes (Plate 112, see plate section), although this finding is not specific of SPLTCL.[215] Karyorrhexis and necrosis are commonly found. Vascular invasion (angiocentricity) has been reported. A variable proportion of reactive histiocytes, often showing features of active phagocytosis (hemophagocytosis or presence of lipid vacuoles) may be seen, in particular in areas of necrosis. Extension of the infiltrate towards the dermis (Plate 113, see plate section) and even epidermis is typically not seen in $\alpha\beta$ SPLTCL , but is relatively frequent in $\gamma\delta$ CTCL.[208,214]

The cytologic atypia might be minimal especially in the early stages, when the lesion may be misdiagnosed as benign

Table 39.3 Differential diagnosis of hepatosplenic T cell lymphoma: major distinguishing features

Lymphoma type	Clinical features	Cytology	Cell type	Phenotype	Cytotoxic profile	Bone marrow	Spleen	Liver	Genetics
Hepatosplenic T cell lymphoma	Splenomegaly, B symptoms, cytopenia	Medium sized, monomorphic	T $\gamma\delta$ (>T $\alpha\beta$)	CD3+, CD5−, CD4−/CD8−, CD56+	Nonactivated (TIA1+, GrB−)	Hypercellular, sinusal infiltrate	Red pulp (cords and sinuses)	Sinusoidal (predominant)	Iso 7q ± trisomy 8
Aggressive NK cell leukemia	B symptoms, splenomegaly, HPS, leukemia, cytopenia	Medium/large	NK (>T $\alpha\beta$)	CD3e+, CD5−, CD56+, CD4−/CD8−	Activated (TIA1+, GrB+)	Histiocytes + hemophagocytosis, interstitial, diffuse	Red pulp, mild, wall vessels	Sinusoidal and portal	6q deletion EBV association
LGL leukemia	Indolent, neutropenia, autoimmune manifestations	Lymphocytes with azurophilic granules (LGL)	T $\alpha\beta$ (NK, T $\gamma\delta$)	CD3+, CD8+, CD57+	Activated (TIA1+, GrB+)	Interstitial + sinusal infiltrate often subtle, maturation arrest	Red pulp, mild	Sinusoidal and portal	?
Splenic marginal zone lymphoma	Splenomegaly (mild), slight lymphocytosis	Small lymphocytes, ± villous	B	CD20+, CD5−	−	Sinusal infiltrate, often with nodules	Primary expansion of white pulp (MZ), infiltration of red pulp	Sinusoidal and portal	7q21 deletion
Hairy cell leukemia	Splenomegaly, cytopenia	Hairy cells	B	CD20+, CD25+, CD103+	−	Dense, diffuse ('leukemic'), fibrosis	Red pulp (sinus and cords), red cell 'lakes'	Sinusoidal (predominant)	?

EBV, Epstein–Barr virus; HPS, hemophagocytic syndrome; LGL, large granular lymphocyte; MZ, marginal zone.
Note: Aggressive NK cell leukemia remains the major differential diagnosis with hepatosplenic T cell lymphoma.

Table 39.4 Comparison of the main clinical, histopathologic and phenotypic of $\alpha\beta$ subcutaneous panniculitis-like T cell lymphomas ($\alpha\beta$ SPLTCL) and $\gamma\delta$ cutaneous T cell lymphomas ($\gamma\delta$ CTCL)

	$\alpha\beta$ SPLTCL	$\gamma\delta$ CTCL
Clinical features	Non-ulcerated nodule(s) Rare HPS Relatively indolent course 80% 5-year survival	Disseminated plaques, ulceronecrotic nodules HPS more common Very aggressive course
Histopathology	Panniculitis-like lesions Restricted to subcutis	Panniculitis-like lesions With frequent extension to dermis, even epidermis
Phenotype	CD8+, CD56− Activated cytotoxic TIA-1+, Gr B +, Perf +	Most cases CD4−/CD8− CD56+, CD5− Activated cytotoxic TIA-1+, Gr B+/Perf+
EBV	Absent	Absent

EBV, Epstein–Barr virus; HPS, hemophagocytic syndrome.

panniculitis. In such cases, immunostaining for CD3, CD8 and cytotoxic molecules is essential for a correct diagnosis. These stainings highlight the cytologic atypia and enhance the panniculitis-like distribution, therefore helping to distinguish SPLTCL from other types of non-Hodgkin lymphoma with preferential involvement of the subcutaneous tissue, and above all from benign causes of panniculitis such as lupus profundus and indeterminate lymphocytic lobular panniculitis. It is noteworthy that subsequent biopsies often show cytologic progression with features more typical for lymphoma.

Phenotype/genotype

The tumor cell phenotype is that of activated cytotoxic T cells, i.e. CD3+, CD2+, TIA1+, granzyme B+ and perforin+. The expression of these proteins which mediate cytotoxicity and apoptosis has been proposed to be responsible for the features of karyorrhexis and necrosis which are often observed in SPLTCL.[133] There is a striking phenotypic dichotomy between $\alpha\beta$ and $\gamma\delta$ cases. $\alpha\beta$ SPLTCL are usually CD8+, CD56− (Plate 112C) whereas $\gamma\delta$ CTCL (Plate 113, see plate section) have a common CD4−/CD8− (more rarely CD8+), CD56+ phenotype without expression of CD5. The latter disclose clonal rearrangements of both γ and δ chains of the $\gamma\delta$ receptor and have been reported to derive from the Vδ2 subset.[199] In the $\alpha\beta$ SPLTCL, the cells show clonal rearrangement of the γ gene whereas the β chain may be either deleted or rearranged, following the unproductive rearrangement of the gene as observed in some $\gamma\delta$ hepatosplenic T cell lymphomas.

Genetics and pathogeny

$\alpha\beta$ SPLTCL and $\gamma\delta$ CTCL probably represent the entities that have been less will studied from the molecular point of view among T cell lymphomas. Notably, we are aware of no data regarding karyotypic studies. This might be explained by the fact that diagnosis is often done on small-sized skin

biopsies, often showing marked degrees of necrosis, and is also explained by the rarity of the disease.

The serine protease granzyme M is usually not expressed in CD56− $\alpha\beta$ cases, suggesting that most of these cases are derived from mature $\alpha\beta$ cytotoxic T cells not belonging to the innate immune system.[170] No clear viral association has been reported. In rare cases (six out of 61 studied patients in the literature), the presence of EBV was detected in tissue biopsies by PCR or FISH.[216–219] However, five of the six patients with EBV found in tumor tissues resided in Asia whereas only one of 45 patients residing outside of Asia (two percent) was positive for EBV infection. Cytokines and chemokines, such as interferon-γ and MIP-1α which have been reported to be secreted by neoplastic cells, might explain the frequently observed hemophagocytic syndrome.

In conclusion, despite some common features including the presence of an infiltration of the subcutaneous tissue in both situations, there is evidence for significant differences in terms of histopathology, phenotype and clinical outcome between cases of $\alpha\beta$ and $\gamma\delta$ origin.[214] This dichotomy was first introduced in the WHO/EORTC classification of cutaneous lymphomas[207] which separates cases with an $\alpha\beta$ genotype – referred to as SPLTCL – as a single entity, and groups $\gamma\delta$ cases among a new '$\gamma\delta$ cutaneous' T cell lymphoma category and has been taken into consideration in the updated WHO classification of hematopoietic neoplasms.[5] Future molecular investigations in well-characterized cases are warranted to genetically support this distinction which appears clinically important.

CUTANEOUS AND MUCOSAL $\gamma\delta$ T CELL LYMPHOMAS

Besides hepatosplenic $\gamma\delta$ T cell lymphoma which constitutes the prototype of peripheral T cell lymphoma expressing the $\gamma\delta$ T cell receptor and represents the large proportion of the so far reported cases of $\gamma\delta$ T cell lymphoma, it appears that the latter can also occur in other extranodal sites – i.e. mainly skin and mucosa – and display a marked heterogeneity in terms of clinical presentation and histologic features. Although this matter is still debated, it has been proposed that these 'nonhepatosplenic $\gamma\delta$ T cell lymphomas' constitute a subset of cytotoxic lymphomas with mucosal or skin localization.

Cutaneous $\gamma\delta$ T cell lymphomas

The majority of primary cutaneous $\gamma\delta$ T cell lymphomas show clinical and histologic features reminiscent of subcutaneous panniculitis-like T cell lymphomas, despite some differences with the classical $\alpha\beta$ subtype (see the previous section and Table 39.4). A small proportion of patients with $\gamma\delta$ T cell lymphomas occurring primarily in the skin present with plaques, patches or tumors and show histologic features resembling mycosis fungoides, with perivascular or dermic infiltrate containing atypical irregular small lymphoid cells associated with marked epidermotropism. Some of these that show extreme epidermotropism are reported as pagetoid reticulosis. In contrast to 'classical' mycosis fungoides, which are CD4 positive, mycosis fungoides-like $\gamma\delta$ T cell lymphomas are CD4 and CD8 double negative.[207]

Mucosal $\gamma\delta$ T cell lymphomas

It has been shown in recent years that $\gamma\delta$ T cell lymphomas may develop initially in different mucosal tissues such as the nasopharyngeal region, the intestine, as well as occasionally in the thyroid, larynx, lung, breast or testis.[132,166] Clinically, $\gamma\delta$ T cell lymphomas originating in the nasopharyngeal region usually present as destructive nasal lesions or midline facial tumors such as classical nasal NK cell lymphomas. Those arising in the gastrointestinal tract display localized or multifocal lesions of the gut, which can even be revealed by peritonitis due to perforation. Pathologic features of mucosal $\gamma\delta$ T cell lymphomas are not specific with most often tumors composed of predominantly medium-sized to large cells. Necrosis, angiocentrism and angioinvasion are lesions especially but not exclusively observed in the EBV-positive nasopharyngeal lymphomas. Neoplastic cells express CD3 and CD2 whereas CD5 is commonly lost, CD7 being variable. Most cases are CD4−/CD8−. CD56 is inconsistent. They show an activated cytotoxic phenotype (TIA1+, granzyme B+, perforin+). In view of the clinical and immunomorphologic resemblance of the nasopharyngeal $\gamma\delta$ T cell lymphomas with usual nasal NK cell lymphomas and their EBV association, it has been proposed to lump together all lymphomas occurring in this region and expressing T cell markers as well as EBV association into one category termed 'nasal-type NK/T cell lymphoma'.[5] Gluten-sensitive enteropathy has been documented in at least one case of gastrointestinal $\gamma\delta$ T cell lymphoma which was shown to express the CD103 molecule and to occur in a patient with celiac sprue,[132] thus being indistinguishable from 'enteropathy-associated T cell lymphoma', an observation in accordance with the fact that $\gamma\delta$ T cells account for a significant proportion of intraepithelial lymphocytes, that are activated and increased in celiac disease.

Overall, the distribution of these lymphomas strongly reflects the preferential localization in the skin and different epithelia of normal $\gamma\delta$ T lymphocytes. In view of the known role of $\gamma\delta$ T cells in host mucosal and epithelial immune responses, it is remarkable that some mucosal $\gamma\delta$ T cell lymphomas are described in the context of chronic antigenic stimulation and/or prolonged immune suppression.

KEY POINTS

- Peripheral T cell lymphomas are tumors derived from a wide variety of T cell populations. They are rare, accounting for less than 15 percent of non-Hodgkin lymphomas in most Western countries.
- Peripheral T cell lymphomas globally share a poor prognosis.
- HTLV1-related adult leukemia/lymphomas are probably derived from regulatory T cells. They appear after a long period of viral infection, which is usually acquired at birth or during childhood. Their geographic distribution is related to that of HTLV1 infection. Four distinct clinicobiologic forms are recognized.
- Angioimmunoblastic T cell lymphomas are derived from follicular helper T cells. The diagnosis is based on a characteristic clinical and histopathologic presentation. Immunohistochemistry is helpful to recognize the diagnostic pathological features and molecular techniques are required in difficult cases, specially with benign conditions.
- The term 'peripheral T cell lymphoma, not otherwise specified' groups all types of lymphomas which cannot be classified inside any 'specified' entity among T cell lymphomas. These diseases have a wide variety of clinical presentation and histopathological features, probably reflecting a vast array of cellular origins and pathophysiological mechanisms.
- Three main distinct entities are recognized among extranodal peripheral T cell lymphomas: enteropathy-associated T cell lymphoma, which is related to celiac disease; hepatosplenic T cell lymphoma (mostly of $\gamma\delta$ T cell origin); and subcutaneous T cell lymphoma. The latter entity is derived from CD8+ $\alpha\beta$ T cells and needs to be distinguished from $\gamma\delta$ cutaneous T cell lymphomas, which can also infiltrate the subcutis but have distinct clinical features with a poorer outcome.

REFERENCES

● = Key primary paper
◆ = Major review article

●1. Armitage J, Vose J, Weisenburger D. International peripheral T-cell and natural killer/T-cell lymphoma study: pathology findings and clinical outcomes. *J Clin Oncol* 2008; **26**: 4124–30.

●2. A clinical evaluation of the International Lymphoma Study Group classification of non-Hodgkin's lymphoma. The non-Hodgkin's lymphoma classification project. *Blood* 1997; **89**: 3909–18.

3. Rüdiger T, Weisenburger DD, Anderson JR *et al.* Peripheral T-cell lymphoma (excluding anaplastic large-cell lymphoma): results from the non-Hodgkin's lymphoma classification project. *Ann Oncol* 2002; **13**: 140–9.

◆4. Harris NL, Jaffe ES, Stein H *et al.* A revised European-American classification of lymphoid neoplasms: a proposal from the International Lymphoma Study Group. *Blood* 1994; **84**: 1361–92.

5. Swerdlow SH, Campo E, Harris NL *et al.* (eds) *WHO classification of tumours of haematopoietic and lymphoid tissues.* Lyon: IARC Press, 2008.

6. Shimoyama M. Diagnostic criteria and classification of clinical subtypes of adult T-cell leukaemia-lymphoma. A report from the Lymphoma Study Group (1984–87). *Br J Haematol* 1991; **79**: 428–37.

7. Shirono K, Hattori T, Takatsuki K. A new classification of clinical stages of adult T-cell leukemia based on prognosis of the disease. *Leukemia* 1994; **8**: 1834–7.

◆8. Bazarbachi A, Ghez D, Lepelletier Y *et al.* New therapeutic approaches for adult T-cell leukaemia. *Lancet Oncol* 2004; **5**: 664–72.

9. Ohshima K, Suzumiya J, Kato A *et al.* Clonal HTLV-I-infected CD4+ T-lymphocytes and non-clonal non-HTLV-I-infected giant cells in incipient ATLL with Hodgkin-like histologic features. *Int J Cancer* 1997; **72**: 592–8.

10. Manel N, Kim FJ, Kinet S *et al.* The ubiquitous glucose transporter GLUT-1 is a receptor for HTLV. *Cell* 2003; **115**: 449–59.

11. Ghez D, Lepelletier Y, Lambert S *et al.* Neuropilin-1 is involved in human T-cell lymphotropic virus type 1 entry. *J Virol* 2006; **80**: 6844–54.

12. Grassmann R, Aboud M, Jeang KT. Molecular mechanisms of cellular transformation by HTLV-1 Tax. *Oncogene* 2005; **24**: 5976–85.

◆13. Mortreux F, Gabet AS, Wattel E. Molecular and cellular aspects of HTLV-1 associated leukemogenesis in vivo. *Leukemia* 2003; **17**: 26–38.

14. Gatza ML, Watt JC, Marriott SJ. Cellular transformation by the HTLV-I tax protein, a jack-of-all-trades. *Oncogene* 2003; **22**: 5141–9.

15. Asquith B, Bangham CR. The role of cytotoxic T lymphocytes in human T-cell lymphotropic virus type 1 infection. *J Theor Biol* 2000; **207**: 65–79.

16. Arnulf B, Thorel M, Poirot Y *et al.* Loss of the ex vivo but not the reinducible CD8+ T-cell response to Tax in human T-cell leukemia virus type 1-infected patients with adult T-cell leukemia/lymphoma. *Leukemia* 2004; **18**: 126–32.

17. Hanon E, Hall S, Taylor GP *et al.* Abundant tax protein expression in CD4+ T cells infected with human T-cell lymphotropic virus type I (HTLV-I) is prevented by cytotoxic T lymphocytes. *Blood* 2000; **95**: 1386–92.

18. Yamada Y, Hatta Y, Murata K *et al.* Deletions of p15 and/or p16 genes as a poor-prognosis factor in adult T-cell leukemia. *J Clin Oncol* 1997; **15**: 1778–85.

19. Sasaki H, Nishikata I, Shiraga T *et al.* Overexpression of a cell adhesion molecule, TSLC1, as a possible molecular marker for acute-type adult T-cell leukemia. *Blood* 2005; **105**: 1204–13.

20. Taylor GP, Matsuoka M. Natural history of adult T-cell leukemia/lymphoma and approaches to therapy. *Oncogene* 2005; **24**: 6047–57.

21. Karube K, Ohshima K, Tsuchiya T *et al.* Expression of FoxP3, a key molecule in CD4CD25 regulatory T cells, in adult T-cell leukaemia/lymphoma cells. *Br J Haematol* 2004; **126**: 81–4.

22. Roncador G, Garcia JF, Maestre L *et al.* FOXP3, a selective marker for a subset of adult T-cell leukaemia/lymphoma. *Leukemia* 2005; **19**: 2247–53.

23. Ishida T, Iida S, Akatsuka Y *et al.* The CC chemokine receptor 4 as a novel specific molecular target for immunotherapy in adult T-cell leukemia/lymphoma. *Clin Cancer Res* 2004; **10**: 7529–39.

●24. Gisselbrecht C, Gaulard P, Lepage E *et al.* Prognostic significance of T-cell phenotype in aggressive non-Hodgkin's lymphomas. Groupe d'Etudes des Lymphomes de l'Adulte (GELA). *Blood* 1998; **92**: 76–82.

25. Lukes RJ, Tindle BH. Immunoblastic lymphadenopathy. A hyperimmune entity resembling Hodgkin's disease. *N Engl J Med* 1975; **292**: 1–8.

26. Lennert K. Nature, prognosis and nomenclature of angioimmunoblastic lymphadenopathy (lymphogranulomatosis X or T-zone lymphoma. *Dtsch Med Wochenschr* 1979; **104**: 1246–7.

27. Frizzera G, Moran EM, Rappaport H. Angio-immunoblastic lymphadenopathy with dysproteinaemia. *Lancet* 1974; **1**: 1070–3.

28. Shimoyama M, Minato K, Saito H. Immunoblastic lymphadenopathy (IBL)-like T-cell lymphoma. *Jpn J Clin Oncol* 1979; **9**(Suppl): 347–56.

29. Stansfeld AG, Diebold J, Noel H *et al.* Updated Kiel classification for lymphomas. *Lancet* 1988; **1**: 292–3.

30. Pautier P, Devidas A, Delmer A *et al.* Angioimmunoblastic-like T-cell non Hodgkin's lymphoma: outcome after chemotherapy in 33 patients and review of the literature. *Leuk Lymphoma* 1999; **32**: 545–52.

31. Aozasa K, Ohsawa M, Fujita MQ *et al.* Angioimmunoblastic lymphadenopathy. Review of 44 patients with emphasis on prognostic behavior. *Cancer* 1989; **63**: 1625–9.

32. Lachenal F, Berger F, Ghesquieres H et al. Angioimmunoblastic T-cell lymphoma: clinical and laboratory features at diagnosis in 77 patients. *Medicine (Baltimore)* 2007; **86**: 282–92.

33. Mourad N, Mounier N, Briere J et al. Clinical, biological and pathological features in 157 patients with angioimmunoblastic T-cell lymphoma treated within the Groupe d'Etude des Lymphomes de l'Adulte (GELA) trials. *Blood* 2008; **111**: 4463–70.

34. Siegert W, Nerl C, Agthe A et al. Angioimmunoblastic lymphadenopathy (AILD)-type T-cell lymphoma: prognostic impact of clinical observations and laboratory findings at presentation. The Kiel Lymphoma Study Group. *Ann Oncol* 1995; **6**: 659–64.

35. Siegert W, Agthe A, Griesser H et al. Treatment of angioimmunoblastic lymphadenopathy (AILD)-type T-cell lymphoma using prednisone with or without the COPBLAM/IMVP-16 regimen. A multicenter study. Kiel Lymphoma Study Group. *Ann Intern Med* 1992; **117**: 364–70.

36. Ascani S, Zinzani PL, Gherlinzoni F et al. Peripheral T-cell lymphomas. Clinico-pathologic study of 168 cases diagnosed according to the R.E.A.L classification. *Ann Oncol* 1997; **8**: 583–92.

37. Lopez-Guillermo A, Cid J, Salar A et al. Peripheral T-cell lymphomas: initial features, natural history, and prognostic factors in a series of 174 patients diagnosed according to the R.E.A.L classification. *Ann Oncol* 1998; **9**: 849–55.

38. Savage KJ, Chhanabhai M, Gascoyne RD et al. Characterization of peripheral T-cell lymphomas in a single North American institution by the WHO classification. *Ann Oncol* 2004; **15**: 1467–75.

◆39. Dogan A, Attygalle AD, Kyriakou C. Angioimmunoblastic T-cell lymphoma. *Br J Haematol* 2003; **121**: 681–91.

40. Willenbrock K, Renne C, Gaulard P, Hansmann ML. In angioimmunoblastic T-cell lymphoma, neoplastic T cells may be a minor cell population. A molecular single-cell and immunohistochemical study. *Virchows Arch* 2005; **446**: 15–20.

41. Attygalle A, Al-Jehani R, Diss TC et al. Neoplastic T cells in angioimmunoblastic T-cell lymphoma express CD10. *Blood* 2002; **99**: 627–33.

42. Ree HJ, Kadin ME, Kikuchi M et al. Angioimmunoblastic lymphoma (AILD-type T-cell lymphoma) with hyperplastic germinal centers. *Am J Surg Pathol* 1998; **22**: 643–55.

43. Patsouris E, Noël H, Lennert K. Angioimmunoblastic lymphadenopathy–type of T-cell lymphoma with a high content of epithelioid cells. Histopathology and comparison with lymphoepithelioid cell lymphoma. *Am J Surg Pathol* 1989; **13**: 262–75.

44. Lee SS, Rüdiger T, Odenwald T et al. Angioimmunoblastic T cell lymphoma is derived from mature T-helper cells with varying expression and loss of detectable CD4. *Int J Cancer* 2003; **103**: 12–20.

45. Attygalle AD, Kyriakou C, Dupuis J et al. Histologic evolution of angioimmunoblastic T-cell lymphoma in consecutive biopsies: clinical correlation and insights into natural history and disease progression. *Am J Surg Pathol* 2007; **31**: 1077–88.

46. Lome-Maldonado C, Canioni D, Hermine O et al. Angio-immunoblastic T cell lymphoma (AILD-TL) rich in large B cells and associated with Epstein-Barr virus infection. A different subtype of AILD-TL? *Leukemia* 2002; **16**: 2134–41.

47. Zettl A, Lee SS, Rüdiger T et al. Epstein-Barr virus-associated B-cell lymphoproliferative disorders in angioimmunoblastic T-cell lymphoma and peripheral T-cell lymphoma, unspecified. *Am J Clin Pathol* 2002; **117**: 368–79.

48. Ortonne N, Dupuis J, Plonquet A et al. Characterization of CXCL13+ neoplastic t cells in cutaneous lesions of angioimmunoblastic T-cell lymphoma (AITL). *Am J Surg Pathol* 2007; **31**: 1068–76.

49. Dogan A, Morice WG. Bone marrow histopathology in peripheral T-cell lymphomas. *Br J Haematol* 2004; **127**: 140–54.

◆50. Brüggemann M, White H, Gaulard P et al. Powerful strategy for polymerase chain reaction-based clonality assessment in T-cell malignancies Report of the BIOMED-2 Concerted Action BHM4 CT98–3936. *Leukemia* 2007; **21**: 215–21.

51. Lipford EH, Smith HR, Pittaluga S et al. Clonality of angioimmunoblastic lymphadenopathy and implications for its evolution to malignant lymphoma. *J Clin Invest* 1987; **79**: 637–42.

52. Willenbrock K, Roers A, Seidl C et al. Analysis of T-cell subpopulations in T-cell non-Hodgkin's lymphoma of angioimmunoblastic lymphadenopathy with dysproteinemia type by single target gene amplification of T cell receptor-β gene rearrangements. *Am J Pathol* 2001; **158**: 1851–7.

53. Smith JL, Hodges E, Quin CT et al. Frequent T and B cell oligoclones in histologically and immunophenotypically characterized angioimmunoblastic lymphadenopathy. *Am J Pathol* 2000; **156**: 661–9.

54. Lorenzen J, Li G, Zhao-Höhn M et al. Angioimmunoblastic lymphadenopathy type of T-cell lymphoma and angioimmunoblastic lymphadenopathy: a clinicopathological and molecular biological study of 13 Chinese patients using polymerase chain reaction and paraffin-embedded tissues. *Virchows Arch* 1994; **424**: 593–600.

55. Bräuninger A, Spieker T, Willenbrock K et al. Survival and clonal expansion of mutating 'forbidden' (immunoglobulin receptor-deficient) Epstein–Barr virus-infected B cells in angioimmunoblastic T cell lymphoma. *J Exp Med* 2001; **194**: 927–40.

56. Dupuis J, Boye K, Martin N et al. Expression of CXCL13 by neoplastic cells in angioimmunoblastic T-cell lymphoma (AITL): a new diagnostic marker providing evidence that AITL derives from follicular helper T cells. *Am J Surg Pathol* 2006; **30**: 490–4.

57. Quintanilla-Martinez L, Fend F, Moguel LR et al. Peripheral T-cell lymphoma with Reed–Sternberg-like cells of B-cell

phenotype and genotype associated with Epstein–Barr virus infection. *Am J Surg Pathol* 1999; **23**: 1233–40.

58. Jones D, Jorgensen JL, Shahsafaei A *et al*. Characteristic proliferations of reticular and dendritic cells in angioimmunoblastic lymphoma. *Am J Surg Pathol* 1998; **22**: 956–64.

59. Troxell ML, Schwartz EJ, van de Rijn M *et al*. Follicular dendritic cell immunohistochemical markers in angioimmunoblastic T-cell lymphoma. *Appl Immunohistochem Mol Morphol* 2005; **13**: 297–303.

60. Takagi N, Nakamura S, Ueda R *et al*. A phenotypic and genotypic study of three node-based, low-grade peripheral T-cell lymphomas: angioimmunoblastic lymphoma, T-zone lymphoma, and lymphoepithelioid lymphoma. *Cancer* 1992; **69**: 2571–82.

61. Boulland ML, Kanavaros P, Wechsler J *et al*. Cytotoxic protein expression in natural killer cell lymphomas and in $\alpha\beta$ and $\gamma\delta$ peripheral T-cell lymphomas. *J Pathol* 1997; **183**: 432–9.

62. Lee PS, Lin CN, Chuang SS. Immunophenotyping of angioimmunoblastic T-cell lymphomas by multiparameter flow cytometry. *Pathol Res Pract* 2003; **199**: 539–45.

63. Yuan CM, Vergilio JA, Zhao XF *et al*. CD10 and BCL6 expression in the diagnosis of angioimmunoblastic T-cell lymphoma: utility of detecting CD10+ T cells by flow cytometry. *Hum Pathol* 2005; **36**: 784–91.

64. Baseggio L, Berger F, Morel D *et al*. Identification of circulating CD10 positive T cells in angioimmunoblastic T-cell lymphoma. *Leukemia* 2006; **20**: 296–303.

65. Chen W, Kesler MV, Karandikar NJ *et al*. Flow cytometric features of angioimmunoblastic T-cell lymphoma. *Cytometry B Clin Cytom* 2006; **70**: 142–8.

66. Cook JR, Craig FE, Swerdlow SH. Benign CD10-positive T cells in reactive lymphoid proliferations and B-cell lymphomas. *Mod Pathol* 2003; **16**: 879–85.

67. Ree HJ, Kadin ME, Kikuchi M *et al*. Bcl-6 expression in reactive follicular hyperplasia, follicular lymphoma, and angioimmunoblastic T-cell lymphoma with hyperplastic germinal centers: heterogeneity of intrafollicular T-cells and their altered distribution in the pathogenesis of angioimmunoblastic T-cell lymphoma. *Hum Pathol* 1999; **30**: 403–11.

♦68. Vinuesa CG, Tangye SG, Moser B *et al*. Follicular B helper T cells in antibody responses and autoimmunity. *Nat Rev Immunol* 2005; **5**: 853–65.

69. Chtanova T, Tangye SG, Newton R *et al*. T follicular helper cells express a distinctive transcriptional profile, reflecting their role as non-Th1/Th2 effector cells that provide help for B cells. *J Immunol* 2004; **173**: 68–78.

70. Kim CH, Lim HW, Kim JR *et al*. Unique gene expression program of human germinal center T helper cells. *Blood* 2004; **104**: 1952–60.

71. Dorfman DM, Shahsafaei A. CD69 expression correlates with expression of other markers of Th1 T cell differentiation in peripheral T cell lymphomas. *Hum Pathol* 2002; **33**: 330–4.

72. Jones D, O'Hara C, Kraus MD *et al*. Expression pattern of T-cell-associated chemokine receptors and their chemokines correlates with specific subtypes of T-cell non-Hodgkin lymphoma. *Blood* 2000; **96**: 685–90.

73. Tsuchiya T, Ohshima K, Karube K *et al*. Th1, Th2, and activated T-cell marker and clinical prognosis in peripheral T-cell lymphoma, unspecified: comparison with AILD, ALCL, lymphoblastic lymphoma, and ATLL. *Blood* 2004; **103**: 236–41.

74. Grogg KL, Attygalle AD, Macon WR *et al*. Angioimmunoblastic T-cell lymphoma: a neoplasm of germinal-center T-helper cells? *Blood* 2005; **106**: 1501–2.

75. Grogg KL, Attygale AD, Macon WR *et al*. Expression of CXCL13, a chemokine highly upregulated in germinal center T-helper cells, distinguishes angioimmunoblastic T-cell lymphoma from peripheral T-cell lymphoma, unspecified. *Mod Pathol* 2006; **19**: 1101–7.

76. Krenacs L, Schaerli P, Kis G *et al*. Phenotype of neoplastic cells in angioimmunoblastic T-cell lymphoma is consistent with activated follicular B helper T cells. *Blood* 2006; **108**: 1110–11.

77. Roncador G, Garcia Verdes-Montenegro JF, Tedoldi S *et al*. Expression of two markers of germinal center T cells (SAP and PD-1) in angioimmunoblastic T-cell lymphoma. *Haematologica* 2007; **92**: 1059–66.

78. Dorfman DM, Brown JA, Shahsafaei A *et al*. Programmed death-1 (PD-1) is a marker of germinal center-associated T cells and angioimmunoblastic T-cell lymphoma. *Am J Surg Pathol* 2006; **30**: 802–10.

●79. de Leval L, Rickman DS, Thielen C *et al*. The gene expression profile of nodal peripheral T-cell lymphoma demonstrates a molecular link between angioimmunoblastic T-cell lymphoma (AITL) and follicular helper T (TFH) cells. *Blood* 2007; **109**: 4952–63.

●80. Piccaluga PP, Agostinelli C, Califano A *et al*. Gene expression analysis of angioimmunoblastic lymphoma indicates derivation from T follicular helper cells and vascular endothelial growth factor deregulation. *Cancer Res* 2007; **67**: 10703–10.

81. Ottaviani G, Bueso-Ramos CE, Seilstad K *et al*. The role of the perifollicular sinus in determining the complex immunoarchitecture of angioimmunoblastic T-cell lymphoma. *Am J Surg Pathol* 2004; **28**: 1632–40.

82. de Leval L, Savilo E, Longtine J *et al*. Peripheral T-cell lymphoma with follicular involvement and a CD4+/bcl-6+ phenotype. *Am J Surg Pathol* 2001; **25**: 395–400.

83. Gesk S, Martin-Subero JI, Harder L *et al*. Molecular cytogenetic detection of chromosomal breakpoints in T-cell receptor gene loci. *Leukemia* 2003; **17**: 738–45.

84. Leich E, Haralambieva E, Zettl A *et al*. Tissue microarray-based screening for chromosomal breakpoints affecting the T-cell receptor gene loci in mature T-cell lymphomas. *J Pathol* 2007; **213**: 99–105.

85. Schlegelberger B, Feller A, Gödde E *et al*. Stepwise development of chromosomal abnormalities in

angioimmunoblastic lymphadenopathy. *Cancer Genet Cytogenet* 1990; **50**: 15–29.

86. Thorns C, Bastian B, Pinkel D *et al.* Chromosomal aberrations in angioimmunoblastic T-cell lymphoma and peripheral T-cell lymphoma unspecified: a matrix-based CGH approach. *Genes Chromosomes Cancer* 2007; **46**: 37–44.

87. Zhou Y, Attygalle AD, Chuang SS *et al.* Angioimmunoblastic T-cell lymphoma: histological progression associates with EBV and HHV6B viral load. *Br J Haematol* 2007; **138**: 44–53.

88. Weiss LM, Jaffe ES, Liu XF *et al.* Detection and localization of Epstein-Barr viral genomes in angioimmunoblastic lymphadenopathy and angioimmunoblastic lymphadenopathy-like lymphoma. *Blood* 1992; **79**: 1789–95.

89. Kawano R, Ohshima K, Wakamatsu S *et al.* Epstein-Barr virus genome level, T-cell clonality and the prognosis of angioimmunoblastic T-cell lymphoma. *Haematologica* 2005; **90**: 1192–6.

90. Foss HD, Anagnostopoulos I, Herbst H *et al.* Patterns of cytokine gene expression in peripheral T-cell lymphoma of angioimmunoblastic lymphadenopathy type. *Blood* 1995; **85**: 2862–9.

91. Ohshima KS, Suzumiya J, Kawasaki C *et al.* Cytoplasmic cytokines in lymphoproliferative disorders: multiple cytokine production in angioimmunoblastic lymphadenopathy with dysproteinemia. *Leuk Lymphoma* 2000; **38**: 541–5.

92. Foss HD, Araujo I, Demel G *et al.* Expression of vascular endothelial growth factor in lymphomas and Castleman's disease. *J Pathol* 1997; **183**: 44–50.

93. Zhao WL, Mourah S, Mounier N *et al.* Vascular endothelial growth factor-A is expressed both on lymphoma cells and endothelial cells in angioimmunoblastic T-cell lymphoma and related to lymphoma progression. *Lab Invest* 2004; **84**: 1512–19.

●94. Ballester B, Ramuz O, Gisselbrecht C *et al.* Gene expression profiling identifies molecular subgroups among nodal peripheral T-cell lymphomas. *Oncogene* 2006; **25**: 1560–70.

95. Petit B, Leroy K, Kanavaros P *et al.* Expression of p53 protein in T- and natural killer-cell lymphomas is associated with some clinicopathologic entities but rarely related to p53 mutations. *Hum Pathol* 2001; **32**: 196–204.

96. Morito N, Yoh K, Fujioka Y *et al.* Overexpression of c-Maf contributes to T-cell lymphoma in both mice and human. *Cancer Res* 2006; **66**: 812–19.

97. Murakami YI, Yatabe Y, Sakaguchi T *et al.* c-Maf expression in angioimmunoblastic T-cell lymphoma. *Am J Surg Pathol* 2007; **31**: 1695–702.

98. Feller AC, Lennert K, Zwingers T. Peripheral T-cell lymphomas. *Histopathology* 1991; **19**: 481–4.

99. Ansell SM, Habermann TM, Kurtin PJ *et al.* Predictive capacity of the International Prognostic Factor Index in patients with peripheral T-cell lymphoma. *J Clin Oncol* 1997; **15**: 2296–301.

100. Pellatt J, Sweetenham J, Pickering RM *et al.* A single-centre study of treatment outcomes and survival in 120 patients with peripheral T-cell non-Hodgkin's lymphoma. *Ann Hematol* 2002; **81**: 267–72.

101. Sonnen R, Schmidt WP, Müller-Hermelink HK, Schmitz N. The International Prognostic Index determines the outcome of patients with nodal mature T-cell lymphomas. *Br J Haematol* 2005; **129**: 366–72.

102. Kim K, Kim WS, Jung CW *et al.* Clinical features of peripheral T-cell lymphomas in 78 patients diagnosed according to the Revised European-American lymphoma (REAL) classification. *Eur J Cancer* 2002; **38**: 75–81.

103. Zaja F, Russo D, Silvestri F *et al.* Retrospective analysis of 23 cases with peripheral T-cell lymphoma, unspecified: clinical characteristics and outcome. *Haematologica* 1997; **82**: 171–7.

104. Armitage JO, Weisenburger DD. New approach to classifying non-Hodgkin's lymphomas: clinical features of the major histologic subtypes. Non-Hodgkin's lymphoma classification project. *J Clin Oncol* 1998; **16**: 2780–95.

105. Kojima H, Hasegawa Y, Suzukawa K *et al.* Clinicopathological features and prognostic factors of Japanese patients with 'peripheral T-cell lymphoma, unspecified' diagnosed according to the WHO classification. *Leuk Res* 2004; **28**: 1287–92.

106. Au WY, Ma SY, Chim CS *et al.* Clinicopathologic features and treatment outcome of mature T-cell and natural killer-cell lymphomas diagnosed according to the World Health Organization classification scheme: a single center experience of 10 years. *Ann Oncol* 2005; **16**: 206–14.

107. Dupuis J, Emile JF, Mounier N *et al.* Prognostic significance of Epstein-Barr virus in nodal peripheral T-cell lymphoma, unspecified: a Groupe d'Etude des Lymphomes de l'Adulte (GELA) study. *Blood* 2006; **108**: 4163–9.

●108. Gallamini A, Stelitano C, Calvi R *et al.* Peripheral T-cell lymphoma unspecified (PTCL-U): a new prognostic model from a retrospective multicentric clinical study. *Blood* 2004; **103**: 2474–9.

109. Suchi T, Lennert K, Tu LY *et al.* Histopathology and immunohistochemistry of peripheral T cell lymphomas: a proposal for their classification. *J Clin Pathol* 1987; **40**: 995–1015.

110. Barry TS, Jaffe ES, Sorbara L *et al.* Peripheral T-cell lymphomas expressing CD30 and CD15. *Am J Surg Pathol* 2003; **27**: 1513–22.

111. Falini B, Pileri S, Zinzani PL *et al.* ALK+ lymphoma: clinico-pathological findings and outcome. *Blood* 1999; **93**: 2697–706.

112. Gascoyne RD, Aoun P, Wu D *et al.* Prognostic significance of anaplastic lymphoma kinase (ALK) protein expression in adults with anaplastic large cell lymphoma. *Blood* 1999; **93**: 3913–21.

113. Savage KJ, Harris NL, Vose JM *et al.* ALK- anaplastic large-cell lymphoma is clinically and immunophenotypically different from both ALK+ ALCL and peripheral T-cell lymphoma, not otherwise specified: report from the

International Peripheral T-Cell Lymphoma Project. *Blood* 2008; **111**: 5496–504.

114. Yamashita Y, Nakamura S, Kagami Y *et al.* Lennert's lymphoma: a variant of cytotoxic T-cell lymphoma? *Am J Surg Pathol* 2000; **24**: 1627–33.

115. Geissinger E, Odenwald T, Lee SS *et al.* Nodal peripheral T-cell lymphomas and, in particular, their lymphoepithelioid (Lennert's) variant are often derived from CD8(+) cytotoxic T-cells. *Virchows Arch* 2004; **445**: 334–43.

116. Patsouris E, Noël H, Lennert K. Histological and immunohistological findings in lymphoepithelioid cell lymphoma (Lennert's lymphoma). *Am J Surg Pathol* 1988; **12**: 341–50.

117. Rüdiger T, Ichinohasama R, Ott MM *et al.* Peripheral T-cell lymphoma with distinct perifollicular growth pattern: a distinct subtype of T-cell lymphoma? *Am J Surg Pathol* 2000; **24**: 117–22.

118. Bacon C, Paterson J, Liu H *et al.* Peripheral T-cell lymphoma with a follicular growth pattern: derivation from follicular helper T cells and relationship to angioimmunoblastic T-cell lymphoma. *Br J Haematol* 2008; **143**: 439–41.

119. Ikonomou IM, Tierens A, Troen G *et al.* Peripheral T-cell lymphoma with involvement of the expanded mantle zone. *Virchows Arch* 2006; **449**: 78–87.

120. Jiang L, Jones D, Medeiros LJ *et al.* Peripheral T-cell lymphoma with a 'follicular' pattern and the perifollicular sinus phenotype. *Am J Clin Pathol* 2005; **123**: 448–55.

121. Macon WR, Williams ME, Greer JP *et al.* Paracortical nodular T-cell lymphoma. Identification of an unusual variant of peripheral T-cell lymphoma. *Am J Surg Pathol* 1995; **19**: 297–303.

●122. Streubel B, Vinatzer U, Willheim M *et al.* Novel t(5;9)(q33;q22) fuses ITK to SYK in unspecified peripheral T-cell lymphoma. *Leukemia* 2006; **20**: 313–18.

123. Huang YL, Moreau A, Dupuis J *et al.* Peripheral T-cell lymphomas with a follicular growth pattern are derived from follicular helper T cells (TFH): and may show overlapping features with angioimmunoblastic T-cell lymphomas. *Am J Surg Pathol* 2009; **33**: 682–90.

●124. Went P, Agostinelli C, Gallamini A *et al.* Marker expression in peripheral T-cell lymphoma: a proposed clinical-pathologic prognostic score. *J Clin Oncol* 2006; **24**: 2472–9.

125. Geissinger E, Bonzheim I, Krenács L *et al.* Identification of the tumor cells in peripheral T-cell lymphomas by combined polymerase chain reaction-based T-cell receptor β spectrotyping and immunohistological detection with T-cell receptor β chain variable region segment-specific antibodies. *J Mol Diagn* 2005; **7**: 455–64.

126. Felgar RE, Macon WR, Kinney MC *et al.* TIA-1 expression in lymphoid neoplasms. Identification of subsets with cytotoxic T lymphocyte or natural killer cell differentiation. *Am J Pathol* 1997; **150**: 1893–900.

127. de Bruin PC, Kummer JA, van der Valk P *et al.* Granzyme B-expressing peripheral T-cell lymphomas: neoplastic equivalents of activated cytotoxic T cells with preference for mucosa-associated lymphoid tissue localization. *Blood* 1994; **84**: 3785–91.

128. Ohshima K, Suzumiya J, Sugihara M *et al.* Clinical, immunohistochemical and phenotypic features of aggressive nodal cytotoxic lymphomas, including α/β, γ/δ T-cell and natural killer cell types. *Virchows Arch* 1999; **435**: 92–100.

129. Asano N, Suzuki R, Kagami Y *et al.* Clinicopathologic and prognostic significance of cytotoxic molecule expression in nodal peripheral T-cell lymphoma, unspecified. *Am J Surg Pathol* 2005; **29**: 1284–93.

130. Theodorou I, Raphaël M, Bigorgne C *et al.* Recombination pattern of the TCR γ locus in human peripheral T-cell lymphomas. *J Pathol* 1994; **174**: 233–42.

131. Gaulard P, Bourquelot P, Kanavaros P *et al.* Expression of the alpha/beta and gamma/delta T-cell receptors in 57 cases of peripheral T-cell lymphomas. Identification of a subset of gamma/delta T-cell lymphomas. *Am J Pathol* 1990; **137**: 617–28.

132. Arnulf B, Copie-Bergman C, Delfau-Larue MH *et al.* Nonhepatosplenic γδ T-cell lymphoma: a subset of cytotoxic lymphomas with mucosal or skin localization. *Blood* 1998; **91**: 1723–31.

●133. Jaffe ES, Krenács L, Raffeld M. Classification of cytotoxic T-cell and natural killer cell lymphomas. *Semin Hematol* 2003; **40**: 175–84.

134. Ishida T, Inagaki H, Utsunomiya A *et al.* CXC chemokine receptor 3 and CC chemokine receptor 4 expression in T-cell and NK-cell lymphomas with special reference to clinicopathological significance for peripheral T-cell lymphoma, unspecified. *Clin Cancer Res* 2004; **10**: 5494–500.

135. Ohshima K, Karube K, Kawano R *et al.* Classification of distinct subtypes of peripheral T-cell lymphoma unspecified, identified by chemokine and chemokine receptor expression: analysis of prognosis. *Int J Oncol* 2004; **25**: 605–13.

136. Schlegelberger B, Himmler A, Gödde E *et al.* Cytogenetic findings in peripheral T-cell lymphomas as a basis for distinguishing low-grade and high-grade lymphomas. *Blood* 1994; **83**: 505–11.

137. Lepretre S, Buchonnet G, Stamatoullas A *et al.* Chromosome abnormalities in peripheral T-cell lymphoma. *Cancer Genet Cytogenet* 2000; **117**: 71–9.

138. Chen CY, Yao M, Tang JL *et al.* Chromosomal abnormalities of 200 Chinese patients with non-Hodgkin's lymphoma in Taiwan: with special reference to T-cell lymphoma. *Ann Oncol* 2004; **15**: 1091–6.

●139. Zettl A, Rüdiger T, Konrad MA *et al.* Genomic profiling of peripheral T-cell lymphoma, unspecified, and anaplastic large T-cell lymphoma delineates novel recurrent chromosomal alterations. *Am J Pathol* 2004; **164**: 1837–48.

140. Martinez-Delgado B, Meléndez B, Cuadros M *et al.* Expression profiling of T-cell lymphomas differentiates peripheral and lymphoblastic lymphomas and defines survival related genes. *Clin Cancer Res* 2004; **10**: 4971–82.

141. Martinez-Delgado B, Cuadros M, Honrado E *et al.* Differential expression of NF-κB pathway genes among peripheral T-cell lymphomas. *Leukemia* 2005; **19**: 2254–63.

142. Cuadros M, Dave SS, Jaffe ES *et al.* Identification of a proliferation signature related to survival in nodal peripheral T-cell lymphomas. *J Clin Oncol* 2007; **25**: 3321–9.

●143. Piccaluga PP, Agostinelli C, Califano A *et al.* Gene expression analysis of peripheral T cell lymphoma, unspecified, reveals distinct profiles and new potential therapeutic targets. *J Clin Invest* 2007; **117**: 823–34.

144. Moller MB, Gerdes AM, Skjodt K *et al.* Disrupted p53 function as predictor of treatment failure and poor prognosis in B- and T-cell non-Hodgkin's lymphoma. *Clin Cancer Res* 1999; **5**: 1085–91.

145. Pescarmona E, Pignoloni P, Puopolo M *et al.* p53 over-expression identifies a subset of nodal peripheral T-cell lymphomas with a distinctive biological profile and poor clinical outcome. *J Pathol* 2001; **195**: 361–6.

146. Hoshida Y, Hongyo T, Nakatsuka S *et al.* Gene mutations in lymphoproliferative disorders of T and NK/T cell phenotypes developing in renal transplant patients. *Lab Invest* 2002; **82**: 257–64.

147. Jung JT, Kim DH, Kwak EK *et al.* Clinical role of Bcl-2, Bax, or p53 overexpression in peripheral T-cell lymphomas. *Ann Hematol* 2006; **85**: 575–81.

148. Jones JF, Shurin S, Abramowsky C *et al.* T-cell lymphomas containing Epstein-Barr viral DNA in patients with chronic Epstein-Barr virus infections. *N Engl J Med* 1988; **318**: 733–41.

149. d'Amore F, Johansen P, Houmand A *et al.* Epstein-Barr virus genome in non-Hodgkin's lymphomas occurring in immunocompetent patients: highest prevalence in nonlymphoblastic T-cell lymphoma and correlation with a poor prognosis. Danish Lymphoma Study Group, LYFO. *Blood* 1996; **87**: 1045–55.

150. Ko YH, Cho EY, Kim JE *et al.* NK and NK-like T-cell lymphoma in extranasal sites: a comparative clinicopathological study according to site and EBV status. *Histopathology* 2004; **44**: 480–9.

151. Mori A, Takao S, Pradutkanchana J *et al.* High tumor necrosis factor-α levels in the patients with Epstein–Barr virus-associated peripheral T-cell proliferative disease/lymphoma. *Leuk Res* 2003; **27**: 493–8.

152. Lay JD, Tsao CJ, Chen JY *et al.* Upregulation of tumor necrosis factor-α gene by Epstein–Barr virus and activation of macrophages in Epstein–Barr virus-infected T cells in the pathogenesis of hemophagocytic syndrome. *J Clin Invest* 1997; **100**: 1969–79.

◆153. Jaffe ES, Chan JK, Su IJ *et al.* Report of the workshop on nasal and related extranodal angiocentric T/natural killer cell lymphomas. Definitions, differential diagnosis, and epidemiology. *Am J Surg Pathol* 1996; **20**: 103–11.

154. Swinson CM, Slavin G, Coles EC *et al.* Coeliac disease and malignancy. *Lancet* 1983; **1**: 111–15.

155. Isaacson P, Wright DH. Origin of intestinal lymphomas. *Lancet* 1978; **1**: 984–5.

156. Isaacson PG, O'Connor NT, Spencer J *et al.* Malignant histiocytosis of the intestine: a T-cell lymphoma. *Lancet* 1985; **2**: 688–91.

157. Green PH, Fleischauer AT, Bhagat G *et al.* Risk of malignancy in patients with celiac disease. *Am J Med* 2003; **115**: 191–5.

158. Gale J, Simmonds PD, Mead GM *et al.* Enteropathy-type intestinal T-cell lymphoma: clinical features and treatment of 31 patients in a single center. *J Clin Oncol* 2000; **18**: 795–803.

159. Wöhrer S, Chott A, Drach J *et al.* Chemotherapy with cyclophosphamide, doxorubicin, etoposide, vincristine and prednisone (CHOEP) is not effective in patients with enteropathy-type intestinal T-cell lymphoma. *Ann Oncol* 2004; **15**: 1680–3.

160. Cellier C, Delabesse E, Helmer C *et al.* Refractory sprue, coeliac disease, and enteropathy-associated T-cell lymphoma. French coeliac disease study group. *Lancet* 2000; **356**: 203–8.

161. Schmitt-Gräff A, Hummel M, Zemlin M *et al.* Intestinal T-cell lymphoma: a reassessment of cytomorphological and phenotypic features in relation to patterns of small bowel remodelling. *Virchows Arch* 1996; **429**: 27–36.

162. Chott A, Dragosics B, Radaszkiewicz T. Peripheral T-cell lymphomas of the intestine. *Am J Pathol* 1992; **141**: 1361–71.

163. Chott A, Haedicke W, Mosberger I *et al.* Most CD56+ intestinal lymphomas are CD8+CD5-T-cell lymphomas of monomorphic small to medium size histology. *Am J Pathol* 1998; **153**: 1483–90.

164. Cellier C, Patey N, Mauvieux L *et al.* Abnormal intestinal intraepithelial lymphocytes in refractory sprue. *Gastroenterology* 1998; **114**: 471–81.

◆165. Isaacson PG. Relation between cryptic intestinal lymphoma and refractory sprue. *Lancet* 2000; **356**: 178–9.

◆166. Gaulard P, Belhadj K, Reyes F. $\gamma\delta$ T-cell lymphomas. *Semin Hematol* 2003; **40**: 233–43.

167. Inagaki N, Asaoka D, Mori KL *et al.* Enteropathy-type T-cell lymphoma expressing NK-cell intraepithelial lymphocyte (NK-IEL) phenotype. *Leuk Lymphoma* 2004; **45**: 1471–4.

168. Dukers DF, Vermeer MH, Jaspars LH *et al.* Expression of killer cell inhibitory receptors is restricted to true NK cell lymphomas and a subset of intestinal enteropathy-type T cell lymphomas with a cytotoxic phenotype. *J Clin Pathol* 2001; **54**: 224–8.

169. Haedicke W, Ho FC, Chott A *et al.* Expression of CD94/NKG2A and killer immunoglobulin-like receptors in NK cells and a subset of extranodal cytotoxic T-cell lymphomas. *Blood* 2000; **95**: 3628–30.

170. Krenács L, Smyth MJ, Bagdi E *et al.* The serine protease granzyme M is preferentially expressed in NK-cell, $\gamma\delta$ T-cell, and intestinal T-cell lymphomas: evidence of origin from lymphocytes involved in innate immunity. *Blood* 2003; **101**: 3590–3.

171. Verkarre V, Asnafi V, Lecomte T *et al.* Refractory coeliac sprue is a diffuse gastrointestinal disease. *Gut* 2003; **52**: 205–11.

172. Green PH, Jabri B. Coeliac disease. *Lancet* 2003; **362**: 383–91.

173. Mention JJ, Ben Ahmed M, Bègue B *et al.* Interleukin 15: a key to disrupted intraepithelial lymphocyte homeostasis and lymphomagenesis in celiac disease. *Gastroenterology* 2003; **125**: 730–45.

174. Verkarre V, Romana SP, Cellier C *et al.* Recurrent partial trisomy 1q22-q44 in clonal intraepithelial lymphocytes in refractory celiac sprue. *Gastroenterology* 2003; **125**: 40–6.

175. Zettl A, Ott G, Makulik A *et al.* Chromosomal gains at 9q characterize enteropathy-type T-cell lymphoma. *Am J Pathol* 2002; **161**: 1635–45.

176. Baumgärtner AK, Zettl A, Chott A *et al.* High frequency of genetic aberrations in enteropathy-type T-cell lymphoma. *Lab Invest* 2003; **83**: 1509–16.

177. Cejkova P, Zettl A, Baumgärtner AK *et al.* Amplification of NOTCH1 and ABL1 gene loci is a frequent aberration in enteropathy-type T-cell lymphoma. *Virchows Arch* 2005; **446**: 416–20.

178. Obermann EC, Diss TC, Hamoudi RA *et al.* Loss of heterozygosity at chromosome 9p21 is a frequent finding in enteropathy-type T-cell lymphoma. *J Pathol* 2004; **202**: 252–62.

179. Quintanilla-Martinez L, Lome-Maldonado C, Ott G *et al.* Primary non-Hodgkin's lymphoma of the intestine: high prevalence of Epstein-Barr virus in Mexican lymphomas as compared with European cases. *Blood* 1997; **89**: 644–51.

180. Gaulard P, Zafrani ES, Mavier P *et al.* Peripheral T-cell lymphoma presenting as predominant liver disease: a report of three cases. *Hepatology* 1986; **6**: 864–8.

181. Kanavaros P, Farcet JP, Gaulard P *et al.* Recombinative events of the T cell antigen receptor delta gene in peripheral T cell lymphomas. *J Clin Invest* 1991; **87**: 666–72.

182. Weidmann E. Hepatosplenic T cell lymphoma. A review on 45 cases since the first report describing the disease as a distinct lymphoma entity in 1990. *Leukemia* 2000; **14**: 991–7.

●183. Belhadj K, Reyes F, Farcet JP *et al.* Hepatosplenic $\gamma\delta$ T-cell lymphoma is a rare clinicopathologic entity with poor outcome: report on a series of 21 patients. *Blood* 2003; **102**: 4261–9.

184. Wu H, Wasik MA, Przybylski G *et al.* Hepatosplenic gamma-delta T-cell lymphoma as a late-onset posttransplant lymphoproliferative disorder in renal transplant recipients. *Am J Clin Pathol* 2000; **113**: 487–96.

185. Navarro JT, Ribera JM, Mate JL *et al.* Hepatosplenic T-gammadelta lymphoma in a patient with Crohn's disease treated with azathioprine. *Leuk Lymphoma* 2003; **44**: 531–3.

186. Weidmann E, Hinz T, Klein S *et al.* Cytotoxic hepatosplenic gammadelta T-cell lymphoma following

acute myeloid leukemia bearing two distinct gamma chains of the T-cell receptor. Biologic and clinical features. *Haematologica* 2000; **85**: 1024–31.

187. Kraus MD, Crawford DF, Kaleem Z *et al.* T γ/δ hepatosplenic lymphoma in a heart transplant patient after an Epstein-Barr virus positive lymphoproliferative disorder: a case report. *Cancer* 1998; **82**: 983–92.

188. Rosh JR, Gross T, Mamula P *et al.* Hepatosplenic T-cell lymphoma in adolescents and young adults with Crohn's disease: a cautionary tale? *Inflamm Bowel Dis* 2007; **13**: 1024–30.

189. Cooke CB, Krenacs L, Stetler-Stevenson M *et al.* Hepatosplenic T-cell lymphoma: a distinct clinicopathologic entity of cytotoxic $\gamma\delta$ T-cell origin. *Blood* 1996; **88**: 4265–74.

190. de Wolf-Peeters C, Achten R. $\gamma\delta$ T-cell lymphomas: a homogeneous entity? *Histopathology* 2000; **36**: 294–305.

191. Vega F, Medeiros LJ, Bueso-Ramos C *et al.* Hepatosplenic gamma/delta T-cell lymphoma in bone marrow. A sinusoidal neoplasm with blastic cytologic features. *Am J Clin Pathol* 2001; **116**: 410–19.

192. Aldinucci D, Poletto D, Zagonel V *et al.* In vitro and in vivo effects of 2'-deoxycoformycin (Pentostatin) on tumour cells from human $\gamma\delta+$ T-cell malignancies. *Br J Haematol* 2000; **110**: 188–96.

193. Grigg AP. 2'-Deoxycoformycin for hepatosplenic gammadelta T-cell lymphoma. *Leuk Lymphoma* 2001; **42**: 797–9.

194. Farcet JP, Gaulard P, Marolleau JP *et al.* Hepatosplenic T-cell lymphoma: sinusal/sinusoidal localization of malignant cells expressing the T-cell receptor $\gamma\delta$. *Blood* 1990; **75**: 2213–19.

195. Charton-Bain MC, Brousset P, Bouabdallah R *et al.* Variation in the histological pattern of nodal involvement by gamma/delta T-cell lymphoma. *Histopathology* 2000; **36**: 233–9.

196. Gaulard P, Kanavaros P, Farcet JP *et al.* Bone marrow histologic and immunohistochemical findings in peripheral. T-cell lymphoma: a study of 38 cases. *Hum Pathol* 1991; **22**: 331–8.

197. Morice WG, Macon WR, Dogan A *et al.* NK-cell-associated receptor expression in hepatosplenic T-cell lymphoma, insights into pathogenesis. *Leukemia* 2006; **20**: 883–6.

198. Dommann-Scherrer CC, Kurer SB, Zimmermann DR *et al.* Occult hepatosplenic T-gamma delta lymphoma. Value of genotypic analysis in the differential diagnosis. *Virchows Arch* 1995; **426**: 629–34.

199. Przybylski GK, Wu H, Macon WR *et al.* Hepatosplenic and subcutaneous panniculitis-like γ/δ T cell lymphomas are derived from different Vδ subsets of γ/δ T lymphocytes. *J Mol Diagn* 2000; **2**: 11–19.

200. Lai R, Larratt LM, Etches W *et al.* Hepatosplenic T-cell lymphoma of alphabeta lineage in a 16-year-old boy presenting with hemolytic anemia and thrombocytopenia. *Am J Surg Pathol* 2000; **24**: 459–63.

201. Suarez F, Wlodarska I, Rigal-Huguet F *et al.* Hepatosplenic $\alpha\beta$ T-cell lymphoma: an unusual case with clinical,

histologic, and cytogenetic features of $\gamma\delta$ hepatosplenic T-cell lymphoma. *Am J Surg Pathol* 2000; **24**: 1027–32.

202. Macon WR, Levy NB, Kurtin PJ *et al.* Hepatosplenic $\alpha\beta$ T-cell lymphomas: a report of 14 cases and comparison with hepatosplenic $\gamma\delta$ T-cell lymphomas. *Am J Surg Pathol* 2001; **25**: 285–96.

203. Wlodarska I, Martin-Garcia N, Achten R *et al.* Fluorescence in situ hybridization study of chromosome 7 aberrations in hepatosplenic T-cell lymphoma: isochromosome 7q as a common abnormality accumulating in forms with features of cytologic progression. *Genes Chromosomes Cancer* 2002; **33**: 243–51.

204. Francois A, Lesesve JF, Stamatoullas A *et al.* Hepatosplenic gamma/delta T-cell lymphoma: a report of two cases in immunocompromised patients, associated with isochromosome 7q. *Am J Surg Pathol* 1997; **21**: 781–90.

205. Bordessoule D, Gaulard P, Mason DY. Preferential localisation of human lymphocytes bearing $\gamma\delta$ T cell receptors to the red pulp of the spleen. *J Clin Pathol* 1990; **43**: 461–4.

206. Gonzalez CL, Medeiros LJ, Braziel RM *et al.* T-cell lymphoma involving subcutaneous tissue. A clinicopathologic entity commonly associated with hemophagocytic syndrome. *Am J Surg Pathol* 1991; **15**: 17–27.

207. Willemze R, Jaffe ES, Burg G *et al.* WHO-EORTC classification for cutaneous lymphomas. *Blood* 2005; **105**: 3768–85.

208. Go RS, Wester SM. Immunophenotypic and molecular features, clinical outcomes, treatments, and prognostic factors associated with subcutaneous panniculitis-like T-cell lymphoma: a systematic analysis of 156 patients reported in the literature. *Cancer* 2004; **101**: 1404–13.

209. Guizzardi M, Hendrickx IA, Mancini LL *et al.* Cytotoxic γ/δ subcutaneous panniculitis-like T-cell lymphoma: report of a case with pulmonary involvement unresponsive to therapy. *J Eur Acad Dermatol Venereol* 2003; **17**: 219–22.

210. Moriki T, Wada M, Takahashi T *et al.* Pleural effusion cytology in a case of cytophagic histiocytic panniculitis (subcutaneous panniculitic T-cell lymphoma). A case report. *Acta Cytol* 2000; **44**: 1040–4.

211. Romero LS, Goltz RW, Nagi C *et al.* Subcutaneous T-cell lymphoma with associated hemophagocytic syndrome and terminal leukemic transformation. *J Am Acad Dermatol* 1996; **34**: 904–10.

212. Toro JR, Liewehr DJ, Pabby N *et al.* Gamma-delta T-cell phenotype is associated with significantly decreased survival in cutaneous T-cell lymphoma. *Blood* 2003; **101**: 3407–12.

213. Massone C, Chott A, Metze D *et al.* Subcutaneous, blastic natural killer (NK), NK/T-cell, and other cytotoxic lymphomas of the skin: a morphologic, immunophenotypic, and molecular study of 50 patients. *Am J Surg Pathol* 2004; **28**: 719–35.

◆214. Willemze R, Jansen PM, Cerroni L *et al.* Subcutaneous panniculitis-like T-cell lymphoma: definition, classification, and prognostic factors: an EORTC Cutaneous Lymphoma Group Study of 83 cases. *Blood* 2008; **111**: 838–45.

215. Lozzi GP, Massone C, Citarella L *et al.* Rimming of adipocytes by neoplastic lymphocytes: a histopathologic feature not restricted to subcutaneous T-cell lymphoma. *Am J Dermatopathol* 2006; **28**: 9–12.

216. Harada H, Iwatsuki K, Kaneko F. Detection of Epstein-Barr virus genes in malignant lymphoma with clinical and histologic features of cytophagic histiocytic panniculitis. *J Am Acad Dermatol* 1994; **31**: 379–83.

217. Cho KH, Oh JK, Kim CW *et al.* Peripheral T-cell lymphoma involving subcutaneous tissue. *Br J Dermatol* 1995; **132**: 290–5.

218. Iwatsuki K, Harada H, Ohtsuka M *et al.* Latent Epstein-Barr virus infection is frequently detected in subcutaneous lymphoma associated with hemophagocytosis but not in nonfatal cytophagic histiocytic panniculitis. *Arch Dermatol* 1997; **133**: 787–8.

219. Craig AJ, Cualing H, Thomas G *et al.* Cytophagic histiocytic panniculitis – a syndrome associated with benign and malignant panniculitis: case comparison and review of the literature. *J Am Acad Dermatol* 1998; **39**: 721–36.

PRESENTING FEATURES, DIAGNOSIS AND STAGING

40

Presenting features of lymphoid neoplasms

S MONTOTO AND TA LISTER

ORGAN INFILTRATION

Lymphadenopathy

The overwhelming majority of patients with Hodgkin disease (HD) present with lymph node involvement at diagnosis,[1] whereas in one of the first and most complete large series analyzing the clinical data on non-Hodgkin lymphoma (NHL)[2] lymphadenopathy was found to be the presenting symptom of 'lymphosarcoma' – which mainly included what would nowadays be classified as follicular lymphoma, diffuse large B cell lymphoma and small lymphocytic lymphoma – in 63.5 percent of patients. The percentage of patients with lymph node enlargement at diagnosis varies among different subsets of NHL. In patients with diffuse large cell lymphoma (DLCL), it is the presenting symptom in 84 percent,[3] whereas in patients with follicular lymphoma, the commonest type of 'indolent' lymphoma, it is present in 90–95 percent,[3] the nodes possibly having fluctuated in size for some time prior to the diagnosis.[4] More than 90 percent of chronic lymphocytic leukemia/small lymphocytic lymphoma (CLL/SLL) present with lymph node enlargement at diagnosis.[3] In contrast, this feature is rarely seen in patients with B prolymphocytic leukemia (B-PLL)[5] or in hairy cell leukemia

(HCL).[6] In the latter the presence of abdominal lymphadenopathy is associated with large immature hairy cells and a worse prognosis related to a relative resistance to treatment, suggesting transformation into a more aggressive disease.[7] Anecdotally, lymph node enlargement has been reported to be found in about 10 percent of patients with IgD multiple myeloma.[8] Lymph node enlargement can also be found in acute lymphoblastic leukemia (ALL) and other chronic lymphoproliferative disorders.

In lymphoid malignancies the lymphadenopathy tends to be firm or rubbery in consistency, non-tender and, initially often unilateral.[2] In the Rosenberg series the commonest site of lymph node involvement was the neck, cervical adenopathy representing the initial manifestation in around 40 percent of the patients, followed by the inguinal and the axillary areas.[2] Of note, inguinal involvement was more frequent in 'giant follicle lymphosarcoma' than in other subtypes ('reticulum cell sarcoma' and 'small cell lymphosarcoma'), with a fifth of the patients presenting inguinal adenopathies as the initial manifestation of lymphoma. Mediastinal or hilar involvement was found in only 3 percent of patients in the Rosenberg series[2] and around 20 percent in more recent series,[9,10] probably reflecting more sophisticated imaging technique. The percentage of mediastinal involvement varies from 4 percent in diffuse mixed lymphoma to 64 percent in lymphoblastic lymphoma, but for most subtypes is approximately 20 percent.[10] In contrast, more than half the patients with HD have mediastinal lymphadenopathy at diagnosis[9,11] (Fig. 40.1). In HD mediastinal masses typically present surface lobulation, contrasting with T lymphoblastic lymphoma (T-LL) or primary mediastinal large cell lymphoma (PMLCL).[12] In spite of the fact that bulky mediastinal disease is found in a considerable proportion of patients with HD at

diagnosis, it usually does not cause superior vein cava obstruction (SVCO), because of the slow pace of growth. In contrast, a bulky mediastinal mass causing SVCO at diagnosis is characteristic of T-LL and PMLCL. Thus, in a series of patients with mediastinal lymphoma, radiologic signs of complete obstruction of the superior vena cava were found in 3 percent of patients with HD, 13 percent of patients with T-LL and 19 percent of patients with PMLCL.[12] In contrast with the pattern of dissemination in HD, in which a contiguous spreading is the rule,[13] 40 percent of patients with follicular lymphomas have cervical/supraclavicular and paraaortic involvement without mediastinal lymphadenopathy.[9] The presence of abdominal lymph node enlargement is frequent in patients with NHL, especially in those with follicular lymphoma. Likewise, abdominal involvement, both affecting nodal and extranodal structures, is characteristic of sporadic Burkitt lymphoma (Table 40.1).[14]

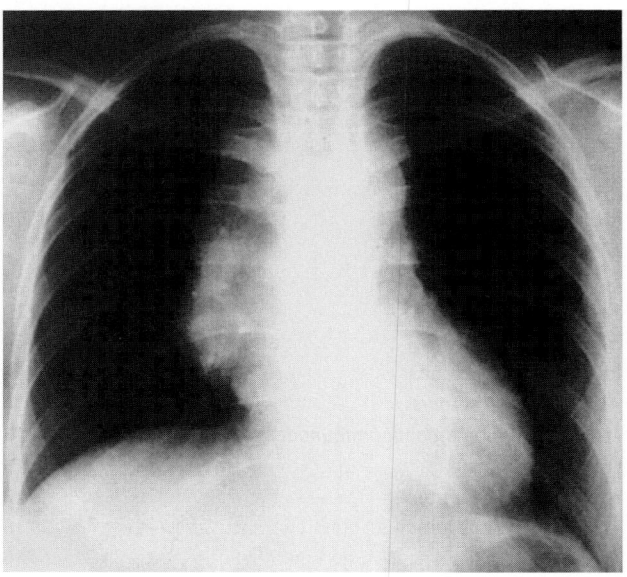

Figure 40.1 Mediastinal mass in a patient with Hodgkin disease. (Reproduced with permission of Taylor and Francis from Husband JE, Reznek RH. *Imaging in Oncology*, 2nd ed., 2004, Figure 32.12, page 831.)

Bone marrow involvement/peripheral blood involvement

Infiltration of the bone marrow is found at diagnosis in 3–31 percent of patients with HD.[11,15,16] The pattern of infiltration is characterized by the presence of typical Reed–Sternberg cells or Reed–Sternberg variants among a background of reactive cells with lymphocytes, plasma cells, eosinophils, neutrophils, dendritic cells and histiocytes.[16] In NHL, the percentage of patients with bone marrow involvement at diagnosis depends on the subtype, being less frequent in 'aggressive' than in 'indolent' lymphomas. Thus, more than half the patients with follicular lymphoma and around 70 percent of patients with SLL present with advanced stage at diagnosis due to bone marrow infiltration,[17–19] whereas it

Table 40.1 Prevalence (in percent) of clinical features in Hodgkin disease and non-Hodgkin lymphoma

	Hodgkin disease	Diffuse large cell lymphoma	Mantle cell lymphoma	Follicular lymphoma	Mucosa-associated lymphoid tissue
B symptoms	24	41	11–50	20–30	
Lymph nodes					
Cervical	60–80	40			
Mediastinal	60–80	20–40[a]			
Retroperitoneal	25–35	55			
Bone marrow	3–31	16–22	80	70	
Bone marrow pattern	Reed–Sternberg cells + reactive cells	Nodular and/or diffuse	Nodular non-paratrabecular	Paratrabecular	Nodular non-paratrabecular
Liver	24	3	25	24	–
Spleen	30	13	45	22	–
Gastrointestinal tract	<1	18	15[b]	4	50
CNS	<1	2–5[c]		<1	
Skin	–	6	3	5	12

[a]64 percent in lymphoblastic lymphoma.
[b]40–80 percent if upper and lower gastrointestinal endoscopy is performed.
[c]7 percent and 13 percent in acute lymphoblastic leukemia and Burkitt lymphoma, respectively.

is found in 16–22 percent of patients with DLCL[17,20] and in 33–36 percent of peripheral T-NHL.[17,21] Nonetheless, there are specific subtypes of NHL with a tendency to infiltrate extranodal structures, such as mantle cell lymphoma (MCL), in which bone marrow involvement can be seen in 80 percent of the patients.[22,23] Different patterns of infiltration can be characteristic of specific subtypes of NHL. Thus, in follicular lymphoma the involvement is typically paratrabecular, whereas in DLCL the infiltration is diffuse or nodular effacing the marrow space.[16] In fact, the finding of a paratrabecular infiltration characteristic of follicular lymphoma in a patient with DLCL is considered as evidence of a previously existent 'indolent' lymphoma and has been termed 'downgraded' lymphoma.[16]

Bone marrow involvement is an absolute diagnostic criterion in ALL, and one of the criteria for multiple myeloma and some lymphoproliferative disorders with or without leukemic expression, i.e. CLL, PLL and HCL. It is relevant that in CLL, the leukemic phase of SLL, the pattern of infiltration correlates with the prognosis of the patients, a diffuse infiltration being related to a worse outcome.[24] The presence of circulating lymphoma cells can be detected by conventional morphology in 12–26 percent of patients with 'indolent' lymphoma.[25,26] The use of more sensitive tools such as flow cytometry allows the detection of lymphoma cells in a higher proportion of cases.[27] In contrast, the presence of a leukemic phase is less frequent in 'aggressive' lymphomas, with the exception of specific subtypes of NHL with a high affinity for extranodal involvement such as MCL, where peripheral blood involvement can be seen at diagnosis in up to 60 percent of the patients.[23] The presence of circulating plasma cells can be detected as *de novo* plasma cell leukemia (PCL), representing around 2 percent of patients with plasma cell malignancies,[28] or during the evolution of a plasma cell disorder, which happens in 1 percent of the patients with multiple myeloma.[8] In any case, the diagnosis of PCL, either primary or secondary, is associated with adverse prognostic factors both clinical (more frequent renal impairment and marrow failure, higher levels of β_2-microglobulin) and biologic (chromosome 13 monosomy found in 85 percent of patients), and thus it confers a dismal prognosis to the patients with this complication.[28]

Bone marrow involvement is usually manifest by infiltration detected on aspiration or biopsy. Cytopenia is relatively uncommon, although it is more of a problem later in the disease. This is more obvious in follicular lymphoma. Despite the fact that most patients with follicular lymphoma present with marrow involvement at diagnosis, anemia and thrombocytopenia are found in less than 10 percent of the patients.[18,29,30] These complications are detected in 10 percent of the patients with DLCL and in 11–23 percent of patients with lymphoblastic lymphoma.[3] In particular, one or more cytopenias manifested as anemia, bleeding or infections secondary to neutropenia can be found at diagnosis in more than three-quarters of patients with HCL.[6] Likewise, the presenting symptoms in

ALL are related to bone marrow failure in the majority of the patients.[31] Anemia is a common complaint in patients with multiple myeloma. It is reported in 62 percent at diagnosis and can be secondary to bone marrow infiltration, erythropoietin deficiency due to renal impairment and, less frequently, hemodilution in the setting of a very high monoclonal component, most often of IgM type.[32,33]

Finally, although an uncommon complication, bone marrow infiltration and subsequently peripheral blood involvement can cause a leukostatic syndrome manifested as neurologic symptoms and respiratory distress if the white cell count is very high. This is unusual in mature leukemias/lymphomas in leukemic phase but can be seen in children with ALL and hyperleukocytosis. Thus, at St Jude's hospital 8 percent of the children presented with an initial leukocyte count $>200 \times 10^9$/L, of whom 9 percent had neurologic symptoms and 6 percent pulmonary leukostasis.[34]

Infiltration of other organs

Hepatosplenic involvement is relatively frequent in lymphoid malignancies. Splenic involvement has been demonstrated by laparotomy in around 30 percent of patients with HD[13] whereas in more recent series spleen *enlargement* is detected either on examination or by computed tomography (CT) scan in 11–50 percent of patients with HD.[35] The real significance of this is unclear as there is not a clear relation between the size of the spleen and the histologic confirmation.[35] With regard to NHL, splenic enlargement is detected in 13 percent of patients with DLCL,[20] 63 percent in T-LL,[12] around 45 percent in MCL[22,23,36] and in 22 percent of patients with follicular lymphoma.[37] Of note, the presence of splenomegaly in patients with MCL has been associated with a poorer prognosis.[22,23] The presence of splenomegaly is the presenting symptom in a large number of patients with HCL, PLL and, obviously, splenic marginal zone lymphoma.[5,6] In these cases massive splenomegaly may cause symptoms due to hypersplenism and splenic infarction.

Liver infiltration is 'documented' at presentation in 30 percent of patients with advanced stage HD,[11] but the diagnosis of liver infiltration is not straightforward.[38] Specifically, according to the Ann Arbor classification,[39] clinical enlargement is not adequate to classify the patient as having liver involvement: on the other hand, the presence of cholestasis is equivocal and does not always correspond to liver infiltration. Thus, it can be secondary to extrinsic compression due to lymph node enlargement, liver infiltration or vanishing bile duct syndrome, a rare disorder characterized by the disappearance of intrahepatic bile ducts, without evidence of HD infiltration, secondary to a variety of causes including immunologic phenomena.[40] Liver enlargement in NHL varies between 11 percent and 83 percent,[3,20] however, the detection of a palpable liver does not always correlate with liver infiltration.[2,23] Sans *et al.* reported that when liver infiltration was assessed by laparoscopy-assisted liver biopsy, this feature was demonstrated in 24.5 percent and 8 percent of patients with NHL and HD, respectively.[41] Of note, computed tomography (CT) scan showed liver enlargement in 33 percent and 18 percent of patients with and without liver infiltration, respectively. Likewise, transaminitis and cholestasis was found in 22 percent and 17 percent of patients with liver involvement versus 9 percent and 10 percent of patients without liver infiltration, none of these differences being statistically significant.[41] In ALL liver involvement is uncommon at diagnosis.

Infiltration of the gastrointestinal tract is relatively frequent in specific types of NHL whereas it is unusual in patients with HD. In fact, the gastrointestinal tract was the commonest site of extranodal infiltration among 2031 patients with DLCL included in the International Non-Hodgkin's Lymphoma Prognostic Factors Project, this complication being detected in 16–18 percent of patients.[17,20] In 'indolent' lymphomas, with the exception of marginal zone B cell lymphoma, mucosa-associated lymphoid tissue (MALT) type, gastrointestinal infiltration is not a frequent feature.[17] The most frequent sites of involvement in patients with NHL in old series were the stomach and small intestine followed by the large intestine.[2,9] More recently the frequency of colonic involvement has been recognized, specifically in two distinct entities, MCL and MALT lymphoma.[42] When upper and lower gastrointestinal endoscopy is performed as part of the initial staging in patients with MCL, colonic and gastroduodenal involvement is demonstrated in 88 percent and 43 percent of patients, respectively, in spite of normal macroscopical findings in the majority of them and the fact that only 26 percent of patients present with gastrointestinal symptoms at diagnosis.[36] In MCL, as well as in MALT lymphoma and other subtypes, colonic infiltration can be manifested as lymphomatous polyposis appearing as polypoid accumulations of malignant cells in a nodular pattern within the submucosa.[43] The frequency of this finding with the frequency of multiorgan involvement in MALT lymphoma has prompted some authors to recommend an extended staging in patients with this subtype of lymphoma.[44] In contrast, other authors have suggested that, in view of the advanced stage at diagnosis of most patients with MCL, gastrointestinal endoscopy is not required as part of the initial staging as it does not change the management in the majority of the patients.[36] A different situation occurs with primary gastrointestinal lymphomas in which the gastrointestinal tract is the initial site of infiltration. In a review of 175 patients with primary gastrointestinal lymphoma, the most frequent sites of involvement were bowel (most frequently in the ileum) in 54 percent of patients, and stomach in 45 percent of patients. The most frequent histologic subtypes were DLCL and MALT lymphoma,[45] the latter being related in a high percentage of cases to infection by *Helicobacter pylori*, and potentially curable with antibiotics. With regard to primary intestinal lymphoma, the majority of primary lymphomas arising in the colon and rectum tend to be of B cell type,[46] whereas T cell lymphomas are more frequent in the

small bowel, with a substantial proportion of them being enteropathy associated.[47]

Thoracic disease other than mediastinal lymph nodes, that is, lung or pleural infiltration, is frequently detected in patients with HD, especially in those with a mediastinal mass in which the lung/pleura involvement is due to contiguous infiltration or due to lymphatic obstruction in pleural effusions, and can be seen in about a third.[12,48] This can also be the mechanism of lung or pleural 'involvement' in other NHL presenting with bulky mediastinal masses as PMLCL and T-LL, where lung or pleural disease can be diagnosed in 22–57 percent of the patients.[12,49–52] Lung infiltration is more frequently seen in patients with HD than in T-LL and PMLCL, whereas pleural effusions are more common in T-LL and PMLCL.[12] The analysis of the pleural fluid shows an exudate with presence of lymphomatous cells in up to 88 percent of patients with NHL and pleural effusion.[48] However, it should be mentioned that the diagnosis of pleural infiltration may be hampered by the scarcity of cells in the pleural fluid and, in 'indolent' lymphomas, the difficulty in distinguishing malignant lymphocytes from reactive lymphocytes and, hence, the importance of including the immunophenotype and molecular analysis of the fluid when suspecting a lymphomatous effusion.[48] Lung or pleural infiltration is rarely seen in other lymphoid malignancies although sporadic case reports have been published.[22,53,54] As the initial and main site of disease, lung infiltration is detected in patients with a chronic history of bronchiectasis or other disorders resulting in chronic antigenic stimulation as a manifestation of MALT lymphoma.[55–57] Recently, primary effusion lymphomas, a new entity that infiltrates the pleural cavity or other body cavities as the principal site of disease, have been described.[48] This is an unusual type of lymphoma related to human herpes virus 8 (HHV-8)/Kaposi sarcoma herpes virus (KSHV) and most commonly seen in immunocompromised patients.

Central nervous system (CNS) infiltration is rarely seen at diagnosis of patients with lymphoid malignancies, other than specific subtypes of NHL with a CNS tropism such as ALL/lymphoblastic lymphoma and Burkitt lymphoma. In these subtypes CNS disease is diagnosed in 7 percent and 13 percent of the patients, respectively.[58] In DLCL this complication is detected at diagnosis in around 2–5 percent of the patients,[3,20] whereas in other lymphoid malignancies the frequency of CNS involvement is much lower. Secondary CNS lymphoma is usually characterized by meningeal infiltration and, hence, it is manifest from a clinical point of view by the presence of subtle symptoms such as mental status changes, headaches or cranial nerves palsies.[59] The diagnosis of suspected CNS lymphoma should be based on the finding of lymphoma cells on a cerebrospinal fluid (CSF) cytospin or on a compatible radiologic image on magnetic resonance imaging (MRI) (Fig. 40.2). The former, however, is not always possible and in spite of a high suspicion of CNS infiltration it is not unusual to fail to demonstrate lymphoma cells in the cytospin even with radiologic evidence of leptomeningeal disease, as reported by

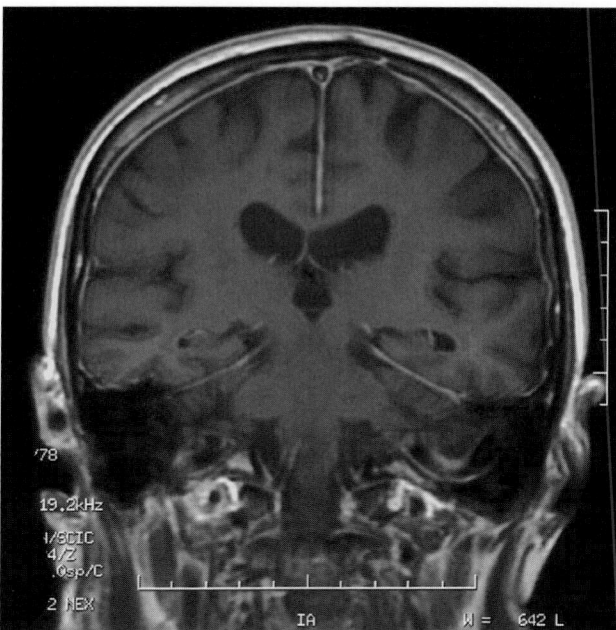

Figure 40.2 Magnetic resonance image showing meningeal involvement in a patient with diffuse large cell lymphoma.

Bishop.[60] In this regard, recently it has been suggested that patients with a high suspicion of CNS infiltration should be investigated with flow cytometry of the CSF in addition to conventional cytology.[61] Less frequently, CNS infiltration presents with parenchymal lesions. This is more typical of PMLCL than of other subtypes of lymphoma.[60] Anecdotal reports of CNS infiltration in multiple myeloma,[62] CLL[63] and HD[64] have been published. In addition to the obvious primary central nervous system lymphoma (PCNSL), another specific subtype with a tendency to infiltrate the CNS as one of the main sites of disease is the intravascular large B cell lymphoma. In a recent review of this uncommon lymphoma, neurological manifestations – which included a wide spectrum of symptoms from vertigo to seizures – were found in 34 percent of patients at diagnosis and CNS infiltration was confirmed in 39 percent of patients.[65]

Infiltration of other non-lymphatic organs is unusual in the majority of lymphoid malignancies, although it can be detected in some subtypes of NHL. Other relatively frequent sites of extranodal involvement include the skin, bone and testes. Primary cutaneous lymphoma is a heterogeneous group of different entities that represents the second commonest type of extranodal NHL. Contrasting with non-cutaneous NHL the majority of the cases are of T cell origin.[66,67] The clinical manifestations can vary from the presence of patches or infiltrated plaques in mycosis fungoides to generalized erythroderma in Sézary syndrome[66] (Plate 113, see plate section). Secondary cutaneous infiltration can be seen in around 5 percent of patients with DLCL or FL[3] whereas it is more frequent in lymphomas with extranodal spread such as ATLL where it is found in about 40 percent of patients[68] and intravascular lymphoma, with

39 percent of patients presenting cutaneous lesions at diagnosis.[65] Apart from these uncommon types of lymphoma, anaplastic large cell lymphoma (ALCL), an aggressive subtype of NHL with extensive extraganglionar disease at diagnosis but with a very good prognosis, can present with cutaneous lesions in 21 percent of patients at diagnosis.[69] Once again, sporadic cases of skin involvement in CLL and HD have been reported.[70,71] Bone infiltration can be seen in 'aggressive' lymphomas. Thus, involvement of the bones affecting the maxilla or mandible is the typical presentation of endemic Burkitt lymphoma[72] whereas in the series reported by Rosenberg et al., bone infiltration was found in 21 percent of patients with large cell lymphoma.[2] The diagnosis and, especially, the reassessment after treatment can be difficult as residual radiologic abnormalities are frequent. Diffuse large cell lymphoma is the commonest subtype with testicular infiltration at diagnosis, either as the only site of disease or in the context of disseminated lymphoma.[73] Testicular involvement can also be found as the primary site of infiltration in testicular large cell follicular lymphoma, a disease that has been considered by some authors as an specific entity due to its differential characteristics with classical follicular lymphoma such as its presentation in children and the lack of *BCL2/IgH* rearrangement.[74] Primary mediastinal large cell lymphoma is a subtype of NHL with a special tropism to involve unusual extranodal areas such as the kidneys and adrenal cortex.[52] Other organs less frequently infiltrated by lymphoma or other lymphoid neoplasms are parotid, thyroid, conjunctiva, ovary and breasts. The majority of these involvements are seen in patients with MALT-type lymphoma with a chronic condition triggering the immune system, but can also be found in other types of lymphoma. Notwithstanding the rarity of other sites of involvement, almost every part of the body has been reported to be infiltrated by lymphoma.[75]

SYSTEMIC SYMPTOMS

B symptoms

B symptoms, defined according to the Ann Arbor classification[39] (weight loss of more than 10 percent of the body weight in the previous 6 months, unexplained persistent or recurrent fever above 38°C during the previous month, drenching night sweats during the previous month) are present at diagnosis in 24 percent of patients with HD[13] and in around 10 percent of patients with NHL,[2] although the percentage of patients with these presenting symptoms is extremely variable in different subtypes of NHL. Thus, in 'indolent' lymphomas such as FL, MALT or SLL/CLL just a small proportion of patients, around 20–30 percent, present with B symptoms at diagnosis.[17,37] In contrast, this percentage is higher among patients with 'aggressive' lymphoma. B symptoms can be found in 41 percent of patients with DLCL,[20] 54 percent in T-NHL[21] and 11–50 percent in MCL.[22,23,36]

Asthenia

Fatigue is a nonspecific, although common, symptom at diagnosis in patients with cancer[76] and, as such, can also be seen frequently in patients with lymphoid malignancies. Although it can be one of the symptoms of anemia, this complaint can also be present without a decrease in the hemoglobin level, its pathogenesis not being clear. The nonspecific nature of this symptom makes it difficult to assess, and it is not reported in the majority of the series. However, in the Rosenberg *et al.* series this was one of the initial manifestations of lymphosarcoma in 8.2 percent of the patients.[2]

Pruritus

Pruritus is a common complaint in patients with HD, present in 10–31 percent at diagnosis.[77,78] This symptom may precede the diagnosis for a long time; in fact, the clinical picture of a young woman with long-standing pruritus before being diagnosed with HD is not unusual.[79] Some authors have suggested the inclusion of this symptom as one of the B symptoms as in some series it has been associated with a poorer outcome,[77] although according to other authors pruritus is only related to a poor prognosis when associated with B symptoms.[78] Despite being regarded as a classic symptom of HD, it also can be found in other lymphoid malignancies, such as NHL. Hence, it was detected at diagnosis in around 2 percent of the patients with lymphosarcoma in Rosenberg's series.[2]

COMPRESSION SYMPTOMS

Superior vena cava obstruction

Superior vena cava obstruction can be seen in patients with bulky mediastinal disease with a rapid growth. It is characterized by a short history of progressive breathlessness, cough, facial and/or upper extremities swelling and dilated collateral veins over the neck and chest.[10] This complication is rarely seen in patients with HD in spite of the presence of bulky disease, given the slow pace of growth allowing the development of collateral circulation. In contrast, SVCO is a common way of presentation in PMLCL and in T-LL; 52–57 percent of patients with PMLCL present with this complication at diagnosis[52,80] whereas it is the presenting problem in 21 percent of patients with T-LL.[10] In a series of 205 patients with lymphoma and mediastinal involvement, SVCO was diagnosed in 36 of them, all of the patients with this complication being diagnosed with lymphoblastic lymphoma, DLCL and follicular lymphoma. Of note, the only patient with follicular lymphoma and SVCO was a patient with a follicular large cell lymphoma.[10] Nonetheless, SVCO has also been reported in other indolent lymphoid malignancies such as CLL.[53]

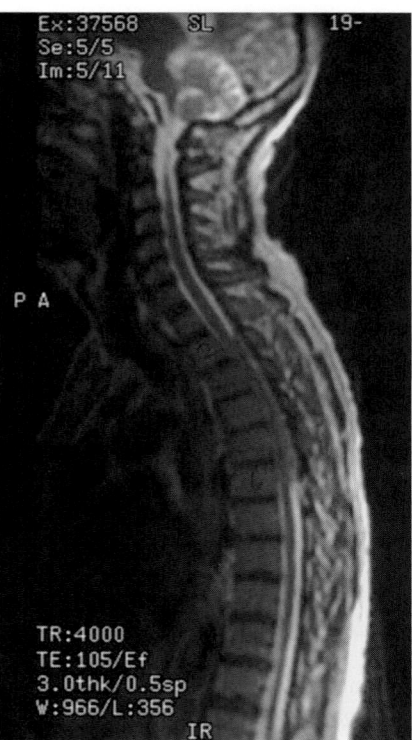

Figure 40.3 Magnetic resonance image showing extradural disease causing cord compression in a patient with diffuse large cell lymphoma.

Cord compression

Cord compression secondary to a vertebral fracture is a common presentation in patients with multiple myeloma. In fact, this is the initial manifestation of disease in 6–24 percent of the patients and is characterized by back pain, incontinence, lower limbs weakness, and sensory levels.[81] It also can be caused by the presence of a spinal plasmocytoma either in patients with solitary plasmocytoma or in the context of systemic disease in multiple myeloma. Less frequently, cord compression can also be seen in patients with other lymphoid malignancies such as NHL caused by an epidural mass, most frequently in the thoracic region.[75] Epidural involvement can be detected as the site of presentation in 3–4 percent of patients with NHL[82] (Fig. 40.3). Although this complication is more common in patients with 'aggressive' NHL it also can be seen in patients with 'indolent' lymphoma.[2,82,83]

Deep venous thrombosis

Deep venous thrombosis (DVT) as a result of compression due to bulky abdominal disease is a potential complication in patients with NHL. In a series of 593 patients with 'high-grade' NHL, DVT or pulmonary embolism (PE) was found in about 7 percent of the patients either at diagnosis or during the evolution of the disease.[84] In the majority of the cases lower limb and/or abdomino-pelvic veins were the site of thrombosis, vein compression being considered the cause of thrombosis in more than half the patients, without an obvious thrombophilic status being detected in laboratory tests.

Hydronephrosis

Likewise, the presence of a bulky mass in the abdomen can cause hydronephrosis, contributing to the pre-treatment azotemia in some patients with NHL.[85,86] As with other compression symptoms they tend to occur more frequently in patients with rapidly growing disease, which does not allow time for the development of compensating mechanisms. Hence, these syndromes are rarely seen in patients with HD or 'indolent' lymphoma, although sporadic cases have been reported.[87–89]

METABOLIC COMPLICATIONS

Hypercalcemia

Hypercalcemia is one of the classic symptoms, either at diagnosis or during the evolution of the disease in patients with multiple myeloma – 15–30 percent present at diagnosis with symptomatic hypercalcemia, manifested by anorexia, nausea, vomiting, polyuria, polydipsia, constipation, weakness, confusion or stupor.[32,90] Although it can be present in all types of multiple myeloma, it is more frequent in IgD subtype and PCL.[8] Another lymphoid malignancy that typically can present with hypercalcemia is ATLL. In fact, serum calcium level higher than 2.74 mmol/L (10.96 mg/dL) is found in almost a third of patients with ATLL and, specifically, in 50 percent of patients with the acute subtype.[68] This disease, similarly to multiple myeloma, is characterized by the presence of osteolytic lesions in about a third of the patients. Finally, hypercalcemia can also be found in 5 percent of patients with HD and in up to 15 percent of patients with NHL, especially in those with 'aggressive' subtypes.[91] A recent report showed an incidence of hypercalcemia of 7 percent in patients with 'high-grade' lymphoma, most of them diagnosed with DLCL.[92] In fact, if hypercalcemia is detected in a patient with an 'indolent' lymphoma, transformation into an 'aggressive' NHL should be suspected as, although not frequent, the association of hypercalcemia and Richter syndrome in patients with CLL or transformation of an 'indolent' lymphoma to an 'aggressive' one has been reported in the literature.[93,94] Of note, in the majority of these patients the underlying skeletal lesion is diffuse osteopenia rather than lytic lesions. The pathogenic mechanisms of hypercalcemia might vary in different lymphoid malignancies. Thus, most cases of hypercalcemia in HD have been associated with dysregulated production of calcitriol, contrasting with humoral hypercalcemia

mediated by parathyroid hormone-related protein (PTHrP) in solid cancers, whereas the latter mechanism has been implicated in some cases of hypercalcemia in NHL, multiple myeloma and ATLL[91,95] The distinction among the different pathogenic mechanisms is not merely an academic one as it can influence the therapeutic management of hypercalcemia.[91] Finally, the possibility of coincidental primary hyperparathyroidism should be taken into account as the prognosis and management differ from those in malignant hypercalcemia.[95]

Tumor lysis syndrome

Tumor lysis syndrome is characterized by an array of metabolic disorders caused by the rapid destruction of malignant cells and the subsequent release of cellular metabolites into the bloodstream. This results in hyperuricemia, hyperphosphatemia, hyperkalemia and hypocalcemia and can lead to life-threatening complications such as renal failure, cardiac arrhythmias, and seizures.[96] Although tumor lysis syndrome is more frequently triggered by the initiation of chemotherapy, a high uric acid level or other laboratory data of tumor lysis can be detected at diagnosis, before starting any chemotherapy, in lymphoid malignancies with a very rapid turnover such as Burkitt lymphoma or with a large tumor burden as in ALL with a very high white cell count. In these two entities azotemia can be found in 20–24 percent of patients at presentation,[85,86] whereas in Rosenberg and coworkers' report, 52 percent of patients with NHL presented a higher than normal uric acid level at diagnosis.[2] A review of 102 patients with 'intermediate' or 'high-grade' lymphoma distinguished laboratory tumor lysis (evidence of metabolic changes requiring no specific therapy) from clinical tumor lysis that resulted in a life-threatening emergency, the former being found in 42 percent of patients contrasting with 6 percent of patients with clinical tumor lysis.[97]

Renal failure

One of the most characteristic manifestations at diagnosis in patients with multiple myeloma is renal failure. Some degree of renal impairment (i.e. creatinine level $\geqslant$176.8 μmol/L [2 mg/dL]) can be found in 20–50 percent of the patients at diagnosis,[32,98] whereas renal failure requiring hemodialysis is seen in 9 percent of the patients.[99] The mechanism of renal failure is usually secondary to the so-called 'myeloma kidney' due to light chain deposition in association with a precipitating factor such as hypercalcemia, fluid depletion, concomitant infections or use of nephrotoxic drugs. This complication is more frequently found in Bence Jones myeloma, IgD multiple myeloma and in PCL than in the other subtypes of plasma cell dyscrasia.[8] It confers a poor prognosis to patients presenting with this feature at diagnosis, the median overall survival being 8.6 months in comparison with 34.5 months for patients without renal impairment.[98] Recovery of renal function, both in patients needing hemodialysis and those not requiring it, is seen in a small proportion of the patients.[98,99] Renal findings at necropsy were analyzed in a series of 77 patients with multiple myeloma undergoing autopsy examination, the most common finding being light chain cast nephropathy.[100]

Renal failure might also be detected in other aggressive lymphoid malignancies such as ATLL, in which 24 percent of patients present with high creatinine level at diagnosis[68] and, as mentioned above, can also be seen in patients with lymphoma and a bulky, rapidly growing abdominal mass causing hydronephrosis such as in Burkitt lymphoma.

Hyperviscosity

In patients with Waldenström macroglobulinemia, the presence of a monoclonal component of IgM subtype can lead to hyperviscosity syndrome in 10–30 percent of patients,[101] especially when the serum IgM concentration is very high. This is characterized by somnolence, headaches, blurred vision, dizziness, vertigo, anemia and a bleeding tendency. It is more frequent in patients with IgM plasma cell dyscrasia than in other subtypes given the high molecular weight as a result of its pentameric structure and the high carbohydrate content of this molecule. Although the blood viscosity does not correlate directly with the clinical symptoms, patients with a blood viscosity less than 4 cp are usually asymptomatic.[102] Likewise, there is not a linear relation between the amount of the monoclonal component and the blood viscosity; however, hyperviscosity symptoms are rarely seen in patients with a monoclonal band lower than 30 g/L.[101] The presence of a high-molecular-weight protein in blood causes an increase in the osmotic pressure with an increase in the resistance to blood flow and, subsequently, impairment in the microcirculation. In addition, monoclonal IgM can also increase the internal viscosity of red blood cells and reduce their deformability, which exacerbates hyperviscosity. Another of the consequences of the presence of the IgM component in blood is the prolongation of the bleeding and clotting times due to two mechanisms: on the one hand by interacting with several circulating proteins such as coagulation factors, and, on the other hand, by coating platelets.[102]

IMMUNE COMPLICATIONS

Autoimmune disorders

The classic example, although not the only one, of a lymphoid malignancy that is accompanied by autoimmune cytopenias is CLL/SLL, the mechanisms leading to autoimmunity not being completely clarified. The commonest cause of secondary autoimmune hemolytic anemia is

CLL/SLL.[103] A positive Coombs test was found in 5 percent of patients at diagnosis in Brittinger and coworkers' series,[3] whereas in a more recent series autoimmune hemolytic anemia was diagnosed in 1.6 percent of patients at diagnosis and in 3 percent of untreated patients.[104] The finding of a positive Coombs test without autoimmune hemolytic anemia is not uncommon. In Kyasa and coworkers' series at least one positive Coombs test was found in 16 of 89 patients (18 percent) at some point during the clinical course, of whom less than half of them had autoimmune hemolytic anemia.[103] These results may be an underestimate as not all patients with CLL/SLL have a Coombs test as part of the initial study. Less frequently, patients with CLL can present autoimmune thrombocytopenia, which can be found in 1–3 percent patients with CLL during the course of the disease.[103] The diagnosis of autoimmune thrombocytopenia, however, is complicated by the lack of a reliable antiplatelet antibody test, most of which have high false-positive rates in CLL/SLL, making the diagnosis of autoimmune thrombocytopenia a diagnosis of exclusion in most of the cases. The presence of autoimmune cytopenias does not seem to influence the prognosis of patients with CLL in several studies.[103,104] Actually, in spite of the fact that neither Rai nor Binet classifications distinguish an autoimmune cytopenia from the cytopenia due to bone marrow involvement, some authors have reported a better prognosis for patients with autoimmune cytopenias than for those with infiltrative cytopenias.[103] Pure red cell aplasia is another autoimmune disorder than can be detected in about 1 percent of patients with CLL.[103] It is characterized by reticulocytopenia and an absence of red blood precursors in the bone marrow and can be associated with parvovirus B19 infection. Other lymphoid malignancies that used to present with a monoclonal component can also display autoimmune disorders. An example of this is the so-called 'immunocytoma' in the Kiel classification, which presented with a monoclonal gammopathy and a Coomb's positive test in 29 percent and 13 percent of the patients, respectively.[3] A monoclonal component of IgM subtype can also behave as an autoantibody. Thus, in Waldenström macroglobulinemia, the IgM component may act as an antibody against the myelin-associated glycoprotein causing peripheral neuropathy, against polyclonal IgG in type II cryoglobulinemia, and can react with erythrocytes resulting in cold agglutinin disease.[102] Autoimmune phenomena can also be found in other lymphoid malignancies. In a 2002 review of 517 patients with NHL (excluding SLL and angioimmunoblastic), autoimmune hemolytic anemia was diagnosed in 3 percent of the patients, and preceded the diagnosis of NHL in more than half of the patients.[105] In this study the presence of autoimmune hemolytic anemia was associated with a poor outcome. Of note, the diagnosis of autoimmune anemia was more frequent among patients with T-NHL than among those with B-NHL. In line with this, one of the characteristic presenting features in patients with angioimmunoblastic lymphoma, an uncommon, aggressive type of T cell malignancy, is the presence of autoimmune anemia.[106] Finally, autoimmune phenomena, frequently in the form of thrombocytopenia, can also be detected in patients with HD. In these cases the behavior of the autoimmune phenomena is more aggressive than in idiopathic cases, being frequently resistant to steroids.

Hypogammaglobulinemia/immunodeficiency

Patients with lymphoid malignancies have an increased tendency to present infectious complications, even before the onset of a myelotoxic treatment, due to several mechanisms. Thus, hypogammaglobulinemia is a common finding in CLL and in multiple myeloma, this feature being seen in 26 percent and 9 percent of patients at diagnosis, respectively.[3,32] This might contribute to a higher susceptibility to infections, especially those due to encapsulated bacteria such as *Streptococcus pneumoniae* and other respiratory pathogens,[107] the most frequent sites of infection in multiple myeloma being the respiratory tract, followed by the urinary tract.[108] The administration of prophylactic immunoglobulins and pneumococcal and *Haemophilus* vaccines has been recommended for these patients, although the results of both strategies have been discouraging, especially those of vaccination due to a poor response to immunization.[108,109] In both diseases, as well as in other hematologic malignancies, there might be other mechanisms that can contribute to increase the risk of infections, such as hyposplenism and neutropenia or lymphopenia (either numerical or 'functional').[110] In a recent report analyzing the risk factors for the development of infections in patients with CLL, hypogammaglobulinemia did not emerge as an important predictive factor for infectious complications, even in untreated patients.[111] Herpetic infections are not uncommon in patients with CLL or HD,[111] whereas some opportunistic infections that are currently regarded as typical of the immunodeficiency linked to human immunodeficiency virus (HIV) infection, i.e. progressive multifocal leukoencephalopathy were initially described in patients with CLL and HD.[112] Subsequently, this complication has been reported in association with profound immunosuppression in patients heavily pretreated or those receiving fludarabine.[113–115] HCL is another lymphoid malignancy that typically may present with repeated infections.[6] This is frequently either the presenting feature or the reason to initiate chemotherapy in patients managed expectantly. The mechanisms for the increased risk of infections in this case can be cytopenias due to bone marrow infiltration or hyposplenism. Finally, it is also characteristic of patients with ATLL to present with opportunistic infectious at diagnosis, which is secondary to the existence of a T immunodeficiency induced by HTLV-1 infection. As a result of this, more than a quarter of the patients present with some infection at the time of diagnosis of ATLL.[68]

OTHER SYMPTOMS

Bone pain

Bone pain is one of the most frequent symptoms at diagnosis in patients with multiple myeloma. It can be found in 68 percent of patients, whereas radiological skeletal abnormalities are seen in 79 percent of them (Fig. 40.4).[32] Likewise, bone pain is a common symptom in other neoplasms infiltrating the bones such as ATLL or primary bone lymphoma. Finally, patients with ALL can present with bone pain due to bone marrow infiltration.[31]

Paraneoplastic syndromes

In spite of the fact that paraneoplastic syndromes are rarely seen in patients with lymphoid malignancies, some of them are more commonly associated with hematological neoplasms than with solid tumors.[116] The pathogenesis of these syndromes is not completely understood, although some cases are considered to be caused by the presence of autoantibodies against a number of cell surface proteins.[116–118] There are several mechanisms to explain the existence of these autoantibodies in association with cancer, such as dysregulation of the immune system or the presence of tumor antigens that cross-react with cell surface proteins.[116] There is not a parallel course of the paraneoplastic syndrome and the neoplasm but the diagnosis of the paraneoplastic syndrome can precede the diagnosis of the hematological malignancy by several months or it can appear in patients in remission.[118] The most frequent types of paraneoplastic syndromes related to lymphomas are cutaneous or neurologic. Thus, paraneoplastic pemphigus, a disorder characterized by the presence of oral ulceration

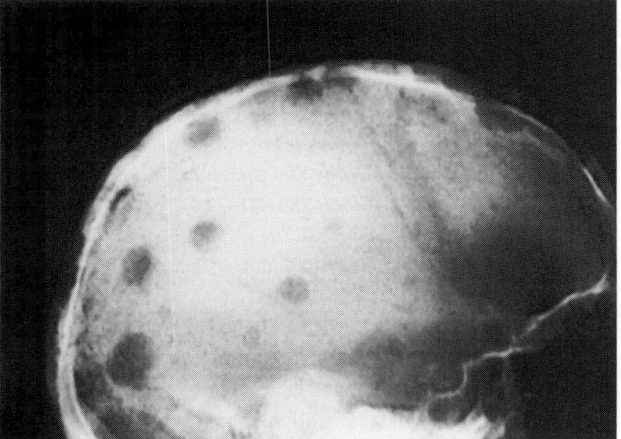

Figure 40.4   Multiple lytic deposits in a patient with multiple myeloma. (Reproduced with permission of Taylor and Francis from Husband JE, Reznek RH. *Imaging in Oncology*, 2nd ed., 2004, Figure 33.1, page 878.)

with or without cutaneous blisters and erosions, is associated in the majority of the cases with lymphoid malignancies,[116] whereas HD is the third commonest cause of paraneoplastic cerebellar degeneration.[118]

KEY POINTS

- Lymphoid malignancies are a heterogeneous group of diseases with a wide spectrum of clinical manifestations.
- The most frequent symptoms are due to organ infiltration, either of lymphoid or extranodal sites.
- Lymph node enlargement is the commonest presenting feature in HD and NHL.
- Extranodal infiltration is more common in NHL than in other lymphoid malignancies.
- Patients with lymphoid neoplasms can also present symptoms secondary to compression of other organs, systemic symptoms and immune or metabolic complications.
- The initial features of patients with multiple myeloma are rather specific for this disease, with symptoms such as bone pain, renal impairment and hypercalcemia.

REFERENCES

● = Key primary paper
◆ = Major review article

1. Weber AL, Rahemtullah A, Ferry JA. Hodgkin and non-Hodgkin lymphoma of the head and neck: clinical, pathologic, and imaging evaluation. *Neuroimaging Clin N Am* 2003; **13**: 371–92.
●2. Rosenberg SA, Diamond HD, Jaslowitz B, Craver LF. Lymphosarcoma: a review of 1269 cases. *Medicine (Baltimore)* 1961; **40**: 31–84.
3. Brittinger G, Bartels H, Common H et al. Clinical and prognostic relevance of the Kiel classification of non-Hodgkin lymphomas results of a prospective multicenter study by the Kiel Lymphoma Study Group. *Hematol Oncol* 1984; **2**: 269–306.
●4. Horning SJ, Rosenberg SA. The natural history of initially untreated low-grade non-Hodgkin's lymphomas. *N Engl J Med* 1984; **311**: 1471–5.
5. Melo JV, Catovsky D, Galton DA. The relationship between chronic lymphocytic leukaemia and prolymphocytic leukaemia, I. Clinical and laboratory features of 300 patients and characterization of an intermediate group. *Br J Haematol* 1986; **63**: 377–87.
◆6. Goodman GR, Bethel KJ, Saven A. Hairy cell leukemia: an update. *Curr Opin Hematol* 2003; **10**: 258–66.
7. Mercieca J, Puga M, Matutes E et al. Incidence and significance of abdominal lymphadenopathy in hairy cell leukaemia. *Leuk Lymphoma* 1994; **14**(Suppl 1): 79–83.

8. Blade J, Kyle RA. Nonsecretory myeloma, immunoglobulin D myeloma, and plasma cell leukemia. *Hematol Oncol Clin North Am* 1999; **13**: 1259–72.
9. Jones SE, Fuks Z, Bull M et al. Non-Hodgkin's lymphomas. IV. Clinicopathologic correlation in 405 cases. *Cancer* 1973; **31**: 806–23.
10. Perez-Soler R, McLaughlin P, Velasquez WS et al. Clinical features and results of management of superior vena cava syndrome secondary to lymphoma. *J Clin Oncol* 1984; **2**: 260–6.
●11. Hasenclever D, Diehl V. A prognostic score for advanced Hodgkin's disease. International prognostic factors project on advanced Hodgkin's disease. *N Engl J Med* 1998; **339**: 1506–14.
12. Tateishi U, Muller NL, Johkoh T et al. Primary mediastinal lymphoma: characteristic features of the various histological subtypes on CT. *J Comput Assist Tomogr* 2004; **28**: 782–9.
13. Mauch PM, Kalish LA, Kadin M et al. Patterns of presentation of Hodgkin disease. Implications for etiology and pathogenesis. *Cancer* 1993; **71**: 2062–71.
14. Blum KA, Lozanski G, Byrd JC. Adult Burkitt leukemia and lymphoma. *Blood* 2004; **104**: 3009–20.
15. Levis A, Pietrasanta D, Godio L et al. A large-scale study of bone marrow involvement in patients with Hodgkin's lymphoma. *Clin Lymphoma* 2004; **5**: 50–5.
◆16. Viswanatha D, Foucar K. Hodgkin and non-Hodgkin lymphoma involving bone marrow. *Semin Diagn Pathol* 2003; **20**: 196–210.
●17. Armitage JO, Weisenburger DD. New approach to classifying non-Hodgkin's lymphomas: clinical features of the major histologic subtypes. Non-Hodgkin's lymphoma classification project. *J Clin Oncol* 1998; **16**: 2780–95.
18. Federico M, Vitolo U, Zinzani PL et al. Prognosis of follicular lymphoma: a predictive model based on a retrospective analysis of 987 cases. Intergruppo Italiano Linfomi. *Blood* 2000; **95**: 783–9.
19. Perea G, Altes A, Montoto S et al. International and Italian prognostic indices in follicular lymphoma. *Haematologica* 2003; **88**: 700–4.
●20. A predictive model for aggressive non-Hodgkin's lymphoma. The International non-Hodgkin's Lymphoma Prognostic Factors Project. *N Engl J Med* 1993; **329**: 987–94.
21. Lopez-Guillermo A, Cid J, Salar A et al. Peripheral T-cell lymphomas: initial features, natural history, and prognostic factors in a series of 174 patients diagnosed according to the REAL classification. *Ann Oncol* 1998; **9**: 849–55.
22. Norton AJ, Matthews J, Pappa V et al. Mantle cell lymphoma: natural history defined in a serially biopsied population over a 20-year period. *Ann Oncol* 1995; **6**: 249–56.
23. Bosch F, Lopez-Guillermo A, Campo E et al. Mantle cell lymphoma: presenting features, response to therapy, and prognostic factors. *Cancer* 1998; **82**: 567–75.
24. Rozman C, Montserrat E, Rodriguez-Fernandez JM et al. Bone marrow histologic pattern – the best single prognostic parameter in chronic lymphocytic leukemia: a

multivariate survival analysis of 329 cases. *Blood* 1984; **64**: 642–8.

25. Romaguera JE, McLaughlin P, North L *et al.* Multivariate analysis of prognostic factors in stage IV follicular low-grade lymphoma: a risk model. *J Clin Oncol* 1991; **9**: 762–9.

26. Lopez-Guillermo A, Montserrat E, Bosch F *et al.* Applicability of the International Index for aggressive lymphomas to patients with low-grade lymphoma. *J Clin Oncol* 1994; **12**: 1343–8.

27. Hanson CA, Kurtin PJ, Katzmann JA *et al.* Immunophenotypic analysis of peripheral blood and bone marrow in the staging of B-cell malignant lymphoma. *Blood* 1999; **94**: 3889–96.

28. Garcia-Sanz R, Orfao A, Gonzalez M *et al.* Primary plasma cell leukemia: clinical, immunophenotypic, DNA ploidy, and cytogenetic characteristics. *Blood* 1999; **93**: 1032–7.

29. Obeso G, Sanz ER, Rivas C *et al.* B-cell follicular lymphomas: clinical and biological characteristics. *Leuk Lymphoma* 1994; **16**: 105–11.

30. Wood LA, Coupland RW, North SA, Palmer MC. Outcome of advanced stage low grade follicular lymphomas in a population-based retrospective cohort. *Cancer* 1999; **85**: 1361–8.

31. Redaelli A, Laskin BL, Stephens JM *et al.* A systematic literature review of the clinical and epidemiological burden of acute lymphoblastic leukaemia (ALL). *Eur J Cancer Care (Engl)* 2005; **14**: 53–62.

●32. Kyle RA. Multiple myeloma: review of 869 cases. *Mayo Clin Proc* 1975; **50**: 29–40.

33. MacLennan IC, Drayson M, Dunn J. Multiple myeloma. *BMJ* 1994; **308**: 1033–6.

34. Lowe EJ, Pui CH, Hancock ML *et al.* Early complications in children with acute lymphoblastic leukemia presenting with hyperleukocytosis. *Pediatr Blood Cancer* 2004; **45**: 10–15.

35. Vinnicombe SJ, Reznek RH. Computerised tomography in the staging of Hodgkin's disease and non-Hodgkin's lymphoma. *Eur J Nucl Med Mol Imaging* 2003; **30**(Suppl 1): s42–55.

36. Romaguera JE, Medeiros LJ, Hagemeister FB *et al.* Frequency of gastrointestinal involvement and its clinical significance in mantle cell lymphoma. *Cancer* 2003; **97**: 586–91.

●37. Solal-Celigny P, Roy P, Colombat P *et al.* Follicular lymphoma international prognostic index. *Blood* 2004; **104**: 1258–65.

38. Sutcliffe SB, Wrigley PF, Smyth JF *et al.* Intensive investigation in management of Hodgkin's disease. *Br Med J* 1976; **ii**: 1343–7.

●39. Lister TA, Crowther D, Sutcliffe SB *et al.* Report of a committee convened to discuss the evaluation and staging of patients with Hodgkin's disease: Cotswolds meeting. *J Clin Oncol* 1989; **7**: 1630–6.

40. de Medeiros BC, Lacerda MA, Telles JE *et al.* Cholestasis secondary to Hodgkin's disease: report of 2 cases of vanishing bile duct syndrome. *Haematologica* 1998; **83**: 1038–40.

41. Sans M, Andreu V, Bordas JM *et al.* Usefulness of laparoscopy with liver biopsy in the assessment of liver involvement at diagnosis of Hodgkin's and non-Hodgkin's lymphomas. *Gastrointest Endosc* 1998; **47**: 391–5.

42. Romaguera J, Hagemeister FB. Lymphoma of the colon. *Curr Opin Gastroenterol* 2005; **21**: 80–4.

43. Isaacson PG, MacLennan KA, Subbuswamy SG. Multiple lymphomatous polyposis of the gastrointestinal tract. *Histopathology* 1984; **8**: 641–56.

44. Raderer M, Vorbeck F, Formanek M *et al.* Importance of extensive staging in patients with mucosa-associated lymphoid tissue (MALT)-type lymphoma. *Br J Cancer* 2000; **83**: 454–7.

●45. Morton JE, Leyland MJ, Vaughan Hudson G *et al.* Primary gastrointestinal non-Hodgkin's lymphoma: a review of 175 British national lymphoma investigation cases. *Br J Cancer* 1993; **67**: 776–82.

46. Shepherd NA, Hall PA, Coates PJ, Levison DA. Primary malignant lymphoma of the colon and rectum. A histopathological and immunohistochemical analysis of 45 cases with clinicopathological correlations. *Histopathology* 1988; **12**: 235–52.

47. Domizio P, Owen RA, Shepherd NA *et al.* Primary lymphoma of the small intestine. A clinicopathological study of 119 cases. *Am J Surg Pathol* 1993; **17**: 429–42.

◆48. Alexandrakis MG, Passam FH, Kyriakou DS, Bouros D. Pleural effusions in hematologic malignancies. *Chest* 2004; **125**: 1546–55.

49. Rohatiner AZ, Whelan JS, Ganjoo RK *et al.* Mediastinal large-cell lymphoma with sclerosis (MLCLS). *Br J Cancer* 1994; **69**: 601–4.

●50. Abou-Elella AA, Weisenburger DD, Vose JM *et al.* Primary mediastinal large B-cell lymphoma: a clinicopathologic study of 43 patients from the Nebraska lymphoma study group. *J Clin Oncol* 1999; **17**: 784–90.

51. Zinzani PL, Martelli M, Bertini M *et al.* Induction chemotherapy strategies for primary mediastinal large B-cell lymphoma with sclerosis: a retrospective multinational study on 426 previously untreated patients. *Haematologica* 2002; **87**: 1258–64.

52. Lazzarino M, Orlandi E, Paulli M *et al.* Primary mediastinal B-cell lymphoma with sclerosis: an aggressive tumor with distinctive clinical and pathologic features. *J Clin Oncol* 1993; **11**: 2306–13.

53. Liu DT, Fan DS, Chan WM *et al.* Challenging problems in malignancy: case 3. Chronic lymphocytic leukemia with ocular complications and superior vena cava obstruction. *J Clin Oncol* 2004; **22**: 3830–2.

54. Chee YC, Chea E. IgA myeloma with primary pleural involvement. *Eur J Respir Dis* 1984; **65**: 136–8.

55. Ahmed S, Kussick SJ, Siddiqui AK *et al.* Bronchial-associated lymphoid tissue lymphoma: a clinical study of a rare disease. *Eur J Cancer* 2004; **40**: 1320–6.

56. Kurtin PJ, Myers JL, Adlakha H *et al.* Pathologic and clinical features of primary pulmonary extranodal marginal zone B-cell lymphoma of MALT type. *Am J Surg Pathol* 2001; **25**: 997–1008.

57. Zinzani PL, Tani M, Gabriele A et al. Extranodal marginal zone B-cell lymphoma of MALT-type of the lung: single-center experience with 12 patients. Leuk Lymphoma 2003; 44: 821–4.

58. Sandlund JT, Murphy SB, Santana VM et al. CNS involvement in children with newly diagnosed non-Hodgkin's lymphoma. J Clin Oncol 2000; 18: 3018–24.

59. Bashir RM, Bierman PJ, Vose JM et al. Central nervous system involvement in patients with diffuse aggressive non-Hodgkin's lymphoma. Am J Clin Oncol 1991; 14: 478–82.

60. Bishop PC, Wilson WH, Pearson D et al. CNS involvement in primary mediastinal large B-cell lymphoma. J Clin Oncol 1999; 17: 2479–85.

61. Hegde U, Filie A, Little RF et al. High incidence of occult leptomeningeal disease detected by flow cytometry in newly diagnosed aggressive B-cell lymphomas at risk for central nervous system involvement: the role of flow cytometry versus cytology. Blood 2005; 105: 496–502.

62. Fassas AB, Muwalla F, Berryman T et al. Myeloma of the central nervous system: association with high-risk chromosomal abnormalities, plasmablastic morphology and extramedullary manifestations. Br J Haematol 2002; 117: 103–8.

63. Akintola-Ogunremi O, Whitney C, Mathur SC, Finch CN. Chronic lymphocytic leukemia presenting with symptomatic central nervous system involvement. Ann Hematol 2002; 81: 402–4.

64. Biagi J, MacKenzie RG, Lim MS et al. Primary Hodgkin's disease of the CNS in an immunocompetent patient: a case study and review of the literature. Neuro-oncol 2000; 2: 239–43.

65. Ferreri AJ, Campo E, Seymour JF et al. Intravascular lymphoma: clinical presentation, natural history, management and prognostic factors in a series of 38 cases, with special emphasis on the 'cutaneous variant'. Br J Haematol 2004; 127: 173–83.

●66. Willemze R, Kerl H, Sterry W et al. EORTC classification for primary cutaneous lymphomas: a proposal from the cutaneous lymphoma study group of the European Organisation for Research and Treatment of Cancer. Blood 1997; 90: 354–71.

67. Fink-Puches R, Zenahlik P, Back B et al. Primary cutaneous lymphomas: applicability of current classification schemes (European Organisation for Research and Treatment of Cancer, World Health Organization) based on clinicopathologic features observed in a large group of patients. Blood 2002; 99: 800–5.

68. Shimoyama M. Diagnostic criteria and classification of clinical subtypes of adult T-cell leukaemia-lymphoma. A report from the lymphoma study group (1984–87). Br J Haematol 1991; 79: 428–37.

◆69. Stein H, Foss HD, Durkop H et al. CD30(+) anaplastic large cell lymphoma: a review of its histopathologic, genetic, and clinical features. Blood 2000; 96: 3681–95.

70. Agnew KL, Ruchlemer R, Catovsky D et al. Cutaneous findings in chronic lymphocytic leukaemia. Br J Dermatol 2004; 150: 1129–35.

71. Erkilic S, Erbagci Z, Kocer NE et al. Cutaneous involvement in Hodgkin's lymphoma: report of two cases. J Dermatol 2004; 31: 330–4.

●72. Burkitt D. A sarcoma involving the jaws in African children. Br J Surg 1958; 46: 218–23.

73. Ferry JA, Harris NL, Young RH et al. Malignant lymphoma of the testis, epididymis, and spermatic cord. A clinicopathologic study of 69 cases with immunophenotypic analysis. Am J Surg Pathol 1994; 18: 376–90.

74. Pileri SA, Sabattini E, Rosito P et al. Primary follicular lymphoma of the testis in childhood: an entity with peculiar clinical and molecular characteristics. J Clin Pathol 2002; 55: 684–8.

◆75. Young GA. Lymphoma at uncommon sites. Hematol Oncol 1999; 17: 53–83.

76. Curt G, Johnston PG. Cancer fatigue: the way forward. Oncologist 2003; 8(Suppl 1): 27–30.

77. Gobbi PG, Attardo-Parrinello G, Lattanzio G et al. Severe pruritus should be a B-symptom in Hodgkin's disease. Cancer 1983; 51: 1934–6.

78. Cavalli F. Rare syndromes in Hodgkin's disease. Ann Oncol 1998; 9(Suppl 5): s109–13.

79. Omidvari SH, Khojasteh HN, Mohammadianpanah M et al. Long-term pruritus as the initial and sole clinical manifestation of occult Hodgkin's disease. Indian J Med Sci 2004; 58: 250–2.

80. Todeschini G, Ambrosetti A, Meneghini V et al. Mediastinal large-B-cell lymphoma with sclerosis: a clinical study of 21 patients. J Clin Oncol 1990; 8: 804–8.

81. Barosi G, Boccadoro M, Cavo M et al. Management of multiple myeloma and related-disorders: guidelines from the Italian Society of Hematology (SIE), Italian Society of Experimental Hematology (SIES) and Italian Group for Bone Marrow Transplantation (GITMO). Haematologica 2004; 89: 717–41.

82. Chahal S, Lagera JE, Ryder J, Kleinschmidt-DeMasters BK. Hematological neoplasms with first presentation as spinal cord compression syndromes: a 10-year retrospective series and review of the literature. Clin Neuropathol 2003; 22: 282–90.

83. Lyons MK, O'Neill BP, Marsh WR, Kurtin PJ. Primary spinal epidural non-Hodgkin's lymphoma: report of eight patients and review of the literature. Neurosurgery 1992; 30: 675–80.

84. Ottinger H, Belka C, Kozole G et al. Deep venous thrombosis and pulmonary artery embolism in high-grade non Hodgkin's lymphoma: incidence, causes and prognostic relevance. Eur J Haematol 1995; 54: 186–94.

85. Cohen LF, Balow JE, Magrath IT et al. Acute tumor lysis syndrome. A review of 37 patients with Burkitt's lymphoma. Am J Med 1980; 68: 486–91.

86. Tsokos GC, Balow JE, Spiegel RJ, Magrath IT. Renal and metabolic complications of undifferentiated and lymphoblastic lymphomas. Medicine (Baltimore) 1981; 60: 218–29.

87. Loening S, Carson CC 3rd, Faxon DP, Morin LJ. Ureteral obstruction from Hodgkin's disease. J Urol 1974; 111: 345–9.

88. Talreja D, Slater LM, Dara P et al. Multiple myeloma complicated by myelomatous obstructive uropathy. Cancer 1980; 46: 1893–5.

89. Maeda Y, Nawa Y, Tanimoto K et al. Ureteric obstruction by retroperitoneal lymphoplasmacytic lymphoma. Am J Hematol 2002; 71: 238.

90. Kyle RA. Update on the treatment of multiple myeloma. Oncologist 2001; 6: 119–24.

91. Seymour JF, Gagel RF. Calcitriol: the major humoral mediator of hypercalcemia in Hodgkin's disease and non-Hodgkin's lymphomas. Blood 1993; 82: 1383–94.

92. Majumdar G. Incidence and prognostic significance of hypercalcaemia in B-cell non-Hodgkin's lymphoma. J Clin Pathol 2002; 55: 637–8.

93. Briones J, Cervantes F, Montserrat E, Rozman C. Hypercalcemia in a patient with chronic lymphocytic leukemia evolving into Richter's syndrome. Leuk Lymphoma 1996; 21: 521–3.

94. Beaudreuil J, Lortholary O, Martin A et al. Hypercalcemia may indicate Richter's syndrome: report of four cases and review. Cancer 1997; 79: 1211–15.

95. Firkin F, Seymour JF, Watson AM et al. Parathyroid hormone-related protein in hypercalcaemia associated with haematological malignancy. Br J Haematol 1996; 94: 486–92.

96. Cairo MS, Bishop M. Tumour lysis syndrome: new therapeutic strategies and classification. Br J Haematol 2004; 127: 3–11.

97. Hande KR, Garrow GC. Acute tumor lysis syndrome in patients with high-grade non-Hodgkin's lymphoma. Am J Med 1993; 94: 133–9.

98. Blade J, Fernandez-Llama P, Bosch F et al. Renal failure in multiple myeloma: presenting features and predictors of outcome in 94 patients from a single institution. Arch Intern Med 1998; 158: 1889–93.

99. Torra R, Blade J, Cases A et al. Patients with multiple myeloma requiring long-term dialysis: presenting features, response to therapy, and outcome in a series of 20 cases. Br J Haematol 1995; 91: 854–9.

100. Herrera GA, Joseph L, Gu X et al. Renal pathologic spectrum in an autopsy series of patients with plasma cell dyscrasia. Arch Pathol Lab Med 2004; 128: 875–9.

101. Dimopoulos MA, Panayiotidis P, Moulopoulos LA et al. Waldenstrom's macroglobulinemia: clinical features, complications, and management. J Clin Oncol 2000; 18: 214–26.

♦102. Dimopoulos MA, Kyle RA, Anagnostopoulos A, Treon SP. Diagnosis and management of Waldenstrom's macroglobulinemia. J Clin Oncol 2005; 23: 1564–77.

103. Kyasa MJ, Parrish RS, Schichman SA, Zent CS. Autoimmune cytopenia does not predict poor prognosis in chronic lymphocytic leukemia/small lymphocytic lymphoma. Am J Hematol 2003; 74: 1–8.

104. Mauro FR, Foa R, Cerretti R et al. Autoimmune hemolytic anemia in chronic lymphocytic leukemia: clinical, therapeutic, and prognostic features. Blood 2000; 95: 2786–92.

105. Sallah S, Sigounas G, Vos P et al. Autoimmune hemolytic anemia in patients with non-Hodgkin's lymphoma: characteristics and significance. Ann Oncol 2000; 11: 1571–7.

106. Sallah S, Gagnon GA. Angioimmunoblastic lymphadenopathy with dysproteinemia: emphasis on pathogenesis and treatment. Acta Haematol 1998; 99: 57–64.

107. Cesana C, Nosari AM, Klersy C et al. Risk factors for the development of bacterial infections in multiple myeloma treated with two different vincristine-adriamycin-dexamethasone schedules. Haematologica 2003; 88: 1022–8.

108. Hargreaves RM, Lea JR, Griffiths H et al. Immunological factors and risk of infection in plateau phase myeloma. J Clin Pathol 1995; 48: 260–6.

109. Winkelstein A, Jordan PS. Immune deficiencies in chronic lymphocytic leukemia and multiple myeloma. Clin Rev Allergy 1992; 10: 39–58.

110. Paradisi F, Corti G, Cinelli R. Infections in multiple myeloma. Infect Dis Clin North Am 2001; 15: 373–84, vii–viii.

111. Hensel M, Kornacker M, Yammeni S et al. Disease activity and pretreatment, rather than hypogammaglobulinaemia, are major risk factors for infectious complications in patients with chronic lymphocytic leukaemia. Br J Haematol 2003; 122: 600–6.

112. Astrom KE, Mancall EL, Richardson EP Jr. Progressive multifocal leuko-encephalopathy; a hitherto unrecognized complication of chronic lymphatic leukaemia and Hodgkin's disease. Brain 1958; 81: 93–111.

113. Gonzalez H, Bolgert F, Camporo P, Leblond V. Progressive multifocal leukoencephalitis (PML) in three patients treated with standard-dose fludarabine (FAMP). Hematol Cell Ther 1999; 41: 183–6.

114. Cid J, Revilla M, Cervera A et al. Progressive multifocal leukoencephalopathy following oral fludarabine treatment of chronic lymphocytic leukemia. Ann Hematol 2000; 79: 392–5.

115. Daibata M, Hatakeyama N, Kamioka M et al. Detection of human herpesvirus 6 and JC virus in progressive multifocal leukoencephalopathy complicating follicular lymphoma. Am J Hematol 2001; 67: 200–5.

116. Kimyai-Asadi A, Jih MH. Paraneoplastic pemphigus. Int J Dermatol 2001; 40: 367–72.

117. Anhalt GJ, Kim SC, Stanley JR et al. Paraneoplastic pemphigus. An autoimmune mucocutaneous disease associated with neoplasia. N Engl J Med 1990; 323: 1729–35.

118. Hammack J, Kotanides H, Rosenblum MK, Posner JB. Paraneoplastic cerebellar degeneration, II. Clinical and immunologic findings in 21 patients with Hodgkin's disease. Neurology 1992; 42: 1938–43.

41

The art of histologic diagnosis

BHARAT N NATHWANI, SEBASTIAN J SASU, ARSHAD N AHSANUDDIN, ANTONIO M HERNANDEZ AND
MILTON R DRACHENBERG

INTRODUCTION

Technology has extensively permeated all medical specialties, including diagnostic anatomic pathology, where innovative new tools are being used with increasing frequency to make accurate diagnoses and provide meaningful biologic information for prognosis and treatment.

In this setting of rapidly emerging scientific knowledge, it is necessary to ask why anatomic pathology should continue to keep microscopic histologic examination as a part of the diagnostic armamentarium. This question has gained further importance, for two specific reasons:

- Many studies have shown that the typical and overt cases of the most common lymphoma entities have characteristic gene expression profiles (signatures) that may also provide more reproducible diagnoses and clinical relevance than histologic and immuno-histologic evaluation of tissue sections.[1–20]

- Morphology has many limitations: it is subjective, diagnostic accuracy is directly proportional to whether the pathologist is a subspecialist, their degree of experience and the daily volume of case material seen.[21–23] Quantitative measurements, such as accurate and reproducible enumeration of cells, are also difficult.[21–23]

Our answer is that histologic examination, as an independent method, provides specific types of diagnostic information that cannot be obtained by any other methodology and

BOX 41.1: The art of histological diagnosis

1. Basic assumptions for forming a differential diagnosis
2. Consequences of the inherent limitations in anatomic pathology and other difficulties in fulfilling the basic assumptions for forming a differential diagnosis:
   - specific knowledge requirements
   - inherent problems associated with histologic evaluation
   - extraneous problems related to artifacts of fixation, processing, cutting and staining that result in cytologic variability and lead to diagnostic errors
   - requirement of image imprinting in the memory for future instant image recall to automatically initiate the differential diagnosis
   - cognizance and understanding of the limitations of individual knowledge and experience
   - relating to the explosion of rapidly evolving new scientific knowledge, technologies, changing concepts and criteria and their application to daily practice
   - imprecise clinical information
3. Reasons why making a histologic diagnosis is an art and not a science:
   - the cardinal skill required to initiate a differential diagnosis is to accurately identify pathologic processes
   - identification of pathologic processes is markedly facilitated by identifying cells based on their colors and/or tinctorial properties seen at low magnification
   - morphologic manifestations of pathologic processes and their recognition
   - different types of pathologic processes
   - methods of identifying pathologic processes and distinguishing them from normal
4. The diagnostic significance of pathologic processes that form distinctive patterns
5. The inherent role of histology:
   - the global importance of morphology, and its value as part of a systematic approach to diagnosis
   - the importance of morphology in the diagnosis of benign lymphoid diseases
   - distinguishing benign from malignant lymphoid proliferations
   - the importance of morphologic patterns and cytologic features in the World Health Organization (WHO) classification of Hodgkin and non-Hodgkin lymphomas
   - naming of lymphomas in the WHO classification after morphologic patterns
   - naming of lymphomas in the WHO classification according to cytologic features, which often also have distinctive morphologic patterns
   - naming of lymphomas in the WHO classification according to eponyms
   - correlation between morphologic patterns, immunohistochemistry and cytogenetics of lymphomas
   - correlation of interobserver reproducibility of lymphomas with and without distinctive patterns with immunophenotyping
   - importance of cell typing in grading and prognosis of lymphomas
   - the relative merits of incisional/excisional biopsies versus fine needle biopsies

that this information is clinically valuable and irreplaceable. Because of these simple facts, histologic diagnosis continues to be the most important first step in making an accurate diagnosis in any new patient subjected to a biopsy.[24]

In a recent, detailed, companion review paper in 2007, we discussed not only the fundamental role that histology plays in establishing a correct diagnosis, but also how its value is enhanced by immunophenotype analysis by flow cytometry, immunohistochemical staining, and molecular techniques in this era of genomics and proteomics, taking into account the limitations of these technologies.[24] The purpose of this chapter is to present an outline of values and limitations in histologic diagnosis as obtained from the published data and our personal experience. We also provide strong justification to continue the practice, with fervor and conviction, of the art of histologic diagnosis, because it is necessary today and in the foreseeable future.

Towards this end, Box 41.1 provides an overview of our chapter.

BASIC ASSUMPTIONS FOR FORMING A DIFFERENTIAL DIAGNOSIS

Before we address in detail some of the inherent problems faced when making a morphologic diagnosis in anatomic and/or lymph node pathology, we briefly summarize the prerequisites for forming a proper differential diagnosis. When making a histologic diagnosis, three basic assumptions are made:[25–33]

- The known diseases have criteria on the basis of which they can be separated from each other,[29,33] requiring specific knowledge of these diseases.

- The diseases can be recognized by the presence/absence of different types of histologic features that can be estimated or quantified,[29,33] requiring specific skills for such recognition.
- The histologic features of disease can be correlated with clinical information, and when available, immunophenotypic and molecular information, and can be synthesized into a logical histologic differential diagnosis,[25–33] requiring the ability to integrate such information.

The intellectual task of integrating information from diverse sources to form a differential diagnosis requires utilizing different types of knowledge and skills. The strategies involved in forming a diagnosis vary from one case to another, and may vary within each slide or between different slides from the same case.[25–33]

In the next section, we present the inherent limitations in the discipline of histopathology, and other problems that are encountered while reviewing histologic sections, which further compound the diagnostic difficulties in making accurate diagnoses.

CONSEQUENCES OF THE INTRINSIC LIMITATIONS IN ANATOMIC PATHOLOGY COUPLED WITH OTHER DIFFICULTIES IN FULFILLING THE ABOVE BASIC ASSUMPTIONS FOR FORMING A DIFFERENTIAL DIAGNOSIS

Specific knowledge requirements

- *Exhaustive knowledge is necessary regarding histologic, immunophenotypic and genotypic criteria for diagnosis of various diseases*

In anatomic pathology, there are currently more than 5000 individual disease entities.[21] Each of these present with different histologic features and at different stages, with their own repertoire of morphologic, immunologic and genetic characteristics. The knowledge regarding different diseases is available in the form of text information, which is considered as passive or theoretical or *a priori* knowledge. This passive textual knowledge is independent of the knowledge obtained from experience. It is impossible for a single pathologist to remember all of this information, especially because it continues to rapidly evolve and change.

- *Dynamic lymph node physiology may markedly but reversibly alter cytologic and architectural features in specific compartments, leading to diagnostic errors*

The histologic examination of lymph node sections is difficult because the lymph node is a unique and dynamic organ. The interaction of lymphoid cells of different types, together with the stromal cells of different types, results in the generation of numerous complex immune responses/functions. These lymphoid cells may change dramatically in size and appearance, and often migrate from one compartment to another in response to endogenous or exogenous stimuli, or to neoplastic transformation. Importantly, because cells and cellular changes are dynamic and occur within different compartments (follicular, mantle zone, marginal zone, paracortical, interfollicular, and medullary) it is therefore natural to find subtle to profound histologic changes in one or more compartments, simultaneously or over time, and these changes often lead to interpretive difficulties and diagnostic errors, especially in the absence of extensive experience.

Inherent problems associated with histologic evaluation

- *Normal and abnormal cells within the same compartment may exhibit a wide histologic spectrum and overlapping histologic features*

There are numerous benign and malignant lymphoid diseases, and their histologic features may overlap, requiring the pathologist to use judgment and experience to accurately recognize them and form a proper diagnosis. Similar to the rest of surgical pathology, diagnosis of lymphoid diseases frequently relies on accurate pattern recognition. Thus, architectural features such as the size, shape and density of lymph node compartments, their relationship to each other, and the various colors that correspond to different cell types, are all examined at low magnification and a rapid differential diagnosis is formed.

The knowledge required for accurate identification of cells and patterns involves recognition, processing information and storage of histologic images in the mind, and it only comes from experiential reinforcement.[21] This experience-based knowledge often is called empirical or *posteriori* or heuristic knowledge. To acquire this type of knowledge and use it effectively in the daily practice of making histologic diagnoses requires time, special effort and undivided concentration. This type of knowledge can only be obtained by continuous, specific, hands-on, one-on-one training, from highly experienced pathologists, preferably with subspecialty training. Thus, it is impossible for one histopathologist to be proficient in interpreting biopsy specimens from all organ systems.

- *Accurate quantification of different types of cells is very difficult*

Often, a differential diagnosis will require quantification of one or more cell populations. Unfortunately, most of the time it is almost impossible to achieve this with great precision, and the inter- and intra-observer agreement tends to be in the 20 percent range and often higher, thus leading to significant disagreements among pathologists and promoting communication and diagnostic errors.[22,23]

- *A well-defined and systematic vocabulary and/or dictionary is not available*

To make a proper histologic diagnosis, a histopathologist requires in-depth knowledge of the wide spectrum of histologic features. However, a universal, systematically organized nomenclature of histologic descriptors is not currently available, nor are there reference materials such as textbooks and/or illustrated texts that outline guidelines for the use of such descriptors. In the real world, histopathologists have to recognize and quantify histologic features to form a proper differential diagnosis, but again with very few exceptions,[29,33] large collections of well-organized, interactive digital libraries of photomicrographs of histologic features and diseases are not available for instant use in daily histopathology practice, which has made the task of histopathologists difficult, especially in conveying to other pathologists what they mean, and in teaching what they have seen or diagnosed.

- *Inadequate sampling of tissue and non-representative specimens are common*

Morphologic evaluation is the first step towards determining specimen adequacy. In an age of core needle biopsies and fine needle aspirations, in which the material submitted for pathologic evaluation has become smaller and smaller, inadequate sampling becomes inevitable and can compound the diagnostic difficulties and lead to errors, especially in the case of inexperienced pathologists. The size of the available specimen is further reduced by taking material for genetic, molecular and other studies. In these cases, experience will also allow the pathologist to decide how 'far to go', i.e. to decide whether he or she is dealing with an adequate or inadequate specimen. These issues are also important in the setting of lesions that may be focal or multifocal, as seen frequently with immunocompromised patients, with coexisting lesions within the same lymph node, or with fibrotic and inflamed, infectious or noninfectious, backgrounds. Importantly, benign diseases typically show multifocal pathologic processes, changes or abnormalities. Lymphomas occasionally may have focal or multifocal distinctive features, or may show focal or multifocal histologic progression. They may also exhibit a prominent benign component, as in Hodgkin lymphoma and mucosa-associated lymphoid tissue (MALT) lymphoma. For these reasons, generous and representative biopsies are necessary.

Extraneous problems related to artifacts of fixation, processing, cutting and staining that result in cytologic variability and lead to diagnostic errors

Good quality of generous histologic sections received for evaluation is of paramount importance for making an accurate morphologic diagnosis. Occasionally, artifacts can be so extensive that they may preclude interpretation of the findings.

It is common to see in one hematoxylin and eosin (H&E)-stained slide, one or more artifacts such as cracking, tearing, wrinkling, crumpling, shattering, dry earth,

peripheral drying, moth-eaten and Venetian blind appearances. Also, the nuclei may be shrunken, muddy or bubbly (Table 41.1).[34,35] These artifacts can occur after a surgical biopsy has been performed, during specimen transportation, slicing of tissue by pathologist, tissue fixative used, duration of tissue fixation, processing, paraffin embedding of tissue, cutting of paraffin blocks, staining of cut slides from paraffin blocks, and cover slipping the slides. There is an excellent correlation between the artifacts seen and their underlying cause, and steps that can be taken to prevent them or the procedures that can be adopted to remove these artifacts. While most of the above-mentioned artifacts are common and readily identified, those that relate to inadequate or poor fixation and the fixative used *are often not recognized and can readily lead to diagnostic errors*, therefore we mention them below.

Lymphoid cells are fragile and prone to significant cytologic distortion of their nuclear chromatin pattern, amount of cytoplasm and immunohistochemical properties (i.e. availability of cell surface antigens). Inadequate fixation can lead to a subtle, yet significant change in the nuclear-to-cytoplasmic ratio due to shrinkage of nuclei and an artificial increase in the amount and staining quality of the cytoplasm. Poorly fixed areas can be recognized by the increased space between lymphoid cells and the artificial clearing that surrounds individual cells, and interpretation of such areas should be avoided. Shrinkage of nuclei can also result in pseudo-condensation of nuclear chromatin, making distinction between 'mature' and 'immature' lymphoid cells very difficult. It should be noted that cautery artifact, introduced by the surgeon, results in smudging that cannot be reversed by good fixation. Thus, extreme care should be exercised when choosing the areas appropriate for histologic evaluation in an inadequately fixed specimen.

Another major problem that is often not well appreciated is that different fixatives create different sets of changes and artifacts in tissue samples. For example, lymphoid cells fixed in B5 appear approximately 15–20 percent smaller than the same cells fixed in formalin. The B5-fixed lymphoid cells also have a finer chromatin pattern and better-defined nuclear and cytoplasmic borders. Formalin-fixed lymphoid cells, in contrast, are larger and may show vesicular chromatin due to ballooning artifact, and their borders may be ill defined. Frozen tissue introduces an artifact that appears to flatten out or blur cytologic features and cannot be reversed (moreover, prior freezing alters antigenicity and thus affects immunohistochemistry). The lack of understanding or appreciation for these changes often leads to errors.

Requirement of image imprinting in the mind for instant image recall to automatically initiate the differential diagnosis

The basis of histologic diagnosis is recognition of morphologic patterns and cytologic features. One of the most

Table 41.1   Problems encountered by pathologists in routine sections and their causes

Problems/artifact seen	Underlying cause of the artifact
Dehydration	
Tissue shrunken, dry and hard results in cracks during sectioning; sections may be both thick and thin	Dehydration; acetone used as dehydrant
Sections crumbled, torn or 'exploded'	Contamination of absolute alcohol with water or other hydrating substance, leading to incomplete dehydration
May exhibit 'dry earth effect' (small irregular cracks throughout)	
Cells are 'muddy'	
Clearing	
Tissue hard and brittle	Excessively prolonged clearing time in xylene
Sections crack and may be both thick and thin	Chloroform used as clearing agent on tissue processor
Sections compressed, wrinkled, will not ribbon	Contamination of xylene by alcohol leading to poor infiltration of paraffin
Infiltration	
Tissue shrunken and hard. Cracks during sectioning, and sectioning may be both thick and thin	Infiltration paraffin too hot
Stain 'muddy' and homogeneous	
Embedding	
Air spaces around tissue in paraffin block make sectioning difficult	Delay in embedding after removal from paraffin bath
Blocks crack and are either impossible to section or yield cracked sections	Water used to cool blocks too cold
Sectioning	
Sections compressed and wrinkled, may fall off slides, will not ribbon, may be cracked	Blunt knife
Linear knife marks, scratches and splits	Knife rough and uneven (even if sharp)
Sections compressed, wrinkled thick and thin (Venetian blind effect)	Loose block or knife
Sections both thick and thin	Blade not angled enough
Sections cracked	Blade angled too much
Punched out areas (Swiss cheese or moth-eaten effect)	Inadequate facing of block after rough-cutting
Cracked circular areas with central shrunken, over stained tissue	Failure to remove air bubbles while picking sections up on slides from water bath (bubbles were produced while layering ribbon on flotation bath)
Hematoxylin and eosin (H&E) staining	
Too much eosinophilic color in the H&E stain (acid formaldehyde, hematin, formalin fixative)	Formation of acid formalin
Randomly distributed brown to black crystalline deposits (mercuric chloride crystals, Zenker and B5 fixatives)	Failure to process tissue from mercury-containing fixatives through iodine and hypo
Results variable, with any sections overstained	Poor differentiation of Harris hematoxylin
Excess eosin appears 'muddy' and obscures detail	Passage through alcohols after eosin staining too rapid
Cover slip	
Air bubbles, excess or insufficient media	Poor technique
Sections appear cloudy	Defective media
Media may form bubbles with time	
Tissue appears dry	Delay between removal from xylol and cover slipping

important facts, which is often not understood or appreciated by many pathologists and clinicians, is that for an image to be retained in long-term memory and for it to be accessible instantly through recall, it must be seen repeatedly, with high frequency. Once so-called 'imprinting'[21,36] of the image has occurred into long-term memory, when encountered or seen in the future, it will be automatically

summoned to instantly and intuitively form a differential diagnosis for the pathologist. Because different entities may exhibit a wide histologic spectrum, for imprinting of images to occur, it is essential for the pathologist to see daily as many cases as possible. To achieve a level of expertise necessary for this process requires the study of thousands of lymph node biopsies each year at a rate of 5–10 cases daily. However, this is very difficult for the general surgical pathologist who typically sees just a few cases of uncommon diseases, such as lymphomas, every year. These facts strongly underscore the need for sub-specialty-based practice in anatomic pathology.

Cognizance and understanding of the limitations of individual knowledge and experience

The vast spectrum of existing benign and malignant diseases and the amount of new data continuously becoming available over a short period of time makes it almost impossible for a single pathologist to be intimately familiar with the diagnostic criteria and subtleties of every single entity. Most critical is the interpretation and integration of all information pertaining to a specific patient, in an ever-changing pathologic context, which needs to be filtered through a thorough understanding of the pathologist's own limitations and experience. In other words, we do not know what we do not know. We see what we know, and the more we know, the more we see. Also, what we recognize is greatly influenced by our training, concepts, criteria, approach and methods used in diagnostic practice.[21,24,36]

Relating to the explosion of rapidly evolving new knowledge, technologies and changing concepts and their application to daily practice

The rapid emergence of techniques, methods and instrument platforms for immunophenotype analysis by flow cytometry, high-resolution conventional cytogenetics, fluorescent *in situ* hybridization, microdissection, and the subsequent development of molecular techniques such as polymerase chain reaction (PCR), genomics and proteomics, have initiated great surges of discovery that have increased our knowledge of the genotypic and phenotype aspects of lymphoid disease by leaps and bounds. For example, the February 2008 research product catalog of Santa Cruz Biotechnology (Santa Cruz, CA) lists over 33,500 primary antibodies, which is an increase of 2100 antibodies within three months. Consequently, it has become more and more difficult for the histopathologist to keep up to date with all the new developments in the field and to determine what can be useful in daily practice. Thus, the daily diagnostic tasks are often overwhelming and may promote diagnostic errors.

Imprecise clinical information

The provision of inaccurate clinical data such as wrong age and wrong site can lead to devastating errors. Also, not providing prior clinical history of lymphoma and type of treatment increases the risk of errors. Such information cannot be gleaned from the histologic material and therefore can lead to misdiagnosis.

HISTOLOGIC DIAGNOSIS AS AN ART RATHER THAN A SCIENCE, AND A DISSECTION AND EXPLANATION OF THIS ART

From the preceding discussions, it is clear to us that in this new scientific world, it is often forgotten by many that making an accurate histologic diagnosis is an art and not a science, and because this art is irreplaceable and indispensable, it is necessary to practice it proficiently. The dictionary definition of the word 'art' is 'skill, dexterity or the power of performing certain actions acquired by experience, study or observation', and highlights several essential attributes. Practicing this art well requires a thorough understanding of why histologic diagnosis is considered an art, what the common problems encountered when practicing this art, how to recognize these problems and solve them, and what is required to become skillful at practicing it. Below, we attempt to address several of these key issues.

The cardinal skill required to initiate a differential diagnosis is to accurately identify pathologic processes

In contrast to normal states, by definition, the pathologic processes are abnormal and recognized by focal or multi-focal changes at a cellular or architectural level, that may be subtle or overt, and well to poorly defined. The pathologic processes can be distinctly different from the normal and thus readily recognizable, especially when they are a prominent or predominant finding and/or diffusely present throughout the node. However, when these processes are multifocal and/or are not well defined, they may be more difficult to recognize and differentiate from normal.[21,36]

When dealing with an abnormal or pathologic area, it is worthwhile to ask whether there is more than one abnormality, what are their locations and the types of abnormalities, and whether more than one diagnosis is required to explain their presence.

Some of the important issues pertaining to the sampling, appearance and recognition of pathologic processes and their etiology, and the variables that affect them are presented in Box 41.2. It is beyond the scope of this chapter to go into great detail about these issues, but rather we attempt to highlight the difficulties and the experience required to recognize them and to integrate all the information pertaining to the pathologic processes. An understanding of all the nuances and subtleties related to the pathologic processes brings a profound realization that making accurate histologic diagnoses consistently is an intricate art, and that it requires special 'hands-on' training with exposure to large volumes of material, and that it cannot be substituted by subspecialty texts and atlases, or by doing diagnostic work only occasionally.

BOX 41.2: Morphologic features and factors influencing the appearance of pathologic processes

Pathologic processes

- Type: similar and/or dissimilar
- Number: one or several
- Size: small, medium, large, mixed
- Shape: any
- Margins: sharp and/or vague
- Cellular constituents: lymphoid cell types, accessory cells, matrix, vessels, etc.
- Relationship of pathologic processes to each other and to normal tissue
- Type and number of compartments involved

Variables affecting the appearance of the pathologic process

- Anatomic site: lymph node, spleen, bone marrow, mucosa, viscera, soft tissue, etc.
- Adequate sampling of the specimen:
  (i) Clinical history of the size of the lesion(s) biopsied
  (ii) Type of biopsy: incisional, excisional, needle core, fine needle aspirate
  (iii) Size of the biopsy specimen
- Gross appearance of the biopsy specimen
- Etiology of the pathologic process: infection, trauma, autoimmunity, neoplasm, etc.
- Findings in step sections: small lesions disappear and new lesions appear in deeper sections
- Changes due to prior treatment and type
- Follow-up biopsy: progression or regression or no change, etc.

Identification of pathologic processes is markedly facilitated by identifying cells based on their colors and/or tinctorial properties seen at low magnification

At high magnification, cells such as eosinophils, epithelioid cells, starry-sky histiocytes, histiocytes, transformed lymphoid cells of medium or large size, blastic cells, small lymphocytes, plasma cells, lacunar and other variants of Sternberg–Reed (S-R) cells, large mummified cells, necrosis, etc., are distinctly different from each other regarding their size, shape, chromatin structure and amount and staining quality of cytoplasm. Because of these distinct differences, when these cells occur in small and/or large clusters and islands, irrespective of whether or not they are confluent or in sheets, they assume distinctive colors and/or tinctorial properties at low magnification.[21,36,37]

Learning, remembering and imprinting of these colors in long-term memory, and their correlation with cell types

as evident at low magnification, permits rapid identification of these cells, regardless of the compartment in which they may be located. With knowledge of the relationship of these colors to each other, awareness of where these colors (cell types) are normally supposed to occur, including their location and distribution in different diseases, most pathologic processes can be recognized at low magnification.[21,36,37]

Once recognized, these pathologic processes can be correlated with each other and integrated into one or more unifying diagnoses. Based on the presence of colors seen in different compartments at low magnification, the pathologist can recognize clusters, islands, and sheets of different cell types very quickly and form a proper and narrow differential diagnosis, which has to be confirmed or clarified or refined or changed by further study at high magnification.[21,36,37] In other words, the differential diagnosis formed at low magnification tells the pathologist what to do next at high magnification. The histologic features observed at high magnification then dictate what should be done next, that is, to review the slide further at high magnification or to go back to 2× magnification or 10× magnification, whichever is most efficient and/or necessary to reach a final diagnosis.[21–23] This evaluation precedes immunohistochemical evaluation.

This iterative approach, based on our longstanding experience in learning and teaching, is one of the most useful and reproducible arts of diagnostic pathology that only comes with dedicated in-depth study, continuous practice and experience. Unfortunately, only a minority of pathologists learn to recognize cells of different types at low magnification based on the colors observed.

Morphologic manifestations of pathologic processes and their recognition

Pathologic cellular interactions occur in one or more compartments of the lymph node, and thus these changes can usually be recognized histologically at low magnification by the presence of one or more of the following findings in one or more compartments.[21–23] First, there could be absence or obliteration of one or more compartments normally seen in the lymph node. Second, the normal compartments could be greatly exaggerated or highly distorted. Third, there may be the presence of pathologic processes or features (patterns) that do not have a normal counterpart and thus their presence is clearly abnormal. Fourth, there may be fusion, distortion, disintegration, colonization of compartments. Fifth, there may be the presence of one or more cell types in a compartment where they are not normally found, or conversely, the absence of cells from a compartment in which they are normally present. Sixth, markedly hyper- or hypo-cellular areas within compartments, focally or multifocally, with an abnormal appearance as compared with adjacent areas are useful in recognizing abnormalities.

Different types of pathologic processes

As abnormalities or pathologic areas occur within compartments, pathologists have usually named them after the compartment in which they occur or from which they arise, and these abnormalities are labeled as patterns that are described in the next section on patterns.[21,36,37] A specific type of pattern(s) may be focal, multifocal or diffuse, and well defined or poorly defined. Also, multiple patterns often coexist and one pattern may predominate.[21] However, the predominating pattern may *not* have major diagnostic relevance, or the pattern that may be focally present may have pathognomonic significance. Thus, the knowledge and experience that is required pertains not only to recognizing patterns accurately, but also to understanding the diagnostic relevance of each pattern.[21,26,37]

Methods of identifying pathologic processes and distinguishing them from normal

Box 41.3 lists the specific methods that are useful for identifying abnormal or pathologic foci.[21] Identifying the pathologic areas requires practice and commitment, and once learnt, the methods come intuitively and naturally to the experienced pathologist to instantaneously or rapidly form narrow and proper differential diagnoses.

DIAGNOSTIC SIGNIFICANCE OF PATHOLOGIC PROCESSES THAT FORM DISTINCTIVE PATTERNS

The lymph node is a unique and dynamic organ. Due to its central role in various types of immunity, it is involved in a myriad of complex immune cellular interactions and functions that occur within the several distinct compartments of the lymph node which have to be critically examined.

Each lymph node is surrounded by a capsule. The subcapsular sinus penetrates the lymph node cortex and branches into the trabecular sinuses, which in turn drain into the medullary sinuses located in the lymph node medulla adjacent to the hilum. The cortex contains primary follicles that transform into secondary follicles upon contact with antigen. The secondary follicles consist of a follicular center surrounded by a second outer layer composed of mantle zones. In secondary follicles, a marginal zone may usually partially surround the mantle zones as a third outer layer. Different types of T cells are present in the follicles, paracortex, and in the interfollicular areas where T cell regulation and differentiation occurs. These architectural structures represent distinct compartments through which migration and trafficking of different cell types occurs and in which complex and dynamic physiologic as well as pathologic interactions occur.

In various disease states, due to initiating events such as infection, trauma, autoimmunity or neoplasia, cellular

---

BOX 41.3: Methods for identifying pathologic processes

- Sequential step-wise examination of each lymph node compartment one at a time, at low and high magnification, with identification of specific histologic features
- Recognition at low magnification of cells of different types, based on their colors and tinctorial properties, and subsequently, comparison of colors present in different compartments in order to identify the presence of abnormal populations and track the migratory pathways of these cells
- Comparison of similar compartments: follicular centers, mantle zones, marginal zones, interfollicular areas and sinuses
- Comparison of adjacent compartments: follicular centers with mantle zones, follicular centers with marginal zones and follicles with interfollicular areas
- Assessment of the density of the lymphoid cellular populations

---

interactions, events, and changes occur in different compartments resulting in their exaggeration, fusion, distortion and/or obliteration. The ensuing result is subtle or overt shifts and changes in one or more compartments, which are recognized under the microscope as pathologic processes which are usually described and recognized as specific patterns.[21,36,37] These patterns are either well described and understood and thus reproducibly recognized, or alternatively, because they are infrequent, poorly understood, and often subtle or vague, they may pose great difficulty in their recognition and/or interpretation.

The accurate recognition and interpretation of these patterns at low magnification is important to formulate a narrow and proper differential diagnosis, and they also aid in preventing erroneous diagnoses. The patterns recognized at low power dictate what one should look for next at high magnification.[21–23] Box 41.4 lists the different types of pattern observed in lymphoid diseases.[24] For each pattern there is a differential diagnosis, which includes benign and/or malignant diseases.[21,36,37]

Box 41.5 summarizes the most important reasons why pattern recognition is of fundamental importance. The WHO classification[38] has recognized the importance of patterns and has named most B cell lymphomas after patterns. We discuss this value of patterns further at length in the next section.

The same pattern approach to diagnosis is used when examining sections of spleen, liver, bone marrow, skin, mucosal sites, soft tissue and other sites. However, because these sites do not have the same precise lymphoid architecture as the lymph node, specific local factors such as function, local architecture and microenvironment also influence the appearance of patterns seen, and therefore,

BOX 41.4: Different types of pattern

Spherical structures

- Follicular pattern
- Mantle zone pattern
- Marginal zone pattern
- Inverse follicular pattern
- Pseudofollicular pattern
- Mantle cell nodules
- Marginal zone (monocytoid) B cell nodules
- Follicular colonization
- Paracortical nodular T zone hyperplasia with and without mottling
- Progressive transformation of germinal centers
- L and H nodular pattern
- Fibrous nodular pattern

Other patterns (non-spherical structures)

- Sinus pattern
- Interfollicular pattern
- Mottled pattern
- Lennert pattern
- Starry sky pattern
- Vascular pattern
- Diffuse pattern
- 'Mass effect'
- Necrosis pattern
- Multiple patterns
- Miscellaneous patterns

BOX 41.5: Reasons why pattern recognition is important

- Most lymphomas and benign diseases have distinctive patterns
- Accurately identifying patterns allows a pathologist to remember and convey the most important diagnostic information with maximum efficiency
- Many lymphomas, such as follicular, mantle cell and marginal zone lymphomas, are named after patterns and can accurately be diagnosed on the basis of morphologic features alone
- 99 percent of nodal small lymphocytic lymphoma/chronic lymphocytic leukemia (CLL) has a pseudofollicular pattern (proliferation centers), which is pathognomonic for this entity
- Diffuse large B cell lymphoma represents a heterogeneous category and not a single disease entity, but by definition it requires the presence of a diffuse pattern
- Nodular lymphocyte-predominant Hodgkin lymphoma and nodular lymphocyte-rich classical Hodgkin lymphoma both require the presence of a nodular pattern
- Nodular sclerosing classical Hodgkin lymphoma requires the presence of at least one fibrous nodule for the diagnosis
- Most distinctive benign entities and diseases have one or more characteristic patterns
- Pattern can be focal or multifocal, subtle or overt, well or poorly defined, and there can be multiple concurrent patterns. Familiarity with subtleties and variant patterns can provide indispensable diagnostic information
- Pattern recognition may aid in resolving diagnostic conflicts with other specimens and/or with results obtained from ancillary techniques such as immunohistochemistry, flow cytometry and molecular studies.

these factors have to be kept in mind while interpreting lymphoid patterns at an extranodal site.

THE INHERENT ROLE OF HISTOLOGY

Morphologic observations correlated with clinical information have resulted in the development of specific clinicopathologic entities, which have then been validated or clarified into distinct entities by immunophenotypic, cytogenetic and molecular techniques much later. A few examples are offered below of the contribution of morphology in the last century:

- The normal MALT and the marginal zone lymphoma of MALT type were first described in 1983 by Issacson and Wright.[39] Based on these seminal morphologic observations, a vast and very useful body of knowledge pertaining to their immunoprofile, cytogenetic abnormalities, molecular biology and clinical correlates has subsequently established that MALT lymphomas are distinct clinicopathologic entities. Furthermore, the involvement of the benign follicular centers by the

marginal zone lymphoma cells (follicular colonization) was morphologically described before being confirmed by immunohistochemistry.[40,41]
- Angioimmunoblastic T cell lymphoma was first defined as a clinical and histopathologic syndrome as angioimmunoblastic lymphadenopathy in 1974 by Frizzera,[42,43] and as immunoblastic lymphadenopathy by Lukes in 1975.[44] This distinct entity has continued to be refined by the addition of morphologic and clinical criteria in the intervening years. For example, the finding of clear cell clusters of malignant T cells was associated with a progressive course and death, confirming the morphologic criteria as valid.[45] Subsequent contributions of immunohistochemistry and *in situ* hybridization have added greatly to our understanding of this disease, and have served to more

precisely define this lymphoma as a distinct disease entity.

- Anaplastic large cell lymphoma of the T cell type was originally described as a morphologic entity termed 'malignant histiocytosis' in 1939 by Scott and Robb-Smith.[46] Immunohistochemistry, cytogenetics and molecular studies later defined this lymphoma as a disease entity by its immunophenotype and characteristic genetic alterations.

These are only a few of the historical examples of histological diagnoses that have held up to close scrutiny over the past several decades. Lymphocytic and histiocytic nodular Hodgkin lymphoma, nodular sclerosing Hodgkin lymphoma, lymphoblastic lymphoma, small lymphocytic lymphoma, follicular lymphoma and large cell lymphomas have been recognized by their morphological characteristics for quite some time. These morphologic observations were then correlated with the natural history of the disease, treatment responses and survival characteristics, which established these associations as distinct entities. Over the past 30–40 years, immunohistochemistry and molecular studies have determined that these associations truly define unique diseases, which were codified in the Revised European–American Lymphoma (REAL) classification,[47] and later in the WHO classification.[48–50]

FUNDAMENTAL IMPORTANCE OF MORPHOLOGY, AND ITS VALUE AS PART OF A SYSTEMATIC APPROACH TO DIAGNOSIS

Lymphoid diseases, especially B cell lymphomas, arise from specific nodal and extranodal locations/compartments, such as follicular centers, mantle zones and marginal zones. Underscoring their fundamental importance, many lymphomas are named after these sites in the WHO classification. From these locations/compartments, the neoplastic cells often spread according to specific signaling, cross-talk, differentiation or transforming events. The microenvironment in all compartments, particularly the interplay between neoplastic and non-neoplastic cellular components present, plays a dynamic role in determining whether or not the host immune response is able to control the spread of neoplastic cells.[51–53] For example, in follicular lymphoma, the gene expression profiles of the background T cells may provide more prognostic information than those of the neoplastic cells.[11,54]

In the current systematic approach to the diagnosis of lymphoid diseases at nodal and extranodal sites, microscopy serves as the first step in the evaluation of a tissue sample. Morphologic examination can confirm adequacy of sampling and it can reveal the presence of a pathologic process by its effect on the specific tissue components, compartments and cell types that are normal and abnormal. Thus, histology can serve simultaneously as the foundation for a differential diagnosis and as a method of quality assurance, especially when evaluating small samples, crush artifacts and the presence of normal or non-representative tissue.[24]

Even though histologic examination is subjective, it generates a recordable observation that serves as a common language among pathologists and consultants. The pathology report, along with the microscopic description, is a record of what the pathologist saw, and the diagnosis thus derived is a record that is valuable for legal purposes as well as clinical care, research and teaching. Furthermore, histological diagnostic qualifiers used in pathology reports such as 'worrisome for', 'suggestive of', 'suspicious for' or 'consistent with' indicate limitations in morphologic criteria or limitations in the sample quality, and thus serve as triggers for additional biopsies and laboratory studies.[24]

The responsibility of the diagnostic histopathologist is to accurately recognize, record and report the important morphologic features of a specimen, which then form the basis for a differential diagnosis. The differential diagnosis guides the selection of subsequent ancillary studies that are undertaken to further characterize and precisely classify a disease process. Once the results of these ancillary studies become available, it is the responsibility of the pathologist to correlate all available data with the clinical information, and based on these data, to arrive at an accurate final diagnosis and offer prognostic and therapeutic information. This integrative approach requires a thorough understanding of the limitations of each test to achieve this end, and we reviewed this extensively in 2007.[24]

This archival material of paraffin blocks and H&E-stained slides has been most useful for histologic comparisons with subsequent biopsies to ascertain whether there is regression, progression or transformation of disease and can be accessed through histological reports. Archival material has also been most useful for research studies and equally importantly for the teaching and training of future pathologists who will be involved in patient care activities. Furthermore, the pathologist becomes the guardian and classifier of the paraffinized tissue by providing morphologic assessment and correlations.[24]

Last, but not least, morphological evaluation and diagnosis often serves as a benchmark against which results of newer tests are validated, which usually takes many years to complete. Based on such extensive comparisons, the limitations and values of morphology, as well as those of other tests that are being compared and evaluated, can be better determined and defined. This process of comparison is necessary, because it has improved not only morphologic criteria and diagnosis, but also the quality of newer tests, teaching and focused clinical and basic research, leading to more accurate diagnoses, proper staging and superior treatment of patients. In the end, making precise differential diagnoses is the first prerequisite for adequate management of patients, teaching and research.[24]

IMPORTANCE OF MORPHOLOGY IN THE DIAGNOSIS OF BENIGN LYMPHOID DISEASES

Benign lymphoid diseases frequently have non-specific immunohistochemical and flow cytometric phenotypes. Therefore histologic examination is indispensable for an accurate diagnosis.

The fundamental value of morphology is further underscored by the lack of sensitivity and specificity of the various antibodies used in the diagnosis of lymphomas, as we recently summarized.[24] Moreover, all flow cytometry and molecular reports contain a disclaimer that states that they should always be correlated with clinical, morphologic and other findings. For these reasons, morphology is very valuable in distinguishing benign lymphoid proliferations from each other.

It is beyond the scope of this chapter to go into the details of resolving a differential diagnosis involving benign diseases. However, we wish to emphasize that morphologic examination, in many cases, is able to differentiate benign disease from malignant.

Benign lymphoid diseases that show distinctive morphologic patterns are:[21]

- dermatopathic lymphadenitis (paracortical nodular T zone hyperplasia)
- infectious mononucleosis/viral lymphadenitis (interfollicular, mottling, intravascular)
- toxoplasmosis (follicular, interfollicular, sinus)
- cat-scratch disease (*Bartonella henselae*) (interfollicular, mottling, necrosis)
- benign, histiocytic, necrotizing lymphadenitis (Kikuchi–Fujimoto disease) (interfollicular, mottling, necrosis)
- sinus histiocytosis with massive lymphadenopathy (Rosai–Dorfman disease) (sinus)
- giant lymph node hyperplasia (Castleman disease) (mantle zone, hyaline vascular)
- Langerhans cell histiocytosis (sinus, interfollicular)
- human immunodeficiency virus (HIV) infection, early stage (follicular, sinus, mottling).

DISTINGUISHING BENIGN FROM MALIGNANT LYMPHOID PROLIFERATIONS

Benign and malignant lymphoid proliferations occur throughout the body at both nodal and extranodal sites and distinguishing between them is a common problem.

As indicated above, distinguishing benign from malignant lymphoid proliferations involves identification and recognition of the pathologic process(es), which includes determining what patterns are present, which compartments are abnormal or involved and whether or not the findings present and absent can be made to fit a specific diagnosis. For each pattern seen, there is a list of differential diagnoses, which includes specific benign and malignant lymphoid proliferations of different types.[21,36,37]

The histologic criteria that are used to distinguish nodal benign diseases that are distinct entities are well known and have been previously well described.

At extranodal sites, differentiating benign from malignant lymphoid proliferations is difficult for several reasons. First and most important, extranodal biopsy specimens are small, often superficial, contain fibroadipose and connective tissue, and are often crushed. Thus, it is easy to make an erroneous diagnosis. Second, at extranodal sites, the lymphoid infiltrates are not surrounded by a capsule, as seen in a lymph node. Third, specific benign lymphoid diseases that are encountered at extranodal sites usually do *not* occur in the lymph nodes, and have specific histologic criteria. Fourth, several specific, benign, non-infectious diseases that primarily involve the lymph node, rarely involve extranodal sites secondarily. Fifth, the normal mucosal extranodal lymphoid tissue (MALT) is found essentially in Peyer's patches and tonsils.[39] Otherwise, it is acquired lymphoid tissue that is secondary to antigenic stimulation, such as seen in the acquired MALT that occurs in the stomach, thyroid and salivary glands, for example. At extranodal sites such as the skin, lung, liver and gastrointestinal tract, non-neoplastic lymphoid infiltrates are more common than primary malignant lymphomas. However, many benign lymphoid diseases at these sites may closely resemble marginal zone B cell lymphomas of MALT type, and indeed in the past, many cases of this lymphoma were diagnosed as pseudo-lymphomas, because follicular hyperplasia is a hallmark of this lymphoma and admixed polyclonal plasmacytosis is common. Sixth, the incidence of various lymphomas at different extranodal sites varies considerably, and is different from those in the lymph nodes. Also, the immunophenotypic and molecular criteria may be different.

In general, the histologic features that strongly favor the diagnosis of typical examples of a nodal non-Hodgkin lymphoma are:

1. Complete obliteration of all sinuses, pericapsular infiltration, a diffuse pattern, and a markedly hypercellular proliferation of large nucleolated lymphoid cells. This is indicative of a large cell lymphoma. In very rare instances, acute infectious mononucleosis can also have this histologic appearance.
2. Similar to item 1, with almost all medium-sized lymphoid cells with multiple nucleoli, is diffuse small centroblastic lymphoma, i.e. a Burkitt lymphoma.
3. Same as item 2, but with medium-sized cells and a blastic chromatin structure, is suggestive of a lymphoblastic lymphoma or perhaps a blastic mantle cell lymphoma.
4. The presence of proliferation centers is indicative of small lymphocytic lymphoma.
5. Complete obliteration of sinuses, pericapsular infiltration, poorly defined follicles without mantle zones or with incomplete or thin mantle zones, and a back-to-back pattern of follicles would be indicative of a follicular lymphoma.

BOX 41.6: Lymphomas that may be mistaken for a benign proliferation and benign diseases that may be mistaken for lymphoma

(A) *Lymphomas that may be mistaken for a benign proliferation because they exhibit a predominant inflammatory component and few malignant cells*

- Hodgkin lymphoma, mixed cellularity type, showing extensive proliferation of epithelioid cells, Langhans and foreign-body giant cells (Hodgkin granuloma)
- Nodular lymphocyte-predominant Hodgkin lymphoma with exuberant proliferation of epithelioid cells and/or histiocytes
- Nodular lymphocyte-rich classical Hodgkin lymphoma
- Peripheral T cell lymphoma, Lennert variant
- Angioimmunoblastic T cell lymphoma with marked plasmacytosis, exuberant epithelioid cells, eosinophils and marked vascular proliferation
- Anaplastic large cell lymphoma, histiocyte and neutrophil-rich variant
- Marginal zone B cell lymphoma (nodal and extranodal) with follicular hyperplasia and polyclonal plasmacytosis
- Extranodal NK/T cell lymphoma with extensive necrosis, degeneration and inflammation
- T cell- and/or histiocyte-rich large B cell lymphoma
- Lymphomatoid granulomatosis

(B) *Benign diseases that may be mistaken for lymphoma because they show a prominent component of benign large cells*

- Florid infectious mononucleosis and other viral lymphadenitis
- Necrotizing lymphadenitis with florid large cell proliferation
- Kikuchi–Fujimoto disease, proliferative stage
- Autoimmune lymphoproliferative syndrome
- Human immunodeficiency virus (HIV) infection, early stage
- Multicentric Castleman disease with IgM-λ and human herpes virus 8 (HHV8)-positive plasmablasts
- Germinotropic lymphoproliferative disorder with HHV8-positive plasmablasts in HIV-negative patients

---

6. Complete obliteration of sinuses, prominent mantle zones, fusion of adjacent mantle zones and mantle cell nodules, as well as follicular colonization, would be indicative of a mantle cell lymphoma.

7. The presence of prominent marginal zone and/or an inverse follicular pattern produced by cells that have features of marginal zone B cells, which also produce follicular colonization, interfollicular and a sinus pattern, is typical of a marginal zone B cell lymphoma.

8. Interfollicular and sinusoid patterns and perivascular rosettes by large cells, some of which have features of hallmark cells, is indicative of an anaplastic large cell lymphoma.

In contrast, the architectural histologic features that generally favor the diagnosis of a benign disease are: the presence of scattered follicles, patent or partially preserved sinuses and no or mild pericapsular infiltration. The cytologic features that favor the diagnosis of a benign proliferation include: a heterogeneous cellular infiltration in interfollicular areas, including benign-appearing plasma cells, plasmacytoid cells and large cells, clusters of benign monocytoid B cells which may be seen in the sinuses, clusters of epithelioid cells, focal areas of necrosis, moderate vascular proliferation and low to moderate mitotic activity in between follicles.

In addition, the absence of any of the typical histologic features of the examples of lymphoma described above favor the diagnosis of a benign disease. Furthermore, the presence of typical histologic features found in the classical examples of specific benign diseases would enable the pathologist to make a diagnosis of specific benign diseases.

The majority of the above histologic criteria that are used for nodal diseases can also be used at extranodal sites. It should be stressed that many times there can be overlap in morphologic features between benign and malignant diseases. For example, florid infectious mononucleosis and a few other benign diseases may have a prominent benign large cell proliferation that can be readily mistaken for lymphoma (Box 41.6). Conversely, certain lymphomas such as Hodgkin and other lymphomas may have a prominent inflammatory component, which may be misinterpreted as a benign process (Box 41.6).

IMPORTANCE OF MORPHOLOGIC PATTERNS AND CYTOLOGIC FEATURES IN THE WHO CLASSIFICATION OF HODGKIN AND NON-HODGKIN LYMPHOMAS

General considerations

Acknowledging the importance and value of the advances of the preceding 25 years in the fields of flow cytometry, immunohistochemistry, cytogenetics, fluorescent *in situ*

Table 41.2 Correlation of frequency of distinctive patterns present in different types of lymphomas with overall incidence of these lymphomas and the terminology used in the World Health Organization (WHO) classification

Patterns of lymphomas		Lymphoma types	
Type	Frequency of association (percent)	WHO terminology	Incidence of lymphomas (percent)
Follicular	100	Follicular lymphoma	35[a]
Diffuse	100	Diffuse large B cell	30[a]
Nodular	100	Nodular lymphocyte-predominant Hodgkin lymphoma	5–10[b]
		Nodular lymphocyte-rich classical Hodgkin lymphoma	4[b]
Nodular sclerosing	100	Nodular sclerosing Hodgkin lymphoma	50[b]
Pseudofollicular (proliferation centers)	99	Small lymphocytic lymphoma/chronic lymphocytic leukemia	8[a]
Mantle zone	Overall 70	Mantle cell	8[a]
Mantle cell nodular			
Follicular colonization			
Marginal zone	Overall 90	Marginal zone	10[a]
Inverse follicular			
Follicular colonization			
Sinus			
Interfollicular			

[a]Percent of non-Hodgkin lymphoma.
[b]Percent of Hodgkin lymphoma.

hybridization and molecular genetics, the WHO published in 2001 the first worldwide consensus classification of malignant lymphomas.[38] This consensus opinion of nearly 100 international experts in the field stressed that 'there is no one gold standard'[55] for reaching a definitive diagnosis. This expert panel recommended an integrated approach to diagnosis, which utilizes clinical, morphologic, immunophenotypic and molecular information to reach an accurate final diagnosis. Moreover, in the introduction to the WHO classification,[55] Dr Nancy L Harris also stressed that it was *not* necessary to obtain information from all of these sources to make an accurate diagnosis, and she emphasized that 'morphology is always important, and some diseases are primarily defined by morphology'.

Specific examples

Histologic patterns represent the interaction of the underlying genetic profile, protein expression, signaling pathways, and trafficking of the malignant lymphoid cells and their associated host accessory/stromal cells, as well as the host immune response. As such, these patterns play a fundamental role in forming a differential diagnosis and often help in reaching a specific diagnosis. According to the WHO classification, the nomenclature of each lymphoma depends on the most useful information necessary to reach a final accurate diagnosis. Table 41.2 outlines in the WHO classification,[38] the frequency of the most commonly encountered patterns and the entities they are most commonly associated with.

NAMING OF LYMPHOMAS IN THE WHO CLASSIFICATION AFTER MORPHOLOGIC PATTERNS

The incidence of B cell lymphomas is much higher than that of T cell lymphomas, particularly in the Western world. Approximately 90 percent of B cell and Hodgkin lymphomas have characteristic architectural patterns that are reflected in their names as delineated below:

- Non-Hodgkin lymphomas:
  - Follicular lymphoma (follicular pattern)
  - Mantle cell lymphoma (mantle zone, mantle cell nodular, follicular colonization patterns)
  - Marginal zone lymphoma (marginal zone, inverse follicular, sinusoidal, interfollicular, and follicular colonization patterns)
  - Small lymphocytic lymphoma (pseudofollicular pattern/proliferation centers)
  - Diffuse large B cell lymphoma (diffuse pattern)
- Hodgkin lymphoma
  - Nodular lymphocyte-predominant Hodgkin lymphoma (nodular pattern)
  - Nodular lymphocyte-rich classical Hodgkin lymphoma (nodular pattern)
  - Nodular sclerosing Hodgkin lymphoma (fibrous nodular pattern)

NAMING OF LYMPHOMAS IN THE WHO CLASSIFICATION ACCORDING TO CYTOLOGIC FEATURES, WHICH OFTEN ALSO HAVE DISTINCTIVE MORPHOLOGIC PATTERNS

Although many lymphomas are named according to specific cytologic features, many of them also show distinctive patterns as delineated below:

- Non-Hodgkin lymphomas
  - Lymphoplasmacytic lymphoma (patent sinuses)
  - Lymphoblastic lymphoma (B or T) (interfollicular pattern, extensive pericapsular and vascular invasion, single file arrangement, crush artifact, starry sky)
  - Hairy cell leukemia (sinusoidal pattern, vascular lakes and pseudosinus formation)
  - Angioimmunoblastic T cell lymphoma (burnt out germinal centers, abnormal hyperplastic follicles, intra- and extravascular clusters of clear cells, marked vascular proliferation)
  - Anaplastic large cell lymphoma (sinus and interfollicular pattern)
  - Langerhans' cell histiocytosis (sinus and interfollicular patterns)
  - Mastocytosis (sinus and interfollicular patterns)
- Hodgkin lymphomas
  - Mixed cellularity Hodgkin lymphoma (interfollicular, mantle cell nodular, 'Lennert' patterns)
  - Lymphocyte-depleted Hodgkin lymphoma (diffuse pattern, fibrosis)

NAMING OF LYMPHOMAS IN THE WHO CLASSIFICATION ACCORDING TO EPONYMS

- Burkitt lymphoma (starry sky and diffuse patterns)
- Mycosis fungoides and Sézary syndrome (exocytosis, epidermotropism, Pautrier microabscesses, lichenoid band-like infiltrate in the upper dermis)

Correlation between morphologic patterns, immunohistochemistry and cytogenetics of lymphomas

That the distinctive histologic patterns described for the lymphomas listed above are real and valuable in diagnostic practice is underscored by the fact that immunohistochemical staining on such cases confirms and highlights the pattern(s) seen in histologic sections. Moreover, there is also an excellent correlation with the specific underlying recurrent balanced translocations, such as t(14;18) in follicular lymphoma, t(11;14) in mantle cell lymphoma, t(11;18) in MALT lymphoma, etc., which further underscore the fundamental value of accurately recognizing patterns.[56–58]

CORRELATION OF INTEROBSERVER REPRODUCIBILITY OF LYMPHOMAS WITH AND WITHOUT DISTINCTIVE PATTERNS WITH IMMUNOPHENOTYPING

Most B cell lymphomas with distinctive patterns can be classified on the basis of morphology alone[59] (Table 41.3), with minimal contribution of immunophenotypic analysis for confirmation or resolution of a differential diagnosis. Furthermore, Table 41.3 also shows that the contribution of immunophenotype analysis is considerably less in the case of lymphomas with distinctive histologic patterns than those that show distinctive cytologic features alone.[59] In other words, *cytologic features for certain diseases may be less specific than histologic patterns*.

IMPORTANCE OF CELL TYPING IN GRADING AND PROGNOSIS OF LYMPHOMAS

In the WHO classification, the cell type and grade of lymphoma are usually established by histologic examination alone or sometimes in conjunction with immunostains.[38]

As a general rule, in those lymphomas that are discrete disease entities, the most important histologic features that suggest aggressive clinical behavior are: (i) the presence of blastic/blastoid chromatin structure, (ii) the number of medium and large lymphoid cells with multiple distinct nucleoli and (iii) increased mitotic activity. For example, in mantle cell lymphoma, patients whose malignant mantle cells have round nuclei often have a relatively good prognosis. But blastic or blastoid forms of mantle cell lymphoma have the most aggressive natural history. The presence of a higher mitotic activity confers a poorer prognosis, which has been confirmed by gene expression profile studies.[5]

With reference to follicular lymphomas, they are graded on the basis of the number of small and large centroblasts into grades 1, 2, 3a and 3b. Grades 3a and 3b are separated on the basis of the proportion of large centroblasts and the presence or absence of centrocytes. However, the grading into 3a or 3b can also be done solely on the basis of the number of small centroblasts and absence of admixed centrocytes. In rare cases, follicular lymphomas with blastoid morphology have been reported and they have an aggressive natural history.

Marginal zone B cell lymphoma that shows transformed large cells (nucleolated cells) in clusters and/or islands have an aggressive natural history and were classified as transformation to a diffuse large B cell lymphoma.[60] Also, if the large cells did not form clusters and/or islands, but represented more than 6–20 percent of malignant cells, they had a more aggressive natural history than those with less than 6 percent large cells. Those that had more than 20 percent large cells were classified as progressed to a diffuse large B cell lymphoma. In addition, in marginal zone B cell lymphoma, patients whose marginal zone B-cells are proliferating as determined by the Ki-67 stain have a more aggressive natural history than those patients whose marginal zone

Table 41.3   Comparison of the value of immunophenotype analysis in lymphomas having distinctive patterns versus those with distinctive cytologic features

Consensus diagnosis of lymphoma	Diagnosis of lymphomas with distinctive patterns (percent)		
	Morphology alone	Morphology with immunophenotyping	Contribution of immunophenotyping
Follicular – overall	93	94	1
Follicular grade 1	72	73	1
Follicular grade 2	61	61	0
Follicular grade 3	60	61	1
Marginal zone B cell of MALT type	84	86	2
Small lymphocytic	84	87	3
Marginal zone nodal	55	63	8
Mantle cell	77	87	10
Diffuse large B cell	73	87	14
	Diagnosis of lymphomas with distinctive cytologic features (percent)		
Lymphoplasmacytoid	53	56	3
High-grade Burkitt-like	47	53	6
Primary mediastinal large B	51	58	7
Precursor T lymphoblastic	52	87	35
Anaplastic large T/null cell	46	85	39
Peripheral T cell, all types	41	86	45

B cells are generally not proliferating (K Muller-Hermelink, personal communication).

In a small lymphocytic lymphoma, increased numbers of prolymphocytes or transformed cells (>30 percent) outside the proliferation centers are associated with an aggressive clinical course. Transformation to blastic, Hodgkin or Hodgkin-like lymphoma is detected by histological examination. In chronic lymphocytic leukemia, the number of prolymphocytes seen in the smears (<10 percent, 10–55 percent, >55 percent) directly correlates with clinical behavior and prognosis. Also, blastic chromatin structure on the smears is associated with an aggressive natural history in CLL.

Peripheral T cell lymphoma, unspecified, with more than 70 percent large transformed cells had a poorer prognosis than those with less than 70 percent.[61] In other rare, specific types of peripheral T cell lymphoma disease entities, such as subcutaneous panniculitis-like T cell lymphoma and enteropathy-type T cell lymphoma, the greater the number of transformed medium- and large-sized cells, the more aggressive the natural history and poorer the prognosis.

In classical Hodgkin lymphoma, nodular sclerosis, grade 2, at least 20 percent of the nodules contain the Hodgkin cells in the form of multiple, confluent clusters and islands. Patients with these features have a more aggressive clinical course than those who do not have this histologic feature.[62]

RELATIVE MERITS OF INCISIONAL/ EXCISIONAL BIOPSIES VERSUS FINE NEEDLE BIOPSIES

As stated before, to form a proper histologic differential diagnosis requires identification of pathologic processes, which *necessitates* accurate detection of architectural distortions and recognition of architectural patterns. Thus, the amount of tissue sent to the pathologist for histologic review directly correlates with diagnostic accuracy. Therefore, the cliché, 'the more, the better', is most fitting.

In our daily practice, we recommend that whenever feasible, an excisional biopsy should be done. If the mass, lesion or lymph node is too large to be excised, a generous incisional biopsy should be performed and labeled as such. When ample tissue is sent to the histopathologist, it can be cryopreserved and/or distributed to the other laboratories for ancillary studies such as flow cytometry, cytogenetics and molecular studies.

Fine needle biopsies can be performed with a full understanding that the material submitted to the pathologist is 'minimal' and it may not be representative of the lesion and may be non-diagnostic. Also, the risk of an erroneous, incomplete, and/or misleading diagnosis is high in this setting.

Clinical indications of a fine needle aspiration biopsy are the presence of deep-seated masses such as those seen in the mediastinum and abdomen. A common problem with these specimens is that the biopsy material is scant and often contains fibrosclerosis and hyalinized tissue with crush artifacts, which further reduce the amount of 'diagnostic tissue' available to the pathologist for review. The biopsy procedure may also sample surrounding fatty and normal tissue, further compounding the diagnostic difficulty.

In the mediastinum, metastatic carcinomas, germ cell tumors and thymomas of different types are common, and Castleman disease has to always be kept in mind as an additional differential diagnosis. There is the possibility that the specimen could represent an infectious disease.

In our practice, unless the biopsy material has diagnostic information, we do not make an unequivocal diagnosis, but ask for an open biopsy specimen.

Fine needle aspiration smears have no architectural features or patterns and thus most lymphomas cannot be classified or accurately diagnosed. Cells in smears are dispersed and frequently their origin cannot be established with accuracy. In general, and with rare exceptions, in any new patient, if a diagnosis of lymphoma has been made on fine needle aspiration material, it is likely that there will be a high diagnostic error rate.[63]

A SUMMARY OF OUR SYSTEMATIC APPROACH TOWARDS ACCURATE HISTOLOGICAL DIAGNOSIS

Box 41.7 briefly summarizes our approach to accurate histologic diagnosis,[24] which is more extensively described elsewhere.[21,36,37,64]

To quote from our November 2007 review:[24]

In this era of cost containment, patients, physicians and insurers demand both cost-effective and accurate diagnoses. It is impossible to perform all tests on all patients. Therefore, a logical, well-defined, standardized and cost-effective approach to diagnosis becomes essential, in order to avoid an inefficient competition between advocates of morphology, immunophenotyping, genomics, proteomics and future technologies. Each of these modalities may provide diagnostic, therapeutic and prognostic information; however, the relative utility of each must be weighed carefully in choosing which tests to pursue in order to generate the most relevant clinical information.

Morphology is still the first and most important step towards establishing an accurate diagnosis, and it must be used appropriately and precisely. In the hands of well-trained histopathologists, careful morphologic evaluations as part of an integrative diagnostic approach can help reduce diagnostic errors.

Frequently, morphologic, clinical, immunologic and molecular information obtained may be in disagreement. To resolve any discordance, pathologists with in-depth knowledge and experience in the field must decide how to weigh criteria to arrive at the most accurate diagnosis.

BOX 41.7: Summary of our approach to forming a differential diagnosis

Methodical diagnostic approach
Prerequisites for making an accurate diagnosis:

- Optimal specimen (size, quality, accurate description of site, fixation, paraffinization, sectioning and staining)
- Adequate microscope (scanning lens, continuous rheostat to modulate light)
- Adequate time allotted for detailed review

Knowledge prerequisites:

- Uniqueness of lymph node and migration of cells between compartments
- Familiarity with histological spectrum (normal, benign diseases, lymphomas)
- Specific criteria for each disease

Recognition of pathologic processes
Low magnification appearance of pathologic processes
Methods for identifying pathologic processes:

- Sequential examination of each compartment
- Recognizing cell types in each compartment based on colors, e.g. plasma cells (purple), small lymphocytes (dark blue) and eosinophils (brick red), etc.
- Comparing similar compartments with each other
- Comparing adjacent compartments with each other
- Assessing cellularity of various compartments (hyper-, normo-, hypocellularity)
- Recognizing patterns accurately:
  ○ Diagnostic/prognostic importance of patterns
  ○ Methods for distinguishing patterns
  ○ Difficulties in identifying similar, multiple and subtle patterns

Formulating a differential diagnosis
Integrated diagnosis

- Clinical correlation
- Immunostains
- Flow cytometry
- Cytogenetic/molecular techniques

We end this chapter on the art of making a histologic diagnosis by using a quote that we often use in our teaching activities:[21,36]

Making an accurate histologic diagnosis correlates directly with experience. The more we know, the more we see, and the more we see the more we know. In other words, we don't know what we don't know, and we see (recognize) only what we know. Also, what we see is influenced by our training criteria, our concepts and methods we use in our diagnostic practice.

KEY POINTS

- Lymphoid infiltrates occur at every site in the human body.
- Extranodal lymphomas comprise about 40 percent of the malignant lymphomas.
- Benign lymphoid infiltrates are more common at extranodal sites such as the skin, gastrointestinal tract, lungs and liver, than malignant lymphomas at these sites. These benign infiltrates may be specific benign diseases or they may be non-specific infiltrates and they may have to be distinguished histologically and immuno-histochemically from malignant lymphomas occurring at these sites.
- In any given new patient who is subjected to biopsy, a precise histologic diagnosis is necessary because it dictates the additional strategies that have to be used to reach a definite diagnosis, which may include immunohistochemical studies, flow cytometry or molecular studies. Lymphoma 'chips' will be available soon for diagnostic use, though their precise role will have to be established.
- In the meantime, it should be recognized that making a histologic diagnosis is an art and not a science, and to become proficient in this art requires extensive training and experience.
- Every attempt should be made to obtain as large a biopsy specimen as possible and it should be properly cut, fixed, processed and stained to avoid diagnostic errors.
- H&E-stained slides must be carefully reviewed at low magnification to study colors, architectural features and patterns that permit formation of a proper differential diagnosis, which in turn dictates to the pathologist what next to do at high magnification to further refine the differential diagnosis.
- This iterative process from low to high magnification permits the pathologist to reach a diagnosis, which should not be rendered unless careful clinical correlation has been made.
- If immunohistochemical studies are ordered, they should be done for the purpose of resolving a differential diagnosis rather than ordering large panels, because of the lack of specificity and sensitivity associated with them.
- In summary, we strongly urge the pathologists to continue to follow the integrative approach to diagnosis recommended in the WHO Classification.

REFERENCES

- ● = Key primary paper
- ◆ = Major review article

●1. Alizadeh A, Eisen M, Davis RE et al. The lymphochip: a specialized cDNA microarray for the genomic-scale analysis of gene expression in normal and malignant lymphocytes. Cold Spring Harb Symp Quant Biol 1999; 64: 71–8.

2. Alizadeh AA, Eisen MB, Davis RE et al. Distinct types of diffuse large B-cell lymphoma identified by gene expression profiling. Nature 2000; 403: 503–11.

●3. Rosenwald A, Wright G, Chan WC et al. The use of molecular profiling to predict survival after chemotherapy for diffuse large-B-cell lymphoma. N Engl J Med 2002; 346: 1937–47.

●4. Rosenwald A, Wright G, Leroy K et al. Molecular diagnosis of primary mediastinal B cell lymphoma identifies a clinically favorable subgroup of diffuse large B cell lymphoma related to Hodgkin lymphoma. J Exp Med 2003; 198: 851–62.

5. Rosenwald A, Wright G, Wiestner A et al. The proliferation gene expression signature is a quantitative integrator of oncogenic events that predicts survival in mantle cell lymphoma. Cancer Cell 2003; 3: 185–97.

6. Savage KJ, Monti S, Kutok JL et al. The molecular signature of mediastinal large B-cell lymphoma differs from that of other diffuse large B-cell lymphomas and shares features with classical Hodgkin lymphoma. Blood 2003; 102: 3871–9.

7. Tzankov A, Zimpfer A, Pehrs AC et al. Expression of B-cell markers in classical Hodgkin lymphoma: a tissue microarray analysis of 330 cases. Mod Pathol 2003; 16: 1141–7.

◆8. Chan WC, Fu K. Molecular diagnostics on lymphoid malignancies. Arch Pathol Lab Med 2004; 128: 1379–84.

●9. Thieblemont C, Nasser V, Felman P et al. Small lymphocytic lymphoma, marginal zone B-cell lymphoma, and mantle cell lymphoma exhibit distinct gene-expression profiles allowing molecular diagnosis. Blood 2004; 103: 2727–37.

10. Dybkaer K, Iqbal J, Zhou G, Chan WC. Molecular diagnosis and outcome prediction in diffuse large B-cell lymphoma and other subtypes of lymphoma. Clin Lymphoma 2004; 5: 19–28.

●11. Dave SS, Wright G, Tan B et al. Prediction of survival in follicular lymphoma based on molecular features of tumor-infiltrating immune cells. N Engl J Med 2004; 351: 2159–69.

12. Schmechel SC, LeVasseur RJ, Yang KH et al. Identification of genes whose expression patterns differ in benign lymphoid tissue and follicular, mantle cell, and small lymphocytic lymphoma. Leukemia 2004; 18: 841–55.

●13. Staudt LM, Dave S. The biology of human lymphoid malignancies revealed by gene expression profiling. Adv Immunol 2005; 87: 163–208.

●14. Monti S, Savage KJ, Kutok JL et al. Molecular profiling of diffuse large B-cell lymphoma identifies robust subtypes including one characterized by host inflammatory response. *Blood* 2005; **105**: 1851–61.

15. Rubio-Moscardo F, Climent J, Siebert R *et al.* Mantle-cell lymphoma genotypes identified with CGH to BAC microarrays define a leukemic subgroup of disease and predict patient outcome. *Blood* 2005; **105**: 4445–54.

16. Thompson MA, Stumph J, Henrickson SE *et al.* Differential gene expression in anaplastic lymphoma kinase-positive and anaplastic lymphoma kinase-negative anaplastic large cell lymphomas. *Hum Pathol* 2005; **36**: 494–504.

●17. Fu K, Weisenburger DD, Greiner TC *et al.* Cyclin D1-negative mantle cell lymphoma: a clinicopathologic study based on gene expression profiling. *Blood* 2005; **106**: 4315–21.

●18. Dave SS, Fu K, Wright GW *et al.* Molecular diagnosis of Burkitt's lymphoma. *N Engl J Med* 2006; **354**: 2431–42.

19. Hummel M, Bentink S, Berger H *et al.* A biologic definition of Burkitt's lymphoma from transcriptional and genomic profiling. *N Engl J Med* 2006; **354**: 2419–30.

20. Harris NL, Horning SJ. Burkitt's lymphoma – the message from microarrays. *N Engl J Med* 2006; **354**: 2495–8.

◆21. Nathwani BN, Hernandez AM, Drachenberg MR. Diagnostic significance of morphologic patterns of lymphoid proliferations in lymph nodes. In: Knowles DM (ed.) *Neoplastic hematopathology*, 2nd ed. Philadelphia: Lippincott Williams and Wilkins, 2001: 507–36.

22. Metter GE, Nathwani BN, Burke JS *et al.* Morphological subclassification of follicular lymphoma: variability of diagnoses among hematopathologists, a collaborative study between the repository center and pathology panel for lymphoma clinical studies. *J Clin Oncol* 1985; **3**: 25–38.

23. Nathwani BN, Metter GE, Miller TP *et al.* What should be the morphologic criteria for the subdivision of follicular lymphomas? *Blood* 1986; **68**: 837–45.

◆24. Nathwani BN, Sasu SJ, Ahsanuddin AN *et al.* The critical role of histology in an era of genomics and proteomics: a commentary and reflection. *Adv Anat Pathol* 2007; **14**: 375–400.

25. Horvitz EJ, Heckerman DE, Nathwani BN, Fagan LM. Diagnostic strategies in the hypothesis-directed pathfinder system. *IEEE Computer Society Press* 1984: 630–6.

26. Horvitz EJ, Heckerman DE, Nathwani BN, Fagan LM. The use of a heuristic problem-solving hierarchy to facilitate the explanation of hypothesis-directed reasoning. In: Salamon R, Blum B, Jorgense M (eds) *MEDINFO 86*. North-Holland: Elsevier Science, 1986: 27–31.

27. Nathwani BN, Heckerman DE, Horvitz EJ, Fagan LM. *The pathfinder project: computer-aided diagnosis of lymph node diseases. The International Colloquium on Lymphoid Malignancy*. Philadelphia: Field and Wood, 1989: 81–7.

28. Horvitz EJ, Heckerman DE, Ng KC, Nathwani BN. Heuristic abstraction in the decision-theoretic pathfinder system. *IEEE Computer Society Press* 1989: 178–82.

◆29. Nathwani BN, Heckerman DE, Horvitz EJ, Lincoln TL. Integrated expert systems and videodisc in surgical pathology: an overview. *Hum Pathol* 1990; **21**: 11–27.

30. Heckerman DE, Horvitz EJ, Nathwani BN. *Toward normative expert systems: part I of the pathfinder project. Methods of information in medicine*. Stuttgart: Schattauer, 1992.

31. Heckerman DE, Nathwani BN. An evaluation of the diagnostic accuracy of pathfinder. *Comput Biomed Res* 1992; **25**: 56–74.

32. Heckerman DE, Nathwani BN. *Toward normative expert systems: part II probability-based representations for efficient knowledge acquisition and inference. Methods of information in medicine*. Stuttgart: Schattauer, 1992.

●33. Nathwani BN, Clarke K, Lincoln T *et al.* Evaluation of an expert system on lymph node pathology. *Hum Pathol* 1997; **28**: 1097–110.

34. Bowling MC. Lymph node specimens: achieving technical excellence. *Lab Med* 1979; **10**: 467–76.

●35. Beard C, Nabers K, Bowling MC. Achieving technical excellence in lymph node specimens: an update. *Lab Med* 1985; **16**: 468–75.

36. Nathwani BN. Diagnostic significance of morphologic patterns in lymph node proliferations. In: Knowles DM (ed.) *Neoplastic hematopathology*, 1st ed. Baltimore: Williams and Wilkins, 1992: 407–25.

37. Nathwani BN, Burke JS, Winberg CD. Architectural features of normal, neoplastic, and non-neoplastic lymph nodes: a practical diagnostic approach. In: Murphy FG, Mihm MC Jr (eds) *Lymphoproliferative disorders of the skin*. Boston: Butterworths, 1986: 73–119.

38. Jaffe ES, Harris NL, Stein H, Vardiman JW (eds) *World Health Organization classification of tumours. Pathology and genetics of tumours of haematopoietic and lymphoid tissues*. Lyon: IARC Press, 2001.

●39. Isaacson P, Wright DH. Malignant lymphoma of mucosa-associated lymphoid tissue. A distinctive type of B-cell lymphoma. *Cancer* 1983; **52**: 1410–16.

40. Isaacson PG, Wotherspoon AC, Diss T, Pan LX. Follicular colonization in B-cell lymphoma of mucosa-associated lymphoid tissue. *Am J Surg Pathol* 1991; **15**: 819–28.

41. Hernandez AM, Nathwani BN, Nguyen D *et al.* Nodal benign and malignant monocytoid B cells with and without follicular lymphomas: a comparative study of follicular colonization, light chain restriction, bcl-2, and t(14;18) in 39 cases. *Hum Pathol* 1995; **26**: 625–32.

42. Frizzera G, Moran EM, Rappaport H. Angio-immunoblastic lymphadenopathy. Diagnosis and clinical course. *Am J Med* 1975; **59**: 803–18.

43. Frizzera G, Moran EM, Rappaport H. Angio-immunoblastic lymphadenopathy with dysproteinaemia. *Lancet* 1974; **1**: 1070–3.

44. Lukes RJ, Tindle BH. Immunoblastic lymphadenopathy. A hyperimmune entity resembling Hodgkin's disease. *N Engl J Med* 1975; **292**: 1–8.

45. Nathwani BN, Rappaport H, Moran EM *et al.* Malignant lymphoma arising in angioimmunoblastic lymphadenopathy. *Cancer* 1978; **41**: 578–606.

46. Scott RB, Robb-Smith AHT. Histiocytic medullary reticulosis. *Lancet* 1939; **2**: 194–8.

47. Harris NL, Jaffe ES, Stein H *et al*. A revised European-American classification of lymphoid neoplasms: a proposal from the International Lymphoma Study Group. *Blood* 1994; **84**: 1361–92.

48. Stein H. Hodgkin lymphomas: introduction. In: Jaffe ES, Harris NL, Stein H, Vardiman JW (eds) *World Health Organization classification of tumours: pathology and genetics of tumours of haematopoietic and lymphoid tissues.* Lyon: IARC Press, 2001: 239.

49. Harris NL. Mature B-cell neoplasms: introduction. In: Jaffe ES, Harris NL, Stein H, Vardiman JW (eds) *World Health Organization classification of tumours: pathology and genetics of tumours of haematopoietic and lymphoid tissues.* Lyon: IARC Press, 2001: 121–6.

50. Jaffe ES, Ralfkiaer E. Mature T-cell and NK-cell neoplasms: introduction. In: Jaffe ES, Harris NL, Stein H, Vardiman JW (eds) *World Health Organization classification of tumours: pathology and genetics of tumours of haematopoietic and lymphoid tissues.* Lyon: IARC Press, 2001: 191–4.

●51. Kuppers R. Prognosis in follicular lymphoma – it's in the microenvironment. *N Engl J Med* 2004; **351**: 2152–3.

●52. Zhou J, Mauerer K, Farina L, Gribben JG. The role of the tumor microenvironment in hematological malignancies and implication for therapy. *Front Biosci* 2005; **10**: 1581–96.

53. Liotta LA, Kohn EC. The microenvironment of the tumour-host interface. *Nature* 2001; **411**: 375–9.

●54. de Jong D. Molecular pathogenesis of follicular lymphoma: a cross talk of genetic and immunologic factors. *J Clin Oncol* 2005; **23**: 6358–63.

55. Harris NL, Jaffe ES, Vardiman JW *et al*. WHO classification of tumours of haematopoietic and lymphoid tissues: introduction. In: Jaffe ES, Harris NL, Stein H, Vardiman JW (eds) *World Health Organization classification of tumours: pathology and genetics of tumours of* *haematopoietic and lymphoid tissues.* Lyon: IARC Press, 2001: 12–13.

56. Campo E, Raffeld M, Jaffe ES. Mantle-cell lymphoma. *Semin Hematol* 1999; **36**: 115–27.

◆57. Isaacson PG, Du MQ. Gastrointestinal lymphoma: where morphology meets molecular biology. *J Pathol* 2005; **205**: 255–74.

58. Zha H, Raffeld M, Charboneau L *et al*. Similarities of prosurvival signals in Bcl-2-positive and Bcl-2-negative follicular lymphomas identified by reverse phase protein microarray. *Lab Invest* 2004; **84**: 235–44.

59. A clinical evaluation of the international lymphoma study group classification of non-Hodgkin's lymphoma. The non-Hodgkin's lymphoma classification project. *Blood* 1997; **89**: 3909–18.

60. Nathwani BN, Drachenberg MR, Anderson JR *et al*. Prognostic factors in marginal zone B-cell lymphoma, extranodal, mucosa-associated lymphoid tissue (MALT) type. Leiden: European Society for Haematopathology, 1998 (abstract).

61. Weisenburger DD, Armitage JO, Vose JM. Peripheral T-cell lymphoma, not otherwise specified: a clinicopathologic study of 340 cases from the International T-cell Project. *Ann Oncol* 2008; **19** (Suppl 4): abstract 113.

●62. MacLennan KA, Bennett MH, Vaughan HB, Vaughan HG. Diagnosis and grading of nodular sclerosing Hodgkin's disease: a study of 2190 patients. *Int Rev Exp Pathol* 1992; **33**: 27–51.

●63. Hehn ST, Grogan TM, Miller TP. Utility of fine-needle aspiration as a diagnostic technique in lymphoma. *J Clin Oncol* 2004; **22**: 3046–52.

64. Nathwani BN. Classifying non-Hodgkin's lymphomas. In: Berard CW, Dorfman RF, Kaufman N (eds) *Malignant lymphoma*, 1st ed. Baltimore: Williams and Wilkins, 1987: 18–80.

42

Immunophenotyping as a diagnostic and prognostic tool

E MATUTES

INTRODUCTION

There have been significant advances in the immunophenotypic characterization of lymphoid neoplasms and this, in turn, has resulted in a better understanding of the normal lymphoid differentiation and maturation. Essentially, lymphoid neoplasms derive from B and T lymphocytes at various stages of maturation or activation. The immunophenotypic profile in most of these malignancies, to some extent, mimics that of the corresponding normal lymphoid counterpart albeit with some deviations which, at present, are not fully understood. In addition, although major efforts have been undertaken to identify the cell origin and/or the stage of differentiation of the neoplastic cell in the various lymphomas, it is apparent that there is heterogeneity within a disease when considering molecular features such as immunoglobulin heavy chain (*IGHV*) gene somatic mutations and gene profile expression. This has made it difficult to assign the neoplastic cell to a normal cell counterpart.

The application of new immunologic techniques has had a major impact not only on the diagnosis of chronic lymphoid leukemias and lymphomas but also has provided insights into their pathogenesis and proved to be relevant for the detection of small numbers of residual leukemia or lymphoma cells. Further to the diagnostic role of the immunologic markers, the expression of certain molecules

has been shown to have a prognostic impact. In addition, some chimeric monoclonal antibodies (MAbs) such as those recognizing the CD20, CD25 and CD52 antigens are used 'in vivo' as therapeutic tools and thus, their detection in the neoplastic cells is a relevant clinical issue.

In parallel to the development and refinement of the immunologic methods, there has been an increasing number of MAbs that identify antigens in lymphoid cells; these recognize molecules that are expressed either in most B and T cells regardless of the stage of differentiation, or their expression is restricted to a certain level of maturation and/or linked to cell activation.

Broadly, currently two approaches are applied to the immunophenotyping of lymphoid neoplasms: flow cytometry on cell suspensions and immunohistochemistry (IHC) on paraffin-embedded tissue. These techniques should be considered complementary. For instance, in cases presenting with a frank leukemic picture, whether primary leukemias or lymphomas in leukemic phase, flow cytometry analysis of the circulating neoplastic cells will provide useful information. Immunohistochemistry on bone marrow trephine biopsy sections and in the lymphoid tissues affected will provide additional relevant information. Indeed, the latter is a key investigation in patients with lymphomas, whether or not they present with leukemia.

Although the diagnostic role of immunophenotyping by flow cytometry or IHC is well recognized in lymphoid malignancies, results should always be combined with clinical features, cell morphology, histology on hematoxylin–eosin-stained sections and other relevant laboratory information such as molecular genetics.

This chapter focuses on the value and use of flow cytometry and IHC as diagnostic tools in lymphoid neoplasms together with the prognostic impact of these assays in patients with lymphoid malignancies and briefly reviews the principles and methodology of both these techniques. The following will be described:

- basic principles and general guidelines of the methodologies used for immunophenotyping in cell suspensions and tissue sections
- panels of MAbs useful for disease classification, the immunophenotypic profiles characteristic of the various lymphoid neoplasms and strategies for detecting small numbers of residual malignant cells (minimal residual disease)
- prognostic value of the immunophenotyping.

METHODOLOGY

Flow cytometry

Flow cytometry is a method that allows detection of antigens in cells in suspension. The principle of flow cytometry is that cells or particles, once labeled with a fluorochrome, flow in a fluid stream through a laser light beam and the light scattering and color fluorescence is measured. Essentially, flow cytometry differentiates cells on the basis of size, granularity and whether they carry fluorescent molecules.[1]

At present it is possible to:

- detect both, membrane and intracellular (cytoplasmic or nuclear) antigens, the latter in cells which have been fixed and stabilized with suitable reagents.[2,3] This is relevant when considering that some molecules are only expressed in the cytoplasm or in the nucleus but not in the membrane of the lymphocytes. Examples include the detection of cytoplasmic Ig, of light chains in multiple myeloma or plasma cell dyscrasias and of the nuclear enzyme TdT, a key test to distinguish lymphoblastic lymphomas from mature lymphoid neoplasms
- analyze whole blood or bone marrow specimens without requiring the isolation of mononuclear cells
- quantify precisely the number of antigens/molecules expressed at a single cell level.[4,5] This may also be useful for minimal residual disease (MRD) detection. In addition to this, the availability of new fluorochrome dyes and advances in the hardware and software have resulted in the routine use of multicolor and multiparametric flow cytometry allowing more accurate measurements of MRD and detection of certain molecules that are not expressed in non-neoplastic mature B cells such as ZAP70.

Specimens suitable for flow cytometry analysis are peripheral blood, bone marrow, body fluids such as pleural or cerebrospinal fluid and tissue cells obtained from fine needle aspirates. In addition, tissue samples (e.g. lymph node, spleen) can also be analyzed by flow cytometry once the tissue is placed in culture medium and finely minced to release the cells to be analyzed into the medium. Analysis of lymphoid tissues by flow cytometry complements, but should not replace, that of tissue sections by IHC. Regarding sample storage and transportation, it should be noted that cell viability in the specimen needs to be optimal at the time of processing. Ideally the sample should be processed within 24 hours, particularly when dealing with body fluids.

Flow cytometry analysis is carried out on isolated mononuclear cells or in whole blood and bone marrow specimens after treatment with lysing solutions. The latter are hypotonic erythrocyte lysing reagents which are commercially available. The time of incubation with the lysing reagent is important as prolonged exposure may influence the forward and side light scatter (FSC/SSC) patterns while a brief exposure may leave red cells in the medium and result in excess debris and inaccurate results.

Immunophenotyping for detection of membrane antigens is performed on unfixed viable cells while the cells should be previously fixed and stabilized for the detection of cytoplasmic and nuclear antigens. There are several commercially available kits that contain two solutions: the fixing agent based on a paraformaldehyde solution and the stabilizing agent based on a combination of a lysing solution and a detergent to fix and stabilize cells to detect the cytoplasmic and/or nuclear antigens. Overall, these reagents have little effect on the light scatter pattern although their reliability and consistency for detecting a particular nuclear and cytoplasmic antigen may vary.[2,3,6]

Whether the assay is aimed at detection of membrane or intracellular antigens, a direct immunofluoresence method with a fluorochrome conjugated MAb is the standard technique. It is also possible to assess the expression of several antigens, both membrane and intracellular, simultaneously. In such a case, the first step will involve immunostaining for detecting the membrane antigen on unfixed cells and this will be followed by cytoplasmic or nuclear antigen staining.[6]

Immunohistochemistry

In the early 1980s, detection of antigens in tissue sections was only possible in frozen material as the number of antibodies which could be applied to paraffin-embedded sections was very limited. Thus, interpretation of the findings was often difficult due to the poor morphologic preservation in the frozen sections. However, in the 1990s, a large panel of MAb suitable for use on fixed paraffin-embedded material became available and are now applied in a routine practice. As in flow cytometry, it is important in IHC to take into account a number of technical considerations to avoid pitfalls. In order to have antigen preservation, the tissues require optimal processing, particularly in regard to the fixation conditions such as the type of fixative, usually formalin based or B5, and the length of fixation. B5-fixed tissue results in good preservation of cytoplasmic and membrane antigens while it is not optimal for the detection of nuclear antigens. In addition, detection of some antigens may require a prior step that it is called 'antigen retrieval'. This is a method that allows unmasking of antigens bound by formaldehyde fixation. Antigen retrieval can be achieved by protein digestion with various enzymes, e.g. trypsin, pepsin or proteases and heating in a warm bath, microwave or autoclave.

The most commonly used immunohistochemical methods are indirect techniques with unconjugated MAbs and an immunoperoxidase or alkaline phosphatase anti-alkaline phosphatase (APAAP) method using peroxidase or alkaline phosphatase, respectively, as substrates. The reaction is visualized by the appropiate chromogen such as diaminobenzidine (DBA) for peroxidase. Among others, the ABC (avidin-biotin-conjugate) and the APAAP are the most frequently used.[7,8]

Interpretation of the results, as in flow cytometry, needs to be done in the light of the morphology and histology on the corresponding hematoxylin–eosin-stained sections.

MONOCLONAL ANTIBODY PANELS AND IMMUNOLOGIC PROFILES IN LYMPHOID DISORDERS

A relatively large number of MAbs can be routinely used in both flow cytometry and IHC. However, some of these reagents are informative and/or only give reliable results when investigated by one or other of these methods. This is due to the fact that some molecules, such as the antigen recognized by the MAb FMC7 or CD103 can only be detected by flow cytometry but not on paraffin-embedded sections, whereas others such as CD30 (Ki-1), ALK, BCL6 or CD21 (detects follicular dendritic cells and B cells), will give useful information in tissue sections by IHC. For this reason the panels which are useful in the flow cytometry and IHC settings for the diagnosis and classification of lymphoid malignancies will be described separately and the characteristic immunologic profiles of the various malignancies outlined.

Flow cytometry

LYMPHOID NEOPLASMS OF PRECURSOR LYMPHOID CELLS

The panel of MAbs should be tailored according to whether a diagnosis of a precursor lymphoid neoplasm or a mature lymphoid neoplasm is suspected. In the first instance, the set of MAbs to be used is that applied for the diagnosis of acute leukemias recommended by the European Group of Immunologic Classification of Leukemias (EGIL).[9]

Table 42.1 Classification of acute lymphoblastic leukemias/lymphoblastic lymphomas (ALL)

B cell lineage	TdT+, CD19+ and/or CD79a+ and/or CD22+
Pro-B-ALL	CD10−, cytoplasmic IgM−, SmIg−
Common ALL	CD10+, cytoplasmic IgM−, SmIg−
Pre-B-ALL	Cytoplasmic IgM+
T cell lineage	TdT+, CD7+, cytoplasmic CD3+
Pro-T-ALL	CD2−, CD5−, CD4−, CD8−, CD1a−
Pre-T-ALL	CD2+ and/or CD5+ and/or CD8+, CD1a−
Cortical T-ALL	CD1a+, membrane CD3−
Mature T-ALL	Membrane CD3+, CD1a−

TdT, terminal deoxynucleotidyl transferase; SmIg, surface immunoglobulin.

This is primarily addressed to distinguish acute lymphoblastic leukemias/lymphoblastic lymphomas (ALL/LbLy) from acute myeloid leukemias, to differentiate B from T cell precursor ALL and define the level of differentiation of the neoplastic cell. This panel comprises MAb that detect antigens in B cell precursors (CD19, CD10, cytoplasmic CD79a and CD22), T lymphoid precursors (CD2, CD7, cytoplasmic CD3), myeloid cells (CD13, CD33, anti-MPO and CD117) and precursor cells (TdT, CD34). Additional MAb may be tested according to whether the results with the above set of markers are indicative of a B cell derived, T cell derived or acute myeloid leukemia. A number of considerations need to be taken into account as follows:

- the great majority of ALL/LbLy will express TdT in the nucleus and hence this marker is essential and should be used to distinguish them from mature lymphoid neoplasms
- close to a third of the ALL/LbLy cases may be positive with myeloid associated but not specific markers such as CD13 and CD33. These cases are designated myeloid antigen positive (My+) ALL and should be distinguished from biphenotypic acute leukemias
- CD10 and CD79a, both of them B cell markers, may be weakly expressed in T cell lineage ALL/LbLy.

Table 42.1 summarizes the characteristic immunophenotypic profiles in B and T cell lineage ALL according to the EGIL and the World Health Organization (WHO).

LYMPHOID NEOPLASMS OF MATURE LYMPHOID CELLS

On a routine basis, the diagnosis of a leukemic mature B or T cell neoplasm requires a small panel of MAbs. From the practical point of view, it is recommended to apply a two-step procedure with the first panel of MAb applicable to all cases.[10,11] The rationale behind this is that the most common mature/chronic lymphoid neoplasm evolving with leukemia is chronic lymphocytic leukemia (CLL). A second panel may then be used and this will be tailored

Table 42.2 Panel of monoclonal antibodies for the diagnosis of lymphoid disorders

	B cell	T cell
First line	SmIg (κ/λ), CD19, CD20, CD23, FMC7, mCD79b, mCD22, CD5[a]	CD2 or CD3
Second line	CD11c, CD25, CD103, CD123, CD38, CD138, cytIg	CD3, anti-TCR β/γ, CD4, CD7, CD8, CD25, NK markers,[b] KIRs

[a]Expressed also on T cells.
[b]NK (natural killer) associated markers, CD16, CD56, CD57 and CD11b.
CyIg, cytoplasmic immunoglobulin; SmIg, surface immunoglobulin; KIR, killer immunoglobulin receptor.

Table 42.3 Scoring system for the diagnosis of chronic lymphocytic leukemia[a]

Marker	Points	
	1	0
CD5	Positive	Negative
CD23	Positive	Negative
FMC7	Negative	Positive
SmIg[b]	Weak	Moderate/strong
CD22/CD79b[b]	Weak	Moderate/strong

[a]Scores range from 0 to 5 (score $\geq$ 3, typical of CLL; score $<$ 3 typical of other B cell disorders).
[b]Membrane expression.
SmIg, surface immunoglobulin.

on the basis of the results with the first panel and the suspected diagnosis by the clinical manifestations and/or cell morphology (Table 42.2).

The first panel of markers is used to:

- distinguish B from T cell lymphoid disorders and to demonstrate clonality by Ig light chain restriction in the case of B cell disorders
- confirm or establish the diagnosis of CLL
- rule out diagnosis of another B cell neoplasm.

This first panel of markers comprises:

- MAb against the Ig light chains (anti-κ and anti-λ)
- CD2 or CD3, two T cell markers expressed in most normal and leukemic mature T lymphocytes, to exclude T cell diseases
- CD5, a MAb positive in T cells and in a small fraction of normal B cells involved in autoimmunity and characteristically, but not exclusively, expressed in certain B cell neoplasms such as CLL and mantle cell lymphomas (MCL)
- a set of MAbs that detect antigens in B cell subsets or are pan-B cell markers that are differentially expressed in B cell disorders. This last set of markers comprises MAb against CD22, CD23, FMC7 and CD79b, the latter identifying a component (the β chain) of the B cell receptor.

B CELL NEOPLASMS

When analyzing the expression of certain antigens and in order to be able to differentiate CLL from other B cell malignancies, it is important to estimate the fluorescence intensity and not only the proportion of positive cells. This is the case for surface Ig (SmIg), CD22 and CD79b. Cells in CLL express these three antigens weakly at the cell surface or may even lack expression of CD79b and CD22, whereas all these antigens are strongly expressed in cells from the other B cell neoplasms.[12,13] Although no single marker is specific for CLL, when the results obtained with the first

line panel of MAbs are combined into a scoring system (Table 42.3)[14–16] this makes it possible to establish the diagnosis of CLL, including cases in which the morphology is atypical, such as those with increased numbers of prolymphocytes (CLL/PL) and lymphoplasmacytic/cleaved cells (atypical CLL), and to exclude the diagnosis of other B cell neoplasms such as B cell prolymphocytic leukemia (B-PLL) and B cell lymphomas in leukemic phase (Fig. 42.1). The immunologic profile typical of CLL is: weak expression of SmIg, CD5+, CD23+, FMC7– and weak or negative CD79b and CD22 (Table 42.3).[16] Since FMC7 has been shown to recognize an epitope of the CD20 multimeric complex, it had been suggested that this MAb could be replaced by CD20 in the diagnostic scoring system for CLL. However, our data show that substitution of FMC7 by CD20 results in a significant decrease in the sensitivity of the diagnostic score as most CLL cases express weak CD20 unlike FMC7, which is weakly positive in less than 20 percent of CLL.[17] Nevertheless, although CD20 is not a useful discriminatory marker, it needs to be included into the panel of markers for the study of chronic/mature lymphoid disorders as it is increasingly used as a therapeutical tool in the management of patients with these neoplasms.

When results with the first line panel of markers indicate a clonal B cell with a phenotype which is not typical of CLL (scores $<$ 3), a second step applying other markers is needed for diagnostic purposes. This panel should be tailored in the light of the clinical features, morphology of the circulating lymphocytes or bone marrow infiltrating cells, and/or some other laboratory features[6,10] (Table 42.2). For example, in B cell disorders with circulating villous or 'hairy' lymphocytes, estimation of the cell reactivity with MAbs that are expressed in activated normal B cells and/or at late stages of differentiation should be carried out in order to establish a precise diagnosis. These markers include MAb against CD11c, CD25 (anti-α chain of the interleukin (IL)-2 receptor), CD103, HC2 and CD123 (anti-β chain of the IL-3 receptor). When applying this combination of markers it is possible to distinguish hairy cell leukemia (HCL) from the other two conditions with circulating villous cells which

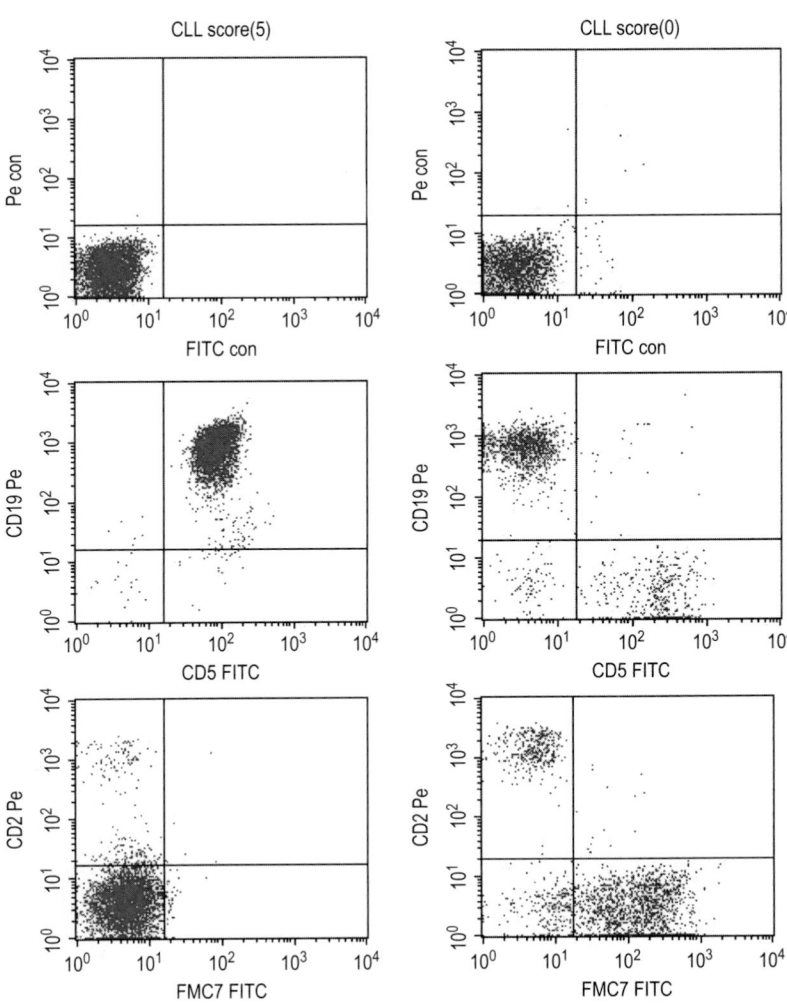

Figure 42.1 Flow cytometry dot plots on a case of chronic lymphocytic leukemia (CLL; left) and a follicular lymphoma in leukemic phase (right). The figures on the left illustrate that the majority of CLL cells are CD19/CD5 positive, express CD23, are weakly positive with anti-Ig λ, CD79b and CD20 while they are negative with FMC7 and CD22 (CLL score 5). The figures on the right show that most follicular lymphoma cells are CD19+, FMC7+, express with strong intensity Ig λ chain, CD79b and CD20 while they are CD5 and CD23 negative (CLL score 0).

may be misdiagnosed as HCL namely, splenic lymphoma with villous lymphocytes (SLVL) or splenic marginal zone lymphoma (SMZL) and the variant form of HCL (HCLv).[18-21] Cells from the majority of HCL cases express four or five of the markers outlined above whereas SLVL/SMZL and cells from HCLv are positive with one, or at most two, of these markers. The least specific MAb to distinguish these three conditions is CD11c as this antigen is expressed in the majority. In contrast, CD123 is extremely useful to differentiate HCL from the other two diseases with villous cells. In HCL, CD123 is consistently positive while cells from the HCLv and SLVL are, as a rule, CD123 negative.[21] Furthermore, another MAb that identifies normal memory B cells and clustered under CD27 has become available. CD27 is a member of the tumor necrosis factor receptor family and, although not systematically used in the context of the differential diagnosis of these diseases, may well be of great value to distinguish SLVL/SMZL from HCL. Thus, CD27 is consistently expressed in the few normal marginal zone circulating B cells and in SLVL as well as in other mature B cell neoplasms[22] while it is negative in HCL. There is no information on the cell reactivity with this antibody in cells from the variant form of HCL. A summary

of the most common immunologic profiles in leukemic B cell disorders is shown in Table 42.4.

RARER B CELL NEOPLASMS

Some scenarios that need to be taken into account in the setting of the differential diagnosis of the mature B cell malignancies are the following:

- unusual plasma cell dyscrasias
- polyclonal B cell lymphocytosis
- large cell lymphomas in leukemic phase.

Concerning plasma cell dyscrasias, although most cases present with a typical clinical picture of multiple myeloma, in a few patients the disease evolves as a primary leukemia with either poorly differentiated circulating blasts, mature plasma cells or a mixture of both. These patients pose diagnostic problems as the circulating neoplastic cells, like normal plasma cells, lack reactivity with most pan-B cell MAbs and do not express Ig in the cell membrane. However, they express cytoplasmic Ig with light chain restriction and are CD138+, CD38+, often CD79a+ and may have aberrant

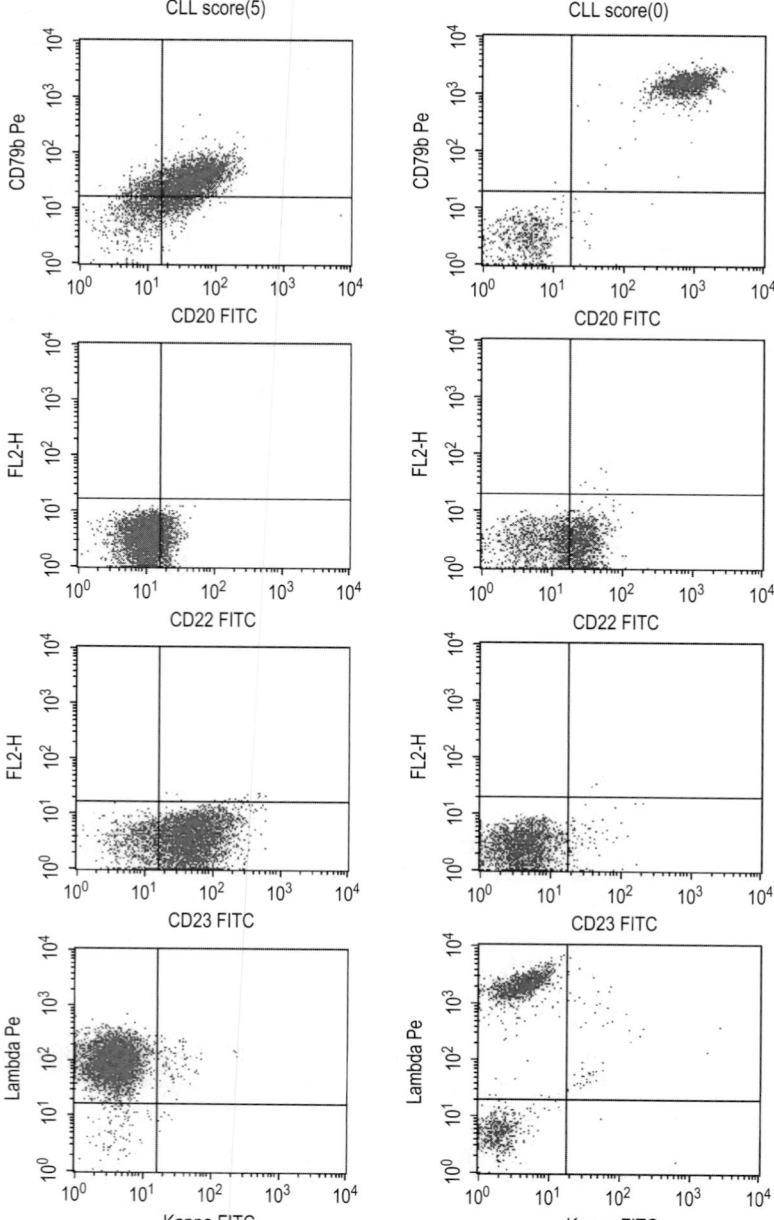

Figure 42.1   Continued

expression of other antigens such as CD56, CD117 and CD10 (Fig. 42.2). The second diagnostic problem is that of polyclonal B cell lymphocytosis. Such patients are usually asymptomatic and are investigated because of an absolute lymphocytosis and/or moderate splenomegaly. Most of the circulating lymphocytes display an atypical morphology resembling lymphoma cells, and are often FMC7 and CD20 positive. However, unlike lymphomas and leukemias, a proportion of lymphocytes in this condition express the κ Ig light chain and a proportion express the λ Ig light chain. Clonality cannot be established by membrane markers or by Southern blot for the Ig heavy-chain gene. Despite this, cytogenetic findings in a proportion of cases will show the iso3q abnormality. The outcome for these patients seems to be favorable as most of them have a stable course without evolving into a lymphoma. An extremely rare situation is that concerning patients with a high-grade/large cell lymphoma that essentially manifests with a leukemic picture where the majority of cells are poorly differentiated blasts, heavy bone marrow infiltration and absence of organomegaly. The clinical picture thus mimics an acute leukemia. Immunophenotyping using a broad panel of MAbs against B and T cell lymphoid antigens in conjunction with myeloid markers is essential to disclose the nature of the neoplastic cells.[23]

T CELL DISORDERS

When the first line panel of MAbs suggests a T cell phenotype (CD2+, CD3+/−, CD5+/−), a battery of MAbs

Table 42.4 Immunological markers in mature B cell disorders (CD19+, CD2−)

Disease	SmIg	CD5	CD23	FMC7	CD22	CD79b
CLL	Weak	++	++	−/+	Weak/−	Weak/−
B-PLL	Strong	−/+	−	++	+	++
HCL	Strong	−	−	++	++	+
HCL-variant	Strong	−	−	++	++	+
SLVL	Strong	−/+	−/+	++	++	++
FL	Strong	−/+	−/+	++	++	++
Mantle cell	Strong	++	−	++	++	++
Large cell	Strong	−/+	−/+	++	++	++
PCL[a]	Negative	−	−	−	−	−

[a]Express cytoplasmic Ig (light chain restricted), CD38, CD138, CD79a.
Scoring: (−), negative or positive in less than 10 percent of cases; (−/+), positive in 10–25 percent of cases; (+), positive in 25–75 percent of cases; (++), positive in more than 75 percent of cases.
B-PLL, B-prolymphocytic leukemia; CLL, chronic lymphocytic leukemia; FL, follicular lymphoma; HCL, hairy cell leukemia; PCL, plasma cell leukemia; SLVL, splenic lymphoma with villous lymphocytes.

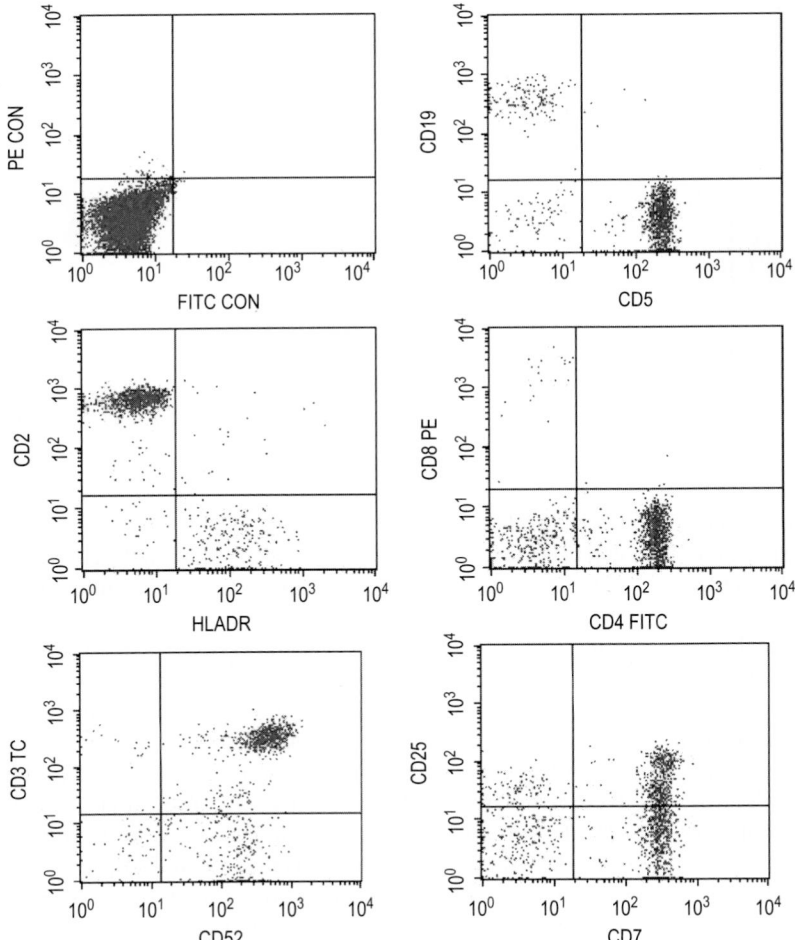

Figure 42.2 Flow cytometry dot plots on cells from a case with T cell prolymphocytic leukemia illustrating that most lymphocytes express CD5, CD2, CD3, CD7, CD4 and CD52 (Campath-1H) and are CD8 negative.

against the T cell receptor (TCR) β/γ chain genes, those identifying the two main T cell subsets (CD4 and CD8), natural killer (NK) cells and others expressed in activated T cells needs to be applied. This approach will help to disclose the origin of the neoplastic cell; whether it is a T cell, NK cell and/or more rarely a plasmacytoid dendritic cell (see below). Regarding T cell proliferations, and unlike in B cell disorders, there is no unique phenotype that establishes the diagnosis of a particular condition. Nevertheless, some immunophenotypes are more commonly seen in

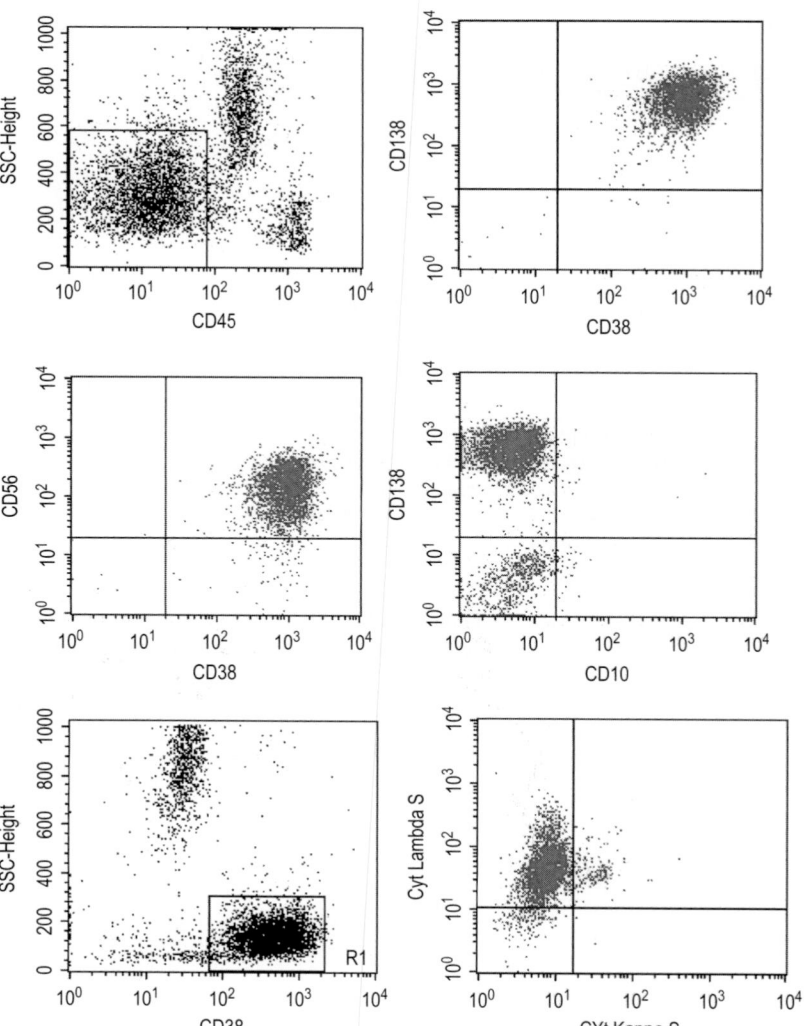

Figure 42.3 Flow cytometry dot plots from a case with multiple myeloma showing strong expression of CD38, CD138 and cytoplasmic λ chain in the CD45-negative gated population. In addition the cells have an aberrant expression of CD56 and are CD10 negative.

certain disorders. Thus, a CD4+/CD8− immunophenotype, coexpression of CD4 and CD8 and strong expression of CD7 are frequent in T cell prolymphocytic leukemia (T-PLL) (Fig. 42.3) while a CD8+/ CD4−, often CD57+, CD16+ is common in large granular lymphocyte (LGL) T cell proliferations and strong expression of CD25 in CD4+ adult T cell leukemia lymphoma (ATLL) cells.[24,25] Loss or lack of expression of some pan-T cell antigens in the lymphoma/leukemia T cells is not uncommon. For instance, ATLL cells are usually CD7 negative and this antigen is also absent from around half of the Sézary syndrome and T cell LGL leukemia cases.

Although in the past assessment of T cell clonality was only possible by cytogenetics or molecular analysis investigating the configuration of the TCR chain genes by Southern blot or by the polymerase chain reaction (PCR), it is now feasible to assess the clonal nature of the T cell population by flow cytometry. This is achieved by immunostaining with MAbs that identify the different variable regions of the TCR β chains. Unlike in reactive T cell lymphocytosis in which different proportions of

T cells will stain with the various MAbs, in clonal T cell expansions the lymphocytes will show a 'clonal' repertoire pattern. This is reflected by an exclusive or preferential stain with one of the MAbs against the TCRVβ family. Since the anti-TCR MAbs cover around 80 percent of the TCRV-β repertoire a negative result ('defective' pattern) can be interpreted as indicative of clonality.[26,27] Although this assay is more cumbersone than PCR molecular analysis for the TCR chain genes and clonality assessment in the B cell neoplasms by flow cytometry, as it requires the use of a large number of antibodies, it may have some role in those laboratories without molecular facilities. In addition, clonality can also be assessed by analyzing the expression of killer immunoglobulin receptors (KIRs), lectine receptors and NK receptors.[28,29] A range of MAbs against KIRs and clustered under CD158 may be expressed in a proportion of T cell LGL leukemias while they are negative in normal CD3+/CD57+ cytotoxic T cells. Therefore the aberrant expression of one or more KIRs is indicative of clonality. Similarly, the lectin-like receptors, CD94 and CD161, absent in normal LGL cells, when positive, may be helpful

Table 42.5 Immunological markers in mature T cell disorders (CD2+, CD19−)

Marker	T–PLL	LGLL	ATLL	SS	T–NHL
CD3	++	++	++	++	+
CD7	++	+	−/+	+	+
CD4+, CD8−	+	−	++	++	+
CD4+, CD8+	−/+	−	−	−/+	+
CD4−, CD8+	−/+	++	−	−	+
CD4−, CD8−	−	−/+[a]	−	−	+
CD25	+	−/+	++	+	+

[a]A proportion of cases are CD3 negative and have a natural killer phenotype, CD56+, CD16+.
Scoring: (−), negative or positive in less than 10 percent of cases; (−/+), positive in 10–25 percent of cases; (+), positive in 25–75 percent of cases; (++), positive in more than 75 percent of cases.
ATLL, adult T cell leukemia lymphoma; LGLL, large granular lymphocyte leukemia; SS, Sézary syndrome; T-NHL, post-thymic T cell lymphoma; T-PLL, T-prolymphocytic leukemia.

Table 42.6 Panel of monoclonal antibodies for the diagnosis of lymphoid neoplasms by immunohistochemistry

	B cell	T cell/NK cell	Others
First line	CD10, CD20, CD79a, CD21, CD23, CD24	CD5[a], CD3, CD43	BCL2, BCL6, Cyclin D1, CD45
Second line		CD4, CD8, TCR β/γ, TIA1, CD56, CD57, granzyme B	ALK, CD15, LMP1, EBERs, EMA, CD30, MYC, Ki-67, TdT

CD21 and CD23 to identify the follicular dendritic cells in addition to B cells.
[a]Reactive with a subset of B cells.
EMA, epithelial membrane antigen; LMP1, EBV latent membrane protein; EBERs, EBV early RNA sequences; ALK, anaplastic lymphoma kinase.

too. A summary of the most common immunophenotypes in the leukemic T cell disorders is shown in Table 42.5.

NK/DENDRITIC CELL DISORDERS

In addition to the B and T cell neoplasms, there are infrequent types of leukemias which represent clonal expansions of NK cells or rarely the neoplastic cells appear to derive from plasmacytoid dendritic cells. Although in the WHO classification, the NK neoplasms are not considered as a single entity but included under different designations such as aggressive NK cell leukemias and blastoid NK cell lymphoma, the immunophenotype is distinct in these diseases and indeed mandatory for the diagnosis.[30–34] Expression of the neural marker CD56 is a hallmark for all these neoplasms. However, by itself, this does not allow a case to be ascribed as an NK neoplasm since this molecule may be expressed in a variety of nonhemopoietic and hemopoietic malignancies such as acute myelomonocytic leukemias. Furthermore, some NK cell disorders may be CD56 negative. In addition to CD56, the cells in the NK cell neoplasms may express other NK-associated markers such as CD16, CD57, CD94 and CD161. T cell lineage specific markers (e.g. CD3) are negative but CD7 and CD2 may be weakly expressed in the neoplastic cells and, in some nasal NK lymphomas, the cells may have cytoplasmic expression of the ε chain of CD3.[31] NK cell neoplasms may be difficult to distinguish from plasmacytoid dendritic cell leukemias as in both of these conditions the neoplastic cells express CD56 and CD123. However, the plasmacytoid dendritic cells are CD4+, HLA-Dr+ and may express CD68[35] while a substantial proportion of NK cell derived lymphomas express CD16/CD57, a feature which is not seen in plasmacytoid dendritic cell leukemias. It is possible that some cases diagnosed in the past as blastoid NK lymphoma/leukemias may well correspond to a plasmacytoid dendritic cell leukemia.

Immunohistochemistry

As outlined above, the panel of MAbs that provides useful information by ICH in the diagnosis of mature lymphoid malignancies is slightly different from that used by flow cytometry although with some overlap. As in flow cytometry, in an IHC setting, a first line panel of markers should be applied essentially aimed at distinguishing B from T cell diseases and to highlight the typical immunologic profiles of the most common lymphomas such as follicular lymphoma and small lymphocytic lymphoma (SLL)/CLL.[36] A second line of markers can then be used when the initial diagnostic workup is different from that seen in FL or SLL or suggests a T cell neoplasm.

B CELL DISORDERS

The first ICH panel of markers, as for FC, should include:

- CD5
- a pan-T cell marker such as CD3 or CD2
- TdT if a precursor lymphoid neoplasm is suspected
- a set of markers against B cells or distinctively expressed in the follicular center-derived neoplasms and/or those which will highlight the dendritic meshwork.

The set of B cell markers comprises: CD10, CD20, CD23, CD24, CD43, CD79a (against the α chain of the B cell receptor), anti-IgM and IgD, anti-BCL2, anti-BCL6, Cyclin D1 and CD21, the latter addressed to identify follicular dendritic cells in addition to B cells (Table 42.6). This panel distinguishes SLL/CLL from mantle cell and follicular lymphomas. In addition, and within the diffuse large B cell lymphomas, it will allow discrimination of cases with or without a germinal center phenotype by the distinct expression of BCL2, BCL6 and CD10, a relevant issue because of the different prognosis.[37] Although strong expression of Cyclin D1 is the hallmark of mantle cell lymphoma,[38] the expression of this cyclin should not be taken in isolation as other lymphoid neoplasms such as HCL, plasma cell discrasias and some lymphoplasmacytic lymphomas may express cyclin D1 as a result or not of the t(11;14).[39]

There is no evidence that SMZL/SLVL or lymphoplasmacytic lymphomas have a distict immunologic profile and therefore immunohistochemical results should be correlated with the morphology on sections stained with hematoxylin–eosin as well as with clinical and other laboratory data. Even markers characteristically expressed in HCL such as DBA-44 may be positive in a minority of SMZL cases; however, in contrast to HCL, SMZL cells do not express Annexin A1. In addition, nodal tissue will be available for diagnosis in only a small proportion of SMZL patients as the main site of involvement in this lymphoma is the spleen while lymphadenopathy is rare. Thus, in a significant proportion of cases the diagnosis will be based on the morphology and immunophenotype of the circulating cells and bone marrow histology. When considering bone marrow histology, although an intrasinusoidal pattern of bone marrow infiltration is very frequently seen in SLVL,[40] it is not unique to this lymphoma and this should not be taken in isolation for diagnosis. Expression of other markers, such as IRFA-1, the product of the marginal zone-related gene, although having pronostic implications, does not distinguish between lymphoplasmacytic lymphomas and SMZL.[41] The immunologic profiles in B cell lymphomas by IHC is summarized in Table 42.7.

When dealing with plasma cell proliferations, staining with CD138 and Ig light chains is indicated; in addition, CD79a, a pan-B cell marker expressed, as a rule, in normal plasma cells will show positivity in most cases of plasma cell dyscrasias.

Table 42.7 Immunological markers in tissue-based B cell neoplasms (CD20+, CD79a+, CD22+, TdT−)

Marker	Mantle cell	Follicular	MZ	MALT	DLCL
CD5	+	−	−	−	−/+
CD10	−/+	+	−	−	−/+
CD21	−/+	+	−/+	+	−/+
CD43	+	−	−/+	−/+	−/+
Cyclin D1	+	−	−	−	−
BCL2	+	+	+	+	−/+
BCL6	−	+	−	−	+
MYC	−	−/+	−	−	−/+

−/+, weak stain or positive in a small fraction of cases.
MZ, marginal zone; MALT, mucosa-associated lymphoid tissue;
DLCL, diffuse large cell lymphoma.

T CELL DISORDERS

When the first line of markers suggests and/or is consistent with a T cell malignancy (CD3+/CD2+/CD5+/−, CD79a−), a second line panel needs to be applied. This will be tailored according to the diagnosis suspected by morphology on the hematoxylin–eosin sections. As for flow cytometry, immunostaining with MAbs recognizing T cell subsets, T cell activation markers, anti-TCR, TIA1, granzyme B, NK associated markers and CD30 (Ki-1) need to be investigated. In addition, if Hodgkin lymphoma is suspected, the epithelial membrane antigen (EMA) and CD15 are recommended to be carried out. Table 42.8 shows the most typical immunologic profiles in T cell lymphomas by IHC.

Table 42.8 Immunological markers on tissue-based T cell lymphomas (TdT−, CD2/CD3+)

Marker	PTCL	Anaplastic[a]	AIL	γδ T-NHL	Intestinal	NK cell[b]
CD4	+	−/+	+	−/+	−/+	−
CD5	−/+	−/+	−/+	−/+	−	−
CD7	−/+	−/+	−/+	−/+	−/+	−/+
CD8	−/+	−	−/+	−/+	−/+	−
CD10	−	−	+[c]	−	−/+	−
CD30	−/+	+	−	−	−/+	−
TIA1	−/+	−/+	−	+	−	−/+
ALK	−	+	−	−	−	−
CD56	−/+	−	−	+	−/+	+
EBV	−/+	−	+/−	−	−/+	+

[a]Anaplastic lymphomas are CD15 and CD25 positive.
[b]NK cell lymphomas may express granzyme B, perforin and the epsilon chain of CD3 in the cytoplasm.
[c]Expressed in the neoplastic T cells.
−/+, expression in a proportion of cases and/or weak stain.
PTCL, peripheral T cell lymphomas; AIL; angioimmunoblastic lymphoma; ALK, anaplastic lymphoma kinase; NK, natural killer; EBV, Epstein–Barr virus.

Examples of ICH staining in tissues from patients with the various lymphoid disorders are illustrated in Plates 114–118, see plate section.

IMMUNOLOGIC MARKERS FOR DETECTION OF MINIMAL RESIDUAL DISEASE

Further to the diagnostic value, immunophenotyping has been shown to be a useful tool to detect small numbers of residual leukemic and lymphoma cells in peripheral blood and bone marrow specimens and/or tissue sections, as such cells cannot be detected by standard morphology or histology. When assessing MRD, it is important to have information of the immunophenotype in the diagnostic sample in order to use the appropriate panel of markers on the follow-up sample. Detection of MRD by flow cytometry can be performed by several approches. One method is to exploit the presence of 'aberrant' phenotypes not present in normal lymphoid cells, using a double, triple or quadruple color immunofluorescent staining with a combination of suitable MAbs. An example of this approach is the estimation of the proportion of CD5+ lymphocytes within the CD19+ cell population in CLL and in MCL[42] or use of a quadruple flow cytometry immunostaining with the MAb CD79b, CD20, CD5 and CD19 in CLL.[43] Similarly, in HCL, it is possible to detect MRD by analyzing the expression of CD123, CD25 or CD103 in the B cell population (CD22+ or CD19+). Another appoach is to perform quantification of antigens when these molecules are expressed at a different density in the leukemic and lymphoma cells compared to normal cells. Immunohistochemistry is also a powerful tool to detect small numbers of residual leukemia/lymphoma cells when using specific MAbs such as DBA-44 staining in HCL.[44] An important issue to consider when investigating MRD is that CD20 expression is downregulated in the B cells from lymphoma and leukemic patients treated with anti-CD20 (rituximab). Therefore, another pan-B marker such as CD79a needs to be used to identify B cells in the follow-up specimens.

PROGNOSTIC MARKERS

Immunologic markers, serologic markers (e.g. lactate dehydrogenase or β_2-microglobulin) and molecular genetics when combined with clinical features have been shown to have predictive value for the outcome (survival and response to treatment) in patients with lymphoid malignancies. The T cell lymphomas, with the exception of ALCL (see below), have an overall less favorable prognosis compared to those with a B cell phenotype.[45] Furthermore, within specific types of lymphoid neoplasms, immunophenotyping allows assessment of the expression of a variety of proteins, such as those involved in cell cycle, apoptosis, cell proliferation or those encoded by genes involved in the pathogenesis of the lymphoma which have a major prognostic impact as outlined below.

Ki-67 and MiB-1

Ki-67 and MiB-1 are markers that allow estimation of the proliferative rate of the tumor. Although they are not useful in the diagnostic workup, they provide information to the clinician regarding prognosis. In patients with aggressive lymphomas, the level of cell proliferation is associated with poor outcome.[46] In chronic lymphoid malignancies, such as CLL, the degree of cell proliferation is generally low but tends to be higher in advanced stages and in association with disease progression[47] (Plate 119, see plate section). In addition, Ki-67 or MiB-1 staining in tissues from some indolent tumors, such as SMZL may highlight the increased cell growth fraction, both in the marginal zone and germinal center.

TP53

Abnormalities (mutations or deletions) of the *TP53* gene localized on the short arm of chromosome 17, have been shown to have a significant prognostic impact in both hemopoietic and nonhemopoietic cancers. The normal *TP53* gene induces apoptosis and/or cell cycle arrest in a damaged cell. Mutations of this gene result in the production of an abnormal TP53 protein that can be detected in the nucleus of the neoplastic cells by IHC or flow cytometry using antibodies specifically directed to p53. In contrast to the aberrant and nonfunctional TP53 which has a prolonged half-life, the normal wild-type TP53 cannot be detected by flow cytometry or IHC due to its rapid clearance. Estimation by flow cytometry requires a prior step of cell fixation.[48] There appears to be a good correlation between TP53 expression, deletion of the gene detected by fluorescence *in situ* hybridization (FISH) and point mutations estimated by gene sequencing.[48] Although abnormalities of *TP53* are more frequently seen in aggressive lymphomas, they can also be detected in low-intermediate grade lymphoid malignancies, particularly during disease evolution.[48-53] In lymphoid malignancies, TP53 expression correlates with disease progression and/or resistance to chemotherapy and radiation therapy, particularly in patients with CLL and other low grade B cell disorders which show chemo-resistance to purine analogs.[48,52]

Other proteins that regulate the cell cycle such as p27 and p21 may influence outcome. For instance downregulation of p21 seems to be associated to a poorer prognosis.

BCL2

BCL2 is an antiapoptotic protein widely expressed in hemopoietic and nonhemopoietic cells. Among other functions

BCL2 inhibits cell death. In the lymphoid system BCL2 is expressed in most B and T lymphocytes, except in cells from the germinal center and cortical thymocytes.[54,55] Follicular lymphoma cells express the protein at a high level compared to B and T lymphocytes and this is associated with the t(14;18) that juxtaposes the *BCL2* gene to the Ig chain gene enhancers. However, BCL2 overexpression is not exclusive of follicular lymphoma and the protein may be overexpressed in a variety of low- and high-grade lymphoid malignancies without an association with the t(14;18).[56,57] In the context of diffuse large cell B-NHL, BCL2 overexpression in the intermediate risk group of patients correlates with a less favorable outcome, which is then similar to that seen in patients with a high risk score.[37]

BCL6

The BCL6 protein is encoded by a gene localized at the 3q27 band and is specifically expressed in germinal center cells.[58] The *BCL6* gene is often disregulated in diffuse large cell lymphomas by a variety of mechanisms including translocations and mutations. Expression of the protein can be easily detected by IHC. Although the prognostic significance of BCL6 alterations had been controversial, recent studies have shown that patients with diffuse large cell lymphoma in whom cells express BCL6 have a better survival than those without expression this protein.[59]

ALK

The expression of ALK usually results from the t(2;5)(p23;q25) that leads to the expression of a chimeric protein due to the fusion of a nucleophosmin gene (5q25) and the *ALK* gene (2p23). Despite the biologic and clinical heterogeneity of ALCL, this lymphoma has an overall favorable outcome when compared with other T cell neoplasms. Further, ALK+ ALCL cases have a significantly superior survival than ALK– cases. Therefore it is important to systematically estimate the expression of this protein in ALCL.[60]

CD38 and ZAP70 expression

These are two markers shown to have a major impact on the prognosis of CLL. Their value in other lymphoid malignancies is uncertain. Although originally it was thought that CD38 expression correlated with *IGHV* mutational status,[61] it has been demonstrated that its expression is independent of the *IGHV* mutational status.[62,63] Most of the studies refer to CD38 staining by flow cytometry but it is also possible to investigate the expression of this antigen in tissue sections; the prognostic relevance of the latter, however, is unknown. This MAb stains a variety of hemopoietic and nonhemopoietic cells from different lineages and therefore, in a flow cytometry setting, it should be estimated by a triple color flow cytometry method on CD19+/CD5+ cells to ensure that its expression is analyzed in the leukemic CLL cells. Although the first reports documented thresholds of 20–30 percent CD38+ CLL cells to consider this marker as positive, it has become apparent that there is an intraclonal diversity within a single case and that a threshold of 7 percent CD38+ CLL cells would be the most reliable and informative in terms of prognosis.[64] In addition, CD38 expression may change during the course of the disease and may become positive in parallel with disease progression.

Another relevant prognostic marker in CLL is ZAP70. ZAP70 encodes for a tyrosine kinase which is expressed in normal T cells, NK cells and a few B cells. Microarray analysis in CLL has shown that the pattern of gene expression is very similar to a normal memory cell without major differences in cases with mutated or unmutated *IGHV* genes.[65] However, discrepancies in the expression of a few genes between these two subgroups of CLL were found. Among these, ZAP70 appeared to be preferentially expressed in CLL with unmutated *IGHV* while ZAP70 was downregulated in those with mutated *IGHV*.[66] It was then suggested that ZAP70 could be a surrogate marker for the mutational status. To date a number of studies have shown the prognostic impact of this marker. The correlation with mutational status ranges from 70 percent to >90 percent. ZAP70 can be estimated by different methods including microarrays, RNA analysis by reverse-transcriptase PCR and flow cytometry. When assessed by flow cytometry, it is important to evaluate the expression in either purified B-CLL cells and/or by a quadruple flow cytometry method that allows assessment of ZAP70 expression in T, NK and CLL cells.[67] At present, there are uncertainities regarding the best method and MAbs to be used and the best threshold (10 percent or 20 percent) of ZAP70+ CLL cells to consider this marker as positive.

BCL10

This is a novel gene which might have a pathogenic and prognostic role in the mucosa-associated lymphomas (MALT). It was identified through one of the recurrent chromosomal abnormalities in this lymphoma, the t(1;14)(p22;q14) that leads to the overexpression of BCL10 in the nucleus of the lymphoma cells. In addition, weak BCL10 staining may be seen in cases harboring the t(11;18)(q21;q21). BCL10 expression in MALT lymphomas has been found to correlate with failure to respond to *Helicobacter pylori* eradication and advanced disease.[68]

KEY POINTS

- Immunophenotypic studies are a robust armamentarium to establish the diagnosis and prognosis of the lymphoid malignancies.
- Studies in cell suspensions by flow cytometry and in tissue sections by immunohistochemistry are complementary.
- Application of adequate MAb panels and interpretation of the findings considering a composite phenotype are essential to establish the diagnosis of the lymphoid neoplasm.
- Immunophenotypic results should be interpreted in the light of clinical features and other laboratory tests.
- Immunophenotyping is a powerful tool to detect residual numbers of leukemia/lymphoma cells (MRD) which cannot be identified by standard morphology and histochemistry.
- Immunophenotyping allows detection of expression of certain proteins involved in the cell cycle and apoptosis and/or others that are encoded by tumor suppressor genes with an impact on prognosis as well as providing some insights into the pathogenesis of the various lymphoid neoplasms.
- The prognostic impact of immunophenotyping should be complemented with that of molecular genetics.

REFERENCES

● = Key primary paper
◆ = Major review article

◆1. McCarthy DA, Macey MG. (eds) *Cytometric analysis of cell phenotype and function.* Cambridge University Press, 2001.
◆2. Groeneveld K, Temarvelde JG, van den Beemd MWM *et al.* Flow cytometry detection of intracellular antigens for immunophenotyping of normal and malignant leukocytes. BTS Technical Report. *Leukemia* 1996; **10**: 1383–9.
◆3. Pizzolo G, Vincenzi C, Nadali G *et al.* Detection of membrane and intracellular antigens by flow cytometry following ORTHO PermeaFix fixation. *Leukemia* 1995; **9**: 226–8.
◆4. Bikoue A, George F, Poncelet LW *et al.* Quantitative analysis of leukocyte membrane antigen expression: normal adult values. *Cytometry* 1996; **26**: 137–47.
◆5. Poncelet P, George F, Papa S *et al.* Quantitation of haemopoietic cell antigens in flow cytometry. *Eur J Histochem* 1996; **40**(Suppl 1): 15–32.

◆6. Matutes E, Morilla R, Catovsky D. Immunophenotyping. In: Lewis SM, Bain BJ, Bates I. (eds) *Practical haematology*, 10th ed. London: Churchill Livingstone, 2006: 335.
◆7. Erber WN, Mynheer LC, Mason DY. APAAP labelling of blood and bone-marrow samples for phenotyping leukaemia. *Lancet* 1986; **1**: 761–5.
◆8. Mason DY, Erber WN. Immunocytochemical labeling of leukemia samples with monoclonal antibodies by the APAAP procedure. In: Catovsky D. (ed.) *The leukemic cell.* Edinburgh: Churchill Livingstone, 1991: 196.
●9. Bene MC, Castoldi G, Knapp W *et al.* European Group for the immunological characterisation of leukemias. Proposals for the immunological classification of acute leukemias. *Leukemia* 1995; **9**: 1783–6.
◆10. Bain BJ, Barnett D, Linch D *et al.* Revised guideline on immunophenotyping in acute leukaemias and chronic lymphoproliferative disorders. *Clin Lab Haematol* 2002; **24**: 1–13.
◆11. Matutes E. New additions to antibody panels in the characterisation of chronic lymphoproliferative disorders. *J Clin Pathol* 2002; **55**: 180–3.
●12. Zomas AP, Matutes E, Morilla R *et al.* Expression of the immunoglobulin associated protein B29 in B-cell disorders with the monoclonal antibody SN8 (CD79b). *Leukemia* 1996; **10**: 1966–70.
●13. Cabezudo E, Morilla R, Carrara P, Matutes E. Quantitative analysis of CD79b, CD5 and CD19 in B-cell lympho-proliferative disorders. *Haematologica* 1999; **84**: 413–18.
●14. Matutes E, Owusu-Ankomah K, Morilla R *et al.* The immunological profile of B-cell disorders and proposal of a scoring system for the diagnosis of CLL. *Leukemia* 1994; **8**: 1640–5.
●15. Moureau EJ, Matutes E, A'Hern RP *et al.* Improvement of the chronic lymphocytic leukemia scoring system with the monoclonal antibody SN8 (CD79b). *Am J Clin Pathol* 1997; **108**: 378–82.
◆16. Matutes E, Polliack A. Morphological and immunophenotypic features of chronic lymphocytic leukemia. *Rev Clin Exp Hematol* 2000; **4**: 22–7.
●17. Delgado J, Matutes E, Morilla A *et al.* Diagnostic significance of CD20 and FMC7 expression in B cell disorders. *Am J Clin Pathol* 2003; **120**: 754–9.
●18. Matutes E. Immunophenotyping and differential diagnosis of hairy cell leukemia. *Hematol Oncol Clin North Am* 2006; **20**: 1051–63.
●19. Matutes E, Morilla R, Owusu-Ankomah K *et al.* The imunophenotype of splenic lymphoma with villous lymphocytes and its relevance to the differential diagnosis with other B-cell disorders. *Blood* 1994; **83**: 1558–62.
●20. Matutes E, Wotherspoon A, Brito-Babapulle V, Catovsky D. The natural history and clinico-pathological features of the variant form of hairy cell leukemia. *Leukemia* 2001; **15**: 184–6.
●21. del Giudice I, Matutes E, Morilla R *et al.* The diagnostic value of CD123 in B-cell disorders with hairy or villous lymphocytes. *Haematologica* 2004; **89**: 303–8.

●22. Forconi F, Raspadori D, Lenoci M, Lauria F. Absence of surface CD27 distinguishes hairy cell leukemia from other leukemic B-cell malignancies. *Haematologica* 2005; **90**: 144–6.

◆23. Bain B, Matutes E, Robinson D *et al*. Leukaemia as a manifestation of large cell lymphoma. *Br J Haematol* 1991; **77**: 301–10.

●24. Matutes E. Chronic T-cell lymphoproliferative disorders. *Rev Clin Exp Hematol* 2003; **6**: 401–20.

●25. Matutes E, Brito-Babapulle V, Swansbury J *et al*. Clinical and laboratory features of 78 cases of T-prolymphocytic leukemia. *Blood* 1991; **78**: 3269–74.

●26. Lima M, Almeida J, Santos AH *et al*. Immunophenotypic analysis of the TCR-Vbeta repertoire in 98 persistent expansions of CD3(+)/TCR-alpha-beta (+) large granular lymphocytes: utility in assessing clonality and insights in the pathogenesis of the disease. *Am J Pathol* 2001; **54**: 565–7.

●27. Langerak AW, van den Beemd R, Wolvers-Tettero IL *et al*. Molecular and flow cytometric analysis of the Vbeta repertoire for clonality assessment in mature TCR alpha/beta T-cell proliferations. *Blood* 2001; **98**: 167–73.

●28. Mourice WG, Kurtin PJ, Leibson PJ *et al*. Demonstration of aberrant T-cell and natural killer-cell antigen expression in all cases of granular lymphocytic leukaemia. *Br J Haematol* 2003; **120**: 1026–36.

●29. Epling-Burnette PK, Painter JS, Chaurasia P *et al*. Dysregulated NK receptor expression in patients with lymphoproliferative disease of granular lymphocytes. *Blood* 2004; **103**: 3431–9.

◆30. Chan JKC, Wong KF, Jaffe ES. Aggressive NK cell leukaemia. In: Jaffe ES, Harris NL, Stein H, Vardiman JW. (eds) *World Health Organization classification of tumours of haemopoietic and lymphoid tissues*. Lyon: IARC Press, 2001: 198–200.

◆31. Chan JKC, Jaffe ES, Ralfkiaer E. Extranodal NK/T cell lymphoma, nasal type. In: Jaffe ES, Harris NL, Stein H, Vardiman JW. (eds) *World Health Organization classification of tumours of haemopoietic and lymphoid tissues*. Lyon: IARC Press, 2001: 204–7.

◆32. Jaffe ES. Classification of natural killer (NK) cell and NK-like T-cell malignancies. *Blood* 1995; **87**: 1207–10.

◆33. Chan JKC, Jaffe ES, Ralfkiaer E. Blastic NK-cell lymphoma. In: Jaffe ES, Harris NL, Stein H, Vardiman JW. (eds) *World Health Organization classification of tumours of haemopoietic and lymphoid tissues*. Lyon: IARC Press, 2001: 214–15.

◆34. Foucart K, Matutes E, Catovsky D. T-cell large granular lymphocyte leukemia, T-prolymphocytic leukemia and aggressive natural killer leukemia. In: Mauch PM, Armitage JO, Coiffier B *et al*. (eds) *Non-Hodgkin's lymphomas*. Philadelphia: Lippincott Williams and Wilkins, 2004: 283–94.

●35. Feulliard J, Jacob MC, Valensi F *et al*. Clinical and biological features of CD4+ CD56+ malignancies. *Blood* 2002; **99**: 1556–63.

◆36. Aoun P, Greiner PC. Immunophenotypic characterisation in lymphoma diagnosis and classification. In: Mauch PM, Armitage JO, Coiffier B *et al*. (eds) *Non-Hodgkin's lymphomas*. Philadelphia: Lippincott Williams and Wilkins, 2004: 59–68.

●37. Barrans SL, Carter I, Owen RG *et al*. Germinal center phenotype and bcl-2 expression combined with the International Prognostic Index improves pateint risk stratification in diffuse large B-cell lymphoma. *Blood* 2002; **99**: 1136–43.

◆38. Swerdlow SH, Berger F, Isaacson PI, Muller-Hermelink HK. Mantle-cell lymphoma. In: Jaffe ES, Harris NL, Stein H, Vardiman JW. (eds) *World Health Organization classification of tumours of haemopoietic and lymphoid tissues*. Lyon: IARC Press, 2001: 168–70.

●39. Zukerberg LR, Yang WI, Arnold A. Cyclin D1 expression in non-Hodgkin's lymphomas. Detection by immunohistochemistry. *J Clin Pathol* 1995; **103**: 756–60.

●40. Franco V, Florena AM, Campesi G. Intrasinusoidal bone marrow infiltration: a possible hallmark of splenic lymphoma. *Histopathology* 1996; **29**: 571–5.

●41. Petit B, Chaury MP, LeClorennec C *et al*. Indolent lymphoplasmacytic and marginal zone B-cell lymphomas: absence of both IRF4 and Ki-67 expression identifies a better prognostic group. *Haematologica* 2005; **90**: 200–6.

●42. Cabezudo E, Matutes E, Ramrattan M *et al*. Analysis of residual disease in chronic lymphocytic leukemia by flow cytometry. *Leukemia* 1997; **11**: 1909–14.

●43. Rawstron AC, Kennedy B, Evans PA *et al*. Quantitation of minimal residual disease levels in chronic lymphocytic leukemia improves the prediction of outcome and can be used to optimize therapy. *Blood* 2001; **98**: 29–35.

●44. Hakimian D, Tallman MS, Peterson L. Detection of minimal residual disease by immunostaining of bone marrow biopsies after 2-chlorodeoxyadenosine for hairy cell leukemia. *Blood* 1993; **82**: 1798–802.

◆45. Melnyk A, Rodriguez A, Pugh W, Cabanillas F. Evaluation of the revised european american lymphoma classification confirms the clinical relevance of immunophenotyping in 560 cases of aggressive non-Hodgkin's lymphoma. *Blood* 1997; **89**: 4514–20.

●46. Miller TP, Grogan TM, Dahlberg S *et al*. Prognostic significance of the Ki-67 associated proliferative antigen in aggressive non-Hodgkin's lymphomas: a prospective Southwest Oncology Group trial. *Blood* 1994; **83**: 1460–6.

●47. Cordone I, Matutes E, Catovsky D. The monoclonal antibody Ki-67 identifies B and T cells in cycle in chronic lymphocytic leukemia: correlation with disease activity. *Leukemia* 1992; **6**: 902–6.

●48. Thornton PD, Gruzka-Westwood AM, Hamoudi RA *et al*. Characterisation of TP53 abnormailities in chronic lymphocytic leukaemia. *Hematol J* 2004; **5**: 47–54.

●49. Gruszka-Westwood AM, Hamoudi RA, Matutes E *et al*. p53 abnormalities in splenic lymphoma with villous lymphocytes. *Blood* 2001; **97**: 3552–8.

●50. Louie DC, Offit K, Jaslow R *et al*. P53 overexpression as a marker of poor prognosis in mantle-cell lymphomas with t(11;14)(q13;q32). *Blood* 1995; **86**: 2892–9.

●51. Lens D, Dyer MJS, Garcia Marco JA *et al.* p53 abnormalities in CLL are associated with excess of prolymphocytes and poor prognosis. *Br J Haematol* 1997; **99**: 848–57.

●52. Dohner H, Fischer K, Bentz M *et al.* p53 gene deletion predicts for poor survival and non-response to therapy with purine analogs in chronic B-cell leukemias. *Blood* 1995; **85**: 1580–9.

●53. Lens D, de Schouner PJJC, Farahat N *et al.* High rate of p53 abnormalities in B-cell prolymphocytic leukemia. *Blood* 1997; **89**: 2015–23.

●54. Krajewski S, Bodrug S, Gascoyne R *et al.* Immunohistochemical analysis of mcl-1 and bcl-2 proteins in normal and neoplastic lymph nodes. *Am J Pathol* 1994; **145**: 515–25.

●55. Fujii Y, Okumura M, Takeuchi Y *et al.* Bcl-2 expression in the thymus and periphery. *Cell Immunol* 1994; **155**: 335–44.

●56. Pezella F, Tse A, Cordell J *et al.* Expression of the bcl-2 oncogene protein is not specific for the 14; 18 chromosomal translocation. *Am J Pathol* 1990; **137**: 225–32.

●57. Monni O, Franssila K, Joensuu H, Knuutila S. bcl-2 overexpression in diffuse large B-cell lymphoma. *Leuk Lymphoma* 1999; **34**: 45–52.

●58. Cattoretti G, Chang CC, Cechova K *et al.* Bcl-6 protein is expressed in germinal center B-cells. *Blood* 1995; **86**: 45–53.

●59. Lossos IS, Jones CD, Warnke R *et al.* Expression of a single gene, bcl-6, strongly predicts survival in patients with diffuse large B-cell lymphoma. *Blood* 2001; **98**: 945–51.

●60. Gayscone RD, Aoun P, Wu D *et al.* Prognostic significance of anaplastic lymphoma kinase (ALK) protein expression in adults with anaplastic large cell lymphoma. *Blood* 1999; **93**: 3913–21.

●61. Damle RN, Wasil T, Fais F *et al.* Immunoglobulin V gene mutation status and CD38 expression as novel prognostic indicators in chronic lymphocytic leukemia. *Blood* 1999; **94**: 1840–7.

●62. Del Poeta G, Maurillo L, Venditti A *et al.* Clinical significance of CD38 expression in chronic lymphocytic leukemia. *Blood* 2001; **99**: 2633–9.

●63. Ibrahim S, Keating M, Do KA *et al.* CD38 as an important prognostic factor in B-cell chronic lymphocytic leukemia. *Blood* 2001; **98**: 181–6.

●64. Thornton PD, Fernandez C, Giustolisi G *et al.* CD38 as a prognostic indicator in chronic lymphocytic leukaemia. *Hematol J* 2004; **5**: 145–51.

●65. Klein U, Tu Y, Stolovitzsky GA *et al.* Gene expression profiling of B-cell chronic lymphocytic leukemia reveals a homogeneous phenotype related to memory B-cells. *J Exp Med* 2001; **194**: 1625–38.

●66. Chen L, Widhopf G, Huynh L *et al.* Expression of ZAP-70 is associated with increased B-cell receptor signaling in chronic lymphocytic leukemia. *Blood* 2002; **100**: 4609–14.

●67. Crespo N, Bosch F, Villamor N *et al.* ZAP-70 expression as a surrogate for Immunoglobulin variable gene region mutations in chronic lymphocytic leukemia. *N Engl J Med* 2003; **348**: 1764–75.

●68. Ye H, Dogan A, Karran L *et al.* Bcl-10 expression in normal and neoplastic tissue. Nuclear localization in MALT lymphoma. *Am J Pathol* 2000; **157**: 1147–54.

43

The utility of molecular genetic studies in the diagnosis, prognostic assessment and monitoring of lymphoid malignancies

DAVID S VISWANATHA

DETERMINATION AND INTERPRETATION OF CLONALITY IN LYMPHOID POPULATIONS

In many, if not most, cases of lymphoid hyperplasia or neoplasia, the morphologic expertise of the hematopathologist supplemented by selective ancillary investigative techniques, is sufficient to establish a conclusive diagnosis. Often, the formal demonstration of monoclonality in a neoplastic lymphoid population is not required for this purpose, such as in the setting of a lymph node biopsy harboring typical diffuse large B cell lymphoma. In practice however, there are seemingly more exceptions than rules in clinical and histopathologic presentations of the lymphoproliferative diseases, and the demonstration of clonality to facilitate the diagnosis of a lymphoid malignancy is an important tool in the hematopathology laboratory. To this end, flow cytometry of cell suspensions, or immunoperoxidase and *in situ* hybridization (ISH) methods on fixed tissue sections, can often successfully delineate restricted immunoglobulin light chain expression by B cell or plasma cell populations in suspect biopsies.

Nonetheless, there exist a number of scenarios in routine hematopathology practice in which the detection of clonal lymphocyte populations can best be achieved by molecular methods (Box 43.1). Of note, standard molecular clonality assays can be supplemented by laboratory investigations for common chromosomal translocations and their corresponding gene fusion abnormalities, which are prevalent in many types of non-Hodgkin lymphomas and lymphoid leukemias. In this way, the molecular hematopathologist has at his or her disposal a formidable set of tools to:

- distinguish between benign and malignant lymphoproliferations
- assist in the accurate subclassification of the lymphoid diseases
- identify markers to monitor therapeutic efficacy and disease recurrence
- provide the technological platforms for incorporating novel advances in the molecular pathogenesis of lymphoid tumors into diagnostic practice.

Principles and techniques for determining B cell and T cell clonality: antigen receptor gene rearrangements and the generation of receptor diversity

The immune receptors present on B and T lymphocytes are generated by a process of somatic rearrangement of the antigen receptor genes, occurring in early precursor B and T cells of the bone marrow and thymus respectively. For B cells, this process is initiated at the immunoglobulin heavy chain locus (*IGH*) located on chromosome 14(q32), in turn leading to production of the heavy chain peptide component of the immunoglobulin molecule.[1,2] Following sequentially, the κ light chain gene (*IGK*) on chromosome 2(p12) is next rearranged, and if these attempts fail at both κ alleles, rearrangement then proceeds at the λ gene (*IGL*) located on chromosome 22(q11). In this way, the hierarchical recombination of the light chain genes ensures only one light chain type is expressed by a given B cell, along with its respective heavy chain. The complete immunoglobulin protein is a tetramer of paired identical heavy and light chains and is displayed on the cell surface as part of the B cell receptor signaling complex. Ordered gene segment recombination also underlies the formation of the heterodimeric T cell receptors, which are of either $\alpha\beta$ or $\gamma\delta$ type. In thymic T cells, rearrangement of the δ gene (*TRD*) on chromosome 14(q11) is initiated in concert with similar activity at the T cell receptor γ gene (*TRG*), located on chromosome 7(p15). However, δ gene rearrangements are seldom productive, thus excluding expression of a complete $\gamma\delta$ surface T cell receptor on the majority of developing T lymphocytes. The cascade of T cell receptor gene rearrangements therefore proceeds nearly synchronously at the alpha (*TRA*) and beta (*TRB*) loci, located on chromosomes 14(q11) and 7(q34), respectively. As the *TRD* gene is in fact embedded within the alpha locus, it is most often deleted in a site-specific manner during rearrangement of the *TRA* gene. The potential for functional alpha and beta T cell receptor gene rearrangements is robust, explaining in part the observed distribution of $\alpha\beta$ T cells (~95 percent) versus $\gamma\delta$ T cells (~5 percent) in humans.

The molecular genetic processes required to produce receptor proteins on B and T cells involve the coordinated scission, splicing and rejoining of DNA coding regions known as V (variable), D (diversity) and J (joining) segments as schematically illustrated for the *IGH* locus in Figure 43.1. This activity is mediated by the recombination activating gene products (RAG1, RAG2) and several proteins involved in DNA repair.[1] While V and J segments are common to all antigen receptor genes, D elements are not present at the *TRA*, *TRG*, and immunoglobulin light chain gene loci. The individual V- (D-) and J segments are selected randomly, but are precisely identified over very large regions of intervening DNA by the placement of recombination signal sequences (RSS), characterized by a 3′ palindromic heptamer sequence separated from a nonamer sequence by 12 or 23 nucleotide spacers.[1] Assembly of the rearranged V-D-J or V-J segment is followed by splicing to a C (constant) region exon, to produce a potential DNA coding sequence for an immunoglobulin or T cell receptor protein. Additional important events in this process include the addition of random, nontemplated nucleotides (N nucleotides) at the junctions of V-(D)-J segments via the action of the enzyme terminal deoxynucleotidyl transferase (TdT), and some degree of 'trimming' of nucleotides at the junctional ends by DNA exonucleases[1] (Fig. 43.1).

The ordered rearrangement of the antigen receptor genes is responsible for much of the remarkable diversity in immunoglobulin and T cell receptor repertoire underpinning the functions of the adaptive immune system. In particular, the random nature of gene segment selection, insertion of nontemplated nucleotides by TdT, and exonuclease trimming of exon junctions, together produce a rich and diverse initial repertoire of possible B cell and T cell receptor proteins. As such, the response to a specific antigenic challenge will engage B and T cells with variable receptor affinity and avidity, which in turn, can become further 'fine-tuned' in secondary lymphoid tissues, as exemplified in B cells by the germinal center-related processes of class switch recombination and somatic hypermutation. Thus, while each lymphoid cell expresses its unique antigen receptor, the collective recruitment of many lymphocytes in an inflammatory or immune response constitutes a polyclonal reaction. In contrast, malignant transformation of a lymphocyte population with subsequent unchecked expansion is characterized by uniformity in the expression of (usually) a single antigen receptor, representing a monoclonal proliferation. At the genomic level, the molecular analysis of antigen receptor gene rearrangements is a highly robust approach for delineating polyclonal from monoclonal lymphocytic populations, made possible by the substantial diversity of nucleotide sequences, in conjunction with some additional serendipitous features of these genetic loci. The subsequent section details the application of molecular genetic methods to determine the clonal status of lymphocytic proliferations.

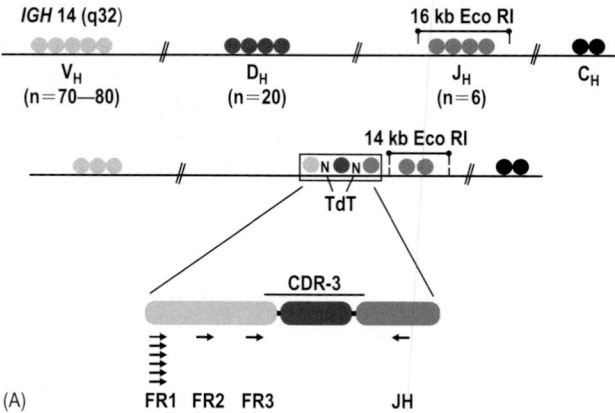

Figure 43.1   Immunoglobulin and T cell receptor gene rearrangements: basic structure and utility in assessment of clonal lymphoid proliferations. (A) Schematic representation of the *IGH* locus demonstrating the process of gene segment recombination to create a functional V-D-J coding cassette. Upper panel depicts germline configuration of the exon regions. Rearrangement of this gene during normal B cell development results from the selection and recombination of individual V-, D- and J-segments (middle panel). Gene segment recombination alters the location of restriction enzyme sites, as shown in this case by EcoRI sites flanking the J_H region (upper and middle panels); these changes are exploited for Southern blot hybridization lymphoid clonality analysis (see part B of figure and text). Exonucleases and the activity of the enzyme terminal deoxynucleotidyl transferase (TdT), which inserts nontemplated random nucleotide (N) bases at the junctions between V-D and D-J segments, together result in a unique hypervariable 'fingerprint' sequence region for the rearranged *IGH* gene in a given B cell (lower panel, expanded). Positions of oligonucleotide primers targeting conserved sequences in the framework (FR) and J-regions (J_H) for PCR-based clonality studies are indicated by horizontal arrows in the lower panel. The rearranged V-D-J segment is subsequently joined to the constant (C) region to complete the coding sequence for the *IGH* heavy chain. A similar sequence of events occurs at the immunoglobulin light chain genes and the T cell receptor genes, although D segments are not present in the light chain and *TRG* loci. (B) Plate 120, see plate section. (C) Plate 121, see plate section.

Techniques used in the determination of lymphoid clonality

In the diagnostic molecular hematology laboratory, two methods are utilized to determine if a lymphoid population represents a polyclonal expansion versus a monoclonal process. Southern blot hybridization (SBH) is a technique that examines relatively large structural rearrangements of genomic DNA via a multistep process involving restriction endonuclease digestion, DNA fragment transfer and immobilization on a charged membrane, and interrogation of the genetic loci of interest with

specific DNA probes.[2-7] Traditionally, probes used in SBH are labeled with a radioactive isotope (i.e. P^{32}) to enable detection on radiographic film, although chemiluminescent methods have also been successfully utilized for this purpose. In the 'germline', or non-rearranged state, the stringent hybridization of complementary probes to enzyme digested DNA fragments produces a particular pattern of fragment sizes or 'bands' characteristic of that locus. If the DNA region in question has been disrupted (e.g. by a gene rearrangement or translocation event), SBH will identify novel sized (non-germline) bands, due to the interposition of new restriction digestion sites or the abolition of native sites within the probed locus (Fig. 43.1). In this way, structural DNA rearrangements deviating from the expected normal band configuration can be unambiguously detected. Thus, in a polyclonal lymphoid proliferation, the large number and diversity of antigen receptor gene rearrangements is expected to produce many different sized nongermline fragments; however, the typical analytic sensitivity of SBH (5–10 percent) is not high enough to detect this polyclonal 'noise' of multiple rearranged bands. The presence of nonlymphoid cells in the analyzed sample allows for the detection of a germline band pattern, which is useful for assessing the quality of the assay. In contrast, a monoclonal lymphoid neoplasm, wherein all cells harbor the same antigen receptor gene rearrangement, will be characterized by the presence of new, clearly defined nongermline DNA fragments, provided the abnormal cell population represents greater than approximately 5–10 percent of total cells. In some cases, the monoclonal band pattern may demonstrate more than one nongermline bands at the antigen receptor locus of interest, denoting a bi-allelic gene rearrangement (i.e. one functional and one nonproductive rearrangement at the respective alleles).

To be successful, SBH requires that interrogated loci are informative relative to the positions of restriction enzyme sites (Fig. 43.1) and that excellent, high molecular weight DNA of adequate quantity is available from a given sample. Considering the former aspect, certain antigen receptor genes are more amenable to analysis by SBH: for B cells, these include the immunoglobulin heavy chain (*IGH*) and the κ light chain (*IGK*) loci; and for T cells, the T cell beta receptor (*TRB*) gene. The remaining antigen receptor genes are generally unfavorable for SBH because of excessive polymorphic variation (i.e. λ light chain, *IGL*); insufficient rearrangement diversity for unequivocally distinguishing polyclonal from monoclonal results (i.e. T cell gamma, *TRG*); or undue structural complexity (i.e. T cell alpha, *TRA*). Limiting factors in the performance of SBH include the requirement of fresh or frozen tissue to supply high-molecular-weight DNA, moderate analytic sensitivity, technical complexity and possible use of radioactive elements. In addition, at least two (and preferably three) different restriction digestions should be employed per locus evaluated, in order to minimize interpretive pitfalls; this concern underscores the need for a sufficient quantity of extracted DNA, which may be problematic with small tissue samples. The analysis of SBH results may also be challenging in certain instances, such as incomplete restriction enzyme digestion, rearranged bands that co-migrate with germline fragments, or improperly sampled lesional tissue. Nevertheless, SBH assessment can be considered a 'gold standard' for the detection of nongermline antigen receptor gene rearrangements and hence the presence of monoclonal B or T cell lymphoid populations, attributed mainly to the ability to visualize relatively large structural changes in DNA. The salient features of SBH technique are summarized in Table 43.1 (see later in Cautions and considerations in data interpretation).

Polymerase chain reaction (PCR) detection of rearranged antigen receptor gene DNA provides a second, powerful method for determining clonality in lymphoid populations.[2–4,7–10] In brief, oligonucleotide primers are chosen to bind to opposite strands of DNA encompassing the antigen receptor genes of interest. In the germline configuration, primer amplification across the large, non-rearranged regions of DNA at the antigen receptor loci cannot occur efficiently and PCR products are not obtained. Conversely, when the antigen receptor genes are rearranged in individual B and T lymphocytes, the flanking primers are brought into a favorable configuration capable of generating specific products during PCR. In a polyclonal lymphocyte population, amplicon fragments of many lengths are obtained, essentially in a normal or Gaussian distribution. The amplified PCR products at a given antigen receptor gene locus in a polyclonal expansion exhibit a predictable size range determined by PCR primer positions and the relative lengths of the rearranging V, (D) and J segments, as well as any additional nucleotide insertions or deletions at segmental junctions. A monoclonal proliferation is, in distinction, characterized by a unique single or double (bi-allelic) amplification product (Fig. 43.1).

The specificity of PCR technique for B and T cell clonality determination is a result of the highly unique nature of the V, (D) and J gene segment recombinations in individual lymphocytes. This feature is exemplified by the complementarity determining region 3 (CDR3) of the rearranged IGH gene in B lymphocytes, encompassing the V-D-J coding region along with a variable number of N-nucleotide insertions at the segmental junctions (Fig. 43.1). Despite the unpredictable nature of heavy chain gene rearrangements in any given B cell, the remarkable utility of the PCR approach relies on the fact that certain sequence regions within V and J segments are relatively conserved, permitting the use of 'consensus' primers that flank this most variable or 'fingerprint' region of the rearranged IGH gene (Fig. 43.1). By situating consensus primers within framework (FR) regions of V and J segments, the vast majority of IGH rearrangements can be amplified by PCR in a B lymphoid population. For T cell proliferations, the T cell receptor γ gene (TRG) is most often assessed by PCR methods. While productive γδ receptors are not made by the majority of T cells, TRG locus rearrangements are retained in nearly all mature T cells, thereby constituting a valuable marker for assessing monoclonality in T cell proliferations. The TRG locus is similarly amenable to evaluation using a multiple consensus primer approach[11] (Fig. 43.1). These two antigen receptor gene loci are thus the most frequently analyzed for the assessment of lymphoid clonality by PCR in clinical molecular diagnostic practice. PCR-based techniques have also been successfully developed to interrogate the κ light chain gene (IGK)[12,13] and, despite more substantial complexity, the beta T cell receptor locus (TRB). PCR products generated by consensus primer amplification are visualized either by gel electrophoresis, or more commonly now by using fluorescently labeled PCR primers and capillary electrophoresis[14,15] (Fig. 43.1).

Cautions and considerations in data interpretation

SBH and PCR can be considered complementary methods in the evaluation of blood or tissue samples for the presence of a clonal lymphoid population. However, the application of each technique is subject to several limitations determined by technical complexity, efficiency, specimen requirements, and clinical and analytic sensitivity (Table 43.1). As indicated, SBH requires a relatively generous amount of high molecular weight and non-degraded DNA. The method is complex and requires substantial technical expertise. Furthermore, results of SBH typically lag behind the tempo of routine hematopathology case evaluation, not infrequently incurring delays in rendering a final diagnosis. PCR in contrast is rapid, analytically sensitive, requires minimal DNA, can be performed using paraffin-embedded sample material, and is technically straightforward. The benefits of PCR analysis are somewhat offset by the finding that not all clonotypic gene rearrangements can be detected by consensus primer strategies (Table 43.1). This feature is most apparent in germinal center-associated B cell lymphomas, in which somatic hypermutation may inhibit the ability of primers to effectively bind to their target sites. Conversely, PCR amplification in certain instances of nonmalignant lymphoid expansions (e.g. in autoimmune disease, or with restricted T cell repertoires encountered in some elderly individuals), may produce skewed rearrangement profiles mimicking an oligoclonal or monoclonal result (i.e. 'pseudoclonality'). The latter phenomenon is sometimes encountered in T cell PCR analysis, owing to the limited V-J segment recombination potential at the TRG locus (Fig. 43.1). For these reasons, SBH retains an important place in many laboratories as the definitive standard for detecting lymphoid clonality. The shortcomings of the PCR approach have been largely mitigated in recent years by the efforts of the Europe Against Cancer (EAC) consortium, culminating in the BIOMED-2 primer protocols for comprehensive B and T cell receptor PCR analysis.[16–20] By first developing reagents with robust

Table 43.1   Comparison of Southern blot hybridization and polymerase chain reaction (PRC) techniques for clonality determination in lymphoid tumors

Parameter	Southern blot	PCR
DNA quantity required	Large (>5 µg per restriction digest)	Small (0.2–1 µg per reaction)
DNA quality	High molecular weight only (fresh/frozen tissue required)	Partly degraded DNA often usable (can use paraffin tissues also)
Assay time	Long, labor intensive (1 week)	Rapid, straightforward (1–2 days)
Analytic sensitivity	Lower (5–10%)	Higher (1–5% with consensus primers)
Interpretive concerns	Partial (incomplete) enzyme digestions, true clonal rearrangements co-migrating with normal germline bands	False-negative results (incomplete primer coverage, somatic hypermutation in immunoglobulin loci) False-positive results (spurious amplifications with minimal lymphocytes in sample, restricted rearrangement repertoire of target locus [e.g. T cell gamma gene, TRG] or with increasing patient age)
Role	'Gold standard' for detecting close to 100% of possible antigen receptor gene rearrangements, but less often performed	Improvements in methods (e.g. BIOMED-2 protocols[16–20]) reduce errors in detection rates, but problematic interpretation (e.g. with *TRG* PCR) remains in some cases

and reproducible characteristics, then accumulating substantial data regarding clinical sensitivity and specificity, this group and others have significantly advanced the capabilities of PCR technique in this area, as well as the parameters for meaningful assay standardization and clinical usage.[21,22]

Several interpretive aspects of lymphoid clonality assessment deserve further mention, particularly regarding PCR technique. Immunoglobulin and T cell receptor gene rearrangements exhibit high fidelity in normal B and T cells respectively; however, lymphoid neoplasms can demonstrate 'cross-lineage' gene rearrangements.[16] This finding is most commonly observed in precursor B cell acute lymphoblastic leukemia/lymphoma, in which aberrant T cell receptor locus rearrangements can be identified in >50 percent of cases. By extension, a monoclonal antigen receptor gene rearrangement cannot be used on its own for the purpose of defining cell lineage in a neoplastic lymphoid proliferation. Such cross-lineage rearrangements can nonetheless serve as important markers for diagnosis and clone-specific minimal residual disease monitoring during therapy.[23,24] Among mature lymphoid tumors, one may also encounter distinct coexisting B and T cell clonal populations by molecular analysis. This situation is noted in some cases of angioimmunoblastic T cell lymphoma (AITL).[25] A thorough knowledge of clinical and histopathological findings is required to correctly interpret gene rearrangement studies in this context. Finally, the occurrence of 'pseudoclonal' PCR results especially with *TRG* assays has been mentioned and can lead to the erroneous diagnosis of a monoclonal (and hence malignant)

T cell process (Table 43.1). T cell PCR studies in particular must be carefully interpreted according to available clinical and pathologic data, as well as semi-objective analytic criteria.[11,26]

DETECTION AND CLINICAL SIGNIFICANCE OF CHROMOSOMAL TRANSLOCATIONS AND OTHER GENETIC ANOMALIES IN THE LYMPHOID NEOPLASMS

Chromosome aberrations are common events in the lymphoid neoplasms and broadly are grouped into numerical and structural changes. Aneuploidy, indicating a deviation from the '2n' modal chromosome number per cell, is well recognized among acute B cell leukemias and non-Hodgkin lymphomas. Insertions, deletions and translocations are the major forms of structural abnormalities. Chromosome translocations notably underlie the pathogenesis of many immature and mature lymphocytic malignancies. The molecular mechanisms responsible for the production of reciprocal chromosome translocations are as yet not fully understood, but may involve susceptible conformations of DNA (e.g. non-B DNA structure), spatial proximity of key genetic loci during cell cycle events, regions prone to DNA double strand breaks, and aberrant activity of RAG recombinase or other DNA breakage/repair proteins.[27,28] The resultant close juxtaposition of two unrelated genes resulting from a chromosomal translocation can result in one of two major consequences. In one instance, a fusion or chimeric gene is produced, resulting in the production of

Table 43.2 Major chromosome translocation abnormalities in the non-Hodgkin lymphomas

Translocation/genetic abnormality	Lymphoma	Molecular consequence	Detection
t(14;18)(q32;q21)/BCL2-IGH	Follicular lymphoma, subset of diffuse large B cell lymphomas	BCL2 overexpression; antiapoptosis phenotype	FISH better than PCR
t(11;14)(q13;q32)/CCND1-IGH	Mantle cell lymphoma	Cyclin D1 overexpression; cell cycle deregulation	FISH better than PCR[a]
BCL6 gene translocations	Large B cell lymphomas	BCL6 overexpression; sustained 'germinal center-like' state	FISH
t(8;14)(q24;q32)/cMYC-IGH	Burkitt lymphoma, some large B cell lymphomas	MYC overexpression; cell proliferation	FISH
t(11;18)(q21;q21)/API2-MALT1	Extranodal marginal zone B cell lymphoma (MALT type)	NFκB pathway activation; cell proliferation, antiapoptosis	FISH, RT-PCR
t(14;18)(q32;q21)/MALT1-IGH	Extranodal marginal zone B cell lymphoma (MALT type)	NFκB pathway activation; cell proliferation, antiapoptosis	FISH
t(2;5)(p23;q35)/NPM-ALK	Anaplastic large T cell lymphoma	ALK tyrosine kinase overexpression; cell proliferation	FISH, RT-PCR[a]
Other ALK gene translocations	Anaplastic large T cell lymphoma	ALK tyrosine kinase overexpression; cell proliferation	FISH[a]

[a]Immunohistochemistry for cyclin D1 and ALK1 protein expression is also typically used for diagnosis of mantle cell lymphoma and anaplastic large cell lymphoma, respectively.
FISH, fluorescence *in situ* hybridization; RT-PCR, recombinant polymerase chain reaction.

a hybrid mRNA and protein. This abnormality is often observed in acute leukemias and is prototypically represented by the *BCR-ABL1* oncogene in chronic myeloid leukemia (CML). Alternatively, a gene that is normally tightly regulated is brought under the control of an actively transcribed locus, resulting in unchecked expression of the former gene. Gene overexpression by this mechanism is more often characteristic of the non-Hodgkin lymphomas, as exemplified by translocations of the *BCL2* or *MYC* genes to the *IGH* locus.

Chromosome translocations (and other genetic anomalies) provide important clues to the pathobiology of lymphoid tumors and are useful in the diagnosis and subclassification of these entities (Table 43.2). Certain markers can also be employed as tumor-specific targets for minimal residual disease detection. Numerical and structural chromosome changes can be identified by classic G-band karyotyping. These standard cytogenetic studies provide a comprehensive survey for many different chromosomal abnormalities in a tumor sample, but are limited by the requirement for fresh sterile cells that will grow adequately in culture. Cytogenetics analysis is also somewhat constrained by the number of metaphases that can be reasonably assessed (typically 20–30). Fluorescence *in situ* hybridization technique (FISH) and PCR are modalities that provide specific and sensitive means for targeted detection of diagnostically relevant genetic abnormalities and these methods are frequently used to supplement the morphologic and immunophenotypic evaluation of the lymphoproliferative disorders.

FISH and PCR techniques for detecting translocations in lymphoid tumors

The FISH technique is based upon the binding of fluorescently labeled DNA probes complementary to specific genomic loci, using intact cell nuclei or metaphase chromosomes.[29] The design of the probes is critical both to produce highly specific and sensitive signals, and to accommodate different analytic strategies germane to the goal of the particular FISH application. Dual color-dual fusion FISH (D-FISH) is commonly employed to identify chromosomal translocations. D-FISH comprises fluorescent DNA probes of two different colors that respectively span the breakpoint regions of the chromosome loci potentially involved in a balanced translocation event. A fusion signal resulting from the colocalization of the DNA probes indicates the presence of the translocation in question. The specificity of D-FISH method is enhanced by the ability to visualize both the target translocation and the reciprocal DNA rearrangement in the same cell. FISH using break-apart probes (BAP) is a second frequently utilized diagnostic approach for evaluating a genetic locus with potentially many translocation partners. The BAP method also relies on a dual color probe set, but the probes are arrayed at a single chromosome locus, giving a fusion signal in the unaltered DNA state. A chromosome translocation involving this site will result in separation of the probes, visualized as split signals. BAP FISH does not identify the exact translocation *per se*, but a positive result indicates that a specific target gene has been involved in such an event. Finally,

Table 43.3   Analytic sensitivity comparison of techniques for detecting genetic abnormalities in lymphomas and lymphoid leukemias

Method	Sensitivity (%)	Utility	Abnormalities detected
Cytogenetics	5	Diagnosis	Numerical and structural anomalies including translocations
Fluorescence *in situ* hybridization	1–5	Diagnosis, selected MRD use	Numerical and structural anomalies including translocations
DNA polymerase chain reaction (PCR)	$1–10^{-3}$	Diagnosis, MRD	Some translocations; antigen receptor gene rearrangements
Reverse transcription (RNA) PCR	$10^{-2}–10^{-4}$	Diagnosis, MRD	Translocations producing fusion (chimeric) mRNA species

MRD, minimal residual disease.

repetitive sequence or enumeration probes (e.g. centromere-specific probes) are commonly employed to identify numerical abnormalities in interphase or metaphase nuclear preparations. FISH offers several powerful advantages for molecular diagnosis including rapidity, the ability to use a variety of tissue types (e.g. nuclei from paraffin-embedded fixed material), and the provision of quantitative results. FISH technique is practically limited by the number of nuclei that can be counted and the presence of degraded sample quality. A large number of DNA probes for various FISH techniques are now commercially available (Vysis, Downers Grove, Illinois, USA).

PCR technique is also useful for the detection of chromosome translocations associated with lymphoid neoplasms. Reverse transcription (RT)-PCR is employed to detect translocation events that produce chimeric mRNA species, commonly encountered in lymphoid and myeloid leukemias. In RT-PCR assays, PCR primers are designed to amplify across the junctional region of the reverse-transcribed hybrid cDNA template in question. RT-PCR is highly sensitive and specific in this regard and forms the basis for quantitative PCR monitoring in several leukemic diseases (e.g. chronic myeloid leukemia, acute promyelocytic leukemia).[30,31] RT-PCR method requires extracted RNA of good quality, thus largely limiting sample sources to fresh or frozen tissues. As indicated, most translocation abnormalities occurring in the non-Hodgkin lymphomas instead result in overexpression or deregulation of a target gene and as such do not form unique mRNA species that would permit detection by RT-PCR. However, PCR with extracted DNA can be used to amplify the genomic region of a specific translocation event using primers placed adjacent to the break-fusion area. For DNA PCR to be successful, the breakpoint region(s) in the involved genes should show relatively tight clustering in the majority of neoplasms with the particular translocation, and primers flanking the fusion site should be physically proximate to permit efficient amplification. While this situation exists for some lymphoma-associated translocations (e.g. the t(14;18)(q32;q21)/*BCL2-IGH*), many others have large intronic breakpoint regions without substantial clustering among individual cases, precluding the routine application of consensus type primers for PCR detection. These features,

in conjunction with the larger and variable amplicon sizes obtained, tend to reduce the utility of DNA PCR for detecting translocations in the lymphomas relative to FISH techniques. DNA PCR continues to be a valuable alternative when inadequate material is available for FISH studies, or for molecular monitoring of a specific genetic translocation during therapy. Table 43.3 outlines the optimum use of FISH and molecular analytic modalities in these different situations. The following section will discuss the lymphoid neoplasms with distinct cytogenetic associations.

Common genetic abnormalities useful in the diagnosis and differential diagnosis of B lineage lymphoid neoplasms

BCL2 GENE TRANSLOCATIONS

The t(14;18)(q32;q21) event is identified in 85 percent of follicular lymphomas and less than one-third of diffuse large B cell lymphomas (DLBCLs). At least for follicular lymphoma, the translocation is thought to occur early in the process of B cell development, possibly due to aberrant recombinase activity at rearrangement prone non-B DNA intermediate structures in the *BCL2* locus.[28] The t(14;18) transfers the *BCL2* gene adjacent to the *IGH* locus on chromosome 14(q32), bringing *BCL2* under control of the powerful *IGH* enhancer element. BCL2 is the prototypic antiapoptotic family member of the intrinsic pathway of apoptosis regulatory proteins and its overexpression is assumed to be a key factor in initiating or sustaining the neoplastic state in many diverse tumors.[32,33] At the molecular level, most breakpoints in the *BCL2* gene occur within or just distal to the noncoding third exon of *BCL2* known as the major breakpoint region (MBR), or less commonly at a locus approximately 20 kilobases (kb) downstream termed the minor cluster region (mcr).[16] In addition, two less well defined breakpoint regions between these sites have been designated the far 3' MBR and 5' mcr, respectively[16,34–36] (Fig. 43.2). The *IGH* break site is invariably located in the JH region. *BCL2* MBR breakpoints comprise nearly 70 percent of *BCL2-IGH* events and, because of substantial breakpoint clustering, these gene fusions are

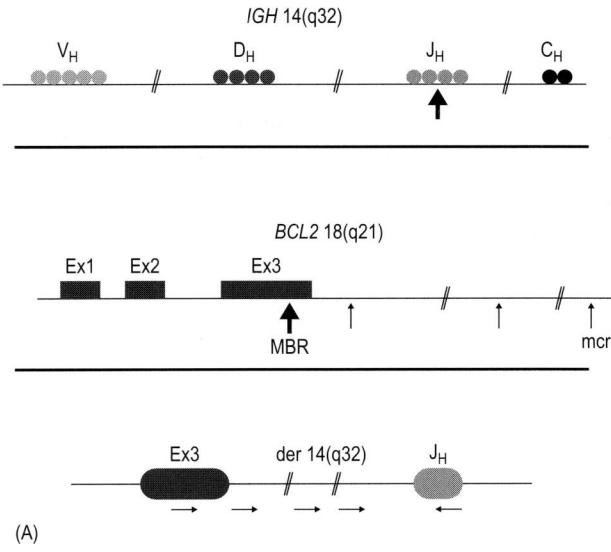

IGH 14(q32)

V_H   D_H   J_H   C_H

BCL2 18(q21)

Ex1 Ex2 Ex3

MBR   mcr

Ex3   der 14(q32)   J_H

(A)

Figure 43.2   Detection of *BCL2* gene translocations in lymphoma. (A) Schematic depicting the breakpoints in the *IGH* and *BCL2* genes as a result of the t(14;18)(q32;q21) event. Break sites in *IGH* involve the JH region, whereas greater heterogeneity is noted in *BCL2*. The majority (two-thirds) of *BCL2* genomic breaks occur in the major breakpoint region (MBR) within exon (Ex) 3, with a small percentage involving the minor cluster region (mcr). Additional vertical arrows indicate other *BCL2* regions with looser clustering of breakpoints (i.e. 3′ MBR and 5′ mcr). The lower panel demonstrates the possible *BCL2-IGH* gene fusions with horizontal arrows indicating placement of PCR primers to detect this translocation event. Comprehensive PCR strategies as indicated can identify the majority of *BCL2-IGH* fusions, but a small number are still undetectable due to breakpoint heterogeneity in *BCL2*; fluorescence *in situ* hybridization (FISH) method is the most clinically sensitive approach in this regard. (B) Plate 122, see plate section.

detectable by DNA PCR using a primer situated just outside the MBR and a reverse consensus primer placed in the JH segment of the *IGH* gene[16,35–40] (Fig. 43.2). The addition of mcr locus PCR primers slightly increases the detection rate for the *BCL2-IGH* abnormality, and primers targeting the 3′MBR and 5′ mcr can further marginally enhance sensitivity.[34–36] In practice, *BCL2-IGH* PCR using paraffin-embedded fixed tissue may be limited by DNA degradation, resulting in an inability to amplify target DNA templates at the larger end of the expected fragment size range.

In addition to standard DNA PCR, long-distance PCR techniques[34,41] have also been described for the comprehensive detection of *BCL2-IGH* fusions; however these methods require high-molecular-weight DNA and more critically optimized PCR conditions. D-FISH analysis is associated with the highest clinical sensitivity for *BCL2-IGH* detection[42] (Fig. 43.2) and can often be performed from fixed tissue material. The identification of the

BCL2-IGH genetic abnormality can be helpful to distinguish follicular lymphoma from atypical follicular hyperplasias or other B cell lymphomas mimicking a follicular histologic pattern (e.g. marginal zone lymphoma, mantle cell lymphoma). Tumor-specific *BCL2-IGH* amplicons or sequences can also be used to sensitively monitor follicular lymphoma patients for recurrence by PCR following curative intent therapy.[43] One molecular diagnostic caveat concerns the small subset of follicular lymphoma lacking the t(14;18). These tumors tend to be of higher cytologic grade and in such cases a negative PCR or D-FISH study should not exclude the diagnosis of follicular lymphoma, if other pathologic findings are supportive. There are perhaps fewer indications for *BCL2-IGH* evaluation in DLBCL, although in some cases of high grade B cell lymphoma, the finding of the *BCL2-IGH* gene fusion helps in the distinction from a true Burkitt lymphoma.[44,45] Of note, while the t(14;18)/*BCL2-IGH* abnormality mechanistically accounts for BCL2 overexpression in most FL and some DLBCL, many other B cell neoplasms can upregulate BCL2 protein levels by non-translocation mechanisms.

CCND1 GENE TRANSLOCATIONS

Mantle cell lymphoma (MCL) is essentially defined by the presence of the t(11;14)(q13;q32) abnormality, resulting in fusion of the *CCND1* gene with the *IGH* locus on 14(q32).[46] *CCND1* encodes the highly regulated protein cyclin D1, a G1 phase cell cycle protein involved along with its cognate cyclin dependent kinases (Cdk4, Cdk6) in promoting the transition from G1 to S-phase of the cell cycle in dividing cells, principally by phosphorylation of the retinoblastoma protein.[47] Overexpression of cyclin D1 as a consequence of juxtaposition with the *IGH* gene is a central factor underlying the proliferative phenotype of MCL. Breakpoints in chromosome 11(q13) occur at the *BCL1* locus, with nearly 50 percent involving the major translocation cluster (MTC) region located approximately 120 kb centromeric to the *CCND1* gene.[46] The remaining break sites in *BCL1* occur over a large expanse of genomic DNA between the MTC and the *CCND1* gene, without significant breakpoint clustering. *IGH* break sites uniformly involve the JH region. The clustering of *BCL1* breakpoints at the MTC allows for a DNA PCR strategy with MTC and JH consensus primers (Fig. 43.3), although this approach will detect slightly less than half of possible *BCL1-IGH* genetic fusions in MCL.[46,48] Improvements in PCR strategy have not been forthcoming, owing to the substantial breakpoint heterogeneity elsewhere in the *BCL1* locus. Thus, while PCR can be used successfully to identify most of the MTC-related *CCND1-IGH* translocation events, D-FISH is the preferable analytic method for the most sensitive detection of this genetic abnormality[49,50] (Fig. 43.3). The very strong association of the *CCND1-IGH* fusion gene with MCL provides a highly specific genetic marker for diagnosis. In addition, some cases of MCL may exhibit a predominantly nodular growth pattern, or features of

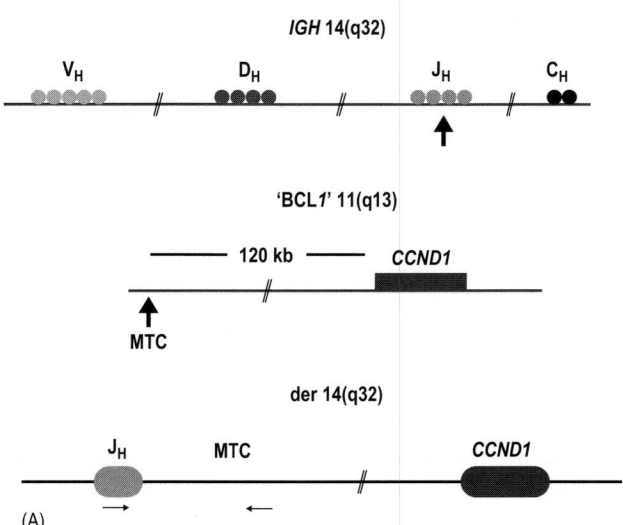

Figure 43.3   Detection of *CCND1* gene translocations in lymphoma. (A) Schematic showing the genomic breakpoints in *IGH* JH region and chromosome 11q13 '*BCL1*' locus arising from the t(11;14)(q13;q32) in mantle cell lymphoma (MCL). The *BCL1* locus is located far upstream of the gene encoding cyclin D1 (*CCND1*), although *CCND1* nonetheless becomes deregulated by the translocation and placement near the actively transcribed *IGH* gene. Approximately one-half of *BCL1* region break sites occur in the major translocation cluster (MTC). PCR primers complementary to MTC and JH sequences can be used to detect most of these events, but overall, the PCR detection rate is below 50 percent for the t(11;14). (B) Plate 123, see plate section.

'monocytoid' differentiation, suggesting a histologic diagnosis of follicular lymphoma or marginal zone B cell lymphoma respectively. In these instances, identification of the *CCND1-IGH* is critical for correct classification. Given the adverse clinical outcome associated with MCL, identification of the *CCND1-IGH* abnormality is clearly of prognostic importance. The diagnostic impact of molecular and FISH evaluation for the *CCND1-IGH* fusion gene has been lessened to some extent by improved immunohistochemical staining for cyclin D1 protein; however, molecular diagnostic assessment remains an important modality in the assessment of MCL. Of note, very rare cases with the phenotypic, morphologic and gene expression features of MCL have been recently described lacking cyclin D1 overexpression and *CCND1-IGH* rearrangement; these tumors are characterized instead by alterations in other D-type cyclins.[51]

MALT1, *BCL10* AND *FOXP1* GENE REARRANGEMENTS IN MARGINAL ZONE B CELL LYMPHOMAS

The molecular biology of extranodal marginal zone B cell lymphomas of mucosa-associated lymphoid tissue (MALT) type has become a fascinating and rapidly progressing area of research. On the one hand, the association of MALT

Table 43.4   Relative frequency and anatomic site distribution of translocation abnormalities in extranodal marginal B cell lymphomas of mucosa-associated lymphoid tissue (MALT) type[a]

Translocation	Tissue/organ sites	Relative frequency (percent)
t(11;18)/API2/MALT1	Stomach	20–25
	Lung	40
	Ocular adnexae	10
	Salivary gland	<5
t(14;18)/MALT1-IGH	Lung	5
	Ocular adnexae	5
t(1;14)/BCL10-IGH	Stomach	5
	Lung	10
t(3;14)/*FOXP1-IGH* (based on limited case numbers)	Thyroid	50
	Ocular adnexae	20
	Skin	10
	Stomach	<5

[a]Adapted from Du.[53]

lymphomas with infectious agents has resulted in the option of antibiotic therapy for some patients, in whom dramatic reversals of low-grade lymphomas have been observed (i.e. *Helicobacter pylori*-associated gastric marginal zone lymphomas).[52] In concert, there has been an exciting realization that several structural genetic anomalies found in the MALT lymphomas share a common pathophysiology converging on abnormal nuclear factor (NF)κB pathway activation.[53] Genetic subclassification of MALT lymphomas thus has diagnostic and therapeutic relevance. A wide range of genetic abnormalities has been identified in the MALT lymphomas, with a subset of cases exhibiting numerical karyotype changes, most often trisomies or additions of chromosomes 3, 12 and 18. Recurrent translocation events characterize a second group of tumors, including the t(11;18)(q21;q21)/*API2-MALT1*, the t(1;14)(p22;q32)/*BCL10-IGH*, and the t(14;18)(q21;q32)/*MALT1-IGH* abnormalities.[53] The frequency and tissue site distribution of these translocations is variable (Table 43.4). The t(11;18)/*API2-MALT1* is relatively common, being found in approximately 20 percent of gastric and up to 40 percent of lung MALT lymphomas, with lower occurrence in other anatomic sites.[53–56] The *API2* gene encodes an apoptosis inhibitor (API2, cIAP2) and becomes fused in proximity to the *MALT1* locus. MALT1 is a paracaspase-like protein that functions in normal NFκB pathway signaling.[57–59] The fusion gene creates a chimeric API2-MALT1 mRNA and protein with altered functionality of both components. A second abnormality, the t(1;14), juxtaposes the *BCL10* gene next to the *IGH* locus, deregulating the expression of the former gene. BCL10 is also involved in NFκB signaling and normal lymphocyte development via interactions with MALT1.[59,60] The *BCL10-IGH* anomaly is rare and mainly occurs in a small number of gastric and lung MALT lymphomas.

The t(14;18) abnormality joins the *MALT1* gene to the *IGH* locus. The *MALT1-IGH* gene fusion is detected in less than 10 percent of lung and ocular adnexal marginal zone lymphomas, but is not prevalent in stomach or other extra-nodal sites. These three translocation events each result in constitutive activation of the NFκB signal transduction pathway, ultimately through degradation of the NFκB regulatory protein IκB.[53] NFκB normally functions as a highly regulated pleiotropic transcription factor targeting genes involved in lymphocyte cell survival, activation and proliferation; aberrant NFκB expression is thus central to the pathophysiology of these lymphomas.[61]

Detection of the *API2-MALT1* and *MALT1-IGH* lesions is best accomplished by D-FISH technique (Plate 124, see plate section). RT-PCR amplification of the chimeric API2-MALT1 mRNA has also been described;[62] however, this approach requires high quality RNA and is technically complicated by substantial breakpoint heterogeneity in both *API2* and *MALT1* genes. Identification of these translocation fusion gene abnormalities, when present, can be helpful for establishing the diagnosis of lymphoma in morphologically challenging small tissue biopsies, or in differentiating marginal zone lymphoma with follicular colonization from true follicular lymphoma. Of note, although the t(14;18) karyotype banding pattern is identical in both marginal zone lymphoma and FL, the *MALT1* gene is situated slightly centromeric to the *BCL2* locus on 18(q21) and these entities can be distinguished with the appropriate application of FISH probes. Perhaps most significantly, recognition of *API2-MALT1* positive gastric marginal zone B cell lymphomas is important, as these tumors do not respond to the broad spectrum antibiotic eradication of *H. pylori*, a therapeutic option which is often successful at inducing tumor regression in a subset of translocation negative cases.[52] Finally, the recent discovery of the t(3;14)(p13;q32)/*FOXP1-IGH* abnormality continues to expand the spectrum of genetic findings in MALT lymphomas.[63] FOXP1, a member of the forkhead family of transcription factors, is involved in regulation of RAG1 and RAG2 protein expression during B cell development.[64] The *FOXP1* gene translocation occurs in subsets of thyroid, ocular adnexa, skin and rare gastric lymphomas, but not in lung lymphoid tumors.

BCL6 GENE ABNORMALITIES

BCL6 is a gene located on chromosome 3(q27) and it encodes a zinc finger transcription factor that is critical for normal germinal center development and T cell dependent antibody responses in B cells.[65,66] BCL6 protein is therefore identified in germinal center B lymphocytes and a subset of mature T cells. BCL6 is rapidly downregulated in B cells upon exit from the germinal center environment. Not surprisingly, BCL6 overexpression is noted in B cell lymphomas associated with germinal center cellular counterparts, namely follicular lymphoma and DLBCL.[67,68]

Rearrangements of the *BCL6* gene occur in a significant number of DLBCL (30–40 percent) and a smaller subset of follicular lymphoma (<20 percent). The *BCL6* gene is more commonly involved in translocations to either the *IGH* or light chain gene loci, although many nonimmunoglobulin translocation gene partners have also been described.[69] An even larger proportion of DLBCL and follicular lymphoma both with and without *BCL6* translocations demonstrate somatic mutations in the 5′ noncoding regions of the gene.[70] Such mutations are also identified in normal memory (postgerminal center) B lymphocytes and are thought to arise during the germinal center-associated somatic hypermutation process.[71] The expression of BCL6 is considered important in the pathogenesis of germinal center-related B cell lymphomas by presumably maintaining the abnormal lymphocytes in a germinal center-like environment, thereby providing protection from proapoptotic stimuli and creating the setting for ongoing cell proliferation and genetic mutation to occur.[72–74] Because *BCL6* translocations and somatic mutations are relatively difficult to detect and at present there is no prognostic value in this regard, molecular diagnostic evaluation of *BCL6* status in B cell lymphomas is infrequently undertaken. Translocation events involving the *BCL6* locus can be determined by BAP FISH methodology.

MYC GENE TRANSLOCATIONS

The *MYC* gene has been extensively studied in models of lymphomagenesis. Most characteristically, translocation of *MYC* to the immunoglobulin genes is a hallmark finding in Burkitt lymphoma.[75,76] The *MYC* gene is also abnormally activated by chromosome translocation in high-grade lymphomas associated with human immunodeficiency virus (HIV) infection/acquired immune deficiency syndrome (AIDS), occasional DLBCL, transformations of indolent lymphomas, and in some monomorphic post-transplant lymphoproliferative disorders. Most commonly, *MYC* is involved in the t(8;14)(q24;q32) abnormality, placing the gene in juxtaposition with the *IGH* locus and its transcriptional enhancer.[75,76] Less frequently, *MYC* translocations can involve the *IGK* and *IGL* loci at 2(p12) or 22(q11) respectively. In each case, *MYC* expression is deregulated, leading to pronounced proliferative consequences in affected lymphocytes. A target of mitogen-stimulated cell signaling events, cMYC is an early response transcription factor that exerts potent effects on cognate genes involved in cell cycle entry and DNA synthesis.[76,77] While *MYC* is considered central to the pathogenesis of Burkitt lymphoma and other high-grade lymphomas, enforced overexpression of the gene is deleterious to the cell and thus additional mechanisms involving protection from apoptosis are likely needed for lymphoma to develop. The molecular events underlying the t(8;14)/*MYC-IGH* abnormality have been extensively studied in Burkitt lymphoma.[76] So-called endemic-type Burkitt lymphoma (associated strongly with Epstein–Barr virus [EBV] infection) show *MYC* break sites distributed far upstream of the gene, and corresponding chromosome 14(q32) breaks in the JH region of *IGH*. In sporadic Burkitt lymphoma, the *MYC* breakpoints occur near or at the 5′ part of the gene, with *IGH* interruptions involving the heavy chain switch region (Sμ). No significant phenotypic or clinical differences appear related to the slightly variant molecular findings in Burkitt lymphoma. Because either heavy or light chain immunoglobulin genes can be involved in translocations with *MYC* and substantial breakpoint heterogeneity in *MYC* precludes the effective placement of oligonucleotide primers for PCR analysis, *MYC* translocations are best identified by FISH techniques.[78] FISH using a BAP strategy at the *MYC* locus can be utilized to initially identify the presence of a gene rearrangement; the presence of *IGH* involvement can subsequently be discerned with a D-FISH approach (Plate 125, see plate section). The use of both FISH techniques is often desirable in assessing the *MYC* locus, because probe signal patterns will be variable based on genomic breakpoint regions and the particular immunoglobulin gene translocation partner utilized in a given case of lymphoma. Detection of *MYC* gene translocation is imperative to establish the diagnosis of BL in cases with strong presumptive clinical and pathologic findings, given that treatment options for these patients are typically more intensive and are often curative. In difficult pathologic presentations for which the cytomorphologic and immunophenotypic differential diagnosis includes Burkitt lymphoma versus a high-grade DLBCL, application of FISH analysis for *MYC*, *BCL2* and possibly *BCL6* gene rearrangements can help to distinguish true Burkitt lymphoma (i.e. with *MYC* translocation only) from 'double hit' high grade DLBCL (e.g. with *MYC* translocation plus a second genetic locus abnormality).[44,45] Among the latter group of DLBCL, the presence of a *MYC* translocation has been associated with aggressive disease and a poor prognosis.[44,45]

Common genetic abnormalities useful in the diagnosis and differential diagnosis of T lineage lymphoid neoplasms

ALK GENE TRANSLOCATIONS

Anaplastic large cell lymphoma (ALCL) is a distinctive morphologic and phenotypic subtype of peripheral T cell lymphoma. The majority of ALCL tumors are characterized by the presence of translocations involving the anaplastic lymphoma kinase gene *ALK*, located on chromosome 2(p23).[79,80] In approximately 75 percent of 'ALK positive' ALCL, the *ALK* gene is involved in a reciprocal translocation with the nucleophosmin (*NPM1*) gene on 5(q35). The hybrid *NPM1-ALK* gene generates a chimeric mRNA and protein. ALK is a tyrosine kinase that is not normally expressed in lymphocytes, but becomes constitutively activated through its fusion with NPM1 resulting from the t(2;5) event.[81,82] NPM1 is a nucleolar shuttle

protein active in ribosome assembly.[83] In turn, the NPM1 moiety directs the ALK component of the fusion protein to an altered subcellular location and promotes autophosphorylation of ALK through dimerization interactions.[79,81,82] Aberrant deregulated ALK activity is a key feature in the pathogenesis of these lymphomas. The abnormal ALK fusion protein can be detected by immunohistochemistry and is observed in a nuclear and nucleolar staining pattern.[80,84] In addition to the t(2;5)/*NPM1-ALK*, other partner genes are involved in translocations with *ALK* including the t(1;2)(q25;p23)/*TPM3-ALK*, t(2;3)(p23;q35)/ *TFG-ALK* and inv(2)(p23q35)/*ATIC-ALK* abnormalities.[80,81] These additional ALK fusions involve partner proteins normally situated in the cytoplasm (e.g. TPM3, tropomyosin-3); a corresponding diffuse cytoplasmic pattern is thus noted by anti-ALK immunohistochemical methods in these lymphoma cases.

Recognition of ALK positive ALCL is important in light of the more favorable treatment response of these tumors relative to ALK negative ALCL.[83–85] Given the range of potential translocation partners, *ALK* gene rearrangements can be comprehensively identified by BAP FISH technique. FISH analysis may be preferable for initial diagnostic assessment, since the actual *ALK* gene fusion type does not appear to significantly influence clinical outcome. The relatively more common *NPM1-ALK* abnormality can also be specifically detected by RT-PCR amplification of the corresponding chimeric mRNA.[86–88] RT-PCR for the NPM1-ALK transcript has been advocated as part of staging bone marrow examinations in pediatric ALCL patients, since molecular positivity more sensitively identifies patients at risk for disease relapse compared to immunophenotyping studies.[89] While *ALK* gene translocations define this distinct group of peripheral T cell lymphomas, rare IgA positive, CD30 negative large B cell lymphomas with plasmablastic or immunoblastic cytology have been described with a t(2;17) anomaly, placing *ALK* next to the clathrin gene *CLTC*.[90–92] The CLTC-ALK fusion protein creates a distinctive immunostaining pattern of granular cell membrane positivity, corresponding to localization within clathrin-coated pits. From the foregoing discussion, it is apparent that immunohistochemistry with an anti-ALK antibody can supplant molecular or molecular cytogenetic studies for the diagnosis of ALK-positive ALCL. The pattern of immunostaining (nuclear, cytoplasmic, or granular membranous) also gives some clues toward the underlying molecular lesion involving the *ALK* gene.[84,92] Nevertheless, molecular genetic investigations are commonly used to help characterize this subset of peripheral T cell lymphomas in many diagnostic hematopathology laboratories.

TCL1 GENE TRANSLOCATIONS

T cell prolymphocytic leukemia (T-PLL) is an uncommon T cell tumor with widespread tissue distribution typically involving blood, bone marrow, spleen and lymph nodes. Most cases of T-PLL express CD4 antigen, although a small number of CD8 positive tumors have also been described. Coexpression of both CD4 and CD8 antigens is considered a characteristic feature of T-PLL, which in conjunction with prolymphocytic cytomorphology, strongly suggests this diagnosis; however, this phenotype is present in a minor subset of cases. In the majority of T-PLL presentations, the differential diagnosis thus broadens to include other subtypes of peripheral T cell neoplasms. The diagnosis of T-PLL is greatly enhanced by detection of translocations involving the *TCL1* gene. Approximately 80 percent of T-PLL harbor either inv14(q11q32) or t(14;14)(q11;q32) rearrangements, placing the *TCL1* gene next to the T cell receptor α (*TRA*) locus.[93,94] A small number of cases of T-PLL are notable for alternative t(X;14)(q28;q11) and t(X;7)(q28;q35) anomalies, involving translocations of the *TCL1*-related gene *MTCP1* to either the *TRA* or T cell β (*TRB*) locus, respectively.[93,95] *TCL1* is an incompletely understood oncogene, but may sustain malignant cell proliferation through the Akt signaling pathway.[93,94] *TCL1* is not normally expressed in mature T cells and is not detected in peripheral T cell neoplasms except for T-PLL, thus providing a relatively specific marker for this tumor.

TCL1 gene rearrangements are best identified by FISH technique, as these abnormalities can be cytogenetically cryptic (Plate 126, see plate section). Standard karyotype studies may nonetheless be helpful for identifying variant translocations involving the *MTCP1* locus in other cases of T-PLL. Immunohistochemical staining for TCL1 protein is also of obvious value in helping to establish the diagnosis of T-PLL in tissue biopsies; however, a small subset of T-PLL may lack both *TCL1* gene rearrangement and expression of TCL1 protein. With the availability of newer therapeutic agents such as alemtuzumab (CAMPATH-1, anti-CD52 antibody) active against T-PLL,[93] the demonstration of TCL1 abnormalities is important for accurate diagnosis in suspected cases, with the caveat that some 'TCL1-negative' T-PLL can rarely occur. Of note, nearly two-thirds of T-PLL cases also show a deletion of chromosome 11q with concomitant mutation of the *ATM* tumor suppressor gene at the remaining allelic locus on 11(q22-q23).[93] The presence of del 11q can also be detected by FISH probe technique as an adjunct to the diagnosis of T-PLL.

ABNORMALITIES OF CHROMOSOME 7q

A variety of other cytogenetic anomalies are correlated with distinct clinicopathologic lymphoid entities, including alterations of the long arm of chromosome 7. Hepatosplenic T cell lymphoma (HSTCL) is an aggressive peripheral T cell neoplasm most commonly derived from $\gamma\delta$ T cells, but is occasionally of $\alpha\beta$ phenotype. In most cases HSTCL is associated with the presence of an isochromosome 7q cytogenetic abnormality.[96,97] Demonstration of the iso 7q by FISH or karyotype analysis confirms this diagnosis and is useful in distinguishing HSTCL from rare occurrences of comparatively indolent $\gamma\delta$ type T cell large granular lymphocyte

chronic leukemia. Among chronic B cell leukemia/lymphomas, splenic marginal zone lymphoma (SMZL) and hairy cell leukemia (HCL) can occasionally show overlapping cytologic and immunophenotypic features. The presence of del 7q, which is observed in approximately one-third of SMZL, favors this diagnosis over HCL in problematic cases.

TUMOR GENETICS, MINIMAL RESIDUAL DISEASE AND PROGNOSIS PREDICTION

The addition of tumor genetic abnormalities has refined the diagnostic classification of hematolymphoid neoplasms, but has also provided prognostic markers generally predictive of disease outcomes. The incorporation of ever-expanding genetic and phenotypic markers into standard diagnostic assessment holds promise for providing the treating physician with more accurate prognostic information concerning individual patients with certain lymphoid malignancies. In a complementary sense, monitoring responses to treatment protocols by measurements of minimal residual disease (MRD) constitutes a second major goal in this field. As a paradigm, the latter issue is best exemplified by the current sophisticated approach to monitoring patients with chronic myeloid leukemia (CML) on imatinib mesylate or related tyrosine kinase inhibitor therapies.[98,99] In the realm of lymphoid tumors, genetic abnormalities and MRD assessment are being integrated into the increasingly tailored management of patients with childhood acute lymphoblastic leukemia and B cell chronic lymphocytic leukemia. Similarly, cytogenetic subclassification has emerged as a major predictor of disease aggressiveness in multiple myeloma. These examples are briefly presented to illustrate the impact of tumor genetics and MRD detection on therapeutic optimization and disease outcomes.

Precursor B lymphoblastic leukemia/lymphoma

Precursor B lymphoblastic leukemia/lymphoma (precursor B cell acute lymphoblastic leukemia), or B-ALL, is the most common childhood hematologic malignancy, but occurs relatively rarely in adults. In addition to this difference in disease incidence, B-ALL in childhood is strikingly distinct in terms of tumor genetic abnormalities (Table 43.5). Approximately 40–50 percent of childhood B-ALL patients are defined by either chromosomal hyperdiploidy, or a small set of recurrent translocations that produce unique chimeric mRNAs and proteins.[100–102] Importantly, the detection of these genetic abnormalities provides a framework for risk-stratifying patients to the most appropriate therapy protocols, an approach currently utilized by some cooperative clinical trials organizations (e.g. Children's Oncology Group).

Among the most common structural genetic changes, analysis of the chimeric mRNA transcripts arising from the

Table 43.5 Major cytogenetic anomalies in precursor B cell acute lymphoblastic leukemias of childhood

Numerical changes	Prognostic significance/ risk for relapse[a]
Hyperdiploidy >52 chromosomes (particularly with +4, +10, +17)	Excellent/low risk
Hypodiploidy	Poor/very high risk
Structural changes	Prognostic significance/ risk for relapse
t(9;22)(q34;q11)/*BCR-ABL1*	Poor/very high risk
t(12;21)(p13;q22)/*ETV6-CBFA*	Good/relatively low risk
t(1;19)(q23;p13)/*E2A-PBX1*	Intermediate/relatively high risk
t(4;11)(q21;q23)/*MLL-AF4* and other *MLL* gene translocations	Poor/high risk

[a]Risk is estimated by a combination of initial clinical and laboratory factors, in conjunction with tumor genetic factors. Minimal residual disease (MRD) measurements typically performed at the end of the induction treatment phase (day 28) add further powerful independent prognostic information concerning relapse risk.

t(9;22)/*BCR-ABL1* (Ph chromosome), t(1;19)/*E2A-PBX1* and t(12;21)/*ETV6-CBFA* (*TEL-AML1*) abnormalities is readily accomplished by RT-PCR methods, although genomic FISH probe analysis is also very useful at diagnosis. With RT-PCR, one must be aware of alternate breakpoint regions in the same locus and alternative splicing events in the primary transcript. The former scenario is encountered with the t(9;22)/*BCR-ABL1*, in which genomic breaks can occur in either the minor or major breakpoint cluster regions of the *BCR* gene, producing one of two possible transcripts in B-ALL (Fig. 43.4). Among pediatric cases, the great majority of break sites in *BCR* occur at the minor breakpoint cluster region (m-BCR), whereas approximately one-third of translocations in adult Ph+ B-ALL are within the major breakpoint region (M-BCR). Primer design in the RT-PCR assay thus needs to account for this variability (Fig. 43.4). Alternative splicing of transcripts is sometimes observed in a single RT-PCR analysis in the form of additional amplified bands lacking one or more exon segments; this phenomenon is observed for example with the *ETV6-CBFA* anomaly. Translocations involving the *MLL* gene on chromosome 11q23 are seen in nearly 70 percent of infants with precursor B cell acute leukemia and also occur at a low frequency in older children with this disease. Detection of *MLL* gene translocations is challenging because of the sheer number (>40) of known possible partner genes.[100] Some of these, such as the t(4;11)/*MLL-AF4*, are more frequently encountered than others, permitting the use of RT-PCR technique to detect specific chimeric transcripts; nonetheless, *MLL* gene translocations are most comprehensively revealed by BAP FISH. Concerning numerical aberrations, hyperdiploid chromosome status in childhood B-ALL can be identified by DNA index (ploidy) analysis, FISH with

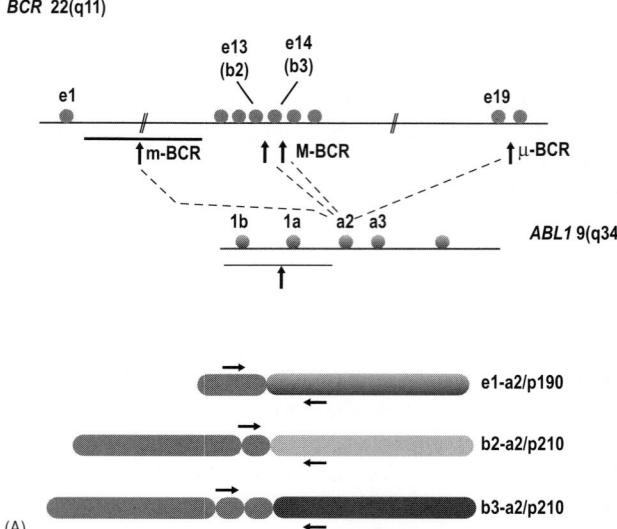

(A)

Figure 43.4 Detection of the t(9;22)/*BCR-ABL1* abnormality in Ph+ precursor B cell acute lymphoblastic leukemia and chronic myeloid leukemia. (A) Upper panel shows schematic of partial genomic maps for the *BCR* and *ABL1* genes. Vertical arrows indicate breakpoint regions in the respective genes. Nearly all cases of chronic myeloid leukemia (CML) are characterized by *BCR* gene breakage in the major breakpoint cluster region (M-BCR); most cases of Ph+ precursor B-lineage acute leukemia (Ph+ B-ALL) have breakpoints in the minor breakpoint region (m-BCR), although a small but significant number of tumors may involve the M-BCR. The rarely involved μ-BCR locus is associated with unusual cases of CML showing complete mature neutrophilic differentiation. With very rare exceptions, *ABL1* breakpoints involve the large intron 1 region of the gene. The lower panel depicts the consequences of both major and minor locus *BCR* fusions to the *ABL1* gene. Break-fusion abnormalities involving the m-BCR generate a transcript known as e1-a2 and a 190 kilodalton BCR-ABL chimeric protein (p190). *BCR* breakpoint events involving M-BCR can utilize either BCR exon 13 (b2) or exon14 (b3), creating an e13(b2)-a2 or e14(b3)-a2 fusion mRNA and a corresponding p210 protein product. Horizontal arrows indicate the general placement of PCR primers to detect these abnormal fusion transcripts in a reverse-transcription PCR analysis with high sensitivity and specificity. A single primer situated in BCR exon 13 (b2) can identify both M-BCR breakpoints (i.e. b3-a2 and b2-a2), but a separate e1 primer is required to detect m-BCR events (e1-a2). (B) Plate 127, see plate section.

repetitive sequence (e.g. centromere-specific) probes, or standard cytogenetics.

The *BCR-ABL1* abnormality is extremely critical to identify in either adult or pediatric B-ALL cases, as its presence dictates a very aggressive disease course and corresponding therapeutic intervention. In contrast, patients with *ETV6-CBFA* positive leukemias appear to have favorable therapeutic responses and overall survival, albeit with some risk for late disease relapse.[103] Hyperdiploidy, especially with karyotypes harboring trisomic changes of chromosomes 4, 10 and 17, has been associated with excellent long-term outcome in childhood B-ALL, but hypodiploid tumor chromosome number is, in contrast, a highly adverse finding in this disease.[104] The presence of *MLL* translocations in infant B-ALL connotes aggressive disease in this already high risk subgroup and appears to confer a worse prognosis in older children as well.[105] These major genetic features of childhood B-ALL are combined with presenting clinical and routine laboratory data (i.e. age, white blood cell count) to provide a rational framework for assigning potential relapse risk to defined groups of patients, and in turn direct individuals to more or less intensive therapies designed to balance toxicity with best outcomes.[106–108]

Despite these advances in pre-treatment stratification for childhood B-ALL, a substantial number of individuals continue to suffer relapse, implying imprecision in the application of tumor genetic markers as surrogate markers of prognosis. Attention has thus turned to the utility of MRD assessment as a measure of disease response to therapy and outcome. Because B-ALL is characterized by clonotypic antigen receptor gene rearrangements (involving both immunoglobulin and cross-lineage T cell receptor loci), and by the presence of recurrent translocation fusion genes in a substantial subset of patients, molecular MRD analyses can be developed to identify low levels of tumor following the institution of chemotherapy. To be useful, MRD assays must be highly specific and sensitive.[23] These requirements are readily met by quantitative real-time PCR (RQ-PCR) platforms represented by either the 'TaqMan' fluorescent probe hydrolysis method (Applied Biosystems, Foster City, California, USA), or the 'LightCycler' dual probe hybridization technique (Roche Diagnostics, Indianapolis, Indiana, USA) based upon fluorescence resonance energy transfer (FRET).[109] Following initial identification and characterization by standard PCR and DNA sequencing, the tumor-specific antigen receptor gene rearrangements involving *IGH*, *IGK*, *TRG*, or *TRB* loci in a given ALL patient sample can be detected at nominal sensitivity levels of 10^{-3}–10^{-4} by specialized DNA-based RQ-PCR analyses.[23,24] One typical RQ-PCR strategy is to use a consensus sequence fluorescent probe in conjunction with patient (allele) specific and consensus PCR primers spanning the region of the unique antigen receptor gene rearrangement.[23] For translocation-positive B-ALL, chimeric mRNA transcripts such as the t(9;22)-associated BCR-ABL1 can be similarly amplified by reverse transcription RQ-PCR with even higher levels of analytic sensitivity (i.e. 10^{-5}–10^{-6}) owing to the essential lack of such aberrant RNA molecules in normal bone marrow or peripheral blood cells[110] (Plate 128, see plate section). Apart from the need to ensure high-quality tissue specimens for optimal nucleic acid extraction, molecular MRD measurements in general are subject to a number of considerations and caveats related to disease type and technical factors. Timing of MRD assessment is of critical

importance, since some post-therapeutic time-points are more informative with respect to tumor response and prognosis than others (e.g. the end of induction phase in childhood B-ALL). The frequency of MRD measurements also provides ongoing data concerning disease levels and fluctuations over time, although more frequent sampling of the patient may be practically limited by morbidity considerations (e.g. multiple bone marrow aspirations). The use of more than one MRD target has been advocated for monitoring pediatric B-ALL in order to maximize detection sensitivity,[23,24] but this may not be possible in some cases. High analytic sensitivity is a cornerstone of MRD analysis, yet uniform inter-laboratory standards are largely lacking in this regard. The concept of sensitivity must include clear definitions of the limit of assay detection, as well as the limit of reproducibility.[24] Finally, a theoretical concern exists for the stochastic detection of antigen receptor gene rearrangements or translocation-associated fusion transcripts in non-leukemic 'bystander' cells. Several studies have demonstrated that translocation gene products (for example BCR-ABL1) can be detected at rather high prevalence but very low abundance in healthy individuals.[111,112] Fortunately, these 'rare events' are detected outside the analytic sensitivity boundaries of typical RQ-PCR assays, which are instead optimized to detect MRD in a clinically relevant range.

Early clinical studies employing antigen receptor gene rearrangement targets and RQ-PCR methodology measured at the end of induction revealed that molecular MRD at levels of 10^{-2}–10^{-3} was associated with a highly unfavorable prognosis in childhood ALL, independent of other known clinical and genetic factors.[113,114] These investigations have been subsequently extended, confirmed and refined, such that end-induction MRD status has become an important component in relapse risk prediction for this disease.[115–121] The addition of end-induction phase MRD evaluation to current risk stratification factors thus provides important information for outcome prediction and moves the clinician closer to the goal of individualized patient prognostication. While molecular MRD methods are indeed powerful tools, the requirement for multiple tumor-specific targets, the labor-intensive delineation of informative antigen receptor gene rearrangements at diagnosis, relative infrequency of fusion gene mRNA abnormalities, and variable target sensitivities together place limitations on these techniques.[122] In turn, flow cytometric immunophenotyping has emerged as an approach with very similar detection sensitivity and the ability to rapidly generate quantitative cellular data with less technical complexity.[123] Flow cytometric MRD relies on the differential expression of aberrant leukemic blast immunophenotypes as compared to normal cells. Phenotypic differences can be manifested as qualitative maturational abnormalities (i.e. aberrant expression of a normally restricted, absent, or temporally regulated surface marker), or quantitative antigen expression changes in the cells of interest.[123] Many studies have demonstrated that such abnormal phenotypic characteristics are present in the vast majority of childhood B-ALL cases, providing the basis for effective MRD monitoring by flow cytometry in these patients.[123–126]

B cell chronic lymphocytic leukemia

B cell chronic lymphocytic leukemia and its nodal manifestation of small lymphocytic lymphoma (B-CLL/SLL) has received substantial attention in recent years, with the recognition that specific tumor biologic parameters subclassify otherwise similar patients into better defined risk groups. Along with phenotypic and functional markers associated with cell activation and proliferation, like CD38 antigen expression and ZAP70 protein kinase positivity respectively, several genetic markers have become incorporated into the initial evaluation of B-CLL/SLL patients[127–129] (Table 43.6). Four common cytogenetic alterations are present in B-CLL/SLL, including deletion (del) of chromosome 13(q14), trisomy 12, del 11(q22–23) and del 17(p13). Each deletion abnormality implicates allelic loss of a tumor suppressor gene: for del 13(q14), the retinoblastoma (RB) locus and two novel microRNA loci (miR-15 and miR-16) are potentially deleted, while del 11(q22–23) results in loss of the ATM gene and del 17(p13) removes one copy of the p53 gene, TP53. Isolated del 13(q14) in B-CLL/SLL has been associated with a favorable prognosis, whereas del 11(q22–23) and del 17(p13) each confer adverse prognosis with significantly shorter survival.[130] With the latter two genetic lesions, inactivation of the remaining allele is thought to result in complete loss of the respective critical tumor suppressor functions. The +12 abnormality on its own confers an intermediate prognosis. Combinations of these cytogenetic aberrations occur less frequently and the overall prognostic significance is generally influenced by the presence of the more deleterious lesion. All of these genetic changes can be readily identified by appropriate FISH probe analyses.

A second key development in the prognostic classification of B-CLL/SLL concerns the presence or absence of somatic hypermutations in the rearranged tumor IGH gene. Long thought to be a B cell neoplasm of 'pregerminal center' or naïve B cells with unmutated IGH gene rearrangements, the discovery of a substantial subset of cases with mutated IGH status has challenged our understanding of the disease pathobiology and provided a remarkably powerful predictor of clinical behavior.[131–133] B-CLL/SLL cases with functional IGH gene rearrangements lacking features of somatic hypermutation (i.e. rearrangements comprised of 'germline sequence' or unmutated V-D-J segments) are associated with an adverse clinical outcome. Conversely, mutated IGH status, defined as >2 percent variation from the expected germline sequence, has been associated with a very favorable prognosis. Mutation status also tends to moderately correlate with other prognostic measures, such as CD38 and ZAP70 expression. Exceptions to the general association of IGH

Table 43.6 Phenotypic and genetic risk factors for B cell chronic lymphocytic leukemia

Abnormality	Clinical correlate[a]
CD38 positivity	Adverse prognosis
ZAP70 positivity	Adverse prognosis
IGH-V mutation status	Mutated: good prognosis; unmutated: adverse prognosis
del 13(q)	Favorable prognosis if sole cytogenetic abnormality
trisomy 12	Intermediate prognosis
del 11(q22)	Adverse prognosis
del 17(p)	Adverse prognosis

[a]Phenotypic and genetic factors are considered in relation to each other and in combination with clinical and laboratory staging to determine risk stratification into low, intermediate and high groups.[128]

mutations and outcome are recognized, such as the high risk mutated VH3–21 genotype,[134] and mutation status is not completely independent of other factors, particularly the influence of the major cytogenetic anomalies. Nevertheless, the evaluation of IGH mutations in de novo B-CLL/SLL is rapidly becoming integrated into the risk assessment for these patients.[127–129] Determination of IGH mutation status by PCR, DNA sequencing and database analysis requires specialized technical and interpretive expertise and is best performed in laboratories with experience and sufficient patient sample volume. With the breadth of cell biologic, cytogenetic and IGH mutation data, patients with B-CLL/SLL can be grouped into low, intermediate and high risk categories.[127–129] While immediate treatment may not be required even for high risk patients at diagnosis, the presence of adverse prognostic factors may eventuate in earlier therapeutic decisions for some individuals. This more refined approach also provides an important tool for evaluating new therapies and reevaluating existing protocols based on tumor biologic factors.[135]

Multiple myeloma

Genetic abnormalities in multiple myeloma have been better characterized through improvements in cytogenetics and FISH methods. In broad terms, cytogenetics can divide multiple myeloma into two groups typified by hyperdiploid karyotype and translocations involving the IGH locus.[136] IGH translocations are intriguing in that the partner genes involved either directly or indirectly deregulate the class of D-type cyclins involved in cell cycle progression.[137,138] The common translocations associated with multiple myeloma include the t(11;14)/CCND1-IGH, t(6;14)/CCND3-IGH, t(4;14)/MMSET-IGH, FGFR3-IGH, and the t(14;16)/MAF-IGH. Of these, hyperdiploidy, the t(11;14) and the t(6;14) are considered 'standard risk' findings, while the t(4;14) and t(14;16) indicate high risk events. Other prognostically relevant abnormalities considered to be of adverse risk in multiple myeloma include hypodiploid karyotype, del 17(p), and the presence of del 13(q) or monosomy 13 (in metaphase preparations).[139] Along with clinical and laboratory parameters for risk stratification, tumor genetics add further value for assessing potential disease aggressiveness in MM.

High-dose chemotherapy with autologous stem cell rescue is a major therapeutic option for multiple myeloma patients and in this regard, MRD evaluation can provide useful information regarding pre-transplant tumor burden and post-transplant relapse risk. RQ-PCR methods detecting tumor-specific clonal *IGH* rearrangements have been developed for this purpose,[141,142] although MRD analysis by multicolor flow cytometry is a significant advance in this area.[142,143]

CONCLUDING REMARKS AND FUTURE DIRECTIONS

The search for and discovery of new genetic markers useful in diagnostic sub-classification and importantly prognostic prediction continues forward at a rapid pace; this chapter clearly represents a synopsis rather than a comprehensive rendering of the subject. Despite these continual scientific and clinical advances, the era of identifying single genetic anomalies associated with specific lymphoid tumor types is becoming modified by the advent of multi-parameter investigative methods examining global gene expression, high-resolution genetic changes, epigenetic alterations, or combinations of these processes. Given the substantial complexity of data arising from high-throughput multi-parameter technologies, defining reliable minimally adequate marker sets for the optimal evaluation of particular tumor sub-types is a key goal in this regard. So-called 'array-based' technologies will thus challenge the current status quo in molecular hematopathology by requiring new approaches to the rational clinical validation and standardization of robust and technically streamlined multiplex assays. An explosion of new knowledge concerning gene transcriptional and translational regulation by microRNAs (miRNAs) and related non-coding RNA species promises to add greater complexity yet, as recently shown for B-CLL/SLL and some other hematologic malignancies.[144–146] In concert, improvements in treatment for hematolymphoid cancers (including therapeutic antibodies, small molecule inhibitors and new chemotherapy agents) continue to impact the clinical course of previously well-understood diseases, converting some entities into relatively stable 'chronic' illnesses. The latter issue indicates that a more expansive role for sensitive and specific measures of MRD is also likely to be expected from the modern molecular hematopathology laboratory.

KEY POINTS

- Illustrate the basic concepts and molecular biology of antigen receptor gene rearrangements underlying the generation of unique immunoglobulin and T-cell receptor proteins on B- and T-cells respectively.
- Introduce and explain the utility of analyzing antigen receptor gene rearrangement patterns in lymphoid populations to identify and distinguish monoclonal (e.g. malignant) from polyclonal (e.g. benign) tissue proliferations.
- Illustrate the two major techniques to evaluate clonal status of a lymphoid population, namely Southern blot hybridization and polymerase chain reaction (PCR). Discuss the technical advantages and limitations of these respective methods, as well as the current status of usage in the molecular hematopathology laboratory.
- Present the concept of recurrent chromosomal translocations in lymphoid neoplasms and the diagnostic utility of detecting these genetic abnormalities. Discuss the major methodologies for identification of translocations, including PCR and fluorescence *in situ* hybridization (FISH), as well as the inherent technical limitations of each modality.
- Discuss the major recurrent cytogenetic and molecular genetic anomalies encountered in lymphoid malignancies and illustrate the importance of molecular techniques in providing accurate diagnosis and sub-classification.
- Examine the current utility of tumor genetic markers for prognosis prediction and minimal disease monitoring using particular lymphoid neoplasms as key examples.

ACKNOWLEDGMENTS

The author would like to gratefully acknowledge the help of the following individuals at Mayo Clinic: RP Ketterling, and RG Meyer for graciously providing images and details of FISH analysis; and SM Franck for superb assistance with manuscript preparation and reference management.

REFERENCES

● = Key primary paper
◆ = Major review article

◆1. Bassing CH, Swat W, Alt FW. The mechanism and regulation of chromosomal V(D)J recombination. *Cell* 2002; **109**(Suppl): s45–55.

2. Macintyre EA, Delabesse E. Molecular approaches to the diagnosis and evaluation of lymphoid malignancies. *Semin Hematol* 1999; **36**: 373–89.

3. Arber DA. Molecular diagnostic approach to non-Hodgkin's lymphoma. *J Mol Diagn* 2000; **2**: 178–90.

4. Medeiros LJ, Carr J. Overview of the role of molecular methods in the diagnosis of malignant lymphomas. *Arch Pathol Lab Med* 1999; **123**: 1189–207.

●5. Langerak AW, Wolvers-Tettero IL, van Dongen JJ. Detection of T cell receptor beta (TCRB) gene rearrangement patterns in T cell malignancies by southern blot analysis. *Leukemia* 1999; **13**: 965–74.

6. Beishuizen A, Verhoeven MA, Mol EJ *et al.* Detection of immunoglobulin heavy-chain gene rearrangements by Southern blot analysis: recommendations for optimal results. *Leukemia* 1993; **7**: 2045–53.

7. Viswanatha DS, Larson RS. Molecular diagnosis of hematopoietic neoplasms. In: McPherson RA, Pincus MR. (eds) *Henry's clinical diagnosis and management by laboratory methods*, 21st ed. Philadelphia: Saunders Elsevier, 2007: 1295–322.

8. Derksen PW, Langerak AW, Kerkhof E *et al.* Comparison of different polymerase chain reaction-based approaches for clonality assessment of immunoglobulin heavy-chain gene rearrangements in B-cell neoplasia. *Mod Pathol* 1999; **12**: 794–805.

9. Segal GH, Jorgensen T, Masih AS, Braylan RC. Optimal primer selection for clonality assessment by polymerase chain reaction analysis: I. Low grade B-cell lymphoproliferative disorders of nonfollicular center cell type. *Hum Pathol* 1994; **25**: 1269–75.

10. Segal GH, Jorgensen T, Scott M, Braylan RC. Optimal primer selection for clonality assessment by polymerase chain reaction analysis: II. Follicular lymphomas. *Hum Pathol* 1994; **25**: 1276–82.

●11. Lawnicki LC, Rubocki RJ, Chan WC *et al.* The distribution of gene segments in T-cell receptor gamma gene rearrangements demonstrates the need for multiple primer sets. *J Mol Diagn* 2003; **5**: 82–7.

12. Pai RK, Chakerian AE, Binder JM *et al.* B-cell clonality determination using an immunoglobulin kappa light chain polymerase chain reaction method. *J Mol Diagn* 2005; **7**: 300–7.

13. van der Velden VH, de Bie M, van Wering ER, van Dongen JJ. Immunoglobulin light chain gene rearrangements in precursor-B-acute lymphoblastic leukemia: characteristics and applicability for the detection of minimal residual disease. *Haematologica* 2006; **91**: 679–82.

14. Beaubier NT, Hart AP, Bartolo C *et al.* Comparison of capillary electrophoresis and polyacrylamide gel electrophoresis for the evaluation of T and B cell clonality by polymerase chain reaction. *Diagn Mol Pathol* 2000; **9**: 121–31.

15. Greiner TC, Rubocki RJ. Effectiveness of capillary electrophoresis using fluorescent-labeled primers in detecting T-cell receptor gamma gene rearrangements. *J Mol Diagn* 2002; **4**: 137–43.

●16. van Dongen JJ, Langerak AW, Bruggemann M *et al.* Design and standardization of PCR primers and protocols for detection of clonal immunoglobulin and T-cell receptor gene recombinations in suspect lymphoproliferations: report of the BIOMED-2 concerted action BMH4-CT98-3936. *Leukemia* 2003; **17**: 2257–317.

●17. van Krieken JH, Langerak AW, Macintyre EA *et al.* Improved reliability of lymphoma diagnostics via PCR-based clonality testing: report of the BIOMED-2 concerted action BHM4-CT98-3936. *Leukemia* 2007; **21**: 201–6.

●18. Bruggemann M, White H, Gaulard P *et al.* Powerful strategy for polymerase chain reaction-based clonality assessment in T-cell malignancies Report of the BIOMED-2 concerted action BHM4 CT98-3936. *Leukemia* 2007; **21**: 215–21.

●19. Evans PA, Pott C, Groenen PJ *et al.* Significantly improved PCR-based clonality testing in B-cell malignancies by use of multiple immunoglobulin gene targets. Report of the BIOMED-2 concerted action BHM4-CT98-3936. *Leukemia* 2007; **21**: 207–14.

●20. Langerak AW, Molina TJ, Lavender FL *et al.* Polymerase chain reaction-based clonality testing in tissue samples with reactive lymphoproliferations: usefulness and pitfalls. A report of the BIOMED-2 concerted action BMH4-CT98-3936. *Leukemia* 2007; **21**: 222–9.

21. McClure RF, Kaur P, Pagel E *et al.* Validation of immunoglobulin gene rearrangement detection by PCR using commercially available BIOMED-2 primers. *Leukemia* 2006; **20**: 176–9.

●22. Liu H, Bench AJ, Bacon CM *et al.* A practical strategy for the routine use of BIOMED-2 PCR assays for detection of B- and T-cell clonality in diagnostic haematopathology. *Br J Haematol* 2007; **138**: 31–43.

◆23. van der Velden VH, Hochhaus A, Cazzaniga G *et al.* Detection of minimal residual disease in hematologic malignancies by real-time quantitative PCR: principles, approaches, and laboratory aspects. *Leukemia* 2003; **17**: 1013–34.

◆24. van der Velden VH, Cazzaniga G, Schrauder A *et al.* Analysis of minimal residual disease by Ig/TCR gene rearrangements: guidelines for interpretation of real-time quantitative PCR data. *Leukemia* 2007; **21**: 604–11.

25. Attygalle AD, Chuang SS, Diss TC *et al.* Distinguishing angioimmunoblastic T-cell lymphoma from peripheral T-cell lymphoma, unspecified, using morphology, immunophenotype and molecular genetics. *Histopathology* 2007; **50**: 498–508.

26. Lee SC, Berg KD, Racke FK *et al.* Pseudo-spikes are common in histologically benign lymphoid tissues. *J Mol Diagn* 2000; **2**: 145–52.

27. Roix JJ, McQueen PG, Munson PJ *et al.* Spatial proximity of translocation-prone gene loci in human lymphomas. *Nat Genet* 2003; **34**: 287–91.

28. Raghavan SC, Lieber MR. DNA structure and human diseases. *Front Biosci* 2007; **12**: 4402–8.

29. Wolff DJ, Bagg A, Cooley LD *et al.* Guidance for fluorescence *in situ* hybridization testing in hematologic disorders. *J Mol Diagn* 2007; **9**: 134–43.

◆30. Grimwade D, Lo Coco F. Acute promyelocytic leukemia: a model for the role of molecular diagnosis and residual disease monitoring in directing treatment approach in acute myeloid leukemia. *Leukemia* 2002; **16**: 1959–73.

●31. Hughes T, Deininger M, Hochhaus A *et al.* Monitoring CML patients responding to treatment with tyrosine kinase inhibitors: review and recommendations for harmonizing current methodology for detecting BCR-ABL transcripts and kinase domain mutations and for expressing results. *Blood* 2006; **108**: 28–37.

◆32. Danial NN, Korsmeyer SJ. Cell death: critical control points. *Cell* 2004; **116**: 205–19.

◆33. Adams JM, Cory S. The Bcl-2 protein family: arbiters of cell survival. *Science* 1998; **281**: 1322–6.

34. Albinger-Hegyi A, Hochreutener B, Abdou MT *et al.* High frequency of t(14;18)-translocation breakpoints outside of major breakpoint and minor cluster regions in follicular lymphomas: improved polymerase chain reaction protocols for their detection. *Am J Pathol* 2002; **160**: 823–32.

●35. Buchonnet G, Jardin F, Jean N *et al.* Distribution of BCL2 breakpoints in follicular lymphoma and correlation with clinical features: specific subtypes or same disease? *Leukemia* 2002; **16**: 1852–6.

36. Buchonnet G, Lenain P, Ruminy P *et al.* Characterisation of BCL2-JH rearrangements in follicular lymphoma: PCR detection of 3′ BCL2 breakpoints and evidence of a new cluster. *Leukemia* 2000; **14**: 1563–9.

37. Horsman DE, Gascoyne RD, Coupland RW *et al.* Comparison of cytogenetic analysis, southern analysis, and polymerase chain reaction for the detection of t(14;18) in follicular lymphoma. *Am J Clin Pathol* 1995; **103**: 472–8.

38. Aster JC, Longtine JA. Detection of BCL2 rearrangements in follicular lymphoma. *Am J Pathol* 2002; **160**: 759–63.

39. Hsi ED, Tubbs RR, Lovell MA *et al.* Detection of bcl-2/J(H) translocation by polymerase chain reaction: a summary of the experience of the molecular oncology survey of the College of American Pathologist. *Arch Pathol Lab Med* 2002; **126**: 902–8.

40. Iqbal S, Jenner MJ, Summers KE *et al.* Reliable detection of clonal IgH/Bcl2 MBR rearrangement in follicular lymphoma: methodology and clinical significance. *Br J Haematol* 2004; **124**: 325–8.

41. Akasaka T, Akasaka H, Yonetani N *et al.* Refinement of the BCL2/immunoglobulin heavy chain fusion gene in t(14;18)(q32;q21) by polymerase chain reaction amplification for long targets. *Genes Chromosomes Cancer* 1998; **21**: 17–29.

42. Vega F, Medeiros LJ. Chromosomal translocations involved in non-Hodgkin lymphomas. *Arch Pathol Lab Med* 2003; **127**: 1148–60.

43. Bowman A, Jones D, Medeiros LJ, Luthra R. Quantitative PCR detection of t(14;18) bcl-2/JH fusion sequences in follicular lymphoma patients: comparison of peripheral blood and bone marrow aspirate samples. *J Mol Diagn* 2004; **6**: 396–400.

●44. McClure RF, Remstein ED, Macon WR *et al.* Adult B-cell lymphomas with burkitt-like morphology are phenotypically and genotypically heterogeneous with aggressive clinical behavior. *Am J Surg Pathol* 2005; **29**: 1652–60.

●45. Haralambieva E, Boerma EJ, van Imhoff GW *et al.* Clinical, immunophenotypic, and genetic analysis of adult lymphomas with morphologic features of Burkitt lymphoma. *Am J Surg Pathol* 2005; **29**: 1086–94.

◆46. Bertoni F, Zucca E, Cotter FE. Molecular basis of mantle cell lymphoma. *Br J Haematol* 2004; **124**: 130–40.

◆47. Sherr CJ. The Pezcoller lecture: cancer cell cycles revisited. *Cancer Res* 2000; **60**: 3689–95.

48. Chibbar R, Leung K, McCormick S *et al.* bcl-1 gene rearrangements in mantle cell lymphoma: a comprehensive analysis of 118 cases, including B-5-fixed tissue, by polymerase chain reaction and southern transfer analysis. *Mod Pathol* 1998; **11**: 1089–97.

●49. Belaud-Rotureau MA, Parrens M, Dubus P *et al.* A comparative analysis of FISH, RT-PCR, PCR, and immunohistochemistry for the diagnosis of mantle cell lymphomas. *Mod Pathol* 2002; **15**: 517–25.

50. Remstein ED, Kurtin PJ, Buno I *et al.* Diagnostic utility of fluorescence *in situ* hybridization in mantle-cell lymphoma. *Br J Haematol* 2000; **110**: 856–62.

51. Fu K, Weisenburger DD, Greiner TC *et al.* Cyclin D1-negative mantle cell lymphoma: a clinicopathologic study based on gene expression profiling. *Blood* 2005; **106**: 4315–21.

52. Du MQ, Isaccson PG. Gastric MALT lymphoma: from aetiology to treatment. *Lancet Oncol* 2002; **3**: 97–104.

◆53. Du MQ. MALT lymphoma: recent advances in aetiology and molecular genetics. *J Clin Exp Hematop* 2007; **47**: 31–42.

54. Remstein ED, James CD, Kurtin PJ. Incidence and subtype specificity of API2-MALT1 fusion translocations in extranodal, nodal, and splenic marginal zone lymphomas. *Am J Pathol* 2000; **156**: 1183–8.

●55. Remstein ED, Kurtin PJ, Einerson RR *et al.* Primary pulmonary MALT lymphomas show frequent and heterogeneous cytogenetic abnormalities, including aneuploidy and translocations involving API2 and MALT1 and IGH and MALT1. *Leukemia* 2004; **18**: 156–60.

56. Ye H, Liu H, Attygalle A *et al.* Variable frequencies of t(11;18)(q21;q21) in MALT lymphomas of different sites: significant association with CagA strains of H pylori in gastric MALT lymphoma. *Blood* 2003; **102**: 1012–18.

57. Ruland J, Duncan GS, Wakeham A, Mak TW. Differential requirement for Malt1 in T and B cell antigen receptor signaling. *Immunity* 2003; **19**: 749–58.

58. Ruefli-Brasse AA, French DM, Dixit VM. Regulation of NF-kappaB-dependent lymphocyte activation and development by paracaspase. *Science* 2003; **302**: 1581–4.

59. Lucas PC, Yonezumi M, Inohara N *et al.* Bcl10 and MALT1, independent targets of chromosomal translocation in malt lymphoma, cooperate in a novel NF-kappa B signaling pathway. *J Biol Chem* 2001; **276**: 19012–19.

●60. Zhou H, Wertz I, O'Rourke K *et al.* Bcl10 activates the NF-kappaB pathway through ubiquitination of NEMO. *Nature* 2004; **427**: 167–71.

◆61. Isaacson PG, Du MQ. MALT lymphoma: from morphology to molecules. *Nat Rev Cancer* 2004; **4**: 644–53.

62. Motegi M, Yonezumi M, Suzuki H *et al.* API2-MALT1 chimeric transcripts involved in mucosa-associated lymphoid tissue type lymphoma predict heterogeneous products. *Am J Pathol* 2000; **156**: 807–12.

63. Streubel B, Vinatzer U, Lamprecht A *et al.* T(3;14)(p14.1;q32) involving IGH and FOXP1 is a novel recurrent chromosomal aberration in MALT lymphoma. *Leukemia* 2005; **19**: 652–8.

64. Hu H, Wang B, Borde M *et al.* Foxp1 is an essential transcriptional regulator of B cell development. *Nat Immunol* 2006; **7**: 819–26.

●65. Dent AL, Shaffer AL, Yu X *et al.* Control of inflammation, cytokine expression, and germinal center formation by BCL-6. *Science* 1997; **276**: 589–92.

●66. Ye BH, Cattoretti G, Shen Q *et al.* The BCL-6 proto-oncogene controls germinal-centre formation and Th2-type inflammation. *Nat Genet* 1997; **16**: 161–70.

67. Onizuka T, Moriyama M, Yamochi T *et al.* BCL-6 gene product, a 92- to 98-kD nuclear phosphoprotein, is highly expressed in germinal center B cells and their neoplastic counterparts. *Blood* 1995; **86**: 28–37.

68. Pittaluga S, Ayoubi TA, Wlodarska I *et al.* BCL-6 expression in reactive lymphoid tissue and in B-cell non-Hodgkin's lymphomas. *J Pathol* 1996; **179**: 145–50.

69. Chen W, Iida S, Louie DC *et al.* Heterologous promoters fused to BCL6 by chromosomal translocations affecting band 3q27 cause its deregulated expression during B-cell differentiation. *Blood* 1998; **91**: 603–7.

70. Migliazza A, Martinotti S, Chen W *et al.* Frequent somatic hypermutation of the 5′ noncoding region of the BCL6 gene in B-cell lymphoma. *Proc Natl Acad Sci U S A* 1995; **92**: 12520–4.

●71. Shen HM, Peters A, Baron B *et al.* Mutation of BCL-6 gene in normal B cells by the process of somatic hypermutation of Ig genes. *Science* 1998; **280**: 1750–2.

72. Saito M, Gao J, Basso K *et al.* A signaling pathway mediating downregulation of BCL6 in germinal center B cells is blocked by BCL6 gene alterations in B cell lymphoma. *Cancer Cell* 2007; **12**: 280–92.

●73. Phan RT, Saito M, Kitagawa Y *et al.* Genotoxic stress regulates expression of the proto-oncogene Bcl6 in germinal center B cells. *Nat Immunol* 2007; **8**: 1132–9.

74. Ohno H. Pathogenetic role of BCL6 translocation in B-cell non-Hodgkin's lymphoma. *Histol Histopathol* 2004; **19**: 637–50.

◆75. Blum KA, Lozanski G, Byrd JC. Adult Burkitt leukemia and lymphoma. *Blood* 2004; **104**: 3009–20.

76. Hecht JL, Aster JC. Molecular biology of Burkitt's lymphoma. *J Clin Oncol* 2000; **18**: 3707–21.

77. Amati B, Brooks MW, Levy N *et al.* Oncogenic activity of the c-Myc protein requires dimerization with Max. *Cell* 1993; **72**: 233–45.

●78. Haralambieva E, Schuuring E, Rosati S *et al.* Interphase fluorescence *in situ* hybridization for detection of 8q24/MYC breakpoints on routine histologic sections: validation in Burkitt lymphomas from three geographic regions. *Genes Chromosomes Cancer* 2004; **40**: 10–18.

◆79. Kutok JL, Aster JC. Molecular biology of anaplastic lymphoma kinase-positive anaplastic large-cell lymphoma. *J Clin Oncol* 2002; **20**: 3691–702.

80. Stein H, Foss HD, Durkop H *et al.* CD30(+) anaplastic large cell lymphoma: a review of its histopathologic, genetic, and clinical features. *Blood* 2000; **96**: 3681–95.

◆81. Chiarle R, Voena C, Ambrogio C *et al.* The anaplastic lymphoma kinase in the pathogenesis of cancer. *Nat Rev Cancer* 2008; **8**: 11–23.

82. Amin HM, Lai R. Pathobiology of ALK+ anaplastic large-cell lymphoma. *Blood* 2007; **110**: 2259–67.

◆83. Falini B, Nicoletti I, Bolli N *et al.* Translocations and mutations involving the nucleophosmin (NPM1) gene in lymphomas and leukemias. *Haematologica* 2007; **92**: 519–32.

84. Falini B. Anaplastic large cell lymphoma: pathological, molecular and clinical features. *Br J Haematol* 2001; **114**: 741–60.

●85. Gascoyne RD, Aoun P, Wu D *et al.* Prognostic significance of anaplastic lymphoma kinase (ALK) protein expression in adults with anaplastic large cell lymphoma. *Blood* 1999; **93**: 3913–21.

86. Yee HT, Ponzoni M, Merson A *et al.* Molecular characterization of the t(2;5) (p23; q35) translocation in anaplastic large cell lymphoma (Ki-1) and Hodgkin's disease. *Blood* 1996; **87**: 1081–8.

87. Lamant L, Meggetto F, al Saati T *et al.* High incidence of the t(2;5)(p23;q35) translocation in anaplastic large cell lymphoma and its lack of detection in Hodgkin's disease. Comparison of cytogenetic analysis, reverse transcriptase-polymerase chain reaction, and P-80 immunostaining. *Blood* 1996; **87**: 284–91.

88. Downing JR, Shurtleff SA, Zielenska M *et al.* Molecular detection of the (2;5) translocation of non-Hodgkin's lymphoma by reverse transcriptase-polymerase chain reaction. *Blood* 1995; **85**: 3416–22.

89. Mussolin L, Pillon M, d'Amore ES *et al.* Prevalence and clinical implications of bone marrow involvement in pediatric anaplastic large cell lymphoma. *Leukemia* 2005; **19**: 1643–7.

90. Reichard KK, McKenna RW, Kroft SH. ALK-positive diffuse large B-cell lymphoma: report of four cases and review of the literature. *Mod Pathol* 2007; **20**: 310–19.

●91. De Paepe P, Baens M, van Krieken H *et al.* ALK activation by the CLTC-ALK fusion is a recurrent event in large B-cell lymphoma. *Blood* 2003; **102**: 2638–41.

●92. Gascoyne RD, Lamant L, Martin-Subero JI *et al.* ALK-positive diffuse large B-cell lymphoma is associated with Clathrin-ALK rearrangements: report of 6 cases. *Blood* 2003; **102**: 2568–73.

◆93. Krishnan B, Matutes E, Dearden C. Prolymphocytic leukemias. *Semin Oncol* 2006; **33**: 257–63.

94. Pekarsky Y, Hallas C, Croce CM. The role of TCL1 in human T-cell leukemia. *Oncogene* 2001; **20**: 5638–43.

95. De Schouwer PJ, Dyer MJ, Brito-Babapulle VB *et al*. T-cell prolymphocytic leukaemia: antigen receptor gene rearrangement and a novel mode of MTCP1 B1 activation. *Br J Haematol* 2000; **110**: 831–8.

96. Vega F, Medeiros LJ, Gaulard P. Hepatosplenic and other gammadelta T-cell lymphomas. *Am J Clin Pathol* 2007; **127**: 869–80.

97. Belhadj K, Reyes F, Farcet JP *et al*. Hepatosplenic gammadelta T-cell lymphoma is a rare clinicopathologic entity with poor outcome: report on a series of 21 patients. *Blood* 2003; **102**: 4261–9.

●98. Druker BJ, Guilhot F, O'Brien SG *et al*. Five-year follow-up of patients receiving imatinib for chronic myeloid leukemia. *N Engl J Med* 2006; **355**: 2408–17.

99. Faderl S, Hochhaus A, Hughes T. Monitoring of minimal residual disease in chronic myeloid leukemia. *Hematol Oncol Clin North Am* 2004; **18**: 657–70, ix–x.

100. Armstrong SA, Look AT. Molecular genetics of acute lymphoblastic leukemia. *J Clin Oncol* 2005; **23**: 6306–15.

◆101. Pui CH, Relling MV, Downing JR. Acute lymphoblastic leukemia. *N Engl J Med* 2004; **350**: 1535–48.

102. Harrison CJ. The detection and significance of chromosomal abnormalities in childhood acute lymphoblastic leukaemia. *Blood Rev* 2001; **15**: 49–59.

103. Ford AM, Fasching K, Panzer-Grumayer ER *et al*. Origins of 'late' relapse in childhood acute lymphoblastic leukemia with TEL-AML1 fusion genes. *Blood* 2001; **98**: 558–64.

104. Heerema NA, Nachman JB, Sather HN *et al*. Hypodiploidy with less than 45 chromosomes confers adverse risk in childhood acute lymphoblastic leukemia: a report from the children's cancer group. *Blood* 1999; **94**: 4036–45.

105. Pui CH, Chessells JM, Camitta B *et al*. Clinical heterogeneity in childhood acute lymphoblastic leukemia with 11q23 rearrangements. *Leukemia* 2003; **17**: 700–6.

◆106. Pieters R, Carroll WL. Biology and treatment of acute lymphoblastic leukemia. *Pediatr Clin North Am* 2008; **55**: 1–20, ix.

107. Schultz KR, Pullen DJ, Sather HN *et al*. Risk- and response-based classification of childhood B-precursor acute lymphoblastic leukemia: a combined analysis of prognostic markers from the Pediatric Oncology Group (POG) and Children's Cancer Group (CCG). *Blood* 2007; **109**: 926–35.

108. Maloney KW, Shuster JJ, Murphy S *et al*. Long-term results of treatment studies for childhood acute lymphoblastic leukemia: Pediatric Oncology Group studies from 1986–1994. *Leukemia* 2000; **14**: 2276–85.

109. Eckert C, Scrideli CA, Taube T *et al*. Comparison between TaqMan and LightCycler technologies for quantification of minimal residual disease by using immunoglobulin and T-cell receptor genes consensus probes. *Leukemia* 2003; **17**: 2517–24.

●110. Gabert J, Beillard E, van der Velden VH *et al*. Standardization and quality control studies of 'real-time' quantitative reverse transcriptase polymerase chain reaction of fusion gene transcripts for residual disease detection in leukemia-a Europe Against Cancer program. *Leukemia* 2003; **17**: 2318–57.

111. Bose S, Deininger M, Gora-Tybor J *et al*. The presence of typical and atypical BCR-ABL fusion genes in leukocytes of normal individuals: biologic significance and implications for the assessment of minimal residual disease. *Blood* 1998; **92**: 3362–7.

112. Biernaux C, Loos M, Sels A *et al*. Detection of major bcr-abl gene expression at a very low level in blood cells of some healthy individuals. *Blood* 1995; **86**: 3118–22.

●113. Cave H, van der Werff ten Bosch J, Suciu S *et al*. Clinical significance of minimal residual disease in childhood acute lymphoblastic leukemia. European Organization for research and treatment of cancer – childhood leukemia cooperative group. *N Engl J Med* 1998; **339**: 591–8.

●114. van Dongen JJ, Seriu T, Panzer-Grumayer ER *et al*. Prognostic value of minimal residual disease in acute lymphoblastic leukaemia in childhood. *Lancet* 1998; **352**: 1731–8.

115. Cazzaniga G, Biondi A. Molecular monitoring of childhood acute lymphoblastic leukemia using antigen receptor gene rearrangements and quantitative polymerase chain reaction technology. *Haematologica* 2005; **90**: 382–90.

116. Szczepanski T, Flohr T, van der Velden VH *et al*. Molecular monitoring of residual disease using antigen receptor genes in childhood acute lymphoblastic leukaemia. *Best Pract Res Clin Haematol* 2002; **15**: 37–57.

117. Nyvold C, Madsen HO, Ryder LP *et al*. Precise quantification of minimal residual disease at day 29 allows identification of children with acute lymphoblastic leukemia and an excellent outcome. *Blood* 2002; **99**: 1253–8.

118. Coustan-Smith E, Sancho J, Hancock ML *et al*. Clinical importance of minimal residual disease in childhood acute lymphoblastic leukemia. *Blood* 2000; **96**: 2691–6.

119. Panzer-Grumayer ER, Schneider M, Panzer S *et al*. Rapid molecular response during early induction chemotherapy predicts a good outcome in childhood acute lymphoblastic leukemia. *Blood* 2000; **95**: 790–4.

120. Borowitz MJ, Devidas M, Hunger SP *et al*. Children's Oncology Group. Clinical significance of minimal residual disease in childhood acute lymphoblastic leukemia and its relationship to other prognostic factors: a Children's Oncology Group study. *Blood* 2008; **111**: 5477–85.

121. Campana D. Status of minimal residual disease testing in childhood haematological malignancies. *Br J Haematol* 2008; **143**: 481–9.

●122. Szczepanski T. Why and how to quantify minimal residual disease in acute lymphoblastic leukemia? *Leukemia* 2007; **21**: 622–6.

◆123. Campana D, Coustan-Smith E. Minimal residual disease studies by flow cytometry in acute leukemia. *Acta Haematol* 2004; **112**: 8–15.

124. Borowitz MJ, Pullen DJ, Winick N *et al.* Comparison of diagnostic and relapse flow cytometry phenotypes in childhood acute lymphoblastic leukemia: implications for residual disease detection: a report from the children's oncology group. *Cytometry B Clin Cytom* 2005; **68**: 18–24.

●125. Borowitz MJ, Pullen DJ, Shuster JJ *et al.* Minimal residual disease detection in childhood precursor-B-cell acute lymphoblastic leukemia: relation to other risk factors. A children's oncology group study. *Leukemia* 2003; **17**: 1566–72.

126. Bjorklund E, Mazur J, Soderhall S, Porwit-MacDonald A. Flow cytometric follow-up of minimal residual disease in bone marrow gives prognostic information in children with acute lymphoblastic leukemia. *Leukemia* 2003; **17**: 138–48.

◆127. Hamblin TJ. Prognostic markers in chronic lymphocytic leukaemia. *Best Pract Res Clin Haematol* 2007; **20**: 455–68.

◆128. Zent CS, Call TG, Hogan WJ *et al.* Update on risk-stratified management for chronic lymphocytic leukemia. *Leuk Lymphoma* 2006; **47**: 1738–46.

129. Seiler T, Dohner H, Stilgenbauer S. Risk stratification in chronic lymphocytic leukemia. *Semin Oncol* 2006; **33**: 186–94.

●130. Shanafelt TD, Witzig TE, Fink SR *et al.* Prospective evaluation of clonal evolution during long-term follow-up of patients with untreated early-stage chronic lymphocytic leukemia. *J Clin Oncol* 2006; **24**: 4634–41.

131. Oscier DG, Gardiner AC, Mould SJ *et al.* Multivariate analysis of prognostic factors in CLL: clinical stage, IGVH gene mutational status, and loss or mutation of the p53 gene are independent prognostic factors. *Blood* 2002; **100**: 1177–84.

132. Hamblin TJ, Davis Z, Gardiner A *et al.* Unmutated Ig V(H) genes are associated with a more aggressive form of chronic lymphocytic leukemia. *Blood* 1999; **94**: 1848–54.

133. Damle RN, Wasil T, Fais F *et al.* Ig V gene mutation status and CD38 expression as novel prognostic indicators in chronic lymphocytic leukemia. *Blood* 1999; **94**: 1840–7.

134. Thorselius M, Krober A, Murray F *et al.* Strikingly homologous immunoglobulin gene rearrangements and poor outcome in VH3–21-using chronic lymphocytic leukemia patients independent of geographic origin and mutational status. *Blood* 2006; **107**: 2889–94.

135. Zenz T, Mertens D, Döhner H, Stilgenbauer S. Molecular diagnostics in chronic lymphocytic leukemia — Pathogenetic and clinical implications. *Leuk Lymphoma* 2008; **49**: 864–73.

136. Higgins MJ, Fonseca R. Genetics of multiple myeloma. *Best Pract Res Clin Haematol* 2005; **18**: 525–36.

137. Chng WJ, Glebov O, Bergsagel PL, Kuehl WM. Genetic events in the pathogenesis of multiple myeloma. *Best Pract Res Clin Haematol* 2007; **20**: 571–96.

◆138. Fonseca R. Strategies for risk-adapted therapy in myeloma. *Hematology Am Soc Hematol Educ Program* 2007; **2007**: 304–10.

●139. Dewald GW, Therneau T, Larson D *et al.* Relationship of patient survival and chromosome anomalies detected in metaphase and/or interphase cells at diagnosis of myeloma. *Blood* 2005; **106**: 3553–8.

140. Sarasquete ME, Garcia-Sanz R, Gonzalez D *et al.* Minimal residual disease monitoring in multiple myeloma: a comparison between allelic-specific oligonucleotide real-time quantitative polymerase chain reaction and flow cytometry. *Haematologica* 2005; **90**: 1365–72.

141. Fenk R, Ak M, Kobbe G *et al.* Levels of minimal residual disease detected by quantitative molecular monitoring herald relapse in patients with multiple myeloma. *Haematologica* 2004; **89**: 557–66.

●142. Rawstron AC, Orfao A, Beksac M *et al.* Report of the European Myeloma Network on multiparametric flow cytometry in multiple myeloma and related disorders. *Haematologica* 2008; **93**: 431–8.

●143. Morice WG, Hanson CA, Kumar S *et al.* Novel multi-parameter flow cytometry sensitively detects phenotypically distinct plasma cell subsets in plasma cell proliferative disorders. *Leukemia* 2007; **21**: 2043–6.

◆144. Lawrie CH. MicroRNAs and haematology: small molecules, big function. *Br J Haematol* 2007; **137**: 503–12.

145. Zhang W, Dahlberg JE, Tam W. MicroRNAs in tumorigenesis: a primer. *Am J Pathol* 2007; **171**: 728–38.

◆146. Shivdasani RA. MicroRNAs: regulators of gene expression and cell differentiation. *Blood* 2006; **108**: 3646–53.

44

Radiological, ultrasound and magnetic resonance imaging

JEAN-NOËL BRUNETON, SÉBASTIEN NOVELLAS, PATRICK CHEVALLIER,
ANNE GRIMAUD AND NICOLAS AMORETTI

INTRODUCTION

The frequent involvement of a broad range of extranodal sites in the non-Hodgkin lymphomas (NHLs) necessitates a correspondingly broad range of imaging studies, if the extent of disease at the time of diagnosis and the response to treatment are to be accurately assessed.[1–4] Extranodal involvement was observed in 44 percent of NHL patients by Scutellari[5] and was most prevalent in the gastrointestinal tract and respiratory sites.

The purposes of pretreatment imaging are twofold:

- To determine whether disease is localized or widespread, and to estimate tumor bulk. This information has important implications for therapy and prognosis, and is essential for meaningful evaluation of the results of clinical trials.
- To provide a baseline against which treatment response (or lack of response) can be measured. This information is essential to the overall management of the patient, including the choice of salvage therapy, should there be disease progression or recurrence at some point.

While the mainstay of imaging studies in the 1980s was computed tomographic (CT) scanning of the chest and abdomen,[6–8] regardless of the age of the patient and the histologic subtype of the lymphoma, in the 1990s much more account was taken of the type of lymphoma in determining the anatomic regions to be imaged, while technological progress permitted more accurate determination of the extent of disease. For example, in children, T cell lymphoblastic lymphomas predominantly involve the chest, and abdominal spread is usually absent or of minor degree, while B cell tumors nearly always involve the abdomen.[9,10] In adults, primary stomach lymphomas of the mucosa-associated lymphoid tissue (MALT) type tend to remain localized to the stomach, draining lymph nodes or other mucosal sites, but uncommonly spread to more distant sites. Thus histologic information determines, to a considerable extent, the focus of imaging studies.

The 1990s saw the development of two other areas of research:

- use of MRI for specific disease sites (central nervous system [CNS], bone marrow) and the evaluation of residual masses
- the association of immunosuppression and NHL, and the problems encountered for differential diagnosis from infectious pathologies.

Since 2000, although CT has remained the primary imaging modality for NHL,[11] numerous literature reports have described two emerging techniques:

- positron emission tomography (PET), and, more recently, PET-CT,[12] two techniques that may replace CT for both initial disease staging and post-therapy follow-up. PET is more specific than CT[13] and can differentiate responders from nonresponders at an early point during therapy. However, the current absence of generally accepted cut-off values for optimum differentiation of responders and nonresponders hampers routine use of this modality.[14]
- imaging-guided (ultrasound, CT) percutaneous core-needle biopsy instead of surgical biopsy, performed with 18–22 gauge needles.[15,16] Percutaneous biopsy is a safe procedure that, for Agid et al.,[15] accurately diagnosed 82.5 percent of lymphomas; moreover, in this last study, repeat CT biopsy had a success rate of 73.9 percent following failure of the initial biopsy procedure. Biopsy is often sufficient for immunophenotyping,[17] and is indicated for all deep-seated lesions in the trunk (lungs, liver, pancreas, retroperitoneum) as well as for superficial lesions.[18–22]

In this chapter we shall discuss the value of ultrasound, CT and MRI for the staging and follow-up of patients with NHL. We shall also address the issue of the evaluation of residual masses, and pay particular attention to the problems that arise in evaluating patients with immunodeficiency-associated lymphomas. Finally, the role of non-radionuclide imaging for post-therapy follow-up shall be reviewed, even though PET-CT will most probably alter current strategies. Generally speaking, the current consensus calls for use of a single imaging technique whenever possible.

ULTRASONOGRAPHY

Nodal examination

Exploration of the abdominal and pelvic regions by ultrasound is often hampered by abdominal gas. The definition of nodal involvement is, therefore, based solely on size (diameter over 1.5 cm), but NHL in these regions is frequently bulky. In our experience, detection of superficial adenopathies is improved by the use of high-frequency transducers providing better quantitative analysis and treatment monitoring; subclinical superficial nodal recurrences have also been successfully visualized.[23] Ultrasound is more accurate than CT or MRI, which should be reserved for exploration of the deep regions of the trunk.

Ultrasound of superficial adenopathies is more accurate than physical examination for the diagnosis of lymphoproliferative disorders. Depending on the anatomic region, physical examination has a false-negative rate of 20–30 percent; physical examination of the supraclavicular and axillary regions involves the most difficulties.[24]

Lymphomatous nodes tend to be confluent and strongly hypoechoic, sometimes with posterior reinforcement (cyst-like); a displaced large arborized hilum is sometimes visualized. Color Doppler shows an abundant hilar flow pattern (Plate 129, see plate section)); the vascular resistance index may be normal or slightly increased.[25–27]

Extranodal examination

Ultrasound can permit visualization of abnormalities in the spleen, liver and kidney. Morphologic findings range from a normal appearance, despite subclinical involvement, to homogeneous hypertrophy, hypoechoic multinodular disease, or a solitary tumor mass (which may be a primary lymphoma).[6,28,29]

Ultrasound of the liver reveals hypoechoic nodules more often than focal tumoral involvement (Fig. 44.1). These multiple lesions are not specific, though, and, in the absence of a known context of NHL, suggest hepatic metastases.[30] Lymphomatous nodules of the liver are not enhanced by ultrasound contrast medium[31] and its use does not appear beneficial for the staging of NHL. The frequency of benign liver lesions can, however, involve diagnostic difficulties for determination of the etiology during pretherapy work-up. For Civardi et al.,[32] 58 percent of all hepatic lesions discovered during initial NHL staging were benign while 39 percent corresponded to lymphoma. In contrast, in that study, 74 percent of all focal lesions or multiple hepatic anomalies detected during follow-up corresponded to NHL.

Certain superficial disease sites are excellent indications for ultrasound: the thyroid,[33] the ocular region[34] and the testis.[35] The ultrasound appearance may even be highly suggestive of the diagnosis, as in testicular lymphoma, where hypoechoic striations may be visualized radiating out from the hypoechoic mediastinum testis (owing to infiltration of the intratesticular lymphatics).

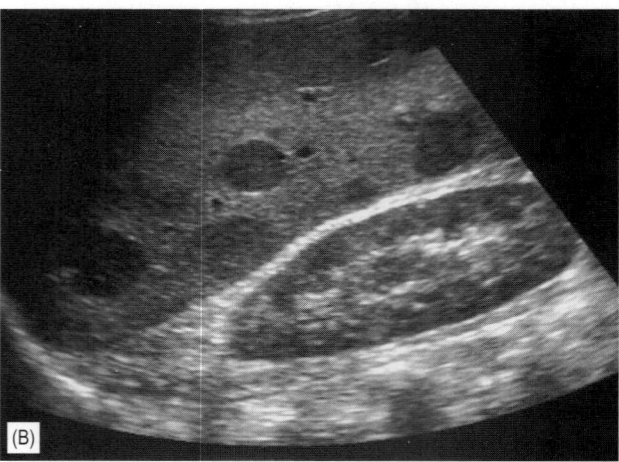

Figure 44.1   Ultrasound of hepatic lymphoma. (A) Plate 130, see plate section. (B) Multinodular secondary involvement.

Gastric endosonography

Gastric endosonography is a particularly valuable technique because, although gastric lymphoma accounts for less than 5 percent of all gastrointestinal tract tumors,[36] it is the main gastrointestinal site of NHL.[6] Primary gastric NHL is relatively rare compared to the frequency of subclinical secondary gastric involvement. This has been demonstrated by gastroscopic studies with systematic multiple biopsies of all nongastrointestinal lymphomas. Seitz et al.,[37] for example, demonstrated gastric involvement in 21 percent of cases. Primary B cell gastric lymphoma is often of MALT origin,[38] and complete excision is possible in 63 percent of cases.[36] The accuracy of endoscopy has improved over recent years; the method currently has a sensitivity of 98 percent for the diagnosis of malignancy and 64 percent for definitive diagnosis.[39]

Endosonography can readily detect involvement of the second and third layers of the gastric wall, and the presence of mucosal ulcerations.[40] Irregular, hypoechoic thickening of the submucosa with complete destruction of the layers of the stomach wall is a typical finding.[41] In addition to this infiltrative form of gastric lymphoma, Palazzo et al.[42] described two other ultrasound patterns: superficial involvement, sometimes with a polypoid or nodular form; and a tumoral mass, which cannot be distinguished from adenocarcinoma using ultrasound.

The classification of Schuder et al.,[41] derived from the TNM classification for gastric cancer, describes the extent of both tumor infiltration (ES T_L 1: confined to the submucosa; ES T_L 2: confined to the muscularis propria or the subserosa; ES T_L 3: through the entire gastric wall; ES T_L 4: involvement of neighboring structures) and the extent of nodal involvement (N_L 0: lymph nodes not involved; N_L 1: nodal involvement).

The diagnostic accuracy of endosonography varies from 80 percent to 95 percent, depending on the location of the tumor, while the sensitivity for the detection of nodal involvement is between 44 percent and 100 percent. Inflammatory nodes are responsible for numerous false-positive errors.[41,42] The major limitation of endosonography is underestimation of the degree of superficial tumoral spread, which occurs in 37.5 percent of all low-grade lymphomas.[42]

Endosonography can be used to guide fine-needle aspiration, permitting flow cytometry and immunocytochemistry studies, and has a sensitivity of 74 percent, a specificity of 93 percent, and an accuracy of 81 percent[43] for the diagnosis of lymphoma.[43] It is, of course, also useful for post-treatment surveillance.[40]

COMPUTED TOMOGRAPHY

Computed tomography has several advantages over ultrasound. The technique is reproducible (which is important for monitoring), the short imaging time improves patient tolerance, and the results are not operator-dependent, and are accessible to radiologists and clinicians who did not perform the study. Drawbacks of the method include the associated irradiation and the use of iodinated contrast agents (oral and intravenous).

Nodal examination

Computed tomography is currently the 'gold standard' for thoracic and abdominal imaging of lymphomas (Fig. 44.2). The indications listed in the literature for thoracic CT for NHL vary, whereas chest CT is of undisputed value for pretherapy staging of Hodgkin disease (HD).[44] Some authors favor systematic thoraco-abdominal CT as part of pretherapy NHL staging[35,45] whereas others[2,46] consider chest radiology sufficient because thoracic NHL generally presents as stage III disease from the outset, with both cervical and abdominal lymphadenopathy and standard chest radiographs often normal. Further, CT of the chest rarely leads to modification of staging or treatment because pulmonary involvement is unlikely. Nevertheless, CT is unquestionably indicated when an abnormality consistent with neoplasia (particularly lymphadenopathy) is seen on the chest radiograph, since this is associated with an increased risk of pulmonary disease. This applies even more so when the patient would otherwise have stage 1 disease. Computed tomography is also more valuable than standard plain films for post-therapy follow-up.

Computed tomography has replaced lymphography for exploration of the abdomen, but CT, like abdominal ultrasound, relies solely on volumetric data, i.e. the presence of enlarged nodes or abnormal masses. Lymph nodes are considered to be pathologically enlarged when intraperitoneal or retroperitoneal nodes have a transverse diameter of over 1 cm, when there are multiple nodes, or over 1.5 cm for a solitary mass. Diffuse disease corresponds to intraperitoneal and/or retroperitoneal lymphomatous masses that appear as a conglomerate of soft tissue masses with a bulky appearance. Such masses, in the presence of bowel that has been well filled by oral contrast, do not normally present diagnostic difficulties. When bowel loops are not filled with contrast, however, it may sometimes be difficult to discern whether a given image represents unopacified bowel or a lymphomatous mass. In addition, since CT is limited to providing volumetric data, it is not possible to determine whether small lesions are benign or malignant. Computed tomography cannot provide information, as lymphography can, on architectural (i.e. intranodal) abnormalities of lymph nodes, chronic granulomatous involvement, or lymphoid hyperplasia.

Morphologic nodal analysis by CT can, however, provide interesting information. Saito et al.[47] reported extensive spontaneous necrosis before the start of treatment in 25 percent of NHL patients; these anomalies were associated with stage II or higher disease, an International Prognostic Index greater than or equal to 2, and a serum lactate dehydrogenase level higher than in patients without necrosis.

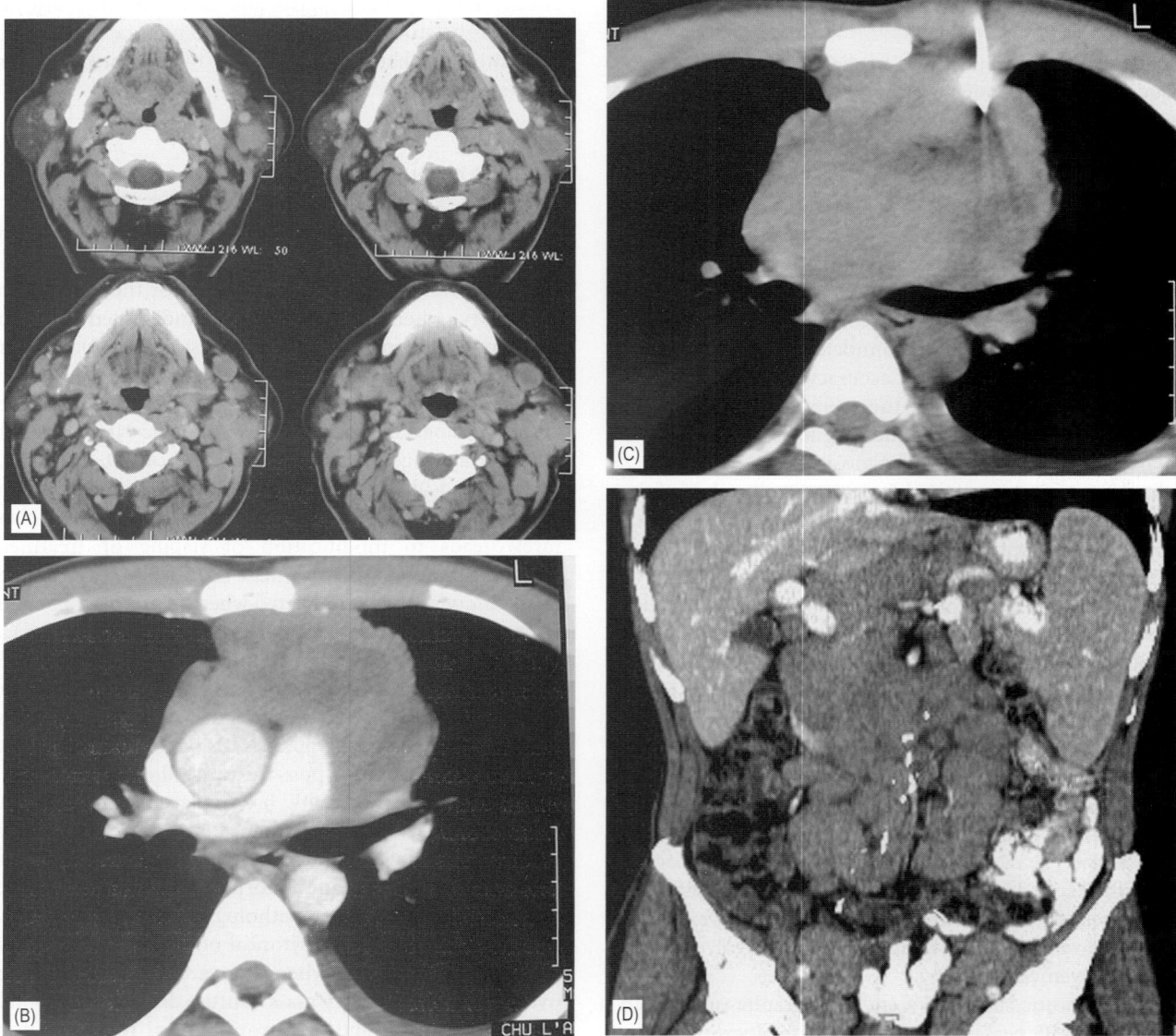

Figure 44.2 CT of nodal localizations. (A) Cervical site. (B) Mediastinal site. (C) CT-guided biopsy (same patient as in B). (D) Coronal reconstruction showing massive intraperitoneal nodal involvement.

Visceral localizations

The imaging features of visceral localizations of NHL were described by a number of authors in the 1990s (Fig. 44.3). Matsumoto *et al.*[48] described the differences, as visualized by CT, between NHL and squamous cell carcinoma of the maxillary sinus. NHL tends to present as a bulky tumor without any aggressive bone destruction, as opposed to carcinoma, which is locally invasive.

Similarly, morphologic differences have been demonstrated in the lung, especially during transformation from low- to high-grade lymphoma.[49] In a series of pulmonary lymphomas, Lewis *et al.*[50] described the most common features encountered, in decreasing order of frequency, as peribronchial thickening, multiple nodules and pleural

effusion. Other less suggestive appearances have also been reported, including stretched and irregularly narrowed bronchi and an unusual appearance of the 'angiogram sign' (intact vascular network within consolidated lung of low attenuation on CT), which is usually seen in bronchiolo-alveolar lobar cancers.[51,52]

The increased number of reports on CT evaluation of renal NHL has helped to define the CT feature of these malignancies. We now know that multiple renal masses or perirenal masses should prompt a search for NHL even in the absence of lymphadenopathy,[53] and that CT is more accurate than ultrasound for the imaging of renal lymphoma in both adults and children.[54] More specific CT studies have investigated NHL subtypes in an attempt to define their main visceral sites or their morphologic particularities.

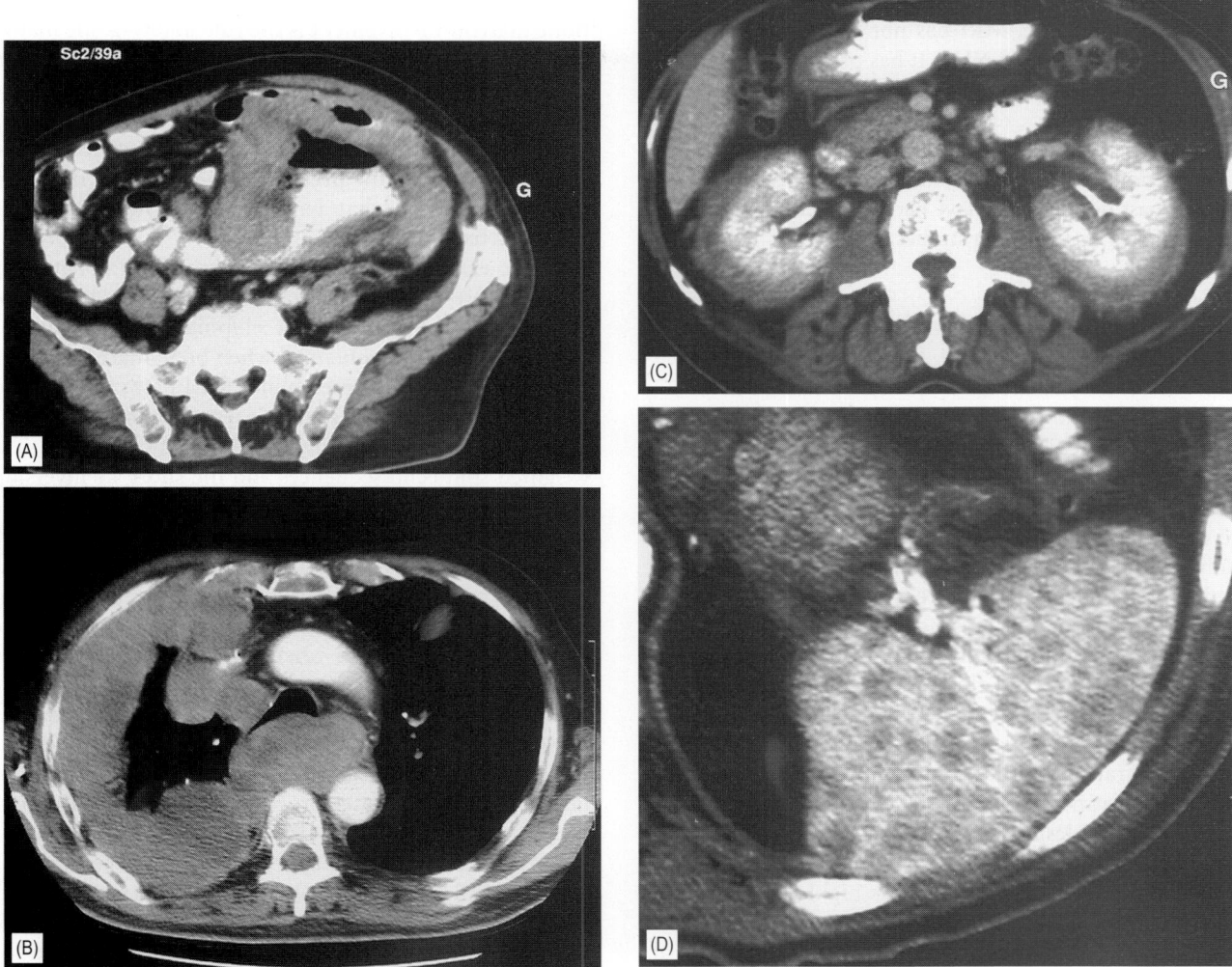

Figure 44.3   CT of visceral localizations. (A) Small bowel: pseudoaneurysmal pattern. (B) Pleural lesion. (C) Bilateral perirenal involvement. (D) Multinodular splenic involvement.

Mantle cell lymphoma is characterized by gastrointestinal tract involvement manifesting as multiple polyps in the small bowel and the colon that range in size from 0.1 cm to 4 cm. Other possible features include wall thickening, a tumor mass, or enlarged lymph nodes; retroperitoneal involvement is frequent.[55]

Mediastinal nodal calcifications are a rare pretreatment finding (0.84 percent of cases for Apter *et al.*)[56] seen during the course of aggressive lymphomas. Mucosa-associated lymphoid tissue lymphomas predominantly affect the stomach, the lung, the ocular region, and the salivary glands.[57] Multiple pulmonary lesions, consisting in an association of masses or mass-like areas of consolidation and pulmonary nodules, occur in 79 percent of patients.[58]

The limitations of CT are currently well recognized, the most prominent being disease detection in a normal-sized node and assessment of the spleen and the bone marrow.[59] Computed tomography is still used for the staging and

follow-up of NHL,[11] but will undoubtedly be replaced by PET, either alone or combined with CT, for all or, more likely, for some of these same indications.[60,61]

MAGNETIC RESONANCE IMAGING

The advantages of MRI include multiplane exploration (coronal scans are especially useful for exploration of the chest, providing satisfactory analysis of the aortopulmonary window and the subcarinal region, while sagittal scans are indicated for adequate examination of the subclavicular region), the absence of an obligatory need for contrast medium injection, and a potential for tissue characterization, permitting the diagnosis of fibrosis. The drawbacks include motion-related artifacts, the classic contraindications of MRI (especially synchronous pacemaker and cerebral aneurysm clips), a high cost compared with CT, a current availability that is always inferior to CT, and a longer imaging time than for CT scans.

Generally speaking, MRI has not replaced CT for the staging and follow-up of NHL. It has proven complementary for certain disease sites and is more effective than CT for the head and neck region and for assessment of bone marrow infiltration. Despite the numerous studies aimed at improving the efficacy of MRI techniques performed over the past decade, they have had no practical impact on the indications for imaging studies.

Current applications of magnetic resonance imaging

Lymphomatous nodal tissue appears hypointense relative to fat and discretely hypointense relative to muscle on T1-weighted sequences, but isointense to fat and hyperintense to muscle on T2-weighted images. These appearances are the same regardless of the grade of NHL.[62] The first studies of the value of MRI for disease staging were focused on the abdomen[63] and the entire trunk.[64]

Magnetic resonance imaging has been found complementary to, or more effective than CT for evaluation of bone sites of NHL, and this rare localization illustrates the difficulties encountered when selecting an imaging technique. For Krishnan et al.,[65] MRI after standard plain radiographs was more helpful than CT for diagnosis and post-treatment follow-up: a solitary, permeative meta-diaphyseal lesion with a layered periosteal reaction on plain radiographs and a soft tissue mass on MR images in a patient older than 30 is highly suggestive of lymphoma.[65]

Late surveillance does not require MRI; CT can reveal images of bone remodeling that resemble Paget disease of the bone.[66] Similarly, for NHL of the head and neck, the exact role of MRI compared to CT has yet to be defined. Some authors[67,68] advocate MRI instead of CT, especially for diffuse large cell NHL or lymphoma involving the nasopharynx and palatine tonsils, as MRI reportedly reveals zones of necrosis better than CT.[68] Weber et al.[69] emphasized the value of MRI for evaluation of disease extension to the fascial spaces (parapharyngeal space, masticator space, infratemporal fossa, tongue and nasopharynx), but recommended CT for aggressive lymphomas (i.e. Burkitt lymphoma, diffuse large B cell lymphoma, NK/T cell lymphomas) for assessment of bone destruction (base of the skull, paranasal sinuses, mandible, maxilla).

Magnetic resonance imaging can exclude a diagnosis of atypical lymphocytic infiltrates of the orbit. A lesion that is hyperintense compared to the extraocular muscles on T1-weighted images both before and after contrast injection is suggestive of orbital lymphoma. Bilateral disease and lacrimal duct involvement are seen only in NHL.[70]

Bone marrow, MRI and cytologic studies have been performed for over 10 years by a number of teams[71,72] that biopsied all pelvic sites suspected, on the basis of

MRI, to be positive (Fig. 44.4). Magnetic resonance imaging is useful, regardless of the histologic type of NHL. Bone marrow involvement is the rule in low-grade malignancies, reflecting the systemic nature of the disease. In high-grade malignancies, however, bone marrow involvement is an indicator of poor prognosis and reflects dissemination of disease. On T1-weighted sequences, yellow (fatty) marrow presents a more or less homogeneous signal such that lymphomatous involvement is readily detectable.

Thus, examination of the pelvis can be improved by accurate pre-biopsy localization of probable sites of involvement by MRI, which eliminates the numerous false-negative results obtained when bone marrow aspiration biopsies are performed blind. Al Mulhim[73] confirmed the utility of MRI in this setting in a study comparing bilateral iliac crest bone marrow biopsies and coronal T1-T2-weighted spin echo sequences and the short T1 inversion recovery technique. Prior to treatment, MRI revealed bone marrow infiltration in 56.7 percent of patients versus 30 percent by biopsy. The most frequent MR appearance was the scattered pattern, followed by uniform and nodular patterns. During post-treatment surveillance, persistence of MRI anomalies, even when not confirmed by biopsy, corresponds to relapse.[73]

Bone regions containing hematopoietic red marrow, however, present diagnostic difficulties. This problem is therefore greater in younger age groups, since the amount of red marrow decreases progressively with age. Fat suppression sequences (STIR [short tau inversion recovery]) or chemical shift imaging appear to improve the performances of MRI, because bone appears black and tumoral areas exhibit a high-intensity signal on images obtained with these techniques. Magnetic resonance imaging is effective for the detection of marrow involvement in high-grade lymphomas, but seems less useful for low-grade lymphomas, where medullary involvement is moderate. This is not a major problem, though, as most patients with low-grade lymphomas have bone marrow involvement. The detection of areas of signal attenuation, however, is not synonymous with tumor infiltration, since decreased signal intensity of bone marrow has a number of possible causes, including tumoral infiltration, myelofibrosis, or recolonization by hematopoietic cells, i.e. areas of active hematopoiesis.[74] Difficulties can be encountered with interpretation in patients who are anemic, particularly after bleeding, since regions of red marrow may extend and the signal pattern may be altered. To surmount the problem of varying amounts of red and yellow marrow in different age groups, a reference map showing the topographic distribution of the red marrow as a function of age has been advocated,[75] but diagnostic dilemmas unrelated to this require histologic adjudication.

Magnetic resonance imaging is superior to CT for the identification of lymphoma in the CNS, a topic discussed in the section on immunodeficient subjects. Post-treatment follow-up by MRI is discussed in the section on residual masses.

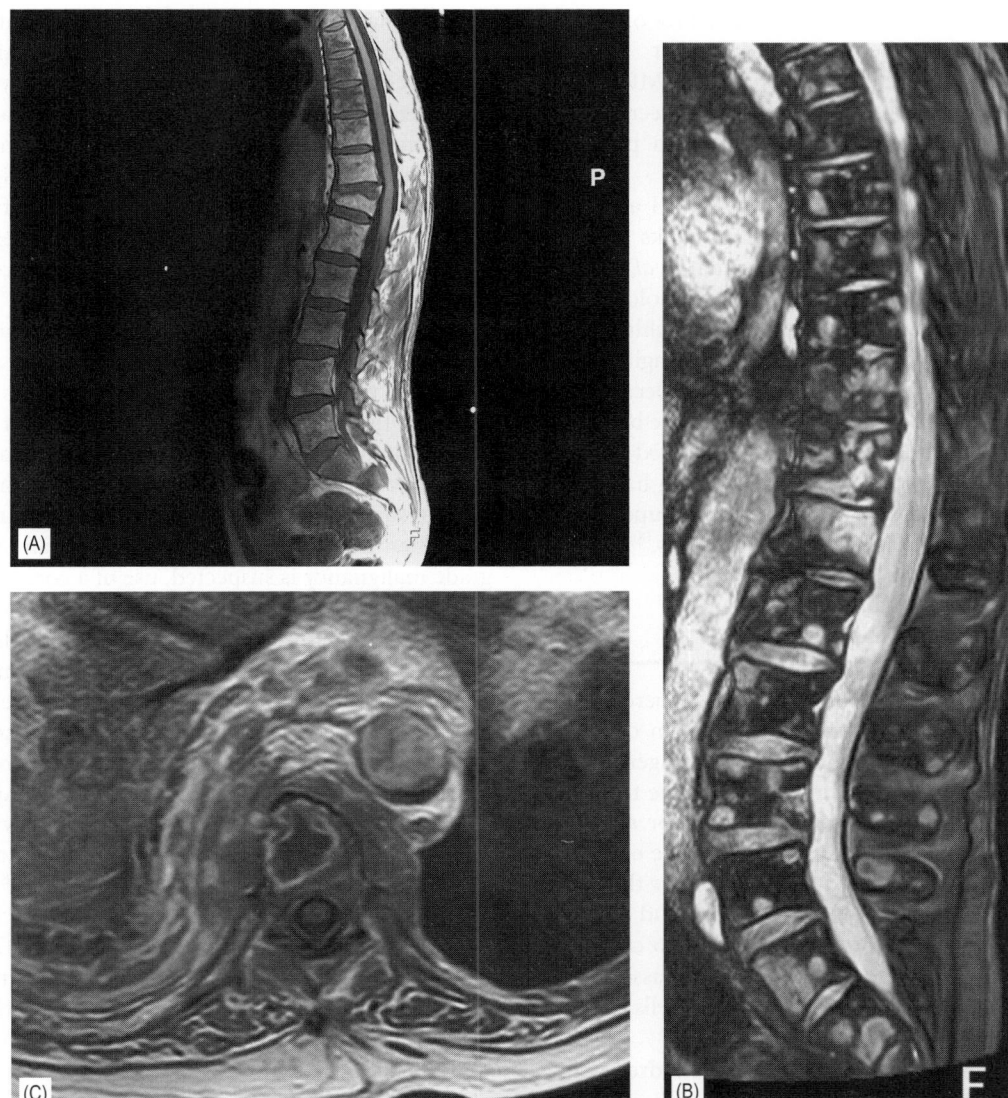

Figure 44.4 Bone marrow MRI. (A) Infiltration of the spine (T1-weighted sequence). (B) Infiltration of the spine (T2-weighted sequence). (C) Infiltration of the dorsal spine with involvement of the adjacent soft tissues (gadolinium-enhanced, T1-weighted STIR [short tau inversion recovery] image).

Newer magnetic resonance imaging techniques

Numerous studies have been conducted since the introduction of MRI, but they have not always had any practical impact on the management of lymphomas, i.e. MR spectroscopy, MR simulation for radiation therapy, and specific contrast agents.[76–79] Even the most recent studies often have yet to show any practical application despite their theoretical interest.

Comparison of the maximum contrast index (CI) of NHL and squamous cell carcinoma of the head and neck using dynamic contrast-enhanced MRI has shown a statistically significant difference in the time needed to reach the maximum CI, and 70.6 percent of NHL show CIs of less than 2.0.[67] Characterization of head and neck lesions by calculation of the apparent depression coefficient (ADC)

from depression-weighted echo-planar MRI has revealed that the mean ADC of malignant lymphomas is significantly smaller than that of carcinoma and that of benign lymphomas.[80] This technique could prove helpful for the assessment of residual masses.

Practical application of other investigative techniques appears more difficult. For example, *in vivo* proton MR spectroscopy of cervical lymph nodes has demonstrated significant differences in the Cho/Cr and Cho/water ratios of NHl and squamous cell carcinoma,[81] but, in practice, a biopsy remains obligatory.

Use of supramagnetic iron oxide as a contrast agent is not new,[82,83] but recent studies have confirmed its value for splenic imaging, thanks to improved detection of lymphomatous lesions,[84,85] and for nodal opacification.[86] Neuwelt *et al.*[87] evaluated the outcome of patients with primary CNS NHL in complete remission who presented post-therapy abnormalities that did not enhance on post-contrast scans; the authors concluded that neither enhanced chemotherapy delivery nor changes in MR imaging T2 signal intensity were associated with a decrease in cognitive function in primary CNS lymphoma patients who achieved a complete response.

Finally, one of the more promising new MRI applications is whole-body MRI, in particular thanks to the improved rapidity of data acquisition. Laffan et al.[88] proposed this imaging modality for all diffuse pathologies in children. Kellenberger et al.[89] emphasized the highly sensitive character of fast-STIR whole-body MR imaging, but also cited its lack of specificity for bone marrow, because an abnormal post-therapy signal cannot differentiate between disease recurrence and residual or therapy-induced abnormalities. In the adult, whole-body MRI imaging has been advocated owing the rapidity of imaging and its superiority over 67 Ga scintigraphy for bone marrow analysis.[90,91]

RESIDUAL MASSES

A persistent residual mass is noted in 20–40 percent of patients after treatment; this raises the problem of their nosology and the most appropriate management.[50] Computed tomography can accurately determine the volume of the residual mass, and define targets for surveillance or for aspiration biopsy. Depending on the context, mere surveillance by CT or aspiration biopsy were the only alternatives before the introduction of MRI and PET.[92] However, size assessment alone is insufficient to confirm complete absence of viable tumor, because masses that have regressed in size may still contain tumoral cells refractory to chemotherapy.[93]

The high frequency of residual masses in children with abdominal Burkitt lymphoma (20.6 percent of cases) has been clearly demonstrated. Karmazyn et al.[94] have proposed expectant watching for these young patients in the absence of any other clinical or paraclinical anomaly.

In the 1990s, several studies compared modifications in the MRI signal with changes in tumor size.[60,93,95] Although no linear relationship exists between size regression and a decrease in tumor signal intensity on T2-weighted sequences, an association of these two findings is highly suggestive of residual fibrous scarring. Persistence of a high-intensity signal on T2-weighted sequences remains a controversial finding. In its early stages, fibrosis consists mainly of fibroblasts and endothelial cells, and is often edematous and rich in mobile protons. This may explain the high-intensity signal observed on T2-weighted sequences. In addition to inflammatory or necrotic reorganization, fat deposits can also increase the signal intensity on T2-weighted sequences, making a fat suppression sequence indispensable. These factors necessitate cautious interpretation of follow-up MRI scans, which should preferably be obtained at least 6 months after the start of therapy, if CT has not demonstrated any recurrence in the meantime. Fibrosis will

be more mature and less likely to give a high-intensity signal on T2-weighted sequences. Lymphomas in which there is a fibrotic element, which may be extensive, may also lead to interpretation difficulties. Lymph nodes that are predominantly composed of fibrous tissue and contain little tumor show minimal reduction in size and T2-weighted signal immediately following treatment. The use of gadolinium can be helpful for masses that enhance after treatment, because such enhancement reflects the presence of tumoral tissue, whereas fibrous masses do not enhance.[96]

The value of percutaneous biopsy performed under ultrasound or CT guidance was mentioned earlier, with emphasis placed on the value of multiple biopsies to improve the accuracy of cytologic diagnosis (Fig. 44.5). The limitations of fine-needle aspiration include false-negative errors related to inadequate tissue samples, sometimes resulting from the presence of fibrosis. In such cases, and when transformation from a low-grade to a higher-grade malignancy is suspected, use of a core biopsy needle or surgical biopsy is indicated.

One of the limitations of non-radionuclide imaging is determination of the etiology of residual masses, a frequent situation for which PET may prove useful. Reske,[97] in a review of 15 studies, emphasized the superiority of $[^{18}F]$2-fluoro-2-deoxy-D-glucose (FDG) PET over CT, as it has a sensitivity of 71–100 percent and a specificity of 69–100 percent. This recognized superiority will undoubtedly be reinforced by the association of PET and CT, but cannot rule out minimal residual disease.[98] Additional studies are required to evaluate the value of PET-CT for correction of the false-positive errors of FDG uptake for benign pathologies (i.e. infection, drug toxicity, granulocyte colony-stimulating factor therapy, radiation therapy, post-operative or post-biopsy changes, etc.).

NON–HODGKIN LYMPHOMA AND IMMUNODEFICIENCY

Non-Hodgkin lymphoma is more frequent in transplant recipients than in the general population, in particular following the administration of high doses of ciclosporin. Acquired immunodeficiency syndrome (AIDS) patients also have a markedly higher incidence of high-grade lymphoma. In such patients, NHL is more common than HD, and particularly aggressive forms of NHL predominate, namely Burkitt lymphoma and large cell immunoblastic lymphoma. Extranodal manifestations are the rule, and there is a predilection for the CNS and digestive tract. These lymphomas, in the context of human immunodeficiency virus (HIV) infection, have a poor prognosis and tend to recur early.[99,100]

Central nervous system lymphoma is much more prevalent in AIDS patients (more than 14 times) than in the general population.[101] The main diagnostic difficulty is differentiation from cerebral abscesses and toxoplasmosis (Fig. 44.6).

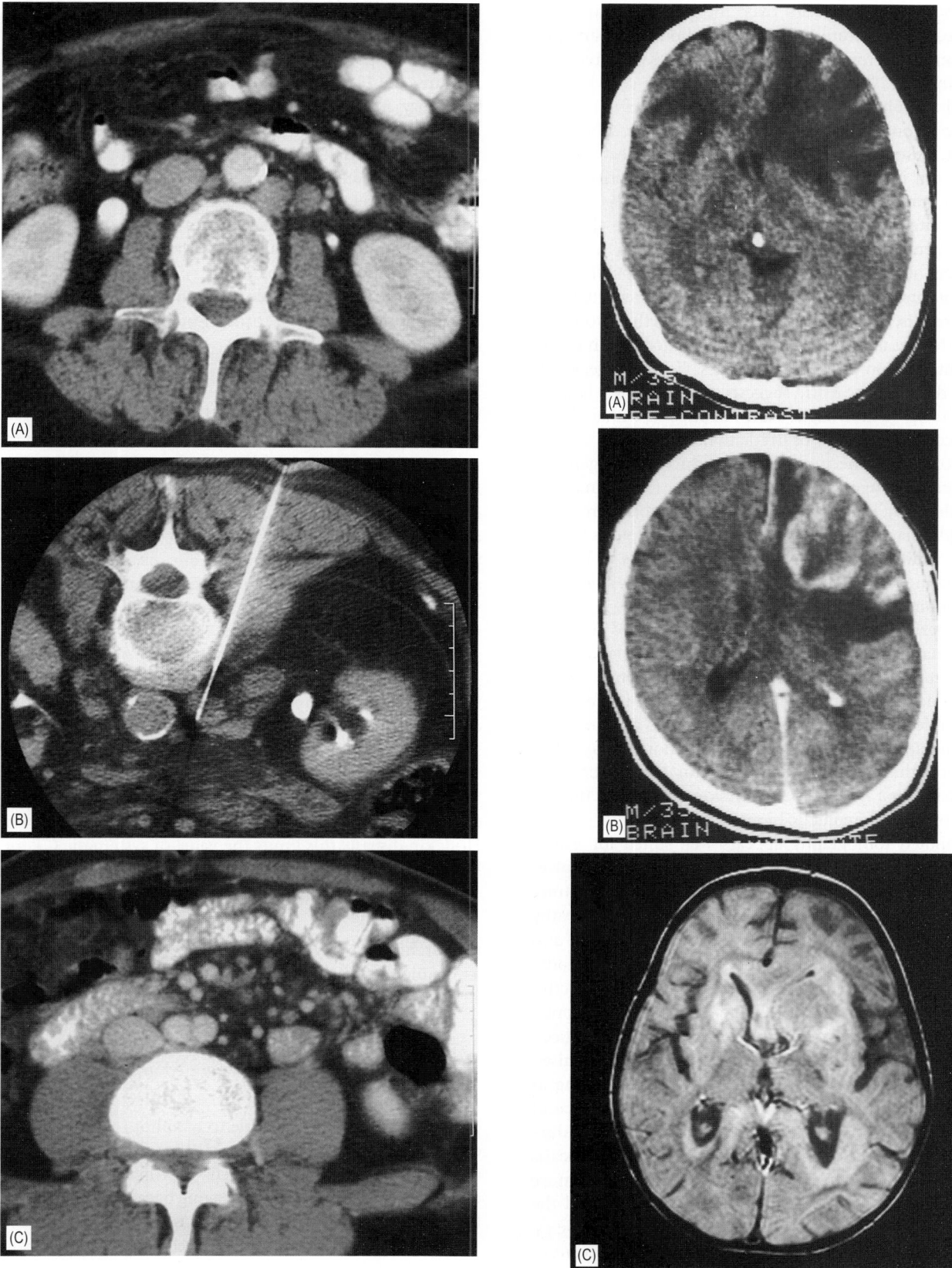

Figure 44.5 CT of residual masses. (A) Enlarged residual nodes in the retroperitoneum. (B) CT-guided biopsy of a residual adenopathy. (C) Multiple post-therapy adenopathies.

Figure 44.6 Cerebral lymphoma in immunocompromised patients. (A) Nonenhanced CT appearance. (B) Post-contrast tumor enhancement (same patient as A). (C) Paraventricular lesion (T2-weighted image).

Numerous investigators over the past 15 years have described the MRI features of CNS lymphomas, in particular in immunocompromised patients. Kim and Kim[102] reported that primary CNS involvement is essentially seen in cases of T cell lymphoma, and associates the following features: multiple lesions more often than a solitary mass, subcortical location, absence of leptomeningeal involvement, iso- to low-T1 and iso- to slightly high T2 signal intensity to the adjacent gray matter, rim enhancement in 71.4 percent of patients after gadolinium injection, hemorrhage (high T1 signal intensity) and necrosis (cystic areas) in less than 20 percent of patients. Similar results have been published by other authors.[103,104] Coulon et al.,[105] however, reported conflicting results, as 80 percent of the patients in their study had solitary lesions and only 40 percent presented a high tumor signal intensity on T2-weighted images. Hemorrhage, which is well detected by MRI, suggests toxoplasmosis because NHL is rarely hemorrhagic, except in patients with a history of corticosteroid therapy or irradiation.[106]

Gadolinium injection may produce homogeneous enhancement suggestive of lymphoma. Occasionally, a ring-enhancing lesion, typical of toxoplasmosis, proves to be lymphoma, although the wall of lymphomatous lesions is thick, while it is thin in case of toxoplasmosis.[107] Finally, irregular and sinuous contrast uptake is strongly suggestive of lymphoma.

The variability of imaging features observed for CNS lymphomas highlights the fact that even spontaneous hemorrhage, a nonenhancing lesion or diffuse white matter changes do not exclude lymphoma in immunocompromised patients.[108] Evaluation of response to antitoxoplasmosis therapy requires a repeat examination 10 days after treatment; this interval is sufficient for the detection of progression in a lymphomatous lesion and such a finding should prompt stereotactic biopsy.[106,109]

Computed tomography appears well suited for exploration of the abdomen, and often reveals visceral involvement, particularly in the liver, spleen, kidneys or omentum. The demonstration of deep abdominal lymphadenopathy should suggest not only the possibility of NHL but also of Kaposi's sarcoma or a mycobacterial infection. Nodes smaller than 15 mm merely reflect nonspecific reactive hyperplasia in the context of AIDS and do not require biopsy.

Secondary hepatic involvement is frequent, having been observed in 25–50 percent of immunocompromised patients with diffuse large B cell NHL. In this setting as well, where findings include a low T1 signal, absence of arterial uptake, and a slight increase in signal intensity during the late venous phase,[110] the differential diagnosis is infection. Diagnostic evaluation of the chest is much more difficult owing to the nonspecificity of CT signs and the frequent association of several intercurrent pathologies. For example, Kaposi's sarcoma affects up to 20 percent of AIDS patients and is often contemporary with a *Pneumocystis carinii* infection.[111] Thoracic lymphadenopathy in the context of AIDS may be indicative of Kaposi sarcoma, NHL or a mycobacterial infection. Patients who are HIV positive often present enlarged mediastinal nodes greater than or equal to 1 cm in size; 55 percent of such nodes correspond to an infection (mycobacterial disease accounts for 78 percent of these infections).[112]

Biopsy may therefore prove necessary to establish a definitive diagnosis in immunodeficient patients if an infectious pathology cannot be established by bronchiolo-alveolar lavage and/or endobronchial biopsy (69–91 percent vs 17–60 percent).[113] The definitive diagnosis of chest masses in immunodeficient patients is, thus, dependent on a constellation of clinical, radiologic, bacteriologic, and histologic findings. In particularly difficult cases, only alterations in the appearance of lesions after anti-infectious or lymphoma-specific treatment lead to the establishment of a diagnosis.

POST–TREATMENT IMAGING

Imaging is required both to monitor response to treatment for lymphoma and to search for late complications (noncancerous complications and secondary cancers).[114] In addition, certain pathologies have a potential for lymphomatous change and therefore also necessitate systematic surveillance. The risk of relapse is greatest the first two years following therapy.[20] The frequency of follow-up CT studies is dictated by the type of NHL: once every two months for forms with a poor prognosis, only after completion of induction chemotherapy (i.e. after 3 or 4 cycles) for other types of lymphoma. Simpler CT studies (without contrast injection or gastrointestinal tract opacification, scans obtained every 2 cm) can also be scheduled during the course of therapy.[115,116]

Patients with high-grade lymphomas are considered cured if they remain relapse-free for 5 years; as for Hodgkin disease, this limits the value of systematic CT for late surveillance.

MRI is indicated in the following cases:

- search for CNS lymphoma in HIV-positive patients
- histologic types of lymphoma with a risk of bone marrow involvement
- analysis of residual masses (the follow-up examination performed 12 months after treatment should reveal a low intensity signal on T2-weighted images).

Those organs most susceptible to lymphoproliferative disorders warrant specific studies: MRI for the bone marrow, echoendoscopy for the stomach. Low-grade lymphomas do not necessitate systematic imaging because no definitive treatment is available in case of relapse.

The criteria used for evaluation of response to treatment are as follows:[117]

- Complete remission (CR): complete disappearance of detectable radiographic and clinical evidence of disease; regression of all lymph nodes to normal size; regression in size of liver and spleen if previously enlarged; complete regression of focal lesions in any organ; normalization of bone marrow involvement.

- Complete remission, unconfirmed (CRU): same criteria as for CR, but 75 percent regression of volume of lymph nodes/masses; indeterminate bone marrow.
- Partial remission (PR): 50 percent regression of the six largest (dominant) lymph nodes; no increase in size of lymph nodes, no new sites; regression or constant size of splenic and hepatic nodules, and bone marrow involvement.
- Stable disease (SD): same criteria as PR but less regression; no new lesions.
- Progressive disease (PD, nonresponders): new lesions; 50 percent reduction in diameters of lymph nodes previously larger than 1 cm diameter.

In patients with high-grade NHL who remain relapse-free for 10 years, the risk of a malignancy or late toxicity is greater than that of relapse. Surveillance of such patients must be re-oriented towards search for a cardiac pathology, for example, or a new cancer. Early detection of such anomalies is often difficult because they do not occur until 5–20 years after curative treatment of the lymphoma. Certain nonmalignant complications, such as infertility, do not require any surveillance by imaging.

More than 50 percent of all cardiac complications correspond to myocardial infarction; pericarditis, cardiac insufficiency, and cardiomyopathy are less frequent. An electrocardiogram and a cardiac sonogram are indicated every 5 years. The risk of cardiac pathologies has decreased since the cumulative doses of anthracycline used have been reduced.

Mention should also be made of postradiation pulmonary complications and those induced by bleomycin, and postradiation hypothyroidism. The majority of studies on the risk of developing a secondary cancer concern Hodgkin's disease; no study to date on NHL allows proposals for use of a particular imaging surveillance schedule. Certain pathologies have a risk of evolution to NHL and probably merit specific surveillance.

Celiac disease is associated with a high risk of enteropathy-associated T cell lymphomas, including both nodal and extranodal sites. These T cell lymphomas are often multifocal, and the many ulcerative lesions explain the elevated risk of perforation.[118] If CT alone proves insufficient, its value can be improved by associated enteroclysis.[119]

Patients with Sjögren syndrome are at risk of developing NHL; the risk remains poorly evaluated to date, but is not correlated with the duration or the severity of the syndrome. Extranodal lymphomatous involvement essentially affects the salivary glands, and 78 percent of patients have adenopathies; cervical surveillance by ultrasound or CT is thus recommended.[120] Finally, the natural course of Hashimoto disease includes a risk of development of NHL,

and any nodule appearing in lesions of chronic thyroiditis warrants biopsy; regular ultrasound surveillance is thus justified.[121,122]

CONCLUSIONS

- The purpose of the pretreatment imaging is to determine the localization and the extension of the disease and to provide a baseline in order to appreciate the treatment response.
- Ultrasonography is more accurate in the detection of the superficial adenopathies than physical examination by showing confluent and strongly hypoechoic nodules. It can also permit visualization of visceral abnormalities.
- Computed tomography remains the primary imaging modality for NHL by showing the deep regions of the trunk with a high reproducibility. In the visceral localizations, NHL is often described as a bulky tumor without local aggressive destruction.
- MRI has been found to be complementary to CT in evaluation of bone sites of NHL and in the head and neck regions. This examination can especially localize the probable site of involvement of the pelvic bone and eliminate the false-negative results of blinded biopsies. Newer MRI techniques such as MR spectroscopy, MR simulation and specific contrast agent could improve detection of lymphomatous lesion.
- A persistent residual mass is frequently noted and should be evaluated by using MRI with intravenous gadolinium injection. Percutaneous biopsies and PET-CT can be useful in the determination of the etiology of residual masses. Post-treatment imaging is also required to search for late complications including a new cancer or a cardiac complication.

KEY POINTS

- Although PET-CT appears to be the most accurate imaging modality, CT remains the basic imaging technique for the staging and the follow-up of NHL.
- MRI is required for CNS and bone marrow involvement.
- Imaging-guided (CT, ultrasound) percutaneous core-needle biopsy is increasingly used instead of surgical biopsy.

ACKNOWLEDGMENT

The authors wish to thank Nancy Reed for translation of the manuscript.

REFERENCES

● = Key primary paper
◆ = Major review article

1. Castellino RA. The non-Hodgkin lymphomas: practical concepts for the diagnostic radiologist. *Radiology* 1991; **178**: 315–21.

2. Frija J, D'Agay MF, Brice P. Imagerie des lymphomes. *Rev Immunol Med* 1993; **5**: 457–68.

◆3. Kumar R, Maillard I, Schuster SJ, Alavi A. Utility of fluorodeoxyglucose–PET imaging in the management of patients with Hodgkin's and non-Hodgkin's lymphomas. *Radiol Clin North Am* 2004; **42**: 1083–100.

◆4. Zinzani PL. Lymphoma: diagnosis, staging, natural history, and treatment strategies. *Semin Oncol* 2005; **32**(Suppl 1): s4–10.

5. Scutellari PN, Borgatti L, Spanedda R. Non-Hodgkin's lymphomas of extranodal localization. Strategies for imaging diagnosis. *Radiol Med (Torino)* 2000; **100**: 262–72.

6. Bruneton JN, Schneider M. *Radiology of lymphomas.* Berlin: Springer Verlag, 1986.

7. Jing BS. Diagnostic imaging of abdominal and pelvic lymph nodes in lymphoma. *Radiol Clin North Am* 1990; **28**: 801–31.

8. Shirkhoda A, Ros PR, Farah J, Staab EV. Lymphoma of the solid abdominal viscera. *Radiol Clin North Am* 1990; **28**: 785–99.

9. Cohen MD, Siddiqui A, Weetman R *et al.* Hodgkin disease and non-Hodgkin lymphomas in children: utilization of radiological modalities. *Radiology* 1986; **158**: 499–505.

10. White L, Siegel SE, Quah TC. Non-Hodgkin's lymphomas in children, I. Patterns of disease and classification. *Crit Rev Oncol Hematol* 1992; **13**: 55–71.

11. Tsang RW, Gospodarowicz MK, O'Sullivan B. Staging and management of localized non-Hodgkin's lymphomas: variations among experts in radiation oncology. *Int J Radiat Oncol Biol Phys* 2002; **52**: 643–51.

●12. Freudenberg LS, Antoch G, Schutt P *et al.* FDG–PET/CT in re-staging of patients with lymphoma. *Eur J Nucl Med Mol Imaging* 2004; **31**: 325–9.

●13. Depas G, De Barsy C, Jerusalem G *et al.* 18 F-FDG PET in children with lymphomas. *Eur J Nucl Med Mol Imaging* 2005; **32**: 31–8.

●14. Avril ME, Weber WA. Monitoring response to treatment in patients utilizing PET. *Radiol Clin North Am* 2005; **43**: 189–204.

●15. Agid R, Sklair-Levy M, Bloom AI *et al.* CT-guided biopsy with cutting-edge needle for the diagnosis of malignant lymphoma: experience of 267 biopsies. *Clin Radiol* 2003; **58**: 143–7.

●16. Lieberman CS, Libson E, Maly B *et al.* Imaging-guided percutaneous splenic biopsy using a 20- or 22-Gauge cutting-edge core biopsy needle for the diagnosis of malignant lymphoma. *AJR Am J Roentgenol* 2003; **181**: 1025–7.

17. Chen L, Kuriakose P, Hawley RC *et al.* Hematologic malignancies with primary retroperitoneal presentation: clinicopathologic study of 32 cases. *Arch Pathol Lab Med* 2005; **129**: 655–60.

18. Appelbaum L, Lederman R, Agid R, Libson E. Hepatic lymphoma: an imaging approach with emphasis on image-guided needle biopsy. *Isr Med Assoc J* 2005; **7**: 19–22.

19. Arcari A, Anselmi E, Bernuzzi P *et al.* Primary pancreatic lymphoma. Report of five cases. *Haematologia* 2005; **90**: ECR09.

20. Chiou HJ, Chou YH, Chiou SY *et al.* High-resolution ultrasonography of primary peripheral soft tissue lymphoma. *J Ultrasound Med* 2005; **24**: 77–86.

21. Deng LP, Hu HJ, Zhang SZ *et al.* Radiological features of primary pulmonary non-Hodgkin lymphoma: report of three cases. *Zhonghua Jie He He Hu Xi Za Zhi* 2003; **26**: 223–6.

22. Woolridge JE, Lin KB. Post-treatment surveillance of patients with lymphoma treated with curative intent. *Semin Oncol* 2003; **30**: 375–81.

23. Bruneton JN, Normand F, Balu-Maestro C *et al.* Lymphomatous superficial lymph nodes: US detection. *Radiology* 1987; **165**: 233–5.

24. Gobbi PG, Broglia C, Carnevale Matte G *et al.* Lymphomatous superficial nodes; limitations of physical examinations for accurate staging and response assessment. *Haematologica* 2002; **87**: 1151–6.

25. Ahuja A, Ying M, King A, Yuen HY. Lymph node hilus: gray scale and power Doppler sonography of cervical nodes. *J Ultrasound Med* 2001; **20**: 987–92.

26. Brnic Z. Doppler ultrasonography of superficial lymph nodes. *Lijec Vjesn* 2004; **126**: 185–93.

27. Giovagnorio F, Galluzzo M, Andreoli C *et al.* Color Doppler sonography in the evaluation of superficial lymphomatous lymph nodes. *J Ultrasound Med* 2002; **21**: 403–8.

28. Goerg C, Schwerk WB. Ultrasound of extranodal abdominal lymphoma. A review. *Clin Radiol* 1991; **44**: 92–7.

29. Soyer P, Van Beers B, Teillet-Thiebaud F *et al.* Hodgkin's and non-Hodgkin's hepatic lymphoma: Sonographic findings. *Abdom Imaging* 1993; **18**: 339–43.

30. Rizzi EB, Schinina V, Cristofaro M *et al.* Non-Hodgkin's lymphoma of the liver in patients with AIDS: sonographic, CT, and MRI findings. *J Clin Ultrasound* 2001; **29**: 125–9.

31. D'Onofrio M, Rozzanigo U, Masinielli BM *et al.* Hypoechoic focal liver lesions: characterization with contrast enhanced ultrasonography. *J Clin Ultrasound* 2005; **33**: 164–72.

32. Civardi G, Vallisa D, Berte R *et al.* Focal liver lesions in non-Hodgkin's lymphoma: investigation of their prevalence, clinical significance and the role of Hepatitis C virus infection. *Eur J Cancer* 2002; **38**: 2382–7.

33. Kasagi K, Hatabu H, Tokuda Y *et al.* Lymphoproliferative disorders of the thyroid gland: radiological appearances. *Br J Radiol* 1991; **64**: 569–75.

34. Peterson K, Gordon KB, Heinemann MH, De Angelis IM. The clinical spectrum of ocular lymphoma. *Cancer* 1993; **72**: 843–9.

35. Tweed CS, Peck RJ. A sonographic appearance of testicular lymphoma. *Clin Radiol* 1991; **43**: 341–2.

36. Morton JE, Leyland MJ, Vaughan Hudson G *et al.* Primary gastrointestinal non-Hodgkin's lymphoma: a review of 175 British National Lymphoma Investigation cases. *Br J Cancer* 1993; **67**: 776–82.

37. Seitz JF, Giovannini M, Monges G *et al.* Intérêt de la fibroscopie digestive haute dans le bilan d'extension initial des lymphomes malins non hodgkiniens extra-digestifs. Résultats chez 101 patients. *Gastroenterol Clin Biol* 1990; **14**: 961–5.

38. Seifert E, Schulte F, Weismuller J *et al.* Endoscopic and biopsic diagnosis of malignant non-Hodgkin's lymphoma of the stomach. *Endoscopy* 1993; **25**: 497–501.

39. Schwarz RJ, Conners JM, Schmidt N. Diagnosis and management of stage IE and stage IIE gastric lymphomas. *Am J Surg* 1993; **165**: 561–5.

40. Hoepffner N, Lahme T, Gilly J *et al.* Value of endosonography in diagnostic staging of primary gastric lymphoma (MALT type). *Med Klin (Munich)* 2003; **98**: 313–17.

41. Schuder G, Hildebrandt V, Kreifler-Haag D *et al.* Role of endosonography in the surgical management of non-Hodgkin's lymphoma of the stomach. *Endoscopy* 1993; **25**: 509–12.

42. Palazzo L, Roseau G, Ruskone-Fourmestraux A *et al.* Endoscopic ultrasonography in the local staging of primary gastric lymphoma. *Endoscopy* 1993; **25**: 502–8.

43. Ribeiro A, Vazquez-Sequeiros E, Wiersema LM *et al.* EUS-guided fine-needle aspiration combined with flow cytometry and immunocytochemistry in the diagnosis of lymphoma. *Gastrointest Endosc* 2001; **53**: 485–91.

44. North LB, Libshitz HI, Lorigan JG. Thoracic lymphoma. *Radiol Clin North Am* 1990; **28**: 745–62.

45. Khoury MB, Godwin JD, Halvorsen R *et al.* Role of chest CT in non-Hodkgin lymphoma. *Radiology* 1986; **158**: 659–62.

46. Zagoria RJ, Muss HB, Wolfman NT *et al.* Computed tomography versus chest radiography: impact on management of patients with lymphoma. *Cancer Invest* 1990; **8**: 357–64.

47. Saito A, Takashima S, Takayama F *et al.* Spontaneous extension necrosis in non-Hodgkin lymphoma: prevalence and clinical significance. *J Comput Assist Tomogr* 2001; **25**: 482–6.

48. Matsumoto S, Shibuya H, Tatera S *et al.* Comparison of CT findings in non-Hodgkin lymphoma and squamous cell carcinoma of the maxillary sinus. *Acta Radiol* 1992; **33**: 523–7.

49. Cordier JF, Chailleux E, Lauque D *et al.* Primary pulmonary lymphomas. A clinical study of 79 cases in nonimmunocompromised patients. *Chest* 1993; **103**: 201–8.

50. Lewis ER, Caskey CI, Fishmann EK. Lymphoma of the lung: CT findings in 31 patients. *AJR Am J Roentgenol* 1991; **156**: 711–14.

51. Bosanko CM, Korobkin M, Fantone JC *et al.* Lobar primary pulmonary lymphoma: CT findings. *J Comput Assist Tomogr* 1991; **15**: 679–82.

52. Vincent JM, Ng YY, Norton AJ, Armstrong P. CT 'angiogram sign' in primary pulmonary lymphoma. *J Comput Assist Tomogr* 1992; **16**: 829–31.

53. Cohan RH, Dunnick NR, Leder RA, Baker ME. Computed tomography of renal lymphoma. *J Comput Assist Tomogr* 1990; **14**: 933–8.

54. Weinberger E, Rosenbaum DM, Pendergrass TW. Renal involvement in children with lymphoma: comparison of CT with sonography. *AJR Am J Roentgenol* 1990; **155**: 347–9.

55. Chung HH, Kim YH, Kim JH *et al.* Imaging findings of mantle cell lymphoma involving gastrointestinal tract. *Yonsei Med J* 2003; **44**: 49–57.

56. Apter S, Avigdor A, Gayer G *et al.* Calcification in lymphoma occurring before therapy: CT features and clinical correlation. *AJR Am J Roentgenol* 2002; **178**: 935–8.

57. Rodallec M, Guermazi A, Brice P *et al.* Imaging of MALT lymphomas. *Eur Radiol* 2002; **12**: 348–56.

●58. King LJ, Padley SP, Wotherspoon AC, Nicholson AG. Pulmonary MALT lymphoma: imaging findings in 24 cases. *Eur Radiol* 2000; **10**: 1932–8.

◆59. Vinnicombe SJ, Reznek RH. Computerised tomography in the staging of Hodgkin's disease and non-Hodgkin's lymphoma. *Eur J Nucl Med Mol Imaging* 2003; **30**(Suppl 1): s42–55.

60. Hermann S, Wormanns D, Pixberg M *et al.* Staging in childhood lymphoma: differences between FDG-PET and CT. *Nuklearmedizin* 2005; **44**: 1–7.

◆61. Schaefer NG, Hany TF, Taverna C *et al.* Non-Hodgkin lymphoma and Hodgkin disease: coregistered FDG PET and CT at staging and restaging. Do we need contrast-enhanced CT? *Radiology* 2004; **232**: 823–9.

62. Negendank WG, Al Katib AM, Karanes C, Smith MR. Lymphomas: MRI contrast characteristics with clinical-pathologic correlations. *Radiology* 1990; **177**: 209–16.

63. Skillings JR, Bramwell V, Nicholson RL *et al.* A prospective study of MRI in lymphoma staging. *Cancer* 1991; **67**: 1838–43.

64. Tesoro-Tess JD, Balzarini L, Ceglia E *et al.* MRI in the initial staging of Hodgkin's disease and non-Hodgkin lymphoma. *Eur J Radiol* 1991; **12**: 81–90.

65. Krishnan A, Shirkhoda A, Tehranzadeh J *et al.* Primary bone lymphoma: radiographic – MR imaging correlation. *Radiographics* 2003; **23**: 1371–83.

66. Mengiardi B, Honegger H, Hodler J *et al.* Primary lymphoma of bone: MRI and CT characteristics during and after successful treatment. *AJR Am J Roentgenol* 2005; **184**: 185–92.

67. Asaumi J, Yanagi Y, Konouchi H et al. Application of dynamic contrast-enhanced MRI to differentiate malignant lymphoma from squamous cell carcinoma in the head and neck. Oral Oncol 2004; **40**: 579–84.

●68. King AD, Lei KI, Ahuja AT. MRI of neck nodes in non-Hodgkin's lymphoma of the head and neck. Br J Radiol 2004; **77**: 111–15.

69. Weber AL, Rahemtullah A, Ferry JA. Hodgkin and non-Hodgkin lymphoma of the head and neck: clinical, pathologic, and imaging evaluation. Neuroimaging Clin North Am 2003; **13**: 371–92.

70. Akansel G, Hendrix L, Erickson BA et al. MRI patterns in orbital malignant lymphoma and atypical lymphocytic infiltrates. Eur J Radiol 2005; **53**: 175–81.

71. Assoun J, Poey C, Attal M. Envahissement médullaire au cours des lymphomes. Corrélation biopsie ostéo-médullaire et IRM. Rev Immunol Med 1993; **5**: 15–21.

72. Guckel F, Semmler W, Dohner H et al. Kernspintomographische darstellung von knochen markinfiltrationen bei malignen Lymphomen. Rofo 1989; **150**: 26–31.

73. Al Mulhim FA. Magnetic resonance imaging of pelvic and femoral bones for detection of bone marrow infiltration in patients with non-Hodgkin's lymphoma. Saudi Med J 2005; **26**: 31–6.

74. Smith SR, Williams CE, Davies JM, Edwards RH. Bone marrow disorders: characterization with quantitative MR imaging. Radiology 1989; **172**: 805–10.

75. Weinreb JC. MR imaging of bone marrow: a map could help. Radiology 1990; **177**: 23–4.

76. Flentje M, Zierhut D, Schraube P, Wannanmacher M. Integration of coronal MRI into radiation treatment planning of mediastinal tumors. Strahlenther Onkol 1993; **169**: 351–7.

77. Kaiser WA, Kombos T, Traber F et al. Erste Ergebnisse der in-vivo-31 P-NMR-Spektroskopie der Milz bei Patienten mit Splenomegalie. Rofo Fortschr Geb Rontgenstr Neuren Bildgeb Verfarhr 1993; **159**: 180–6.

78. Lonnemark M, Hemmingsson A, Bach-Gansmo T et al. Superparamagnetic particles as oral contrast medium in MR imaging of malignant lymphoma. Acta Radiol 1991; **32**: 232–8.

79. Smith SR, Martin PA, Davies JM, Stevens AN. The assessment of treatment response in non-Hodgkin's lymphoma by image guided 31P MR spectroscopy. Br J Cancer 1990; **61**: 485–90.

80. Wang J, Takashima S, Takayama F et al. Head and neck lesions: characterization with diffusion-weighted echo-planar MR imaging. Radiology 2001; **220**: 621–30.

81. King AD, Yeung DK, Ahuja AT et al. Human cervical lymphadenopathy: evaluation with in vivo H-MRS at 1.5 T. Clin Radiol 2005; **60**: 592–8.

82. Seneterre E, Weissleder R, Jaramillo D et al. Bone marrow: ultrasmall superparamagnetic iron oxide for MR imaging. Radiology 1991; **179**: 529–33.

83. Weissleder R, Elizondo G, Wittenberg J. Ultrasmall superparamagnetic iron oxide: an intravenous contrast agent for assessing lymph nodes with MR imaging. Radiology 1990; **175**: 494–8.

84. Gaffke G, Stroszczynski C, Gnauck M et al. Differential diagnosis of intra and periilienal tumors by use of a RES-specific MRI contrast agent. Rontgenpraxis 2004; **55**: 192–9.

85. Harisinghani MG, Saini S, Weissleder R et al. Splenic imaging with ultrasmall superparamagnetic iron oxide ferumoxtran-10 (AMI-7227): preliminary observations. J Comput Assist Tomogr 2001; **25**: 770–6.

◆86. Golder WA. Lymph node diagnosis in oncologic imaging: a dilemma still writing to be solved. Onkologie 2004; **27**: 194–9.

●87. Neuwelt EA, Guastadisegni PE, Varallyay P, Doolittle ND. Imaging changes and cognitive outcome in primary CNS lymphoma after enhanced chemotherapy delivery. AJNR Am J Neuroradiol 2005; **26**: 258–65.

88. Laffan EE, O'Connor R, Ryan SS, Donoghue VB. Whole-body magnetic resonance imaging: a useful additional sequence in paediatric imaging. Pediatr Radiol 2004; **34**: 472–80.

●89. Kellenberger CJ, Epelman M, Miller SF, Babyn PS. Fast STIR whole-body MR imaging in children. Radiographics 2004; **24**: 1317–30.

90. Iizuka-Mikami M, Nagai K, Yoshida K et al. Detection of bone marrow and extramedullary involvement in patients with non-Hodgkin's lymphoma by whole-body MRI: comparison with bone and 67 Ga scintigraphies. Eur Radiol 2004; **14**: 1074–81.

91. Leng S, Fischer S, Kotter I et al. Possibilities of whole-body MRI for investigating musculoskeletal diseases. Radiologe 2004; **44**: 844–53.

●92. Whelan JS, Reznek RH, Daniell SJ et al. CT and US guided core biopsy in the management of non-Hodgkin's lymphoma. Br J Cancer 1991; **63**: 460–2.

93. Rahmouni A, Tempany C, Jones R et al. Lymphoma: monitoring tumor size and signal intensity with MR imaging. Radiology 1993; **188**: 445–51.

94. Karmazyn B, Ash S, Goshen Y et al. Significance of residual abdominal masses in children with abdominal Burkitt's lymphoma. Pediatr Radiol 2001; **31**: 801–5.

95. Lee JKT, Glazer HS. Controversy in the MR imaging appearance of fibrosis. Radiology 1990; **177**: 21–2.

96. Rahmouni A, Divine M, Lepage E et al. Mediastinal lymphomas: quantitative changes in Gadolinium enhancement at MR imaging after treatment. Radiology 2001; **219**: 621–8.

◆97. Reske SN. PET and restaging of malignant lymphoma including residual masses and relapse. Eur J Nucl Med Mol Imaging 2003; **30**(Suppl 1): s80–96.

98. Kazama T, Faria SC, Varavithya V et al. FDG-PET in the evaluation of treatment for lymphoma: clinical usefulness and pitfalls. Radiographics 2005; **25**: 191–207.

99. Hennessy BT, Hanrahan EO, Daly PA. Non-Hodgkin lymphoma: an up-date. Lancet Oncol 2004; **5**: 341–53.

100. Little RF. AIDS-related non-Hodgkin's lymphoma: etiology, epidemiology, and impact of highly active antiretroviral therapy. Leuk Lymphoma 2003; **44**(Suppl 3): s63–8.

101. Ioachim HL, Dorsett B, Cronin W *et al.* AIDS-associated lymphomas: clinical, pathologic, immunologic, and viral characteristics of 111 cases. *Hum Pathol* 1991; **22**: 659–73.

102. Kim EY, Kim SS. Magnetic resonance findings of primary central nervous system T-cell lymphoma in immunocompetent patients. *Acta Radiol* 2005; **46**: 187–92.

◆103. Guinto G, Felix I, Arechiga N *et al.* Primary central nervous system lymphomas in immunocompetent patients. *Histol Histopathol* 2004; **19**: 963–72.

104. Suwanwela N, Tantanatrakool B, Suwanwela NC. Intracranial lymphoma: CT and MR findings. *J Med Assoc Thai* 2001; **84**(Suppl 1): s228–43.

●105. Coulon A, Lafitte F, Huong-Xuan K *et al.* Radiographic findings in 37 cases of primary CNS lymphoma in immunocompetent patients. *Eur Radiol* 2002; **12**: 329–40.

106. Cordoliani YS, Derosier C, Pharaboz C *et al.* Primary cerebral lymphoma in patients with AIDS: MR findings in 17 cases. *J Radiol* 1992; **73**: 367–76.

107. Dina TS. Primary central nervous system lymphoma versus toxoplasmosis in AIDS. *Radiology* 1991; **179**: 823–8.

108. Thurnher MM, Rieger A, Kleibl-Popov C *et al.* Primary central nervous system lymphoma in AIDS: a wider spectrum of CT and MRI findings. *Neuroradiology* 2001; **43**: 29–35.

109. Levy RM, Russel E, Yungbluth M *et al.* The efficacy of image-guided stereotactic brain biopsy in neurologically symptomatic acquired immunodeficiency syndrome patients. *Neurosurgery* 1992; **30**: 186–9.

110. Coenegrachts K, Vanbeckevoort D, Deraedt K, Van Steenbergen W. MRI findings in primary non-Hodgkin's lymphoma of the liver. *JBR-BTR* 2005; **88**: 17–19.

111. Herts BR, Megibow AJ, Birnbaum BA *et al.* High-attenuation lymphadenopathy in AIDS patients: significance of findings at CT. *Radiology* 1992; **185**: 777–81.

112. Fishman JE, Sagar M. Thoracic lymphadenopathy in HIV patients: spectrum of disease and differential diagnosis. *AIDS Patient Care STDS* 1999; **13**: 645–9.

113. Janzen DL, Padley SPG, Adler BD, Muller NL. Acute pulmonary complications in immunocompromised non-AIDS patients: comparison of diagnostic accuracy of CT and chest radiography. *Clin Radiol* 1993; **47**: 159–65.

114. Bruneton JN, Stines J, Padovani A *et al.* *Imagerie et surveillance post-thérapeutique en oncologie.* Paris: Masson, 2000.

115. Sandrasegaran K, Robinson PJ, Selby P. Staging of lymphomas in adults. *Clin Radiol* 1994; **49**: 149–61.

116. Thomas JL, Barnes PA, Bernardino ME, Hagemeister FB. Limited CT studies in monitoring treatment of lymphomas. *AJR Am J Roentgenol* 1982; **138**: 537–9.

117. Cheson BD, Horning SJ, Coiffier B *et al.* Report of an international workshop to standardize response criteria for non-Hodgkin's lymphomas. NCI Sponsored International Working Group. *J Clin Oncol* 1999; **17**: 1244–53.

118. Meijer JW, Mulder CJ, Goerres MG *et al.* Coeliac disease and (extra) intestinal T-cell lymphomas: definition, diagnosis and treatment. *Scand J Gastroenterol Suppl* 2004; **241**: 78–84.

119. Boudiaf M, Jaff A, Soyer P *et al.* Small-bowel diseases: prospective evaluation of multi-detector row helical CT enteroclysis in 107 consecutive patients. *Radiology* 2004; **233**: 338–44.

120. Tonami H, Matoba M, Kuginuki Y *et al.* Clinical and imaging findings of lymphoma in patients with Sjogren Syndrome. *J Comput Assist Tomogr* 2003; **27**: 517–24.

121. Di Cataldo A, Sgroi AV, Occhipinti R *et al.* Rare malignant tumors of the thyroid. *G Chir* 2004; **25**: 420–3.

122. Kim HC, Han MH, Kim KH *et al.* Primary thyroid lymphomas: CT findings. *Eur J Radiol* 2003; **46**: 233–9.

45

Radionuclide imaging

JORGE A CARRASQUILLO, RONALD E WEINER, DOROTHEA McAREAVEY AND RONALD D NEUMANN

INTRODUCTION

The nuclear medicine tests available for staging and post-treatment evaluation of lymphoma patients are generally most useful when they are used to survey the patient for unsuspected sites of disease and/or to evaluate a physiologic or biochemical parameter to determine whether a suspected site or lesion found by an anatomic structural imaging test, such as computed tomography (CT) or magnetic resonance imaging (MRI), represents viable tumor tissue. Nuclear medicine tests are notable for relatively high sensitivity in detecting active disease but these tests often have low specificities. The multiplicity of possible disease locations in lymphomas and the wide variety of clinical presentations preclude a simple scheme for using nuclear medicine tests in the evaluation of each and every patient. We will thus discuss briefly some of the nuclear medicine tests available, their likely application, and give an indication of effectiveness. We shall begin with the most widely used of these, 2-[^{18}F] fluoro-2-deoxyglucose (^{18}F-FDG) positron emission tomography (PET), which has widespread application in lymphoma patient evaluation and is now generally available.

POSITRON EMISSION TOMOGRAPHY USING ^{18}F-FDG

An expanding area of oncology imaging is the use of PET with short-lived radiopharmaceuticals for physiological imaging of most tumors including lymphomas. The advantage of PET derives from the nature of positron tomography, which allows for more precise quantification of radioactivity in tumors. In addition to positron-emitting isotopes of gallium, there are a number of metabolic-analogue radiopharmaceuticals such as ^{18}F-FDG which have shown potential as agents to permit improved PET imaging of lymphomas. Recent papers have even stated that in patients with untreated lymphomas (Hodgkin and various grade NHL) the degree to which their tumors accumulated ^{18}F-FDG is correlated with the host patient's prognosis.

The reason for the ^{18}F-FDG PET test's success derives from its underlying mechanisms. By taking advantage of a lymphocyte's normal and/or its malignant-phenotype's carbohydrate metabolism one can 'label' specific cells using a radionuclide-carrying sugar analogue as the radiopharmaceutical. For the typical clinical PET ^{18}F-FDG study, 2-[^{18}F] fluoro-2-deoxyglucose is given intravenously to patients after a multi-hour period of fasting. ^{18}F-FDG initially follows the same metabolic pathway as glucose. It is carried via the circulation to the interstitial fluid from which cells accumulate ^{18}F-FDG via the same system of cell-membrane glut transport proteins that are used for glucose uptake. Intracellularly, ^{18}F-FDG is phosphorylated by hexokinase, forming 2-[^{18}F] fluoro-2-deoxyglucose 6-phosphate. But while glucose 6-phoshate can then isomerize to fructose 6-phosphate, the radiopharmaceutical is blocked because it lacks an oxygen atom at the C2 position. Moreover, the ^{18}F-FDG 6-phosphate cannot rapidly leave the cell; effectively radiolabelling the cell with fluorine-18. Because malignant cells often have an increased rate of glycolysis, they have also an increased uptake of glucose. The ^{18}F-FDG radiopharmaceutical uptake is thus proportionately increased in malignant cells as compared to most 'resting' normal cells.

The radiopharmaceutical is enhanced through high-specific-activity labeling with ^{18}F (i.e. most of the FDG molecules carry a radioactive fluorine 'tag' which will decay during the test to produce a measurable radiodecay event) thus identifying the cell with the radiopharmaceutical uptake. PET cameras, now equipped for better anatomic localization with an attached CT instrument, are basically very sensitive external detectors of the photons produced from ^{18}F radiodecay. ^{18}F radiodecay produces a positron (B+) which immediately fuses with an electron nearby to produce two 511 keV photons emitted in nearly opposite trajectories. The multi-ring PET detector's crystals produce scintillations upon photon impact which are then mathematically recorded as to origin. The PET system's sensitivity characteristics allow one to inject only nanomolar amounts of the sugar analog FDG so as not to perturb the glucose metabolism pathways being imaged. This test is a classic example of the radiotracer principle used clinically.

The precise role for ^{18}F-FDG PET studies in the management of patients with lymphomas is not yet conclusively studied. ^{18}F-FDG studies are now used in the initial staging of patients, for treatment evaluations, and in 'long-term' follow-up. However, the accuracies for the test in each application remain unclear because ^{18}F-FDG PET studies were introduced widely into clinical practice without prior comprehensive randomized trials, especially the so-called 'double-blinded' trials, to assess the utility of this test when it was first made available. Unfortunately a similar pattern of insufficient testing before introduction into clinical practice seems to be the history for many new imaging tests.

A second confounder in determining this test's accuracy is the myriad of histologically characterized subtypes of lymphoma. Because there is not necessarily a direct relationship between the pathologist's diagnosis of lymphoma subtype and a tumor's glucose metabolism, complete data for each subtype have been slow coming into publication. There is also an overlap between the ^{18}F-FDG uptake of so-called 'reactive' lymphocytes and the truly malignant lymphocyte. For example, lymphoid follicular cells have a

strong expression of GLUT transporters in instances of follicular hyperplasia. This results in increased ^{18}F-FDG uptake by these cells which can mimic the PET images presented by low-grade malignancies.[1]

Another of the most frequent causes of 'false-positive' ^{18}F-FDG studies is the presence of focal inflammation.[2] That discussion is beyond the scope of this chapter, but it suffices to say that both functioning inflammatory response cells and pathogens may use glucose as an energy source. Thus, ^{18}F-FDG uptake in such foci will also be enhanced.

Fluorodeoxyglucose imaging of lymphoma patients

PATIENT PREPARATION AND IMAGE ACQUISITION

Patients should be fasted for 4–6 hours prior to injection of the ^{18}F-FDG in order to minimize the potential competition at the tumor cell membrane from elevated blood sugar. In addition, in the post-prandial state, the increase in insulin levels stimulates an increase in GLUT-4, which drives ^{18}F-FDG and glucose into muscles, thus degrading imaging. After an intravenous injection of ^{18}F-FDG, an uptake period of about 60 minutes is allowed in which the patient is resting quietly to minimize any physiologic uptake in muscles due to patient use. Because ^{18}F-FDG accumulation in most tumors increases with time, to a point, the uptake period should be consistent in any follow-up studies.[3]

The emission images obtained from the ^{18}F need to be corrected for tissue attenuation in order to be quantitative. Older PET scanners accomplished this by using a radionuclide transmission source that circled stepwise around the patient. Newer PET cameras often have an attached CT instrument that allows the use of the CT data to correct for attenuation; and, in addition, the CT images obtained permit co-registration of ^{18}F-FDG uptake with anatomic structures.[4]

In addition to a simple visual interpretation of the ^{18}F-FDG distribution in the PET images, there are several ways in which quantitive uptake can be expressed.[5] The simplest method is called a standardized uptake value (SUV = uptake in tumor (mCi/g)/injected dose (mCi)/patient weight (g)).[6] Some modifications of this method to account for body surface area or lean body mass are also often applied.[5] Alternatively, metabolic rates can be determined,[5] but typically these determinations are more time consuming; such calculations are usually limited to a single area of interest, cannot be obtained over the whole body, and are thus most often used in the research setting.

^{18}F-FDG PET versus other imaging tests (staging and restaging)

At this moment the staging of Hodgkin disease and non-Hodgkin lymphoma (NHL) is based on the Ann Arbor system originally developed for Hodgkin disease,[7] which relies on determining the sites of nodal and extranodal tumor involvement. Radiographic staging is thus an integral part of the evaluation of these patients because the location, number, and size of lesions has prognostic implications.[8] Most oncologists utilize CT scanning to stage and follow patients, relying on size and morphology for detection of nodal involvement. Nonetheless, it is known that small nodes may harbor lymphoma cells while large nodes may be functionally benign.[9] Numerous studies have evaluated the role of ^{18}F-FDG imaging in Hodgkin disease and NHL.[10,11] Because many studies deal with both Hodgkin disease and NHL, and because the ^{18}F-FDG results are generally similar, we will include data for both Hodgkin disease and NHL in this chapter without discrete presentations.

^{18}F-FDG PET is of value in the staging and restaging of both Hodgkin disease and NHL. In most series, ^{18}F-FDG PET has been found to be superior to traditional imaging tests. The sensitivity and specificity of ^{18}F-FDG PET ranges from 79 percent to 100 percent and 92 percent to 100 percent, respectively.[12–17] In contrast, the sensitivity and specificity for CT have generally been lower and numbers from 81 percent to 100 percent, and 23 percent to 100 percent, respectively have been reported.[12–15,17] In most of these reports where ^{18}F-FDG PET was compared to CT scans, the PET study was superior in both sensitivity and specificity. The high sensitivity for disease detection holds true for peripheral, thoracic and abdominal nodes.[15,18] In addition to better individual lesion detection, most studies comparing the staging of Hodgkin disease and NHL have also found that ^{18}F-FDG PET is more accurate in disease staging than other imaging modalities.[12,14–16,19]

[67]Ga scanning, both planar and single photon emission computed tomography (SPECT), has almost completely been supplanted by ^{18}F-FDG PET in well-funded hospitals for the evaluation of lymphoma patients. Among the advantages of ^{18}F-FDG PET over ^{67}Ga SPECT are the higher tumor to background ratios, same day test completion, and better lesion quantitation. Furthermore, multiple studies have shown both a higher sensitivity and specificity for ^{18}F-FDG PET lymphoma detection and staging than for ^{67}Ga SPECT in both Hodgkin disease and NHL.[20–23] Rini et al. compared ^{18}F-FDG PET and ^{67}Ga in 32 children and young adults.[24] While no significant differences were seen in the accuracy in the supradiagphragmatic region, the ^{18}F-FDG PET was more accurate than ^{67}Ga for detecting splenic involvement (0.91 vs 0.61), infradiaphragmatic (0.89 vs 0.75), and also all disease sites combined (0.95 vs 0.91). Furthermore, ^{18}F-FDG PET-determined stage agreed with clinical stage in 79 percent of patients compared with 71 percent for ^{67}Ga scintigraphy. Other studies have also shown higher sensitivity of ^{18}F-FDG PET for detecting nodal and extranodal sites, including bone and mediastinum.[23,25,26] Of course, these comparisons are akin to comparisons of apples and oranges; i.e., ^{18}F-FDG marks glucose metabolism while ^{67}Ga traces cellular iron metabolism. PET also is inherently a more sensitive technique than planar scintigraphy or single photon emission tomography (SPECT).

Evaluation of residual masses post–therapy

A dilemma that commonly arises following treatment of patients with lymphomas is the persistence of a residual tissue mass at a site of previous lymphoma involvement. Although up to 64 percent of lymphoma patients may have residual masses after completion of therapy, only 18 percent reportedly relapsed.[27] The presence of a residual mass is more frequent when bulky disease is present initially, and is more frequent with Hodgkin disease than NHL.[28] Computed tomography and MRI readily identify these residual masses, but cannot distinguish between residual viable tumor and tissue fibrosis. Magnetic resonance imaging has been reported to have a sensitivity of 45 percent, specificity of 90 percent, positive predictive value (PPV) of 71 percent and a negative predictive value (NPV) of 75 percent for detection of residual tumor.[29] ^{18}F-FDG PET has been shown to be a better predictor of residual disease than traditional radiographic techniques. Persistent accumulation of ^{18}F-FDG in a residual mass following treatment correlates with a 80–95 percent incidence of relapse or local recurrence.[30–33] In contrast, only 0–20 percent of patients with a residual mass negative for ^{18}F-FDG uptake will have recurrent disease; and even then the recurrence is often outside of the residual mass.[31,32] Yet Masiey et al., however, reported much lower sensitivity and specificity distinguishing between viable tumor and fibrosis with ^{18}F-FDG in both Hodgkin disease and NHL patients. These results may be explained by the particular imaging instrumentation used, and therefore may not otherwise be relevant.[34]

Extranodal lymphoma detection

The stomach is the most common extranodal site of primary NHL. Two reports have evaluated the role of ^{18}F-FDG in gastric lymphoma.[35,36] The ability of ^{18}F-FDG to detect gastric lymphoma varies according to the histology. In a series of 10 patients with extranodal marginal zone B-cell lymphoma of mucosa-associated lymphoid tissue (MALT type) of the stomach, Hoffman et al. noted that ^{18}F-FDG scans were invariably negative. This apparent lack of sensitivity for detection of MALT-type lymphoma may be related to the indolent biology of this particular tumor.[36] In contrast, Rodriguez et al.[35] were able to demonstrate increased ^{18}F-FDG uptake in 86 percent of the patients with primary gastric NHL of other histologies (not MALT type). Beat et al. retrospectively reviewed 42 cases that had an initial staging evaluation with ^{18}F-FDG PET. In 34 patients (81 percent), focal, abnormal ^{18}F-FDG accumulation was noted. Although some of these patients had disease outside the stomach, 6/10 patients with gastric lymphoma were positive.[37] Care is necessary not to confuse physiologic ^{18}F-FDG uptake in the stomach wall from the pathologic uptake of gastric lymphoma.[38] The stomach contains smooth muscle, which uses glucose. Whereas the sensitivity of detecting follicular lymphoma in lymph nodes has been good, primary gastrointestinal follicular lymphoma in the duodenum failed to accumulate ^{18}F–FDG in one small report.[39] All gastrointestinal tract organs use glucose; peristalsis of smooth muscle in the gastrointestinal tract can thus be a confounder in trying to interpret ^{18}F–FDG PET images of the abdomen and pelvis.

Bone marrow involvement is present in 5–14 percent of patients with Hodgkin disease, whereas in NHL it has a higher prevalence with estimates ranging from 25 percent to 80 percent.[40] Frequently, bilateral iliac bone marrow biopsies are performed to assess involvement. The difference when single versus bilateral bone marrow biopsies are performed ranges from 10 percent to 50 percent, indicating the variability in such sampling. Some reports suggest that ^{18}F–FDG PET may be useful in evaluating tumor involvement of the bone marrow.[41,42] Unfortunately, the criteria used for 'abnormal' marrow accumulation of ^{18}F–FDG vary. They include ^{18}F–FDG uptake that is greater or equal to that in the liver and higher uptake compared with the surrounding 'normal' bone marrow. In addition, areas of moderate uptake can also be considered positive, depending on their shape, size and asymmetry. Although ^{18}F–FDG accumulates in the normal marrow, the accumulation is minimal and nearly homogeneous with relatively low SUV ($\sim$1.6) when no treatment with growth factors has occurred.[43] However, bone marrow growth factor administration, such as granulocyte-colony stimulating factor (G-CSF), often results in diffusely increased ^{18}F–FDG accumulation in the bone marrow.[44–46] Some papers addressing ^{18}F–FDG bone marrow uptake have only evaluated patients prior to such treatment, and thus do not contend with the increase ^{18}F–FDG uptake frequently seen after growth factors are administered. Moog *et al.* prospectively evaluated 78 consecutive patients with untreated NHL and Hodgkin disease where bone marrow biopsies were used as the gold standard.[42] In 73 percent of the patients the findings were concordantly negative, in 9 percent they were concordantly positive; and in 5 percent the bone marrow biopsy was positive and the ^{18}F–FDG scan was negative. In 12 percent (10 patients) where ^{18}F–FDG data were thought to be falsely positive, directed evaluation of the site confirmed bone marrow lymphoma in 8/10 patients. This paper, and that of Carr *et al.*[47] underscores the difficulties in confirming abnormalities detected by ^{18}F–FDG in the bone marrow; particularly if the results do not make a difference in the patient's management in which case marrow biopsies are usually not performed. Thus, it is hard to find studies with biopsy-confirmed proof of all false-positive or false-negative findings.[47] A metaanalysis of data from 587 patients, including the reports described above and several others with small numbers of patients, when bone marrow status was determined showed an estimated sensitivity of 51 percent and specificity of 92 percent.[48] Subgroup analysis of this series found a higher detection rate for Hodgkin disease than NHL, and a better detection rate of marrow involvement with the more aggressive lymphoma subtypes than for the

less aggressive. In some reports, at least half of ^{18}F–FDG positive sites that had initial negative biopsies were found to be positive on redirected biopsies.[15,42] Based on these inconclusive findings, patients with abnormal ^{18}F–FDG accumulation in the bone marrow that suggests lymphoma involvement which would result in alteration in patient management probably should be evaluated further with tissue biopsy methods.

Several imaging tests have been used to evaluate lymphoma involvement of the skeletal bone.[49] In contrast to plain X-rays that require at least 50 percent bone mineral loss for detection of a bone lesion, traditional ^{99m}technetium-MDP bone scintigraphy is much more sensitive,[50] and thus is generally used to evaluate bone involvement. Moog *et al.* performed a comparison of ^{18}F–FDG and conventional bone scintigraphy in 56 consecutive patients with Hodgkin disease and NHL.[51] In 60 percent of patients, the ^{18}F–FDG PET and a bone scan were concordantly negative. In 21 percent, of the patients the studies were concordantly positive, although ^{18}F–FDG PET showed 10 additional sites not seen on conventional bone scintigraphy. Three of five patients with a positive ^{18}F–FDG scan and a negative bone scan had confirmed bone lymphoma, whereas two were unconfirmed. Three of five patients with a positive bone scan and a negative ^{18}F–FDG scan were confirmed to be false positives, due to benign bone abnormalities. Two remained unconfirmed. The recent availability of PET/CT instruments is likely to improve the ability to correctly assign abnormal foci of ^{18}F–FDG uptake to the bone marrow, or bone. Whereas ^{18}F–FDG PET done without CT coregistration has little anatomic information and often makes this distinction impossible.

Changes in patient management

Given the generally higher sensitivity, specificity and accuracy of ^{18}F–FDG PET than traditional anatomic imaging tests, it is not surprising that the use of ^{18}F–FDG PET will result in changes in patient staging that often translate into changes in patient management. Such changes can result in both upstaging and downstaging of patients. When added to traditional methods for staging, ^{18}F–FDG PET resulted in changes in patient staging in 8 percent to 28 percent of patients.[15,18,51–55] Even when ^{18}F–FDG PET may not result in a stage change, changes in patient management can occur, such as modifications to the geometry of a radiation therapy plan.[55] A preliminary cost analysis review suggested that ^{18}F–FDG PET may be thus more cost effective than staging using CT[56] in the traditional lymphoma staging workup of these patients.

Monitoring treatment response

^{18}F–FDG PET is a useful test in evaluating response to treatment (Fig. 45.1); and studies suggest that it may have

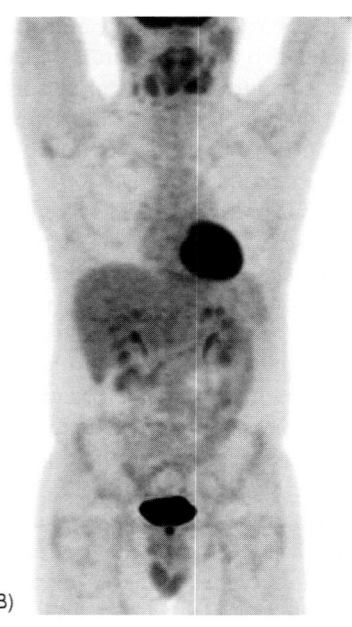

(A)   (B)

Figure 45.1   A patient who presented with non-Hodgkin lymphoma. 2-[^{18}F] fluoro-2-deoxyglucose (FDG) positron emission tomography (PET) at baseline (A) show hypermetabolic, abnormal, bilateral cervical nodes and right inguinal adenopathy. Follow-up ^{18}F-FDG PET post-therapy shows complete disappearance of the nodal disease (B).

prognostic value in distinguishing patients who will respond to chemotherapy from those responders at high risk of relapse. Several papers evaluated the ability of sequential ^{18}F-FDG scans to predict response or relapse following chemotherapy. Abnormal ^{18}F-FDG uptake after therapy is a bad prognostic sign.[57–61] Kaplan–Meier survival plots of disease-free survival from 32 patients with Hodgkin disease studied retrospectively showed a better disease-free survival of ^{18}F-FDG negative than ^{18}F-FDG positive patients.[62] Similar findings have been reported by Guay *et al.*, who found the sensitivity and specificity of ^{18}F-FDG PET to predict relapse in a group of patients with Hodgkin disease to be 79 percent and 97 percent, respectively.[17] The positive predictive value and negative predictive value were both equal to 92 percent.[17] Furthermore, the diagnostic accuracy of ^{18}F-FDG PET (92 percent) was significantly higher than that of CT (56 percent). These finding were in concurrence with those of Filmont *et al.*[62] Most patients with positive ^{18}F-FDG uptake after two or more cycles of chemotherapy never achieved a complete remission (CR) or relapsed.[57–61] In a series of 93 patients with NHL, de Wit *et al.* found that all 26 patients with post-chemotherapy positive FDG scans relapsed.[63] In contrast, of the 67 patients with no ^{18}F-FDG uptake on their follow-up scans, only 11 (16 percent) relapsed.[61] These findings were similar to those of Cremerius *et al.*[57] In a small series evaluating ^{18}F-FDG or ^{67}Ga lesion uptake after two chemotherapy regimens, the lack of uptake of either agent correlated well with remission; high uptake predicted treatment failure, and faint uptake heralded variable outcomes.[58]

Some reports have tried to correlate response or survival with the degree of reduction in ^{18}F-FDG uptake after

a few cycles of chemotherapy in patients with Hodgkin disease or NHL.[64–67] Jerusalem *et al.* showed that patients with NHL who underwent chemotherapy and had persistent ^{18}F-FDG uptake after 2 or more cycles of chemotherapy all relapsed, with four never achieving a CR.[60] Kostakoglu *et al.* also found that ^{18}F-FDG uptake after a single cycle of chemotherapy correlated well with progression-free survival in 30 patients with Hodgkin disease and NHL.[68] While ^{18}F-FDG PET results at the end of therapy also correlated positively with progression-free survival, they found that ^{18}F-FDG uptake decrease after a single cycle was a better predictor, with five of the six discordant cases that were ^{18}F-FDG positive early but negative at completion who went on to relapse.[68] In a prospective study evaluating 'early PET' after 2 cycles of chemotherapy, a negative ^{18}F-FDG PET correlated with better progression-free and overall survival; with 83 percent of ^{18}F-FDG negative achieving a CR compared to only 58 percent of those who were ^{18}F-FDG positive.[64] These findings were irrespective of whether patients were in low- or high-risk groups. In a group of Hodgkin disease and NHL patients who had failed prior chemotherapy, but were shown to be chemosensitive to second-line induction chemotherapy and who went on to receive myeloablative therapy and autologous stem cell transplant, the ^{18}F-FDG PET findings after 2 cycles correlated with disease-free survival and ultimate outcome.[69] In these patients, improved progression-free survival was noted in those with an intensity reduction in ^{18}F-FDG uptake of 90 percent. In those with >90 percent reduction, only 33 percent of patients relapsed compared to 74 percent in those with <90 percent reduction. Therefore, there may be a role for ^{18}F-FDG PET in the early assessment of response that may allow one to change therapy before a complete course is given. But because false positives can occur with ^{18}F-FDG PET, consideration of biopsy may be necessary prior to proceeding with salvage therapy.

Several published studies suggest a prognostic role for ^{18}F-FDG PET following induction chemotherapy and prior to bone marrow transplant. Both progression-free survival and overall survival is higher in patients that have negative ^{18}F-FDG scans prior to receiving stem cell transplants.[70–72] When patients had negative ^{18}F-FDG scans prior to transplant, only 3 of 25 recurred; whereas 26 of 30 with positive ^{18}F-FDG scans had progression.[72] In these studies, ^{18}F-FDG PET had a better predictive value than the conventional international prognostic index.

Several groups have shown that glucose metabolic pathway responses can occur very quickly after chemotherapy is given, including intervals as short as 1 day.[58,59,73] Yamane et al. evaluated 12 patients with NHL at baseline and 1 and 20 days after chemotherapy.[73] They showed a rapid glucose uptake response to chemotherapy with a mean change in ^{18}F-FDG SUV at baseline of 10.7 that fell to 5.8 one day after therapy, and a progressive drop at 20 days. Others have shown that 1 week after treatment, a mean drop in SUV of 60 percent occurs, with a further drop to 79 percent of baseline at 6 weeks.[59] In these patients, it was the later scan that best predicted ultimate response. These studies suggest that a baseline ^{18}F-FDG PET assessment should be performed prior to any treatment because of the rapid effect of therapy on ^{18}F-FDG uptake by lymphomas.

There is no generally agreed standard as to how to use ^{18}F-FDG uptake as a measure of treatment response. Although most investigators consider complete disappearance of uptake in all lesions as a complete response and the appearance of new lesions as progression, quantitative increases or decreases in individual tumors are difficult to interpret. Weber et al., in patients with a variety of different cancers, showed that the quantitative reproducibility of the SUV from ^{18}F-FDG PET without treatments was approximately 10 percent.[74] Preliminary criteria have been put forward by the European Organisation for Research and Treatment of Cancer (EORTC) working group[75] and still other groups have used semiquantitative visual or SUV criteria for assessing response.[70,71] Several multi-institutional studies that the National Cancer Institute has been supporting are supposed to produce more comprehensive guidelines to incorporate into clinical trials.

Proliferation indices and grade of lymphomas

There appears to be some associations between ^{18}F-FDG uptake, histological grade and a lymphoma's cellular proliferation rate. Several reports have shown that ^{18}F-FDG uptake is somewhat related to a large S fraction, aneuploidy and proliferation activity based on a mitotic count.[76] In these papers they found that the higher histologic grades had the highest ^{18}F-FDG uptake. In addition,

there was also an association between a high S-phase fraction and high ^{18}F-FDG uptake.[76,77] Similarly, other investigators have found higher SUVs in patients with high-grade lymphoma compared with those with low and intermediate grade disease.[78,79] But many investigators have found an 'overlap' in ^{18}F-FDG accumulation values between the different grades of NHL.[19,80] Hoffman et al., when evaluating extranodal marginal zone lymphomas (mucosa-associated lymphoid tissue [MALT]) versus nodal marginal zone lymphomas showed that the former were ^{18}F-FDG negative and the latter ^{18}F-FDG avid.[81] Nevertheless, this result did not correlate with Ki-67 scores; and the patient with the lymphoma having the highest Ki-67 score was ^{18}F-FDG negative. Similarly, in patients with follicular lymphoma of the duodenum that were all negative on ^{18}F-FDG PET, there was no correlation with lymphoma grade or proliferative activity.[39]

Summary

^{18}F-FDG PET is an emerging test to stage lymphoma patients at initial presentation, and to use during follow-up when checking for disease response and recurrent disease. ^{18}F-FDG PET has a higher sensitivity and specificity for detecting nodal and extranodal disease when compared to traditional anatomic radiographic tests in both Hodgkin disease and NHL patients. In addition, ^{18}F-FDG PET is useful in following the patient's response to therapy if the initial study was positive, and may even provide prognostic predictions. Abnormal ^{18}F-FDG uptake following at least 2 cycles of therapy gives a very poor prognosis. In the difficult cases where residual masses persist after treatment, ^{18}F-FDG PET results can be used to separate patients into a bad prognostic group with residual active disease and high incidence of relapse and a good prognostic group with a much lower risk of recurrence. At present ^{18}F-FDG PET is used to complement CT scanning, but in the future with the spread of PET/CT instruments, and as more exact criteria for evaluating treatment response with ^{18}F-FDG PET become available, we will probably see a greater reliance on ^{18}F-FDG PET as the primary imaging test for evaluation of lymphoma patients.

GALLIUM SCINTIGRAPHY FOR DETECTION OF MALIGNANT LYMPHOMAS

[67]Ga citrate, introduced more than three decades ago,[82] still remains a clinically useful, cost-effective radiopharmaceutical in the management of patients with certain neoplastic diseases. There have been numerous investigations into how this radionuclide localizes in both normal and malignant cells in order to improve the ^{67}Ga imaging techniques. The main point of contention has been the role of transferrin receptors (TFR), originally proposed by Larson et al.,[83] as the rate-limiting factor governing ^{67}Ga cellular

incorporation.[84] Others have suggested that alternatively, TF-independent pathways were more important in ^{67}Ga localization. More details of this transport system have emerged to explain its role in iron metabolism. In addition, with the intense interest in labeled monoclonal antibodies as tumor detection agents, there has been a variety of studies on endothelial transport of macromolecules. This is particularly relevant to ^{67}Ga localization because this radionuclide can easily shift between low molecular weight (mw) and fast endothelial transport and a high molecular weight form with slower transport. All this new information has been integrated to reconcile conflicting sets of data. We will attempt to illustrate the role a mechanistic understanding can fulfill to aid in the utilization of ^{67}Ga in imaging tests as well as for therapies, which use the non-radioactive isotopes of gallium.

Gallium as an iron analog

In the early 1970s, it was first demonstrated that ^{67}Ga in serum was bound tightly to the iron-transport protein transferrin (TF; molecular weight 80 kDa).[84] TF also stimulated ^{67}Ga incorporation into cultured tumor cells; and many iron-binding molecules, desferrioxamine (DEF), lactoferrin and ferritin, all bound ^{67}Ga with high affinity. This led to the thesis that ^{67}Ga was handled as an iron analog, i.e. similarly to iron.[85] However, animal[86] and human[87] studies showed that ^{59}Fe localized in hemopoietic tissue and red blood cells (RBCs) but not in tumor tissue. In contrast, ^{67}Ga had a great affinity for tumor tissue but low affinity for RBCs and marrow. Hoffer[85] originally suggested that this pronounced difference was related to the unique oxidation-reduction properties of each element. For iron to be eventually incorporated into hemoglobin and other essential proteins, requires iron to cycle between its two physiologically stable states, Fe^{2+} and Fe^{3+}.[88,89] In contrast, $^{67}Ga^{3+}$, under physiological conditions, cannot be reduced to Ga^{2+}; and thus cannot follow metabolic pathways where reduction is necessary.[90] More recent evidence[84,90] suggests that the aqueous solubility of the two metals is much more important in determining their biodistribution. In a physiological environment, and at trace levels (222 MBq/3 L, [~50 pM]), ^{67}Ga, as the gallate, $[Ga(OH)_4]^-$, is soluble whereas iron is not. Therefore iron, not ^{67}Ga, absolutely requires a chelate of some type, e.g. TF, for *in vivo* transport. In addition, gallium binding to TF is particularly sensitive to *in vivo* conditions, TF bicarbonate concentration and pH.[90] While these conditions in blood are optimal for ^{67}Ga binding to TF, if any are changed in the blood or at the tumor site, hydroxyl ions could effectively compete with TF for the radionuclide and form more gallate. In patients with normal TF concentration and iron saturation, the gallate concentration is only 1 percent of the total injected activity.[84] However, if, for example, the concentration of iron-free TF is lowered from $40\,\mu M$ to $5\,\mu M$ by an increase in TF-iron-saturation, this would increase ^{67}Ga-gallate concentration to 7 percent and increase the amount of the gallate that could pass out in the urine.

Transferrin receptors as ^{67}Ga transporters

Larson and coworkers, based on careful studies in both *in vivo*[91,92] and *in vitro*[83,92] model systems, extended the iron analog concept to specifically include TF receptors (TFR). They proposed that TFR is responsible for gallium incorporation in certain neoplasms. This hypothesis was consistent with what was known about the TFR system. With the normal concentration of iron complexed with TF (Fe*TF) in the blood, the TFR are saturated with Fe*TF and cells must upregulate the number of TFR to increase iron uptake.[88] TFR is regulated mainly to meet specific iron needs of DNA synthesis and specifically, ribonucleotide reductase.[93] This is a nonheme iron enzyme, which catalyzes the rate-limiting step in DNA synthesis, conversion of ribonucleotides to deoxyribonucleotides.[93] In rapidly proliferating tumor cells with a high level of DNA synthesis, upregulation of the surface TFR would also lead to increased ^{67}Ga uptake. An increased number of TFR was detected on a variety of tumor cells.[84,89]

In the early 1980s, a number of studies appeared to contradict Larson's suggestion. Fully saturating the TF with iron in the blood had no effect on tumor uptake in animal tumor models.[94,95] To explain this apparent conflict with the TFR hypothesis, Sephton[96] suggested that extravascular TF, i.e. the TF in fluid that was in direct contact with the tumor cell, was really responsible for ^{67}Ga uptake. For ^{67}Ga tumor uptake, it was necessary for the blood [67]Ga*TF to penetrate the endothelium and exchange with TF in the extravascular fluid. This is known to be a slow (15–24 h) process.[97] However, ^{67}Ga could easily equilibrate with extravascular TF, since the low-molecular-weight gallate could rapidly penetrate the endothelium. Uptake would be also dependent on kidney excretion, which would also be increased. The outflow of the gallate from the kidney would reduce the concentration gradient driving the ^{67}Ga into the tumor and other tissues. Therefore, the tumor uptake in these model studies was critically dependent on the amount of TF saturation in these experiments at the time of injection and the time necessary for saturation to return to normal. Tumor uptake could remain the same, be slightly increased or be decreased.

The importance of ^{67}Ga scintigraphy as a diagnostic tool lies in its ability to differentiate viable tumor from nonviable tumor and/or nontumor tissues and predict long-term clinical outcomes. Thus, data that link ^{67}Ga uptake to cell viability and DNA synthesis are critical. Iosilevsky *et al.*[98] showed that both ^{67}Ga and deoxyglucose uptake in a tumor model had a parallel decline after chemotherapy and radiation therapy. Also, inhibiting tumor ATP production caused a similar decline in ^{67}Ga incorporation.[99] When the response to radiotherapy was monitored in a tumor model using metabolic tracers for glucose metabolism, DNA, RNA and protein synthesis, ^{67}Ga could not detect early response to treatment.[100] However the DNA synthesis indicator and ^{67}Ga could differentiate between tumor with small foci of recurrence and nonviable tumor, whereas the glucose metabolic indicator could not. [67]Ga and Fe uptake in synchronized mouse tumor cells both peaked at G2 in the cell cycle which precedes mitosis.[101] Nonradioactive gallium interferes with DNA synthesis by the specific inhibition of ribonucleotide reductase.[102,103]

Such data from model systems provide useful insights but there are also data from patient studies that imply a correlation exists between ^{67}Ga uptake, TFR and cell proliferation. For example, Ga nitrate shows its greatest effect as a therapeutic agent in large cell lymphomas which frequently express large numbers of TFR.[104,105] In a study of 29 patients with NHL, all cases identified as 'low grade' were TFR negative; 'high grade' had up to 28 percent TFR-positive cells and 'intermediate grade' had 10–15 percent.[106] In an immunohistochemical study of tumor tissue from patients with hepatocellular carcinomas (a ^{67}Ga-avid tumor), 33 of 34 samples were TFR positive and more intensely stained than surrounding liver parenchyma.[107] In patients with NHL and Hodgkin lymphoma,[108] and with lung cancers (squamous cell and adenocarcinomas)[109] when the tumor tissue was positive for TFR, the ^{67}Ga scan was positive, and a negative ^{67}Ga scan was found when tumors were negative for TFR. Lastly, DNA content and proliferative indices of thyroid tumor tissue (adenocarcinomas, anaplastic carcinomas and malignant lymphomas) obtained from patients with ^{67}Ga-positive scans were significantly greater than the same factors obtained from patients with ^{67}Ga-negative scans.[99]

Finally, TF plays a pivotal role in delivering ^{67}Ga to normal tissue. When the available ^{67}Ga binding sites on TF were reduced in animals by a variety of techniques, the normal tissue (liver, spleen, bone marrow) uptake of ^{67}Ga was depressed, whole body excretion is enhanced and activity in bone was unaffected or increased.[84] These data closely parallel results from patient studies.[84,110] Chen et al.[111] showed that the small intestine was the major contributor (60 percent) of ^{67}Ga excretion into gastrointestinal tract, and bile made a 20 percent contribution. Increasing the TF saturation, thus reducing the unsaturated iron binding capacity, substantially reduced ^{67}Ga in the gastrointestinal tract. Excess iron is also excreted via the small intestine.[88]

The use of gallium positron–emitting radionuclides in lymphoma patient PET

The increasing availability and utilization of PET imaging for oncology has led to the exploration of additional positron-emitting radionuclides. At present ^{18}F is the predominate radionuclide in labeled FDG. [68]Ga presents an attractive alternative, particularly for utilization in the management of NHL. It is one of the few positron-emitters that are available from a radionuclide generator, which means it is available at all times similar to [99m]Tc. This is particularly relevant with the development of a newer more user-friendly ^{68}Ga generator.[112] Ga-68 has a short $T_{1/2}$ (68 min), and thus requires rapid target localization and fast blood clearance to achieve high target to background ratios. Its physical characteristics are very good; i.e. 90 percent of the decays are B$^+$ (^{18}F; 97 percent) and its maximum energy is 1.9 MeV.[113] This high energy B$^+$ allows the particle to travel farther than [18]F (0.6 MeV) but this, unfortunately, reduces intrinsic PET camera resolution. [66]Ga, another positron emitter, is not as attractive alternative.[114] It is cyclotron-produced with a $T_{1/2}$ of 9.5 h, has only 56 percent B$^+$, and has a very high maximum energy (4.2 MeV) which again reduces intrinsic resolution.

Since ^{67}Ga has been used from the early 1970s, the chemistry of gallium is well established, and this should promote ^{68}Ga radiopharmaceutical development. Ga-67 citrate is well established as a tumor viability indicator in lymphoma management; it might be anticipated that ^{68}Ga citrate could be a direct replacement. A somatostatin analogue labeled with ^{68}Ga has already been used to provide high resolution (lesion size 7–8 mm) PET images for patients with neuroendocrine tumors.[115] However, in vitro data from Aloj et al.[116] implied that ^{68}Ga localizes too slowly (>6 h) to be useful for lymphoma patient lesion detection. Therefore, the unadorned radionuclide may not be accepted in routine patient management imaging as is ^{18}F-FDG.[117] But a ^{68}Ga-labeled radiopharmaceutical, once developed, might be useful detecting lesions in patients with 'low grade' NHL, since there is a reported lower sensitivity of FDG in this subset of patients.[117] The gallium-based PET radiopharmaceutical could also give information about a second metabolic pathway in lymphoma cells, namely iron requirements.

BONE SCINTIGRAPHY

Bone scintigraphy with ^{99m}Tc-MDP (methylene diphosphonate) is the best and least expensive method for performing a skeletal survey to detect bone involvement by neoplasms. Bone scintigraphy is also readily repeated at appropriate intervals to assess the effect of therapeutic regimens, especially in the first few years following diagnosis. Bone abnormalities detected by scintigraphy must sometimes be further evaluated with a CT, because although scintigraphy is a very sensitive procedure it does not always provide specificity in determining the cause of altered skeletal radionuclide uptake. Not all abnormal sites in the scintigram will necessarily be caused by lymphoma; degenerative disease, trauma, benign bone lesions, etc. can all give false-positive indications of skeletal lymphoma. Comparison of directed CTs and ^{18}F FDG-PET or ^{67}Ga citrate scintigrams can often be helpful in determining the exact etiology of abnormal sites. Patterns of more diffusely increased radionuclide uptake in the long bones, and particularly increased uptake in the region of the metaphyses, can indicate bone marrow involvement by lymphoma and/or the effects of bone-marrow stimulation therapy.

Sites of previous marrow biopsy will frequently show increased ^{99m}Tc-MDP activity for variable periods after the biopsy procedures and should not be misinterpreted. Those patients receiving treatment regimens which include steroids are sometimes at increased risk for avascular necrosis, which will be apparent in a bone scintigram; but the pattern of altered bone uptake will change with evolution of the bone necrosis. Finally, areas of bone included in radiation therapy treatments can show increased or decreased uptake of skeletal-seeking radiopharmaceuticals – both ^{99m}Tc-MDP and ^{67}Ga – so that knowledge of the skeletal areas which received irradiation is essential for accurate interpretation of subsequent bone scintigrams.[118]

RADIOLABELED ANTIBODIES FOR TARGETING LYMPHOMA

Since the discovery of a method to generate monoclonal antibodies (MAbs) by Kohler and Milstein,[119] a large number of MAbs have been generated recognizing a variety of tumor-associated antigens. These, in turn, have led to numerous clinical trials which have resulted in approval of several MAbs for clinical applications in benign diseases, solid tumors and hematological malignancies. Following the first successful reports of the use of a MAb for therapy of a hematologic malignancy,[120,121] a large number of MAbs have been evaluated as therapeutic and diagnostic agents in lymphoma, and two have been approved in the USA by the Food and Drug Administration (FDA) for radioimmunotherapy (RIT) applications (ibritumomab tiuxetan, tositumomab). In this chapter we will focus on radiolabeled MAbs utilized for imaging (typically for dosimetry estimates), and only briefly mention these for therapy of lymphoma.

Target antigens

Numerous tumor-associated antigens have been described on lymphoma and leukemia cells. These antigens are complex structures, many of whose functions have not been fully elucidated. Clinical trials in B cell malignancies have targeted antibody binding to B cell antigens, including idiotypes, CD20, CD21, CD22, CD37 and human leukocyte antigen (HLA) Dr.[120,122–125] In T cell malignancies, antigens targeted include CD5 and CD25.[126–130] Hodgkin-associated antigens, such as ferritin and CD30, have also been probed.[131–133] While most antigens are not tumor-specific, their altered presence in various lymphomas may allow targeting. Various clinical trials testing both Hodgkin lymphoma and

Table 45.1 Antigens targeted with radiolabeled monoclonal antibodies in patients with lymphomas

Target antigen	Antibody	Radionuclide	References
CD 37	MB-1	I-131	134–136
HLA-Dr	Lym-1	I-123/I-131/Cu-67	137–144
CD19	Anti-CD19	Tc-99m	145
CD20	Anti-B1/ 1F5/2B8	I-131/In-111/Y-90	135,146–158
CD21	OKB-7	I-131	159,160
CD22	LL2	I-131/Tc-99m/Y-90	161–165
CD5	T101	In-111.Y-90/I-131	166–169
CD25	Anti-Tac	In-111/Y-90	170–172
CD30	HRS-1/HRS-3/ Ber-H2/Ki-4	I-131	133, 173–175

NHL have been performed and selected references with the antigen targeted are shown in Table 45.1.

Radiolabeling

The major criteria for selecting a radionuclide for labeling antibodies used for imaging or therapy are:

- acceptable physical properties
- the labeling procedure should preserve the immunoreactivity of the antibody
- the radionuclide should be firmly bound chemically to the antibody.

When MAbs are used for imaging purposes, it is preferable to have only γ emissions that can be detected with a γ camera or PET instruments, and limit the radiation dose to normal tissue. For therapeutic purposes, β emitters have been the reagents of choice and a number are available that have various β particle path lengths for use in different situations.[176] In some cases, the radionuclide may have both γ and β emissions, allowing both imaging and therapy. Examples include ^{131}I or ^{177}Lu. Other isotopes that emit α particles such as Bi-213 or Auger electron emitters such as ^{111}In and ^{125}I have also been considered for therapy.

A variety of methods have been used to radiolabel antibodies for tumor imaging.[177–181] These methods can be grossly divided into direct labeling, where the radionuclide is directly attached to the antibody, typically via one of its amino acids,[177] or an indirect labeling method that typically uses a chelating agent to bind radiometals such as ^{111}In or ^{90}Y.[180,181] ^{131}I is among the most frequently used radionuclides for imaging and therapy because of its availability, well-established and simple labeling procedures (Chloramine T and Iodogen), and low cost. Because of problems frequently encountered with dehalogenation and release of radionuclide from the tumor site, other iodination methods which are thought to produce a more stable chemical bond have been used.[182–184] [111]In is a cyclotron-produced radiometal that has been used extensively for radiolabeling antibodies. Its γ ray emissions, although somewhat higher than the ideal, are superior to those of ^{131}I, and can be detected efficiently by existing planar and SPECT γ cameras.

One of the main goals of radiolabeled MoAb imaging studies is to determine the pharmacokinetics and optimize the delivery methodology of antibody to tumor so that therapeutic trials may be undertaken. For this reason, investigators have pursued the concept of a 'matched-pair' of radionuclides, where one radionuclide with good characteristics for imaging is used for detection and pharmacokinetic analysis; then either the same radionuclide (at a higher dose) or a second radionuclide with similar chemistry is substituted for therapeutic purposes. This is exemplified best in studies where ^{131}I at low doses is used for diagnostic studies (or ^{123}I could be used) and large doses of ^{131}I are used for therapy. Other matched pairs are ^{111}In and ^{90}Y, and ^{99m}Tc and [186]Re or [189]Re.

Human applications of radiolabeled MAbs

The majority of the studies with radiolabeled MAbs in lymphomas have been performed as a part of therapeutic trials which required imaging for dosimetry calculations. Only two antibodies to date have been approved for radioimmunotherapy: Bexxar (^{131}I-tositumomab) and Zevalin (^{111}In/^{90}Y ibritumomab). Both are directed against the CD20 antigen present in lymphomas. CD20 was first characterized as a B cell associated antigen and termed B1.[185,186] Its desirable characteristics as a target include that it is present on the cell surface of most of B cell associated malignancies, and its lack of internalization. It is not expressed in B lymphoid stem cells but does appear relative early in B cell development, and is present on normal B cells and >90 percent of B cell lymphomas. While its function is not completely understood, it is thought to be involved in calcium channels and appears to be important in B cell activation, regulation, proliferation and differentiation. When CD20 is targeted with MABs such as tositumomab, antitumor effects are observed, possibly due to induction of apoptosis, complement dependent cytotoxicity, and antibody-dependent cytotoxicity.[185,187]

Most of the studies using MAbs in lymphoma are thus now aimed at using imaging for the purpose of dosimetry calculations or as a surrogate of dosimetry prior to a therapeutic administration. With the availability of positron-emitting radionuclides that result in better image quality than single photon emitters such as ^{99m}Tc, ^{111}In and ^{131}I, it is possible that we may be able to take advantage of the specificity of targeting of intact and genetically engineered antibodies for tumor imaging. Nonetheless given that ^{18}F-FDG imaging is readily available, has high sensitivity, provides quantitative results, and does not depend on

specific surface antigens, it seems likely that future research will continue to mainly focus on using diagnostic doses of radiolabeled antibodies as a prelude to therapy.

^{99m}Tc–SESTAMIBI SCINTIGRAPHY APPLICABLE TO LYMPHOMA LOCALIZATIONS

[99m]Tc-sestamibi (hexakis(2-methoxyisobutylisonitrile) is a myocardial perfusion agent which has also been used for imaging various tumors. This cationic, lipophilic compound accumulates passively in cells, driven by negative membrane potentials generated across plasma and mitochondrial membranes.[188–190] Mechanisms of efflux from cells for this compound are not yet fully understood, but one route appears to involve the energy-dependent, multidrug-resistance, membrane proteins for which ^{99m}Tc-sestamibi is a substrate.[191]

In vitro, studies have demonstrated increased ^{99m}Tc-sestamibi uptake in carcinoma cells compared to nontransformed cell lines.[192] This is probably due to the higher negative mitochondria membrane potentials maintained by malignant cells.[193–195] *In vivo*, ^{99m}Tc-sestamibi has also been used to image both primary and metastatic tumors.[170,196–198] Visualization of tumors of the lung,[170,199] breast,[199,200] thyroid,[173,201] kidneys,[173] bone,[197,198] and Burkitt lymphoma[173] have been reported.

Several case reports of ^{99m}Tc-sestamibi tumor visualization in patients with NHL have appeared in the literature. These include a primary cardiac lymphoma[202] and a primary thyroid lymphoma.[203] Lastly, in a report by Aktolun *et al.*,[199] sestamibi was successful in imaging NHL in lymph nodes in one of two patients.

Given its ideal imaging characteristics, dosimetry, ease of preparation, and the ability to image soon after injection, ^{99m}Tc-sestamibi may become a useful agent in the detection and monitoring of the multidrug resistance proteins; however, further studies are needed to define its sensitivity and specificity in these applications.

EVALUATION OF MYOCARDIAL FUNCTION DURING AND AFTER CHEMOTHERAPY

Several chemotherapeutic agents used to treat human solid tumors, leukemias and some lymphomas cause or predispose to cardiotoxicity. The best known are anthracyclines that can cause dose-related myocardial damage either acutely, subacutely or chronically, the latter being a function of the peak plasma concentration and cumulative dose received.[204,205] Cardiotoxicity may often be the single factor limiting treatment for patients who might otherwise benefit from continuation of chemotherapy. There is also concern that chemotherapy-induced cardiomyopathy leads to a reduction in lifespan following otherwise successful cancer treatment. The ability to predict and prevent chemotherapy-induced myocardial toxicity could enhance effective use of these agents in the treatment of tumors.

It is now apparent that there is a continuous relationship between anthracycline dose and incident heart failure.[206] Although early data suggested that the maximum tolerated dose of anthracycline was 550 mg/m^2;[206] recent analyses suggest that 26 percent of patients given this dose would experience heart failure during a 4-year follow-up.[207] Histopathologic evidence of myocardial injury can occur with as little as 60 mg/m^2;[208,209] and so, current standard breast cancer regimens have been further restricted to 240 mg/m^2. Other coadministered agents such as paclitaxel and trastuzumab may enhance cardiac injury,[204] and the myocardium may be more vulnerable to injury if there is prior anthracycline use or mediastinal radiation therapy. Dexrazoxane may have a role in ameliorating myocardial damage caused by chemotherapy.[210,211]

The incidence and rate of chronic decline in cardiac function is unknown but early asymptomatic myocardial insult can lead to activation of a cascade of ventricular remodeling pathways, ultimately progresses to left ventricular dilatation and contractile dysfunction,[212,213] sometimes many years after initial treatment.[214–216] The prognosis for chemotherapy-induced cardiomyopathy is worse than for other cardiomyopathies.[217]

It is very important to have a sensitive, reliable and reproducible technique to provide serial assessments of cardiac function. Available methods provide equivalent results and include radionuclide angiography, echocardiography and cardiac MRI.[218,219] Echocardiographic assessment of ejection fraction is dependent on assumptions regarding cardiac geometry and is time consuming. Although cardiac MRI provides excellent imaging quality, it is not yet routinely widely available, and it is not suitable for some patients. The method of cardiac assessment is dependent on local resources but radionuclide angiography is still the most widely available method.

The most widely used radionuclide for multiple-gated cardiac blood pool (MUGA) scintigraphy is ^{99m}Tc. To allow acquisition of images, it is essential that the radionuclide remains in the intravascular space. This is achieved by *in vivo* labeling of autologous red blood cells. An aliquot of the patient's own erythrocytes is prelabeled by direct intravenous injection of a reducing agent, stannous pyrophosphate. After a 15–20 minute incubation, an appropriate dose of ^{99m}Tc pertechnetate is injected and binds to the stannous pyrophosphate which is already bound to erythrocytes. This method provides an excellent radionuclide intravascular signal which does not leak into the interstitial space for several hours. There are other *in vitro* labeling methods, but the labeling efficiency for each method is equivalent at about 90 percent.[220–222] The unbound portion of the ^{99m}Tc dose clears rapidly from the body via renal excretion, thus providing a good image of the intravascular blood pool. Because ^{99m}Tc has a physical half-life of only 6 hours, a patient's radiation dose is within an acceptable range, permitting repeated studies over the lifetime of the patients without discernible harm.

The MUGA study is performed with a single head γ camera placed in one or more positions, but typically in a left anterior oblique view. The camera must have sufficient sensitivity and resolution to provide optimal imaging of quantitative images of the cardiac blood pool during the cardiac cycle. The electrocardiogram is used as a signal occurring at a fixed time in relation to the mechanical activity of the heart to trigger or gate the scintillation counts, thus permitting repetitive sampling of each specific phase of the cardiac cycle from each of the many cycles until a statistically significant scintillation count density is recorded. Typically there should be 150–200 K counts per movie frame to allow accurate visual assessment and statistically stable quantitative calculations. The study can usually be completed in 10–15 minutes. Most cameras divide the collected images into a fixed number of frames (typically 24–32) from which the ejection fraction is calculated. These data are analyzed to produce a quantitative evaluation of both global and regional ventricular function, by measuring the changes in either the activity or volume of the ventricular chamber from systole to diastole. An attempt to further increase the sensitivity of this test by adding an exercise-induced stress to the work of the left ventricle has not been widely accepted; probably because of the resultant decrease in the specificity of the test, even though the sensitivity was improved.

Usually a baseline MUGA study is obtained prior to initial chemotherapy, followed by serial studies in the intervals between treatments. As the toxic effects of chemotherapeutic agents have been increasingly understood, even small doses of anthracycline can be associated with subclinical toxicity or idiosyncratic reactions. Significant decreases in left ventricular ejection fraction (LVEF) are sensitive indicators of impending congestive heart failure. In general, cardiotoxicity is mild if the ejection fraction decreases by 10 percent, without signs of heart failure, and moderate if the decline is 15 percent, still without signs of heart failure. In our laboratory, a fall in LVEF to <45 percent is predictive of subsequent clinical heart failure, and severe cardiotoxicity is observed with signs of heart failure if the LVEF is less than 30 percent. These absolute values must be transposed for the normal LVEF range as determined by the technique used in one's own reference nuclear cardiology laboratory. For patients with a baseline decreased LVEF, the risk/benefit ratio of anthracycline use should be weighed carefully.

Radionuclide angiography provides a reliable serial assessment of myocardial function in patients with malignancies undergoing chemotherapy with potentially cardiotoxic agents. The technique is well accepted, easy to perform and time-efficient. Within the next few years, it is likely that cardiac MRI or two- or three-dimensional echocardiography will become more widely available for routine serial assessment of cardiac function.

KEY POINTS

- PET, using ^{18}F-FDG, is the current standard test.
- Gallium scintigraphy for detection of malignant lymphomas has declined in use.
- Bone scintigraphy can be helpful in discriminating skeletal metastases.
- Radiolabeled antibodies for targeting lymphoma are in use mainly for therapy.
- ^{99m}Tc-sestamibi scintigraphy is applicable to lymphoma localizations in an experimental approach.
- Evaluation of myocardial function during and after chemotherapy is important in order to detect and to reduce the risk of treatment-induced cardiotoxicity.

REFERENCES

● = Key primary paper

◆ = Major review article

●1. Chung JH, Cho KJ, Lee SS et al. Overexpression of Glut1 in lymphoid follicles correlates with false-positive F-FDG PET results in lung cancer staging. J Nucl Med 2004; 45: 999–1003.

●2. Strauss LG. Fluorine-18 deoxyglucose and false-positive results: a major problem in the diagnostics of oncological patients. Eur J Nucl Med 1996; 23: 1409–15.

●3. Hamberg LM, Hunter GJ, Alpert NM et al. The dose uptake ratio as an index of glucose metabolism: useful parameter or oversimplification? J Nucl Med 1994; 35: 1308–12.

●4. Kinahan PE, Townsend DW, Beyer T, Sashin D. Attenuation correction for a combined 3D PET/CT scanner. Med Phys 1998; 25: 2046–53.

◆5. Hoekstra CJ, Paglianiti I, Hoekstra OS et al. Monitoring response to therapy in cancer using [F-18]-2-fluouo-2-deoxy-D-glucose and positron emission tomography: an overview of different analytical methods. Eur J Nucl Med 2000; 27: 731–43.

●6. Huang SC. Anatomy of SUV. Nucl Med Biol 2000; 27: 643–6.

◆7. Carbone PP, Kaplan HS, Musshoff K et al. Report of the committee on Hodgkin's disease staging classification. Cancer Research 1971; 31: 1860–1.

●8. Shipp MA. Prognostic factors in aggressive non-Hodgkins-lymphoma – who has high-risk disease. Blood 1994; 83: 1165–73.

●9. Castellino RA, Hoppe RT, Blank N et al. Computed-tomography, lymphography, and staging laparotomy – correlations in initial staging of Hodgkin disease. AJR Am J Roentgenol 1984; 143: 37–41.

◆10. Gambhir SS, Czernin J, Schwimmer J et al. A tabulated summary of the FDG PET literature. J Nucl Med 2001; 42: s1–93.

●11. Delbeke D. Oncological applications of FDG PET imaging. J Nucl Med 1999; 40: 1706–15.

●12. Tatsumi M, Kitayama H, Sugahara H et al. Whole-body hybrid PET with F-18-FDG in the staging of non-Hodgkin's lymphoma. J Nucl Med 2001; 42: 601–8.

●13. Cremerius U, Fabry U, Kroll U et al. [Clinical value of FDG PET for therapy monitoring of malignant lymphoma – results of a retrospective study in 72 patients]. Nuklearmedizin 1999; 38: 24–30.

●14. Stumpe KD, Urbinelli M, Steinert HC et al. Whole-body positron emission tomography using fluorodeoxyglucose for staging of lymphoma: effectiveness and comparison with computed tomography. Eur J Nucl Med 1998; 25: 721–8.

●15. Buchmann I, Reinhardt M, Elsner K et al. 2-(Fluorine-18)fluoro-2-deoxy-D-glucose positron emission tomography in the detection and staging of malignant lymphoma – a bicenter trial. Cancer 2001; 91: 889–99.

●16. Mikosch P, Gallowitsch HJ, Zinke-Cerwenka W et al. Accuracy of whole-body F-18-FDP-PET for restaging malignant lymphoma. Acta Medica Austriaca 2003; 30: 41–7.

◆17. Guay C, Lepine M, Verreault J, Benard F. Prognostic value of PET using F-18-FDG in Hodgkin's disease for posttreatment evaluation. J Nucl Med 2003; 44: 1225–31.

●18. Jerusalem G, Beguin Y, Fassotte MF et al. Whole-body positron emission tomography using F-18-fluorodeoxyglucose compared to standard procedures for staging patients with Hodgkin's disease. Haematologica 2001; 86: 266–73.

◆19. Moog F, Bangerter M, Diederichs CG et al. Lymphoma: role of whole-body 2-deoxy-2-[F-18]fluoro-D-glucose (FDG) PET in nodal staging. Radiology 1997; 203: 795–800.

◆20. Paul R. Comparison of fluorine-18-2-fluorodeoxyglucose and gallium-67 citrate imaging for detection of lymphoma. J Nucl Med 1987; 28: 288–92.

●21. Kostakoglu L, Leonard JP, Kuji I et al. Comparison of fluorine-18 fluorodeoxyglucose positron emission tomography and Ga-67 scintigraphy in evaluation of lymphoma. Cancer 2002; 94: 879–88.

●22. Bar-Shalom R, Yefremov N, Haim N et al. Camera-based FDG PET and Ga-67 SPECT in evaluation of lymphoma: comparative study. Radiology 2003; 227: 353–60.

●23. Shen YY, Kao A, Yen RF. Comparison of 18F-fluoro-2-deoxyglucose positron emission tomography and gallium-67 citrate scintigraphy for detecting malignant lymphoma. Oncol Rep 2002; 9: 321–5.

●24. Rini JN, Nunez R, Nichols K et al. Coincidence-detection FDG-PET versus gallium in children and young adults with newly diagnosed Hodgkin's disease. Pediatr Radiol 2005; 35: 169–78.

◆25. Lin P, Chu J, Kneebone A et al. Direct comparison of F-18-fluorodeoxyglucose coincidence gamma camera tomography with gallium scanning for the staging of lymphoma. Intern Med J 2005; 35: 91–6.

●26. Wirth A, Seymour JF, Hicks RJ et al. Fluorine-18 fluorodeoxyglucose positron emission tomography, gallium-67 scintigraphy, and conventional staging for Hodgkin's disease and non-Hodgkin's lymphoma. *Am J Med* 2002; **112**: 262–8.

◆27. Canellos GP. Residual mass in lymphoma may not be residual disease. *J Clin Oncol* 1988; **6**: 931–3.

◆28. Surbone A, Longo DL, Devita VT *et al.* Residual abdominal masses in aggressive non-Hodgkins lymphoma after combination chemotherapy – significance and management. *J Clin Oncol* 1988; **6**: 1832–7.

●29. Hill M, Cunningham D, Macvicar D *et al.* Role of magnetic-resonance-imaging in predicting relapse in residual masses after treatment of lymphoma. *J Clin Oncol* 1993; **11**: 2273–8.

●30. Jerusalem G, Beguin Y, Fassotte MF *et al.* Whole-body positron emission tomography using 18F-fluorodeoxy-glucose for posttreatment evaluation in Hodgkin's disease and non-Hodgkin's lymphoma has higher diagnostic and prognostic value than classical computed tomography scan imaging. *Blood* 1999; **94**: 429–33.

●31. Mikhaeel NG, Timothy AR, O'Doherty MJ *et al.* 18-FDG-PET as a prognostic indicator in the treatment of aggressive non-Hodgkin's lymphoma-comparison with CT. *Leuk Lymphoma* 2000; **39**: 543–53.

◆32. Zinzani PL, Magagnoli M, Chierichetti F *et al.* The role of positron emission tomography (PET) in the management of lymphoma patients [see comments]. *Ann Oncol* 1999; **10**: 1181–4.

◆33. de Wit M, Bumann D, Beyer W *et al.* Whole-body positron emission tomography (PET) for diagnosis of residual mass in patients with lymphoma. *Ann Oncol* 1997; **8**(Suppl 1): 57–60.

●34. Maisey NR, Hill ME, Webb A *et al.* Are fluorodeoxyglucose positron emission tomography and magnetic resonance imaging useful in the prediction of relapse in lymphoma residual masses? *Eur J Cancer* 2000; **36**: 200–6.

●35. Rodriguez M, Ahlstrom H, Sundin A *et al.* [18F] FDG PET in gastric non-Hodgkin's lymphoma. *Acta Oncol* 1997; **36**: 577–84.

●36. Hoffmann M, Kletter K, Diemling M *et al.* Positron emission tomography with fluorine-18-2-fluoro-2-deoxy-D-glucose (F18-FDG) does not visualize extranodal B-cell lymphoma of the mucosa-associated lymphoid tissue (MALT)-type. *Ann Oncol* 1999; **10**: 1185–9.

●37. Beat KP, Yeung HW, Yahalom J. FDG-PET scanning for detection and staging of extranodal marginal zone lymphomas of the MALT type: a report of 42 cases. *Ann Oncol* 2005; **16**: 473–80.

●38. Koga H, Sasaki M, Kuwabara Y *et al.* An analysis of the physiological FDG uptake pattern in the stomach. *Ann Nucl Med* 2003; **17**: 733–8.

●39. Hoffmann M, Chott A, Puspok A *et al.* 18F-fluorodeoxyglucose positron emission tomography (18F-FDG-PET) does not visualize follicular lymphoma of the duodenum. *Ann Hematol* 2004; **83**: 276–8.

●40. McKenna RW, Hernandez JA. Bone-marrow in malignant-lymphoma. *Hematol Oncol Clin North Am* 1988; **2**: 617–35.

●41. Jerusalem G, Warland V, Najjar F *et al.* Whole-body 18F-FDG PET for the evaluation of patients with Hodgkin's disease and non-Hodgkin's lymphoma. *Nucl Med Commun* 1999; **20**: 13–20.

●42. Moog F, Bangerter M, Kotzerke J *et al.* 18-F-fluorodeoxyglucose-positron emission tomography as a new approach to detect lymphomatous bone marrow. *J Clin Oncol* 1998; **16**: 603–9.

●43. Dobert N, Menzel C, Hamscho N *et al.* Atypical thoracic and supraclavicular FDG-uptake in patients with Hodgkin's and non-Hodgkin's lymphoma. *Q J Nucl Med Mol Imaging* 2004; **48**: 33–8.

●44. Yao WJ, Hoh CK, Hawkins RA *et al.* Bone-marrow glucose metabolic response to GMCSF by quantitative FDG pet imaging. *J Nucl Med* 1994; **35**: 8.

◆45. Wahl RL, Fisher SJ. FDG uptake into normal bone-marrow is markedly increased by recombinant colony-stimulating factors G-CSF and GM-CSF. *J Nucl Med* 1993; **34**: 245.

●46. Bautovich G, Angelides S, Lee FT *et al.* Detection of deep venous thrombi and pulmonary embolus with technetium-99m-DD-3B6/22 anti-fibrin monoclonal antibody Fab' fragment [see comments]. *J Nucl Med* 1994; **35**: 195–202.

●47. Carr R, Barrington SF, Madan B *et al.* Detection of lymphoma in bone marrow by whole-body positron emission tomography. *Blood* 1998; **91**: 3340–6.

◆48. Pakos EE, Fotopoulos AD, Ioannidis JPA. F-18-FDG PET for evaluation of bone marrow infiltration in staging of lymphoma: a meta-analysis. *J Nucl Med* 2005; **46**: 958–63.

●49. Ferrant A, Rodhain J, Michaux JL *et al.* Detection of skeletal involvement in Hodgkin's disease: a comparison of radiography, bone scanning, and bone marrow biopsy in 38 patients. *Cancer* 1975; **35**: 1346–53.

●50. Schechter JP, Jones SE, Woolfenden JM *et al.* Bone scanning in lymphoma. *Cancer* 1976; **38**: 1142–8.

◆51. Moog F, Bangerter M, Diederichs CG *et al.* Extranodal malignant lymphoma: detection with FDG PET versus CT. *Radiology* 1998; **206**: 475–81.

●52. Hueltenschmidt B, Sautter ML, Lang O *et al.* Whole body positron emission tomography in the treatment of Hodgkin disease. *Cancer* 2001; **91**: 302–10.

●53. Partridge S, Timothy A, O'Doherty MJ *et al.* 2-Fluorine-18-fluoro-2-deoxy-D glucose positron emission tomography in the pretreatment staging of Hodgkin's disease: Influence on patient management in a single institution. *Ann Oncol* 2000; **11**: 1273–9.

◆54. Montravers F, McNamara D, Landman-Parker J *et al.* F-18 FDG in childhood lymphoma: clinical utility and impact on management. *Eur J Nucl Med Mol Imaging* 2002; **29**: 1155–65.

●55. Foo SS, Mitchell PL, Berlangieri SU *et al.* Positron emission tomography scanning in the assessment of patients with lymphoma. *Intern Med J* 2004; **34**: 388–97.

●56. Klose T, Leidl R, Buchmann I *et al.* Primary staging of lymphomas: cost-effectiveness of FDG-PET versus computed tomography. *Eur J Nucl Med* 2000; **27**: 1457–64.

●57. Cremerius U, Fabry U, Neuerburg J *et al.* Positron emission tomography with 18F-FDG to detect residual disease after therapy for malignant lymphoma. *Nucl Med Commun* 1998; **19**: 1055–63.

●58. Hoekstra OS, van Lingen A, Ossenkoppele GJ *et al.* Early response monitoring in malignant lymphoma using fluorine-18 fluorodeoxyglucose single-photon emission tomography. *Eur J Nucl Med* 1993; **20**: 1214–17.

●59. Romer W, Hanauske AR, Ziegler S *et al.* Positron emission tomography in non-Hodgkin's lymphoma: assessment of chemotherapy with fluorodeoxyglucose. *Blood* 1998; **91**: 4464–71.

◆60. Jerusalem G, Beguin Y, Fassotte MF *et al.* Persistent tumor F-18-FDG uptake after a few cycles of polychemotherapy is predictive of treatment failure in non-Hodgkin's lymphoma. *Haematologica* 2000; **85**: 613–18.

●61. Spaepen K, Stroobants S, Dupont P *et al.* Prognostic value of positron emission tomography (PET) with fluorine-18 fluorodeoxyglucose ([F-18]FDG) after first-line chemotherapy in non-Hodgkin's lymphoma: is [F-18]FDG-PET a valid alternative to conventional diagnostic methods? *J Clin Oncol* 2001; **19**: 414–19.

●62. Filmont JE, Yap CS, Ko F *et al.* Conventional imaging and 2-deoxy-2 F-18 fluoro-D-glucose positron emission tomography for predicting the clinical outcome of patients with previously treated Hodgkin's disease. *Mol Imaging Biol* 2004; **6**: 47–54.

●63. de Wit M, Bohuslavizki KH, Buchert R *et al.* FDG-PET following treatment as valid predictor for disease-free survival in Hodgkin's lymphoma. *Ann Oncol* 2001; **12**: 29–37.

◆64. Haioun C, Itti E, Rahmouni A *et al.* F-18 fluoro-2-deoxy-D-glucose positron emission tomography (FDG-PET) in aggressive lymphoma: an early prognostic tool for predicting patient outcome. *Blood* 2005; **106**: 1376–81.

●65. Hutchings M, Loft A, Hansen M *et al.* FDG-PET after two cycles of chemotherapy predicts treatment failure and progression-free survival in Hodgkin lymphoma. *Blood* 2006; **107**: 52–9.

●66. Hutchings M, Mikhaeel NG, Fields PA *et al.* Prognostic value of interim FDG-PET after two or three cycles of chemotherapy in Hodgkin lymphoma. *Ann Oncol* 2005; **16**: 1160–8.

●67. Mikhaeel NG, Hutchings M, Fields PA *et al.* FDG-PET after two to three cycles of chemotherapy predicts progression-free and overall survival in high-grade non-Hodgkin lymphoma. *Ann Oncol* 2005; **16**: 1514–23.

●68. Kostakoglu L, Coleman M, Leonard JP *et al.* PET predicts prognosis after 1 cycle of chemotherapy in aggressive lymphoma and Hodgkin's disease. *J Nucl Med* 2002; **43**: 1018–27.

◆69. Schot B, van Imhoff G, Pruim J *et al.* Predictive value of early F-18-fluoro-deoxyglucose positron emission tomography in chemosensitive relapsed lymphoma. *Br J Haematol* 2003; **123**: 282–7.

●70. Becherer A, Mitterbauer M, Jaeger U *et al.* Positron emission tomography with F-18 2-fluoro-D-2-deoxyglucose (FDG-PET) predicts relapse of malignant lymphoma after high-dose therapy with stem cell transplantation. *Leukemia* 2002; **16**: 260–7.

●71. Cremerius U, Fabry U, Wildberger JE *et al.* Non-Hodgkin's lymphoma – pre-transplant positron emission tomography (PET) using fluorine-18-fluoro-deoxyglucose (FDG) predicts outcome in patients treated with high-dose chemotherapy and autologous stem cell transplantation for non-Hodgkin's lymphoma. *Bone Marrow Transplant* 2002; **30**: 103–11.

●72. Spaepen K, Stroobants S, Dupont P *et al.* Prognostic value of pretransplantation positron emission tomography using fluorine 18-fluorodeoxyglucose in patients with aggressive lymphoma treated with high-dose chemotherapy and stem cell transplantation. *Blood* 2003; **102**: 53–9.

●73. Yamane T, Daimaru S, Ito S *et al.* Decreased F-18-FDG uptake 1 day after initiation of chemotherapy for malignant lymphomas. *J Nucl Med* 2004; **45**: 1838–42.

◆74. Weber WA, Ziegler SI, Thodtmann R *et al.* Reproducibility of metabolic measurements in malignant tumors using FDG PET. *J Nucl Med* 1999; **40**: 1771–7.

◆75. Young H, Baum R, Cremerius U *et al.* Measurement of clinical and subclinical tumour response using F-18-fluorodeoxyglucose and positron emission tomography: review and 1999 EORTC recommendations. *Eur J Cancer* 1999; **35**: 1773–82.

●76. Lapela M, Leskinen S, Minn HR *et al.* Increased glucose metabolism in untreated non-Hodgkin's lymphoma: a study with positron emission tomography and fluorine-18-fluorodeoxyglucose. *Blood* 1995; **86**: 3522–7.

●77. Okada J, Oonishi H, Yoshikawa K *et al.* FDG-PET for predicting the prognosis of malignant lymphoma. *Ann Nucl Med* 1994; **8**: 187–91.

●78. Rodriguez M, Rehn S, Ahlstrom H *et al.* Predicting malignancy grade with PET in non-Hodgkin's lymphoma. *J Nucl Med* 1995; **36**: 1790–6.

●79. Leskinenkallio S, Ruotsalainen U, Nagren K *et al.* Uptake of carbon-11-methionine and fluorodeoxyglucose in non-Hodgkins-lymphoma – a PET study. *J Nucl Med* 1991; **32**: 1211–18.

●80. Newman JS, Francis IR, Kaminski MS, Wahl RL. Imaging of lymphoma with PET with 2-[F-18]-fluoro-2-deoxy-D-glucose: correlation with CT. *Radiology* 1994; **190**: 111–16.

◆81. Hoffmann M, Kletter K, Becherer A *et al.* F-18-fluorode-oxyglucose positron emission tomography (F-18-FDG-PET) for staging and follow-up of marginal zone B-cell lymphoma. *Oncology* 2003; **64**: 336–40.

◆82. Edwards CL, Hayes RL. Tumor scanning with 67Ga citrate. *J Nucl Med* 1969; **10**: 103–5.

●83. Larson SM, Rasey JS, Allen DR *et al.* Common pathway for tumor cell uptake of gallium-67 and iron-59 via a transferrin receptor. *J Natl Cancer Inst* 1980; **64**: 41–53.

●84. Weiner RE. The mechanism of 67Ga localization in malignant disease. *Nucl Med Biol* 1996; **23**: 745–51.

●85. Hoffer P. Gallium: mechanisms. *J Nucl Med* 1980; **21**: 282–5.

●86. Sephton RG, Hodgson GS, De Abrew S, Harris AW. Ga-67 and Fe-59 distributions in mice. *J Nucl Med* 1978; **19**: 930–5.

●87. Logan KJ, Ng PK, Turner CJ *et al*. Comparative pharmacokinetics of 67 Ga and 59 Fe in humans. *Int J Nucl Med Biol* 1981; **8**: 271–6.

●88. Crichton RR, Ward RJ. Iron metabolism – new perspectives in view. *Biochemistry* 1992; **31**: 11255–64.

●89. Gomme PT, McCann KB, Bertolini J. Transferrin: structure, function and potential therapeutic actions. *Drug Discov Today* 2005; **10**: 267–73.

●90. Weiner RE, Thakur M. Chemistry of gallium and indium radiopharmaceuticals. In: Welch MaR C. (ed.) *Handbook of radiopharmaceuticals: radiochemistry and applications*. Chicester: John Wiley, 2003: 363–99.

●91. Larson SM, Rasey JS, Allen DR, Grunbaum Z. A transferrin-mediated uptake of gallium-67 by EMT-6 sarcoma, II. Studies *in vivo* (BALB/c mice): concise communication. *J Nucl Med* 1979; **20**: 843–6.

●92. Larson SM, Rasey JS, Nelson NJ. The kinetics of uptake and macormolecular binding of ^{67}Ga and ^{59}Fe by the EMT-6 sarcoma-like tumor of Balb/c mice. In: Sorensen J. (ed.) *Radiopharmaceuticals II: proceedings of the 2nd International Symposium on Radiopharmaceuticals*. New York: Society of Nuclear Medicine, 1979: 277–308.

●93. Taetle R. The role of transferrin receptors in hemopoietic cell growth. *Exp Hematol* 1990; **18**: 360–5.

●94. Sephton R. *Factors affecting* ^{67}Ga *distribution*. Frontiers in nuclear medicine. New York: Springer-Verlag, 1980: 154–61.

●95. Hayes RL, Rafter JJ, Byrd BL, Carlton JE. Studies of the *in vivo* entry of Ga-67 into normal and malignant tissue. *J Nucl Med* 1981; **22**: 325–32.

●96. Sephton R. Relationships between the metabolism of 67 Ga and iron. *Int J Nucl Med Biol* 1981; **8**: 323–31.

●97. Morgan EH. Exchange of iron and transferrin across endothelial surfaces in the rat and rabbit. *J Physiol* 1963; **169**: 339–52.

●98. Iosilevsky G, Front D, Bettman L *et al*. Uptake of gallium-67 citrate and [2–3H]deoxyglucose in the tumor model, following chemotherapy and radiotherapy. *J Nucl Med* 1985; **26**: 278–82.

●99. Higashi T, Kobayashi M, Wakao H, Jinbu Y. The relationship between 67Ga accumulation and ATP metabolism in tumor cells *In vitro*. *Eur J Nucl Med* 1989; **15**: 152–6.

●100. Kubota K, Ishiwata K, Kubota R *et al*. Tracer feasibility for monitoring tumor radiotherapy: a quadruple tracer study with fluorine-18-fluorodeoxyglucose or fluorine-18-fluorodeoxyuridine, L-[methyl-14C]methionine, [6-3H]thymidine, and gallium-67. *J Nucl Med* 1991; **32**: 2118–23.

●101. Higashi T, Wakao H, Yamaguchi M, Suga K. The relationship between Ga-67 accumulation and cell cycle in malignant tumor cells *In vitro*. *Eur J Nucl Med* 1988; **14**: 155–8.

●102. Chitambar CR, Matthaeus WG, Antholine WE *et al*. Inhibition of leukemic HL60 cell growth by transferrin-gallium: effects on ribonucleotide reductase and demonstration of drug synergy with hydroxyurea. *Blood* 1988; **72**: 1930–6.

●103. Hedley DW, Tripp EH, Slowiaczek P, Mann GJ. Effect of gallium on DNA synthesis by human T-cell lymphoblasts. *Cancer Res* 1988; **48**: 3014–18.

◆104. Chitambar CR. Gallium compounds as antineoplastic agents. *Curr Opin Oncol* 2004; **16**: 547–52.

●105. Straus DJ. Gallium nitrate in the treatment of lymphoma. *Semin Oncol* 2003; **30** (2 Suppl 5): 25–33.

●106. Das Gupta A, Shah VI. Correlation of transferrin receptor expression with histologic grade and immunophenotype in chronic lymphocytic leukemia and non-Hodgkin's lymphoma. *Hematol Pathol* 1990; **4**: 37–41.

●107. Sciot R, Paterson AC, van Eyken P *et al*. Transferrin receptor expression in human hepatocellular carcinoma: an immunohistochemical study of 34 cases. *Histopathology* 1988; **12**: 53–63.

●108. Feremans W, Bujan W, Neve P *et al*. CD71 phenotype and the value of gallium imaging in lymphomas. *Am J Hematol* 1991; **36**: 215–16.

●109. Tsuchiya Y, Nakao A, Komatsu T *et al*. Relationship between gallium 67 citrate scanning and transferrin receptor expression in lung diseases. *Chest* 1992; **102**: 530–4.

●110. Leong LC, Ho YY. Suppressed soft tissue uptake of Ga-67 after blood transfusion and chemotherapy. *Clin Nucl Med* 2005; **30**: 128–30.

●111. Chen DC, Scheffel U, Camargo EE, Tsan MF. The source of gallium-67 in gastrointestinal contents: concise communication. *J Nucl Med* 1980; **21**: 1146–50.

●112. Breeman WA, de Jong M, de Blois E *et al*. Radiolabelling DOTA-peptides with 68Ga. *Eur J Nucl Med Mol Imaging* 2005; **32**: 478–85.

●113. Patton J. *Basic physics of nuclear medicine*, 4th ed. Baltimore, Maryland, Lippincott, Williams and Wilkins, 2003.

●114. Ugur O, Kothari PJ, Finn RD *et al*. Ga-66 labeled somatostatin analogue DOTA-DPhe1-Tyr3-octreotide as a potential agent for positron emission tomography imaging and receptor mediated internal radiotherapy of somatostatin receptor positive tumors. *Nucl Med Biol* 2002; **29**: 147–57.

●115. Henze M, Schuhmacher J, Hipp P *et al*. PET imaging of somatostatin receptors using [68GA]DOTA-D-Phe1-Tyr3-octreotide: first results in patients with meningiomas. *J Nucl Med* 2001; **42**: 1053–6.

●116. Aloj L, Jogoda E, Lang L *et al*. Targeting of transferrin receptors in nude mice bearing A431 and LS174T xenografts with [18F]holo-transferrin: permeability and receptor dependence. *J Nucl Med* 1999; **40**: 1547–55.

◆117. Bar-Shalom R, Mor M, Yefremov N, Goldsmith SJ. The value of Ga-67 scintigraphy and F-18 fluorodeoxyglucose positron emission tomography in staging and monitoring the response of lymphoma to treatment. *Semin Nucl Med* 2001; **31**: 177–90.

●118. King MA, Weber DA, Casarett GW *et al.* A study of irradiated bone. Part II. changes in Tc-99m pyrophosphate bone imaging. *J Nucl Med* 1980; **21**: 22–30.

◆119. Kohler G, Milstein C. Continuous cultures of fused cells secreting antibody of predefined specificity. *Nature* 1975; **256**: 495–7.

●120. Nadler LM, Stashenko P, Hardy R *et al.* Serotherapy of a patient with a monoclonal antibody directed against a human lymphoma-associated antigen. *Cancer Res* 1980; **40**: 3147–54.

●121. Miller RA, Maloney DG, Warnke R, Levy R. Treatment of B-cell lymphoma with monoclonal anti-idiotype antibody. *N Engl J Med* 1982; **306**: 517–22.

●122. Link MP, Bindl J, Meeker TC *et al.* A unique antigen on mature B cells defined by a monoclonal antibody. *J Immunol* 1986; **137**: 3013–18.

●123. Epstein AL, Marder RJ, Winter JN *et al.* Two new monoclonal antibodies, Lym-1 and Lym-2, reactive with human B-lymphocytes and derived tumors, with immunodiagnostic and immunotherapeutic potential. *Cancer Res* 1987; **47**: 830–40.

●124. Pawlak-Byczkowska EJ, Hansen HJ, Dion AS, Goldenberg DM. Two new monoclonal antibodies, EPB-1 and EPB-2, reactive with human lymphoma. *Cancer Res* 1989; **49**: 4568–77.

●125. Leonard JP, Coleman M, Ketas JC *et al.* Epratuzumab, a humanized anti-CD22 antibody, in aggressive non-Hodgkin's lymphoma: phase I/II clinical trial results. *Clin Cancer Res* 2004; **10**: 5327–34.

●126. Royston I, Majda JA, Baird SM *et al.* Human T cell antigens defined by monoclonal antibodies: the 65,000-dalton antigen of T cells (T65) is also found on chronic lymphocytic leukemia cells bearing surface immunoglobulin. *J Immunol* 1980; **125**: 725–31.

●127. Robb RJ, Greene WC, Rusk CM. Low and high affinity cellular receptors for interleukin 2. Implications for the level of Tac antigen. *J Exp Med* 1984; **160**: 1126–46.

●128. Ledbetter JA, Frankel AE, Herzenberg LA, Herzenberg HA. Human Leu T-cell differentiation antigen: quantitative expression on normal lymphoid cells and cell lines. In: Hammerling G, Hammerling U, Kearney J. (eds) *Monoclonal antibodies and T-cell hybridomas: perspectives and technical notes.* New York: Elsevier/North Holland, 1981: 16–22.

◆129. Waldmann TA, White JD, Carrasquillo JA *et al.* Radioimmunotherapy of interleukin-2R alpha-expressing adult T-cell leukemia with Yttrium-90-labeled anti-Tac. *Blood* 1995; **86**: 4063–75.

●130. Junghans RP, Carrasquillo JA, Waldmann TA. Impact of antigenemia on the bioactivity of infused anti-Tac antibody: implications for dose selection in antibody immunotherapies. *Proc Natl Acad Sci U S A* 1998; **95**: 1752–7.

●131. Pfreundschuh M, Mommertz E, Meissner M *et al.* Hodgkin and Reed-Sternberg cell associated monoclonal antibodies HRS-1 and HRS-2 react with activated cells of lymphoid and monocytoid origin. *Anticancer Res* 1988; **8**: 217–24.

●132. Order SE, Porter M, Hellman S. Hodgkin's disease: evidence for a tumor-associated antigen. *N Engl J Med* 1971; **285**: 471–4.

●133. Carde P, Manil L, da Costa L *et al.* Hodgkin's disease immunoscintigraphy: use of the anti Reed-Stemberg cells H-RS-I monoclonal antibody in 9 patients. *Proc Annu Meet Am Assoc Cancer Res* 1988; **7**: 227.

●134. Bernstein ID, Eary JF, Badger CC *et al.* High dose radiolabeled antibody therapy of lymphoma. *Cancer Res* 1990; **50** (3 Suppl): 1017s–21s.

●135. Press OW, Eary JF, Badger CC *et al.* Treatment of refractory non-Hodgkin's lymphoma with radiolabeled MB-1 (anti-CD37) antibody. *J Clin Oncol* 1989; **7**: 1027–38.

◆136. Kaminski MS, Fig LM, Zasadny KR *et al.* Imaging, dosimetry, and radioimmunotherapy with iodine 131-labeled anti-CD37 antibody in B-cell lymphoma. *J Clin Oncol* 1992; **10**: 1696–711.

●137. DeNardo SJ, DeNardo GL, O'Grady LF *et al.* Treatment of a patient with B cell lymphoma by I-131 LYM-1 monoclonal antibodies. *Int J Biol Markers* 1987; **2**: 49–53.

◆138. DeNardo S, DeNardo G, O'Grady L *et al.* Pilot studies of radioimmunotherapy of B cell lymphoma and leukemia using I-131 Lym-1 monoclonal antibody. *Antibody Immunoconjugates Radiopharmacy* 1988; **1**: 17–33.

●139. DeNardo S, DeNardo G, O'Grady L *et al.* Treatment of B cell malignancies with I-131 Lym-1 monoclonal antibodies. *Int J Cancer* 1988; **3**: 96–101.

●140. Deshpande SV, DeNardo SJ, Meares CF, *et al.* Copper-67-labeled monoclonal antibody Lym-1, a potential radiopharmaceutical for cancer therapy: labeling and biodistribution in RAJI tumored mice. *J Nucl Med* 1988; **29**: 217–25.

●141. DeNardo GL, DeNardo SJ, Meares CF *et al.* Pharmacokinetics of Copper-67 conjugated Lym-1, a potential therapeutic radioimmunoconjugate, in mice and in patients with lymphoma. *Antibody Immunoconjugates and Radiopharmaceuticals* 1991; **4**: 777–85.

●142. Meredith R, Khazacli MB, Plott G *et al.* Comparison of diagnostic and therapeutic doses of I-131 Lym-1 in patients with non-Hodgkin's lymphoma. *Antibody Immunoconjugates and Radiopharmaceuticals* 1993; **6**: 1–11.

●143. DeNardo GL, DeNardo SJ, Kukis DL *et al.* Maximum-tolerated dose, toxicity, and efficacy of I-131-Lym-1 antibody for fractionated radioimmunotherapy of non-Hodgkin's lymphoma. *J Clin Oncol* 1998; **16**: 3246–56.

●144. DeNardo GL, O'Donnel RT, Shen S *et al.* Radiation dosimetry for Y-90-2IT-BAD-Lym-1 extrapolated from pharmacokinetics using In-111-2IT-BAD-Lym-1 in patients with non-Hodgkin's lymphoma. *J Nucl Med* 2000; **41**: 952–8.

●145. Vervoordeldonk SF, Heikens J, Goedemans WT *et al.* Tc-99m-CD19 monoclonal antibody is not useful for imaging of B cell non-Hodgkin's lymphoma. *Cancer Immunol Immunother* 1996; **42**: 291–6.

●146. Press OW, Eary JF, Appelbaum FR *et al.* Radiolabeled-antibody therapy of B-cell lymphoma with autologous bone-marrow support. *N Engl J Med* 1993; **329**: 1219–24.

●147. Knox SJ, Goris ML, Trisler K et al. Yttrium-90-labeled anti-CD20 monoclonal antibody therapy of recurrent B-cell lymphoma. Clin Cancer Res 1996; 2: 457.

●148. Wiseman GA, Kornmehl E, Leigh B et al. Radiation dosimetry results and safety correlations from Y-90-ibritumomab tiuxetan radioimmunotherapy for relapsed or refractory non-Hodgkin's lymphoma: Combined data from 4 clinical trials. J Nucl Med 2003; 44: 465–74.

◆149. Kaminski MS, Zasadny KR, Moon S et al. Initial clinical radioimmunotherapy results with 131-i-anti-b1 (anti-cd20) in refractory B-cell lymphoma. Antibody Immunoconjugates and Radiopharmaceuticals 1982; 5: 345.

●150. Kaminski MS, Zasadny KR, Francis IR et al. Radioimmunotherapy of B-cell lymphoma with [131I]anti-B1 (anti-CD20) antibody. N Engl J Med 1993; 329: 459–65.

●151. Press OW, Eary JF, Applebaum FR et al. Radiolabeled antibody therapy of lymphoma. Cancer Treat Res 1993; 66: 127–45.

●152. Press OW, Eary J, Badger CC et al. High-dose radioimmunotherapy of lymphomas. Cancer Treat Res 1993; 68: 13–22.

●153. Press OW, Eary JF, Appelbaum FR et al. Radiolabeled-antibody therapy of B-cell lymphoma with autologous bone marrow support [see comments]. N Engl J Med 1993; 329: 1219–24.

●154. Kaminski et al. Radioimmunotherapy of refractory B-cell lymphoma with 131-I- Anti-B1 (Anti-Cd20) antibody. Clin Res 1994; 42: A405.

●155. GrilloLopez AJ et al. Phase I study of IDEC-Y2B8: 90-yttrium labeled anti-CD20 monoclonal antibody therapy of relapsed non-Hodgkin's lymphoma. Blood 1995; 86: 207.

●156. McLaughlin P et al. IDEC-C2B8 anti-CD20 antibody: Final report on a phase III pivotal trial in patients (PTS) with relapsed low-grade or follicular lymphoma (LG/F NHL). Blood 1996; 88: 349.

●157. Wiseman GA, Leigh BR, Dunn WL et al. Additional radiation absorbed dose estimates for Zevalin (TM) radioimmunotherapy. Cancer Biother Radiopharm 2003; 18: 253–8.

●158. Wiseman GA, Leigh BR, Erwin WD et al. Radiation dosimetry results front a phase II trial of ibritumomab tiuxetan (Zevalin (TM)) radioimmunotherapy for patients with non-Hodgkin's lymphoma and mild thrombocytopenia. Cancer Biother Radiopharm 2003; 18: 165–78.

●159. Scheinberg DA, Straus DJ, Yeh SD et al. A phase I toxicity, pharmacology, and dosimetry trial of monoclonal antibody OKB7 in patients with non-Hodgkin's lymphoma: effects of tumor burden and antigen expression. J Clin Oncol 1990; 8: 792–803.

●160. Czuczman MS, Straus DJ, Divgi CR et al. Phase-I dose-escalation trial of Iodine 131-labeled monoclonal-antibody Okb7 in patients with non-Hodgkins-lymphoma. J Clin Oncol 1993; 11: 2021–9.

●161. Behr TM, Wörmann B, Gramatzki M et al. Low- versus high-dose radioimmunotherapy with humanized anti-CD22 or chimeric anti-CD20 antibodies in a broad spectrum of B cell-associated malignancies. Clin Cancer Res 1999; 5: 3304S–14S.

●162. Goldenberg DM, Horowitz JA, Sharkey RM et al. Targeting, dosimetry, and radioimmunotherapy of B-cell lymphomas with Iodine-131-labeled LI2 Monoclonal-antibody. J Clin Oncol 1991; 9: 548–64.

◆163. Baum RP, Niesen A, Hertel A et al. Initial clinical results with technetium-99m-labeled LL2 monoclonal antibody fragment in the radioimmunodetection of B-cell lymphomas. Cancer, 1994; 73 (3 Suppl): 896–9.

●164. Blend MJ, Hyun H, Kozloff M et al. Improved staging of B-cell non-Hodgkin's lymphoma patients with 99mTc-labeled LL2 monoclonal antibody fragment. Cancer Res 1995; 55 (23 Suppl): 5764s–70s.

●165. Juweid ME, Stadtmauer E, Hajjar G et al. Pharmacokinetics, dosimetry, and initial therapeutic results with I-131- and In-111-/Y-90-labeled humanized LL2 anti-CD22 monoclonal antibody in patients with relapsed, refractory non-Hodgkin's lymphoma. Clin Cancer Res 1999; 5: 3292S–303S.

●166. Bunn PA, Carrasquillo JA, Keenan AM et al. Imaging of T-cell lymphoma by radiolabelled monoclonal antibody [letter]. Lancet 1984; 2: 1219–21.

●167. Carrasquillo JA, Bunn PA Jr, Keenan AM et al. Radioimmunodetection of cutaneous T-cell lymphoma with In-111 labeled T101 monoclonal antibody. N Engl J Med 1986; 315: 673–80.

●168. Carrasquillo JA, Mulshine JL, Bunn PA Jr et al. Indium-111 T101 monoclonal antibody is superior to iodine-131 T101 in imaging of cutaneous T-cell lymphoma. J Nucl Med 1987; 28: 281–7.

●169. Foss FM, Raubitscheck A, Mulshine JL et al. Phase I study of the pharmacokinetics of a radioimmunoconjugate, Y-90-T101, in patients with CD5- expressing leukemia and lymphoma. Clin Cancer Res 1998; 4: 2691–700.

◆170. Waldmann TA, White JD, Carrasquilla JA et al. Radioimmunotherapy of interleukin-2R alpha-expressing adult T-cell leukemia with Yttrium-90-labeled anti-Tac. Blood 1995; 86: 4063–75.

●171. Carrasquillo JA, White JD, Carrasquillo JA et al. Biodistribution of In-111 vs Y-90 labeled anti-Tac monoclonal antibody. J Nucl Med 1996; 37: 1055–5.

●172. Junghans RP, Dobbs D, Brechbiel MW et al. Pharmacokinetics and bioactivity of 1,4,7,10-tetra-azacylododecane, N″,N‴-tetraacetic acid (DOTA)-bismuth-conjugated anti-Tac antibody for alpha-emitter (212Bi) therapy. Cancer Res 1993; 53: 5683–9.

●173. da Costa L, Carde P, Lumbroso JD et al. Immunoscintigraphy in Hodgkin's disease and anaplastic large cell lymphomas: results in 18 patients using the iodine radiolabeled monoclonal antibody HRS-3. Ann Oncol 1992; 3 (Suppl 4): 53–7.

●174. Falini B, Flenghi L, Fedeli L et al. In vivo targeting of Hodgkin and Reed-Sternberg cells of Hodgkins-disease with monoclonal-antibody Ber-H2 (Cd30) – Immunohistological evidence. Br J Haematol 1992; 82: 38–45.

●175. Schnell R, Dietlein M, Staak JO *et al.* Treatment of refractory Hodgkin's lymphoma patients with an iodine-131-labeled murine anti-CD30 monoclonal antibody. *J Clin Oncol* 2005; **23**: 4669–78.

●176. Odonoghue JA, Bardies M, Wheldon TE. Relationships between tumor size and curability for uniformly targeted therapy with beta-emitting radionuclides. *J Nucl Med* 1995; **36**: 1902–9.

●177. Eary JF, Krohn KA, Kishore R, Nelp WB. Radiochemistry of halogenated antibodies. In: Zalutsky M. (ed.) *Antibodies in radiodiagnosis and therapy.* Boca Raton: CRC Press, 1989: 84–102.

●178. Eckelman WC, Paik CH. Labeling antibodies with metals using bifunctional chelates. In: Zalutsky MR. (ed.) *Antibodies in radiodiagnosis and therapy.* Boca Raton: CRC Press, 1989: 103–428.

●179. Rhodes BA. Direct labeling of proteins with 99mTc. *Int J Rad Appl Instrum B* 1991; **18**: 667–76.

●180. Meares CF, Moi MK, Diril H *et al.* Macrocyclic chelates of radiometals for diagnosis and therapy. *Br J Cancer* 1990; **62**(Suppl): 21–6.

181. Gansow OA. Newer approaches to the radiolabeling of monoclonal antibodies by use of metal chelates. *Int J Rad Appl Instrum B* 1991; **18**: 369–81.

182. Wilbur DS, Hadley SW, Hylarides MD *et al.* Development of a stable radioiodinating reagent to label monoclonal antibodies for radiotherapy of cancer. *J Nucl Med* 1989; **30**: 216–26.

183. Garg PK, Slade SK, Harrison CL, Zalutsky MR. Labeling proteins using aryl iodide acylation agents: influence of meta vs para substitution on *in vivo* stability. *Int J Rad Appl Instrum [B]* 1989; **16**: 669–73.

184. Pittman RC, Carew TE, Glass CK *et al.* A radioiodinated, intracellularly trapped ligand for determining the sites of plasma protein degradation *in vivo. Biochem J* 1983; **212**: 791–800.

185. Stashenko P, Nadler LM, Hardy R, Schlossman SF. Characterization of a human lymphocyte-B-specific antigen. *J Clin Immunol* 1980; **125**: 1678–85.

186. Nadler LM, Ritz J, Hardy R *et al.* A unique cell surface antigen identifying lymphoid malignancies of B cell origin. *J Clin Invest* 1981; **67**: 134–40.

187. Cardarelli PM, Quinn M, Buckman D *et al.* Binding to CD20 by Anti-B1 Antibody or F(ab') is sufficient for induction of apoptosis in B-cell lines. *Cancer Immunol Immunother* 2002; **51**: 15–24.

188. Chiu ML, Kronauge JF, Piwnica-Worms D. Effect of mitochondrial and plasma membrane potentials on accumulation of hexakis (2-methoxyisobutylisonitrile) technetium(I) in cultured mouse fibroblasts. *J Nucl Med* 1990; **31**: 1646–53.

189. Piwnica-Worms D, Kronauge JF, Chiu ML. Uptake and retention of hexakis (2-methoxyisobutyl isonitrile) technetium(I) in cultured chick myocardial cells. Mitochondrial and plasma membrane potential dependence. *Circulation* 1990; **82**: 1826–38.

190. Piwnica-Worms D, Kronauge JF, Chiu ML. Enhancement by tetraphenylborate of technetium-99m-MIBI uptake kinetics and accumulation in cultured chick myocardial cells. *J Nucl Med* 1991; **32**: 1992–9.

191. Piwnica-Worms D, Chiu ML, Budding M *et al.* Functional imaging of multidrug-resistant P-glycoprotein with an organotechnetium complex. *Cancer Res* 1993; **53**: 977–84.

192. Delmon-Moingeon LI, Piwnica-Worms D, Van den Abbeele AD *et al.* Uptake of the cation hexakis(2-methoxyisobutylisonitrile)-technetium-99m by human carcinoma cell lines *In vitro. Cancer Res* 1990; **50**: 2198–202.

193. Summerhayes IC, Lampidis TJ, Bernal SD *et al.* Unusual retention of rhodamine 123 by mitochondria in muscle and carcinoma cells. *Proc Natl Acad Sci U S A* 1982; **79**: 5292–6.

194. Davis S, Weiss MJ, Wong JR *et al.* Mitochondrial and plasma membrane potentials cause unusual accumulation and retention of rhodamine 123 by human breast adenocarcinoma-derived MCF-7 cells. *J Biol Chem* 1985; **260**: 13844–50.

195. Chen LB. Mitochondrial membrane potential in living cells. *Annu Rev Cell Biol* 1988; **4**: 155–81.

196. Caner B, Kitapci M, Aras T *et al.* Increased accumulation of hexakis (2-methoxyisobutylisonitrile)technetium(I) in osteosarcoma and its metastatic lymph nodes. *J Nucl Med* 1991; **32**: 1977–8.

197. Caner B, Kitapci M, Erbengi G *et al.* Increased accumulation of Tc-99m MIBI in undifferentiated mesenchymal tumor and its metastatic lung lesions. *Clin Nucl Med* 1992; **17**: 144–5.

198. Caner B, Kitapcl M, Unlu M *et al.* Technetium-99m-MIBI uptake in benign and malignant bone lesions: a comparative study with technetium-99m-MDP. *J Nucl Med* 1992; **33**: 319–24.

199. Aktolun C, Bayhan H, Kir M. Clinical experience with Tc-99m MIBI imaging in patients with malignant tumors. Preliminary results and comparison with Tl-201. *Clin Nucl Med* 1992; **17**: 171–6.

200. Campeau RJ, Kronemer KA, Sutherland CM. Concordant uptake of Tc-99m sestamibi and Tl-201 in unsuspected breast tumor. *Clin Nucl Med* 1992; **17**: 936–7.

201. O'Driscoll CM, Baker F, Casey MJ, Duffy GJ. Localization of recurrent medullary thyroid carcinoma with technetium-99m-methoxyisobutylnitrile scintigraphy: a case report. *J Nucl Med* 1991; **32**: 2281–3.

202. Medolago G, Virotta G, Piti A *et al.* Abnormal uptake of technetium-99m hexakis-2-methoxyisobutylisonitrile in a primary cardiac lymphoma. *Eur J Nucl Med* 1992; **19**: 222–5.

203. Scott AM, Kostakoglu L, O'Brien JP *et al.* Comparison of technetium-99m-MIBI and thallium-201-chloride uptake in primary thyroid lymphoma. *J Nucl Med* 1992; **33**: 1396–8.

204. Ewer MS, Martin FJ, Henderson C *et al.* Cardiac safety of liposomal anthracyclines. *Semin Oncol* 2004; **31**(6 Suppl 13): 161–81.

205. Petit T. Anthracycline-induced cardiotoxicity. *Bull Cancer* 2004; **91**(Suppl 3): 159–65.

206. Von Hoff DD, Layard MW, Basa P *et al*. Risk factors for doxorubicin-induced congestive heart failure. *Ann Intern Med* 1979; **91**: 710–17.

207. Swain SM, Whaley FS, Ewer MS. Congestive heart failure in patients treated with doxorubicin: a retrospective analysis of three trials. *Cancer* 2003; **97**: 2869–79.

208. Bristow MR, Mason JW, Billingham ME, Daniels JR. Doxorubicin cardiomyopathy: evaluation by phonocardiography, endomyocardial biopsy, and cardiac catheterization. *Ann Intern Med* 1978; **88**: 168–75.

209. Carrio I, Lopez-Pousa A, Estorch M *et al*. Detection of doxorubicin cardiotoxicity in patients with sarcomas by indium-111-antimyosin monoclonal antibody studies. *J Nucl Med* 1993; **34**: 1503–7.

210. Cvetkovic RS, Scott LJ. Dexrazoxane: a review of its use for cardioprotection during anthracycline chemotherapy. *Drugs* 2005; **65**: 1005–24.

211. Iarussi D, Indolfi P, Casale F *et al*. Recent advances in the prevention of anthracycline cardiotoxicity in childhood. *Curr Med Chem* 2001; **8**: 1649–60.

212. Jensen BV, Skovsgaard T, Nielsen SL. Functional monitoring of anthracycline cardiotoxicity: a prospective, blinded, long-term observational study of outcome in 120 patients. *Ann Oncol* 2002; **13**: 699–709.

213. Lipshultz SE, Lipsitz SR, Sallan SE *et al*. Long-term enalapril therapy for left ventricular dysfunction in doxorubicin-treated survivors of childhood cancer. *J Clin Oncol* 2002; **20**: 4517–22.

214. Lishner M, Elis A, Ravid M. Late doxorubicin cardiotoxicity. *Anticancer Drugs* 1992; **3**: 367–9.

215. Steinherz LJ, Steinherz PG, Tan C. Cardiac failure and dysrhythmias 6–19 years after anthracycline therapy: a series of 15 patients. *Med Pediatr Oncol* 1995; **24**: 352–61.

216. Lipshultz SE, Colan SD, Gelber RD *et al*. Late cardiac effects of doxorubicin therapy for acute lymphoblastic leukemia in childhood. *N Engl J Med* 1991; **324**: 808–15.

217. Felker GM, Thompson RE, Hare JM *et al*. Underlying causes and long-term survival in patients with initially unexplained cardiomyopathy. *N Engl J Med* 2000; **342**: 1077–84.

218. Vourvouri EC, Poldermans D, Bax JJ *et al*. Evaluation of left ventricular function and volumes in patients with ischaemic cardiomyopathy: gated single-photon emission computed tomography versus two-dimensional echocardiography. *Eur J Nucl Med* 2001; **28**: 1610–15.

219. Sierra-Galan LM, Ingkanisorn WP, Rhoads KL *et al*. Qualitative assessment of regional left ventricular function can predict MRI or radionuclide ejection fraction: an objective alternative to eyeball estimates. *J Cardiovasc Magn Reson* 2003; **5**: 451–63.

220. Hegge FN, Hamilton GW, Larson SM *et al*. Cardiac chamber imaging: a comparison of red blood cells labeled with Tc-99m *In vitro* and *in vivo*. *J Nucl Med* 1978; **19**: 129–34.

221. Pavel DG, Zimmer M, Patterson VN. *In vivo* labeling of red blood cells with 99mTc: a new approach to blood pool visualization. *J Nucl Med* 1977; **18**: 305–8.

222. Thrall JH, Freitas JE, Swanson D *et al*. Clinical comparison of cardiac blood pool visualization with technetium-99m red blood cells labeled *in vivo* and with technetium-99m human serum albumin. *J Nucl Med* 1978; **19**: 796–803.

46

Staging systems and staging investigations at presentation

LENA SPECHT

DEFINITION AND PURPOSE OF STAGING

Staging is the process of defining the extent and aggressiveness of a malignant disease within a given patient. A valid and universally accepted staging classification for the lymphomas is of paramount importance for the following reasons:

- The stage of the disease should provide important prognostic information, aiding the clinician in predicting, with some accuracy, the outcome of the disease for a patient or a group of patients, thus defining risk groups.
- The results of the staging investigations should assist the clinician in selecting and planning the most appropriate therapeutic program for the individual patient. Depending on the estimated prognosis decisions are made as to how aggressive or conservative treatment should be for a particular patient. Moreover, the investigations should provide information about all potential complications, which may necessitate prompt action. Involvement of certain sites may require specially designed treatment. If local treatment, i.e. radiotherapy or surgery, is contemplated, precise anatomic delineation of the disease is needed for planning radiotherapy or

determining feasibility and extent of surgical procedures.
- The staging classification should assist in the evaluation of treatment results. In the context of clinical trials the stage of the disease may be used beforehand to define eligibility and stratification criteria, and afterwards in the statistical analysis to allow adjustments for more valid comparisons.
- The staging classification should provide a widely accepted descriptive system facilitating the exchange of information among different institutions and, ultimately, assisting in the comparison of groups of cases, particularly with regard to the results of different therapeutic programs.

STAGING SYSTEMS

The current standard staging system

The Tumor, Node, Metastasis (TNM) classification employed for other malignancies is not a workable staging system for the lymphomas, because the site of origin of the disease is often unclear, and there is no way to differentiate between T, N and M.[1,2] Since no other convincing and tested overall staging system is yet available, the Ann Arbor

Table 46.1   Ann Arbor staging classification[3]

Stage	Characteristics
I	Involvement of a single lymphatic region (I), or localized involvement of a single extralymphatic organ or site (IE)
II	Involvement of two or more lymphatic regions on the same side of the diaphragm (II), or localized involvement of a single extralymphatic organ or site and of one or more lymphatic regions on the same side of the diaphragm (IIE). An optional recommendation is that the number of lymphatic regions involved should be indicated by a subscript (e.g. II$_3$)
III	Involvement of lymphatic regions on both sides of the diaphragm (III), which may also be accompanied either by localized involvement of an extralymphatic organ or site (IIIE), or by involvement of the spleen (IIIS), or by both (IIIE+S)
IV	Diffuse or disseminated involvement of one or more extralymphatic organs with or without associated lymphatic involvement. The organs involved should be identified by a symbol: H for liver, L for lung, M for bone marrow, P for pleura, O for bone, D for skin.

The absence or presence of unexplained fever, night sweats and/or unexplained weight loss of more than 10 percent of the usual body weight in the 6 months prior to diagnosis is denoted by the suffix letters A or B, respectively.

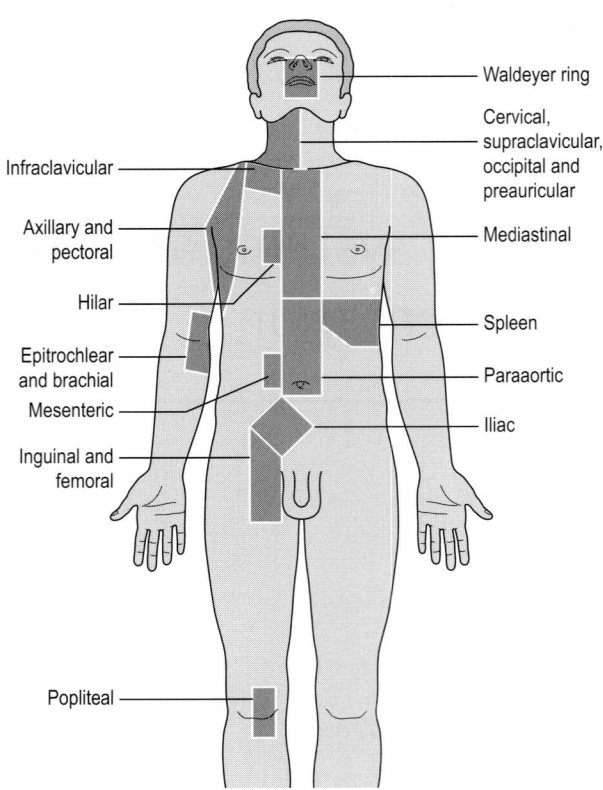

Figure 46.1   The lymph node regions as defined in the Ann Arbor staging system. (Reproduced, by permission, from Kaplan and Rosenberg.[4])

staging classification, originally designed for Hodgkin lymphoma, is widely used and recommended for the staging classification of lymphomas in general.[3]

The Ann Arbor staging system is summarized in Table 46.1. It reflects the number of sites of involvement and their relation to the diaphragm, the existence of B symptoms, and the presence of extralymphatic involvement. Lymphatic structures are lymph nodes, spleen, thymus, Waldeyer ring, appendix and Peyer patches. Lymph node regions as defined in the Ann Arbor staging system are shown in Figure 46.1.[4] Involvement of other structures is regarded as extralymphatic disease. Extralymphatic disease may be either localized or diffuse. Localized involvement of an extralymphatic site, a so-called E-lesion, is usually interpreted as a lesion which, although extralymphatic, can be sensibly contained in a curative radiation field, as initially described by Musshoff.[5] In practice, however, there is considerable disagreement among clinicians as to what does and what does not constitute a localized extralymphatic lesion.[6]

In the original Ann Arbor staging classification patients were assigned a clinical stage based on the initial biopsy and subsequent nonsurgical staging examinations. A pathologic stage was designated based on all clinical examinations as well as subsequent surgical staging procedures such as bone marrow biopsy, staging laparotomy and splenectomy. However, bone marrow biopsy is now a routine examination in most lymphoma patients, whereas staging laparotomy and splenectomy is no longer performed. Consequently, the designation of clinical and pathologic stages has been abandoned. The methods employed to determine the extent of disease in lymphomas are rapidly evolving and changing. Hence, the precise staging investigations employed in different studies should always be clearly delineated.

PROBLEMS WITH THE ANN ARBOR CLASSIFICATION

The Ann Arbor system has proved valuable for Hodgkin lymphoma, for which it was originally established. However, even in Hodgkin lymphoma it has been recognized that the Ann Arbor staging system is inadequate for the evaluation of patients, and is even less satisfactorily for other lymphoma types. There are several reasons for this:

- The Ann Arbor stage is not a sensitive indicator of prognosis in lymphomas. The extent of disease may vary considerably in stages other than stage I, and the volume of disease in individual regions is not taken into account. At a meeting in the

Table 46.2   Stage distribution of 14 308 cases of Hodgkin lymphoma from 20 institutions in eleven countries reported in the International Database on Hodgkin's Disease,[50] and in 1213 cases of lymphoma (excluding Hodgkin lymphoma) from nine institutions in eight countries which were reviewed by the Non-Hodgkin's Lymphoma Classification Project[49]

	Stage (%)					
Histological subtype	I	IE	II	IIE	III	IV
Hodgkin lymphoma	19	2	37	5	23	13
Diffuse large B cell lymphoma	12	13	13	16	13	33
Follicular lymphoma	16	2	11	4	16	51
Small lymphocytic lymphoma	4	0	2	3	8	83
Mantle cell lymphoma	10	3	6	1	9	71
Peripheral T cell lymphoma	1	7	6	6	15	65
Marginal zone B cell lymphoma, MALT type	0	39	0	28	2	31
Primary mediastinal large G cell lymphoma	10	0	34	22	3	31
Anaplastic large T/null-cell lymphoma	16	3	22	10	10	39
Lymphoblastic lymphoma (T/B)	0	0	11	0	14	75
Burkitt-like lymphoma	19	7	4	22	7	41
Marginal zone B cell lymphoma, nodal type	13	0	13	0	34	40
Lymphoplasmacytic lymphoma	7	0	0	13	7	73
Burkitt lymphoma	25	12	13	12	0	38

Cotswolds region of England in 1988, a modification of the Ann Arbor staging system for Hodgkin lymphoma was devised to incorporate a designation for number of sites and bulk.[7] However, the recommendations of the Cotswolds meeting have not been universally adopted. In many types of non-Hodgkin's lymphoma there is often little difference in prognosis between stage III disease and stage IV disease, nor even between these and stage II disease. Consequently, numerous studies have investigated other prognostic factors in the lymphomas. The important prognostic factors have in the vast majority of studies proved to be surrogate measures of the total tumor burden (e.g. number of nodal and extranodal sites, size of tumor masses, percent bone marrow involvement, hemoglobin, lymphocyte count, serum albumin, erythrocyte sedimentation rate (ESR), serum lactate dehydrogenase (LDH), serum β_2-microglobulin, B symptoms) or the physiologic reserve of the patient (e.g. age, performance status).[8–48]

- The distribution of patients in the different stages is not even and varies from subtype to subtype. Some lymphoma types, e.g. Hodgkin lymphoma and diffuse large B cell lymphoma, present reasonably frequently in all different stages, whereas other types are seen predominantly in either early stages, e.g. MALT lymphomas, or advanced stages, e.g. follicular lymphomas, mantle cell lymphomas, or peripheral T cell lymphomas. This pattern is obvious from the relationship between histologic subtype and stage, which was demonstrated in the International Database on Hodgkin's Disease and the Non-Hodgkin's

Lymphoma Classification Project, as shown in Table 46.2.[49,50] B symptoms occur in varying proportions of patients, from less than 20 percent in MALT lymphomas and lymphoplasmacytic lymphomas to 40–50 percent in more aggressive subtypes.[49,50]

- Unlike Hodgkin lymphoma, many other lymphoma types have a propensity to originate in extranodal sites.[51–55] This is particularly true in children, where lymphomas are more often extranodal than nodal and have a tendency to spread hematogenously early in their course.[56, 57] The Ann Arbor staging system is not well suited for the classification of predominantly extranodal disease.

- Lymphomas are a diverse group of diseases with differing patterns of involvement and spread. It cannot be realistically expected that a single system will be satisfactory as a staging classification for all the different subgroups of lymphomas.

PROPOSED NEWER STAGING SYSTEMS

The need for better staging systems for the lymphomas has been widely recognized and has led to the proposal of a number of alternative staging classifications for some of the lymphoma types.

Hodgkin lymphoma

For Hodgkin lymphoma a modification of the Ann Arbor classification incorporating some indication of number of sites and bulk was proposed at the meeting in the

Table 46.3 Proposed divisions of Hodgkin lymphoma into early, intermediate and advanced disease

EORTC[58]	
Early	Stage I or II without risk factors
Intermediate	Stage I or II with risk factors (age >50, 4+ nodal sites, ESR >50 mm/h or B symptoms and ESR >30 mm/h, bulky mediastinum)
Advanced	Stage III or IV
GHSG[59]	
Early	Stage I or II without risk factors
Intermediate	Stage I or II with risk factors (large mediastinal mass, extranodal involvement, elevated ESR, >2 involved lymph node areas)
Advanced	Stage IIB with large mediastinal mass and/or extranodal involvement, Stage III and IV
NLG[60]	
Early	Stage IA, IB or IIA without risk factors
Intermediate	Stage IA, IB or IIA with risk factors (large mediastinal mass, node or nodal mass >10 cm, >2 involved lymph node areas, ESR >50)
Advanced	Stage IIB, III or IV

EORTC, European Organisation for Research and Treatment of Cancer; GHSG, German Hodgkin Study Group; NLG, Nordic Lymphoma Group; ESR, erythrocyte sedimentation rate.

Cotswolds, UK, mentioned above.[7] It proposes to add the subscript X if bulky disease is present, bulky disease being defined as a node or nodal mass of 10 cm or greater or a mediastinal mass greater than one-third of the internal transverse diameter of the thorax at the level of T5/6. Furthermore, stage III may be subdivided into stage III_1 (spleen, splenic hilar, celiac or portal node involvement) and stage III_2 (para-aortic, iliac or mesenteric node involvement). More recently, divisions into early, intermediate and advanced disease based on stage and other prognostic factors have been proposed by different centers and groups (Table 46.3). For advanced disease an International Prognostic Score (IPS) has been developed which incorporates seven risk factors: age ≥45 years, male sex, stage IV disease, hemoglobin <105 g/L, serum albumin <40 g/L, leukocytosis ≥15 × 10^9/L, and lymphocytopenia <0.6 × 10^9/L or <8 percent of white blood cell count.[45] Patients are divided according to the number of risk factors.

Non–Hodgkin lymphoma

For intermediate- and high-grade non-Hodgkin lymphomas in adults combinations of prognostic factors defining risk groups or 'stages' have been proposed both for early stage disease[28,31,40,43] and for advanced disease.[12,16,25,27,33,36,37,41,42,61] The International Non-Hodgkin's Lymphoma Prognostic Factors Project analyzed clinical features in 3273 patients

from centers in Europe and America with aggressive lymphomas, a term which included a number of different histologic types of the present WHO lymphoma classification.[8] An International Prognostic Index (IPI) for all patients and an age-adjusted IPI for younger patients (≤60 years) were constructed (Table 46.4). The prognostic factors employed in the IPI and the earlier proposals do not differ greatly. Most of them are tumor-related, based on measures of tumor mass and tumor dissemination ultimately reflecting the total tumor burden, or based on biological factors (lactate dehydrogenase [LDH], β_2-microglobulin), in turn reflecting the total tumor burden and possibly also the growth characteristics of the tumor. In some of the proposals other factors are included which are not tumor related, but which must rather be defined as patient features determining tolerance to treatment (e.g. age, performance status).[8,11,17,25,65,66] Although both types of prognostic factors, tumor related and patient related, are clearly important for prognosis, it would seem advisable to keep them clearly separate. Staging aims to define the extent and aggressiveness of the disease within the patient. Neither age nor performance status contributes to this objective. Moreover, if it is decided to rely on the staging classification for selecting patients for more intensive treatment, all prognostic factors that indicate patients with particularly poor-prognosis tumors should be used. It would hardly be justified to use factors that select patients who are characterized by being barely able to tolerate standard treatment. Nevertheless, the IPI has gained wide international acceptance. Numerous publications have shown that the IPI is indeed prognostic in aggressive lymphomas, but also that other prognostic factors, in particular new biomarkers, have independent significance.[67–87]

The IPI was constructed mainly based on advanced cases of diffuse large B cell lymphoma. A modified index for early stage disease was proposed by Miller *et al.* (see Table 46.4).[62] This stage modified index has been shown to work in localized disease.[88,89]

With the acceptance of the World Health Organization (WHO) classification it has become clear that the lymphomas previously grouped into intermediate- and high-grade consist of different disease entities with varying presentations and prognosis. Efforts are now being made to devise staging classification systems for each of the well-defined entities in the WHO classification.

Follicular lymphoma

In the follicular lymphomas proposals for new staging systems have also been put forward.[10,22,34,90] The essential parameters are not very different from those found to be important in intermediate- and high-grade lymphomas, again largely reflecting tumor burden.[91] The IPI works in follicular lymphomas, but not as well as in aggressive lymphomas.[92,93] An international cooperative study analyzed 4167 cases and proposed a prognostic index specifically designed for follicular lymphomas (the so-called FLIPI) (see

Table 46.4   Risk groups for aggressive lymphomas proposed by the International Non-Hodgkin's Lymphoma Prognostic Factors Project (IPI and age-adjusted IPI),[8] for early stage aggressive lymphomas,[62] for peripheral T cell lymphomas unspecified[63] and for follicular lymphomas.[64]

International Prognostic Index (IPI)

Risk factors	Ann Arbor stage III-IV, >1 extranodal site, high LDH, age >60 years, performance status ≥2 (ECOG)
Low risk	0–1 risk factors
Low intermediate risk	2 risk factors
High intermediate risk	3 risk factors
High risk	4–5 risk factors

Age-adjusted IPI

Risk factors	Ann Arbor stage III-IV, high LDH, performance status ≥2 (ECOG)
Low risk	0 risk factors
Low intermediate risk	1 risk factor
High intermediate risk	2 risk factors
High risk	3 risk factors

Modified IPI for early stage disease

Risk factors	Age >60 years, stage II disease, high LDH, performance status ≥2 (ECOG)
Low risk	0–1 risk factors
Low intermediate risk	2 risk factors
High intermediate risk	3 risk factors
High risk	4 risk factors

Prognostic index for peripheral T cell lymphoma unspecified (PIT)

Risk factors	Age >60 years, performance status ≥2 (ECOG), high LDH, bone marrow involvement
Group 1	0 risk factors
Group 2	1 risk factor
Group 3	2 risk factors
Group 4	3–4 risk factors

Follicular lymphoma international prognostic index (FLIPI)

Risk factors	Age ≥60 years, Ann Arbor stage III-IV, hemoglobin <120 g/L, high LDH, number of nodal sites >4
Low risk	0–1 risk factors
Intermediate risk	2 risk factors
High risk	≥3 risk factors

ECOG, Eastern Co-operative Oncology Group; LDH, lactate dehydrogenase.

Table 46.4).[64] The prognostic value of the FLIPI has been confirmed also in relapsing patients.[94] New histological parameters (cyclin D1, sCD27) would seem to provide additional prognostic information in this subtype as well.[95,96]

For some of the rarer lymphoma subtypes the IPI has been shown to be applicable too.[49,83,97–102] However, when large patient materials with these subtypes have been collected and analyzed specifically designed prognostic indices for each subtype may well in the future turn out to be more informative.

Extranodal lymphoma

Ann Arbor stage is not well suited for localized extranodal lymphomas. Proposals have been made for special staging systems for particular localizations of extranodal lymphomas in order to achieve more informative staging. For lymphomas in the nasal cavity, paranasal sinuses and the Waldeyer ring, the TNM staging classification for solid tumors has been advocated because it better reflects tumor burden and prognosis.[103–105]

For gastrointestinal lymphomas the extent of disease is the most important prognostic factor. The modification of the Ann Arbor staging system proposed by Musshoff,[106] distinguishing in stage II between local nodal involvement of gastric or mesenteric nodes (stage II1E) and distant nodal involvement of other abdominal nodes (stage II2E), has proved significant,[107,108] and is, in addition, also useful for primary intestinal lymphomas. Tumor diameter >5 cm and penetration of the gastric wall and invasion of adjacent structures have also been associated with a poor prognosis. On this basis it has been proposed employing the TNM classification designed for gastric carcinomas[108–111] or a modification called the Manchester system which takes penetration into adjacent organs or perforation into account.[112] Consensus was reached at a workshop in Lugano in 1993 to propose the following system for gastric lymphoma:[113]

- Stage I: Lymphoma confined to stomach (single or multiple lesions)
- Stage II1: Involvement of local (paragastric lymph nodes)
- Stage II2: Involvement of distant (celiac or retroperitoneal) lymph nodes
- Stage IIE: Penetration into adjacent organs or tissues
- Stage IV: Disseminated extranodal involvement or gastric lesions with supradiaphragmatic nodal involvement

T cell lymphoma

Peripheral T cell lymphoma unspecified is the most common type of the peripheral T cell lymphomas. Although their clinical course is generally much worse than that of the aggressive B cell lymphomas, the IPI works in this entity as well.[97,114–117] However, a prognostic index specifically designed for peripheral T cell lymphoma unspecified (the so-called PIT) works even better (see Table 46.4).[63]

Cutaneous T cell lymphomas

Cutaneous lymphomas pose particular problems with regard to staging because of the concept of diffuse or disseminated involvement and because of the highly variable clinical course of the many different subtypes. For mycosis fungoides a tumor-node-metastasis-blood (TNMB) staging system has proved useful.[1,118] For other cutaneous lymphomas modifications of the Ann Arbor system distinguishing between localized and disseminated cutaneous disease are commonly used.[119,120]

Pediatric lymphoma

The highly aggressive lymphomas are more common in children than in adults. In childhood lymphomas it has long been recognized that the Ann Arbor system is inadequate, and other systems have been proposed.[57,121–123] The St Jude system, applicable to all histological types of childhood lymphomas, is now the most widely used (Table 46.5).[57,122] This system is modified from the Ann Arbor staging system, from which it differs in that it does not differentiate between primary nodal and extranodal disease, and it recognizes the poor prognosis of bone marrow and central nervous system (CNS) involvement. It separates patients with small tumor burdens, i.e. one or two masses on the same side of the diaphragm, excluding all primary intrathoracic tumors (which are nearly always bulky), from patients with large tumor burdens, i.e. masses on both sides of the diaphragm, primary intrathoracic tumors, or unresectable intraabdominal disease. This staging system is, however, insufficient for stratifying patients for therapy, mainly because each stage may encompass patients with a wide range of tumor burdens. Hence, patients are divided into risk groups using stage and additional factors for different protocols.[56]

Table 46.5 The St Jude staging system for childhood lymphomas[57,122]

Stage	Characteristics
I	A single tumor (extranodal) or single anatomic area (nodal), excluding mediastinum or abdomen
II	A single tumor (extranodal) with regional node involvement
	Two or more nodal areas on same side of diaphragm
	Two single (extranodal) tumors with or without regional node involvement on same side of diaphragm
	A primary gastrointestinal tract tumor (usually ileocecal) with or without associated mesenteric node involvement, grossly completely resected
III	Two single (extranodal) tumors on both sides of diaphragm
	Two or more nodal areas on both sides of diaphragm
	All primary intrathoracic tumors (mediastinal, pleural, thymic)
	All extensive (unresectable) primary intra-abdominal disease
	All paraspinal or epidural tumors regardless of other sites
IV	Any of the above with initial central nervous system or bone marrow involvement

The prognostic indices and risk groups outlined above for some of the more common lymphoma types are all based on common clinical variables. They perform well in many cases. Other, less common histological subtypes of lymphomas have been defined. Their clinical characteristics and important prognostic factors are not yet fully established. Clearly, the lymphomas are a highly diverse group of neoplasms with remarkably different clinical presentations, prognoses and responses to therapy. Ideally, for each clinicopathological entity a separate staging system should be devised, specifically tailored to that particular entity. As indicated above, this has as yet been achieved only for the most common subgroups. Consequently, the Ann Arbor staging classification, despite its shortcomings, remains, for the time being, the most commonly used staging system for the lymphomas. However, an improved understanding of the biology of the lymphomas and consequent development of biomarkers that can be combined with the clinical variables will most likely significantly improve the prognostic models. In particular, gene expression profiles[69,84,86,124] and immunohistochemistry, demonstrating the expression of the relevant proteins, will probably be incorporated in the current prognostic models allowing us to move beyond the clinically based prognostic indices.[125,126]

STAGING INVESTIGATIONS

Staging procedures required for all patients

The exact histopathologic diagnosis, including subtype, must be established by securing an adequate surgical biopsy, which must be reviewed by an experienced hematopathologist. Repeat biopsies are sometimes necessary. The staging procedures should establish the extent and aggressiveness of the disease to enable for the rational planning of treatment, estimation of prognosis and evaluation of response. A number of staging procedures (listed in Box 46.1) are required for all patients, regardless of histology and initial presentation. Under certain circumstances supplementary or alternative staging procedures may be indicated (listed in Table 46.6).

A careful history is important. Risk factors for lymphoma (e.g. immune deficiency or autoimmune disease) should be determined. The date that a mass was first observed and its subsequent growth rate should be ascertained. The presence and duration of the different B symptoms of the Ann Arbor classification should be noted. Focal symptoms suggesting an obstructing nodal mass in the thorax or abdomen (e.g. cough, superior vena caval syndrome, obstructive uropathy, abdominal discomfort) and symptoms suggesting extralymphatic involvement (e.g. bone pain, gastrointestinal complaints, neurological symptoms, cardiopulmonary symptoms, cutaneous involvement) should be enquired into and, if confirmed, should lead to further investigations in order to establish whether they are due to lymphoma. Performance status has prognostic value and, together with information on comorbid illness, predicts the patients' tolerance of treatment.

The physical examination should include a careful evaluation of all lymph node regions, including the preauricular, occipital, epitrochlear, femoral and popliteal nodes. If there is uncertainty about involvement of lymph nodes in a peripheral region, ultrasonography may be helpful.[127] The site and size of abnormal lymph nodes should be recorded, preferably on a schematic drawing of the body,

---

BOX 46.1: Required staging procedures for all patients

- History, including risk factors for lymphoma, duration and growth rate of lymph node enlargement, presence or absence of B symptoms, symptoms suggesting obstructing nodal masses or extralymphatic involvement, performance status, comorbid illness
- Physical examination, including evaluation of all lymph node regions, recording site and size of all abnormal lymph nodes, inspection of the Waldeyer ring, evaluation of the presence or absence of hepatosplenomegaly, inspection of the skin and detection of palpable masses
- Laboratory studies:
  - complete blood count
  - serum LDH and β_2-microglobulin levels
  - ESR in patients with Hodgkin lymphoma
  - evaluation of renal function (serum creatinine, uric acid, electrolytes including calcium)
  - evaluation of liver function (liver enzymes, bilirubin, and serum alkaline phosphatase)
  - serum protein electrophoresis
  - viral serologies (human immunodeficiency virus [HIV], hepatitis B and C, Epstein–Barr virus [EBV])
- Radiological studies:
  - standard posteroanterior and lateral chest radiographs
  - chest CT scan
  - abdominopelvic CT scan
- Bilateral posterior iliac crest bone marrow biopsies and peripheral blood smear

---

Table 46.6 Supplementary or alternative staging procedures

Evaluation of peripheral nodal regions	Ultrasound
Evaluation of the chest	FDG-PET scan
	Gallium scintigraphy
Evaluation of the abdomen	FDG-PET scan
	Ultrasound
	MRI
Evaluation of the bone marrow	MRI or FDG-PET scan
Evaluation of the central nervous system	MRI
Evaluation of the testes	Ultrasound

MRI, magnetic resonance imaging; FDG-PET, [^{18}F]2-fluoro-2-deoxy-D-glucose-positron emission tomography.

which often gives a better description of initial involvement for later comparison than a verbal description. The Waldeyer ring should be inspected either by indirect laryngoscopy or by direct fiberoptic examination; the latter is preferable for viewing the nasopharynx. Examination of the Waldeyer ring is particularly important in patients with involvement of high neck nodes or thyroid, testis or gastrointestinal tract. Hepatosplenomegaly should be noted, although the correlation with tumor involvement is not very strong.[128–133] Inspection of the skin and biopsy of suspicious lesions should be performed. Palpable masses, e.g. in salivary glands, thyroid, breast, abdomen, testicles or bones should be detected. A general physical examination to detect comorbid illness should also be undertaken.

Laboratory studies should include a complete blood count. The blood count does not correlate very well with bone marrow involvement,[134–137] but it provides baseline pre-treatment values. Lactate dehydrogenase and β_2-microglobulin are important because they are indirect measures of the total tumor burden and hence of great prognostic value.[8,12,16,27,33,37,41–43] For patients with Hodgkin lymphoma, the ESR is an important prognostic factor.[138] Serum creatinine, uric acid and electrolytes (including calcium) are important for identifying patients with hypercalcemia or those at risk for the development of tumor lysis syndrome. Impaired renal function may also suggest ureteric obstruction from retroperitoneal tumor, which may necessitate temporary urinary diversion before treatment of the lymphoma is initiated. Liver function tests, particularly the alkaline phosphatase, may be abnormal, but correlate poorly with hepatic involvement.[129,139,140] An isolated elevation in alkaline phosphatase would suggest skeletal involvement. A serum protein electrophoresis may detect monoclonal gammopathy. Viral serologies may be performed according to the risk pattern of the environment, in most locations tests for HIV, hepatitis B and C and EBV are carried out routinely.

Standard posteroanterior and lateral chest radiographs will detect mediastinal and/or hilar adenopathy in 18–25 percent of patients with non-Hodgkin lymphomas and even more in patients with Hodgkin lymphoma.[130,131,141,142] Pleural effusion is found in 8–10 percent, usually associated with mediastinal adenopathy.[130,141,143,144] However, pleural effusion requires pathologic verification, as it quite often consists of a transudate without malignant cells. Parenchymal lung involvement is seen in 3–8 percent.[141,142,144]

Computed tomography (CT) of the thorax delineates more precisely the anatomic extent of lymphadenopathy in the mediastinum and involvement of the chest wall or pericardium than conventional chest radiographs or tomography.[142,145–148] Chest CT will regularly identify disease which was not seen on chest radiograph, and even in cases where the chest radiograph was unremarkable.[142,146] Hence, chest CT is now routinely employed in the staging of lymphomas.

Abdominopelvic CT scan is now the standard test for evaluation of the abdomen. Previously, staging laparotomies were performed and provided valuable information on the anatomical distribution of disease.[128,131,132,149–155] However, the improvements in imaging and the present treatment strategies with widespread use of chemotherapy have rendered staging laparotomies obsolete. Lymphangiography has also been replaced by CT scanning because it only visualizes retroperitoneal lymph nodes up to the level of the renal vessels, and none of the other abdominal structures. CT scanning is able to detect involvement of lymph nodes provided they are enlarged. Involvement of the liver and spleen is frequently diffuse with tumor deposits often less than 1 cm in size, and such lesions are usually not detectable with CT scan (or any other currently available imaging technique). Organ size is an unreliable predictor of involvement. Overall, the accuracy of abdominopelvic CT scan compared with laparotomy for detecting intraabdominal disease is over 80 percent, a figure which is not surpassed by any other noninvasive technique.[156–158]

An adequate abdominal ultrasound examination is able to detect abdominal disease with about the same accuracy as a CT scan.[159] However, technical difficulties such as the presence of gas or bone often preclude examination of all abdominal and pelvic structures. The quality of ultrasound examination is, moreover, highly dependent on the ultrasonographer. The images generated by ultrasound are generally considered difficult to understand for clinicians and they cannot easily be used in the planning of radiation fields. Ultrasound may, however, be very useful in patients, typically children, with little retroperitoneal fat, where CT scans cannot delineate lymph nodes properly. Ultrasound may also be extremely helpful in situations where the abdominal CT scan is difficult to interpret, because segments of the bowel do not fill with contrast and may be mistaken for lymphoma. Radionuclide liver/spleen scans have not generally proved useful.[159,160]

The role of magnetic resonance imaging (MRI) in staging is limited, although is seems to be equal to CT in detecting chest or abdominal disease.[161–166] MRI is more costly and less available than CT, and the imaging time is longer. However, in cases where the radiation exposure from CT is important, e.g. young children or pregnant women, MRI would seem to be a good alternative. For the detection of bone disease or marrow involvement MRI is more sensitive than other modalities.[162,163,165,167–172] For the detection of central nervous system disease MRI is superior to CT.

Functional imaging with gallium-67 scintigraphy has been used in many centers to detect viable lymphoma tissue. With modern technique using higher doses of gallium and more advanced technology the sensitivity is high in aggressive lymphomas but less so in indolent lymphomas.[173–181] However, the use of functional imaging with [^{18}F]2-fluoro-2-deoxy-D-glucose positron emission tomography (FDG-PET) is now gaining widespread acceptance; FDG-PET can visualize both indolent and aggressive lymphomas, including Hodgkin lymphoma, and several studies suggest that it is more sensitive than CT scans.[182–196]

Exceptions seem to be extranodal marginal zone lymphomas and small lymphocytic lymphomas, which are not well visualized by FDG-PET.[197,198] This modality seems superior to bone scan for the detection of osseous involvement,[199,200] and may also be of value in detecting bone marrow involvement.[198,201,202] Several studies show that PET-FDG is more sensitive than gallium-67 scintigraphy.[203–209] The use of FDG-PET for staging of lymphomas is increasing rapidly, and it is recommended, although not mandatory, in routine staging for many types of lymphoma.[210–212]

Bone marrow involvement is common in certain types of lymphomas, e.g. follicular, mantle cell and small lymphocytic lymphomas, but uncommon in other types, e.g. diffuse large B cell, anaplastic large T/null cell and Hodgkin lymphoma.[50,98] Bone marrow examination is mandatory in the staging of lymphoma patients. Marrow biopsy is necessary as marrow aspiration is inferior in identifying marrow involvement.[135,213] Bilateral posterior iliac crest biopsy has been recommended, because marrow involvement is usually focal, and doing more than one biopsy may increase the detection of involvement by up to 30 percent.[128,130,135,214,215] However, for most patients unilateral biopsy is considered sufficient provided the size of the sample is adequate (minimal total length of 2.0 cm).[216,217] Newer techniques such as flow cytometry, Southern blot analysis, and polymerase chain reaction are far more sensitive than conventional morphologic assessment and can detect lymphoma cells in blood and bone marrow in a much larger proportion of patients.[218–226] However, whether the results of these highly sensitive analyses should, in future, influence staging and treatment of patients is as yet unknown. Hence, these techniques may still be regarded primarily as research tools.[210,216,219,227,228] MRI seems to be very sensitive for the detection of bone marrow involvement.[167,169–171,229–231] FDG-PET also seems to be sensitive for bone marrow involvement.[201,202] In patients, where marrow involvement is suspected in spite of negative random biopsies, and where a positive marrow would change treatment strategy, an MRI or FDG-PET may be used to identify focal areas of involvement.[201,232] However, the specificity of MRI or FDG-PET for detection of marrow involvement is questionable, and suspicious areas should be biopsied for histologic confirmation.

Procedures indicated in patients with specific symptoms

In addition to the staging procedures required in all patients to establish the extent of the disease, additional procedures may be indicated in the individual patient if certain specific symptoms are present. The more common of these additional procedures are listed in Table 46.7. These procedures are not indicated in asymptomatic patients because the yield of positive results is too low.

Table 46.7 Procedures indicated in patients with specific symptoms

General central nervous system dysfunction or cranial nerve abnormalities	CT or MRI of brain Lumbar puncture with examination of cerebrospinal fluid
Spinal cord dysfunction	MRI of spinal cord (or myelography) Lumbar puncture with examination of cerebrospinal fluid
Visual symptoms	Ophthalmologic evaluation, including slit-lamp examination MRI (or CT) of orbits and brain Lumbar puncture with examination of cerebrospinal fluid
Bone pain or swelling	FDG-PET, MRI or bone scan
Gastrointestinal complaints	Gastroscopy Barium studies
Abnormal liver function tests	Percutaneous liver biopsy
Cardiac symptoms	Echocardiogram

CT, computed tomography; MRI, magnetic resonance imaging; FDG-PET, [^{18}F]2-fluoro-2-deoxy-D-glucose-positron emission tomography.

Neurological symptoms should always prompt careful examination. General CNS dysfunction or cranial nerve abnormalities may be caused by leptomeningeal involvement or less commonly by intraparenchymal lesions.[233–245] Contrast enhanced CT or MRI scanning and lumbar puncture with examination of the cerebrospinal fluid (CSF) should be carried out. MRI may sometimes show lesions not visible on CT scan. If these tests are negative in spite of continued symptoms, additional lumbar punctures must be carried out. Immunohistochemical stains may demonstrate a monoclonal population of cells in the CSF even if they appear cytologically benign.[238] Elevated tumor markers (LDH and β_2-microglobulin) in the CSF may provide circumstantial evidence for lymphomatous invasion of the CNS.[244,246]

Symptoms of spinal cord dysfunction, most often caused by compression from epidural lesions,[239,240,244,247] should also be promptly evaluated. MRI of the spinal cord, or alternatively myelography (or CT scan) after intrathecal contrast injection, should establish the diagnosis. Epidural lesions frequently coexist with leptomeningeal involvement, and examination of the CSF should also be carried out.[243,244] Visual symptoms may be caused by ocular involvement (vitreous, retina or choroid), by involvement of extraocular orbital structures, or by leptomeningeal or parenchymal brain involvement. Examinations should include a careful ophthalmologic evaluation, including ophthalmoscopy and slit-lamp examination, CT or MRI scans of the orbits and brain, and a lumbar puncture with examination of the CSF.[235,248–251]

A patient with bone pain and swelling or isolated elevation of alkaline phosphatase should undergo further studies. Radionuclide bone scans are highly sensitive as an indicator of bone involvement,[252,253] and MRI and FDG-PET may even be superior.[200,254] However, findings are not as specific as conventional radiographs, and positive areas should be confirmed by plain radiographs or, if more complicated bone structures such as the facial bones show up positive, by CT scans (and biopsied if needed). Bone involvement is found in less than 10 percent of patients without specific symptoms,[131] and a bone scan is not recommended as a routine staging procedure.

Patients with gastrointestinal complaints should undergo endoscopy and barium studies of the gastrointestinal tract. The abdominal CT scan is not very sensitive for detection of intrinsic bowel involvement, and the routine staging procedures cannot be relied on to rule out gastrointestinal involvement. Although gastrointestinal involvement is a fairly common extranodal manifestation,[51,255] virtually all patients with gastrointestinal involvement have signs or symptoms leading to further investigations, and routine barium studies on all patients are therefore not warranted.[141,256,257] If liver function tests are abnormal with no clear explanation a percutaneous liver biopsy should be performed. Finally, patients with cardiac symptoms should be evaluated with echocardiogram to detect cardiac and pericardial involvement.

Procedures indicated for patients with specific histologic subtypes and/or disease localizations

Lymphomas can involve virtually any organ or tissue. However, different subtypes have differing patterns of spread and involvement of nodal or extranodal areas. These differences reflect the biologic characteristics of the tumor cells. The WHO classification of the lymphomas delineates different disease entities with characteristic clinical features, and in comparison with earlier lymphoma classifications it provides a much improved basis for the rational evaluation of patients.[258,259] However, the site of origin probably also affects the biologic characteristics of the lymphoma.[125] For most patients the routine staging procedures and procedures prompted by specific symptoms are sufficient. In a number of situations patients with specific histologic subtypes and/or specific disease localizations should undergo additional studies (listed in Table 46.8).

Patients with lymphoblastic lymphoma or Burkitt lymphoma have a high probability of developing leptomeningeal disease, in most series around 25 percent, and lumbar puncture with examination of the cerebrospinal fluid (CSF) is mandatory in all such patients.[23,56,239,241,243,244,260–262] Patients with large cell lymphomas and involvement of bone marrow, testis, bone, orbit, nose/paranasal sinus, or epidural space or who have involvement of more than one extranodal site

Table 46.8   Procedures indicated for patients with specific histological subtypes and/or specific disease localizations

Lymphoblastic lymphoma (all)	Lumbar puncture with examination of cerebrospinal fluid
Burkitt lymphoma (all)	
Large cell lymphoma with involvement of bone marrow, testis, bone, orbit, nose/ paranasal sinus or epidural space	
Large cell lymphoma with more than one extranodal site or elevated LDH	
Brain or ocular structures	MRI (or CT) of brain and orbits
	Lumbar puncture with examination of cerebrospinal fluid
	Ophthalmologic evaluation, including split-lamp examination
Nasal cavity, nasopharynx, paranasal sinuses, orbit	MRI (or CT) of the head and neck
	Lumbar puncture with examination of cerebrospinal fluid
Waldeyer's ring	Gastroscopy
	Barium studies of the GI tract
Stomach	Endoscopic ultrasound
	Test for *H. pylori* (MALT lymphomas)
Bone	FDG-PET, MRI or bone scan
Breast	Bilateral mammogram
Testis	Testicular ultrasound
	Examination of Waldeyer's ring and skin
	Lumbar puncture (see above)

CT, computed tomography; MRI, magnetic resonance imaging; FDG-PET, [^{18}F]2-fluoro-2-deoxy-D-glucose-positron emission tomography; LDH, lactate dehydrogenase.

or/and elevated LDH also have an increased risk in the order of 20 percent of developing leptomeningeal disease, and a lumbar puncture as part of the staging procedures is recommended.[241–243,245,260,263–265]

Primary brain lymphomas are usually parenchymal lesions, which are multifocal in roughly half of immunocompetent patients and in nearly all AIDS patients.[235,249] Patients should be evaluated with contrast-enhanced MRI (preferred) or CT of the brain and orbits, preferably before corticosteroids are instituted since corticosteroids can cause contrast-enhancing lesions to shrink or disappear. At least one-third of patients have positive CSF, and a lumbar puncture with examination of the CSF should be part of the staging procedure for all such patients except in cases where it is not considered safe. The eye, being a direct extension of the central nervous system, is reported to be involved in 20 percent of patients with primary brain lymphomas at diagnosis, if carefully examined.[266] Typically,

the vitreous, retina or choroid are involved. The initial evaluation of patients with primary brain lymphomas should therefore include a careful ophthalmologic evaluation including slit-lamp examination. Patients diagnosed initially with lymphomas of the ocular structures (as opposed to the extraocular orbital structures) should be examined in the same way as patients with primary brain lymphomas. Patients presenting with primary CNS lymphomas will rarely have systemic lymphoma at the time of diagnosis, hence the routine staging procedures would be expected to be negative in these patients and should not delay treatment.[267]

Patients with lymphomas involving the nasal cavity, nasopharynx, paranasal sinuses and extraocular orbital structures have a high risk of spread to the CNS.[268–270] They should have a lumbar puncture with analysis of the CSF, and should be examined with MRI (preferred) or CT of the relevant area to define the anatomic extent of the disease including possible invasion of bony structures. This is important for the planning of radiation portals and for follow-up. Patients with involvement of the Waldeyer ring have an increased risk of involvement of the gastrointestinal tract either at presentation or at relapse. In most series the risk is around 10 percent.[271–275] Gastroscopy and barium studies of the gastrointestinal tract are therefore recommended as part of the staging of these patients. The reverse may also be true; hence patients with gastrointestinal lymphomas should be carefully examined for involvement of the Waldeyer ring.[273] Gastric lymphoma is the single most common extranodal lymphoma.[51,276] Patients with gastric lymphoma are increasingly being managed after endoscopic biopsy and non-invasive staging procedures.[257,277,278] In order to assess the degree of invasion of the gastric wall and to identify patients at high risk of bleeding or perforation without performing a laparotomy, the technique of endoscopic ultrasound may be helpful.[279–282] Gastric mucosa-associated lymphoid tissue (MALT) lymphomas are related to *Helicobacter pylori* infection, hence biopsies should be examined accordingly. A third of patients with primary lymphoma of bone have involvement of more than one bone.[283] FDG-PET, MRI or radionuclide bone scans are highly sensitive for the detection of bone involvement and should be included in the staging investigations for patients with lymphoma of bone. Positive areas should be confirmed by plain radiographs.

Extranodal lymphomas in paired organs, e.g. orbital adnexae, salivary glands, breasts, ovaries, testes, have a propensity to spread to the contralateral organ.[243,263,264,273,284] Particular care should therefore be taken to examine the contralateral organ. For breast lymphomas this involves bilateral mammogram, for testicular lymphomas ultrasound of the contralateral testis. Patients with testicular lymphomas should be examined for CNS involvement as mentioned above, and also for involvement of the Waldeyer ring and skin, since the risk of involvement of either of these is about 10 percent.[264]

KEY POINTS

- The results of the staging investigations provide the basis for the rational management of the individual patient.
- The histologic subtype and the anatomic extent and localization of the disease are the factors deciding the treatment modalities to be employed. Additional prognostic factors, mostly reflecting the total tumor burden, the aggressiveness of the disease and the patient's tolerance to treatment, will influence treatment intensity. The staging investigations outlined in this chapter will provide the information needed to classify a patient in the currently used staging systems.
- The staging investigations provide information indicating whether immediate treatment of impending serious complications is needed. Some of these investigations may be prompted by specific symptoms, e.g. neurologic, cardiac or pulmonary. However, the staging procedures routinely performed in all patients may well disclose conditions which, although asymptomatic, require instant vigorous treatment, e.g. renal failure, ureteral obstruction, metabolic and electrolyte derangements.
- If radiotherapy is envisaged as part of the treatment, special procedures must be observed already at the time of the initial staging investigations, even if radiotherapy is to be administered at a later point in time after chemotherapy. For the optimal planning of radiation portals precise anatomic delineation of lymphomatous involvement before chemotherapy is necessary in order to encompass the entire initially involved area within the target volume. To this end, supplementary investigations, e.g. CT, MRI or FDG-PET scans of the relevant areas, may have to be carried out as part of the initial staging procedure.
- The staging investigations provide baseline information for comparison in later follow-up. With this purpose in mind it is important to anticipate situations in which evaluation of response to treatment may be difficult. This may be the case with large tumor masses or infiltration into neighboring structures, which are sometimes encountered, e.g. in the mediastinum. In these situations residual masses of unknown significance may pose problems after treatment. Supplementary CT, MRI or radionuclide scans may thus be indicated as part of the initial staging procedures, to be repeated after treatment for the evaluation of response.

REFERENCES

● = Key primary paper
◆ = Major review article

1. Greene FL, Page DL, Fleming ID et al. AJCC Cancer Staging Handbook, 6th ed. New York, Springer, 2004.
2. Sobin LH, Wittekind C. (eds) TNM classification of malignant tumours, 6th ed. New York, Wiley-Liss, 2002.
●3. Carbone PP, Kaplan HS, Musshoff K et al. Report of the committee on Hodgkin's disease staging classification. Cancer Res 1971; 31: 1860–1.
4. Kaplan HS, Rosenberg SA. The treatment of Hodgkin's disease. Med Clin North Am 1966; 50: 1591–610.
5. Musshoff K. Therapy and prognosis of two different forms of organ involvement in cases of malignant lymphoma (Hodgkin's disease, reticulum cell sarcoma, lymphosarcoma) as well as a report about stage division in these diseases. Klin Wochenschr 1970; 48: 673–8.
6. Connors JM, Klimo P. Is it an E lesion or stage IV? An unsettled issue in Hodgkin's disease staging. J Clin Oncol 1984; 2: 1421–3.
●7. Lister TA, Crowther D, Sutcliffe SB et al. Report of a committee convened to discuss the evaluation and staging of patients with Hodgkin's disease: Cotswolds meeting. J Clin Oncol 1989; 7: 1630–6.
●8. A predictive model for aggressive non-Hodgkin's lymphoma. The international non-Hodgkin's lymphoma prognostic factors project. N Engl J Med 1993; 329: 987–94.
9. Anderson T, DeVita VT Jr, Simon RM et al. Malignant lymphoma, II. Prognostic factors and response to treatment of 473 patients at the National Cancer Institute. Cancer 1982; 50: 2708–21.
10. Bastion Y, Berger F, Bryon PA et al. Follicular lymphomas: assessment of prognostic factors in 127 patients followed for 10 years. Ann Oncol 1991; 2(Suppl 2): 123–9.
11. Cabanillas F, Burke JS, Smith TL et al. Factors predicting for response and survival in adults with advanced non-Hodgkin's lymphoma. Arch Intern Med 1978; 138: 413–18.
12. Coiffier B, Gisselbrecht C, Vose JM et al. Prognostic factors in aggressive malignant lymphomas: description and validation of a prognostic index that could identify patients requiring a more intensive therapy. The Groupe d'Etudes des Lymphomes Agressifs. J Clin Oncol 1991; 9: 211–19.
13. Coiffier B, Shipp MA, Cabanillas F et al. Report of the first workshop on prognostic factors in large-cell lymphomas. Ann Oncol 1991; 2(Suppl 2): 213–17.
14. Cowan RA, Jones M, Harris M et al. Prognostic factors in high and intermediate grade non-Hodgkin's lymphoma. Br J Cancer 1989; 59: 276–82.
15. D'Amore F, Brincker H, Christensen BE et al. Non-Hodgkin's lymphoma in the elderly. A study of 602 patients aged 70 or older from a Danish population-based registry. The Danish LYFO-Study Group. Ann Oncol 1992; 3: 379–86.

16. Danieu L, Wong G, Koziner B, Clarkson B. Predictive model for prognosis in advanced diffuse histiocytic lymphoma. *Cancer Res* 1986; **46**: 5372–9.

17. Dixon DO, Neilan B, Jones SE *et al*. Effect of age on therapeutic outcome in advanced diffuse histiocytic lymphoma: the Southwest Oncology Group experience. *J Clin Oncol* 1986; **4**: 295–305.

18. Federico M, Vitolo U, Zinzani PL *et al*. Prognosis of follicular lymphoma: a predictive model based on a retrospective analysis of 987 cases. Intergruppo Italiano Linfomi. *Blood* 2000; **95**: 783–9.

19. Fisher RI, DeVita VT Jr, Johnson BL *et al*. Prognostic factors for advanced diffuse histiocytic lymphoma following treatment with combination chemotherapy. *Am J Med* 1977; **63**: 177–82.

20. Fisher RI, Hubbard SM, DeVita VT *et al*. Factors predicting long-term survival in diffuse mixed, histiocytic, or undifferentiated lymphoma. *Blood* 1981; **58**: 45–51.

21. Goldwein JW, Coia LR, Hanks GE. Prognostic factors in patients with early stage non-Hodgkin's lymphomas of the head and neck treated with definitive irradiation. *Int J Radiat Oncol Biol Phys* 1991; **20**: 45–51.

22. Gospodarowicz MK, Bush RS, Brown TC, Chua T. Prognostic factors in nodular lymphomas: a multivariate analysis based on the Princess Margaret Hospital experience. *Int J Radiat Oncol Biol Phys* 1984; **10**: 489–97.

23. Haddy TB, Adde MA, Magrath IT. CNS involvement in small noncleaved-cell lymphoma: is CNS disease per se a poor prognostic sign? *J Clin Oncol* 1991; **9**: 1973–82.

24. Horwich A, Catton CN, Quigley M *et al*. The management of early-stage aggressive non-Hodgkin's lymphoma. *Hematol Oncol* 1988; **6**: 291–8.

25. Hoskins PJ, Ng V, Spinelli JJ *et al*. Prognostic variables in patients with diffuse large-cell lymphoma treated with MACOP-B. *J Clin Oncol* 1991; **9**: 220–6.

26. Jacobs JP, Murray KJ, Schultz CJ *et al*. Central lymphatic irradiation for stage III nodular malignant lymphoma: long-term results. *J Clin Oncol* 1993; **11**: 233–8.

27. Jagannath S, Velasquez WS, Tucker SL *et al*. Tumor burden assessment and its implication for a prognostic model in advanced diffuse large-cell lymphoma. *J Clin Oncol* 1986; **4**: 859–65.

28. Kaminski MS, Coleman CN, Colby TV *et al*. Factors predicting survival in adults with stage I and II large-cell lymphoma treated with primary radiation therapy. *Ann Intern Med* 1986; **104**: 747–56.

29. Litam P, Swan F, Cabanillas F *et al*. Prognostic value of serum beta-2 microglobulin in low-grade lymphoma. *Ann Intern Med* 1991; **114**: 855–60.

30. Magrath I, Lee YJ, Anderson T *et al*. Prognostic factors in Burkitt's lymphoma: importance of total tumor burden. *Cancer* 1980; **45**: 1507–15.

31. Mauch P, Leonard R, Skarin A *et al*. Improved survival following combined radiation therapy and chemotherapy for unfavorable prognosis stage I–II non-Hodgkin's lymphomas. *J Clin Oncol* 1985; **3**: 1301–8.

32. Paryani SB, Hoppe RT, Cox RS *et al*. The role of radiation therapy in the management of stage III follicular lymphomas. *J Clin Oncol* 1984; **2**: 841–8.

33. Rodriguez J, Cabanillas F, McLaughlin P *et al*. A proposal for a simple staging system for intermediate grade lymphoma and immunoblastic lymphoma based on the 'tumor score'. *Ann Oncol* 1992; **3**: 711–17.

34. Romaguera JE, McLaughlin P, North L *et al*. Multivariate analysis of prognostic factors in stage IV follicular low-grade lymphoma: a risk model. *J Clin Oncol* 1991; **9**: 762–9.

35. Shimoyama M, Ota K, Kikuchi M *et al*. Chemotherapeutic results and prognostic factors of patients with advanced non-Hodgkin's lymphoma treated with VEPA or VEPA-M. *J Clin Oncol* 1988; **6**: 128–41.

36. Shipp MA, Yeap BY, Harrington DP *et al*. The m-BACOD combination chemotherapy regimen in large-cell lymphoma: analysis of the completed trial and comparison with the M-BACOD regimen. *J Clin Oncol* 1990; **8**: 84–93.

37. Simon R, Durrleman S, Hoppe RT *et al*. Prognostic factors for patients with diffuse large cell or immunoblastic non-Hodgkin's lymphomas: experience of the non-Hodgkin's Lymphoma Pathologic Classification Project. *Med Pediatr Oncol* 1990; **18**: 89–96.

38. Steward WP, Crowther D, McWilliam LJ *et al*. Maintenance chlorambucil after CVP in the management of advanced stage, low-grade histologic type non-Hodgkin's lymphoma. A randomized prospective study with an assessment of prognostic factors. *Cancer* 1988; **61**: 441–7.

39. Sullivan KM, Neiman PE, Kadin ME *et al*. Combined modality therapy of advanced non-Hodgkin's lymphoma: an analysis of remission duration and survival in 95 patients. *Blood* 1983; **62**: 51–61.

40. Sutcliffe SB, Gospodarowicz MK, Bush RS *et al*. Role of radiation therapy in localized non-Hodgkin's lymphoma. *Radiother Oncol* 1985; **4**: 211–23.

41. Swan F Jr, Velasquez WS, Tucker S *et al*. A new serologic staging system for large-cell lymphomas based on initial beta 2-microglobulin and lactate dehydrogenase levels. *J Clin Oncol* 1989; **7**: 1518–27.

42. Velasquez WS, Jagannath S, Tucker SL *et al*. Risk classification as the basis for clinical staging of diffuse large-cell lymphoma derived from 10-year survival data. *Blood* 1989; **74**: 551–7.

43. Velasquez WS, Fuller LM, Jagannath S *et al*. Stages I and II diffuse large cell lymphomas: prognostic factors and long-term results with CHOP-bleo and radiotherapy. *Blood* 1991; **77**: 942–7.

44. Gobbi PG, Broglia C, Di Giulio G *et al*. The clinical value of tumor burden at diagnosis in Hodgkin lymphoma. *Cancer* 2004; **101**: 1824–34.

●45. Hasenclever D, Diehl V. A prognostic score for advanced Hodgkin's disease. International prognostic factors project on advanced Hodgkin's disease. *N Engl J Med* 1998; **339**: 1506–14.

46. Specht L. Prognostic factors in Hodgkin's disease. *Cancer Treat Rev* 1991; **18**: 21–53.

47. Specht L. Tumour burden as the main indicator of prognosis in Hodgkin's disease. *Eur J Cancer* 1992; **28A**: 1982–5.

◆48. Specht L. Hodgkin lymphoma. In: Gospodarowicz MK, O'Sullivan B, Sobin LH. (eds) *Prognostic factors in cancer*, 3rd ed. New Jersey, Wiley-Liss, 2006: 281–4.

●49. Armitage JO, Weisenburger DD. New approach to classifying non-Hodgkin's lymphomas: clinical features of the major histologic subtypes. Non-Hodgkin's Lymphoma Classification Project. *J Clin Oncol* 1998; **16**: 2780–95.

50. Henry-Amar M, Aeppli DM, Anderson J *et al.* Workshop statistical report. In: Somers R, Henry-Amar M, Meerwaldt YH, Carde P (eds) *Treatment strategies in Hodgkin's disease*. London: INSERM/John Libby Eurotext. 1990; 169–425.

51. D'Amore F, Christensen BE, Brincker H *et al.* Clinicopathological features and prognostic factors in extranodal non-Hodgkin lymphomas. Danish LYFO Study Group. *Eur J Cancer* 1991; **27**: 1201–8.

52. Freeman C, Berg JW, Cutler SJ. Occurrence and prognosis of extranodal lymphomas. *Cancer* 1972; **29**: 252–60.

53. Gurney KA, Cartwright RA. Increasing incidence and descriptive epidemiology of extranodal non-Hodgkin lymphoma in parts of England and Wales. *Hematol J* 2002; **3**: 95–104.

54. Krol AD, le Cessie S, Snijder S *et al.* Primary extranodal non-Hodgkin's lymphoma (NHL): the impact of alternative definitions tested in the Comprehensive Cancer Centre West population-based NHL registry. *Ann Oncol* 2003; **14**: 131–9.

55. Moller MB, Pedersen NT, Christensen BE. Diffuse large B-cell lymphoma: clinical implications of extranodal versus nodal presentation – a population-based study of 1575 cases. *Br J Haematol* 2004; **124**: 151–9.

56. Magrath IT. Malignant non-Hodgkin's lymphomas in children. In: Pizzo PA, Poplack DG. (eds) *Principles and practice of pediatric oncology*, 4th ed. Philadelphia, Lippincott Williams & Wilkins, 2002: 661–705.

●57. Murphy SB. Classification, staging and end results of treatment of childhood non-Hodgkin's lymphomas: dissimilarities from lymphomas in adults. *Semin Oncol* 1980; **7**: 332–9.

58. Noordijk EM, Carde P, Mandard AM *et al.* Preliminary results of the EORTC-GPMC controlled clinical trial H7 in early-stage Hodgkin's disease. EORTC Lymphoma Cooperative Group. Groupe Pierre-et-Marie-Curie. *Ann Oncol* 1994; **5** (Suppl 2): 107–12.

◆59. Diehl V, Thomas RK, Re D. Part II: Hodgkin's lymphoma – diagnosis and treatment. *Lancet Oncol* 2004; **5**: 19–26.

60. Glimelius B, Specht L, Nome O, Tuurpeenniemi-Hujanen T. Treatment in adult patients with early stages of Hodgkin's disease. Nordic Lymphoma Group. Uppsala, Regionalt Onkologiskt Centrum Örebroregionen, 1999.

61. Shipp MA, Harrington DP, Klatt MM *et al.* Identification of major prognostic subgroups of patients with large-cell lymphoma treated with m-BACOD or M-BACOD. *Ann Intern Med* 1986; **104**: 757–65.

62. Miller TP, Dahlberg S, Cassady JR *et al.* Chemotherapy alone compared with chemotherapy plus radiotherapy for localized intermediate- and high-grade non-Hodgkin's lymphoma. *N Engl J Med* 1998; **339**: 21–6.

63. Gallamini A, Stelitano C, Calvi R *et al.* Peripheral T-cell lymphoma unspecified (PTCL-U): a new prognostic model from a retrospective multicentric clinical study. *Blood* 2004; **103**: 2474–9.

●64. Solal-Celigny P, Roy P, Colombat P *et al.* Follicular lymphoma international prognostic index. *Blood* 2004; **104**: 1258–65.

65. Jones SE, Miller TP, Connors JM. Long-term follow-up and analysis for prognostic factors for patients with limited-stage diffuse large-cell lymphoma treated with initial chemotherapy with or without adjuvant radiotherapy. *J Clin Oncol* 1989; **7**: 1186–91.

66. Vose JM, Armitage JO, Weisenburger DD *et al.* The importance of age in survival of patients treated with chemotherapy for aggressive non-Hodgkin's lymphoma. *J Clin Oncol* 1988; **6**: 1838–44.

67. Adida C, Haioun C, Gaulard P *et al.* Prognostic significance of survivin expression in diffuse large B-cell lymphomas. *Blood* 2000; **96**: 1921–5.

68. Alici S, Bavbek SE, Kaytan E *et al.* Prognostic factors in localized aggressive non-Hodgkin's lymphoma. *Am J Clin Oncol* 2003; **26**: 1–5.

69. Alizadeh AA, Eisen MB, Davis RE *et al.* Distinct types of diffuse large B-cell lymphoma identified by gene expression profiling. *Nature* 2000; **403**: 503–11.

70. Banham AH, Connors JM, Brown PJ *et al.* Expression of the FOXP1 transcription factor is strongly associated with inferior survival in patients with diffuse large B-cell lymphoma. *Clin Cancer Res* 2005; **11**: 1065–72.

71. Barrans SL, Carter I, Owen RG *et al.* Germinal center phenotype and bcl-2 expression combined with the International Prognostic Index improves patient risk stratification in diffuse large B-cell lymphoma. *Blood* 2002; **99**: 1136–43.

72. Biasoli I, Morais JC, Scheliga A *et al.* CD10 and Bcl-2 expression combined with the International Prognostic Index can identify subgroups of patients with diffuse large-cell lymphoma with very good or very poor prognoses. *Histopathology* 2005; **46**: 328–33.

73. Conconi A, Zucca E, Roggero E *et al.* Prognostic models for diffuse large B-cell lymphoma. *Hematol Oncol* 2000; **18**: 61–73.

74. Goto H, Tsurumi H, Takemura M *et al.* Serum-soluble interleukin-2 receptor (sIL-2R) level determines clinical outcome in patients with aggressive non-Hodgkin's lymphoma: in combination with the International Prognostic Index. *J Cancer Res Clin Oncol* 2005; **131**: 73–9.

75. Hans CP, Weisenburger DD, Greiner TC *et al.* Confirmation of the molecular classification of diffuse large B-cell lymphoma by immunohistochemistry using a tissue microarray. *Blood* 2004; **103**: 275–82.

76. Jerkeman M, Anderson H, Dictor M et al. Assessment of biological prognostic factors provides clinically relevant information in patients with diffuse large B-cell lymphoma – a Nordic Lymphoma Group study. *Ann Hematol* 2004; **83**: 414–19.

77. Juszczynski P, Kalinka E, Bienvenu J et al. Human leukocyte antigens class II and tumor necrosis factor genetic polymorphisms are independent predictors of non-Hodgkin lymphoma outcome. *Blood* 2002; **100**: 3037–40.

78. Leroy K, Haioun C, Lepage E et al. p53 gene mutations are associated with poor survival in low and low-intermediate risk diffuse large B-cell lymphomas. *Ann Oncol* 2002; **13**: 1108–15.

79. Lorand-Metze I, Pereira FG, Costa FP, Metze K. Proliferation in non-Hodgkin's lymphomas and its prognostic value related to staging parameters. *Cell Oncol* 2004; **26**: 63–71.

80. Lossos IS, Jones CD, Warnke R et al. Expression of a single gene, BCL-6, strongly predicts survival in patients with diffuse large B-cell lymphoma. *Blood* 2001; **98**: 945–51.

81. Lossos IS, Alizadeh AA, Rajapaksa R et al. HGAL is a novel interleukin-4-inducible gene that strongly predicts survival in diffuse large B-cell lymphoma. *Blood* 2003; **101**: 433–40.

82. Lossos IS, Czerwinski DK, Alizadeh AA et al. Prediction of survival in diffuse large-B-cell lymphoma based on the expression of six genes. *N Engl J Med* 2004; **350**: 1828–37.

83. Raty R, Franssila K, Joensuu H et al. Ki-67 expression level, histological subtype, and the International Prognostic Index as outcome predictors in mantle cell lymphoma. *Eur J Haematol* 2002; **69**: 11–20.

84. Rosenwald A, Wright G, Chan WC et al. The use of molecular profiling to predict survival after chemotherapy for diffuse large-B-cell lymphoma. *N Engl J Med* 2002; **346**: 1937–47.

85. Saez AI, Saez AJ, Artiga MJ et al. Building an outcome predictor model for diffuse large B-cell lymphoma. *Am J Pathol* 2004; **164**: 613–22.

86. Shipp MA, Ross KN, Tamayo P et al. Diffuse large B-cell lymphoma outcome prediction by gene-expression profiling and supervised machine learning. *Nat Med* 2002; **8**: 68–74.

87. Terol MJ, Tormo M, Martinez-Climent JA et al. Soluble intercellular adhesion molecule-1 (s-ICAM-1/s-CD54) in diffuse large B-cell lymphoma: association with clinical characteristics and outcome. *Ann Oncol* 2003; **14**: 467–74.

88. Moller MB, Christensen BE, Pedersen NT. Prognosis of localized diffuse large B-cell lymphoma in younger patients. *Cancer* 2003; **98**: 516–21.

89. Cortelazzo S, Rossi A, Oldani E et al. The modified International Prognostic Index can predict the outcome of localized primary intestinal lymphoma of both extranodal marginal zone B-cell and diffuse large B-cell histologies. *Br J Haematol* 2002; **118**: 218–28.

90. Soubeyran P, Eghbali H, Bonichon F et al. Low-grade follicular lymphomas: analysis of prognosis in a series of 281 patients. *Eur J Cancer* 1991; **27**: 1606–13.

91. Coiffier B. How should prognostic factors influence therapy in follicular lymphomas? *Ann Oncol* 1991; **2**: 619–20.

92. Maartense E, le Cessie S, Kluin-Nelemans HC et al. Age-related differences among patients with follicular lymphoma and the importance of prognostic scoring systems: analysis from a population-based non-Hodgkin's lymphoma registry. *Ann Oncol* 2002; **13**: 1275–84.

93. Perea G, Altes A, Montoto S et al. International and Italian prognostic indices in follicular lymphoma. *Haematologica* 2003; **88**: 700–4.

94. Montoto S, Lopez-Guillermo A, Altes A et al. Predictive value of Follicular Lymphoma International Prognostic Index (FLIPI) in patients with follicular lymphoma at first progression. *Ann Oncol* 2004; **15**: 1484–9.

95. Bjorck E, Ek S, Landgren O et al. High expression of cyclin B1 predicts a favorable outcome in patients with follicular lymphoma. *Blood* 2005; **105**: 2908–15.

96. Kok M, Bonfrer JM, Korse CM et al. Serum soluble CD27, but not thymidine kinase, is an independent prognostic factor for outcome in indolent non-Hodgkin's lymphoma. *Tumour Biol* 2003; **24**: 53–60.

97. Lopez-Guillermo A, Cid J, Salar A et al. Peripheral T-cell lymphomas: initial features, natural history, and prognostic factors in a series of 174 patients diagnosed according to the R.E.A.L. Classification. *Ann Oncol* 1998; **9**: 849–55.

●98. A clinical evaluation of the International Lymphoma Study Group classification of non-Hodgkin's lymphoma. The Non-Hodgkin's Lymphoma Classification Project. *Blood* 1997; **89**: 3909–18.

99. Falini B, Pileri S, Zinzani PL et al. ALK+ lymphoma: clinico-pathological findings and outcome. *Blood* 1999; **93**: 2697–706.

100. Gascoyne RD, Aoun P, Wu D et al. Prognostic significance of anaplastic lymphoma kinase (ALK) protein expression in adults with anaplastic large cell lymphoma. *Blood* 1999; **93**: 3913–21.

101. Hermans J, Krol AD, Van Groningen K et al. International Prognostic Index for aggressive non-Hodgkin's lymphoma is valid for all malignancy grades. *Blood* 1995; **86**: 1460–3.

102. Nola M, Pavletic SZ, Weisenburger DD et al. Prognostic factors influencing survival in patients with B-cell small lymphocytic lymphoma. *Am J Hematol* 2004; **77**: 31–5.

103. Robbins KT, Fuller LM, Vlasak M et al. Primary lymphomas of the nasal cavity and paranasal sinuses. *Cancer* 1985; **56**: 814–19.

104. Shirato H, Tsujii H, Arimoto T et al. Early stage head and neck non-Hodgkin's lymphoma. The effect of tumor burden on prognosis. *Cancer* 1986; **58**: 2312–19.

105. Tran LM, Mark R, Fu YS et al. Primary non-Hodgkin's lymphomas of the paranasal sinuses and nasal cavity. A report of 18 cases with stage IE disease. *Am J Clin Oncol* 1992; **15**: 222–5.

106. Musshoff K. Klinische stadieneinteilung der nicht-Hodgkin-lymphome. *Strahlentherapie* 1977; **153**: 218–21.

107. Azab MB, Henry-Amar M, Rougier P et al. Prognostic factors in primary gastrointestinal non-Hodgkin's lymphoma. A multivariate analysis, report of 106 cases, and review of the literature. Cancer 1989; 64: 1208–17.

108. Weingrad DN, Decosse JJ, Sherlock P et al. Primary gastrointestinal lymphoma: a 30-year review. Cancer 1982; 49: 1258–65.

109. Gospodarowicz MK, Bush RS, Brown TC, Chua T. Curability of gastrointestinal lymphoma with combined surgery and radiation. Int J Radiat Oncol Biol Phys 1983; 9: 3–9.

110. Hockey MS, Powell J, Crocker J, Fielding JW. Primary gastric lymphoma. Br J Surg 1987; 74: 483–7.

111. Lim FE, Hartman AS, Tan EG et al. Factors in the prognosis of gastric lymphoma. Cancer 1977; 39: 1715–20.

112. Blackledge G, Bush H, Dodge OG, Crowther D. A study of gastro-intestinal lymphoma. Clin Oncol 1979; 5: 209–19.

●113. Rohatiner A, D'Amore F, Coiffier B et al. Report on a workshop convened to discuss the pathological and staging classifications of gastrointestinal tract lymphoma. Ann Oncol 1994; 5: 397–400.

114. Ansell SM, Habermann TM, Kurtin PJ et al. Predictive capacity of the International Prognostic Factor Index in patients with peripheral T-cell lymphoma. J Clin Oncol 1997; 15: 2296–301.

115. Gisselbrecht C, Gaulard P, Lepage E et al. Prognostic significance of T-cell phenotype in aggressive non-Hodgkin's lymphomas. Groupe d'Etudes des Lymphomes de l'Adulte (GELA). Blood 1998; 92: 76–82.

116. Reiser M, Josting A, Soltani M et al. T-cell non-Hodgkin's lymphoma in adults: clinicopathological characteristics, response to treatment and prognostic factors. Leuk Lymphoma 2002; 43: 805–11.

117. Savage KJ, Chhanabhai M, Gascoyne RD, Connors JM. Characterization of peripheral T-cell lymphomas in a single North American institution by the WHO classification. Ann Oncol 2004; 15: 1467–75.

●118. Bunn PA Jr, Lamberg SI. Report of the committee on staging and classification of cutaneous T-cell lymphomas. Cancer Treat Rep 1979; 63: 725–8.

119. Horwitz SM, Duncan LM, Kim YH, Hoppe RT. Cutaneous B-cell lymphomas. In: Mauch PM, Armitage JO, Coiffier B et al. (eds) Non-Hodgkin's lymphomas. Philadelphia: Lippincott Williams & Wilkins, 2004: 319–31.

120. Kadin ME, Liu HL, Kim YH, Hoppe RT. CD30+ cutaneous lymphoproliferative disease (anaplastic large-cell lymphoma) and lymphomatoid papulosis. In: Mauch PM, Armitage JO, Coiffier B et al. (eds) Non-Hodgkin's lymphomas. Philadelphia: Lippincott Williams & Wilkins, 2004: 333–43.

121. Anderson JR, Jenkin RD, Wilson JF et al. Long-term follow-up of patients treated with COMP or LSA2L2 therapy for childhood non-Hodgkin's lymphoma: a report of CCG-551 from the Children's Cancer Group. J Clin Oncol 1993; 11: 1024–32.

122. Murphy SB, Fairclough DL, Hutchison RE, Berard CW. Non-Hodgkin's lymphomas of childhood: an analysis of the histology, staging, and response to treatment of 338 cases at a single institution. J Clin Oncol 1989; 7: 186–93.

123. Wollner N, Burchenal JH, Lieberman PH et al. Non-Hodgkin's lymphoma in children. A comparative study of two modalities of therapy. Cancer 1976; 37: 123–34.

124. Ramaswamy S, Golub TR. DNA microarrays in clinical oncology. J Clin Oncol 2002; 20: 1932–41.

125. Armitage JO. Defining the stages of aggressive non-Hodgkin's lymphoma – a work in progress. N Engl J Med 2005; 352: 1250–2.

◆126. Gascoyne RD. Emerging prognostic factors in diffuse large B cell lymphoma. Curr Opin Oncol 2004; 16: 436–41.

127. Bruneton JN, Normand F, Balu-Maestro C et al. Lymphomatous superficial lymph nodes: US detection. Radiology 1987; 165: 233–5.

128. Bitran JD, Golomb HM, Ultmann JE et al. Non-Hodgkin's lymphoma, poorly differentiated lymphocytic and mixed cell types: results of sequential staging procedures, response to therapy, and survival of 100 patients. Cancer 1978; 42: 88–95.

129. Chabner BA, Johnson RE, Chretien PB et al. Percutaneous liver biopsy, peritoneoscopy and laparotomy: an assessment of relative merits in the lymphomata. Br J Cancer 1975; 31(Suppl 2): 242–7.

130. Chabner BA, Johnson RE, DeVita VT et al. Sequential staging in non-Hodgkin's lymphoma. Cancer Treat Rep 1977; 61: 993–7.

131. Goffinet DR, Warnke R, Dunnick NR et al. Clinical and surgical (laparotomy) evaluation of patients with non-Hodgkin's lymphomas. Cancer Treat Rep 1977; 61: 981–92.

132. Lotz MJ, Chabner B, DeVita VT Jr et al. Pathological staging of 100 consecutive untreated patients with non-Hodgkin's lymphomas: extramedullary sites of disease. Cancer 1976; 37: 266–70.

133. Moran EM, Ultmann JE, Ferguson DJ et al. Staging laparotomy in non-Hodgkin's lymphoma. Br J Cancer 1975; 31(Suppl 2): 228–36.

134. Bloomfield CD, McKenna RW, Brunning RD. Significance of haematological parameters in the non-Hodgkin's malignant lymphomas. Br J Haematol 1976; 32: 41–6.

135. Coller BS, Chabner BA, Gralnick HR. Frequencies and patterns of bone marrow involvement in non-Hodgkin lymphomas: observations on the value of bilateral biopsies. Am J Hematol 1977; 3: 105–19.

136. Conlan MG, Armitage JO, Bast M, Weisenburger DD. Clinical significance of hematologic parameters in non-Hodgkin's lymphoma at diagnosis. Cancer 1991; 67: 1389–95.

137. Stein RS, Ultmann JE, Byrne GE Jr et al. Bone marrow involvement in non-Hodgkin's lymphoma: implications for staging and therapy. Cancer 1976; 37: 629–36.

138. Specht L, Hasenclever D. Prognostic factors in Hodgkin lymphoma. In: Hoppe RT, Mauch PM, Armitage JO et al. (eds) Hodgkin lymphoma. Philadelphia: Lippincott Williams & Wilkins, 2007: 157–74.

139. Belliveau RE, Abt AB, Wiernik PH. Hepatic enzymes in Hodgkin's and non Hodgkin's lymphoma. *Tumori* 1979; **65**: 215–19.

140. Veronesi U, Musumeci R, Pizzetti F *et al.* Proceedings: the value of staging laparotomy in non-Hodgkin's lymphomas (with emphasis on the histiocytic type). *Cancer* 1974; **33**: 446–59.

141. Castellino RA, Goffinet DR, Blank N *et al.* The role of radiography in the staging of non-Hodgkin's lymphoma with laparotomy correlation. *Radiology* 1974; **110**: 329–38.

142. Castellino RA, Blank N, Hoppe RT, Cho C. Hodgkin disease: contributions of chest CT in the initial staging evaluation. *Radiology* 1986; **160**: 603–5.

143. Celikoglu F, Teirstein AS, Krellenstein DJ, Strauchen JA. Pleural effusion in non-Hodgkin's lymphoma. *Chest* 1992; **101**: 1357–60.

144. Filly R, Bland N, Castellino RA. Radiographic distribution of intrathoracic disease in previously untreated patients with Hodgkin's disease and non-Hodgkin's lymphoma. *Radiology* 1976; **120**: 277–81.

145. Castellino RA, Hilton S, O'Brien JP, Portlock CS. Non-Hodgkin lymphoma: contribution of chest CT in the initial staging evaluation. *Radiology* 1996; **199**: 129–32.

146. Khoury MB, Godwin JD, Halvorsen R *et al.* Role of chest CT in non-Hodgkin lymphoma. *Radiology* 1986; **158**: 659–62.

147. Romano M, Libshitz HI. Hodgkin disease and non-Hodgkin lymphoma: plain chest radiographs and chest computed tomography of thoracic involvement in previously untreated patients. *Radiol Med Torino* 1998; **95**: 49–53.

148. Salonen O, Kivisaari L, Standertskjold-Nordenstam CG *et al.* Chest radiography and computed tomography in the evaluation of mediastinal adenopathy in lymphoma. *Acta Radiol* 1987; **28**: 747–50.

149. Castellani R, Bonadonna G, Spinelli P *et al.* Sequential pathologic staging of untreated non-Hodgkin's lymphomas by laparoscopy and laparotomy combined with marrow biopsy. *Cancer* 1977; **40**: 2322–8.

150. Chabner BA, Johnson RE, Young RC *et al.* Sequential nonsurgical and surgical staging of non-Hodgkin's lymphoma. *Cancer* 1978; **42**: 922–5.

151. British National Lymphoma Investigation. The value of laparotomy and splenectomy in the management of early Hodgkin's disease. A report from the British National Lymphoma Investigation. *Clin Radiol* 1975; **26**: 151–7.

152. Castellino RA, Marglin SI. Imaging of abdominal and pelvic lymph nodes: lymphography or computed tomography? *Invest Radiol* 1982; **17**: 433–43.

153. Heifetz LJ, Fuller LM, Rodgers RW *et al.* Laparotomy findings in lymphangiogram-staged I and non-Hodgkin's lymphomas. *Cancer* 1980; **45**: 2778–86.

154. Kaplan HS, Dorfman RF, Nelsen TS, Rosenberg SA. Staging laparotomy and splenectomy in Hodgkin's disease: analysis of indications and patterns of involvement in 285 consecutive, unselected patients. *Natl Cancer Inst Monogr* 1973; **36**: 291–301.

155. Piro AJ, Hellman S, Moloney WC. The influence of laparotomy on management decisions in Hodgkin's disease. *Arch Intern Med* 1972; **130**: 844–8.

156. Best JJ, Blackledge G, Forbes WS *et al.* Computed tomography of abdomen in staging and clinical management of lymphoma. *Br Med J* 1978; **2**: 1675–7.

157. Breiman RS, Castellino RA, Harell GS *et al.* CT-pathologic correlations in Hodgkin's disease and non-Hodgkin's lymphoma. *Radiology* 1978; **126**: 159–66.

158. Lee JK, Stanley RJ, Sagel SS, Levitt RG. Accuracy of computed tomography in detecting intraabdominal and pelvic adenopathy in lymphoma. *AJR Am J Roentgenol* 1978; **131**: 311–15.

159. Neumann CH, Parker BR, Castellino RA. Hodgkin's disease and the non-Hodgkin lymphomas. In: Bragg DG, Rubin P, Youker JE. (eds) *Oncologic imaging.* New York: Pergamon Press, 1985: 477–500.

160. Mellor JA, Simmons AV, Barnard DL, Cartwright SC. A retrospective evaluation of mediastinal tomograms, isotope liver scans, and isotope bone scans in the staging and management of patients with lymphoma. *Cancer* 1983; **52**: 2227–9.

161. Hoane BR, Shields AF, Porter BA, Borrow JW. Comparison of initial lymphoma staging using computed tomography (CT) and magnetic resonance (MR) imaging. *Am J Hematol* 1994; **47**: 100–5.

162. Jung G, Heindel W, Bergwelt-Baildon M *et al.* Abdominal lymphoma staging: is MR imaging with T2-weighted turbo-spin-echo sequence a diagnostic alternative to contrast-enhanced spiral CT? *J Comput Assist Tomogr* 2000; **24**: 783–7.

163. Kellenberger CJ, Miller SF, Khan M *et al.* Initial experience with FSE STIR whole-body MR imaging for staging lymphoma in children. *Eur Radiol* 2004; **14**: 1829–41.

164. Skillings JR, Bramwell V, Nicholson RL *et al.* A prospective study of magnetic resonance imaging in lymphoma staging. *Cancer* 1991; **67**: 1838–43.

165. Tesoro-Tess JD, Balzarini L, Ceglia E *et al.* Magnetic resonance imaging in the initial staging of Hodgkin's disease and non-Hodgkin lymphoma. *Eur J Radiol* 1991; **12**: 81–90.

166. Weinreb JC, Brateman L, Maravilla KR. Magnetic resonance imaging of hepatic lymphoma. *AJR Am J Roentgenol* 1984; **143**: 1211–14.

167. Altehoefer C, Blum U, Bathmann J *et al.* Comparative diagnostic accuracy of magnetic resonance imaging and immunoscintigraphy for detection of bone marrow involvement in patients with malignant lymphoma. *J Clin Oncol* 1997; **15**: 1754–60.

168. Hermann G, Klein MJ, Abdelwahab IF, Kenan S. MRI appearance of primary non-Hodgkin's lymphoma of bone. *Skeletal Radiol* 1997; **26**: 629–32.

169. Hoane BR, Shields AF, Porter BA, Shulman HM. Detection of lymphomatous bone marrow involvement with magnetic resonance imaging. *Blood* 1991; **78**: 728–38.

170. Porter BA, Shields AF, Olson DO. Magnetic resonance imaging of bone marrow disorders. *Radiol Clin North Am* 1986; **24**: 269–89.

171. Shields AF, Porter BA, Churchley S *et al.* The detection of bone marrow involvement by lymphoma using magnetic resonance imaging. *J Clin Oncol* 1987; **5**: 225–30.

172. White LM, Schweitzer ME, Khalili K *et al.* MR imaging of primary lymphoma of bone: variability of T2-weighted signal intensity. *AJR Am J Roentgenol* 1998; **170**: 1243–7.

173. Anderson KC, Leonard RC, Canellos GP *et al.* High-dose gallium imaging in lymphoma. *Am J Med* 1983; **75**: 327–31.

174. Andrews GA, Hubner KF, Greenlaw RH. Ga-67 citrate imaging in malignant lymphoma: final report of cooperative group. *J Nucl Med* 1978; **19**: 1013–19.

175. Brown ML, O'Donnell JB, Thrall JH *et al.* Gallium-67 scintigraphy in untreated and treated non-hodgkin lymphomas. *J Nucl Med* 1978; **19**: 875–9.

176. Front D, Bar-Shalom R, Israel O. The continuing clinical role of gallium 67 scintigraphy in the age of receptor imaging. *Semin Nucl Med* 1997; **27**: 68–74.

177. Glass RB, Fernbach SK, Conway JJ, Shkolnik A. Gallium scintigraphy in American Burkitt lymphoma: accurate assessment of tumor load and prognosis. *AJR Am J Roentgenol* 1985; **145**: 671–6.

178. Nejmeddine F, Raphael M, Martin A *et al.* 67Ga scintigraphy in B-cell non-Hodgkin's lymphoma: correlation of 67Ga uptake with histology and transferrin receptor expression. *J Nucl Med* 1999; **40**: 40–5.

179. Sandrock D, Lastoria S, Magrath IT, Neumann RD. The role of gallium-67 tumour scintigraphy in patients with small, non-cleaved cell lymphoma. *Eur J Nucl Med* 1993; **20**: 119–22.

180. Tumeh SS, Rosenthal DS, Kaplan WD *et al.* Lymphoma: evaluation with Ga-67 SPECT. *Radiology* 1987; **164**: 111–14.

181. Turner DA, Fordham EW, Ali A, Slayton RE. Gallium-67 imaging in the management of Hodgkin's disease and other malignant lymphomas. *Semin Nucl Med* 1978; **8**: 205–18.

182. Bangerter M, Kotzerke J, Griesshammer M *et al.* Positron emission tomography with 18-fluorodeoxyglucose in the staging and follow-up of lymphoma in the chest. *Acta Oncol* 1999; **38**: 799–804.

183. Buchmann I, Moog F, Schirrmeister H, Reske SN. Positron emission tomography for detection and staging of malignant lymphoma. *Recent Results Cancer Res* 2000; **156**: 78–89.

184. Buchmann I, Reinhardt M, Elsner K *et al.* 2-(fluorine-18) fluoro-2-deoxy-D-glucose positron emission tomography in the detection and staging of malignant lymphoma. A bicenter trial. *Cancer* 2001; **91**: 889–99.

185. Depas G, De Barsy C, Jerusalem G *et al.* 18F-FDG PET in children with lymphomas. *Eur J Nucl Med Mol Imaging* 2004; **32**: 31–8.

◆186. Hutchings M, Eigtved AI, Specht L. FDG-PET in the clinical management of Hodgkin lymphoma. *Crit Rev Oncol Hematol* 2004; **52**: 19–32.

187. Jerusalem G, Beguin Y, Fassotte MF *et al.* Whole-body positron emission tomography using 18F-fluorodeoxyglucose compared to standard procedures for staging patients with Hodgkin's disease. *Haematologica* 2001; **86**: 266–73.

188. Jerusalem GH, Beguin YP. Positron emission tomography in non-Hodgkin's lymphoma (NHL): relationship between tracer uptake and pathological findings, including preliminary experience in the staging of low-grade NHL. *Clin Lymphoma* 2002; **3**: 56–61.

189. Menzel C, Dobert N, Mitrou P *et al.* Positron emission tomography for the staging of Hodgkin's lymphoma – increasing the body of evidence in favor of the method. *Acta Oncol* 2002; **41**: 430–6.

190. Moog F, Bangerter M, Diederichs CG *et al.* Lymphoma: role of whole-body 2-deoxy-2-[F-18]fluoro-D-glucose (FDG) PET in nodal staging. *Radiology* 1997; **203**: 795–800.

191. Moog F, Bangerter M, Diederichs CG *et al.* Extranodal malignant lymphoma: detection with FDG PET versus CT. *Radiology* 1998; **206**: 475–81.

192. Najjar F, Hustinx R, Jerusalem G *et al.* Positron emission tomography (PET) for staging low-grade non-Hodgkin's lymphomas (NHL). *Cancer Biother Radiopharm* 2001; **16**: 297–304.

193. Rini JN, Leonidas JC, Tomas MB, Palestro CJ. 18F-FDG PET versus CT for evaluating the spleen during initial staging of lymphoma. *J Nucl Med* 2003; **44**: 1072–4.

194. Schaefer NG, Hany TF, Taverna C *et al.* Non-Hodgkin lymphoma and Hodgkin disease: coregistered FDG PET and CT at staging and restaging – do we need contrast-enhanced CT? *Radiology* 2004; **232**: 823–9.

◆195. Schiepers C, Filmont JE, Czernin J. PET for staging of Hodgkin's disease and non-Hodgkin's lymphoma. *Eur J Nucl Med Mol Imaging* 2003; **30**(Suppl 1): s82–88.

196. Stumpe KD, Urbinelli M, Steinert HC *et al.* Whole-body positron emission tomography using fluorodeoxyglucose for staging of lymphoma: effectiveness and comparison with computed tomography. *Eur J Nucl Med* 1998; **25**: 721–8.

197. Hoffmann M, Kletter K, Becherer A *et al.* 18F-fluorodeoxyglucose positron emission tomography (18F-FDG-PET) for staging and follow-up of marginal zone B-cell lymphoma. *Oncology* 2003; **64**: 336–40.

198. Jerusalem G, Beguin Y, Najjar F *et al.* Positron emission tomography (PET) with 18F-fluorodeoxyglucose (18F-FDG) for the staging of low-grade non-Hodgkin's lymphoma (NHL). *Ann Oncol* 2001; **12**: 825–30.

199. Lee J, Park CH, Kim HC, Kim HS. Dichotomy between Tc-99m MDP bone scan and fluorine-18 fluorodeoxyglucose coincidence detection positron emission tomography in patients with non-Hodgkin's lymphoma. *Clin Nucl Med* 2000; **25**: 532–5.

200. Moog F, Kotzerke J, Reske SN. FDG PET can replace bone scintigraphy in primary staging of malignant lymphoma. *J Nucl Med* 1999; **40**: 1407–13.

201. Carr R, Barrington SF, Madan B et al. Detection of lymphoma in bone marrow by whole-body positron emission tomography. Blood 1998; 91: 3340–6.

202. Moog F, Bangerter M, Kotzerke J et al. 18-F-fluorodeoxyglucose-positron emission tomography as a new approach to detect lymphomatous bone marrow. J Clin Oncol 1998; 16: 603–9.

203. Bar-Shalom R, Mor M, Yefremov N, Goldsmith SJ. The value of Ga-67 scintigraphy and F-18 fluorodeoxyglucose positron emission tomography in staging and monitoring the response of lymphoma to treatment. Semin Nucl Med 2001; 31: 177–90.

204. Even-Sapir E, Israel O. Gallium-67 scintigraphy: a cornerstone in functional imaging of lymphoma. Eur J Nucl Med Mol Imaging 2003; 30(Suppl 1): s65–81.

205. Friedberg JW, Fischman A, Neuberg D et al. FDG-PET is superior to gallium scintigraphy in staging and more sensitive in the follow-up of patients with de novo Hodgkin lymphoma: a blinded comparison. Leuk Lymphoma 2004; 45: 85–92.

206. Kostakoglu L, Goldsmith SJ. Fluorine-18 fluorodeoxyglucose positron emission tomography in the staging and follow-up of lymphoma: is it time to shift gears? Eur J Nucl Med 2000; 27: 1564–78.

207. Kostakoglu L, Leonard JP, Kuji I et al. Comparison of fluorine-18 fluorodeoxyglucose positron emission tomography and Ga-67 scintigraphy in evaluation of lymphoma. Cancer 2002; 94: 879–88.

208. Sasaki M, Kuwabara Y, Koga H et al. Clinical impact of whole body FDG-PET on the staging and therapeutic decision making for malignant lymphoma. Ann Nucl Med 2002; 16: 337–45.

209. Wirth A, Seymour JF, Hicks RJ et al. Fluorine-18 fluorodeoxyglucose positron emission tomography, gallium-67 scintigraphy, and conventional staging for Hodgkin's disease and non-Hodgkin's lymphoma. Am J Med 2002; 112: 262–8.

210. Cheson BD, Pfistner B, Juweid ME et al. Revised response criteria for malignant lymphoma. J Clin Oncol 2007; 25: 579–86.

211. Hutchings M, Specht L. PET/CT in the management of haematological malignancies. Eur J Haematol 2008; 80: 369–80.

212. Seam P, Juweid ME, Cheson BD. The role of FDG-PET scans in patients with lymphoma. Blood 2007; 110: 3507–16.

213. Jones SE, Rosenberg SA, Kaplan HS. Non-Hodgkin's lymphomas, I. Bone marrow involvement. Cancer 1972; 29: 954–60.

214. Brunning RD, Bloomfield CD, McKenna RW, Peterson LA. Bilateral trephine bone marrow biopsies in lymphoma and other neoplastic diseases. Ann Intern Med 1975; 82: 365–6.

215. Juneja SK, Wolf MM, Cooper IA. Value of bilateral bone marrow biopsy specimens in non-Hodgkin's lymphoma. J Clin Pathol 1990; 43: 630–2.

216. Cheson BD, Horning SJ, Coiffier B et al. Report of an international workshop to standardize response criteria for non-Hodgkin's lymphomas. NCI Sponsored International Working Group. J Clin Oncol 1999; 17: 1244.

217. Luoni M, Declich P, De Paoli A et al. Bone marrow biopsy for the staging of non-Hodgkin's lymphoma: bilateral or unilateral trephine biopsy? Tumori 1995; 81: 410–13.

218. Berliner N, Ault KA, Martin P, Weinberg DS. Detection of clonal excess in lymphoproliferative disease by kappa/lambda analysis: correlation with immunoglobulin gene DNA rearrangement. Blood 1986; 67: 80–5.

219. Duggan PR, Easton D, Luider J, Auer IA. Bone marrow staging of patients with non-Hodgkin lymphoma by flow cytometry: correlation with morphology. Cancer 2000; 88: 894–9.

220. Gribben JG, Freedman A, Woo SD et al. All advanced stage non-Hodgkin's lymphomas with a polymerase chain reaction amplifiable breakpoint of bcl-2 have residual cells containing the bcl-2 rearrangement at evaluation and after treatment. Blood 1991; 78: 3275–80.

221. Gulley ML, Dent GA, Ross DW. Classification and staging of lymphoma by molecular genetics. Cancer 1992; 69: 1600–6.

222. Horning SJ, Galili N, Cleary M, Sklar J. Detection of non-Hodgkin's lymphoma in the peripheral blood by analysis of antigen receptor gene rearrangements: results of a prospective study. Blood 1990; 75: 1139–45.

223. Lambrechts AC, de Ruiter PE, Dorssers LC, 't Veer MB. Detection of residual disease in translocation (14;18) positive non-Hodgkin's lymphoma, using the polymerase chain reaction: a comparison with conventional staging methods. Leukemia 1992; 6: 29–34.

224. Lee MS, Chang KS, Cabanillas F et al. Detection of minimal residual cells carrying the t(14;18) by DNA sequence amplification. Science 1987; 237: 175–8.

225. Smith BR, Weinberg DS, Robert NJ et al. Circulating monoclonal B lymphocytes in non-Hodgkin's lymphoma. N Engl J Med 1984; 311: 1476–81.

226. Stetler-Stevenson M, Braylan RC. Flow cytometric analysis of lymphomas and lymphoproliferative disorders. Semin Hematol 2001; 38: 111–23.

227. Hanson CA, Kurtin PJ, Katzmann JA et al. Immunophenotypic analysis of peripheral blood and bone marrow in the staging of B-cell malignant lymphoma. Blood 1999; 94: 3889–96.

228. Naughton MJ, Hess JL, Zutter MM, Bartlett NL. Bone marrow staging in patients with non-Hodgkin's lymphoma: is flow cytometry a useful test? Cancer 1998; 82: 1154–9.

229. Takagi S, Tsunoda S, Tanaka O. Bone marrow involvement in lymphoma: the importance of marrow magnetic resonance imaging. Leuk Lymphoma 1998; 29: 515–22.

230. Tardivon AA, Vanel D, Munck JN, Bosq J. Magnetic resonance imaging of the bone marrow in lymphomas and leukemias. Leuk Lymphoma 1997; 25: 55–68.

231. Tsunoda S, Takagi S, Tanaka O, Miura Y. Clinical and prognostic significance of femoral marrow magnetic

resonance imaging in patients with malignant lymphoma. *Blood* 1997; **89**: 286–90.

232. Tardivon AA, Munck JN, Shapeero LG *et al.* Can clinical data help to screen patients with lymphoma for MR imaging of bone marrow? *Ann Oncol* 1995; **6**: 795–800.

233. Bunn PA, Schein PS, Banks PM, DeVita VT. Central nervous system complications in patients with diffuse histiocytic and undifferentiated lymphoma: leukemia revisited. *Blood* 1976; **47**: 3–10.

234. Colocci N, Glantz M, Recht L. Prevention and treatment of central nervous system involvement by non-Hodgkin's lymphoma: a review of the literature. *Semin Neurol* 2004; **24**: 395–404.

♦235. DeAngelis LM, Hormigo A. Treatment of primary central nervous system lymphoma. *Semin Oncol* 2004; **31**: 684–92.

236. Dubuisson A, Kaschten B, Lenelle J *et al.* Primary central nervous system lymphoma report of 32 cases and review of the literature. *Clin Neurol Neurosurg* 2004; **107**: 55–63.

237. Feugier P, Virion JM, Tilly H *et al.* Incidence and risk factors for central nervous system occurrence in elderly patients with diffuse large-B-cell lymphoma: influence of rituximab. *Ann Oncol* 2004; **15**: 129–33.

238. Hegde U, Filie A, Little RF *et al.* High incidence of occult leptomeningeal disease detected by flow cytometry in newly diagnosed aggressive B-cell lymphomas at risk for central nervous system involvement: the role of flow cytometry versus cytology. *Blood* 2005; **105**: 496–502.

239. Herman TS, Hammond N, Jones SE *et al.* Involvement of the central nervous system by non-Hodgkin's lymphoma: the Southwest Oncology Group experience. *Cancer* 1979; **43**: 390–7.

240. Levitt LJ, Dawson DM, Rosenthal DS, Moloney WC. CNS involvement in the non-Hodgkin's lymphomas. *Cancer* 1980; **45**: 545–52.

241. Liang R, Chiu E, Loke SL. Secondary central nervous system involvement by non-Hodgkin's lymphoma: the risk factors. *Hematol Oncol* 1990; **8**: 141–5.

242. Litam JP, Cabanillas F, Smith TL *et al.* Central nervous system relapse in malignant lymphomas: risk factors and implications for prophylaxis. *Blood* 1979; **54**: 1249–57.

243. MacKintosh FR, Colby TV, Podolsky WJ *et al.* Central nervous system involvement in non-Hodgkin's lymphoma: an analysis of 105 cases. *Cancer* 1982; **49**: 586–95.

244. Recht LD. Neurologic complications of systemic lymphoma. *Neurol Clin* 1991; **9**: 1001–15.

245. Young RC, Howser DM, Anderson T *et al.* Central nervous system complications of non-Hodgkin's lymphoma. The potential role for prophylactic therapy. *Am J Med* 1979; **66**: 435–43.

246. Lossos IS, Breuer R, Intrator O, Lossos A. Cerebrospinal fluid lactate dehydrogenase isoenzyme analysis for the diagnosis of central nervous system involvement in hematooncologic patients. *Cancer* 2000; **88**: 1599–604.

247. Chahal S, Lagera JE, Ryder J, Kleinschmidt-DeMasters BK. Hematological neoplasms with first presentation as spinal cord compression syndromes: a 10-year retrospective series and review of the literature. *Clin Neuropathol* 2003; **22**: 282–90.

248. Chan CC, Wallace DJ. Intraocular lymphoma: update on diagnosis and management. *Cancer Control* 2004; **11**: 285–95.

249. Hochberg FH, Miller DC. Primary central nervous system lymphoma. *J Neurosurg* 1988; **68**: 835–53.

250. Hoffman PM, McKelvie P, Hall AJ *et al.* Intraocular lymphoma: a series of 14 patients with clinicopathological features and treatment outcomes. *Eye* 2003; **17**: 513–21.

251. Hormigo A, DeAngelis LM. Primary ocular lymphoma: clinical features, diagnosis, and treatment. *Clin Lymphoma* 2003; **4**: 22–9.

252. Anderson KC, Kaplan WD, Leonard RC *et al.* Role of 99mTc methylene diphosphonate bone imaging in the management of lymphoma. *Cancer Treat Rep* 1985; **69**: 1347–51.

253. Schechter JP, Jones SE, Woolfenden JM *et al.* Bone scanning in lymphoma. *Cancer* 1976; **38**: 1142–8.

254. Stroszczynski C, Oellinger J, Hosten N *et al.* Staging and monitoring of malignant lymphoma of the bone: comparison of 67Ga scintigraphy and MRI. *J Nucl Med* 1999; **40**: 387–93.

255. D'Amore F, Brincker H, Gronbaek K *et al.* Non-Hodgkin's lymphoma of the gastrointestinal tract: a population-based analysis of incidence, geographic distribution, clinicopathologic presentation features, and prognosis. Danish Lymphoma Study Group. *J Clin Oncol* 1994; **12**: 1673–84.

256. Brooks JJ, Enterline HT. Primary gastric lymphomas. A clinicopathologic study of 58 cases with long-term follow-up and literature review. *Cancer* 1983; **51**: 701–11.

257. Taal BG, Burgers JM, Van Heerde P *et al.* The clinical spectrum and treatment of primary non-Hodgkin's lymphoma of the stomach. *Ann Oncol* 1993; **4**: 839–46.

258. Harris NL, Jaffe ES, Diebold J *et al.* World Health Organization classification of neoplastic diseases of the hematopoietic and lymphoid tissues: report of the Clinical Advisory Committee meeting-Airlie House, Virginia, November 1997. *J Clin Oncol* 1999; **17**: 3835–49.

♦259. Jaffe ES, Harris NL, Stein H, Vardiman JW. (eds) *World Health Organization classification of tumours. Pathology and genetics of tumours of haematopoietic and lymphoid tissues.* Lyon: IARC Press, 2001.

260. Ersboll J, Schultz HB, Thomsen BL *et al.* Meningeal involvement in non-Hodgkin's lymphoma: symptoms, incidence, risk factors and treatment. *Scand J Haematol* 1985; **35**: 487–96.

261. Nathwani BN, Diamond LW, Winberg CD *et al.* Lymphoblastic lymphoma: a clinicopathologic study of 95 patients. *Cancer* 1981; **48**: 2347–57.

262. Picozzi VJ Jr, Coleman CN. Lymphoblastic lymphoma. *Semin Oncol* 1990; **17**: 96–103.

263. Crellin AM, Hudson BV, Bennett MH *et al.* Non-Hodgkin's lymphoma of the testis. *Radiother Oncol* 1993; **27**: 99–106.

264. Doll DC, Weiss RB. Malignant lymphoma of the testis. *Am J Med* 1986; **81**: 515–24.

265. van Besien K, Ha CS, Murphy S *et al.* Risk factors, treatment, and outcome of central nervous system recurrence in adults with intermediate-grade and immunoblastic lymphoma. *Blood* 1998; **91**: 1178–84.

266. DeAngelis LM. Primary CNS lymphoma: treatment with combined chemotherapy and radiotherapy. *J Neurooncol* 1999; **43**: 249–57.

267. O'Neill BP, Dinapoli RP, Kurtin PJ, Habermann TM. Occult systemic non-Hodgkin's lymphoma (NHL) in patients initially diagnosed as primary central nervous system lymphoma (PCNSL): how much staging is enough? *J Neurooncol* 1995; **25**: 67–71.

268. Frierson HF Jr, Mills SE, Innes DJ Jr. Non-Hodgkin's lymphomas of the sinonasal region: histologic subtypes and their clinicopathologic features. *Am J Clin Pathol* 1984; **81**: 721–7.

269. Juman S, Robinson P, Balkissoon A, Kelly K. B-cell non-Hodgkin's lymphoma of the paranasal sinuses. *J Laryngol Otol* 1994; **108**: 263–5.

270. Logsdon MD, Ha CS, Kavadi VS *et al.* Lymphoma of the nasal cavity and paranasal sinuses: improved outcome and altered prognostic factors with combined modality therapy. *Cancer* 1997; **80**: 477–88.

271. Banfi A, Bonadonna G, Ricci SB *et al.* Malignant lymphomas of Waldeyer's ring: natural history and survival after radiotherapy. *Br Med J* 1972; **3**: 140–3.

272. Brugere, Schlienger M, Gerard-Marchant R *et al.* Non-Hodgkin's malignant lymphomata of upper digestive and respiratory tract: natural history and results of radiotherapy. *Br J Cancer* 1975; **31**(Suppl 2): 435–40.

273. Gospodarowicz MK, Sutcliffe SB, Brown TC *et al.* Patterns of disease in localized extranodal lymphomas. *J Clin Oncol* 1987; **5**: 875–80.

274. Jacobs C, Hoppe RT. Non-Hodgkin's lymphomas of head and neck extranodal sites. *Int J Radiat Oncol Biol Phys* 1985; **11**: 357–64.

275. Saul SH, Kapadia SB. Primary lymphoma of Waldeyer's ring. Clinicopathologic study of 68 cases. *Cancer* 1985; **56**: 157–66.

◆276. Gospodarowicz MK, Sutcliffe SB. The extranodal lymphomas. *Semin Radiat Oncol* 1995; **5**: 281–300.

277. Maor MH, Velasquez WS, Fuller LM, Silvermintz KB. Stomach conservation in stages IE and IIE gastric non-Hodgkin's lymphoma. *J Clin Oncol* 1990; **8**: 266–71.

278. Rossi A, Lister TA. Primary gastric non-Hodgkin's lymphoma: a therapeutic challenge. *Eur J Cancer* 1993; **29A**: 1924–6.

279. Caletti GC, Ferrari A, Bocus P *et al.* Endoscopic ultrasonography in gastric lymphoma. *Schweiz Med Wochenschr* 1996; **126**: 819–25.

280. Fujishima H, Misawa T, Maruoka A *et al.* Staging and follow-up of primary gastric lymphoma by endoscopic ultrasonography. *Am J Gastroenterol* 1991; **86**: 719–24.

281. Tio TL, Hartog Jager FC, Tijtgat GN. Endoscopic ultrasonography of non-Hodgkin lymphoma of the stomach. *Gastroenterology* 1986; **91**: 401–8.

282. Tio TL, Hartog Jager FC, Tytgat GN. Endoscopic ultrasonography in detection and staging of gastric non-Hodgkin lymphoma. Comparison with gastroscopy, barium meal, and computerized tomography scan. *Scand J Gastroenterol Suppl* 1986; **123**: 52–8.

283. Ostrowski ML, Unni KK, Banks PM *et al.* Malignant lymphoma of bone. *Cancer* 1986; **58**: 2646–55.

284. Zucca E, Conconi A, Mughal TI *et al.* Patterns of outcome and prognostic factors in primary large-cell lymphoma of the testis in a survey by the International Extranodal Lymphoma Study Group. *J Clin Oncol* 2003; **21**: 20–7.

47

Special aspects of diagnosis in developing countries

KIKKERI N NARESH

INTRODUCTION

In recent years, there has been great progress in the understanding, classification and management of lymphoid neoplasms. In 1994, the International Lymphoma Study Group published a new classification scheme named the Revised European–American Lymphoma (REAL) classification, and this was followed by the World Health Organization (WHO) classification in 2001.[1,2] The new systems have incorporated immunophenotyping/immunohistochemistry, cytogenetics and molecular genetics into the classification, which is an improvement over previous classifications that only used morphology and clinical parameters and sometimes immunophenotypic features. However, this technology-intense approach to classification, although providing a more objective and precise lymphoma diagnosis, may have a deleterious impact on clinical practice, particularly in countries with limited sources, because of its need of additional facilities, knowledge and skills.

The term 'developing countries' usually includes most nations in Africa, most nations in Asia except Japan, Hong Kong, South Korea, Taiwan and Singapore, and most nations of South America, Central America and the Caribbean. It should be noted that these countries have large differences in ethnicity, lifestyle and environment.

INCIDENCE OF LYMPHOID NEOPLASMS IN THE DEVELOPING WORLD

There are major differences in the incidence of non-Hodgkin lymphoma (NHL) across the world as noted in the data from Globocan 2002 of IARC.[3] Age-standardized incidence rates are the highest in North America, recording 21.8 per 100 000 per year in men and 17.2 in women. In Europe, the rates are 10.3–11 in men and 11.8–13.8 in women. In contrast, the incidence rates in the rest of the world is 5.0 or less. Incidence rates for specific lymphoma subtypes from the developing world are currently not available. In fact, barring few exceptions, such data are not available even from developed countries. Recently, data from 12 separate US population-based cancer registries on lymphoma cases diagnosed during 1992–2001, and classified by the new WHO classification has been published. A comparison of incidence rates between the white, black and Asian population shows that ethnicity impacts on the incidence of lymphoma and the lymphoma subtype distribution. The age-adjusted incidence rates for all lymphoid neoplasms (including Hodgkin lymphoma and myeloma) in white, black and Asian men are 44.01, 41.09 and 25.38 per 100 000 population per year, respectively. Similar rates for white, black and Asian women are

42.56, 26.53 and 16.76 per 100 000 population per year, respectively. However, it should be noted that 'Asian' population is ethnically diverse, and contains a mix of people from China and South East Asia, Middle East and the Indian subcontinent.[4]

GEOGRAPHIC VARIATION IN LYMPHOMA SUBSETS

It is currently possible to look at differences in the proportions of various lymphoma subtypes from different regions within the developing world and compare with other developing nations and also the developed world. The WHO classification of lymphoid neoplasia, published in 2001, is widely publicized and read across the world. It is based predominantly on morphologic and immunohistochemical characteristics and to a lesser extent on molecular genetic and cytogenetic findings.[2] Recently, the panel of antibodies that can be used on paraffin sections has widened considerably, and classifying lymphoid neoplasms according to the WHO criteria has become easier. The use of fixed tissue avoids the need for frozen material and even makes possible the retesting of archived material. This has made it possible for pathologists to use the WHO lymphoma classification in retrospect, or with the aid of expert review, so that diagnosis and comparisons of the relative frequency of lymphoma subtypes can be explored across the world.[5,6]

The differences in the major subtypes are summarized in Tables 47.1 and 47.2.

Table 47.1 Distribution (in percent) of major non-Hodgkin lymphoma (NHL) subtypes according to the World Health Organization classification in different parts of the world

Subtypes	North America[7]	Europe[7]	South Africa[7]	Egypt[6]	Middle East[6,12,13]	Pakistan[6,11]	India[5]	Oriental countries[6-10]
B cell lymphomas								
Chronic lymphocytic leukemia	7	5–11	8	6	1–4	4	5	1–3
Follicular lymphoma	32	11–28	33	5	7–11	3	15	6–8
Mantle cell lymphoma	7	7–14	1	4	0	0	5	1–3
Marginal zone B cell lymphoma, all types	6	3–13	4	5	2–4	1	4	10–21
Diffuse large B cell lymphoma	28	27–36	28	49	51–59	38–75	35	36–47
Burkitt and Burkitt-like lymphomas	2–5	3–4	2	7	4–13	1	4	1–2
T cell lymphomas								
Precursor T lymphoblastic lymphoma	2	0–1	2	5	3–4	3	7	1–4
Peripheral T cell lymphoma, unspecified and angioimmunoblastic T cell lymphoma	3	4–8	8	4	2–5	1	5	9–10
Anaplastic large cell lymphoma	2	0–3	3	2	2–7	1	4	1–4
Extranodal natural killer (NK)/T cell lymphoma, nasal type	0	0–2	0	0	0	<1	<1	3–9

Table 47.2 Distribution (in percent) of major non-Hodgkin lymphoma subtypes in pediatric age group in different parts of the world

Subtypes	Europe[15,16]	Egypt[6]	Middle East[6]	Pakistan[6]	India[14]	Oriental countries[6]
B cell lymphomas						
Precursor B lymphoblastic lymphoma	3–4	0	5	13	3	8
Diffuse large B cell lymphoma	4–10	17	12	16	25	3
Burkitt and Burkitt-like lymphomas	21–44	39	68	12	11	9
Unclassified high-grade B cell lymphoma	4–18	0	0	13	8	17
T cell lymphomas						
Precursor T lymphoblastic lymphoma	19–21	21	8	8	32	24
Anaplastic large cell lymphoma	8–15	4	2	0	10	8

B cell neoplasms

B cell lymphomas from the developing world apart from South East Asia form about 82–88 percent of all the NHLs. This is not very different to the proportion of B cell neoplasms seen in the West.

Precursor B cell neoplasms

Estimating the proportion of lymphoblastic lymphoma among all NHLs is difficult because the distinction between lymphoblastic lymphoma and acute lymphoblastic leukaemia (ALL) is rather arbitrary. ALL is usually defined as 25 percent or more blast cells in the bone marrow, and to a certain extent, this may depend upon the time from first symptoms to diagnosis, because in places where treatment and medical attention is delayed, LL may present already in a leukemic phase as ALL. This would be particularly relevant to the developing world.

Mature B cell neoplasms

The proportions of chronic lymphocytic leukemia (CLL)/small lymphocytic lymphoma (SLL) (4–6 percent), mantle cell lymphoma (MCL) (3–5 percent), and plasmacytoma (2–4 percent) are similar among the different countries within the developing world. It appears that CLL/SLL accounts for a lower proportion (approximately one-half) of lymphoid neoplasms as compared with the West. In South East Asia, the frequency of CLL/SLL is even lower (1–3 percent). Similarly, MCL accounts for less than half of that seen in the West (7–14 percent of NHLs in the West).[7–10] Within the developing world, there is a significant variation in the proportion of follicular lymphoma, which accounts for about 15 percent in India and Kuwait, as compared with less than 5 percent in Pakistan and Egypt.[6] On the other hand, the proportion of follicular lymphoma in the West varies between 17 percent and 32 percent.[5] The derived incidence rates of follicular lymphoma in the West vary between 2.4 and 3.5 per 100 000 population per year. Similar rates in developing world are less than 0.3 per 100 000 population per year. Going by these figures, the follicular lymphoma incidence would be 8–10 times higher in the West as compared with the developing world.[17] However, the incidence rates of follicular lymphoma among white and Asian men in the USA are 3.85 and 1.89 per 100 000 population per year, respectively, and those of white and Asian women in the USA are 3.31 and 1.37 per 100 000 population per year, respectively; a ratio of 2–2.5:1.[4] These studies suggest that while ethnic differences may account, to a certain extent, for the differences in the incidence of follicular lymphoma, environmental factors also probably have an important role to account for the huge difference in the incidence rates of follicular lymphoma seen between the developing world and the West.

Diffuse large B cell lymphoma (DLBCL) accounts for about 35 percent of cases in India, and for more than half of all the NHLs in other developing countries like Pakistan, Egypt and Kuwait. The proportion of DLBCL in India is similar to the West (25–36 percent) and to the developed South East Asian countries, such as Japan and Hong Kong (36 percent).[5–8] In contrast with India, DLBCL accounts for over 75 percent of all adult NHLs in Pakistan.[11] Given the fact that the population of India and Pakistan are ethnically similar, this is of particular interest. It is not clear whether these differences can be accounted for by differences in environmental factors or referral patterns.

These apparent differences in the proportions of follicular lymphoma and DLBCL are particularly noteworthy and account for most of the variations in proportions of the lymphoma subtypes. Because follicular lymphoma can evolve into DLBCL, one possible explanation for the variability in the follicular lymphoma/DLBCL ratio is that environmental or genetic factors determine the time of transformation of follicular lymphoma into DLBCL and that a greater proportion of 'follicular lymphoma' patients present rather 'later' in countries such as Egypt and Pakistan. Such progression could occur at a stage when follicular lymphoma is subclinical, or before the patient has presented to a major hospital. In such instances it may be difficult to discern, in the absence of follicular component, whether the tumor presented is a *de novo* DLBCL or a DLBCL transformed from a follicular lymphoma.

The marginal zone B cell lymphoma (MZL) of nodal and mucosa-associated lymphoid tissue (MALT) types accounts for 5 percent or less of NHLs in most countries from the developing world. In contrast, MZLs amount to 3–13 percent in the West and 10–21 percent of all NHLs in South East Asia.[7–10] Because the MZLs can also progress to DLBCL, the prevalence of MZL could also be relevant to differences in the proportions of follicular lymphoma and DLBCL, as well as the proportions of DLBCL that are nodal or extranodal.[18]

A common feature of lymphomas in the Middle East is the occurrence of a high proportion of extranodal lymphomas, and in a published series from the United Arab Emirates, 29 percent of all NHLs were extranodal.[12,13] Of relevance to the above issue is the occurrence of a high proportion of DLBCL in Kuwait, a higher proportion of which are extranodal cases. Extranodal DLBCL may be less likely to have evolved from follicular lymphoma, which is almost always nodal in origin and the higher proportion of observed extranodal DLBCLs in the Middle East may represent transformed forms of MZLs.

In most Asian countries, when lymphomas at all ages are considered, the proportion of Burkitt lymphoma is similar to the West, varying between 1 percent and 4 percent. Egypt, however, has a higher overall frequency (7 percent). Among patients in the pediatric age group (≤14 years), Burkitt lymphoma has a lower frequency of 9–12 percent in India, Pakistan, and Shanghai as compared with the West, where it varies between 21 percent and 44 percent.

In contrast, in the pediatric age group, Burkitt lymphoma accounts for 68 percent and 39 percent of cases in Saudi Arabia and Egypt, respectively. There is clear evidence that the incidence of Burkitt lymphoma varies markedly throughout the world, being particularly high in equatorial Africa, most probably because of early infection by Epstein–Barr virus (EBV) and chronic exposure to malaria. EBV association in Burkitt lymphoma varies in different geographic areas between 25 percent and 80 percent. The association is strongest in equatorial Africa and weakest in the West. In most developing countries, the association is intermediate between the non-endemic Burkitt lymphoma of the West and endemic Burkitt lymphoma.[6,19,20]

T/natural killer cell neoplasms

PRECURSOR T CELL NEOPLASMS

The proportion of precursor T cell lymphoblastic lymphoma (T-LL) as a fraction of all NHLs is higher in India (6–7 percent) as compared with the other countries. It is higher than the proportion noted in Europe, North America, and other parts of Asia (0–4 percent).[5,7,9,10,12,21,22] The proportion of T-LL in India is higher even in the first two decades of life as compared with the rest of the developing world (32 percent vs 19–21 percent).[14–16,23] The higher frequency of lymphoblastic lymphoma in India is unlikely to be due to the inclusion of cases of ALL involving lymph nodes. This is suggested by another study from India on lymphomas in childhood and adolescents that had exclusion criteria of 5 percent or more blasts in the bone marrow. In this study, lymphoblastic lymphoma accounted for 50 percent of all cases.[24]

PERIPHERAL T/NATURAL KILLER CELL NEOPLASMS

In most of the developing world, peripheral T/natural killer (NK) cell neoplasms account for only about 12–18 percent of all NHLs, which is not dissimilar to that seen in the West. It contrasts with figures from South East Asia, where peripheral T/NK NHLs account for about 20–45 percent of all NHLs. This is particularly so in regions where HTLV-1 is prevalent.[7–10,25] It is not clear, whether this perceived difference could be due to relative infrequency of other lymphomas and a particular paucity of B cell NHLs, an actual increased incidence of T cell NHLs, or a combination of both. Apart from South East Asia, in the rest of the developing world, the proportion of nodal peripheral T cell lymphomas (PTCLs) (unspecified and angioimmunoblastic subtypes) is similar to the West (3–5 percent). Similarly, in most of the developing world, NK/T cell lymphoma is rare (<1 percent). In contrast, the proportion of nodal PTCLs and NK/T cell lymphoma in South East Asia is in the range of 9–14 percent and 3–9 percent, respectively.[7–10,25] The great majority of NK/T cell lymphomas are EBV associated.

HODGKIN LYMPHOMA

The incidence rates of Hodgkin lymphoma vary widely and there are major differences between the developing world and developed countries. As per the Globocan 2002 of IARC, the age-standardized incidence rates are the highest in North America, recording 3.5 per 100 000 per year in men and 2.6 per 100 000 per year in women. In contrast, the incidence rates are 0.3–1.2 in Asian men and 0.1–0.5 in Asian women, and 0.5–1.5 in African men and 0.2–0.7 in African women. The rates are intermediate in Europe and the Middle East.[3] The ratio of the incidence of NHL:Hodgkin lymphoma in the European Union is 4.47. It is highest in the UK (6.33) and lowest in Austria (1.22).[26] Furthermore, within a country, the ratio of NHL:Hodgkin lymphoma is related to ethnicity. In contrast to the overall figures from UK, the ratio among South Asian males and females residing in England is 2.8 and 4.0, respectively.[27] The ratio of NHL:Hodgkin lymphoma in India is 2.19. However, this ratio varies within India, being highest in the western (6.28) as compared with either southern (1.26) or northern (2.27) parts of India.[28]

Since the criteria and definition of Hodgkin lymphoma subtypes has been refined in recent times, it is difficult to compare published data from the past for the purposes of subtype distribution. In many earlier studies from the developing world, mixed cellularity was thought to be the most common subtype and was reported to account for 40–80 percent of cases. However, using the current criteria, data from India suggest that mixed cellularity subtype accounts for about for 37 percent, which is not very different from the nodular sclerosis subtype that accounts for about 46 percent of cases. It is likely that the reported differences between literature of the past and the more recent do not depict a true change in the pattern of Hodgkin lymphoma but rather represent a shift in the criteria for diagnosis and subtyping Hodgkin lymphoma.[28]

There has been a strong association between EBV and Hodgkin lymphoma. It is relatively easy to study EBV association employing immunohistochemistry using LMP1 antibody or in situ hybridization using EBER1 probe. Geographic differences in the EBV association also exist. While in the developing countries 70–100 percent of Hodgkin lymphoma are EBV associated, only 30–50 percent of Hodgkin lymphomas in the developed countries show such an association. In the Oriental population from China and Hong Kong, the association is about 65 percent.[29–35] Within Hodgkin lymphoma, the association varies with the subtype, and the mixed cellularity subtype has a stronger association as compared to the nodular sclerosis subtype.[36,37]

The EBV association is particularly strong among children in the developing world, and in some countries almost all pediatric cases are EBV associated. Furthermore, in the developing world, even the nodular lymphocyte predominant subtype of Hodgkin lymphoma, which is usually not associated with EBV may show an association in the pediatric age group.[29,38,39] Similarly, the association is said to be stronger among elderly patients.[31,32,37] The stronger

EBV association in these subsets of patients might be related to either environmental factors or to the patient's lowered immune status. In the developing world, it is likely that EBV is acquired at an earlier age. Furthermore, a lower socioeconomic status might play a role in altering the immune status of the EBV-infected children. The EBV association is significantly higher among Hispanics than whites from similar geographic locations.[35] Thus, age, ethnicity and the physiologic effects of poverty may function as biologic modifiers.[30,31,33,40] The impact of economic conditions effected through population density and immune status can be observed by the fact that EBV association is much lower in countries such as Saudi Arabia, where it is reported to be about 29 percent, which is no different than the EBV association seen in the West.[41]

HIV-ASSOCIATED NEOPLASMS

The human immunodeficiency virus (HIV) epidemic has had a significant impact on the developing world. In most of the developing world, the exact proportion of individuals who are HIV positive or have lymphomas that are HIV associated is not currently known. Patients with acquired immune deficiency syndrome (AIDS) have a 150- to over 250-fold higher relative risk (RR) for developing NHL compared with the general population. While the RR for high grade B cell NHLs is about 400, the RR for low grade B-NHLs and T cell NHLs is about 15. The risk of developing classical Hodgkin lymphoma (RR 7.6–10) and plasmacytoma (RR 2–5) is also higher in HIV-positive individuals than in the general population. Furthermore, within the HIV-NHLs, the RR for different lymphoma types varies. In the developing world, especially Africa, the RR for developing NHL is said to be about 10 times less than that in the more developed countries. It could well be that a higher proportion of patients succumb to infective complications before they develop HIV-associated malignancies. Following the introduction of highly active antiretroviral therapy (HAART) there has been a decline in the incidence of some lymphoma types of NHL, primary central nervous system lymphoma (PCNSL) being the prime example.[42,43]

The HIV-associated lymphoid proliferations include Burkitt lymphoma, DLBCL of centroblastic subtype, DLBCL of immunoblastic subtype, primary central nervous system (CNS) DLBCL and classic Hodgkin lymphoma that may be EBV associated. Other rarer lymphoid proliferations include primary effusion lymphoma, oral plasmablastic lymphoma, and multicentric Castleman disease with or without associated plasmablastic microlymphoma or plasmablastic lymphoma. This latter group shows an association with HHV-8, and primary effusion lymphoma shows association with both EBV and HHV-8. As compared with the West, HIV-NHLs from the developing world differ by:[44–46]

- immunoblastic DLBCLs being more common
- lymph nodal presentation being more common

- rarity of PCNSL
- almost complete absence of HHV-8 associated HIV-NHLs.

T cell lymphomas are rare in the HIV/AIDS setting and large studies have shown that only about 3 percent of HIV lymphomas are of T cell type.[47] In a more recent publication from Peru, 27 percent of the HIV lymphomas were of T cell type.[48]

HIV-Hodgkin lymphoma shows a male predilection, and mixed cellularity and lymphocyte-depleted subtypes are more common. Furthermore, bone marrow involvement and, at times, bone marrow as the primary site of presentation is well known. In contrast to patients with multiple myeloma in the general population, HIV-plasmacytoma patients are younger and they present with extramedullary or solitary osseous lesions.[49]

PRACTICE OF LYMPHOMA DIAGNOSTICS IN THE DEVELOPING WORLD

While there may be lack of skilled human resources in some of the developing countries, if expertise is nurtured and developed, and as long as histologic material is properly fixed and sectioned, it would appear that the WHO classification could be effectively employed, at least in major centers in the developing world, to obtain accurate information both for routine diagnostic purposes and also for purposes of comparison with other series.[21]

Many studies have shown that interobserver disagreements in classifying NHL exist even between expert hematopathologists, and a certain degree of intraobserver variability (lack of reproducibility by the same pathologist) also exists.[22] This has been adequately addressed by five expert hematopathologists of the NHL Classification Project who have travelled to several countries around the world including developing countries over the past 10 years. In some of the studies involving their site visits, they have addressed the questions:

- Within the limitation of the prevailing conditions in a developing country, can the WHO classification of NHL be practiced to acceptable standards?
- How would the diagnosis made by a well-trained lymphoma expert in a developing country with recourse to technology compared with that of expert hematopathologists from the developed world?
- In what proportion of cases would further work-up by a reference laboratory in a developed country be necessary to arrive at a definitive diagnosis?[5]

In one such study from the developing world, the mean agreement of the expert hematopathologists with their consensus diagnosis (as defined as at least four of five experts agreeing with a diagnosis) was 82 percent (76–88 percent).

The mean agreement of the expert hematopathologists was slightly lower than the 85 percent agreement that they had achieved in their earlier studies performed on material accrued in developed countries. Among the cases reviewed, in about 10 percent of cases a specific histologic subtype as defined in the WHO classification could not be assigned. The minor drop in agreement and a considerably higher proportion of cases of NHL without a specific subtype was thought to be due to: (1) suboptimal quality of the tissue in many of the cases; (2) less than optimal workup of some of the cases, in terms of immunostains and molecular studies.[5,22]

The agreement of the diagnoses offered by the host pathologist from the developing world (82 percent) with the consensus diagnoses was not different from that of the experts. This suggests that, if well-trained and experienced hematopathologists are available and expertise can be nurtured, the WHO classification of NHL can be practiced nearly as accurately as in the developed world.[5] In the same study, additional studies were redone in an institute from the developed world in 10 percent of cases. However, the repeated investigations led to a specific diagnosis in only one-third of cases. The technical hurdles included small biopsy size, inadequate tissue fixation and suboptimal processing, thus leading to suboptimal hematoxylin and eosin (H&E)-stained sections. Furthermore, in such cases, poor antigen preservation posed problems for some of the critical immunostains required for precise subtyping.[5]

High-quality lymphoma diagnosis is dependent on high-quality H&E-stained sections and immunohistochemistry. Furthermore, centralization of specialized immunohistochemistry and molecular genetic studies, which are important adjuncts to lymphoma diagnosis, could promote high standards and good quality assurance in the developing world. Suboptimal antigen preservation in paraffin blocks is a major problem in the developing world. This is compounded by a lack of automation and the use of conventional immunohistochemical detection systems that are far less sensitive than those often employed in the developed countries. These issues could be short lived. With improvements in economy, improved laboratory budgets and reduction in costs, it is likely that the problems can be overcome. Immunohistochemical staining procedures for cyclin D1, CD5, CD10 and CD15 are some of the more common procedures that may have lower sensitivity in the developing world.

With some lymphoma entities, achieving an acceptable interobserver concordance may be difficult even in developed countries. For example, differentiating PTCL-unspecified and angio-immunoblastic T cell lymphoma can pose problems even in the developed world. In the NHL classification study, the diagnostic reliability improved from 33 percent to 72 percent after detailed immunophenotyping results were available, but did not improve further with the addition of detailed clinical data.[50] In recent times, CD10 has been recognized as a marker that could help distinguish angioimmunoblastic T cell lymphomas from the PTCL-unspecified category.[51] Currently, robust antibodies are available for CD10, and this would possibly improve the interobserver concordance.

PERIPHERAL BLOOD AND BONE MARROW BASED LYMPHOPROLIFERATIVE DISORDERS

This group of disorders is very likely to be under-diagnosed or wrongly diagnosed for various reasons. Patients with many chronic lymphoproliferative disorders remain asymptomatic for many years, and such diseases are clinically under-reported in the developing world. Even among symptomatic patients, these patients require assessment by flow cytometry, high-quality bone marrow trephine histology, a very wide panel of immunohistochemistry on bone marrow trephine sections and, in many cases, cytogenetics and molecular biology to arrive at a specific diagnosis. Just as there has been an attempt for technical improvement in lymphoma histology across the world, there is need for improving the quality of bone marrow trephine examination worldwide.[52]

BENIGN MIMICS OF LYMPHOMAS THAT CAUSE PARTICULAR CONCERN IN THE DEVELOPING WORLD

Owing to the suboptimal quality of histologic material and nonavailability of a wide array of immunohistochemistry, some reactive or non-neoplastic lymphoid lesions are at special risk of being labeled lymphomas. These entities include:

- toxoplasmosis
- autoimmune lymphoproliferative syndrome
- Kikuchi–Fujimoto disease or histiocytic necrotizing lymphadenitis, particularly in its so-called early lymphoproliferative phase
- Rosai–Dorfman disease, especially in its extranodal presentation
- Castleman disease.

Toxoplasma lymphadenitis histologically shows the triad of follicular hyperplasia, expansion of monocytoid B cells and presence of small clusters of epithelioid cells within, and close to, the germinal centres. When monocytoid B cell/marginal zone expansion is florid, a misdiagnosis of marginal zone lymphoma is possible. Some of the cases of toxoplasma lymphadenitis have scattered larger immunoblasts. Though classical Reed–Sternberg cells are not seen, a misdiagnosis of interfollicular Hodgkin lymphoma remains a possibility.[53]

Autoimmune lymphoproliferative syndrome (ALPS) is an uncommon disease, but can cause major problems in diagnosis. Young patients usually present with generalized lymphadenopathy, hepatosplenomegaly, hypergammaglobulinemia, B cell lymphocytosis and autoimmune manifestations such as hemolytic anemia, idiopathic thrombocytopenic purpura, urticarial rash, glomerulonephritis and Guillain–Barré syndrome. The lymph nodes characteristically show a paracortical expansion of double negative T cells (CD4 and CD8 negative). In addition, there is an infiltrate of plasma cells, small lymphocytes and immunoblasts. Florid follicular hyperplasia, follicle changes akin to Castleman disease and progressive transformation of germinal centers may be seen. The lymphoid proliferation is related to an impairment of apoptosis as a consequence of inherited heterozygous mutations in the Fas, Fas ligand or caspase 10 genes. Some of these patients later develop nodular lymphocyte-predominant Hodgkin lymphoma or a T cell-rich B cell lymphoma.[54–56]

Kikuchi–Fujimoto disease was first described by two Japanese pathologists, Kikuchi and Fujimoto in 1972. It involves predominantly cervical lymph nodes of young South East Asian women (mean age of 25–29 years), though it can affect patients of any age, gender or ethnicity. The female:male ratio is usually about 4:1. Among the Japanese population, there is a significant association with certain human leukocyte antigen (HLA) class II alleles – DPA1*01 and DPB1*0202. The lymphadenopathy may be painful. Lymph nodes outside of the cervical region may be involved, and in a small subset the process can involve extranodal sites such as skin, internal organs and bone marrow. Most patients are asymptomatic. Kikuchi–Fujimoto disease is a self-limiting disorder that resolves spontaneously within months, and may rarely persist up to a year.[54,57,58]

Early in the evolution of Kikuchi–Fujimoto disease, in the so-called lymphoproliferative phase, there is a predominance of atypical mononuclear cells along with a large number of mitoses and apoptosis. At this stage, classic fibrinoid necrosis is lacking. This lesion, in inexperienced hands with suboptimal morphology and inadequate recourse to immunohistochemistry can be misdiagnosed as a high grade NHL. Helpful clues to the diagnosis include:[54,58–60]

- patchy paracortical involvement of the lymph node
- presence of more than one cell type that includes unusual histiocytes with crescentic or C-shaped nuclei, immunoblasts, plasmacytoid monocytes, and small lymphoid cells
- absence of granulocytes and plasma cells
- rest of the lymph node showing 'reactive' features with foci of paracortical hyperplasia having a 'mottled' appearance.

On immunostaining, the lymphoid component consists predominantly of T cells with an admixture of CD8-positive and CD4-positive cells, with CD8-positive cells coexpressing cytotoxic molecules (TIA1, perforin and granzyme B). B cells are scanty. The histiocytes express the usual histiocytic markers – CD11c, CD68 (KP1), CD68 (PGM-1), Mac-387 and lysozyme. In addition, they also express myeloperoxidase (Plate 131, see plate section). The plasmacytoid monocytes in addition express CD123 and CD10. The Ki-67 expression is usually very high among the T cells.[58,60]

Some patients who are initially diagnosed as having Kikuchi–Fujimoto disease have positive laboratory investigations for systemic lupus erythematosus (SLE) and some go on to later develop full-blown SLE. Serological testing for infectious agents, including those for different viruses is usually negative. In a minority of patients, positive serology for EBV, parvovirus B19, HTLV-I, *Yersinia enterocolitica*, *Toxoplasma* and *Brucella* has been obtained.

Rosai Dorfman disease or sinus histiocytosis with massive lymphadenopathy (SHML) is a disease that often presents with massively enlarged lymph nodes in the cervical region or other peripheral sites. Diagnosis of lymph node disease does not usually pose major problems. Typical sinusoidal expansion with characteristic histiocytic cells showing emperipolesis is diagnostic. However, in as many as 40 percent, patients can present with exclusive extranodal disease involving skin and subcutis, sinonasal areas, orbit and other sites. In extranodal SHML, features are subtle – the sinusoidal pattern is absent or less obvious, and emperipolesis is less appreciable. Such lesions can be misdiagnosed, on some occasions as lymphomas. The histiocytic cells that are always present, apart from expressing CDC-68, are also positive for S-100 protein and this is a helpful feature in diagnosis.[54]

UNDERDIAGNOSIS OF LYMPHOMA IN THE DEVELOPING WORLD

Underdiagnosis of lymphomas often stems from suboptimal sample quality and inadequate personnel training. In certain lymphoid neoplasms, where features may be subtle, cases may not be referred from a 'general' histopathologist to a specialist hematopathologist. This aspect may not be entirely limited to the developing world, and can happen even in the affluent countries. Prime examples are marginal zone lymphoma, follicular lymphomas, MCLs (especially those with a nodular pattern) and Hodgkin lymphoma of nodular lymphocyte predominant subtype. These entities may be underdiagnosed as 'reactive' lymph nodes, only to be revisited when the patient presents with recurrent disease. On some occasions 'high-grade' lymphomas may be wrongly labeled as one of the 'indolent' lymphomas due to suboptimal tissue processing and sectioning, and inadequate immunohistochemical workup. Lymphoblastic lymphoma and extranodal DLBCL being underdiagnosed as CLL or MALT lymphoma, respectively, are typical examples. Using Tdt or Ki-67 immunostains can help avert such mistakes even in poorly processed samples. Similarly, peripheral T cell lymphomas can be underdiagnosed as 'reactive' lesions. Since epithelioid cells form a major reactive component of some of the neoplasms such as Hodgkin lymphoma and PTCLs, underdiagnosis as granulomatous diseases is not uncommon. Suboptimal morphology, lack of adequate immunohistochemical support and inadequate experience can result in both overdiagnosis and underdiagnosis of lymphoid neoplasms.[61]

DOUBLE PATHOLOGIES

Since some infections affecting lymph nodes, especially tuberculosis, are extremely common in the developing world, lymph nodes and other sites involved by lymphoid neoplasms may in higher frequencies also harbor tuberculosis or other infective pathologies. This infective component may overshadow the neoplastic component and cause problems not only in diagnosis but also in management.[62,63] The coexistence of metastasis and indolent lymphomas in lymph nodes is less common than in the West.

ROLE OF FINE NEEDLE ASPIRATION IN THE DIAGNOSIS OF LYMPHOID LESIONS

Fine needle aspiration (FNA) is a simple and inexpensive procedure. Its role in the work-up of lymphoid lesions has been highly debated. It is definitely the preferred first procedure in screening patients with peripheral lymphadenopathy. It is very useful in the management of specific infective conditions such as tuberculosis (especially in places with a high prevalence) and in planning treatment in patients with metastasis. However, its role in the diagnosis of primary lymphoid lesions needs better definition. While attempting to classify lymphoid lesions, a considerable proportion of false-positives or false-negatives are encountered.[64,65] However, there are reports which claim higher success rates.[66] Combining FNA with immunohistochemistry, flow cytometry, fluorescence *in situ* hybridization techniques or other molecular tools might improve the accuracy, but problems of sampling and errors associated with lack of architectural assessment in lymphoid lesions remain. Furthermore, in those parts of the developing world where there are inadequate facilities for performing a formal biopsy, these expensive and sophisticated supplementary techniques are often impractical. Even in most developed countries, unless under exceptional circumstances, patients are rarely subjected to treatment based solely on FNA diagnosis. In some countries such as Sweden, however, patients are said to be treated on FNA diagnosis alone without undergoing surgical biopsy.[67] In the developing world, a cautious approach is needed towards the practice of FNA, taking into consideration the ease of performing FNA and the popularity of the technique.

GAPS IN IMPROVEMENTS ACHIEVED IN MANAGEMENT STRATEGIES AND DIAGNOSTIC FACILITIES

The advances in treatment strategies that occur in developed countries have percolated to the developing world at a faster pace than various aspects related to diagnosis and pathology.[68,69] This is especially true for protocols that do not require marrow transplant. This is partly due to the relative ease with which training can be imparted in instituting treatment protocols, interest shown by the international community in initiating more effective treatments in the developing world, and partly due to the enthusiasm of the pharmaceutical industry. Though not all patients in the developing world are treated the same as patients in the West, a proportion who can afford it, do receive treatment protocols similar to those in more developed countries. Hence, the know-how to deliver complex treatments does exist in the developing world. On the contrary however, improvements in diagnostic infrastructure involve extended training of histopathologists and other technologists, improvements in tissue accrual at all levels, developing good laboratories and training personnel in cytogenetics and molecular biology. In the developing world, these facilities may be limited to few institutions (and may not exist at all in some countries), in contrast to the clinical expertise available.

SOME SUGGESTIONS FOR DEVELOPING A QUALITY LYMPHOMA SERVICE IN THE DEVELOPING WORLD

The main ingredients for a successful lymphoma service is the presence of a hematopathologist with high expertise (histopathologist with expertise in lymphomas), an adequate number of cases to hone and maintain skills, a good immunohistochemistry set-up and recourse to molecular biology in a proportion of cases where required. Developing a competent and reliable hematopathologist involves identifying a histopathologist with profound interest and dedication toward lymphomas and providing specific training in lymphomas, preferably at a center of excellence so that there is a proper transfer of concepts. Having an adequate number of lymphoma samples is extremely important. However, it is difficult to specify what numbers could be considered 'adequate'. One would suspect that in the developing world, an expert lymphoma pathologist would have to see at least 1000 cases annually to maintain good skills. This is particularly so in the developing world because the spectrum of lymphomas seen in the developing world is smaller than in the West. Having an excellent immunohistochemistry facility is a must. One might be able to function with a relatively limited panel of immunostains, but the results need to be absolutely reliable. Developing a limited molecular pathology service within the hemtopathologists' arena with facilities for polymerase chain reaction (PCR), reverse transcriptase-PCR (RT-PCR) and FISH-based studies should be encouraged. To achieve all these, a certain amount of centralization and a planned referral pattern need to be developed. Such a center should have a fast turnaround time for diagnosis and the links between referring institutions and the referral center need to strong and cordial.

SOME PRACTICAL SUGGESTIONS FOR PLANNING IMMUNOHISTOCHEMISTRY IN THE DEVELOPING WORLD

Owing to limitations on resources, the panels of antibodies available are often limited, and even where available hematopathologists in the developing world could be under pressure to employ as few immunostains per case as possible. Table 47.3 provides a guide for working-up lymphomas when confronted with such difficulties. In the West, the high costs of immunostaining are related to the sensitive detection systems and automation involved, and the high costs of

Table 47.3   Essential/desirable diagnostic panel of antibodies for more common lymph nodal lymphomas in centers with limited resources

Hematoxylin and eosin staining diagnosis	Diagnosis on first panel of immunostains	Immunohistochemistry panel
Suspected 'indolent' lymphoma		CD20, CD3, Ki-67, CD21, BCL2
	Suspected FL	BCL6, CD10
	FL vs MCL	CD5, CD10, BCL6, cyclin D1
	CLL vs MCL	CD5, CD23, cyclin D1
	Suspected MZL or MALT lymphoma	CD10, CD5, CD23, BCL6, cyclin D1, keratin (MALT lymphoma)
	Lymphomaplasmacytic lymphoma	CD10, CD5, CD23, BCL6, cyclin D1, light chains, heavy chains
Monomorphic 'large' cell proliferations		CD20, CD3, Ki-67, CD21
	DLBCL	–
	Burkitt lymphoma	CD10, BCL6, BCL2
	Negative for CD20 and CD3; suspicious of metastasis	Keratins, CD45 (LCA)
	Negative for CD20 and CD3; suspicious of ALCL	CD45 (LCA), CD43, CD5, CD30, ALK, EMA
	Negative for CD20 and CD3; suspicious of plasmacytoma	CD45 (LCA), CD138, CD79a, light chains
	Negative for CD20 and CD3; suspicious of myeloid sarcoma	Work-up like blastic malignancy
Monomorphic blastic malignancy		CD20, CD3, Ki-67, Tdt, CD10, CD43
	T-LL	–
	CD20-positive B-LL	–
	CD10 and Tdt positive but negative for CD20, CD3 and CD43	CD79a, PAX5, myeloperoxidase, CD34 and CD117.
	Suspicious of myeloid sarcoma	CD79a, PAX5, myeloperoxidase, CD34 and CD117.
Classical Hodgkin lymphoma		CD45 (LCA), CD20, CD3, CD15, CD30
	Classical Hodgkin lymphoma vs T cell rich B cell lymphoma	CD79a, IgD, IgM, CD4, CD8, OCT2, BOB.1
	Classical Hodgkin lymphoma vs anaplastic large cell lymphoma	CD79a, PAX5, ALK, CD4, CD8, CD43, CD5, EBV-LMP1
Hodgkin lymphoma, nodular lymphocyte predominant type		CD45 (LCA), CD20, CD3, CD15, CD30, CD21, EMA
	Hodgkin lymphoma, nodular lymphocyte predominant type vs classical Hodgkin lymphoma	CD57, OCT2, BOB.1, BCL6, MUM1, EBV-LMP1, J-chain
Polymorphous proliferation; suspicious of a peripheral T cell lymphoma		CD20, CD3, Ki-67, CD21, CD30, CD4, CD8, CD10
	PTCL vs classical Hodgkin lymphoma	CD5, CD15, CD45 (LCA), IgD, IgM, light chains
	PTCL vs T cell rich B cell lymphoma	CD5, CD2, CD7, light chains
	PTCL vs anaplastic large cell lymphoma	ALK, EMA

CLL, chronic lymphocylic leukemia; FL, follicular lymphoma; MCL, mantle cell lymphoma; MZL, marginal zone B cell lymphoma; MALT, mucosa-associated lymphoid tissue; DLBCL, diffuse large B cell lymphoma; ALCL, anaplastic large cell lymphoma; T-LL, T lymphoblastic lymphoma; B-LL, B lymphoblastic lymphoma; PTCL, peripheral T cell lymphomas.

the personnel employed, rather than the primary antibodies. In the DW, personnel costs are low, and hence employing additional technical staff would be preferable to automation, though automation does bring in a better standardization of procedures. Furthermore, if reliable detection systems are made available locally at relatively lower costs, a much wider panel of immunohistochemistry can be administered.

NEED FOR STUDYING LYMPHOMAS FROM THE DEVELOPING WORLD WITH PRECISION

Information relating to the distribution of lymphoma subtypes in different geographic regions and ethnic groups could prove to be invaluable in developing a better understanding of causal or predisposing factors to lymphomas, and potentially, to providing information relevant to treatment outcome. Of course, this would require the uniform and expert use of a single, widely accepted classification scheme. If the WHO classification cannot be used prospectively on a case by case basis, the cases, especially those that are on clinical trials can be analyzed in batches with some help from other centers. Whether tissue arrays (with 50–500 samples arrayed on one paraffin block) can be used in this setting for classifying lymphomas retrospectively, needs to be addressed. This could be an alternative method to investigate large volumes of cases, in a standardized way, using a wide panel of immunohistochemistry at a low cost.

KEY POINTS

- There is a significant variation in the incidence of lymphoma across different geographic regions in the world. Similarly, the proportions of various lymphoma subtypes also vary.
- Though there may be a lack of skilled human resources in some of the developing countries, if expertise is nurtured and developed, and as long as histologic material is properly fixed and sectioned, the WHO classification can be employed, at least in major centers in the developing world.
- Due to the suboptimal quality of histologic material and nonavailability of a wide array of immunohistochemistry, some non-neoplastic lymphoid lesions are at special risk of being labelled as lymphomas.
- Underdiagnosis of lymphomas often stems from suboptimal sample quality and inadequate personnel training.
- FNA is the preferred first procedure in *screening* patients with peripheral lymphadenopathy.
- In the developing world, a high standard of lymphoma practice can be achieved through a certain amount of centralization and a planned referral practice.

REFERENCES

● = Key primary paper
◆ = Major review article

◆1. Harris NL, Jaffe ES, Stein H *et al.* A revised European-American classification of lymphoid neoplasms: a proposal from the International Lymphoma Study Group. *Blood* 1994; **84**: 1361–92.

2. Jaffe ES, Harris NL, Stein H *et al. World Health Organization of tumours, pathology and genetics. Tumours of haematopoietic and lymphoid tissues.* Lyon: IARC Press, 2001.

3. Ferlay J, Bray F, Pisani P, Parkin DM. *GLOBOCAN 2002: cancer incidence, mortality and prevalence worldwide.* Lyon: IARC Press, 2004.

4. Morton LM, Wang SS, Devesa SS *et al.* Lymphoma incidence patterns by WHO subtype in the United States, 1992–2001. *Blood* 2006; **107**: 265–76.

5. Naresh KN, Agarwal B, Nathwani BN *et al.* Use of the World Health Organization (WHO) classification of non-Hodgkin's lymphoma in Mumbai, India: a review of 200 consecutive cases by a panel of five expert hematopathologists. *Leuk Lymphoma* 2004; **45**: 1569–77.

◆6. Naresh KN, Advani S, Adde M *et al.* Report of an International Network of Cancer Treatment and Research workshop on non-Hodgkin's lymphoma in developing countries. *Blood Cells Mol Dis* 2004; **33**: 330–7.

●7. Anderson JR, Armitage JO, Weisenburger DD. Epidemiology of the non-Hodgkin's lymphomas: distributions of the major subtypes differ by geographic locations. Non-Hodgkin's Lymphoma Classification Project. *Ann Oncol* 1998; **9**: 717–20.

●8. The World Health Organization classification of malignant lymphomas in Japan: incidence of recently recognized entities. Lymphoma Study Group of Japanese Pathologists. *Pathol Int* 2000; **50**: 696–702.

●9. Ko YH, Kim CW, Park CS *et al.* REAL classification of malignant lymphomas in the Republic of Korea: incidence of recently recognized entities and changes in clinicopathologic features. Hematolymphoreticular Study Group of the Korean Society of Pathologists. Revised European-American lymphoma. *Cancer* 1998; **83**: 806–12.

●10. Chuang SS, Lin CN, Li CY. Malignant lymphoma in southern Taiwan according to the revised European-American classification of lymphoid neoplasms. *Cancer* 2000; **89**: 1586–92.

11. Abid MB, Nasim F, Anwar K, Pervez S. Diffuse large B cell lymphoma (DLBCL) in Pakistan: an emerging epidemic? *Asian Pac J Cancer Prev* 2005; **6**: 531–4.

12. Castella A, Joshi S, Raaschou T, Mason N. Pattern of malignant lymphoma in the United Arab Emirates – a histopathologic and immunologic study in 208 native patients. *Acta Oncol* 2001; **40**: 660–4.

13. Baker H, Al-Jarallah M, Manguno H *et al.* Clinical characteristics and pathological classification of non-Hodgkin's lymphoma in Kuwait. Results of a

collaborative study with the International Lymphoma Study Group (ILSG). *Leuk Lymphoma* 2004; **45**: 1865–71.

●14. Srinivas V, Soman CS, Naresh KN. Study of the distribution of 289 non-Hodgkin lymphomas using the WHO classification among children and adolescents in India. *Med Pediatr Oncol* 2002; **39**: 40–3.

15. Wright D, McKeever P, Carter R. Childhood non-Hodgkin lymphomas in the United Kingdom: findings from the UK Children's Cancer Study Group. *J Clin Pathol* 1997; **50**: 128–34.

16. Samuelsson BO, Ridell B, Rockert L *et al.* Non-Hodgkin lymphoma in children: a 20-year population-based epidemiologic study in western Sweden. *J Pediatr Hematol Oncol* 1999; **21**: 103–10.

●17. Biagi JJ, Seymour JF. Insights into the molecular pathogenesis of follicular lymphoma arising from analysis of geographic variation. *Blood* 2002; **99**: 4265–75.

18. Barth TF, Bentz M, Leithauser F *et al.* Molecular-cytogenetic comparison of mucosa-associated marginal zone B-cell lymphoma and large B-cell lymphoma arising in the gastro-intestinal tract. *Genes Chromosomes Cancer* 2001; **31**: 316–25.

19. Magrath IT. African Burkitt's lymphoma. History, biology, clinical features, and treatment. *Am J Pediatr Hematol Oncol* 1991; **13**: 222–46.

20. Rao CR, Gutierrez MI, Bhatia K *et al.* Association of Burkitt's lymphoma with the Epstein–Barr virus in two developing countries. *Leuk Lymphoma* 2000; **39**: 329–37.

●21. Naresh KN, Srinivas V, Soman CS. Distribution of various subtypes of non-Hodgkin's lymphoma in India: a study of 2773 lymphomas using R.E.A.L. and WHO Classifications. *Ann Oncol* 2000; **11**(Suppl 1): 63–7.

●22. A clinical evaluation of the International Lymphoma Study Group classification of non-Hodgkin's lymphoma. The non-Hodgkin's Lymphoma Classification Project. *Blood* 1997; **89**: 3909–18.

23. Lee SH, Su IJ, Chen RL *et al.* A pathologic study of childhood lymphoma in Taiwan with special reference to peripheral T-cell lymphoma and the association with Epstein–Barr viral infection. *Cancer* 1991; **68**: 1954–62.

24. Advani S, Pai S, Adde M *et al.* Preliminary report of an intensified, short duration chemotherapy protocol for the treatment of pediatric non-Hodgkin's lymphoma in India. *Ann Oncol* 1997; **8**: 893–7.

25. Ohshima K, Suzumiya J, Kikuchi M. The World Health Organization classification of malignant lymphoma: incidence and clinical prognosis in HTLV-1-endemic area of Fukuoka. *Pathol Int* 2002; **52**: 1–12.

26. Ferlay J, Bray F, Sankila R, Parkin DM. *EUCAN: cancer incidence, mortality and prevalence in the European Union 1996*, version 3.1 ed. Lyon: IARC Press, IARC Cancer Base No. 4, 1999.

27. Winter H, Cheng KK, Cummins C *et al.* Cancer incidence in the south Asian population of England (1990–92). *Br J Cancer* 1999; **79**: 645–54.

28. Naresh KN, Agarwal B, Sangal BC *et al.* Regional variation in the distribution of subtypes of lymphoid neoplasms in India. *Leuk Lymphoma* 2002; **43**: 1939–43.

●29. Naresh KN, Johnson J, Srinivas V *et al.* Epstein–Barr virus association in classical Hodgkin's disease provides survival advantage to patients and correlates with higher expression of proliferation markers in Reed-Sternberg cells. *Ann Oncol* 2000; **11**: 91–6.

30. Glaser SL, Lin RJ, Stewart SL *et al.* Epstein–Barr virus-associated Hodgkin's disease: epidemiologic characteristics in international data. *Int J Cancer* 1997; **70**: 375–82.

●31. Jarrett AF, Armstrong AA, Alexander E. Epidemiology of EBV and Hodgkin's lymphoma. *Ann Oncol* 1996; **7**(Suppl 4): 5–10.

32. Huh J, Park C, Juhng S *et al.* A pathologic study of Hodgkin's disease in Korea and its association with Epstein–Barr virus infection. *Cancer* 1996; **77**: 949–55.

33. Chan JK, Yip TT, Tsang WY *et al.* Detection of Epstein–Barr virus in Hodgkin's disease occurring in an Oriental population. *Hum Pathol* 1995; **26**: 314–18.

34. Belkaid MI, Briere J, Djebbara Z *et al.* Comparison of Epstein–Barr virus markers in Reed-Sternberg cells in adult Hodgkin's disease tissues from an industrialized and a developing country. *Leuk Lymphoma* 1995; **17**: 163–8.

●35. Gulley ML, Eagan PA, Quintanilla-Martinez L *et al.* Epstein–Barr virus DNA is abundant and monoclonal in the Reed-Sternberg cells of Hodgkin's disease: association with mixed cellularity subtype and Hispanic American ethnicity. *Blood* 1994; **83**: 1595–602.

36. Zarate-Osorno A, Roman LN, Kingma DW *et al.* Hodgkin's disease in Mexico. Prevalence of Epstein–Barr virus sequences and correlations with histologic subtype. *Cancer* 1995; **75**: 1360–6.

37. Razzouk BI, Gan YJ, Mendonca C *et al.* Epstein–Barr virus in pediatric Hodgkin disease: age and histiotype are more predictive than geographic region. *Med Pediatr Oncol* 1997; **28**: 248–54.

38. Chang KC, Khen NT, Jones D, Su IJ. Epstein–Barr virus is associated with all histological subtypes of Hodgkin lymphoma in Vietnamese children with special emphasis on the entity of lymphocyte predominance subtype. *Hum Pathol* 2005; **36**: 747–55.

39. De Matteo E, Baron AV, Chabay P *et al.* Comparison of Epstein–Barr virus presence in Hodgkin lymphoma in pediatric versus adult Argentine patients. *Arch Pathol Lab Med* 2003; **127**: 1325–9.

●40. Armstrong AA, Alexander FE, Paes RP *et al.* Association of Epstein–Barr virus with pediatric Hodgkin's disease. *Am J Pathol* 1993; **142**: 1683–8.

41. Al-Kuraya K, Narayanappa R, Al-Dayel F *et al.* Epstein–Barr virus infection is not the sole cause of high prevalence for Hodgkin's lymphoma in Saudi Arabia. *Leuk Lymphoma* 2006; **47**: 707–13.

42. Goedert JJ. The epidemiology of acquired immunodeficiency syndrome malignancies. *Semin Oncol* 2000; **27**: 390–401.

43. Dal Maso L, Franceschi S. Epidemiology of non-Hodgkin lymphomas and other haemolymphopoietic neoplasms in people with AIDS. *Lancet Oncol* 2003; **4**: 110–19.

44. Agarwal B, Ramanathan U, Lokeshwas N *et al.* Lymphoid neoplasms in HIV-positive individuals in India. *J Acquir Immune Defic Syndr* 2002; **29**: 181–3.

◆45. Knowles DM. Etiology and pathogenesis of AIDS-related non-Hodgkin's lymphoma. *Hematol Oncol Clin North Am* 2003; **17**: 785–820.

◆46. Knowles DM, Chamulak GA, Subar M *et al.* Lymphoid neoplasia associated with the acquired immunodeficiency syndrome (AIDS). The New York University Medical Center experience with 105 patients (1981–1986). *Ann Intern Med* 1988; **108**: 744–53.

47. Arzoo KK, Bu X, Espina BM *et al.* T-cell lymphoma in HIV-infected patients. *J Acquir Immune Defic Syndr* 2004; **36**: 1020–7.

48. Collins JA, Hernandez AV, Hidalgo JA *et al.* High proportion of T-cell systemic non-Hodgkin lymphoma in HIV-infected patients in Lima, Peru. *J Acquir Immune Defic Syndr* 2005; **40**: 558–64.

49. Gold JE, Schwam L, Castella A *et al.* Malignant plasma cell tumors in human immunodeficiency virus-infected patients. *Cancer* 1990; **66**: 363–8.

●50. Rudiger T, Weisenburger DD, Anderson JR *et al.* Peripheral T-cell lymphoma (excluding anaplastic large-cell lymphoma): results from the non-Hodgkin's Lymphoma Classification Project. *Ann Oncol* 2002; **13**: 140–9.

●51. Attygalle AD, Diss TC, Munson P *et al.* CD10 expression in extranodal dissemination of angioimmunoblastic T-cell lymphoma. *Am J Surg Pathol* 2004; **28**: 54–61.

52. Naresh KN, Lampert I, Hasserjian R *et al.* Optimal bone marrow trephine biopsy processing – the Hammersmith protocol. *J Clin Pathol* 2006; **59**: 903–11.

53. Pai SA, Naresh KN. Toxoplasma lymphadenitis is mistaken for malignant lymphoma in India. *Natl Med J India* 1997; **10**: 48.

54. Greiner T, Armitage JO, Gross TG. Atypical lymphoproliferative diseases. *Hematology Am Soc Hematol Educ Program* 2000: 133–46.

55. Sneller MC, Wang J, Dale JK *et al.* Clinical, immunologic, and genetic features of an autoimmune lymphoproliferative syndrome associated with abnormal lymphocyte apoptosis. *Blood* 1997; **89**: 1341–8.

●56. Lim MS, Straus SE, Dale JK *et al.* Pathological findings in human autoimmune lymphoproliferative syndrome. *Am J Pathol* 1998; **153**: 1541–50.

57. Brown JR, Skarin AT. Clinical mimics of lymphoma. *Oncologist* 2004; **9**: 406–16.

58. Onciu M, Medeiros LJ. Kikuchi-Fujimoto lymphadenitis. *Adv Anat Pathol* 2003; **10**: 204–11.

59. Pai SA, Naresh KN, Soman CS, Borges AM. Pseudolymphomatous phase of Kikuchi-Fujimoto disease. *Indian J Cancer* 1998; **35**: 119–28.

60. Bosch X, Guilabert A, Miquel R, Campo E. Enigmatic Kikuchi-Fujimoto disease: a comprehensive review. *Am J Clin Pathol* 2004; **122**: 141–52.

61. Ahmed Z, Yaqoob N, Muzaffar S *et al.* Diagnostic surgical pathology: the importance of second opinion in a developing country. *J Pak Med Assoc* 2004; **54**: 306–11.

62. Khan H, Pervez S. Coexistence of caseating granulomas with lymphoma: a diagnostic and clinical dilemma. *J Coll Physicians Surg Pak* 2006; **16**: 540–2.

63. Centkowski P, Sawczuk-Chabin J, Prochorec M, Warzocha K. Hodgkin's lymphoma and tuberculosis coexistence in cervical lymph nodes. *Leuk Lymphoma* 2005; **46**: 471–5.

64. Thomas JO, Adeyi D, Amanguno H. Fine-needle aspiration in the management of peripheral lymphadenopathy in a developing country. *Diagn Cytopathol* 1999; **21**: 159–62.

65. Zhang JR, Raza AS, Greaves TS, Cobb CJ. Fine-needle aspiration diagnosis of Hodgkin lymphoma using current WHO classification – re-evaluation of cases from 1999–2004 with new proposals. *Diagn Cytopathol* 2006; **34**: 397–402.

66. Young NA, Al-Saleem T. Diagnosis of lymphoma by fine-needle aspiration cytology using the revised European-American classification of lymphoid neoplasms. *Cancer* 1999; **87**: 325–45.

67. Skoog L, Tani E. Diagnosis of lymphoma by fine-needle aspiration cytology using the revised European-American classification of lymphoid neoplasms. *Cancer* 2000; **90**: 320–3.

68. Biswas G, Parikh PM, Nair R *et al.* Rituximab (anti-CD20 monoclonal antibody) in lymphoproliferative malignancies: Tata Memorial experience. *J Assoc Phys India* 2006; **54**: 29–33.

69. Hesseling PB, Broadhead R, Molyneux E *et al.* Malawi pilot study of Burkitt lymphoma treatment. *Med Pediatr Oncol* 2003; **41**: 532–40.

48

Imaging lymphomas in developing countries

ALI NAWAZ KHAN

INTRODUCTION

The World Health Organization (WHO) has identified aging, infections, cancer and mental health as the four major health issues that confront the global population this century. In 2002 there were an estimated 11 million new cancers diagnosed in the world and the International Agency for Research on Cancer (IARC) predicts an increase to 16 million by 2020, with some 60 percent occurring in the less developed parts of the world. They project that regions with traditionally low numbers of cancer deaths could see significant increases in mortality. North Africa, Western Asia, South America, the Caribbean, and South East Asia, could face increases of 75 percent in the number of cancer deaths compared with 2000. However, most developing countries are not well equipped to deal with such an increase in the incidence of cancer.

In the developed world, the role of diagnostic imaging in the diagnosis and management of malignancy is well recognized and the evolution of cross-sectional and functional imaging over the past two decades has had a profound effect on the practice of oncology. In these countries, a high proportion of deaths already occur as a result of cancer (see Table 48.1). In contrast, in developing countries the imaging facilities and skills are generally much scarcer relative to the populations to be served. In part, this reflects different patterns of disease; in countries which still suffer high mortality from communicable disease and where life expectancy is relatively low, cancers are less prevalent. But in absolute terms there is still a large number of cancer cases in developing countries (Table 48.1) and over time this number is likely to rise as populations grow, incomes increase and life expectancy improves.

Table 48.1 Deaths from malignant neoplasms, 2002, by country income level group

Country group	Number of deaths from malignant neoplasms	
	Thousands	As a percentage of total deaths in country group
High income	2059	26.2
Upper middle income	592	17.4
Lower middle income	2670	15.5
Low income	1797	6.3

Source: World Health Organization. *Global burden of disease data, deaths by age, sex and cause for the year 2002.* Geneva: WHO. Available at: www.who.int/healthinfo/statistics/gbdincomelevelmortality2002.xls (accessed 18 August 2007).

CHOICE OF IMAGING TECHNIQUE

With a plethora of imaging techniques available, what role should imaging lymphomas play in developing countries? Answering the question is difficult because of the high costs of imaging technologies coupled with the fact that in developing countries expenditure on health is much lower than in developed countries (see Table 48.2), so financial resources available are very much more limited.

Table 48.2 Health expenditure per capita, 2003 (US$) by country income level group

Country group	Health expenditure per capita (US$)
High income	3449
Upper middle income	275
Lower middle income	76
Low income	30

Source: World Bank. HNPStats. Available at: www.devdata.worldbank.org/hnpstats (accessed 18 August 2007).

The choice of imaging modality to improve lymphoma management will typically be made in the context of wider decisions about priorities for imaging and for health service provision. These wider decisions reflect many different factors, which vary between countries, including disease patterns and how health services are financed. The WHO diagnostic imaging website provides useful guidance.

In taking decisions about imaging technologies, it is important to take due account of local expertise, operational arrangements, diagnostic advantage and therapeutic options.

Local expertise

Effective imaging services require not only equipment but also staff skilled in operating it and interpreting the results. There are about 500 radiologists in South Africa, for a population of 42 million people and an estimated 700 radiologists in all of sub-Saharan Africa, the majority of whom work in the private sector.[1] But training radiologists is costly and some developing countries have found it difficult to retain sufficient trained staff where they are needed; once trained they may migrate, even internationally, to work where employment conditions are better. Investment in equipment needs to be matched by investment in staff training.

Operational arrangements

In many developing countries, imaging equipment (especially advanced technology) cannot be used to its full potential because of suboptimal operational arrangements, often reflecting shortages of funding. It may be difficult to provide and sustain an appropriate environment, in terms of electricity or water supply or air conditioning. There may be supply problems with peripheral software and contrast media. Maintenance services, radiation protection and quality control may be weak, particularly if there is a shortage of specially trained staff. So choice of equipment, and securing funding for investment in equipment (even if this is in the form of an external aid grant), should not be separated from ensuring sound arrangements for its operation.

Diagnostic advantage

Evidence-based medical practice recognizes that sophisticated imaging is not always diagnostically superior to simpler technologies. *Conventional radiology*, which includes chest radiographs, skeletal X-rays, barium studies and intravenous urography, are more readily available in developing countries and easily read by nonradiologists, and still offer valuable diagnostic information. A good example is the role of a chest X-ray in the management of Hodgkin disease, which commonly appears as intrathoracic disease, and can readily be diagnosed and monitored by plain chest images in all but those cases with very subtle abnormalities.

In addition, findings by Wernecke et al. indicate that for monitoring patients with mediastinal lymphomas ultrasound is clearly superior to chest radiographs and comparable to CT.[2] And in primary bone lymphoma, plain radiographs of the affected skeleton combined with physical and laboratory examination can achieve a fairly reliable diagnosis and staging.

It is generally recognized that the best technique currently available for diagnosis, staging and follow-up of malignant lymphoma is chest-abdomen computed tomography (CT). Scutellari et al.[3] studied 134 patients with early non-Hodgkin lymphoma (NHL) to evaluate the flow charts proposed by the International Union against Cancer (UICC) for diagnosis and staging of lymphomas in developed and developing countries (1998), based on the histology of lymph node biopsy material and on imaging techniques such as CT, magnetic resonance imaging (MRI) and positron emission tomography (PET). Their study not only confirmed that CT was the most valuable imaging modality but also concluded that in developing countries, lymph node biopsy was the preferred examination because it is the most easily available, while imaging should focus on chest radiography and abdominal ultrasound.

Most, if not all, conventional radiographic studies are useful and can be fruitfully combined with ultrasound, a thorough physical examination and other laboratory tests to arrive at a fairly accurate diagnosis. However, some lymphomas such as primary cerebral lymphomas would remain elusive as they do require a cranial CT or MRI.

Therapeutic options

The value of sophisticated imaging of lymphomas is reduced when options for treating them are limited, as will often be the case in developing countries. For instance, detection of residual disease is less valuable if there is little prospect of access to salvage therapy. And the frequency of follow-up investigations needs also to take account of how much value is added by imaging when other assessments, such as clinical examination, provide clear evidence of disease progression or failure to respond to treatment.

IMAGING SERVICES IN DEVELOPING COUNTRIES

The factors affecting decisions about imaging technology discussed above suggest that in many developing country settings, aiming to replicate exactly the imaging services seen in the richest countries would lead to disappointing results in terms of enhanced clinical outcomes. It would be more appropriate to develop imaging services using some of the following options, which can be mutually reinforcing: strengthening low cost services, making greater use of radiologically guided biopsies, adopting appropriate training strategies, and making more systematic use of teleradiology.

Strengthen low cost services

Compared with sophisticated imaging, basic X-ray units and ultrasound machines are comparatively cheap, generally reliable, and easier to use and maintain. The results can also be more easily read by nonradiologists, such as nurses and technologists. Currently a large proportion of the world's population has no access even to the most basic imaging equipment such as conventional chest radiography. Strengthening the use of these services in a large number of smaller hospitals is in line with the objectives of the WHO Basic Radiological System (and its upgraded version, the World Health Imaging System for Radiology).[4] The Jefferson Ultrasound Research and Education Institute has established a program called 'Teaching the Trainers Initiative for Ultrasound Training in Africa', which provides physicians from several African countries with ultrasound training and also instructs them to train others. A two-pronged approach will be appropriate in many countries; alongside efforts to strengthen low-cost imaging services, complementary investment in higher technology such as CT and MRI can be made in a limited number of secondary referral centres, for instance attached to medical schools.

Make greater use of radiologically guided biopsies

Interventional radiology procedures are becoming increasingly important in the management of lymphomas and other cancers. Imaging can help save costs when it is used for radiologically guided biopsies. These are low technology procedures which are cheaper than some more invasive alternatives, such as laparotomy. Mediastinal, pleural and deeper visceral lesions can be effectively biopsied using ultrasound guidance and intra-thoracic and osseous lesions can be biopsied using conventional fluoroscopy.

Thomas et al.[5] reviewed the use of fine needle aspirates (FNA) in investigating peripheral lymphadenopathy as an alternative to the expensive surgical excision biopsy. They reviewed all lymph node aspirates done in the FNA clinic at the Department of Pathology, University College Hospital, Ibadan, Nigeria, between 1995 and 1997. The aspirates were obtained using 21- or 22-gauge needles with a 5 mL or 10 mL disposable plastic syringe, smeared on standard microscopic slides and stained with Giemsa and/or Papanicolaou stains. The sensitivity and specificity of lymph node FNA in the diagnosis of tuberculosis were 79.5 percent and 100 percent, respectively. The overall accuracy rate of lymph node aspiration was 89.5 percent. They concluded that FNA was a simple, cost-effective and well-tolerated procedure that offered a reliable method of diagnosis in distinguishing reactive lymphadenopathy, tuberculosis and malignant conditions.

To determine the effectiveness of interventional radiological techniques in diagnosing specific haematological malignancies in children, Garrett et al.[6] undertook 25 percutaneous biopsies, 6 fluid aspirations, 3 catheter drainages, and 1 needle localization in 22 patients (16 male, 6 female; median age, 13 years) for diagnosing suspected hematologic malignancy. They found percutaneous biopsy of lymphoma is usually diagnostic. Drainage or aspiration of a fluid collection associated with NHL or leukemia is often diagnostic and is less invasive than biopsy. These procedures are minimally invasive and effective for diagnosing pediatric hematologic malignancies.

Ben-Yehuda et al.[7] evaluated 1500 CT-guided core-needle biopsies performed at their institute during the period 1989–1994. Non-Hodgkin lymphoma was diagnosed in 71 patients, and 29 had Hodgkin disease. Among the NHL patients, 17 (24 percent) had proven lymphoma diagnosed before the biopsy was performed; in 54 (76 percent) core-needle biopsy was performed as the first diagnostic procedure. Of 29 Hodgkin disease patients, nine (31 percent) were already established cases of Hodgkin disease, and in 20 (69 percent) core-needle biopsy was the first diagnostic procedure attempted. The biopsies were performed under CT control using a 20- or 18-gauge Turner biopsy needle. They concluded that image-guided core-needle biopsies provide sufficient information for the diagnosis of and subsequent therapeutic decision to treat most cases of lymphoma. It is reasonable to suppose that similar success could be achieved with biopsies carried out using simple fluoroscopy and/or ultrasound guidance.

Adopt appropriate training strategies

It is expensive to train engineers, radiographers and radiologists. Staff training for imaging services in developing countries needs to be cost-effective and adapted to the working conditions trainees will face. In June 1999, the WHO established a Global Steering Group for Education and Training in Diagnostic Imaging and its policy is to 'train the trainers' in regional centers of excellence for education and training (in Africa, Asia, Latin America and the Western Pacific), rather than sending people to train in institutions in the developed world. Other elements of their approach include developing generic training materials and practical manuals that can be translated into local languages and will be more appropriate and user-friendly than textbooks. The WHO is also supporting the training of senior radiographers to help improve diagnostic decision-making where no radiologist is available. There is also growing scope for countries to use internet-based materials for 'tele-learning' in medical education. For example, MyPACS Enterprise, partly funded by the National Institute of Health, provides free access to a large library of images and case reports for reference, training and decision-support. MyPACS is an efficient browser-based application which runs on standard PC hardware and can be used by radiologists round the world to create their own electronic teaching files and to exchange information with each other. It has been endorsed by several prestigious institutions including the International Society of Radiology and the American College of Radiology.

Make systematic use of teleradiology[8,9]

As radiology is an image-based specialty and depends highly on pattern recognition, the development of the internet has led to the emergence of 'teleradiology'. This involves images from basic radiography, ultrasound or CT, together with consultative text, being electronically transmitted from one location to another. It permits hospitals with limited medical resources to consult expert opinion even if it is hundreds or thousands of miles away from the patient. In countries where there are few radiologists, this can assist diagnosis and patient management. Teleradiology services depend on high speed telecommunications, allowing rapid transmission of digital images without loss of content or resolution. Although teleradiology entails some risks, such as virus or worm infections of electronic patient data, this way of working is expanding fast in developing countries, including in Latin America, Asia and sub-Saharan Africa, and this can be expected to continue as internet access and security improves.

KEY POINTS

(A) In taking decisions about imaging technologies in developing countries, costs will continue to be a major obstacle and so it is important to take due account of:

- local availability of staff with the required expertise
- suitability and sustainability of operational arrangements for the equipment
- diagnostic advantage (if any) of the more sophisticated techniques
- therapeutic options which are available.

(B) In expanding imaging services in developing countries, options which are likely to have value include:

- strengthening low-cost services such as ultrasound and conventional radiography, in line with the WHO Basic Radiological System
- making greater use of radiologically guided biopsies which are less invasive and cheaper than surgical procedures such as laparotomy or excision biopsy
- adopting appropriate training strategies, including 'training the trainers', delivering training in-country, and using locally appropriate training materials and user manuals
- making more systematic use of teleradiology as a means of obtaining specialist opinion regarding diagnosis and patient management.

REFERENCES

● = Key primary paper
◆ = Major review article

●1. The Global Face of Radiology. Round Table 2003. Available at: www.diagnosticimaging.com/roundtable2003 (accessed 18 August 2007).
2. Wernecke K, Peters P, Galanski M. Mediastinal tumors. Evaluation with suprasternal US. *Radiology* 1986; **159**: 405–9.
3. Scutellari PN, Borgatti L, Spanedda R. Non-Hodgkin's lymphomas of extra nodal localization. Strategies for imaging diagnosis. *Radiol Med (Torino)* 2000; **100**: 262–72.
4. World Health Organization website: www.who.int
5. Thomas JO, Adeyi D, Amanguno H. Fine-needle aspiration in the management of peripheral lymphadenopathy in a developing country. *Diagn Cytopathol* 1999; **21**: 159–62.
6. Garrett KM, Hoffer FA, Behm FG *et al.* Interventional radiology techniques for the diagnosis of lymphoma or leukemia. *Pediatr Radiol* 2002; **32**: 653–62.
7. Ben-Yehuda D, Polliack A, Okon E *et al.* Image-guided core-needle biopsy in malignant lymphoma: experience with 100 patients that suggests the technique is reliable. *J Clin Oncol* 1996; **14**: 2415–16.
●8. Edworthy SM. Telemedicine in developing countries. *BMJ* 2001; **323**: 524–5.
●9. Rigby M. And into the 21st century: telecommunications and the global clinic. In: Rigby M, Roberts R, Thick M. (eds) *Taking health telematics into the 21st century.* Abingdon: Radcliffe Medical Press, 2000: 187–206.

GENERAL PRINCIPLES OF MANAGEMENT

49

Emergency management in lymphoid malignancies

AZIZA T SHAD AND AMAL M ABU-GHOSH

INTRODUCTION

With the continuing rise in the incidence of cancer (including leukemia, lymphoma, and multiple myeloma) and the current trend of treating malignancies more aggressively, an increasing number of patients are at risk for complications arising from either the disease itself or unwanted side effects of treatment. Many of these complications present as oncologic emergencies, and carry with them considerable morbidity and mortality. Thus, the successful management of the lymphoid neoplasms, as for all other cancers, not only involves the administration of specific therapy, but the treatment of these complications, which may arise either acutely, i.e., before or during therapy, or later, i.e., months or years after the completion of treatment.

Complications frequently encountered during cancer management can be divided into two broad categories, each of which can be further subdivided into various subcategories as shown in Tables 49.1 and 49.2. These categories are:

1. *Tumor-related complications.* These include
   (a) complications that arise as a result of the physical encroachment of tumor masses on vital structures or from the large bulk of tumor at diagnosis: for example, airway obstruction, superior and inferior vena caval obstruction, pleural and pericardial effusions, cardiac tamponade or arrhythmias, raised intracranial pressure, spinal cord compression, and pulmonary embolism; (b) metabolic complications including the tumor lysis syndrome, hypercalcemia, hypo/hyperglycemia, and syndrome of inappropriate antidiuretic hormone secretion (SIADH); (c) complications related to lymphomatous involvement of the gastrointestinal tract, such as intestinal obstruction, hemorrhage, and fistulae; (d) complications such as cardiac arrest, associated with the administration of anesthetics in patients with large mediastinal masses; and (e) cytokine-mediated complications, such as cancer cachexia and fever.

2. *Treatment-related complications.* This broad category includes common and frequently expected complications such as fever and neutropenia, nausea and vomiting, anemia, thrombocytopenia, and mucositis, along with serious, and at times, life-threatening emergencies such as typhlitis/neutropenic enterocolitis, perforation of a viscus, gastrointestinal bleeding, seizures following chemotherapy, drug extravasation, and severe neuropathy. Less common complications such as methotrexate-associated encephalopathy, myelopathy following intrathecal drugs, dermatological problems such as palmar-plantar dyskinesia and pigmentation, and some cytokine-related effects also fall into this category.

Table 49.1 Common complications and emergencies associated with the management of lymphoid neoplasms

1. Tumor-related complications

1.1 Complications related to space-occupying lesions
  a. Superior vena cava syndrome and superior mediastinal syndrome
  b. Spinal cord compression and other neurological emergencies
  c. Pleural and pericardial effusions
  d. Obstructive uropathy
1.2 Metabolic complications
  a. Tumor lysis syndrome
  b. Hypercalcemia
1.3 Gastrointestinal complications
  a. Gastrointestinal bleeding, fistulae, intestinal obstruction
1.4 Complications associated with massive mediastinal disease
  a. Anesthetic problems; cardiac arrest
1.5. Hematological complications
  a. Bone marrow infiltration
  b. Autoimmune cytopenias

Table 49.2 Common complications and emergencies associated with the management of lymphoid neoplasms

2. Treatment-related complications

2.1 Myelosuppression
  a. Fever and neutropenia
  b. Anemia and thrombocytopenia
2.2 Abdominal emergencies
  Typhlitis/neutropenic enterocolitis
2.3 Neurological complications following chemotherapy
  a. Seizures and/or acute encephalopathy
  b. Myelopathy following administration of intrathecal therapy
  c. Cranial nerve palsies/peripheral neuropathy
2.4 Metabolic complications
  a. Hyperglycemia
  b. Syndrome of inappropriate antidiuretic hormone secretion
2.5 Cardiac complications
2.6 Nausea and vomiting
2.7 Mucositis
2.8 Central line-related complications
  a. Infection
  b. Thrombosis and embolism

In this chapter we will only discuss the most frequent, life-threatening complications that either present at the time of diagnosis of a lymphoid neoplasm or occur acutely in association with treatment.

TUMOR-RELATED COMPLICATIONS

Complications related to space-occupying lesions

An important characteristic of most intermediate- and high-grade lymphomas is the rapidity with which they grow, which often leads to the acute onset and rapid progression of complications arising from space-occupying lesions. Since these lymphomas can arise in essentially any organ or tissue, early treatment is essential, and all attempts should be made to establish the diagnosis as soon as possible, particularly in the presence of a tumor mass adjacent to vital structures such as in the mediastinum or central nervous system (CNS). It is critical that an adequate tumor sample be obtained for diagnostic purposes prior to commencing emergency treatment (except in life-threatening situations), since a rapid response to therapy could result in an uninterpretable histological picture, even within the space of 48 hours,[1] and consequently deprive the patient of optimal (histology based) therapy. Loeffler et al., for example, reported a series of 19 patients who received emergency prebiopsy irradiation for a mediastinal mass. In eight of these patients the biopsy was reported as uninterpretable.[2]

As far as possible, an attempt should be made to establish a diagnosis by biopsying or aspirating accessible sites of disease (i.e., lymph nodes, subcutaneous tumors, serous effusions, bone marrow, and cerebrospinal fluid [CSF]). Risky surgical procedures such as a mediastinal biopsy under general anesthesia in a patient with a large mediastinal mass and compromised airway should be avoided.

SUPERIOR VENA CAVA SYNDROME AND SUPERIOR MEDIASTINAL SYNDROME

Superior vena cava syndrome (SVCS) is the clinical presentation of superior vena cava (SVC) obstruction or compression which results in severe reduction of venous return from the head, neck, and upper extremities. When accompanied by tracheal compression, the condition is known as superior mediastinal syndrome (SMS). Adults tend to present with signs of SVC obstruction alone, whereas in children, tracheal compression and respiratory embarrassment are usually accompanying features of SVCS because of the softness and small size of the trachea.[3]

Since the first description of SVCS by William Hunter in 1757[4] the underlying etiology has changed from predominantly infectious, particularly tuberculosis and syphilitic aortic aneurysm, to predominantly malignant in more recent reports.[5–7]

In adults, lymphoma is the third most frequent malignant cause of SVC obstruction, accounting for 12 percent of cases, following non-small-cell carcinoma and small cell lung cancer, which account for 50 percent and 22 percent of malignant causes, respectively.[7,8] In addition, with the increasing use of intravascular devices and pacemakers, 35 percent of adult SVCS cases are reported due to nonmalignant conditions.[9]

Superior vena cava syndrome is rare in the pediatric population, occurring in 12 percent of patients with malignant mediastinal tumors.[10,11] Non-Hodgkin lymphoma (NHL) continues to head the list as the most common malignant cause of SVC obstruction in children. An extensive review of the literature by Issa et al.[12] in 1983 revealed 150 reported cases of SVCS in childhood. Of these, only 24 (16 percent) were neoplastic in origin, 16 of them resulting from NHL and one from Hodgkin lymphoma (HL). In another study, Pokorny and Sherman[10] described 109 children with mediastinal masses, including 24 with lymphoma. Superior vena cava syndrome occurred in three (20 percent) of 15 children with NHL and in none of nine with HL. In another review of the 121 children with mediastinal masses who presented to the Royal Children's Hospital, Melbourne, the commonest cause found was NHL (36 cases).[13] These studies reiterate the fact that NHL is still the most frequent neoplastic cause of SVC obstruction in children.

The anatomy of the SVC, with its thin wall and close apposition to the vertebral column, makes it particularly vulnerable to compression or invasion by malignancies arising in the mediastinum. It is surrounded by lymph nodes that drain the right and lower-left sides of the chest, and by the thymus in the anterior, superior mediastinum. Thus, involvement of the thymus or adjacent lymph nodes by tumor can cause compression of the SVC. Prolonged compression and/or invasion frequently results in intraluminal thrombosis (which may be exacerbated by the low pressure flow within the SVC) and complete occlusion of the vein, although lymphomas, being less invasive and more rapidly growing than carcinomas, more often cause compression without thrombosis.[14] The trachea and right main-stem bronchus, although relatively rigid when compared to the SVC, can also be easily compressed by tumor in children. The small intraluminal diameter of the trachea in children compared to adults can only accommodate minimal edema, thus symptoms of respiratory obstruction often occur rapidly. The degree and rapidity of obstruction that occurs secondary to compression, clotting, and edema determines the severity of the symptoms and signs. Collateral vessels enlarge in compensation, but fail to adequately relieve the obstruction in most instances.

The severity of clinical symptoms is dependent on the rate and degree of SVC obstruction. Rapidly developing obstruction results in more severe symptoms compared to slowly developing obstruction that allows sufficient time for the formation of collateral circulation. More severe clinical symptoms are also seen when obstruction occurs below the level of the azygous vein. Both adults and children with SVC obstruction can present with a wide range of clinical symptoms, which commonly include cough, hoarseness, chest pain, dyspnea, and orthopnea. Respiratory distress and hoarseness were the prominent symptoms in

all 11 children with T cell lymphoma who presented to the Chaim Sheba Medical Center, Israel.[15] Armstrong et al.[7] found that dyspnea, often associated with swelling of the trunk or extremities, was the most common presenting symptom in both bronchogenic carcinomas and lymphomas. Other less common but more sinister symptoms suggesting cerebral edema are those of dizziness, headache, anxiety, epistaxis, distorted vision, altered mental status, and syncope, the latter often aggravated by bending.[1,14,16–18] Signs of SVCS include swelling, plethora and cyanosis of the face, neck, and arms with prominence of collateral veins, diaphoresis, wheezing, and stridor. There may be associated pleural or pericardial effusions. The presence of a pleural effusion may indicate simultaneous obstruction of the thoracic duct, although direct involvement of the pleura is also likely. The presence of laryngeal and/or cerebral edema has often been stated to indicate a poor prognosis in patients with SVC obstruction,[6,16] but these complications are rare and have not been clearly shown to be an immediate consequence of SVC obstruction – they may be more likely caused by direct compression of airways, or invasion of the brain by tumor.[19] An unusual finding, not reported in children but sometimes seen in adults in association with SVCS, is spinal cord compression.[20] This again probably relates most often to direct compression by tumor rather than venous congestion or infarction. In adults, the onset of SVCS caused by malignant tumor is often insidious (depending on the histology) with symptoms developing over a period of a few weeks, in contrast to children and adolescents, in whom symptoms may rapidly progress in a few days.

In a patient who presents with clinical evidence of SVC obstruction, an efficient radiological workup can help to establish the diagnosis, guide attempts at pathologic confirmation, and aid in management decisions.[21] Routine studies with demonstrable ability include chest x-rays, ultrasound, computed tomography (CT) and magnetic resonance imaging (MRI) scans, venography, and nuclear studies. A chest x-ray can usually be obtained expeditiously and almost always demonstrates a right-sided mediastinal mass or mediastinal widening. Armstrong et al.[7] found a superior mediastinal mass in 59 percent of all patients with an SVCS, with a right-sided hilar mass in an additional 19 percent. Pleural and pericardial effusions, hilar adenopathy, and evidence of tracheal compression may also be seen on chest x-ray. Ultrasonography of the neck, subclavian, and brachial veins is noninvasive and can identify the presence of a thrombus. A CT scan of the chest with contrast has the advantage of providing more accurate information on the location of the obstruction and is useful for guiding subsequent attempts at biopsy via mediastinoscopy, bronchoscopy, or percutaneous fine needle aspiration. A peripheral venogram may be helpful in determining the patency of the venous system as well as the establishment and efficiency of collateral circulation,[22,23] but this is a more invasive procedure and is only used if surgery or a stent placement is planned. Magnetic resonance imaging of the mediastinum has several advantages over a CT scan, including the ability to image in several different planes and to directly visualize blood flow without the use of iodinated contrast material.[24,25] However, it has some disadvantages such as the lengthy time needed for scanning (which may not be ideal in a patient with SVCS and respiratory distress) and high cost. Positron emission tomography-CT may distinguish malignant from nonmalignant mediastinal lesions although chronic thrombosis may show 2-fluoro-2-deoxy-D-glucose (FDG) uptake.[26]

A histological diagnosis of malignancy is essential prior to initiation of antineoplastic therapy. However, it is wise to avoid biopsy of a large mediastinal mass if possible, because of its relative inaccessibility and the potential for complications.[27] Children with SVCS or SMS tolerate invasive diagnostic procedures poorly. Patients with large mediastinal masses are at increased risk for developing complications during the induction of anesthesia[1] (primarily because of airway obstruction) or during the surgical procedure itself. Difficulty in intubation, acute cardiac arrest, as well as increased bleeding from engorged mediastinal veins have been described.[19,28] If tracheal intubation is performed (either as an emergency procedure for respiratory arrest, or electively for diagnostic purposes) it may be difficult to extubate the patient until significant reduction in the size of the mediastinal mass has been achieved. In consequence, some authors have recommended therapy with corticosteroids (which may induce only minimum shrinkage) or mediastinal radiation therapy before performing a biopsy.[19] This course should only be undertaken when there is no alternative to mediastinal biopsy, and the latter is considered to be too risky to undertake.

Clearly, because of the risks associated with anesthesia, the least invasive procedure likely to establish a diagnosis of a lymphoid neoplasm should be chosen in patients with a mediastinal mass. A simple blood count may show evidence of leukemia, or a fine needle aspiration or biopsy of an enlarged peripheral lymph node under local anesthesia may provide the diagnosis. Detailed characterization of cells from a pleural effusion (including immunophenotyping), if present, should be performed and the bone marrow should always be examined for involvement prior to a surgical procedure. If the tumor is confined to the mediastinum, however, then biopsy via CT or ultrasound guidance, mediastinoscope or parasternal mediastinotomy, median sternotomy, video-assisted thoracoscopy, or conventional thoracotomy is warranted, if deemed safe. Mediastinoscopy provides better access to paratracheal masses than mediastinotomy, which is the procedure of choice for anterior mediastinal tumors.[14] It has been reported to be a safe and effective technique for establishing a histological diagnosis in SVCS when less invasive techniques have been unsuccessful.[29] A major concern is the risk of bleeding with mediastinoscopy in the presence of SVCS, but data from several published series suggest that this is an uncommon problem.[5,30] An alternative method to establish the diagnosis in patients with advanced

SVCS is ultrasound-guided transthoracic needle aspiration biopsy. The diagnostic yield using this method in 41 patients with advanced SVCS was approximately 83 percent. None of the patients was reported to have had any complications.[31]

Clearly, in patients with lymphoma causing SVC obstruction, it is appropriate to institute treatment expeditiously.[8] It is worth pointing out, however, that the presence of SVC obstruction itself does not appear to be life threatening. It is the accompanying tracheal compression and respiratory embarrassment that prompts emergency management.[32,33] Fatalities due to venous obstruction *per se* have not been indisputably demonstrated in the literature and patients have survived for as long as 28 years with unrelieved SVC obstruction.[19] These observations suggest that emergency treatment is not indicated simply because of the presence of SVC obstruction, and that an uncomplicated SVCS does not represent sufficient grounds for immediate irradiation without the establishment of a pathological diagnosis. Chemotherapy can bring about rapid resolution of SVC obstruction caused by NHL and is emerging as the treatment of choice in this situation. This is already the case in aggressive, high-grade lymphomas, where a considerable reduction of tumor bulk can be achieved with a single cycle of chemotherapy, and is particularly relevant in children where the commonest NHL causing SVC obstruction is lymphoblastic lymphoma, in which overall survival is not improved by the addition of mediastinal radiation to chemotherapy.[17] In fact, in younger patients, radiation may cause additional problems such as tracheal edema, resulting in postirradiation respiratory embarrassment, and significantly increase the risk of late pulmonary or cardiac toxicity. Radiation therapy should thus be reserved for tumors that are less likely to respond quickly to chemotherapy.

When radiation therapy is utilized, the field usually includes all gross tumors plus a tumor-free margin. The mediastinal, hilar, and supraclavicular lymph nodes are also usually irradiated, but this will depend upon plans for subsequent chemotherapy.[18] Although the total radiation dose and rate of administration are dependent on the type of tumor, the patient's condition, and the degree of local disease extension, relatively low-dose therapy is preferable when radiation is being used purely as emergency therapy (e.g., to a total of 1200 cGy) to avoid local complications such as esophagitis, including recall esophagitis with subsequent chemotherapy. Irradiation of a large volume of bone marrow may also significantly impair the ability to deliver subsequent chemotherapy effectively. Anthracyclines, usually an important component of leukemia and lymphoma treatment, enhance radiation damage, so that the risk of added toxicity, especially esophagitis, pericarditis, and myocardial damage, is significantly increased if mediastinal irradiation is used. Tumors such as lymphoblastic lymphoma, which are extremely radioresponsive, can undergo rapid dissolution with doses as low as 200 cGy. Almost 75 percent of patients with SVCS who receive radiation experience symptomatic relief within 3–4 days after initiation of treatment, while 90 percent are symptom free by the end of the first week.[27] In the 10 percent of patients whose symptoms do not improve within the first week of therapy, one should either reconsider the diagnosis or suspect thrombosis and consider treatment with anticoagulants.

The presence of a documented thrombosis in patients with SVCS requires treatments that may include thrombectomy using tissue plasminogen activator (tPA), streptokinase, or urokinase.[34] The use of stents with or without anticoagulants to reopen the occluded SVC has also been reported with response rates of greater than 90 percent.[8,35]

Rarely, a patient may need other emergency measures such as a decompressive SVC bypass. It is recommended that an SVC bypass be considered early in the occasional patient who presents with profound cerebral or laryngeal edema, extensive thrombosis of the SVC, or severe hypertension and in whom a tissue diagnosis requires a mediastinal exploration.[33]

NEUROLOGICAL EMERGENCIES – SPINAL CORD COMPRESSION

Involvement of the CNS by malignancy, especially leukemia and lymphoma, has been well described, its overall incidence ranging between 5 and 11 percent, for example, in patients with NHL.[32,36–40] The most frequent type of neurological involvement reported is meningeal infiltration, followed by spinal cord compression,[36,41] the latter also seen as a presenting feature in multiple myeloma, although some series report the opposite.[42] Central nervous system involvement can either be a presenting feature or occur at relapse (in isolation or accompanied by systemic disease). Prior to the advent of CNS prophylaxis, cerebral and meningeal disease frequently occurred in patients who had achieved clinical remission, as shown by Levitt et al.[32] in their series of 30 patients, 12 of whom relapsed within 9 months of the initiation of therapy. Risk factors for the development of CNS involvement include a histological diagnosis of leukemia, high-grade lymphoma (82 percent of patients described by Young et al. had diffuse histology as compared to 3 percent with nodular lymphoma[36]), advanced disease at presentation, and associated bone marrow involvement.

Leukemic or lymphomatous infiltration or compression of nervous tissue by a mass can occur in any part of the nervous system including the leptomeninges, cranial nerves, brain, spinal cord, and peripheral nerves, resulting in neurological emergencies such as paraplegia, cranial nerve or nerve plexus palsies, meningeal infiltration, and intracerebral tumor. Lymphomatous masses arising from extradural locations (e.g., skull, orbit, nasopharynx, paraspinal) may also impinge upon adjacent nervous tissue. Radicular and spinal cord compression are the commonest severe neurological complications seen in NHL and multiple myeloma.[38]

The signs and symptoms of nervous system involvement can therefore be extremely diverse and include relatively nonspecific though potentially serious symptoms such as headache, backache, or seizures. The single most common presenting sign seen in patients with malignant leptomeningitis is cranial nerve palsies, particularly involving the facial, oculomotor, or abducent nerves.[32,36] Sometimes, more definite features of raised intracranial pressure such as papilledema, bradycardia, and vomiting are present, and localizing signs such as motor weakness and sensory changes may also be observed. Occasionally, patients may present with signs and symptoms indicative of a localized radiculopathy only, as reported by Levitt et al.[32] In their series of 24 patients who had CNS involvement at presentation, five had features confined only to involvement of the lumbosacral (three cases) or brachial plexus (two cases). All five patients had negative myelograms, positive CSF cytologies, and lymphomatous infiltration of root and plexus documented at postmortem.

Spinal cord compression

Spinal cord compression is a relatively rare presentation of NHL and multiple myeloma, occurring in about 0.1–10.2 percent of patients as reported in different series.[38–40,43,44] It is most commonly caused by extradural disease, either due to an isolated deposit within the spinal canal or by extension from an adjacent nodal mass or bone involvement. Less commonly, in the case of NHL, it may arise subdurally or within the spinal cord, when the disease may behave like a primary cerebral lymphoma, recurring within the CNS. The most frequent site of extradural compression appears to be the lower thoracic spine (T7–T12) followed by the lumbar and cervical spine and sacrum.[37–40,45]

Extradural presentations of lymphoma have been described in all age groups, including childhood, but tend to cluster in the fifth to sixth decades.[37,40,45]

In spite of the rarity of its occurrence, malignant lymphoma is still one of the most common causes of spinal cord compression. This complication has been reported as a late manifestation of NHL but is more often a presenting feature.[39,40,45,46] Patients may have rapidly or more slowly progressive symptoms, depending upon the growth rate of the lymphoma. Back pain is one of the commonest symptoms of spinal cord compression, and may precede the onset of myelopathy by a few days to a few months.[38–40,45] Any patient with proven or suspected cancer and unexplained back pain should be considered to have spinal cord compression and evaluated without delay. Other presenting symptoms include paresthesias and/or weakness of the lower extremities, with complete paralysis and bladder dysfunction occurring in the most severe cases. On physical examination, the most common findings include a discrete sensory level, hyperreflexia, and paraparesis or paraplegia.[39] Aggressive, rapidly growing lymphoid neoplasms can result in painless paraplegia within hours; hence it is imperative that suspected paraspinal disease be evaluated and treated immediately in order to avoid irreversible neurological damage. Occasionally, infarction of the cord may occur, due to compression of the spinal arteries, and such patients are unlikely to recover full function.

Plain films of the spine are usually unremarkable, and lack of bony involvement on plain film or CT scan can provide an important clue to diagnosis; thus, extradural compression of the cord in the presence of normal radiographs should immediately arouse suspicion of a lymphoid neoplasm.[47] Occasionally, lytic bony lesions and paraspinal lymphomatous masses may be detected on plain films. Magnetic resonance imaging is the method of choice today for accurate determination of the level of spinal cord block and has virtually replaced contrast myelography. In the absence of other sites of tumor, a laminectomy may be required to establish a histological diagnosis.

Current treatment of spinal cord compression consists of a combination of steroids and chemotherapy/radiation therapy to the spine (Table 49.3). A decision to utilize decompressive surgery should be made after taking into consideration factors such as the degree of paresis, histology of the lymphoid malignancy, and whether the spinal cord compression is a manifestation of initial presentation or relapse. If the history is suggestive of rapidly progressive spinal cord dysfunction, high-dose steroids (dexamethasone) should be given immediately to try and reduce local edema and lessen the degree of compression, besides exerting a lympholytic effect. A laminectomy may be indicated in patients who present with spinal cord compression secondary to recurrence, particularly when it presents in a previously irradiated region.[48] Chemotherapy should be thought of as a primary therapeutic option for the treatment of spinal cord compression[37,43] and is probably more effective than radiation therapy in highly chemosensitive tumors such as Burkitt lymphoma (which is also relatively radioresistant), lymphoblastic lymphoma, and intermediate-grade lymphomas. The avoidance of radiation, where possible, has the advantages of not adding to myelosuppression because of irradiation of vertebral bone marrow or increasing the risk of severe esophagitis and cardiac or pulmonary toxicity when compression is in the thoracic spine. This is not a minor consideration in tumors where chemotherapy provides the only real chance of a cure.

PLEURAL AND PERICARDIAL EFFUSIONS

Pleural involvement

Lymphoid neoplasms that present with mediastinal involvement are usually associated with malignant pleural or pericardial effusions that may be clinically silent and only detectable on a chest x-ray or CT scan, or large enough to cause significant respiratory distress. Leukemias and lymphomas account for approximately 13 percent of malignant pleural effusions, while 16 percent of patients with lymphoma are said to develop a pleural effusion in the course of their disease.[49] Thoracocentesis is indicated for confirmation of diagnosis, relief from respiratory distress, or, occasionally, for elimination of a potential reservoir for drugs such as methotrexate which are used early on in the treatment of high-grade lymphoma.[50] Pleural effusions provide an excellent source of malignant cells for cytological and immunophenotypic diagnosis.[51]

The most effective therapy for a malignant effusion is treatment of the underlying malignancy. In a newly diagnosed patient with respiratory distress, it may be sufficient to remove fluid just once, since the initiation of specific therapy should prevent reaccumulation. However, an existing pleural effusion can be exacerbated by the hydration necessary for prevention of tumor lysis in patients with extensive disease or prior to the institution of chemotherapy, especially with agents such as cyclophosphamide and methotrexate. Thus, repeated therapeutic thoracentesis or an indwelling chest tube may sometimes become necessary for symptomatic relief while awaiting response to chemotherapy. Because rapid response to therapy is the rule, pleurodesis with a sclerosing agent[52–54] after complete drainage of the pleural fluid is only indicated for palliation of tumors refractory to chemotherapy. A metaanalysis of pleurodesis studies showed that two-thirds of patients respond to pleurodesis and the most effective agents were tetracyclines, bleomycin, and talc.[55] For patients with loculated pleural effusions, the use of urokinase followed by minocycline pleurodesis in responders was successful.[56]

Table 49.3 Evaluation and management of back pain in a patient with suspected or proven malignancy

Obtain complete history followed by a detailed neurological exam

1. **Evidence of rapidly progressive, severe neurological deficit indicative of cord or conus involvement**
   1.1 Immediate institution of high-dose steroids (dexamethasone)
   1.2 Emergency x-ray of the spine, MRI, and/or metrizamide myelogram
   1.3 If evidence of spinal cord compression: treat with surgery, radiation therapy, or chemotherapy as appropriate[a]
2. **Stable neurological exam with mild deficits indicative of cauda involvement**
   2.1 Immediate institution of steroids (dexamethasone)
   2.2 X-ray of the spine, MRI, and/or metrizamide myelogram within 24 hours
   2.3 Treat with chemotherapy or radiation therapy, as appropriate
3. **Normal neurological exam with no evidence of neurological deficits**
   3.1 X-ray of the spine, bone scan, CT scan/MRI within 48–96 hours
   3.2 Treat with chemotherapy once diagnosis has been obtained

Any patient with cancer and back pain should be considered to have spinal cord compression until proven otherwise

[a]The therapeutic modality used will depend upon factors such as type of malignancy, clinical situation (primary vs relapse), etc.
MRI, magnetic resonance imaging; CT, computed tomography.

Rarely, patients do not respond to the above measures and surgical options are considered such as the placement of a pleuroperitoneal shunt or surgical pleurectomy.[57]

Pericardial involvement

Pericardial effusion can occur either through hematogenous spread or as a result of direct extension from adjacent lymph nodes. Although less common than pleural effusions, it is a far more serious complication of lymphoma because of the risk of life-threatening cardiac tamponade (the inability of the left ventricle to maintain output, usually because of extrinsic pressure, or rarely because of an intrinsic mass). Pericardial effusion is a rare complication of multiple myeloma and, when it does occur, is usually due to malignant infiltration of the pericardium by plasma cells.[58] Thus, suspicion of a malignant pericardial effusion mandates rapid evaluation and, depending on the duration and severity of symptoms, urgent treatment. In those cases where gradual accumulation of fluid occurs within the pericardial sac, symptoms of cough and dyspnea develop slowly and tamponade is less likely. However, the rapid accumulation of even a few hundred milliliters can cause tamponade and result in symptoms resembling heart failure, namely, the sudden onset of cough, chest pain, dyspnea, orthopnea, and nonspecific abdominal pain.[27,50]

M-mode or two-dimensional echocardiography – which demonstrates two echoes, one from the cardiac muscle and the other from the pericardium – is probably the most useful test for determining the presence and severity of both a pericardial effusion and cardiac tamponade.[27,50] It should be performed whenever a pericardial effusion is suspected because of the symptoms described above, or in the presence of a pericardial rub, characteristic low-voltage QRS complexes with ST segment elevation and T wave flattening or inversion on an electrocardiogram, or because of suggestive radiological findings of cardiomegaly with the typical 'waterbag shadow.' When there are signs of cardiac tamponade such as pulsus paradoxus, hypotension, and elevated venous pressure, pericardiocentesis should be performed without delay. This procedure both relieves tamponade and provides fluid for diagnostic cytology. As with pleural effusions caused by lymphoma, pericardial fluid usually stops accumulating after the initiation of chemotherapy. Radiation therapy should be avoided, if possible, because of the potential for cardiac damage, particularly if an anthracycline is included in the planned drug regimen. Continuous drainage of the pericardium with a catheter or surgical construction of a pericardial window may be necessary while awaiting a response to chemotherapy if reaccumulation of fluid is rapid after pericardiocentesis, or for palliation in patients with refractory lymphoma or myeloma. In the latter circumstance, the instillation of tetracycline into the pericardial sac has successfully prevented the accumulation of pericardial fluid without causing constrictive pericarditis, as seen in 30 of 33 and 15 of 22 patients described by Davis et al.[52] and Shepherd et al.,[53] respectively.

OBSTRUCTIVE UROPATHY

A frequently encountered complication of large intra-abdominal and pelvic lymphomas is obstruction of the ureters and urinary bladder, resulting in acute or subacute urinary retention. It may also be seen rarely in multiple myeloma that presents with a large retroperitoneal myelomatous mass.[59] Renal ultrasound is the simplest test to document obstructive uropathy, and the size of the kidney, extent of hydronephrosis, and the amount of residual renal cortex are extremely helpful in determining the potential for restoration of renal function, which is usually very high in this situation.[27,50] A CT scan may be required to determine the actual site of obstruction, which is often not well defined on renal ultrasound.

Once diagnosed, an effort should be made to relieve the obstruction as soon as possible. Ureteric obstruction can best be managed by hemodialysis (to normalize serum electrolyte, uric acid, urea, and creatinine levels) followed by appropriate chemotherapy. Placement of ureteral stents or nephrostomy tubes is not normally recommended because of the risk of perforation or leakage, thus increasing the risk of infection and delaying chemotherapy.[60] However, in circumstances where hemodialysis is not available, e.g., in developing countries, this may be a reasonable course of action. Peritoneal dialysis, even in the presence of abdominal lymphoma, has also been used with success.

Metabolic complications

HYPERURICEMIA AND TUMOR LYSIS SYNDROME

Hyperuricemia is a well-recognized occurrence at presentation in patients with extensive hemopoietic neoplasms, particularly NHLs, and leukemias that present with high white cell counts. Along with other metabolic complications, it occurs predominantly in the B cell lymphomas and, to a lesser extent, in lymphoblastic lymphomas, all of which have a high growth fraction.[61–63] Rapid turnover of these tumor cells, rich in nucleic acids, especially DNA, leads to an increase in the solute burden on the kidneys, resulting in renal complications that include oliguric acute renal failure prior to treatment, an exacerbation after the initiation of chemotherapy, and, sometimes, sudden death.[64–67] Both hyperuricemia and hyperuricosuria (from two to five times the normal rate) can occur.[68,69] In particular, as the concentration of uric acid increases, crystal formation and deposition in renal tubules increases leading to uric acid nephropathy. This process can ultimately lead to renal failure and, furthermore, it correlates directly with the tumor burden[65–67,70–72] and therefore to prognosis.

Tumor lysis syndrome (TLS) is an oncologic emergency that results from the rapid degradation of malignant cells. It is a consequence of the release of intracellular contents, such as nucleic acids, phosphorous, and potassium, into systemic circulation. The release of these breakdown products exceeds the capacity of normal homeostatic mechanisms and results in hyperuricemia, hyperphosphatemia, hypocalcemia, hyperkalemia, and uremia (Fig. 49.1). Intrinsic tumor-related factors and extrinsic host-related factors play a role in the propensity of an individual patient to develop TLS. Tumor-related factors include sensitivity to chemotherapeutic agents, tumor burden (extent of dissemination), lactate dehydrogenase (LDH) levels, and cell proliferation and turnover rate. Host-related factors relate to hydration status and baseline renal function.

Although TLS has long been recognized as a set of metabolic abnormalities associated with treatment of tumors with rapid cell turnover and growth rates, only in recent years has a more comprehensive system of grading and classification been developed. Cairo and Bishop[73] recently modified a system of classification originally developed by Hande and Garrow.[66] According to their classification schema, TLS can be divided into two classes – laboratory TLS and clinical TLS. Specifically, this system differentiates between patients who merely have laboratory findings and those displaying symptoms as a result of abnormal laboratory findings. Cairo and Bishop[73] took the basic premise of laboratory versus clinical TLS and refined its inclusion criteria and created a grading scheme for TLS. According to their definition, laboratory TLS is present if two or more serum values of uric acid, potassium, phosphorous, or calcium are abnormal at presentation or if they change by 25 percent within 3 days before or 7 days after the initiation of treatment. In clinical TLS, not only must laboratory TLS be present, but also one or more of the following clinical complications: renal insufficiency (creatinine), cardiac arrhythmias/sudden death, and seizures. The grading system is related to clinical TLS and is based on maximal clinical manifestation (renal, cardiac, neurologic) (Table 49.4).[66,73]

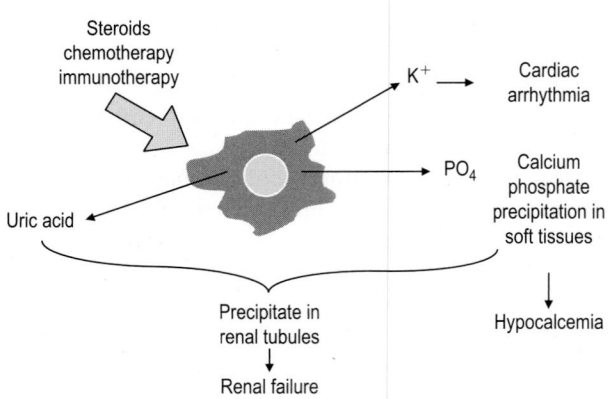

Figure 49.1 Diagrammatic depiction of tumor lysis syndrome and associated metabolic abnormalities. Adapted with permission from Wetzstein GA. *Clin Oncol Special Ed* 2001; **4**: 123–6.

Table 49.4. Cairo–Bishop grading classification of tumor lysis syndrome

	Grade 0[a]	Grade I	Grade II	Grade III	Grade IV	Grade V
Laboratory tumor lysis syndrome (LTLS)	–	+	+	+	+	+
Creatinine[b,c]	≤1.5 × ULN	1.5 × ULN	>1.5–3.0 × ULN	>3.0–6.0 × ULN	>6.0 ULN	Death[d]
Cardiac arrhythmia[c]	None	Intervention not indicated	Non-urgent medical intervention indicated	Symptomatic and incompletely controlled, medically or controlled with device (e.g. defibrillator)	Life-threatening (e.g. arrhythmia associated with CHF, hypotension, syncope, shock)	Death[d]
Seizure[c]	None	–	One brief generalized seizure; seizure(s) well controlled by anticonvulsants or infrequent focal motor seizures not interfering with ADL	Seizure in which consciousness is altered; poorly controlled seizure disorder; with breakthrough generalized seizures despite medical intervention	Seizure of any kind which is prolonged, repetitive or difficult to control (e.g. status epilepticus, intractable epilepsy)	Death[d]

Clinical tumor lysis syndrome (CTLS) requires one or more clinical manifestations along with criteria for LTLS.
Maximal CTLS manifestation (renal, cardiac, neurologic) defines the grade.

[a]No LTLS.

[b]Creatinine levels: patients will be considered to have elevated creatinine if their serum creatinine is 1.5 times greater than the ULN below age/gender defined ULN. If not specified by an institution, age/sex ULN creatinine may be defined as: > 1 < 12 years, both male and female, 61.6 μmol/L; ≥12 < 16 years, both male and female, 88 μmol/L; ≥16 years, female, 105.6 μmol/L; ≥16 years, male 114.4 μmol/L.

[c]Not directly or probably attributable to a therapeutic agent (e.g. rise in creatinine after amphotericin administration).

[d]Attributive probably or definitely to CTLS.

UNL, upper limit of normal; CHF, congestive heart failure; ADL, activities of daily living.

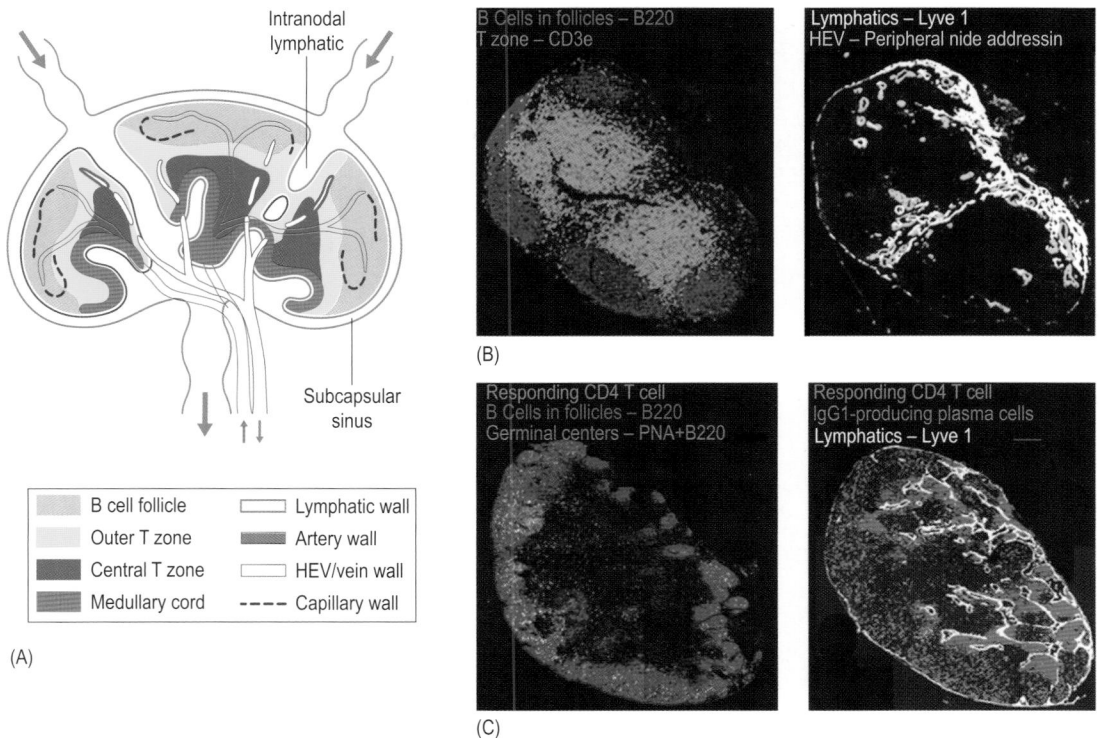

Plate 1 The structure of lymph nodes (LN). (A) LN vasculature and different LN compartments. (B) Confocal microscopy of a popliteal LN from a nonimmunized mouse. The follicles and T zone are delineated in the left photomicrograph by B220 expression (blue) and CD3 expression (green), respectively. An adjacent section from the same node (right) shows the relationship between lymphatic channels (white) and high endothelial venules (HEV) (yellow). An intranodal lymphatic is clearly seen. The medullary cords appear as compacted lymphatic tissue at the base of the photomicrograph; there were few if any plasma cells in this node (not shown). (C) Further popliteal node sections from a mouse 8 days after immunization with the T-dependent antigen, alum-precipitated ovalbumin, given in the foot. Inflated lymphatics are shown in white (right photomicrograph) surrounded by IgG1-switched plasmacytoid cells (red). Ovalbumin-specific CD4 T cells in both sections are stained green. These T cells derive from small numbers of ovalbumin-specific transgenic CD4 T cells transferred into the mouse before immunization. Magenta-colored germinal centers (left panel) result from double staining for PNA-binding (red) and B220 expression (blue). Anti-Lyve-1 antibody was a kind gift from Dr David Jackson of the Weatherall Institute, Oxford.[121]

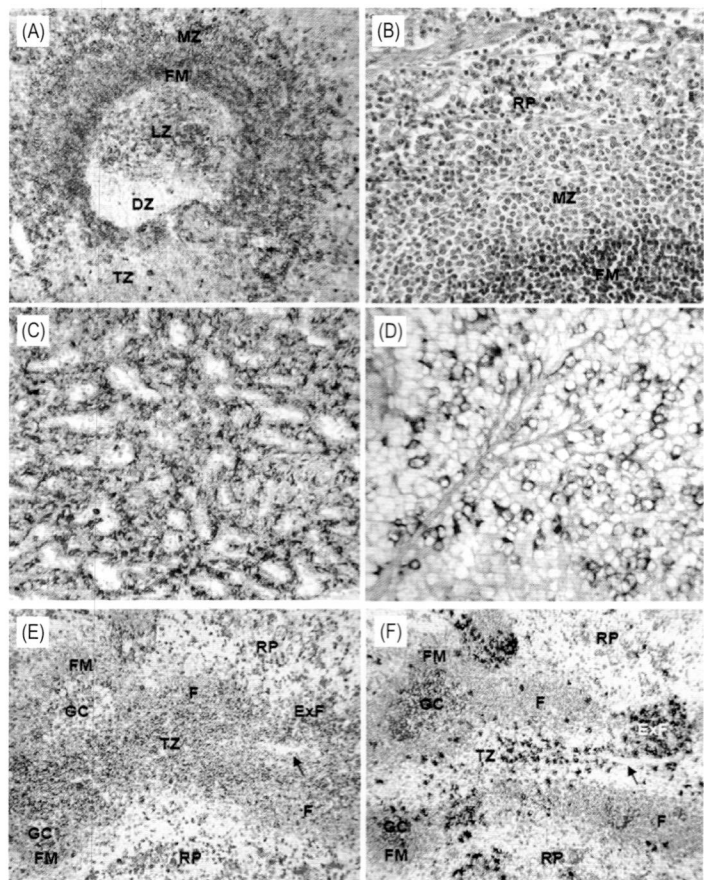

Plate 2 Microanatomy of the spleen. (A), (B), (C) Photomicrographs of 'healthy' human spleen. (A) Micrograph shows IgM expression in brown and nuclei pale blue. The follicular mantle (FM) and marginal zone (MZ) contain IgM$^+$ B cells; the more condensed chromatin of the follicular mantle cells gives the FM a darker appearance. A prominent germinal center (GC) is seen within the FM. The lymphocytes in the GC are IgM$^-$. A dense follicular dendritic cell (FDC) network in the upper part of the GC – the light zone (LZ) – stains brown through bound antigen:IgM complex. The dark zone (DZ) at the bottom of the GC lacks FDCs and is IgM$^-$. The T zone (TZ) is also shown. (B) Conventional hematoxylin and eosin staining of FM, MZ, and red pulp (RP). Note the less-condensed chromatin of the MZ B cells. The fixation used preserves some of the red cells; these mark blood sinusoids in the red pulp and outer portion of the MZ. (C) Macrophages on the cords of Billroth (stained brown by their α-naphthyl acetate esterase activity). Nuclei are stained with methyl green. (D) Photomicrograph of mouse spleen 3 weeks after immunization with a T-dependent antigen shows antigen-specific plasmacytoid cells (blue) on red pulp stroma. IgM is stained brown. (E), (F) Sections from the spleen of a mouse 4 days after secondary immunization with a T-dependent antigen. Cells with red nuclear staining are in S phase of the cell cycle (22); these are mainly GC B cells, plasmablasts in an extrafollicular focus (ExF), and hemopoietic cells in the red pulp (RP). IgD$^+$ follicular mantle B cells are brown. Blue cells in (E) are CD3$^+$ T cells; blue cells in (F) are antigen-specific B blasts and plasmacytoid cells. Arrows mark central arterioles.

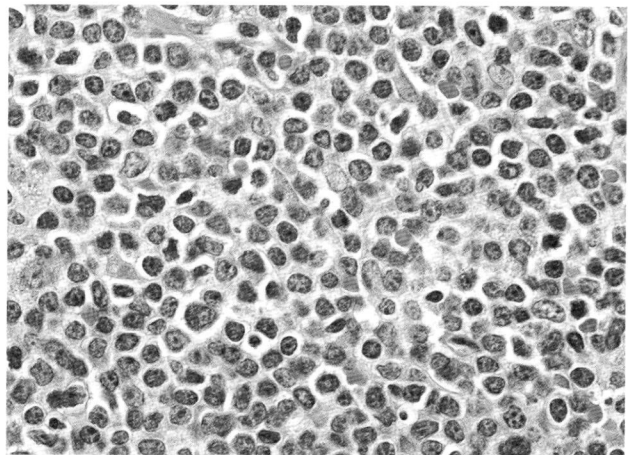

Plate 3 Small B cell lymphoma showing a uniform population of small lymphocytes similar to those of the normal mantle zone. There are few mitotic figures, apoptotic bodies, or tingible body macrophages.

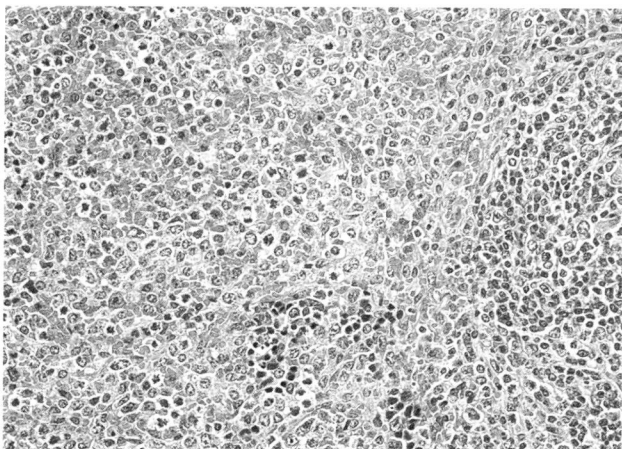

Plate 5 Splenic marginal zone lymphoma. The marginal zone is replaced by neoplastic lymphocytes adjacent to atrophic white pulp. Cells retain the features of normal marginal zone cells with an ovoid nucleus featuring fine chromatin, small, often inconspicuous nucleoli, and plentiful cytoplasm.

Plate 4 Splenic marginal zone lymphoma. Note atrophic white pulp and a halo of normal-appearing marginal zone lymphoid cells fingering out into the red pulp. Mitoses and apoptotic bodies are uncommon at this stage.

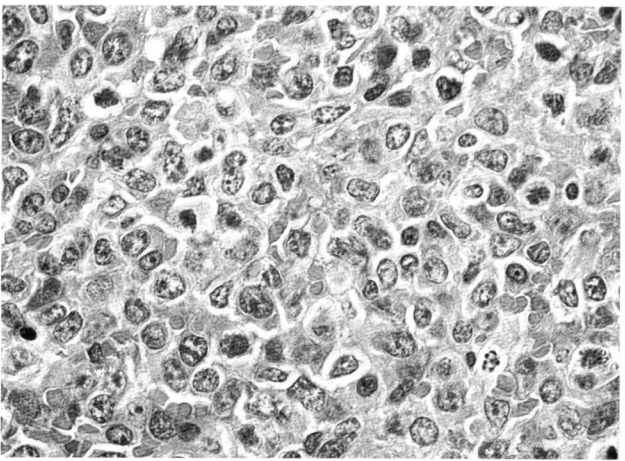

Plate 6 Marginal zone lymphoma with pleiomorphic population of lymphocytes with moderate amount of eosinophilic cytoplasm.

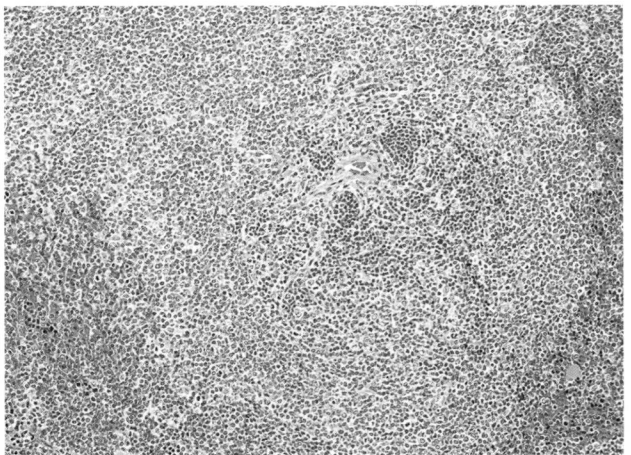

Plate 7 Follicular lymphoma. Depletion of normal darker T lymphocytes in the periarteriolar lymphoid sheath and replacement of white pulp by lymphoma.

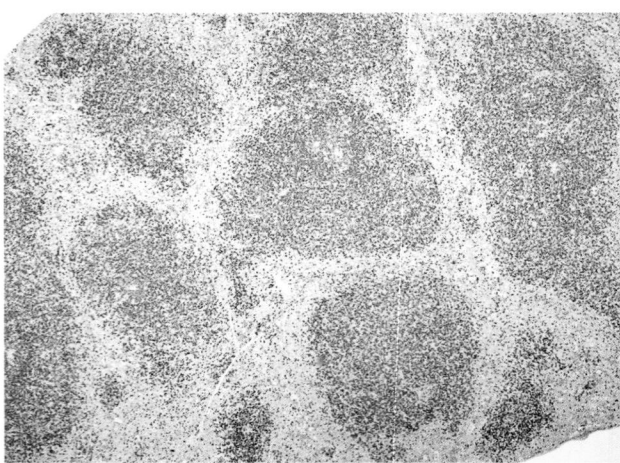

Plate 9 Immunohistochemistry of follicular lymphoma B cells expressing CD45R(B220) on the cell surface.

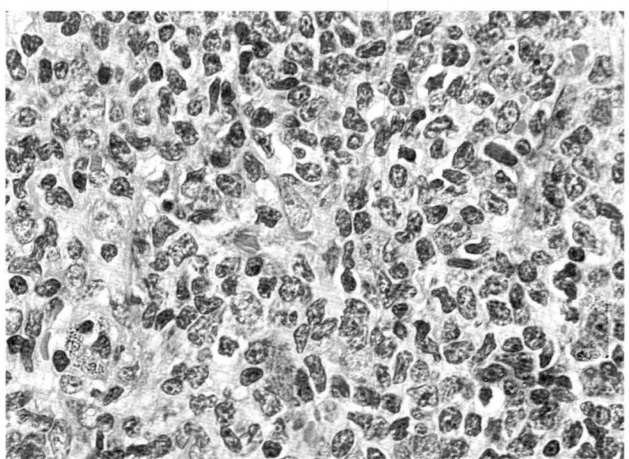

Plate 8 Follicular lymphoma showing a pleiomorphic population of centroblasts and centrocytes. Centrocytes feature irregularly shaped, often elongated, relatively dense nuclei with little cytoplasm. Centroblasts are marked by larger, vesicular nuclei with more prominent nucleoli, often with two appended to the nuclear membrane.

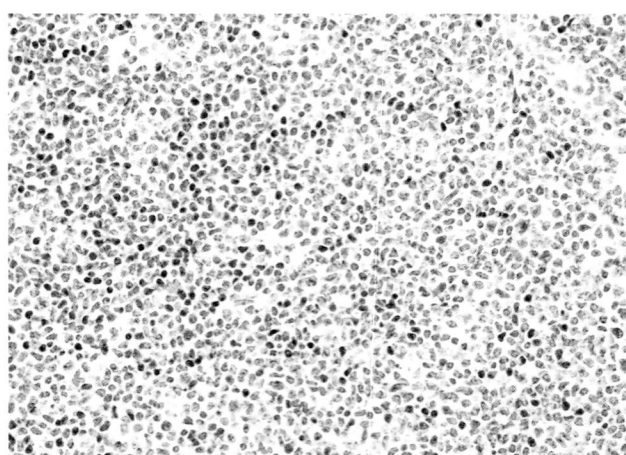

Plate 10 Immunohistochemistry of follicular lymphoma expressing PAX5 (B cell lineage specific activator protein; BSAP) at high levels in the nucleus of lymphoma cells.

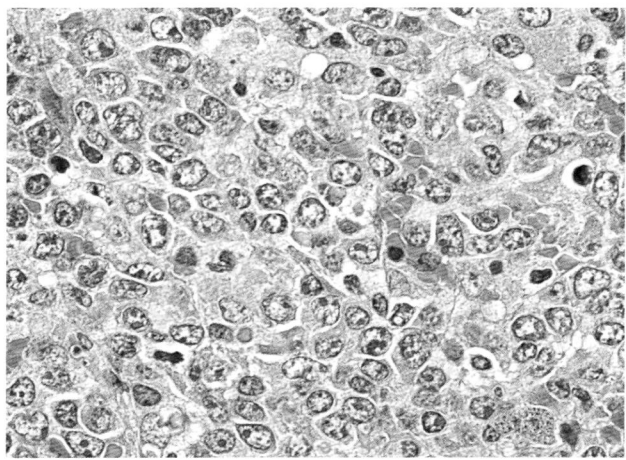

Plate 11 Diffuse large B cell lymphoma (DLBCL), centroblastic. Centroblasts have chromatin along the nuclear membrane and prominent nucleoli.

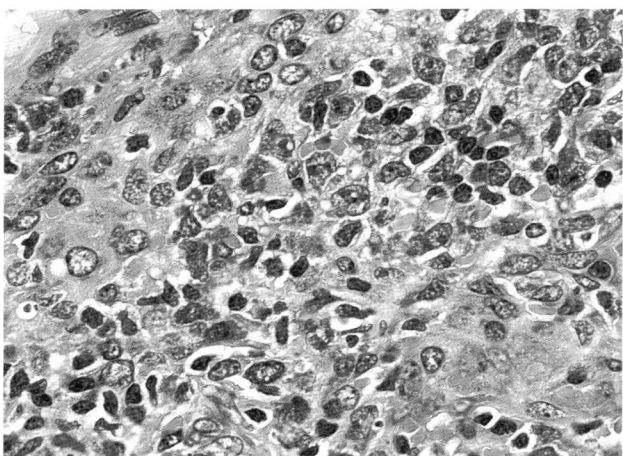

Plate 13 Diffuse large B cell lymphoma (DLBCL), histiocyte-associated, showing large eosinophilic histiocytes in association with large blastic B lymphoma cells and normal erythroid cells with small dark nucleoli. The B cell component is most often centroblastic or follicular, but cases with malignant immunoblasts, plasma cells, marginal zone B cells or, rarely, small B cells, are seen.

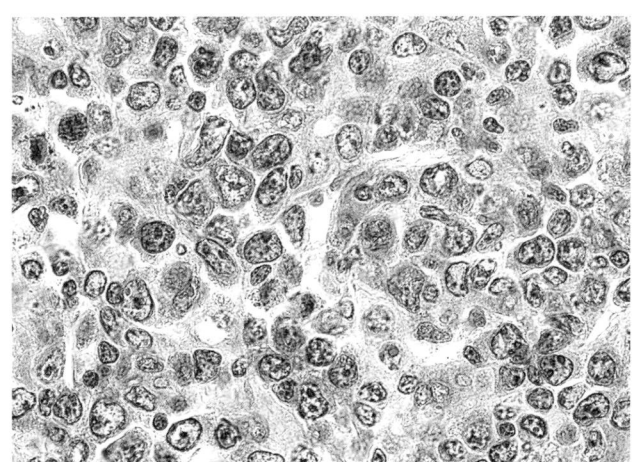

Plate 12 Diffuse large B cell lymphoma (DLBCL), centroblastic-immunoblastic. Central nucleoli can be seen in some of the large blast cells. Immunoblasts often have large, magenta, bar-shaped nucleoli appended to the nuclear membrane on one side.

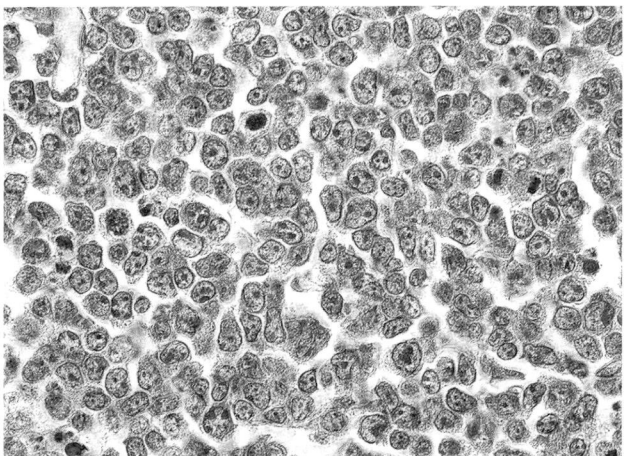

Plate 14 Diffuse high-grade lymphoblastic lymphoma of mature B cells. Cells are of intermediate size with scant cytoplasm and often having a prominent central nucleolus. Mitoses and apoptotic bodies are common and tingible body macrophages in many cases can give a starry-sky appearance.

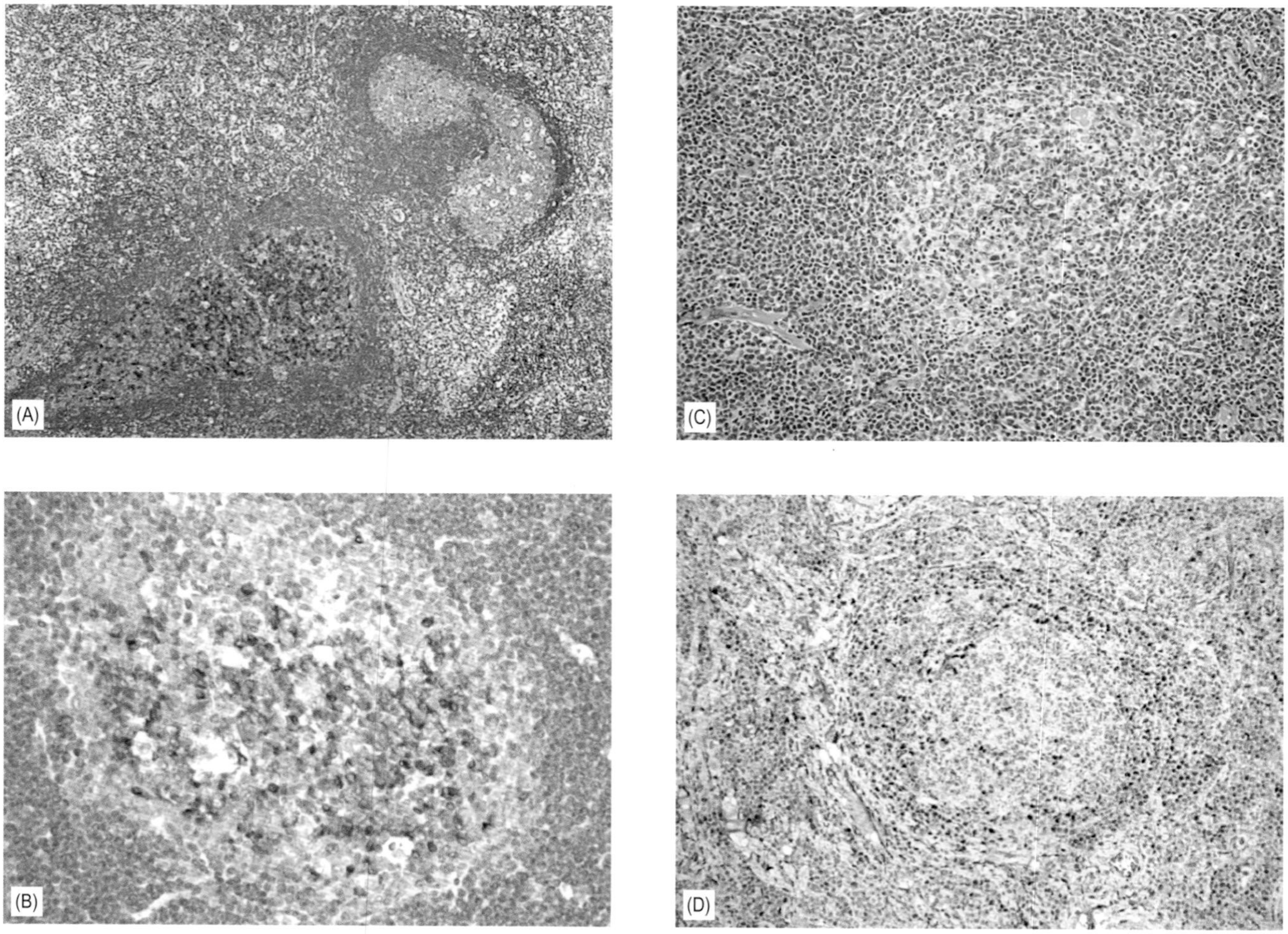

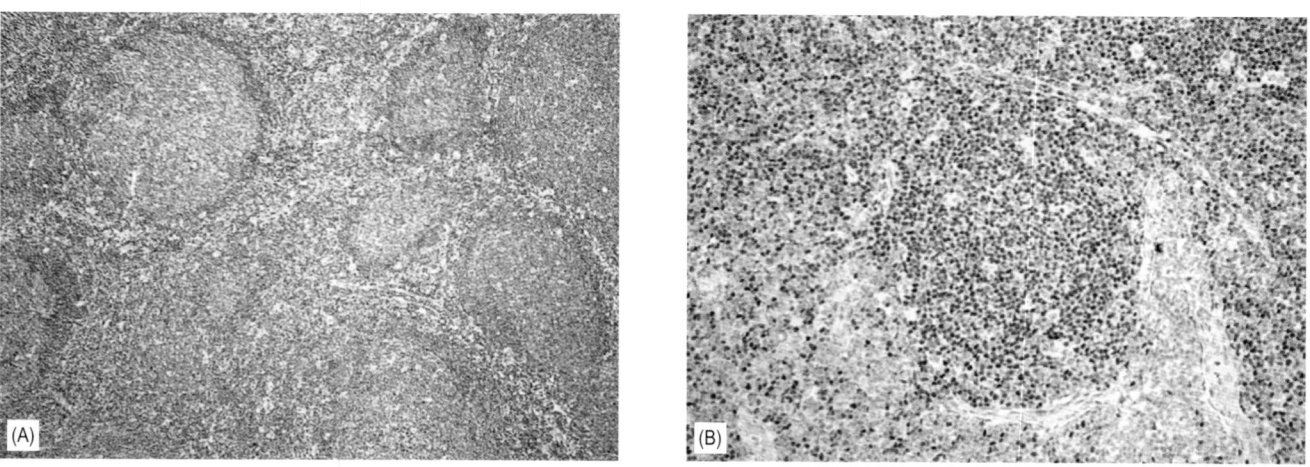

Plate 15 (A) and (B) illustrate '*in situ*' follicular lymphoma, BCL2 immunostaining.[20] Note the colonization of reactive follicles with BCL2-positive lymphoma cells. '*In situ*' mantle cell lymphoma[21] is represented in (C) with hematoxylin and eosin and (D) by cyclin D1 immunohistochemistry. A discrete population of lymphoid cells with aberrant cyclin D1 overexpression is observed in mantle zones (D) of lymph node with follicular hyperplasia.

Plate 16 Chronic lymphocytic leukemia mimicking follicular lymphoma. (A) In a routine stain, a typical pattern of follicular lymphoma is seen (Giemsa; 25×). (B) Nuclear overexpression of cyclin D1 proves a mantle cell lymphoma (CCND1 immunostain, 100×).

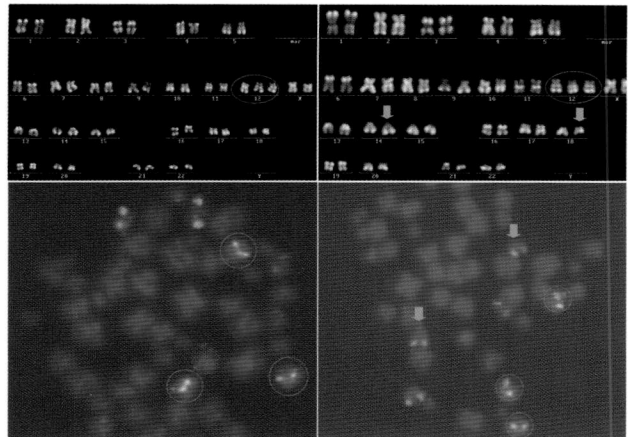

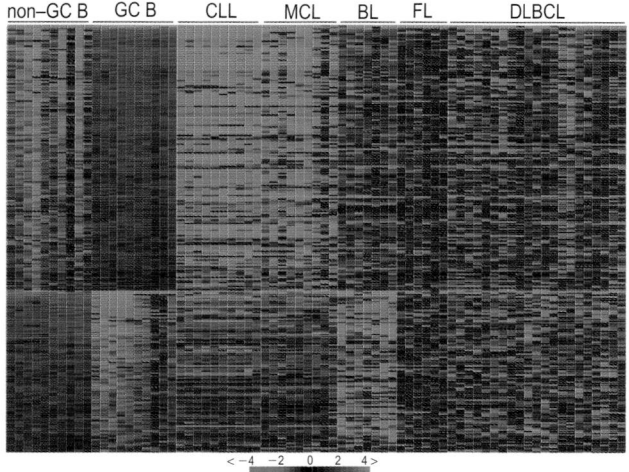

Plate 17 t(14;18)(q32;q21) leading to *IGH-BCL2* fusion as secondary chromosomal aberration in chronic lymphocytic leukemia (CLL). Two different cases of CLL with clonal trisomy 12 and subclonal t(14;18)(q32;q21). Representative reverse-banded karyogram of the first case is shown in the upper panel. The lower panel shows FISH analysis of the second case using commercially available probes for the *IGH* locus in 14q32 (green signal), the *BCL2* locus in 18q21 (red signal) (LSI IGH/BCL2, Vysis/Abbott), and a mixed red/green probe for the CHOP locus in 12q13 (LSI CHOP, Vysis/Abbott). Metaphase counterstained with DAPI. Trisomy 12 is indicated by a red circle, t(14;18)/*IGH-BCL2* fusion is indicated by green arrows.

Plate 18 Identification of the histological derivation of B cell malignancies. Genes differentially expressed between normal B cell subpopulations, namely germinal center (GC) B cells (GC B) and non-GC B cells (non-GC B), were identified by supervised pattern discovery analysis (left). The matrix shows the expression level of those signature genes in different subtypes of B cell malignancies (right). The relatedness of the tumor cases to either the GC B cells or non-GC B cells is visible from the color-coded expression values and can be quantitatively expressed by statistical analysis (not shown). Upregulated genes are identified by red, downregulated genes by green color. Columns represent individual samples, rows correspond to genes. DLBCL, diffuse large B cell lymphoma; FL, follicular lymphoma; MCL, mantle cell lymphoma; CLL, B cell chronic lymphocytic leukemia; BL, Burkitt lymphoma.

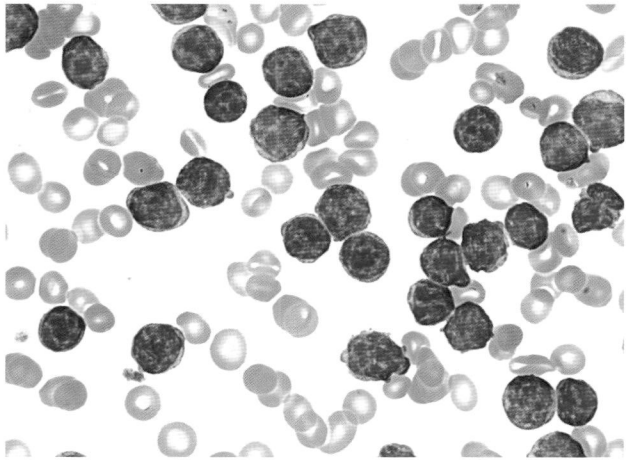

Plate 19 Peripheral blood smear morphology of typical chronic lymphocytic leukemia (1000×). Small lymphocytes with condensed and clumped chromatin ('soccer ball' pattern) are present with round nuclei.

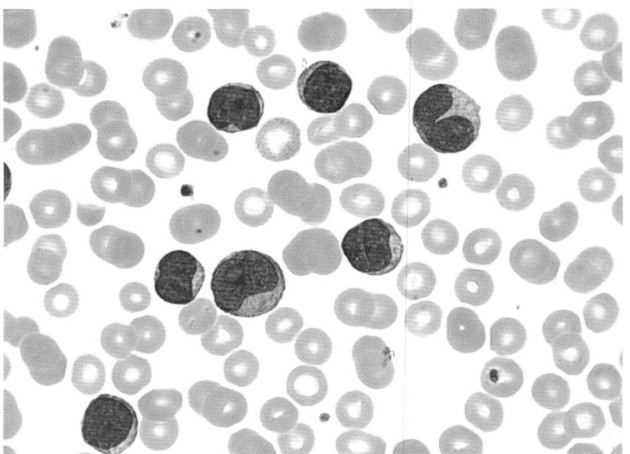

Plate 20 Peripheral blood smear morphology of chronic lymphocytic leukemia (1000×). Compared with Plate 19, some cells have irregular or clefted nuclear contours. Prolymphocytes are seen (with nucleoli) but less than 55 percent are needed to qualify as prolymphocytic leukemia.

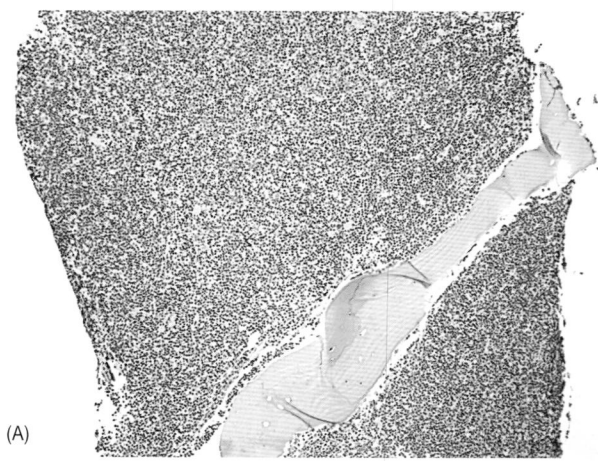

(A)

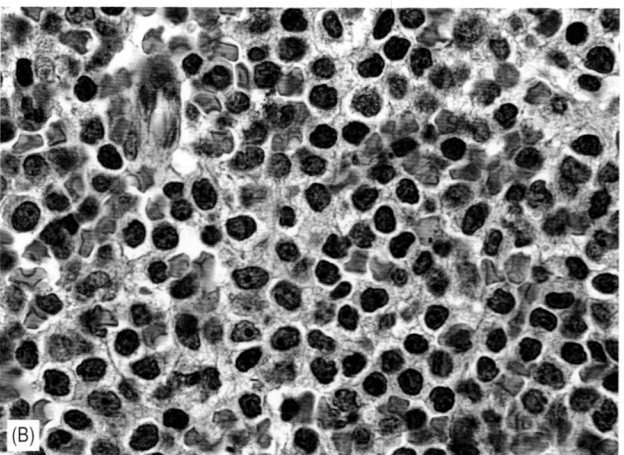

(B)

Plate 21 (A) Bone marrow biopsy with extensive and diffuse involvement by chronic lymphocytic leukemia. There is loss of the normal fat pattern of bone marrow and replacement of the hematopoietic elements by leukemia (40×). (B) Bone marrow biopsy, the cells are small with clumped chromatin. An occasional prolymphocyte (nucleated) is present.

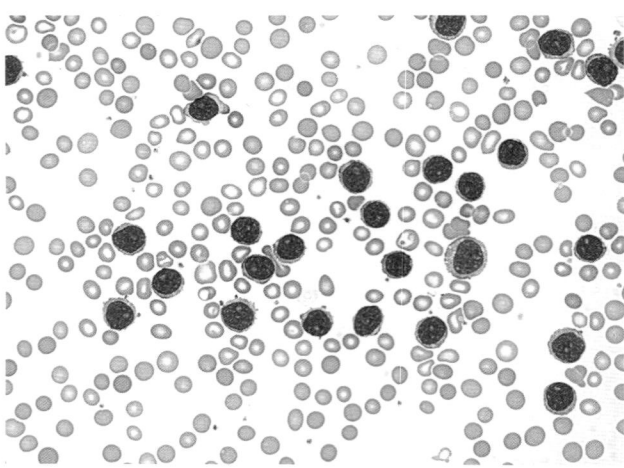

Plate 22 B prolymphocytic leukemia. Peripheral blood smear with numerous prolymphocytes (1000×). Note the slightly less condensed chromatin compared with chronic lymphocytic leukemia and the presence of nucleoli.

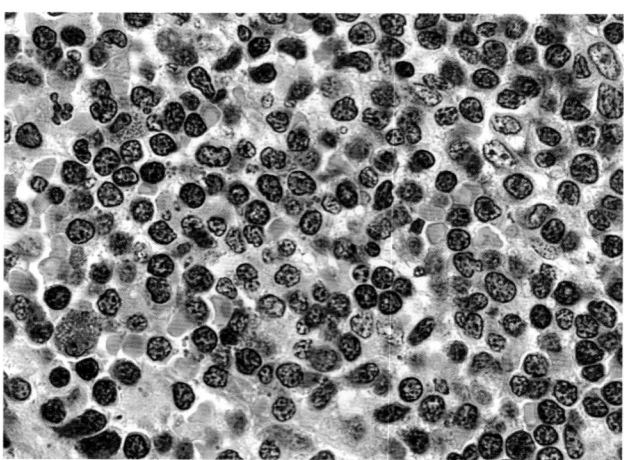

Plate 23 B prolymphocytic leukemia. Bone marrow trephine (1000×) with lymphoid infiltrate (same patient as in Plate 22).

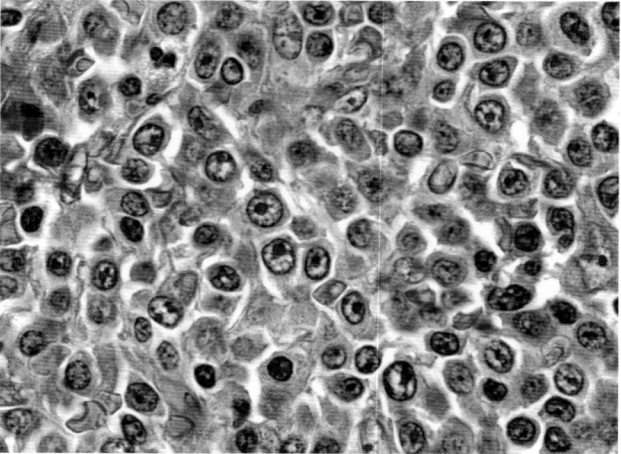

Plate 24 Splenic involvement by B prolymphocytic leukemia (1000×). Sheets of round intermediate-sized cells with central nucleoli similar to paraimmunoblasts seen in small lymphocytic lymphoma.

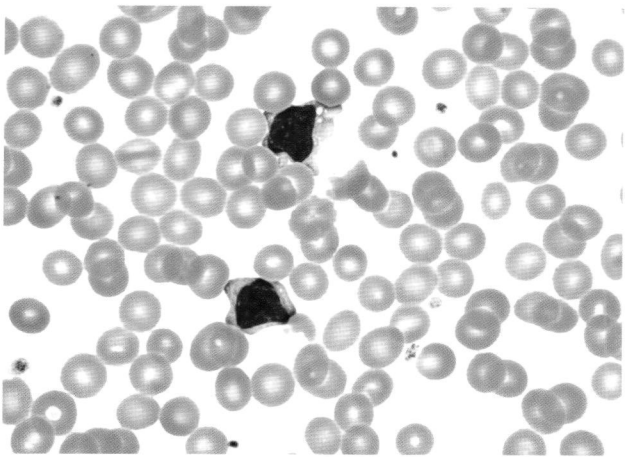

Plate 25 Peripheral blood smear from a patient with T cell large granular lymphocyte leukemia (T-LGL). The lymphocytes resemble normal T-LGLs with abundant pale cytoplasm. Granules are variably present and in this case are not prominent.

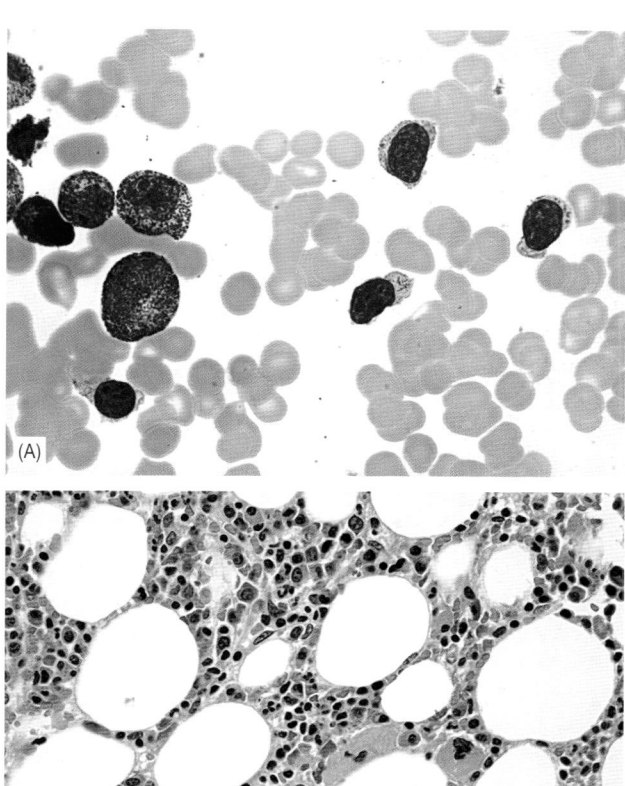

Plate 26 (A) Bone marrow aspirate smear from a patient with T cell large granular lymphocyte leukemia (T-LGL). Cytoplasmic granules are seen in the lymphocytes on the right side. Note the toxic granulation of the granulocytic precursors. This patient was neutropenic as a result of the T-LGL and was being treated with granulocyte colony stimulating factor. (B) Bone marrow clot section. A lymphoid infiltrate is difficult to appreciate on routine staining.

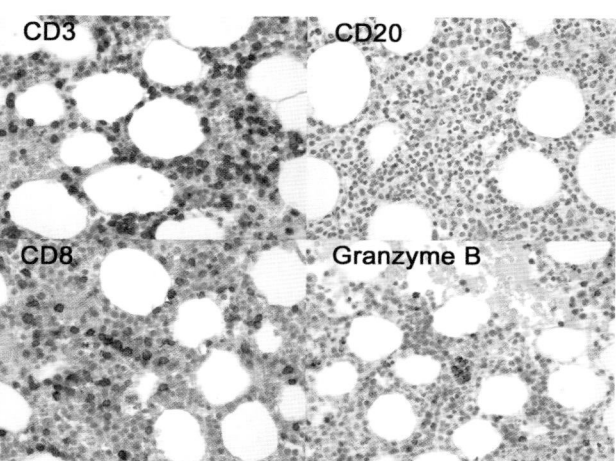

Plate 27 Immunostaining of the clot section in Figure 28.8B shows the infiltrate is composed of T cells expressing CD3, CD8, CD20 and granzyme B. The latter is a cytotoxic marker.

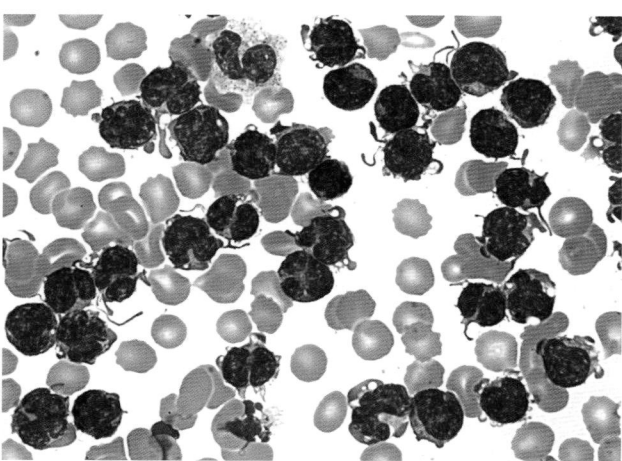

Plate 28 Peripheral blood smear with involvement by T prolymphocytic leukemia (1000×). Cells show marked nuclear irregularity and indistinct nucleoli.

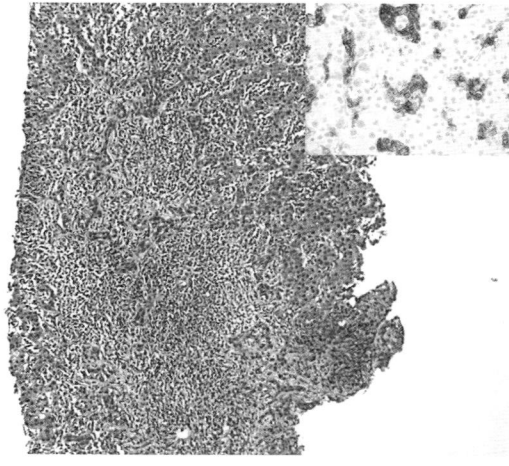

Plate 29 Liver involvement by T prolymphocytic leukemia. Note sinusoidal involvement which is highlighted by CD8 immunostain (inset).

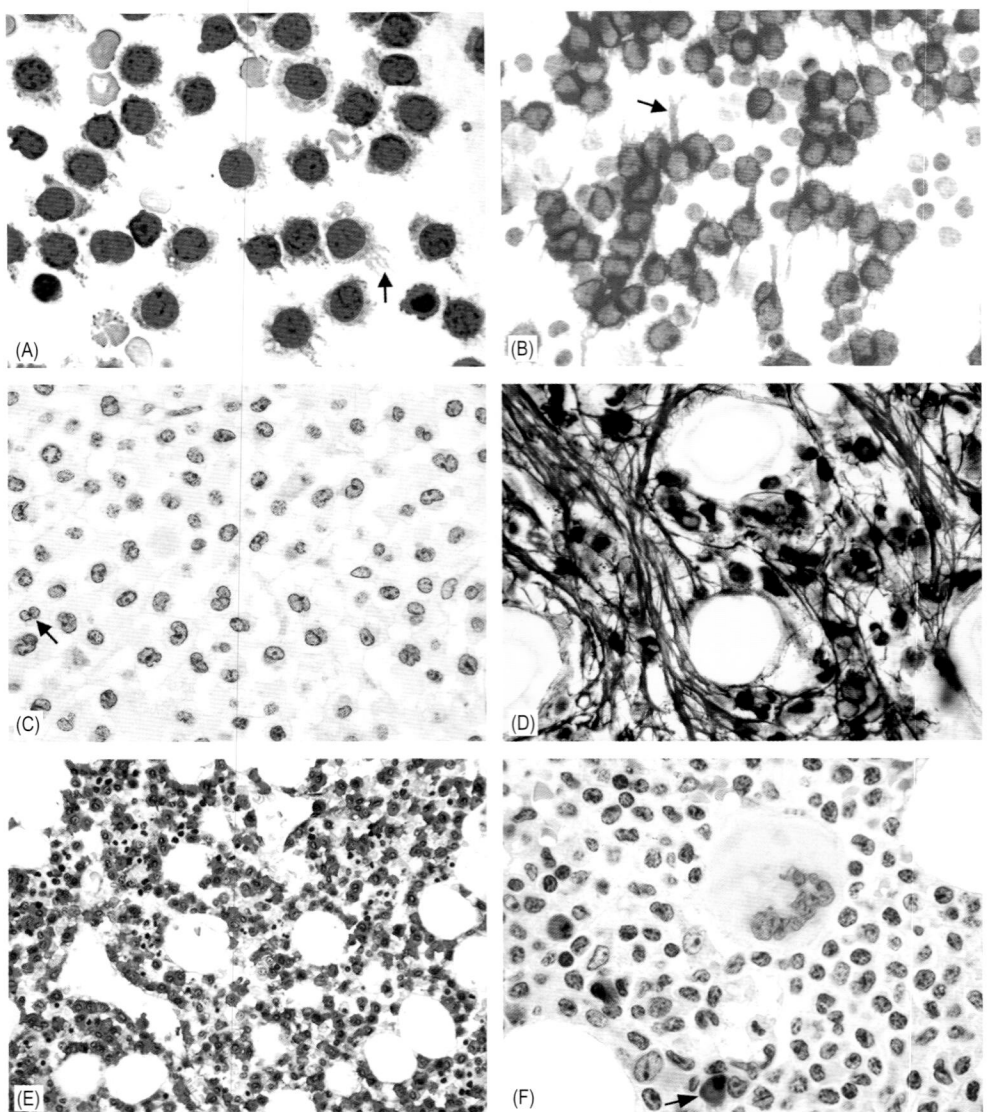

Plate 30 Peripheral and bone marrow involvement in hairy cell leukemia (HCL). (A) Typical 'hairy' appearance of HCL cells (peripheral blood cytospin); the arrow indicates surface projections of the leukemic cells. (B) CD22 expression in HCL cells (peripheral blood cytospin); the arrow indicates surface projections. (Reproduced from Falini B. *et al.*, 'Selection of a panel of monoclonal antibodies for monitoring minimal residual disease in peripheral blood and bone marrow of interferon-treated hairy cell leukemia patients'. *British Journal of Haematology*, 1990, vol. 76, pp. 460–8, Figure 1a, by copyright permission of Blackwell Publishing, Oxford, UK.) (C) Typical 'fried-egg' histologic pattern in bone marrow biopsy from HCL. Because of the wide cytoplasm, tumor cell nuclei are distant from each other; the arrow indicates a leukemic cell with bean-shaped nucleus. (D) Marked increase in reticulin fibers in HCL bone marrow biopsy (Silver stain). (E) DBA44 positivity of HCL cells in paraffin section (bone marrow biopsy). (F) HCL cells are MUM1/IRF4 negative; the arrow indicates a residual MUM1+ plasma cell.

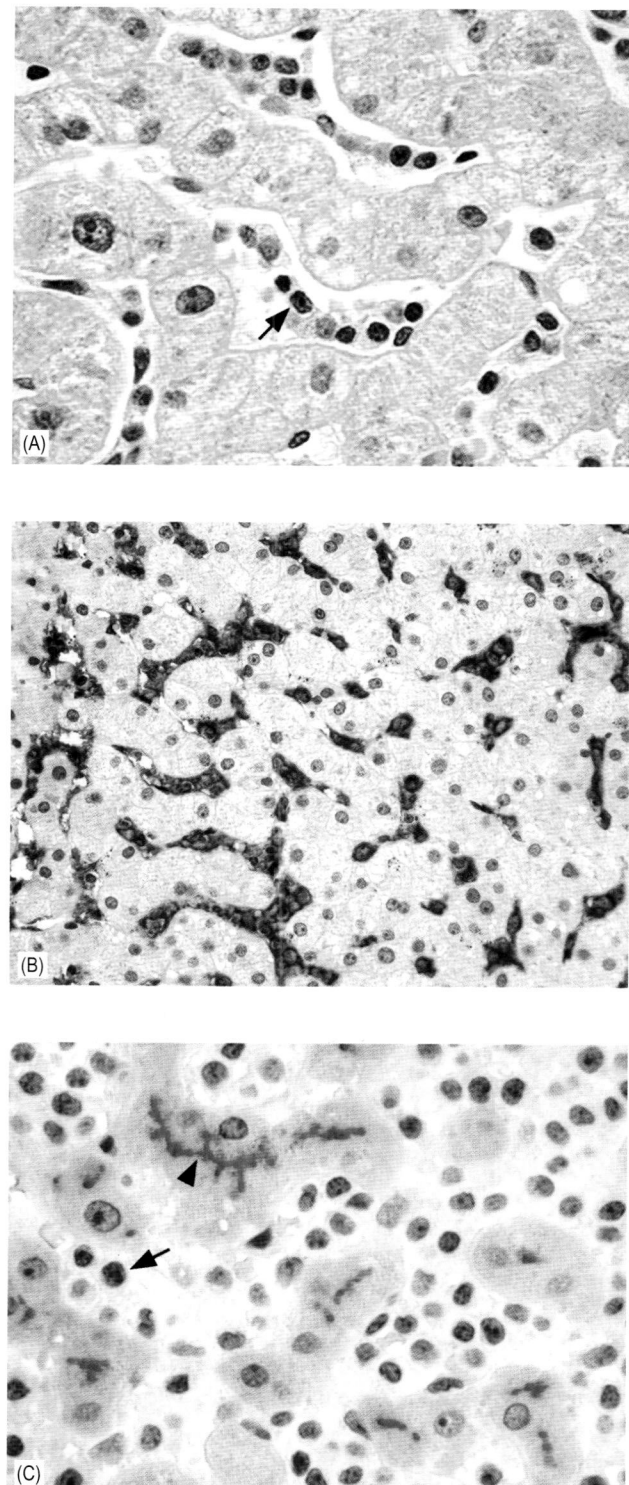

Plate 31 Liver involvement in hairy cell leukemia (HCL). (A) Typical involvement of hepatic sinusoids by HCL (hematoxylin and eosin; liver paraffin section). (B) HCL cells within hepatic sinusoids are CD20-positive (APAAP immunostaining; liver paraffin section). (C) HCL cells within hepatic sinusoids are CD10-negative; the arrow indicates CD10-positive bile duct canaliculi. (APAAP immunostaining; liver paraffin section.)

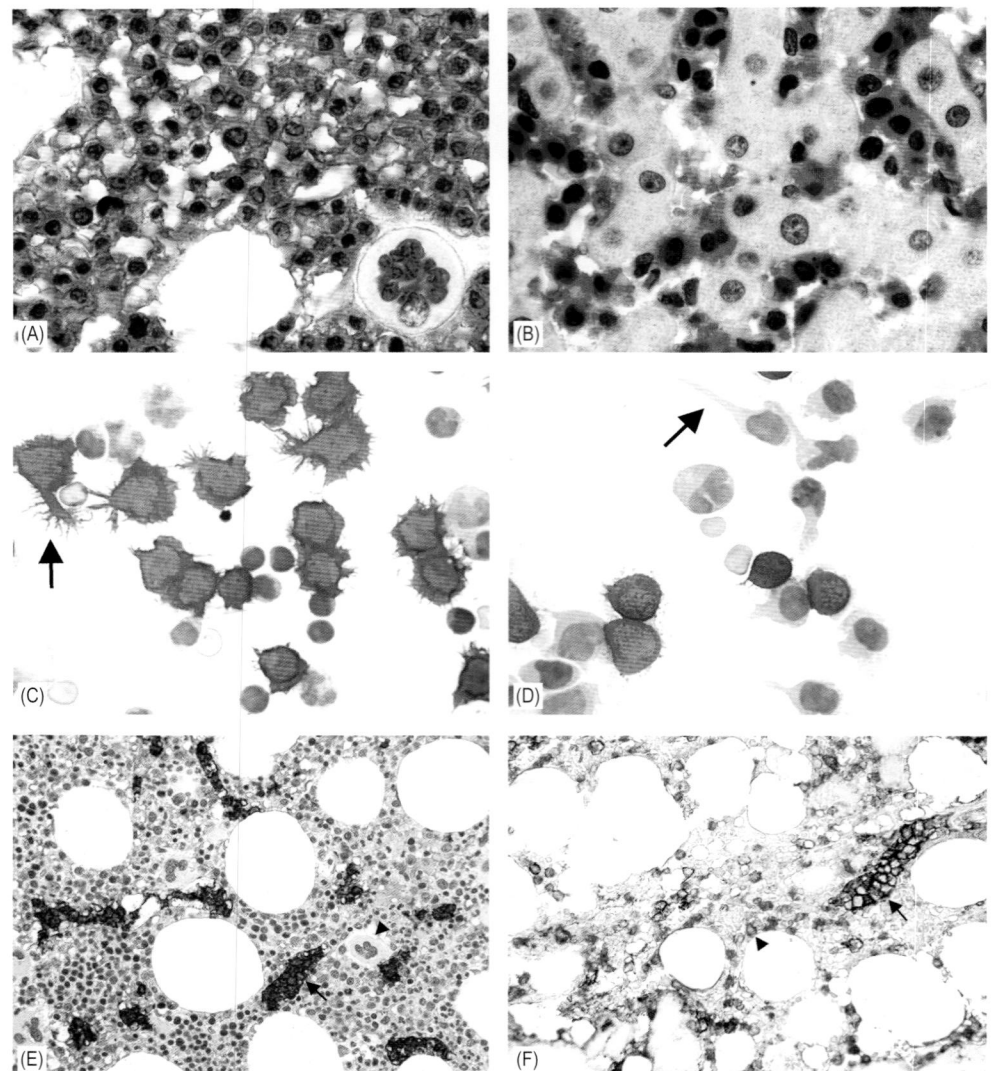

Plate 32 Annexin A1 (ANXA1) expression in hairy cell leukemia (HCL) and splenic lymphoma with villous lymphocytes (SLVL). (A) HCL cells in the bone marrow biopsy are strongly annexin A1-positive (APAAP technique; paraffin section). (B) HCL cells in the hepatic sinusoids are strongly annexin A1-positive (APAAP technique; paraffin section). (C) SLVL tumor cells are strongly DBA44-positive; the arrow indicates the polar projection of a leukemic cell (APAAP technique; peripheral blood cytospin). (D) SLVL tumor cells are annexin A1-negative; the arrow indicates the polar projection of a negative tumor cell. Positivity for annexin A1 is observed in normal monocytes and T cells (APAAP technique; peripheral blood cytospin). (E) Typical intrasinusoidal pattern in bone marrow biopsy indicating involvement by SLVL; the arrow indicates a cluster of intrasinusoidal CD20-positive tumor cells; the arrowhead indicates a CD20-negative megakaryocyte (APAAP technique; paraffin section). (F) Double staining for CD20 (brown) and annexin A1 (blue) in bone marrow biopsy from a patient with SLVL. Labeling is mutually exclusive: SLVL cells in the marrow sinusoids are positive for CD20 (arrow) but negative for annexin A1 that only stains residual hemopoietic cells (arrowhead). (Immunoperoxidase/APAAP double staining; no counterstain.)

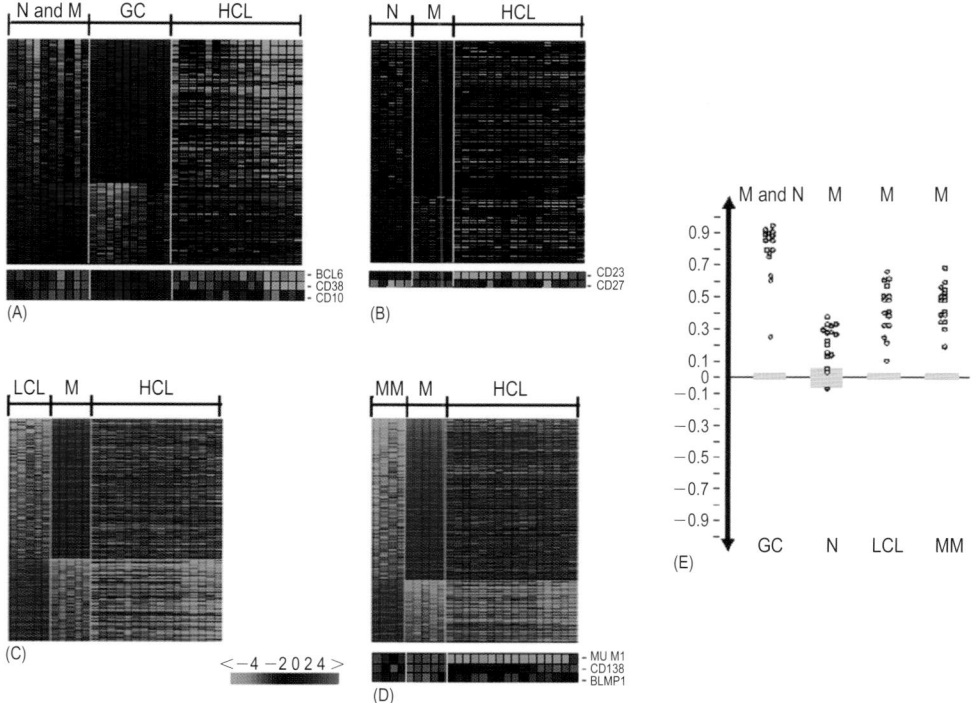

Plate 33 Relatedness of the gene expression profile of HCL to normal B cell population, and lymphoblastoids (LCLs) and multiple myeloma (MM) cell lines. A supervised analysis is used to identify the gene differentially expressed between two groups of samples. (A) Naïve and memory B cells (N and M) are compared with germinal center (GC) centroblasts and centrocytes. (B) Naïve B cells (N) are compared with memory B cells (M). (C) Epstein–Barr virus (EBV)-transformed LCLs, representing immunoblasts, are compared with memory B cells (M). (D) MM cell lines representing transformed plasma cells, are compared with memory B cells (M). The expression of the selected genes is investigated in HCL represented on the right side of each matrix (A–D). The expression of specific GC (BCL6, CD38 and CD10), naïve (CD23), memory B cell (CD27), and plasma cell (MUM1, CD138 and BLIMP1) markers are highlighted (A–D, bottom). The supervised analyses are shown in the matrices, where each row represents a gene and each column represents a sample. Genes are ranked according to the z score (mean expression difference of the gene between the phenotype group and the control group/standard deviation). The color change in each row represents the gene expression relative to the mean across the samples. Values are visualized according to the scale bar that represents the difference in the score (expression difference/standard deviation) relative to the mean. (E) A cell-type classification is used to measure the relatednesss of HCL to memory and naïve B cells or LCL cell lines and to memory B cells and MM cell lines. The gray area marks 95 percent of confidence: the P value decreases with increasing distance from the X axis. (Reproduced from Basso K. *et al.*, 'Gene expression profiling of hairy cell leukemia reveals a phenotype related to memory B cells with altered expression of chemokine and adhesion receptors', *The Journal of Experimental Medicine*, 2004, vol. 199, pp. 59–68, Figure 2, by copyright permission of the Rockfeller University Press.)

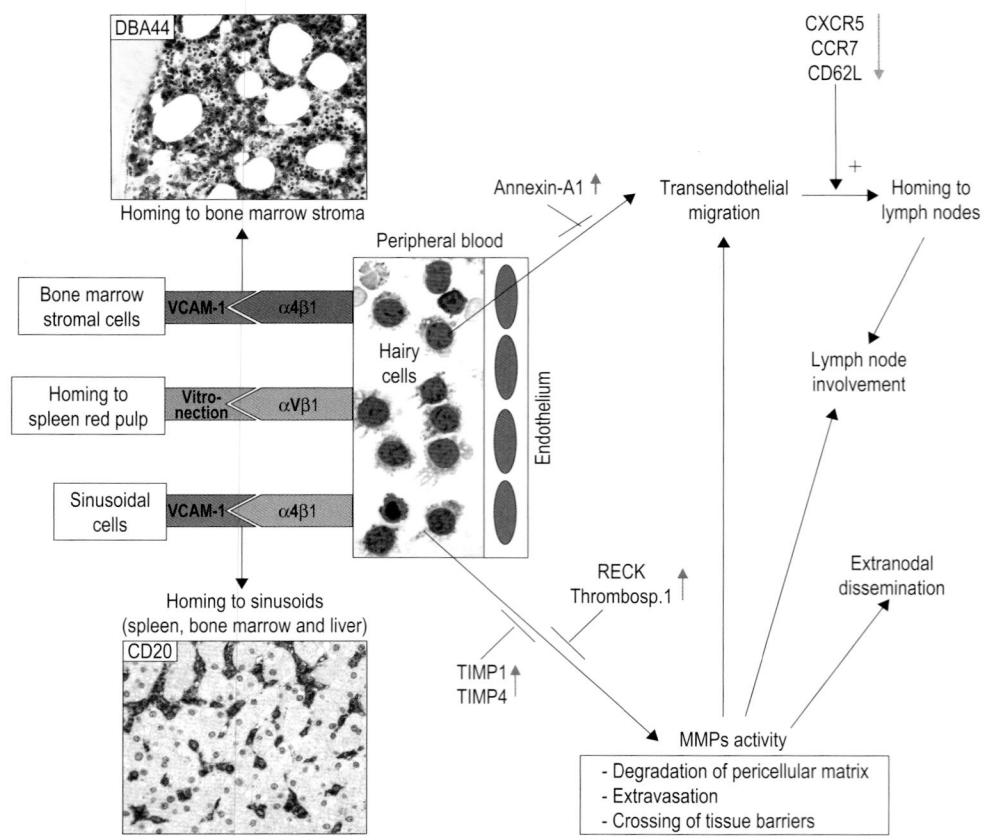

Plate 34 Hairy cell leukemia (HCL) homing and dissemination properties. Hypothetical scheme of tumor dissemination in hairy cell leukemia. Leukemic cells home to bone marrow stroma (upper box) and liver sinusoids (lower box) by expressing integrins which interact with their ligands on stromal and sinusoidal cells. The right side of the schema illustrates other molecules which may contribute to the unique homing properties of HCL cells. MMPs, metalloproteinases.

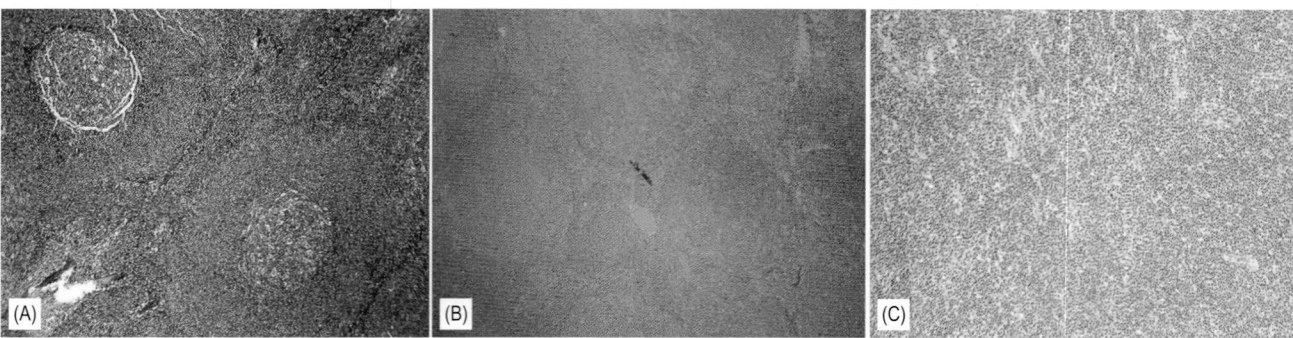

Plate 35 Architectural patterns in mantle cell lymphoma. (A) Mantle zone pattern: the tumor cells expand the mantle cell cuff surrounding a reactive germinal center. (B) Nodular pattern: the nodules are composed of tumor cells without evidence of residual germinal centers. (C) Diffuse pattern: the lymph node is diffusely infiltrated by tumor cells. (Hematoxylin and eosin stain.)

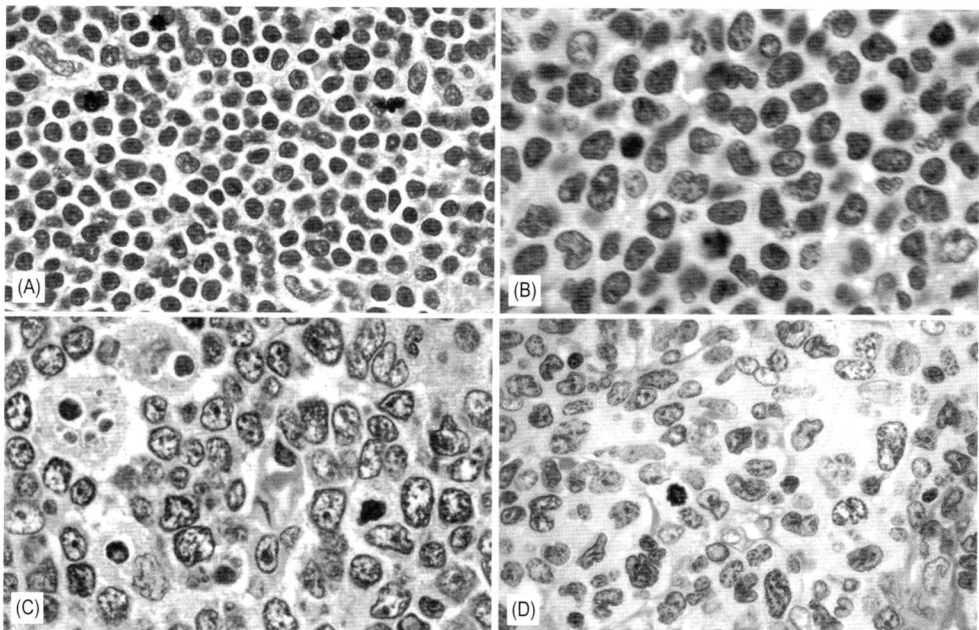

Plate 36 Cytologic variants of mantle cell lymphoma (MCL). (A) Small cell variant is composed of small lymphocytes with rounded nuclei simulating chronic lymphocytic leukemia. However, prolymphocytes and paraimmunoblasts are absent. (B) Typical or classical MCL is characterized by small- to medium-sized lymphocytes with irregular nuclei, condensed chromatin and scant cytoplasm. (C) Blastic variant. The tumor cells are medium-sized lymphocytes with rounded nuclei and finely distributed chromatin, inconspicuous or very small nuclei, and high mitotic index. (D) Pleomorphic variant. These cases have large cells with very irregular nuclei. (Hematoxylin and eosin stain).

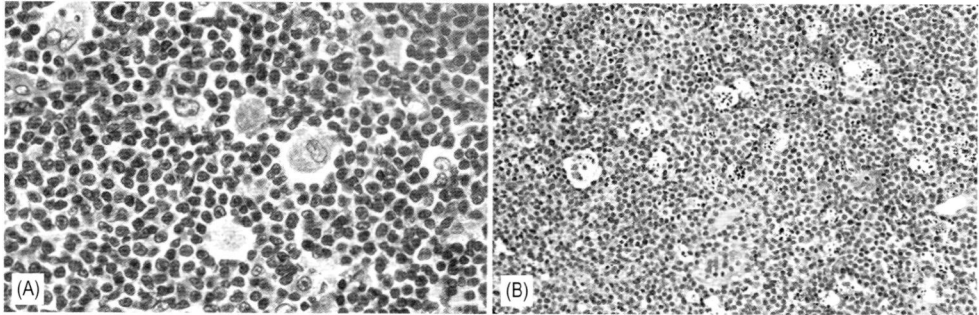

Plate 37 (A) Typical variant of mantle cell lymphoma with scattered histiocytes with eosinophilic cytoplasm. (B) 'Starry sky' pattern with histiocytes and tingible bodies in a blastic mantle cell lymphoma. (Hematoxylin and eosin stain.)

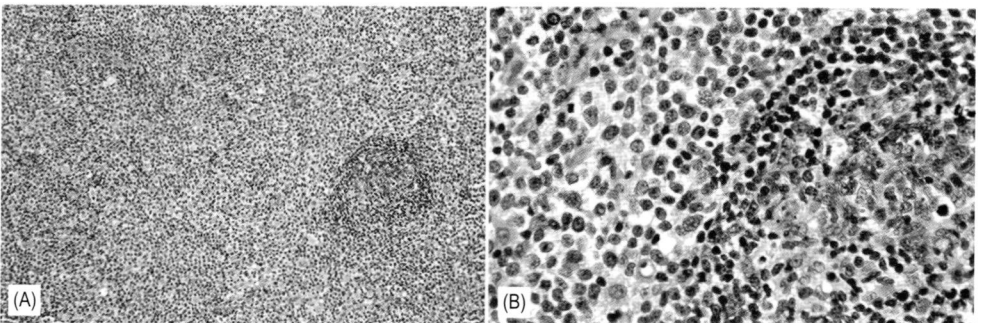

Plate 38 Mantle cell lymphoma with marginal zone pattern. (A) Tumor cells expand the marginal zone area outside an apparent preserved mantle cuff. (B) Tumor cells in the marginal zone area have abundant and pale cytoplasm resembling 'monocytoid' cells.

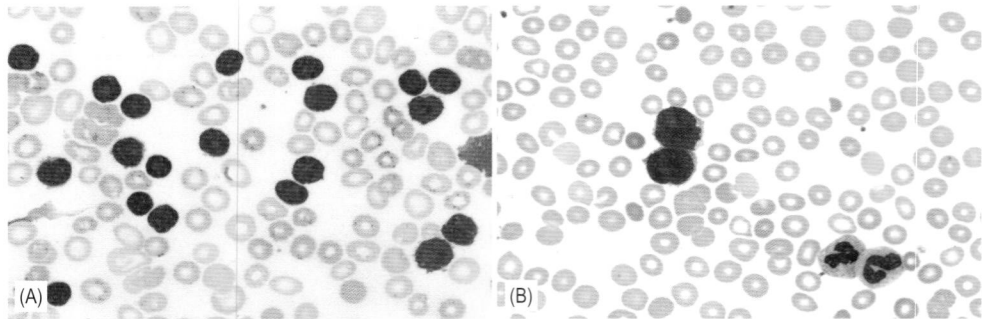

Plate 39 Cytological spectrum of tumor cells in peripheral blood smears in leukemic mantle cell lymphoma. (A) The tumor cells in typical variants are small-sized lymphocytes with slightly indented or cleaved nuclei, condensed chromatin and scant cytoplasm. (B) Blastoid variants show larger cells with finely dispersed chromatin and evident nucleoli. (Giemsa stain.)

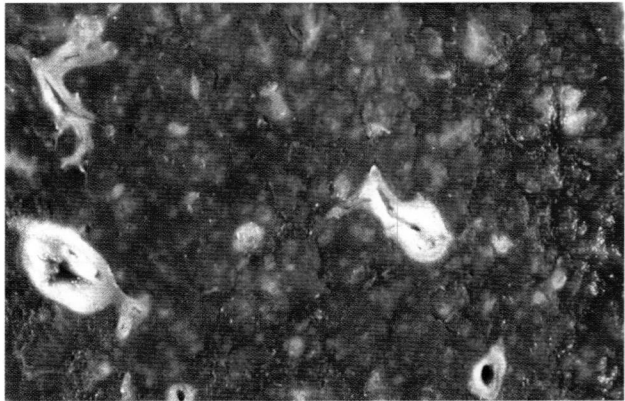

Plate 40 Mantle cell lymphoma involving the spleen, showing generalized micronodular pattern.

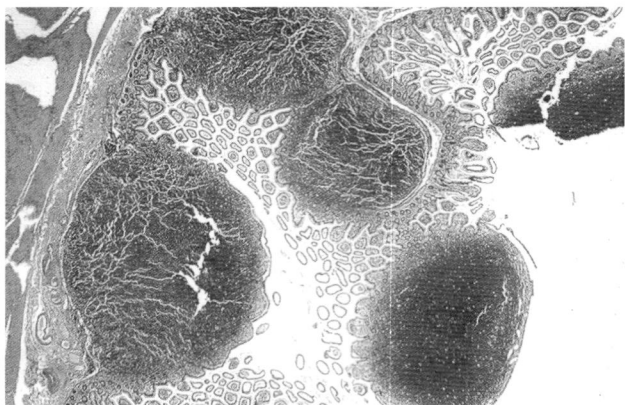

Plate 41 Mantle cell lymphoma involving intestine with multiple lymphomatous polyposis. Polyps correspond to a nodular expansion of atypical lymphoid cells.

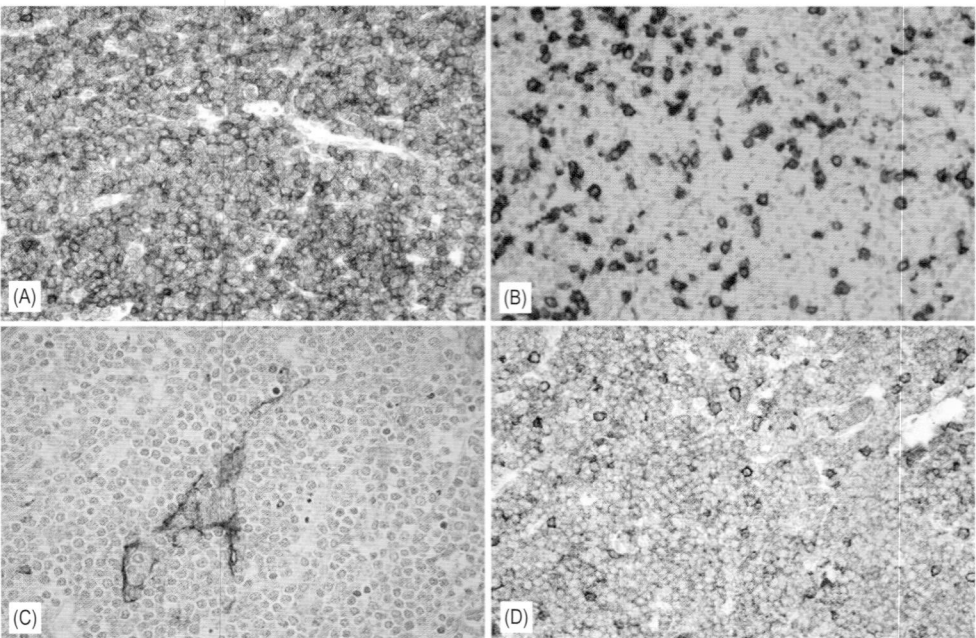

Plate 42 Mantle cell lymphoma immunophenotype. Tumor cells are strongly positive for CD20 (A), with coexpression of CD5 (D). CD3 is only positive in scattered reactive T cells (B). CD23 is negative in tumoral cells, showing positivity in some residual dendritic cells (C). (Immunoperoxidase stain.)

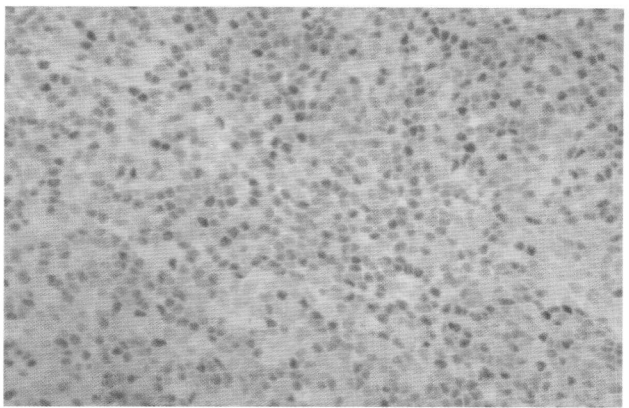

Plate 43 Cyclin D1 in MCL is expressed in the nucleus of the cells with variable intensity. (Immunoperoxidase stain.)

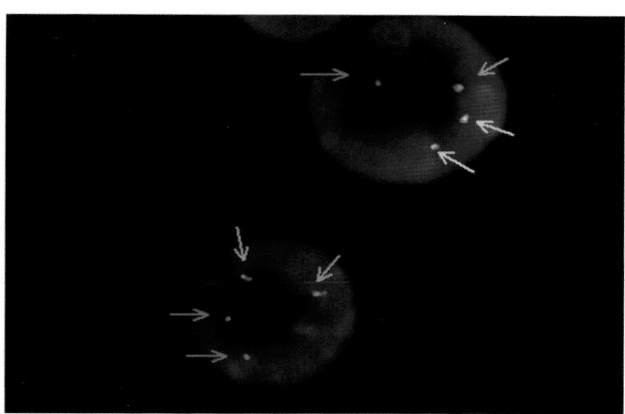

Plate 44 Fluorescent *in situ* hybridization (FISH) for t(11;14) translocation. CCND1 locus at 11q13 is labeled in green whereas the IgH locus at 14q32 is labeled in red. Yellow arrows show presence of the translocation in upper right cell, red and green arrows show derivatives of chromosomes 11 and 14. The cell at the low part of the picture shows no CCND1/IgH translocation.

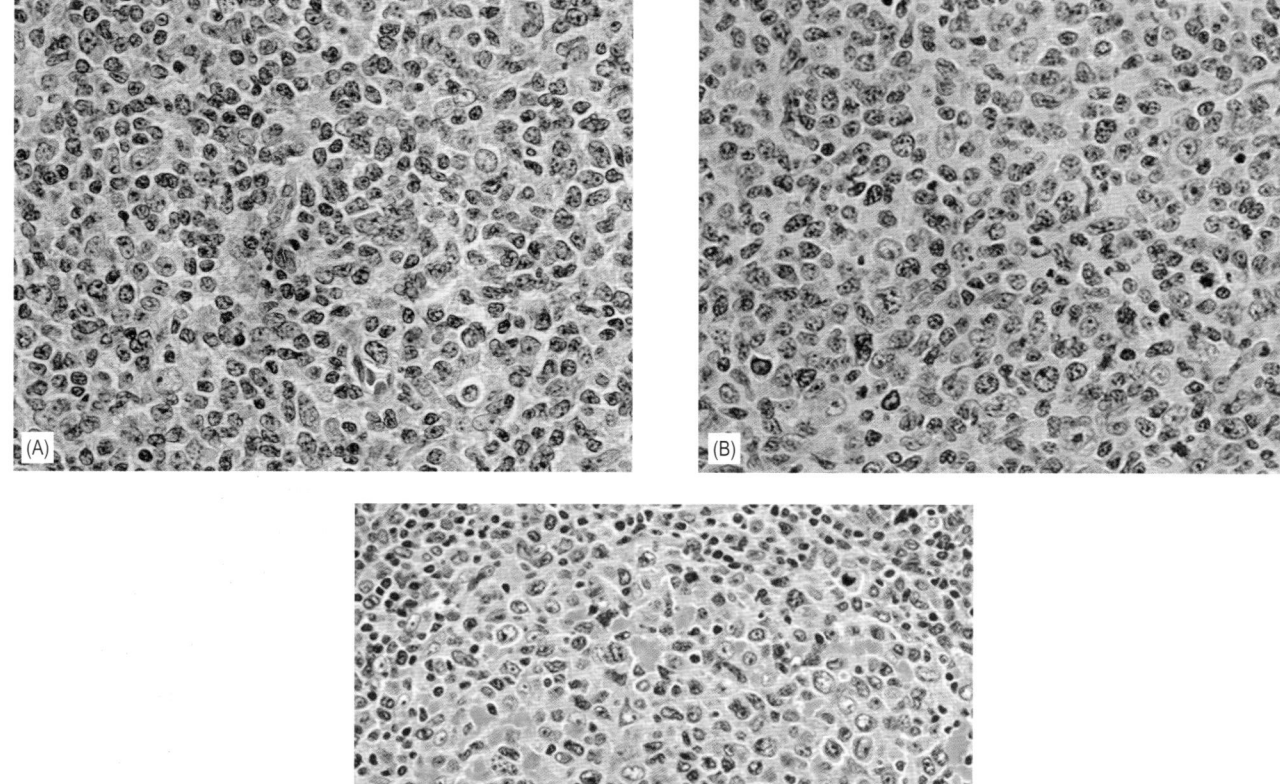

Plate 45 Typical cytologic composition of (A) grade 1, (B) grade 2 and (C) grade 3a follicular lymphoma.

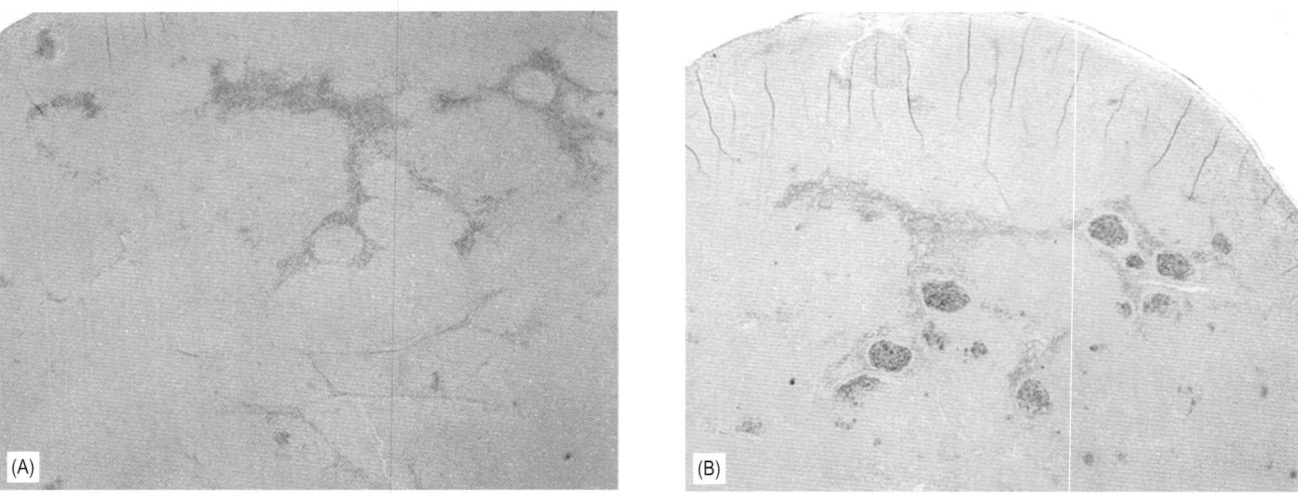

Plate 46   Grade 3b follicular lymphoma with (A) diffuse areas and corresponding CD21 stain showing (B) a small number of neoplastic follicles in an otherwise diffuse infiltrate.

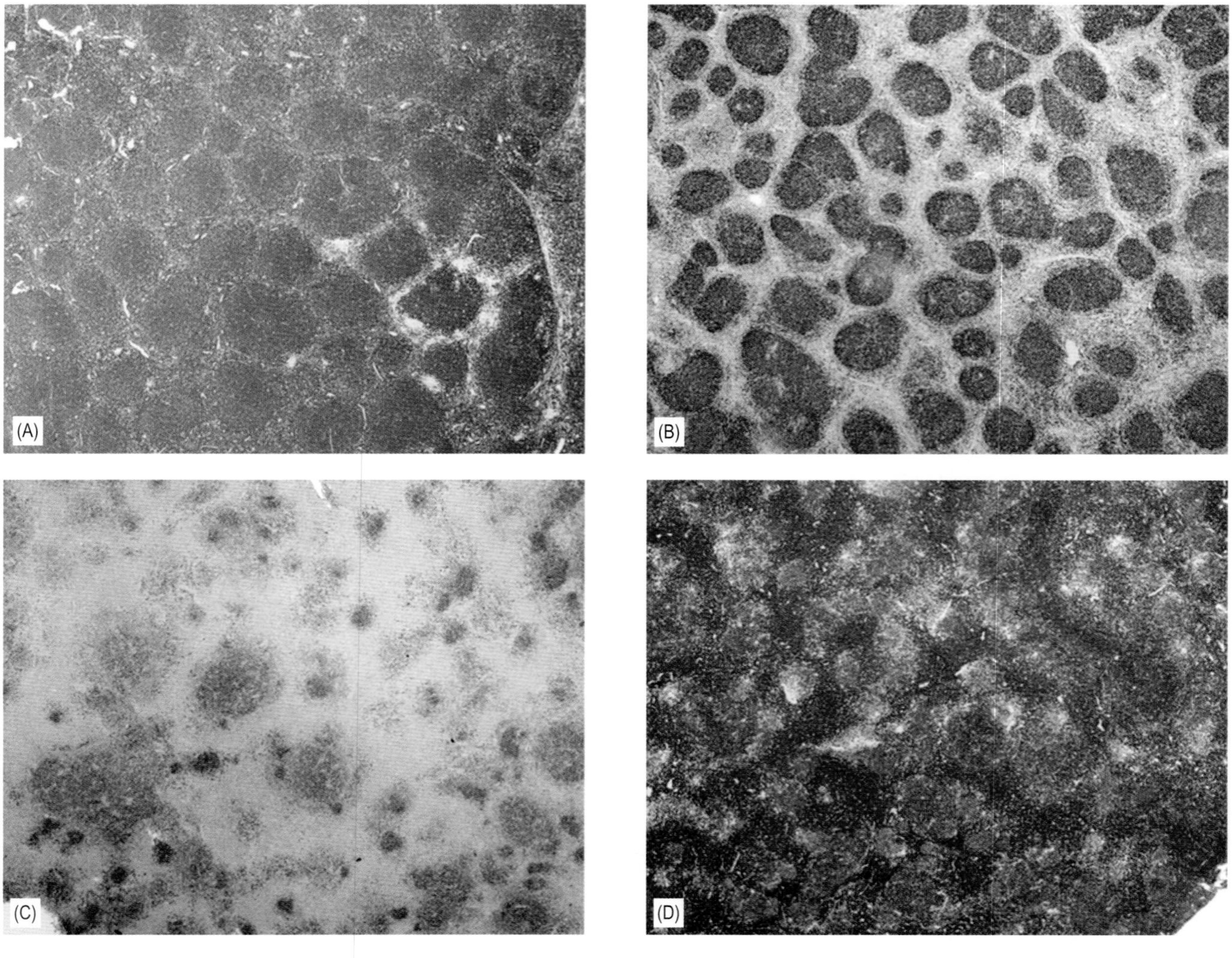

Plate 47   Typical immunophenotype of follicular lymphoma with neoplastic cells expressing (A) CD20, (B) BCL2, (C) BCL6 and (D) CD10.

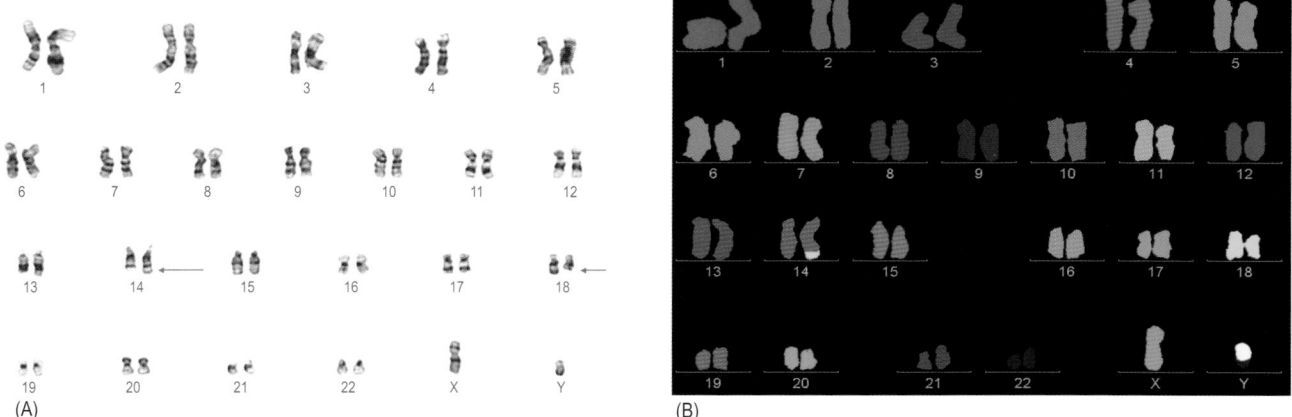

Plate 48 (A) Karyotype of FL with isolated t(14;18) and (B) multicolor fluorescence *in situ* hybridization showing the t(14;18) as the sole abnormality. Note that the small piece of chromosome 14 that is translocated to the derivative chromosome 18 is not visible, while the derivative 14 does show a piece of chromosome 18 (yellow) on the end of the derivative chromosome 14.

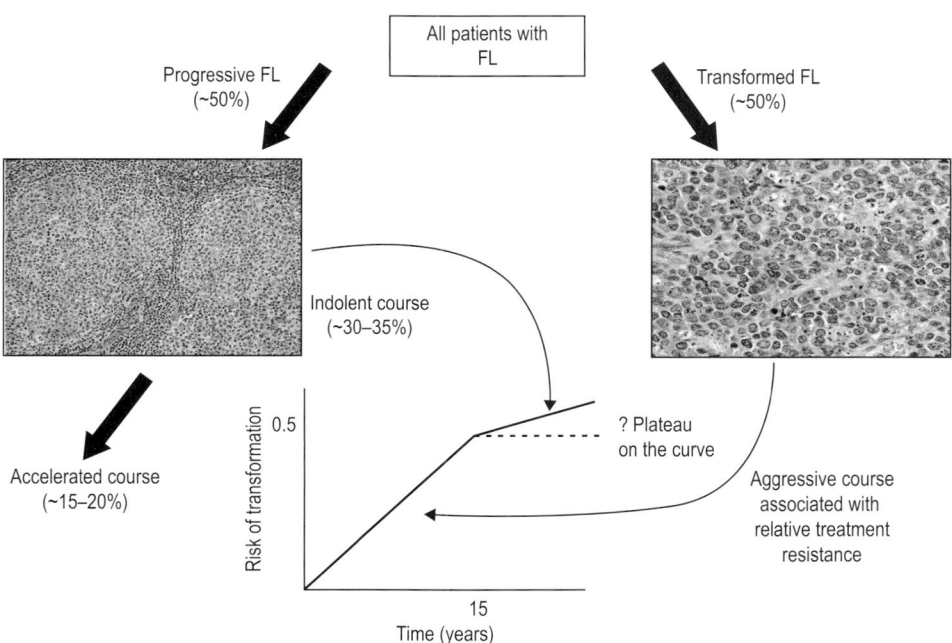

Plate 49 Proposed schematic linking pathogenesis to clinical behavior in follicular lymphoma (FL). Two major subgroups of FL may be distinguished based on the risk of transformation. The group on the left of the figure may not be at risk to transform. A proportion of these patients will experience aggressive behavior and may die from rapidly progressive FL. This could result from increased macrophage numbers at diagnosis or the presence of a *MYC* oncogene rearrangement. Many, however, relapse and remit and may experience a prolonged course, possibly contributing to a possible plateau on the overall survival curve. The group on the right side of the figure experiences transformation at a steady rate of approximately 3 percent per year. Many of these patients die following the transformation event due to treatment-resistant diffuse large B cell lymphoma.

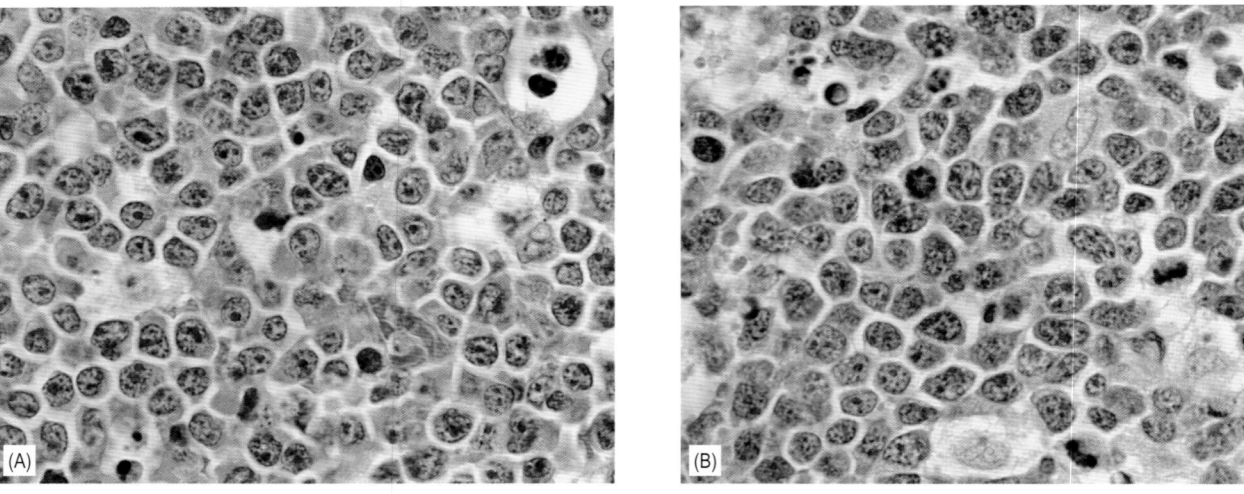

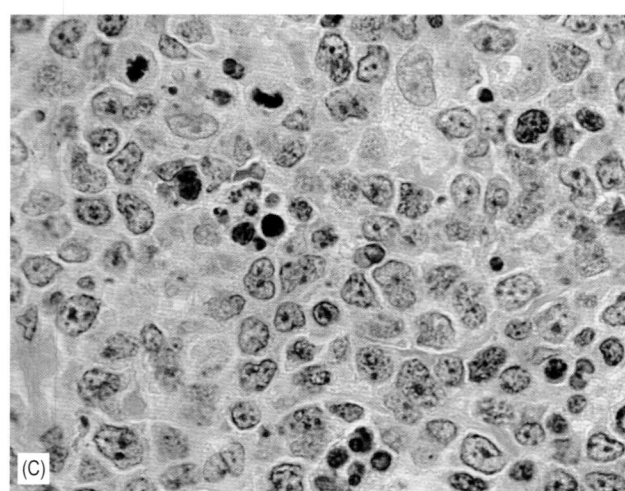

Plate 50 Range of histologic appearances of tumors with a Burkitt lymphoma (BL) molecular profile. All diffusely infiltrate the tissue of involvement, and never have a follicular appearance. All express pan-B cell markers including CD19, CD20, CD22 and CD79a, although not all are always present, particularly in diffuse large B cell lymphoma (DLBCL). The vast majority of BLs and Burkitt-like lymphoma (BLL) express surface IgM, rarely, IgG or IgA. The latter Ig classes are more often seen in DLBCL, although IgM is still the most frequent. TdT is negative. Images kindly provided by Dr R Gascoyne. (A) A classic case of Burkitt lymphoma harboring a *MYC* translocation. The cells show the characteristic squaring-off of the cytoplasm. These cells expressed CD20, BCL6 and CD10 and had a proliferative rate ~100 percent. They lacked expression of BCL2 protein. (B) Similar morphology as in (A) with a modest degree of nuclear irregularity and slight variability in cell size. These cells were confirmed to have a *MYC* translocation and a t(14;18), a so-called dual-translocation lymphoma. These cells expressed BCL2 protein. The case was classified as Burkitt-like lymphoma. (C) A diffuse large cell lymphoma. The low-power appearance revealed a starry-sky pattern and the proliferative rate was ~100 percent. The immunophenotype was identical to classic Burkitt lymphoma and fluorescence *in situ* hybridization studies confirmed the presence of a *MYC* gene rearrangement.

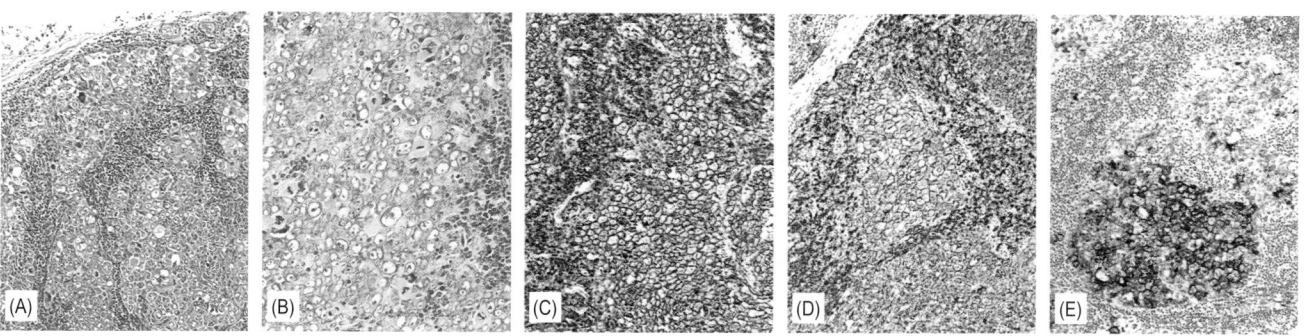

Plate 51 Diffuse large B cell lymphoma (DLBCL), anaplastic variant. (A) The anaplastic variant of DLBCL typically displays sinusoidal infiltration (×100). (B) This lymphoma is composed of large pleomorphic cells forming cohesive sheets (×200). The lymphoma cells are positive for (C) CD45 and (D) CD20, (E) and frequently coexpress CD30 (immunoperoxidase, ×100). Despite morphologic and phenotypic overlap with anaplastic large cell lymphoma of T or null type, ALK expression and translocations involving the *ALK* gene have never been demonstrated in anaplastic large B cell lymphoma; and the two entities are biologically unrelated.

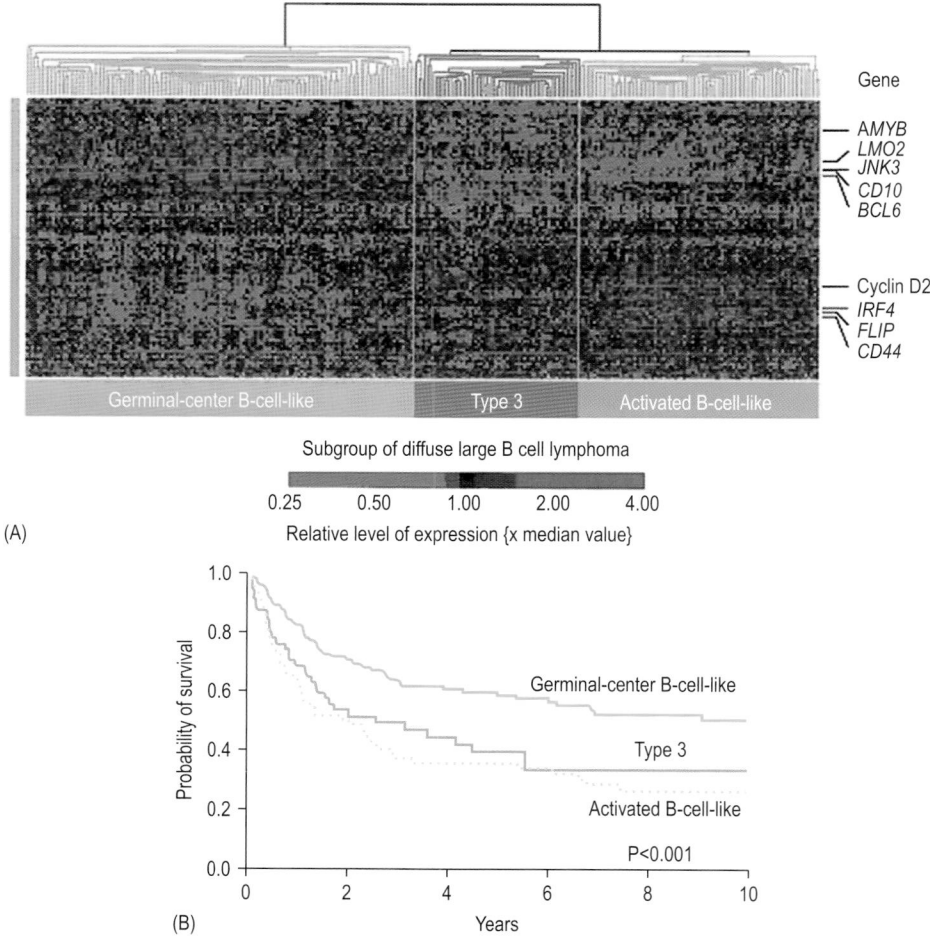

Plate 52 Subgroups of diffuse large B cell lymphomas (DLBCLs) according to gene expression profiles. (A) Hierarchical clustering of DLBCL from 274 patients (240 patients with untreated disease and 34 patients who had been previously treated or had a preexisting low-grade lymphoma) according to the level of expression of 100 genes. Red areas indicate increased expression and green areas indicate decreased expression. Each column represents a single DLBCL patient and each row represents a single gene. The dendrogram at the top shows the degree to which each DLBCL is related to the others with respect to their gene expression profile. Genes that are characteristically expressed in GCB-DLBCL and ABC-DLBCL are indicated. Relative expression levels for each gene are presented according to the color scale. (B) Kaplan–Meier estimates of overall survival of DLBCL patients after chemotherapy among the 240 previously untreated patients, according to the gene expression subgroup. (Reproduced with permission from Rosenwald A, Wright G, Chan WC *et al.*, for the Lymphoma/Leukemia Molecular Profiling Project. The use of molecular profiling to predict survival after chemotherapy for diffuse large-B-cell lymphoma. *N Engl J Med* 2002; **346**: 1937–47.)

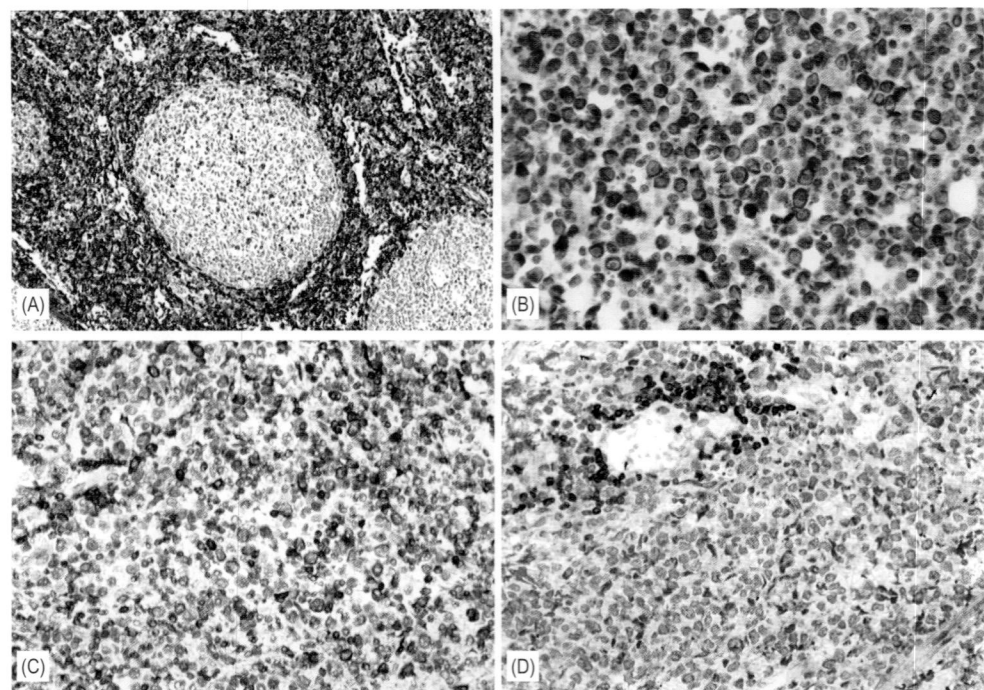

Plate 53 Patterns of BCL2 expression in reactive lymphoid tissue (A) and in diffuse large B cell lymphomas (DLBCLs) (B–D). In (A) reactive tonsils, BCL2 is strongly expressed in most cells except germinal center B cells (immunoperoxidase, ×100). In DLBCL, BCL2 expression is variable: (B) is an example of a case in which most lymphoma cells are strongly positive; (C) lymphoma cells display heterogeneous BCL2 positivity; (D) lymphoma cells are negative for BCL2, in contrast to reactive T cells (immunoperoxidase, ×400). (Reproduced with permission from: de Leval L, Harris NL. Variability in immunophenotype in diffuse large B cell lymphoma and its clinical relevance. *Histopathology* 2003; **43**: 509–28.)

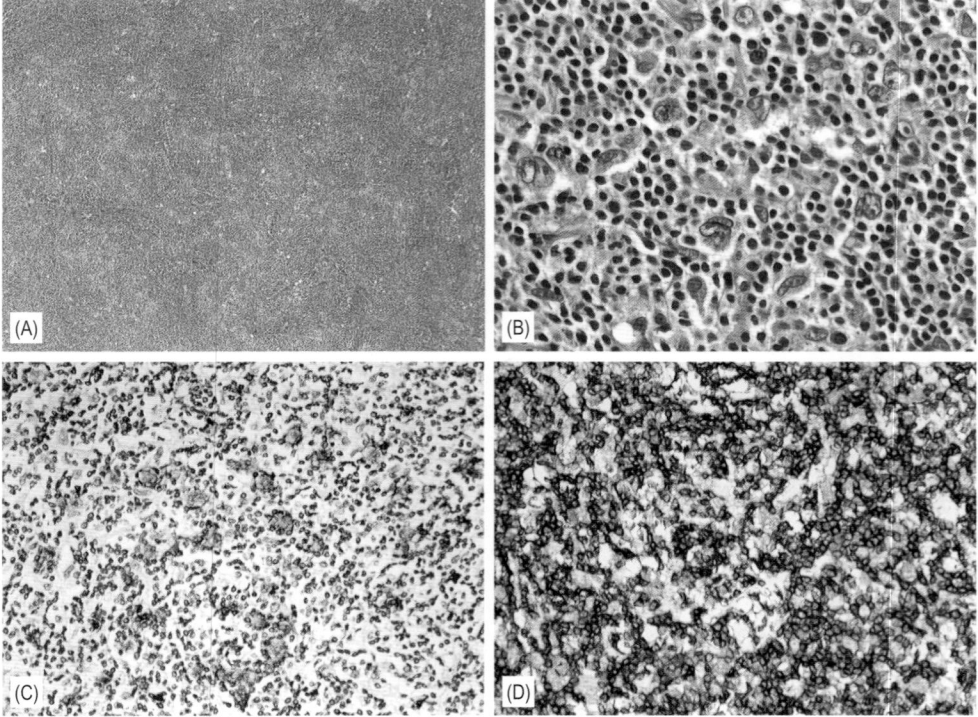

Plate 54 T cell/histiocyte-rich large B cell lymphoma (THRLBCL). (A) THRLBCL consists of a diffuse infiltrate predominantly composed of small lymphoid cells with scattered histiocytes (×50); (B) there are few large neoplastic cells with variable cytologic appearance (×400); (C) the large neoplastic cells are CD20-positive while (D) the small cell stain for CD3 (immunoperoxidase, ×200).

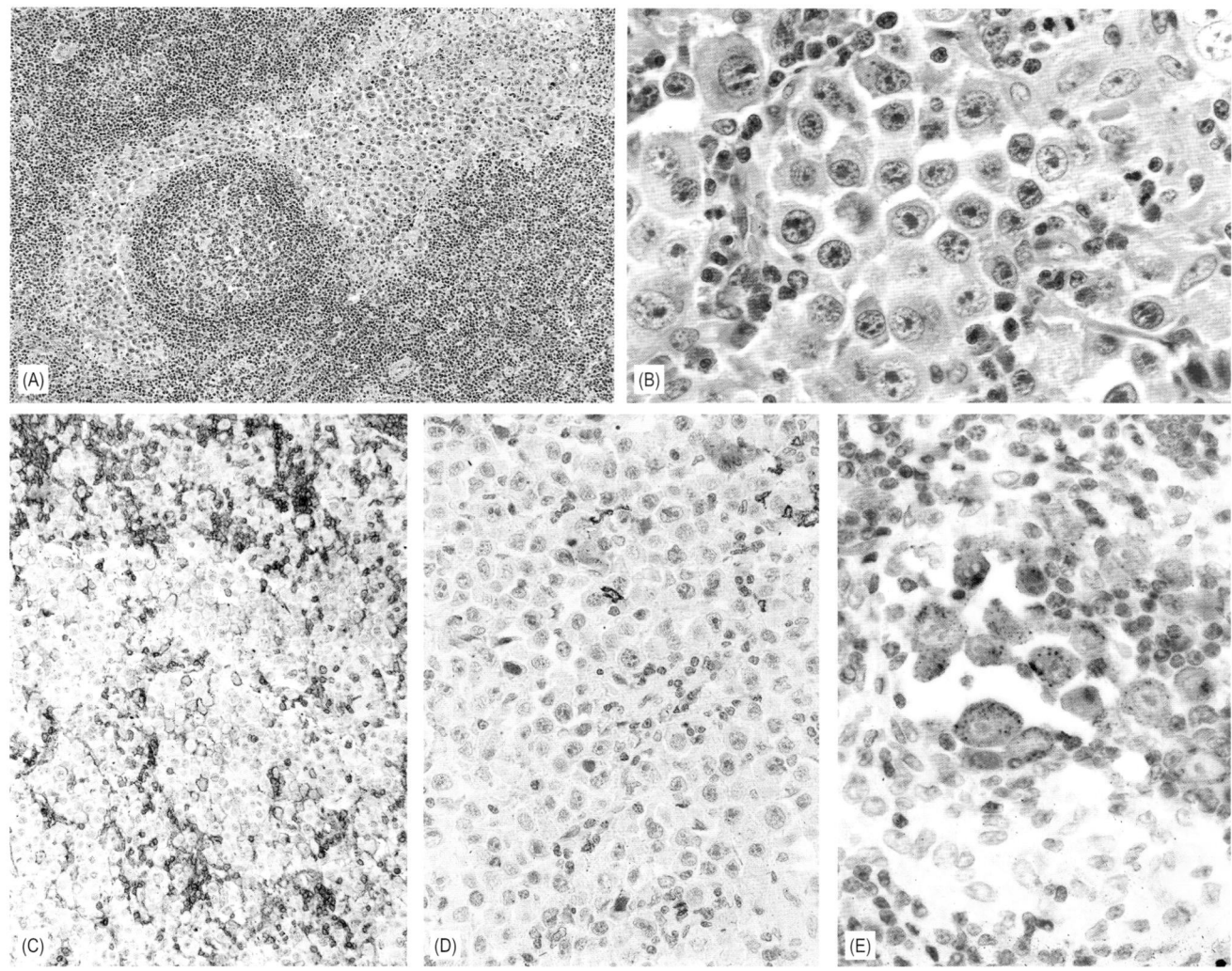

Plate 55 Anaplastic lymphoma kinase-positive DLBCL. (A) The tumor shows a sinusoidal growth pattern (×40). (B) The neoplastic cells show immunoblastic and plasmablastic features (×800). (C) The lymphoma cells are negative or faintly positive for CD45 (×100). (D) They are negative for CD20 (×100). (E) ALK immunostain reveals fine granular cytoplasmic localization of the ALK protein (×800).

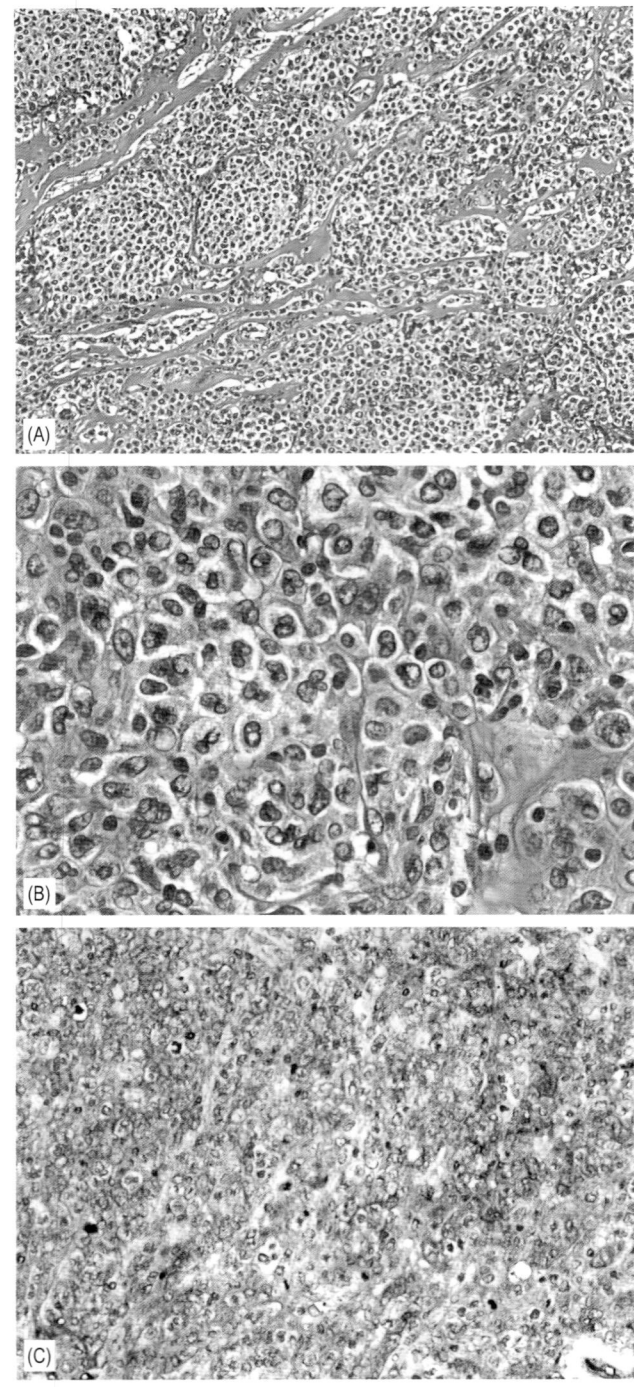

Plate 56 Primary mediastinal large B cell lymphoma (PMLBCL). (A) PMLBCL typically appears as a diffuse proliferation of lymphoid cells associated with fine compartmentalizing sclerosis (×100). (B) The cells have abundant clear cytoplasm and multilobulated nuclei (×400). (C) A subset of PMLBCL express CD30 (immunoperoxidase, ×200).

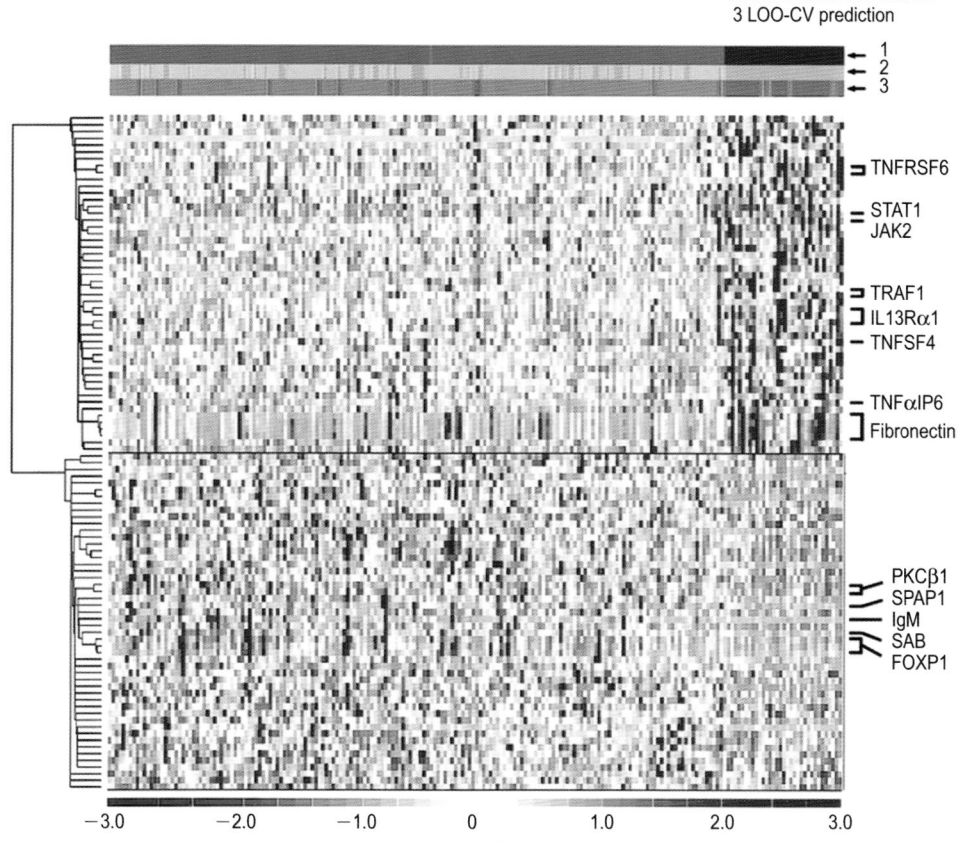

Plate 57 Gene expression profile of diffuse large B cell lymphoma (DLBCL) and primary mediastinal large B cell lymphoma (MLBCL). Comparative gene expression profiles of DLBCL and MLBCL. At the top, the actual clinical/pathologic diagnosis of DLBCL versus MLBCL (green versus red), presence or absence of mediastinal disease (pink versus light green), and molecular prediction of DLBCL versus MLBCL (green versus red) are compared. The top 50 genes that were expressed at higher levels in MLBCL are shown in the upper half of the figure and the top 50 that were more abundant in DLBCL are shown in the lower half of the figure. Red indicates high relative expression; blue, low expression. Color scale at the bottom indicates relative expression in standard deviations from the mean. Each column is a sample and each row is a gene. Genes are clustered using hierarchical clustering. Expression profiles of 176 DLBCLs are on the left; profiles of the 34 MLBCLs are on the right. (Reproduced with permission from Savage KJ, Monti S, Kutok JL *et al.* The molecular signature of mediastinal large B cell lymphoma differs from that of other diffuse large B cell lymphomas and shares features with classical Hodgkin lymphoma. *Blood* 2003; **102**: 3871–9.)

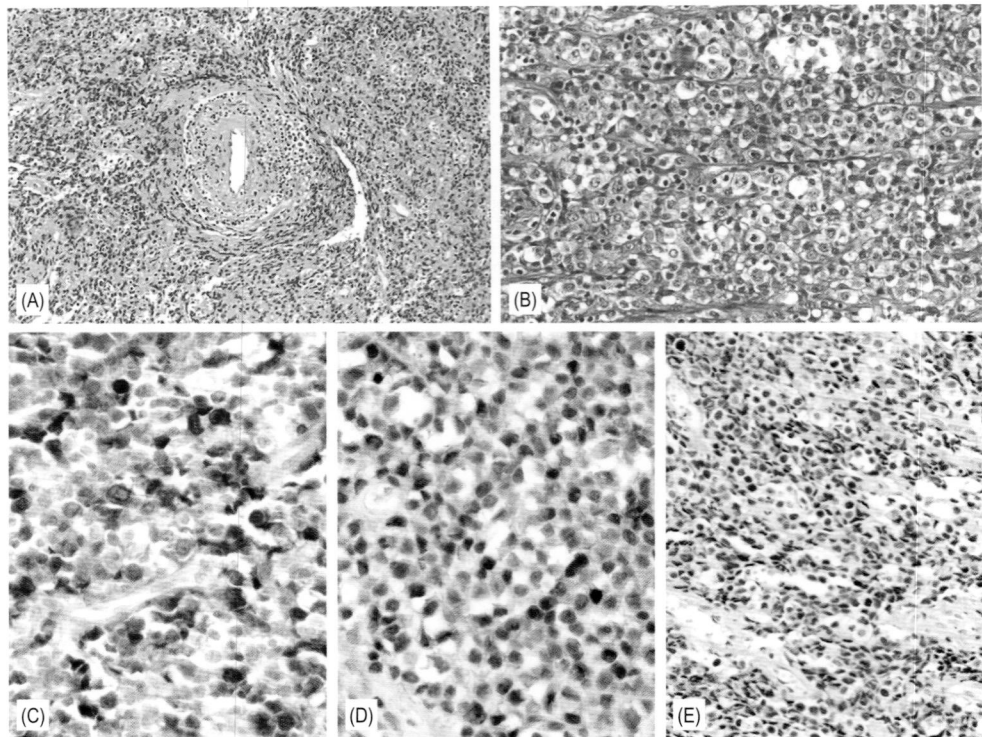

Plate 58 Pyothorax-associated lymphoma (PAL). (A) Low-power view of a PAL case illustrates the angiocentric features of this neoplasm (×100). (B) The tumor consists of diffuse sheets of large lymphoid cells with immunoblastic features (×250). (C) CD79a expression is typically heterogeneous (×400). (D) Virtually all cases strongly express MUM1 (×400). (E) EBV has a type III latency pattern with EBNA2 expression (×250). (Courtesy of Professor Philippe Gaulard, Hôpital Henri Mondor, Créteil, France.)

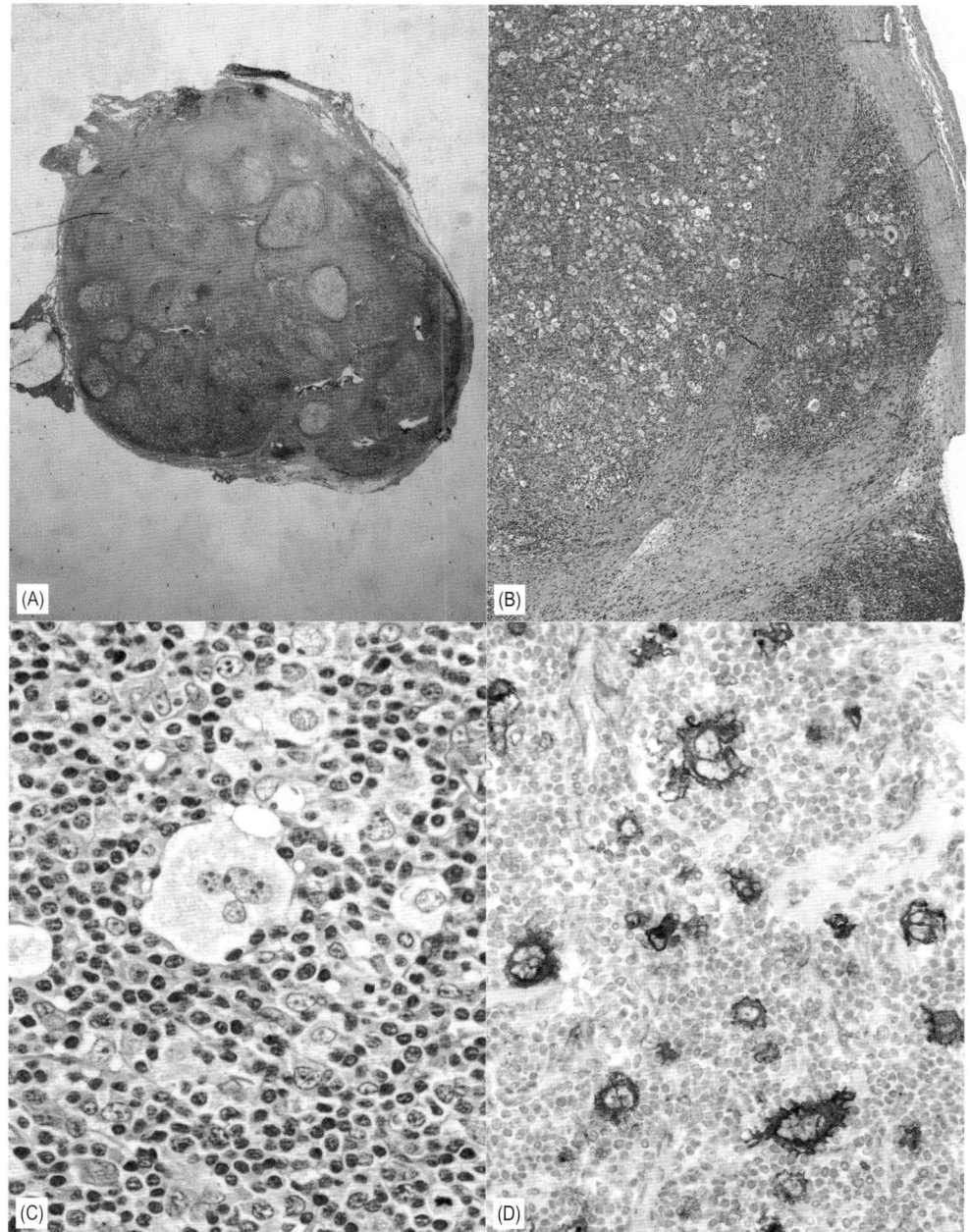

Plate 59 Histology of nodular sclerosis Hodgkin lymphoma (NSHL). (A) Low magnification of a lymph node involved by NSHL. Multiple nodules surrounded by sclerotic bands are visible (hemalan–eosin staining). (B) Many pale cells (lacunar cells) are visible in the nodules surrounded by sclerotic bands of a case of NSHL. (C) In the center of the picture a large lacunar cell is visible. Smaller lacunar cells with pale cytoplasm are seen in the neighborhood. The centrally located lacunar cell shows a broad pale cytoplasm and a small rim (lacuna) in the periphery of the cell. The nucleus is lobulated and has some medium-sized nucleoli. Several lymphocytes are visible in the cytoplasm (emperipolesis). The tumor cells are surrounded by small lymphocytes and histiocytes (hemalaun–eosin staining). (D) CD30-positive HRS cells in NSHL. HRS and lacunar cells show a strong membrane-bound and intracytoplasmic immunoreaction for CD30 (alkaline phosphatase immunoreaction).

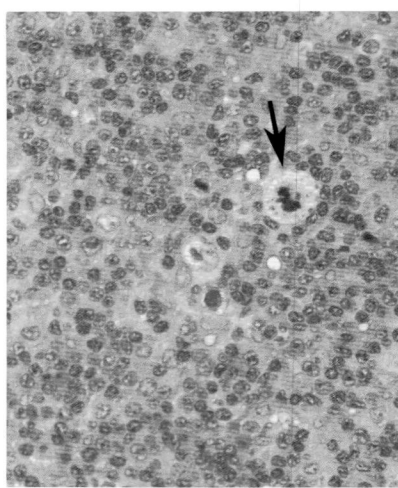

Plate 60 Histology of mixed cellularity Hodgkin lymphoma. In the center of the picture a Hodgkin cell with an irregularly shaped nucleolus and a prominent nucleolus is visible. Beside the Hodgkin cell a so-called 'mummified' cell. In addition, an atypical mitosis is visible (arrow). Several eosinophilic granulocytes are intermingled with small lymphocytes and histiocytes (hemalaun–eosin staining).

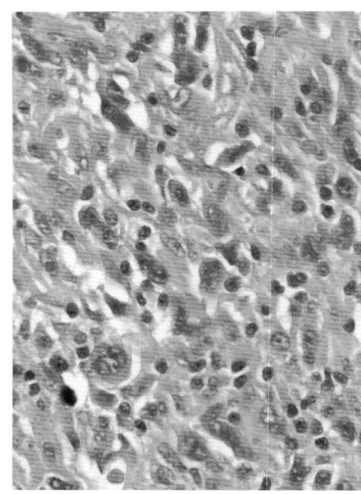

Plate 62 HRS cells in lymphocyte-depleted Hodgkin lymphoma (LDHL). This picture shows many large tumor cells in a case of LDHL. Some of them showing features of HRS cells. Only a few lymphocytes are seen (hemalaun–eosin staining).

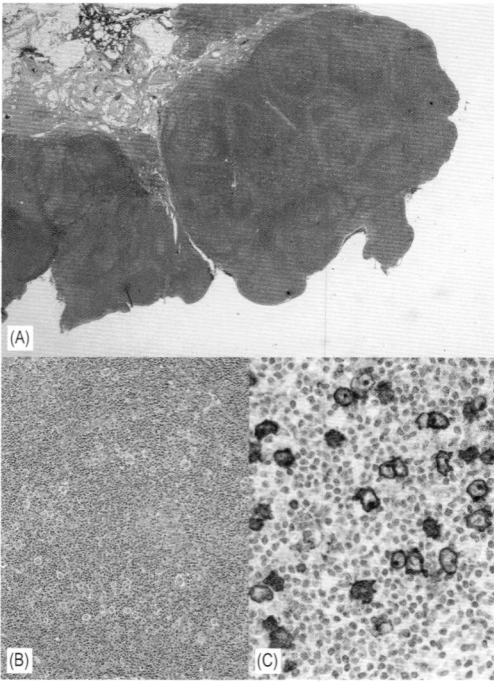

Plate 61 Histology of lymphocyte-rich classical Hodgkin lymphoma (LRCHL). (A) Low magnification of a lymph node involved by LRCHL (hemalaun–eosin staining). Many nodules are seen. In contrast to NSHL, no sclerotic bands are visible. Morphologic distinction between this type of HL and NLPHL is not possible. (B) A weakly nodular appearing infiltrate of LRCHL is seen. Many large cells with round or slightly irregularly shaped nuclei and relatively pale cytoplasm (Hodgkin cells) can be found in a background of small lymphocytes. (C) Hodgkin and Reed–Sternberg (HRS) cells in LRCHL. The tumor cells of LRCHL are strongly immunostained with CD30 (immuno alkaline phosphatase reaction).

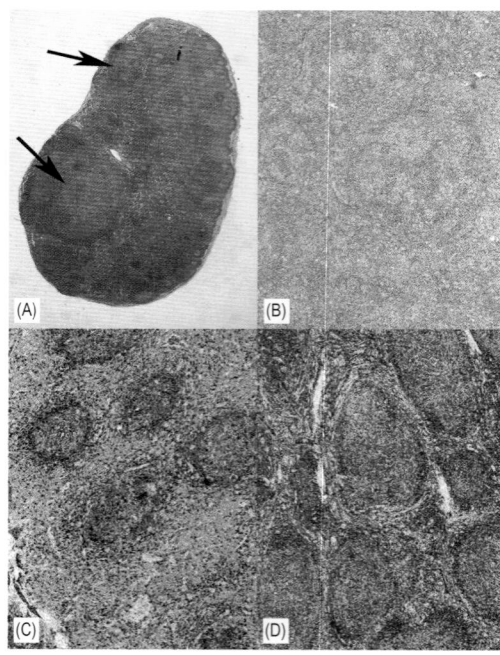

Plate 63 Histology of nodular lymphocyte-predominant Hodgkin lymphoma (NLPHL). (A) Low magnification of lymph node partially involved by NLPHL. Two tumor nodules are visible (arrows). The remaining lymph node shows reactive features mainly preserved GCs and pulp areas. (B) Nodular infiltrate by a NLPHL showing a 'mottled' appearance (Giemsa staining). (C) The nodular infiltrates of NLPHL are composed of many B lymphocytes (CD20 immunostaining). (D) Numerous T cells can be found inside and outside the nodules of NLPHL (CD3 staining, alkaline phosphatase reaction).

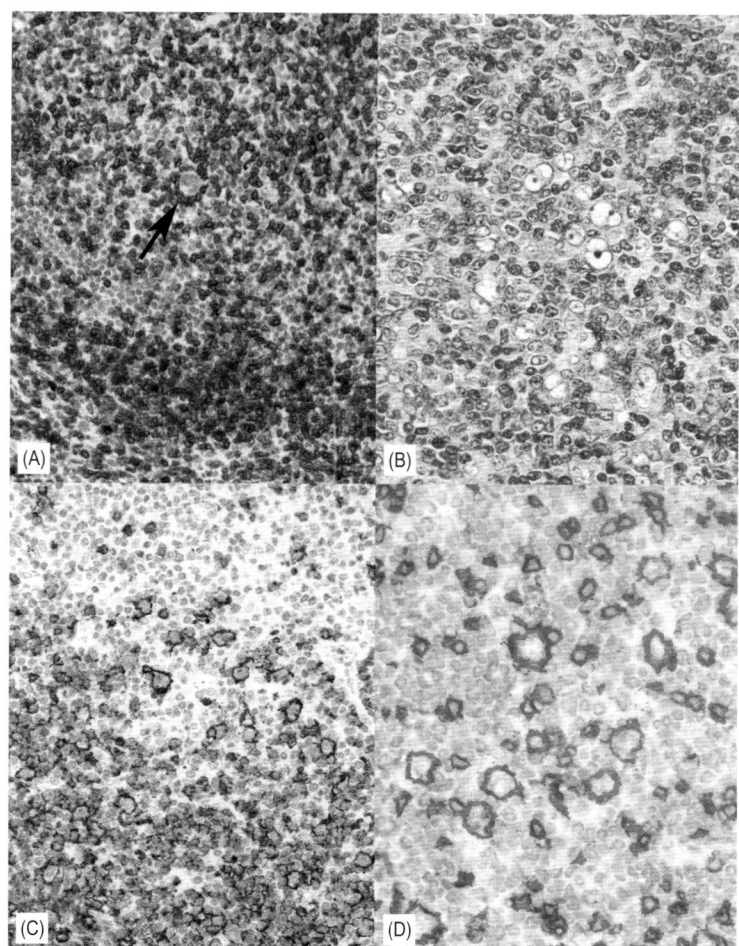

Plate 64 Histology of nodular lymphocyte-predominant Hodgkin lymphoma (NLPHL). (A) Part of a nodular infiltrate immunostained with CD3 showing a T cell rosette around a LP cell (arrow) (alkaline phosphatase reaction); (B) LP cells of a NLPHL in the center of the picture. These cells show round or lobulated nuclei with medium sized nucleoli and a broad cytoplasm. Small lymphocytes are dominating (Giemsa staining); (C) CD20 expression in NLPHL. CD20 reacts with large blastic cells (LP cells) as well as the small B lymphocytes in a lymph node infiltrated by NLPHL (L26 antibody, alkaline phosphatase reaction); (D) CD20 expression by LP cells in NLPHL. CD20 localized mainly on the cell membrane of LP cells showing large nuclei. Only a few B lymphocytes are visible. This picture shows a mainly diffuse infiltrate of NLPHL (alkaline phosphatase immunoreaction).

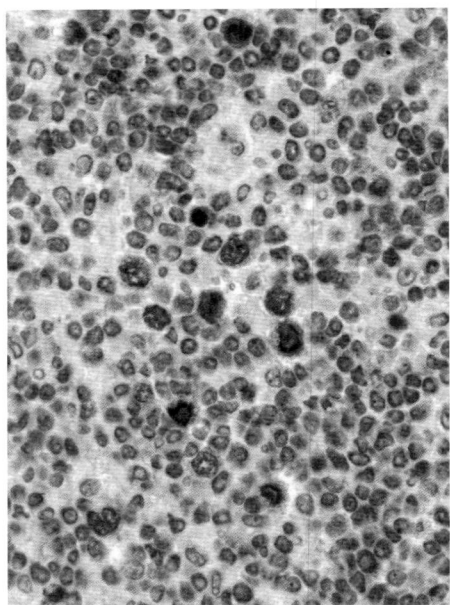

Plate 65 PAX5 expression in NLPHL. An antibody detecting PAX5 shows an immunoreaction localized mainly in the nucleus of several LP cells in a case of NLPHL (alkaline phosphatase immunoreaction).

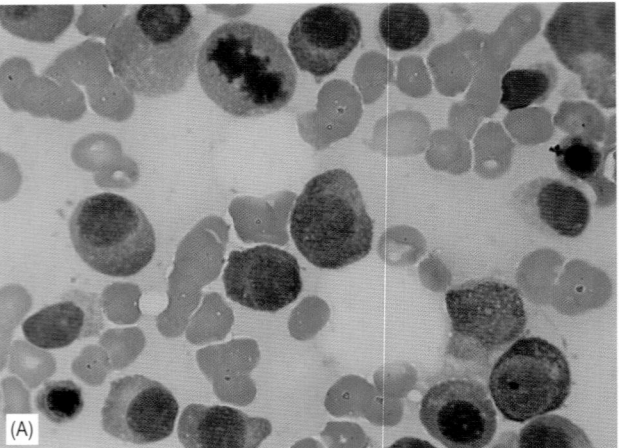

(A)

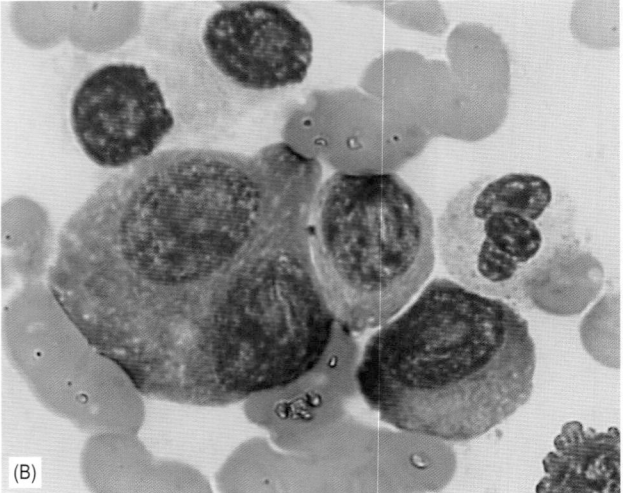

(B)

Plate 66 Bone marrow aspirate in multiple myeloma. (A) Mature plasma cells are demonstrated with oval cytoplasm, eccentric nuclei and a perinuclear hof. A mitotic figure is demonstrated. Note background rouleaux formation (MGG, ×400) (B) A cluster of plasma cells including a binucleate form (MGG, ×400).

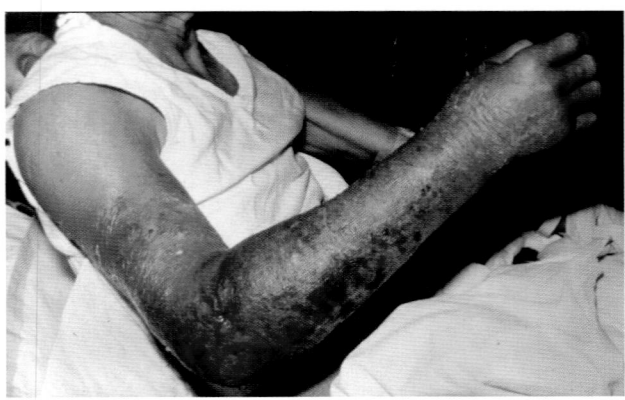

Plate 67 Nasal NK/T cell lymphoma. The disease relapses in the skin, causing swelling of the right arm and forearm. The skin shows scaling, brownish induration and areas of necrosis.

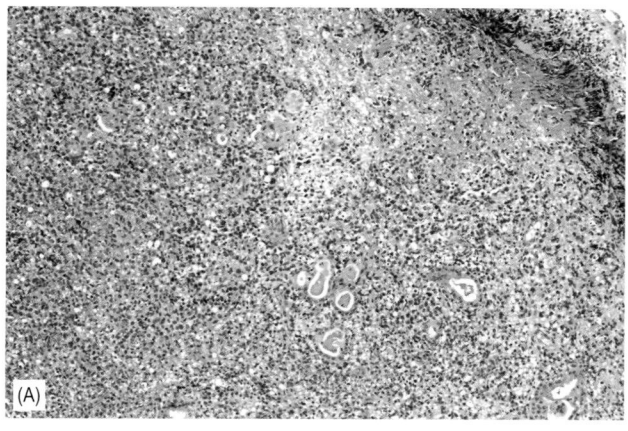

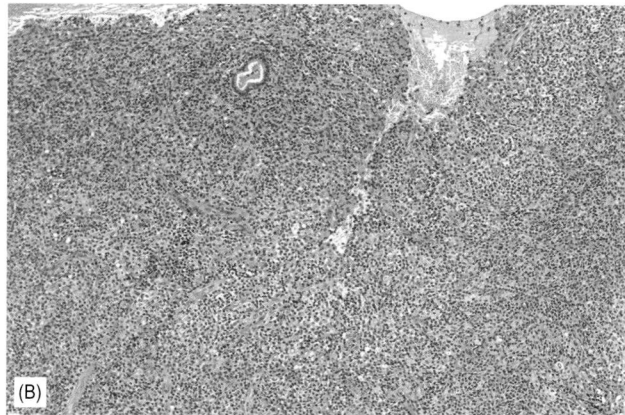

Plate 68 Nasal NK/T cell lymphoma. (A) The nasal biopsy shows a dense infiltrate of lymphoid cells, with ulceration and areas of necrosis. (B) Less commonly, the nasal mucosa does not show ulceration. The dense lymphomatous infiltrate causes marked loss of mucosal glands (with only a single residual gland seen in the left upper field).

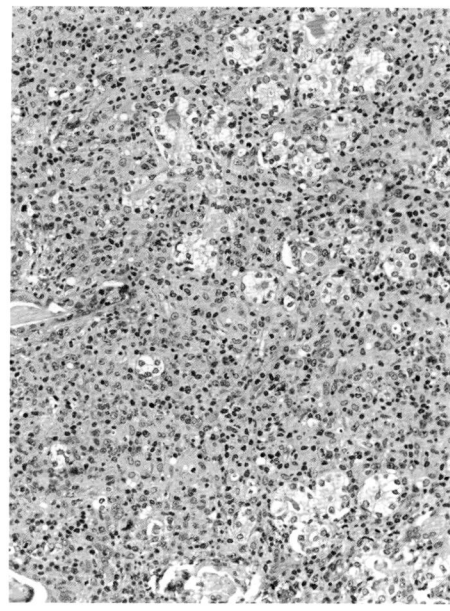

Plate 70 Nasal NK/T cell lymphoma. The lymphomatous infiltrate pushes the mucosal glands apart. In this case, the glandular epithelium shows cytoplasmic clearing.

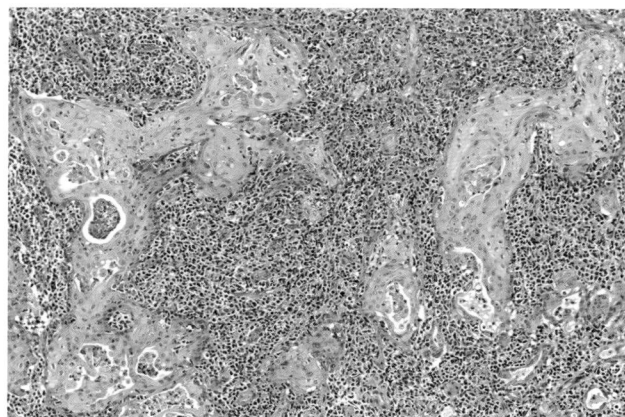

Plate 69 Nasal NK/T cell lymphoma accompanied by remarkable pseudoepitheliomatous hyperplasia, which may lead to a misdiagnosis of squamous cell carcinoma.

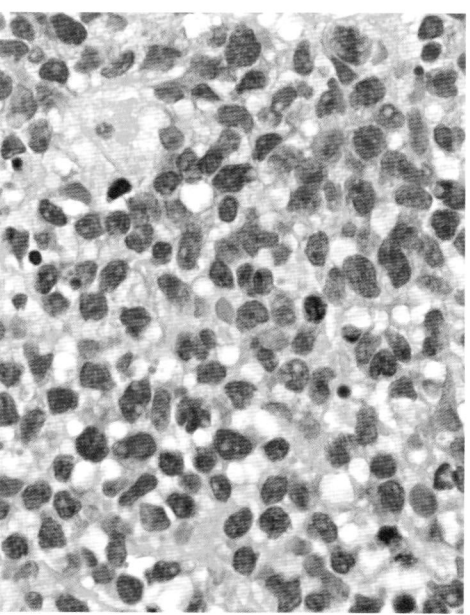

Plate 71 Nasal NK/T cell lymphoma. Most commonly the lymphoma cells are medium sized, and exhibit irregular nuclear foldings.

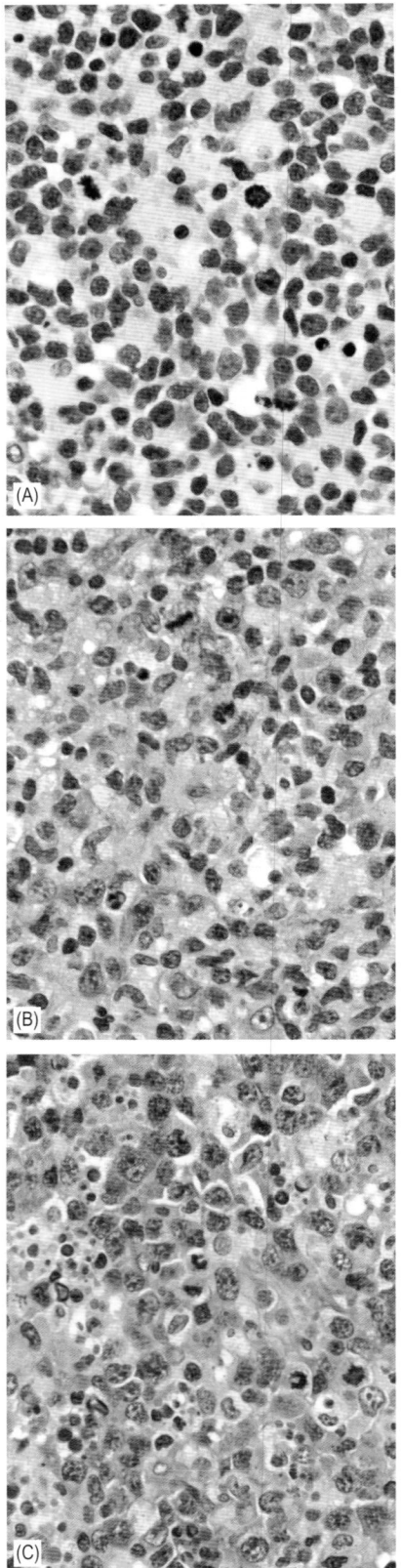

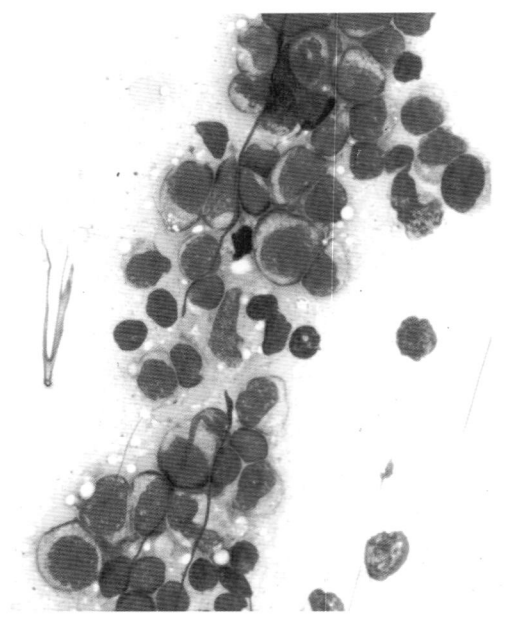

Plate 73 Nasal NK/T cell lymphoma: Giemsa-stained touch preparation. The lymphoma cells possess pale-staining cytoplasm that contain fine azurophilic granules.

Plate 72 Nasal NK/T cell lymphoma: the cytologic spectrum. (A) This case is dominated by small cells with irregularly folded nuclei. (B) This case shows a mixture of small, medium-sized and large cells. (C) This case is dominated by large cells. Note the abundance of admixed karyorrhectic debris.

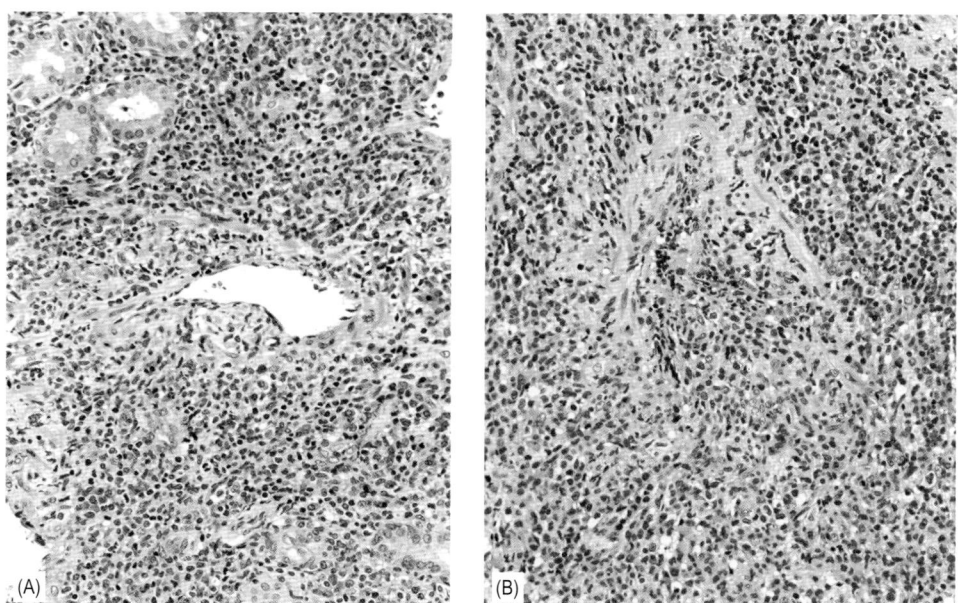

Plate 74 Nasal NK/T cell lymphoma: angioinvasion. (A) The vessel wall shows infiltration by lymphoma cells. (B) The blood vessel is completely obliterated by lymphoma cells.

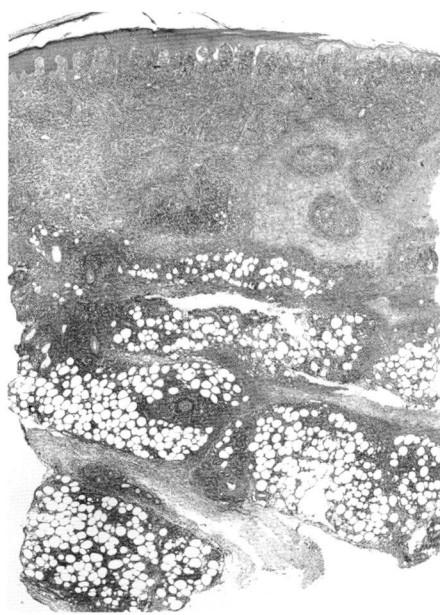

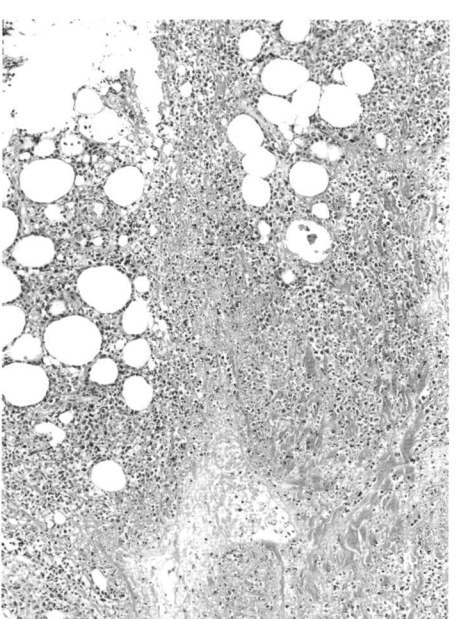

Plate 75 Extranasal NK/T cell lymphoma involving skin. The lymphoma infiltrates the dermis and subcutaneous tissue. Note focal necrosis of the epidermis (right upper field) and the dermis. Angioinvasion is also evident in the subcutaneous tissue.

Plate 76 Extranasal NK/T cell lymphoma involving skin. Note the characteristic presence of necrosis (right lower field).

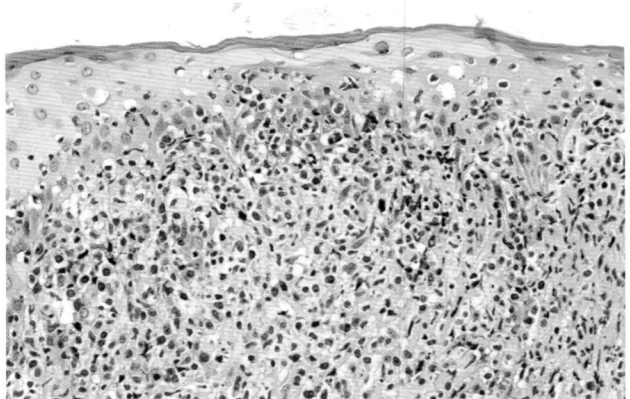

Plate 77 Extranasal NK/T cell lymphoma involving skin, showing epidermotropism.

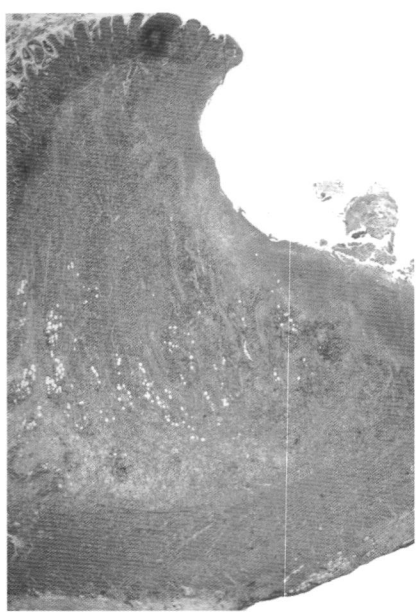

Plate 79 Extranasal NK/T cell lymphoma involving the small intestine. There is transmural lymphomatous infiltration. Necrotic tissue lines the perforation site (right field).

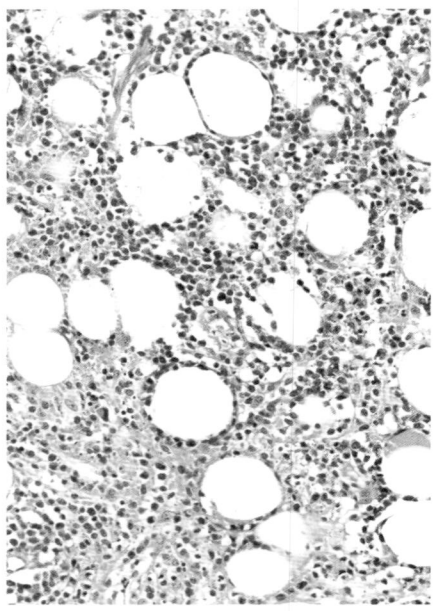

Plate 78 Extranasal NK/T cell lymphoma involving skin. The lymphoma cells show interstitial infiltration in the subcutaneous tissue. The rimming of fat vacuoles results in a picture simulating subcutaneous panniculitis-like T cell lymphoma.

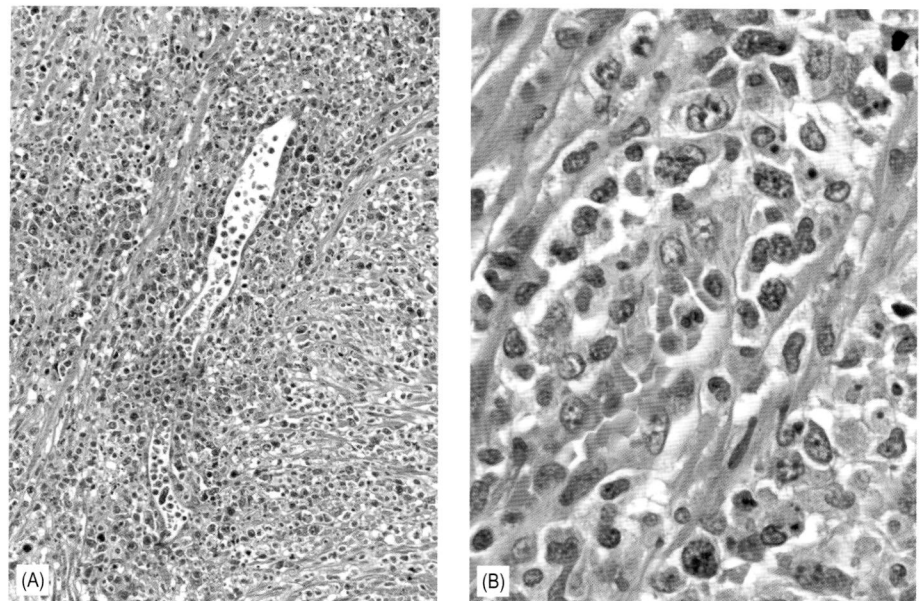

Plate 80 Extranasal NK/T cell lymphoma involving the small intestine. (A) Angiocentric growth is evident. The lymphoma cells are admixed with fibrinous exudates and karyorrhectic debris. (B) The lymphoma cells are medium sized to large, and exhibit granular chromatin.

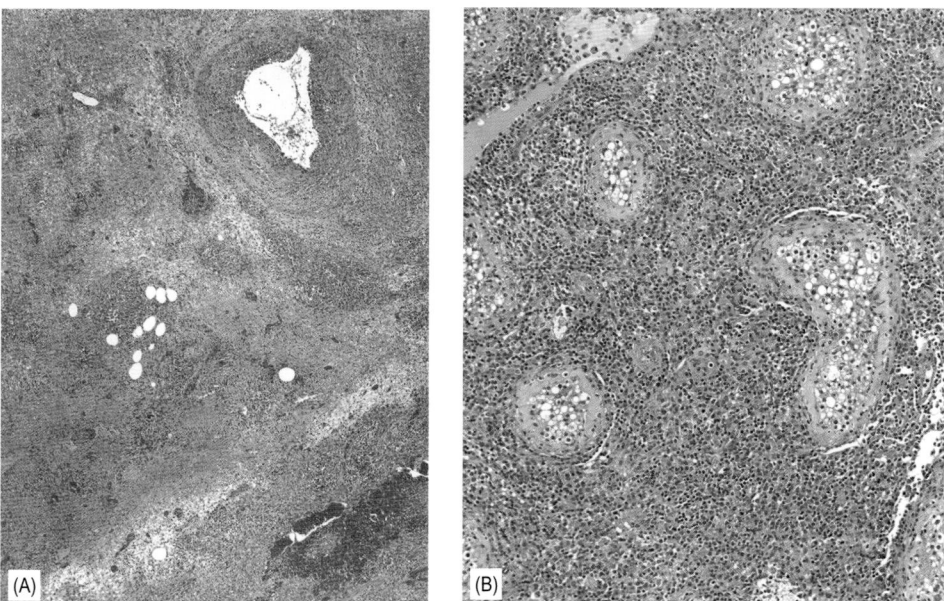

Plate 81 Extranasal NK/T cell lymphoma involving the testis. (A) There is extensive replacement of the testicular tissue by lymphomatous infiltrate. Angioinvasion and necrosis are evident. (B) The interstitium between the seminiferous tubules is markedly expanded by the lymphomatous infiltrate.

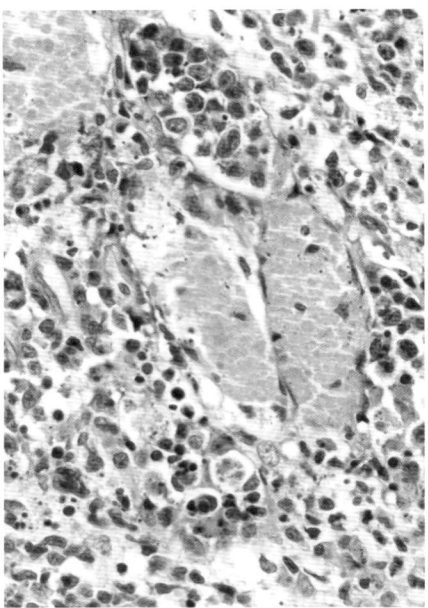

Plate 82   Extranasal NK/T cell lymphoma involving skeletal muscle. There is marked destruction of the skeletal muscle fibers. In the upper field, the lymphoma cells 'colonize' a necrotic muscle fiber.

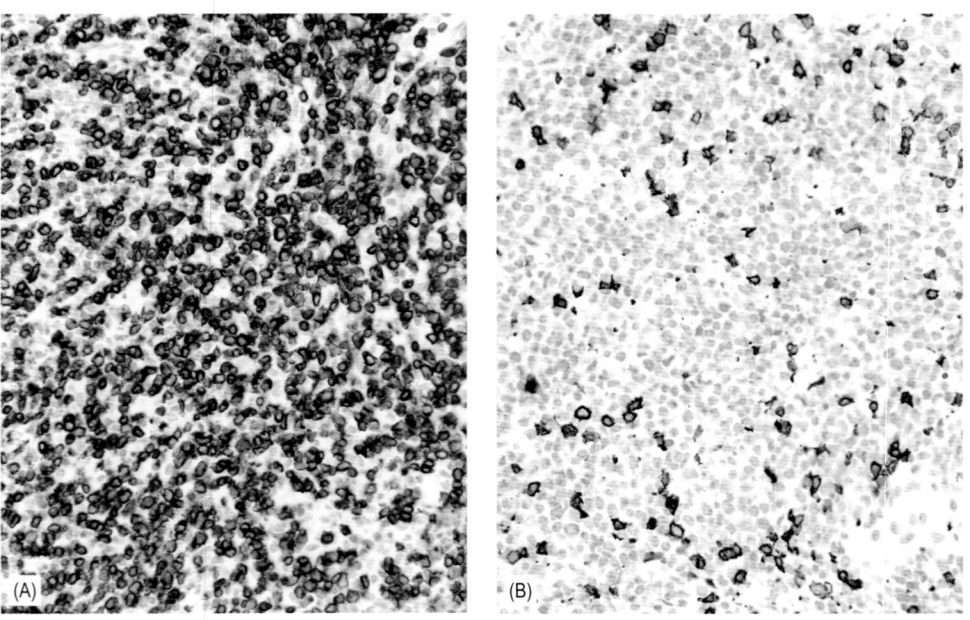

Plate 83   Nasal NK/T cell lymphoma: immunohistochemical staining. (A) The lymphoma cells show positive staining for cytoplasmic CD3ε. (B) On the other hand, CD5 is typically negative.

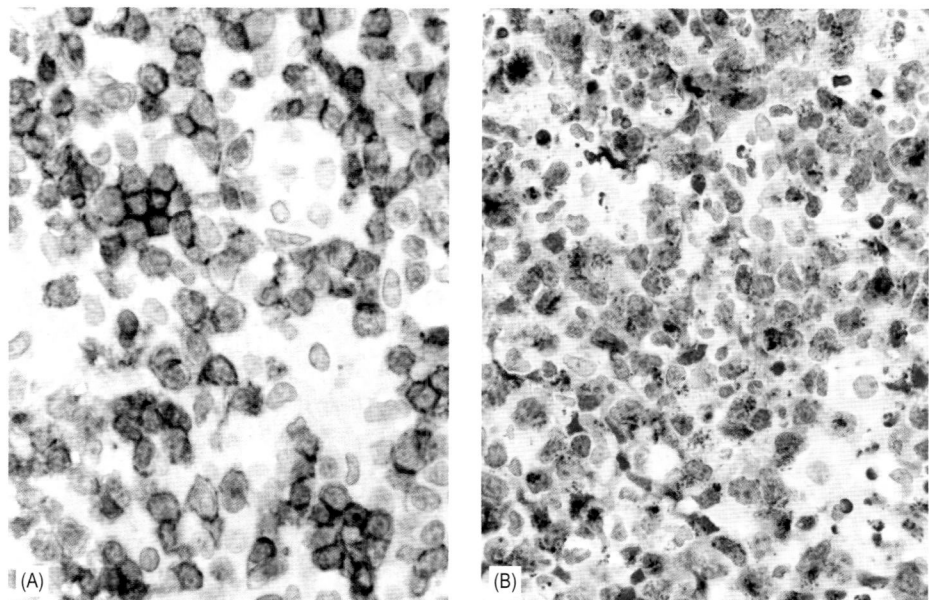

Plate 84   Nasal NK/T cell lymphoma: immunohistochemical staining. (A) The lymphoma cells show positive staining for CD56. (B) There is granular staining for granzyme B.

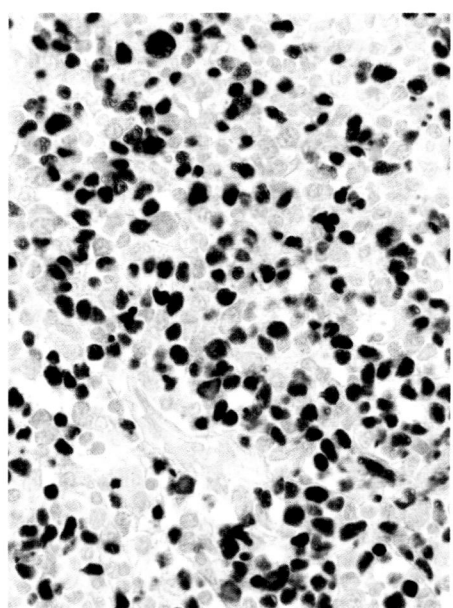

Plate 85   Nasal NK/T cell lymphoma: *in situ* hybridization for EBER. Most of the lymphoma cells show nuclear labeling for EBER.

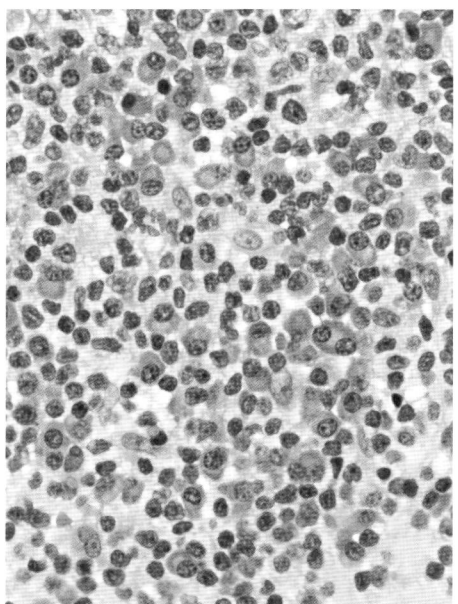

Plate 86   Nasal NK/T cell lymphoma: difficult case mimicking an inflammatory lesion. This case is difficult to diagnose because the lymphoma cells are small, resembling normal small lymphocytes, and there are numerous admixed reactive plasma cells.

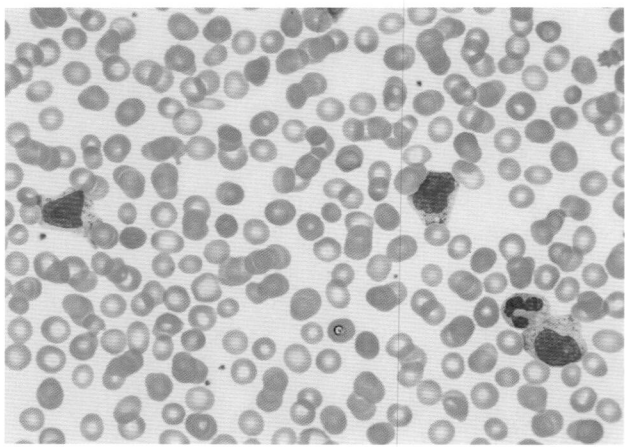

Plate 87 Aggressive NK cell leukemia: peripheral blood smear stained with Giemsa. The circulating neoplastic cells resemble normal large granular lymphocytes, with fine azurophilic granules in the cytoplasm. However, the chromatin is less condensed, and nucleoli are sometimes seen (cell in right lower field).

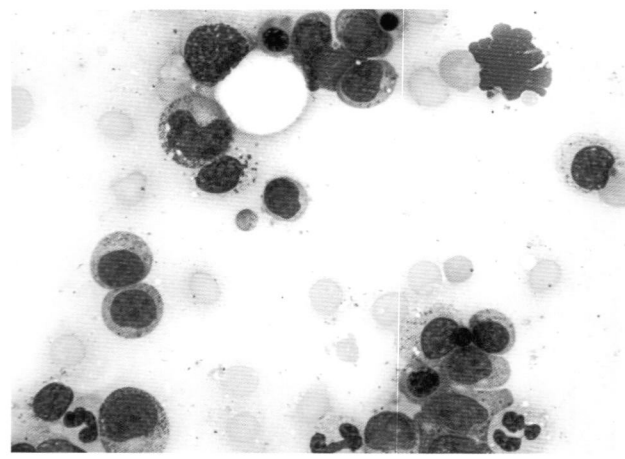

Plate 89 Aggressive NK cell leukemia: marrow smear stained with Giemsa. In contrast to the usual leukemias, the bone marrow is usually not completely overrun by neoplastic cells, and there are still intermingled hematopoietic cells. The neoplastic cells have round nuclei and fine to coarse azurophilic granules.

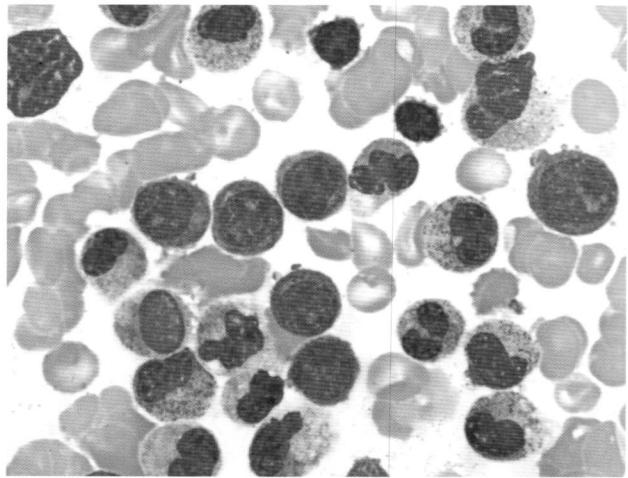

Plate 88 Aggressive NK cell leukemia: buffy coat smear stained with Giemsa. This case comprises neoplastic cells that are even more atypical. The chromatin is open, and there are multiple distinct nucleoli. Fine azurophilic granules are evident in the lightly basophilic cytoplasm.

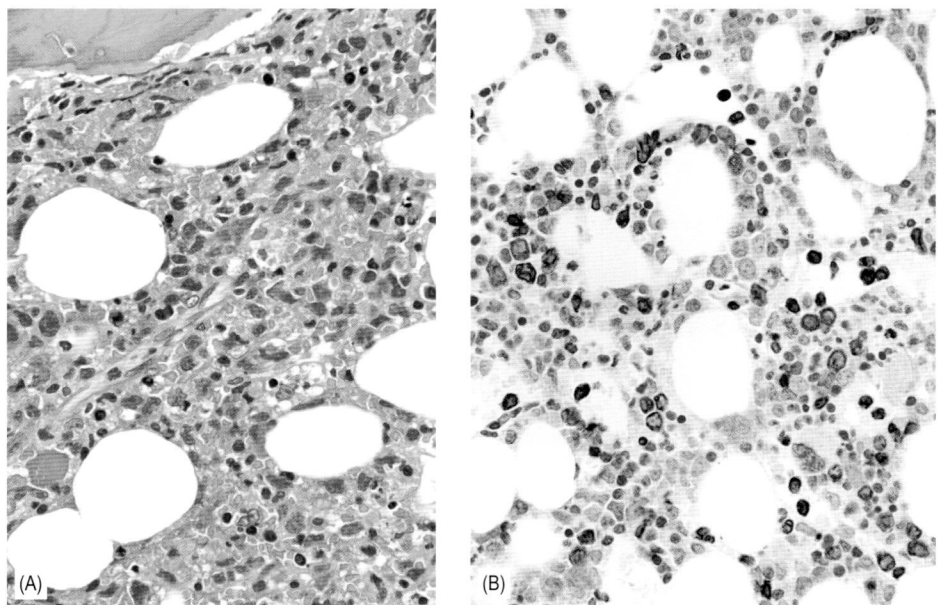

Plate 90 Aggressive NK cell leukemia: bone marrow biopsy. (A) The neoplastic cells are scattered among the hematopoietic cells. (B) They are highlighted by immunostaining for cCD3ε.

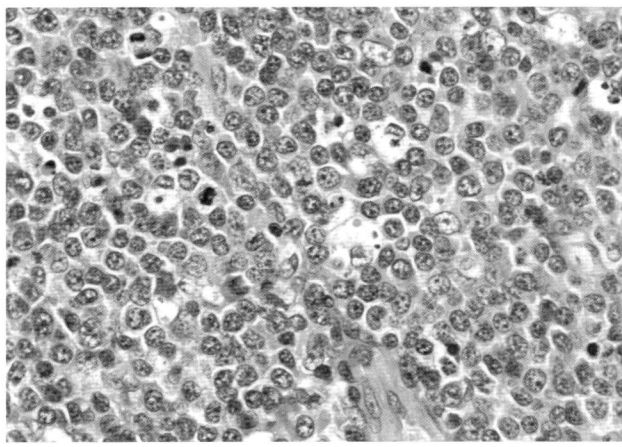

Plate 91 Aggressive NK cell leukemia with lymph node involvement. There is a monotonous infiltrate of medium-sized cells with round nuclei. There are admixed apoptotic bodies.

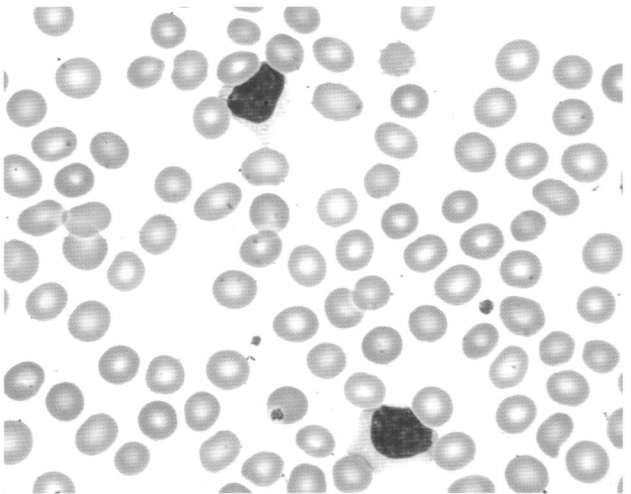

Plate 92 Chronic lymphoproliferative disorder of NK cells: peripheral blood smear stained with Giemsa. There is an increase in circulating normal-looking large granular lymphocytes.

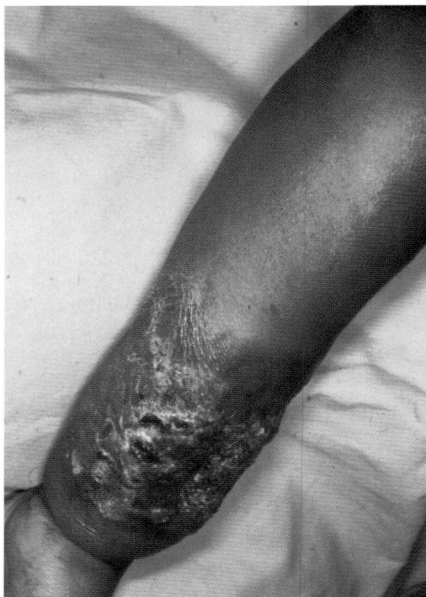

Plate 93   Blastic plasmacytoid dendritic cell neoplasm involving the skin of the forearm. The lesion is raised, and has a crusted surface.

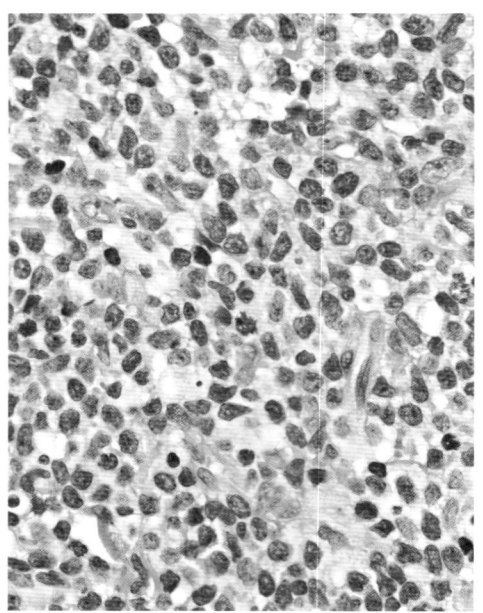

Plate 95   Blastic plasmacytoid dendritic cell neoplasm involving the skin. The neoplastic cells are medium-sized cells and show irregular nuclear foldings and fine chromatin. Usually the nuclei do not appear as crowded as in lymphoblastic lymphoma. Mitotic figures are evident.

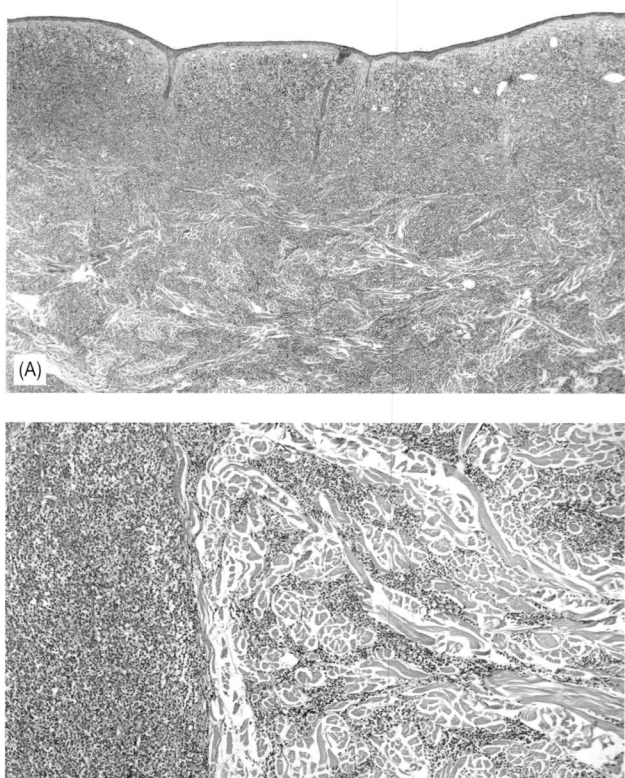

Plate 94   Blastic plasmacytoid dendritic cell neoplasm involving the skin. (A) There is characteristically a diffuse and dense dermal infiltrate without coagulative necrosis. (B) There is permeative infiltration of the collagen fibers at the edge of the lesion.

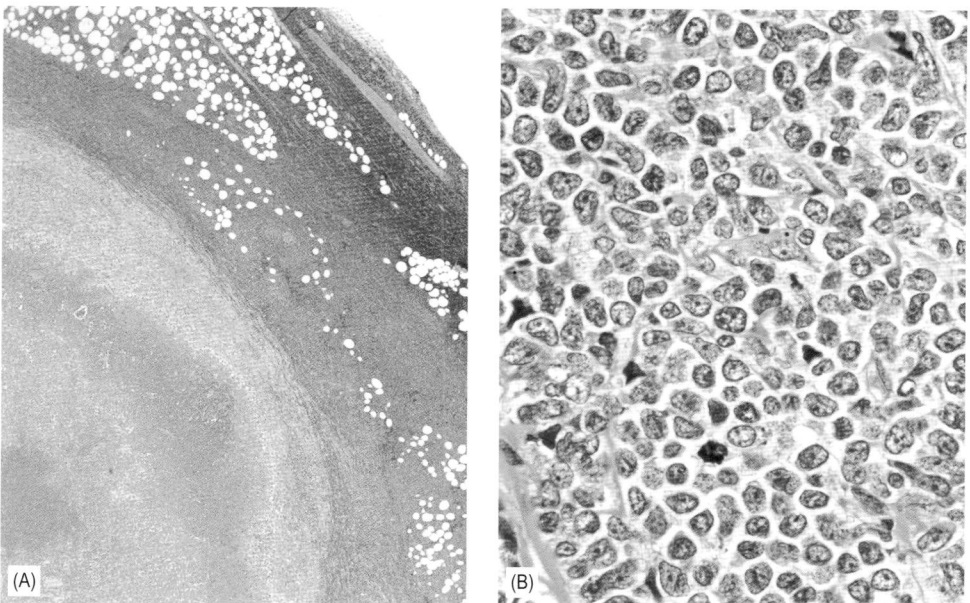

Plate 96 Blastic plasmacytoid dendritic cell neoplasm involving lymph node. (A) The lymph node architecture is totally effaced by neoplastic cells, and there is perinodal involvement. The necrosis seen in the left field represents post-fine needle aspiration infarction rather than coagulative necrosis as commonly seen in extranodal NK/T cell lymphoma. (B) The neoplastic cells are medium-sized, with thin nuclear membranes, irregular nuclear foldings and fine chromatin.

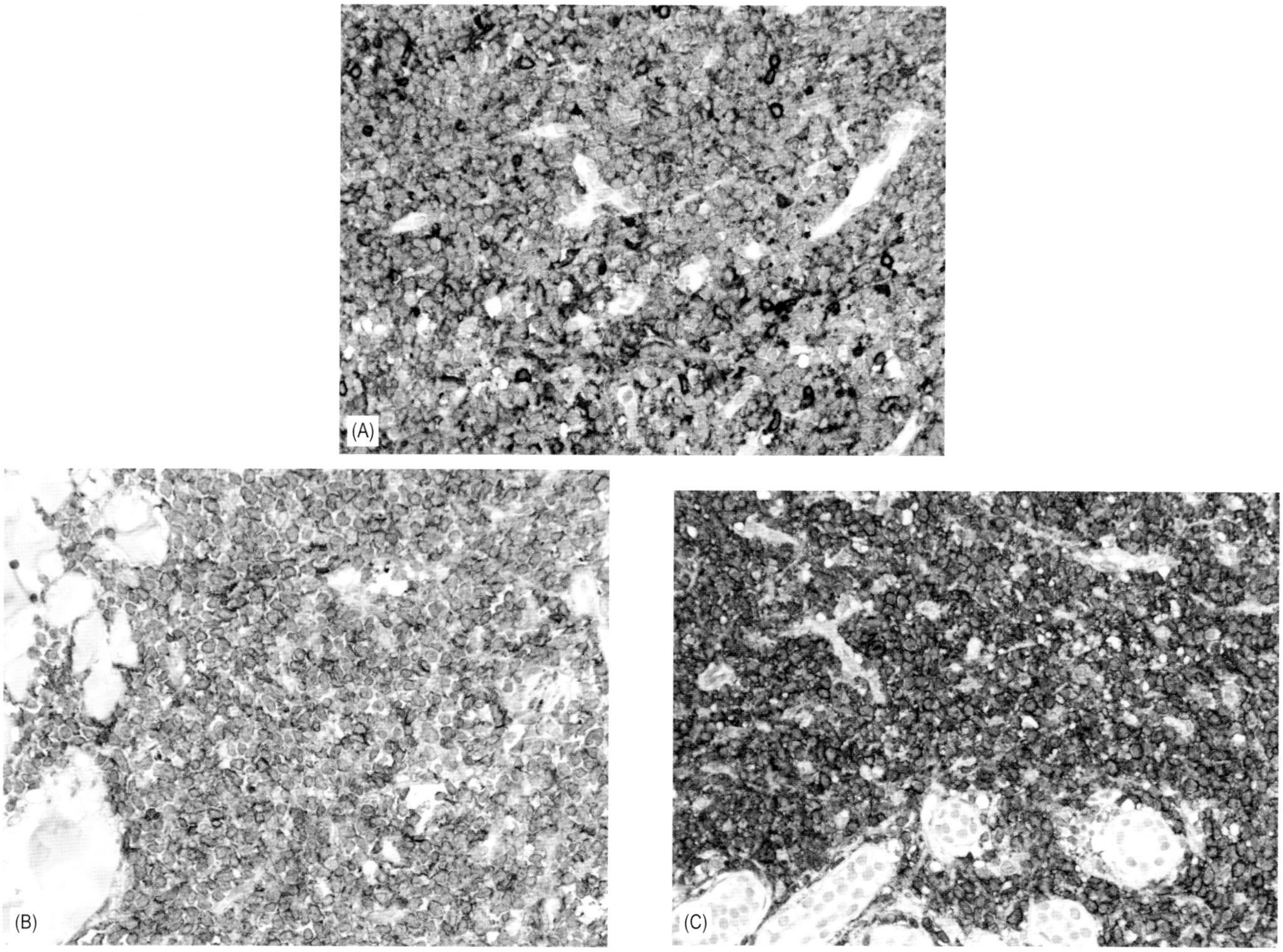

Plate 97 Blastic plasmacytoid dendritic cell neoplasm involving the skin: immunohistochemical staining. (A) Positive staining for CD4. (B) Positive staining for CD56. (C) Positive staining for CD123.

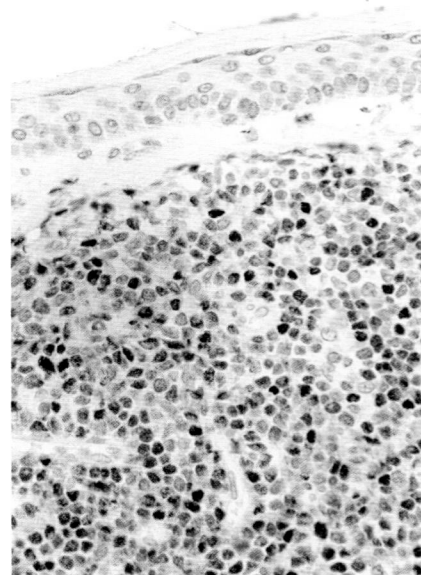

Plate 98 Blastic plasmacytoid dendritic cell neoplasm involving the skin: immunohistochemical staining. There is positive staining for TdT.

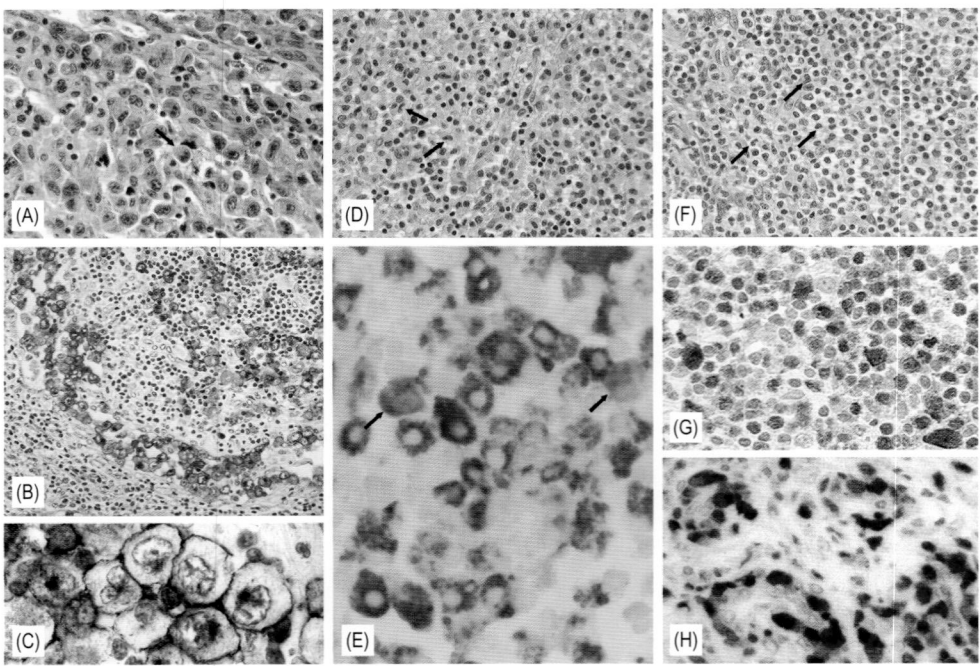

Plate 99 Morphologic features and immunostainings of anaplastic large cell lymphomas (ALCLs) A–C. ALCL common type: (A) Predominant population of large cells with irregular nuclei. Note large 'hallmark cells' showing eccentric kidney-shaped nuclei (arrow) (hematoxylin and eosin). (B) Tumor cells in the subcapsular sinus of a lymph node strongly positive for CD30. (C) Higher power view showing the characteristic CD30 membrane staining associated with a paranuclear dot. ALCL lymphohistiocytic variant: (D, E) Rare malignant cells (arrows) are admixed with a predominant population of non-neoplastic histiocytes (hematoxylin and eosin). (E) Double immunostaining with CD68/KP1 (brown staining of histiocytes) and ALK1 (blue) confirms the paucity of malignant cells (arrows) (blue nuclear staining). ALCL small cell variant: (F) Predominant population of small cells with dark irregular nuclei and clear cytoplasm associated with scattered 'hallmark cells' with kidney-shaped nucleus (arrows). (G) In the small variant of ALCL associated with the t(2;5) (p23;q35) translocation (NPM-ALK), the ALK staining is frequently restricted to nuclei. Note the cytoplasmic and nuclear staining of scattered large-sized cells. (H) Characteristically neoplastic cells often cluster around blood vessels. This perivascular pattern is highlighted by immunostaining using antibodies to CD30 or ALK1 as illustrated here. Such a perivascular pattern is also observed in ALCL lymphohistiocytic variant.

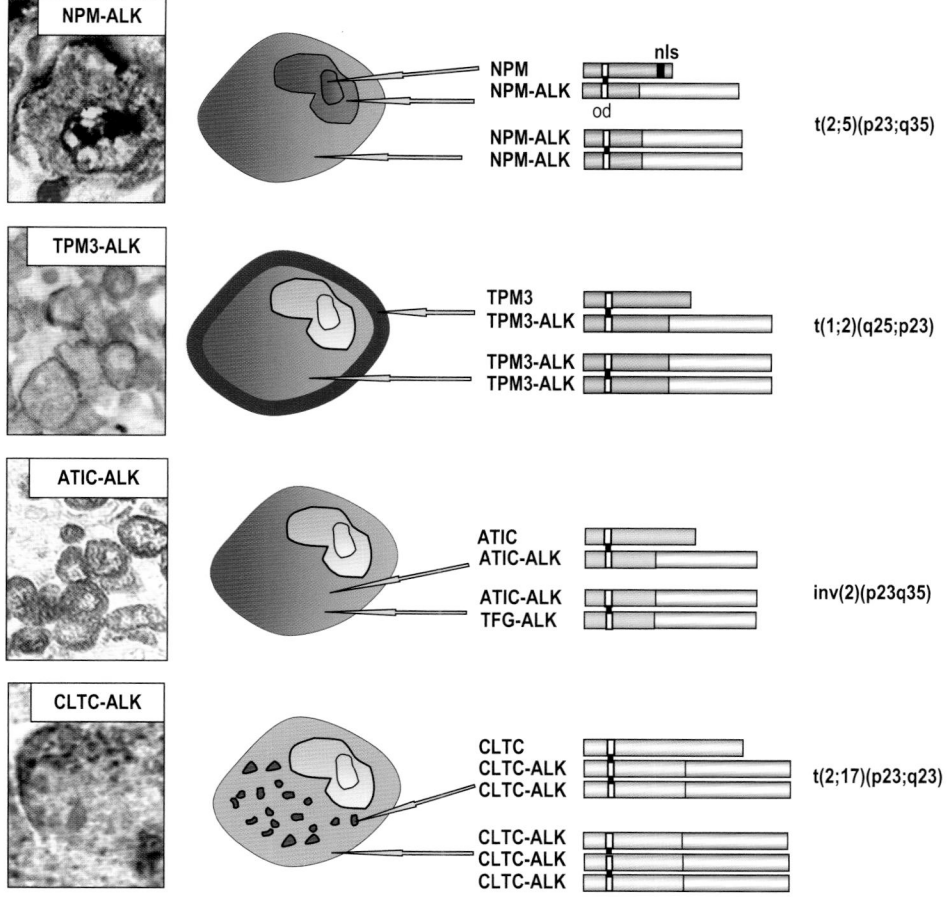

Plate 100 Schematic representation of the most frequent translocations involving *ALK* gene at 2p23 and the resultant fusion proteins. The t(2;5)(p23;q35) translocation fuses part of the nucleophosmin (*NPM*) gene to a portion of the *ALK* kinase gene on chromosome 2p23, resulting in expression of the chimeric NPM-ALK protein (80 KD). Malignant cells carrying the t(2;5)(p23;q35) translocation show both cytoplasmic, nuclear and nucleolar staining with antibodies (e.g. ALK1, ALKc) recognizing the ALK tyrosine kinase domain. Such an ALK staining pattern appears to be due to oligomer formation with wild-type NPM and subsequent transport from the cytoplasm to the nucleus directed by nuclear localization signals (nls) in the wild-type NPM molecule.[46,47] On the other hand, the formation of NPM-ALK homodimers using oligomerization domains (od) at the N-terminus of NPM mimics ligand binding and is responsible for the activation of the ALK catalytic domain, i.e. autophosphorylation of the tyrosine kinase domain of ALK that is responsible for the oncogenic properties of the ALK protein. In approximately 30 percent of ALK-positive anaplastic large cell lymphomas (ALCLs), the staining is restricted to the cytoplasm. In 15–20 percent of these cases, malignant cells carry a variant t(1;2)(q25;p23) translocation and express the TPM3-ALK protein. ALK staining is restricted to the cytoplasm of malignant cells but, in virtually all cases, a stronger staining on the cell membrane is observed. Two percent to 5 percent of ALCLs are associated with the inv(2)(p23q35) which involves *ATIC* gene (formerly known as *pur-H*) encoding the 5-aminomidazole-4-carboxamide-ribonucleotide transformylase-IMP cyclohydrolase (ATIC), known to play a key role in the *de novo* purine biosynthesis pathway.[49] Rare cases of ALCLs show a unique granular ALK cytoplasmic staining pattern.[50] In these cases, associated with the t(2;17)(p23;q23), the *ALK* gene is fused to *CLTC* gene encoding the clathrin heavy polypeptide which is the main structural protein of coated vesicles. In the CLTC-ALK positive ALCLs, the implication of the clathrin heavy polypeptide in the hybrid protein accounts for the granular cytoplasmic staining pattern since the CLTC-ALK hybrid protein is involved in the formation of the clathrin coat on the surface of vesicles. Moreover, the process of clathrin coat formation mimics ligand binding and this would allow the autophosphorylation of the carboxy-terminal domain of ALK protein.

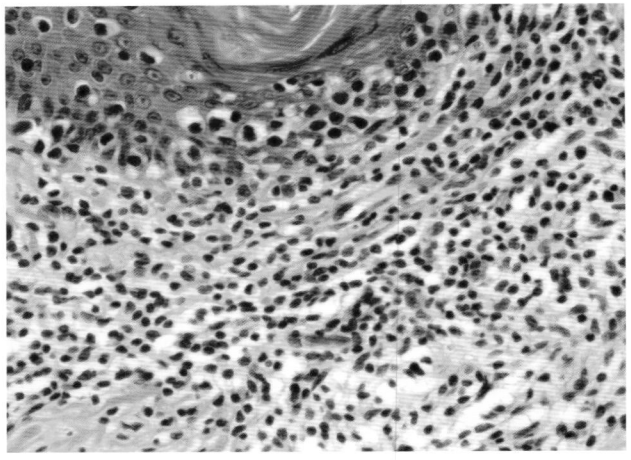

Plate 101 Lymphocytes within the epidermis that are larger than those within the dermis are indicative of mycosis fungoides.

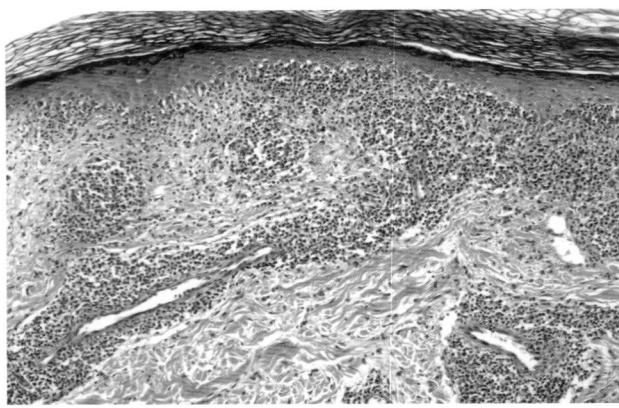

Plate 104 Plaque stage mycosis fungoides typically shows features of patch stage disease but also involves the reticular dermis.

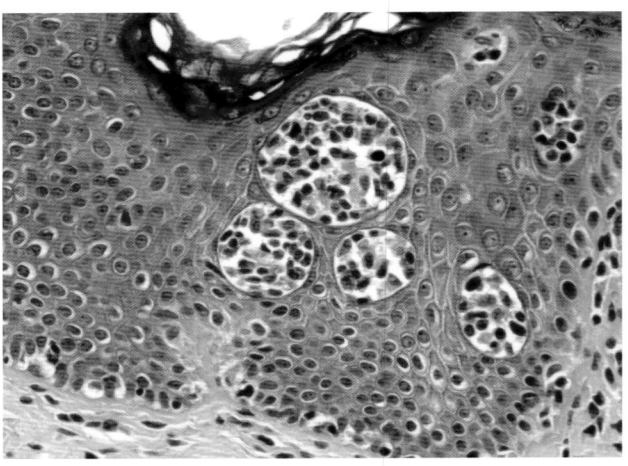

Plate 102 Pautrier microabscesses, comprised of neoplastic lymphocytes, are a relatively specific feature of mycosis fungoides.

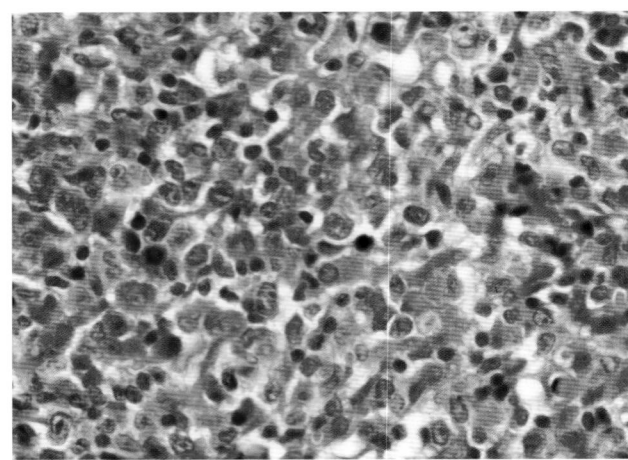

Plate 105 Adult T cell leukemia/lymphoma (HTLV1-positive): at a high magnification, histopathology shows that neoplastic cells are medium to large lymphoid cells with irregular nuclei.

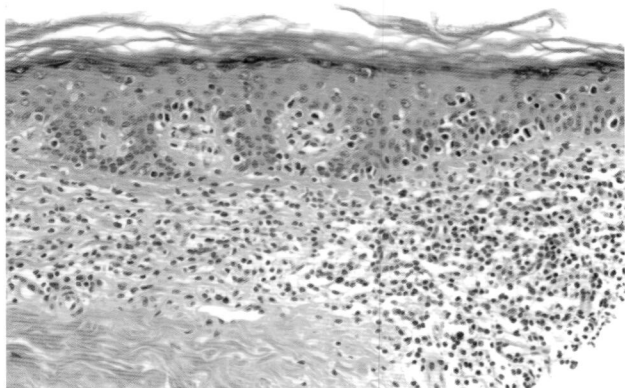

Plate 103 Intraepidermal lymphocytes whose nuclei approximate the width of basal keratinocyte nuclei are indicative of mycosis fungoides.

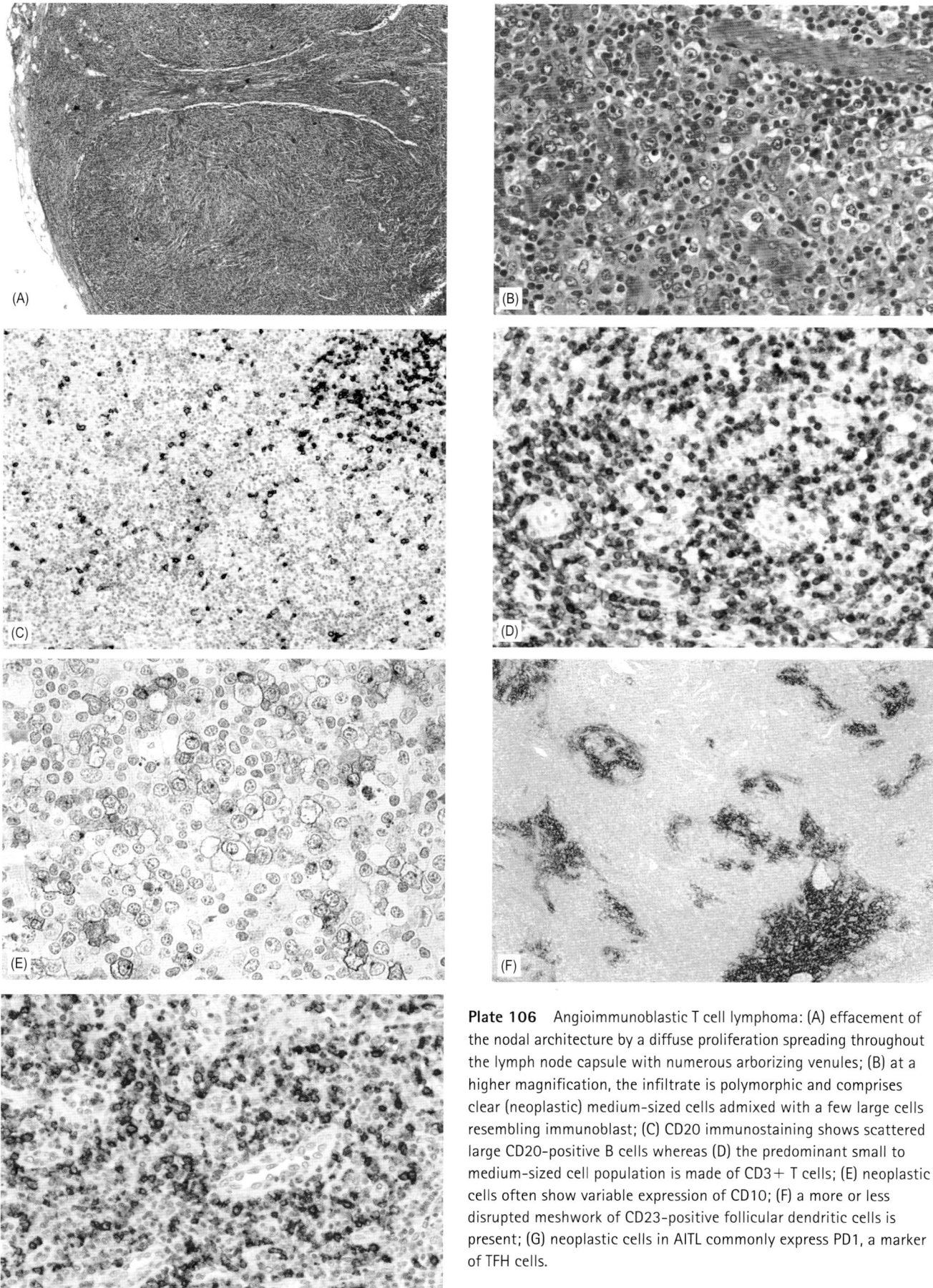

Plate 106 Angioimmunoblastic T cell lymphoma: (A) effacement of the nodal architecture by a diffuse proliferation spreading throughout the lymph node capsule with numerous arborizing venules; (B) at a higher magnification, the infiltrate is polymorphic and comprises clear (neoplastic) medium-sized cells admixed with a few large cells resembling immunoblast; (C) CD20 immunostaining shows scattered large CD20-positive B cells whereas (D) the predominant small to medium-sized cell population is made of CD3+ T cells; (E) neoplastic cells often show variable expression of CD10; (F) a more or less disrupted meshwork of CD23-positive follicular dendritic cells is present; (G) neoplastic cells in AITL commonly express PD1, a marker of TFH cells.

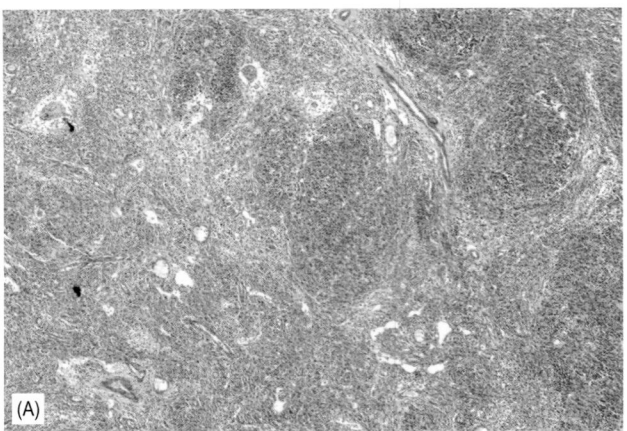
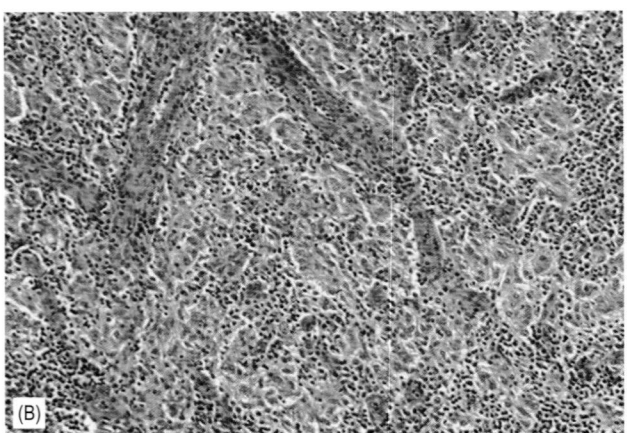

Plate 107 Morphological spectrum of angioimmunoblastic T cell lymphoma: (A) a case showing hyperplastic germinal centers without a clear mantle zone; and (B) an example of AITL with numerous clusters of epithelioid cells.

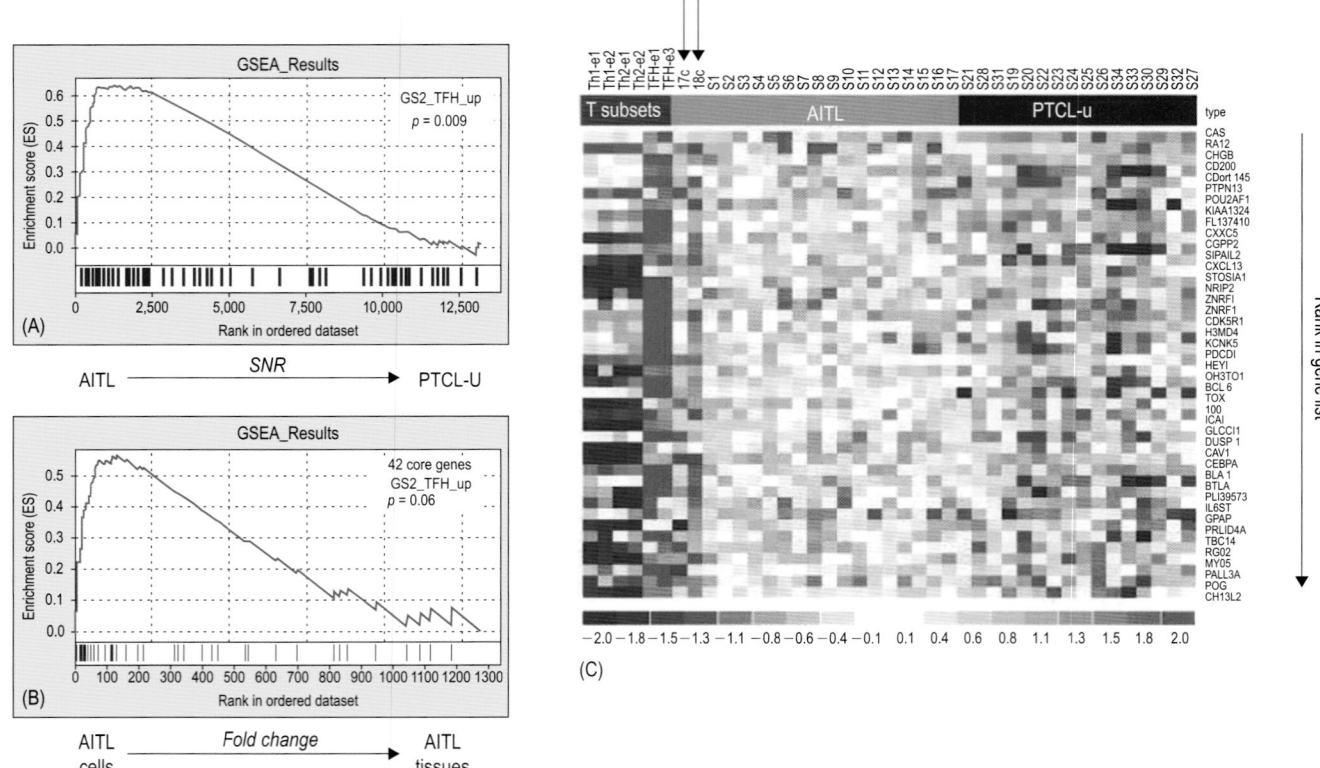

Plate 108 Gene expression profiling of angioimmunoblastic T cell lymphoma (AITL). In this molecular profiling study of 18 AITL and 16 peripheral T cell lymphoma, unspecified (PTCL-U) samples, gene set enrichment analyses (GSEA) were performed by using sets of genes representative of distinct normal T cell subsets, in order to compare the molecular signature of the tumor samples. (A) and (B) show the enrichment score (ES) curves generated by such analyses. (A) shows genes discriminant between AITL and PTCL/NOS were ranked (according to the signal to noise ratio) from left to right, and GSEA was performed by using a set of 100 genes overexpressed in normal follicular B helper T cells (T$_{FH}$); the ES curve is significant, meaning that the AITL samples display significant enrichment in the T$_{FH}$ signature, as compared to PTCL/NOS. In (B), two AITL samples consisting of purified tumor cell suspensions are compared with 16 AITL tissue samples, and GSEA showed a significant enrichment of the tumor cell suspensions in the set of the 42 core genes (accounting for the enrichment in (A). Finally the finding that the imprint of the TFH signature was stronger in purified AITL tumor cells samples compared to AITL tissues validates that the molecular link with T$_{FH}$ cells was related to the neoplastic cells. (C) shows the associated heatmap of these 42 core genes. Expression data from normal T cell subsets, 2 AITL tumor cell suspension samples (arrows), 16 AITL tissue samples and 16 PTCL/NOS samples are represented. Standardized expression ranges from −2.0 (blue) to 2.0 (red). (Adapted with persmission from de Leval L, *et al.* The gene expression profile of nodal peripheral T-cell lymphoma demonstrates a molecular link between angioimmunoblastic T-cell lymphoma (AITL) and follicular helper T (TFH) cells. *Blood* 2007; **109**: 4952–63.)

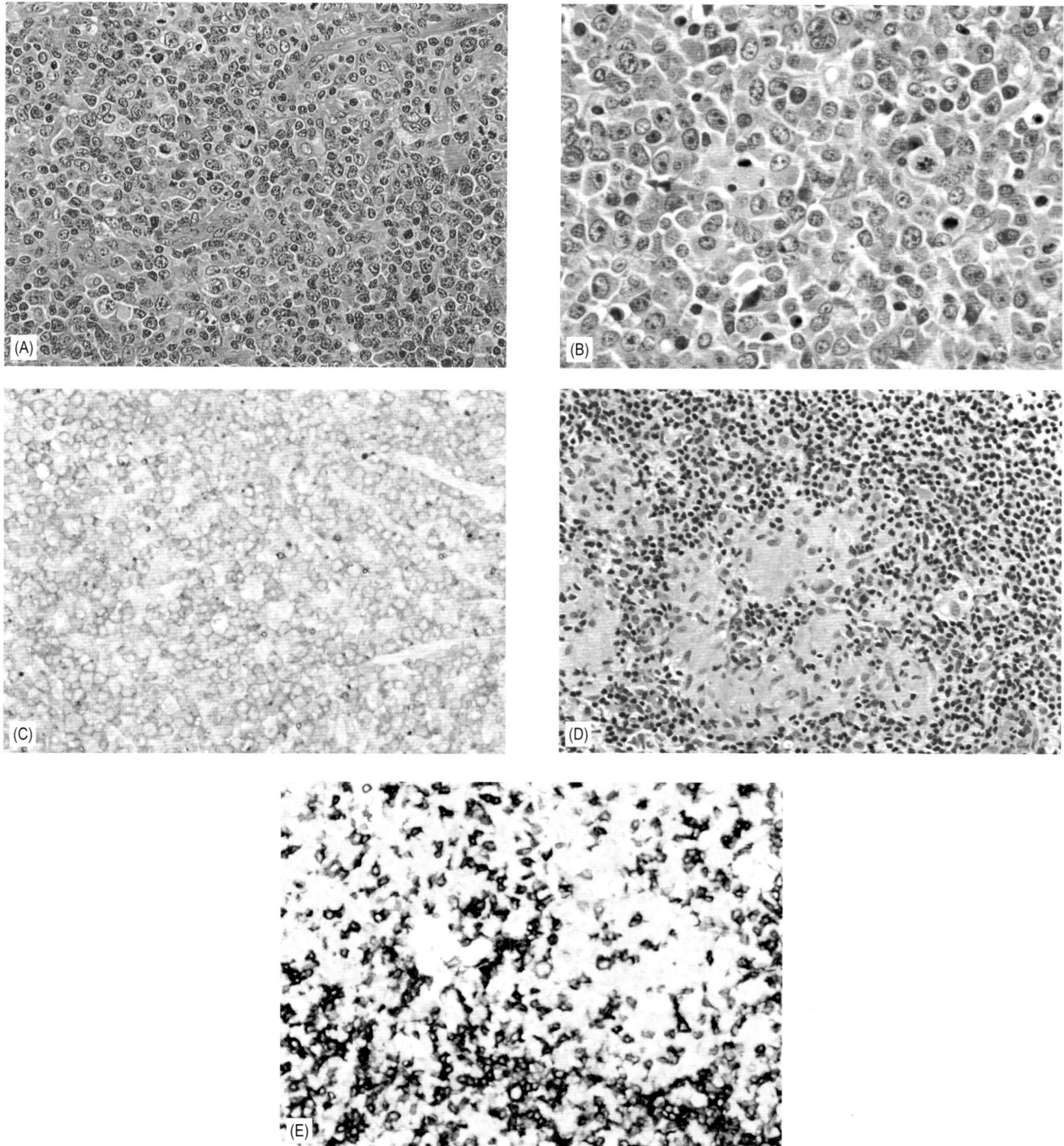

Plate 109 Peripheral T cell lymphoma, not otherwise specified (PTCL, NOS): (A) a case composed of a pleomorphic population of medium and almost large tumor cells, (B) a case composed of uniformly large tumor cells with regular often round nuclei; in this latter case, note that most tumor cells express CD30 (C), but are negative for epithelial membrane antigen, anaplastic lymphoma kinase and cytotoxic molecules; (D) example of a so-called Lennert lymphoma composed of small to medium-sized lymphoid cells admixed with clusters of epithelioid cells; and (E) neoplastic cells in this latter case have a cytotoxic CD8 phenotype.

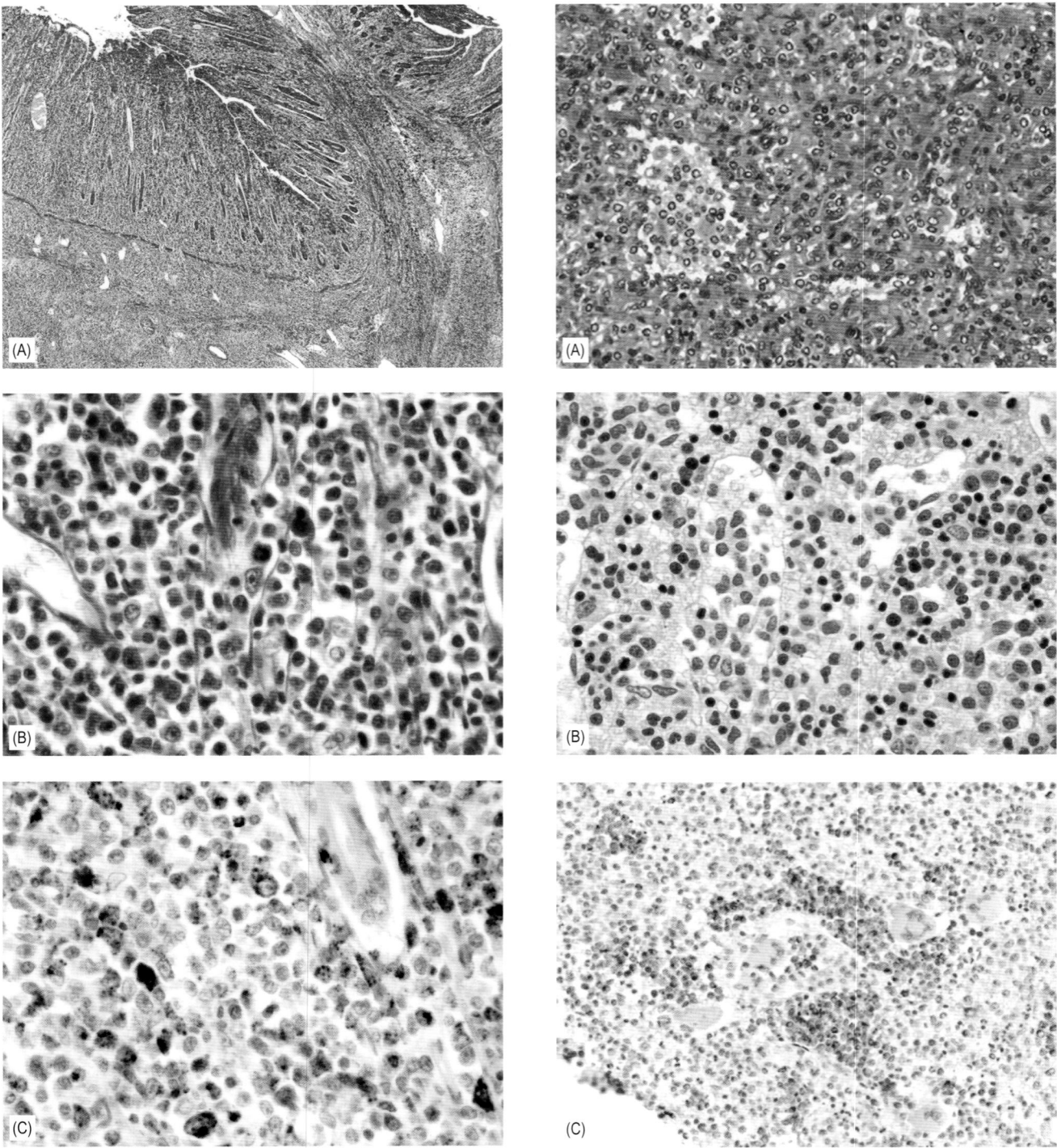

Plate 110 Enteropathy-associated T cell lymphoma: (A) the wall of the intestine including mucosa is densely infiltrated by a lymphoid proliferation (B) made of atypical predominantly large cells which, on immunostaining, are T cells with an activated cytotoxic profile as shown by (C) strong granular cytoplasmic granzyme B expression.

Plate 111 Hepatosplenic T cell lymphoma: (A) in the spleen, the neoplastic monomorphic medium-sized cells infiltrate the red cords and the sinuses of the red pulp; (B) in the bone marrow, the infiltrate is also confined to the sinuses; (C) in this case, note that the marrow sinusal distribution is emphasized by TIA1 immunostaining.

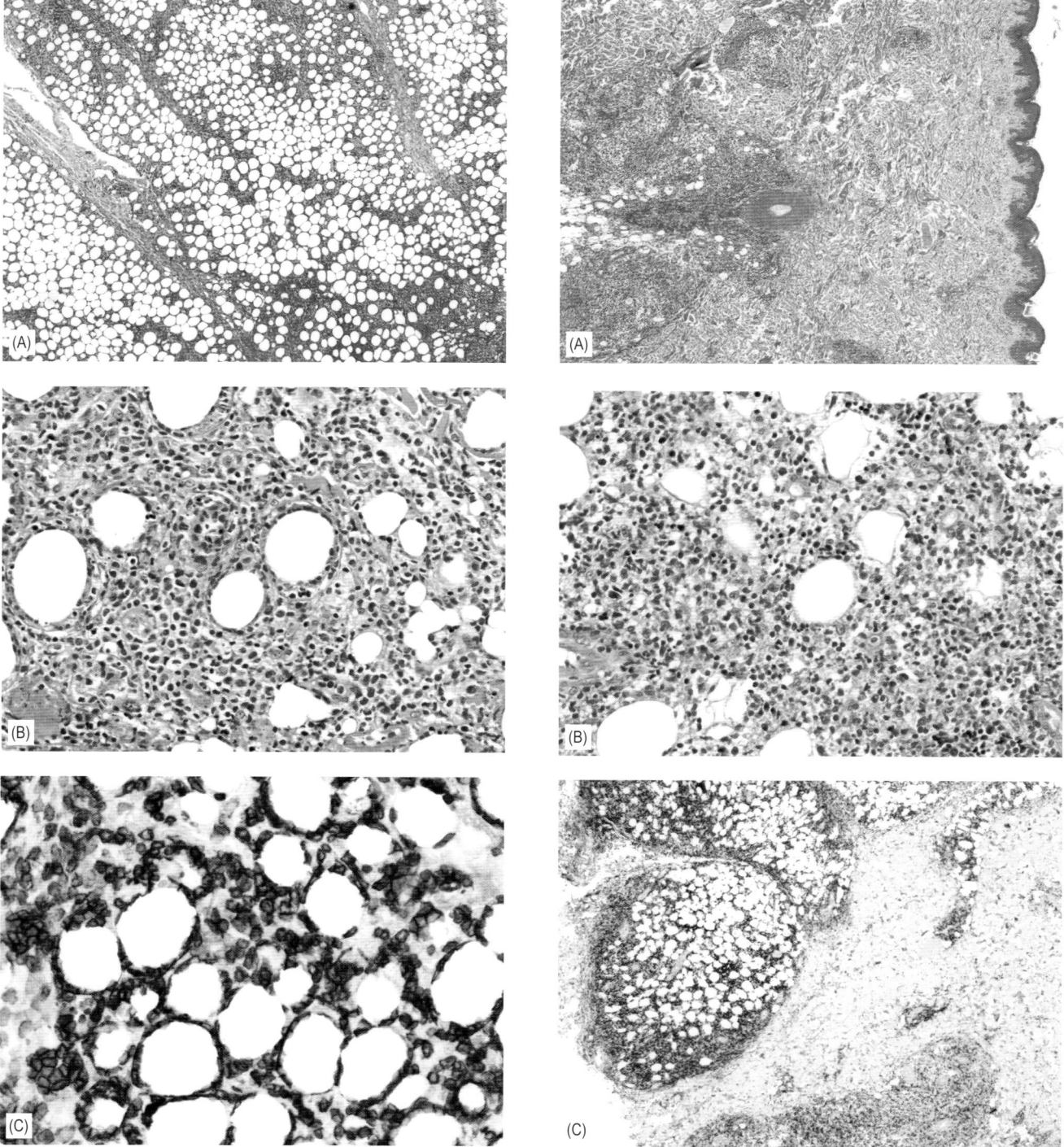

Plate 112 Subcutaneous panniculitis-like T cell lymphoma: (A) at a low magnification, the neoplastic cellular infiltrate extends diffusely throughout the subcutaneous fat tissue simulating a panniculitis; (B) at a higher magnification, the population is composed of a predominance of slightly atypical small to medium lymphoid cells which often adopt a rimming configuration around adipocytes; (C) these cells have a cytotoxic CD8+ phenotype.

Plate 113 Cutaneous $\gamma\delta$ T cell lymphoma: (A) at a low magnification, the cellular infiltrate extends towards the dermis; (B) neoplastic medium-sized cells also infiltrate the subcutaneous tissue, but have a CD4$-$/CD8$-$ and CD56+ (C) phenotype.

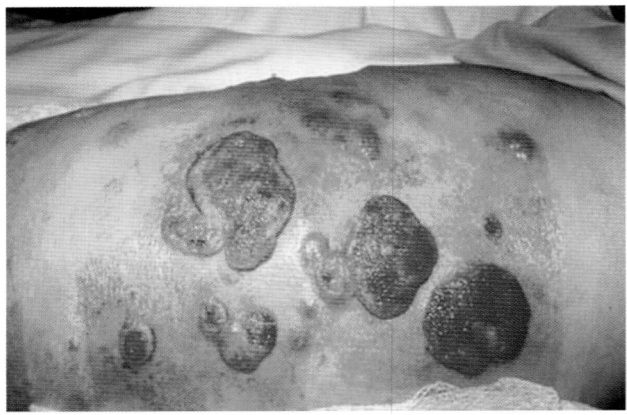

Plate 114 Cutaneous infiltration in a patient with Sézary syndrome. (Reproduced with permission of *Fondo de imágenes de la Asociación Española de Hematología y Hemoterapia.*)

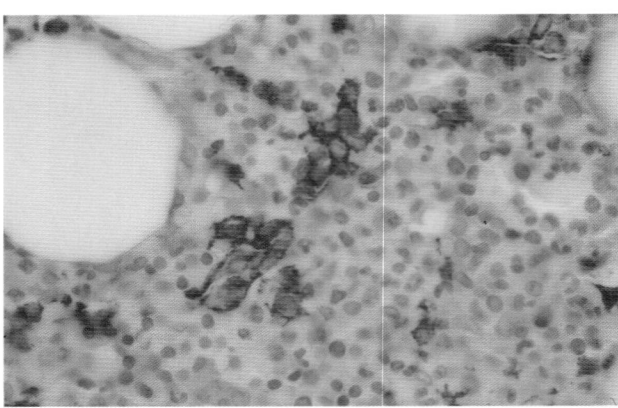

Plate 117 Bone marrow section from a patient with hairy cell leukemia with mild infiltration highlighted by the immunostaining with the antibody DBA-44 (APAAP technique).

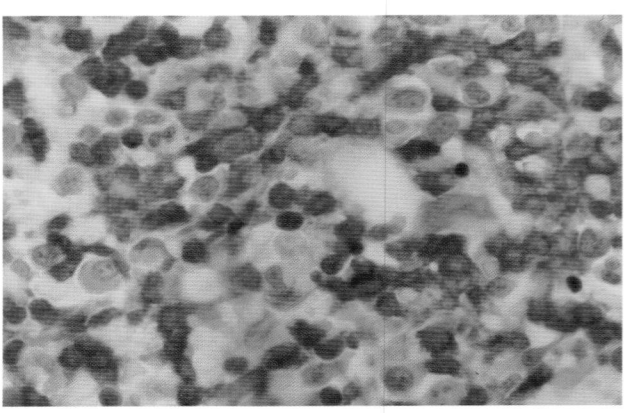

Plate 115 Immunohistochemistry of a spleen section from a patient with mantle cell lymphoma showing diffuse infiltration by lymphoid cells strongly positive with CD20 (APAAP technique).

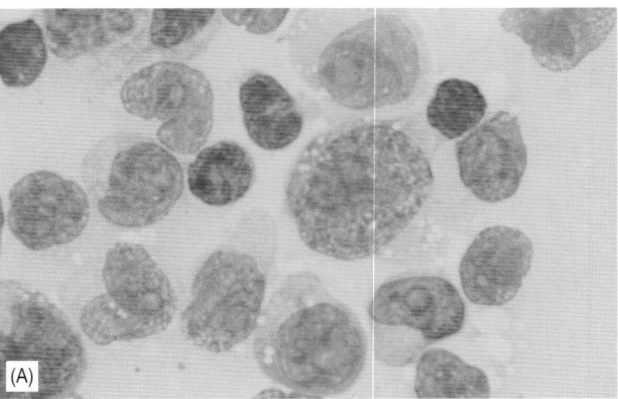

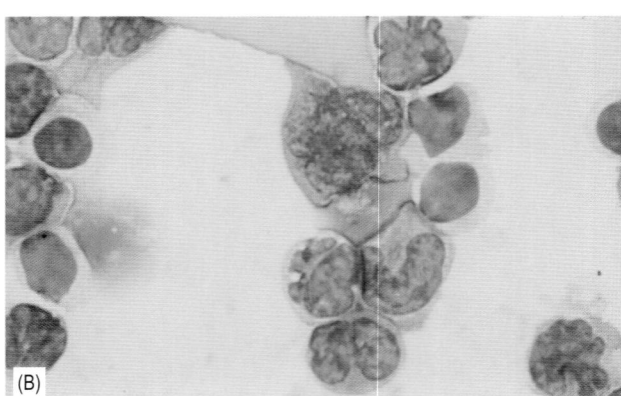

Plate 118 (A, B) Lymph node imprint from a patient with HTLV-I+ adult T cell leukemia lymphoma showing the presence of large poorly differentiated lymphoid cells (A: hematoxylin–eosin) which express CD25 (B: immunoperoxidase technique).

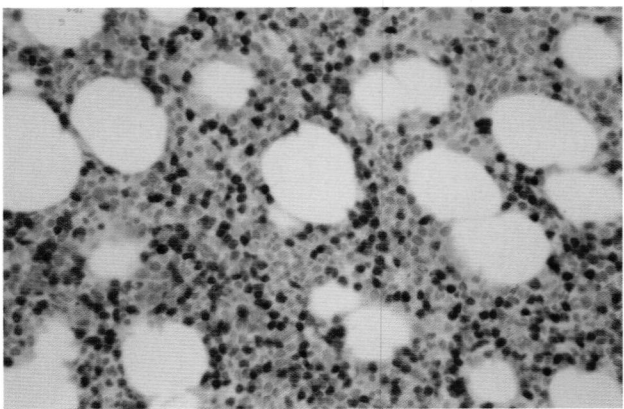

Plate 116 Immunostaining with a CD79a MAb on a bone marrow section from a patient with B cell lymphoma showing an interstitial infiltrate (APAAP technique).

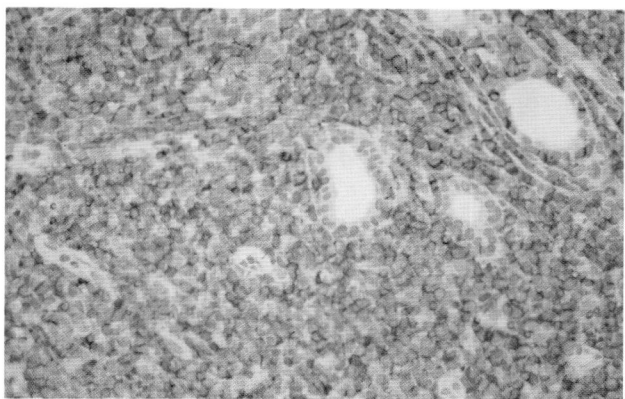

Plate 119 Expression of the NK antigen CD56 in a case of nasal NK/T cell lymphoma (immunoperoxidase technique).

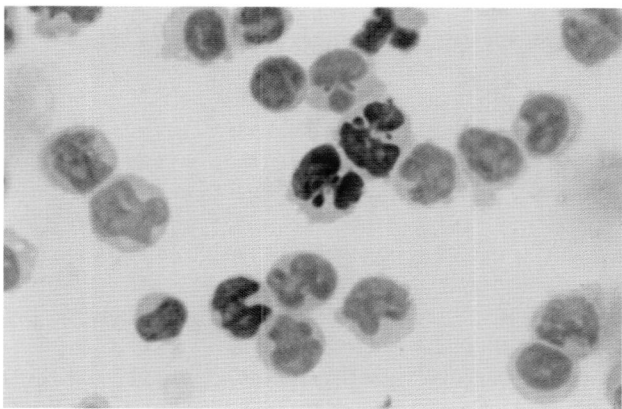

Plate 120 Cytospin of blood lymphocytes from a patient with B cell prolymphocytic leukemia illustrating a dense nuclear staining with the McAb Ki-67 (immunoperoxidase technique).

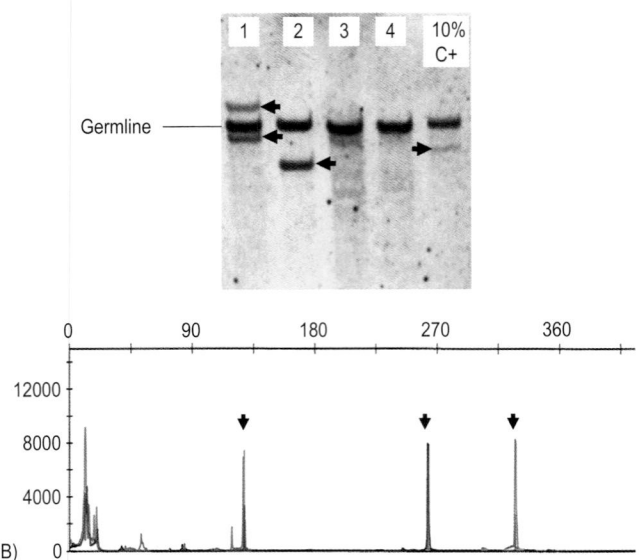

Plate 121   Immunoglobulin and T cell receptor gene rearrangements: basic structure and utility in assessment of clonal lymphoid proliferations. (B) Upper image demonstrates Southern blot hybridization (SBH) result. In the germline (non-rearranged) state, digestion of high molecular weight DNA by an appropriate restriction enzyme (e.g. EcoRI) produces a fragment of defined length revealed by stringent hybridization with a probe complementary to the target region of DNA (e.g. *IGH* J-region). Following V-(D)-J-rearrangement in lymphoid cells, the location of particular restriction sites is altered, resulting in different sized fragments after enzyme digestion. In a monoclonal B cell proliferation, all lymphocytes harbor the same (monoclonal) V-(D)-J rearrangement and this abnormality can be detected as a new band distinct from the germline size by SBH. Lanes 1–4 are patient DNA samples. Lane indicated by '10% C+' represents a 10 percent dilution of a positive control lymphoma cell line. Non-germline rearranged bands are detected in samples 1 and 2 (short horizontal arrows). Germline bands are also identified in the samples with a positive SBH rearrangement result, due to the presence of DNA from nonlymphoid cells. In the case of sample 1, the presence of two distinct rearranged bands is consistent with bi-allelic *IGH* locus rearrangements in this lymphoid neoplasm. Because a uniform quantity of DNA is used for each digestion (e.g. 5 μg), the intensities of the rearranged bands are representative of the relative amount of clonal disease in the sample. Of note, the numerous individual gene rearrangements present in polyclonal lymphocyte populations are typically not detected at the nominal sensitivity of SBH (about 5–10 percent). The lower panel shows results of a positive *IGH* PCR assay using fluorescently labeled primers and analyzed by capillary electrophoresis. As depicted in part A of this figure, the most hypervariable region of the *IGH* rearrangement is known as the complementarity determining region 3 (CDR3), comprised of the 3′ end of the V-segment, along with N-D-N-J sequence. Each CDR3 in a polytypic B cell population is essentially unique, resulting in a spectrum or range of possible sequences and nucleotide lengths. In contrast, each cell of a monoclonal proliferation contains the same CDR3 sequence and rearrangement size, as shown in this panel. In this case, positive monoclonal peaks (short vertical arrows) were obtained with consensus primers situated in FR1, FR2 and FR3 regions and a reverse J_H primer. Detection of B cell clonality can be further enhanced by targeting the *IGK* locus (not shown). The use of multiple primers is advisable to ensure high detection sensitivity in polymerase chain reaction (PCR)-based methods. Similar strategies are used to target the *TRG* locus for determination of T cell lymphoid clonality. (C) PCR interpretation examples of *TRG* clonality analysis. Upper panel demonstrates multiple primer set amplifications targeting the *TRG* locus in a case of a polyclonal T cell expansion, with numerous normally distributed peak populations observed. The middle panel shows a monoclonal result with two prominent peaks, likely indicating a bi-allelic rearrangement. The lower panel illustrates the pitfalls in *TRG* PCR interpretation: a relatively prominent peak is identified in one reaction, but it is of modest intensity with accompanying polyclonal rearrangements. While this result could represent the detection of a true monoclonal T cell subset in a polyclonal T cell background, similar 'pseudoclonal' results can also occur because of restricted T cell repertoires in benign conditions (e.g. autoimmune disease) or with normal aging, thus emphasizing the risk of potential false-positive interpretations with *TRG* PCR in particular.

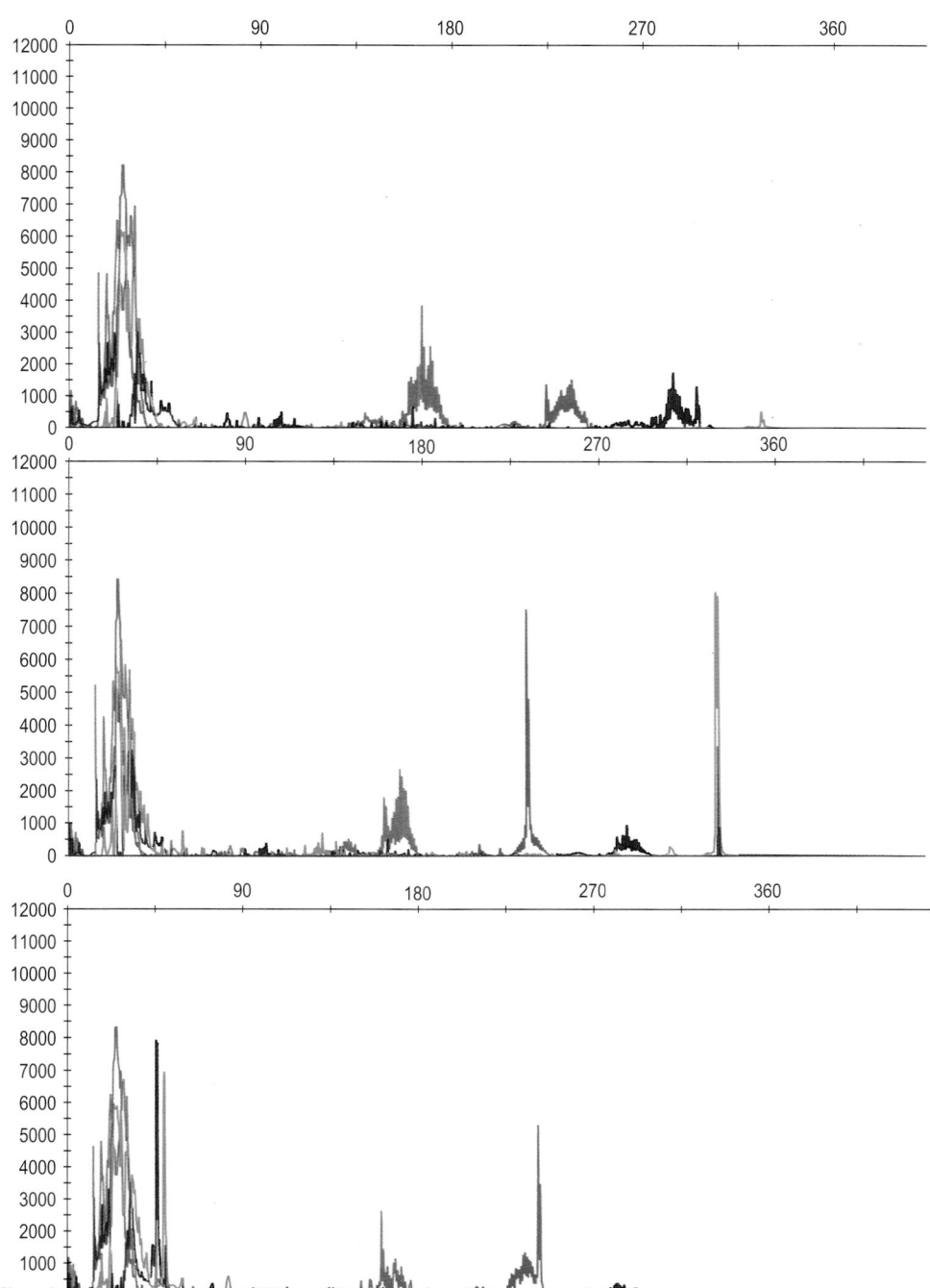

Plate 121 Continued

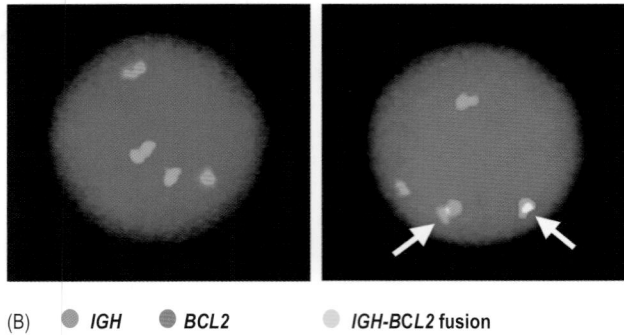

(B) ● IGH ● BCL2 ○ IGH-BCL2 fusion

Plate 122   Detection of *BCL2* gene translocations in lymphoma. (B) Interphase FISH analysis for the t(14;18)/*BCL2-IGH* abnormality using a dual fusion/dual color strategy. Left side image demonstrates red labeled fluorescent probes targeting both *BCL2* alleles at 18q21 and green probes hybridized to the *IGH* loci at 14q32. Right side image in the case of a follicular lymphoma with the t(14;18) indicates two abnormal fusion signals (co-localized red-green and more typically yellow) representing both the *BCL2-IGH*, and the reciprocal consequence of the translocation (arrows). Nuclei are counterstained with 4′,6-diamidino-2-phenylindole (DAPI).

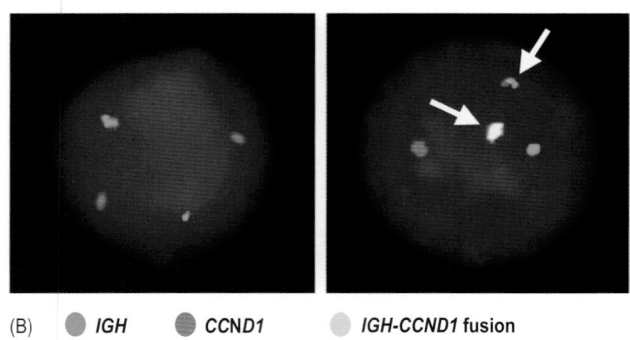

(B) ● IGH ● CCND1 ○ IGH-CCND1 fusion

Plate 123   Detection of *CCND1* gene translocations in lymphoma. (B) Interphase FISH analysis for the t(11;14)/*BCL1-IGH* abnormality using a dual fusion/dual color strategy. Left side image demonstrates red labeled fluorescent probes targeting both *BCL1* alleles at 11q13 and green probes hybridized to the *IGH* loci at 14q32. Right side image in the case of MCL with the t(11;14) indicates two abnormal fusion signals representing both the *BCL1-IGH*, and the reciprocal consequence of the translocation (arrows). Nuclei are counterstained with 4′,6-diamidino-2-phenylindole (DAPI).

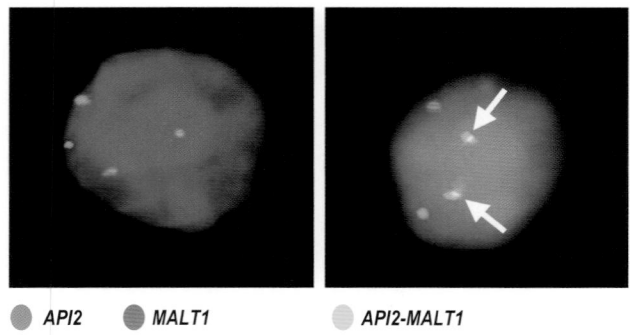

● API2 ● MALT1 ○ API2-MALT1

Plate 124   Detection of the *API2–MALT1* gene translocation in lymphoma. Interphase FISH analysis for the t(11;18)(q21;q21)/*API2-MALT1* abnormality using a dual fusion/dual color strategy. Left side image demonstrates red labeled fluorescent probes targeting both *MALT1* alleles at 18q21 and green probes hybridized to the *API2* loci at 11q21. Right side image in the case of a gastric extranodal marginal zone B cell lymphoma with the t(11;18) indicates two abnormal fusion signals (co-localized red-green and more typically yellow) representing both the *API2–MALT1*, and the reciprocal consequence of the translocation (arrows). Nuclei are counterstained with 4′,6-diamidino-2-phenylindole (DAPI).

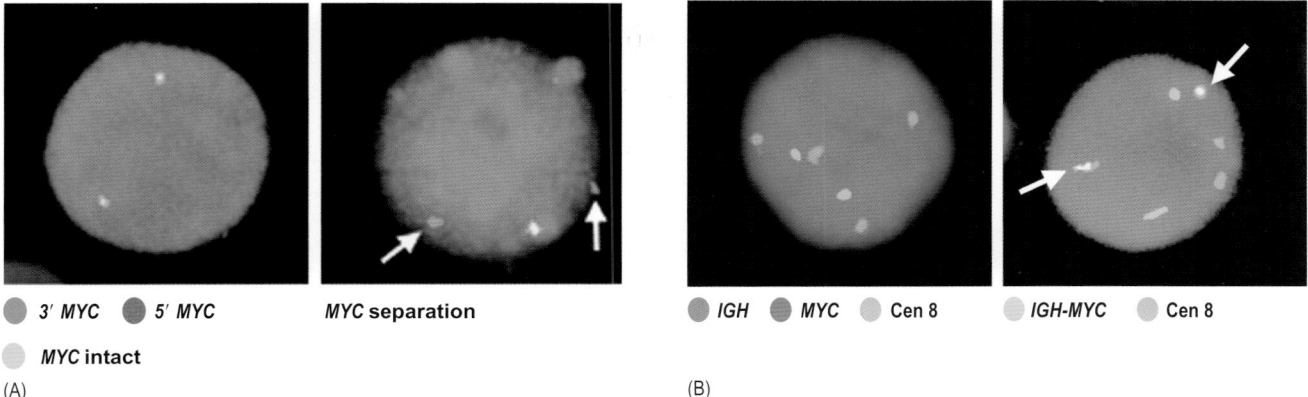

3′ MYC **5′ MYC** **MYC separation**

MYC intact

(A)

IGH **MYC** **Cen 8** **IGH-MYC** **Cen 8**

(B)

Plate 125 Detection of *MYC* gene translocations in lymphoma. (A) Interphase FISH analysis detecting alteration of the *MYC* gene using a break-apart (BAP) strategy. Left image demonstrates two fusion signals (yellow) in a normal cell, indicating intact *MYC* genes at 8q24. Right image reveals splitting of one fusion signal into separate red (5′ *MYC*) and green (3′ *MYC*) signals in a case of Burkitt lymphoma. The presence of a split signal only indicates disruption of one *MYC* locus, but does not confirm the specific translocation event. Nuclei are counterstained with 4′,6-diamidino-2-phenylindole (DAPI). (B) Interphase fluorescence *in situ* hybridization (FISH) analysis for the t(8;14)/*MYC-IGH* abnormality using a dual fusion/dual color strategy. Left side image demonstrates red labeled fluorescent probes targeting both *MYC* alleles at 8q24 and green probes hybridized to the *IGH* loci at 14q32. The aqua color signal is a centromere-specific probe for chromosome 8 (Cen 8). Right side image in a case of Burkitt lymphoma with the t(8;14) indicates two abnormal fusion signals representing both the *MYC-IGH*, and the reciprocal consequence of the translocation (arrows). The Cen 8 probe is useful in conjunction with the *MYC* probe to demonstrate *MYC* gene amplification in some lymphoid tumors lacking the t(8;14). Most cases of Burkitt lymphoma are characterized by *MYC-IGH* fusions, although a smaller number may involve *MYC* translocations to either of the immunoglobulin light chain gene loci. Nuclei are counterstained with 4′,6-diamidino-2-phenylindole (DAPI).

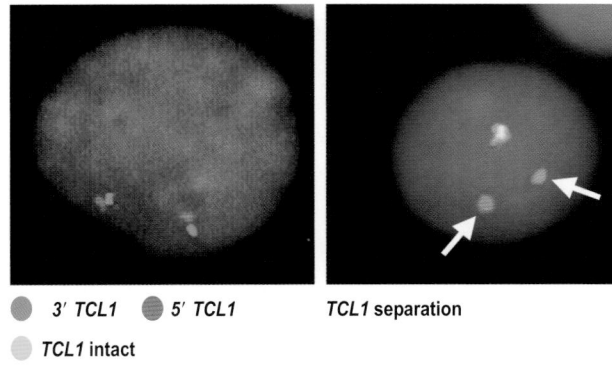

3′ TCL1 **5′ TCL1** **TCL1 separation**

TCL1 intact

Plate 126 Detection of *TCL1* gene rearrangements in T cell prolymphocytic leukemia. Interphase FISH analysis detecting alteration of the *TCL1* gene using a break-apart (BAP) strategy. Left image demonstrates two fusion signals (red–green juxtaposition) in a normal cell, indicating intact *TCL1* genes at 14q32. Right image reveals splitting of one fusion signal into separate red (5′ *TCL1*) and green (3′ *TCL1*) signals in a case of T-PLL. *TCL1* gene rearrangement with resultant gene overexpression is highly characteristic of T-PLL and helps to exclude other types of peripheralizing mature T cell leukemia/lymphoma. Nuclei are counterstained with 4′,6-diamidino-2-phenylindole (DAPI).

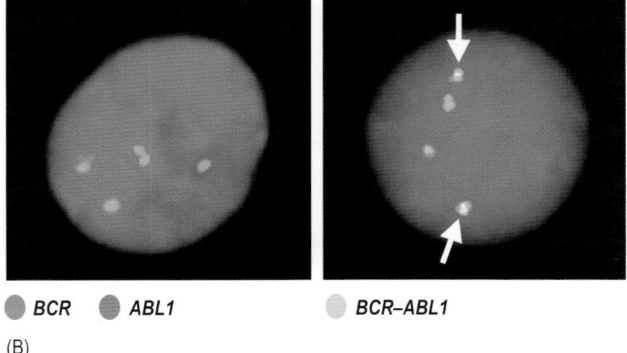

BCR **ABL1** **BCR–ABL1**

(B)

Plate 127 Detection of the t(9;22)/*BCR–ABL1* abnormality in Ph+ precursor B cell acute lymphoblastic leukemia and chronic myeloid leukemia. (B) Interphase FISH analysis for the t(9;22)/*BCR–ABL1* abnormality using a dual fusion/dual color strategy. Left side image demonstrates green labeled fluorescent probes targeting both *BCR* alleles at 22q11 and red probes hybridized to the *ABL1* loci at 9q34. Right side image in the case of a Ph+ precursor B cell ALL indicates 2 abnormal fusion signals representing both the *BCR-ABL1*, and the reciprocal consequence of the translocation (arrows). Nuclei are counterstained with 4′,6-diamidino-2-phenylindole (DAPI).

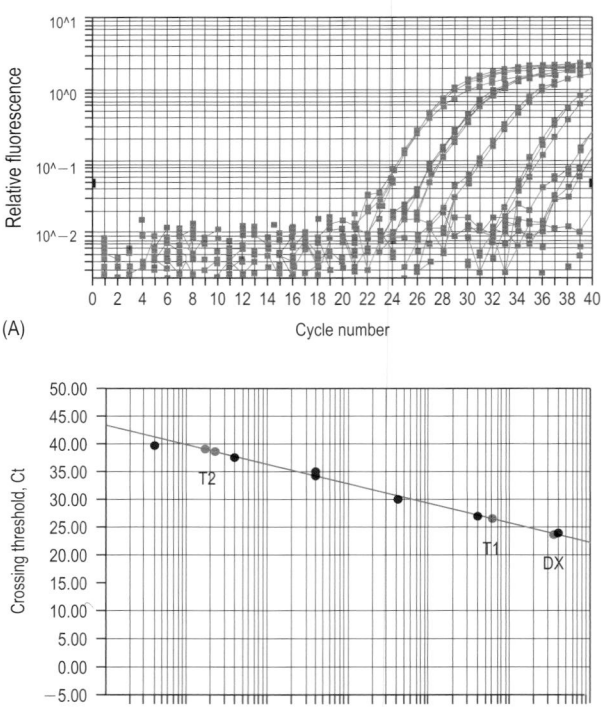

(A)

(B)

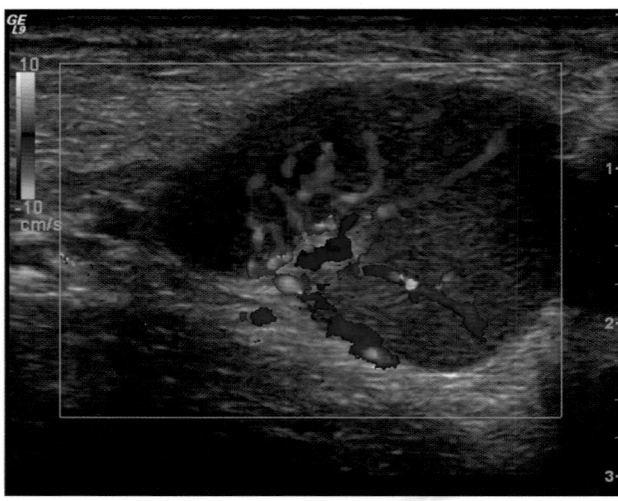

Plate 129 Color Doppler study demonstrating a lymphomatous node with abundant hilar flow.

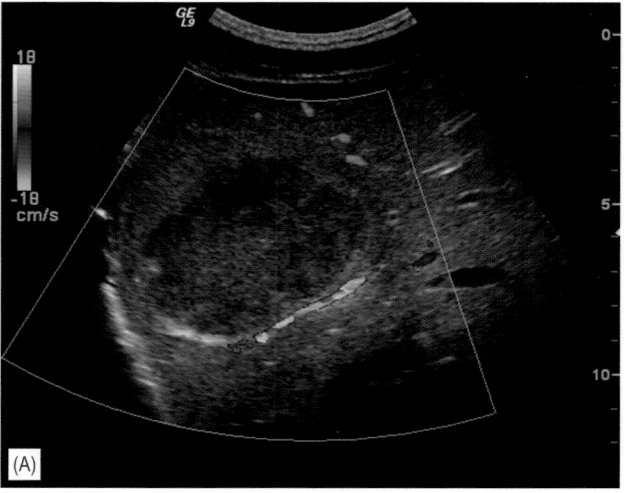

Plate 128 Real-time quantitative polymerase chain reaction (RQ-PCR) analysis for minimal residual disease (MRD) detection of the t(9;22)/*BCR–ABL1* abnormality in Ph+ precursor B cell acute lymphoblastic leukemia. (A) Data from a 'TaqMan' or 5′ fluorescent nuclease automated real time quantitative PCR analysis. Red tracings represent 10-fold dilutions of plasmid standards containing the e1-a2 *BCR–ABL1* fusion cDNA. The early exponential phase of PCR amplification, denoted the crossing threshold (Ct), is related to the quantity of starting template. The aqua, blue and purple tracings represent bone marrow RNA samples from a patient with Ph+ B-ALL at diagnosis and two sequential post-therapy time-points respectively; the three specimens are analyzed together for comparison purposes in this figure. (B) Standard curve plot of Ct versus starting amount of BCR–ABL1. Black dots represent the standard dilutions in part (A). A linear relationship between the Ct value and quantity is present. This measurement is highly reproducible, provided sample quality, reverse transcription efficiency and technical variability factors (e.g. pipetting errors) are optimized. Unknown sample quantities can be derived from the standard curve, shown as red dots at the three time points corresponding to the patient's diagnostic (Dx) and two post-therapy samples (T1, T2). This type of quantitative analysis can be used as a powerful surrogate to evaluate the relative extent of disease reduction and (over serial measurement intervals) the rate of decreasing tumor burden, provided that specific tumor genetic markers are available.

Plate 130 Ultrasound of hepatic lymphoma. (A) Color Doppler demonstration of an avascular primary tumor.

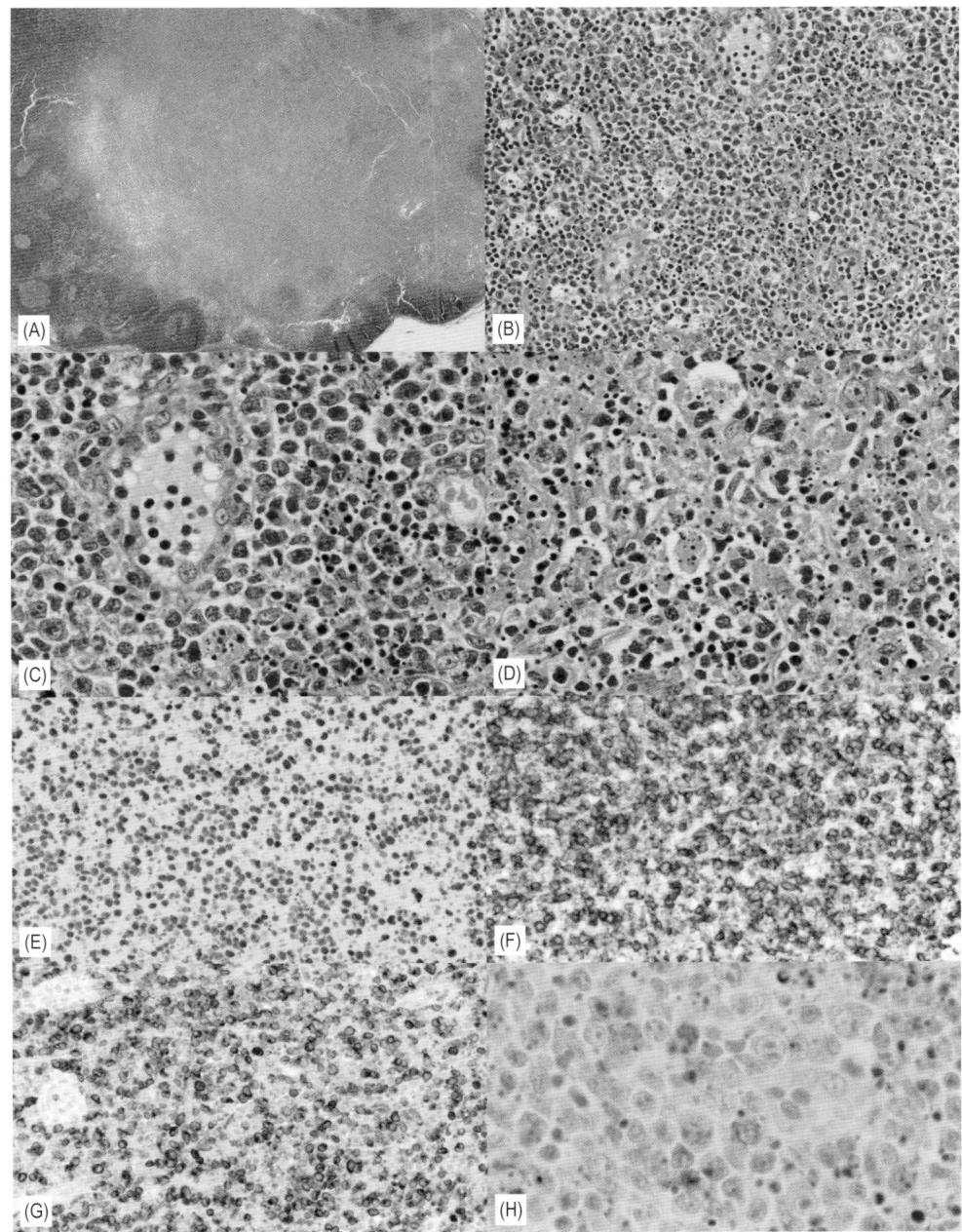

Plate 131 Kikuchi–Fujimoto disease showing: (A) patchy paracortical involvement of the lymph node, (B–D) presence of more than one cell type that includes unusual histiocytes with crescentic or C-shaped nuclei, immunoblasts, plasmacytoid monocytes and small lymphoid cells. On immunostaining, there is a high proliferation rate, as noted by Ki-67 expression (E) and the lymphoid component consists predominantly of CD8-positive T cells (F) coexpressing perforin (G). Occasional cells express myeloperoxidase (H).

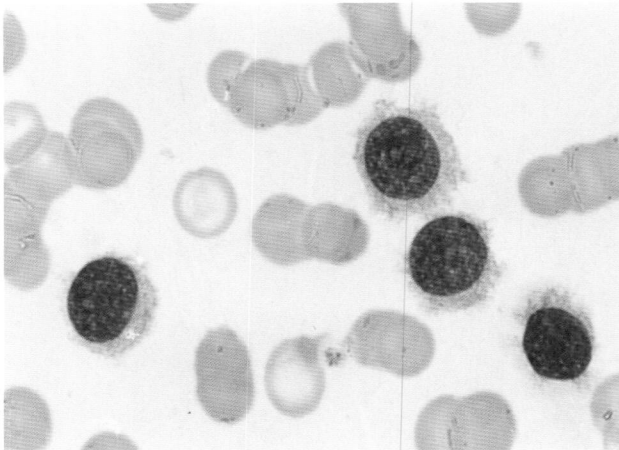

Plate 132 May-Grünwald-Giemsa (MGG)-stained peripheral blood film showing typical hairy cells with oval slightly eccentric nucleus and abundant pale cytoplasm with cytoplasmic projections.

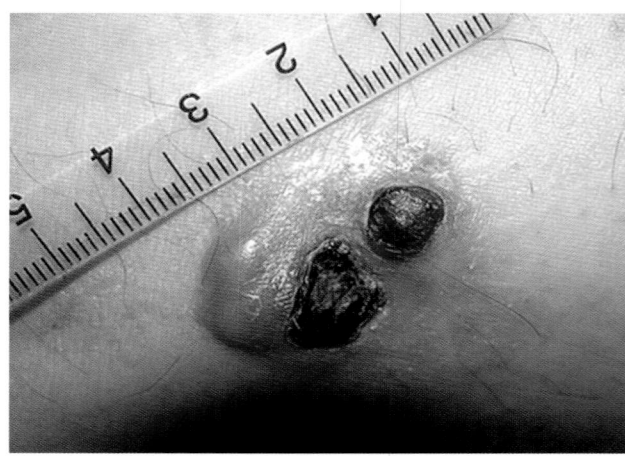

Plate 133 Cutaneous anaplastic large cell lymphoma; solitary ulcerated nodule of the skin.

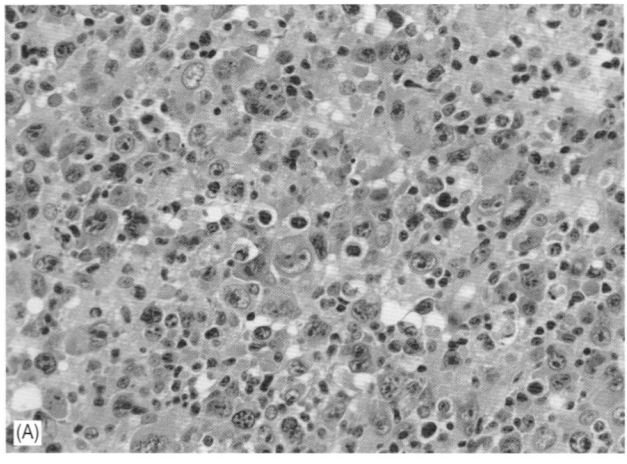

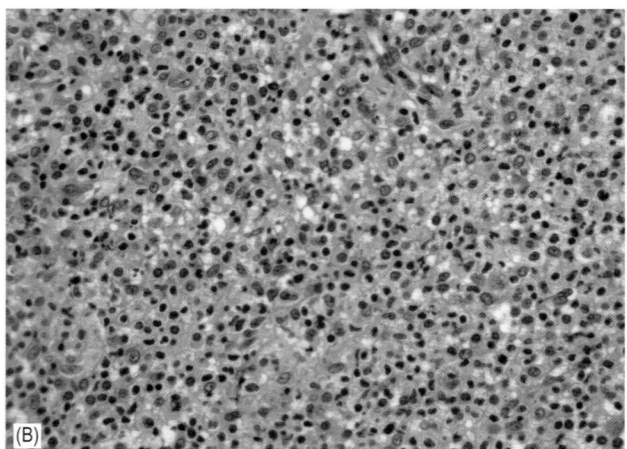

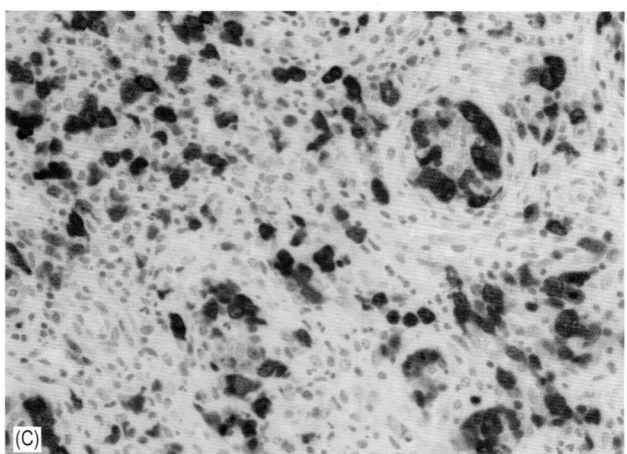

Plate 134 Histologic and molecular analysis of anaplastic large cell lymphoma (ALCL). (A) Classic ALCL. Note the pleomorphic cells with some embryoid nuclei. (B) Small cell variant: monomorphic small cells with slightly atypical nuclei. (C) Nuclear and cytoplasmic reaction to ALK-1 antibody. Note the perivascular arrangement of some neoplastic cells.

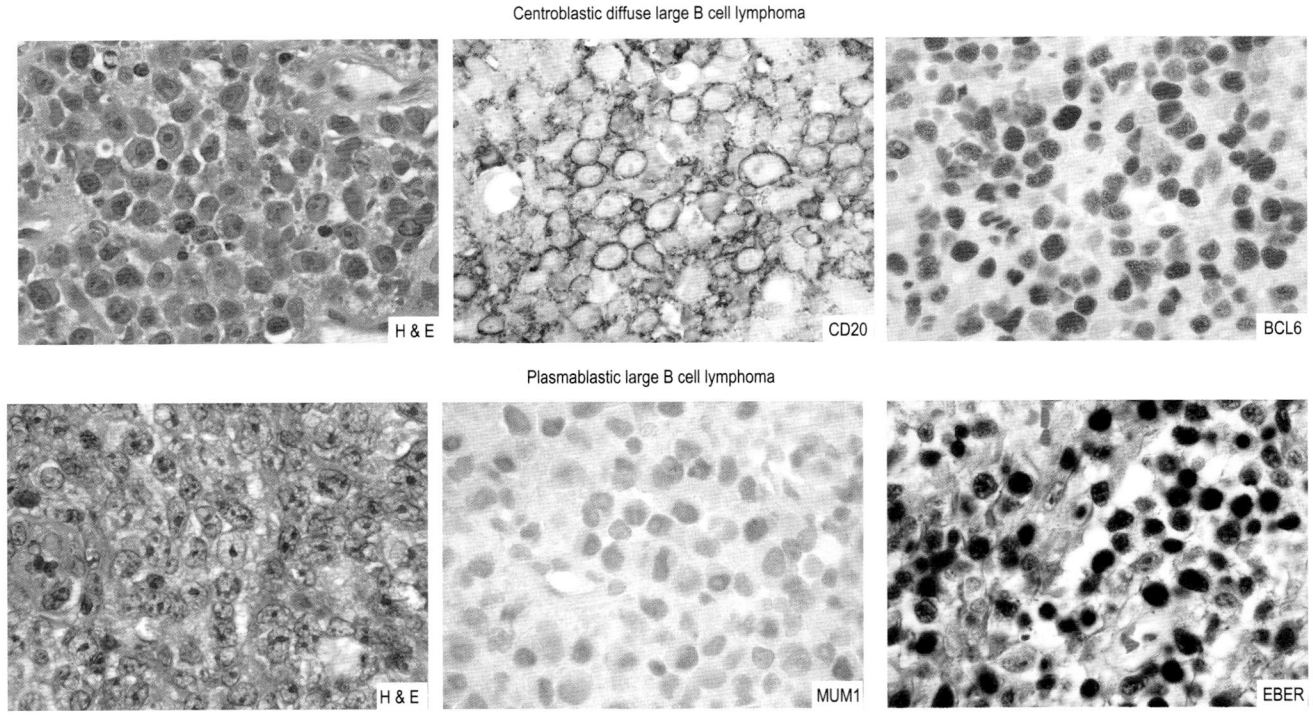

Plate 135 Subtypes of diffuse large B cell lymphoma (DLBCL) identified by gene expression profiling of biopsies from 274 cases of untreated DLBCL.[53] Based on this analysis, DLBCL can be divided into two subtypes, one derived from germinal center B cells (GCB) and one from post-germinal center B cells that have an activated B cell (ABC) genotype. A third group lacking an ABC or GCB genotype was identified and likely reflects a mixture of 'subtypes' that occur at low frequency. Expression of discriminating genes is shown on the right, and likelihood a sample belongs to the ABC or GCB subtype is displayed on top. Immunoblastic or centroblastic histologic features most likely correspond to the ABC and GCB subtypes, respectively.[52]

Plate 136 Histology and immunophenotype of centroblastic and plasmablastic large B cell lymphomas. Immunophenotype of centroblastic lymphoma is usually CD20 and BCL6 positive, consistent with germinal center origin. Immunophenotype of plasmablastic lymphoma is usually MUM1 positive, consistent with a post-germinal center origin, and is Epstein–Barr virus (EBV) positive as detected by EBV encoded small RNA (EBER) *in situ* hybridization.

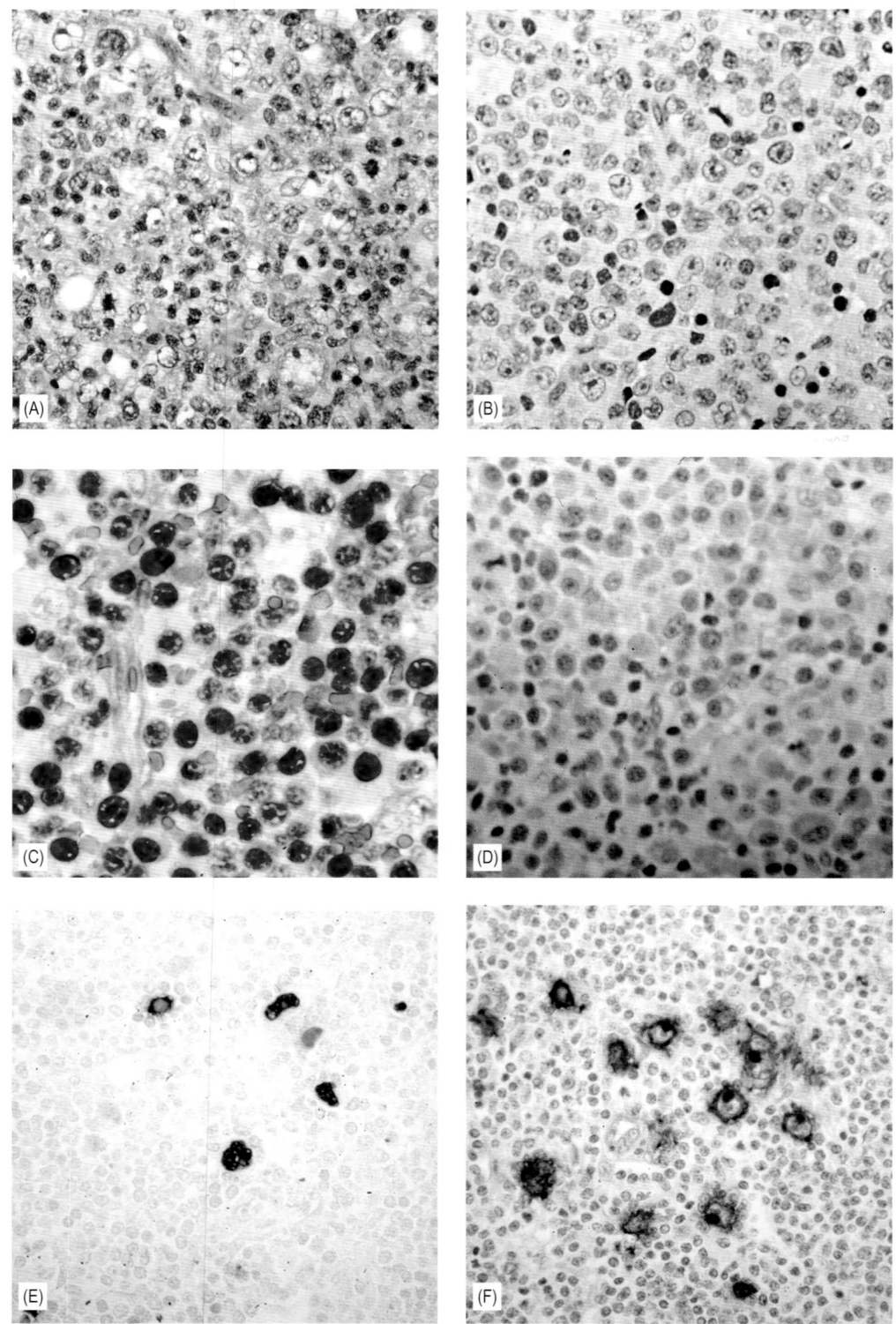

Plate 137   Histology and immunohistology of lymphomas in immunodeficiency. (A, B) Hematoxylin and eosin staining of (A) polymorphic and (B) monomorphic diffuse large B cell lymphoma. (C, D) Epstein–Barr virus encoded small nuclear RNA (EBER) staining of a myelomatous form of post-transplant lymphoproliferative disease with (C) fast red staining of most nuclei and (D) hematoxylin and eosin staining of the same. (E, F) EBER staining of Hodgkin disease (HD) in immunodeficiency with (E) diaminobenzidine (DAB) nickel staining of infrequent HD and Reed–Sternberg cells and (F) CD15 staining of the same.

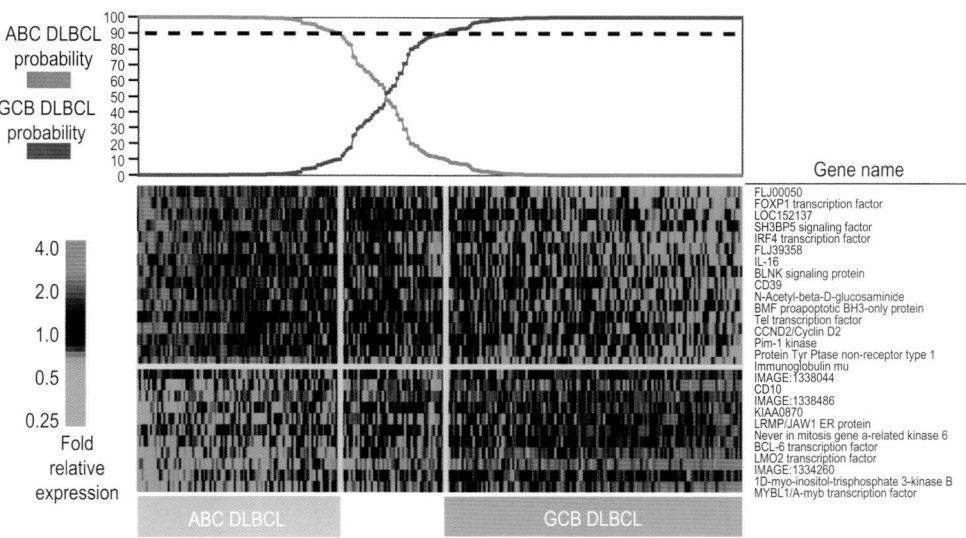

Plate 138 Diffuse large B cell lymphoma (DLBCL) can be separated into the germinal center B cell (GCB) and activated B cell (ABC) types by using Bayesean algorithm. A small number of cases cannot be classified into either of the subgroups. Reprinted with permission: Wright G *et al. Proc Natl Acad Sci* 2003; **100**: 9991–6, Figure 1A.

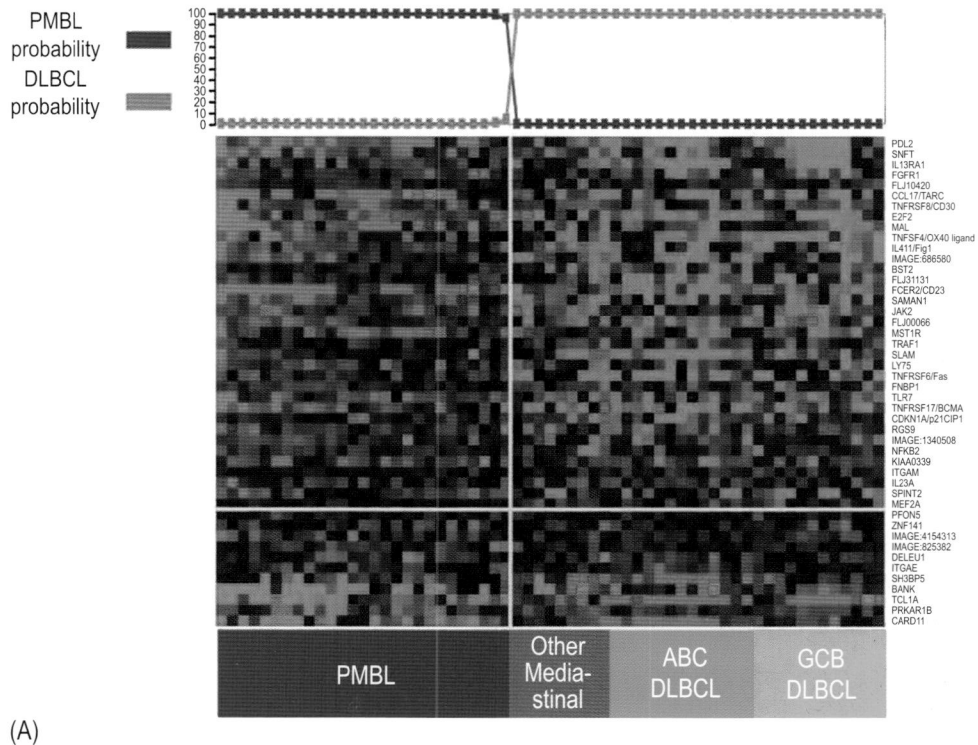

(A)

Plate 139 (A) Primary mediastinal large B cell lymphoma (PMBL) has a distinct gene expression signature that can separate it from other types of diffuse large B cell lymphoma (DLBCL) including those that happen to occur in the anterior mediastinum. Reprinted with permission: Rosenwald A *et al. J Exp Med* 2003; **198**: 851–62, Figure 2A and Figure 3A.

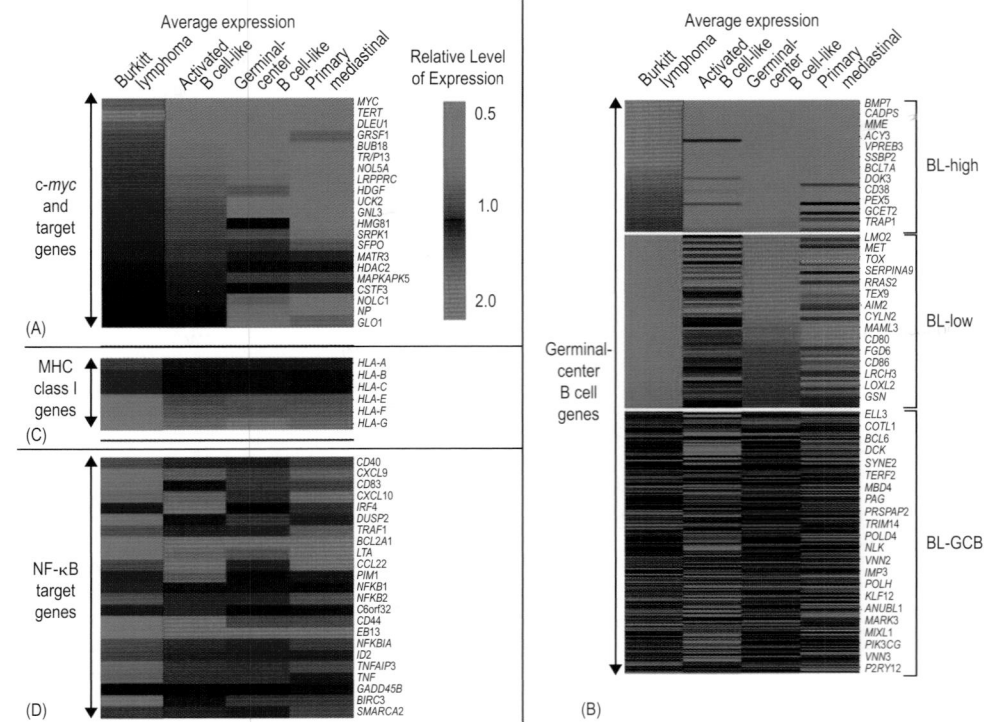

Plate 140 Burkitt lymphoma (BL) is characterized by the low expression of nuclear factor κB (NF-κB) target genes and major histocompatibility complex (MHC) class I genes and the high expression of *MYC* target genes. The expression profile of the germinal center signature is distinguishable from that of germinal center B cell type diffuse large B cell lymphoma (GCB DLBCL). Reprinted with permission: Dave SS *et al. N Engl J Med* 2006; **354**: 2431–42.

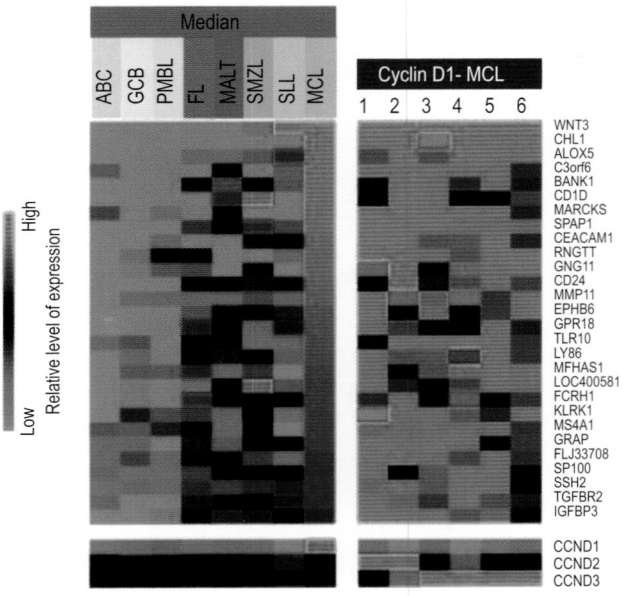

Plate 141 Mantle cell lymphoma (MCL) has a distinctive gene expression signature. Using this signature, rare cases of tumors that resemble mantle cell lymphoma morphologically and immunophenotypically but lack cyclin D1 expression and t(11;14) can be identified as cyclin D1-negative mantle cell lymphoma. ABC, activated B cell; GCB, germinal center B cell; PMBL, primary mediastinal large B cell lymphoma; FL, follicular lymphoma; MALT, mucosal-associated lymphoid tissue; SMZL, splenic marginal zone lymphoma; SLL, small lymphocytic lymphoma. Reprinted with permission: Fu K *et al. Blood* 2005; **106**: 4315–21, Figure 1.

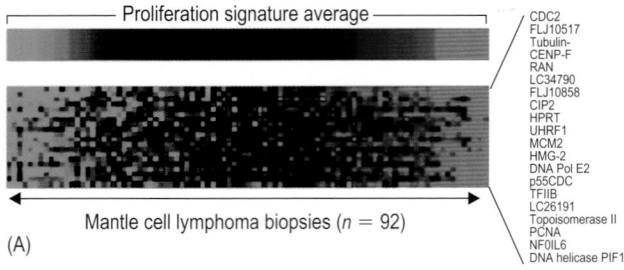

Plate 142 (A) Mantle cell lymphoma can be arranged according to the proliferation signature score. Reprinted with permission: Rosenwald A *et al. Cancer Cell* 2002; **3**: 185–97, Figure 2A and Figure 2B.

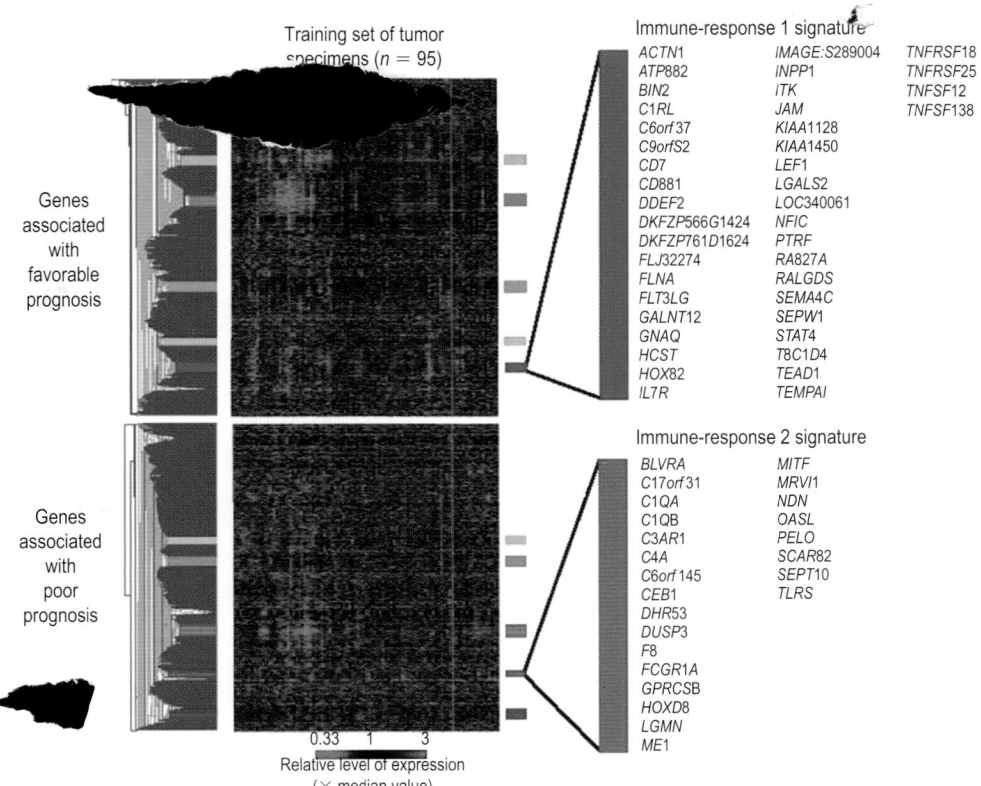

Training set of tumor specimens (n = 95)

Genes associated with favorable prognosis

Genes associated with poor prognosis

0.33 1 3
Relative level of expression
(× median value)

Immune-response 1 signature

ACTN1	IMAGE:S289004	TNFRSF18
ATP882	INPP1	TNFRSF25
BIN2	ITK	TNFSF12
C1RL	JAM	TNFSF138
C6orf37	KIAA1128	
C9orfS2	KIAA1450	
CD7	LEF1	
CD881	LGALS2	
DDEF2	LOC340061	
DKFZP566G1424	NFIC	
DKFZP761D1624	PTRF	
FLJ32274	RA827A	
FLNA	RALGDS	
FLT3LG	SEMA4C	
GALNT12	SEPW1	
GNAQ	STAT4	
HCST	T8C1D4	
HOX82	TEAD1	
IL7R	TEMPAI	

Immune-response 2 signature

BLVRA	MITF
C17orf31	MRVI1
C1QA	NDN
C1QB	OASL
C3AR1	PELO
C4A	SCAR82
C6orf145	SEPT10
CEB1	TLRS
DHR53	
DUSP3	
F8	
FCGR1A	
GPRCSB	
HOXD8	
LGMN	
ME1	

Plate 143 This figure shows the two gene expression signatures from the training set of follicular lymphoma that are synergistic in predicting survival of the patients. Both sets of transcripts reflect gene expression of infiltrating host cells and stromal elements. Reprinted with permission: Dave SS et al. N Engl J Med 2004; **351**: 2159–69, Figure 1.

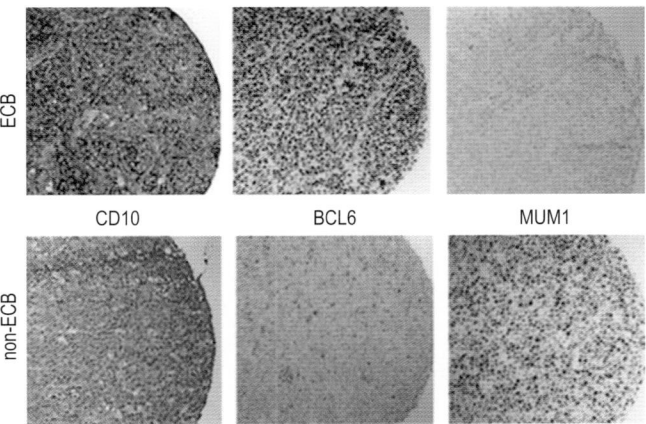

Plate 144 (A) Using antibodies to stain for CD10, BCL6, and MUM1, Hans and coworkers derived an algorithm that is useful in distinguishing germinal center B cell type diffuse large B cell lymphoma (GCB DLBCL) from non-GCB DLBCL in archival tissues. Reprinted with permission: Hans CP et al. Blood 2004; **103**: 275–82, Figure 2 and Figure 3A.

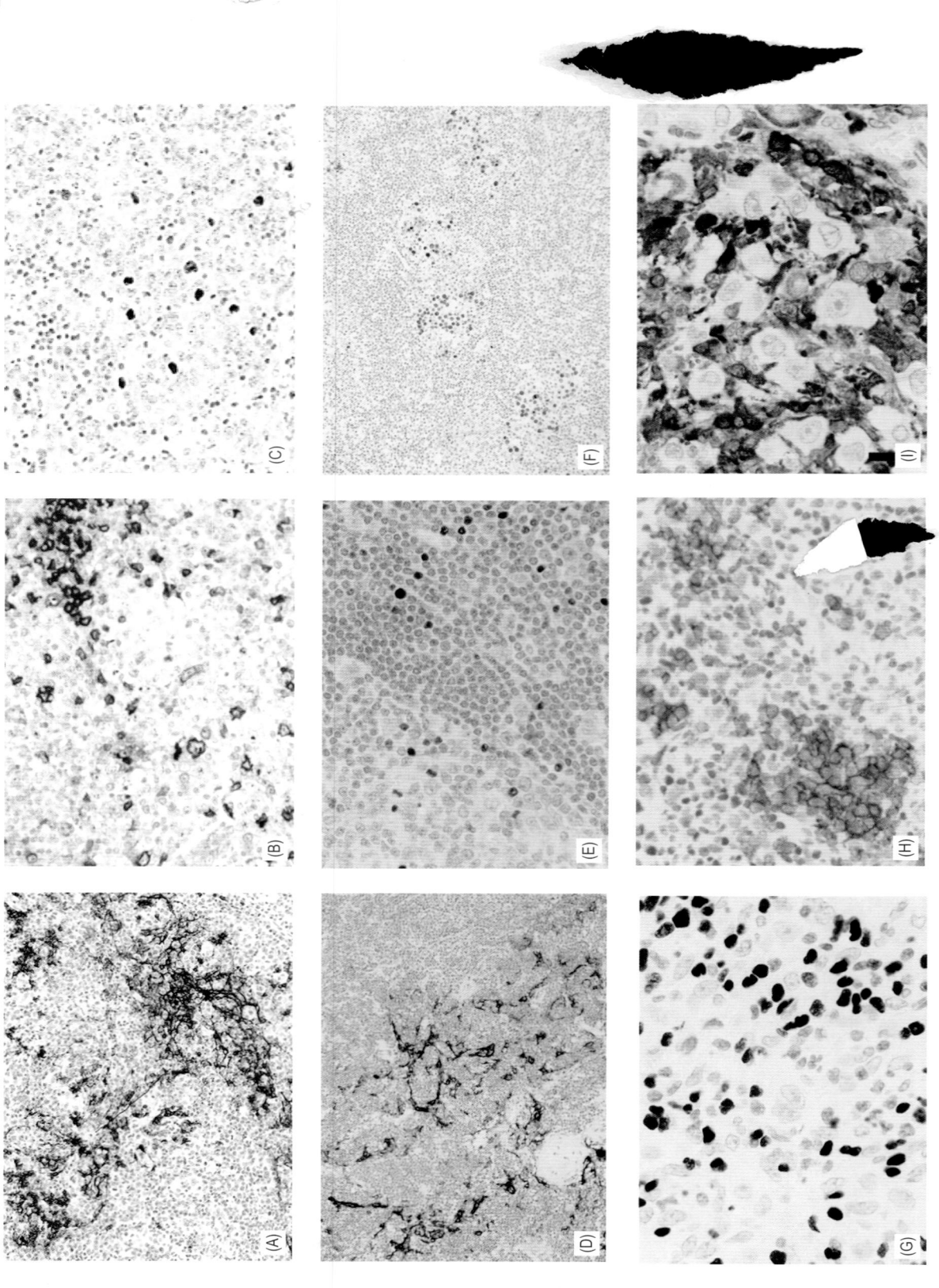

Plate 145 Non-tumoral cell populations. An infiltrate composed of multiple types of immune cells is regularly present in numerous lymphoma types. (A), (B), and (C) correspond to angioimmunoblastic T cell lymphoma (AITL). Staining is of (A) follicular dendritic cells, (B) CD20$^+$ B cells, and (C) Epstein–Barr virus (EBV)$^+$ cells. (D) Follicular dendritic cell network observed in a mantle cell lymphoma. (E) Regulatory T cells stained for FOXP3 in a reactive lymphoid follicle. (F) Germinocentric lymphoproliferative disorder. Human herpesvirus 8 (HHV-8)$^+$ cells within the germinal center. (G) CD123$^+$ plasmacytoid dendritic cells in cutaneous marginal zone lymphoma. (H) and (I) represent Hodgkin lymphoma. (H) T regulatory cells (FOXP3$^+$) surrounding Hodgkin and Reed–Sternberg (H–RS) cells. (I) Macrophages are stained for STAT1. STAT1 becomes nuclear in activated macrophages. A ring of STAT1$^+$ macrophages surrounds H–RS cells.

Whereas it is important to initiate specific therapy as soon as possible, starting chemotherapy in the presence of hyperuricemia and an impaired urinary output without corrective measures is likely to result in the death of the patient secondary to hyperkalemia. This is likely because potassium released from tumor cells cannot be excreted efficiently in the absence of an adequate urine flow. As such, biochemical abnormalities must be corrected before the initiation of specific therapy (although this by no means guarantees that a TLS will not occur). This period of biochemical correction should not normally exceed 24 to 48 hours. In a review of 37 patients with advanced stage Burkitt lymphoma who were treated with induction chemotherapy, renal failure was present at the outset in eight of the patients, two of whom required dialysis for uric acid nephropathy before chemotherapy could be instituted.[70] When hemodialysis is instituted, chemotherapy is normally commenced after the completion of a period of hemodialysis, when biochemical parameters are close to normal. Since further dialysis is unlikely to be required for at least a few hours, the possibility of removing drugs (e.g., cyclophosphamide) by dialysis is, in this way, minimized.

In general, it is advisable to manage patients at highest risk for developing TLS initially in a critical care unit because of the intensive monitoring required. Vigorous hydration with half normal saline (or patient-appropriate hydration fluids) in the region of 2–3 L/m^2 of body surface area every 24 hours and liberal use of diuretics where necessary (e.g., intravenous furosemide, 2–3 mg every 2–3 hours) should be commenced immediately in this group of patients in order to maintain high urine flow (as much as 80–100 mL/m^2/hour or even more in patients at highest risk) for the first few days after the initiation of chemotherapy (Table 49.5). These measures are taken to ensure that the high solute load created by tumor lysis (primarily composed of phosphates and oxypurines) is accommodated without the onset of hyperkalemia or acute renal failure.

Urine alkalinization has been used in the treatment of TLS,[74] as an alkaline urine promotes the solubility of uric acid. However, at urine pH of ⩾6.5 the solubility of xanthine and hypoxanthine is significantly reduced causing the development of xanthine crystals and subsequent obstructive uropathy. In addition, phosphates are poorly soluble in alkaline urine, which can also lead to intratubular deposits. Thus it is preferable to maintain the urine pH at about 7 and not to administer bicarbonate during chemotherapy. In the recently published guidelines by Coiffier et al., alkalinization was only indicated for patients with metabolic acidosis; urine alkalinization was not recommended for patients using rasburicase.[75]

In addition to the above measures, blocking the conversion of xanthines and hypoxanthine to uric acid with the administration of allopurinol is important to prevent TLS. Both allopurinol and its metabolite oxypurinol are strong inhibitors of the enzyme xanthine oxidase, and markedly reduce the conversion of xanthines and hypoxanthine to uric acid. This results in the excretion of purines in three forms that are independently soluble in urine (Fig. 49.2).[67] Alkalinization of the urine to a pH of about 7 increases the solubility of uric acid and xanthines. At this pH, uric acid is 10 to 12 times more soluble,[76] and xanthines more than twice as soluble, than at pH 5. The solubility of hypoxanthine differs little at either pH. High-dose allopurinol ensures that a significant proportion of purine metabolites are excreted as xanthines and hypoxanthine, but if urate production is totally inhibited, there is an increased risk of xanthine nephropathy.[77]

Recent pharmacological advances have led to the development of nonrecombinant and recombinant forms of urate oxidase (rasburicase), an enzyme that promotes the catabolism of uric acid to allantoin, which is five to ten

Table 49.5 Characteristics of renal failure associated with tumor lysis syndrome

	Type of nephropathy		
	Uric acid	Phosphate	Xanthine
Hyperkalemia	++	+	+/−
Uricosemia	++	+	+
Hyperphosphatemia	+	++	+
Predisposing factors	Aciduria	Alkaluria	Allopurinol
Time of onset	Before and after starting therapy	Within 48 hours after starting therapy	After starting allopurinol
Prevention	Hydration Alkalinization Allopurinol	Hydration	Hydration

+, increase in potassium, urate, and phosphate levels in plasma.

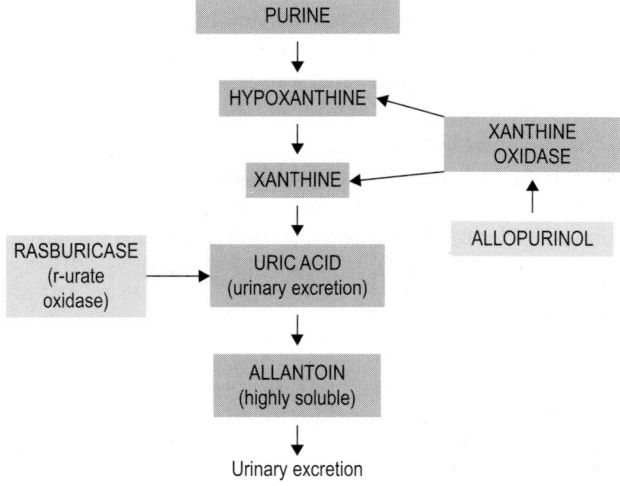

Figure 49.2 Uricosuric agents and their mechanism of action.

times more soluble in urine.[78] The nonrecombinant form of urate oxidase has been effective in reducing uric acid levels in patients at risk of TLS.[79] The recombinant form of urate oxidase (rasburicase) has been recently developed. Pui *et al.* reported a significant reduction of uric acid levels within 4 hours of administration.[80] An established dose of 0.15–0.2 mg/kg of rasburicase is effective at decreasing uric acid levels significantly at 4 h after administration and to undetectable levels within 48 h of initiation.[80] Compared to allopurinol, rasburicase demonstrated a more rapid control and lower uric acid levels in patients at high risk of TLS.[81] Rasburicase has demonstrated excellent tolerability and is potentially cost effective in patients at high risk for TLS.[73,80,82] Rasburicase is a safe and effective hypouricemic agent for both adults and children at high risk for TLS and should be considered the uricolytic agent of choice in these patients. In Europe, some protocols (e.g., the COP regimen in the LMB81 protocol of the Société Francaise d'Oncologie Pédiatrique [SFOP]) call for the use of a 'pre-phase'; that is, low-dose chemotherapy and uricase given a week before initiation of the major induction regimen, to lessen the risk of tumor lysis.[83]

Under physiological conditions, the solubility product for total calcium and phosphate is 4.6×10^{-6} mol/L.[67,83,84] When this product is exceeded (as mentioned above), calcium phosphate salts may be precipitated in the renal parenchyma and other soft tissues. Hyperphosphatemia, which may give rise to hypocalcemia and renal failure, occurs within 48 hours of the onset of chemotherapy, is maximal on the second and third days, and may last for up to 7 days.[85] For this reason, hypocalcemia should not be treated unless symptomatic (presenting with tetany or cardiac arrhythmias), and intravenous calcium chloride should be given with great caution, if at all. Rarely, hemodialysis may be required for symptomatic hypocalcemia.

Tumor lysis syndrome was originally recognized because of sudden death occurring as a direct consequence of hyperkalemia, which may occur within hours of starting therapy. Thus, potassium supplements should be avoided shortly before and during the first few days of therapy, except in exceptional circumstances. Ideally, the patient should be mildly hypokalemic prior to the start of chemotherapy. Hyperkalemia is most unlikely to occur in the presence of a high urine output, and in fact urine flow is the key to the management of the TLS. As long as a high urine flow can be maintained, other interventions are unlikely to be needed. If this is not the case, rapid progression of biochemical abnormalities will occur, necessitating emergency hemodialysis.

HYPERCALCEMIA OF MALIGNANCY

Hypercalcemia is defined as a serum calcium level greater than 2.6 mmol/L (10.5 mg/dL). Levels above 3.0 mmol/L (12.0 mg/dL) may cause transitional disturbances in virtually every organ system, while those above 5.0 mmol/L (20.0 mg/dL) can be fatal.[50] Hypercalcemia is the most common life-threatening metabolic disorder associated with cancer, especially multiple myeloma, usually occurring in about 10–20 percent of patients with advanced malignancy.[86] It is, however, an uncommon complication of leukemia and malignant lymphoma, and is generally encountered only in human T cell lymphotrophic virus 1 (HTLV-1)-associated adult T cell lymphomas and some childhood NHLs such as Burkitt lymphoma (rarely) and lymphoblastic lymphoma widely metastatic to bone.[87,88]

Humoral hypercalcemia, which accounts for 80 percent of cases, is due to excessive paracrine production of parathyroid hormone-related peptide (PTHrP), which results in increased bone turnover and calcium release, increased intestinal calcium uptake, and reduced renal calcium excretion. Osteoclastic bony metastases as seen in multiple myeloma and certain lymphomas account for approximately 20 percent of cases. Other causes, such as ectopic parathyroid hormone secretion and vitamin D-secreting lymphomas, account for fewer than 1 percent of the cases.[89]

Hypercalcemia most often occurs in patients with large tumor burdens and may be precipitated by dehydration or immobilization. Once the plasma calcium level rises, homeostatic mechanisms are activated to normalize the serum calcium level. If these mechanisms cannot keep up with the rapidly rising serum calcium, the hypercalcemia itself begins to causes renal dysfunction, with a decrease in the glomerular filtration rate and concentrating ability of the kidneys, resulting in dehydration and consequent worsening of the hypercalcemia. Anorexia and vomiting, a direct effect of hypercalcemia, cause further volume depletion. As a result, there is decrease in the urinary output and, unless aggressively treated, a hypercalcemic crisis can ensue rapidly.[90]

There is little correlation beween serum calcium levels and the severity of signs and symptoms of hypercalcemia. However, a relationship has been noted between clinical manifestations and the rate of rise of the calcium level,[86] the presence of other metabolic abnormalities, and the extent of the patient's underlying debility from cancer.[27] Effects of hypercalcemia can be seen on the gastrointestinal, renal, cardiovascular, neurologic, and skeletal systems (Table 49.6). Gastrointestinal symptoms include nausea, vomiting, constipation, and abdominal pain, while CNS symptoms are initially vague, being manifested as weakness, somnolence, and lethargy, a symptom complex which can be mistaken for intracerebral involvement by lymphoma. Polyuria, precipitation of calcium phosphate in the renal tubules, and stones can occur.[86] Hypercalcemia of any degree can cause some increase in myocardial contractility and irritability, but serum calcium levels over 4.0 mmol/L (16 mg/dL) can result in fatal cardiac arrhythmias.[86,91] Bony symptoms, in the form of bone pain, fractures, and skeletal deformities, are often found in the presence of hypercalcemia.[92]

Treatment of hypercalcemia secondary to a lymphoid malignancy must include specific therapy for the hypercalcemia in addition to treatment for the underlying

Table 49.6 Hypercalcemia of malignancy

Signs and symptoms

Gastrointestinal
 Anorexia, nausea, vomiting, constipation, abdominal pain, and ileus
Cardiovascular
 Bradycardia, arrhythmias, bundle branch block
Renal
 Polyuria, nocturia, dehydration, calcium phosphate stones
Central nervous system
 Lethargy, apathy, depression, psychoses, stupor, and coma
Musculoskeletal
 Hypotonia, bone pain, fractures

Treatment
 Vigorous hydration with saline diuresis
 Thyrocalcitonin
 Mithramycin
 Bisphosphonates
 Gallium nitrate
 Corticosteroids

lymphoma (Table 49.6). Aggressive hydration followed by a potent bisphosphonate (pamidronate [90 mg], ibandronate [4 mg], or zolendronate [4 mg] given intravenously as a single infusion) is the mainstay of treatment for malignant hypercalcemia today.[89,93] In 80 percent of patients, the calcium level is restored to normal within 5 days. A serum calcium level of more than 3.5 mmol/L (14 mg/dL) should be considered a medical emergency and treated in an intensive care unit with close cardiac monitoring. In patients with a serum calcium level less than 3.5 mmol/L (14 mg/dL), saline repletion with standard furosemide (1 mg/kg) diuresis usually provides adequate control while definitive treatment for the lymphoma is being initiated. With higher serum calcium levels, a more vigorous forced diuresis is recommended for adults, using volumes of normal saline up to three times the maintenance requirement with furosemide (2–3 mg/kg) every 2–3 hours, with the goal of achieving a urine output of at least 500 mL/h.[94] Urine output, electrolytes, and magnesium should be closely monitored during therapy as almost half the patients with hypercalcemia are hypokalemic at presentation, and require potassium and magnesium replacement during saline diuresis.

There are a number of pharmacological agents available for the treatment of hypercalcemia that does not respond to the above measures. In an acute crisis, agents such as thyrocalcitonin (3–8 MRC units/kg intravenously) can be administered in conjunction with the saline diuresis. The calcitonin acts within 1–2 hours to reduce serum calcium by inhibiting bone resorption. However, almost 25 percent of patients may not respond and resistance has been noted with repeated administration.[86,95] Gallium nitrate, another potent osteoclast inhibitor, is used less often.[96–98]

Corticosteroids may have a role in steroid-responsive lymphomas. Rarely, hemodialysis may be necessary in unresponsive cases.

Gastrointestinal complications

Primary gastrointestinal lymphomas can present as a medical or surgical emergency resulting from mechanical obstruction, hemorrhage, or perforation of the involved viscus. Presenting symptoms include unexplained abdominal masses, intestinal obstruction, intussusception, and an 'acute abdomen.'[99] The most frequent site of involvement varies with age and histology. In the first two decades of life, B cell lymphomas (small noncleaved cell and diffuse large cell) commonly involve the small bowel, particularly the terminal ileum and the cecum. The average age of the 92 patients with NHL who were treated at the National Institutes of Health between 1977 and 1994 was 16 years; 80 percent of these patients had abdominal disease at presentation.[99] The B cell lymphomas of childhood sometimes present with bowel obstruction, either by obliteration of the bowel lumen, or by serving as the nidus for an ileo-ileal or ileocolic intussusception. A high index of suspicion for NHL should be entertained in any child who develops an intussusception after the first year of life. Most patients undergo emergency laparotomy, at which time the diagnosis is made. The tumor can be completely resected in about 25 percent of patients, and such patients have an excellent prognosis.[60] Definitive chemotherapy should be given within days of surgery since regrowth can be rapid and the advantage of reduction of tumor bulk may quickly be lost.

Complications commonly associated with gastric lymphomas, particularly in older patients with atherosclerotic vessels, include massive gastrointestinal bleeding and perforation. Treatment of these lymphomas remains controversial, with some oncologists recommending up-front chemotherapy without surgical resection, and others advocating surgery only or up-front surgery followed by chemotherapy[100–102] to try and avoid these complications. Although it is generally felt that the approach utilizing surgery followed by chemotherapy can better avoid these complications while producing excellent results, it is important to bear in mind that not all patients are amenable to surgery, and in some series the mortality rate of surgery is as high as 18 percent.[101,102]

It is now possible to predict by endoscopic examination, and where possible by selective angiography, which patients are more likely to develop massive hemorrhage or perforation when chemotherapy is commenced (e.g., extent of involvement of the stomach wall, degree of ulceration and necrosis), and recent results suggest that a similar rate of overall survival may be obtained by using intensive chemotherapy either with no surgery or with surgery in selected patients only, e.g., those with very large (over 10 cm diameter) but resectable tumors, or those considered at high risk for massive hemorrhage or perforation.[101,102]

Complications associated with massive mediastinal disease

ANESTHETIC COMPLICATIONS

The preoperative diagnosis of a large, anterior mediastinal mass should alert both the oncologist and anesthesiologist to a potential life-threatening situation, as severe respiratory and cardiovascular complications have been described in this group of patients.[1,15,21,28,50,103,104] In the pediatric population, the mediastinum is the primary site of involvement in approximately one-third of Hodgkin disease and NHLs.[1] The risks associated with general anesthesia in these patients are widely recognized. Tracheal or bronchial obstruction can arise unexpectedly at any time during anesthesia and surgery, including induction, intubation, positioning, or extubation.[28,103,104] In addition, despite patency of the airway, there is the risk of profound hypoxemia following compression of the pulmonary vessels.[28]

Taking into account these risks, controversy often arises in the management of a patient with SVC obstruction as to the need for pathological confirmation of malignancy prior to initiating therapy.[1,103] As mentioned earlier (in the section on SVCS) every effort should be made to establish a diagnosis prior to starting therapy, preferably from sites other than the mediastinum (such as peripheral lymph nodes, pleural effusion, or bone marrow) and, as far as possible, under local anesthesia.

In the patient with a large mediastinal mass in whom diagnosis remains inconclusive, and where biopsy of either a lymph node or the mass itself needs to be performed under general anesthesia, one should proceed with great caution. A preoperative CT scan of the chest should be obtained to determine the degree of bronchial obstruction, along with upright and supine echocardiography and a pulmonary flow volume loop study.[50,103] Patients who demonstrate abnormalities on any of these tests should not be subjected to general anesthesia.[28] Ferrari et al. and Neuman et al. recommend the following measures be undertaken in patients who do undergo operative procedures under general anesthesia: preservation of spontaneous ventilation whenever possible; induction of anesthesia with the patient in the sitting or lateral semi-Fowler position; secure intravenous access in a lower extremity; rapid change in the patient's position at the first sign of cardiorespiratory arrest; and the availability of a functioning bronchoscope and bronchoscopist at all times during the procedure.[28,103,104]

Hematologic complications

BONE MARROW INFILTRATION

Quantitative disorders of platelets, leukocytes, and red cells are frequently seen in association with bone marrow infiltration in leukemia and lymphomas. In fact, in some patients, thrombocytopenia with its accompanying purpura and/or overt bleeding may be one of the presenting features at the time of diagnosis. Marrow replacement by blasts resulting in decreased synthesis of megakaryocytes and leukocyte and red cell precursors can be confirmed by a bone marrow examination. Blood products and/or antibiotics are usually needed through the period of chemotherapy for the underlying lymphoid malignancy.

AUTOIMMUNE CYTOPENIAS

In addition to anemia and thrombocytopenia, the diagnosis of lymphoma is sometimes made when a patient presents with either an autoimmune hemolytic anemia or idiopathic thrombocytopenia (the mechanism of which still remains unknown).[105,106]

The incidence of hemolytic anemia is highest in diseases of the lymphatic and reticuloendothelial system. It is most commonly associated with NHL and chronic lymphatic leukemia, but may also be seen with adenocarcinomas, autologous bone marrow transplantation (BMT), ABO-incompatible allogeneic BMT, cyclosporine therapy, and infections.

The most common presenting symptom is anemia. Laboratory evidence of accelerated red cell destruction is demonstrated by a low hematocrit, schistocytes on a blood smear, decreased haptoglobin level, and elevated serum LDH. The degree of anemia at presentation is variable, and occasionally the patient may present with severe hemolysis or a hemolytic uremic syndrome. The presence of a Coombs-positive hemolytic anemia is considered a sign of disseminated NHL.[106]

Idiopathic thrombocytopenia in association with NHL is not as frequently seen as autoimmune hemolytic anemia; however, in the few reported cases, it always occurred either at the time of, or subsequent to, the diagnosis.[105]

Treatment of these disorders is primarily by treatment of the underlying malignancy. However, corticosteroids, intravenous gamma globulin, and anti-prostaglandin agents have been used with varying success.[105,106]

TREATMENT-RELATED COMPLICATIONS

Fever and neutropenia

Perhaps the most common oncologic emergency encountered today is febrile neutropenia (FN). Infection due to neutropenia is associated with significant morbidity and, sometimes, mortality in patients receiving chemotherapy. Neutropenia is likely to be more severe and prolonged in patients with bone marrow infiltration or following previous irradiation of a large volume of bone marrow.

Although neutropenia (defined as an absolute neutrophil count of less than 500 per mm^3) is the single most important risk factor for infection, other factors can increase the risk as well. These include the degree of neutropenia (patients with an absolute neutrophil count of less than

Table 49.7 Guidelines for the management of neutropenic patients

1. Evaluation of the patient daily or every other day while the neutrophil counts are falling
2. Instructions to the patient to seek medical help in case of a temperature above 38°C or development of new symptomatology in the absence of a fever
3. Prompt institution of broad-spectrum antibiotic therapy (after blood cultures drawn[a]) when a neutropenic patient becomes febrile (single elevation in oral temperature to >38.5°C or three elevations to >38°C in a 24-hour period) or presents with new onset of symptoms. Consider use of colony-stimulating factors
4. In the presence of an indwelling intravenous catheter, daily blood cultures to be obtained from all lumens, along with peripheral cultures, while the patient is still febrile
5. Careful monitoring of the patient for secondary infections requiring modification of the initial antibiotic regimen
6. Addition of antifungal therapy to the existing antibiotic regimen in case of persistent fever (more than 5 days) and continuing neutropenia
7. Discontinuation of antibiotic therapy when the neutrophil count rises above 500 per mm^3 in a patient with no documented focus of infection. Prolonged therapy may be necessary in a patient with a residual focus of infection (e.g., pneumonia, catheter site infection, or hepatosplenic candidiasis)
8. In carefully selected cases where the fever has defervesced, patient has been afebrile for >48 hours, cultures are negative, clinical evidence of infection has resolved, and the neutrophil count is showing recovery, patients may be converted from intravenous antibiotics to an oral antibiotic. The choice of the antibiotic would depend on the sensitivity of the organism (in the case of an initial positive culture) or, if cultures are negative, a fluoroquinolone for at least 7 days

[a]At presentation, a febrile neutropenic patient must have a complete workup which should include at least blood cell counts, electrolytes, peripheral and central blood cultures, urine culture, stool for *Clostridium difficile* toxin, and a chest x-ray. Other tests should be dictated by the clinical findings.

100 per mm^3 are at the highest risk); duration of neutropenia (the more prolonged the period of neutropenia, the greater the risk of infection); phagocyte function (this can be impaired by the lymphoma or by the chemotherapy used to treat it); the status of the patient's cellular or humoral immunity; alteration of physical defense barriers (secondary either to mucositis, following the administration of chemotherapeutic agents such as methotrexate and anthracyclines, or to the insertion of an indwelling central venous catheter); the patient's endogenous microflora; and the acquisition of organisms due to a prolonged stay in the hospital.[93,107,108]

In the late 1960s and 1970s, the organisms predominantly responsible for life-threatening infections in neutropenic hosts included both Gram-negative (*Pseudomonas aeruginosa*, *Escherichia coli*, and *Klebsiella pneumoniae*) and Gram-positive (*Staphylococcus* and *Streptococcus* species) bacteria.[109,110] Over the past couple of decades, infections with Gram-positive organisms, particularly coagulase-positive and coagulase-negative staphylococci, alpha-hemolytic streptococci, and *Enterococcus* species, have become predominant.[111] Possible explanations (in addition to those mentioned above) include the widespread use of prophylactic antibiotics, particularly the quinolones,[112] and the increased use of proton pump inhibitors.[113] Repeated use of antibiotics in neutropenic patients along with the increasing use of chemotherapeutic agents such as methotrexate and doxorubicin are resulting in an increased frequency of infections such as *Clostridium difficile*-associated pseudomembranous enterocolitis. In addition, organisms such as *Clostridium septicum* and *Clostridium tertium* are also being more frequently encountered in cases of neutropenic enterocolitis and perianal cellulitis. Patients with prolonged neutropenia are also at risk for acquiring herpesvirus infections (especially herpes simplex, varicella-zoster, and cytomegalovirus [CMV]) and invasive mycoses (*Candida* species or *Aspergillus fumigatus*).

All patients who have received chemotherapy in the preceding 3–6 weeks and are neutropenic, whether febrile or not, should be kept under close surveillance.[93] Prompt institution of broad-spectrum antibiotics is crucial to the successful management of neutropenic patients who present with fever or may be afebrile but have other presenting complaints such as abdominal pain or cough, etc. Patients on corticosteroids, those infected by organisms such as *Pseudomonas aeruginosa* or *Clostridium septicum*, or patients presenting in septic shock may also have a blunted inflammatory response.[114] Outlined in Table 49.7 are some guidelines for the management of neutropenic patients.

Current Infectious Diseases Society of America (IDSA) guidelines stipulate that a thorough physical examination, with particular attention to sites of occult infection such as the oral cavity and perianal area, be the first step in the evaluation of a febrile neutropenic patient.[114] The initial workup should include a complete blood count, renal and hepatic profiles, at least two sets of blood cultures (one from a peripheral vein and the other from an indwelling central catheter, if present), a specimen for urine culture, and a radiograph of the chest (pick-up is low in the absence of symptoms, but detection of an early infiltrate in a small fraction of patients makes the study worthwhile).[108,115] Depending on the presenting symptoms and findings on physical examination, other investigations such as chest CT, oral culture for herpetic infection, stool for rotavirus and bacteria including *Clostridium difficile*, and a needle aspiration or biopsy of any potential source of infection should also be performed. In spite of all these investigations, it may not be possible to identify the cause of fever in the majority of patients.[116]

For coverage of the most likely pathogens, an aminoglycoside (gentamicin) plus an anti-pseudomonal penicillin (piperacillin-tazobactam), cephalosporin (ceftazidime), or carbopenem (imipenem or meropenem) are recommended.[117,118] Monotherapy with a cephalosporin (ceftazidime, cefepime) may be equally effective in most cases.[118,119] Recently, however, there has been an increase in the number of infections caused mainly by the *Enterobacter* species, and to a lesser extent by *Citrobacter* and *Serratia* species, all of which have the property of developing resistance rapidly to cephalosporins and penicillins. This information must be kept in mind when deciding on an antibiotic regimen in a neutropenic febrile patient.

With the reemergence of Gram-positive infections in immunocompromised patients, there has been considerable debate about whether vancomycin should be part of the initial empirical antibiotic regimen.[107] It is currently recommended that vancomycin be only added for bacteriologic or serologic evidence of methicillin-resistant *Staphylococcus aureus* (MRSA) infection, such as severe mucositis, catheter-related sepsis, and hypotension, since early combined use of vancomycin confers no advantage and increases resistance and the risk of adverse reactions.[117]

However, in the final analysis, the selection of any antibiotic or combination regimen must be based on the antimicrobial sensitivity of the major isolates of the institution concerned and economics.

Regardless of the initial choice of antibiotics, the key to successful treatment of a febrile neutropenic episode is frequent, thorough physical examinations of the patient throughout the neutropenic period and prompt modification of the original regimen in the face of continuing fever and prolonged neutropenia (more than 5–7 days).[118,120] This is important because the original regimen may not be effective against all the organisms responsible for the infection, the organisms may have become resistant to the regimen, or the patient may have acquired an infection with other non-bacterial pathogens such as herpesviruses or invasive fungi.

Recently, considerable attention has been paid to 'risk stratification' – that is, to attempt to identify the subgroup of patients who might be safely managed with a more simplified, oral regimen (quinolone based or amoxicillin/clavulanate) that could be monitored on an outpatient basis. The challenge lies in the identification of this 'low risk' patient. Two major models – the Talcott[121] and the Multinational Association for Supportive Care in Cancer (MASCC)[122] – have attempted to do this; however, there are still limitations to this approach. Other innovative developments in this area include the evaluation of inflammatory markers and early-phase reactant proteins as adjunctive information in risk assessment. C-reactive protein, interleukin-6 (IL-6), IL-8, and procalcitonin are all hopeful candidate markers.[123–125]

Hematopoietic growth factors such as granulocyte and granulocyte-macrophage colony-stimulating factors (G-CSF and GM-CSF) have been shown to reduce the duration and severity of neutropenia following chemotherapy and therefore allow delivery of dose-intense therapy. With the increasing use of CHOP (cyclophosphamide, doxorubicin, vincristine, and prednisone) and CHOP-R (CHOP plus rituximab) chemotherapy for intermediate and high-grade lymphoma, the risk of developing fever and neutropenia in the absence of G-CSF is close to 50 percent. Current guidelines published by the American Society of Clinical Oncology (ASCO), National Comprehensive Cancer Network (NCCN), and European Organization for Research and Treatment of Cancer (EORTC) recommend that G-CSF should be used routinely when the following are likely: (1) a predicted overall FN risk of $\geq$20 percent; (2) a predicted overall FN risk of 10–20 percent in the presence of other factors, such as age greater than 65 years, previous FN, or advanced malignancy; (3) to maintain or escalate dose intensity; or (4) in the presence of severe sepsis.[126–128]

The role of prophylactic antibiotics in preventing fever and neutropenia remains controversial. The current IDSA guidelines caution strongly against their use, citing antibiotic resistance and colonization with fungi and other bacteria as major concerns.[117] However, two recently published, randomized controlled clinical trials assessing levofloxacin prophylaxis have shown a trend toward decrease in overall mortality without an increased rate of colonization or infection with resistant organisms.[129,130]

A significant decrease in the incidence of herpetic gingivostomatitis, pneumocystis pneumonia, CMV infection, and candidal infections has been demonstrated with the prophylactic use of antiviral, antiparasitic, and antifungal agents (namely acyclovir, trimethoprim-sulfamethoxazole, ganciclovir, and fluconazole) in neutropenic patients,[131–133] and in particularly intensive chemotherapy protocols or following bone marrow transplantation.

Anemia and thrombocytopenia

Chemotherapy-related temporary aplasia of the bone marrow is the most common cause of anemia in a patient with lymphoid malignancy. This anemia is further exaggerated by ongoing external blood losses that occur either in association with thrombocytopenia (epistaxis or occult gastrointestinal tract bleeding) or secondary to repeated sampling for diagnostic tests. Additionally, cancer patients usually have a component of the anemia of chronic disease as well, which is characterized by defective iron reutilization and diminished serum concentrations of erythropoietin.[134] Treatment of chemotherapy-associated anemia is usually with packed red cell transfusions, not only for symptomatic patients but also for those who have borderline hemoglobin (close to 8 g/dL) and have just received an intensive cycle of chemotherapy. Irradiated blood products are preferred to minimize the risk of transfusion-associated graft-versus-host disease. An alternative to blood transfusion that is currently being investigated is the use of the erythropoiesis-stimulating agents (ESAs).[135,136] Data from randomized, double-blind, placebo-controlled studies with epoetin alpha (150–300 units/kg three times weekly or 40 000–60 000 units once weekly) showed that epoetin alpha can effectively and safely achieve anemia treatment goals for the majority of patients with lymphoid malignancies. Data from clinical trials of darbopoietin, which has a longer half-life than epoetin alpha, also showed that it is effective in increasing hemoglobin level, reducing transfusions, and improving quality of life in patients with lymphoid malignancies.[137] A recently published systematic review of the literature by Shehata et al.[138] demonstrated that ESAs reduced transfusion requirements in patients with hematological malignancies. However, the data were not sufficient to assess the quality of life or confirm the inferior survival associated with ESAs.

Chemotherapy-associated bone marrow ablation is also the commonest cause of thrombocytopenia in a cancer patient. Severe thrombocytopenia (a count of less than 10 000 platelets/mm^3) puts patients at high risk for hemorrhage and must be treated with prophylactic platelet transfusions. These transfusions are not without risk and problems with refractoriness, transfusion reactions, alloimmunization, and hepatitis constantly have to be dealt with in patients who are undergoing chemotherapy. Several hematopoietic growth factors such as thrombopoietin, IL-3, IL-6, and IL-11 have been investigated.[139] The use of IL-1, IL-3, and IL-6 was abandoned due to toxicity and/or limited effectiveness. Clinical trials with the first generation of thrombopoietic growth factors – recombinant human thrombopoietin (TPO) and PEGylated recombinant human megakaryocyte growth and development factor – were promising in reducing thrombocytopenia following chemotherapy, but studies were also stopped due to the development of neutralizing antibodies to megakaryocyte growth and development factor.[140] New nonimmunogenic peptides and nonpeptide TPO agonists have entered clinical trials and appear to be promising: romiplostim, a peptibody already approved for clinical use in the USA; and eltrombopag, an oral nonpeptide agonist of the thrombopoietic receptor.[141] Eltrombopag was effective in increasing the platelet count in healthy subjects, in patients with relapsed or refractory immune thrombocytopenia, and in patients with hepatitis C virus infection and cirrhosis. Side effects were similar between both the eltrombopag and placebo arms.[142–144]

Typhlitis/neutropenic enterocolitis

Typhlitis is a life-threatening gastrointestinal complication of aggressive chemotherapy, most often associated with leukemia or lymphoma.[145] Typhlitis, from the Greek word typhlon, meaning cecum, is a necrotizing inflammation of the cecum, sometimes extending into the ileum and ascending colon. Other terms used for typhlitis include neutropenic enterocolitis, necrotizing enterocolitis, and ileocecal syndrome. Bacterial invasion of the mucosa is responsible for the inflammation, which can rapidly progress to infarction and perforation. Various organisms, alone or in combination, have been identified in surgical specimens and peritoneal fluid, including Clostridium septicum (most commonly implicated) followed by Pseudomonas aeruginosa, other Gram-negative rods, Gram-positive cocci, enterococci, Candida, and CMV.[146–148] Clostridium difficile toxin is occasionally detected in the stools.[148]

Typhlitis occurs specifically in immunodeficient patients, usually in the setting of severe neutropenia. Initially described as a complication of leukemia,[147,149,150] it has subsequently been associated with lymphoma,[149] aplastic anemia,[151] immunosuppression following renal transplantation,[152] the use of aggressive chemotherapy in patients with solid tumors,[153,154] and in association with the acquired immune deficiency syndrome.[155] The pathogenesis of typhlitis is multifactorial. Implicating factors (besides those just mentioned) include intramural hemorrhage and massive bacterial invasion.[146,147,150,154] However, severe neutropenia and the microbiologic environment of the colon are the two most essential predisposing conditions necessary for the development of typhlitis. The cecum seems to be the most vulnerable site compared to other parts of the large intestine because of its unique properties, namely, decreased vascular perfusion, decreased lymphatic drainage, and greater distensibility and wall tension.[147,149] Direct cytotoxicity to the cecal mucosa from aggressive chemotherapy, utilizing drugs such as cytosine arabinoside (Ara-C), doxorubicin, methotrexate, prednisone, and taxol etc., results in breaks in the cecal mucosa, which then serve as portals of entry for bacteria.[147,153,154]

Typhlitis is defined clinically as fever with abdominal pain, usually in the right lower quadrant, in the setting of grade 4 neutropenia (absolute neutrophil count less than 500 per mm^3). It has, however, been seen to present in the absence of fever.[156] Other accompanying findings include nausea and vomiting, abdominal distension, diarrhea, rebound tenderness, and occult blood in the stool.[153] The diagnosis is usually confirmed by ultrasound[157] or CT scan.[158] Ultrasound findings of the characteristic 'target' or 'halo' sign of a solid mass with an echogenic center (collapsed mucosa and intestinal contents) and hypoechoic periphery (thickened bowel wall) in the setting of abdominal pain in a neutropenic patient is diagnostic of typhlitis. Computed tomography findings in typhlitis usually include symmetric bowel wall thickening, pericecal inflammation, and, if perforation has occurred, a pericecal soft tissue mass. Recently, bowel wall thickening has been shown to be an important diagnostic and prognostic marker for typhlitis.[159] Demonstration of bowel wall thickening of more than 4 mm by ultrasound or CT scan in association with fever and abdominal pain is considered diagnostic for typhlitis; if greater than 10 mm, it may be predictive of increased mortality.[159]

The management of neutropenic enterocolitis is controversial, especially with regard to the necessity and timing of surgical intervention.[150,160] However, in recent years, initial conservative management has become more acceptable.[153] Mortality is high, in the range of 50 percent to almost 100 percent, with either surgical intervention or conservative treatment. If diagnosed early, a majority of patients can be managed medically with bowel rest, nasogastric suction, total parenteral nutrition, and broad-spectrum antibiotics, including anaerobic coverage (clindamycin, metronidazole, imipenem) to cover for Gram-negative pathogens and gastrointestinal anaerobes. Granulocyte colony-stimulating factor has been recommended to hasten recovery of cell counts which would promote bowel wall healing.[148] Surgery is indicated in the face of clinical deterioration in spite of intensive medical management, massive bleeding, or perforation.

Patients who do not fit the description of typhlitis but have signs and symptoms of enterocolitis may have antibiotic-related pseudomembranous or clostridial enterocolitis.

Neurological complications following chemotherapy

Neurological complications in the form of transient seizures, encephalopathy, and ascending myelopathy have been described in patients following the systemic or intrathecal administration of chemotherapeutic agents such as methotrexate, Ara-C, cisplatin, and ifosfamide, all of which are extremely effective drugs for the treatment of various high-grade lymphomas and leukemias.[161–164] Methotrexate and Ara-C continue to remain the two most commonly implicated drugs. However, these complications are uncommon, being seen in fewer than 3 percent of the patients receiving these agents.[161,164] More recently, rituximab-associated hyperammonemic encephalopathy has been described.[165]

Seizures, in most instances, occur as a result of the direct effect of the drug on the CNS. They can be seen either following the use of systemic high-dose chemotherapy (in particular, methotrexate, Ara-C, or ifosfamide) with or without associated intrathecal therapy, or following chemotherapy in patients who have received a prior insult such as previous cranial irradiation.[50,162] Focal or generalized seizures can also occur as a result of metabolic abnormalities, such as SIADH or other electrolyte disturbances, after the administration of drugs such as vincristine, cyclophosphamide, and cisplatin. Most chemotherapy-related seizures are usually transient in nature, may be associated with temporary abnormalities on CT or MRI scans, and, once controlled, seldom require antiseizure medication for more than a few months.

Much more serious neurological complications are acute encephalopathy following the use of high-dose methotrexate and/or Ara-C, and myelopathy following the intrathecal administration of the same drugs, either together or separately.[161–164] Myelopathy is the most frequently cited serious neurological complication of intrathecal Ara-C and methotrexate therapy. Prolonged drug clearance as a result of leptomeningeal tumor, the presence of preservatives in these chemotherapeutic agents (e.g., benzyl alcohol), total cumulative intrathecal dose, and other causes of reduced CSF flow have also been implicated as being contributory.[161,162,166] Patients with this syndrome characteristically present within a few days to a week after the administration of chemotherapy with symptoms of radicular or back pain, weakness of the extremities, numbness, paresthesias, or sphincter dysfunction, which can rapidly progress in some cases to paraplegia or quadriplegia. If there is associated encephalopathy, cranial nerve palsies, ataxia, visual impairment, seizures, and coma may also ensue. A CT scan of the brain may initially be normal, but the more sensitive MRI scan may show swelling of the thoracic or lumbar spinal cord or the presence of other transient abnormalities such as 'venous infarcts.' Cerebrospinal fluid examination is usually significant for an elevation of the total protein, with a marked elevation in the level of the myelin basic protein content (which is barely detectable in the CSF of normal subjects). Rising levels of this protein are found to correlate with disease progression.[167] In most cases, the patient's neurological symptoms improve after the initial event and there is a corresponding fall in the myelin basic protein level. However, there are several reports of fatal outcomes and irreversible neurological damage.[161–164,166,167]

Subacute or acute myeloencephalopathy is a rare, serious neurological side effect, the mechanism of which is poorly understood. Thus it is difficult to make recommendations for its prevention. However, it has been suggested that an interval of 48–72 hours between successive doses of intrathecal therapy,[162,163] along with serial determination of CSF myelin basic protein, in patients at risk for developing treatment-related neurotoxicity[167] may help lower the chances of developing this complication.

Another set of neurological complications seen in patients receiving vincristine includes peripheral neuropathy and cranial nerve palsies. The neuropathy is usually confined to the hands and feet (glove and stocking pattern), but may be more severe at times.[168] Severe vincristine neuropathy may also manifest as palatal palsy, rarely vocal cord paralysis, and ptosis.[169] A complete neurological examination should be performed on every patient prior to administration of each dose of vincristine.

Metabolic complications

Treatment of the underlying leukemia or lymphoma can result in certain metabolic complications such as SIADH and hyperglycemia. Both these complications are drug related and easily correctable. The most common cause of SIADH in oncology is the administration of chemotherapeutic agents such as vincristine, cyclophosphamide, or morphine.[170] SIADH usually coincides with severe vincristine neurotoxicity, suggesting a direct effect on the supraoptic nuclei, while cyclophosphamide reduces free water clearance. This effect of cyclophosphamide is especially difficult to manage in the face of the aggressive hydration needed to prevent hemorrhagic cystitis.

Fluid restriction is all that is needed in patients who are asymptomatic and have a serum sodium concentration of more than 120 mEq/L. With fluid restriction, imperceptible water losses lead to equilibration of the serum osmolality and sodium concentration. In patients who present with seizures or coma and have a serum sodium concentration of less than 120 mEq/L, fluid restriction along with furosemide and intravenous administration of hypertonic saline (200–300 mL of 3 percent NaCl) infused over several hours can correct the situation in about 6 hours. However, the serum sodium level should be monitored carefully to ensure that it does not increase by more than 1 mEq/L/hour, as a rapid rise can lead to central pontine myelinolysis. In the occasional patient who is unresponsive to fluid restriction, demeclocycline may be necessary. Demeclocycline in a dose of 200–300 mg 2–3 times per day causes dose-dependent, reversible, nephrogenic diabetes insipidus, which counteracts the effect of vasopressin on the kidney.

Hyperglycemia is another troublesome treatment-related complication that is frequently encountered in practice. It usually occurs as a result of the administration of steroids (either for the treatment of the lymphoid malignancy or prevention of emesis) alone, or in conjunction with dextrose-containing intravenous fluids and other chemotherapeutic agents such as asparaginase. The hyperglycemia can usually be controlled by a reduction in the dose of the steroid; rarely, insulin may be required where a dose reduction is not possible or is ineffective.

Cardiac complications

Most treatment protocols for leukemia and lymphomas today (including CHOP) utilize anthracycline antibiotics such as doxorubicin and daunorubicin. Clinical use of these agents can be associated with both an acute and a chronic cardiomyopathy that is often debilitating and not infrequently fatal.[171] It is hypothesized that one of the mechanisms of cardiac toxicity is the result of anthracycline activation by the cardiac mitochondria, causing the anthracyclines to release toxic free radicals which are cardiotoxic.[172,173] Factors that can increase the risk of cardiomyopathy in patients receiving anthracyclines include mediastinal radiation therapy, uncontrolled hypertension, administration of individual doses of anthracyclines more than 50 mg/m^2 every 3–4 weeks, cumulative dose of doxorubicin greater than 200 mg/m^2, age greater than 65 years,

and the coadministration of other chemotherapeutic agents such as cyclophosphamide in high doses.[171,173]

Acutely, patients may present with arrhythmias and conduction abnormalities, which can range in severity from benign supraventricular tachycardia to complete heart block. Another manifestation of acute toxicity sometimes seen within a short interval of anthracycline administration is the 'myocarditis-pericarditis syndrome' which, in its most severe form, is characterized by the onset of florid congestive heart failure and pericarditis. Patients who develop this syndrome present with an acute and steep decline in their left ventricular function (documented by radionuclide cineangiography multiple-gated acquisition [MUGA]), which in most cases is transient. Near-complete recovery is usually seen although, in the rare case, death may ensue rapidly.[173]

Since anthracycline-induced cardiomyopathy is a direct consequence of reduced myocardial contractility, it is important to measure the change in contractility at periodic intervals while the patient is on therapy. Although no method by itself is 100 percent accurate, the commonly used tests include echocardiography (which measures the shortening fraction) and MUGA (which measures the ejection fraction). Guidelines for stopping anthracyclines include an ejection fraction of less than 45 percent, a shortening fraction of 30 percent or less, or a drop of greater than 15 percent in the ejection fraction from pretreatment values.

Nausea and vomiting

Nausea and vomiting are two of the most distressing side effects of cancer chemotherapy encountered today, and when severe and prolonged can result in pronounced physiological debilitation and psychological distress.

Numerous chemotherapeutic agents used in the treatment of lymphoid malignancies can cause nausea and vomiting. A list of the emetogenic potential of various chemotherapeutic agents is presented in Table 49.8.

Various different antiemetic regimens have been evaluated over the years. In randomized, comparative clinical trials, high and repeated doses of corticosteroids have been consistently shown to be effective and well tolerated.[174,175] In patients undergoing moderately emetogenic chemotherapy, dexamethasone and methylprednisolone have been found to be superior to the phenothiazines.[176] The development of the highly effective antiemetogenic agents – the serotonin (5-hydroxytryptamine [5-HT]) 5-HT3 receptor antagonists – in the 1990s was one of the most significant advances in the management of this problem. Recently, ASCO, NCCN, and MASCC updated their antiemetic guidelines to include, in addition to the above-mentioned agents, aprepitant, the first drug in another class of antiemetics – the neurokinin-1 receptor antagonists.[177] Table 49.9 outlines some of the commonly used antiemetic agents/regimens.

Table 49.8 Emetogenic potential of selected chemotherapeutic agents and time course of the nausea and vomiting

	Onset (h)	Duration (h)
I. Very high emetogenic potential (>90%)		
Cisplatin	1–4	12–96
Cyclophosphamide	6–8	8–24
Cytarabine	1–3	3–8
Dacarbazine	1–2	2–4
II. High emetogenic potential (60%–90%)		
Carboplatin	2–6	1–48
Carmustine	2–6	4–6
Dactinomycin	2–5	4–24
Daunorubicin	1–3	4–24
Doxorubicin	1–3	4–24
III. Moderate emetogenic potential (30%–60%)		
Ifosfamide	2–3	12–72
Etoposide	2–3	8–12
Epirubicin	1–3	4–24
Asparaginase	2–4	8–24
IV. Low emetogenic potential (0%–30%)		
Methotrexate	–	–
6-Mercaptopurine	–	–
Vincristine	–	–

Mucositis

Oropharyngeal mucositis is a major complication of intensive chemotherapy regimens, radiation to the head and neck area, and bone marrow transplantation.[178–180] Not only can it be severe enough to cause debilitating pain and interfere with swallowing, speech, and nutrition, it can also be a site of bleeding (especially in the severely thrombocytopenic patient) or portal of entry for systemic infection.

Normally, the oral mucosa is regenerated every 7–14 days. Both chemotherapy and radiation therapy can interfere with cellular mitosis and reduce the ability of the oral mucosa to regenerate. Oral complications can begin as early as 3 days following the administration of chemotherapy or radiation and typically include dryness (xerostomia), generalized mucosal erythema with associated pain and dysphagia (mucositis), gingival bleeding, and discrete oral ulcerations (stomatitis).

Stomatitis is most frequently associated with the cell cycle-specific agents – that is, the antibiotics, antimetabolites, and alkylating agents such as daunorubicin, doxorubicin, bleomycin, dactinomycin, 5-fluorouracil, methotrexate, and melphalan. Oral problems due to radiation therapy are the result of local tissue changes from direct radiation to the head and neck, and the severity of mucositis depends on the type of

ionizing radiation, the volume of irradiated tissue, the dose per day, and the cumulative dose.

To assess the severity of the mucositis, both in terms of pain and the ability of the patient to maintain adequate nutritional intake, a mucositis grading system can be helpful. Commonly used grading systems include the National Cancer Institute scale for oral mucositis and the Oral Mucositis Assessment Scale (OMAS) shown in Table 49.10.[179,181]

There is no standardized approach for the prevention and treatment of chemotherapy- and radiation-induced mucositis. Effective prevention of mucositis requires a comprehensive oral examination of the patient (preferably prior to or soon after commencement of chemotherapy) to identify problems such as poor oral hygiene, peridontal disease, dental caries, orthodontic appliances, ill-fitting prostheses, and any other potential source of infection. Other prophylactic measures usually employed at the onset of chemotherapy include chlorhexidine (Peridex), saline and sodium bicarbonate rinses, and, at some centers, oral acyclovir and nystatin/fluconazole for herpetic or fungal infections.

Regimens frequently used (with varying degrees of success) for the treatment of mucositis and its associated pain include (either alone or in combination) a local anesthetic such as lidocaine or Dyclone, Maalox or Mylanta, diphenhydramine, nystatin, or sucralfate. Other less commonly used agents include allopurinol, topical capsaicin, vitamin E mouthwash, prostaglandins, and antibiotics. Prolonged administration of oral and parenteral narcotics is required in cases of severe mucositis. Targeted approaches to prevent mucositis include the development of promising agents such as palifermin, a human recombinant keratinocyte growth factor[181] currently in clinical trials, and repifermin and velafermin, two other human growth factors.[182]

Central line-related complications

Indwelling temporary central venous catheters and long-term silastic venous catheters, such as Hickman and Broviac catheters, have become ubiquitous with the treatment of cancer today. However, these devices are not free of complications; the frequently encountered complications in association with these catheters include infection, thrombosis, and SVCS. Only the first two of these complications will be discussed briefly in this section as SVCS has been discussed in detail previously.

Although Gram-positive bacteria (particularly coagulase-negative staphylococci and *Staphylococcus aureus*) are the commonest causes of catheter-related infections, other organisms such as resistant corynebacteria (CDC-JK), *Bacillus* species, atypical mycobacteria, Gram-negative organisms (especially *Acinetobacter* species, *Pseudomonas*, *Enterobacter*, *Klebsiella*, and *Stenotrophomonas*), and fungi can occasionally be the offending agents as well.[108,183]

The majority of catheter-related bacteremias, especially those associated with coagulase-negative staphylococci, can usually be treated with appropriate antibiotics

Table 49.9 Commonly prescribed antiemetic agents

Drug	Indication	Side effects
Serotonin antagonists Dolasetron (Anzemet) Granisetron (Kytril) Ondansetron (Zofran) Palonosetron (Aloxi)	Acute and delayed emesis	Headache, fatigue, constipation
NK–1 antagonist Aprepitant (Emend)	Acute and delayed emesis	Drug interactions with corticosteroids, warfarin

Corticosteroids
Dexamethasone (Decadron)
Methylprednisolone
   (Solumedrol)
	Acute and delayed emesis	Aprepitant increases the AUC of dexamethasone
		Best used in combination with other antiemetic
		   agents, e.g., ondansetron and metoclopramide

Dopamine antagonists Droperidol (Inapsine) Haloperidol (Haldol) Metoclopramide (Reglan) Prochlorperazine (Compazine) Promethazine (Phenargan)	Breakthrough emesis	Drowsiness, dizziness, extrapyramidal side effects, anticholinergic side effects

Miscellaneous medications
Dronabinol (Marinol)
Lorazepam (Ativan)
Olanzepine (Zyprexa)
	Refractory emesis
	Breakthrough emesis
	Acute, delayed,
	   breakthrough emesis
		Sedation, dizziness, confusion, euphoria
		Sedation, respiratory depression
		Sedation, extrapyramidal side effects,
		   hyperglycemia

Adjunctive agents Diphenhydramine (Benadryl)	Breakthrough emesis	Use with Reglan and Phenargan to prevent extrapyramidal side effects

Modified with permission. Jordan K, Sippel C, Schmoll HJ. Guidelines for antiemetic treatment of chemotherapy-induced nausea and vomiting: past, present, and future recommendations. *Oncologist* 2007; 12: 1143–50.
NK, neurokinin; AUC, area under the curve.

Table 49.10 National Cancer Institute grading system for oral mucositis

Grade 0	No mucositis
Grade 1	Painless ulcers, erythema, or mild soreness
Grade 2	Painful erythema, edema, or ulcers; can eat
Grade 3	Painful erythema, edema, or ulcers; cannot eat
Grade 4	Patient requires parenteral or enteral support

(e.g., vancomycin) and do not necessitate catheter removal from patients. It is recommended, though, that the antibiotic infusions be rotated amongst the different ports in a multilumen catheter for complete eradication of the organism.[108] However, in the face of bacteremia lasting more than 48 hours, the catheter should be removed. *Bacillus* species and *Candida albicans* are more difficult to eradicate with antibiotics alone, and when they are isolated, the catheter should be removed promptly. Other infections that necessitate line removal include exit-site infections and bacteremia with Gram-negative bacteria (e.g., *Stenotrophomonas, Pseudomonas aeruginosa*), mycobacteria (e.g., *Mycobacterium cheloneii*), and fungi (*Aspergillus*), and tunnel infections.[184]

Thrombosis of the central veins is a recognized complication of central venous catheters.[185,186] The incidence of clinical thrombosis associated with catheters is reported to be anywhere from 4 to 12 percent[185] and recombinant tissue plasminogen activator or urokinase are routinely recommended to clear this thrombo-occlusion.[186] Deep venous thrombosis of the arm has also been reported in patients with central indwelling catheters.[187] As the risk of pulmonary embolism is high in this situation, anticoagulants should be instituted as soon as the diagnosis is established (with the help of venography and CT scan with contrast media) in order to minimize clot propagation, allow collateral channels to remain open, and reduce the risk of pulmonary embolism. Good results have been reported when thrombolytic agents are given together with anticoagulants in the early stages.[188] Another frequently encountered complication in immunosuppressed patients in intensive care units is that of septic venous thrombosis (the simultaneous occurrence of central venous catheter infection, central venous thrombosis, and ongoing bacteremia after removal of the catheter). Therapy for this serious complication includes a prolonged course of intravenous antibiotics and full-dose heparinization after prompt removal of the catheter.[189]

KEY POINTS

- With the current trend of treating lymphoid malignancies more aggressively, an increasing number of patients are at risk for complications arising either from the disease itself or as unwanted side effects of treatment.

- Successful management of lymphoid malignancies therefore involves not only the administration of specific therapy, but the treatment of these complications, which may occur before or during treatment, or years later.

- These complications can therefore be categorized as either tumor-related complications or treatment-related complications.

- Among the tumor-related complications, superior vena cava syndrome (SVCS), spinal cord compression, acute gastrointestinal bleeding and tumor lysis syndrome are some of the acute oncological emergencies that can prove to be life threatening unless recognized and treated promptly.

- Fever and neutropenia still remains the leading treatment-related complication associated with significant morbidity and mortality receiving chemotherapy.

- In this chapter, we have attempted to provide an updated overview of the most common disease or treatment-related complications that oncologists encounter in their practice. New advance in the management of complications such as tumor lysis syndrome, febrile neutropenia, and nausea and vomiting have been discussed in detail.

REFERENCES

● = Key primary paper
◆ = Major review article

1. Halpern S, Chatten J, Meadows AT *et al.* Anterior mediastinal masses: anesthesia hazards and other problems. *J Pediatr* 1983; **102**: 407–10.

2. Loeffler JS, Leopold KA, Recht A *et al.* Emergency prebiopsy radiation for mediastinal masses: impact on subsequent pathologic diagnosis and outcome. *J Clin Oncol* 1986; **4**: 716–21.

3. Ostler PJ, Clarke DP, Watkinson AF, Gaze MN. Superior vena cava obstruction: a modern management strategy. *Clin Oncol (R Coll Radiol)* 1997; **9**: 83–9.

4. Hunter W. History of aneurysm in the aorta with some remarks on aneurysm in general. *Med Obser Inq* 1757; **1**: 323–57.

5. Chen JC, Bongard F, Klein SR. A contemporary perspective on superior vena cava syndrome. *Am J Surg* 1990; **160**: 207–11.

6. Parish JM, Marschke RF Jr, Dines DE, Lee RE. Etiologic considerations in superior vena cava syndrome. *Mayo Clin Proc* 1981; **56**: 407–13.

7. Armstrong BA, Perez CA, Simpson JR, Hedermn MA. Role of irradiation in the management of superior vena cava syndrome. *Int J Radiat Oncol Biol Phys* 1987; **13**: 531–9.

8. Wilson LD, Detterbeck FC, Yahalom J. Clinical practice. Superior vena cava syndrome with malignant causes. *N Engl J Med* 2007; **356**: 1862–9.

●9. Rice TW, Rodriguez RM, Light RW. The superior vena cava syndrome: clinical characteristics and evolving etiology. *Medicine (Baltimore)* 2006; **85**: 37–42.

10. Pokorny WJ, Sherman JO. Mediastinal masses in infants and children. *J Thorac Cardiovasc Surg* 1974; **68**: 869–75.

11. King RM, Telander RL, Smithson WA *et al.* Primary mediastinal tumors in children. *J Pediatr Surg* 1982; **17**: 512–20.

12. Issa PY, Brihi ER, Janin Y, Slim MS. Superior vena cava syndrome in childhood: report of ten cases and review of the literature. *Pediatrics* 1983; **71**: 337–41.

13. Simpson I, Campbell PE. Mediastinal masses in childhood: a review from a paediatric pathologist's point of view. *Prog Pediatr Surg* 1991; **27**: 92–126.

14. Nieto AF, Doty DB. Superior vena cava obstruction: clinical syndrome, etiology, and treatment. *Curr Probl Cancer* 1986; **10**: 441–84.

15. Yellin A, Mandel M, Rechavi G *et al.* Superior vena cava syndrome associated with lymphoma. *Am J Dis Child* 1992; **146**: 1060–63.

16. Lochridge SK, Knibbe WP, Doty DB. Obstruction of the superior vena cava. *Surgery* 1979; **85**: 14–24.

17. O'Brien RT, Matlak ME, Condon VR, Johnson DG. Superior vena cava syndrome in children. *West J Med* 1981; **135**: 143–7.

18. Levitt SH, Jones TK Jr, Kilpatrick SJ Jr, Bogardus CR Jr. Treatment of malignant superior vena caval obstruction. A randomized study. *Cancer* 1969; **24**: 447–51.

19. Ahmann FR. A reassessment of the clinical implications of the superior vena caval syndrome. *J Clin Oncol* 1984; **2**: 961–9.

20. Carabell G. Superior vena cava syndrome. In: Devita MS, Rosenberg VT Jr. (eds) *Principles and practice of oncology.* New York: Lippincott, 1985: 1855–60.

21. Abner A. Approach to the patient who presents with superior vena cava obstruction. *Chest* 1993; **103**(4 Suppl): 394S–7S.

22. Stanford W, Doty DB. The role of venography and surgery in the management of patients with superior vena cava obstruction. *Ann Thorac Surg* 1986; **41**: 158–63.

23. Stanford W, Jolles H, Ell S, Chiu LC. Superior vena cava obstruction: a venographic classification. *AJR Am J Roentgenol* 1987; **148**: 259–62.

24. Webb WR, Sostman HD. MR imaging of thoracic disease: clinical uses. *Radiology* 1992; **182**: 621–30.

25. Khimji T, Zeiss J. MRI versus CT and US in the evaluation of a patient presenting with superior vena cava syndrome. Case report. *Clin Imaging* 1992; **16**: 269–71.

26. Lin EC, Quaife RA. FDG uptake in chronic superior vena cava thrombus on positron emission tomographic imaging. *Clin Nucl Med* 2001; **26**: 241–2.

27. Markman M. Common complications and emergencies associated with cancer and its therapy. *Cleve Clin J Med* 1994; **61**: 105–14; quiz 162.

28. Northrip DR, Bohman BK, Tsueda K. Total airway occlusion and superior vena cava syndrome in a child with an anterior mediastinal tumor. *Anesth Analg* 1986; **65**: 1079–82.

29. Jahangiri M, Taggart DP, Goldstraw P. Role of mediastinoscopy in superior vena cava obstruction. *Cancer* 1993; **71**: 3006–8.

30. Yellin A, Rosen A, Reichert N, Lieberman Y. Superior vena cava syndrome. The myth–the facts. *Am Rev Respir Dis* 1990; **141**: 1114–8.

31. Ko JC, Yang PC, Yuan A *et al.* Superior vena cava syndrome. Rapid histologic diagnosis by ultrasound-guided transthoracic needle aspiration biopsy. *Am J Respir Crit Care Med* 1994; **149**: 783–7.

32. Levitt LJ, Dawson DM, Rosenthal DS, Moloney WC. CNS involvement in the non-Hodgkin's lymphomas. *Cancer* 1980; **45**: 545–52.

33. Baker GL, Barnes HJ. Superior vena cava syndrome: etiology, diagnosis, and treatment. *Am J Crit Care* 1992; **1**: 54–64.

34. Gauden SJ. Superior vena cava syndrome induced by bronchogenic carcinoma: is this an oncological emergency? *Australas Radiol* 1993; **37**: 363–6.

35. Nicholson AA, Ettles DF, Arnold A *et al.* Treatment of malignant superior vena cava obstruction: metal stents or radiation therapy. *J Vasc Interv Radiol* 1997; **8**: 781–8.

36. Young RC, Howser DM, Anderson T *et al.* Central nervous system complications of non-Hodgkin's lymphoma. The potential role for prophylactic therapy. *Am J Med* 1979; **66**: 435–43.

37. Eeles RA, O'Brien P, Horwich A, Brada M. Non-Hodgkin's lymphoma presenting with extradural spinal cord compression: functional outcome and survival. *Br J Cancer* 1991; **63**: 126–9.

38. Correale J, Monteverde DA, Bueri JA, Reich EG. Peripheral nervous system and spinal cord involvement in lymphoma. *Acta Neurol Scand* 1991; **83**: 45–51.

39. Lyons MK, O'Neill BP, Marsh WR, Kurtin PJ. Primary spinal epidural non-Hodgkin's lymphoma: report of eight patients and review of the literature. *Neurosurgery* 1992; **30**: 675–80.

40. Perry JR, Deodhare SS, Bilbao JM *et al.* The significance of spinal cord compression as the initial manifestation of lymphoma. *Neurosurgery* 1993; **32**: 157–62.

41. Lewis DW, Packer RJ, Raney B *et al.* Incidence, presentation, and outcome of spinal cord disease in children with systemic cancer. *Pediatrics* 1986; **78**: 438–43.

42. Aysun S, Topçu M, Günay M, Topaloğlu H. Neurologic features as initial presentations of childhood malignancies. *Pediatr Neurol* 1994; **10**: 40–3.

43. Oviatt DL, Kirshner HS, Stein RS. Successful chemotherapeutic treatment of epidural compression in non-Hodgkin's lymphoma. *Cancer* 1982; **49**: 2446–8.

44. Spiess JL, Adelstein DJ, Hines JD. Multiple myeloma presenting with spinal cord compression. *Oncology* 1988; **45**: 88–92.

45. Laing RJ, Jakubowski J, Kunkler IH, Hancock BW. Primary spinal presentation of non-Hodgkin's lymphoma. A reappraisal of management and prognosis. *Spine* 1992; **17**: 117–20.

46. Haddad P, Thaell JF, Kiely JM *et al.* Lymphoma of the spinal extradural space. *Cancer* 1976; **38**: 1862–6.

47. Botterell EH, Fitzgerald GW. Spinal cord compression produced by extradural malignant tumours; early recognition, treatment and results. *Can Med Assoc J* 1959; **80**: 791–6.

48. Friedman M, Kim TH, Panahon AM. Spinal cord compression in malignant lymphoma. Treatment and results. *Cancer* 1976; **37**: 1485–91.

49. McKenna RJ Jr, Ali MK, Ewer MS, Frazier OH. Pleural and pericardial effusions in cancer patients. *Curr Probl Cancer* 1985; **9**: 1–44.

50. Lange B, D'Angio GJ. Oncologic emergencies. In: Pizzo PA, Poplack DG. (eds) *Principles and practice of pediatric oncology.* Philadelphia: JB Lippincott, 1993: 951–72.

51. Salyer WR, Eggleston JC, Erozan YS. Efficacy of pleural needle biopsy and pleural fluid cytopathology in the diagnosis of malignant neoplasm involving the pleura. *Chest* 1975; **67**: 536–9.

52. Davis S, Rambotti P, Grignani F. Intrapericardial tetracycline sclerosis in the treatment of malignant pericardial effusion: an analysis of thirty-three cases. *J Clin Oncol* 1984; **2**: 631–6.

53. Shepherd FA, Ginsberg JS, Evans WK *et al.* Tetracycline sclerosis in the management of malignant pericardial effusion. *J Clin Oncol* 1985; **3**: 1678–82.

54. Spain RC, Whittlesey D. Respiratory emergencies in patients with cancer. *Semin Oncol* 1989; **16**: 471–89.

55. Walker-Renard PB, Vaughan LM, Sahn SA. Chemical pleurodesis for malignant pleural effusions. *Ann Intern Med* 1994; **120**: 56–64.

●56. Hsu LH, Soong TC, Feng AC, Liu MC. Intrapleural urokinase for the treatment of loculated malignant pleural effusions and trapped lungs in medically inoperable cancer patients. *J Thorac Oncol* 2006; **1**: 460–67.

●57. Fiocco M, Krasna MJ. The management of malignant pleural and pericardial effusions. *Hematol Oncol Clin North Am* 1997; **11**: 253–65.

58. Haddad R, Paul P. Pericardial effusion: a rare complication of multiple myeloma. Presented at 37th Annual Meeting of the American Society of Clinical Oncology, San Francisco, CA, 2001; abstract 2692.

59. Talreja D, Slater LM, Dara P *et al.* Multiple myeloma complicated by myelomatous obstructive uropathy. *Cancer* 1980; **46**: 1893–5.

◆60. Shad AT, Magrath I. Diagnosis and treatment of NHL in childhood. In: Wernik P. (ed.) *Neoplastic diseases of the blood.* Edinburgh: Churchill Livingstone, 1995: 925–62.

61. Braylan RC, Jaffe ES, Triche TJ *et al.* Structural and functional properties of the 'hairy' cells of leukemic reticuloendotheliosis. *Cancer* 1978; **41**: 210–27.

62. Lynch EC. Uric acid metabolism in proliferative diseases of the marrow. *Arch Intern Med* 1962; **109**: 639–53.

63. Murphy SB, Melvin SL, Mauer AM. Correlation of tumor cell kinetic studies with surface marker results in childhood non-Hodgkin's lymphoma. *Cancer Res* 1979; **39**: 1534–8.

64. Chasty RC, Liu-Yin JA. Acute tumour lysis syndrome. *Br J Hosp Med* 1993; **49**: 488–92.

65. Fleming DR, Doukas MA. Acute tumor lysis syndrome in hematologic malignancies. *Leuk Lymphoma* 1992; **8**: 315–8.

66. Hande KR, Garrow GC. Acute tumor lysis syndrome in patients with high-grade non-Hodgkin's lymphoma. *Am J Med* 1993; **94**: 133–9.

67. Veenstra J, Krediet RT, Somers R, Arisz L. Tumour lysis syndrome and acute renal failure in Burkitt's lymphoma. Description of 2 cases and a review of the literature on prevention and management. *Neth J Med* 1994; **45**: 211–6.

68. Hande K. Hyperuricemia uric acid nephropathy–the tumor lysis syndrome. In: Mckinney T. (ed.) *Renal complications of neoplasia*. New York: Praeger Scientific, 1986: 134–56.

69. Primikirios N, Stutzman L, Sandberg AA. Uric acid excretion in patients with malignant lymphomas. *Blood* 1961; **17**: 701–18.

70. Cohen LF, Balow JE, Magrath IT *et al*. Acute tumor lysis syndrome. A review of 37 patients with Burkitt's lymphoma. *Am J Med* 1980; **68**: 486–91.

71. Krakoff IH, Meyer RL. Prevention of hyperuricemia in leukemia and lymphoma: use of alopurinol, a xanthine oxidase inhibitor. *JAMA* 1965; **193**: 1–6.

72. Tsokos GC, Balow JE, Spiegel RJ, Magrath IT. Renal and metabolic complications of undifferentiated and lymphoblastic lymphomas. *Medicine (Baltimore)* 1981; **60**: 218–29.

♦73. Cairo MS, Bishop M. Tumour lysis syndrome: new therapeutic strategies and classification. *Br J Haematol* 2004; **127**: 3–11.

74. Ten Harkel AD, Kist-Van Holthe JE, Van Weel M, Van der Vorst MM. Alkalinization and the tumor lysis syndrome. *Med Pediatr Oncol* 1998; **31**: 27–8.

♦75. Coiffier B, Altman A, Pui CH *et al*. Guidelines for the management of pediatric and adult tumor lysis syndrome: an evidence-based review. *J Clin Oncol* 2008; **26**: 2767–78.

76. Hande KR, Hixson CV, Chabner BA. Postchemotherapy purine excretion in lymphoma patients receiving allopurinol. *Cancer Res* 1981; **41**: 2273–9.

77. Ablin A, Stephens BG, Hirata T *et al*. Nephropathy, xanthinuria, and orotic aciduria complicating Burkitt's lymphoma treated with chemotherapy and allopurinol. *Metabolism* 1972; **21**: 771–8.

78. Brogard JM, Coumaros D, Franckhauser J *et al*. Enzymatic uricolysis: a study of the effect of a fungal urate-oxydase. *Rev Eur Etud Clin Biol* 1972; **17**: 890–95.

●79. Patte C, Sakiroglu C, Ansoborlo S *et al*. Urate-oxidase in the prevention and treatment of metabolic complications in patients with B-cell lymphoma and leukemia, treated in the Societe Francaise d'Oncologie Pediatrique LMB89 protocol. *Ann Oncol* 2002; **13**: 789–95.

●80. Pui CH, Mahmoud HH, Wiley JM *et al*. Recombinant urate oxidase for the prophylaxis or treatment of hyperuricemia in patients With leukemia or lymphoma. *J Clin Oncol* 2001; **19**: 697–704.

●81. Goldman SC, Holcenberg JS, Finklestein JZ *et al*. A randomized comparison between rasburicase and allopurinol in children with lymphoma or leukemia at high risk for tumor lysis. *Blood* 2001; **97**: 2998–3003.

♦82. Cairo MS. Recombinant urate oxidase (rasburicase): a new targeted therapy for prophylaxis and treatment of patients with hematologic malignancies at risk of tumor lysis syndrome. *Clin Lymphoma* 2003; **3**: 233–4.

83. Patte C, Philip T, Rodary C *et al*. High survival rate in advanced-stage B-cell lymphomas and leukemias without CNS involvement with a short intensive polychemotherapy: results from the French Pediatric Oncology Society of a randomized trial of 216 children. *J Clin Oncol* 1991; **9**: 123–32.

84. Hebert LA, Lemann J Jr, Petersen JR, Lennon EJ. Studies of the mechanism by which phosphate infusion lowers serum calcium concentration. *J Clin Invest* 1966; **45**: 1886–94.

85. Macher MA, Loirat C, Pillion G, Maisin A. Acute kidney failure caused by hyperphosphoremia in tumor lysis. *Arch Fr Pediatr* 1988; **45**: 271–4.

●86. Bajorunas DR. Clinical manifestations of cancer-related hypercalcemia. *Semin Oncol* 1990; **17**(2 Suppl 5): 16–25.

87. Leblanc A, Caillaud JM, Hartmann O *et al*. Hypercalcemia preferentially occurs in unusual forms of childhood non-Hodgkin's lymphoma, rhabdomyosarcoma, and Wilms' tumor. A study of 11 cases. *Cancer* 1984; **54**: 2132–6.

88. Spiegel A, Greene M, Magrath I *et al*. Hypercalcemia with suppressed parathyroid hormone in Burkitt's lymphoma. *Am J Med* 1978; **64**: 691–5.

♦89. Lumachi F, Brunello A, Roma A, Basso U. Medical treatment of malignancy-associated hypercalcemia. *Curr Med Chem* 2008; **15**: 415–21.

90. Besarab A, Caro JF. Mechanisms of hypercalcemia in malignancy. *Cancer* 1978; **41**: 2276–85.

91. Bull F. Hypercalcemia in cancer. In: *Oncologic emergencies*. Yarbro J, Bornstein R. (eds) New York: Grune and Stratton, 1981: 197–214.

92. Pimentel L. Medical complications of oncologic disease. *Emerg Med Clin North Am* 1993; **11**: 407–19.

93. Walji N, Chan AK, Peake DR. Common acute oncological emergencies: diagnosis, investigation and management. *Postgrad Med J* 2008; **84**: 418–27.

94. Suki WN, Yium JJ, Von Minden M *et al*. Acute treatment of hypercalcemia with furosemide. *N Engl J Med* 1970; **283**: 836–40.

95. Ralston SH, Gallacher SJ, Patel U *et al*. Cancer-associated hypercalcemia: morbidity and mortality. Clinical experience in 126 treated patients. *Ann Intern Med* 1990; **112**: 499–504.

●96. Bilezikian JP. Management of acute hypercalcemia. *N Engl J Med* 1992; **326**: 1196–203.

97. Gucalp R, Ritch P, Wiernik PH *et al*. Comparative study of pamidronate disodium and etidronate disodium in the treatment of cancer-related hypercalcemia. *J Clin Oncol* 1992; **10**: 134–42.

98. Warrell RP Jr, Israel R, Frisone M *et al.* Gallium nitrate for acute treatment of cancer-related hypercalcemia. A randomized, double-blind comparison to calcitonin. *Ann Intern Med* 1988; **108**: 669–74.

99. Kemeny MM, Magrath IT, Brennan MF. The role of surgery in the management of American Burkitt's lymphoma and its treatment. *Ann Surg* 1982; **196**: 82–6.

100. Fleming ID, Mitchell S, Dilawari RA. The role of surgery in the management of gastric lymphoma. *Cancer* 1982; **49**: 1135–41.

101. Paulson S, Sheehan RG, Stone MJ, Frenkel EP. Large cell lymphomas of the stomach: improved prognosis with complete resection of all intrinsic gastrointestinal disease. *J Clin Oncol* 1983; **1**: 263–9.

102. Sheridan WP, Medley G, Brodie GN. Non-Hodgkin's lymphoma of the stomach: a prospective pilot study of surgery plus chemotherapy in early and advanced disease. *J Clin Oncol* 1985; **3**: 495–500.

103. Ferrari LR, Bedford RF. General anesthesia prior to treatment of anterior mediastinal masses in pediatric cancer patients. *Anesthesiology* 1990; **72**: 991–5.

104. Neuman GG, Weingarten AE, Abramowitz RM *et al.* The anesthetic management of the patient with an anterior mediastinal mass. *Anesthesiology* 1984; **60**: 144–7.

105. Rabinowe SN, Soiffer RJ, Tarbell NJ *et al.* Hemolytic-uremic syndrome following bone marrow transplantation in adults for hematologic malignancies. *Blood* 1991; **77**: 1837–44.

106. Sierra RD. Coombs-positive hemolytic anemia in Hodgkin's disease: case presentation and review of the literature. *Mil Med* 1991; **156**: 691–2.

◆107. Ellis M. Febrile neutropenia. *Ann N Y Acad Sci* 2008; **1138**: 329–50.

●108. Pizzo PA. Management of fever in patients with cancer and treatment-induced neutropenia. *N Engl J Med* 1993; **328**: 1323–32.

109. Ladisch S, Pizzo PA. *Staphylococcus aureus sepsis* in children with cancer. *Pediatrics* 1978; **61**: 231–4.

110. Schimpff SC, Young VM, Greene WH *et al.* Origin of infection in acute nonlymphocytic leukemia. Significance of hospital acquisition of potential pathogens. *Ann Intern Med* 1972; **77**: 707–14.

111. Viscoli C, Castagnola E. Factors predisposing cancer patients to infection. *Cancer Treat Res* 1995; **79**: 1–30.

112. Wisplinghoff H, Seifert H, Wenzel RP, Edmond MB. Current trends in the epidemiology of nosocomial bloodstream infections in patients with hematological malignancies and solid neoplasms in hospitals in the United States. *Clin Infect Dis* 2003; **36**: 1103–10.

113. Viscoli C, Castagnola E. Treatment of febrile neutropenia: what is new? *Curr Opin Infect Dis* 2002; **15**: 377–82.

◆114. Rolston KV. The Infectious Diseases Society of America 2002 guidelines for the use of antimicrobial agents in patients with cancer and neutropenia: salient features and comments. *Clin Infect Dis* 2004; **39**(Suppl 1): S44–8.

115. Feusner J, Cohen R, O'Leary M, Beach B. Use of routine chest radiography in the evaluation of fever in neutropenic pediatric oncology patients. *J Clin Oncol* 1988; **6**: 1699–702.

116. Pizzo PA. Evaluation of fever in the patient with cancer. *Eur J Cancer Clin Oncol* 1989; **25**(Suppl 2): S9–16.

117. Hughes WT, Armstrong D, Bodey GP *et al.* 2002 guidelines for the use of antimicrobial agents in neutropenic patients with cancer. *Clin Infect Dis* 2002; **34**: 730–51.

●118. Pizzo PA, Hathorn JW, Hiemenz J *et al.* A randomized trial comparing ceftazidime alone with combination antibiotic therapy in cancer patients with fever and neutropenia. *N Engl J Med* 1986; **315**: 552–8.

119. Paul M, Silbiger I, Grozinsky S *et al.* Beta lactam antibiotic monotherapy versus beta lactam-aminoglycoside antibiotic combination therapy for sepsis. *Cochrane Database Syst Rev* 2006; (1): CD003344.

120. Pizzo PA. After empiric therapy: what to do until the granulocyte comes back. *Rev Infect Dis* 1987; **9**: 214–9.

121. Talcott JA, Siegel RD, Finberg R, Goldman L. Risk assessment in cancer patients with fever and neutropenia: a prospective, two-center validation of a prediction rule. *J Clin Oncol* 1992; **10**: 316–22.

◆122. Klastersky J, Paesmans M, Rubenstein EB *et al.* The Multinational Association for Supportive Care in Cancer risk index: A multinational scoring system for identifying low-risk febrile neutropenic cancer patients. *J Clin Oncol* 2000; **18**: 3038–51.

123. Persson L, Söderquist B, Engervall P *et al.* Assessment of systemic inflammation markers to differentiate a stable from a deteriorating clinical course in patients with febrile neutropenia. *Eur J Haematol* 2005; **74**: 297–303.

124. Tromp YH, Daenen SM, Sluiter WJ, Vellenga E. The predictive value of interleukin-8 (IL-8) in hospitalised patients with fever and chemotherapy-induced neutropenia. *Eur J Cancer* 2009; **45**: 596–600.

125. von Lilienfeld-Toal M, Dietrich MP, Glasmacher A *et al.* Markers of bacteremia in febrile neutropenic patients with hematological malignancies: procalcitonin and IL-6 are more reliable than C-reactive protein. *Eur J Clin Microbiol Infect Dis* 2004; **23**: 539–44.

◆126. Aapro MS, Cameron DA, Pettengell R *et al.* EORTC guidelines for the use of granulocyte-colony stimulating factor to reduce the incidence of chemotherapy-induced febrile neutropenia in adult patients with lymphomas and solid tumours. *Eur J Cancer* 2006; **42**: 2433–53.

◆127. Lyman GH. Guidelines of the National Comprehensive Cancer Network on the use of myeloid growth factors with cancer chemotherapy: a review of the evidence. *J Natl Compr Canc Netw* 2005; **3**: 557–71.

◆128. Smith TJ, Khatcheressian J, Lyman GH *et al.* 2006 update of recommendations for the use of white blood cell growth factors: an evidence-based clinical practice guideline. *J Clin Oncol* 2006; **24**: 3187–205.

129. Bucaneve G, Micozzi A, Menichetti F *et al.* Levofloxacin to prevent bacterial infection in patients with cancer and neutropenia. *N Engl J Med* 2005; **353**: 977–87.

130. Cullen M, Steven N, Billingham L et al. Antibacterial prophylaxis after chemotherapy for solid tumors and lymphomas. N Engl J Med 2005; **353**: 988–98.

●131. Goodman JL, Winston DJ, Greenfield RA et al. A controlled trial of fluconazole to prevent fungal infections in patients undergoing bone marrow transplantation. N Engl J Med 1992; **326**: 845–51.

132. Hughes WT, Rivera GK, Schell MJ et al. Successful intermittent chemoprophylaxis for Pneumocystis carinii pneumonitis. N Engl J Med 1987; **316**: 1627–32.

133. Saral R, Burns WH, Laskin OL et al. Acyclovir prophylaxis of herpes-simplex-virus infections. N Engl J Med 1981; **305**: 63–7.

134. Spivak JL. Recombinant human erythropoietin and the anemia of cancer. Blood 1994; **84**: 997–1004.

135. Case DC Jr, Bukowski RM, Carey RW et al. Recombinant human erythropoietin therapy for anemic cancer patients on combination chemotherapy. J Natl Cancer Inst 1993; **85**: 801–6.

136. Henry DH, Abels RI. Recombinant human erythropoietin in the treatment of cancer and chemotherapy-induced anemia: results of double-blind and open-label follow-up studies. Semin Oncol 1994; **21**(2 Suppl 3): 21–8.

137. Henry DH. Guidelines and recommendations for the management of anaemia in patients with lymphoid malignancies. Drugs 2007; **67**: 175–94.

138. Shehata N, Walker I, Meyer R et al. The use of erythropoiesis-stimulating agents in patients with non-myeloid hematological malignancies: a systematic review. Ann Hematol 2008; **87**: 961–73.

139. Vose JM, Armitage JO. Clinical applications of hematopoietic growth factors. J Clin Oncol 1995; **13**: 1023–35.

140. Ciurea SO, Hoffman R. Cytokines for the treatment of thrombocytopenia. Semin Hematol 2007; **44**: 166–82.

141. Rodeghiero F, Ruggeri M. Chronic immune thrombocytopenic purpura. New agents. Hamostaseologie 2009; **29**: 76–9.

142. Bussel JB, Cheng G, Saleh MN et al. Eltrombopag for the treatment of chronic idiopathic thrombocytopenic purpura. N Engl J Med 2007; **357**: 2237–47.

143. McHutchison JG, Dusheiko G, Shiffman ML et al. Eltrombopag for thrombocytopenia in patients with cirrhosis associated with hepatitis C. N Engl J Med 2007; **357**: 2227–36.

144. Jenkins JM, Williams D, Deng Y et al. Phase 1 clinical study of eltrombopag, an oral, nonpeptide thrombopoietin receptor agonist. Blood 2007; **109**: 4739–41.

●145. Wagner ML, Rosenberg HS, Fernbach DJ, Singleton EB. Typhlitis: a complication of leukemia in childhood. Am J Roentgenol Radium Ther Nucl Med 1970; **109**: 341–50.

146. Hopkins DG, Kushner JP. Clostridial species in the pathogenesis of necrotizing enterocolitis in patients with neutropenia. Am J Hematol 1983; **14**: 289–95.

◆147. Paulino AF, Kenney R, Forman EN, Medeiros LJ. Typhlitis in a patient with acute lymphoblastic leukemia prior to the administration of chemotherapy. Am J Pediatr Hematol Oncol 1994; **16**: 348–51.

●148. Sloas MM, Flynn PM, Kaste SC, Patrick CC. Typhlitis in children with cancer: a 30-year experience. Clin Infect Dis 1993; **17**: 484–90.

149. Amromin GD, Solomon RD. Necrotizing enteropathy: a complication of treated leukemia or lymphoma patients. JAMA 1962; **182**: 23–9.

150. Shamberger RC, Weinstein HJ, Delorey MJ, Levey RH. The medical and surgical management of typhlitis in children with acute nonlymphocytic (myelogenous) leukemia. Cancer 1986; **57**: 603–9.

151. Mulholland MW, Delaney JP. Neutropenic colitis and aplastic anemia: a new association. Ann Surg 1983; **197**: 84–90.

152. Foucar E, Mukai K, Foucar K et al. Colon ulceration in lethal cytomegalovirus infection. Am J Clin Pathol 1981; **76**: 788–801.

153. Keidan RD, Fanning J, Gatenby RA, Weese JL. Recurrent typhlitis. A disease resulting from aggressive chemotherapy. Dis Colon Rectum 1989; **32**: 206–9.

154. Pestalozzi BC, Sotos GA, Choyke PL et al. Typhlitis resulting from treatment with taxol and doxorubicin in patients with metastatic breast cancer. Cancer 1993; **71**: 1797–800.

155. Balthazar EJ, Megibow AJ, Fazzini E et al. Cytomegalovirus colitis in AIDS: radiographic findings in 11 patients. Radiology 1985; **155**: 585–9.

156. Karp JE, Merz WG, Hendricksen C et al. Infection management during antileukemia treatment-induced granulocytopenia: the role for oral norfloxacin prophylaxis against infections arising from the gastrointestinal tract. Scand J Infect Dis Suppl 1986; **48**: 66–78.

157. Merine D, Nussbaum AR, Fishman EK, Sanders RC. Sonographic observations in a patient with typhlitis. Clin Pediatr (Phila) 1989; **28**: 377–9.

158. Merine DS, Fishman EK, Jones B et al. Right lower quadrant pain in the immunocompromised patient: CT findings in 10 cases. AJR Am J Roentgenol 1987; **149**: 1177–9.

159. Cartoni C, Dragoni F, Micozzi A et al. Neutropenic enterocolitis in patients with acute leukemia: prognostic significance of bowel wall thickening detected by ultrasonography. J Clin Oncol 2001; **19**: 756–61.

160. Moir CR, Scudamore CH, Benny WB. Typhlitis: selective surgical management. Am J Surg 1986; **151**: 563–6.

●161. Bates SE, Raphaelson MI, Price RA et al. Ascending myelopathy after chemotherapy for central nervous system acute lymphoblastic leukemia: correlation with cerebrospinal fluid myelin basic protein. Med Pediatr Oncol 1985; **13**: 4–8.

162. Resar LM, Phillips PC, Kastan MB et al. Acute neurotoxicity after intrathecal cytosine arabinoside in two adolescents with acute lymphoblastic leukemia of B-cell type. Cancer 1993; **71**: 117–23.

163. Schiff D, Wen P. Central nervous system toxicity from cancer therapies. Hematol Oncol Clin North Am 2006; **20**: 1377–98.

164. Werner RA. Paraplegia and quadriplegia after intrathecal chemotherapy. *Arch Phys Med Rehabil* 1988; **69**: 1054–6.

165. Nott L, Price TJ, Pittman K *et al.* Hyperammonaemic encephalopathy associated with rituximab-containing chemotherapy. *Intern Med J* 2008; **38**: 800–3.

166. García-Tena J, López-Andreu JA, Ferrís J *et al.* Intrathecal chemotherapy-related myeloencephalopathy in a young child with acute lymphoblastic leukemia. *Pediatr Hematol Oncol* 1995; **12**: 377–85.

167. Gangji D, Reaman GH, Cohen SR *et al.* Leukoencephalopathy and elevated levels of myelin basic protein in the cerebrospinal fluid of patients with acute lymphoblastic leukemia. *N Engl J Med* 1980; **303**: 19–21.

♦168. Weintraub M, Adde MA, Venzon DJ *et al.* Severe atypical neuropathy associated with administration of hematopoietic colony-stimulating factors and vincristine. *J Clin Oncol* 1996; **14**: 935–40.

169. Mohamad I, Abdullah B. Unilateral vocal cord palsy following chemotherapy for lymphoma. *Pak J Med Sci* 2008; **24**: 612–13.

170. Harlow PJ, DeClerck YA, Shore NA *et al.* A fatal case of inappropriate ADH secretion induced by cyclophosphamide therapy. *Cancer* 1979; **44**: 896–8.

171. Limat S, Demesmay K, Voillat L *et al.* Early cardiotoxicity of the CHOP regimen in aggressive non-Hodgkin's lymphoma. *Ann Oncol* 2003; **14**: 277–81.

●172. Doroshow JH, Locker GY, Myers CE. Enzymatic defenses of the mouse heart against reactive oxygen metabolites: alterations produced by doxorubicin. *J Clin Invest* 1980; **65**: 128–35.

173. Myers CE. Cardiac and pulmonary toxicity. In: Devita VT, Hellman S. (eds) *Cancer: practice and principles of oncology.* Philadelphia, PA: JB Lippincott, 1985: 2022–32.

174. Del Favero A, Roila F, Tonato M. Reducing chemotherapy-induced nausea and vomiting. Current perspectives and future possibilities. *Drug Saf* 1993; **9**: 410–28.

175. Markman M, Sheidler V, Ettinger DS *et al.* Antiemetic efficacy of dexamethasone. Randomized, double-blind, crossover study with prochlorperazine in patients receiving cancer chemotherapy. *N Engl J Med* 1984; **311**: 549–52.

176. Dexamethasone, granisetron, or both for the prevention of nausea and vomiting during chemotherapy for cancer. The Italian Group for Antiemetic Research. *N Engl J Med* 1995; **332**: 1–5.

♦177. Jordan K, Sippel C, Schmoll HJ. Guidelines for antiemetic treatment of chemotherapy-induced nausea and vomiting: past, present, and future recommendations. *Oncologist* 2007; **12**: 1143–50.

178. Berger A, Henderson M, Nadoolman W *et al.* Oral capsaicin provides temporary relief for oral mucositis pain secondary to chemotherapy/radiation therapy. *J Pain Symptom Manage* 1995; **10**: 243–8.

179. Weisdorf DJ, Bostrom B, Raether D *et al.* Oropharyngeal mucositis complicating bone marrow transplantation: prognostic factors and the effect of chlorhexidine mouth rinse. *Bone Marrow Transplant* 1989; **4**: 89–95.

180. Wright WE. Periodontium destruction associated with oncology therapy. Five case reports. *J Periodontol* 1987; **58**: 559–63.

181. Spielberger R, Stiff P, Bensinger W *et al.* Palifermin for oral mucositis after intensive therapy for hematologic cancers. *N Engl J Med* 2004; **351**: 2590–98.

182. Hofmeister CC, Stiff PJ. Mucosal protection by cytokines. *Curr Hematol Rep* 2005; **4**: 446–53.

183. Hanna H, Afif C, Alakech B *et al.* Central venous catheter-related bacteremia due to gram-negative bacilli: significance of catheter removal in preventing relapse. *Infect Control Hosp Epidemiol* 2004; **25**: 646–9.

184. Boktour M, Hanna H, Ansari S *et al.* Central venous catheter and Stenotrophomonas maltophilia bacteremia in cancer patients. *Cancer* 2006; **106**: 1967–73.

185. Ross AH, Griffith CD, Anderson JR, Grieve DC. Thromboembolic complications with silicone elastomer subclavian catheters. *JPEN J Parenter Enteral Nutr* 1982; **6**: 61–3.

186. Schwartzberg LS, Holbert JM. Hemorrhagic and thrombotic abnormalities of cancer. *Crit Care Clin* 1988; **4**: 107–28.

187. Hung SS. Deep vein thrombosis of the arm associated with malignancy. *Cancer* 1989; **64**: 531–5.

188. Menzoian JO, Sequeira JC, Doyle JE *et al.* Therapeutic and clinical course of deep vein thrombosis. *Am J Surg* 1983; **146**: 581–5.

189. Glynn MF, Langer B, Jeejeebhoy KN. Therapy for thrombotic occlusion of long-term intravenous alimentation catheters. *JPEN J Parenter Enteral Nutr* 1980; **4**: 387–90.

50

Systemic therapy of lymphoma

APAR KISHOR GANTI AND JAMES O ARMITAGE

INTRODUCTION

Lymphoproliferative disorders are disseminated in nature and hence therapy for the lymphoid malignancies has shown an increasing shift away from local therapy and toward systemic therapy. For a long time, cytotoxic chemotherapy has been the mainstay of systemic therapy for the lymphoid malignancies, but increasing knowledge about the basic molecular biology of these illnesses has resulted in the increasing use of agents targeted against key metabolic pathways responsible for carcinogenesis. In this chapter we will discuss the basic principles of action of the various individual chemotherapeutic agents, the rationale of combining two or more individual agents together, the concepts of high-dose chemotherapy with stem cell support, the newer targeted agents including monoclonal antibodies and small molecules that affect key intracellular pathways, and finally look at agents that are currently being investigated.

CYTOTOXIC CHEMOTHERAPY

History

The observation that mustard gas led to bone marrow and lymphoid hypoplasia during World War II led to the initial clinical trials using nitrogen mustard in patients with hematologic malignancies. The dramatic response with this agent heralded a new era in cancer chemotherapy and led to the screening and subsequent introduction of other agents for the management of cancer, especially hematologic malignancies. In 1955, the United States Congress appropriated funds for a national effort, and the National Cancer Institute undertook a National Chemotherapy program devoted to testing chemicals that might be effective against cancer. This effort led to landmark studies that demonstrated that combination chemotherapy could cure advanced stage Hodgkin disease and diffuse large cell lymphoma.[1,2] Scientific discoveries have led to an increased knowledge of cell mechanisms and the immune system, leading to the development of new technologies such as genetic engineering and production of synthetic antibodies in the past two decades.

Pharmacology of individual agents

A list of cytotoxic chemotherapeutic agents used in the treatment of lymphoid malignancies, along with their major adverse effects, is presented in Table 50.1. The discussion below focuses on the mechanism of action of each individual class of agents.

Table 50.1 Cytotoxic chemotherapeutic agents used in the treatment of lymphoid neoplasms

Agent	Pharmacokinetics	Indications	Important adverse effects
Alkylating agents (nitrogen mustards)			
Mechlorethamine	Intracellular transport	Hodgkin disease	Myelosuppression, nausea, vomiting, thrombophlebitis, infertility, secondary malignancy
Chlorambucil	Hepatic metabolism	CLL, Waldenstrom macroglobulinemia, NHL	Myelosuppression, neurologic toxicity, rash, infertility with increased doses, pulmonary fibrosis, secondary malignancy
Melphalan	Renal clearance	Multiple myeloma, conditioning agent for HSCT	Myelosuppression, mucositis, secondary malignancy
Cyclophosphamide	Converted to phosphoramide mustard (active) and acrolein (toxic)	NHL, ALL, mycosis fungoides, conditioning agent for HSCT	Myelosuppression, nausea, vomiting, hemorrhagic cystitis, SIADH, infertility, alopecia, stomatitis
Ifosfamide	Similar to cyclophosphamide	Relapsed lymphoma, ALL, CLL	Nephrotoxicity, alopecia, nausea, vomiting, hemorrhagic cystitis, encephalopathy
Busulfan	Hepatic metabolism	CML, conditioning agent for HSCT	Myelosuppression, infertility, secondary malignancy, hyperpigmentation, hepatic veno-occlusive disease, pulmonary interstitial fibrosis
Carmustine (BCNU)	Rapid entry into CSF; renal excretion	Hodgkin disease, conditioning agent for HSCT	Hypotension, dizziness, ataxia, nausea, vomiting, delayed myelosuppression, burning at injection site, retinal hemorrhages, increased liver enzymes, pulmonary fibrosis, renal failure, arrhythmias, encephalopathy, hepatic veno-occlusive disease
Alkylating agents (platinum compounds)			
Cisplatin	Renal excretion	Relapsed lymphoma, conditioning agent for HSCT	Nausea, vomiting (acute and delayed), renal failure, alopecia, peripheral neuropathy, elevated liver enzymes, myelosuppression
Carboplatin	Renal excretion	Relapsed lymphoma, conditioning agent for HSCT	Thrombocytopenia, nausea, vomiting, stomatitis, elevated liver enzymes, hearing loss, renal failure
Alkylating agents (methylating agents)			
Dacarbazine	Hepatic metabolism, renal excretion	Hodgkin disease, conditioning agent for HSCT	Myelosuppression, nausea, vomiting, pain at injection site, flu-like syndrome, hepatic vein thrombosis, photosensitivity
Procarbazine	Hepatic and renal metabolism	Hodgkin disease, conditioning agent for HSCT	Myelosuppression, peripheral neuropathy, psychosis, nausea, vomiting, nystagmus, pleural effusion
Antimetabolites (folate analogs)			
Methotrexate	Excreted unchanged by the kidney	ALL, NHL, CNS lymphoma and leukemia	Neutropenia, mucositis, rash, alopecia, renal failure, demyelinating encephalopathy (intrathecal)
Antimetabolites (pyrimidine analogs)			
Cytarabine	Rapid deamination in blood and various organs	ALL, CLL, meningeal leukemia, NHL, MDS, conditioning agent for HSCT	Myelosuppression, nausea, vomiting, anorexia, diarrhea, metallic taste, conjunctivitis, keratitis, pulmonary edema, pericarditis, cerebellar dysfunction, arachnoiditis (intrathecal)
Gemcitabine	Hepatic metabolism, renal excretion	Relapsed/refractory lymphoma	Nausea, vomiting, fever, myelosuppression, rash, alopecia, pain, elevated liver enzymes
Azacytidine	Renal excretion	MDS, AML	Nausea, vomiting, leukopenia, diarrhea, alopecia, rash, transient azotemia

(Continued)

Table 50.1   Continued

Agent	Pharmacokinetics	Indications	Important adverse effects
Antimetabolites (purine analogs)			
Fludarabine	Extensively bound to tissues, renal excretion	CLL, low-grade lymphomas, mycosis fungoides, Waldenstrom macroglobulinemia	Myelosuppression, nausea, vomiting, increased risk of opportunistic infections
6-mercaptopurine	Hepatic metabolism	ALL	Myelosuppression, hepatic dysfunction
6-thioguanine	Renal excretion	AML, CML	Myelosuppression, hepatotoxicity (including veno-occlusive disease)
Cladribine	Renal excretion, enters CSF	Hairy cell leukemia, CLL, CML, NHL	Myelosuppression, fever and infections, transient blindness and sensorimotor neuropathy
Pentostatin	Renal excretion	Hairy cell leukemia, NHL, cutaneous T cell lymphoma, conditioning agent for nonmyeloablative HSCT	Myelosuppression, opportunistic infections, nephrotoxicity, lethargy, fatigue, nausea, vomiting, keratoconjunctivitis
Ribonucleotide reductase inhibitors			
Hydroxyurea	Hepatic metabolism, renal excretion	CML, emergent treatment of AML	Myelosuppression, stomatitis, nausea, diarrhea, constipation, acute alveolitis, leg ulcers
Antitumor antibiotics			
Bleomycin	Renal excretion	Hodgkin disease	Raynaud phenomenon, hyperpigmentation, pain at tumor site, stomatitis, interstitial pneumonitis, pulmonary fibrosis, fever, anaphylactoid reactions
Antitumor antibiotics (anthracyclines)			
Daunorubicin	Hepatic metabolism to active metabolite, fecal excretion	AML, ALL	Alopecia, red discoloration of urine, heart failure (max. lifetime dose [550 mg/m^2]), darkening of skin, GI ulceration, myelosuppression, local reactions (vesicant), elevation in liver enzymes, myocarditis, pericarditis
Doxorubicin	Hepatic metabolism to active metabolite, fecal excretion	AML, ALL, Hodgkin disease, NHL	Heart failure (max. lifetime dose [550 mg/m^2]), alopecia, nausea, vomiting, ulceration and necrosis of the colon, red discoloration of urine, myelosuppression, local reaction (vesicant), radiation recall
Idarubicin	Hepatic metabolism to active metabolite	AML, ALL, CML (blast crisis)	Heart failure (max. lifetime dose [540 mg/m^2]), headache, alopecia, radiation recall, nausea, vomiting, diarrhea, myelosuppression, elevated liver enzymes, local reaction (vesicant), seizures, hyperuricemia
Antitumor antibiotics (anthracenediones)			
Mitoxantrone	Hepatic metabolism, extensive protein binding	AML, ALL, CML	Nausea, constipation, diarrhea, mucositis, stomatitis, seizure, increased liver enzymes, allergic reactions, local reaction (vesicant), interstitial pneumonitis
Epipodophyllotoxins			
Etoposide	Hepatic metabolism, extensive protein binding	Relapsed lymphoma, AML, conditioning agent for HSCT	Alopecia, severe mucositis (high dose), neurotoxicity, myelosuppression, hypotension, toxic hepatitis (high dose)
Teniposide	Hepatic metabolism, urinary excretion	Relapsed ALL	Mucositis, diarrhea, nausea, vomiting, anorexia, myelosuppression, hypotension peripheral neuropathy

(Continued)

Table 50.1   Continued

Agent	Pharmacokinetics	Indications	Important adverse effects
Vinca alkaloids			
Vinblastine	Hepatic metabolism to active metabolite	Hodgkin disease, NHL, mycosis fungoides, CML (blast crisis)	Alopecia, SIADH, severe bone marrow suppression, hypertension, Raynaud phenomenon, hyperuricemia, constipation, paralytic ileus, stomatitis, urinary retention, bronchospasm, hemorrhagic colitis, neurotoxicity, rectal bleeding
Vincristine	Hepatic metabolism to active metabolite	ALL, Hodgkin disease, NHL, multiple myeloma	Alopecia, seizure, CNS depression, cranial nerve paralysis, constipation and possible paralytic ileus, oral ulceration, vesicant, peripheral neuropathy, photophobia, SIADH, symptomatic hyponatremia
Vinorelbine	Hepatic metabolism, triphasic elimination	Hodgkin disease	Fatigue, nausea, constipation, vomiting, diarrhea, severe bone marrow suppression, elevated liver enzymes, vesicant, peripheral neuropathy, anaphylaxis, angioedema, DVT/PE, hemorrhagic cystitis, SIADH, pancreatitis, pulmonary edema, radiation recall
Camptothecin analogs			
Topotecan	Rapid plasma metabolism	Relapsed lymphoma	Myelosuppression, headache, fatigue, fever, pain, alopecia, nausea, vomiting, diarrhea, constipation, elevated liver enzymes, allergic reactions, anaphylactoid reactions, angioedema
Enzymes			
L-asparaginase	Systemically degraded	ALL	Hallucinations, agitation, hyperglycemia, nausea, vomiting, anorexia, abdominal cramps, acute pancreatitis, hypofibrinogenemia, decreased clotting factors V and VIII, elevated liver enzymes, allergic reactions, anaphylaxis, azotemia, diabetes, ketoacidosis, DVT/PE, parkinsonism
Corticosteroids			
Prednisone, dexamethasone, methylprednisone	Hepatic metabolism, renal excretion	ALL, CLL, NHL, multiple myeloma	Insomnia, tachycardia, hyperglycemia, increased gastric acidity, proximal muscle weakness, mania, immunosuppression

CLL, chronic lymphocytic leukemia; NHL, Non-Hodgkin lymphoma; HSCT, hematopoietic stem cell transplantation; ALL, acute lymphoblastic leukemia; SIADH, syndrome of inappropriate antidiuretic hormone secretion; CML, chronic myeloid leukemia; AML, acute myeloid leukemia; MDS, myelodysplastic syndrome; DVT/PE, deep venous thrombosis/pulmonary embolism; CSF, cerebrospinal fluid; CNS, central nervous system; GI, gastrointestinal.

ALKYLATING AGENTS

Nitrogen mustards

The alkylating agents can be transformed to intermediates that are strongly electrophilic in nature. These intermediates then alkylate the various nucleophilic moieties of the DNA bases and form covalent linkages. The 7-nitrogen (N^7) atom of guanine is particularly susceptible to the alkylating effects of these agents. This results in the formation of a modified guanine residue that can mispair with thymine residues resulting in the substitution of an adenine:thymine base pair with a guanine:cytosine base pair (Fig. 50.1). Another consequence of the alkylation of the guanine residue is that it results in the formation of an unstable guanine that is very susceptible to cleavage by DNA repair enzymes. Either of these effects seriously damages the DNA molecule. Certain agents like mechlorethamine

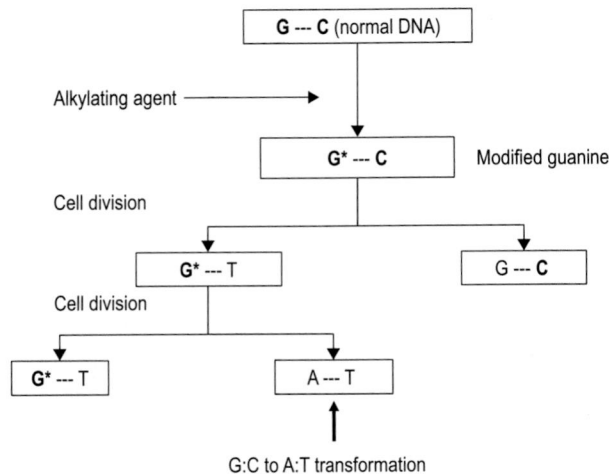

Figure 50.1   Mechanism of action of alkylating agents (schematic).

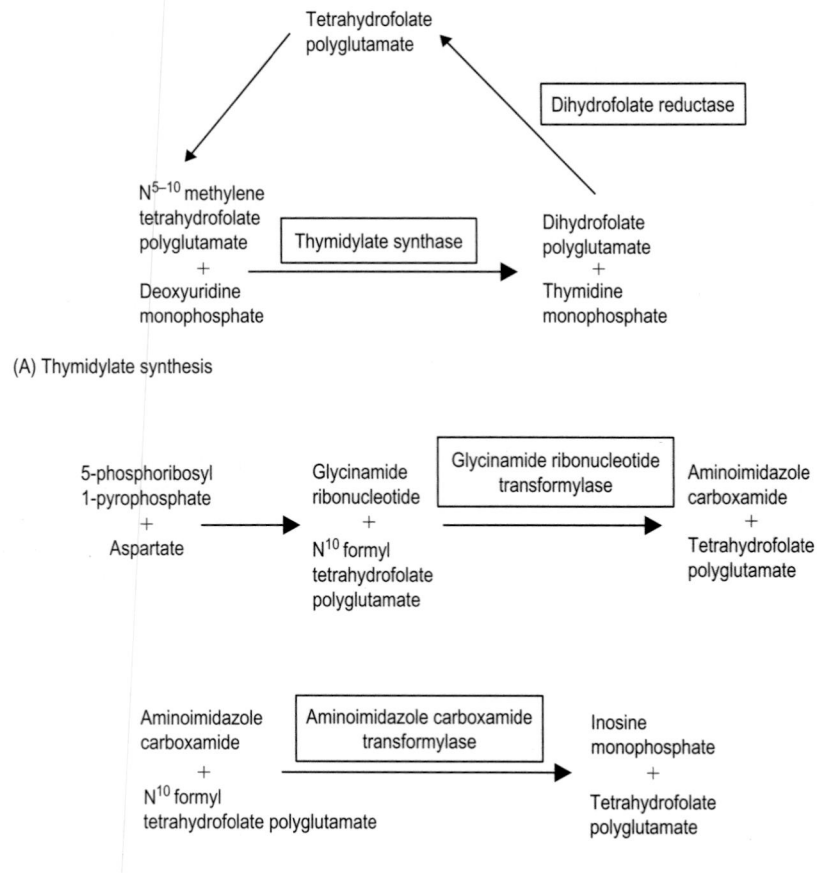

Figure 50.2   Mechanism of action of methotrexate.

can alkylate two such guanine residues simultaneously and lead to the formation of crosslinkages between two nucleic acid chains and cause a major disruption of nucleic acid function. The DNA damage eventually leads to cell death.[3]

The ability of these agents to interfere with DNA integrity and functioning in rapidly proliferating tissues forms the basis for their use in cancer therapy. Although their activity is most pronounced in proliferating tissues in which a large proportion of cells are in cell division, they can alkylate non-dividing cells as well thereby leading to their toxicity.

Platinum coordination complexes

The platinum coordination complexes – cisplatin and carbo-platin – enter cells by diffusion and react with the DNA forming both intrastrand and interstrand complexes. The N^7 of guanine is highly reactive and platinum can form crosslinks between adjacent guanine bases and also between adenine and guanine residues. These DNA adducts inhibit DNA replication and transcription thereby leading to strand breaks and miscoding. The repair of these adducts involves excision of the affected base, insertion of a new base, and relegation of the affected strand.[3] The cisplatin-DNA adduct is believed to produce a bend in the DNA helix that is recognized by certain proteins that are believed to inhibit the repair process.[4]

ANTIMETABOLITES

Methotrexate

Methotrexate exerts its action by inhibiting the enzyme dihydrofolate reductase (DHFR), which is involved in the synthesis of purines and thymidylate, an essential component of DNA (Fig. 50.2). The inhibition of DHFR leads to accumulation of methotrexate polyglutamates and dihydrofolate polyglutamates that then inhibit folate-dependent enzymes of purine metabolism, namely glycinamide ribonucleotide transformylase and aminoimidazole carboxamide transformylase.

The toxicity of methotrexate can be ameliorated by leucovorin, a reduced form of folic acid that enters the cells via a specific carrier-mediated transport system and supplies the necessary cofactor blocked by methotrexate.[5]

Pyrimidine analogues (cytarabine, azacytidine, gemcitabine)

These are S phase-specific agents that have to be activated by conversion to the 5′-monophosphate form. This compound then activates the appropriate nucleotide kinases to form the di- and triphosphate nucleotides. The accumulation of the triphosphate nucleotide analogues causes inhibition of the DNA chain elongation and eventually leads to the inhibition of DNA synthesis. These compounds also act by inducing differentiation in tumor cells.[3,6] It is believed that continued inhibition of DNA synthesis for at least one cell cycle is necessary to expose cells to these agents during the S phase of the cell cycle. The exact mechanism of cell death caused by these agents is uncertain, but fragmentation of DNA has been observed and there is cytological and biochemical evidence of apoptosis in treated cells.[7]

Purine analogues

6-Mercaptopurine and 6-thioguanine are converted by the enzyme hypoxanthine-guanine phosphoribosyltransferase (HGPRT) to 6-thioIMP and 6-thioGMP, respectively. 6-thioIMP accumulates in the cell and inhibits several vital steps in the synthesis of adenine and guanine nucleotides. 6-thioGMP, on the other hand, is converted to 6-thioGTP that is then incorporated into the nucleic acids. In addition, accumulation of 6-thioGMP and 6-thioIMP and other monophosphate derivatives of purine analogues can cause a negative feedback, inhibiting the initial steps in the *de novo* pathway of purine synthesis.

Fludarabine and cladribine are converted to their respective triphosphate derivatives and subsequently incorporated in the DNA, producing strand breaks and depletion of ATP. Fludarabine also inhibits key enzymes responsible for DNA synthesis, including ribonucleotide reductase, DNA polymerase, and DNA primase.

Pentostatin inhibits the enzyme adenosine deaminase, leading to accumulation of adenosine and deoxyadenosine nucleotides that inhibit DNA synthesis. It is also phosphorylated to its triphosphate derivative, which is incorporated into the DNA. It also inhibits the enzyme S-adenosyl homocysteine hydrolase leading to the accumulation of S-adenosyl homocysteine, which is directly toxic to lymphocytes.

ANTITUMOR ANTIBIOTICS

Bleomycin

Bleomycin exerts its cytotoxic effects by reacting with oxygen in the presence of ferrous iron to produce active oxygen species that then cause DNA scission. Bleomycin causes cells to accumulate in the G2 phase of the cell cycle and a large proportion of these cells display chromosomal aberrations (chromatid breaks, gaps, fragments, and translocations).[8]

Anthracyclines (daunorubicin, doxorubicin, idarubicin)

Anthracyclines react with cytochrome P450 reductase leading to the production of oxygen free radicals that are destructive to cells. They also intercalate with DNA leading to single- and double-strand breaks and sister chromatid exchange. The exact mechanism of DNA scission is unclear but may involve either the topoisomerase II enzyme or the formation of oxygen free radicals. In addition, these agents have the capability to interact with the cell membrane and alter cell membrane function; this latter mechanism is thought to play an important role in the cardiotoxicity of these agents.[3]

Anthracenediones (mitoxantrone)

Mitoxantrone intercalates with the DNA leading to strand breaks mediated by topoisomerase II. However, it has a limited capacity to produce free radicals and causes less cardiotoxicity as compared to the anthracyclines.

EPIPODOPHYLLOTOXINS (ETOPOSIDE, TENIPOSIDE)

Cells in the S and G2 phases of the cell cycle are most sensitive to the effects of the epipodophyllotoxins, etoposide and teniposide. These compounds form a ternary complex with DNA and topoisomerase II leading to strand breaks. However, the strand passage and resealing of the DNA are inhibited by the presence of the drug. There is accumulation of DNA breaks eventually leading to cell death.

VINCA ALKALOIDS (VINBLASTINE, VINCRISTINE, VINORELBINE)

The vinca alkaloids are cell cycle-specific agents that block cells in mitosis. They bind specifically to tubulin and block its ability to polymerize into microtubules. In the absence of a mitotic spindle, chromosomes disperse throughout the cytoplasm. The inability to correctly segregate chromosomes during mitosis leads to cell death.[7]

CAMPTOTHECIN ANALOGUES (TOPOTECAN)

The camptothecins are S phase-specific drugs, because ongoing DNA synthesis is a necessary condition to induce cytotoxicity. These agents bind to and stabilize the DNA-topoisomerase I complex.[9] Although the drug does not affect the initial cleavage action of topoisomerase I, the religation step that is necessary for DNA repair is inhibited, leading to the accumulation of single-strand breaks in the DNA. Similar to the epipodophyllotoxins, collision of the DNA replication fork with the ternary drug-enzyme-DNA complex produces an irreversible double-strand break that ultimately leads to cell death.[10]

ENZYMES (L-ASPARAGINASE)

L-asparaginase catalyzes the hydrolysis of circulating asparagine to aspartic acid and ammonia and deprives the acute lymphoblastic leukemic cells of asparagine necessary for protein synthesis thereby leading to activation of apoptosis and cell death.[3]

CORTICOSTEROIDS

The predominant role of glucocorticoids in the management of lymphoproliferative disorders is due their direct lymphotoxicity.[11] This effect seems to be mediated by binding to specific corticosteroid receptors on the surface of lymphoid cells, leading rapidly to apoptosis.[12] In addition, the glucocorticoids also block the effects of lymphokines and cytokines that mediate many of the B symptoms associated with the lymphoproliferative disorders.

Combination chemotherapy

RATIONALE

1. The incidence of initial resistance to any given drug is frequent even in the most sensitive tumors.
2. Drug exposure leads to the rapid development of resistance to that agent (probably due to the selection of naturally resistant clones from a heterogeneous tumor cell population).
3. The selection of multiple agents, each with a different mechanism of action, allows independent cell killing by each agent, thereby overcoming the problem of drug resistance, at least in part.
4. Drugs with nonoverlapping toxicities, if combined, can provide improved efficacy with acceptable toxicity.[13]

PRINCIPLES

For years, a set of principles have guided our efforts to develop optimal combination chemotherapy regimens for the treatment of cancer in general and hematologic malignancies in particular.[14]

1. Only drugs that have demonstrated antitumor activity against the disease to be treated should be employed in combination.
2. Drugs to be used in the combination chemotherapy regimen should be administered at their optimal doses and schedules. A natural corollary of this is that ideally the drugs chosen for inclusion in a combination should have nonoverlapping toxicities.
3. Only drugs that have different mechanisms of action or different mechanisms of resistance should be selected for inclusion in the combination.
4. The drug combination should be given in the shortest possible interval that allows for recovery of the normal tissue, which is the dose-limiting toxicity.

However, the recent development of therapies that do not necessarily have single-agent antitumor activity, but improve the efficacy of cytotoxic agents, has cast a shadow of doubt over the utility of these principles in this era of targeted agents. Even so, these principles have contributed in large part to the development of effective combinations, especially in the treatment of the hematologic malignancies, and are still valid.

The combinations that are commonly used for the treatment of lymphoid malignancies, for initial therapy and relapsed disease, are described in Table 50.2.

BIOLOGIC THERAPY

Introduction

Despite the availability of potent cytotoxic agents for the treatment for lymphoid malignanices, drug resistance is still a major problem. Also, the long-term toxicities of the cytotoxic chemotherapeutic agents have fueled the research into less-toxic agents for the treatment of these potentially curable diseases. Improved understanding of the biology of the lymphoid malignancies has led to great progress in the development of biologic therapies targeted toward key molecules or pathways responsible for carcinogenesis. This section will discuss the various biologic therapies used currently, including interferon and monoclonal antibodies, both unlabeled and radiolabeled. The biologic approaches that are currently being evaluated will be discussed at the end of this chapter.

Interferon

MECHANISM OF ACTION

Interferons (IFNs) are naturally occurring polypeptides produced by eukaryotic cells in response to various stimuli. In 1957, Isaacs and Lindemann named interferons based on their ability to 'interfere' with viral replication in infected cells.[15] Since then a variety of immunomodulatory and cytostatic effects of IFNs have been demonstrated, and currently three major types of IFN (IFNα, IFNβ, IFNγ) are commercially available for clinical use. Of these, IFNα has been extensively studied in the therapy of lymphomas.

EFFICACY IN LYMPHOID MALIGNANCIES

Interferon was initially found to be active in L1210 leukemia[16] and AKR lymphoma[17] models, although the mechanism of action was unclear. This led to the introduction, in the early 1980s, of recombinant IFNα into clinical studies for indolent lymphomas (especially follicular lymphoma [FL]) in an effort to improve survival. Phase I studies demonstrated that approximately 50 percent of patients (including those who had been previously treated with combination cytotoxic chemotherapy) with low-grade lymphoma achieved an objective clinical response with recombinant IFNα2b.[18] Interferon has been tried alone and in combination with cytotoxic chemotherapy for the treatment of advanced FL with mixed results (Table 50.3). In an Eastern Cooperative Oncology Group (ECOG) study that compared combination chemotherapy (cyclophosphamide, doxorubicin, vincristine, and prednisone) with and without IFNα2a, Smalley et al. found that patients randomized to receive IFN had a prolonged time to treatment failure (TTF) (2.4 vs 1.6 years).[19] They also found a statistically nonsignificant prolongation of overall survival by IFN (7.8 vs 5.7 years). A subset analysis, based on disease histology, revealed a significant prolongation of TTF by IFN in patients with either low-grade or FL but not intermediate-grade lymphoma.[19]

Table 50.2   Combinations effective in the treatment of lymphoid malignanices

No.	Acronym	Agents	Disease
1.	Linker regimen	Daunorubicin, vincristine, prednisone, L-asparaginase alternating with teniposide and cytarabine; followed by high-dose methotrexate	ALL – induction
2.	Larson regimen	Cyclophosphamide, daunorubicin, vincristine, prednisone, L-asparaginase followed by early intensification with methotrexate (IT), cyclophosphamide, 6-mercaptopurine, cytarabine, vincristine, L-asparaginase	ALL – induction
3.	R-CHOP	Rituximab, cyclophosphamide, doxorubicin, vincristine, prednisone	NHL
4.	R-CVP	Rituximab, cyclophosphamide, vincristine, prednisone	NHL
5.	FCR	Fludarabine, rituximab, cyclophosphamide	CLL/SLL
6.	R-HyperCVAD	Rituximab, hyperfractionated cyclophosphamide, vincristine, doxorubicin, dexamethasone; alternating with high-dose methotrexate and cytarabine	Mantle cell lymphoma, ALL – induction
7.	R-CNOP	Rituximab, cyclophosphamide, mitoxantrone, vincristine, prednisone	NHL
8.	FND	Fludarabine, mitoxantrone, dexamethasone	NHL
9.	EPOCH	Etoposide, prednisone, vincristine, cyclophosphamide, doxorubicin	NHL
10.	Magrath regimen	Rituximab, cytarabine (IT), vincristine, doxorubicin, methotrexate (IT and IV), cyclophosphamide; alternating cytarabine, rituximab, methotrexate (IT), ifosfamide, etoposide	Burkitt lymphoma
11.	VAD	Vincristine, doxorubicin, dexamethasone	Multiple myeloma
12.	MP	Melphalan, prednisone (non-transplant candidate)	Multiple myeloma
13.	DVD	Pegylated doxorubicin, thalidomide, dexamethasone	Multiple myeloma
14.	ABVD	Doxorubicin, bleomycin, vinblastine, dacarbazine	Hodgkin disease
15.	MOPP	Mechlorethamine, vincristine, procarbazine, prednisone	Hodgkin disease
16.	Stanford V	Mechlorethamine, doxorubicin, vinblastine, vincristine, bleomycin, etoposide, prednisone	Hodgkin disease
17.	BEACOPP	Cyclophosphamide, doxorubicin, etoposide, vincristine, bleomycin, procarbazine, prednisone	Hodgkin disease
18.	ESHAP	Etoposide, methylprednisolone, cisplatin, cytarabine	NHL – salvage
19.	R-ICE	Rituximab, ifosfamide, carboplatin, etoposide, mesna	NHL – salvage
20.	DHAP	Cisplatin, dexamethasone, cytarabine	NHL – salvage
21.	MINE	Ifosfamide, mitoxantrone, etoposide, mesna	NHL – salvage

AML, acute myeloid leukemia; APL, acute promyelocytic leukemia, NHL, non-Hodgkin lymphoma; CLL, chronic lymphocytic leukemia; SLL, small lymphocytic lymphoma; ALL, acute lymphoblastic leukemia; IT, intrathecal; IV, intravenous.

Table 50.3   Randomized trials of interferon (IFN) in advanced (stage III or IV) follicular lymphoma

Reference	No. of patients	Regimens	Result
Brice et al. 1997[23]	193	Prednimustine vs. IFNα2b	Similar RR and OS rates
Price et al. 1991[24]	124	Chlorambucil ± IFNα2b	IFN improved remission duration. No effect on OS
Chisesi et al. 1991[25]	63	Chlorambucil ± IFNα2b	IFN decreased relapse rate
Solal-Celigny et al. 1993[26]	242	CHVP ± IFNα2b	IFN improved RR, median EFS, and OS at 3 years
Ozer et al. 1994[27]	105	Cyclophosphamide ± IFNα2b	Similar RR
Solal-Celigny et al. 1998[28]	268	CHVP ± IFNα2b	Increased PFS and OS with IFN
Coiffier et al. 1999[29]	131	CHVP + IFNα2b vs. fludarabine	Combination – higher RR, longer TTP, and a longer survival, but less well tolerated
Rohatiner et al. 2001[30]	204	Chlorambucil ± IFNα2b	Similar RR, TTP, OS
Neri et al. 2001[31]	55	COPP ± IFN	IFN improved EFS but not OS

RR, response rate; OS, overall survival; CHVP, cyclophosphamide, doxorubicin, teniposide, and prednisone; EFS, event-free survival; PFS, progression-free survival; TTP, time to progression; COPP, cyclophosphamide, vincristine, prednisone, and procarbazine.

In an effort to clarify the issue, Rohatiner *et al.* conducted a metaanalysis of the phase III trials.[20] They found that the addition of IFNα2 to initial chemotherapy did not significantly influence response rate, but did show a survival benefit in favor of IFNα2. This survival advantage was most appreciable when IFN was given in conjunction with relatively intensive initial chemotherapy, at higher doses, and in combination with chemotherapy rather than as maintenance therapy.[20] However, the side effects of interferon, notably fatigue, preclude its routine usage in clinical practice despite evidence to suggest that the benefits of concomitant IFN can significantly offset the associated toxic effects.[21]

Interferonα has been studied extensively in multiple myeloma with similar results. A large metaanalysis suggested that IFNα has a moderate effect on relapse-free survival and only a marginal beneficial effect on overall survival in patients with multiple myeloma.[22]

In addition to indolent lymphomas and multiple myeloma, interferon has been indicated for the palliative management of advanced or refractory mycosis fungoides, mantle cell lymphoma, and post-transplant lymphoproliferative disorders.

ADVERSE EFFECTS

Flu-like symptoms are the most common adverse event seen with interferon, occurring in over 90 percent of patients administered the drug. Other less common but significant side effects include chest pain, edema, hypertension, psychiatric disturbances (including depression and suicidal behavior/ideation), fatigue, headache, dizziness, irritability, insomnia, somnolence, lethargy, confusion, rash, elevated liver enzymes, anorexia, nausea, vomiting, diarrhea, abdominal pain, myelosuppression, arthralgia, and myalgia.

Monoclonal antibodies

Immunologic interventions have been particularly appealing in the search for effective, nontoxic therapies for the lymphoproliferative disorders because they use existing components of the normal human immune system to selectively eradicate malignant cells without affecting normal nonmalignant cells. Although Paul Ehrlich is credited with developing the idea of therapeutic anticancer antibodies in the late nineteenth century, Pressman and Korngold showed for the first time in 1953 that antibodies could specifically target cancer cells.[32] There were, however, no major developments in the field until 1975, when Kohler and Milstein described the mouse hybridoma method that enabled a continuous supply of monoclonal antibodies that targeted specific antigens,[33] and in 1980, Nadler treated the first patient with a monoclonal antibody.[34] Since then there has been great progress in the development of monoclonal antibodies, especially in the treatment of lymphoproliferative disorders. There are, however, various obstacles to the development of monoclonal antibodies including identification of tumor-specific antigens, varying expression/density of

antigen on the tumor cells, internalization of antigen-antibody complex, poor access of antibody to bulky tumors, rapid clearance of antibody by circulating tumor cells, inability to produce cell death, and induction of human anti-mouse antibody responses.[35]

There are three major types of cytotoxic monoclonal antibodies currently being developed, namely

1. Unconjugated antibodies, where the antibody itself mediates cell killing, e.g., rituximab (anti-CD20), alemtuzumab (anti-CD52);
2. Antibody conjugated to a radioisotope, e.g., iodine-131-labeled (^{131}I)-tositumomab, yttrium-90-labeled (^{90}Y)-ibritumomab tiuxetan;
3. Antibody conjugated to a potent drug or a toxin, e.g., gemtuzumab ozogamicin (used for refractory myeloid leukemias).

This section will discuss the first two classes of monoclonal antibodies, since they have been approved for the treatment of non-Hodgkin lymphoma (NHL) and chronic lymphocytic leukemia (CLL).

RITUXIMAB

Introduction

Rituximab is a molecularly engineered chimeric murine/human anti-CD20 antibody that has a human gamma-1-kappa antibody with variable regions isolated from a murine anti-CD20 monoclonal antibody. It has been approved by the US Food and Drug Administration (FDA) for use in patients with NHL. Rituximab is among the most widely studied and available of the therapeutic monoclonal antibodies for the treatment of NHL.

The CD20 antigen is nearly an ideal target for unconjugated monoclonal antibody therapy because it is not expressed on precursor B cells or stem cells, but is found in high density on mature B cells (normal and malignant) except plasma cells.[36] The antigen is not shed and does not appear to undergo modulation in response to antibody binding.

Mechanism of action

After binding to the CD20 antigen, the Fc portion of rituximab binds to Fc receptors on effector cells (e.g., cytotoxic T cells, natural killer [NK] cells) and triggers a lytic reaction leading to cell death. Rituximab-CD20 complex also leads to activation of the complement cascade, resulting in cell lysis. In addition to these mechanisms, CD20 is probably involved in regulation of calcium channel activity in the cell membrane. Binding with the anti-CD20 antibody leads to high intracellular calcium levels, which keeps the cell in the G1 phase, resulting in maturation arrest and apoptosis.[37] This would therefore decrease reliance on host complement-dependent cytotoxicity or antibody-dependent cell-mediated cytotoxicity for antitumor activity. This third mechanism probably best explains the synergism seen with rituximab and cytotoxic chemotherapeutic agents.[38]

Table 50.4 Rituximab monotherapy in indolent lymphoproliferative disorders

Reference	Disease	No. of patients	Response rates	
			CR (%)	PR (%)
Colombat et al. 2001[44]	Newly diagnosed follicular NHL with low tumor burden	49	26	47
Witzig et al. 2002[45]	Newly diagnosed follicular NHL	37	25	36
Conconi et al. 2001[46]	Newly diagnosed and relapsed extranodal marginal zone (MALT-type) lymphoma	35	49	25
Foran et al. 2000[47]	Newly diagnosed and relapsed SLL, immunocytoma, mantle cell NHL	120	8	22
Treon et al. 2001[48]	Newly diagnosed and relapsed/refractory Waldenstrom macroglobulinemia	30	27	33
Foran et al. 2000[49]	Relapsed/refractory follicular NHL	70	3	43
McLaughlin et al. 1998[39]	Relapsed/refractory follicular NHL	166	6	42
Walewski et al. 2001[50]	Recurrent indolent lymphoma	34	24	35
Davis et al. 1999[51]	Relapsed/refractory low-grade NHL with bulky disease	31	3	36
Huhn et al. 2001[52]	Relapsed/refractory CLL	30	0	23

CR, complete response; PR, partial response; NHL, non-Hodgkin lymphoma; MALT, mucosal-associated lymphoid tissue; CLL, chronic lymphocytic leukemia.

Efficacy in lymphoproliferative disorders

Based on phase I/II clinical trials that demonstrated an acceptable toxicity profile and an objective response in a significant number of patients, the dose of rituximab was standardized at 375 mg/m^2 administered intravenously weekly for 4 weeks. In a phase II trial, 166 patients with relapsed low-grade or follicular lymphoma were treated with rituximab using the above schedule with a 48 percent response rate and a median time to progression of 13 months in responders. The common adverse events included infusion reactions, namely fever and chills.[39] Subset analyses revealed lower response rates in patients with small lymphocytic lymphoma (12 percent overall), and patients with chemotherapy-resistant disease had decreased response rates as compared to patients who had previously undergone high-dose chemotherapy and stem cell transplant (78 percent vs 43 percent).

Rituximab has been tried as a single agent in a number of low-grade lymphomas, both as first-line therapy and in the setting of recurrent disease, with varying response rates (Table 50.4). The best response rates have been seen in the setting of FL, both newly diagnosed and relapsed, whereas the response rates to small lymphocytic lymphoma/chronic lymphocytic leukemia (SLL/CLL) have been much lower.

Given the demonstration of synergism between rituximab and cytotoxic chemotherapy *in vitro*, several trials have been conducted using rituximab in combination with cytotoxic chemotherapy in lymphoid malignancies (Table 50.5).

The Groupe d'Etude des Lymphomes de l'Adulte (GELA) conducted a randomized clinical trial of combination chemotherapy using cyclophosphamide, doxorubicin, vincristine, and prednisone (CHOP) for 8 cycles with or without rituximab in 400 elderly patients (60–80 years old) with previously untreated diffuse large B cell lymphoma.[40] A higher proportion of patients who received the combination treatment achieved a complete response (CR) as compared to those treated with CHOP alone (76 percent vs 63 percent) ($P < 0.005$). Also, with a median follow-up of 2 years, both median event-free survival (EFS) and overall survival (OS) were significantly longer in patients treated with rituximab plus CHOP compared with CHOP alone. This has subsequently been confirmed in other multi-institutional settings.[41–43]

Adverse reactions

Rituximab is generally well tolerated by most patients. However, the initial infusion may cause a syndrome of fever, chills, and occasional hypotension and dyspnea. Patients with preexisting cardiac or pulmonary conditions and those with a high tumor burden may be at a higher risk for developing these infusion reactions. Less commonly, tumor lysis syndrome and severe mucocutaneous reactions including paraneoplastic pemphigus, Stevens-Johnson syndrome, and toxic epidermal necrolysis have been reported.[64]

ALEMTUZUMAB

Introduction

Alemtuzumab is a humanized therapeutic monoclonal antibody that recognizes the CD52 antigen expressed on normal and malignant lymphocytes, monocytes, and NK cells. It has been approved by the US FDA for the treatment of relapsed B cell CLL following alkylating agents and fludarabine.

Mechanism of action

After ligation and crosslinking of T cell CD52, alemtuzumab has been shown to induce signal transduction via the T cell receptor. Alemtuzumab can cause cell lysis using a host effector mechanism such as complement-dependent cytolysis and antibody-dependent cellular cytotoxicity.

Table 50.5   Rituximab in combination with cytotoxic chemotherapy in lymphoproliferative disorders

Reference	Disease	Regimen	No. of patients	Response rates (%)
Coiffier et al. 2002[40]	Newly diagnosed DLBCL in elderly patients	CHOP × 8	202	69
		R-CHOP × 8	197	82
Hiddeman et al. 2002[53]	Newly diagnosed follicular, mantle cell NHL, or immunocytomas	CHOP	272	85
		R-CHOP		95
Hiddeman et al. 2002[53]	Relapsed/refractory follicular, mantle cell NHL, or immunocytomas	FCM	94	58
		R-FCM		83
Howard et al. 2002[54]	Newly diagnosed mantle cell NHL	R-CHOP × 6	40	96
Vose et al. 2002[55]	Newly diagnosed advanced, aggressive NHL	R-CHOP × 6	33	97
Czuczman et al. 2001[56]	Newly diagnosed and relapsed/refractory low-grade B cell lymphoma	R-CHOP × 6	38	95
Rodriguez et al. 2002[57]	Newly diagnosed aggressive NHL	R-CHOP × 6–8 (liposomal vincristine)	66	100
Boue et al. 2002[58]	HIV-related high-grade NHL	R-CHOP × 6	50	88
Wilson et al. 2002[59]	Newly diagnosed or relapsed/refractory aggressive NHL	R-EPOCH	34	85
Czuczman et al. 2002[60]	Newly diagnosed or relapsed/refractory low-grade lymphoma	Rituximab (single infusion) followed by FR × 6	30	93
Schulz et al. 2002[61]	Newly diagnosed or relapsed/refractory CLL (anthracycline and fludarabine naïve)	RF × 4	31	87
Keating et al. 2002[62]	Newly diagnosed CLL	FCR × 6	135	85
Byrd et al. 2001[63]	Newly diagnosed CLL	Concurrent FR	104	90
		Sequential F, R		77

R, rituximab; CHOP, cyclophosphamide, doxorubicin, vincristine, and prednisone; FCM, fludarabine, cyclophosphamide, and mitoxantrone; EPOCH, etoposide, vincristine, doxorubicin, cyclophosphamide, and prednisone; HIV, human immunodeficiency virus; NHL, non-Hodgkin lymphoma; CLL, chronic lymphocytic leukemia.

There is also evidence to suggest that alemtuzumab may trigger apoptosis, both caspase-dependent and caspase-independent. Alemtuzumab plus complement was rapidly cytotoxic for cultured CLL cells.[65]

Efficacy

Alemtuzumab has been shown to be highly effective in patients with pretreated CLL. In the first study to demonstrate efficacy, Osterborg et al. treated 27 patients with alemtuzumab at a dose of 30 mg three times a week for 12 weeks and obtained a 43 percent response rate, including one patient with a complete response.[66] Keating et al. investigated the efficacy of alemtuzumab in 93 patients who had been previously treated with alkylating agents and fludarabine and found similar responses (CR 2 percent, partial response [PR] 31 percent).[67]

These and other similar results have spurred an interest in the use of alemtuzumab as first-line therapy for the treatment of CLL. In a pilot phase II study, Lundin et al. treated 38 patients with alemtuzumab as first-line therapy for CLL.[68] They obtained an overall response rate of 87 percent with a 19 percent CR rate. Currently, phase III studies comparing alemtuzumab with chlorambucil for the first-line treatment of CLL are underway.[68] Alemtuzumab has been shown to increase the efficacy of fludarabine both in combination and sequential therapy in small phase II studies. However, as will be discussed below, the increased

incidence of infections with alemtuzumab, make it less attractive for the treatment of CLL.

Adverse reactions

Infusion reactions including a flu-like syndrome, rigors, fever, nausea, vomiting, skin rash, urticaria, dyspnea, and hypotension are frequent events associated with alemtuzumab. These symptoms are a consequence of cytokine release, mainly by NK cells. Subcutaneous administration may be associated with a decreased incidence and severity of infusion reactions. Alemtuzumab can cause myelosuppression, especially in heavily pretreated patients. Lymphopenia can be profound and prolonged thereby increasing susceptibility to opportunistic infections. In the pivotal study performed by Keating et al.,[67] 51 (55 percent) of 93 pretreated patients with CLL experienced one or more infections, and 25 had severe or life-threatening infections. Of these, 14 patients (15 percent) developed septicemia, while 11 developed opportunistic infections (cytomegalovirus, seven patients; Herpes simplex, six patients; Herpes zoster, four patients).[67] Due to the risk of these infections, antimicrobial prophylaxis is mandatory while administering alemtuzumab. Cardiac toxicity, in the form of angina, arrhythmias, and congestive heart failure, has been reported with alemtuzumab. The exact mechanism is unknown, but may be related to cytokine release or a direct effect on the cardiac myocytes.

Radioimmunotherapy

MECHANISM OF ACTION

Radioimmunotherapy (RIT) is a novel treatment modality that combines the benefits of radiation therapy and immunotherapy. Monoclonal antibodies directed against tumor-specific antigens (CD20, most commonly) are used to target radioactive particles to the surface of lymphoma cells. Once the radioisotope is bound to the target cell, radiolysis is induced in neighboring tumor cells, including antigen-negative cells and cells to which the antibody is unable to gain access. The major advantages of RIT include its potential activity in disease that has already developed resistance to targeted immunotherapy directed against the same antigen and its ability to treat multiple sites of disease simultaneously, while minimizing toxicity to uninvolved tissues.

Radioimmunotherapy using radiolabeled anti-CD20 antibodies has been explored most extensively in FL and FL that has transformed to a higher grade. Currently, two radiolabeled anti-CD20 antibodies are approved by the US FDA for clinical use in the USA: ^{90}Y-ibritumomab tiuxetan and ^{131}I-tositumomab.

^{90}Y-IBRITUMOMAB TIUXETAN

Introduction

^{90}Y-ibritumomab tiuxetan was the first RIT approved for the treatment of patients with advanced relapsed NHL. It is a murine IgG1 kappa anti-CD20 monoclonal antibody (ibritumomab) covalently bound to tiuxetan, which chelates the radioisotope ^{90}Y. The advantages of using ^{90}Y include:

- Elution of ^{90}Y from the antibody is negligible, resulting in highly effective targeting of radioactivity to the tumor;
- ^{90}Y emits pure therapeutic beta radiation for which no special isolation or protection procedures are required, thus permitting outpatient treatment;
- The physical half-life of ^{90}Y and the biological half-life of the antibody are similar, therefore limiting the potential for irradiation of uninvolved tissues due to freely circulating isotope;
- The radiation crossfire with ^{90}Y is effective over a radius of approximately 100–200 cells, which is particularly advantageous in the treatment of bulky disease.[69]

Efficacy

Witzig et al. compared ^{90}Y-ibritumomab tiuxetan with rituximab in 143 patients with relapsed or refractory low-grade, follicular, or transformed CD20(+) transformed NHL in a randomized phase III trial and found that patients receiving ^{90}Y-ibritumomab tiuxetan had a siginficantly higher overall response rate (80 percent vs 56 percent) and CR rate (30 percent vs 16 percent) as compared to those receiving rituximab.[70] In a phase II study, Wiseman and associates evaluated the safety and efficacy of a reduced dose of ^{90}Y-ibritumomab tiuxetan

in 30 patients with mild thrombocytopenia who had advanced, relapsed, or refractory, low-grade, follicular, or transformed B cell NHL. They achieved an overall response rate of 83 percent with a 43 percent CR rate thereby demonstrating that reduced-dose ^{90}Y-ibritumomab tiuxetan is safe, efficacious, and well tolerated.[71]

^{90}Y-ibritumomab tiuxetan has been shown to be efficacious even in patients who are refractory to rituximab. In a multicenter study, Witzig and colleagues used ^{90}Y-ibritumomab tiuxetan in 54 patients with FL who had failed rituximab, and obtained an overall response rate of 74 percent (CR 15 percent).[72] In a phase I trial Vose et al. treated 16 patients, who had relapsed after high-dose chemotherapy and autologous stem cell transplantation, with ^{90}Y-ibritumomab. They found an overall response rate of 45 percent (CR two patients, PR three patients) thereby showing that this agent can be effective even in the post-transplant setting.[73] Preliminary data suggest that multiple doses of ^{90}Y-ibritumomab could be administered safely.

Current investigations are evaluating the potential benefits for patients with aggressive lymphoma. Current trials include single-agent therapy with ^{90}Y-ibritumomab tiuxetan for patients with diffuse large B cell lymphoma not eligible for transplantation, and consolidation treatment for low-grade lymphoma patients after first-line chemotherapy.

Adverse effects

The major toxicity of ^{90}Y-ibritumomab is myelosuppression, which usually has a nadir at about 7–9 weeks after treatment and recovers within 1–4 weeks. The myelosuppression seems to be greater in patients who have bone marrow involvement at baseline. Major infectious complications following ^{90}Y-ibritumomab are seen in approximately 5 percent of patients. Approximately 1 percent of patients developed secondary myelodysplastic syndrome/acute myeloid leukemia following treatment with ^{90}Y-ibritumomab.

^{131}I-TOSITUMOMAB

Introduction

^{131}I-Tositumomab is a murine IgG2a anti-CD20 monoclonal antibody radiolabeled with ^{131}I. The advantages of using ^{131}I include:

- The γ-emission of ^{131}I allows the use of noninvasive imaging to follow the pharmacokinetics and dosimetry of the tracer used for therapy;
- Chemistry and biodistribution and potential toxicities of free ^{131}I are well understood;
- Free iodine is substantially excreted through the kidneys in patients on thyroid blockade;
- The β-particle path-length of ^{131}I is relatively short ($\sim$1 mm); thus small foci of tumor can be treated more effectively;
- Free ^{131}I does not bind to bone cortex;
- The half-life of ^{131}I (8 days) matches with the retention of the radiolabeled antibody at tumor sites and the clearance of background normal tissue radioactivity.[74]

Efficacy

In a phase I/II single-center study conducted at the University of Michigan, Kaminski and colleagues treated 59 relapsed or refractory patients treated with ^{131}I-tositumomab and achieved a response rate of 71 percent (CR 34 percent). Sixteen patients were retreated on progression, and of these nine responded (CR in five patients).[75] This study included 14 patients with transformed low-grade lymphoma and the overall response rate in this subgroup of patients was 79 percent (CR 50 percent). These results were confirmed in a multicenter study that compared the efficacy of ^{131}I-tositumomab to the patients' last qualifying chemotherapy (LQC) regimens. Sixty patients who had not responded or progressed within 6 months after their LQC were treated with a single course of ^{131}I-tositumomab. The response rates (65 percent vs 28 percent), CR rates (20 percent vs 3 percent), and median duration of response (6.5 months vs 3.4 months) were higher after ^{131}I-tositumomab compared with their LQC.[76]

^{131}I-tositumomab has been studied in previously untreated FL with similar results. A recent Southwest Oncology Group (SWOG) protocol treated 90 patients with 6 cycles of CHOP followed by tositumomab/^{131}I-tositumomab. The overall response rate to the entire treatment regimen was 90 percent, including a CR rate of 67 percent. Fifty-seven percent of the patients who achieved less than a CR with CHOP improved their status after RIT. At a median follow-up of 2.3 years, the estimated 2-year progression-free survival (PFS) and overall survival were excellent (81 percent and 97 percent, respectively).[77]

Current studies directed toward using RIT in the setting of a myeloablative stem cell transplant show promising preliminary results.

Adverse effects

^{131}I-tositumomab has predictable myelosuppressive effects, the severity of which increase with the extent of the prior therapy the patient may have received. Myelodysplastic syndromes and acute myeloid leukemia have been observed in a small proportion of patients, similar to that seen after cytotoxic chemotherapy for lymphoma. Although patients are given thyroid blockade with a saturated solution of potassium iodide to prevent the development of hypothyroidism, elevated thyroid-stimulating hormone levels have been observed in a fraction of patients. Infusion reactions have been observed.

HIGH-DOSE CHEMOTHERAPY WITH STEM CELL TRANSPLANTATION

History

Hematologic malignancies show a dose-dependent response to increasing doses of cytotoxic agents, but the major dose-limiting toxicity of these agents is myelosuppression. The concept of hematopoietic stem cell transplantation (HSCT) was initially developed in order to allow patients to receive extremely high doses of cytotoxic chemotherapy without the complications of bone marrow toxicity. Since its first introduction into clinical practice, HSCT has developed to an increasingly important role in the treatment of hematologic malignancies. In the 1950s, stem cell transplantation by intravenous infusion of allogeneic bone marrow was attempted for the treatment of advanced hematologic malignancies, but initial attempts resulted in only transient engraftment. These transplants were performed prior to the development of histocompatibility typing, which could explain the poor outcomes. The first sustained engraftment occurred in 1965 in a patient with acute lymphoblastic leukemia (ALL).[78] The first successful trial was reported in 1977 on a group of 100 patients with end-stage leukemia.[79] The encouraging results from this study helped the concept of high-dose chemotherapy followed by stem cell transplantation gain momentum and led to its widespread application in the last two decades of the twentieth century.

High-dose chemotherapy

The two purposes of the preparative chemotherapeutic regimen (conditioning regimen) for HSCT are to eradicate the endogenous bone marrow to allow complete engraftment of the stem cells being infused, and to eradicate the tumor either completely or to a sufficient degree to allow the complete eradication by an immune response directed against the residual tumor.

The first agent used for HSCT for malignancy was total-body irradiation (TBI) alone. However, though TBI was successful in eradicating the endogenous bone marrow, it was insufficient to eradicate the leukemia being treated. High-dose cyclophosphamide was also initially used as a single agent but did not consistently eradicate either the bone marrow or the leukemia. The combinations of high-dose cyclophosphamide plus TBI, or high-dose cyclophosphamide plus the alkylating agent, busulfan, soon became the two most common regimens used for HSCT.[80] However, with the widespread use of HSCT, multiple other agents and their combinations have been investigated for conditioning, but there were no differences in outcome seen with the various regimens (Table 50.6). Consistent with the principles of combination chemotherapy described above, the selection of agents for use in combination for high-dose therapy in conjunction with HSCT should be based on the following:

- Nonoverlapping spectrums of toxicity.
- The major toxicity of all the agents at the doses used should be hematopoietic toxicity.
- Synergistic, or at least additive, effects of the agents being used against the tumor being treated.
- Lack of cross-resistance of the different agents.

Methods of collection of hematopoietic stem cells

Since the bone marrow is the most reliable source of hematopoietic stem cells, the original stem cell transplants were performed by harvesting the bone marrow. This

Table 50.6 Myeloablative conditioning regimens for hematopoietic stem cell transplantation

No.	Regimen	Doses
1.	Cyclophosphamide + TBI	120 mg/kg; 1200 cGy
2.	Etoposide + TBI	60 mg/kg; 1320 cGy
3.	Cyclophosphamide + etoposide + TBI (autologous)	100 mg/kg; 60 mg/kg; 1200 cGy
4.	Cyclophosphamide + etoposide + TBI (allogeneic)	60 mg/kg; 60 mg/kg; 1320 cGy
5.	Melphalan + TBI	200 mg/kg; 1200 cGy
6.	Busulfan + cyclophosphamide	16 mg/kg; 120 mg/kg
7.	Busulfan + etoposide	16 mg/kg; 60 mg/kg
8.	Cyclophosphamide + carmustine + etoposide	6–7.2 g/m^2; 300–500 mg/m^2; 600–2400 mg/m^2
9.	Cyclophosphamide + carmustine + etoposide + cisplatin	6 g/m^2; 600 mg/m^2; 1200 mg/m^2; 150 mg/m^2
10.	Carmustine + etoposide + cytarabine + melphalan	300 mg/m^2; 400–800 mg/m^2; 800–1600 mg/m^2; 140 mg/m^2
11.	Lomustine + cyclophosphamide + etoposide	15 mg/kg; 100 mg/kg; 60 mg/kg
12.	Busulfan + melphalan + thiotepa	12 mg/kg; 100 mg/kg; 450–500 mg/m^2
13.	Cyclophosphamide + anti-thymocyte globulin	50 mg/kg/d × 4d; 30 mg/kg/d × 3d
14.	Cyclophosphamide + thiotepa	1.5 g/m^2/d × 4d; 200 mg/m^2/d × 4d
15.	Cyclophosphamide + cisplatin + carmustine	1875 mg/m^2/d × 3d; 55 mg/m^2/d × 3d; 600 mg/m^2
16.	Cyclophosphamide + cisplatin + melphalan	5625 mg/m^2; 165 mg/m^2; 40 mg/m^2
17.	Cyclophosphamide + thiotepa + carboplatin	6 g/m^2; 500 mg/m^2; 800 mg/m^2
18.	Carmustine + etoposide + cytarabine + cyclophosphamide	300 mg/m^2; 300 mg/m^2; 800 mg/m^2; 6 g/m^2
19.	Melphalan + etoposide	140–180 mg/m^2; 60 mg/kg
20.	Carmustine + melphalan + etoposide	500 mg/m^2; 80–140 mg/m^2; 300 mg/m^2
21.	Melphalan + cytarabine	140 mg/m^2; 12 g/m^2
22.	Melphalan + mitoxantrone	180 mg/m^2; 60 mg/m^2
23.	Melphalan + mitoxantrone + carboplatin	160 mg/m^2; 50 mg/m^2; 1400 mg/m^2
24.	Melphalan + mitoxantrone + paclitaxel	180 mg/m^2; 60–90 mg/m^2; 500–700 mg/m^2
25.	Carmustine + amsacrine + cytarabine + etoposide	800 mg/m^2; 450 mg/m^2; 900 mg/m^2; 450 mg/m^2

TBI, total-body irradiation.

involves repeated aspiration of bone marrow from the posterior iliac crest, preferably under general anesthesia, until a sufficient number of nucleated marrow cells have been collected. However, with the discovery that an increased number of stem cells could be found in the peripheral blood during recovery from myelosuppressive chemotherapy or following growth factor administration, the use of peripherally collected stem cells has gained popularity. The peripheral blood stem cells (PBSC) are collected by apheresis, concentrated using various techniques, cryopreserved, and infused following myeloablative chemotherapy. In addition to quicker engraftment, and economic advantages, some studies have shown an increase in disease-free survival when PBSC were compared to marrow transplantation.[78]

Source of stem cells

Although the initial HSCTs were performed using donor cells (allogeneic transplants), current strategies involve using either donor cells or the patient's own cells for reconstitution of the bone marrow (autologous transplants).

ALLOGENEIC STEM CELL TRANSPLANTATION

Allogeneic HSCT involves the transplantation of a donor's stem cells after the administration of the conditioning regimen to the recipient. This is done using a HLA-identical sibling donor if possible in order to minimize the incidence of graft-versus-host disease (GVHD). This method offers the advantage of a tumor-free graft and also seems to provide a donor immune cell-mediated tumor eradication (graft versus malignancy). As the donor stem cells are not genetically identical, the donor cells occasionally mount an immune response against the recipient tissues. Although this can affect any host tissue, skin, gastrointestinal, and liver effects predominate.

Patients who develop GVHD also seem to develop a more potent graft-versus-tumor response, as multiple studies have demonstrated that patients affected with GVHD have a lower relapse rate than patients not so affected.[81] Not surprisingly, this effect seems to be most prominent when there are a small number of residual tumor cells. Donor T lymphocytes are postulated to play a major role in the graft-versus-tumor response, although NK cells could also mediate such a response.

Patients who do not have a HLA-matched sibling could receive a transplant from a matched unrelated donor (MUD), although this is associated with increased incidence and severity of GVHD and consequently a higher transplant-related mortality. However, the graft-versus-tumor effect is very potent in these situations and this procedure may provide better long-term disease-free survival in younger patients who can tolerate the increased toxicity.

Syngeneic transplantation can be performed in certain uncommon situations, when the donor and recipient are identical twins and therefore genetically identical. This offers a tumor-free source of stem cells that are genetically identical to those of the host. A major advantage of this is the absence of GVHD, but this also means an absence of the graft-versus-malignancy effect and, as a consequence, relapse rates are higher than in allogeneic transplants.[82]

The major disadvantages of allogeneic HSCT include the increased transplant-related mortality (20–50 percent), most of which is associated with GVHD. Older patients tend to be affected more by this and hence patients more than 55 years old are generally not considered candidates for allogeneic HSCT.

Currently attempts are underway to diminish transplant-related morbidity and possibly mortality by administering relatively nontoxic, nonmyeloablative doses of chemotherapy or radiation therapy prior to allogeneic transplantation, thus permitting the treatment of older patients and patients with medical comorbidities, who would not have otherwise been candidates for HSCT. The main aim of this new strategy of nonmyeloablative HSCT is to create a state in the patient in which the host's and the donor's hematopoietic systems coexist (mixed chimerism). The induction of mixed chimerism, moreover, may serve as a platform for the development of a graft-versus-tumor effect. A nonmyeloablative conditioning regimen should fulfill the following criteria:

- It should be sufficiently immunosuppressive to allow engraftment of allogeneic hematopoietic stem cells;
- In the event of graft failure, it should allow for autologous hematopoietic recovery without stem cell support;
- It should induce hematopoietic mixed chimerism following the engraftment of donor stem cells.

AUTOLOGOUS STEM CELL TRANSPLANTATION

Autologous transplantation involves infusion of the patient's own stem cells after treatment with a myeloablative conditioning regimen. This procedure is associated with less toxicity due to the absence of GVHD, and the procedure-related mortality associated with autologous HSCT is much lower than in allogeneic HSCT and comparable to standard chemotherapy in most centers.

However, the success of an autologous transplant is completely dependent on ablation of the malignancy with chemotherapy, in the absence of a graft-versus-tumor effect. Therefore, although an autologous HSCT is relatively safe and efficacious in chemotherapy-sensitive disease, this approach has very little benefit in chemotherapy-refractory disease. Another potential problem is the contamination of the graft with tumor. Chemotherapeutic agents or monoclonal antibodies have been used in an attempt to remove any residual tumor cells present in the graft, by a process known as

purging. However, despite the theoretical attractiveness of purging, current evidence does not indicate a clinical benefit from the use of purged grafts and further studies utilizing better purging techniques are needed to evaluate this issue further.

Efficacy

ACUTE LYMPHOBLASTIC LEUKEMIA

Acute lymphoblastic leukemia has a much poorer prognosis in adults, with a cure rate of only 30–40 percent, as opposed to children in whom the cure rate is approximately 75 percent. A French study compared allogeneic HSCT to other postremission therapy in 257 patients. Although this study did not demonstrate any benefit in the 5-year overall survival rate for allogeneic HSCT, a subgroup analysis indicated an overall and progression-free survival advantage for allogeneic HSCT for patients with high-risk features (Philadelphia chromosome positive, undifferentiated ALL, age greater than 35 years, high presenting white blood cell count, time to achieve complete remission more than 4 weeks).[83]

Autologous and MUD HSCT have been studied in patients with ALL who do not have a matched sibling donor. Although the overall survival rates appear to be similar between the autologous and allogeneic HSCT groups, the autologous HSCT patients tend to relapse early.[84] Matched unrelated donor transplantation, on the other hand, does decrease the risk of relapse when compared to autologous SCT, but is associated with higher treatment-related mortality.[85]

MULTIPLE MYELOMA

Autologous HSCT has been shown to be beneficial in prolonging survival in patients with multiple myeloma and is currently the standard of care for younger patients, who are otherwise healthy. The Intergroupe Francois du Myelome (IFM) demonstrated an increased event-free survival and overall survival when autologous SCT was compared to a standard chemotherapy regimen.[86]

Given the success of autologous HSCT in increasing the number of patients with CR, double autologous HSCT is currently being studied in an attempt to increase the number of complete remissions. A recent randomized study by the IFM showed an improvement in event-free, relapse-free, and overall survival following double HSCT as compared to a single HSCT. A subgroup analysis showed that the majority of this benefit was restricted to patients who did not have either a CR or a good PR after the first transplant.[87]

While autologous transplantation has been successful in prolonging survival, most if not all of these patients relapse and long-term survival rates are low. Allogeneic HSCTs have been attempted to overcome this, but are complicated by increased toxicity. In an attempt to minimize toxicity, nonmyeloablative allogeneic transplantation is being studied currently. The follow-up on these studies, however, is relatively short and long-term outcomes are unknown at this time.

LYMPHOMA

Hematopoietic stem cell transplantation has been used extensively over the last 15–20 years in an attempt to improve the prognosis for patients with both Hodgkin disease and non-Hodgkin lymphoma.

Although the cure rate for Hodgkin disease with conventional chemotherapy is approximately 80 percent, patients who fail to enter a complete remission do very poorly. Autologous stem cell transplantation improves the outcome of these patients significantly. Moskowitz et al. treated patients with biopsy-proven primary refractory Hodgkin disease with cytoreductive chemotherapy followed by high-dose therapy and autologous HSCT.[88] At a median follow-up of 10 years, progression-free survival and overall survival were 49 percent and 48 percent, respectively. Autologous stem cell transplantation has also been shown to be superior to conventional second-line chemotherapy in patients who have relapsed Hodgkin disease.[89,90] Although the results are variable in patients who have a prolonged first CR, patients who relapse early seem to definitely benefit from autologous HSCT.

Autologous HSCT has been utilized in an attempt to lengthen the duration of remission in patients with diffuse large B cell lymphoma. The PARMA study randomized patients who responded to two courses of standard chemotherapy to either further chemotherapy or autologous transplant.[91] They found that both event-free and overall survival rates were superior in the group that received HSCT. When patients were classified according to the age-adjusted international prognostic index (IPI), patients with an IPI >0 showed a benefit with HSCT. Autologous HSCT for relapsed aggressive NHL has become standard therapy based on the results of this trial. A transplant in first complete remission has been proposed in high-risk patients, but the results are more controversial at this stage.

Definite conclusions about autologous HSCT in follicular lymphoma are more difficult, as although HSCT improved disease-free survival rates compared to historical controls, an overall survival advantage has not been consistently demonstrated. The randomized European CUP trial of relapsed follicular lymphoma patients did, however, show an improved progression-free survival and overall survival with both purged and unpurged autologous transplant when compared to further chemotherapy.[92] The German low-grade lymphoma study group compared the effect of myeloablative radiochemotherapy followed by autologous stem cell transplantation versus IFNα maintenance therapy in first remission. They found that the 5-year progression-free survival was significantly better in the group that underwent the transplant. However, the results for overall survival are not sufficiently mature to

make any conclusions about the efficacy of HSCT in prolonging overall survival in follicular lymphoma.[93]

As mentioned previously, allogeneic transplantation is associated with a significantly higher morbidity and mortality, but offers the benefit of a tumor-free graft as well as a potential graft-versus-lymphoma effect. Studies comparing autologous and allogeneic HSCT have consistently demonstrated decreased relapse rates with allogeneic transplantation; this is offset by the higher transplant-related mortality and, consequently, there is no survival advantage. Protocols using nonmyeloablative doses of chemotherapy in an attempt to minimize mortality of allogeneic transplantation are currently being investigated.

CHRONIC LYMPHOCYTIC LEUKEMIA

Standard chemotherapy regimens have not been able to extend survival in patients with CLL. Although studies investigating utilization of autologous transplant as both a primary and salvage regimen for CLL have shown a reasonable response, whether they offer a benefit over standard chemotherapy is unknown.

Allogeneic transplantation has been attempted, but its use is quite limited due to the advanced age of most patients and increased transplant-related mortality.[94] While relapse rates do seem to plateau, it remains hard to recommend a procedure with such a high mortality rate for this indolent disease. Better definition of prognostic factors and longer follow-up of nonmyeloablative protocols may improve these outcomes in the future.

MISCELLANEOUS THERAPIES

Thalidomide and its analogues

INTRODUCTION

Thalidomide is a glutamic acid derivative first introduced in 1954 for treating the morning sickness of pregnancy, due to its sedative and antiemetic effects; but, it was soon found to be teratogenic, causing phocomelia, and was therefore withdrawn from the market in 1961. Continuing research, however, led to the discovery of multiple mechanisms of action that led to a resurrection of the drug.

MECHANISM OF ACTION

Thalidomide has multiple mechanisms of action including:

1. Inhibition of angiogenesis: thalidomide attenuates the activity of proangiogenic factors like tumor necrosis factor α (TNFα), vascular endothelial growth factor (VEGF), and interleukin 6 (IL-6).
2. Inhibition of tumor growth: thalidomide reduces the concentration of growth-stimulating factors like IL-6, insulin-like growth factor 1 (IGF-1), and fibroblast

growth factor (FGF). It also increases the susceptibility of tumor cells to apoptosis by affecting both the intrinsic and extrinsic apoptotic pathways.

3. Stimulation of immune responses: thalidomide stimulates cytotoxic T cell proliferation and induces the secretion of IFNγ and IL-2. It also induces cytokine production by T helper (TH) cell type 2 and concomitantly inhibits TH1 cytokine production.

4. Attenuation of metastatic potential: thalidomide downregulates TNFα-induced expression of adhesion molecules and abrogates adhesion of tumor cells to surrounding stroma.[95]

EFFICACY

Multiple studies have confirmed the efficacy of thalidomide alone and in combination with other agents in multiple myeloma, with a single-agent response rate of 25–35 percent and median response duration of ~12 months,[96] both in the setting of newly diagnosed and relapsed disease.

Preliminary results of a phase III ECOG trial, comparing thalidomide with or without dexamethasone as induction therapy for multiple myeloma, suggest an improved response for the combination.[97]

Thalidomide has also been investigated in the treatment of Waldenström macroglobulinemia, amyloidosis, and non-Hodgkin lymphoma, but the results are preliminary and long-term data are needed before it can be recommended for routine use.

TOXICITY

Side effects associated with thalidomide seem to be dose related and include sedation, fatigue, constipation, tremor, dizziness, bradycardia, and skin rashes. These effects, although mild, could affect the patient's quality of life and lead to the discontinuation of treatment. Peripheral neuropathy also limits prolonged administration. Deep venous thrombosis is usually observed, especially in combination with dexamethasone or other cytotoxic agents, particularly doxorubicin. Side effects are typically reversible and disappear after decreasing the dose and/or suspending drug use.

Use of thalidomide in myeloma is experimental in all countries except Australia. Because of the problem of teratogenicity, participating patients, physicians, and pharmacies in the United States must adhere to FDA-approved restrictions regarding its use, and must register with the 'System for Thalidomide Education and Prescribing Safety' (STEPS) program.

THALIDOMIDE ANALOGUES (LENALIDOMIDE)

Lenalidomide (CC-5013) is an immunomodulatory derivative of thalidomide with significantly greater *in vitro* activity. A randomized phase II study in relapsed refractory myeloma using two dose levels of lenalidomide demonstrated partial responses in 24 percent of 83 evaluable patients.[98] Two large phase III studies using lenalidomide with or without dexamethasone have been stopped by their data and safety monitoring boards due to superior response rates with the combination.

The most common adverse effects were thrombocytopenia and neutropenia. Adverse effects commonly observed with thalidomide such as sedation, constipation, and neuropathy, have not been seen so far.

Proteasome inhibitors (bortezomib)

INTRODUCTION

Bortezomib (PS 341) is a boronic acid derivative that is a highly selective, potent, reversible proteasome inhibitor.

MECHANISM OF ACTION

The proteasome is a multienzyme complex present in all eukaryotic cells that degrades proteins regulating cell-cycle progression and thereby causes proteolysis of the endogenous inhibitor of nuclear factor κB (NF-κB). Proteasome inhibition leads to the accumulation of a number of cell-cycle regulatory proteins and sensitizes these cells to apoptosis. Malignant cells are much more sensitive to proteasomal inhibition, probably to a differential effect on the cell-cycle regulatory proteins.[99]

EFFICACY

Early results of a randomized phase III multicenter trial comparing bortezomib with high-dose dexamethasone in 669 patients with relapsed/refractory myeloma found that patients receiving bortezomib demonstrated a benefit in time to progression and overall survival.[100] Bortezomib was approved by the US FDA and the European Union in 2005 as a second-line treatment of patients with multiple myeloma.

O'Connor *et al.* administered bortezomib to 26 previously treated patients with relapsed or refractory indolent lymphomas. They found an overall response rate of 58 percent, but the response was not uniform in the subtypes of lymphoma studied, with follicular and mantle cell lymphoma showing most benefit.[101] In a multicenter prospective phase II study of 155 patients with recurrent mantle cell lymphoma an overall response rate of 33 percent (8 percent complete or unconfirmed complete response) was seen with bortezomib.[102] Based on the results of these and other similar studies, the United States FDA approved bortezomib for the treatment of patients with mantle cell lymphoma who have received at least one prior therapy.

TOXICITY

Bortezomib has been generally well tolerated, with some patients experiencing low-grade fever and/or fatigue after several cycles. Thrombocytopenia has also been reported, but no patient had supportive transfusions. Other major adverse effects include neutropenia, low-grade diarrhea, which may be prevented with prophylactic loperamide, and peripheral neuropathy.

NEWER APPROACHES

Vaccines

The B cell lymphomas express a tumor-specific clonal immunoglobulin (idiotype [Id]). This is composed of the unique antigenic determinants in the variable regions of the clonal immunoglobulin (Ig) expressed by the tumor cells. This can be recognized by the immune system and can serve as a target for active immunotherapy.

Newer monoclonal antibodies

The success of the monoclonal antibody rituximab and the radioimmunoconjugates, tositumomab and ibritumomab, has spurred research into the development of newer targeted therapies. Epratuzumab is a humanized monoclonal antibody directed against the CD22 determinant RFB4, which is present on 75 percent of B lymphocytes. Apolizumab (Hu1D10) is a humanized IgG1 monoclonal antibody that binds to a variant of the HLA-DR B chain. Hu1D10 induces antibody-dependent cellular cytoxicity and complement-mediated lysis in lymphoma cell lines. Galiximab is a macaque-human chimeric antibody directed against CD80, an immune costimulatory molecule expressed on the surface of a wide variety of hematologic malignancies.

Antisense therapy

The BCL-2 gene is commonly overexpressed in NHL. More than 85 percent of patients with follicular lymphoma and t(14;18) translocation overexpress BCL-2. This leads to resistance to apoptosis thereby promoting tumorigenesis. Phase I studies have shown that antisense therapy targeting BCL-2 is feasible and potentially effective in treating NHL.

Cytosine–phosphorothioate–guanine (CpG) oligonucleotides

Bacterial DNA and synthetic oligodeoxynucleotides containing unmethylated cytosine-guanine dinucleotides known as cytosine-phosphorothioate-guanine (CpG) oligodeoxynucleotides can activate immune-cell subsets, including cells that participate in antibody-dependent cell-mediated cytotoxicity, and therefore potentially augment the antitumor effects of monoclonal antibodies.

KEY POINTS

- Combination chemotherapy is the backbone of the chemotherapy of non-Hodgkin lymphoma.
- Interferon therapy although effective is not commonly used due to the side effects associated with its usage.
- The advent of rituximab and other monoclonal antibodies, both naked and radiolabeled, has revolutionized the therapy of non-Hodgkin lymphoma.
- High-dose chemotherapy with stem cell support is an important option in patients with relapsed or refractory lymphoma.
- Thalidomide and its analogues are now the standard of care for the treatment of multiple myeloma.
- Newer approaches, like vaccines and antisense are currently being investigated.

REFERENCES

● = Key primary paper
◆ = Major review article

1. Devita VT Jr, Serpick AA, Carbone PP. Combination chemotherapy in the treatment of advanced Hodgkin's disease. *Ann Intern Med* 1970; **73**: 881–95.
2. DeVita VT Jr, Canellos GP, Chabner B *et al.* Advanced diffuse histiocytic lymphoma, a potentially curable disease. *Lancet* 1975; **1**: 248–50.
3. Chabner BA, Allegra CJ, Curt GA, Calabresi P. Antineoplastic agents. In: Hardman JG, Limbird LE, Molinoff PB, Ruddon RW, Gilman AG. (eds) *The pharmacological basis of therapeutics*, 9th Edn. New York: McGraw Hill, 1996: 1233–89.
4. Huang JC, Zamble DB, Reardon JT *et al.* HMG-domain proteins specifically inhibit the repair of the major DNA adduct of the anticancer drug cisplatin by human excision nuclease. *Proc Soc Natl Acad Sci U S A* 1994; **91**: 10394–8.
5. Boarman DM, Baram J, Allegra CJ. Mechanism of leucovorin reversal of methotrexate cytotoxicity in human MCF-7 breast cancer cells. *Biochem Pharmacol* 1990; **40**: 2651–60.
6. Storniolo AM, Allerheiligen SR, Pearce HL. Preclinical, pharmacologic, and phase I studies of gemcitabine. *Semin Oncol* 1997; **24** (2 Suppl 7): S7-2-7.
7. Smets LA. Programmed cell death (apoptosis) and response to anti-cancer drugs. *Anticancer Drugs* 1994; **5**: 3–9.
8. Twentyman PR. Bleomycin-mode of action with particular reference to the cell cycle. *Pharmacol Ther* 1983; **23**: 417–41.
9. Hsiang YH, Liu LF. Identification of mammalian DNA topoisomerase I as an intracellular target of the anticancer drug camptothecin. *Cancer Res* 1988; **48**: 1722–6.

10. Tsao YP, Russo A, Nyamuswa G et al. Interaction between replication forks and topoisomerase I-DNA cleavable complexes: studies in a cell-free SV40 DNA replication system. Cancer Res 1993; **53**: 5908–14.

11. Claman HN. Corticosteroids and lymphoid cells. N Engl J Med 1972; **287**: 388–97.

12. Lippman ME, Yarbro GK, Leventhal BG. Clinical implications of glucocorticoid receptors in human leukemia. Cancer Res 1978; **38**: 4251–6.

13. Chabner BA. Clinical strategies for cancer treatment: the role of drugs. In: Chabner BA, Collins JM. (eds) Cancer chemotherapy: principles and practice. Philadelphia, PA: JB Lippincott Company, 1990: 1–16.

14. DeVita VT, Schein PS. The use of drugs in combination for the treatment of patients with cancer. Rationale and results. N Engl J Med 1973; **288**: 998–1006.

15. Isaacs A, Lindemann J. Virus interference. I. The interferon. Proc R Soc Lond B Biol Sci 1957; **147**: 258–73.

16. Gresser I, Brouty-Boye D, Thomas M-T et al. Interferon and cell division, I: Inhibition of the multiplication of mouse leukaemia L1210 cells in vitro by an interferon preparation. Proc Natl Acad Sci U S A 1970; **66**: 1052–8.

17. Gresser I, Maury C, Tovey MG. Interferon and murine leukaemia VII: Therapeutic effect of interferon preparations after diagnosis of lymphoma in AKR mice. Int J Cancer 1976; **17**: 647–51.

18. Foon KA, Sherwin SA, Abrams PG et al. Treatment of advanced non-Hodgkin's lymphoma with recombinant leukocyte A interferon. N Engl J Med 1984; **311**: 1148–52.

19. Smalley RV, Weller E, Hawkins MJ et al. Final analysis of the ECOG I-COPA trial (E6484) in patients with non-Hodgkin's lymphoma treated with interferon alfa (IFN-alpha2a) plus an anthracycline-based induction regimen. Leukemia 2001; **15**: 1118–22.

●20. Rohatiner AZ, Gregory WM, Peterson B et al. Meta-analysis to evaluate the role of interferon in follicular lymphoma. J Clin Oncol 2005; **23**: 2215–23.

21. Cole BF, Solal-Celigny P, Gelber RD et al. Quality-of-life-adjusted survival analysis of interferon alfa-2b treatment for advanced follicular lymphoma: an aid to clinical decision making. J Clin Oncol 1998; **16**: 2339–44.

22. Kirkwood J. Cancer immunotherapy: the interferon-alpha experience. Semin Oncol 2002; **29**: 18–26.

23. Brice P, Bastion Y, Lepage E et al. Comparison in low-tumor-burden follicular lymphomas between an initial no-treatment policy, prednimustine, or interferon alfa: a randomized study from the Groupe d'Etude des Lymphomes Folliculaires. Groupe d'Etude des Lymphomes de l'Adulte. J Clin Oncol 1997; **15**: 1110–17.

24. Price CG, Rohatiner AZ, Steward W et al. Interferon alfa-2b in addition to chlorambucil in the treatment of follicular lymphoma: preliminary results of a randomized trial in progress. Eur J Cancer 1991; **27**(Suppl 4): S34–6.

25. Chisesi T, Congiu M, Contu A et al. Randomized study of chlorambucil (CB) compared to interferon (alfa-2b) combined with CB in low-grade non-Hodgkin's lymphoma: an interim report of a randomized study. Non-Hodgkin's Lymphoma Cooperative Study Group. Eur J Cancer 1991; **27**(Suppl 4): S31–3.

26. Solal-Celigny P, Lepage E, Brousse N et al. Recombinant interferon alfa-2b combined with a regimen containing doxorubicin in patients with advanced follicular lymphoma. Groupe d'Etude des Lymphomes de l'Adulte. N Engl J Med 1993; **329**: 1608–14.

27. Ozer H, Anderson JR, Peterson BA et al. Combination trial of subcutaneous recombinant alpha 2 b interferon and oral cyclophosphamide in follicular low-grade non-Hodgkin's lymphoma. Med Pediatr Oncol 1994; **22**: 228–35.

28. Solal-Celigny P, Lepage E, Brousse N et al. Doxorubicin-containing regimen with or without interferon alfa-2b for advanced follicular lymphomas: final analysis of survival and toxicity in the Groupe d'Etude des Lymphomes Folliculaires 86 Trial. J Clin Oncol 1998; **16**: 2332–8.

29. Coiffier B, Neidhardt-Berard EM, Tilly H et al. Fludarabine alone compared to CHVP plus interferon in elderly patients with follicular lymphoma and adverse prognostic parameters: a GELA study. Groupe d'Etudes des Lymphomes de l'Adulte. Ann Oncol 1999; **10**: 1191–7.

30. Rohatiner A, Radford J, Deakin D et al. A randomized controlled trial to evaluate the role of interferon as initial and maintenance therapy in patients with follicular lymphoma. Br J Cancer 2001; **85**: 29–35.

31. Neri N, Aviles A, Cleto S et al. Chemotherapy plus interferon-alpha2b versus chemotherapy in the treatment of follicular lymphoma. J Hematother Stem Cell Res 2001; **10**: 669–74.

32. Pressman D, Korngold L. The in vivo localization of anti-Wagner osteogenic sarcoma antibody. Cancer 1953; **6**: 619–23.

33. Kohler G, Milstein C. Continuous cultures of fused cells secreting antibody of predefined specificity. Nature 1975; **256**: 495–97.

34. Nadler LM, Stashenko P, Hardy R et al. Serotherapy of a patient with a monoclonal antibody directed against a human lymphoma-associated antigen. Cancer Res 1980; **40**: 3147–54.

35. Countouriotis A, Moore TB, Sakamoto KM. Cell surface antigen and molecular targeting in the treatment of hematologic malignancies. Stem Cells 2002; **20**: 215–29.

36. Anderson KC, Bates MP, Slaughenhoupt BL et al. Expression of human B cell-associated antigens on leukemias and lymphomas: A model of human B cell differentiation. Blood 1984; **63**: 1424–33.

37. Maloney DG, Smith B, Appelbaum FR. The anti-tumor effect of monoclonal anti-CD20 antibody (mAb) therapy includes direct antiproliferative activity and induction of apoptosis in CD20 positive non-Hodgkin's lymphoma (NHL) cell lines. Blood 1996; **8**: A2535 (abstract).

◆38. Hainsworth JD. Monoclonal antibody therapy in lymphoid malignancies. Oncologist 2000; **5**: 376–84.

39. McLaughlin P, Grillo-Lopez AJ, Link BK et al. Rituximab chimeric anti-CD20 monoclonal antibody therapy for relapsed indolent lymphoma: half of patients respond to a four-dose treatment program. J Clin Oncol 1998; **16**: 2825–33.

●40. Coiffier B, Lepage E, Briere J et al. CHOP chemotherapy plus rituximab compared with CHOP alone in elderly patients with diffuse large-B-cell lymphoma. N Engl J Med 2002; 346: 235–42.

41. Pfreundschuh MG, Ho A, Wolf M et al. Treatment results of CHOP-21, CHOEP-21, MACOP-B and PMitCEBO with and without rituximab in young good-prognosis patients with aggressive lymphomas: rituximab as an 'equalizer' in the MINT (Mabthera International Trial Group) study. J Clin Oncol 2005; 23: abstract 6529.

42. Haberman TM, Weller EA, Morrison VA et al. Phase III trial of rituximab-CHOP vs. CHOP with a second randomization to maintenance rituximab or observation in patients 60 years of age and older with diffuse large B cell lymphoma. Blood 2003; 102: 6a.

43. Sehn LH, Donaldson J, Chhanabhai M et al. Introduction of combined CHOP plus rituximab therapy dramatically improved outcome of diffuse large B-cell lymphoma in British Columbia. J Clin Oncol 2005; 23: 5027–33.

44. Colombat P, Salles G, Brousse N et al. Rituximab (anti-CD20 monoclonal antibody) as single first-line therapy for patients with follicular lymphoma with a low tumor burden: clinical and molecular evaluation. Blood 2001; 97: 101–6.

45. Witzig TE, Vukov AM, Habermann TM et al. Rituximab therapy for patients with newly diagnosed, asymptomatic advanced-stage follicular grade I non-Hodgkin's lymphoma (NHL): a phase II trial in the North Central Cancer Treatment Group (NCCTG). Blood 2002; 100: 361a (abstract).

46. Conconi A, Thiéblemont C, Martinelli G et al. Activity of rituximab in extranodal marginal zone lymphomas (MALT-type). Blood 2001; 98: 807a (abstract).

47. Foran JM, Rohatiner AZ, Cunningham D et al. European phase II study of rituximab (chimeric anti-CD20 monoclonal antibody) for patients with newly diagnosed mantle-cell lymphoma and previously treated mantle-cell lymphoma, immunocytoma, and small B-cell lymphocytic lymphoma. J Clin Oncol 2000; 18: 317–24.

48. Treon SP, Agus TB, Link B et al. CD20-directed antibody-mediated immunotherapy induces responses and facilitates hematologic recovery in patients with Waldenstrom's macroglobulinemia. J Immunother 2001; 24: 272–9.

49. Foran JM, Gupta RK, Cunningham D et al. A UK multicentre phase II study of rituximab (chimaeric anti-CD20 monoclonal antibody) in patients with follicular lymphoma, with PCR monitoring of molecular response. Br J Haematol 2000; 109: 81–8.

50. Walewski J, Kraszewska E, Mioduszewska O et al. Rituximab (Mabthera, Rituxan) in patients with recurrent indolent lymphoma: evaluation of safety and efficacy in a multicenter study. Med Oncol 2001; 18: 141–8.

51. Davis TA, White CA, Grillo-Lopez AJ et al. Single-agent monoclonal antibody efficacy in bulky non-Hodgkin's lymphoma: results of a phase II trial of rituximab. J Clin Oncol 1999; 17: 1851–7.

●52. Huhn D, von Schilling C, Wilhelm M et al. Rituximab therapy of patients with B-cell chronic lymphocytic leukemia. Blood 2001; 98: 1326–31.

53. HiddemannW, Unterhalt M, Dreyling M et al. The addition of rituximab (R) to combination chemotherapy (CT) significantly improves the treatment of mantle cell lymphomas (MCL): results of two prospective randomized studies by the German Low Grade Lymphoma Study Group (GLSG). Blood 2002; 100: 92a (abstract).

54. Howard OM, Gribben JG, Neuberg DS et al. Rituximab and CHOP induction therapy for newly diagnosed mantle-cell lymphoma: molecular complete responses are not predictive of progression-free survival. J Clin Oncol 2002; 20: 1288–94.

55. Vose JM, Link BK, Grossbard ML et al. Long-term follow-up of a phase II study of rituximab in combination with CHOP chemotherapy in patients with previously untreated aggressive non-Hodgkin's lymphoma (NHL). Blood 2002; 100: 361a (abstract).

56. Czuczman M. Progression free survival (PFS) after six years (median) follow-up of the first clinical trial of rituximab/CHOP chemoimmunotherapy. Blood 2001; 98: 601a (abstract).

57. Rodriguez MA, Sarris A, East K et al. A phase II study of liposomal vincristine in CHOP with rituximab for patients with untreated aggressive B cell non-Hodgkin's lymphoma (NHL): a safe and effective combination. Blood 2002; 100: 92a (abstract).

58. Boue F, Gabarre J, Gisselbrecht C et al. CHOP chemotherapy plus rituximab in HIV patients with high grade lymphoma–results of an ANRS trial. Blood 2002; 100: 470a (abstract).

59. Wilson WH, Gutierrez M, O'Connor P et al. The role of rituximab and chemotherapy in aggressive B cell lymphoma: a preliminary report of dose-adjusted EPOCH-R. Semin Oncol 2002; 29: 41–7.

60. Czuczman MS, Fallon A, Mohr A et al. Rituximab in combination with CHOP or fludarabine in low-grade lymphoma. Semin Oncol 2002; 29: 36–40.

61. Schulz H, Klein SK, Rehwald U et al. Phase 2 study of a combined immunochemotherapy using rituximab and fludarabine in patients with chronic lymphocytic leukemia. Blood 2002; 100: 3115–20.

●62. Keating M, Manshouri T, O'Brien S et al. A high proportion of molecular remission can be obtained with a fludarabine, cyclophosphamide, rituximab combination (FCR) in chronic lymphocytic leukemia (CLL). Blood 2002; 100: 205a (abstract).

63. Byrd JC, Peterson BL, Park K et al. Concurrent rituximab and fludarabine has a higher complete response rate than sequential treatment in untreated chronic lymphocytic lymphoma (CLL) patients: results from CALGB 9712. Blood 2001; 98: 772a (abstract).

64. Rastetter W, Molina A, White CA. Rituximab: expanding role in therapy for lymphomas and autoimmune diseases. Annu Rev Med 2004; 55: 477–503.

◆65. Robak T. Alemtuzumab in the treatment of chronic lymphocytic leukemia. BioDrugs 2005; 19: 9–22.

66. Osterborg A, Dyer MJ, Bunjes D et al. Phase II multicenter study of human CD52 antibody in previously treated

chronic lymphocytic leukemia. *J Clin Oncol* 1997; **15**: 1567–74.

•67.   Keating MJ, Flinn I, Jain V *et al.* Therapeutic role of alemtuzumab (Campath-1H) in patients who have failed fludarabine: results of a large international study. *Blood* 2002; **99**: 3554–61.

68.   Lundin J, Kimby E, Bjorkholm M *et al.* Phase II trial of subcutaneous anti CD52 monoclonal antibody alemtuzumab (Campath-1H) as first-line treatment for patients with B-cell chronic lymphocytic leukemia (B-CLL). *Blood* 2002; **100**: 768–73.

69.   Hagenbeek A. Radioimmunotherapy for NHL: experience of 90Y-ibritumomab tiuxetan in clinical practice. *Leuk Lymphoma* 2003; **44**(Suppl 4): S37–47.

70.   Witzig TE, Gordon LI, Cabanillas F *et al.* Randomized controlled trial of yttrium-90-labeled ibritumomab tiuxetan radioimmunotherapy versus rituximab immunotherapy for patients with relapsed or refractory low-grade, follicular, or transformed B-cell non-Hodgkin's lymphoma. *J Clin Oncol* 2002; **20**: 2453–63.

71.   Wiseman GA, Gordon LI, Multani PS *et al.* Ibritumomab tiuxetan radioimmunotherapy for patients with relapsed or refractory non-Hodgkin lymphoma and mild thrombocytopenia: a phase II multicenter trial. *Blood* 2002; **99**: 4336–42.

72.   Witzig TE, Flinn IW, Gordon LI *et al.* Treatment with ibritumomab tiuxetan radioimmunotherapy in patients with rituximab-refractory follicular non-Hodgkin's lymphoma. *J Clin Oncol* 2002; **20**: 3262–9.

73.   Vose JM, Bierman PJ, Lynch JC *et al.* Phase I clinical trial of Zevalin (90Y-ibritumomab) in patients with B-cell non-Hodgkin s lymphoma (NHL) with relapsed disease following high-dose chemotherapy and autologous stem cell transplantation (ASCT). *Blood* 2003; **102**: 30a.

74.   Wahl RL. Tositumomab and (131)I therapy in non-Hodgkin's lymphoma. *J Nucl Med* 2005; **46**(Suppl 1): 128S–40S.

75.   Kaminski MS, Estes J, Zasadny KR *et al.* Radioimmunotherapy with iodine (131)I tositumomab for relapsed or refractory B-cell non-Hodgkin lymphoma: updated results and long-term follow-up of the University of Michigan experience. *Blood* 2000; **96**: 1259–66.

76.   Kaminski MS, Zelenetz AD, Press OW *et al.* Pivotal study of iodine I 131 tositumomab for chemotherapy-refractory low-grade or transformed low-grade B-cell non-Hodgkin's lymphomas. *J Clin Oncol* 2001; **19**: 3918–28.

77.   Press OW, Unger JM, Braziel RM *et al.* A phase 2 trial of CHOP chemotherapy followed by tositumomab/iodine I 131 tositumomab for previously untreated follicular non-Hodgkin lymphoma: Southwest Oncology Group Protocol S9911. *Blood* 2003; **102**: 1606–12.

♦78.   Archuleta TD, Devetten MP, Armitage JO. Hematopoietic stem cell transplantation in hematologic malignancy. *Panminerva Med* 2004; **46**: 61–74.

79.   Thomas ED, Buckner CD, Banaji M *et al.* One hundred patients with acute leukemia treated by chemotherapy, total body irradiation, and allogeneic marrow transplantation. *Blood* 1977; **49**; 511–33.

80.   Colvin OM, Petros W. Pharmacologic strategies for high-dose therapy. In: Armitage JO, Antman KH. (eds) *High-dose cancer therapy: Pharmacology, hematopoietins, stem cells*, 3rd Edn. Philadelphia, PA: Lippincott Williams & Wilkins, 2000: 3–14.

81.   Weiden PL, Sullivan KM, Flournoy N *et al.* Antileukemic effect of chronic graft-versus-host disease: contribution to improved survival after allogeneic marrow transplantation. *N Engl J Med* 1981; **304**; 1529–33.

82.   Gale RP, Horowitz MM, Ash RC *et al.* Identical twin bone marrow transplants for leukemia. *Ann Intern Med* 1994; **120**; 646–52.

83.   Sebban C, Lepage E, Vernant JP *et al.* Allogeneic bone marrow transplantation in adult acute lymphoblastic leukemia in first complete remission: a comparative study. French Group of Therapy of Adult Acute Lymphoblastic Leukemia. *J Clin Oncol* 1994; **12**: 2580–7.

84.   Kersey JH, Weisdorf D, Nesbit ME *et al.* Comparison of autologous and allogeneic bone marrow transplantation for treatment of high-risk refractory acute lymphoblastic leukemia. *N Engl J Med* 1987; **317**: 461–7.

85.   Weisdorf DJ, Billett AL, Hannan P *et al.* Autologous versus unrelated donor allogeneic marrow transplantation for acute lymphoblastic leukemia. *Blood* 1997; **90**: 2962–8.

•86.   Attal M, Harousseau JL, Stoppa AM *et al.* A prospective, randomized trial of autologous bone marrow transplantation and chemotherapy in multiple myeloma. Intergroupe Francais du Myelome. *N Engl J Med* 1996; **335**: 91–7.

•87.   Attal M, Harousseau JL, Facon T *et al.* Single versus double autologous stem-cell transplantation for multiple myeloma. *N Engl J Med* 2003; **349**: 2495–502.

88.   Moskowitz CH, Kewalramani T, Nimer SD *et al.* Effectiveness of high dose chemoradiotherapy and autologous stem cell transplantation for patients with biopsy-proven primary refractory Hodgkin's disease. *Br J Haematol* 2004; **124**: 645–52.

89.   Schmitz N, Pfistner B, Sextro M *et al.* Aggressive conventional chemotherapy compared with high-dose chemotherapy with autologous haemopoietic stem-cell transplantation for relapsed chemosensitive Hodgkin's disease: a randomised trial. *Lancet* 2002; **359**: 2065–71.

•90.   Bierman PJ, Anderson JR, Freeman MB *et al.* High-dose chemotherapy followed by autologous hematopoietic rescue for Hodgkin's disease patients following first relapse after chemotherapy. *Ann Oncol* 1996; **7**: 151–6.

91.   Blay J, Gomez F, Sebban C *et al.* The International Prognostic Index correlates to survival in patients with aggressive lymphoma in relapse: analysis of the PARMA trial. Parma Group. *Blood* 1998; **92**: 3562–8.

•92.   Schouten HC, Qian W, Kvaloy S *et al.* High-dose therapy improves progression-free survival and survival in relapsed follicular non-Hodgkin's lymphoma: results from the randomized European CUP trial. *J Clin Oncol* 2003; **21**: 3918–27.

93.   Lenz G, Dreyling M, Schiegnitz E *et al.* German Low-Grade Lymphoma Study Group. Myeloablative radiochemotherapy

followed by autologous stem cell transplantation in first remission prolongs progression-free survival in follicular lymphoma: results of a prospective, randomized trial of the German Low-Grade Lymphoma Study Group. *Blood* 2004; **104**: 2667–74.

94. Dreger P, Montserrat E. Autologous and allogeneic stem cell transplantation for chronic lymphocytic leukemia. *Leukemia* 2002; **16**: 985–92.

95. Ribatti D, Vacca A. Therapeutic renaissance of thalidomide in the treatment of haematological malignancies. *Leukemia* 2005; **19**: 1525–31.

◆96. Dimopoulos MA, Anagnostopoulos A, Weber D. Treatment of plasma cell dyscrasias with thalidomide and its derivatives. *J Clin Oncol* 2003; **21**: 4444–54.

97. Rajkumar SV, Blood E, Vesole DH *et al.* Thalidomide plus dexamethasone versus dexamethasone alone in newly diagnosed multiple myeloma (E1A00): Results of a phase III trial coordinated by the Eastern Cooperative Oncology Group. *Blood* 2004; **104**: 63a.

98. Richardson P, Jagannath S, Schlossman R *et al.* A multi-center, randomized, phase 2 study to evaluate the efficacy

and safety of 2 CDC-5013 dose regimens when used alone or in combination with dexamethasone (Dex) for the treatment of relapsed or refractory multiple myeloma (MM) (abstract). *Blood* 2003; **102**: 235a.

◆99. Adams J, Kauffman M. Development of the proteasome inhibitor Velcade (Bortezomib). *Cancer Invest* 2004; **22**: 304–11.

100. Richardson PG, Sonneveld P, Schuster MW *et al.* Assessment of Proteasome Inhibition for Extending Remissions (APEX) Investigators. Bortezomib or high-dose dexamethasone for relapsed multiple myeloma. *N Engl J Med* 2005; **352**: 2487–98.

101. O'Connor OA, Wright J, Moskowitz C *et al.* Phase II clinical experience with the novel proteasome inhibitor bortezomib in patients with indolent non-Hodgkin's lymphoma and mantle cell lymphoma. *J Clin Oncol* 2005; **23**: 676–84.

102. Fisher RI, Bernstein SH, Kahl BS *et al.* Multicenter phase II study of bortezomib in patients with relapsed or refractory mantle cell lymphoma. *J Clin Oncol* 2006; **24**: 4867–74.

51

Role of radiation therapy

RICHARD T HOPPE

HISTORICAL REVIEW

Radiation therapy was first used for the treatment of lymphoma more than a century ago, within just a few years of the discovery of x-rays by Roentgen. The first reports included patients with Hodgkin disease and the non-Hodgkin lymphomas.[1,2] The responses to x-ray exposure at times were described as 'almost magical' and early radiologists recognized that curative treatment programs for these diseases might be developed. However, they also appreciated a need for a better understanding of the disease entities and better radiation therapy technology to achieve these goals.

By the early 1930s, improved equipment was available and clinicians had begun to recognize that many lymphomas, especially Hodgkin disease, had a propensity to spread to other lymph node regions, often contiguous with initial sites of disease. This led the Swiss radiotherapist Rene Gilbert to first test the concepts of extended field treatment.[3] His concepts were later adapted by Peters[4] and Kaplan,[5] both of whom had the advantage of improved diagnostic imaging and advanced treatment technologies with the cobalt machine or linear accelerator.

Until the late 1960s, the only systemic chemotherapy that had been identified to be useful in the lymphomas was nitrogen mustard. For that reason, radiation therapy was often relied upon as the sole initial treatment for patients with lymphoma, with nitrogen mustard used for relapse or for advanced disease presentations. At about that time, classification systems for the lymphomas became more accurate and reproducible and entities with predictable outcomes could be identified. As new systemic agents were identified, treatment plans could be defined for individual disease entities that incorporated radiation therapy, chemotherapy, or combined modalities.

Developments in radiation therapy were closely linked to advances in diagnostic imaging. Relying heavily on initial staging evaluations to identify sites of disease, radiation treatment plans could become more precise with the introduction of imaging modalities such as lymphography, planar tomography, computed tomographic scanning, magnetic resonance imaging, gallium scanning, and positron emission tomography. As computer applications saw their way into imaging and treatment, three-dimensional treatment planning, intensity-modulated radiation therapy, and image-guided radiation therapy have been introduced.

Radiation therapy for the lymphomas has evolved into a complex discipline. Many curative treatment programs for the lymphomas require careful integration of both chemotherapy and irradiation. Although radiation fields became large following Gilbert's work, they have become smaller and more precise as programs of combined modality therapy have been introduced, as functional imaging has helped us to identify sites of active disease more precisely, and as clinicians have come to appreciate the potential late risks of treatment in these patients who often live for several decades after their treatment.

PRINCIPLES OF RADIATION THERAPY

Methods of radiation treatment delivery

In general, radiation treatment may be delivered through external or internal sources. Most commonly, for lymphoma, treatment is delivered by external beam radiation therapy using a linear accelerator or cobalt machine. Radiation therapy may be delivered internally by radioactive implants (brachytherapy) or unsealed sources (radioisotope injections).

THE LINEAR ACCELERATOR

The linear accelerator is the most common device used in developed countries to administer external beam radiation therapy. Technology used in radar development during World War II was adapted in the UK at the Hammersmith hospital and in the USA at Stanford in the late 1950s to develop the first medical linear accelerators. Essentially, the linear accelerator consists of a wave guide into which electrons are injected and then accelerated. At the end of the wave guide the electrons interact with a tungsten target, producing high-energy x-rays. X-rays produced by linear accelerators generally have energies of 4–20 MV. If the target is withdrawn, the electron beam may also be used for therapy. This requires diffusion of the pencil-thin electron beam. Effective electron energies are usually in the range of 6–20 MeV. Most modern linear accelerators have a choice of multiple x-ray and electron energies for therapy.

COBALT MACHINE

The cobalt machine was developed in Canada in the early 1950s. It relies on an artificially produced source of radioactive cobalt-60 (^{60}Co). As the ^{60}Co source decays, it emits gamma rays with energies of 1.173 and 1.332 MV that may then be used for therapy. In developed countries, the cobalt machine has largely been supplanted by the linear accelerator.

UNSEALED SOURCES

Unsealed sources are radioisotopes that are injected intravenously. Unsealed sources are used commonly for diagnostic purposes (e.g., thyroid scans, bone scans, etc.). With respect to lymphoma therapy, the most common use of unsealed sources is in applications of radioimmunotherapy. Radioimmunotherapy (RIT) is treatment with radiolabeled antibodies. Both iodine-131 (^{131}I) and yttrium-90 (^{90}Y) have been linked to anti-CD20 antibodies for therapy of B cell lymphomas. The ^{131}I-labeled agent is known as tositumomab (Bexxar) and the ^{90}Y-labeled agent is known as ibritumomab tiuxetan (Zevalin).

BRACHYTHERAPY

Brachytherapy consists of the temporary or permanent implantation of radioactive sources into or close to a tumor. Temporary implants may be with radioactive sources of iridium, californium, or cesium. Permanent implants are generally with radioactive iodine seeds. Brachytherapy has its primary applications in the treatment of solid tumors such as prostate cancer, breast cancer, and gynecological cancer. It is almost never employed as a component of treatment for lymphoma.

Types of ionizing irradiation

PHOTONS/X-RAYS/GAMMA RAYS

Photons refer to the x-rays produced by a linear accelerator or the gamma rays produced by a decaying source of ^{60}Co. The characteristics of photons are dependent upon their energy, not the device by which they are produced. The dose gradient of photons as they pass through tissue is proportional to the square of the distance that the photons have passed from their source (or target in a linear accelerator) – i.e., the 'inverse square law' – and also by the energy of the photons. For example, for a 10 × 10 cm square field, at a depth of 10 cm in tissue, the relative dose is 57.8 percent of the maximum for ^{60}Co, 67 percent of the maximum for 6 MV x-rays, and 80.1 percent of maximum for 10 MV x-rays. However, there will always be some 'exit dose' since any thickness of normal tissue will fail to attenuate the beam completely. Shielding normal tissues in the primary path of the beam requires a thickness of $\approx$10 cm of lead-equivalent.

High-energy photon beams are also characterized by a small amount of 'skin sparing,' so that the maximum dose is not at the actual skin surface. For ^{60}Co, the maximum dose occurs at 0.5 cm depth, for 6 MV x-rays it is at 1.5 cm depth, and for 10 MV x-rays it is at 2.0 cm depth. The therapeutic implications are clear. The higher-energy beams will provide more sparing of the superficial tissues, which is usually, but not always, desirable. Skin sparing may be avoided by the placement of a tissue-equivalent bolus material on the skin surface, which then raises the depth of the maximum dose by the same amount as the thickness of the bolus material.

ELECTRONS

Electrons are negatively charged particles. For the energies that are usually employed for therapy, the 'depth dose' characteristics for electrons are substantially different from photons. The attenuation in tissue is much more rapid and electron beams in the therapeutic range will usually be attenuated completely in normal tissue. In general, the effective depth of penetration of electrons in centimeters is equivalent to one-third of the electron energy in MeV. Beyond that depth, the dose falls off rapidly. So, the effective depth of penetration of 6 MeV electrons is 2 cm (6/3) and the effective depth of penetration of 20 MeV electrons is just under 7 cm. There is little deposition of dose deep to the effective range of the electrons. This makes electrons suitable for the treatment of superficially located disease and a common modality employed for the treatment of cutaneous lymphomas.

OTHER FORMS OF IONIZING RADIATION

Other forms of external beam ionizing radiation include neutrons, protons, alpha particles, and heavy ions. All of these forms have been used for cancer treatment, but only protons may prove to have advantages for lymphoma therapy.[6]

The radioactive decay of radionuclides is another form of radiation that may be used for therapeutic purposes. The most common forms of ionizing irradiation resulting from such decay are beta particles and gamma rays. Beta particles are equivalent to electrons and have an effective path length that is reflective of their energy. For example, the majority of the beta particles from ^{131}I decay have an energy of 606 KeV and a maximum range in tissue of 2.4 mm. The beta particles of ^{90}Y have an energy of 2.29 MeV and a range of 1.19 cm. However, the radiation protection concerns are greater for ^{131}I, since there is also a component of gamma ray production associated with ^{131}I decay. These gamma rays have an energy of 3.64 KeV, which requires shielding for personnel. An advantage of ^{131}I is that this energy of gamma emission permits imaging.

Radiation fields

The definition of radiation fields is quite confusing. Concepts of 'involved' or 'extended' field irradiation are linked to the Ann Arbor staging system and its definition of lymphoid regions.[7,8] However, other terminology has

often been employed to describe particular configurations of fields, such as the 'mantle,' 'inverted-Y,' 'Waldeyer' field, and so on. Definitions may be quite variable and the following sections are meant to emphasize this variability.

INVOLVED FIELD

The definition of involved field arose in the context of patients being treated with radiation therapy alone for lymphoma and was originally defined as treatment to the entire lymphoid region as defined in the Ann Arbor staging description.[7] In many instances, when radiation therapy alone was employed, the definition was expanded in its application to certain regions. For example, when treating an involved mediastinum, the uninvolved bilateral hila or uninvolved supraclavicular areas may also have been included.

As programs of combined modality therapy have evolved, there has tended to be a reduction in the involved field definition. For example, in order to minimize morbidity secondary to irradiation, the upper cervical region may be excluded from treatment when only the supraclavicular area is involved; the contralateral tonsil may be excluded from the Waldeyer region when there is only unilateral tonsilar involvement, and so forth.

In the context of treating an extranodal lymphoma, involved field irradiation implies treatment to the affected site plus adequate margin to account for microscopic spread.

INVOLVED NODE RADIATION THERAPY

As functional imaging techniques have become more widely utilized for the initial evaluation of patients, there has been increased confidence that, in combination with computed tomography (CT), all sites of clinical disease have been identified. This has led to the recommendation to treat only very focal involved fields, ignoring the traditional definitions entirely, in the context of combined modality therapy.[9] Involved node radiation therapy describes treatment fields that include only those lymph nodes that are abnormal by size (CT criteria) or are 2-fluoro-2-deoxy-D-glucose (FDG)-avid. Criteria are being developed to help define the margins to place around the involved nodes in order to ensure their adequate coverage.[10] Involved node radiation therapy may only be considered in the context of combined modality treatment programs. It would have been inappropriate for treatment programs utilizing radiation therapy alone.

REGIONAL FIELDS

Regional fields would generally include anything beyond involved fields, but less than 'total lymphoid.'

EXTENDED FIELD

The original definition of extended field was to treat the involved lymphoid region plus each region contiguous to the involved region(s). For example, the regions contiguous to the mediastinum include the bilateral cervical/supraclavicular, bilateral hilar, and paraaortic. The regions contiguous to the cervical/supraclavicular include the contralateral cervical/supraclavicular, the Waldeyer region, the mediastinum, and ipsilateral axillary/infraclavicular. However, this definition is rarely applied in its strict form. Sometimes extended fields have been defined as extensions beyond immediately adjacent sites, but restricted to one side of the diaphragm. At other times, the definition has been applied whenever there is extension of the treatment field to the *other* side of the diaphragm!

MANTLE

The mantle field is a classical radiation field, originally described by Kaplan.[5] It was defined to include all of the major supradiaphragmatic lymph node regions – the mediastinal and bilateral cervical/supraclavicular, infraclavicular, axillary, and pulmonary hilar regions. The term 'minimantle' was used to define a mantle in which the mediastinal/hilar areas were shielded.

INVERTED-Y

The inverted-Y field was also defined by Kaplan. The inverted-Y includes all of the major subdiaphragmatic lymphoid regions – the paraaortic, bilateral iliac, and inguinal-femoral nodes, as well as the spleen (unless there has been a splenectomy). The term 'spade' has been used to define an inverted-Y field in which the external and common iliac and bilateral inguinal-femoral nodes are blocked. The term 'lower mantle' has been used by some authors as synonymous with inverted-Y. This is a misnomer. The term 'lower mantle' is inappropriate in this context, and equally inappropriate is the term 'upper mantle' to describe the classical supradiaphragmatic mantle field.

CRANIOSPINAL IRRADIATION

Craniospinal irradiation may be used occasionally in the treatment of lymphoma that involves the central nervous system (CNS). More commonly, it is used for medulloblastoma or for leukemia involving the CNS. It includes treatment to the entire brain by opposed lateral fields. This field is matched to a spine field, which is usually treated posteriorly. The matching of these fields requires careful attention to detail in order to minimize the risk of overlapping radiation doses.

TOTAL LYMPHOID IRRADIATION/TOTAL NODAL IRRADIATION

Total lymphoid irradiation (TLI) includes sequential treatment to the major lymph node regions both above and below the diaphragm. However, the details vary significantly. The Waldeyer region may or may not be included.

The whole abdomen, not simply the paraaortic nodes with or without the spleen, may be treated in some instances. Subtotal lymphoid irradiation/subtotal nodal irradiation has been used to define TLI in which the pelvic lymph nodes are blocked. Total lymphoid irradiation is rarely used any longer in the treatment of lymphoma, but low-dose TLI has been incorporated into some protocols for immunosuppression to prevent or treat organ graft rejection or to enhance transplantation tolerance in hematopoietic cell transplantation studies. Another term that has been used to describe fields similar to TLI is 'central lymphatic irradiation.'

TOTAL BODY IRRADIATION

Low-dose total body irradiation (TBI) was used in the past for selected patients with indolent lymphoma. Currently, the primary role for TBI is as a component of high-dose therapy for patients who are undergoing programs of autologous or allogeneic hematopoietic cell transplantation. The techniques of TBI vary widely. Generally, the treatments are fractionated, administered over a period of 3 to 4 days, with the lungs shielded for a portion of the dose.

TOTAL SKIN IRRADIATION

Total skin irradiation is used for the management of diffuse cutaneous lymphoma, most commonly mycosis fungoides. This treatment is accomplished with electrons, taking advantage of their superficial depth of penetration, sparing the deeper tissues entirely. Special treatment considerations are required to ensure treatment of the entire skin surface.[11]

Radiation dose

The unit of radiation absorbed dose is the Gray (Gy). One Gy is equivalent to 100 rad. Lymphomas, in general, are quite radiosensitive. This may be due to the intrinsic radiosensitivity of lymphocytes, which die an interphase death, secondary to apoptosis, after exposure to low doses of radiation. This radiosensitivity is manifest also in the lymphoid neoplasms. However, among the lymphomas, there is a variation in sensitivity. The more responsive lymphomas include follicular lymphoma, mucosal-associated lymphoid tissue (MALT) lymphomas, mycosis fungoides, small lymphocytic lymphoma, and mantle cell lymphoma. Among the less radiosensitive is diffuse large B cell lymphoma. Hodgkin disease is intermediate in its radiosensitivity.

The radiation dose prescribed for individual patients will vary as a function of diagnosis, treatment goal (palliation or cure), and whether radiation is to be used as a single modality or in a combined modality program. For example, some palliative treatment programs for follicular lymphoma utilize doses as low as 2 Gy times two (4 Gy total)[12] while curative treatment programs for follicular lymphoma generally employ doses of 30–36 Gy.[13] When treating Hodgkin disease with radiation alone, doses of 36–40 Gy are generally employed, while in combined modality settings the dose is 20–30 Gy, as recommended by the Clinical Practice Guidelines of the National Comprehensive Cancer Network (www.nccn.org).

Another important concept related to dose is fractionation, i.e., the individual daily dose. The usual daily dose for conventional fractionated treatments is 1.5–2.5 Gy. However, daily doses lower or higher than this may be appropriate in some situations. For example, if the entire abdomen and pelvis are being treated, the daily dose may be decreased to 1.20–1.25 Gy in order to minimize nausea. If a treatment volume is small and a brief course of treatment is indicated, daily doses as high as 3 Gy may be used.

The fractionation schedule for TBI is unique. The use of irradiation in this setting serves multiple purposes, including ablation of the bone marrow, immunosuppression (for allogeneic transplantation), and as a component of antilymphoma (or antileukemia) therapy. Common dose/fractionation programs include 2 Gy times six, with treatment twice a day, for a total dose of 12 Gy over 3 days, and 1.2 Gy times ten or eleven, with treatment two or three times a day to a total dose of 12 or 13.2 Gy. In these programs, the lungs are shielded from at least a portion of the dose. Single fraction TBI is less common in high-dose therapy programs, but generally the dose has been 8 Gy. Recently, nonablative transplants have incorporated a single fraction of 2 Gy as a component of the preparative procedure.

Radiation treatment planning

Proper radiation therapy treatment requires careful planning. Patients are generally 'simulated' in the treatment position and conventional planar or computed tomographic images are taken to assist in design of the treatment fields. For some simple treatments, external anatomic landmarks may be utilized to design the treatment fields. More commonly, the imaging studies are used to design the configuration of treatment fields that will provide the best coverage of the volume to be treated. In the management of lymphomas, treatment fields are often treated from 180 degree opposed directions – i.e., 'opposed lateral' or 'anterior-posterior/posterior-anterior opposed' fields.

More advanced, computerized treatment-planning systems incorporate three-dimensional treatment planning. This permits a more complex field design, with the possibility of incorporating treatment from multiple different directions. This may be especially useful in treating lymphomas in extranodal sites. However, even when three-dimensional planning results in the use of opposed fields, the planning process permits a more precise conformation of dose to the tumor volume.

A more recent advance in radiation therapy planning and treatment delivery is intensity-modulated radiation therapy (IMRT). Intensity-modulated radiation therapy combines a computerized inverse planning algorithm with computer-controlled treatment delivery defined by multileaf collimators on the linear accelerator to achieve a very refined dose distribution that exposes the tumor volume to a high dose while severely limiting the dose to adjacent sensitive organs. Intensity-modulated radiation therapy is not widely employed in treating lymphoma, since the doses required for tumor treatment are modest, but may be useful in some extranodal sites where sensitive tissues are present. For example, it is possible to provide better sparing of the salivary glands when treating extranodal lymphomas of the head and neck using IMRT techniques, compared to conventional or three-dimensional treatment planning.

HODGKIN DISEASE

Radiation therapy has a long history in the management of Hodgkin disease and improvements in the cure of Hodgkin disease during the mid-twentieth century can largely be attributed to irradiation. It has curative potential in early stage disease and contributes to improved control of bulky disease in more advanced stages.

Favorable presentations of stage I–II

Favorable presentations of stage I–II include patients with stage I–II who do not have systemic symptoms or large mediastinal adenopathy. In some series, patients with an elevated erythrocyte sedimentation rate (ESR; $\geqslant$50 mm/h), numerous sites of disease (more than three), or older age (greater than 50 years) are also excluded and treated according to algorithms for 'intermediate prognosis.' Historically, patients with favorable presentations of stage I–II Hodgkin disease were candidates for treatment with radiation therapy alone, with curative intent and expectations. Treatment volume generally included the mantle and paraaortic fields, as well as the spleen. Results in single-institution and cooperative group trials included 10-year survival of 90 percent and freedom from relapse of 80 percent.[14] These results are excellent, but the appearance of late risks of radiation therapy has resulted in a shift of management to the use of combined modality therapy. The major concerns include the risks of secondary neoplasia, especially breast cancer in women, and an increased risk of cardiovascular disease after mediastinal irradiation.[15]

The current treatment of choice for these patients is with abbreviated chemotherapy and limited (involved field) irradiation. Representative trials have included the Milan trial of adriamycin, bleomycin, vinblastine, and dacarbazine (ABVD) times four plus 36 Gy involved field irradiation (IFRT),[16] the British trial of vinblastine, adriamycin, prednisone, etoposide, cyclophosphamide, and bleomycin (VAPEC-B) for 4 weeks followed by 30–40 Gy IFRT,[17] and the Stanford trial of 8 weeks of Stanford V chemotherapy followed by 30 Gy IFRT.[18]

Important issues that have been addressed in clinical trials include the duration of chemotherapy and the dose of irradiation. In the HD10 trial of the German Hodgkin Study Group (GHSG), patients with favorable characteristics (normal ESR, no E-lesions, less than three involved regions) were randomized to two versus four cycles of ABVD and 20 versus 30 Gy IFRT.[19] Thus far, there have been no differences in survival or freedom from treatment failure among the four groups, suggesting that as little as 2 months of chemotherapy and 20 Gy IFRT may be sufficient in this setting.

Trials that have eliminated radiation therapy entirely have been inconclusive. The National Cancer Institute Canada (NCIC) HD6 trial included arms of ABVD alone, but the comparison arms included subtotal lymphoid irradiation alone for the patients with favorable presentations (age less than 40 years, lymphocyte predominance or nodular sclerosis histology, ESR less than 50 mm/h, and fewer than four involved regions) and 2 months of ABVD followed by subtotal lymphoid irradiation for patients with presentations with any unfavorable characteristics. Although neither radiation therapy-containing arm would currently be considered appropriate management, the freedom from progression in the two radiation-containing arms of the trial was superior to that of ABVD alone (93 percent vs 87 percent, $P = 0.006$).[20] There were no survival differences. In addition, the European Organization for Research and Treatment in Cancer (EORTC) H9 trial treated patients with epirubicin, bleomycin, vinblastine, and prednisone (EBVP) chemotherapy and randomized those who achieved a complete response to no further therapy or IFRT (20 vs 36 Gy). This study included patients who were aged younger than 50 years, had an ESR less than 50 mm/h (or less than 30 mm/h in the presence of B symptoms), and fewer than four sites of involvement. The 4-year event-free survival among patients treated with EBVP alone was an unacceptably low 70 percent and that arm of the study was closed early.[21]

Based on consensus data, the most commonly employed treatment for favorable presentations of stage I–IIA Hodgkin disease is combined modality therapy with chemotherapy and involved field irradiation. Selected patients may be treated with chemotherapy alone if radiation therapy is contraindicated and the increased risk for relapse is acceptable. Results of selected studies using combined modality therapy with involved field irradiation are displayed in Table 51.1.

The use of radiation therapy alone has a long history in the successful treatment of early stage Hodgkin disease, but has largely been abandoned due to the long-term risks of treatment, as noted above. It remains a good option for patients in whom there is a contraindication to chemotherapy. A specific scenario in which radiation therapy alone is the preferred management for early stage Hodgkin disease is the treatment of patients with stage I–II lymphocyte predominance Hodgkin disease. In this setting, IFRT to a dose of 30–36 Gy has achieved excellent freedom from relapse and long-term survival.[22] There does not appear to be any benefit from the addition of chemotherapy in this setting.

Unfavorable presentations of stage I–II

Patients who have unfavorable presentations of stage I–II Hodgkin disease, usually by virtue of a large mediastinal mass, routinely receive radiation therapy to sites of bulky disease. There is abundant experience with 3 to 6 months of chemotherapy followed by 30–40 Gy radiation therapy achieving an excellent outcome. Similar issues remain unanswered as for the favorable presentations, i.e., the duration of chemotherapy and the dose of radiation therapy. The GHSG HD11 trial for patients with intermediate prognosis randomized the chemotherapy to BEACOPP versus ABVD and the radiation therapy dose to 20 versus 30 Gy. Thus far, no difference in outcome has been reported.[23] However, this trial was not limited to patients with large mediastinal adenopathy and included patients with other adverse factors, including an elevated ESR, the

Table 51.1 Representative trials of combined modality therapy (chemotherapy plus involved field irradiation) for patients with 'favorable' presentations of stage I–II Hodgkin disease

Institution/group	Exclusions	n	Chemotherapy	Radiation dose	FFP (years)	OS (years)
Stanford G4 trial[18]	B symptoms LMA	87	Stanford V × 8 weeks	30 Gy	96% (8)	98% (8)
Milan[16]		70	ABVD × 4	36 Gy	94% (12)	94% (12)
German Hodgkin study group HD10 trial[19]	B symptoms Elevated ESR LMA E-lesion ≥3 sites	1131	ABVD × 2 versus ABVD × 4	20 Gy versus 30 Gy	97%[a] (2)	99%[a] (2)

[a]Pooled results from all four arms of the HD10 trial

N, number; FFP, freedom from progression; OS, overall survival; LMA, large mediastinal adenopathy.

Table 51.2 Representative trials of combined modality therapy (chemotherapy plus involved field irradiation) for patients with 'unfavorable' presentations of stage I–II Hodgkin disease

Institution/group	Inclusion criteria	n	Chemotherapy	Involved field radiation dose	FFP (years)	OS (years)
Stanford G2 trial[18]	LMA	61	Stanford V × 12 weeks	36 Gy	92% (8)	92% (8)
German Hodgkin study group HD11 trial[23]	B symptoms or Elevated ESR or LMA or E-lesion or ≥3 sites	1363	ABVD × 4 versus BEACOPP × 4	20 Gy versus 30 Gy	90%[a] (2)	97% (2)
EORTC H9U trial[21]	Age ≥50 or IIA, ESR >50 or IIB, ESR >30 or ≥4 sites or LMA	808	ABVD × 4 versus ABVD × 6 versus BEACOPP × 4	30 Gy	91–94%[b] (4)	93–96% (4)

[a]Freedom from treatment failure, range of results from the three arms of the H9U Trial.
[b]Event-free survival.
N, number; FFP, freedom from progression, pooled results from all four arms of the HD 11 Trial; OS, overall survival; LMA, large mediastinal adenopathy; BEACOPP, BEACOPP baseline.

Table 51.3 Summary results of the EORTC 20884 trial for patients with stage III–IV Hodgkin disease[24]

Treatment	Remission status	Consolidation therapy	n	5-year EFS	5-year OS
MOPP-ABV × 6–8	CR	None	161	84%	91%
MOPP-ABV × 6–8	CR	IFRT 24 Gy	172	79%	85%
MOPP-ABV × 8	PR	IFRT 30 Gy	250	79%	87%

N, number; CR, complete response; PR, partial response; IFRT, involved field radiation therapy, EFS, event-free survival; OS, overall survival.

presence of extranodal disease, and three or more sites of involvement. An analysis has not been performed restricted to patients with large mediastinal masses. Table 51.2 displays selected results using combined modality therapy for patients with unfavorable presentations of stage I–II Hodgkin disease.

Stage III–IV

Several trials have addressed the role of IFRT in stage III–IV Hodgkin disease. The largest and most convincing is the EORTC 20884 trial.[24] In this trial, patients were treated with six to eight cycles of nitrogen mustard, vincristine, procarbazine, prednisone, adriamycin, bleomycin, and vinblastine (MOPP-ABV) chemotherapy and those who achieved a complete response (CR) were randomized to no further therapy versus 25 Gy IFRT. No differences in free-dom from treatment failure (FFTF) or overall survival were identified. However, in that same trial, patients who achieved only a partial response (PR) all received 30 Gy

IFRT. The subsequent FFTF and survival for this group closely paralleled the outcome for patients who had achieved a CR, suggesting a value to adding IFRT after only a PR has been achieved. Table 51.3 summarizes the results of the EORTC 20884 trial.

Although the EORTC 20884 trial failed to support the routine use of IFRT after patients achieve a CR to a full course of conventional chemotherapy, there are programs of attenuated chemotherapy in which radiation therapy is retained. The Stanford V program includes only 12 weeks of chemotherapy, with very attenuated total doses of some of the drugs. Radiation therapy (36 Gy) is routinely added to initially bulky (greater than 5 cm) sites of disease, as well as to macroscopic splenic involvement. The results of this approach have been excellent.[25] The 12-year freedom from progression is 83 percent and the 12-year survival is 95 percent, with only minimal late complications of therapy. However, the radiation therapy component is essential, since a study that did not employ the same guidelines for radiation therapy resulted in a much worse outcome.[26]

Table 51.4   Local irradiation as a component of high-dose salvage treatment in relapsed Hodgkin disease[27]

Patient characteristics	n	3-year FFR		3-year EFS		3-year OS	
		RT	No RT	RT	No RT	RT	No RT
Relapse stage I–III	62	100%	69%	85%	54%	85%	67%
No prior RT	39	85%	57%	79%	52%	93%	55%

N, number; FFR, freedom from relapse; EFS, event-free survival; OS, overall survival; RT, radiation therapy.

Relapsed disease

There may be a role for radiation therapy in programs of high-dose therapy for 'salvage' after relapse. High-dose chemotherapy and autologous hematopoietic cell rescue is the standard treatment for these patients. Since radiation therapy is so effective in the treatment of Hodgkin disease, there is compelling reason to incorporate it into these programs, especially if sites of relapse have not been irradiated previously. This has been done in the form of localized irradiation[27] and total lymphoid irradiation.[28] Although randomized trials have not been performed, retrospective data suggest a benefit to the incorporation of radiation therapy (see Table 51.4).[27]

FOLLICULAR LYMPHOMA

This section deals with follicular lymphoma, grade 1–2. Patients with follicular lymphoma, grade 3, are usually treated in the same fashion as those with diffuse large B cell lymphoma.

Stage I–II

The follicular lymphomas (FL), grade 1–2, are quite radiosensitive and there is a significant experience using primary radiation therapy in early stage FL. However, since stage I–II FL is uncommon, accounting for less than 20 percent of patients with FL, only a few reports include a large number of patients. The treatment of choice for these patients is IFRT, although fields are sometimes extended somewhat beyond the sites of involvement.

Large experiences in the management of patients with stage I–II FL have been reported from several centers and the results are detailed in Table 51.5.[29–33] The long-term (greater than 10 years) freedom from relapse is generally 40–60 percent and survival is 60–70 percent. Most patients who relapse do so in unirradiated lymph node regions. Based on this relapse pattern, the use of more extensive radiation fields has been evaluated in several series.[29,32,34] In general, although the freedom from relapse may be improved with more extended fields, there is no improvement in survival.

Table 51.5   Results of treatment with radiation therapy alone for stage I–II follicular lymphoma

Institution/ group	n	Stage	FFR/DFS (years)	Survival (years)
Princess Margaret[31]	460	I–II	41% (10)	62% (10)
BNLI[30]	208	I	49% (10)	64% (10)
Stanford[29]	177	I–II	44% (10)	64% (10)
German multicenter[33]	60	I	74% (7)	
	40	II	56% (7)	
MD Anderson[32]	80	I–II	41% (15)	43% (15)

N, number; FFR, freedom from relapse; DFS, disease-free survival; OS, overall survival; BNLI, British National Lymphoma Investigation.

The use of combined modality therapy in this setting also has not proved to be superior to radiation therapy alone in randomized trials. The single prospective randomized trial with reasonable patient numbers to test this concept was conducted by the British National Lymphoma Investigation (BNLI) and the chemotherapy employed was single-agent chlorambucil.[30] No improvement was reported in 10-year survival or freedom from relapse for the combined modality regimen. Another randomized trial, incorporating 30–36 Gy IFRT with or without cyclophosphamide, vincristine, and prednisone (CVP) chemotherapy, is being conducted by the Trans-Tasman Radiation Oncology Group (TROG). This trial, TROG 99.03, is still accruing patients. A nonrandomized trial from the MD Anderson hospital, however, reported a 10-year survival of 80 percent and freedom from relapse of 72 percent for patients treated with cyclophosphamide, vincristine, and prednisone (COP) or cyclophosphamide, adriamycin, vincristine, prednisone, and bleomycin (CHOP-Bleo) plus IFRT, suggesting a value to the combined modality approach.[35]

Finally, there has been a trial combining low-dose fractionated total body irradiation (FTBI) with involved field irradiation.[36] Low-dose FTBI has been used previously in advanced disease (see below). In this trial for patients with stage I–II FL, 0.15 Gy times ten FTBI was followed by 40 Gy IFRT; however, the 5-year survival and freedom from relapse did not appear superior to treatment with IFRT alone.

An untested concept for patients with stage I–II FL is the potential value of combined treatment with rituximab and radiation therapy, with or without conventional chemotherapy.

Stage III–IV

There is limited experience treating patients with stage III follicular lymphoma using total lymphoid or central lymphatic irradiation.[37,38] However, this scenario of disease presentation is extremely uncommon. The general experience reports an overall survival of 45 percent and freedom from relapse of 35 percent at 10 years. Selected patients who have relatively few sites of nonbulky disease and are without systemic symptoms have long-term survival and freedom-from-relapse rates nearly as good as patients with stage II FL.[35] Alternatively, patients may be treated with combined modality therapy, including cyclophosphamide, adriamycin, vincristine, and prednisone (CHOP) and IFRT, with reported 5-year survival of 75 percent and relapse-free survival 52 percent.[39]

Patients with stage IV disease generally do not receive radiation therapy as a component of primary management. However, historically these patients were sometimes treated with low-dose fractionated TBI, for example 0.1 Gy three times a week to a total dose of 1.5 Gy.[40] Involved field irradiation was sometimes added to the involved lymphoid regions. Given the radiosensitivity of FL, it is not surprising that excellent responses were often observed. However, few patients remained free of disease and the hematologic toxicity was significant. This program is no longer employed.

Palliation

Patients with follicular lymphoma, especially in stage III–IV presentations, are often considered to be incurable; however, their median survival is long – more than 10 years in many large series. Many of these patients undergo repeated courses of systemic therapy; but, not infrequently, they develop local regional progression of disease that requires palliation. Radiation therapy can be extremely effective in this situation. Relatively low doses of radiation, 20–25 Gy, have been utilized with excellent palliation. More recently, programs of very-low-dose palliative irradiation have been tested. A total dose of 4 Gy (generally 2 Gy times two) is associated with an overall response rate of 92 percent and a complete response rate of 61 percent.[12]

MARGINAL ZONE, INCLUDING MALT LYMPHOMAS

Extranodal marginal zone lymphomas commonly present as stage IE disease and are often managed with radiation therapy alone. The most common extranodal marginal zone lymphoma is gastric MALT lymphoma. Gastric lymphomas that are associated with *Helicobacter pylori*

infection are treated initially with histamine H_2 receptor blockers and antibiotic therapy. However, stage IE gastric MALT lymphomas that are not associated with *H. pylori* or that persist after an adequate trial of antibiotic therapy may be treated quite effectively with local radiation therapy. The appropriate treatment is involved field irradiation, including the entire stomach and perigastric lymph nodes. A dose of 30 Gy has been associated with an event-free survival of 100 percent.[41]

The second most common site of MALT lymphoma is the ocular adnexal tissues, including the conjunctiva, lacrimal gland, and retro-orbital tissues. These lymphomas almost always present as stage IE disease. Local (involved field) irradiation is the treatment of choice. Relatively complex configurations of treatment fields are often necessary, sometimes including combinations of photons and electrons, in order to spare the lens, which is very radiosensitive. Fortunately, doses of only 25–30 Gy are required to achieve excellent long-term local control. Although local control is very close to 100 percent, as many as 30–40 percent of patients will have a relapse, usually located in other common MALT lymphoma sites, including the contralateral orbit.[42,43]

Other common primary sites of MALT lymphoma include the salivary glands and thyroid. Local control is generally achieved with a dose of 30 Gy. Distant failure is unusual for thyroid MALT, but occurs in as many as 20 percent of patients with salivary gland presentations.[43]

Palliative irradiation for MALT lymphoma can be very effective. Programs of very-low-dose irradiation (2 Gy times two) have been utilized for some patients.[12]

LARGE B CELL LYMPHOMA

Stage I–II

Radiation therapy plays a significant role in the management of diffuse large B cell lymphoma (DLBCL). Historically, radiation therapy alone was used in the management of this disease, at a time when it was referred to as 'diffuse histiocytic lymphoma.' Although results were not spectacular by current standards, some series reported long-term freedom-from-relapse rates as high as 60 percent in stage I and 40 percent in stage II.[44] With the introduction of programs of adriamycin-containing chemotherapy, patients began to be treated systemically, often to the exclusion of radiation.

Two important trials in the USA addressed the question of chemotherapy alone with cyclophosphamide, adriamycin, vincristine, and prednisone (CHOP) versus CHOP plus IFRT. In the Southwest Oncology Group (SWOG) 8736 trial, patients with stage I–II nonbulky disease were randomized to eight cycles of CHOP versus three cycles of CHOP plus 30–40 Gy IFRT.[45] The complete response rates were 73 percent and 75 percent, the 5-year progression-free survival rates were 67 percent and 76 percent ($P = 0.03$), and the overall survival rates were 74 percent and 82 percent ($P = 0.01$), favoring the combined modality

Table 51.6   The ECOG EST 1484 and SWOG 8736 trials for stage I–II DLBCL[45,46,49]

Trial	Randomization	n	Exclusions	Treatments	RT dose	PFS/DFS (years)	OS (years)
SWOG 8736[45,49]	Pretreatment	401	Bulky stage II (>10 cm)	CHOP × 8		67%[a] (5)	74%[a]
				CHOP × 3 + IFRT	40–50 Gy	76%[a] (5)	82%[a]
ECOG EST 1484[46]	Post-CR	352	Minimal bulk Nodal stage I	CHOP × 8		55%[a] (6)	73% (5)
				CHOP × 8 + IFRT	30 Gy	69%[a] (6)	87% (5)
	Nonrandomized PR patients	71		CHOP × 8 + IFRT	40–50 Gy	63% (6)	69% (5)

[a] $P < 0.05$ favoring combined modality therapy over CHOP alone.

N, number; IF, involved field; RT, radiation therapy; PFS, progression-free survival; DFS, disease-free survival; OS, overall survival; CR, complete response; PR, partial response.

approach over chemotherapy alone. These data are summarized in Table 51.6.

In the Eastern Cooperative Oncology Group (ECOG) EST 1484 trial, patients with stage I–II disease, excluding stage I peripheral presentations, were all treated with eight cycles of CHOP.[46] Those who achieved a complete response were then randomized to no further therapy versus 30 Gy IFRT. The 6-year progression-free survival rates were 53 percent and 69 percent ($P = 0.04$) and the 5-year overall survival rates were 73 percent and 87 percent ($P = 0.24$), again both favoring the combined modality approach. Based upon the results of these two trials, combined modality therapy is considered the standard of care in the USA.[13] Neither of these studies stratified patients according to the International Prognostic Index (IPI),[47] so a question remains whether the patients with the most favorable presentation see a benefit from combined modality therapy compared to CHOP alone. In addition, neither of these trials included rituximab, which is now generally administered to this population of patients.

In Europe, a trial was reported by the Groupe d'Etude des Lymphomes de l'Adulte (GELA) (LNH 93-1) in which patients with IPI = 0 were treated with chemotherapy alone versus combined modality therapy.[48] This trial has been interpreted by some to contradict the SWOG and ECOG studies; however, it was of substantially different design. Patients treated with chemotherapy alone received three cycles of adriamycin, cyclophosphamide, vindesine, bleomycin, and prednisone (ACVBP) chemotherapy followed by consolidation with methotrexate, ifosfamide, etoposide, and cytosine arabinoside chemotherapy. In the combined modality arm, the systemic therapy was only three cycles of CHOP plus IFRT! This clearly was imbalanced with respect to the systemic component of treatment and did not really address the question of the potential benefit of adjunctive IFRT. In addition, the outcome of patients treated with CHOP plus IFRT on the GELA study was quite inferior to the outcome of patients treated either with CHOP alone or CHOP plus IFRT on the SWOG study. The 5-year survival of patients with 'stage-modified' IPI = 0 in the SWOG study was 94 percent (both arms combined),[49] whereas in the GELA study the 5-year survival for patients

with 'age-adjusted' IPI = 0 was only 84 percent after CHOP plus IFRT and only 90 percent after ACVBP.

Given the historical role of radiation therapy in DLBCL, the question also remains whether some patients with stage I–II disease could be managed effectively with radiation therapy alone. Three series bear on this issue. Investigators at the Princess Margaret Hospital reviewed their experience in treating stage I–II large cell lymphoma with 40 Gy IFRT alone.[50] Based on their results they identified three prognostic categories of patients. The most favorable category was patients who were younger than 60 years, had no more than two contiguous sites of disease, were asymptomatic, and had no bulk exceeding 5 cm. In this group of patients, the freedom from treatment failure was 77 percent. Furthermore, in a series of patients reported by the Japanese Lymphoma Radiotherapy Group, patients with stage I–II who had no site of disease exceeding 3 cm had a 5-year event-free survival of 78 percent.[51] Finally, the BNLI group reported a 10-year cause-specific survival of about 74 percent for patients younger than 60 years with stage I aggressive lymphoma treated with local radiation therapy alone.[52] The 10-year cause-specific survival for patients with stage II disease was about 64 percent. The excellent results reported in these series would suggest that IFRT should be considered in very selected patients who may not be able to tolerate a course of conventional chemotherapy. The administration of rituximab in this setting would likely improve the results even further.

Stage III–IV

There are very few data regarding the role of radiation therapy in stage III–IV DLBCL. The ECOG conducted a trial comparing three adriamycin-containing chemotherapy regimens with an additional randomization to IFRT (25–30 Gy to nodal sites, 15 Gy to extranodal sites) for patients who achieved a complete response to the chemotherapy. Although an early report of this trial suggested a benefit for patients with stage III disease, a later publication indicated no benefit.[53]

In another study, from the National Medical Center in Mexico, 801 patients with stage IV diffuse large cell lymphoma were treated with cyclophosphamide, vincristine, etoposide, prednisone, and bleomycin (CVEP-bleo) chemotherapy. The 341 patients who had bulky disease in any site greater than 10 cm were then randomized to no further therapy or to 40–50 Gy delivered to the initially bulky sites. The 5-year event-free survival rates (55 percent vs 82 percent, $P < 0.001$) and 5-year survival rates (66 percent vs 87 percent, $P < 0.01$) both favored consolidative irradiation.[54]

Salvage therapy

Radiation therapy may be a useful adjunct in the salvage setting. First, there are patients who fail to achieve a complete response to initial chemotherapy. In the ECOG EST 1484 trial for patients with stage I–II disease cited above, when patients achieved only a partial response to eight cycles of CHOP, they were assigned to be treated with 40 Gy IFRT.[46] The long-term survival and freedom from treatment failure among these patients were similar to those who had achieved a CR. This suggests a role for IFRT in converting partial responses to CRs.

Patients who have a relapse of DLBCL after primary therapy are usually candidates for high-dose therapy and autologous hematopoietic cell salvage. Although TBI has been used in some programs as part of the preparatory regimen, this is not an appealing way to use radiation. Diffuse large B cell lymphoma is not as radiosensitive as the follicular lymphomas and the dose employed in TBI is unlikely to be an effective cytoreductive agent. However, the use of local field radiation therapy in this setting may be beneficial. Although there are no data that bear specifically on this point, in the 'Parma trial' that tested the concept of high-dose therapy for patients in first relapse of intermediate- or high-grade lymphoma, patients with relapse sites of 5 cm or greater were selected to receive IFRT to those sites. This was not a random assignment; however, the patients who had bulky disease and received IFRT had a subsequent relapse risk of only 36 percent, versus 55 percent in the patients with nonbulky disease who received no radiation therapy.[55]

PRIMARY MEDIASTINAL LARGE B CELL LYMPHOMA

Primary mediastinal large B cell lymphoma (MLBCL) is a distinct subtype of diffuse large B cell lymphoma. There is a female prevalence and an aggressive local behavior leading to intrathoracic and respiratory symptoms and complications. In addition to evidence supporting the use of more intensive chemotherapy for MLBCL compared to conventional DLBCL, there is a very strong indication for the early use of radiation therapy, even in patients who have stage III–IV disease.[56,57] Following completion of chemotherapy, mediastinal irradiation is initiated with a prescribed dose of 30–40 Gy.

MANTLE CELL LYMPHOMA

Although mantle cell lymphoma (MCL) is a relatively radiosensitive disease, the role of radiation therapy in its management is limited, since nearly all patients with MCL present with advanced disease. For patients with stage III–IV, fractionated total body irradiation may be incorporated in programs of high-dose therapy as either primary or salvage management. For the few patients with stage I–II disease, the same principles of management are employed as for stage I–II DLBCL. No prospective trials restricted to stage I–II MCL have been reported. However, limited experience indicates that radiation therapy is an important component of therapy for patients with stage I–II disease. In a report from Vancouver, British Columbia, a superior progression-free and overall survival was associated with the use of radiation in stage I–II MCL.[58] The optimal treatment for these patients is likely to be CHOP chemotherapy with rituximab (R-CHOP) plus IFRT.

PLASMA CELL NEOPLASMS

Solitary plasmacytoma is a 'solid tumor' manifestation of multiple myeloma. Solitary plasmacytomas may occur in the soft tissue sites (extramedullary) or bone (osseous) and, by definition, are not associated with bone marrow involvement. M protein may be detected in the serum or urine in one-third to one-half of patients with solitary plasmacytoma. Solitary plasmacytomas account for only 2–5 percent of plasma cell tumors.

Osseous plasmacytomas account for 70 percent of solitary plasmacytomas. They arise most commonly in the vertebrae, pelvis, ribs, sternum, scapula, and femurs. Appropriate staging studies include bone marrow biopsy and skeletal survey, to rule out generalized myeloma. In addition, magnetic resonance imaging of the spine may reveal subtle myeloma involvement.

The treatment of choice for solitary plasmacytoma of bone is radiation therapy. The treatment volume includes the involved bone and adjacent soft tissue extension, if present, with generous margin. For example, when treating an involved vertebral body, at least one additional vertebra should be included above and below the involved vertebra. The prescribed dose is at least 40 Gy in 2 Gy fractions. The local control rate after radiation therapy alone is 85–95 percent.[59–61] If myeloma protein is present, the likelihood of its disappearance after radiation therapy is 25–30 percent. The actuarial risk of progression to myeloma is greater than 50–60 percent at 10 years, and ultimately more than 80 percent of patients progress to myeloma. The risk of progression is greater if there is persistence of abnormal protein following radiation therapy. The overall median survival is about 10 years following diagnosis.

Extramedullary plasmacytomas are less common than plasmacytomas of bone; 80 percent occur in the upper aerodigestive tract, including the nasal cavity and maxillary sinus, and may be associated with bony destruction. Again, radiation therapy is the treatment of choice and the recommended dose is 50 Gy in 2 Gy fractions. The volume should include the entire tumor with reasonable margin. Regional nodes may be included in treatment of plasmacytomas of nonsinus head and neck sites. Local control is reported in 85–95 percent of patients[62] and the presence of bony erosion is not necessarily an adverse factor. In contrast to osseous plasmacytomas, the actuarial risk of progression to myeloma is only 10–30 percent.

Radiation therapy has frequent application in the palliation of painful bony lesions affected by multiple myeloma. Rapid fractionation schemes such as 8 Gy in a single dose are sometimes used, but more commonly the dose fractionation is 30 Gy in 3 Gy fractions. The palliative effects are excellent.

BURKITT LYMPHOMA

Burkitt lymphoma is an aggressive, often systemic disease. Large abdominal or mediastinal masses are often encountered. The African variety presents with large jaw tumors. There is a modest risk for central nervous system involvement. The role of radiation therapy in this disease is limited. Due to its high proliferation index, hyperfractionated irradiation (two- or three-times-a-day treatment) has been suggested as appropriate if there is an indication for irradiation;[63] however, there is no evidence to support its routine use in primary patient management, even for patients with large tumor masses.[64] Cranial or cranial-spinal irradiation may be employed for patients with central nervous system involvement.

LYMPHOBLASTIC LYMPHOMA/LEUKEMIA

Lymphoblastic lymphoma/leukemia (LL/L) is a very radiosensitive lymphoma. However, due to the systemic nature of this disease and its responsiveness to chemotherapy, radiation therapy is not commonly employed in its management, even for consolidation of complete responses in cases of bulky mediastinal disease. Although some data suggest that consolidative irradiation to the mediastinum may decrease the risk for mediastinal recurrence among patients who achieve a CR to chemotherapy, this does not translate into a survival benefit.[65] Due to the propensity of this lymphoma to involve the CNS, most treatment protocols incorporate a component of CNS prophylaxis. This may be either with intrathecal chemotherapy alone or with a combination of intrathecal chemotherapy and whole brain irradiation. The dose employed in these situations is 18–24 Gy, with 1.5–1.8 Gy fractions.[66]

NATURAL KILLER/T CELL LYMPHOMA, NASAL TYPE

The natural killer (NK)/T cell lymphomas, nasal type, are most prevalent among people of Asian, South American, or Central American ethnicity and are Epstein–Barr virus positive in the majority of cases. This disease presents most commonly in the nasal cavity, and is locally aggressive with frequent extension into the paranasal sinuses. Regional lymphatics may also be involved. Unlike many other lymphomas, NK/T cell lymphoma is relatively resistant to systemic management[67] and higher doses of radiation are required to reliably achieve local control.[68]

The general principle of management is to use combined modality therapy. In patients who have stage IE disease, radiation therapy may be employed initially in order to achieve local control. The involved region plus 1.5–2 cm of adjacent tissue is normally included in the primary treatment field, modifying the field and dose as appropriate for important structures such as the optic chiasm. Three-dimensional treatment planning or IMRT is essential to devise an optimal treatment plan. An initial dose of 50–54 Gy is prescribed, followed by adjuvant systemic therapy.

For patients with stage IIE disease (lymph node involvement), systemic therapy may be administered first, followed by irradiation to the primary site and involved nodes. Even patients with stage III–IV may benefit from the use of local irradiation following the completion of systemic therapy, since local recurrence is such a common problem in these patients if chemotherapy alone is used in their management. The 5-year survival of patients with stage IE–IIE disease is approximately 40 percent.

ANAPLASTIC LARGE CELL LYMPHOMA

There is little in the literature relevant to the role of radiation therapy for anaplastic large cell lymphoma. Generally, treatment programs for this disease are similar to those for diffuse large B cell lymphoma, with the exception that rituximab is not included as a component of the systemic management (unless it is a CD30-positive variant).

PERIPHERAL T CELL LYMPHOMA

There is little in the literature relevant to the role of radiation therapy for peripheral T cell lymphoma. Generally, this disease has a worse prognosis than equivalent stage B cell lymphoma. The treatment programs for peripheral T cell lymphoma may be similar to those for diffuse large B cell lymphoma, at other times more intensive chemotherapy is utilized. Of course, rituximab is not included as a component of the systemic management. Consolidative irradiation is reasonable for the occasional patient who has only stage I–II disease.

THE PRIMARY CUTANEOUS LYMPHOMAS

Mycosis fungoides

Mycosis fungoides (MF), a T cell lymphoma, is the most common cutaneous lymphoma. Radiation therapy is a very effective agent in treating this disease.[69] Patients with MF commonly present with generalized skin involvement, consisting of patches and plaques. Topical therapies such as nitrogen mustard or corticosteroids, phototherapy such as narrow band UVB, and radiation therapy may all be used for patients with generalized skin disease. Radiation therapy achieves the highest complete response rates. When cutaneous tumors are present, radiation has a far greater ability to eradicate disease than any other modality.

For patients with generalized skin involvement, a special technique of irradiation has been developed – total skin electron beam therapy (TSEBT) – that permits treatment to the entire skin. Patients are treated in the standing position and must assume several different 'poses,' or else they may be treated on a rotating table, in order to expose the entire skin surface to the treatment.[11] Electrons are chosen as the form of ionizing irradiation because they will penetrate to only a finite depth. Therefore, despite the entire skin surface being treated, there is no effect of the irradiation beyond a centimeter or so of depth. The energy of electrons commonly used in this situation is 9 MeV. The dosimetry is complex due to the intersection of multiple beams at oblique angles to the skin surface. The 80 percent depth dose – i.e., the depth at which the dose of irradiation is degraded to 80 percent of its maximum – occurs at 0.7–0.8 cm. Each treatment fraction is generally small, e.g., 1 Gy. The total dose delivered is generally 30–36 Gy.

The overall results of TSEBT are excellent. For stage IB–IIA disease (generalized patch/plaque disease), the overall response rate is nearly 100 percent and the complete response rate is 56–81 percent in large series. For patients with stage IIB (cutaneous tumors), the complete response rate is 24–53 percent.[70] Complications include hair loss, temporary effects on ability to sweat, occasional skin atrophy or telangiectasia, and an increased risk of squamoproliferative lesions. Because of those risks, the treatment is generally not used for patients with stage IA (limited patch/plaque). In addition, it is not often used in stage IIIA (erythroderma), since the atrophic skin of those patients does not tolerate irradiation very well.

Although TSEBT has a high likelihood of clearing the skin entirely, disease will often recur, and the major benefit of treatment is its important palliative effect and ability to decrease the disease 'burden.' Other therapies, such as topical nitrogen mustard or phototherapy, may then be used in an attempt to maintain the skin clearance.

Occasional patients present with 'unilesional MF.' When this disease presents as a solitary patch or plaque, the likelihood of eradicating it completely and permanently with a single course of local electron beam therapy is excellent.[71] Doses of 25–35 Gy have been used in this setting, treating the primary lesion and including 2 cm margins of apparently normal skin.

Local irradiation is also very useful as a palliative therapy for patients with cutaneous tumors or plaques that are refractory to other therapies. Doses of 15–35 Gy may be used, depending upon the site of involvement and rapidity of response.

Patients with extracutaneous MF may also benefit from the use of irradiation. Lymph node involvement, especially when localized, can be treated with involved field irradiation in a fashion analogous to that used for other lymphomas.

Follicle center cell lymphoma

The second most common type of primary cutaneous lymphoma is follicle center cell lymphoma (FCCL), a B cell disease. This includes many lymphomas classified previously as follicular lymphoma or diffuse large B cell lymphoma. Follicle center cell lymphoma often presents as a solitary lesion. Local irradiation is usually successful in achieving long-term local control.[72] Doses of 30–40 Gy, depending upon location and size of disease, are usually employed. Margins of uninvolved skin should be 1.5–2 cm. Although the local control rates are excellent, about 20 percent of patients will have a relapse of disease in a remote skin site. Recurrent disease may again be treated with irradiation.

Marginal zone lymphoma

Marginal zone lymphoma (MZL) of the skin is as responsive to irradiation as MZL in other sites. In some instances, there may be a solitary lesion, in which case local irradiation to a dose of 25–35 Gy may achieve excellent local control and freedom from treatment failure. When there are multiple lesions, they may still be irradiated; however, the risk of subsequent relapse is much greater.

Anaplastic large cell lymphoma

Anaplastic large cell lymphoma (ALCL) is part of the spectrum of CD30-positive lymphoproliferative diseases of the skin. It may occur in the previous setting of mycosis fungoides, lymphomatoid papulosis, or even Hodgkin disease. Local irradiation is the treatment of choice; however, the response to treatment is variable, and doses in the range of 35–55 Gy may be used, depending upon the rapidity of the response.

Other primary cutaneous lymphomas

Other cutaneous lymphomas may include peripheral T cell lymphoma, NK/T cell lymphoma, diffuse large cell lymphoma (leg type), and other miscellaneous entities. Radiation therapy may be employed for these patients, especially when the lesions are solitary; however, most commonly these are treated with combined modality therapy, including local irradiation.

KEY POINTS

- Radiation therapy has broad applications in the management of patients with lymphoma.
- Involved field irradiation is often a curative treatment for patients with stage I–II nodular lymphocyte-predominant Hodgkin disease.
- Involved field irradiation is an important component of curative combined modality therapy programs for stage I–II classical Hodgkin lymphoma, especially for patients with large mediastinal adenopathy.
- The role of radiation therapy in stage III–IV Hodgkin lymphoma is debatable, but essential in some programs, such as the Stanford V regimen
- Involved field irradiation is often a curative treatment for patients with stage I–II follicular lymphoma (grade 1–2).
- Low-dose radiation ($2\,\mathrm{Gy} \times 2$) is often an effective palliative therapy for patients with follicular or marginal zone lymphoma.
- Involved field irradiation is often a curative treatment for patients with stage IE–IIE marginal zone lymphoma.
- Involved field irradiation is an important component of curative combined modality therapy programs for stage I–II diffuse large B cell lymphoma and other aggressive lymphomas.

REFERENCES

● = Key primary paper
◆ = Major review article

1. Pusey WE. Cases of sarcoma and of Hodgkin's disease treated by exposures to x-rays – a preliminary report. *JAMA* 1902; **38**: 166–9.
2. Senn N. *New York Medical Journal* 1903; **77**: 665–8.
3. Gilbert R, Babaiantz L. Notre methode de roentgentherapie de la lymphogranulomatose (Hodgkin): resultats eloignes. *Acta Radiol* 1931; **12**: 523–9.
4. Peters M, Middlemiss K. A study of Hodgkin's disease treated by irradiation. *Am J Roentgenol Radium Ther Nucl Med* 1958; **79**: 114–21.
5. Kaplan HS. The radical radiotherapy of regionally localized Hodgkin's disease. *Radiology* 1962; **78**: 553–61.
6. Mendenhall NP, Yeung D. Potential role of proton therapy in the management of lymphoma. In: Delaney TF, Kooy HM (eds) *Proton and charged particle therapy*. Philadelphia: Lippincott Williams & Wilkins, 2008: 262–66.
7. Carbone PP, Kaplan HS, Musshoff K *et al.* Report of the committee on Hodgkin's disease staging classification. *Cancer Res* 1971; **31**: 1860–1.
8. Kaplan HS, Rosenberg S. The treatment of Hodgkin's disease. *Med Clin North Am* 1966; **50**: 1591–1610.
●9. Girinsky T, van der Maazen R, Specht L *et al.* Involved-node radiotherapy (INRT) in patients with early Hodgkin lymphoma: concepts and guidelines. *Radiother Oncol* 2006; **79**: 270–7.
10. Girinsky T, Ghalibafian M, Bonniaud G *et al.* Is FDG-PET scan in patients with early stage Hodgkin lymphoma of any value in the implementation of the involved-node radiotherapy concept and dose painting? *Radiother Oncol* 2007; **85**: 178–86.
◆11. Hoppe RT, Fuks Z, Bagshaw MA. Radiation therapy in the management of cutaneous T-cell lymphomas. *Cancer Treat Rep* 1979; **63**: 625–32.
●12. Haas RL, Poortmans P, deJong D *et al.* High response rates and lasting remissions after low-dose involved field radiotheray in indolent lymphomas. *J Clin Oncol* 2003; **21**: 2474–80.
◆13. NCCN: NCCN Treatment Guidelines for Hodgkin's Disease. www.nccn.org
14. Hoppe RT, Coleman CN, Cox RS *et al.* The management of stage I–II Hodgkin's disease with irradiation alone or combined modality therapy: the Stanford experience. *Blood* 1982; **59**: 455–65.
15. Hoppe RT. Hodgkin's disease: complications of therapy and excess mortality. *Ann Oncol* 1997; **8**(Suppl 1): 115–8.
16. Bonadonna G, Bonfante V, Viviani S *et al.* ABVD plus subtotal nodal versus involved-field radiotherapy in early-stage Hodgkin's disease: long-term results. *J Clin Oncol* 2004; **22**: 2835–41.
17. Moody AM, Pratt J, Hudson GV *et al.* British National Lymphoma Investigation: pilot studies of neoadjuvant chemotherapy in clinical stage Ia and IIa Hodgkin's disease. *Clin Oncol (R Coll Radiol)* 2001; **13**: 262–8.
18. Horning S, Hoppe RT, Advani R *et al.* Efficacy and late effects of Stanford V chemotherapy and radiotherapy in untreated Hodgkin's disease: Mature data in early and advanced stage patients. *Blood* 2004; **104**: abstract 308.
19. Diehl V, Brillant C, Engert A *et al.* HD10: Investigating reduction of combined modality treatment intensity in early stage Hodgkin's lymphoma. Interim analysis of a randomized trial of the German Hodgkin Study Group (GHSG). *J Clin Oncol* 2005; **23**(16 Suppl I): 6506 (abstract).
●20. Meyer RM, Gospodarowicz M, Connors JM *et al.* Randomized comparison of ABVD chemotherapy with a strategy that includes radiation therapy in patients with

limited-stage Hodgkin's lymphoma: National Cancer Institute of Canada Trials Group and the Eastern Cooperative Oncology Group. *J Clin Oncol* 2005; **23**: 4634–42.

21. Noordijk E, Thomas J, Ferme C *et al.* First results of the EORTC-GELA H9 randomized trials: the H9-F trial (comparing 3 radiation dose levels) and H9-U trial (comparing 3 chemotherapy schemes) in patients with favorabe or unfavorable early stage Hodgkin's lymphoma (HL). *J Clin Oncol* 2005; **23**(16 Suppl I): 6505 (abstract).

22. Wirth A, Chao M, Corry J *et al.* Mantle irradiation alone for clinical stage I–II Hodgkin's disease: long-term follow-up and analysis of prognostic factors in 261 patients. *J Clin Oncol* 1999; **17**: 230–40.

23. Klimm B, Engert C, Brillant C *et al.* Comparison of BEACOPP and ABVD chemotherapy in intermediate stage Hodgkin's lymphoma: results of the fourth interim analysis of the HD 11 trial of the GHSG. *J Clin Oncol* 2005; **23**(16 Suppl I): 6507 (abstract).

●24. Aleman BM, Raemakers JM, Tirelli U *et al.* Involved field radiotherapy for advanced Hodgkin's lymphoma. *N Engl J Med* 2003; **348**: 2396–406.

25. Horning S, Hoppe R, Advani R *et al.* Efficacy and late effects of Stanford V chemotherapy and radiotherapy in untreated Hodgkin's disease: mature data in early and advanced stage patients. *Blood* 2004; **104**: 308.

26. Federico M, Levis S, Luminari S *et al.* ABVD vs Stanford V (SV) vs MOPP-EBV-CAD (MEC) in advanced Hodgkin's lymphoma. Final results of the IIL HD9601 randomized trial. *J Clin Oncol* 2004; **22**: 559s.

●27. Poen JC, Hoppe RT, Horning SJ. High-dose therapy and autologous bone marrow transplantation for relapsed/refractory Hodgkin's disease: the impact of involved field radiotherapy on patterns of failure and survival [see comments]. *Int J Radiat Oncol Biol Phys* 1996; **36**: 3–12.

28. Moskowitz CH, Kewalramani T, Nimer SD *et al.* Effectiveness of high dose chemoradiotherapy and autologous stem cell transplantation for patients with biopsy-proven primary refractory Hodgkin's disease. *Br J Haematol* 2004; **124**: 645–52.

●29. MacManus MP, Hoppe RT. Is radiotherapy curative for stage I and II low-grade follicular lymphoma? Results of a long-term follow-up study of patients treated at Stanford University. *J Clin Oncol* 1996; **14**: 1282–90.

30. Vaughan HB, Vaughan HG, MacLennan K *et al.* Clinical stage 1 non-Hodgkin's lymphoma: longterm followup of patients treated by the British National Lymphoma Investigation with radiotherapy alone as inital therapy. *Br J Cancer* 1994; **69**: 1088–93.

31. Gospodarowicz M, Lippuner T, Pintilie M *et al.* Stage I and II follicular lymphoma: longterm outcome and pattern of failure following treatment with involved field radiation therapy alone. *Int J Radiat Oncol Biol Phys* 1999; **45**: 217a.

32. Wilder RB, Jones K, Tucker SL. Longterm results with radiotherapy of Stage I–II follicular lymphomas. Radiation therapy after a partial response to CHOP chemotherapy for aggressive lymphomas: preliminary report of toxicity following 3D radiation therapy for prostate cancer on 3DOG/RTOG 9406. *Int J Radiat Oncol Biol Phys* 2001; **51**: 1219–27.

33. Stuschke M, Hoederath A, Sack H *et al.* Extended field and total central lymphatic radiotherapy in the treatment of early stage lymph node centroblastic-centrocytic lymphomas: results of a prospective multicenter study. Study Group NHL-fruhe Stadien. *Cancer* 1997; **80**: 2273–84.

34. Pendlebury S, El Awadi M, Ashley S *et al.* Radiotherapy results in early stage low grade nodal non-Hodgkin's lymphoma. *Radiother Oncol* 1995; **36**: 167–71.

35. Seymour JF, Pro B, Fuller LM *et al.* Longterm follow-up of a prospective study of combined modality therapy for Stage I–II indolent non-Hodgkin's lymphoma. *J Clin Oncol* 2003; **21**: 2115–22.

36. Richaud PM, Soubeyran P, Eghbali H *et al.* Place of low-dose total body irradiation in the treatment of localized follicular non-Hodgkin's lymphoma: results of a pilot study. *Int J Radiat Oncol Biol Phys* 1998; **40**: 387–90.

37. Murtha AD, Knox SJ, Hoppe RT *et al.* Long-term follow-up of patients with Stage III follicular lymphoma treated with primary radiotherapy at Stanford University. *Int J Radiat Oncol Biol Phys* 2001; **49**: 3–15.

38. Ha CS, Kong JS, Tucker SL *et al.* Central lymphatic irradiation for Stage I–III follicular lymphoma: report from a single-institutional prospective study. *Int J Radiat Oncol Biol Phys* 2003; **57**: 316–20.

39. Ha CS, Kong JS, McLaughlin P *et al.* Stage III follicular lymphoma: longterm followup and patterns of failure. *Int J Radiat Oncol Biol Phys* 2003; **57**: 748–54.

40. Hoppe RT, Kushlan P, Kaplan HS *et al.* The treatment of advanced stage favorable histology non-Hodgkin's lymphoma: a preliminary report of a randomized trial comparing single agent chemotherapy, combination chemotherapy, and whole body irradiation. *Blood* 1981; **58**: 592–8.

41. Schechter NR, Portlock CS, Yahalom J. Treatment of mucosa-associated lymphoid tissue lymphoma of the stomach with radiation alone. *J Clin Oncol* 1998; **16**: 1916–21.

42. Le QT, Eulau SM, George TI *et al.* Primary radiotherapy for localized orbital MALT lymphoma. *Int J Radiat Oncol Biol Phys* 2002; **52**: 657–63.

●43. Tsang RW, Gospodarowicz MK, Pintilie M *et al.* Localized mucosa-associated lymphoid tissue lymphoma treated with radiation therapy has excellent clinical outcome. *J Clin Oncol* 2003; **21**: 4157–64.

44. Kaminski MS, Coleman CN, Colby TV *et al.* Factors predicting survival in adults with Stage I and II large-cell lymphoma treated with radiation therapy. *Ann Intern Med* 1986; **104**: 747–56.

●45. Miller TP, Dahlberg S, Cassady JR *et al.* Chemotherapy alone compared with chemotherapy plus radiotherapy for localized intermediate-and high grade non-Hodgkin's lymphoma. *N Engl J Med* 1998; **339**: 21–6.

●46. Horning S, Weller E, Kim K *et al.* Chemotherapy with or without radiotherapy in limited-stage diffuse aggressive non-Hodgkin's lymphoma: Eastern Cooperative Oncology Group study 1484. *J Clin Oncol* 2004; **22**: 3032–8.

47. Shipp MA, Harrington DP, Anderson JR *et al.* A predictive model for aggressive non-Hodgkin's lymphoma. The International Non-Hodgkin's Lymphoma Prognostic Factors Project. *N Engl J Med* 1993; **329**: 987–94.

48. Reyes F, Lepage E, Ganem G *et al.* ACVBP versus CHOP plus radiotherapy for localized aggressive lymphoma. *N Engl J Med* 2005; **352**: 1197–205.

49. Miller TP, LeBlanc M, Spier C *et al.* CHOP alone compared to CHOP plus radiotherapy for early stage aggressive non-Hodgkin's lymphomas: update of the Southwest Oncology Group (SWOG) randomized trial. *ASH abstract* 2001; **98**: 3024.

50. Sutcliffe SB, Gospodarowicz MK, Bush RS *et al.* Role of radiation therapy in localized non-Hodgkin's lymphoma. *Radiother Oncol* 1985; **4**: 211–23.

51. Oguchi M, Ikeda H, Isobe K *et al.* Tumor bulk as a prognostic factor for the management of localized aggressive non-Hodgkin's lymphoma: a survey of the Japan Lymphoma Radiation Therapy Group. *Int J Radiat Oncol Biol Phys* 2000; **48**: 161–8.

52. Spicer J, Smith PJ, Maclennan K *et al.* Long-term follow-up of patients treated with radiotherapy alone for early-stage histologically aggressive non-Hodgkin's lymphoma. *Br J Cancer* 2004; **90**: 1151–5.

53. O'Connell MJ, Harrington DP, Earle JD *et al.* Prospectively randomized clinical trial of three intensive chemotherapy regimens for the treatment of advanced unfavorable histology non-Hodgkin's lymphoma. *J Clin Oncol* 1987; **5**: 1329–39.

54. Aviles A, Fernandez R, Perez F *et al.* Adjuvant radiotherapy in stage IV diffuse large cell lymphoma improves outcome. *Leuk Lymphoma* 2004; **45**: 1385–9.

55. Philip T, Guglielmi C, Hagenbeek A *et al.* Autologous bone marrow transplantation as compared with salvage chemotherapy in relapses of chemotherapy-sensitive non-Hodgkin's lymphoma. *N Engl J Med* 1995; **333**: 1540–5.

●56. Zinzani PL, Martelli M, Bertini M *et al.* Induction chemotherapy strategies for primary mediastinal large B-cell lymphoma with sclerosis: a retrospective multinational study on 426 previously untreated patients. *Haematologica* 2002; **87**: 1238–9.

57. Todeschini G, Secchi S, Morra E *et al.* Primary mediastinal large B-cell lymphoma (PMLBCL): long-term results from a retrospective multicentre Italian experience in 138 patients treated with CHOP or MACOP-B/VACOP-B. *Br J Cancer* 2004; **90**: 372–6.

58. Leitch HA, Gascoyne RD, Chhanabhai M *et al.* Limited stage mantle cell lymphoma. *Ann Oncol* 2003; **14**: 1555–61.

59. Chak LY, Cox RS, Bostwick DG *et al.* Solitary plasmacytoma of bone: treatment, progression, and survival. *J Clin Oncol* 1987; **5**: 1811–5.

60. Bolek T, Marcus R, Mendenhall NP. Solitary plasmacytoma of bone and soft tissue. *Int J Radiat Oncol Biol Phys* 1996; **36**: 329–33.

61. Liebross R, Ha C, Cox J *et al.* Solitary bone plasmacytoma: outcome and prognostic factors following radiotherapy. *Int J Radiat Oncol Biol Phys* 1998; **41**: 1063–7.

62. Liebross R, Ha CS, Cox J *et al.* Clinical course of solitary extramedullary plasmacytoma. *Radiother Oncol* 1999; **52**: 245–9.

63. Norin T, Onyango DMRT. Radiotherapy in Burkitt's lymphoma - conventional or superfractionated regime - early results. *Int J Radiat Oncol Biol Phys* 1977; **2**: 399–406.

64. Bernstein JI, Coleman CN, Strickler JG *et al.* Combined modality therapy for adults with small noncleaved cell lymphoma (Burkitt's and non-Burkitts's types). *J Clin Oncol* 1986; **4**: 847–58.

65. Dabaja BS, Ha CS, Thomas DA *et al.* The role of local radiation therapy for mediastinal disease in adults with T-cell lymphoblastic lymphoma. *Cancer* 2002; **94**: 2738–44.

66. Coleman CN, Picozzi VJ, Jr., Cox RS *et al.* Treatment of lymphoblastic lymphoma in adults. *J Clin Oncol* 1986; **4**: 1628–37.

67. Li CC, Tien HF, Tang JL *et al.* Treatment outcome and pattern of failure in 77 patients with sinonasal natural killer/T-cell or T-cell lymphoma. *Cancer* 2004; **100**: 366–75.

68. Koom WS, Chung EJ, Yang WI *et al.* Angiocentric T-cell and NK/T-cell lymphomas: radiotherapeutic viewpoints. *Int J Radiat Oncol Biol Phys* 2004; **59**: 1127–37.

◆69. Hoppe R. Mycosis fungoides: radiation therapy. *Dermatol Ther* 2003; **16**: 347–54.

70. Jones GW, Hoppe RT, Glatstein E. Electron beam treatment for cutaneous T-cell lymphoma. *Hematol Oncol Clin North Am* 1995; **9**: 1057–76.

71. Micaily B, Miyamoto C, Kantor G *et al.* Radiotherapy for unilesional mycosis fungoides. *Int J Radiat Oncol Biol Phys* 1998; **42**: 361–4.

●72. Grange F, Hedelin G, Joly P *et al.* Prognostic factors in primary cutaneous lymphomas other than mycosis fungoides and the Sezary syndrome. The French Study Group on Cutaneous Lymphomas. *Blood* 1999; **93**: 3637–42.

52

Response assessment and follow-up of the patient with malignant lymphoma

BRUCE D CHESON

PRETREATMENT ASSESSMENT

One of the most critical elements in response assessment and follow-up of the patient with lymphoma begins early in the clinical course, with appropriate pretreatment diagnostic and staging studies. Excisional biopsy with immunohistochemical and flow cytometric analysis will ensure the correct diagnosis. A fine needle aspiration should be discouraged because of the extremely high rate of false-negative results.[1] Core biopsies may be adequate for nodes in areas inaccessible for excision and at the time of a suspected relapse.

A comprehensive history and physical examination provide the basis for subsequent assessment. The presence or absence of constitutional symptoms should be noted – fevers greater than 38°C, night sweats, and/or unintentional weight loss of greater than 10 percent of body weight during the 6 months prior to the time of diagnosis – since their recurrence may herald a relapse. Other lymphoma-related complaints, including pruritus and, in Hodgkin lymphoma (HL), alcohol-induced pain or other symptoms in an involved node-bearing area, should be similarly noted.[2] At the time of the physical examination, notation of the location and size of all lesions should be recorded by accurate two-dimensional measurements as a baseline against which to compare subsequent determinations. The extent of the liver and spleen below their respective costal margins should also be noted.

Baseline laboratory studies include a complete blood count with careful examination of the peripheral blood smear to evaluate for the presence of circulating lymphoma cells, liver chemistries, a lactate dehydrogenase (LDH) as an indicator of tumor mass, and a serum uric acid. A unilateral bone marrow aspirate and a biopsy with a goal of at least 2 cm in length are necessary.[3,4] Not only should the marrow be classified as being involved with lymphoma or not, but, if involved, the histologic subtype of lymphoma should be noted, because of the possibility of a discordant histology.

Imaging studies should include computed tomography (CT) scans of the neck, chest, abdomen, and pelvis. Positron emission tomography (PET) scanning is currently not included in determining patient stage since the initial therapy is altered only in a small proportion of patients on the basis of PET scan results.[5–7] In a metaanalysis of ^{18}F-fluorodeoxyglucose (FDG)-PET in staging of patients with lymphoma,[8] the pooled sensitivity for 14 studies with patient-based data was 90.9 percent (95 percent confidence interval [CI], 88.0–93.4) with a false-positive rate of 10.3 percent (95 percent CI, 7.4–13.8). The maximum joint sensitivity and specificity was 87.8 percent (95 percent CI, 85.0–90.7) with an apparently higher sensitivity and false-positive rate in patients with HL compared with non-Hodgkin lymphoma (NHL). The pooled sensitivity for seven studies with lesion-based data was 95.6 percent (95 percent CI, 93.9–97.0) with a false-positive rate of only 1.0 percent (95 percent CI, 0.6–1.3). The maximum sensitivity and specificity was 95.6 percent (95 percent CI, 93.1–98.1). Thus, PET detects more occult lymphomatous sites than contrast-enhanced CT and bone marrow biopsy.[5,6,9–13] Although PET identifies more lesions than CT, PET alone cannot replace CT for pretreatment staging.[11,14–16]

Moreover, the frequency of a positive PET scan at diagnosis varies with the histologic subtype.[17–19] There appears to be a greater likelihood of aggressive B cell lymphomas being PET positive than low-grade lymphomas, with an especially high false-negative rate in extranodal marginal zone lymphomas and small lymphocytic lymphoma.[6,18,19] Several investigators have examined the role of PET in identifying bone marrow involvement as part of staging; however, bone marrow biopsy remains an essential part of patient evaluation.[10,20]

RESPONSE ASSESSMENT

Response in patients with lymphomas is generally assessed by quantifying the regression in size and number of enlarged lymph nodes, confluent lymph node masses, or organ involvement. Considerable controversy surrounds the size of a 'normal' lymph node. Based on CT scanning and autopsy series, the upper limit of lymph node size in normal individuals is approximately 10 mm in the short axis. However, this threshold varies with anatomic location.[21–28] The upper limits of normal mediastinal nodes ranges from 5 mm to 12 mm in the short axis, with greater variation in the long axis. The size of abdominal nodes on CT scans in patients with either blunt trauma or diseases other than lymphoma varies by region from 8 mm to 11 mm; however, normal nodes in the pelvis may be as large as 15 mm. A lymph node that is either larger than 10 mm in its short transverse diameter or hard to palpation should be considered suspicious for involvement by lymphoma. Moreover, smaller nodes, but more numerous than expected or in unusual sites, should also be considered suspicious for involvement. Since different radiologists will likely review the pretreatment and posttreatment scans, consistent indicator lesions should be identified and measured to minimize interobserver variability.

The criterion of a node less than 15 mm in transverse diameter has been adopted as normal for Hodgkin lymphoma.[29] Nodes that are ≤15 mm but are considered to be abnormal should decrease to ≤10 mm to be considered normal in size. Using the longest transverse diameter appears to provide a more accurate assessment of response than the short axis in patients with NHL.[30] Incrementally reducing the bidimensional requirement from 20 mm × 20 mm to 15 mm × 15 mm, and 10 mm × 10 mm, does not appear

to reduce the overall response rate in patients with follicular lymphoma, but it does result in a significant decrease in the complete remission (CR) rate.[30]

Lymph nodes may be completely or only partially involved by lymphoma. Thus, as tumor-involved nodes shrink in size following treatment, fibrosis, necrosis, or inflammation may result in a persistent enlargement of a node that is histologically uninvolved by tumor.[31] Therefore, persistence of residual masses following chemotherapy does not necessarily indicate residual disease.[32–35] Indeed, as many as 30 percent to 50 percent of patients with a large intraabdominal mass at presentation may have a residual mass following therapy.[32,34] In a comparison of ProMACE/MOPP with ProMACE/CytaBOM conducted at the National Cancer Institute (NCI), restaging laparotomy was abandoned because 95 percent of residual abdominal masses did not contain lymphoma.[35]

This finding has resulted in confusion in clinical trials. In some series, responses in patients with residual masses were classified retrospectively, depending on the subsequent behavior of the mass.[36,37] The proportion of decrease of a mass to qualify for a CR has varied from more than 50 percent to more than 75 percent, given the absence of any other measurable disease.[34–40] In other studies, a complete remission required a return of all nodes to less than 1 cm, unless larger nodes were histologically negative.[41] In an attempt to standardize the assessment of such residual masses, the International Working Group (IWG) recommended the term complete remission unconfirmed (CRu) to designate a mass that had decreased by at least 75 percent but was still detectable by imaging studies.[42]

The increasing availability of PET scans has reduced the confusion surrounding the persistent mass.[43,44] Positron emission tomography not only has totally replaced gallium scanning,[45,46] but it is more predictive of outcome than CT.[47] Nevertheless, PET and CT appear to provide complementary information.[48] Fusion scans appear to be more accurate than either modality alone.[49] Where CT/PET scans are available, the role of an additional CT scan is less clear. Raanani et al.[50] reported 103 patients studied retrospectively in whom PET/CT upstaged NHL in 31 percent of patients and downstaged 1 percent with an alteration in therapy in 25 percent; in those with HL, upstaging occurred in 32 percent and downstaging in 15 percent with an alteration in therapy in 45 percent of patients.

RESPONSE CRITERIA IN MALIGNANT LYMPHOMA

Standardized response criteria help to promote the reporting of uniform endpoints, allow for comparisons among studies, and, as a result, facilitate the identification of new and more effective therapies. They also assist in the evaluation and regulatory approval of new chemotherapeutic and biologic agents. In 1999, an IWG composed of lymphoma investigators published the first standardized response criteria for

NHL. These recommendations included definitions for complete remission, complete remission unconfirmed (CRu), partial remission, stable disease, relapsed disease, and progressive disease.[42] A complete remission required the absence of clinical, imaging, or other evidence of disease or disease-related symptoms. Lymph nodes were required to regress to 'normal' size using 1.5 cm as the cutoff. The spleen and liver were to be normal in size by physical examination, with a histologically normal bone marrow. A CRu included all of the features of a CR except either a single residual node mass of greater than 1.5 cm that regressed by more than 75 percent or residual nodes that were previously confluent that regressed by more than 75 percent but were still detectable by clinical or imaging techniques, or a bone marrow that was considered to be indeterminate. A partial response required a 50 percent or greater decrease in the size of lymph nodes or other lesions. Follow-up included a patient history, physical examination, and routine blood tests (e.g., serum LDH), with other studies as clinically indicated.

However, after the IWG recommendations were widely adopted and used extensively in clinical trials, a number of limitations became apparent. Certain features were unclear and subject to misinterpretations, most notably in the application of the term CRu which, while intended to designate those large masses that decreased and were still present but were likely scar or fibrosis, often included partial remissions (PR) of more than 75 percent decrease in the sum of the products of the diameters as a CRu, thus inflating CR rates. These criteria depended on inadequate methods of assessment such as physical examination, which is complicated by inter- and intraobserver variability and poor reproducibility. Imaging studies that were recommended were limited to those that were routinely available at the time, including chest radiographs, CT scans, and magnetic resonance imaging (MRI), which are not able to distinguish viable residual tumor from masses of fibrosis and necrosis. Single photon emission computed tomography (SPECT) gallium scans were recommended; however, this test is less sensitive than current PET scans and is no longer widely used.[45] Finally, a visual bone marrow evaluation was recommended, which is unable to identify small populations of residual lymphoma cells. The guidelines were designed for NHL but were adopted for Hodgkin lymphoma. They were also developed for adults but were adopted for pediatric patients.

There is now ample rationale for integrating FDG-PET or PET/CT into the IWG response criteria.[43] This technology is now more widely available, it is superior to CT in differentiating viable tumor from scar or fibrotic tissue, and the results of PET can predict clinical outcome[47,51–54] even better than standard prognostic scoring systems (Fig. 52.1).[54] The impact of integrating PET into the IWG was first evaluated by Juweid et al.,[43] who reported 54 patients with diffuse large B cell NHL, treated with an anthracycline-based regimen. Not only was the number of CRs increased from 17 to 35, but CRus were eliminated. Moreover, use of PET significantly improved the discrimination between CR and PR in progression-free survival.

However, there are a number of problems with PET scans. There are false-negative and false-positive results, and points of controversy as to what should be called a positive study. There is also marked variability among histologies in FDG avidity.[18,19]

Revised response criteria

As a result of these new developments, revisions of the IWG criteria were warranted based largely on the incorporation of PET. Thus, to ensure transparency among clinical trials groups in their assessment of response in malignant lymphomas, an International Harmonization Project was convened to review the existing response criteria and to present the rationale for new response criteria based on advances in pathology and genetics as well as the increased use of PET scans.[4] A number of working groups were organized to focus on pathology/genetics, clinical features, imaging, and endpoints for clinical trials. The two major outcomes of the International Harmonization Project were a standardization of performance and interpretation of PET in lymphoma clinical trials[55] and new response criteria incorporating PET as well as bone marrow immunohistochemistry.[4] A positive scan was defined as focal or diffuse FDG uptake above background in a location incompatible with normal anatomy or physiology. Exceptions include mild and diffusely increased FDG uptake at the site of moderate- or large-sized masses with an intensity that is lower than or equal to the mediastinal blood pool, hepatic or splenic nodules of at least 1.5 cm in diameter with FDG uptake lower than the surrounding liver/spleen uptake, and diffusely increased bone marrow uptake within weeks following treatment.[55] Areas of necrosis may be FDG avid within an otherwise negative residual mass and a follow-up scan in a few months is often indicated to confirm this clinical impression. Residual masses ≥2 cm in greatest transverse diameter (GTD) with FDG activity visually exceeding that of mediastinal blood pool structures are considered PET positive whereas residual masses 1.1–1.9 cm are considered PET positive only if their activity exceeds surrounding background activity. Visual assessment is currently considered adequate for determining whether a PET scan is positive, and using the standardized uptake value (SUV) is not necessary.[55] What percentage reduction in SUV correlates with response is being evaluated in clinical trials. However, the numerous causes of false-positive scans must be ruled out including sarcoidosis, infection, or inflammation.[56]

RECOMMENDED TIMING OF PET OR PET/CT SCANS IN LYMPHOMA CLINICAL TRIALS

Pretreatment assessment

For histologic subtypes of malignant lymphoma that are routinely FDG-avid and curable, such as diffuse large B cell NHL (DLBCL), Hodgkin lymphoma, a pretreatment PET

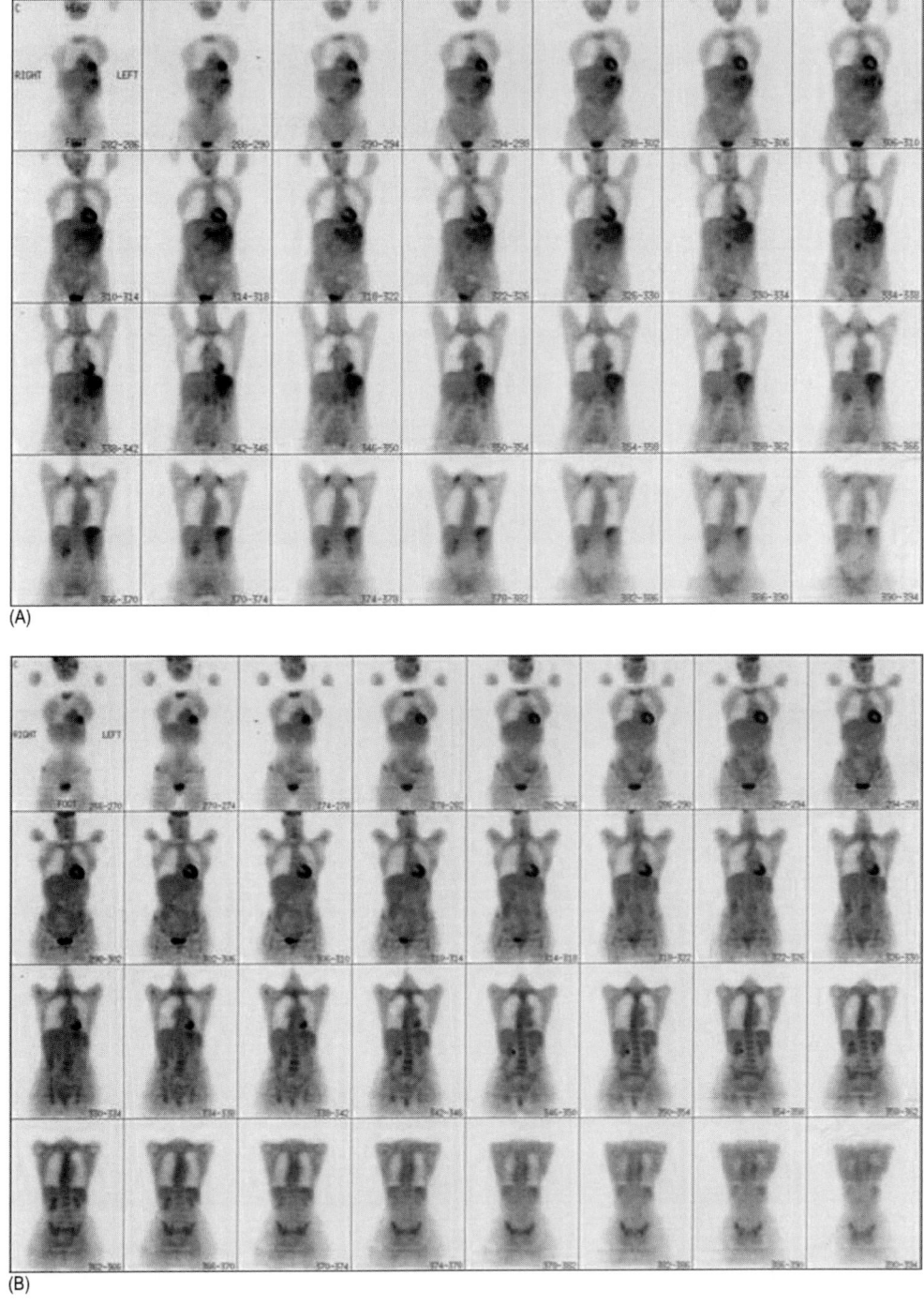

(A)

(B)

Figure 52.1   Pretreatment, midtreatment, and posttreatment positron emission tomography (PET) scan on a patient with subdiaphragmatic diffuse large B cell non-Hodgkin lymphoma (NHL). Although there was rapid resolution of the PET scan finding, new disease in the chest was detected. Biopsy made the diagnosis of sarcoidosis and the patient is alive and without recurrence of her lymphoma for almost 3 years.

scan is strongly recommended to better characterize the extent of disease. For the other aggressive and indolent NHLs, a pretreatment PET scan should only be performed if complete response is a major study endpoint (Table 52.1).

Response assessment during therapy

It is important to assess patients during the course of therapy. Clearly, if a regimen fails to produce a response after two to three cycles, an alternate approach should be

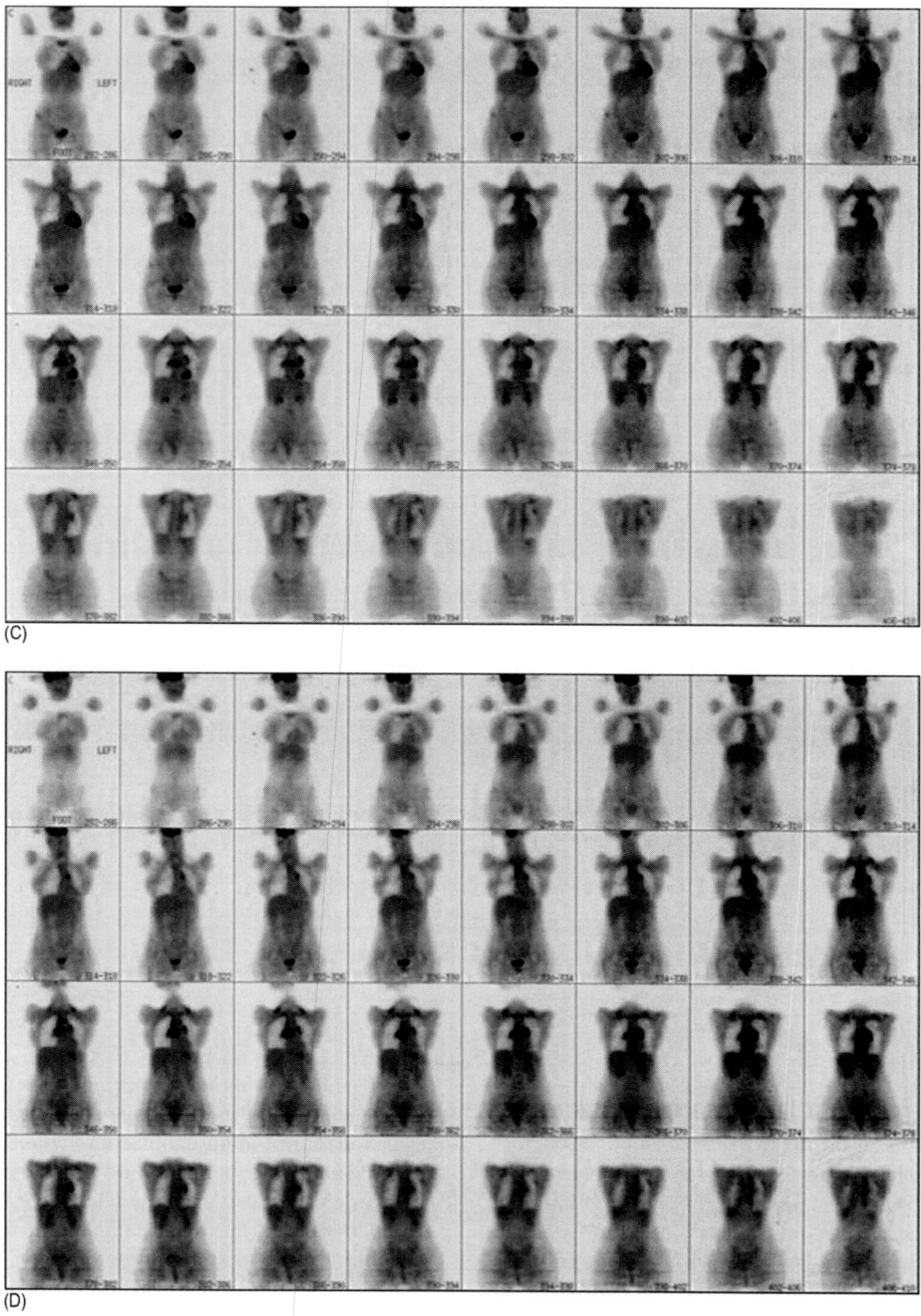

Figure 52.1   Continued

considered. Physical examination and CT scans are the standard approach for interim evaluation. Nevertheless, a large body of data now supports the predictive value of PET scanning. Römer et al.[57] performed PET scans in 11 patients with a variety of histologies of NHL, mostly but not all aggressive, at baseline and at weeks 1 and 6 after chemotherapy was initiated. During the follow-up period of a median of 16 months, six of the patients remained in

remission, and these tended to be those with a lower day 7 metabolic rate of FDG, which improved in predictability at day 42. Spaepen et al.[58] evaluated 70 patients with aggressive NHL who underwent a PET scan after three or four cycles of treatment. None of the 33 patients showing a positive scan sustained a durable remission compared with 31 of the 37 patients who had a negative scan and remained in remission at 1107 days. Haioun et al.[52] conducted a

Table 52.1   Recommendations for PET (PET/CT) scans in lymphoma clinical trials[4]

Histology	Pretreatment	Midtreatment	Response assessment	Posttreatment surveillance
DLBCL	Yes[a]	Clinical trial	Yes	No
Hodgkin	Yes[a]	Clinical trial	Yes	No
Follicular NHL	No[b]	Clinical trial	No[b]	No
MCL	No[b]	Clinical trial	No[b]	No
Other aggressive NHLs	No[b]	Clinical trial	No[b,c]	No
Other indolent NHLs	No[b]	Clinical trial	No[b,c]	No

[a]Strongly recommended.
[b]Only if response is a primary study endpoint.
[c]Only if PET + pretreatment.
DLBCL, diffuse large B cell lymphoma; NHL, non-Hodgkin lymphoma; MCL, mantle cell lymphoma; PET, positron emission tomography; CT, computed tomography.

prospective evaluation of PET prior to therapy and after two cycles of combination chemotherapy in 90 patients with aggressive NHL. Early PET was interpreted as negative in 54 patients and positive in 36. After therapy, 83 percent of those patients who had been PET negative had attained a complete remission compared with 58 percent of the PET-positive patients. More importantly, the 2-year estimated event-free and overall survival rates were 82 percent and 90 percent, respectively, for those who had been PET negative compared with 43 percent and 61 percent for PET-positive patients. These differences were detected regardless of International Prognostic Index (IPI) risk group. Hutchings et al.[59] prospectively assessed the value of PET prior to therapy and after two, four, and six cycles of chemotherapy in 77 patients with previously untreated HL. Eleven of the 16 patients with a positive PET scan progressed compared with three of the 61 with a negative PET scan. Early PET was more predictive of progression-free survival than PET performed later during treatment. The impact of early PET scanning has also been reported in the salvage setting.[51,60]

Despite the large number of studies demonstrating that a PET scan performed after one to four courses of therapy can predict time to progression and patient survival, no currently available data show a beneficial effect on outcome of altering therapy on the basis of the PET scan. Thus, a midtreatment PET scan is not indicated unless it is part of an objective of a clinical research trial. This position is supported by a recent metaanalysis.[61,62]

Assessment posttreatment

The clearest role for PET is in posttreatment assessment, especially in patients with diffuse large B cell NHL and Hodgkin lymphoma.[63] The recommended time point to measure response is 6–8 weeks, or longer, after therapy, depending on the type of treatment. Jerusalem et al.[47] reported on 54 patients with intermediate- or high-grade NHL or Hodgkin lymphoma. Residual masses were identified by CT in 13 of 19 patients with Hodgkin lymphoma

and 11 of 35 with NHL. Of the 24 patients with residual masses on CT, five had a positive PET scan compared with only one of 30 without a residual mass. All six patients who were PET positive relapsed compared with five of 19 (26 percent) patients with a mass on CT but a negative PET scan, and three of 29 patients with negative CT and PET scans. Patients with a positive PET scan had a 1-year progression-free survival of 0 percent versus 86 percent in patients with a negative PET scan, with an overall survival of 50 percent versus 92 percent. Spaepen et al.[64] studied 93 patients with various lymphomas who underwent PET after treatment and were followed for at least a year. Of the 67 patients with a normal PET scan, 56 of 67 remained in CR for a median follow-up of 653 days. The 26 patients who were PET-positive all relapsed at a median of 73 days. Zinzani et al.[65] reported on 44 patients with HL or aggressive NHL presenting with abdominal disease, which was bulky in 41 percent. Following therapy, none of those with a negative PET and CT scan relapsed, yet all of those who had a positive CT and PET scan relapsed. One patient of 24 who was positive by CT but negative by PET relapsed. The 2-year relapse-free survival for those with a positive PET scan was 0 percent compared with 95 percent for those who were PET-negative.

In patients with follicular lymphoma and mantle cell lymphoma, a posttreatment PET scan should only be performed if complete and overall response rates are major study endpoints. However, in general, time-dependent endpoints such as progression-free survival or overall survival are more relevant. For the other histologies, a posttreatment PET scan is only indicated if a PET scan was positive prior to treatment and if response is the primary endpoint of interest.

INTERNATIONAL HARMONIZATION PROJECT RECOMMENDATIONS FOR RESPONSE IN MALIGNANT LYMPHOMAS

The currently recommended response criteria[4] include the following definitions.

Complete remission

Complete remission requires:

1. Complete disappearance of all clinical evidence of disease and disease-related symptoms.
2. (a) Typically FDG-avid lymphoma. In patients with no pretreatment PET scan or when the FDG-PET scan was positive prior to therapy, a posttreatment residual mass of any size is permitted as long as it is PET negative. (b) Variably FDG-avid lymphomas/FDG avidity unknown. In patients without a pretreatment PET scan, or if a pretreatment PET scan was negative, all lymph nodes and nodal masses must have regressed on CT to normal size (≤1.5 cm in their GTD for nodes >1.5 cm prior to therapy). Previously involved nodes that were 1.1–1.5 cm in their long axis and >1.0 cm in their short axis prior to treatment must have decreased to ≤1.0 cm in their short axis after treatment.
3. The spleen and/or liver, if considered enlarged prior to therapy on the basis of a physical examination or CT scan, should not be palpable on physical examination and should be considered normal size by imaging studies, and nodules related to lymphoma should disappear. However, determination of splenic involvement is not always reliable as a spleen considered normal in size may still contain lymphoma, whereas an enlarged spleen may reflect variations in anatomy, blood volume, the use of hematopoietic growth factors, or other causes rather than lymphoma.
4. If the bone marrow was involved by lymphoma prior to treatment, the infiltrate must have cleared on repeat bone marrow biopsy. The biopsy sample on which this determination is made must be adequate (with a goal of ≥20 mm unilateral core). If the sample is indeterminate by morphology, it should be negative by immunohistochemistry. A sample that is negative by immunohistochemistry but demonstrating a small population of clonal lymphocytes by flow cytometry will be considered a CR until data become available demonstrating a clear difference in patient outcome.

Complete remission unconfirmed

Using the above definition for CR and that below for PR eliminates the category of CRu.

Partial remission

Partial remission requires all of the following:

1. At least 50 percent decrease in sum of the product of the diameters (SPD) of up to six of the largest dominant nodes or nodal masses. These nodes or masses should be selected according to all of the following: (a) they should be clearly measurable in at least two perpendicular dimensions; (b) if possible, they should be from disparate regions of the body; (c) they should include mediastinal and retroperitoneal areas of disease whenever these sites are involved.
2. No increase in the size of other nodes, liver, or spleen.
3. Splenic and hepatic nodules must regress by ≥50 percent in their SPD or, for single nodules, in the GTD.
4. With the exception of splenic and hepatic nodules, involvement of other organs is usually evaluable and not measurable disease.
5. Bone marrow assessment is irrelevant for determination of a PR if the sample was positive prior to treatment. However, if positive, the cell type should be specified, e.g., large cell lymphoma or small neoplastic B cells. Patients who achieve a complete remission by the above criteria, but who have persistent morphologic bone marrow involvement, will be considered partial responders.

   In cases where the bone marrow was involved prior to therapy that resulted in a clinical CR, but with no bone marrow assessment following treatment, patients should be considered partial responders.
6. No new sites of disease.
7. Typically FDG-avid lymphoma. For patients with no pretreatment PET scan or if the PET scan was positive prior to therapy, the posttreatment PET scan should be positive in at least one previously involved site.
8. Variably FDG-avid lymphomas/FDG avidity unknown. For patients without a pretreatment PET scan, or if a pretreatment PET scan was negative, CT criteria should be used.

Stable disease

1. Failing to attain the criteria needed for a CR or PR, but not fulfilling those for progressive disease (see below).
2. Typically FDG-avid lymphomas. The FDG-PET scan should be positive at prior sites of disease with no new areas of involvement on the posttreatment CT or PET scan.
3. Variably FDG-avid lymphomas/FDG avidity unknown. For patients without a pretreatment PET scan or if the pretreatment PET scan was negative, there must be no change in the size of the previous lesions on the posttreatment CT scan.

Relapsed disease (after CR)/progressive disease (after PR, stable disease)

Lymph nodes should be considered abnormal if the long axis is more than 1.5 cm regardless of the short axis. If a lymph node has a long axis of 1.1–1.5 cm it should only be considered abnormal if its short axis is more than 1.0 cm.

Lymph nodes ≤1.0 cm by ≤1.0 cm will not be considered as abnormal for relapse or progressive disease.

1. Appearance of any new lesion more than 1.5 cm in any axis during or at the end of therapy, even if others are decreasing in size. Increased FDG uptake in a previously unaffected site should only be considered relapsed or progressive disease after confirmation with other modalities. In patients with no prior history of pulmonary lymphoma, new lung nodules identified by CT are mostly benign. Thus, a therapeutic decision should not be made solely on the basis of the PET scan without histologic confirmation.
2. At least 50 percent increase from nadir in the SPD of any previously involved nodes, or in a single involved node, or the size of other lesions (e.g., splenic or hepatic nodules). To be considered progressive disease, a lymph node with a diameter of the short axis of less than 1.0 cm must increase by ≥50 percent and to a size of 1.5 cm by 1.5 cm or more than 1.5 cm in the long axis.
3. At least 50 percent increase in the longest diameter of any single previously identified node more than 1 cm in its short axis.
4. Lesions should be PET positive if a typical FDG-avid lymphoma or one that was PET positive prior to therapy unless the lesion is too small to be detected with current PET systems (less than 1.5 cm in its long axis by CT).

A PET scan should be used and interpreted in conjunction with patient history, physical examination, and CT scans. False-positive results have been reported with infection, inflammation, sarcoidosis, or thymic hyperplasia following therapy. Thus, treatment decisions should not be based on a PET scan alone. Depending on the clinical circumstances, either a biopsy should be performed or a repeat PET scan obtained 2–3 months later before initiating treatment.

BONE MARROW ASSESSMENT

In patients with bone marrow involvement prior to therapy, residual lymphoid nodules may persist following treatment. However, whether these represent residual disease has been difficult to determine by morphology alone.

Immunohistochemistry can reduce the number of indeterminate bone marrow assessments by distinguishing lymphomatous nodules from benign residual lymphoid nodules. On the other hand, for a bone marrow that is morphologically negative, the clinical significance of a small population of clonal cells identified only by flow cytometry is controversial. Treatment decisions should not yet be based on such findings.

ENDPOINTS

Whereas response rates are of interest in phase II studies of new agents, they are generally not the most important endpoint in phase I studies, where toxicity is identified, or phase III trials, where efficacy endpoints are more important. In phase III trials, the major endpoints of interest should include progression-free survival, event-free survival (time to treatment failure), response duration, and overall survival. Overall survival and failure-free survival are measured from entry onto a trial until death from any cause, or until death or progression of disease, respectively. Progression-free survival for all patients is taken from the time of entry onto study until disease progression or death from NHL. This endpoint is more important in aggressive NHL, where it correlates better with survival than in follicular NHL. Secondary endpoints such as disease-free survival or cause-specific survival may also be included, but only when the other endpoints have been reported. Disease-free survival for patients in CR is measured from the first assessment that documents that response to the date of disease progression. An endpoint that has become increasingly popular is time to next treatment. However, unless the indications for treatment are clearly specified, there can be considerable bias in these determinations. For phase III trials, an intent-to-treat analysis should be used in which all patients entered onto the study are included. Subsequent planned subset analysis of various groups may be considered, such as only patients eligible for the study or only those treated according to the arm to which they are assigned.

FOLLOW-UP

Good clinical judgment and a careful history and physical examination are the most important components of monitoring patients after treatment. The manner in which patients are followed will vary considerably between a clinical trial and clinical practice, and depending on whether treatment is initiated and, if so, with curative or palliative intent. For example, patients with a follicular or low-grade NHL who are being managed with a 'watch-and-wait' approach need to be observed for the development of disease-related symptoms or signs of organ involvement. No consensus regarding the frequency of follow-up of such patients exists. Routine imaging studies (e.g., CT scans) may be considered to assess whether there is sufficient progression of disease to warrant initiation of therapy.

There is little indication for regular surveillance CT or PET scans. Weeks et al.[66] assessed the role of conventional screening for relapse in patients with NHL. The authors concluded that follow-up strategies based on standard radiographic procedures and blood tests were not effective in detecting preclinical relapse patients with large cell lymphoma. They recommended that screening studies should not be site specific and the frequency of study should be determined by the patient's risk for relapse and whether there is a potentially curative salvage therapy. Oh et al.[67] studied 328 patients with previously untreated stage I follicular NHL, 78 of whom relapsed and were part of the study. They had received a variety of treatments. At a median follow-up of 101 months, only 14 percent of relapses were identified by CT scans, and just 4.3 percent benefited from the CT results. The number of relapses identified by physical examination was similar to CT scans. Minimum testing at follow-up visits should include history, physical examination for lymphadenopathy, abdominal masses, or organomegaly, and blood tests including a complete blood count and serum chemistries, including LDH. Additional blood tests and imaging studies may be added for relevant clinical indications. Routine surveillance by CT, PET, or PET/CT is not recommended because of the lack of evidence for clinical benefit. More than 80 percent of the time it is the patient or the physician who detects relapse.[68] Jerusalem et al.[69] reported a series of 36 patients who underwent PET following therapy and every 4–6 months thereafter. There were five events detected by PET, one in a patient with known residual disease. Two of the four patients whose relapse 5–24 months following treatment was identified by PET already had developed disease-related symptoms. In addition, there were six false-positive studies. Zinzani et al.[70] conducted a prospective evaluation of 160 patients with Hodgkin lymphoma and 261 patients with indolent or aggressive non-Hodgkin lymphoma who underwent PET at 6, 12, 18, and 24 months post-therapy. The likelihood of relapse was negligible after 12 months for the Hodgkin lymphoma patients, and after 18 months for aggressive non-Hodgkin lymphomas. There was a continuous risk of relapse for the indolent non-Hodgkin lymphomas. Patients with suspected relapse were biopsied and more than 40 percent of those with a positive PET scan but negative CT scan had a negative biopsy. The authors concluded that there was no benefit from continued surveillance studies after 18 months.

In a clinical trial, uniformity of reassessment is necessary to ensure comparability among studies with respect to the major endpoints of event-free survival, disease-free survival, and progression-free survival. It is obvious, for example, that a protocol requiring extensive reevaluation every 2 months will produce different apparent intervals for those endpoints compared to one requiring the same testing annually, even if the true times to events are the same. One recommendation has been to assess patients on clinical trials after completion of treatment at a minimum of every 3 months for 2 years, then every 6 months for 3 years, and then annually for at least 5 years.[42] Few recurrences occur beyond that point for patients with large cell NHL. However, there is a continuous risk of relapse for patients with lymphoma with a follicular histology. These intervals may vary with specific treatments, protocols, or unique drug characteristics.

CONCLUSIONS

There has been considerable recent interest in using FDG-PET and other imaging modalities to measure early response

to therapy to facilitate new drug development in a variety of tumor types, including lymphomas. Thus, PET is being considered a potential early surrogate endpoint for clinical benefit[71,72] that can potentially facilitate the development of new and more effective therapies. Further study of the role of FDG-PET in staging, response assessment, and risk-adapted therapy could improve outcome for patients with lymphomas.

KEY POINTS

- Standardized response criteria are essential to compare data among clinical trials.
- FDG-PET is more sensitive and specific than CT scans and helps distinguish scar/fibrosis from active lymphoma.
- FDG-PET is limited by the number of false-positive and false-negative results.
- FDG-PET use should be limited to specific histologic subtypes (e.g., diffuse large B cell NHL, Hodgkin lymphoma) and certain clinical indications where its use is supported by data demonstrating clinical benefit.

REFERENCES

● = Key primary paper
◆ = Major review article

1. Hehn ST, Grogan TM, Miller TP. Utility of fine-needle aspiration as a diagnostic technique in lymphoma. *J Clin Oncol* 2004; **22**: 3046–52.
2. Cheson BD. Hodgkin's disease, alcohol and vena caval obstruction. *JAMA* 1978; **239**: 23–4.
3. Cheson BD, Bennett JM, Kantarjian H *et al.* Report of an international working group to standardize response criteria for myelodysplastic syndromes. *Blood* 2000; **96**: 3671–4.
●4. Cheson BD, Pfistner B, Juweid ME *et al.* Revised response criteria for malignant lymphoma. *J Clin Oncol* 2007; **25**: 579–86. (The revised response criteria for lymphoma incorporating FDG-PET and bone marrow immunohistochemistry.)
5. Buchmann I, Reinhardt M, Elsner K *et al.* 2-(fluorine-18) fluoro-2-deoxy-D-glucose positron emission tomography in the detection and staging of malignant lymphoma. A bicenter trial. *Cancer* 2001; **91**: 889–99.
6. Jerusalem G, Beguin Y, Najjar F *et al.* Positron emission tomography (PET) with 18F-fluorodeoxyglucose (18F-FDG) for the staging of low-grade non-Hodgkin's lymphoma (NHL). *Ann Oncol* 2001; **12**: 825–30.
7. Munker R, Glass J, Griffeth LK *et al.* Contribution of PET imaging to the initial staging and prognosis of patients with Hodgkin's disease. *Ann Oncol* 2004; **15**: 1699–704.

8. Isasi CR, Lu P, Blaufox MD. A metaanalysis of ^{18}F-2-deoxy-2-fluoro-D-glucose positron emission tomography in the staging and restaging of patients with lymphoma. *Cancer* 2005; **104**: 1066–74.

9. Moog F, Bangerter M, Diederichs CG *et al.* Extranodal malignant lymphoma: detection with FDG PET versus CT. *Radiology* 1998; **206**: 475–81.

10. Moog F, Bangerter M, Kotzerke J *et al.* 18-F-fluorodeoxyglucose-positron emission tomography as a new approach to detect lymphomatous bone marrow. *Blood* 1998; **16**: 603–9.

11. Naumann R, Beuthien-Baumann B, Reiss A *et al.* Substantial impact of FDG PET imaging on the therapy decision in patients with early-stage Hodgkin's lymphoma. *Br J Cancer* 2004; **90**: 620–5.

12. Hutchings M, Loft A, Hansen M *et al.* Positron emission tomography with or without computed tomography in the primary staging of Hodgkin's lymphoma. *Haematologica* 2006; **91**: 482–9.

13. Schaefer NG, Hany TF, Taverna C *et al.* Non-Hodgkin lymphoma and Hodgkin disease: coregistered FDG PET and CT at staging and restaging – do we need contrast-enhanced CT? *Radiology* 2004; **232**: 823–9.

14. Bangerter M, Moog F, Buchmann I *et al.* Whole-body 2-[18F]-fluoro-2-deoxy-D-glucose positron emission tomography (FDG-PET) for accurate staging of Hodgkin's disease. *Ann Oncol* 1998; **9**: 1117–22.

15. Jerusalem G, Beguin Y, Fassotte MF *et al.* Whole-body positron emission tomography using 18F-fluorodeoxyglucose compared to standard procedures for staging patients with Hodgkin's disease. *Haematologica* 2001; **86**: 266–73.

16. Weihrauch MR, Re D, Bischoff S *et al.* Whole-body positron emission tomography using 18F-fluorodeoxyglucose for initial staging of patients with Hodgkin's disease. *Ann Hematol* 2002; **81**: 20–5.

17. Najjar F, Hustinx R, Jerusalem G *et al.* Positron emission tomography (PET) for staging low-grade non-Hodgkin's lymphomas (NHL). *Cancer Biother Radiopharm* 2001; **16**: 297–304.

18. Hoffmann M, Kletter K, Diemling M *et al.* Positron emission tomography with fluorine-18-2-fluoro-2-deoxy-D-glucose (F18-FDG) does not visualize extranodal B-cell lymphoma of the mucosa-associated lymphoid tissue (MALT)-type. *Ann Oncol* 1999; **10**: 1185–9.

19. Elstrom R, Guan L, Baker G *et al.* Utility of FDG-PET scanning in lymphoma by WHO classification. *Blood* 2003; **101**: 3875–6.

20. Carr R, Barrington SF, Madan B *et al.* Detection of lymphoma in bone marrow by whole-body positron emission tomography. *Blood* 1998; **91**: 3340–6.

21. Dorfman RE, Alpern MB, Gross BH *et al.* Upper abdominal lymph nodes: criteria for normal size determined with CT. *Radiology* 1991; **180**: 319–22.

22. Einstein DM, Singer AA, Chilcote WA *et al.* Abdominal lymphadenopathy: spectrum of CT findings. *Radiographics* 1991; **11**: 457–72.

23. Glazer GM, Gross BH, Quint LE *et al.* Normal mediastinal lymph nodes: number and size according to American Thoracic Society mapping. *AJR Am J Roentgenol* 1985; **144**: 261–5.

24. Hopper KD, Kasales CJ, Van Slyke MA *et al.* Analysis of interobserver and intraobserver variability in CT tumor measurements. *AJR Am J Roentgenol* 1996; **187**: 851–4.

25. Kiyono K, Sone S, Sakai F *et al.* The number and size of normal mediastinal lymph nodes: a postmortem study. *AJR Am J Roentgenol* 1988; **150**: 771–6.

26. Steinkamp HJ, Hosten N, Richter C *et al.* Enlarged cervical lymph nodes at helical CT. *Radiology* 1994; **191**: 795–8.

27. van den Brekel MWM, Castelijns JA, Snow GB. Detection of lymph node metastases in the neck: radiologic criteria. *Radiology* 1994; **192**: 617–18.

28. Genereux GP, Howie JL. Normal mediastinal lymph node size and number: CT and anatomic study. *AJR Am J Roentgenol* 1984; **142**: 1095–100.

29. Lister TA, Crowther D, Sutcliffe SB *et al.* Report of a committee convened to discuss the evaluation and staging of patients with Hodgkin's disease: Cotswolds Meeting. *J Clin Oncol* 1989; **7**: 1630–6.

30. Grillo-López AJ, Cheson B, Horning S *et al.* Response criteria for NHL: importance of 'normal' lymph node size and correlations with response rates. *Ann Oncol* 2000; **11**: 399–408.

31. Lewis E, Bernardino ME, Salvador PG *et al.* Post-therapy CT-detected mass in lymphoma patients: is it viable tissue? *J Comput Assist Tomogr* 1982; **6**: 792–5.

32. Fuks JZ, Aisner J, Wiernik PH. Restaging laparotomy in the management of the non-Hodgkin lymphomas. *Med Ped Oncol* 1982; **10**: 429–38.

33. Stewart FM, Williamson BR, Innes DJ *et al.* Residual tumor masses following treatment for advanced histiocytic lymphoma. *Cancer* 1085; **55**: 620–3.

34. Surbone A, Longo DL, DeVita VT Jr *et al.* Residual abdominal masses in aggressive non-Hodgkin's lymphoma after combination chemotherapy: significance and management. *J Clin Oncol* 1988; **6**: 1832–7.

35. Longo DL, DeVita VT Jr, Duffey PL *et al.* Superiority of ProMACE-CytaBOM over ProMACE-MOPP in the treatment of advanced diffuse aggressive lymphoma: Results of a prospective randomized trial. *J Clin Oncol* 1991; **9**: 25–38.

36. Waits TM, Greco FA, Greer JP *et al.* Effective therapy for poor-prognosis non-Hodgkin's lymphoma with 8 weeks of high-dose-intensity combination chemotherapy. *J Clin Oncol* 1993; **11**: 943–9.

37. Coiffier B, Gisselbrecht C, Herbrecht R *et al.* LNH-84 regimen: a multicenter study of intensive chemotherapy in 737 patients with aggressive malignant lymphoma. *J Clin Oncol* 1989; **7**: 1018–26.

38. Zuckerman KS, LoBuglio AF, Reeves JA. Chemotherapy of intermediate- and high-grade non-Hodgkin's lymphomas with a high-dose doxorubicin-containing regimen. *J Clin Oncol* 1990; **8**: 248–56.

39. Chopra R, Goldstone AH, Pearce R *et al.* Autologous versus allogeneic bone marrow transplantation for non-Hodgkin's

lymphoma: A case-controlled analysis of the European Bone Marrow Transplant Group Registry data. *J Clin Oncol* 1992; **10**: 1690–5.

40. Zuckerman KS, Case DC Jr, Gams RA *et al.* Chemotherapy of intermediate- and high-grade non-Hodgkin's lymphomas with an intensive epirubicin-containing regimen. *Blood* 1993; **82**: 3564–73.

41. Meyer RM, Quirt IC, Skillings JR *et al.* Escalated as compared with standard doses of doxorubicin in BACOP therapy for patients with non-Hodgkin's lymphoma. *New Engl J Med* 1993; **329**: 1770–6.

42. Cheson BD, Horning SJ, Coiffier B *et al.* Report of an International Workshop to standardize response criteria for non-Hodgkin's lymphomas. *J Clin Oncol* 1999; **17**: 1244–53.

●43. Juweid M, Wiseman GA, Vose JM *et al.* Response assessment of aggressive non-Hodgkin's lymphoma by integrated International Workshop criteria (IWC) and 18F-fluorodeoxyglucose positron emission tomography (PET). *J Clin Oncol* 2005; **23**: 4652–61.

◆44. Juweid M, Cheson BD. Positron emission tomography (PET) in post-therapy assessment of cancer. *New Engl J Med* 2006; **354**: 496–507. (Review of the indications for use of PET scans in the management of patients with cancer.)

45. Van Den Bossche B, Lambert B, De Winter F *et al.* 18FDG PET versus high-dose 67Ga scintigraphy for restaging and treatment follow-up of lymphoma patients. *Nuc Med Comm* 2002; **23**: 1079–83.

46. Kostakoglu L, Leonard JP, Kuji I *et al.* Comparison of fluorine-18 fluorodeoxyglucose positron emission tomography and Ga-67 scintigraphy in evaluation of lymphoma. *Cancer* 2002; **94**: 879–88.

47. Jerusalem G, Beguin Y, Fassotte MF *et al.* Whole-body positron emission tomography using 18F-fluorodeoxyglucose for posttreatment evaluation in Hodgkin's disease and non-Hodgkin's lymphoma has higher diagnostic and prognostic value than classical computed tomography scan imaging. *Blood* 1999; **94**: 429–33.

48. Freudenberg LS, Antoch G, Schütt P *et al.* FDG-PET/CT in re-staging of patients with lymphoma. *Eur J Nucl Med Mol Imaging* 2004; **31**: 325–9.

49. Tatsumi M, Cohade C, Nakamoto Y *et al.* Direct comparison of FDG PET and CT findings in patients with lymphoma: initial experience. *Radiology* 2005; **237**: 1038–45.

50. Raanani P, Shasha Y, Perry C *et al.* Is CT scan still necessary for staging in Hodgkin and nonHodgkin lymphoma patients in the PET/CT era? *Ann Oncol* 2006; **17**: 117–22.

51. Spaepen K, Stroobants S, Dupont P *et al.* Prognostic value of pretransplantation positron emission tomography using fluorine 18-fluorodeoxyglucose in patients with aggressive lymphoma treated with high-dose chemotherapy and stem cell transplantation. *Blood* 2003; **102**: 53–9.

●52. Haioun C, Itti E, Rahmouni A *et al.* [^{18}F]fluoro-2-deoxy-D-glucose positron emission tomography (FDG-PET) in aggressive lymphoma: an early prognostic tool for

predicting patient outcome. *Blood* 2005; **106**: 1376–81. (PET performed after 2 cycles of R-CHOP chemotherapy predicted patients who would have an excellent outcome versus those with a poorer outcome with treatment.)

53. Kostakoglu L, Goldsmith SJ, Leonard JP *et al.* FDG-PET after 1 cycle of therapy predicts outcome in diffuse large cell lymphoma and classic Hodgkin disease. *Cancer* 2006; **107**: 2678–87.

●54. Gallamini A, Hutchings M, Rigacci L *et al.* Early interim 2-[18F]fluoro-2-D-glucose positron emission tomography is prognostically superior to international prognostic score in advanced stage Hodgkin's lymphoma: a report from a joint Italian-Danish study. *J Clin Oncol* 2007; **25**: 3746–52. (A demonstration of the prognostic strength of the PET scan in patients with Hodgkin lymphoma, being a more powerful predictor of outcome than the International Prognostic Score.)

●55. Juweid ME, Stroobants S, Hoekstra OS *et al.* Use of positron emission tomography for response assessment of lymphoma: consensus recommendations of the Imaging Subcommittee of the International Harmonization Project in Lymphoma. *J Clin Oncol* 2007; **25**: 571–8. (The report of the International Harmonization Project that standardized the conduct and interpretation of PET scanning.)

56. Castellucci P, Nanni C, Farsad M *et al.* Potential pitfalls of ^{18}F-FDG PET in a large series of patients treated for malignant lymphoma: prevalence and scan interpretation. *Nuc Med Comm* 2005; **26**: 689–94.

57. Römer W, Hahauske A-R, Zieger S *et al.* Positron-emission tomography in non-Hodgkin's lymphoma: assessment of chemotherapy with fluorodeoxyglucose. *Blood* 1998; **91**: 4464–71.

58. Spaepen K, Stroobants S, Dupont P *et al.* Early restaging positron emission tomography with 18F-fluorodeoxyglucose predicts outcome in patients with aggressive non-Hodgkin's lymphoma. *Ann Oncol* 2002; **13**: 1356–63.

59. Hutchings M, Loft A, Hansen M *et al.* FDG-PET after two cycles of chemotherapy predicts treatment failure and progression-free survival in Hodgkin lymphoma. *Blood* 2006; **107**: 52–9.

60. Schot B, van Imhoff G, Pruim J *et al.* Predictive value of early 18F-deoxyglucose positron emission tomography in chemosensitive relapsed lymphoma. *Br J Haematol* 2003; **123**: 282–7.

61. Terasawa T, Lau J, Bardet S, *et al.* Fluorine-18-fluorodeoxyglucose positron emission tomography for interim response assessment of advanced-stage Hodgkin's lymphoma and diffuse large B-cell lymphoma: a systematic review. *J Clin Oncol* 2009; **27**: 1906–14.

62. Cheson BD. The case against heavy Peting. *J Clin Oncol* 2009; **27**: 1742–3.

63. de Wit M, Bohuslavizki KH, Buchert R *et al.* 18FDG-PET following treatment as valid predictor for disease-free

survival in Hodgkin's lymphoma. *Ann Oncol* 2001; **12**: 29–37.

64. Spaepen K, Stroobants S, Dupont P *et al.* Prognostic value of positron emission tomography (PET) with fluorine-18 fluorodeoxyglucose ([^{18}F]FDG) after first-line chemotherapy in non-Hodgkin's lymphoma: Is [^{18}F]FDG-PET a valid alternative to conventional diagnostic methods? *J Clin Oncol* 2001; **19**: 414–19.

65. Zinzani PL, Magagnoli M, Chierichetti F *et al.* The role of positron emission tomography (PET) in the management of lymphoma patients. *Ann Oncol* 1999; **10**: 1181–4.

66. Weeks JC, Yeap BY, Canellos GP *et al.* Value of follow-up procedures in patients with large-cell lymphoma who achieve a complete remission. *J Clin Oncol* 1991; **9**: 1196–203.

67. Oh YK, Ha CS, Samuels BI *et al.* Stages I-III follicular lymphoma: Role of CT of the abdomen and pelvis in follow-up studies. *Radiology* 1999; **210**: 483–6.

68. Foltz LM, Song KW, Connors JM. Who actually detects relapse in Hodgkin lymphoma: patient or physician. *Blood* 2004; **104**: 853–4a (abstract 3124).

69. Jerusalem G, Beguin Y, Fassotte MF *et al.* Early detection of relapse by whole-body positron emission tomography in the follow-up of patients with Hodgkin's disease. *Ann Oncol* 2003; **14**: 123–30.

●70. Zinzani PL, Stefoni V, Tani M et al. Role of [^{18}F]fluorodeoxyglucose positron emission tomography scan in the follow-up of lymphoma. *J Clin Oncol* 2009; **27**: 1781–7.

71. Kelloff GJ, Hoffman JM, Johnson B *et al.* Progress and promise of FDG-PET imaging for cancer patient management and oncologic drug development. *Clin Cancer Res* 2005; **11**: 2785–808.

72. Kelloff GJ, Krohn KA, Larson SM *et al.* The progress and promise of molecular imaging probes in oncologic drug development. *Clin Cancer Res* 2005; **15**: 7967–85.

53

Prognostic factors and risk adaptation

JEREMY G FRANKLIN

AIMS AND PRINCIPLES OF PROGNOSTIC FACTORS

A prognostic factor is a measurement or classification of an individual patient, usually determined at or soon after diagnosis, which gives information on the likely outcome of the disease. This information will generally be phrased in terms of probabilities – for instance, the probability of cure for various values of a prognostic factor – or in terms of expected length of survival. It may be used for informing the patient, or in the context of clinical trials for defining or describing the study population or adjusting the data analysis. However, for the clinician the most important role of the prognostic factor is to help choose an appropriate treatment strategy.

As noted by Windeler,[1] an understanding of the interaction between prognostic factors, treatment, and prognosis is crucial in order to use prognostic factors to choose the optimal treatment. The important comparison for treatment selection is between treatment options for the patient concerned, not between different categories of patient. A frequent assumption is that a poorer prognosis justifies a more intensive treatment. The basis for this assumption is that the greater potential benefit of treatment intensification for a patient with poor prognosis outweighs the disadvantages of increased toxicity or cost. This may often be true, but only a comparison of outcome (including effectiveness and toxicities) between the treatment options for poor and good prognosis patients, respectively, can provide reliable evidence. Ultimately, therefore, controlled (if possible, randomized) comparisons are needed to inform treatment choice for prognostically characterized patients – see, for example, analyses by Byar and Corle[2] and Byar and Green.[3]

INVESTIGATION OF PROGNOSTIC FACTORS

Prognostic factors may be proposed theoretically or discovered through biological research or clinical observation.

They must, however, be confirmed, evaluated, and validated through statistical analysis of the characteristics, treatment, and outcomes of large cohorts of comparable patients. Hypotheses should be formulated in advance. Ideally, the study should be prospective, but this is rare in the field of prognostic factors.

Usually, a new factor is useful only if it provides prognostic information additional to that provided by the known factors, i.e., it has an independent effect on prognosis when the effects of the known factors are accounted for. (Failing this, advantages of availability or ease of measurement might nevertheless justify the use of a new factor.)

For statistical precision there must be large numbers of uniformly treated patients, but for generalizability the major relevant treatment options must be represented. In order to avoid confounding, the patients receiving the various treatment options must be comparable with each other, ideally through randomization. Thus, large randomized controlled trials provide an optimal basis for the evaluation of prognostic factors and their relationship to treatment.

Simon and Altman[4] provide a useful guide to critical methodological aspects of prognostic factor studies. Generally accepted standards for such studies are lacking, and the results of comparable investigations are sometimes inconsistent. These authors emphasize the importance of the following:

- Precise hypotheses to be stated in advance, or failing this the statement that the study is exploratory;
- Care in defining the study population and need for an adequate sample size;
- Need for a strategy to deal with missing data;
- Need for multivariate analysis in order to establish prognostic value beyond other known factors;
- Problems with and avoidance of stepwise regression methods;
- Appropriate tests for differences between subgroups.

A prognostic model derived using data from one or more cohorts of patients needs to be validated by testing its predictive ability in one or more further, independent data sets. The issue of validation is described by Altman and Royston[5] and Royston et al.[6]

In order to combine the prognostic information from relevant prognostic factors in a form applicable to treatment selection, a prognostic score or prognostic classification may be derived. Begg et al.[7] discuss how rival classifications may be compared. If the result is to help make treatment decisions then the values of the score or the prognostic classes must be linked to specific treatment options.

TYPES OF PROGNOSTIC FACTORS AND THEIR INTERRELATIONSHIP

The prognosis of a patient suffering from a lymphoid neoplasm is largely directly dependent on the characteristics of the tumor or malignant cells: size of tumor or number of malignant cells, location of tumor, growth rate, and dispersion rate. These tumor characteristics are influenced by the microenvironment surrounding the tumor or cells, which includes both (a) the physiologic microenvironment and (b) the local impact of therapy (drug concentrations, local radiation dose, etc.). Thus, prognostic factors must be associated with one or more of these aspects, i.e., tumor characteristics, tumor microenvironment, or intensity of treatment to tumor.

A prognostic factor may relate in various ways to the tumor aspects. It may:

- Measure a tumor aspect directly ('measurement'), e.g., determination of initial tumor burden via imaging techniques;
- Influence a tumor aspect ('causal' factor). For instance, the gene product BCL2 blocks apoptosis of malignant lymphocytes and thereby supports proliferation. Thus, higher levels of BCL2 correlate with more rapid proliferation. Lowering BCL2 levels by intervention would tend to retard proliferation (this principle has been tested clinically using 'BCL2 antisense therapy'[8]);
- Merely be associated with a tumor aspect and thus indicate its likely state ('indicator' factor). For instance, anemia is associated with poorer prognosis in Hodgkin lymphoma (HL), but it is not necessarily causal, in the sense that treatment of the anemia would not necessarily improve the prognosis concerning HL.

A given factor may relate to tumor aspects in more than one way; poor performance status, for instance, may indicate (be caused by) extensive or aggressive tumor, but it may also tend to lead to incomplete treatment and thus lower dose to tumor.

The diagram in Figure 53.1 attempts to depict schematically the interrelationships between tumor aspects, prognostic factors, and treatment parameters. Unfortunately, the causal or indicator mechanisms for many prognostic factors are still poorly or incompletely understood. Thus, in this diagram the prognostic factors have been divided into three broad types, namely, general patient factors, clinical factors, and immunologic factors. The diagram shows the presumably most prevalent causal relationships between these broad categories, treatment, the tumor microenvironment, and the tumor itself.

In the following sections, prognostic factors recognized for lymphoid neoplasms in adults will be described under the three broad categories, with an account of their mechanisms if known.

GENERAL PATIENT FACTORS

Age

Advanced age is recognized as an adverse prognostic factor for all lymphoid neoplasms.[9–12] The definition of what

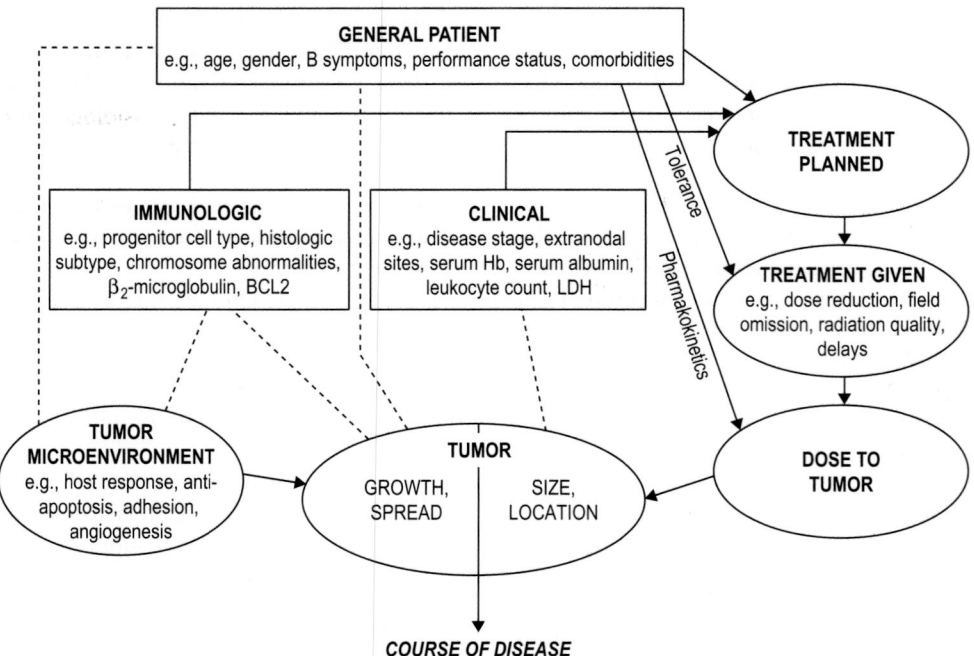

Figure 53.1 Schematic depiction of the presumably most prevalent relationships between tumor parameters, prognostic factors, and treatment. Broad categories of prognostic factors are shown as rectangles, while tumor and treatment aspects are shown as ellipses. Arrows portray causal effects and dashed lines show other associations (indicator variables). Hb, hemoglobin; LDH, lactate dehydrogenase.

constitutes 'advanced' varies, according to the age-incidence spectrum of the disease, among the entities concerned, from 45 years and above for HL[9] to 65 or even 80 years and above for multiple myeloma (MM).[13] Several different mechanisms have been proposed to account for the relationship between age and prognosis. First, life expectancy in the general population obviously decreases markedly with increasing age above 60–70 years, so that the survival curves of older patients will inevitably be lower. This mechanism has nothing to do with the disease itself. Second, older patients more frequently have comorbidities and acute treatment toxicities (such as severe infections) which can be fatal, and even if not fatal can limit the administration of therapy.[10–12] Thus, older patients typically receive a dose-reduced and/or delayed treatment, which in general will be less effective. Even if first-line treatment is administered according to protocol, aggressive salvage treatment is often severely limited in older patients. Furthermore, certain life-threatening, treatment-related diseases such as second malignancies are more frequent in older patients.[12] These mechanisms apply generally to all these diseases. Third, for specific entities the typical characteristics of the disease may vary with age: for instance, in HL the relative frequency of the various histologic subtypes is age dependent; in adult acute lymphocytic leukemia (ALL) older patients more frequently have Philadelphia-positive disease.[11,12] Fourth, it has been speculated that older patients may have a blunted host immune response to their disease.[10]

Gender

Male patients have a slightly worse prognosis than females in certain lymphoid neoplasms (HL, chronic lymphocytic leukemia [CLL]) but this effect has not been established for other entities. There seems to be no consensus on the mechanism of this relationship. In the general population, males have a somewhat shorter life expectancy than females. Further, drug metabolism appears to differ according to gender. This may explain why females suffer more severe hematologic toxicities during chemotherapy.[14–16] A correlation between more severe treatment toxicity and better prognosis has been demonstrated for HL patients.[15,16] Finally, the typical disease characteristics may differ between males and females, e.g., the relative frequencies of the histologic subtypes in HL.

Performance status

Performance status is a further general prognostic factor in, for instance, aggressive non-Hodgkin lymphoma (NHL)[10] and relapsed HL.[17] Patients may have reduced performance status due to more severe disease characteristics, less tolerance of disease-related morbidity, or due to comorbidities; each of these factors may clearly lead to a poorer prognosis, either directly or due to poorer prospects of complete administration of therapy. In MM, physical functioning as measured using a quality-of-life questionnaire completed by the patients prior to treatment was shown to correlate both with World Health Organization (WHO) performance status and with survival.[18]

Systemic symptoms

The so-called B symptoms, comprising weight loss, unexplained fever, and night sweats, are recognized for the staging of HL and NHL. There is strong evidence that these symptoms are caused by abnormal production of cytokines by tumor or bystander cells.[19,20] The presence of one or more B symptoms is associated with poorer prognosis in both of these diseases. In HL, there is evidence that fever has the greatest prognostic value while night sweats contribute little or nothing. The presence of B symptoms in HL is correlated with total tumor burden, and they lose their prognostic significance if precise tumor burden has been accounted for. Therefore, the usual prognostic value of B symptoms may be due to their providing additional information on tumor burden beyond the usual staging examinations. In CLL, the presence of B symptoms may be taken to indicate disease requiring immediate treatment.

CLINICAL FACTORS

Results of staging examinations, i.e., the location and size of tumors, blood cell counts, and organ abnormalities as well as further clinical parameters are considered here.

Tumor location and size

Extent of tumor is the main determinant of stage in HL and NHL. It is mainly assessed using physical examination and imaging techniques such as computed tomography, x-rays, sonography, positron emission tomography (PET), gallium scan, nuclear magnetic resonance (NMR) imaging, or bone or bone marrow scintigraphy. Additionally, biopsies of the bone marrow or liver, or in certain cases laparotomy and/or splenectomy, may be performed. Prognostic aspects of tumor extent, as systematized in the Ann Arbor staging definitions, include the number of involved nodal sites, the involvement of sites above, below, or on both sides of the diaphragm, the size of tumor in certain locations (such as the mediastinal mass), the extension of nodal involvement into extranodal tissue (E-lesions), and the involvement of extranodal organs. However, there is no consistent evidence that the involvement of particular anatomic sites is associated with worse prognosis in HL or NHL. In MM, the number of bone lesions is associated with prognosis. All these features constitute aspects of total tumor burden and therefore reflect the amount of 'work' to be accomplished by the therapy. Further, they will usually be correlated with tumor aggressiveness, since large tumor burden will usually be a result of recent rapid

growth. In addition, organ involvement in HL or aggressive NHL[10] is associated with poor prognosis, whereas the prognostic significance of particular locations of involvement such as E-lesions or infradiaphragmatic sites in early stage HL is controversial. Since no imaging or other technique fully reveals the extent of tumor involvement, it is possible that indirect indications of tumor burden may show independent prognostic value (see below).

Hematologic parameters

The levels of various serum constituents and other hematologic parameters are correlated with prognosis. Anemia predicts poorer prognosis in advanced stage HL,[9] aggressive NHL,[10] follicular NHL,[21] CLL,[22] and MM.[23] Low serum albumin has been identified as prognostic in HL[9] and MM.[24] Elevated serum lactate dehydrogenase (LDH) level has established prognostic value in NHL[10,21] and MM,[25] and possibly a prognostic role in HL.[26,27] Thrombocytopenia is recognized to define advanced stage in CLL.

Hemoglobin and serum albumin are correlated with each other and with extent of disease, B symptoms, and other serum parameters in HL. Both of these factors have been identified as independently prognostic in advanced stage HL; when these two factors are accounted for, further correlated factors such as elevated erythrocyte sedimentation rate (ESR) and serum alkaline phosphatase level lose their prognostic value.[9] Probably, all these factors are indicators of tumor burden and activity.

Leukocyte counts

An elevated white blood cell count (leukocytosis) predicts poorer prognosis in both advanced stage HL[9] and ALL.[11,28] In HL, leukocytosis is associated with lymphocytopenia (either absolute or as a percentage of leukocytes). In ALL, it is correlated with a high percentage of circulating blasts, which also shows independent prognostic value.

IMMUNOLOGIC FACTORS

The progression of lymphoid neoplasms is closely influenced by the immune system from which they originate and in which they are embedded. Tumor cell proliferation, apoptosis, adhesion, dissemination, angiogenesis, and the host response to the tumor are causal factors which may be associated with measurable immunologic parameters. Other parameters may indicate tumor burden.

Tumor subtype

T cell as opposed to B cell tumor origin may be associated with poorer prognosis in both aggressive NHL[10] and

ALL.[11] However, under modern therapies for ALL this difference seems to have disappeared, and only particular subtypes (pre-T cell ALL, pro-B ALL) continue to do worse than others. In CLL, the poorer prognosis associated with unmutated immunoglobulin (Ig) V_H genes may be due to derivation from a pre-germinal cell naïve B cell as opposed to a germinal or post-germinal center memory B cell.[29] In HL, mixed cellularity subtype has sometimes been regarded as adverse compared to the prevailing nodular sclerosis subtype, while the lymphocyte-predominant subtype is now recognized as a distinct entity and is associated with a more favorable prognosis[30] after mild therapy.

Tumor cell proliferation

Measurement of proliferation using flow cytometric DNA assessment and thymidine uptake has been related to prognosis in aggressive NHL.[31,32] Thymidine kinase activity in the serum of CLL patients has been demonstrated as an independent prognostic factor, helping to distinguish between 'smoldering' disease and disease prone to rapid progression.[33] Furthermore, the presence of nuclear proliferation antigen Ki-67 in aggressive NHL has been shown to correlate with shorter overall survival.[34]

Apoptosis

The gene product BCL2 blocks apoptosis in B lymphocytes, and increased expression of BCL2 has been shown to predict poorer prognosis in NHL[10] and HL.[35] The protein p53 has also been shown to be involved in induction of apoptosis and to be correlated with prognosis in HL[36] (although this is controversial[37]), NHL,[38,39] and CLL.[40] Further, serum interleukin-10 (IL-10) causes an increase in the BCL2 level and has been shown by several groups to be independently prognostic in HL.[41,42]

Finally, the activation of caspase-3 constitutes the final step in the process of apoptosis.[35] The level of activated caspase-3 was associated with prognosis in HL, independently of BCL2 and conventional factors.

Adhesion

Adhesion molecules influence the binding of lymphocytes or their malignant counterparts. The lymphocyte homing receptor CD44 facilitates binding to high endothelial venules and thus enables lymphocytes to migrate into nodal areas.[43] CD44 is associated in NHL with advanced stage, greater risk of dissemination, and worse prognosis.[44,45] In HL, intercellular and vascular cell adhesion molecules (ICAM, VCAM) often show elevated serum levels; their competitive inhibition of receptor-ligand mechanisms may facilitate the dissemination and metastasis of the malignant cells. Both these molecules have proved to be independent prognostic factors in HL.[46]

Host immune response to tumor

A poor host response has been measured in aggressive NHL using the count of $CD8^+$ T tumor-infiltrating lymphocytes,[47] and low counts have been shown to correlate with the lack of class I or II major histocompatibility complex (MHC) molecules. Further, both lack of MHC molecules and low counts of $CD8^+$ T tumor-infiltrating lymphocytes have been demonstrated to correlate with shorter survival in NHL.[48]

In NHL, CLL, and MM patients (and possibly in HL), elevated serum levels of β_2-microglobulin are associated with poorer prognosis (and greater tumor burden).[24,35,49,50] β_2-microglobulin is noncovalently associated with the α chain of the class I MHC.

Angiogenesis

To date, a prognostic role for angiogenesis-related factors has not been reliably established for the lymphoid neoplasms. The tissue expression of metalloproteinases 2 and 9 is possibly correlated with prognosis in HL.[51]

Other immunologic factors

The above six categories of immunologic factors are neither definitive nor all-encompassing. Further factors for which prognostic value has been demonstrated include

HL: serum CD30, IL-1 receptor antagonist (IL-1RA);

NHL: other chromosome abnormalities;

CLL: CD38, Zap70, serum CD23;

MM: C-reactive protein, monosomy 13/13q, serum immunoglobulins, other chromosome abnormalities;

ALL: CD34.

Table 53.1 summarizes the information on those prognostic factors which are relevant to more than one lymphoid neoplasm disease. Considerable overlap in prognostic associations among these diseases is demonstrated.

RISK ADAPTATION

The following steps are required to establish a risk-adapted treatment strategy:

First, a standard treatment is recognized for a certain indication.

Second, prognostic factors are demonstrated to identify (two or more) subgroups of patients within this indication with differing prognoses, as defined by a relevant outcome.

Third, alternative treatments are proposed for the identified prognostic groups. This may involve, for instance, an intensified treatment scheme for the poor prognosis group(s), while the remainder continue to receive the standard treatment, or a treatment of reduced intensity for the good prognosis group(s), or both. In certain cases the allocation

Table 53.1 Prognostic factors relevant to more than one lymphoid neoplasm

Prognostic factor	HL	NHL	CLL	MM	ALL
General patient					
Age	>45 years	>60 years	Older	>65 years	Older
Gender	Male	Male	Male		(Male)
B symptoms	Yes		Yes		
Clinical					
Extranodal involvement	Yes	>1 site			
Hemoglobin	<10.5 g/dL	Low	Low	Low	
Serum albumin	Low			Low	
Serum LDH	(High)	High	(High)	High	
Leukocyte count	High				High
Immunologic					
Tumor subtype	non-LP	(T cell)			Naïve B cell
Tumor cell proliferation		High; Ki-67+	High thym. kinase		
BCL2	High	High			
p53	High	High	High		
β_2-microglobulin		High	High	High	
Genetic abnormalities		Various	Various	Various	Various

Entries in the body of the table indicate adverse characteristics (in parentheses: prognostic value uncertain).
HL, Hodgkin lymphoma; NHL, non-Hodgkin lymphoma; CLL, chronic lymphocytic leukemia; MM, multiple myeloma; ALL, acute lymphoblastic lymphoma; LDH, lactate dehydrogenase; thym. kinase, thymidylate kinase; non-LP, non-lymphocyte predominant.

of a new treatment scheme may be equivalent to 'shifting the boundaries' separating the indication in question from neighboring groups: for instance, use of the 'risk factors' large mediastinal mass and extranodal lesions to locate patients with stage II HL in the advanced stage group with the consequence of more intensive treatment.

Fourth, the alternative treatment allocated to any subgroup must be confirmed as superior, in terms of effectiveness, toxicity, etc., to the standard in that subgroup by means of a randomized controlled trial.

Further optimization of risk adaptation will involve testing the optimality of both the subgroup definition (which prognostic factors, which cutpoints) and the respective treatment schemes in each subgroup.

An example of the risk adaptation process is provided by the development of adapted treatment within early stage Hodgkin lymphoma by the European Organization for Research and Treatment in Cancer (EORTC).[52,53] In the 1960s and 1970s, patients suffering from stage I–II (early stage) Hodgkin lymphoma received radiation to the extended or total nodal field, without chemotherapy, as standard treatment. The EORTC analyzed the results of its first two clinical trials in this area, H1 and H2, which recruited from 1963 to 1976 and prescribed mantle field irradiation with or without extension to the paraaortic field as initial therapy. They concluded that four prognostic factors were relevant to identify patients with relatively poor prognosis:

- Age ≥40 years;
- ESR ≥70 mm/h;

- Histologic subtype (mixed cellularity [MC] or lymphocyte depleted [LD]);
- Stage II *without* mediastinal involvement.

These factors were employed in the subsequent trial, H5 (1977–82), to define two prognostic groups within the early stages. Laparotomy-negative patients without any of the above factors ('favorable' group) were treated with radiation alone as previously, while patients with at least one adverse factor ('unfavorable' group) were randomized between total nodal irradiation (TNI) alone and TNI sandwiched between 3 + 3 cycles of mechlorethamine, vincristine, procarbazine, and prednisone (MOPP) chemotherapy. Superior results in the combined modality arm led to the adoption of this treatment as EORTC standard for unfavorable early stage HL. The definition of this group was refined following further prognostic factor analyses, resulting in the following factors:

- Age ≥40 years;
- ≥2 lymph node areas;
- ESR ≥50 mm/h (without B symptoms) or ESR ≥70 mm/h (with B symptoms);
- Large mediastinal mass (ratio mediastinal mass:thorax ≥0.5).

Subsequent EORTC trials used these factors to define unfavorable disease and employed 6 cycles of chemotherapy plus extensive irradiation as standard treatment. Further refinement to these prognostic factors adjusted the critical age to 50 years, the critical number of nodal areas to four, and the critical mediastinal mass:thorax ratio to 0.35.

The following sections describe, for each entity, the most important prognostic factors, prognostic classification schemes, and risk adaptation as practised or proposed by the major clinical trials groups.

HODGKIN LYMPHOMA

In HL, patients are divided into two or three basic prognostic groups, chiefly according to stage and B symptoms but also taking various other factors into account. Patients with stage IIIB or IV ('advanced stages') are associated with the poorest prognosis and are assigned an intensive chemotherapy protocol, sometimes followed by adjuvant radiation therapy. Further prognostic factors are often used to assign certain stage IIIA or stage IIB patients to the advanced stage group. Among the remaining patients ('early stages'), who had previously received extended field radiation therapy alone, 'favorable' and 'unfavorable' subgroups are defined on the basis of stage, B symptoms, and/or further prognostic factors. Early stage patients in unfavorable subgroups are currently given combined modality therapy; patients in favorable subgroups may still receive radiation alone, but are increasingly receiving mild chemotherapy followed by radiation. Each group is thus associated with a typical standard treatment strategy:

- Early stages, favorable: mild chemotherapy (typically 2–4 cycles) plus radiation (or extended-field radiation alone);
- Early stages, unfavorable: moderate chemotherapy (typically 4–6 cycles) plus radiation;
- Advanced stages: extensive chemotherapy (typically 8 cycles) with or without consolidatory (usually local) radiation.

Figure 53.2 displays the prognostic divisions used by some major study groups and institutions.

Chemotherapy usually consists of doxorubicin, bleomycin, vinblastine, and dacarbazine (ABVD) or a similar anthracycline-containing multidrug regimen, although for advanced stage patients more dose-intensive regimens are often used.

In the above scheme, two divisions between the three prognostic groups must be defined, each division possibly defined by a different set of factors. Furthermore, the attempt has been made to identify advanced stage patients with a particularly high risk of failure for intensified therapy, e.g., early high-dose chemotherapy with stem cell support.[54]

In the following sections, recognized prognostic factors will be described for early stage and for advanced stage HL patients, respectively, who are clinically staged and treated with combined modality according to the above scheme.

(1) EORTC		Stage	
		I, II	III, IV
Risk factors	None	Early favorable	Advanced*
	ESR ≥50 mm/h (with B symptoms: ≥30)		
	Large mediastinal mass	Early unfavorable	
	Age ≥50 years		

* Trial 20012 is restricted to patients with IPS ≥ 3

(2) GHSG		Stage		
		I, IIA	IIB	III, IV
Risk factors	None	Early		
	ESR ≥50 mm/h (with B symptoms: ≥30)			Advanced
	≥3 nodal areas	Intermediate		
	Large mediastinal mass			
	E-lesions			

(3) Stanford*		Stage		
		IA, IIA	IB, IIB	III, IV
Risk factors	None	Early favorable		
	≥2 E-lesions	Early unfavorable		
	Large mediastinal mass			Advanced

* Lymphocyte predominant HL is excluded from this scheme

Figure 53.2 Risk adaptation employed in recent clinical trials for Hodgkin lymphoma (HL) patients. (1) Lymphoma Group of the European Organization for Research and Treatment of Cancer (EORTC), trials H9F, H9U, and #20012; (2) German Hodgkin Study Group (GHSG), trials HD13, HD14, HD15; (3) Stanford University, trials G5 and E2496. IPS, International Prognostic Score; HL, Hodgkin lymphoma; ESR, erythrocyte sedimentation rate.

Prognostic factors for early stages (CSI–II)

The main adverse factors currently recognized for assignment of patients to a prognostic group and hence treatment selection are as follows.

- Advanced age
- Male sex
- Histologic subtype mixed cellularity (MC)
- Stage II
- B symptoms
- Large mediastinal mass (LMM) or bulky disease
- Many involved nodal regions
- Elevated ESR
- Anemia
- Low serum albumin

The above factors have been identified and confirmed in retrospective analyses of large data sets from patients treated in (mainly multicenter) clinical trials or single institutions.[52,55]

These factors are relevant to the decision as to which stage I–II patients should be classed as having 'unfavorable' disease and receive more (or more intensive) chemotherapy. If patients with 'favorable' disease are still being treated with radiation alone, then prognostic factors must be evaluated specifically for this treatment option, but in general the list of recognized factors in early stage HL does not depend on the treatment modality. Major study groups have employed the criteria described below.

The EORTC defines CSI–II (supradiaphragmatic only) patients as in an unfavorable group if they have any of the following factors: age over 50 years, asymptomatic with ESR greater than 50 mm/h, B symptoms with ESR greater than 30 mm/h, and LMM. The development of these criteria was described above (see under 'Risk adaptation'). Patients in favorable groups have been treated with radiation therapy either alone or following mild chemotherapy, whereas patients in unfavorable groups have received more intensive chemotherapy with radiation therapy.

The German Hodgkin Study Group (GHSG) has, since 1988, assigned treatment with four chemotherapy cycles plus radiation therapy to 'intermediate stage' CSI–II patients with any of the following adverse factors: LMM, three or more involved regions, high ESR ($\geqslant$50 mm/h if B symptoms absent, $\geqslant$30 mm/h if B symptoms present), localized extranodal infiltration (*E-lesions*), or massive splenic involvement; other 'early stage' CSI–II patients received 2–4 cycles of chemotherapy plus involved field (IF) radiation therapy (or, until 1994, extended field [EF] radiation therapy alone).[56]

Stanford began in 1980 to give combined modality treatment to CSI–II patients with LMM or multiple E-lesions. The current Stanford phase III trial, G5, administers risk-adapted chemotherapy plus involved field radiation to 'favorable' group, early stage patients, i.e., those without LMM or multiple E-lesions.

The EORTC has investigated the use of localized radiation therapy in a 'very favorable' subgroup of early stage patients. Inclusion criteria were stage IA female under 40 years, nodular sclerosing (NS) or lymphocyte predominant (LP) histology, without elevated ESR or LMM. However, a 30 percent long-term failure rate was observed and this policy was not continued.

These same factors are relevant to the decision as to which stage II patients should be classed as advanced stage and receive extensive chemotherapy (usually 6–8 cycles). The EORTC has included stages III and IV only in its advanced stage cohorts, without regard to other factors (although the current trial 20012 is restricted to stages III–IV with an International Prognostic Index of at least 3). The US National Cancer Institute and several US cooperative groups similarly equate 'advanced stage' with stages III–IV. In the GHSG, stage IIB with LMM or E-lesions is also included in the 'advanced' group. Certain other trial groups treat further stage I–II patients as 'advanced,' for instance IB and IIB or bulky stage II disease.[57]

Prognostic factors for advanced stages

The more uniform treatment modality and the greater frequency of treatment failure events have permitted more conclusive and generally applicable results for prognostic factor analyses for the advanced stages, compared with early stages. The results of the International Prognostic Factor Project,[9] while not necessarily including all possible factors, can be taken as reliable. Seven adverse factors contribute to the resulting International Prognostic Score (IPS):

- Age 45 years or more
- Male sex
- Ann Arbor stage IV
- Anemia (hemoglobin <10.5 g/dL)
- Low serum albumin (<4 g/dL)
- Leukocytosis ($\geqslant$15 000/mm^3)
- Lymphocytopenia (<600/mm^3 and/or <8 percent of white blood cell [WBC] count)

All these factors were highly significant in the multivariate analysis of data from 5141 patients treated in 25 centers, and their prognostic power was confirmed in an independent sample. Note that the first five factors are also recognized for early stage patients. All seven factors were associated with similar relative risks of between 1.26 and 1.49. Therefore, Hasenclever and Diehl recommended combining these factors into a single score by simply counting the number of adverse factors, giving an integer prognostic score between 0 and 7. However, even patients with five or more factors (7 percent of cases) had a 5-year failure-free rate of over 40 percent. The best failure-free rate was close to 80 percent for those with at most one factor (29 percent of cases), suggesting that a group of advanced stage patients with a relatively favorable prognosis could be recognized.

A recent analysis of patients at unfavorable early stage in the French GELA trials[58] identified a subset of prognostic factors for these patients closely similar to the IPS for advanced HL, with the factor 'stage IV' replaced by extranodal disease. The IPS together with the factor 'extranodal disease' has also been shown to be prognostic for patients at unfavorable early stage in a GHSG trial.[59] These results suggest that it may be possible to harmonize prognostic factors over all stages of HL based on the IPS.

Certain study groups consider other recognized adverse factors for treatment selection, such as large mediastinal mass, bulky disease, or serum LDH.

Factors relevant to advanced stage patients may be used to identify patients either for treatment intensification or for treatment reduction. Reduction can be achieved by creating a modified protocol or by including these patients in the (unfavorable) early stage group.

Concerning intensification, various investigators have treated a poor prognosis subset of advanced stage patients, who had attained a remission by conventional chemotherapy, with high-dose chemotherapy accompanied by hematologic stem cell support.[54,60] Proctor et al.[60] constructed a continuous numerical index for this purpose as a weighted sum of the variables age, stage, lymphocyte count, hemoglobin, and presence of bulky disease, and included patients with an index greater than 0.5 in the poor prognosis subset. Federico *et al.* included patients with two or more of the factors high LDH, very large mediastinal mass, two or more extranodal sites, inguinal involvement, and low hematocrit.[61] However, none of these methods could consistently select a subset with a failure rate of less than 40 percent with conventional therapy (see also Lee *et al.*[62]). This means that the early high-dose approach is unlikely to show a clinically relevant long-term survival benefit compared with conventional treatment.[63]

Concerning treatment reduction, the short-duration, reduced-dose Stanford V chemotherapy regimen with or without radiation therapy is currently being tested in patients with bulky stage II or advanced stage disease having at most two IPS adverse factors.[64] However, Stanford V is not merely a reduction of therapy but rather a rescheduling with lower total doses but greater dose intensities.

In conclusion, the three-level scheme of division into early favorable, early unfavorable, and advanced stage cases remains valid according to current knowledge. Separation of very favorable early or high-risk advanced stage patients for especially mild or intensive therapy, respectively, does not appear justified. Several prognostic factors, other than clinical stage, are employed in the divisions between favorable, unfavorable, and advanced cases and no universally valid set of factors has been determined. Nevertheless, the list of reliably confirmed, independently prognostic factors given above encompasses most of those used by the major institutions and study groups. For early and advanced stages receiving radiation therapy or chemotherapy, or both, the set of relevant factors is fairly similar. Additional prognostic value has been indicated for several immunologic factors directly related to tumor burden, growth, and microenvironment,[42] but such factors have not yet been integrated into treatment strategies.

AGGRESSIVE LYMPHOMAS

Unlike HL, the non-Hodgkin lymphomas are a biologically heterogeneous collection of diseases, each with its own distinguishing features, relevant treatment strategies, and prognosis. This fact hampers the investigation of prognostic factors in NHL. Nevertheless, the International Prognostic Index established in 1993 (IPI)[65] has been shown to classify both patients with diffuse aggressive lymphoma as a whole[65] and specifically those with nodal mature T cell lymphomas[66] into relatively good and relatively poor prognostic groups. The IPI is based on the presence/absence of five adverse factors:

- Age 60 years or more
- Ann Arbor stage III–IV
- Serum LDH above normal range
- Performance status $\geqslant 2$
- Extranodal involvement in more than one site

The motto 'worse prognosis justifies more intensive treatment' referred to in the introductory sections is implicit in the aims of the IPI (as also seen in the context of the IPS for HL). The factor 'age more than 60 years' clearly does not lend itself to this approach, since older patients are less able to tolerate intensified treatment – indeed, their poor tolerance is an important mechanism to explain their poorer prognosis. Therefore, the prognostic index was reevaluated separately for patients up to 60 years old. The resulting, so-called 'age-adjusted' IPI includes only the three factors stage, LDH, and performance status.

The main prognostic division used for treatment selection within aggressive lymphomas is that between limited stage and advanced stage disease. Limited stage means Ann Arbor stage I or non-bulky stage II. These patients typically receive 3–4 cycles of an anthracycline-containing chemotherapy (usually cyclophosphamide, vincristine, doxorubicin, and prednisolone [CHOP]) followed by radiation therapy (usually involved field). Although the IPI can distinguish relatively good and poor subsets within limited stage disease, treatment choice is usually independent of IPI for these patients.

Patients with bulky stage II disease are generally treated as advanced stage patients (stages III–IV), for whom 6–8 cycles of CHOP plus rituximab (R-CHOP) is currently standard treatment. R-CHOP seems to be more effective than CHOP alone in both high- and low-risk groups as defined by the IPI.[67] Thus, to date there is no firm basis for distinct treatment selection within the advanced stages according to the IPI. However, there is some evidence that the addition of rituximab to CHOP benefits BCL2-positive but not BCL2-negative patients.[68]

In Germany, the German High Grade Non-Hodgkin's Lymphoma Study Group (DSHNHL) distinguishes between younger (18–60 years) and elderly (61–80 years) patients, reserving dose-escalated (Hi-CHOEP [etoposide added to CHOP]) chemotherapy with granulocyte colony-stimulating factor (G-CSF) support and high-dose chemotherapy (Mega-CHOEP) with autologous stem cell transplantation (ASCT) for younger patients. The latest protocols (2003-1 and 2003-2) also distinguish between CD20+ B-NHL and T-NHL. Certain trial populations are limited to IPI scores of 0 to 3.

The EORTC separates patients mainly according to age and stage. Currently, patients aged 18–70 years in stage II–IV are given 8 cycles of CHOP with/without gemcitabine, whereas those aged above 70 receive 4 (stage I–II) or 6 (stage III–IV) cycles of CHOP or CHOEP. Recent protocols tested high-dose chemotherapy (HDCT)/ASCT additional to conventional chemotherapy for younger stage II–IV patients (age up to 60 years).

Current Southwest Oncology Group (SWOG) protocols employ age (cutpoint 60 years), stage, and IPI for assigning patients to protocols. Trials specify CHOP plus rituximab for younger patients with IPI score 0–1 and for older patients with bulky stage II or stage III–IV. CHOP plus involved field radiation therapy (IFRT) (plus monoclonal antibody) is used for localized (stage I and non-bulky II) disease in older patients. Early HDCT/ASCT is tested against CHOP in patients with bulky stage II or stage III–IV and a high-intermediate or high-risk IPI score.

Currently, attempts are being made to define biological subsets of aggressive lymphoma using genetic profiling. Prognostic differences independent of the IPI have been demonstrated.[69] It is hoped to use these results to develop new treatments targeted to critical cell pathways.

INDOLENT LYMPHOMAS

As with aggressive NHL, a basic division into early stage (I, II) and advanced stage disease influences treatment selection. For early stage patients, involved field radiation therapy is standard. It may be possible to defer treatment until symptoms or other indications for therapy appear. The possible benefit of additional chemotherapy is also being tested. Advanced stage patients are standardly treated with single or multiagent chemotherapy. Treatment may be delayed until the appearance of symptoms or signs of progression without impairing survival.[70] Phase II investigations of the use of rituximab, immunotherapy, or even high-dose chemotherapy with stem cell transplantation in advanced stage low-grade lymphomas are currently in progress.

Therefore, prognostic models may potentially be used to help in the following treatment decisions.

- Immediate treatment or watch and wait
- Radiation therapy or systemic therapy
- For advanced stages: whether to use a new strategy such as immunotherapy or high-dose chemotherapy with stem cell transplantation

Several large-scale investigations have identified and confirmed a number of prognostic factors in low-grade lymphoma.[71,72] The International Prognostic Index developed for aggressive lymphomas has been shown to have prognostic power in low-grade lymphoma, although few such patients are allocated to poor-risk groups.[73,74] Most recently, an international cooperative study in follicular lymphoma[21] recommended a prognostic score based on the number of adverse factors.

- Age 60 years or more
- Ann Arbor stage III–IV
- Anemia (hemoglobin <120 g/L)
- >4 nodal areas involved
- Serum LDH above normal range

This score, named Follicular Lymphoma International Prognostic Index (FLIPI), shares several factors with the IPI developed for aggressive lymphomas. Compared with the IPI and with the index developed by the Intergruppo Italiano Linfomi,[72] the FLIPI identified a larger proportion of high-risk patients.[75] Prognostic capacity of the FLIPI has also been demonstrated for mantle cell lymphoma.[76]

As yet, prognostic factors other than stage are not widely formally employed in treatment selection. Solal-Céligny et al.[21] recommend the formation of three prognostic groups. Those with zero to one adverse factor are candidates for radiation therapy (localized disease) or watch and wait (disseminated disease). Those with two factors should receive conventional chemotherapy. Those with three or more factors are candidates for an experimental approach (see above). These recommendations have yet to be confirmed in phase III clinical trials.

In the German Low Grade Lymphoma Study Group (GLSG) trials, entry criteria are defined mainly by stage and age. For stage III–IV disease, patients receive between four and eight chemotherapy cycles according to early remission criteria. Younger patients (less than 60 years) with stage III–IV mantle cell lymphoma or those requiring treatment (due to B symptoms, bulky disease, progressive disease, or further criteria) are randomized after four or six CHOP (+ rituximab) cycles to HDCT/ASCT or interferon maintenance therapy.

The EORTC protocols distinguish between stage I–II disease, assigned to radiation therapy (IF or total-body irradiation [TBI]), and stage III–IV disease, assigned to combination chemotherapy (cyclophosphamide, vincristine, and prednisone; CVP) or single-agent fludarabine. No further risk adaptation is employed.

The Eastern Cooperative Oncology Group (ECOG) trial E4402 for indolent lymphoma selects advanced stage (III–IV) patients with *low tumor burden* for treatment with rituximab alone, defined as follows.

- No nodal or extranodal mass ≥7 cm
- Less than three nodal masses >3 cm
- No systemic symptoms
- No splenomegaly >16 cm in computed tomography
- No evidence of risk of ureteral or epidural compression
- No leukemic phase with >5000/mm^3 circulating malignant cells
- No leukocytopenia, thrombocytopenia, or anemia

CHRONIC LYMPHOCYTIC LEUKEMIA

Staging according to the systems of Binet or Rai are still currently used to divide patients into broad prognostic groups (early, intermediate, and advanced stage) and to determine treatment strategy. Prognosis concerns mainly the risk of progression and thus the desirability of immediate treatment versus a watch-and-wait strategy. However, the course of disease within these broad categories remains very heterogeneous, particularly within the early stages which comprise around 80 percent of CLL. Therefore, further prognostic factors are needed to help choose the appropriate treatment.

The recently closed German CLL Study Group trial CLL1 treated early stage CLL (Binet A) with a risk-adapted approach based on the following adverse factors.

- Predicted lymphocyte doubling time <12 months
- Unfavorable molecular cytogenetics
- Serum thymidine kinase >10 U/L
- Unmutated Ig V_H gene (homology ≥98 percent)

In the successor trial CLL7 it is planned to incorporate V_H mutation status and genetic aberrations into risk adaptation.

Patients are assigned to the high-risk group if they exhibit at least two of the above adverse factors. While low-risk patients receive no immediate treatment, high-risk patients are randomized to immediate fludarabine-cyclophosphamide-rituximab versus watch and wait. Thus, these four prognostic factors are used to define a subset of early stage patients who may benefit from immediate therapy.

For intermediate and advanced stage patients, the German CLL Study Group has started the CLL8 trial. Here, immediate treatment with 6 cycles of fludarabin and cyclophosphamide is given, according to randomization with or without rituximab. The trial is limited to patients requiring treatment, defined as those with one or more of the following.

- B symptoms
- Lymphocyte doubling time <6 months AND lymphocyte count >50 G/L
- Progressive anemia and/or thrombocytopenia
- Massive, progressive, or painful splenomegaly, massive lymph nodes, and/or hyperviscosity problems

These factors include symptoms requiring urgent alleviation and may not necessarily be prognostic in the long term.

The EORTC now defines advanced stage disease using the concept of total tumor burden (TTM). TTM is based on the blood lymphocyte count, the largest nodal diameter, and the size of the spleen. Advanced stage disease is that with one or more of the features TTM greater than 9, TTM doubling time less than 12 months, or bone marrow failure (defined using hemoglobin level and platelet count). Such patients are treated with single-agent chemotherapy.

For symptomatic CLL patients, Byrd and Stilgenbauer[77] recommended the following risk adaptation based on the following factors.

- Genomic aberrations (using fluorescence in situ hybridization [FISH])
- CD38
- Zap70
- Ig mutational status

Low-risk group: Minimally toxic treatment using rituximab, chlorambucil, or fludarabine
Intermediate-risk group: Nucleoside analogue combination regimens using fludarabine plus cyclophosphamide and/or rituximab
High-risk group: Consider an autologous or allogeneic bone-marrow transplantation

In view of the advanced age of many CLL patients, the toxicity of treatment, and the rarity of cure, the choice of therapeutic strategy must depend strongly on the patient's general condition and life expectancy. Herishanu and Polliack[22] recommend a watch-and-wait approach for patients older than 65 years, unless they show clear signs of progressive disease or exhibit several adverse prognostic factors. On the other hand, due to the increased effectiveness of modern therapies, the immediate treatment of younger patients with even early stage disease has been suggested.[78] These recommendations, however, have yet to be confirmed or corrected by evidence from clinical trials.

MULTIPLE MYELOMA

An initial decision in the management of newly diagnosed MM patients is whether to treat immediately or to watch and wait in the case of indolent, asymptomatic disease. Factors associated with indolent disease include absence of lytic bone lesions, absence of hypercalcemia, absence of renal disease, normal hemoglobin levels, and low β_2-microglobulin. Thalidomide is the only treatment which is sometimes given to delay progression of indolent MM to symptomatic disease.

Symptomatic disease may be treated by conventional chemotherapy or by HDCT with stem cell support. The commonly recognized prognostic factors in MM treated by conventional chemotherapy include serum albumin, serum creatinine, serum β_2-microglobulin, and C-reactive protein. Recently, an international pooled prognostic factor analysis based on 10750 patients recommended classification according to the two factors serum β_2-microglobulin and serum albumin.[24] However, such factors account for only a small fraction of the heterogeneity in outcome. Newer, genetic factors include the presence of abnormal karyotypes, hypodiploidy, and certain translocations other than t(11;14). All the above factors are potentially relevant to the decision as to which patients would benefit most from HDCT. However, reliable evidence as to the benefit (or lack of benefit) of HDCT relative to conventional chemotherapy for prognostic subgroups of MM is still limited. Child et al.[79] showed in a large randomized trial of conventional chemotherapy versus HDCT in patients under 65 years that the improvement in overall survival due to HDCT was significantly greater in the group with unfavorable (>8 mg/L) serum β_2-microglobulin, although both groups benefited.

Amongst patients treated with HDCT, similar prognostic factors have been found to those treated with conventional chemotherapy: β_2-microglobulin, C-reactive protein, LDH, and albumin; newer factors include hypodiploidy and cytogenetic abnormalities. Resulting poor-prognosis subgroups may be candidates for even more intensive strategies such as double transplantation. Attal et al.[80] performed a randomized trial to compare single and double transplantation in patients under 60 years. Double transplantation improved overall survival in most prognostic subgroups as defined by β_2-microglobulin, LDH, Durie-Salmon stage, and age. No significant differences in benefit between subgroups were reported. However, the benefit due to double transplantation was higher in those patients who had a less favorable response to the first transplantation, indicating a possible 'late' prognostic factor for selection of patients for double transplantation.

The Durie-Salmon staging system is used in the EORTC trials to select untreated patients for immediate chemotherapy with/without HDCT/ASCT (stage III and aggressive stage I–II), while stage I patients are enrolled for a randomized study of biphosphonate therapy versus watch and wait.

ACUTE LYMPHOCYTIC LEUKEMIA

Adult ALL patients are typically treated with four distinct phases of therapy, namely:

1. An induction chemotherapy using mildly hematotoxic drugs, aiming to induce a complete remission
2. A more intensive consolidation regimen
3. Maintenance therapy for approximately 2 years
4. CNS prophylaxis concurrently to (1) and/or (2)

Most patients (about 75 percent) now achieve remission through induction, but many subsequently relapse; therefore, the favored risk adaptation strategy is to adapt post-remission treatment (especially the consolidation therapy) to prognostic factors available at the time of remission.

A report of multivariate prognostic factor analyses in ALL in 1988[28], confirmed by subsequent analyses, led to the establishment of five accepted adverse factors.

- Elevated WBC count (at diagnosis)
- Advanced age
- Leukemic cell immunophenotype of the type 'mature B cell'
- Philadelphia-positive (Ph^+) disease
- Time to achieve complete remission (CR) more than 4–5 weeks ('late' factor)

The identification of some of the above prognostic factors in the German GMALL multicenter trial[28] led to risk adaptation through definition of low, high, and highest risk groups. The high-risk group was subsequently treated with HDCT/ASCT.

In one recent EORTC trial (EORTC-06861), high-risk patients were defined following induction and consolidation treatment as those with at least one of the factors AUL/B-ALL subtype, Philadelphia-positive subtype, age over 35 years, elevated WBC, or no early CR. These high-risk patients were then randomized to HDCT/ASCT or maintenance chemotherapy. However, in another such trial (EORTC-06951) ALL patients receive similar treatment strategies irrespective of prognostic factors.

FACTORS MEASURED AFTER STARTING TREATMENT

We have mainly been concerned with prognostic factors ascertained prior to starting initial treatment, which can be used to guide the choice of initial treatment strategy. Factors observed at a later point in time can only be used to guide the subsequent course of treatment, for example:

- Patients who attain complete remission early during initial chemotherapy (early response) may be spared part of the subsequent treatment plan
- Laboratory measurements or the results of imaging examinations done after completion of initial treatment may indicate patients with a high risk of relapse who thus require further, preemptive therapy
- The length of remission prior to a relapse, or patient or disease characteristics at relapse (such as performance status, stage, hematologic parameters), may influence selection of salvage therapy

It is important to distinguish clearly between factors observed at different time points to avoid invalid conclusions as to which factors are predictive for which management decisions. Outcome measures must be defined solely on the basis of events occurring *after* observation of the prognostic factor concerned. The so-called landmark method[81] has been developed to permit valid prognostic factor analysis of, for example, early response. With this method, a 'landmark' time point (e.g., 6 months after start of initial therapy) must be chosen *a priori*. The occurrence (or otherwise) of the predictive event (e.g., early response) *before* the landmark constitutes the prognostic factor for the course of disease (e.g., progression-free survival) *subsequent to* the landmark. Thus, the defined predictive factor is clearly separated from the defined outcome. Several investigators[82–84] have used the landmark method in prognostic studies of lymphoid neoplasms. Alternatively, the predictive observation may be modeled as a time-dependent covariate (the Mantell-Byar method[81]). This technique avoids the need for an arbitrary definition of landmark time, which may introduce bias, and uses the data more efficiently.

Hodgkin lymphoma

Various studies have investigated the possibility to reduce subsequent treatment in patients achieving an early CR.[85,86] The EORTC trial for advanced stage HL[85] concluded that additional radiation therapy is not beneficial for patients in CR after 6–8 cycles of MOPP/ABV (mechlorethamine, vincristine, procarbazine, prednisone, doxorubicin, bleomycin, and vinblastine) chemotherapy. All patients in partial remission (PR) after 8 cycles were assigned additional radiation therapy and had a similar overall survival to those attaining CR. Thus, the adequacy of six chemotherapy cycles alone is demonstrated for patients with early CR and the adequacy of eight chemotherapy cycles plus IFRT for PR patients. However, the role of early CR as a prognostic factor is not strictly proven, since PR patients might conceivably have done equally well without radiation therapy. More recently, [^{18}F]2-fluoro-2-deoxy-D-glucose positron emission tomography (FDG-PET) has been increasingly employed for determination of response to treatment. Various investigators have demonstrated that the outcome of FDG-PET during chemotherapy (after 2–4 cycles) is an independent predictor of progression-free survival in HL patients, and have suggested a corresponding reduction or intensification of subsequent treatment.[87,88]

More severe acute hematologic toxicity during first-line chemotherapy has been shown to predict superior long-term outcome in advanced HL.[15,16] The authors hypothesize that this effect is due to pharmacokinetic heterogeneity among patients resulting in higher dose-to-tumor and thus greater toxicity and efficacy in a subset of patients. They suggest individual adaptation of treatment in intermediate stage HL according to observed hematologic toxicity by dose escalation for low-toxicity patients, a concept which has not yet been tried.

An investigation of prognostic factors at early progression of HL[82] revealed three significant adverse factors for overall survival after progression: age over 50 years and poor performance status (both at time of progression) are clearly related to ability to tolerate salvage treatment; failure to have attained temporary remission on first-line therapy may be associated with aggressively resistant disease and indicate the need for more intensive salvage therapy. At relapse, the same group[17] identified time to relapse, relapse stage, and anemia at relapse as prognostic for overall survival and freedom from second treatment failure after relapse. Other investigators have demonstrated prognostic power at relapse after first-line chemotherapy for the following further factors: extranodal versus nodal relapse; number of involved sites, B symptoms, histology, age, and performance status (all at relapse); and stage IV at original presentation.[89] Specifically for patients receiving HDCT/ASCT as salvage therapy, a number of factors have been associated with poor prognosis.[90–92] Factors such as response to initial therapy and time to relapse indicate chemosensitivity of the tumor, while other factors such as stage, B symptoms, bulky disease, and extranodal disease, all prior to transplantation, indicate disease burden. Bierman et al.[92] identified four of the seven IPS factors proposed for newly diagnosed advanced HL[9] as prognostic for event-free and overall survival at entry to HDCT/ASCT.

Non–Hodgkin lymphoma

Time to achievement of a complete remission with first-line therapy, preferably established using gallium imaging, is recognized as strongly prognostic in aggressive lymphomas.[10,93,94] Positron emission tomography after two to three chemotherapy cycles has been shown to predict overall and progression-free survival in high-grade NHL patients.[95] The International Prognostic Index[10] developed for untreated aggressive lymphomas has been shown to predict the outcome of HDCT/ASCT for relapsed or refractory DLCL[96] and intermediate-grade lymphomas.[97]

Chronic lymphocytic leukemia

Currently, prognostic factors play a role only at diagnosis of CLL or at the first appearance of symptomatic disease requiring treatment.

Multiple myeloma

Response to first-line treatment has been shown to predict longer survival in MM patients,[98] but these authors did not find any prognostic impact for early versus late response.

As mentioned in the multiple myeloma section above, an unfavorable response to HDCT/ASCT is associated with greater benefit from a second transplantation.[80] Measurement of the number of residual tumor cells in the bone marrow following HDCT/ASCT may also allow prediction of progression-free survival and thus identify patients in need of further treatment.[99]

For disease refractory to or progressive after initial therapy, the German trials group prescribes HDCT/ASCT for those patients progressing with stage II–III disease after at least two cycles of chemotherapy or progressing after salvage therapy for relapsed disease.

Acute lymphocytic leukemia

Early response to induction therapy has been shown to predict attainment of complete remission in ALL patients.[28,100] The German GMALL group used assessment of minimal residual disease (MRD) to define prognostic groups after 12 months of treatment with conventional chemotherapy in patients lacking those standard adverse prognostic factors at diagnosis which would already indicate the need for HDCT/ASCT. In the current trial, GMALL 07/2003, patients with low MRD risk receive no further treatment, those with intermediate MRD risk receive intensive maintenance therapy, and those with high MRD risk receive ASCT and maintenance therapy.

SUMMARY AND OUTLOOK

The investigation and application of prognostic factors in the management of patients with lymphoid neoplasms must be performed in close cooperation with the evaluation of alternative treatment strategies. The primary aim is to define patient subgroups and assign a treatment strategy to each subgroup so as to optimize treatment results for each individual patient. The prognostic relevance of a given factor may depend upon the definition of the patient population in which it is evaluated, the other factors accounted for, and the treatment administered. Similarly, the relative efficacy of treatment alternatives may depend upon the definition of the patient population in terms of prognostic and other factors. Thus, the optimization process comprises a series of steps alternating between risk group definition and treatment evaluation. Given the low incidence of lymphoid malignancies and the long-term nature of outcome measures such as overall and progression-free survival, the process is slow. New immunologic and genetic techniques and new therapeutic possibilities have recently set new demands and targets for the optimization process.

Reliable prognostic factors based upon general and clinical characteristics have been identified for all the main categories of lymphoid malignancies. Many important factors (see Table 53.1) are common to several diseases. Many of these factors have been incorporated into established prognostic indices. Appropriate treatment strategies have been established for many so-defined risk groups. However, new immunologic and genetic factors have been shown to have prognostic value, in some cases outdoing the established clinical factors. Again, some influential factors (such as β_2-microglobulin and BCL2) apply to various types of lymphoid malignancy. Reliable multivariate analyses of these new factors based on large, homogeneously treated populations are lacking, such that they have still not been incorporated into systematic risk adaptation, which remains largely based upon the conventional clinical factors and staging systems.

Furthermore, some new treatment techniques such as monoclonal antibodies are applicable to very specific types of disease, while others such as HDCT/ASCT may be feasible only for younger patients in good general condition. Therefore, several considerations including treatment efficacy, treatment tolerance, and prognostic factors must be accounted for when selecting treatment.

It is hoped that detailed insights into the mechanisms of tumor growth and therapeutic effect will replace the traditional 'black box' approach for identification and investigation of prognostic factors. Nevertheless, the traditional clinical study and analysis methods will still be needed for an objective assessment of future risk adaptation schemes.

KEY POINTS

- The influence of prognostic factors and treatment options upon prognosis must be assessed together in order to identify optimal treatment strategies for individual patients.
- Large cohorts of comparable patients, an external validation cohort, and suitable multivariate analysis techniques are required for confirmation

- evaluation of prognostic factors and prognostic indices.
- Many of the prognostic factors applying to lymphoid neoplasms are common to several of these diseases.
- For each disease, a number of important prognostic factors are widely recognized and employed for risk adaptation by many study groups.
- Recent developments have identified new immunologic factors and corresponding biologic mechanisms which have yet to be confirmed and incorporated into management schemes.

REFERENCES

● = Key primary paper

◆ = Major review article

●1. Windeler J. Prognosis – what does the clinician associate with this notion? *Stat Med* 2000; **19**: 425–30.

2. Byar DP, Corle DK. Selecting optimal treatment in clinical trials using covariate information. *J Chronic Dis* 1977; **30**: 445–59.

3. Byar DP, Green SB. The choice of treatment for cancer patients based on covariate information. *Bull Cancer* 1980; **67**: 477–90.

◆4. Simon R, Altman DG. Statistical aspects of prognostic factor studies in oncology. *Br J Cancer* 1994; **69**: 979–85.

5. Altman DG, Royston P. What do we mean by validating a prognostic model? *Stat Med* 2000; **19**: 453–73.

6. Royston P, Parmar MKB, Sylvester R. Construction and validation of a prognostic model across several studies, with an application in superficial bladder cancer. *Stat Med* 2004; **23**: 907–26.

7. Begg CB, Cramer LD, Venkatraman ES, Rosai J. Comparing tumour staging and grading systems: a case study and a review of the issues, using thymoma as a model. *Stat Med* 2000; **19**: 1977–2014.

8. Chanan-Khan A, Czuczman MS. Bcl-2 antisense therapy in B-cell malignant proliferative disorders. *Curr Treat Options Oncol* 2004; **5**: 261–7.

●9. Hasenclever D, Diehl V. A prognostic score for advanced Hodgkin's disease. *N Engl J Med* 1998; **339**: 1506–14.

●10. Shipp MA. Prognostic factors in aggressive non-Hodgkin's lymphoma: who has 'high-risk' disease? *Blood* 1994; **83**: 1165–73.

11. Thomas X, Le Q-H. Prognostic factors in adult acute lymphoblastic leukemia. *Hematology* 2003; **8**: 233–42.

12. Houot R, Tavernier E, Le Q-H *et al*. Philadelphia chromosome-positive acute lymphoblastic leukemia in the elderly: prognostic factors and treatment outcome. *Hematology* 2004; **9**: 369–76.

13. Garcia-Sanz R, Gonzalez-Fraile MI, Mateo G *et al.* Proliferative activity of plasma cells is the most relevant prognostic factor in elderly multiple myeloma patients. *Int J Cancer* 2004; **112**: 884–9.

14. Janssen-Heijnen MLG, van Spronsen DJ, Lemmens VEPP *et al.* A population-based study of severity of comorbidity among patients with non-Hodgkin's lymphoma: prognostic impact independent of International Prognostic Index. *Br J Haematol* 2005; **129**: 597–606.

15. Brosteanu O, Hasenclever D, Loeffler M, Diehl V. German Hodgkin's lymphoma Study Group. Low acute hematological toxicity during chemotherapy predicts reduced disease control in advanced Hodgkin's disease. *Ann Hematol* 2004; **83**: 176–82.

16. Klimm B, Reineke T, Haverkamp H *et al.* Role of hematotoxicity and sex in patients with Hodgkin's lymphoma: an analysis from the German Hodgkin Study Group. *J Clin Oncol* 2005; **23**: 8003–11.

17. Josting A, Franklin J, May M *et al.* New prognostic score based on treatment outcome of patients with relapsed Hodgkin's lymphoma registered in the database of the German Hodgkin's Lymphoma Study Group. *J Clin Oncol* 2001; **20**: 221–30.

18. Wisloff F, Hjorth M. Health-related quality of life assessed before and during chemotherapy predicts for survival in multiple myeloma. *Br J Haematol* 1997; **97**: 29–37.

19. Kurzrock R, Redman J, Cabanillas F *et al.* Serum interleukin 6 levels are elevated in lymphoma patients and correlate with survival in advanced Hodgkin's disease and with B symptoms. *Cancer Res* 1993; **53**: 2118–22.

20. Gorschlueter M, Bohlen H, Hasenclever D *et al.* Serum cytokine levels correlate with clinical parameters in Hodgkin's disease. *Ann Oncol* 1995; **6**: 477–82.

●21. Solal-Céligny P, Roy P, Colombat P *et al.* Follicular lymphoma international prognostic index. *Blood* 2004; **104**: 1258–65.

22. Herishanu Y, Polliack A. Chronic lymphocytic leukemia: a review of some new aspects of the biology, factors influencing prognosis and therapeutic options. *Transfus Apher Sci* 2005; **32**: 85–97.

23. San Miguel JF, Sanchez J, Gonzalez M. Prognostic factors and classification in multiple myeloma. *Br J Cancer* 1989; **59**: 113–18.

●24. Greipp PR, San Miguel J, Durie BJM *et al.* International staging system for multiple myeloma. *J Clin Oncol* 2005; **23**: 3412–20.

25. Dimopoulos MA, Barlogie B, Smith TL, Alexanian R. High serum lactate dehydrogenase level as a marker for drug resistance and short survival in multiple myeloma. *Ann Intern Med* 1991; **115**: 931–5.

26. Straus DJ, Gaynor JJ, Myers J *et al.* Prognostic factors among 185 adults with newly diagnosed advanced Hodgkin's disease treated with alternating potentially noncross-resistant chemotherapy and intermediate-dose radiation therapy. *J Clin Oncol* 1990; **8**: 1173–86.

27. Ferme C, Bastion Y, Brice P *et al.* Prognosis of patients with advanced Hodgkin's disease: evaluation of four prognostic models using 344 patients included in the Groupe d'Etudes des Lymphomes de l'Adulte study. *Cancer* 1997; **80**: 1124–33.

●28. Hoelzer D, Thiel E, Löffler H *et al.* Prognostic factors in a multicenter study for treatment of acute lymphoblastic leukemia in adults. *Blood* 1988; **71**: 123–31.

29. Kröber A, Seiler T, Benner A *et al.* V_H mutation status, CD38 expression level, genomic aberrations, and survival in chronic lymphocytic leukemia. *Blood* 2002; **100**: 1410–16.

30. Nogová L, Reineke T, Brillant C *et al.* Lymphocyte-predominant and classical Hodgkin's lymphoma: a comprehensive analysis from the German Hodgkin Study Group. *J Clin Oncol* 2008; **26**: 434–9.

31. Bauer KD, Merkel DE, Winter JN *et al.* Prognostic implication of ploidy and proliferative activity in diffuse large cell lymphomas. *Cancer Res* 1986; **46**: 3173–8.

32. Del Bino G, Silvestrini R, Costa A *et al.* Morphological and clinical significance of cell kinetics in non-Hodgkin's lymphomas. *Basic Appl Histochem* 1986; **30**: 197–202.

◆33. Montillo M, Hamblin T, Hallek M *et al.* Chronic lymphocytic leukemia: novel prognostic factors and their relevance for risk-adapted therapeutic strategies. *Haematologica* 2005; **90**: 391–9.

34. Grogan TM, Lippman SM, Spier CM *et al.* Independent prognostic significance of a nuclear proliferation antigen in diffuse large cell lymphomas as determined by the monoclonal antibody Ki-67. *Blood* 1988; **71**: 1157–60.

◆35. Vassilakopoulos TP, Pangalis GA. Biological prognostic factors in Hodgkin's lymphoma. *Haema* 2004; **7**: 147–64.

36. Montalban C, Garcia JF, Abraira V *et al.* Influence of biologic markers on the outcome of Hodgkin's lymphoma: a study by the Spanish Hodgkin's Lymphoma Study Group. *J Clin Oncol* 2004; **22**: 1664–73.

37. Spector N, Milito CB, Biasoli I, Morais JC. P53 expression as a prognostic factor in Hodgkin's lymphoma (Letter). *J Clin Oncol* 2004; **23**: 3158–9.

38. Stokke T, Galteland E, Holte H *et al.* Oncogenic aberrations in the p53 pathway are associated with a high S phase fraction and poor patient survival in B-cell Non-Hodgkin's lymphoma. *Int J Cancer* 2000; **89**: 313–24.

39. Moller MB, Gerdes A-M, Skjodt K *et al.* Disrupted p53 function as predictor of treatment failure and poor prognosis in B- and T-cell non-Hodgkin's lymphoma. *Clin Cancer Res* 1999; **5**: 1085–91.

40. Del Principe MI, del Poeta G, Venditti A *et al.* Clinical significance of soluble p53 protein in B-cell chronic lymphocytic leukemia. *Haematologica* 2004; **89**: 1568–75.

41. Sarris AH, Kliche KO, Pethambaram P *et al.* Interleukin-10 levels are often elevated in serum of adults with Hodgkin's disease and are associated with inferior failure-free survival. *Ann Oncol* 1999; **10**: 433–40.

42. Axdorph U, Sjoberg J, Grimfors G *et al.* Biological markers may add to prediction of outcome achieved by the International Prognostic Score in Hodgkin's disease. *Ann Oncol* 2000; **11**: 1405–11.

43. Stoolman LM. Adhesion molecules controlling lymphocyte migration. *Cell* 1989; **56**: 907–10.

44. Pals ST, Horst E, Ossekoppele GH *et al.* Expression of lymphocyte homing receptor as a mechanism of dissemination in non-Hodgkin's lymphoma. *Blood* 1989; **73**: 885–8.

45. Jalkanen S, Joensuu H, Klemi P. Prognostic value of lymphocyte homing receptor and S-phase fraction in non-Hodgkin's lymphoma. *Blood* 1990; **75**: 1549–56.

46. Christiansen I, Sundstrom C, Enblad G, Tötterman TH. Soluble vascular cell adhesion molecule-1 (sVCAM-1) is an independent prognostic marker in Hodgkin's disease. *Br J Haematol* 1998; **102**: 701–9.

47. List AF, Spier CM, Miller TP, Grogan TM. Deficient tumor-infiltrating T-lymphocyte response in malignant lymphoma: relationship to HLA expression and host immunocompetence. *Leukemia* 1993; **7**: 398–403.

48. Miller TP, Lippman SM, Spier CM *et al.* HLA-DR (Ia) immune phenotype predicts outcome for patients with diffuse large cell lymphoma. *J Clin Invest* 1988; **82**: 370–2.

49. Swan F, Velasquez WS, Tucker S *et al.* A new serologic staging system for large-cell lymphomas based on initial β_2-microglobulin and lactate dehydrogenase levels. *J Clin Oncol* 1989; **7**: 1518–27.

50. Hallek M, Wanders I, Ostwald M *et al.* Serum beta(2)-microglobulin and serum thymidine kinase are independent predictors of progression-free survival in chronic lymphocytic leukemia and immunocytoma. *Leuk Lymphoma* 1996; **22**: 439–47.

51. Kuittinen O, Soini Y, Turpeenniemi-Hujanen T. Diverse role of MMP-2 and MMP-9 in the clinicopathological behavior of Hodgkin's lymphoma. *Eur J Haematol* 2002; **69**: 205–12.

●52. Tubiana M, Henry-Amar M, van der Werf-Messing B *et al.* A multivariate analysis of prognostic factors in early stage Hodgkin's disease. *Int J Radiat Oncol Biol Phys* 1985; **11**: 23–30.

●53. Carde P, Burgers JM, Henry-Amar M *et al.* Clinical stages I and II Hodgkin's disease: a specifically tailored therapy according to prognostic factors. *J Clin Oncol* 1988; **6**: 239–52.

54. Goldstone A. The case for and against high-dose therapy with stem cell rescue for early poor prognosis Hodgkin's disease in first remission. *Ann Oncol* 1998; **9**(Suppl 5): S83–5.

55. Horwich A, Easton D, Nogueira-Costa R *et al.* An analysis of prognostic factors in early stage Hodgkin's disease. *Radiother Oncol* 1986; **7**: 95–106.

56. Loeffler M, Pfreundschuh M, Rühl U *et al.* Risk factor adapted treatment of Hodgkin's lymphoma: strategies and perspectives. *Recent Results Cancer Res* 1989; **117**: 142–62.

57. Viviani S, Bonadonna G, Santoro A *et al.* Alternating versus hybrid MOPP and ABVD combinations in advanced Hodgkin's disease: ten-year results. *J Clin Oncol* 1996; **14**: 1421–30.

58. Gisselbrecht C, Mounier N, Andre M *et al.* How to define intermediate stage in Hodgkin's lymphoma? *Eur J Haematol Suppl* 2005; **66**: 111–14.

59. Franklin J, Paulus U, Lieberz D *et al.* Is the international prognostic index for advanced stage Hodgkin's disease

applicable to early stage patients. *Ann Oncol* 2000; **11**: 617–23.

●60. Proctor S, Taylor P, Mackie M *et al.* A numerical prognostic index for clinical use in identification of poor-risk patients with Hodgkin's disease at diagnosis. The Scotland and Newcastle Lymphoma Group (SNLG) Therapy Working Party. *Leuk Lymphoma* 1992; **7**(Suppl 17): 17–20.

61. Federico M, Bellei M, Brice P *et al.* High-dose therapy and autologous stem-cell transplantation versus conventional therapy for patients with advanced Hodgkin's lymphoma responding to front-line therapy. *J Clin Oncol* 2003; **21**: 2320–5.

62. Lee SM, Radford JA, Ryder WDJ *et al.* Prognostic factors for disease progression in advanced Hodgkin's disease: an analysis of patients aged under 60 years showing no progression in the first 6 months after starting primary chemotherapy. *Br J Cancer* 1997; **75**: 110–15.

63. Hasenclever D, Schmitz N, Diehl V. Is there a rationale for high-dose chemotherapy as first line treatment of advanced Hodgkin's disease? German Hodgkin's Lymphoma Study Group (GHSG). *Leuk Lymphoma* 1995; **15**(Suppl 1): 47–9.

64. Horning SJ, Yahalom J, Tesch H. Treatment of stage III–IV Hodgkin's disease. In: Mauch PM, Armitage JO, Diehl V, Hoppe RT, Weiss LM. (eds) *Hodgkin's disease*. Philadelphia: Lippincott Williams and Wilkins, 1999: 483–506.

●65. The International Non-Hodgkin's Lymphoma Prognostic Factors Project. A predictive model for aggressive non-Hodgkin's lymphoma. *N Engl J Med* 1993; **329**: 987–94.

66. Sonnen R, Schmidt W-P, Mueller-Hermelink H-K, Schmitz N. The international prognostic index determines the outcome of patients with nodal T-cell lymphomas. *Br J Haematol* 2005; **129**: 366–72.

67. Coiffier B, Lepage E, Briere J *et al.* CHOP chemotherapy plus rituximab compared with CHOP alone in elderly patients with diffuse large-B-cell lymphoma. *N Engl J Med* 2002; **346**: 235–42.

68. Mounier N, Briere J, Gisselbrecht C *et al.* Rituximab plus CHOP (R-CHOP) overcomes bcl-2-associated resistance to chemotherapy in elderly patients with diffuse large B-cell lymphoma (DLBCL). *Blood* 2003; **101**: 4279–84.

69. Rosenwald A, Wright G, Chan WC *et al.* The use of molecular profiling to predict survival after chemotherapy for diffuse large-B-cell lymphoma. *N Engl J Med* 2002; **346**: 1937–47.

70. Ardeshna KM, Smith P, Norton A *et al.* Long-term effect of a watch and wait policy versus immediate systemic treatment for asymptomatic advanced-stage non-Hodgkin lymphoma: a randomised controlled trial. *Lancet* 2003; **362**: 516–22.

●71. Decaudin D, Lepage E, Brousse N *et al.* Low-grade stage III–IV follicular lymphoma: multivariate analysis of prognostic factors in 484 patients – a study of the Groupe d'Etude des Lymphomes de l'Adulte. *J Clin Oncol* 1999; **17**: 2499–505.

●72. Federico M, Vitolo U, Zinzani PL *et al.* Prognosis of follicular lymphoma: a predictive model based on a retrospective analysis of 987 cases. *Blood* 2000; **95**: 783–9.

73. Lopez-Guillermo A, Montserrat E, Bosch F *et al*. Applicability of the International Index for aggressive lymphomas to patients with low-grade lymphoma. *J Clin Oncol* 1994; **12**: 1343–8.

74. Foussard C, Desablens B, Sensebe L *et al*. Is the International Prognostic Index for aggressive lymphomas useful for low-grade lymphoma patients? Applicability to stage III–IV patients. The GOELAMS Group, France. *Ann Oncol* 1997; **8**(Suppl 1): 49–52.

75. Perea G, Altés A, Montoto S *et al*. Prognostic indices in follicular lymphoma: a comparison of different prognostic systems. *Ann Oncol* 2005; **16**: 1508–13.

76. Moller MB, Pedersen NT, Christensen BE. Mantle cell lymphoma: prognostic capacity of the Follicular Lymphoma Prognostic Index. *Br J Haematol* 2006; **133**: 43–9.

◆77. Byrd JC, Stilgenbauer S, Flinn IW. Chronic lymphocytic leukemia. *Hematology Am Soc Hematol Educ Program* 2004: 163–83.

78. Polliack A. Current therapeutic options for subgroups of chronic lymphocytic leukemia. Planning risk-adapted treatment according to recognized prognostic factors. *Haematologica* 2003; **88**: 726–9.

79. Child JA, Morgan GJ, Davies FE *et al*. High-dose chemotherapy with hematopoietic stem-cell rescue for multiple myeloma. *N Engl J Med* 2003; **348**: 1875–83.

80. Attal M, Harousseau JL, Facon T *et al*. Single versus double stem-cell transplantation for multiple myeloma. *N Engl J Med* 2003; **349**: 2495–502.

81. Anderson JR, Cain KC, Gelber RD. Analysis of survival by tumor response. *J Clin Oncol* 1983; **1**: 710–19.

82. Josting A, Rueffer U, Franklin J *et al*. Prognostic factors and treatment outcome in primary progressive Hodgkin lymphoma: a report from the German Hodgkin Lymphoma Study Group. *Blood* 2000; **96**: 1280–6.

83. DeNardo GL, Lamborn KR, Goldstein DS *et al*. Increased survival associated with radiolabeled Lym-1 therapy for non-Hodgkin's lymphoma and chronic lymphocytic leukemia. *Cancer* 1997; **80**: 2706–11.

84. Wisloff F, Hjorth M. Health-related quality of life assessed before and during chemotherapy predicts for survival in multiple myeloma. *Br J Haematol* 1997; **97**: 29–37.

85. Aleman BMP, Raemaekers JMM, Tirelli U *et al*. Involved-field radiotherapy for advanced Hodgkin's lymphoma. *N Engl J Med* 2003; **348**: 2396–406.

86. Bjorkholm M, Axdorph U, Grimfors G *et al*. Fixed versus response-adapted MOPP/ABVD chemotherapy in Hodgkin's disease. A prospective randomized trial. *Ann Oncol* 1995; **6**: 895–9.

87. Hutchings M, Mikhaeel NG, Fields PA *et al*. Prognostic value of interim FDG-PET after two or three cycles of chemotherapy in Hodgkin's lymphoma. *Ann Oncol* 2005; **16**: 1160–8.

88. Hutchings M, Loft A, Hansen M *et al*. FDG-PET after two cycles of chemotherapy predicts treatment failure and progression-free survival in Hodgkin's lymphoma. *Blood* 2006; **107**: 52–9.

◆89. Specht L, Hasenclever D. Prognostic factors of Hodgkin's disease. In: Mauch PM, Armitage LO, Diehl V, Hoppe RT, Weiss LM. (eds) *Hodgkin's disease*. Philadelphia: Lippincott Williams and Wilkins, 1999: 295–325.

90. Brice P, Bouabdallah R, Moreau P *et al*. Prognostic factors for survival after high-dose therapy and autologous stem cell transplantation for patients with relapsing Hodgkin's disease: analysis of 280 patients from the Frech registry. Societe Franciase de Greffe de Moelle. *Bone Marrow Transplant* 1997; **20**: 21–6.

91. Horning SJ, Chao NJ, Negrin RS *et al*. High-dose therapy and autologous hematopoietic progenitor cell transplantation for recurrent or refractory Hodgkin's disease: analysis of the Stanford University results and prognostic indices. *Blood* 1997; **89**: 801–13.

92. Bierman PJ, Lynch JC, Bociek RG *et al*. The International Prognostic Factors Project score for advanced Hodgkin's disease is useful for predicting outcome of autologous hematopoietic stem cell transplantation. *Ann Oncol* 2002; **13**: 1370–7.

93. Armitage JO, Weisenberger DD, Hutchins M *et al*. Chemotherapy for diffuse large cell lymphoma – rapidly responding patients have more durable remissions. *J Clin Oncol* 1986; **4**: 160–4.

94. Engelhard M, Meusers P, Brittinger G *et al*. Prospective multi-center trial for the response-adapted treatment of high-grade malignant non-Hodgkin's lymphomas: updated results of the COP-BLAM/IMVP-16 protocol with randomised adjuvant radiotherapy. *Ann Oncol* 1991; **2**(Suppl 2): 177–80.

95. Mikhaeel NG, Hutchings M, Fields PA *et al*. FDG-PET after two or three cycles of chemotherapy predicts progression-free and overall survival in high-grade non-Hodgkin lymphoma. *Ann Oncol* 2005; **16**: 1514–23.

96. Hamlin PA, Zelenetz AD, Kewalramani T *et al*. Age-adjusted International Prognostic Index predicts autologous stem cell transplantation outcome for patients with replases or primary refractory diffuse large B-cell lymphoma. *Blood* 2003; **102**: 1989–96.

97. Moskowitz CH, Nimer SD, Glassman JR *et al*. The International Prognostic Index predicts for outcome following autologous stem cell transplantation in patients with relapsed and primary refractory intermediate-grade lymphoma. *Bone Marrow Transplant* 1999; **23**: 561–7.

98. Blade J, Lopez-Guillermo A, Bosch F *et al*. Impact of response to treatment on survival in multiple myeloma: results in a series of 243 patients. *Br J Haematol* 1994; **88**: 117–21.

99. Bakkus MHC, Bouko Y, Samson D *et al*. Post-transplantation tumour load in bone tumour, as assessed by quantitative ASO-PCR, is a prognostic parameter in multiple myeloma. *Br J Haematol* 2004; **126**: 665–74.

100. Dombret H, Gabert J, Boiron J-M *et al*. Outcome of treatment in adults with Philadelphia chromosome-positive acute lymphoblastic leukemia – results of the prospective multicenter LALA-94 trial. *Blood* 2002; **100**: 2357–66.

54

Second-line therapy for lymphoid neoplasms

CHRISTIAN GISSELBRECHT AND NICOLAS MOUNIER

INTRODUCTION

Progress in the treatment of lymphoid malignancies obtained with multiagent chemotherapy has been dramatic for almost all the different histologic subtypes. By combining chemotherapy and monoclonal antibodies complete remission (CR) with disease disappearance can now be achieved in 50 percent to 90 percent of the patients, with the percentage variation reflecting histology and stage. However, two different situations induce treatment modifications and use of a salvage regimen: resistant disease, which is characterized as having a dismal or ephemeral response at the end of first-line therapy, or relapses after CR and then fails to respond to salvage therapy; and partial response (PR), which is defined as an objective response less than CR. The time at which the response is evaluated varies from one lymphoma subtype to another and, for chronic lymphoproliferative disorders, achieving a measurable PR could be the initial goal. In many situations in younger patients, salvage treatment in a chemosensitive patient is followed by high-dose therapy (HDT) and autologous stem cell transplantation (ASCT). Thus, the reported outcomes of salvage treatment have included two entities: efficacy of alternative treatment and the impact of HDT with ASCT.

Lymphoid malignancies are among the few neoplastic diseases for which salvage therapy can significantly prolong survival. The choice of which regimen should be administered for relapsing lymphoid malignancies depends on the type of disease (chronic or acute), prognostic factors at the time of relapse, and the general strategy according to age and whether or not the patient is eligible for stem cell transplantation. Numerous old and new drugs are available to treat patients and their efficacies have mostly been evaluated in nonrandomized studies. Obviously, the difficulty of obtaining a cure or a prolonged disease-free period with salvage conventional chemotherapy can explain the numerous phase II studies. The response rate is assessed within 30 days of completing treatment according to the International Harmonization Project criteria, which were recently revised to include the use of positron emission tomography (PET) scanning.[1] Moreover, very often results are reported only in abstracts and not followed by peer-reviewed publications. More recently, the addition of monoclonal antibodies – radiolabeled or not – has brought new insights into the design of salvage treatments. Amazingly, the benefits of the chemotherapy-immunotherapy combinations were demonstrated in first-line randomized trials before the completion of studies on relapsing patients. One of the main goals for the future is to identify those patients in relapse who will benefit from additional monoclonal antibody treatments after prior exposure to such products. More patients are now being treated beyond their first relapses and cumulative doses or toxicities must be considered in the management of these patients. This problem can be crucial for patients with chronic lymphoproliferative disorders who can survive more than 10 years and whose treatments will expose them to enhanced risk of developing second cancers, solid tumors, or myelodysplastic syndromes. This risk also exists for patients with high potential cure rates such as those with Hodgkin lymphoma, who, at 15 years, run equal risks of dying of Hodgkin lymphoma or late adverse effects of therapy. Due to the wide spectrum of diseases, salvage regimens are reviewed disease by disease and questions of general or specific approaches are raised at that time. This chapter does not deal with ongoing experimental studies and is restricted to the wide variety of agents already registered or well on their way to being approved.

AGGRESSIVE LYMPHOMA

Aggressive lymphoma patients who relapse or fail to achieve a CR have a life expectancy of 3–4 months. Since less than 10 percent of these patients obtain long-term disease-free survival[2] with a salvage regimen alone, it has long been established that salvage chemotherapy should, whenever possible, be followed in a chemosensitive patient by consolidation with HDT and then ASCT. Consequently, outcomes of salvage regimens are generally expressed as response rates and the possibility of collecting stem cells for ASCT. Survival data very often represent a mixture of transplanted patients and those not eligible for transplantation. Obviously, the response rate is affected by other parameters such as age, time to progression (less than 1 year or not), and secondary International Prognostic Index (IPI)[3,4] and now prior exposure to rituximab has been added. The long-term analysis of rituximab combined with cyclophosphamide, doxorubicin, vincristine, and prednisone (R-CHOP), in the LNH 98-5 trial demonstrated that relapsing patients randomized to receive R-CHOP did worse than patients given CHOP only.[5] For patients who have previously undergone ASCT in first-line treatment, salvage was more difficult because of enhanced toxicity and more refractory disease, and survival was shorter after relapse.[6]

Second-line treatment before the rituximab era

First attempts to modify the poor outcome of relapses initially combined ifosfamide, etoposide, and methotrexate, and later added mitoguazone (MIME); CR rates of 24–37 percent were reported, but long-term remission remained a rare event.[7] Later, better results were reported by the same investigators, who combined cisplatin with high-dose Ara-C

(cytarabine) and dexamethasone (DHAP),[8] one of the most popular salvage regimens used worldwide. Further improvement was obtained by adding etoposide (VP16)[9,10] and, finally, by the development of a regimen alternating MINE and ESHAP (Table 54.1).[11]

Some of the most widely investigated salvage regimens in recent years have contained ifosfamide and etoposide. The combination of ifosfamide, etoposide, cytarabine, and methotrexate (IVAM) was investigated in 31 patients with relapsed or refractory aggressive non-Hodgkin lymphoma (NHL).[12] After two chemotherapy cycles, CR and PR rates were 61 percent and 26 percent, respectively. Ifosfamide, epirubicin, and etoposide were prescribed as salvage therapy for 51 patients with relapsed or refractory aggressive NHL, and achieved an objective response rate of 77 percent with 32 percent CR.[13] A regimen combining teniposide, ifosfamide, mitoxantrone, mitoguazone, high-dose methotrexate, high-dose cytarabine, and prednisolone prior to ASCT gave a 72 percent response rate in 71 patients with refractory or relapsing aggressive NHL, with CR in 45 percent of the patients.[14]

One second-line ICE (ifosfamide, carboplatin, and etoposide) chemotherapy regimen is currently widely used to improve response rates in relapsed patients. This regimen was initially evaluated in 163 transplant-eligible patients with relapsed or primary refractory aggressive NHL.[15] The overall response rate was 66 percent and 89 percent (96/108) of the responders underwent HDT and ASCT. Results accumulated from successive studies conducted at the Memorial Sloan-Kettering Cancer Center showed that a 72 percent response rate was obtained in more than 400 patients given ICE chemotherapy after failure of first-line anthracycline-based therapy.[16]

An effective doxorubicin regimen consisting of continuous infusion of etoposide, prednisone, oncovin, cyclophosphamide, and adriamycin (EPOCH) was developed with the goal of improving efficacy by reducing drug resistance by prolonged exposure.[17] Among the 100 patients with aggressive de novo histology, induction failure, or relapses, 36 percent achieved CR with a 70 percent response rate. Notably, 65 percent of the patients who had failed on induction therapy responded to EPOCH. The response was not associated with the number of prior exposures to EPOCH drugs. Among 33 patients who did not undergo ASCT, 18 percent were event-free at five years.

Second-line treatment with rituximab

The addition of rituximab to CHOP chemotherapy has significantly improved the CR rate and event-free and overall survival rates compared to CHOP alone, as first-line treatment of aggressive NHL, without increasing toxicity.[18] Thus, the combination of rituximab with ICE (R-ICE), one of the most effective salvage regimens, has been given to patients with relapsed/refractory disease. Interim results from the first 36 assessable patients who had relapsed

Table 54.1 Salvage regimens in relapsing/refractory aggressive lymphoma

Authors	Regimen	No. of patients	CR (%)	Objective response (%)
Alkylants + etoposide				
Cabanillas et al.[9]	IFMVP16	52	18 (35)	32 (62)
Cabanillas et al.[7]	MIME	208	50 (24)	125 (60)
Haim et al.[105]	DVIP	30	10 (33)	19 (63)
Herbrecht et al.[106]	VIM	24	10 (42)	14 (58)
Chao et al.[107]	CEPP(B)	75	21 (28)	43 (57)
Bosly et al.[2]	CV	65	15 (23)	33 (51)
	All	**454**	**124 (27)**	**266 (59)**
Alkylants + etoposide + anthracyclines or platin				
Bosly et al.[2]	MIV	40	13 (33)	28 (70)
Rodriguez et al.[11]	MINE	48	10 (21)	23 (48)
Hopfinger et al.[108]	VIM	33	8 (24)	15 (45)
Garay et al.[109]	MIZE	54	25 (46)	39 (72)
Moskowitz[16]	ICE	137	32 (23)	87 (64)
Gutierrez et al.[17]	EPOCH	125	28 (22)	72 (57)
	All	**437**	**116 (26)**	**264 (64)**
Ara-C + platin + etoposide				
Velasquez et al.[8]	DHAP	90	28 (31)	50 (56)
Press et al.[110]	DHAP	39	9 (23)	26 (67)
Philip et al.[111]	DHAP	48	7 (15)	28 (58)
Velasquez et al.[10]	ESHAP	122	45 (37)	78 (64)
Philip et al.[112]	DHAP	215	53 (25)	125 (58)
Soussain et al.[113]	ESHAP	63	17 (27)	39 (62)
	All	**577**	**159 (28)**	**346 (60)**
Ara-C + anthracyclines				
Ho et al.[114]	NOAC	51	17 (33)	29 (57)
Ruit et al.[115]	CAMP	30	8 (27)	14 (47)
Dufour et al.[116]	Ida-Ara-C	32	13 (41)	14 (44)
Brusamolino et al.[117]	ICA	30	6 (20)	18 (60)
	All	**143**	**44 (31)**	**75 (52)**
Ara-C + anthracyclines + alkylants + etoposide				
Rodriguez et al.[118]	MINE/ESHAP	92	44 (48)	63 (69)
Stamatoullas et al.[12]	IVAM	31	19 (61)	27 (87)
Caballero et al.[119]	Mini-BEAM/ESHAP	28	7 (25)	11 (39)
Plantier-Colcher et al.[14]	VIM$_3$ Ara-C	71	32 (45)	51 (72)
	All	**222**	**102 (46)**	**152 (68)**
Rituximab + chemotherapy				
Kewalramani[19]	RICE	36	19 (53)	28 (78)

CR, complete remission; Ara-C, cytarabine. IFMVP16: ifosfamide, VP16; MIME: ifosfamide, etoposide, methotrexate, mitoguazone; DVIP: dexamethasone, etoposide, ifosfamide, cisplatin; VIM (MIV): ifosfamide, etoposide mitoxantrone; CEPP(B): cyclophosphamide, etoposide, procarbazine, prednisone (bleomycine); CV: cyclophosphamide, VP16; MINE: mesna, ifosfamide, mitoxantrone, etoposide; MIZE: mesna, ifosfamide, idarubicin, etoposide; ICE: ifosfamide, carboplatin and etoposide; RICE: ICE + rituximab; EPOCH: etoposide, prednisone, oncovin, cyclophosphamide, adriamycin; DHAP: cisplatin in combination with high-dose Ara-C and dexamethasone; ESHAP: cisplatin in combination with high-dose Ara-C, etoposide, and dexamethasone; NOAC: mitoxantrone, high-dose Ara-C; CAMP: lomustine, cytarabine, mitoxantrone, prednisone; Ida-Ara-C: idarubicin, high-dose Ara-C; ICA: idarubicin, cytarabine; IVAM: ifosfamide, etoposide, cytarabine, methotrexate; Mini-BEAM: carmustine, etoposide, Ara-C, melphalan, dexamethasone; VIM$_3$ Ara-C: teniposide, ifosfamide, mitoxantrone, mitoguazone, high-dose methotrexate, high-dose cytarabine, and prednisolone.

($n = 23$) or refractory ($n = 13$) disease following a single standard anthracycline-based treatment for diffuse large B cell lymphoma (DLBCL) have been reported.[19,20] The overall response rate was 78 percent and the CR rate 53 percent (Table 54.1). The CR rate was significantly higher for patients receiving R-ICE than historical controls, with a similar second-line IPI given ICE ($P = 0.006$). Patients with relapsed disease had a significantly higher overall response rate than those who had primary refractory disease (96 percent vs 46 percent; $P = 0.01$).

Thus, adding rituximab to ICE appears to double the CR rate compared with ICE alone. There are ongoing prospective randomized trials further exploring the potential benefits associated with the addition of rituximab to platinum-based salvage regimens. In the study conducted by the HOVON group, 239 patients with relapsed or refractory DLBCL received a salvage regimen consisting of DHAP-VIM-DHAP $\pm$ rituximab followed by ASCT. Analysis of 225 evaluable patients showed that after two courses of chemotherapy, PR/CR was obtained in 54 percent of the patients in the DHAP arm and 75 percent in the R-DHAP arm ($P \leqslant 0.01$; intention-to-treat analysis). Post-transplantation PR or CR was obtained in 50 percent and 73 percent of the patients, respectively ($P = 0.003$). A marked difference in favor of the R-DHAP arm was observed at 24 months for failure-free survival (50 percent vs 24 percent; $P < 0.001$) but not for overall survival (52 percent vs 59 percent; $P = 0.15$). Cox regression analysis demonstrated a significant effect of rituximab treatment on failure-free survival (FFS) and overall survival (OS) when adjusted for time since upfront treatment, age, performance status, and secondary age-adjusted IPI.[21]

However, one question remains – what is the optimal chemotherapy regimen to combine with rituximab as salvage therapy for DLBCL? The ongoing CORAL trial comparing R-DHAP versus R-ICE induction followed by HDT and ASCT with or without post-transplantation rituximab maintenance in patients with relapsed/refractory aggressive NHL was designed to answer this question. An interim analysis was planned based on the first 200 patients enrolled in this study – six patients did not receive any treatment and therefore the intention-to-treat analysis was conducted on 194 patients. The overall response rate was 68 percent with 41 percent CR rate, and toxicity was similar to that expected with intensive therapy. In univariate analysis, the response rate was significantly ($P < 0.0001$) adversely affected by the following parameters: early relapse (within 12 months) or not achieving a CR after first-line treatment, IPI >1 at second-line treatment, and prior exposure to rituximab. Ninety-seven patients were treated in first-line therapy with rituximab combination chemotherapy. Characteristics of this patient group revealed that 79 patients had early relapses within 12 months and had poor adverse prognostic factors at diagnosis. The response rate was 54 percent and was markedly inferior to the 82 percent response rate seen in patients not previously exposed to rituximab. However, in a logistic regression model, only early relapse and secondary IPI >1 remained significant for response rate, but not rituximab. Intention-to-treat 2-year event-free survival (EFS) and OS rates were 50 percent and 69 percent, respectively. Two-year EFS was significantly adversely affected by early relapse (within 12 months) or not achieving a CR after first-line treatment ($P < 0.0001$), IPI >1 at second-line treatment ($P = 0.03$), and prior treatment with rituximab ($P = 0.0001$).[22]

Rituximab and other chemotherapy regimens

Not all patients are candidates for transplantation, because of age, previous transplantation, and/or comorbidity. Therefore, effective and well-tolerated salvage therapies with minimal toxicities are still needed.

More recently, oxaliplatin and gemcitabine have also been shown to be active separately against relapsed or refractory NHL. A study on 24 patients assessed the efficacy and safety of oxaliplatin replacement of cisplatin in the DHAP regimen for patients with relapsed or refractory NHL.[23] The objective response rate was 77 percent for patients treated at first relapse, and there was no major renal or neurotoxicity.

In hematologic malignancies, gemcitabine alone had some degree of efficacy against aggressive NHL.[24] The combination of rituximab with platinum and gemcitabine (GEMOX) seems promising and is currently being evaluated. In a single-arm study involving 46 patients with aggressive B-NHL who received up to eight cycles of rituximab, gemcitabine, and oxaliplatin in combination (R-GEMOX), 38 patients (83 percent) responded after four cycles and 50 percent were in CR or CR unconfirmed (Cru) by the end of treatment.[25] With a median follow-up of 27 months, the 2-year and overall survival rates were 53 percent and 66 percent, respectively. The estimated median time to progression (TTP) was 20 months (range 1.6 to more than 33.5 months) and median duration of response (DR) was 18 months (range 0.5 to more than 31.4 months).

In addition, this platform was chosen to investigate the combination of chemotherapy and enzastaurin. Enzastaurin is a potent, selective inhibitor of protein kinase C (PKC) and phosphatidylinositol 3-kinase (PI3K)/protein kinase 3 (AKT) pathways known to promote tumor-induced angiogenesis, as well as tumor cell survival and proliferation.[26] A phase II trial with oral enzastaurin plus GEMOX is ongoing. Oral enzastaurin is also being tested as maintenance after the end of chemotherapy.

At present, no real 'gold standard' treatment exists for relapsed aggressive NHL. Because the goal of salvage therapy for aggressive NHL is CR, and because the major breakthrough in the treatment of B cell malignancies was the addition of rituximab to chemotherapy for front-line treatment, most physicians are in favor of including rituximab in salvage chemotherapy regimens.

Monoclonal antibodies in aggressive lymphoma

Rituximab, a humanized monoclonal anti-CD20 antibody, has been used alone initially and to treat relapses of DLBCL patients. The overall response rate was 37 percent but the CR rate was only 9 percent.[27] In studies *in vitro*, the addition of rituximab to standard anticancer drugs increased cell lysis, even of chemoresistant cell lines. Its action blocks the interleukin-10 (IL-10) loop and therefore limits BCL2 oncoprotein expression.[28] The results of the GELA trial on elderly patients with DLBCL demonstrated an *in vivo* chemosensitization effect. Indeed, R-CHOP was significantly more effective in terms of survival in patients overexpressing BCL2.[29] It remains to be determined whether this mechanism is found in relapsed patients resistant to chemotherapy.

Radioimmunotherapy

Few data are available on the efficacy of yttrium-90-labeled ibritumomab tiuxetan (Zevalin) against aggressive lymphoma relapses. A phase II study on 104 relapsing or refractory patients with DLBCL achieved an overall response rate of 44 percent.[30] The response rate was 52 percent for the primary refractory disease, 40 percent for patients relapsing after less than 1 year, and 58 percent for those relapsing after more than 1 year, and their respective median durations of progression-free survival (PFS) were 5.9, 2.3, and 6.2 months, respectively. Among 28 patients previously treated with chemotherapy and rituximab, 37 percent were refractory to R-CHOP and the response rate was 19 percent. As for all radioimmunoconjugates, Zevalin is administered in a single injection. Consolidation by radioimmunotherapy after cytoreductive treatment might be an option to study in patients not eligible for stem cell transplantation. Randomized studies are in progress with conventional doses after front-line chemotherapy.

Concomitant chemoradiotherapy

The place of radiation therapy in treating aggressive lymphoma remains a matter of debate even for localized stages.[31] It is accepted that radiation therapy alone is often unsuccessful in chemoresistant patients, but is very helpful for local control of the disease. However, concomitant chemoradiotherapy is widely used to treat various solid tumors and a number of randomized trials have demonstrated its superiority over radiation alone. Chemoradiotherapy can also be presented for refractory lymphoma to obtain local control in patients with life-threatening tumor masses. Adjunction of radiosensitizing chemotherapeutic agents, such as cisplatin and etoposide, was used in 21 refractory lymphoma patients with bulky disease. The response rate was 70 percent with 20 percent CR rate. Three patients with localized disease were still alive and disease-free at 16, 33, and 48 months after multimodality treatment.[32]

FOLLICULAR LYMPHOMA

Follicular lymphoma and other indolent lymphomas cannot be cured by conventional therapeutic approaches and are characterized by a high initial response rate to chemotherapy followed by recurrence. These lymphomas retain their sensitivity to chemotherapy over a prolonged period before becoming resistant or transforming into high-grade lymphomas. Predicting the outcome of these lymphomas is not easy and different prognostic indexes have been described. Notably, in a joint effort, the Follicular Lymphoma International Prognostic Index (FLIPI) was established[33] for use at diagnosis. It has also been shown that the duration of response after the first relapse was shorter after each subsequent progression or relapse.[34] Patients relapsing with a low tumor burden might remain asymptomatic for a prolonged period. Therefore, a watch-and-wait policy should be considered for asymptomatic patients. This approach should not be extended in the case of progression after an early recurrence, indicating the biological aggressiveness of the disease. The choice of treatment depends on several parameters: age; 'prognostic factors'; extent of the disease; prior therapy, with special attention given to the cumulative drug doses and bone marrow reserve; and, finally, if the patient is a candidate for stem cell transplantation. In the latter case, drugs reducing stem cell mobilization should be avoided whenever possible. Every effort should be made to treat patients with histologic transformation like others with DLBCL. As for first-line treatment, several competing options are available; no consensus has yet been reached on a standardized chemotherapy regimen, and the integration of rituximab into chemotherapy regimens has changed most of the outcomes. In practice, relapsing patients are either given the same chemotherapy as initially or one of the known effective regimens not yet taken with rituximab. Salvage regimens described for DLBCL are generally effective, especially DHAP. It remains to be decided whether ASCT is recommended, and to establish a general strategy.

According to country or cooperative group, patients are treated with the alkylating agents chlorambucil or cyclophosphamide alone, or repeated cycles of CVP (cyclophosphamide, vincristine, and prednisone). A purine analogue, fludarabine, as a subsequent line of therapy for relapsed or refractory indolent lymphoma has been studied in several clinical trials. One randomized study[35] compared fludarabine monotherapy to CVP and demonstrated that fludarabine significantly prolonged PFS (10.9 vs 9.2 months; $P = 0.03$). Regimens combining fludarabine with cyclophosphamide or mitoxantrone achieved objective response rates up to 70 percent.[36–38]

Adding rituximab to chemotherapy yielded higher remission rates. A randomized study comparing 465 patients receiving CHOP or R-CHOP followed by observation or 2 years of maintenance with rituximab (in 334 patients) demonstrated the advantage of adding rituximab with chemotherapy and as maintenance. There was a significant increase of median PFS with maintenance for patients responding to CHOP (11.6 months with observation vs 37.5 months with rituximab, $P < 0.0001$) or R-CHOP induction (22.1 months with observation vs 51.9 months with rituximab, $P = 0.0071$).[39] In a comparison of FCM versus R-FCM (rituximab, fludarabine, cylophosphamide, and mitoxantrone) activity against relapsed follicular or mantle cell lymphoma in 65 follicular lymphoma patients, a more beneficial effect of R-FCM versus FCM was shown in terms of CR rates (40 percent vs 23 percent, respectively). Median PFS for the R-FCM group had not been reached at 3 years, but was 21 months for the FCM group ($P = 0.01$).[40]

Since rituximab chemotherapy regimens have become standard first-line chemotherapy, it remains to be seen if patients previously exposed to this antibody are still responsive to retreatment. On the other hand, maintenance with rituximab after achieving at least a partial response has been shown to improve clinical outcome of relapsed/resistant follicular non-Hodgkin lymphoma in patients both with and without rituximab during induction.[39]

In addition, a recent paper on single-agent bendamustine therapy demonstrated durable objective responses (35 percent CR, 7 months median disease-free survival [DFS]) with acceptable toxicity in heavily pretreated patients with rituximab-refractory, indolent NHL.[41] These findings are promising and will serve for future clinical trials in this novel patient population.

Monoclonal antibodies in low-grade lymphoma

The anti-CD20 monoclonal antibody rituximab has been registered based on the results of a phase II study on 166 patients with relapsed low-grade or follicular lymphoma after a median of two prior chemotherapies. About 50 percent of the patients responded with 6 percent CR and a median duration of response of 1 year. In a subsequent analysis, follicular lymphoma patients appeared to have a similar response duration after rituximab alone in comparison to the last effective chemotherapy regimen.[42] Moreover, the duration of the response can be prolonged by either maintenance therapy with rituximab[43,44] or retreatment at progression. The probability of a second response is approximately 40 percent.[45] Moreover, rituximab is able to induce clearance of BCL2 gene rearrangement-expressing cells in both bone marrow and blood. This disappearance is associated with a longer time to progression.

Nevertheless, as stated previously, the maximum impact of rituximab is in combination with chemotherapy, but this well-tolerated drug can be proposed for use alone in elderly patients or those refusing to undergo chemotherapy. In addition, new anti-CD20 or anti-CD22 monoclonal antibodies demonstrate promising biological and clinical activity.[46,47]

Radiation therapy and radioimmunotherapy in low-grade lymphoma

Lymphomas are sensitive to radiation and one of the particular features of low-grade lymphoma is to be very sensitive to a low dose of radiation therapy. It has been shown that local control could be observed in 92 percent of cases with only 4 Gy.[48] It allows treatment of local relapse and even multiple local relapses with long-term duration in elderly patients and does not prevent subsequent treatment. In conjunction with a monoclonal antibody, such as anti-CD20, it enables targeted radiation therapy. Radiation is delivered to the cells reached by the antibody as well as surrounding cells. Two radionuclides are mainly used for labeling antibodies: iodine-131 (^{131}I) and yttrium-90 (^{90}Y). Iodine-131 was the first radioisotope to be tested and it was linked to the murine anti-CD20 antibody tositumomab (Bexxar). Because it emits both beta and gamma particles, patients have to be admitted to a nuclear medicine department for several days, according to legislation in most European countries. Yttrium-90 was conjugated to the antibody ibritumomab, the murine anti-CD20, to make Zevalin. Yttrium-90 is a pure beta emitter and can be administered on an outpatient basis depending on national legislation. Most of the studies were performed on patients with relapsed or refractory indolent or transformed lymphoma.

The efficacy of ^{90}Y-ibritumomab (Zevalin) was demonstrated in two studies.[49,50] The first, a randomized study, compared a single dose of Zevalin (0.4 mCi/kg) to standard rituximab (375 mg/m^2) given once a week for four consecutive weeks to patients with relapsed or refractory low-grade follicular or transformed lymphomas who had not previously been treated with rituximab.[49] Of the 143 patients randomized, the overall response rate was 80 percent for the 73 patients treated with Zevalin compared to 56 percent for the 70 patients given rituximab alone ($P = 0.002$). The CR rate was also significantly higher for the Zevalin arm (30 percent vs 16 percent, respectively; $P = 0.04$). Moreover, Zevalin was responsible for a significantly different median response duration; 14.2 months versus 12.1 months, respectively. The second study concerned 54 rituximab-refractory follicular lymphoma patients, who achieved a 74 percent response rate and 15 percent CR rate.[51] The main toxicity was hematological with late thrombocytopenia, and the potential for bone marrow depletion of stem cells must be closely monitored. This agent is not recommended for patients with massive bone marrow involvement or those with low platelet counts.

A similar response was obtained with ^{131}I-tositumomab (Bexxar). In the pivotal study[52] on 60 patients with refractory or transformed (38 percent of patients) follicular or low-grade lymphomas who received one injection of ^{131}I-tositumomab, 65 percent responded including 20 percent CR with a median response duration of 6.5 months. The response lasted significantly longer than the last effective chemotherapy. However, the response rate was only 39 percent for patients with transformed lymphoma in contrast to 81 percent for other low-grade lymphomas. Toxicity was also primarily hematological. One of the concerns about radioimmunotherapy is the risk of increasing myelodysplastic syndromes in these heavily treated patients. Careful follow-up of the population is ongoing and so far no excess of myelodysplastic syndromes has been observed with either radiolabeled agent.[53]

These treatments might be better placed at the end of salvage chemotherapy as consolidation, or when the clinician considers that one short treatment is enough to control or stabilize the disease.

MANTLE CELL LYMPHOMA

Mantle cell lymphoma can be viewed as having one of the worst prognoses of all lymphoma forms, with a low CR rate and a continuous relapse rate. Fewer than 20 percent of the patients treated with a CHOP regimen survive more than 5 years. Mantle cell lymphoma patients are candidates for innovative therapy to be evaluated at relapse. Rituximab has been used alone with a response rate of 37 percent[54] and produced some long-lasting responses. A rituximab-chemotherapy combination prolonged the response and several regimens other than CHOP are recommended; mainly adding rituximab to a fludarabine-based regimen or to high-dose cytosine arabinoside. These combinations are often non-cross resistant and can be used as first- or second-line therapy. One example of the sensitivity to cytarabine was provided by the use of CHOP first, followed by DHAP,[55] which increased objective response rate up to 90 percent. Another major advance was intensive chemotherapy such as HyperCVAD (fractionated cyclophosphamide, doxorubicin, vincristine, and dexamethasone) alternating with high-dose cytarabine and methotrexate,[56] or treatment incorporating HDT and ASCT.[57,58] However, as a consequence, the treatment of relapses might be more difficult because patients will have poorer bone marrow reserves. Obviously, no standard therapy exists for this type of patient and innovative second-line treatments should be encouraged. For the elderly, a single nonmyelotoxic drug, such as chlorambucil, should retard disease progression.

The proteasome inhibitor bortezomib (Velcade) can act through multiple mechanisms to arrest tumor growth, tumor spread, and angiogenesis. In two early phase II studies, lymphoma patients with various histologies were treated with bortezomib.[59,60] In the first study, 33 patients with relapsed or refractory mantle cell lymphoma received intravenous bortezomib. These mantle cell lymphoma patients had a median of 2.1 prior therapies and seven of them had prior ASCT; they achieved a response rate of 53 percent. Response duration nonetheless exceeded 7 months. Bortezomib alone showed promising activity against mantle cell lymphoma with a response rate of 50 percent, but responses were also observed in other types of lymphoma. New combinations with other agents are under investigation, in particular with cytarabine and rituximab.

CHRONIC LYMPHOCYTIC LEUKEMIA AND SMALL LYMPHOCYTIC LYMPHOMA

As for other B cell hematologic malignancies, rapid progress has been made by simultaneously incorporating new drugs for relapses and front-line treatment. The first was fludarabine, alone and then in combination with chemotherapy, as is now being done with monoclonal antibodies. Fludarabine induces higher remission rates than conventional chemotherapy in randomized studies,[61] particularly in patients with disease resistant to alkylating agents.[62] However, all patients eventually relapse and the overall prognosis of advanced chronic lymphocytic leukemia (CLL) remains poor. Several phase II studies have combined fludarabine and chemotherapy (e.g., cyclophosphamide).[63] The response rate was close to 90 percent but with only 15 percent CR and a median response duration close to 24 months. However, hematologic malignancies previously exposed to fludarabine are generally resistant to new treatment with it and enhanced hematotoxicity precludes its prolonged administration. Combining fludarabine, cyclophosphamide, and mitoxantrone achieved a higher CR rate in patients with resistant or relapsed CLL.[64]

Although rituximab alone is weakly effective against CLL, it might perform better at a higher dose.[65] The combination of fludarabine, cyclophosphamide, and rituximab (FCR)[66] looks promising. A single-arm study using FCR as the initial therapy for 224 patients demonstrated a 70 percent CR rate with no flow cytometry-detectable disease for 30–50 percent of responding patients. Prolongation of survival has not yet been demonstrated but comparison with historical controls suggests a significant benefit of FCR. Prolonged survival was observed even in patients previously treated with fludarabine and an alkylating agent, but only ongoing randomized studies comparing the efficacy against relapses of fludarabine plus cyclophosphamide versus FCR as front-line therapy will confirm these findings.

Patients relapsing with a low tumor burden might remain asymptomatic for a prolonged period. Therefore, a watch-and-wait policy can be instituted in elderly asymptomatic patients. Although most of the patients in the near future will be treated upfront with highly effective fludarabine combinations, treatment of relapses might be even more difficult because cumulative toxicity will develop rapidly under retreatment with fludarabine. Moreover, it will diminish the possibility of consolidation with ASCT, as most of the patients will have poor bone marrow reserve. Hence, old treatments such as chlorambucil, or cyclophosphamide, doxorubicin, and prednisone (CAP) or CHOP regimens, will emerge again.

Monoclonal antibodies

Alemtuzumab (Campath-1H) is a humanized anti-CD52 monoclonal antibody that has been approved for the treatment of fludarabine-refractory CLL. In an early phase II study[67] on 29 patients with relapsed or chemotherapy-refractory CLL, the response rate was 42 percent, including 4 percent CR, and CLL cells were rapidly cleared from the blood. A pivotal study[68] included 93 patients, 76 percent with stage II or IV disease, whose median time since the previous therapy was 4.1 months. The response rate was 33 percent with a median time to response of 1.5 months and median response duration of 8.7 months. Clonal lymphocytes decreased by week 4. Alemtuzumab is associated with moderate myelosuppression and immunosuppression. Antimicrobial prophylaxis is strongly recommended. Impressive activity of alemtuzumab against T cell prolymphocytic leukemia has also been reported,[69–71] with response rates ranging between 51 percent and 76 percent, and CR rates of 40 percent to 60 percent. Although median response duration was about 8 months, some long-term responses persisted for as long as 2 years. The potential of this monoclonal antibody needs to be investigated further with different doses and administration schedules to reduce toxicity.

Rituximab has been included in broad phase II and III trials for indolent lymphoma including small lymphocytic lymphoma and CLL. Given alone[42,65] for relapses or refractory disease, the response rate was lower than for the other types of indolent lymphomas. Better results were obtained in treatment-naïve patients or with a higher dose and, above all, when combined with chemotherapy.

Rituximab has successfully treated complications of CLL or its therapy, including pure red-cell aplasia, immune thrombocytopenia, or immune hemolytic anemia.[72] The rituximab and alemtuzumab combination has been studied by several groups. Among 47 patients, 53 percent responded, including CR in 9 percent, but more than half of the patients experienced infectious complications.[73] Emerging data seem to indicate that antiangiogenic agents like thalidomide may induce tumor response in progressive CLL.[74]

LYMPHOPLASMACYTOID LYMPHOMA AND WALDENSTRÖM MACROGLOBULINEMIA

The diagnosis of Waldenström macroglobulinemia is based on high serum monoclonal immunoglobulin M and bone marrow infiltration by lymphoplasmacytoid lymphoma as defined by the World Health Organization (WHO) criteria.[75] Most patients diagnosed with Waldenström macroglobulinemia have symptoms attributable to tumor infiltration and/or high serum monoclonal protein concentrations. However, some patients are completely asymptomatic and do not require any treatment. A consensus panel on therapeutics considered retaining three main treatment options for patients with relapsed or refractory disease:[76] alkylating agents, purine analogues, and the monoclonal antibody rituximab for systemic primary treatment of symptomatic patients. An alternate first-line agent is reasonable for patients with refractory or relapsing disease; and for patients potentially eligible for ASCT, further exposure to stem cell-damaging agents should be avoided. Use of rituximab is perhaps a better option to preserve the possibility to harvest stem cells. More experience has been accumulated with fludarabine, and approximately one-third of patients respond to fludarabine. Its activity was confirmed in a randomized trial that compared salvage treatment with either fludarabine or CAP; 28 percent of fludarabine-treated patients responded versus 11 percent of CAP-treated

patients ($P = 0.019$).[77] Rituximab at a standard dose may induce major responses in approximately 30 percent to 40 percent of previously treated patients,[75] with a median time to treatment failure of approximately 8 months. Prolonging treatment is likely to increase the duration of the response for as long as 29 months.[78,79] Combining rituximab with chemotherapy is likely to improve the response rate, as was seen for previously untreated patients. For patients relapsing from unsustained remission, readministration of the same agent has a high likelihood of being active. For patients who develop resistance to all three classes of agents, limited experience suggests a modest benefit with thalidomide and alemtuzumab. Preliminary data suggest that bortezomib has some activity and its evaluation is ongoing.[59] As new treatments are able to achieve good responses, intensification with HDT and ASCT has to be considered for younger patients in relapse, applying the same guidelines as those established for other low-grade lymphomas.

MARGINAL ZONE LYMPHOMA

Splenic marginal zone lymphoma is a well-characterized B cell neoplasm with splenomegaly and involvement of various organs, especially the bone marrow.[80] To date, no definitive standard treatment for splenic marginal zone lymphoma has been established. Similarly to other chronic lymphoproliferative disorders, one-third of the patients are asymptomatic and will never require treatment. A general consensus considers splenectomy the best first-line therapy, but no univocal convergence has been reached as to when and how to use chemotherapy, and it is generally given after post-splenectomy progression. The role of alkylating agents, such as chlorambucil or cyclophosphamide, is marginal. Patients may achieve a good response but seldom CR. Purine analogues can be used and CR has been reported.[81] Many drugs with different schemes have been administered. In general, the response to chemotherapy is not as complete as for many other low-grade lymphoma subtypes. This situation has prompted investigators to try rituximab in combination with chemotherapy, as for other low-grade lymphomas expressing CD20, and higher response rates were observed more frequently. One particular presentation is splenic lymphoma associated with large villous lymphocytes and hepatitis C virus infection, which responds to interferon-alpha alone or in combination with ribavirin.[82]

HODGKIN LYMPHOMA

Most patients with Hodgkin lymphoma can be cured with chemotherapy alone or in combination with radiation therapy. Depending on the initial treatment, different treatment options are available for patients who relapse after achieving CR, including radiation therapy for localized

Table 54.2 Salvage regimens for relapsed Hodgkin lymphoma

Authors	Regimen	No. of patients	CR (%)	PR (%)
Josting et al.[91]	DHAP	102	21	68
Linch et al.[120]	Mini-BEAM	55	31	29
Schmitz et al.[83]	Dexa-BEAM	44	32	52
Rodriguez et al.[90]	ASHAP	56	34	36
Moskowitz et al.[121]	ICE	65	26	59
Fermé et al.[88]	MIME	100	34	39
Hagemeister et al.[87]	MINE	47	23	40

CR, complete remission; PR, partial response; DHAP: cisplatin in combination with high-dose Ara-C and dexamethasone; Mini-BEAM, Dexa-BEAM: carmustine, etoposide, Ara-C, melphalan, dexamethasone; ASHAP: adriamycin, solumedrol, high-dose Ara-C, cisplatin; ICE: ifosfamide, carboplatin, etoposide; MINE: ifosfamide, etoposide, navelbine, mitoguazone; MIME: mitoguazone, ifosFamide, methotrexate, etoposide.

disease and conventional salvage chemotherapy. However, patients who fail to achieve an initial CR and those who relapse within the first year after CR have a poor outcome. Salvage chemotherapy regimens with HDT and ASCT are associated with higher response rates and longer progression-free survival[83] when compared to Dexa-BEAM (dexamethasone and carmustine, etoposide, cytarabine, and melphalan) combination chemotherapy. Several studies have attempted to better characterize prognostic factors at relapse and to facilitate the choice of treatment.[84,85] Relapse within 1 year, disseminated stages, B symptoms, anemia, and age are the main prognostic factors described. The 4-year probability of survival ranged from 83 percent for patients without any unfavorable factors to 27 percent for patients with three risk factors.[85] Consequently, patients without risk factors with late localized relapse in a nonirradiated area can be treated with combined chemo-radiotherapy. The choice of salvage regimen is based on several considerations, such as cumulative toxicity with prior exposure to doxorubicin or use of non-cross resistant drugs. Patients who had progressive disease after MOPP (mechlorethamine, vincristine, procarbazine, and prednisone) were treated with ABVD (doxorubicin, bleomycin, vinblastine, and dacarbazine) and a second remission was achieved in 35 percent, whereas only 61 percent of those who suffered relapse after ABVD responded to MOPP.[86] Consequently, a number of salvage protocols have been developed during the last decade as shown in Table 54.2.

As all the patients are exposed to anthracycline derivatives, there is a need to develop an effective combination without cardiotoxic drugs. After the results obtained with the MIME (mitoguazone, ifosfamide, methotrexate, and etoposide) regimen,[87] where a 23 percent CR rate was observed in heavily pretreated patients, we undertook a prospective trial to test an intensive regimen followed, in chemosensitive patients, by HDT and ASCT. The MINE regimen was derived from MIME and comprised mitoguazone, ifosfamide, vinorelbine, and etoposide.[88] Among the 100 patients included in the study, the overall response rate was 75 percent, with a 35 percent CR rate. Response rates were 92.5 percent for patients with untreated relapse and

53 percent for those with resistant relapse or induction failure. Platinum-based combinations (DHAP, ASHAP, ESHAP) have been investigated in patients with relapsed and refractory Hodgkin lymphoma.[89,90] The overall response rate for patients after two cycles of DHAP was 88 percent (21 percent CR and 67 percent PR). The results were comparable in patients with late relapse, early relapse, and multiple relapse. In contrast, the response rate in patients with progressive disease was only 65 percent (CR 12 percent, PR 53 percent).[91] In addition, gemcitabine alone[92] or in combination with cisplatin and dexamethasone[93] or ifosfamide and etoposide (IGEV)[94] was described as being effective. Overall response rates to salvage therapy were high, reaching 60–80 percent, but only 20–35 percent of patients achieved CR. Long-term follow-up data on these newer regimens are not yet available because most of the patients who achieved CR and PR went on to receive HDT and ASCT.

The anti-CD30 monoclonal antibodies are under evaluation, and show limited efficacy when used as a single agent. The association of yttrium-90 to the anti-CD30 antibody has produced a response rate of 27 percent in 22 heavily treated patients.[95] It should be kept in mind that salvage radiation therapy in nonirradiated areas provides an alternative strategy for patients with localized disease not able to receive chemotherapy. A subset of patients with limited-stage late relapses, without B symptoms, and with good performance status could be candidates for a conservative approach. The 5-year freedom from second failure and overall survival rates were 28 percent and 51 percent, respectively.[89]

T CELL LYMPHOMA

The WHO classification recognizes numerous entities with different clinical presentations and outcomes. The non-cutaneous forms can be divided into nodal peripheral T cell lymphoma, anaplastic and nonanaplastic, in terms of prognosis.[96] Anaplastic lymphomas expressing the anaplastic lymphoma kinase (ALK) protein have a better prognosis and relapses can be managed like other aggressive lymphomas with common salvage chemotherapy regimens before stem cell transplantation. The other subtypes – angioimmunoblastic lymphoma, unspecified T cell lymphoma, or extranodal T cell lymphoma – are more difficult to treat. Despite sensitivity to corticosteroids, they are usually chemoresistant to conventional salvage treatment and very few patients become eligible for stem cell transplantation. In small phase II studies different agents such as gemcitabine,[97] interferon alpha,[98] or alemtuzumab[99] have shown some activity. Unfortunately, combined chemotherapy and alemtuzumab was associated with increased toxicity and severe immunodepression, making the design of any further studies dangerous. Pertinently, natural killer/T cell lymphoma responded to L-asparaginase, which warrants further evaluation.[100] New agents and regimens are needed in the light of the poor prognosis of patients. A recent paper showed that pralatrexate, a novel class of antifol with high affinity for the reduced folate carrier-type 1, produces marked complete and durable remissions in a diversity of chemotherapy-refractory cases of T cell lymphoma.[101]

CUTANEOUS T CELL LYMPHOMA

Cutaneous T cell lymphomas (CTCL) are a group of lymphoproliferative disorders characterized by localization of neoplastic T lymphocytes homing to the skin. Although mycosis fungoides represents the majority of these diseases, there are many distinct entities which can have dissimilar presentations, prognoses, and treatments. It is imperative that clinicians appreciate these differences to provide appropriate management of these patients, especially those with presentation corresponding to a cutaneous localization of peripheral unspecified T cell lymphoma.[102]

The easiest treatment of primary anaplastic CD30[+] cutaneous lymphoma is generally radiation therapy. However, this entity has a tendency to relapse in the skin and, again, radiation therapy is the first treatment of choice if the lesion is accessible. There is no specific chemotherapy for this type of lymphoma; classical treatment can be tried for disseminated disease and usually has transient activity.

Mycosis fungoides management is more complex because no treatment is curative. Treatments are generally tailored to the stage of disease, with many patients progressing inexorably through the panoply of immunomodulatory or cytotoxic therapies. The treatment goal is to modulate symptoms and prevent rapid disease progression and complications. Because many patients become refractory to the currently available treatments, new therapies are needed.

Alemtuzumab has been proposed for treating patients refractory to conventional treatment. In a phase II study, 22 patients received the monoclonal antibody and 50 percent responded with 32 percent in CR.[103] Larger trials are warranted, with special attention paid to prophylaxis and diagnosis of opportunistic and other severe infections, as CTCL patients are already severely immunocompromised.

Denileukin diftitox, a fusion protein that combines the cytotoxic diphtheria toxin with recombinant IL-2, targets cells that express the IL-2 receptor CD25. Among 71 CTCL patients treated with denileukin diftitox, 30 percent responded (including 10 percent CR), and some durable responses were obtained.[104] Clinical benefit is evident after the first or second injection. Because myelosuppression is an uncommon effect, it may be useful in patients with limited bone marrow reserves.

FUTURE DIRECTIONS

Dramatic progress has been made with salvage therapies, often derived empirically according to the level of biotechnological development. Ongoing microarray and proteomic studies on novel agents are discovering molecular mechanisms of drug sensitivity and drug resistance. Those studies will generate more selective therapies for validation in animal models and subsequent introduction to the bedside in clinical trials. Furthermore, gene microarray and proteomic analyses of tumors from patients treated with novel agents in clinical trials will identify *in vivo* targets and provide the framework for the development of more selective, potent, and, hopefully, less toxic targeted therapies.

KEY POINTS

- Lymphoid neoplasms can be salvaged by second-line treatment with a curative intent.
- Second-line therapy should be integrated in a therapeutic strategy.
- Stem cell transplantation – autologous or allogeneic – is the natural option after second-line treatment in most young patients.
- Rituximab associated to chemotherapy has dramatically changed outcome in B cell malignancies.
- Multiple retreatments are likely to occur in chronic lymphoid neoplasms.
- Cumulative toxicity must be weighted when deciding second-line treatment.
- T cell lymphomas remained poorly salvaged.

REFERENCES

● = Key primary paper
◆ = Major review article

●1. Cheson BD, Pfistner B, Juweid ME *et al*. Revised response criteria for malignant lymphoma. *J Clin Oncol* 2007; **25**: 579–86.
2. Bosly A, Coiffier B, Gisselbrecht C *et al*. Bone marrow transplantation prolongs survival after relapse in

aggressive-lymphoma patients treated with the LNH-84 regimen. *J Clin Oncol* 1992; **10**: 1615–23.

3. Guglielmi C, Gomez F, Philip T *et al.* Time to relapse has prognostic value in patients with aggressive lymphoma enrolled onto the Parma trial. *J Clin Oncol* 1998; **16**: 3264–9.

4. Blay J, Gomez F, Sebban C *et al.* The International Prognostic Index correlates to survival in patients with aggressive lymphoma in relapse: analysis of the PARMA trial. Parma Group. *Blood* 1998; **92**: 3562–8.

5. Feugier P, Van Hoof A, Sebban C *et al.* Long-term results of the R-CHOP study in the treatment of elderly patients with diffuse large B-cell lymphoma: a study by the Groupe d'Etude des Lymphomes de l'Adulte. *J Clin Oncol* 2005; **23**: 4117–26.

6. Gisselbrecht C, Lepage E, Molina T *et al.* Shortened first-line high-dose chemotherapy for patients with poor-prognosis aggressive lymphoma. *J Clin Oncol* 2002; **20**: 2472–9.

7. Cabanillas F, Hagemeister FB, McLaughlin P *et al.* Results of MIME salvage regimen for recurrent or refractory lymphoma. *J Clin Oncol* 1987; **5**: 407–12.

●8. Velasquez WS, Cabanillas F, Salvador P *et al.* Effective salvage therapy for lymphoma with cisplatin in combination with high-dose Ara-C and dexamethasone (DHAP). *Blood* 1988; **71**: 117–22.

9. Cabanillas F, Velasquez WS, McLaughlin P *et al.* Results of recent salvage chemotherapy regimens for lymphoma and Hodgkin's disease. *Semin Hematol* 1988; **25**(2 Suppl 2): 47–50.

10. Velasquez WS, McLaughlin P, Tucker S *et al.* ESHAP – an effective chemotherapy regimen in refractory and relapsing lymphoma: a 4-year follow-up study. *J Clin Oncol* 1994; **12**: 1169–76.

11. Rodriguez MA, Cabanillas FC, Velasquez W *et al.* Results of a salvage treatment program for relapsing lymphoma: MINE consolidated with ESHAP. *J Clin Oncol* 1995; **13**: 1734–41.

12. Stamatoullas A, Fruchart C, Bastit D *et al.* Ifosfamide, etoposide, cytarabine, and methotrexate as salvage chemotherapy in relapsed or refractory aggressive non-Hodgkin's lymphoma. *Cancer* 1996; **77**: 2302–7.

13. Zinzani PL, Tani M, Molinari AL *et al.* Ifosfamide, epirubicin and etoposide regimen as salvage and mobilizing therapy for relapsed/refractory lymphoma patients. *Haematologica* 2002; **87**: 816–21.

14. Plantier-Colcher I, Dupriez B, Simon M *et al.* The VIM3-AraC regimen followed by autologous stem cell transplantation in refractory or relapsing aggressive non-Hodgkin's lymphoma. A prospective study of 71 consecutive cases. *Leukemia* 1999; **13**: 282–8.

●15. Moskowitz CH, Bertino JR, Glassman JR *et al.* Ifosfamide, carboplatin, and etoposide: a highly effective cytoreduction and peripheral-blood progenitor-cell mobilization regimen for transplant-eligible patients with non-Hodgkin's lymphoma. *J Clin Oncol* 1999; **17**: 3776–85.

16. Moskowitz C. Risk-adapted therapy for relapsed and refractory lymphoma using ICE chemotherapy. *Cancer Chemother Pharmacol* 2002; **49**(Suppl 1): S9–12.

17. Gutierrez M, Chabner BA, Pearson D *et al.* Role of a doxorubicin-containing regimen in relapsed and resistant lymphomas: an 8-year follow-up study of EPOCH. *J Clin Oncol* 2000; **18**: 3633–42.

●18. Coiffier B, Lepage E, Briere J *et al.* CHOP chemotherapy plus rituximab compared with CHOP alone in elderly patients with diffuse large-B-cell lymphoma. *N Engl J Med* 2002; **346**: 235–42.

●19. Kewalramani T, Zelenetz AD, Nimer SD *et al.* Rituximab and ICE as second-line therapy before autologous stem cell transplantation for relapsed or primary refractory diffuse large B-cell lymphoma. *Blood* 2004; **103**: 3684–8.

20. Zelenetz AD, Hamlin P, Kewalramani T *et al.* Ifosfamide, carboplatin, etoposide (ICE)-based second-line chemotherapy for the management of relapsed and refractory aggressive non-Hodgkin's lymphoma. *Ann Oncol* 2003; **14**(Suppl 1): i5–10.

21. Vellenga E, van Putten WL, van't Veer MB *et al.* Rituximab improves the treatment results of DHAP-VIM-DHAP and ASCT in relapsed/progressive aggressive CD20+ NHL: a prospective randomized HOVON trial. *Blood* 2008; **111**: 537–43.

22. Gisselbrecht C, Schmitz N, Mounier N *et al.* R-ICE versus R-DHAP in relapsed patients with CD20 diffuse large B-cell lymphoma (DLBCL) followed by stem cell transplantation and maintenance treatment with rituximab or not: first interim analysis on 200 patients. CORAL Study. *Blood* 2007; **110**: 159a (abstract).

23. Chau I, Webb A, Cunningham D *et al.* An oxaliplatin-based chemotherapy in patients with relapsed or refractory intermediate and high-grade non-Hodgkin's lymphoma. *Br J Haematol* 2001; **115**: 786–92.

24. Fossa A, Santoro A, Hiddemann W *et al.* Gemcitabine as a single agent in the treatment of relapsed or refractory aggressive non-Hodgkin's lymphoma. *J Clin Oncol* 1999; **17**: 3786–92.

25. El Gnaoui T, Dupuis J, Belhadj K *et al.* Rituximab, gemcitabine and oxaliplatin: an effective salvage regimen for patients with relapsed or refractory B-cell lymphoma not candidates for high-dose therapy. *Ann Oncol* 2007; **18**: 1363–8.

26. Robertson MJ, Kahl BS, Vose JM *et al.* Phase II study of enzastaurin, a protein kinase C beta inhibitor, in patients with relapsed or refractory diffuse large B-cell lymphoma. *J Clin Oncol* 2007; **25**: 1741–6.

27. Coiffier B, Haioun C, Ketterer N *et al.* Rituximab (anti-CD20 monoclonal antibody) for the treatment of patients with relapsing or refractory aggressive lymphoma: a multicenter phase II study. *Blood* 1998; **92**: 1927–32.

●28. Jazirehi AR, Bonavida B. Cellular and molecular signal transduction pathways modulated by rituximab (rituxan, anti-CD20 mAb) in non-Hodgkin's lymphoma: implications in chemosensitization and therapeutic intervention. *Oncogene* 2005; **24**: 2121–43.

●29. Mounier N, Briere J, Gisselbrecht C *et al.* Rituximab plus CHOP (R-CHOP) overcomes Bcl-2 associated resistance to chemotherapy in elderly patients with diffuse large B-cell lymphoma (DLBCL). *Blood* 2003; **101**: 4279–84.

30. Morschhauser F, Illidge T, Huglo D *et al.* Efficacy and safety of yttrium-90 ibritumomab tiuxetan in patients with relapsed or refractory diffuse large B-cell lymphoma not appropriate for autologous stem-cell transplantation. *Blood* 2007; **110**: 54–8.

●31. Reyes F, Lepage E, Ganem G *et al.* ACVBP versus CHOP plus radiotherapy for localized aggressive lymphoma. *N Engl J Med* 2005; **352**: 1197–205.

32. Girinsky T, Lapusan S, Ribrag V *et al.* Phase II study of concomitant chemoradiotherapy in bulky refractory or chemoresistant relapsed lymphomas. *Int J Radiat Oncol Biol Phys* 2005; **61**: 476–9.

●33. Solal-Celigny P, Roy P, Colombat P *et al.* Follicular lymphoma international prognostic index. *Blood* 2004; **104**: 1258–65.

●34. Johnson PW, Rohatiner AZ, Whelan JS *et al.* Patterns of survival in patients with recurrent follicular lymphoma: a 20-year study from a single center. *J Clin Oncol* 1995; **13**: 140–7.

●35. Klasa RJ, Meyer RM, Shustik C *et al.* Randomized phase III study of fludarabine phosphate versus cyclophosphamide, vincristine, and prednisone in patients with recurrent low-grade non-Hodgkin's lymphoma previously treated with an alkylating agent or alkylator-containing regimen. *J Clin Oncol* 2002; **20**: 4649–54.

36. McLaughlin P, Hagemeister FB, Romaguera JE *et al.* Fludarabine, mitoxantrone, and dexamethasone: an effective new regimen for indolent lymphoma. *J Clin Oncol* 1996; **14**: 1262–8.

37. Santini G, Nati S, Spriano M *et al.* Fludarabine in combination with cyclophosphamide or with cyclophosphamide plus mitoxantrone for relapsed or refractory low-grade non-Hodgkin's lymphoma. *Haematologica* 2001; **86**: 282–6.

38. Lazzarino M, Orlandi E, Montillo M *et al.* Fludarabine, cyclophosphamide, and dexamethasone (FluCyD) combination is effective in pretreated low-grade non-Hodgkin's lymphoma. *Ann Oncol* 1999; **10**: 59–64.

39. van Oers MH, Klasa R, Marcus RE *et al.* Rituximab maintenance improves clinical outcome of relapsed/resistant follicular non-Hodgkin lymphoma in patients both with and without rituximab during induction: results of a prospective randomized phase 3 intergroup trial. *Blood* 2006; **108**: 3295–301.

●40. Forstpointner R, Dreyling M, Repp R *et al.* The addition of rituximab to a combination of fludarabine, cyclophosphamide, mitoxantrone (FCM) significantly increases the response rate and prolongs survival as compared with FCM alone in patients with relapsed and refractory follicular and mantle cell lymphomas: results of a prospective randomized study of the German Low-Grade Lymphoma Study Group. *Blood* 2004; **104**: 3064–71.

41. Friedberg JW, Cohen P, Chen L *et al.* Bendamustine in patients with rituximab-refractory indolent and transformed non-Hodgkin's lymphoma: results from a phase II multicenter, single-agent study. *J Clin Oncol* 2008; **26**: 204–10.

42. McLaughlin P, Grillo-Lopez AJ, Link BK *et al.* Rituximab chimeric anti-CD20 monoclonal antibody therapy for relapsed indolent lymphoma: half of patients respond to a four-dose treatment program. *J Clin Oncol* 1998; **16**: 2825–33.

●43. Ghielmini M, Schmitz SF, Cogliatti SB *et al.* Prolonged treatment with rituximab in patients with follicular lymphoma significantly increases event-free survival and response duration compared with the standard weekly × 4 schedule. *Blood* 2004; **103**: 4416–23.

44. Hainsworth JD, Litchy S, Morrissey LH *et al.* Rituximab plus short-duration chemotherapy as first-line treatment for follicular non-Hodgkin's lymphoma: a phase II trial of the minnie pearl cancer research network. *J Clin Oncol* 2005; **23**: 1500–6.

45. Davis TA, Grillo-Lopez AJ, White CA *et al.* Rituximab anti-CD20 monoclonal antibody therapy in non-Hodgkin's lymphoma: safety and efficacy of re-treatment. *J Clin Oncol* 2000; **18**: 3135–43.

46. Coiffier B, Lepretre S, Pedersen LM *et al.* Safety and efficacy of ofatumumab, a fully human monoclonal anti-CD20 antibody, in patients with relapsed or refractory B-cell chronic lymphocytic leukemia: a phase 1–2 study. *Blood* 2008; **111**: 1094–100.

47. Leonard JP, Goldenberg DM. Preclinical and clinical evaluation of epratuzumab (anti-CD22 IgG) in B-cell malignancies. *Oncogene* 2007; **26**: 3704–13.

48. Haas RL, Poortmans P, de Jong D *et al.* High response rates and lasting remissions after low-dose involved field radiotherapy in indolent lymphomas. *J Clin Oncol* 2003; **21**: 2474–80.

●49. Witzig TE, Gordon LI, Cabanillas F *et al.* Randomized controlled trial of yttrium-90-labeled ibritumomab tiuxetan radioimmunotherapy versus rituximab immunotherapy for patients with relapsed or refractory low-grade, follicular, or transformed B-cell non-Hodgkin's lymphoma. *J Clin Oncol* 2002; **20**: 2453–63.

50. Witzig TE, Flinn IW, Gordon LI *et al.* Treatment with ibritumomab tiuxetan radioimmunotherapy in patients with rituximab-refractory follicular non-Hodgkin's lymphoma. *J Clin Oncol* 2002; **20**: 3262–9.

51. Witzig TE. Efficacy and safety of 90^Y ibritumomab tiuxetan (Zevalin) radioimmunotherapy for non-Hodgkin's lymphoma. *Semin Oncol* 2003; **30**(6 Suppl 17): 11–16.

●52. Kaminski MS, Zelenetz AD, Press OW *et al.* Pivotal study of iodine I-131 tositumomab for chemotherapy-refractory low-grade or transformed low-grade B-cell non-Hodgkin's lymphomas. *J Clin Oncol* 2001; **19**: 3918–28.

53. Czuczman MS, Emmanouilides C, Darif M *et al.* Treatment-related myelodysplastic syndrome and acute

myelogenous leukemia in patients treated with ibritumomab tiuxetan radioimmunotherapy. *J Clin Oncol* 2007; **25**: 4285–92.

54. Foran JM, Rohatiner AZ, Cunningham D *et al.* European phase II study of rituximab (chimeric anti-CD20 monoclonal antibody) for patients with newly diagnosed mantle-cell lymphoma and previously treated mantle-cell lymphoma, immunocytoma, and small B-cell lymphocytic lymphoma. *J Clin Oncol* 2000; **18**: 317–24.

55. Lefrere F, Delmer A, Suzan F *et al.* Sequential chemotherapy by CHOP and DHAP regimens followed by high-dose therapy with stem cell transplantation induces a high rate of complete response and improves event-free survival in mantle cell lymphoma: a prospective study. *Leukemia* 2002; **16**: 587–93.

●56. Khouri IF, Romaguera J, Kantarjian H *et al.* Hyper-CVAD and high-dose methotrexate/cytarabine followed by stem-cell transplantation: an active regimen for aggressive mantle-cell lymphoma. *J Clin Oncol* 1998; **16**: 3803–9.

57. Gianni AM, Magni M, Martelli M *et al.* Long-term remission in mantle cell lymphoma following high-dose sequential chemotherapy and in vivo rituximab-purged stem cell autografting (R-HDS regimen). *Blood* 2003; **102**: 749–55.

●58. Dreyling M, Lenz G, Hoster E *et al.* Early consolidation by myeloablative radiochemotherapy followed by autologous stem cell transplantation in first remission significantly prolongs progression-free survival in mantle-cell lymphoma: results of a prospective randomized trial of the European MCL Network. *Blood* 2005; **105**: 2677–84.

59. Goy A, Younes A, McLaughlin P *et al.* Phase II study of proteasome inhibitor bortezomib in relapsed or refractory B-cell non-Hodgkin's lymphoma. *J Clin Oncol* 2005; **23**: 667–75.

60. O'Connor OA, Wright J, Moskowitz C *et al.* Phase II clinical experience with the novel proteasome inhibitor bortezomib in patients with indolent non-Hodgkin's lymphoma and mantle cell lymphoma. *J Clin Oncol* 2005; **23**: 676–84.

●61. Leporrier M, Chevret S, Cazin B *et al.* Randomized comparison of fludarabine, CAP, and CHOP in 938 previously untreated stage B and C chronic lymphocytic leukemia patients. *Blood* 2001; **98**: 2319–25.

◆62. Chun HG, Leyland-Jones B, Cheson BD. Fludarabine phosphate: a synthetic purine antimetabolite with significant activity against lymphoid malignancies. *J Clin Oncol* 1991; **9**: 175–88.

63. Hallek M, Schmitt B, Wilhelm M *et al.* Fludarabine plus cyclophosphamide is an efficient treatment for advanced chronic lymphocytic leukaemia (CLL): results of a phase II study of the German CLL Study Group. *Br J Haematol* 2001; **114**: 342–8.

64. Bosch F, Ferrer A, Lopez-Guillermo A *et al.* Fludarabine, cyclophosphamide and mitoxantrone in the treatment of resistant or relapsed chronic lymphocytic leukaemia. *Br J Haematol* 2002; **119**: 976–84.

65. O'Brien SM, Kantarjian H, Thomas DA *et al.* Rituximab dose-escalation trial in chronic lymphocytic leukemia. *J Clin Oncol* 2001; **19**: 2165–70.

66. Keating MJ, O'Brien S, Albitar M *et al.* Early results of a chemoimmunotherapy regimen of fludarabine, cyclophosphamide, and rituximab as initial therapy for chronic lymphocytic leukemia. *J Clin Oncol* 2005; **23**: 4079–88.

67. Osterborg A, Dyer MJ, Bunjes D *et al.* Phase II multicenter study of human CD52 antibody in previously treated chronic lymphocytic leukemia. European Study Group of CAMPATH-1H Treatment in Chronic Lymphocytic Leukemia. *J Clin Oncol* 1997; **15**: 1567–74.

●68. Keating MJ, Flinn I, Jain V *et al.* Therapeutic role of alemtuzumab (Campath-1H) in patients who have failed on fludarabine: results of a large international study. *Blood* 2002; **99**: 3554–61.

69. Pawson R, Dyer MJ, Barge R *et al.* Treatment of T-cell prolymphocytic leukemia with human CD52 antibody. *J Clin Oncol* 1997; **15**: 2667–72.

70. Dearden CE, Matutes E, Cazin B *et al.* High remission rate in T-cell prolymphocytic leukemia with CAMPATH-1H. *Blood* 2001; **98**: 1721–6.

71. Keating MJ, Cazin B, Coutre S *et al.* Campath-1H treatment of T-cell prolymphocytic leukemia in patients for whom at least one prior chemotherapy regimen has failed. *J Clin Oncol* 2002; **20**: 205–13.

72. Hegde UP, Wilson WH, White T, Cheson BD. Rituximab treatment of refractory fludarabine-associated immune thrombocytopenia in chronic lymphocytic leukemia. *Blood* 2002; **100**: 2260–2.

73. Faderl S, Thomas DA, O'Brien S *et al.* Combined use of Alemtuzumab and Rituximab in patients with relapsed and refractory chronic lymphoid malignancies – an update of the MD Anderson experience. *Blood* 2002; **100**: 775 (abstract).

74. Morotti A, Cilloni D, Parvis G *et al.* Thalidomide-induced partial stable remission in a case of refractory progressive B Cell Chronic Lymphoid Leukemia. *Leuk Res* 2008; **32**: 506–7.

◆75. Dimopoulos MA, Kyle RA, Anagnostopoulos A, Treon SP. Diagnosis and management of Waldenstrom's macroglobulinemia. *J Clin Oncol* 2005; **23**: 1564–77.

76. Gertz MA, Anagnostopoulos A, Anderson K *et al.* Treatment recommendations in Waldenstrom's macroglobulinemia: consensus panel recommendations from the Second International Workshop on Waldenstrom's Macroglobulinemia. *Semin Oncol* 2003; **30**: 121–6.

77. Leblond V, Levy V, Maloisel F *et al.* Multicenter, randomized comparative trial of fludarabine and the combination of cyclophosphamide-doxorubicin-prednisone in 92 patients with Waldenstrom's Macroglobulinemia in first relapse or with primary refractory disease. *Blood* 2001; **98**: 2640–4.

78. Treon SP, Emmanouilides C, Kimby E *et al.* Extended rituximab therapy in Waldenstrom's Macroglobulinemia. *Ann Oncol* 2005; **16**: 132–8.

79. Gertz MA, Rue M, Blood E et al. Multicenter phase 2 trial of rituximab for Waldenstrom's Macroglobulinemia (WM): an Eastern Cooperative Oncology Group Study (E3A98). Leuk Lymphoma 2004; 45: 2047–55.

◆80. Franco V, Florena AM, Iannitto E. Splenic marginal zone lymphoma. Blood 2003; 101: 2464–72.

81. Bolam S, Orchard J, Oscier D. Fludarabine is effective in the treatment of splenic lymphoma with villous lymphocytes. Br J Haematol 1997; 99: 158–61.

82. Hermine O, Lefrere F, Bronowicki JP et al. Regression of splenic lymphoma with villous lymphocytes after treatment of hepatitis C virus infection. N Engl J Med 2002; 347: 89–94.

●83. Schmitz N, Pfistner B, Sextro M et al. Aggressive conventional chemotherapy compared with high-dose chemotherapy with autologous haemopoietic stem-cell transplantation for relapsed chemosensitive Hodgkin's disease: a randomised trial. Lancet 2002; 359: 2065–71.

84. Brice P, Bastion Y, Divine M et al. Analysis of prognostic factors after the first relapse of Hodgkin's disease in 187 patients. Cancer 1996; 78: 1293–9.

85. Josting A, Franklin J, May M et al. New prognostic score based on treatment outcome of patients with relapsed Hodgkin's lymphoma registered in the database of the German Hodgkin's lymphoma study group. J Clin Oncol 2002; 20: 221–30.

●86. Canellos GP, Anderson JR, Propert KJ et al. Chemotherapy of advanced Hodgkin's disease with MOPP, ABVD, or MOPP alternating with ABVD. N Engl J Med 1992; 327: 1478–84.

87. Hagemeister FB, Tannir N, McLaughlin P et al. MIME chemotherapy (methyl-GAG, ifosfamide, methotrexate, etoposide) as treatment for recurrent Hodgkin's disease. J Clin Oncol 1987; 5: 556–61.

88. Fermé C, Bastion Y, Lepage E et al. The MINE regimen as intensive salvage chemotherapy for relapsed and refractory Hodgkin's disease. Ann Oncol 1995; 6: 543–9.

89. Josting A, Nogova L, Franklin J et al. Salvage radiotherapy in patients with relapsed and refractory Hodgkin's lymphoma: a retrospective analysis from the German Hodgkin Lymphoma Study Group. J Clin Oncol 2005; 23: 1522–9.

90. Rodriguez J, Rodriguez MA, Fayad L et al. ASHAP: a regimen for cytoreduction of refractory or recurrent Hodgkin's disease. Blood 1999; 93: 3632–6.

●91. Josting A, Rudolph C, Mapara M et al. Cologne high-dose sequential chemotherapy in relapsed and refractory Hodgkin's lymphoma: results of a large multicenter study of the German Hodgkin's Lymphoma Study Group (GHSG). Ann Oncol 2005; 16: 116–23.

92. Santoro A, Bredenfeld H, Devizzi L et al. Gemcitabine in the treatment of refractory Hodgkin's disease: results of a multicenter phase II study. J Clin Oncol 2000; 18: 2615–19.

93. Baetz T, Belch A, Couban S et al. Gemcitabine, dexamethasone and cisplatin is an active and non-toxic chemotherapy regimen in relapsed or refractory Hodgkin's

disease: a phase II study by the National Cancer Institute of Canada Clinical Trials Group. Ann Oncol 2003; 14: 1762–7.

94. Magagnoli M, Sarina B, Balzarotti M et al. Mobilizing potential of ifosfamide/vinorelbine-based chemotherapy in pretreated malignant lymphoma. Bone Marrow Transplant 2001; 28: 923–7.

95. Schnell R, Dietlein M, Staak JO et al. Treatment of refractory Hodgkin's lymphoma patients with an iodine-131-labeled murine anti-CD30 monoclonal antibody. J Clin Oncol 2005; 23: 4669–78.

●96. Gisselbrecht C, Gaulard P, Lepage E et al. Prognostic significance of T-cell phenotype in aggressive non-Hodgkin's lymphomas. Groupe d'Etudes des Lymphomes de l'Adulte (GELA). Blood 1998; 92: 76–82.

97. Zinzani PL, Baliva G, Magagnoli M et al. Gemcitabine treatment in pretreated cutaneous T-cell lymphoma: experience in 44 patients. J Clin Oncol 2000; 18: 2603–6.

98. Armitage JO, Coiffier B. Activity of interferon-alpha in relapsed patients with diffuse large B-cell and peripheral T-cell non-Hodgkin's lymphoma. Ann Oncol 2000; 11: 359–61.

99. Enblad G, Hagberg H, Erlanson M et al. A pilot study of alemtuzumab (anti-CD52 monoclonal antibody) therapy for patients with relapsed or chemotherapy-refractory peripheral T-cell lymphomas. Blood 2004; 103: 2920–4.

100. Matsumoto Y, Nomura K, Kanda-Akano Y et al. Successful treatment with Erwinia L-asparaginase for recurrent natural killer/T cell lymphoma. Leuk Lymphoma 2003; 44: 879–82.

101. O'Connor OA, Hamlin PA, Portlock C et al. Pralatrexate, a novel class of antifol with high affinity for the reduced folate carrier-type 1, produces marked complete and durable remissions in a diversity of chemotherapy refractory cases of T-cell lymphoma. Br J Haematol 2007; 139: 425–8.

◆102. Siegel RS, Pandolfino T, Guitart J et al. Primary cutaneous T-cell lymphoma: review and current concepts. J Clin Oncol 2000; 18: 2908–25.

●103. Lundin J, Hagberg H, Repp R et al. Phase 2 study of alemtuzumab (anti-CD52 monoclonal antibody) in patients with advanced mycosis fungoides/Sezary syndrome. Blood 2003; 101: 4267–72.

104. Olsen E, Duvic M, Frankel A et al. Pivotal phase III trial of two dose levels of denileukin diftitox for the treatment of cutaneous T-cell lymphoma. J Clin Oncol 2001; 19: 376–88.

105. Haim N, Rosenblatt E, Wollner M et al. Salvage therapy for non-Hodgkin's lymphoma with a combination of dexamethasone, etoposide, ifosfamide, and cisplatin. Cancer Chemother Pharmacol 1992; 30: 243–4.

106. Herbrecht R, Damonte JC, Dufour P et al. Etoposide, ifosfamide, and methotrexate combination chemotherapy for aggressive non-Hodgkin's lymphomas after failure of the LNH 84 regimen. Semin Oncol 1992; 19(1 Suppl 1): 7–10.

107. Chao NJ, Rosenberg SA, Horning SJ. CEPP(B): an effective and well-tolerated regimen in poor-risk, aggressive non-Hodgkin's lymphoma. Blood 1990; 76: 1293–8.

108. Hopfinger G, Heinz R, Koller E *et al.* Ifosfamide, mitoxantrone and etoposide (VIM) as salvage therapy of low toxicity in non-Hodgkin's lymphoma. *Eur J Haematol* 1995; **55**: 223–7.

109. Garay G, Dupont J, Dragosky M *et al.* Combination salvage chemotherapy with MIZE (ifosfamide-mesna, idarubicin and etoposide) for relapsing or refractory lymphoma. *Leuk Lymphoma* 1997; **26**: 595–602.

110. Press OW, Livingston R, Mortimer J *et al.* Treatment of relapsed non-Hodgkin's lymphomas with dexamethasone, high-dose cytarabine, and cisplatin before marrow transplantation. *J Clin Oncol* 1991; **9**: 423–31.

111. Philip T, Chauvin F, Armitage J *et al.* Parma international protocol: pilot study of DHAP followed by involved-field radiotherapy and BEAC with autologous bone marrow transplantation. *Blood* 1991; **77**: 1587–92.

●112. Philip T, Guglielmi C, Hagenbeek A *et al.* Autologous bone marrow transplantation as compared with salvage chemotherapy in relapses of chemotherapy-sensitive non-Hodgkin's lymphoma. *N Engl J Med* 1995; **333**: 1540–5.

113. Soussain C, Souleau B, Gabarre J *et al.* Intensive chemotherapy with hematopoietic cell transplantation after ESHAP therapy for relapsed or refractory non-Hodgkin's lymphoma. Results of a single-centre study of 65 patients. *Leuk Lymphoma* 1999; **33**: 543–50.

114. Ho AD, Del Valle F, Engelhard M *et al.* Mitoxantrone/high-dose Ara-C and recombinant human GM-CSF in the treatment of refractory non-Hodgkin's lymphoma. A pilot study. *Cancer* 1990; **66**: 423–30.

115. Ruit JB, Lowenberg B, Hagenbeek A *et al.* Phase II study of lomustine, cytarabine, mitoxantrone, and prednisone (CAMP) combination chemotherapy for doxorubicin-resistant intermediate- and high-grade malignant non-Hodgkin's lymphoma. *Semin Oncol* 1990; **17**(6 Suppl 10): 24–7.

116. Dufour P, Mors R, Berthaud P *et al.* Idarubicin and high dose cytarabine: a new salvage treatment for refractory or relapsing non-Hodgkin's lymphoma. *Leuk Lymphoma* 1996; **22**: 329–34.

117. Brusamolino E, Passamonti F, Pagnucco G *et al.* Efficacy of a combination of idarubicin, etoposide and intermediate-dose cytosine arabinoside as salvage therapy in relapsing or resistant unfavorable lymphoma. *Haematologica* 1998; **83**: 323–8.

118. Rodriguez MA, Cabanillas FC, Hagemeister FB *et al.* A phase II trial of mesna/ifosfamide, mitoxantrone and etoposide for refractory lymphomas. *Ann Oncol* 1995; **6**: 609–11.

119. Caballero MD, Amigo ML, Hernandez JM *et al.* Alternating mini-BEAM/ESHAP as salvage therapy for refractory non-Hodgkin's lymphomas. *Ann Hematol* 1997; **74**: 79–82.

120. Linch DC, Winfield D, Goldstone AH *et al.* Dose intensification with autologous bone-marrow transplantation in relapsed and resistant Hodgkin's disease: results of a BNLI randomised trial. *Lancet* 1993; **341**: 1051–4.

●121. Moskowitz CH, Nimer SD, Zelenetz AD *et al.* A 2-step comprehensive high-dose chemoradiotherapy second-line program for relapsed and refractory Hodgkin's disease: analysis by intent to treat and development of a prognostic model. *Blood* 2001; **97**: 616–23.

55

High-dose therapy with stem cell rescue

JOHN W SWEETENHAM

INTRODUCTION

High-dose therapy (HDT) and stem cell transplantation (SCT) has been in widespread use in the treatment of Hodgkin (HL) and non-Hodgkin lymphomas (NHLs) for more than 20 years. Despite this, the impact of this treatment on remission duration and overall survival for patients with these diseases remains poorly defined. High-dose therapy with autologous stem cell transplantation (ASCT) is now regarded as the standard of care for certain patients with relapsed and refractory HL or relapsed aggressive B cell NHL. This is supported by results from prospective, randomized clinical trials. The role of HDT and ASCT as a component of first-line therapy for certain 'high risk' patients with HL and NHL is also being better defined as results emerge from recently completed randomized studies.

Despite recent progress, however, many uncertainties persist concerning the use of SCT in lymphoma. Interpretation of studies addressing the role of HDT and SCT in these diseases has been limited by study design. Relatively few randomized studies have been performed until recently, and much of the data on which current transplant practice is based are from retrospective studies from single institutions

or from transplant registries. Such studies have many potential biases. Most report outcomes from the date of SCT. They therefore do not provide information on the potential selection of patients which took place prior to (and after) referral to a transplant center and do not include a denominator for the overall population from which the transplanted patients were selected. Additionally, most retrospective studies do not analyze survival by intent to treat. These problems are accentuated in studies of allogeneic transplantation, in which issues of patient selection are likely to be more complex. This is partly because of the increased regimen-related toxicity of this approach, and partly because of the potential biases introduced as patients with very early relapses are 'selected out' of transplant series in view of the time taken to find a suitable donor.

For most subtypes of lymphoma, the optimal timing of SCT remains uncertain, as does the best high-dose regimen, the preferred stem cell source, and the optimal regimen for pre-transplant cytoreductive therapy. The existence of a 'graft-versus-lymphoma' effect has been reported from many *in vitro*, animal model, and clinical studies, but its true impact on outcome for patients undergoing allogeneic SCT for lymphoma is poorly defined.

The emergence of new, highly effective therapies for lymphoma over the last 5 to 10 years has posed new questions about the role of SCT, even for indications previously regarded as 'standard.' In particular, the advent of new, highly effective combination chemotherapy regimens for HL has resulted in lower relapse rates and a smaller number of patients requiring SCT. Recent data suggest that standard SCT approaches may not produce effective salvage for patients who relapse after these intensive chemotherapy regimens. New transplant (or other) strategies may therefore be required. The introduction of monoclonal antibody therapy (unlabeled and radio-labeled) in the treatment of B cell NHL has improved the effectiveness of first-line therapy. This poses questions concerning the ability of high-dose strategies to 'salvage' patients who relapse after these regimens. Additionally, questions regarding the role of SCT as a first-line therapy will need to be revisited for certain types of B cell NHL, for which rituximab/chemotherapy combinations have become a new standard in recent years.

Despite these uncertainties, new data are beginning to define the impact of SCT in the lymphomas more clearly. Clinical trials have identified patients for whom SCT probably does and probably does not offer a survival or progression-free survival advantage compared with standard therapy. New studies are exploring novel treatment approaches including the incorporation of radioimmunotherapy into transplant regimens, and manipulation of the immune system in the peri-and post-transplant settings to reduce relapse.

HODGKIN LYMPHOMA

Relapsed Hodgkin lymphoma

Results of conventional-dose salvage therapy for patients with HL who relapse after initial chemotherapy have been poor. Studies in patients whose disease relapsed after MOPP (mechlorethamine, vincristine, procarbazine, and prednisone) chemotherapy demonstrated that MOPP was able to induce second complete remissions in about 50 percent of patients, with a median duration of 21 months.[1] Patients with an initial remission duration of less than 12 months had a significantly worse progression-free and overall survival than those with longer initial remissions. However, the long-term outcome was poor for all patients, irrespective of the duration of remission. Patients with an initial remission of less than 12 months duration had a second complete remission (CR) rate of 29 percent compared with 93 percent of those with an initial remission lasting more than 12 months. Even in the latter group, only 17 percent were alive at 20 years of follow up.

The ABVD[2] (doxorubicin, bleomycin, vinblastine, and dacarbazine) regimen, now widely accepted as standard first-line therapy, was initially developed as a salvage regimen and later compared to MOPP and MOPP/ABVD as

first-line therapy in a randomized trial by the Cancer and Leukemia Group B (CALGB).[3] Patients who relapsed after initial therapy with ABVD and were retreated with MOPP had a 5-year failure-free survival rate of 31 percent, compared with only 15 percent for those receiving ABVD for relapse after first-line MOPP.

Early retrospective studies reported superior results for patients treated with HDT and ASCT. Long-term disease-free survival rates between 40 percent and 65 percent were observed for patients receiving ASCT at first relapse.[4–7] In a matched analysis from Stanford University, the outcome for 60 patients with relapsed/refractory Hodgkin lymphoma receiving HDT and ASCT was compared with a group receiving conventional-dose salvage therapy.[5] Four-year event-free survival (EFS) and freedom from progression (FFP) were higher in the ASCT group (53 percent vs 27 percent, for EFS; 62 percent vs 27 percent, for FFP). Four-year actuarial overall survival was not significantly different between the two groups (54 percent for high dose vs 47 percent for conventional dose), but a difference in favor of high-dose therapy was observed for the subset of patients relapsing within 12 months of initial chemotherapy.

In a study from the European Group for Blood and Marrow Transplantation (EBMT), 45 percent of 139 patients undergoing ASCT at first relapse were in continuing second remission at 5 years.[8]

Two randomized trials have compared HDT and ASCT with conventional-dose salvage therapy for relapsed HL with similar results. In a study from the British National Lymphoma Investigation (BNLI), 40 patients in first or subsequent relapse were randomized to receive HDT with BEAM (carmustine, etoposide, cytarabine, and melphalan) or conventional-dose therapy, using lower doses of the same drugs ('mini-BEAM').[9] Event-free survival was superior in patients receiving BEAM (3-year EFS: 53 percent for BEAM vs 10 percent for mini-BEAM, $P = 0.025$). No overall survival difference was observed. However, since some patients who relapsed after mini-BEAM crossed over to receive BEAM and ASCT, the effect of high-dose therapy on overall survival is difficult to interpret.

In a randomized study by the German Hodgkin Lymphoma Study Group, 161 patients with relapsed HL were initially treated with two cycles of Dexa-BEAM (dexamethasone, carmustine [BCNU], etoposide, cytarabine, and melphalan). Responding patients were randomized between two further cycles of Dexa-BEAM or HDT and ASCT.[10] Three-year freedom from treatment failure (FFTF) was improved in the SCT arm (55 percent vs 34 percent, $P = 0.019$) but overall survival (OS) was similar in both treatment arms (71 percent vs 65 percent, $P = 0.331$). Again, the failure to demonstrate an OS difference related to the 'crossover' of patients who relapsed on the conventional-dose arm who were salvaged by ASCT. In a recent update of this study, with 83 months median follow up, the 7-year FFTF rate was higher in the SCT arm (32 percent vs 49 percent).[11] No overall survival difference was observed (56 percent for Dexa-BEAM vs 57 percent for ASCT at 7 years).

High-dose therapy and ASCT is now regarded as the standard of care for patients with relapsed HL after a prior chemotherapy regimen such as MOPP or ABVD.

The emergence of dose-dense and dose-intensive chemotherapy regimens for initial treatment of advanced HL raises new question regarding the effectiveness of HDT and ASCT at relapse. The Stanford V and escalated BEACOPP (bleomycin, etoposide, doxorubicin, cyclophosphamide, vincristine, procarbazine, and prednisone) regimens both result in high rates of remission and disease-free survival in advanced HL.[12,13] The 5-year actuarial progression-free and overall survival rates were 89 percent and 96 percent, respectively, in the initial phase II study of Stanford V. Sixteen of the 142 patients treated with this regimen subsequently relapsed, of whom 11 underwent high-dose therapy and ASCT.[12] The freedom from second relapse in the entire group of 16 patients was 69 percent at 5 years.

The German Hodgkin Lymphoma Study Group has recently reported that salvage rates were equivalent for all patients treated on the HD9 study, irrespective of the treatment allocated at randomization. However, there was an apparent trend for those who relapsed after baseline or escalated BEACOPP to be less readily salvaged by HDT and ASCT than those relapsing after COPP/ABVD (cyclophosphamide, vincristine, procarbazine, prednisone/doxorubicin, bleomycin, vinblastine, and dacarbazine). This will require continued follow up.

If these results are confirmed in future studies, the role of HDT and ASCT after dose-intensive first-line therapy will need to be reexamined. Randomized trials are likely to prove difficult to conduct since the number of patients with relapsed HL will continue to decline as intensive regimens gain widespread use.

Refractory Hodgkin lymphoma

Primary refractory Hodgkin lymphoma is associated with a poor prognosis. The use of conventional-dose second-line regimens in this situation results in response rates of 40 percent to 50 percent, but very few patients achieve long-term disease-free survival.[1,2] A study from Stanford University reported 4-year overall survival for 38 percent of patients, with a 4-year progression-free survival (PFS) of 19 percent.[5]

The role of HDT and ASCT for primary refractory HL has been reported in some retrospective studies. Data from randomized trials are not available in view of the rarity of this situation. In a matched analysis from Stanford, the 4-year overall and freedom-from-progression rates were 44 percent and 52 percent, respectively, after ASCT.[5] These results were significantly superior to the historical group who received conventional-dose salvage therapy. In a study of 46 patients with primary refractory disease

treated with BEAM and ASCT at University College Hospital, London, the 6-year actuarial progression-free survival rate was 33 percent, similar to results reported from Memorial Sloan Kettering Cancer Center.[7,14] The EBMT has reported results from patients treated with ASCT after failure of first-line therapy with 5-year actuarial overall and progression-free survival rates of 36 percent and 32 percent, respectively.[15] Similar results were reported from the Autologous Blood and Marrow Transplant Registry of North America (ABMTR).[16] The definition of refractory disease in the ABMTR study required either biopsy proof of persistent disease or clear radiologic or clinical evidence of disease progression for eligibility. The other retrospective series described above have used less stringent criteria for definition of refractory disease.

The apparent improvement in outcome with the use of high-dose therapy and ASCT must be interpreted in the context of differing definitions of refractory disease, which continue to change. Assessment of response in HL can be difficult, particularly in patients with extensive disease in the mediastinum. The failure to achieve a complete clinical and radiologic remission after induction therapy does not necessarily imply that active disease is still present within the residual mass although eligibility for some earlier studies of refractory disease was based purely on failure to achieve an early and complete radiologic remission.

Patients who have minimally responsive disease after induction therapy may not have active disease within the residual mass and are distinct from those patients who have obvious disease progression during induction therapy. Recent studies of the use of 'early' [^{18}F]2-fluoro-2-deoxy-D-glucose positron emission tomography (FDG-PET) scanning after two cycles of chemotherapy in patients with advanced stage Hodgkin lymphoma have shown that this can be highly predictive of subsequent outcome.[17] Future studies of primary refractory HL are therefore likely to use functional imaging to define refractory disease, establishing a new paradigm for the investigation of salvage strategies. The role of high-dose therapy and ASCT in this context will therefore require evaluation in prospective studies.

Prognostic factors after HDT and ASCT for Hodgkin lymphoma

Prognostic factors for relapsed and refractory HL patients undergoing SCT have been published from several groups, based on retrospective analyses.[18–21] Few consistent factors have emerged, primarily because of the relative small sample size in each of the published series. Most studies have identified B symptoms at the time of ASCT, short remission duration after initial chemotherapy, extent of disease at the time of ASCT, and extent of prior therapy as adverse factors for subsequent disease-free and overall survival.

The group from Vancouver reported 20-year follow-up of 100 patients undergoing HDT and ASCT for relapsed and refractory HL.[22] Prior therapy with at least two chemotherapy regimens was the only adverse predictive factor in the entire patient population. For those patients undergoing ASCT in first relapse, extranodal disease at the time of relapse was also predictive.

The use of pre-transplant functional imaging may have prognostic value for outcome after transplantation. The group at Memorial Sloan Kettering Cancer Center has reported results for 152 patients with relapsed or refractory Hodgkin lymphoma who were treated with ICE (ifosfamide, carboplatin, and etoposide)[23] at the time of relapse. All of the patients reported responded to this chemotherapy. Functional imaging was performed after completion of their salvage therapy, prior to high-dose therapy and ASCT. The functional imaging modality changed during the period of the study from gallium scanning in the mid to late 1990s to FDG-PET for more recent patients. The 5-year EFS for patients with negative and positive functional imaging results were 74 percent and 29 percent, respectively, suggesting that this approach might provide a new tool for selection of patients most likely to benefit from ASCT after salvage therapy. Perhaps more importantly, it may help to identify a group of patients in whom ASCT is unlikely to be beneficial, and who may be considered for experimental strategies. Prospective evaluation of FDG-PET in this context is in progress.

Hodgkin lymphoma in first remission

Most recent studies of first-line therapy for patients with advanced Hodgkin lymphoma report long-term disease-free survival rates of 80 percent to 90 percent. However, 'poor risk' patients have been identified who have lower survival rates after conventional first-line regimens. The most widely used method for risk stratification is the International Prognostic Factors Project on Advanced Hodgkin's Disease, which identified seven adverse clinical prognostic factors.[24] Freedom from progression at 5 years was noted to be lower according to the number of adverse factors present. Patients with no adverse factors had a 5-year FFP rate of 84 percent compared with 42 percent for those with four or more risk factors.

The use of high-dose therapy and ASCT for patients with 'poor risk' Hodgkin lymphoma has been reported by several groups, although the definition or poor risk has varied and none of these studies used the International Prognostic Score (IPS) criteria. In the largest of these studies, from Europe, 163 patients with poor-risk disease (defined according to criteria reported from Memorial Sloan Kettering Cancer Center) received initial therapy with four cycles of ABVD or similar chemotherapy.[25] Those patients achieving a complete or partial response were randomized to high-dose therapy and ASCT (83 patients) or four further cycles of chemotherapy. After a median follow-up of 4 years, the 5-year failure-free survival rates were 75 percent for the transplant arm, compared with 82 percent for the conventional therapy arm ($P = 0.4$). The overall survival rates were 88 percent versus 88 percent ($P = 0.99$), respectively.

There is no established role for the 'early' use of high-dose therapy and ASCT in advanced Hodgkin lymphoma. The introduction of new dose-dense and dose-intensive regimens such as BEACOPP in advanced HL may have improved response and disease-free survival rates and appears to have overcome the prognostic significance of the adverse factors identified in the IPS.[13]

It is possible that future studies including 'early' functional imaging (see above), gene expression profiling, or proteomic studies may identify patients with HL with poor-risk disease at presentation. If so, the potential use of early high-dose therapy in this group may merit further investigation, although this is likely to be a small minority of patients with HL.

NON–HODGKIN LYMPHOMA

Relapsed diffuse large B cell lymphoma

The PARMA randomized trial established high-dose therapy and ASCT as the standard of care for patients with relapsed diffuse large B cell lymphoma (DLBCL) and some other types of diffuse aggressive lymphoma.[26] Two hundred fifteen patients with relapsed aggressive NHL (mostly DLBCL) were included in this study, all of whom had achieved an initial complete remission after adriamycin-based chemotherapy. At study entry, patients were treated with 2 cycles of DHAP (dexamethasone, high-dose cytosine arabinoside, and cisplatin) and responding patients were randomized to receive further DHAP chemotherapy, or to proceed to high-dose therapy with BEAC (carmustine, etoposide, cytarabine, and cyclophosphamide) and autologous bone marrow transplantation. Patients over 60 years of age as well as those with bone marrow or central nervous system involvement were excluded. The 5-year event-free survival (46 percent vs 12 percent, $P = 0.0001$) and overall survival (53 percent vs 32 percent, $P = 0.038$) rates were superior for patients receiving ASCT compared with those receiving conventional-dose salvage therapy.

Although widely regarded as a landmark study that established ASCT as the standard of care in this setting, there are many aspects of the trial design which limit its relevance to the current therapy of DLBCL and other aggressive NHLs. The response rate to the initial DHAP therapy was 56 percent and largely as a result of this, only 109 of the original 215 patients were randomized. All analyses were restricted to this group of patients, and no intent-to-treat analysis was performed. The trial was closed because of slow accrual and it is not clear that the study was adequately powered for the primary endpoints of event-free and overall survival. An updated analysis of this study has never been published.

Improved peri-transplant management, particularly the use of peripheral blood progenitor cells (PBPCs), has reduced the transplant-related morbidity and extended use of transplantation to patients up to 70 or 75 years old. The use of PBPCs has also reduced the necessity for an uninvolved bone marrow at the time of harvesting. Patients receiving ASCT now are more heterogeneous than those included in the PARMA study. Although the PARMA trial is generally regarded as the landmark study for patients with relapsed DLBCL, it included patients with various histologies including some with peripheral T cell lymphoma.

The emergence of new first-line treatments, particularly rituximab, added to combination chemotherapy regimens, has improved disease-free and overall survival in DLBCL.[27,28] It is unclear if patients who suffer relapses after one of these regimens can be salvaged as effectively as those not receiving antibody-containing therapy. One recent retrospective comparison of patients receiving first-line CHOP or CHOP-rituximab who subsequently underwent ASCT for relapsed disease has been reported from the University of Nebraska.[29] No difference in event-free or overall survival following ASCT was observed according to initial therapy. A similar study from the Cleveland Clinic has reported comparable results.[30]

High response and survival rates have been reported for dose-dense and dose-intensive regimens for DLBCL, including CHOP-14 and dose-adjusted EPOCH-R (etoposide, prednisone, vincristine, cyclophosphamide, doxorubicin, and rituximab).[28,31] Whether high-dose therapy and ASCT will be effective second-line therapy for patients who relapse after these regimens is uncertain. A recent study of dose-adjusted EPOCH-R as initial therapy for DLBCL reported 2-year progression-free survival in 83 percent of patients with an overlapping overall survival curve, suggesting that patients who relapsed after this highly active regimen are unlikely to be salvaged with a standard transplant approach.[31]

High-dose therapy and ASCT remains the standard of care for patients with relapsed DLBCL which is sensitive to second-line chemotherapy.

Further evaluation of the role of HDT and ASCT in this context is unlikely, although ongoing studies are addressing the optimal pre-transplant salvage therapy and the potential role of rituximab in this context. Additionally, the use of FDG-PET scanning as a method to assess response to pre-transplant salvage and identify patients unlikely to benefit from ASCT is under investigation.

Prognostic factors for relapsed DLBCL

The age-adjusted International Prognostic Index (aaIPI) has been shown to have predictive value in a follow-up report of the PARMA study.[32] Data were available for 204 of the original 215 patients at the time of study entry. Patients with an aaIPI score of 0 had an overall response rate of 77 percent compared to 42 percent for patients with three adverse factors. The aaIPI was predictive of overall survival for the entire patient cohort.

For the subset of patients who were randomized, the aaIPI was predictive for those on the DHAP arm, but not in those on the ASCT arm. No difference in overall or progression-free survival was observed according to randomized arm for patients with an aaIPI score of 0, although a difference remained for those with scores of 1 to 3.

Hamlin et al. have reported 150 patients with relapsed/refractory DLBCL receiving ICE chemotherapy followed by high-dose therapy and ASCT.[33] This study showed that the aaIPI had predictive value in this context. When analyzed by intent to treat, patients with a score of 2 or 3 at the time of relapse had 4-year progression-free and overall survival rates of 16 percent and 18 percent, respectively, compared with 70 percent and 74 percent for those with a score of 0. The same group has also analyzed the prognostic significance of cell of origin of DLBCL as determined by immunohistochemistry using tissue microarrays.[34] Unlike previous studies investigating cell of origin in the context of initial therapy, there was no evidence of a difference in outcome according to germinal center-derived or non-germinal center phenotype.

Diffuse large B cell and other aggressive B cell lymphomas in first remission

Response rates of 70 percent to 80 percent for patients with advanced DLBCL, and long-term disease-free survival (DFS) rates of 45 percent to 60 percent, are reported after CHOP and related chemotherapy regimens. The addition of rituximab to CHOP and similar regimens has improved these results. However, a significant proportion of patients will relapse after this therapy, or will never achieve an initial complete response. Many centers have investigated the incorporation of ASCT into first-line therapy, particularly for patients identified as having 'poor risk' disease according to various risk models. Results from many trials are available.[35–39]

The Groupe d'Etude des Lymphomes de l'Adulte (GELA) in France conducted a prospective, randomized trial in 916 patients with diffuse aggressive NHL, all aged less than 55 years and defined as high risk according to factors which pre-dated the development of the aaIPI. Four hundred sixty four of these patients achieved a CR and were randomized to conventional-dose sequential consolidation or high-dose therapy and ASCT.[40] The 3-year DFS was 52 percent for the ASCT arm, compared with 59 percent for the sequential arm. The corresponding overall survival rates were 71 percent versus 69 percent. A retrospective subset analysis, for patients with high or high-intermediate-risk disease according to the aaIPI, reported an 8-year DFS and OS of 55 percent and 64 percent, respectively, for the ASCT

Table 55.1   Results of high-dose therapy (HDT) and autologous stem cell transplantation (ASCT) in first remission for diffuse large B cell lymphoma and other aggressive non-Hodgkin lymphomas

Reference	n	Randomization	DFS (conventional chemotherapy vs SCT)	OS (conventional chemotherapy vs SCT)
Haioun et al.[35]	464	Sequential chemotherapy vs HDT and ASCT in patients in CR after induction chemotherapy	52% vs 59% at 3 years ($P = 0.46$)	71% vs 69% at 3 years ($P = 0.6$)
Santini et al.[36]	124	VACOP-B vs VACOP-B plus HDT and ASCT for responding patients	60% vs 80% at 6 years ($P = 0.1$)	65% vs 65% at 6 years ($P = 0.5$)
Kluin-Nelemans et al.[37]	194	CHVmP/BV vs CHVmP/BV plus HDT and ASCT for responding patients	56% vs 61% at 5 years ($P = 0.712$)	77% vs 68% at 5 years ($P = 0.336$)
Gianni et al.[38]	98	MACOP-B vs high dose sequential therapy including HDT and ASCT	49% vs 76% at 7 years ($P = 0.004$)	55% vs 81% at 7 years ($P = 0.09$)
Gisselbrecht et al.[39]	370	ACVBP and sequential consolidation versus intensive induction chemotherapy plus HDT and ASCT	76% vs 58% at 5 years ($P = 0.004$)	60% vs 46% at 5 years ($P = 0.007$)
Milpied et al.[41]	207	CHOP vs intensive induction chemotherapy plus HDT and ASCT	37% vs 55% at 5 years ($P = 0.037$)	44% vs 74% at 5 years ($P = 0.001$)

VACOP-B: etoposide, doxorubicin, cyclophosphamide, vincristine, prednisone, and bleomycin; CHVmP/BV: cyclophosphamide, doxorubicin, teniposide, and prednisone, with bleomycin and vincristine added mid-cycle; MACOP-B: methotrexate, doxorubicin, cyclophosphamide, vincristine, prednisone, and bleomycin; ACVBP: doxorubicin, cyclophosphamide, vindesine, bleomycin, and prednisone; CHOP: cyclophosphamide, doxorubicin, vincristine, and prednisone; DFS, disease-free survival; OS, overall survival; CR, complete remission; SCT, stem cell transplantation.

arm compared with 39 percent and 49 percent for the conventional-dose arm.

Many prospective studies have been conducted since the publication of this study, most of which have defined eligibility according to the aaIPI, most commonly including only those patients with high or high-intermediate-risk disease (Table 55.1). Most studies have shown equivalent long-term DFS and OS rates for conventional versus high-dose consolidation therapy in this setting.

In contrast to most of these studies, a recent French trial compared 8 cycles of CHOP chemotherapy with 2 cycles of a dose-intensive first-line regimen, followed by high-dose therapy and ASCT in advanced diffuse aggressive NHL.[41] Eligible patients were aged less than 60 years old and had a maximum of two adverse risk factors according to the aaIPI (low, low-intermediate, or high-intermediate-risk disease).

An intent-to-treat analysis was used in this study, which included 207 patients. When all randomized patients were analyzed, there was a higher EFS in the ASCT arm (55 percent vs 37 percent, $P = 0.037$), but no difference in OS. On subset analysis, a difference in OS was seen in the patients with high-intermediate-risk disease ($P = 0.001$). The results of this study are intriguing, but must be interpreted cautiously since the study was conducted prior to the introduction of rituximab. In view of the improved response and survival rates seen when first-line chemotherapy is combined with rituximab, it is not clear that the apparent benefit of ASCT will be maintained.

A metaanalysis of HDT and ASCT as a component of first-line therapy of diffuse aggressive NHL included

3079 patients from 15 randomized trials for toxicity, and 2018 patients from 13 trials for outcome.[42] A significantly higher CR rate was reported for ASCT, but no differences in EFS or OS were seen. No differences in outcome could be detected according to IPI risk group, conditioning regimen, or histologic subtype.

Based on these results, inclusion of ASCT in first-line therapy for patients with diffuse aggressive lymphoma (including DLBCL) should not be considered a standard of care, even for those with poor-risk disease according to the IPI. Most of the studies reported above were completed before the advent of rituximab or dose-dense chemotherapy regimens. The relevance of these studies to the current treatment of diffuse aggressive NHL in general, and DLBCL in particular, is uncertain. The results of the Southwest Oncology Group 9704 study in the USA will be helpful in resolving this. In this study, patients with DLBCL aged 60 years or less with high-intermediate or high-risk disease according to the aaIPI were randomized to 8 cycles of CHOP-rituximab therapy alone, or the same therapy for 5 cycles followed by ASCT. This study originally used CHOP chemotherapy alone, but was modified to incorporate rituximab early in its accrual.

Diffuse aggressive NHL which is 'slow' to enter remission

'Slow' response to chemotherapy was identified as a possible adverse prognostic factor in early studies in diffuse aggressive lymphomas, with patients whose disease was not

Table 55.2 Results of studies of high-dose therapy (HDT) and autologous stem cell transplantation (ASCT) in 'slowly responding' patients with DLBCL and other aggressive non-Hodgkin lymphomas

Reference	n	Randomization	DFS (conventional chemotherapy vs SCT)	OS (conventional chemotherapy vs SCT)
Verdonck et al.[44]	65	CHOP vs HDT and ASCT if in PR after 3 initial cycles of CHOP	85% vs 56% at 4 years (NS)	72% vs 72% at 4 years (NS)
Martelli et al.[45]	49	DHAP vs HDT and ASCT after PR to F-MACHOP or MACOP-B	52% vs 73% at 3 years (NS)	59% vs 73% at 3 years (NS)

DLBCL, diffuse large B cell lymphoma; DFS, disease-free survival; OS, overall survival; SCT, stem cell transplantation; PR, partial response; CHOP: cyclophosphamide, doxorubicin, vincristine, and prednisone; DHAP: dexamethasone, cisplatin, and cytarabine; F-MACHOP: fluorouracil, methotrexate, cytarabine, cyclophosphamide, doxorubicin, vincristine, and prednisone; MACOP-B: methotrexate, leucovorin, doxorubicin, cyclophosphamide, vincristine, prednisone, and bleomycin; NS, not significant.

in clinical CR after 3 or 4 cycles of chemotherapy having a poor outcome compared with those already in remission. Several studies have investigated the 'early' use of early high-dose therapy and ASCT in these patients.[43–45] Results are summarized in Table 55.2, and show no evidence that 'early' ASCT improves outcome in this group.

Results of PET scanning after 1 or 2 cycles of chemotherapy have been shown to be predictive of subsequent relapse-free and overall survival in some recent studies.[46–48] Phase II studies are now in progress in DLBCL in which patients who have disease that is FDG-avid after 1 or 2 cycles of rituximab-CHOP or similar chemotherapy proceed directly to high-dose therapy and ASCT. Mature results from these studies are not yet available.

Follicular lymphoma in first remission

Results from retrospective studies based on registry and single-center experience have suggested a potential improvement in outcome for patients with low-grade follicular lymphoma undergoing ASCT as a component of first-line therapy (Table 55.3). Interpretation of these studies is difficult in view of their retrospective nature and the potential for referral and selection bias.[49–52]

Three prospective randomized trials have now been reported which investigate the role of first-remission ASCT in follicular lymphoma. In a study from the German Low-Grade Lymphoma Study Group (GLSG), 375 patients were randomized, after 2 cycles of CHOP or CHOP-like induction therapy, between ASCT and interferon alpha (IFNα) maintenance.[53] They then received a further two to four cycles of induction therapy prior to their assigned treatment according to randomization. Of the 375 patients entered, 279 initiated consolidation therapy. The remainder did not receive their assigned treatment either because of ineligible histology, or failure to respond to the first-line treatment. Higher progression-free survival was observed in the ASCT arm compared with the IFNα arm (64.7 percent vs 33.3 percent at 5 years, $P = 0.0001$). Overall survival was not reported in view of the short follow-up

Table 55.3 Results of retrospective studies of high-dose therapy (HDT) and autologous stem cell transplantation (ASCT) for follicular lymphoma in first remission

Reference	n	DFS	OS	Follow-up (years)
Horning et al.[49]	37	86%	97%	10
Freedman et al.[50]	77	66%	89%	3
Ladetto et al.[51]	92	67%	84%	4
Colombat et al.[52]	27	55% (RFS)	64%	6

DFS, disease-free survival; OS, overall survival; RFS, relapse-free survival.

duration. Unfortunately, because the survival analyses were conducted from completion of induction therapy, rather than at study entry, no intent-to-treat analysis is available. More than 90 percent of the patients had IPI low-risk or low-intermediate-risk disease. Comparable PFS rates have been reported for this group using less-intensive first-line therapies.

The GELA has reported a randomized trial in which 401 untreated patients with follicular lymphoma with high tumor burden were randomized between CHVP (cyclophosphamide, doxorubicin, teniposide, and prednisone) plus IFNα or 4 cycles of CHOP followed by high-dose therapy and ASCT.[54] Intent-to-treat analyses were conducted. Although longer overall survival was seen in the transplant arm, which just achieved statistical significance (7-year OS: 74 percent for chemotherapy arm vs 84 percent for transplant arm, $P = 0.05$), there was no difference in 7-year EFS rates, which were 45 percent for the ASCT arm and 36 percent for the chemotherapy/interferon arm ($P = 0.5$). The apparent discrepancy between the results for OS and EFS is probably explained by the duration of therapy in the conventional chemotherapy arm.

The GOELAMS study group has investigated the use of consolidation with ASCT in a randomized study in which 170 patients were randomized to receive either chemoimmunotherapy with CHVP plus interferon or VCAP (cyclophosphamide, doxorubicin, prednisone, and vincristine) and

IMVP16 (ifosfamide, methotrexate, and VP16) followed by ASCT.[55] A higher response rate was observed in the ASCT arm (69 percent vs 81 percent, $P = 0.045$). Five-year EFS rate was also higher in the transplant arm at 48 percent vs 60 percent ($P = 0.05$), but only for patients with high-risk disease according to the Follicular Lymphoma International Prognostic Index (FLIPI). Overall survival was equivalent in both arms of the study, mainly because of an excess of second malignancies in the ASCT arm. Excessive rates of second malignancy have been a concern in the use of early ASCT in follicular lymphoma. Results from the three studies above give rates of second malignancy ranging from 0 percent to 8.5 percent.

The use of first-remission ASCT needs to be evaluated in the context of antibody-based therapy as first-line treatment in follicular lymphoma. Various rituximab-chemotherapy combinations have now been assessed in first-line therapy of follicular lymphoma, with long remissions reported.[56–58] Additionally, the use of radiolabeled monoclonal antibodies such as iodine-131 (^{131}I)-tositumomab both alone and in combination with chemotherapy has been shown to produce high rates of disease-free survival.[59] The use of high-dose therapy and ASCT will therefore need to be reevaluated in the setting of these new and highly effective first-line regimens and should not be regarded as standard of care.

Relapsed follicular lymphoma

Most of the published experience documenting the use of ASCT in relapsed follicular lymphoma has been based on single center or collaborative group retrospective studies including selected patients with respect to age, responsiveness to conventional-dose chemotherapy prior to ASCT, and the requirement for a minimal residual disease state to have been attained prior to ASCT.[59–63] Intent-to-treat analyses have not been performed. Results of these studies are summarized in Table 55.4. Although most of these studies have reported encouraging disease-free and overall survival rates, they are difficult to interpret in view of the highly selected patient populations.

More recently, combined long-term follow-up data from the Dana Farber Cancer Institute and St Bartholomew's Hospital, London, have been reported for 121 patients transplanted in second or subsequent remission.[64] With median follow-up of 13.5 years, the 5-year and 10-year overall survival rates were 71 percent and 54 percent, respectively. The relapse-free survival curve shows an apparent plateau at 48 percent from 12 years onward.

A small randomized trial compared CHOP with high-dose therapy and ASCT in 89 patients with relapsed follicular lymphoma who responded to 2 cycles of initial salvage therapy with CHOP.[65] Relapsed patients were initially treated with CHOP or a similar regimen and responding patients were randomized between continuing CHOP, ASCT with an unmanipulated stem cell product, or ASCT with 'purging' of the stem cell product. This study showed a

Table 55.4 Results of retrospective studies of high-dose therapy (HDT) and autologous stem cell transplantation (ASCT) for relapsed and refractory follicular lymphoma

Reference	n	DFS	OS	Follow-up (years)
Freedman et al.[60]	153	42%	66%	8
Bierman et al.[61]	100	44%	65%	4
Apostolides et al.[62]	99	63% (FFR)	69%	5
Van Besien et al.[63]	597	31%	55%	5

DFS, disease-free survival; OS, overall survival; FFR, freedom from recurrence.

relapse-free and overall survival advantage to the use of high dose – compared with conventional dose – salvage therapy. Interpretation of these results is limited by the small sample size and imbalances in clinical factors between the three arms of the trial. Further studies are required to clarify the role of transplant strategies in relapsed follicular NHL.

Mantle cell lymphoma

High-dose therapy and ASCT for mantle cell lymphoma (MCL) has been investigated by several groups as a component of first-line therapy, and for patients with relapsed or refractory disease. Results of these studies are summarized in Table 55.5.[66–68] These series are variable with respect to previous treatment, high-dose regimen, and disease status at the time of transplant. Since some series did not include routine central histologic review, the reliability of diagnosis in some of the earlier studies is doubtful. The small patient numbers and heterogeneous populations limit comparisons with non-transplant series, particularly in view of the probable selection and reporting bias in these small series. There is no standard of care for the first-line therapy or second-line therapy of MCL, and therefore no regimen against which these results can be compared.

The use of high-dose therapy and ASCT as a component of first-line therapy in MCL has been evaluated in phase II and more recently phase III trials. The MD Anderson Cancer Center has reported results in patients treated with HyperCVAD (fractionated cyclophosphamide, doxorubicin, vincristine, and dexamethasone) alternating with high-dose methotrexate and cytarabine, followed by high-dose therapy with autologous or allogeneic SCT for responding patients.[69] Three-year EFS and OS rates of 72 percent and 92 percent, respectively, were reported. Whether the apparently encouraging results of this regimen are related to higher effectiveness of HyperCVAD, first-remission SCT, or patient selection is unclear.

A randomized trial from the European MCL Network has investigated the role of ASCT in first remission in MCL.[70] In this study 230 eligible patients with MCL were randomized to receive either 6 to 8 cycles of CHOP-like chemotherapy followed by IFNα maintenance, or 4 to 6

Table 55.5 Results of retrospective studies of high-dose therapy (HDT) and autologous stem cell transplantation (ASCT) for relapsed and refractory mantle cell lymphoma

Reference	n	EFS	OS	Follow-up
Vandenberghe et al.[66]	150	30%	48%	3
Freedman et al.[67]	28	31%	62%	4
Ganti et al.[68]	80	39%	47%	5
Khouri et al.[69]	20	17%	25%	N/A

EFS, event-free survival; OS, overall survival; N/A, not available.

cycles of CHOP-like chemotherapy followed by high-dose therapy with ASCT. Patients on the ASCT arm had longer PFS (median PFS 39 months vs 17 months for the conventional-dose arm, $P = 0.0108$), but no difference in overall survival. All survival analyses in this study were calculated from the date of completion of induction therapy, with no intent-to-treat analysis. None of the patients in this study received rituximab as a component of induction therapy, which also makes the results difficult to interpret in the current context.

Burkitt lymphoma and atypical Burkitt lymphoma

Transplant strategies have been evaluated in Burkitt lymphoma (BL) and atypical or Burkitt-like lymphoma as postinduction therapy and for the treatment of relapsed and refractory disease. Interpretation of results of ASCT in this disease is complicated by the varying classification of Burkitt lymphoma and, more recently, Burkitt-like or atypical Burkitt lymphoma. The largest series investigating the role of ASCT in these diseases was reported by the EBMT,[71] comprising a retrospective analysis of 117 patients with Burkitt and Burkitt-like lymphoma. The reported 3-year overall survival rate was 72 percent for patients undergoing ASCT in first complete remission. Since recent studies of dose-intensive first-line chemotherapy regimens for BL have reported superior results, there is no apparent role for ASCT in this setting.

The EBMT series reported a 37 percent 3-year overall survival rate for patients with BL transplanted in chemosensitive relapse. Previous reports from single centers using conventional-dose salvage therapy have shown very poor results in this situation, suggesting that ASCT should be considered standard of care for patients with chemosensitive relapse of their disease. For those with chemoresistant relapse, the 3-year overall survival rate was only 7 percent indicating that there is no role for a transplant approach in this setting.

Peripheral T cell lymphomas

The use of ASCT in patients with peripheral T cell lymphomas (PTCLs) has been reported in only a few, relatively

small series. Interpretation of these data is difficult in view of the heterogeneity of PTCL, and the relative rarity of these diseases. Vose et al. reported outcomes for 41 patients with recurrent aggressive NHL, of whom 17 had T cell disease.[72] No difference in 2-year OS or EFS was observed according to immunophenotype. Single-institution studies of ASCT for PTCL have reported results generally comparable to those reported for aggressive B cell lymphomas.[73,74] In a study from MD Anderson Cancer Center, 36 patients with relapsed or refractory PTCL underwent SCT (29 autologous and seven allogeneic SCT).[75] They reported 3-year OS and PFS rates of 36 percent and 28 percent, respectively. Comparable results were reported recently for 77 patients with PTCL undergoing ASCT either at relapse or in first remission. The 5-year actuarial OS and DFS were 49 percent and 44 percent, respectively. For those transplanted in first CR, the 5-year OS was 80 percent.

The use of ASCT in anaplastic large cell lymphoma has recently been reported from some groups.[76–78] For patients with anaplastic lymphoma kinase (ALK)-1-positive disease, high long-term DFS rates have been reported for patients transplanted in first remission. However, in view of the favorable prognosis of this disease, there is no clear role for ASCT as a component of first-line therapy. The use of ASCT in the salvage setting is recommended, although recent series have reported poor long-term DFS after ASCT for patients with ALK-1-negative disease.

A recent report of ASCT for PTCL from the Cleveland Clinic comprised 32 patients, 21 of whom had T anaplastic large cell lymphoma.[79] Median 5-year overall and relapse-free survival rates were 34 percent and 18 percent, respectively.

Overall, results in this disease suggest that the use of ASCT is associated with a poor outcome, and novel treatment approaches are needed.

Precursor T cell and B cell lymphoblastic leukemia/lymphoma

Autologous and allogeneic SCT have been used in first remission for patients with these diseases. Retrospective series from registries and single institutions have reported long-term OS rates of 50 percent to 80 percent for patients receiving SCT in first remission.[80–83] These results have been comparable to those reported for conventional chemotherapy protocols. A small randomized trial comparing ASCT with conventional chemotherapy in adult lymphoblastic lymphoma showed no OS advantage for the transplant arm.[84] For patients with relapsed or refractory disease after conventional-dose first-line therapy, ASCT produces long-term DFS in around 40 percent and 20 percent of patients, respectively.

Although these results are poor, they are superior to results reported for conventional-dose salvage regimens and the use of ASCT in this situation is widely regarded as a standard approach.

ALLOGENEIC STEM CELL TRANSPLANTATION IN LYMPHOMAS

Graft-versus-tumor effects in lymphoma

Allogeneic SCT has theoretical advantages compared with autologous SCT for patients with lymphoma. The risk of contamination of the donor bone marrow with malignant cells is eliminated and the donor marrow will not have been exposed to previous chemotherapy. The presence of a 'graft-versus-lymphoma effect' has, however, been the major stimulus to investigate the role of allogeneic SCT in these diseases.

Evidence for a graft-versus-lymphoma (GvL) effect in lymphoid malignancies has been largely anecdotal and includes the apparent effectiveness of reduction of immunosuppressive therapy,[85] responses to donor lymphocyte infusions,[86] and the reported responses to nonmyeloablative conditioning regimens with allogeneic SCT.[87]

Evidence for GvL effects in lymphoma is based partly on studies comparing autologous and allogeneic SCT. These have mostly been registry based, comparing matched patients undergoing allogeneic and autologous SCT, and have reported lower relapse rates in patients receiving allogeneic transplants, suggesting that GvL effects may account for this lower relapse rate. The lower relapse rates have often been accompanied by higher transplant-related mortality in allogeneic recipients, and overall survival has been comparable between the two groups.[88]

In a recent study from the IBMTR and EBMT[89] the outcome for patients undergoing syngeneic transplantation was compared with that for patients receiving allogeneic transplants (both T cell depleted and T cell replete). No differences in relapse, disease-free survival, or overall survival rates were seen in any NHL subtype. No evidence for a clinically significant GvL effect was observed.

Results of studies of allogeneic SCT in lymphoma are prone to major selection bias. The regimen-related mortality of allogeneic SCT has restricted its use primarily to patients below age 50 years. No studies have analyzed outcomes of allogeneic SCT by intent to treat. There is potential bias in transplant series to include only patients with sufficiently durable remissions to complete the donor selection and evaluation process, which can take several months. Patients with very aggressive disease may be 'selected out' by relapsing during that time.

Hodgkin lymphoma

Early studies using myeloablative regimens in patients with relapsed and refractory Hodgkin lymphoma, with related-donor transplants, reported high transplant-related mortality rates of approximately 50 percent to 60 percent (Table 55.6),[89–92] with long-term disease-free survival observed in 15 percent to 20 percent. Comparative analyses of allogeneic versus autologous SCT failed to show a survival advantage for allogeneic transplantation.

Recent studies have investigated the use of reduced-intensity allogeneic transplantation for patients with refractory and relapsed HL. In a study from MD Anderson Cancer Center, 40 patients with relapsed or refractory HL were treated with reduced-intensity conditioning followed by related ($n = 20$) or matched unrelated ($n = 20$) donor transplantation.[93] The median follow up was only 13 months but the 18-month actuarial PFS and OS were 32 percent and 61 percent, respectively.

The use of allogeneic SCT in HL should still be regarded as experimental and should only be performed in a clinical trial context.

Diffuse large B cell and other diffuse aggressive non–Hodgkin lymphomas

Very limited data exist assessing the role of allogeneic transplantation in these diseases. A study from the EBMT compared outcomes for patients with diffuse aggressive NHL undergoing allogeneic and autologous transplantation.[88] Although the study was case matched, only limited matching was possible and there was a higher proportion of patients with chemoresistant disease in the allogeneic population (31 percent vs 18 percent for the autologous group). No differences in disease-free or overall survival were observed. Data for the use of reduced-intensity conditioning regimens and allogeneic transplantation in these diseases are summarized in Table 55.7.[93–98]

In many cases, patients have been treated with these regimens after relapse or disease progression following

Table 55.6   Results of studies of allogeneic stem cell transplantation with myeloablative conditioning regimens in patients with relapsed and refractory Hodgkin lymphoma

Reference	n	TRM	DFS
Gajewski et al.[90]	100	61% at 3 years	15% at 3 years
Milpied et al.[91]	45	48% at 4 years	15% at 4 years
Anderson et al.[92]	53	49% at 5 years	18% at 5 years
Akpek et al.[93]	53	32% at 10 years	26% at 10 years

TRM, treatment-related mortality; DFS, disease-free survival.

Table 55.7   Results of studies of allogeneic stem cell transplantation with reduced-intensity conditioning regimens in diffuse large B cell lymphoma

Reference	n	TRM	PFS	OS
Nagler et al.[97]	8	63% at 2 years	13% at 2 years	13% at 2 years
Spitzer et al.[98]	20	0 at 100 days	25% (follow-up not provided)	N/A

TRM, treatment-related mortality; PFS, progression-free survival; OS, overall survival; N/A, not available.

autologous SCT. Interpretation of these studies is difficult since many pre-date the introduction of the Revised European American Lymphoma/World Health Organization (REAL/WHO) classification and the populations may be highly heterogeneous with respect to histologic subtype of aggressive NHL.

The use of allogeneic transplant strategies in DLBCL and other diffuse aggressive lymphomas should be considered experimental and limited to prospective clinical trials.

Indolent B cell non–Hodgkin lymphoma

Early studies of allogeneic transplantation in indolent NHL used myeloablative regimens in patients who were not considered eligible for autologous SCT mainly because of the presence of bone marrow involvement. Low relapse rates were observed in some of these studies but high treatment-related mortality was also reported such that overall survival rates were comparable with ASCT. A retrospective IBMTR study reported results for 904 patients with follicular NHL undergoing SCT between 1990 and 1999.[63] One hundred seventy six of these patients underwent allogeneic SCT with myeloablative regimens, and outcomes were compared with patients undergoing purged ($n = 131$) or unpurged ($n = 597$) autologous transplants. The 5-year relapse rate was lower in patients undergoing allogeneic SCT (21 percent) compared with ASCT (43 percent for purged ASCT and 58 percent for unpurged ASCT). However, the high treatment-related mortality in allogeneic recipients (30 percent at 5 years) resulted in comparable overall survival in all three groups (51 percent, 62 percent, and 55 percent, respectively, at 5 years).

A recently initiated study from the BMT Clinical Trials Network in the USA, comparing autologous SCT with reduced-intensity allogeneic SCT for patients with relapsed follicular lymphoma, will help to clarify the role of allogeneic SCT in this situation.

Published series of patients treated with myeloablative transplants for chronic lymphocytic leukemia (CLL) are summarized in Table 55.8.[99–101]

Table 55.8 Results of studies of allogeneic stem cell transplantation with myeloablative conditioning regimens in chronic lymphocytic leukemia

Reference	n	TRM	PFS	OS
Pavletic et al.[99]	23	17% at 100 days	62% at 5 years	65% at 5 years
Doney et al.[100]	25	N/A	N/A	32% at 5 years
Khouri et al.[101]	28	11% at 100 days	42% at 5 years	45% at 5 years

TRM, treatment-related mortality; PFS, progression-free survival; OS, overall survival; N/A, not available.

Encouraging outcomes have been reported from many of these series, although they have included selected, younger CLL patients. Further investigation of this approach is merited, although a recent report of the use of unrelated donor transplantation with myeloablative regimens in CLL suggests that the treatment-related mortality of this approach may be prohibitive.[102]

Mantle cell lymphoma

There is limited experience in the use of allogeneic SCT in MCL, partly because of the relative rarity and advanced median age of patients with this disease. A study from the EBMT reported 22 patients with a 2-year OS and PFS of 62 percent and 50 percent, respectively.[66] Khouri et al. reported similar results in 16 patients with a median age of 52 years undergoing donor transplants for relapsed or refractory MCL or, in five cases, for patients in first CR.[103]

The same group has reported experience with reduced-intensity transplantation in 18 patients with MCL.[104] Sibling donors were used for 13 of the patients, the rest receiving matched unrelated transplants. Progression-free survival was 82 percent at 3 years. Maris et al. recently reported experience with 33 patients with relapsed or refractory MCL undergoing related ($n = 16$) or unrelated ($n = 17$) donor transplants after reduced-intensity conditioning. Two-year PFS and OS rates were 60 percent and 64 percent, respectively.[105]

Other aggressive non–Hodgkin lymphoma subtypes

There are no comparative data that demonstrate a benefit for allogeneic compared with autologous SCT for patients with Burkitt, Burkitt-like, or lymphoblastic lymphoma.[106] Comparative studies have shown no survival benefit, and the clinically aggressive nature of these diseases suggests that they are unlikely to be susceptible to graft-versus-lymphoma effects. Very limited data are available for peripheral T cell lymphomas and cutaneous T cell lymphomas, and the use of allogeneic SCT for these diseases is still largely anecdotal.[107]

KEY POINTS

- High-dose therapy and autologous SCT is the standard of care for patients with relapsed and refractory Hodgkin lymphoma. Functional imaging is emerging as a prognostic factor which may allow selection of patients most likely to benefit from this approach

- There is no proven role for first remission transplantation in Hodgkin lymphoma, even in patients considered to be 'poor risk.'
- A single randomized trial has demonstrated that high-dose therapy and autologous SCT improves survival compared with conventional dose therapy in relapsed DLBCL.
- There is no proven role for high-dose therapy and autologous SCT in first remission in DLBCL, even in 'poor risk' patients.
- High-dose therapy and autologous SCT may induce long remissions in patients with relapsed follicular lymphoma but has no proven curative role.
- Although a graft-versus-lymphoma effect has been observed after allogeneic SCT in several lymphoma subtypes, this approach should still be considered experimental.

REFERENCES

● = Key primary paper
◆ = Major review article

1. Longo DL, Duffey PL, Young RC et al. Conventional-dose salvage combination chemotherapy in patients relapsing with Hodgkin's disease after combination chemotherapy: the low probability of cure. *J Clin Oncol* 1992; **10**: 210–18.
2. Bonfante V, Santoro A, Viviani S et al. Outcome of patients with Hodgkin's disease failing MOPP-ABVD. *J Clin Oncol* 1997; **15**: 528–34.
3. Canellos GP, Anderson JR, Propert KJ et al. Chemotherapy of advanced Hodgkin's disease with MOPP, ABVD or MOPP alternating with ABVD. *N Engl J Med* 1992; **327**: 1478–84.
4. Horning SJ, Chao NJ, Negrin RS et al. High-dose therapy and autologous hematopoietic progenitor cell transplantation for recurrent or refractory Hodgkin's disease: Analysis of the Stanford University results and prognostic indices. *Blood* 1997; **89**: 801–13.
5. Yuen AR, Rosenberg SA, Hoppe RT et al. Comparison between conventional salvage therapy and high-dose therapy with autografting for recurrent or refractory Hodgkin's disease. *Blood* 1997; **89**: 814–22.
6. Reece DE, Connors JM, Spinelli JJ et al. Intensive therapy with cyclophosphamide, carmustine, etoposide ± cisplatin, and autologous bone marrow transplantation for Hodgkin's disease in first relapse after combination chemotherapy. *Blood* 1994; **83**: 1193–9.
7. Chopra R, McMillan AK, Linch DC et al. The place of high-dose BEAM therapy and autologous bone marrow transplantation in poor-risk Hodgkin's disease. A single center eight-year study of 155 patients. *Blood* 1993; **81**: 1137–45.
8. Sweetenham JW, Taghipour G, Milligan D et al. High-dose therapy and autologous stem cell rescue for patients with Hodgkin's disease in first relapse after chemotherapy: results from the EBMT. *Bone Marrow Transplant* 1997; **20**: 745–52.
●9. Linch DC, Winfield D, Goldstone AH et al. Dose intensification with autologous bone marrow transplantation in relapsed and resistant Hodgkin's disease: results of a BNLI randomized trial. *Lancet* 1993; **341**: 1051–4.
●10. Schmitz N, Pfistner B, Sextro M et al. Aggressive conventional chemotherapy compared with high-dose chemotherapy with autologous haemopoietic stem-cell transplantation for relapsed chemosensitive Hodgkin's disease: a randomized trial. *Lancet* 2002; **359**: 2065–71.
11. Schmitz N, Haverkamp H, Josting A et al. Long term follow up in relapsed Hodgkin's disease (HD): Updated results of the HD-R1 study comparing conventional chemotherapy (cCT) to high-dose chemotherapy (HDCT) with autologous haemopoietic stem cell transplantation (ASCT) of the German Hodgkin's Study Group (GHSG) and the Working Party Lymphoma of the European Group for Blood and Marrow Transplantation (EBMT). *J Clin Oncol* 2005; **23**: 562s (abstract).
12. Horning SJ, Hoppe RT, Breslin S et al. Stanford V and radiotherapy for locally extensive and advanced Hodgkin's disease: mature results of a prospective clinical trial. *J Clin Oncol* 2002; **20**: 630–7.
13. Diehl V, Franklin J, Pfreundschuh M et al. Standard and increased-dose BEACOPP chemotherapy compared with COPP-ABVD for advanced Hodgkin's disease. *N Engl J Med* 2003; **348**: 2386–95.
14. Yahalom J, Gulati S, Toia M et al. Accelerated hyperfractionated total lymphoid irradiation, high-dose chemotherapy and autologous bone marrow transplantation for refractory and relapsing patients with Hodgkin's disease. *J Clin Oncol* 1993; **11**: 1062–70.
●15. Sweetenham JW, Carella AM, Taghipour G et al. High-dose therapy and autologous stem cell transplantation for adult patients with Hodgkin's disease who do not enter complete remission after induction chemotherapy: Results in 175 patients reported to the European Group for Blood and Marrow Transplantation. *J Clin Oncol* 1999; **17**: 3101–9.
●16. Lazarus HM, Rowlings PA, Zhang M-J et al. Autotransplants for Hodgkin's disease in patients never achieving remission: A report from the Autologous Blood and Marrow Transplant Registry. *J Clin Oncol* 1999; **17**: 534–45.
17. Gallamini A, Hutchings M, Rigacci L et al. Early interim 2-[18F]fluoro-2-deoxy-D-glucose positron emission tomography is prognostically superior to international prognostic score in advanced-stage Hodgkin's lymphoma: a report from a joint Italian-Danish study. *J Clin Oncol* 2007; **25**: 3746–52.

18. Wheeler C, Eickhoff C, Elias A *et al.* High-dose cyclophosphamide, carmustine and etoposide with autologous transplantation in Hodgkin's disease: A prognostic model for treatment outcomes. *Biol Blood Marrow Transplant* 1997; **3**: 98–106.

19. Bierman PJ, Lynch JC, Bociek RG *et al.* The International Prognostic Factors Project score for advanced Hodgkin's disease is useful for predicting outcome of autologous hematopoietic stem cell transplantation. *Ann Oncol* 2002; **13**: 1370–7.

20. Reece DE, Barnett MJ, Shepherd JD *et al.* High-dose cyclophosphamide, carmustine (BCNU), and etoposide (VP16-213) with or without cisplatin (CVB±P) and autologous transplantation for patients with Hodgkin's disease who fail to enter a complete remission after combination chemotherapy. *Blood* 1995; **86**: 451–6.

21. Josting A, Franklin J, May M *et al.* New prognostic score based on treatment outcome of patients with relapsed Hodgkin's lymphoma registered in the database of the German Hodgkin's lymphoma study group. *J Clin Oncol* 2002; **20**: 221–30.

22. Lavoie JC, Connors JM, Phillips GL *et al.* High-dose chemotherapy and autologous stem cell transplantation for primary refractory or relapsed Hodgkin lymphoma: long-term outcome in the first 100 patients treated in Vancouver. *Blood* 2005; **106**: 1473–8.

23. Moskowitz CH, Zelenetz AD, Nimer SD *et al.* Risk-adapted two-step high dose chemoradiotherapy salvage (ASCT (HDT) program for Hodgkin's disease. *Ann Oncol* 2002; **13**(Suppl 2): 62 (abstract).

24. Hasenclever D, Diehl V, Armitage JO *et al.* A prognostic score for advanced Hodgkin's disease. *N Engl J Med* 1998; **339**: 1506–14.

●25. Federico M, Bellei M, Brice P *et al.* High-dose therapy and autologous stem cell transplantation versus conventional therapy for patients with advanced Hodgkin's lymphoma responding to front-line therapy. *J Clin Oncol* 2003; **21**: 2320–5.

●26. Philip T, Guglielmi C, Hagenbeek A *et al.* Autologous bone marrow transplantation as compared with salvage chemotherapy in relapses of chemotherapy-sensitive non-Hodgkin's lymphoma. *N Engl J Med* 1995; **333**: 1540–5.

27. Coiffier B, Lepage E, Briere J *et al.* CHOP chemotherapy plus rituximab compared with CHOP alone in elderly patients with diffuse large B-cell lymphoma. *N Engl J Med* 2002; **346**: 235–42.

28. Pfreundschuh M, Trumper L, Kloess M *et al.* Two-weekly or 3-weekly CHOP chemotherapy with or without etoposide for the treatment of elderly patients with aggressive lymphomas: results of the NHL-B2 trial of the DSHNHL. *Blood* 2004; **104**: 634–41.

29. Vose JM, Bierman PJ, Lynch JC *et al.* Autologous transplant event-free survival (EFS) following failure of CHOP-rituximab (CHOP-R) for diffuse large B-cell lymphoma (DLBCL) is the same as the EFS following failure of CHOP alone. *Blood* 2004; **104**; 254a (abstract).

30. Thakkar S, Sweetenham JW, Rybicki L *et al.* Prior therapy with rituximab (R) in patients (pts) with diffuse large B-cell lymphoma (DLBCL) does not affect disease free survival (DFS) or overall survival (OS) following high dose therapy (HDT) and autologous stem cell transplantation (ASCT). *Blood* 2006; **108**: 869a (abstract).

31. Wilson WH, Porcu P, Hurd D *et al.* Phase II study of dose-adjusted EPOCH-R in untreated de novo CD20+ diffuse large B-cell lymphoma (DLBCL) – CALGB 50103. *J Clin Oncol* 2005; **23**: 567s (abstract).

32. Blay J-Y, Gomez F, Sebban C *et al.* The international prognostic index correlates to survival in patients with aggressive lymphoma in relapse: analysis of the PARMA trial. *Blood* 1998; **92**: 3562–8.

33. Hamlin PA, Zelenetz AD, Kewalramani T *et al.* Age-adjusted international prognostic index predicts autologous stem cell transplantation outcome for patients with relapsed or primary refractory diffuse large B-cell lymphoma. *Blood* 2003; **102**: 1989–96.

●34. Moskowitz CH, Zelenetz AD, Kewalramani T *et al.* Cell of origin, germinal center versus nongerminal center, determined by immunohistochemistry on tissue microarray, does not correlate with outcome in patients with relapsed and refractory DLBCL. *Blood* 2005; **106**: 3383–5.

●35. Haioun C, Lepage E, Gisselbrecht C *et al.* Survival benefit of high-dose therapy in poor risk aggressive non-Hodgkin's lymphoma: final analysis of the prospective LNH87-2 protocol – a groupe d'etudes des lymphomas de l'adulte study. *J Clin Oncol* 2000; **18**: 3025–30.

36. Santini G, Salvagno L, Leoni P *et al.* VACOP-B versus VACOP-B plus autologous bone marrow transplantation for advanced diffuse non-Hodgkin's lymphoma: Results of a prospective randomized trial by the non-Hodgkin's Lymphoma Co-operative Study Group. *J Clin Oncol* 1998; **18**: 2796–802.

37. Kluin-Nelemans HC, Zagonel V, Anastsopoulou A *et al.* Standard chemotherapy with or without high-dose chemotherapy for aggressive non-Hodgkin's lymphoma: randomized phase III EORTC study. *J Natl Cancer Inst* 2001; **93**: 22–30.

38. Gianni A, Bregni M, Siena S *et al.* High-dose chemotherapy and autologous bone marrow transplantation compared with MACOP-B in aggressive B-cell lymphoma. *N Engl J Med* 1997; **336**: 1290–7.

●39. Gisselbrecht C, Lepage E, Molina T *et al.* Shortened first-line high-dose chemotherapy for patients with poor-prognosis aggressive lymphoma. *J Clin Oncol* 2002; **20**: 2472–9.

●40. Haioun C, Lepage E, Gisselbrecht C *et al.* Comparison of autologous bone marrow transplantation with sequential chemotherapy for intermediate-grade and high-grade non-Hodgkin's lymphoma in first complete remission: A study of 464 patients. *J Clin Oncol* 1994; **12**: 2543–51.

41. Milpied N, Deconinck E, Gaillard F *et al.* Initial treatment of aggressive lymphoma with high-dose chemotherapy and autologous stem-cell support. *N Engl J Med* 2004; **350**: 1287–95.

42. Greb A, Schiefer DH, Bohlius J *et al.* High-dose chemotherapy with autologous stem cell support is not superior to conventional-dose chemotherapy in the first-line treatment of aggressive non-Hodgkin's lymphoma–Results of a comprehensive meta-analysis. *Blood* 2004; **104**: 263a (abstract).

43. Vose JM, Zhang M-J, Rowlings PA *et al.* Autologous transplantation for diffuse aggressive non-Hodgkin's lymphoma patients never achieving remission: a report from the Autologous Blood and Marrow Transplant Registry. *J Clin Oncol* 2001; **19**: 406–13.

44. Verdonck LF, van Putten WLJ, Hagenbeek A *et al.* Comparison of CHOP chemotherapy with autologous bone marrow transplantation for slowly responding patients with aggressive non-Hodgkin's lymphoma. *N Engl J Med* 1995; **332**: 1045–51.

45. Martelli M, Vignetti M, Zinzani P *et al.* High-dose chemotherapy followed by autologous bone marrow transplantation versus dexamethasone, cisplatin and cytarabine in aggressive non-Hodgkin's lymphoma with partial response to front-line chemotherapy: a prospective randomized Italian multicenter study. *J Clin Oncol* 1996; **14**: 534–42.

46. Kostakoglu L, Coleman M, Leonard JP *et al.* PET predicts prognosis after one cycle of chemotherapy in aggressive lymphoma and Hodgkin's disease. *J Nucl Med* 2002; **43**: 1018–27.

47. Haioun C, Itti E, Rahmouni A *et al.* [^{18}F]fluoro-2-deoxy-D-glucose positron emission tomography (FDG-PET) in aggressive lymphoma: an early prognostic tool for predicting patient outcome. *Blood* 2005; **106**: 1376–81.

48. Juweid ME, Wiseman GA, Vose JM *et al.* Response assessment of aggressive non-Hodgkin's lymphoma by integrated International Workshop Criteria and fluorine-18-fluorodeoxyglucose positron emission tomography. *J Clin Oncol* 2005; **23**: 4653–61.

49. Horning SJ, Negrin RS, Hoppe RT *et al.* High-dose therapy and autologous bone marrow transplantation for follicular lymphoma in first complete or partial remission: results of a phase II clinical trial. *Blood* 2001; **97**: 404–9.

50. Freedman AS, Gribben JG, Neuberg D *et al.* High-dose therapy and autologous bone marrow transplantation in patients with follicular lymphoma during first remission. *Blood* 1996; **88**: 2780–6.

51. Ladetto M, Corrandini P, Vallet S *et al.* High rate of clinical and molecular remissions in follicular lymphoma patients receiving high-dose sequential chemotherapy and autografting at diagnosis: a multicenter, prospective study by the Gruppo Italiano Trapianto Midollo Osseo (GITMO). *Blood* 2002; **100**: 1559–65.

52. Colombat P, Cornillet P, Deconinck E *et al.* Value of autologous stem cell transplantation with purged bone marrow as first line therapy for follicular lymphoma with high tumor burden: a GOELAMS phase II study. *Bone Marrow Transplant* 2000: **26**: 971–7.

53. Lenz G, Dreyling M, Schiegnitz E *et al.* Myeloablative radiochemotherapy followed by autologous stem cell transplantation in first remission prolongs progression-free survival in follicular lymphoma – results of a prospective randomized trial of the German Low-Grade Lymphoma Study Group. *Blood* 2004; **104**: 2667–74.

54. Sebban C, Belanger C, Brousse N *et al.* Comparison of CHVP + interferon with CHOP followed by autologous stem cell transplantation with a TBI conditioning regimen in untreated patients with high tumor burden follicular lymphoma: results of the randomized GELF94 trial (GELA Study Group). *Blood* 2003; **102**: 104a (abstract).

55. Deconinck E, Foussard C, Milpied N *et al.* High-dose therapy followed by autologous purged stem-cell transplantation and doxorubicin-based chemotherapy in patients with advanced follicular lymphoma: a randomized multicenter study by GOELAMS. *Blood* 2005; **105**: 3817–23.

56. Czuczman MS, Weaver R, Alkuzweny B *et al.* Prolonged clinical and molecular remission in patients with low-grade or follicular non-Hodgkin's lymphoma treated with rituximab plus CHOP chemotherapy: 9-year follow up. *J Clin Oncol* 2004; **22**: 4711–16.

57. Marcus R, Imrie K, Belch A *et al.* CVP chemotherapy plus rituximab compared with CVP as first-line treatment for advanced follicular lymphoma. *Blood* 2005; **105**: 1417–23.

58. Hainsworth JD, Burris HA 3rd, Morrissey LH *et al.* Rituximab monoclonal antibody as initial systemic therapy for patients with low grade non-Hodgkin's lymphoma. *Blood* 2000; **95**: 3052–6.

59. Kaminski MS, Tuck M, Estes J *et al.* ^{131}I-tositumomab therapy as initial treatment for follicular lymphoma. *N Engl J Med* 2005; **352**: 441–9.

60. Freedman AS, Neuberg D, Mauch P *et al.* Long-term follow up of autologous bone marrow transplantation in patients with relapsed follicular lymphoma. *Blood* 1999; **94**: 3325–33.

61. Bierman PJ, Vose JM, Anderson JR *et al.* High-dose therapy with autologous hematopoietic rescue for follicular low-grade non-Hodgkin's lymphoma. *J Clin Oncol* 1997; **15**: 445–50.

62. Apostolidis J, Gupta RK, Grenzelias D *et al.* High-dose therapy with autologous bone marrow support as consolidation of remission in follicular lymphoma: long-term clinical and molecular follow-up. *J Clin Oncol* 2000; **18**: 527–36.

63. Van Besien K, Loberiza FR, Bajorunaite R *et al.* Comparison of autologous and allogeneic hematopoietic stem cell transplantation for follicular lymphoma. *Blood* 2003; **102**: 3521–9.

●64. Rohatiner AZ, Nadler L, Davies AJ *et al.* Myeloablative therapy with autologous bone marrow transplantation for follicular lymphoma at the time of second or subsequent remission: long-term follow-up. *J Clin Oncol* 2007; **25**: 2554–9.

●65. Schouten HC, Qian W, Kvaloy S *et al.* High-dose therapy improves progression free survival and survival in relapsed follicular non-Hodgkin's lymphoma: results from the randomized European CUP trial. *J Clin Oncol* 2003; **21**: 3918–27.

66. Vandenberghe E, Ruiz de Elvira C, Loberiza FR *et al.* Outcome of autologous transplantation for mantle cell lymphoma: a study by the European Blood and Bone Marrow and Autologous Blood and Marrow Transplant Registries. *Br J Haematol* 2003; **120**: 793–800.

67. Freedman AS, Neuberg D, Gribben JG *et al.* High-dose chemoradiotherapy and anti-B-cell monoclonal antibody-purged autologous bone marrow transplantation in mantle cell lymphoma: no evidence for long-term remission. *J Clin Oncol* 1998; **16**: 13–18.

68. Ganti AK, Bierman PJ, Lynch JC *et al.* Hematopoietic stem cell transplantation in mantle cell lymphoma. *Ann Oncol* 2005; **16**: 618–24.

69. Khouri IF, Romaguera J, Kantarjian H *et al.* Hyper-CVAD and high-dose methotrexate/cytarabine followed by stem cell transplantation: an active regimen for aggressive mantle cell lymphoma. *J Clin Oncol* 1998; **16**: 3803–9.

●70. Dreyling M, Lenz G, Hoster E *et al.* Early consolidation by myeloablative radiochemotherapy in first remission significantly prolongs progression-free survival in mantle-cell lymphoma: results of a prospective randomized trial of the European MCL Network. *Blood* 2005; **105**: 2677–84.

71. Sweetenham JW, Pearce R, Taghipour G *et al.* Adult Burkitt's and Burkitt-like non-Hodgkin's lymphoma – outcome for patients treated with high-dose therapy and autologous stem cell transplantation in first remission or at relapse: results from the European group for Blood and Marrow Transplantation. *J Clin Oncol* 1996; **14**: 2465–72.

72. Vose JM, Peterson C, Bierman PJ *et al.* Comparison of high-dose therapy and autologous bone marrow transplantation for T-cell and B-cell non-Hodgkin's lymphomas. *Blood* 1990; **76**: 424–31.

73. Blystad AK, Enblad G, Kvaloy S *et al.* High-dose therapy with autologous stem cell transplantation in patients with peripheral T-cell lymphomas. *Bone Marrow Transplant* 2001; **27**: 711–16.

74. Rodriguez J, Caballero MD, Gutierrez A *et al.* High-dose chemotherapy and autologous stem cell transplantation in peripheral T-cell lymphoma: the GEL-TAMO experience. *Ann Oncol* 2003; **14**: 1768–75.

75. Rodriguez J, Munsell M, Yazji S *et al.* Impact of high-dose chemotherapy on peripheral T-cell lymphomas. *J Clin Oncol* 2001; **19**: 3766–70.

76. Fanin R, Silvestri F, Geromin A *et al.* Primary systemic CD30 (Ki-1)-positive anaplastic large cell lymphoma of the adult: sequential intensive treatment with F-MACHOP regimen (± radiotherapy) and autologous bone marrow transplantation. *Blood* 1996; **87**: 1243–8.

77. Deconinck E, Lamy T, Foussard C *et al.* Autologous stem cell transplantation for anaplastic large cell lymphomas: results of a prospective trial. *Br J Haematol* 2000; **109**: 736–42.

78. Zamkoff KW, Matulis MD, Mehta AC *et al.* High dose therapy and autologous stem cell transplantation does not

result in long term disease-free survival in patients with recurrent, chemosensitive ALK-negative anaplastic-large cell lymphoma. *Bone Marrow Transplant* 2004; **33**: 635–8.

79. Smith SD, Bolwell BJ, Rybicki LA *et al.* Autologous hematopoietic stem cell transplantation in peripheral T-cell lymphoma using a uniform high-dose regimen. *Bone Marrow Transplant* 2007; **40**: 239–43.

80. Bouabdallah R, Xerri L, Bardou V-J *et al.* Role of induction chemotherapy and bone marrow transplantation in adult lymphoblastic lymphoma: A report on 62 patients from a single center. *Ann Oncol* 1998; **9**: 619–25.

81. Jost LM, Jacky E, Dommann-Scherrer C *et al.* Short-term weekly chemotherapy followed by high dose therapy with autologous bone marrow transplantation for lymphoblastic and Burkitt's lymphomas in adult patients. *Ann Oncol* 1995; **6**: 445–51.

82. Verdonck LF, Dekker AW, deGast GC *et al.* Autologous bone marrow transplantation for adult poor risk lymphoblastic lymphoma in first remission. *J Clin Oncol* 1992; **4**: 644–6.

83. Sweetenham JW, Liberti G, Pearce R *et al.* High-dose therapy and autologous bone marrow transplantation for adult patients with lymphoblastic lymphoma: Results from the European Group for Bone Marrow Transplantation. *J Clin Oncol* 1994; **12**: 1358–65.

●84. Sweetenham JW, Santini G, Qian W *et al.* High-dose therapy and autologous stem-cell transplantation versus conventional dose consolidation/maintenance therapy as post-remission therapy for adult patients with lymphoblastic lymphoma: Results of a randomized trial of the European Group for Blood and Marrow Transplantation and the United Kingdom Lymphoma Group. *J Clin Oncol* 2001; **19**: 2927–36.

85. van Besien K, De Lima M, Giralt S *et al.* Management of lymphoma recurrence after allogeneic transplantation: the relevance of the graft-versus-lymphoma effect. *Bone Marrow Transplant* 1997; **19**: 977–82.

86. Rondon G, Giralt S, Huh Y *et al.* Graft-versus-leukemia after allogeneic bone marrow transplantation for chronic lymphocytic leukemia. *Bone Marrow Transplant* 1996; **18**: 669–72.

87. Escalon MP, Champlin RE, Saliba RM *et al.* Non-myeloablative allogeneic hematopoietic transplantation: a promising salvage therapy for patients with non-Hodgkin's lymphoma whose disease has failed a prior autologous transplant. *J Clin Oncol* 2004; **22**: 2419–23.

●88. Peniket AJ, Ruiz de Elvira MC, Taghipour G *et al.* An EBMT registry matched study of allogeneic stem cell transplants for lymphoma: allogeneic transplantation is associated with a lower relapse rate but a higher procedure-related mortality rate than autologous transplantation. *Bona Marrow Transplant* 2003; **31**: 667–78.

●89. Bierman PJ, Sweetenham JW, Loberiza FR *et al.* Syngeneic hematopoietic stem cell transplantation for non-Hodgkin's lymphoma: A comparison with allogeneic and autologous transplantation. *J Clin Oncol* 2003; **21**: 3744–53.

90. Gajewski JL, Phillips GL, Sobconski KA *et al.* Bone marrow transplants from HLA-identical siblings in advanced Hodgkin's disease. *J Clin Oncol* 1996; **14**: 572–8.

91. Milpied N, Fielding AK, Pearce R *et al.* Allogeneic bone marrow transplant is not better than autologous transplant for patients with relapsed Hodgkin's disease. *J Clin Oncol* 1996; **14**: 1291–6.

92. Anderson JE, Litzow MR, Appelbaum FR *et al.* Allogeneic syngeneic and autologous marrow transplantation for Hodgkin's disease: the 21-year Seattle experience. *J Clin Oncol* 1993; **11**: 2342–50.

93. Akpek G, Ambinder RF, Piantodosi S *et al.* Long-term results of blood and marrow transplantation for Hodgkin's lymphoma. *J Clin Oncol* 2001; **19**: 4314–21.

●94. Anderlini P, Saliba R, Acholonu S *et al.* Reduced-intensity allogeneic stem cell transplantation in relapsed and refractory Hodgkin's disease: low transplant-related mortality and impact of intensity of conditioning regimen. *Bone Marrow Transplant* 2005; **35**: 943–51.

95. Dhedin N, Giraudier S, Gaulard P *et al.* Allogeneic bone marrow transplantation in aggressive non-Hodgkin's lymphoma (excluding Burkitt and lymphoblastic lymphoma): a series of 73 patients from the SFGM database. Societe Francaise de Graffe de Moelle. *Br J Haematol* 1999; **107**: 154–61.

96. Chopra R, Goldstone AH, Pearce R *et al.* Autologous versus allogeneic transplantation for non-Hodgkin's lymphoma: a case-controlled analysis of the European Bone Marrow Transplant Group registry data. *J Clin Oncol* 1992; **10**: 1690–95.

97. Nagler A, Slavin S, Varadi G *et al.* Allogeneic peripheral blood stem cell transplantation using a fludarabine-based low intensity conditioning regimen for malignant lymphoma. *Bone Marrow Transplant* 2000; **25**: 1021–8.

98. Spitzer TR, McAfee SL, Dey BR *et al.* Durable progression free survival (PFS) following non-myeloablative bone marrow transplantation (BMT) for chemorefractory diffuse large B cell lymphoma (B-LCL) *Blood* 2001; **98**: 672a (abstract).

99. Pavletic ZS, Arrowsmith ER, Bierman PJ *et al.* Outcome of allogeneic stem cell transplantation for B cell chronic lymphocytic leukemia. *Bone Marrow Transplant* 2000; **25**: 717–22.

100. Doney KC, Chauncey T, Appelbaum FR. Allogeneic related donor hematopoietic stem cell transplantation for treatment of chronic lymphocytic leukemia. *Bone Marrow Transplant* 2002; **29**: 817–23.

101. Khouri IF, Keating MJ, Saliba RM, Champlin RE. Long-term follow-up of patients with CLL treated with allogeneic hematopoietic transplantation. *Cytotherapy* 2002; **4**: 217–21.

102. Pavletic SZ, Khouri IF, Haagenson M *et al.* Unrelated donor marrow transplantation for B-cell chronic lymphocytic leukemia after myeloablative conditioning: results from the Center for International Blood and Marrow Transplant Research. *J Clin Oncol* 2005; **23**: 5788–94.

103. Khouri IF, Lee MS, Romaguera J *et al.* Allogeneic hematopoietic transplantation for mantle cell lymphoma: molecular remissions and evidence of graft-versus-malignancy. *Ann Oncol* 1999; **10**: 1293–9.

104. Khouri IF, Lee MS, Saliba RM *et al.* Non-ablative allogeneic stem-cell transplantation for advanced/recurrent mantle cell lymphoma. *J Clin Oncol* 2003; **21**: 4407–12.

105. Maris MB, Sandmaier BM, Storer BE *et al.* Allogeneic hematopoietic cell transplantation after fludarabine and 2 Gy total body irradiation for relapsed and refractory mantle cell lymphoma. *Blood* 2004; **104**: 3535–42.

106. Levine JE, Harris RE, Loberiza FR *et al.* A comparison of allogeneic and autologous bone marrow transplantation for lymphoblastic lymphoma. *Blood* 2003; **101**: 2476–82.

107. Corradini P, Dodero A, Zallio F *et al.* Graft-versus-lymphoma effect in relapsed peripheral T-cell non-Hodgkin's lymphomas after reduced-intensity conditioning followed by allogeneic transplantation of hematopoietic cells. *J Clin Oncol* 2004; **22**: 2172–6.

56

Management of lymphoid neoplasia during pregnancy

IRFAN MAGHFOOR AND ADNAN EZZAT

Although cancer is the leading cause of death in females of childbearing age,[1] there is no evidence that incidence of cancers is higher during pregnancy. The incidence of cancer in pregnancy is estimated to be about 0.1 percent or approximately 1 in 1000 pregnancies.[2,3] The most common malignancies diagnosed during pregnancy are those of breast, cervix, lymphoma, leukemia, cervix, ovary, and thyroid.[4,5] Since most of the literature regarding cancer in pregnancy exists in the form of case reports, case series, or literature reviews, the important questions of effects of maternal cancer or effects of staging studies and therapy on fetus are not clearly answered. Whether pregnancy alters presentation, course, or prognosis of cancer in the mother is also largely unclear.

Various issues complicate this situation of maternal-fetal conflict where maternal interest may lie in immediate termination of pregnancy, while continuation of pregnancy is in the best interest of fetus, thus causing delay in institution of appropriate therapy resulting in an adverse outcome for the mother. The issue of pregnancy adversely affecting the prognosis of cancer remains unsettled[6,7] with some authors reporting no adverse outcome of the maternal cancer diagnosed during pregnancy[8] while others report a higher incidence of malignancies with poor prognostic features during pregnancy.[9,10]

The ethical and moral issues surrounding this complicated situation are largely unclear and may differ among cultures, religions, and even among physicians. Legal status of the fetus as a separate human is yet to be clearly defined. Despite all these difficulties, it is the professional and ethical responsibility of the treating physician to closely involve the mother in the decision-making process. While it is important to ensure that the maternal cancer is diagnosed and treated in the most expeditious way, it is equally important to remember the safety of the fetus. In this regard, the knowledge of potential harmful effects of continued presence of uncontrolled malignancy in the mother, various diagnostic and staging procedures, pharmacokinetics of pregnancy, and finally the effect of the various treatment modalities – particularly those of chemotherapeutic agents on the fetus – is of utmost importance before a decision regarding management of the pregnancy and that of malignancy is made. It is imperative that a multidisciplinary approach is adopted where obstetrician, medical and radiation oncologists, social workers, and ethicist (where available) are all involved along with the mother in the decision-making process so that legal and moral rights of both the mother and fetus are protected.[11]

LYMPHOMA IN PREGNANCY

Lymphoproliferative disorders including Hodgkin and non-Hodgkin lymphomas constitute the fourth most common malignancy diagnosed during pregnancy.[12] The incidence of Hodgkin lymphoma during pregnancy is at best uncertain but has been estimated to range from 1 in 1000 to 1 in 6000 pregnancies.[5,13] The incidence of non-Hodgkin lymphoma complicating pregnancy is unknown. Among women of childbearing age, the incidence of Hodgkin and non-Hodgkin lymphoma is similar at 2–6 per 100 000 for Hodgkin lymphoma and 1–8 per 100 000 for non-Hodgkin lymphoma.[13] While the peak incidence of Hodgkin lymphoma is at 20 years of age, that of non-Hodgkin lymphoma occurs at an older age and steadily increases with advancing age. With the rising incidence of non-Hodgkin lymphoma during recent past decades, as well as increasing maternal age at first pregnancy, it is anticipated that the coexistence of non-Hodgkin lymphoma and pregnancy is likely to increase.[12,13]

HODGKIN LYMPHOMA

Although it is thought that presentation of Hodgkin lymphoma during pregnancy may not differ significantly from that in the nonpregnant state,[14–16] studies have reported a higher proportion of advanced stage disease at diagnosis among pregnant females compared to nonpregnant women, suggesting a possible masking of the early symptoms and signs of lymphoma by pregnancy.[14] A Swedish study has recently reported a lower-than-expected incidence during pregnancy and a higher-than-expected incidence in the first 6 months postpartum, again suggesting a masking effect by pregnancy.[16]

Conversely, several studies have reported that pregnancy had no influence on outcome of Hodgkin lymphoma, and vice versa.[17,18] In an older study, Barry et al. reported on a series of 84 pregnant women with Hodgkin lymphoma and found no influence of pregnancy on outcome of Hodgkin lymphoma with regard to response rates and survival when compared to nonpregnant women with the same lymphoma.[17] The studies by Barry et al. and Hennessey and Rottino did not find any survival difference among women who underwent therapeutic abortion and those who did not.[17,18] Similar conclusions have been reported in more recent studies.[14,19] A study by Lishner et al. reported on 50 pregnancies in 48 patients and compared them with a control group matched for age, stage, and year of diagnosis. Twenty-two were diagnosed with Hodgkin lymphoma before or during pregnancy and 27 after delivery or termination of pregnancy (data were not available on one pregnancy). No statistically significant difference was identified in stage at diagnosis or outcome of maternal malignancy and that of pregnancy between these women and the control group.[15]

A study by Gelb et al. reported the outcome of 17 pregnancies associated with Hodgkin lymphoma.[20] The diagnosis of Hodgkin lymphoma was made at a median of 24 weeks (range 4–30 weeks) of gestation. Only three patients were diagnosed during the first trimester. Three patients had therapeutic abortions and one had spontaneous abortion, while three women delivered before start of therapy. Ten patients received radiation therapy either alone or as part of combined modality therapy, while nine patients received chemotherapy either alone or with radiation therapy. The timing of chemotherapy was not specified except in those who had either had an abortion or had delivered. No fetal malformations were identified. There were three premature deliveries. At a median follow-up of 35 months (range 6–79 months) 15 of the 17 women were in continued remission.

In a large review of the literature, Ebert et al. identified 24 women with Hodgkin lymphoma diagnosed during pregnancy.[21] Fifteen of these women who received combination chemotherapy consisting of COPP (cyclophosphamide, vincristine, procarbazine, and prednisone; $n = 1$), MOPP (nitrogen mustard, vincristine, procarbazine, and prednisone; $n = 4$), ABVD (adriamycin, bleomycin, vinblastine, and dacarbazine; $n = 7$), or MOPP/ABV ($n = 3$) beginning in the first ($n = 5$), second ($n = 8$), and third ($n = 2$) trimester delivered normal offspring who were healthy at a median follow-up of 9 years (range 0–17 years). Nine other women had adverse outcomes of their pregnancies after receiving chemotherapy and/or radiation therapy during pregnancy. Three women underwent therapeutic abortion after starting therapy with chemotherapy and/or radiation therapy in the first trimester. All three fetuses had multiple congenital anomalies. One woman had a therapeutic abortion at 15 weeks of gestation after initiation of ABVD chemotherapy. Two women had spontaneous abortion after starting therapy in the first trimester. One of these fetuses had multiple anomalies. Two women delivered after initiating chemotherapy in the first trimester. One delivered an infant with hydrocephalus who died 4 hours after birth and the other delivered an infant with multiple anomalies. Finally, a woman who received chemotherapy beginning in week 25 of gestation delivered an infant with atrial septal defect who died 2 days after birth. It is thus obvious that administration of antineoplastic therapy for Hodgkin lymphoma during the first trimester of pregnancy carries a grave prognosis for the developing fetus.

Spread to placenta or fetus of maternal Hodgkin lymphoma is rare and only two cases have been reported.[12] In one of these there was placental involvement by Hodgkin lymphoma with delivery of a normal infant, while the other case was that of possible fetal spread of maternal Hodgkin lymphoma.[22]

NON-HODGKIN LYMPHOMA

Most patients who develop non-Hodgkin lymphoma during pregnancy have aggressive histologies and present with advanced stage disease.[13,23] This could be due to delay in diagnosis caused by masking of the early symptoms of lymphoma by pregnancy or, conversely, may be due to the biology of lymphoma in younger patients. Moore and Taslimi in their review of 37 patients noted that the majority of the patients presented with unusual features and a delay in diagnosis.[24] Extranodal sites were involved by lymphoma in 28 of these women. A correct diagnosis was established at a median of 17 days after presentation and in 20 percent of these women there were delays of more than 3 months before a correct diagnosis was established. Another interesting finding in this review was of an unusually high incidence of involvement of breast, ovary, uterus, and cervix by lymphoma.[25–30] Although the mechanism for this predilection for the lymphoma to involve these sites in pregnant women is not understood, it is thought to be either due to increased blood flow to these organs during pregnancy or hormonal changes of pregnancy.[13]

Although it has been thought that spread of maternal non-Hodgkin lymphoma to placenta and fetus is as uncommon as for Hodgkin lymphoma,[13] recent reports suggest that it occurs more frequently compared to Hodgkin lymphoma.[31–36] Vertical transmission of maternal lymphoma to the fetus has been clearly documented in two cases,[37,38] one of these being a natural killer T cell lymphoma[37] while the other was a B cell non-Hodgkin lymphoma.[38] This fact should, therefore, be clearly considered when management is being planned for maternal non-Hodgkin lymphoma.

The effect of maternal non-Hodgkin lymphoma on outcome of pregnancy is unclear. It has been suggested that the presence of lymphoma may adversely affect the outcome of pregnancy due mainly to maternal death caused by lymphoma.[23] Conversely, others have concluded no increased rates of spontaneous abortions or premature birth in pregnant women diagnosed with non-Hodgkin lymphoma.[3,39] Similarly, what effect pregnancy might have on the presentation, course, and prognosis of lymphoma is unknown. While some reports suggest essentially no effect of pregnancy on the course of lymphoma, others have reported a relatively stable course during pregnancy followed by a rapidly worsening course after delivery, suggesting that hormonal changes of pregnancy may somehow stabilize the lymphoma.[13,23,40]

Approximately 100 cases of non-Hodgkin lymphoma occurring during pregnancy have been reported by Pohlman et al.[41] Diffuse large B cell or immunoblastic histology accounted for 36 percent of these. The rest were small noncleaved cell (23 percent), lymphoblastic (11 percent), or diffuse small-cleaved cell or diffuse mixed (10 percent) histologies. Histologic subtype was unknown in 20 percent of cases. Despite limited staging workup, 60 percent of cases were found to have advanced stage, i.e., stage III or IV, while stage was not known in 20 percent of cases.[13] This may represent an underestimation of advanced presentation of non-Hodgkin lymphoma associated with pregnancy due to the limited staging workup.

Outcome was known for 90 women: only 39 were disease-free at a median of 21 months of follow-up, four were alive with disease, and 47 had died at a median of 6 months after delivery.[13] The prognosis was particularly adverse in patients with Burkitt lymphoma, with only one patient out of 19 remaining alive after being diagnosed with stage I disease in the third trimester and receiving a bone marrow transplant. Prognosis was better in those who were diagnosed in the third trimester compared to the first and second trimester and in those who presented with early stage compared to advanced disease.[13] The prognosis did not seem to be better for those who initiated therapy during pregnancy compared to those in whom therapy was delayed until after delivery. Another histologic subtype that appears to be associated with poor prognosis when diagnosed during pregnancy is T cell/natural killer cell lymphoma. In a report of four patients diagnosed with T cell/natural killer cell lymphoma during pregnancy, three mothers died within 6.5 months of diagnosis and only one was alive at a follow-up of 17 months.[40] Aviles et al. have reported outcome of pregnancy and lymphoma in 19 pregnancies.[42] All patients received anthracycline-based therapy including eight who received chemotherapy in the first trimester. Three mothers and their babies died during induction. Sixteen of these 19 patients delivered normal, healthy infants either spontaneously or by cesarean section. Eight of these sixteen mothers were in complete remission 4–9 years after delivery, while seven died of lymphoma and one was lost to follow-up.

Long-term follow-up of the babies has been reported separately and 15 of these babies were alive and healthy at 3–11 years after delivery.[43] One had died at 5 years of age in an automobile accident. None of the offspring developed leukemia or other malignancies and they were reported to have normal learning abilities and educational performance. Based on these findings, the authors recommend full-dose combination chemotherapy even during first trimester of pregnancy when cure is the likely outcome.[43]

STAGING

Staging workup for both non-Hodgkin and Hodgkin lymphoma includes a completed history and physical examination, chest x-ray, computed tomographic scans of chest, abdomen, and pelvis, bone marrow aspiration and biopsy, and in the case of Hodgkin lymphoma a functional imaging study like gallium scan or, more recently, positron emission tomography (PET).[44] In the past, bipedal lymphangiography has been used extensively in the staging evaluation of Hodgkin lymphoma, with a reported accuracy of up to 90 percent.[45] It is, however, rarely performed these days since it is technically cumbersome and difficult to interpret. In addition, several groups have reported that it may not provide any additional information over a computed tomography (CT) scan,[46,47] Sombeck et al. from the University of Florida also concluded that gallium scan might not provide additional staging information over a CT scan. It is, however, well recognized that a gallium scan or PET scan may predict treatment failure or detect recurrence in addition to being helpful in cases where CT findings are equivocal. These scans can therefore be safely excluded in the staging workup of a pregnant female.

The initial staging workup of a nonpregnant female should include a complete history and physical examination, chest x-ray, CT scans of chest, abdomen, and pelvis, bone marrow aspirates, and trephine biopsy. In pregnant females, staging workup (Table 56.1) should include a two-view chest x-ray performed with abdominal shielding with negligible exposure of the fetus. Because of the potential radiation hazard to the fetus, CT scans, lymphangiography, and radioisotope scans (i.e., gallium and PET scans) are contraindicated.[44] For completion of staging, magnetic resonance imaging (MRI) of chest, abdomen, and pelvis

Table 56.1 Recommendations for evaluation of newly diagnosed lymphoma patients with and without pregnancy

	Nonpregnant	Pregnant
Confirmation of diagnosis		
Must include excision of a lymph node with interpretation by an expert hematopathologist including immunophenotyping	Mandatory	Mandatory
General overview		
Careful history with special emphasis on history of B symptoms,[a] history of pruritis in case of Hodgkin lymphoma, and physical examination with special emphasis on lymph node–bearing areas, size of liver and spleen	Mandatory	Mandatory
Laboratory studies		
Complete blood counts, serum chemistries to include liver and kidney function tests, serum lactate dehydrogenase, erythrocyte sedimentation rate, serum albumin, alkaline phosphatase	Mandatory	Mandatory
Radiologic evaluation		
Chest x-ray	Mandatory	If shielding available
CT scan of chest	Mandatory	No[b]
CT scan of addomen and pelvis	Mandatory	No[b]
US abdomen	Not needed	Mandatory
MRI scan replace US	Not needed	May
Gallium/PET	If indicated	No[b]
Bone marrow aspiraton and trephine biopsy	Mandatory	Mandatory

[a]B symptoms include unexplained weight loss of greater than 10% of baseline body weight, drenching night sweats, and fever of greater than 101°F.
[b]Contraindicated due to fetal exposure to ionizing radiation.
CT, computed tomography; US, ultrasound; MRI, magnetic resonance imaging; PET, positron emission tomography.

can be performed with no danger to the fetus.[48] It has the added advantage of assessing the bone marrow and splenic involvement that may be undetectable on CT scan.[49] These are, however, expensive techniques and may not be readily available. Gross disease in the abdomen can be identified with an ultrasound scan and cardiac function may be assessed with an echocardiogram rather than radionuclide scans.

RADIATION THERAPY DURING PREGNANCY

At the cellular level, the effects of ionizing radiation range from no harmful effect to mutagenesis, carcinogenesis, and cell death. In humans, harmful effects of *in utero* exposure to ionizing radiation depend on dose as well as stage of fetal development. Greskovich and Macklis, in their excellent review, point out that effects of ionizing radiation on a developing fetus may include (1) prenatal or neonatal death, (2) congenital anomalies, (3) severe mental retardation, (4) temporary or permanent growth retardation, (5) carcinogenesis, (6) sterility, and (7) germ cell mutations (Table 56.2).[50]

Ionizing radiation exposure between 0 and 3 weeks postconception may not result in severe congenital anomalies but a majority of the embryos may be aborted or resorbed.[12,50,51] Severe congenital anomalies result from ionizing radiation exposure between 4 and 11 weeks postconception, while radiation exposure between 11 and 16 weeks postconception results in few anomalies of eyes and skeletal and genital organs, as well as microcephaly and mental retardation.[51] Radiation exposure between 16 and 20 weeks postconception may result in mild microcephaly, mental retardation, and stunted growth. Radiation exposure after 30 weeks may not cause any structural abnormalities but may result in functional anomalies, i.e., sterility as well as genetic defects and/or malignancies.[12]

Current radiobiology data available from animal studies, as well as other studies, place a fetal exposure threshold

Table 56.2 Adverse effects of *in utero* exposure to ionizing radiation according to stage of fetal development

Effect	Stage of fetal development	Gestational age
Prenatal death	Preimplantation	Day 0 to day 8
Neonatal death	Organogenesis	Day 9 to week 8
Congenital anomalies	Organogenesis	Day 9 to week 8
Severe mental retardation	Fetal stage (early to mid fetal)	Week 8 to week 25
Permanent growth retardation	Fetal stage	Week 9 to term
Temporary growth retardation	Organogenesis	Day 9 to week 8
Carcinogenesis	Organogenesis/fetal	Day 9 to term
Sterility	Fetal (late fetal)	Week 26 to term
Germ cell mutations	Fetal (late fetal)	Week 26 to term

at 10 cGy.[12,52] Should radiation therapy become necessary in a pregnant woman, it is important to estimate the fetal dose before start of therapy.[53–55] The predicted growth of the fetus during the period of radiation exposure must also be taken into account. Fetal dose can be further reduced by modifications in radiation technique as well as application of appropriate shielding, but at all costs must be calculated to be below the threshold value of 10 cGy.

CHEMOTHERAPY DURING PREGNANCY

The majority of cancer chemotherapy drugs interfere with cell division and kill rapidly dividing cells. This is accomplished via a variety of mechanisms that may include alteration of DNA, RNA, protein synthesis or function, and assembly of microtubules leading to arrest of cell division or cell death. The majority of these agents are nonspecific and in addition to their effect on cancer cells may damage normal tissues. Normal tissues most susceptible to the deleterious effects of antineoplastic agents are rapidly dividing cells of the bone marrow, lining of the gastrointestinal tract, and hair follicles. Since the fetus is composed of rapidly diving cells, its development can be severely affected by exposure to these agents.

PHARMACOKINETICS IN PREGNANCY

Several physiologic changes occur during pregnancy that may alter the efficacy and safety of antineoplastic agents. In addition, placenta and fetus may take part in drug elimination. The biochemical structure of the drug may or may not facilitate entry of drug into the fetal circulation. All these effects may lead to hazardous exposure of the fetus to antineoplastic drugs or their metabolites.[11]

Plasma volume expansion during pregnancy[56,57] leads not only to dilution of the drug but also results in increased volume of distribution and may result in changes in efficacy as well as toxicity.[58] In addition, serum albumin concentration decreases leading to an increase in the concentration of free and active drugs that are normally protein bound, leading to an increase in their biologic effect.[59] Hepatic metabolism and renal excretion are both enhanced during pregnancy leading to alterations in drug metabolism and excretion.[58,60,61] Late in pregnancy, the expanding uterus may cause slowing of gastric emptying leading to altered bioavailability of antineoplastic agents. These physiologic changes of pregnancy may alter the drug metabolism, excretion, and efficacy resulting in potentially deleterious effects on the developing fetus.[11]

The placenta acts as a barrier to passage of harmful substances from the maternal circulation to the fetus. In addition, the placenta may also be the site of metabolism as well as route of excretion for some of these agents. Drugs that have low molecular weight, are highly lipid soluble, and are loosely bound to plasma proteins may easily cross the placenta and enter the fetal circulation.[58–60]

Fetal liver and kidneys are immature and therefore metabolism and elimination of drugs may be abnormal in the fetus. In addition, amniotic fluid may act as physiologic third space where drugs such as methotrexate may accumulate resulting in prolonged fetal exposure.[62] Once inside the fetal circulation, drugs may be excreted in the urine into the amniotic fluid and ingested by the fetus again, thereby prolonging the exposure of the fetus to potentially harmful effects of chemotherapeutic agents.

EFFECTS OF CHEMOTHERAPY ON THE DEVELOPING FETUS

The deleterious effects of exposure to antineoplastic therapy on the developing fetus are critically dependent upon the stage of fetal development at the time of exposure.[11,63–67] During the initial stages of gestation from conception to implantation of the embryo in the uterus, exposure to chemotherapeutic agents probably results in an 'all-or-nothing' phenomenon. This means that the embryo will either abort or may develop normally.[11] During the period of organogenesis (first trimester) when all major organs and organ systems are developing, exposure to antineoplastic therapy may result in severe teratogenic effects or result in abortion. The majority of the congenital malformations observed after chemotherapy administered during pregnancy result from fetal exposure during this period. Although most organ systems are fully developed by the end of the first trimester, the central nervous system, eyes, and respiratory system continue to develop throughout gestation and may be vulnerable to the effects of chemotherapy. In the second and third trimesters, the majority of the organ systems continue to grow and mature. Exposure to cancer chemotherapy during this period may result in growth retardation and low birth weight (Table 56.3).

Table 56.3 Adverse effects of chemotherapeutic agents on the developing fetus

Immediate

First trimester exposure	Second trimester and later exposure
Spontaneous abortion	Spontaneous abortion
Congenital anomalies	Premature birth
Premature birth	Low birth weight
	Organ toxicity
	Pancytopenia

Delayed

Retarded mental development
Retarded physical development
Sterility
Carcinogenesis
Gene mutations
Second-generation carcinogenesis

Although teratogenic effects of cancer chemotherapy are well documented in animals, it is not always possible to extrapolate from animal data since drugs that are harmless to animals may be teratogenic in humans, and vice versa. A well-known example is that of thalidomide, which appears harmless in animals but has been clearly documented to cause fetal anomalies in humans. Conversely, aspirin appears harmless in humans but may be teratogenic in animals.[11]

The consequences of cancer chemotherapy on the fetus may depend upon dose and schedule of administration, gestational age at the time of exposure, duration of chemotherapy, as well as the type of chemotherapy used. Additional factors that can affect fetal development may include maternal immune suppression from chemotherapy leading to infection in the fetus, as well as nutritional deficiencies resulting from anorexia, nausea, and vomiting during pregnancy. In addition, synergistic teratogenic interactions may occur with combination chemotherapy[67] as well as with combination of chemotherapy and radiation therapy.[68] Individual and genetic susceptibility may be other important determinants of teratogenic effects of antineoplastic agents.[69] All these factors need to be taken into account when chemotherapy is to be delivered during pregnancy and an individualized and multidisciplinary approach is essential.

MANAGEMENT

Appropriate management of lymphomas requires complete staging workup, which includes a thorough history and physical examination, histologic confirmation of diagnosis with immunohistochemistry as well as cytogenetic and molecular studies where needed, bone marrow aspiration and biopsy, and CT scans of chest, abdomen, and pelvis. Additional investigations may include gallium or PET scans and/or lumbar puncture with cerebrospinal fluid cytologic analysis, depending upon clinical situation. In a pregnant female, the majority of these staging procedures cannot be

Table 56.4 Important issues to be addressed in a pregnant female with malignancy

Maternal issues

Stage of maternal cancer
Optimal therapy for maternal cancer
Prognosis for mother with optimal therapy if instituted immediately
Prognosis for mother in case of delaying optimal therapy
Social, cultural, and religious beliefs of mother

Fetal issues

Stage of fetal development
Prognosis for fetus if immediate delivery was carried out
Effect of maternal cancer on fetus
Effect of therapy (chemotherapy and/or radiation therapy) on fetus
Methods to enhance fetal maturity if available
Monitoring facilities for fetus and neonate
Optimum time and method of delivery

carried out due to risk of fetal exposure to ionizing radiation. The staging should therefore be limited to history and physical examination, a chest x-ray with abdominal shielding, and an ultrasound scan of the abdomen. Magnetic resonance imaging scans of chest, abdomen, and pelvis can be carried out for complete staging workup without risk of fetal exposure of ionizing radiation, but are expensive and may not be readily available. A bone marrow aspiration and biopsy can be safely carried out under local analgesia whereas all radioisotope imaging studies including gallium and PET scans are contraindicated during pregnancy. Cardiac function should be assessed with an echocardiogram rather than a nuclear multiple-gated acquisition (MUGA) scan.

The decision to institute therapy immediately or adopt a watch-and-wait policy should be made with a multidisciplinary approach in which patient, oncologist, obstetrician, neonatologist, social workers, and ethicists (if available) should be involved. Issues that need consideration include prognosis for the mother, prognosis for fetus should the delivery be carried out immediately, prognosis for fetus if therapy is instituted for maternal cancer, risk of spread of maternal cancer to the fetus, ways to enhance fetal maturity (i.e., use of steroids to enhance fetal lung maturity), and potential harmful effects of different diagnostic and therapeutic modalities on the fetus (Table 56.4).[11]

The management of individual lymphomas clearly depends upon the biology of the disease, individual patient stage of disease, and stage of pregnancy at diagnosis.

THERAPEUTIC ABORTION

The decision to terminate pregnancy is always a difficult one. Therapeutic abortion can generally be recommended early in pregnancy, i.e., before the end of the first trimester, and even then it may not be required in every patient. Most authorities are of the opinion that in cases where treatment can be safely deferred until term or at least until the end of the first trimester, pregnancy may be allowed to continue.

Therapeutic abortion may be recommended when there is an urgent need to institute therapy during the first trimester of pregnancy and there is risk to the fetus from exposure to chemotherapy or ionizing radiation from staging procedures or therapeutic radiation therapy. Thus termination of pregnancy may be recommended in the first trimester when the mother is diagnosed with an aggressive non-Hodgkin lymphoma, indolent lymphoma with bulky abdominal or mediastinal adenopathy, systemic symptoms and/or cytopenias, and in advanced stage Hodgkin lymphoma.[12,13]

Regardless of the reasons why it is recommended to terminate the pregnancy, the decision should be achieved with utmost care and in consultation with the patient and her family along with the medical and radiation oncologists, obstetrician, and social worker.

MANAGEMENT OF HODGKIN LYMPHOMA

Available literature suggests that individual patients have been successfully treated with a variety of different modalities during pregnancy. Management, however, depends upon several factors that include presentation of disease, stage, associated symptoms, stage of pregnancy, and anticipated harm to mother as well as fetus. For the purpose of management, the issues that need to be considered include: (1) management during early versus late pregnancy, especially indications for a therapeutic abortion; (2) management of localized supradiaphragmatic disease; (3) management of subdiaphragmatic disease; and (4) management of disseminated disease (Fig. 56.1).

Several investigators have reported on their experience with management of Hodgkin lymphoma during pregnancy. Thomas *et al.* from the Royal Marsden Hospital, UK,

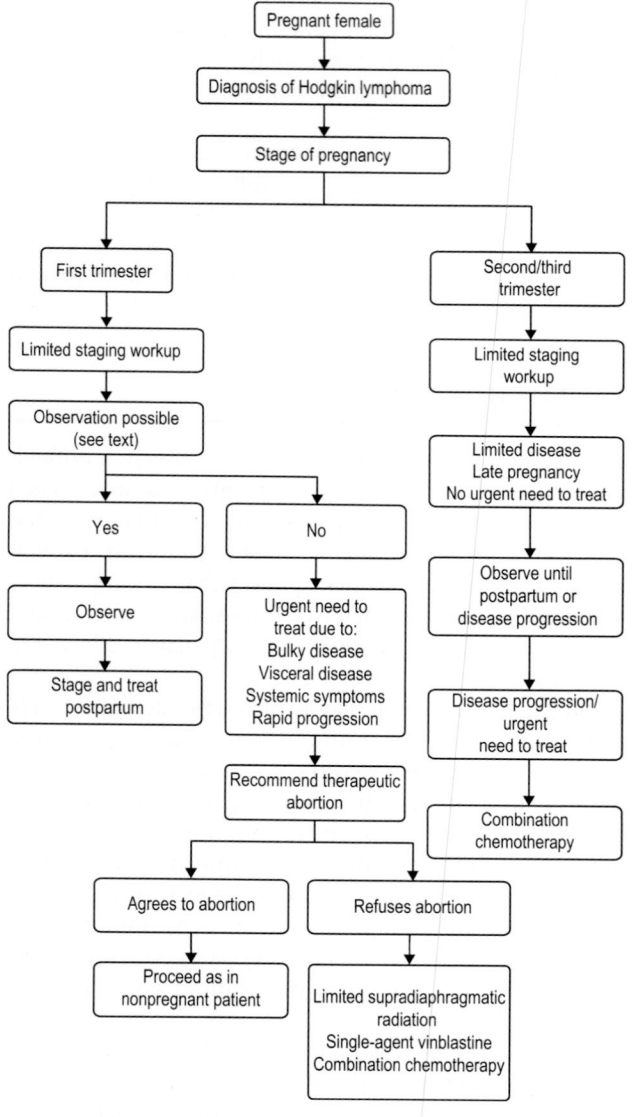

Figure 56.1 Guidelines for management of Hodgkin lymphoma during pregnancy.

reported on 19 pregnancies in 15 patients with Hodgkin lymphoma.[70] Seven of these patients were managed with supradiaphragmatic radiation (2550 cGy to 4000 cGy) during pregnancy (first to third trimesters). All delivered normal infants. Six of these patients were in complete remission at the time of report, though two required salvage chemotherapy. Seven patients were managed with deferment of therapy until postpartum. Two patients underwent therapeutic abortion; one patient underwent resection of a pulmonary nodule with continuation of pregnancy. Two patients had become pregnant while on chemotherapy for Hodgkin lymphoma. One of these elected to continue pregnancy with ongoing chemotherapy, delivering an immature baby who died of respiratory distress syndrome.

Similarly, investigators from Stanford University[22] and Memorial Sloan Kettering Hospital[19] have reported on 15 and 17 patients, respectively, diagnosed with Hodgkin lymphoma and pregnancy. Of the nine patients in the Stanford group who developed Hodgkin lymphoma during pregnancy, three underwent therapeutic abortion and achieved complete remission with radiation therapy. Of the remaining six patients, four received supradiaphragmatic radiation for localized disease during pregnancy and additional radiation therapy postpartum and achieved prolonged disease-free status. One patient received supradiaphragmatic radiation only during pregnancy and combination chemotherapy on relapse. The last patient who continued her pregnancy was treated after delivery and achieved complete remission. One patient relapsed with Hodgkin lymphoma during pregnancy, delayed her therapy, and died postpartum without any treatment. In the Stanford series, five patients became pregnant while on therapy for Hodgkin lymphoma. Three patients underwent therapeutic abortion, two of which remained in complete remission. One patient had spontaneous abortion while receiving breast irradiation. The fifth patient continued her pregnancy on chlorambucil therapy, delivered a normal infant, and achieved complete remission with combination chemotherapy.

Of the 17 patients reported by Memorial Sloan Kettering, 15 presented with Hodgkin lymphoma during pregnancy while two became pregnant while on chemotherapy for Hodgkin lymphoma. Six of these patients underwent therapeutic abortion to avoid treatment delay because of the presence of systemic symptoms or visceral disease. Four of these patients remained in complete remission. Two with advanced disease died after failing chemotherapy. Nine patients presented with clinical stage IA or IIA. Seven of these were treated with irradiation during pregnancy (one patient received radiation therapy during the first trimester and one patient during the third trimester). All seven women delivered normal infants after limited supradiaphragmatic radiation to sites of disease. All these patients underwent completion of staging with bipedal lymphangiogram postpartum and then received additional therapy with radiation with or without chemotherapy. Five of these patients were in complete remission at a follow-up ranging from 10 months to 11 years. One patient presented with Hodgkin lymphoma at 18 weeks of gestation and was treated with single-agent vinblastine to term, following which she completed her staging workup and achieved a complete remission with total nodal irradiation. Another patient presented at 32 weeks gestation and was treated with radiation therapy postpartum and remained in complete remission after a successful salvage therapy for a relapse. One patient became pregnant twice while on single-agent vinblastine and delivered normal infants on both occasions, while another patient became pregnant while on radiation therapy following chemotherapy. Radiation was discontinued and the patient delivered a normal infant and remained in complete clinical remission. Based on these data and observations, management of Hodgkin lymphoma may be considered separately according to the period of pregnancy in which it is diagnosed – i.e., early pregnancy (first trimester) versus middle or late pregnancy (second trimester or later).

Management of Hodgkin lymphoma in early pregnancy

For a newly diagnosed pregnant patient with Hodgkin lymphoma, management may be necessary during the first trimester. However, if the pregnancy has to be continued, therapy should be avoided if at all possible during the first trimester. If delay in institution of therapy is not possible, for example for those with subdiaphragmatic disease, then most authorities recommend a therapeutic abortion followed by adequate staging, as in a nonpregnant patient, followed by standard management.[22] In general, since both chemotherapy and radiation therapy during first trimester may cause congenital malformations, intrauterine growth retardation, or other unforeseen delayed effects, patients unwilling to accept these risks should undergo therapeutic abortion. If the fetus is exposed inadvertently to chemotherapy or radiation therapy in excess of 10 cGy during the first trimester, the patient should undergo therapeutic abortion. After the termination of pregnancy, the patients should be staged and treated as for nonpregnant patients. A possible exception to this rule could be a patient with non-bulky stage IA disease presenting in the neck, which may be treated with modified field and dose radiation during pregnancy followed by completion of staging and treatment after delivery.

Not all investigators recommend therapeutic abortion for patients with Hodgkin lymphoma diagnosed during the first trimester. Investigators from Memorial Sloan Kettering Hospital recommend that therapeutic abortions should be reserved for those with infradiaphragmatic disease requiring pelvic irradiation, those with systemic symptoms or visceral disease requiring chemotherapy, those with diagnosis in the first 10 weeks of pregnancy when delay in starting therapy is unacceptable, those who have been exposed to more than 10 cGy of radiation or potentially teratogenic chemotherapy during the first trimester, and patients with bulky adenopathy requiring combination of chemotherapy and radiation therapy.[19]

Management of Hodgkin lymphoma presenting after the first trimester

For patients presenting with Hodgkin lymphoma in the second or third trimesters, a therapeutic abortion is generally not an option. Such patients may undergo limited staging with history and physical examination, ultrasound examination of abdomen, and possibly a chest x-ray with abdominal shielding, except for late third trimester when the uterus has moved into the abdominal cavity and fetal exposure may occur despite adequate shielding.

Management decisions during the later half of pregnancy depend upon the stage and location of disease. Most authorities believe that Hodgkin lymphoma presenting with localized disease in the latter half of pregnancy may be observed without therapy until after delivery.[71] The patients, however, should be followed closely and therapy may be instituted if progression of disease threatens mother or fetus.[13] Should therapy be needed, localized supradiaphragmatic disease in the latter half of pregnancy may be managed with modified field and dose radiation therapy, with adequate shielding to limit fetal exposure to less than 10 cGy, deferring the definitive therapy until after accurate staging is completed postpartum.[19,22] Radiation therapy cannot be recommended for supradiaphragmatic disease in the third trimester of pregnancy when the uterus has moved into the abdominal cavity and it may be impossible to limit fetal exposure despite adequate shielding.[72] Some investigators, on the other hand, believe chemotherapy to be safer during the second trimester and later compared to radiation therapy.[73]

It is unsafe to delay therapy in those patients presenting with advanced stage disease, systemic symptoms, visceral disease, bulky mediastinal adenopathy, or subdiaphragmatic disease later in the pregnancy. These patients are primarily treated with chemotherapy. Although chemotherapy has been used safely during the second and third trimesters without an increase in the incidence of congenital malformations, other possible adverse effects on the fetus include intrauterine growth retardation and spontaneous abortion. Chemotherapy use in this situation has been variable, ranging from single-agent vinblastine to combination chemotherapy consisting of adriamycin, bleomycin, vinblastine, and dacarbazine (ABVD). Although several authors recommend use of single-agent chemotherapy primarily consisting of vinblastine with completion of staging and appropriate therapy postpartum,[19,74] others have strongly criticized this approach and recommend full-dose combination chemotherapy to avoid compromising the outcome for the mother.[23,75] In our review of 213 patients exposed to chemotherapy during the second and third trimesters of pregnancy, the incidence of congenital malformations was 1.4 percent, which is no higher than the incidence in offspring not exposed *in utero* to chemotherapy.[11] Combination chemotherapy may therefore be recommended to patients with advanced disease requiring therapy in the latter half of pregnancy. Use of dacarbazine and procarbazine should, however, be avoided.[11,13]

While there may be little consensus on how to manage Hodgkin lymphoma during pregnancy, it is generally agreed that therapy should be individualized, the patient should be fully informed and involved in the decision making, investigations that may expose the fetus to ionizing radiation should be avoided, therapy during the first trimester of pregnancy should be avoided if possible, and offspring should be delivered as early as possible. Patients in whom treatment is delayed should be observed closely to monitor signs of disease progression as well as to aid decisions regarding timing of delivery.

Development of Hodgkin lymphoma during early pregnancy should not necessarily lead to therapeutic abortion, as evidenced in case series published to date. The indications for therapeutic abortion include accidental exposure to teratogenic chemotherapy during the first trimester and fetal exposure to ionizing radiation with estimated fetal exposure of 10 cGy or more.[74] In addition, if watchful waiting is undesirable due to infradiaphragmatic disease that is difficult to follow, bulky disease, presence of systemic symptoms, visceral involvement, or rapid progression of disease, therapeutic abortion may be recommended. Those patients who can be treated with modified dose and field radiation to a limited supradiaphragmatic disease with calculated fetal exposure of less than 10 cGy may be an exception to this recommendation. Should there be an urgent indication to treat and the mother elects to continue the pregnancy, published data suggest that adequate disease control may be achieved with single-agent vinblastine.[11,23] Treatment should, however, be delayed to beyond the first trimester if at all possible.[13] Once the period of organogenesis is past, the treatment may be switched to combination chemotherapy or radiation therapy in case of supradiaphragmatic disease. It should be kept in mind that chemotherapy may not be entirely safe during the second and third trimesters, with risks of spontaneous abortion, intrauterine growth retardation, and other unknown side effects of *in utero* exposure to chemotherapy. Alternatively, single-agent vinblastine may be continued until delivery and then followed by full staging and appropriate therapy. Patients who undergo a therapeutic abortion should be managed similarly to nonpregnant patients.

Pregnant patients with relapsed and refractory disease who have previously been exposed to the ABVD regimen may be treated with MOPP in the latter half of pregnancy. Since combinations containing procarbazine may result in an unacceptably high incidence of congenital malformations,[11] procarbazine should be omitted from these regimens. Due to the relatively higher incidence of secondary myelodysplasia and acute leukemia with MOPP,[76–78] our preference in this situation is a MOPP-like regimen, i.e., COPP.

MANAGEMENT OF NON–HODGKIN LYMPHOMA

The literature is scanty regarding the management of lymphoma during pregnancy. Ward and Weiss were the first authors to publish recommendations for management of non-Hodgkin lymphoma during pregnancy.[23] The experience of managing lymphoma during pregnancy is limited. It appears that the majority of non-Hodgkin lymphomas diagnosed during pregnancy are aggressive.[13] Indolent lymphomas comprise a minority of patients presenting during pregnancy. It is well known that a vast majority of indolent lymphomas present with disseminated disease and may not require treatment unless causing symptoms. Management of non-Hodgkin lymphoma during pregnancy can therefore be considered according to biologic behavior of the disease – i.e., indolent versus aggressive (Fig. 56.2).

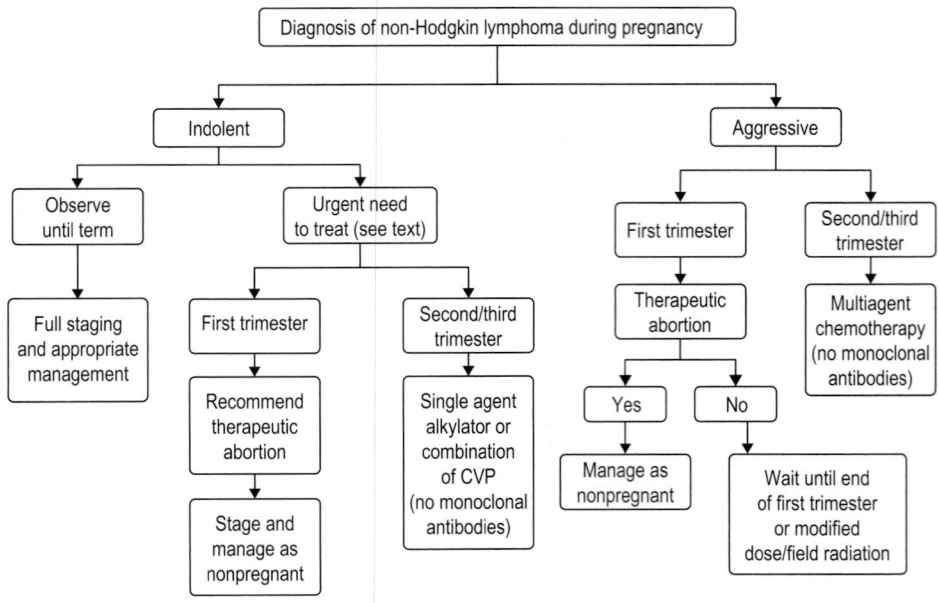

Figure 56.2 Guidelines for management of non-Hodgkin lymphoma during pregnancy. CVP, cyclophosphamide, vincristine, and prednisone. Adapted from Pavlidis,[12] Greskovich and Macklis,[50] and Debakan.[51]

Management of indolent lymphomas during pregnancy

In their review of 42 patients, Ward and Weiss did not find any report of indolent lymphomas presenting during pregnancy.[23] Other reviews have reported similar findings. It therefore appears that indolent lymphomas are rare during pregnancy. As alluded to above, a vast majority of indolent lymphomas present with disseminated disease and are not curable with currently available modalities. Rare exceptions are those that present with truly localized disease (stage IA) where local radiation therapy can be curative. Such patients could be offered potentially curative radiation therapy even during pregnancy provided the disease is supradiaphragmatic and fetal exposure can be limited to less than 10 cGy with appropriate shielding.[23] Practically, this can only be achieved during the first trimester and by keeping the total radiation dose below 3500 cGy. It should be pointed out, however, that it is impossible to diagnose such a scenario during pregnancy due to restrictions on the staging workup in this situation. Therefore it is prudent to adopt a policy of watchful waiting in this case until after delivery, when full staging workup can be carried out and the patient managed accordingly.[13,74]

Therapy may, however, be indicated in those patients with bulky adenopathy, systemic symptoms, or evidence of bone marrow failure. Management in these cases consists of chemotherapy and is best delayed until after the period of organogenesis. Chemotherapy can be in the form of single alkylating agent or in combination with vincristine and prednisone (CVP) with minimal risk of teratogenesis. However, the patients should be fully informed of the risks of premature birth, spontaneous abortion, and intrauterine growth retardation.[11]

Little is known about effects of the presence of maternal lymphoma on the fetus and a therapeutic abortion may be indicated if the mother is not willing to accept any possibility of fetal harm from lymphoma or therapy.[23] Other indications for therapeutic abortion include progressive disease, bulky abdominal disease, and urgent need to institute therapy during the first trimester with chemotherapy or radiation therapy with an expected fetal exposure of greater than 10 cGy.[13,23]

Management of aggressive lymphomas during pregnancy

Patients presenting with unfavorable histologies (diffuse large cell, peripheral T cell, Burkitt, lymphoblastic, etc.) need urgent institution of therapy.[79] In their review of 96 patients with non-Hodgkin lymphoma during pregnancy, Pohlman et al. reported that the majority (60 percent) of these patients were diagnosed with stage III or IV disease, and the stage was unknown in 20 percent. Outcome was known for only 90 women; only 39 were alive and disease-free at a median of 21 months after delivery, while four were alive with disease. Forty-seven had died. Those diagnosed with early stage disease or diagnosed late in pregnancy (third trimester) appeared to have a better prognosis. Prognosis was particularly poor for those with Burkitt lymphoma. Nineteen patients were reported to be diagnosed with Burkitt lymphoma and only one diagnosed with early stage disease during the third trimester survived following bone marrow transplantation. Those who started therapy during pregnancy did not fare better than those in whom therapy was delayed until after delivery.

It therefore appears that prognosis for women diagnosed with non-Hodgkin lymphoma during pregnancy may be worse than for stage-matched nonpregnant females. Those who are diagnosed with an aggressive lymphoma during the first trimester should be recommended to undergo a therapeutic abortion followed by complete staging and appropriate therapy.[13,74] Those patients who are diagnosed with an aggressive lymphoma and localized disease during the first trimester and refuse to undergo a therapeutic abortion may be observed until the end of the first trimester or offered modified field and dose radiation therapy. Those who are observed may start therapy with combination chemotherapy after the first trimester.

Patients who are diagnosed during the second and third trimesters of pregnancy with aggressive lymphomas should start multiagent chemotherapy without delay.[79] Standard management of aggressive non-Hodgkin lymphomas with localized disease is three to eight cycles of chemotherapy with CHOP (cyclophosphamide, adriamycin, vincristine, and prednisone) or a CHOP-like regimen followed by involved field radiation therapy.[80] The standard management for those with advanced stage aggressive lymphoma consists of six to eight cycles of CHOP chemotherapy.[81] Patients with limited stage aggressive lymphoma presenting in the later half of pregnancy may complete their chemotherapy, and undergo radiation treatment after delivery.

Several randomized trials reported recently have shown improved outcome with the addition of anti-CD20 antibody (rituximab) to standard CHOP or CHOP-like regimens in all age groups and this regimen is thus considered to be standard in the management of patients with aggressive B cell lymphomas.[82,83] Although use of rituximab during pregnancy has been reported to be without harmful effects on the fetus, experience with its use during pregnancy as well as knowledge of its adverse effects on the fetus are extremely limited.[84,85] Therefore use of rituximab during pregnancy cannot be recommended at this time.

Patients diagnosed with Burkitt lymphoma during pregnancy have a particularly poor prognosis. The majority of chemotherapy regimens for Burkitt lymphoma include high doses of antimetabolites, especially methotrexate which is associated with an extremely high risk of congenital malformations.[11] Delaying therapy or administration of chemotherapy for Burkitt lymphoma during the first trimester is therefore not an option. Thus, patients diagnosed with Burkitt lymphoma during the first trimester should undergo immediate therapeutic abortion and institution of appropriate therapy.[13] Those diagnosed with Burkitt lymphoma during the second or third trimester should be treated with full-dose combination chemotherapy.[23] Patients diagnosed with lymphoblastic lymphoma need to be managed similarly to acute lymphoblastic leukemia.

MANAGEMENT OF LYMPHOMA RELAPSE DURING PREGNANCY

No data exist for those patients who relapse with non-Hodgkin or Hodgkin lymphoma during pregnancy. In several centers, standard management of Hodgkin lymphoma relapsing after multiagent chemotherapy is salvage chemotherapy followed by high-dose chemotherapy and stem cell rescue.[86–89] The same is true for relapsed non-Hodgkin lymphoma, provided chemotherapy sensitivity can be documented with a salvage regimen.[90–94] Relapsed lymphoma is also thought to be more aggressive than at initial diagnosis. Thus, observation and delay in institution of therapy is not considered a sound strategy. Thus for patients in whom a cure or long-term survival is a realistic possibility, management should not be compromised due to pregnancy. For those women who relapse during the first trimester of pregnancy, therapeutic abortion followed by full staging workup followed by salvage chemotherapy should be recommended. For those who relapse during the second or third trimester, salvage chemotherapy may be initiated and continued until delivery, following which those eligible may undergo high-dose chemotherapy and stem cell transplantation. The fetal effects of salvage chemotherapy are generally unknown; therefore no specific recommendations can be made.

KEY POINTS

- Although uncommon, the coexistence of pregnancy and lymphoid neoplasia, especially non-Hodgkin lymphoma, is expected to increase in the future.
- The ethical, moral, and legal issues concerning a concurrent diagnosis of pregnancy and malignancy are largely unclear.
- It is of paramount importance to involve the mother in all decision making regarding staging, continuation of pregnancy, and therapy.
- It may be wise to advise or recommend therapeutic abortion to those diagnosed with a malignancy during the first trimester.
- Use of ionizing radiation is contraindicated during pregnancy. Therefore no radionuclide scans or CT scans should be done during pregnancy.

- Magnetic resonance imaging scans and ultrasound scans may be used to assess the extent of disease during pregnancy.
- Antineoplastic therapy, i.e., radiation therapy or chemotherapy, should be avoided during the period of organogenesis (first trimester).
- Radiation with modified dose and field to supradiaphragmatic disease may be used in the second trimester using appropriate abdominal shielding.
- Although single agent and combination chemotherapy may be used after the period of organogenesis, i.e., first trimester, it is not entirely safe and may cause spontaneous abortion and intrauterine growth retardation.

REFERENCES

● = Key primary paper
◆ = Major review article

1. Jemal A, Murray T, Ward E et al. Cancer Statistics, 2005. CA Cancer J Clin 2005; **55**: 10–30.
◆2. Donegan WL. Cancer and pregnancy. CA Cancer J Clin 1983; **33**: 194–214.
3. Antonelli NM, Dotters DJ, Katz VL et al. Cancer in pregnancy: a review of the literature. Part II. Obstet Gynecol Surv 1996; **51**: 135–42.
4. Lutz M, Underwood P, Rozier J et al. Genital malignancy in pregnancy. Am J Obstet Gynecol 1977; **129**: 536–42.
●5. Haas JF. Pregnancy in association with a newly diagnosed cancer: a population-based epidemiologic assessment. Int J Cancer 1984; **34**: 229–35.
●6. Petrek J, Dukoff R, Rogatko A. Prognosis of pregnancy-associated breast cancer. Cancer 1991; **67**: 869–72.
●7. Guinee V, Olsson H, Miller T et al. Effect of pregnancy on prognosis for young women with breast cancer. Lancet 1994; **343**: 1587–9.
●8. Ezzat A, Raja M, Berry J et al. Impact of pregnancy on non-metastatic breast cancer: a case control study. Clin Oncol (R Coll Radiol) 1996; **8**: 367–70.
●9. Anderson B, Petrek J, Byrd D et al. Pregnancy influences breast cancer stage at diagnosis in women 30 years of age and younger. Ann Surg Oncol 1996; **3**: 204–11.
●10. Bonnier P, Romain S, Dilhuydy J et al. Influence of pregnancy on the outcome of breast cancer: a case-control study. Societe Francaise de Senologie et de Pathologie Mammaire Study Group. Int J Cancer 1997; **72**: 720–7.
11. Maghfoor I, Doll D. Chemotherapy in pregnancy. In: Perry MC. (ed.) Chemotherapy sourcebook, 3rd Edn. Philadelphia: Lippincott Williams and Wilkins, 2001: 537–46.
◆12. Pavlidis N. Coexistence of pregnancy and malignancy. Oncologist 2002; **7**: 279–87.
◆13. Pohlman B, Macklis RM. Lymphoma and pregnancy. Semin Oncol 2000; **27**: 657–66.

●14. Gobbi PG, Attardo-Parrinello A, Danesino M *et al.* Hodgkin's disease and pregnancy. *Haematologica* 1984; **69**: 336–41.

●15. Lishner M, Zemlickis D, Degendorfer P *et al.* Maternal and foetal outcome following Hodgkin's disease in pregnancy. *Br J Cancer* 1992; **65**: 114–7.

●16. Lambe M, Ekbom A: Cancers coinciding with childbearing: delayed diagnosis during pregnancy? *BMJ* 1995; **311**: 1607–8.

●17. Barry R, Diamond HD, Graver L. Influence of pregnancy on the course of Hodgkin's disease. *Am J Obstet Gynecol* 1962; **84**: 445–54.

◆18. Hennessy J, Rottino A. Hodgkin's disease and pregnancy. *Haematologica* 1963; **87**: 851–3.

●19. Nisce LZ, Tome MA, He S *et al.* Management of coexisting Hodgkin's disease and pregnancy. *Am J Clin Oncol* 1986; **9**: 146–51.

●20. Gelb AB, van de Rijn M, Warnke RA *et al.* Pregnancy-associated lymphomas. A clinicopathologic study. *Cancer* 1996; **78**: 304–10.

◆21. Ebert U, Loffler H, Kirch W. Cytotoxic therapy and pregnancy. *Pharmacol Ther* 1997; **74**: 207–20.

●22. Jacobs C, Donaldson SS, Rosenberg SA *et al.* Management of the pregnant patient with Hodgkin's disease. *Ann Intern Med* 1981; **95**: 669–75.

◆23. Ward FT, Weiss RB. Lymphoma and pregnancy. *Semin Oncol* 1989; **16**: 397–409.

24. Moore D, Taslimi M. Non-Hodgkin's lymphoma in pregnancy: a diagnostic dilemma. Case report and review of the literature. *J Tenn Med Assoc* 1992; **85**: 467–9.

25. Armon P. Burkitt's lymphoma of the ovary in association with pregnancy. Two case reports. *Br J Obstet Gynaecol* 1976; **83**: 169–72.

26. Roumen F, de Leeuw J, van der Linden P *et al.* Non-Hodgkin lymphoma of the puerperal uterus. *Obstet Gynecol* 1990; **75**: 527–9.

27. Armitage J, Feagler J, Skoog D. Burkitt lymphoma during pregnancy with bilateral breast involvement. *JAMA* 1977; **237**: 151.

28. Tunca J, Reddi P, Shah S *et al.* Malignant non-Hodgkin's-type lymphoma of the cervix uteri occurring during pregnancy. *Gynecol Oncol* 1979; **7**: 385–93.

29. Bucciarelli E, Cavaliere A, Sidoni A *et al.* Bilateral primary malignant lymphoma of the breast. A case report. *Tumori* 1988; **74**: 587–91.

30. Kirkpatrick AW, Bailey DJ, Weizel HA. Bilateral primary breast lymphoma in pregnancy: a case report and literature review. *Can J Surg* 1996; **39**: 333–5.

31. Kurtin P, Gaffey T, Habermann T. Peripheral T-cell lymphoma involving the placenta. *Cancer* 1992; **70**: 2963–8.

32. Meguerian-Bedoyan Z, Lamant L, Hopfner C *et al.* Anaplastic large cell lymphoma of maternal origin involving the placenta: case report and literature survey. *Am J Surg Pathol* 1997; **21**: 1236–41.

33. Nishi Y, Suzuki S, Otsubo Y *et al.* B-cell-type malignant lymphoma with placental involvement. *J Obstet Gynaecol Res* 2000; **26**: 39–43.

34. Pollack R, Sklarin N, Rao S *et al.* Metastatic placental lymphoma associated with maternal human immunodeficiency virus infection. *Obstet Gynecol* 1993; **81**: 856–7.

35. Rothman L, Cohen C, Astarloa J. Placental and fetal involvement by maternal malignancy: a report of rectal carcinoma and review of the literature. *Am J Obstet Gynecol* 1973; **116**: 1023–34.

36. Tsujimura T, Matsumoto K, Aozasa K. Placental involvement by maternal non-Hodgkin's lymphoma. *Arch Pathol Lab Med* 1993; **117**: 325–7.

37. Catlin EA, Roberts JD Jr, Erana R *et al.* Transplacental transmission of natural-killer-cell lymphoma. *N Engl J Med* 1999; **341**: 85–91.

38. Maruko K, Maeda T, Kamitomo M *et al.* Transplacental transmission of maternal B-cell lymphoma. *Am J Obstet Gynecol* 2004; **191**: 380–1.

●39. Zuazu J, Julia A, Sierra J *et al.* Pregnancy outcome in hematologic malignancies. *Cancer* 1991; **67**: 703–9.

40. Kato M, Ichimura K, Hayami Y *et al.* Pregnancy-associated cytotoxic lymphoma: a report of 4 cases. *Int J Hematol* 2001; **74**: 186–92.

41. Pohlman B, Lyons J, Macklis R. Lymphoma in pregnancy. In: Trimble E, Trimble C. (eds) *Cancer obstetrics and gynecology*. Philadelphia, PA: Lippincott Williams and Wilkins, 1999: 209–38.

●42. Aviles A, Diaz-Maqueo JC, Torras V *et al.* Non-Hodgkin's lymphomas and pregnancy: presentation of 16 cases. *Gynecol Oncol* 1990; **37**: 335–7.

●43. Aviles A, Neri N. Hematological malignances and pregnancy: a final report of 84 children who received chemotherapy in utero. *Clin Lymphoma* 2001; **2**: 173–7.

◆44. Nicklas A, Baker M. Imaging strategies in the pregnant cancer patient. *Semin Oncol* 2000; **27**: 623–32.

45. Castellino R, Billingham M, Dortman R. Lymphangiographic accuracy in Hodgkin's disease and malignant lymphoma with a note on the 'reactive' lymph node as a cause of most false-positive lymphograms. *Invest Radiol* 1990; **25**: 412–22.

●46. Sombeck M, Mendenhall N, Kaude J *et al.* Correlation of lymphangiography, computed tomography, and laparotomy in the staging of Hodgkin's disease. *Int J Radiat Oncol Biol Phys* 1993; **25**: 425–9.

●47. North L, Wallace S, Lindell M *et al.* Lymphography for staging lymphomas: is it still a useful procedure? *AJR Am J Roentgenol* 1993; **151**: 867–9.

●48. Hoane B, Shields A, Porter B *et al.* Comparison of initial lymphoma staging using computed tomography (CT) and magnetic resonance (MR) imaging. *Am J Hematol* 1994; **47**: 100–5.

●49. Hoane B, Shields A, Porter B *et al.* Detection of lymphomatous bone marrow involvement with magnetic resonance imaging. *Blood* 1991; **78**: 728–38.

◆50. Greskovich JF Jr., Macklis RM. Radiation therapy in pregnancy: risk calculation and risk minimization. *Semin Oncol* 2000; **27**: 633–45.

◆51. Debakan A. Abnormalities in children exposed to x-radiation during various stages of gestation: Tentative timetable of radiation to the human fetus. *Int J Nucl Med* 1968; **9**: 471–7.

●52. Becker M, Hyman G. Management of Hodgkin's disease coexistant with pregnancy. *Radiology* 1965; **85**: 725–8.

●53. Zucali R, Marchesini R, De Palo G. Abdominal dosimetry for supradiaphragmatic irradiation of Hodgkin's disease in pregnancy. Experimental data and clinical considerations. *Tumori* 1981; **67**: 203–8.

●54. Sharma SC, Williamson JF, Khan FM *et al.* Measurement and calculation of ovary and fetus dose in extended field radiotherapy for 10 MV x rays. *Int J Radiat Oncol Biol Phys* 1981; **7**: 843–6.

●55. Wong PS, Rosemark PJ, Wexler MC *et al.* Doses to organs at risk from mantle field radiation therapy using 10 MV x-rays. *Mt Sinai J Med* 1985; **52**: 216–20.

●56. Pirani B, Campbell D, MacGillivray I. Plasma volume in normal first pregnancy. *J Obstet Gynaecol Br Commonw* 1973; **80**: 884–7.

●57. Prichard J. Changes in blood volume during pregnancy and delivery. *Anesthesiology* 1965; **26**: 393.

◆58. Redmond G. Physiologic changes during pregnancy and their implications for pharmacological treatment. *Clin Invest Med* 1985; **8**: 317–22.

◆59. Muchlow I. The fate of drugs in pregnancy. *Clin Obstet Gynecol* 1986; **13**: 161–75.

60. Koren G. Changes in drug disposition during pregnancy and their clinical implications. In: Koren G, Lishner M, Farine D. (eds) *Cancer in pregnancy. Maternal and fetal risks.* Cambridge: Cambridge University Press, 1996: 27–37.

◆61. Powis G. Anticancer drug pharmacodynamics. *Cancer Chemother Pharmacol* 1985; **14**: 177–83.

●62. Wan S, Huffman D, Azarnoff D *et al.* Effect of route of administration and effusionson methotrexate pharmacokinetics. *Cancer Res* 1974; **34**: 3487–91.

◆63. Sokal J, Lessman E. Effects of cancer chemotherapeutic agents on the human fetus. *JAMA* 1960; **172**: 1765–71.

◆64. Nickolson H. Cytotoxic drugs in pregnancy: review of reported cases. *J Obstet Gynaecol Br Commonw* 1968; **75**: 307–12.

◆65. Barber H. Fetal and neonatal effects of cytotoxic agents. *Obstet Gynecol* 1981; **58**: 41S–47S.

◆66. Gilliland J, Weinstein L. The effects of cancer chemotherapeutic agents on the developing fetus. *Obstet Gynecol Surv* 1983; **38**: 6–13.

●67. Mulvihill J, McKeen E, Rosner F *et al.* Pregnancy outcome in cancer patients. *Cancer* 1987; **60**: 1143–50.

68. Toledo T, Harper R, Moser R. Fetal effects during cyclophosphamide and irradiation therapy. *Ann Intern Med* 1971; **74**: 87–91.

●69. Zemlickis D, Lishner M, Erlich R *et al.* Teratogenecity and carcinogenecity in a twin exposed in utero to cyclophosphamide. *Teratog Carcinog Mutagen* 1993; **13**: 139–43.

◆70. Thomas PR, Biochem D, Peckham MJ. The investigation and management of Hodgkin's disease in the pregnant patient. *Cancer* 1976; **38**: 1443–51.

71. Doll D, Ringenberg Q, Yarbro J. Management of cancer during pregnancy. *Arch Intern Med* 1988; **148**: 2058–64.

72. D'Angio G, Nisce L. Problems with the irradiation of children and pregnant patients. *JAMA* 1973; **223**: 171–3.

73. Sutcliffe S, Chapman R. Lymphomas and leukemias. In: Allen H, Nisker J. (eds) *Cancer in Pregnancy.* Mt Kisco: Futura, 1986: 135–89.

74. Dhedin N, Coiffier B. Lymphoma in the elderly and in pregnancy. In: Canellos G, Lister T, Skalr J. (eds) *The lymphomas.* Philadelphia: Saunders, 1998: 549–56.

75. Chapman R, Crosby W. Hodgkin's disease and the pregnant patient. *Ann Intern Med* 1982; **96**: 681–2.

●76. Kaldor JM, Day NE, Clarke EA *et al.* Leukemia following Hodgkin's disease. *N Engl J Med* 1990; **322**: 7–13.

●77. Blayney DW, Longo DL, Young RC *et al.* Decreasing risk of leukemia with prolonged follow-up after chemotherapy and radiotherapy for Hodgkin's disease. *N Engl J Med* 1987; **316**: 710–14.

●78. Longo DL, Young RC, Wesley M *et al.* Twenty years of MOPP therapy for Hodgkin's disease. *J Clin Oncol* 1986; **4**: 1295–306.

◆79. Lishner M, Zemlickis D, Sutcliffe S. Non-Hodgkin's lymphoma and pregnancy. *Leuk Lymphoma* 1994; **14**: 411–13.

●80. Miller T, Dahlberg S, Cassady R *et al.* Chemotherapy alone compared with chemotherapy plus radiotherapy for localized intermediate- and high-grade non-Hodgkin's lymphoma. *N Engl J Med* 1998; **339**: 21–6.

●81. Fisher R, Gaynor K, Dahlberg S *et al.* Comparison of a standard regimen (CHOP) with three intensive chemotherapy regimens for advanced non-Hodgkin's lymphoma. *N Engl J Med* 1993; **328**: 1002–6.

●82. Coiffier B, Lepage E, Briere J *et al.* CHOP chemotherapy plus rituximab compared with CHOP alone in elderly patients with diffuse large-B-cell lymphoma. *N Engl J Med* 2002; **346**: 235–42.

●83. Pfreundschuh M, Trumper L, Ma D *et al.* Randomized intergroup trial of first line treatment for patients ⩽60 years with diffuse large B-cell non-Hodgkin's lymphoma (DLBCL) with a CHOP-like regimen with or without the anti-CD20 antibody rituximab – early stopping after the first interim analysis. In: Grunberg SM. (ed.) 2004 ASCO Annual Meeting Proceedings. New Orleans, LA, 2004: 558s.

◆84. Kimby E, Sverrisdottir A, Elinder G. Safety of rituximab therapy during the first trimester of pregnancy: a case history. *Eur J Haematol* 2004; **72**: 292–5.

85. Herold M, Schnohr S, Bittrich H. Efficacy and safety of a combined rituximab chemotherapy during pregnancy. *J Clin Oncol* 2001; **19**: 3439.

◆86. Canellos GP, Nadler L, Takvorian T. Autologous bone marrow transplantation in the treatment of malignant lymphoma and Hodgkin's disease. *Semin Hematol* 1988; **25**: 58–65.

●87. Linch DC, Winfield D, Goldstone AH *et al.* Dose intensification with autologous bone-marrow transplantation in relapsed and resistant Hodgkin's disease: results of a BNLI randomised trial. *Lancet* 1993; **341**: 1051–4.

●88. Gribben JG, Linch DC, Singer CR *et al*. Successful treatment of refractory Hodgkin's disease by high-dose combination chemotherapy and autologous bone marrow transplantation. *Blood* 1989; **73**: 340–4.

●89. Carella AM, Congiu AM, Gaozza E *et al*. High-dose chemotherapy with autologous bone marrow transplantation in 50 advanced resistant Hodgkin's disease patients: an Italian study group report. *J Clin Oncol* 1988; **6**: 1411–16.

●90. Kessinger A, Armitage JO, Smith DM *et al*. High-dose therapy and autologous peripheral blood stem cell transplantation for patients with lymphoma. *Blood* 1989; **74**: 1260–5.

●91. Philip T, Armitage JO, Spitzer G *et al*. High-dose therapy and autologous bone marrow transplantation after failure of conventional chemotherapy in adults with intermediate-grade or high-grade non-Hodgkin's lymphoma. *N Engl J Med* 1987; **316**: 1493–8.

●92. Takvorian T, Canellos GP, Ritz J *et al*. Prolonged disease-free survival after autologous bone marrow transplantation in patients with non-Hodgkin's lymphoma with a poor prognosis. *N Engl J Med* 1987; **316**: 1499–505.

●93. Vose JM, Anderson JR, Kessinger A *et al*. High-dose chemotherapy and autologous hematopoietic stem-cell transplantation for aggressive non-Hodgkin's lymphoma. *J Clin Oncol* 1993; **11**: 1846–51.

●94. Petersen FB, Appelbaum FR, Hill R *et al*. Autologous marrow transplantation for malignant lymphoma: a report of 101 cases from Seattle. *J Clin Oncol* 1990; **8**: 638–47.

57

Management of lymphoid malignancies in the infant

ZOANN E DREYER AND GREGORY H REAMAN

INTRODUCTION

Malignancy in the first year of life is a rare yet biologically intriguing event. Lymphomas, such as Hodgkin disease and non-Hodgkin lymphoma, are essentially nonexistent; thus, in infancy, acute lymphoid leukemia is by far the most common lymphoid malignancy. Infantile acute lymphoid leukemia (ALL) represents only 4 percent of childhood ALL with an annual incidence of 20 per one million infants at risk and a slight predominance of girls.[1-4,5] The incidence of ALL is nearly double that of acute nonlymphoid leukemia during the first year of life.[6,7] Acute lymphoid leukemia in infancy differs significantly from ALL in older children, not only in presentation but also in prognostic factors, response to therapy, and outcome.

ACUTE LYMPHOID LEUKEMIA IN INFANCY

Acute lymphoid leukemia in infants presents a therapeutic challenge and represents a form of ALL which has been far more difficult to treat and cure than that in any other age group. The event-free survival (EFS) for older children with ALL approaches 70–75 percent while in infant ALL published 5-year EFS ranges from 17 percent to 43 percent. In the early 1980s, most infants were treated on the high-risk, more intensive arms of *pediatric* ALL protocols with dismal outcomes characterized by short-term disease control, early relapse, and 5-year EFS in the range of 20 percent.[8-10] Subsequently, many groups have developed intensified, *infant-specific* therapy with some improvement, increasing average EFS to 30–45 percent.[1,11-15] In one report of consecutive trials in a single institution, EFS reached 54 percent.[16] Dosing regimens vary, with many protocols utilizing infant dose reductions based on age and weight rather than delivering more intensive therapy by dosed body surface area (BSA).

In infant ALL, first remission is easily attained with complete remission rates of 94–95 percent, mirroring rates obtained for older children. The most common cause of failure is marrow relapse followed much less frequently by central nervous system (CNS) and testicular failure. In a review of the literature by Pieters, 318 of 593 patients failed, for a 54 percent relapse rate.[17] Although CNS relapses are less frequent than marrow relapses, rate of CNS relapse for infants exceeds that of older children despite equivalent preventive therapy. Eighty percent of failures were marrow, 30 percent CNS, and 8 percent testicular. Combined relapse represented 19 percent of the total relapses observed, with 14 percent being combined marrow and CNS relapses. Time to relapse was early in all studies, with two-thirds of relapses occurring within 6–12 months after initial diagnosis.[1,9,11] Toxic death or death in remission occurred on average in 4–5 percent of infants[1,11–13] though it reached 14–15 percent in two trials.[10,16]

Infantile ALL is characterized by hyperleukocytosis and extreme organomegaly; evidence of tumor lysis syndrome with hyperuricemia and renal compromise are much more common complications at presentation in infants compared with older children with ALL. Presenting white blood cell (WBC) counts are greater than $50\,000 \times 10^9$/L in two-thirds of infants and greater than $100\,000 \times 10^9$/L in more than half.[17] In the very young infant, WBC counts greater than $1\,000\,000 \times 10^9$/L may be seen.

Historically, risk factors associated with a poorer prognosis in infant ALL appear interrelated and include evidence of the *MLL* gene rearrangement,[1,11,15,18–24] absence of CD10,[1,10,11,17,18] coexpression of myeloid antigens,[19,25] higher WBC counts (greater than $50–100\,000 \times 10^9$/L),[1,10–12,16,26,27] organomegaly,[11] and younger age (less than 3–6 months) at presentation.[1,10–12,19] In general, 90 percent of infants with CD10-negative ALL have the *MLL* gene rearrangement; 80 percent of infants with germ-line *MLL* are CD10 positive and at least two-thirds of infants who have *MLL* rearrangements are less than 6 months of age.[20,21] Unlike in older children, gender is not prognostic in infant ALL.[1,10,12,16,21]

PROGNOSTIC FACTORS

Cytogenetics

Acute lymphoid leukemia in infancy is characterized by a high incidence of nonrandom structural abnormalities within the chromosomal makeup of the leukemic blast population. These translocations affect the 11q23 region involving the *MLL* gene and result in rearrangements which can be detected using molecular analysis in more than 70 percent of patients.[18,20–24,28–35] In older children, deletions and inversions in the 11q23 region are seen but balanced translocations are not nearly as common and the *MLL* gene is typically not rearranged.[28] The exact function of the *MLL* gene, also known as *ALL-1* or *HRX*, is unknown. Its role in leukemogenesis is also unclear.[36] However, its frequency and role as a poor prognostic factor have been well studied.[4,19,20,23,37] The *MLL* gene rearrangement, historically a high-risk feature in infant ALL, has been associated with a variety of 11q23 abnormalities, though t(4;11) is observed in 60–70 percent of cases. Translocations t(11;19) and t(9;11) are much less common.[17,37,38] There is evidence to suggest that leukemogenesis and response to therapy in infants with *MLL* gene rearrangements may differ depending on the fusion partner gene, in particular *MLL-AF4*, the most prevalent subtype of the 11q23/*MLL* rearrangement.[24,36,37,39] In older children, t(4;11) has widely been accepted as the 11q23 abnormality associated with the worst overall outcome, yet in infants outcomes are not as variable within the group of 11q23 translocations. Pui *et al.* reviewed the outcome in 497 infants and children with ALL characterized by 11q23 rearrangements; among infants less than 1 year of age, any category of 11q23 abnormality conferred a dismal prognosis whereas in older children t(4;11) and t(9;11) were associated with a worse outcome.[40] Cytogenetic findings in older children with ALL, such as t(12;21), t(1;19), and t(9;22), are extremely rare in infants.

Immunophenotype

The immunophenotypic patterns observed in infantile ALL also vary considerably from the typical patterns seen in older children with ALL. The majority of infants have B precursor ALL yet nearly two-thirds are CD10 negative[41–43] unlike B-lineage ALL in older children. T cell ALL in infancy is uncommon and mature B cell ALL is extremely rare.[9] The presence of myeloid-associated antigens on blasts, which is rare in older children, is not uncommon in infants with ALL.[19,25,41] In a small number of infants, classification can be difficult due to a lack of lineage-specific markers or expression of both myeloid and lymphoid markers in biphenotypic or mixed leukemia.[9,11,12] In a review of the major infant ALL studies published to date,[1,9–17,44] event-free survival ranges by risk factor are as follows:

Risk factor	EFS
Age <6 months	10–30%
Age >6 months	40–60%
CD10 negative	20–30%
CD10 positive	50–60%
MLL rearranged	5–25%
MLL germ line	40–60%[a]

[a]Up to 90% in one study.[15,45]

Encouraging improvements in EFS are being observed in recent studies. In the European infant leukemia trial, Interfant 99, preliminary analysis demonstrated that the 2-year EFS in a small group of prednisone good responders who did not have the *MLL* rearrangement exceeded 80 percent.[46] In the Children's Cancer Group (CCG) study, CCG-1953, a concurrent pilot with POG 9407, infants less than 90 days of age at diagnosis did unexpectedly well with EFS of 41 percent compared with historical controls in CCG-1883 of 9.5 percent.[47] In POG 9407, the prognostic factor of greatest relevance to outcome was age less than 90 days at presentation, in which patients EFS was 17 percent – more typical of that in most previous infant studies.[48]

Early response

Clinical response has been accepted by several groups to be an additional prognostic factor of importance. Reaman *et al.*[11]

demonstrated a threefold excess risk of failure in infants who had not achieved an M1 status by day 14, which persisted after correction for age, WBC count, and *MLL* rearrangement. In CCG-1953, infants with the *MLL* rearrangement who were early responders had a 46 percent EFS compared with 29 percent in the predecessor study, CCG-1883.[47]

In the Berlin-Frankfurt-Munster (BFM) trials, clinical response to a 7-day prednisone prophase was the strongest predictor of EFS (53 percent vs 14.7 percent) with *MLL* rearrangement losing its predictive strength in multivariate analysis with prednisone response.[1] Based on these data, prednisone response was used as the only stratification in the European Intergroup infant ALL trial, Interfant 99. When receiving therapy according to Interfant 99, prednisone response was shown to be predictive in infants with *MLL* rearranged ALL with good responders having a 4-year EFS of 56 percent versus 30 percent in poor responders.[46]

TREATMENT PROTOCOLS FOR INFANT ACUTE LYMPHOID LEUKEMIA

It remains difficult to compare outcomes from protocol to protocol and thus selecting the optimal treatment strategy for infants remains challenging. Some reports of infant outcome incorporate analysis of consecutive trials,[1,8,10,11,13,14,16,44] which improves patient numbers, while others report outcome in a smaller number of patients treated on a single-arm protocol (Table 57.1).[9,12] The reproducibility of outcomes observed in a population with a small sample can be quite difficult using similar therapy in a large patient population. Several larger trials of single-arm therapy (CCG-1953, POG 9407) have recently been completed.[47,48]

To date, there have been few randomized trials of infant therapy, largely due to the limited number of patients diagnosed annually. In the BFM consecutive trials, patients were stratified by prednisone response.[1] In a Japanese trial, infants were assigned to differing arms of therapy based on the presence or absence of the *MLL* gene rearrangement.[15] While risk is typically therapy dependent, utilizing risk-based therapy in the future for infant ALL is an ideal strategy.

The intensity of therapy offered to infants with ALL has evolved over time, resulting in improved EFS. Infant therapy now typically includes intermediate-, high-, and very high-dose methotrexate (IDM, HDM, and VHMTX, respectively) ranging from 100 mg/kg/dose to as high as 33.6 g/m^2/dose, high-dose cytosine arabinoside (HDAra-C) ranging from 100 mg/kg/dose to 3 g/m^2/dose, cyclophosphamide (CTX), or ifosfamide (Ifos) in many protocols. The steroid chosen varies between prednisone and dexamethasone (Table 57.2).

In the early POG trials, which accrued patients between 1984 and 1990, approximately 2.5 years of therapy were delivered without exposure to HDAra-C, dexamethasone, or ifosfamide. Cranial irradiation was excluded from both protocols either for treatment of overt CNS disease

at diagnosis or prophylaxis. Eighty-two infants were treated on POG 8493, in which prolonged maintenance was intensified with pulses of low-dose CTX, vincristine, prednisone, and cytosine arabinoside (Ara-C).[12] Intensive triple intrathecal therapy appeared adequate and compared favorably to earlier studies, which incorporated far more toxic cranial irradiation as prophylaxis. Event-free survival was 27 percent at 4 years. In the POG pilot study, thirty-three infants received 12 intensive treatments of alternating pairs of IDM–6-mercaptopurine, Ara-C–daunorubicin, and Ara-C–teniposide administered in 30 weeks following induction. This earlier intensive therapy did not result in improved EFS.[9]

In the largest group reported to date of similarly treated infants, the CCG studies CCG-107 and CCG-1883 registered 99 and 135 infants, respectively, with 4-year EFS of 33 percent and 39 percent.[11] Boys received therapy for 3 years and girls for 2 years after beginning interim maintenance. These CCG studies further confirmed that cranial irradiation for CNS treatment or prophylaxis was not necessary in the face of intensified systemic therapy including HDAra-C, CTX, intensified L-asparaginase, HDM, and intrathecal therapy with methotrexate and Ara-C.

Consecutive trials for ALL patients of all ages in the BFM studies registered 105 infants between 1983 and 1995 with an overall 6-year EFS of 43 percent.[1] Patients were stratified based on early prednisone response thus resulting in a higher proportion of infants on the higher-risk arms of therapy. Cranial irradiation was used in a subgroup of infants. Similar results were achieved in the European Organization for Research and Treatment in Cancer–Children's Leukemia Cooperative Group (EORTC-CLCG) using a modified BFM approach, which also included cranial irradiation for a subgroup of patients. Twenty-eight patients were treated between 1982 and 1989.[13]

In a large, consecutive trial conducted in the United Kingdom (MRC UKALL), 88 infants received therapy including HDM, HDAra-C, and intrathecal therapy without cranial irradiation. L-asparaginase was given only during induction. The 4-year EFS was only 25 percent and the rate of death in remission was uncommonly high at 14 percent.[10] Recently, the MRC UKALL trial reported the outcomes of 126 infants treated on two consecutive trials between 1987 and 1999. All patients received high-dose chemotherapy and the later trial allowed stem cell transplantation in first remission. Four-year EFS ranged from 22 percent in the earlier trial to 33 percent in the later trial.[14]

Although in a small study, the Dana-Farber Cancer Institute (DFCI) was able to demonstrate significant improvement in EFS through intensification of therapy on three consecutive protocols.[16] Twenty-three infants registered on these studies between 1985 and 1995 had an overall 4-year EFS of 54 percent compared with an EFS of 9 percent prior to 1985. Therapy included HDM, HDAra-C, intensified anthracycline, L-asparaginase, and cranial irradiation. While EFS was better than previously reported in

Table 57.1 Published treatment results for infant acute lymphoid leukemia

Protocol/ years Tx	Age eligibility	No. of infant patients	CR no./ total (%)	11q23 abn (%)	CNS+ at Dx (%)	% ≤6 mo at Dx	WBC at Dx >50 000/ 100 000%	SCT in CR1 on protocol	Outcome (%)	Relapse or second malignancy (%)	Death in remission no./ total (%)	CNS prophylaxis Tx
DFCI Consortium 73–01, 77–01, 81–01, 1985–95[16]	All	23	22/23 (96)	40%	13%	35%	78/57	None	4-yr EFS, 54 ± 11	6/23 (26) 3 BM, 2 BM + CNS 1–2nd malignancy	3/23 (13)	ITM/CRXRT at age 1 yr
POG 8493 1984–90[12]	Inf	82	76/82 (93)	42%	26%	41%	57/39	None	4-yr EFS, 27 ± 6	50/82 (61) 35 BM, 8 BM+CNS, 5 CNS, 1 BM + CNS + testis, 1 BM + testis (3 BMT pts censored)	4/82 (5)	TIT
POG Pilot 1984–90[9]	All	33	31/33 (94)	58%	12%	61%	67/55	None	5-yr EFS, 17 ± 8	24/33 (73) 13 BM, 3 BM + CNS, 3 CNS, 4 testis, 4 CNS + testis (1 BMT pt censored)	1/33 (3)	TIT
CCG-107 1984–87[11]	Inf	99	94/99 (94)	55%	7%	48%	None	None	4-yr EFS, 33 ± 11	59/99 (59) 35 BM, 7 BM + CNS, 8 CNS, 4 BM + testis, 2 testis, 3 other	2/99 (2)	ITM IT Ara-C
CCG-1883 1988–93[11]	Inf	135	131/ 135 (97)	58%	14%	42%	61/NA	None	4-yr EFS, 39 ± 4	74/135 (55) 55 BM, 7 BM + CNS, 4 CNS, 4 BM + testis, 2 testis, 2 other	5/135 (4)	ITM IT Ara-C
ALL-BFM 83, 86, 90, 1983–95[1]	All	105	100/ 105 (95)	49%	24%	47%	NA/52	None	6-yr EFS, 43 ± 5	50/105 (48) 26 BM, 10 BM + CNS, 9 CNS, 3 testis, 1 BM + testis 1–2nd malignancy	4/105 (4)	ITM+CR XRT at age 1yr if >6 mo at dx; ITM only if <6 mo at Dx
EORTC-CLCG 58831, 58832 1982–89[13]	All	28	24/28 (86)	40%	22%	54%	NA	None	4-yr EFS, 43 ± 19	11/28 (39) 7 BM, 3 BM + CNS, 1 CNS	1/28 (4)	ITM+CR XRT; after 1988 ITM only
MRC–UKALL VIII, X, pilot 1985–90[10]	All	88	81/88 (92)	56%	8%	43%	67/51	11/88	5-yr EFS, ~25	44/88 (50) 23 BM, 14 CNS, 6 BM + CNS, 1 testis	12/88 (14)	ITM

(Continued)

Table 57.1 Continued

Protocol/ years Tx	Age eligibility	No. of infant patients	CR no./ total (%)	11q23 abn (%)	CNS+ at Dx (%)	% ≤6 mo at Dx	WBC at Dx >50 000/ 100 000%	SCT in CR1 on protocol	Outcome (%)	Relapse or second malignancy (%)	Death in remission no./ total (%)	CNS prophylaxis Tx
Japanese MLL 9601 (MLL+) 1995–98[15]	Inf	42	38/42 (90)	100% MLL+	25%	Median age 4 mo	Median WBC 234 K	19/42	3-yr EFS, 34 ± 8	11/42 prior to SCT (26); 2/9 post SCT (10%); 2/8 on maint chemo relapse type NA	6/42 (14%) all post SCT (25%);	TIT
Japanese MLL 9602 (MLL−) 1995–98[15]	All	13	13/13 (100)	0%	NA	Median age 9 mo	Median WBC 21K	None	3-yr EFS, 92 ± 7	1/13 (7) 1 BM	0/13	TIT
CCG-1953 1996–2000[47]	Inf	115	90/113 (80)	69%	16%	53%	67/NA	38/115	5-yr EFS, 48	24/115 19 BM, 1 CNS, 2 testis, 2 BM + other	25/115 (22)	TIT
POG 9407 cohort 1+2 1996–2000[48]	Inf	71	53/53 (100) 17/70 (not evaluated for CR)	70%	30%	56%	85/61	15/71	5-yr EFS, 47 all 24 ≤ 90 days 56 > 90 days	13/17 9 BM, 3 CNS, 1 extramedullary	6/71 (8)	TIT
Interfant 99 1999–2004[46]	Inf	482	445/482 (92)	65%	9%	48%	NA/44	41/482	47/4 yr	163/445 122 BM, 12 CNS, 23 BM + other, 5 miscellaneous	25/482 (5)	ITM IT Ara-C

Tx, treatment; Dx, diagnosis; CR, complete remission; abn, abnormal; WBC, white blood cells; EFS, event-free survival; BM, bone marrow; BMT, bone marrow transplant; CNS, central nervous system; DFCI, Dana-Farber Cancer Institute; POG, Pediatric Oncology Group; CCG, Children's Cancer Group; BFM, Berlin–Frankfurt–Munster; EORTC-CLCG, European Organization for Research and Treatment of Cancer – Children's Leukemia Cooperative Group; MRC–UKALL, Medical Research Council – United Kingdom, ALL trials; Age eligibility: All (all pediatric ages), Inf (infant); NA, not available; SCT, stem cell transplant; CR1, first remission; IT, intrathecal; ITM, IT methotrexate; TIT, triple intrathecal; CR XRT, cranial radiotherapy; mo, months; yr, years; maint chemo, maintenance chemotherapy.

Table 57.2   Treatment advances in infant acute lymphoid leukemia (published studies)

Study	Treatment advance
DFCIC[16]	Intensive anthracycline/L-Asp; many late sequelae of therapy and L-Asp; many late sequelae of therapy and cranial irradiation
POG 8493[12]	No significant improvement
POG pilot[9]	Postinduction intensification with alternating drug pairs
CCG[11]	HD Ara-C/cyclo consolidation
−107	HD MTX/IT MTX/Ara-C; decreased CNS relapse rate; normal development outcomes
−1883	
BFM[1]	
83	Delayed intensification[a]
86	Prednisone response: 5-yr EFS 53 ± 6 vs 14% ± 7% for good vs poor responders[b]
90	
EORTC-CLCG[13]	Cyclo/Ara-C consolidation; HD (2.5 g/m^2) MTX; sequelae of cranial irradiation
MRC-UKALL VIII/X[10]	Ara-C/etoposide consolidation; HD Ara-C/mitoxantrone reinduction allo/auto BMT
MLL 9601[15]	Age <6 months or CNS disease at diagnosis were independent predictors of very poor outcome
MLL 9602[15]	This standard high risk B-lineage ALL therapy was adequate for germ-line *MLL* infants
CCG-1953[47]	MLL/11q23 rearrangement, CD10 expression, age <6 months important prognostic factors; 11q23 translocation partners not prognostic
POG 9407[48]	Age <90 days most important prognostic factor; traditional extended maintenance no advantage over this shortened, intensified therapy
Interfant 99[46]	Addition of late intensification did not offer a survival advantage though did add toxicity

POG, Pediatric Oncology Group; EORTC-CLCG, European Organization for the Research and Treatment of Cancer – Children's Leukemia Cooperative Group; MRC-UKALL, Medical Research Council, United Kingdom, ALL trials; DFCIC, Dana-Farber Cancer Institute Consortium; CCG, Children's Cancer Group; BFM, Berlin-Frankfurt-Munster Group; EFS, event-free survival; Cyclo, cyclophosphamide; HD, high dose; IT, intrathecal; Ara-C, cytarabine; MTX, methotrexate; allo/auto BMT, allogeneic/autologous bone marrow transplantation; L-Asp, L-asparaginase; CNS, central nervous system; ALL, acute lymphoid leukemia; AML, acute myeloid leukemia.
[a]Includes all three BFM studies.
[b]BFM-86/90.

other trials, fewer than half of this small number of infants were CD10 negative or had evidence of the *MLL* gene rearrangement. Three of the 23 infants died in remission. As a result of the cranial irradiation and intensified anthracycline therapy, the late effects observed in survivors were extreme.

In the most recent publication of outcomes on a collaborative group protocol, the Japanese group have reported the EFS for 55 infants registered on two different trials between 1995 and 1998.[15] Of those infants, 42 were found to have the *MLL* gene rearrangement and were treated on infant-specific, intensive systemic therapy, with stem cell transplantation for patients with a suitable donor. Three-year EFS was 34 percent overall, though was only 20 percent in those less than 6 months of age at diagnosis, and for those with CNS disease at diagnosis the EFS was particularly dismal at 10 percent. In patients without the *MLL* rearrangement treated for 2.5 years with systemic therapy for high-risk B cell ALL, 3-year EFS was 89 percent in one trial and 5-year EFS 95 percent in a subsequent trial.[49] The EFS in this small group was higher than previously reported for infants with germ-line *MLL* disease. In follow-up, 44 infants with *MLL* rearranged

ALL diagnosed between 1998 and 2002 underwent stem cell transplantation (SCT) and had a 3-year EFS reported of 43 percent.[50] Again, patients less than 6 months of age at diagnosis or with CNS disease at diagnosis had very poor outcomes, with 3-year EFS of 10 percent and 9 percent, respectively.

Two concurrent, recently completed North American pilot studies, CCG-1953[47] and POG 9407,[48] shared an identical 3-week induction followed immediately by induction intensification. This intensification was designed to address the pattern of early relapse typical of infant ALL. Induction intensification included 2 weeks of HDM (4 g/m^2/dose) and a 5-day cycle of cyclophosphamide and etoposide. Remission was assessed at that point followed by a 3-week reinduction. After completion of reinduction, infants on the CCG pilot with *MLL* rearrangements were to undergo SCT (matched related donor [MRD]/matched unrelated donor [MUD]) while SCT was optional for infants on the POG pilot. In an effort to further intensify therapy, all dosages, with the exception of vincristine, daunomycin, and triple intrathecal therapy, were delivered based on BSA without an age or weight reduction traditionally used in previous infant protocols.

Therapy following reinduction diverged, with the CCG infants receiving four courses of VHMTX at $33.6\,g/m^2$/dose and approximately 2 years of maintenance therapy. Reinduction was followed on POG 9407 with consolidation similiar to induction intensification with an additional cycle of HDAra-C. Maintenance therapy was short, lasting only from weeks 18 to 46.

On CCG-1953, in rank order of significance, CD10 negativity, age less than 6 months, and MLL rearrangement all had a negative impact on prognosis. On POG 9407, the prognostic factor of greatest relevance to outcome was age less than 90 days at presentation, in which patients EFS was 17 percent – typical of that in most previous infant studies. In children more than 90 days of age at diagnosis, presenting WBC count (greater or less than $300\,000 \times 10^9$/L) and the presence or absence of an MLL rearrangement within the blasts had far less impact on EFS than in previous studies: 52 percent versus 56 percent for WBC count and 52 percent versus 65 percent for MLL status, respectively. Early relapse at less than 6–9 months post-diagnosis, typical of relapse patterns in previous infant protocols, was nearly eliminated on this therapy incorporating early intensification. Extended maintenance on the CCG trial did not offer an EFS advantage for either the MLL rearranged or germ-line MLL infants when compared with the shorter therapy on POG 9407.

Both studies, however, were associated with high toxic death rates related to bacterial, viral, and fungal infections, particularly during the dexamethasone-based induction. Nearly two-thirds of events in both studies were toxic deaths. In the successor Children's Oncology Group Infant ALL study, P9407, a change in induction steroid to prednisone, the only change in therapy from the original POG pilot, resulted in a dramatic reduction in toxic deaths, offering a better opportunity to assess the impact of this shortened, intensified therapy on outcome.[51]

Interfant 99 included infants from 22 countries treated by 17 study groups. Patients were stratified for risk by peripheral blood response to a 7-day prednisone prophase and later randomized to establish the value of a late intensification course. Overall EFS was 47 percent with 37 percent EFS for those with MLL rearranged ALL and 74 percent for those without the MLL rearrangement. While prednisone good responders did better than poor responders, addition of late intensification did not improve overall survival though it did add significant grade 3–4 toxicity.[46]

ROLE OF STEM CELL TRANSPLANTATION IN INFANT ACUTE LYMPHOID LEUKEMIA

As in older children with ALL, it is widely accepted that SCT offers an advantage for infants in their second complete remission (CR2). Stem cell transplantation is rarely used in first remission (CR1) in older children with the exception of those with very-high-risk ALL, such as those with t(9;22), those with induction failure, or those with extreme hypodiploidy. However, the role of SCT in CR1 in infants is controversial.[14,52–57] Critically evaluating outcomes with SCT versus aggressive systemic chemotherapy in CR1 is dependent on comparing characteristics of the infant population including age, WBC count, the presence of the MLL gene rearrangement, presence of extramedullary disease, donor source, preparative regimen, and disease status at time of transplant.

As transplant techniques become more refined in infant ALL, with a reduction of both acute and long-term toxicity as well as improved disease control, it is possible that a randomized trial might show an advantage for SCT over intensive chemotherapy in CR1. However, given the relatively small numbers of patients as well as investigator bias – both for and against SCT in CR1 – there have been no randomized trials to date. A number of small studies, both retrospective and prospective, have been reported (Table 57.3); however, the results certainly do not clear up the controversy surrounding SCT and its role in CR1. In the early 1990s, Ferster et al.[13] reported a single successful transplant and Chessells et al. reported two toxic deaths and one relapse in three transplanted infants.[10] A subsequent report by Chessells et al.[14] described 21 infants in CR1 who underwent either autologous (seven infants) or allogeneic matched related or unrelated transplant (14 infants) following intensive chemotherapy. No advantage for SCT following high-dose chemotherapy was demonstrated over chemotherapy alone, with an EFS of only 30 percent overall at 4 years. On CCG-1883, 12 infants in CR1 underwent SCT off protocol. Two infants survived without experiencing an event, five died in remission post-transplant, and five relapsed.[11] Pirich et al. described seven infants who received either matched related or cord blood transplants following a preparative regimen including total body irradiation (TBI), cyclophosphamide, and etoposide.[54] Of those seven infants, four were leukemia free at a median of 775 days post-transplant. Marco et al. described ten infants with ALL who underwent autologous or allogeneic transplants.[57] Of those infants, five had either MLL rearranged and/or CD10-negative ALL, with eight in CR1. Four of the ten infants relapsed, with the remaining six alive and well at a median of 32 months post-transplant. An interval of less than 4 months between remission and SCT was the only significant factor associated with greater disease-free survival. The Japanese group reported a 3-year EFS of 64 percent for 29 MLL rearranged infants in CR1 who underwent transplant with a variety of donor sources (20 unrelated cord blood; four related marrow; three unrelated marrow; two related stem cell) and preparative regimens. Time to transplant was not a prognostic variable in this study although patients in CR1 did better than those who had relapsed prior to SCT.[50] Furthermore, in a comprehensive analysis of 497 children with ALL and 11q23 abnormalities treated between 1983 and 1995 by 11 cooperative groups, SCT did not demonstrate a superior outcome in any age group.[40]

Table 57.3 Stem cell therapy in infant acute lymphoid leukemia in first complete remission

Author/ year published	No. of patients	No. MLL+ (if reported)	Donor type	Prep	Outcome	Authors' conclusion
Reaman 1999[11] (CCG–1883)	12		Allo-varied	Varied Chemo ± TBI	5 death in CR; 5 relapse; 2 disease-free	Varied SCT performed off protocol; no definite conclusion
Pirich 1999[54]	7	4/7	Allo, MR/cord	Chemo/TBI	4 disease-free median 775 days	Allo transplant is an alternative to chemo if suitable donor available
Marco 2000[57]	8	4/8	Allo/auto	Chemo (7); Chemo/TBI (1)	5 disease-free 3 relapse	Time to transplant important in outcome; early SCT outcome better and can be a valid option
Chessells 2002[14] (MRC–UKALL, VIII, X, pilot)	21		7 Auto 14 Allo (MUD; MR)	Chemo/no TBI	4-yr EFS 30%	SCT no advantage over intensive chemo
Kosata 2004[50] MLL 98	29	29	Allo-varied	Varied Chemo ± TBI	3-yr EFS 64%	SCT in CR1 may improve survival in MLL+ infant ALL
Sanders 2005[58]	17	14/17	Allo-varied	Chemo/TBI	3-yr EFS 76%	SCT may improve outcome in CR1; MLL status not and prognostic; neuropsychological endocrine late effects common
Dreyer 2007[59] (POG 9407/ CCG-1953)	48	48	Allo-varied	Varied Chemo ± TBI	3-yr EFS 55%	SCT no advantage over MLL+ controls receiving intensified chemo alone (EFS 55% vs 60%)

Additional comment:

Pui 2002[40]						Infants with 11q23 abnormality undergoing SCT in 11 collaborative group trials had poorer DFS and overall survival than those treated with chemo alone even after adjusting for age at diagnosis, WBC count, or time to SCT

Chemo, chemotherapy; CR, complete remission; CR1, first complete remission; SCT, stem cell transplant; Allo, allogeneic; Auto, autologous; MR, matched related; MUD, matched unrelated donor; TBI, total body irradiation; EFS, event-free survival; MRC–UKALL, Medical Research Council – United Kingdom, ALL trials; CCG, Children's Cancer Group; POG, Pediatric Oncology Group; DFS, disease-free survival; WBC, white blood cell.

In a recently reported study of SCT in infants with ALL, Sanders described a disease-free survival of 76 percent at 3 years in 17 infants in CR1 transplanted between 1982 and 2003.[58] Phase of disease, remission, or relapse, but not the presence of the *MLL* rearrangement, was predictive of outcome. Patients transplanted in second/third complete remission or in relapse had 3-year disease-free survival rates of 43 percent and 6 percent, respectively. All patients received TBI as part of their preparative regimen. In 16 survivors who underwent neuropsychological testing, three were normal, six had speech delay, three had developmental delay (motor ± language), and four had slight fine and gross motor delay.

The influence of donor source (MRD vs MUD) on transplant outcome in children less than 18 months of age with acute leukemia in CR1 was evaluated using data from the Center for International Blood and Marrow Transplant Research and the New York Blood Placenta Program. In this patient population, transplant from a MRD did not show an advantage over transplant from a MUD, suggesting MUD transplants are safe and efficacious in CR1 and should not be reserved solely for patients in CR2 (personal communication, M. Eapen).

The efficacy of transplant for *MLL* rearranged infants (CCG-1953/POG 9407) and prednisone poor responders (Interfant 99) is under evaluation internationally. After completing identical prior therapy on the concurrent CCG/POG pilot studies, 48 infants underwent SCT in CR1 – the largest SCT study in infants in CR1. Twenty-two patients were treated according to protocol guidelines for transplant preparative regimen and graft-versus-host disease (GVHD) prophylaxis. The remaining 26 patients underwent transplants off protocol with a variety of preparative regimens and GVHD prophylaxis. Preliminary results of this collaborative CCG-POG study demonstrated that in infants transplanted both on and off protocol compared with the control *MLL* rearranged infants, who received chemotherapy only, there was no advantage for SCT over the intensified chemotherapy delivered on protocol.[59]

PHARMACOLOGY OF INFANT DOSING

Infants present a chemotherapeutic challenge based on the unique aspects of infant pharmacology. Infants experience rapid changes in the relative volume of fluid compartments after birth, decreased efficiency of renal excretion, decreased protein binding, different rates of hepatic metabolism, increased volume of cerebrospinal fluid, brain, and spinal cord tissue relative to BSA, and increased permeability of the blood–brain barrier.[60] Based on concerns that the total body water in infants is relatively much greater than in adults and because most chemotherapeutic agents are distributed in the total body water, chemotherapy delivered to infants has traditionally been dosed based on an age- and weight-based infant dose reduction rather than on BSA, especially in infants weighing less than 6 kg.

The formula typically used in many infantile cancers has been to multiply the dose in milligrams per 1 m^2 by the weight in kilograms divided by 30, with a resultant decrease in dose of approximately 50 percent in a 6 kg infant. The resultant dose reductions may explain the high rate of treatment failure in many past infant protocols. While such dose reductions have been necessary in other malignancies seen in infants, infants with ALL treated on CCG-1953, POG 9407, and COG P9407 appear to have tolerated dosing based on BSA for most agents, with the exception of vincristine and daunorubicin. No doubt delivery of this much more intensively dosed therapy is responsible in large part for the success of these treatment protocols.

Pharmacokinetic (PK) evaluations of the principal agents used to treat infant ALL are critical for defining appropriate dosing in these very young children. Studies of drug metabolism in infants may better help us understand optimal dosing of these chemotherapeutic agents. Pharmacokinetic analyses in infants are underway for several widely used antileukemia agents including vincristine, daunorubicin, and etoposide. Pharmacokinetic analysis of methotrexate in infants demonstrated that the clearance for infants greater than 3 months of age was very similar to that reported in older children 1–19 years of age.[61,62] Analysis of methotrexate PK in infants less than 3 months of age is ongoing. Ideally, PK analyses of agents used to treat infants with cancer should be incorporated into all ongoing studies.

EPIDEMIOLOGY OF INFANT LEUKEMIA

Why infants should develop lymphoid malignancies within the first year, or even the first few days of life, remains unclear. However, there is epidemiologic and molecular genetic evidence that suggests most, perhaps all, cases of infant leukemia arise *in utero*.[52] A minimum of two mutational events are thought necessary for the development of leukemia, thus in infantile leukemia at least one, if not both, events may take place *in utero*. Genetic evidence for mutational events *in utero* includes the fact that infant leukemias exhibit fetal-type DJ_H joining sequences in the immunoglobin gene[63] and cases diagnosed within the first few days of life typically have 11q23 chromosomal rearrangements suggesting a prenatal leukemogenic event.[64] Molecular studies of identical twins with leukemia with *ALL1/MLL/HRX* rearranged genes support the suggestion that such rearrangements are acquired *in utero* and likely spread through the monochorionic placenta from one twin to the other.[49,65–68] One report of fetal death due to acute myeloid leukemia (AML) with the *ALL1/MLL/HRX* rearrangement offers further direct evidence for oncogenesis *in utero*.[69] In children diagnosed up to 14 years of age with T cell or B precursor ALL with *TEL-AML1*, and in babies diagnosed from age 5 months to 2 years with ALL with *ALL1/MLL/HRX-AF4* genomic fusion patterns, the same clonotypic patterns have been found upon examination of the patients' neonatal blood spots (Guthrie cards).[70,71] These findings suggest that in many cases of infantile leukemia, at least one mutagenic event occurs *in utero* while additional genetic or postnatal events are also required.[52]

The leukemogenic potential of *in utero* exposures can be better studied in infants than in older children. Maternal exposures associated with development of infantile AML include marijuana use[72] and alcohol, there being a dose-dependent relationship to maternal alcohol consumption.[73,74] Higher birth weight correlates with a higher incidence of infant ALL and AML[75–78] perhaps associated with high levels of insulin-like growth factor 1.[79]

Exposure to topoisomerase II inhibitors, such as the epipodophyllotoxins, has been associated with the development of secondary leukemias characterized by MLL gene rearrangements.[80] Thus, it has been postulated that, given the very high incidence of *MLL* rearrangements in infant leukemia, exposure to topoisomerase II inhibitors, such as flavonoids (fruits and vegetables), soybeans, quinolone antibiotics, catechins (tea and wine), podophylline resin, benzene metabolites, and estrogens in pregnant women may play a role in leukemogenesis in infants.[81–84] The risk of postnatal dietary intake of soy-based infant formulas is also under investigation.[82,84]

The frequencies of single and double glutathione-S-transferase (GST) gene deletions in studies of *GST* gene polymorphisms are higher in parents of infants with leukemia than expected. This suggests a possible role of parental genetic susceptibility factors in modulating parental exposure to carcinogens and leukemogenesis in infants.[85]

Lastly, the effect of parental exposure to radiation on leukemogenesis *in utero* is controversial. Neither the German study[86] nor the European Childhood Leukemia-Lymphoma Incidence Study[87] demonstrated an increase in childhood leukemia following the Chernobyl accident, while a Greek study did suggest an increased incidence.[88]

LATE EFFECTS IN INFANT ACUTE LYMPHOID LEUKEMIA

It is anticipated that infants cured of their malignancies will experience a normal life span. For that reason, this population presents unique challenges to the pediatric oncologist. To maintain a normal, physically healthy and psychologically sound life, it is critical that infant survivors are followed closely for delayed effects of their therapy. Inherent in that challenge is the need to work to design therapies that are successful yet which avoid exposure to toxic therapies that we know present the greatest risks, such as excessive anthracyclines and radiation therapy.

It is only since the late 1990s that survival rates in infant ALL have begun to improve to the point that a substantial number of infants are surviving. Currently, the overall 4-year EFS ranges from 40 percent to 45 percent in the larger studies published to date, although encouraging

improvements in EFS are on the horizon in three of the larger infant ALL studies which have recently completed accrual. In certain subgroups on Interfant 99 and the collaborative protocols POG 9407/CCG-1953, 4-year EFS exceeds 55 percent, even in some of the higher-risk populations.[46–48] The study of late effects in infant survivors has been hampered not only by the historically poor EFS but also by the rarity of the disease resulting in a very limited number of patients available for study. Teenagers who are survivors of infant ALL are indeed rare.

The use of radiation therapy both as prophylaxis and treatment for CNS disease and as part of the preparative regimen for patients undergoing SCT presents the greatest hazard for infant survivors. On consecutive CCG protocols, 115 infants were treated between 1972 and 1982.[11] Seventy-five infants received cranial irradiation in addition to intrathecal therapy. Of the eight infants who survived more than 1 year post-treatment, five had significant late effects including severe hypogammaglobulinemia in one patient and severe neurotoxicity in four, including chronic encephalopathy and severe retardation with seizures in one each and seizures and ataxia in two patients. All had received cranial irradiation. Subsequently, both the CCG and POG eliminated cranial irradiation for both treatment and prophylaxis of CNS disease in infants with ALL.

Infants treated with cranial irradiation on the DFCI infant protocol between 1985 and 1995 experienced significant late effects.[16] These delayed effects included speech and/or learning disabilities in nine of 11 infants tested, cataracts in six of nine tested, growth delay or obesity in five of 11 screened, and thee of ten patients had modest cardiac abnormalities.

Leung *et al.* reported the incidence of late effects in survivors of infant ALL (19 infants) and AML (15 infants) treated on a variety of protocols between 1970 and 1994, some of which included cranial radiation therapy or TBI prior to SCT.[89] The most frequently observed late effects included problems with growth (66 percent), learning (50 percent), hypothyroidism (15 percent), and delayed puberty (12 percent). Cataract, cardiac, and hearing abnormalities were less common, occurring in only 6 percent of patients. Only 24 percent of infants survived without any late effects. In comparison to patients who did not receive radiation therapy, the incidence of having at least one late effect was significantly higher; there was a greater decrease in height Z score and a higher incidence of academic difficulties. The estimated odds of academic difficulties increased by 18 percent for each month younger a patient was at the time of radiation.

In 30 infants treated on CCG-107 with systemic VHMTX and intrathecal Ara-C and methotrexate but no cranial irradiation, no neuropsychological abnormalities were detected.[90] In a smaller study of 18 long-term survivors who did not receive radiation therapy or SCT, only one had severe developmental delay and a seizure disorder. The remaining 17 had normal neurological function and school performance.[12]

Sanders *et al.* evaluated 17 infants, who underwent SCT between 1982 and 2003 and who survived in complete remission for more than 1 year post-transplant, at a median of 6.1 years after SCT.[58] All but one infant had received TBI as part of the preparative regimen prior to SCT. In this group, all had gradually decreasing height score and 12 of 14 patients evaluated for growth hormone (GH) production had biochemical GH deficiency; five of 17 tested showed compensated hypothyroidism; two of three teenagers tested for pubertal development were diagnosed with precocious puberty; six of 17 screened had mild cataracts; seven of eight evaluated with panographic dental films had abnormalities detected; and four of seven screened with dual energy x-ray absorptiometry (DEXA) scans showed osteopenia with a median Z-score of -1.48. Importantly, in 15 patients who had no evidence of developmental delay prior to SCT, comprehensive neuropsychological screening was performed. Three patients were normal while the remaining 12 had some degree of delay in motor skills, speech, and/or language.

While all organs in the rapidly growing and developing infant are potentially at risk from high-dose therapy, which includes potential cardiotoxins (anthracyclines), renal and hepatotoxins (methotrexate, cyclophosphamide, ifosfamide), pulmonary toxins (TBI) and neurotoxins (vincristine, high-dose methotrexate, high-dose Ara-C, intrathecal chemotherapy, and cranial irradiation/TBI), the most striking and severe late effects are those associated with radiation therapy delivered to the developing brain. Based on these debilitating late effects, the POG and CCG studies lead the way in the elimination of cranial radiation for infant ALL, despite high incidence rates of CNS disease at diagnosis averaging 25 percent. CCG-107 and CCG-1883 proved that intensive systemic and intrathecal therapy were adequate to prevent CNS relapse (relapse rates of 9 percent and 3 percent, respectively)[11] compared with historical controls with CNS relapse rates as high as 20 percent.[8] Similar findings were observed in the POG study and of the five of 82 patients who did experience CNS relapse, none had CNS disease at diagnosis.[12] These studies and others have subsequently proven that with intensive systemic therapy including high-dose methotrexate and high-dose Ara-C as well as intrathecal therapy with various combinations of methotrexate, Ara-C, and hydrocortisone, cranial irradiation can be successfully avoided.[46–48]

SUPPORTIVE CARE

The increasing success rates associated with more intensive systemic therapy to treat infant ALL mandates aggressive supportive care to ensure continued gains in EFS. Infants with ALL frequently present with very elevated WBC counts which not uncommonly reach $250\,000–500\,000 \times 10^9$/L. Occasionally, infants present with WBC counts greater than $1\,000\,000 \times 10^9$/L. Although no controlled studies have been performed, it is strongly recommended that infants with presenting WBC counts greater than $200\,000 \times 10^9$/L be considered for exchange transfusion to avoid life-threatening complications such as acute renal failure and metabolic derangements as a result of tumor lysis syndrome, central nervous system complications including thrombosis and hemorrhage, as well as pulmonary leukostasis. Correction of coagulation abnormalities such as disseminated intravascular coagulation, extreme thrombocytopenia, and the coagulation deficiencies observed in very young infants as a result of immature hepatic functioning and reduced production of liver-dependent coagulation factors plays an important role in maintaining the infant's ability to safely tolerate therapy. Blood product support should be provided using leukocyte-reduced, irradiated products with cytomegalovirus (CMV)-negative blood products as available, particularly for infants less than 6 months of age.

The immunosuppression and myelosuppression associated with agents used to treat infant ALL today may be extreme. For these reasons, it is imperative that the treating physician respond immediately and aggressively to febrile illnesses. Rapidly instituting broad-spectrum antibiotic coverage in the face of a febrile, neutropenic event may be the difference between life and death. Early addition of empiric antifungal coverage for persistent fever is of equal importance. Many protocols now mandate not only *Pneumocystis carinii* prophylaxis but fungal prophylaxis as well. Though not proven in randomized trials, the use of empiric intravenous immunoglobulin for infants with low levels of immunoglobulin G may be an important aspect of infection prevention and warrants prospective evaluation. Infants who develop viral infections such as respiratory syncytial virus should be treated aggressively with antiviral therapy.

High-dose methotrexate and the anthracyclines pose additional problems for the infantile gut. Mucositis and perineal breakdown are not uncommon. In addition, intestinal irritation including a picture similar to necrotizing enterocolitis (NEC) may have a relatively subtle presentation, followed by rapid deterioration including perforation and death. Infants presenting with gastrointestinal symptoms such as pain, ileus, or bloody diarrhea should be considered at high risk for this NEC-like picture. Surgical intervention may even be necessary dependent on the clinical picture.

For infants who are unable to take adequate calories to maintain growth and healthy tissue, supplemental nutrition in the form of total parenteral nutrition (TPN) via intravenous central catheter or milk drip therapy via gastrosomy or naso-duodenal tube should be instituted.

FUTURE DIRECTIONS

Continued improvement in EFS in infant ALL is dependent on better use of existing therapies as well as developing targeted therapies directed at the unique features present in the blasts of infants with ALL. Maximizing conventional agents through pharmacologically based dosing will avoid undertreatment and untoward toxicity. Screening *in vivo* of new agents as well as screening existing agents using an *in vitro* drug resistance assay (MTT assay) can determine dosing as well as projected efficacy of potential therapeutic agents.[91,92]

Aggressive efforts to pilot novel agents targeted at infant blasts will perhaps play one of the most significant roles in successfully treating infant ALL. Encouraging results are now being reported using the FMS-like tyrosine kinase 3 (FLT3) inhibitor, CEP-701, in ALL cell lines and marrow samples from infants and children with various subtypes of ALL.[93] FLT3 has been implicated in the pathogenesis of infant and childhood ALL, with gene expression analyses demonstrating some of the highest levels of FLT3 expression in infants and children with the *MLL* rearrangement.[94,95] Clinical testing of CEP-701 as a novel, molecularly targeted agent is ongoing in a randomized setting in infants currently being treated on Children's Oncology Group study AALL0631.

Identifying prognostic features of greatest impact on outcome will allow the development of risk-based therapy. The outcomes of CCG-1953, POG 9407, and P9407 are the basis for the development of risk-based therapy in the COG infant ALL successor study to P9407. In light of improved EFS in some infant groups including children greater than 3 months of age regardless of *MLL* rearrangement, many now agree that the role of SCT in CR1 should be restricted to those groups with EFS less than 40 percent.

As molecular technologies improve, it is likely that evidence of slow early response and minimal residual disease postinduction may define the highest risk group of all.[96,97] While neither of these factors has been used to modify therapy in any infant trials to date, it is anticipated that both will be used widely in upcoming protocol development.

As in older children with ALL, the ability to complete randomized trials in a reasonable period of time with adequate statistical power is key. Though limited by available patient numbers in the past, international collaborative trials may permit randomized studies in the future.

KEY POINTS

- Acute lymphoid leukemia (ALL) is by far the most common lymphoid neoplasm in infancy.
- Infant ALL is a biologically different disease from ALL in older children:
  - Approximately 80 percent of infants with ALL have leukemic blasts which are common ALL antigen (CALLA) negative and have translocations of the 11q23 region of the *MLL* gene (*MLL* gene rearrangement).
  - Historically, event-free survival (EFS) has been quite poor with cure rates ranging from 20 percent to 40 percent in those infants with leukemic blasts having the *MLL* gene rearrangement.
  - Early relapse less than 6–12 months after diagnosis is common.
- Prognostic factors associated with a poor outcome in infant ALL include younger age (less than 3–6 months at diagnosis), the presence of the *MLL* gene rearrangement in the leukemic blasts, and poor early response.
- Recent infant-specific treatment protocols have improved the EFS by markedly intensifying the therapy delivered.
- The role of stem cell transplantation, particularly in first remission, is uncertain.
- Infants who receive radiation therapy either as part of primary central nervous system prophylaxis or treatment, or as part of a transplant preparative regimen, are at high risk for late effects including neurocognitive sequelae and growth disturbances.
- The etiology of infant ALL remains unclear though investigations continue to explore the leukemogenic potential of *in utero* exposures, exposure during infancy to topoisomerase II inhibitors such as flavinoids and soy products, and parental genetic susceptibility factors which may play a role in modulating parental exposure to carcinogens.
- The future direction of therapy for infant ALL includes development of novel, targeted agents directed at the leukemic blasts.

REFERENCES

● = Key primary paper
◆ = Major review article

●1. Dordelmann M, Reiter A, Borkhardt A *et al.* Prednisone response is the strongest predictor of treatment outcome in infant acute lymphoblastic leukemia. *Blood* 1999; **94**: 1209–17.

●2. van Wering ER, Kamps WA. Acute leukemia in infants. A unique pattern of acute nonlymphocytic leukemia. *Am J Pediatr Hematol Oncol* 1986; **8**: 220–4.

●3. Schorin MA, Blattner S, Gelber RD *et al.* Treatment of childhood acute lymphoblastic leukemia: results of Dana Farber Cancer Institute/Children's Hospital Acute Lymphoblastic Leukemia Consortium Protocol 85-01. *J Clin Oncol* 1994; **12**: 740–7.

●4. Pui CH, Riberiro RC, Campana D *et al.* Prognostic factors in the acute lymphoid and myeloid leukemias of infants. *Leukemia* 1996; **10**: 952–6.

●5. Birch JM, Blair V. The epidemiology of infant cancers. *Br J Cancer* 1992; **18**: 52–4.

●6. Ross JA, Davies SM, Potter JD, Robison LL. Childhood leukemia with a focus on infants. *Epidemiol Rev* 1994; **16**: 243–72.

●7. Gurney JG, Severson RK, Davis S, Robison LL. Incidence of cancer in children in the United States: sex-, race-, and 1-year age-specific rates for histologic types. *Cancer* 1995; **75**: 2186–95.

●8. Reaman GH, Zeltzer P, Bleyer WA *et al.* Acute lymphoblastic leukemia in infants less than one year of age: a cumulative experience of the Childrens Cancer Study Group. *J Clin Oncol* 1985; **3**: 1513–21.

●9. Lauer SJ, Camitta BM, Leventhal BG *et al.* Intensive alternating drug pairs after remission induction for treatment of infants with acute lymphoblastic leukemia: a Pediatric Oncology Group pilot study. *J Pediatr Hematol Oncol* 1998; **20**: 229–33.

●10. Chessells JM, Eden OB, Bailey CC *et al.* Acute lymphoblastic leukaemia in infancy: experience in MRC UKALL trials. Report from the Medical Research Council Working Party on Childhood Leukaemia. *Leukemia* 1994; **8**: 1275–9.

●11. Reaman GH, Sposto R, Sensel MG *et al.* Treatment outcome and prognostic factors for infants with acute lymphoblastic leukemia treated on two consecutive trials of the Children's Cancer Group (see comments). *J Clin Oncol* 1999; **17**: 445–55.

●12. Frankel LS, Ochs J, Shuster JJ *et al.* Therapeutic trial for infant acute lymphoblastic leukemia: the Pediatric Oncology Group experience (POG 8493). *J Pediatr Hematol Oncol* 1997; **19**: 35–7.

●13. Ferster A, Bertrand Y, Benoit Y *et al.* Improved survival for acute lymphoblastic leukaemia in infancy: Experience of EORTC-Childhood Leukaemia Cooperative Group. *Br J Haematol* 1994; **86**: 284–90.

●14. Chessells JM, Harrison CJ, Kempski H *et al.* Clinical features, cytogenetics and outcome in acute lymphoblastic and myeloid leukaemia of infancy: report from the MRC Childhood Leukaemia working party. *Leukemia* 2002; **16**: 776–84.

●15. Isoyama K, Eguchi M, Hibi S *et al.* Risk-directed treatment of infant acute lymphoblastic leukaemia based on early assessment of MLL gene status: results of the Japan Infant Leukaemia Study (MLL96). *Br J Haematol* 2002; **118**: 999–1010.

●16. Silverman LB, McLean TW, Gelber RD *et al.* Intensified therapy for infants with acute lymphoblastic leukemia – results from the Dana Farber Cancer Institute Consortium. *Cancer* 1997; **80**: 2285–95.

●17. Pieters R. Biology and treatment of infant leukemias. In: Ching-Hon Pui. (ed.) *Current clinical oncology: treatment of acute leukemias: new directions for clinical research.* Totowa, NJ: Humana Press Inc., 2003: 61–73.

●18. Taki T, Ida K, Bessho F *et al.* Frequency and clinical significance of the MLL gene rearrangements in infant acute leukemia. *Leukemia* 1996; **10**: 1303–7.

●19. Pui CH, Behm FG, Downing JR *et al.* 11q23/MLL rearrangement confers a poor prognosis in infants with acute lymphoblastic leukemia. *J Clin Oncol* 1994; **12**: 909–15.

●20. Hilden JM, Frestedt JL, Moore RO *et al.* Molecular analysis of infant acute lymphoblastic leukemia: MLL gene rearrangement and reverse transcriptase-polymerase chain reaction for t(4;11)(q21;q23). *Blood* 1995; **86**: 3876–82.

●21. Cimino G, Rapanotti MC, Rivolta A *et al.* Prognostic relevance of ALL-1 gene rearrangement in infant acute leukemias. *Leukemia* 1995; **9**: 391–5.

●22. Chen CS, Sorensen PH, Domer PH *et al.* Molecular rearrangements on chromosome 11q23 predominate in infant acute lymphoblastic leukemia and are associated with specific biologic variables and poor outcome. *Blood* 1993; **81**: 2386–93.

●23. Rubnitz JE, Link MP, Shuster JJ *et al.* Frequency and prognostic significance of HRX rearrangements in infant acute lymphoblastic leukemia: A Pediatric Oncology Group study. *Blood* 1994; **84**: 570–3.

●24. Heerema NA, Arthur DC, Sather H *et al.* Cytogenetic features of infants less than 12 months of age at diagnosis of acute lymphoblastic leukemia: impact of the 11q23 breakpoint on outcome: a report of the Children's Cancer Group. *Blood* 1994; **83**: 2274–84.

●25. Basso G, Putti MC, Cantu-Bajnoldi A. The immunophenotype in infant acute lymphoblastic leukemia: correlation with clinical outcome. An Italian multicentre study (AIEOP). *Br J Haematol* 1992; **81**: 184–91.

●26. Ishii E, Okamura J, Tsuchida M *et al.* Infant leukemia in Japan: clinical and biological analysis of 48 cases. *Med Pediatr Oncol* 1991; **19**: 28–32.

●27. Pui CH. Acute leukemia in children. *Curr Opin Hematol* 1996; **3**: 249–58.

●28. Behm FG, Raimondi SC, Frestedt JL *et al.* Rearrangement of the MLL gene confers a poor prognosis in childhood acute lymphoblastic leukemia, regardless of presenting age. *Blood* 1996; **87**: 2870–7.

●29. Greaves MF. Infant leukaemia biology, aetiology and treatment. *Leukemia* 1996; **10**: 372–7.

●30. Pui C-H, Kane JR, Crist WM. Biology and treatment of infant leukemias. *Leukemia* 1995; **9**: 762–9.

●31. Chen CS, Sorensen PHB, Domer PH *et al.* Molecular rearrangements on chromosome 11q23 predominate in infant acute lymphoblastic leukemia and are associated with specific biologic variables and poor outcome. *Blood* 1993; **81**: 2386–93.

●32. Cimino G, Lo Coco F, Biondi A *et al.* ALL-1 gene at chromosome 11q23 is consistently altered in acute leukemia of early infancy. *Blood* 1993; **82**: 544–6.

●33. Johansson B, Moorman AV, Haas OA *et al.* Hematologic malignancies with t(4;11)(q21;q23) – a cytogenetic, morphologic, immunophenotypic and clinical study of 183 cases. European 11q23 Workshop participants. *Leukemia* 1998; **12**: 779–87.

●34. Rubnitz JE, Camitta BM, Mahmoud H *et al.* Childhood acute lymphoblastic leukemia with the MLL-ENL fusion and t(11;19)(q23;p13.3). *J Clin Oncol* 1999; **17**: 191–6.

●35. Cimino G, Rapanotti MC, Sprovieri T, Elia L. ALL 1 gene alterations in acute leukemia: biological and clinical aspects. *Haematologica* 1998; **83**: 350–7.

●36. Hilden JM, Kersey JH. The MLL (11q23) and AF-4 (4q21) genes disrupted in t(4;11) acute leukemia: molecular and clinical studies. *Leuk Lymphoma* 1994; **14**: 189–95.

37. Heerema NA, Sather HN, Ge J *et al.* Cytogenetic studies of infant acute lymphoblastic leukemia: poor prognosis of infants with t(4;11) – a report of the Children's Cancer Group. *Leukemia* 1999; **13**: 679–86.

38. Pui C-H. Acute lymphoblastic leukemia in infants. *J Clin Oncol* 1999; **17**: 438–40.

39. Li Q, Frestedt JL, Kersey JH. AF4 encodes a ubiquitous protein that in both natve and MLL-AF4 fusion types localizes to subnuclear compartments. *Blood* 1998; **92**: 3841–7.

40. Pui C-H, Gaynon PS, Boyett JM *et al.* Outcome of treatment in childhood acute lymphoblastic leukaemia with rearrangements of the 11q23 chromosomal region. *Lancet* 2002; **359**: 1909–15.

41. Basso G, Rodelli R, Covezzoli A. The role of immunophenotype in acute lymphoblastic leukemia of infant age. *Leuk Lymphoma* 1994; **15**: 51–60.

42. Ludwig W-D, Bartram CR, Harbott J *et al.* Phenotypic and genotypic heterogeneity in infant acute lymphoblastic leukemia. *Leukemia* 1989; **3**: 431–9.

43. Felix CA, Reaman GH, Korsmeyer SJ *et al.* Immunoglobulin and T cell receptor gene configuration in acute lymphoblastic leukemia in infancy. *Blood* 1987; **70**: 536–41.

44. Jabali Y, Stary J, Hak J *et al.* Acute lymphoblastic leukemia in infants: A decade of experience in the Czech Republic. *Med Pediatr Oncol* 2000; **34**: 493–5.

45. Nagayama J, Tomizawa D, Koh K *et al.* Infants with acute lymphoblastic leukemia and a germline MLL gene are highly curable with use of chemotherapy alone: results from the Japan Infant Leukemia Study Group. *Blood* 2006; **107**: 4663–5.

46. Pieters R, Schrappe M, De Lorenzo P *et al.* A treatment protocol for infants younger than 1 year with acute lymphoblastic leukemia (Interfant-99): an observational study and multicentre randomized trail. *Lancet* 2007; **370**: 240–50.

47. Hilden JM, Dinndorf PA, Meerbaum SO *et al.* Analysis of prognostic factors of acute lymphoblastic leukemia in infants: report on CCG 1953 from the Children's Oncology Group. *Blood* 2006; **108**: 441–51.

48. Dreyer Z, Dinndorf PA, Sather H *et al.* Shortened intensified therapy in infant ALL: a Pediatric Oncology Group study. Presented at 20th Annual Meeting of the American Society of Pediatric Hematology/Oncology, Toronto, Canada, 2007.

49. Campbell M, Cabrera ME, Legues ME *et al.* Discordant clinical presentation and outcome in infant twins sharing a common clonal leukaemia. *Br J Haematol* 1996; **93**: 166–9.

50. Kosata Y, Koh K, Kinukawa N *et al.* Infant acute lymphoblastic leukemia with MLL gene rearrangements: outcome following intensive chemotherapy and hematopoietic stem cell transplantation. *Blood* 2004; **104**: 3527–34.

51. Dreyer Z, Dinndorf PA, Hilden JM *et al.* Unexpected toxicity with intensified induction in infant ALL. *Blood* 2007; **110**: 261a (abstract).

52. Biondi A, Cimino G, Pieters R, Pui C-H. Biological and therapeutic aspects of infant leukemia. *Blood* 2000; **96**: 24–33.

53. Emminger W, Emminger-Schmidmeier W, Haas OA *et al.* Treatment of infant leukemia with busulfan, cyclophosphamide ± etoposide and bone marrow transplantation. *Bone Marrow Transplant* 1992; **9**: 313–18.

54. Pirich L, Haut P, Morgan E *et al.* Total body irradiation, cyclophosphamide, and etoposide with stem cell transplant as treatment for infants with acute lymphoblastic leukemia. *Med Pediatr Oncol* 1999; **32**: 1–6.

55. von Bueltzingsloewen A, Esperou-Bourdeau H, Souillet G *et al.* Allogeneic bone marrow transplantation following a busulfan-based conditioning regimen in young children with acute lymphoblastic leukemia: a cooperative study of the Societe Francaise de Greffe de Molle. *Bone Marrow Transplant* 1995; **16**: 521–7.

56. Saarinen UM, Mellander L, Nysom K *et al.* Allogeneic bone marrow transplantation in first remission for children with very high-risk acute lymphoblastic leukemia: a retrospective case-control study in the Nordic countries. *Bone Marrow Transplant* 1996; **17**: 357–63.

57. Marco F, Bureo E, Ortega JJ *et al.* High survival rate in infant acute leukemia treated with early high-dose chemotherapy and stem-cell support. *J Clin Oncol* 2000; **18**: 3256–61.

58. Sanders JE, Im HJ, Hoffmeister PA *et al.* Allogeneic hematopoietic cell transplantation for infants with acute lymphoblastic leukemia. *Blood* 2005; **105**: 3749–56.

59. Dreyer Z, Dinndorf PA, Sather H *et al.* Hematopoietic stem cell transplant (HSCT) versus intensive chemotherapy in infant acute lymphoblastic leukemia (ALL). *J Clin Oncol* 2007; **25**: 9514.

60. Siegel SE, Moran RG. Problems in the chemotherapy of cancer in the neonate. *Am J Pediatr Hematol Oncol* 1981; **3**: 287.

61. Thompson P, Dreyer ZE, Blaney S *et al.* Pharmacokinetics of methotrexate in infants with acute lymphoblastic leukemia. *Clin Pharmacol Ther* 2004; **75**: P47.

62. Thompson PA, Murray DJ, Rosner GL *et al.* Methotrexate pharmacokinetics in infants with acute lymphoblastic leukemia. *Cancer Chemother Pharmacol* 2007; **59**: 847–53.

63. Wasserman R, Galili N, Ito Y *et al.* Predominance of fetal type DJ_H joining in young children with B precursor lymphoblastic leukemia as evidence for an in utero transforming event. *J Exp Med* 1992; **176**: 1577–81.

64. Sansone R, Negri D. Cytogenetic features of neonatal leukemias. *Cancer Genet Cytogenet* 1992; **63**: 56–61.

65. Ford AM, Ridge SA, Cabrera ME *et al.* In utero rearrangements in the trithorax-related oncogene in infant leukaemias. *Nature* 1993; **363**: 358–60.

66. Gill Super HJ, Rothberg PG, Kobayashi F *et al.* Clonal, nonconstitutional rearrangements of the MLL gene in infant twins with the acute lymphoblastic leukemia: in utero chromosome rearrangement of 11q23. *Blood* 1994; **83**: 641–4.

67. Mahmoud HH, Ridge SA, Behm FG *et al.* Intrauterine monoclonal origin of neonatal concordant acute lymphoblastic leukemia in monozygotic twins. *Med Pediatr Oncol* 1995; **24**: 77–81.

●68. Richkind KE, Loew T, Meisner L et al. Identical cytogenetic clones and clonal evolution in pediatric monozygotic twins with acute myeloid leukemia: presymptomatic disease detection by interphase fluorescence in situ, hybridization and review of the literature. *J Pediatr Hematol Oncol* 1998; **20**: 264–7.

●69. Hunger SP, McGavran L, Meltesen L et al. Oncogenesis in utero: fetal death due to acute myelogenous leukaemia with an MLL translocation. *Br J Haematol* 1998; **103**: 539–42.

●70. Gale KB, Ford AM, Repp R et al. Backtracking leukemia to birth: identification of clonotypic gene fusion sequences in neonatal blood spots. *Proc Natl Acad Sci U S A* 1997; **94**: 13950–4.

●71. Wiermels JL, Cazzaniga G, Daniotti M et al. Prenatal origin of acute lymphoblastic leukaemia in children. *Lancet* 1999; **354**: 1499–503.

●72. Shu XO, Ross JA, Pendergrass TW et al. Parental alcohol consumption, cigarette smoking, and risk of infant leukemia: a Children's Cancer Group study. *J Natl Cancer Inst* 1996; **88**: 24–31.

●73. Severson RK, Buckley JD, Woods WG et al. Cigarette smoking and alcohol consumption by parents of children with acute myeloid leukemia: an analysis within morphological subgroups – a report from Children's Cancer Group. *Cancer Epidemiol Biomarkers Prev* 1993; **5**: 433–9.

●74. van Duijin CM, van Steensel-Moll HA, Coebergh JW, van Zanen GE. Risk factors for childhood acute non-lymphocytic leukemia: an association with maternal alcohol consumption during pregnancy? *Cancer Epidemiol Biomarkers Prev* 1994; **3**: 457–60.

●75. Ross JA, Potter JD, Shu XO et al. Evaluating the relationships among maternal reproductive history, birth characteristics, and infant leukemia: a report from the Children's Cancer Group. *Ann Epidemiol* 1997; **7**: 172–9.

●76. Westergaard T, Andersen PK, Pedersen JB et al. Birth characteristics, sibling patterns and acute leukemia risk in childhood: a population-based cohort study. *J Natl Cancer Inst* 1997; **89**: 939–47.

●77. Wertelecki W, Mantel N. Increased birthweight in leukemia. *Pediatr Res* 1973; **7**: 132–8.

●78. Cnattingius S, Zack MM, Ekbom A et al. Prenatal and neonatal risk factors for childhood lymphatic leukemia. *J Natl Cancer Inst* 1995; **87**: 908–14.

●79. Ross JA, Perentesis JP, Robison LL, Davies SM. Big babies and infant leukemia: a role for insulin-like growth factor-1? *Cancer Causes Control* 1996; **7**: 553–9.

●80. Pui CH, Relling MV, Rivera GK et al. Epipodophyllotoxin-related acute myeloid leukemia: a study of 35 cases. *Leukemia* 1995; **9**: 1990–6.

●81. Ross JA, Potter JD, Reaman GH et al. A preliminary investigation examining maternal exposure to potential DNA topoisomerase II inhibitors and infant leukemia: a report from the Children's Cancer Group. *Cancer Causes Control* 1996; **7**: 581–90.

●82. Setchell KDR, Zimmer-Nechemias L, Cai J, Heubi JE. Exposure of infants to photo-oestrogens from soy-based infant formula. *Lancet* 1997; **350**: 23–7.

●83. Cimino G, Rapanotti MC, Biondi A et al. Infant acute leukemias show the same biased distribution of ALL1 gene breaks as topoisomerase II related secondary acute leukemias. *Cancer Res* 1997; **57**: 2879–83.

●84. Ross JA. Dietary flavonoids and the MLL gene: A pathway to infant leukemia? *Proc Natl Acad Sci U S A* 2000; **97**: 4411–13.

●85. Biondi A, Garte S, Crosti F et al. Parental exposure and susceptibility factors in the etiology of infant leukemia. *Blood* 1998; **92**: 391a.

●86. Michaelis J, Kaletsch U, Burkart W, Grosche B. Infant leukemia after the Chernobyl accident. *Nature* 1997; **387**: 246.

●87. Parkin DM, Clayton D, Black RJ et al. Childhood leukaemia in Europe after Chernobyl: 5 year follow-up. *Br J Cancer* 1996; **73**: 1006–12.

●88. Petridou E, Trichopoulos D, Dessypris N et al. Infant leukaemia after in utero exposure to radiation from Chernobyl. *Nature* 1996; **382**: 352–3.

●89. Leung W, Hudson M, Zhu Y et al. Late effects in survivors of infant leukemia. *Leukemia* 2000; **14**: 1185–90.

●90. Kaleita TA, Reaman GH, MacLean WE et al. Neurodevelopmental outcome of infants with acute lymphoblastic leukemia: a Children's Cancer Group report. *Cancer* 1999; **85**: 1859–65.

●91. Pieters R, Kaspers GJL, Huismans DR et al. Cellular drug resistance profiles that might explain the prognostic value of immunophenotype and age in childhood acute lymphoblastic leukemia. *Leukemia* 1993; **7**: 392–7.

●92. Pieters R, den Boer ML, Durian M et al. Relation between age, immunophenotype and in vitro drug resistance in 395 children with acute lymphoblastic leukemia implications for treatment of infants. *Leukemia* 1998; **12**: 1344–8.

●93. Brown P, Levis M, Shurtleff S et al. FLT3 inhibition selectively kills childhood acute lymphoblastic leukemia cells with high levels of FLT3 expression. *Blood* 2005; **105**: 812–20.

●94. Armstrong SA, Staunton JE, Silverman LB et al. MLL translocations specify a distinct gene expression profile that distinguishes a unique leukemia. *Nat Genet* 2002; **30**: 41–7.

●95. Yeoh EJ, Ross ME, Shurtleff SA et al. Classification, subtype discovery, and prediction of outcome in pediatric acute lymphoblastic leukemia by gene expression profiling. *Cancer Cell* 2002; **1**: 133–43.

●96. Cimino G, Elia L, Rapanotti MC et al. A prospective study of residual-disease monitoring of the ALL1/AF4 transcript in patients with t(4;11) acute lymphoblastic leukemia. *Blood* 2000; **95**: 96–101.

●97. Laughton SJ, Ashton LJ, Kwan E et al. Early responses to chemotherapy of normal and malignant hematologic cells are prognostic in children with acute lymphoblastic leukemia. *J Clin Oncol* 2005; **23**: 2264–71.

58

Management of lymphoid neoplasms in the elderly

JOSEPH M CONNORS

Clinicians caring for patients with lymphoid cancers need to appreciate two long-term trends unfolding throughout the world: first, the median age of the populations of most countries is steadily increasing; second, the incidence of lymphoma in the elderly continues to rise, a robust trend that has continued for more than 50 years.[1–7] In addition, physicians caring for elderly patients with lymphoma also need to take into consideration the physiologic changes that accompany aging and the impact of lifestyle choices and effects of long-term medication for other conditions. In the public health sphere, policy planners must anticipate the increased demands these patients will impose on the medical care system. Characterization of these trends and a description of the progress that has been made in the classification and treatment of lymphoid cancers in general should prove helpful for both individual patient care and population health-care planning.

AGING OF THE POPULATION AND LYMPHOMA INCIDENCE: SYNERGISTIC TRENDS

It is reasonable to anticipate that the proportion of the population over the age of 65 years throughout much of the world will double from approximately 10 percent to 20 percent over the next two decades.[3] Since more than half of all lymphomas are seen in the minority of the population over the age of 65 years[5–7] clinicians and health-care planners should expect an increase of at least

70 percent in the absolute numbers of lymphoma patients solely on the basis of demographics. If lymphomas were rare in the elderly this change would have only a modest consequence. However, the opposite is true. In the developed countries of the world the lymphoid cancers, in aggregate, are now the fourth most common human neoplasm in incidence[5,6] comprising more than 5 percent of all newly diagnosed cancers. Thus, any increase in the number of the elderly will cause disproportionate increases in the number of new lymphomas. This impact of demographic shifts now underway will, all by itself, translate into a challenge for physicians and health-care planners.

A second trend will synergistically interact with the increase in new lymphomas caused by aging of the population: wherever reliable statistics are available, the incidence of lymphoma has been rising at a rate of approximately 3 percent per year and has been doing so for more than 50 years, suggesting a robust trend that will continue.[3–6] Further, other than modest contributions due to increased incidence secondary to the acquired immune deficiency syndrome (AIDS) epidemic, wider use of immunosuppressant medications, and increased frequency of infection with hepatitis C and human T cell lymphotrophic virus type 1 (HTLV-1), most of the increased incidence of lymphoma is occurring in the elderly,[3–6] independent of these other causes of lymphoma. Thus, we are witnessing the cumulative impact of multiple trends: the numbers of the elderly, the subgroup within the general population who disproportionately develop lymphoma, are increasing;

the incidence of lymphoma in general is rising; and the greatest rise in incidence is occurring in the elderly. As has been seen for at least the past several decades, clinicians and health-care planners should expect more than a doubling of the absolute numbers of patients with lymphoma who are over the age of 65 years during the next two decades. To be adequately addressed, these trends must be anticipated and planned for now.

CLASSIFICATION AND STAGING OF LYMPHOMA IN THE ELDERLY

Classification

Through the 1990s the most widely used classification scheme for the malignant lymphomas was the Working Formulation.[8] This scheme was very useful because most of its subtypes were reproducibly recognizable and had consistent behavior in terms of sites of presentation, natural

history, response to treatment, and prognosis. However, the identification of distinct new subtypes, the need to integrate the classification systems used in Europe and North America, and the recognition that emerging new diagnostic techniques added valuable information led to proposals to adopt a new scheme with more subtypes, clearer linkage to immunophenotype, and a better incorporation of insights from molecular biology and cytogenetics. In the later 1990s a new classification scheme entitled the Revised European American Lymphoma (REAL) classification[9] was proposed and then modified, by consensus among international experts in lymphoma pathology and treatment, into the current, widely accepted World Health Organization (WHO) classification system.[10] Table 58.1 lists the entities from the WHO classification in a fashion relevant to clinical management, segregating the lymphomas into subgroups that must be considered separately when planning therapy.

A number of clinically relevant improvements have been made in the transition from the Working Formulation

Table 58.1 The World Health Organization classification of the lymphomas, adapted for clinical application

	B cell	T cell
Indolent lymphomas		
	Small lymphocytic lymphoma/ chronic lymphocytic leukemia	Mycoses fungoides
	Lymphoplasmacytic lymphoma	Cutaneous CD30-associated lymphoproliferative disease
	Follicular lymphoma grades 1,2,3	
	Marginal zone lymphoma	
	Nodal	
	Splenic	
	Mucosal-associated (MALT)	
Aggressive lymphomas		
	Mantle cell lymphoma	Peripheral T cell lymphoma, unspecified
	Diffuse large B cell lymphoma	Anaplastic large cell lymphoma
		Angioimmunoblastic lymphoma
		Nasal T/NK type lymphoma
		Enteropathy-associated T cell lymphoma
		Subcutaneous panniculitic type lymphoma
		$\gamma\delta$ hepatosplenic type
Special lymphomas		
	Lymphoblastic B cell lymphoma	Lymphoblastic T cell lymphoma
	Burkitt lymphoma	
Virus-induced lymphomas		
	Primary effusion lymphoma (HHV-8)	HTLV-1 lymphoma/leukemia (HTLV-1)
Hodgkin lymphomas		
	Nodular lymphocyte predominant	
	Classical Hodgkin lymphoma	
	Nodular sclerosing	
	Mixed cellularity	
	Lymphocyte rich	
	Lymphocyte depleted	

MALT, mucosal-associated lymphoid tissue; NK, natural killer; HHV-8, human herpesvirus 8; HTLV-1, human T cell lymphotrophic virus.

to the WHO classification. All the follicular lymphomas, grade 1 (follicular small cleaved cell), grade 2 (follicular mixed large and small cell), and grade 3 (follicular large cell) are collapsed into a single subtype, follicular lymphoma. Several new B cell entities are recognized. Marginal zone lymphoma, which includes nodal and splenic types and the mucosal-associated lymphoid type (MALT) variant, is a type of small B cell lymphoma distinct from the small lymphocytic lymphoma/chronic lymphocytic leukemia type in terms of sites of presentation, lesser tendency to disseminate, and, in the case of MALT lymphoma of the stomach, a unique association with antecedent infection with *Helicobacter pylori*. Mantle cell lymphoma, which, before its recent recognition, was usually called diffuse small cleaved cell lymphoma, is a B cell lymphoma with relatively poor prognosis, little evidence of curability, and an often relentless course with short-duration responses and rapid relapses. Primary effusion lymphoma has been recognized as one of the rare virus-induced lymphomas, in this case associated with human herpesvirus type 8 (HHV-8) and is usually, but not always, seen in association with human immunodeficiency virus (HIV) infection.

Although important new types of lymphoma are recognized among the B cell lymphomas in the WHO classification[10] the greatest number of new entities is among the T cell lymphomas. These include cutaneous CD30-positive lymphoproliferative disease, angioimmunoblastic lymphoma, anaplastic large cell lymphoma, nasal T/natural killer (NK) type lymphoma, enteropathy-associated T cell lymphoma, subcutaneous panniculitic type lymphoma, $\gamma\delta$ hepatosplenic type lymphoma, and the catchall category, peripheral T cell lymphoma, not otherwise specified. All but the first of this new list of T cell lymphomas are aggressive diseases requiring measures similar to those used for diffuse large B cell lymphoma if they are to be cured or even temporarily controlled.

The purpose of a classification scheme for lymphomas, as for any disease, is to separate subtypes with clinically relevant differences and group together subtypes with similar overall natural histories and responses to treatment. Ideally, subtypes should be unique and uniform in terms of sites of presentation, natural history, response to treatment, and prognosis and at the same time be readily and reproducibly identifiable. The scheme shown in Table 58.1 shows a practical way to divide the lymphomas that can readily guide therapeutic decisions. The overall approach to management of elderly patients with lymphoma should start from this classification.

Staging

The stage indicates the extent of dissemination of the malignant lymphoma for the purpose of designing treatment and strongly influences prognosis. Table 58.2 shows the standard diagnostic and staging evaluations which all patients should undergo unless the tests are precluded by frailty. Additional radiographs and scans, radionucleotide studies, samples of pleural or peritoneal effusions, and directed biopsies should be obtained to clarify suspicious lesions, always remembering, however, that additional testing is only necessary insofar as it will alter the therapeutic plan. The role of positron emission tomographic (PET) scanning, although clearly the most innovative imaging technique to be developed in the last decade, remains unclear for staging purposes. For most patients it is unlikely to lead to alteration of the therapeutic plan and is, therefore, unnecessary.

The staging criteria for malignant lymphoma were developed specifically for Hodgkin lymphoma, a disease with an orderly and predictable pattern of spread. However, their ready application, familiarity, and prognostic relevance have led to use for all lymphomas. These Ann Arbor

Table 58.2 Standard diagnostic and staging evaluations for patients with lymphoma, including the elderly, and their justification

Test	Reason
Histopathologic review by experienced hematopathologist	Subclassification requires special experience and techniques and is a crucial determinant of treatment and prognosis
History searching for B symptoms[a] or localized new abnormalities	B symptoms indicate advanced disease
Physical exam searching for lymphadenopathy, masses, or hepatosplenomegaly	Additional potential disease sites may be detected
CBC, serum creatinine, serum liver enzymes, LDH	Bone marrow, renal, and hepatic reserve affect choice and dosing of treatments; LDH is a strong prognostic indicator
Serum protein electrophoresis	A lymphoma-associated monoclonal paraprotein may be detected
Chest radiograph	To detect intrathoracic disease
Computed tomographic scan of thorax, abdomen, and pelvis	To detect otherwise-unsuspected areas of involvement
Bone marrow biopsy	To detect involvement in this frequent site of disease

[a]B symptoms: weight loss >10% of baseline, persistent fever, night sweats.
CBC, complete blood count; LDH, lactate dehydrogenase.

Table 58.3   Ann Arbor staging criteria

Stage	Criteria
I	One area of nodal or extranodal disease
II	Two or more nodal sites of disease of nodal and proximate extranodal sites on the same side of the diaphragm
III	Two or more nodal sites of disease or nodal and proximate extranodal sites of disease on both sides of the diaphragm
IV	Disseminated extranodal with or without nodal sites of disease
	A No constitutional symptoms
	B Constitutional symptoms
	Weight loss >10% of baseline
	Night sweats
	Persistent fever

Table 58.4   Lymphoma staging simplified for treatment planning

Limited stage	Advanced stage
Ann Arbor I or II	Ann Arbor stage III or IV
and	or
No B symptoms	B symptoms
and	or
Greatest single tumor diameter <10 cm	Diameter ≥10 cm

criteria[11] are summarized in Table 58.3. In theory, eight different stages ranging from IA to IVB are possible but in practice these can be collapsed into two broad categories of limited and advanced disease. Because large bulk connotes a high tumor burden equivalent to that of advanced stage disease most authorities include tumor bulk in the staging and choice of therapy.[12] Consideration of Ann Arbor stage, symptomatic state, and tumor bulk allows assignment of the patient to one of two stage groups as shown in Table 58.4. This simplified stage grouping is useful across all the different types of lymphoma and directly indicates the appropriate choices for treatment planning.

SPECIAL CONSIDERATIONS FOR TREATMENT OF LYMPHOMA IN THE ELDERLY

Factors that may affect the results of treatment in the elderly population are of two types: those which are independent of the lymphoma and those intrinsic to it. Factors unrelated to the lymphoma include comorbid illnesses; cumulative consequences of long-term use or abuse of tobacco, alcohol, or medications; alterations in host immunologic integrity; loss of reserve in organs that may now be additionally damaged

by chemotherapy or irradiation; alteration in absorption, distribution, activation, detoxification, metabolism, and clearance of drugs, altering their pharmacodynamics and pharmacokinetics; and reduced emotional or physiological tolerance for invasive procedures and toxic therapies. Several of these factors may be present in the same patient, reducing his or her ability to tolerate treatments and leading to reduction in delivered doses or intensity of treatment. Furthermore, in elderly patients the participation that is needed from the patient's own immune, inflammatory, phagocytic, and other systems to help deal with the disease may be suboptimal.

The lymphomas seen in the elderly differ intrinsically from those seen in the younger population. Carbone and coworkers[13] found a striking preponderance of diffuse (85 percent) over nodular (15 percent) subtypes in the elderly. Other studies[14,15] and our own results from the province of British Columbia (data not shown) confirm this same shift. These data indicate that there is a clinically relevant shift to the more aggressive subtypes of lymphoma seen with advancing age. Another indicator of their altered biology is the tendency of lymphomas in the elderly to involve extranodal sites more commonly. Several series have documented this increased likelihood of extranodal disease, especially to sites such as the gastrointestinal tract, brain, and testes.[13,16–18] It seems reasonable to speculate that the lymphomas seen in the elderly have had more time to accumulate cytogenetic abnormalities and mutational events. These genetic changes may then, in turn, account for a more aggressive phenotype. Thus, both host-related factors and changes intrinsic to the lymphomas predict for more aggressive tumor behavior and reduced tolerance for treatment in the elderly when they are treated for lymphoma. This may help to explain the generally poorer outcomes seen in older patients even when attempts have been made to give treatment equal in potency to that given to younger patients.

SPECIFIC LYMPHOMAS

The development of the WHO classification system for the lymphoid cancers,[10] by relating basic biology to individual diseases, represents a major step forward in our understanding of these diverse diseases. This system, however, presents the clinician with an unwieldy large number of separate types, far more than we have different treatment strategies. Fortunately, it is possible to group the lymphomas into clinically relevant subsets based on their pretreatment behavior and typical natural history. Table 58.1 is arranged using such a grouping. The indolent lymphomas usually present with widely disseminated disease, progress slowly, and threaten the patient's life over time usually measured in years. The aggressive lymphomas may present with either localized or widely disseminated disease, have a predisposition to involve extranodal tissue, and, if unaltered by treatment, threaten survival in a matter of months. The special lymphomas share many characteristics with adult acute leukemia. They present with, or rapidly develop, widespread dissemination; frequently involve the bone marrow and central nervous system; threaten the patient's survival in weeks or even days; and require intensified therapy combined with central nervous system treatment to be cured reliably. Finally, the viral lymphomas are quite rare outside of a few endemic areas such as Japan and may be associated with quite variable presentations and natural histories but are reasonably grouped because of their etiologic connection with a specific causative pathogen. The approach to treatment of the lymphomas can be most sensibly described by starting with these broad subgroups – indolent, aggressive, special, and viral – and then noting exceptions.

INDOLENT LYMPHOMA

Follicular lymphoma is the most common type of indolent lymphoma, constituting approximately 25 percent of all lymphomas seen in Western countries and about 60 percent of the indolent variety.[10,19] There are few detailed reports of treatment of indolent lymphoma purely focused on the elderly. Such patients are often included in series with younger patients. A few lessons can be drawn from the available literature. Patients with limited stage indolent lymphoma only constitute about 10 percent of patients with indolent disease but can be treated, regardless of age, with involved region irradiation.[20] It is reasonable to hope to cure at least 50 percent of such patients[20] and many elderly patients can live out the rest of their lives free of lymphoma after such treatment. The treatment approach to the special case of mucosal-associated lymphoid tissue (MALT) lymphoma of the stomach, which is seen in association with *H. pylori*[21–23] in most cases, also applies regardless of age. Patients with gastric MALT lymphoma confined to the stomach should have the *H. pylori* organism eradicated with antibiotics. In many patients durable regression of the MALT lymphoma will ensue.[22,23] If the lymphoma does not regress, the possibility of coincident presence of more aggressive lymphoma should be pursued with appropriate biopsies. If no aggressive-type lymphoma is present, conventional irradiation or single-agent chemotherapy are reasonable choices for persistent gastric MALT lymphoma after effective anti-*Helicobacter pylori* antibiotics fail to induce remission.

Advanced stage indolent lymphoma has not been systematically evaluated in the elderly. One randomized prospective trial of modest size ($n = 142$) found that FM (fludarabine and mitoxantrone) produced a superior response rate and failure-free survival but did not alter overall survival when compared to CHVP (cyclophosphamide, doxorubicin, vindesine, and prednisone).[24] Lacking studies specifically focused on the elderly we must rely on the lessons available from series including patients of all ages. Given their shorter life expectancy and greater potential for treatment-related toxicity many elderly patients

are reluctant to embark on an invasive staging evaluation or toxic treatments. An approach of watchful waiting and intervention with chemotherapy when symptomatic or threatening disease develops is appropriate for such patients.[25] Judicious use of involved region irradiation can also provide very helpful palliation. With the demonstration that multiagent chemotherapy plus the monoclonal anti-CD20 antibody rituximab produces substantially superior progression-free survival for patients of all ages with follicular lymphoma compared to chemotherapy alone,[26,27] such an approach has become the standard of care for patients with symptomatic indolent lymphoma. Both CVP (cyclophosphamide, vincristine, and prednisone) and CHOP (cyclophosphamide, doxorubicin, vincristine, and prednisone) produce superior response rates and progression-free survival when combined with rituximab.[26,27] Given a lack of evidence that the doxorubicin is necessary, the former combination is preferable for most elderly patients allowing reduced toxicity and potentially safer, but equally effective, treatment.

AGGRESSIVE LYMPHOMA

Although many different histologic subtypes can be included in the aggressive lymphoma category (Table 58.1), by far the most common is B cell large cell lymphoma.[10] Almost 50 percent of all lymphomas seen in the elderly fall into this single subgroup. About one-third of elderly patients with diffuse large cell lymphoma present with limited stage disease. Curative treatment can usually be given with excellent results. A large study conducted by the Southwest Oncology Group showed that a brief course of chemotherapy with CHOP followed by involved region irradiation is at least as effective as prolonged chemotherapy alone and less toxic.[28] We have used this brief chemotherapy-based approach at the British Columbia Cancer Agency (BCCA) since 1981 and have found it routinely well tolerated by patients even well into their ninth decade of life.[29] Although the results for those over the age of 70 years in the SWOG study and in our BCCA experience (Table 58.5) are not quite as good as those for younger patients they are still excellent. Recently the need for the radiation therapy has been questioned based on results achieved using intensified chemotherapy alone, either with CHOP administered every 2 weeks with neutrophil growth factor support[30] or with a special intensified regimen ACVBP (doxorubicin, cyclophosphamide, vindesine, bleomycin, and prednisone).[31] However, both of these approaches are difficult to deliver to the elderly, are considerably more expensive and toxic, and take longer to complete than treatment with brief chemotherapy and involved field radiation. In addition, preliminary data with new combinations adding rituximab to CHOP indicate that the efficacy of brief chemotherapy plus radiation can be improved with that maneuver without increasing either the toxicity or length of treatment (personal communication, Dr Thomas

Miller, 2005). Thus, the best approach to treat limited stage aggressive lymphoma in the elderly remains brief chemotherapy, now with the addition of rituximab for those with B cell disease, followed by involved field radiation. For uncommon presentations in which the radiation may be potentially more toxic, such as those involving the mouth or upper throat, more extended chemotherapy plus rituximab without radiation is a reasonable alternative.

Most clinical research into lymphomas seen in the elderly population has focused on advanced stage diffuse large B cell lymphoma. Until recently only a few randomized trials were designed specifically for the elderly. Table 58.6 lists the findings from selected representative phase II trials that have been published[32–39] and Table 58.7 shows the results from the randomized prospective studies.[30,40–45] Although all the results shown in these tables reflect relatively short follow-up, the completion of several large, well-designed,

prospective randomized trials since 2002 allows us to draw firm conclusions.

The overall survivals achieved in the phase II trials range from 21 percent to 49 percent and the variation is more likely due to patient selection and immature follow-up than differences in efficacy of the tested regimens. None of these trials produced compelling evidence of superiority

Table 58.6 Results of phase II studies of elderly patients with advanced stage diffuse large cell lymphoma

Regimen	n	Age (years)	Overall survival (%)	Reference
TP + EP	66	>70	21	32
VMP	52	>0	25	33
LD-ACOP-B	40	65–85	38	34
VABE	32	65–85	43	34
DOCE	63	65–85	45	35
BECALM	26	>64	36	36
CHOP	81	>64	32	37
P-VEBEC	67	65–80	40	38
VNCOP-B	350	>60	49	39

TP + EP: teniposide, prednimustine, etoposide; VMP: etoposide, mitoxantrone, prednimustine; LD-ACOP-B: doxorubicin, cyclophosphamide, vincristine, prednisone, bleomycin; VABE: etoposide, doxorubicin, bleomycin, vincristine, prednisone; DOCE: doxorubicin, vincristine, cyclophosphamide, etoposide, prednisone; BECALM: bleomycin, etoposide, cyclophosphamide, doxorubicin, methotrexate, leucovorin; CHOP: cyclophosphamide, doxorubicin, vincristine, prednisone; P-VEBEC: prednisone, vincristine, etoposide, bleomycin, epirubicin, cyclophosphamide; VNCOP-B: cyclophosphamide, mitoxantrone, vincristine, etoposide, bleomycin, prednisone.

Table 58.5 Results of treatment of limited stage diffuse large cell lymphoma with brief chemotherapy and involved region irradiation analyzed by age at diagnosis

Age (years)	n	Survival	
		10–year overall (%)[a]	10–year disease specific (%)[a]
16–69	197	76	85
>70	100	38	73

[a]Overall survival includes all deaths from any cause; disease-specific survival censors patients at the time of death if it is unrelated to disease or toxicity and better reflects ability to cure the lymphoma.

Table 58.7 Results of randomized phase III trials of treatment of elderly patients with advanced stage diffuse large cell lymphoma

Regimens	Median age (years)	n	EFS (%)	OS (%)	p (for OS)	Reference
ld-CHOP	74	77		(3 yr) 43	NS	40
MCOP		78		41		
CHOP	72	192	(5 yr) 18	(5 yr) 22	NS	41
CHOP + G-CSF		197	17	24		
ld-CHOP	74	~160		(5 yr) ~30	NS	42
THP-COP		~160		~30		
THP-COPE		~160		~30		
CHOP	71	72		(3 yr) 42	0.029	43
CNOP		76		26		
CHOP	71	205	(3 yr) 40	(3 yr) 61	<0.001	44
CNOP		203	19	33		
CHOP	69	197	(5 yr) 29	(5 yr) 58	0.0073	45
CHOP + rituximab		202	47	45		
CHOP	~68	178	(5 yr) 33	(5 yr) 41	<0.001	30
CHOP-14 + G-CSF		172	44	53		

EFS, event-free survival; OS, overall survival; NS, not significant; ld-CHOP: low-dose cyclophosphamide, doxorubicin, vincristine, prednisone; MCOP: mitoxantrone, cyclophosphamide, vincristine, prednisone; CHOP: standard dose-CHOP; CHOP + G-CSF: CHOP plus filgrastim; THP-COP: pararubicin, cyclophosphamide, vincristine, prednisone; THP-COPE: pararubicin, cyclophosphamide, vincristine, prednisone, etoposide; CNOP: cyclophosphamide, mitoxantrone, vincristine, prednisone; CHOP-14: standard-dose CHOP delivered every 14 days plus filgrastim.

of the tested regimen compared to standard CHOP primarily because of lack of a randomized control. Hence, by default and consensus, the standard of care remained CHOP despite the promise shown by several of the new regimens in these and other phase II trials.

The results of the randomized trials demonstrate several important lessons. First, achieving a reduction in toxicity by using less than the standard doses in CHOP reduces effectiveness. Low-dose versions of CHOP are inferior to standard CHOP.[40,42] Second, substitution of less-toxic agents in the CHOP regimen may reduce side effects but at the price of effectiveness. CNOP, using mitoxantrone instead of doxorubicin, reduced toxicity compared to CHOP but also produced inferior results.[40,43,44] Third, using neutrophil growth factors to ensure full dosing of standard CHOP ensures closer adherence to the planned protocol without increased infectious complications but does not improve survival.[41,44] Finally, introduction of novel agents at the expense of full dosing of the agents in standard CHOP does not increase efficacy.[40,42–44,46]

Progress in improving on the effectiveness of standard-dose CHOP for the treatment of aggressive lymphomas in the elderly was not achieved until recently. Two landmark studies have now established a new standard of care. The addition of rituximab to standard CHOP improved the response rates, event-free survival, and overall survival, reducing the likelihood of dying from lymphoma by at least 30 to 40 percent.[45,47,48] Intensifying the dosing of CHOP by giving treatment every 14 days with neutrophil growth factor support also produced approximately the same degree of benefit.[30] Whether one or the other of these two new approaches is superior is currently being tested in prospective trials. Until their results are available, the less-toxic approach employing rituximab has emerged as the new standard of care. It is gratifying to have these major steps forward in the treatment of patients of all ages with diffuse large B cell lymphoma achieved by well-conceived and efficiently executed trials specifically targeted at the elderly population.

SPECIAL LYMPHOMAS

The special or leukemia-like lymphomas are rare overall and especially uncommon in the elderly. Some types, such as T cell lymphoblastic and Burkitt lymphoma, are only anecdotally encountered in those over 65 to 70 years of age. Thus, it is not surprising that there are no substantial reports of treatment outcomes for these most aggressive lymphomas in populations confined to the elderly. The types of intensive chemotherapy required to eradicate lymphoblastic lymphoma and Burkitt lymphoma in young patients are ill-suited to the elderly and usually beyond their tolerance. All but the most exceptionally vigorous patients in this age range should be treated with palliative intent pending identification of better, less-toxic treatments than are now available.

HODGKIN LYMPHOMA

Curative treatments for Hodgkin lymphoma have steadily improved over the last 50 years.[49] This has been achieved through a combination of better imaging techniques, technical advances in radiation therapy, and development of combination chemotherapy, initially MOPP (mechlorethamine, vincristine, procarbazine, and prednisone) and later ABVD (doxorubicin, bleomycin, vinblastine, and dacarbazine). However, studies of prognostic factors in Hodgkin lymphoma have regularly shown that elderly patients have a worse outcome.[50–60] For patients younger than 65 years of age, the 5-year overall survival rate exceeds 80 percent, while it is less than 50 percent for those older than 65 years.[61] Various reasons for this difference have been postulated including less favorable histology,[53,61] more advanced stage in the elderly,[53,61] comorbid diseases, delay in diagnosis,[59] incomplete staging,[53] inadequate adherence to protocol, and failure to maintain dose intensity.[53,55] In virtually every study in which it has been examined, age greater than 50 years is an important negative prognostic factor.

The one aspect of treatment under the partial control of the treating oncologist is treatment intensity. In reported series of elderly Hodgkin lymphoma patients examined for adequacy of treatment delivery, those who had similar doses to younger patients had equivalent outcomes,[55,59] whereas those who had dose reductions had a worse outcome.[53,55,59] For example, a study of all patients treated for Hodgkin lymphoma from three counties in Sweden from 1979 to 1982 revealed that patients older than 60 years received less than 40 percent of the planned chemotherapy doses.[54]

Attempts to improve the outcome for elderly patients with Hodgkin lymphoma have focused on two aspects. First, the steps taken in diagnosing and staging the lymphoma have been made equivalent to those employed for younger patients. Second, full dosing of standard chemotherapy has been attempted or special regimens have been designed hoping for better tolerance and therefore better maintenance of dose intensity. Thus, investigators have reported on the use of MOPP-type, ABVD, or MOPP/ABVD hybrids for elderly patients (older than 60 years) with the observation of 5-year overall survival of approximately 50 percent.[51] Innovative regimens such as ODBEP (vincristine, doxorubicin, bleomycin, etoposide, and prednisone),[62] CVP/CEP (chlorambucil, vinblastine, procarbazine, cyclophosphamide, etoposide, and prednisone),[63] and VEPEMB (vinblastine, cyclophosphamide, procarbazine, etoposide, mitoxantrone, and bleomycin)[64] produced somewhat encouraging results with lower toxicity and increased dose intensity of at least some of the agents but in the end have not produced compellingly better outcomes. None has been widely adopted. Only one randomized trial targeting elderly patients with Hodgkin lymphoma has been reported,[65] comparing BEACOPP (bleomycin, etoposide, doxorubicin, cyclophosphamide, vincristine, procarbazine, and prednisone) with alternating COPP/ABVD (cyclophosphamide, vincristine, procarbazine, prednisone, and ABVD). It reached the modest conclusion that the new regimen, BEACOPP, did not improve on the results that can be achieved with standard chemotherapy.

Without clear evidence of superiority for any of the phase II regimens that have been tested for elderly patients with Hodgkin lymphoma there is no justification to employ such regimens outside of clinical trials. The best approach is to use standard ABVD, with its well-understood spectrum of toxicity and known efficacy, supported by neutrophil growth factors to enable safe delivery of full but not escalated doses. For patients with preexisting pulmonary or cardiac disease it may be necessary to reduce or eliminate bleomycin or doxorubicin, respectively. There is no satisfactory substitute for bleomycin but etoposide can be substituted for the doxorubicin in ABVD. Whether removing the bleomycin or substituting etoposide for the doxorubicin compromises treatment outcome is unknown. It appears likely that improvements in the treatment of Hodgkin lymphoma in elderly patients will await identification of novel agents that can be added to the basic ABVD regimen without increasing toxicity. Clinical trials in this patient population should emphasize novel agents that minimize hematologic, pulmonary, and cardiac toxicity.

CONCLUSION

Many elderly patients with lymphoma can expect to tolerate currently available treatments with nearly as good an outcome as can be achieved in patients who are younger. This includes patients with limited stage indolent lymphoma; initially asymptomatic patients with advanced stage indolent lymphoma; patients with *Helicobacter pylori*-associated gastric MALT lymphoma; and patients with limited stage large B cell lymphoma. Such patients should be evaluated and treated the same as younger patients.

Although elderly patients with advanced stage aggressive lymphoma do not have as good a prognosis as younger patients they can still frequently be cured. Such patients should be given CHOP, with rituximab if they have a B cell lymphoma. However, patients presenting with marked frailty, major symptomatic comorbid illnesses, or substantial organ compromise should not be subjected to the toxicity of multiagent chemotherapy. If at the outset or during treatment it becomes clear that they will not be able to complete the planned treatment, the focus should shift away from attempting to cure the lymphoma to controlling its symptoms and offering supportive palliation. This choice between aggressive and palliative treatment requires careful clinical judgment and an informed choice on the part of the physician, patient, and family.

Some elderly patients with lymphoma should be approached with palliative intent from the time of diagnosis. In addition to the already mentioned frail, ill, and organ-compromised groups there are those whose lymphoma cannot be cured within the bounds of tolerable treatment.

This includes patients with lymphoblastic or Burkitt lymphoma. Such patients are much better served by a caring but realistic explanation of their disease, judicious use of single-agent chemotherapy and local irradiation, and the best available supportive and palliative care.

During the decades up to the 1990s many patients with lymphoma were enrolled in clinical trials in Europe and North America but very few were from the elderly population. Despite the fact that nearly one-half of all patients with lymphoma are over the age of 65 years such elderly patients constituted only a small minority of those included in clinical trials. Encouragingly that pattern of neglect has recently been reversed. Inspired by a need to craft treatments specifically suited for elderly patients and, even more importantly, the availability of potent hematologic growth factors and, more recently, effective agents such as rituximab that can be added to standard treatment regimens without increasing major toxicity, clinical investigators have successfully completed trials focused specifically on the elderly. These investigations have identified new, more effective regimens such as CHOP plus rituximab and CHOP-14 with neutrophil growth factor support as superior to our previous standard regimens. These successes confirm that this group of patients needs focused clinical investigation specifically designed to increase treatment effectiveness within the bounds of tolerable toxicity. Gratifyingly, progress in this area of oncology has occurred directly in proportion to the willingness of investigators and clinicians to test novel approaches in well-organized, interpretable, prospective clinical trials.

KEY POINTS

- Lymphoma incidence increases 2–3 percent per year.
- Half of all lymphomas occur in the 10–12 percent of the population over 65 years of age.
- The median age of the general population is steadily rising.
- These trends will lead to a doubling of numbers of lymphoma cases every 20 years.
- Lymphomas in elderly patients are more often of aggressive histologic types.
- Factors affecting elderly patients' tolerance for antilymphoma treatment include
  - comorbid illnesses
  - cumulative consequences of long-term use of tobacco, alcohol, or medications
  - alterations in host immunologic integrity
  - loss of physiologic reserve in organs
  - alteration in absorption, distribution, activation, detoxification, metabolism, and clearance of drugs
  - reduced emotional or physiological tolerance.

REFERENCES

● = Key primary paper
◆ = Major review article

1. SEER cancer statistics review: 1973–1994. In: Reis LAG, Kosary CL, Hankey BF et al. (eds) NIH publication no. 97-2789. Bethesda: National Cancer Institute; 1997: 196–206.

2. Muir CS, Fraumeni JF Jr, Doll R. The interpretation of time trends. *Cancer Surv* 1994; **19–20**: 5–21.

3. Kennedy BJ. Aging and cancer. *Oncology (Williston Park)* 2000; **14**: 1731–3, discussion 1734, 1739–40.

4. Zheng T, Mayne ST, Boyle P et al. Epidemiology of non-Hodgkin lymphoma in Connecticut. 1935–1988. *Cancer* 1992; **70**: 840–9.

5. Non-Hodgkin's lymphoma: Canadian Cancer Statistics, 2003. http://www.cancer.ca/ccs/internet/standard/0,3182,3172_367655_194217223_langId-en,00.html

6. Jemal A, Murray T, Ward E et al. Cancer statistics, 2005. *CA Cancer J Clin* 2005; **55**: 10–30.

●7. Baranovsky A, Myers MH. Cancer incidence and survival in patients 65 years of age and older. *CA Cancer J Clin* 1986; **36**: 26–41.

8. National Cancer Institute sponsored study of classifications of non-Hodgkin's lymphomas: summary and description of a working formulation for clinical usage. The Non-Hodgkin's Lymphoma Pathologic Classification Project. *Cancer* 1982; **49**: 2112–35.

9. Harris NL, Jaffe ES, Stein H et al. A revised European-American classification of lymphoid neoplasms: a proposal from the International Lymphoma Study Group. *Blood* 1994; **84**: 1361–92.

●10. Jaffe ES, Harris NL, Stein H, Vardiman JW. (eds) *Pathology and genetics of tumours of haematopoietic and lymphoid tissues.* Lyon: IARC Press, 2001.

11. Carbone PP, Kaplan HS, Musshoff K et al. Report of the Committee on Hodgkin's Disease Staging Classification. *Cancer Res* 1971; **31**: 1860–1.

12. Lister TA, Crowther D, Sutcliffe SB et al. Report of a committee convened to discuss the evaluation and staging of patients with Hodgkin's disease: Cotswolds meeting. *J Clin Oncol* 1989; **7**: 1630–6.

13. Carbone A, Volpe R, Gloghini A et al. Non-Hodgkin's lymphoma in the elderly. I. Pathologic features at presentation. *Cancer* 1990; **66**: 1991–4.

14. Barnes N, Cartwright RA, O'Brien C et al. Variation in lymphoma incidence within Yorkshire Health Region. *Br J Cancer* 1987; **55**: 81–4.

15. Jones SE, Fuks Z, Bull M et al. Non-Hodgkin's lymphomas. IV. Clinicopathologic correlation in 405 cases. *Cancer* 1973; **31**: 806–23.

16. Hancock BW, Aitken M, Ross CM, Dunsmore IR. Non-Hodgkin's lymphoma in Sheffield 1971–1980. *Clin Oncol* 1983; **9**: 109–19.

17. Foucar K, Armitage JO, Dick FR. Malignant lymphoma, diffuse mixed small and large cell. A clinicopathologic study of 47 cases. *Cancer* 1983; **51**: 2090–9.

18. Otter R, Gerrits WB, vd Sandt MM et al. Primary extranodal and nodal non-Hodgkin's lymphoma. A survey of a population-based registry. *Eur J Cancer Clin Oncol* 1989; **25**: 1203–10.

●19. A clinical evaluation of the International Lymphoma Study Group classification of non-Hodgkin's lymphoma. The Non-Hodgkin's Lymphoma Classification Project. *Blood* 1997; **89**: 3909–18.

20. MacManus MP, Hoppe RT. Is radiotherapy curative for stage I and II low-grade follicular lymphoma? Results of a long-term follow-up study of patients treated at Stanford University. *J Clin Oncol* 1996; **14**: 1282–90.

21. Isaacson PG. Primary gastric lymphoma. *Br J Biomed Sci* 1995; **52**: 291–6.

22. Chen LT, Lin JT, Shyu RY et al. Prospective study of *Helicobacter pylori* eradication therapy in stage I(E) high-grade mucosa-associated lymphoid tissue lymphoma of the stomach. *J Clin Oncol* 2001; **19**: 4245–51.

23. Tursi A, Cammarota G, Papa A et al. Long-term follow-up of disappearance of gastric mucosa-associated lymphoid tissue after anti-*Helicobacter pylori* therapy. *Am J Gastroenterol* 1997; **92**: 1849–52.

24. Foussard C, Colombat P, Maisonneuve H et al. Long-term follow-up of a randomized trial of fludarabine-mitoxantrone, compared with cyclophosphamide, doxorubicin, vindesine, prednisone (CHVP), as first-line treatment of elderly patients with advanced, low-grade non-Hodgkin's lymphoma before the era of monoclonal antibodies. *Ann Oncol* 2005; **16**: 466–72.

●25. Ardeshna KM, Smith P, Norton A et al. Long-term effect of a watch and wait policy versus immediate systemic treatment for asymptomatic advanced-stage non-Hodgkin lymphoma: a randomised controlled trial. *Lancet* 2003; **362**: 516–22.

26. Marcus R, Imrie K, Belch A et al. CVP chemotherapy plus rituximab compared with CVP as first-line treatment for advanced follicular lymphoma. *Blood* 2005; **105**: 1417–23.

27. Hiddemann W, Dreyling M, Unterhalt M. Rituximab plus chemotherapy in follicular and mantle cell lymphomas. *Semin Oncol* 2003; **30**: 16–20.

●28. Miller TP, Dahlberg S, Cassady JR et al. Chemotherapy alone compared with chemotherapy plus radiotherapy for localized intermediate- and high-grade non-Hodgkin's lymphoma. *N Engl J Med* 1998; **339**: 21–6.

29. Shenkier TN, Voss N, Fairey R et al. Brief chemotherapy and involved-region irradiation for limited-stage diffuse large-cell lymphoma: an 18-year experience from the British Columbia Cancer Agency. *J Clin Oncol* 2002; **20**: 197–204.

●30. Pfreundschuh M, Trumper L, Kloess M et al. Two-weekly or 3-weekly CHOP chemotherapy with or without etoposide for the treatment of elderly patients with aggressive lymphomas: results of the NHL-B2 trial of the DSHNHL. *Blood* 2004; **104**: 634–41.

31. Reyes F, Lepage E, Ganem G et al. ACVBP versus CHOP plus radiotherapy for localized aggressive lymphoma. *N Engl J Med* 2005; **352**: 1197–205.

32. Tirelli U, Carbone A, Zagonel V et al. Non-Hodgkin's lymphomas in the elderly: prospective studies with specifically devised chemotherapy regimens in 66 patients. Eur J Cancer Clin Oncol 1987; 23: 535–40.

33. Tirelli U, Zagonel V, Errante D et al. A prospective study of a new combination chemotherapy regimen in patients older than 70 years with unfavorable non-Hodgkin's lymphoma. J Clin Oncol 1992; 10: 228–36.

34. O'Reilly S, Klimo P, Connors JM. Low-dose ACOP-B and VABE: weekly chemotherapy for elderly patients with advanced-stage diffuse large-cell lymphoma. J Clin Oncol 1991; 9: 741–7.

35. O'Reilly SE, Connors JM, Howdle S et al. In search of an optimal regimen for elderly patients with advanced-stage diffuse large-cell lymphoma: results of a phase II study of P/DOCE chemotherapy. J Clin Oncol 1993; 11: 2250–7.

36. McMaster ML, Johnson DH, Greer JP et al. A brief-duration combination chemotherapy for elderly patients with poor-prognosis non-Hodgkin's lymphoma. Cancer 1991; 67: 1487–92.

37. Dixon DO, Neilan B, Jones SE et al. Effect of age on therapeutic outcome in advanced diffuse histiocytic lymphoma: the Southwest Oncology Group experience. J Clin Oncol 1986; 4: 295–305.

38. Bertini M, Freilone R, Vitolo U et al. The treatment of elderly patients with aggressive non-Hodgkin's lymphomas: feasibility and efficacy of an intensive multidrug regimen. Leuk Lymphoma 1996; 22: 483–93.

39. Zinzani PL, Storti S, Zaccaria A et al. Elderly aggressive-histology non-Hodgkin's lymphoma: first-line VNCOP-B regimen experience on 350 patients. Blood 1999; 94: 33–8.

40. Bessell EM, Burton A, Haynes AP et al. A randomised multicentre trial of modified CHOP versus MCOP in patients aged 65 years and over with aggressive non-Hodgkin's lymphoma. Ann Oncol 2003; 14: 258–67.

41. Doorduijn JK, van der Holt B, van Imhoff GW et al. CHOP compared with CHOP plus granulocyte colony-stimulating factor in elderly patients with aggressive non-Hodgkin's lymphoma. J Clin Oncol 2003; 21: 3041–50.

42. Mori M, Kitamura K, Masuda M et al. Long-term results of a multicenter randomized, comparative trial of modified CHOP versus THP-COP versus THP-COPE regimens in elderly patients with non-Hodgkin's lymphoma. Int J Hematol 2005; 81: 246–54.

43. Sonneveld P, de Ridder M, van der Lelie H et al. Comparison of doxorubicin and mitoxantrone in the treatment of elderly patients with advanced diffuse non-Hodgkin's lymphoma using CHOP versus CNOP chemotherapy. J Clin Oncol 1995; 13: 2530–9.

●44. Osby E, Hagberg H, Kvaloy S et al. CHOP is superior to CNOP in elderly patients with aggressive lymphoma while outcome is unaffected by filgrastim treatment: results of a Nordic Lymphoma Group randomized trial. Blood 2003; 101: 3840–8.

●45. Feugier P, Van Hoof A, Sebban C et al. Long-term results of the R-CHOP study in the treatment of elderly patients with diffuse large B-cell lymphoma: a study by the Groupe d'Etude des Lymphomes de l'Adulte. J Clin Oncol 2005; 23: 4117–26.

46. Zinzani PL, Gherlinzoni F, Storti S et al. Randomized trial of 8-week versus 12-week VNCOP-B plus G-CSF regimens as front-line treatment in elderly aggressive non-Hodgkin's lymphoma patients. Ann Oncol 2002; 13: 1364–9.

●47. Coiffier B, Lepage E, Briere J et al. CHOP chemotherapy plus rituximab compared with CHOP alone in elderly patients with diffuse large-B-cell lymphoma. N Engl J Med 2002; 346: 235–42.

48. Sehn LH, Donaldson J, Chhanabhai M et al. Introduction of combined CHOP-rituximab therapy dramatically improved outcome of diffuse large B-cell lymphoma in British Columbia. J Clin Oncol 2004; 23: 5027–33.

◆49. Connors JM. State of the Art Therapeutics: Hodgkin lymphoma. J Clin Oncol 2005; 19: 6400–8.

50. Vaughan Hudson B, MacLennan KA, Easterling MJ et al. The prognostic significance of age in Hodgkin's disease: examination of 1500 patients (BNLI report no. 23). Clin Radiol 1983; 34: 503–6.

51. Rossi Ferrini P, Bosi A, Casini C et al. Hodgkin's disease in the elderly: a retrospective clinicopathologic study of 61 patients aged over 60 years. Acta Haematol 1987; 78(Suppl 1): 163–70.

52. Specht L, Nissen NI. Hodgkin's disease and age. Eur J Haematol 1989; 43: 127–35.

53. Walker A, Schoenfeld ER, Lowman JT et al. Survival of the older patient compared with the younger patient with Hodgkin's disease. Influence of histologic type, staging, and treatment. Cancer 1990; 65: 1635–40.

54. Enblad G, Glimelius B, Sundstrom C. Treatment outcome in Hodgkin's disease in patients above the age of 60: a population-based study. Ann Oncol 1991; 2: 297–302.

55. Erdkamp FL, Breed WP, Bosch LJ et al. Hodgkin disease in the elderly. A registry-based analysis. Cancer 1992; 70: 830–4.

56. Kennedy BJ, Loeb V Jr, Peterson V et al. Survival in Hodgkin's disease by stage and age. Med Pediatr Oncol 1992; 20: 100–4.

57. Bennett JM, Andersen JW, Begg CB, Glick JH. Age and Hodgkin's disease: the impact of competing risks and possibly salvage therapy on long term survival: an E.C.O.G. study. Leuk Res 1993; 17: 825–32.

58. Diaz-Pavon JR, Cabanillas F, Majlis A, Hagemeister FB. Outcome of Hodgkin's disease in elderly patients. Hematol Oncol 1995; 13: 19–27.

59. Proctor SJ, Rueffer JU, Angus B et al. Hodgkin's disease in the elderly: current status and future directions. Ann Oncol 2002; 13: 133–7.

60. Stark GL, Wood KM, Jack F et al. Hodgkin's disease in the elderly: a population-based study. Br J Haematol 2002; 119: 432–40.

61. Medeiros LJ, Greiner TC. Hodgkin's disease. *Cancer* 1995; **75**: 357–69.

62. Macpherson N, Klasa RJ, Gascoyne R *et al.* Treatment of elderly Hodgkin's lymphoma patients with a novel 5-drug regimen (ODBEP): a phase II study. *Leuk Lymphoma* 2002; **43**: 1395–402.

63. Levis A, Depaoli L, Bertini M *et al.* Results of a low aggressivity chemotherapy regimen (CVP/CEB) in elderly Hodgkin's disease patients. *Haematologica* 1996; **81**: 450–6.

64. Levis A, Anselmo AP, Ambrosetti A *et al.* VEPEMB in elderly Hodgkin's lymphoma patients. Results from an Intergruppo Italiano Linfomi (IIL) study. *Ann Oncol* 2004; **15**: 123–8.

●65. Ballova V, Ruffer JU, Haverkamp H *et al.* A prospectively randomized trial carried out by the German Hodgkin Study Group (GHSG) for elderly patients with advanced Hodgkin's disease comparing BEACOPP baseline and COPP-ABVD (study HD9elderly). *Ann Oncol* 2005; **16**: 124–31.

59

Management of lymphomas at extranodal locations

FRANCO CAVALLI, ANNARITA CONCONI AND EMANUELE ZUCCA

INTRODUCTION

Nodal versus extranodal lymphomas

Approximately one-third of non-Hodgkin lymphomas (NHL) arise from sites other than lymph nodes, spleen, or the bone marrow and even from sites which normally contain no native lymphoid tissue.[1,2] The exact designation of extranodal lymphoma is controversial, particularly in the presence of both nodal and extranodal disease. Different criteria for the diagnosis of primary extranodal lymphoma have been proposed, most of them initially made for the gastrointestinal lymphomas and later extrapolated to extranodal localizations in general.

The first definition was proposed by Dawson for gastrointestinal lymphomas,[3] and later refined by Lewin[4] and Herrmann.[5] The original Dawson criteria defined primary gastrointestinal lymphoma, a presentation with main disease manifestation in the gastrointestinal tract, with regional lymph node involvement only, with no peripheral lymph node involvement, and no liver or spleen involvement. Later these criteria were relaxed to allow for contiguous involvement of other organs (e.g., liver, spleen) and for distant nodal disease, providing that the extranodal lesion was the presenting site and constituted the predominant disease bulk. More recently, it has been proposed to operationally designate as extranodal those lymphomas where, after routine staging procedures, there is either no or only 'minor' nodal involvement along with a clinically 'dominant' extranodal component, to which primary treatment must often be directed.[6] The choice of a strict or a liberal definition of extranodal lymphoma inevitably introduces a selection bias. A study from a population-based lymphoma registry in the Netherlands showed that the frequency of extranodal NHL fluctuated from 20 percent to 34 percent depending on the adopted definition criteria.[7]

Another area of controversy is designation of extranodal versus extralymphatic site. This may affect taxonomy in extranodal lymphomas since the Ann Arbor staging system recognizes tonsils and Waldeyer's ring, thymus, spleen, appendix, and Peyer's patches of the small intestine as lymphatic tissues. However, most clinicians use the extranodal definition as indicating any presentation outside lymph node areas.

Epidemiology and etiopathogenesis

The incidence of NHL in Western countries has increased substantially in the last 40 years. This increase appears to be higher in extranodal rather than nodal disease and cannot be completely explained by the acquired immune deficiency syndrome (AIDS) epidemics in the 1980s.[8–10] This rise may in part be due to improved diagnostic procedures (particularly in brain and gastrointestinal lymphomas) and changes in classification, but much of the change is real and the reasons for it have been the subject of much debate.

Extranodal presentations of lymphoma account for between 24 percent and 58 percent of new lymphoma cases and often present as localized disease. Variation in the proportion of NHL presenting at extranodal sites in different countries has been reported: USA 24 percent, Canada 27 percent, Israel 36 percent, Lebanon 44 percent, Denmark 37 percent, Holland 41 percent, Greece 46 percent, Turkey 45 percent, Italy 48 percent, Jordan 30 percent, Thailand 58 percent, Taiwan 55 percent, Kuwait 45 percent, and Hong Kong 29 percent.[1,11–16] The reasons for these discrepancies include variable reporting criteria with diverse definitions of primary extranodal disease, variable inclusion of mycosis fungoides and other T cell lymphomas, variable inclusion of Waldeyer's ring lymphomas, and different types of data source (referral cancer centers vs population-based tumor registry series). However, there are also true geographic differences in the incidence of extranodal lymphomas; for example, the higher incidence of Epstein–Barr virus (EBV)- and human T cell lymphotrophic virus 1 (HTLV-1)-associated T cell lymphomas and the lower incidence of follicular and small lymphocytic lymphoma in Asia affect the frequency of extranodal presentations. Table 59.1 shows the geographic variations in the frequency of the different histologic subtypes in extranodal lymphomas.

Despite this relative prominence of extranodal presentations, the outcomes of extranodal lymphomas are difficult to ascertain; the literature on many of the specific types and sites is scant and often contradictory. This is primarily because these tumors, numerous when considered together, are distributed so widely throughout the body that it is difficult to assemble adequate series of any given site.

Histologic subtypes at different sites

The extranodal lymphomas represent a frequent challenge in routine lymphoma diagnosis due to the diversity of morphologies, molecular abnormalities, and clinical pictures that can be present. The literature on extranodal lymphomas lacks uniformity in histopathological classification; many historical series were published before the recognition of mucosal-associated lymphoid tissue (MALT) as the origin of many extranodal lymphomas, and the older classification of NHL did not take into account peculiar histogenetic features of primary extranodal lymphomas. The first attempt to eliminate this problem was made in 1994 with the proposal of the Revised European-American Lymphoma (REAL) classification[17] and afterwards with the World Health Organization (WHO) classification.[18]

According to the population-based cancer registries of the SEER (Surveillance, Epidemiology, and End Results) Program of the National Cancer Institute, approximately 27 percent of all NHL cases diagnosed in the USA during the period from 1978 through 1995 were extranodal.[10] For the majority of the histologic subtypes, this fraction ranged between 21 percent and 33 percent, with two notable exceptions: 82 percent of peripheral T cell NHL cases were extranodal, almost all of which involved the skin, and only 9 percent of follicular NHL cases were extranodal. Nearly 50 percent of all extranodal NHL cases were of diffuse large cell histology. About one-third of extranodal NHL were found in the gastrointestinal tract and most of the extranodal presentations were concentrated in just four sites: skin (18 percent), stomach (17 percent), brain (10 percent), and small intestine (7 percent).[10]

The histologic spectrum of extranodal lymphomas comprises some site-specific T cell lymphomas (such as mycosis fungoides, enteropathy-associated T cell lymphoma, nasal natural killer [NK]/T cell lymphomas), and the extranodal marginal zone B cell lymphomas of mucosal-associated lymphoid tissue (MALT lymphoma). Regulation of lymphocyte trafficking and homing may play a major role in the biology of primary extranodal lymphomas of the skin and gastrointestinal tract.[19] These lymphomas show a striking tendency to spread or recur in the skin or at mucosal (gastrointestinal) sites, respectively. In gastric MALT lymphoma cells, the finding of the integrin $\alpha_4\beta_7$, a mucosal homing receptor that binds to the adhesion molecule MAdCAM-1, a vascular recognition addressin selectively expressed on mucosal endothelium, supports the unique character of gastrointestinal (GI) and other MALT lymphomas,[20,21] suggesting that lymphocyte homing

Table 59.1   Distribution of histologic subtypes in extranodal lymphomas according to the REAL-WHO classification, in recent series from different countries

NHL type	Canada, 2006[24] n = 709	Jordan, 2005[11] n = 99	Taiwan, 2004[14] n = 96	Kuwait, 2004[16] n = 821	The Netherlands, 2003[7] n = 389
B cell lymphomas					
Lymphoblastic	–	4%	0	<1%	1%
DLCL	64%	40%	30%	59%	50%
Burkitt lymphoma	–	15%	2%	4%	3%
Follicular	10%	7%	0	5%	7%
Small lymphocytic	<1%	0	0	1%	11%
Lymphoplasmacytic	<1%	0	2%	–	4%
Mantle cell	2%	2%	2%	<1%	2%
Splenic marginal zone	–	1%	–	<1%	–
MALT type	17%	9%	19%	10%	7%
Other/unclassifiable	6%	9%	19%	–	11%
T cell lymphomas					
Lymphoblastic	–	0	0	<1%	0%
Peripheral T cell	–	3%	4%	1.50%	2%
NK/T cell, nasal type	–	3%	12.50%	–	–
Enteropathy-type T cell	–	2%	1%	2%	–
Mycosis fungoides	–	10%	13.50%	14%	–
Anaplastic large T cell (ALCL)	–	2%	4%	2%	<1%
Cutaneous ALCL	–	–	5%	–	–
Subcutaneous panniculitis-like					
T cell	–	–	4%	–	–
Hepatosplenic $\gamma\delta$	–	1%	–	–	–

REAL-WHO, Revised European-American Lymphoma–World Health Organization; NHL, non-Hodgkin lymphoma; DLCL, diffuse large cell lymphoma; MALT, mucosal-associated lymphoid tissue; NK, natural killer; ALCL, anaplastic large cell lymphoma.

properties can be implicated in the determination of the specific location of extranodal forms.

With respect to histologic classification, aggressive subtypes are predominant in NHL of the central nervous system (CNS), testis, bone, and liver, while in other sites, for example in the GI tract, a large spectrum of histologic disease entities can be seen.[1,2] Certain extranodal sites appear to have characteristic patterns of either B or T cell disease (e.g., nearly all primary lymphoma of the bone are of B cell origin, while cutaneous lymphoma clearly comprises a wide range of lymphomas of T cell origin with only a minority of B cell cases) (Table 59.2).

Histologic type is the main predictor of prognosis in either nodal or extranodal lymphomas. However, the specific presenting site is also of importance in extranodal lymphomas. For example, in spite of the other factors being equal, the prognosis of diffuse large cell lymphoma in the brain or testis is different from that of gastric or bone lymphoma (Table 59.3). The pronounced heterogeneity of outcome of the various primary extranodal presentations is one of the main justifications for a detailed consideration of the different sites of origin of these lymphomas. Furthermore, some specific disease localizations can require specific staging procedures, which are summarized in Table 59.4.

Clinical characteristics and outcome

Extranodal lymphomas can arise in almost every organ. Table 59.5 summarizes the frequency of site-specific primary extranodal lymphomas in different countries. Gastrointestinal localizations, about one-third of all cases in most series, represent the most common form of extranodal lymphoma. If tonsils and Waldeyer's ring are still included, head and neck localizations are the second most frequent site of involvement, averaging about one-fifth of all cases. In the classic report by Freeman et al. of the SEER experience from 1950 through 1964, stomach lymphoma was most common, followed by intestine, tonsil, and skin.[22] More recent SEER reports found stomach, skin, intestine, and brain to be the most common sites of extranodal lymphoma.[8,10] In a population-based study from Denmark, stomach, intestine, skin, and bone were the most frequent sites. Referral patterns may affect institutional experience with primary extranodal lymphoma.[6] In the series from the Princess Margaret Hospital of Toronto[19,23] and from the British Columbia Cancer Agency of Vancouver,[24] Waldeyer's ring lymphoma (mostly tonsil) and stomach lymphoma were consistently the most common extranodal sites over the last two decades.

Table 59.2 Histologic subtypes (according to the WHO classification) in primary noncutaneous extranodal non-Hodgkin lymphoma with preferential involvement sites

WHO classification lymphoma subtype	Preferred extranodal sites
B cell	
Follicular lymphoma	Waldeyer's ring, GI tract, parotid, ocular adnexa, breast, Waldeyer's ring
Lymphoplasmacytic lymphoma	Waldeyer's ring
Mantle cell lymphoma	GI tract (multiple polyposis), Waldeyer's ring
Extranodal marginal zone lymphoma (MALT type)	Stomach, intestine, salivary glands, lungs, thyroid, ocular adnexa (and many others)
Diffuse large cell lymphoma	GI tract, Waldeyer's ring, testis, breast, CNS, bone, oral cavity (plasmablastic variant)
Lymphoblastic lymphoma	Waldeyer's ring, paranasal sinuses
Burkitt lymphoma	Ileocecal area, ovary, Waldeyer's ring, jaw
Extramedullary plasmacytoma	Head and neck area
T cell	
Peripheral T cell lymphoma, unspecified	Waldeyer's ring
NK/T cell, nasal-type lymphoma	Nose, palate, skin, paranasal sinuses, orbit, GI tract
Hepatosplenic T cell lymphoma	Liver, spleen, skin and subcutaneous, nasal region, intestine
Lymphoblastic lymphoma	Waldeyer's ring, paranasal sinuses

WHO, World Health Organization; MALT, mucosal-associated lymphoid tissue; NK, natural killer; GI, gastrointestinal; CNS, central nervous system.

Table 59.3 Outcome of lymphomas with diffuse large B cell histology at different primary extranodal presentations in recent series

Localization	Author	Patient numbers	Long-term survival (5-yr OS)
Stomach	Cortelazzo, 1999[84]	312	75%
	Ibrahim, 1999[82]	185	68%
	Koch, 2005[75]	194	87%
Intestine	Ibrahim, 2001[83]	66	58%
	Cortelazzo, 2002[85]	87	68%
	Daum, 2003[214]	18	94%
Bone	Christie, 1999[185]	70	59%
	Zinzani, 2003[184]	52	68%
	Beal, 2006[183]	65	88%
Head and neck area	Aviles, 1996[121]	316	56–90% (Waldeyer's ring only)
	Cortelazzo, 2005[215]	309	72%
Breast	Aviles, 2005[179]	95	50–76%
	Ryan, 2005[180]	204	63%
Testis	Fonseca, 2000[106]	62	38%
	Zucca, 2003[30]	373	48%
Prostate	Botswick, 1998[112]	22	33%
CNS	Ferreri, 2002[161]	370	24%
	Abrey, 2006[156]	388	37%

5-yr OS, 5-year overall survival.

Distinct primary extranodal lymphoma sites include other head and neck sites (thyroid, salivary gland, paranasal sinus lymphoma, gingiva, nose), orbit (lacrimal gland, conjunctiva, eyelids, orbital soft tissues), breast, lung, female genital tract (ovary, cervix, uterus), genitourinary tract (testis, bladder, prostate), liver, spleen, and soft tissue lymphomas. The least common lymphoma sites include heart, muscle, kidney, pleura, adrenal gland, and dura. The distributions by age and gender of nodal and extranodal NHL are very similar.[1,2]

In general, patients with extranodal lymphomas tend to present B symptoms less often than do patients suffering from lymphomas arising in the nodal regions.[6] Signs and symptoms at presentation depend largely on the localization and usually do not differ significantly from those of other malignancies affecting that specific organ. Gastric lymphomas present typically with symptoms of peptic disease, bowel lymphomas with diarrhea or obstruction, and bone lymphoma usually with fractures or pain. Especially in the absence of nodal involvement, primary extranodal lymphoma is often not suspected and most often is clinically indistinguishable from a carcinoma arising in the same site. Histologic diagnosis with immunophenotypic and histochemical analysis is therefore particularly important.

Whether or not extranodal lymphomas have an overall survival similar to that of nodal cases as a whole remains a matter of controversy. However, considering the many variables which influence site-specific outcome in extranodal lymphomas, it is questionable whether such an overall difference has clinical relevance. In a survey of 382 patients with diffuse large B cell lymphoma, 42 percent were primary extranodal and patients with Waldeyer's ring or GI lymphomas showed a significantly better outcome than patients with nodal or other extranodal sites of disease.[25] Indeed, as shown in Table 59.3, survival rates vary among all of the specific sites of primary extranodal lymphomas. In fact, in addition to the histologic subtype, the primary organ of origin represents the most significant prognostic factor among extranodal lymphomas. This is

Table 59.4   Specific staging procedures for specific extranodal localizations

Stomach:
– Gastroduodenal endoscopy with multiple gastric biopsies
– Endoscopic ultrasound
– Histologic and histochemical examination for *H. pylori*
– Careful examination of Waldeyer's ring

Small intestine:
– Endoscopy
– Small bowel series; *Campylobacter jejuni* search in IPSID

Large intestine:
– Colonoscopy

Waldeyer's ring:
– Gastroduodenal endoscopy with multiple gastric biopsies

Nasal cavity, nasopharynx, paranasal sinus, orbit:
– CT scan or MRI of the head and neck

Salivary gland, tonsils, parotid:
– ENT examination and echography

Thyroid:
– Echography ± CT scan of the neck and thyroid function tests

Ocular adnexa:
– MRI (or CT scan) and ophthalmologic examination
– *Chlamydia psittaci* in the tumor biopsy and blood mononuclear cells

Central nervous system:
– MRI with gadolinium
– Stereotaxic biopsy
– Lumbar puncture with examination of cerebrospinal fluid
– Ophthalmological examination with slit-lamp
– Spinal MRI with gadolinium (when appropriate)

Testis:
– Clinical and ultrasonographic examination of the scrotum
– Lumbar puncture with examination of cerebrospinal fluid

Breast:
– Bilateral mammography and MRI (or CT scan)

Bone:
– MRI

Heart:
– Echocardiogram

Lung:
– Bronchoscopy + bronchoalveolar lavage

IPSID, immunoproliferative small intestinal disease; CT, computed tomography; MRI, magnetic resonance imaging; ENT, ear, nose and throat.

partially due to differences in natural history, but mainly to differences in management strategy which are related to organ-specific problems.

Testis and thyroid lymphomas are seen almost exclusively in patients more than 50 years of age, while a significantly higher incidence of hepatic and intestinal lymphomas is related to younger age. Salivary gland and thyroid lymphomas are significantly more common in females, while intestinal and pulmonary lymphomas are more often found in males.[6] Non-Hodgkin lymphomas of the stomach, salivary glands, and thyroid are more frequently localized, whereas extranodal lymphomas of the lungs, liver, bones, and testes are often widespread.[6,26]

APPROACH TO MANAGEMENT OF EXTRANODAL LYMPHOMAS

PATIENT ASSESSMENT

For lymphomas with primary extranodal presentation the assessment of tumor extent is similar to that for nodal disease. All patients should be evaluated by recording clinical history with documentation of B symptoms, and performing complete physical examination, complete blood count and lactate dehydrogenase (LDH), computed tomography (CT) examination of neck, chest, abdomen, and pelvis, and bone marrow biopsy. A positron emission tomography (PET)

scan is useful in aggressive histologies while its role in MALT lymphoma is at present less clear. Specific tests to define local disease extent in the presenting extranodal site and in high-risk areas for potential occult disease are often indicated (Table 59.4). Specifically, it is very important to image the head and neck region with CT or magnetic resonance imaging (MRI) to define disease extent in extranodal lymphomas presenting in the head and neck region; MRI is very useful for primary bone lymphoma, or extranodal lymphomas involving soft tissue. Endoscopy should be used to define local disease extent in airways, GI tract, and urinary tract. Endoscopic ultrasonography provides relevant prognostic information in defining the local extent of primary GI lymphomas. In *Helicobacter pylori*-associated gastric lymphomas, C14 breath test or assessment of *H. pylori* stool antigen are useful to diagnose infection and ascertain its eradication after therapy. Cerebrospinal fluid (CSF) cytology is an essential part of the assessment of primary CNS lymphomas. It is also recommended in the assessment of lymphomas involving parameningeal sites such as extradural or paranasal sinus lymphomas, as well as in primary testis and breast lymphomas because of their peculiar pattern of relapse.[1,2] Data supporting the increased sensitivity of assessment of occult leptomeningeal disease by flow cytometry have been reported.[27]

Anatomic disease extent is described using Ann Arbor stage or specific staging systems for peculiar extranodal locations.[28] The Ann Arbor classification does not directly address the issue of stage designation in cases with demonstrated

Table 59.5 Frequency (%) and sites of non-Hodgkin lymphomas presenting with extranodal involvement in different countries

	USA 1961[1]	USA 1972[22]	Hong Kong 1984[1]	The Netherlands 1989[26]	Denmark[a] 1991[6]	Canada[b] 1992[23]	Pakistan 1992[1]	Egypt 1994[1]	Switzerland 1997[1]	Turkey 2004[15]	Taiwan 2004[14]	Jordan 2005[11]	Kuwait 2004[16]	Canada[b] 2006[24]
Gastrointestinal tract	19	37	63	35	30	24	37	21	51	67	30	32	35	25
Waldeyer's ring	22	14	8	16	–[c]	19	17	22	15	9	5	11	9	15
Nose, sinus	1	2	9	1	3	–	1	<1	–	–	11	6	–	4
Orbit	3	2	1	3	1	4	<1	<1	5	–	–	–	–	8
Thyroid gland	<1	3	4	2	5	6	–	–	1	–	–	3	3	5
Other head and neck sites	10	2	1	4	<1	9	–	–	3	–	–	2	6	–
CNS	0	2	–	6	7	10	2	1	1	5	4	1	4	–
Lung	3	4	–	5	5	1	–	–	1	–	1	3	1	2
Bone	16	5	4	3	9	4	2	11	3	3	1	8	7[e]	6
Soft tissue	–	9	3	2	3	5	–	–	1	–	17	6	–	–
Breast	1	2	–	2	1	2	–	–	3	–	–	–	0.5	2
Skin (other than mycosis fungoides)	21[d]	8	3	2	11	4	8	4	6	3	28[d]	17[d]	18	5
Testis	2	1.5	–	2	3	–	12	–	3	2	–	–	2	5
Genitourinary tract	<1	0	4	1	2	4	–	6	<1	–	–	–	2	–
Gynecologic tract	<1	1	4	<1	1	1	–	–	1	2	–	1	2	–

[a]Population-based tumor registry.
[b]Only stage I and II included.
[c]Waldeyer's ring considered as nodal site.
[d]Including mycosis fungoides.
[e]Bone and soft tissue.
CNS, central nervous system.

bilateral involvement of paired organs but there is some agreement in considering these cases as expression of localized disease.

PRINCIPLES OF TREATMENT

As for primary nodal disease, in the field of extranodal lymphomas the treatment intent – i.e., the choice between a curative or palliative therapeutic approach – depends on the patient's clinical conditions, the extent and/or location of the disease, and the histologic type. However, tumor location and pattern of disease should also be considered. Exact disease extent has to be established prior to treatment start in order to precisely define the quality of response and correctly plan involved field radiation therapy when required.

The principles of management of patients with extranodal lymphomas are in general analogous to those of the nodal lymphomas. In addition to histology, factors known to influence the outcome in patients with extranodal lymphomas include stage, local tumor bulk, number of extranodal sites, LDH, performance status, and the International Prognostic Index (IPI). The presenting extranodal site may by itself carry an adverse prognosis as seen, for example, in CNS lymphoma[29] and in testis lymphoma.[30] In stage I and II disease, with low tumor burden, local therapy is a relevant option, both for cure and local control. However, the recognition of occult distant disease and risk of relapse mandate the use of chemotherapy in patients with large cell or mantle cell lymphomas. In advanced stage disease, systemic therapy in terms of chemotherapy, immunotherapy, or a combination of both is required. Local treatment is not routinely used, although it may still have a role for sites of bulky disease or incomplete response, particularly in locations where local control is important (e.g., extradural space).

Surgery

The role of surgery in the management of extranodal lymphoma is poorly defined. Stage I primary indolent extranodal NHL may be cured with surgery alone, but surgical cure is an infrequent event. However, resection of the primary tumor may be diagnostic and helpful in obtaining local control of the tumor, e.g., in localized intestinal disease and testis lymphoma.[30] Nevertheless, for aggressive histologic types, due to the high risk of distant recurrence, combination of both radiation therapy and chemotherapy is required; therefore aggressive surgical approaches with esthetic and functional compromise are not useful nor indicated. Specifically, there is no need for amputation in bone lymphoma, mastectomy in breast lymphoma, cystectomy in bladder lymphoma, abdominoperineal resection in rectal lymphoma, or radical surgical resection of parotid lymphoma. Accordingly,

an accurate preoperative or intraoperative diagnosis is essential.

Radiation therapy

Local disease control is an important consideration in extranodal lymphoma as presentation with bulky disease is common, organ function may be at risk, and tumor may compress vital structures, e.g., spinal cord or airways. These factors and the observation that lymphomas in sanctuary sites (brain, testis) are not adequately controlled with chemotherapy alone underline the relevant role of radiation therapy in the management of extranodal lymphomas. Involved field radiation therapy, which is most commonly used, implies treatment to the extranodal site and its immediate lymph node drainage area. The dose of radiation therapy required to achieve local control varies depending upon histologic type and tumor bulk. There are no prospective randomized trials designed to determine the optimal dose when irradiation is used as single therapy or in combination with chemotherapy and a survey of expert radiation oncologists showed significant variation within a range of 30–45 Gy.[31,32]

Chemotherapy and combined modality therapy (chemotherapy/radiation therapy)

Distant failure has been well documented in localized disease treated with radiation therapy alone.[33] Chemotherapy has been documented to cure patients with diffuse large cell lymphoma. A combined modality approach has been shown to improve local control over that obtained with irradiation alone, and to reduce distant relapse rates. It is important to note that in cases where no response or only partial response to chemotherapy is observed, the radiation therapy dose may have to be increased.[34] In patients with localized MALT, follicular, and other small cell lymphomas, although distant failure is common, there is no evidence that addition of chemotherapy improves survival and radiation therapy is standard treatment in most instances of localized disease.[35]

Management of relapse

The assessment of response includes all sites of initial lymphoma involvement and should follow well-defined general and organ-specific criteria.[36] Treatment at relapse in general is similar to that of nodal disease, usually involves chemotherapy, and must take into account the histologic type, the relapse site, and its extent. In patients who relapse with localized disease, retreatment with chemotherapy and radiation may offer a higher chance of prolonged disease control. In selected circumstances of follicular lymphoma or MALT lymphoma with localized small bulk recurrence, radiation therapy alone may offer prolonged disease control.

GASTROINTESTINAL TRACT LYMPHOMA

Epidemiology and classification

The GI tract is the most frequently involved extranodal localization, representing 30–40 percent of extranodal lymphomas[22,26,37] and 4–20 percent of all NHL cases.[5,38]

In Western countries, the most common location is the stomach (approximately 50–60 percent), followed by the small intestines (30 percent) and the large intestine (around 10 percent) (Table 59.6). Involvement of the esophagus is very rare. These proportions can differ geographically, with small intestinal lymphomas being more common in the Middle East. With respect to gastric involvement, NHL represents the most frequent tumor following adenocarcinoma.[39]

The most common histologic subtype in localized GI presentations is diffuse large B cell lymphoma, which is present in approximately 60 percent of the gastric and 70 percent of the intestinal cases. MALT lymphoma represents about 35 percent of primary gastric lymphoma but fewer than 10 percent of the intestinal cases. Follicular lymphomas are very rare in the stomach but have been reported in up to 17 percent of intestinal cases. The other histologic subtypes are much less common and taken together comprise approximately 5 percent of the cases;[24,40] they include T cell lymphomas, Burkitt lymphoma, and mantle cell lymphomas (which in the GI tract often present as a multiple lymphomatous polyposis).

An epidemiologic study carried out in comparable demographic areas in the UK and northern Italy showed a higher incidence of gastric NHL in the northeastern regions of Italy (13.2×10^5/year vs 1×10^5/year). This suggests the existence of geographic variations, perhaps correlated to the rate of chronic gastritis caused by *H. pylori* in the regions under examination.[41] Less consistent epidemiologic information is available on intestinal NHL. Numerous studies have reported on the significant association between celiac disease and the otherwise uncommon enteropathy-associated or enteropathy-type T cell lymphoma (ETL). Aberrant clonal intraepithelial T cell populations can be found in patients with refractory celiac sprue and the patients with celiac disease have an increased risk of developing ETL[42] and perhaps also intestinal lymphoma of other histologic types.[43]

Diagnosis and staging procedures

Regardless of histologic type, the presenting symptoms are generally due to the local lesion (abdominal pain, dyspepsia, nausea and vomiting, anorexia, obstruction, hemorrhage). Fever and night sweats are uncommon and if they do occur are more often associated with a T cell phenotype and/or intestinal localization.[38]

Compared to nodal lymphomas, fewer patients with gastric lymphoma present with bone marrow involvement or elevated LDH levels.[44] Weight loss, however, is common, although this is more often a consequence of the localization of the primary lymphoma rather than a constitutional symptom of the disease.[45] Gastrointestinal bleeding

Table 59.6 Anatomic distribution (frequency) of gastrointestinal lymphomas in different geographic areas

Country	Total number of GI tract cases	Stomach	Intestine (small and large)	Small bowel	Colon and rectum
Austria 1985[216]	133	79%	21%[a]	10%	6%
Canada 2006[24]	176	48%	52%	–	–
Denmark 1991[6]	139	63%	37%	–	–
Hong Kong 1987[217]	425	56%	–	31%	12%
Italy 1993[218]	135	73%	27%[a]	15%	9%
Japan 2003[219]	455	75%	25%[b]		
Kuwait 2004[16]	290	56%	–	28%	16%
Saudi Arabia 1994[220]	185	51%	49%	–	–
Southern Switzerland 1997[1]	103	68%	–	24%	7%
The Netherlands 1989[26]	96	56%	44%[c]	13%	16%
Turkey 2004[15]	145	43%	–	50%	7%
UK 1993[221]	175	45%	54%[a]	33%	15%
USA 1972[22]	538	64%	–	20%	15%
USA 1988[222]	87	60%	–	26%	14%

[a]Including cases (approximately 3–5 percent of all cases) with multifocal gastrointestinal involvement.
[b]Including cases (approximately 4 percent of all cases) with concomitant gastric and intestinal involvement.
[c]Mesenterial localization was considered as primary intestinal and cases with multifocal GI tract involvement were also included.
GI, gastrointestinal.

may occur at presentation in 20–30 percent of patients, while gastric occlusion and perforation are quite uncommon.[40,46–49]

There is no consensus concerning classification and staging of GI NHL and a variety of staging systems are currently in use.[28,50,51]

In the past, surgery was considered an essential component of the diagnostic workup in view of the fact that it provided adequate tumor specimens for diagnosis. However, sufficient material for diagnosis is nowadays obtained in more than 90 percent of cases by endoscopic biopsy and diagnostic surgery, at least in gastric lymphomas, is not needed anymore. Imaging techniques have also significantly improved and, in the past decade, the introduction of endoscopic ultrasonography has been proven to be useful in assessing the depth of the stomach wall infiltration and the presence of perigastric lymph nodes, and in identifying patients at high risk of bleeding and/or perforation.[52–57] In MALT lymphomas, deep infiltration of the gastric wall is associated with a greater risk of lymph node positivity and a smaller chance of response to antibiotics only.[58–60]

In all GI lymphomas, a CT scan of the chest and abdomen is recommended in order to exclude systemic, lymph node extension and/or infiltration of the adjacent structures. The usefulness of a PET scan has been clearly documented only for diffuse large B cell lymphomas (whatever their site) and is controversial for MALT lymphomas.[61] An ear, nose, and throat (ENT) examination is also often recommended in gastric lymphomas in order to exclude concomitant involvement of Waldeyer's ring, occasionally associated with a gastric presentation.[62]

Clinical management

As previously mentioned, surgical resection with postoperative radiation therapy and/or chemotherapy has been widely used in the past. Surgery alone employing partial or total gastrectomy has been reported to cure a proportion of patients, mostly those with low-grade lymphomas.[63,64] A retrospective review of the Danish Lymphoma Study Group experience found that patients with gastric lymphoma who received irradiation as part of their therapy had a reduced risk of relapse.[38] The benefit of low-dose (20–25 Gy) postoperative radiation therapy in patients with stage IA and IIA gastric lymphoma was also shown in the series from the Princess Margaret Hospital of Toronto, which reported an 86 percent 10-year relapse-free survival.[65–67] Others have shown good results in patients with complete resection of tumor followed by chemotherapy alone or combined modality therapy.[68] It has been shown by several studies that chemotherapy alone or chemotherapy followed by radiation therapy may produce similar results and that gastrectomy is thus redundant.[69–72] Taal and colleagues reported a 5-year relapse-free survival of 85 percent in stage I and 58 percent in stage II patients treated with chemotherapy and radiation therapy or radiation therapy alone without prior tumor resection.[73,74] In a

recent large German study, 393 patients with localized primary gastric lymphoma were treated with radiation therapy and/or chemotherapy only or additional surgery. The survival rate at 42 months for patients treated with surgery was 86 percent compared with 91 percent for patients without surgery.[75]

Hence, the need for surgery for diagnostic purposes has disappeared, at least for the gastric tumors, and the assumption of an increased risk of perforation and bleeding associated with front-line chemotherapy, for which 'debulking surgery' was carried out preventatively, has not been confirmed in modern series. Indeed, the presence of a bulky mass is sometimes itself an obstacle to surgical intervention and surgery does not necessarily prevent these complications, as episodes of bleeding or perforation have also been reported to occur despite surgical resection. On the contrary, several studies have reported a high degree of postsurgical complications that resulted in a delay in the start of chemotherapy[71,75–77] and surgical resection has been replaced by conservative therapeutic approaches for gastric lymphomas.[40,48,75,78–80] For primary intestinal lymphoma, however, there are no studies clearly demonstrating that surgery is unnecessary.

Even though there is a dearth of randomized studies comparing surgery alone with the addition of adjuvant chemotherapy and/or radiation therapy, combined modality treatment is nowadays considered the procedure of choice for patients with primary intestinal lymphoma.[23,81] With such an approach, primary gastric and intestinal lymphomas appear to have similar outcomes if they are comparable with respect to histology and prognostic index; in the past, the prognosis for intestinal localization was considered to be generally worse.[38] Recently, retrospective studies proposed modifications of the IPI to effectively identify subsets of patients with primary GI diffuse large B cell lymphoma with significantly different outcomes.[82–85] Optimal treatment of GI lymphomas depends mainly on the histologic type but also on the site and the stage of the disease. The different situations will therefore be discussed separately.

Diffuse large B cell lymphoma of the stomach

Diffuse large B cell lymphoma (DLBCL) represents the most common histologic type among GI lymphomas. Locally advanced or disseminated aggressive GI lymphomas appear to behave in the same manner as other advanced lymphomas with comparable histology and prognostic factors.[70] Therefore, treatment of disseminated DLBCL is today based on chemotherapy combined with the anti-CD20 monoclonal antibody rituximab. In general, the same guidelines followed for nodal DLBCL can also be applied to GI lymphomas with aggressive histologies (i.e., 3–4 cycles of CHOP-rituximab [cyclophosphamide, doxorubicin, vincristine, and prednisone with rituximab] followed by involved field radiation therapy for localized stages, and 6–8 cycles of CHOP-rituximab for disseminated disease).

Analogous to MALT lymphomas, some recent studies have demonstrated possible regression of diffuse large B cell localized lymphomas following anti-*Helicobacter pylori* therapy.[86–88] This suggests that an antigenic drive may remain present in a subset of aggressive gastric lymphomas, especially those where a MALT lymphoma component can be detected. It is our opinion that when an existing or a previous *H. pylori* infection is documented, antibiotics could be added to chemotherapy at a clinician's discretion. Nevertheless, before an antibiotic therapy alone can be considered 'standard' in the treatment of localized diffuse large B cell gastric lymphoma, these results must be validated by prospective, wider-scale studies.

Marginal zone B cell lymphomas of the gastrointestinal tract

GASTRIC MALT LYMPHOMA

A detailed discussion of these lymphomas including the management of those localized in the stomach is presented in Chapter 66 and only a brief outline is given here. Gastric MALT lymphoma is often multimodal within the stomach but is characterized by an indolent natural history and prolonged confinement to the site of origin in most cases. Epidemiologic evidence of a plausible etiologic correlation between gastric MALT lymphomas and chronic *H. pylori* infection has been found; clinical studies demonstrated histologic regressions of gastric MALT lymphoma after eradication of *H. pylori* in the majority of the patients who received antibiotic therapy. Nowadays, it is generally accepted that eradication of *H. pylori* with antibiotics should be the sole initial treatment of MALT lymphomas confined to the gastric wall.[89] No definite guidelines exist for the management of the subset of *H. pylori*-negative cases and for the patients who fail antibiotic therapy. A choice can be made between conventional oncologic modalities but there are no published randomized studies to help the decision. Very good disease control using radiation therapy has been reported by several institutions. Surgery has been widely and successfully used in the past, but the precise role for surgical resection should be redefined in view of the excellent results achieved with conservative approaches.[90] Patients with systemic disease should be considered for systemic treatment but only a few anticancer compounds and chemotherapy regimens have been tested specifically in MALT lymphomas. Rituximab is also very active and may represent an additional option for the treatment of systemic disease.

IMMUNOPROLIFERATIVE SMALL INTESTINAL DISEASE

Immunoproliferative small intestinal disease (IPSID), alpha heavy chain disease, and Mediterranean lymphoma all refer to the same condition, which is presently considered a MALT lymphoma variant characterized by a diffuse lymphoplasmacytic/plasmacytic infiltrate in the small intestine.[91,92] Most of the cases have been described in the

Middle East, especially in the Mediterranean area where the disease is endemic, affecting young adults. Patients usually present with poor performance status and severe malabsorption. Remissions have been described following chemotherapy but frequently the patients cannot tolerate standard therapy and a poor prognosis was described in most published reports. Nevertheless, the most recent data suggest that anthracycline-containing regimens, combined with nutritional support plus antibiotics to control diarrhea and malabsorption, may offer concrete chances of cure to most patients. Treatment with antibiotics can produce clinical, histologic, and immunologic remissions in early stages, but only in 2004 did Lecuit and colleagues demonstrate the presence of a specific pathogen, *Campylobacter jejuni*, linked to this lymphoma.[93] Further information on this condition, can be found in Chapter 66.

Primary intestinal lymphomas

In this category, small bowel lymphoma is by far the most common presentation, with large bowel or rectal lymphoma being less frequent. Presenting symptoms vary from a feeling of abdominal fullness, nausea, diarrhea, and abdominal pain to bowel obstruction and perforation. Because of these nonspecific presenting symptoms many patients require laparotomy for diagnosis and have resection of bowel lesions at diagnosis.

The majority of primary intestinal lymphomas are large cell tumors of B cell lineage, but distinct histologic presentations can include intestinal MALT lymphoma or IPSID, enteropathy-associated T cell lymphoma, mantle cell lymphoma, or follicular lymphoma, underscoring the importance of skilled histologic diagnosis.[94,95]

The management of large B cell lymphoma is usually with surgery followed by chemotherapy (which is today usually combined with rituximab).[19] The outcome reported in the literature varies depending on the extent of disease and histology. In a large series of intestinal lymphoma cases, a 60–75 percent 5-year survival for patients with B cell lymphomas is reported[83,85,96] and only a 25 percent 5-year survival for those with T cell tumors.[96]

Rectal presentations are less common than for other sites in the lower intestinal tract. Treatment usually includes immunochemotherapy and radiation therapy (30–40 Gy in 1.5–2 Gy daily fractions) for patients presenting with DLBCL. Involved field radiation therapy alone (30–35 Gy in 1.5–1.75 Gy daily fractions) has been successful in providing long-term disease control for MALT lymphoma of the rectum. There is no evidence that abdominoperineal resection can improve local control or survival.

MULTIPLE LYMPHOMATOUS POLYPOSIS

This is a peculiar type of lymphoma presenting with multiple lymphomatous polyps of the GI tract. In most cases it represents the intestinal form of mantle cell lymphoma. The prognosis is quite poor in spite of aggressive chemotherapy, similar to its nodal counterpart.[1] In rare instances multiple polyposis appears as a clinical syndrome produced by different histologic subtypes other than mantle cell, especially follicular lymphoma.[97] Thus, the term multiple lymphomatous polyposis should not be used to define a histopathologic entity.

ENTEROPATHY-TYPE T CELL LYMPHOMA

According to the WHO classification, enteropathy-type T cell lymphoma (ETL) is a tumor of intraepithelial T lymphocytes, usually composed of large monomorphic $CD3^+$ $CD7^+$ $CD8^{-/+}$ $CD4^-$ $CD103^+$ cells that contain cytotoxic granule-associated proteins.[98] As stated previously, patients with celiac disease (gluten-sensitive enteropathy) have an increased risk of developing intestinal lymphoma. Enteropathy-type T cell lymphoma usually develops following a longstanding history of celiac disease and most patients show the HLA DQA1*0501, DQB1*0201 genotype that characterizes celiac disease.[99] It occurs most often in the sixth or seventh decades of life but there have been sporadic reports of cases in young adults. Abdominal pain and/or exacerbation of enteropathy-associated symptoms are the most common presentation features. Approximately 25 percent of cases present with an intestinal perforation. The clinical course is often very unfavorable. A variety of combination chemotherapy regimens have been proposed, but responses to the therapy (which is often poorly tolerated because of the malnourished state of most patients) are in general scarce and brief.[1] Death usually results from multifocal intestinal perforations due to relapsing/refractory ulcerating lymphoma.

GASTROINTESTINAL BURKITT LYMPHOMA

Sporadic Burkitt lymphoma, a common childhood lymphoma but very rare in adults, often presents with abdominal pain and intussusception. The ileocecal region is a very common site of involvement and 60 percent of cases are primarily intestinal.[1,100] The primary treatment modality is intensive combination chemotherapy. Local and locoregional therapy (i.e., surgery and radiation therapy) does not provide adequate treatment, even for patients with localized disease. Surgery remains important for establishing the diagnosis and, in certain circumstances, surgical resection may be beneficial (acute abdominal emergencies, resection of intussuscepted bowel). Moreover, in some geographic areas (e.g., Africa) where intensive chemotherapy is not readily available, complete surgical resection may improve clinical outcome and should always be considered in the presence of a completely resectable mass.

GENITOURINARY TRACT LYMPHOMA

Genitourinary lymphomas constitute less than 5 percent of all extranodal NHL.[1] Testicular lymphomas comprise the vast majority of genitourinary lymphomas, with all other sites being very rare; however, not uncommon is a secondary involvement of genitourinary sites in advanced lymphoma.

Testis lymphoma

Primary malignant lymphoma of the testis is a rare disease that represents approximately 5 percent of all testicular tumors and only 1–2 percent of all NHL. Lymphoma, however, is still the most common testis tumor in men older than 60 years of age and the large majority of patients with testis lymphoma are older than 60 years.[1]

The large majority (80–90 percent) of cases are of diffuse large B cell histology but isolated cases of other histologic subtypes have been described, such as Burkitt and Burkitt-like lymphomas, mainly in human immunodeficiency virus (HIV)-infected patients, and, very rarely, T cell lymphoma or follicular lymphomas.[101]

Peculiar histologic and molecular features have been described in DLBCL of the testis, including plasmacytoid differentiation and somatic hypermutation of the immunoglobulin heavy chain gene, suggesting a possible antigen-driven stimulation, analogous to that seen in extranodal B cell marginal zone lymphoma of the MALT type.[102] In addition, lack of adhesion molecules mediating cell–cell and cell–matrix interaction has been shown in testis DLBCL; moreover, tumor cells appear to express the molecules mediating intravasation or extravasation. This expression profile of adhesion molecules is suggestive of a high metastatic potential and may contribute to the early and rapid dissemination that is often seen in these lymphomas.[103] Moreover, the structural loss of HLA class I and II expression with extensive genetic alterations of HLA region described in testis lymphomas may provide the tumor cells with a mechanism to escape from the immune system.[104]

The most common clinical presentation is a unilateral, painless scrotal swelling. Bilateral testicular involvement may be present at diagnosis or, more frequently, contralateral involvement may develop years later and has been observed in up to 35 percent of cases. Over 50 percent of patients present with stage I disease limited to testis and approximately 20 percent present with stage II disease.[19,30,105]

Ultrasound scan of the testis is the initial investigation of choice and then the assessment of the patient with testis lymphoma is similar to that for other lymphomas. However, in addition to the routine tests, staging investigations should include CSF cytology and in some centers brain imaging is recommended.[19]

Orchiectomy is both diagnostic and therapeutic, providing local tumor control, but it is nearly always not curative. Indeed, primary testicular lymphoma has been recognized as a highly lethal disease, with overall 5-year survival rates ranging from 16 percent to 50 percent. The characteristic pattern of failure is mostly distant with a high proportion of relapses in extranodal sites, including skin, lung, pleura, soft tissues, and Waldeyer's ring. Central nervous system relapse is frequent as is recurrence in the contralateral testis.[19,30,105] Many CNS failures occur in brain parenchyma rather than meninges and some also occur several years after the initial presentation.[30,106,107]

Failure in the contralateral testis is well documented and occurs in 5–35 percent of patients. Low-dose radiation therapy (25–30 Gy) to the contralateral testis carries little morbidity in this typically elderly patient population and has been shown to eliminate the risk of failure at this site.[30] Retroperitoneal irradiation in stage I disease has largely been abandoned; however, patients with stage II disease usually receive radiation therapy as part of a combined modality approach recommended for stage II diffuse large cell lymphoma presenting in other sites.

The International Extranodal Lymphoma Study Group (IELSG) conducted a large retrospective survey of 373 patients with a diagnosis of primary testicular diffuse large cell lymphoma.[30] The median age at presentation in this study was 66 years. Approximately 80 percent of patients presented with Ann Arbor stage I–II and low or low-intermediate risk according to the IPI. Systemic chemotherapy was given to 75 percent of cases. In addition, 34 percent of patients received prophylactic scrotal radiation therapy, but only 18 percent had prophylactic intrathecal chemotherapy, and only 8 percent had high-dose methotrexate. The 5-year survival was 48 percent and the 10-year survival was 27 percent, the survival curves showing no clear evidence of a substantial proportion of cured patients. The outcome of patients who received anthracycline-based chemotherapy was better than for those who did not receive it.[30] Multivariate analysis of prognostic factors showed that a favorable IPI, no B symptoms, anthracycline-containing regimens, and prophylactic scrotal radiation therapy were significantly associated with longer survival. However, even for patients with stage I disease and favorable IPI, the outcome appears worse than that reported for diffuse large cell lymphoma at other sites. At a median follow-up of 7.6 years, 195 patients had relapsed. Extranodal recurrence was reported in 140 cases. A continuous risk of recurrence in the contralateral testis was seen in patients not receiving prophylactic scrotal radiation therapy. Relapses/progressions in the CNS were detected in 15 percent of patients and appeared continuously up to 10 years following the initial presentation. Prophylactic intrathecal chemotherapy was associated with an improved progression-free survival. High-dose intravenous methotrexate apparently did not improve the outcome but was given only to a very small subset of patients. The limited number of cases (9 percent) in this series who had received systemic CHOP-like chemotherapy together with prophylactic intrathecal chemotherapy and prophylactic scrotal irradiation appeared to have a better outcome with a 3-year overall survival of 88 percent.[30]

There are very few published data regarding the benefit of prophylactic cranial irradiation in testis lymphoma. Based on the results of the retrospective series, the IELSG

evaluated the feasibility and efficacy of a treatment program comprising prophylactic radiation therapy to the contralateral testis and intrathecal methotrexate in addition to rituximab plus CHOP chemotherapy in a prospective single-arm trial. The preliminary analysis of this study showed a complete remission (CR) rate of 98 percent at a median follow-up of 28 months; 3-year overall survival and 3-year event-free survival were 86 percent and 77 percent, respectively. Lymphoma relapses were seen either at nodal or extranodal sites, including the CNS, but no contralateral testis relapses were observed.[108] In comparison with historical retrospective series, scrotal radiation therapy seems to have eliminated testicular relapses and prophylactic intrathecal methotrexate seems to have reduced, but not eliminated, CNS relapses. More effective treatment to prevent CNS relapses needs, therefore, to be devised. Intrathecal chemotherapy may decrease the risk of meningeal failure while prevention of parenchymal brain relapse can be addressed with the use of high-dose systemic methotrexate, but this is not always feasible in elderly patients where even the delivery of standard intrathecal chemotherapy is often problematic.

Lymphoma of the kidney

Functional renal impairment has been described as a paraneoplastic syndrome in both NHL and Hodgkin disease; however, primary lymphoma of the kidney is very rare.[1] Many cases are represented by diffuse large B cell lymphoma but MALT-type lymphomas have also been described.[1] Several cases with bilateral disease have been reported and may have a poorer survival.[109] Flank pain and renal insufficiency are the commonest clinical features at presentation. Given the limited radiation tolerance of the kidney, combination chemotherapy (in association with rituximab) is the indicated treatment, even in cases of apparently localized renal lymphoma.

Lymphoma of the bladder, urethra, and prostate

Primary lymphoma of the bladder is very rare, accounting for less than 1 percent of all bladder neoplasms,[1] but a number of small series of patients have been reported. Patients commonly present with dysuria and, sporadically, hematuria. Cystoscopic examination shows a submucosal mass with an edematous and friable mucosa. Primary extranodal marginal zone lymphoma of MALT type, frequently arising on a background of chronic cystitis, is the most common primary bladder lymphoma and is associated with an excellent prognosis.[110] Treatment has traditionally involved partial cystectomy and/or radiation therapy to the pelvis. The prognosis is related to histologic type and extent of tumor. As in other extranodal lymphomas, small cell lymphomas may be managed with radiation therapy alone, but large cell lymphomas should be treated with anthracycline-based chemotherapy followed by local radiation therapy. Repeat cystoscopy is very important for follow-up.[111] Primary prostate lymphomas have been reported very rarely,[112] although secondary involvement, mainly in low-grade lymphoma, might be more frequent than is clinically evident.[1] Very few cases of primary lymphoma arising in the urethra have been reported, most commonly in female patients.[113]

Primary lymphomas of the female genital tract

The female genital lymphomas are extremely rare conditions accounting for less than 0.5 percent of gynecologic cancers and for 1.5 percent of all NHL.[114] The adnexa are the most frequent site, followed by the uterus; vagina and vulva localization is unusual.[114,115] Occasionally, two or more adjacent genital organs can be involved. The majority of cases are diffuse large B cell lymphomas, followed by Burkitt lymphoma and follicular lymphoma. Marginal zone lymphoma and lymphoplasmacytic lymphoma have also been described.[115]

LYMPHOMA OF THE OVARY

This is a very rare form of primary extranodal lymphoma. Patients present with abdominal pain or finding of an asymptomatic abdominal mass. Diffuse large B cell lymphomas are most common, but the ovary is one of the known sites of Burkitt lymphoma.[116] Treatment with chemotherapy alone may preserve gonadal and hormonal function, but for localized diffuse large cell lymphoma, combined modality therapy is recommended. As lymphomas of the ovary are most commonly of the diffuse large B cell type and clearly are most commonly associated with extensive dissemination, the initial treatment approach must include chemotherapy. Chemotherapy alone showed promising results and a conservative management based on exclusive chemotherapy in localized lymphoma may be considered in patients desiring future pregnancy.[114] Radiation therapy may be useful in the circumstance of a localized residual disease postsurgery or following definitive chemotherapy. Local control is, however, a less important issue given the usual resection of the presenting lesion and the common pattern of failure being systemic progression.

LYMPHOMA OF THE UTERUS AND VAGINA

Lymphomas of uterus, cervix, and vagina usually present in middle-aged women although presentations at a younger age can occur. Symptoms commonly involve vaginal bleeding. The standard therapy for patients with stage IE lesions has usually comprised radiation therapy with or without antecedent surgery. There is no evidence that radical surgery is necessary and, indeed, there is no strong indication

for more than a diagnostic biopsy with subsequent detailed staging evaluation. Radiation therapy alone for localized MALT or follicular lymphoma offers a very high probability of local control. Combined chemotherapy and radiation therapy for diffuse large B cell tumors is appropriate and, given the impact of radiation therapy on ovarian function in those in the reproductive age range, the use of chemotherapy alone has been recommended with some clinical justification. Favorable long-term outcome has been reported for patients with stage IE disease. Important prognostic factors include stage and histology. Local failure is very uncommon following surgery and radiation therapy for endometrial, cervical, or vaginal lymphoma.[117]

LYMPHOMA PRESENTING IN THE HEAD AND NECK REGION

It is evident that considering all the lymphomas arising in the head and neck region as a single group is simply the heritage of a historical topographical distinction, related to the fact that this anatomic region is the second most common site of localized extranodal presentation of NHL. However, different lymphoma entities can arise within the head and neck area. The tonsils are the most common site, followed by nasopharynx, oral cavity, salivary glands, paranasal sinuses, and base of tongue. The signs and symptoms of a NHL may be similar to those of a head and neck squamous cancer and only histologic examination can distinguish them. Long-term outcomes of patients with extranodal lymphomas in the head and neck area may vary, mostly depending on the histologic type but also, to some degree, on the site of presentation.

Waldeyer's ring lymphoma

Despite controversy as to whether tonsils and Waldeyer's ring in general should be considered as nodal or extranodal sites, most authors consider Waldeyer's ring lymphomas as extranodal lymphomas. The tonsil resembles MALT in its relation to the pharyngeal epithelium and its lack of afferent lymphatics, but its overall structure, lack of prominent marginal zone, and predominant immunoglobulin (Ig) G as opposed to IgA secretion by its resident plasma cells are more characteristic of peripheral lymph nodes and from this perspective the Waldeyer's ring may be considered as the point of contact between the gastrointestinal MALT and the peripheral lymphoid tissue of the lymph nodes.[118] Tonsils are the most common site of lymphoma involvement in Waldeyer's ring; the other sites include nasopharynx and base of the tongue. A wide spectrum of histology with follicular, MALT, and other small cell lymphomas is seen. However, the commonest histologic type is diffuse B cell large cell lymphoma.[119,120]

Patients may present with dysphagia, airway obstruction, or a mass lesion in the throat. An important aspect of the natural history of Waldeyer's ring lymphoma is the possible concomitant GI tract involvement.[62,121] Therefore, GI tract investigations belong to the recommended staging procedure.

Historical literature reports high local control rates for localized disease with sole radiation therapy but the description of distant failures with this approach indicates a high risk of occult systemic disease. Aviles *et al.* showed the superiority of a combined modality approach including anthracycline-containing chemotherapy and radiation therapy in a prospective randomized trial. The 5-year failure-free survival was 48 percent for radiation therapy, 45 percent for chemotherapy alone, and 83 percent for the combined modality arm.[121] Combined modality therapy has become the standard approach to the management of localized Waldeyer's ring diffuse large cell lymphoma.[119–121]

Thyroid lymphoma

Primary thyroid lymphoma is uncommon, accounting for only 1–5 percent of thyroid neoplasms and less than 2 percent of extranodal lymphomas, and usually affects elderly women.[2] Different histologic subtypes are described in this clinical setting.[122–124] The large majority of cases are represented by MALT lymphomas and by diffuse large B cell lymphomas with or without a marginal zone B cell lymphoma component.[118] The occurrence of a primary thyroid MALT lymphoma is generally considered the late result of the acquisition of intrathyroid lymphoid tissue in the context of autoimmune thyroid disease such as Hashimoto thyroiditis.[122] Patients usually present with a painless, rapidly growing neck mass (rarely, with compression of surrounding structures) and symptoms such as dysphagia and/or dyspnea. Frequent involvement of the GI tract has been reported in cases presenting with disseminated disease.[122] Central nervous system involvement is rare. Surgery is a diagnostic procedure and is not considered a definitive intervention for thyroid lymphoma, although historical series reported optimal clinical control after radical thyroidectomy in localized MALT lymphomas. Exceptionally, tracheostomy is required to relieve airway obstruction at diagnosis. For localized primary thyroid MALT lymphomas, locoregional radiation therapy to a moderate dose of 30 Gy achieves excellent local control.[125] For diffuse large cell lymphoma, with or without a MALT component – given the high distant relapse rates with radiation therapy alone[124] – chemotherapy alone or chemotherapy and radiation therapy have become the standard treatment approaches.

Salivary gland lymphoma

Salivary gland lymphomas account for 5–10 percent of all salivary gland tumors and somewhat less than 5 percent of lymphomas at all sites. The vast majority of salivary gland lymphomas are located in the parotid. The spectrum of histologic subtypes most frequently observed in this clinical setting includes B cell neoplasms: MALT lymphomas and, less frequently, diffuse large cell lymphomas *de novo* or on the basis of transformation from indolent lymphomas. Other histotypes rarely occur as primary salivary gland disease. In an IELSG survey concerning MALT lymphomas arising in nongastric sites, salivary glands were the most common primary site of disease.[126] MALT lymphomas more often arise from the lymphoid tissue acquired in the context of the autoimmune chronic inflammation of myoepithelial sialoadenitis (MESA) typically observed in Sjögren syndrome. MALT lymphomas have generally an indolent course and tend to remain localized for prolonged periods of time. Patients usually present with a painless mass in the parotid or submandibular gland.[127] Bilateral presentations are frequent. A recent study of marginal zone B cell lymphoma of the parotid glands showed a 90 percent 5-year overall survival and 100 percent CR rate. No advantage in remission rate or time to treatment failure was seen for combined modality treatment over radiation therapy alone.[128] The role of surgery should be limited to excisional biopsy. Therapy has to be tailored to stage and especially to the histologic subtype: radiation therapy is an option for localized indolent lymphomas; doxorubicin-containing chemotherapy or a combined modality approach is the standard treatment for diffuse large B cell lymphomas. Chemotherapy not containing anthracyclines has a role in the treatment of indolent advanced stage disease and cases associated with Sjögren syndrome, in which patients the radiation therapy may aggravate preexisting xerostomia. Rituximab[129] has clinical activity in this as in other locations of MALT lymphomas but its role in the treatment of this entity has still to be ascertained.

Lymphoma of the ocular adnexa (orbital lymphoma)

The definition of orbital lymphomas applies to lymphomatous lesions primarily involving any orbital and ocular adnexal tissue, i.e., the conjunctiva, eyelids, lacrimal glands, or retro-orbital soft tissues. Bilateral involvement is observed in 10–15 percent of cases, mostly in conjunctival forms. MALT lymphomas represent the commonest histologic subtype, followed by follicular lymphomas, while aggresssive histologic subtypes are less common in the ocular adnexal area.[130,131] This entity is more frequent than the intraocular lymphoma, or lymphoma of the eye, which represents a subset of primary CNS lymphomas and has aggressive histology and different natural history. The clinical picture depends greatly on the structures compromised.[132] The lymphomas of ocular adnexa usually present as anterior lesions, small nodules or in the conjunctiva, with a typical 'salmon red patch' appearance sometimes with symptoms of blurred vision. The posterior lesions present with swelling and proptosis. Pain is uncommon, but with increasing bulk of the lesion pressure and diplopia may occur. Histology is usually extranodal marginal zone B cell lymphoma of MALT type. Treatment is directed at cure, while preserving vision and the integrity of the orbit. Extensive surgery should be avoided as it is entirely unnecessary. Conventional treatment of localized lesions consists of low to moderate doses of radiation therapy with local control rate in excess of 95 percent[35,133,134] for indolent lymphomas. Conjunctiva lesions may be treated with direct photon beams, sparing orbital structures. For patients with large B cell tumors and for patients with bulky tumors, where the cornea cannot be adequately protected, short-duration chemotherapy (e.g., R-CHOP for three courses) followed by radiation therapy may be used. The tolerance radiation therapy dose of the lacrimal gland is 40 Gy in 20 daily fractions. The complications of radiation therapy, commonly seen when doses of 40 Gy or more are used, include cataract formation, keratitis, and dry eye. Damage to the optic nerve and retina should not be observed with a dose of 40 Gy or less.[135]

The overall actuarial 10-year survival rates for orbital lymphomas reported in the literature are 75–80 percent. The most common site of relapse is the contralateral orbit but generalized disease is occasionally seen.

The development of ocular adnexal MALT lymphoma is frequently associated with chronic conjunctivitis, a recently recognized cause of which is infection by *Chlamydia*.[132] Evidence for an association between *Chlamydia psittaci* infection and ocular adnexal MALT lymphoma was first observed in a series of patients from northern Italy.[136] A subsequent epidemiologic study has shown a possible real increase in the incidence of ocular adnexal lymphomas, suggesting *C. psittaci* or another microorganism as possible causative agents.[137] *Chlamydia psittaci* appears to be variably associated with ocular adnexal MALT lymphoma in different geographic regions with an incidence ranging from 0 to 87 percent of ocular adnexal lymphoma in the published series.[138] Thus, our understanding of the role of *C. psittaci* is far from complete. Nevertheless, antilymphoma activity of antibiotic therapy (with doxycycline) directed against *C. psittaci* has been reported in MALT lymphomas of the ocular adnexa, similar to what was observed in treatment of patients with gastric lymphomas for *H. pylori* infection.[139] Its safety profile and its activity in pretreated patients, including those with relapses in previously irradiated areas,[139] might make doxycycline a valid therapeutic alternative to conventional chemotherapy and radiation therapy in orbital MALT lymphomas. However, at present, until more cumulative experience is gained from prospective trials, this approach should be considered investigational.

Paranasal sinuses and nasal cavity lymphoma

Lymphomas of the sinonasal region are exceedingly rare in Western countries, where they usually show a B cell phenotype, but in Asian countries they represent the second-largest group of extranodal lymphomas after GI localizations, and most of them are located in the nasal cavity[140] and have a NK/T cell phenotype.[141] Lymphomas of paranasal sinuses present most commonly in the maxillary sinus and usually have a B cell phenotype.

The clinical presentation varies upon the histologic subtype. Indolent lymphomas present with a sinonasal mass associated with obstructive symptoms. The aggressive histotypes are more likely to present with aggressive signs and symptoms including nonhealing ulcer, cranial nerve manifestations, facial swelling, epistaxis, or pain. Diffuse large B cell lymphomas may present with soft tissue or bone destruction, particularly of the orbit with associated proptosis, whereas the T cell lymphomas are associated with nasal septal perforation and/or destruction.[142] Natural killer/T cell tumors are more commonly associated with angioinvasion, necrosis, and bone erosion. Because of the destructive features, sinonasal lymphomas were historically named as lethal midline granuloma; in the WHO classification the extranodal NK/T cell lymphoma, nasal type is recognized as a distinct clinic pathologic entity highly associated with EBV infection.[143] These tumors are not exclusively confined in the nasal cavity but may arise in the nasopharynx, in the palate, and in a variety of other extranodal sites, most commonly in the skin, soft tissue, and GI tract.[143] Natural killer/T cell lymphoma of nasal type arising outside the upper aero-digestive tract seems usually to have a particularly high aggressive clinical behaviour.[144]

The prognosis of sinonasal lymphomas is variable and depends upon the histologic type and the anatomic extent of the tumor.[144,145]

The clinical course of nasal NK/T cell lymphoma is highly aggressive and the optimal treatment remains uncertain. Prolonged remission after aggressive chemotherapy combined with irradiation can be achieved only in cases with very localized disease. Disseminated disease has a very poor outcome despite aggressive therapy and the clinical outcome does not seem to be improved significantly by the use of doxorubicin-containing chemotherapeutic regimens in addition to radiation therapy.[143,146] In a Chinese study of 175 patients, mostly stage IE NK/T cell, nasal type, the overall 5-year survival was 65 percent. The 5-year overall survival for limited stage IE lesions (i.e., confined to the nasal cavity) was 90 percent compared with 57 percent for extensive stage IE (i.e., presenting with extension beyond the nasal cavity) lesions. The addition of chemotherapy to radiation in stage IE did not result in a significant survival benefit.[147]

In a small series of 16 patients with paranasal sinus lymphomas (10 B cell, four T cell, and two NK cell) treated at Stanford University with combined modality therapy and CNS prophylaxis, the overall survival at 5 years was 29 percent with a median survival of 18 months. All T and NK cell patients relapsed or were dead by 6 months. The authors concluded that sinus lymphoma is an aggressive disease characterized by distant relapse and early mortality.

Combined modality therapy with CNS prophylaxis is recommended but prognosis remains poor, especially in patients with NK/T-lineage lymphoma who might benefit from early intensification.[148]

It is not surprising that aggressive lymphomas of the face and the base of the skull have a tendency to CNS dissemination. In a French series of 14 patients, treated with a CHOP or CHOP-like program, four of seven relapses involved the CNS.[149] The MD Anderson group reported a series of 70 patients with lymphoma of the nasal cavity and paranasal sinuses. They appeared to have a more favorable prognosis when treated with combined modality therapy compared with radiation therapy alone. Failure in the CNS after initial therapy was very rare in this series. The local extent of disease was the strongest prognostic factor for patients treated with radiation therapy alone, while the IPI was the most significant predictor of outcome for patients also receiving chemotherapy.[145]

In general, a significant proportion of patients presenting with B cell lymphomas may be cured with combined modality therapy (with CHOP-type chemotherapy associated with rituximab followed by involved field radiation therapy). The role of CNS prophylaxis is controversial, but it is in general recommended and appears to reduce the risk of CNS relapse.[150]

Nasal NK/T cell lymphoma is a highly aggressive tumor. Aggressive chemotherapy associated with radiation therapy achieves long-term disease control only in a minority of patients. Locally advanced or disseminated disease is associated with poorer prognosis and the clinical usefulness of early treatment intensification with high-dose chemotherapy and autologous or allogeneic stem cell support is being tested in clinical trials.[151]

Plasmablastic lymphoma of the oral cavity

This tumor represents a variant of diffuse large B cell lymphoma initially described as a HIV-associated entity, usually EBV-positive, presenting in the oral cavity, and characterized by immunoblastic morphology and a plasma cell phenotype.[152] The clinical course is often aggressive with poor response to chemotherapy and short survival. Diffuse large B cell lymphomas with plasmablastic differentiation may also arise at other sites and appear to represent a clinically heterogeneous group of neoplasms with different clinicopathological characteristics that may correspond to distinct entities.[153]

Primary lymphomas of the upper airways

Tracheal involvement usually occurs with disseminated lymphoma. Primary tracheal lymphoma is a rare entity. Reported histologies are varied, with a predominance of indolent subtypes, including lymphomas of MALT type.[118] The therapeutic approach for localized disease should comprise combined chemoradiotherapy.[2] Primary laryngeal lymphomas are also very rare and may arise from the MALT.[118]

PRIMARY CENTRAL NERVOUS SYSTEM LYMPHOMA

Primary CNS lymphoma (PCNSL) is a rare subtype of NHL that is characterized by the primary and exclusive involvement of the brain, spinal cord, leptomeninges, and eyes. From the 1970s to the 1990s the incidence of PCNSL increased steadily, partly in association with the AIDS epidemic. Indeed, immunodeficiency is the only established risk factor and patients with HIV infection have a significantly increased risk of developing PCNSL. However, highly active antiretroviral therapy (HAART) has changed the clinical and immunological course of HIV infection and is probably the reason for a recent slight decline in PCNSL incidence.[29] In immunocompetent patients the disease incidence has also been increasing over recent past decades and occurs mostly in the sixth and seventh decades of life.

The large majority of PCNSLs in immunocompetent individuals are diffuse large B cell lymphomas that show morphologic and immunophenotypic characteristics similar to nodal diffuse large B cell lymphomas. In CNS lymphoma of immunocompetent patients, EBV infection is usually absent, while it is frequently detected in the large B cell lymphomas of HIV-infected patients. In this latter group, PCNSLs can also present with histologic features of classic or atypical Burkitt lymphoma. Rare cases of small lymphocytic, lymphoplasmacytic, and T cell lymphoma similar to those seen outside the CNS have been also reported.

The clinical presentation is dominated by neurological symptoms, their nature depending on the disease location: focal deficits, neuropsychiatric symptoms, seizures, and manifestations of increased intracranial pressure. The contemporary involvement of the eyes, often bilateral, has been reported in 20 percent of cases.[29]

The International PCNSL Collaborative Group (IPCG) has indicated guidelines for standardized baseline evaluation in newly diagnosed PCNSL.[154] The baseline clinical examination should include a comprehensive physical and neurological examination. Particular attention should be paid to examination of peripheral lymph nodes and testicular examination in men over the age of 65 years. Evaluation of cognitive function is important at baseline and follow-up assessments are critical to estimate the benefit of therapy and to monitor for treatment-related neurocognitive decline, but at present there is no standard battery of neuropsychological testing. The best tool in defining the tumor extent is contrast-enhanced brain MRI. The initial staging should also include a lumbar puncture (with cytologic evaluation, flow cytometry, cell count, protein, and glucose dosing in CSF) and an ophthalmology evaluation with slit-lamp examination. A CT scan of thorax, abdomen, and pelvis, together with a bone marrow biopsy, should also be planned. In men, the ultrasound examination of the testis can exclude a primary testicular lymphoma localization at high risk of subsequent CNS spread. No defined role for positron emission tomography has been identified in the initial workup of PCNSL.

A large retrospective study of the IELSG devised a five-point scoring system based on five prognostic variables: age older than 60 years, Eastern Cooperative Oncology Group (ECOG) performance status higher than 1, elevated LDH level, high CSF total protein concentration, and involvement of deep regions of the brain (periventricular regions, basal ganglia, brainstem, and/or cerebellum). Patients with zero or one risk factor had a 2-year overall survival of 80 percent, patients with four or five adverse risk factors had a 2-year overall survival of 15 percent.[155] Another prognostic score has been proposed by the Memorial Sloan-Kettering Cancer Center and is based only on age and Karnofsky performance status: patients younger than 50 years had significantly improved outcome with regard to both overall and failure-free survival compared with older patients. Patients older than 50 years with Karnofsky performance score below 70 have the poorest outcome while those of age more than 50 years but with good performance status (Karnofsky score greater than 70) have an intermediate prognosis.[156]

Surgical debulking does not result in any survival benefit. In immunocompetent patients treatment options include corticosteroids, radiation therapy, and chemotherapy. The use of sole corticosteroid therapy, although active in a relevant proportion of patients, is invariably followed by early relapse. Whole brain radiation therapy (WBRT), required because of the multifocal nature of PCNSL, has been associated with a median survival of 12 months.[157] Current therapeutic strategies in PCNSL result from a limited number of small nonrandomized phase II trials and metaanalyses of retrospective series. Even though it has not been confirmed in a randomized trial, there is a consensus that combined chemoradiotherapy is superior to radiation therapy alone. High-dose systemic methotrexate is necessary for adequate CSF penetration, and doses from 1 to 8 g/m^2 are commonly administered.[158] The optimal dose of methotrexate has not been defined.[159] Data from retrospective series indicate that high-dose methotrexate (HDM)-based chemotherapy followed by WBRT should be preferred over radiation therapy alone. Methotrexate-based chemotherapy combined with WBRT is associated with radiographic responses in more than 50 percent of patients with PCNSL and a 2-year survival of 40–70 percent.[159] However, even with this strategy, the 5-year survival rate remains approximately 20–25 percent, and it is not known whether more intensive combined treatment will improve outcome. Combining high-dose methotrexate and WBRT increases disease control but it also presents an increased likelihood of treatment-related neurotoxicity, mostly in patients older than 60 years.[159] Some authors suggest delaying WBRT in this subset of patients.[160]

Although a large, multicenter, retrospective study by Ferreri et al.[161] showed that WBRT did not improve survival in patients in complete remission after high-dose methotrexate, withholding WBRT in younger patients is more controversial because it may jeopardize the long-term disease control.[162]

High-dose chemotherapy supported by autologous stem cell transplantation has been used to intensify the treatment in younger patients with newly diagnosed or relapsed PCNSL. Theoretically, this strategy can be used to replace WBRT in an effort to avoid treatment-related neurotoxicity, but despite some encouraging results[162–164] its role remains to be defined.

Whole brain radiation therapy (if not delivered in first-line therapy), autologous bone marrow transplantation, combinations of drugs crossing the blood-brain barrier, or retreatment with high-dose methotrexate, as well as phase II studies of novel treatment strategies, represent options for relapsed disease.

Primary ocular lymphoma

Primary ocular lymphoma (i.e., restricted to the globe, usually the vitreous, retina, and choroids) is an exceedingly rare subset of CNS lymphomas.[165,166] Ocular involvement can often be bilateral and is usually associated with brain lymphoma or precedes it.[2] Chemotherapy combined with ocular irradiation seems effective in the control of ocular disease but does not necessarily prevent CNS progression. Patients whose ocular disease is identified and treated before CNS progression have a better survival.

Primary leptomeningeal lymphoma

In rare instances, malignant lymphoma presents as a localized leptomeningeal disease, in the absence of parenchymal brain involvement, with symptoms of raised intracranial pressure or cranial or spinal polyradiculopathies.[167] Diagnosis is commonly made on the basis of positive CSF cytology or meningeal biopsy; detection of a monoclonal lymphocytic population by flow cytometry studies is helpful.[27] Treatment options include irradiation and intrathecal or systemic chemotherapy.

A completely different type of primary meningeal lymphoma is the primary MALT lymphoma of the dura, which, in contrast to other types of CNS lymphomas, has a very good prognosis with minimally aggressive treatment.[168]

Primary extradural lymphoma

Primary extradural lymphoma represents approximately 1 percent of all localized NHLs; it most often presents with spinal cord compression. Diffuse large B cell lymphoma is the most common histologic type. Magnetic resonance imaging is the examination of choice; CSF study results are negative at diagnosis. Data on pattern of relapse are discordant, but CNS relapses seem to be rare. Primary spinal epidural lymphoma usually has a relatively good prognosis.[169,170] Combined modality treatment appears to be superior to radiation therapy alone.[171]

PRIMARY EXTRANODAL LYMPHOMAS AT OTHER SITES

Primary cutaneous lymphomas

Primary cutaneous lymphomas represent T and B cell neoplasms primarily arising in the skin with no evidence of extracutaneous disease at the time of diagnosis. The skin is one of the most common sites of extranodal non-Hodgkin lymphoma, with an estimated annual incidence of 1 in 100 000.[10]

A consensus was recently achieved for a common WHO-EORTC (European Organization for Research and

Treatment in Cancer) classification of cutaneous lymphomas, overcoming previous discrepancies between the EORTC and WHO classifications, in particular the controversies on definition and terminology of B cell neoplasms. The WHO-EORTC classification of cutaneous lymphomas comprises mature T cell and NK cell neoplasms, mature B cell neoplasms, and immature hematopoietic malignancies (Table 59.7). This classification reflects the unique features of primary cutaneous lymphoproliferative diseases and is, as much as possible, compatible with the concept of the WHO classification for nodal lymphomas and the EORTC classification of cutaneous lymphomas.[172]

The group of T and NK cell lymphomas account for up to 75–80 percent of all cutaneous lymphomas. Each one of the most common subtypes – mycosis fungoides, Sézary syndrome, cutaneous anaplastic large cell lymphoma, and lymphomatoid papulosis – has unique biologic and clinical features, all but Sézary syndrome being part of the group of indolent entities. Among B cell lymphomas two main entities with indolent clinical behavior have been

Table 59.7 WHO-EORTC classification of cutaneous lymphomas with primary cutaneous manifestations (with relative frequency and outcome according to the Dutch and Austrian Cutaneous Lymphoma Group registries 1986–2002)

Entity	Frequency	Clinical behavior	Disease-specific 5-year survival
Cutaneous T cell and NK cell lymphomas			
Mycosis fungoides (MF)	44%	Indolent	88%
MF variants and subtypes			
– Folliculotropic MF	4%	Indolent	80%
– Pagetoid reticulosis	<1%	Indolent	100%
– Granulomatous slack skin	<1%	Indolent	100%
Sézary syndrome	3%	Aggressive	24%
Adult T cell leukemia/lymphoma (ATLL)	NR	Aggressive	NR
Primary cutaneous CD30$^+$ lymphoproliferative disorders			
– Primary cutaneous anaplastic large cell lymphoma	8%	Indolent	95%
– Lymphomatoid papulosis	12%	Indolent	100%
Subcutaneous panniculitis-like $\alpha\beta$ T cell lymphoma	1%	Indolent	82%
Extranodal NK/T cell lymphoma, nasal type	<1%	Aggressive	Median survival <12 months
Primary cutaneous peripheral T cell lymphoma, unspecified	2%	Aggressive	16%
– Primary cutaneous aggressive epidermotropic CD8$^+$ T cell lymphoma (provisional)	<1%	Aggressive	18%
– Cutaneous $\gamma\delta$ T cell lymphoma (provisional)	<1%	Aggressive	NR
– Primary cutaneous CD4$^+$small/medium-sized pleomorphic T cell lymphoma (provisional)	2%	Indolent	75%
Cutaneous B cell lymphomas			
Primary cutaneous marginal zone B cell lymphoma	7%	Indolent	99%
Primary cutaneous follicle center lymphoma	11%	Indolent	95%
Primary cutaneous diffuse large B cell lymphoma, leg type	4%	Intermediate	55%
Primary cutaneous diffuse large B cell lymphoma, other	<1%	Intermediate	50%
– Intravascular large B cell lymphoma	<1%	Intermediate	65%
Precursor hematologic neoplasm			
CD4$^+$/CD56$^+$hematodermic neoplasm (blastic NK cell lymphoma, early plasmacytoid dendritic cell leukemia/lymphoma)	NR	AggressiveMedian survival 14 months	

WHO-EORTC, World Health Organization–European Organization for Research and Treatment in Cancer; NK, natural killer.

identified: primary cutaneous marginal zone B cell lymphoma and primary cutaneous follicle center lymphoma. The peculiar clinical-pathologic and genetic features recognized to the primary cutaneous large B cell lymphoma, leg of the EORTC classification[173–175] led to the additional identification in the WHO-EORTC classification of primary cutaneous large B cell lymphoma, leg type as a distinct disease entity with intermediate clinical behavior.

Since the skin is a relatively common site of dissemination of many nodal non-Hodgkin lymphomas, especially those of T cell phenotype, proper staging procedures are important in any patient who presents with lymphomatous skin infiltration. The Ann Arbor staging system is largely inadequate for staging primary cutaneous lymphomas and a modified TNM (tumor, node, metastases) system devised for the staging of mycosis fungoides and Sézary syndrome is widely used and recommended.[176]

The spectrum of treatment tools available for primary cutaneous T cell lymphomas is wide. Depending on disease extent, mycosis fungoides can be treated with skin-targeted therapies such as photo- (chemo-) therapy, topical nitrogen mustard, chlormustine, radiation therapy including total skin electron beam irradiation, or bexarotene gel, or with systemic therapy such as bexarotene capsules, interferon α, receptor-targeted cytotoxic fusion proteins (e.g., denileukin diftitox), extracorporeal photoapheresis, or alemtuzumab. The exact role of these treatments, either as single agents or in combination with other therapies, remains to be established[177] and details on the treatment of the main cutaneous lymphoma entities are given elsewhere in this book.

Serology for *Borrelia burgdorferi* should be part of the staging procedures in primary cutaneous marginal zone B cell lymphomas due to the suggested pathogenetic relationship between *B. burgdorferi* and this entity. In fact, anecdotal regression of cases of cutaneous marginal zone B cell lymphomas has been reported following eradication of *B. burgdorferi* infection.[178]

Localized cutaneous indolent B cell lymphomas can be successfully treated with radiation therapy alone; systemic treatment, chemotherapy, and/or anti-CD20 immunotherapy is reserved for patients with multiple cutaneous or subcutaneous localizations. Anthracycline-containing chemotherapy may be required for primary cutaneous diffuse large B cell lymphoma, leg type.

Breast lymphoma

Breast is an uncommon primary site of lymphoma localization, comprising only 2 percent of localized extranodal NHL presentations. Only a few hundred cases have been reported, most in small retrospective series with only one small prospective study identified.[179] This sparse information prevents the definition of prognosis and patterns of failure of patients with primary breast NHL, with wide variations in outcomes and prognostic factors reported.

However, some common features have been described: predominant diffuse large B cell histology (although follicular and MALT lymphomas and Burkitt lymphomas have also been reported), prognosis poorer than anticipated by stage, significant risk of contralateral breast involvement, and tendency to CNS relapse. In a retrospective IELSG survey of more than 200 cases of primary localized diffuse large cell lymphoma of the breast, peculiar clinical features and characteristic patterns of relapse have been identified. The contralateral breast and other extranodal sites were major sites of relapse. The CNS relapse rate was lower than anticipated from literature series, despite the lack of CNS prophylaxis in the large majority of patients. In this patient population, receiving chemotherapy in 80 percent of cases (mainly with anthracycline-containing regimens) and in a relevant proportion a combination strategy of both chemotherapy and radiation therapy, median overall survival was 8.0 years, with 5- and 10-year overall survival rates of 63 percent and 47 percent, respectively; median progression-free survival was 5.5 years.[180] Based on these data, referring to a pre-rituximab era, the combination of anthracycline-containing chemotherapy and locoregional radiation therapy seems adequate, following a diagnostic surgical biopsy. Addition of rituximab has never been studied but is likely to be beneficial.

Primary lymphoma of the bone

A primary bone localization of NHL is a rare entity with peak incidence in the fifth decade of life and a slight male preponderance. Symptoms at presentation usually consist of localized bone pain, in some cases with soft tissue swelling, and possibly pathologic fractures. Polyostotic presentations may occur. Diffuse large B cell lymphoma represents the most frequent histology[181] but indolent lymphomas with a primary osseous presentation have also been reported. In this peculiar clinical setting the exact definition of tumor staging is quite problematic: MRI has a relevant role in revealing extension of disease not visualized by routine x-rays or bone scan. Data showing the usefulness of a PET scan in evaluation of lymphomatous bone lesion have been reported.[182] Historical cases of surgical cure of primary bone lymphoma have been reported but solely surgery is no longer considered an appropriate therapy and should be limited to the open biopsy often required to make the diagnosis. With radiation therapy, 5- and 10-year overall survival rates of 58 percent and 53 percent, respectively, are reported for solitary bone lesions. Key issues relating to local control are the intramedullary and soft tissue extent of disease in relation to radiation therapy volume. Treatment approaches using radiation therapy alone have unacceptable rates of local or marginal failure (20 percent) probably related to underestimation of tumor extent and bulk, and a systemic failure rate approaching 50 percent. A treatment strategy including chemotherapy and radiation therapy produces in retrospective series the best clinical results.[183–186] A better outcome for patients treated with a combination of CHOP chemotherapy and rituximab over sole CHOP treatment has been suggested[181] but prospective multicenter studies are required in order to define the role of radiation therapy in patients treated with R-CHOP.

Primary lymphoma of the lung

While lung is frequently involved by disseminated lymphoma, isolated pulmonary lymphoma is rare, accounting for less than 1 percent of all extranodal localized disease. The peak incidence is in the sixth decade of life, with a slight predominance in men. The prognosis of most primary pulmonary lymphomas is favorable in comparison with other lung tumors and does not depend on disease resectability. Therefore it is important that clinicians and pathologists consider the possibility in the diagnostic workup of any new pulmonary tumor in order to avoid unnecessary invasive procedures. Primary NHL of the lung is a heterogeneous disease. A variety of histologic subtypes have been reported including B and T cell lymphomas. Most cases appear to derive from acquired MALT lymphoma developed in the lung as a consequence of chronic inflammatory conditions. They are relatively rare, but the diagnostic procedure of lung opacities should take them into account because their management is different from lung cancer. Histology is the main prognostic factor that directs the treatment choice. Difficulties with safe delivery of irradiation to the lungs often lead to individualized therapy. Treatment of the aggressive subtypes must be based on aggressive chemotherapy (plus rituximab for large B cell tumors). There are several therapeutic options for the management of MALT lymphomas, including single-agent chemotherapy, anti-CD20 antibodies, radiation therapy, and surgery, with no data from randomized studies to help the decision.[187]

Lymphomas arising from the thymus

The inclusion of mediastinal lymphomas in the group of extranodal lymphomas is clearly arguable. Nevertheless, primary mediastinal large B cell lymphoma with sclerosis may derive from a special thymic medullary B cell population. This view is based mainly on the location and on the frequent persistence of thymic epithelial structure. It should not be surprising that the major organ of T cell development may be the site of a B cell lymphoma, since recent evidence has shown the presence of a significant B cell population in the thymus.[2] The WHO classification of tumors of the hematopoietic and lymphoid systems recognizes primary mediastinal B cell lymphoma (PMBL) as a distinct entity.[18] It comprises less than 5 percent of all lymphomas and tends to occur in a younger population than the other diffuse large B cell lymphomas. The median age

at diagnosis is 30 years and the disease shows a (slight) preponderance among females. It is characterized clinically by a rapidly progressive anterior mediastinal mass, often with local invasion and compressive syndromes, and unusual extranodal sites of spread, such as the liver, kidneys, and CNS, among those for whom initial therapy is not successful.[188] Involvement of the bone marrow is unusual. The outcomes of therapy for patients with PMBL are probably better than those seen in the rest of the diffuse large B cell lymphomas, partly as a result of their younger age and earlier stage at presentation. Previous series of PMBL reported long-term progression-free survival rates which ranged from 38 percent to 88 percent.[188] In the IELSG study of 426 patients, the largest study reported to date, the 10-year progression-free survival was projected as 62 percent with overall survival 65 percent.[189] The optimum chemotherapy schedule is unclear; the retrospective IELSG study suggested that outcomes were better in patients treated with more intensive chemotherapy regimens in comparison with conventional CHOP.[189] The role of mediastinal radiation therapy is controversial. Retrospective series suggest that the best outcomes are seen where consolidation radiation therapy is given to the mediastinum, particularly in patients with a residual tumor at the completion of chemotherapy.[189] In addition, very few cases of primary MALT lymphoma have been reported in the thymus, some of them preceded by a history of Sjögren syndrome.[2]

Other uncommon primary extranodal sites

SEROUS CAVITY LYMPHOMAS

Serous cavities can represent sites of disease spread in a number of different histologic subtypes of primary nodal and extranodal non-Hodgkin lymphomas. Primary effusion lymphoma (PEL) is a rare entity, accounting for about 3 percent of all aggressive non-Hodgkin lymphomas and is recognized as a distinct disease entity in the WHO classification of lymphoid neoplasms.[190]

Human herpesvirus 8 (HHV-8) infection of the tumor clone is considered a condition *sine qua non* for PEL diagnosis with a critical role in its pathogenesis. A liquid growth in fluid-filled body spaces represents a unique feature of this entity, which is characterized by a close link with underlying immunodeficiency status: it is related to HIV infection, post-transplant immunosuppression, or older age. Primary effusion lymphoma has both anaplastic and immunoblastic morphologic features and a non-B non-T phenotype with aspects of plasma cell differentiation. In most series, a poor prognosis with median overall survival of 6 months is reported.[191,192] Anthracycline-containing chemotherapy produces unsatisfactory results. Interesting data relate to the antilymphoma activity of HAART-induced immunologic reconstitution in HIV-positive patients and antilymphoma activity of cidofovir, an antiviral therapy directed against HHV-8 infection.[190–193]

Pyothorax-associated lymphoma represents an EBV-positive B cell lymphoma, nearly always related to an iatrogenic pneumothorax or a tuberculous pleuritis. Pyothorax-associated lymphoma consistently presents with a tumor mass localized in the body cavities and only rarely gives rise to a lymphomatous effusion.[194]

INTRAVASCULAR (ANGIOTROPIC) LYMPHOMA

Primary intravascular lymphoma is a rare disease and a large number of cases reported postmortem attests the difficulty in obtaining the correct diagnosis.[195] Most cases are of diffuse large B cell type but there are a few with T cell phenotype. Neoplastic cells typically grow trapped within small arteries, veins, and capillaries and only rarely extravasate.[196] It is an aggressive and usually disseminated disease that predominantly affects elderly patients. Most patients have impaired performance status, high LDH levels, and B symptoms. Anemia is also common at presentation.[197] Presenting clinical features are varied, often comprising bizarre neurological symptoms and nonspecific cutaneous manifestations. In a retrospective international series of 38 patients, brain and skin were the most common sites of disease. In contrast to previous reports, hepatosplenic involvement and bone marrow infiltration were found to be quite common, while nodal disease was confirmed as rare.[197] Anthracycline-based chemotherapy is the standard treatment for intravascular lymphoma; however, survival is disappointing (about 30 percent at 3 years). Addition of rituximab appears to offer a relevant clinical benefit.[198,199] Chemotherapy combinations containing drugs with high CNS bioavailability are needed in cases with brain involvement.[200] Patients with disease limited to the skin ('cutaneous variant'; approximately one quarter of cases) are most frequently females and seem to have a significantly better outcome.[197]

PRIMARY LYMPHOMA OF THE LIVER AND SPLEEN

Liver involvement by lymphoma is relatively common and usually indicates advanced disease. However, primary lymphoma of the liver is exceedingly rare.[201] A possible pathogenetic role of hepatitis viruses has been proposed. Primary liver lymphoma typically occurs in the fifth decade of life with a male predominance. The majority of cases have diffuse large B cell histologies but peripheral T cell lymphomas and primary low-grade MALT lymphomas have also been reported. Presentation may mimic hepatocellular carcinoma since primary liver lymphoma may present as single or multiple masses or even as a diffuse infiltration that may manifest itself as various liver diseases, or very occasionally as fulminant hepatic failure. The disease is often associated with several poor-prognosis characteristics, i.e., advanced age, bulky disease, and aggressive histology.

The spleen is frequently involved by Hodgkin and non-Hodgkin lymphomas of nodal type and by acute and chronic leukemias during the course of these diseases. About 20 percent of nodal non-Hodgkin lymphomas show evidence of spleen involvement at presentation.[2] However, primary lymphomas of the spleen are quite uncommon. Most cases of primary splenic lymphoma have the characteristics of the so-called splenic marginal zone B cell lymphoma, which is described in another chapter of this book. Together with the liver, the spleen is the primary site of involvement of the rare hepatosplenic $\gamma\delta$ T cell lymphoma. This disease affects young patients who present with marked hepatosplenomegaly, commonly with bone marrow involvement and without lymphadenopathy or significant peripheral blood lymphocytosis. The clinical course is usually very aggressive, with a median survival of less than 1 year despite the possibility of an initial response to combination chemotherapy.[202,203]

PRIMARY CARDIAC LYMPHOMA

Primary malignant lymphomas of the heart are extremely rare in immunocompetent patients.[204] They account for about 1 percent of the primary cardiac tumors and less than 1 percent of the extranodal lymphomas.[205] These tumors present with a variety of clinical manifestations and very rarely are diagnosed antemortem.[2]

PRIMARY LYMPHOMAS OF THE PANCREAS, GALLBLADDER, AND BILIARY DUCTS

Primary pancreatic lymphoma accounts for less than 3 percent of all pancreatic tumors. It usually presents with symptoms and radiological findings similar to those of a carcinoma of the pancreatic head. Preoperative or intraoperative histologic or cytologic diagnosis should be obtained because there is no indication for radical surgery. Treatment is usually chemotherapy or combined modality therapy.[206–208] Primary malignant lymphoma of the gallbladder is exceedingly rare; fewer than 20 well-documented cases have been reported in the literature. The histology can be variable and occasional cases of MALT lymphomas have been reported.[209] The possible growth of malignant lymphoma in the biliary ducts has also been described.[210]

PRIMARY LYMPHOMA OF THE ESOPHAGUS

Although lymphoma may involve any part of the gastrointestinal tract, either primarily or secondarily, esophageal involvement is exceedingly rare. Clinical and endoscopic findings are unspecific and the diagnosis is generally biopsy related.[211] No exact therapeutic rules have been established but combined radiation therapy and chemotherapy seems advisable.

PRIMARY ADRENAL LYMPHOMA

Adrenal involvement in disseminated lymphoma is a relatively common occurrence; however, involvement of the adrenal glands as the sole manifestation of lymphoma is very rare. The true incidence of this neoplasm is not known.

Most of the cases appear to be of B cell origin with diffuse large cell histology. The disease is often bilateral. Patients are most commonly older men. The presenting symptoms are nonspecific and may be related to lymphoma or to an associated adrenal insufficiency, which may be a lethal complication. Long delays between the onset of symptoms and the diagnosis are frequent. In clinically silent cases, adrenal insufficiency may be latent and the disease is revealed as an adrenal mass incidentally discovered by diagnostic imaging. Unresolved therapeutic issues include the optimal chemotherapy regimen (with vs without monoclonal antibody), the role of bilateral adrenalectomy and/or adjuvant radiation therapy, and the need for CNS prophylaxis, given recent reports that raise the possibility of a high risk of parenchymal or meningeal relapse.[212]

PRIMARY LYMPHOMA OF SOFT TISSUES

Non-Hodgkin lymphomas, usually diffuse large B cell lymphoma, have been described in some soft tissues. This localization is very rare, however, with an incidence not exceeding 2 percent of all soft tissue tumors. In differential diagnosis, undifferentiated metastatic carcinomas and round-cell sarcomas have to be considered, and immunohistochemistry studies are often decisive for the final diagnosis.[2] Intermuscular tissue is the most common localization but primary skeletal muscle involvement is also well described.[213]

> ## KEY POINTS
>
> - The epidemiology of extranodal lymphomas.
> - The clinicopathologic distinctiveness of lymphomas primarily arising at extranodal sites.
> - General principles concerning the clinical management of extranodal lymphomas.
> - Detailed information on the specific clinical problems posed by the most common extranodal lymphomas.
> - Limited information on the less common presentations or on those already covered in detail in other chapters.

REFERENCES

● = Key primary paper
◆ = Major review article

1. Zucca E, Roggero E, Bertoni F, Cavalli F. Primary extranodal non-Hodgkin's lymphomas. Part 1: Gastrointestinal, cutaneous and genitourinary lymphomas. *Ann Oncol* 1997; **8**: 727–37.

2. Zucca E, Roggero E, Bertoni F *et al*. Primary extranodal non-Hodgkin's lymphomas. Part 2: Head and neck, central nervous system and other less common sites. *Ann Oncol* 1999; **10**: 1023–33.

3. Dawson IM, Cornes JS, Morson BC. Primary malignant lymphoid tumours of the intestinal tract. Report of 37 cases with a study of factors influencing prognosis. *Br J Surg* 1961; **49**: 80–9.

4. Lewin KJ, Ranchod M, Dorfman RF. Lymphomas of the gastrointestinal tract: a study of 117 cases presenting with gastrointestinal disease. *Cancer* 1978; **42**: 693–707.

●5. Herrmann R, Panahon AM, Barcos MP *et al*. Gastrointestinal involvement in non-Hodgkin's lymphoma. *Cancer* 1980; **46**: 215–22.

●6. d'Amore F, Christensen BE, Brincker H *et al*. Clinicopathological features and prognostic factors in extranodal non-Hodgkin lymphomas. Danish LYFO Study Group. *Eur J Cancer* 1991; **27**: 1201–8.

●7. Krol AD, le Cessie S, Snijder S *et al*. Primary extranodal non-Hodgkin's lymphoma (NHL): the impact of alternative definitions tested in the Comprehensive Cancer Centre West population-based NHL registry. *Ann Oncol* 2003; **14**: 131–9.

8. Devesa SS, Fears T. Non-Hodgkin's lymphoma time trends: United States and international data. *Cancer Res* 1992; **52**: 5432s–40s.

9. Chiu BC, Weisenburger DD. An update of the epidemiology of non-Hodgkin's lymphoma. *Clin Lymphoma* 2003; **4**: 161–8.

●10. Groves FD, Linet MS, Travis LB, Devesa SS. Cancer surveillance series: non-Hodgkin's lymphoma incidence by histologic subtype in the United States from 1978 through 1995. *J Natl Cancer Inst* 2000; **92**: 1240–51.

11. Haddadin WJ. Malignant lymphoma in Jordan: a retrospective analysis of 347 cases according to the World Health Organization classification. *Ann Saudi Med* 2005; **25**: 398–403.

12. Sukpanichnant S. Analysis of 1983 cases of malignant lymphoma in Thailand according to the World Health Organization classification. *Hum Pathol* 2004; **35**: 224–30.

13. Economopoulos T, Asprou N, Stathakis N *et al*. Primary extranodal non-Hodgkin's lymphoma in adults: clinicopathological and survival characteristics. *Leuk Lymphoma* 1996; **21**: 131–6.

14. Chang KC, Huang GC, Jones D *et al*. Distribution and prognosis of WHO lymphoma subtypes in Taiwan reveals a low incidence of germinal-center derived tumors. *Leuk Lymphoma* 2004; **45**: 1375–84.

15. Isikdogan A, Ayyildiz O, Buyukcelik A *et al*. Non-Hodgkin's lymphoma in southeast Turkey: clinicopathologic features of 490 cases. *Ann Hematol* 2004; **83**: 265–9.

16. Temmim L, Baker H, Amanguno H *et al*. Clinicopathological features of extranodal lymphomas: Kuwait experience. *Oncology* 2004; **67**: 382–9.

17. Harris NL, Jaffe ES, Stein H *et al*. A revised European-American classification of lymphoid neoplasms: a

proposal from the International Lymphoma Study Group. *Blood* 1994; **84**: 1361–92.

18. Jaffe ES, Harris NL, Stein H, Vardiman JW. (eds) *World Health Organization classification of tumours. Pathology and genetics of tumours of haematopoietic and lymphoid tissues.* Lyon: IARC Press, 2001.

19. Gospodarowicz MK, Ferry JA, Cavalli F. Unique aspects of primary extranodal lymphomas. In: Mauch PM, Armitage JO, Harris NL, Dalla-Favera R, Coiffier B. (eds) *Non-Hodgkin's lymphomas.* Philadelphia, PA: Lippincott Williams and Wilkins, 2003: 685–707.

●20. Dogan A, Du M, Koulis A *et al.* Expression of lymphocyte homing receptors and vascular addressins in low-grade gastric B-cell lymphomas of mucosa-associated lymphoid tissue. *Am J Pathol* 1997; **151**: 1361–9.

●21. Drillenburg P, van der Voort R, Koopman G *et al.* Preferential expression of the mucosal homing receptor integrin alpha 4 beta 7 in gastrointestinal non-Hodgkin's lymphomas. *Am J Pathol* 1997; **150**: 919–27.

22. Freeman C, Berg JW, Cutler SJ. Occurrence and prognosis of extranodal lymphomas. *Cancer* 1972; **29**: 252–60.

23. Sutcliffe SB, Gospodarowicz MK. Localized extranodal lymphomas In: Keating A, Armitage J, Burnett A, Newland A. (eds) *Hematological oncology.* Cambridge: Cambridge University Press, 1992: 189–222.

24. Shenkier TN, Connors JM. Primary extranodal non-Hodgkin's lymphomas In: Canellos GP, Lister TA, Young BD. (eds) *The lymphomas,* 2nd Edn. Philadelphia, PA: Saunders Elsevier, 2006: 325–47.

●25. Lopez-Guillermo A, Colomo L, Jimenez M *et al.* Diffuse large B-cell lymphoma: clinical and biological characterization and outcome according to the nodal or extranodal primary origin. *J Clin Oncol* 2005; **23**: 2797–804.

26. Otter R, Gerrits WB, vd Sandt MM *et al.* Primary extranodal and nodal non-Hodgkin's lymphoma. A survey of a population-based registry. *Eur J Cancer Clin Oncol* 1989; **25**: 1203–10.

27. Hegde U, Filie A, Little RF *et al.* High incidence of occult leptomeningeal disease detected by flow cytometry in newly diagnosed aggressive B-cell lymphomas at risk for central nervous system involvement: the role of flow cytometry versus cytology. *Blood* 2005; **105**: 496–502.

●28. Rohatiner A, d'Amore F, Coiffier B *et al.* Report on a workshop convened to discuss the pathological and staging classifications of gastrointestinal tract lymphoma. *Ann Oncol* 1994; **5**: 397–400.

29. Batchelor T, Loeffler JS. Primary CNS lymphoma. *J Clin Oncol* 2006; **24**: 1281–8.

●30. Zucca E, Conconi A, Mughal TI *et al.* Patterns of outcome and prognostic factors in primary large-cell lymphoma of the testis in a survey by the International Extranodal Lymphoma Study Group. *J Clin Oncol* 2003; **21**: 20–27.

●31. Tsang RW, Gospodarowicz MK, O'Sullivan B. Staging and management of localized non-Hodgkin's lymphomas: variations among experts in radiation oncology. *Int J Radiat Oncol Biol Phys* 2002; **52**: 643–51.

32. Shenkier TN, Voss N, Fairey R *et al.* Brief chemotherapy and involved-region irradiation for limited-stage diffuse large-cell lymphoma: an 18-year experience from the British Columbia Cancer Agency. *J Clin Oncol* 2002; **20**: 197–204.

33. Gospodarowicz MK, Sutcliffe SB, Brown TC *et al.* Patterns of disease in localized extranodal lymphomas. *J Clin Oncol* 1987; **5**: 875–80.

34. Aref A, Yudelev M, Mohammad R *et al.* Neutron and photon clonogenic survival curves of two chemotherapy resistant human intermediate-grade non-Hodgkin lymphoma cell lines. *Int J Radiat Oncol Biol Phys* 1999; **45**: 999–1003.

●◆35. Tsang RW, Gospodarowicz MK. Radiation therapy for localized low-grade non-Hodgkin's lymphomas. *Hematol Oncol* 2005; **23**: 10–17.

●36. Cheson BD, Pfistner B, Juweid ME *et al.* Revised response criteria for malignant lymphoma. *J Clin Oncol* 2007; **25**: 579–86.

37. Otter R, Willemze R. Extranodal non-Hodgkin's lymphoma. *Neth J Med* 1988; **33**: 49–51.

38. d'Amore F, Brincker M, Gronbaek K *et al.* Non-Hodgkin's lymphoma of the gastrointestinal tract: a population-based analysis of incidence, geographic distribution, clinicopathologic presentation features, and prognosis. *J Clin Oncol* 1994; **12**: 1673–84.

39. Hockey MS, Powell J, Crocker J, Fielding JW. Primary gastric lymphoma. *Br J Surg* 1987; **74**: 483–7.

●40. Koch P, del Valle F, Berdel WE *et al.* Primary gastrointestinal non-Hodgkin's lymphoma: I. anatomic and histologic distribution, clinical features, and survival data of 371 patients registered in the German multicenter study GIT NHL 01/92. *J Clin Oncol* 2001; **19**: 3861–73.

41. Doglioni C, Wotherspoon AC, Moschini A *et al.* High incidence of primary gastric lymphoma in northeastern Italy. *Lancet* 1992; **339**: 834–5.

●42. Catassi C, Bearzi I, Holmes GK. Association of celiac disease and intestinal lymphomas and other cancers. *Gastroenterology* 2005; **128**: S79–86.

43. Smedby KE, Akerman M, Hildebrand H *et al.* Malignant lymphomas in coeliac disease: evidence of increased risks for lymphoma types other than enteropathy-type T cell lymphoma. *Gut* 2005; **54**: 54–9.

44. Krol AD, Hermans J, Kramer MH *et al.* Gastric lymphomas compared with lymph node lymphomas in a population-based registry differ in stage distribution and dissemination patterns but not in patient survival. *Cancer* 1997; **79**: 390–97.

45. Zucca E, Cavalli F. Gut lymphomas. *Baillieres Clin Haematol* 1996; **9**: 727–41.

46. Raderer M, Vorbeck F, Formanek M *et al.* Importance of extensive staging in patients with mucosa-associated lymphoid tissue (MALT)-type lymphoma. *Br J Cancer* 2000; **83**: 454–7.

47. Radaszkiewicz T, Dragosics B, Bauer P. Gastrointestinal malignant lymphomas of the mucosa-associated

lymphoid tissue: factors relevant to prognosis. *Gastroenterology* 1992; **102**: 1628–38.

●48. Koch P, del Valle F, Berdel WE *et al.* Primary gastrointestinal non-Hodgkin's lymphoma: II. Combined surgical and conservative or conservative management only in localized gastric lymphoma – results of the prospective German multicenter study GIT NHL 01/92. *J Clin Oncol* 2001; **19**: 3874–83.

●49. Cogliatti SB, Schmid U, Schumacher U *et al.* Primary B-cell gastric lymphoma: a clinicopathological study of 145 patients. *Gastroenterology* 1991; **101**: 1159–70.

●50. Ruskone-Fourmestraux A, Dragosics B, Morgner A *et al.* Paris staging system for primary gastrointestinal lymphomas. *Gut* 2003; **52**: 912–3.

51. de Jong D, Aleman BM, Taal BG, Boot H. Controversies and consensus in the diagnosis, work-up and treatment of gastric lymphoma: an international survey. *Ann Oncol* 1999; **10**: 275–80.

52. Eidt S, Stolte M, Fischer R. Factors influencing lymph node infiltration in primary gastric malignant lymphoma of the mucosa-associated lymphoid tissue. *Pathol Res Pract* 1994; **190**: 1077–81.

53. Taal BG, Boot H, van Heerde P *et al.* Primary non-Hodgkin lymphoma of the stomach: endoscopic pattern and prognosis in low versus high grade malignancy in relation to the MALT concept. *Gut* 1996; **39**: 556–61.

●54. Nakamura S, Matsumoto T, Suekane H *et al.* Predictive value of endoscopic ultrasonography for regression of gastric low grade and high grade MALT lymphomas after eradication of *Helicobacter pylori*. *Gut* 2001; **48**: 454–60.

55. Caletti G, Zinzani PL, Fusaroli P *et al.* The importance of endoscopic ultrasonography in the management of low-grade gastric mucosa-associated lymphoid tissue lymphoma. *Aliment Pharmacol Ther* 2002; **16**: 1715–22.

56. Fischbach W, Goebeler-Kolve ME, Greiner A. Diagnostic accuracy of EUS in the local staging of primary gastric lymphoma: results of a prospective, multicenter study comparing EUS with histopathologic stage. *Gastrointest Endosc* 2002; **56**: 696–700.

57. Fusaroli P, Buscarini E, Peyre S *et al.* Interobserver agreement in staging gastric malt lymphoma by EUS. *Gastrointest Endosc* 2002; **55**: 662–8.

58. Sackmann M, Morgner A, Rudolph B *et al.* Regression of gastric MALT lymphoma after eradication of *Helicobacter pylori* is predicted by endosonographic staging. MALT Lymphoma Study Group. *Gastroenterology* 1997; **113**: 1087–90.

59. Steinbach G, Ford R, Glober G *et al.* Antibiotic treatment of gastric lymphoma of mucosa-associated lymphoid tissue. An uncontrolled trial. *Ann Intern Med* 1999; **131**: 88–95.

60. Ruskone-Fourmestraux A, Lavergne A, Aegerter PH *et al.* Predictive factors for regression of gastric MALT lymphoma after anti-*Helicobacter pylori* treatment. *Gut* 2001; **48**: 297–303.

◆61. Ferrucci PF, Zucca E. Primary gastric lymphoma pathogenesis and treatment: what has changed over the past 10 years? *Br J Haematol* 2007; **136**: 521–38.

62. Bertoni F, Sanna P, Tinguely M *et al.* Association of gastric and Waldeyer's ring lymphoma: a molecular study. *Hematol Oncol* 2000; **18**: 15–19.

63. Thirlby RC. Gastrointestinal lymphoma: a surgical perspective. *Oncology* 1993; **7**: 29–32.

64. Sano T. Treatment of primary gastric lymphoma: experience in the National Cancer Center Hospital, Tokyo. *Recent Results Cancer Res* 2000; **156**: 104–7.

65. Gospodarowicz MK, Bush RS, Brown TC, Chua T. Curability of gastrointestinal lymphoma with combined surgery and radiation. *Int J Radiat Oncol Biol Phys* 1983; **9**: 3–9.

66. Gospodarowicz MK, Sutcliffe SB, Clark RM *et al.* Outcome analysis of localized gastrointestinal lymphoma treated with surgery and postoperative irradiation. *Int J Radiat Oncol Biol Phys* 1990; **19**: 1351–5.

67. Gospodarowicz MK, Pintilie M, Tsang R *et al.* Primary gastric lymphoma: brief overview of the recent Princess Margaret Hospital experience. *Recent Results Cancer Res* 2000; **156**: 108–15.

68. Shepherd FA, Evans WK, Kutas G *et al.* Chemotherapy following surgery for stages IE and IIE non-Hodgkin's lymphoma of the gastrointestinal tract. *J Clin Oncol* 1988; **6**: 253–60.

69. Maor MH, Velasquez WS, Fuller LM, Silvermintz KB. Stomach conservation in stages IE and IIE gastric non-Hodgkin's lymphoma. *J Clin Oncol* 1990; **8**: 266–71.

●70. Salles G, Herbrecht R, Tilly H *et al.* Aggressive primary gastrointestinal lymphomas: review of 91 patients treated with the LNH-84 regimen. A study of the Groupe d'Etude des Lymphomes Agressifs. *Am J Med* 1991; **90**: 77–84.

71. Gobbi PG, Ghirardelli ML, Cavalli C *et al.* The role of surgery in the treatment of gastrointestinal lymphomas other than low-grade MALT lymphomas. *Haematologica* 2000; **85**: 372–80.

●72. Gobbi PG, Dionigi P, Barbieri F *et al.* The role of surgery in the multimodal treatment of primary gastric non-Hodgkin's lymphomas. A report of 76 cases and review of the literature. *Cancer* 1990; **65**: 2528–36.

73. Taal BG, Burgers JM, van Heerde P *et al.* The clinical spectrum and treatment of primary non-Hodgkin's lymphoma of the stomach. *Ann Oncol* 1993; **4**: 839–46.

74. Taal BG, Burgers JM. Primary non-Hodgkin's lymphoma of the stomach: endoscopic diagnosis and the role of surgery. *Scand J Gastroenterol* 1991; **188**: 33–7.

●75. Koch P, Probst A, Berdel WE *et al.* Treatment results in localized primary gastric lymphoma: data of patients registered within the German multicenter study (GIT NHL 02/96). *J Clin Oncol* 2005; **23**: 7050–9.

76. Ferreri AJ, Cordio S, Ponzoni M, Villa E. Non-surgical treatment with primary chemotherapy, with or without radiation therapy, of stage I-II high-grade gastric lymphoma. *Leuk Lymphoma* 1999; **33**: 531–41.

77.　Schmidt WP, Schmitz N, Sonnen R. Conservative management of gastric lymphoma: the treatment option of choice. *Leuk Lymphoma* 2004; **45**: 1847–52.

78.　Raderer M, Chott A, Drach J *et al.* Chemotherapy for management of localised high-grade gastric B-cell lymphoma: how much is necessary? *Ann Oncol* 2002; **13**: 1094–8.

79.　Aviles A, Nambo MJ, Neri N *et al.* The role of surgery in primary gastric lymphoma: results of a controlled clinical trial. *Ann Surg* 2004; **240**: 44–50.

80.　Yoon SS, Coit DG, Portlock CS, Karpeh MS. The diminishing role of surgery in the treatment of gastric lymphoma. *Ann Surg* 2004; **240**: 28–37.

81.　Tondini C, Balzarotti M, Santoro A *et al.* Initial chemotherapy for primary resectable large-cell lymphoma of the stomach. *Ann Oncol* 1997; **8**: 497–9.

82.　Ibrahim EM, Ezzat AA, Raja MA *et al.* Primary gastric non-Hodgkin's lymphoma: clinical features, management, and prognosis of 185 patients with diffuse large B-cell lymphoma. *Ann Oncol* 1999; **10**: 1441–9.

83.　Ibrahim EM, Ezzat AA, El-Weshi AN *et al.* Primary intestinal diffuse large B-cell non-Hodgkin's lymphoma: clinical features, management, and prognosis of 66 patients. *Ann Oncol* 2001; **12**: 53–8.

84.　Cortelazzo S, Rossi A, Roggero F *et al.* Stage-modified international prognostic index effectively predicts clinical outcome of localized primary gastric diffuse large B-cell lymphoma. International Extranodal Lymphoma Study Group (IELSG). *Ann Oncol* 1999; **10**: 1433–40.

85.　Cortelazzo S, Rossi A, Oldani E *et al.* The modified International Prognostic Index can predict the outcome of localized primary intestinal lymphoma of both extranodal marginal zone B-cell and diffuse large B-cell histologies. *Br J Haematol* 2002; **118**: 218–28.

86.　Chen LT, Lin JT, Tai JJ *et al.* Long-term results of anti-*Helicobacter pylori* therapy in early-stage gastric high-grade transformed MALT lymphoma. *J Natl Cancer Inst* 2005; **97**: 1345–53.

87.　Montalban C, Santon A, Boixeda D, Bellas C. Regression of gastric high grade mucosa associated lymphoid tissue (MALT) lymphoma after *Helicobacter pylori* eradication. *Gut* 2001; **49**: 584–7.

88.　Morgner A, Miehlke S, Fischbach W *et al.* Complete remission of primary high-grade B-cell gastric lymphoma after cure of *Helicobacter pylori* infection. *J Clin Oncol* 2001; **19**: 2041–8.

89.　Zucca E, Cavalli F. Are antibiotics the treatment of choice for gastric lymphoma? *Curr Hematol Rep* 2004; **3**: 11–16.

◆90.　Bertoni F, Zucca E. State-of-the-art therapeutics: marginal-zone lymphoma. *J Clin Oncol* 2005; **23**: 6415–20.

◆91.　Al-Saleem T, Al-Mondhiry H. Immunoproliferative small intestinal disease (IPSID): a model for mature B-cell neoplasms. *Blood* 2005; **105**: 2274–80.

●92.　Isaacson PG, Muller-Hermelink HK, Piris MA *et al.* Extranodal marginal zone B-cell lymphoma of mucosa-associated lymphoid tissue (MALT lymphoma). In: Jaffe ES, Harris NL, Stein H, Vardiman JW. (eds) *World Health Organization classification of tumours. Pathology and genetics of tumours of haematopoietic and lymphoid tissues.* Lyon: IARC Press, 2001: 157–60.

●93.　Lecuit M, Abachin E, Martin A *et al.* Immunoproliferative small intestinal disease associated with *Campylobacter jejuni. N Engl J Med* 2004; **350**: 239–48.

94.　Foss HD, Stein H. Pathology of intestinal lymphomas. *Recent Results Cancer Res* 2000; **156**: 33–41.

95.　Isaacson PG. Gastrointestinal lymphomas of T- and B-cell types. *Mod Pathol* 1999; **12**: 151–8.

96.　Domizio P, Owen RA, Shepherd NA *et al.* Primary lymphoma of the small intestine: A clinicopathological study of 119 cases. *Am J Surg Pathol* 1993; **17**: 429–42.

97.　Hashimoto Y, Nakamura N, Kuze T *et al.* Multiple lymphomatous polyposis of the gastrointestinal tract is a heterogenous group that includes mantle cell lymphoma and follicular lymphoma: analysis of somatic mutation of immunoglobulin heavy chain gene variable region. *Hum Pathol* 1999; **30**: 581–7.

98.　Isaacson PG, Wright DH, Ralfkiaer E, Jaffe ES. Enteropathy-type T-cell lymphoma. In: Jaffe ES, Harris NL, Stein H, Vardiman JW. (eds) *World Health Organization classification of tumours. Pathology and genetics of tumours of haematopoietic and lymphoid tissues.* Lyon: IARC Press, 2001: 208–9.

99.　Howell WM, Leung ST, Jones DB *et al.* HLA-DRB, -DQA, and -DQB polymorphism in celiac disease and enteropathy-associated T-cell lymphoma. Common features and additional risk factors for malignancy. *Hum Immunol* 1995; **43**: 29–37.

◆100.　Ferry JA. Burkitt's lymphoma: clinicopathologic features and differential diagnosis. *Oncologist* 2006; **11**: 375–383.

101.　Ferry JA, Harris NL, Young RH *et al.* Malignant lymphoma of the testis, epididymis, and spermatic cord. A clinicopathologic study of 69 cases with immunophenotypic analysis. *Am J Surg Pathol* 1994; **18**: 376–90.

102.　Hyland J, Lasota J, Jasinski M *et al.* Molecular pathological analysis of testicular diffuse large cell lymphomas. *Hum Pathol* 1998; **29**: 1231–9.

103.　Horstmann WG, Timens W. Lack of adhesion molecules in testicular diffuse centroblastic and immunoblastic B cell lymphomas as a contributory factor in malignant behaviour. *Virchows Arch* 1996; **429**: 83–90.

104.　Jordanova ES, Riemersma SA, Philippo K *et al.* Hemizygous deletions in the HLA region account for loss of heterozygosity in the majority of diffuse large B-cell lymphomas of the testis and the central nervous system. *Genes Chromosomes Cancer* 2002; **35**: 38–48.

105.　Shahab N, Doll DC. Testicular lymphoma. *Semin Oncol* 1999; **26**: 259–69.

106.　Fonseca R, Habermann TM, Colgan JP *et al.* Testicular lymphoma is associated with a high incidence of extranodal recurrence. *Cancer* 2000; **88**: 154–61.

107.　Seymour JF, Solomon B, Wolf MM *et al.* Primary large-cell non-Hodgkin's lymphoma of the testis: a retrospective analysis of patterns of failure and prognostic factors. *Clin Lymphoma* 2001; **2**: 109–15.

108. Vitolo U, Zucca E, Martelli M *et al.* Primary diffuse large B-cell lymphoma of the testis (PTL): a prospective study of rituximab (R)-CHOP with CNS and contralateral testis prophylaxis. Results of the IELSG 10 study. *Blood* 2006; **108**: 65a (abstract 208).

109. Okuno SH, Hoyer JD, Ristow K, Witzig TE. Primary renal non-Hodgkin's lymphoma. An unusual extranodal site. *Cancer* 1995; **75**: 2258–61.

110. Kempton CL, Kurtin PJ, Inwards DJ *et al.* Malignant lymphoma of the bladder: evidence from 36 cases that low-grade lymphoma of the MALT-type is the most common primary bladder lymphoma. *Am J Surg Pathol* 1997; **21**: 1324–33.

111. Hughes M, Morrison A, Jackson R. Primary bladder lymphoma: management and outcome of 12 patients with a review of the literature. *Leuk Lymphoma* 2005; **46**: 873–7.

112. Bostwick DG, Iczkowski KA, Amin MB *et al.* Malignant lymphoma involving the prostate: report of 62 cases. *Cancer* 1998; **83**: 732–8.

113. Hofmockel G, Dammrich J, Manzanilla Garcia H *et al.* Primary non-Hodgkin's lymphoma of the male urethra. A case report and review of the literature. *Urol Int* 1995; **55**: 177–80.

114. Signorelli M, Maneo A, Cammarota S *et al.* Conservative management in primary genital lymphomas: the role of chemotherapy. *Gynecol Oncol* 2007; **104**: 416–21.

◆115. Kosari F, Daneshbod Y, Parwaresch R *et al.* Lymphomas of the female genital tract: a study of 186 cases and review of the literature. *Am J Surg Pathol* 2005; **29**: 1512–20.

116. Dimopoulos MA, Daliani D, Pugh W *et al.* Primary ovarian non-Hodgkin's lymphoma: outcome after treatment with combination chemotherapy. *Gynecol Oncol* 1997; **64**: 446–50.

117. Stroh EL, Besa PC, Cox JD *et al.* Treatment of patients with lymphomas of the uterus or cervix with combination chemotherapy and radiation therapy. *Cancer* 1995; **75**: 2392–9.

118. Isaacson PG, Norton AJ. *Extranodal lymphomas.* Edinburgh: Churchill Livingstone, 1994.

119. Ezzat AA, Ibrahim EM, El Weshi AN *et al.* Localized non-Hodgkin's lymphoma of Waldeyer's ring: clinical features, management, and prognosis of 130 adult patients. *Head Neck* 2001; **23**: 547–58.

120. Krol AD, Le Cessie S, Snijder S *et al.* Waldeyer's ring lymphomas: a clinical study from the Comprehensive Cancer Center West population based NHL registry. *Leuk Lymphoma* 2001; **42**: 1005–13.

121. Aviles A, Delgado S, Ruiz H *et al.* Treatment of non-Hodgkin's lymphoma of Waldeyer's ring: radiotherapy versus chemotherapy versus combined therapy. *Eur J Cancer B Oral Oncol* 1996; **32B**: 19–23.

122. Thieblemont C, Mayer A, Dumontet C *et al.* Primary thyroid lymphoma is a heterogeneous disease. *J Clin Endocrinol Metab* 2002; **87**: 105–11.

123. Skacel M, Ross CW, Hsi ED. A reassessment of primary thyroid lymphoma: high-grade MALT-type lymphoma as a distinct subtype of diffuse large B-cell lymphoma. *Histopathology* 2000; **37**: 10–18.

124. Doria R, Jekel JF, Cooper DL. Thyroid lymphoma. The case for combined modality therapy. *Cancer* 1994; **73**: 200–6.

●125. Tsang RW, Gospodarowicz MK, Pintilie M *et al.* Localized mucosa-associated lymphoid tissue lymphoma treated with radiation therapy has excellent clinical outcome. *J Clin Oncol* 2003; **21**: 4157–64.

●126. Zucca E, Conconi A, Pedrinis E *et al.* Nongastric marginal zone B-cell lymphoma of mucosa-associated lymphoid tissue. *Blood* 2003; **101**: 2489–95.

127. Ambrosetti A, Zanotti R, Pattaro C *et al.* Most cases of primary salivary mucosa-associated lymphoid tissue lymphoma are associated either with Sjoegren syndrome or hepatitis C virus infection. *Br J Haematol* 2004; **126**: 43–9.

128. Aviles A, Delgado S, Huerta-Guzman J. Marginal zone B cell lymphoma of the parotid glands: results of a randomised trial comparing radiotherapy to combined therapy. *Eur J Cancer B Oral Oncol* 1996; **32B**: 420–2.

129. Conconi A, Martinelli G, Thieblemont C *et al.* Clinical activity of rituximab in extranodal marginal zone B-cell lymphoma of MALT type. *Blood* 2003; **102**: 2741–5.

130. Coupland SE, Krause L, Delecluse HJ *et al.* Lymphoproliferative lesions of the ocular adnexa. Analysis of 112 cases. *Ophthalmology* 1998; **105**: 1430–41.

131. Bardenstein DS. Ocular adnexal lymphoma: classification, clinical disease, and molecular biology. *Ophthalmol Clin North Am* 2005; **18**: 187–97, x.

◆132. Ferreri AJM, Dolcetti R, Du MQ *et al.* Ocular adnexal MALT lymphoma: an intriguing model for antigen-driven lymphomagenesis and microbial-targeted therapy. *Ann Oncol* 2008; **19**: 835–46.

133. Lee SW, Suh CO, Kim GE *et al.* Role of radiotherapy for primary orbital lymphoma. *Am J Clin Oncol* 2002; **25**: 261–5.

134. Stafford SL, Kozelsky TF, Garrity JA *et al.* Orbital lymphoma: radiotherapy outcome and complications. *Radiother Oncol* 2001; **59**: 139–44.

135. Bessell EM, Henk JM, Whitelocke RA, Wright JE. Ocular morbidity after radiotherapy of orbital and conjunctival lymphoma. *Eye* 1987; **1**: 90–96.

●136. Ferreri AJ, Guidoboni M, Ponzoni M *et al.* Evidence for an association between *Chlamydia psittaci* and ocular adnexal lymphomas. *J Natl Cancer Inst* 2004; **96**: 586–94.

137. Moslehi R, Devesa SS, Schairer C, Fraumeni JF Jr. Rapidly increasing incidence of ocular non-Hodgkin lymphoma. *J Natl Cancer Inst* 2006; **98**: 936–9.

138. Zucca E, Bertoni F. Chlamydia or not Chlamydia, that is the question: which is the microorganism associated with MALT lymphomas of the ocular adnexa? *J Natl Cancer Inst* 2006; **98**: 1348–9.

139. Ferreri AJ, Ponzoni M, Guidoboni M *et al.* Bacteria-eradicating therapy with doxycycline in ocular adnexal MALT lymphoma: a multicenter prospective trial. *J Natl Cancer Inst* 2006; **98**: 1375–82.

140. Hatta C, Ogasawara H, Okita J et al. Non-Hodgkin's malignant lymphoma of the sinonasal tract – treatment outcome for 53 patients according to REAL classification. *Auris Nasus Larynx* 2001; **28**: 55–60.

141. Jaffe ES, Chan JK, Su IJ et al. Report of the workshop on nasal and related extranodal angiocentric T/natural killer cell lymphomas. Definitions, differential diagnosis, and epidemiology. *Am J Surg Pathol* 1996; **20**: 103–11.

142. Abbondanzo SL, Wenig BM. Non-Hodgkin's lymphoma of the sinonasal tract. A clinicopathologic and immunophenotypic study of 120 cases. *Cancer* 1995; **75**: 1281–91.

143. Chan JKC, Jaffe ES, Ralfkiaer E. Extranodal NK-/T-cell lymphoma, nasal type. In: Jaffe ES, Harris NL, Stein H, Vardiman JW. (eds) *World Health Organization classification of tumours. Pathology and genetics of tumours of haematopoietic and lymphoid tissues.* Lyon: IARC Press, 2001: 204–7.

144. Lee J, Park YH, Kim WS et al. Extranodal nasal type NK/T-cell lymphoma: elucidating clinical prognostic factors for risk-based stratification of therapy. *Eur J Cancer* 2005; **41**: 1402–8.

145. Logsdon MD, Ha CS, Kavadi VS et al. Lymphoma of the nasal cavity and paranasal sinuses: improved outcome and altered prognostic factors with combined modality therapy. *Cancer* 1997; **80**: 477–88.

146. Liang R, Todd D, Chan TK et al. Treatment outcome and prognostic factors for primary nasal lymphoma. *J Clin Oncol* 1995; **13**: 666–70.

147. Li YX, Coucke PA, Li JY et al. Primary non-Hodgkin's lymphoma of the nasal cavity: prognostic significance of paranasal extension and the role of radiotherapy and chemotherapy. *Cancer* 1998; **83**: 449–56.

148. Hausdorff J, Davis E, Long G et al. Non-Hodgkin's lymphoma of the paranasal sinuses: clinical and pathological features, and response to combined-modality therapy. *Cancer J Sci Am* 1997; **3**: 303–11.

149. Oprea C, Cainap C, Azoulay R et al. Primary diffuse large B-cell non-Hodgkin lymphoma of the paranasal sinuses: a report of 14 cases. *Br J Haematol* 2005; **131**: 468–71.

150. Laskin JJ, Savage KJ, Voss N et al. Primary paranasal sinus lymphoma: natural history and improved outcome with central nervous system chemoprophylaxis. *Leuk Lymphoma* 2005; **46**: 1721–7.

151. Au WY, Lie AK, Liang R et al. Autologous stem cell transplantation for nasal NK/T-cell lymphoma: a progress report on its value. *Ann Oncol* 2003; **14**: 1673–6.

152. Delecluse HJ, Anagnostopoulos I, Dallenbach F et al. Plasmablastic lymphomas of the oral cavity: a new entity associated with the human immunodeficiency virus infection. *Blood* 1997; **89**: 1413–20.

153. Colomo L, Loong F, Rives S et al. Diffuse large B-cell lymphomas with plasmablastic differentiation represent a heterogeneous group of disease entities. *Am J Surg Pathol* 2004; **28**: 736–47.

●154. Abrey LE, Batchelor TT, Ferreri AJ et al. Report of an international workshop to standardize baseline evaluation and response criteria for primary CNS lymphoma. *J Clin Oncol* 2005; **23**: 5034–43.

155. Ferreri AJ, Blay JY, Reni M et al. Prognostic scoring system for primary CNS lymphomas: the International Extranodal Lymphoma Study Group experience. *J Clin Oncol* 2003; **21**: 266–72.

156. Abrey LE, Ben-Porat L, Panageas KS et al. Primary central nervous system lymphoma: the Memorial Sloan-Kettering Cancer Center prognostic model. *J Clin Oncol* 2006; **24**: 5711–5.

157. Nelson DF, Martz KL, Bonner H et al. Non-Hodgkin's lymphoma of the brain: can high dose, large volume radiation therapy improve survival? Report on a prospective trial by the Radiation Therapy Oncology Group (RTOG): RTOG 8315. *Int J Radiat Oncol Biol Phys* 1992; **23**: 9–17.

158. Deangelis LM, Iwamoto FM. An update on therapy of primary central nervous system lymphoma. *Hematology Am Soc Hematol Educ Program* 2006: 311–16.

159. Ferreri AJ, Abrey LE, Blay JY et al. Summary statement on primary central nervous system lymphomas from the Eighth International Conference on Malignant Lymphoma, Lugano, Switzerland, June 12 to 15, 2002. *J Clin Oncol* 2003; **21**: 2407–14.

●160. Batchelor T, Carson K, O'Neill A et al. Treatment of primary CNS lymphoma with methotrexate and deferred radiotherapy: a report of NABTT 96–07. *J Clin Oncol* 2003; **21**: 1044–9.

161. Ferreri AJ, Reni M, Pasini F et al. A multicenter study of treatment of primary CNS lymphoma. *Neurology* 2002; **58**: 1513–20.

●162. Gavrilovic IT, Hormigo A, Yahalom J et al. Long-term follow-up of high-dose methotrexate-based therapy with and without whole brain irradiation for newly diagnosed primary CNS lymphoma. *J Clin Oncol* 2006; **24**: 4570–4.

163. Illerhaus G, Marks R, Ihorst G et al. High-dose chemotherapy with autologous stem-cell transplantation and hyperfractionated radiotherapy as first-line treatment of primary CNS lymphoma. *J Clin Oncol* 2006; **24**: 3865–70.

164. Colombat P, Lemevel A, Bertrand P et al. High-dose chemotherapy with autologous stem cell transplantation as first-line therapy for primary CNS lymphoma in patients younger than 60 years: a multicenter phase II study of the GOELAMS group. *Bone Marrow Transplant* 2006; **38**: 417–20.

●165. Hormigo A, Abrey L, Heinemann MH, DeAngelis LM. Ocular presentation of primary central nervous system lymphoma: diagnosis and treatment. *Br J Haematol* 2004; **126**: 202–8.

●166. Ferreri AJ, Blay JY, Reni M et al. Relevance of intraocular involvement in the management of primary central nervous system lymphomas. *Ann Oncol* 2002; **13**: 531–8.

♦167. Shenkier TN. Unusual variants of primary central nervous system lymphoma. *Hematol Oncol Clin North Am* 2005; **19**: 651–64, vi.

168. Rottnek M, Strauchen J, Moore F, Morgello S. Primary dural mucosa-associated lymphoid tissue-type

lymphoma: case report and review of the literature. *J Neurooncol* 2004; **68**: 19–23.

169. Lyons MK, O'Neill BP, Kurtin PJ, Marsh WR. Diagnosis and management of primary spinal epidural non-Hodgkin's lymphoma. *Mayo Clin Proc* 1996; **71**: 453–7.

170. Rathmell AJ, Gospodarowicz MK, Sutcliffe SB, Clark RM. Localized extradural lymphoma: survival, relapse pattern and functional outcome. The Princess Margaret Hospital Lymphoma Group. *Radiother Oncol* 1992; **24**: 14–20.

171. Monnard V, Sun A, Epelbaum R *et al*. Primary spinal epidural lymphoma: patients' profile, outcome, and prognostic factors: a multicenter Rare Cancer Network study. *Int J Radiat Oncol Biol Phys* 2006; **65**: 817–23.

●172. Willemze R, Jaffe ES, Burg G *et al*. WHO-EORTC classification for cutaneous lymphomas. *Blood* 2005; **105**: 3768–85.

173. Smith BD, Glusac EJ, McNiff JM *et al*. Primary cutaneous B-cell lymphoma treated with radiotherapy: a comparison of the European Organization for Research and Treatment of Cancer and the WHO classification systems. *J Clin Oncol* 2004; **22**: 634–9.

174. Grange F, Bekkenk MW, Wechsler J *et al*. Prognostic factors in primary cutaneous large B-cell lymphomas: a European multicenter study. *J Clin Oncol* 2001; **19**: 3602–10.

175. Hoefnagel JJ, Dijkman R, Basso K *et al*. Distinct types of primary cutaneous large B-cell lymphoma identified by gene expression profiling. *Blood* 2005; **105**: 3671–8.

176. Siegel RS, Pandolfino T, Guitart J *et al*. Primary cutaneous T-cell lymphoma: review and current concepts. *J Clin Oncol* 2000; **18**: 2908–25.

177. Rosen ST, Querfeld C. Primary cutaneous T-cell lymphomas. *Hematology Am Soc Hematol Educ Program* 2006: 323–30.

178. Roggero E, Zucca E, Mainetti C *et al*. Eradication of *Borrelia burgdorferi* infection in primary marginal zone B-cell lymphoma of the skin. *Hum Pathol* 2000; **31**: 263–8.

179. Aviles A, Delgado S, Nambo MJ *et al*. Primary breast lymphoma: results of a controlled clinical trial. *Oncology* 2005; **69**: 256–60.

●180. Ryan G, Martinelli G, Kuper-Hommel M *et al*. Primary diffuse large B-cell lymphoma of the breast: prognostic factors and outcomes of a study by the International Extranodal Lymphoma Study Group. *Ann Oncol* 2008; **19**: 233–41.

181. Ramadan KM, Shenkier T, Sehn LH *et al*. A clinicopathological retrospective study of 131 patients with primary bone lymphoma: a population-based study of successively treated cohorts from the British Columbia Cancer Agency. *Ann Oncol* 2007; **18**: 129–35.

182. Schaefer NG, Strobel K, Taverna C *et al*. Bone involvement in patients with lymphoma: the role of FDG-PET/CT. *Eur J Nucl Med Mol Imaging* 2007; **34**: 60–7.

183. Beal K, Allen L, Yahalom J. Primary bone lymphoma: treatment results and prognostic factors with long-term follow-up of 82 patients. *Cancer* 2006; **106**: 2652–6.

184. Zinzani PL, Carrillo G, Ascani S *et al*. Primary bone lymphoma: experience with 52 patients. *Haematologica* 2003; **88**: 280–5.

185. Christie DR, Barton MB, Bryant G *et al*. Osteolymphoma (primary bone lymphoma): an Australian review of 70 cases. Australasian Radiation Oncology Lymphoma Group (AROLG). *Aust N Z J Med* 1999; **29**: 214–9.

186. Fairbanks RK, Bonner JA, Inwards CY *et al*. Treatment of stage IE primary lymphoma of bone. *Int J Radiat Oncol Biol Phys* 1994; **28**: 363–72.

187. Wannesson L, Cavalli F, Zucca E. Primary pulmonary lymphoma: current status. *Clin Lymphoma Myeloma* 2005; **6**: 220–7.

188. van Besien K, Kelta M, Bahaguna P. Primary mediastinal B-cell lymphoma: a review of pathology and management. *J Clin Oncol* 2001; **19**: 1855–64.

189. Zinzani PL, Martelli M, Bertini M *et al*. Induction chemotherapy strategies for primary mediastinal large B-cell lymphoma with sclerosis: a retrospective multinational study on 426 previously untreated patients. *Haematologica* 2002; **87**: 1258–64.

190. Gaidano G, Carbone A. Primary effusion lymphoma: a liquid phase lymphoma of fluid-filled body cavities. *Adv Cancer Res* 2001; **80**: 115–46.

191. Conconi A, Spina M, Ascoli V *et al*. An IELSG International Survey of Primary Effusion Lymphoma (PEL). *Blood* 2004; **104**: Abstract 3265.

192. Boulanger E, Gerard L, Gabarre J *et al*. Prognostic factors and outcome of human herpesvirus 8-associated primary effusion lymphoma in patients with AIDS. *J Clin Oncol* 2005; **23**: 4372–80.

193. Luppi M, Trovato R, Barozzi P *et al*. Treatment of herpesvirus associated primary effusion lymphoma with intracavity cidofovir. *Leukemia* 2005; **19**: 473–6.

194. Nakatsuka S, Yao M, Hoshida Y *et al*. Pyothorax-associated lymphoma: a review of 106 cases. *J Clin Oncol* 2002; **20**: 4255–60.

195. Sanna P, Bertoni F, Roggero E *et al*. Angiotropic (intravascular) large cell lymphoma: case report and short discussion of the literature. *Tumori* 1997; **83**: 772–5.

196. Ponzoni M, Ferreri AJ. Intravascular lymphoma: a neoplasm of 'homeless' lymphocytes? *Hematol Oncol* 2006; **24**: 105–12.

●197. Ferreri AJ, Campo E, Seymour JF *et al*. Intravascular lymphoma: clinical presentation, natural history, management and prognostic factors in a series of 38 cases, with special emphasis on the 'cutaneous variant'. *Br J Haematol* 2004; **127**: 173–83.

198. Shimada K, Matsue K, Yamamoto K *et al*. Retrospective analysis of intravascular large B-cell lymphoma treated with rituximab-containing chemotherapy as reported by the IVL study group in Japan. *J Clin Oncol* 2008; **26**: 3189–95.

199. Ferreri AJ, Dognini GP, Bairey O. The addition of rituximab to anthracycline-based chemotherapy significantly improves outcome in 'Western' patients with intravascular

large B-cell lymphoma. *Br J Haematol* 2008 Aug 10 [Epub ahead of print].

200. Ferreri AJ, Campo E, Ambrosetti A *et al*. Anthracycline-based chemotherapy as primary treatment for intravascular lymphoma. *Ann Oncol* 2004; **15**: 1215–21.

201. Salmon JS, Thompson MA, Arildsen RC, Greer JP. Non-Hodgkin's lymphoma involving the liver: clinical and therapeutic considerations. *Clin Lymphoma Myeloma* 2006; **6**: 273–80.

202. Belhadj K, Reyes F, Farcet JP *et al*. Hepatosplenic gammadelta T-cell lymphoma is a rare clinicopathologic entity with poor outcome: report on a series of 21 patients. *Blood* 2003; **102**: 4261–9.

203. Armitage JO, Liang RHS, Sweetenham JW *et al*. Mature nodal and extranodal T-cell and Non-Hodgkin-Cell Lymphomas (Peripheral T-cell, Angioimmunoblastic, Nasal Natural Killer/T-cell, Hepatosplenic T-cell, Enteropathy-Type T-cell, and Subcutaneous Panniculitis-Like T-cell lymphomas) In: Mauch PM, Armitage J, Coiffier B *et al*. (eds) *Non-Hodgkin's lymphomas*. Philadelphia, PA: Lippincott Williams and Wilkins, 2004: 405–26.

204. Sanna P, Bertoni F, Zucca E *et al*. Cardiac involvement in HIV-related non-Hodgkin's lymphoma: a case report and short review of the literature. *Ann Hematol* 1998; **77**: 75–8.

205. Gowda RM, Khan IA. Clinical perspectives of primary cardiac lymphoma. *Angiology* 2003; **54**: 599–604.

206. Saif MW. Primary pancreatic lymphomas. *JOP* 2006; **7**: 262–73.

207. Nishimura R, Takakuwa T, Hoshida Y *et al*. Primary pancreatic lymphoma: clinicopathological analysis of 19 cases from Japan and review of the literature. *Oncology* 2001; **60**: 322–9.

208. Arcari A, Anselmi E, Bernuzzi P *et al*. Primary pancreatic lymphoma. A report of five cases. *Haematologica* 2005; **90**: ECR09.

209. Jelic TM, Barreta TM, Yu M *et al*. Primary, extranodal, follicular non-Hodgkin lymphoma of the gallbladder: case report and a review of the literature. *Leuk Lymphoma* 2004; **45**: 381–7.

210. Chiu KW, Changchien CS, Chen L et al. Primary malignant lymphoma of common bile duct presenting as acute obstructive jaundice: report of a case. *J Clin Gastroenterol* 1995; **20**: 259–61.

211. Gupta NM, Goenka MK, Jindal A *et al*. Primary lymphoma of the esophagus. *J Clin Gastroenterol* 1996; **23**: 203–6.

212. Grigg AP, Connors JM. Primary adrenal lymphoma. *Clin Lymphoma* 2003; **4**: 154–60.

213. Gill SI, Gibbs SD, Hicks RJ, Seymour JF. Primary skeletal muscle marginal zone lymphoma with persistent tissue tropism and PET-avidity. *Leuk Lymphoma* 2006; **47**: 117–20.

214. Daum S, Ullrich R, Heise W *et al*. Intestinal non-Hodgkin's lymphoma: a multicenter prospective clinical study from the German Study Group on Intestinal non-Hodgkin's Lymphoma. *J Clin Oncol* 2003; **21**: 2740–6.

215. Cortelazzo s, Rossi A, Federico M *et al*. The Stage-Modified IPI (MIPI), histology and a combined treatment influence the clinical outcome of 401 patients with primary extranodal head and neck B-cell lymphomas (PHNBCL) (IELSG 23). *Blood* 2005; **106**: Abstract 927.

216. Dragosics B, Bauer P, Radaszkiewicz T. Primary gastrointestinal non-Hodgkin's lymphomas. A retrospective clinicopathologic study of 150 cases. *Cancer* 1985; **55**: 1060–73.

217. Liang R, Todd D, Chan TK *et al*. Prognostic factors for primary gastrointestinal lymphoma. *Hematol Oncol* 1995; **13**: 153–63.

218. Tondini C, Giardini R, Bozzetti F *et al*. Combined modality treatment for primary gastrointestinal non-Hodgkin's lymphoma: the Milan Cancer Institute experience. *Ann Oncol* 1993; **4**: 831–7.

•219. Nakamura S, Matsumoto T, Iida M *et al*. Primary gastrointestinal lymphoma in Japan: a clinicopathologic analysis of 455 patients with special reference to its time trends. *Cancer* 2003; **97**: 2462–73.

220. Amer MH, el-Akkad S. Gastrointestinal lymphoma in adults: clinical features and management of 300 cases. *Gastroenterology* 1994; **106**: 846–58.

221. Morton JE, Leyland MJ, Vaughan Hudson G *et al*. Primary gastrointestinal non-Hodgkin's lymphoma: a review of 175 British National Lymphoma Investigation cases. *Br J Cancer* 1993; **67**: 776–82.

222. List AF, Greer JP, Cousar JC *et al*. Non-Hodgkin's lymphoma of the gastrointestinal tract: an analysis of clinical and pathologic features affecting outcome. *J Clin Oncol* 1988; **6**: 1125–33.

60

Special aspects of management of lymphomas in developing countries

REETU JAIN AND SH ADVANI

INTRODUCTION

Medical oncology is witnessing an exciting era in terms of better understanding of biology of disease process at the molecular level, improved diagnostics, and better treatment strategies, including biological therapies. This has translated to better quality of life and improved survival. However, there is a vast discrepancy in the overall patient survival in the developed nations as against the developing ones.

Despite a lower cancer incidence, developing countries bear more than half of the global cancer burden because 75 percent of the world population lives in these countries.[1] Due to population overgrowth, aging, urbanization, changing dietary habits, better control of infections, and increased tobacco consumption, developing countries are anticipated to bear even greater cancer burden, including lympho-hemopoietic malignancies.[2]

The discrepancy in survival rates in the developing nations can be attributed to the following:

1. Epidemiologic differences (race or geography)
2. Patterns of presentation

3. Childhood variations
4. Presence of retroviral or other infections
5. Management programs
6. Limitations of human, physical, and financial resources
7. Limitations in supportive care, comorbidities (hepatitis, malnutrition)
8. Abandonment of therapy and lost to follow-up

Key points are **developing nations**, **resources**, **epidemiology**, **biology**, and **infection**.

MAGNITUDE OF PROBLEM

Epidemiologic differences

There are notable differences in the demography between populations. Published data from the developed world for Hodgkin lymphoma (HL) show little variation when geographic areas are compared. There are two well-defined age peaks in the United States and in other developed countries – the first at 25 years and the other at 70 years[4–6] – while in India the peak is in the first and second decade of life.[7,8] The early peak in Indians may reflect exposure to infections in early childhood. Incidence rates are highest in whites, followed by blacks and Hispanics, and lower in Asians. Acute leukemias are the tenth commonest cancer in men and twelfth in women and constitute 3 percent of the total global cancer burden.[10] North America, Australia, and New Zealand have the highest incidence of leukemias, while sub-Saharan Africa has the lowest.[10]

Lymphoid leukemias have the highest incidence in Canada-Yukon (males 9.6/100 000, females 11.1/100 000), whereas New Zealand Maoris (males 6.7/100 000, females 4.5/100 000) have the highest incidence for myeloid leukemia.[10] In India, in rural areas (Barshi) the incidence for myeloid leukemia is 0.8/100 000, while in urban areas (Delhi) it has been reported to be as high as 5/100 000.[11] Non-Hodgkin lymphoma (NHL) accounts for 5 percent of new cancer in men and 4 percent in women each year in the USA. The US annual age-adjusted rate (AAR) was 15.5 per 100 000 in 1996.[12] The highest incidence of NHL is reported in the USA, Europe, and Australia and the lowest from Asia.[13]

For multiple myeloma, the annual AAR from the USA is 4.8 and 3.3 per 100 000 per year for males and females, respectively.[13] It is lower in Africans and Caucasians,[9] and in India it is reported as 1.9 and 1.3 per 100 000 for males and females, respectively.

The annual incidence of chronic myeloid leukemia (CML) in the USA is about 1–2 per 100 000 population and it accounts for 7–15 percent of adult leukemias.[14,15] However, data from hospital-based studies from different parts of India indicate that CML constitutes 30–50 percent of all cases of leukemia in adults.[16–18] From the five population-based registries in India, the incidence of CML varies from 0.8 to 2.2 per 100 000 population in males and 0.6 to 1.6 per 100 000 population in females.[11] A similar pattern has been observed in China, Singapore, and Japan.[19]

Similar observations have been made for chronic lymphocytic leukemia (CLL). Western countries have reported CLL as the commonest form of leukemia in adults. In the USA, CLL accounts for about 30 percent of all cases whereas it is infrequently observed in Japan, China, and other Asian countries. In India, the incidence reported is 1.95–8.8 percent and the median age at presentation is 55 years, a decade earlier in contrast to Western countries.[20] Lower incidence of CLL may not be due entirely to lower life expectancy in India and other developing countries as incidence of CLL is also lower in Japan, where life expectancy is the highest.

The pattern of cancer in developing countries differs from that in richer countries. Diego Serraino, an epidemiologist from the Italian National Institute for Infectious Diseases, says that this variation makes it all the more important to collect information about cancer incidence and cancer mortality. In the Nordic countries, population-based cancer registries cover almost 100 percent of the population. In Italy the figure is 20 percent. In Africa,

registries cover less than 5 percent of the population and there are not even accurate data on cancer deaths. Thus '**cancer registration in developing countries is a public health priority.**' The eighth edition of *Cancer Incidence in Five Continents*, published in 2002 by the International Agency for Research on Cancer, reflects this weakness. It has data from North America and from 27 European countries, but only from 14 countries in Central and South America, 12 in Asia, and just nine in Africa.

Thus epidemiologic differences do exist pertaining to race and geographic region in the different parts of the world. The epidemiologic data are not comparable (if environmental factors are not considered) to the incidences as reported by the West. This can be attributed to various factors; for example, a lack of cancer-based registries and trained personnel, a lesser number of epidemiologists, delay in seeking medical attention, underreporting, and lack of uniform reporting policies. For example, in India (which has 16 percent of the world's total population), under the national cancer control program there are only 17 regional cancer centers.[21] Population-based and hospital-based cancer registries cover only 0.3 percent of the total Indian population. Population-based data on the incidence on hematolymphoid malignancies and other cancers in the developing world are neither consistently available nor reliable due to under registration and absence of organized cancer registries.[22]

Patterns of presentation of differences in the biology of the disease

Patients in the underdeveloped nations access health care late. Differences in biology of the disease have been observed which can influence both disease stage and treatment outcome. In Hodgkin lymphoma, groups from India have reported as many as 65 percent of patients presenting at advanced stage, 42–73 percent having B symptoms, with mixed cellularity (MC) as the commonest histologic subtype (50–70 percent).[8,23,24] Studies from Asia, Africa, and South America have also shown MC as the predominant histologic subtype[25–27] whereas data from the West report nodular sclerosis (NS) and lymphocyte predominant (LP) as the commonest subtypes, MC constituting 15–30 percent of cases.[5,28] Why this predominance of MC in developing countries occurs is not clear. One possible explanation is that viral illness in early life may predispose individuals. Epstein–Barr virus (EBV) is the leading viral candidate for Hodgkin lymphoma causation;[29] EBV positivity rate is lower in the NS subtype (15–30 percent) and higher in the MC subtype (60–70 percent).[30]

The association of EBV with HL in developing countries is 70–100 percent whereas in developed countries it is 30–50 percent; in an oriental population from China and Hong Kong, the association was intermediate (65 percent).[31] Patients with MC histology tend to have advanced stage disease.[8]

Thus poor prognostic histology and advanced stage at presentation seems to be a feature of HL in developing nations. This probably results in lower overall survival rate. In the West, reported 5-year survival rate in early stage disease is 90 percent.[32] However, in Eastern European countries it is 45 percent[13] (for patients diagnosed over 65 years of age). In India, the 7-year event-free and actual survival rates were reported in 1996 as 73 percent and 64 percent, respectively;[7] essentially similar data were reported from the same institution a decade later.[33]

The US annual AAR for NHL was 19 per 100 000 population in 2001[34] and 56 390 NHL cases were estimated to be diagnosed in the USA in 2005.[35] Internationally, NHL incidence rates vary from eight- to ten-fold[36,37] with higher rates observed in Western countries. Rates are high in North America, Australia, Italy, and Switzerland, and lower in Asian countries.[10,13] Rates in South America are intermediate between those in Asia and North America.[38] In children, high incidence rates have been noted in Egypt, among non-Kuwaitis in Kuwait, in Portugal, in Spain, and among US blacks.[39] Excluding Burkitt lymphoma, the NHL pattern mirrors that for HL: lowest in Asian countries, intermediate in developed countries of North America and Europe, and highest in developing countries in Latin America and the Middle East.

Geographic variations in histologic subtypes

Examples of geographic variation include higher rates of gastric lymphoma in northern Italy, endemic form of Burkitt lymphoma in children in the Middle East, and adult T cell leukemia/lymphoma (ATLL) in southern Japan and the Caribbean.[40] Similar observations have been made for leukemias. The incidences of leukemia are highest in North America and Australia/New Zealand and lowest in sub-Saharan Africa. Ramot and Magrath[41] reported predominance of T cell subtype in economically underprivileged nations and incidence of common acute lymphoblastic leukemia antigen (C-ALL; CD10 positive) increasing with prosperity and industrialization of nations. In underdeveloped countries like Nigeria, Kenya, Israel (Tel Aviv), and South Africa, the incidence of C-ALL is relatively low, while developed nations like the UK, USA, and Japan have reported increases in C-ALL in the years corresponding to industrialization of these nations. India, at an intermediate stage of development, has shown an increase in C-ALL despite T cell acute lymphoblastic leukemia (T-ALL) incidence remaining high.[42] Advani and colleagues[43] reported frequencies of C-ALL and T-ALL as 31 percent and 33 percent, respectively, whereas a later study by the same group showed figures of 68.6 percent and 20.7 percent, respectively, indicating a trend of increasing C-ALL.[44] In the same study, this group reported presence of lymphadenopathy as the most significant risk factor associated with a worse event-free survival (53 percent vs 77 percent).[43]

While environmental factors may be responsible for the variability in ALL subtypes, genetic alterations influence the susceptibility of the leukemic cell population to drugs. In a study from India, T cell receptor β gene rearrangement was seen in 58 percent of children with B-ALL,[45] 45 percent higher than the 15–29 percent reported from the USA[46] but closer to the 40 percent reported from Egypt.[47] T cell receptor β gene rearrangement is associated with a higher mean age at presentation, lower mean platelet count, and poorer disease-free survival (DFS). *TEL-AML1* translocation, which is seen in 25 percent of patients from the West and is associated with better outcome, occurs less frequently in Indian patients.[48]

Thus differences in environment and lifestyle, as well as potential genetic differences, influence not only the incidence of ALL, but also its biology. Such differences in biology can influence both disease extent and ultimately the treatment outcome and patient survival. These differences in the biologic features indicate that in order to improve the survival of patients with hematolymphoid malignancies it is of utmost necessity to conduct research into the biological response to treatment and prognostic factors in the developing nations themselves. This geographic inequality in cancer treatment poses challenges that have only just begun to be addressed.[49,50]

Presence of retroviral infections and other infections

Human immunodeficiency virus (HIV) infection is associated with aggressive, systemic NHL presenting with widespread disease and extranodal involvement with poor prognosis.[51] Pediatric HIV infection and acquired immune deficiency syndrome (AIDS) remain a critical health priority in sub-Saharan Africa. Epstein–Barr virus is present in essentially all cases of endemic Burkitt lymphoma, which occurs in children where malaria is endemic.[52,53] It is the most common pediatric cancer in tropical Africa, accounting for 50 percent of childhood cancer.[54] Human T cell lymphotrophic virus 1 (HTLV-1) is a major risk factor for ATLL in endemic areas of southern Japan, the Caribbean basin, West Africa, the Middle East, South America, and Malaysia.[55]

With the introduction of highly active antiretroviral therapy (HAART), incidence of AIDS-related NHL has declined from 6.2 to 3.6 per 1000 person-years in the Western world;[56] however, in sub-Saharan Africa it remains a critical health priority and accounts for two million deaths per year in Africa. This can be attributed to nonaccessibility to health care.

The way the above variables (epidemiology, biology of disease, patterns of presentation, presence of retroviral or other infections) exert their influence has led to a perspective of poorly nourished people who delay seeking medical attention for prolonged periods of time and, consequently, appear with extensive disease. Also, there is a lack of disciplined protocol management, except in a few centers where first-world standards prevail. These circumstances combine to generate figures for emerging nations that range from appallingly poor response and survival rates to those commensurate with developed countries.

LIMITATIONS IN 'THE LESS ECONOMICALLY SOUND OR PRIVILEGED NATIONS'

Financial resources

The term 'less economically sound or privileged nations' has been applied to the developing nations recently. These nations, although poor by Western economic standards, are rich in human and cultural resources.[57]

Given the allocation of already scarce access to health care, and other pressing needs such as family planning, nutrition, and prevention of infectious diseases, the task for managing cancer patients appears Herculean. The majority of the budgetary allocation in the developing nations is directed towards preventing millions of deaths by focusing on strategies for combating infectious diseases. Noncommunicable diseases are not among the priorities. The World Health Organization (WHO) and international charities have also committed resources to reducing mortality from infectious disease by two-thirds in the next decade. Not surprisingly, the survival rates even in childhood ALL in the developing nations are not comparable with those of the developed nations. The extent of resource constraints can be studied from this model. In a country like India, which is intermediate between a developing and developed country, the total government expenditure on health care per person per year is about US $55, and in the private sector is US $16. (These were $2 and $6, respectively, in 1989.[58]) If a child with ALL is treated with a moderately intensive chemotherapy protocol for 2 years, the cost escalates to US $500–2000, depending on treatment at government or private hospitals. This highlights that resources are just not available to manage even curable malignancies like childhood ALL.

At the Shanghai Children's Medical Center, which serves the only Chinese city in which health insurance for catastrophic disease is offered, 234 children with ALL were admitted for treatment between October 1998 and June 2003.[59] According to Dr JY Tang of the Medical Center, therapy for 66 of these children (most of whom did not live in Shanghai) had to be abandoned, apparently for financial reasons, and another 52 children died of leukemia from treatment-related complications, leaving only 116 in continuous complete remission. In the rural areas, problems are much worse; only 10 percent of Chinese children younger than 14 years of age received protocol-based therapy. This highlights the urgent need for proper budgetary allocations. A second issue apart from financial constraint is the uneven distribution of

resources. Chandy[60] has proposed three profiles or categories of population with regard to income, educational status, and motivation to undergo treatment. Within many countries there is a contrast between services available to the poor and the rich.

Profile 1: Illiterate, laborer parents with a family income of less than US $20 per month and no motivation to obtain adequate treatment for a cancer-stricken child constitute 70 percent of the population of the developing world.

Profile 2: Literate parents with a monthly family income of around US $50–100 and good motivation to obtain treatment but a lack of necessary resources constitute 25 percent of the developing world's population.

Profile 3: Elite, educated parents from cities with monthly family incomes above US $1000 who can use their own resources for the best possible treatment constitute less than 5 percent of the population in the developing world.

With capitation and market forces ruling the world economy, the heterogeneity in the population with regard to income, educational status, and motivation is a uniform feature of all developing countries, with the proportion of the population in each of the above categories differing among such countries.

Many Latin American countries are trying to expand coverage to the population that traditionally has not been able to afford care. Countries like Chile, Cuba, Uruguay, and Brazil all offer 100 percent public care for those who cannot afford to pay, while Bolivia only has an equivalent of US $74 per person per year to spend on health care, but still manages to enrol patients into phase I and phase II studies.[60]

Other factors apart from finances

In the developing nations, other nonfinancial factors exist that woefully join the inadequate government and family monetary resources to hinder the availability of adequate health services.[61] These are educational and sociocultural barriers. Lower literacy rates inhibit awareness of cancer in general. Dissemination of information, efficient communication, and education of masses is consequently slow and difficult. Then there are social mores, traditional cultural beliefs which compound with economic backwardness and lack of education. These beliefs form major deterrents to proper community utilization of health services. As reported by Chandy,[60] even in childhood leukemia motivation of the family to obtain treatment is not always forthcoming.

A combination of the above realities results in a majority of patients availing treatment in an advanced stage, thereby minimizing the chances of physicians administering curative treatment. Poor compliance with the treatment prescribed is the other consequence of the interplay of the financial and social factors and accounts for the overall poor survival.

To address these complex social challenges is a Herculean task which cannot be tackled by medical personnel alone. These nations have to adopt a behavioral, social, and economic mode of change and uplift.

Another important factor that hinders the administration of intensive protocol-based chemotherapy, as done in the developed nations, is the relatively lower nutritional status of patients. As a result of poor nutritional status, patients experience more drug toxicities. Nutritional factors and prevalent infectious disease are likely to be among the most important environmental factors influencing treatment outcome and survival in the developing nations.[62–65] Poor nutritional status in a child undergoing treatment is associated with higher numbers of toxic deaths.[66] A high prevalence of hepatitis B viral infections among oncology patients in developing countries warrants a special mention: it leads not only to greater morbidity and toxic deaths but also unmeasured effects on survival from repeated interruptions in treatment.[64,65,67]

Availability of drugs

Another major issue in treating patients in developing countries is the availability of the newer drugs and targeted therapies. The newer drugs are not freely available due to many factors such as governmental policies, higher cost of the drugs, and governmental approval. In countries where the patient bears the cost of his or her treatment, affordability becomes a major issue. In these countries, it is the richer class, or profile 3 patients described by Chandy,[60] that can avail the best possible treatment, while 80 percent of patients cannot avail the best treatment. Thus urgent measures are required to address this issue.

Minimal requirements for diagnosis

Apart from the economic, social, and cultural issues, another issue is of early detection and early treatment. Lack of awareness at the patient level and at the primary physician's level leads to late diagnosis and delayed referral to the oncologist. Minimal diagnostic facilities like morphology, cytochemistry, and immunophenotyping should be made available and should be accessible to the hematopathologist. Apart from the issues of infrastructure and availability of the above, there is an urgent need for trained hematologists, histopathologists, and oncopathologists for early precise diagnosis. These services should be available at the district/community hospital, the primary point of patient referral. Once these basics for minimal diagnosis are available, study of molecular mechanisms, genetics, pharmacogenomics, and pharmacokinetics can be embarked on.

Thus to diagnose patients at an early stage of disease, a high level of clinical suspicion and immediate detailed evaluation is required so that patients can be referred early to a specialist; this will break the vicious cycle of late diagnosis, advanced stage of disease at presentation, more drug resistance, and decreased survival.

REQUIREMENTS FOR SUPPORTIVE CARE

The improved survival in hematolymphoid malignancies can be attributed, apart from improved diagnostics, to improvement in supportive care: growth factors, blood components, and better antibiotics and antifungal drugs. Newer aggressive protocols in conjunction with better supportive care have led to improvements in survival in the Western world.

The scenario in the developing world is different. The facilities for providing supportive care are often lacking, leading to toxic deaths.[68,69] High levels of antimicrobial resistance in developing countries, due to poor sanitation, contributes to higher rates of fatal sepsis.[70] Blood component therapy is available only in a few tertiary centers. Blood transfusion facilities are inadequate. Thus institution of aggressive chemotherapy or the choice of a chemotherapeutic protocol must be based on the available supportive care services and facilities. Improved supportive care can reduce mortality caused by infection remarkably and can also improve disease-free survival rates.[71]

TREATMENT STRATEGIES

Due to improvement in diagnostics, patients with hematolymphoid malignancies are being carefully assessed for risk of failure. This has translated to high-risk patients receiving aggressive treatment protocols and low-risk patients receiving less-toxic therapy. However, as discussed in the earlier part of the chapter, differences in the biology of the disease are now being documented. Hence, whether the risk stratification, criteria, or definitions hold true for populations in developing countries remains to be determined. Therefore a uniform assessment policy should be followed by the treating oncologists so that the importance of different prognostic variables becomes clear.

At present the treatment protocols of the developed nations are being followed by developing nations. This may not be cost effective and also each aspect of the protocol has to be considered carefully. An example is the protocols of treating childhood ALL; omission of L-asparaginase from the dexamethasone, vincristine, and anthracyclines in remission/induction to decease costs,[72] continued triple intrathecal therapy in standard-risk ALL in lieu of central nervous system (CNS) radiation,[73] and use of vincristine and dexamethasone pulses during maintenance therapy to decrease the risk of CNS relapse[72] have been incorporated into protocols. Such information should be optimally utilized to design tailored protocols for individual patients. At present, there are no standard protocols that can be uniformly recommended for use in the developing countries.

MANAGEMENT OF HEMATOLYMPHOID DISEASE – HOW TO PROCEED?

There are two fundamental aspects to better management for patients in underprivileged nations. First is provision of easily available and affordable comprehensive oncology services for treatment; second is ensuring proper community utilization of these services and increasing the access to care for the large majority of the population. Making the treatment cost effective is the major hurdle to overcome. The previous half of this chapter has described the resources constraint on all fronts. These nations simply cannot afford to provide the care required for all newly diagnosed patients. What should the strategies be to address such a grim situation? They can be addressed through the following.

Establishment of comprehensive cancer care units or teaching hospitals

The establishment of cancer teaching hospitals or comprehensive cancer care centers is the first step. This will help to concentrate specialists, increase interdisciplinary cooperation, make optimal use of resources, develop supportive care, and ensure training, data management, and follow-up.[74,75]

In 1991 an International Society of Paediatric Oncology (SIOP) committee recommended requirements for a pediatric cancer unit (PCU). A PCU model with the required staff, facilities, and resources obtained from the state, insurance, or private sector for ensuring a favorable outcome in a child with cancer is shown in Figure 60.1.

A PCU will consist of at least a full-time pediatric oncologist and specialist willing to cooperate within the frame of the PCU. Pediatric cancer units are essential for providing optimal pediatric oncology care for children and adolescents with cancer within the framework of available resources

and for the training of pediatric oncology specialists at all levels.

Similar principles can be applied for development of comprehensive cancer care centers all across the underprivileged nations. These can function efficiently provided they have a good hematology, microbiology, and histopathology laboratory, good surgical and radiation facilities, dedicated oncology nursing personnel, plus drugs, blood products, and minimum facilities for data management and follow-up. Standardization (adjusted to the local conditions) of initial investigations, treatment, supportive care, and evaluation of toxicities and treatment results is essential in order to make progress.[76] These PCUs in developing countries have responsibilities to establish 'standards of care' minimum diagnostic criteria, tailored effective protocols that are both affordable and practical, and structured supportive care guidelines relevant to the existing local situations.

Shared care model

EXPANDING ACCESS TO HEALTH CARE

The shared care model aims to ensure early referrals and early diagnosis as well as participation in follow-up care. The concept of shared care with peripheral participation would be beneficial to both the patients and the crowded hospitals. The challenge to make health care accessible to all, can be met by working collaboratively with policy makers and the community and by reorganization of existing services through a tight linkage of primary, secondary, and tertiary care services (Fig. 60.2).

This model involves early referrals by a physician or pediatric specialist at district level or primary level to the cancer care unit. Thus, decentralization of the treatment

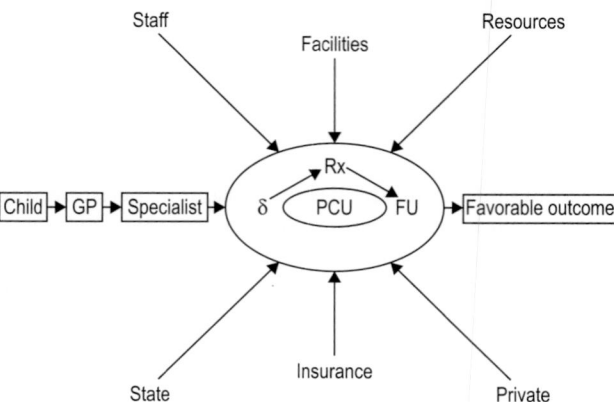

Figure 60.1 Pediatric cancer unit (PCU) model for the provision of a comprehensive pediatric cancer care unit. GP, general practitioner; FU, follow-up; δ, diagnosis; Rx, reaction.

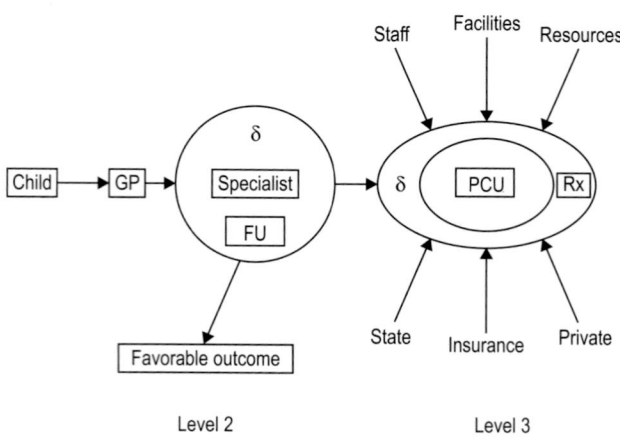

Figure 60.2 Shared-care pediatric cancer unit (PCU) model. This strategy would help to ensure early referrals and early diagnosis, as well as adequate follow-up care of children with leukemia in underprivileged nations. FU, follow-up; GP, general practitioner; δ, diagnosis; Rx, reaction.

process by a shared management approach would decrease the workload on the PCU. More patients can gain access to treatment and treatment will be more acceptable to patients as there would be reduced direct and indirect costs (traveling expenses, time, and loss of wages). This is of prime importance for poor families who have no 'buffer funds.' Lessons can be learnt from Brazil. Howard et al.[77] established a pediatric oncology program in a resource-poor area in the city of Recife, Brazil. In the report of their collaborative program, they noted that in the 1980s there was no dedicated pediatric oncology program in Recife, where the mean annual per capita income is only US $1049. In the last 15 years, systematic improvements have been made in all aspects of pediatric oncology care despite little change in the region's economy and rate of infant mortality (85 per 1000 live births in 1991 vs 74 in 2000).[78] The 5-year event-free survival improved steadily in childhood ALL from 32 percent in the 1980s to 47 percent during the period 1994 to 1997, and to 63 percent in the period from 1997 to 2000. The abandonment of therapy (16 percent in the 1980s) was brought down to 0.5 percent in the period from 1997 to 2000. Similar results have been achieved in El Salvador and other countries with limited resources.[79–82]

This success they attribute to uniform protocol-based therapy, reliable supply of drugs, training of nurses, 24-hour on-site physician coverage, ready access to intensive care, written evidence-based supportive care guidelines, and improved identification and treatment of comorbid conditions (e.g., malnutrition, infection) at diagnosis.[80–83] By training and exchanging staff with peripheral hospitals and dispensaries and establishing contacts with practitioners, PCUs could contribute to earlier detection and referral of cancer patients. Thus sharing of treatment responsibilities would make therapy accessible to all and minimize the logistic, economic, and psychological problems.

Agarwal and Dalvi[84] have proposed a reorganization of the existing health care infrastructure in developing countries. This will be customized and tailor-made for each country. This is shown in Table 60.1.

Training of professionals and health care community workers

In developing nations, because of scarce resources and the perception of cancer being incurable, people do not want to 'waste' resources. Even health care professionals, due to ignorance, have this negative approach that influences the patients to avail minimal or symptomatic treatment only. Thus education of professionals regarding permanent cures and the natural history of malignancy is a priority. These nations also lack trained oncologists. As reported by Peter McIntyre, in Nigeria there are fewer than 100 practising oncologists catering to a population of 120 million people, with limited supply of drugs and imaging equipment.[61] Hence young doctors need to be encouraged to take up oncology as a specialty. A well-planned global professional educational program needs to be directed toward physicians, pediatricians, surgeons, and nurses, and toward ancillary paramedical staff.

Another approach is by training doctors, nurses, and ancillary paramedical staff at Western institutions. However, according to Dr Magrath of the International Network for Cancer Treatment and Research (INCTR), a non-governmental organization founded by the International Union Against Cancer (UICC) and Institut Pasteur in Brussels, this can be counterproductive. Many never return home while others are demoralized on their return by lack of resources. Hence it is essential for countries to build the capacity of cancer services to break a vicious cycle in which governments give a low priority to cancer treatment and patients present with advanced disease and die with acceptable care.

Twinning program

Twinning is a global, long-lasting cooperation between a pediatric cancer center in a developing country and a center from a developed country. The training of PCU personnel in underprivileged nations is best promoted

Table 60.1 Levels of care. Guidelines for pediatric oncology practice. Organization of services with distribution of responsibilities within the existing health care infrastructure of developing countries (Indian model)

Level of health system		Responsibilities	
Facility	Unit	Lab Services	Therapeutics
Regional cancer center	PCU	IP/IHC molecular assays	Chemotherapy, radiation therapy, BMT
Medical college, department of pediatrics	PCU	Hematology, imaging, histopathology	Initial chemotherapy, blood component
District headquarters hospital	Outreach center	CBC, biochemistry, microbiology	Chemotherapy with follow-up

PCU, Pediatric Cancer Unit: IP/IHC, immunophenotyping/immunohistochemistry; CBC, complete blood count; BMT, bone marrow transplantation.

through this strategy. The success of this strategy can be seen in El Salvador, where the partnership program started in 1994 in childhood ALL has resulted in a 4-year event-free survival of 40 percent in a high-risk group and 69 percent in the standard-risk group.[85]

The La Mascota ALL twinning programme between La Mascota pediatric hospital in Managua, Nicaragua, and hospitals in Monza and Milan, Italy, has clearly demonstrated how intellectual, organizational, and financial resources can be generated by a dedicated twinning program.[86]

According to Masera et al.,[86] cooperation in twinning was not an exercise of transferability of established diagnostic and therapeutic protocols, but a research effort aimed at adaptation and assessment of the protocols in the specific local conditions of Nicaragua. However, Franco Cavalli, president elect of the UICC favors twinning programs between countries, so long as they build local expertise and do not promote inappropriate high-technology solutions. The aim should be to create conditions for independence, rather than dependency, and encourage a 'research-minded attitude.' Individual countries must find their own solutions to the problem of resource generation, independent of the West.

Therapeutic alliances

Masera et al.[87] have described the role of a therapeutic alliance. This is a collaboration (alliance) of the medical staff with the parents of children with cancer and with community volunteers. This is a realistic means to sensitize society and mobilize resources and energies at national and international levels. Strong and viable support groups are essential when resources are scarce and the economic psychosocial needs of families are unmet.

This strategy has worked remarkably well in pediatric cancer within the therapeutic alliance program in Monza, Italy[88] with the Tettamanti Foundation and the parent's association Comitato ML Verga. GRAACC, a support group for children and adolescents with cancer in Sao Paulo, Brazil, in collaboration with the university of Sao Paulo and community volunteers, parents, and the physicians, was successful within 3 years in constructing a modern 11-floor pediatric oncology hospital for supporting more than 200 low-income new pediatric oncology patients each year.

Creating national cooperative groups

Variability of presentation of most of the cancers due to geography, race, and biology is well documented. Most of the therapeutic protocols practised by oncologists in developing nations are based on Western literature and trials. However, to formulate treatment guidelines and protocols, developing nations should conduct clinical research in their own respective countries. Evidence from Europe and the USA is used to develop guidelines for these nations,

assuming the disease is the same but that the genetics and lifestyles are different. Hence to address these issues, original research work needs to be done within these nations. This can be done by forming cooperative groups of like-minded practitioners in these countries. This will not only help to formulate guidelines, but will also train the younger generation of physicians.

Research opportunities

There is still a considerable gap between the exciting scientific developments in the field of medicine and what is readily available to the underserved segments of society.[89] It is essential for the world community to realize the vital role of social and environmental factors in determining both the disease pattern and the approach to health care in developing countries. Effective but low-cost scientific intervention needs to be developed separately for the developing world in order to achieve universal success. Initiatives through training programs such as INCTR's outreach programs should ensure that collaboration does not simply result in the transfer of established diagnostic and therapeutic protocols but rather promotes research aimed at adaptation and assessment of the protocols in a specific cultural and economic condition.

Research activities should be relevant to these countries. The transferability of therapies, a critical evidence-based assessment of what is essential, and the cost-benefit profile of any proposed research are not only fundamental aspects of oncology in the developing (South) countries but are also important in the developed North. Research in the developing nations should be conducted by investigators from these nations, on their own people, for the good of the people. Close interplay is needed between the North and South in drawing up research methods and mobilizing resources to conduct investigations.

CONCLUSIONS

The treatment of hematolymphoid malignancies in the underprivileged nations is beset with multiple hurdles. The difference in survival of cancer patients in developed and developing countries (North and South) is a reminder of wider truth: the asymmetry between the global regions, with respect to the basic right to life, is at the same time both total and avoidable. Given the meager resources and other constraints in these developing countries, together with the apparent differences in biology of disease, hope does not seem to be in sight. The North-South asymmetry will remain. However, lessons have been learnt by training or professional adoption in pediatric acute lymphoblastic leukemia. Collaborative projects or therapeutic alliances are already providing impressive results by mobilizing intellectual, cultural, and financial resources. Thus small and consistent steps will improve survival in these less fortunate nations.

KEY POINTS

- Epidemiologic, racial, geographic and histologic differences exist in lymphomas in developing nations.
- Limitations in finances, a lack of skilled, trained manpower and awareness, the relative inaccessibility of health care and a lack of proper diagnostic facilities are the major hindrances.
- Unequal budgetary allocation policies for health care in developing nations is another major hindrance.
- Establishing comprehensive cancer care units and expanding access to health care and the training of professionals and health care community workers can help improve survival in these underdeveloped nations.
- Creating national cooperative groups and fostering twinning programs and therapeutic alliances with developed nations will help to improve survival.

REFERENCES

● = Key primary paper

◆ = Major review article

●1. WHO. *Health situation in the South East Asia region 1994–1997*. New Delhi: Regional Office for SEAR, 2000.

●2. Magrath I, Liluak J. Cancer in developing countries: Opportunity and challenges. *J Natl Cancer Inst* 1993; **85**: 862–74.

●3. Hartge P, Devessa SS, Froumeri JF. Hodgkin's and Non Hodgkin's lymphoma. In: Dell R, Froumer J, Muir CL. (eds) *Trends in cancer, incidence and mortality cancer surveys.* New York: Cold Spring Harbor Laboratory Press, 1994: 423–53.

●4. Kennedy BJ, Fremgen AM, Merck HR. National Cancer Data Base report for 1985–89 and 1990–94. *Cancer* 1998; **83**: 1041–7.

◆5. Roy P, Vaughan Hudson G, Vaughan Hudson B *et al.* Long-term survival in Hodgkin's disease patients. A comparison of relative survival in patients in trials and those recorded in population-based cancer registries. *Eur J Cancer* 2000; **36**: 384–9.

◆6. Lorraine L. Hodgkin's disease in black Zimbabweans. *Cancer* 1988; **61**: 189–94.

◆7. Kapoor G, Advani SH, Dinshaw K *et al.* Treatment results of Hodgkin's disease in Indian children. *Pediatr Hematol Oncol* 1996; **14**: 1442–6.

◆8. Chandi L, Kumar L, Kochupillai V *et al.* Hodgkin's disease: A retrospective analysis of 15 years experience at a large referral centre. *Natl Med J India* 1998; **11**: 212–7.

●9. Ries LAG, Eisner MP, Kosary CL *et al.* (eds) *SEER cancer statistics review 1975–2001*. Bethesda, MD: National Cancer Institute, 2004.

●10. Parkin DM, Whelam SL, Ferloy J *et al.* (eds) *Cancer incidence in five continents.* Vol VII. IARC scientific publications no. 143. Lyon: International Agency for Research on Cancer, 1997: 804–913.

●11. National Cancer Registry programme. *Consolidated report of the population based cancer registries 1990–1996, incidence and distribution of cancer.* New Delhi: Indian Council of Medical Research, 2001.

●12. Greenlee RT, Murray T, Bolden S, Wingo PA. Cancer statistics, 2000. *CA Cancer J Clin* 2000; **50**: 7–33.

●13. Ries LAG, Kosary CL, Hankey BF *et al.* (eds) *SEER cancer statistic review, 1973–1996*. Bethesda, MD: National Cancer Institute, 1999.

●14. WHO. World Health report 1999, making a difference. Report of the Director General WHO, 1999.

●15. Morrison VA. Chronic leukemias. *CA Cancer J Clin* 1994; **44**: 353–77.

◆16. Kumar L, Sagar TG, Maitreyan V *et al.* Chronic granulocytic leukemia, a study of 160 cases. *J Assoc Physicians India* 1990; **38**: 899–902.

◆17. Prabhu M, Kochupillai V, Sharma S *et al.* Prognostic assessment of various parameters in chronic myeloid leukemia cancer. 1986; **58**: 1357–60.

◆18. Bhaduri S, Gupta RC, Chawla SP. Chronic granulocytic leukemia. A study of 177 cases. *Indian J Cancer* 1979; **16**: 1–7.

◆19. Wells R, Lau KS. Incidence of leukemia in Singapore and rarity of CLL in Chinese. *Br Med J* 1960; **1**: 759–63.

◆20. Nair NC, Chougule A, Dhond S *et al.* Trisomy 12 in chronic lymphocytic leukemia – geographical variation. *Leuk Res* 1998, **22**: 313–17.

●21. Park K. (ed.) *Parks textbook of preventive and social medicine.* 16th Edn. Jabalpur: Banarsidas Bhanot, 2000: 305–18.

●22. Reading R. Poverty and the health of children and adolescents. *Arch Dis Child* 1997; **76**: 463–7.

◆23. Dinshaw KA, Advani SH, Gopal R *et al.* Management of Hodgkin's disease in western India. *Cancer* 1984; **54**: 1276–82.

◆24. Shanta V, Sastri DV, Sagar TG *et al.* A review of Hodgkin's disease at the Cancer Institute, Madras. *Clin Oncol* 1982; **8**: 5–15.

◆25. Hassan YA, Ezzeldin MI. Hodgkin's disease in adults in Saudi Arabia. *Int J Cancer* 1991; **47**: 822–6.

◆26. Larraine L. Hodgkin's lymphoma in black Zimbabweans. *Cancer* 1988; **61**: 189–94.

◆27. Evans AS, Kirchhaff LV, Pannuti CS, Carvaltio RPS. A case controlled study of Hodgkin's disease in Brazil. Seroepidemiologic studies in cases and family members. *Am J Epidemiol* 1980; **112**: 609–18.

●28. Kennedy BJ, Fremgen AM, Merck HR. The National Cancer Data Base report on Hodgkin's disease for 1985–1989 and 1990–1994. *Cancer* 1998; **83**: 1041–7.

◆29. Knecht H, Odermann BF, Bachmann F *et al.* Frequent detection of Epstein–Barr virus DNA by the polymerase chain reaction in lymph node biopsies from patients with Hodgkin's disease without genomic evidence of B or T cell clonality. *Blood* 1991; **78**: 760–7.

◆30. Brousset P, Chittal S, Schlaifer D *et al.* Detection of Epstein-Barr virus messenger RNA in Reed-Sternberg cells of Hodgkin's disease by in situ hybridization with biotinylated probes on specially processed modified acetone methyl benzoate xylene (ModAMex) sections. *Blood* 1991; **77**: 1781–6.

●31. Jarrett AF, Armstrong AA, Alexander E. Epidemiology of EBV and Hodgkin's lymphoma. *Ann Oncol* 1996; **7**(Suppl 4): 11–17.

●32. Kennedy BJ, Loeb V, Peterson VM *et al.* National survey of patterns of care for Hodgkin's disease. *Med Pediatr Oncol* 1985; **56**: 2547–56.

◆33. Laskar S, Gupta T, Vimal S *et al.* Consolidation radiation after complete remission in Hodgkin's disease following six cycles of doxorubicin, bleomycin, vinblastine and dacarbazine chemotherapy: is there a need? *J Clin Oncol* 2004; **22**: 62–5.

●34. Jemal A, Murray T, Ward E *et al.* Cancer statistics, 2005. *CA Cancer J Clin* 2005; **55**: 10–30.

●35. Ries LAG, Eisner MP, Kosary CL *et al.* (eds) *SEER cancer statistics, 1975–2001.* Bethesda, MD: National Cancer Institute, 2004.

●36. Waterhouse J, Shanmugaratnam K *et al.* Cancer incidence in five continents, Vol IV. IARC scientific publications no. 42. Lyon: International Agency for Research on Cancer, 1982.

●37. Muir C, Waterhouse J, Mack T *et al.* Cancer incidence in five continents, Vol V. IARC scientific publication no. 42: Lyon: International agency for Research on Cancer, 1987.

●38. Devesa SS, Fears T. Non-Hodgkin's Lymphoma time trends: United States and International data. *Cancer Res* 1992; **52** (Suppl 19): 5432S–40S.

●39. Parkin DM, Kramarova E, Draper GJ *et al.* (eds) International incidence of childhood cancer, Vol II. IARC scientific publication no. 144. Lyon: International Agency for Research on Cancer, 1998.

●40. Armitage JO, Naugh PM, Harris NL, Bierman P. Non Hodgkin's lymphoma. In: Devita VT, Hellman S, Rosenberg SA. (eds) *Cancer principles and practice of oncology*, 6th Edn. Philadelphia, PA: Lippincott Williams and Wilkins, 2001: 2256–316.

◆41. Ramot B, Magrath I. Hypothesis: the environment is a major determinant of the immunological subtype of lymphoma and acute lymphoblastic leukemia in children. *Br J Haematol* 1982; **52**: 183–9.

◆42. Bhargava M, Kumar R, Karak A *et al.* Immunological subtypes of acute lymphoblastic leukemia in north India. *Leuk Res* 1988; **12**: 673–8.

◆43. Kamat DM, Gopal R, Advani SH, Nair CN. Pattern of subtypes of acute lymphoblastic leukemia in India. *Leuk Res* 1985; **9**: 927–34.

◆44. Advani SH, Pai S, Venzon D *et al.* Acute lymphoblastic leukemia in India: an analysis of prognostic factors using a single treatment regimen. *Ann Oncol* 1999; **10**: 167–76.

◆45. Sazawal S, Bhatia K, Gurbaxani S *et al.* Pattern of immunoglobulin (Ig) and T cell receptor (TCR) gene rearrangements in childhood acute lymphoblastic leukemia in India. *Leuk Res* 2000; **24**: 575–82.

◆46. Tama A, Bendict SH, Gelfand EW. Rearrangement of T cell receptor chain gene in childhood acute lymphoblastic leukemia. *Blood* 1984; **70**: 1933–9.

◆47. Hamdy N, Bhatia K, Shaker H *et al.* Molecular epidemiology of acute lymphoblastic leukemia in Egypt. *Leukemia* 1995; **9**: 194–202.

◆48. Inamdar N, Kumar SA, Banavali SD *et al.* Comparative incidence of the rearrangement of TEL/AML1 and ALL 1 genes in pediatric precursor B acute lymphoblastic leukemia in India. *Int J Oncol* 1988; **13**: 1319–22.

●49. Pui CH, Schrappe M, Masera G *et al.* Ponte di Legno Working Group: Statement on the right of children with leukemia to have full access to essential treatment and report on the Sixth International Childhood Acute Lymphoblastic Leukemia Workshop. *Leukemia* 2004; **18**: 1043–53.

●50. Pui CH, Ribeiro RC. International collaboration on childhood leukemia. *Int J Hematol* 2003; **78**: 383–9.

◆51. Cote TR, Bigger RJ, Rosenberg P *et al.* Non Hodgkin's Lymphoma among people with AIDS. Incidence, presentation and public health burden. *Int J Cancer* 1997; **73**: 645–50.

◆52. De-Thé G, Geser A, Day NE *et al.* Epidemiological evidence for causal relationship between Epstein-Barr virus and Burkitt's lymphoma from Ugandan prospective study. *Nature* 1978; **274**: 756–61.

●53. Burkitt DP. The discovery of Burkitt's lymphoma. *Cancer* 1983; **51**: 1776–86.

●54. Carbone A, Canzonieri V, Gloghini A *et al.* Burkitt's lymphoma historical background and recent insights into classification and pathogenesis. *Ann Otol Rhinol Laryngol* 2000; **109**: 693–702.

◆55. Hisada M, Stuver SO, Okayama A *et al.* Persistent paradox of natural history of human T-lymphotropic virus type I. Parallel analyses of Japanese and Jamaican carriers. *J Infect Dis* 2004; **190**: 1605–9.

◆56. International collaboration on HIV and cancer. Highly active antiretroviral therapy and incidence of cancer in human immunodeficiency virus infected adults. *J Natl Cancer Inst* 2000; **92**: 1823–30.

●57. Williams C. Teaching pediatrics for the developing world. *Arch Dis Child* 1998; **78**: 484–7.

●58. Tognani G. North-south asymmetry. *Ann Oncol* 1993: **4**: 7–8.

●59. Ribeiro R, Pui C. Saving the children. Improving childhood cancer treatment in developing countries. *N Engl J Med* 2005; **352**: 2158–60.

●60. Chandy M. Childhood acute lymphoblastic leukemia in India: an approach to management in a three-tier society. *Med Pediatr Oncol* 1995; **25**: 197–203.

●61. McIntyre P. Rising to the challenge in the developing world. *Cancer World* 2005; 44–8.

●62. Agarwal B. Hemophilia control in the LES nations. Problems and priorities: a personal view. *Hemophilia* 1995; **1**: 222–6.

●63. Lobato Mendizabal E, Ruiz-Arguelles GI, Marine-Lopez A. Leukemia and nutrition. Malnutrition is an adverse prognostic factor in the outcome of treatment of patients with standard risk acute lymphoblastic leukemia. *Leuk Res* 1989; **13**: 899–906.

●64. Vianna MB, Murao M, Rames G *et al.* Malnutrition as a prognostic factor in lymphoblastic leukemia: a multivariate analysis. *Arch Dis Child* 1994; **71**: 304–10.

●65. Dutta U, Raina R, Garg PK *et al.* A prospective study on the incidence of hepatitis B and C infections amongst patients with lymphoproliferative disorders. *Indian J Med Res* 1998; **107**: 78–82.

◆66. Nag S, Vaidya S, Pais *et al.* Hepatis B viral infection in ALL. *Ind J Hematol Blood Trans* 1995; **13**: 150–3.

◆67. Advani SH, Pai SK, Venzon D *et al.* Acute lymphoblastic leukemia in India: an analysis of prognostic factors using a single treatment regimen. *Ann Oncol* 1999; **10**: 167–76.

◆68. Iyer RS, Rao S, Gujra S *et al.* Childhood acute lymphoblastic leukemia: MCP 841 protocol. In: Proceedings of the 32nd Annual Conference of the India Society of Hematology and Blood Transfusion, 1991: 15.

◆69. Appaji L. Acute lymphoblastic leukemia – KM10 experience. In: Proceedings of the 32nd Annual Conference of the Indian Society of Hematology and Blood Transfusion, 1991: 13.

◆70. Amyes SGB, Tait S, Thomson CJ *et al.* The incidence of antibiotic resistance in aerobic faecal flora in south India. *J Antimicrob Chemother* 1992; **29**: 415–25.

◆71. Kurkure P, *et al.* Impact of improved supportive care on treatment outcome in Acute Lymphoblastic Leukemia – an Indian experience. *Med Pediatric Oncol* 1995; **25**: 261

◆72. Veerman AJP, Wahlen K, Kamps WA *et al.* High cure rate with a moderately intensive treatment regimen in non high risk childhood acute lymphoblastic leukemia: results of protocol ALL-V1 from the Dutch Childhood Leukemia study group. *J Clin Oncol* 1996; **14**: 911–18.

◆73. Conter V, Arico M, Vaselserchi MG *et al.* Extended intrathecal methotrexate may replace cranial irradiation for prevention of CNS relapse in children with intermediate risk acute lymphoblastic leukemia treated with Berlin-Frankfurt-Munster based intensive therapy. *J Clin Oncol* 1995; **13**: 2497–502.

●74. Magrath IT, Shad A, Epelman S *et al.* Pediatric oncology in countries in limited resources. In: Pizzo PA, Poplack DG. (eds) *Principles and practice of pediatric oncology*, 3rd Edn. Philadelphia, PA: Lipppincott-Raven, 1997: 1395–1420.

●75. SIOP committee on standards of care and training in pediatric oncology. Requirements for the training of a pediatric hematologist/oncologist and recommendations for the organization of a pediatric cancer unit (PCU). Amsterdam: SIOP, 1991.

●76. Wagner HP, Antic V. The problems of pediatric malignancies in the developing world. Challenges and opportunities in pediatric oncology. *Ann NY Acad Sci* 1998; **842**: 193–204.

◆77. Howard S, Pedrosa M, Lins M *et al.* Establishment of a pediatric oncology program and outcomes of childhood acute lymphoblastic leukemia in a resource-poor area. *JAMA* 2004; **291**: 2471–5.

78. World Health Organization statistical information available at: http//www3.who.int/whosis/menu.cfm.

◆79. Metzger ML, Howard SC, Fu LC *et al.* Outcome of childhood acute lymphoblastic leukemia in resource-poor countries. *Lancet* 2003; **362**: 706–8.

●80. Wilimas JA, Donahue N, Chammas G *et al.* Training subspecialty nurses in developing countries. Methods, outcome and cost. *Med Pediatr Oncol* 2003; **41**: 136–40.

●81. Wilimas JA, Ribeiro RC. Pediatric hematology oncology outreach for developing countries. *Hematol Oncol Clin North Am* 2001; **15**: 775–87.

●82. Pui CH, Ribeiro RC. International collaboration on childhood leukemia. *Int J Hematol* 2003; **78**: 383–9.

◆83. Pedrosa F, Bonilla M, Lin A *et al.* Effect of malnutrition at the time of diagnosis on the survival of children treated for cancer in El Salvador and Northern Brazil. *J Pediatr Hematol Oncol* 2000; **22**: 502–5.

●84. Agarwal B, Dalvi R. Treatment of childhood leukemias in underprivileged countries. In: Ching-Hon Pui. (ed.) *Current clinical oncology: treatment of acute leukemias: new directions of clinical research*. Humana Press, Totowa, New Jersey, USA. 2003: 321–9.

●85. Wilimas JA, Marina N, Crist W *et al.* Developing a pediatric hematology/oncology partnership program (PHOPP) in El Salvador. *Blood* 1999; **94**: 367a.

●86. Masera G, Baez F, Biondi A *et al.* North South training in pediatric hemato-oncology: The La Mascota programme, Nicaragua. *Lancet* 1998; **352**: 1923–6.

◆87. Masera G, Spinetta JJ, Jankovic M *et al.* Guidelines for a therapeutic alliance between families and staff. A report of the SIOP working committee on psychological issues in pediatric oncology. *Med Pediatr Oncol* 1988; **30**: 183–6.

●88. Sergio P. Result of University, private institutions and community alliances, fighting pediatric cancer in Brazil. In: Proceedings of the symposium on development of an alliance of stakeholders, parents and health professionals world wide: investing in the future. Joint annual meeting of SIOP and ASPHO, Montreal, 1999: 8.

●89. Bellamy C. *The state of the World's children*. New York: UNICEF, 2000:1–120.

61

Late effects of cancer treatment and quality of life

SADHNA SHANKAR AND SMITA BHATIA

Cancer survival rates have shown a steady and remarkable improvement over the past four decades. While only one in five individuals with cancer was expected to survive 5 or more years from diagnosis in 1930, presently one in two persons is expected to survive for greater than 5 years.[1,2] Significant improvements in survival have been evidenced in breast, ovarian, prostate, and colorectal cancer as well as hematologic malignancies including Hodgkin lymphoma (HL), non-Hodgkin lymphoma (NHL), and leukemia,[2] with survival rates as high as 80 percent reported after HL and NHL.[2] As a result of these improvements, in January 2004 there were an estimated 10.8 million cancer survivors in the United States of America (USA).[3] Sixty percent of these survivors are over 60 years of age. While most of them are less than 5 years from their diagnosis, 14 percent have lived for more than 20 years from their initial diagnosis.

Within the pediatric population, the success story is even more dramatic, where use of risk-based therapy has resulted in an overall 5-year survival rate approaching 80 percent.[4] In 1997, there were an estimated 270 000 survivors of childhood cancer, of whom more than two-thirds were older than 20 years of age.[5] This translates into approximately 1 in 810 individuals under the age of 20 being a childhood cancer survivor, and 1 in 640 individuals between the ages 20 and 39 years having successfully survived childhood cancer.

Improvement in survival has shifted the focus of attention to the quality of survival and issues relating to late treatment-related sequelae. The term 'late effect' refers to a late-occurring or chronic outcome – either physical or psychological – that persists or develops beyond 5 years from the diagnosis of cancer. Among the childhood cancer survivors, approximately two out of every three survivors will experience at least one late effect[6–9] and about one in four will experience a late effect that is severe or life threatening.[10,11] Recognizing that large cohorts of survivors are needed to evaluate the effects of multiple therapies on individuals treated for a variety of neoplasms at different ages, the Childhood Cancer Survivor Study (CCSS)[12] and the Bone Marrow Transplant Survivor Study (BMTSS)[13] were established with funding from the National Cancer Institute. In this chapter, we will focus on a general discussion of selected late effects of cancer treatment used for treating hematologic malignancies, and the health-related quality of life of the cancer survivors.

CARDIOTOXICITY

Chronic cardiotoxicity is a serious complication of cancer therapy, most commonly associated with exposure to anthracyclines in a dose-dependent fashion. In a retrospective review, the incidence of congestive heart failure (CHF) and cardiomyopathy rose from 4 percent at a cumulative dose of 500–550 mg of doxorubicin per square meter to 18 percent at 551–600 mg/m^2 and 36 percent for cumulative doses greater than 600 mg/m^2.[14] While a lower cumulative dose of anthracyclines may place children at increased risk for cardiac compromise,[15] a cumulative dose greater than 300 mg/m^2, when compared with a lower dose, was associated with an increased risk of CHF (relative risk 11.8).[15]

In fact, the use of anthracyclines, one of the most effective groups of anticancer drugs, is limited by the increased risk of development of delayed, life-threatening, dilated and restrictive cardiomyopathy.[14] Recovery from anthracycline-induced CHF is rare with symptomatic management,[14,16,17] and mortality in excess of 50 percent within 2 years from diagnosis is seen in patients with New York Heart Association (NYHA) class III/IV CHF.[16]

Several factors including older age (over 70 years), female gender, combination therapy with other agents (cyclophosphamide, dactinomycin, mitomycin C, and bleomycin), mediastinal radiation (previous or concomitant), previous cardiac disease (coronary, valvular, or myocardial), hypertension, hyperthermia, and liver disease are associated with increased risk for cardiomyopathy.[18,19] In addition to overt CHF, subclinical cardiomyopathy characterized by asymptomatic decrease in fractional shortening (FS) or left ventricular ejection fraction (LVEF) or abnormal left ventricular wall motion has also been associated with anthracyclines.[20] Male gender, older age, higher dose of doxorubicin, association with other anthracyclines, radiation therapy, and being overweight were identified as risk factors for subclinical cardiomyopathy in this group of patients.

Among children, 23 percent to 75 percent of children treated with a median cumulative dose of doxorubicin of 330–450 mg/m^2 (range 200–1275) have been reported to have echocardiographic abnormalities at a median of 7 years after therapy.[21,22] Pathology specimens have shown myocyte hypertrophy. Doxorubicin administered in childhood may result in acute asymptomatic loss of myocytes, which, in turn, results in hypertrophy of the remaining myocytes with inadequate left ventricular mass and secondary heart disease later in life.[22] The long-term evolution of subclinical cardiotoxicity is not known and no treatment recommendations can be made at this time. However, appropriate cardiac follow-up with serial echocardiography is recommended.[23]

These studies and others emphasize that cardiomyopathy can occur many years (15 to 20 years) after completion of therapy and that the onset may be spontaneous or coincide with exertion or pregnancy. During the third trimester of pregnancy the cardiac volume increases, increasing the cardiac workload, leading to overt symptomatology in women with left ventricular dysfunction.[24,25]

Prevention of cardiotoxicity is a primary focus of investigation. Certain analogues of doxorubicin and daunomycin and liposomal anthracyclines, which appear to have decreased cardiotoxicity with equivalent antitumor activity, are being explored. The anthracyclines chelate iron and the anthracycline–iron complex catalyzes the formation of hydroxyl radicals. Agents such as dexrazoxane that are able to remove iron from the anthracyclines have been investigated as cardioprotectants. The large majority of the reports regarding the use of these agents are in the setting of patients with breast cancer.[26] Currently, the American Society of Clinical Oncology recommends dexrazoxane use to be considered for patients with breast cancer who receive more than 300 mg/m^2 of doxorubicin if they have various risk factors including age over 65 years, hypertension, history of myocardial infarction, or previous mediastinal radiation therapy.[27] Additionally, clinical trials of dexrazoxane have been conducted in children, with encouraging evidence of short-term cardioprotection,[28,29] although the long-term avoidance of cardiotoxicity with the use of this agent needs to be determined. Lower doses of anthracyclines and reduced port sizes of radiation therapy may also help in decreasing the incidence of cardiomyopathy. The role of angiotensin-converting enzyme inhibitors in management of subclinical cardiomyopathy among cancer survivors remains controversial.[30,31]

Mediastinal radiation is associated with cardiac toxicity in the form of constrictive pericarditis, valvular heart disease, coronary artery disease, and conduction defects.[32,33] Approximately 5 percent of patients have been shown to have symptomatic heart disease 10 years following mediastinal radiation therapy for HL.[34] It has been shown that up to 29 percent of irradiated patients have a clinically asymptomatic but significant degree of valve disease for which endocarditis prophylaxis should be considered.[35] Clinically significant valvular disease was noted in 6.2 percent of patients at a median of 22 years after radiation and aortic stenosis was the most common lesion. Symptomatic coronary artery disease has been reported in 10 percent of patients at a median of 9 years after mediastinal radiation, and 7.4 percent of patients developed carotid and subclavian artery stenosis at a median of 17 years after irradiation.[36] Higher doses of radiation to the heart and the presence of other known risk factors for coronary artery disease were associated with development of coronary artery disease following mediastinal radiation. Deaths related to myocardial infarction were significantly higher than expected in a large cohort of British HL survivors (standardized mortality ratio: 2.5; 95 percent confidence interval 2.1 to 2.9).[37] The increased risk of mortality related to myocardial infarction persisted for up to 25 years after initial therapy in this cohort. Treatment with supradiaphragmatic radiation therapy, anthracyclines, and vincristine was statistically significantly and independently associated with increased risk of mortality related to myocardial infarction in this study. The association with vincristine has not been previously described and will need further evaluation.[37]

Table 61.1 summarizes guidelines for follow-up of patients at risk for cardiovascular disease after completion of therapy for cancer. These guidelines are derived from the Long-Term Follow-Up Guidelines developed by the Children's Oncology Group (COG).[38]

PULMONARY DYSFUNCTION

Pulmonary fibrosis and pneumonitis can result from pulmonary radiation and is most often observed in patients with HL. Asymptomatic radiographic findings or restrictive

Table 61.1   Monitoring for cardiovascular disease after cancer therapy

Therapeutic agent	Adverse event	Risk factors	Recommendation
Anthracyclines	Cardiomyopathy	Children: – <5 years of age – Cumulative dose >350 mg/m^2 – Mediastinal radiation Adults: – Cumulative dose >550 mg/m^2 – Mediastinal radiation – Hypertension	1. Annual history and physical exam 2. Periodic echocardiography or MUGA with the frequency dependent on the cumulative dose of anthracyclines and presence of other risk factors
Mediastinal radiation	– Valvular disease – CAD	– Higher dose of radiation – Other risk factors for CAD (smoking, hypertension, family history, hypercholesterolemia)	1. Periodic echocardiography 2. Bacterial endocarditis prophylaxis if valve dysfunction present 3. Periodic stress test/stress echocardiography to assess for coronary disease 4. Advise about weight management, healthy diet, control of hypertension, exercise and avoid smoking
Neck radiation	– Carotid stenosis – Subclavian artery stenosis – Stroke	– High doses of radiation	1. Consider carotid Doppler for carotid stenosis several years after therapy

MUGA, multiple-gated acquisition scan; CAD, coronary artery disease.

changes on pulmonary function testing have been reported in more than 30 percent of such individuals.[39] Clinically apparent pneumonitis with cough, fever, or dyspnea occurs in only 5 percent to 15 percent of patients and is generally limited to those who received more than 30 Gy in standard fractions to more than 50 percent of the lung.[40] Obstructive changes have also been reported after conventional radiation therapy.

Radiation-related pulmonary injuries in older patients are likely mediated by cytokine production, which stimulates septal fibroblasts, increasing collagen production and resulting in pulmonary fibrosis.[41] It is important to note that the basis for respiratory damage in young children appears to be different from that in the adult or adolescent. Restrictive lung changes after lower doses of whole-lung radiation (11–14 Gy) have been reported in several studies of children with various malignancies.[42] Some investigators have suggested that children younger than 3 years old at the time of therapy experience more chronic toxicity.[42]

Following hematopoietic stem cell transplantation (HSCT), both restrictive and obstructive lung diseases including bronchiolitis obliterans are well described.[43] Children seem to be at less risk for significant late pulmonary dysfunction than adults,[44] although both restrictive and obstructive pulmonary changes have been described in children following HSCT.

The incidence of radiation-induced late pulmonary toxicity has dramatically decreased in the last decade secondary to refined techniques of radiation therapy. In a published study of patients with stage I and IIA HL treated with radiation alone (40–45 Gy to involved fields), the late pulmonary effects observed were minimal.[45] Use of more modest radiation doses may contribute to further decrease in pulmonary toxicity.[46]

Bleomycin toxicity is the prototype for chemotherapy-related lung injury. Although interstitial pneumonitis and pulmonary fibrosis have been reported in children,[47] clinically apparent bleomycin pneumopathy is most frequent in older adults. The chronic lung toxicity usually follows persistence or progression of abnormalities developing within 3 months of therapy. Like the acute toxicity, it is dose dependent above a threshold cumulative dose of 400 units/m^2 and is exacerbated by concurrent or previous radiation therapy.[48] Above 400 units, in the absence of other risk factors, 10 percent of patients experience fibrosis.[48] At lower doses, fibrosis occurs sporadically in fewer than 5 percent of patients, with a 1 percent to 2 percent mortality rate. Bleomycin pulmonary toxicity has been shown to significantly decrease the overall survival in HL. Age of 40 years or older, higher total dose of bleomycin, and impaired renal function substantially increase the risk of pulmonary toxicity.[49] In some reports, bleomycin toxicity was anticipated on the basis of carbon monoxide diffusing capacity (DLCO) abnormalities. More recently, 2-fluoro-2-deoxy-D-glucose positron emission tomography (FDG-PET) scan has also been noted to be a useful modality for early diagnosis of bleomycin-induced pneumonitis.[50]

Carmustine (BCNU)- and lomustine (CCNU)-related pulmonary toxicity is dose related. Cumulative BCNU

Table 61.2   Monitoring for pulmonary disease after cancer therapy

Therapeutic agent	Adverse event	Risk factors	Recommendations

Lung radiation
Total body radiation
Bleomycin
BCNU/ CCNU
Busulphan
	– Interstitial pneumonitis
	– Pulmonary fibrosis
	– Restrictive/obstructive
	  lung disease
		– Higher cumulative dose of
		  therapeutic exposure
		– Combined modality therapy
		– Cigarette smoking
			1. Annual history and physical exam
			2. Smoking cessation
			3. Periodic pulmonary function tests, DLCO,
			   and chest radiograph
			4. Influenza and pneumococcal vaccinations

DLCO, carbon monoxide diffusing capacity.

doses greater than $600\,mg/m^2$ result in a 50 percent incidence of symptoms.[51] Pulmonary fibrosis has also been observed in 16 percent to 40 percent of transplant recipients treated with cytotoxic conditioning agents including BCNU at doses of 500 to $600\,mg/m^2$; the incidence of fibrosis declines considerably when doses are limited to less than 300 to $450\,mg/m^2$.[52,53] Female patients are at a higher risk for this complication. Cyclophosphamide, melphalan, and busulfan have also been associated with delayed-onset pulmonary fibrosis.[54]

Additional factors contributing to chronic pulmonary toxicity include superimposed infection, underlying pneumopathy (e.g., asthma), exposure to cigarette smoke, chronic graft-versus-host disease, and the effects of chronic pulmonary involvement by tumor or reaction to tumor. Increased oxygen concentrations associated with general anesthesia or SCUBA diving also have been found to exacerbate pulmonary fibrosis.[55,56]

The best approach to chronic pulmonary toxicity of anticancer therapy is preventive, and includes respecting cumulative dosage restrictions of bleomycin and alkylators, limiting radiation dosage and port sizes, and avoiding primary or second-hand smoke. Patients with risk factors for lung disease are discouraged from SCUBA diving. Monitoring guidelines for pulmonary consequences of cancer therapy are derived from the COG Long-Term Follow-Up Guidelines and are summarized in Table 61.2.[38]

SUBSEQUENT MALIGNANCIES

Approximately 85 percent of patients with HL are expected to survive beyond 5 years from diagnosis.[4] Subsequent malignancies are now one of the leading causes of death in long-term survivors of HL.[57] Second or higher-order malignancies constitute approximately 16 percent of incident cancers reported to the National Cancer Institute's Surveillance, Epidemiology, and End Results Program.[4] Several studies have demonstrated a significantly increased incidence of therapy-related myelodysplasia (t-MDS) and acute myeloid leukemia (t-AML), as well as solid tumors involving breast, uterine cervix, skin, salivary glands, colon, esophagus, stomach, small intestine, lung, and thyroid tissue, among survivors of HL.[58–60] Data from a recently published population-based study show an actuarial

risk of developing a solid tumor 25 years after treatment for HL to be 21.9 percent.[58] For several solid tumor sites, such as esophagus, stomach, colon, female breast, and urinary bladder, risks do not increase until 10 years after diagnosis and remain elevated for at least a decade. This temporal pattern is suggestive of a radiation-induced process. Increased risk for other cancers such as bone and connective tissue, acute leukemia, NHL, and melanoma is noted both in early as well as later years of follow-up after HL. Such a pattern of occurrence may suggest that chemotherapy and radiation play a role in these cancers.

Breast cancer is the most frequent solid tumor among female survivors of HL. Breast tissue at young ages is known to have increased sensitivity to ionizing radiation and breast cancer risk is inversely related to age at treatment, with largest risk (6–15-fold) reported among women treated at age 30 years or younger.[59,61] The risk of breast cancer increases with higher doses of radiation while ovarian damage secondary to alkylating agents reduces it.[60] Increased risk for breast cancer persists for 25 or more years following the diagnosis of HL.[62] The rate of bilateral lesions is also reported to be high in this population.[63] A recent study using individualized dosimetry data to model the risk of radiation-induced second cancer predicts a significant reduction of 20-year excess relative risk for breast and lung cancer with contemporary involved field radiation therapy as compared to mantle field radiation.[64]

Radiation therapy for several primary cancers, including HL, acute lymphoblastic leukemia, and after total-body irradiation (TBI) for HSCT, has been associated with thyroid cancer.[65–67] The risk of thyroid cancer was reported to be 18-fold that of the general population among 1791 5 year survivors of HL followed as part of the CCSS cohort.[68] Thyroid cancer has also been reported among patients receiving radiation to the craniospinal axis for acute lymphoblastic leukemia.[65]

The risk of lung cancer is significantly increased in survivors of HL, with a mean relative risk of 2.6–7.0 in various studies.[69] Both chemotherapy and chest radiation contribute to the risk. Chemotherapy-related risk is highest in the first 10 years after therapy while radiation-associated lung cancer is reported up to 25 years after treatment. Exposure to alkylating agents such as procarbazine, chlorambucil, dacarbazine, mechlorethamine, and nitrosoureas has been associated with increased risk of lung cancer.[70,71] The risk is known to be higher among smokers, and appears to expand with increasing length of follow-up of survivors.[70] Among survivors of HL, the risk escalates with increasing dose of radiation and is much greater among the patients who smoked after the diagnosis of HL.[72] Lung cancer has the largest absolute excess risk among patients with HL diagnosed between 40 and 60 years of age. In one study, the cumulative incidence of lung cancer 25 years after diagnosis of HL was 6 percent for males and 3 percent for females.[58] Significantly increased risk of lung cancer has been reported 1 to 4 years after initial treatment with alkylating agents. Although uncommon, radiation-associated pleural mesothelioma has been reported, usually occurring 20 to 24 years after radiation, developing in the absence of exposure to asbestos.[73]

Cancers of the gastrointestinal tract, including that of the esophagus, stomach, colon, and rectum, have been reported to occur at a cumulative incidence of 5 percent at 25 years after HL. Radiation therapy and combined modality therapy are associated with increased risk for such cancers.[58] Increased risk of cancer of urinary bladder has also been reported following HL and is considered to be secondary to exposure to inverted-Y field of radiation as well as cyclophosphamide.[58] Children receiving cranial radiation have increased risk of developing brain tumors and meningiomas.

Alkylating agents[74] and topoisomerase II inhibitors[75] have been associated with the development of therapy-related myelodysplasia and acute myeloid leukemia (t-MDS/AML). A dose-dependent relationship is noted with alkylating agents, which typically cause leukemia after latencies of 5 to 10 years. Abnormalities of chromosomes 5 or 7 are found in t-MDS/AML associated with alkylating agents. Topoisomerase II inhibitor-associated t-AML classically has a shorter latency, no preceding dysplastic phase, and cytogenetic abnormalities involving chromosome 11q23. Older age (over 40 years), combined modality therapy including alkylating agent exposure, advanced stage disease, and splenectomy or splenic irradiation increase risk of t-MDS/AML in survivors of HL.[76,77] Genetic polymorphisms of enzymes capable of metabolic activation or detoxification of anticancer drugs, such as NAD(P)H:quinone oxidoreductase 1 (NQO1), glutathione-S-transferase (GST) M1 and T1, and CYP3A4, have been examined for their role in the development of t-MDS/AML. These studies indicate that NQO1 polymorphism and CYP3A4-W genotype is significantly associated with the genetic risk of t-MDS/AML.[78] The incidence of t-MDS/AML has been estimated at 5–20 percent at 10 years after autologous HSCT for HL or NHL.[79] Specific risk factors include older age, low stem cell dose, use of peripheral blood stem cells, prior radiation therapy, extent and type of prior chemotherapy, conditioning with total body irradiation, and use of etoposide for stem cell priming.[79–81] Survival following development of t-MDS/AML is generally poor. One recent study showed that median survival after development of t-MDS/AML in patients treated for HL was only

0.4 years and 5-year survival was 4.9 percent (0.0–14.2 percent).[82]

Alcohol consumption has been shown to be a risk factor for oral, esophageal, and liver cancers occurring as second cancers.[83] The associations between other important environmental exposures and lifestyle factors and subsequent adult-onset cancers are not known. The suggested recommendations for screening for second malignancies in cancer survivors are in Table 61.3.[38]

NEUROCOGNITIVE IMPAIRMENT

Neurocognitive impairment is seen in childhood cancer survivors as a consequence of radiation to the whole brain, systemic therapy with high-dose methotrexate or cytarabine, or with intrathecal methotrexate and other agents. Children with a history of acute lymphoblastic leukemia or NHL are most likely to be affected. Risk factors include increasing radiation dose, young age at the time of therapy, treatment with both cranial radiation and systemic or intrathecal chemotherapy, and female gender.[84] Severe deficits are most frequently noted in children who were younger than 5 years of age at the time of treatment.

Neurocognitive deficits usually become evident within 1 to 2 years following radiation and are progressive in nature. Children affected may experience information-processing deficits resulting in academic difficulties. These children are particularly prone to problems with receptive and expressive language, attention span, and visual and perceptual motor skills. They most often experience academic difficulties in the areas of reading, language, and mathematics. Children in the younger age groups may experience significant drops in IQ scores, with irradiation- or chemotherapy-induced destruction in normal white matter partially explaining intellectual and academic achievement deficits.[85]

Cognitive deficits associated with cancer treatment have also been recognized as one of the major challenges facing survivors of adult-onset cancers.[86] A growing number of studies have demonstrated that adults with cancer experience cognitive deficits associated with a variety of treatments including cranial radiation, conventional chemotherapy, high-dose chemotherapy, HSCT, and biologic response modifiers.[87,88] A study of long-term survivors, who were 5 years from diagnosis and disease-free of breast cancer and lymphoma, showed that patients treated with systemic chemotherapy had significantly lower scores on a battery of neuropsychological tests compared with those treated with local therapy only.[88] Verbal memory and psychomotor functioning were most affected. The significant overall effect of treatment across domains suggests that the effect is relatively diffuse. The cognitive deficits have been identified as long as 10 years after therapy, suggesting that these effects may persist indefinitely. Neuropsychological performance index of this group of patients was generally within the normal range. Thus the

Table 61.3 Monitoring for second malignant neoplasms after cancer therapy

Therapeutic agent	Adverse event	Risk factors	Recommendation
Alkylating agents topoisomerase II inhibitors	t-MDS/AML	– Autologous peripheral blood stem cell transplantation	1. Annual complete blood count for 10–15 years
Radiation to following sites – Mantle – Mediastinal – Whole lung	Breast cancer	– Higher dose of radiation – Exposure before 30 years of age – Ovarian suppression reduces risk	1. Monthly self breast exam 2. Every 6 month clinical breast exam 3. Annual mammography starting 8 years after or at age 25 years (whichever is later)
Radiation to following sites – Mantle – Mediastinal – Whole lung	Lung cancer	– Smoking	1. Annual physical exam 2. Smoking cessation
Radiation to following sites – Neck – Total body radiation	Thyroid cancer	– Younger age at treatment – Female gender	1. Palpation of neck at annual physical examination 2. Ultrasound if any thyroid nodule
Radiation to following sites – Abdominal/pelvic	Colorectal cancer		1. Fecal occult blood annually 2. Colonoscopy every 10 years or flexible sigmoidoscopy every 5 years starting at age 35 years or 15 years after therapy (whichever is later)
Radiation to any site	Skin cancer/ soft tissue sarcoma	Sunburn	1. Careful annual physical examination of skin and soft tissues in radiation field 2. Advice about sunscreen and avoiding sunburn
Transfusion-associated chronic viral hepatitis	Hepatocellular carcinoma		1. Annual serum alpha feto-protein, liver ultrasound in patients with cirrhosis

t-MDS/AML, therapy-related myelodysplasia and acute myeloid leukemia.

effects of chemotherapy, although important to the individual, are generally subtle.

The pathogenesis of radiation-induced central nervous system damage is only partially understood and evidence suggests that direct effects on intracranial endothelial cells and brain white matter, as well as immunologic mechanisms, play a role. A spectrum of clinical syndromes may occur, including radionecrosis, necrotizing leukoencephalopathy, and mineralizing microangiopathy with dystrophic calcification, cerebellar sclerosis, and spinal cord dysfunction.[89] Mulhern et al. have shown an association between full scale IQ and the volume of white matter loss determined by quantitative neuroimaging,[85,90] providing a model to better predict neurocognitive outcomes and identify those at higher risk.

The mechanism of chemotherapy-related cognitive changes is not known. Some of the possible mechanisms include direct neurotoxic effects leading to atrophy of cerebral gray matter and/or demyelination of white matter fibers, secondary immunologic responses causing inflammatory reactions, and microvascular injury. Altered neurotransmitter levels and metabolites could constitute an additional mechanism related to neurotoxic effects.[91] Advanced brain-imaging techniques such as morphometric magnetic resonance imaging (MRI), functional MRI (fMRI), diffusion

tensor imaging (DTI), and MR spectroscopy (MRS) can directly or indirectly assess many of these mechanisms, but to date there has been very limited application of these tools.

Recognition of cognitive deficits among survivors is important as cognitive rehabilitation approaches, which have been shown to improve functioning of other types of patients with subtle cognitive deficits, may be effective for cancer patients experiencing deficits secondary to chemotherapy and radiation.

GROWTH

Severe growth retardation, defined as a standing height below the fifth percentile, has been observed in 10 percent to 15 percent of children treated for cancer.[92,93] One major risk factor for short stature is whole-brain irradiation, especially in doses exceeding 18 Gy.[94] Treatment with 18 Gy affects the final height to a lesser degree.[95] Survivors of acute lymphoblastic leukemia treated with 24 Gy cranial irradiation have a decrease in median height of about five to ten centimeters.[93,96] The effects of cranial irradiation are age related, and the consensus is that children younger than 5 years at the time of therapy are particularly susceptible to its growth-inhibiting properties. One recent study identified age less than 8 years at the time of cranial irradiation as a risk factor for adult height below the third percentile.[92] Young girls may be at greatest risk, [93,94,97] although this observation has not been universal.[92] The precise mechanism by which cranial irradiation induces short stature is not clear. Growth hormone deficiency, early onset of puberty in girls with acute lymphoblastic leukemia – also reported as a consequence of cranial irradiation – and direct inhibition of vertebral growth by spinal irradiation may contribute to loss of final height.

Among children with acute lymphoblastic leukemia who received abdominal irradiation (12 Gy) in addition to 18 to 24 Gy of craniospinal irradiation, almost 30 percent had standing heights less than the fifth percentile.[93] This result may have been due to irradiation of the gonads or thyroid, scatter radiation to the femoral heads, or both. When lower doses (10–25 Gy) have been given to ports including part or all of the spine, patients – although not necessarily short – have reduced sitting heights (measured from crown to rump).[98] Such is the case for as many as 40 percent of long-term survivors of HL. This problem has been seen particularly in children who are either younger than 6 years old or who are undergoing their adolescent growth spurt at the time of radiation therapy. Thoraco-abdominal preparative radiation in the setting of HSCT also has been associated with short stature.[99] Fractionation of TBI appears to decrease growth retardation.[100] The pathogenesis of short stature in these children includes factors other than radiation, notably graft-versus-host disease and its therapy. Treatment with growth hormone prior to closure of epiphyses in patients with documented growth hormone deficiency usually results in near-normalization of final height, unless the spinal axis has also been irradiated.

Growth hormone also has an important physiological role in adulthood.[101] Growth hormone deficiency after radiation-induced damage to the hypothalamic-pituitary axis is one of the few evolving forms of growth hormone deficiency; i.e., the growth hormone production continues to decline over time.[102] Deficiency of growth hormone in adults can cause abnormalities of metabolism, body composition, and bone mineralization.[103] Impaired cardiac muscle function as well as central obesity and unfavorable lipid profile has been reported in adults with growth hormone deficiency.[103–105] Furthermore, growth hormone deficiency may have profound effects on psychosocial well-being and quality of life.[106]

Growth hormone therapy during childhood is often stopped after attainment of final height. However, it is now known that continuation of growth hormone therapy is necessary in patients with severe growth hormone deficiency to maintain a favorable body composition and bone mass.[107,108] The biochemical criteria for growth hormone deficiency in childhood differ from those used in adults. While children with all degrees of growth hormone (GH) deficiency from severe to mild (GH <6.7 ng/mL; 1 ng/mL = 3 mU/L) are considered for growth hormone replacement, only adults with severe growth hormone deficiency (GH <3 ng/mL) receive replacement therapy.[109] Growth hormone deficiency in the absence of any significant effect

on final height has been found in young adult survivors of childhood acute lymphoblastic leukemia who received cranial radiation.[110] Growth hormone deficiency has been reported occasionally following chemotherapy without exposure to cranial radiation.[111]

THYROID FUNCTION

Hypothyroidism is a common late effect and almost always is due to radiation to the neck for a nonthyroid malignancy. At a mean of 7 years after radiation doses of 15 to 70 Gy, laboratory evidence of primary hypothyroidism (increased serum thyrotropin [TSH] with normal or low thyroxine [T4] levels) has been demonstrated in 30 percent to 90 percent of patients with HL and NHL[68,112,113] and in as many as 50 percent of children after HSCT for hematologic malignancy.[114]

The likelihood of abnormalities depends on radiation dose. Children treated with less than 20 Gy have a less than 20 percent incidence of hypothyroidism. In the CCSS study, among patients treated with radiation doses exceeding 45 Gy, the actuarial risk of hypothyroidism at 20 years was 50 percent.[68] Within the pediatric age range, adolescents may experience more severe abnormalities, with higher TSH levels than those seen in young children. Other factors that may contribute to the development of hypothyroidism in survivors of cancer include female gender, hemithyroidectomy, and use of iodide-containing contrast material, as in lymphangiography. In some instances, hypothyroidism has been reversible after as long as 3 years, even without replacement therapy.[112] The risk of thyroid nodules has been reported to be 27-fold that of sibling controls, occurring at a mean latency of 14 years after treatment.[68] Female gender and radiation dose exceeding 25 Gy are independent risk factors. About 7 percent of nodules have been found to be malignant. Significant thyrotoxicity from antileukemic chemotherapy and MOPP (mechlorethamine, vincristine, procarbazine, and prednisone) for HL without radiation is notably absent.[112] Secondary hypothyroidism with low TSH and T4 levels appears to be uncommon after radiation to the head or neck.[98] Hyperthyroidism has been described in about 5 percent of patients after radiation for HL[68,113] or other nonthyroid neoplasms of the neck[115] and after TBI for HSCT.[116]

Radiation therapy to the neck increases the risk for developing thyroid carcinoma. The risk of thyroid cancer has been shown to increase with increasing dose of radiation up to 20–29 Gy. However, the risk decreases at higher doses with about 95 percent reduction in excess relative risk at doses of 40 Gy or higher. Age less than 10 years at time of diagnosis is associated with increased risk.[117]

Careful shielding of the thyroid during irradiation, elimination of radiation, or the use of lower doses and avoidance of the concurrent use of radiation and iodide-containing contrast materials should help to decrease the incidence of thyroid abnormalities. Patients who have received direct radiation to the neck should be routinely screened indefinitely for thyroid abnormalities by physical examination, since nodules may be late appearing. Recommendations as per the COG Long-Term Follow-Up Guidelines[38] for monitoring are described in Table 61.4.

GONADAL FUNCTION

Male gonadal function

All therapeutic modalities (radiation, surgery, or chemotherapy) can cause germ-cell depletion as well as abnormalities of gonadal endocrine function among male cancer survivors. Radiation to the testes is known to result in germinal loss with decreases in testicular volume and sperm production and increases in follicle-stimulating hormone (FSH). These effects are dose dependent, following fractionated exposures of 0.1 to 6 Gy.[118] All males treated with inverted-Y radiation for HL at a cumulative testicular dose of 1.4 to 3.0 Gy become azoospermic without recovery after 2–40 months of follow-up, despite lead shielding of the scrotum.[119] At doses of 4–6 Gy, azoospermia may persist for at least 3–5 years, and at doses above 6 Gy usually appears to be irreversible.[120,121] Monitoring of gonadal function in a large group of male patients who were past puberty at the time of TBI at a dose of 10 Gy delivered in a single fraction, has revealed azoospermia to be universal, although two of 41 patients had recovery of sperm production 6 years after HSCT.[116]

Prepubertal testicular germ cells also appear to be radiosensitive, although tubular damage may be difficult to assess until the patient progresses through puberty.[122] Data on gonadal function in boys treated with radiation alone for HL[123] or with TBI for acute myeloid leukemia[114] before puberty are limited, but they are consistent with data from older patients. Transplantation of the testes to the thigh or abdomen during radiation appears to spare the prepubertal testis.[124]

Radiation therapy may also be toxic to Leydig cells, although at doses higher than those which are toxic to germ cells. As summarized by Sklar,[125] Leydig cell damage is dose dependent and inversely related to age at treatment. Boys treated prepubertally or peripubertally with ≥20 Gy for testicular leukemia, in addition to suffering germ-cell depletion, are at high risk of delayed sexual maturation associated with decreased testosterone levels, despite increased luteinizing hormone (LH) levels. Fractionated doses of less than 12 Gy to the prepubertal testis are compatible with normal pubertal maturation in most patients, although often at the expense of compensated Leydig cell failure (normal testosterone levels with elevated LH levels).[125] Adolescent and young adult male testes are relatively radioresistant, and fractionated doses greater than 30 Gy to the testes may induce Leydig cell failure in only about 50 percent of cases.[126]

Alkylating agents decrease spermatogenesis in a dose-dependent fashion. At doses below 7.5 g/m^2 or 200 mg/kg, as used in HSCT, the damage may be reversible in up to 70 percent of patients after an interval of several years.[127] Germ-cell depletion occurs as an acute toxicity in younger patients as well.[128] Among pubertal or adult males treated for HL, azoospermia is found in 80–100 percent of patients treated with five or six cycles of MOPP. Exposure to more than three cycles of MOPP conveys a risk of azoospermia.[129] This effect is reversible in only about 20 percent of cases, even 7 years after completion of therapy. After doxorubicin (adriamycin), bleomycin, vinblastine, and dacarbazine (ABVD), the incidence of azoospermia appears to be lower (36 percent) and the incidence of recovery higher (100 percent) than after MOPP.[130]

Azoospermia or oligospermia is also common in survivors of acute lymphoblastic leukemia in childhood or adolescence treated on Berlin-Frankfurt-Munster (BFM) regimens.[131] Cyclophosphamide has replaced mechlorethamine in many HL protocols in an effort to reduce the risk of azoospermia. In contrast to their prominent effects on germ-cell epithelium, chemotherapy effects are less striking on slowly dividing Leydig cells, and may be age related. Normal pubertal development and testosterone levels are seen following MOPP in prepubertal boys. Gynecomastia with low testosterone and increased LH has been reported in patients treated during adolescence, and compensated Leydig cell failure (increased LH with low normal testosterone levels or exaggerated FSH and LH responses to LH-releasing hormone) without gynecomastia is common in adults.[129,132,133] Compensated Leydig cell failure has been found at the time of diagnosis in almost half of men with HL.[134] Decline in libido without impotence may be a common problem and does not correlate with testosterone levels. The reversibility of these abnormalities has not been addressed in the literature.

The effects of surgery on the gonads include impotence or retrograde ejaculation after bilateral retroperitoneal lymph node dissection. Hydroceles have been seen in long-term survivors of HL[135] after surgery or radiation therapy.

The gonadal toxicities, although not life threatening, are of serious concern to patients and their families. Although many men with HL have lower-than-expected sperm counts and decreased sperm motility at the time of diagnosis, discussion of sperm banking with adolescent male patients and their parents is advisable. Recommendations for screening for gonadal dysfunction are described in Table 61.4. Conversely, reminders about contraception should be given in light of the potential for recovery of spermatogenesis and interpatient variations in gonadal toxicity.

Female gonadal function

In contrast to what occurs in male survivors, germ-cell failure and loss of ovarian endocrine function usually occur concomitantly in females. Following radiation therapy, manifestations are both age and dose dependent. In women older than 40 years at the time of treatment, irreversible ovarian failure (amenorrhea, increased LH and FSH levels with or without symptoms of menopause, and loss of libido) is an almost universal result of 4 Gy to 7 Gy conventionally fractionated radiation delivered to both ovaries (as in whole-abdomen irradiation).[136] Prepubertal ovaries are relatively radioresistant.[137] When secondary amenorrhea results, it appears to be reversible within several months to 4 years in 50–60 percent of patients.[138] In some series, TBI (10 Gy single fraction) has been associated with primary amenorrhea and absent secondary sexual characteristics in most patients treated as young girls and followed for as long as 10 years.[114] However, others have reported normal pubertal progression, although with elevated FSH levels following TBI during early childhood.[139] As with standard radiation, increasing age at the time of TBI has been found to predict ovarian failure.[140] Premature menopause has also been reported in the setting of HSCT.[114] The effect of ovarian scatter from craniospinal radiation is less clear.

Ovarian failure secondary to chemotherapy is most frequently described with single alkylating agents (cyclophosphamide, busulfan, nitrogen mustard) and MOPP.[141,142] As with radiation therapy, chemotherapy results in dose- and age-dependent toxicity. Women older than 40 years may develop amenorrhea with as little as one to four cycles of MOPP. In contrast, 30 percent of women younger than 35 years of age require 3 to 12 cycles to become amenorrheic.[141] Young girls treated with conventional doses of single alkylating agents or MOPP generally are capable of normal puberty,[129,142] although they may have biopsy-proven or transient clinical evidence of ovarian failure.[142,143] Moreover, measurement of serum anti-Mullerian hormone and inhibin levels, and sonographic measurement of ovarian size, suggest that subclinical abnormalities of ovarian function may occur despite normal menses and gonadotropin levels.[144]

Based on results of the Five Center Study, the incidence of premature menopause in women who had been treated prior to puberty is not greatly in excess of controls.[145] Following myeloablative doses of alkylating agents, including busulfan and cyclophosphamide, permanent ovarian failure can be expected at all ages.[146] Unilateral oophorectomy does not appear to compromise gonadal function,[147] although long-term follow-up data regarding onset of menopause have not been reported.

In an attempt to prevent gonadal failure, some investigators have studied the use of oral contraceptives to suppress ovulation and thus prevent loss of ova.[148] Harvesting and freezing of ova prior to therapy that is likely to cause premature ovarian failure is under investigation.[149] Survivors with concerns regarding fertility are urged to seek consultation with reproductive endocrinologists. Table 61.4 summarizes

Table 61.4 Monitoring for neurocognitive and endocrine dysfunction after cancer therapy

Therapeutic agent	Adverse event	Risk factors	Recommendations
Cranial radiation	Neurocognitive deficits	High dose of systemic or intrathecal – Methotrexate – Cytarabine Higher dose of radiation Younger age at exposure Female gender	1. Consider neuropsychological evaluation at end of therapy 2. Assess educational and vocational progress annually
Cranial radiation Total body irradiation	Growth hormone deficiency	Younger age at exposure Higher dose of radiation	1. Monitor height, weight, BMI, Tanner staging every 6 months until growth is complete 2. Consult endocrinology if drop in percentile, growth velocity, lack of pubertal growth 3. Evaluate thyroid function in any poorly growing child
Radiation to the neck	Hypothyroidism	Higher dose of radiation Older age Female gender	1. Annual thyroid exam 2. Free T4 and TSH annually
Alkylating agents Radiation to gonads	Infertility Delayed sexual maturation Premature menopause	Postpubertal age Higher dose of alkylators Radiation to gonads/brain	1. Annual physical examination for sexual maturation, Tanner staging, gynecomastia in boys 2. History of primary/secondary amenorrhea, difficulty conceiving 3. Check LH, FSH, testosterone and estradiol at 11 years of age and repeat annually until puberty achieved 4. In adults enquire about libido and sexual dysfunction

BMI, body mass index; T4, thyroxine; TSH, thyrotropin; LH, luteinizing hormone; FSH, follicle-stimulating hormone.

the recommendations for monitoring for gonadal failure, which are adapted from the COG Long-Term Follow-Up Guidelines.[38]

QUALITY OF LIFE

Improved survival from childhood cancer has placed increasing emphasis on the health status and health-related quality of life (HRQL) among survivors. Numerous studies have shown that cancer and its treatment predispose individuals to late morbidity and increase the risk of mortality in long-term childhood cancer survivors.[150,151] Studies of psychosocial functioning of adult survivors of childhood cancer have shown that 10–20 percent of individuals show signs of psychological maladjustment in the form of mood disturbances, behavioral problems, and somatic distress.[150–152] Most of these studies focus on adult survivors of childhood cancer and indicate that the general health as perceived by adult survivors of childhood cancer is very good, with only a small proportion of patients reporting fair or poor health. Survivors of HL and NHL are significantly more likely than sibling controls to report symptoms of depression and somatic distress. Female gender, lower level of educational attainment, and lower socioeconomic status increase the risk for adverse health status and symptomatic levels of depression and somatic distress.[153,154]

Some studies have reported a better HRQL among off-therapy survivors when compared with healthy controls. These findings were most notable among younger survivors.[155,156] A possible explanation is that these survivors may have been too young to experience negative psychosocial impacts of cancer and its treatment.

Studies of HRQL among survivors of adult-onset HL have shown that in comparison with healthy controls, the survivors have more restrictions in physical functioning and lower perceived overall health. The survivors also have been found to have problems with sexual functioning and are less satisfied with their sexual lives. They have greater difficulty in obtaining personal loans and life insurance and have a higher rate of health-related unemployment.[157] Furthermore, several studies have demonstrated the positive coping strategies and processes used by cancer survivors and the ways that quality of life may be enhanced rather than diminished by the experience of having faced a potentially fatal disease and toxic and painful treatments.[158]

Fatigue is a common symptom in survivors of HL and NHL.[159] No significant associations have been found between treatment characteristics and fatigue. Fatigue is also very prevalent among patients with NHL who have undergone autologous HSCT. Females were more likely to be fatigued in this population and many had gonadal dysfunction.[160]

Health-related quality of life has been shown to be adversely affected in survivors of HSCT in several studies.[161,162] In general, the overall HRQL in this group of patients was significantly reduced in the first year after autologous HSCT and improved with interval from transplant, reaching the level of the general population after 4 years. The recipients of allogeneic HSCT have been found to have worse HRQL than autologous recipients. Older age at HSCT, more advanced disease, and lower level of education were associated with poorer HRQL.

DELIVERING SURVIVORSHIP CARE

Providing appropriate health care for survivors of cancer is emerging as one of the major challenges in medicine. Several key components are required for optimal survivorship care.[163] These include: (1) longitudinal care utilizing a comprehensive multidisciplinary team approach; (2) continuity with a single health-care provider coordinating needed services; and (3) an emphasis on the whole person, with sensitivity to the cancer experience and its impact on the entire family. Providing comprehensive risk-based care that is readily accessible to survivors is a significant challenge. Therefore, finding ways to educate local health-care providers regarding necessary follow-up is a priority.

The Children's Oncology Group recently released risk-based, exposure-related guidelines (*Long-Term Follow-Up Guidelines for Survivors of Childhood, Adolescent, and Young Adult Cancers*) specifically designed to direct follow-up care for patients who were diagnosed and treated for pediatric malignancies.[38] These guidelines represent a set of comprehensive screening recommendations that are clinically relevant and can be used to standardize and direct the follow-up care for this group of cancer survivors with specialized health-care needs. The entire set of guidelines, with associated Health Links, can be downloaded from www.survivorshipguidelines.org

SUMMARY

This review has detailed selected topics relating to the late effects of therapy in patients with hematologic malignancies. Within the spectrum of potential late effects for this ever-increasing population of cancer survivors, there are other important outcomes that clearly can have a significant impact on subsequent quality of life. Examples of other outcomes include musculoskeletal effects (e.g., osteoporosis and avascular necrosis); dental complications (e.g., developmental defects of tooth enamel and roots); compromise of the ocular function (e.g., Sjögren syndrome, cataracts, glaucoma); reproduction (e.g., fertility, pregnancy outcomes, health of offspring); and hematologic and immunologic function (e.g., bone marrow reserve, cell-mediated immunity).

Most of the available information relates to outcomes within the first decade following treatment and only minimal data address the longer-term outcomes that may occur many years after cancer treatment. It is critical that we understand the potential long-term impact of cancer therapy if we are to effectively counsel survivors and offer effective intervention strategies to prevent or minimize the impact of adverse late effects.

KEY POINTS

- Improvement in survival is resulting in a growing population of cancer survivors, currently estimated to be 10.8 million.
- The term 'late effects' refers to a late-occurring or chronic outcome – either physical or psychological – that persists or develops beyond 5 years from the diagnosis of cancer.
- Long-term consequences include organ dysfunction (cardiopulmonary, endocrine), neurocognitive impairment, second malignancies, impaired quality of life, and premature mortality.
- There is a well-defined association of these late effects with therapeutic exposures, thus leading to identification of 'high risk' groups of survivors.
- There is urgent need for follow-up of long-term survivors utilizing standardized recommendations that are determined by therapeutic exposures, such as those developed by the Children's Oncology Group (Long-Term Follow-Up Guidelines for Survivors of Childhood, Adolescent, and Young Adult Cancers, available at www.survivorshipguidelines.org
- Ongoing research is needed to identify new late effects with the constantly changing landscape of new therapeutic modalities.

REFERENCES

● = Key primary paper
◆ = Major review article

1. Ganz P. *Abolishing the myths: the facts about cancer.* Mount Vernon, NY: Consumers Union, 1990.
2. Parker SL, Tong T, Bolden S, Wingo PA. Cancer statistics, 1997. *CA Cancer J Clin* 1997; **47**: 5–27.
3. Estimated number of cancer survivors in the United States from 1971 to 2004. *National Cancer Institute* 2008. http://dccps.nci.nih.gov/ocs/prevalence/prevalence.html# survivor
4. Ries LAG, Melbert D, Krapcho M *et al.* (eds) *SEER Cancer Statistics Review, 1975–2004.* Bethesda, MD: National Cancer Institute. Based on 2006 SEER data submission. http://seer.cancer.gov/csr/1975_2004
5. Hewitt MWS, Simone JV. (eds) *Childhood cancer survivorship: improving care and quality of life.* Washington, DC: National Academies Press, 2003.

6. Garre ML, Gandus S, Cesana B *et al.* Health status of long-term survivors after cancer in childhood. Results of an uninstitutional study in Italy. *Am J Pediatr Hematol Oncol* 1994; **16**: 143–52.
7. Oeffinger KC, Eshelman DA, Tomlinson GE *et al.* Grading of late effects in young adult survivors of childhood cancer followed in an ambulatory adult setting. *Cancer* 2000; **88**: 1687–95.
●8. Stevens MC, Mahler H, Parkes S. The health status of adult survivors of cancer in childhood. *Eur J Cancer* 1998; **34**: 694–8.
9. Vonderweid N, Beck D, Caflisch U *et al.* Standardized assessment of late effects in long-term survivors of childhood cancer in Switzerland: results of a Swiss Pediatric Oncology Group (SPOG) pilot study. *Int J Pediatr Hematol Oncol* 1996; **3**: 483–90.
●10. Oeffinger KC, Mertens AC, Sklar CA *et al.* Chronic health conditions in adult survivors of childhood cancer. *N Engl J Med* 2006; **355**: 1572–82.
●11. Geenen MM, Cardous-Ubbink MC, Kremer LC *et al.* Medical assessment of adverse health outcomes in long-term survivors of childhood cancer. *JAMA* 2007; **297**: 2705–15.
12. Robison LL, Mertens AC, Boice JD Jr *et al.* Study design and cohort characteristics of the Childhood Cancer Survivor Study: a multi-institutional collaborative project. *Med Pediatr Oncol* 2002; **38**: 229–39.
13. Bhatia S, Robison LL, Francisco L *et al.* Late mortality in survivors of autologous hematopoietic-cell transplantation: report from the Bone Marrow Transplant Survivor Study. *Blood* 2005; **105**: 4215–22.
14. Lefrak EA, Pitha J, Rosenheim S, Gottlieb JA. A clinicopathologic analysis of adriamycin cardiotoxicity. *Cancer* 1973; **32**: 302–14.
●15. Kremer LCM, van Dalen EC, Offringa M *et al.* Anthracycline-induced clinical heart failure in a cohort of 607 children: long-term follow-up study. *J Clin Oncol* 2001; **19**: 191–6.
16. Ryberg M, Nielsen D, Skovsgaard T *et al.* Epirubicin cardiotoxicity: an analysis of 469 patients with metastatic breast cancer. *J Clin Oncol* 1998; **16**: 3502–8.
◆17. Singal PK, Iliskovic N. Doxorubicin-induced cardiomyopathy. *N Engl J Med* 1998; **339**: 900–5.
18. Von Hoff DD, Rozencweig M, Layard M *et al.* Daunomycin-induced cardiotoxicity in children and adults. A review of 110 cases. *Am J Med* 1977; **62**: 200–8.
19. Pihkala J, Saarinen UM, Lundstrom U *et al.* Myocardial function in children and adolescents after therapy with anthracyclines and chest irradiation. *Eur J Cancer* 1996; **32A**: 97–103.
20. Hequet O, Le QH, Moullet I *et al.* Subclinical late cardiomyopathy after doxorubicin therapy for lymphoma in adults. *J Clin Oncol* 2004; **22**: 1864–71.
●21. Steinherz LJ, Steinherz PG, Tan CT *et al.* Cardiac toxicity 4 to 20 years after completing anthracycline therapy. *JAMA* 1991; **266**: 1672–7.

●22. Lipshultz SE, Colan SD, Gelber RD *et al.* Late cardiac effects of doxorubicin therapy for acute lymphoblastic leukemia in childhood. *N Engl J Med* 1991; **324**: 808–15.

23. Wang TJ, Levy D, Benjamin EJ, Vasan RS. The epidemiology of 'asymptomatic' left ventricular systolic dysfunction: implications for screening. *Ann Intern Med* 2003; **138**: 907–6.

24. Pan PH, Moore CH. Doxorubicin-induced cardiomyopathy during pregnancy: three case reports of anesthetic management for cesarian and vaginal delivery in two kyphoscoliotic patients. *Anesthesiology* 2002; **97**: 513–15.

25. Hinkle AS, Proukou CB, Deshpande SS *et al.* Cardiovascular complications: Cardiotoxicity caused by chemotherapy. In: Wallace H, Green DM. (eds) *Late effects of childhood cancer.* New York: Oxford University Press, 2004.

26. Swain SM, Whaley FS, Gerber MC *et al.* Cardioprotection with dexrazoxane for doxorubicin-containing therapy in advanced breast cancer. *J Clin Oncol* 1997; **15**: 1318–32.

◆27. Hensley ML, Schuchter LM, Lindley C *et al.* American Society of Clinical Oncology clinical practice guidelines for the use of chemotherapy and radiotherapy protectants. *J Clin Oncol* 1999; **17**: 3333–55.

28. Bu'Lock FA, Gabriel HM, Oakhill A *et al.* Cardioprotection by ICRF187 against high dose anthracycline toxicity in children with malignant disease. *Br Heart J* 1993; **70**: 185–8.

●29. Lipshultz SE, Rifai N, Dalton VM *et al.* The effect of dexrazoxane on myocardial injury in doxorubicin-treated children with acute lymphoblastic leukemia. *N Engl J Med* 2004; **351**: 145–53.

30. Lipshultz SE, Lipsitz SR, Sallan SE *et al.* Long-term enalapril therapy for left ventricular dysfunction in doxorubicin-treated survivors of childhood cancer. *J Clin Oncol* 2002; **20**: 4517–22.

●31. Silber JH, Cnaan A, Clark BJ, *et al.* Design and baseline characteristics for the ACE Inhibitor After Anthracycline (AAA) study of cardiac dysfunction in long-term pediatric cancer survivors. *Am Heart J* 2001; **142**: 577–85.

32. Hancock SL, Tucker MA, Hoppe RT. Factors affecting late mortality from heart disease after treatment of Hodgkin's disease. *JAMA* 1993; **270**: 1949–55.

33. Slama MS, Le Guludec D, Sebag C *et al.* Complete atrioventricular block following mediastinal irradiation: a report of six cases. *Pacing Clin Electrophysiol* 1991; **14**: 1112–18.

34. Lund MB, Ihlen H, Voss BM *et al.* Increased risk of heart valve regurgitation after mediastinal radiation for Hodgkin's disease: an echocardiographic study. *Heart* 1996; **75**: 591–5.

●35. Heidenreich PA, Hancock SL, Lee BK *et al.* Asymptomatic cardiac disease following mediastinal irradiation. *J Am Coll Cardiol* 2003; **42**: 743–9.

●36. Hull MC, Morris CG, Pepine CJ, Mendenhall NP. Valvular dysfunction and carotid, subclavian, and coronary artery disease in survivors of Hodgkin lymphoma treated with radiation therapy. *JAMA* 2003; **290**: 2831–7.

●37. Swerdlow AJ, Higgins CD, Smith P *et al.* Myocardial infarction mortality risk after treatment for Hodgkin disease: a collaborative British cohort study. *J Natl Cancer Inst* 2007; **99**: 206–14.

38. Landier W, Bhatia S, Eshelman DA *et al.* Development of risk-based guidelines for pediatric cancer survivors: the Children's Oncology Group Long-Term Follow-Up Guidelines from the Children's Oncology Group Late Effects Committee and Nursing Discipline. *J Clin Oncol* 2004; **22**: 4979–90.

●39. Horning SJ, Adhikari A, Rizk N. Effect of treatment for Hodgkin's disease on pulmonary function: results of a prospective study. *J Clin Oncol* 1994; **12**: 297–305.

40. Wara WM, Phillips TL, Margolis LW, Smith V. Radiation pneumonitis: a new approach to the derivation of time-dose factors. *Cancer* 1973; **32**: 547–52.

41. Kikkawa Y, Smith F. Cellular and biochemical aspects of pulmonary surfactant in health and disease. *Lab Invest* 1993; **49**: 122–39.

42. Miller RW, Fusner JE, Fink RJ *et al.* Pulmonary function abnormalities in long-term survivors of childhood cancer. *Med Pediatr Oncol* 1986; **14**: 202–7.

43. Griese M, Rampf U, Hofmann D *et al.* Pulmonary complications after bone marrow transplantation in children: twenty-four years of experience in a single pediatric center. *Pediatr Pulmonol* 2000; **30**: 393–401.

44. Quigley PM, Yeager AM, Loughlin GM. The effects of bone marrow transplantation on pulmonary function in children. *Pediatr Pulmonol* 1994; **18**: 361–7.

45. Villani F, Viviani S, Bonfante V *et al.* Late pulmonary effects in favorable stage I and IIA Hodgkin's disease treated with radiotherapy alone. *Am J Clin Oncol* 2000; **23**: 18–21.

46. Salloum E, Tanoue LT, Wackers FJ *et al.* Assessment of cardiac and pulmonary function in adult patients with Hodgkin's disease treated with ABVD or MOPP/ABVD plus adjuvant low-dose mediastinal irradiation. *Cancer Invest* 1999; **17**: 171–80.

47. Eigen H, Wyszomierski D. Bleomycin lung injury in children: pathophysiology and guidelines for management. *Am J Pediatr Hematol Oncol* 1985; **7**: 71–8.

48. Samuels ML, Johnson DE, Holoye PY, Lanzotti VJ. Large-dose bleomycin therapy and pulmonary toxicity: a possible role of prior radiotherapy. *JAMA* 1976; **235**: 1117–20.

●49. Martin WG, Ristow KM, Habermann TM *et al.* Bleomycin pulmonary toxicity has a negative impact on the outcome of patients with Hodgkin's lymphoma. *J Clin Oncol* 2005; **23**: 7614–20.

50. Buchler T, Bomanji J, Lee SM. FDG-PET in bleomycin-induced pneumonitis following ABVD chemotherapy for Hodgkin's disease – a useful tool for monitoring pulmonary toxicity and disease activity. *Haematologica* 2007; **92**: e120–1.

51. Aronin PA, Mahaley MS Jr, Rudnick SA *et al.* Prediction of BCNU pulmonary toxicity in patients with malignant gliomas: an assessment of risk factors. *N Engl J Med* 1980; **303**: 183–8.

52. Wheeler C, Antin JH, Churchill WH *et al.*
     Cyclophosphamide, carmustine, and etoposide with
     autologous bone marrow transplantation in refractory
     Hodgkin's disease and non-Hodgkin's lymphoma: a dose-
     finding study. *J Clin Oncol* 1990; **8**: 648–56.

53. Rubio C, Hill ME, Milan S *et al.* Idiopathic pneumonia
     syndrome after high-dose chemotherapy for relapsed
     Hodgkin's disease. *Br J Cancer* 1997; **75**: 1044–8.

54. Bauer KA, Skarin AT, Balikian JP *et al.* Pulmonary
     complications associated with combination chemotherapy
     programs containing bleomycin. *Am J Med* 1983;
     74: 557–63.

55. Goldiner PL, Schweizer O. The hazards of anaesthesia
     and surgery in bleomycin-treated patients. *Semin Oncol*
     1979; **6**: 121–4.

56. Schwerzmann M, Seiler C. Recreational scuba diving,
     patent foramen ovale and their associated risks. *Swiss
     Med Wkly* 2001; **131**: 365–74.

◆57. Hoppe RT. Hodgkin's disease: complications of therapy and
      excess mortality. *Ann Oncol* 1997; **8** (Suppl 1): 115–18.

●58. Dores GM, Metayer C, Curtis RE *et al.* Second malignant
      neoplasms among long-term survivors of Hodgkin's
      disease: a population-based evaluation over 25 years.
      J Clin Oncol 2002; **20**: 3484–94.

●59. Bhatia S, Robison LL, Oberlin O *et al.* Breast cancer and
      other second neoplasms after childhood Hodgkin's
      disease. *N Engl J Med* 1996; **334**: 745–51.

●60. Travis LB, Hill DA, Dores GM *et al.* Breast cancer following
      radiotherapy and chemotherapy among young women
      with Hodgkin disease. *JAMA* 2003; **290**: 465–75.

61. Hancock SL, Tucker MA, Hoppe RT. Breast cancer after
     treatment of Hodgkin's disease. *J Natl Cancer Inst* 1993;
     85: 25–31.

62. Travis LB, Hill D, Dores GM *et al.* Cumulative absolute
     breast cancer risk for young women treated for Hodgkin
     lymphoma. *J Natl Cancer Inst* 2005; **97**: 1428–37.

63. Cutuli B, Dhermain F, Borel C *et al.* Breast cancer in
     patients treated for Hodgkin's disease: clinical and
     pathological analysis of 76 cases in 63 patients. *Eur J
     Cancer* 1997; **33**: 2315–20.

●64. Hodgson DC, Koh ES, Tran TH *et al.* Individualized
      estimates of second cancer risks after contemporary
      radiation therapy for Hodgkin lymphoma. *Cancer* 2007;
      110: 2576–86.

65. Neglia JP, Meadows AT, Robison LL *et al.* Second
     neoplasms after acute lymphoblastic leukemia in
     childhood. *N Engl J Med* 1991; **325**: 1330–6.

66. Tucker MA, Jones PH, Boice JD Jr *et al.* Therapeutic
     radiation at a young age is linked to secondary thyroid
     cancer. The Late Effects Study Group. *Cancer Res* 1991;
     51: 2885–8.

67. Acharya S, Sarafoglou K, LaQuaglia M *et al.* Thyroid
     neoplasms after therapeutic radiation for malignancies
     during childhood or adolescence. *Cancer* 2003; **97**:
     2397–403.

68. Sklar C, Whitton J, Mertens A *et al.* Abnormalities of the
     thyroid in survivors of Hodgkin's disease: data from the

     Childhood Cancer Survivor Study. *J Clin Endocrinol Metab*
     2000; **85**: 3227–32.

◆69. Lorigan P, Radford J, Howell A, Thatcher N. Lung cancer
      after treatment for Hodgkin's lymphoma: a systematic
      review. *Lancet Oncol* 2005; **6**: 773–9.

●70. Travis LB, Gospodarowicz M, Curtis RE *et al.* Lung cancer
      following chemotherapy and radiotherapy for Hodgkin's
      disease. *J Natl Cancer Inst* 2002; **94**: 182–92.

71. Gilbert ES, Stovall M, Gospodarowicz M *et al.* Lung cancer
     after treatment for Hodgkin's disease: focus on radiation
     effects. *Radiat Res* 2003; **159**: 161–73.

72. Van Leeuwen FE, Klokman WJ, Stovall M *et al.* Roles of
     radiotherapy and smoking in lung cancer following
     Hodgkin's disease. *J Natl Cancer Inst* 1995; **87**:
     1530–7.

73. Kramer G, Gans S, Rijnders A, Leer J. Long term survival of
     a patient with malignant pleural mesothelioma as a late
     complication of radiotherapy for Hodgkin's disease treated
     with 90yttrium-silicate. *Lung Cancer* 2000; **27**: 205–8.

74. Bhatia S, Ramsay NKC, Steinbuch M *et al.* Malignant
     neoplasms following bone marrow transplantation. *Blood*
     1996; **87**: 3633–9.

75. Smith MA, Rubinstein L, Anderson JR *et al.* Secondary
     leukemia or myelodysplastic syndrome after treatment
     with epipodophyllotoxins. *J Clin Oncol* 1999; **17**: 569–77.

76. Henry-Amar M. Second cancer after the treatment for
     Hodgkin's disease: a report from the International
     Database on Hodgkin's Disease. *Ann Oncol* 1992;
     3 (Suppl 4): 117–28.

77. Dietrich PY, Henry-Amar M, Cosset JM *et al.* Second
     primary cancers in patients continuously disease-free
     from Hodgkin's disease: a protective role for the spleen?
     Blood 1994; **84**: 1209–15.

78. Naoe T, Takeyama K, Yokozawa T *et al.* Analysis of genetic
     polymorphism in NQO1, GST-M1, GST-T1, and CYP3A4
     in 469 Japanese patients with therapy-related
     leukemia/myelodysplastci syndrome and de novo acute
     myeloid leukemia. *Clin Cancer Res* 2000; **6**: 4091–5.

79. Darrington DL, Vose JM, Anderson JR *et al.* Incidence and
     characterization of secondary myelodysplastic syndrome
     and acute myelogenous leukemia following high-dose
     chemoradiotherapy and autologous stem-cell
     transplantation for lymphoid malignancies. *J Clin Oncol*
     1994; **12**: 2527–34.

●80. Krishnan A, Bhatia S, Slovak ML *et al.* Predictors of
      therapy-related leukemia and myelodysplasia following
      autologous transplantation for lymphoma: an assessment
      of risk factors. *Blood* 2000; **95**: 1588–93.

●81. Brown JR, Yeckes H, Friedberg JW *et al.* Increasing
      incidence of late second malignancies after conditioning
      with cyclophosphamide and total-body irradiation and
      autologous bone marrow transplantation for non-
      Hodgkin's lymphoma. *J Clin Oncol* 2005; **23**: 2208–14.

●82. Ng AK, Bernardo MV, Weller E, *et al.* Second malignancy
      after Hodgkin disease treated with radiation therapy with
      or without chemotherapy: long-term risks and risk
      factors. *Blood* 2002; **100**: 1989–96.

83. Rothman K, Keller AZ. The effect of joint exposure to alcohol and tobacco on risk of cancers of the mouth and pharynx. *J Chronic Dis* 1972; **25**: 711–16.

84. Brown RT, Sawyer MB, Antoniou G *et al.* A 3-year follow-up of the intellectual and academic functioning of children receiving central nervous system prophylactic chemotherapy for leukemia. *J Dev Behav Pediatr* 1996; **17**: 392–8.

85. Mulhern RK, Reddick WE, Palmer SL *et al.* Neurocognitive deficits in medulloblastoma survivors and white matter loss. *Ann Neurol* 1999; **46**: 834–41.

86. Ahles TA, Saykin A. Cognitive effects of standard-dose chemotherapy in patients with cancer. *Cancer Invest* 2001; **19**: 812–20.

87. Brezden CB, Phillips KA, Abdolell M *et al.* Cognitive function in breast cancer patients receiving adjuvant chemotherapy. *J Clin Oncol* 2000; **18**: 2695–701.

88. Ahles TA, Saykin AJ, Furstenberg CT *et al.* Neuropsychologic impact of standard-dose systemic chemotherapy in long-term survivors of breast cancer and lymphoma. *J Clin Oncol* 2002; **20**: 485–93.

●89. Packer RJ, Meadows AT, Rorke LB *et al.* Long-term sequelae of cancer treatment on the central nervous system in childhood. Med Pediatr Oncol 1987; **15**: 241–53.

90. Reddick WE, White HA, Glass JO *et al.* Developmental model relating white matter volume to neurocognitive deficits in pediatric brain tumor survivors. *Cancer* 2003; **97**: 2512–19.

◆91. Saykin AJ, Ahles TA, McDonald BC. Mechanisms of chemotherapy-induced cognitive disorders: neuropsychological, pathophysiological, and neuroimaging perspectives. *Semin Clin Neuropsychiatry* 2003; **8**: 201–16.

92. Noorda EM, Somers R, van Leeuwen FE. Dutch Late Effects Study Group. Adult height and age at menarche in childhood cancer survivors. *Eur J Cancer* 2001; **37**: 605–12.

93. Robison LL, Nesbit ME Jr, Sather HN *et al.* Height of children successfully treated for acute lymphoblastic leukemia: a report from the Late Effects Study Committee of Childrens Cancer Study Group. *Med Pediatr Oncol* 1985; **13**: 14–21.

●94. Sklar C, Mertens A, Walter A *et al.* Final height after treatment for childhood acute lymphoblastic leukemia: comparison of no cranial irradiation with 1800 and 2400 centigrays of cranial irradiation. *J Pediatr* 1993; **123**: 59–64.

95. Melin AE, Adan L, Leverger G *et al.* Growth hormone secretion, puberty and adult height after cranial irradiation with 18 Gy for leukaemia. *Eur J Pediatr* 1998; **157**: 703–7.

96. Schriock EA, Schell MJ, Carter M *et al.* Abnormal growth patterns and adult short stature in 115 long-term survivors of childhood leukemia. *J Clin Oncol* 1991; **9**: 400–5.

◆97. Livesey EA, Hindmarsh PC, Brook CG *et al.* Endocrine disorders following treatment of childhood brain tumours. *Br J Cancer* 1990; **61**: 622–5.

98. Oberfield SE, Allen JC, Pollack J *et al.* Long-term endocrine sequelae after treatment of medulloblastoma: prospective study of growth and thyroid function. *J Pediatr* 1986; **108**: 219–23.

99. Cohen A, Duell T, Socie G *et al.* Nutritional status and growth after bone marrow transplantation (BMT) during childhood: EBMT Late-Effects Working Party retrospective data. European Group for Blood and Marrow Transplantation. *Bone Marrow Transplant* 1999; **23**: 1043–7.

100. Cohen A, Rovelli A, Bakker B *et al.* Final height of patients who underwent bone marrow transplantation for hematological disorders during childhood: a study by the Working Party for Late Effects-EBMT. *Blood* 1999; **93**: 4109–15.

●101. Carroll PV, Christ ER, Bengtsson BA *et al.* Growth hormone deficiency in adulthood and the effects of growth hormone replacement: a review. Growth Hormone Research Society Scientific Committee. *J Clin Endocrinol Metab* 1998; **83**: 382–95.

102. Toogood AA, Ryder WD, Beardwell CG, Shalet SM. The evolution of radiation-induced growth hormone deficiency in adults is determined by the baseline growth hormone status. *Clin Endocrinol (Oxf)* 1995; **43**: 97–103.

●103. Talvensaari KK, Lanning M, Tapanainen P, Knip M. Long-term survivors of childhood cancer have an increased risk of manifesting the metabolic syndrome. *J Clin Endocrinol Metab.* 1996; **81**: 3051–5.

104. Amato G, Carella C, Fazio S *et al.* Body composition, bone metabolism, and heart structure and function in growth hormone (GH)-deficient adults before and after GH replacement therapy at low doses. *J Clin Endocrinol Metab* 1993; **77**: 1671–6.

105. Link K, Moell C, Garwicz S *et al.* Growth hormone deficiency predicts cardiovascular risk in young adults treated for acute lymphoblastic leukemia in childhood. *J Clin Endocrinol Metab* 2004; **89**: 5003–12.

106. Rosen T, Wiren L, Wilhelmsen L *et al.* Decreased psychological well-being in adult patients with growth hormone deficiency. *Clin Endocrinol (Oxf)* 1994; **40**: 111–16.

107. Drake WM, Carroll PV, Maher KT *et al.* The effect of cessation of growth hormone (GH) therapy on bone mineral accretion in GH-deficient adolescents at the completion of linear growth. *J Clin Endocrinol Metab* 2003; **88**: 1658–63.

108. Shalet SM, Shavrikova E, Cromer M *et al.* Effect of growth hormone (GH) treatment on bone in postpubertal GH-deficient patients: a 2-year randomized, controlled, dose-ranging study. *J Clin Endocrinol Metab* 2003; **88**: 4124–9.

109. Gleeson HK, Gattamaneni HR, Smethurst L *et al.* Reassessment of growth hormone status is required at final height in children treated with growth hormone replacement after radiation therapy. *J Clin Endocrinol Metab* 2004; **89**: 662–6.

110. Jarfelt M, Bjarnason R, Lannering B. Young adult survivors of childhood acute lymphoblastic leukemia: spontaneous GH secretion in relation to CNS radiation. *Pediatr Blood Cancer* 2004; **42**: 582–8.

◆111. Rose SR, Schreiber RE, Kearney NS *et al.* Hypothalamic dysfunction after chemotherapy. *J Pediatr Endocrinol Metab* 2004; **17**: 55–66.

112. Devney RB, Sklar CA, Nesbit ME Jr *et al.* Serial thyroid function measurements in children with Hodgkin disease. *J Pediatr* 1984; **105**: 223–7.

●113. Hancock SL, Cox RS, McDougall IR. Thyroid diseases after treatment of Hodgkin's disease. *N Engl J Med* 1991; **325**: 599–605.

114. Liesner RJ, Leiper AD, Hann IM, Chessells JM. Late effects of intensive treatment for acute myeloid leukemia and myelodysplasia in childhood. *J Clin Oncol* 1994; **12**: 916–24.

115. Wasnich RD, Grumet FC, Payne RO, Kriss JP. Grave's ophthalmopathy following external neck irradiation for nonthyroidal neoplastic disease. *J Clin Endocrinol Metab* 1973; **37**: 703–13.

116. Sanders J. Late effects after bone marrow transplantation. In: Ruccione KS. (ed.) *Survivors of childhood cancer: assessment and management.* St. Louis: Mosby-Yearbook, 1994: 293–318.

117. Sigurdson AJ, Ronckers CM, Mertens AC *et al.* Primary thyroid cancer after a first tumour in childhood (the Childhood Cancer Survivor Study): a nested case-control study. *Lancet* 2005; **365**: 2014–23.

118. Rowley MM, Leach DR, Warner GA, Heller CG. Effect of graded doses of ionizing radiation on the human testes. *Radiat Res.* 1974; **59**: 665–78.

119. Speiser B, Rubin P, Casarett G. Aspermia following lower truncal irradiation in Hodgkin's disease. *Cancer* 1973; **32**: 692–8.

120. Hahn EW, Feingold SM, Simpson L, Batata M. Recovery from aspermia induced by low dose radiation in seminoma patients. *Cancer* 1982; **50**: 337–40.

121. Clifton DK, Bremner WJ. The effect of testicular x-irradiation on spermatogenesis in man. *J Androl* 1983; **4**: 387–92.

122. Shalet SM, Beardwell CG, Jacobs HS, Pearson D. Testicular function following irradiation of the human prepubertal testes. *Clin Endocrinol (Oxf)* 1978; **9**: 483–90.

123. Green DM, Brecher ML, Lindsay AN *et al.* Gonadal function in pediatric patients following treatment for Hodgkin disease. *Med Pediatr Oncol* 1981; **9**: 235–44.

124. Heyn R, Raney RB Jr, Hays DM *et al.* Late effects of therapy in patients with paratesticular rhabdomyosarcoma. Intergroup Rhabdomyosarcoma Study Committee. *J Clin Oncol* 1992; **10**: 614–23.

125. Sklar C. Reproductive physiology and treatment-related loss of sex hormone production. *Med Pediatr Oncol* 1999; **33**: 2–8.

126. Izard MA. Leydig cell function and radiation: a review of the literature. *Radiother Oncol* 1995; **34**: 1–8.

127. Meistrich ML, Wilson G, Brown BW *et al.* Impact of cyclophosphamide on long-term reduction in sperm count in men treated with combination chemotherapy for Ewing and soft tissue sarcomas. *Cancer* 1992; **70**: 2703–12.

128. Lendon M, Hann IM, Palmer MK *et al.* Testicular histology after combination chemotherapy in childhood for acute lymphoblastic leukaemia. *Lancet* 1978; **2**: 439–41.

129. Whitehead E, Shalet SM, Jones PH *et al.* Gonadal function after combination chemotherapy for Hodgkin's disease in childhood. *Arch Dis Child* 1982; **57**: 287–91.

130. Santoro A, Bonadonna G, Valagussa P *et al.* Long-term results of combined chemotherapy-radiotherapy approach in Hodgkin's disease: superiority of ABVD plus radiotherapy versus MOPP plus radiotherapy. *J Clin Oncol* 1987; **5**: 27–37.

131. Humpl T, Schramm P, Gutjahr P. Effects of cancer treatment on male fertility. *Proceedings of the 5th International Conference on Long-term Complications of Treatment of Children and Adolescents for Cancer* Niagara-on-the-Lake, 1998.

132. Sherins RJ, DeVita VT. Effect of drug treatment for lymphoma on male reproductive capacity. *Ann Intern Med* 1973; **79**: 216–20.

133. Sherins RJ, Olweny CLM, Ziegler JL. Gynecomastia and gonadal dysfunction in adolescent boys treated with combination chemotherapy for Hodgkin's disease. *N Engl J Med* 1978; **299**: 12–16.

●134. Chapman RM, Sutcliffe SB, Malpas JS. Male gonadal dysfunction in Hodgkin's disease: a prospective study. *JAMA* 1981; **245**: 1323.

135. Duffey P, Campbell EW, Wiernik PH. Hydrocele following treatment for Hodgkin's disease. *Cancer* 1982; **50**: 305–7.

136. Lushbaugh CC, Casarett GW. The effects of gonadal irradiation in clinical radiation therapy: a review. *Cancer* 1976; **37**(2 Suppl): 1111–25.

137. Stillman RJ, Schinfeld JS, Schiff I *et al.* Ovarian failure in long-term survivors of childhood malignancy. *Am J Obstet Gynecol* 1981; **139**: 62–6.

●138. Ortin TTS, Shostak CA, Donaldson SS. Gonadal status and reproductive function following treatment for Hodgkin's disease in childhood: the Stanford experience. *Int J Radiat Oncol Biol Phys* 1990; **19**: 873–80.

139. Matsumoto M, Shinohara O, Ishiguro H *et al.* Ovarian function after bone marrow transplantation performed before menarche. *Arch Dis Child* 1999; **80**: 452–4.

●140. Couto-Silva AC, Trivin C, Thibaud E *et al.* Factors affecting gonadal function after bone marrow transplantation during childhood. *Bone Marrow Transplant* 2001; **28**: 67–75.

141. Chapman RM, Sutcliffe SB, Malpas JS. Cytotoxic-induced ovarian failure in women with Hodgkin's disease. *JAMA* 1979; **242**: 1877–81.

142. Siris ES, Leventhal BG, Vaitukaitis JL. Effects of childhood leukemia and chemotherapy on puberty and reproductive function in girls. *N Engl J Med* 1976; **294**: 1143–6.

143. Nicosia SV, Matus-Ridley M, Meadows AT. Gonadal effects of cancer therapy in girls. *Cancer* 1985; **55**: 2364–72.

144. Bath LE, Wallace WH, Shaw MP *et al*. Depletion of ovarian reserve in young women after treatment for cancer in childhood: detection by anti-Mullerian hormone, inhibin B and ovarian ultrasound. *Hum Reprod* 2003; **1811**: 2368–74.

145. Byrne J. Infertility and premature menopause in childhood cancer survivors. *Med Pediatr Oncol* 1999; **33**: 24–8.

146. Sanders JE, Buckner CD, Leonard JM *et al*. Late effects on gonadal function of cyclophosphamide, total-body irradiation, and marrow transplantation. *Transplantation* 1983; **36**: 252–5.

147. Brewer M, Gershenson DM, Herzog CE *et al*. Outcome and reproductive function after chemotherapy for ovarian dysgerminoma. *J Clin Oncol* 1999; **17**: 2670–5.

148. Chapman RM, Sutcliffe SB. Protection of ovarian function by oral contraceptives in women receiving chemotherapy for Hodgkin's disease. *Blood* 1981; **58**: 849–51.

149. Wallace WH, Anderson R, Baird D. Preservation of fertility in young women treated for cancer. *Lancet Oncol* 2004; **5**: 269–70.

150. Green DM, Hyland A, Chung CS *et al*. Cancer and cardiac mortality among 15-year survivors of cancer diagnosed during childhood or adolescence. *J Clin Oncol* 1999; **17**: 3207–15.

151. Hudson MM, Jones D, Boyett J *et al*. Late mortality of long-term survivors of childhood cancer. *J Clin Oncol* 1997; **15**: 2205–13.

152. Mertens AC, Yasui Y, Neglia JP *et al*. Late mortality experience in five-year survivors of childhood and adolescent cancer: the Childhood Cancer Survivor Study. *J Clin Oncol* 2001; **19**: 3163–72.

153. Hudson MM, Mertens AC, Yasui Y *et al*. Health status of adult long-term survivors of childhood cancer: a report from the Childhood Cancer Survivor Study. *JAMA* 2003; **290**: 1583–92.

154. Zebrack BJ, Zeltzer LK, Whitton J *et al*. Psychological outcomes in long-term survivors of childhood leukemia, Hodgkin's disease, and non-Hodgkin's lymphoma: a report from the Childhood Cancer Survivor Study. *Pediatrics* 2002; **110**: 42–52.

●155. Elkin TD, Phipps S, Mulhern RK, Fairclough D. Psychological functioning of adolescent and young adult survivors of pediatric malignancy. *Med Pediatr Oncol* 1997; **29**: 582–8.

156. Shankar S, Robison L, Jenney ME *et al*. Health-related quality of life in young survivors of childhood cancer using the Minneapolis-Manchester Quality of Life-Youth Form. *Pediatrics* 2005; **115**: 435–42.

157. Loge JH, Abrahamsen AF, Ekeberg O, Kaasa S. Reduced health-related quality of life among Hodgkin's disease survivors: a comparative study with general population norms. *Ann Oncol* 1999; **10**: 71–7.

158. Gotay CC, Muraoka MY. Quality of life in long-term survivors of adult-onset cancers. *J Natl Cancer Inst* 1998; **90**: 656–67.

159. Loge JH, Abrahamsen AF, Ekeberg O, Kaasa S. Hodgkin's disease survivors more fatigued than the general population. *J Clin Oncol* 1999; **17**: 253–61.

160. Knobel H, Loge JH, Nordoy T *et al*. High level of fatigue in lymphoma patients treated with high dose therapy. *J Pain Symptom Manage* 2000; **19**: 446–56.

161. Andrykowski MA, Bishop MM, Hahn EA *et al*. Long-term health-related quality of life, growth, and spiritual well-being after hematopoietic stem-cell transplantation. *J Clin Oncol* 2005; **23**: 599–608.

162. Kopp M, Holzner B, Meraner V *et al*. Quality of life in adult hematopoietic cell transplant patients at least 5 yr after treatment: a comparison with healthy controls. *Eur J Haematol* 2005; **74**: 304–8.

163. Oeffinger KC. Longitudinal risk-based health care for adult survivors of childhood cancer. *Curr Probl Cancer* 2003; **27**: 143–67.

PART **8**

MANAGEMENT OF SPECIFIC DISEASES

62

Lymphoblastic lymphoma and leukemia in children

HELMUT GADNER, GEORG MANN AND ANDISHE ATTARBASCHI

INTRODUCTION

Lymphoblastic diseases represent nearly one-third of all malignancies diagnosed in childhood and adolescence. Acute lymphoblastic leukemia (ALL) is the most common and accounts for approximately a quarter of all cancers in this age group.[1–3] In contrast, non-Hodgkin lymphoma (NHL) represents the third most frequent malignancy in childhood, with the precursor lymphoblastic subtypes making up about 30 percent of cases.[4–6]

Lymphoblastic lymphomas (LBL) are histologically and morphologically indistinguishable from ALL, as both disorders are derived from immature precursor B or T cells. The distinction of ALL from LBL is based on the number of blasts in the bone marrow, patients with more than 25 percent blasts in the bone marrow being classified as having ALL, whereas those with fewer than 25 percent blasts in the bone marrow are classified as having LBL. Although lymphoblastic leukemia and lymphoma appear grossly identical on a morphological level and respond very well to identical treatment, sophisticated molecular-genetic studies are necessary to reveal whether they are also biologically identical disorders.

The development of intensive multiagent chemotherapeutic regimens during the last 30 years, together with important principles of diagnostic workup at diagnosis and during treatment, have all contributed to the excellent outcome and high cure rates in children, for lymphoblastic neoplasms being around 70–80 percent.[7–12]

EPIDEMIOLOGY

The incidence of ALL in Western Europe and the United States is 3–4 cases per year, among 100 000 children less than 15 years old. The peak incidence of ALL occurs at age 2–5 years and the male to female ratio is 1.2:1.[13] The higher prevalence of the male gender is particularly seen in T cell ALL, whilst in infant leukemia there is a female preponderance. The incidence of LBL is around 0.2–0.3 cases per year (among 100 000 children less than 15 years old).[14] The median age at diagnosis is 8.1 and 9.8 years for precursor T cell and B cell LBL, respectively.[4] With a male to female ratio of 1.8:1, precursor T cell LBL shows a male preponderance, whereas in precursor B cell LBL, the ratio is 1:1.4.[4]

Intriguingly, there appear to be geographic differences in the incidence of ALL and NHL – e.g., in North Africa and the Middle East, ALL is rarely seen and Epstein–Barr virus (EBV)-related Burkitt lymphoma is the most frequent cancer. Furthermore, the incidence of ALL is twice as high in Germany, Australia, Costa Rica, and in white children from the United States than in India, China, Kuwait, Cuba, and in black children from the United States. The explanation for these differences remains obscure, but may in part be due to socioeconomic influences and possibly reflects an underdiagnosis of ALL in developing countries.

ETIOLOGY

Genetics

The etiologies of ALL and NHL are not yet fully clarified. However, in a small proportion of patients, inborn genetic factors are presumed to play a significant role in leukemogenesis/lymphomagenesis. Children with specific constitutional genetic defects have a proven risk of developing lymphoid neoplasms – e.g., the risk of developing leukemia (transient myeloproliferative disease of the newborn, acute myeloid leukemia [AML] in infancy and early childhood, ALL in early and late childhood) is increased 20-fold in children with constitutional trisomy 21 compared with children with a normal karyotype.[2,13] Moreover, Klinefelter syndrome and Turner syndrome are both also associated with an increased risk of childhood leukemia.

Disorders such as Fanconi anemia, neurofibromatosis type 1, Shwachman-Diamond syndrome, Kostmann syndrome, dyskeratosis congenita, and Bloom syndrome represent other genetic predispositions for the development of acute leukemia.[2] In addition, inherited conditions associated with immunodeficiency such as ataxia telangiectasia, Wiskott-Aldrich syndrome, X-linked lymphoproliferative syndrome, or the Nijmegen breakage syndrome are also associated with an increased prevalence of NHL and leukemia.[5,14] Children with acquired immunodeficiency, for example following organ or stem cell transplantation, and those with acquired immunodeficiency syndrome are also particularly prone to the development of lymphomas. However, such NHLs are mostly Burkitt lymphoma and anaplastic large cell lymphoma, while LBL is rarely observed.[15]

The role of genetic factors in the etiology of lymphoid neoplasms is further outlined by the observation of familial leukemia/lymphoma, a higher incidence of leukemia in identical twins, and the detection of specific karyotypic abnormalities in the vast majority of cases. The genetic plasticity of naïve cells with lymphatic determination, together with a high proliferative capacity, makes the lymphatic system at specific risk to undergo mutations. Results of sophisticated molecular-genetic studies, particularly in twins and triplets, together with retrospective analysis of neonatal blood spots on Guthrie cards, have demonstrated that at least in a few leukemia subtypes such as TEL/AML1+ ALL, the initiating chromosomal events occur at an early stage of fetal development.[16–18] However, due to nonconcordant onset of an otherwise molecularly concordant ALL in pairs of identical twins, additional postnatal factors appear to be necessary to trigger the development of overt leukemia. Exposure to infections in early childhood has been extensively discussed as playing a role in this setting, causing secondary chromosomal mutations (e.g., TEL deletion in TEL/AML1+ ALL) which may then pave the way to manifestation of clinical disease.[16] This so-called 'two- or multi-hit' hypothesis is also supported by recent findings that specific leukemic translocations can be found in cord bloods of healthy newborns at a 100-fold higher frequency than would be expected from the actual incidence of acute leukemia.

Environmental factors and infections

Several environmental factors such as exposure to ionizing radiation or electromagnetic fields, diagnostic or therapeutic irradiation, chemicals (e.g., benzene), and nutrition have been controversially discussed as possibly being associated with the development of leukemia.[19] Exposure to ionizing radiation is now a very-well-documented risk factor, as proven by the high incidence of acute leukemia among survivors of the atomic bomb blasts in Japan during World War II. There is also substantial evidence that chemotherapy, particularly alkylating agents (e.g., cyclophosphamide) or DNA topoisomerase II inhibitors (e.g., etoposide), may increase the risk of secondary leukemia.[20,21] However, the varying incidence of secondary leukemia (mainly MLL-rearranged AML M4 or M5) reported from the United States and European study groups may relate to a different scheduling of the epipodophyllotoxins within different treatment protocols. Epipodophyllotoxins given once- or twice-weekly for extended periods seem to significantly increase the risk for secondary leukemias, which usually present 4–6 years from initial therapy. Furthermore, transplacental exposure to DNA topoisomerase II inhibitors (e.g., flavonoids in fruits and vegetables) may also play a critical role in the development of leukemia, especially in the occurrence of infant MLL-rearranged cases.[22]

Other investigations have revealed that maternal smoking, advanced maternal age, high birth weight, and reproductive history may also represent risk factors for ALL – e.g., the report of one or more fetal losses increased the risk of ALL 5–25-fold.[2,3,13] This observation may reflect either a genetic predisposition (mutations of germ-line cells) or chronic exposure to environmental factors or unidentified infections.

At the moment, there is no clear evidence that pre- or postnatal infections play a significant role in leukemogenesis, although nonconcordant onset of a molecularly concordant ALL in pairs of identical twins suggests that viral infections in early childhood may be involved, causing a deranged response of the immune system which triggers the development of acute leukemia.

CLASSIFICATION

Cytomorphology/cytochemistry

The morphologic diagnosis of ALL (bone marrow, peripheral blood) and LBL (tumor touch imprints, bone marrow, and/or malignant effusions) is performed according to the French-American-British (FAB) classification system (L1, L2, L3).[23] In light of the development of novel technologies such as immunophenotyping with multicolor flow cytometry techniques and elegant molecular-genetic methods (e.g., fluorescence *in situ* hybridization), which together define the leukemia, the morphologic distinction of the ALL subtypes L1 and L2 has lost its former significance. However, cytomorphologic analysis of May-Grünwald-Giemsa (Pappenheim)-stained bone marrow (BM) and blood smears is still the easiest and most rapid and cost-effective way to diagnose ALL.[24] If the BM aspirate fails ('dry tap'), the histologic results of a trephine biopsy should help in establishing a definite diagnosis. Furthermore, cytochemical reactions are still useful in differentiating lymphoblastic (periodic acid Schiff and acid phosphatase reaction [T cell blasts]) from myeloid cells (myeloperoxidase, Sudan Black, nonspecific esterase reaction [monoblasts]).[24] Notably, the recognition of FAB L3 blasts has important therapeutic implications as this leukemia subtype is not only closely related to but is also treated in studies as for Burkitt lymphoma.

Immunophenotype

In the 1980s, leukemic blast cells were analyzed microscopically by standard indirect immunofluorescence assays with a panel of monoclonal antibodies directed against lymphoid- and myeloid-associated antigens. The advent of flow cytometry in the 1990s enabled the establishment of a reliable classification system for acute leukemias.[24–26] In Europe, it follows the guidelines of the European Group for the Immunological Characterization of Leukemias (EGIL) (Table 62.1).[27] As some ALLs coexpress myeloid markers such as MPO (myeloperoxidase), CD13, CD33, CD15, or CDw65, a strict scoring system has been created in order to describe these biphenotypic leukemias precisely (Table 62.2).[27]

Several standardized antibody combinations are usually used to screen ALL samples at diagnosis for leukemia-associated phenotypic aberrations.[24–26,28] The arbitrarily chosen criteria for immunophenotypic marker positivity are expression on 20 percent or more of blasts for cell-surface markers and on 10 percent or more of blasts for intracytoplasmic and intranuclear markers. Finally, the introduction of multicolor flow cytometry into a standard diagnostic workup has not only contributed to the immunophenotypic characterization and classification of acute leukemias and other myeloproliferative diseases, but is also a promising tool for the assessment of minimal residual disease during the course of therapy.[29–32]

Table 62.1 Immunophenotypic classification of ALL according to the EGIL criteria

ALL subtype	Immunophenotypic profile
Precursor B cell ALL	At least two of the three following markers: CD19$^+$ and/or CD22$^+$ and/or CD79a$^+$; often TdT$^+$, CD34$^+$, and HLA-DR$^+$
Pro-B-ALL (B-I)	No further B cell differentiation marker
Common ALL (B-II)	CD10$^+$
Pre-B-ALL (B-III)	Cytoplasmic IgM$^+$, CD10$^{+/-}$
Mature B AL (B-IV)	Ig$^+$ (cytoplasmic or surface) or sIgκ^+ or sIgλ^+
Precursor T cell ALL	Cytoplasmic or surface CD3$^+$; often TdT$^+$, HLA-DR$^+$, and CD34$^-$
Pro-T-ALL (T-I)	CD7$^+$
Pre-T-ALL (T-II)	CD2$^+$ and/or CD5$^+$ and/or CD8$^+$
Cortical T-ALL (T-III)	CD1a$^+$
Mature T-ALL (T-IV)	Surface CD3$^+$, CD1a$^-$
$\alpha\beta^+$ T-ALL	Anti-TCRα/β^+
$\gamma\delta^+$ T-ALL	Anti-TCRγ/δ^+
ALL with myeloid markers (My$^+$)	CD13$^+$ and/or CD33$^+$ and/or CDw65$^+$

ALL, acute lymphoblastic leukemia; EGIL, European Group for the Immunological Characterization of Leukemias; Ig, immunoglobulin; AL, acute leukemia; TCR, T cell receptor; TdT, terminal deoxynucleotidyl transferase.

Table 62.2 Scoring system for biphenotypic leukemias according to the EGIL criteria

Points	B cell marker	T cell marker	Myeloid marker
2	CD79a cyIgM cyCD22	cyCD3 or sCD3 anti-TCRα/β anti-TCRγ/δ	anti-MPO
1	CD19, CD10, CD20	CD2, CD5, CD8, CD10	CD13, CD33, CD65, CD117
0.5	TdT, CD24	TdT, CD7, CD1a	CD14, CD15, CD64

Biphenotypic leukemia: total scores must be >2 points for the myeloid and >1 point for the lymphoid markers.
EGIL, European Group for the Immunological Characterization of Leukemias; cy, cytoplasmic; s, surface; TCR, T cell receptor; MPO, myeloperoxidase; TdT, terminal deoxynucleotidyl transferase.

Histology

The cytomorphologic diagnosis of leukemia has been established for many decades, whereas the diagnosis of the lymphomatous counterparts (LBL, Burkitt lymphoma) traditionally requires histopathologic confirmation.[33] Most LBLs have a precursor T cell immunophenotype (75 percent), whereas only a small proportion is of precursor B cell origin (25 percent). Lymphoblastic lymphomas have a uniform appearance with a diffuse and monotonous growth pattern. The histologic features indicative of LBL are medium-sized cells with a narrow and pale cytoplasm and round or convoluted nuclei, with poorly discernible nucleoli and a finely stippled chromatin. The tumor cells are cytologically indistinguishable from the blast cells of ALL and are thus classified as either FAB L1 or L2.[23] Immunophenotypic subgrouping is performed according to the EGIL criteria (Table 62.1).[27]

Cytogenetic and molecular–genetic analysis

Chromosomal aberrations in number and structure can now be identified in the vast majority of childhood leukemia cases and possess diagnostic and prognostic significance.[34,35] In contrast, in childhood LBL, genetic results have not yet contributed to treatment because the abnormalities seen are more heterogeneous and found in only one-third of the patients.[4,14] In precursor T cell LBL, for example, most translocations involve the gene locus of the $\alpha\delta$-chain of the T cell receptor (TCR) on chromosome 14q11 or the gene locus of the β-chain of the TCR on chromosome 7q35. However, the fusion gene partners vary considerably. They are often protooncogenes encoding for a transcription factor (Table 62.3). In precursor B cell LBL, no consistent cytogenetic abnormalities have been recognized.

With the development of improved chromosomal banding techniques and molecular-genetic methods such as fluorescence *in situ* hybridization (FISH) analysis and reverse transcription polymerase chain reaction (RT-PCR), chromosomal abnormalities can be found in 70–80 percent of ALL cases, whereas the remaining 20–30 percent of ALL cases display a normal karyotype. Nevertheless, it is generally believed that the blast cells of the latter ALL patients may also carry genetic aberrations, which, however, are not detectable with current methods. A former example for this hypothesis is the most common genetic rearrangement in precursor B cell ALL, namely the translocation t(12;21)(p13,q22) with its genetic counterpart, the *TEL/AML1* fusion gene.[36,37] As this aberration is virtually undetectable with conventional cytogenetic techniques, the two preferred screening methods are RT-PCR and FISH.[38–41] The latter technology has the advantage that it enables the identification and quantification of the most common and, probably, most relevant secondary changes [*TEL* deletion, +21, +der(21)] at a single-cell level in a rapid, reliable, and economically efficient manner.[38]

Most patients with ALL have structural chromosomal abnormalities, mostly balanced nonrandom translocations (Table 62.3), while deletions [e.g., del(12p); del(6q);

Table 62.3   Genetic abnormalities in childhood ALL and LBL: incidence, association with immunophenotypes, and prognosis

Aberration	Molecular genetics	Immunophenotype	Incidence	Prognosis
t(1;19)(q23;p13)	*E2A/PBX1*	Pre-B-ALL	5%	Good
t(4;11)(q21;23)	*MLL/AF4*	Pro-B-ALL and CD10⁻ pre-B-ALL	4%	Poor
t(11;19)(q23;p13)	*MLL/ENL*	Pro-B-ALL and CD10⁻ pre-B-ALL	1%	Intermediate
t(9;22)(q34;q11)	*BCR/ABL*	Common ALL	3%	Poor
t(12;21)(p13;q22)	*TEL/AML1*	Common ALL	22%	Good
t(8;14)(q24;q32)	*MYC/IgH*	Mature B AL, Burkitt lymphoma	3%	Good
t(8;22)(q24;q11)	*MYC/Igλ*	Mature B AL, Burkitt lymphoma	3%	Good
t(2;8)(p12;q24)	*Igκ/MYC*	Mature B AL, Burkitt lymphoma	3%	Good
High-hyperdiploidy	–	Common ALL	25%	Good
Near-tetraploidy	–	Common ALL, T-ALL	1%	Unclear
Near-triploidy	–	Pre-B-ALL	<1%	Unclear
14q11-aberration	*TCRα/δ*	T-ALL, T-LBL	5–10%	Intermediate
t(11;14)(p13;q11)	*TTG2*			
t(10;14)(q24;q11)	*HOX11*			
t(8;14)(q24;q11)	*MYC*			
t(1;14)(p32;q11)	*TAL1*			
t(7;19)(q35;p13)	*TCRβ/LYL1*	T-LBL		Unclear
t(1;7)(p34;q34)	*TCRβ/LCK*	T-LBL		Unclear

ALL, acute lymphoblastic leukemia; LBL, lymphoblastic lymphoma; Ig, immunoglobulin; AL, acute leukemia; TCR, T cell receptor.

del(9p)], inversions, point mutations (e.g., *FLT3*), and amplifications (e.g., *AML1*; *ABL*) account for a comparatively small number of cases.[34,35,42–44] The most important translocations which possess prognostic and/or therapeutic implications are the following: t(12;21)(p13;q22), t(4;11)(q21;q23), t(9;22)(q34;q11), t(1;19)(q23;p13), and t(11;19)(q23,p13). Chromosomal abnormalities such as del(12p), del(6q), or del(9p) are so-called secondary aberrations that are rarely found alone but most often occur with any of the aforementioned specific translocations. They may lead to genomic imbalances and are considered to play a significant role in leukemia progression.

The ploidy and DNA content of leukemic blast cells also represent well-established genetic hallmarks in ALL.[34,35,44] Only two have clinical relevance. Patients with high-hyperdiploidy (51–65 chromosomes) account for approximately 25 percent of cases and are usually associated with a good prognosis, whereas hypodiploidy (fewer than 46 chromosomes) has an increased risk of relapse with conventional treatment.[45–47] The incidence and prognostic relevance of the most frequent chromosomal abnormalities in ALL and LBL and their association with specific immunophenotypes are shown in Table 62.3.

Clinical features at diagnosis

The clinical symptoms of a patient with ALL usually depend on the extent of BM involvement and of the extramedullary disease spread.[1,2] The history is often very short, although patients with a 2–3-month history of nonspecific symptoms, with variable bone or joint pain, recurrent infections, and increasing fatigue, are occasionally seen. The failure of normal hematopoiesis results in neutropenia, anemia, and thrombocytopenia. The clinical consequences are fever, pallor, fatigue, headache, bruises, and petechiae.

Bone pain, particularly affecting the long bones, is another leading symptom in childhood ALL, reflecting the leukemic infiltration of the bone and periosteum. Children also often suffer from arthralgias, with or without swelling of the joints, and may present with a limp or refuse to walk. This situation may mimic a variety of nonmalignant diseases such as osteomyelitis or juvenile rheumatoid arthritis. Other diseases that may share symptoms of childhood ALL include infectious mononucleosis, idiopathic thrombocytopenic purpura, and aplastic anemia. Childhood ALL must also be differentiated from myelodysplastic syndromes and solid tumors with BM involvement such as neuroblastoma, rhabdomyosarcoma, or retinoblastoma.

Symptoms of extramedullary disease usually include hepatomegaly and/or splenomegaly, generalized or localized painless lymphadenopathy (mostly cervical lymph nodes), and a unilateral indolent swelling of the testicles. Symptoms and signs of central nervous system (CNS) disease are rarely observed at initial diagnosis, but may include headache, neck rigidity, impaired vision, or cranial nerve palsies. In children with a high white cell count, kidney enlargement due to leukemic infiltration may be present, so that an ultrasound and detailed laboratory workup is obligatory before initiation of treatment.

Patients with T cell lymphoblastic disease often have serious complications at initial presentation due to local tumor effects or tumor lysis syndrome. Most cases present with a mediastinal mass consisting of thymic enlargement and/or mediastinal lymphadenopathy. The mediastinal tumor may displace the trachea and esophagus causing cough, pain, dyspnea, or dysphagia, and compress the mediastinal vessels leading to life-threatening superior vena caval obstruction. The presence of pleural and pericardial effusions may further worsen the patient's clinical condition.

The abdomen is not usually a site of involvement in children with ALL or LBL, in contrast to the situation with Burkitt lymphoma and leukemia. Other rare sites of manifestation are the orbits, skin, gingiva, lungs, heart, and salivary glands (Mikulicz syndrome). Radiologically visible skeletal manifestations without clinical symptoms may be observed but have no prognostic relevance.

While precursor T cell LBL and T cell ALL have similar clinical characteristics at initial presentation, clinical features of the rare cases of precursor B cell LBL vary considerably, with peripheral lymph nodes, BM, and skin being the preferential sites of involvement.[10] The differential diagnoses of NHL include nonmalignant, mostly infectious, and other malignant disorders (Table 62.4). A detailed history, the duration of symptoms, the clinical appearance of the involved lymph nodes (localized vs generalized, size, pain, signs of inflammation, consistency, mobility), and a thorough clinical evaluation are often helpful in distinguishing lymphoma from nonmalignant diseases.

Table 62.4   Differential diagnosis of childhood non-Hodgkin lymphoma

Nonmalignant diseases
EBV, CMV, HIV infection
Kawasaki syndrome
Streptococcal or staphylococcal infections
Tularemia
Toxoplasmosis
Tuberculosis, atypical tuberculosis
Leishmaniasis, brucellosis
Cat scratch disease
Histoplasmosis
Storage disorders

Malignant diseases
ALL, AML
Hodgkin disease
Langerhans cell histiocytosis
Metastases of neuroblastoma or rhabdomyosarcoma

EBV, Epstein–Barr virus; CMV, cytomegalovirus; HIV, human immunodeficiency virus; ALL, acute lymphoblastic leukemia; AML, acute myeloid leukemia.

DIAGNOSIS

The diagnosis of ALL and LBL is based on a set of parameters including clinical evaluation, laboratory workup, and imaging studies (Table 62.5).[1,2,4,5] Nevertheless, the primary goal is to avoid and adequately treat life-threatening complications at presentation. As children with certain subtypes of ALL and LBL have a high initial tumor burden (e.g., infant or Philadelphia+ ALL, T cell lymphoid neoplasms), serious complications due to spontaneous tumor lysis syndrome or local tumor effects may be observed. On the other hand, since early initiation of specific therapy will help avoid early death or persistent impairment, physicians have to perform a balancing act between stabilizing a critically ill patient and getting a reliable diagnosis as soon as possible. For example, when general anesthesia – needed to perform a BM puncture and/or tumor biopsy – has to be avoided due to airway obstruction from a mediastinal mass, cytologic examination of blood smears or cytospin preparations of malignant effusions is often sufficient to obtain a diagnosis and start specific treatment. Nevertheless, diagnosis of ALL or LBL must be confirmed by a BM aspirate within the first 1–3 days after initiation of therapy.

In Europe (at least within the 'Berlin-Frankfurt-Münster [BFM] family'), there is an international consensus on the minimal requirements for the diagnosis of ALL, which was published in 1992.[24] The definitive diagnosis of ALL requires a BM aspirate. The diagnosis of LBL should be established by the least invasive method, preferentially by the cytomorphologic and immunophenotypic analysis of cytospin preparations of malignant effusions (pleural and pericardial effusions, ascites) or BM smears. However, in some cases, surgical procedures such as a peripheral lymph node biopsy are necessary to obtain the diagnosis. Time-consuming radical surgical debulking or mutilating interventions should be definitely avoided. Preparation of tumor touch imprints may allow a rapid diagnosis and start of effective therapy. Although fine-needle aspirates of tumor masses are not generally recommended, they may be justified in exceptional cases with otherwise inaccessible tumors in critically ill patients.

Distinction between leukemia and lymphoma

As mentioned above, lymphoblastic lymphoma is morphologically indistinguishable from ALL, as both diseases arise from precursor B or T cells. The arbitrarily defined distinction is based on the number of blast cells in the BM. Patients with more than 25 percent blasts in the BM have ALL, whereas cases with fewer than 25 percent blasts in the BM have LBL. This traditional method is evidently not based on either biological or clinical differences.

Basic diagnostic issues

The basic laboratory parameters that need to be obtained at initial diagnosis of ALL or LBL include the hemoglobin, white cell (with differential) and platelet counts, and the serum concentrations of sodium, potassium, calcium, phosphorus, lactate dehydrogenase, uric acid, and creatinine (Table 62.5). In most patients, neutropenia, anemia,

Table 62.5   Initial diagnostic workup in acute lymphoblastic leukemia and lymphoblastic lymphoma

Acute lymphoblastic leukemia	Lymphoblastic lymphoma
Clinical examination (liver, spleen, lymph nodes, testicles, CNS, signs of infection and bleeding)	In addition: evaluation of B symptoms; inspection of the ear, nose, and throat region
Laboratory (electrolytes, P, Ca, Mg, uric acid, LDH, creatinine, BUN, liver transaminases, immunoglobulins, CRP, clotting tests)	
Blood group, optional: TPMT, APCR	
Virology (toxoplasmosis)	
Ultrasound of the abdomen, eventually of the mediastinum	In addition: abdominal MRI or CT in case of equivocal results
X-ray of the thorax, local x-ray in case of symptomatic disease EKG, echocardiography, EEG	Chest CT in case of a mediastinal mass
Ophthalmologic examination	
Cranial CT	Cranial MRI in case of head and neck lymphoma
Craniospinal MRI in case of neurologic symptoms	
Differential blood count, PB smears for morphology	
BM smears for morphology	
BM with heparin for cytogenetics, molecular genetics, immunology, and minimal residual disease	
CSF for cytospin preparations (morphology)	
Malignant effusions for cytospin preparations (morphology) and with heparin for cytogenetics, molecular genetics, immunology	In addition: tumor touch imprints for morphology

CNS, central nervous system; LDH, lactate dehydrogenase; BUN, blood urea nitrogen; CRP, C-reactive protein; TPMT, thiopurine methyl transferase; APCR, activated protein C resistance; MRI, magnetic resonance imaging; CT, computed tomography; EKG, electrocardiography; EEG, electroencephalography; BM, bone marrow; PB, peripheral blood; CSF, cerebrospinal fluid.

and thrombocytopenia are present. Neutropenia may be associated with leukocytosis, but occasionally also with leukopenia. In all cases, the diagnosis of ALL has to be confirmed by a BM aspirate. Patients with T cell ALL often present with a high white cell count, but may not have a very low hemoglobin level and platelet count. Reasons to explain this typical blood count constellation may be that the leukemic blasts primarily originate in the thymus and secondarily invade the BM. This would be expected to spare relatively more stem cells than a disease originating in the BM. It may also be speculated that the high proliferation rate of T cell leukemias leads to a diagnosis before complete depletion of the normal BM can occur. As the platelet count is rarely less than 10 000/μL, severe hemorrhage is a rare event in ALL and LBL, but its likelihood may increase in the presence of infection or coagulation disturbances which may be present with high initial leukocyte counts. All other biochemical parameters mostly reflect the leukemic cell burden, the extramedullary disease spread, and the degree of proliferation and spontaneous apoptosis of the blast cells. In patients with LBL, determination of the extent of disease, which is the most important prognostic factor and used for risk stratification, is done according to the St. Jude's (Murphy) staging system (Table 62.6).[48]

Diagnosis of central nervous system disease

Whilst involvement of the liver, spleen, and testicles is established by clinical examination of the patient, diagnosis of CNS disease not only includes a clinical neurological evaluation, but also a lumbar puncture to obtain cerebrospinal fluid (CSF), which has to be examined after cytocentrifugation. According to an international consensus, the definition of CNS disease in ALL and LBL is based on the following criteria: CNS-1 status: no blast cells; CNS-2 status: <5 white blood cells/μL with unequivocally

identifiable blast cells; and CNS-3 status: $\geq$5 white blood cells/μL with unequivocally identifiable blast cells.[24] In almost all clinical trials, patients with CNS-3 status are defined as having true CNS disease, which means that they need intensified intrathecal chemotherapy and therapeutic cranial irradiation. However, controversies exist about the relevance of blasts in ALL patients with CNS-2 status. Several studies have demonstrated a higher incidence of CNS relapse, while others have documented an outcome similar to patients with CNS-1 status.[49]

In case of a traumatic lumbar puncture (blood contamination of the CSF), a thorough counting of the number of blast cells, leukocytes, and red cells in the CSF and peripheral blood usually helps to reveal or rule out CNS-3 status. Patients with cranial nerve palsies, infiltration of the retina, and cerebral infiltrates on cranial computed tomographic scans or magnetic resonance imaging are defined as having CNS disease.

PROGNOSTIC FACTORS

Acute lymphoblastic leukemia

The delineation of prognostic features both at initial diagnosis and during treatment has become an essential element in the design and conduct of clinical trials.[50] As childhood ALL comprises many different biologic subsets with different prognoses, adjustment of treatment according to the risk of treatment failure is an important goal in most clinical trials. However, even in specific biologic subgroups, the patients' prognoses are varied, as shown by their different early response to treatment and its influence on event-free survival (EFS).[51,52] Most study groups are challenged to refine their stratification criteria to find a low-risk group with a nearly 100 percent cure rate using a treatment with a limited potential for late adverse sequelae.

Table 62.6 St. Jude's (Murphy) staging system for childhood non-Hodgkin lymphoma

Stage	Definition	Distribution of LBL
Stage I	A single tumor (extranodal) or single anatomical area (nodal) with the exclusion of the mediastinum or abdomen	5%
Stage II	A single tumor (extranodal) with regional lymph node involvement	6%
	Two or more nodal areas on the same side of the diaphragm	
	Two single (extranodal) tumors with or without regional lymph node involvement on the same side of the diaphragm	
	A primary gastrointestinal tract tumor, usually in the ileocecal area, with or without involvement of associated mesenteric lymph nodes only, completely resected	
Stage III	Two single tumors (extranodal) on both sides of the diaphragm	65%
	Two or more nodal areas on both sides of the diaphragm	
	All the primary intrathoracic tumors (mediastinal, thymic, pleural)	
	All extensive primary abdominal tumors, not resectable	
	All paraspinal or epidural tumors	
Stage IV	Any of the above with initial BM (<25%) and/or CNS involvement	24%

LBL, lymphoblastic lymphoma; BM, bone marrow; CNS, central nervous system.

It is equally important to identify high-risk patients for whom augmentation of therapy is necessary. Prognostic markers in childhood ALL mostly include clinical and biological parameters assessed at the time of initial diagnosis (Table 62.7), while some study groups also incorporate estimates of initial treatment response into their stratification system. However, treatment itself still is the most important prognostic factor, as the relevance of virtually all other factors is associated with the type and intensity of the treatment administered.

Due to the fact that therapy varies between different study groups and hence comparison of prognostic factors and treatment results is therefore difficult, participants of a workshop held in Rome in 1985 (sponsored by the National Cancer Institute [NCI]) developed a uniform approach to risk stratification in childhood ALL, taking into account age and white blood cell (WBC) count at initial diagnosis.[53] These so-called NCI or Rome Criteria defined two risk groups for precursor B cell ALL (standard-risk group: WBC count <50 000/μL and age 1–9 years; high-risk group: WBC count ≥50 000/μL and age ≥10 years). Patients with infant ALL and T cell ALL were not included in the classification.

Besides age and WBC count at diagnosis, a list of other parameters with potential prognostic relevance has been identified in several studies, including gender, race, organomegaly, CNS status, immunophenotype, genetic abnormalities, and early response to treatment as assessed by the number of blasts in the BM and peripheral blood (PB) or by minimal residual disease.[7,50,52,54–60]

Clinical features at diagnosis

Age and WBC count at diagnosis have consistent prognostic relevance in most clinical trials, retaining their significance after adjustment for other criteria. In general, infants have the worst outcome (EFS ~50 percent).[61,62] However, this observation reflects the association with a high tumor load at diagnosis and the unfavorable pro-B-ALL phenotype that is accompanied by *MLL* rearrangements (mostly *MLL/AF4*) in about 70–80 percent of cases.[51,56] Patients with an intermediate age (between 1 and 10 years) have the best prognosis, in particular patients between 2 and 5 years old, who comprise approximately 60 percent of the entire ALL population. Adolescents with ALL have a relatively poor prognosis.[63] This association seems to be related to a greater constellation of high-risk features in this age group as shown by the increasing incidence of the T cell and pro-B-ALL phenotype and of the Philadelphia translocation. In contrast, the *TEL/AML1* rearrangement or high-hyperdiploid karyotypes are rarely observed in adolescents. Intriguingly, a French study demonstrated that patients aged between 15 and 20 years had a significantly better outcome when treated with intensive protocols for children than within adult ALL trials.[64] This

Table 62.7 Clinical features at initial diagnosis of ALL with their corresponding EFS rates (according to the results of trial ALL-BFM 90[69])

	Patients	Distribution (%)	6-year EFS (% ± SE)	P (log-rank)
All patients	2178	100	78 ± 1	
Male	1261	57.9	75 ± 1	0.0001
Female	917	42.1	82 ± 1	
Age (years)				
<1	59	2.7	50 ± 7	0.0001
1–5	1316	60.4	83 ± 1	
6–9	417	19.2	74 ± 2	
10–13	245	11.2	66 ± 3	
14–18	141	6.5	64 ± 4	
Leukocytes(×10³/μL)				
<10	1000	45.9	85 ± 1	0.0001
10–19	343	15.8	80 ± 2	
20–49	350	16.1	81 ± 2	
50–199	358	16.4	66 ± 3	
≥200	127	5.8	36 ± 5	
CNS disease	54	2.5	48 ± 7	0.0001
Mediastinal mass	171	8.1	64 ± 4	0.0001
Hepatosplenomegaly				
Liver >4 cm*	673	30.9	71 ± 2	0.0001
Spleen >4 cm*	589	27.0	68 ± 2	0.0001

*Below the costal margin.
ALL, acute lymphoblastic leukemia; EFS, event-free survival; BFM, Berlin-Frankfurt-Münster; SE, standard error; CNS, central nervous system.

discrepancy was interpreted as being due to the more condensed use and higher dosages of important ALL drugs in the pediatric protocols such as corticosteroids, L-asparaginase (L-ASP), and etoposide and by the observation that patients treated according to adult protocols had a significant treatment delay between remission and the first postremission course (7 days in the adult vs 2 days in the pediatric trial).

The leukemic cell mass as reflected by the initial WBC count and the extent of organomegaly still has overriding prognostic relevance in most clinical trials. Overall, there is a clear correlation between the initial WBC count and outcome. Children with high WBC counts have the poorest prognosis. Taking this fact into consideration, the combination of age and WBC count was used to establish the NCI criteria. Moreover, in the BFM group trials ALL-BFM 81 and ALL-BFM 83, risk stratification was merely based on the so-called BFM risk factor, including the peripheral blast cell count and size of liver and spleen at diagnosis.[58]

The prognostic relevance of a mediastinal mass in patients with T cell ALL has been controversial, but recent analyses have demonstrated that neither its presence nor its response to treatment has prognostic implications when children are treated according to their risk of treatment failure (e.g., prednisone response).[65,66] Since most study groups consider their patients with T-lineage ALL *per se* at a higher risk of relapse and treat them accordingly, survival rates are now comparable with those of children with precursor B cell ALL.[7,67]

The worse prognosis of boys with ALL as compared to girls is another consistent finding of most studies. It cannot be explained by a higher incidence of testicular relapse, as the frequency of this has dramatically dropped with the introduction of higher dosages of intravenous methotrexate. However, analysis of recent ALL-BFM studies showed that boys more often showed a poor response to prednisone as compared to girls.[7,66]

Patients with initial CNS disease have a dismal prognosis without adequate treatment. Analysis of the ALL-BFM 95 study demonstrated that children with CNS-3 status more often had associated characteristics for an unfavorable prognosis such as age $\geqslant$10 years, high WBC counts, T cell phenotype, and a poor response to prednisone.[49] It was also shown that CNS-3 status and a traumatic lumbar puncture were poor prognostic markers, whereas CNS-2 status, although also associated with unfavorable features at diagnosis, had a similarly good outcome to CNS-1 status.

Immunophenotype

Patients with pro-B-ALL and T cell ALL have a worse prognosis as compared to the largest group of children with common ALL (cALL). For the pro-B-ALL patients, the relatively dismal prognosis may be due to the association with *MLL* rearrangements, high incidence of infant ALL, and its poor early response to treatment.[7,51,68] In T cell ALL cases, the poor prognosis is mainly related to the higher proportion of prednisone poor responders rather than to the association with a

mediastinal mass or high WBC counts at diagnosis.[66,69] As T cell blasts accumulate fewer methotrexate polyglutamates, the steadily improving prognosis of T-lineage ALL within the ALL-BFM trials could be attributed to the introduction of higher dosages of methotrexate from study ALL-BFM 86 onward, which may overcome this relative resistance. Several other trials have also demonstrated that sensitivity to L-ASP may in part be responsible for the improved prognosis.[67]

The common and pre-B-ALL cases represent the most favorable ALL subtypes. Most good-risk genetic features such as the *TEL/AML1* fusion gene or high-hyperdiploid karyotypes can be found among these cases.[36,40,47] The prognostic relevance of the coexpression of myeloid markers on lymphoid blast cells is a controversial issue which has been discussed for many years. However, more recent studies have shown that outcome for myeloid marker-positive ALL is similar to that of typical precursor B cell ALL.[26,66,69–71]

Cytogenetic abnormalities

Due to their major prognostic relevance, cytogenetic abnormalities are used for risk stratification in almost all contemporary protocols. Patients with high-hyperdiploid karyotypes have a favorable outcome with antimetabolite-based chemotherapy.[47] Gain of chromosomes 4, 10, and 17 seems to identify a specific subset with EFS rates greater than 90 percent.[45] High-hyperdiploid leukemic cells have a marked propensity to undergo spontaneous apoptosis, which together with the high sensitivity to chemotherapy may account for the high survival rates.[72] Moreover, they exhibit a higher expression level of the methotrexate uptake transporter RFC (reduced folate carrier), which may explain the higher accumulation of methotrexate polyglutamates in the blasts, as compared to other ALL subsets.[73] In contrast, hypodiploidy has been reported to have a worse treatment outcome. However, a recent intergroup study demonstrated that the prognosis is not uniformly poor and that patients with 44 chromosomes had significantly better results than patients with fewer than 44 chromosomes (mostly 25–29 chromosomes).[74]

The cryptic translocation t(12;21) confers an extremely good prognosis. The *TEL/AML1* rearrangement is usually associated with a favorable age and WBC count at diagnosis, a cALL phenotype with coexpression of myeloid markers, and a rapid early response to treatment.[38,40,44] Conversely, the translocation t(9;22) has a worse outcome and is often associated with high WBC counts and a poor early response to prednisone. In patients with Philadelphia$^+$ ALL, treatment is usually intensified with myeloablative therapy followed by stem cell transplantation.[52,75]

As recent collaborative studies have shown marked clinical heterogeneity among 11q23/*MLL*-rearranged ALL, requiring distinct treatment approaches for different age groups and different 11q23/*MLL* translocations, it seems absolutely essential to screen for *MLL* abnormalities and their fusion partners in childhood ALL.[56,68] According to a large collaborative analysis in 497 11q23/*MLL*-rearranged patients, infants with a t(4;11) translocation appeared to have the worst prognosis.[68]

Assessment of early response to treatment

It is now very well established that estimates of early response are strong predictors for treatment outcome. Several study groups have evaluated a variety of methods to assess early response to therapy such as the reduction of blasts in BM and PB at different time points in induction therapy.

The easiest method for early response evaluation is determination of the blast cell count in the PB after a 7-day therapy with prednisone and one intrathecal dose of methotrexate on day 1. The BFM group has used this so-called 'prednisone response' since 1986 as the basis for patient stratification.[7] In the original ALL-BFM 83 study, the *in vivo* response to prednisone was prospectively proven to have a significant impact on survival, because patients with ≥1000 blasts/μL had a significantly inferior outcome compared to patients with <1000 blasts/μL on day 8 of treatment.[76] Moreover, in study ALL-BFM 90, it was shown that patients with <1000 blasts/μL at diagnosis did not have a different outcome from true 'prednisone good responders' with ≥1000 blasts/μL at initial diagnosis.[77] However, it remains unknown whether patients with very high initial WBC counts and an impressive cell reduction after 7 days of prednisone (but still ≥1000 blasts/μL on day 8) are subject to subsequent overtreatment or not. Based on the accumulating experience with a significant population of patients, the prednisone response has retained its strong prognostic significance over the years, defining a group of patients with a good prognosis and one with a poor prognosis (Fig. 62.1).[7,69] Intriguingly, among specific leukemia subsets such as infant and Philadelphia+ ALL, the prednisone response also

emerged as an independent prognostic factor.[51,52] This finding suggests that genetic abnormalities do not predict outcome *per se* and that the *in vivo* response to chemotherapy is an overriding prognostic factor. It not only reflects the propensity of the blasts to undergo apoptosis but also the interpatient variability in pharmacodynamics. In addition, studies from the St. Jude Children's Hospital have also shown that the presence of circulating blasts after 1 week of multi-agent chemotherapy is an adverse prognostic indicator.[78]

Other methodologies for evaluation of early response to treatment include cytological analysis of the BM on days 7 and 14 as used by the Children's Cancer Group (CCG).[59,79,80] The BM is usually rated M1, M2, or M3. M1 is defined by less than 5 percent residual blasts and signs of recovering hematopoesis, M2 refers to 5–25 percent blasts, and M3 describes a BM with ≥25 percent blasts. At both time points M1 indicates a good prognosis, whereas patients with M2 or M3 BM on day 7 can be further separated according to their risk for relapse by using the BM on day 14. Patients with a M2 or M3 BM on day 14 have a poor prognosis. The BFM group also utilized BM status on day 15 to assess early treatment response. (This specific time point is now being used for risk stratification in the ALL Intercontinental-BFM 2002 trial.)[81] Although the prednisone response more accurately separates patients with different prognoses as compared to the BM status on day 15 (Fig. 62.2), the BM status on day 15 may add some extra information regarding risk groups – e.g., patients with a poor prednisone response and a M3 BM on day 15 have an extremely dismal prognosis and thus are candidates for stem cell transplantation. In summary, blood and BM cytology reliably identifies patients with an inadequate early response to treatment who have a very high risk of relapse, but the majority of patients who will relapse are in fact not defined by this conventional method.

Assessment of the kinetics of minimal residual disease (MRD) beyond the optical limit of detection during

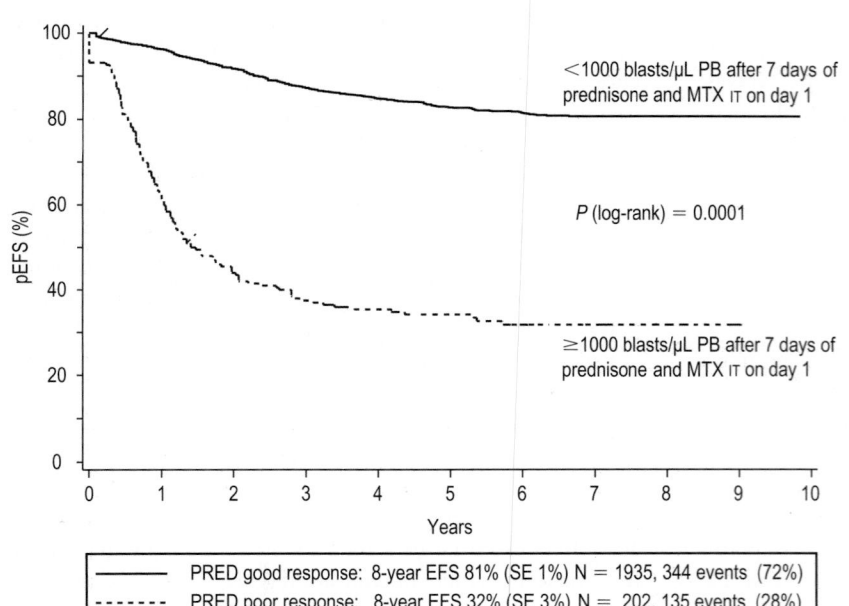

Figure 62.1 Probability of event-free survival (pEFS) in precursor B cell ALL according to the response in peripheral blood (PB) after a 7-day prephase with prednisone (PRED) and one intrathecal (IT) dose of methotrexate (MTX) on day 1 (study ALL-BFM 90). SE, standard error.

treatment by investigation of clone-specific immunoglobulin (Ig) and TCR gene rearrangements, leukemia-specific fusion genes, or immunophenotypes further improved the accuracy of risk allocation.[28,31,32,82–85] This new concept is based on the fact that modern technologies like RT-PCR or flow cytometry can detect as low as one residual leukemic cell in 10 000 BM cells and are therefore more accurate methods for defining response than morphologic examination of the BM. The problem with genetic markers such as the *TEL/AML1*, *BCR/ABL*, or *MLL/AF4* rearrangements is that fewer than 40 percent of patients carry such defined translocations and the majority of relapses occur in patients with normal or undetectable cytogenetic aberrations. However, clone-specific Ig or TCR rearrangements or leukemia-associated phenotypic aberrations are detectable in nearly all patients with ALL. Flow cytometric MRD analysis is relatively inexpensive, can be done very quickly, and has an adequate sensitivity of one leukemic cell in 1000–10 000 nucleated BM cells. However, the use and interpretation of fluorescence-activated cell sorting (FACS) is highly dependent on the experience of the investigators. On the other hand, PCR-based methods used to identify clone-specific Ig or TCR rearrangements require more intensive laboratory workup and are therefore also more expensive.

The BFM group introduced assessment of MRD as the general stratification factor [besides prednisone response and translocations t(9;22) and t(4;11)] in its ongoing trial ALL-BFM 2000, using clone-specific Ig and TCR gene rearrangements. The risk group classification is based on the data of an international trial performed at the beginning of the 1990s that proved that using two time points for evaluation of MRD (5 and 12 weeks after initiation of therapy) can identify three distinct risk groups with completely different prognoses (Fig. 62.3).[85] Children without detectable MRD at

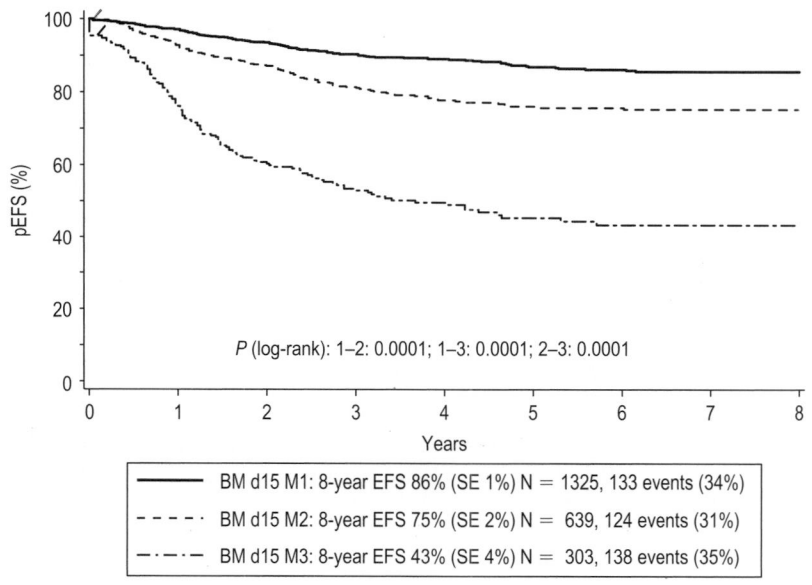

Figure 62.2 Probability of event-free survival (pEFS) in precursor B cell ALL according to the morphologic response in bone marrow (BM) after 14 days of induction therapy (study ALL-BFM 90). d15, day 15; SE, standard error.

P (log-rank): 1–2: 0.0001; 1–3: 0.0001; 2–3: 0.0001

— BM d15 M1: 8-year EFS 86% (SE 1%) N = 1325, 133 events (34%)
- - - BM d15 M2: 8-year EFS 75% (SE 2%) N = 639, 124 events (31%)
-·-·- BM d15 M3: 8-year EFS 43% (SE 4%) N = 303, 138 events (35%)

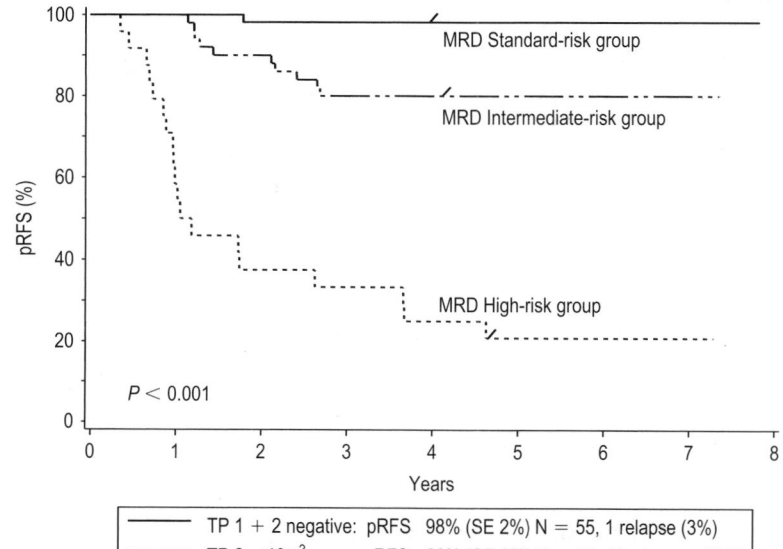

Figure 62.3 Probability of relapse-free survival (pRFS) according to minimal residual disease (MRD) after 5 and 12 weeks of therapy as well as the prednisone response on day 8 (PPR, prednisone poor response).[85] TP, time point; SE, standard error.

MRD Standard-risk group

MRD Intermediate-risk group

MRD High-risk group

P < 0.001

— TP 1 + 2 negative: pRFS 98% (SE 2%) N = 55, 1 relapse (3%)
-·-·- TP 2 <10^{-3}: pRFS 80% (SE 6%) N = 50, 10 relapses (33%)
- - - TP 2 ≥10^{-3}/PPR: pRFS 21% (SE 8%) N = 24, 19 relapses (64%)

both time points had a chance of cure almost equivalent to 100 percent and are now allocated to the standard-risk group (40 percent of all patients). High-risk patients with a MRD level $\geq 10^{-3}$ (≥ 1 leukemic cell in 10^3 mononuclear cells) at time points 1 and 2 included approximately two-thirds of relapses if the prednisone response was also taken into consideration (20 percent of all patients). The remaining intermediate-risk patients (approximately one-third to one-half of the patients) who had an MRD level $<10^{-3}$ at time point 2 had an EFS of 75–80 percent.

In general, most ongoing studies rely on the MRD level at the end of induction therapy and some further subdivide patients using a second time point.[29–32] However, as the protocols differ in most clinical trials, the overall prognostic value and the feasibility of evaluating MRD in large multicenter trials has first to be confirmed prospectively by the different study groups.

Lymphoblastic lymphoma

Since the early 1980s it has been well established that the choice of initial treatment in pediatric NHL depends on whether the disease is localized or disseminated and whether the histologic subtype is lymphoblastic or nonlymphoblastic (B cell NHL, anaplastic large cell lymphoma).[4,5,12,86–88] Patients with LBL are usually treated with a protocol similar or identical to that for ALL and risk stratification is merely based on stage of disease.[11,89] To date, no study group has succeeded in finding any other stable prognostic factor other than stage. Since response to treatment is well established to be an overriding prognostic factor in childhood ALL, enabling intensification of treatment for early poor responders, it seems probable that intensified regimens would cure comparable patients with slowly responding NHL.

While a reliable assessment for minimal disseminated and residual disease in the BM or PB of children with LBL has not yet been established, the dimensions of the mediastinal tumor currently appear to be the only disease marker to quantify treatment response. While the persistence of a large tumor mass after induction therapy (less than 70 percent regression on day 33 in the NHL-BFM trials) is usually regarded as treatment failure and has been used to upgrade patients into high-risk therapy arms, the significance of a small residual mass is not yet completely clear. Trial NHL-BFM 90 revealed that local recurrence in the mediastinum was indeed mostly responsible for treatment failure, but it did not show that patients with a persistent tumor at day 33 (incomplete regression, but greater than 70 percent) or after completion of early intensification (day 63, any residual tumor) had a significantly worse prognosis compared with those whose tumor vanished completely.[11] Local recurrences were diagnosed with a comparable frequency in patients with and without a residual tumor at both time points. However, a British study reported that children with a persistent mediastinal mass after 60 days of therapy had a dismal prognosis.[90] This discrepancy between the two studies might be due to differences in intensity or combinations of chemotherapy; the British protocols did not include high-dose methotrexate or cyclophosphamide.

TREATMENT OF ACUTE LYMPHOBLASTIC LEUKEMIA

With cure rates around 80 percent, treatment results achieved with chemotherapy in childhood ALL serve as a model of successful anticancer treatment (Table 62.8).[7–9] Modern ALL therapy is divided into four components: (1) remission induction therapy; (2) consolidation and extra-compartment therapy; (3) delayed reintensification or reinduction therapy; and (4) maintenance therapy.

Remission induction

The initial aim of ALL therapy is induction of remission. Remission is a condition defined by the absence of clinical symptoms and signs of disease, absence of blast cells in PB and CSF, and a BM with less than 5 percent blast cells. The induction protocol usually lasts 4–6 weeks and includes three to four drugs. The basic three-drug regimen comprises corticosteroids (prednisone, in a few trials dexamethasone), vincristine, and L-ASP.[69,91–93] The BFM group and others

Table 62.8 Five-year event-free survival rates achieved in childhood ALL (all patients, precursor B cell, and precursor T cell ALL) by 12 different study groups[7–9]

Trial	Patients	All	Precursor B cell	Precursor T cell
DFCI 91-01	377	83%	84%	79%
BFM 90	2178	78%	80%	61%
NOPHO 92-98	1143	78%	79%	61%
POG 86-94	4267	n.a.	71%	51%
COALL 92	538	77%	78%	71%
STJCH 13A	165	77%	80%	61%
CCG 89-95	5121	75%	75%	73%
DCLSG ALL8	467	73%	73%	71%
CLCG-EORTC 58881	2065	71%	72%	64%
AIEOP 91	1194	71%	75%	40%
UKALL XI	2090	63%	65%	51%
Tokyo 92-13	347	63%	63%	59%

ALL, acute lymphoblastic leukemia; DFCI, Dana-Farber Cancer Institute Consortium; BFM, Berlin-Frankfurt-Münster; NOPHO; Nordic Society of Pediatric Hematology and Oncology; POG, Pediatric Oncology Group; COALL, Cooperative ALL Group; STJHC, St. Jude Children's Hospital; CCG, Children's Cancer Group; DCLSG, Dutch Childhood Leukemia Study Group; CLCG-EORTC, Children Leukemia Cooperative Group from EORTC (European Organization for Research and Treatment in Cancer); AIEOP, Italian Association of Pediatric Hematology and Oncology; UK, United Kingdom; Tokyo, Tokyo Children's Cancer Study Group; n.a., not available.

have added an anthracycline (e.g., daunorubicin) as a fourth drug.[7,69] However, due to a possible increase in both acute and long-term toxicity, several study groups avoid anthracyclines in patients with a low risk for relapse.[93,94] Moreover, there are other small differences in the composition of the induction protocol used by the different study groups. For example, the Cooperative ALL study group postpones L-ASP to consolidation in order to avoid thromboembolic side effects during induction therapy.[95]

The choice of the corticosteroid in induction treatment is a matter of controversial discussion.[96,97] There is some evidence that dexamethasone has a stronger antileukemic efficacy *in vitro* and a better penetration into the CSF than prednisone, but it may also be associated with a greater risk of toxicity when combined with vincristine, anthracyclines, and L-ASP.[98] Some study groups are currently performing randomized trials in order to definitively establish whether patients with ALL benefit from substituting dexamethasone for prednisone with respect to prevention of CNS relapse and achievement of better EFS rates.

Another aspect concerning induction therapy is dose intensity, which may have a significant impact on the results.[69,76] Using a three- to four-drug induction treatment, more than 95 percent of patients will achieve remission. The remaining patients eventually die from disease- or treatment-related complications or suffer from resistant disease (slow responders or nonresponders). In order to measure the prednisone response, the BFM induction protocol (protocol I, phase a) traditionally starts with a 7-day prephase of prednisone and one intrathecal dose of methotrexate on day 1 (Fig. 62.4). This window is also particularly helpful in avoiding early complications due to severe tumor lysis. The first 5 weeks of induction therapy are then followed by an early 4-week intensification phase (protocol I, phase b) including cyclophosphamide, cytarabine (Ara-C), intrathecal methotrexate, and oral 6-mercaptopurine (Fig. 62.4).

Consolidation and sanctuary sites

Consolidation and 'extracompartment' therapy aim to kill residual leukemic cells residing in sanctuary sites such as the CNS and testicles. This part of the treatment relies mainly on methotrexate (intravenous and intrathecal) and oral 6-mercaptopurine. Intensification of consolidation for intermediate-risk patients by the addition of high-dose L-ASP or high-dose Ara-C in recent randomized ALL-BFM studies has not shown any benefit with respect to disease-free survival.

Prophylactic cranial radiation therapy (usually timed after reinduction therapy) given in high dosages during the 1960s and 1970s largely contributed to the improvement in overall treatment results. However, due to acute and especially long-term toxicity (development of secondary malignancies, neuropsychological and hormonal deficits) associated with cranial radiation therapy, reduction and finally elimination of the irradiation seemed mandatory in view of the high cure rates in ALL (around 70–80 percent) with contemporary chemotherapeutic regimens.[99,100] Along with the use of more CNS-directed chemotherapy and intensified intrathecal therapy, it is now possible to omit prophylactic cranial irradiation altogether for the vast majority of patients.

In trial ALL-BFM 81, it was shown that intermediate-dose methotrexate (four cycles of $0.5\,g/m^2/24$ hours) can reliably protect the testicles from relapse but not avoid CNS relapses when cranial irradiation is omitted.[57,101] With the introduction of four cycles of high-dose methotrexate ($5\,g/m^2$) during consolidation therapy in trial ALL-BFM 86 and its successors, it was demonstrated that despite a stepwise reduction of cranial radiation therapy, patients could be adequately protected from CNS relapse.[7,66,69] This appeared to be particularly due to the cytotoxic steady-state concentrations of methotrexate in the CSF after a 24-hour

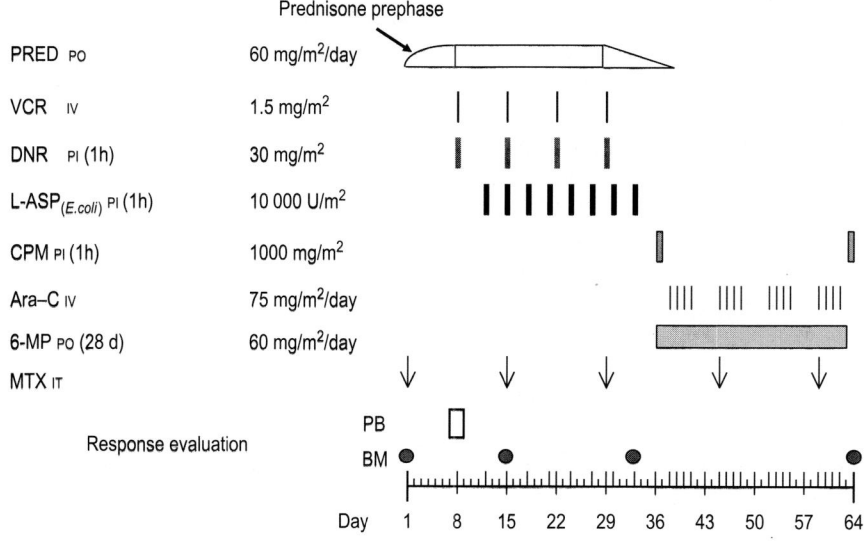

Figure 62.4 Outline of induction therapy (protocol I, phase a) and early intensification treatment (protocol I, phase b) according to trial ALL-BFM 90 (including time points of response evaluation in peripheral blood [PB] and bone marrow [BM]). PO, oral; IV, intravenous; PI, per infusion; IT, intrathecal; PRED, prednisone; VCR, vincristine; DNR, daunorubicin; L-ASP, L-asparaginase; CPM, cyclophosphamide; Ara-C, cytarabine; 6-MP, 6-mercaptopurine; MTX, methotrexate.

infusion. Finally, in trial ALL-BFM 95, CNS prophylaxis with 12 Gy cranial irradiation was only given to patients with T cell and high-risk ALL and older than 12 months, which proved to be efficient in prevention of CNS recurrences after adequate long-term follow-up.[102]

As the prognosis of patients with T cell ALL improved dramatically following the introduction of high-dose methotrexate and extended use of L-ASP, the use of prophylactic cranial radiation therapy in this particular subset of patients was questioned in several studies. Intriguingly, an intergroup study in patients with intermediate-risk T cell ALL showed that replacement of cranial radiation therapy by triple intrathecal chemotherapy (prednisone, cytarabine, methotrexate) given during maintenance therapy (study ALL-Italian Association of Pediatric Hematology and Oncology [AIEOP] 91) was less efficient in prevention of systemic and CNS relapses than 12 Gy prophylactic cranial irradiation in identical patients treated in trial ALL-BFM 90.[103] Another study performed by the CCG, however, found that intensified chemotherapy including a delayed intensification phase, together with extended intrathecal treatment, is as effective in preventing CNS relapse as cranial radiation therapy.[104] This observation suggests that prevention of CNS recurrence largely depends on the underlying systemic chemotherapy.

Reintensification (reinduction) therapy

Reintensification therapy uses similar drugs to those used in the induction protocol and is normally given 2–3 weeks after consolidation therapy. In the treatment protocol (protocol II or III, phase a) used by the ALL-BFM studies, dexamethasone is substituted for prednisone and doxorubicin is used instead of daunorubicin. Vincristine and L-ASP are given as in induction therapy. The reintensification regimen also includes a second 2-week phase with

cyclophosphamide, Ara-C, intrathecal methotrexate, and oral 6-thioguanine (protocol II or III, phase b).

An important milestone in recognizing that reinduction or delayed reintensification could significantly improve EFS was trial ALL-BFM 76, in which it was shown that high-risk patients had a 10-year EFS of 70 percent using a delayed reintensification (protocol II), as compared to 60 percent with an intensification phase given shortly after induction and 38 percent with no reinduction therapy.[92] In trial ALL-BFM 83 it was clearly proven that reintensification is of benefit with regard to the frequency of both systemic and CNS relapses.[76] In an attempt to decrease therapy-related toxicity, low-risk patients were randomized to receive reintensification therapy (protocol III) or not. Protocol III is very similar to protocol II, but includes only two doses of vincristine and doxorubicin instead of four. None of the patients underwent prophylactic cranial irradiation. Although the number of isolated CNS relapses was low in both groups, the number of combined CNS and BM relapses as well as of isolated systemic relapses was particularly high in patients without reintensification (Fig. 62.5). Similar results were found in trial ALL-BFM 86, in which standard-risk patients fared worse without a delayed reintensification (protocol II), as reflected by the occurrence of more systemic relapses.[66] The value of reintensification was finally confirmed by the CCG and AIEOP study groups in high-risk patients in a trial which showed an improvement in EFS consequent upon using two delayed reintensification phases.[105,106]

Maintenance therapy

The principle aim of maintenance therapy is to sustain remission by reducing the pool of residual leukemic cells while sparing the normal BM. Maintenance therapy is

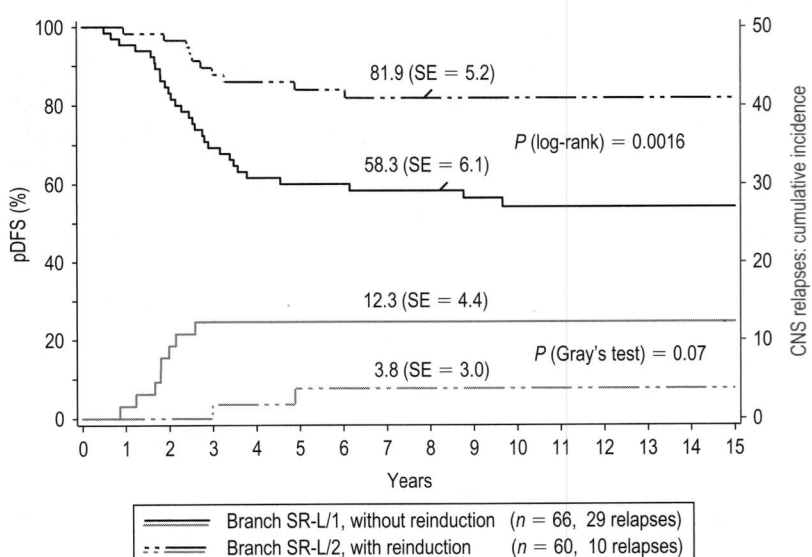

Figure 62.5 Influence of reinduction therapy on disease-free survival (DFS) and the cumulative incidence of CNS relapses in low-risk patients of trial ALL-BFM 83[76]. CNS, central nervous system; SE, standard error.

mainly based on daily oral 6-mercaptopurine and weekly oral methotrexate. Several study groups suggest the additional use of monthly pulses of vincristine accompanied by an oral glucocorticoid.[107] However, at the moment, there is no clear evidence that the addition of such pulses may translate into improved EFS. It is generally accepted that maintenance therapy for up to 2 years has an unequivocal place in ALL treatment as most attempts to reduce its duration to less than 2 years have resulted in an increased frequency of leukemic relapse.[7] Maintenance therapy seems to have particular value in the treatment of precursor B cell ALL as compared to T cell ALL, which may be explained by the different relapse pattern in patients with T cell ALL, who tend to relapse very early. The role of extended maintenance therapy in boys (3 years vs 2 years for girls) as used by the CCG or trial ALL-BFM 95 (standard-risk group) will be clarified when long-term follow-up data become available.

Treatment failures and relapses

There are four ways in which treatment can fail: (1) in a small proportion of patients (~1 percent) the disease is resistant to standard induction therapy; (2) 2–3 percent of patients die during induction therapy or in complete remission due to severe adverse events; (3) 1–2 percent of patients develop a secondary malignancy; and (4) 15–20 percent of children suffer from a relapse – patients with recurrent ALL account for one of the most common malignancies diagnosed in childhood.

Patients who relapse whilst on chemotherapy are less likely to attain a second remission and most often have shorter remission durations than patients with disease recurrence after cessation of therapy.[108–110] Thus, regarding prognosis of ALL relapse, most study groups distinguish between very early (<18 months after initial diagnosis), early (between 18 and 30 months after initial diagnosis), and late relapses (≥6 months after the end of first-line therapy).[111] Besides duration of first remission, site of relapse has also been consistently referred to as an important prognostic factor.[108–110] Recently, the widespread clinical impression that BM relapse is associated with a worse prognosis has been confirmed (10-year EFS 15 percent for isolated BM and 34 percent for combined BM relapse) as compared to extramedullary relapses (CNS, testicles, or other focal relapses; 10-year EFS 44 percent).[110,112,113] The best prognosis is associated with extramedullary relapses when not accompanied by a systemic relapse. In addition to the duration of first remission and relapse site, other factors like age at diagnosis, immunophenotype, cytogenetic or molecular-genetic abnormalities, WBC or blast cell count, as well as gender and previous treatment may influence the patient's prognosis;[111] for example, poor-risk features are T cell phenotypes, age <1 or ≥10 years at diagnosis, and translocations t(9;22) and t(4;11).[114,115] In contrast, good-risk features comprise the *TEL/AML1* rearrangement (mainly

due to late recurrence) and low or undetectable MRD levels early during second remission induction therapy.[116,117]

Approximately 85 percent of patients achieve a second remission, but half of them will finally succumb to further recurrent disease when treated by conventional chemotherapy alone.[111] Similar to the common trend in the management of newly diagnosed ALL, biological and clinical risk factors have been used as a basis for the prospective stratification of relapsed patients into different risk groups. The BFM group was the first to address the effect of this concept systematically in five consecutive multicenter studies (ALL-REZ BFM 83–96).[118] By considering only risk factors with independent influence on outcome (time, site, and phenotype of relapse) four treatment groups could be identified (Table 62.9).

Chemotherapy in all types of relapsed ALL is based on reinduction, postinduction/consolidation, and maintenance chemotherapy, relying on antileukemic drugs that have already been used during initial treatment. The BFM strategy consists of rotating 7-day treatment blocks and also includes triple intrathecal chemotherapy for prophylactic and therapeutic CNS therapy. Although there is controversy as to whether or not a patient should be included in a BM transplantation program, patients with a particularly high risk for subsequent relapse (risk groups S3/S4) all proceed to a myeloablative allograft.

Children with CNS relapse additionally receive cranial irradiation (18 Gy), but the dose of radiation has to be modified according to previous radiation therapy and the interval to second irradiation. The ALL-REZ BFM group also demonstrated that patients with isolated BM relapse profit from prophylactic cranial irradiation (12 Gy).[119] In unilateral testicular disease, the clinically affected testis may be removed and the remaining one irradiated (15–18 Gy according to the results of biopsy). In cases of clinical unilateral or bilateral testicular involvement and no resection, local irradiation with 24 Gy is recommended.

Table 62.9 Risk groups for relapsed childhood acute lymphoblastic leukemia

Therapy group	Patients	pEFS
S1	All patients with late extramedullary relapse	77%
S2	All patients with very early and early extramedullary relapse, all combined (early and late) non-T-ALL relapses, and all late non-T-ALL BM relapses	35%
S3	All patients with early isolated non-T-ALL BM relapses	4%
S4	All patients with very early combined and isolated BM relapses, and all patients with T cell ALL BM relapses	0%

ALL, acute lymphoblastic leukemia; pEFS, probability of event-free survival; BM, bone marrow.

Hematopoietic stem cell transplantation

Allogeneic stem cell transplantation is a widely accepted treatment option for defined ALL patients resistant to initial therapy with a very high risk of relapse and recurrent disease.[108,110,111,120,121] The efficacy of this procedure relates to further intensification of therapy as performed by the conditioning regimen and to the graft-versus-leukemia effect. As approximately 75 percent of patients lack a HLA-matched sibling, who would be the preferred donor, transplantation from HLA-matched unrelated donors has emerged as an alternative for the highest-risk patients. Improvements in supportive care, HLA typing and matching by high-resolution techniques, development of granulocyte colony-stimulating factor (G-CSF)-stimulated blood stem cell harvests, and effective methods for stem cell selection have resulted in this approach being recommended more frequently. Transplantation from mismatched, unrelated, or haploidentical donors and cord blood transplantation are less often advocated due to a significantly higher treatment-related mortality, in the range of 25 percent as compared to 10 percent with HLA-identical sibling donors.

As a result of the experience with a significant number of patients during the last 20 years, the BFM group recently established a protocol including explicit indications for stem cell transplantation in first and second remission of childhood ALL.[122] For newly diagnosed patients, the indications for BM transplantation from a HLA-identical sibling are: Philadelphia[+] ALL, t(4;11)[+] ALL, induction failure, MRD level $\geqslant 10^{-3}$ after 12 weeks of therapy, and prednisone poor response with either pro-B-ALL, T cell ALL, WBC count $\geqslant 100\,000/\mu L$, or a M3 BM on day 15. The conditioning regimen for patients older than 2 years comprises fractionated total-body irradiation and etoposide. Patients younger than 2 years receive busulfan, cyclophosphamide, and etoposide. For relapsed ALL cases stratified into therapy group S2, the MRD level after two induction blocks is used to enrol the patient into a transplantation setting or not, whereas for poor-risk patients in category S3/S4, all available donors are considered for the transplant procedure, except for autologous grafts which can be recommended only in patients with isolated CNS involvement.

TREATMENT OF LYMPHOBLASTIC LYMPHOMA

An increase in the cure rate for children and adolescents with LBL, from 10 percent in the 1950s to 80 percent currently, has been gained with modern chemotherapeutic regimens.[11,88,89,123] A first major step was the introduction of multiagent chemotherapy by Wollner et al. in the 1970s with the LSA$_2$-L$_2$ protocol consisting of elements known to be effective against LBL and ALL.[124] The ten-drug combination comprising induction, consolidation, and maintenance therapy was given for a total treatment duration of 3 years. Intrathecal methotrexate was added in all phases. Most patients underwent radiation therapy to the local tumor but no prophylactic cranial irradiation. The program was superior to more classical pulse-like therapies as proven in randomized studies.[87] Finally, it became the gold standard and was applied worldwide with several modifications.

At the same time, the BFM protocol for ALL was developed and used in its unchanged form for LBL.[125] The main difference from the LSA$_2$-L$_2$ protocol was a lower cumulative dosage of drugs with a risk of long-term adverse sequelae, for example the alkylating agents (which harbor the risk of secondary malignancies and infertility) and the potentially cardiotoxic anthracyclines. Additionally, as foreseen in the BFM protocol, no routine local irradiation was given to the mediastinum, inferring the life-long increased risk of secondary malignancies in that region. From the beginning, systemic methotrexate was part of the BFM regimen and was soon escalated to four cycles of 5 g/m^2/24 hours given as consolidation therapy.[11,88,125] Prior to consolidation, the NHL-BFM regimen includes a 5-week induction and early 4-week intensification therapy (protocol I, phase a and b; Fig. 62.4). Patients with stage III/IV disease also undergo a delayed intensification phase (protocol II). For all patients, maintenance treatment with 6-mercaptopurine and methotrexate is scheduled for a total treatment duration of 2 years. Until recently, all patients with stage III/IV disease received prophylactic cranial irradiation (12 Gy). Finally, trial NHL-BFM 90 for T cell LBL resulted in an EFS rate of 90 percent (Fig. 62.6).[11] Precursor B cell LBL patients included in trials NHL-BFM 86 and 90 had an EFS of 73 percent.[10]

Although LBLs are radiosensitive malignancies, local irradiation as a routine measure has been abandoned since the introduction and use of highly effective chemotherapy. However, there is a lack of sufficient information to define the role of local radiation therapy in patients with an inadequate early response of the mediastinal tumor to chemotherapy. With respect to the high cure rates, omission of prophylactic cranial radiation therapy in children receiving

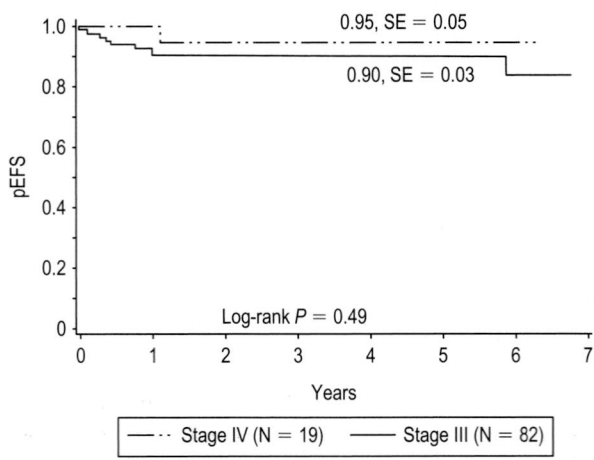

Figure 62.6 Event-free survival (EFS) of T cell LBL patients with stage III and IV disease enrolled into trial NHL-BFM 90[69] (therapy group I for LBL).

highly active, CNS-directed systemic and intrathecal chemotherapy is now being evaluated within the BFM studies, whereas therapeutic irradiation for the rare patients with CNS disease at diagnosis seems indicated. The role of surgery is confined to diagnostic procedures, which should be restricted to the least invasive interventions to gain sufficient tumor material.

Relapse of lymphoblastic lymphoma

Patients with relapsed LBL (mostly local disease recurrences with or without BM and/or CNS involvement) are usually treated with protocols used for relapsed or high-risk ALL, consisting of alternating pulse-like chemotherapy courses based on similar drugs used during initial therapy. In patients with T cell LBL, the interval between initial response and subsequent relapse is usually brief and cure rates with various retrieval chemotherapy regimens are extremely low. Intriguingly, patients with precursor B cell LBL may have a greater chance to achieve a second complete remission. However, the role of hematopoietic stem cell transplantation as second-line treatment of patients with relapsed LBL is as yet unclear and remains to be evaluated in larger cohorts of children within an international cooperation.

ACUTE AND LONG-TERM COMPLICATIONS

The most common acute complications of treatment of childhood lymphoid diseases are infections and the necessity to give blood products due to pancytopenia.[7] Another relevant complication at the time of initial diagnosis and, particularly, at the beginning of chemotherapy is the acute tumor cell lysis syndrome (hyperleukocytosis) that is characterized by electrolyte imbalances, hyperuricemia, and subsequent uric acid nephropathy. The prevention and treatment of infectious complications has largely contributed to the increasing long-term EFS rates. However, regarding prevention of infection, only the use of cotrimoxazole as prophylaxis against *Pneumocystis carinii* pneumonia is well established. The cumulative incidence of early mortality in the ALL-BFM trials 83–90 ranged from 0.3 to 1.7 percent, with the main cause of treatment-related deaths being neutropenic sepsis.[7] With the overall increase in survival, long-term side effects have become the major complication of treatment for childhood lymphoid neoplasms. They include secondary leukemias after etoposide- and alkylating agent-based treatment, radiation therapy-associated brain tumors, cardiomyopathy after therapy including anthracyclines, and avascular necrosis of bone after intensive use of corticosteroids.[21,99,100,126]

FUTURE PERSPECTIVES

In view of the high cure rates, clinical research is now concentrated on three major tasks: to more precisely define patients at risk, to further develop treatment strategies for them, and to reduce the acute and long-term treatment-related toxicity for children with a high probability of cure.

The rate of disease reduction during treatment has a high predictive power to define cohorts with different risks of relapse. Monitoring MRD kinetics during treatment is carried out by many groups.[31,83] Currently, in trial ALL-BFM 2000, a randomized controlled reduction in treatment is being studied in patients with negative MRD results after 5 weeks of therapy, whereas treatment is intensified for those with an MRD level $\geqslant 10^{-3}$ after 12 weeks of therapy. Whether MRD results at different time points have different prognostic significance for biologic subentities (e.g., T cell ALL) is also a matter of ongoing investigation. MLL/AF4$^+$, TEL/AML1$^+$, or hyperdiploid leukemias can be traced back to birth using Guthrie cards, in which samples the respective cytogenetic alterations were already present.[17,127] Whether these preleukemic cell clones escape treatment of full-blown leukemia and detection of MRD as a prognostic factor remains to be elucidated.

Refinement of genetic diagnostic procedures might further highlight the role of gene alterations in leukemogenesis, offering the chance for targeting therapy. Antagonizing the BCR/ABL tyrosine kinase with imatinib mesylate in Philadelphia$^+$ ALL is the first example of a successful translation of this concept into clinical practice.[128] The Fms-like tyrosine kinase 3 (FLT3) expressed in MLL-rearranged or hyperdiploid ALL is another example, in which FLT3 inhibitors may offer a therapeutic option.[129] Moreover, gene expression profiling is on the way to not only reproducing known, biologically different subsets but can also be a tool for detecting new entities. Evaluation of gene polymorphisms or different gene expression in the patient, e.g., those involved in purine or folate metabolism, could allow adaptation of antimetabolite treatment on an individual basis.[73,130]

Treatment with the anti-CD20 antibody rituximab has been shown to be successful in nonlymphoblastic B cell NHL and in adult lymphoproliferative diseases. Its role in pediatric mature B cell lymphoid neoplasms is currently under investigation. Responses of CD20$^+$ ALLs have already been reported, stimulating the design of prospective trials, but since only some precursor B cell ALLs express CD20 at a high level, other epitopes such as CD19 or CD22 are candidates for treatment with monoclonal antibodies.[131]

Halogenized nucleoside analogues such as cladribine and gemcitabine are currently being investigated in phase I and II trials in children with ALL. The latest product of this series, clofarabine, seems to have the most promising activity.[132] A liposomal preparation of intrathecal cytarabine with prolonged activity in the CSF is also now available and might offer improved antileukemic activity and reduce the frequency of lumbar punctures.[133] The polyethylene glycol conjugate of *Escherichia coli*-derived L-ASP (PEG-ASNase) has been found to have protracted activity with respect to asparagine depletion in PB and to be less immunogenic than the native drug.[134] However, it appears to be less active in the CSF and its optimal use and impact on long-term survival remain to be evaluated.

Regarding new prognostic markers in LBL, analysis of minimal disseminated disease at diagnosis and its response kinetics, by using flow cytometry to reveal lymphoma-associated phenotypes, or RT-PCR-based methods to monitor specific rearrangements (e.g., *SIL/TAL*), may allow better risk stratification and identification of patients at risk early during the disease course. A European intergroup collaboration is now evaluating the prognostic significance of MRD and early local tumor regression in LBL patients treated with a BFM backbone. A matter of concern is the nature of a residual mass. Possibly, positron emission tomography will not only allow better monitoring of response but may also differentiate between residual active disease and inert residual masses.[135] As there are still relatively few but increasing data describing the genetic nature of LBL, there is realistic hope that the future will bring less toxic and more risk-adapted treatment regimens designed according to the specific biology of the disease and the patient.

KEY POINTS

- The diagnosis of ALL is based on the cytomorphologic analysis of bone marrow and peripheral blood smears, but the inclusion of immunophenotyping and molecular genetics is needed for the definite diagnosis of biologic subentities. The diagnosis of LBL is traditionally based on the histologic results of a tumor biopsy, but in experienced hands, cytomorphologic and immunophenotypic analyses of freshly obtained tumor cell material are reliable tools to establish a preliminary diagnosis.
- Clinical and laboratory features at diagnosis of ALL are used to adapt treatment to the risk of relapse. However, evaluation of early *in vivo* response to treatment with conventional (morphology of bone marrow and peripheral blood) or submicroscopic methods (clone-specific immunoglobulin and T cell receptor gene rearrangements, leukemia-specific fusion genes, or immunophenotypes) is performed to refine risk group stratification. In LBL, risk group allocation is based on the stage of disease.
- Early response to prednisone is an independent prognostic parameter in different biologic leukemia subentities, suggesting that genetic abnormalities do not predict outcome *per se* and that the *in vivo* response to chemotherapy is a highly important prognostic factor. It not only reflects the propensity of the blasts to undergo apoptosis but also the interpatient variability of pharmacodynamics.

- The prognostic value of minimal residual disease at different time points in ALL therapy depends on the structure and composition of each treatment protocol. Thus, its overriding relevance first has to be proven prospectively by different study groups.
- Multiagent chemotherapy, including more continuous drug exposure, together with repetitive intrathecal therapy, is the hallmark of treatment in ALL and LBL. Cure rates of around 80–90 percent have been achieved in specific subgroups of ALL and for the distinct subgroup of T cell LBL. However, therapy results remain to be improved for high-risk patients and for those with recurrent disease.
- All patients with ALL and LBL need prophylactic CNS therapy. However, with the development of highly effective CNS-directed systemic and intrathecal chemotherapy, cranial radiation therapy is now restricted to ALL patients with initial CNS disease, high-risk features (e.g., poor early response to prednisone), and T cell phenotype.
- A small subgroup of patients with high-risk ALL in first remission (e.g., Philadelphia⁺ ALL, induction failure) but the vast majority of patients in second remission (e.g., very early and early isolated bone marrow relapses) are candidates for hematopoietic stem cell transplantation.

REFERENCES

● = Key primary paper
◆ = Major review article

1. Schrappe M, Harbott J, Riehm H. Acute lymphoblastic leukemia. In: Gadner H, Gaedicke G, Niemeyer C, Ritter J. (eds) *Pediatric hematology and oncology*, 1st Edn. Heidelberg: Springer Medizin Verlag, 2005: 656–79.
2. Margolin J, Poplack D. Acute lymphoblastic leukemia. In: Pizzo P, Poplack D. (eds) *Principles and practice of oncology*, 3rd Edn. Philadelphia: Lippincott-Raven, 1997: 409–62.
3. Niemeyer C, Sallan S. Acute lymphoblastic leukemia. In: Nathan D, Oski F. (eds) *Hematology of infancy and childhood*, 4th Edn. Philadelphia: WB Saunders Company, 1993: 1249–87.
4. Reiter A, Mann G, Parwaresch R. Non-Hodgkin's lymphoma. In: Gadner H, Gaedicke G, Niemeyer C, Ritter J. (eds) *Pediatric hematology and oncology*, 1st Edn. Heidelberg: Springer Medizin Verlag, 2005: 732–51.
5. Shad A, Magrath I. Malignant Non-Hodgkin's lymphoma. In: Pizzo P, Poplack D. (eds) *Principles and practice of*

oncology, 3rd Edn. Philadelphia: Lippincott-Raven, 1997: 545–88.

6. Link M, Donaldson SS. The lymphomas and lymphadenopathy. In: Nathan D, Oski F. (eds) *Hematology of infancy and childhood*, 4th Edn. Philadelphia: WB Saunders Company, 1993: 1319–53.

●7. Schrappe M, Reiter A, Zimmermann M *et al.* Long-term results of four consecutive trials in childhood ALL performed by the ALL-BFM study group from 1981 to 1995. Berlin-Frankfurt-Munster. *Leukemia* 2000; **14**: 2205–22.

8. Pui CH, Boyett JM, Rivera GK *et al.* Long-term results of total therapy studies 11, 12 and 13A for childhood acute lymphoblastic leukemia at St Jude children's research hospital. *Leukemia* 2000; **14**: 2286–94.

9. Gaynon PS, Trigg ME, Heerema NA *et al.* Children's cancer group trials in childhood acute lymphoblastic leukemia: 1983–1995. *Leukemia* 2000; **14**: 2223–33.

10. Neth O, Seidemann K, Jansen P *et al.* Precursor B-cell lymphoblastic lymphoma in childhood and adolescence: clinical features, treatment, and results in trials NHL-BFM 86 and 90. *Med Pediatr Oncol* 2000; **35**: 20–7.

●11. Reiter A, Schrappe M, Ludwig WD *et al.* Intensive ALL-type therapy without local radiotherapy provides a 90% event-free survival for children with T-cell lymphoblastic lymphoma: a BFM group report. *Blood* 2000; **95**: 416–21.

●12. Mora J, Filippa DA, Qin J, Wollner N. Lymphoblastic lymphoma of childhood and the LSA$_2$-L$_2$ protocol: the 30-year experience at Memorial-Sloan-Kettering cancer center. *Cancer* 2003; **98**: 1283–91.

13. Smith OP, Hann I. Pathology of leukaemia. In: Pinkerton CR, Plowman PN, Pieters R. (eds) *Paediatric oncology*, 3rd Edn. London: Arnold, 2004: 83–100.

14. Gupta J, McCarthy KP. Pathology of lymphoma. In: Pinkerton CR, Plowman PN, Pieters R. (eds) *Paediatric oncology*, 3rd Edn. London: Arnold, 2004: 101–14.

15. Seidemann K, Tiemann M, Henze G *et al.* Therapy for non-Hodgkin lymphoma in children with primary immunodeficiency: analysis of 19 patients from the BFM trials. *Med Pediatr Oncol* 1999; **33**: 536–44.

●16. Greaves MF, Maia AT, Wiemels JL, Ford AM. Leukemia in twins: lessons in natural history. *Blood* 2003; **102**: 2321–33.

17. Maia AT, van der Velden VH, Harrison CJ *et al.* Prenatal origin of hyperdiploid acute lymphoblastic leukemia in identical twins. *Leukemia* 2003; **17**: 2202–6.

18. Wiemels JL, Xiao Z, Buffler PA *et al. In utero* origin of t(8;21) *AML1-ETO* translocations in childhood acute myeloid leukemia. *Blood* 2002; **99**: 3801–5.

◆19. Greaves MF. Aetiology of acute leukaemia. *Lancet* 1997; **349**: 344–9.

20. Pui CH, Relling MV. Topoisomerase II inhibitor-related acute myeloid leukaemia. *Br J Haematol* 2000; **109**: 13–23.

21. Sandoval C, Pui CH, Bowman LC *et al.* Secondary acute myeloid leukemia in children previously treated with alkylating agents, intercalating topoisomerase II inhibitors, and irradiation. *J Clin Oncol* 1993; **11**: 1039–45.

22. Alexander FE, Patheal SL, Biondi A *et al.* Transplacental chemical exposure and risk of infant leukemia with *MLL* gene fusion. *Cancer Res* 2001; **61**: 2542–6.

23. Bennett JM, Catovsky D, Daniel MT *et al.* Proposals for the classification of the acute leukaemias. French-American-British (FAB) co-operative group. *Br J Haematol* 1976; **33**: 451–8.

●24. van der Does-van den Berg A, Bartram CR, Basso G *et al.* Minimal requirements for the diagnosis, classification, and evaluation of the treatment of childhood acute lymphoblastic leukemia (ALL) in the 'BFM Family' cooperative group. *Med Pediatr Oncol* 1992; **20**: 497–505.

25. Pui CH, Behm FG, Crist WM. Clinical and biologic relevance of immunologic marker studies in childhood acute lymphoblastic leukemia. *Blood* 1993; **82**: 343–62.

26. Ludwig WD, Teichmann JV, Sperling C *et al.* Incidence, clinical markers and prognostic significance of immunologic subtypes of acute lymphoblastic leukemia (ALL) in children: experiences of the ALL-BFM 83 and 86 studies. *Klin Padiatr* 1990; **202**: 243–52.

27. Bene MC, Castoldi G, Knapp W *et al.* Proposals for the immunological classification of acute leukemias. European Group for the Immunological Characterization of Leukemias (EGIL). *Leukemia* 1995; **9**: 1783–6.

28. Dworzak MN, Froschl G, Printz D *et al.* Prognostic significance and modalities of flow cytometric minimal residual disease detection in childhood acute lymphoblastic leukemia. *Blood* 2002; **99**: 1952–8.

29. Dworzak MN, Panzer-Grumayer ER. Flow cytometric detection of minimal residual disease in acute lymphoblastic leukemia. *Leuk Lymphoma* 2003; **44**: 1445–55.

30. Campana D, Coustan-Smith E, Janossy G. The immunologic detection of minimal residual disease in acute leukemia. *Blood* 1990; **76**: 163–71.

●31. Cave H, van der Werff ten Bosch J, Suciu S *et al.* Clinical significance of minimal residual disease in childhood acute lymphoblastic leukemia. European organization for research and treatment of cancer – childhood leukemia cooperative group. *N Engl J Med* 1998; **339**: 591–8.

32. Coustan-Smith E, Behm FG, Sanchez J *et al.* Immunological detection of minimal residual disease in children with acute lymphoblastic leukaemia. *Lancet* 1998; **351**: 550–4.

33. Harris NL, Jaffe ES, Diebold J *et al.* The world health organization classification of neoplasms of the hematopoietic and lymphoid tissues: report of the clinical advisory committee meeting–Airlie House, Virginia, November, 1997. *Hematol J* 2000; **1**: 53–66.

34. Pui CH, Crist WM, Look AT. Biology and clinical significance of cytogenetic abnormalities in childhood acute lymphoblastic leukemia. *Blood* 1990; **76**: 1449–63.

35. Raimondi SC. Current status of cytogenetic research in childhood acute lymphoblastic leukemia. *Blood* 1993; **81**: 2237–51.

36. Borkhardt A, Cazzaniga G, Viehmann S *et al.* Incidence and clinical relevance of *TEL/AML1* fusion genes in children with acute lymphoblastic leukemia enrolled in

the German and Italian multicenter therapy trials. Associazione Italiana ematologia oncologia pediatrica and the Berlin-Frankfurt-Munster study group. *Blood* 1997; **90**: 571-7.

●37. Romana SP, Le Coniat M, Berger R. t(12;21): a new recurrent translocation in acute lymphoblastic leukemia. *Genes Chromosomes Cancer* 1994; **9**: 186-91.

38. Attarbaschi A, Mann G, Konig M *et al*. Incidence and relevance of secondary chromosome abnormalities in childhood *TEL/AML1+* acute lymphoblastic leukemia: an interphase FISH analysis. *Leukemia* 2004; **18**: 1611-16.

39. Harbott J, Viehmann S, Borkhardt A *et al*. Incidence of *TEL/AML1* fusion gene analyzed consecutively in children with acute lymphoblastic leukemia in relapse. *Blood* 1997; **90**: 4933-7.

40. Loh ML, Rubnitz JE. *TEL/AML1*-positive pediatric leukemia: prognostic significance and therapeutic approaches. *Curr Opin Hematol* 2002; **9**: 345-52.

41. Romana SP, Mauchauffe M, Le Coniat M *et al*. The t(12;21) of acute lymphoblastic leukemia results in a *tel-AML1* gene fusion. *Blood* 1995; **85**: 3662-70.

42. Barber KE, Martineau M, Harewood L *et al*. Amplification of the *ABL* gene in T-cell acute lymphoblastic leukemia. *Leukemia* 2004; **18**: 1153-6.

43. Robinson HM, Broadfield ZJ, Cheung KL *et al*. Amplification of *AML1* in acute lymphoblastic leukemia is associated with a poor outcome. *Leukemia* 2003; **17**: 2249-50.

44. Harbott J, Ritterbach J, Ludwig WD *et al*. Clinical significance of cytogenetic studies in childhood acute lymphoblastic leukemia: experience of the BFM trials. *Recent Results Cancer Res* 1993; **131**: 123-32.

45. Sutcliffe MJ, Shuster JJ, Sather HN *et al*. High concordance from independent studies by the Children's Cancer Group (CCG) and Pediatric Oncology Group (POG) associating favorable prognosis with combined trisomies 4, 10, and 17 in children with NCI Standard-Risk B-precursor Acute Lymphoblastic Leukemia: a Children's Oncology Group (COG) initiative. *Leukemia* 2005; **19**: 734-40.

46. Harrison CJ, Moorman AV, Broadfield ZJ *et al*. Three distinct subgroups of hypodiploidy in acute lymphoblastic leukaemia. *Br J Haematol* 2004; **125**: 552-9.

47. Trueworthy R, Shuster J, Look T *et al*. Ploidy of lymphoblasts is the strongest predictor of treatment outcome in B-progenitor cell acute lymphoblastic leukemia of childhood: a pediatric oncology group study. *J Clin Oncol* 1992; **10**: 606-13.

48. Murphy SB. Classification, staging and end results of treatment of childhood non-Hodgkin's lymphomas: dissimilarities from lymphomas in adults. *Semin Oncol* 1980; **7**: 332-9.

●49. Burger B, Zimmermann M, Mann G *et al*. Diagnostic cerebrospinal fluid examination in children with acute lymphoblastic leukemia: significance of low leukocyte counts with blasts or traumatic lumbar puncture. *J Clin Oncol* 2003; **21**: 184-8.

◆50. Pui CH, Evans WE. Acute lymphoblastic leukemia. *N Engl J Med* 1998; **339**: 605-15.

51. Dordelmann M, Reiter A, Borkhardt A *et al*. Prednisone response is the strongest predictor of treatment outcome in infant acute lymphoblastic leukemia. *Blood* 1999; **94**: 1209-17.

●52. Schrappe M, Arico M, Harbott J *et al*. Philadelphia chromosome-positive (Ph+) childhood acute lymphoblastic leukemia: good initial steroid response allows early prediction of a favorable treatment outcome. *Blood* 1998; **92**: 2730-41.

●53. Smith M, Arthur D, Camitta B *et al*. Uniform approach to risk classification and treatment assignment for children with acute lymphoblastic leukemia. *J Clin Oncol* 1996; **14**: 18-24.

54. Pui CH, Boyett JM, Relling MV *et al*. Sex differences in prognosis for children with acute lymphoblastic leukemia. *J Clin Oncol* 1999; **17**: 818-24.

55. Pui CH, Sandlund JT, Pei D *et al*. Results of therapy for acute lymphoblastic leukemia in black and white children. *JAMA* 2003; **290**: 2001-7.

56. Pui CH, Chessells JM, Camitta B *et al*. Clinical heterogeneity in childhood acute lymphoblastic leukemia with 11q23 rearrangements. *Leukemia* 2003; **17**: 700-6.

57. Schrappe M, Beck J, Brandeis WE *et al*. Treatment of acute lymphoblastic leukemia in childhood and adolescence: results of the multicenter therapy study ALL-BFM 81. *Klin Padiatr* 1987; **199**: 133-50.

58. Langermann HJ, Henze G, Wulf M, Riehm H. Estimation of tumor cell mass in childhood acute lymphoblastic leukemia: prognostic significance and practical application. *Klin Padiatr* 1982; **194**: 209-13.

59. Gaynon PS, Desai AA, Bostrom BC *et al*. Early response to therapy and outcome in childhood acute lymphoblastic leukemia: a review. *Cancer* 1997; **80**: 1717-26.

60. Moricke A, Zimmermann M, Reiter A *et al*. Prognostic impact of age in children and adolescents with acute lymphoblastic leukemia: data from the trials ALL-BFM 86, 90, and 95. *Klin Padiatr* 2005; **217**: 310-20.

61. Reaman GH, Sposto R, Sensel MG *et al*. Treatment outcome and prognostic factors for infants with acute lymphoblastic leukemia treated on two consecutive trials of the children's cancer group. *J Clin Oncol* 1999; **17**: 445-55.

62. Borkhardt A, Wuchter C, Viehmann S *et al*. Infant acute lymphoblastic leukemia – combined cytogenetic, immunophenotypical and molecular analysis of 77 cases. *Leukemia* 2002; **16**: 1685-90.

63. Nachman J. Clinical characteristics, biologic features and outcome for young adult patients with acute lymphoblastic leukaemia. *Br J Haematol* 2005; **130**: 166-73.

64. Boissel N, Auclerc MF, Lheritier V *et al*. Should adolescents with acute lymphoblastic leukemia be treated as old children or young adults? Comparison of the French FRALLE-93 and LALA-94 trials. *J Clin Oncol* 2003; **21**: 774-80.

65. Attarbaschi A, Mann G, Dworzak M *et al.* Mediastinal mass in childhood T-cell acute lymphoblastic leukemia: significance and therapy response. *Med Pediatr Oncol* 2002; **39**: 558–65.

66. Reiter A, Schrappe M, Ludwig WD *et al.* Chemotherapy in 998 unselected childhood acute lymphoblastic leukemia patients. Results and conclusions of the multicenter trial ALL-BFM 86. *Blood* 1994; **84**: 3122–33.

67. Amylon MD, Shuster J, Pullen J *et al.* Intensive high-dose asparaginase consolidation improves survival for pediatric patients with T cell acute lymphoblastic leukemia and advanced stage lymphoblastic lymphoma: a pediatric oncology group study. *Leukemia* 1999; **13**: 335–42.

68. Pui CH, Gaynon PS, Boyett JM *et al.* Outcome of treatment in childhood acute lymphoblastic leukaemia with rearrangements of the 11q23 chromosomal region. *Lancet* 2002; **359**: 1909–15.

69. Schrappe M, Reiter A, Ludwig WD *et al.* Improved outcome in childhood acute lymphoblastic leukemia despite reduced use of anthracyclines and cranial radiotherapy: results of trial ALL-BFM 90. German-Austrian-Swiss ALL-BFM study group. *Blood* 2000; **95**: 3310–22.

70. Uckun FM, Sather HN, Gaynon PS *et al.* Clinical features and treatment outcome of children with myeloid antigen positive acute lymphoblastic leukemia: a report from the children's cancer group. *Blood* 1997; **90**: 28–35.

71. Baruchel A, Cayuela JM, Ballerini P *et al.* The majority of myeloid-antigen-positive (My$^+$) childhood B-cell precursor acute lymphoblastic leukaemias express TEL-AML1 fusion transcripts. *Br J Haematol* 1997; **99**: 101–6.

72. Ito C, Kumagai M, Manabe A *et al.* Hyperdiploid acute lymphoblastic leukemia with 51 to 65 chromosomes: a distinct biological entity with a marked propensity to undergo apoptosis. *Blood* 1999; **93**: 315–20.

73. Kager L, Cheok M, Yang W *et al.* Folate pathway gene expression differs in subtypes of acute lymphoblastic leukemia and influences methotrexate pharmacodynamics. *J Clin Invest* 2005; **115**: 110–17.

74. Gadner H, Masera G, Schrappe M *et al.* The eighth international childhood acute lymphoblastic leukemia workshop ('Ponte di Legno meeting') report: Vienna, Austria, April 27–28, 2005. *Leukemia* 2006; **20**: 9–17.

●75. Arico M, Valsecchi MG, Camitta B *et al.* Outcome of treatment in children with Philadelphia chromosome-positive acute lymphoblastic leukemia. *N Engl J Med* 2000; **342**: 998–1006.

●76. Riehm H, Reiter A, Schrappe M *et al.* Corticosteroid-dependent reduction of leukocyte count in blood as a prognostic factor in acute lymphoblastic leukemia in childhood (therapy study ALL-BFM 83). *Klin Padiatr* 1987; **199**: 151–60.

77. Lauten M, Stanulla M, Zimmermann M *et al.* Clinical outcome of patients with childhood acute lymphoblastic leukaemia and an initial leukaemic blood blast count of less than 1000 per microliter. *Klin Padiatr* 2001; **213**: 169–74.

78. Gajjar A, Ribeiro R, Hancock ML *et al.* Persistence of circulating blasts after 1 week of multiagent chemotherapy confers a poor prognosis in childhood acute lymphoblastic leukemia. *Blood* 1995; **86**: 1292–5.

79. Steinherz PG, Gaynon PS, Breneman JC *et al.* Cytoreduction and prognosis in acute lymphoblastic leukemia – the importance of early marrow response: report from the childrens cancer group. *J Clin Oncol* 1996; **14**: 389–98.

80. Gaynon PS, Bleyer WA, Steinherz PG *et al.* Day 7 marrow response and outcome for children with acute lymphoblastic leukemia and unfavorable presenting features. *Med Pediatr Oncol* 1990; **18**: 273–9.

◆81. Schrappe M, Reiter A, Riehm H. Cytoreduction and prognosis in childhood acute lymphoblastic leukemia. *J Clin Oncol* 1996; **14**: 2403–6.

82. Fronkova E, Madzo J, Zuna J *et al.* TEL/AML 1 real-time quantitative reverse transcriptase PCR can complement minimal residual disease assessment in childhood ALL. *Leukemia* 2005; **19**: 1296–7.

83. Campana D, Neale GA, Coustan-Smith E, Pui CH. Detection of minimal residual disease in acute lymphoblastic leukemia: the St Jude experience. *Leukemia* 2001; **15**: 278–9.

84. Pongers-Willemse MJ, Seriu T, Stolz F *et al.* Primers and protocols for standardized detection of minimal residual disease in acute lymphoblastic leukemia using immunoglobulin and T cell receptor gene rearrangements and TAL1 deletions as PCR targets: report of the BIOMED-1 CONCERTED ACTION: investigation of minimal residual disease in acute leukemia. *Leukemia* 1999; **13**: 110–18.

●85. van Dongen JJ, Seriu T, Panzer-Grumayer ER *et al.* Prognostic value of minimal residual disease in acute lymphoblastic leukaemia in childhood. *Lancet* 1998; **352**: 1731–8.

◆86. Sandlund JT, Downing JR, Crist WM. Non-Hodgkin's lymphoma in childhood. *N Engl J Med* 1996; **334**: 1238–48.

87. Hvizdala EV, Berard C, Callihan T *et al.* Lymphoblastic lymphoma in children – a randomized trial comparing LSA$_2$-L$_2$ with the A-COP+ therapeutic regimen: a pediatric oncology group study. *J Clin Oncol* 1988; **6**: 26–33.

88. Reiter A, Schrappe M, Parwaresch R *et al.* Non-Hodgkin's lymphomas of childhood and adolescence: results of a treatment stratified for biologic subtypes and stage – a report of the Berlin-Frankfurt-Munster group. *J Clin Oncol* 1995; **13**: 359–72.

89. Patte C, Kalifa C, Flamant F *et al.* Results of the LMT81 protocol, a modified LSA$_2$L$_2$ protocol with high dose methotrexate, on 84 children with non-B-cell (lymphoblastic) lymphoma. *Med Pediatr Oncol* 1992; **20**: 105–13.

90. Shepherd SF, A'Hern RP, Pinkerton CR. Childhood T-cell lymphoblastic lymphoma – does early resolution of mediastinal mass predict for final outcome? The United Kingdom Children's Cancer Study Group (UKCCSG). *Br J Cancer* 1995; **72**: 752–6.

●91. Riehm H, Gadner H, Welte K. The west-Berlin therapy study of acute lymphoblastic leukemia in childhood – report after 6 years (author's translation). *Klin Padiatr* 1977; **189**: 89–102.

92. Henze G, Langermann HJ, Bramswig J *et al.* The BFM 76/79 acute lymphoblastic leukemia therapy study (author's translation). *Klin Padiatr* 1981; **193**: 145–54.

93. Tubergen DG, Gilchrist GS, O'Brien RT *et al.* Improved outcome with delayed intensification for children with acute lymphoblastic leukemia and intermediate presenting features: a childrens cancer group phase III trial. *J Clin Oncol* 1993; **11**: 527–37.

94. Arico M, Conter V, Valsecchi MG *et al.* Treatment reduction in highly selected standard-risk childhood acute lymphoblastic leukemia. The AIEOP ALL-9501 study. *Haematologica* 2005; **90**: 1186–91.

95. Mauz-Korholz C, Junker R, Gobel U, Nowak-Gottl U. Prothrombotic risk factors in children with acute lymphoblastic leukemia treated with delayed *E. coli* asparaginase (COALL-92 and 97 protocols). *Thromb Haemost* 2000; **83**: 840–3.

96. Mitchell CD, Richards SM, Kinsey SE *et al.* Benefit of dexamethasone compared with prednisolone for childhood acute lymphoblastic leukaemia: results of the UK medical research council ALL97 randomized trial. *Br J Haematol* 2005; **129**: 734–45.

97. Bostrom BC, Sensel MR, Sather HN *et al.* Dexamethasone versus prednisone and daily oral versus weekly intravenous mercaptopurine for patients with standard-risk acute lymphoblastic leukemia: a report from the children's cancer group. *Blood* 2003; **101**: 3809–17.

98. Kaspers GJ, Veerman AJ, Popp-Snijders C *et al.* Comparison of the antileukemic activity *in vitro* of dexamethasone and prednisolone in childhood acute lymphoblastic leukemia. *Med Pediatr Oncol* 1996; **27**: 114–21.

99. Loning L, Zimmermann M, Reiter A *et al.* Secondary neoplasms subsequent to Berlin-Frankfurt-Munster therapy of acute lymphoblastic leukemia in childhood: significantly lower risk without cranial radiotherapy. *Blood* 2000; **95**: 2770–5.

100. Relling MV, Rubnitz JE, Rivera GK *et al.* High incidence of secondary brain tumours after radiotherapy and antimetabolites. *Lancet* 1999; **354**: 34–9.

101. Dordelmann M, Reiter A, Zimmermann M *et al.* Intermediate dose methotrexate is as effective as high dose methotrexate in preventing isolated testicular relapse in childhood acute lymphoblastic leukemia. *J Pediatr Hematol Oncol* 1998; **20**: 444–50.

102. Schrappe M. Evolution of BFM trials for childhood ALL. *Ann Hematol* 2004; **83**(Suppl 1): S121–3.

103. Conter V, Schrappe M, Arico M *et al.* Role of cranial radiotherapy for childhood T-cell acute lymphoblastic leukemia with high WBC count and good response to prednisone. Associazione Italiana Ematologia Oncologia Pediatrica and the Berlin-Frankfurt-Munster groups. *J Clin Oncol* 1997; **15**: 2786–91.

104. Tubergen DG, Gilchrist GS, O'Brien RT *et al.* Prevention of CNS disease in intermediate-risk acute lymphoblastic leukemia: comparison of cranial radiation and intrathecal methotrexate and the importance of systemic therapy: a Childrens Cancer Group report. *J Clin Oncol* 1993; **11**: 520–6.

105. Arico M, Valsecchi MG, Conter V *et al.* Improved outcome in high-risk childhood acute lymphoblastic leukemia defined by prednisone-poor response treated with double Berlin-Frankfurt-Muenster protocol II. *Blood* 2002; **100**: 420–6.

106. Nachman JB, Sather HN, Sensel MG *et al.* Augmented post-induction therapy for children with high-risk acute lymphoblastic leukemia and a slow response to initial therapy. *N Engl J Med* 1998; **338**: 1663–71.

107. Riehm H, Gadner H, Henze G *et al.* Results and significance of six randomized trials in four consecutive ALL-BFM studies. *Haematol Blood Transfus* 1990; **33**: 439–50.

◆108. Gaynon PS. Childhood acute lymphoblastic leukaemia and relapse. *Br J Haematol* 2005; **131**: 579–87.

109. Chessells JM. Relapsed lymphoblastic leukaemia in children: a continuing challenge. *Br J Haematol* 1998; **102**: 423–38.

110. von Stackelberg A, Henze G. Relapse of acute lymphoblasticlLeukemia. In: Gadner H, Gaedicke G, Niemeyer C, Ritter J. (eds) *Pediatric hematology and oncology*, 1st Edn. Heidelberg: Springer Medizin Verlag, 2005: 680–9.

111. Gadner H, Mann G, Peters C. Treatment of relapsed acute lymphoblastic leukemia. In: Pui CH. (ed.) *Treatment of acute leukemias: new directions for clinical research*, 1st Edn. Totowa, NJ: Humana Press, 2003: 183–97.

112. Gaynon PS, Qu RP, Chappell RJ *et al.* Survival after relapse in childhood acute lymphoblastic leukemia: impact of site and time to first relapse – the Children's Cancer Group Experience. *Cancer* 1998; **82**: 1387–95.

113. Buhrer C, Hartmann R, Fengler R *et al.* Superior prognosis in combined compared to isolated bone marrow relapses in salvage therapy of childhood acute lymphoblastic leukemia. *Med Pediatr Oncol* 1993; **21**: 470–6.

114. Beyermann B, Agthe AG, Adams HP *et al.* Clinical features and outcome of children with first marrow relapse of acute lymphoblastic leukemia expressing BCR-ABL fusion transcripts. BFM Relapse Study Group. *Blood* 1996; **87**: 1532–8.

115. Buhrer C, Hartmann R, Fengler R *et al.* Peripheral blast counts at diagnosis of late isolated bone marrow relapse of childhood acute lymphoblastic leukemia predict response to salvage chemotherapy and outcome. Berlin-Frankfurt-Munster Relapse Study Group. *J Clin Oncol* 1996; **14**: 2812–17.

116. Eckert C, Biondi A, Seeger K *et al.* Prognostic value of minimal residual disease in relapsed childhood acute lymphoblastic leukaemia. *Lancet* 2001; **358**: 1239–41.

117. Seeger K, von Stackelberg A, Taube T *et al.* Relapse of *TEL-AML1*-positive acute lymphoblastic leukemia in childhood: a matched-pair analysis. *J Clin Oncol* 2001; **19**: 3188–93.

118. Henze G, Fengler R, Hartmann R *et al.* Six-year experience with a comprehensive approach to the treatment of recurrent childhood acute lymphoblastic leukemia (ALL-REZ BFM 85). A relapse study of the BFM group. *Blood* 1991; **78**: 1166–72.

119. Buhrer C, Hartmann R, Fengler R *et al.* Importance of effective central nervous system therapy in isolated bone marrow relapse of childhood acute lymphoblastic leukemia. BFM (Berlin-Frankfurt-Munster) relapse study group. *Blood* 1994; **83**: 3468–72.

120. Chessells JM, Bailey C, Wheeler K, Richards SM. Bone marrow transplantation for high-risk childhood lymphoblastic leukaemia in first remission: experience in MRC UKALL X. *Lancet* 1992; **340**: 565–8.

●121. Barrett AJ, Horowitz MM, Pollock BH *et al.* Bone marrow transplants from HLA-identical siblings as compared with chemotherapy for children with acute lymphoblastic leukemia in a second remission. *N Engl J Med* 1994; **331**: 1253–8.

●122. Peters C, Schrauder A, Schrappe M *et al.* Allogeneic haematopoietic stem cell transplantation in children with acute lymphoblastic leukaemia: the BFM/IBFM/EBMT concepts. *Bone Marrow Transplant* 2005; **35**(Suppl 1): S9–11.

123. Eden OB, Hann I, Imeson J *et al.* Treatment of advanced stage T cell lymphoblastic lymphoma: results of the United Kingdom Children's Cancer Study Group (UKCCSG) protocol 8503. *Br J Haematol* 1992; **82**: 310–16.

●124. Wollner N, Exelby PR, Lieberman PH. Non-Hodgkin's lymphoma in children: a progress report on the original patients treated with the LSA$_2$-L$_2$ protocol. *Cancer* 1979; **44**: 1990–9.

125. Muller-Weihrich S, Beck J, Henze G *et al.* BFM study 1981/83 of the treatment of highly malignant non-Hodgkin's lymphoma in children: results of therapy stratified according to histologic immunological type and clinical stage. *Klin Padiatr* 1984; **196**: 135–42.

126. Burger B, Beier R, Zimmermann M *et al.* Osteonecrosis: a treatment related toxicity in childhood acute lymphoblastic leukemia (ALL) – experiences from trial ALL-BFM 95. *Pediatr Blood Cancer* 2005; **44**: 220–5.

127. Wiemels JL, Cazzaniga G, Daniotti M *et al.* Prenatal origin of acute lymphoblastic leukaemia in children. *Lancet* 1999; **354**: 1499–503.

128. Buchdunger E, Zimmermann J, Mett H *et al.* Inhibition of the Abl protein-tyrosine kinase *in vitro* and *in vivo* by a 2-phenylaminopyrimidine derivative. *Cancer Res* 1996; **56**: 100–4.

129. Armstrong SA, Mabon ME, Silverman LB *et al. FLT3* mutations in childhood acute lymphoblastic leukemia. *Blood* 2004; **103**: 3544–6.

130. Stanulla M, Schaeffeler E, Flohr T *et al.* Thiopurine methyltransferase (TPMT) genotype and early treatment response to mercaptopurine in childhood acute lymphoblastic leukemia. *JAMA* 2005; **293**: 1485–9.

131. Gokbuget N, Hoelzer D. Treatment with monoclonal antibodies in acute lymphoblastic leukemia: current knowledge and future prospects. *Ann Hematol* 2004; **83**: 201–5.

132. Jeha S, Gandhi V, Chan KW *et al.* Clofarabine, a novel nucleoside analog, is active in pediatric patients with advanced leukemia. *Blood* 2004; **103**: 784–9.

133. Bomgaars L, Geyer JR, Franklin J *et al.* Phase I trial of intrathecal liposomal cytarabine in children with neoplastic meningitis. *J Clin Oncol* 2004; **22**: 3916–21.

134. Muller HJ, Beier R, da Palma JC *et al.* PEG-asparaginase (Oncaspar) 2500 U/m^2 BSA in reinduction and relapse treatment in the ALL/NHL-BFM protocols. *Cancer Chemother Pharmacol* 2002; **49**: 149–54.

135. Amthauer H, Furth C, Denecke T *et al.* FDG-PET in 10 children with Non-Hodgkin's lymphoma: initial experience in staging and follow-up. *Klin Padiatr* 2005; **217**: 327–33.

63

Acute lymphoblastic leukemia and lymphoma in adults

ANJALI S ADVANI, HETTY E CARRAWAY, JUDITH E KARP AND IVAN D HORAK

Almost 5500 cases of acute lymphoblastic leukemia (ALL) were predicted to be diagnosed in 2008 in the United States,[1] approximately one-third of which would be in adults. Acute lymphoblastic leukemia is a heterogeneous group of potentially curable lymphoid disorders that results from monoclonal proliferation and accumulation of lymphoblasts in the bone marrow, peripheral blood, and other organs. Acute lymphoblastic leukemia is a sharply contrasting disease in pediatric and adult populations. Excellent medical progress in the therapy of childhood ALL has been made, with steady improvement over the past five decades; combination chemotherapy and central nervous system (CNS) prophylaxis have improved the cure rate of ALL in children from 5 percent in 1950 to 85 percent in 2000.[2] Following the lead from the pediatric experience, dose-intense multiagent regimens administered to adult patients with ALL now achieve remission rates exceeding 80 percent but with 5-year survival of only around 40 percent.[3] Current therapy for adults with ALL has become increasingly dependent on patient- and disease-specific characteristics. Therefore, proper diagnostic workup with leukemic-cell phenotyping, cytogenetics, and molecular diagnosis, including identification of the *BCR-ABL* fusion gene, is critical for prognostication and for guiding appropriate therapeutic choice. Progress has been made in moving toward tailored treatment that is more age specific and biologically relevant. Recent results suggest that applying age- and risk-adopted therapeutic strategies using several components of complex pediatric protocols may lead to improved outcome in adult patients with ALL. Participation in well-designed clinical trials is critical for future progress in the management of adult patients with ALL.

EPIDEMIOLOGY

Acute lymphoblastic leukemia has a bimodal distribution, with the first peak between 2 and 5 years of age, with an incidence of 4 to 5 per 100 000; a second steady increase begins at approximately 50 years of age, with a peak incidence of about 2 per 100 000.[4] The age-specific annual incidence of ALL in the United States is only 0.4 to 0.6 cases per 100 000 individuals between age 25 and 50 years old, and is two- to three-fold higher in individuals above the age of 60 years, with a second peak in the age group above 85 years.[5] The incidence of ALL is higher in whites than in blacks. Almost 5500 patients with ALL were predicted to be diagnosed in the United States in 2008, and approximately two-thirds would be children and adolescents.[1] Thus, adult ALL represents approximately 20 percent of all adult acute leukemias. Approximately 15 percent of pediatric patients with ALL will be diagnosed between 10 and 20 years of age. The worldwide incidence of ALL can be estimated as up to 100 000 patients per year based on the incidence of pediatric malignancies.[6]

ETIOLOGY

Genetic predisposition

Genetic factors seem to play a more important role in pediatric ALL than in adult patients with ALL, but generally the cause of ALL remains unknown. A small minority (less than 5 percent) of ALL occurs in patients with known predisposing genetic conditions, which include certain deoxyribonucleic acid (DNA) repair defect syndromes. Autosomal recessive genetic diseases associated with increased chromosomal fragility and predisposition to ALL include ataxia teleangiectasia, Nijmegen breakage syndrome, and Bloom syndrome. Children with Down syndrome have a 10- to 20-fold increased risk of leukemia, but acute myeloid leukemia (AML) is more common than ALL.

Environmental factors

The incidence of acute leukemias, mainly AML, but also ALL, was increased almost 20-fold in survivors of the atomic bomb explosions (>1 Gy exposure) in Japan, with a peak incidence occurring 6 to 7 years after the radiation exposure.[7] Exposure to chemical agents such as benzene, or some chemotherapy agents (e.g., cyclophosphamide, epidophyllotoxins, topoisomerase II inhibitors, and, rarely, anthracyclines), can be associated with an increased risk of ALL.[8,9] Although there is no direct evidence that a virus causes ALL in children or adults, viral involvement is strongly associated with two lymphoid neoplasms: the Epstein–Barr virus is involved in the development of an African type of Burkitt lymphoma, and human T cell leukemia virus I has been shown to be an etiologic agent for adult T cell leukemia and lymphomas.

APPROACH TO DIAGNOSIS

Classification of ALL requires traditional morphologic and cytochemical evaluations, immmunophenotyping, cytogenetic analysis, and more recently introduced molecular profiling. Traditional morphologic assessment together with cytochemical reactions are the initial tools in distinguishing between ALL and AML.

Lymphoblasts in ALL tend to be smaller than blasts in AML. Using the French-American-British (FAB) criteria, ALL can be classified into L1, L2, and L3 subgroups.[10] L1 blasts are uniform in size, with homogenous nuclear chromatin, indistinct nucleoli, and scanty cytoplasm with few, if any, granules. L1 blasts are more common in pediatric ALL. L2 blasts, which are more common in adult ALL, are larger and more variable in size and may have nucleoli. L3 blasts, which are observed in up to 5 percent of adult patients with ALL, are distinct, with prominent nucleoli and deeply basophilic cytoplasm with vacuoles. Acute lymphoblastic leukemia with L3 blasts indicates a mature B cell ALL, which currently requires a therapeutic strategy similar to the management of Burkitt lymphoma, and therefore should be confirmed by surface-antigen analysis (e.g., fluorescence-activated cell sorting [FACS]). L3 (Burkitt) is characterized by the MYC translocation; this is detailed further in Chapter 32. According to the World Health Organization classification,[11,12] ALL is grouped together with lymphoblastic lymphoma as either a precursor B cell or T cell neoplasm.

Combined use of morphologic, immunohistochemical, and immunologic methods frequently can accurately diagnose ALL and AML. Acute lymphoblastic leukemia can be distinguished from AML based on the gene expression profiles.[13] A recently described class of micro-ribonucleic acids (miRNAs) seems to play an important regulatory role in development, cell proliferation, differentiation, and apoptosis. Furthermore, there is emerging evidence that miRNAs can function as oncogenes and tumor suppressors. In a study of 18 patients with ALL and 54 patients with AML, the expression signature of as few as two miRNAs could accurately discriminate ALL from AML.[14] To support the routine use of miRNA in the diagnosis of ALL and AML, confirmation in a prospective study of a large group of patients will be required.

Immunologic classification of acute lymphoblastic leukemia

Specific ALL phenotype, such as B or T cell lineage disease, can be identified by using only immunophenotyping by FACS analysis, which provides a rapid and accurate method to characterize lymphoblasts. Acute lymphoblastic leukemia is divided into subtypes based on the presence of B or T cell lineage-specific differentiation antigens detected on the surface of leukemic blast cells. B cell precursor ALL (B-ALL) is the most common (approximately 70 percent to 80 percent) subtype in adults.[15] T cell ALL (T-ALL) has been diagnosed in up to 25 percent of adult patients with ALL.[15] Immature subtypes, pro-B-ALL and early T-ALL, occur more frequently in adults than in children. In about 25 percent of patients with ALL, the blast cells express myeloid antigens.[15]

B–LINEAGE ALL

Pro-B-ALL, also known as pre-pre-B-ALL or early pre-B, lacks B, T, and pre-B cell markers but expresses the HLA-DR, terminal deoxynucleotidyl transferase (TdT), and CD19 and has rearranged immunoglobulin genes. CD19 is the earliest B-lineage-specific antigen presently known. CD19 precedes the appearance of HLA-DR, CD10, CD20, and CD22 as well as other B cell-specific antigens. Lack of reactivity with CD19 rules out a B-lineage leukemia.[16] CD22, a B cell surface antigen, is highly expressed in more than 90 percent of cases of childhood B-precursor ALL,[17] but the level of expression is not well documented in adult ALL. Cytoplasmic CD22 and weak surface CD22 expression is common, and CD20 is present on a minor proportion of blast cells. Pro-B-ALL occurs in approximately 11 percent of adults with ALL.[15]

Common ALL is characterized by the presence of CD10 and positivity for CD19 and TdT. Common ALL is the most frequently identified immunologic subtype of ALL in adults (i.e., up to 50 percent of adults with ALL have the common ALL subtype). CD10 is a very sensitive marker for early detection of leukemia, and the level of expression correlates with some chromosomal abnormalities.[16]

Pre-B-ALL is characterized by the presence of cytoplasmic immunoglobulins, which are absent in common ALL. Pre-B-ALL is detected in up to 15 percent of adults with ALL.[15]

Mature B cell ALL is found in approximately 4 percent of adults with ALL.[15] The blast cells express mature B cell surface antigens, including surface membrane immunoglobulins. Mature B cell ALL is characterized by L3 morphology according to FAB classification. Cells express CD19, CD22m, CD20, and frequently CD10 and CD23.

Aberrant antigen expression in B-ALL has been found in approximately 30 percent to 45 percent of children and adults with B-ALL.[16] Myeloid surface antigens are more common than T-lineage antigens and are more frequently identified in pediatric patients than in adults with B-ALL. The prognostic significance of myeloid antigen expression is unclear.

T–LINEAGE ALL

Approximately 15 percent to 25 percent of adults with ALL have blast cells characterized by the T cell phenotype.[15] Flow cytometric diagnosis of T-ALL is more challenging than that of B-ALL. Clinically, most patients are older males who present with high peripheral blast counts and mediastinal masses. CD7 is the most sensitive marker for T-ALL (95 percent to 100 percent), and blast cells may express other T cell antigens (e.g., CD2, CD1, CD3, CD4) according to their degree of T cell differentiation.[18] A minority of T-ALL blast cells also may express CD10 together with T cell-specific antigens. Because of this high incidence of CD7 positivity in T-ALL, a diagnosis of this type of leukemia should not be made in the absence of

CD7-positive cells.[16] Since CD7 positivity can be detected in B cell ALL and AML, the diagnosis of T-ALL should be made in the presence of CD7 together with other T cell markers (e.g., CD2, CD3, and CD5). T cell ALL can be divided into three groups according to immunophenotypic differentiation: pre-T-ALL, thymic T-ALL, and mature T-ALL. Pre-T-ALL constitutes up to 7 percent of adult ALL. Thymic T-ALL accounts for approximately 13 percent of adult ALL and is characterized by the presence of CD1a expression. Mature T-ALL is diagnosed in approximately 7 percent of adult ALL, and blast cells express surface CD3.[19] T cell ALL can be further classified according to the subtypes of T cell receptor (TCR). The clinical significance of the immunophenotype in adult ALL is more controversial than in the pediatric patient population, and no difference in remission duration and survival has been documented.[20]

Cytogenetic and molecular genetics of acute lymphoblastic leukemia

In childhood ALL numerous good-risk and high-risk cytogenetic subgroups have been identified and are regularly used to stratify patients to particular therapy. Over the last two decades, the presence (Ph[+]) or absence (Ph[−]) of Philadelphia chromosome was the primary focus of cytogenetic studies in adult patients with ALL. Other recurrent chromosomal abnormalities have been infrequently described, and their prognostic relevance was unclear. The rarity of adults with ALL and the less than 10 percent incidence of other chromosomal abnormalities are the main obstacles to assessing prognostic value of cytogenetic abnormalities in patients with Ph[−] ALL in a randomized prospectively designed study.

Recurrent abnormalities in ALL can be divided into aberrations of chromosome number (ploidy) and abnormalities of chromosome structure. Cytogenetic abnormalities are independent prognostic factors for predicting the outcome of ALL in adults.[21] Sixty percent to 85 percent of adults with ALL have detectable clonal chromosomal abnormalities.[22] Chromosomal translocations are a frequent type of structural abnormality in ALL. Cytogenetic analysis using karyotype and fluorescence *in situ* hybridization (FISH) are the current standard methods used in clinic.

ABNORMALITIES OF CHROMOSOME NUMBER (PLOIDY)

Ploidy can be assessed by chromosome number or flow cytometry using DNA index. Hypodiploidy is diagnosed in approximately 2 percent to 8 percent of adults with ALL and is associated with an adverse prognosis.[21] Hyperdiploidy occurs in about 10 percent of adult patients with Ph[−] ALL, and is significantly less common than in pediatric ALL (25 percent to 30 percent). These patients tend to be younger and have a lower white blood cell (WBC) count.

According to a recently published study, event-free survival (EFS) and overall survival (OS) were significantly improved for patients with high hyperdiploidy compared with other patients in the cohort ($P \leq 0.015$).[22]

PRE-B-ALL ABNORMALITIES OF CHROMOSOME STRUCTURE

The t(9;22) translocation was the first recurrent chromosomal abnormality identified in human cancer, in association with chronic myelocytic leukemia (CML).[23] This translocation, known as Philadelphia chromosome (Ph+), is an essential criterion in the diagnosis of CML and the cytogenetic abnormality most frequently identified in adults with ALL,[24] occurring in 25 percent of the adult population. The frequency of Ph+ ALL increases markedly with age; in adults over the age of 60 years, up to 50 percent of precursor-B-ALL is Ph+.[25] Compared to patients with Ph− ALL, patients with Ph+ ALL have a tendency to be older and to have a higher WBC count.

The Philadelphia chromosome is formed by in-frame fusion of the 5′ portion of the breakpoint cluster region (BCR) on chromosome 22 to the 3′ portion of the protein tyrosine kinase (PTK) C-ABL on chromosome 9, a critical protooncogene. The fusion protein possesses increased PTK activity. Two main fusion proteins with different BCR breakpoints can be detected. Most adults with Ph+ leukemias have a 190 kDa protein, known as p190, similar to pediatric ALL, and approximately 25 percent of adult patients have a 210 kDa protein known as p210. It has been suggested that the p190 protein arises in *de novo* ALL, whereas p210 protein may represent the blast crisis of previously undiagnosed CML. To define other lesions that cooperate with BCR-ABL, a genome-wide analysis of 304 patients with ALL was performed.[26] Surprisingly, the transcription factor Ikaros, essential for B cell differentiation, was deleted in 76 percent of pediatric patients with Ph+ ALL and 91 percent of adult patients with Ph+ ALL but not in the chronic phase of CML (Table 63.1); however, this lesion was acquired during blast transformation of CML. Due to the differential expression of multiple isoforms in various leukemias, Ikaros provides a unique tool to study post-transcriptional regulation in leukemogenesis and acquisition of resistance to targeted therapies.[27] Thus, treatment of Ph+ ALL has been revolutionized by one protein tyrosine kinase inhibitor (PTKI), imatinib mesylate, also known as Gleevec®.[28]

Before the introduction of PTKIs, the presence of Ph+ ALL had been an important adverse prognostic marker and was associated with a significantly lower rate of complete remission (CR), more frequent and earlier relapse, and poorer OS.[29] Therefore, these patients have traditionally received an allogeneic bone marrow transplant in first CR, if they are appropriate candidates.[30] At MD Anderson Cancer Center, remission rates after receiving standard hyper-CVAD (cyclophosphamide, vincristine, adriamycin, and dexamethasone) induction for patients with Ph+ ALL

Table 63.1 Transcription factors implicated in B cell acute lymphoblastic leukemia

Transcription factor	Gene	Association with human B cell malignancies
Ikaros	*IKZF1*	Deletion (pediatric Ph+ ALL 76%; adult Ph+ ALL 91%)
		Differential expression of isoforms in Ph+ ALL
E2A	*TSFE2A*	Translocation in approximately 6% of B-ALL
EBF1	*EBF1*	Monoallelic deletion; cryptic translocations and point mutations
PAX5	*PAX5*	Monoallelic loss in approximately 30% of B-ALL
Aiolos	*IKZF3*	Deletion
Lef1	*LEF1*	Deletion

ALL, acute lymphoblastic leukemia; B-ALL, B cell ALL; Ph+, Philadelphia chromosome positive.

are comparable to remission rates for patients with Ph− ALL, but the remissions are brief, with a median CR duration of 16 months.[31]

Results from a recent study provide new evidence of a possible link between the expression of oncogenic Ikaros isoforms (Ik6) and the resistance of Ph+ ALL to both PTKIs imatininb and desatinib.[32] Overall, mutations in gene-encoding regulators of B cell development and differentiation can be identified in approximately 40 percent of B-ALL. The most common targets of these gene alterations (*EFB1*, *PAX5*, and *IKZF1*) play critical roles in the physiologic development of B cells (Table 63.1).[33] The role of *IKZF1* has been studied in a cohort of 221 children with high-risk B-ALL; genetic alteration of *IKZF1* was associated with a very poor outcome and therefore should be considered for evaluation before treatment initiation.[34] Ph+ ALL is discussed in further detail later in this chapter.

MLL, 11q23 REARRANGEMENTS

MLL gene rearrangements located at 11q23 occur in approximately 10 percent of adults with ALL,[35] and most have t(4;11). The involved gene on chromosome 11 is named *MLL* for 'mixed-lineage leukemia.' The *MLL* gene is fused to the AF-4 gene located on chromosome 4. Patients with this cytogenetic abnormality have a tendency to have a high WBC count and inferior EFS and OS compared with other patients with Ph− ALL.[22]

T-ALL/T CELL LYMPHOBLASTIC LYMPHOMA

T cell ALL/T cell lymphoblastic lymphoma occurs most often in adolescents and young adults (AYA) (second to third decade) and is an aggressive disease, frequently presenting with an extremely high WBC, CNS involvement (5 percent to 10 percent), a mediastinal mass (60 percent to 70 percent), marked lymphadenopathy (60 percent to 80 percent), hepatosplenomegaly, and bone marrow involvement (approximately 20 percent).[36] Central nervous system recurrence is common in the absence of adequate CNS prophylaxis. Although intensive chemotherapy has significantly improved the outcome of patients with T-ALL, up to 30 percent of pediatric patients and approximately 50 percent of adult patients will relapse.[37]

Similar to recent advancements in the molecular biology of B cell ALL, progress has been made in the molecular biology of T-ALL. Mammalian NOTCH1 was discovered because of its involvement in the (7;9) chromosomal translocation identified in T-ALL. Subsequent studies have elucidated the critical role of NOTCH1 in the normal development of T cells.[38] NOTCH signaling is critical for T cell development and leukemogenesis as well. The NOTCH pathway regulates critical processes that control cellular transformation, cell-cycle progression, and apoptosis. The key role of NOTCH is documented by its activation in 60 percent of T-ALL.[39] The precise mechanism of NOTCH1-associated T cell transformation is not clear; activation of downstream genes (e.g., MYC) or pathways (e.g., phosphatidylinositol 3-kinase [PI3K]/AKT) may play an important role.[37] Due to the central role the NOTCH signaling pathway plays in leukemogenesis, it appears to be a very attractive novel target for therapeutic intervention.[40] Gamma-secretase inhibitors (GSI) block activation of NOTCH1 in T-ALL. Severe gastrointestinal toxicity has limited clinical use of this class of agents. Thus, results of a recent study in a preclinical model indicate that combining glucocorticoids with GSI can improve antileukemic effects of GSI and reduce their gastrointestinal toxicity.[41] The role of dexamethasone in the treatment of T-ALL is supported by the results of a recent study.[42] The outcome of T-ALL in adults is clearly heterogeneous, and cytogenetic markers have been of limited help in dissecting this subset.[43]

The leukemogenic event in T-ALL typically involves overexpression of an unaltered protooncogene, rather than generation of a novel fusion protein, due to a translocation placing the protooncogene under control of a TCR promoter or enhancer, most often TCR-β or TCR-α/δ. Genetic abnormalities involving basic helix-loop-helix genes (e.g., TAL1, TAL2, LUL1, MYC), cysteine-rich LIM domain-containing genes (e.g., LMO1, LMO2), or homodomain genes (e.g., HOX11/TLX1, HOX11L2/TLX3, the HOXA gene cluster) can participate in the transformation of normal thymocytes by blocking differentiation.[37] Aberrant TAL1 expression via a variety of mechanisms occurs in over 60 percent of T-ALL.[44] In a systematic review of 67 adult patients with T-ALL at a single institution, 33 percent of patients had blasts expressing at least one myeloid-associated antigen, and abnormal karyotypes were identified in almost one-third of patients.[45] Complete remission was achieved in 88 percent of patients, with a 74 percent CR rate in patients with blasts expressing at least one myeloid-associated antigen. No prognostic factors were identified in this study. The Cancer and Leukemia Group B (CALGB) in collaboration

with the Eastern Cooperative Oncology Group (ECOG)[46] as well as a large German study[47] demonstrated that overexpression of HOX11 confers a good outcome for adult patients with T-ALL and, therefore, this patient population should not undergo stem cell transplantation (SCT) in the first remission.[43] Increased self-renewal or impaired response to extracellular signals may be associated with a different group of genes (e.g., RAS, JAK2, FLT3, ABL1, or LCK).[48]

Early trials of T cell lymphoblastic lymphoma used chemotherapy regimens designed for less aggressive non-Hodgkin lymphoma (NHL). Therefore, a low CR rate (24 percent) with fewer than 10 percent of patients alive at 5 years was not a surprise.[49–51] The introduction of complex chemotherapy protocols with intensive CNS prophylaxis has changed the outcome of patients with T cell NHL. Most of these studies induced CR in 77 to 93 percent of patients and have reported long-term disease-free survival (DFS) rates between 40 to 60 percent.[52]

DETECTION OF GENETIC AND MOLECULAR ABNORMALITIES

Recent developments

The last decade has been characterized by development of several new strategies to more precisely characterize genetic abnormalities in patients with ALL. Development of array-based comparative genome hybridization and single nucleotide polymorphism genotyping has enabled genome-wide detection of copy number with a significantly improved sensitivity than provided by cytogenetics.[53] Recent data showed that cryptic genetic changes are present in close to 100 percent of adult and adolescent patients with ALL, similar to the incidence in the pediatric ALL patient population.[54] Intrachromosomal deletions of genes involved in B lymphopoiesis and cell-cycle regulation occur with high frequency in ALL.[54] Results of a recent study of a monochorionic twin pair, one preleukemic and one with overt leukemia, support a 'second-hit' theory that at least two hits will be required for progression to frank leukemia.[55]

Microarray-based analysis of gene expression patterns is a powerful tool that has been increasingly used over the past few years to provide better understanding of ALL biology and to identify potential novel targets for therapeutic intervention (e.g., BCR-ABL). Gene expression can be used as an important predictor of early response and outcome in high-risk childhood and adult ALL.[24,56,57] Single nucleotide polymorphism (SNP) arrays provide an opportunity to assess genome-wide analysis of DNA, copy number abnormalities (CNAs), and loss of heterozygosity (LOH). These types of studies may provide new insights into the pathogenesis of newly diagnosed ALL and identify potential targets for therapy of recurrent ALL.[58] Transcription factors in concert with the cytokine-regulated signaling pathway play a key role in a highly regulated multistep process in which pluripotent hematopoietic stem cells differentiate to produce mature B cells.[59] Therefore, it is not surprising that high-resolution SNP arrays and genomic DNA sequencing of 242 pediatric patients with ALL revealed deletion, amplification, point mutation, and structural rearrangements in genes encoding principal regulators of B cell development and differentiation in 40 percent of B cell ALL (Table 63.2).[33] Full integration of a high-resolution genome-wide platform to detect CNAs and regions of LOH, coupled with methods to accurately and quantitatively assess the total transcriptome of leukemia cells, into the prognostic assessment of patients with newly diagnosed ALL will provide an opportunity to more effectively introduce risk- and subgroup-adapted therapy to improve the outcome for adult patients with B-ALL and T-ALL.[61]

Minimal residual disease (MRD)

Detection of molecular abnormalities in ALL has important implications for the initial risk assessment as well as disease monitoring (MRD) of ALL. The classical definition of CR requires fewer than 5 percent lymphoblasts in the bone marrow by morphologic examination. Tracing residual leukemic blasts during induction and consolidation provides important prognostic information. Newer molecular definitions of remission based on the absence of MRD are far more sensitive in identifying patients at risk for relapse or ultimate outcome of disease (Table 63.3).[62] Optimal MRD techniques should provide sensitivity to at least 10^{-4} (i.e., one malignant cell among 10 000 normal cells), should be feasible, and should be highly reproducible. Quantification with multiparameter flow cytometry phenotyping following at least two leukemia-specific immunophenotypes has been recommended to prevent false-negative results. Minimal residual disease also can be measured by four–six color FACS and by reverse transcription polymerase chain reaction (RT-PCR), and sensitivity ranges from 10^{-3} to 10^{-6} (Table 63.2).[2,60,63]

Numerous pediatric studies have demonstrated negative prognostic significance of MRD positivity during induction independent of other risk factors. The prognostic value of MRD was analyzed in more than 2100 pediatric patients treated in a study conducted by the Children's Oncology Group (COG).[64] The presence of MRD in Day-8 blood and Day-29 marrow was associated with shorter EFS in all risk groups. Conversely, rapid achievement of MRD negativity before the end of induction has been associated with excellent prognosis. Therefore, assessment of MRD during induction therapy, as well as kinetics to achieve MRD clearance, can lead to early adjustment of therapy (i.e., standard therapy for patients with fast disappearance of MRD and intensification of therapy for slow responders). A recent study has confirmed the prognostic value of real-time quantitative PCR (RQ-PCR) and/or FACS method for assessment of MRD kinetics.[65]

Minimal residual disease studies have been limited in adults with ALL. Pediatric studies use MRD for risk stratification, but MRD is not routinely used for adults with ALL. The prognostic impact of MRD has been demonstrated, and MRD will probably be used in future studies of adult ALL. Adult patients with ALL tend to have higher levels of MRD positivity during induction therapy.[66,67] More frequent and more prolonged duration of MRD positivity has been detected in significantly more adult patients than pediatric patients with ALL. Nevertheless, MRD does appear to have independent predictive value in the adult population as well.[68] After consolidation treatment, most adult patients with standard-risk ALL will have an MRD level below the detection limit, and about 30 percent of these patients ultimately relapse.[69] In German Multicenter Study Group for ALL (GMALL) Studies 06/99 and 07/03 in patients with standard-risk ALL, the median time from MRD positivity to clinical relapse was 9.5 months. Only 6 percent of patients relapsed after continuous MRD negativity.[69] In study GMALL 05/93, 188 adult patients with standard-risk ALL (GMALL 06/99) were prospectively studied to determine the clinical relevance of MRD kinetics.[70] The MRD quantification during the treatment identified prognostic subgroups within an otherwise homogenous population of adult patients with standard-risk ALL. For future trials in adults with ALL, it will probably be important to evaluate MRD to determine the appropriate treatment in this patient population and possibly to select which patients should receive a transplant.

CLINICAL MANIFESTATIONS

Most adult patients with ALL initially present with clinical symptoms related to bone marrow failure. Physical findings related to symptoms such as pallor, tachycardia, and fatigue are attributable to anemia; hemorrhagic manifestations are associated with thrombocytopenia; and neutropenia may lead to severe infections. Common sites of extramedullary involvement in patients diagnosed with ALL include the liver, spleen, and lymph nodes. Bone pain and arthralgia may be caused by leukemic infiltration but are rarely observed in adult patients with ALL, in contrast to pediatric patients. Symptoms related to hyperleukocytosis are rarely diagnosed in patients with ALL.

In two consecutive German multicenter trials, one-third of patients had infection or fever and hemorrhagic episodes at presentation.[19] Approximately half of the patients presented at the diagnosis with lymphadenopathy, splenomegaly, and hepatomegaly. A small fraction of patients had hilar lymphadenopathy or a thymic mass documented by chest radiographs or computed tomography scans. At presentation, fewer than 10 percent of patients with ALL had CNS involvement diagnosed by leukemic cells in the cerebrospinal fluid (CSF), but only 4 percent of these patients had CNS signs and symptoms such as headache, vomiting, lethargy, nuchal rigidity, and cranial nerve or peripheral nerve impairment.

In a large prospective study of 1508 adult patients with ALL (MRC UKALL XII/ECOG E2993), 5 percent of patients

Table 63.2 Characteristics of methods currently used for minimal residual disease detection in patients with acute lymphoblastic leukemia

	Morphology	Multiparameter FACS	PCR analysis of chromosomal aberrations	PCR analysis of immunoglobulin/TCR
Sensitivity	1–5%	0.01–0.1%	0.0001–0.001%	0.0001–0.001%
Applicability to:				
B-ALL	Not applicable	>95%	40–45%	90–95%
T-ALL		>95%	15–35%	90–95%
Advantages	Applicable to all patients	Applicable to most patients	Relatively easy and cheap	Applicable to virtually all patients
		Relatively cheap	Rapid (2–3 days)	Sensitive
		Rapid (1–2 days)	Suitable for monitoring of uniform patient groups (e.g., Ph⁺ ALL)	Patient specific
				Rapid during follow-up (2–3 days)
Disadvantages	Lack of sensitivity and inability to distinguish normal and malignant clone	Need preferably two aberrant immunophenotype per patient	Useful in minority of patients	Time consuming at diagnosis to identify junctional regions
		Drug-induced modulation of the phenotype might impact sensitivity	False-positive results due to contamination of PCR product	Relatively expensive
				Need for two PCR targets per patient
Recent developments		≥6-color cytometry promises increased sensitivity and specificity; currently under development in the European EuroFlow Consortium	Largely standardized due to pan-European collaboration within the BIOMED-1 and EAC project	Target identification standardized within European BIOMED-1 and BIOMED-2 networks (European Study Group for MRD detection in ALL)

Modified from Bailey et al. 2008[2] and Szczepanski 2007.[60]
ALL, acute lymphoblastic leukemia; B-ALL, B cell ALL; EAC, Europe Against Cancer; FACS, fluorescence-activated cell sorting; MRD, minimal residual disease; PCR, polymerase chain reaction; Ph⁺, Philadelphia chromosome positive; T-ALL, T cell ALL; TCR, T cell receptor.

Table 63.3   Unfavorable clinical and biological factors predicting clinical outcome in the first-line therapy of adults with acute lymphoblastic leukemia

Older age (>35 years, although clearly a continuum)
High WBC count (>30 000/µL in B cell ALL and >100 000/µL in T cell ALL)
Cytogenetics [t(9;22) *BCR-ABL*, del (7) + (8), t(4;11)]
Non-T cell immunophenotype
Longer time to achieve complete remission (>4 weeks)
Slow kinetics to negative MRD (>10^{-3} after induction)

ALL, acute lymphoblastic leukemia; MRD, minimal residual disease; WBC, white blood cell.

were diagnosed with CNS leukemia at presentation, and 90 percent of patients achieved CR.[71] The 5-year OS rate was 29 percent in patients with CNS involvement at diagnosis versus 38 percent for those without ($P = 0.03$). Testicular involvement at the time of ALL diagnosis is rare and, with the advent of modern treatment regimens, the incidence of recurrent testicular disease at the time of relapse remains low.

LABORATORY EVALUATION

More than 50 percent of patients present with an increased WBC count, and one-quarter of patients present with leukopenia. Almost all patients have blasts cells detected in the peripheral blood smear. Therefore, initial traditional microscopic evaluation of blood smears is critical for further diagnostic workup. In a study of 938 adult patients with ALL, elevated WBC count (>100 000 × 10^6/L) was observed in fewer than 20 percent of patients.[19] In general, a high WBC is found more frequently in patients with T-ALL than with B-ALL. In patients with T-ALL, almost one-quarter of patients have severe neutropenia or thrombocytopenia at the presentation.[72]

Bone marrow biopsy and a quality aspiration are critical for the diagnosis of ALL, and can be obtained from most patients. Dry taps on aspiration may be due to densely packed bone marrow with blast cells and less commonly due to fibrosis or inadequate technique. Most patients have more than 50 percent of blast cells in the bone marrow at the time of presentation.

For patients with disease confined to mass lesions (e.g., lymphadenopathy) and having ≤25 percent blasts in the bone marrow, the diagnosis of lymphoblastic lymphoma is used.[73,74] Lymphoblastic lymphoma may be confirmed by a biopsy of a lymph node or mass lesion.

Lumbar puncture should be performed to complete the evaluation of patients with ALL. The identification of leukemic cells in the CSF using conventional cytopathologic examination of Papanicolaou-stained cytospin preparation has a significant incidence of false-negative results. Therefore, immunophenotyping analysis of CSF specimens may provide

the true incidence of leptomeningeal disease in adult patients with ALL.[75]

Metabolic abnormalities such as increased serum uric acid level and lactate dehydrogenase may be associated with rapid destruction of blast cells. Elevated liver function tests may be due to leukemic infiltration. Abnormal coagulation is rarely present at the time of diagnosis of ALL.

DIFFERENTIAL DIAGNOSIS

The differentiation of ALL from AML can be made by morphologic evaluation of bone marrow aspirate/bone marrow biopsy, using cytochemistry assessment and immunologic characterization of leukemic cells using FACS scan analysis. Acute lymphoblastic leukemia lymphoblasts are negative for myeloperoxidase and Sudan Black B stains. Periodic acid-Schiff reaction and nonspecific esterase may be positive.[76] Terminal deoxynucleotidyl transferase also is positive in most cases of ALL. Coexpression of myeloid and lymphoid surface markers can be documented in almost one-third of patients with ALL. By convention, the degree of blast infiltration of bone marrow (>25 percent) distinguishes ALL from lymphoblastic lymphoma.

THERAPY

Supportive therapy

Initial complete physical examination is critical for successful outcome of induction therapy. Spontaneous or treatment-induced tumor lysis syndrome (TLS) can cause significant morbidity and potential mortality. Vigorous hydration (approximately 100 mL/hour), alkalinization, and inhibition of uric acid synthesis with allopurinol (300 mg/day to 600 mg/day will effectively block xanthine oxidase) are the most frequently used methods for treatment and prevention of TLS. If concomitant use of allopurinol with 6-mercaptopurine (6-MP) is planned, the dose of 6-MP has to be reduced. However, this approach fails to prevent renal insufficiency in up to 25 percent of high-risk patients.[77] With the increased intensity and efficacy of antileukemic therapies, novel approaches for the management of TLS are needed. Unlike allopurinol, urate oxidase promptly reduces the existing uric acid pool, prevents accumulation of xanthine and hypoxanthine, and does not require alkalinization, thereby facilitating phosphorus excretion. A recombinant form of urate oxidase, rasburicase, is now registered for the treatment and prevention of TLS in children and adolescents.[78,79] Results from a prospective, randomized, phase III study in adult patients with hematologic malignancies, presented at the 2008 American Society of Hematology (ASH) meeting, indicate that rasburicase was superior to allopurinol in normalization of serum uric acid, with a faster effect in adult patients at risk for TLS.[77]

Infection management

The intensification of induction therapy in adult patients with ALL has been associated with an increased CR rate and a higher frequency of infection-associated morbidity and mortality. Several decades ago, long-term neutropenia was recognized as one of the most important risk factors for severe infections. Over the past two decades, substantial progress has been made regarding the management of patients with febrile neutropenia. However, the ever-changing patterns of infection, ecology, and antibiotic-resistance trends prevent the development of universal treatment guidelines. Hence, each institution's predominant pathogens and resistance patterns should guide the empirical choice of antimicrobials. Prompt initiation of broad-spectrum antimicrobial therapy remains the gold standard. Monotherapy with the newer broad-spectrum antimicrobials has tended to replace the classic combination therapy. Empirical administration of glycopeptides, such as vancomycin, without documentation of a Gram-positive infection has not been favored in recent years. The initiation of empiric antifungal therapy in persistently febrile neutropenic patients has become common practice, especially recently, since the introduction of new, effective, less toxic antifungal drugs. It is hoped that the development of new non-culture-based diagnostic methods (e.g., PCR based) will facilitate the early detection of invasive fungal infections and, thus, the replacement of empiric antifungal therapy with pathogen-specific, preemptive therapy.[80]

Hematopoietic growth factors, such as a granulocyte colony-stimulating factor (G-CSF), have been broadly used in patients with ALL. Prophylactic administration of G-CSF significantly accelerates neutrophil recovery, as well as reduces febrile neutropenia and severe infections in adult patients with ALL, but does not significantly alter disease outcome.[81,82]

Chemotherapy

Treatment programs in adult ALL have evolved around two different philosophies. Over several decades, adult leukemia experts treated adult ALL using different protocols than those used for pediatric ALL. Frequently, adult patients were treated with high-dose-intensive chemotherapy, exemplified by the hyper-CVAD regimen pioneered at MD Anderson Cancer Center.[83] Over the last decade, a different approach has been developed based on the successful treatment strategies for pediatric patients with ALL.[84] Completed contemporary trials in adults with ALL or lymphoma are listed in Table 63.4. For adults, two approaches have been constructed: a chemotherapy-based regimen for patients with standard-risk ALL and a transplantation-based regimen for patients with Ph+ ALL.

Preliminary results from a few contemporary studies have demonstrated an encouraging CR rate (90 percent) and respectable EFS rates (60 percent to 70 percent)[94–97] with application of the above approach. Stratification according to various prognostic factors at the time of diagnosis and MRD-based stratification also may allow us to select patients who may benefit from allogeneic SCT.[69,70,85]

All current regimens incorporate multiple active agents into complex regimen-specific sequential therapies. Although there is no standard therapy for adult patients with ALL, two regimen modifications (German Berlin-Munster-Frankfurt [BFM][98] and hyper-CVAD[90]) in combination with CNS prophylaxis and long-term maintenance are commonly used. Contemporary ALL treatment programs have been constructed from a

Table 63.4 Completed contemporary large clinical trials in adults with acute lymphoblastic leukemia/lymphoma

Study	Year	Median age (years)	n	CR rate (%)	Early mortality (%)	Survival (%)	Reference
MRC XII/ECOG E2993	2005	31 (15–64)	1521	91	5	38 (5-year)	85
GIMEMA 0496	2005	16–60	450	80	Not reported	33 (5-year)	86
PETHEMA ALL-93	2005	27 (15–50)	222	82	6	34 (5-year)	87
PALG 4-2002	2008	26 (17–60)	131	90	Not reported	43 (3-year)	88
LALA-94	2004	33 (15–55)	922	84	4	37 (3-year)	89
MD Anderson	2004	40 (15–92)	288	92	5	38 (5-year)	90
EORTC ALL-3	2004	33 (14–79)	340	74	Not reported	36 (6-year)	91
GOELAL02	2004	33 (15–59)	198	86	2	41 (6-year)	92
GMALL 04/89 and 06/53 (T-ALL)	2002	45 (15–61)	45	93	2	48 (7-year)	52
LALA-94 (Ph+ ALL)	2002	42 (17–56)	154	53	2	35 (3-year)	93
JALSG ALL202 (Ph+ ALL)	2004	41 (15–64)	24	94 (Imatinib)	0.5	89 (1-year)	28

ALL, acute lymphoblastic leukemia; CR, complete remission; ECOG, Eastern Cooperative Oncology Group; EORTC, European Organisation for Research and Treatment of Cancer; GIMEMA, Gruppo Italiano Malattie Ematologiche dell'Adulto; GMALL, German Multicenter Study Group for ALL; GOELAL, Groupe Ouest Est des Leucémies Aiguës Lymphoblastiques; JALSG , Japan Adult Leukemia Study Group; LALA, Leucémie Aiguë Lymphoblastique de l'Adulte; MRC, Medical Research Council; PALG, Polish Adult Leukemia Group; PETHEMA, Programa para el Estudio y la Terapéutica de las Hemopatías Malignas; Ph+, Philadelphia chromosome positive; T-ALL, T cell ALL.

template that generally includes four phases: induction, intensification/consolidation, maintenance treatment, and CNS prophylaxis. The objective of induction therapy is to rapidly eliminate leukemic cells from the bone marrow, as assessed by morphologic criteria (CR). In the future, studies in adults with ALL are more likely to incorporate MRD measurement after induction therapy.

The overall results of clinical trials for adult patients with ALL have been less encouraging than those trials conducted in the pediatric patient population. Complete response rates range between 74 percent and 93 percent and OS rates between 27 percent and 48 percent.[15] As discussed later in this chapter, younger adults have demonstrated superior outcomes.

INDUCTION

Remission induction therapy, which aims at the rapid induction of CR and restoration of normal hematopoiesis, incorporates a combination of various doses and schedules of nonmyelosuppressive agents, vincristine, corticosteroid (mostly prednisone and prednisolone), asparaginase (primarily used in pediatric and AYA patients), and anthracyclines (mostly daunorubicin).

Asparaginase

Asparagine-depletion therapy using polyethylene glycol (PEG)-asparaginase (PEGylated) or native asparaginase is an important component of all contemporary treatment protocols for childhood ALL.[99] An asparagine-depletion agent(s) has been only recently added to the initial therapy of adult patients with ALL; furthermore, pediatric patients have received more extensive asparaginase exposure than adults. A number of asparaginase products are in clinical use, but only two *Escherichia coli* (*E. coli*) products have been approved by the Food and Drug Administration (FDA) in the United States: native and PEGylated asparaginase. PEGylated asparaginase has been approved by the FDA for the front-line therapy of ALL.[100] Native *E. coli*-derived asparaginase is dosed from $10\,000\,IU/m^2$ semiweekly to $5000\,IU/m^2$ biweekly administered intramuscularly. PEGylated *E. coli*-derived asparaginase has been used at $2500\,IU/m^2$ administered intravenously every 2 weeks.

Addition of asparaginase to the induction regimen has increased the CR rate to 95 percent and has had an even greater impact on early bone marrow response and end-induction disease burden or MRD in pediatric patients with ALL.[99] In Dana–Farber Cancer Institute (DFCI) study DFCI-77-01, addition of more doses of asparaginase therapy during postinduction treatment was shown to improve long-term EFS.[101] This observation was confirmed by multiple studies in the United States and Europe.[102,103] In DFCI and European Organisation for Research and Treatment of Cancer (EORTC) studies, *Erwinia*-derived asparaginase achieved an inferior EFS compared with *E. coli* asparaginase when used at the same dose and schedule in the presence of multiagent therapy.[104,105] In the CCG-1962 study

in 100 children with ALL, EFS at 3 years was 85 percent for patients treated with PEGylated *E. coli* asparaginase and 78 percent for those who received native *E. coli* asparaginase. Results from this study led to replacement of native asparaginase with PEGylated asparaginase in current Children's Oncology Group trials. Therefore, careful monitoring of safety and avoiding premature discontinuation of PEGylated asparaginase is very important.[99]

Asparaginase also plays an important role in the treatment of recurrent ALL. Although asparaginase is not myelosuppressive, it has a unique side-effect profile: pancreatitis, hyperglycemia, hyperbilirubinemia, elevated liver enzymes, hypoalbuminemia, decreased clotting factors, and decreased antithrombin III, as well as an increased incidence of thrombosis, lethargy, and somnolence especially in older adults.[106] Ongoing studies are evaluating asparaginase in pediatric and adult patients with ALL to define the optimal dose and intensity of asparagine-depletion therapy. For example, an ongoing study, Total Therapy XVI, is being conducted at St. Jude Cancer Institute to evaluate regimens using the standard dose ($2500\,IU/m^2$) of PEGylated *E. coli* asparaginase compared to an increased dose ($3500\,IU/m^2$).

Asparaginase is a bacterial protein and therefore is immunogenic. Patients may develop an allergic reaction with urticaria, wheezing, or hypotension, or they may develop neutralizing antibodies. PEGylated asparaginase may be less immunogenic, and intravenous (IV) administration may provide additional benefit (e.g., less immunogenic and more convenient) over intramuscular administration. Historically, adults with ALL have received less asparaginase than children, principally due to safety concerns. Experience at DFCI suggests that the asparaginase-related toxicity in patients aged 18 to 50 years is very similar to that of children aged 10 to 18 years.[95,107] These results were confirmed by a second study.[106,108] Several ongoing phase II and phase III studies (Table 63.5) are being conducted to identify the optimal dose, schedule, and intensity of asparagine-depletion therapy in pediatric patients with ALL (e.g., Total XVI), in adult patients with ALL (e.g., DFCI), and in geriatric patients with ALL (e.g., GMALL).

Asparaginase therapy also should be considered in the context of other drugs given in a particular regimen. In some pediatric programs, replacement of prednisone with dexamethasone was associated with a decreased CNS relapse rate and improved survival,[109] but dexamethasone was not extensively studied in adult patients with ALL.[110] Hypoalbuminemia associated with administration of an asparagine-depleting agent may be associated with lower dexamethasone-apparent clearance.[111,112] Increased incidence of primarily aseptic osteonecrosis observed in the new high-risk protocol for children with ALL led to dose modification of dexamethasone, and close monitoring of long-term safety will be required before broad clinical use for adult patients with ALL. In adult ALL protocols, asparagine-depletion therapy is used much less in post-remission phase and for shorter duration when compared to pediatric protocols.[113]

Table 63.5 Ongoing phase II–IV studies in Ph− acute lymphoblastic leukemia

Study group	Country	Clinicaltrials.gov #	Study name	Age range (years)	Study phase	Main goal
Phase II–IV (antibody-based therapy)						
GMALL	Germany	NCT00198978	GMALL02	>55	IV	Reduced-dose chemotherapy plus rituximab
GMALL	Germany	NCT00199004	GMALL03	15–65	IV	Intensified chemotherapy plus rituximab
GRAALL	France	NCT00327678	GRAALL 2005	18–59	III	Chemotherapy plus rituximab
MRC	United Kingdom		UKALL14/ECOG 2907	20–65	III	Rituximab, epratuzumab, or combination with chemotherapy
GMALL	Germany		GMALL–07/2003 +	18–65	III	Stratification by MRD and CD20 for rituximab therapy
NCRI	United Kingdom		MARALL	20–65	II	Rituximab, epratuzumab plus chemotherapy in relapsed ALL
Phase IV (BMT)						
PETHEMA	Spain		LAL-AR-03	30–60	IV	High-risk ALL treated with chemotherapy or allogeneic HSCT in first CR
Phase II–IV (MRD adjusted)						
GMALL	Germany	NCT00198991	GMALL01	15–65	IV	MRD-based tailored therapy
NILG	Italy	NCT00222612	09/00	15–65	IV	Postremission dose modification according to MRD
NCRI	United Kingdom	NCT00222612	UKALL 2003	1–24	III	MRD-based randomization to more dose-intensive therapy
PALG	Poland		PALG 5-2007	16–60	III	Individualized MRD-based therapy
SWOG	United States	NCT00109837	SWOG S0333	18–64	II	Prognostic value of MRD
Phase II (AYA)						
JALSG	Japan	NCT00131053	ALL202-U	15–24	II	Feasibility of pediatric-based regimen in AYA
DFCI	United States	NCT00476190	06-254	18–50	II	Safety and efficacy of pediatric-based regimen including PEG-L-asparaginase
CALGB/ECOG/SWOG	United States	NCT00558519	CALGB 10403	16–29	II	Safety and efficacy of pediatric-based regimen
Phase II–IV (asparagine-depletion strategy)						
DFCI	United States	NCT00400946	DFCI-05001	1–17	III	Safety and efficacy of PEG-asparaginase and native asparaginase in patients with standard-risk ALL
DFCI	United States	NCT00476190	DFCI-06254	18–50	II	Safety and efficacy of high-risk pediatric ALL protocol in adult patients
MDACC	United States	NCT00506597	2007-0183	No restrictions	II	Safety of *Erwinia* asparaginase in patients with allergy to *E. coli*–derived asparaginase
COG	United States	NCT00671034	AALL07P4	1–30	III	Safety and efficacy of PEGylated asparaginase versus new formulation in patients with high-risk ALL
NCCC	United States	NCT00184041	96-0-1	18–55	II	Safety and efficacy of PEGylated asparaginase
NOPHO	Denmark	NCT00192673	2004-41-4276	1–14	II	Safety and immunogenicity of PEGylated asparaginase
COG	United States	NCT00537030	AALL07P2	1–30	II	Safety and PK in patents allergic to PEGylated *E. coli*-derived asparaginase
SJCRH	United States	NCT00549848	Total XVI	1–18	III	Safety and efficacy of high dose versus standard dose of PEGylated asparaginase

ALL, acute lymphoblastic leukemia; AYA, adolescents and young adults; BMT, bone marrow transplant; CALGB, Cancer and Leukemia Group B; COG, Children's Oncology Group; CR, complete remission; DFCI, Dana-Farber Cancer Institute; ECOG, Eastern Cooperative Oncology Group; *E. coli*, *Escherichia coli*; GMALL, German Multicenter Study Group for ALL; GRAALL, Group for Research on Adult Acute Lymphoblastic Leukemia; HSCT, hematopoietic stem cell transplant; JALSG, Japan Adult Leukemia Study Group; MARALL, monoclonal antibodies in relapsed acute lymphoblastic leukemia; MDACC, MD Anderson Cancer Center; MRC, Medical Research Council; MRD, minimal residual disease; NCCC, Norris Comprehensive Cancer Center; NCRI, National Cancer Research Institute; NILG, Northern Italy Leukemia Group; NOPHO, Nordic Society for Pediatric Hematology and Oncology; PALG, Polish Adult Leukemia Group; PEG, polyethylene glycol; PETHEMA, Programa para el Estudio y la Terapéutica de las Hemopatías Malignas; Ph−, Philadelphia chromosome negative; PK, pharmacokinetics; SJCRH, St. Jude Children's Research Hospital; SWOG, Southwest Oncology Group.

Additional chemotherapeutics

Another agent extensively studied in the induction therapy of ALL is daunorubicin. The most frequent dosage of daunorubicin is 30 to 60 mg/m^2 for 2 or 3 days.[114] Intensive anthracycline therapy may be associated with higher mortality during induction, and therefore intensive prophylactic and supportive therapy are required.[25]

Using contemporary chemotherapy regimens, the CR rate in ALL is 85 percent to 90 percent.[115] Therefore, it is difficult to increase the CR rate further. However, several approaches have been explored during the induction phase. A randomized study by the Italian Gruppo Italiano Malattie Ematologiche dell'Adulto (GIMEMA) group compared a three-drug induction regimen with and without cyclophosphamide (CY) and did not demonstrate an improvement in CR rates (81 percent versus 82 percent).[116] High-dose cytarabine (1 to 3 g/m^2 for up to 12 doses) also did not increase CR rates.[117] A high-dose chemotherapy regimen (hyper-CVAD), has been introduced at the MD Anderson Cancer Center.[118] The key component of this regimen consists of alternating cycles of CY, high-dose methotrexate (HD MTX), and cytarabine with intensive CNS prophylaxis followed by 2 years of maintenance with 6-MP, MTX, vincristine, and prednisone (POMP). Using hyper-CVAD, the overall CR rate was 92 percent with the 5-year DFS of 38 percent. A recent update regarding the use of hyper-CVAD in AYA patients age 13 to 21 years with de novo ALL (92 patients) and lymphoblastic lymphoma (10 patients) was presented at ASH 2008.[119] Very commendable efficacy has been achieved in the single-center study in the AYA group of patients; the CR rate was 97 percent, and 3-year EFS and OS rates were 65 percent and 70 percent, respectively. Long-term follow-up in this study and experience in a multicenter trial will be needed before

broader application of this strategy. In the Group for Research on Adult Acute Lymphoblastic Leukemia (GRAALL)-2003 study, the reported 42-month EFS and OS rates for 225 patients with de novo ALL age 15 to 60 years (median 31 years) were 55 percent and 60 percent, respectively; median follow-up was 37 months.[120] A similar cohort of patients treated with the hyper-CVAD regimen included 385 patients with a slightly older median age of 35 years. Median follow-up was 62 months (range, 1 to 180 months). Event-free survival and OS rates for the entire cohort were 50 percent and 55 percent, respectively. For patients younger than 35 years, these rates improved to 55 percent and 67 percent. It is not surprising that, even with intensive chemotherapy approaches, age remains a prognostic factor. Outcomes with the hyper-CVAD regimens appear to more closely resemble those of the pediatric approaches than the conventional regimens.

Progress in the outcome of adult patients with ALL has been mainly due to intensification and optimization of chemotherapy, risk-adapted use of stem-cell transplantation, and improved supportive care. However, results for adult patients with ALL are still considerably inferior to those for pediatric patients with ALL (Tables 63.4 and 63.6).

In a multicenter phase II study that extended the pediatric treatment approach to older adults up to 50 years of age, 89 adult patients with newly diagnosed ALL received a dose-intensified pediatric induction regimen (DFCI) consisting of doxorubicin, prednisone, vincristine, HD MTX, L-asparaginase, and triple intrathecal (IT) therapy.[126] Ten 3-week courses of doxorubicin, vincristine, dexamethasone, and 6-MP and 30 weeks of L-asparaginase were used for intensification. Maintenance therapy of 3-week courses of vincristine, dexamethasone, MTX, and 6-MP were used for 2 years from the time CR was achieved. Median follow-up

Table 63.6 Adolescent acute lymphoblastic leukemia outcome according to treatment protocol

Study	Year	Median age (years)	n	CR rate (%)	Early mortality (%)	Survival (%)	Reference
CCG	2008	16–20	197	90	Not reported	67 (7-year)	113
CALGB	2008	16–20	124	90	Not reported	46 (7-year)	113
FRALLE 93	2003	15–20	77	94		78 (5-year)	121
LALA-94	2003	15–20	100	83		45 (5-year)	121
DCOG	2004	15–18	47	98	Not reported	71 (5-year)	122
HOVON	2004	15–18	44	91	Not reported	37 (5-year)	122
MRC ALL97	2007	15–17	61			65 (5-year)	123
UKALLXII	2007	15–17	67			49 (5-year)	123
NOPHO-92	2006	15–18	36	99	1	74 (5-year)	124
Swedish Adult ALL	2006	15–20	21	90	2	39 (5-year)	124
AIEOP	2006	14–18	150	94	Not reported	80 (2-year)	125
GIMEMA	2006	14–18	95	89	Not reported	71 (2-year)	125

AIEOP, Associazione Italiana Ematologia Oncologia Pediatrica; ALL, acute lymphoblastic leukemia; CALGB, Cancer and Leukemia Group B; CCG, Children's Cancer Group; CR, complete remission; DCOG, Dutch Childhood Oncology Group; FRALLE, French Acute Lymphoblastic Leukaemia Group; GIMEMA, Gruppo Italiano Malattie Ematologiche dell'Adulto; HOVON, Dutch-Belgian Hemato-Oncology Cooperative Study Group; LALA, Leucémie Aiguë Lymphoblastique de l'Adulte; MRC, Medical Research Council; NOPHO, Nordic Society of Pediatric Hematology and Oncology.

was 15 months. Complete remission was 84 percent with a very respectable 2-year EFS rate of 73 percent and OS rate of 77 percent; the safety profile was acceptable (i.e., nine patients developed pancreatitis, two osteonecrosis, and 14 thrombosis/embolism).

Up to 50 percent of adult and elderly patients with ALL test positive for the Philadelphia chromosome. Early introduction of a BCR-ABL targeting agent (imatinib) in combination with chemotherapy may be associated with improved CR rate and long-term outcome of Ph+ ALL. Preliminary results from a short-term follow-up study show that 25 of 26 patients (96 percent) achieved CR with a median time to response of 21 days; the 2-year DFS rate was 87 percent for the hyper-CVAD imatinib combination compared with 28 percent for hyper-CVAD alone.[127] An update regarding imatinib in combination with hyper-CVAD in adult patients with Ph+ ALL was presented at ASH 2007.[128] Of the 39 treated patients, 92 percent achieved CR after the first course and 8 percent after the second course; the median time to CR was 21 days. Treatment was well tolerated. Imatinib has been used in combination chemotherapy during induction and consolidation therapy in patients with de novo Ph+ ALL (GRAAPH-2003 study); the overall CR rate was 96 percent, but RQ-PCR negativity was achieved in only 29 percent of patients.[129] Further refinement of the therapy of de novo Ph+ ALL is needed. The role of the next generation of PTKIs (dasatinib and nilotinib) currently is being evaluated (Table 63.7).

Immunochemotherapy

Introduction of novel nonmyelosuppressive agents, noncross-resistant with currently used therapeutics, may provide an opportunity to increase clearance of MRD and to improve EFS and OS as well. The increased use of complex pediatric protocols and adoption of a risk-tailored approach in conjunction with the introduction of novel targeted therapies (e.g., naked or drug-conjugated monoclonal antibodies [mAbs], and PTKIs) may improve the outcome of adults with ALL without additional toxicities. Acute lymphoblastic leukemia blast cells express a variety of specific antigens (e.g., CD19, CD20, CD22, CD33, and CD52) that may serve as targets for therapeutic intervention.[17,130,131] Of these approaches, the most experience is available for the anti-CD20 antibody, rituximab.

Frequent expression of high levels of CD22 antigen in ALL has been well documented. In a study of 54 children and AYAs, CD22 was expressed at 68 percent to 99 percent in patients with more than 20 percent of leukemic blasts; CD20 expression was positive in 54 percent of patients.[132] Therefore, expression of CD22 on precursor-B-ALL blasts from children and AYAs supports its consideration as a target for immunotherapy approaches in high-risk or relapsed disease.

In the MRC UKALLXII/ECOG2993 Intergroup Trial, ECOG's reference laboratories centrally characterized the ALL for 613 (91 percent) patients, and 505 had B cell lineage ALL.[133] Expression of 32 antigens, including nine myeloid-associated antigens, was determined by multiparameter flow cytometry on gated blasts, both as percentage of antigen-expressing blasts and intensity of antibody staining (equivalent of antigen density). To test for the potential therapeutic use of mAbs such as rituximab, epratuzumab, alemtuzumab, or gemtuzumab in future trials, expression of antigens for these antibodies (CD20, CD22, CD52, or CD33, respectively) was determined. The results confirmed frequent expression of high-density CD22.[133]

In ALL, rituximab is combined with chemotherapy mainly in mature B-ALL and Burkitt lymphoma, and interim results are promising. In adults with Burkitt or Burkitt-type lymphoma or ALL, rituximab in combination with hyper-CVAD was well tolerated with no induction deaths; the 3-year OS, EFS, and DFS rates were 89 percent, 80 percent, and 88 percent, respectively.[134] In another study, patients younger than 60 years with ALL or lymphoblastic lymphoma were treated with a modified hyper-CVAD in combination with rituximab (if ≥20 percent of the leukemic blasts expressed CD20) in induction, and POMP.[135] Of the 190 patients who were treated, 91 percent achieved CR. Fifteen AYA patients with newly diagnosed ALL were treated with rituximab in combination with hyper-CVAD, and the combination was well tolerated.[119] Several recent studies with rituximab also have been initiated in precursor-B-ALL (Table 63.5).

CD22 is another B cell-specific marker that is frequently detected in B cell ALL. There has been significant experience with a CD22-targeted antibody, epratuzumab, in patients with indolent and aggressive B cell NHL.[136–139] The COG recently published data from a phase I study in which epratuzumab (humanized anti-CD22 antibody) was administered alone and in combination with reinduction chemotherapy in children with relapsed ALL.[17] Fifteen patients (12 fully assessable for toxicity) with first or later CD22-positive ALL marrow relapse enrolled in the feasibility portion of the study from December 2005 to June 2006. Two dose-limiting toxicities occurred: one grade 4 seizure of unclear etiology and one asymptomatic grade 3 alanine aminotransferase (ALT) elevation. In all but one patient, surface CD22 was not detected by flow cytometry on peripheral blood leukemic blasts within 24 hours of drug administration, indicating effective targeting of leukemic cells by epratuzumab. A CR after chemoimmunotherapy was achieved by nine patients, seven of whom were MRD negative. Treatment with epratuzumab plus standard reinduction chemotherapy is feasible and acceptably tolerated in children with relapsed CD22-positive ALL. Subsequent studies should determine the role of epratuzumab in the armamentarium of novel anti-ALL agents.

Monoclonal antibody conjugated with toxin may further enhance antitumor activity. This strategy has been used with limited success with gemtuzumab (anti-CD33 antibody conjugated to calicheamicin) in patients with AML. A similar approach was used in a phase I study that evaluated anti-CD22 antibody (inotuzumab ozogamicin, CMC-544) administered every 28 days to patients with

Table 63.7 Ongoing phase II–IV studies in Ph[+] acute lymphoblastic leukemia

Study group	Country	Clinicaltrials.gov #	Study name	Age range (years)	Study phase	Main goal
Phase II–IV (hyper-CVAD based)						
MDACC	United States	NCT00390793	2006-0478	18–64	II	Hyper-CVAD with desatinib
GRAALL	France		GRAAPhO2/2015	15–59	III	Hyper-CVAD/standard imatinib versus 'imatinib-based'
Phase II–IV (BMT)						
European Intergroup (Rennes University Hospital Ministry of Health)	France	NCT00287105	ESPHALL	1–17	II/III	Risk stratification
CALGB/NCI	United States	NCT00039377	CALGB 10001		II	Chemotherapy and imatinib followed by BMT
SWOG/NCI	United States	NCT00792948	S0805	18–50	II	Desatinib in combination with chemotherapy and SCT
Phase II (imatinib or desatinib based)						
EWALL	Pan-European		EWALLPh	>65	II	Desatinib with low-dose chemotherapy
GIMEMA	Italy	NCT00391989[a]	LAL1205	≥15	II	Desatinib as induction therapy
GMALL	Germany		Imatinib/MRD/01/01	≥15	II	Imatinib in induction
GMALL	Germany	NCT00199186	GMALL ST1571-ELDERLY- 01/02	≥55	II	Safety and efficacy of single-agent imatinib
JALSG	Japan		Ph[+]ALL2008	18–64	II	Intensified imatinib and chemotherapy in postremission therapy
COG-NCI	United States	NCT00720109	AALL0622	1–30	II	Feasibility and toxicity of desatinib in combination with intensified chemotherapy in newly diagnosed patients
GIMEMA	Italy	NCT00376467	LAL0201	18–60	II	Imatinib in combination with chemotherapy
GIMEMA	Italy	NCT00475280	LAL1104	>60	II	Assessment adapted therapy in geriatric patients
GIMEMA	Italy	NCT00458848	GIMEMA-LAL0904	15–60	II	Imatinib added to chemotherapy, postremission intensification, MRD monitoring
MDACC	United States	NCT00390793	2006-0478	>18	II	Hyper-CVAD in combination in combination with desatinib

[a]Trial was recently completed.

ALL, acute lymphoblastic leukemia; BMT, bone marrow transplant; CALGB, Cancer and Leukemia Group B; COG, Children's Oncology Group; EWALL, European Working Group on Adult Acute Lymphoblastic Leukemia; GIMEMA, Gruppo Italiano Malattie Ematologiche dell'Adulto; GMALL, German Multicenter Study Group for ALL; GRAALL, Group for Research on Adult Acute Lymphoblastic Leukemia; JALSG , Japan Adult Leukemia Study Group; MDACC, MD Anderson Cancer Center; MRD, minimal residual disease; NCI, National Cancer Institute; Ph[+], Philadelphia chromosome positive; SCT, stem cell transplant; SWOG, Southwest Oncology Group.

NHL; a favorable safety profile was reported at ASH 2008.[140] In a phase I/II study of inotuzumab ozogamicin in combination with rituximab in patients with B cell NHL, preliminary data confirm good safety and preliminary efficacy.[141] It is very likely that due to the excellent safety and efficacy profile of unconjugated and drug-conjugated antibodies,[140–142] these immunochemotherapeutics will be studied in patients with high-risk ALL and recurrent disease as well. Other potential therapeutic targets include the B cell-specific antigen, CD19, which is highly expressed in leukemic blasts. The safety and efficacy of anti-CD52 and anti-CD33 antibodies in the treatment of ALL have been evaluated in small clinical studies. Overall, mAb therapy in ALL represents a promising treatment approach. However, further investigation of this approach is needed.[131]

INTENSIFICATION/CONSOLIDATION THERAPY

Although induction CR rates are around 90 percent in many series of adult patients with ALL, the long-term DFS over the last decade remains 25 percent to 48 percent (Table 63.4), and therefore there is need to optimize postremission therapy in adult patients with ALL. Intensification/consolidation/reinduction therapy refers to the introduction or use of multiple new, preferentially non-cross-resistant agents, agents used during induction therapy, or high-dose chemotherapy. The primary purpose of the intensification phase is the further elimination of MRD and prevention of appearance of resistant clones. Intensive consolidation is standard in pediatric and AYA protocols (Table 63.6), but its benefit in the management of patients older than 50 years with ALL remains to be confirmed.[116,143] Intensification therapy may include teniposide, etoposide, mitoxantrone, idarubicin, and high-dose cytarabine and intermediate or HD MTX. The optimal dose and schedule of high-dose cytarabine is not clear; the dosage may range from 1 g/m^2 to 3 g/m^2 administered every 12 hours for 3 to 5 days. High-dose cytarabine and HD MTX may provide additional benefit in the prophylaxis and treatment of CNS leukemia, but there is a potential for significant toxicities, primarily in patients older than 50 years. High-dose MTX has been studied extensively in pediatric patients.

REINDUCTION

Periodic reintroduction of agents used during initial induction therapy, called reinduction or late intensification, is very common in pediatric and AYA protocols.

MAINTENANCE THERAPY

In contrast to the management of aggressive AML and Burkitt lymphoma, for which long-term chemotherapy is not routinely used, maintenance therapy administered for 2 years or longer after completion of induction and consolidation is standard for patients with ALL. Extension of maintenance treatment beyond 3 years has not shown additional benefits, but omission of maintenance therapy has been associated with shorter DFS in children.[144,145] Orally administered 6-MP and IV (or oral) administration of MTX constitute the backbone of maintenance therapy. The dose of these agents is aimed to keep the WBC count below $3000/\mu L$ during maintenance therapy to achieve optimal outcome.[62] Contemporary ALL protocols may tailor dose intensity based on the presence of MRD and other well-defined characteristics of ALL (e.g., presence of Ph^+ may lead to introduction of PTKI). Based on experience with AYA, the outcome of adult patients with ALL may be improved with the introduction of protocols with designs that resemble the designs of complex pediatric trials. Strict adherence to the optimal schedule and dose intensity of multiple agents, avoidance of dose reduction due to toxicities, and improved compliance may enhance the outcome of adult patients with ALL.[84,106,146]

PROPHYLAXIS OF CENTRAL NERVOUS SYSTEM LEUKEMIA

Central nervous system leukemia may be discovered in a small fraction (1 percent to 10 percent) of patients at the time of diagnosis, with a higher incidence in patients with T-ALL (8 percent) and mature B-ALL (13 percent).[147] Prophylactic therapy of CNS leukemia must be an integral part of therapy, as lack of CNS-targeted therapy is associated with a high incidence of CNS relapse (up to one-third of patients).[147] Prophylactic therapy may consist of IT application of MTX alone or in combination with cytarabine and prednisone. Similar agents may be administered via Ommaya reservoir. Systemic administration of HD MTX or high-dose cytarabine may further reduce the rate of CNS relapse. Prophylactic CNS irradiation (24 Gy) has been used to prevent or treat CNS leukemia. Today, almost no protocols include CNS irradiation, unless the patient has T cell ALL or active CNS disease, because of the neurocognitive defects. Some studies have demonstrated no increase in CNS relapse rate with this approach; however, it has been important to use high-dose systemic therapy with agents such as MTX or cytarabine, which cross the blood–brain barrier.[148] A combined modality approach to CNS prophylaxis further decreased the incidence of CNS relapse rate. Future clinical studies in adult patients with ALL may test the role of risk-adapted CNS prophylaxis.[149] The role of liposomal cytarabine for IT therapy may improve patient compliance due to the reduced number of IT applications; thus, integration of this agent in complex regimens should be prospectively assessed to evaluate the safety profile.[15,150]

AGE–ADAPTED THERAPY

Survival is significantly less favorable for adults with ALL than for the pediatric patient population. The reason for this disparity may be multifactorial and has been thought to include physician experience in managing ALL (e.g., AML is significantly more common in the adult leukemia practice), more experience and rigid adherence to complex protocols by pediatric hematologists/oncologists and staff, difference in treatment protocols, and a different biology of ALL (i.e., high incidence of Ph$^+$ ALL and other changes such as gene expression profiles). On the other hand, adult patients may be less compliant and may not tolerate therapy as well (e.g., HD MTX and high-dose cytarabine) due to comorbid medical conditions in the aging population.[94]

Therapy for adolescents and young adults

The outcome of AYA patients significantly improves if they are treated in pediatric clinical trials.[84,106,146] Adolescent patients are less likely to be referred to a COG institution, and consequently are potentially exposed to a worse outcome.[151] Several retrospective analyses have unveiled some striking differences in the outcome of AYA patients, depending on the enrollment in pediatric versus adult clinical trials.

Results from retrospective studies focused on patients aged 15 to 21 years indicate that AYA treated with adult ALL protocols have a poorer outcome than a similar group of patients treated with pediatric protocols.[125,152] Five-year EFS rates for AYA treated with pediatric and adult protocols range from 64 percent to 69 percent and 34 percent to 49 percent, respectively.[153–156] The outcome for AYA with ALL was retrospectively analyzed according to treatment programs between 1988 and 2001 at Children's Cancer Group (CCG) and CALGB.[113] Although CR rate (90 percent) was identical for CALGB and CCG AYA, EFS and OS rates at 7 years were significantly higher in CCG studies (63 percent and 67 percent for CCG versus 34 percent and 46 percent for CALGB)

(Table 63.6). Comparison of the regimens demonstrated that CCG AYA received earlier and more intensive CNS prophylaxis and higher doses of nonmyelosuppressive agents (e.g., vincristine, steroids, and asparagine-depletion agents). Based on these observations, prospective clinical trials using regimens to treat AYA up to 30 to 50 years with standard-risk ALL have been initiated. These observations led to the launch of an important intergroup study (CALGB/ECOG/Southwest Oncology Group [SWOG] 10403) for patients age 16 years to less than 30 years (Table 63.5). The purpose of this study, which is being conducted in collaboration with the COG group and the AALL0232 study, is to assess the outcomes (i.e., CR rate, EFS, DFS, and OS) of AYA patients with newly diagnosed ALL treated with a pediatric chemotherapy regimen by adult hematologists/oncologists.

Pediatric protocols contain significantly higher cumulative doses of nonmyelosuppressive drugs, including prednisone, vincristine, and asparagine-depleting agent (e.g., native or PEG-L-asparaginase), which may contribute to the superior outcome of AYA patients treated with these regimens[121] (Table 63.6). Furthermore, more frequent and protracted CNS prophylaxis also may contribute to improved survival.[113] A recently initiated (November 2007) intergroup phase II study (CALGB 10403) will prospectively explore safety and efficacy of a pediatric protocol (AALL0232) in AYA patients treated by adult hematologists/oncologists (Table 63.5). See Table 63.8 for selected ongoing phase III studies in AYA or adult ALL.

Table 63.8   Selected ongoing phase III studies in adolescents and young adults or adult acute lymphoblastic leukemia

Study group	Country	Clinicaltrials.gov #	Study name	Age range (years)	Study phase	Main goal
JALSG	Japan	NCT00131027	JALSG ALL202-O	25–64	III	HD versus intermediate-dose MTX
MDACC	United States	NCT00501826	2006-0328	No restrictions	II	Hyper-CVAD with nelarabine in previously untreated T–ALL and T-lymphoblastic lymphoma
NILG	Italy	NCT00795756	NILG-ALL 10/07	18–65	II	A randomized study on CNS prophylaxis with liposome-encapsulated cytarabine in association with a lineage-targeted and MRD-oriented postremission strategy in adult ALL
COG/NCI	United States	NCT00408005	COG-AALL0434	1–30	III	Safety and efficacy of combination chemotherapy in patients with T-ALL
COG/NCI	United States	NCT00075725	COG-AALL-03B1	1–30	III	Safety and efficacy of dexamethasone versus prednisone in high-risk B-ALL
NOPHO (Rigshospitalet)	Denmark	NCT00548431	NOPHO ALL-2008	1–18	II	Safety and efficacy of dose-adjusted 6-MP, HD MTX, and PEGylated asparaginase
GER (Universitätsklinikum Hamburg-Eppendorf)	Germany	NCT00343369	GER-COALL-07-03	1–18	III	Safety and efficacy of intensive chemotherapy in patients with standard risk ALL (B- and T-ALL)

ALL, acute lymphoblastic leukemia; B-ALL, B cell ALL; CNS, central nervous system; COG, Children's Oncology Group; HD, high dose; JALSG, Japan Adult Leukemia Study Group; MDACC, MD Anderson Cancer Center; 6-MP, 6-mercaptopurine; MRD, minimal residual disease; MTX, methotrexate; NCI, National Cancer Institute; NILG, Northern Italy Leukemia Group; NOPHO, Nordic Society for Pediatric Hematology and Oncology; PEG, polyethylene glycol; T-ALL, T cell ALL.

Therapy for elderly patients

According to the United States Census Bureau, one-fifth of the population in 2050 will be older than 65 years, and the fastest-growing segment of the elderly population is 85 years and older. It has been estimated that up to 31 percent of ALL will be diagnosed in patients 60 years and older.[5] In addition, the incidence of Ph$^+$ ALL rapidly increases with age – up to 50 percent for patients older than 56 years;[157] similar results were obtained in a series of GMALL studies.[158] With very few exceptions, elderly patients have been excluded from clinical trials, and most studies limit the age of participants to 60 or 65 years. In a CALGB study of 759 adult patients with ALL treated between 1988 and 2002, the CR rate decreased from 90 percent for patients less than 30 years, to 81 percent for those between 30 and 59 years, and to 57 percent for patients 60 years and older. Not surprisingly, the OS rate at 3 years followed a similar pattern: 58 percent for patients less than 30 years, 38 percent for those 30 to 59 years, and only 12 percent for patients older than 60 years. Similar results have been reported by other large cooperative groups.[5] Results for 94 patients in a GMALL study show a CR rate of 48 percent but with a very poor long-term survival of 10 percent.[159]

Comorbid conditions, potential for drug–drug interactions, and baseline functional reserve of key organs (e.g., liver, kidney, and heart) may profoundly impact the pharmacokinetics and therapeutic index of agents commonly used in the management of ALL. Therefore, it is not likely that dose intensification would be appropriate for biologically aged patients (i.e., a specific age limit may not be appropriate). Introduction of new targeted agents (e.g., monoclonal antibodies and PTKIs) may improve efficacy without increasing treatment-related mortality. Thus, it is possible that adjusting the dose and schedule of drugs with proven efficacy in patients with ALL, as well as addition of targeted agents with a novel mechanism of action, may improve the outcome of biologically aged patients with ALL. To ensure progress in this fast-growing segment of the patient population, it is imperative that large cooperative groups initiate studies specifically designed for biologically aged patients.

The efficacy and safety of antileukemic drugs are determined by the interplay of numerous gene products that will influence pharmacokinetics and pharmacodynamics. Genetic makeup may influence the therapeutic index of several antileukemic drugs (e.g., thiopurines, methotrexate, glucocorticosteroids, and asparagines). Therefore, pharmacogenomics has the potential to optimize the use of antileukemic agents.[160]

Transplantation

ROLE OF DOSE INTENSIFICATION USING STEM CELL TRANSPLANTATION

Significant challenges remain for improving the treatment outcome for most adults with ALL. Another strategy to further eliminate MRD and consequently improve survival of adult patients with ALL is the introduction of SCT. Several prognostic factors have been applied to identify low- and high-risk categories for DFS. This stratification may help to identify the group of patients who may benefit from intensification therapy using SCT.

HISTORY OF ALLOGENEIC TRANSPLANTATION IN ALL

Allogeneic bone marrow transplantation (allo-BMT) was first employed as a method to permit delivery of high-dose chemotherapy. However, it was subsequently discovered that the donor cells exerted a graft-versus-leukemia (GvL) effect. Graft-versus-leukemia effect was first recognized in animal models.[161,162] In 1979, GvL effects were reported in patients with ALL. Patients undergoing allo-BMT who developed $\geq$ grade 2 acute graft-versus-host-disease (GVHD) had a lower relapse rate than patients with grade 1 or no GVHD or those who underwent syngeneic transplant.[161,163,164] T cell depletion was associated with a high relapse rate.[165,166] Allogeneic bone marrow transplantation exerts the most potent antileukemic effect in ALL; however, its place in the therapeutic armamentarium must be balanced against its treatment-related mortality (20 percent to 30 percent in most series).[167]

CONDITIONING REGIMENS

Total body irradiation (TBI)-based conditioning regimens, which provide additional CNS prophylaxis, generally have been preferred for the treatment of ALL.[168] Davies *et al.* demonstrated improved overall and leukemia-free survival in patients with ALL less than 20 years of age who received CY/TBI compared to busulfan/CY.[169]

ALLOGENEIC BONE MARROW TRANSPLANTATION

Allo-BMT for standard-risk ALL in first complete remission

Only one-third of adults with ALL (excluding Burkitt) are disease-free survivors at 5 years. The question is whether allo-BMT, given its potent antileukemic effect, can improve clinical outcome for patients with ALL in the first CR. There has been reluctance to use this approach due to the substantial treatment-related mortality associated with allo-BMT. The MRC UKALL XII/ECOG 2993 trial was initiated in 1993 to prospectively define the role of allo-BMT, autologous BMT (auto-BMT), and chemotherapy in almost 2000 adult patients age 15 up to 64 years with Ph$^-$ and Ph$^+$ ALL.[30] Patients received induction chemotherapy, and those with an HLA-matched sibling donor received allo-BMT as postremission therapy. High-risk patients were defined by: age greater than 35 years, high WBC count ($>$30 000/μL for B-ALL or $>$100 000/μL for T-ALL), time to CR greater than 4 weeks, or specific cytogenetic abnormalities. Standard-risk patients with an HLA-matched sibling donor had a significantly superior OS to those without a donor (5-year OS rate 53 percent versus 45 percent, $P = 0.01$) because of a substantially lower relapse rate in the allo-BMT group ($P \leqslant 0.001$).[30] This is the largest randomized study to address the question of allo-BMT in ALL; however, there are some caveats. The average age of the patients was young (mid-30s), making these results difficult to extrapolate to older adults with ALL. In older patients, the treatment-related mortality abrogated the benefit, and the age limit in the trial was decreased. In addition, the outcome of AYA patients with ALL with pediatric therapeutic regimens has been similar, and recent experience at DFCI with AYA patients up to the age of 25 years or older might in 2007 achieve better outcomes with pediatric protocols.[156] Therefore, introduction of novel prognostic tools (e.g., molecular profiling and MRD kinetics), which may improve prognostication of patients with adult ALL, together with incorporation of targeted agents in the contemporary multiagent protocols, will likely play a role in the future in deciding which patients should proceed to allo-BMT.[168]

Allo–BMT for Ph+ ALL and ALL with high-risk features in first complete remission

Patients with pre-B cell ALL and high-risk features have a poor prognosis with standard therapy, and allo-BMT in first CR should be considered. High-risk features include poor-risk cytogenetics, greater than 4 weeks to achieve CR, and WBC count greater than 30 000/μL.[98,170] Patients with at least one risk factor have a 5-year DFS rate less than 30 percent.[171] Slow MRD kinetics or detection of MRD during postinduction course of treatment defines high-risk patients and also is associated with impending relapse.[172]

Allo–BMT for Ph+ ALL in first complete remission

The advent of PTKIs has complicated the decision for allo-BMT in patients with Ph+ ALL in the first CR; however, preliminary data suggest that PTKIs in combination with chemotherapy are unlikely to be curative, secondary to the presence of new mutations, in preventing inhibition of tyrosine kinase.[173] Therefore, an allo-BMT from a matched related donor or matched unrelated donor (MUD) is generally recommended in the first CR. In the ECOG/MRC trial, where 167 patients with Ph+ ALL were treated in the first CR, the EFS and OS rates were higher in the allo-BMT arm (36 percent and 42 percent, respectively) compared with the rates for patients not receiving an allo-BMT (17 percent and 19 percent).[174] Similar results have been published by the Leucémie Aiguë Lymphoblastique de l'Adulte (LALA) group (LALA-94).[93]

Allo–BMT for high-risk ALL in first complete remission

For patients with high-risk ALL in the LALA-87 trial, patients receiving an allo-BMT had a significantly higher 10-year OS than the control group (44 percent versus 11 percent, $P = 0.009$).[175] In the ECOG/MRC trial, patients with Ph– high-risk ALL had no survival advantage with an allo-BMT at 5 years (41 percent and 35 percent; $P = 0.2$), despite a much-reduced relapse rate for high-risk patients (63 percent versus 37 percent at 5 years; $P \leqslant 0.001$), reflecting that transplant-related mortality was unacceptably high and abrogated all benefit of improved relapse rates.[30] Two major differences in these studies that may account for these divergent results are a younger population in the LALA-87 study (age 15 to 40 years) versus age 15 to 55 years in the ECOG/MRC study (which likely led to a lower treatment-related mortality), and the inclusion of Ph+ patients in the high-risk group in the LALA-87 study.

Allo–BMT for relapsed ALL

Allogeneic bone marrow transplantation is the only curative treatment for patients with relapsed or refractory ALL. The outcome is worse when patients with more advanced disease receive a transplant. The decision to proceed ultimately depends on patient age, donor availability, disease status, performance status, and comorbidities.[176] Fewer than one-third of patients will have a matched related donor.[165] Because of the substantial time required to find a MUD, a donor search should be initiated at the time of diagnosis. The outcome after transplantation depends on disease status, duration of the first CR, disease biology/cytogenetics, and development of GVHD.[161,165,177] The MRC/ECOG trial evaluated 609 patients with relapsed ALL.[176] The 5-year OS rate was significantly higher in patients undergoing a matched related donor or MUD BMT (16 percent and 23 percent, respectively) compared to chemotherapy (4 percent), but only 25 percent of patients were able to proceed to BMT.[176] The reasons were not explored in this trial; however, many patients did not have sibling donors. In addition, only half of all patients will achieve CR with salvage chemotherapy,[176] and the outcome with BMT is dismal in the setting of refractory disease.[168] As novel agents are developed and a higher CR rate is achieved with salvage therapy, the number of patients who may benefit from BMT and the outcomes of BMT may improve as well. Currently, even with BMT, the results in the relapsed setting are dismal, raising the question of whether BMT should be moved up front in the treatment course.

AUTOLOGOUS BONE MARROW TRANSPLANTATION

The place of auto-BMT in the treatment of ALL in the first CR also was examined in the MRC UKALL XII/ECOG E2993 trial. Patients without a sibling-matched donor were randomized to standard chemotherapy versus an auto-BMT. Among 456 patients randomized to chemotherapy versus auto-BMT, patients who received chemotherapy had a higher 5-year OS (46 percent) than those randomized to auto-BMT (37 percent; $P = 0.03$). Therefore, there is no evidence that auto-BMT can replace consolidation/maintenance chemotherapy.[30]

ALTERNATIVES SOURCES OF MARROW AND OTHER TYPES OF BONE MARROW TRANSPLANTATION

Alternative sources of bone marrow including unrelated, haploidentical, and umbilical cord transplants have been explored; but most series are small and have evaluated hematologic malignancies together (rather than just ALL). Given the dismal outcome with chemotherapy alone in the setting of relapsed ALL or high-risk ALL, physicians should consider these alternative sources if a matched-related donor is not available. Nonmyeloablative transplants also have been evaluated. This strategy utilizes the potent antileukemic effect of BMT, while decreasing transplant-related mortality and morbidity. Since many patients with ALL are older and have high-risk features such as Ph$^+$ chromosome, such a strategy may expand the number of patients receiving BMT. The proposed intergroup/MRC trial will evaluate this approach: nonmyeloablative BMT in the first CR for patients older than 40 years with a matched sibling and nonmyeloablative BMT in the first CR with an unrelated donor for patients older than 40 years with other high-risk features.

Treatment algorithm

Participation of adult patients with ALL in clinical trials is critical to improve the outcome for this population. Adolescents and young adult patients should be treated in pediatric ALL protocols for adolescents with high-risk ALL. A recently opened intergroup trial by the CALGB, SWOG, and ECOG will treat patients younger than 30 years with the regimen currently used for children with high-risk ALL. The ECOG continues to explore the benefit of allo-SCT for younger patients in first remission. Common expression of CD22 and CD20 antigens on B-ALL leukemic cells,[133] together with excellent preliminary safety and efficacy data of epratuzumab in pediatric patients with recurrent ALL,[17] support the prospective study of the role of mAbs in the treatment of adult patients with newly diagnosed B cell ALL as it has been considered for the new MRC/ECOG phase IIII study.

Therapy for recurrent and resistant acute lymphoblastic leukemia

The most important predictor for long-term outcome of recurrent ALL is the duration of the initial CR. Patients with remission lasting more than 18 months have a higher CR rate and longer duration of second remission.[178,179] Therapeutic strategy should take into account the duration of first remission, age, and therapeutic options such as SCT. The outcome of patients with early relapse may require a more aggressive and innovative strategy.

NOVEL AGENTS FOR ADULT ACUTE LYMPHOBLASTIC LEUKEMIA: A PROSPECTIVE LOOK

Despite high CR rates, the long-term DFS rate of adult patients with ALL remains approximately 40 percent.[180] In addition to early mortality (5 percent to 10 percent) during induction, approximately 10 percent to 25 percent of patients have resistant or refractory disease.[98,114,143,181] Most adult patients with ALL will relapse, often within 2 years after achieving CR. Management of patients with resistant or refractory ALL poses a great challenge. To significantly impact the outcome for adult ALL, novel agents (or combinations of agents) that are safe as well as non-cross-resistant with existing therapies, account for the adult phenotypes, and have an associated low morbidity need further investigation. Novel purine nucleoside analogues, inhibitors of receptor and non-receptor PTKIs (e.g., Src family), and inhibitors of angiogenesis, including angiogenesis factors and modulators of gene expression (i.e., epigenetic therapies), represent a spectrum of agents that are currently under preclinical and clinical development. Below we discuss selected agents that target one or more of these mechanisms.

Purine nucleoside analogues

The rationale, pharmacology, and clinical experience to date with three novel purine nucleoside analogues in the treatment of patients with refractory acute leukemia are reviewed, with a highlight on ALL.[182]

CLOFARABINE

Clofarabine is a purine nucleoside analogue that exerts its cytotoxicity through multiple mechanisms of action, with a major effect on ribonucleotide reductase inhibition and incorporation into DNA followed by inhibition of DNA polymerases. Additionally, effects on mitochondrial membrane polarization and disruption with resultant cytochrome c release and apoptosis induction have been reported. Clofarabine has demonstrated clinical activity as a single agent and in combination with cytosine arabinoside against refractory and relapsed ALL in phase I and II studies.[183–186] In adult patients with ALL, the overall response rates (ORRs) to single-agent clofarabine were low (16 percent) with a median survival of 7 months. However, response rates were about 30 percent in the pediatric population, and this clinical response eventually led to improvements in OS since some of these patients could make the transition to SCT. In 2004, the FDA granted accelerated approval for clofarabine for use in pediatric patients (age 1 to 21 years) with relapsed and refractory ALL. Because clofarabine is a potent inhibitor of ribonucleotide reductase and has shown activity against acute leukemia, the hypothesis that clofarabine could potentiate the activity of cytarabine has been evaluated based on *in vitro* synergy. A phase II trial through the SWOG evaluating the combination of clofarabine and cytarabine recently has completed accrual, and the results are expected soon. The addition of clofarabine in combination with CY appears to enhance DNA damage in acute myeloid and lymphoid leukemias.[187] The ORR in this phase I study for the six adult patients with ALL was 67 percent (three CRs and one partial response). Correlative work demonstrated increased DNA damage, as measured by phosphorylation of γ-H2AX. We await results from these ongoing studies that are attempting to validate this combination as well as the correlative work for the mechanism of enhanced DNA damage.

NELARABINE

Agents such as nelarabine are likely to be important for adult T cell leukemia and show promising response rates in phase II studies, with an ORR of 33 percent to 60 percent, a CR of 31 percent to 47 percent, and a median response duration of 5 months, and overall 1-year survival rate of 28 percent in adults.[182,188,189] Nelarabine recently has been approved for T-ALL and T cell lymphoblastic lymphoma (T-LBL) based on two clinical studies conducted by the COG (pediatric patients) and CALGB (adult patients) in patients with T-ALL and T-LBL whose disease had not responded to or had relapsed following treatment with at least two chemotherapy regimens.[190]

FORODESINE

Forodesine is the most recent novel agent, with a unique mechanism that has shown single-agent activity in relapsed and refractory T and B cell leukemias and cutaneous lymphomas.[182] Although clinical experience is limited, treatment-related toxicities appear to be mild.

Signal transduction inhibitors

The prototype PTKI, imatinib, has made a profound impact on the management of Ph+ ALL. Continued studies, incorporating this and other BCR-ABL-directed agents in upfront therapy in combination with chemotherapy[191] and maintenance therapy, will determine their added benefit versus late toxicities. To date, numerous international studies have demonstrated feasibility and efficacy when imatinib was added to multiagent induction chemotherapy.[28,191–193] The primary toxicities included cytopenias, liver function abnormalities, and nausea. In young patients with Ph+ ALL, imatinib has been used as maintenance therapy as a bridge to BMT.[194] Additionally, imatinib has been used in conjunction with prednisone for elderly (older than 60 years) patients with Ph+ ALL.[195] Ultimately, the likelihood that resistance to imatinib will emerge for most patients underscores the need for non-cross-resistant BCR-ABL-directed agents such as nilotinib or dual inhibitors such as dasatinib or bosutinib that are directed against Src as well as BCR-ABL. In this regard, a phase II study of dasatinib for patients with

Ph+ ALL who were refractory to imatinib demonstrated hematologic and cytogenetic responses as well as tolerability in this patient cohort.[196] Currently, the optimal doses and schedules for incorporating PTKIs into the paradigm for ALL therapy are being evaluated, although concurrent use appears to be substantiated.[28,127] Due to disappointing long-term survival of patients with Ph+ ALL, several strategies are being tested in ongoing clinical studies, including hyper-CVAD-based approaches, postinduction use of BMT, and imatinib- or desatinib-based therapies (Table 63.7).

Src inhibitors

The Src family consists of a group of non-receptor PTKs and includes Src, Lyn, Hck, Yes, Lck, Fgr, and Fyn.[197] These kinases are critically involved in diverse cellular processes, including cell survival, proliferation, motility, adhesion, and transformation.[198,199] Aberrant activation of Src is commonly observed in epithelial tumors, most notably in colon and breast cancer, but also can occur in other tumor types.[200] Activated Src proteins translocate from the cytoplasm to the cell membrane, where they interact with selected receptor PTKs such as the epidermal growth factor receptor (EGFR) family, focal adhesion kinase, and steroid hormone receptors to trigger downstream activation of multiple signal pathways. While rarely mutated, these proteins can be overexpressed or activated in a broad spectrum of epithelial and hematologic malignancies and are linked to the processes of metastasis, angiogenesis, and drug resistance.[198,199,201] Activated Src kinases abrogate the function of the critical negative regulator phosphatase and tensin homolog (PTEN), thereby permitting activation of the PI3K/AKT pathway[201] which, in turn, leads to inhibition of apoptosis pathways and results in net cellular survival and drug resistance.

The targeting of Src may have a special role in Ph+ leukemias. First, the Abl portion of the Ph+ chromosome-encoded Bcr-Abl kinase is closely related to the Src family. Second, the Src family kinase Lyn is expressed by B lymphocytes and myeloid cells, with growth factor-driven overexpression in AML and with constitutive activation by the Bcr-Abl fusion protein.[198] Furthermore, Lyn may be overexpressed in Ph+ leukemic cells independent of Bcr-Abl activity and may confer imatinib resistance without concomitant Bcr-Abl mutations.[202–204] These findings plus the notable conformational similarities between activated Abl and activated Lyn[205,206] have led to the design of dual-specific inhibitors of both Abl and Src that can bind to both the activated and inactivated forms of Abl and Lyn.[207–209] As noted above, the dual inhibitor dasatinib has major clinical activity with induction of hematologic and cytogenetic responses in imatinib-resistant Ph+ ALL.[196] Continuing development of Src and dual Src-Abl inhibitors should explore the ability of these agents to circumvent resistance of both Ph+ and Ph− ALLs to conventional cytotoxic drugs, with design of combination modalities for clinical testing.

Antiangiogenesis agents

Data obtained from animal models and partially confirmed in preclinical studies have provided clear evidence of the importance of angiogenesis for the growth of solid tumors. Acute leukemia cells also use angiogenic growth factor signaling pathways, namely those activated by vascular endothelial growth factor (VEGF), in both an autocrine and paracrine fashion. Stimulation of VEGF results in cell proliferation, increased cell survival, and migration. The observation that leukemia progression might be accompanied by an increase in bone marrow vascularization was first demonstrated by Judah Folkman's laboratory, when increased blood vessel content in the bone marrow from patients with ALL was seen as compared to their normal counterparts.[210] Additionally, urine and peripheral blood samples from patients with ALL contained elevated levels of pro-angiogenic growth factors, namely basic fibroblast growth factor and VEGF, which correlated with an increase in bone marrow angiogenesis.[209–212] Furthermore, plasma and serum VEGF have been shown to correlate with disease progression in AML.[213]

Vascular endothelial growth factor expression is regulated by a plethora of intrinsic and extrinsic factors including hypoglycemia, hypoxia (via hypoxia-inducible factor 1α [HIF-1α] to a hypoxic response element, located in the VEGF promoter),[214] and cytokines (i.e., fibroblast growth factor 4, tumor necrosis factor α, and transforming growth factor β). Inactivation of tumor suppressors is another mechanism that leads to overexpression of VEGF, such as mutations in TP53 and von Hippel-Lindau genes.[215,216] Genetic control of angiogenesis has been demonstrated in CML, where the oncoprotein BCR-ABL induces VEGF and HIF-1α gene expression through PI3Ks and mammalian target of rapamycin (mTOR), and may contribute to leukemic pathogenesis.[217] Clarification of these pathways and their biological ramifications could lead to improved understanding of Ph$^+$ ALL, and potentially offer therapeutic approaches not yet identified.

Several studies have shown that VEGF/VEGF receptor expression and activation is necessary for normal hematopoietic function.[218] In hematopoietic malignancies such as acute leukemia, constitutive or inducible activation of this pathway may represent a mechanism whereby malignant cells survive at particular stages of disease. Stimulation of the microenvironment results in increased angiogenesis and thus an augmented and perhaps a lineage-specific, hematopoietic growth factor production. Such changes in the cytokine milieu ultimately induce cellular and biochemical changes within the bone marrow and therefore provide a survival advantage for leukemia cells.

Several groups have been focusing on treatment of acute leukemia cells with VEGF to better understand the molecular basis for their biological effects. Pretreatment of acute leukemia cells using VEGF before chemotherapy resulted in an increase of viable cells, suggesting that VEGF inhibited chemotherapy-induced apoptosis.[219] Several groups have demonstrated that VEGF stimulation activates the mitogen-activated protein kinase signaling pathway and increases heat shock protein-90 (Hsp-90) with a resulting increased expression of BCL2.[220–222] Specifically, VEGF produced by stromal cells has been shown to directly upregulate BCL2 phosphorylation in ALL cell lines, protecting them from chemotherapy exposure.[222]

Vascular endothelial growth factor receptors (VEGFR-1, -2, -3) are expressed primarily on vascular endothelial cells. VEGFR-1 is expressed on hematopoietic stem cells (HSC), leukemic blasts, vascular smooth muscle cells, and monocytes. The ability of VEGF to have a multifunctional impact on angiogenesis and HSC survival, in combination with the prevalence of VEGFR expression on leukemic blasts, suggests that the VEGF pathway may have a pivotal role in leukemia evolution and disease progression. In fact, VEGFR-1 activation appears to modulate ALL distribution in the bone marrow, determining leukemia survival and onset of extramedullary disease.[223]

Ultimately, the contributions of angiogenesis may be detected through the molecular changes that result from shifts in cytokine balance within the bone marrow, and may allow for better prediction of leukemia progression or prognosis. Given these preclinical data, therapeutic approaches designed to block angiogenesis in ALL could affect clinical outcome, and should be explored. Agents such as bevacizumab (recombinant humanized immunoglobulin G [IgG] mAb directed against VEGF), SU5416/Sugen (small-molecule VEGFR inhibitor), PTK787/ZK222584/vatalanib (oral PTKI that binds to the adenosine triphosphate binding sites of VEGFR), ZD6474 (VEGFR-2 PTKI), GW786034 (oral pan-VEGFR inhibitor), and sorafenib (Raf kinase inhibitor that indirectly inhibits VEGFR) could all yield interesting and promising results in ALL. An ORR of 48 percent was seen in patients with refractory AML who received bevacizumab plus chemotherapy.[224] Corresponding decreases in microvessel density on the day 15 bone marrow biopsy in more than 70 percent of patients was appreciated and underscores the importance for further investigation of angiogenesis inhibitors in treatment of leukemia. Future clinical studies need to be designed to better understand the impact of antiangiogenic agents on ALL pathogenesis as well as on chemotherapy-resistant disease.

Epigenetic therapy

Although chromosomal abnormalities are a hallmark of pathogenesis of ALL, evidence suggests that they must act in concert with additional genetic lesions to induce overt leukemia. Deletions of *p15* and *p16* genes are known to occur in patients with ALL.[225,226] Aberrant epigenetic lesions, particularly DNA methylation of promoter-associated CpG islands, are common in ALL.[227] DNA methylation resulting in silencing of these same genes, as well as other key tumor suppressor genes (*MDR1*, *ER*, *TP73*, *p57^KIP2*), also have been shown to occur in patients with *de novo* and relapsed ALL.[228–232] *p57^KIP2* is a cyclin-dependent kinase inhibitor that is aberrantly methylated in several ALL-derived cell lines (Jurkat, CCRF-CEM, BALL1, CCRF-HSB2, Malt4, SupT1, PEER, TALL1). Gene silencing of these methylated cell lines has been demonstrated, as well as gene reexpression post-exposure to decitabine. Additionally, $p57^{KIP}$ was methylated in 50 percent of patients with newly diagnosed and relapsed ALL.[228] No association was found between $p57$ methylation alone and OS or DFS, or of any clinical or biologic characteristics. However, methylation of at least two genes from the ten-gene panel identified patients with Ph⁻ ALL with a worse prognosis. More recent studies have focused on epigenetic silencing of genes in the Wnt pathway that appear to constitutively activate the Wnt pathway and lead to the pathogenesis of ALL.[231] Hebert and colleagues tested more than 260 samples of primary neoplastic cells from patients with ALL and found that presence of multiple simultaneous methylated genes was an independent factor for poor prognosis in both childhood and adult ALL in terms of DFS and OS.[226]

The data in cell lines and in patient samples help to support the notion that epigenetic agents may be beneficial for the treatment of patients with ALL.[232,233] A phase I study of the DNA methyltransferase inhibitor decitabine (5-aza-2′-deoxycytidine) in patients with diverse hematologic malignancies (mainly myeloid) yielded an ORR of 34 percent, with 65 percent of those responses occurring at the low dose and long duration of drug exposure (15 mg/m² for 10 days).[233] A phase II study combining decitabine with one of two anthracyclines was tested in patients with relapsed acute leukemias including relapsed ALL, with response rates ranging from 16 percent to 60 percent.[234]

Other epigenetic agents such as histone deacetylases (HDACs) also are important regulators of chromatin-involved silencing of tumor suppressor genes. Inhibitors of histone deacetylases can induce apoptosis in ALL cells *in vitro*[235,236] as well as *in vivo* in clinical treatment for cutaneous T cell lymphomas and other lymphoproliferative malignancies.[237,238] An open chromatin structure can be accomplished by preventing deacetylation of histones with HDAC inhibitors. Agents such as entinostat, vorinistat, and LBH589 have been evaluated in phase I and II clinical trials for patients with refractory leukemias, including small numbers of patients with ALL.[239–241] Optimal combinations of epigenetic therapies currently are being investigated in patients with ALL. Thoughtful laboratory correlative work is imperative to investigate the mechanism of action of these agents (i.e., reversal of methylation, DNA damage, etc.), and answers to these questions will offer improved ability for clinical investigators to develop sound rationale for combinations and sequencing of agents.

SUMMARY AND FUTURE DIRECTIONS

The survival of adults with ALL will likely improve with a number of changes, including strict adherence to complex clinical regimens as well as development of novel agents. Purine nucleoside analogues such as clofarabine and nelarabine may have much to offer in the treatment of adult ALL but need further investigation, likely with combined chemotherapy regimens. Protein tyrosine kinase inhibitors will improve outcome for those patients with Ph⁺ disease, and alternatives exist when resistance emerges. Further understanding of use of PTKIs in induction and maintenance will become clearer. Src and angiogenesis inhibitors are on the frontline of investigation, with a significant amount of preclinical data to warrant clinical exploration. Epigenetic therapy is well tolerated and may offer a feasible option for elderly patients as well as an option along with combination cytotoxic therapy. Introduction of naked or drug-conjugated antibody in the induction regimens may accelerate elimination of MRD without overlapping toxicities. The effective and timely evaluation of several sound hypotheses in well-designed clinical trials is imperative for the advancement of treatment for adults with ALL.

KEY POINTS

- Acute lymphoblastic leukemia (ALL) is a sharply contrasting disease in the pediatric and adult populations.
- Proper diagnostic workup involving immunologic classification, as well as cytogenetic and molecular genetics of ALL, is crucial for prognostication and for appropriate treatment.
- Current therapy for adults with ALL is based on patient- and disease-specific characteristics.
- Asparaginase is a critical component of multiagent front-line therapy for pediatric and adult patients with ALL.
- Application of age- and risk-adopted therapeutic strategies using several components of complex pediatric protocols may lead to improved outcome in adult patients with ALL, including elderly patients.
- Stratification by prognostic factors for low- and high-risk categories for disease-free survival may help to identify the group of patients who may benefit from intensification therapy using stem cell transplantation.
- Novel agents for adult ALL include purine nucleoside analogues (clofarabine, nelarabine, and forodesine), naked and drug-conjugated monoclonal antibodies, signal transduction inhibitors, Src inhibitors, antiangiogenesis agents, and epigenetic therapy.
- Participation in well-designed clinical studies is critical for future advances in the management of adult patients with ALL.

REFERENCES

● = Key primary paper

◆ = Major review article

1. Jemal A, Siegel R, Ward E *et al.* Cancer statistics, 2008. *CA Cancer J Clin* 2008; **58**: 71–96.

2. Bailey LC, Lange BJ, Rheingold SR, Bunin NJ. Bone-marrow relapse in paediatric acute lymphoblastic leukemia. *Lancet Oncol* 2008; **9**: 873–83.

3. Faderl S, Thomas DA, Kantarjian HM. ALL therapy: review of the MD Anderson Program. In: Estey EH, Faderl SH, Katarjian HM. (eds) *Hematologic malignancies – acute leukemias.* New York: Springer Berlin Heidelberg, 2008: 161–6.

◆4. Faderl S, Jeha S, Kantarjian HM. The biology and therapy of adult acute lymphoblastic leukemia. *Cancer* 2003; **98**: 1337–54.

◆5. Larson RA. Acute lymphoblastic leukemia: older patients and newer drugs. *Hematology Am Soc Hematol Educ Program* 2005; 131–6.

6. Katikireddi V. 100 000 children die needlessly from cancer every year. *BMJ* 2004; **328**: 422.

7. Heath CW. Leukemogenesis and low-dose exposure to radiation and chemical agents. In: Yohn DS, Blakeslee JR. (eds) *Advances in comparative leukemia research.* Amsterdam: Elsevier Biomedical, 1982: 23.

8. Pui CH, Ribeiro RC, Hancock ML *et al.* Acute myeloid leukemia in children treated with epipodophyllotoxins for acute lymphoblastic leukemia. *N Engl J Med* 1991; **325**: 1682–7.

9. Zuna J, Cavé H, Eckert C *et al.* Childhood secondary ALL after ALL treatment. *Leukemia* 2007; **21**: 1431–5.

10. Bennett JM, Catovsky D, Daniel MT *et al.* Proposals for the classification of the acute leukemias. French-American-British (FAB) co-operative group. *Br J Haematol* 1976; **33**: 451–8.

11. Harris NL, Jaffe ES, Diebold J *et al.* World Health Organization classification of neoplastic diseases of the hematopoietic and lymphoid tissues: report of the Clinical Advisory Committee meeting-Airlie House, Virginia, November 1997. *J Clin Oncol* 1999; **17**: 3835–49.

12. Swerdlow SH, Campo E, Harris NL *et al. WHO classification of tumours of haematopoietic and lymphoid tissue,* 4th Edn. Lyon, France: International Agency for Research on Cancer, 2008.

13. Golub TR, Slonim DK, Tamayo P *et al.* Molecular classification of cancer: class discovery and class prediction by gene expression monitoring. *Science* 1999; **286**: 531–7.

14. Mi S, Lu J, Sun M *et al.* MicroRNA expression signatures accurately discriminate acute lymphoblastic leukemia from acute myeloid leukemia. *Proc Natl Acad Sci U S A* 2007; **104**: 19971–6.

◆15. Gökbuget N, Hoelzer D. Treatment of adult acute lymphoblastic leukemia. *Hematology Am Soc Hematol Educ Program* 2006; 133–41.

16. Riley RS, Massey D, Jackson-Cook C *et al.* Immunophenotypic analysis of acute lymphocytic leukemia. *Hematol Oncol Clin North Am* 2002; **16**: 245–99.

17. Raetz EA, Cairo MS, Borowitz MJ *et al.* Chemoimmunotherapy reinduction with epratuzumab in children with acute lymphoblastic leukemia in marrow relapse: a Children's Oncology Group pilot study. *J Clin Oncol* 2008; **26**: 3756–62.

◆18. Huh YO, Ibrahim S. Immunophenotypes in adult acute lymphocytic leukemia. Role of flow cytometry in diagnosis and monitoring of disease. *Hematol Oncol Clin North Am* 2000; **4**: 1251–65.

◆19. Hoelzer D, Gökbuget N. Acute lymphocytic leukemia in adults. In: Abeloff MD, Armitage JO, Niederhuber JE *et al.* (eds) *Abeloff's clinical oncology,* 4th Edn. Philadelphia: Churchill Livingstone Elsevier, 2008: 2191–213.

20. Roper M, Crist WM, Metzgar R *et al.* Monoclonal antibody characterization of surface antigens in childhood T-cell lymphoid malignancies. *Blood* 1983; **61**: 830–7.

◆21. Faderl S, Kantarjian HM, Talpaz M, Estrov Z. Clinical significance of cytogenetic abnormalities in adult acute lymphoblastic leukemia. *Blood* 1998; **91**: 3995–4019.

●22. Moorman AV, Harrison CJ, Buck GA *et al.* Karyotype is an independent prognostic factor in adult acute lymphoblastic leukemia (ALL): analysis of cytogenetic data from patients treated on the Medical Research Council (MRC) UKALLXII/Eastern Cooperative Oncology Group (ECOG) 2993 trial. *Blood* 2007; **109**: 3189–97.

23. Novell PC, Hungerford DA. A minute chromosome in human granulocytic leukemia. *Science* 1960; **132**: 1497.

●24. Mancini M, Scappaticci D, Cimino G *et al.* A comprehensive genetic classification of adult acute lymphoblastic leukemia (ALL): analysis of the GIMEMA 0496 protocol. *Blood* 2005; **105**: 3434–41.

◆25. Larson S, Stock W. Progress in the treatment of adults with acute lymphoblastic leukemia. *Curr Opin Hematol* 2008; **15**: 400–7.

26. Mullighan CG, Miller CB, Radtke I *et al.* BCR-ABL1 lymphoblastic leukaemia is characterized by the deletion of Ikaros. *Nature* 2008; **453**: 110–14.

27. Tonnelle C, Calmels B, Maroc C *et al.* Ikaros gene expression and leukemia. *Leuk Lymphoma* 2002; **43**: 29–35.

●28. Towatari M, Yanada M, Usui N *et al.* Combination of intensive chemotherapy and imatinib can rapidly induce high-quality complete remission for a majority of patients with newly diagnosed BCR-ABL-positive acute lymphoblastic leukemia. *Blood* 2004; **104**: 3507–12.

29. Ottmann OG, Wassmann B. Treatment of Philadelphia chromosome-positive acute lymphoblastic leukemia. *Hematology Am Soc Hematol Educ Program* 2005; 118–22.

●30. Goldstone AH, Richards SM, Lazarus HM *et al.* In adults with standard-risk acute lymphoblastic leukemia, the greatest benefit is achieved from a matched sibling allogeneic transplantation in first complete remission, and an autologous transplantation is less effective than conventional consolidation/maintenance chemotherapy in all patients: final results of the International ALL Trial (MRC UKALL XII/ECOG E2993). *Blood* 2008; **111**: 1827–33.

●31. Faderl S, Kantarjian HM, Thomas DA *et al.* Outcome of Philadelphia chromosome-positive adult acute lymphoblastic leukemia. *Leuk Lymphoma* 2000; **36**: 263–73.

32. Iacobucci I, Lonetti A, Messa F *et al.* Expression of spliced oncogenic Ikaros isoforms in Philadelphia-positive acute lymphoblastic leukemia patients treated with tyrosine kinase inhibitors: implications for a new mechanism of resistance. *Blood* 2008; **112**: 3847–55.

33. Mullighan CG, Goorha S, Radtke I *et al.* Genome-wide analysis of genetic alterations in acute lymphoblastic leukaemia. *Nature* 2007; **446**: 758–64.

34. Mullighan CG, Su X, Zhang J *et al.* Deletion of *IKZF1* and prognosis in acute lymphoblastic leukaemia. *N Engl J Med* 2009; **360**: 470–80.

35. Pui CH, Relling MV, Downing JR. Acute lymphoblastic leukemia. N Engl J Med 2004; **350**: 1535–48.

●36. Sweetenham JW, Santini G, Qian W *et al.* High-dose therapy and autologous stem-cell transplantation versus conventional-dose consolidation/maintenance therapy as postremission therapy for adult patients with lymphoblastic lymphoma: results of a randomized trial of the European Group for Blood and Marrow Transplantation and the United Kingdom Lymphoma Group. *J Clin Oncol* 2001; **19**: 2927–36.

37. Pui CH. T cell acute lymphoblastic leukemia: NOTCHing the way toward a better treatment outcome. *Cancer Cell* 2009; **15**: 85–7.

38. Pear WS, Aster JC. T cell acute lymphoblastic leukemia/lymphoma: a human cancer commonly associated with aberrant NOTCH1 signaling. *Curr Opin Hematol* 2004; **11**: 426–33.

39. Armstrong F, Brunet de la Grange P, Gerby B *et al.* NOTCH is a key regulator of human T-cell acute leukaemia initiating cell activity. *Blood* 2009; **113**: 1730–40.

40. Demarest RM, Ratti F, Capobianco AJ. It's T-ALL about Notch. *Oncogene* 2008; **27**: 5082–91.

41. Real PJ, Tosello V, Palomero T *et al.* γ-secretase inhibitors reverse glucocorticoid resistance in T cell acute lymphoblastic leukemia. *Nat Med* 2009; **15**: 50–8.

42. Schrappe M, Zimmermann M, Möricke A *et al.* Dexamethasone in induction can eliminate one third of all relapses in childhood acute lymphoblastic leukemia (ALL): results of an international randomized trial in 3655 patients (Trial AIEOP-BFM ALL 2000). *Blood* 2007; **112**: 7 (abstract).

43. Bloomfield CD, Mrózek K, Caligiuri MA. Cancer and Leukemia Group B Leukemia Correlative Science Committee: major accomplishments and future directions. *Clin Cancer Res* 2006; **12**: 3564s–71s.

44. Bash RO, Hall S, Timmons CF *et al.* Does activation of the TAL1 gene occur in a majority of patients with T-cell acute lymphoblastic leukemia? A pediatric oncology group study. *Blood* 1995; **86**: 666–76.

45. Al Khabori M, Samiee S, Fung S *et al.* Adult precursor T-lymphoblastic leukemia/lymphoma with myeloid-associated antigen expression is associated with a lower complete remission rate following induction chemotherapy. *Acta Haematol* 2008; **120**: 5–10.

46. Ferrando AA, Neuberg DS, Dodge RK *et al.* Prognostic importance of TLX1 (HOX11) oncogene expression in adults with T-cell acute lymphoblastic leukaemia. *Lancet* 2004; **363**: 535–6.

47. Baak U, Gökbuget N, Orawa H *et al.* Thymic adult T-cell acute lymphoblastic leukemia stratified in standard- and high-risk group by aberrant HOX11L2 expression: experience of the German multicenter ALL study group. *Leukemia* 2008; **22**: 1154–60.

◆48. Pui CH, Robison LL, Look AT. Acute lymphoblastic leukemia. *Lancet* 2008; **371**: 1030–43.

49. Nathwani BN, Diamond LW, Winberg CD *et al.* Lymphoblastic lymphoma: a clinicopathologic study of 95 patients. *Cancer* 19891; **48**: 2347–57.

50. Voakes JB, Jones SE, McKelvey EM. The chemotherapy of lymphoblastic lymphoma. *Blood* 1981; **57**: 186–8.

51. Kaiser U, Uebelacker I, Havemann K. Non-Hodgkin's lymphoma protocols in the treatment of patients with Burkitt's lymphoma and lymphoblastic lymphoma: a report on 58 patients. *Leuk Lymphoma* 1999; **36**: 101–8.

●52. Hoelzer D, Gökbuget N, Digel W *et al.* Outcome of adult patients with T-lymphoblastic lymphoma treated according to protocols for acute lymphoblastic leukemia. *Blood* 2002; **99**: 4379–85.

53. Pinkel D, Albertson DG. Array comparative genomic hybridization and its applications in cancer. *Nat Genet* 2005; **37**(Suppl): S11–17.

54. Paulsson K, Cazier JB, Macdougall F *et al.* Microdeletions are a general feature of adult and adolescent acute lymphoblastic leukemia: Unexpected similarities with pediatric disease. *Proc Natl Acad Sci U S A* 2008; **105**: 6708–13.

55. Hong D, Gupta R, Ancliff P *et al.* Initiating and cancer-propagating cells in TEL-AML1-associated childhood leukemia. *Science* 2008; **319**: 336–9.

56. Bhojwani D, Kang H, Menezes RX *et al.* Gene expression signatures predictive of early response and outcome in high-risk childhood acute lymphoblastic leukemia: A Children's Oncology Group Study. *J Clin Oncol* 2008; **26**: 4376–84.

57. Bhojwani D, Moskowitz N, Raetz EA, Carroll WL. Potential of gene expression profiling in the management of childhood acute lymphoblastic leukemia. *Paediatr Drugs* 2007; **9**: 149–56.

58. Mullighan CG, Phillips LA, Su X *et al.* Genomic analysis of the clonal origins of relapsed acute lymphoblastic leukemia. *Science* 2008; **322**: 1377–80.

59. Wang H, Lee CH, Qi C *et al.* IRF8 regulates B-cell lineage specification, commitment, and differentiation. *Blood* 2008; **112**: 4028–38.

60. Szczepański T. Why and how to quantify minimal residual disease in acute lymphoblastic leukemia? *Leukemia* 2007; **21**: 622–6.

◆61. Mullighan CG, Downing JR. Global genomic characterization of acute lymphoblastic leukemia. *Semin Hematol* 2009; **46**: 3–15.

◆62. Pui CH, Evans WE. Treatment of acute lymphoblastic leukemia. *N Engl J Med* 2006; **354**: 166–78.

63. Hoelzer D, Gökbuget N, Ottmann O *et al.* Acute lymphoblastic leukemia. *Hematology Am Soc Hematol Educ Program* 2002: 162–92.

64. Borowitz MD, Devidas M, Hunger SP *et al.* Clinical significance of minimal residual disease in childhood acute lymphoblastic leukemia and its relationship to other prognostic factors: a Children's Oncology Group study. *Blood* 2008; **111**: 5477–85.

65. Ryan J, Quinn F, Meunier A *et al.* Minimal residual disease detection in childhood acute lymphoblastic leukaemia patients at multiple time-points reveals high levels of concordance between molecular and immunophenotypic approaches. *Br J Haematol* 2009; **144**: 107–15.

◆66. Foroni L, Hoffbrand AV. Molecular analysis of minimal residual disease in adult acute lymphoblastic leukemia. *Best Pract Res Clin Haematol* 2002; **15**: 71–90.

●67. Spinelli O, Peruta B, Tosi M *et al.* Clearance of minimal residual disease after allogeneic stem cell transplantation and the prediction of the clinical outcome of adult patients with high-risk acute lymphoblastic leukemia. *Haematologica* 2007; **92**: 612–18.

68. Rabin KR, Margolin J, Poplack DG. Molecular genetics of ALL. In: Mendelson J, Howley PM, Israel MA *et al.* (eds) *The molecular basis of cancer*, 3rd Edn. Philadelphia: Saunders Elsevier, 2008: 361–70.

●69. Raff T, Gökbuget N, Lüschen S *et al.* Molecular relapse in adult standard-risk ALL patients detected by prospective MRD monitoring during and after maintenance treatment: data from the GMALL 06/99 and 07/03 trials. *Blood* 2007; **109**: 910–15.

●70. Brüggemann M, Raff T, Flohr T *et al.* Clinical significance of minimal residual disease quantification in adult patients with standard-risk acute lymphoblastic leukemia. *Blood* 2006; **107**: 1116–23.

●71. Lazarus HM, Richards SM, Chopra R *et al.* Central nervous system involvement in adult acute lymphoblastic leukemia at diagnosis: results from the international ALL trial MRC UKALL XII/ECOG E2993. *Blood* 2006; **108**: 465–72.

●72. Ludwig WD, Rieder H, Bartram CR *et al.* Immunophenotypic and genotypic features, clinical characteristics, and treatment outcome of adult pro-B acute lymphoblastic leukemia: results of the German multicenter trials GMALL 03/87 and 04/89. *Blood* 1998; **92**: 1898–909.

73. Murphy SB. Childhood non-Hodgkin's lymphoma. *N Engl J Med* 1978; **299**: 1446–8.

74. Morton LM, Turner JJ, Cerhan JR *et al.* Proposed classification of lymphoid neoplasms for epidemiologic research from the Pathology Working Group of the International Lymphoma Epidemiology Consortium (InterLymph). *Blood* 2007; **110**: 695–708.

75. Schinstine M, Filie AC, Wilson W *et al.* Detection of malignant hematopoietic cells in cerebral spinal fluid previously diagnosed as atypical or suspicious. *Cancer* 2006; **108**: 157–62.

76. Brunning RD *et al.* In: Jaffe ES, Harris NL, Stein H, Vardiman JW (eds) *World Health Organization classification of tumours. Pathology and genetics of tumours of haematopoietic and lymphoid tissues.* Lyon, France: IARC Press, 2001: 181.

77. Cortes J, Seiter K, Maziarz RT *et al.* Superiority of rasburicase versus allopurinol on serum uric acid control in adult patients with hematological malignancies at risk of developing tumor lysis syndrome: results of a randomized comparative phase III study. *Blood* 2008; **112**: 919 (abstract).

78. Pui CH, Jeha S, Irwin D, Camitta B. Recombinant urate oxidase (rasburicase) in the prevention and treatment of malignancy-associated hyperuricemia in pediatric and adult patients: results of a compassionate-use trial. *Leukemia* 2001; **15**: 1505–9.

79. Coiffier B, Riouffol C. Management of tumor lysis syndrome in adults. *Expert Rev Anticancer Ther* 2007; **7**: 233–9.

80. Sipsas NV, Bodey GP, Kontoyiannis DP. Perspectives for the management of febrile neutropenic patients with cancer in the 21st century. *Cancer* 2005; **103**: 1103–13.

●81. Geissler K, Koller E, Hubmann E *et al.* Granulocyte colony-stimulating factor as an adjunct to induction chemotherapy for adult acute lymphoblastic leukemia–a randomized phase-III study. *Blood* 1997; **90**: 590–6.

82. Ozer H, Armitage JO, Bennett CL *et al.* 2000 update of recommendations for the use of hematopoietic colony-stimulating factors: evidence-based, clinical practice guidelines. American Society of Clinical Oncology Growth Factors Expert Panel. *J Clin Oncol* 2000; **18**: 3558–85.

◆83. Garcia-Manero G, Kantarjian HM. The hyper-CVAD regimen in adult acute lymphoblastic leukemia. *Hematol Oncol Clin North Am* 2000; **6**: 1381–96.

◆84. Larson RA. What determines the outcome for adolescents and young adults with acute lymphoblastic leukemia? *Am J Hematol Oncol* 2007; **6**(4 Suppl 5): 17–19.

●85. Rowe JM, Buck G, Burnett AK *et al.* Induction therapy for adults with acute lymphoblastic leukemia: results of more than 1500 patients from the international ALL trial: MRC UKALL XII/ECOG E2993. *Blood* 2005: **106**; 3760–7.

86. Gökbuget N, Hoelzer D. Risk-adapted therapy of acute lymphoblastic leukaemia. *Hematology Education: the education program for the annual congress of the European Haematology Association* 2008; **2**: 64–70.

87. Ribera JM, Oriol A, Bethencourt C *et al.* Comparison of intensive chemotherapy, allogeneic or autologous stem cell transplantation as post-remission treatment for adult patients with high-risk acute lymphoblastic leukemia. Results of the PETHEMA ALL-93 trial. *Haematologica* 2005; **90**: 1346–56.

88. Holowiecki J, Krawczyk-Kulis M, Giebel S *et al.* Status of minimal residual disease after induction predicts outcome in both standard and high-risk Ph-negative adult acute lymphoblastic leukaemia. The Polish Adult Leukemia Group ALL 4-2002 MRD Study. *Br J Haematol* 2008; **142**: 227–37.

89. Thomas X, Boiron JM, Huguet F *et al.* Outcome of treatment in adults with acute lymphoblastic leukemia: analysis of the LALA-94 trial. *J Clin Oncol* 2004; **22**: 4075–86.

90. Kantarjian H, Thomas D, O'Brien S *et al.* Long-term follow-up results of hyperfractionated cyclophosphamide, vincristine, doxorubicin, and dexamethasone (Hyper-CVAD), a dose-intensive regimen, in adult acute lymphocytic leukemia. *Cancer* 2004; **101**: 2788–801.

91. Labar B, Suciu S, Zittoun R *et al.* Allogeneic stem cell transplantation in acute lymphoblastic leukemia and non-Hodgkin's lymphoma for patients ≤50 years old in first complete remission: results of the EORTC ALL-3 trial. *Haematologica* 2004; **89**: 809–17.

92. Hunault M, Harousseau JL, Delain M *et al.* Better outcome of adult acute lymphoblastic leukemia after early genoidentical allogeneic bone marrow transplantation (BMT) than after late high-dose therapy and autologous BMT: a GOELAMS trial. *Blood* 2004; **104**: 3028–37.

●93. Dombret H, Gabert J, Boiron JM *et al.* Outcome of treatment in adults with Philadelphia chromosome-positive acute lymphoblastic leukemia–results of the prospective multicenter LALA-94 trial. *Blood* 2002; **100**: 2357–66.

●94. Ribera JM, Oriol A, Sanz MA *et al.* Comparison of the results of the treatment of adolescents and young adults with standard-risk acute lymphoblastic leukemia with the Programa Español de Tratamiento en Hematología pediatric-based protocol ALL-96. *J Clin Oncol* 2008; **26**: 1843–9.

●95. DeAngelo DJ, Silverman LB, Couban S *et al.* A multicenter phase II study using a dose intensified pediatric regimen in adults with untreated acute lymphoblastic leukemia. *Blood* 2006; **108**: 1858 (abstract).

●96. Storring JM, Brandwein J, Gupta V *et al.* Treatment of adult acute lymphoblastic leukemia (ALL) with a modified DFCI pediatric regimen – The Princess Margaret Experience. *Blood* 2006; **108**: 1875 (abstract).

●97. Huguet F, Leguay T, Raffoux E *et al.* Pediatric-inspired therapy in adults with Philadelphia chromosome-negative acute lymphoblastic leukemia: The GRAALL-2003 study. *J Clin Oncol* 2009; **27**: 911–18.

●98. Hoelzer D, Theil E, Löffler H *et al.* Prognostic factors in a multicenter study for treatment of acute lymphoblastic leukemia in adults. *Blood* 1988; **71**: 123–31.

99. Gaynon PS. 40 years of asparaginase therapy in childhood acute lymphoblastic leukemia. *Am J Hematol Oncol* 2007; **6**(4 Suppl 5): 8–14.

100. Dinndorf PA, Gootenberg J, Cohen MH *et al.* FDA drug approval summary: pegaspargase (Oncaspar®) for the first-line treatment of children with acute lymphoblastic leukemia (ALL). *Oncologist* 2007; **12**: 991–8.

101. Sallan SE, Hitchcock-Bryan S, Gelber R *et al.* Influence of intensive asparaginase in the treatment of childhood non-T-cell acute lymphoblastic leukemia. *Cancer Res* 1983; **43**: 5601–7.

102. Riehm H, Gadner H, Henze G *et al.* Results and significance of six randomized trials in four consecutive ALL-BFM studies. *Haematol Blood Transfus* 1990; **33**: 439–50.

103. Nachman JB, Sather HN, Sensel MG *et al.* Augmented post-induction therapy for children with high-risk acute lymphoblastic leukemia and a slow response to initial therapy. *N Engl J Med* 1998; **338**: 1663–71.

104. Moghrabi A, Levy DE, Asselin B *et al.* Results of the Dana-Farber Cancer Institute ALL Consortium Protocol 95-01 for children with acute lymphoblastic leukemia. *Blood* 2007; **109**: 896–904.

105. Duval M, Suciu S, Ferster A *et al.* Comparison of Escherichia coli-asparaginase with Erwinia-asparaginase in the treatment of childhood lymphoid malignancies: results of a randomized European Organisation for Research and Treatment of Cancer–Children's Leukemia Group phase 3 trial. *Blood* 2002; **99**: 2734–9.

◆106. Douer D. Asparaginase in the treatment of young adults with acute lymphoblastic leukemia. *Am J Hematol Oncol* 2007; **6**(4 Suppl 5): 20–3.

107. Sallan SE. The evolving role of asparaginase therapy–what does the future hold? *Am J Hematol Oncol* 2007; **6**(4 Suppl 5): 15–16.

◆108. Douer D. Is asparaginase a critical component in the treatment of acute lymphoblastic leukemia? *Best Pract Res Clin Haematol* 2008; **21**: 647–58.

109. Mitchell CD, Richards SM, Kinsey SE *et al.* Benefit of dexamethasone compared with prednisolone for childhood acute lymphoblastic leukaemia: results of the UK Medical Research Council ALL97 randomized trial. *Br J Haematol* 2005; **129**: 734–45.

●110. O'Brien S, Thomas DA, Ravandi F *et al.* Results of the hyperfractionated cyclophosphamide, vincristine, doxorubicin, and dexamethasone regimen in elderly patients with acute lymphocytic leukemia. *Cancer* 2008; **113**: 2097–101.

111. Yang L, Panetta JC, Cai X *et al.* Asparaginase may influence dexamethasone pharmacokinetics in acute lymphoblastic leukemia. *J Clin Oncol* 2008; **26**: 1932–9.

112. Adamson PC, Barrett JS. All dex'ed out with nowhere to go? *J Clin Oncol* 2008; **26**: 1917–18.

●113. Stock W, La M, Sanford B *et al.* What determines the outcomes for adolescents and young adults with acute lymphoblastic leukemia treated on cooperative group protocols? A comparison of Children's Cancer Group and Cancer and Leukemia Group B studies. *Blood* 2008; **112**: 1646–54.

114. Larson RA, Dodge RK, Linker CA *et al.* A randomized controlled trial of filgrastim during remission induction and consolidation chemotherapy for adults with acute lymphoblastic leukemia: CALGB study 9111. *Blood* 1998; **92**: 1556–64.

115. Apostolidou E, Swords R, Alvarado Y, Giles FJ. Treatment of acute lymphoblastic leukaemia: a new era. *Drugs* 2007; **67**: 2153–71.

●116. Annino L, Vegna ML, Camera A *et al*. Treatment of adult acute lymphoblastic leukemia (ALL): long-term follow-up of the GIMEMA ALL 0288 randomized study. *Blood* 2002; **99**: 863–71.

●117. Gökbuget N, Hoelzer D. The role of high-dose cytarabine in induction therapy for adult ALL. *Leuk Res* 2002; **26**: 473–6.

●118. Kantarjian HM, O'Brien S, Smith TL *et al*. Results of treatment with hyper-CVAD, a dose-intensive regimen, in adult acute lymphocytic leukemia. *J Clin Oncol* 2000; **18**: 547–61.

119. Thomas DA, O'Brien S, Rytting M *et al*. Acute lymphoblastic leukemia (ALL) or lymphoblastic lymphoma (LL) after frontline therapy with hyper-CVAD regimens. *Blood* 2008; **112**: 1930 (abstract).

●120. Huguet F, Leguay T, Raffoux E *et al*. Pediatric–inspired therapy in adults with Philadelphia chromosome-negative acute lymphoblastic leukemia: the GRALL-2003 study. *J Clin Oncol* 2009; **27**: 911–18.

●121. Boissel N, Auclerc MF, Lhéritier V *et al*. Should adolescents with acute lymphoblastic leukemia be treated as old children or young adults? Comparison of the French FRALLE-93 and LALA-94 trials. *J Clin Oncol* 2003; **21**: 760–1.

●122. de Bont JM, Holt B, Dekker AW *et al*. Significant difference in outcome for adolescents with acute lymphoblastic leukemia treated on pediatric vs adult protocols in the Netherlands. *Leukemia* 2004; **18**: 2032–5.

●123. Ramanujachar R, Richards S, Hann I *et al*. Adolescents with acute lymphoblastic leukaemia: outcome on UK national paediatric (ALL97) and adult (UKALLXII/E2993) trials. *Pediatric Blood Cancer* 2007; **48**: 254–61.

●124. Hallböök H, Gustafsson G, Smedmyr B *et al*. Treatment outcome in young adults and children >10 years of age with acute lymphoblastic leukemia in Sweden: a comparison between a pediatric protocol and an adult protocol. *Cancer* 2006; **107**: 1551–61.

●125. Testi AM, Valsecchi MG, Conter V *et al*. Difference in outcome of adolescents with acute lymphoblastic leukemia (ALL) enrolled in pediatric (AIEOP) and adult (GIMEMA) protocols. *Blood* 2004; **104**: 1954 (abstract).

●126. DeAngelo DJ, Dahlberg S, Silverman LB *et al*. A multicenter phase II study using a dose intensified pediatric regimen in adults with untreated acute lymphoblastic leukemia. *Blood* 2007; **110**: 587 (abstract).

127. Thomas DA, Faderl S, Cortes J *et al*. Treatment of Philadelphia chromosome-positive acute lymphocytic leukemia with hyper-CVAD and imatinib mesylate. *Blood* 2004; **103**: 4396–407.

128. Thomas DA, Kantarjian HM, Ravandi F *et al*. Long-term follow-up after frontline therapy with the hyper-CVAD and imatinib mesylate regimen in adults with Philadelphia (Ph) positive acute lymphocytic leukemia (ALL). *Blood* 2007; **110**: 9 (abstract).

129. de Labarthe A, Rousselot P, Huguet-Rigal F *et al*. Imatinib combined with induction or consolidation chemotherapy in patients with de novo Philadelphia chromosome-positive acute lymphoblastic leukemia: results of the GRAAPH-2003 study. *Blood* 2007; **109**: 1408–13.

130. Stock W, Yu D, Sanford B *et al*. Incorporation of alemtuzumab into front-line therapy of adult acute lymphoblastic leukemia (ALL) is feasible: a phase I/II study from the Cancer and Leukemia Group B (CALGB 10102). *Blood* 2005; **106**: 145 (abstract).

131. Gökbuget N, Hoelzer D. Novel antibody-based therapy for acute lymphoblastic leukaemia. *Best Pract Res Clin Haematol* 2006; **19**: 701–13.

●132. Rayburg MS, Marmer D, Mo J *et al*. Prevalence and clinical characterization of CD20 and CD22 expression in pediatric precursor B-cell acute lymphoblastic leukemia. *Blood* 2008; **112**: 4872 (abstract).

●133. Paietta E, Li X, Richards S *et al*. Implications for the use of monoclonal antibodies in future adult ALL trials: analysis of antigen expression in 505 B-lineage (B-Lin) ALL patients (pts) on the MRC UKALLXII/ECOG2993 Intergroup trial. *Blood* 2008; **112**: 1907 (abstract).

●134. Thomas DA, Faderl S, O'Brien S *et al*. Chemoimmunotherapy with hyper-CVAD plus rituximab for the treatment of adult Burkitt and Burkitt-type lymphoma or acute lymphoblastic leukemia. *Cancer* 2006; **106**: 1569–80.

●135. Thomas DA, Kantarjian H, Faderl S *et al*. Update of the modified hyper-CVAD regimen with or without rituximab as frontline therapy of adults with acute lymphocytic leukemia (ALL) or lymphoblastic lymphoma (LL). *Blood* 2007; **110**: 2824 (abstract).

136. Leonard JP, Schuster SJ, Emmanouilides C *et al*. Durable complete responses from therapy with combined epratuzumab and rituximab: final results from an international multicenter, phase 2 study in recurrent, indolent, non-Hodgkin lymphoma. *Cancer* 2008; **113**: 2714–23.

137. Leonard JP, Coleman M, Ketas JC *et al*. Phase I/II trial of epratuzumab (humanized anti-CD22 antibody) in indolent non-Hodgkin's lymphoma. *J Clin Oncol* 2003; **21**: 3051–9.

138. Leonard JP, Coleman M, Ketas JC *et al*. Epratuzumab, a humanized anti-CD22 antibody, in aggressive non-Hodgkin's lymphoma: phase I/II clinical trial results. *Clin Cancer Res* 2004; **10**: 5327–34.

139. Leonard JP, Coleman M, Ketas J *et al*. Combination antibody therapy with epratuzumab and rituximab in relapsed or refractory non-Hodgkin's lymphoma. *J Clin Oncol* 2005; **23**: 5044–51.

140. Tobinai K, Ogura M, Hatake K *et al*. Phase I and pharmacokinetic study of inotuzumab ozogamicin (CMC-544) as a single agent in Japanese patients with follicular lymphoma retreated with rituximab. *Blood* 2008; **112**: 1565 (abstract).

141. Fayad L, Patel H, Verhoef G *et al*. Safety and clinical activity of the anti-CD22 immunoconjugate inotuzumab ozogamicin (CMC-544) in combination

with rituximab in follicular lymphoma or diffuse large B-cell lymphoma: preliminary report of a phase 1/2 study. *Blood* 2008; **112**: 266 (abstract).

142. Kreitman RJ, Wilson WH, Stetler-Stevenson M *et al.* Interim phase I results of recombinant immunotoxin HA22 in patients with hairy cell and chronic lymphocytic leukemias. *Blood* 2008; **112**: 3160 (abstract).

143. Takeuchi J, Kyo T, Naito K *et al.* Induction therapy by frequent administration of doxorubicin with four other drugs, followed by intensive consolidation and maintenance therapy for adult acute lymphoblastic leukemia: the JALSG-ALL93 study. *Leukemia* 2002; **16**: 1259–66.

144. Childhood ALL Collaborative Group. Duration and intensity of maintenance chemotherapy in acute lymphoblastic leukaemia: overview of 42 trials involving 12 000 randomised children. *Lancet* 1996; **347**: 1783–8.

●145. Dekker AW, van't Veer MB, Sizoo W *et al.* Intensive postremission chemotherapy without maintenance therapy in adults with acute lymphoblastic leukemia. Dutch Hemato-Oncology Research Group. *J Clin Oncol* 1997; **15**: 476–82.

146. Albritton K. Introduction. *Am J Hematol Oncol* 2007; **6**(4 Suppl 5): 5–7.

147. Gökbuget N, Hoelzer D. Meningeosis leukaemia in adult acute lymphoblastic leukaemia. *J Neurooncol* 1998; **38**: 167–80.

●148. Rytting M, Thomas D, Franklin A *et al.* Young adults with acute lymphoblastic leukemia (ALL) treated with adapted augmented Berlin-Frankfurt-Munster (ABFM) therapy. *Blood* 2008; **112**: 3957 (abstract).

149. Cortes J, O'Brien SM, Pierce S *et al.* The value of high-dose systemic chemotherapy and intrathecal therapy for central nervous system prophylaxis in different risk groups of adult acute lymphoblastic leukemia. *Blood* 1995; **86**; 2091–7.

150. Sancho JM, Morgades M, Arranz R *et al.* Practice of central nervous system prophylaxis and treatment in acute leukemias in Spain. Prospective registry study. *Med Clin (Barc)* 2008; **131**: 401–5.

151. Howell DL, Ward KC, Austin HD *et al.* Access to pediatric cancer care by age, race, and diagnosis, and outcomes of cancer treatment in pediatric and adolescent patients in the state of Georgia. *J Clin Oncol* 2007; **25**: 4610–15.

◆152. Ramanujachar R, Richards S, Hann I, Webb D. Adolescents with acute lymphoblastic leukaemia: emerging from the shadow of paediatric and adult treatment protocols. *Pediatr Blood Cancer* 2006; **47**: 748–56.

◆153. Schiffer CA. Differences in outcome in adolescents with acute lymphoblastic leukemia: a consequence of better regimens? Better doctors? Both? *J Clin Oncol* 2003; **21**: 760–1.

◆154. DeAngelo DJ. The treatment of adolescents and young adults with acute lymphoblastic leukemia. *Hematology Am Soc Hematol Educ Program* 2005; 123–30.

◆155. Sallan SE. Myths and lessons from the adult/pediatric interface in acute lymphoblastic leukemia. *Hematology Am Soc Hematol Educ Program* 2006; 128–32.

◆156. Barry E, DeAngelo DJ, Neuberg D *et al.* Favorable outcome for adolescents with acute lymphoblastic leukemia treated on Dana-Farber Cancer Institute Acute Lymphoblastic Leukemia Consortium Protocols. *J Clin Oncol* 2007; **25**: 813–19.

◆157. Appelbaum FR. Impact of age on the biology of acute leukemia. *ASCO Educational Book* 2005; 528–32.

●158. Gökbuget N, Hoelzer D, Arnold R *et al.* Subtypes and treatment outcome in adult acute lymphoblastic leukemia less than or greater than 55 years. *Hematol J* 2001; **1**(Suppl 1): 186.

●159. Hoelzer D, Gökbuget N, Beck J *et al.* Subtype adjusted therapy improves outcome of elderly patients with acute lymphoblastic leukemia. *Blood* 2004; **104**(Suppl 1): 2732 (abstract).

◆160. Cheok MH, Pottier N, Kager L, Evans WE. Pharmacogenetics in acute lymphoblastic leukemia. *Semin Hematol* 2009; **46**: 39–51.

161. Avivi I, Rowe JM. Acute lymphocytic leukemia: role of hematopoietic stem cell transplantation in current management. *Curr Opin Hematol* 2003; **10**: 463–8.

162. Chester SJ, Esparaza AR, Flinton LJ *et al.* Further development of a successful protocol of graft versus leukemia without fatal graft-versus-host disease in AKR mice. *Cancer Res.* 1977; **37**: 3794–6.

●163. Doney K, Fisher L, Appelbaum FR *et al.* Treatment of adult acute lymphoblastic leukemia with allogeneic bone marrow transplantation: multivariate analysis of factors affecting graft-versus-host disease, relapse, and relapse-free survival. *Bone Marrow Transplant* 1991; **7**: 453–9.

164. Horowitz MM, Gale RP, Sondel PM *et al.* Graft-versus-leukemia reactions after bone marrow transplantation. *Blood* 1990; **75**: 555–62.

165. Avivi I, Rowe JM, Goldstone AH. Stem cell transplantation in adult ALL patients. *Best Pract Res Clin Haematol* 2002; **15**: 653–74.

166. Vettenranta K, Saarinen-Pihkala UM, Cornish J *et al.* Pediatric marrow transplantation for acute leukemia using unrelated donors and T-replete or -depleted grafts: a case-matched analysis. *Bone Marrow Transplant* 2000; **25**: 395–9.

◆167. Martin TG, Gajewski JL. Allogeneic stem cell transplantation for acute lymphocytic leukemia in adults. *Hematol Oncol Clin North Am* 2001; **15**: 97–120.

◆168. Rowe JM, Goldstone AJ. How I treat acute lymphocytic leukemia in adults. *Blood* 2007; **110**: 2268–75.

169. Davies SM, Ramsey NK, Klein JP *et al.* Comparison of preparative regimens in transplants for children with acute lymphoblastic leukemia. *J Clin Oncol* 2000; **18**: 340–7.

170. Bloomfield CD, Goldman AI, Alimena G *et al.* Chromosomal abnormalities identify high-risk and low-risk patients with acute lymphoblastic leukemia. *Blood* 1986; **67**: 415–20.

171. Gaynor J, Chapman D, Little C *et al.* A cause-specific hazard rate analysis of prognostic factors among 199 adults with acute lymphoblastic leukemia: The Memorial Hospital experience since 1969. *J Clin Oncol* 1988; **6**: 1014–30.

●172. Mortuza FY, Papaioannou M, Moreira IM *et al.* Minimal residual disease tests provide an independent predictor of clinical outcome in adult acute lymphoblastic leukemia. *J Clin Oncol* 2002; **20**: 1094–104.

173. Pfeifer H, Wassmann B, Pavlova A *et al.* Kinase domain mutations of BCR-ABL frequently precede imatinib-based therapy and give rise to relapse in patients with de novo Philadelphia-positive acute lymphoblastic leukemia (Ph$^+$ ALL). *Blood* 2007; **110**: 727–34.

174. Avivi I, Goldstone AH. Bone marrow transplant in Ph$^+$ ALL patients. *Bone Marrow Transplant* 2003; **31**: 623–32.

●175. Sebban C, Lepage E, Vernant JP *et al.* Allogeneic bone marrow transplantation in adult acute lymphoblastic leukemia in first complete remission: a comparative study French Group of Therapy of Adult Acute Lymphoblastic Leukemia. *J Clin Oncol* 1994; **12**: 2580–7.

●176. Fielding AK, Richards SM, Chopra R *et al.* Outcome of 609 adults after relapse of acute lymphoblastic leukemia (ALL): an MRC UKALL12/ECOG 2993 study. *Blood* 2007; **109**: 944–50.

177. Garcia-Manero G, Thomas DA. Salvage therapy for refractory or relapsed acute lymphocytic leukemia. *Hematol Oncol Clin North Am* 2001; **15**: 163–205.

●178. Giona F, Testi AM, Annino L *et al.* Treatment of primary refractory and relapsed acute lymphoblastic leukaemia in children and adults: the GIMEMA/AIEOP experience. Gruppo Italiano Malattie Ematologiche Maligne dell'Adulto. Associazione Italiana Ematologia ed Ocologia Pediatrica. *Br J Haematol* 1994; **86**: 55–61.

●179. Freund M, Diedrich H, Ganser A *et al.* Treatment of relapsed or refractory adult acute lymphocytic leukemia. *Cancer* 1992; **69**: 709–16.

●180. Hoelzer D, Gökbuget N. New approaches to acute lymphoblastic leukemia in adults: where do we go? *Semin Oncol* 2000; **27**: 540–59.

●181. Larson RA, Dodge RK, Burns CP *et al.* A five-drug remission induction regimen with intensive consolidation for adults with acute lymphoblastic leukemia: Cancer and Leukemia Group B study 8811. *Blood* 1995; **85**: 2025–37.

182. Larson RA. Three new drugs for acute lymphoblastic leukemia: nelarabine, clofarabine, and forodesine. *Semin Oncol* 2007; **34**(6 Suppl 5): S13–20.

183. Jeha S, Gandhi V, Chan KW *et al.* Clofarabine, a novel nucleoside analog, is active in pediatric patients with advanced leukemia. *Blood* 2004; **103**: 784–9.

●184. Jeha S, Gaynon PS, Razzouk BI *et al.* Phase II study of clofarabine in pediatric patients with refractory or relapsed acute lymphoblastic leukemia. *J Clin Oncol* 2006; **24**: 1917–23.

185. Kantarjian H, Gandhi V, Cortes J *et al.* Phase 2 clinical and pharmacologic study of clofarabine in patients with refractory or relapsed acute leukemia. *Blood* 2003; **102**: 2379–86.

186. Kantarjian HM, Gandhi V, Kozuch P *et al.* Phase I clinical and pharmacology study of clofarabine in patients with solid and hematologic cancers. *J Clin Oncol* 2003; **21**: 1167–73.

●187. Karp JE, Ricklis RM, Balakrishnan K *et al.* A phase 1 clinical-laboratory study of clofarabine followed by cyclophosphamide for adults with refractory acute leukemias. *Blood* 2007; **110**: 1762–9.

●188. DeAngelo DJ, Yu D, Johnson JL *et al.* Nelarabine induces complete remissions in adults with relapsed or refractory T-lineage acute lymphoblastic leukemia or lymphoblastic lymphoma: Cancer and Leukemia Group B study 19801. *Blood* 2007; **109**: 5136–42.

189. Goekbuget N, Arnold R, Atta J *et al.* Compound GW506U78 has high single-drug activity and good feasibility in heavily pretreated relapsed T-lymphoblastic leukemia (T-ALL) and T-lymphoblastic lymphoma (T-LBL) and offers the option for cure with stem cell transplantation (SCT). *Blood* 2005; **106**: 150 (abstract).

190. Cohen MH, Johnson JR, Justice R, Pazdur R. FDA drug approval summary: nelarabine (Arranon®) for the treatment of T-cell lymphoblastic leukemia/lymphoma. *Oncologist* 2008; **13**: 709–14.

191. Yanada M, Takeuchi J, Sugiura I *et al.* High complete remission rate and promising outcome by combination of imatinib and chemotherapy for newly diagnosed BCR-ABL-positive acute lymphoblastic leukemia: a phase II study by the Japan Adult Leukemia Study Group. *J Clin Oncol* 2006; **24**: 460–6.

192. Wassmann B, Pfeifer H, Goekbuget N *et al.* Alternating versus concurrent schedules of imatinib and chemotherapy as front-line therapy for Philadelphia-positive acute lymphoblastic leukemia (Ph$^+$ ALL). *Blood* 2006; **108**: 1469–77.

193. Lee S, Kim DW, Kim YJ *et al.* Minimal residual disease-based role of imatinib as a first-line interim therapy prior to allogeneic stem cell transplantation in Philadelphia chromosome-positive acute lymphoblastic leukemia. *Blood* 2003; **102**: 3068–70.

●194. Lee S, Kim YJ, Min CK *et al.* The effect of first-line imatinib interim therapy on the outcome of allogeneic stem cell transplantation in adults with newly diagnosed Philadelphia chromosome-positive acute lymphoblastic leukemia. *Blood* 2005; **105**: 3449–57.

195. Vignetti M, Fazi P, Cimino G *et al.* Imatinib plus steroids induces complete remissions and prolonged survival in elderly Philadelphia chromosome-positive patients with acute lymphoblastic leukemia without additional chemotherapy: results of the Gruppo Italiano Malattie Ematologiche dell'Adulto (GIMEMA) LAL0201-B protocol. *Blood* 2007; **109**: 3676–8.

●196. Ottmann O, Dombret H, Martinelli G *et al.* Dasatinib induces rapid hematologic and cytogenetic responses in adult patients with Philadelphia chromosome positive acute lymphoblastic leukemia with resistance or intolerance to imatinib: interim results of a phase 2 study. *Blood* 2007; **110**: 2309–15.

197. Bolen JB, Thompson PA, Eiseman E, Horak ID. Expression and interactions of the Src family of tyrosine protein kinases in T lymphocytes. *Adv Cancer Res* 1991; **57**: 103–49.

◆198. Summy JM, Gallick GE. Src family kinases in tumor progression and metastasis. *Cancer Metastasis Rev* 2003; **22**: 337–58.

199. Ishizawar R, Parsons SJ. c-Src and cooperating partners in human cancer. *Cancer Cell* 2004; **6**: 209–14.

200. Lutz MP, Eßer IBS, Flossmann-Kast BBM *et al.* Overexpression and activation of the tyrosine kinase Src in human pancreatic carcinoma. *Biochem Biophys Res Commun* 1998; **243**: 503–8.

201. Lu Y, Yu Q, Liu JH *et al.* Src family protein-tyrosine kinases alter the function of PTEN to regulate phosphatidylinositol 3-kinase/AKT cascades. *J Biol Chem* 2003; **278**: 40057–66.

202. Dai Y, Rahmani M, Corey SJ *et al.* A Bcr/Abl-independent, Lyn-dependent form of imatinib mesylate (STI-571) resistance is associated with altered expression of Bcl-2. *J Biol Chem* 2004; **279**: 34227–39.

203. Donato NJ, Wu JY, Stapley J *et al.* BCR-ABL independence and LYN kinase overexpression in chronic myelogenous leukemia cells selected for resistance to STI571. *Blood* 2003; **101**: 690–8.

204. Lombardo LJ, Lee FY, Chen P *et al.* Discovery of N-(2-chloro-6-methyl-phenyl)-2-(6-(4-(2-hydroxyethyl)-piperazin-1-yl)-2methylpyrimidin-4-ylamino) thiazole-5-carboxamide (BMS-354825), a dual Src/Abl kinase inhibitor with potent antitumor activity in preclinical assays. *J Med Chem* 2004; **47**: 6658–61.

205. Nagar B, Hantschel O, Young MA *et al.* Structural basis for the autoinhibition of c-Abl tyrosine kinase. *Cell* 2003; **112**: 859–71.

206. Plattner R, Kadlec L, DeMali KA *et al.* c-ABL is activated by growth factors and Src family kinases and has a role in the cellular response to PDGF. *Genes Dev* 1999; **13**: 2400–411.

207. Kimura S, Naito H, Segawa H *et al.* NS-187, a potent and selective dual Bcr-Abl/Lyn tyrosine kinase inhibitor is a novel agent for imatinib-resistant leukemia. *Blood* 2005; **106**: 3948–54.

208. Shah NP, Tran C, Lee FY *et al.* Overriding imatinib resistance with a novel ABL kinase inhibitor. *Science* 2004; **305**: 399–401.

209. Warmuth M, Simon N, Mitina O *et al.* Dual-specific Src and Abl inhibitors, PP1 and CGP76030, inhibit growth and survival of cells expression imatinib mesylate-resistant Bcr-Abl kinases. *Blood* 2003; **101**: 664–72.

210. Perez-Atayde AR, Sallan SE, Tedrow U *et al.* Spectrum of tumor angiogenesis in the bone marrow of children with acute lymphoblastic leukemia. *Am J Pathol* 1997; **150**: 815–21.

211. Yetgin S, Yenicesu I, Cetin M, Tuncer M. Clinical importance of serum vascular endothelial and basic fibroblast growth factors in children with acute lymphoblastic leukemia. *Leuk Lymphoma* 2001; **42**: 83–8.

212. Koomagi R, Zintl F, Sauerbrey A, Volm M. Vascular endothelial growth factor in newly diagnosed and recurrent childhood acute lymphoblastic leukemia as measured by real-time quantitative polymerase chain reaction. *Clin Cancer Res* 2001; **7**: 3381–4.

213. Aguayo A, Estey E, Kantarjian H *et al.* Cellular vascular endothelial growth factor is a predictor of outcome in patients with acute myeloid leukemia. *Blood* 1999; **94**: 3717–21.

214. Wang GL, Semenza GL. Purification and characterization of hypoxia-inducible factor 1. *J Biol Chem* 1995; **270**: 1230–7.

215. Narendran A, Ganjavi H, Morson N *et al.* Mutant p53 in bone marrow stromal cells increases VEGF expression and supports leukemia cell growth. *Exp Hematol* 2003; **31**: 693–701.

216. Iliopoulos O, Levy AP, Jiang C *et al.* Negative regulation of hypoxia-inducible genes by the von Hippel-Lindau protein. *Proc Natl Acad Sci U S A* 1996; **93**: 10595–9.

217. Mayerhofer M, Valent P, Sperr WR *et al.* BCR/ABL induces expression of vascular endothelial growth factor and its transcriptional activator, hypoxia inducible factor-1α, through a pathway involving phosphoinositide 3-kinase and the mammalian target of rapamycin. *Blood* 2002; **100**: 3767–75.

218. Gerber HP, Malik AK, Solar GP *et al.* VEGF regulates haematopoietic stem cell survival by an internal autocrine loop mechanism. *Nature* 2002; **417**: 954–8.

219. Katoh O, Takahashi T, Oguri T *et al.* Vascular endothelial growth factor inhibits apoptotic death in hematopoietic cells after exposure to chemotherapeutic drugs by inducing MCL1 acting as an antiapoptotic factor. *Cancer Res* 1998; **58**: 5565–9.

220. Dias S, Choy M, Alitalo K, Rafii S. Vascular endothelial growth factor (VEGF)-C signaling through FLT-4 (VEGFR-3) mediates leukemic cell proliferation, survival, and resistance to chemotherapy. *Blood* 2002; **99**: 2179–84.

221. Dias S, Shmelkov SV, Lam G, Rafii S. VEGF(165) promotes survival of leukemic cells by Hsp90-mediated induction of Bcl-2 expression and apoptosis inhibition. *Blood* 2002; **99**: 2532–40.

222. Wang L, Chen L, Benincosa J *et al.* VEGF-induced phosphorylation of Bcl-2 influences B lineage leukemic cell response to apoptotic stimuli. *Leukemia* 2005; **19**: 344–53.

223. Fragoso R, Pereira T, Wu Y *et al.* VEGFR-1 (FLT-1) activation modulates acute lymphoblastic leukemia localization and survival within the bone marrow, determining the onset of extramedullary disease. *Blood* 2006; **107**: 1608–16.

●224. Karp JE, Gojo I, Pili R *et al.* Targeting vascular endothelial growth factor for relapsed and refractory adult acute myelogenous leukemias: therapy with sequential 1-β-d-arabinofuranosylcytosine, mitoxantrone, and bevacizumab. *Clin Cancer Res* 2004; **10**: 3577–85.

225. Ogawa S, Hangaishi A, Miyawaki S et al. Loss of the cyclin-dependent kinase 4-inhibitor (p16; MTS1) gene is frequent in and highly specific to lymphoid tumors in primary human hematopoietic malignancies. *Blood* 1995; **86**: 1548–56.

226. Hebert J, Cayuela JM, Berkeley J, Sigaux F. Candidate tumor-suppressor genes MTS1 (p16INK4A) and MTS2 (p15INK4B) display frequent homozygous deletions in primary cells from T- but not from B-cell lineage acute lymphoblastic leukemias. *Blood* 1994; **84**: 4038–44.

◆227. Garcia-Manero G, Yang H, Kuang SQ et al. Epigenetics of acute lymphoblastic leukemia. *Semin Hematol* 2009; **46**: 24–32.

228. Shen L, Toyota M, Kondo Y et al. Aberrant DNA methylation of p57KIP2 identifies a cell-cycle regulatory pathway with prognostic impact in adult acute lymphocytic leukemia. *Blood* 2003; **101**: 4131–6.

●229. Garcia-Manero G, Bueso-Ramos C, Daniel J et al. DNA methylation patterns at relapse in adult acute lymphocytic leukemia. *Clin Cancer Res* 2002; **8**: 1897–903.

●230. Garcia-Manero G, Daniel J, Smith TL et al. DNA methylation of multiple promoter-associated CpG islands in adult acute lymphocytic leukemia. *Clin Cancer Res* 2002; **8**: 2217–24.

231. Roman-Gomez J, Jimenez-Velasco A, Cordeu L et al. WNT5A, a putative tumour suppressor of lymphoid malignancies, is inactivated by aberrant methylation in acute lymphoblastic leukaemia. *Eur J Cancer* 2007; **43**: 2736–46.

●232. Román-Gómez J, Cordeu L, Agirre X et al. Epigenetic regulation of Wnt-signaling pathway in acute lymphoblastic leukemia. *Blood* 2007; **109**: 3462–9.

233. Issa JP, Garcia-Manero G, Giles FJ et al. Phase 1 study of low-dose prolonged exposure schedules of the hypomethylating agent 5-aza-2′-deoxycytidine (decitabine) in hematopoietic malignancies. *Blood* 2004; **103**: 1635–40.

234. Willemze R, Suciu S, Archimbaud E et al. A randomized phase II study on the effects of 5-Aza-2′-deoxycytidine combined with either amsacrine or idarubicin in patients with relapsed acute leukemia: an EORTC Leukemia Cooperative Group phase II study (06893). *Leukemia* 1997; **11**(Suppl 1): S24–7.

235. Tsapis M, Lieb M, Manzo F et al. HDAC inhibitors induce apoptosis in glucocorticoid-resistant acute lymphatic leukemia cells despite a switch from the extrinsic to the intrinsic death pathway. *Int J Biochem Cell Biol* 2007; **39**: 1500–509.

236. Scuto A, Kirschbaum M, Kowolik C et al. The novel histone deacetylase inhibitor, LBH589, induces expression of DNA damage response genes and apoptosis in Ph– acute lymphoblastic leukemia cells. *Blood* 2008; **111**: 5093–100.

237. Duvic M, Talpur R, Ni X et al. Phase 2 trial of oral vorinostat (suberoylanilide hydroxamic acid, SAHA) for refractory cutaneous T-cell lymphoma (CTCL). *Blood* 2007; **109**: 31–9.

238. Younes A, Wedgwood A, McLaughlin P et al. Treatment of relapsed or refractory lymphoma with the oral isotype-selective histone deacetylase inhibitor MGCD0103; interim results from a Phase II study. *Blood* 2007; **110**: 2571 (abstract).

●239. Gojo I, Jiemjit A, Trepel JB et al. Phase 1 and pharmacologic study of MS-275, a histone deacetylase inhibitor, in adults with refractory and relapsed acute leukemias. *Blood* 2007; **109**: 2781–90.

●240. Garcia-Manero G, Yang H, Bueso-Ramos C et al. Phase 1 study of the histone deacetylase inhibitor vorinostat (suberoylanilide hydroxamic acid [SAHA]) in patients with advanced leukemias and myelodysplastic syndromes. *Blood* 2008; **111**: 1060–6.

241. Giles F, Fischer T, Cortes J et al. A phase I study of intravenous LBH589, a novel cinnamic hydroxamic acid analogue histone deacetylase inhibitor, in patients with refractory hematologic malignancies. *Clin Cancer Res* 2006; **12**: 4628–35.

64

Small B cell lymphomas and leukemias including hairy cell leukemia

CLAIRE DEARDEN

INTRODUCTION

Small B cell lymphoproliferative disorders comprise a variety of disease entities, the commonest of which is chronic lymphocytic leukemia (CLL). Rarer primary B cell leukemias include B prolymphocytic leukemia (PLL) and hairy cell leukemia (HCL). In addition, clonal B cells may appear in the peripheral blood originating from a primary non-Hodgkin lymphoma (NHL).

The B NHLs that most frequently have a leukemic phase are splenic marginal zone lymphoma (SMZL), mantle cell lymphoma (MCL), and follicular lymphoma. These may be distinguished from one another and from CLL by clinical features, morphology, immunophenotype, and, in some cases, cyto/molecular genetics.

CHRONIC LYMPHOCYTIC LEUKEMIA

Chronic lymphocytic leukemia is a neoplasm of mono-clonal B cells which express CD19, CD5, and CD23. These small, mature B lymphocytes can be found in the peripheral blood, bone marrow, and lymph nodes, where they may be associated with prolymphocytes and paraimmunoblasts. Small lymphocytic lymphoma (SLL) is defined within the World Health Organization (WHO) classification[1] of lymphoid malignancies as the tissue counterpart of CLL, where the cellular morphology and immunophenotype is identical to that of CLL but without the presence of B cells circulating in the peripheral blood. There is considerable clinical heterogeneity. In some patients, CLL is identified on routine blood tests and they may survive for many years without therapy, eventually dying with, rather than from, CLL. Others may have a rapidly fatal disease despite intensive treatments. Over the past decade, improved understanding of the underlying biology of the disease has gone some way toward explaining this clinical diversity and allowing the subclassification of CLL into various prognostic groups. This not only assists in predicting future outcome but also helps to direct treatment decisions. In parallel with these advances, progress has also been made in the development of new therapies and treatment strategies, together with the ability to better assess response to therapy (with detection of minimum disease levels). It is therefore possible now to deliver and monitor complete morphologic and, in some cases, molecular remissions. Such remissions are associated with improved disease-free and overall survival and have led to a shift in the goal of treatment in CLL from that of palliation to cure.

EPIDEMIOLOGY

In Western countries, CLL is the commonest leukemia in adults, with an incidence of 3–4 per 100 000 per year. It appears to be relatively infrequent in Africa and Asia.[2] It is a disease of older adults with a median age at presentation of 69 years and is twice as frequent in males as in females. Unlike acute leukemia and chronic myeloid leukemia, CLL has not been associated with exposure to radiation and there is little evidence to support specific environmental causal factors. However, evidence from epidemiologic and family studies strongly suggests the possibility that genetic or familial factors may predispose to CLL.[3,4] There is an inherited susceptibility to CLL in 10 percent of patients, with first-degree relatives exhibiting a 2–7-fold excess risk over the general population. Family studies have shown the phenomenon of anticipation, with earlier onset and more severe disease in successive generations.[5] Linkage analysis using single nucleotide polymorphisms to identify and characterize susceptibility genes is currently being undertaken. A further observation to support a familial susceptibility is that of finding low levels of monoclonal CLL-like B cell lymphocytes in 12–18 percent of healthy relatives.[6] The risk of finding such clones is particularly significant in those aged below 40 years, where it is 17 times higher than in an age-matched population.

The incidence of second malignancies is increased in both treated and untreated CLL.

DIAGNOSIS

By classical definition, CLL has a lymphocytosis of $>5 \times 10^9$/L in the peripheral blood and at least 40 percent lymphoid infiltrate in the bone marrow.[7] Lymph node histology is not required for the diagnosis of typical CLL but may be necessary to exclude transformation in patients presenting with bulky nodes. A diagnosis of SLL can be made histologically without involvement of either the blood or bone marrow. Morphology and immunophenotype (Table 64.1) are characteristic and enable CLL to be readily distinguished from other B cell leukemias and lymphomas in leukemic phase.[8,9] In typical CLL, 79 percent of cells are small or medium-sized lymphocytes with clumped chromatin, indistinct nucleoli, and scanty cytoplasm. In 15 percent of patients the morphology is atypical with either more than 10 percent of prolymphocytes (CLL/PL)

or more than 15 percent of cells having lymphoplasmacytoid features. There is no consistent cytogenetic or molecular genetic abnormality such as seen in follicular and mantle cell lymphomas to confirm the diagnosis. Recently the diagnostic criteria have been challenged by the use of sensitive multiparameter flow cytometry, which allows the detection of very low numbers of CLL cells in the peripheral blood. Indeed, using this technique it has been possible to identify subclinical CLL clones in up to 3 percent of individuals who have otherwise normal lymphocyte counts.[6] This has been termed clonal lymphocytosis of uncertain significance (CLUS) or monoclonal B cell lymphocytosis (MBL), somewhat analogous to the monoclonal gammopathy seen in plasma cell disorders. The significance of this finding is unclear and as yet there have been no longitudinal studies to establish the risk of subsequent evolution into clinical CLL.

CLINICAL FEATURES

In more than half of patients with CLL the diagnosis is made as an incidental finding on a routine full blood count. Patients may present with B symptoms, infections, or autoimmune complications. Lymphadenopathy, hepatosplenomegaly, or involvement of extranodal sites may be present at diagnosis or develop over the course of the disease. Patients with advanced disease may present with anemia or thrombocytopenia due to bone marrow failure. Infections are a particular problem during the clinical course for patients with CLL. This is due to a combination of marrow failure, immunosuppression, and hypogammaglobulinemia. This infection risk increases in severity with advancing disease and may be compounded by the effects

Table 64.1 Immunophenotypic differentiation of B cell chronic lymphocytic leukemia from other chronic lymphoproliferative disorders

Antigen/marker	CLL	MCL	SLVL	B-PLL
SmIg intensity	Weak/+	++	++	+++
CD19/CD20	Weak/+	+/+	+/+	+/+
CD5	+	+	−/+	−/+
CD23	+	−	−/+	−
CD11c	−/+	−	+/−	−
FMC7	−	+	+	+
CD79b	−/weak	+	+/−	+
CD22	−	+/−	+	+
CLL score[a]	3–5	<3	<3	<3

[a]CLL score: 1 point for weak SmIg and weak CD79b or CD22; 1 each for positive CD5 and CD23, and negative FMC7; total of 5 points for typical CLL.[8,9]
CLL, chronic lymphocytic leukemia; MCL, mantle cell lymphoma/leukemia; SLVL, splenic lymphoma with villous lymphocytes; B-PLL, B cell prolymphocytic leukemia.

of therapy. Patients with advanced refractory CLL have an incidence of serious infections of around 98 percent and this is associated with a high mortality.[10] Hypogammaglobulinemia may be present in up to 10 percent of patients at diagnosis, increasing to two-thirds of patients later in the course of the disease. Usually all three immunoglobulin (Ig) classes (IgG, IgA, and IgM) are decreased. A minority of patients (fewer than 10 percent) may also have low-level monoclonal bands, usually IgM.

CLINICAL STAGING AND PROGNOSTIC MARKERS

The natural history of CLL is extremely variable, with a survival time from initial diagnosis that ranges from 2 to 20 years and a median survival of approximately 10 years. The underlying mechanisms promoting initiation and progression of CLL remain largely unknown. The traditional model was of the accumulation of immature immune-incompetent B cells with an inherent failure of apoptosis.[11] In the past decade this model has been challenged by evidence suggesting that CLL arises from mature antigen-stimulated B cells which survive and proliferate in response to signals received from the surrounding environment.[12]

Clinical staging systems

Clinically, about one-third of patients will have prolonged survival and never require treatment, another third may have initially indolent disease followed by progression, and the remaining third present with symptomatic disease requiring immediate treatment and often following an aggressive course. Some 25 years ago, two systems of clinical staging (the Binet and Rai staging systems, Table 64.2)

were developed for CLL to separate patients into three prognostic groups.[13,14] These still form the basis for decisions regarding initiation of therapy and have also been important in the design of clinical trials.[15] It is important to exclude hemolysis or other causes of anemia before assigning a patient to a Binet stage C or Rai stage III.

Traditional prognostic markers

In addition to clinical stage, factors such as age, gender,[16] pattern of bone marrow infiltration,[17] lymphocyte morphology, and rate of proliferation[18] all influence prognosis (Table 64.3). The superior survival for women has been shown consistently in a number of studies. This is partly due to a higher proportion of women having stage A disease but additionally females requiring therapy fare better. Morphologically atypical lymphocytes and increased numbers of prolymphocytes are both associated with poorer prognosis. Lymphocyte doubling time is defined as the time required for an increase in absolute lymphocyte count in the blood to twice the baseline value in untreated patients. If this is longer than 12 months the prognosis is better than if it is less than 12 months.[18] Nodular or interstitial bone marrow infiltration is associated with a better prognosis compared to diffuse infiltration.[17] There are also a number of serum markers such as lactate dehydrogenase (LDH),[19] β_2-microglobulin,[20] thymidine kinase,[21] and soluble serum CD23[22] levels, which correlate with increased disease activity and poorer survival but have not been validated in prospective studies. However, these staging systems and parameters are limited in their ability to predict progression and outcome accurately for individuals presenting with CLL. Over the past decade there have been major advances in the identification of novel prognostic

Table 64.2 Binet[13] and Rai[14] clinical staging systems for chronic lymphocytic leukemia

Binet stage		Rai stage		Prognosis	Survival (years)	% of patients
Stage	Characteristics	Stage	Characteristics			
A	Hb >10 g/dL, platelets >100 × 10⁹/L, <3 lymph node areas involved	Rai 0	Lymphocytosis alone, Hb >11 g/dL, platelets >100 × 10⁹/L	Good	>10	6%
B	Hb >10 g/dL, platelets >100 × 10⁹/L, ≥3 lymph node areas involved	Rai I	Lymphocytosis + lymphadenopathy, Hb >11 g/dL, platelets >100 × 10⁹/L	Intermediate	5–7	30%
		Rai II	Lymphocytosis + splenomegaly and/or hepatomegaly, Hb >11 g/dL, platelets >100 × 10⁹/L			
C	Hb <10 g/dL or platelets <100 × 10⁹/L	Rai III	Lymphocytosis + Hb <11 g/dL	Poor	1.5–3	10%
		Rai IV	Lymphocytosis + platelets <100 × 10⁹/L			

Lymph node areas: (1) head and neck (including Waldeyer's ring; unilateral or bilateral); (2) axillary (unilateral or bilateral); (3) inguinal (unilateral or bilateral); (4) splenomegaly; (5) hepatomegaly.
Hb, hemoglobin.

Table 64.3 Prognostic markers in chronic lymphocytic leukemia

Characteristic	Favorable	Poor
Clinical stage	Binet A, Rai 0/I	Binet C, Rai III/IV
Gender	Female	Male
Lymphocyte morphology	Typical	'Atypical,' increased prolymphocytes
Lymphocyte doubling time	>12 months	<12 months
Bone marrow biopsy	Nodular/interstitial	Diffuse
Serum markers (β_2M, LDH, thymidine kinase, CD23)	Normal	Raised
Cytogenetic abnormalities	None, 13q del (sole)	11q del, 17p del
IGHV genes	Mutated	Unmutated
CD38	<30%	>30%
ZAP70	<20%	>20%

β_2M, β_2-microglobulin; LDH, lactate dehydrogen ase; IGHV, immunoglobulin heavy chain.

Table 64.4 Genomic aberrations in chronic lymphocytic leukemia.[32] Interphase FISH results – 82% abnormal

Abnormality	Number of patients (%)	Characteristics
17p deletion	7%	CLL/PL
		Poor response to treatment
		Richter transformation
11q 23 deletion	18%	Younger age
		Male
		Lymphadenopathy
		Shortened survival
Trisomy 12q	15%	CLL/PL
		Disease progression
		High proliferative rate
13q deletion (sole)	36%	Good prognosis
6q21 deletion	5%	

CLL/PL, chronic lymphocytic leukemia with more than 10% of prolymphocytes.
FISH, fluorescence *in situ* hybridization.

variables which not only provide new information about the underlying pathophysiology of CLL but also add to the traditional staging methods in order to predict prognosis more precisely (Table 64.3).

New prognostic markers

Data published in 1999 suggested that CLL patients could be divided into two groups according to the number of mutations in the variable segments of the immunoglobulin heavy chain genes (*IGHV*) of the tumor cell clone.[23,24] The two groups are defined as mutated, with at least a 2 percent difference from the germ line, and unmutated, with less than 2 percent difference. There is a significant difference in disease progression and survival between the two groups, with shorter survival for the patients with unmutated *IGHV* genes. This difference is also seen in the group of patients with Binet stage A disease, with a median survival of 8 years for patients with unmutated *IGHV* genes compared to 24 years for those whose genes are mutated.[23] *IGHV* gene usage also appears to be selective in CLL and use of certain genes, such as *IGHV3–21* is associated with more aggressive disease.[25] The observation that patients either had mutated or unmutated genes initially raised the question of whether CLL might be two separate diseases. However, microarray analysis has shown that overall gene expression profiles are the same for the two groups and readily distinguish CLL from other B lymphoid malignancies. There are about 20 genes that are differentially expressed between the mutated and unmutated subtypes.[26] One of the best discriminating genes was shown to be a tyrosine kinase inhibitor, zeta-associated protein 70 (ZAP70). This protein is important in

normal T cell signaling but is not usually expressed in B lymphocytes. More recently, antibodies to this protein have been developed which can be used in cell suspension and tissue sections to detect surface expression of ZAP70. This has been shown to be a good (about 80 percent), but not exact, surrogate marker for mutational status.[27–29] Most discordance is seen in the group with IGHV3–21 usage who have mutated IGHV genes but high ZAP70 expression. It also appears to be a strong independent prognostic marker, with high expression (more than 20 percent) being associated with progressive disease and shortened survival.[27–29] An additional antigen that also has independent prognostic significance is CD38.[30] Again, this was initially thought to correlate strongly with *IGHV* mutation status but in this case the concordance is less good and, furthermore, expression of CD38 can change over time during the course of the disease.

Conventional cytogenetic analysis only yields results in about 50 percent of patients. On the basis of this, Juliusson *et al.* were able to demonstrate that the presence of chromosomal abnormalities was associated with poorer prognosis.[31] The use of fluorescence *in situ* hybridization (FISH) analysis has enabled detection of genomic aberrations in around 80 percent of patients.[32] These aberrations provide insight into the pathogenesis of the disease through the identification of candidate genes and also identify subgroups of patients with distinct clinical features and outcome (Table 64.4). Five genomic changes have emerged as significant in CLL patients both in frequency of occurrence and in association with prognosis. These are abnormalities of 13q, 12q, 11q22–23, 6q, and 17p. The latter have enabled a hierarchical model of prognostic relevance to be developed, with 13q deletion as a single abnormality being seen as favorable, whilst 11q and

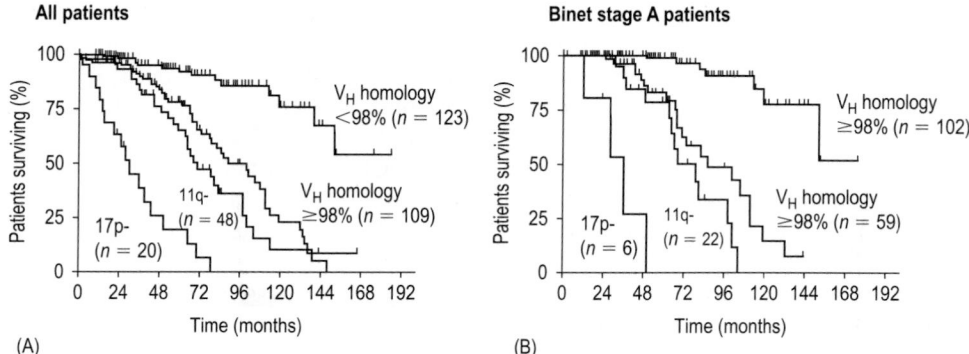

Figure 64.1 Survival probabilities among patients with the following genetic abnormalities: 17p deletion (irrespective of heavy chain gene [V_H][a] mutation status), 11q deletion (irrespective of V_H mutation status), unmutated immunoglobulin (Ig) V_H, and mutated Ig V_H. (A) Survival for all patients and (B) for Binet stage A patients only. Irrespective of clinical stage, patients with 17p deletion have median survival of $\leq$3 years compared to patients with mutated Ig V_H genes in whom median survival has not been reached. (From Krober *et al.* VH Mutation status, CD38 expression level, genomic aberrations, and survival in chronic lymphocytic leukaemia. *Blood* 2002; **100**: 1410–16 [with permission])
[a]*IGHV*

17p deletions are associated with the poorest prognosis.[32] 17p deletions usually involve loss of the *TP53* tumor suppression gene. Loss or mutation of *TP53* has been shown to be associated with primary resistance to conventional treatments such as alkylating agents and purine analogues.[33,34]

Three recent multivariate analyses, which included assessment of genetic abnormalities, CD38 expression, and *IGHV* gene status, showed that only *IGHV* gene status and loss or mutation of the *TP53* gene had independent prognostic significance (Fig. 64.1).[35–37] The next goal will be to develop a prognostic scoring index for CLL. This will allow a risk stratification for patients which can then be validated in prospective clinical trials.

TREATMENT

There have been major changes in the approach to treatment of CLL over the past 20 years. Historically, the goal of therapy was palliation, achieved by the use of intermittent single alkylating agents such as chlorambucil to reduce the level of lymphocytosis and improve symptoms. In the twenty-first century there are now not only new ways of evaluating disease and response to treatment but also a number of new agents already in clinical use and additional therapies in preclinical studies. The challenge over the next decade will be to integrate these treatments into effective management strategies.

Pretreatment evaluation

The first decision to be made in CLL is whether the patient requires therapy at the time of initial diagnosis. Stage A patients who have a hemoglobin level in excess of 10 g/dL and lymphocyte count of $<30 \times 10^9$/L with minimal or no

Table 64.5 National Cancer Institute Working Group (NCI-WG):[7] indications to initiate treatment for chronic lymphocytic leukemia

- Constitutional symptoms referable to CLL ($>$10% weight loss, fever, sweats, fatigue)[a]
- Progressive marrow failure (worsening anemia[a] and/or thrombocytopenia)
- Rapid lymphocyte doubling time ($<$6 months)
- Massive ($>$6 cm) or progressive splenomegaly
- Massive ($>$10 cm) or progressive lymphadenopathy
- Autoimmune cytopenias poorly responsive to corticosteroids

[a]It is important to exclude other causes.
CLL, chronic lymphocytic leukemia.

lymphadenopathy and a lymphocyte doubling time of more than 12 months have an 80 percent chance of being alive at 10 years and only 15 percent are likely to require treatment. A number of large studies were conducted in the 1980s in Europe and the USA addressing the question of whether stage A patients benefited from early treatment intervention.[38–41] The treatment given in these trials was chlorambucil, either alone or together with prednisone. No survival benefit was observed in any of the trials for patients receiving early treatment. New information regarding the impact of unfavorable prognostic markers within the group of stage A patients enables us to more readily predict those patients who will progress and require treatment. There are therefore a number of trials currently underway reexamining the question of whether early treatment may benefit this subset of stage A patients with unfavorable prognostic markers.

The National Cancer Institute (NCI) has developed guidelines for initiation of therapy (Table 64.5).[7] Patients with progressive stage A disease have a similar life expectancy to those presenting with stage B disease and therefore usually require treatment. However, some patients with stable low-level stage B disease may not require immediate therapy. Patients presenting with autoimmune complications such as autoimmune hemolytic anemia and/or thrombocytopenia in the absence of disease progression should be treated for the immune phenomenon but this is not necessarily an indication for cytoreductive therapy. Similarly, although marked hypogammaglobulinemia generally occurs in the setting of advanced progressive disease, it is not in itself an indication for therapy. Those patients not requiring initial therapy should be monitored at appropriate intervals, watching for evidence of disease progression and/or complications.

Other pretreatment considerations include patient factors such as age, performance status, comorbidities, and patient choice, together with disease-related factors such as severity of symptoms, speed of progression, and prognostic factors (especially the presence of *TP53* deletions or mutations). There may be particular contraindications regarding the use of specific agents and ever-increasing concern regarding the cost of therapy.

Criteria for response and minimal residual disease

Comparison of data from different clinical trials has been hampered by a lack of uniformity in response assessment (e.g., some trials have not evaluated bone marrow response) and this needs to be addressed for the future. The NCI working group criteria for response require bone marrow biopsy evaluation as well as maintenance of remission beyond 2 months (Table 64.6).[7] The presence or absence of nodules in the bone marrow can only be evaluated on a good-quality trephine biopsy, allowing definition of the category 'nodular partial remission.' Immunostaining of these nodules is important since occasionally these are found to be composed of reactive T lymphocytes rather than residual CLL. The presence of residual nodular CLL is associated with a shortened time to disease progression.

In the same way that criteria for diagnosis have been challenged by the introduction of sensitive flow cytometry techniques, this has also been applied to definition of response. Rawstron *et al.* have developed a sensitive four-color flow cytometric method (based on expression of CD19/CD5/CD20 and CD79b) that has a level of detection of 1 in 10^5 white cells.[42] They have been able to use this methodology to detect residual disease and demonstrate a progressive increase in levels of residual B-CLL cells on follow-up after treatment. Other groups have used less-sensitive flow cytometry techniques incorporating CD5 and CD19 with or without kappa and lambda expression. With the increasing use of therapeutic monoclonal antibodies such as rituximab, new combinations of antigens have been developed for minimal residual disease (MRD) detection, since CD20 no longer has utility in this setting as antigen is blocked. There is now an international consensus on the methodology, which will allow for better comparisons between trial data.[43] Flow cytometry has the advantage of being rapid, applicable to all patients without the need for a prior sample, and readily available to most clinicians.

Evaluation and monitoring of MRD may also be achieved using molecular techniques, with the most sensitive of these being real-time quantitative allele-specific oligonucleotide polymerase chain reaction (PCR).[44] These techniques, however, are more time consuming, expensive, less reproducible, and also require pretreatment samples versus flow cytometry.

Minimal residual disease monitoring has been shown in the transplant context, both after autograft and allograft, to be of clinical relevance in predicting duration of response and survival outcome.[45] With the advent of more intensive chemotherapy and chemoimmunotherapy regimens this has now become a relevant endpoint in nontransplant treatment strategies. Studies have shown that those patients achieving MRD negativity, measured using sensitive flow cytometry or PCR, have prolonged survival compared with those patients who still have detectable disease at the end of treatment.[46–49] This therefore sets a new standard for

Table 64.6   National Cancer Institute Working Group (NCI-WG) response criteria for chronic lymphocytic leukemia[7]

Parameter	CR[a]	PR[a]
Symptoms	None	
Lymph nodes (liver/spleen)	No palpable disease	$\geqslant$50% reduction
Lymphocytes	$\leqslant$4 $\times$ 10^9/L	$\geqslant$50% reduction
Neutrophils	$\geqslant$1.5 $\times$ 10^9/L	$\geqslant$1500/μL or $\geqslant$50% improvement from baseline
Platelets	>100 $\times$ 10^9/L	>100 000/μL or $\geqslant$50% improvement from baseline
Hemoglobin	>11 g/dL	>11 g/dL or $\geqslant$50% improvement from baseline
Bone marrow aspirate	<30% lymphocytes	
Bone marrow trephine	No interstitial or nodular infiltrate	$\pm$ Nodules

[a] $\geqslant$2 months' duration.
Progressive disease = new nodes/organ enlargement or >50% increase in size, and/or >50% increase in lymphocytosis.
CR, complete response; PR, partial response.

response assessment and monitoring of duration of response, which is likely to be included in future studies. The methodology and thresholds, however, need to be validated in prospective, randomized clinical trials.

First-line therapy

CHLORAMBUCIL

For more than four decades chlorambucil has been the standard therapy for CLL, given either on a low-dose continuous basis or according to an intermittent schedule. Reported overall response (OR) rates have varied from 45 percent to 86 percent depending on the schedule and dose used, but complete responses (CR), where evaluated, were less than 10 percent.[40,50–54] Two studies by the UK MRC CLL Trials group have shown no advantage for the addition to chlorambucil of prednisone (MRC CLL 2)[40] or epirubicin (MRC CLL 3).[50] In addition, no survival benefit has been shown for combination treatment such as COP (cyclophosphamide, vincristine, prednisone)[51–53] or modified CHOP (with addition of low-dose doxorubicin)[54,55] when compared with chlorambucil used alone (Table 64.7). Furthermore, the addition of steroids or anthracyclines increases the incidence of infection.[56]

A study evaluating a higher dose of chlorambucil (15 mg/day) demonstrated higher overall response rates and median survival when compared to CHOP, but because nonstandard response criteria were used it is difficult to compare this with results from new trials.[54]

PURINE ANALOGUES

In the 1980s, pentostatin, fludarabine, and cladribine were developed and found to have considerable activity in lymphoid malignancies. These purine deoxynucleotide analogues block crucial metabolic pathways for nucleic acid synthesis resulting in inhibition of DNA repair. As a result they have cytotoxicity against both resting and dividing lymphocytes and are likely to be synergistic with agents that cause DNA damage.

Fludarabine has been the most extensively studied purine analogue in CLL following initial studies which showed significant activity in patients with advanced refractory disease.[57–59] A number of studies evaluating fludarabine as initial therapy in previously untreated patients with CLL have shown overall response rates of 63–79 percent, with complete remission rates of 20–40 percent.[60–62] One of these studies[60] tested the addition of prednisone, which was not shown to improve response rate over fludarabine alone. Long-term follow-up of treatment-naïve patients with CLL who had received fludarabine treatment showed a significant improvement in median survival for patients achieving a complete remission or nodular partial remission of around 90 months, compared with 48 months for partial responders and 36 months for patients in whom therapy failed.[61] A series of prospective randomized studies comparing fludarabine with chlorambucil or alkylator-based combinations (CAP [cyclophosphamide, doxorubicin, and prednisone] or CHOP) as initial treatments of CLL[63–66] have been consistent in showing higher remission rates and disease-free interval with fludarabine but have been unable to demonstrate any differences in overall survival (Table 64.8). A large intergroup trial in the USA compared fludarabine to chlorambucil and showed a 63 percent versus 37 percent overall response rate and a 20 percent versus 4 percent complete response rate, respectively.[63] This study included a crossover design and although 46 percent of patients who did not respond to chlorambucil benefited from fludarabine subsequently, only 7 percent of patients in whom fludarabine treatment failed responded to chlorambucil. Although there was a significant difference in duration of response and progression-free survival (PFS) in favor of fludarabine, because of the trial design there was no difference in overall survival, with a median for both groups of around 5 years. The French Cooperative Group showed complete response rates of 40 percent for fludarabine versus 30 percent for CHOP and 15 percent for CAP.[64] Furthermore,

Table 64.7 Randomized studies of alkylating agent-based combination chemotherapy in previously untreated chronic lymphocytic leukemia

Regimen	*n*	CR (%)	PR (%)	Survival (months)
COP vs Chl[51]	291	28/20	41/46	57/58
COP vs Chl-PRD[52]	122	23/25	59/47	45/56
ChOP vs HD-Chl[54]	228	30/60	42/28	47/68
ChOP vs Chl-PRD[55]	287	24/14	46/38	ND

COP, cyclophosphamide, vincristine, and prednisone; CHOP, cyclophosphamide, doxorubicin, vincristine, and prednisone; Chl, chlorambucil; PRD, prednisone; CR, complete response; PR, partial response; ND, no difference; HD, high dose. ChOP, Binet modified CHOP (doxorubicin 25 mg/m²).

Table 64.8 Randomized studies of fludarabine compared with alkylator-based therapy in previously untreated chronic lymphocytic leukemia

Regimen	*n*	CR (%)	PR (%)	Survival (months)
F vs Chl[63]	509	20/4	43/33	66/56
F vs ChOP vs CAP[64]	938	40/15/30	31/43/42	69/70/67
F vs CAP[65]	100	23/17	48/43	NA

F, fludarabine; ChOP, Binet modified CHOP (doxorubicin 25 mg/m²); CAP, cyclophosphamide, doxorubicin, and prednisone; CHOP, cyclophosphamide, doxorubicin, vincristine, and prednisone; Chl, chlorambucil; CR, complete response; PR, partial response; NA, not available.

fludarabine was better tolerated in this study. The German CLL study group has reported the results of a randomized phase III study of fludarabine versus chlorambucil in patients over the age of 65 years.[66] Again, fludarabine induced higher overall and complete remission rates and this was associated with prolonged PFS and improved quality of life, but no survival benefit. A European Organization for Research and Treatment of Cancer (EORTC) study comparing fludarabine with high-dose chlorambucil has reported similar OR rates, response duration, and survival.[67]

More recently, fludarabine has been studied in combination with alkylating agents, based on the knowledge that both are effective single-agent therapies in CLL and synergism between the two agents had been demonstrated in vitro.[68,69] Response rates in previously untreated patients rose to over 80 percent with the fludarabine and cyclophosphomide (FC) combination, with an increase in complete response rates to 40 percent.[70–72] Two large (>200 patients), prospective randomized trials have compared fludarabine and FC.[73,74] The German study group looked at patients under the age of 65 years and were able to show a superior OR rate (94 percent compared with 85 percent) and CR rate (21 percent versus 9 percent) with improved time to treatment failure of more than 28 months versus 19 months in favor of the combination.[73] Although more neutropenia was seen with the FC combination, there was no difference between the two study arms in infectious complications. The US Intergroup trial showed lower-than-expected OR and CR rates for both study arms although, again, superiority was demonstrated for the FC combination versus fludarabine alone (70.4 percent vs 49.6 percent OR and 22.4 percent vs 5.8 percent CR, respectively).[74] The median PFS was significantly prolonged for FC (41 months) compared with fludarabine (17.7 months). The results of the UK LRF CLL 4 study comparing chlorambucil to fludarabine with or without the addition of cyclophosphamide in nearly 800 patients, also showed superior response rates and PFS for the FC combination, which was evident across all age groups (one-third of patients more than 70 years of age) and risk groups.[75]

The group from Barcelona have recently reported results of fludarabine, cyclophosphamide, and mitoxantrone (FCM) given to younger (less than 65 years of age) previously untreated CLL patients.[76] An overall response rate of 91 percent with 50 percent CR (27 percent MRD negative) was seen, making this one of the most effective regimens in CLL; 55 percent of patients remained in remission at 36 months. Notably, no patient with a 17p deletion responded.

Oral fludarabine[77,78] given at an equivalent dose either alone or in combination with cyclophosphamide appears to achieve comparable remission rates to intravenous (IV) administration, although this has not been evaluated in a randomized study.

Pentostatin (2-deoxycoformycin) was the first purine analogue to be tested in clinical trials, having been developed as a tight binding inhibitor of adenosine deaminase, a key enzyme in the purine degradation pathway.[79] Response rates in refractory CLL are significantly lower than those seen with fludarabine in the same patient group, with OR rates ranging from 18 percent to 29 percent and CR rates of 0–8 percent.[80] Recently, interest has been revived in the use of pentostatin in combination with alkylating agents. Response rates of 74 percent with 17 percent CR have been seen in previously treated (including fludarabine-refractory) patients receiving pentostatin in combination with cyclophosphamide.[81] One of the advantages of pentostatin in these combination strategies is that it is regarded as less myelosuppressive than the other purine analogues.

Cladribine has also been investigated in both refractory and previously untreated patients.[82–85] In the latter group, response rates as high as 80 percent with 38 percent CR have been seen.[84] A phase III randomized study comparing cladribine and prednisone with chlorambucil and prednisone reported a higher OR rate, CR rate, and PFS for patients receiving cladribine but no overall survival advantage.[86] A randomized study has also demonstrated the advantage of adding cyclophosphamide with or without mitoxantrone compared to cladribine alone.[87] However, of the three purine analogues, cladribine is probably the most myelosuppressive and this may limit its use in combination regimens.

MONOCLONAL ANTIBODIES

Over the past decade therapeutic monoclonal antibodies which target lineage-specific antigens have played a key role in advancing treatment for hematopoietic malignancies. In CLL two monoclonal antibodies, rituximab and alemtuzumab, are now in routine clinical use.

Rituximab is a chimeric antibody targeting CD20 and has been shown to have significant activity in the treatment of non-Hodgkin lymphomas.[88] However, as a single agent in both CLL and SLL, whether used first-line or in previously treated patients, less favorable response rates have been observed (Table 64.9).[89–93] Overall (51 percent) and complete response rate (4 percent) when rituximab is used as first-line therapy are similar to rates seen with

Table 64.9 Single-agent rituximab in chronic lymphocytic leukemia/small lymphocytic lymphoma

Study	n	OR (%)	CR (%)
McLaughlin et al.[88]	30	13	0
Winkler et al.[89]	10	10	0
Nguyen et al.[90]	12	0	0
Huhn et al.[91]	28	25	0
Hainsworth[93a]	44	52[a]	4

[a]Previously untreated.
OR, overall response; CR, complete response.

chlorambucil.[93] Even in studies where the dose of rituximab has been increased or it has been administered in a more frequent schedule (three times a week) there has only been a modest increase in response rates.[94,95] This may be related to the weak expression of the CD20 antigen on CLL/SLL lymphocytes and/or the presence of neutralizing serum CD20 antigen in patients with CLL.[96] However, when the antibody is combined with purine analogues such as fludarabine, with or without the addition of cyclophosphamide, there appears to be a significant improvement in response rates for the chemoimmunotherapy combination compared with chemotherapy alone. The Cancer and Leukemia Group B (CALGB) group in the USA examined the use of rituximab together with fludarabine in more than 100 previously untreated patients with CLL.[97] In this study, patients were randomized to receive the two agents either sequentially (fludarabine for 6 months followed by rituximab) or concurrently (fludarabine and rituximab given together). Responses in both groups were superior to historical controls receiving fludarabine alone; OR of 84 percent compared to 63 percent.[98] Interestingly, OR and, in particular, CR rates were improved when fludarabine and rituximab were given concurrently, with CR rates of 47 percent compared to only 28 percent when rituximab was given following fludarabine induction. This suggests the possibility of synergism between the two agents, and is supported by in vitro experiments which have shown that rituximab enhances the cytotoxicity of both fludarabine and cyclophosphamide.[99] These observations have been attributed to the downregulation of complement defense proteins (CD55 and CD59) by fludarabine, which may enhance rituximab efficacy, coupled with the effect that rituximab has in modulating antiapoptotic proteins associated with fludarabine resistance, thus enhancing the activity of DNA-damaging agents.[100] This has provided the rationale for combining rituximab with both fludarabine and cyclophosphamide, which has resulted in OR and CR rates higher than have ever previously been documented in CLL. The MD Anderson Cancer Center has reported results of FCR (fludarabine, cyclophosphamide, and rituximab) in 224 previously untreated CLL patients, showing an OR rate of 95 percent with 70 percent complete remission and 15 percent nodular partial response.[101] Two-thirds of the patients in this single-arm study had Rai stage I or II disease, which is higher than in most other reported studies for CLL. Using a two-color flow cytometry method (CD5/CD19), 71 percent of patients achieved fewer than 1 percent of CLL cells in the bone marrow. This subgroup of patients had a significantly lower relapse rate (3.6 percent) than patients who had greater than 1 percent or greater than 5 percent tumor cells by flow cytometry (20 percent and 43 percent, respectively). This study also showed that flow cytometry negativity correlated with improved overall survival. This and other studies are providing consistent evidence that achieving MRD-negative remission is associated with a decreased risk of relapse and superior survival. However,

prospective randomized studies using sensitive quantitative assays for MRD will be needed to determine the threshold that predicts disease relapse.

Pentostatin has also been used in chemoimmunotherapy combinations for both previously untreated and relapsed refractory patients.[102,103] Ninety-seven percent of 33 previously untreated patients with CLL achieved a response with pentostatin, cyclophosphamide, and rituximab; 40 percent achieved complete remission and nine out of these 11 patients had fewer than 1 percent CD5/CD19-positive cells in the bone marrow.[103] This patient group was considered high risk, with 80 percent having unmutated IGHV genes. Myelosuppression appears to be reduced compared with fludarabine-based therapy. However, follow-up data are required to evaluate time to progression and overall survival with this regimen.

Alemtuzumab is a fully humanized IgG monoclonal antibody directed against the CD52 antigen that is highly expressed on both normal and malignant B and T lymphocytes. Two studies, including one phase III randomized trial, have evaluated this antibody as a single agent in newly diagnosed patients with symptomatic CLL.[104,105] In the first study, the antibody was administered subcutaneously three times a week for 18 weeks and resulted in an OR rate of 87 percent with durable remissions lasting more than 18 months.[104] In this setting, infectious complications were manageable, although cytomegalovirus (CMV) reactivation was seen in around 10 percent of patients. In a prospective, international, randomized phase III trial (CAM307) comparing alemtuzumab with chlorambucil as first-line therapy in patients with progressive CLL,[105] 297 patients were randomized to IV alemtuzumab 30 mg three times weekly for up to 12 weeks or chlorambucil 40 mg/m^2 orally, once every 28 days for up to 12 cycles. The OR rate was 83 percent in the alemtuzumab arm compared to 50 percent in the chlorambucil arm, with CR rates of 24 percent and 2 percent, respectively. This translated into a 43 percent lower risk of the combined end point of progression or death in those treated with alemtuzumab. Responses in high-risk patients, notably those with deletion of 17p, were markedly superior in the alemtuzumab arm (64 percent OR compared to 26 percent in the chlorambucil arm). Based on this trial, alemtuzumab has now been licensed for first-line treatment for CLL.

In relapsed patients alemtuzumab has been shown to be very effective in clearing disease from peripheral blood and bone marrow but less so in the setting of bulky nodal disease (Table 64.10).[48,106–110] This has provided the rationale for a number of studies looking at using alemtuzumab to consolidate responses achieved using purine analogue-based initial treatment with the intention of eliminating any residual disease (particularly from bone marrow).[111–114] It has been possible to demonstrate improvement in responses in up to 50 percent of patients (e.g., from partial response to CR) including MRD negativity following alemtuzumab consolidation.

Table 64.10 Single-agent alemtuzumab in chronic lymphocytic leukemia

Study	Disease phase	n	OR (%)	CR (%)
Österborg et al.[106]	Alkylating agent refractory	29	42	3
Keating et al.[107] (pivotal)	Fludarabine refractory	93	33	2
Rai et al.[108]	Fludarabine refractory	152	43	5
Moreton et al.[48]	Chemotherapy refractory	91	55	35
Lozanski et al.[109]	Chemotherapy refractory	36	31	6
Kröber et al.[110a]	Fludarabine refractory	44	36	2
Lundin et al.[104a]	Previously untreated	41	87	19
Hillmen et al.[105b]	Previously untreated	149	83	24

[a]Subcutaneous administration.
[b]In a randomized trial compared to chlorambucil.
OR, overall response; CR, complete response.

Table 64.11 Purine analogue-based combination therapy for chronic lymphocytic leukemia

Treatment	Previously untreated patients			Relapsed patients		
	n	OR (%)	CR (%)	n	OR (%)	CR (%)
FC[70]	34	80	35	94	80	12
FCM[47,76]	57	91	50	37	78	50
FR (concurrent)[97]	51	90	47			
FCR[49,101]	224	95	70	177	73	25
FluCam[119]				37	83	30
PC[81]				23	74	17
PR[102]				64	33	5.5
PCR[103,116]	33	97	40	32	75	25

F/Flu, fludarabine; P, pentostatin; C, cyclophosphamide; R, rituximab; Cam, alemtuzumab; M, mitoxantrone.
OR, overall response; CR, complete response.

The German CLL study group has reported results of the only randomized study evaluating consolidation with alemtuzumab.[114] Twenty-one patients who had completed treatment with either fludarabine or fludarabine and cyclophosphamide and had achieved a partial response or better, proceeded to randomization between observation alone or alemtuzumab consolidation. This study was suspended because of the increased incidence of infection seen in the group receiving alemtuzumab. However, follow-up of the randomized patients showed a significant improvement in PFS for those patients receiving alemtuzumab. This study has now been reopened using a different schedule of alemtuzumab, with a lower dose delivered after an interval following induction treatment, to allow for bone marrow recovery. Results from larger randomized studies are awaited.

In summary, the treatment paradigm for CLL has changed considerably over the last decade; first with the ability to risk-stratify patients according to new prognostic markers, and second with the demonstration that chemoimmunotherapy combinations can achieve high rates of hematologic, flow cytometric, and molecular responses in CLL (Table 64.11). Although curative therapy may not yet exist for this disease, it is now apparent that more aggressive therapy can yield PFS of significant duration, which may also translate into a survival advantage for patients. This lays the foundation for further clinical research into combination treatment approaches in CLL. As newer monoclonal antibodies and other novel agents become available, the challenge will be to incorporate these optimally into purine analogue- and alkylator-based regimens. Current clinical trials are also likely to give additional information concerning differential response to treatment according to genetic subsets leading to a more refined 'targeted' treatment approach.

Treatment at relapse

There have been no large randomized studies compari[ng] treatments for patients with relapsed or refractory C[LL.] The results of some treatment regimens used as sa[lvage] therapy in CLL are summarized in Table 64.11. In p[atients] who have achieved prolonged responses with f[ludarabine]

therapy it is reasonable to retreat at relapse with the same agent, either alone or in combination. However, the quality and duration of response is usually inferior to that obtained with initial treatment. Regimens such as COP and CHOP have induced responses in 13–27 percent of patients refractory to chlorambucil, and in 38 percent of patients unresponsive to fludarabine.[64] Two-thirds of patients who have responded to single-agent fludarabine given as initial therapy will have a second response. The regimens FC and FCR have been reported as achieving overall response rates of 56 percent (39 percent for fludarabine-refractory patients)[70] and 72 percent, respectively.[49] The FCM combination is effective in relapsed refractory CLL.[47,115] One study has shown overall response rates of 78 percent, with 50 percent complete remissions, including 10 of 37 patients with MRD negativity.[47] The median survival of patients achieving complete remission was 5 years and was not reached at 4 years for the MRD-negative group. Cladribine does not appear to be effective in the treatment of patients refractory to fludarabine.[85] However, the combination of pentostatin and cyclophosphamide (PC) induces response in 74 percent (17 percent CR) of relapsed patients including those who were refractory to fludarabine.[81] The addition of rituximab to PC increased the CR rate to 25 percent (OR 75 percent).[116]

ALEMTUZUMAB

Patients who are refractory to fludarabine have a very poor prognosis, with a median survival of only 10–12 months.[117] Rituximab-based regimens (FR and FCR) have shown markedly inferior response rates when administered to patients who are fludarabine refractory compared with those who have previously been sensitive to fludarabine. Alemtuzumab has been investigated as a novel salvage therapy for this group of patients. Whether administered intravenously or subcutaneously, responses are seen in one-third to one-half of patients, predominantly those without bulky nodal disease (Table 65.10).[48,106–110] A study of alemtuzumab in 91 patients with relapsed refractory CLL, of whom half were refractory to fludarabine, showed an overall response rate of 53 percent, with 36 percent achieving a complete remission.[48] Eighteen of the 91 patients had no detectable CLL at the end of alemtuzumab monotherapy as assessed by a sensitive four-color flow cytometric method of MRD assessment. This subgroup of patients was shown to have improved progression-free and overall survival compared with the patients who had MRD-positive remissions at the end of therapy. This is further evidence to support the hypothesis that achieving MRD negativity may translate into improved overall survival for patients. Again in this study, bulky lymphadenopathy (>5 cm) predicted for poor response to single-agent alemtuzumab. One strategy to overcome this would be to 'debulk' disease with an alternative regimen such as high-dose methylprednisolone or CHOP and to then proceed with alemtuzumab to clear residual bone marrow

infiltration with the objective of achieving an MRD-negative remission. An alternative strategy is to use fludarabine and alemtuzumab (FluCam) in combination. An early pilot study demonstrated that this combination was active in patients who had previously failed monotherapy with either agent.[118] The German CLL study group has gone on to evaluate this combination in 37 patients with relapsed refractory CLL.[119] They have used a modified regimen, giving alemtuzumab only on 3 consecutive days of each 4-week cycle at the same time as fludarabine. The overall response rate was 83 percent with 11 out of 37 patients achieving CR and 19 patients achieving a partial response. Forty-seven percent of patients became MRD negative in the peripheral blood or bone marrow as measured by four-color flow cytometry. Freedom from treatment failure for responding patients was 12.8 months and the median OS was 35.6 months. The regimen was very well tolerated with modest thrombocytopenia and neutropenia but few serious infections. Based on these results, an ongoing phase II study is being conducted to evaluate the combination of fludarabine, cyclophosphamide (FC), and alemtuzumab. In addition, a prospective randomized phase III trial has been initiated to confirm the efficacy of the FluCam combination in CLL patients with first relapse. The combination of rituximab and alemtuzumab has been evaluated at the MD Anderson Cancer Center in relapsed refractory CLL patients, again showing that this combination may overcome some of the limitations of single-agent antibody therapy and salvage a proportion of patients with refractory disease.[120] The combination of FCR plus alemtuzumab is also being tested in a prospective trial.

Of particular note is the efficacy of alemtuzumab in the subset of patients who have *TP53* deletions or mutations, which result in resistance to standard purine analogue- and alkylator-based therapies.[109,121,122] Although fewer than 10 percent of patients receiving first-line therapy will have *TP53* abnormalities, up to 50 percent of patients will acquire such genetic changes later in the course of their disease. Responses, usually partial, are seen in this group of patients with alemtuzumab and also with high-dose methylprednisolone[123] when other therapies appear to be ineffective. Studies are ongoing to examine the combination of alemtuzumab with methylprednisolone in patients with *TP53* dysfunction.

HIGH-DOSE METHYLPREDNISOLONE

Steroids have been widely used in the treatment of CLL although there are few published data regarding efficacy. Certainly, in first-line therapy, steroids have not been shown to add value to standard alkylating agent or purine analogue when evaluated in randomized trials. A study of high-dose methylprednisolone ($1 g/m^2$/day for 5 days repeated every month) in 25 relapsed refractory patients with CLL showed an overall response rate of 77 percent including 18 percent of patients who achieved a nodular partial response.[123] Interestingly, responses were seen in five out of 10 patients with loss and/or mutation of the *TP53* gene. Median response duration was 9 months with significant improvement in event-free and overall survival for responders compared with nonresponders. This may therefore be a useful agent, providing palliation in advanced refractory disease and in particular for those patients with *TP53* dysfunction.

RADIATION THERAPY

Chronic lymphocytic leukemia is a very radiosensitive disease. However, because of its systemic nature, radiation therapy has only played a limited role in the management of CLL. Prior to the advent of systemic chemotherapy, splenic irradiation was frequently given as palliative treatment. It may still be useful in patients with symptomatic splenomegaly who are resistant to chemotherapy and in whom splenectomy is contraindicated; 50–90 percent of patients will obtain symptomatic relief and around one-third will have improvement in hematologic parameters following this modality.[124] With the advent of newer, more effective chemoimmunotherapy regimens, this approach has largely fallen out of fashion. Comparatively low doses of radiation can achieve good palliation for bulky nodal masses with overall responses of up to 80 percent.[125]

SPLENECTOMY

Splenectomy may still be indicated in selected patients who have symptomatic massive splenomegaly resistant to systemic chemotherapy and/or refractory cytopenias, including those with an autoimmune pathogenesis.[126] The operative mortality is low (less than 10 percent) but infectious complications, both early and delayed, may occur in up to 50 percent of cases. There have been no randomized studies comparing splenectomy with other treatments for CLL.

Stem cell transplantation

The traditional palliative approach to treatment of CLL has meant that experience in the field of transplantation in this disease has been relatively limited. Clearly, the majority of patients with CLL, who may be elderly and have relatively benign, good-risk disease, do not merit such an approach. However, CLL remains 'incurable' with traditional alkylator- and purine analogue-based therapies and the one-third of patients who are under the age of 60 years and have advanced CLL and/or poor prognostic factors may have a survival of less than 3 years. It is therefore important to consider potentially curative stem cell transplantation (SCT) options in this group. Furthermore, as new transplant strategies develop and the associated mortality and morbidity decreases, this treatment modality may become more accessible for suitable patients. It is critical that transplants, whether autologous or allogeneic, should be

Table 64.12 Stem cell transplantation in chronic lymphocytic leukemia

Study	No. of patients	TRM (%)	EFS (%)	OS (%)
Autograft				
EBMT[128]	370	10		69 (at 4 y)
UK Pilot[129]	117	2	52 (at 5 y)	77 (at 5 y)
German[130]	77	4	69 (at 4 y)	94 (at 4 y)
Esteve[46]	124	6	37 (at 4 y)	65 (at 4 y)
Conventional Allograft				
EBMT[133]	209	40		55 (at 3 y)
Reduced–intensity allograft				
UK[134]	13		69 (at 2 y)	69 (at 2 y)
MDACC[135]	17	6 (at 1 y)	60 (at 2 y)	80 (at 2 y)
German[136]	42	6	72 (at 3 y)	84 (at 3 y)

TRM, transplant-related mortality; EFS, event-free survival; OS, overall survival; EBMT, European Blood and Marrow Transplantation; MDACC, MD Anderson Cancer Center; y, years.

conducted within appropriate clinical trials, in order to evaluate the long-term benefit. Results from a selection of retrospective and prospective series are summarized in Table 64.12.

AUTOLOGOUS STEM CELL TRANSPLANTATION

The principle underlying autograft in CLL is that there is a dose–response relationship to chemotherapy, but that dose escalation is limited by stem cell toxicity. Collection and storage of stem cells that can later be returned to restore bone marrow function allows delivery of high-dose chemotherapy. A number of studies conducted in the 1990s demonstrated the feasibility of this approach, with transplant-related mortality (TRM) of 2–10 percent using, in most cases, a cyclophosphamide and total body irradiation (TBI) conditioning regimen.[127–131] The key finding from these studies was that although the majority of patients achieve complete remission and over half may be negative for MRD by PCR, relapse appears to be inevitable, with no plateau on the survival curve. However, disease-free survival was improved compared with historical controls who did not proceed to autograft. A German study showed increased benefit for patients who had mutated *IGHV* gene status compared to those with unmutated *IGHV* genes.[131] But even for those patients with unmutated *IGHV* genes there was prolonged survival compared to risk-matched patients receiving conventional treatment. Two concerns have been raised from these studies. First, the difficulty of mobilizing peripheral progenitor cells following induction treatment, particularly with fludarabine or fludarabine-based therapies.[129,132] In the MRC pilot study, fludarabine was used alone as initial treatment and one-third of patients failed to mobilize adequate numbers of stem cells.[129] Second, transplant-related myelodysplasia and acute myeloid leukemia (MDS/AML) has been reported as a late complication, and the relationship of this to induction chemotherapy and/or conditioning for autologous stem cell transplantation is yet to be established.[129] The optimal timing of autologous transplantation remains uncertain. There is currently a European prospective randomized study comparing immediate versus deferred autograft which will help to address many of the issues and evaluate whether or not autograft offers any advantage over the new chemoimmunotherapy regimens.

ALLOGENEIC STEM CELL TRANSPLANTATION

This approach, using conventional conditioning regimens, adds to dose intensification the potential advantage of achieving a graft-versus-leukemia (GvL) effect from donor-derived immune cells. Although this has resulted in improved disease control, with a plateau emerging on the survival curve at about 40 percent, this has been at the expense of greater toxicity, with TRM approaching 50 percent.[133] In addition, the age and comorbidities of most patients with CLL preclude the use of allogeneic transplantation with a standard preparative regimen. However, MRD negativity is more likely to be achieved with allo- than autograft.[45,46] Since much of the benefit for CLL patients is mediated through the GvL effect, reduced-intensity conditioning (RIC) regimens have been developed which aim to maximize the benefits whilst reducing the TRM. Although this is a relatively new approach, data are emerging that suggest that TRM is significantly reduced using a RIC regimen (TRM 18 percent)[134,135] with durable remissions, including molecular remission, even in *IGHV* unmutated CLL patients[136] and those with *TP53* deletion. There is now a consensus agreement from the European Group for Blood and Marrow Transplantation (EBMT) on indications for allograft in CLL.[137] As yet there are insufficient data on long-term follow-up to know whether this strategy may result in cure for some patients.

New therapies

Many new treatments are currently in clinical trials for CLL including new purine analogues such as clofarabine. One of the most promising of the novel therapies is the cyclin-dependent kinase inhibitor flavopiridol, which was shown to have significant activity against CLL *in vitro* but gave rather surprisingly poor responses *in vivo* in initial phase I/II studies.[138] More recently it has been reintroduced in clinical trials using a modified schedule of administration resulting in improved clinical responses.

A large number of monoclonal antibodies are being developed including engineered anti-CD20 antibodies and a range of antibodies directed against other antigens, such as HLA-DR, CD40, CD22, and interleukin-2 (IL-2) and TRAIL receptors. In some cases these have been conjugated to immunotoxins.[139] In addition, a number of small inhibitory molecules targeting important intracellular processes and signaling pathways have been developed that are likely to have application across a wide range of malignancies via their effects on cellular proliferation and apoptosis. These include immunomodulatory drugs (IMiDs; thalidomide, revlimid), histone deacetylase inhibitors, hypomethylating agents, proteasome inhibitors, and HSP90 inhibitors. Of these, revlimid (lenalidomide) has already demonstrated significant efficacy in relapsed refractory CLL[140] and is now being tested in combination regimens and in front-line treatment. Research programs investigating vaccines and gene therapies are ongoing.

The challenge over the next few years will be to develop treatment regimens incorporating a number of these novel agents together with established chemotherapy to further improve responses in this disease.

Richter large cell transformation

Richter syndrome[141] is reported to occur in 3–5 percent of CLL cases, although this may be an underestimation since not all patients undergo lymph node biopsies at the time of disease progression. Clinically, this syndrome is associated with systemic B symptoms and rapid lymph node enlargement, usually at a single site, which may be intraabdominal. Transformation can also take place in the bone marrow and, rarely, also in the central nervous system. Histologically, the cells show features of large cell lymphoma or, when circulating in the peripheral blood, may resemble the blast cells of acute leukemia. However, the cells retain an immunophenotype consistent with CLL, although there may be some subtle changes such as increased expression of surface membrane immunoglobulin. Richter transformation is usually associated with a rise in serum LDH. Monoclonal proteins and hypercalcemia may be found in association with transformation, although the latter does occur in the advanced stages of CLL without transformation. Methods to demonstrate clonality have indicated that approximately half of Richter syndrome cases occur as a result of evolution of the CLL clone, whereas the remainder represent new malignancies unrelated to the CLL clone.[142] Acquisition of new genetic abnormalities such as *TP53* deletion and/or mutation are relatively common in association with Richter transformation. A few reports have suggested that transformation may be precipitated by immunosuppressive therapy such as fludarabine. In 15–20 percent of these cases, reactivation of Epstein–Barr virus (EBV) has been implicated in the pathogenesis.[143]

Treatment for Richter syndrome has been largely unsatisfactory using conventional cytotoxic chemotherapy. The standard has been to use a CHOP-like regimen with, more recently, the addition of rituximab. Remissions may be seen in up to 30 percent of patients but these remissions are not prolonged. Radiation therapy may play a role in the palliation of bulky nodal sites. Use of high-dose therapy and SCT (particularly allogeneic SCT) improves survival and should be offered to eligible patients.[144] In cases where the transformation histologically resembles Hodgkin lymphoma, treatment with standard therapy (doxorubicin, bleomycin, vinblastine, and dacarbazine; ABVD) results in a response rate of 40 percent and survival of 12–18 months.[145] The prognosis for patients who have undergone Richter transformation is poor with death usually within 1 year; median survival in one series was 5 months.[146]

Management of complications

AUTOIMMUNE CYTOPENIA

The mechanism of the immune complications in CLL is still poorly understood. The direct antiglobulin test (DAT) may be positive at some time during the course of the illness in up to 35 percent of cases, but overt autoimmune hemolytic anemia (AIHA) only occurs in about 11 percent of cases.[147] Immune thrombocytopenic purpura (ITP) is much less common, occurring in around 1–2 percent of patients.[148] The incidence of immune pure red cell aplasia (PRCA) is similar, but less well recognized, and may be secondary to parvovirus infection. Patients with AIHA or ITP should be treated according to guidelines for idiopathic AIHA or ITP; namely prednisone at 1 mg/kg body weight per day for 2–4 weeks, tapering off over several weeks. Intravenous immunoglobulin may be used where there is steroid refractoriness or an urgent requirement, such as preparation for surgery. Other treatments include splenectomy, cyclosporine A, and rituximab.[149] Rituximab and alemtuzumab have both been reported as effective in reversing PRCA.

Based on a number of anecdotal reports, there was some concern regarding the risk of precipitating AIHA in patients (with or without a positive DAT) receiving purine analogue therapy. The UK LRF CLL4 trial is the largest prospective trial in CLL to examine the risk of developing both a positive DAT and AIHA during treatment.[150] In this study, 777 patients were randomized to receive chlorambucil or fludarabine, alone or with cyclophosphamide (FC). The incidence of a positive DAT was 14 percent and AIHA 10 percent. The DAT correctly predicted the development, or not, of AIHA after therapy in 83 percent of cases. The approximate risk of a patient with a positive DAT developing AIHA was 1 in 3. Patients treated with chlorambucil or fludarabine were more than twice as likely to develop AIHA as those receiving FC. Four deaths were attributed to AIHA after first-line treatment, all on fludarabine monotherapy. In addition, a positive DAT status at the time of initiation of therapy and development of AIHA during therapy were associated with reduced PFS and OS. It remains clear that close monitoring of hemoglobin, DAT, and reticulocyte count should be carried out on all patients whatever therapy they may be receiving. Furthermore, if patients have developed overt hemolysis

whilst receiving a particular agent this should probably be avoided in future treatment.

INFECTIONS

Infectious complications are common in patients with CLL, mostly comprising bacterial infections in a variety of sites (e.g., pneumococcal pneumonia, *Haemophilus influenzae*, *Staphylococcus*), accounting for up to 50 percent of CLL-related deaths. The risk of infections is greatest in the elderly, those with advanced disease, and those undergoing treatment. Susceptibility is multifactorial, including hypogammaglobulinemia, neutropenia, impaired T and natural killer (NK) cell function, and defective complement activity.[151] Also, since the advent of newer therapies – notably the purine analogues, alemtuzumab, and methylprednisolone – fungal, viral, and opportunistic infections are becoming more common. The prolonged T cell depletion seen with purine analogues and alemtuzumab has led to the introduction of routine prophylaxis against *Pneumocystis carinii* and in many cases also herpesviruses. The duration of such prophylaxis needs to be extended following completion of treatment, as CD4 count recovery may not occur for 6–12 months. Patients receiving high-dose steroid therapy should receive *Candida* prophylaxis.

Reactivation of CMV is a complication of alemtuzumab treatment and has resulted in the recommendation of routine monitoring for CMV reactivation by PCR, with preemptive treatment when this occurs. Interestingly, since CMV monitoring has become much more commonplace in CLL, it is clear that CMV is occasionally reactivated in patients receiving other therapies also. Bacterial prophylaxis is not recommended apart from exceptional cases and in those patients with persistent prolonged neutropenia. Patients with recurrent severe infections and documented hypogammaglobulinemia may benefit from regular infusions of intravenous immunoglobulin (IV Ig). Randomized studies have shown a significant reduction of bacterial infections in those patients receiving IV Ig but no effect on the incidence of viral or fungal infections or on overall survival.[152,153]

Immunization in patients with CLL is also controversial. The efficacy of administering vaccines to patients with CLL remains unproven since they have a reduced ability to mount an adequate immune response to such a strategy, particularly to unconjugated vaccines. There are few data documenting antibody levels achieved following vaccination in this patient group. Nevertheless, the recommendation remains that patients should receive pneumococcal and annual influenza vaccinations as at least some patients will derive benefit from this.

OTHER SUPPORTIVE CARE

The role of growth factors, granulocyte colony-stimulating factor (G-CSF), and erythropoietin has not been systematically evaluated in CLL. However, with the advent of newer, more intensive treatment regimens and the increased risk of developing treatment-associated neutropenia, G-CSF is more regularly used now to support patients through treatment cycles.[154] Blood products transfused to patients who have received purine analogues or alemtuzumab should be irradiated to prevent the risk of transfusion-associated graft-versus-host disease.

B CELL PROLYMPHOCYTIC LEUKEMIA

This extremely rare leukemia, comprising approximately 1 percent of lymphocytic leukemias, was first recognized as a distinct entity in the 1970s.[155] It was not until a decade later, however, that it was possible to differentiate between the T and B cell subtypes, which otherwise had much clinical and morphological overlap. Most patients with B cell prolymphocytic leukemia (B-PLL) are over the age of 60 with a median age of 70 years and male predominance (male/female ratio of 1.6). Patients typically present with marked splenomegaly and very high white cell counts, usually over 100×10^9/L. Peripheral lymphadenopathy is much less common. Examination of the peripheral blood reveals characteristic prolymphocytes: medium-sized cells with a round nucleus, moderately condensed nuclear chromatin, and a prominent nucleolus. These cells must exceed 55 percent of lymphoid cells to distinguish this condition from CLL with increased prolymphocytes, although generally prolymphocytes exceed 90 percent.[156] The cytoplasm is usually less basophilic and without the characteristic protrusions seen in T-PLL.

IMMUNOPHENOTYPE AND CYTOGENETICS

The membrane immunophenotype of the B prolymphocytes is distinct from that of CLL, with strong expression of surface immunoglobulin, usually IgM and/or IgD, and other B cell antigens (CD19, CD20, CD22, CD79a, and FMC7). Although CD5 may be present in up to one-third of cases, CD23 is typically negative.

There is no hallmark mutation in B-PLL. Using interphase FISH, Lens *et al.* described in their series of 18 B-PLL patients 13q14 deletions in 55 percent and monoallelic 11q23 deletions in 39 percent of the cases.[157] Other abnormalities described include 6q−, t(6;12), and structural aberrations of 1p and 1q.[158] The translocation t(11;14) should be absent to discriminate between this leukemia and mantle cell lymphoma in leukemic phase.[159] Mutations of the *TP53* gene are seen in over 50 percent of cases of B-PLL and this is the highest reported level among all subtypes of B cell malignancies.[160] This may explain the frequent chemoresistance encountered in this disease. The abnormalities of *TP53* are distinct from those seen in CLL.

CLINICAL COURSE AND MANAGEMENT

B cell prolymphocytic leukemia is characterized by refractoriness to conventional chemotherapy and an aggressive clinical course, with a median survival of approximately 3 years. Splenectomy or splenic irradiation may be beneficial in relieving symptoms, improving peripheral blood counts, reducing transfusion requirement, and allowing leukopharesis to control rising white cell counts.[161]

There are few published data on successful chemotherapy regimens in B-PLL. Single-agent chemotherapy with purine analogue or alkylating agents, as has been used in CLL, is less likely to be effective. Most patients receive treatment with combination regimens such as CHOP or purine analogue (fludarabine, cladribine)-based therapies.[162] Even in those patients who achieve a remission, these tend to be short-lived remissions. In a phase II trial of combination chemotherapy with fludarabine and cyclophosphamide in B-PLL, an overall response rate of 50 percent was achieved with a median survival of 32 months.[163] With the increasing success of anti-CD20 (rituximab) and anti-CD52 (alemtuzumab) monoclonal antibody therapy in CLL and the poor response to conventional therapy in B-PLL, it seems reasonable to advocate a combination of chemotherapy and monoclonal antibody. A pilot study with bendamustine, mitoxantrone, and rituximab (BMR) in patients with B lymphoid malignancies reported an overall response of 99 percent with CR in 41 percent.[164] However, this series of patients included only a single case of B-PLL. Bowen *et al.*[165] reported complete remission in a patient with B-PLL following subcutaneous alemtuzumab three times a week for 6–12 weeks. Because of age and comorbidities, relatively few patients are eligible for stem cell transplantation procedures although in younger patients this should be considered.

HAIRY CELL LEUKEMIA

Hairy cell leukemia is a rare B cell neoplasm first described by Bouroncle in 1958[166] and accounts for approximately 2 percent of all lymphoid leukemias. It is a disease affecting predominantly middle-aged men, with a median age younger than that of CLL, at 55 years, and a male:female ratio of 5:1. Patients commonly present with splenomegaly and pancytopenia which may be associated with unusual infections.[167] Lymphadenopathy is rare, although occasional cases have been reported of bulky abdominal nodes in association with a more aggressive disease progression.[168] Osteolytic bone lesions can occur in around 5 percent of patients. Unusual skin manifestations such as vasculitis, pyoderma gangrenosum, and cutaneous infections have also been reported.[169]

MORPHOLOGY AND IMMUNOPHENOTYPE

Diagnosis rests on the identification of the characteristic B lymphocytes in blood, bone marrow, or spleen. Hairy cells are small to medium-sized lymphoid cells with an oval or bean-shaped nucleus and stippled chromatin (Plate 132, see plate section). The abundant pale blue/gray cytoplasm has fine, hairy projections. The number of circulating hairy cells in the peripheral blood may be low and there is often not a lymphocytosis. Characteristically, there is an absolute monocytopenia. The bone marrow may be difficult to aspirate and the most helpful test for diagnostic purposes is a high-quality trephine biopsy. The infiltrate may be patchy or diffuse but does not show the nodular or paratrabecular patterns seen in other lymphoid malignancies. The nuclei appear widely spaced from one another, surrounded by areas of empty pale cytoplasm. Invariably there is increased reticulin and this may be very marked. The spleen, which is enlarged in about 80 percent of patients, has very characteristic involvement, predominantly in the red pulp with development of congested 'angiomatous lakes.'

The tumor cells are surface-immunoglobulin positive and express common B cell-associated antigens such as CD19, CD20, CD22, and CD79A. They are typically CD5, CD10, and CD23 negative. They express CD11c, CD25, CD103, and CD123, all markers that are generally negative in other B cell leukemias.[170] Tartrate-resistant acid phosphatase (TRAP) is present in most cases and can be detected in tissue biopsies using an antibody.[171] In addition, in tissue sections the monoclonal antibody DBA44 gives strong staining of hairy cells, although this is not specific.[172] Most studies have shown that the immunoglobulin heavy chain gene is mutated, consistent with a post-germinal center B cell phenotype.[173–175] There are no specific cytogenetic abnormalities described in hairy cell leukemia.

TREATMENT

There have been major advances in the therapy of hairy cell leukemia over the past 20 years with the advent first of interferon alpha followed by the purine analogues pentostatin and cladribine. Prior to this, splenectomy was the only effective therapy, with very little benefit achieved using conventional lymphoma chemotherapy.

Splenectomy

Although splenectomy has no effect on the bone marrow involvement, blood counts return to normal in 40–70 percent of patients and this response may be maintained for many years.[176] However, with the advent of more effective therapies, splenectomy is now only performed in a minority of cases.

Interferon alpha

Interferon alpha was introduced in the early 1980s and was shown to induce high overall response rates of 75–90 percent,[177–179] the majority of which were partial (normalization of peripheral blood counts but residual bone marrow infiltration). As a result, relapse is inevitable following cessation of therapy. A randomized trial showed that interferon alpha was superior to splenectomy both in response rate and time to treatment failure.[180]

Pentostatin

Pentostatin was the first agent found to induce a significant complete remission rate in hairy cell leukemia. Overall responses of 98 percent and complete remission rates in excess of 80 percent have been reported in a large number of patients in various studies conducted since the mid-1980s.[181–186] These responses are durable with a median disease-free survival of 15 years in one large study. Overall survival curves are comparable to an age-matched population with 10-year survival of >80 percent (Fig. 64.2). A large, prospective randomized study conducted by the US Cooperative Oncology Groups showed that CR rates and relapse-free survival for pentostatin were significantly better than with interferon alpha.[187]

Cladribine

The first series of cladribine (2-chlorodeoxyadenosine; 2-CdA) treatment of hairy cell leukemia was reported by Piro *et al.* in 1990.[188] Again, a number of subsequent studies have confirmed the very high overall response rates (around 98 percent) and CR rates of 85 percent.[189–192] These results have been achieved in most cases with a single 7-day cycle of treatment allowing delivery of a quick, effective, and relatively nontoxic treatment. The efficacy of cladribine and pentostatin appears to be identical and there has never been a randomized trial comparing the two purine analogues.[193]

Treatment at relapse

Although the majority of patients treated with either purine analogue (cladribine or pentostatin) will achieve prolonged remissions, 20–40 percent of patients will relapse and require additional therapy.[194] The overall response rates for second- and third-line purine analogue treatment remain the same at 95–100 percent, although the proportion of complete responses declines with second- and third-line therapy. In addition, there is a very small number of patients who will be resistant to purine analogue treatment. Over the past 5 years, monoclonal antibody therapy has been evaluated in such cases.

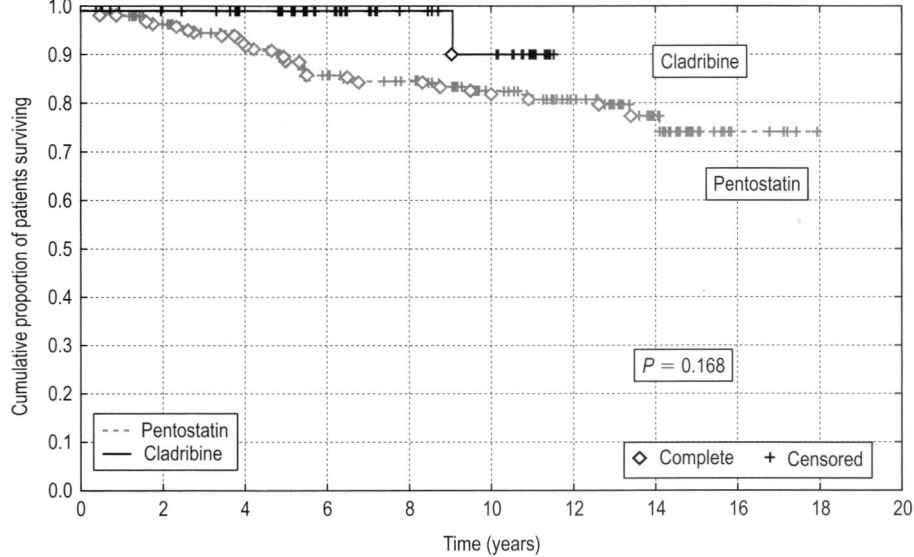

Figure 64.2   Overall survival in previously untreated patients with hairy cell leukemia treated with pentostatin or cladribine, showing no difference between them.

Rituximab has been shown to induce responses in patients who either failed to respond to purine analogue or had an early relapse.[195–197] This may prove to be a valuable addition to therapy either in combination with purine analogues in resistant cases[198] and/or to purge residual bone marrow disease[199] following purine analogue induction treatment. Two immunotoxins have been developed combining *Pseudomonas* exotoxin with either anti-CD22 or anti-CD25 monoclonal antibodies.[200,201] Both of these have been shown to have activity in patients in whom purine analogue therapy has failed and studies continue at the NCI.

HAIRY CELL LEUKEMIA VARIANT

Hairy cell leukemia variant is a very rare disease in which bone marrow and spleen histology are the same as in classical hairy cell leukemia but the circulating cells are morphologically and phenotypically distinct.[202,203] Patients often present with a high white blood cell count and the monocytopenia, so typical of hairy cell leukemia, is absent. Morphologically the cells have a round or oval nucleus with a prominent nucleolus and less abundant, more basophilic villous cytoplasm. These are B lymphocytes but usually lack expression of CD25, CD103, and TRAP. This variant is much less responsive to treatment than classical hairy cell leukemia and consequently the prognosis is less good. Because of the rarity there have been few clinical trials exploring effective therapy for this subgroup of patients.

KEY POINTS

- Chronic lymphocytic leukemia is a clinically heterogeneous disorder with a wide variation in prognosis. Although traditional clinical staging systems (Binet and Rai) still form the foundation for decisions about treatment, newer prognostic variables (*IGHV* mutation status, *ZAP*70, molecular cytogenetics) are becoming increasingly important in predicting outcome for patients and thus for selecting specific therapies.
- Purine analogues developed in the 1980s, particularly fludarabine, form the backbone of treatment in combination with alkylating agents (cyclophosphamide). These combinations have been shown to give superior response rates and progression-free survival compared with single-agent therapy.
- The addition of monoclonal antibodies (rituximab and alemtuzumab), given either concurrently or sequentially with fludarabine-based regimens, has demonstrated that higher rates of hematologic, flow cytometric, and molecular responses in CLL can be achieved. The challenge in the future will be to determine the optimal manner in which these and other novel agents may be incorporated into treatment strategies with the goal of achieving prolonged survival, and potentially cure, for patients with CLL.
- Response criteria are being revised to incorporate the more sensitive methods (multicolor flow

cytometry and PCR) to assess minimal residual disease and monitor for early relapse.

- Stem cell transplantation, either autologous or allogeneic, may be used to consolidate responses achieved using chemotherapy or chemoimmunotherapy and prolong remissions. The most promising of these approaches is reduced-intensity allogeneic transplantation, which has acceptable TRM and may result in long-term remissions. Although still an experimental approach with as-yet short-term follow-up, this should be considered for suitable patients with high-risk disease.
- With an ever-increasing number of new agents and treatment strategies it is critical that these are examined prospectively in well-conducted clinical trials.
- Hairy cell leukemia is one of the most successfully treated hematopoietic malignancies with the majority of patients (greater than 90 percent) achieving long-term survival with single-agent purine analogue therapy.

REFERENCES

● = Key primary paper
◆ = Major review article

◆1.   Jaffe ES, Harris N, Stein H et al. Tumours of haematopoietic and lymphoid tissues. World health organization classification of tumours. Lyon, France: IARC Press, 2001.

2.   Boggs DR, Chen SC, Zhang ZN et al. Chronic lymphocytic leukemia in China. Am J Hematol 1987; 25: 349–54.

3.   Conley CL, Misiti J, Laster AJ. Genetic factors predisposing to chronic lymphocytic leukemia and to autoimmune disease. Medicine 1980; 59: 323–34.

4.   Linet MS, Van Natta ML, Brookmeyer R et al. Familial cancer history and chronic lymphocytic leukemia. A case-control study. Am J Epidemiol 1989; 130: 655–64.

5.   Houlston RS, Sellick G, Yuille M et al. Causation of chronic lymphocytic leukemia: insights from familial disease. Leuk Res 2003; 27: 871–6.

6.   Rawstron AC, Yuille MR, Fuller J et al. Inherited predisposition to CLL is detectable as subclinical monoclonal B-lymphocyte expansion. Blood 2002; 100: 2289–90.

◆7.   Cheson BD, Bennett JM, Grever M et al. National cancer institute-sponsored working group guidelines for chronic lymphocytic leukemia: revised guidelines for diagnosis and treatment. Blood 1996; 87: 4990–7.

8.   Matutes E, Owusu-Ankomah K, Morilla R et al. The immunological profile of B-cell disorders and proposal

of a scoring system for the diagnosis of CLL. Leukemia 1994; 8: 1640–5.

9.   Moreau EJ, Matutes E, A'Hern RP et al. Improvement of the chronic lymphocytic leukemia scoring system with the monoclonal antibody SN8 (CD79b). Am J Clin Pathol 1997; 108: 378–82.

10.   Perkins JG, Flynn JM, Howard RS et al. Frequency and type of serious infections in fludarabine-refractory B-cell chronic lymphocytic leukemia and small lymphocytic lymphoma: implications for clinical trials in this patient population. Cancer 2002; 94: 2033–9.

11.   Damashek W. Chronic lymphocytic leukaemia-an accumulative disease of immunologically incompetent lymphocytes. Blood 1967; 29: 566–84.

12.   Chiorazzi N, Rai KR, Ferrarini M. Chronic lymphocytic leukemia. N Engl J Med 2005; 352: 804–15.

●13.   Binet JL, Auguier A, Dighiero G et al. A new prognostic classification of CLL derived from a multivariate survival analysis. Cancer 1981; 48: 198–206.

●14.   Rai KR, Sawitsky A, Cronkite EP et al. Clinical staging of chronic lymphocytic leukaemia. Blood 1975; 46: 219–34.

15.   International Workshop on CLL (IWCLL). Chronic lymphocytic leukemia: proposal for a revised prognostic staging system. Ann Intern Med 1981; 48: 365–7.

16.   Catovsky D, Fooks J, Richards S. Prognostic factors in CLL: the importance of age, sex and response to treatment in survival. A report from the URC CLL I trial. MRC Working Party on Leukaemia in Adults. Br J Haematol 1989; 72: 141–9.

17.   Mauro FR, DeRossi G, Bmgio VL et al. Prognostic value of bone marrow histology in CLL: a study of 335 untreated cases from a single institution. Haematologica 1994; 79: 334–41.

18.   Montserrat E, Sanchez-Bisono J, Vinolas N et al. Lymphocyte doubling time in chronic lymphocytic leukaemia: analysis of its prognostic significance. Br J Haematol 1986; 62: 567–75.

19.   Lee JS, Dixon DO, Kantarjian HM et al. Prognosis of CLL: multivariate regression analysis of 325 untreated patients. Blood 1987; 69: 929–36.

20.   Di Giovanni S, Valentini G, Carducci P et al. Beta-2-microglobulin is a reliable tumor marker in chronic lymphocytic leukemia. Acta Haematol 1989; 81: 181–5.

21.   Hallek M, Langenmayer I, Ned C et al. Elevated serum thymidine kinase levels identify a subgroup at high risk of disease progression in early non-smoldering CLL. Blood 1999; 93: 1732–7.

22.   Molica S, Levato D, Dell'Olio M et al. Cellular expression and serum circulating levels of CD23 in B-cell CLL: implications for prognosis. Haematologica 1996; 81: 428–33.

●23.   Hamblin TJ, Davis Z, Gardiner A et al. Unmutated Ig V(H) genes are associated with a more aggressive form of chronic lymphocytic leukemia. Blood 1999; 94: 1848–54.

●24. Damle RN, Wasil T, Fais F *et al.* Ig V gene mutation status and CD38 expression as novel prognostic indicators in chronic lymphocytic leukemia. *Blood* 1999; **94**: 1840–7.

25. Tobin G, Thunberg U, Johnson A *et al.* Somatically mutated Ig V(H)3-21 genes characterized a new subset of chronic lymphocytic leukaemia. *Blood* 2002; **99**: 2262–4.

●26. Rosenwald A, Alizadeh AA, Widhopf G *et al.* Relation of gene expression phenotype to immunoglobulin mutation genotype in B cell chronic lymphocytic leukaemia. *J Exp Med* 2001; **194**: 1639–47.

●27. Crespo M, Bosch F, Villamor N *et al.* ZAP-70 expression as a surrogate for immunoglobulin-variable-region mutations in chronic lymphocytic leukemia. *N Engl J Med* 2003; **348**: 1764–75.

28. Orchard JA, Ibbotson RE, Davis Z *et al.* ZAP-70 expression and prognosis in chronic lymphocytic leukaemia. *Lancet* 2004; **363**: 105–11.

29. Rassenti LZ, Hytna L, Toy TL *et al.* ZAP-70 compared with immunoglobulin heavy-chain gene mutation status as a predictor of disease progression in chronic lymphocytic leukaemia. *N Engl J Med* 2004; **351**: 893–901.

30. Hamblin TJ, Orchard JA, Ibbotson RE *et al.* CD38 expression and immunoglobulin variable region mutations are independent prognostic variables in chronic lymphocytic leukemia, but CD38 expression may vary during the course of the disease. *Blood* 2002; **99**: 1023–9.

31. Juliusson G, Oscier DG, Fitchett M *et al.* Prognostic subgroups in B-cell chronic lymphocytic leukaemia defined by specific chromosomal abnormalities. *N Engl J Med* 1990; **323**: 720–4.

●32. Dohner H, Stilgenbauer S, Benner A *et al.* Genomic aberrations and survival in chronic lymphocytic leukemia. *N Engl J Med* 2000; **343**: 1910–16.

33. Cordone I, Masi S, Mauro FR *et al.* Tp53 expression in B-cell chronic lymphocytic leukemia: a marker of disease progression and poor prognosis. *Blood* 1998; **91**: 4342–9.

34. Dohner H, Fischer K, Bentz M *et al.* Tp53 gene deletion predicts for poor survival and non-response therapy with purine analogues in chronic B-cell leukaemias. *Blood* 1995; **85**: 1580–9.

●35. Krober A, Seiler T, Benner A *et al.* VH Mutation status, CD38 expression level, genomic aberrations, and survival in chronic lymphocytic leukemia. *Blood* 2002; **100**: 1410–16.

36. Oscier DG, Gardiner AC, Mould SJ *et al.* Multivariate analysis of prognostic factors in CLL: clinical stage, IGVH gene mutational status, and loss or mutation of the Tp53 gene are independent prognostic factors. *Blood* 2002; **100**: 1110–11.

37. Lin K, Sherrington PD, Dennis M *et al.* Relationship between Tp53 dysfunction, CD38 expression, and IgV(H) mutation in chronic lymphocytic leukemia. *Blood* 2002; **100**: 1404–9.

38. French Cooperative Group on Chronic Lymphocytic Leukemia. Effects of chlorambucil and therapeutic decision in initial forms of chronic lymphocytic leukemia (stage A): results of a randomized clinical trial on 612 patients. *Blood* 1990; **75**: 1414–21.

●39. Dighiero G, Maloum K, Desablens B *et al.* Chlorambucil in indolent chronic lymphocytic leukemia. French Cooperative Group on Chronic Lymphocytic Leukemia. *N Eng J Med* 1998; **338**: 1506–14.

40. Catovsky D, Fooks J, Richards S. The UK Medical Research Council CLL trials 1 and 2. *Nouv Rev Fr Hematol* 1988; **30**: 423–7.

41. CLL Trialists' Collaborative Group. Chemotherapeutic options in chronic lymphocytic leukemia: a meta-analysis of the randomized trials. CLL Trialists' Coliaborative Group. *J Natl Cancer Inst* 1999; **91**: 861–8.

●42. Rawstron AC, Kennedy B, Evans PA *et al.* Quantitation of minimal disease levels in chronic lymphocytic leukemia using a sensitive flow cytometric assay improves the prediction of outcome and can be used to optimize therapy. *Blood* 2001; **98**: 29–35.

43. Rawstron A, Villamor N, Ritgen M *et al.* International standardized approach for flow cytometric residual disease monitoring in chronic lymphocytic leukaemia. *Leukemia* 2007; **21**: 956–64.

44. Pfitzner T, Reiser M, Barth S *et al.* Quantitative molecular monitoring of residual tumour cells in chronic lymphocytic leukaemia. *Ann Hematol* 2002; **81**: 258–66.

45. Provan D, Bartlett-Pandite L, Zwicky C *et al.* Eradication of polymerase chain reaction-detectable chronic lymphocytic leukemia cells is associated with improved outcome after bone marrow transplantation. *Blood* 1996; **88**: 2228–35.

46. Esteve J, Villamor N, Colomer D *et al.* Stem cell transplantation for chronic lymphocytic leukemia: different outcome after autologous and allogeneic transplantation and correlation with minimal residual disease status. *Leukemia* 2001; **15**: 445–51.

47. Bosch F, Ferrer A, Lopez-Guillermo A. Fludarabine, cyclophosphomide and mitoxantrone in the treatment of resistant or relapsed chronic lymphocytic leukaemia. *Br J Haematol* 2002; **119**: 976–84.

●48. Moreton P, Kennedy B, Lucas G *et al.* Eradication of minimal residual disease in B-cell chronic lymphocytic leukaemia after alemtuzumab therapy is associated with prolonged survival. *J Clin Oncol* 2005; **23**: 2971–9.

●49. Weirda W, O'Brien S, Wen Sijin *et al.* Chemoimmunotherapy with fludarabine, cyclophosphamide, and rituximab for relapsed and refractory chronic lymphocytic leukemia. *J Clin Oncol* 2005; **23**: 4070–8.

50. Catovsky D, Hamblin T, Richards S. Preliminary results of UK MRC trial in chronic lymphocytic leukemia CLL3. In: Proceedings of the 27th Congress of the International Society of Haematology (ISH-EHA). *Br J Haematol* 1998; **102**: 278, abstract 114.

51. French Cooperative Group on Chronic Lymphocytic Leukemia. A randomized clinical trial of chlorambucil

versus COP in stage B chronic lymphocytic leukemia. *Blood* 1990; **75**: 1422–5.

52. Montserrat E, Alcala A, Parody R *et al.* Treatment of chronic lymphocytic leukemia in advanced stages. A randomized trial comparing chlorambucil plus prednisone versus cyclophosphamide, vincristine, and prednisone. *Cancer* 1985; **56**: 2369–75.

53. Raphael B, Andersen JW, Silber R *et al.* Comparison of chlorambucil and prednisone versus cyclophosphamide, vincristine, and prednisone as initial treatment for chronic lymphocytic leukemia: long-term follow-up of an Eastern Cooperative Oncology Group randomized clinical trial. *J Clin Oncol* 1991; **9**: 770–6.

54. Jaksic B, Brugiatelli M, Krc I *et al.* High dose chlorambucil versus Binet's modified cyclophosphamide, doxorubicin, vincristine, and prednisone regimen in the treatment of patients with advanced B-cell chronic lymphocytic leukemia. Results of an international multicenter randomized trial. International Society for Chemo-Immunotherapy, Vienna. *Cancer* 1997; **79**: 2107–14.

◆55. French Cooperative Group on CLL. Is the CHOP regimen a good treatment for advanced CLL? Results from two randomized clinical trials. French Cooperative Group on Chronic Lymphocytic Leukemia. *Leuk Lymphoma* 1994; **13**: 449–56.

56. Keating MJ, Scouros M, Murphy S *et al.* Multiple agent chemotherapy (POACH) in previously treated and untreated patients with chronic lymphocytic leukemia. *Leukemia* 1988; **2**: 157–64.

57. Keating MJ, Kantarjian H, Talpaz M *et al.* Fludarabine: a new agent with major activity against chronic lymphocytic leukemia. *Blood* 1989; **74**: 19–25.

58. Sorensen JM, Vena DA, Fallavollita A *et al.* Treatment of refractory chronic lymphocytic leukemia with fludarabine phosphate via the group C protocol mechanism of the National Cancer Institute: five-year follow-up report. *J Clin Oncol* 1997; **15**: 458–65.

59. Robertson LE, O'Brien S, Kantarjian H *et al.* A 3-day schedule of fludarabine in previously treated chronic lymphocytic leukemia. *Leukemia* 1995; **9**: 1444–9.

60. O'Brien S, Kantarjian H, Beran M *et al.* Results of fludarabine and prednisone therapy in 264 patients with chronic lymphocytic leukaemia with multivariate analysis-derived prognosis model for response to treatment. *Blood* 1993; **82**: 1695–700.

●61. Keating MJ, O'Brien S, Learner S *et al.* Long-term follow-up of patients with chronic lymphocytic leukaemia (CLL) receiving fludarabine regimens as initial therapy. *Blood* 1998; **92**: 1165–71.

62. Clavio M, Miglino M, Spirano M *et al.* First line fludarabine treatment of symptomatic chronic lymphoproliferative diseases: clinical results and molecular analysis of minimal residual disease. *Eur J Haematol* 1998; **61**: 197–203.

●63. Rai KR, Peterson BL, Appelbaum FR *et al.* Fludarabine compared with chlorambucil as primary therapy for chronic lymphocytic leukemia. *N Engl J Med* 2000; **343**: 1750–7.

●64. Leporrier M, Chevret S, Cazin B *et al.* Randomized comparison of fludarabine, CAP, and CHOP in 938 previously untreated stage B and C chronic lymphocytic leukemia patients. *Blood* 2001; **98**: 2319–25.

65. Johnson S, Smith AG, Loffler H *et al.* Multicentre prospective randomised trial of fludarabine versus cyclophosphamide, doxorubicin, and prednisone (CAP) for treatment of advanced-stage chronic lymphocytic leukaemia. The French Cooperative Group on CLL. *Lancet* 1996; **347**: 1432–8.

66. Eichhorst BF, Busch R, Stauch M *et al.* No significant clinical benefit of first line therapy with fludarabine (F) in comparison to chlorambucil (CLb) to elderly patients (pts) with advanced chronic lymphocytic leukemia (CLL): results of a phase III study of the German CLL Study Group (GCLLSG). *Blood* 2007; **110**: abstract 629.

67. Jaksic B, Brugiatelli M, Suciu S. Fludarabine versus high-dose continuous chlorambucil in untreated patients with B-CLL: Results of CLL1 EORTC randomized trial. *Haematol Cell Ther* 2000; **42**.

68. Koehl ULL, Nowak B, Ruiz van Haperen V *et al.* Fludarabine and cyclophosphamide: synergistic cytotoxicity associated with inhibition of interstrand crosslink removal. *Proc Am Assoc Cancer Res* 1997; **38**: 10.

69. Bellosillo B, Villamor N, Colomer D *et al.* In vitro evaluation of fludarabine in combination with cyclophosphamide and/or mitoxantrone in B-cell chronic lymphocytic leukaemia. *Blood* 1999; **94**: 2836–43.

●70. O'Brien SM, Kantarjian HM, Cortes J *et al.* Results of the fludarabine and cyclophosphamide combination regimen in chronic lymphocytic leukemia. *J Clin Oncol* 2001; **19**: 1414–20.

71. Flinn JW, Byrd JC, Morrison C *et al.* Fludarabine and cyclophosphamide with filgrastim support in patients with previously untreated indolent lymphoid malignancies. *Blood* 2000; **96**: 71–5.

72. Hallek M, Schmitt B, Wilhelm M *et al.* Fludarabine plus cyclophosphamide is an efficient treatment for advanced chronic lymphocytic leukaemia (CLL): results of a phase II study of the German CLL Study Group. *Br J Haematol* 2001; **114**: 342–8.

73. Eichhorst BF, Busch R, Hopfinger G *et al.* Fludarabine plus cyclophosphamide versus fludarabine alone in first-line therapy of younger patients with chronic lymphocytic leukaemia. *Blood* 2006; **107**: 885–91.

74. Flinn IW, Neuberg DS, Grever MR *et al.* Phase III trial of fludarabine and cyclophosphamide compared with fludarabine for patients with previously untreated CLL: US Intergroup Trial E2997. *J Clin Oncol* 2007; **25**: 793–8.

75. Catovsky D, Richards S, Matutes E *et al.* Assessment of fludarabine plus cyclophosphamide for patients with chronic lymphocytic leukaemia (the LRF CLL 4 Trial): A randomised controlled trial. *Lancet* 2007; **370**: 230–9.

76. Bosch F, Ferrer A, Villamor N *et al.* Fludarabine, cyclophosphamide and mitoxantrone as initial therapy of CLL: high response rate and disease eradication. *Clin Cancer Res* 2008; **14**: 155–61.

77. Boogaerts MA, Van Hoof A, Catovsky D *et al.* Activity of oral fludarabine phosphate in previously treated chronic lymphocyte leukaemia. *J Clin Oncol* 2001; **19**: 4252–8.

78. Cazin BF, Malourm K, Cretcil MD *et al.* Oral fludarabine phosphate and cyclophosphamide in previously untreated CLL: final response and follow-up in 75 patients. *Blood* 2003; **102**: 1598a (abstract).

79. Grever MR, Leiby JM, Kraut EH *et al.* Low-dose deoxycoformycin in lymphoid malignancy. *J Clin Oncol* 1985; **3**: 1196–201.

80. Dillman RO, Mick R, Mcintyre OR. Pentostatin in chronic lymphocytic leukemia: a phase II trial of cancer and leukemia group B. *J Clin Oncol* 1989; **7**: 433–8.

81. Weiss MA, Maslak PO, Iureic IG *et al.* Pentostatin and cyclophosphamide: an effective new regimen in previously treated patients with chronic lymphocytic leukemia. *J Clln Oncol* 2003; **21**: 1278–84.

82. Byrd JC, Peterson B, Piro L *et al.* A phase II study of cladribine treatment for fludarabine refractory B cell chronic lymphocytic leukemia: results from CALGB study 9211. *Leukemia* 2003; **17**: 323–7.

83. Juliusson G, Elmhorn-Rosenborg A. Liliemark I. Response to 2-chlorodeoxyadenosine in patients with B-cell chronic lymphocytic leukemia resistant to fludarabine. *N Engl J Med* 1992; **327**: 1056–61.

84. Robak T, Blasinka-Morawiec M, Krykowski E *et al.* Intermittent 2-hour intravenous infusions of 2-chlorodeoxyadenosine in the treatment of 110 patients with refractory or previously untreated B-cell chronic lymphocytic leukemia. *Leuk Lymphoma* 1996; **22**: 509–14.

85. O'Brien S, Kantaljian H, Estey E *et al.* Lack of effect of 2 chlorodeoxyadenosine therapy in patients with chronic lymphocytic leukemia refractory to fludarabine therapy. *N Engl J Med* 1994; **330**: 319–22.

86. Robak T, Blonski JZ, Kasznicki M *et al.* Cladribine with prednisone versus chlorambucil with prednisone as first-line therapy in chronic lymphocytic leukemia: report of a prospective, randomized, multicenter trial. *Blood* 2000; **96**: 2723–9.

87. Robak T, Blonski J Z, Gora-Tybor J *et al.* Cladribine alone and in combination with cyclophosphamide or cyclophosphamide plus mitoxantrone in the treatment of progressive chronic lymphocytic leukemia: report of a prospective multicenter randomised trial of the Polish Adult Leukemia Group (PALG CLL2). *Blood* 2006; **108**: 473–9.

●88. McLaughlin P, Grillo-Lopez AH, Link BK *et al.* Rituximab chimeric anti-CD20 monoclonal antibody therapy for relapsed indolent lymphoma: half of patients respond to a four-dose treatment program. *J Clin Oncol* 1998; **16**: 2825–33.

89. Winkler U, Jensen M, Manzke O *et al.* Cytokine-release syndrome in patients with B-cell chronic lymphocytic leukaemia and high lymphocyte counts after treatment with an anti-CD20 monoclonal antibody (rituximab, IDEC-C2B*). *Blood* 1999; **94**: 2217–24.

90. Nguyen DT, Amess JA, Doughty H *et al.* IDEC-C2B8 anti-CD20 (rituximab) immunotherapy in patients with low-grade non-Hodgkin's lymphoma and lymphoproliferative disorders: evaluation of response on 48 patients. *Eur J Haematol* 1999; **62**: 76–82.

91. Huhn D, von Schilling C, Wilhelm M *et al.* German Chronic Lymphocytic Leukaemia Study Group. Rituximab therapy of patients with B-cell chronic lymphocytic leukaemia. *Blood* 2001; **98**: 1326–31.

92. Thomas DA, Giles Fl, Cortes I *et al.* Single agent rituxan in early stage chronic lymphocytic leukemia (CLL). *Blood* 2001; **98**: 364a.

●93. Hainsworth JD, Litchy S, Barton JH *et al.* Single-agent rituximab as first-line and maintenance treatment for patients with chronic lymphocytic leukemia or small lymphocytic lymphoma: a phase II trial of the minnie pearl cancer research network. *J Clin Oncol* 2003; **21**: 1746–51.

94. O'Brien SM, Kantaijian H, Thomas DA *et al.* Rituximab dose-escalation trial in chronic lymphocytic leukemia. *J Clin Oncol* 2001; **19**: 2165–70.

●95. Byrd JC, Murphy T, Howard RS *et al.* Rituximab using a thrice weekly dosing schedule in B-cell chronic lymphocytic leukemia and small lymphocytic lymphoma demonstrates clinical activity and acceptable toxicity. *J Clin Oncol* 2001; **19**: 2153–64.

96. Manshouri T, Do KA, Wang X *et al.* Circulating CD20 is detectable in the plasma of patients with chronic lymphocytic leukaemia and is of prognostic significance. *Blood* 2003; **101**: 2507–13.

●97. Byrd JC, Peterson B, Morrison VA *et al.* Randomized phase 2 study of fludarabine with concurrent versus sequential treatment with rituximab in symptomatic, untreated patients with B-cell chronic lymphocytic leukemia: results from Cancer and Leukemia Group B 9712 (CALGB 9712). *Blood* 2003; **101**: 6–14.

98. Byrd JC, Rai K, Peterson BL *et al.* Addition of rituximab to fludarabine may prolong progression free survival and overall survival of patients with previously untreated chronic lymphocytic leukaemia: an updated retrospective comparative analysis of CALGB 9712 and CALGB 9011. *Blood* 2005; **105**: 49–53.

99. Demiden A, Iam T, Alas S *et al.* Chimeric anti-CD20 (DEC-C2B8) monoclonal antibody sensitizes a B-cell lymphoma cell line to cell killing by cytotoxic drugs. *Cancer Biother Radiopharm* 1997; **12**: 177–86.

100. Golay J, Zaffaroni L, Vaccari T *et al.* Biologic response of B lymphoma cells to anti-Cd20 monoclonal antibody rituximab in vitro: CD55 and CD59 regulate complement-mediated cell lysis. *Blood* 2000; **95**: 3900–8.

●101. Keating MJ, O'Brien S, Albitar M *et al.* Early results of a chemo-immunotherapy regimen of fludarabine, cyclophosphamide and rituximab as initial therapy for chronic lymphocytic leukaemia. *J Clin Oncol* 2005; **23**: 4079–88.

102. Drapkin R. Pentostatin and rituximab in the treatment of patients with B-cell malignancies. *Oncology (Williston Park)* 2000; **14** (6 Suppl 2): 25–9.

103. Kay NE, Geyer SM, Call TG *et al.* Combination chemoimmunotherapy with pentostatin, cyclophosphamide and rituximab shows significant clinical activity with low accompanying toxicity in previously untreated B-chronic lymphocytic leukaemia. *Blood* 2007; **109**: 405–11.

●104. Lundin K, Kimby E, Bjorkholm M *et al.* Phase II trial of subcutaneous anti-CD52 monoclonal antibody alemtuzumab (Campath-1H) as first-line treatment for patients with B-cell chronic lymphocytic leukaemia (B-CLL). *Blood* 2002; **100**: 768–73.

●105. Hillmen P, Skotnicki AB, Robak T *et al.* Alemtuzumab compared with chlorambucil as first-line therapy for chronic lymphocytic leukaemia. *J Clin Oncol* 2007; **25**: 5616–23.

106. Osterborg A, Dyer MJ, Bunjes D *et al.* Phase II multicentre study of human CD52 antibody in previously treated chronic lymphocytic leukaemia. *J Clin Oncol* 1997; **15**: 1567–74.

●107. Keating MJ, Flinn I, Iain V *et al.* Therapeutic role of alemtuzumab (Campath-IH) in patients who have failed fludarabine: results of a large international study. *Blood* 2002; **99**: 3554–61.

108. Rai KR, Freter CE, Mercier RJ *et al.* Alemtuzumab in previously treated chronic lymphocytic leukaemia patients who also had received fludarabine. *J Clin Oncol* 2002; **23**: 3891–7.

●109. Lozanski G, Heerema NA, Flinn JW *et al.* Alemtuzumab is an effective therapy for chronic lymphocytic leukemia with Tp53 mutations and deletions. *Blood* 2004; **103**: 3278–81.

110. Kröber A, Kienle D, Hallek M *et al.* Subcutaneous Campath-1H (Alemtuzumab) in fludarabine refractory CLL: Interim analysis of the CLL2h study of the German CLL study group (GCLLSG). *Blood* 2004; **104**: abstract 478.

111. Montillo M, Tedeschi A, Miqueleiz S *et al.* Alemtuzumab as consolidation after a response to fludarabine is effective in purging residual disease in patients with chronic lymphocytic leukaemia. *J Clin Oncol* 2006; **24**: 2337–42.

112. O'Brien SM, Kantarjian HM, Thomas DA *et al.* Alemtuzumab as treatment for residual disease after chemotherapy in patients with chronic lymphocytic leukemia. *Cancer* 2005; **98**: 2657–63.

113. Rai KR, Byrd JC, Peterson BI *et al.* A phase II trial of fludarabine followed by alemtuzumab (Campath-1H) in previously untreated chronic lymphocytic leukaemia (CII) patients with active disease: cancer and leukaemia group B (CALGB) study 19901. *Blood* 2002; **100**: 772 (abstract).

●114. Schweighofer CD, Ritgen M, Eichhorst BF, *et al.* Consolidation with alemtuzumab improves progression-free survival in patients with chronic lymphocytic leukaemia (CLL) in first remission – long-term follow-up of phase III trial of the German CLL Study Group (GCLLSG). *Br J Haematol* 2009; **144**: 95–8.

115. Hendry L, Bowen A, Matutes E *et al.* Fludarabine, cyclophosphamide and mitoxantrone in relapsed or refractory chronic lymphocytic leukaemia and low-grade non-Hodgkin's lymphoma. *Leuk Lymphoma* 2004; **45**: 945–50.

116. Lamanna N, Kalayeio M, Maslak P *et al.* Pentostatin, cyclophosphamide and rituximab is an active, well tolerated regimen for patients with previously treated chronic lymphocytic leukaemia. *J Clin Oncol* 2006; **24**: 1575–81.

117. Keating MJ, O'Brien S, Kontoyiannis D *et al.* Results of first salvage therapy for patients refractory to a fludarabine regimen in chronic lymphocytic leukaemia. *Leuk Lymphoma* 2002; **43**: 1755–62.

118. Kennedy B, Rawstron A, Carter C *et al.* Campath-1H and fludarabine in combination are highly active in refractory chronic lymphocytic leukemia. *Blood* 2002; **99**: 2245–7.

119. Elter T, Borchmann P, Schulz H *et al.* Fludarabine in combination with alemtuzumab is effective and feasible in patients with relapsed or refractory B-cell chronic lymphocytic leukaemia: results of a phase II trial. *J Clin Oncol* 2005; **23**: 7024–31.

120. Faderl S, Thomas DA, O'Brien S *et al.* Experience with alemtuzumab plus rituximab in patients with relapsed and refractory lymphoid malignancies. *Blood* 2003; **101**: 3413–15.

121. Stilgenbauer S, Dohner H. Campath-1H-induced complete remission of chronic lymphocytic leukemia despite Tp53 gene mutation and resistance to chemotherapy. *N Engl J Med* 2002; **347**: 452–3.

122. Osuji N, Del Giudice I, Matutes E *et al.* The efficacy of alemtuzumab for refractory chronic lymphocytic leukaemia in relation to cytogenetic abnormalities of Tp53. *Haematologica* 2005; **90**: 1435–6.

123. Thornton PD, Hamblin M, Treleaven JG *et al.* High dose methyl prednisolone can induce remissions in CLL patients with Tp53 abnormalities. *Ann Haematol* 2003; **82**: 759–65.

124. Catovsky D, Richards S, Fooks J *et al.* CLL Trials in the United Kingdom. The Medical Research Council CLL Trials 1,2 3. *Leuk Lymphoma Suppl* 1991; 105–7.

125. Girinsky T, Guillot-Vals D, Koscielny S *et al.* A high and sustained response rate in refractory or relapsing low-grade lymphoma masses after low-dose radiation: analysis of predictive parameters of response to treatment. *Int J Radiat Oncol Biol Phys* 2001; **91**: 115–18.

126. Seymour JF, Cusack JD, Lerner SA *et al.* Case control study of the role of splenectomy in chronic lymphocytic leukaemia. *J Clin Oncol* 1997; **15**: 52–60.

127. Rabinowe SN, Soiffer RJ, Gribben JG *et al.* Autologous and allogeneic bone marrow transplantation for poor prognosis patients with B-cell chronic leukemia. *Blood* 1993; **82**: 1366–76.

◆128. Michallet M, Thiebaut A, Dreger P *et al.* Peripheral blood stem cell (PBSC) mobilization and transplantation after fludarabine therapy in chronic lymphocytic leukaemia (CLL): a report of the European Blood and Marrow

Transplantation (EBMT) CLL subcommittee on behalf of the EBMT Chronic Leukaemias Working Party (CLWP). *Br J Haematol* 2000; **108**: 595–601.

●129. Milligan DW, Fernandes S, Dasgupta R *et al.* Autografting for younger patients with chronic lymphocytic leukaemia is safe and achieves a high percentage of molecular responses. Results of the MRC pilot study. *Blood* 2004; **105**: 397–404.

130. Dreger P, Montserrat E. Autologous and allogeneic stem cell transplantation for chronic lymphocytic leukemia. *Leukemia* 2002; **16**: 985–92.

●131. Dreger P, Stilgenbauer S, Benner A *et al.* The prognostic impact of autologous stem cell transplantation in patients with chronic lymphocytic leukemia: a risk-matched analysis based on the VH gene mutational status. *Blood* 2004; **103**: 2850–8.

132. Micallef IN, Apostolidis J, Rohatiner AZ *et al.* Factors which predict unsuccessful mobilisation of peripheral blood progenitor cells following G-CSF alone in patients with non-Hodgkin's lymphoma. *Hematol J* 2000; **1**: 367–73.

●133. Michallet M, Archimbaud E, Bandini G *et al.* HLA-identical sibling bone marrow transplantation in younger patients with chronic lymphocytic leukemia. European group for blood and marrow transplantation and the international bone marrow transplant registry. *Ann Intern Med* 1996; **96**: 311–15.

134. Faulkner RD, Craddock C, Byrne JL *et al.* BEAM-alemtuzumab reduced intensity allogeneic stem cell transplantation for lymphoproliferative diseases: GVHD, toxicity and survival in 65 patients. *Blood* 2004; **103**: 428–34.

135. Khouri IF, Lee MS, Saliba RM *et al.* Non-ablative allogeneic stem cell transplantation for chronic lymphocytic leukaemia: *Exp Haematol* 2004; **32**: 28–35.

136. Ritgen M, Stilgenbauer S, von Neuhoff N *et al.* Graft-versus leukemia activity may overcome therapeutic resistance of chronic lymphocytic leukemia with unmutated immunoglobulin variable heavy chain gene status: implications of minimal residual disease measurement with quantitative PCR. *Blood* 2004; **104**: 2600–2.

137. Dreger P, Corradini P, Kimby E *et al.* Indications for allogeneic stem cell transplant in chronic lymphocytic leukaemia: the EBMT transplant consensus. *Leukemia* 2007; **21**: 12–17.

138. Byrd JC, Shinn C, Waselenko JK *et al.* Flavopiridol induces apoptosis in chronic lymphocytic leukaemia cells via activation of caspase-3 without evidence of bcl-2 modulation or dependence on functional Tp53. *Blood* 1998; **92**: 3804–16.

139. Frankel AE, Fleming DR, Hall PD *et al.* A phase II study of DT fusion protein denileukin diftitox in patients with fludarabine-refractory chronic lymphocytic leukaemia. *Clin Cancer Res* 2003; **9**: 3555–61.

140. Chanan-Khan A, Miller KC, Musial L *et al.* Clinical efficacy of lenalidomide in patients with relapsed or refractory chronic lymphocytic leukemia: results of a phase II study. *J Clin Oncol* 2006; **24**: 5343–9.

141. Richter MN. Generalized reticular cell sarcoma of lymph nodes associated with lymphocytic leukemia. *Am J Pathol* 1928; **4**: 285–92.

142. Foon KA, Thiruvengadam R, Saven A *et al.* Genetic relatedness of lymphoid malignancies. Transformation of chronic lymphocytic leukemia as a model. *Ann Intern Med* 1993; **119**: 63–73.

143. Thornton PD, Bellas C, Santon A *et al.* Richter's transformation of chronic lymphocytic leukaemia. The possible role of Epstein-Barr virus in its pathogenesis. *Leuk Res* 2005; **29**: 389–95.

144. Tsimberidou AM, Keating MJ. Richter syndrome: biology, incidence, and therapeutic strategies. *Cancer* 2005; **103**: 216–28.

145. Giles FJ, O'Brien SM, Keating MJ. Chronic lymphocytic leukaemia in (Richter's) transformation. *Semin Oncol* 1998; **25**: 57–65.

●146. Robertson LE, Pugh W, O'Brien S *et al.* Richter's syndrome: a report on 39 patients. *J Clin Oncol* 1993; **11**: 1985–9.

●147. Mauro FR, Foa R, Cerretti R *et al.* Autoimmune hemolytic anemia in chronic lymphocytic leukemia: clinical, therapeutic, and prognostic features. *Blood* 2000; **95**: 2786–92.

148. Hamblin TJ, Oscier DG, Young BJ. Autoimmunity in chronic lymphocytic leukaemia. *J Clin Pathol* 1986; **39**: 731–6.

149. Ahrens N, Kingreen D, Seltsam *et al.* Treatment for refractory autoimmune haemolytic anaemia with anti-CD20 (rituximab). *Br J Haematol* 2001; **114**: 241–2.

●150. Dearden C, Wade R, Else M. The prognostic significance of a positive direct antiglobulin test in chronic lymphocytic leukemia: a beneficial effect of the combination of fludarabine and cyclophosphamide on the incidence of hemolytic anemia. *Blood* 2008; **111**: 1820–6.

151. Molica S. Infections in chronic lymphocytic leukaemia: risk factors, impact on survival and treatment. *Leuk Lymphoma* 1994; **13**: 203–14.

152. Chapel H, Dicato M, Gamm H *et al.* Immunoglobulin replacement in patients with chronic lymphocytic leukaemia: a comparison of two dose regimens. *Br J Haematol* 1994; **88**: 209–12.

153. Weeks JC, Tierney MR, Weinstein MC. Cost effectiveness of prophylactic intravenous immune globulin in chronic lymphocytic leukaemia. *N Engl J Med* 1991; **325**: 81–6.

154. O'Brien S, Kantarjian H, Beran M *et al.* Fludarabine and granulocyte colony stimulating factor (G-CSF) in patients with chronic lymphocytic leukaemia. *Leukemia* 1997; **11**: 1631–5.

◆155. Galton DAG, Goldman JM, Wiltshaw E *et al.* Prolymphocytic leukaemia. *Br J Haematol* 1974; **27**: 7–23.

156. Melo N, Catovsky D, Galton DAG. The relationship between chronic lymphocytic leukaemia and pro lymphocytic leukaemia: I. Clinical and laboratory features of 300 patients and characterization of an intermediate group. *Br J Haematol* 1986; **63**: 377–87.

157. Lens D, Matutes E, Catovsky D *et al.* Frequent deletions at 11q23 and 13q14 in B cell prolymphocytic leukaemia. *Leukemia* 2000; **14**: 427–30.

158. Solé F, Woessner S, Espinet B *et al.* Cytogenetic abnormalities in three patients with B-cell prolymphocytic leukemia. *Cancer Genet Cytogenet* 1998; **103**: 43–5.

159. Ruchlemer R, Parry-Jones N, Brito-Babapulle V *et al.* B-Prolymphocytic leukaemia with t(11,14) revisited: a splenomegalic form of mantle cell lymphoma evolving with leukaemia. *Br J Haematol* 2004; **125**: 330–6.

160. Lens D, De Schouwer PJJ, Hamoudi RA *et al.* Tp53 abnormalities in B-Cell prolymphocytic leukaemia. *Blood* 1997; **89**: 2015–23.

161. Oscier DG, Catovsky D, Errington D *et al.* Splenic irradiation in B-prolymphocytic leukaemia. *Br J Haematol* 1981; **48**: 577–84.

162. Saven A, Lee T, Shultz M *et al.* Major activity of cladribine in patients with de novo B cell prolymphocytic leukaemia. *J Clin Oncol* 1997; **15**: 37–43.

163. Herold M, Spohn C, Schlag R *et al.* Fludarabine/cyclophosphamide chemotherapy for B – Prolymphocytic Leukaemia. *Blood* 2003; **102**: 2499 (abstract).

164. Weide R, Pandorf A, Heymanns J, Köppler H. Bendamustine/Mitoxantrone/Rituximab (BMR): a very effective, well tolerated outpatient chemo-immunotherapy for relapsed and refractory CD20-positive indolent malignancies. Final results of a pilot study. *Leuk Lymphoma* 2004; **45**: 2445–9.

165. Bowen AL, Zomas A, Emmett E *et al.* Subcutaneous CAMPATH-1H in fludarabine-resistant/relapsed chronic lymphocytic and B-prolymphocytic leukaemia. *Br J Haematol* 1997; **96**: 617–19.

◆166. Bouroncle B. Leukemic reticuloendotheliosis. *Blood* 1958; **13**: 609–30.

167. Flandrin G, Sigaux F, Sebahouns S *et al.* Hairy cell leukemia: Clinical presentation and follow-up of 211 patients. *Semin Oncol* 1984; **11** (Suppl 2): 458–71.

168. Mercieca J, Puga M, Matutes E *et al.* Incidence and significance of abdominal lymphadenopathy in hairy cell leukaemia. *Leuk Lymphoma* 1994; **14** (Suppl): 79–83.

169. Van den Neste E, Ravoet C, Delannoy A. Unusual manifestations of hairy cell leukaemia. In: Tallman M, Polliack A. (eds) *Hairy cell leukemia*. The Netherlands: Harwood Academic Publishers, 2000: 85–106.

●170. Matutes E, Morilla R, Owusu-Ankomah K *et al.* The immunophenotype of HCL: Proposal for a scoring system to distinguish HCL from B cell disorders with hairy or villous lymphocytes. *Leuk Lymphoma* 1994; **14**: 57–61.

171. Yam LT, Li CY, Lam KW. Tartrate-resistant acid phosphatase isoenzyme in the reticulum cells of leukemic reticuloendotheliosis. *N Engl J Med* 1971; **284**: 357–60.

172. Hounieu H, Chittal S, Al Saati T *et al.* Hairy cell leukemia. Diagnosis of bone marrow involvement in sections with monocloncal antibody DBA 44. *Am J Clin Pathol* 1992; **98**: 26–33.

173. Maloum K, Magnac C, Azgui Z *et al.* VH gene expression in hairy cell leukaemia. *Br J Haematol* 1998; **101**: 171–8.

174. Vanhenterikj V, Tierens A, Wlodarska I *et al.* V(H) gene analysis of hairy cell leukaemia reveals a homogeneous mutation status and suggests its marginal zone B-cell origin. *Leukemia* 2004; **18**: 1729–32.

175. Thorsélius K, Walsh SH, Thunberg U *et al.* Heterogeneous somatic hypermutation status confounds the cell of origin in hairy cell leukaemia. *Leuk Res* 2005; **29**: 153–8.

176. Golomb HM, Vardiman W. Response to splenectomy in 65 patients with hairy cell leukemia. An evaluation of spleen weight and bone marrow involvement. *Blood* 1983; **61**: 349–52.

●177. Quesada JR, Reuben J, Manning T *et al.* Alpha interferon for induction of remission in hairy cell leukemia. *N Engl Med* 1984; **310**: 15–18.

178. Golomb HM. Jacobs A, Fefer A *et al.* Alpha-2 interferon therapy for hairy-cell leukemia. A multicenter study of 64 patients. *J Clin Oncol* 1986; **4**: 900–5.

179. Ratain MJ, Golomb HM, Bardawil RG *et al.* Durability of responses to interferon alpha 2b in advanced hairy cell leukemia. *Blood* 1987; **69**: 872–7.

180. Smalley RV, Connors J, Tuttle RL *et al.* Splenectomy vs alpha interferon: a randomized study in patients with previously untreated hairy cell leukemia. *Am J Hematol* 1992; **41**: 13–18.

181. Ho AD, Thaler J, Mandelli F *et al.* Response to pentostatin in hairy-cell leukemia refractory to interferon-alpha. The European Organization for Research and Treatment of Cancer Leukemia Cooperative Group. *J Clin Oncol* 1989; **7**: 1533–8.

182. Kraut EH, Bouroncle BA, Grever MR. Pentostatin in the treatment of advanced hairy cell leukemia. *J Clin Oncol* 1989; **7**: 168–72.

183. Golomb HM, Dodge R, Mick R *et al.* Pentostatin treatment for hairy cell leukemia patients who failed initial therapy with recombinant alpha-interferon: a report of CALGB study 8515. *Leukemia* 1994; **8**: 2037–40.

●184. Dearden CE, Matutes E, Hilditch BL *et al.* Long-term follow-up of patients with hairy cell leukaemia after treatment with pentostatin or cladribine. *Br J Haematol* 1999; **106**: 515–19.

185. Flinn IW, Kopecky KJ, Foucar MK *et al.* Long-term follow-up of remission duration, mortality, and second malignancies in hairy cell leukemia patients treated with pentostatin. *Blood* 2000; **96**: 2981–6.

186. Maloisel F, Benboubker L, Gardembas M *et al.* Long-term outcome with pentostatin treatment in hairy cell leukemia patients. A French retrospective study of 238 patients. *Leukemia* 2003; **17**: 45–51.

●187. Grever M, Kopecky K, Foucar MK *et al.* A randomized comparison of pentostatin vs alpha-interferon in previously untreated patients with hairy cell leukaemia: an international group study. *J Clin Oncol* 1995; **13**: 974–82.

●188. Piro LD, Carrera CJ, Carson DA *et al.* Lasting remissions in hairy-cell leukemia induced by a single infusion of 2-chlorodeoxyadenosine. *N Engl J Med* 1990; **322**: 1117–21.

189. Cheson BD, Sorensen JM, Vena DA *et al.* Treatment of hairy cell leukemia with 2-chlorodeoxyadenosine via the Group C protocol mechanism of the National Cancer Institute: a report of 979 patients. *J Clin Oncol* 1998; **16**: 3007–15.

190. Hoffman MA, Janson D, Rose E *et al.* Treatment of hairy-cell leukemia with cladribine: response, toxicity, and long-term follow-up. *J Clin Oncol* 1997; **15**: 1138–42.

191. Saven A, Burian C, Koziol JA *et al.* Long-term follow-up of patients with hairy cell leukemia after cladribine treatment. *Blood* 1998; **92**: 1918–26.

192. Jehn U, Bartl R, Dietzfelbinger H *et al.* An update: 12-year follow-up of patients with hairy cell leukemia following treatment with 2chlorodeoxyadenosine. *Leukemia* 2004; **18**: 1476–81.

193. Else M, Ruchlemer R, Osuji N *et al.* Long remissions in hairy cell leukemia with purine analogs: a report of 219 patients with a median follow-up of 12.5 years. *Cancer* 2005; **104**: 2442–8.

194. Tallman MS, Hakimian D, Kopecky KJ *et al.* Minimal residual disease in patients with hairy cell leukemia in complete remission treated with 2-chlorodeoxyadenosine or 2-deoxycoformycin and prediction of early relapse. *Clin Cancer Res* 1999; **5**: 1665–70.

195. Hagberg H, Lundholm L. Rituximab, a chimeric anti-CD20 monoclonal antibody, in the treatment of hairy cell leukaemia. *Br J Haematol* 2001; **115**: 609–11.

196. Lauria F, Lenoci M, Annino L *et al.* Efficacy of anti-CD20 monoclonal antibodies (Mabthera) in patients with progressed hairy cell leukemia. *Haematologica* 2001; **86**: 1046–50.

197. Thomas DA, O'Brien S, Bueso-Ramos C *et al.* Rituximab in relapsed or refractory hairy cell leukemia. *Blood* 2003; **102**: 3906–11.

198. Else M, Osuji N, Forconi F *et al.* The role of rituximab in combination with pentostatin or cladribine for the treatment of recurrent/refractory hairy cell leukemia. *Cancer* 2007; **110**: 2240–7.

199. Cervetti G, Galimberti S, Andreazzoli F *et al.* Rituximab as treatment for minimal residual disease in hairy cell leukaemia. *Eur J Haematol* 2004; **73**: 412–17.

200. Kreitman RJ, Wilson WH, Robbins D *et al.* Responses in refractory hairy cell leukemia to a recombinant immunotoxin. *Blood* 1999; **94**: 3340–8.

●201. Kreitman RJ, Wilson WH, Bergeron K *et al.* Efficacy of the anti-CD22 recombinant immunotoxin BL22 in chemotherapy resistant hairy-cell leukemia. *N Engl J Med* 2001; **345**: 241–7.

202. Catovsky D, O'Brien M, Melo J *et al.* Hairy cell leukemia (HCL) variant: An intermediate disease between HCL and B prolymphocytic leukemia. *Semin Oncol* 1984; **11**: 362–9.

◆203. Matutes E, Wotherspoon A, Catovsky D. The natural history and clinico-pathological features of the variant form of hairy cell leukaemia. *Leukaemia* 2001; **15**: 184–6.

65

Mantle cell lymphoma

MARTIN DREYLING, GEORG LENZ AND WOLFGANG HIDDEMANN

INTRODUCTION

Mantle cell lymphoma (MCL) is molecularly characterized by the chromosomal translocation t(11;14)(q13;q32), which results in a juxtaposition of the *BCL1* gene locus to the immunoglobulin (Ig) heavy chain promoter and the subsequent overexpression of the cell cycle regulator protein cyclin D1. Accordingly, MCL has been recognized as a distinct subentity of non-Hodgkin lymphoma (NHL) in the previous Revised European–American Lymphoma (REAL) and the current World Health Organization (WHO) classification.[1,2] The incidence of MCL is approximately 2–3/100 000 per year, representing only 5–10 percent of all NHL cases.[3–5] The disease is diagnosed mainly in advanced Ann Arbor stages III/IV and characterized by an aggressive clinical course and poor prognosis with virtually no long-term survivors.[6] Conventional chemotherapy has failed to substantially alter the natural course of the disease and remains a palliative approach. However, several randomized trials clearly demonstrated recently the superiority of a combined immunochemotherapy containing the anti-CD20 antibody rituximab in first-line therapy as well as in relapsed disease.[7,8] In addition, a randomized trial of the European MCL Network showed that myeloablative radiochemotherapy followed by autologous stem cell transplantation significantly improved the progression-free survival in patients up to 65 years of age as compared to conventional therapy.[9] However, even after such an intensified approach, the vast majority of patients with MCL will eventually relapse. Thus, new strategies such as new molecular targeting agents (e.g., proteasome inhibitors

or radiolabeled antibodies) or allogeneic transplantation after dose-reduced conditioning ('mini-transplantation') are currently being investigated to improve the dismal prognosis of MCL.

CLINICAL PRESENTATION

Median age of MCL patients at diagnosis is 65 years with a male to female ratio of 3–4:1. The majority of cases are diagnosed in advanced Ann Arbor stages III or IV, often with splenomegaly and generalized lymphadenopathy.[6] In addition, extranodal manifestations are found in approximately 90 percent of patients, including bone marrow infiltration (50–80 percent), liver (25 percent), and gastrointestinal tract (10–25 percent).[10–14] Less common are skin, lung, breast, or soft tissue involvement. Leukemic expression of MCL cells is diagnosed in approximately 20 percent of cases, whereas central nervous system involvement is found in up to 20 percent of relapsed MCL cases.[15] B symptoms are described in less than 50 percent of patients.

PROGNOSTIC FACTORS

Numerous studies have investigated the value of several prognostic factors in MCL. Thus, clinical as well as biological prognostic factors can be identified which are able to predict outcome in MCL patients.

Clinical prognostic factors

Clinical features that are associated with adverse prognosis of MCL patients are advanced stage disease, the occurrence of B symptoms, and a poor performance status.[6,12,16] In contrast, younger age (less than 65 years), normal lactate dehydrogenase (LDH) serum levels, as well as normal β_2-microglobulin seem to be associated with a better outcome.[6,12]

The value of the International Prognostic Index (IPI) is interpreted differently. Several groups claimed that a high-risk profile according to the IPI is associated with an adverse outcome in MCL.[6,16] However, this finding could not be confirmed in the retrospective as well as prospective analyses by the European MCL Network, in which a significant overlap of the survival curves of the different IPI groups was observed.[10,17] Thus, the IPI is only of limited additional impact in predicting outcome of MCL patients. In contrast, an MCL-specific prognostic score has been recently established which incorporates performance status, age, leukocyte count, and LDH (MCL International Prognostic Index, MIPI).[17]

The value of minimal residual disease (MRD) is interpreted differently. A recent study by Pott et al. indicates that MRD is a strong prognostic factor predicting an improved progression-free survival in MCL patients following high-dose therapy and autologous stem cell transplantation.[18] In contrast, in the study of Howard et al., MRD was not associated with outcome, as the progression-free survival of patients who achieved molecular remission after a combined immunochemotherapy of CHOP (cyclophosphamide, doxorubicin, vincristine, and prednisone) and rituximab was similar to those without molecular remission (16.5 vs 18.8 months).[19] Thus, the role of MRD has not yet been fully elucidated and therefore has to be further determined in future prospective studies.

Biological prognostic factors

Several biological prognostic factors such as growth pattern, histology, or cytology have been investigated by different groups.[12,16,17,20–22] However, the published results regarding the prognostic impact on the overall survival of MCL patients vary substantially and thus the role of these prognostic factors remains not fully elucidated. In contrast, the poor outcome of patients with TP53 gene mutations was confirmed by several analyses. The study of Greiner et al. detected TP53 gene mutations in 15 percent (8 out of 53) of MCL patients with a rather short median survival of only 1.3 years as compared to 5.1 years for cases with germ-line TP53.[23] These results were confirmed by two other studies by Hernandez et al. and Zoldan et al.[24,25]

However, an even more important prognostic factor is the proliferation rate determined by the Ki-67 staining index or the number of mitoses. Bosch and colleagues showed that patients with >2.5 mitoses/high power field (HPF) had a

median survival of only 24 months as compared to patients with ≤2.5 mitoses/HPF who showed an overall survival of 50 months.[12] Similarly, in a large retrospective study of 350 patients, different proliferation indices represented the most powerful prognostic marker, clearly superior to cytomorphology and clinical parameters.[21] These results were confirmed in a study of Rosenwald et al., in which 101 MCL cases were investigated by gene expression profiling.[26] In this analysis, determination of tumor cell proliferation identified subgroups of patients that differed in median overall survival by more than 5 years.

CLINICAL MANAGEMENT

With a median survival of only 3–4 years and a high degree of primary and secondary treatment resistances, MCL remains the lymphoma subtype with the poorest long-term outcome.[5,16,21] Thus, MCL represents a major challenge to clinicians and researchers. This section summarizes the knowledge on the different therapeutic approaches in the treatment of MCL with special focus on recent improvements.

Radiation in early stages

Mantle cell lymphoma is usually diagnosed in advanced Ann Arbor stage III or IV. Patients with limited disease potentially may be cured by extended or involved field radiation. However, the data available on the efficacy of radiation in MCL are limited and thus several studies are currently being performed to evaluate the activity of radiation therapy in MCL more precisely.

A recent study of Leitch et al. suggested an advantage of sequential radiochemotherapy.[27] In contrast, in advanced stage III–IV, the benefit of radiation is not proven. Thus radiation therapy should only be applied in clinical trials.

Chemotherapeutic approaches

INDUCTION THERAPY

Due to the aggressive clinical course and the poor prognosis, various attempts have been performed to overcome limitations by implementing several drug combinations including alkylating agents, anthracyclines, or purine analogues. However, they all failed to substantially alter the long-term outcome, achieving overall response rates of approximately 60–80 percent with complete remissions in only 20–30 percent of cases.[6,28] Thus, conventional chemotherapy remains a noncurative approach. Due to the aggressive course, a 'watch and wait' strategy should be pursued only in very selected cases and therapy should be initiated as soon as possible after diagnosis.

The efficacy of anthracycline-containing regimens was evaluated in various studies (Table 65.1). However, in the

Table 65.1   Anthracyclines in the treatment of advanced stage mantle cell lymphoma

Author	n	Disease status	Regimen	CR/OR (%/%)	PFS (mo)	OS (mo)
Meusers et al. 1989[29]	37	First-line therapy	COP	41/84	10	32
	26		CHOP	58/89	7	37
Unterhalt et al. 1996[80]	20	First-line therapy	COP	5/80	NA	NA
	19		PmM	27/80		
Zinzani et al. 2000[33]	18	First-line therapy	Fludarabine/idarubicin	33/61	NA	NA
	11		Fludarabine	27/73		
Nickenig et al. 2006[30]	90	First-line therapy	CHOP	15/87	21	NA
			MCP	20/73	15	NA
Lenz et al. 2005[7]	60	First-line therapy	CHOP	7/75	19	Median not reached

COP: cyclophosphamide, vincristine, and prednisone; CHOP: cyclophosphamide, doxorubicin, vincristine, and prednisone; PmM: prednimustine, mitoxantrone; MCP: mitoxantrone, chlorambucil, and prednisone; n, number of patients; CR, complete remission; OR, overall response; PFS, progression-free survival; mo, months; OS, overall survival; NA, not available.

Table 65.2   Efficacy of fludarabine in the treatment of mantle cell lymphoma

Author	Regimen	n	Disease status	CR/OR (%/%)
Decaudin et al. 1998[32]	Fludarabine 25 mg/m^2/d × 5	15	Untreated and relapsed	0/33
Foran et al. 1999[31]	Fludarabine 25 mg/m^2/d × 5	17	Untreated	29/41
McLaughlin et al. 1996[35]	Fludarabine 25 mg/m^2/d × 3 Mitoxantrone 10 mg/m^2/d × 1 Dexamethasone 20 mg/d × 5	5	Relapsed	20/80
Flinn et al. 2000[36]	Fludarabine 20 mg/m^2/d × 5 Cyclophosphamide 600 mg/m^2/d × 1	10	Untreated	40/80
Cohen et al. 2001[37]	Fludarabine 20–25 mg/m^2/d × 3 Cyclophosphamide 600 mg/m^2/d × 1	30	Untreated and relapsed	30/63
Seymour et al. 2002[38]	Fludarabine 30 mg/m^2/d × 2 Cisplatin 25 mg/m^2/d × 4 Cytarabine 500 mg/m^2/d × 2	8	Relapsed	88 (OR)

n, number of patients; CR, complete remission; OR, overall response.

only randomized trial, no advantage of the anthracycline-containing CHOP regimen (cyclophosphamide, doxorubicin, vincristine, and prednisone) in comparison to a non-anthracycline combination (COP: cyclophosphamide, vincristine, and prednisone) was detectable.[29] The overall response rate (84 percent after COP vs 89 percent after CHOP), the relapse-free survival (10 vs 7 months), as well as the overall survival (32 vs 37 months) were not significantly different in the two study arms. These results were confirmed by a retrospective analysis by Weisenburger et al.[16] In contrast, in a retrospective study, Zucca and colleagues showed the superiority of anthracycline-containing regimens in MCL patients with low and low-intermediate risk profile according to the IPI.[6] Similarly, a recent prospective trial detected a borderline advantage of a CHOP regimen.[30] Thus, although clinical trials could not uniformly prove the superiority of anthracycline-containing combinations, many clinicians favor CHOP-like regimens as MCL is characterized by an aggressive course (Table 65.1).

The use of purine analogues (e.g., fludarabine, cladribine) has been investigated in various studies (Table 65.2).[11,31–33]

Fludarabine, which has high activity in follicular lymphoma and in chronic lymphocytic leukemia, showed only moderate efficacy in MCL when applied as a single agent with overall response rates of approximately 30–40 percent (Table 65.2). In contrast, based on an in vitro synergism,[34] combinations with either alkylating agents (e.g., cyclophosphamide) or anthracyclines (e.g., mitoxantrone, idarubicin) are able to achieve significantly higher remission rates (Table 65.2).[35–38] In the study of Cohen et al., the combination of fludarabine and cyclophosphamide was highly effective in newly diagnosed and relapsed or refractory disease.[37] Previously untreated patients had an overall response rate of 100 percent (70 percent complete and 30 percent partial remissions) with a progression-free survival of 28.1 months (Table 65.2). The use of cladribine has been investigated in a multicenter phase II study in combination with mitoxantrone.[39] This combination showed high activity, achieving an overall response rate of 100 percent and a complete remission rate of 44 percent with a median duration of remission of 24 months. However, the number of investigated patients was rather small and efficacy

Table 65.3   Combined immunochemotherapy in mantle cell lymphoma

Author	*n*	Regimen	CR/OR (%/%)	PFS (mo)	OS (mo)
Howard *et al.* 2002[19]	40	R-CHOP	48/96	17	NA
Forstpointner *et al.* 2004[8]	24	R-FCM	33/62[a]	8	Median not reached
Lenz *et al.* 2005[7]	62	R-CHOP	34/94[a]	19	Median not reached
Herold *et al.* 2004[81]	44	R-MCP	32/71	20	Median not reached
Rummel *et al.* 2005[82]	16[b]	R-Bendamustine	50/75	18	Not available
Romaguera *et al.* 2005[83]	97	R-HyperCVAD	87/97	64 (3 years)	82 (3 years)

[a]Significant improvement in comparison to chemotherapy alone; [b]relapsed disease.
R-CHOP: rituximab, cyclophosphamide, doxorubicin, vincristine, and prednisone; R-FCM: rituximab, fludarabine, cyclophosphamide, mitoxantrone; R-MCP: rituximab, mitoxantrone, chlorambucil, and prednisone; *n*, number of patients; CR, complete remission; OR, overall response; PFS, progression-free survival; mo, months; OS, overall survival; NA, not available; [b] relapsed disease.

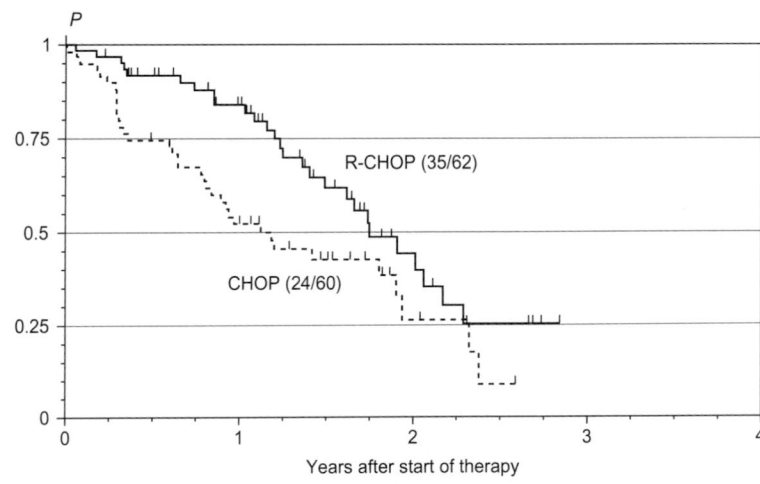

Figure 65.1   Time to treatment failure (TTF) after initiation of CHOP and R-CHOP.[7] Patients assigned to R-CHOP experienced a significantly longer TTF ($P = 0.0131$). Values shown in parentheses are number of censored patients/total number of patients.

has to be confirmed in additional trials. Another alternative approach, especially in medically nonfit patients, is bendamustine because of its comparable response rates but limited side effects.

Various other studies investigated the efficacy of high-dose cytarabine (Ara-C), reporting very promising results. In the study of Lefrere *et al.*, more than 80 percent of patients obtained a complete remission following a sequential CHOP-DHAP regimen (dexamethasone, high-dose cytarabine, and cisplatin).[40] Similarly, high response rates of more than 90 percent could be demonstrated by the MD Anderson Cancer Center applying an alternating regimen of hyper-CVAD (fractionated cyclophosphamide, vincristine, doxorubicin, and dexamethasone) with high-dose cytarabine and methotrexate in elderly patients not suitable for stem cell transplantation.[41] As these data suggest a high efficacy of high-dose cytarabine in MCL, the European MCL Network is currently testing this concept in a phase III trial.[42]

MONOCLONAL ANTIBODIES

Another encouraging approach is represented by the anti-CD20 antibody rituximab. Rituximab is a chimeric murine/human monoclonal antibody which binds the B cell-specific antigen CD20. *In vitro* studies demonstrated that rituximab lyzes $CD20^+$ cells by complement activation or antibody-dependent cell-mediated cytotoxicity.[43,44] The high expression of CD20 makes MCL an attractive target for rituximab treatment. However, response rates of only 20–35 percent could be achieved by a rituximab monotherapy in relapsed or refractory disease.[45–47] In contrast, based on a proposed *in vitro* synergism, a combined immunochemotherapy of rituximab and CHOP (R-CHOP) achieved high overall and complete remission rates (96 percent/48 percent) in a recent phase II study (Table 65.3).[19] Based on these promising results, the German Low Grade Lymphoma Study Group (GLSG) initiated a randomized trial comparing the combination of rituximab and CHOP to CHOP alone in previously untreated patients with advanced stage MCL.[7] R-CHOP was significantly superior to CHOP in terms of overall response rate (94 percent vs 75 percent; $P = 0.0054$), complete remission rate (34 percent vs 7 percent; $P = 0.00024$; Tables 65.2 and 65.3), and time to treatment failure (TTF; median 21 vs 14 months; $P = 0.0131$; Fig. 65.1). However, no differences were observed for the progression-free survival. Thus, R-CHOP might represent a new baseline regimen for advanced stage MCL which needs to be further improved by novel strategies in remission.

Table 65.4   Autologous stem cell transplantation in the treatment of mantle cell lymphoma

Author	n	Disease status	PFS	OS
Dreger *et al.* 2000[64]	34	First-line therapy	77% (2 years)	100% (2 years)
	12	Relapsed/refractory	30% (2 years)	54% (2 years)
Dreyling *et al.* 2005[9]	62	First-line therapy	54% (3 years)	83% (3 years)
Andersen *et al.* 2003[61]	27	First-line therapy	15% (4 years)	51% (4 years)
Vandenberghe *et al.* 2003[62]	195	First-line therapy/relapsed/refractory	55% (2 years)	76% (2 years)
Geisler *et al.*[84]	160	First-line therapy	66% (6 years)	70% (6 years)

n, number of patients; PFS, progression-free survival; OS, overall survival.

In elderly patients in particular, the combination of bendamustine and rituximab has shown high efficiency paired with favorable side effects.

In patients with relapsed or refractory MCL who were treated with the combination of rituximab and the FCM regimen (fludarabine, cyclophosphamide, and mitox-antrone), an improved overall response rate (58 percent vs 46 percent) and even more importantly an improved overall survival could be achieved in comparison to FCM chemotherapy alone (Table 65.3).[8]

Consolidation

INTERFERON α

Two phase III studies investigated the value of interferon α (IFNα) maintenance following conventional induction therapy.[48,49] Both trials demonstrated a tendency toward a prolonged progression-free survival in MCL patients receiving IFNα in comparison to observation alone. However, the number of patients was too low to definitely answer the question of to what extent IFNα may be of benefit.

RITUXIMAB MAINTENANCE

Besides promising results in phase II trials, a small randomized trial (*n* = 48) detected a significant benefit of rituximab maintenance after initial salvage immuno-chemotherapy in relapsed MCL.[50,51] After 3 years of follow-up, all patients in the control arm relapsed whereas after ritxuimab maintenance 30 percent of patients were still in ongoing remission. Currently this concept is being tested in first-line treatment of MCL.[42]

RADIOIMMUNOTHERAPY

An innovative approach is the application of radio-labeled (iodine-131 or yttrium-90) anti-CD20 antibodies. Myeloablative regimens achieved a high rate of and long-lasting remissions in relapsed or refractory MCL patients whereas conventional-dose regimens resulted in only rather short remissions.[52,53] Gopal and colleagues investigated the efficacy of the iodine-131-labeled anti-CD20 antibody tositumomab in pretreated patients with MCL in combination with high-dose chemotherapy followed by autologous stem cell transplantation.[52] High overall response rates of 100 percent with 91 percent complete remissions were reported with an estimated 3-year overall survival of 93 percent. In contrast, conventional-dose radioimmunotherapy (RIT) delivered varying results with 36 percent overall response and rapid progresses resulting in a median progression-free survival of 3 months only in relapsed disease.[53] Thus, the concept of a radioimmunotherapy is currently being evaluated as consolidation after chemotherapy induction. In a phase II trial, MCL patients received conventional-dose RIT after 4 cycles of R-CHOP.[54] Complete remission rate increased from 13 percent to 55 percent after RIT, translating to a median progression-free survival of 33 months.

AUTOLOGOUS STEM CELL TRANSPLANTATION

Encouraging results were also obtained by different phase II studies exploring the potential of consolidation by myeloablative therapy followed by autologous stem cell transplantation (ASCT) to eliminate residual lymphoma cells after conventional chemotherapy (Table 65.4).[55–64] In order to define the impact of this approach more precisely, the European MCL Network performed a randomized trial comparing myeloablative radiochemotherapy followed by ASCT as consolidation in first remission to IFNα maintenance in 122 patients up to 65 years of age.[9] Patients in the ASCT arm experienced a significantly longer progression-free survival with a median of 39 months compared to only 17 months for patients in the IFNα study arm (*P* = 0.0108; Fig. 65.2). After a longer follow-up, median overall survival was 7.5 years after ASCT versus 5.4 years in the IFNα group. Thus, myeloablative radiochemotherapy followed by ASCT represents one of the most effective therapeutic approaches in first remission. In contrast, efficacy in advanced relapsed disease seems to be limited.[65]

However, even after such a dose-intensified consolidation, the vast majority of patients with MCL will eventually relapse. One major obstacle of stem cell transplantation

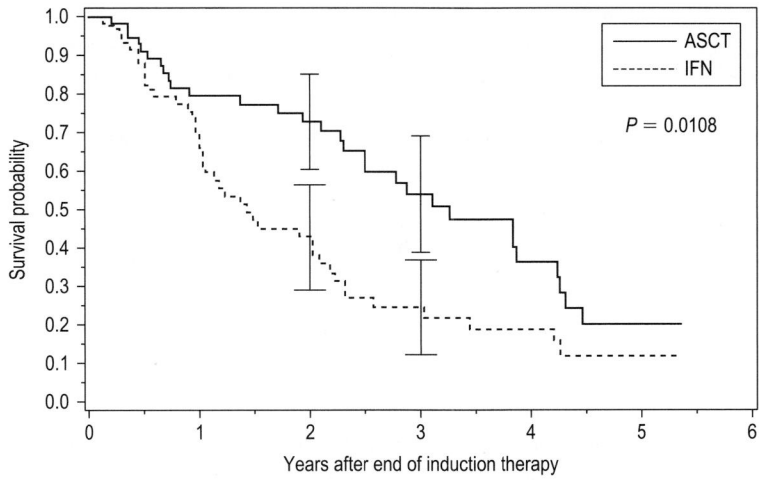

Figure 65.2 Progression-free survival after high-dose radiochemotherapy followed by autologous stem cell transplantation (ASCT) and interferon α (IFN) maintenance in mantle cell lymphoma. Patients assigned to stem cell transplantation experience significantly longer progression-free survival (log rank-test).[9] Vertical bars indicate 95% confidence intervals for progression-free survival.

is the contamination of the harvested stem cells with circulating lymphoma cells. Thus, *in vitro* as well as *in vivo* purging procedures have been introduced to eliminate residual lymphoma cells.[66,67] Antibody-based *in vivo* purging, especially, seems to be a very efficient approach. In previously untreated MCL patients, Gianni *et al.* reported an overall survival of 89 percent at 54 months following an *in vivo* purging with rituximab and subsequent high-dose consolidation.[66]

Allogeneic transplantation

Allogeneic bone marrow or stem cell transplantation is still the only curative approach in patients with advanced stage MCL. A graft-versus-lymphoma effect has been suggested which is capable of inducing long-lasting complete remissions even in patients with relapsed or refractory MCL.[68–70] However, transplantation-related mortality is relatively high and especially graft-versus-host disease and infectious complications are common. Thus, allogeneic transplantation in first complete remission should not be applied outside of clinical trials.[71]

New innovative approaches

A new molecular targeting agent is the proteasome inhibitor bortezomib (Velcade®) which showed high activity in the therapy of relapsed multiple myeloma. Very promising results have also been reported in various phase II studies in relapsed MCL patients.[72–74] Approximately 30–40 percent of previously heavily pretreated patients responded to bortezomib therapy at a dose of 1.3 mg/m^2. Thus, various phase III studies are currently evaluating the efficacy of a combined approach of bortezomib and conventional chemotherapy.[75]

Another molecular targeting agent in the treatment of MCL is the cyclin-dependent kinase inhibitor flavopiridol. First studies showed only moderate efficacy in the treatment of MCL which was significantly improved after pharmacokinetic modulation of the application scheme.[76,77] As cell culture experiments suggest a chemosensitizing effect, flavopiridol might be even more effective in combination with chemotherapy.

Immunomodulatory agents (IMiDs) have been also proven to be highly effective in MCL. Thalidomide in combination with rituximab achieved responses in 13 out of 16 predominantly rituximab-naïve patients.[78] Most patients required a dose reduction of thalidomide due to anticipated toxicities of somnolence, fatigue, and constipation. Even more encouraging are the response rates of up to 50 percent of lenalidomide in relapsed MCL, paired with a more favorable toxicity profile.

Finally, in a small phase II study ($n = 34$), the mammalian target of rapamycin (mTOR) inhibitor temsirolimus (CCI-7709) achieved sustained remissions in 38 percent of patients.[79]

SUMMARY AND PERSPECTIVES

Mantle cell lymphoma represents a rare lymphoma subentity which mainly occurs in elderly men. It is characterized by an aggressive clinical course and poor prognosis with a median survival of only 3–4 years. Whereas conventional chemotherapy represents a noncurative approach only, promising results have been achieved recently by a combined immunochemotherapy with the anti-CD20 antibody rituximab in first-line therapy as well as in relapsed disease. Additionally, high-dose therapy followed by autologous stem cell transplantation proved to be an effective consolidation strategy. However, the majority of patients will eventually relapse and allogeneic transplantation is still the only curative treatment option. Thus, new therapeutic agents are currently being evaluated to improve the long-term perspectives of MCL patients.

KEY POINTS

- Histology: varying morphology, detection of cyclin D1 overexpression essential.
- Prognostic factors: cell proliferation (Ki67 [MIB-1], M1P1).
- Clinical presentation: advanced stage, male preponderance, extranodal involvement.
- Clinical course: short remissions after conventional regimens, 5 years median survival.
- Dose intensification achieves prolonged remissions.
- Molecular approaches: proteasome inhibitors, IMIDS, mTOR inhibitors.

REFERENCES

● = Key primary paper
◆ = Major review article

1. Harris NL, Jaffe ES, Stein H et al. A revised European-American classification of lymphoid neoplasms: a proposal from the International Lymphoma Study Group. Blood 1994; **84**: 1361–92.
2. Swerdlow SH, Campo E, Harris NL et al. (eds) WHO classification of tumours of haematopoietic and lymphoid tissues. Lyon: IARC Press, 2008.
3. Meusers P, Hense J, Brittinger G. Mantle cell lymphoma: diagnostic criteria, clinical aspects and therapeutic problems. Leukemia 1997; **11**(Suppl 2): S60–4.
4. Weisenburger DD, Armitage JO. Mantle cell lymphoma – an entity comes of age. Blood 1996; **87**: 4483–94.
5. Dreyling M, Weigert O, Hiddemann W. Current treatment standards and future strategies in mantle cell lymphoma. Ann Oncol 2008; **19**(Suppl 4): iv41–4.
6. Zucca E, Roggero E, Pinotti G et al. Patterns of survival in mantle cell lymphoma. Ann Oncol 1995; **6**: 257–62.
●7. Lenz G, Dreyling M, Hoster E et al. Immuno-chemotherapy with rituximab and CHOP significantly improves response and time to treatment failure but not long-term outcome in patients with previously untreated mantle cell lymphoma – results of a prospective randomized trial of the German Low Grade Lymphoma Study Group (GLSG). J Clin Oncol 2005; **23**: 1984–92.
8. Forstpointner R, Dreyling M, Repp R et al. The addition of rituximab to a combination of fludarabine, cyclophosphamide, mitoxantrone (FCM) significantly increases the response rate and prolongs survival as compared to FCM alone in patients with relapsed and refractory follicular and mantle cell lymphomas – results of a prospective randomized study of the German Low Grade Lymphoma Study Group (GLSG). Blood 2004; **104**: 3064–71.
●9. Dreyling M, Lenz G, Hoster E et al. Early consolidation by myeloablative radiochemotherapy followed by autologous stem cell transplantation in first remission significantly prolongs progression-free survival in mantle cell lymphoma – results of a prospective randomized trial of the European MCL Network. Blood 2005; **105**: 2677–84.
10. Dreyling MH, Hiddemann W, for the European MCL Study Group. Prognostic factors in mantle cell lymphoma: Clinical characteristics, pathology and cell proliferation. J Clin Oncol 1999; **18**: 3a (abstract).
11. Samaha H, Dumontet C, Ketterer N et al. Mantle cell lymphoma: a retrospective study of 121 cases. Leukemia 1998; **12**: 1281–7.
◆12. Fernandez V, Hartmann E, Ott G et al. Pathogenesis of mantle-cell lymphoma: all oncogenic roads lead to dysregulation of cell cycle and DNA damage response pathways. J Clin Oncol 2005; **23**: 6364–9.
13. Pittaluga S, Wlodarska I, Stul MS et al. Mantle cell lymphoma: a clinicopathological study of 55 cases. Histopathology 1995; **26**: 17–24.
14. Velders GA, Kluin-Nelemans JC, De Boer CJ et al. Mantle-cell lymphoma: a population-based clinical study. J Clin Oncol 1996; **14**: 1269–74.
15. Ferrer A, Bosch F, Villamor N et al. Central nervous system involvement in mantle cell lymphoma. Ann Oncol 2008; **19**: 135–41.
16. Weisenburger DD, Vose JM, Greiner TC et al. Mantle cell lymphoma. A clinicopathologic study of 68 cases from the Nebraska Lymphoma Study Group. Am J Hematol 2000; **64**: 190–6.
●17. Hoster E, Dreyling M, Klapper W et al. A new prognostic index (MIPI) for patients with advanced stage mantle cell lymphoma. Blood 2008; **111**: 558–65.
18. Pott C, Schrader C, Gesk S et al. Quantitative assessment of molecular remission following high-dose therapy with autologous stem cell transplantation predicts long term remission in mantle cell lymphoma. Blood 2006; **107**: 2271–8.
19. Howard OM, Gribben JG, Neuberg DS et al. Rituximab and CHOP induction therapy for newly diagnosed mantle-cell lymphoma: molecular complete responses are not predictive of progression-free survival. J Clin Oncol 2002; **20**: 1288–94.
◆20. Jares P, Colomer D, Campo E. Genetic and molecular pathogenesis of mantle cell lymphoma: perspectives for new targeted therapeutics. Nat Rev Cancer 2007; **7**: 750–62.
●21. Tiemann M, Schrader C, Klapper W et al. Histopathology, cell proliferation indices and clinical outcome in 304 patients with mantle cell lymphoma (MCL): a clinicopathological study from the European MCL Network. Br J Haematol 2005; **131**: 29–38.
22. Norton AJ, Matthews J, Pappa V et al. Mantle cell lymphoma: natural history defined in a serially biopsied population over a 20-year period. Ann Oncol 1995; **6**: 249–56.

23. Greiner TC, Moynihan MJ, Chan WC *et al.* *p53* mutations in mantle cell lymphoma are associated with variant cytology and predict a poor prognosis. *Blood* 1996; **87**: 4302–10.

24. Hernandez L, Fest T, Cazorla M *et al.* *p53* gene mutations and protein overexpression are associated with aggressive variants of mantle cell lymphomas. *Blood* 1996; **87**: 3351–9.

25. Zoldan MC, Inghirami G, Masuda Y *et al.* Large-cell variants of mantle cell lymphoma: cytologic characteristics and *p53* anomalies may predict poor outcome. *Br J Haematol* 1996; **93**: 475–86.

●26. Rosenwald A, Wright G, Wiestner A *et al.* The proliferation gene expression signature is a quantitative integrator of oncogenic events that predicts survival in mantle cell lymphoma. *Cancer Cell* 2003; **3**: 185–97.

27. Leitch HA, Gascoyne RD, Chhanabhai M *et al.* Limited stage mantle cell lymphoma. *Ann Oncol* 2003; **10**: 1555–61.

28. Vandenberghe E, De Wolf-Peeters C, Vaughan Hudson G *et al.* The clinical outcome of 65 cases of mantle cell lymphoma initially treated with non-intensive therapy by the British National Lymphoma Investigation Group. *Br J Haematol* 1997; **99**: 842–7.

29. Meusers P, Engelhard M, Bartels H *et al.* Multicentre randomized therapeutic trial for advanced centrocytic lymphoma: anthracycline does not improve the prognosis. *Hematol Oncol* 1989; **7**: 365–80.

30. Nickenig C, Dreyling M, Hoster E *et al.* CHOP improves response rates but not survival and has a lower hematologic toxicity as compared to MCP in follicular and mantle cell lymphomas – results of a prospective randomized trial of the German Low Grade Lymphoma Study Group (GLSG). *Cancer* 2006; **107**: 1014–22.

31. Foran JM, Rohatiner AZ, Coiffier B *et al.* Multicenter phase II study of fludarabine phosphate for patients with newly diagnosed lymphoplasmacytoid lymphoma, Waldenstrom's macroglobulinemia, and mantle-cell lymphoma. *J Clin Oncol* 1999; **17**: 546–53.

32. Decaudin D, Bosq J, Tertian G *et al.* Phase II trial of fludarabine monophosphate in patients with mantle-cell lymphomas. *J Clin Oncol* 1998; **16**: 579–83.

33. Zinzani PL, Magagnoli M, Moretti L *et al.* Randomized trial of fludarabine versus fludarabine and idarubicin as frontline treatment in patients with indolent or mantle-cell lymphoma. *J Clin Oncol* 2000; **18**: 773–9.

34. Koehl U, Li L, Nowak B *et al.* Fludarabine and cyclophosphamide: synergistic cytotoxicity associated with inhibition of interstrand cross-link removal. *Proceedings of the American Society of Clinical Oncology (ASCO)* 1997; **38**: A10 (abstract).

35. McLaughlin P, Hagemeister FB, Romaguera JE *et al.* Fludarabine, mitoxantrone, and dexamethasone: an effective new regimen for indolent lymphoma. *J Clin Oncol* 1996; **14**: 1262–8.

36. Flinn IW, Byrd JC, Morrison C *et al.* Fludarabine and cyclophosphamide with filgrastim support in patients with previously untreated indolent lymphoid malignancies. *Blood* 2000; **96**: 71–5.

37. Cohen BJ, Moskowitz C, Straus D *et al.* Cyclophosphamide/fludarabine (CF) is active in the treatment of mantle cell lymphoma. *Leuk Lymphoma* 2001; **42**: 1015–22.

38. Seymour JF, Grigg AP, Szer J *et al.* Cisplatin, fludarabine, and cytarabine: a novel, pharmacologically designed salvage therapy for patients with refractory, histologically aggressive or mantle cell non-Hodgkin's lymphoma. *Cancer* 2002; **94**: 585–93.

39. Rummel M, Chow K, Karakas T *et al.* Reduced-dose cladribine (2-CdA) plus mitoxantrone is effective in the treatment of mantle-cell and low-grade non-Hodgkin's lymphoma. *Eur J Cancer* 2002; **38**: 1739–46.

40. Lefrere F, Delmer A, Suzan F *et al.* Sequential chemotherapy by CHOP and DHAP regimens followed by high-dose therapy with stem cell transplantation induces a high rate of complete response and improves event-free survival in mantle cell lymphoma: a prospective study. *Leukemia* 2002; **16**: 587–93.

41. Romaguera JE, Khouri IF, Kantarjian HM *et al.* Untreated aggressive mantle cell lymphoma: results with intensive chemotherapy without stem cell transplant in elderly patients. *Leuk Lymphoma* 2000; **39**: 77–85.

42. Dreyling M, Hoster E, Hermine O *et al.* European MCL Network: An update on current first line trials. *Blood* 2007; **110**: 388.

43. Manches O, Lui G, Chaperot L *et al.* In vitro mechanisms of action of rituximab on primary non-Hodgkin lymphomas. *Blood* 2003; **101**: 949–54.

44. Smith MR. Rituximab (monoclonal anti-CD20 antibody): mechanisms of action and resistance. *Oncogene* 2003; **22**: 7359–68.

45. Ghielmini M, Schmitz Hsu S-F, Cogliatti S *et al.* Effect of single-agent rituximab given at the standard schedule or as prolonged treatment in patients with mantle cell lymphoma: a study of the Swiss Group for Clinical Cancer Research (SAKK). *J Clin Oncol* 2005; **23**: 705–11.

46. Foran JM, Cunningham D, Coiffier B *et al.* Treatment of mantle-cell lymphoma with Rituximab (chimeric monoclonal anti-CD20 antibody): analysis of factors associated with response. *Ann Oncol* 2000; **11**: 117–21.

47. Tobinai K. Monoclonal antibody therapy for B-cell lymphoma: clinical trials of an anti-CD20 monoclonal antibody for B-cell lymphoma in Japan. *Int J Hematol* 2002; **76**: 411–19.

48. Hiddemann W, Unterhalt M, Herrmann R *et al.* Mantle-cell lymphomas have more widespread disease and a slower response to chemotherapy compared with follicle-center lymphomas: results of a prospective comparative analysis of the German Low-Grade Lymphoma Study Group. *J Clin Oncol* 1998; **16**: 1922–30.

49. Teodorovic I, Pittaluga S, Kluin-Nelemans JC *et al.* Efficacy of four different regimens in 64 mantle-cell lymphoma cases: clinicopathologic comparison with 498 other non-Hodgkin's lymphoma subtypes. European Organization for the Research and Treatment of Cancer

Lymphoma Cooperative Group. *J Clin Oncol* 1995; **13**: 2819–26.

50. Kahl BS, Longo WL, Eickhoff JC *et al*. Maintenance rituximab following induction chemoimmunotherapy may prolong progression-free survival in mantle cell lymphoma: a pilot study from the Wisconsin Oncology Network. *Ann Oncol* 2006; **17**: 1418–23.

51. Forstpointner R, Unterhalt M, Dreyling M. Maintenance therapy with rituximab leads to a significant prolongation of response duration after salvage therapy with a combination of rituximab, fludarabine, cyclophosphamide and mitoxantrone (R-FCM) in patients with relapsed and refractory follicular and mantle cell lymphomas – results of a prospective randomized study of the German Low Grade Lymphoma Study Group (GLSG). *Blood* 2006; **108**: 4003–8.

52. Gopal AK, Rajendran JG, Petersdorf SH *et al*. High-dose chemo-radioimmunotherapy with autologous stem cell support for relapsed mantle cell lymphoma. *Blood* 2002; **99**: 3158–62.

53. Weigert O, Jurczak W, von Schilling C *et al*. Efficacy of radioimmunotherapy with (^{90}Y) ibritumomab tiuxetan is superior as consolidation in relapsed or refractory mantle cell lymphoma: results of two phase II trials of the European MCL Network and the PLSG. *J Clin Oncol* 2006; **24**(18 Suppl): 7502 (abstract).

54. Smith MR, Zhang L, Gordon LI *et al*. Phase II study of R-CHOP followed by 90Y-ibritumomab tiuxetan in untreated mantle cell lymphoma: Eastern Cooperative Oncology Group Study E1499. *Blood (ASH Annual Meeting Abstracts)* 2007; **110**: 389 (abstract).

55. Stewart DA, Vose JM, Weisenburger DD *et al*. The role of high-dose therapy and autologous hematopoietic stem cell transplantation for mantle cell lymphoma. *Ann Oncol* 1995; **6**: 263–6.

56. Ketterer N, Salles G, Espinouse D *et al*. Intensive therapy with peripheral stem cell transplantation in 16 patients with mantle cell lymphoma. *Ann Oncol* 1997; **8**: 701–4.

57. Haas R, Brittinger G, Meusers P *et al*. Myeloablative therapy with blood stem cell transplantation is effective in mantle cell lymphoma. *Leukemia* 1996; **10**: 1975–9.

58. Khouri IF, Romaguera J, Kantarjian H *et al*. Hyper-CVAD and high-dose methotrexate/cytarabine followed by stem-cell transplantation: an active regimen for aggressive mantle-cell lymphoma. *J Clin Oncol* 1998; **16**: 3803–9.

59. Milpied N, Gaillard F, Moreau P *et al*. High-dose therapy with stem cell transplantation for mantle cell lymphoma: results and prognostic factors, a single center experience. *Bone Marrow Transplant* 1998; **22**: 645–50.

60. Freedman AS, Neuberg D, Gribben JG *et al*. High-dose chemoradiotherapy and anti-B-cell monoclonal antibody-purged autologous bone marrow transplantation in mantle-cell lymphoma: no evidence for long-term remission. *J Clin Oncol* 1998; **16**: 13–18.

61. Andersen NS, Pedersen L, Elonen E *et al*. Primary treatment with autologous stem cell transplantation in mantle cell lymphoma: outcome related to remission pretransplant. *Eur J Haematol* 2003; **71**: 73–80.

62. Vandenberghe E, Ruiz de Elvira C, Loberiza FR *et al*. Outcome of autologous transplantation for mantle cell lymphoma: a study by the European Blood and Bone Marrow Transplant and Autologous Blood and Marrow Transplant Registries. *Br J Haematol* 2003; **120**: 793–800.

63. Mangel J, Leitch HA, Connors JM *et al*. Intensive chemotherapy and autologous stem-cell transplantation plus rituximab is superior to conventional chemotherapy for newly diagnosed advanced stage mantle-cell lymphoma: a matched pair analysis. *Ann Oncol* 2004; **15**: 283–90.

64. Dreger P, Martin S, Kuse R *et al*. The impact of autologous stem cell transplantation on the prognosis of mantle cell lymphoma: a joint analysis of two prospective studies with 46 patients. *Hematol J* 2000; **1**: 87–94.

65. Dreger P, Martin S, Kroger N *et al*. The impact of early stem cell transplantation on the prognosis of mantle cell lymphoma. *Blood* 1999; **94**: 750 (abstract).

66. Gianni AM, Magni M, Martelli M *et al*. Long-term remission in mantle cell lymphoma following high-dose sequential chemotherapy and in vivo rituximab-purged stem cell autografting (R-HDS regimen). *Blood* 2003; **102**: 749–55.

67. Magni M, Di Nicola M, Devizzi L *et al*. Successful in vivo purging of CD34-containing peripheral blood harvests in mantle cell and indolent lymphoma: evidence for a role of both chemotherapy and rituximab infusion. *Blood* 2000; **96**: 864–9.

68. Grigg A, Bardy P, Byron K *et al*. Fludarabine-based non-myeloablative chemotherapy followed by infusion of HLA-identical stem cells for relapsed leukemia and lymphoma. *Bone Marrow Transplant* 1999; **23**: 107–10.

69. Adkins D, Brown R, Goodnough LT *et al*. Treatment of resistant mantle cell lymphoma with allogeneic bone marrow transplantation. *Bone Marrow Transplant* 1998; **21**: 97–9.

70. Khouri IF, Lee MS, Saliba RM *et al*. Nonablative allogeneic stem-cell transplantation for advanced/recurrent mantle-cell lymphoma. *J Clin Oncol* 2003; **21**: 4407–12.

71. Robinson SP, Goldstone AH, Mackinnon S *et al*. Chemoresistant or aggressive lymphoma predicts for a poor outcome following reduced-intensity allogeneic progenitor cell transplantation: an analysis from the Lymphoma Working Party of the European Group for Blood and Bone Marrow Transplantation. *Blood* 2002; **100**: 4310–16.

72. Goy A, Hart S, Pro B *et al*. Report of a phase II study of proteasome inhibitor bortezomib (Velcade) in patients with relapsed or refractory indolent or aggressive lymphomas. *J Clin Oncol* 2005; **23**: 657–8.

73. O'Connor OA, Wright J, Moskowitz C *et al*. Phase II clinical experience with the novel proteasome inhibitor bortezomib in patients with indolent non-Hodgkin's lymphoma and mantle cell lymphoma. *J Clin Oncol* 2005; **23**: 676–84.

•74. Fisher RI, Bernstein SH, Kahl BS *et al.* Multicenter phase II study of bortezomib in patients with relapsed or refractory mantle cell lymphoma. *J Clin Oncol* 2006; **24**: 4867–74.

75. Weigert O, Pastore A, Rieken M *et al.* Sequence-dependent synergy of the proteasome inhibitor bortezomib and cytarabine in mantle cell lymphoma. *Leukemia* 2007; **21**: 524–8.

76. Kouroukis CT, Belch A, Crump M *et al.* Flavopiridol in untreated or relapsed mantle-cell lymphoma: results of a phase II study of the National Cancer Institute of Canada Clinical Trials Group. *J Clin Oncol* 2003; **21**: 1740–5.

77. Byrd JC, Lin TS, Dalton JT *et al.* Flavopiridol administered as a pharmacologically-derived schedule demonstrates marked clinical activity in refractory, genetically high risk, chronic lymphocytic leukemia (CLL). *Blood* 2004; **104**: 101a (abstract).

78. Kaufmann H, Raderer M, Wohrer S *et al.* Antitumor activity of rituximab plus thalidomide in patients with relapsed/refractory mantle cell lymphoma. *Blood* 2004; **104**: 2269–71.

79. Witzig TE, Geyer SM, Ghobrial I *et al.* Phase II trial of single-agent temsirolimus (CCI-779) for relapsed mantle cell lymphoma. *J Clin Oncol* 2005; **23**: 5347–56.

80. Unterhalt M, Herrmann R, Tiemann M *et al.* Prednimustine, mitoxantrone (PmM) vs cyclophosphamide, vincristine, prednisone (COP) for the treatment of advanced low-grade non-Hodgkin's lymphoma. German Low-Grade Lymphoma Study Group. *Leukemia* 1996; **10**: 836–43.

81. Herold M, Pasold R, Srock S *et al.* Results of a prospective randomised open label phase III study comparing rituximab plus mitoxantrone, chlorambucile, prednisolone chemotherapy (R-MCP) versus MCP alone in untreated advanced indolent non-Hdogkin's lymphoma (NHL) and mantle cell lymphoma (MCL). *Blood* 2004; **104**: 168a (abstract).

•82. Rummel MJ, Al-Batran SE, Kim SZ *et al.* Bendamustine plus rituximab is effective and has a favourable toxicity profile in the treatment of mantle cell and low-grade non-Hodgkin's lymphoma. *J Clin Oncol* 2005; **23**: 3383–9.

•83. Romaguera JE, Fayad L, Rodriguez MA *et al.* High rate of durable remissions after treatment of newly diagnosed aggressive mantle-cell lymphoma with rituximab plus hyper-CVAD alternating with rituximab plus high-dose methotrexate and cytarabine. *J Clin Oncol* 2005; **23**: 7013–23.

•84. Geisler CH, Kolstad A, Laurell A *et al.* Long-term progression-free survival of mantle cell lymphoma after intensive front-line immunochemotherapy with in vivo-purged stem cell rescue: a nonrandomized phase 2 multicenter study by the Nordic Lymphoma Group. *Blood* 2008; **112**: 2687–93.

66

Marginal zone lymphomas

EMANUELE ZUCCA AND FRANCO CAVALLI

DEFINITION AND CLASSIFICATION OF MARGINAL ZONE LYMPHOMAS

In the World Health Organization (WHO) classification of tumors of hematopoietic and lymphoid tissues, the group of marginal zone lymphomas (MZL) comprises three different subtypes, namely the *extranodal marginal zone B cell lymphoma of mucosa-associated lymphoid tissue* (previously defined as 'low-grade B cell lymphoma of MALT type' and currently named MALT lymphoma), the *nodal marginal zone B cell lymphoma* (previously known as monocytoid lymphoma), and the *splenic marginal zone B cell lymphoma* (corresponding to the splenic lymphoma with villous lymphocytes of the French-American-British (FAB) classification.[1]

The term MZL relates to the fact that extranodal MZL, nodal MZL, and splenic MZL are believed to derive from B cells normally present in the marginal zone, which is the outer part of the mantle zone of B cell follicles. The marginal zone is more prominent in lymphoid organs which are presented with a high flow of antigens, such as the spleen, Peyer's patches, and the mesenteric lymph nodes.[2–5]

The most common B cells resident in the marginal zone are naïve B cells, with a restricted immunoglobulin (Ig) repertoire, that are involved in the T cell-independent early immune response. Post-germinal center memory B cells necessary for T cell-dependent immune responses are also localized in the marginal zone, as well as plasma cells, macrophages, T cells, and granulocytes.

While splenic and nodal MZL are quite rare, each comprising less than 1 percent of lymphomas, the extranodal MZL of MALT type is relatively common. Each entity is addressed separately.

EXTRANODAL MARGINAL ZONE LYMPHOMA OF MUCOSAL-ASSOCIATED LYMPHOID TISSUE (MALT LYMPHOMA)

GENERAL DESCRIPTION

Extranodal MZL can arise in a variety of extranodal sites and occur most often in organs where lymphocytes are normally absent and MALT is the result of chronic inflammatory events, in response to either infectious conditions such as *Helicobacter pylori*-associated chronic gastritis, or autoimmune disorders like Hashimoto thyroiditis and myoepithelial sialadenitis. Within these conditions, in the context of continual antigenic stimulation, abnormal B cell clones acquiring successive genetic abnormalities can progressively replace the normal B cell population of the inflammatory tissue giving rise to the lymphoma. The acquisition of MALT is induced by a series of agents which are likely to be different in each organ.

Helicobacter pylori was identified as an etiologic factor in gastric MALT lymphomas following the demonstration, in the early 1990s, of tumor regressions in early stage cases treated with anti-*Helicobacter* antibiotic therapy and this tumor then became a popular model of the pathogenetic link between chronic inflammation and lymphoma development.[6–8] Recognition of the driving source of the antigenic stimulation in different tissues may therefore have important therapeutic implications. Indeed, other bacterial infections have since been found to be possibly implicated in the pathogenesis of MZL arising in the skin (*Borrelia burgdorferi*),[9] in the ocular adnexa (*Chlamydia psittaci*),[10] and in the small intestine (*Campylobacter jejuni*).[11]

Although this lymphoma occurs in many different anatomic locations, the gastrointestinal (GI) tract is the most common site, encompassing half of all cases.[12] Within the GI tract, the disease is most common (85 percent) in the stomach, where MALT lymphomas comprise up to 50 percent of all primary lymphomas.[13,14] Primary intestinal involvement is typical of a special subtype of MALT lymphoma, the immunoproliferative small intestinal disease (IPSID).[15] Extranodal MZL may also arise in a variety of non-GI organs, mucosal or not, such as the salivary gland, thyroid, upper respiratory tract, lung, ocular adnexa (lachrymal gland, conjunctiva, eyelid, orbital soft tissue), skin, breast, liver, bladder, kidney, prostate, thymus, and even in the intracranial dura.[16]

In a survey of more than 1400 non-Hodgkin lymphomas from nine institutions in the USA, Canada, the UK, Switzerland, France, Germany, South Africa, and Hong Kong, this entity represented approximately 8 percent of the total number of cases, including both the most common GI and the less usual non-GI localizations.[17]

The highest prevalence of gastric cases has been reported in northeastern Italy (13.2 per 100 000/year, which is 13 times higher than in corresponding UK communities), suggesting the existence of important geographic variations likely related to variations in the incidence of *H. pylori*.[14] Indeed, *H. pylori* infection can be found in 70–90 percent of patients with primary MALT lymphoma of the stomach.[18,19] In the USA, the incidence of gastric MALT lymphoma has been estimated to be between 1:30 000 and 1:80 000 among the *H. pylori*-infected population.[20]

As detailed in another chapter of this book (Chapter 30), four main recurrent chromosomal translocations have been associated with the pathogenesis of MALT lymphomas: t(11;18)(q21;q21), t(1;14)(p22;q32), t(14;18)(q32;q21), and t(3;14)(p14.1;q32).[21,22] Interestingly, these four recurrent chromosomal translocations seem to be mutually exclusive and demonstrate site specificity in terms of their incidence. The latter translocation is the most recently described[23] and its pathogenetic relevance is still unclear.[21,22] The other three seemingly disparate translocations, despite involving different genes, all appear to affect the same signaling pathway, resulting in the activation of nuclear factor κB (NF-κB), a transcription factor with a central role in immunity, inflammation, and apoptosis.[21,22] The most common is the translocation t(11;18)(q21;q21), which results in a fusion of the cIAP2 region on chromosome 11q21 with the *MALT1* gene on chromosome 18q21 and is present in more than one-third of cases. The frequency of this translocation is site related: it is common in the GI tract and lung, rare in conjunctiva and orbit, and almost absent in salivary glands, thyroid, liver, and skin. It can be speculated that there are site-specific pathogenetic pathways; however, whether the presence of different infections at different sites can lead not only to chronic B cell proliferation but also to the specific translocations that characterize most MALT lymphomas remains unclear. Nevertheless, these translocations may carry significant clinical relevance. For instance, the t(11;18) translocation is present in only 10 percent of tumors confined to the gastric wall but is common in those disseminated beyond the stomach. Moreover, the presence of this translocation can predict a poor therapeutic response of gastric MALT lymphoma to *H. pylori* eradication[24] but not necessarily to other therapeutic approaches.[25,26]

CLINICAL FEATURES

Mucosa-associated lymphoid tissue lymphoma is a tumor of adults, with a median age at presentation near 60 years and a slightly higher proportion of females.[12,17] The clinical features and presenting symptoms are mainly related to the primary location[7,16,27] but some collective characteristics can be described.[12,28,29] Few patients present with elevated lactate dehydrogenase (LDH) or β_2-microglobulin levels. Constitutional B symptoms are extremely uncommon. MALT lymphoma usually remains localized for a prolonged period within the tissue of origin, but dissemination to multiple sites is not uncommon, being reported in up to one-quarter of cases, with either synchronous or metachronous involvement of multiple mucosal sites or nonmucosal sites such as spleen, bone marrow, or liver; regional lymph nodes can also be infiltrated.[12,28,30,31] The frequency of early multiorgan involvement appears to be lower in Japanese patients than in European patients.[32] Bone marrow involvement is reported in up to 20 percent of cases.[33]

Within the stomach, MALT lymphoma is often multifocal and this may explain the report of relapses in the gastric stump after surgical excision.[7] Gastric MALT lymphoma can often disseminate to the small intestine[34] and to the splenic marginal zone.[35] Concomitant GI and non-GI

Table 66.1   Main clinical features at diagnosis and outcome according to the primary extranodal site[27,28]

Extranodal site	Female	Elevated LDH	Nodal involvement	Stage I	B symptoms	Bone marrow involvement	5-year overall survival (95% CI)	5-year progression-free survival (95% CI)
GI localization								
Stomach	50%	2%	4%	88%	1%	8%	82% (67–91)	67% (51–79)
Intestine	67%	11%	44%	56%	11%	0	100%	63% (24–87)
Non-GI localization								
Skin	50%	9%	0	82%	0	9%	100%	53% (22–77)
Ocular adnexa[a]	60%	26%	10%	84%	3%	13%	94% (77–98)	57% (27–79)
Salivary glands	68%	17%	11%	83%	2%	9%	97% (81–100)	67% (48–81)
Lung	47%	27%	27%	60%	0	7%	100%	75% (41–91)
Upper airways	58%	42%	33%	50%	0	33%	46% (7–80)	0
Breast	100%	33%		100%	0	0	100%	33% (1–77)
Thyroid	60%	10%	40%	60%	0	0	100%	100%
Urinary tract	50%	0	0	100%	0	0	100%	0
Liver	63%		50%	0	17%	33%	0	0
Multiorgan[b]	67%	26%	45%	Not applicable	5%	33%	77% (43–93)	25% (3–58)

[a]Recalculated from the published[28] split data on orbital and conjuntival MALT lymphomas.
[b]Patients with multiple mucosal-associated lymphoid tissue (MALT) sites with or without nodal and/or bone marrow (or both) involvement.
GI, gastrointestinal; LDH, lactate dehydrogenase; CI, confidence interval.

involvement can be detected in approximately 10 percent of cases. Disseminated disease appears to be more common in non-GI MALT lymphomas.[16] It has been postulated that dissemination of MALT lymphoma may be due to specific expression of homing receptors or adhesion molecules on the surface of most B cells of MALT, either normal or transformed.[36–38]

Most patients with MALT lymphoma have a favorable outcome with prolonged overall survival (usually higher than 85 percent at 5 years).[12,28,31] There are no significant differences in overall survival between GI and non-GI lymphoma. Patients at high risk according to the International Prognostic Index (IPI) and those with lymph node or bone marrow involvement at presentation, but not those with involvement of multiple mucosal sites, may have a worse prognosis. If initially localized, the disease is generally slow to disseminate. Recurrences may involve either extranodal or nodal sites. The median time to progression is apparently better for GI compared to non-GI lymphomas (9 vs 5 years, respectively).[29] Localization may also have prognostic relevance because of organ-specific clinical problems, which result in particular management strategies but, as different genetic lesions have been reported at different anatomic locations, it is also possible that different sites have a distinct natural history. In a radiation therapy study from Toronto, gastric and thyroid MALT lymphomas had the best outcome, whereas distant failures were more common for other sites.[39] In the multicenter series from the International Extranodal Lymphoma Study Group, patients with disease initially presenting in the upper

airways appeared to have a slightly poorer outcome (Table 66.1), but the small number of patients prevented any definitive conclusion.[7] In general, despite frequent relapses, MALT lymphomas most often maintain an indolent course. Histologic transformation to large cell lymphoma is reported in about 10 percent of cases, usually late during the course of the disease and independently from dissemination.[12]

Recommended staging procedures

The finding that patients presenting with lymphoma disseminated at multiple mucosal sites have a favorable outcome, with survival curves similar to those of patients with localized disease, makes using the traditional Ann Arbor staging system problematic. The Ann Arbor system is mainly based on extent of nodal disease and can be misleading in MALT lymphomas. Alternative staging systems (Table 66.2) for extranodal lymphomas have been proposed,[40] but a general consensus has not been achieved.

The main problem in staging patients with MALT lymphoma is the number of extranodal sites to be explored at diagnosis. The finding of asymptomatic dissemination in patients with apparently localized disease,[34] as well as the above-mentioned relatively high proportion of patients with early dissemination,[12,28,30,31] have been considered valid reasons to suggest extensive staging procedures in all patients with MALT lymphoma.[30]

Table 66.2 Staging systems for gastrointestinal tract lymphoma

Ann Arbor stage[48]	Musshof staging[40]	Lugano staging system for gastrointestinal lymphomas[49]	Adapted TNM[a] staging system[53]	Lymphoma extension
I$_E$	I$_{E1}$	Stage I = confined to GI tract (single primary or multiple, noncontiguous)	T1 N0 M0	Mucosa, submucosa
I$_E$	I$_{E2}$		T2 N0 M0	Muscolaris propria
I$_E$			T3 N0 M0	Serosa
II$_E$	II$_{E1}$	Stage II = extending into abdomen	T1-3 N1 M0	Perigastric lymph nodes
II$_E$	II$_{E2}$	II$_1$ = local nodal involvement	T1-3 N2 M0	More distant regional lymph nodes
		II$_2$ = distant nodal involvement		
I$_E$	I$_E$	Stage II$_E$ = penetration of serosa to involve adjacent organs or tissues	T4 N0 M0	Invasion of adjacent structures
III$_E$	III$_E$	Stage IV = disseminated extranodal	T1-4 N3 M0	Lymph nodes on both sides of the
IV$_E$	IV$_E$	involvement or concomitant supradiaphragmatic nodal involvement	T1-4 N0-3 M1	diaphragm, and/or distant metastases (e.g., bone marrow or additional extranodal sites)

[a]The European Gastro-Intestinal Lymphoma Study Group (EGILS) has proposed in 2003 a novel TNM-derived system named the 'Paris staging system.'[125] This system is aimed to improve the accuracy of the description of local tumor extent. The main modifications include the addition of the T1m and T1sm categories to separate the tumors confined to the mucosa from those confined to the submucosa, the definition of N3 as spread to extraabdominal lymph node, the distinction of M1 referring to noncontiguous involvement of separate sites in the gastrointestinal (GI) tract (e.g., stomach and rectum) from M2, that describes the involvement of non-GI tract tissues (including the serosae) and organs. Moreover, to describe the bone marrow infiltration, the B category was introduced with three subgroups: BX (bone marrow not assessed), B0 (bone marrow not involved), and B1 (lymphoma infiltration of the bone marrow).

TNM, Tumor, nodes, metastases.

On the other hand, however, patients with disseminated disease seem to have the same long-term outcome as those with localized disease. Moreover, in retrospective comparisons of different therapeutic approaches, in spite of higher complete response rates with surgery, no difference in survival was found between subsets (local treatment with surgery or radiation therapy vs systemic treatment with chemotherapy vs combined modality treatment).[27,41]

Thus, outside of clinical trials, aggressive staging procedures should be tailored to the individual patient according to the clinical condition (site of presentation, age, intended treatment, performance status, and symptoms). Staging procedures for all locations of MALT lymphoma should comprise a complete clinical history and physical examination, with careful evaluation of all lymph node regions, inspection of the upper airways and tonsils, thyroid examination, and clinical evaluation of the size of liver and spleen. Standard posteroanterior and lateral chest radiographs and a computed tomography (CT) scan of thorax, abdomen, and pelvis should be performed. Bone marrow biopsy must be performed at diagnosis. Laboratory tests should include complete blood count with cytologic examination, LDH and β_2-microglobulin levels, evaluation of renal and liver function, and hepatitis C virus (HCV) and human immunodeficiency virus (HIV) serology (Table 66.3). Utility of positron emission tomography (PET) scanning is controversial.[42-44]

Since the stomach is the most common and best-studied site,[7] the main clinical aspects of diagnosis, staging, and treatment of gastric MALT lymphoma are discussed separately from other localizations.

Diagnosis and staging of gastric MALT lymphoma

The most common presenting symptoms of gastric MALT lymphoma are nonspecific upper GI complaints (dyspepsia, epigastric pain, nausea, and chronic manifestations of GI bleeding such as anemia) often leading to an endoscopy that usually reveals nonspecific gastritis or peptic ulcer, with mass lesions being unusual. Diagnosis is based on the histopathologic evaluation of gastric biopsies.[7,16] In addition to routine histology and immunohistochemistry, fluorescence *in situ* hybridization (FISH) analysis for detection of t(11;18) may be useful for identifying cases that are unlikely to respond to antibiotic therapy.[45,46]

The best staging system for GI tract lymphoma is still controversial.[16,47] As mentioned above, the Ann Arbor staging system[48] routinely used for non-Hodgkin lymphomas is not adequate for the specific problems posed by GI tract lymphomas. A variety of alternative systems has therefore been proposed, and those most commonly used are summarized in Table 66.2. We have largely used the modification of the Blackledge staging system known as the 'Lugano staging system.'[49] However, this system was proposed before the widespread use of endoscopic ultrasound and does not accurately describe the depth of infiltration in the gastric wall, a parameter that is highly predictive for the response to anti-*Helicobacter* therapy. Indeed, there is a general consensus that initial staging procedures should include a gastroduodenal endoscopy with multiple biopsies from each region of the stomach, duodenum, and gastro-esophageal junction, and from any

Table 66.3 Staging procedures for MALT lymphoma

All sites:
- History (duration and presence of local or systemic symptoms)
- Physical examination (careful evaluation of all lymph node regions, inspection of the upper airways and tonsils, clinical evaluation of thyroid, liver and spleen, detection of palpable masses)
- Laboratory tests, including complete blood counts with peripheral blood smear, LDH, β_2-microglobulin, serum electrophoresis, HCV and HIV serology, evaluation of renal and liver function
- Bone marrow biopsy
- Standard posteroanterior and lateral chest radiographs and/or chest CT scan
- Abdominal and pelvic CT scan

Additional investigations by site of involvement:
- *Stomach*: Gastroduodenal endoscopy with multiple gastric biopsies from all the visible lesions and the noninvolved areas with a complete mapping. Histologic and histochemical examination for *H. pylori* (Genta stain or Warthin-Starry stain of antral biopsy specimen) and serology studies if histology results are negative. FISH for the t(11;18) translocation. Endoscopic ultrasound
- *Small intestine (IPSID)*: Endoscopy. Small bowel series (double-contrast x-ray examination of the small intestine). *Campylobacter jejuni* search in the tumor biopsy by PCR, immunohistochemistry, or *in situ* hybridization
- *Large intestine*: Colonoscopy
- *Lung*: Bronchoscopy + bronchoalveolar lavage
- *Salivary gland, tonsils, parotid*: ENT examination and echography
- *Thyroid*: echography ± CT scan of the neck and thyroid function tests
- *Ocular adnexa*: MRI (or CT scan) and ophthalmologic examination. *Chlamydia psittaci* in the tumor biopsy and blood mononuclear cells by PCR
- *Breast*: Mammography and MRI (or CT scan)
- *Skin*: *Borrelia burgdorferi* in the tumor biopsy by PCR

MALT, mucosal-associated lymphoid tissue; LDH, lactate dehydrogenase; HCV, hepatitis C virus; HIV, human immunodeficiency virus; CT, computed tomography; FISH, fluorescence *in situ* hybridization; PCR, polymerase chain reaction; ENT, ear nose throat; MRI, magnetic resonance imaging; IPSID, Immunoproliferative small intestinal disease.

abnormal-appearing site. Fresh biopsy and washings material should be available for cytogenetic studies in addition to routine histology and immunohistochemistry.

The presence of active *H. pylori* infection must be determined by histochemistry (Genta stain or Warthin-Starry stain) and breath test; serology studies are recommended when the results of histology are negative. Endoscopic ultrasound is recommended in the initial follow-up for evaluation of depth of infiltration and presence of perigastric lymph nodes. Indeed, deep infiltration of the gastric wall is associated with a higher risk of lymph node involvement and a lower response rate with antibiotic therapy.[50–53] Although the disease usually remains localized to the stomach, systemic dissemination and bone marrow involvement should be excluded at presentation since the prognosis is worse with advanced stage disease or with an unfavorable IPI score.[7]

Staging procedures in nongastric MALT lymphoma

Presentation with multiple MALT localizations is more frequent in patients with non-GI lymphoma. Workup studies should include complete blood count, basic biochemical studies (including LDH and β_2-microglobulin, see above), CT scan of the chest, abdomen, and pelvis, and

a bone marrow biopsy. Then, depending on the particular clinical presentation, the investigations should focus on the specific organs suspected of being involved, as summarized in Table 66.3. Particular attention should be paid to the demonstration of certain chronic infections that may have a pathogenetic role; i.e., *Borrelia burgdorferi* in cutaneous localizations,[9] *Chlamydia psittaci* in the ocular adnexae,[10] and *Campylobacter jejuni* in the small intestine.[11]

MANAGEMENT AND FOLLOW-UP

Helicobacter pylori eradication in gastric MALT lymphoma

Eradication of *H. pylori* with antibiotics as the sole initial treatment of localized (i.e., confined to the gastric wall) MALT lymphoma is at present the best-studied therapeutic approach, with more than 20 reported (nonrandomized) studies.[6,54–56]

Regression of gastric MALT lymphoma after antibiotic eradication of *H. pylori* was first reported in 1993 by Wotherspoon and colleagues, who described histologically proven regression following anti-*Helicobacter* therapy in five of six patients with superficially invasive gastric MALT

Table 66.4 Comparison of the Wotherspoon and the GELA scoring systems for the histologic evaluation of gastric MALT lymphoma endoscopic biopsies

Score	Description	Histologic features
Wotherspoon's score for diagnosis and posttreatment evaluation		
0	Normal	Scattered plasma cells in LP
1	Chronic active gastritis	Small clusters of lymphocytes in LP, no lymphoid follicles; no LEL
2	Chronic active gastritis with lymphoid follicles	Prominent lymphoid follicles with surrounding mantle zone and plasma cells; no LEL
3	Suspicious lymphoid infiltrate, probably reactive	Lymphoid follicles surrounded by small lymphocytes that infiltrate diffusely in LP and occasionally into epithelium
4	Suspicious lymphoid infiltrate, probably lymphoma	Lymphoid follicles surrounded by centrocyte-like cells that infiltrate diffusely in LP and into epithelium in small groups
5	Low-grade MALT lymphoma	Dense diffuse infiltrate of centrocyte-like cells in LP with prominent LEL
GELA grading system for posttreatment evaluation		
CR	Complete histologic remission	Normal or empty LP and/or fibrosis with absent or scattered plasma cells and small lymphoid cells in the LP, no LEL
pMRD	Probable minimal residual disease	Empty LP and/or fibrosis with aggregates of lymphoid cells or lymphoid nodules in the LP/MM and/or SM, no LEL
rRD	Responding residual disease	Focal empty LP and/or fibrosis with dense, diffuse, or nodular lymphoid infiltrate, extending around glands in the LP, focal LEL or absent
NC	No change	Dense, diffuse, or nodular lymphoid infiltrate, LEL usually present

Modified from Wotherspoon *et al.* 1993[57] and from Copie-Bergman *et al.* 2003.[65]
MALT, mucosal-associated lymphoid tissue; GELA, Groupe d'Etude des Lymphomes de l'Adulte; LEL, lymphoepithelial lesions; LP, lamina propria; MM, muscolaris mucosa; SM, submucosa.

lymphoma.[57] A long-term follow-up report of these six patients, published in 1999, confirmed the achievement of prolonged remissions and described the occurrence of transient histologic and molecular relapses, suggesting that the neoplastic clone can again temporarily expand but that without the growth stimulus from *H. pylori,* this may remain a self-limiting event.[58]

Several groups thereafter confirmed the achievement of durable remissions in 60–100 percent of patients with localized *H. pylori*-positive gastric MALT lymphoma treated with antibiotics.[27,50,51,53,59–61] Histologic remission can usually be documented within 6 months from the start of *H. pylori* eradication but sometimes the period required is more prolonged and the therapeutic response may be delayed for up to or more than 1 year.[7] Several effective anti-*H. pylori* programs are available.[62] The choice should be based on the epidemiology of the infection in the country concerned, taking into account the locally expected antibiotic resistance. The most commonly used regimen is triple therapy with a proton pump inhibitor (e.g., omeprazole, lansoprazole, pantoprazole, or esomeprazole), in association with amoxicillin and clarithromycin. Metronidazole can be substituted for amoxicillin in penicillin-allergic individuals. Other regimens that include bismuth or histamine H_2-receptor antagonists (rather than proton pump inhibitors) with antibiotics are also effective.

Anti-*Helicobacter* therapy in diffuse large B cell lymphoma of the stomach

A subset of gastric large cell lymphoma cases may derive from a MALT lymphoma, therefore anti-*Helicobacter* therapy may be of benefit in some patients. Antibiotics may eliminate a residual low-grade component that can be responsible for tumor recurrence following antigen stimulation. Cases of regression of high-grade lesions after anti-*H. pylori* therapy have been reported, suggesting that high-grade transformation is not necessarily associated with the loss of *H. pylori* dependence.[63,64] At present, however, the sole use of antibiotic therapy for gastric large cell lymphoma cannot be advised outside of clinical trials until large-scale prospective studies have validated its use as first-line therapy.

Posttreatment histologic evaluation

Interpretation of a residual lymphoid infiltrate in posttreatment gastric biopsies can be very difficult and there are no uniform criteria for the definition of histologic remission. The Wotherspoon score[57] reported in Table 66.4 can be very useful to express the degree of confidence in the MALT lymphoma diagnosis on small gastric biopsies; however, it is difficult to apply in the evaluation of response to therapy and other criteria have been proposed.[59] The lack of standard reproducible criteria can affect comparison of the results of different clinical trials. A novel histologic grading system has been proposed by Copie-Bergman and colleagues[65] with the aim of providing clinically relevant information. This system, summarized in Table 66.4, may become a useful tool if its reproducibility is confirmed by further testing on larger series.

Factors predicting response to *Helicobacter pylori* eradication

Endoscopic ultrasound can be useful in predicting response to *H. pylori* eradication. Several studies have shown that there is a significant difference between the response rates of lymphomas restricted to the gastric mucosa and those with less superficial lesions. The response rate is highest for the mucosa-confined lymphomas (approximately 70–90 percent) and then decreases markedly for tumors infiltrating the submucosa, the muscularis propria, and the serosa. In cases with documented nodal involvement, response is very unlikely.[51,53,66]

Liu *et al.* have shown that the t(11;18) translocation is present in only 10 percent of tumors confined to the gastric wall but in 78 percent of those disseminated beyond the stomach.[24] As stated above, the presence of the t(11;18) translocation can predict for therapeutic response to *H. pylori* eradication[24,45,46,67] but not necessarily to other therapeutic approaches.[25,26]

Clinical and molecular follow-up

A number of molecular follow-up studies have shown that postantibiotic histologic and endoscopic remission does not necessarily equate with cure. The long-term persistence of monoclonal B cells after histologic regression of the lymphoma has been reported in about one-half of cases, suggesting that *H. pylori* eradication suppresses but does not eradicate the lymphoma clones.[61,68,69] The clinical relevance of the detection of monoclonal B cells by molecular methods remains unclear. In the long-term follow-up of some cases with minimal residual disease, neither clinical progression nor histologic transformation were documented despite persistent clonality, suggesting that a watch-and-wait policy could be feasible and safe.[70] On the other hand, recurrence of lymphoma following *H. pylori* reinfection has been reported, suggesting that residual dormant tumor cells can be present despite histologic remission.[59] Relapses have also been documented in the absence of *H. pylori* reinfection, indicating the presence of B cell lymphoma clones that may have escaped the antigenic drive,[59] and histologic transformation into diffuse large B cell lymphoma (DLBCL) has also been described.[27,71] Strict

follow-up is strongly advised and histologic evaluation of repeated biopsies continues to be the fundamental follow-up procedure, despite the reproducibility problems previously discussed. We perform a breath test two months after treatment to document *H. pylori* eradication, and repeat posttreatment endoscopies with multiple biopsies every 6 months for 2 years, and then annually.

Management of *Helicobacter pylori*-negative or antibiotic-resistant cases

No definite guidelines exist for the management of the subset of *H. pylori*-negative cases and for the patients in whom antibiotic therapy fails. There are no published randomized studies to help make the choice of treatment. In two retrospective series of patients with gastric low-grade MALT lymphoma, no statistically significant difference in survival was apparent between patients who received different initial treatments (including chemotherapy alone, surgery alone, surgery with additional chemotherapy or radiation therapy, or antibiotics against *H. pylori*).[27,41]

Excellent disease control using radiation therapy has been reported by several institutions, supporting the approach that modest dose, involved field radiation therapy (30 Gy given in 4 weeks to the stomach and perigastric nodes) is the treatment of choice for patients with stage I–II MALT lymphoma of the stomach without evidence of *H. pylori* infection or with persistent lymphoma after antibiotics.[39,72,73] Surgery has also been widely and successfully used in the past, but the precise role for surgical resection should nowadays be redefined in view of the promising results of a conservative approach.[7]

Patients with systemic disease should be considered for systemic treatment (i.e., chemotherapy and/or immunotherapy with anti-CD20 monoclonal antibodies).[6,74] In the presence of disseminated or advanced disease, chemotherapy is an obvious choice, but only a few compounds and regimens have been tested specifically in MALT lymphomas. Oral alkylating agents (either cyclophosphamide or chlorambucil, used for 1 year) can result in a high rate of disease control.[66,75] More recent phase II studies have demonstrated some antitumor activity for the purine analogues fludarabine[76] and cladribine (2-CDA).[77] The latter might, however, be associated with an increased risk of secondary myelodysplastic syndrome.[78] A combination regimen of chlorambucil, mitoxantrone, and prednisone has also been used.[79] Aggressive anthracycline-containing chemotherapy should be reserved for patients with a high tumor burden (bulky masses, high IPI score).[80]

The activity of the anti-CD20 monoclonal antibody rituximab has also been shown in a phase II study (with a response rate of about 70 percent), and may represent an additional option for the treatment of systemic disease.[25,81,82] The efficacy of the combination of rituximab with chemotherapy is being explored in a randomized study of the International Extranodal Lymphoma Study Group (IELSG).

Management of MALT lymphomas at other sites

Nongastric MALT lymphomas have been difficult to characterize because these tumors, numerous when considered together, are distributed so widely throughout the body that it is difficult to assemble adequate series for any given site. At least a quarter of non-GI MALT lymphomas have been reported to present with involvement of multiple mucosal sites, with or without the participation of nonmucosal sites such as bone marrow and lymph nodes.[12,28,29] Non-GI MALT lymphomas, despite presenting with stage IV disease more often than the gastric variant, usually have a quite indolent course regardless of treatment type. In a multicenter retrospective survey of 180 nongastric cases observed over a long period, patients were treated according to the current policy of each institution at the time of diagnosis, and the presence of organ-specific problems presumably had a role in the choice of treatment. This study showed no evidence of a clear advantage for any type of therapy and, despite the high proportion of cases with disseminated disease, which should require a systemic approach, no clear advantage was associated with a chemotherapy program.[28]

In general, the considerations previously described regarding the treatment of *H. pylori*-negative cases can be applied to nongastric MALT lymphomas. Radiation therapy is the best-studied approach and is the treatment of choice for localized lesions.[39,73,83] The optimal management of disseminated MALT lymphomas is less clearly defined. The treatment choice should be 'patient tailored,' taking into account the site, stage, and clinical characteristics of disease for the individual patient. The finding that *C. psittaci* is associated with MALT lymphoma of the ocular adnexa may provide the rationale for antibiotic treatment of localized lesions, and preliminary encouraging results have been reported, but this approach remains investigational and will need to be confirmed by larger clinical studies.

Immunoproliferative small intestinal disease

This condition, known in the past as alpha heavy chain disease or Mediterranean lymphoma, is nowadays considered a special variant of MALT lymphoma.[15,84] It is characterized by a diffuse lymphoplasmacytic/plasmacytic infiltrate in the proximal small intestine.[85] The distinguishing feature of IPSID is the synthesis of alpha heavy chain that is secreted and is detectable in the serum, urine, saliva, and duodenal fluid in approximately two-thirds of cases; in the remaining cases, the protein is demonstrable by immunohistochemistry but is not secreted. Most of the cases have been described in the Middle East, especially in the Mediterranean area where the disease is endemic, affecting young men and women, but predominantly males.[86] A few cases have been reported from industrialized Western countries, usually among immigrants from the endemic area.[84,86] The natural course of IPSID is usually prolonged, often over many years, and includes a potentially reversible early phase, with the disease usually confined to the abdomen. If untreated, it degenerates, with high-grade transformation into large B cell lymphoma.[85] Since the histology of mucosal lesions and mesenteric lymph nodes can be discordant, with a higher grade in the latter, staging laparoscopy or laparotomy can be useful in the evaluation of mesenteric nodal involvement; however, surgery has no therapeutic role because intestinal involvement is generally diffuse.

Since the 1970s it was known that in the early phases of IPSID, durable remissions could be obtained with sustained treatment with antibiotics (such as tetracycline or metronidazole and ampicillin for at least 6 months), but only in 2004 did Lecuit and colleagues demonstrate the presence of a specific pathogen, linking this lymphoma to *Campylobacter jejuni*.[11] Indeed, the presence of *Campylobacter* species may be demonstrated in tumor sections and, at an early stage, antibiotic treatment directed against *Campylobacter* may lead to lymphoma regression.[11] However, there is no clear evidence that antibiotics alone are of benefit in the advanced phases. Although the early studies reported that aggressive chemotherapy is not well tolerated by patients with advanced disease and severe malabsorption, who have poor survival rates, more recent data suggest that anthracycline-containing regimens, combined with nutritional support plus antibiotics to control diarrhea and malabsorption, may offer the best chance of cure, with 5-year survival rates as high as 70 percent.[87–89]

PRIMARY SPLENIC MARGINAL ZONE LYMPHOMA (WITH OR WITHOUT CIRCULATING VILLOUS LYMPHOCYTES)

GENERAL DESCRIPTION

Splenic MZL is a very rare disorder comprising less than 1 percent of all lymphomas.[17] Up to two-thirds of patients present with circulating villous lymphocytes with characteristic fine, short, cytoplasmic polar projections. When these constitute more than 20 percent of the lymphocyte count, the term 'splenic lymphoma with villous lymphocytes' is commonly used.[90] Despite relevant geographic variations, HCV seems to be involved in lymphomagenesis.[4,91–97] Very interesting is the observation that some patients with splenic lymphoma with villous lymphocytes and HCV infection obtain a complete remission after treatment with interferon α.[98] In contrast, interferon treatment has no antitumor effect on HCV-negative splenic MZL. These data, also confirmed by other groups,[97] suggest a pathogenetic relationship between HCV and splenic MZL. An association with malaria and with Epstein–Barr virus (EBV) infection (both strong polyclonal B cell activators) and with malarial splenomegaly has been shown in tropical Africa, especially in Ghana.[99,100] Tropical splenic lymphoma appears to be a form of splenic MZL, characterized by a high percentage of circulating villous lymphocytes.

CLINICAL FEATURES

Most patients with primary splenic MZL are aged over 50 years, and there is a similar incidence in males and females.[101] The disease usually presents with massive splenomegaly, which produces abdominal discomfort and pain. Diagnosis is often made at splenectomy performed to establish the cause of unexplained splenic enlargement. B symptoms are present in 25–60 percent of cases; anemia, thrombocytopenia, or leukocytosis are reported in approximately 25 percent of cases. Autoimmune hemolytic anemia is not uncommon, being found in up to 15 percent of patients. The splenic hilar lymph nodes appear involved in about one-quarter of cases and approximately one-third have liver involvement.[102–106]

According to the WHO classification, peripheral lymph node involvement is typically absent,[101] but some reports refer to splenic MZL even with some evidence of peripheral nodal or extranodal involvement.[105] Patients with disseminated MZL can be observed in advanced stages of splenic MZL, nodal MZL, or extranodal MZL[107] and a precise diagnosis can be very difficult in cases presenting with concomitant splenic, extranodal, and nodal involvement. In a retrospective French series of 124 patients from Lyon with non-MALT type MZL,[104] four clinical subtypes were observed: splenic (48 percent of cases), nodal (30 percent), disseminated (splenic and nodal, 16 percent), and leukemic (neither splenic nor nodal, 6 percent). Even when the data are restricted to cases presenting with splenomegaly, nearly all patients have bone marrow involvement, often accompanied by involvement of peripheral blood (defined as the presence of an absolute lymphocytosis of more than 5 percent).[105] Because of the high frequency of bone marrow or liver involvement, about 95 percent of cases are classified as Ann Arbor stage IV. Serum paraproteinemia is observed in about 10–25 percent of cases and is most frequently of IgM type, posing the problem of the differential diagnosis with lymphoplasmacytic lymphoma or Waldenstrom macroglobulinemia.[103–105,108] These diseases often present with similar clinical features (splenomegaly, bone marrow infiltration, anemia), but marked hyperviscosity and hypergammaglobulinemia are uncommon in splenic MZL.[104,109] The clinical course of splenic MZL is

most usually indolent, with 5-year overall survival ranging from 65 percent to 80 percent. In the above-mentioned study from Lyon,[104] the subgroup of patients with splenic lymphoma had a more favorable outcome with a median survival of more than 9 years. Histologic transformation is rare and often associated with B symptoms, disease dissemination, and poorer outcome.[80]

MANAGEMENT

The largest reported series[103,105,106] show that most patients can be initially managed with a watch-and-wait policy and they do not seem to have a worse outcome.[102,104,107] When treatment is needed, it is usually because of symptomatic splenomegaly or cytopenia. Splenectomy appears to be the treatment of choice, resulting in a reduction/disappearance of circulating tumor lymphocytes and recovery of the lymphoma-associated cytopenia.[102,103,106,107,110] The benefit of splenectomy often persists for several years and time to next treatment can be longer than 5 years. Adjuvant chemotherapy after splenectomy may result in a higher rate of complete responses; however, there is no evidence of a survival benefit.[107]

Chemotherapy alone may be considered for patients who require treatment but have a contraindication to splenectomy and for those with clinical progression after splenectomy. Alkylating agents (chlorambucil or cyclophosphamide) have been reported to be active and can be used as single agents or in combination (as in the CVP [cyclophosphamide, vincristine, prednisone] and CHOP [cyclophosphamide, doxorubicin, vincristine, prednisone] regimens). Among the purine analogues, fludarabine has been shown to be effective;[111,112] curiously, cladribine seems not to be.[113] The anti-B cell monoclonal antibody rituximab, alone or in combination with chemotherapy, is capable – according to a few case reports – of inducing good responses in cases refractory to standard chemotherapy.[107,114,115]

The reported association with HCV infection led Hermine and colleagues to treat this infection in a series of nine patients with splenic lymphoma with villous lymphocytes and HCV infection. Treatment consisted of interferon α alone or in combination with ribavirine. Of the nine patients who received interferon α, seven had a complete remission of the lymphoma and loss of detectable HCV RNA. The other two patients had a partial and a complete remission after the addition of ribavirine and loss of detectable HCV RNA. One patient relapsed when HCV RNA became detectable again in the blood. No HCV-negative patient had a response to interferon therapy.[98] Analogous to the *H. pylori* infection in gastric MZL, it appears that HCV may be responsible for an antigen-driven stimulation of the lymphoma clone. This report suggests that all cases should be tested for HCV infection and antiviral therapy should be considered in positive cases before any decision about more aggressive therapeutic approaches.

NODAL MARGINAL ZONE LYMPHOMA (MONOCYTOID LYMPHOMA)

GENERAL DESCRIPTION

In contrast with mucosa-based extranodal MALT lymphoma, nodal MZL is typically lymph node-based. This type of lymphoma is exceedingly rare, accounting for less than 10 percent of all MZL and less than 1 percent of all non-Hodgkin lymphomas.[17,80] It has also been associated with HCV infection in some epidemiologic studies.[4,91–93,95–97] Clinical data are sparse and have been largely drawn from pathologic series rather than clinical series.[116,117] Nodal MZL is a disease of older people, with the median age at presentation in the sixth decade, and affects both sexes with a slight female predominance.

CLINICAL FEATURES

A common presenting feature is localized lymphadenopathy – most often in the neck. Concurrent extranodal involvement, most often of the salivary gland, is not rare, and some patients have a history of Sjögren syndrome or other autoimmune diseases, suggesting a possible overlap with extranodal MALT lymphomas.[118,119] Many patients present with generalized adenopathy. The bone marrow is involved at presentation in fewer than half of cases. Transformation to high-grade lymphoma has been described in some cases.

MANAGEMENT

There is at present no consensus about the best treatment, individual cases being managed differently according to site and stage of disease. In a study published by the Southwest Oncology Group (SWOG), comparing different low-grade lymphomas presenting with advanced disease (stage III–IV) and uniformly treated with the standard CHOP regimen, 21 patients with nodal MZL (monocytoid B cell lymphoma) and 19 with extranodal MZL (MALT lymphoma) were identified. Advanced stage MALT lymphoma appeared to carry a worse prognosis than nodal MZL (10-year actuarial survival of 21 percent versus 53 percent, respectively).[120] All nodal MZL patients were given full-dose CHOP and showed a survival pattern superimposable on that of advanced follicular lymphoma, but it remains unclear how they would have responded to other treatment strategies frequently used in low-grade lymphomas (such as 'watchful waiting,' single alkylating agents, purine analogues, or rituximab).

The international validation of the Revised European–American Lymphoma (REAL) classification, which included patients of any stage treated with heterogeneous modalities, showed 5-year survival of 57 percent for marginal zone B cell lymphoma (MZBCL) and 74 percent for MALT lymphomas.[17] This discrepancy with the results of the SWOG study might at least in part be due to the higher incidence of advanced disease in the nodal MZBCL group (82 percent vs 44 percent in the extranodal MALT-type group).[116,121] In the above-mentioned Lyon series of non-MALT type marginal zone B cell lymphomas,[104] four clinical subtypes were identified: splenic, nodal, disseminated (splenic and nodal), and leukemic (not splenic nor nodal). The nodal cases comprised 30 percent of patients and showed a more aggressive behavior. Nodal and disseminated subtypes had shorter median time to progression (about 1 year) in comparison with the splenic and leukemic subtypes (median time to progression longer than 5 years). The cases with disseminated disease more often presented with poor prognostic parameters (high LDH and β_2-microglobulin, poor performance status, bulky disease) and might represent the end-stage of the other subtypes.[104,107] However, in all subsets – even if the median time to progression was short – prolonged survival was observed (splenic 9 years, nodal 5.5 years, disseminated 15 years, and leukemic 7 years).

Many cases with nodal or disseminated disease presented with more than 50 percent of large cells or sheets of large B cells. These patients may be considered as having a 'transformed' lymphoma at diagnosis or a composite lymphoma with aspects of MZL and features of DLBCL. Cases with a high proportion of large cells are definitely less common in the splenic subsets. This finding may at least partially explain the observed differences in outcome between different subsets.

The retrospective nature of the published studies precludes any conclusions being made about optimal treatment, and treatment decisions should be based on the histologic and clinical features of disease in the individual patient.[4,122] Conservative treatment is recommended for leukemic and splenic subtypes, whilst in the nodal and disseminated subtypes front-line chemotherapy may be considered. Treatment options include single-agent chlorambucil or fludarabine, or combination chemotherapy regimens (such as CVP or CHOP). Rituximab may also have some efficacy[123] and can be combined with chemotherapy.[80] Anti-HCV treatment may induce lymphoma regression in some HCV-infected patients.[124] Autologous transplantation has been used in younger patients with adverse prognostic factors or an increased number of large cells.[104]

KEY POINTS

- The marginal zone lymphomas comprise three separate entities believed to derive from the marginal zone B cells, namely the extranodal marginal zone B cell lymphoma of mucosal-associated lymphoid tissue (MALT lymphoma), the nodal marginal zone B cell lymphoma, and the splenic marginal zone B cell lymphoma.

- Splenic and nodal marginal zone lymphomas are quite rare, each comprising less than 1 percent of lymphomas, but MALT lymphoma is relatively common and constitutes about 8 percent of all non-Hodgkin lymphomas.
- MALT lymphoma can arise in a variety of extranodal sites in association with chronic infections, such as *Helicobacter pylori* in the stomach. Other bacterial infections possibly implicated in its pathogenesis are *Borrelia burgdorferi* in the skin, *Chlamydia psittaci* in the ocular adnexa, and *Campylobacter jejuni* in the small intestine.
- *H. pylori* eradication is the best-studied therapeutic approach in gastric MALT lymphoma, with several studies showing achievement of durable remissions in most patients with localized *H. pylori*-positive gastric MALT lymphoma treated with antibiotics.
- Radiation therapy (or chemotherapy or immunotherapy) can be effective in localized *H. pylori*-negative cases or in failures after antibiotics, as well as in nongastric cases. Chemotherapy or immunotherapy can be employed in advanced stage MALT lymphoma.

REFERENCES

● = Key primary paper
◆ = Major review article

1. Jaffe ES, Harris NL, Stein H, Vardiman JW. (eds) *World Health Organization classification of tumours. Pathology and genetics of tumours of haematopoietic and lymphoid tissues.* Lyon: IARC Press, 2001.
2. Lopes-Carvalho T, Kearney JF. Development and selection of marginal zone B cells. *Immunol Rev* 2004; **197**: 192–205.
3. Martin F, Kearney JF. Marginal-zone B cells. *Nat Rev Immunol* 2002; **2**: 323–35.
4. Arcaini L, Paulli M, Boveri E *et al.* Marginal zone-related neoplasms of splenic and nodal origin. *Haematologica* 2003; **88**: 80–93.
5. Sagaert X, De Wolf-Peeters C. Classification of B-cells according to their differentiation status, their micro-anatomical localisation and their developmental lineage. *Immunol Lett* 2003; **90**: 179–86.
6. Zucca E, Cavalli F. Are antibiotics the treatment of choice for gastric lymphoma? *Curr Hematol Rep* 2004; **3**: 11–16.
◆7. Zucca E, Bertoni F, Roggero E, Cavalli F. The gastric marginal zone B-cell lymphoma of MALT type. *Blood* 2000; **96**: 410–19.
◆8. Isaacson PG. The MALT lymphoma concept updated. *Ann Oncol* 1995; **6**: 319–20.
●9. Roggero E, Zucca E, Mainetti C *et al.* Eradication of *Borrelia burgdorferi* infection in primary marginal zone B-cell lymphoma of the skin. *Hum Pathol* 2000; **31**: 263–8.
●10. Ferreri AJ, Guidoboni M, Ponzoni M *et al.* Evidence for an association between *Chlamydia psittaci* and ocular adnexal lymphomas. *J Natl Cancer Inst* 2004; **96**: 586–94.
●11. Lecuit M, Abachin E, Martin A *et al.* Immunoproliferative small intestinal disease associated with *Campylobacter jejuni. N Engl J Med* 2004; **350**: 239–48.
●12. Thieblemont C, Berger F, Dumontet C *et al.* Mucosa-associated lymphoid tissue lymphoma is a disseminated disease in one third of 158 patients analyzed. *Blood* 2000; **95**: 802–6.
13. Radaszkiewicz T, Dragosics B, Bauer P. Gastrointestinal malignant lymphomas of the mucosa-associated lymphoid tissue: factors relevant to prognosis. *Gastroenterology* 1992; **102**: 1628–38.
14. Doglioni C, Wotherspoon AC, Moschini A *et al.* High incidence of primary gastric lymphoma in northeastern Italy. *Lancet* 1992; **339**: 834–5.
◆15. Isaacson PG, Muller-Hermelink HK, Piris MA *et al.* Extranodal marginal zone B-cell lymphoma of mucosa-associated lymphoid tissue (MALT lymphoma). In: Vardiman JW. (ed) *World Health Organization classification of tumours. Pathology and genetics of tumours of haematopoietic and lymphoid tissues.* Lyon: IARC Press, 2001: 157–60.
◆16. Thieblemont C, Coiffier B. MALT lymphoma: Sites of presentations, clinical features and staging procedures. In: Bertoni F. (ed) *MALT lymphomas.* Georgetown, TX: Landes Bioscience/Kluwer Academic, 2004: 60–80.
17. The Non-Hodgkin's Lymphoma Classification Project. A clinical evaluation of the International Lymphoma Study Group classification of non-Hodgkin's lymphoma. *Blood* 1997; **89**: 3909–18.
18. Nakamura S, Yao T, Aoyagi K *et al.* Helicobacter pylori and primary gastric lymphoma. A histopathologic and immunohistochemical analysis of 237 patients. *Cancer* 1997; **79**: 3–11.
●19. Wotherspoon AC, Ortiz-Hidalgo C, Falzon MR, Isaacson PG. *Helicobacter pylori*-associated gastritis and primary B-cell gastric lymphoma. *Lancet* 1991; **338**: 1175–6.
20. Zaki M, Schubert ML. *Helicobacter pylori* and gastric lymphoma. *Gastroenterology* 1995; **108**: 610–12.
21. Bertoni F, Zucca E. Delving deeper into MALT lymphoma biology. *J Clin Invest* 2006; **116**: 22–6.
◆22. Farinha P, Gascoyne RD. Molecular pathogenesis of mucosa-associated lymphoid tissue lymphoma. *J Clin Oncol* 2005; **23**: 6370–8.
23. Streubel B, Vinatzer U, Lamprecht A *et al.* T(3;14)(p14.1;q32) involving IGH and FOXP1 is a novel recurrent chromosomal aberration in MALT lymphoma. *Leukemia* 2005; **19**: 652–8.
24. Liu H, Ye H, Dogan A *et al.* T(11;18)(q21;q21) is associated with advanced mucosa-associated lymphoid tissue lymphoma that expresses nuclear BCL10. *Blood* 2001; **98**: 1182–7.

25. Martinelli G, Laszlo D, Ferreri AJ *et al.* Clinical activity of rituximab in gastric marginal zone non-Hodgkin's lymphoma resistant to or not eligible for anti-*Helicobacter pylori* therapy. *J Clin Oncol* 2005; **23**: 1979–83.

26. Streubel B, Ye H, Du MQ *et al.* Translocation t(11;18)(q21;q21) is not predictive of response to chemotherapy with 2CdA in patients with gastric MALT lymphoma. *Oncology* 2004; **66**: 476–80.

●27. Pinotti G, Zucca E, Roggero E *et al.* Clinical features, treatment and outcome in a series of 93 patients with low-grade gastric MALT lymphoma. *Leuk Lymphoma* 1997; **26**: 527–37.

●28. Zucca E, Conconi A, Pedrinis E *et al.* Nongastric marginal zone B-cell lymphoma of mucosa-associated lymphoid tissue. *Blood* 2003; **101**: 2489–95.

29. Thieblemont C, Bastion Y, Berger F *et al.* Mucosa-associated lymphoid tissue gastrointestinal and nongastrointestinal lymphoma behavior: analysis of 108 patients. *J Clin Oncol* 1997; **15**: 1624–30.

30. Raderer M, Vorbeck F, Formanek M *et al.* Importance of extensive staging in patients with mucosa-associated lymphoid tissue (MALT)-type lymphoma. *Br J Cancer* 2000; **83**: 454–7.

31. Zinzani PL, Magagnoli M, Galieni P *et al.* Nongastrointestinal low-grade mucosa-associated lymphoid tissue lymphoma: analysis of 75 patients. *J Clin Oncol* 1999; **17**: 1254.

32. Yoshino T, Ichimura K, Mannami T *et al.* Multiple organ mucosa-associated lymphoid tissue lymphomas often involve the intestine. *Cancer* 2001; **91**: 346–53.

33. Cavalli F, Isaacson PG, Gascoyne RD, Zucca E. MALT Lymphomas. *Hematology (Am Soc Hematol Educ Program)* 2001; 241–58.

34. Du MQ, Xu CF, Diss TC *et al.* Intestinal dissemination of gastric mucosa-associated lymphoid tissue lymphoma. *Blood* 1996; **88**: 4445–51.

35. Du MQ, Peng HZ, Dogan A *et al.* Preferential dissemination of B-cell gastric mucosa-associated lymphoid tissue (MALT) lymphoma to the splenic marginal zone. *Blood* 1997; **90**: 4071–7.

36. Dogan A, Du M, Koulis A *et al.* Expression of lymphocyte homing receptors and vascular addressins in low-grade gastric B-cell lymphomas of mucosa-associated lymphoid tissue. *Am J Pathol* 1997; **151**: 1361–9.

37. Drillenburg P, van der Voort R, Koopman G *et al.* Preferential expression of the mucosal homing receptor integrin alpha 4 beta 7 in gastrointestinal non-Hodgkin's lymphomas. *Am J Pathol* 1997; **150**: 919–27.

38. Drillenburg P, Pals ST. Cell adhesion receptors in lymphoma dissemination. *Blood* 2000; **95**: 1900–10.

●39. Tsang RW, Gospodarowicz MK, Pintilie M *et al.* Localized mucosa-associated lymphoid tissue lymphoma treated with radiation therapy has excellent clinical outcome. *J Clin Oncol* 2003; **21**: 4157–64.

40. Musshoff K. Clinical staging classification of non-Hodgkin's lymphomas (author's translation). *Strahlentherapie* 1977; **153**: 218–21.

41. Thieblemont C, Dumontet C, Bouafia F *et al.* Outcome in relation to treatment modalities in 48 patients with localized gastric MALT lymphoma: a retrospective study of patients treated during 1976–2001. *Leuk Lymphoma* 2003; **44**: 257–62.

42. Beal KP, Yeung HW, Yahalom J. FDG-PET scanning for detection and staging of extranodal marginal zone lymphomas of the MALT type: a report of 42 cases. *Ann Oncol* 2005; **16**: 473–80.

43. Elstrom R, Guan L, Baker G *et al.* Utility of FDG-PET scanning in lymphoma by WHO classification. *Blood* 2003; **101**: 3875–6.

44. Hoffmann M, Kletter K, Becherer A *et al.* 18F-fluorodeoxyglucose positron emission tomography (18F-FDG-PET) for staging and follow-up of marginal zone B-cell lymphoma. *Oncology* 2003; **64**: 336–40.

●45. Liu H, Ruskon-Fourmestraux A, Lavergne-Slove A *et al.* Resistance of t(11;18) positive gastric mucosa-associated lymphoid tissue lymphoma to *Helicobacter pylori* eradication therapy. *Lancet* 2001; **357**: 39–40.

46. Liu H, Ye H, Ruskone-Fourmestraux A *et al.* T(11;18) is a marker for all stage gastric MALT lymphomas that will not respond to *H. pylori* eradication. *Gastroenterology* 2002; **122**: 1286–94.

●47. de Jong D, Aleman BM, Taal BG, Boot H. Controversies and consensus in the diagnosis, work-up and treatment of gastric lymphoma: an international survey. *Ann Oncol* 1999; **10**: 275–80.

48. Carbone PP, Kaplan HS, Musshoff K *et al.* Report of the Committee on Hodgkin's Disease Staging Classification. *Cancer Res* 1971; **31**: 1860–1.

49. Rohatiner A, d'Amore F, Coiffier B *et al.* Report on a workshop convened to discuss the pathological and staging classifications of gastrointestinal tract lymphoma. *Ann Oncol* 1994; **5**: 397–400.

●50. Sackmann M, Morgner A, Rudolph B *et al.* Regression of gastric MALT lymphoma after eradication of *Helicobacter pylori* is predicted by endosonographic staging. MALT Lymphoma Study Group. *Gastroenterology* 1997; **113**: 1087–90.

●51. Ruskone-Fourmestraux A, Lavergne A, Aegerter PH *et al.* Predictive factors for regression of gastric MALT lymphoma after anti-*Helicobacter pylori* treatment. *Gut* 2001; **48**: 297–303.

52. Eidt S, Stolte M, Fischer R. Factors influencing lymph node infiltration in primary gastric malignant lymphoma of the mucosa-associated lymphoid tissue. *Pathol Res Pract* 1994; **190**: 1077–81.

53. Steinbach G, Ford R, Glober G *et al.* Antibiotic treatment of gastric lymphoma of mucosa-associated lymphoid tissue. An uncontrolled trial. *Ann Intern Med* 1999; **131**: 88–95.

54. Stolte M, Bayerdorffer E, Morgner A *et al.* Helicobacter and gastric MALT lymphoma. *Gut* 2002; **50**(Suppl 3): III19–24.

55. Ahmad A, Govil Y, Frank BB. Gastric mucosa-associated lymphoid tissue lymphoma. *Am J Gastroenterol* 2003; **98**: 975–86.

56. Conconi A, Cavalli F, Zucca E. Gastric MALT lymphomas: The role of antibiotics. In: Zucca E. (ed.) *MALT lymphomas*. Georgetown, TX: Landes Bioscience/Kluwer Academic, 2004: 81–90.

●57. Wotherspoon AC, Doglioni C, Diss TC *et al.* Regression of primary low-grade B-cell gastric lymphoma of mucosa-associated lymphoid tissue type after eradication of *Helicobacter pylori*. *Lancet* 1993; **342**: 575–7.

●58. Isaacson PG, Diss TC, Wotherspoon AC *et al.* Long-term follow-up of gastric MALT lymphoma treated by eradication of *H. pylori* with antibodies. *Gastroenterology* 1999; **117**: 750–1.

59. Neubauer A, Thiede C, Morgner A *et al.* Cure of *Helicobacter pylori* infection and duration of remission of low-grade gastric mucosa-associated lymphoid tissue lymphoma. *J Natl Cancer Inst* 1997; **89**: 1350–5.

●60. Nakamura S, Matsumoto T, Suekane H *et al.* Predictive value of endoscopic ultrasonography for regression of gastric low grade and high grade MALT lymphomas after eradication of *Helicobacter pylori*. *Gut* 2001; **48**: 454–60.

●61. Bertoni F, Conconi A, Capella C *et al.* Molecular follow-up in gastric mucosa-associated lymphoid tissue lymphomas: early analysis of the LY03 cooperative trial. *Blood* 2002; **99**: 2541–4.

62. Howden CW, Hunt RH. Guidelines for the management of *Helicobacter pylori* infection. Ad Hoc Committee on Practice Parameters of the American College of Gastroenterology. *Am J Gastroenterol* 1998; **93**: 2330–8.

63. Chen LT, Lin JT, Shyu RY *et al.* Prospective study of *Helicobacter pylori* eradication therapy in stage I(E) high-grade mucosa-associated lymphoid tissue lymphoma of the stomach. *J Clin Oncol* 2001; **19**: 4245–51.

64. Chen LT, Lin JT, Tai JJ *et al.* Long-term results of anti-*Helicobacter pylori* therapy in early-stage gastric high-grade transformed MALT lymphoma. *J Natl Cancer Inst* 2005; **97**: 1345–53.

●65. Copie-Bergman C, Gaulard P, Lavergne-Slove A *et al.* Proposal for a new histological grading system for post-treatment evaluation of gastric MALT lymphoma. *Gut* 2003; **52**: 1656.

66. Levy M, Copie-Bergman C, Traulle C *et al.* Conservative treatment of primary gastric low-grade B-cell lymphoma of mucosa-associated lymphoid tissue: predictive factors of response and outcome. *Am J Gastroenterol* 2002; **97**: 292–7.

67. Alpen B, Neubauer A, Dierlamm J *et al.* Translocation t(11;18) absent in early gastric marginal zone B-cell lymphoma of MALT type responding to eradication of *Helicobacter pylori* infection. *Blood* 2000; **95**: 4014–15.

●68. Thiede C, Wundisch T, Alpen B *et al.* Persistence of monoclonal B cells after cure of *Helicobacter pylori* infection and complete histologic remission in gastric mucosa-associated lymphoid tissue B-cell lymphoma. *J Clin Oncol* 2001; **19**: 1600–9.

69. Wotherspoon AC, Savio A. Molecular follow-up in gastric MALT lymphomas. In: Zucca E. (ed.) *MALT lymphomas*. Georgetown, TX: Landes Bioscience/Kluwer Academic, 2004: 91–8.

70. Fischbach W, Goebeler-Kolve M, Starostik P *et al.* Minimal residual low-grade gastric MALT-type lymphoma after eradication of *Helicobacter pylori*. *Lancet* 2002; **360**: 547–8.

71. Montalban C, Manzanal A, Castrillo JM *et al.* Low grade gastric B-cell MALT lymphoma progressing into high grade lymphoma. Clonal identity of the two stages of the tumour, unusual bone involvement and leukemic dissemination. *Histopathology* 1995; **27**: 89–91.

●72. Schechter NR, Portlock CS, Yahalom J. Treatment of mucosa-associated lymphoid tissue lymphoma of the stomach with radiation alone. *J Clin Oncol* 1998; **16**: 1916–21.

◆73. Gospodarowicz M, Tsang R. Radiation therapy of mucosa-associated lymphoid tissue (MALT) lymphomas. In: Zucca E. (ed.) *MALT lymphomas*. Georgetown, TX: Landes Bioscience/Kluwer Academic, 2004: 104–29.

74. Conconi A, Cavalli F, Zucca E. MALT lymphomas: The role of chemotherapy. In: Zucca E. (ed.) *MALT lymphomas*. Georgetown, TX: Landes Bioscience/Kluwer Academic, 2004: 99–103.

75. Hammel P, Haioun C, Chaumette MT *et al.* Efficacy of single-agent chemotherapy in low-grade B-cell mucosa-associated lymphoid tissue lymphoma with prominent gastric expression. *J Clin Oncol* 1995; **13**: 2524–9.

76. Zinzani PL, Stefoni V, Musuraca G *et al.* Fludarabine-containing chemotherapy as frontline treatment of nongastrointestinal mucosa-associated lymphoid tissue lymphoma. *Cancer* 2004; **100**: 2190–4.

77. Jager G, Neumeister P, Brezinschek R *et al.* Treatment of extranodal marginal zone B-cell lymphoma of mucosa-associated lymphoid tissue type with cladribine: a phase II study. *J Clin Oncol* 2002; **20**: 3872–7.

78. Jager G, Hofler G, Linkesch W, Neumeister P. Occurence of a myelodysplastic syndrome (MDS) during first-line 2-chloro-deoxyadenosine (2-CDA) treatment of a low-grade gastrointestinal MALT lymphoma. Case report and review of the literature. *Haematologica* 2004; **89**: ECR01.

79. Wohrer S, Drach J, Hejna M *et al.* Treatment of extranodal marginal zone B-cell lymphoma of mucosa-associated lymphoid tissue (MALT lymphoma) with mitoxantrone, chlorambucil and prednisone (MCP). *Ann Oncol* 2003; **14**: 1758–61.

80. Thieblemont C. Clinical presentation and management of marginal zone lymphomas. *Hematology (Am Soc Hematol Educ Program)* 2005; 307–13.

●81. Conconi A, Martinelli G, Thieblemont C *et al.* Clinical activity of rituximab in extranodal marginal zone B-cell lymphoma of MALT type. *Blood* 2003; **102**: 2741–5.

82. Raderer M, Jager G, Brugger S *et al.* Rituximab for treatment of advanced extranodal marginal zone B cell lymphoma of the mucosa-associated lymphoid tissue lymphoma. *Oncology* 2003; **65**: 306–10.

83. Schechter NR, Yahalom J. Low-grade MALT lymphoma of the stomach: a review of treatment options. *Int J Radiat Oncol Biol Phys* 2000; **46**: 1093–103.

◆84. Al-Saleem T, Al-Mondhiry H. Immunoproliferative small intestinal disease (IPSID): a model for mature B-cell neoplasms. *Blood* 2005; **105**: 2274–80.

85. Zucca E, Roggero E, Bertoni F, Cavalli F. Primary extranodal non-Hodgkin's lymphomas. Part 1: Gastrointestinal, cutaneous and genitourinary lymphomas. *Ann Oncol* 1997; **8**: 727–37.

86. Salem P, el-Hashimi L, Anaissie E *et al.* Primary small intestinal lymphoma in adults. A comparative study of IPSID versus non-IPSID in the Middle East. *Cancer* 1987; **59**: 1670–6.

87. Ben-Ayed F, Halphen M, Najjar T *et al.* Treatment of alpha chain disease. Results of a prospective study in 21 Tunisian patients by the Tunisian-French intestinal Lymphoma Study Group. *Cancer* 1989; **63**: 1251–6.

88. el Saghir NS, Jessen K, Mass RE *et al.* Combination chemotherapy for primary small intestinal lymphoma in the Middle East. *Eur J Cancer Clin Oncol* 1989; **25**: 851–6.

89. Akbulut H, Soykan I, Yakaryilmaz F *et al.* Five-year results of the treatment of 23 patients with immunoproliferative small intestinal disease: a Turkish experience. *Cancer* 1997; **80**: 8–14.

90. Isaacson PG, Matutes E, Burke M, Catovsky D. The histopathology of splenic lymphoma with villous lymphocytes. *Blood* 1994; **84**: 3828–34.

91. Gisbert JP, Garcia-Buey L, Pajares JM, Moreno-Otero R. Prevalence of hepatitis C virus infection in B-cell non-Hodgkin's lymphoma: systematic review and meta-analysis. *Gastroenterology* 2003; **125**: 1723–32.

92. Chan CH, Hadlock KG, Foung SK, Levy S. V(H)1-69 gene is preferentially used by hepatitis C virus-associated B cell lymphomas and by normal B cells responding to the E2 viral antigen. *Blood* 2001; **97**: 1023–6.

93. Karavattathayyil SJ, Kalkeri G, Liu HJ *et al.* Detection of hepatitis C virus RNA sequences in B-cell non-Hodgkin lymphoma. *Am J Clin Pathol* 2000; **113**: 391–8.

94. Zucca E, Roggero E, Maggi-Solca N et al. Prevalence of *Helicobacter pylori* and hepatitis C virus infections among non-Hodgkin's lymphoma patients in Southern Switzerland. *Haematologica* 2000; **85**: 147–53.

95. Thalen DJ, Raemaekers J, Galama J, Cooreman MP. Absence of hepatitis C virus infection in non-Hodgkin's lymphoma. *Br J Haematol* 1997; **96**: 880–1.

96. Luppi M, Negrini R. MALT lymphoma: epidemiology ad infectious agents. In: Zucca E. (ed.) *MALT lymphomas*. Georgetown, TX: Landes Bioscience/Kluwer Academic, 2004: 1–16.

97. Arcaini L, Paulli M, Boveri E *et al.* Splenic and nodal marginal zone lymphomas are indolent disorders at high hepatitis C virus seroprevalence with distinct presenting features but similar morphologic and phenotypic profiles. *Cancer* 2004; **100**: 107–15.

●98. Hermine O, Lefrere F, Bronowicki JP *et al.* Regression of splenic lymphoma with villous lymphocytes after treatment of hepatitis C virus infection. *N Engl J Med* 2002; **347**: 89–94.

99. Bates I, Bedu-Addo G, Jarrett RF *et al.* B-lymphotropic viruses in a novel tropical splenic lymphoma. *Br J Haematol* 2001; **112**: 161–6.

100. Bedu-Addo G, Bates I. Causes of massive tropical splenomegaly in Ghana. *Lancet* 2002; **360**: 449–54.

101. Isaacson PG. Splenic marginal zone B cell lymphoma. In: Harris NL. (ed.) *Human lymphoma: clinical implications of the REAL classification*. London: Springer-Verlag, 1999: 7.1–7.6.

102. Catovsky D, Matutes E. Splenic lymphoma with circulating villous lymphocytes/splenic marginal-zone lymphoma. *Semin Hematol* 1999; **36**: 148–54.

103. Troussard X, Valensi F, Duchayne E *et al.* Splenic lymphoma with villous lymphocytes: clinical presentation, biology and prognostic factors in a series of 100 patients. Groupe Francais d'Hematologie Cellulaire (GFHC). *Br J Haematol* 1996; **93**: 731–6.

●104. Berger F, Felman P, Thieblemont C *et al.* Non-MALT marginal zone B-cell lymphomas: a description of clinical presentation and outcome in 124 patients. *Blood* 2000; **95**: 1950–6.

●105. Chacon JI, Mollejo M, Munoz E *et al.* Splenic marginal zone lymphoma: clinical characteristics and prognostic factors in a series of 60 patients. *Blood* 2002; **100**: 1648–54.

106. Thieblemont C, Felman P, Berger F *et al.* Treatment of splenic marginal zone B-cell lymphoma: an analysis of 81 patients. *Clin Lymphoma* 2002; **3**: 41–7.

◆107. Thieblemont C, Felman P, Callet-Bauchu E *et al.* Splenic marginal-zone lymphoma: a distinct clinical and pathological entity. *Lancet Oncol* 2003; **4**: 95–103.

108. Berger F, Isaacson PG, Piris MA *et al.* Lymphoplasmacytic lymphoma/Waldenstroem macroglobulinemia. In: Jaffe ES, Harris NL, Stein H, Vardiman JW. (eds) *World Health Organization classification of tumours. Pathology and genetics of tumours of haematopoietic and lymphoid tissues*. Lyon: IARC Press, 2001: 135–7.

109. Mollejo M, Menarguez J, Lloret E *et al.* Splenic marginal zone lymphoma: a distinctive type of low-grade B-cell lymphoma. A clinicopathological study of 13 cases. *Am J Surg Pathol* 1995; **19**: 1146–57.

110. Mulligan SP, Matutes E, Dearden C, Catovsky D. Splenic lymphoma with villous lymphocytes: natural history and response to therapy in 50 cases. *Br J Haematol* 1991; **78**: 206–9.

111. Lefrere F, Hermine O, Belanger C *et al.* Fludarabine: an effective treatment in patients with splenic lymphoma with villous lymphocytes. *Leukemia* 2000; **14**: 573–5.

112. Bolam S, Orchard J, Oscier D. Fludarabine is effective in the treatment of splenic lymphoma with villous lymphocytes. *Br J Haematol* 1997; **99**: 158–61.

113. Lefrere F, Hermine O, Francois S *et al.* Lack of efficacy of 2-chlorodeoxyadenoside in the treatment of splenic lymphoma with villous lymphocytes. *Leuk Lymphoma* 2000; **40**: 113–17.

114. Arcaini L, Orlandi E, Scotti M *et al.* Combination of rituximab, cyclophosphamide, and vincristine induces

complete hematologic remission of splenic marginal zone lymphoma. *Clin Lymphoma* 2004; **4**: 250–2.

115. Paydas S, Yavuz S, Disel U *et al.* Successful rituximab therapy for hemolytic anemia associated with relapsed splenic marginal zone lymphoma with leukemic phase. *Leuk Lymphoma* 2003; **44**: 2165–6.

●116. Nathwani BN, Anderson JR, Armitage JO *et al.* Marginal zone B-cell lymphoma: A clinical comparison of nodal and mucosa-associated lymphoid tissue types. Non-Hodgkin's lymphoma classification project. *J Clin Oncol* 1999; **17**: 2486–92.

117. Sheibani K, Burke JS, Swartz WG *et al.* Monocytoid B-cell lymphoma. Clinicopathologic study of 21 cases of a unique type of low-grade lymphoma. *Cancer* 1988; **62**: 1531–8.

118. Royer B, Cazals-Hatem D, Sibilia J *et al.* Lymphomas in patients with Sjogren's syndrome are marginal zone B-cell neoplasms, arise in diverse extranodal and nodal sites, and are not associated with viruses. *Blood* 1997; **90**: 766–75.

119. Shin SS, Sheibani K, Fishleder A *et al.* Monocytoid B-cell lymphoma in patients with Sjogren's syndrome: a clinicopathologic study of 13 patients. *Hum Pathol* 1991; **22**: 422–30.

120. Fisher RI, Dahlberg S, Nathwani BN *et al.* A clinical analysis of two indolent lymphoma entities: mantle cell lymphoma and marginal zone lymphoma (including the mucosa-associated lymphoid tissue and monocytoid B-cell subcategories): a Southwest Oncology Group study. *Blood* 1995; **85**: 1075–82.

121. Nathwani BN, Drachenberg MR, Hernandez AM *et al.* Nodal monocytoid B-cell lymphoma (nodal marginal-zone B-cell lymphoma). *Semin Hematol* 1999; **36**: 128–38.

122. Berger F, Traverse-Glehen A, Salles G. Nodal marginal zone B-cell lymphoma. In: Harris NL. (ed.) *Non-Hodgkin's lymphomas.* Philadelphia, PA: Lippincott Williams and Wilkins, 2004: 361–5.

123. Koh LP, Lim LC, Thng CH. Retreatment with chimeric CD 20 monoclonal antibody in a patient with nodal marginal zone B-cell lymphoma. *Med Oncol* 2000; **17**: 225–8.

124. Vallisa D, Bernuzzi P, Arcaini L *et al.* Role of anti-hepatitis C virus (HCV) treatment in HCV-related, low-grade, B-cell, non-Hodgkin's lymphoma: A multicenter Italian experience. *J Clin Oncol* 2005; **23**: 468–73.

125. Ruskone-Fourmestraux A, Dragosics B, Morgner A *et al.* Paris staging system for primary gastrointestinal lymphomas. *Gut* 2003; **52**: 912–13.

67

Follicular lymphoma

AZS ROHATINER

BACKGROUND

Follicular lymphoma is the second most common histologic subtype of non-Hodgkin lymphoma (NHL) worldwide.[1] The World Health Organization (WHO) Lymphoma Classification[2] is based on cell of origin and the pathophysiological behavior of the lymphoma. Follicular lymphoma is derived from germinal center B cells and, in terms of gene expression profiling,[3] maintains the molecular features of this stage in B cell ontogeny. Occurring with a frequency of approximately 2:100 000 in the Western world,[2] its incidence varies with geographic location and amongst different ethnic groups, being seen less often in Asia and developing countries than in Europe and the United States.[4] This difference is reflected in the fact that the risk of developing the illness is also lower in first-generation immigrants from China and Japan than for subsequent generations living in the United States.[5]

The etiology of the illness remains obscure, although in 85 percent of patients, the t(14;18) translocation, which results in rearrangement of *BCL2*, contributes to its pathogenesis. The incidence of the *BCL2* rearrangement is the same amongst normal individuals from Asian countries as in the West;[6] however, the t(14;18) translocation is less often associated with follicular lymphoma occurring

in Asian patients than in those developing the disease in Western countries.[6]

The clinical course of follicular lymphoma is changing. For over 30 years, the median survival of patients with the illness was approximately 10 years,[7–11] despite many attempts to alter its clinical course. It is now becoming apparent that with developments in treatment, the median survival is improving. Recent analyses from the USA[12,13] and from Europe[14] confirm data from the Surveillance, Epidemiology and End Results (SEER) Registry published in 2003,[15] which have shown a definitive, albeit small change in outcome in recent years.

This chapter will discuss the new approaches that have contributed to this improvement. It will address the pragmatic, clinical questions faced by physicians and their patients and review current treatment options at the time of diagnosis and recurrence.

There is no established treatment of choice for newly diagnosed patients or at recurrence. Until recently, the illness was considered incurable because no plateau on the survival curves was demonstrable. Since more intensive, for example, anthracycline-containing treatment did not improve survival (as compared to the results achieved with oral, alkylating agent chemotherapy alone),[16] the aim of treatment has been to maintain as good a quality of life as possible, for as long as possible. Therapy has been started only when symptoms supervene. With this overall strategy, although there is great variability in the clinical behavior of the illness, the average person with follicular lymphoma will receive treatment several times over a 10-year period. The first remission is likely to be longer than subsequent ones,[17] but death as a consequence of the illness (or of treatment for it) is virtually inevitable, irrespective of whether transformation to diffuse large B cell (DLBC) pathology has occurred.

Historical perspective

Follicular lymphoma is first alluded to in the German literature by Becker in 1917[18] and subsequently, as 'generalised giant lymph follicle hyperplasia of lymph nodes and spleen' in the *Journal of the American Medical Association* in 1925.[19] In 1938, Symmers reported a series of patients with 'giant follicular lymphadenopathy with or without splenomegaly'[20] describing an illness very similar to follicular lymphoma as seen in clinical practice today. Patients presented with generalized lymph node enlargement and the spleen was often enlarged. In some, the illness progressed quickly (presumably the equivalent of transformation); occasionally, spontaneous regression was noted but the illness was invariably fatal. Radiation therapy, the only treatment available, was effective in temporarily reducing the size of lymph nodes and spleen.

Patients treated at the Massachusetts General Hospital formed the basis of two reports in which the histologic subtype of lymphoma was described as 'follicular' on the basis of lymph node biopsy or postmortem material.[21,22] A further contribution to the description of the pathology made the distinction between follicular hyperplasia and its 'malignant' counterpart, follicular lymphoma, on account of the follicles in the latter having a different cellular composition.[23] A subsequent description of what is termed 'giant follicle lymphosarcoma' refers to an illness with a median age at diagnosis of 50 years. Most of the patients had generalized lymphadenopathy at presentation but were well. The median survival, however, was only 5 years, death occurring from progressive disease.[24] Apart from survival being shorter, the only other difference between these early descriptions and more recent ones is that the incidence of *follicular* lymphoma (as compared to other subtypes of NHL) was apparently lower than now. In the pathological series published in 1941, it accounted for only 9 percent of cases;[21] in the description by Rosenberg *et al.* in 1961[24] it was 13 percent, as opposed to 22 percent in 1997.[1]

Pathology

MORPHOLOGY

Follicular lymphomas are a group of B cell malignancies of follicle center cells, characterized by two cell types that are present in the follicle centers of normal lymph nodes. Centrocytes (small, cleaved cells) predominate amongst variable numbers of centroblasts (large, noncleaved cells). Degrees of follicularity may coexist with diffuse areas, being reported as follows: predominantly follicular (more than 75 percent follicular), follicular and diffuse (25–75 percent follicular), and predominantly diffuse (less than 25 percent follicular).[2] By definition, the normal lymph node structure is effaced by the neoplastic follicles and between these there may be areas of sclerosis (Chapter 31).

The WHO classification[2] defines three subgroups of follicular lymphoma, termed grades 1, 2, and 3, based on the number of centroblasts per high-power field, using the cell counting method of Mann and Berard;[25] more than 15 centroblasts per high-power field defines grade 3. The latter is in turn subclassified into grades 3a and 3b, representing in the former an admixture of centrocytes and centroblasts, whereas in grade 3b there are just sheets of centroblasts. However, the three grades are parts of a continuum, reflecting the clinical behavior of the illness. The pathological appearance may change from one grade to another, the direction of change usually (but not always) being toward an increasing number of large cells, often culminating in transformation to DLBC pathology. The heterogeneity within grade 3 also correlates with differences in antigenic profile and clinical behavior. Thus, whilst patients with grade 1 and 2 follicular lymphoma are treated in a similar way to those with grade 3a disease, in those with grade 3b the illness behaves like DLBC lymphoma and therefore should be treated as such.[26]

There are also, very rarely, cases of diffuse lymphoma which consist largely of centrocytes, with some centroblasts but with no recognizable follicular structure. The term 'follicle center lymphoma, diffuse' has therefore been retained as a separate category within the WHO classification,[2] the diagnosis usually being made when there is some additional indicator of follicle center derivation, such as the *BCL2* rearrangement or CD10 expression.[27] Further variations include the presence of monocytoid B cells[28] or plasmacytoid differentiation. Apart from the diffuse variant, the WHO classification also describes *primary cutaneous* follicular lymphoma in which both centrocytes and centroblasts are present in a partially follicular pattern. Almost always, the cells are BCL2 negative.[2]

THE IMPORTANCE OF REPEAT BIOPSY

Recognition of the changing histologic pattern within the spectrum referred to above can only be made with stringent attention to re-biopsy at each progression or recurrence. This is essential with regard to transformation to DLBC pathology because at this point the illness behaves quite differently and the treatment used for follicular lymphoma will not be effective. Thus, re-biopsy is not just an academic exercise: it has real implications for therapy (see below). Whilst clinical progression is mostly accompanied by histologic progression from grade 1 or 2 through grade

3a to grade 3b or transformation, this is by no means always the case. Following transformation and successful treatment for it – for example, high-dose therapy with autologous peripheral blood progenitor cell (PBPC) support – 'reversion' to a follicular pattern may occur. Again, re-biopsy is very important in this situation because of the implications for treatment.

IMMUNOPHENOTYPE

As B cells, the cells of follicular lymphoma express surface immunoglobulin (Ig), most often IgM, although IgD, IgG, and IgA can also be found (in decreasing frequency).[2] The cells express B cell antigens (CD19, CD20, CD22, CD79a, and CD79b) and variably CD10,[2] the latter being seen less often in cases of higher histologic grade,[29] in contrast to the situation with BCL6, which is more frequently found in this group.[30] The cells are usually CD5 negative, but not always CD23 negative. CD43 is only expressed in grade 3 follicular lymphoma,[31] BCL2 in the majority.[32]

t(14;18) CHROMOSOMAL TRANSLOCATION

Eighty-five percent of cases are associated with the t(14;18) (q32;q21) translocation,[33,34] but often this is not the only chromosomal abnormality.[35] Rearrangement of the *BCL2* gene results in overexpression of the antiapoptotic protein BCL2, which is presumed to allow accumulation of centrocytes.[36–38] The translocation is thought to occur at an early stage of B cell development during immunoglobulin gene rearrangement.[39]

Polymerase chain reaction (PCR) analysis has demonstrated the presence of the *IGH/BCL2* rearrangement in a proportion of healthy blood donors but at low levels.[40,41] Thus, dysregulation of BCL2 expression in the presence of the *IGH/BCL2* rearrangement clearly does not necessarily lead to the development of follicular lymphoma, suggesting that a further 'event' is required for genesis of the disease. Further evidence for this comes from BCL2 transgenic mice which develop polyclonal follicular hyperplasia. After a period of time, this *may* progress to monoclonal immunoblastic lymphoma.[42] Moreover, in a minority of patients, the illness is not associated with a t(14;18) translocation, suggesting an alternative mechanism.

MOLECULAR REMISSION

Use of PCR methodology has made it possible to detect very low levels of *IGH/BCL2* rearrangement-containing cells, which in turn has led to the concept of 'molecular remission.' The term was originally used to describe absence of *BCL2* rearrangement-containing cells at the molecular level, at a time when such results were described as either positive or negative. With the advent of quantitative, so-called 'real-time' PCR, it is now possible to quantify the 'copy number' of *BCL2* rearrangement-containing cells to a level of one abnormal cell in 10^5 normal cells.[41]

The presence or absence of such cells in blood or bone marrow has therefore been used as a surrogate marker of disease activity and, as such, has been applied as a measure of efficacy following various treatment modalities. The concept was first used in relation to high-dose treatment supported by autologous bone marrow transplantation (ABMT), and later to fludarabine and antibody-based treatments.

MOLECULAR PATHOLOGY

The advent of microarray methodology has shown that the gene expression pattern at the time of presentation can determine outcome of patients with follicular lymphoma (see Chapter 31). Furthermore, recent data[3] have also demonstrated the role of the 'nonmalignant' cellular component of the microenvironment in determining outcome. Thus, survival correlates not only with the gene expression signature of the lymphoma cells but also with genes derived from T cells, dendritic cells, and macrophages, suggesting that the immune response to the presence of lymphoma also contributes to prognosis (see Chapter 31).

CLINICAL CONSIDERATIONS

Presenting symptoms

Follicular lymphoma is generally an illness of middle-aged and older people, virtually equal numbers of men and women being affected. The majority of patients consult a doctor because of painless lymph node enlargement. Most present with already advanced stage disease, discernible on computed tomography (CT) scans as intrathoracic, intraabdominal, or pelvic lymph node enlargement; the bone marrow is usually involved. Presentation in the leukemic phase may be seen but extranodal sites are less frequently involved than in DLBC lymphoma.

The clinical features at presentation for more than 4000 patients with follicular lymphoma, from which the Follicular Lymphoma International Prognostic Index (FLIPI) was derived,[43] are representative of patients diagnosed between 1985 and 2002 (Table 67.1). Their laboratory parameters at the time of presentation are shown in Table 67.2.

Making the diagnosis

BIOPSY

The diagnosis of any lymphoma should be made by an experienced histopathologist, on the basis of an excision biopsy of a lymph node. Where there is not an accessible peripheral node, core needle biopsy performed under control of ultrasound or CT scan is safe and effective;[44] fine needle aspiration is not helpful. If possible, in addition to performing standard pathological and immunocytochemical analyses, fresh tissue should be frozen for potential future investigations.

Sometimes, in addition to peripheral lymph nodes, biopsy of which shows follicular lymphoma (grade 1, 2, or 3a), there may be another, often larger, intraabdominal mass. It is important, whether at first presentation or at the time of recurrence, that a separate, additional biopsy of this mass is done, because it may show discordant pathology; that is, follicular lymphoma in the peripheral node but 'transformation' in the abdominal mass. The choice of treatment will clearly be influenced by this, so again, it should not be regarded as a 'research biopsy.'

STAGING

As for any illness, a clear medical history together with an accurate physical examination will point to specific areas for further investigation. The following are mandatory: a full blood count and examination of the blood film, tests of kidney and liver function, uric acid and lactate dehydrogenase (LDH), together with a unilateral bone marrow

Table 67.1 Clinical characteristics of follicular lymphoma at presentation

Feature	Proportion (%)
Gender male:female	51:49
Age <60:≥ 60 years	63:37
Stage I + I:III + IV	22:78
B symptoms absent:present	81:19
Performance status ECOG 0–1:ECOG >1	88:12
Number of nodal sites <4:≥ 4	65:35
Splenic involvement negative:positive	78:22
Bone marrow negative:positive	52:48
Histology small cell:mixed pattern:large cell	50:41:9

After Solal-Celigny et al.[43]
ECOG, Eastern Cooperative Oncology Group.

Table 67.2 Laboratory findings in follicular lymphoma at presentation

Features		Proportion (%)
Hemoglobin (g/dL)	≥12:<12	82:18
Lymphocyte count × 10^9/L	≥1:<1	80:20
Platelet count × 10^9/L	≥150:<50	88:12
ESR (mm/h)	≤40:>40	89:11
Serum LDH	≤ULN:>ULN	79:21
Serum β_2-microglobulin	≤ULN:>ULN	59:41
Serum albumin (g/L)	≥3.5:<3.5	90:10

After Solal-Celigny et al.[43]
ESR, erythrocyte sedimentation rate; LDH, lactate dehydrogenase; ULN, upper limit of normal.

aspirate and trephine biopsy. Computed axial tomography scans are essential to provide a baseline against which response to treatment can be evaluated, or if treatment is not indicated and the patient is being observed in the first instance, to monitor the rate of progression.

Positron emission tomography (PET) scanning is included in the revised guidelines for management and outcome assessment of 'aggressive' lymphomas.[45] It has been less extensively studied in follicular lymphoma but PET scanning demonstrates 94 percent sensitivity and 100 percent specificity in this illness.[46] At present, it is not used routinely in follicular lymphoma, but the emergence of areas of intense uptake should raise the suspicion of transformation to DLBC pathology.

Natural history

Unusually in a malignancy for which numerous different treatment modalities exist, it is possible to comment on the true 'natural history' of the illness (as opposed to the clinical course, when the latter is modified by treatment), since not all patients are treated from the outset. The rationale for observation (so-called 'watchful waiting' or a 'watch-and-wait approach,' otherwise termed 'expectant management'), is based on three randomized studies.[47–49] These show no difference in survival between patients in whom treatment was started at the time of diagnosis and those in whom intervention was deliberately postponed until there was an indication to start treatment. This strategy was originally advocated at Stanford University Medical Center, where it was demonstrated that the survival of patients managed with 'no initial therapy' was the same as that of historical control patients who received immediate therapy.[50] The original series describes 83 patients, 62 with advanced stage follicular lymphoma (the remainder having small lymphocytic lymphoma). The outcome over a 20-year period can be summarized as follows: a degree of spontaneous regression was observed in 16 patients; at the time of publication, 51 of the original 83 patients had required treatment, mostly for increasing lymphadenopathy, extranodal involvement, systemic symptoms, or a combination of these.[50]

Another retrospective analysis has since been conducted (also at Stanford University) in 43 patients presenting with stage I or II follicular lymphoma, in whom no initial therapy was given. At a median follow-up of just over 7 years, 27 patients (63 percent) had not required treatment; the median time to specific therapy in the remainder was 22 months. Nine patients died during the observation period, six due to progressive lymphoma. In four patients, there was transformation to DLBC pathology. The estimated survival at 5, 10, and 20 years was 97 percent, 85 percent, and 22 percent, respectively.[51] The other group of patients for whom information is available is those with no evidence of disease following an excision biopsy (so-called 'stage I_0' disease). With a median follow-up of 6 years,

13 out of 26 patients not given specific therapy postoperatively were reported to be well and without disease progression.[52] Thus, it is acceptable to observe patients in this situation in the first instance.

Clinical course

In most patients, the illness responds to treatment repeatedly but further recurrence is virtually inevitable. Despite responsiveness to chemotherapy, irradiation, and to biologic therapies, death almost always supervenes as a consequence of the illness (or of complications of treatment), irrespective of transformation to DLBC pathology. This pattern of repeated response but inexorable recurrence results in the characteristic survival curve of patients with follicular lymphoma[8–11,43] shown in Figure 67.1 (overall survival) and Figure 67.2 (survival according to stage) for patients treated at St. Bartholomew's Hospital (SBH) in London.[53]

Remissions in follicular lymphoma are usually incomplete and not durable, both the response rate and duration of remission tending to decrease with time.[17] Duration of first to fifth remission in patients with follicular lymphoma treated with chlorambucil or cyclophosphamide, vincristine, and prednisolone (CVP) at SBH is shown in Figure 67.3.[53]

HISTOLOGIC TRANSFORMATION

Histologic transformation of the illness to DLBC pathology (or, rarely, to Burkitt lymphoma) changes the prognosis dramatically. In a recent analysis from SBH,[54] as shown in Figure 67.4, the median survival from the time of transformation was only 1.2 years. There is much variation in the reported frequency of transformation, ranging from 16 percent to 60 percent.[54–62] To some extent, this reflects the length of follow-up and the strategy regarding repeat biopsy at the time of recurrence. It also depends on the definition of transformation, which can occur early in the course of the illness, after several recurrences, many years after the diagnosis, or never. In the SBH series,[54] with a median follow-up of 15 years and a repeat biopsy rate of 70 percent, the risk of transformation was 28 percent at 10 years, and it was not

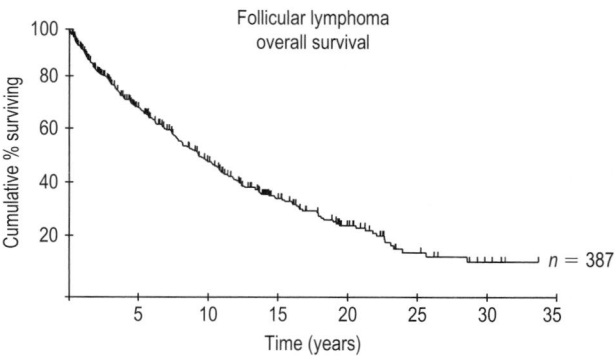

Figure 67.1   Overall survival of newly diagnosed patients with follicular lymphoma presenting to St. Bartholomew's Hospital, London.[53]

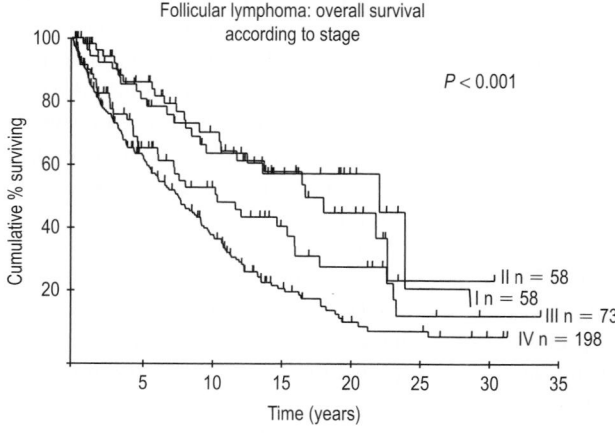

Figure 67.2   Overall survival according to stage for patients with follicular lymphoma presenting to St. Bartholomew's Hospital, London.[53]

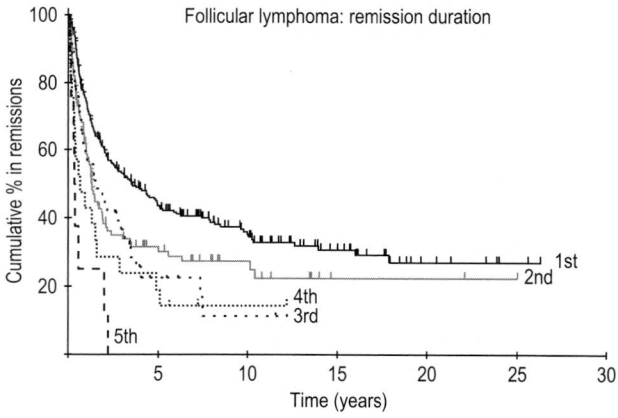

Figure 67.3   Remission duration of patients with follicular lymphoma treated at St. Bartholomew's Hospital, London.[17, 253]

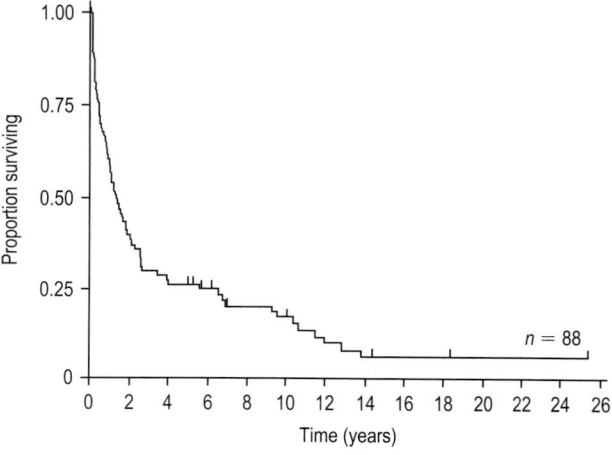

Figure 67.4   Survival from transformation in 88 patients in whom histologic transformation was documented.[53]

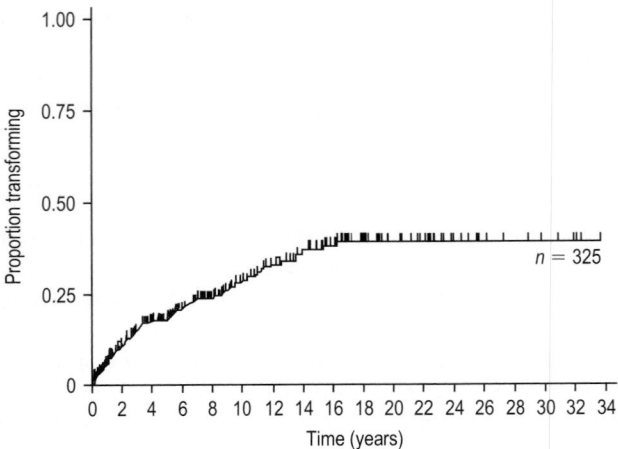

Figure 67.5 Cumulative incidence of transformation in 325 patients with follicular lymphoma.[53]

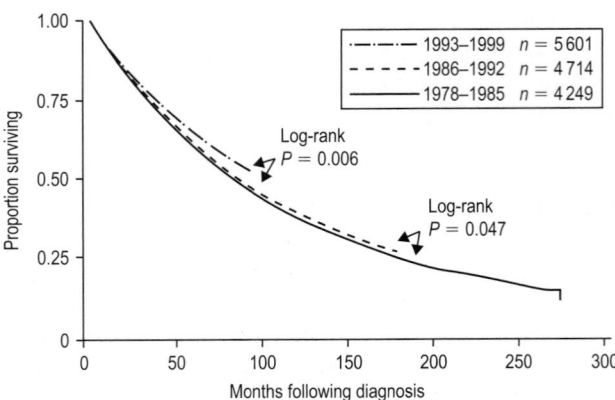

Figure 67.6 Changes in survival of patients with follicular lymphoma over three time periods.[15]

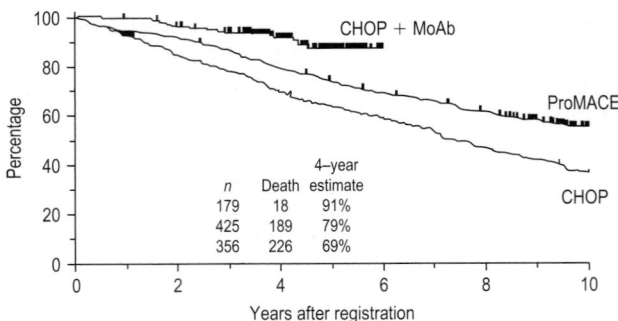

Figure 67.7 Changes in survival of patients with follicular lymphoma in Southwest Oncology Group studies.[12] CHOP, cyclophosphamide, doxorubicin, vincristine, and prednisone; MoAb, monoclonal antibody; ProMACE, prednisone, methotrexate, doxorubicin, cyclophosphamide, and etoposide.

observed beyond 16.2 years (Fig. 67.5). Importantly, patients with transformation at any point had a significantly shorter overall survival than those in whom it did not occur.

The pathological change is often associated with changes in the clinical behavior of the illness, most patients describing rapid enlargement of lymph nodes and the development of systemic symptoms. In the SBH series, clinical correlates of biopsy-proven transformation in a lymph node *at the time of first recurrence* were older age, low hemoglobin level, high LDH, and a 'high-risk' FLIPI or International Prognostic Index (IPI) score.[43]

The sequence of molecular events associated with transformation is now beginning to be elucidated (see Chapter 31) and may lead to new therapeutic targets being identified. If transformation could be prevented or treated more effectively when it occurs, significant therapeutic progress would have been made.

SURVIVAL

The pattern of illness described above is based on numerous observations over a 40-year period. However, in contrast to results published from Stanford University for patients treated in sequential studies between 1960 and 1991,[7] in which the overall survival remained the same, it is now becoming apparent that the survival of patients with follicular lymphoma is changing. The SEER data from the United States,[15] based on a survival analysis for more than 14 000 patients treated during three consecutive time periods, demonstrate an improvement in survival between each of three eras (Fig. 67.6); the change was seen, however, only in white patients.

The improvement reflects a similar change in outcome reported from two other sources in the United States. At MD Anderson Cancer Center,[13] overall survival (OS) and failure-free survival (FFS) were analyzed for 580 patients treated in five consecutive studies. All but the first involved combination chemotherapy followed by interferon; the last

also included rituximab. At 5 years (a relatively short follow-up for follicular lymphoma), OS had improved from 64 percent to 95 percent and FFS from 29 percent to 60 percent. An unexpected finding was an apparent plateau on the FFS curve. In the second study, outcome for patients treated in the context of Southwest Oncology Group (SWOG) trials was analyzed.[12] Three sequential treatment approaches were evaluated: (1) cyclophosphamide, doxorubicin, vincristine, and prednisolone (CHOP) ± nonspecific immunostimulants; (2) a more complex, third-generation chemotherapy regimen ± interferon; and (3) CHOP followed by rituximab or iodine-131 (^{131}I)-tositumomab (radiolabeled anti-CD20). The progression-free survival (PFS) curves for the first two chemotherapy regimens overlapped, with 4-year PFS estimates of 46 percent and 48 percent, respectively, but for the studies using chemotherapy followed by antibody, this improved to 61 percent. Furthermore, the estimates of OS were 69 percent for CHOP, 79 percent for the third-generation regimen, and 91 percent for the antibody-containing regimen (Fig. 67.7). These results remained the same after adjusting for differences in prognostic factors between the study groups.

The results differ, partly because the SEER data are from a population-based cancer registry whereas the latter two data sets represent selected patients treated in clinical trials. Two things, however, are common to all three: the overall pattern of survival has not changed but the median has improved over time. It is concluded that this is due to the development of new treatment options, either given as initial therapy or later in the course of the illness. For the SEER data, the improvement predates the introduction of rituximab.

Support for the suggestion that rituximab has, to some extent at least, contributed to the improvement comes from analysis of two consecutive generations of studies run by the German Low-Grade Lymphoma Study Group (GLGLSG) over a 10-year period. The analysis was adjusted for risk factors such as FLIPI score and type of initial chemotherapy, which was given with or without rituximab.[14] In more than 1300 patients with stage III or IV follicular lymphoma, deemed to be in need of treatment, the use of rituximab was associated with a significantly improved response rate and overall survival. However, it is not the only factor responsible. Data from SBH also show an improvement in survival, probably in part attributable to a strategy of consolidating second remission with high-dose treatment.

MANAGEMENT

To treat or not to treat?

The current standard treatment approach for patients with localized (that is, stage I or II, grade 1 or 2) follicular lymphoma is to give radiation therapy with curative intent, and for patients with advanced disease to start treatment only when there is a specific indication to do so. This strategy is based on the fact that a proportion of people with localized disease will unquestionably be cured with radiation therapy and that for those presenting with advanced disease, it has been shown that treatment can be deferred without compromising survival, provided that specific criteria are fulfilled. Two groups of criteria are in clinical use, put forward by the Groupe pour l'Etude de Lymphome Folliculaire (GELF)[48] and the British National Lymphoma Investigation (BNLI)[49] (Table 67.3). Viewed separately or as being complementary, they constitute useful guidelines for management. With increasing use of the FLIPI, it is becoming apparent that patients in the low-risk group may not need treatment immediately, whilst those in the high-risk group should be treated straightaway, and on clinical grounds this is indeed often the case. For clinical trials currently being designed for newly diagnosed patients, stratification on the basis of the FLIPI score is being proposed.

It is possible to argue that perhaps the time has come to question the traditional, conservative viewpoint. In Europe, a randomized phase III study in patients considered to be not in need of treatment is currently in progress.

Table 67.3   Criteria for treatment of follicular lymphoma

BNLI criteria for starting treatment[49]
Absence of all of the following:

1. Pruritus or B symptoms
2. Rapid generalized disease progression
3. 'Life-endangering' organ involvement
4. Marrow compromise (Hb $\leqslant$100 g/L, WBC <3.0 × 10^9/L or platelets <100 × 10^9/L)
5. Bone lesions
6. Renal infiltration
7. Macroscopic liver involvement

GELF criteria for delaying treatment[48]
All of the following:

1. Maximum diameter of any site of disease <7 cm
2. Fewer than 3 nodal sites with a diameter >3 cm
3. Absence of systemic symptoms
4. No 'substantial' splenic involvement (spleen <16 cm in length based on CT measurement)
5. No significant serious effusions clinically evident or on chest x-ray
6. Absence of risk of local compressive symptoms (epidural, ureteral)
7. No circulating lymphoma cells or peripheral blood cytopenias (Hb >10 g/dL, neutrophils >1.5 × 10^9/L, platelets >100 × 10^9/L).

Using these criteria 36% of consecutive patients diagnosed with follicular lymphoma were considered to have a 'low' tumor burden

BNLI, British National Lymphoma Investigation; GELF, Groupe pour l'Etude de Lymphome Folliculaire; HB, hemoglobin; WBC, white blood cell; CT, computed tomography.

In this study, observation is being compared with the use of rituximab (four infusions or four infusions followed by maintenance rituximab) to determine whether the use of antibody will delay the need for systemic chemotherapy. Quite apart from such considerations, for the newly diagnosed patient with follicular lymphoma it can be extremely difficult to accept that a diagnosis of 'cancer' has been made but that no immediate treatment is being advocated. It is important to explain to the person who is ill that observation does not imply 'doing nothing.' On the contrary, such patients are followed closely, preferably by the same person. At SBH, they are seen every 3 months and a CT scan is performed after 6 months in the first instance, to check for progression. Further scans are not done routinely unless new symptoms are noted by the patient or there is evidence of progression, such as an increase in lymphadenopathy.

OBSERVATION – LOCALIZED DISEASE

In view of the data from France in patients with stage I_0 disease,[52] it is acceptable to observe such patients in the first instance, but this is for the patient and the physician to decide together. The traditional approach is to give involved field radiation therapy (IFRT) to the site from which the original lymph node was excised. Similarly, patients with stage I or II disease are generally treated with IFRT[63–65] but the report from Stanford University for patients with limited disease suggests that it is entirely appropriate to follow such patients closely and to intervene only when necessary.[51]

OBSERVATION – ADVANCED DISEASE

For newly diagnosed patients with advanced stage but *asymptomatic* follicular lymphoma and no indication for immediate treatment, the 'watch-and-wait' policy has been evaluated in three randomized trials. The first compared 'watchful waiting' with combined modality therapy, the chemotherapy regimen being ProMACE-MOPP (prednisone, methotrexate, doxorubicin, cyclophosphamide, etoposide, mechlorethamine, vincristine, and procarbazine),[47] and the second (in patients considered to have a 'low tumor burden' according to GELF criteria) compared no initial treatment with interferon or prednimustine.[48] There was no difference in overall survival. The third, more recent randomized study[49] compared observation with chlorambucil. With a 16-year median follow-up, the median survival was 5.9 years for chlorambucil and 6.7 years for observation. Cause-specific survival was similar in the two study arms.

However, in the United States, at least, practice is changing. The National LymphoCare study[66] prospectively documents presentation features, treatment given, and clinical outcome in newly diagnosed patients with follicular lymphoma. Data collected thus far, for approximately 1500 patients treated at 237 centers, show that 26 percent of those being observed in the first instance had been started on specific treatment after a median of only 2.8 months from diagnosis. Moreover, at 6 months, only 19 percent of patients who had initially been observed remained untreated. Whether this was appropriate is impossible to comment on, but certainly for older patients it is hard to justify starting treatment in this situation knowing that in the BNLI study,[49] deaths from causes other than lymphoma having been censored, 40 percent of patients aged more than 70 years randomized to observation had still not required treatment 10 years later. Regional differences, however, do apply, even within the United States: in the northeast of the country, 31 percent of patients were observed initially in comparison with only 13 percent in southeastern states.[66]

Radiation therapy

STAGE I AND II DISEASE

Radiation is highly effective in follicular lymphoma, a dose–response relationship having been demonstrated.

Recurrences within the radiation field are rare, provided 45 Gy are given,[67] but this is higher than the usual dose administered, which varies between 30 Gy and 40 Gy.[68–77] Most patients are now treated with IFRT; that is, treatment to the lymph node (or extranodal site) and its immediate lymph node drainage area. Results vary but are, in general, excellent. A recent report with long follow-up from the Princess Margaret Hospital in Toronto shows overall survival to be 79 percent and 62 percent at 5 and 10 years, respectively, with disease-free survival being 56 percent and 41 percent, respectively.[78]

STAGE III DISEASE

Three retrospective studies have evaluated the use of extended field radiation therapy (EFRT) in patients with stage III follicular lymphoma.[68,79,80] Patients with less extensive disease (defined as fewer than five sites, tumor masses less than 10 cm in diameter, and no B symptoms) had an excellent outcome (FFS 88 percent at over 23 years follow-up). There is, however, an increased risk of secondary malignancy with the use of EFRT (in comparison with chemotherapy) and it is not now used as first-line treatment.

LOW-DOSE RADIATION

Low-dose total body irradiation (TBI) is also effective in follicular lymphoma but because of the degree and duration of thrombocytopenia associated with this treatment[81–84] it has been abandoned. However, a recent report of very-low-dose IFRT in patients with recurrent 'localized' disease showed the treatment to be virtually devoid of toxicity and this may be appropriate for specific older or otherwise frail patients for whom chemotherapy is not an option.[85]

COMBINED MODALITY TREATMENT

Radiation therapy has also been combined with chemotherapy in patients with advanced disease. However, there is no evidence from randomized studies (comparing radiation therapy followed by adjuvant chemotherapy with radiation therapy alone) to support the use of combined modality treatment.[86,87] Data on combined modality therapy are also available for patients with stage I or II follicular lymphoma considered to have a 'high tumor burden' and to be at 'high risk' (in terms of an IPI score >1). Three phase II studies[88–90] of chemotherapy followed by IFRT (as opposed to the other way round) showed 5-year OS and FFS to be 70–75 percent and 55–65 percent, respectively.

Treatment of advanced disease

NEWLY DIAGNOSED PATIENTS: PERSPECTIVE

Debate and controversy continue as to what constitutes optimal initial therapy for the person 'in need of treatment.'

For a long time, and still today, choice of treatment has varied according to physicians' opinions and the country in which the person lives. Thus in the UK for many years an alkylating agent-based treatment, either chlorambucil[11,17,91–93] or the combination of cyclophosphamide, vincristine, and prednisone (CVP/COP),[93–96] was the treatment of choice. A series of studies (on both sides of the Atlantic) compared chlorambucil or cyclophosphamide with CVP, and whilst the latter resulted in a higher complete response rate and longer duration of remission, no survival advantage was shown for the combination. Nonetheless, it continued to be used. In North America, CHOP[97–102] predominated, despite the fact that in comparison with historical control patients, no survival advantage could be demonstrated for addition of the anthracycline.[16] In France meanwhile, etoposide was added to a CHOP-like regimen (CHVEP),[103] which was usually given with interferon alpha (IFNα).

The use of purine analogues, particularly fludarabine, as treatment for chronic lymphocytic leukemia was soon followed by successful use in follicular lymphoma,[104–110] especially when the oral formulation was shown to have good bioavailability.[111] The publication of results from the MD Anderson Cancer Center showing that 'molecular remission' could be achieved with the combination FMD (fludarabine, mitoxantrone, and dexamethasone) as well as a complete response (CR) rate of almost 80 percent caused much excitement.[112] Concurrently, in Spanish and German centers as well as in the United States, fludarabine-based combinations, such as fludarabine plus cyclophosphamide (in Spain and the USA)[113] and FCM (fludarabine, cyclophosphamide, and mitoxantrone, in Italy and Germany),[114,115] were being used with similarly high response and CR rates.

Opinion has been divided about the use of IFNα probably more than about any other drug for follicular lymphoma. Widely used as part of initial therapy in France and Germany until recently, it was never popular in the United States due to its clinical toxicity. When given in conjunction with doxorubicin-containing chemotherapy, a survival advantage was demonstrated[116–118] and subsequently confirmed in a metaanalysis of ten randomized studies using individual, updated patient information.[119] The metaanalysis showed a survival advantage, but only when the drug was given with relatively intensive chemotherapy, at a dose higher than 5 million units, and at a cumulative dose greater than 36 million units per month. The use of IFNα as maintenance therapy did not improve survival. However, in terms of 'biological therapy,' IFNα has now been superseded by the use of anti-CD20.

The advent of monoclonal antibodies as treatment for B cell malignancies has made 'chemoimmunotherapy' the treatment of choice for newly diagnosed patients in the Western world. The concept of 'antikorp' (antibody) as treatment for cancer was first put forward with remarkable prescience by Ehrlich in 1890.[120] Recognition of the CD20 antigen, originally termed B1,[121] led to the development of

anti-CD20 and the chimeric monoclonal antibody now commercially available as rituximab/Mabthera. Rituximab was first evaluated alone at the somewhat empirical dose of 375 mg/m^2 in part derived from a phase I study.[122] Given weekly for 4 weeks (as in the 'pivotal' phase II study),[123] this has remained the standard dose and schedule. Its use as a single agent in the United States far exceeds that in Europe. It has since been investigated in combination with various chemotherapy regimens and as 'maintenance therapy' (see below).

Specific treatment options

ALKYLATING AGENTS

First shown to be effective in 1955,[91] chlorambucil given alone results in a response rate of more than 75 percent in newly diagnosed patients and most patients will respond again at first and subsequent recurrence.[11,17,91–93] The responses are usually incomplete (CR rate 25 percent) and (as with most other treatments for this illness) not durable. Nonetheless, given the ease with which the treatment can be given, and minimal clinical toxicity other than myelosuppression, it remains a useful treatment option for older patients. At SBH, it is currently being evaluated in combination with rituximab.

Cyclophosphamide has been the mainstay of treatment for follicular lymphoma for many years, as part of the combination CVP, with response rates similar to those seen with chlorambucil but a somewhat higher percentage of complete responses (CR rate 37 percent).[93–96] Readers from the United States will be most familiar with its use as part of the CHOP regimen,[16,97–102] which results in CR being achieved in approximately 64 percent of patients (clearly higher than with chlorambucil or CVP) but no survival advantage.

FLUDARABINE AND FLUDARABINE-BASED COMBINATIONS

The original studies with fludarabine resulted in overall response rates of 30–70 percent, depending on the population of patients being treated[104–110] and in newly diagnosed patients,[124,125] and CR rates of 37 percent and 47 percent, respectively. Subsequent studies of fludarabine in combination with other drugs (on the basis of in vitro evidence of synergy)[126,127] resulted in very high CR rates, ranging from 79 percent to 89 percent in newly diagnosed patients receiving FC (fludarabine plus cyclophosphamide),[113] FND (fludarabine, mitoxantrone, and dexamethasone),[112] and FCM (fludarabine, cyclophosphamide, and mitoxantrone).[114,115] In the latter two studies, a 'molecular' CR was also achieved in 66 percent and 75 percent of patients, respectively (Table 67.4).

Fludarabine-based regimens are highly effective but have to be used with an awareness of the potential short-term

Table 67.4 Outcome for patients who received fludarabine combinations

Treatment	Disease status	CR (%)	PR (%)	Molecular CR (%)	OS	FFS	Reference
FCM	Recurrence	50	7	21	NS	NS	114
FMD	Rec./newly diag.	20	48	23	10 m[a]	30 m[a]	111
FC	Newly diag.	89	11	Not eval.	66%[b]	53%[b]	112
FND	Newly diag.	79	18	66	84%[b]	39%[b]	127
FCM	Newly diag.	80	13	75	90%[c]	76%[c]	113

[a]Median; [b]at 5 years; [c]at 2 years.
CR, complete remission; PR, partial remission; OS, overall survival; FFS, failure-free survival; FCM: fludarabine, cyclophosphamide, mitoxantrone; FMD: fludarabine, mitoxantrone, dexamethasone; FC: fludarabine, cyclophosphamide; FND: fludarabine, mitoxantrone, dexamethasone; Newly diag., newly diagnosed; Rec., recurrence; NS, not stated; Not eval., not evaluated.

and longer-term toxicity. The myelosuppression is profound and, in addition, fludarabine is associated with a specific T cell dysfunction which results in a propensity for opportunistic infections, particularly by *Pneumocystis carinii* and *Listeria monocytogenes*.[128] The use of prophylactic cotrimoxazole usually prevents the former but the possibility of *Listeria* infection (septicemia or meningitis) should be considered when a patient receiving treatment with fludarabine becomes febrile. Other potential problems are hemolysis and longer-term sequelae. In about one-third of patients treated with fludarabine there will be difficulty in collecting sufficient numbers of autologous PBPC[129,130] and in a small proportion of patients who received TBI-containing myeloablative therapy after treatment with fludarabine, there was an increased probability of developing secondary myelodysplasia (MDS).[131]

MONOCLONAL ANTIBODIES – RITUXIMAB ALONE

Most of the original studies were conducted in patients with indolent disease; that is, not necessarily *follicular* lymphoma but, where possible in this review, results will be stated for the latter. Currently, rituximab is licensed by the European Agency for the Evaluation of Medicinal Products[132] and by the Food and Drug Administration (FDA) of the United States[133] for use in three specific situations: (1) in combination with CVP as initial therapy; (2) in patients in whom CVP as first-line treatment has resulted in a complete or partial response or 'stable disease'; and (3) in patients with recurrent or refractory disease.

In the original phase II studies, the response rate for patients with recurrent disease was 50–60 percent[123,134,135] and the median time to progression for responding patients was 13 months.[123] Lower response rates were seen in patients who were refractory to the last previous chemotherapy[123] and in those who had received multiple previous chemotherapy regimens.[135] Patients with large masses did respond but the response rate was lower.[136] Retreatment was effective.[137]

In newly diagnosed patients, the response rate was somewhat higher[138–140] as it was in those with a 'low tumor burden' by GELF criteria, 73 percent.[141] A follow-up analysis

for this group 7 years after treatment shows that a proportion remains disease free and in continuous 'molecular remission,'[142] providing justification for the current European trial in such patients comparing observation with rituximab.

Responses may occur early but can be ongoing for up to 6 months after completion of treatment.[123,134,136] In most patients, the drug is associated with minimal clinical toxicity in the form of fever and rigors although anaphylactic reactions have been described. If clinical toxicity is going to occur, it tends to do so with the first cycle of treatment and not with subsequent ones. Slowing down the rate of infusion generally deals with the problem. The antibody depletes the B cell compartment of cells that express CD20 – both normal and tumor cells. Although extremely rare, there is a propensity for development of progressive multifocal leukoencephalopathy caused by reactivation of latent JC polyomavirus[143] which is almost invariably fatal.

CHEMOIMMUNOTHERAPY

Standard treatment for follicular lymphoma now comprises one of several combination chemotherapy regimens, such as CVP, CHOP, or a fludarabine-based regimen given in conjunction with rituximab, on the basis of randomized trials which have shown benefit for the addition of the antibody (Table 67.5).[144–148] The original observations were made in just 40 patients who received six cycles of CHOP accompanied by six infusions of rituximab. The overall response rate was 95 percent with a CR rate of 55 percent.[149] In another study, which included both newly diagnosed and previously treated patients, rituximab was given in conjunction with fludarabine, resulting in an overall response rate of 90 percent and an unprecedented CR rate of 80 percent.[150]

All of these randomized studies show a significant improvement in time to treatment failure and, most importantly, now, with somewhat longer follow-up, a survival difference in favor of the addition of rituximab. Furthermore, a metaanalysis confirms the findings of the individual trials, both response rate and overall survival being significantly better for the combination.[151] Thus, at least in the West, rituximab has now been incorporated

Table 67.5 Randomized studies comparing chemotherapy alone with chemotherapy plus rituximab

Treatment	Ref.	No. of pts	Median follow-up (months)	OR rate (%) (CR rate)	TTF (months)	OS P[a]
CVP	144	159		57 (10%)	15	0.029
CVP + Rit		162	53	81 (41%)	34	
CHOP	145	205		90 (17%)	29	0.016
CHOP + Rit		223	18	96 (20%)	NR	
MCP	146	96		75 (25%)	26	0.010
MCP + Rit		105	47	92 (50%)	NR	
CHVP + IFN	147	183		73 (63%)	46	0.010
CHVP + IFN + Rit		175	42	84 (79%)	67	

[a]P value for TTF for all four studies = <0.001.
pts, patients; OR, overall response; CR, complete remission; TTF, time to treatment failure; NR, not reached; OS, overall survival; CVP: cyclophosphamide, vincristine, prednisolone; CHOP: cyclophosphamide, doxorubicin, vincristine, prednisone; MCP, mitoxantrone, chlorambucil, prednisone; CHVP: cyclophosphamide, doxorubicin, teniposide, prednisone; IFN, interferon alpha; Rit, rituximab.

into first-line treatment of patients with follicular lymphoma who have an indication for treatment. The obvious problem is the cost of the drug, although a cost-benefit analysis suggests (perhaps surprisingly) that, in view of the greater efficacy of the combination overall, it is actually cost effective.[152]

The value of maintenance therapy *following initial treatment that includes rituximab* is currently unproven. The PRIMA study (conducted in Europe and Canada), in which one of four different chemotherapy regimens was given with rituximab and then, in a second randomization, patients were allocated to maintenance rituximab or to no further treatment, should answer this question. The results are awaited with interest.

MONOCLONAL ANTIBODIES – RITUXIMAB AS MAINTENANCE THERAPY

The concept of 'maintaining' remission in follicular lymphoma is not new, both chlorambucil[153] and interferon[154–162] having been used in this way. Continuing rituximab for 4 weeks beyond the somewhat empirical, conventional 4 weeks – that is, for a total of 8 weeks – results in both a higher response rate and longer duration of response.[163] Several studies in patients with recurrent or refractory follicular lymphoma have also shown prolongation of duration of response in patients receiving 'maintenance' rituximab.[164–166] Indeed, FDA approval of the drug followed demonstration of a survival advantage for patients receiving rituximab 'maintenance,' remission having been achieved with CVP.[164]

'Maintenance' has been given in two different ways, again reflecting a difference between Europe and the United States. In studies from the SAKK Group in Switzerland, patients with recurrent disease received rituximab alone followed by a single monthly dose for 2 years. This resulted in significant prolongation of median

Table 67.6 Studies in progress to evaluate the use of rituximab as maintenance therapy

Study group	Ref.	Diagnoses	Disease status	Initial therapy
ECOG	163	FL, SLL	Newly diagnosed	CVP
SAKK	165	FL, MCL	Newly diagnosed/ recurrent	Rituximab
EORTC	143	FL	Recurrent/ refractory	CHOP/CHOP + R
GLSG	271	FL, MCL	Recurrent/ refractory	FCM/FCM + R
LYM-5	164	FL, SLL	Recurrent/ refractory	Rituximab

ECOG, Eastern Cooperative Oncology Group; SAKK, Swiss Group for Clinical Cancer Research; EORTC, European Organization for Research and Treatment of Cancer; GLSG, German Lymphoma Study Group, LYM-5, Minnie Pearl Cancer Research Network; FL, follicular lymphoma; SLL, small lymphocytic lymphoma; MCL, mantle cell lymphoma; CVP: cyclophosphamide, vincristine, prednisolone; CHOP: cyclophosphamide, doxorubicin, vincristine, prednisone; R, rituximab; FCM: fludarabine, cyclophosphamide, mitoxantrome.

event-free survival from 1 to almost 2 years.[166] In contrast, in the United States, rituximab has been given as four sequential weekly infusions administered every 3 months.[138,165] There are currently no data to favor either approach and a number of studies are in progress (Table 67.6).

ALTERNATIVE ANTIBODIES

Following the demonstration of efficacy for rituximab, other antibodies such as anti-CD22 have been developed and are being tested. Almost completely 'humanized' (as opposed to chimeric) anti-CD20 antibodies are also being tested.[167] CD22 is expressed in a similar pattern and frequency to CD20. The 'humanized' anti-CD22 antibody epratuzumab showed encouraging efficacy when given as a single agent.[168] It was subsequently combined with rituximab in the hope that using antibodies targeted against two different antigens on the same cell might result in additive or even synergistic efficacy. Ten of sixteen patients with 'indolent' lymphoma responded, nine achieving CR or complete remission (unconfirmed; CRu).[169] In a more recent study conducted in Europe, again combining epratuzumab with rituximab in patients with refractory or recurrent lymphoma, 34 patients with follicular lymphoma who had received a median of two prior therapies received both antibodies, weekly, for four consecutive weeks. The therapy was well tolerated without greater toxicity than that to be expected with rituximab alone. The response rate in patients with follicular lymphoma was 64 percent with 24 percent of patients achieving CR/CRu. Patients with a low-risk FLIPI score had a particularly encouraging response rate of 83 percent.[170]

Anti-CD22 has also been evaluated when conjugated to the highly potent anthracycline, calicheamycin (inotuzumab ozogamicin). A phase I/II study showed encouraging results in patients with follicular lymphoma, the main toxicity being thrombocytopenia and reversible liver dysfunction.[171] Further studies are in progress.

Other antibodies are currently being investigated. A fully human, IgG1 monoclonal antibody that triggers apoptosis through interaction with the death receptor DR5 ('Apomab') promotes receptor clustering and stimulates apoptosis by triggering caspase activation.[172] A study is currently in progress comparing its activity when given in conjunction with rituximab against rituximab plus placebo.

RADIOLABELED ANTI-CD20 ANTIBODIES

The concept of conjugating a radioisotope to a monoclonal antibody, to some extent anyway, fulfils the medical oncologists' 'dream' of selectively delivering treatment to targeted tumor cells. Both ^{131}I- and yttrium-90 (^{90}Y)-conjugated anti-CD20 antibodies are commercially available and are very effective. They are highly specific, targeting irradiation to cells that express CD20 but also killing surrounding, antigen-negative cells – the so-called 'crossfire' effect. Other mechanisms of action have also been invoked, such as antibody-dependent cellular cytotoxicity (ADCC), activation of complement, and induction of apoptosis. Both radiolabeled antibodies have been evaluated at recurrence, in newly diagnosed patients, following chemotherapy (as part of sequential treatments), and as part of myeloablative therapy.

Perhaps the main advantage of this approach is the fact that the treatment needs to be given only once. However, it can only be given in a hospital with excellent nuclear medicine facilities and experienced personnel. Administration of Bexxar (^{131}I-labeled tositumomab) in some European countries and a few states in the USA involves admission for a few days to a lead-lined room until the levels of radi-

ation have fallen to those considered 'safe' (but the definition of what is safe varies). The first studies were conducted using Bexxar, which is currently available only in the United States. Subsequent studies have used ^{90}Y chelated to the anti-CD20 antibody, ibritumomab. The latter is now commercially available in the United States and Europe as Zevalin. No direct comparison between the two radiolabeled antibodies has ever been conducted, but there is probably very little difference between them in terms of efficacy. Response data are summarized in Table 67.7.

In practical terms, there are differences in the way that the treatments are given, partly as a consequence of their different physical properties. Iodine-131 emits both gamma and beta radiation. The former makes it possible (as is deemed necessary) to give a 'test dose' of the radioactive antibody prior to the actual treatment dose, to check whether there is favorable biodistribution. The radioisostope ^{90}Y emits only beta radiation and cannot therefore be used for imaging, but it is now apparent that the treatment dose can be based entirely on the patient's weight. The attraction of the ^{90}Y-labeled antibody is therefore that it can be given entirely on an outpatient basis.

For both compounds, infusion of the radioactive antibody is preceded by infusion of unlabeled antibody (tositumomab in the case of Bexxar, rituximab prior to Zevalin) to saturate antigen-containing sites, such as the spleen and thereby improve tumor targeting. A limiting factor of both treatments is the degree of bone marrow infiltration. It is not safe to give either compound to patients with more than 25 percent infiltration of the 'bone marrow space' on a trephine biopsy because of the possibility of prolonged myelosuppression.[173] A further concern is the small but definite incidence of secondary myelodysplasia which has been observed with both Bexxar and Zevalin when given to patients who have received previous chemotherapy.[174]

^{131}I-labeled tositumomab (Bexxar)

The ^{131}I-labeled antibody has been evaluated in patients with follicular lymphoma who have received multiple previous therapies,[175] in newly diagnosed patients,[176] and as retreatment.[177] Not surprisingly, the most impressive responses were observed in those with newly diagnosed follicular lymphoma, in whom the overall response rate was an almost unprecedented 95 percent with an equally very high (75 percent) complete response rate. Furthermore, 80 percent of patients (some of whom might not necessarily have been deemed to be in need of treatment at other centers) became 'PCR negative.'[176] At the time of publication, the median progression-free survival was 6.1 years and, importantly, myelodysplastic syndrome was not seen. Direct comparison of the radioactive antibody with the parent monoclonal antibody[178] showed significantly improved efficacy for the former.

Bexxar has proved useful when conventional chemotherapy has failed. In a phase II study, in which responsiveness to the radioactive antibody was compared with each individual's response to the previous chemotherapy,

Table 67.7 Response data for CD20-directed radioimmunotherapy

Type of study/pt population	No. of pts	Median no. of prior therapies (range)	Overall response rate	CR/CRu	Remission duration	Rem. durn for pts in whom CR/CRu was achieved	Reference
⁹⁰Y ibritumomab (Zevalin)							
Phase I/II Recurrent/refractory	51 (FL 33)	2 (1–7)	All: 73% (FL: 85%)	All: 51% (FL: 57%)	11.7 m	12.4 m	265
Recurrent/refractory	73 (FL 55, Tr. FL 9)	2 (1–6)	80%	34%	14.2 m (for pts with FL18.5 m)	NS	266[a]
Recurrent/refractory	30 (FL 25, Tr. FL 3)	2 (1–9)	83%	44%	11.7 m	NS	267[b]
Rituximab refractory FL	57 (54 FL)	4 (1–9)	FL 74%	FL: 15%	6.4 m	NS	187
Tositumomab and ¹³¹I tositumomab (Bexxar)							
Recurrent/refractory	47 ('low grade' 37, Tr. FL 10)	4 (1–8)	57% ('low grade' 57%)	32% ('low grade' 27%)	9.9 m ('low grade' 8.2 m)	19.9 m ('low grade' 25.5 m)	268
Phase I/II Recurrent/refractory	59 ('low grade' 28, Tr. FL 14)	4 (1–3)	71% ('low grade' 86%)	34% ('low grade' 46%)	PFS 12 m	PFS 20.3 m	269
Pivotal phase II Chemotherapy refractory	60 ('low grade' 36, Tr. FL 23)	4 (2–13)	65% ('low grade' 81%)	28%	6.5 m	NYR (>47 m)	178
1st/2nd recurrence	41 (FL 29, Tr. FL 7)	1 (1–34)	76% (FL 79%)	49% (FL 59%)	15.6 m	36 m	270
Recurrent/refractory	42 ('low grade' 36, Tr. FL 6)	2 (1–4)	55%	33%	14.7 m	NYR	177[c]
Rituximab refractory	40 (FL 28, Tr. FL 10)	4 (1–11)	65% (grade 1/2 FL 86%)	38% (grade 1/2 FL 57%)	PFS 10.4 m (grade 1/2 FL, NYR)	PFS 24.5 m (grade 1/2 FL NYR)	179
Initial therapy	76	0	95%	75%	PFS 73 m	PFS NYR (77% at 5 years)	175

'Low grade' refers to histology as given in the respective publications. (The majority of these patients will have had follicular lymphoma, although this is not stated by authors.)

[a]Randomized study comparing Zevalin to rituximab. Results shown are for RIT arm only; total patient population = 143.

[b]In patients with a platelet count of 100–149 × 10⁹/L, dose of RIT reduced to 0.3 mCi/kg.

[c]Randomized study of tositumomab vs Bexxar. Results shown are for RIT arm only; total patient population = 78.

FL, follicular lymphoma; Tr. FL, transformed FL; pts, patients; RIT, radioimmunotherapy; NYR, not yet reached at time of publication; CR, complete remission; CRu, complete remission unconfirmed; Rem., remission; durn, duration

65 percent of 60 patients who had not responded to the last regimen (or had progressed within 6 months) did respond, CR being achieved in 23 percent.[179] Furthermore, when duration of response was compared with that following the last previous regimen, in 53 percent of patients it lasted longer. Bexxar has also been shown to be effective in patients who have previously received rituximab[180] and following transformation to DLBC pathology.[181] In terms of hematologic toxicity, it is important to recognize that the nadir occurs much later than following chemotherapy; that is, 4–6 weeks posttreatment, recovery of the blood count usually occurring by week 9–10.[174–181]

Small numbers of patients have received Bexxar at myeloablative doses[182–184] or as part of a myeloablative regimen.[185,186] Although the results have been very impressive, the logistics of administering this treatment have to some extent precluded its widespread use. Bexxar has also been given sequentially, following chemotherapy. In a SWOG study, it was administered to newly diagnosed patients with advanced stage follicular lymphoma 1–2 months after the sixth cycle of CHOP. The overall response rate was very high (91 percent), with CR being achieved in 69 percent of patients. At the time of publication (with a short median follow-up of 1.1 years), the estimated 5-year overall survival was 87 percent. The latter represented a more than 20 percent improvement when compared with the use of CHOP alone in previous SWOG studies.[187]

^{90}Y–labeled ibritumonab tiuxetan (Zevalin)

As with other drugs, Zevalin was first evaluated in patients with recurrent and refractory disease. In patients refractory to rituximab, it resulted in an overall response rate of 74 percent with CR being achieved in 15 percent.[188] In a phase III study, direct comparison with rituximab showed an overall response rate of 80 percent for Zevalin compared with 56 percent for the rituximab-treated group. However, response duration and time to progression were not significantly different between the two groups.[189] As with Bexxar, hematologic toxicity was seen, with a nadir at 7–9 weeks after treatment and lasting for 1–4 weeks.[189] Patients treated with Zevalin are able to go on to receive conventional chemotherapy regimens safely afterwards.[190]

More recently, the drug has been investigated in a randomized phase III study as consolidation of first remission in newly diagnosed patients receiving conventional chemotherapy as first-line treatment. With a median follow-up of 3.5 years, PFS for those who received Zevalin was 37 months compared with 13.5 months for the control group. Eighty percent of patients receiving Zevalin in partial remission converted to CR, with prolongation of PFS by 2 years and a favorable toxicity profile.[191] Conversion to CR was associated with PCR negativity for *BCL2* rearrangement-containing cells and this occurred in 90 percent of patients who remained PCR positive following initial chemotherapy. Conversion to PCR negativity was in turn associated with prolongation of PFS.[192]

Thus, these are highly effective treatments which are continuing to be investigated, now, as part of sequential regimens in large, multicenter trials. The main drawback is their cost.

TREATMENT AT RECURRENCE

In an illness in which recurrence is still virtually inevitable, treatment in the context of a clinical trial should be the aim. In practical terms, there is a large range of possibilities which are essentially the same as those for newly diagnosed patients. Thus, recurrence in an asymptomatic person does not in itself necessarily constitute a reason to start treatment. The extent of disease should be evaluated with a CT scan and a bone marrow aspirate and trephine biopsy. Lymph node biopsy is essential to exclude the possibility of transformation to DLBC pathology. If the biopsy shows follicular lymphoma grade 1, 2, or 3a and the person is well with a normal blood count, treatment can be delayed and the person observed. In contrast, if the histology is consistent with grade 3b follicular lymphoma, or if transformation has occurred, treatment needs to be given straightaway, as for DLBC lymphoma, with the aim – at least in younger patients treated at SBH – of proceeding to high-dose therapy supported by autologous peripheral blood progenitor cells (see below).

When treatment is needed, the person's overall situation – age, response to previous therapy and duration of that response, performance status, comorbidities, and, of course, his or her wishes – need to be considered. The overall aim of treatment will also radically influence the choice of treatment. If it is simply to achieve a further response, a combination chemotherapy regimen given in conjunction with rituximab should be considered. A randomized comparison of CHOP plus rituximab (or CHOP followed by rituximab) showed a survival advantage for chemoimmunotherapy as compared to the drug regimen alone. There was further benefit when rituximab was given as subsequent maintenance therapy.[144] In older or more frail patients (and more widely in the United States), rituximab is being given alone, the antibody being a licensed and approved treatment for recurrent follicular lymphoma.

At SBH, younger patients in whom a second remission is achieved are now advised to proceed to high-dose therapy supported by autologous peripheral blood progenitor cells, on the basis of a combined analysis from SBH and the Dana Farber Cancer Institute (DFCI). With a minimum follow-up of now 12 years, this shows a survival advantage for patients treated in second remission when comparison is made with an albeit historical control group treated at SBH prior to the introduction of high-dose treatment (HDT).[193]

With regard to second and subsequent recurrence, again, the range of possibilities remains wide. Participation in clinical trials of new therapies is appropriate. Reduced-intensity allografting should be considered (see below).

High-dose treatment with autologous hematopoietic cell support

The rationale for using myeloablative therapy for follicular lymphoma is based, first, on the fact that improvements in response rate and duration of remission were seen with intensification of initial therapy (although this had no impact on overall survival because of the inherent, seemingly relentless pattern of repeated recurrence). Moreover, promising results were seen with HDT as treatment for recurrent DLBC lymphoma.[194–196] When the first phase II studies of HDT supported by ABMT were undertaken in follicular lymphoma 20 years ago, the treatment was certainly given with curative intent[197–206] and some patients have survived for unexpectedly long periods of time. The best results were achieved when the treatment was given earlier rather than later in the course of the illness. However, with longer follow-up, it became apparent that there was a significant late treatment-related mortality associated with development of secondary MDS and secondary acute myelogenous leukemia (AML) which occurred predominantly in patients who had received a lot of previous treatment and in whom a TBI-containing myeloablative regimen had been used.[131,207–212] At SBH, evaluation using a 'triple fluorescence in situ hybridization (FISH) assay' of frozen, stored samples of bone marrow from patients undergoing HDT who subsequently developed secondary MDS or secondary AML showed that, in fact, clonal chromosomal abnormalities, presumably the consequence of earlier chemotherapy, were present prior to administration of cyclophosphamide and TBI.[213] In general, these involved chromosomes 5 or 7 or represented complex abnormalities. In view of this, currently at SBH, bone marrow from patients being considered for HDT is tested using the 'triple FISH assay.' If a clonal abnormality is detected, the patient does not proceed to HDT.

HIGH-DOSE TREATMENT AS CONSOLIDATION OF FIRST REMISSION

With the change away from TBI-containing regimens to 'drug-only' ones such as 'BEAM' (carmustine, etoposide, cytarabine, and melphalan) because of justifiable concerns about secondary MDS and secondary AML, and encouraging results from (mainly) single-center studies,[197–206] the logical next step was to investigate HDT in the situation in which, theoretically anyway, it was most likely to succeed; that is, as consolidation of first remission. Again, phase II studies were promising,[214,215] although inevitably they were conducted in a somewhat selected group of patients. At about this time, autologous PBPC replaced autologous bone marrow as the source of hematopoetic progenitor cells, and large randomized trials were initiated to evaluate HDT in first remission. These trials have not, however, shown a survival advantage.[216–218] In a study from the GLGLSG, patients aged less than 60 years were randomized to receive CHOP or MCP (mitoxantrone, cyclophosphamide,

and prednisone) followed by a second randomization to either maintenance IFNα or HDT supported by autologous PBPC. The PFS at 5 years for 240 evaluable patients was significantly better for HDT (65 percent versus 33 percent for IFNα, $P < 0.001$) but as yet no survival advantage has emerged.[216]

Two studies have been conducted in France. In the first (Groupe Ouest Est de Leucemie Aigue et des Maladies du Sang, GOELAMS),[217] newly diagnosed patients were randomized to receive either CHVP (cyclophosphamide, doxorubicin, teniposide, and prednisone), given in conjunction with IFNα, or HDT. The response rate (81 percent versus 69 percent, $P < 0.045$) and PFS (not yet reached versus 45 months) were both higher for the group receiving HDT. However, the greater number of patients developing secondary malignancies in the HDT group precluded a better overall survival. The second large French study comparing CHVP given with IFNα to 4 cycles of CHOP followed by HDT (using a TBI-containing regimen) resulted in similar response rates (79 percent and 78 percent). A preliminary analysis suggested a survival advantage for HDT, but with longer follow-up (median 7.5 years) and by 'intention-to-treat' analysis there is now no difference in overall survival between the two study arms ($P = 0.53$) or PFS ($P = 0.11$).[218]

Thus at least as given at present, irrespective of FLIPI score, there is currently no justification for using HDT routinely as consolidation of first remission. That does not mean that this approach should not continue to be investigated, perhaps as part of a sequence of treatments given with curative intent, in the context of clinical trials.

HIGH-DOSE TREATMENT FOLLOWING RECURRENCE

Whilst it is now considered 'standard of care' in patients with recurrent DLBC lymphoma to strive to achieve second complete (or at least partial) remission, with a view to going on to HDT, there is still debate and controversy as to whether this should be the case in follicular lymphoma. The development of new therapeutic approaches, particularly the advent of rituximab, has altered many peoples' perception about the use of HDT. Quite appropriate concerns about the risk of development of secondary MDS or AML[208–213,219] have also deterred many from using it in this situation.

There has only been one randomized study to investigate the role of HDT in recurrent disease.[220] Although it did not accrue the planned number of patients, a PFS and OS advantage in favor of HDT was demonstrated, with OS being 71 percent at 4 years for patients who received HDT compared with 46 percent for those receiving chemotherapy (CHOP) alone. No difference was demonstrated between patients receiving autologous bone marrow (or PBPC) that had been treated in vitro or not. Currently, at SBH, in light of the long-term analysis mentioned above of combined data from SBH and the DFCI,[193] which shows a survival advantage for patients receiving HDT in second (but no later) remission, HDT is being recommended in this situation.

HIGH–DOSE TREATMENT FOLLOWING TRANSFORMATION TO DIFFUSE LARGE B CELL PATHOLOGY

In the past, transformation, even if treated with intensive combination chemotherapy as for DLBC lymphoma, was associated with a universally extremely poor prognosis, the median survival virtually always being less than 18 months.[55–62] However, with the introduction of HDT supported by autologous PBPC, provided that a complete (or at least partial) remission can first be achieved, both single-center studies[221–223] and the European Bone Marrow Transplant Registry results[224] show that in somewhat younger patients (those less than 65 years old) it is worth striving to achieve remission with a view to going on to HDT; 30–40 percent of patients can be cured.

Allogeneic bone marrow transplantation

It has become clear that allogeneic stem cell transplantation dramatically decreases the risk of recurrence of follicular lymphoma and that a proportion of patients can be cured. Data from the International Bone Marrow Transplant Registry[225] and single-center studies[225–231] using myeloablative conditioning regimens suggest that 40–50 percent of patients will survive long term. Clearly they are highly selected people but long-term progression-free survival has been observed even in patients with refractory disease.[229]

There is clear evidence for a graft-versus-lymphoma effect[232,233] on the basis of donor lymphocyte infusions being effective as treatment for recurrence after an allograft. However, the high treatment-related mortality, largely a consequence of graft-versus-host disease (GVHD),[230] has deterred many physicians (and their patients) from pursuing this option, even if an HLA-matched sibling donor is available.

The advent of reduced-intensity allografting (Table 67.8) has certainly made some difference to the probability of death as a consequence of the transplant, and the use of alemtuzumab has been shown to be associated with a lower incidence of GVHD. The original data from the MD Anderson Cancer Center in Houston[233] described 18 patients (median age 51 years) who received fludarabine plus cyclophosphamide as the conditioning regimen; 20 percent developed acute and 64 percent chronic GVHD but the disease-free survival was 84 percent at 2 years. In another study, 28 patients with follicular lymphoma (of a total of 65 patients) received BEAM plus alemtuzumab. The incidence of both acute and chronic GVHD was 17 percent (the latter rising to 38 percent after administration of donor lymphocyte infusion) but the event-free survival was 69 percent at 1 year.[234] A further 29 patients (out of a total of 88),[234] with a median age of 48 years, received an alternative conditioning regimen: fludarabine, melphalan, and alemtuzumab; incidence of acute GVHD was 15 percent but progression-free survival was 65 percent at 3 years.

Thus these results are certainly encouraging and at SBH reduced-intensity allografting is being considered currently in younger patients in third or later remission for whom an HLA-identical donor (sibling or not) is available.

Vaccination

The concept of harnessing the immune response directed against a tumor-specific antigen has for a long time been the 'holy grail' of immunologists striving to develop alternative or additional treatment for follicular lymphoma.

Table 67.8 Results of reduced-intensity (nonmyeloablative) stem cell transplantation in follicular lymphoma

No. of pts (FL/total)	Age	No. of previous treatments	Conditioning regimen	Post-transplant immuno-suppression	GVHD	Graft failure	Outcome	Reference
18/20[a]	51	2	CY + Flu ± Rit	Tacro + MTX	Acute: 20% Chronic: 64%	0	20 CR TRM: 2 DFS: 84% at 2 years	232
26/65	46	2	BEAM + alemtuzumab	CSA + MTX	Acute: 17% Chronic: 17% (38% post DLI)	3	EFS: 69% TRM: 8% at 1 year	233
29/88	48	3	Flu + MEL + alemtuzumab	CSA	Acute: 15% Chronic: 6.8% (28% post DLI)	4	PFS: 65% at 3 years TRM: 11% at 3 years	233

[a]Tacrolimus.

Tacro, tacrolimus; CSA, cyclosporin A; pts, patients; FL, follicular lymphoma; GVHD, graft-versus-host disease; BEAM: carmustine, etoposide, cytarabine, and melphalan; DLI, donor lymphocyte infusion; Flu, fludarabine; MEL, melphalan; MTX, methotrexate; CY + Flu, cyclophosphamide + fludarabine; Rit, rituximab; CR, complete remission; TRM, transplant-related mortality; DFS, disease-free survival; EFS, event-free survival; PFS, progression-free survival.

Two approaches have been evaluated: in the first, 'vaccination' using the idiotype as the antigen to generate a polyclonal response has been the subject of a sequence of studies at Stanford University.[235,236] Both antibody-mediated and cellular responses were demonstrated in patients with B cell lymphoma. Furthermore, patients in whom a specific immunologic response was evoked had longer-lasting remissions. At the National Cancer Institute of the USA 'molecular remissions' were demonstrated in patients given protein idiotype and granulocyte colony-stimulating factor (G-CSF), the latter being used to enhance the immune response when such treatment was given in first remission.[237] An alternative approach has been followed at the University of Southampton in the UK using DNA vaccination,[238,239] again following achievement of remission with conventional chemotherapy.

These ambitious projects have not, however, been widely applied, mainly because of the logistic problems involved. Furthermore, disappointingly, the outcome of a major trial recently reported from Stanford University showed no statistical difference in PFS or time to subsequent antilymphoma therapy following immunization.[240] Patients with newly diagnosed follicular lymphoma received 8 cycles of CVP. Those in whom at least a partial response was maintained for 6 months were randomized to receive 'personalized immunotherapy' consisting of tumor-specific idiotype protein conjugated to keyhole limpet hemocyanin administered in a series of subcutaneous immunizations with granulocyte macrophage colony-stimulating factor (GM-CSF) or control immunotherapy. The PFS in both arms of the study had a plateau at greater than 30 percent at 5 years; a statistically significant improvement in PFS ($P = 0.002$) was seen in patients able to mount an anti-idiotype immune response but overall there was no advantage.

GENERAL CONSIDERATIONS

Follow–up

At SBH, patients being observed (either initially or at recurrence) are seen every 3 months. A clinical examination is carried out, and the blood count and tests of liver and renal function are performed together with measurement of LDH level. Computed tomography scans are not routinely done unless there are symptoms or signs of recurrence or progression. Lymph node biopsy is performed to exclude transformation (either an excision biopsy of a peripheral lymph node or 'Tru-cut' needle biopsy under CT or ultrasound control) if the scans show development of new nodes. If the biopsy shows follicular lymphoma grade I or II, it may well be appropriate to simply continue to observe the person on a regular basis, but it is always better to have done the biopsy and have excluded transformation than not to do it.

Evaluation of response

The 'revised response criteria for malignant lymphoma' published in 2007 are now being used.[45] Clearly, if there is palpable lymphadenopathy, response can easily be assessed as treatment continues. In the absence of palpable lymph nodes, it is appropriate to repeat CT scans midway through treatment. On completion of treatment, all previously abnormal tests are repeated.

Entry into clinical trials

There are sufficient questions to be answered with regard to the optimal treatment for follicular lymphoma that all patients with the illness should at least be given the opportunity to take part in a clinical trial. However, for many patients, the concept of taking part in a study is unacceptable and many simply want their physician to give them good advice as to what is the best treatment available. Equally, there will be patients who are not eligible for a clinical trial although they wish to participate in one.

In the UK, the National Cancer Plan aims to achieve a situation whereby 10 percent of patients with cancer are treated in national clinical trials. Elsewhere, similarly relatively small numbers of patients participate in clinical trials, whether randomized or not. The reasons for this are multiple and complex and will vary from country to country, in addition to potential variations in access to treatment. Thus, published results will reflect selection bias in that patients treated within a clinical trial are a highly selected group, but such results are the only basis upon which progress can be made.

Prognostic factors

In view of the heterogeneity of clinical behavior of patients with follicular lymphoma, several attempts have been made to categorize them according to clinical features that in retrospective analyses have been shown to correlate with outcome. Application of such prognostic indices should, theoretically anyway, lead to selection of better therapy for an individual person. In clinical practice, however, treatment has rarely been allocated according to them. A notable exception is the GELF schema which has been applied in France, allocating patients into groups described as having a 'high' or 'low' tumor burden (see above). It should also be remembered that a prognostic index is to some extent specific to the treatment being given. Its usefulness will also depend upon whether the index applies to prognosis at the time of diagnosis (as is usually the case) or later in the course of the illness at progression or recurrence.

The following prognostic indices have been proposed:

- The GELF schema defines a 'high tumor burden' as: the presence of B symptoms, a high LDH level, a bulky lesion >7 cm in diameter, effusions, involvement of three or more anatomic sites each 3 cm or >3 cm in diameter, circulating lymphoma cells, cytopenias, and splenomegaly.[48]

- The IPI for 'aggressive' lymphoma has been applied to follicular lymphoma and does actually separate patients into three subgroups with significantly different prognoses.[241–243] The main problem is that only a small group of patients fulfil the criteria for being in the high-risk group.
- In the scheme proposed by the BNLI group,[49] number of lymph node sites involved, the presence of B symptoms, splenomegaly, and increasing age were found to have an adverse effect on probability of response and on cause-specific survival.
- The Italian Lymphoma Intergroup (ILI) Index[244] used six variables, namely: age, extranodal involvement, LDH level, presence of B symptoms, male gender, and erythrocyte sedimentation rate (ESR) to classify patients into low-, intermediate-, and high-risk groups, but it has not been widely used outside of Italy.
- The FLIPI,[43] involving a major collaborative effort to analyze 17 pretreatment variables in more than 4000 patients treated between 1985 and 2002, was an attempt to identify patients in whom conventional therapy resulted in a poor prognosis. However, it became clear during the development of the Index that four potentially key factors significant on univariate analysis could not be included, either because of missing data or due to disparities between clinical practice in Europe and North America. Nonetheless, five variables – that is, age >60 years, advanced stage (III–IV), high serum LDH, hemoglobin level <12 g/dL, and number of nodal sites (five or more) – were used to ascribe a prognostic score, which in turn led to identification of three risk groups with considerably different survival patterns at 5 and 10 years. Patients scoring 0–1 were deemed 'low risk' (survival 90.6 percent and 70.7 percent at 5 and 10 years, respectively), score 2 was 'intermediate risk' (77.6 percent and 50.9 percent, respectively), and score >3 equated to 'high risk' (52.2 percent and 35.5 percent, respectively).

Concern has been expressed that the FLIPI, having been developed in a 'pre-rituximab' era, may not be applicable now. However, a recent analysis has shown that it is applicable to patients receiving rituximab-containing initial therapy. The FLIPI is beginning to be used on a routine daily basis and future large multicenter studies are being designed on the basis of it.

In terms of histology, survival appears to be no different for patients with grade 1, 2, and 3a disease at the time of diagnosis, although there is a correlation between histologic grade and freedom from progression following treatment, patients with grade 2 and 3a disease having (perhaps surprisingly) a better outcome than those with grade 1 disease.[245–247] (The latter publications refer to the histology using the previous nomenclature.)

The significance of chromosomal abnormalities has also been evaluated, patients with abnormalities involving 6q23-26 and 17p having a higher risk of transformation to DLBC pathology[33] as do those with deletions of p15 and p16.[248,249] Alterations or mutations of MYC and of TP53[250–252] have also been shown to correlate with a poor prognosis.

Response to treatment at the 'molecular level,' as evidenced by PCR analysis for BCL2 rearrangement-containing cells in the blood or bone marrow, has been shown to correlate with event-free survival. The original publications related to high-dose therapy, those patients becoming PCR negative having a lower probability of recurrence[253–255] and better survival.[256] Since then, molecular response has also been found to correlate with event-free survival in patients receiving anthracycline-containing[257] and fludarabine-containing regimens, with or without rituximab.[258]

Recently, several retrospective analyses have tried to define biological parameters that influence survival. Gene expression profiling suggests that the survival of patients with follicular lymphoma correlates with the molecular features of the nonmalignant 'immune cells,' the so-called 'microenvironment' present in the tumor.[3,259,260] Immunohistochemical analysis has shown the presence of high numbers of FOXP3-positive infiltrating T cells to be associated with improved survival[261] but this has also been questioned.[262] The number of tumor-associated macrophages has also been shown to correlate with survival[263] and a recent study showed that the adverse prognostic significance of high numbers of macrophages could be circumvented by the use of rituximab.[264]

CONCLUSION

Physicians and patients are today faced with an ever-growing range of possible treatments for follicular lymphoma. Clearly the most important thing is to choose the best treatment for the person concerned in the context of circumstances, wishes, and previous treatments. However, with the improvements in survival now being described, there is also an almost unprecedented opportunity to develop curative treatment for this illness. It is an exciting time.

KEY POINTS

- Follicular lymphoma is generally considered to be incurable, although the survival of patients is now improving.
- In 85 percent of patients, the disease is associated with the t(14:18) translocation.

- In a proportion of patients, recurrence/ progression is associated with transformation to diffuse large B cell pathology. Biopsy at each progression/recurrence is therefore mandatory to determine the correct treatment at that point.
- Standard treatment in the Western world is now considered to be a chemotherapy regimen + rituximab, the addition of which has been shown to improve response rate, duration of response and survival.
- Maintenance rituximab appears to prolong the duration of the second remission.
- High-dose treatment supported by autologous peripheral blood progenitor cells and reduced intensity allografting may be appropriate in specific situations.

REFERENCES

● = Key primary paper
◆ = Major review article

●1. A clinical evaluation of the International Lymphoma Study Group classification on non-Hodgkin's Lymphoma. The Non-Hodgkin's Lymphoma Classification Project. *Blood* 1997; **89**: 3909–18.

2. Jaffe ES, Harris NL, Stein H, Vardiman JW. (eds) *World Health Organization classification of tumours. Pathology and genetics of tumours of haematopoietic and lymphoid tissues.* Lyon: IARC Press, 2001.

●3. Dave SS, Wright G, Tan B *et al.* Prediction of survival in follicular lymphoma based on molecular features of tumour-infiltrating immune cells. *N Engl J Med* 2004; **351**: 2159–69.

4. Groves F, Linet M, Travis L *et al.* Cancer surveillance series: non-Hodgkin's lymphoma incidence by histologic subtype in the United States from 1978 through 1995. *J Natl Cancer Inst* 2000; **92**: 1240–51.

5. Herrinton L, Goldoft M, Schwartz S *et al.* The incidence of non-Hodgkin's lymphoma and its histologic subtypes in Asian migrants to the United States and their descendants. *Cancer Causes Control* 1996; **7**: 224–30.

6. Biagi JS. Insights into the molecular pathogenesis of follicular lymphoma arising from analysis of geographic variation. *Blood* 2002; **99**: 4265–75.

◆7. Horning SJ. Natural history of and therapy for the indolent non-Hodgkin's lymphomas. *Semin Oncol* 1993; **20**: 75–88.

8. Jones S, Fuks Z, Bull M *et al.* Non-Hodgkin's lymphoma: IV. Clinicopathologic correlation in 405 cases. *Cancer* 1973; **31**: 806–823.

9. Anderson T, De Vita V, Simon R *et al.* Malignant lymphoma: II. Prognostic factors and response to treatment of 473 patients at the National Cancer Institute. *Cancer* 1982; **50**: 2708–21.

10. Brittinger G, Bartels H, Common H *et al.* Clinical and prognostic revelance of the Kiel classification of non-Hodgkin's lymphomas: Results of a prospective multicentre study of Kiel lymphoma study group. *Hematol Oncol* 1984; **2**: 269–306.

●11. Gallagher CJ, Gregory W, Jones AE *et al.* Follicular lymphoma: prognostic factors for response and survival. *J Clin Oncol* 1986; **4**: 1470–80.

●12. Fisher RI, LeBlanc M, Press OW *et al.* New treatment options have changed the survival of patients with follicular lymphoma. *J Clin Oncol* 2005; **23**: 8447–52.

●13. Liu Q, Fayad L, Hagemeister F *et al.* Stage IV indolent lymphoma: 25 years of treatment progress. *Blood* 2003; **102**: 1446.

14. Hiddemann W, Hoster E, Buske C *et al.* Rituximab is the essential treatment modality that underlies the significant improvement in short and long term outcome of patients with advanced stage follicular lymphoma: a 10 year analysis of GLSG trials. *Blood* 2006; **108**: 483 (abstract).

●15. Swenson W, Wooldridge J, Lynch C *et al.* Improved survival of follicular lymphoma patients in the United States. *J Clin Oncol* 2005; **23**: 5019–26.

16. Dana BW, Dahlberg S, Nathwani BN *et al.* Long-term follow-up of patients with low-grade malignant lymphomas treated with doxorubicin-based chemotherapy or chemoimmunotherapy. *J Clin Oncol* 1993; **11**: 644–51.

●17. Johnson PW, Rohatiner A, Whelan JS *et al.* Patterns of survival in patients with recurrent follicular lymphoma: a 20-year study from a single center. J Clin Oncol 1995; **13**: 140–7.

18. Becker E. Ein Beitag zur lehre von den lymphomen. *Dtsch Med Wochenschr* 1917; **27**: 726–8.

19. Brill NE, Baehr G, Rosenthal N. Generalised giant lymph follicle hyperplasia of lymph nodes and spleen. A hitherto undescribed type. *JAMA* 1925; **2**: 668–71.

20. Symmers D. Giant follicular lymphadenopathy with or without splenomegaly. *Arch Path* 1938; **26**: 603–47.

21. Gall E, Morrison H, Scott A. The follicular type of malignant lymphoma: a survey of 63 cases. *Ann Intern Med* 1941; **14**: 2073.

22. Gall EA, Mallory T. Malignant lymphoma: A clinicopathological survey of 618 cases. *Am J Pathol* 1942; **18**: 381–415.

23. Rappaport H, Winter H, Hicks E. Follicular lymphoma: A re-evaluation of its place in the scheme of malignant lymphoma based on a survey of 253 cases. *Cancer* 1956; **9**: 792.

24. Rosenberg SA, Diamond HD, Craver LF. Lymphosarcoma: survival and the effects of therapy. *Am J Roentgenol Radium Ther Nucl Med* 1961; **85**: 521–32.

25. Mann RB, Berard C. Criteria for the cytologic subclassification of follicular lymphomas: a proposed alternative method. *Hematol Oncol* 1983; **1**: 187–92.

26. Ott G, Katzenberger T, Lohr A *et al.* Cytomorphologic, immunohistochemical and cytogenetic profiles of follicular lymphoma. *Blood* 2002; **99**: 3806–12.

●27. Harris NL, Jaffe ES, Diebold J *et al.* World Health Organization classification of neoplastic diseases of the hematopoietic and lymphoid tissues: report of the Clinical Advisory Committee meeting (Airlie House, Virginia, November 1997). *J Clin Oncol* 1999; **17**: 3835–49.

28. Nathwani BN, Anderson J, Armitage JO *et al.* Clinical significance of follicular lymphoma with monocytoid B cells. Non-Hodgkin's Lymphoma Classification Project. *Hum Pathol* 1999; **30**: 263–8.

29. Eshoa C, Perkins S, Kampalath B *et al.* Decreased CD10 expression in grade III and in interfollicular infiltrates of follicular lymphoma. *Am J Clin Pathol* 2001; **115**: 862–7.

30. Cattoretti G, Chang CC, Cechova K *et al.* BCL-6 protein is expressed in germinal-center B cells. *Blood* 1996; **86**: 45–53.

31. Lai R, Weiss L, Chang KL *et al.* Frequency of CD43 expression in non-Hodgkin's lymphoma. A survey of 742 cases and further characterization of rare CD43+ follicular lymphomas. *Am J Clin Pathol* 1999; **111**: 488–94.

32. Nguyen PL, Zukerberg LR, Benedict WF *et al.* Immunohistochemical detection of P53, BCL-2 and retinoblastoma proteins in follicular lymphoma. *Am J Clin Pathol* 1996; **105**: 538–43.

●33. Yunis JJ, Frizzera G, Oken MM *et al.* Multiple recurrent genomic defects in follicular lymphoma. A possible model for cancer. *N Engl J Med* 1987; **316**: 79–84.

34. Tilly H, Rossi A, Stamatoullas A *et al.* Prognostic value of chromosomal abnormalities in follicular lymphoma. *Blood* 1994; **84**: 1043–9.

35. Horsman DE, Connors JM, Pantzar T *et al.* Analysis of secondary chromosomal alterations in 165 cases of follicular lymphoma with t(14; 18). *Genes Chromosomes Cancer* 2001; **30**: 375–82.

36. Hockenbery DM, Zutter M, Hickey W *et al.* BCL-2 protein in topographically restricted in tissues characterized by apoptotic cell death. *Proc Natl Acad Sci U S A* 1991; **88**: 6961–5.

37. McDonnell TJ, Deane N, Platt FM *et al.* BCL-2 immunoglobulin transgenic mice demonstrate extended B cell survival and follicular lymphoproliferation. *Cell* 1989; **57**: 79–88.

38. Tsujimoto Y, Cossman J, Jaffe E *et al.* Involvement of the BCL-2 gene in human follicular lymphoma. *Science* 1985; **228**: 1440–3.

39. Küppers R, Klein U, Hansmann ML *et al.* Cellular origin of human B-cell lymphomas. *N Engl J Med* 1999; **341**: 1520–9.

40. Dolken G, Illerhaus G, Hirt C *et al.* BCL-2/JH rearrangements in circulating B-cells of healthy blood donors and patients with non-malignant diseases. *J Clin Oncol* 1996; **14**: 1333–44.

41. Summers KE, Goff LK, Wilson AG *et al.* Frequency of the BCL-2/IgH rearrangement in normal individuals: implications for the monitoring of disease in patients with follicular lymphoma. *J Clin Oncol* 2001; **19**: 420–4.

42. McDonnell TJ, Korsmeyer SJ. Progression from lymphoid hyperplasia to high grade malignant lymphoma in mice transgenic for the t(14; 18). *Nature* 1991; **349**: 254–6.

●43. Solal-Celigny P, Roy P, Colombat P *et al.* Follicular lymphoma international prognostic index. *Blood* 2004; **104**: 1258–65.

44. Pappa VI, Hussain H, Reznek RH *et al.* Role of image-guided core-needle biopsy in the management of patients with lymphoma. *J Clin Oncol* 1996; **14**: 2427–30.

●45. Cheson BD, Pfistner B, Juweid ME *et al.* Revised response criteria for malignant lymphoma. *J Clin Oncol* 2007; **25**: 579–86.

46. Karam M, Novak L, Cyriac J *et al.* Role of fluorine-18 fluoro-deoxyglucose positron emission tomography scan in the evaluation and follow-up of patients with low-grade lymphoma. *Cancer* 2006; **107**: 175–83.

47. Young R, Longo D, Glatstein E *et al.* Watchful waiting vs. aggressive combined modality treatment. *Semin Oncol* 1988; **11**: 6.

48. Brice P, Bastion Y, Lepage E *et al.* Comparison in low-tumor-burden follicular lymphomas between an initial no-treatment policy, prednimustine or interferon-alpha: A randomised study from the Groupe d'Etude Lymphomas Folliculaires. *J Clin Oncol* 1997; **15**: 1110–17.

●49. Ardeshna K, Smith P, Norton A *et al.* Long-term effect of a watch and wait policy vs. immediate systemic treatment for asymptomatic advanced stage non-Hodgkin's lymphoma: a randomised controlled trial. *Lancet* 2003; **362**: 516–22.

●50. Horning S, Rosenberg S. The natural history of initially untreated low-grade non-Hodgkin's lymphoma. *N Engl J Med* 1984; **311**: 1471–508.

51. Advani R, Rosenberg S, Horning S. Stage I and II follicular non-Hodgkin's lymphoma: long-term follow-up of no initial therapy. *J Clin Oncol* 2004; **22**: 1454–9.

52. Soubeyran P, Eghbali H, Torjani M *et al.* Is there any place for a wait and see policy in Stage 1_0 follicular lymphoma? A study of 43 consecutive patients in a single centre. *Ann Oncol* 1996; **7**: 713–18.

◆53. Rohatiner AZ, Davies A, Montoto S, Lister TA. Follicular lymphoma. In: Canellos GP, Lister TA, Young B. (eds) *The lymphomas*, 2nd Edn. Philadelphia, PA: Saunders Elsevier, 2006.

●54. Montoto S, Davies AJ, Matthews J *et al.* Risk and clinical implications of transformation of follicular lymphoma to diffuse large B-cell lymphoma. *J Clin Oncol* 2007; **25**: 2426–33.

55. Hubbard S, Chabner B, De Vita D *et al.* Histologic progression in non-Hodgkin's lymphoma. *Blood* 1982; **59**: 258–64.

56. Cullen M, Lister T, Brearley RI *et al.* Histological transformation of non-Hodgkin's lymphoma: a prospective study. *Cancer* 1979; **44**: 645–51.

57. Ostrow S, Digs C, Sutherland J *et al.* Nodular poorly differentiated lymphocytic lymphoma: changes in histology and survival. *Cancer Treat Rep* 1981; **65**: 929–33.

58. Ersboll J, Schultz H, Pederson-Bjergaard J *et al.* Follicular low-grade non-Hodgkin's lymphoma: long-term outcome with or withour tumor progression. *Eur J Haematol* 1989; **42**: 155–63.

59. Armitage J, Dick F, Corder M. Diffuse histiocytic lymphoma after histologic conversion: a poor prognostic variant. *Cancer Treat Rep* 1981; **65**: 413–18.

60. Bastion Y, Sebban C, Berger F *et al*. Incidence, predictive factors and outcome of lymphoma transformation in follicular lymphoma patients. *J Clin Oncol* 1997; **15**: 1587–94.

61. Acker B, Hoppe R, Colby T *et al*. Histologic conversion in the non-Hodgkin's lymphomas. *J Clin Oncol* 1983; **1**: 11–16.

62. Yuen AR, Kamel O, Halpern J *et al*. Long-term survival after histologic transformation of low-grade follicular lymphoma. *J Clin Oncol* 1995; **13**: 1726–33.

63. Vaughan Hudson B, Vaughan Hudson G, MacLennan KA *et al*. Clinical stage 1 non-Hodgkin's lymphoma: long-term follow-up of patients treated by the British National Lymphoma Investigation with radiotherapy alone as initial therapy. *Br J Cancer* 1994; **69**: 1088–93.

64. Besa PC, McLaughlin P, Cox JD *et al*. Long term assessment of patterns of treatment failure and survival in patients with stage I and II follicular lymphoma. *Cancer* 1995; **75**: 2361–7.

65. Pendlebury S, el Awadi M, Ashley S *et al*. Radiotherapy results in early stage low grade nodal non-Hodgkin's lymphoma. *Radiother Oncol* 1995; **36**: 167–71.

66. Friedberg JW, Huang J, Dillon H *et al*. Initial therapeutic strategy in follicular lymphoma: an analysis from the National LymphoCare study. J Clin Oncol 2006; 24: 7527.

67. Fuks Z, Kaplan H. Recurrence rates following radiation therapy of nodular and diffuse malignant lymphomas. *Radiology* 1973; **108**: 675–84.

68. De Los Santos JF, Mendenhall NP, Lynch JW Jr. Is comprehensive lymphatic irradiation for low-grade non-Hodgkin's lymphoma curative therapy? Long-term experience at a single institution. *Int J Radiat Oncol Biol Phys* 1997; **38**: 3–8.

●69. MacManus MP, Hoppe R. Is radiotherapy curative for stage I and II low-grade follicular lymphoma? Results of a long-term follow-up study of patients treated at Stanford University. *J Clin Oncol* 1996; **14**: 1282–90.

70. Chen M, Prosnitz L, Gonzales-Serva A *et al*. Results of radiotherapy in control of stage I and II non-Hodgkin's lymphoma. *Cancer* 1979; **43**: 1245–54.

71. Gomez G, Barcos M, Krishnamsetty R. Treatment of early stage I and II nodular poorly differentiated lymphocytic lymphoma. *Am J Clin Oncol* 1986; **9**: 40–4.

72. Gospodarowicz M, Bush R, Brown T *et al*. Prognostic factors in nodular lymphomas: a multivariate analysis based on the Princess Margaret Hospital experience. *Int J Radiat Oncol Biol Phys* 1984; **10**: 489–97.

73. Paryani S, Hoppe R, Cox R. Analysis of non-Hodgkin's lymphomas with nodular and favourable histologies, stages I and II. *Cancer* 1983; **52**: 2300–7.

74. Reddy S, Saxena V, Pellettiere E *et al*. Stage I and II non-Hodgkin's lymphomas: Long-term results of radiation therapy. *Int J Radiat Oncol Biol Phys* 1989; **16**: 687–92.

75. McLaughlin P, Fuller L, Velasquez W *et al*. Stage I-II follicular lymphoma: Treatment results for 76 patients. *Cancer* 1986; **58**: 1596–602.

76. Richards M, Gregory W, Hall P *et al*. Management of localized non-Hodgkin's lymphoma: The experience at St. Bartholomew's Hospital, 1972–1985. *Hematol Oncol* 1989; **7**: 1–18.

77. MacManus MP, Hoppe R. Overview of treatment of localized low-grade lymphomas. *Hematol Oncol Clin North Am* 1997; **11**: 901–18.

●78. Petersen PM, Gospodarowicz M, Tsang R *et al*. Long-term outcome in stage I and II follicular lymphoma following treatment with involved field radiation therapy alone. *J Clin Oncol* 2004; **22**: 561.

79. Jacobs JP, Murray K, Schultz CJ *et al*. Central lymphatic irradiation for stage III nodular malignant lymphoma: long-term results. *J Clin Oncol* 1993; **11**: 233–8.

80. Murtha AD, Rupnow B, Hansosn J *et al*. Long-term follow-up of patients wih Stage III follicular lymphoma treated with primary radiotherapy at Stanford University. *Int J Radiat Oncol Biol Phys* 2001; **49**: 3–15.

81. Mendenhall N, Noyes W, Million R. Total body irradiation for stage II-IV non-Hodgkin's lymphoma: ten-year follow-up. *J Clin Oncol* 1989; **7**: 67–74.

82. Lybeert M, Meerwaldt J, Deneve W. Long-term results of low dose total body irradiation for advanced non-Hodgkin lymphoma. *Int J Radiat Oncol Biol Phys* 1987; **13**: 1167–72.

83. Chaffey J, Hellman S, Rosenthal D *et al*. Total body irradiation in the treatment of lymphocytic lymphoma. *Cancer Treat Rep* 1977; **61**: 1149–52.

84. Choi N, Timothy A, Kaufman S *et al*. Low dose fractionated total body irradiation in the treatment of non-Hodgkin's lymphoma. *Cancer* 1979; **43**: 1636–42.

85. Haas R, Poortmans P, de Jong D *et al*. High response rates and lasting remissions after low-dose involved field radiotherapy in indolent lymphomas. *J Clin Oncol* 2003; **21**: 2474–80.

86. Carde P, Burgers J, van Glabbeke M *et al*. Combined radiotherapy-chemotherapy for early stages non-Hodgkin's lymphoma: the 1975–1980 EORTC controlled lymphoma trial. *Radiother Oncol* 1984; **2**: 301–12.

87. Monfardini S, Banfi A, Bonadonna G *et al*. Improved five year survival after combined radiotherapy-chemotherapy for stage I-II non-Hodgkin's lymphoma. *Int J Radiat Oncol Biol Phys* 1980; **6**: 125–34.

88. Kamath SS, Marcus JR, Lynch JW *et al*. The impact of radiotherapy dose and other treatment-related and clinical factors on in-field control in stage I and II non-Hodgkin's lymphoma. *Int J Radiat Oncol Biol Phys* 1999; **44**: 563–8.

89. Wilder RB, Jones D, Tucker SL *et al*. Long-term results with radiotherapy for Stage I-II follicular lymphomas. *Int J Radiat Oncol Biol Phys* 2001; **51**: 1219–27.

90. Seymour JF, Pro B, Fuller LM *et al*. Long-term follow-up of a prospective study of combined modality therapy for stage I-II indolent non-Hodgkin's lymphoma. *J Clin Oncol* 2003; **21**: 2115–22.

91. Galton D, Israels L, Nabarro J et al. Clinical trial of p-(dichloroethylamino)-phenylbutyric acid (CB 1348) in malignant lymphoma. Br Med J 1955; **2**: 1172–6.

92. Israels L, Galton D, Till M et al. Clinical evaluation of CB 1348 in malignant lymphoma and related diseases. Ann NY Acad Sci 1958; **68**: 915–25.

93. Lister TA, Cullen M, Beard M et al. Comparison of combined and single agent chemotherapy in non-Hodgkin's lymphoma of favourable histological subtype. Br Med J 1978; **1**: 533–7.

94. Hoogstraten B, Owens A, Lenhard R et al. Combination chemotherapy in lymphosarcoma and reticulum cell sarcoma. Blood 1969; **33**: 370–8.

95. Luce J, Gamble J, Wilson H et al. Combined cyclophosphamide, vincristine and prednisolone therapy for malignant lymphoma. Cancer 1971; **28**: 306–17.

96. Bagley C, Devita V, Berard C et al. Advanced lymphosarcoma: intensive cyclical combination chemotherapy with cyclophosphamide, vincristine and prednisolone. Ann Intern Med 1972; **76**: 227–34.

97. Rodriguez V, Cabanillas F, Burgess M et al. Combination chemotherapy ('CHOP–Bleo') in advanced non-Hodgkin's lymphoma. Blood 1977; **49**: 325–33.

98. McKelvey E, Gottlieb J, Wilson H et al. Hydroxyldaunomycin (Adriamycin) combination chemotherapy in malignant lymphoma. Cancer 1976; **38**: 1484–93.

99. Jones S, Grozea P, Metz E et al. Superiority of adriamycin-containing combination chemotherapy in the treatment of diffuse lymphoma: A Southwest Oncology Group study. Cancer 1979; **43**: 417–25.

100. Kalter S, Holmes L, Cabanillas F. Long-term results of treatment of patients with follicular lymphomas. Hematol Oncol 1987; **5**: 127–38.

101. Petersen B, Anderson J, Frizzera G et al. Nodular mixed lymphoma: A comparative trial of cyclophosphamide and cyclophosphamide, Adriamycin, vincristine, prednisolone and bleomycin. Blood 1985; **66**: 216.

102. Anderson K, Skarin A, Rosenthal D et al. Combination chemotherapy for advanced non-Hodgkin's lymphomas other than diffuse histiocytic or undifferentiated histologies. Cancer Treat Rep 1984; **68**: 1343–50.

103. Carde P, Meerwaldt J, Van Glabbeke M et al. Superiority of second over first generation chemotherapy in a randomized trial for stage III–IV intermediate and high-grade non-Hodgkin's lymphoma (NHL): the 1980–1985 EORTC trial. Ann Oncol 1991; **2**: 431–5.

104. Hochster H, Cassileth P. Fludarabine phosphate therapy of non-Hodgkin's lymphoma. Semin Oncol 1990; **17**(5 Suppl 8): 63–5.

105. Leiby J, Snider K, Kraut E et al. Phase II trial of 9-beta-D-arabinofuranosyl-2-fluoroadenine 5'-monophosphate in non-Hodgkin's lymphoma: prospective comparison of response with deoxycytidine kinase activity. Cancer Res 1987; **47**: 2719–22.

106. Whelan J, Davis C, Rule S et al. Fludarabine phosphate for the treatment of low grade lymphoid malignancy. Br J Cancer 1991; **64**: 120–3.

107. Redman J, Cabanillas F, Velasquez W et al. Phase II trial of fludarabine phosphate in lymphoma: an effective new agent in low-grade lymphoma. J Clin Oncol 1992; **10**: 790–4.

108. Hiddemann W, Unterhalt M, Pott C et al. Fludarabine single-agent therapy for relapsed low-grade non-Hodgkin's lymphomas: a phase II study of the German Low-Grade Non-Hodgkin's Lymphoma Study Group. Semin Oncol 1993; **20**(5 Suppl 7): 28–31.

109. Zinzani P, Lauria F, Rondelli D et al. Fludarabine: an active agent in the treatment of previously treated and untreated low-grade non-Hodgkin's lymphoma. Ann Oncol 1993; **4**: 575–8.

110. Pigaditou A, Rohatiner A, Whelan J et al. Fludarabine in low-grade lymphoma. Semin Oncol 1993; **20**(5 Suppl 7): 24–7.

111. Foran J, Oscier D, Orchard J et al. Pharmacokinetic study of single doses of oral fludarabine phosphate in patients with 'low-grade' non-Hodgkin's lymphoma and B-cell chronic lymphocytic leukemia. J Clin Oncol 1999; **17**: 1574–9.

112. McLaughlin P, Hagemeister F, Romaguera J et al. Fludarabine, mitoxantrone and dexamethasone: an effective new regimen for indolent lymphoma. J Clin Oncol 1996; **14**: 1262–8.

113. Hochster H, Oken M, Winter J et al. Phase I study of fludarabine plus cyclophosphamide in patients with previously untreated low-grade lymphoma: results and long-term follow-up: a report from the Eastern Cooperative Oncology Group. J Clin Oncol 2000; **18**: 987–94.

114. Santini G, Chisesi T, Nati S et al. Fludarabine, cyclophosphamide and mitoxantrone for untreated follicular lymphoma: a report from the Non-Hodgkin's Lymphoma Co-operative Study Group. Leuk Lymph 2004; **45**: 1141–7.

115. Bosch F, Perales M, Cobo F et al. Fludarabine, cyclophos-phamide and mitoxantrone (FCM) therapy in resistant or relapsed chronic lymphocytic leukaemia (CLL) or follicular lymphoma (FL). Blood 1997; **90**: 530.

116. Solal-Celigny P, Lepage E, Brousse N et al. Recombinant interferon alfa-2b combined with a regimen containing doxorubicin in patients with advanced follicular lymphoma. N Engl J Med 1993; **329**: 1608–14.

117. Smalley RV, Anderson JW, Hawkins MJ et al. Interferon alfa combined with cytotoxic chemotherapy for patients with non-Hodgkin's lymphoma. N Engl J Med 1992; **327**: 1336–41.

118. Smalley RV, Weller E, Hawkins MJ et al. Final analysis of the ECOG I-COPA trial (E6484) in patients with non-Hodgkin's lymphoma treated with interferon alfa (IFN-α2a) plus an anthracycline-based induction regimen. Leukemia 2001; **15**: 1118–22.

119. Rohatiner AZ, Gregory WM, Peterson B et al. Meta-analysis to evaluate the role of interferon in follicular lymphoma. J Clin Oncol 2005; **23**: 2215–23.

120. Ehrlich P. On immunity with special reference to cell life. Proc R Soc Lond (Biol) 1890.

121. Nadler LM, Stashenko P, Hardy R et al. Serotherapy of a patient with a monoclonal antibody directed against a

human lymphoma-associated antigen. *Cancer Res* 1980; **40**: 3147–54.

122. Maloney DG, Grillo-Lopez AJ, Bodkin DJ *et al.* IDEC-C2B8: results of a phase I multiple-dose trial in patient with relapsed non-Hodgkin's lymphoma. *J Clin Oncol* 1997; **15**: 3266–74.

●123. McLaughlin P, Grillo-Lopez AJ, Link BK *et al.* Rituximab chimeric anti-CD20 monoclonal antibody therapy for relapsed indolent lymphoma: half of patients respond to a four-dose treatment program. *J Clin Oncol* 1998; **15**: 3266–74.

124. Zinzani PL, Magagnoli M, Moretti L *et al.* Randomized trial of fludarabine versus fludarabine and idarubicin as frontline treatment in patients with indolent or mantle-cell lymphoma. *J Clin Oncol* 2000; **18**: 773–9.

125. Hagenbeek A, Eghbali H, Monfardini S *et al.* Phase III intergroup study of fludarabine phosphate compared with cyclophosphamide, vincristine, and prednisone chemotherapy in newly diagnosed patients with stage III and IV low-grade malignant Non-Hodgkin's lymphoma. *J Clin Oncol* 2006; **24**: 1590–6.

126. Bellosillo B, Villamor N, Colomer D *et al.* In vitro evaluation of fludarabine in combination with cyclophosphamide and/or mitoxantrone in B-cell chronic lymphocytic leukaemia. *Blood* 1999; **94**: 2836–43.

◆127. Johnson S, Thomas W. Therapeutic potential of purine analogue combinations in the treatment of lymphoid malignancies. *Hematol Oncol* 2000; **18**: 141–53.

128. Schilling PJ, Vadhan-Raj S. Concurrent cytomegalovirus and Pneumocystis pneumonia after fludarabine therapy. *N Engl J Med* 1990; **323**: 833–4.

129. Tournilhac O, Cazin B, Lepretre S *et al.* Impact of frontline fludarabine and cyclophosphamide combined treatment on peripheral blood stem cell mobilisation in B-cell chronic lymphocytic leukaemia. *Blood* 2004; **103**: 363–5.

130. Micallef IN, Apostolidis J, Rohatiner AZ *et al.* Factors which predict unsuccessful mobilisation of peripheral blood progenitor cells following G-CSF alone in patients with non-Hodgkin's lymphoma. *Hematol J* 2000; **1**: 367–73.

●131. Micallef IN, Lillington DM, Apostolidis J *et al.* Therapy-related myelodysplasia and secondary acute myelogenous leukemia after high-dose therapy with autologous hematopoietic progentor-cell support for lymphoid malignancies. *J Clin Oncol* 2000; **18**: 947–55.

132. European Medicine Agency. European Public Assessment Report for Mabthera. http://www.emea.eu.int/humandocs/Humans/EPAR/mabthera/mabthera.htm

133. Food and Drug Administration. Draft labeling text for Rituxan (rituximab). http://www.fda.gov/cder/foi/label/2006/103705s5230-s52311bl.pdf

134. Foran JM, Gupta RK, Cunningham D *et al.* A UK multicentre phase II study of rituximab (chimeric anti-CD20 monoclonal antibody) in patients with follicular lymphoma, with PCR monitoring of molecular response. *Br J Haematol* 2000; **109**: 81–8.

135. McLaughlin P, Hagemeister FB, Grillo-Lopez AJ. Rituximab in indolent lymphoma: the single-agent pivotal trial. *Semin Oncol* 1999; **26**: 79–87.

136. Davis TA, White CA, Grillo-Lopez AJ *et al.* Single-agent monoclonal antibody efficacy in bulky non-Hodgkin's lymphoma: results of a phase II trial of rituximab. *J Clin Oncol* 1999; **17**: 1851–7.

137. Davis TA, Grillo-Lopez AJ, White CA *et al.* Rituximab anti-CD20 monoclonal antibody therapy in non-Hodgkin's lymphoma: safety and efficacy of re-treatment. *J Clin Oncol* 2000; **18**: 3135–43.

138. Hainsworth JD, Litchy S, Burris HA *et al.* Rituximab as first-line and maintenance therapy for patients with indolent non-Hodgkin's lymphoma. *J Clin Oncol* 2002; **20**: 4261–7.

139. Hainsworth JD, Burris HA, Morrissey LH *et al.* Rituximab monoclonal antibody as initial systemic therapy for patients with low-grade non-Hodgkin's lymphoma. *Blood* 2000; **95**: 3052–6.

140. Witzig TE, Vukov AM, Habermann TM *et al.* Rituximab therapy for patients with newly diagnosed, advanced-stage, follicular grade I non-Hodgkin's lymphoma: a phase II trial in the North Central Cancer Treatment Group. *J Clin Oncol* 2005; **23**: 1103–8.

141. Colombat P, Salles G, Brousse N *et al.* Rituximab (anti-CD20 monoclonal antibody) as first-line therapy for patients with follicular lymphoma with a low tumor burden: clinical and molecular evaluation. *Blood* 2001; **97**: 101–6.

142. Colombat P, Brousse N, Morschhauser F *et al.* Single treatment with rituximab monotherapy for low-tumor burden follicular lymphoma (FL): survival analyses with extended follow-up of 7 years. *Blood* 2006; **108**: 147a–8a (abstract).

143. Carson KR, Evens AM, Rosen ST *et al.* Progressive multifocal leukoencephalopathy associated with rituximab treatment of B-cell lymphoproliferative disorders: A report of 29 cases from the RADAR project. *Blood* 2007; **110**: 370 (abstract).

●144. van Oers MH, Klasa R, Marcus RE *et al.* Rituximab maintenance improves clinical outcome or relapsed/resistant follicular non-Hodgkin's lymphoma, both in patients with and without rituximab during induction: results of a prospective randomized phase III intergroup trial. *Blood* 2006; **108**: 3295–301.

●145. Marcus R, Imrie K, Belch A *et al.* CVP chemotherapy plus rituximab compared with CVP as first line treatment for advanced follicular lymphoma. *Blood* 2005; **105**: 1417–23.

●146. Hiddemann W, Kneba M, Dreyling M *et al.* Frontline therapy with rituximab added to the combination of cyclophosphamide, doxorubicin, vincristine, and prednisone (CHOP) significantly improves the outcome for patients with advanced-stage follicular lymphoma compared with therapy with CHOP alone: results of a prospective randomized study of the German Low-Grade Lymphoma Study Group. *Blood* 2005; **106**: 3725–32.

●147. Herold M, Haas A, Srock S *et al.* Addition of rituximab to first-line MCP (mitoxantrone, chlorambucil, prednisolone) chemotherapy prolongs survival in advanced follicular lymphoma: 4 year follow-up results of a phase III trial of the East German Study Group Hematology and Oncology (OSHO#39). *Blood* 2006; **108**: 147a (abstract).

148. Foussard C, Mounier N, Van Hoof A *et al.* Update of the FL2000 randomized trial combining rituximab to CHVP-interferon in follicular lymphoma (FL) patients, *J Clin Oncol* 2006; **24**: 7508 (abstract).

●149. Czuczman MS, Grillo-Lopez AJ, White CA *et al.* Treatment of patients with low-grade B-cell lymphoma with the combination of chimeric anti-CD20 monoclonal antibody and CHOP chemotherapy. *J Clin Oncol* 1999; **17**: 268–76.

150. Czuczman MS, Koryzna A, Mohr *et al.* Rituximab in combination with fludarabine chemotherapy in low-grade or follicular lymphoma. *J Clin Oncol* 2005; **23**: 694–704.

151. Schulz H, Bohlius J, Skoetz N *et al.* Combined immunochemotherapy with rituximab improves overall survival in patients with follicular lymphoma: updated meta-analysis results. *Blood* 2006; **108**: 781a (abstract).

152. Millar DR, Lewis G, Marcus RB. Cost effectiveness of rituximab maintenance (R-Maint) vs Autologous Stem Cell Transplant (ASCT) from a UK National Health Service (NHS) perspective. *Blood* 2007; **110**: 3321 (abstract).

153. Steward WP, Crowther D, McWilliam LJ *et al.* Maintenance chlorambucil after CVP in the management of advanced stage, low-grade histologic type non-Hodgkin's lymphoma: a randomized prospective study with an assessment of prognostic factors. *Cancer* 1988; **61**: 441–8.

154. Rohatiner AZS, Richards MA, Barnett MJ *et al.* Chlorambucil and interferon for low grade non-Hodgkin's lymphoma. *Br J Cancer* 1987; **55**: 225–6.

155. Chisesi T, Congiu M, Contu A *et al.* Randomized study of chlorambucil (CB) compared to Interferon (Alfa-2B) combined with CB in low-grade non-Hodgkin's lymphoma: An interim report of a randomized study – Non-Hodgkin's Lymphoma Co-operative Study Group. *Eur J Cancer* 1991; **27**: S31–3.

156. Peterson BA, Petroni GR, Oken MM *et al.* Cyclophosphamide versus cyclophosphamide plus interferon alfa-2b in follicular low-grade lymphomas: An intergroup phase III trial (CALGB 8691 and EST 7486). *Proc Am Soc Clin Oncol* 1997; **16**: 14a.

157. Solal-Celigny P, Lepage E, Brousse N *et al.* Doxorubicin-containing regimen with or without interferon alfa-2b for advanced follicular lymphomas: Final analysis of survival and toxicity in the Groupe d'Etude des Lymphomes Folliculaires 86 trial. *J Clin Oncol* 1998; **16**: 2332–8.

158. Arranz R, Garcia-Alfonso P, Sobrino P *et al.* Role of interferon alfa-2b in the induction and maintenance treatment of low-grade non-Hodgkin's lymphoma: Results from a prospective, multicenter trial with double randomization. *J Clin Oncol* 1998; **16**: 1538–46.

159. Hagenbeck A, Carde P, Meerwaldt JH *et al.* Maintenance of remission with human recombitant interferon alfa-2a in patients with stages III and IV low-grade malignant non-Hodgkin's lymphoma: European Organisation for Research and Treatment of Cancer, Lymphoma Co-operative Group. *J Clin Oncol* 1998; **16**: 41–7.

160. Unterhalt M, Hermann R, Koch P *et al.* Long term interferon alpha maintenance prolongs remission duration in advanced low grade lymphomas and is related to the efficacy of initial cytoreductive chemotherapy. *Blood* 1996; **88**: abstract 1801.

161. Aviles A, Duque G, Talavera A *et al.* Interferon alpha 2b as maintenance therapy in low grade malignant lymphoma improves duration of remission and survival. *Leuk Lymphoma* 1996; **20**: 495–9.

162. Rohatiner AZ, Radford J, Deakin D *et al.* A randomized controlled trial to evaluate the role of interferon as initial and maintenance therapy in patients with follicular lymphoma. *Br J Cancer* 2001; **85**: 29–35.

163. Piro LD, White CA, Grillo-Lopez AJ *et al.* Extended rituximab (anti-CD20 monoclonal antibody) therapy for relapsed or refractory low-grade or follicular non-Hodgkin's lymphoma. *Ann Oncol* 1999; **10**: 655–61.

164. Hochster HS, Weller E, Gascoyne RD *et al.* Maintenance rituximab after CVP results in superior clinical outcome in advanced follicular lymphoma (FL): results of the E1496 phase III trial from the Eastern Cooperative Oncology Group and the Cancer and Leukemia Group B. *Blood* 2005; **106**: 106a (abstract).

165. Hainsworth JD, Litchy S, Shaffer DW *et al.* Maximizing therapeutic benefit of rituximab: maintenance therapy versus re-treatment at progression in patients with indolent non-Hodgkin's lymphoma – a randomized phase II trial of the Minnie Pearl Cancer Research Network. *J Clin Oncol* 2005; **23**: 1088–95.

●166. Ghielmini M, Schmitz SF, Cogliatti SB *et al.* Prolonged treatment with rituximab in patients with follicular lymphoma significantly increases event-free survival and response duration compared with the standard weekly × 4 schedule. *Blood* 2004; **103**: 4416–23.

167. Morschhauser F, Leonard JP, Fayad L *et al.* Rituximab-relapsing patients with non-Hodgkins lymphoma respond even at lower doses of humanized anti-CD20 antibody, IMMU-106 (*ha* 20): Phase I/II results. *Blood* 2006; **108**: 2719 (abstract).

168. Leonard JP, Coleman M, Ketas JC *et al.* Phase I/II trial of epratuzumab (humanized CD22 antibody) in indolent non-Hodgkin's lymphoma. *J Clin Oncol* 2003; **21**: 3051–9.

169. Leonard JP, Coleman M, Ketas J *et al.* Combination antibody therapy with epratuzumab and rituximab in relapsed or refractory non-Hodgkin's lymphoma. *J Clin Oncol* 2005; **23**: 5044–51.

170. Strauss SJ, Morschhauser F, Rech J *et al.* Multicenter phase II trial of immunotherapy with the humanised anti-CD22 antibody, epratuzumab, in combination with rituximab, in refractory or recurrent non-Hodgkin's lymphoma. *J Clin Oncol* 2006; **24**: 3880–6.

171. DiJoseph JF, Dougher MM, Kalyandrug LB *et al.* Antitumor efficacy of a combination of CMC-544 (inotuzumab ozogamicin), a CD22-targeted cytotoxic immunoconjugate of calicheamicin, and rituximab against non-Hodgkin's B-cell lymphoma. *Clin Cancer Res* 2006; **12**: 242–9.

172. Ashkenazi A. Targeting death and decoy receptors of the tumor necrosis factor superfamily. *Nat Rev Cancer* 2002; **2**: 420–30.

●173. Witzig TE, White CA, Gordon LI *et al.* Safety of yttrium-90 ibritumomab tiuxetan radioimmunotherapy for relapsed low-grade, follicular, or transformed non-Hodgkin's lymphoma. *J Clin Oncol* 2003; **21**: 1263–70.

174. Bennett JM, Kaminski MS, Leonard JP *et al.* Assessment of treatment-related myelodysplastic syndromes and acute myeloid leukemia in patients with non-Hodgkin's lymphoma treated with Tositumomab and Iodine I 131 Tositumomab (BEXXAR). *Blood* 2005; **105**: 4576–82.

175. Fisher RI, Kaminski MS, Wahl RL *et al.* Tositumomab and iodine-131 tositumomab produces durable complete remissions in a subset of heavily pretreated patients with low-grade and transformed non-Hodgkin's lymphomas. *J Clin Oncol* 2005; **23**: 7565–73.

●176. Kaminski MS, Tuck M, Estes J *et al.* 131I-tositumomab therapy as initial treatment for follicular lymphoma. *N Engl J Med* 2005; **352**: 441–9.

177. Kaminski MS, Radford JA, Gregory SA *et al.* Re-treatment with I-131 tositumomab in patients with non-Hodgkin's lymphoma who had previously responded to I-131 tositumomab. *J Clin Oncol* 2005; **23**: 7985–93.

178. Davis TA, Kaminski MS, Leonard JP *et al.* The radioisotope contributes significantly to the activity of radioimmunotherapy. *Clin Cancer Res* 2004; **10**: 7792–8.

●179. Kaminski MS, Zelenetz AD, Press OW *et al.* Pivotal study of iodine I 131 tositumomab for chemotherapy-refractory low-grade or transformed low-grade B-cell non-Hodgkin's lymphomas. *J Clin Oncol* 2001; **19**: 3918–28.

180. Horning SJ, Younes A, Jain V *et al.* Efficacy and safety of tositumomab and iodine-131 tositumomab (Bexxar) in B-cell lymphoma, progressive after rituximab. *J Clin Oncol* 2005; **23**: 712–19.

181. Zelenetz AD, Saleh M, Vose JM *et al.* Patients with transformed low-grade lymphoma attain durable responses following outpatient radioimmunotherapy with Tositumomab and Iodine I-131 Tositumomab (Bexxar®). *Blood* 2002; **100**: 357a.

●182. Press OW, Eary JF, Appelbaum FR *et al.* Radiolabeled-antibody therapy of B-cell lymphoma with autologous bone marrow support. *N Engl J Med* 1993; **329**: 1219–24.

183. Press OW, Eary JF, Appelbaum FR *et al.* Phase II trial of 131I-B1 (anti-CD20) antibody therapy with autologous stem cell transplantation for relapsed B cell lymphomas. *Lancet* 1995; **346**: 336–40.

184. Gopal AK, Gooley TA, Maloney DG *et al.* High-dose radioimmunotherapy versus conventional high-dose therapy and autologous hematopoietic stem cell transplantation for relapsed follicular non-Hodgkin's lymphoma: a multivariate cohort analysis. *Blood* 2003; **102**: 2351–7.

●185. Vose JM, Bierman PF, Enke C *et al.* Phase I trial of Iodine-131 Tositumomab with high-dose chemotherapy and autologous stem-cell transplantation for relapsed non-Hodgkin's lymphoma. *J Clin Oncol* 2005; **5**: 461–7.

186. Press OW, Eary JF, Gooley T *et al.* A phase I/II trial of iodine-131-tositumomab (anti-CD20), etoposide, cyclophosphamide, and autologous stem cell transplantation for relapsed B-cell lymphomas. *Blood* 2000; **96**: 2934–42.

187. Press OW, Unger JM, Braziel RM *et al.* Phase II trial of CHOP chemotherapy followed by tositumomab/iodine I-131 tositumomab for previously untreated follicular non-Hodgkin's lymphoma: five-year follow-up of Southwest Oncology Group Protocol S9911. *J Clin Oncol* 2006; **24**: 4143–9.

188. Witzig TE, Flinn IW, Gordon LI *et al.* Treatment with ibritumomab tiuxetan radioimmunotherapy in patients with rituximab-refractory follicular non-Hodgkin's lymphoma. *J Clin Oncol* 2002; **20**: 3262–9.

●189. Witzig TE, Gordon LI, Cabanillas F *et al.* Randomized controlled trial of yttrium-90-labeled ibritumomab tiuxetan radioimmunotherapy versus rituximab immunotherapy for patients with relapsed or refractory low-grade, follicular, or transformed B-cell non-Hodgkin's lymphoma. *J Clin Oncol* 2002; **20**: 2453–63.

190. Ansell SM, Ristow KM, Habermann TM *et al.* Subsequent chemotherapy regimens are well tolerated after radioimmunotherapy with yttrium-90 ibritumomab tiuxetan for non-Hodgkin's lymphoma. *J Clin Oncol* 2002; **20**: 3885–90.

●191. Morschhauser F, Radford J, Van Hoof A *et al.* Phase III trial of consolidation therapy with yttrium-90-ibritumomab tiuxetan compared with no additional therapy after first remission in advanced follicular lymphoma. *J Clin Oncol* 2008; **26**: 5156–64.

192. Goff L, Summers K, Iqbal S *et al.* Radioimmunotherapy with 90Y-Ibritumomab Tiuxetan (Zevalin®) as consolidation of first remission in patients with advanced stage follicular lymphoma: A 'real-time' MBR RQ-PCR analysis. *Blood* 2007; **110**: 3412 (abstract).

●193. Rohatiner AZS, Nadler L, Davies AJ *et al.* Myeloablative therapy with autologous bone marrow transplantation for follicular lymphoma at the time of second or subsequent remission: long-term follow-up. *J Clin Oncol* 2007; **25**: 2554–9.

●194. Phillip T, Armitage JO, Spitzer G *et al.* High-dose therapy and autologous bone marrow transplantation after failure of conventional chemotherapy in adults with intermediate-grade or high-grade non-Hodgkin's lymphoma. *N Engl J Med* 1987; **316**: 1493–8.

195. Philip T, Gugliemi C, Hagenbeek A *et al.* Autologous bone marrow transplantation as compared with salvage chemotherapy in relapses of chemotherapy-sensitive non-Hodgkin's lymphoma. *N Engl J Med* 1995; **333**: 1540–5.

196. Petersen FB, Appelbaum FR, Hill R *et al.* Autologous marrow transplantation for malignant lymphoma: A report of 101 cases from Seattle. *J Clin Oncol* 1990; **8**: 638–47.

197. Schouten H, Bierman P, Vaughan W *et al.* Autologous bone marrow transplantation in follicular non-Hodgkin's lymphoma before and after histologic transformation. *Blood* 1989; **74**: 2579–84.

198. Freedman A, Ritz J, Neuberg D et al. Autologous bone marrow transplantation in 69 patients with a history of low-grade B-cell non-Hodgkin's lymphoma. Blood 1991; 77: 2524–9.

199. Rohatiner AZ, Johnson PW, Price CG et al. Myeloablative therapy with autologous bone marrow transplantation as consolidation therapy for recurrent follicular lymphoma. J Clin Oncol 1994; 12: 1177–84.

200. Berglund A, Enblad G, Carlson K et al. Long-term follow-up of autologous stem cell transplantation in follicular and transformed follicular lymphoma. Eur J Haematol 2000; 65: 17–22.

201. Gonzales-Barca E, Fernandez de Sevilla A, Domingo-Claros A et al. Autologous stem cell transplantation (ASCT) with immunologically purged progenitor cells in patients with advanced stage follicular lymphoma after early partial or complete remission: toxicity, follow-up of minimal residual disease and survival. Bone Marrow Transplant 2000; 26: 1051–6.

202. Ladetto M, Corradini P, Vallet S et al. High rate of clinical and molecular remissions in follicular lymphoma patients receiving high-dose sequential chemotherapy and autografting at diagnosis: multicenter, prospective study by the Gruppo Italiano Trapianto Midollo Osseo (GITMO). Blood 2002; 100: 1559–65.

203. Bierman PJ, Vose JM, Anderson JR et al. High-dose therapy with autologous hematopoietic rescue for follicular low-grade non-Hodgkin's lymphoma. J Clin Oncol 1997; 15: 445–50.

204. Corradini P, Ladetto M, Zallio F et al. Long-term follow-up of indolent lymphoma patients treated with high-dose sequential chemotherapy and autografting evidence that durable molecular and clinical remission frequently can be attained only in follicular subtypes. J Clin Oncol 2004; 22: 1460–8.

205. Pettengell R. Autologous stem cell transplantation in follicular non-Hodgkin's lymphoma. Bone Marrow Transplant 2002; 29: S1–4.

206. Brice P, Simon D, Bouabdallah R et al. High-dose therapy with autologous stem cell transplantation (ASCT) after first progression: Prolonged survival of follicular lymphoma patients included in the prospective GELF 86 protocol. Ann Oncol 2000; 11: 1585–90.

●207. Lenz G, Unterhalt M, Haferlach T et al. Significant increase of secondary myelodysplasia and acute myeloid leukaemia after myeloablative radiochemotherapy followed by autologous stem cell transplantation in indolent lymphoma patients: results of a prospective randomized study for the GLSG. Blood 2003; 102: 986.

208. Miller J, Arthur D, Litz C et al. Myelodysplastic syndrome after autologous bone marrow transplantation: an additional late complication of curative cancer therapy. Blood 1994; 83: 3780–6.

209. Stone R, Neuberg D, Soiffer R et al. Myelodysplastic syndrome as a late complication following autologous bone marrow transplantation for non-Hodgkin's lymphoma. J Clin Oncol 1994; 12: 2535–42.

210. Darrington D, Vose J, Anderson J et al. Incidence and characterization of secondary myelodysplastic syndrome following autologous stem cell transplantation for lymphoid malignancies. J Clin Oncol 1994; 12: 2527–34.

211. Friedberg J, Neuberg D, Stone R et al. Outcome in patients with myelodysplastic syndrome after autologous bone marrow transplantation for non-Hodgkin's lymphoma. J Clin Oncol 1999; 17: 3128–35.

212. Milligan DW, Ruiz De Elvira MC, Kolb HJ et al. Secondary leukaemia and myelodysplasia after autografting for lymphoma: results from the EBMT. EBMT Lymphoma and Late Effects Working Parties. European Group for Blood and Marrow Transplantation. Br J Haematol 1999; 106: 1020–6.

213. Lillington DM, Micallef IN, Carpenter E et al. Detection of chromosome abnormalities pre-high-dose treatment in patients developing therapy-related myelodysplasia and secondary acute myelogenous leukaemia after treatment for non-Hodgkin's lymphoma. J Clin Oncol 2001; 19: 2472–81.

214. Freedman AS, Gribben JG, Neuberg D et al. High dose therapy and autologous bone marrow transplantation in patients with follicular lymphoma during first remission. Blood 1996; 88: 2780–6.

215. Horning SJ, Negrin RS, Hoppe RT et al. High-dose therapy and autologous bone marrow transplantation for follicular lymphoma in first complete or partial remission: results of a phase II clinical trial. Blood 2001; 97: 404–9.

●216. Lenz G, Dreyling M, Schiegnitz E et al. Myeloablative radiochemotherapy followed by autologous stem cell transplantation in first remission prolongs progression-free survival in follicular lymphoma: results of a prospective, randomized trial of German Low-Grade Lymphoma Study Group. Blood 2004; 104: 2667–74.

●217. Deconinck E, Foussard C, Milpied N et al. High-dose therapy followed by autologous purged stem-cell transplantation and doxorubicin-based chemotherapy in patients with advanced follicular lymphoma: a randomized multicenter study by GOELAMS. Blood 2005; 105: 3817–23.

●218. Sebban C, Mounier N, Brousee N et al. Standard chemotherapy with interferon compared with CHOP followed by high-dose therapy with autologous stem cell transplantation in untreated patients with advanced follicular lymphoma: the GELF-94 randomized study from the Groupe d'Etude des Lymphomes de l'Adulte (GELA). Blood 2006; 108: 2540–4.

219. Stone RM. Myelodysplastic syndrome after autologous transplantation for lymphoma: the price of progress? Blood 1994; 83: 3437–40.

220. Schouten HC, Qian W, Kvaloy S et al. High-dose therapy improves progression-free survival and survival in relapsed follicular non-Hodgkin's lymphoma: results from the randomized European CUP trial. J Clin Oncol 2003; 21: 3918–27.

221. Friedberg J, Neuberg D, Gribben J et al. Autologous bone marrow transplantation following histologic

transformation of indolent B cell malignancies. *Biol Blood Marrow Transplant* 1999; **5**: 262–8.

222. Gisselbrecht C, Lepage E, Molina T. Shortened first line high dose chemotherapy for patients with poor prognosis aggressive lymphoma. *J Clin Oncol* 2002; **20**: 2472–9.

●223. Williams C, Harrison C, Lister T *et al.* High dose therapy and autologous stem cell support for chemosensitive transformed low-grade follicular non-Hodgkin's lymphoma: a case-matched study from the European Bone Marrow Transplant Registry. *J Clin Oncol* 2001; **19**: 727–35.

224. Chen C, Crump M, Tsang R *et al.* Autotransplants for histologically transformed follicular non-Hodgkin's lymphoma. *Br J Haematol* 2001; **113**: 202–8.

●225. van Besien K, Loberiza FR Jr, Bajorunatie R *et al.* Comparison of autologous and allogeneic hematopoietic stem cell transplantation for follicular lymphoma. *Blood* 2003; **102**: 3521–9.

226. van Besien KW, Mehra RC, Giralt SA *et al.* Allogeneic bone marrow transplantation for low-grade lymphoma. *Blood* 1998; **92**: 1832–6.

227. Yakoub-Agha I, Fawaz A, Foliot O *et al.* Allogeneic bone marrow transplantation in patients with follicular lymphoma: a single center study. *Bone Marrow Transplant* 2002; **30**: 229–34.

228. Forrest D, Thompson K, Nevill T *et al.* Allogeneic hematopoietic stem cell transplantation for progressive follicular lymphoma. *Bone Marrow Transplant* 2002; **29**: 973–8.

229. Toze C, Barnett M, Connors J *et al.* Long-term disease-free survival of patients with advanced follicular lymphoma after allogeneic bone marrow transplantation. *Br J Haematol* 2004; **127**: 311–21.

230. Hosing C, Saliba RM, McLaughlin P *et al.* Long-term results favor allogeneic over autologous hematopoietic stem cell transplantation in patients with refractory or recurrent indolent non-Hodgkin's lymphoma. *Ann Oncol* 2003; **14**: 737–44.

231. Verdonck L. Allogeneic versus autologous bone marrow transplantation for refractory and recurrent low-grade non-Hodgkin's lymphoma: updated results of Utrecht experience. *Leuk Lymphoma* 1999; **34**: 120–36.

232. Gribben JG, Zahrieh D, Stephans K *et al.* Autologous and allogeneic stem cell transplantations for poor-risk chronic lymphocytic leukaemia. *Blood* 2005; **106**: 4389–96.

●233. Khouri I, Saliba R, Giralt S *et al.* Nonablative allogeneic hematopoietic transplantation as adoptive immunotherapy for indolent lymphoma: low incidence of toxicity, acute graft-versus-host-disease, and treatment-related mortality. *Blood* 2001; **98**: 3595–9.

●234. Morris E, Thomson K, Craddock C *et al.* Outcomes after alemtuzumab-containing reduced-intensity allogeneic bone marrow transplantation regimen for relapsed and refractory non-Hodgkin lymphoma. *Blood* 2004; **104**: 3865–71.

●235. Hsu FJ, Caspar CB, Czerwinski D *et al.* Tumor-specific idiotype vaccines in the treatment of patients with B-cell lymphoma – long-term results of a clinical trial. *Blood* 1997; **89**: 3129–35.

236. Benandi M, Gocke CD, Kobrin CB *et al.* Complete molecular remissions induced by patient-specific vaccination plus granulocyte-monocyte colony-stimulation factor against lymphoma. *Nat Med* 1999; **5**: 1171–7.

237. Timmerman JM, Czerwinski DK, Davis TA *et al.* Idiotype-pulsed dendritic cell vaccination for B-cell lymphoma: clinical and immune responses in 35 patients. *Blood* 2002; **99**: 1517–26.

●238. Stevenson FK, Zhu D, King CA *et al.* Idiotypic DNA vaccines against B-cell lymphoma. *Immunol Rev* 1995; **145**: 211–28.

239. Stevenson FK, Ottenmeier CH, Johnson P *et al.* DNA vaccines to attack cancer. *Proc Natl Acad Sci U S A* 2004; **2**: 14646–52.

240. Levy R, Houot R, Brody J. New immunologic treatments for lymphoma. *Ann Oncol* 2008; **19** (Suppl 4): abstract 139.

241. Foussard C, Desablens B, Sensebe L *et al.* Is the International Prognostic Index for aggressive lymphomas useful for low-grade lymphoma patients? Applicability to stage III-IV patients. The GOELAMS Groups, France. *Ann Oncol* 1997; **1**: 49–52.

242. Lopez-Guillermo A, Montserrat E, Bosch F *et al.* Applicability of the International Index for aggressive lymphomas to patients with low-grade lymphoma. *J Clin Oncol* 1994; **12**: 1343–8.

243. Decaudin D, Lepage E, Brousse N *et al.* Low-grade stage III-IV follicular lymphoma: multivariate analysis of prognostic factors in 484 patients – a study of the Groupe d'Etude des Lymphomes de l'Adulte. *J Clin Oncol* 1999; **17**: 2499–505.

244. Federico M, Vitolo U, Zinzani PL *et al.* Prognosis of follicular lymphoma: a predictive model based on a retrospective analysis of 987 cases. Intergruppo Italiano Linfomi. *Blood* 2000; **95**: 783–9.

245. Longo D, Young R, Hubbard S *et al.* Prolonged initial remission in patients with nodular mixed lymphomas. *Ann Intern Med* 1984; **100**: 651–6.

246. Peterson B, Anderson J, Frizzera G *et al.* Combination chemotherapy prolongs survival in follicular mixed lymphoma (FML). *Proc Am Soc Clin Oncol* 1990; **9**: 259.

247. Glick J, Barnes J, Ezdinli E *et al.* Nodular mixed lymphoma: results of a randomized trial failing to confirm prolonged disease-free survival with COPP chemotherapy. *Blood* 1981; **58**: 920–5.

248. Dreyling MH, Roulston D, Bohlander SK *et al.* Codeletion of CDKN2 and MTAP genes in a subset of non-Hodgkin's lymphoma may be associated with histologic transformation from low-grade to diffuse large B-cell lymphoma. *Genes Chromosomes Cancer* 1998; **22**: 72–8.

249. Pinyol M, Cobo F, Bea S *et al.* p16(INK4a) gene inactivation by deletions, mutations, and hypermethylation is associated with transformed and aggressive variants of non-Hodgkin's lymphomas. *Blood* 1998; **91**: 2977–84.

250. Lo Coco F, Gaidano G, Louie DC et al. p53 mutations are associated with histologic transformation of follicular lymphoma. Blood 1993; 82: 2289–95.

251. Sander CA, Yano T, Clark HM et al. p53 mutation is associated with progression in follicular lymphomas. Blood 1993; 82: 1994–2004.

252. Yano T, Jaffe ES, Longo DL, Raffeld M. MYC rearrangements in histologically progressed follicular lymphomas. Blood 1992; 80: 758–67.

253. Freedman AS, Neuberg D, Mauch P et al. Long-term follow-up of autologous bone marrow transplantation in patients with relapsed follicular lymphoma. Blood 1999; 94: 3325–33.

254. Voso MT, Pantel G, Weis M et al. In vivo depletion of B cells using a combination of high-dose cytosine arabinoside/mitoxantrone and rituximab for autografting in patients with non-Hodgkin's lymphoma. Br J Haematol 2000; 109: 729–35.

255. Ladetto M, Corradini P, Vellet S et al. High rate of clinical and molecular remissions in follicular lymphoma patients recieving high-dose sequential chemotherapy and autografting at diagnosis: a multicenter, prospective study by the Gruppo Italiano Trapianto Midollo Osseo (GITMO). Blood 2002; 100: 1559–65.

256. Apostolidis J, Gupta RK, Grenzelias D et al. High-dose therapy with autologous bone marrow support as consolidation of remission in follicular lymphoma: long-term clinical and molecular follow-up. J Clin Oncol 2000; 18: 527–36.

●257. Rambaldi A, Carlotti E, Oldani E et al. Quantative PCR of bone marrow BCL2/IgH+ cells at diagnosis predicts treatment response and long-term outcome in follicular non-Hodgkin lymphoma. Blood 2005; 105: 3428–33.

●258. Lopez-Guillermo A, Cabanillas F, McLaughlin P et al. The clinical significance of molecular response in indolent follicular lymphomas. Blood 1998; 91: 2955–60.

259. Michels J, Foria V, Mead B et al. Immunohistochemical analysis of the antiapoptotic Mcl-1 and Bcl-2 proteins in follicular lymphoma. Br J Haematol 2006; 132: 743–6.

260. Glas AM, Kersten MJ, Delahaye LJ et al. Gene expression profiling in follicular lymphoma to assess clinical aggressiveness and to guide the choice of treatment. Blood 2005; 105: 301–7.

261. Carreras J, Lopez-Guillermo A, Fox BC et al. High numbers of tumor-infiltrating FOXP3-positive regulatory T cells are associated with improved overall survival in follicular lymphoma. Blood 2006; 108: 2957–64.

262. Lee AM, Clear AJ, Calaminici M et al. Number of CD4+ cells and location of forkhead box protein PS-positive cells in diagnostic follicular lymphoma tissue mircoarrays correlates with outcome. J Clin Oncol 2006; 24: 5052–9.

263. Farinha P, Masoudi H, Skinnider BF et al. Analysis of multiple biomarkers shows that lymphoma-associated macrophage (LAM) content is an independent predictor of survival in follicular lymphoma (FL). Blood 2005; 106: 2169–74.

264. Canioni D, Salles G, Mounier N et al. High numbers of tumor-associated macrophages have an adverse prognostic value that can be circumvented by rituximab in patients with follicular lymphoma enrolled onto the GELA-GOELAMS FL-200 trial. J Clin Oncol 2008; 26: 440–6.

265. Witzig TE, White CA, Wiseman GA et al. Phase I/II trial of IDEC-Y2B8 radioimmunotherapy for treatment of relapsed or refractory CD20(+) B-cell non-Hodgkin's lymphoma. J Clin Oncol 1999; 17: 3793–803.

266. Gordon LI, Molina A, Witzig T et al. Durable responses after ibritumomab tiuxetan radioimmunotherapy for CD20+ B-cell lymphoma: long-term follow-up of a phase 1/2 study. Blood 2004; 103: 4429–31.

267. Wiseman GA, Gordon LI, Multani PS et al. Ibritumomab tiuxetan radioimmunotherapy for patients with relapsed or refractory non-Hodgkin lymphoma and mild thrombo-cytopenia: a phase II multicenter trial. Blood 2002; 99: 4336–42.

268. Vose JM, Wahl RL, Saleh M et al. Multicenter phase II study of iodine-131 tositumomab for chemotherapy-relapsed/refractory low-grade or transformed low-grade B-cell non-Hodgkin's lymphomas. J Clin Oncol 2000; 18: 1316–23.

269. Kaminski MS, Estes J, Zasadny KR et al. Radioimmunotherapy with iodine (131)I tositumomab for relapsed or refractory B-cell non-Hodkin lymphoma: updated results and long-term follow-up of the University of Michigan experience. Blood 2000; 96: 1259–66.

270. Davies AJ, Rohatiner AZ, Howell S et al. Tositumomab and iodine I 131 tositumomab for recurrent indolent and transformed B-cell non-Hodgkin's lymphoma. J Clin Oncol 2004; 22: 1469–79.

271. Forstpointer R, Unterhalt M, Dreyling M et al. Maintenance therapy with rituximab leads to significant prolongation of response duration after salvage therapy with a combination of rituximab, fludarabine, cyclophosphamide, and mtoxantrone (R-FCM) in patients with recurring and refractory follicular and mantle cell lymphomas: results of a prospective randomized study of the German Low-Grade Lymphoma Study Group (GLSG). Blood 2006; 108: 4003–8.

68

Burkitt lymphoma/leukemia in children

C PATTE

INTRODUCTION

Burkitt lymphoma was first described, as indicated by its name, by Dennis Burkitt in 1959, as a rapidly growing facial tumor occurring in black African children, especially males. This tumor seemed to occur preferentially in the subtropical belt and to be related to Epstein–Barr virus (EBV), particles of which were found in the tumor nuclei. Later, the same histologic aspects were found in 'reticulosarcomas' occurring in North American and European children in other sites, especially in the abdomen. Thus they were described the 'endemic' Burkitt lymphoma as described by Burkitt and related to EBV and the 'nonendemic' Burkitt lymphoma occurring in other parts of the world and usually not related to EBV. These two entities present the same histocytologic aspects but have some different clinical and biological features. An important phase in the understanding of the biology of the disease was the description of nonrandom chromosomal translocations involving the protooncogene *MYC* on chromosome 8q24 and one of the heavy μ or light κ or λ chain immunoglobulin constant region genes on chromosome 14q32 (the most frequent), 2p12, or 22q11, respectively.

During the 1970s, in parallel with increased understanding of the lymphoid system, the concept of B cell non-Hodgkin lymphomas (B-NHL) of childhood including Burkitt lymphoma developed on the basis of clinical and biological criteria. The need for specific therapeutic modalities has now become clear and has made differences of practical relevance. In parallel, acute leukemia derived from mature B lymphoblasts (B-ALL) was recognized as an entity distinct from other types of childhood acute lymphoblastic leukemia (ALL), and therapeutic improvements in B-ALL have occured in parallel with those in B-NHL. This is why they are presented together. It is now recognized that Burkitt lymphoma and mature B cell leukemia (L3-ALL) are different forms of the same disease. Lymphoblasts are characterized by similar cytologic features, by the presence of B cell markers (especially CD20) and monoclonal immunoglobulins on their surface, and specific translocations.

The terminology to designate Burkitt lymphoma evolved during the 1980s and 1990s through the different histopathological classifications. Initially called Burkitt lymphoma, it became *undifferentiated* then *small noncleaved lymphoma* in the US classifications[1] and has now reverted to *Burkitt lymphoma*.[2,3] The spectrum of the disease also evolved, being either restricted to the typical forms or including the variants. In the recent World Health Organization (WHO) classification, variants, called atypical/Burkitt-like, are included in the category Burkitt lymphoma if Ki-67 (a marker of proliferation) staining is positive in more than 95 percent of the malignant cells with evidence of a *MYC* rearrangement when cytogenetic analysis is available.[3]

Burkitt lymphoma is characterized by a very high proliferation rate and a short cell-cycle time, by a great propensity to spread from the original site and to invade the central nervous system (CNS), and by early relapse. A patient with a Burkitt NHL or L3-ALL remaining in complete remission for 1 year can be considered as cured.

EPIDEMIOLOGY

Burkitt lymphoma is the most frequent lymphoma in children. The male:female ratio is between 1.5 and 4.5 to 1, depending on the age and the country.[4,5] It is rare before 2 years of age. The median age of occurrence is around 6 years in the endemic regions and 8 years in Europe/North America, but it depends on the upper age limit of the series.[4,5]

The incidence differs greatly in different parts of the world. In the USA, according to the National Cancer Institute's Surveillance, Epidemiology, and End Results (SEER) Program, the average annual incidence rate of Burkitt lymphoma is approximately 3–5 per million in the age group 0–19 years.[6] Burkitt lymphoma represents about 50 percent of all lymphoma in this age group. According to the International Agency for Research on Cancer (IARC) publication considering children below 15 years of age, age-standardized incidence rates per million are between 1 and 5.5, with the incidence decreasing from the South to the North. It is reported to be lower in India and East Asia (Japan, Hong Kong, Singapore).[7] On the contrary, in the so-called endemic regions which include equatorial Africa, the incidence rate was estimated at 5–10 cases per 100 000 children below 16 years of age. Burkitt lymphoma accounts for between 30 percent and 70 percent of all childhood cancer.[7]

It is interesting to note that although all tumors have the MYC/IG translocation, the chromosomal breakpoints differ in different geographic regions, as well as the association with EBV.[8–10] In fact, analysis of the immunoglobulin gene rearrangements suggests that EBV-negative and EBV-positive Burkitt lymphoma may originate from two distinct subsets of B cells, whatever the geographic or human immunodeficiency virus (HIV)-related origin of the tumors.[11]

Burkitt lymphoma also occurs at increased frequency among patients with immunodeficiency and in families with the X-linked lymphoproliferative syndrome.[12–14] The incidence of HIV-related NHL in children greatly decreased with the advent of effective antiviral treatment.

CLINICAL PRESENTATIONS

Burkitt lymphoma can occur in any organ or tissue, although there are preferential sites. There are also clinical differences between the 'nonendemic' form (predominance of abdominal tumors and frequent bone marrow involvement) and the 'endemic' form (younger median age, frequent facial involvement, and paraplegia) as shown in Table 68.1. It is also interesting to note that among endemic Burkitt lymphomas, site is related to age. In the series of endemic Burkitt lymphoma described in Table 68.1, jaw involvement peaked at 3 years (66.7 percent of the cases) and abdominal disease at 14 years (66.7 percent), whilst in adults, abdominal and CNS involvement (39 percent) and HIV positivity predominated.[15]

Table 68.1 Differences between endemic and nonendemic Burkitt lymphoma/mature B cell leukemia

Involvement	Endemic[a]	Nonendemic[b]
Jaw	51.6%	8.5%
Abdomen	25%	63%
Jaw + abdomen	13.8%	
Other sites	9.6%	15%
Central nervous system	16.8%	13%
Bone marrow	25%	34%

[a]From a series of Burkitt lymphoma seen in Kenyan patients.[15]
[b]From the series of Burkitt non-Hodgkin lymphoma/acute lymphoblastic leukemia treated in the LMB 89 protocol.[45]

Most Burkitt lymphomas involve the abdomen, generally originating in the ileocecal region. Acute intussusception revealing a small tumor, which can be easily resected, is infrequent. Most often at the time of diagnosis, the disease has spread to the mesentery. Ascites may be present, as well as involvement of paraaortic lymph nodes and the viscera, such as liver, ovaries, kidney, pancreas, or spleen (Fig. 68.1). The tumor can also originate from other parts of the gut: ileum, duodenum, stomach, and colon. Except for resection of a very localized tumor (those generally revealed by intussusception), aggressive attempts at debulking extensive abdominal disease are contraindicated.[16–18]

Burkitt lymphoma is also common in the head and neck region. It may involve one or several jaw quadrants, typically seen in the endemic forms (Fig. 68.2). In nonendemic head and neck tumors, Waldeyer's ring is most frequently involved (nasopharynx, tonsils), revealed by symptoms related to the tumor, but more often by cervical lymph nodes. Central nervous system involvement is also frequent in patients with involvement of these sites.[19]

Burkitt lymphoma can also originate from other areas, such as superficial nodes, thorax, kidney (Fig. 68.3), bone, orbit, and thyroid. Bone marrow is one of the sites of dissemination, occurring in about 20 percent of nonendemic cases. In the St. Jude's staging system, the arbitrary border with leukemia has been defined by the presence of 25 percent blasts in bone marrow. But it does not always correlate with clinical experience. There are patients presenting as leukemia with clinical symptoms of bone marrow infiltration, often associated with liver, spleen, renal, and lymph node enlargement, but many others present with huge abdominal masses and staging then reveals bone marrow involvement with more than 25 percent blasts.[20] But the relevance of such distinctions has now weakened since Burkitt NHL and L3-ALL are now treated according to the same protocols.

As in lymphoblastic leukemia, there can be testicular involvement. However, this has no prognostic impact and does not require radiation therapy in addition to chemotherapy.[21]

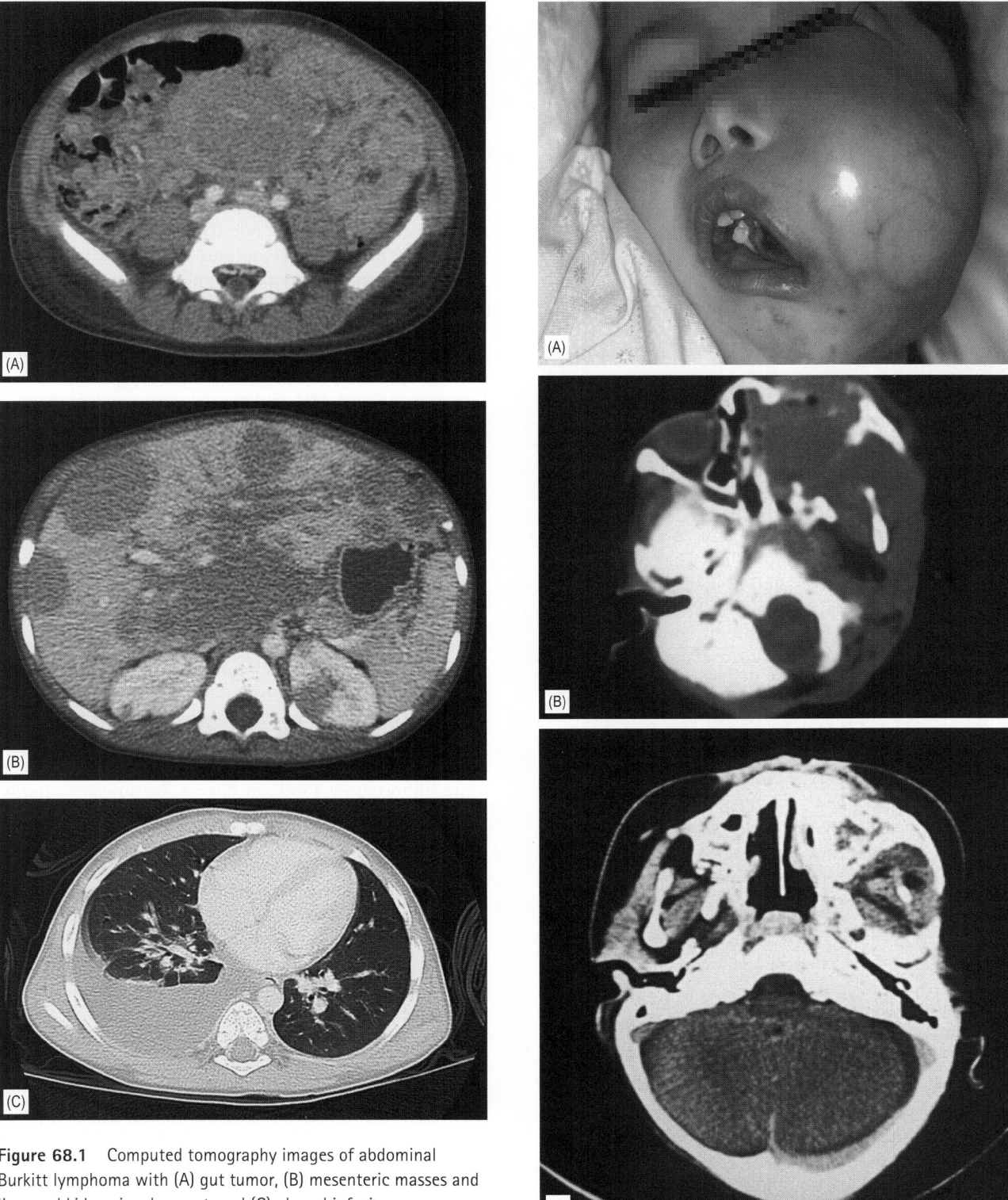

Figure 68.1 Computed tomography images of abdominal Burkitt lymphoma with (A) gut tumor, (B) mesenteric masses and liver and kidney involvement, and (C) pleural infusion.

Central nervous system involvement is the most dreaded site of dissemination because it still has poor prognostic implications. It is defined by the presence of unequivocal malignant cells in a cytocentrifuged specimen of spinal fluid and/or the presence of obvious neurological deficits, such as cranial nerve palsies. Blastic meningitis is

Figure 68.2 Facial Burkitt lymphoma presenting with a rapidly growing tumor of the left maxilla. (A) Clinical presentation and (B) computed tomography scan. Bone marrow involvement and central nervous system involvement, with blasts in the cerebrospinal fluid, were found at the workup. (C) Complete regression of the tumor after two cycles of chemotherapy, i.e., 6 weeks of treatment.

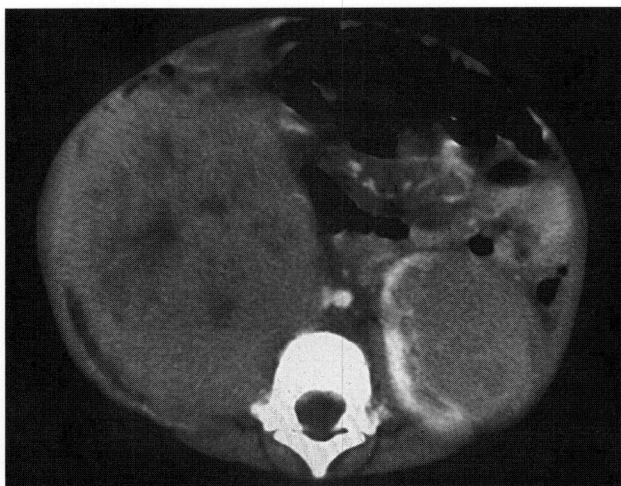

Figure 68.3 Bilateral kidney Burkitt lymphoma in an 18-month-old boy presenting with alteration of the general status, renal function impairment, and blasts in the cerebrospinal fluid.

often asymptomatic. Palsies are not always associated with blasts in the cerebrospinal fluid (CSF). They often involve oculomotor or facial nerves, and rarely peripheral nerves. Paraplegia is common in endemic Burkitt lymphoma, but can also occur in nonendemic Burkitt lymphoma. In the latter situation, if paraplegia is isolated, some will but others will not consider it as CNS involvement. Other questions are discussed below. How should numbness of the chin be considered? It may be caused by compression of the mental branch of the alveolar branch of the facial nerve by a facial tumor, or by involvement of the mandible, but it can also occur independently and is then considered as CNS involvement. How should intracranial extension of parameningeal tumors be considered? If it is huge, invading cerebral structures, protocols designed for CNS-positive patients should be considered. Isolated CNS disease such as an intracerebral mass is extremely rare.[22]

INITIAL WORKUP AND STAGING AND INITIATION OF TREATMENT

Due to the predominance of extranodal primary sites, the usual staging classification used in children is the St. Jude's classification (Table 68.2A).[23] However, it does not take into consideration lactate dehydrogenase (LDH) level, which is recognized to be an accurate reflection of tumor burden, the presence of CNS involvement among patients with stage IV disease, and, to a lesser extent, tumor resection in localized disease. Recent therapeutic stratifications include some of these factors, such as in the Berlin-Frankfurt-Munster (BFM) protocols or LMB (Lymphomes Malins B) protocols of the French Society of Pediatric Oncology (SFOP).

The staging classification is sometimes simplified into localized (stages I and II) and disseminated or advanced stage (stages III, IV, and ALL) disease. A classification taking into consideration facial or abdominal primary site and CNS involvement had been previously developed for endemic Burkitt lymphoma (Table 68.2B).

For staging, the minimal requirements include detailed physical examination, chest x-ray, abdominal ultrasound, two bone marrow aspirates, and CSF examination with a cytospin preparation. Blood count, serum LDH level, blood biochemistry, urea, creatinine, and uric acid are recommended although do not contribute to the staging. Depending on clinical symptoms and tumor sites, computed tomography (CT) and magnetic resonance imaging (MRI) scans, bone x-rays and scintigraphy, and cranial and spinal MRI should be done. In abdominal disease, abdominal ultrasound adequately describes involvement of the different organs, especially in young children who lack retroperitoneal fat, and may be more efficient than CT scanning to detect small gut tumors.[24] It is also useful for following the decrease/disappearance of tumors during treatment. But it relies on the expertise of the ultrasonographer, so CT scanning may be preferred as it can be reviewed secondarily. Computed tomographic scans are also more efficient for exploring the lower pelvis.

Gallium scintigraphy has been used in some countries to provide a whole body screen, but not in others, the specificity and sensitivity not being considered reliable enough. Positron emission tomography (PET) may be more efficient, but this technique has still to be evaluated in children with lymphoma. Besides not being available everywhere, it might not be possible to use it in the frequently seen context of an urgent need to start chemotherapy. In fact, accuracy for determining extent of disease is more important in localized disease, because it would be treated with less-intensive therapy.

Because of its high proliferation rate, Burkitt lymphoma is usually a very fast-growing tumor that requires prompt diagnosis and staging, and treatment is considered a medical emergency. The minimal staging procedures (indicated above) can be done in a few hours. When necessary, diagnosis of Burkitt lymphoma can be established rapidly on cytology smears (of ascitic fluid, pleural effusion, bone marrow, node, or tumor aspirate). Before starting chemotherapy, it is important to evaluate any associated problems, which must be managed before and/or in parallel with chemotherapy. These problems – for example, airway obstruction by a huge Waldeyer's ring tumor, infection, postsurgical complications, or metabolic problems – must be recognized and adequately treated.

Adequate renal function allowing a high urine flow is necessary prior to starting chemotherapy safely.[25] If renal failure is present, its cause must be established (e.g., urate nephropathy, renal infiltration by tumor, or urinary obstruction by a pelvic tumor) in order to start prompt and appropriate treatment. This may include dialysis or urine diversion by a transcutaneous nephrostomy or ureteral endoprothesis.

The commonest complications at presentation are due to metabolic disorders related to the high proliferation rate of

Table 68.2 (A) St. Jude/Murphy's Staging System for childhood non-Hodgkin lymphoma.[23] (B) Classification often used for endemic Burkitt lymphoma.[82,88]

Stage	Description
(A)	
I	A single tumor (extranodal) or a single anatomic area (nodal) with the exclusion of the mediastinum or abdomen
II	A single extranodal tumor with regional node involvement
	Two single extranodal tumors on the same side of the diaphragm with or without regional node involvement
	Two or more nodal areas on the same side of the diaphragm. Primary gastrointestinal tumor with or without involvement of associated mesenteric nodes only, grossly resected
III	Two single extranodal tumors on opposite sides of the diaphragm
	Two or more nodal areas on opposite sides of the diaphragm
	All primary intrathoracic tumors (mediastinal, pleural, thymic)
	All extensive primary intraabdominal disease
	All paraspinal or epidural tumors, regardless of other tumor sites
IV	Any of the above with initial central nervous system (CNS) and/or bone marrow involvement (less than 25% involvement; greater than 25% involvement is defined as mature B cell leukemia [L3-ALL])
(B)	
A or I	A single facial tumor
B or II	Multiple facial tumors or facial tumor and involvement of any site except intraabdominal or CNS
C or III	Intraabdominal tumor (including retroperitoneal) with or without tumor elsewhere except CNS
D or IV	CNS (malignant pleocytosis)

Burkitt lymphoma. The 'tumor lysis syndrome' is due to the sudden release of the products of cell catabolism including potassium, phosphorus, and purines, the end product of which is uric acid. Tumor lysis leads to hyperkalemia with risk of cardiac complications including sudden death; to hyperphosphatemia with risk of phosphate deposition in the tubules, inducing nephropathy and hypocalcemia, with its known muscular complications; and to high levels of uric acid, which precipitates in the kidneys causing nephropathy. The tumor lysis syndrome may be present prior to chemotherapy or may develop during treatment. Its intensity correlates with tumor burden. Patients with advanced stage disease and a high LDH level are at higher risk of developing severe metabolic complications, all the more as the renal function is already impaired.[26] Preventive measures against the tumor lysis syndrome must be instituted before and during the first days of chemotherapy. Treatment to reduce the serum uric acid level (allopurinol, urate oxidase) and hyperhydration ($3 L/m^2$/day or more) to obtain a high urine flow are essential. Allopurinol prevents the conversion of xanthine into uric acid, but xanthine can also precipitate in the kidneys. Urate oxidase converts uric acid into allantoin that is highly soluble in the kidneys. Nonrecombinant urate oxidase (Uricozyme), purified from *Aspergillus flavus* fungus, has been available for some time in France[27] and Italy, but the recombinant product, although more expensive, is now widely available.[28] This drug very efficiently lowers the uric acid in a few hours and consequently preserves/restores normal renal function, allowing better elimination of potassium and phosphorus.[29,30] Urate oxidase is preferable in cases with

a high tumor burden.[31] If allopurinol is used, alkalinization of the urine has to be instituted. It is essential to closely monitor weight, urine flow, blood pressure, and ionic balance several times a day during the critical days; that is, the 2–5 days following start of treatment. In cases with a high tumor burden, it may be preferable to start chemotherapy while having the patient near an intensive care unit. If not adequately handled, tumor lysis syndrome can be fatal. For this reason, both the French LMB and the German BFM protocols start with a 'prephase' with low-dose therapy. This generally induces good tumor regression and allows management of the initial problems without the additional hematologic and mucosal complications of the more-intensive regimens that start 1 week later.

TREATMENT

General considerations

Treatment of Burkitt lymphoma has been a successful story considering the great improvements in cure rates over 20 years. It is now established that Burkitt lymphoma has to be treated differently from lymphoblastic NHL: the first with short intensive pulse treatment, the second with semi-continuous and prolonged leukemia-like regimens.

Surgery is not considered part of the treatment. Initial surgery should be limited to: (1) biopsy for diagnosis when no other means (e.g., examination of ascites or pleural fluid, bone marrow, or CSF) are possible; biopsy should be limited to the sampling necessary for diagnosis and biological studies. Percutaneous fine-needle biopsy may be preferable in cases of deep tumor, thus avoiding a laparotomy; (2) complete removal of localized disease but excluding mutilating surgery;[32] and (3) acute abdominal complications, generally intussusception, and, exceptionally, perforation or bleeding.

With current chemotherapy, it has been clearly demonstrated that there is no advantage in performing major tumor resection or debulking procedures. Extensive surgery is unnecessary and is generally followed by tumor regrowth. It delays and may complicate chemotherapy.[16–18] It should be kept in mind that the good outcome of resected disease (and consequently the possibility of reduced therapy) is a reflection of its having been very localized disease and not that it was resected. During the 1970s it was shown that patients who were treated by resection of a very localized tumor could be cured without any CNS prophylaxis, which was not the case for nonlocalized resected tumors.[33]

Radiation therapy is no longer used. It was shown that in childhood non-Hodgkin lymphomas it gives no advantage over chemotherapy and adds both immediate and long-term toxicity.[34,35] Moreover, clinical experience shows that sensitivity to radiation and hence curability seem lower in Burkitt than in lymphoblastic lymphoma.

Treatment strategies and their evolution

In this section, the major studies will first be summarized, so that guidelines can be drawn, and remaining controversies will be addressed subsequently.

IN 'WESTERN' COUNTRIES

In the late 1970s, it was recognized that Burkitt lymphoma (at least nonlymphoblastic lymphoma) should be treated differently from lymphoblastic lymphoma. This was one of the main conclusions of the randomized Children's Cancer Group (CCG) study indicating that nonlymphoblastic lymphoma benefited more from the COMP (cyclophosphamide, oncovin, low-dose methotrexate, prednisone) regimen compared to the ALL strategy used in the LAS2-L2 regimen.[36] Similar conclusions were drawn from nonrandomized series. The Institut Gustave Roussy (IGR) group had better results with the COPAD regimen (cyclophosphamide, oncovin, prednisone, doxorubicin) in Burkitt lymphoma than in lymphoblastic lymphoma,[37] while the BFM group had quite the opposite experience with the BFM-ALL strategy.[38] At that time, survival improved from less than 10 percent[39,40] to 25–50 percent, depending on the series and stage distribution. It was also shown that complete response rates, relapse frequency, and survival in American patients were similar to the results in Africa.[41]

Since 1981, the largest national studies have taken place in France (LMB protocols)[42–45] and Germany (BFM protocols).[46–50] Considerable improvements have resulted as a consequence of these well-organized multicenter studies.

Other national or institutional studies have also contributed to the improvements in therapy.

LMB studies

Since 1981, the SFOP has conducted several consecutive multicenter 'LMB' studies in France, in two centers in Belgium, and in one in the Netherlands.[42–45] The general scheme of the LMB protocols is the same. Treatment begins with a prephase, called COP, with small doses of vincristine, cyclophosphamide, and prednisone, which induces a good tumor reduction and permits the management of metabolic or other acute problems without myelosuppression. The intensive induction phase starts 1 week later, with two consecutive courses of COPADM based on fractionated high-dose (HD) cyclophosphamide and HD methotrexate (MTX) given in conjunction with vincristine, doxorubicin, and prednisone. The two consolidation courses are based on 5 days of cytarabine (Ara-C) given by continuous intravenous infusion. Central nervous system prophylaxis comprises HD MTX and intrathecal (IT) MTX plus Ara-C. Maintenance therapy, comprising monthly cycles (for 5 days) of the previously used drugs, varied with the studies and was progressively shortened.

The major conclusions of the first LMB studies can be summarized as follows.[42,43] While event-free survival (EFS) of CNS-negative advanced stage disease increased to 75–80 percent for patients treated in the first two LMB 81 and 84 studies, duration of treatment was progressively reduced from 12 to 4 months, and toxicity, especially treatment-related deaths, decreased in parallel with the investigators' experience. Central nervous system prophylaxis with HD MTX ($3 \, g/m^2$ as a 3 h infusion) and IT MTX were effective, with a CNS relapse rate of less than 2 percent. It was shown that partial remission (with documented viable cells in the residual mass) after 3 cycles had a poor outcome, but could be salvaged by treatment intensification,[51] and that absence of tumor reduction after COP was indicative of a poor prognosis (EFS 29 percent). With the introduction of higher doses of MTX ($8 \, g/m^2$ in 4 h), HD Ara-C (CYVE courses[52]), and repeated triple IT therapy in the LMB 86 study, the EFS of patients with initial CNS involvement improved from 19 percent to 75 percent.[44] This intensified strategy also benefited patients with L3-ALL: those without CNS involvement could achieve an EFS rate of around 90 percent.

Based on the results of these studies, the next LMB 89 study was designed (Fig. 68.4).[45] Three risk groups were defined which received treatment of progressive intensity: Group A patients (resected stage I and resected abdominal stage II) received 2 cycles of COPAD; Group B patients (not eligible for inclusion in groups A or C) received a three-and-a-half-month treatment identical to the short arm of the LMB 84 protocol; Group C patients (with CNS involvement and ALL with more than 70 percent of blasts in the bone marrow) received the more intensive 8 cycle treatment similar to that of the LMB 86 protocol. Treatment was further intensified for Group B patients who did not respond to COP and any patient with residual viable cells after the consolidation phase. Event-free survival of the 420 patients with Burkitt lymphoma was 92 percent, similar to that of patients with diffuse large B cell lymphoma (DLBCL) or patients with non-B cell lymphoma, unclassified, who were also included in the study. Results by stage and therapeutic group are shown in Figure 68.5. Prognostic factors remained LDH level in stage III disease, nonresponse to COP (although EFS increased from 29 percent to 70 percent), and CNS disease.

The EFS of the 100 patients with L3-ALL was 88 percent overall, and 92 percent and 83 percent for patients without and with CNS ($n = 35$) involvement, respectively.

The next study, FAB LMB 96 (May 1996–June 2001), was a randomized international trial with the participation of the SFOP, the United Kingdom Children's Cancer Study Group (UKCCSG), and the CCG from the USA.[53–55] It was an attempt to reduce total drug dosage further, especially that of cyclophosphamide, to avoid sterility in boys, to reduce treatment duration, and to obviate the need for cranial irradiation in patients with initial CNS involvement.

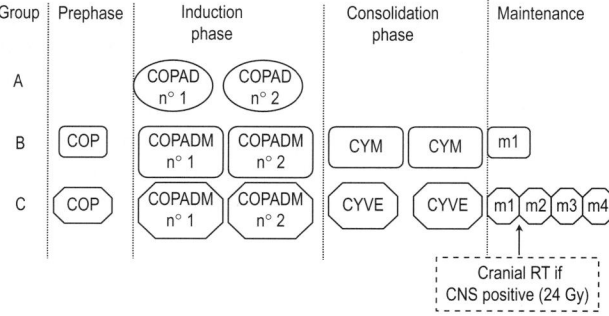

Figure 68.4 Scheme of the protocol for study LMB (Lyphomes Malins B) 89 according to the different therapeutic groups: A, B, and C. With the results of the FAB LMB 96 trial, Group B regimen was reduced (study arm B4: no double dose of cyclophosphamide in COPADM number 2, and no m1 maintenance). Cranial radiation therapy (RT) is no longer included in the LMB studies. Regimen details are as follows (in *italic* is therapy specific to the Group C regimens).[45]

COP Cyclophosphamide: 300 mg/m², day 1 (D1); Oncovin (vincristine): 1 mg/m², D1; prednisone: 60 mg/m²/day, D1 to D7; plus intrathecal methotrexate (IT MTX), D1; (*triple IT D1, D3, D5 in Group C*).

COPADM Cyclophosphamide: 250 mg/m² × 6 q12 h in COPADM1, double dose in COPADM2; oncovin: 2 mg/m², D1; prednisone: 60 mg/m²/day, D1 to D7; doxorubicin (adriamycin): 60 mg/m², D2; high-dose (HD) MTX : 3 g/m² in 3 h infusion in Group B (*8 g/m² in 4 h infusion in Group C*), D1; plus leucovorin rescue starting at 24 h until serum MTX level $<1 \times 10^{-7}$ M plus IT MTX, D2 and D6 (*triple IT D2, D4, D6 in Group C*).

CYM Cytarabine:100 mg/m² by continuous infusion, D2 to D6; IT cytarabine, D6; HD MTX: 3 g/m² in 3 h infusion, D1; plus leucovorin rescue, IT MTX, D2.

CYVE Cytarabine: 50 mg/m² *by continuous infusion over 12 h, D1 to D5; HD cytarabine 3 g/m² in 3 h, D2 to D5; etoposide (VP16): 200 mg/m², D2 to D5.*

m1 Cyclophosphamide: 1 g/m²; oncovin: 2 mg/m², D1; prednisone: 60 mg/m²/day, D1 to D7; doxorubicin: 60 mg/m², D2; HD MTX: 3 g/m² by 3 h infusion in Group B (*8 g/m² in 4 h infusion in Group C*), D1; plus leucovorin rescue starting at 24 h plus IT MTX (*triple IT in Group C*) D2.

m2 and **m4** *50 mg/m² × 2/day subcutaneously D1 to D5; etoposide (VP16) 150 mg/m² D1 to D3.*

m3 *idem m1 without HD MTX or IT administration.*

All IT administrations are with hydrocortisone.

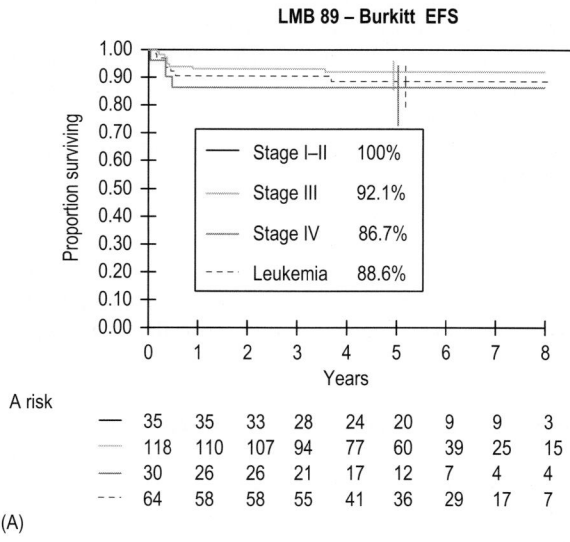

(A)

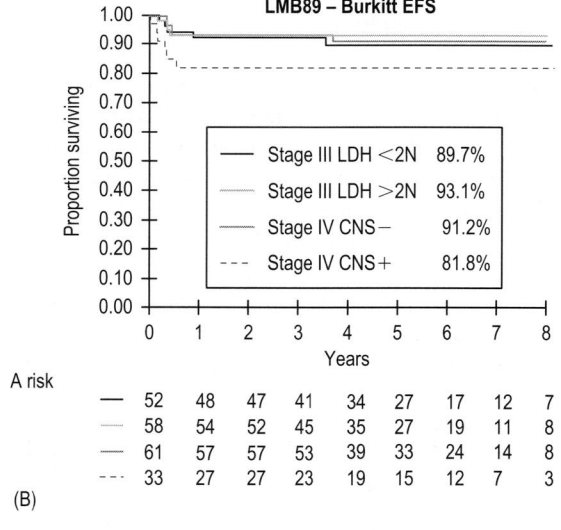

(B)

Figure 68.5 Five-year event-free survival (EFS) of patients with Burkitt non-Hodgkin lymphoma and L3-ALL treated in the LMB 89 study protocol. (A) Event-free survival according to stage. (B) Event-free survival in stage III according to lactate dehydrogenase (LDH) level (less than or more than twice the normal value, N) and in stage IV and ALL according to central nervous system (CNS) involvement (CNS−, no CNS involvement; CNS+, CNS involvement).

Final data confirm the excellent outcome of group A in a larger number of patients.[53] For the patients in Group B, being good responders to COP and in complete remission after the third cycle of chemotherapy, treatment can be decreased to 4 cycles delivering only 3.3 g/m^2 of cyclophosphamide and 120 mg/m^2 of doxorubicin.[54] In Group C, the diminution by one-third of the Ara-C dose, and of the etoposide dose by one-half, led to a decrease of 10 percent in EFS, so the trial was closed after the third interim analysis.[55] An interesting observation in Group B is the prognostic value of the intercycle time between the two induction courses. Patients who started COPADM2 more than 21 days after COPADM1 had a significant 8 percent lower survival rate than those who started within day 21.[56]

In the observational ongoing study, SFOP/SFCE LMB 2001/2003, the possibility of improving the outcome of patients with CNS involvement or those with a poor response to COP is being tested by increasing the duration of the HD MTX infusion from 4 h to 24 h.

BFM studies

The first BFM 81 protocol was based on alternating blocks of treatment consisting of intermediate dose (ID) MTX and cyclophosphamide, with doxorubicin alternating with Ara-C plus VM26 (teniposide).[46] During the three following studies (BFM 83, 86, and 90),[47,48] treatment intensity was progressively increased, with the introduction of corticosteroids, vincristine, HD MTX, ifosfamide, and etoposide, while treatment duration was reduced and CNS irradiation was withdrawn. In the BFM 90 study (1990–1995), treatment was stratified into three risk groups: R1, completely resected; R2, extraabdominal primary tumor only or abdominal tumor and LDH <500 units/L; and R3, abdominal tumor and LDH >500 units/L or bone marrow/CNS/multifocal bone disease.[48] The study consisted of two, four, or six 5-day cycles comprising dexamethasone, methotrexate (0.5 or 5 g/m^2 in the lowest and the highest risk groups, respectively) given by 24 h infusion and intrathecal injections with each cycle, and ifosfamide, cytarabine, and etoposide (course 'A' or 'AA' with MTX 0.5 or 5 g/m^2) alternating with cyclophosphamide and doxorubicin (course 'B' or 'BB'). Patients in partial remission after 2 cycles received additional cycles 'CC' with HD Ara-C/etoposide. The insertion of an Ommaya reservoir was recommended for patients with CNS involvement in order to deliver MTX and Ara-C into the CSF. The 6-year EFS was 89 percent overall for the 413 patients with B cell disease (Burkitt lymphoma and DLBCL): 97 percent, 98 percent, 88 percent, 73 percent, and 74 percent for stages I, II, III, IV, and L3-ALL, respectively. The EFS was 89 percent for the 322 patients with Burkitt NHL/ALL but was not detailed by stage, except for the 56 patients with B-ALL (14 of whom had CNS involvement) whose EFS was 74 percent (standard error [SE] 6 percent). Among the 13 events occurring within the first year, 7 were related to toxicity and 6 to treatment failure.

One of the most remarkable findings is the increase in EFS from 50 percent to 80 percent for patients with stage IV disease and L3-ALL (study 86) and those with abdominal stage 3 and LDH >500 units/L (study 90) when MTX was increased from 0.5 to 5 g/m^2.

In the following BFM 95 study, the duration of the MTX infusion was randomized to 24 h versus 4 h. The dose of MTX was 1 g/m^2 in the low-risk groups (R1, resected; R2, LDH <500 units/L) and 5 g/m^2 in the higher-risk groups (R3, LDH >500–<1000 units/L; R4, LDH >1000 units/L and/or CNS disease).[49] In addition, the 'CC' cycle was given in R3 and R4 (Fig. 68.6). Results showed that the incidence of grade III–IV mucositis was significantly reduced with HD MTX given as a 4 h infusion and that MTX given over 4 h was not inferior to MTX over 24 h for limited stage disease, but not for advanced disease. In addition, the outcome of R3/R4 patients receiving the long-duration infusion was superior to that in BFM 90, probably due to the addition of the extra 'CC' cycle.

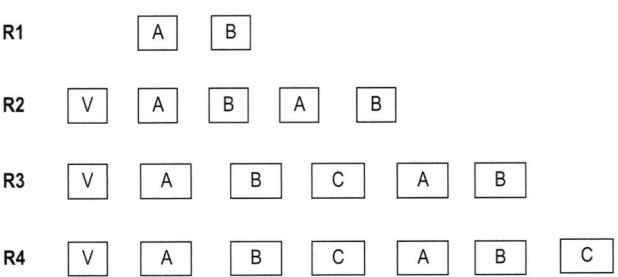

Figure 68.6 Scheme of study protocol BFM 95 according to the different therapeutic groups: R1, R2, R3, and R4, based on tumor resection, lactate dehydrogenase (LDH) level, stage, and central nervous system (CNS) involvement. Regimen details are as follows (in *italic* is therapy specific to AA and BB courses). For more details refer to the publication.[49]

V (prophase) Dexamethasone: 5 mg/m^2, day 1 (D1)–D2, 10 mg/m^2, D3–5; cyclophosphamide: 200 mg/m^2, D1–2; triple intrathecal (TIT), D1.

A(A) Dexamethasone: 10 mg/m^2, D1–5; vincristine: 1.5 mg/m^2, D1; ifosfamide: 800 mg/m^2/day, D1–5; high-dose (HD) methotrexate (MTX): 1 g/m^2 (*AA: 5 g/m^2*), D1; TIT, D2 (*AA: TIT, D2; D5, half dose*); cytarabine 75 mg/m^2 × 2/day, D4–5; etoposide (VP16): 100 mg/m^2/day, D4–5.

B(B) Dexamethasone: 10 mg/m^2, D1–5; vincristine: 1.5 mg/m^2, D1; cyclophosphamide: 200 mg/m^2/day, D1–5; HD MTX: 1 g/m^2 (*BB: 5 g/m^2*), D1; TIT, D2 (*BB: TIT, D2; D5, half dose*); doxorubicin: 25 mg/m^2/day, D4–5.

CC Dexamethasone: 20 mg/m^2, D1–5; vindesine: 3 mg/m^2, D1; cytarabine: 3 g/m^2 × 2/day, D1–2; etoposide (VP16): 100 mg/m^2 × 2/day, D3–4, 100 mg/m^2 D5; TIT, D5.

HD MTX infusion randomized between 4 h or 24 h; leucovorin given at 42 h, 48 h, and 54 h after start of MTX. TIT = MTX plus cytarabine plus prednisone, dose adapted to age and according to the course. If CNS positive, given intraventricularly.

POG protocols

The Pediatric Oncology Group (POG) in the USA performed several studies, generally randomized, for advanced stage Burkitt lymphoma.[57–62] The randomized POG 8615 study for patients with stage III disease showed the total-therapy-B regimen[63] to be more efficient than the previous protocol which did not contain anthracycline and low-dose Ara-C:[58,64] EFS 79 percent (SE 6 percent) versus 64 percent (SE 6 percent).[59] The nonrandomized POG 8617 study for stage IV Burkitt lymphoma and B-ALL showed that replacement of low dose Ara-C by HD Ara-C improved outcome.[60] In the following POG 9317 study, two questions were randomized on the total-therapy-B backbone: (1) administration of Ara-C either as a 48 h infusion or as four HD injections, and (2) the addition of 1 cycle of ifosfamide/etoposide (patients with CNS disease were not randomized and received the ifosfamide/etoposide cycle). Although it was concluded that the use of ifosfamide/etoposide increased EFS of CNS-positive patients (79 percent compared to 64 percent in the previous study),[61] analysis of the second randomization showed that it did not improve EFS of CNS-negative patients (83 ± 4 percent for the 141 patients receiving it vs 79 ± 5 percent for the 136 not receiving it).[62] Results relating to the use of Ara-C administration have not been published.

When the disease was localized (stages I and II), Burkitt lymphomas were included in the same studies as other histologies. It was shown that localized stages of nonlymphoblastic histology could be treated with a 9-week treatment without radiation therapy.[35]

CCG protocols

The CCG developed randomized studies for nonlymphoblastic lymphoma.[65] After the trial showing that COMP was superior to the LSA_2-L_2 regimen,[36] the following trial compared, in patients with stage III disease, the addition of daunorubicin (D-COMP) to the standard COMP regimen.[66] There was no difference in outcome: EFS 57 ± 4.2 percent versus 55 ± 4.3 percent; in patients with Burkitt lymphoma it was 61 ± 3.5 percent. The EFS of patients with stage IV disease who all received D-COMP was 39 ± 5.2 percent. But before concluding that anthracyclines are not efficient in Burkitt lymphoma, it should be noticed that it was daunorubicin and not doxorubicin, and that the regimen was suboptimal.

The other CCG studies for Burkitt lymphoma were pilot studies[67,68] before the CCG participated and provided an important contribution in the international FAB LMB 96 trial.

Single-center original protocols

The National Cancer Institute (NCI) in Bethesda, USA, developed protocols for Burkitt lymphoma in children and adults. The protocol 89-C-41, also called CODOX-M/IVAC, comprises cyclophosphamide, oncovin, doxorubicin, and HD MTX, with IT therapy, alternating with ifosfamide, etoposide, and Ara-C. The results were first published for 41 patients (20 adults and 21 children) with an EFS of 92 percent at 2 years (Fig. 68.7).[69]

The Istituto Nazionale Tumori of Milan in Italy developed a 45-day intensive chemotherapy program with weekly consecutive cycles of vincristine, cyclophosphamide, doxorubicin, and HD MTX, and IT MTX or Ara-C, HD Ara-C, and cisplatin by 4-day infusion, intensified by adding etoposide and escalating MTX doses; 26 of the 29 patients with advanced stage disease survived.[70]

In other European countries

After developing several approaches, especially the intensive MACHO protocol for advanced disease,[71] the UKCCSG adopted the LM89 strategy in parallel to the French study. The EFS rates in study 9002 (Group B) and study 9003 (Group C) were a little lower than in the French study (83 percent and 69 percent, respectively) in part due to the necessity of becoming familiar with a new intensive regimen and to the lack of availability of urate oxidase, which might explain a higher rate of early metabolic complications and toxic deaths, especially in Group C.[72,73] Subsequently, the UKCCSG participated in the FAB LMB96 study.

The AIEOP (the Italian Association of Paediatric Hematology and Oncology) adopted the BFM strategy: the AIEOP LNH92 study was based on the BFM 90 protocol.[74] Similar results were observed, although a little inferior to those of the BFM group, also probably in part due to inexperience with the regimen. The next AIEOP LNH97 study is also based on the BFM strategy, but results are not yet published.

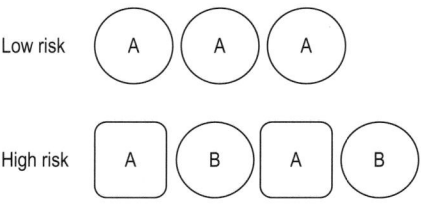

Figure 68.7   Scheme of study protocol 89-C-41.[69] Low-risk patients were defined by a single extraabdominal mass or completely resected abdominal disease with lactate dehydrogenase (LDH) within the normal range. The other patients were defined as high risk. Regimen details are as follows (in *italic* is therapy specific to high-risk patients).
Regimen A = CODOX-M Cyclophosphamide: 800 mg/m^2, day 1 (D1), then 200 mg/m^2/g, D2–5; oncovin (vincristine): 1.5 mg/m^2, D1, D8 (*D15 cycle 3 for high risk*); doxorubicin: 40 mg/m^2, D1; high-dose (HD) methotrexate (MTX): 1200 mg/m^2 over 1 h, then 240 mg/m^2/h during 23 h, D10; plus leucovorin 192 mg/m^2 at 36 h, then 12 mg/m^2 every 6 h until MTX <10^{-8} M; intrathecal (IT) cytarabine: 70 mg (>3 years), D1 (*D3 if high risk*); IT MTX: 12 mg (>3 years), D3 (*D15 if high risk*).
Regimen B = IVAC Ifosfamide: 1.5 g/m^2/day plus mesna, D1–5; etoposide (VP16): 60 mg/m^2/day, D1–5; Ara-C: 2 g/m^2 × 2/d, D1–2; IT MTX, D5.

In other European countries, either the BFM or the LMB strategies have mostly been followed.[75–78]

COUNTRIES WITH ENDEMIC BURKITT LYMPHOMA

Following the description of the disease by Burkitt, data were published about patients in sub-Saharan Africa in the 1960s and 1970s. They showed that facial tumors responded well to chemotherapy and that a certain percentage of children could be cured by single-agent therapy, especially cyclophosphamide.[79–81] In a series of 119 patients treated in Uganda and followed for at least 18 months, survival at 3 years was 73 percent in stage I–II jaw tumors, 50 percent in stage III, and 44 percent in stage IV. All patients were treated with cyclophosphamide, one to six doses at 40 mg/kg.[82] This seemed quite different from what was being observed at the same period of time in the USA and Europe[83]. Another difference was that recurrent disease seemed more curable, including CNS relapse.[82,84,85] Patients with recurrent disease frequently responded to chemotherapy, either cyclophosphamide again or other drugs such as methotrexate, Ara-C, or vincristine, and long-term survival seemed to be possible after one or more relapses.[86] This might be due to the fact that the patients were undertreated and that short-duration, low-dose, or single-agent therapy did not induce resistance, so that the tumor cells remained sensitive to the chemotherapy.

Some studies were done in Uganda and Ghana comparing cyclophosphamide alone to combined treatment adding vinscristine and methotrexate (COM regimen) or Ara-C to cyclophosphamide.[84,87,88] The combined treatment seemed superior, but in one study the toxic deaths rate overcame the improved antitumor effect of the combination and overall survival was not improved.[89] Unfortunately, mainly due to political and economic circumstances, these studies were not continued.

Because of limited facilities and the high cost of chemotherapeutic agents in Africa, therapeutic approaches have not progressed much since that time and few data have been published.

However, recently, endemic Burkitt lymphoma has been the subject of attention and of prospective trials in collaboration with and with help from more economically advanced countries. Three studies are distinguishable: the Malawi projects,[90,91] the FAPOG project, and the International Network for Cancer Treatment and Research (INCTR) program.[92]

It was first demonstrated that the LMB 89 regimen was feasible in South Africa.[93] An overall survival of 79 percent was achieved in 19 patients compared to 25 percent for 24 children who had been treated with COM ± P prior to 1993. Then, with the support of the International Society of Pediatric Oncology (SIOP), trials were initiated in Malawi. In the first study, using a very modified LMB protocol without doxorubicin and with a lower dose of cyclophosphamide, but with HD MTX, EFS was 57 percent at 1 year for all 44 patients, 90 percent for stage I, and

52 percent for stage III.[90] Toxicity contributed to ten deaths and treatment failure to eight. In the following study, Malawi2000, the treatment was less intensive, especially the dose of cyclophosphamide, but the EFS was only 33 percent (50 percent in stage I and II, 25 percent in stage III and IV).[91] A retrospective study of 97 patients treated between 1991 and 1997 with cyclophosphamide alone showed 40 patients to be long-term survivors.[94] A new study was then designed to prospectively investigate cure rate with weekly cyclophosphamide: 40 mg/kg on days 1, 8, and 15 in limited stage disease and a repeated cycle for patients with advanced stage disease. Preliminary results indicated survival of 55 percent, 53 percent, 48 percent, and 10 percent in stages I, II, III, and IV, respectively.[95]

The FAPOG (French-African Pediatric Oncology Group) also conducted a prospective study using a modified LMB 89 protocol. Half of the centers used doxorubicin (MAT regimen) and the other half did not (GFA regimen). The EFS was 61 percent for all 306 patients (39 stage I and II, 209 stage III, and 50 stage IV). Interestingly, EFS increased regularly each year due to increasing experience of the investigators and improvements in supportive care.[96]

OTHER COUNTRIES

In other countries, therapeutic improvements have also been achieved.[97,98] In those with resources and health care infrastructure intermediate between those of Europe and central Africa and where Burkitt lymphoma is frequent, the improved results were achieved as a result of adaptation of therapy to the local environment and to better management of the initial, especially metabolic, problems.[99–106]

General guidelines and controversies

During the last 20 years, major improvements have been achieved in the treatment of B-NHL and B-ALL, with cure rates now ranging from 65 percent to 90 percent, even when the CNS is involved. The biological characteristics of the disease and analysis of the previously reported series allow the following conclusions and questions.

TREATMENT MODALITIES

Burkitt NHL and ALL are characterized by a very high growth fraction (approaching 100 percent in some cases) and a very short doubling time, so treatment must be intensive: short, multiagent chemotherapy given as 3–5-day cycles, with a schedule characterized by fractionation or continuous infusion of drugs. The purpose is to maintain a cytotoxic level of the drug over at least 48 to 72 hours, during which every malignant cell should have a chance to enter the cell cycle. Also, because of the rapid tumor cell doubling time and the potential for tumor regrowth before bone marrow recovery, the cycles have to be administered with the shortest intervals between them. Delays due to toxicity in the UKCCSG 9003 study might explain the inferior results compared to those of the LMB 89 group C protocol.

The necessity of early dose intensity was clearly demonstrated in the FAB LMB 96 study. In Group B, an interval greater than 21 days between the first two induction cycles lowered the EFS rate by 8 percent. In Group C, the diminution of the dose of HD Ara-C and etoposide in the consolidation cycles decreased the EFS by 10 percent.

The time to relapse has not changed with the intensification of treatment. Relapses are still occurring early within the first year of treatment. This is a supplementary argument for not prolonging therapy beyond 6 to 8 months and for not giving maintenance therapy in L3-ALL, in contrast to the other types of ALL. Intensity of treatment must be adapted to the tumor burden and take into account prognostic factors.

LOCALIZED DISEASE

Localized disease needs less intensive treatment. The question is how little. Patients with resected stage I disease and resected abdominal stage II disease have an excellent prognosis and can receive only two cycles of chemotherapy with vincristine, cyclophosphamide, methotrexate, or doxorubicin, with or without prednisone. Central nervous system prophylaxis does not need to be given, at least in localized resected abdominal tumors.[33,45] For other localized, non-resected disease, treatment can also be less intensive and reduced to 3 to 4 cycles, but CNS prophylaxis is needed and EFS should be at least 90 percent.

PROGNOSTIC FACTORS

Since the first therapeutic studies, tumor site, tumor extension, and bone marrow and CNS involvement were recognized as prognostic factors. This was taken into consideration in designing the Ziegler (for endemic Burkitt lymphoma) and the St. Jude's (for nonendemic Burkitt lymphoma) classifications to which treatment intensity was subsequently adapted.

With the development of more effective therapeutic strategies adapted to disease stage, the importance of stage decreased, although it remains discriminating, and new prognostic factors have appeared. Lactate dehydrogenase level has always been found to be prognostic but correlates greatly with stage. However, within the same stage, LDH can distinguish categories with different outcomes.[45,47,65,107] In Germany, where the technique for measuring LDH is well standardized (500 units/L being equivalent to twice the normal value), LDH value was taken into consideration to stratify the risk groups of the BFM 95 study. However, although LDH level was found to be prognostic for the whole population of patients with B cell lymphoma treated

in the LMB 89 study, it was not prognostic for those with Burkitt lymphoma (Fig. 68.5B).

One of the major prognostic factors is treatment and a 'good' treatment adapted to the known prognostic factors should erase the prognostic value of these factors. This is the case for bone marrow involvement in the LMB series. CNS-negative patients with stage IV disease (bone marrow with less than 25 percent of blasts) can be treated successfully in the same risk group as those with stage III disease. CNS-negative L3-ALL (bone marrow with more than 25 percent of blasts) now attain an EFS rate around 90 percent.[45,49]

Central nervous system involvement still defines a group of patients with a worse prognosis[48,49,77,98] and, in the LMB 89 study, it is the only bad prognostic factor in Group C.[45] Is it because it is correlated to more advanced disease,[108–110] or is it a bad prognostic factor *per se*?[111]

Response to chemotherapy is also a prognostic factor in Burkitt lymphoma. Early response and early achievement of remission is important. In the LMB studies, absence of response after 1 week of treatment is a predictor of a poor outcome. Even if EFS increased with early intensification of treatment, response to chemotherapy still remains prognostic.[45]

Until recently, biologic factors were not recognized as prognostic, but recent studies have indicated some clues to their prognostic value. Contrary to the findings for DLBCL, gene expression arrays have not yet contributed to the identification of prognostic factors, but standard cytogenetics analyses have. A review of the cytogenetics studies in the FAB study LMB 96 indicates the prognostic impact of complexity (more than four abnormalities including 8q24 [MYC] rearrangement), of (del)13q and of +7q, but not of +1q.[112]

Patient genotypes may also contribute to the outcome. In the BFM 95 study, it was shown that tumor necrosis factor *TNF –308* (G→A) and the lymphototoxin α *Lt-a +252* (A→G) polymorphisms had a negative impact on the outcome of Burkitt lymphoma. This was not found in the other pediatric lymphomas.[113]

EFFECTIVE DRUGS

Burkitt NHL and ALL are sensitive to many drugs. The single-agent phase II studies were mainly carried out in African Burkitt lymphoma tumors, but nonendemic disease seems to have a similar response to chemotherapeutic agents.[41] In advanced stage NHL and in L3-ALL, high doses of some of these effective drugs seems necessary to obtain better results. From a review of the most successful series, cyclophosphamide, HD MTX, and Ara-C appear to be the three major drugs for treatment.

- **Cyclophosphamide** is one of the oldest drugs with proven efficacy in Burkitt lymphoma and has been used for a long time. It should be given on a fractionated schedule: three to five consecutive days or every 12 hours for six doses, at a minimum dose of 1 g/m^2 per cycle.

- **Methotrexate** has also been shown to be efficacious for systemic disease when given at a low dose as a single agent or in protocols such as COM or COMP, and at high doses as a single agent.[114,115] In advanced stage NHL and in L3-ALL, HD MTX treatment is necessary, as clearly demonstrated by the BFM studies as well as by other successful protocols. But the dose and the duration of infusion is still debated. Dose varies from $1 g/m^2$ to $8 g/m^2$ depending on the protocols. The BFM 95 study is in favor of prolonged (24 h) infusion, at least in advanced stages, although excellent results were also obtained in the LMB protocols with short infusions. However, it can be said that the more advanced the disease, the longer should be the exposure of the tumor cells to the drug. The further point is obtaining a 'therapeutic level' of MTX in the CNS. This depends on infusion duration and the dose. It is generally agreed that the dose should be at least $1 g/m^2$.

- **Ara-C** must be given either in repeated doses, in continuous infusion, or at high doses. In the treatment of B-ALL, the POG 8617 study and the LMB 86 and 89 Group C data demonstrated the superiority of high-dose versus low-dose Ara-C, even in continuous infusion. The necessity of the dose intensity of HD Ara-C was also demonstrated with the failure of the reduced-dose study arm in the FAB LMB 96 Group C study. The introduction of the 'CC' cycle with HD Ara-C in BFM 95 R3 and R4 contributed to the increase in EFS of patients with advanced stages of disease compared to patients in BFM 90.

Among the other drugs effective for treatment are vincristine, doxorubicin, epipodophyllotoxins, corticosteroids, and ifosfamide.

- **Vincristine** was demonstrated to be efficacious for treating Burkitt NHL in an early phase II study, showing a response rate of 81 percent and a CR rate of 48 percent.[81]

- **Doxorubicin** was not tested in a phase II study for Burkitt NHL but it is used in all the successful protocols. Although the randomized CCG study did not show any benefit of adding daunorubicin to the COMP regimen for nonlymphoblastic lymphoma,[66] this drug may have contributed to the superiority of the total-therapy-B regimen over the other regimen in the POG 8615 study.[59]

- The **epipodophyllotoxins** are known to be effective in NHL/ALL in general, but the single-agent phase II studies were done at a time where these lymphomas were not as well characterized as they are now. The epipodophyllotoxins are associated to Ara-C or ifosfamide in most protocols and are generally used for advanced stage disease (LMB 86–89, BFM, and NCI protocols).

- **Corticosteroids** are used in many protocols. However, apart from clinical observations, no clear demonstration has been made of the sensitivity of mature B cell disease to corticosteroids. Should dexamethasone be preferred to prednisone? No study has been done in B cell disease to evaluate this, contrary to B-lineage leukemia.

- **Ifosfamide** has been introduced in some protocols. In phase II studies, it is effective in association with other drugs, especially etoposide (VP16).[116] But there is no demonstration that it has more (or equivalent or non-cross) effectiveness than cyclophosphamide. The recent randomized POG study did not demonstrate a benefit of adding one cycle of ifosfamide/etoposide in advanced stage Burkitt NHL and L3-ALL,[62] although the addition of the IVAC course (ifosfamide and etoposide, but associated with Ara-C) to the CODOX-M course in the NCI protocol improved the outcome in advanced disease stages.[69]

CENTRAL NERVOUS SYSTEM–DIRECTED THERAPY

Intensive CNS-directed therapy with preventive or curative intent is necessary. High-dose MTX and HD Ara-C, in addition to their clear systemic effects, are essential because of their passage into the CNS. Intensive local therapy is also necessary, especially in the case of overt CNS disease. Whether intraventricular therapy, which was used in the BFM 83, 90, and 95 studies and in some patients in the POG 8616 studies, is superior to intrathecal therapy, by delivering higher concentrations of MTX and Ara-C locally to the CNS, has not been demonstrated. Furthermore, the insertion of an Ommaya reservoir might not be easy to achieve at the beginning of treatment, the device could be a source of infection, and use of the device may not be easy to manage at all centers. However, an Ommaya reservoir may remain useful when IT administration is not possible due to technical problems or when repeated injections are no longer accepted by the patient.

There is now general agreement that cranial irradiation is not necessary if the CNS is not involved. It also seems unnecessary in cases of CNS involvement, as its omission in several protocols did not change the outcome.[47,55,117]

Central nervous system involvement is nowadays curable with intensive conventional chemotherapy. However, patients with CNS disease still have the worst outcome. The question remains of how to intensify treatment in the group of patients who have the highest rate of toxic deaths.

SUPPORTIVE CARE

More than in any other NHL or ALL, metabolic complications are a major problem in the initial management of Burkitt NHL/L3-ALL. Due to the short doubling time of the clonal proliferation, the resultant tumor masses are often huge and the tumor lysis syndrome has to be carefully managed. A more generalized use of urate oxidase in more advanced disease should prevent some of the deaths observed in countries where it is not yet available. Urate oxidase may also better preserve renal function, which is essential for the resolution of the tumor lysis syndrome and for the adequate elimination of HD MTX. This then allows for the correct administration of the planned therapy (Table 68.3).

The COP prephase treatment incorporated in the LMB protocols allows management of the tumor lysis syndrome without the other complications of an intensive regimen and its use was not deleterious for patient survival. It is interesting to observe that in the BFM 90 study, the decrease of cyclophosphamide in the cytoreductive phase from $200 \, mg/m^2/day$ during 5 days to 2 days diminished the number of early deaths.[48]

Toxicity-related death is another cause of treatment failure. The most common toxicities encountered in the different chemotherapy regimens are related to myelosuppression and mucositis and need appropriate supportive care. It was disappointing that the randomized studies on granulocyte (macrophage) colony-stimulating factor (G[M]-CSF) did not prove the benefit of using these growth factors.[69,118,119] The necessity for treatment to be intensive to be successful indicates that patients must be treated in specialized centres, that clinicians have to

Table 68.3 Tumor lysis syndrome: definition and recommendations

- Tumor lysis syndrome is characterized by hyperuricemia leading to uratic nephropathy and hyperuremia, hyperphosphatemia, and secondary hypocalcemia and hyperkalemia
- It may exist at presentation and will be provoked by the tumor treatment. Its seriousness is correlated with tumor burden and with renal impairment
- Preventive (or curative) treatment must be initiated before the start of chemotherapy and continued during the lysis phase, generally 3–5 days. It requires:
1. 'Uricolytic' drug:
   - either allopurinol (10 mg/kg/d in three fractions), or
   - urate oxidase. The recommended dose for the recombinant product, rasburicase, is 0.20 mg/kg in one daily IV injection over 30 minutes
2. Hyperhydration in order to achieve a urine output of $125 \, ml/m^2/h$. Alkalization is necessary with allopurinol, not with urate oxidase
   - Renal function (creatininemia, electrolytic balance, diuresis, kidney ultrasound) must be evaluated at diagnosis and corrected if necessary by appropriate measures. Furosemide may be necessary to initiate correct diuresis
   - Metabolic balance, urine flow, weight, and blood pressure must be evaluated 2–4 times per day during the critical period of 2–5 days after initiation of chemotherapy
   - Potassium and bicarbonates should be used very cautiously in the intravenous infusions. Calcium should be introduced only if necessary

acquire experience with a given protocol, and that supportive care must continue to be improved.

HIGH-DOSE THERAPY WITH HEMATOPOIETIC STEM CELL RESCUE

Due to the good results now achievable by use of conventional therapy, there is no indication for high-dose chemotherapy with hematopoietic stem cell graft in first complete remission. Contrary to previous experience showing curability of relapses,[120,121] relapses that now occur following successful chemotherapy protocols have a very poor outcome, and patients are generally resistant to salvage treatments. For these difficult situations, new drugs and new approaches have to be found.

If a second complete remission has been obtained, high-dose chemotherapy with hematopoietic stem cell graft has to be considered. Which regimen should be used? A regimen similar to BACT or BEAM with autologous bone marrow transplantation proved to be effective in relapsed Burkitt lymphoma,[120,121] but it might not be sufficient for relapsed L3-ALL. A regimen with high-dose busulfan associated with high-dose alkylating drugs may be a preferred approach.[122]

In L3-ALL, an allogeneic graft might be preferable, at least in the diseases that primarily involve the bone marrow. However, so far there has been no clear demonstration of a graft-versus-tumor reaction in Burkitt lymphoma. In a series of 71 children and adult patients who received an allogeneic transplant, the presence of a graft-versus-tumor reaction had no impact on survival. The comparison with matched patients who received an autologous transplant showed an equivalent relapse rate and an overall survival superior for the autologous transplantation study arm.[123]

IS THERE A ROLE FOR TUMOR–SPECIFIC TARGETED THERAPY IN BURKITT LYMPHOMA?

The use of monoclonal antibody-targeted therapy for adult B cell lymphomas has produced encouraging results. The anti-CD20 antibody rituximab has been studied in large cohorts of patients. Its efficacy has been proved in follicular lymphoma, in large B cell lymphoma of elderly patients in association with chemotherapy, and, recently, in large B cell lymphoma occurring in younger adults. With the exception of children with post-transplant lymphoproliferative disease, rituximab has not yet been evaluated in pediatric practice;[124,125] neither has it been evaluated in Burkitt lymphoma, regardless of patient age, except in anecdotal observations.[126,127] Demonstrating the effectiveness of rituximab in childhood Burkitt lymphoma might be difficult; due to the currently high survival rates attainable, phase III studies will need a very large number of patients recruited in more than one continent. Phase II studies may also be difficult due to the small number of patients relapsing. The possibility of administering rituximab directly into the CNS is being investigated.[128,129]

CONCLUSION

Burkitt NHL and L3-ALL are now curable diseases in the majority of the cases. Although some questions remain, general guidelines of the initial treatment are now well established and are completely different from those of the other NHL/ALLs. However, treatment is difficult to manage because of the related toxicity. The remaining therapeutic challenges concern relapses for which new approaches have to be found and monoclonal antibody therapy whose place has to be defined in front-line treatment.

SUMMARY

Burkitt NHL is the most frequent NHL in children; L3-ALL is another form of the same disease and they are treated according to the same protocols. Treatment must be a pulse-intensive polychemotherapy regimen of short duration. Treatment intensity is adapted to tumor volume (resection, stage, LDH level, and CNS involvement) and to tumor response during treatment. Cyclophosphamide, HD MTX, and Ara-C are the major drugs used in treatment. Other drugs include vincristine, corticosteroids, epipodophyllotoxins, anthracyclines, and other alkylating agents. Central nervous system-directed therapy is essential. Surgery and radiation therapy no longer have any indication. The LMB, BFM, and other protocols have greatly contributed to an improved cure rate, which now reaches 85–90 percent in the majority of patients. However, treatment is difficult to manage and should be performed in specialized centers. Prevention of the initial metabolic manifestations of the tumor lysis syndrome and supportive care are important parts of the treatment. Relapses are rare and occur early within the first year; they are difficult to cure and are indications for high-dose chemotherapy if a second remission is obtained. The place of monoclonal anti-CD20 antibody (rituximab) in the therapy of Burkitt lymphoma has to be evaluated.

KEY POINTS

- Burkitt lymphoma is the most frequent lymphoma in children. It arises mostly in the abdomen (gut) or in the Waldeyer's ring or facial region and rapidly disseminates regionally, in the bone marrow and/or in the CNS. Its geographic distribution is not homogeneous, with an increased occurrence in subtropical Africa where it is associated with EBV ('endemic' Burkitt lymphoma).
- Burkitt NHL and L3-ALL must be treated with a pulse-intensive polychemotherapy regimen of short duration, the intensity of which is adapted

to tumor volume (resection, stage, LDH level, and CNS involvement) and to tumor response during treatment. Cure rates now reach 80–90 percent.
- Cyclophosphamide, HD MTX, and Ara-C are the major drugs for treatment of Burkitt lymphoma. Central nervous system-directed therapy is essential.
- Prevention of the initial metabolic manifestations of the tumor lysis syndrome (for which use of urate oxidase is important) and supportive care are important parts of the treatment.
- In countries with less medical resource, prospective studies are needed to define the best treatment with the available resources.
- The place of monoclonal anti-CD20 antibody (rituximab) in the therapy of Burkitt lymphoma remains to be evaluated.

REFERENCES

● = Key primary paper
◆ = Major review article

1. National Cancer Institute sponsored study of classifications of non-Hodgkin's lymphomas: summary and description of a working formulation for clinical usage. The Non-Hodgkin's Lymphoma Pathologic Classification Project. *Cancer* 1982; **49**: 2112–35.
2. Harris NL, Jaffe ES, Stein H *et al.* A revised European-American classification of lymphoid neoplasms: a proposal from the International Lymphoma Study Group. *Blood* 1994; **84**: 1361–92.
3. Harris NL, Jaffe ES, Diebold J *et al.* World Health Organization classification of neoplastic diseases of the hematopoietic and lymphoid tissues: report of the Clinical Advisory Committee meeting – Airlie House, Virginia, November 1997. *J Clin Oncol* 1999; **17**: 3835–49.
4. Burkhardt B, Zimmermann M, Oschlies I *et al.* The impact of age and gender on biology, clinical features and treatment outcome of non-Hodgkin lymphoma in childhood and adolescence. *Br J Haematol* 2005; **131**: 39–49.
5. Mwanda OW, Rochford R, Moormann AM *et al.* Burkitt's lymphoma in Kenya: geographical, age, gender and ethnic distribution. *East Afr Med J* 2004; (Suppl 8): S68–77.
6. Percy CL, Smith MA, Linet M *et al.* Lymphomas and reticuloendothelial neoplasms. In: Ries LAG, Smith MA, Gurney JG *et al.* (eds) Cancer incidence and survival among children and adolescents. United States SEER program 1975–1995. Bethesda, MD: National Cancer Institute, 1999: 35–50.
7. IARC Scientific Publications. (ed.) *International incidence of childhood cancer, Vol. II.* Lyon: International Agency for Research Cancer, 1998.

8. Shiramizu B, Barriga F, Neequaye J et al. Patterns of chromosomal breakpoint locations in Burkitt's lymphoma: relevance to geography and Epstein-Barr virus association. *Blood* 1991; **77**: 1516–26.

9. Gutierrez MI, Bhatia K, Barriga F et al. Molecular epidemiology of Burkitt's lymphoma from South America: differences in breakpoint location and Epstein-Barr virus association from tumors in other world regions. *Blood* 1992; **79**: 3261–6.

10. Sandlund JT, Fonseca T, Leimig T et al. Predominance and characteristics of Burkitt lymphoma among children with non-Hodgkin lymphoma in northeastern Brazil. *Leukemia* 1997; **11**: 743–6.

11. Bellan C, Lazzi S, Hummel M et al. Immunoglobulin gene analysis reveals 2 distinct cells of origin for EBV-positive and EBV-negative Burkitt lymphomas. *Blood* 2005; **106**: 1031–6.

12. Granovsky MO, Mueller BU, Nicholson HS et al. Cancer in human immunodeficiency virus-infected children: a case series from the Children's Cancer Group and the National Cancer Institute. *J Clin Oncol* 1998; **16**: 1729–35.

13. Gandemer V, Verkarre V, Quartier P et al. Lymphomas in children infected with HIV-1. *Arch Pediatr* 2000; **7**: 738–44.

14. Strahm B, Rittweiler K, Duffner U et al. Recurrent B-cell non-Hodgkin's lymphoma in two brothers with X-linked lymphoproliferative disease without evidence for Epstein-Barr virus infection. *Br J Haematol* 2000; **108**: 377–82.

15. Mwanda OW. Clinical characteristics of Burkitt's lymphoma seen in Kenyan patients. *East Afr Med J* 2004; (Suppl 8): S78–89.

16. LaQuaglia MP, Stolar CJ, Krailo M et al. The role of surgery in abdominal non-Hodgkin's lymphoma: experience from the childrens cancer study group. *J Pediatr Surg* 1992; **27**: 230–5.

17. Miron I, Frappaz D, Brunat-Mentigny M et al. Initial management of advanced Burkitt lymphoma in children: is there still a place for surgery? *Pediatr Hematol Oncol* 1997; **14**: 555–61.

18. Reiter A, Zimmermann W, Zimmermann M et al. The role of initial laparotomy and second-look surgery in the treatment of abdominal B-cell non-Hodgkin's lymphoma of childhood. A report of the BFM Group. *Eur J Pediatr Surg* 1994; **4**: 74–81.

19. Bergeron C, Patte C, Caillaud JM et al. Clinical, anatomo-pathologic aspects and therapeutic results in 63 malignant ORL non-Hodgkin's lymphomas in children. *Arch Fr Pediatr* 1989; **46**: 583–7.

20. Dayton VD, Arthur DC, Gajl-Peczalska KJ, Brunning R. L3 acute lymphoblastic leukemia. Comparison with small noncleaved cell lymphoma involving the bone marrow. *Am J Clin Pathol* 1994; **101**: 130–9.

21. Dalle JH, Mechinaud F, Michon J et al. Testicular disease in childhood B-cell non-Hodgkin's lymphoma: the French society of pediatric oncology experience. *J Clin Oncol* 2001; **19**: 2397–403.

22. Yang CP, Wan YL, Hung IJ. Successfully treated central nervous system Burkitt's lymphoma with minimal extraneural disease in a child. *J Formos Med Assoc* 1999; **98**: 66–9.

23. Murphy SB. Classification, staging and end results of treatment of childhood non-Hodgkin's lymphomas: dissimilarities from lymphomas in adults. *Semin Oncol* 1980; **7**: 332–9.

24. Leclere J, Ollivier L, Neuenschwander S et al. Ultrasononographic diagnosis of abdominal Burkitt's lymphoma in children (100 cases). *Diagn Interv Radiol* 1991; **3**: 77–83.

25. Stapleton FB, Strother DR, Roy S III et al. Acute renal failure at onset of therapy for advanced stage Burkitt lymphoma and B cell acute lymphoblastic lymphoma. *Pediatrics* 1988; **82**: 863–9.

26. Seidemann K, Meyer U, Jansen P et al. Impaired renal function and tumor lysis syndrome in pediatric patients with non-Hodgkin's lymphoma and B-ALL. Observations from the BFM-trials. *Klin Padiatr* 1998; **210**: 279–84.

•27. Patte C, Sakiroglu C, Ansoborlo S et al. Urate-oxidase in the prevention and treatment of metabolic complications in patients with B-cell lymphoma and leukemia, treated in the societe francaise d'oncologie pediatrique LMB89 protocol. *Ann Oncol* 2002; **13**: 789–95.

•28. Pui CH, Mahmoud HH, Wiley JM et al. Recombinant urate oxidase for the prophylaxis or treatment of hyperuricemia in patients with leukemia or lymphoma. *J Clin Oncol* 2001; **19**: 697–704.

29. Pui CH, Relling MV, Lascombes F et al. Urate oxidase in prevention and treatment of hyperuricemia associated with lymphoid malignancies. *Leukemia* 1997; **11**: 1813–16.

•30. Goldman SC, Holcenberg JS, Finklestein JZ et al. A randomized comparison between rasburicase and allopurinol in children with lymphoma or leukemia at high risk for tumor lysis. *Blood* 2001; **97**: 2998–3003.

31. Wossmann W, Schrappe M, Meyer U et al. Incidence of tumor lysis syndrome in children with advanced stage Burkitt's lymphoma/leukemia before and after introduction of prophylactic use of urate oxidase. *Ann Hematol* 2003; **82**: 160–5.

32. Wakim A, Helardot PG, Sapin E. The surgeon facing malignant non-Hodgkin's lymphoma of the abdomen in children. *Chir Pediatr* 1989; **30**: 197–200.

33. Murphy SB, Hustu HO, Rivera G, Berard CW. End results of treating children with localized non-Hodgkin's lymphomas with a combined modality approach of lessened intensity. *J Clin Oncol* 1983; **1**: 326–30.

34. Murphy SB, Hustu HO. A randomized trial of combined modality therapy of childhood non-Hodgkin's lymphoma. *Cancer* 1980; **45**: 630–7.

•35. Link MP, Donaldson SS, Berard CW et al. Results of treatment of childhood localized non-Hodgkin's lymphoma with combination chemotherapy with or without radiotherapy. *N Engl J Med* 1990; **322**: 1169–74.

36. Anderson JR, Wilson JF, Jenkin DT et al. Childhood non-Hodgkin's lymphoma. The results of a randomized

therapeutic trial comparing a 4-drug regimen (COMP) with a 10-drug regimen (LSA2-L2). *N Engl J Med* 1983; **308**: 559–65.

37.   Patte C, Rodary C, Sarrazin D *et al.* Results of treatment of 178 pediatric non Hodgkin's malignant lymphomas between 1973 and 1978 (author's translation). *Arch Fr Pediatr* 1981; **38**: 321–7.

38.   Muller-Weihrich S, Henze G, Jobke A *et al.* BFM study 1975/81 for treatment of non-Hodgkin lymphoma of high malignancy in children and adolescents. *Klin Padiatr* 1982; **194**: 219–25.

39.   Lemerle M, Gerard-Marchant R, Sancho H, Schweisguth O. Natural history of non-Hodgkin's malignant lymphomata in children. A retrospective study of 190 cases. *Br J Cancer* 1975; **31** (Suppl 2): 324–31.

40.   Murphy SB, Fairclough DL, Hutchison RE, Berard CW. Non-Hodgkin's lymphomas of childhood: an analysis of the histology, staging, and response to treatment of 338 cases at a single institution. *J Clin Oncol* 1989; **7**: 186–93.

41.   Ziegler JL. Treatment results of 54 American patients with Burkitt's lymphoma are similar to the African experience. *N Engl J Med* 1977; **297**: 75–80.

42.   Patte C, Philip T, Rodary C *et al.* Improved survival rate in children with stage III and IV B cell non-Hodgkin's lymphoma and leukemia using multi-agent chemotherapy: results of a study of 114 children from the French pediatric oncology society. *J Clin Oncol* 1986; **4**: 1219–26.

43.   Patte C, Philip T, Rodary C *et al.* High survival rate in advanced-stage B-cell lymphomas and leukemias without CNS involvement with a short intensive polychemotherapy: results from the French pediatric oncology society of a randomized trial of 216 children. *J Clin Oncol* 1991; **9**: 123–32.

44.   Patte C, Leverger G, Perel Y *et al.* Updated results of the LMB86 protocol of the French Society of Pediatric Oncology (SFOP) for B-cell non Hodgkin's lymphoma with CNS involvement and B ALL. *Med Pediatr Oncol* 1990; **18**: 397 (abstract).

●45.   Patte C, Auperin A, Michon J *et al.* The Societe Francaise d'Oncologie Pediatrique LMB89 protocol: highly effective multiagent chemotherapy tailored to the tumor burden and initial response in 561 unselected children with B-cell lymphomas and L3 leukemia. *Blood* 2001; **97**: 3370–9.

46.   Muller-Weihrich S, Beck J, Henze G *et al.* BFM study 1981/83 of the treatment of highly malignant non-Hodgkin's lymphoma in children: results of therapy stratified according to histologic immunological type and clinical stage. *Klin Padiatr* 1984; **196**: 135–42.

47.   Reiter A, Schrappe M, Parwaresch R *et al.* Non-Hodgkin's lymphomas of childhood and adolescence: results of a treatment stratified for biologic subtypes and stage–a report of the Berlin-Frankfurt-Munster Group. *J Clin Oncol* 1995; **13**: 359–72.

●48.   Reiter A, Schrappe M, Tiemann M *et al.* Improved treatment results in childhood B-cell neoplasms with tailored intensification of therapy: a report of the Berlin-Frankfurt-Munster Group Trial NHL-BFM 90. *Blood* 1999; **94**: 3294–306.

●49.   Woessmann W, Seidemann K, Mann G *et al.* The impact of the methotrexate administration schedule and dose in the treatment of children and adolescents with B-cell neoplasms: a report of the BFM Group Study NHL-BFM95. *Blood* 2005; **105**: 948–58.

50.   Reiter A. Therapy of B-cell acute lymphoblastic leukaemia in childhood: the BFM experience. *Baillieres Clin Haematol* 1994; **7**: 321–37.

51.   Philip T, Hartmann O, Biron P *et al.* High-dose therapy and autologous bone marrow transplantation in partial remission after first-line induction therapy for diffuse non-Hodgkin's lymphoma. *J Clin Oncol* 1988; **6**: 1118–24.

52.   Gentet JC, Patte C, Quintana E *et al.* Phase II study of cytarabine and etoposide in children with refractory or relapsed non-Hodgkin's lymphoma: a study of the French society of pediatric oncology. *J Clin Oncol* 1990; **8**: 661–5.

53.   Gerrard M, Cairo MS, Weston C *et al.* Excellent survival following two courses of COPAD chemotherapy in children and adolescents with resected localized B-cell non-Hodgkin's lymphoma: results of the FAB/LMB 96 international study. *Br J Haematol* 2008; **141**: 840–7.

54.   Patte C, Auperin A, Gerrard M *et al.* Results of the randomized international FAB/LMB96 trial for intermediate risk B-cell non-Hodgkin lymphoma in children and adolescents: it is possible to reduce treatment for the early responding patients. *Blood* 2007; **109**: 2773–80.

55.   Cairo MS, Gerrard M, Sposto R *et al.* Results of a randomized international study of high-risk central nervous system B non-Hodgkin lymphoma and B acute lymphoblastic leukemia in children and adolescents. *Blood* 2007; **109**: 2736–43.

56.   Patte C, Gerrard M, Auperin A *et al.* Early treatment intensity has a major prognostic impact in the 'intermediate risk' childhood and adolescent B-cell lymphoma: Results of the international FAB LMB 96 Trial. *Blood* 2003; **102**: 143A (abstract number 491).

57.   Hvizdala EV, Berard C, Callihan T *et al.* Nonlymphoblastic lymphoma in children–histology and stage-related response to therapy: a Pediatric Oncology Group study. *J Clin Oncol* 1991; **9**: 1189–95.

58.   Sullivan MP, Brecher M, Ramirez I *et al.* High-dose cyclophosphamide-high-dose methotrexate with coordinated intrathecal therapy for advanced nonlymphoblastic lymphoma of childhood: results of a pediatric oncology group study. *Am J Pediatr Hematol Oncol* 1991; **13**: 288–95.

59.   Brecher ML, Schwenn MR, Coppes MJ *et al.* Fractionated cylophosphamide and back to back high dose methotrexate and cytosine arabinoside improves outcome in patients with stage III high grade small non-cleaved cell lymphomas (SNCCL): a randomized trial of the pediatric oncology group. *Med Pediatr Oncol* 1997; **29**: 526–33.

60.   Bowman WP, Shuster JJ, Cook B *et al.* Improved survival for children with B-cell acute lymphoblastic leukemia and

stage IV small noncleaved-cell lymphoma: a pediatric oncology group study. *J Clin Oncol* 1996; **14**: 1252–61.

61. Schwenn MR, Mahmoud H, Bowman PW *et al.* Successful treatment of small noncleaved cell lymphoma and B cell ALL with CNS involvement: a Pediatric Oncology Group (POG) study. *J Clin Oncol* 2000; **19** (abstract in Proceedings of the 36th Meeting of the American Society of Clinical Oncology).

62. Schwenn MR, Mahmoud H, Bowman PW *et al.* The addition of VP-Ifosfamide did not improve EFS for CNS negative patients with advanced-stage small noncleaved lymphoma or B-cell ALL: a POG study. *J Clin Oncol* 2001; **21** (abstract in Proceedings of the 37th Meeting of the American Society of Clinical Oncology).

63. Murphy SB, Bowman WP, Abromowitch M *et al.* Results of treatment of advanced-stage Burkitt's lymphoma and B cell (SIg+) acute lymphoblastic leukemia with high-dose fractionated cyclophosphamide and coordinated high-dose methotrexate and cytarabine. *J Clin Oncol* 1986; **4**: 1732–9.

64. Sullivan MP, Ramirez I. Curability of Burkitt's lymphoma with high-dose cyclophosphamide-high-dose methotrexate therapy and intrathecal chemoprophylaxis. *J Clin Oncol* 1985; **3**: 627–36.

65. Cairo MS, Sposto R, Perkins SL *et al.* Burkitt's and Burkitt-like lymphoma in children and adolescents: a review of the children's cancer group experience. *Br J Haematol* 2003; **120**: 660–70.

66. Sposto R, Meadows AT, Chilcote RR *et al.* Comparison of long-term outcome of children and adolescents with disseminated non-lymphoblastic non-Hodgkin lymphoma treated with COMP or daunomycin-COMP: A report from the children's cancer group. *Med Pediatr Oncol* 2001; **37**: 432–41.

67. Finlay JL, Anderson JR, Cecalupo AJ *et al.* Disseminated nonlymphoblastic lymphoma of childhood: a childrens cancer group study, CCG-552. *Med Pediatr Oncol* 1994; **23**: 453–63.

68. Cairo MS, Krailo MD, Morse M *et al.* Long-term follow-up of short intensive multiagent chemotherapy without high-dose methotrexate ('Orange') in children with advanced non-lymphoblastic non-Hodgkin's lymphoma: a children's cancer group report. *Leukemia* 2002; **16**: 594–600.

●69. Magrath I, Adde M, Shad A *et al.* Adults and children with small non-cleaved-cell lymphoma have a similar excellent outcome when treated with the same chemotherapy regimen. *J Clin Oncol* 1996; **14**: 925–34.

70. Spreafico F, Massimino M, Luksch R *et al.* Intensive, very short-term chemotherapy for advanced Burkitt's lymphoma in children. *J Clin Oncol* 2002; **20**: 2783–8.

71. Hann IM, Eden OB, Barnes J, Pinkerton CR. 'MACHO' chemotherapy for stage IV B cell lymphoma and B cell acute lymphoblastic leukaemia of childhood. United Kingdom Children's Cancer Study Group (UKCCSG). *Br J Haematol* 1990; **76**: 359–64.

72. Atra A, Imeson JD, Hobson R *et al.* Improved outcome in children with advanced stage B-cell non-Hodgkin's lymphoma (B-NHL): results of the United Kingdom Children Cancer Study Group (UKCCSG) 9002 protocol. *Br J Cancer* 2000; **82**: 1396–402.

73. Atra A, Gerrard M, Hobson R et al. Improved cure rate in children with B-cell acute lymphoblastic leukaemia (B-ALL) and stage IV B-cell non-Hodgkin's lymphoma (B-NHL)–results of the UKCCSG 9003 protocol. *Br J Cancer* 1998; **77**: 2281–5.

74. Pillon M, Di Tullio MT, Garaventa A *et al.* Long-term results of the first Italian association of pediatric hematology and oncology protocol for the treatment of pediatric B-cell non-Hodgkin lymphoma (AIEOP LNH92). *Cancer* 2004; **101**: 385–94.

75. Vivanco Martinez JL, Lopez PJ, Melero MC *et al.* The treatment results in children diagnosed with non-Hodgkin's lymphomas and acute B-cell lymphoblastic leukemias treated by the BFM protocols. The report of the POGM (Pediatric Oncology Group of Madrid). *An Esp Pediatr* 1998; **49**: 603–8.

76. Kavan P, Kabickova E, Gajdos P *et al.* Treatment of pediatric B-cell non-Hodgkin's lymphomas at the Motol Hospital in Prague, Czech Republic: results based on the NHL BFM 90 protocols. *Pediatr Hematol Oncol* 1999; **16**: 201–12.

77. Marky I, Bjork O, Forestier E *et al.* Intensive chemotherapy without radiotherapy gives more than 85% event-free survival for non-Hodgkin lymphoma without central nervous involvement: a 6-year population-based study from the nordic society of pediatric hematology and oncology. *J Pediatr Hematol Oncol* 2004; **26**: 555–60.

78. Wrobel G, Kazanowska B, Chybicka A *et al.* Progress in the treatment of non-Hodgkin's lymphoma (NHL) in children. The report of polish Pediatric Leukaemia/lymphoma Study Group (PPLLSG)]. *Przegl Lek* 2004; **61** (Suppl 2): 45–8.

79. Burkitt D. Long-term remissions following one and two-dose chemotherapy for African lymphoma. *Cancer* 1967; **20**: 756–9.

80. Oettgen HF, Burkitt D, Burchenal JH. Malignant lymphoma involving the jaw in African children: treatment with Methotrexate. *Cancer* 1963; **16**: 616–23.

81. Burkitt D. African lymphoma. Observations on response to vincristine sulphate therapy. *Cancer* 1966; **19**: 1131–7.

82. Ziegler JL. Chemotherapy of Burkitt's lymphoma. *Cancer* 1972; **30**: 1534–40.

83. Lemerle M, Gerard-Marchant R, Sarrazin D *et al.* Lymphosarcoma and reticulum cell sarcoma in children. A retrospective study of 172 cases. *Cancer* 1973; **32**: 1499–507.

84. Olweny CL, Katongole-Mbidde E, Kaddu-Mukasa A *et al.* Treatment of Burkitt's lymphoma: randomized clinical trial of single-agent versus combination chemotherapy. *Int J Cancer* 1976; **17**: 436–40.

85. Ziegler JL, Bluming AZ. Intrathecal chemotherapy in Burkitt's lymphoma. *Br Med J* 1971; **3**: 508–12.

86. Ziegler JL, Magrath IT, Olweny CL. Cure of Burkitt's lymphoma. Ten-year follow-up of 157 Ugandan patients. *Lancet* 1979; **2**: 936–8.

87. Olweny CL, Katongole-Mbidde E, Otim D *et al*. Long-term experience with Burkitt's lymphoma in Uganda. *Int J Cancer* 1980; **26**: 261–6.

88. Nkrumah FK, Perkins IV. Burkitt's lymphoma: a clinical study of 110 patients. *Cancer* 1976; **37**: 671–6.

89. Nkrumah FK, Perkins IV, Biggar RJ. Combination chemotherapy in abdominal Burkitt's lymphoma. *Cancer* 1977; **40**: 1410–16.

90. Hesseling PB, Broadhead R, Molyneux E *et al*. Malawi pilot study of Burkitt lymphoma treatment. *Med Pediatr Oncol* 2003; **41**: 532–40.

91. Hesseling P, Broadhead R, Mansvelt E *et al*. The 2000 Burkitt lymphoma trial in Malawi. *Pediatr Blood Cancer* 2005; **44**: 245–50.

92. Naresh KN, Advani S, Adde M *et al*. Report of an International Network of Cancer Treatment and Research workshop on non-Hodgkin's lymphoma in developing countries. *Blood Cells Mol Dis* 2004; **33**: 330–7.

93. Hesseling PB. High-dose intense chemotherapy in South African children with B-cell lymphoma: morbidity, supportive measures, and outcome. *Med Pediatr Oncol* 2000; **34**: 143–6.

94. Kazembe P, Hesseling PB, Griffin BE *et al*. Long term survival of children with Burkitt lymphoma in Malawi after cyclophosphamide monotherapy. *Med Pediatr Oncol* 2003; **40**: 23–5.

95. Hesseling P, Molyneux E, McCormick P *et al*. High frequency intravenous cyclophosphamide plus intrathecal methotrexate in endemic Burkitt lymphoma. Analysis of multicentre trial in Malawi, Cameroon and Ghana. *Pediatr Blood Cancer* 2005; **45**: 412–3 (abstract).

96. Harif M, Barsaoui S, Benchekroun S *et al*. Treatment of B-cell lymphoma with LMB modified protocols in Africa. Report of the French-African-Pediatric Oncology group (GFAOP). *Pediatr Blood Cancer* 2008; **50**: 1138–42.

97. Yaniv I, Fischer S, Mor C *et al*. Improved outcome in childhood B-cell lymphoma with the intensified French LMB protocol. *Med Pediatr Oncol* 2000; **35**: 8–12.

98. Horibe K, Akiyama Y, Kobayashi M *et al*. Treatment outcome of AT-B88 regimen for B-cell non-Hodgkin's lymphoma and surface immunoglobulin-positive acute lymphoblastic leukemia in children. *Int J Hematol* 1997; **66**: 89–98.

99. de Andrea ML, de Camargo B, Melaragno R. A new treatment protocol for childhood non-Hodgkin's lymphoma: preliminary evaluation. *J Clin Oncol* 1990; **8**: 666–71.

100. Acquatella G, Insausti CL, Garcia R *et al*. Outcome of children with B cell lymphoma in Venezuela with the LMB-89 protocol. *Pediatr Blood Cancer* 2004; **43**: 580–6.

101. Advani S, Pai S, Adde M *et al*. Preliminary report of an intensified, short duration chemotherapy protocol for the treatment of pediatric non-Hodgkin's lymphoma in India. *Ann Oncol* 1997; **8**: 893–7.

102. Belgaumi AF, Shalaby L, Al Kofide A *et al*. Treatment of a clinically determined lower-risk stage III non-lymphoblastic non-Hodgkin lymphoma with less intensive therapy does not impact negatively on outcome. *Pediatr Blood Cancer* 2006; **46**: 367–71.

103. Chantada GL, Felice MS, Zubizarreta PA *et al*. Results of a BFM-based protocol for the treatment of childhood B-non-Hodgkin's lymphoma and B-acute lymphoblastic leukemia in Argentina. *Med Pediatr Oncol* 1997; **28**: 333–41.

104. Klumb CE, Schramm MT, De Resende LM *et al*. Treatment of children with B-cell non-Hodgkin's lymphoma in developing countries: the experience of a single center in Brazil. *J Pediatr Hematol Oncol* 2004; **26**: 462–8.

105. Madani A, Benhmiddoune L, Zafad S *et al*. Treatment of childhood Burkitt lymphoma according to LMB89 protocol in Casablanca. *Bull Cancer* 2005; **92**: 193–8.

106. Mottl H, Bajciova V, Nemec J *et al*. High survival rate in childhood non-Hodgkin lymphoma without CNS involvement: results of BFM 95 study in Kuwait. *Pediatr Hematol Oncol* 2003; **20**: 103–10.

107. Patte C, Gerrard M, Auperin A *et al*. Prognostic factors in childhood/adolescent B-cell lymphoma: results of the international FAB LMB96 study. *Ann Oncol* 2005; **16** (Suppl 5): v63 (abstract).

108. Gururangan S, Sposto R, Cairo MS *et al*. Outcome of CNS disease at diagnosis in disseminated small noncleaved-cell lymphoma and B-cell leukemia: a children's cancer group study. *J Clin Oncol* 2000; **18**: 2017–25.

109. Haddy TB, Adde MA, Magrath IT. CNS involvement in small noncleaved-cell lymphoma: is CNS disease per se a poor prognostic sign? *J Clin Oncol* 1991; **9**: 1973–82.

110. Sandlund JT, Murphy SB, Santana VM *et al*. CNS involvement in children with newly diagnosed non-Hodgkin's lymphoma. *J Clin Oncol* 2000; **18**: 3018–24.

111. Patte C, Auperin A, Coze C *et al*. CNS involvement in childhood maligancies: is it a bad prognostic factor per se? Experience of the SFOP LMB89 study. *Ann Oncol* 2002; **2** (Suppl 2): 47 (abstract number 147 of the International Conference on Malignant Lymphoma, Lugano).

112. Poirel HA, Cairo MS, Heerema NA *et al*. Specific cytogenetic abnormalities are associated with a significantly inferior outcome in children and adolescents with mature B-cell non-Hodgkin's lymphoma: results of the FAB/LMB 96 international study. *Leukemia* 2008; Nov 20 [Epub ahead of print].

113. Seidemann K, Zimmermann M, Book M *et al*. Tumor necrosis factor and lymphotoxin alfa genetic polymorphisms and outcome in pediatric patients with non-Hodgkin's lymphoma: results from Berlin-Frankfurt-Munster Trial NHL-BFM 95. *J Clin Oncol* 2005; **23**: 8414–21.

114. Djerassi I, Kim JS. Methotrexate and citrovorum factor rescue in the management of childhood lymphosarcoma and reticulum cell sarcoma (non-Hodgkin's lymphomas): prolonged unmaintained remissions. *Cancer* 1976; **38**: 1043–51.

115. Patte C, Bernard A, Hartmann O *et al*. High-dose methotrexate and continuous infusion Ara-C in children's

non-Hodgkin's lymphoma: phase II studies and their use in further protocols. *Pediatr Hematol Oncol* 1986; **3**: 11–18.

116. Magrath I, Adde M, Sandlund J, Jain V. Ifosfamide in the treatment of high-grade recurrent non-Hodgkin's lymphomas. *Hematol Oncol* 1991; **9**: 267–74.

117. Magrath IT, Haddy TB, Adde MA. Treatment of patients with high grade non-Hodgkin's lymphomas and central nervous system involvement: is radiation an essential component of therapy? *Leuk Lymphoma* 1996; **21**: 99–105.

●118. Patte C, Laplanche A, Bertozzi AI *et al.* Granulocyte colony-stimulating factor in induction treatment of children with non-Hodgkin's lymphoma: a randomized study of the French society of pediatric oncology. *J Clin Oncol* 2002; **20**: 441–8.

119. Rubino C, Laplanche A, Patte C, Michon J. Cost-minimization analysis of prophylactic granulocyte colony-stimulating factor after induction chemotherapy in children with non- Hodgkin's lymphoma. *J Natl Cancer Inst* 1998; **90**: 750–5.

120. Hartmann O, Pein F, Beaujean F *et al.* High-dose polychemotherapy with autologous bone marrow transplantation in children with relapsed lymphomas. *J Clin Oncol* 1984; **2**: 979–85.

121. Philip T, Hartmann O, Pinkerton R *et al.* Curability of relapsed childhood B-cell non-Hodgkin's lymphoma after intensive first line therapy: a report from the Societe Francaise d'Oncologie Pediatrique. *Blood* 1993; **81**: 2003–6.

122. Loiseau HA, Hartmann O, Valteau D *et al.* High-dose chemotherapy containing busulfan followed by bone marrow transplantation in 24 children with refractory or relapsed non- Hodgkin's lymphoma. *Bone Marrow Transplant* 1991; **8**: 465–72.

123. Peniket AJ, Ruiz de Elvira MC, Taghipour G *et al.* An EBMT registry matched study of allogeneic stem cell transplants for lymphoma: allogeneic transplantation is associated with a lower relapse rate but a higher procedure-related mortality rate than autologous transplantation. *Bone Marrow Transplant* 2003; **31**: 667–78.

124. Faye A, Quartier P, Reguerre Y *et al.* Chimaeric anti-CD20 monoclonal antibody (rituximab) in post-transplant B-lymphoproliferative disorder following stem cell transplantation in children. *Br J Haematol* 2001; **115**: 112–18.

125. Serinet MO, Jacquemin E, Habes D *et al.* Anti-CD20 monoclonal antibody (Rituximab) treatment for Epstein-Barr virus-associated, B-cell lymphoproliferative disease in pediatric liver transplant recipients. *J Pediatr Gastroenterol Nutr* 2002; **34**: 389–93.

126. Corbacioglu S, Eber S, Gungor T *et al.* Induction of long-term remission of a relapsed childhood B-acute lymphoblastic leukemia with rituximab chimeric anti-CD20 monoclonal antibody and autologous stem cell transplantation. *J Pediatr Hematol Oncol* 2003; **25**: 327–9.

127. de Vries MJ, Veerman AJ, Zwaan CM. Rituximab in three children with relapsed/refractory B-cell acute lymphoblastic leukaemia/Burkitt non-Hodgkin's lymphoma. *Br J Haematol* 2004; **125**: 414–15.

128. Schulz H, Pels H, Schmidt-Wolf I *et al.* Intraventricular treatment of relapsed central nervous system lymphoma with the anti-CD20 antibody rituximab. *Haematologica* 2004; **89**: 753–4.

129. Rubenstein JL, Fridlyand J, Abrey L *et al.* Phase I of intraventricular administration of rituximab in patients with recurrent intra-ocular and CNS lymphoma. *J Clin Oncol* 2007; **25**: 1350–56.

69

Burkitt and Burkitt-like lymphoma/leukemia in adults

GM MEAD

GENERAL DESCRIPTION

Burkitt lymphoma is a well-defined clinicopathological entity.[1–4] This highly aggressive B cell neoplasm occurs in three forms: endemic, an Epstein–Barr virus (EBV)-related lymphoma of African children; acquired immune deficiency syndrome (AIDS)-related, in association with human immunodeficiency virus (HIV); and sporadic, a lymphoma which characteristically occurs in childhood or early adult life, without the above features. This latter group is the subject of this chapter.

Pathologically, this condition has a characteristic (although not specific) appearance on conventional morphology (often described as a 'starry-sky' pattern) and a uniform (although again not specific) immune profile (CD20$^+$ CD3$^-$ CD10$^+$ BCL6$^+$ BCL2$^-$, TP53$^+$, and p21$^-$). All cases are characterized by virtually 100 percent cell division detected using Ki-67 staining. This finding is again uniform but not specific. Finally, and in addition to the above, Burkitt lymphoma (BL) is characterized by chromosomal translocations – typically t(8;14), but occasionally t(2;8) or t(8;22) – associated with *MYC* rearrangement. This precise definition – cytologic, immunophenotypic, high growth fraction, typical translocation, and overexpression of *MYC* – should characterize all new patients.

Whilst this may be a reasonable goal now, it should be noted that cases described as BL in the literature have not necessarily been characterized in this fashion, and almost certainly represent a miscellany of 'high-grade' tumors.

Whilst the diagnosis of BL can be made with considerable precision, this cannot be said of Burkitt-like (non-Burkitt, atypical Burkitt) lymphoma which by contrast is ill defined, probably comprising multiple 'high-grade' lymphomas. At the World Health Organization (WHO) classification meeting[4] it was proposed that this 'high-grade' lymphoma be considered part of diffuse large B cell lymphoma, noting that, in terms of reproducibility, it was the least well defined non-Hodgkin lymphoma subtype, with only 50 percent interpathologist agreement.[5,6] Clinicians, however, won the day, proposing that the definition be used for lymphomas with a very high (greater than 99 percent) proliferative fraction but with greater pleomorphism. The cytogenetics of this condition have not been defined and unsurprisingly the literature relating to it is, at the least, unsatisfactory and in many cases uninterpretable.

A third rare entity should also be mentioned. Occasional cases of follicular lymphoma transform into typical BL as described above.[2] These patients may have had clinical features of follicular lymphoma over a period of months or years, or may present *de novo* with the finding of a dual t(14;18) and t(8;14) translocation indicating the pathogenesis of the lymphoma.

Early clinical series of BL are difficult to analyze. Patient accrual often occurred over many years and the cases were often classified as diffuse, small, noncleaved lymphoma (incorporating both BL and Burkitt-like lymphoma). In addition, many series include patients who are HIV positive, or include both children and adults, rendering separate analysis of adult BL impracticable.

Clinical features

Burkitt lymphoma occurs more commonly in males, who comprise 60–70 percent of cases. The illness can develop at any age, but characteristically occurs in adolescence or early adult life. Burkitt lymphoma is the most rapidly growing cancer described in man, cell division being driven by MYC, which is the underlying explanation of the usual explosive onset.

The most characteristic primary sites are intraabdominal, particularly the ileocecal region, often progressing with time to peritoneal spread with ascites. Spontaneous gastrointestinal perforation through bowel wall lymphoma can occur as a presenting feature. Other common primary sites are the tonsils, small bowel, ovaries, breasts, and bone marrow (with leukemic dissemination). Frequently, it is not possible to define the primary site precisely because of the gross widespread, often intraabdominal, nature of the disease.

Central nervous system (CNS) disease at presentation is found in approximately 10–20 percent of patients. This can manifest as spinal cord compression secondary to extradural spread (which can be the primary site), or presentation with an intracerebral mass, although this is unusual. The most characteristic CNS manifestation is following spread to the meninges. Clinically, these patients usually present with a numb chin or extraocular muscle palsies, although any meningeal site can be affected.

Ureteric, inferior venacaval, or bowel obstruction can occur as a result of rapidly expanding tumor masses. High cell turnover often results in hyperuricemia and occasional patients will present with (or develop after chemotherapy, *vide infra*) uric acid nephropathy and renal failure.

Diagnosis

Burkitt lymphoma should be considered in any young adult with rapid onset (or bulky) lymphoma or leukemia, particularly when involving the extranodal sites described above. Most patients present initially to district or community hospitals, not infrequently to a surgical team as an abdominal emergency. Consequently, pathology samples are frequently obtained out of hours and fixed in formalin.

All lymphomas should be assessed with conventional stains and immunophenotyping but also with Ki-67 (Mib-1),

100 percent staining often providing the initial clue to the underlying diagnosis. Diagnostic delays, however, remain common, often with an incorrect initial diagnosis of diffuse large B cell lymphoma, with a pathological diagnosis of BL first being made at expert pathological review in a regional center.

Increasingly, BL is diagnosed by needle biopsy of an intraabdominal mass, in which event resection is not required. Where complete resection of an ileocecal mass (usually by right hemicolectomy) has been performed, all patients should routinely receive postoperative chemotherapy.

Once a diagnosis of BL has been made, clinical assessment, staging, and treatment should be completed with considerable urgency, aiming to start therapy in advanced cases within 24 to 36 hours of presentation and stabilization.

Staging

All patients should be staged with a full blood count and film, and cytogenetic analysis when leukemic cells are apparent. In addition, an urgent biochemical profile (including uric acid, phosphate, and lactate dehydrogenase [LDH] levels) should be ordered. Whole body computed tomography (CT) scans, including scans of the brain, should be obtained. Magnetic resonance imaging (MRI) scanning is indicated when CNS involvement is suspected. A bone marrow aspirate and trephine should be obtained, with cytogenetics, and within 24 to 48 hours of presentation a diagnostic (and therapeutic, with instillation of methotrexate) lumbar puncture should be obtained, with examination of the cerebrospinal fluid (CSF) for abnormal cytology.

Burkitt lymphoma in childhood has traditionally been staged using the Murphy classification.[7] This preceded modern analysis of prognostic factors in large populations of non-Hodgkin lymphoma (NHL) patients and should now be replaced by a combination of Ann Arbor staging and International Prognostic Index (IPI). Many series also divide patients into two prognostic groups considered to require different levels of treatment intensity or duration in order to achieve cure.

MANAGEMENT

Initial stabilization

Many, although not all, patients with BL present with advanced, rapidly progressive disease. These cases often have a high LDH level and poor performance status. The initial priority is clinical stabilization to allow intensive therapy. Dehydration, renal impairment, infection, and bleeding (particularly in leukemic cases) and viscus obstruction or CNS compression are all common.

All patients require vigorous intravenous (IV) hydration with normal saline, receiving at least 3 L/m^2 for 24 hours, aiming to achieve rehydration and establish a diuresis. In the presence of bulk disease and normokalemia, no potassium should be added to the infusion fluid. Allopurinol should be commenced immediately to reduce the uric acid levels, and antibiotics, blood, and platelets given as necessary. A tunneled IV line is often a useful adjunct to the forthcoming intensive chemotherapy.

Where renal compromise is present it should be established whether this is obstructive (by retroperitoneal or pelvic tumor masses) requiring urgent nephrostomy or stenting, is tumor related because of renal parenchymal replacement by BL, or is metabolic, most commonly secondary to uric acid and/or phosphate nephropathy. Many cases are multifactorial. If uric acid nephropathy is thought to be an important component of renal failure, then rasburicase[8] (recombinant urate oxidase) should be administered as this will reduce uric acid levels within a few hours. If, following rehydration (with relief of urinary tract obstruction where relevant) with correction of uric acid levels, renal failure persists, then hemodialysis should be considered prior to chemotherapy.

Spinal cord compression may be the presenting feature of BL with an initial presentation to neurosurgery. Decompressive surgery and biopsy are then often performed. Where a diagnosis of BL has been confirmed at other sites, then neither surgery nor irradiation are necessary in these cases as disease at this site will be exquisitely sensitive to both steroids and chemotherapy. In such cases, urgent IV hydration and control of uric acid (as above) should precede treatment. Excellent CNS recovery can occur despite advanced loss of power, sensation, or sphincter function.

Patients with oropharyngeal or bowel obstruction should be managed as above. Bowel perforation as a presenting feature should be handled on an individual patient basis, but will require surgical intervention with peritoneal drains.

Younger, fitter patients may request gamete storage. In males, sperm banking on one or two occasions may be reasonable. Caution should be expressed about oocyte or ovarian storage. These techniques take time and there should be concern about occult ovarian infiltration with BL. Clinical experience in fact suggests that modern intensive treatment protocols do not result in permanent male or female infertility and pregnancy can be achieved, if desired, in many cases once treatment has been completed.

Managing early treatment-related complications

Burkitt lymphoma is commonly characterized by widespread bulk disease, often with marrow infiltration and a low performance status. This disease is exquisitely sensitive to steroids and chemotherapy and initial tumor lysis and subsequent profound cytopenias are common with modern chemotherapy regimens.

The best approach to tumor lysis is prevention. Following hydration, allopurinol, and establishment of diuresis, creatinine levels should be checked to confirm normal renal function. Rasburicase (urate oxidase) given intravenously is capable of reducing uric acid levels *in vivo* to virtually undetectable levels within 2 or 3 hours.[8] This drug should be used in all but the least bulky cases, and is generally administered a few hours before chemotherapy. Rasburicase has removed the need for urinary alkalinization prechemotherapy, which was used in the past to reduce uric acid levels.

Following chemotherapy administration, tumor lysis will occur within a few hours. Cell and DNA degradation result in high levels of uric acid and phosphate, either of which can deposit in the renal tubules causing renal failure and resulting, in inadequately managed patients, in hyperkalemia and early death. Rasburicase can prevent uric acid but not phosphate nephropathy. Patients with bulky BL should be intensively monitored with frequent checks on hydration and the adequacy of ongoing diuresis. In addition, potassium and creatinine levels should be checked twice daily. Dialysis may be necessary in rare cases developing oliguria or anuria despite this approach. Tetany has rarely been reported as a result of hypocalcemia in patients with hyperphosphatemia.

Modern chemotherapy regimens will almost always result in short-term grade IV neutropenia and granulocyte colony-stimulating factor (G-CSF) should be considered a standard treatment approach. Anemia and grade IV thrombocytopenia also commonly occur and require appropriate support.

Bowel perforation has been described, either at the site of occult gastrointestinal involvement or at the primary site, commonly the ileocecal area. This usually occurs within one to two weeks, often at a time of peripheral blood count nadir. Emergency surgery will then be necessary, accompanied by appropriate hematologic support.

CHEMOTHERAPY

Before discussing chemotherapy regimens it is important to examine the underlying principles of treatment in BL, which in many cases are derived from management of this disease in childhood (see Chapter 68).

Burkitt lymphoma disseminates rapidly, and in modern practice there is no role for surgery alone and little or no role for radiation therapy. Chemotherapy regimens can generally be delivered at full dose, with subsequent treatment cycles delivered as soon as possible (and certainly, more quickly than a traditional 21-day schedule). Methotrexate is commonly used at intermediate/high dose enabling both midcycle dose intensity (this drug is often given at the time of the chemotherapy-induced blood count nadir) and effective treatment of the CNS. Alternating drug combinations are designed to prevent early drug resistance. Central nervous system prophylaxis is routine, comprising at the very least multiple intrathecal or intraventricular injections of methotrexate and/or cytarabine supplemented by use of high-dose intravenous methotrexate and sometimes cytarabine.

Treatment need not be prolonged and can generally be completed within 2–3 months. There is no evidence of benefit of post-treatment maintenance regimens.

Chemotherapy regimens

As adult BL is rare, no randomized trials have been performed. No chemotherapy regimen can currently be regarded as standard, although national groups have often standardized their approach. It is anticipated that the treatment regimens described in the last five to ten years will have comparable cure rates.

As described previously, caution is necessary in interpreting the historical trial database as few, if any, studies have defined BL using modern diagnostic criteria. Many studies are confined to populations of children and young adults. Clinical experience suggests that older patients with comorbid conditions are frequently insufficiently fit to receive modern intensive treatments, as a result of which they are not included in published studies, and they often have an exceptionally poor prognosis.

Wherever reasonable, patients should be treated from diagnosis with full-dose chemotherapy regimens. Not infrequently, however, either because of misdiagnosis (usually diffuse large B cell lymphoma) or because of threatening presentation with gross advanced disease with renal failure, initial non-BL regimens (usually CHOP [cyclophosphamide, doxorubicin, vincristine, and prednisone] or CVP [cyclophosphamide, vincristine, and prednisone]) may have been given, often at reduced dose. Indeed, this approach is mandated by some trial groups as an initial treatment approach. In these cases, CNS prophylaxis should commence early and commencement of a standard BL-directed regimen should start as soon as possible – usually within 10–20 days of initial treatment.

In the following two sections, the early evolution of the modern chemotherapy approach to BL is described, followed by a detailed appraisal of currently recommended treatments.

Early chemotherapy trials (1984–1990)

In 1984, Magrath et al.[9] described the initial stages in the evolution of the now widely used CODOX-M chemotherapy regimen. This study comprised 65 patients, 34 of whom were adults aged 17–35 years, the remainder were children. Histology was mixed, comprising BL (37 patients) but also 'undifferentiated lymphoma' and lymphoblastic lymphoma. Chemotherapy comprised cyclophosphamide $1.2\,g/m^2$ given with steroids and day 10 methotrexate $(2.7\,g/m^2)$ in cycle 1, with additional doxorubicin $(40\,mg/m^2)$

and vincristine for the remaining cycles. Treatment was restarted on neutrophil recovery for the first 6 cycles and was then given every 28 days. A total of 15 cycles of treatment were given unless the disease was localized or completely resected, when 6 cycles were given. Central nervous system prophylaxis was not initially used but was introduced when isolated CNS relapse proved common.

Adult BL patients were not separately described; however, a number of interesting observations were made. Age had no effect on outcome, which was predominantly related to LDH level, bone marrow involvement, and stage. Overall 3-year survival was 60 percent but patients with bone marrow disease had a survival of only 14 percent.

In 1986 Bernstein,[10] representing Stanford University, described treatment of 18 adults (16 under 45 years of age) with small noncleaved lymphoma (BL and non-Burkitt type). Chemotherapy was similar to that given by Magrath (above) except that this was supplemented with twice-daily irradiation to the abdomen in patients with abdominal masses measuring >10 cm. In addition, all treatment cycles contained doxorubicin and vincristine, with methotrexate at a dose of $3\,g/m^2$.

Overall 2-year survival was 67 percent (60 percent for eight patients with BL). Prognosis was again related to LDH levels, disease bulk, and stage. No clear role for irradiation was seen.

Lessons learnt from pediatric oncology (1990–1995)

This era saw a number of new publications describing successful adaptation of pediatric oncology protocols to an adult population. In many studies it was increasingly appreciated that treatment need not be prolonged to achieve cure.

In a study published in 1990, Lopez et al.[11] from the MD Anderson Cancer Center described treatment of 44 adults (median age 32 years) with small noncleaved cell lymphoma (16 considered BL, 12 HIV positive) with two complex cycling chemotherapy protocols (81-01 and 84-30). Methotrexate was given at a modest dose $(1\,g/m^2)$ in both protocols and no intrathecal therapy was included.

It is difficult to break down subgroups in this paper. However, 5-year survival for HIV-negative patients was 57 percent, with advanced tumor stage and poor performance status being adverse prognostic features.

Strauss et al.[12] reported the Memorial Hospital experience in 1991. Like many adult series, this paper includes data on 29 younger patients (nine HIV positive, age 15–43, median 27 years) treated over a 14-year period with a series of complex, acute leukemia-derived regimens, incorporating high-dose therapy in four cases. The results were consistent with the others described here, with 59 percent of HIV-negative patients apparently cured on prolonged follow-up.

McMaster et al., publishing in 1991[13] with an update in 1993,[14] described a series of 20 patients treated at Vanderbilt with a high-intensity, brief-duration chemotherapy regimen. All patients are described as having small noncleaved lymphoma (with only one case recorded as typical BL); three patients were also HIV positive. Clinically it was clear that this population had highly aggressive lymphoma. Only two chemotherapy cycles were given – cycle 1 incorporated high-dose ($3 \, g/m^2$) cyclophosphamide and etoposide ($1.2 \, g/m^2$), with methotrexate at $200 \, mg/m^2$, and cycle 2 was given with reduced doses of cyclophosphamide and etoposide but with high-dose doxorubicin. Severe myelosuppression was reported with two toxic deaths. A failure-free survival rate of 60 percent was achieved on long-term follow-up.

During this period, a French Collaborative Group[15] described their experience with the pediatric LMB protocols used in a nonprospective study in adults. Sixty-five patients with a median age of 26 years (and maximum age of 65 years) were included in this study. The pathology was described as small noncleaved cell lymphoma and leukemia (L3), but karyotypes obtained in ten patients were all typical of BL. The LMB protocols comprised an initial induction with intravenous cyclophosphamide ($300 \, mg/m^2$), vincristine, and prednisone, followed on day 8 by COPADEM comprising high-dose cyclophosphamide, with vincristine, doxorubicin, methotrexate (variable dose but at least $3 \, g/m^2$), and prednisone. A consolidation and maintenance phase followed, incorporating variable doses of high-dose cytarabine and methotrexate, with cranial irradiation for those with CNS disease. In addition, 13 patients received high-dose chemotherapy with autologous bone marrow rescue.

Whilst this study is complex, and the LMB protocols used were relatively diverse, the results are noteworthy, with a 3-year survival of 74 percent, including a survival of 57 percent of patients presenting with marrow and CNS disease. No role for high-dose therapy was established.

In a useful second French series, Fenaux et al.[16] published their experience of leukemic BL in 18 patients (age 16–66, median 26 years) treated over a 7-year period. Seventeen of the patients had a t(8;14) translocation and a further 15 had CNS disease at presentation, predominantly manifest by mental neuropathy. A variety of complex intravenous/intrathecal protocols supplemented in four cases by high-dose chemotherapy were used. Remarkably, six early deaths occurred including two prior to treatment and two from cerebral hemorrhage of uncertain cause. Six further cases relapsed in the CNS alone or together with bone marrow. No relapsing patients could be salvaged, a theme of this disease. Six patients were in ongoing complete remission at the time of this report.

Approaching consensus (1996–2005)

In the last 10 years, a number of more satisfactory publications have appeared – characterized by larger patient numbers, more uniform treatment protocols, and better

(although far from perfect) definitions of BL as an entity. Older patients remain inadequately represented in most of these series.

CODOX-M/IVAC

Ian Magrath at the National Cancer Institute (NCI) devised this alternating chemotherapy regimen (designated 89-C-41), which was initially evaluated in young adults and children.[17] Subsequent clinical series have simplified and modified the protocol, which is in widespread use today.

CODOX-M comprises a high-dose cyclophosphamide, vincristine, and doxorubicin regimen given over 5 days and intensified on day 10 by administration of methotrexate at a dose of $6.7 \, g/m^2$. Three intrathecal injections are given with each cycle. This regimen results in uniform and severe myelosuppression. Intensive chemotherapy exposure is achieved by restarting chemotherapy, where possible, on the day that the unsupported granulocyte count reaches $1 \times 10^9/L$ with an unsupported platelet count of $50 \times 10^9/L$.

Patients were designated 'low risk' in the presence of a normal LDH level, completely resected abdominal disease, or BL confined to a single extraabdominal site – all other patients were regarded as 'high risk.' Low-risk patients received 3 cycles of CODOX-M as described, and high-risk patients received 2 cycles each of alternative CODOX-M and IVAC – the latter comprising high-dose cytarabine, ifosfamide, and etoposide, again supplemented by a single intrathecal injection of methotrexate.

In the original description of this regimen, 20 adult patients aged 18–59 years (median 26 years) with diffuse small noncleaved cell lymphoma (not otherwise specified) were treated; 15 were regarded 'high risk' and 5 'low risk.' All 20 patients achieved and remained in complete remission, with a minimal follow-up time of 16 months. Essentially all patients suffered grade IV neutrophil toxicity for a median of 12 days, and 46 percent and 89 percent of patients suffered grade IV thrombocytopenia with, respectively, CODOX-M and IVAC. Twenty percent of treatment cycles were complicated by septicemia, and grade III and IV mucositis occurred in 58 percent of the CODOX-M cycles.

High-risk patients in this study were randomized to either receive or not receive granulocyte macrophage colony-stimulating factor (GM-CSF) prophylaxis; G-CSF was not available at this time. GM-CSF appeared to result in no beneficial reduction in neutropenia, but was strongly associated with severe and painful peripheral neuropathy[18] not subsequently described in reports of this regimen.

The next step in the evaluation of CODOX-M/IVAC was its assessment in a multigroup setting. This was achieved by the United Kingdom Lymphoma Group in a study designated LY06.[19] Different criteria were used to allocate patients to 'low-risk'/'high-risk' groups, incorporating data from the International Prognostic Index. The

protocol was slightly modified by omission of day 15 vincristine (to avoid neurotoxicity) and hematologic support
with G-CSF was routinely recommended between treatment cycles. More caution was used when restarting cycles,
with a platelet count of at least 75×10^9/L being required.

All patients' slides were reviewed centrally. Cytogenetic
analysis was not routinely available and BL was diagnosed
on the basis of 100 percent Ki-67 staining in the presence
of characteristic morphology. Despite these imprecise criteria by modern standards, 20 percent of cases entered in
the study were regarded as examples of diffuse large B cell
lymphoma on central review, and were removed from the
analyses. Overall, 52 of 72 patients entered were regarded
as eligible for the study, comprising 11 'low-risk' and 41
'high-risk' patients. Patients in this study were older (aged
15–60, median 35 years). Overall, a 2-year event-free survival (EFS) of 65 percent with survival of 73 percent was
achieved. Results were better in the 'low-risk' than the 'high-
risk' group: 2-year EFS was 83 percent versus 60 percent
and survival was 82 percent versus 60 percent, respectively.
Toxicity was severe and comparable to that described by
Magrath et al.[17] although neuropathy was not a particular
problem. Three toxic deaths occurred. Relapse rates were
strikingly low (0 percent in 'low-risk' vs 10 percent in
'high-risk' patients) with only one patient being salvaged
following disease progression. Limited numbers precluded
accurate identification of prognostic factors. However, a
trend (regarded by the investigators as hypothesis generating) was noted for worsening EFS amongst older patients,
those with poorer IPI scores, and those with bone marrow
involvement.

In a subsequent study (LY10)[20], this collaborative group
continued to treat BL with CODOX-M/IVAC but with a
number of protocol modifications. It was clear from LY06
that the major source of morbidity was that associated with
high-dose methotrexate, used in this study at a dose of
6.7 g/m^2. In the absence of data supporting such a large dose,
LY10 reduced the dose of methotrexate to 3 g/m^2. In addition, and in an attempt to increase accrual, a modified protocol was introduced for patients aged greater than 65 years,
utilizing lower doses of methotrexate and cytarabine.

LY10 was designed as a clinicopathological study. The
entry criterion was not a diagnosis of BL, but rather a diagnosis of a B cell lymphoma with 100 percent Ki-67 staining.
Patients with this pathologic abnormality were treated
with dose-modified CODOX-M/IVAC if fit and consent-
ing or, if not, entered into a 'pathology only' study. All
blocks were reviewed centrally when fluorescence in situ
hybridization (FISH) studies were performed

One hundred twenty-eight patients were eligible for
the study, of whom 58 were considered to have BL based
on the finding of a germinal center phenotype, absent
expression of BCL2, and the presence of MYC as the sole
cytogenetic abnormality. The remaining 70 patients were
considered to have diffuse large B cell lymphoma (DLBCL),
five of whom had not only a MYC rearrangement but
also an atypical immunophenotypic profile and coexisting

t(14;18) translocation indicating underlying follicular
lymphoma.

One hundred ten patients (BL $n = 53$ and DLBCL
$n = 57$) were treated with dose-modified CODOX-M/
IVAC in the trial. The two groups were clinically distinct –
BL patients were younger (median age 37 vs 56 years),
with a higher incidence of bone marrow involvement
(44 percent vs 24 percent) and more frequent B symptoms
(63 percent vs 43 percent). The 2-year progression-free
survival favored BL (64 percent vs 55 percent); overall
survival was 85 percent for low-risk patients treated with
3 cycles of dose-modified CODOX-M and 49 percent
for high-risk patients who were treated with 4 cycles
of dose-modified CODOX-M/IVAC. Results in the older
(>65 years) patients and those with dual translocations
were very poor. Comparison with LY06 suggested reduced
toxicity but comparable survival.

It was concluded that all future studies should use FISH
in conjunction with immunostains to accurately diagnose
BL. There was no convincing evidence that dose-modified
CODOX-M/IVAC was of additional benefit to CHOP-R
in the DLBCL patients and it was recommended that this
highly intensive and toxic therapy be confined to BL patients.

In a small, broadly comparable clinical study, Lacasce
et al.[21] treated 14 patients aged 18–65 (median 47) years
with BL or Burkitt-like lymphoma (not otherwise specified). Interestingly, 10 of 12 evaluable patients had Ki-67
staining of greater than 90 percent. Two other patients
with lower scores had a t(8;14) translocation but also additional translocations involving chromosome 14 implying
an underlying follicular subtype. Minor changes in drug
scheduling and doses were made but notably, as in LY10,
the methotrexate dose was reduced to 3 g/m^2 and doxorubicin dose increased to 50 mg/m^2. Overall, progression-free
survival and survival were comparable with those in LY06,
(64 percent and 71 percent, respectively) but treatment
toxicity, particularly mucositis, was markedly reduced.

CALGB-9251

CALGB-9251,[22] which commenced in 1992, is now a
mature study conducted as two cohorts comprising a total
of 92 patients with a median age of 47 years (range 17–78).
All patients received identical systemic therapy, comprising initial cyclophosphamide (200 mg/m^2 IV daily, days
1–5) and prednisone, followed on day 8 by alternating
intravenous cycles of chemotherapy comprising (i) ifosfamide, methotrexate (2 g/m^2), vincristine, cytarabine,
and etoposide and (ii) cyclophosphamide, methotrexate
(1.5 g/m^2), vincristine, and doxorubicin for a total of 6 cycles.
Dexamethasone was given orally with both treatments,
which were given at 21-day intervals.

The two cohorts differ in the approach to CNS prophylaxis. The earlier cohort (cohort 1) received cranial irradiation to a dose of 24 Gy accompanied by intrathecal
methotrexate, cytarabine, and hydrocortisone on days 1
and 5 of intravenous treatment in cycles 2–7. Undue CNS

toxicity was observed, therefore patients in cohort 2 received only a single intrathecal injection of these three drugs per treatment cycle (in cycles 2–7) with cranial irradiation reserved for patients presenting with bone marrow disease.

Pathologic immunophenotypic data were said to be 'often available,' whilst Ki-67 staining was not. One hundred thirty-five patients were entered into this study, of whom 92 proved pathologically eligible using the limited criteria. Twenty-six patients had a t(8;14) translocation or other typical BL phenotype but many karyotypes were normal or failed to confirm BL.

Treatment toxicity, as with CODOX-M/IVAC, was severe, with universal grade 3 and 4 myelosuppression and seven infection-related deaths. Metabolic, renal, gastrointestinal, and mucosal toxicity were also common. A particularly striking feature of this study was the difference in neurotoxicity between the two cohorts. In cohort 1, CNS toxicity was frequent and severe and included sensory and motor neuropathy, cortical and cerebellar dysfunction, and transverse myelitis in a total of 60 percent of patients, compared with 23 percent of patients in cohort 2.

Considering the adverse nature of this group (63 percent of patients had bone marrow involvement) and the relatively advanced age, the treatment results were good and consistent, with no difference between leukemic and non-leukemic patients, and no significant differences either in progression-free survival, survival, or CNS relapse between cohorts 1 and 2. With a median follow-up of 6.8 years, EFS in cohort 1 was 52 percent and survival 54 percent. With a median follow-up of 4.1 years, EFS was 45 percent in cohort 2 with survival of 50 percent. Comparable results were obtained in the 26 patients with a t(8;14) or other typical Burkitt-like lymphoma (BL-L) karyotype and in those without an abnormal karyotype.

The CALGB group concluded from this study that a reduced CNS prophylaxis regimen was appropriate and in a new, ongoing study have omitted cranial irradiation for all patients except those with positive CSF cytology.

HYPER–CVAD

This regimen was described by the MD Anderson Cancer Center[23] and comprises hyperfractionated cyclophosphamide (300 mg/m^2 IV, 12-hourly for 6 doses), vincristine, doxorubicin, and dexamethasone, alternating with methotrexate (1 g/m^2 intravenously over 24 hours) on day 1, with cytarabine 3 g/m^2 IV, 12-hourly × 4, on days 2 and 3. Cycle 2 and subsequent courses were initiated when the total white cell count was >3 × 10^9/L, with a platelet count of >60 × 10^9/L. Each treatment cycle was administered within a 14–21-day window and was accompanied by an intrathecal injection of methotrexate and cytarabine given on days 2 and 7 of each course. No prophylactic cranial irradiation was used. Twenty-six patients aged 17–79 years (median 58 years) were included in this study. All had leukemic BL. However, only ten had a characteristic

karyotype. Four additional cases had a t(14;18) translocation and seven had terminal deoxynucleotidyl transferase (TdT) positivity, not usually considered typical of BL. Eleven patients had disease spread to the CNS. This was clearly a very adverse group not, as previously described, confined to BL. This was a toxic regimen. Five patients (19 percent) died during induction, four of fungal infection. Four of 12 patients were more than 60 years of age. The estimated 3-year survival rate was 49 percent (77 percent in patients younger than 60 years). Survival appeared best in 'typical' BL and was much worse in patients more than 60 years of age (3-year survival 77 percent vs 17 percent, respectively). Remarkably, nine patients relapsed from complete remission (CR). No second CR was obtained and all these patients died, with a median duration of survival of 1 month. No isolated CNS relapses were seen.

GERMAN STUDIES

In 1996, Hoelzer et al.[24] reported the German experience of L3 leukemia in three sequential protocols running from October 1978 until January 1993. Practically speaking, the third study (B-NHL 86) provided the most useful information, accruing 35 patients between 1989 and 1993. L3 morphology and/or surface immunoglobulin (Ig) with at least 25 percent marrow infiltration were the entry criteria, with patients aged between 15 and 65 years (median 36 years). In 19 cases, cytogenetic analysis was performed which demonstrated a characteristic BL translocation in eight cases, again confirming the heterogeneity of this patient population diagnosed using conventional histologic criteria. Treatment lasted for 19 weeks and comprised initial induction cyclophosphamide (200 mg/m^2 IV daily × 5) and prednisone, followed by an alternating schedule of intravenous vincristine, methotrexate (1.5 g/m^2), ifosfamide, teniposide, and cytarabine, alternating with vincristine, methotrexate (1.5 g/m^2), cyclophosphamide, and doxorubicin. All patients received dexamethasone and triple intrathecal therapy. Supplementary CNS irradiation (whole brain treated to 24 Gy, spinal irradiation in patients with CNS disease) was routinely used. Forty patients were enrolled in this study and 35 were considered evaluable. A CR rate of 74 percent was achieved with 51 percent 4-year survival. All six relapses occurred within 7 months, and five were confined to the bone marrow. Age appeared to have no effect on outcome.

Myelotoxicity and mucositis were the common toxic side effects; perhaps remarkably, no mention was made of CNS toxicity. Central nervous system irradiation did, however, contribute to mucositis and has been omitted from the following protocol (B-ALL 05/93) and substituted by an increase in the methotrexate dose to 3 g/m^2.

NORWEGIAN STUDIES

In a recent paper, Smeland et al.[25] describe the Norwegian Radium Hospital experience of BL and BL-L over a 20-year period. Unfortunately, this study was marred by inadequate histopathologic details relating to the diagnostic criteria used for patient entry. Patient numbers in each of three groups were small (13, 17, and 19) but the lessons learned were worthwhile. The median age of patients in these studies was 30–36 years, with a maximum of 69 years. Median follow-up was a minimum of 4 years.

The initial cohort of 13 patients was treated with 8 cycles of CHOP, supplemented with high-dose intravenous ($2\,g/m^2$) and intrathecal methotrexate in the first 6 cycles. Intrathecal methotrexate was also given with each cycle. The next 17 patients received additional treatment consolidation with routine high-dose therapy with cyclophosphamide and total body irradiation (TBI) supported by autologous bone marrow transplantation. Five-year survival in the first of these two cohorts was only 23 percent, with modest remission rates and multiple relapses in the CNS and periphery. High-dose therapy appeared to improve these results with 71 percent 5-year survival attained. No relapses from CR were seen.

A final cohort of 19 patients was treated with the Berlin-Frankfurt-Münster (BFM) protocol, BFM 90. Patients achieving only a partial remission (PR) were treated, in addition, with BEAM (carmustine, etoposide, cytarabine, and melphalan) and autograft (two patients). Utilizing this approach, a 5-year survival of 65 percent was achieved. No patients relapsed from CR or in the CNS.

The authors concluded that both CHOP/methotrexate with supplemental high-dose therapy or the BFM protocol are effective approaches. The BFM approach was, however, favored as it was considered less likely to cause long-term bone marrow, cardiac, or gonadal damage.

Brief chemotherapy

In a recently reported study from Italy, Di Nicola et al.[26] treated 22 adult BL patients aged 18–76 years (median 36 years) with a brief intensive regimen, achieving good results. This is a well-defined group as all cases had 100 percent Ki-67 staining, and the lymphomas were also well characterized immunophenotypically. Unfortunately, no cytogenetic studies were reported.

The treatment regimen comprised weekly treatment of sequential cyclophosphamide ($1\,g/m^2$ IV in split dose), methotrexate (150 mg/kg), etoposide ($250\,mg/m^2$ IV), methotrexate (250 mg/kg), doxorubicin, and vincristine, then consolidated on day 42 with cytarabine $1\,g/m^2$ by intravenous infusion, daily for 4 days, given with cisplatin $20\,mg/m^2$, also given daily for 4 days by infusion. Treatment was supported with G-CSF and supplemented by alternating intrathecal methotrexate and cytarabine for six doses. Patients achieving less than CR (four patients) were treated with a complex cycling high-dose chemotherapy regimen with stem cell support.

The median age of these patients was 36 years (18–76 years), with seven patients ⩾50 years old. Half the patients

were stage IV using Ann Arbor criteria. Seventeen patients (77 percent) achieved CR, although one of these died from early treatment-related toxicity. One patient died of primary refractory disease, as did the single patient relapsing from CR. All four patients receiving high-dose therapy because of poor response/residual mass achieved complete remission in which they remained. With a median follow-up time of 29 months (6–58) the survival rate was 68 percent and progression-free survival 77 percent. This treatment program lasted only 12 weeks and was given on a largely outpatient basis. Whether the switch to a high-dose salvage regimen in this study was necessary remains to be determined. However, this approach certainly warrants examination in a larger patient population.

High-dose chemotherapy

Many of the publications described above include small numbers of patients treated with high-dose chemotherapy (HDT) with autologous stem cell rescue, either as a part of the initial planned therapy or after achieving partial remission. It is not possible from these publications to determine the effectiveness or otherwise of this approach, particularly as the treatment was often given without histologic evidence of residual disease (which in this author's experience can often be benign).

Sweetenham et al.[27] studied the European Group for Blood and Marrow Transplantation retrospective data set with regard to HDT in adults with BL/BL-L. Local pathology was accepted, with no stringently imposed pathologic criteria or review. No cytogenetic studies were reported. Burkitt lymphoma and BL-L were not separated. A total of 117 patients were included in this study. Data were collected from 54 separate centers. The patients were divided into four groups according to remission status when the HDT was given: (1) first CR (70 patients); (2) second or subsequent CR (15 patients); (3) PR, 'chemosensitive,' response not specified, or untested (18 patients); and (4) primary refractory disease, or refractory relapse (14 patients).

Various induction protocols were used and were not fully documented, although most appeared to be standard treatments for large cell lymphoma. The overall survival of this group was 53 percent at 3 years, with 54 percent progression-free survival. Disease status at HDT determined outcome. Patients transplanted in first CR had a 3-year survival of 72 percent compared with 37 percent for chemosensitive patients and only 7 percent for resistant patients. There were ten transplant-related deaths.

These results should be interpreted with considerable caution. This group is, at best, poorly defined pathologically. The initial treatment regimens were also not well defined but appear to be, in most cases, not BL specific. High-dose chemotherapy as consolidation of a lower-intensity chemotherapy regimen may be necessary and effective, but is not needed using more modern treatment approaches where relapse from complete remission is uncommon. The lack of efficacy of salvage chemotherapy was, however, usefully confirmed.

Allogeneic transplantation has been less widely performed, presumably because of methodological difficulties. However, in a paper by Troussard et al.,[28] nine adult patients with CNS BL in all cases and marrow involvement in seven cases (defined using French-American-British [FAB] criteria) were given conventional lymphoma treatment (although this was not well defined) and then were consolidated with cyclophosphamide and total body irradiation. Remarkably, seven patients appeared to be in long-term remission, but two died of high-dose therapy-related toxicity. The authors recommended a randomized trial but this seems non-credible. However, these results are striking, although difficult to place in the context of the current treatment climate.

In a European Bone Marrow Transplantation (EBMT) registry study, Peniket et al.[29] traced 71 allogeneic transplants for BL and compared them with similar patients receiving an autologous transplant. Patients were treated in CR or first relapse, with 20 percent having chemoresistant disease. Overall survival was reported at 37 percent, with equivalent relapse rates for allogeneic or autologous transplantation but an increased transplant-related mortality when allogeneic transplantation was used.

FOLLOW-UP

Once patients with BL complete chemotherapy, the initially abnormal sites should be reevaluated radiologically or by bone marrow examination as appropriate. Residual tumor masses, particularly in the abdomen and pelvis, are not uncommon. If these are bulky, consideration should be given to positron emission tomography (PET) scanning where available, although it is suggested that positive findings be confirmed by biopsy.

Recommended follow-up is initially at monthly intervals. When CR has been achieved, few relapses are seen, almost always within 9–12 months. Long-term toxicity (including gonadal) is uncommon and most patients resume their previous lifestyle. Follow-up beyond 5 years is almost certainly unnecessary.

BURKITT-LIKE LYMPHOMA AND TRANSFORMED FOLLICULAR LYMPHOMA

As described above, BL-L is an ill-defined and controversial 'high-grade' B cell lymphoma, characterized in the WHO classification by 100 percent Ki-67 staining, but with more pleomorphism. This is not considered a separate entity by many pathologists who prefer to consider this as the top end of the spectrum, in terms of proliferative capacity, of diffuse large B cell lymphoma. Many patients with BL-L are inseparable from BL in the published clinical series. However, two reasonable-sized studies have attempted to look at this entity in isolation. Longo et al., publishing in

1994,[30] described the National Cancer Institute experience of diffuse small noncleaved cell, non-Burkitt lymphoma in adults. Further histologic detail was not given but this is assumed to comprise what is now described at BL-L. Eight patients were treated for localized disease with ProMACE/MOPP chemotherapy (cyclophosphamide, doxorubicin, etoposide, methotrexate with leucovorin, prednisone/mechlorethamine, vincristine, procarbazine, and prednisone) with involved field irradiation. All achieved CR, none relapsed, and a single death occurred from an unrelated condition. A further 25 patients were treated with ProMACE/MOPP, or the flexitherapy variant, or ProMACE/CytaBOM (ProMACE/cytarabine, bleomycin, vincristine, and methotrexate with leucovorin). Central nervous system prophylaxis was provided by the moderate dose of methotrexate incorporated in these regimens although cranial irradiation was given at complete remission to those patients with bone or bone marrow involvement. All patients achieved complete remission, but there were a number of toxic deaths and relapses, with 51 percent long-term survival. In the entire series, 60 percent of patients were long-term survivors.

The Southwest Oncology Group in 2001[31] published a clinicopathologic description of BL-L. This would be considered unsatisfactory today. The mean Ki-67 score was 88 percent and a t(8;14) translocation (in the absence of a t(14;18) translocation) was seen in four out of five cases in which FISH analysis could be performed on snap-frozen archival tissue. As in the previous series, interpathologist variation in allocation of this diagnosis was extreme. Most patients were treated in trials with third-generation doxorubicin-containing chemotherapy regimens. Survival analyses were reported on small numbers (10 patients with BL-L and 37 with diffuse large B cell lymphoma) and the authors concluded that BL-L had an increased early mortality when compared with diffuse large B cell lymphoma, but similar 5-year survival.

A small clinical literature[32–34] describes transformed follicular lymphoma with combined follicular/Burkitt karyotype (i.e., both t(14;18) and t(8;14) translocations). In a particularly instructive series, Macpherson et al.[32] described 39 patients with BL-L with cytogenetic data. Three groups were described: (1) MYC translocation; (2) MYC and BCL2 translocation; and (3) other cytogenetic abnormalities. Poor survival was described in all three groups. However, the 13 patients with MYC and BCL2 translocations had particularly aggressive disease. Six of these patients had a preceding clinical history of follicular NHL. They were an older group (median age 65 years) and all died from aggressive disease in less than 1 year.

FUTURE DEVELOPMENT

Rituximab, a humanized anti-CD20 antibody,[35] is highly active in B cell lymphoma and is likely to be incorporated into all the new treatment protocols for BL.[35,36] A recent report from the MD Anderson Cancer Center[36] describes incorporation of rituximab into the hyper-CVAD regimen in 31 patients with non-HIV BL or BL-L. Apparently improved treatment results were reported, particularly in older patients who were routinely treated in laminar air-flow rooms. Randomized trial evaluation of this drug in this rare neoplasm is not a practical possibility, and it is likely to be incorporated routinely into future trial protocols.

Liposomal cytarabine[37] for intrathecal use supplies sustained levels of this drug over a period of weeks and may have a role in CNS prophylaxis, although more data on its efficacy are needed before it can be routinely recommended for adoption.

Diagnostic PET scanning may also be useful in the future. Since all patients require treatment with intensive systemic therapy, and patients with good-prognosis disease have an excellent outcome with limited chemotherapy, it seems unlikely that PET will have a role here. It is, however, likely that this technique will provide useful data on the viability of tissue in post-chemotherapy residual masses in patients with poor-prognosis disease. However, even in this situation, biopsy proof of abnormal uptake should be considered necessary until more data are available.

New drug use in the management of BL is likely to be slow in uptake as this is a rare and highly curable neoplasm, which at relapse often has a brief and rapidly downhill clinical course. In fact the main impediment to cure in this disease is the gross advanced nature of the lymphoma at presentation in some patients, and earlier diagnosis and treatment are the clue to improved prognosis.

The main hope for the future must be further elucidation of the molecular biology of this tumor, with potential utilization of antibodies or small molecules as tools against cell receptors or intracellular biochemical pathways in a fashion analogous to the use of imatinib in chronic myeloid leukemia.

CONCLUSIONS

Burkitt lymphoma is a fascinating, rare, and potentially highly defined form of non-Hodgkin lymphoma. Burkitt lymphoma usually arises at extranodal sites and spreads with considerable rapidity, often involving the marrow and CNS. Historic literature is scattered and difficult to interpret. What has become apparent is that this is a highly chemosensitive and curable cancer.

Treatment should be given urgently and intensively, incorporating high-dose methotrexate and routine meningeal prophylaxis. There is no defined role for high-dose chemotherapy as a routine part of this treatment and where this treatment approach has been described as successful it has generally been in the context of inadequate induction therapy. Collaborative groups in different nations around the world have, in the last 10 years, developed a variety of comparably effective treatment approaches. Randomized trial comparisons of these regimens are

considered impracticable and not worthwhile. Relapse from CR is relatively uncommon, occurs early (generally in less than 6–9 months), and has a poor prognosis.

Data from new studies incorporating rituximab and perhaps utilizing PET scanning are awaited with interest. Specialist referral is recommended wherever possible as no local treatment center can achieve sufficient experience with this rare cancer type.

Once chemotherapy is completed, patients can almost always return to their former lifestyle with no long-term side effects. There can be few more satisfying scenarios for the clinician than discharging patients to the community 5 years after such a fulminant illness.

KEY POINTS

- Burkitt lymphoma is a rare and rapidly progressive form of non-Hodgkin lymphoma.
- Burkitt lymphoma commonly arises at extranodal sites; spread to nodal sites, the bone marrow, and the CNS is common and occurs early.
- Burkitt lymphoma is curable with intensive chemotherapy. Treatment is highly myelosuppressive, generally comprising combinations including high-dose intravenous cyclophosphamide and methotrexate with intrathecal drugs. Rituximab should be routinely included in induction therapy, although this statement is not satisfactorily evidence based.
- Patients with 'low-risk' disease (variously defined) have a cure rate close to 100 percent. Patients with 'high-risk' disease should have a cure rate of at least 60–70 percent.
- Burkitt-like lymphoma is a less well defined and controversial entity which also appears to be curable with intensive chemotherapy.

REFERENCES

● = Key primary paper
◆ = Major review article

◆1. Diebold J, Jaffe ES, Raphael M. Warnker A. Burkitt lymphoma. In: Jaffe ES, Harris N, Stein H et al. (eds) *World Health Organization Classification of Tumours. Tumours of haematopoietic and lymphoid tissues.* Lyon, France: IARC Press, 2001.

◆2. Hecht JL, Aster JC. Molecular biology of Burkitt's lymphoma. *J Clin Oncol* 2000; **18**: 3707–21.

◆3. Blum KA, Lozanski G, Byrd JC. Adult Burkitt leukemia and lymphoma. *Blood* 2004; **104**: 3009–20.

◆4. Harris NL, Jaffe ES, Diebold J et al. The World Health Organization classification of neoplastic diseases of the hematopoietic and lymphoid tissues. *Ann Oncol* 1999; **10**: 1419–32.

5.   Lones MA, Auperin A, Raphael M *et al*. Mature B cell lymphoma/leukemia in children and adolescents: Intergroup pathologist consensus with the revised European - American lymphoma classification. *Ann Oncol* 2000; **11**: 47–51.

6.   The Non-Hodgkin's Lymphoma Classification Project. A clinical evaluation of the International Lymphoma Study Group classification of non-Hodgkin's lymphoma. *Blood* 1997; **89**: 3909–18.

7.   Murphy SB. Classification, staging and end results of treatment of childhood non-Hodgkin's lymphomas: Dissimilarities from lymphomas in adults. *Semin Oncol* 1980; **7**: 332–9.

8.   Goldman SC, Holcenberg JS, Finklestein JZ *et al*. A randomized comparison between rasburicase and allopurinol in children with lymphoma or leukemia at high risk for tumor lysis. *Blood* 2001; **97**: 2998–3003.

9.   Magrath IT, Edwards BK, Spiegel R *et al*. An effective therapy for both undifferentiated (including Burkitt's) lymphomas and lymphoblastic lymphomas in children and young adults. *Blood* 1984; **63**: 1102–11.

10. Bernstein JI, Coleman CN, Strickler JG *et al*. Combined modality therapy for adults with small noncleaved cell lymphoma (Burkitt's and non-Burkitt's types). *J Clin Oncol* 1986; **4**: 847–58.

11. Lopez TM, Hagemeister B, McLaughlin P *et al*. Small noncleaved cell lymphoma in adults: superior results for stages I–III disease. *J Clin Oncol* 1990; **8**: 615–22.

12. Strauss DJ, Wong GY, Liu J *et al*. Small non-cleaved cell lymphoma (undifferentiated lymphoma, Burkitt's type) in American adults: results with treatment designed for acute lymphoblastic leukaemia. *Am J Med* 1991; **90**: 328–37.

13. McMaster MA, Greer JP, Wolff SN *et al*. Results of treatment with high intensity, brief duration chemotherapy in poor prognosis non-Hodgkin's lymphoma. *Cancer* 1991; **68**: 233–41.

14. Waits TM, Greco FA, Greer J, Hainsworth JD. Treatment of poor prognosis non-Hodgkin's lymphoma with intensive, inpatient combination chemotherapy of brief duration: long-term followup. *Leuk Lymphoma* 1993; **10**: 453–9.

15. Soussain C, Patte C, Ostronoff M *et al*. Small noncleaved cell lymphoma and leukemia in adults. A retrospective study of 65 adults treated with the LMB pediatric protocols. *Blood* 1995; **85**: 664–74.

16. Fenaux P, Lai JL, Miaux O *et al*. Burkitt cell acute leukaemia (L3 ALL) in adults: a report of 18 cases. *Br J Haematol* 1989; **71**: 371–6.

●17. Magrath I, Adde M, Shad A *et al*. Adults and children with small non-cleaved cell lymphoma have a similar excellent outcome when treated with the same chemotherapy regimen. *J Clin Oncol* 1996; **14**: 925–34.

18. Weintrab M, Adde M, Venzon BJ *et al*. Severe atypical neuropathy associated with administration of hematopoietic colony-stimulating factors and vincristine. *J Clin Oncol* 1996; **14**: 935–40.

●19. Mead GM, Sydes MR, Walewski J *et al*. An international evaluation of CODOX-M and CODOX-M alternating with IVAC in adult Burkitt's lymphoma: results of United Kingdom lymphoma group LY06 study. *Ann Oncol* 2002; **13**: 1264–74.

●20. Mead GM, Barrans SL, Qian W *et al*. A prospective clinicopathologic study of dose-modified CODOX-M/IVAC in patients with sporadic Burkitt lymphoma defined using cytogenetic and immunophenotypic criteria (MRC/NCRI LY10 trial). *Blood* 2008; **112**: 2248–60.

21. Lacasce A, Howard O, Li S *et al*. Modified Magrath regimens for adults with Burkitt and Burkitt like lymphomas: Preserved efficacy with decreased toxicity. *Leuk Lymphoma* 2004; **45**: 761–7.

22. Rizzieri DA, Johnson JL, Niedzwiecki D *et al*. Intensive chemotherapy with and without cranial radiation for Burkitt leukemia and lymphoma. *Cancer* 2004; **100**: 1438–48.

●23. Thomas DA, Cortes J, O'Brien S *et al*. Hyper-CVAD program in Burkitt's type adult acute lymphoblastic leukemia. *J Clin Oncol* 1999; **17**: 2461–70.

24. Hoelzer D, Ludwig WD, Thiel E *et al*. Improved outcome in adult B cell acute lymphoblastic leukemia. *Blood* 1996; **87**: 495–508.

25. Smeland S, Blystad AK, Kvaloy SO *et al*. Treatment of Burkitt's/Burkitt-like lymphoma in adolescents and adults: a 20 year experience from the Norwegian radium hospital with the use of three successive regimens. *Ann Oncol* 2004; **15**: 1072–8.

●26. Di Nicola MD, Carolo-Stella C, Mariotti J *et al*. High response rate and manageable toxicity with an intensive, short-term chemotherapy programme for Burkitt's lymphoma in adults. *Br J Haematol* 2004; **126**: 815–20.

27. Sweetenham JW, Pearce R, Taghipour G *et al*. Adult Burkitt's and Burkitt-like non-Hodgkin's lymphoma – outcome for patients treated with high dose therapy and autologous stem-cell transplantation in first remission or at relapse: results from the European Group for Blood and Marrow Transplantation. *J Clin Oncol* 1996; **14**: 2465–72.

28. Troussard X, Leblond V, Kuentz M *et al*. Allogeneic bone marrow transplantation in adults with Burkitt's lymphoma or acute lymphoblastic leukemia in first complete remission. *J Clin Oncol* 1990; **8**: 809–12.

29. Peniket AJ, Ruiz de Elvira MC, Taghipour G *et al*. An EBMT registry matched study of allogeneic stem cell transplants for lymphoma: allogeneic transplantation is associated with a lower relapse rate but a higher procedure-related mortality rate than autologous transplantation. *Bone Marrow Transplant* 2003; **31**: 667–78.

30. Longo DL, Duffey PL, Jaffe ES *et al*. Diffuse small noncleaved-cell, non Burkitt's lymphoma in adults: A high-grade lymphoma responsive to ProMACE-based combination chemotherapy. *J Clin Oncol* 1994; **12**: 2153–9.

31. Braziel RM, Arber DA, Slovak ML *et al*. The Burkitt-like lymphomas: a Southwest Oncology Group study delineating phenotypic, genotypic and clinical features. *Blood* 2001; **97**: 3713–20.

●32. Macpherson N, Lesack D, Klasa R *et al.* Small noncleaved, non-Burkitt's (Burkitt-like) lymphoma: cytogenetics predict outcome and reflect clinical presentation. *J Clin Oncol* 1999; **17**: 1558–67.

33. Ladanyi M, Offit K, Parsa NZ *et al.* Follicular lymphoma with t(8;14) (q24;q32): a distinct clinical and molecular subset of t(8;14)-bearing lymphomas. *Blood* 1992; **79**: 2124–30.

34. De Jong D, Voetdijk BMH, Beverstock GC *et al.* Activation of the c-myc oncogene in a precursor B cell blast crisis of follicular lymphoma, presenting as composite lymphoma. *N Engl J Med* 1988; **318**: 1373–8.

35. Yokohama A, Tsukamoto N, Uchiumi H *et al.* Durable remission induced by rituximab-containing chemotherapy in a patient with primary refractory Burkitt's lymphoma. *Ann Hematol* 2004; **83**: 120–3.

●36. Thomas DA, Faderi S, O'Brien S *et al.* Chemoimmunotherapy with Hyper-CVAD and rituximab for the treatment of adult Burkitt and Burkitt-type lymphoma and acute lymphoblastic leukaemia. *Cancer* 2006; **106**: 1569–80.

37. Glantz MJ, LaFollette S, Jaeckle KA *et al.* Randomized trial of a slow-release versus a standard formulation of cytarabine for the intrathecal treatment of lymphomatous meningitis. *J Clin Oncol* 1999; **17**: 3110–16.

70

Diffuse large B cell lymphoma in children

MARY S HUANG AND HOWARD J WEINSTEIN

INTRODUCTION

The non-Hodgkin lymphomas (NHLs) comprise about 10 percent of all childhood cancers and are typically intermediate compared to 'high-grade' tumors.[1] By immunophenotype, the pediatric NHLs are evenly divided between B and T cell neoplasms.[1] The four major pathologic subtypes of pediatric NHL include Burkitt lymphoma, diffuse large B cell lymphoma (DLBCL), anaplastic large cell lymphoma (ALCL), and lymphoblastic lymphoma. Diffuse large B cell lymphoma is the least common NHL in children and makes up approximately 10–20 percent of cases.[2] However, it is the most common histologic subtype of NHL seen in teenagers.

As in adults, the morphologic variants of DLBCL in children include centroblastic, immunoblastic, T cell/ histiocyte-rich, and anaplastic. In recent studies using the World Health Organization (WHO) or Revised European-American Lymphoma (REAL) classifications, no prognostic significance has been found to be associated with the various morphologic variants of DLBCL.[3] However, immunohistochemical analyses of cell surface antigens, oncogene expression, and gene expression profiling have all demonstrated the heterogeneity of adult DLBCL and have been shown to be powerful predictors of outcome.[4–6] Historically, in terms of determining treatment, pediatric oncologists have grouped DLBCL by immunophenotype with Burkitt lymphomas, or by morphology with other large cell lymphomas such as peripheral T cell lymphomas and ALCL. Advances in clinical staging and a better appreciation of patterns of spread, coupled with improvements in chemotherapy and supportive care, have contributed to an improved outcome for children with DLBCL using

either treatment strategy. During the past 30 years, survival rates for children with NHL of all histologic subtypes have improved from less than 30 percent to approximately 80 percent at 5 years.[2,7] In some groups, such as children with St. Jude stage I and II DLBCL, survival rates approaching 95 percent have been achieved.[8–10] In others, most notably primary mediastinal large B cell lymphoma (PMLBCL), significant challenges to successful therapy remain.[9]

EPIDEMIOLOGY

Little epidemiologic information is available with regard to DLBCL in children. By Surveillance, Epidemiology, and End Results (SEER) data, the average annual incidence of DLBCL in the United States between 1977 and 1995 for patients aged 0–19 years was nine per million. Of these, fewer than 10 percent were in children less than 5 years of age. Greater than 60 percent of cases were in patients aged 15 years and older. The incidence of DLBCL appears to have remained stable from 1975 to 1995 in children younger than 15 years of age. Notably, there has been an increased incidence in 15–19-year-olds, from 10.7 per million in 1975–1979 to 16.3 per million between 1990 and 1995.[7] The reason for this increased incidence is unclear.

There is a slight male predominance of DLBCL with a male to female ratio of 1.4:1.0 in the United States. There is a slightly increased incidence of NHL in white patients, with an incidence 1.3–1.4-fold higher than in black patients younger than 20 years of age.[11] Diffuse large B cell lymphoma and Burkitt lymphoma are the most common subtypes of NHL that are observed with congenital or acquired immunodeficiency syndromes.[12,13] Unlike the experience in adults, DLBCL has rarely been shown to be a progression or transformation arising from a prior lymphoma, such as follicular lymphoma or nodular lymphocyte-predominant Hodgkin lymphoma.[14] Unlike Burkitt and lymphoblastic lymphoma, there does not appear to be marked variation in the incidence of DLBCL in different world regions.[1]

Histopathology/immunophenotype/genetics

Several distinct clinical and pathologic types of DLBCL have been described including primary mediastinal (thymic) large B cell lymphoma and intravascular large B cell lymphoma.[15] The latter has not been reported in children. The immunophenotype of DLBCL in children is similar to that described for adults but there are some differences. Recent analysis of 63 cases of pediatric DLBCL by immunohisto-chemistry and fluorescence *in situ* hybridization suggests that pediatric tumors may be biologically distinct from adult disease.[16] In both children and adults, DLBCL demonstrates a mature B cell phenotype with expression of cell-surface immunoglobulin (Ig) and B cell-specific markers such as CD19, CD20, CD22, and CD79a. About one-half of the cases of pediatric DLBCL are CD10 positive and CD5 is not commonly expressed.[17] It is sometimes difficult to distin-guish Burkitt lymphoma from DLBCL by morphology and immunophenotype. Molecular abnormalities such as *MYC* translocations, overexpression of *BCL2*, and translocations of *BCL6* may not be helpful in distinguishing Burkitt lym-phoma from DLBCL. Gene expression profiling is a promis-ing tool to help classify these difficult cases.[2,17,18]

In the pediatric age range, primary mediastinal large B cell lymphomas are most often diagnosed in adolescents. This unique subtype of DLBCL arises from thymic B cells and shows a diffuse large cell population with a variable amount of sclerosis that compartmentalizes groups of cells. Primary mediastinal large B cell lymphoma is sometimes difficult to distinguish from classical Hodgkin lymphoma, although immunophenotypic analysis (positive for CD45, CD20, and CD79a and lack of surface Ig) is usually suffi-cient to separate these entities.[17]

Unlike the situation in adults, there are no recurrent cytogenetic abnormalities associated with DLBCL in chil-dren; the *BCL2* translocation is rarely seen.[18,19] However, translocations associated with the *MYC* oncogene, such as the t(8;14) translocation, are much more frequently seen in pediatric as compared to adult DLBCL.[20] Structural chro-mosomal abnormalities as well as numerical abnormalities are noted in the majority of cases of DLBCL in children and adolescents.[18,19] *BCL6* gene rearrangements are likely involved in the pathogenesis of DLBCL in adults.[21–23] The incidence of *BCL6* translocations and mutations in pediatric DLBCL is unknown; karotypic abnormalities involving the *BCL6* locus on 3q27 are reported in less than 10 percent of pediatric cases.[18] As mentioned above, gene expression profiling (microarray analysis) has identified the biologic and clinical heterogeneity of adult DLBCL.[4–6] Similar micro-array studies of pediatric DLBCL are under way.

STAGING/WORKUP

The staging classification most widely used in pediatric NHL is the Murphy or St. Jude staging system (Table 70.1). This staging system was designed to take into account common presenting features and patterns of spread of the most common subtypes of NHL in children. The St. Jude staging system has been most useful for Burkitt and lymphoblastic lymphomas. The International Prognostic Index has not been routinely applied to children with any subtype of NHL.

In contrast to adult series, the majority of pediatric patients with DLBCL present with advanced stage disease – stage III by the St. Jude classification.[2] Stage IV disease, defined by bone marrow involvement and central nervous system (CNS) disease, is rare (less than 5 percent); CNS involvement is particularly rare in PMLBCL.[24] Another commonly used staging system for children with B cell lymphomas is the LMB classification. This is similar to the St. Jude classification but includes the outcome of surgery in groups A, B, and C. Other prognostic features used to stratify therapy include lactate dehydrogenase (LDH), early response to therapy, and primary sites of disease (Table 70.2).

The initial evaluation of a child with DLBCL includes imaging and laboratory studies to determine the extent of disease and assign appropriate therapy. In some cases, it also serves to identify risk for oncologic emergencies such as airway compression or superior vena cava syndrome

Table 70.1 St. Jude staging system for non-Hodgkin lymphoma

Stage I

A single tumor (extranodal) or single anatomic area (nodal) with the exclusion of mediastinum or abdomen

Stage II

A single tumor (extranodal) with regional node involvement

Two or more nodal areas on the same side of the diaphragm

Two single (extranodal) tumors with or without regional node involvement on the same side of the diaphragm

A primary gastrointestinal tract tumor, usually in the ileocecal area, with or without involvement of associated mesenteric nodes only[a]

Stage III

Two single tumors (extranodal) on opposite sides of the diaphragm

Two or more nodal areas above and below the diaphragm

All the primary intrathoracic tumors (mediastinal, pleural, and thymic)

All extensive primary intraabdominal disease

All paraspinal or epidural tumors, regardless of other tumor site(s)

Stage IV

Any of the above with initial central nervous system and/or bone marrow involvement[b]

[a]Modified from Murphy, 1980.[45]

[b]If marrow involvement is present initially, the number of abnormal cells must be 25% or less in an otherwise normal marrow aspirate with a normal peripheral blood picture.

Table 70.2   Risk group comparison for BFM, LMB, and POG approaches

	BFM 95[9,29]		SFOP/CCG/UKCCSG[10,36,42]		POG[8,28,35]
Limited stage	R1	Completely resected stage I & II	A	Completely resected stage I Completely resected **abdominal** stage II	Stage I & II
Advanced stage	R2	Unresected stage I & II Stage III with LDH <500	B	All but A or C	Stage III & IV
	R3	Stage III with LDH 500–1000 Stage IV with LDH <1000 CNS negative	C	CNS + BM >25% blasts	
	R4	Stage IV with LDH ≥1000 ± CNS			

LDH, lactate dehydrogenase (units/L); CNS, central nervous system; BM, bone marrow.
BFM, Berlin-Frankfurt-Münster; LMB, Lymphomes Malins B protocols of the Société Francaise d'Oncologie Pédiatrique (French Society of Pediatric Oncology; SFOP); POG, Pediatric Oncology Group; CCG, Children's Cancer Group; UKCCSG, United Kingdom Children's Cancer Study Group.

from an anterior mediastinal mass. The laboratory studies typically include a complete blood cell count and differential, erythrocyte sedimentation rate (ESR) or C-reactive protein (CRP), and serum chemistries including electrolytes, calcium, magnesium, phosphorus, blood urea nitrogen (BUN), and creatinine, as well as liver function tests and LDH. Staging will vary depending on the major sites of disease at diagnosis but should include a computed tomography (CT) scan of the neck, chest, abdomen, and pelvis. A neck and chest CT scan should be obtained before any invasive procedure is undertaken in a child with a mediastinal mass to assess the airway. Biopsy under general anesthesia or deep sedation should be avoided, if at all possible, in the presence of significant airway narrowing (to less than 50 percent of predicted tracheal cross-sectional area) or symptoms of orthopnea.[25] Magnetic resonance imaging (MRI) scans are most useful for evaluating bone abnormalities and CNS sites of disease. Bone scans are not routinely indicated. However, other nuclear medicine scans including gallium or fluorodeoxyglucose positron emission tomography (FDG-PET) scans are routine and helpful both in initial staging and in assessing response to treatment.

Many pediatric oncology centers are replacing gallium scans with PET or PET/CT imaging. The relative ease with which PET imaging can be performed presents advantages over gallium imaging. Positron emission tomography, as in adults with NHL, may also be more sensitive than gallium for both staging and assessing response to therapy.[26,27] Although St. Jude stage IV disease is relatively rare, complete staging includes a bone marrow aspirate/biopsy and diagnostic lumbar puncture. Given the association between DLBCL and primary or acquired immunodeficiency, human immunodeficiency virus (HIV) testing is indicated in all newly diagnosed patients with B cell lymphoma.

CLINICAL FEATURES

In the adult population, up to 40 percent of newly diagnosed DLBCL cases present with extranodal disease, the most common extranodal site being the gastrointestinal tract. Other primary sites include skin, CNS, bone, testis, soft tissue, salivary gland, female genital tract, lung, kidney, liver, Waldeyer's ring, and spleen.[2] Most pediatric series report DLBCL with either other large cell or mature B cell lymphomas. Therefore, it is difficult to establish the specific incidence of primary sites for DLBCL alone. In addition, referral patterns, particularly in the United States, may result in bias with regard to primary sites of presentation, particularly in patients greater than 15 years of age. However, in general, the abdomen is the most common extranodal site of disease for mature B cell NHL in children.

Of 46 pediatric patients with stage I and II large B cell lymphoma compiled from Pediatric Oncology Group (POG) data, the most common primary sites of disease were lymph node (13 patients), gastrointestinal tract (8), bone (8), tonsil (8), and testis (3).[8] In a series of patients from the United States with advanced stage large cell lymphoma, 59 percent presented with peripheral lymphadenopathy, 21 percent had hepatosplenomegaly, 24 percent bone involvement,[28] and 54 percent mediastinal involvement. It is unclear whether the latter figure includes cases not consistent with primary mediastinal involvement, as it is in contrast with reports of PMLBCL comprising only 1.8–3 percent of all childhood NHL in Berlin-Frankfurt-Münster (BFM) series and less than 10 percent of DLBCL.[9,29]

Clinical presentation depends upon both sites of involvement and extent of disease. Low stage disease may present with palpable adenopathy without constitutional symptoms. Abdominal primary lymphomas may present with gastrointestinal bleeding, intussusception, or acute abdomen, mimicking appendicitis; although presentation with ileocecal intussusception is more typical of abdominal Burkitt lymphoma. In the POG series, 36 percent of 75 stage III and IV DLBCL patients presented with B symptoms (fever greater than 101°F or weight loss greater than 10 percent of body weight); 76 percent of patients in this group presented with an elevated LDH.[28]

Primary DLBCL of bone is a relatively rare entity. In the past, primary lymphoma of bone has been reported as 5 percent of NHLs and 7 percent of primary bone tumors.[30]

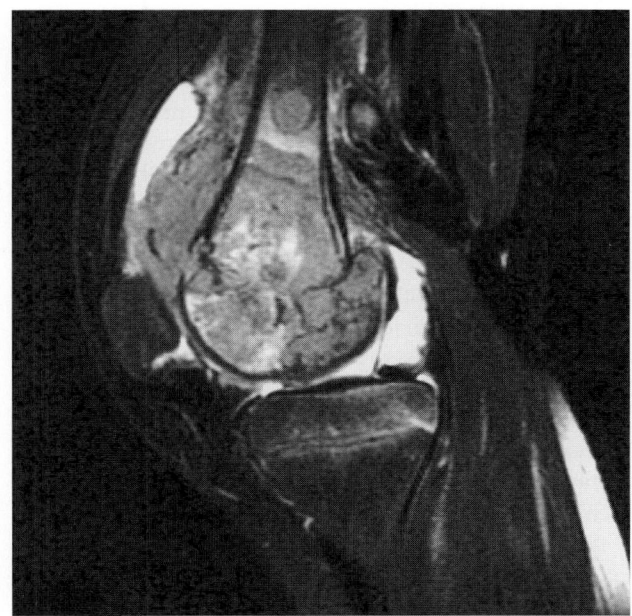

Figure 70.1   Primary diffuse large B cell lymphoma of bone. Sagittal T2 weighted magnetic resonance imaging (MRI) image of the knee, demonstrating primary lymphoma of bone rising from the distal femur.

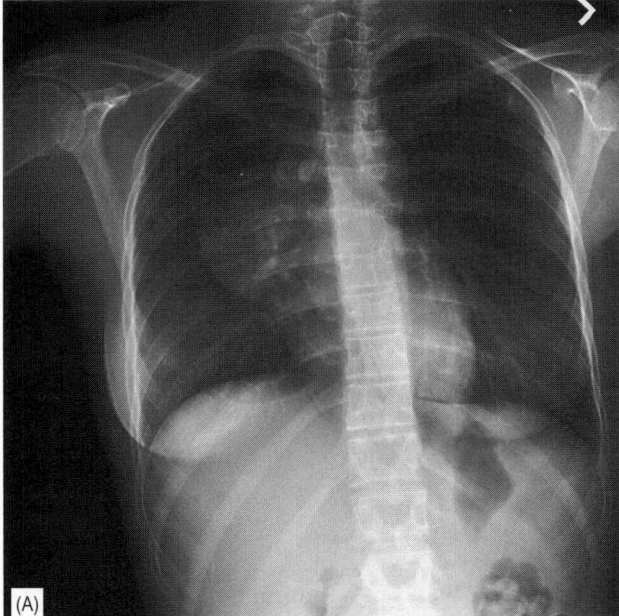

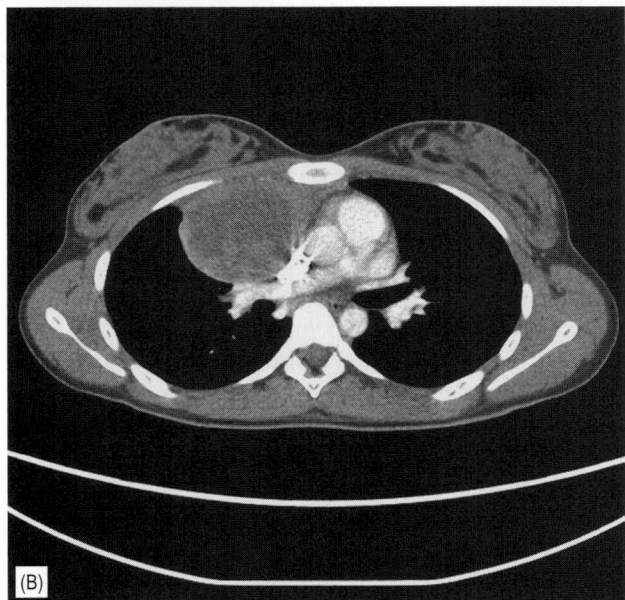

Figure 70.2   Primary mediastinal large B cell lymphoma. (A) Plain radiograph and (B) computed tomography (CT) image of primary mediastinal large B cell lymphoma. (A) Chest radiograph shows a right-sided mediastinal mass. (B) CT confirms a large peripherally enhancing mass with central low density consistent with central necrosis or hemorrhage post-needle biopsy.

Presentation may be that of primary bone tumors, such as Ewing sarcoma, with localized bone pain sometimes accompanied by a palpable mass. Radiographic studies usually demonstrate an osteolytic lesion. Magnetic resonance imaging findings may mimic those of primary bone tumors (Fig. 70.1). The peak incidence of primary lymphoma of bone is in the fifth decade with a male predominance. Approximately one-half of lesions occur in the long bones with pelvic and vertebral lesions accounting for an additional 25 percent of cases.

The Pediatric Oncology Group reported about 5 percent of children with low stage NHL as having bony sites of disease, most commonly reported in the lower extremity. Diffuse large B cell lymphoma was not separated out as a distinct histologic subtype. In 31 cases reported, sites of involvement included nine in the femur, eight in the tibia, five in the mandible, and individual cases involving the mastoid, maxilla, zygomatic arch, rib, clavicle, scapula, ulna, talus, and calcaneum.[31] The Children's Cancer Group (CCG) also reported on 31 cases of primary lymphoma of bone which represented 2 percent of patients enrolled on CCG studies between 1977 and 1996.[30] In general, patients with primary lymphoma of bone did as well as other NHL patients with therapy appropriate for stage and histology.[30,31]

Primary mediastinal large B cell lymphoma represents a distinct clinical and biologic subset of DLBCL and is discussed in more detail in a separate section of this chapter. Patients with mediastinal involvement may present with symptoms of cardiac, vascular, or respiratory compromise related to locally invasive disease. Mass effect, airway compression, and pleural or pericardial effusions may occur. Vascular compromise by compression or thrombosis may cause superior vena cava (SVC) syndrome. Shoulder and arm pain may also be presenting complaints. A chest x-ray will typically demonstrate a mediastinal mass (Fig. 70.2). With primary mediastinal disease, extrathoracic involvement is rare, the most commonly involved distant site being the kidney. Although renal involvement is relatively common (approximately 22 percent in one series), renal impairment, defined as serum creatinine greater than two times normal for age, is rare.[32,33]

MANAGEMENT

Chemotherapy

The cornerstone of treatment for DLBCL in children is chemotherapy, which has resulted in markedly improved long-term event-free survival (EFS) over the course of the past 15–20 years. In the United States, SEER reported significantly improved survival rates in patients 0–19 years of age: between the periods 1975–1979 and 1995–2000, survival rates improved from 42.1 percent to 78.5 percent in males and 57.9 percent to 82.4 percent in females.[7] In some subgroups, cure rates approaching 100 percent have been reported recently.[10] Current therapy focuses on stratifying treatment on the basis of clinical and pathologic features to optimize cure rates, but also to minimize late effects. To this end, relatively shorter courses of more intensive therapy, decreased CNS prophylaxis, and omission of radiation therapy have been used.

Grouping large B cell lymphomas with other mature B cell lymphomas has been the strategy of several groups, including the BFM group as well as the Société Francaise d'Oncologie Pédiatrique (French Society of Pediatric Oncology; SFOP), Italian Association of Pediatric Hematology and Oncology, United Kingdom Children's Cancer Study Group (UKCCSG), and the CCG in the United States. These groups have taken a risk-adapted approach to treatment and modify therapy based upon early response to treatment. Although risk-group definition has differed slightly, the overall strategy is based upon the extent of disease at presentation and overall tumor burden, sometimes as measured by LDH (Table 70.2). The majority of patients entered on these protocols have had Burkitt or Burkitt-like lymphoma, but despite being a distinct disease entity, there has been no significant difference between the outcome of the relatively low number of DLBCL patients and that of the overall group.

The POG took a different approach to large B cell lymphoma, grouping them by histology with other large cell lymphomas. Separate analyses of DLBCL compared with other subtypes are reported, but with relatively small numbers of cases.

For the purposes of further discussion, we focus on studies conducted by three collaborative groups – BFM, SFOP, and POG – because the BFM and SFOP studies, especially, form the 'backbone' for future studies.

LIMITED STAGE DISEASE

It has been demonstrated that a relatively brief course of chemotherapy effectively treats patients in the 'low-risk' category. In study LMB 89 from SFOP, 'low-risk' patients, designated group A (n = 52), had a 5-year EFS of 98 percent.[10] Preliminary data from the subsequent international group trial confirmed a 98.5 percent 3-year EFS in 'low-risk' patients (n = 137) with just two cycles of COPAD (cyclophosphamide, vincristine, prednisone, and doxorubicin).[34] No intrathecal chemotherapy was given.

Study BFM 90 evaluated 71 patients in the 'low-risk' group (group R1), with 100 percent 6-year EFS.[29] These patients also received a short course of intensive chemotherapy with a cytoreductive prephase, followed by two cycles of chemotherapy. In BFM 95, the prephase of treatment was eliminated and dose and duration of delivery of methotrexate were changed while maintaining excellent results; 95–100 percent failure-free survival (FFS) at 1 year.[9] Cycles of chemotherapy were given as closely as 2 weeks apart for a potentially very short total duration of therapy. Intrathecal chemotherapy was administered with each cycle.

Similar to other series, the POG 9219 study reported excellent results, with 98 percent 5-year EFS in 46 patients with St. Jude stage I and II DLBCL who received nine weeks of chemotherapy.[8] The predecessor of this POG study randomly assigned patients with early stage NHL to receive either chemotherapy (vincristine, cyclophosphamide, doxorubicin, prednisone, mercaptopurine, and methotrexate) and irradiation (27 Gy) of the involved field, or chemotherapy alone. The conclusion of this study was that radiation therapy can be safely omitted for such children. It also demonstrated that nine injections of intrathecal methotrexate was sufficient CNS prophylaxis for children with NHL originating in the head and neck region and that other patients did not need CNS prophylaxis. In a follow-up study, it was shown that 9 weeks of CHOP (cyclophosphamide, doxorubicin, vincristine, and prednisone) chemotherapy without any maintenance was sufficient for these children with Burkitt lymphoma and DLBCL.[35]

Chemotherapy comparison

All three regimens described above resulted in excellent EFS (greater than 90 percent) and overall survival (OS; 95 percent). It is difficult to compare their outcomes directly as about one-half of stage I and approximately 60 percent of stage II patients in the BFM and SFOP trials were stratified to the 'intermediate-risk' group and were reported together with patients with advanced stage disease.

An important consideration in choosing the best regimen for future therapy is the potential for late effects. With excellent treatment outcomes, minimizing late toxicity becomes a priority. Exposure to agents which may affect cardiac function, fertility, or risk of second malignancy long term is of concern. One would not predict significant risk of late toxicity based upon total cumulative exposure to anthracyclines and alkylating agents in these regimens (Table 70.3). Study LMB 89 reported no secondary malignancy in 'low-risk' patients. Study BFM 95 reported one second malignancy in a patient in the 'low-risk' group.

Table 70.3 Therapy comparison for POG (CHOP[8] and APO[28]), LMB 89,[10] and BFM 95[9]

Protocol	Agents	Duration	CNS	Dox	Ifos:Cyt	HD–MTX	VP16
POG CHOP	Cyclophosphamide Prednisone Doxorubicin Vincristine	9 weeks	MTX/Ara-C/HC (head/neck only)	120 mg/m^2	NA:2.25 g/m^2	NA	NA
LMB 89 Group A COPAD	Cyclophosphamide Prednisone Doxorubicin Vincristine	6 weeks	NA	120 mg/m^2	NA:3 g/m^2	NA	NA
POG APO	Prednisone Vincristine Mercaptopurine Doxorubicin Methotrexate	1 year	MTX $\times$ 6	300 mg/m^2	NA:NA	NA	NA
LMB 89 Group B	Prednisone Vincristine Cyclophosphamide Doxorubicin Methotrexate Cytarabine	Approx. 13 weeks	MTX/HC $\times$ 8 Ara-C/HC $\times$ 2	120 mg/m^2	NA:4.8 g/m^2	3 g/m^2 $\times$ 5	NA
LMB 89 Group C	Prednisone Vincristine Cyclophosphamide Doxorubicin Methotrexate Cytarabine HD-Cytarabine Etoposide	Approx. 21 weeks	MTX/Ara-C/HC $\times$ 10	240 mg/m^2	NA:6.8 g/m^2	8 g/m^2 $\times$ 3	2.5 g/m^2
BFM 95 Group R1	Dexamethasone Vincristine Ifosfamide Cytarabine Etoposide Methotrexate	4–6 weeks	MTX/Ara-C/Pred $\times$ 2	50 mg/m^2	4 g/m^2:1 g/m^2	1 g/m^2 $\times$ 2	0.2 g/m^2
BFM 95 Group R2	Dexamethasone Vincristine Ifosfamide Cytarabine Etoposide Methotrexate	9–13 weeks	MTX/Ara-C/Pred $\times$ 5	100 mg/m^2	8 g/m^2:2.4 g/m^2	1 g/m^2 $\times$ 4	0.4 g/m^2
BFM 95 Group R3	Dexamethasone Vincristine Vindesine Ifosfamide Cytarabine HD-Cytarabine Etoposide Methotrexate	11–16 weeks	MTX/Ara-C/Pred $\times$ 10	100 mg/m^2	8 g/m^2:2.4 g/m^2	5 g/m^2 $\times$ 4	0.9 g/m^2
BFM 95 Group R4	Dexamethasone Vincristine Vindesine Ifosfamide Cytarabine HD-Cytarabine Etoposide Methotrexate	13–19 weeks	MTX/Ara-C/Pred $\times$ 11	100 mg/m^2	8 g/m^2:2.4 g/m^2	5 g/m^2 $\times$ 4	1.4 g/m^2

CNS, central nervous system; Dox, doxorubicin; MTX, methotrexate; Ifos, ifosfamide; Cyt, Cytotaxan (CTX) or cyclophosphamide; HD-MTX, high-dose methotrexate; VP16, etoposide; Ara-C, cytosine arabinoside (cytarabine); HC, hydrocortisone; NA, not applicable; Pred, prednisone; BFM, Berlin-Frankfurt-Münster; LMB, Lymphomes Malins B protocols of the Société Francaise d'Oncologie Pédiatrique (French Society of Pediatric Oncology; SFOP); POG, Pediatric Oncology Group; CCG, Children's Cancer Group; UKCCSG, United Kingdom Children's Cancer Study Group.

ADVANCED STAGE DISEASE

For patients with higher risk and higher stage disease, it is more difficult to compare treatment outcomes directly as stratification of therapy and subsequent analysis of outcomes were not performed in comparable groups. Both BFM and SFOP used a stepwise approach to stratify therapy based upon extent of disease, with increasing intensity and duration of therapy based upon risk assessment. Of note, there are few data available regarding specific risk group assignment of DLBCL patients in BFM or SFOP reports. However, one would expect the majority of patients to be assigned to the R2, R3 (BFM), and B (SFOP) groups.

Berlin–Frankfurt–Münster studies

In BFM 90, patients with 'intermediate-risk' disease (R2) were treated with 4 cycles of chemotherapy after an initial cytoreductive phase.[29] Patients who had a poor response to therapy, with either residual tumor or persistent bone marrow or CNS involvement after 2 cycles, received intensified therapy. Patients with 'high-risk' disease (R3) were started on a course of 6 cycles of treatment and were similarly upgraded to intensified therapy after 2 cycles if there was not an adequate response.[29] In BFM 95, patients were further stratified to an R4 group. Patients in the R3 group received 5 cycles of chemotherapy, while R4 patients received 6 cycles of treatment. Poor response to initial intensification was considered an indication for further intensification of treatment with high-dose chemotherapy and autologous stem cell rescue.[9]

In BFM 90, patients with 'intermediate-risk' disease, R2 ($n = 167$), had a 6-year EFS of 96 percent ± 2 percent. Of note within this group, 46 patients (28 percent) in the 'intermediate-risk' group had a residual mass present after 2 cycles. In this study, 'second-look' operative procedures were pursued in patients with incomplete radiographic response. Just two of 46 patients with a residual mass after 2 cycles of therapy went on to tumor progression despite intensification of therapy. A small percentage of patients with radiographic complete response at this stage of therapy went on to progress despite an initial excellent response to treatment. Therefore, presence of a residual mass does not predict progressive disease. The initial risk-group assignment predicts risk for failure more reliably than the presence of a residual mass.[29] 'Second-look' operative procedures are not recommended in this group as they subject patients to significant morbidity. Whether there may be a significant role for PET imaging in this setting remains to be determined.[2]

In patients with 'high-risk' disease (R3; $n = 175$), especially those with stage III disease with LDH greater than 500 units/L, a significant improvement in outcome with more intensive therapy was seen in BFM 90 compared to BFM 86. Six-year EFS in that group improved from 43 percent ± 10 percent to 81 percent ± 4 percent. Overall 6-year EFS in 'high-risk' patients was 78 percent ± 3 percent. In the 'high-risk' group, 73 patients

(44 percent) had residual masses present after 2 cycles of therapy; 13 of these patients went on to develop progressive disease. Clearly, the majority of patients at risk to develop progressive disease were stratified to the 'high-risk' group. Amongst that group, a predictor of progression was pretreatment LDH greater than 1000 units/L.[29] This finding was the basis for the further stratification of the R4 group in BFM 95.

Overall in the BFM 90 study, there were 56 patients with DLBCL, including eight with mediastinal disease. Six-year EFS was not significantly different from that of patients with other histologic subtypes at 95 percent ± 3 percent.[29] Because of relatively small numbers of patients, details to assess specific strata of therapy in this group are not available. It is not clear how many patients with DLBCL were represented in each of the risk groups, or whether the stratification was specifically beneficial to these patients.

With the excellent results of BFM 90, BFM 95 focused on retaining efficacy while reducing toxicity by adjusting dose and delivery of methotrexate. In R2 patients, methotrexate dose was decreased from 5 g/m^2 to 1 g/m^2 without a significant detrimental effect on FFS. Significantly decreased oral and intestinal mucositis was seen when the drug was given over 4 hours compared with a 24-hour infusion. Median follow-up was relatively short – 3.3 years (range 0.4–6.3 years) at the time of this report – but showed promising results.[9]

Significantly, randomization for duration of methotrexate infusion was discontinued early in R3 and R4 patients because of inferior results. Failure-free survival at 1 year was 93 ± 3 percent compared with 77 ± 5 percent for patients receiving methotrexate over 24 hours and 4 hours, respectively.[9] This is in contrast to the LMB 89 regimen in which methotrexate infusions are delivered over 3–4 hours.[10] The weighted importance of duration of methotrexate infusions appears to be dependent upon the background of other agents used.

Notably, in BFM 95, an increased percentage of DLBCL was seen: 28 percent compared with 17 percent in BFM 90. Primary mediastinal large B cell lymphoma represented 2 percent of patients in BFM 95 compared with 4 percent in BFM 90. Again there was no significant difference in overall outcome between patients with Burkitt lymphoma and those with DLBCL. However, inferior outcome in PMLBCL was noted. This was primarily attributed to an increased incidence of local failure. Of 15 patients with PMLBCL, the 3-year EFS was 63 ± 13 percent. For all seven patients in whom treatment failed, it did so locally with or without other sites of disease.[9] In contrast, in BFM 90, eight patients with PMLBCL were reported with only one local failure.[29]

French Society of Pediatric Oncology studies

The SFOP LMB 89 trial comprised a much broader group defined as 'intermediate risk' (group B). The total number of patients enrolled was 579. Of note, there was no stratification for LDH. Patients in the 'intermediate-risk' group were evaluated for response after only 1 week of therapy, for potential intensification to the 'high-risk' group treatment arm (group C). An assessment of disease status after 4 cycles of therapy for both 'intermediate' and 'high-risk' patients directed potential intensification to high-dose chemotherapy with autologous stem cell rescue.[10]

Five-year EFS was 92 percent for 'intermediate-risk' patients ($n = 386$) and 84 percent for 'high-risk' patients ($n = 123$). Although this study did not stratify therapy for LDH, results showed a significantly poorer 5-year EFS for patients with LDH elevated to greater than two times the normal value (95 percent versus 87 percent). Other unfavorable prognostic factors identified included age greater than 15 years and 'no response' to the initial week of therapy. Interestingly, 126 patients were identified as having 'residual masses or suspicious images' after 4 cycles of therapy. Of these patients, 13 underwent exploration, 57 biopsy, and 56 complete removal of the residual mass. Only 12 patients had residual viable tumor cells identified. This, again, challenges the utility of 'second-look' surgery. Again, the majority of patients had Burkitt or Burkitt-type lymphoma; 63 patients had large B cell lymphoma. There was no significant difference between the outcomes for these patients compared with those of other histologic subtypes; 5-year EFS was 89 percent overall.[10]

The French-American-British (FAB) LMB 96 study was an international collaborative effort, enrolling patients from COG, SFOP, and UKCCSG. Patients with 'intermediate-risk' disease and rapid response to therapy were randomized to receive reduced therapy; 637 'intermediate-risk' patients were randomized including 145 patients with DLBCL. The 4-year EFS for DLBCL (not mediastinal) was 92.7 percent overall for randomized patients. An inferior outcome (4-year EFS 71.5 percent) for 32 patients with PMLBCL was again noted. Overall, therapy was successfully reduced in patients with rapid response to therapy without detriment to outcome.[36]

Pediatric Oncology Group studies

The POG treated patients with DLBCL as for other large cell lymphomas. Patients with advanced stage disease, St. Jude stage III or IV, recieved treatment for 1 year and were then randomized to receive one of two maintenance regimens: APO alone (doxorubicin, vincristine, prednisone, 6-mercaptopurine, and methotrexate) or APO alternating with intermediate-dose methotrexate and high-dose cytarabine. One hundred eighty patients were enrolled; 75 patients had DLBCL. The 4-year EFS was 63.8 percent for patients with DLBCL. There was no significant difference in outcome between the two maintenance regimens.[28]

Interestingly, in this group, there was no significant difference in outcomes in stage III compared with stage IV patients, or in patients greater than or less than 14 years of age. Although numbers are small, there was also no significant difference in outcome according to whether patients were radiographically in complete remission (CR) or partial remission (PR) after initial induction chemotherapy.

Six patients received radiation therapy for incomplete response to chemotherapy. Four of these patients had biopsy-proven viable tumor. Two received radiation based upon radiographic studies alone.[28]

Primary mediastinal large B cell lymphoma

This subset of DLBCL appears to be clinically and histologically distinct. The tumor is typically associated with sclerosis and represents only a small percentage of DLBCL in pediatric series (2–7 percent).[9,32,33] Primary mediastinal large B cell lymphoma was first described as a unique entity in adults in the early 1980s.[37,38] It is predominantly diagnosed in young female adults with a median age at diagnosis of 28–35 years. Clinically, patients present with bulky mediastinal tumors, frequently with invasion of adjacent structures. Data from immunohistochemistry as well as microarray studies in adult tumors suggest unique biologic features compared with DLBCL in other sites.[39] The molecular signature of PMLBCL has been described as more similar to that of classical Hodgkin lymphoma than to other DLBCL. Limited analysis of DLBCL in pediatric patients suggests distinct molecular features in tissues from pediatric tumors in comparison to adult DLBCL.[19] Primary mediastinal large B cell lymphoma in children has not yet been specifically looked at. Clinical presentation is discussed earlier in this chapter.

As a small percentage of DLBCL in childhood, with relatively few cases being reported, it has been difficult to evaluate PMLBCL as a group with respect to treatment. Historically these patients have been treated identically to other DLBCL patients. As subsets of pediatric series, various results have been reported.

The CCG reported retrospectively on 20 patients with mediastinal lymphoma treated between 1977 and 1993. Age ranged from 4 to 19 years. These cases represented a mix of B cell and T cell tumors. In contrast to adult series, 55 percent of patients were male. All patients achieved CR, having been treated with various chemotherapy regimens with or without radiation therapy. Estimated 5-year EFS was 75 percent ± 10 percent with an OS 85 percent ± 8 percent. These outcomes fell between those of other patients with localized disease (EFS and OS 92 percent ± 3 percent and 97 percent ± 2 percent, respectively) and disseminated disease (EFS and OS 50 percent ± 4 percent and 63 percent ± 4 percent, respectively). Radiation therapy did not appear to be of specific benefit.[33] Other series report comparable results with combination chemotherapy alone.

The BFM group retrospectively reported on PMLBCL in 30 patients treated on three consecutive protocols between 1986 and 1999. These patients represented just under 2 percent of the patients treated on protocol. The patients ranged from 1.4 to 16.7 years of age. Similar to the CCG experience, 50 percent of the reported patients were male. All cases were considered stage III (thoracic tumor without bone marrow or CNS involvement). Compared with other stage III patients, PMLBCL patients fared slightly worse with 5-year pEFS of 75 percent (standard error [SE] 0.08) compared with 85 percent (SE 0.02), although the difference was not statistically significant.[32] More recently in NHL-BFM 95, 15 cases of PMLBCL, or 3 percent of registered patients, were included in the study. The 3-year pEFS was significantly worse for these patients compared with other DLBCL cases (53 percent ± 13 percent). All patients who suffered recurrent disease failed at least locally.[9] As noted above, the recent LMB 96 study also reported inferior outcomes for patients with PMLBCL compared with DLBCL (not mediastinal).[10]

Noted in the CCG report was a relatively slow reduction in size of the primary mass radiographically. This is postulated to be due to prominent fibrosis in the tumor. Slow radiographic response and the common observation of a residual mass are not thought to portend a particularly poor prognosis. Neither 'second-look' surgery nor radiographic CR have reliably predicted the likelihood of relapse.[33] It is possible that new imaging modalities, such as PET imaging, may be more predictive in the future. Although adult data suggest that rapidity of response by PET may be predictive of outcome,[40,41] pediatric data do not yet support a role for modifying therapy based upon rapidity of response in PMLBCL. It is difficult to know whether clinical experience in adults can be reliably extrapolated to pediatric tumors. It is possible that further studies to determine whether PMLBCL in children and adolescents is sufficiently biologically similar to adult tumors will help to guide us. It may also be helpful to foster collaborative efforts with adult oncology to help direct and optimize the therapy of children with this rare subtype of NHL.

Chemotherapy comparison

It is difficult to directly compare regimens described for advanced stage DLBCL as the stratification of patients into risk groups has not been uniform. Overall, outcomes from all reported trials have improved. However, the POG approach yielded lower EFS compared with B cell approaches (SFOP, BFM). Numbers of patients are relatively low, however, and the POG included patients in their low-risk group who would have been stratified to the high-risk group in SFOP or BFM trials. As well, the intermediate-risk group reported by BFM and SFOP included greater than half of their patients with St. Jude stage I and II disease, representing a significant difference from the patients evaluated in the POG study. Regardless, the 3-year EFS reported in the POG study is inferior to those reported for high-risk patients with the SFOP and BFM approaches. Current approaches favor treating patients with DLBCL with therapy directed toward B cell immunophenotype.

In general we recommend that, when available, patients with DLBCL be treated on study to further advance our ability to understand and treat this disease. In the absence of an available clinical trial, we recommend treatment as per established regimens as described above (Table 70.4). Notably, PMLBCL remains a distinct and challenging

Table 70.4   Recommended therapy for diffuse large B cell non-Hodgkin lymphoma

Risk group	Regimen	Event-free survival
Stage I, II	CHOP[1]	90–95%
Group A	COPAD[1]	90–95%
Stage III, IV	APO[2]	65–75%
Group B, C	LMB 96[2]	70–90%

[1,2]CNS prophylaxis: (1) intrathecal methotrexate for head and neck primary only; (2) intrathecal methotrexate.
CHOP, COPAD: cyclophosphamide, vincristine, prednisone, and doxorubicin; APO: doxorubicin, vincristine, prednisone, 6-mercaptopurine, and methotrexate; LMB, Lymphomes Malins B protocols of the Société Francaise d'Oncologie Pédiatrique (French Society of Pediatric Oncology; SFOP).

subset of DLBCL. Future studies focusing on this group of patients will hopefully identify successful new strategies for treatment.

Interestingly, both BFM and SFOP use similar approaches to intensify therapy for 'high-risk' groups with greater duration of therapy, increased use of intrathecal medications, and dose intensification of methotrexate and cytarabine. Total duration of therapy is relatively short, however – typically less than 6 months, and in some cases as short as 4 weeks (Table 70.3). Subtle differences in regimens, however, may be important as recent attempts to incorporate a shorter duration of methotrexate infusion, similar to that used in SFOP, resulted in poorer outcomes in BFM 95.[9]

As noted in the case of treatment for low stage disease, toxicity, both acute and long term, is an important consideration in treatment choice. Again, with good outcomes, toxicity of therapy becomes a significant concern even in advanced stage disease. Recent data from FAB LMB 96 suggest that therapy can be reduced without compromising survival for some 'intermediate-risk' patients.[36] In higher-risk patients, however, decreased intensity of therapy resulted in inferior outcomes overall.[42]

Study BFM 90 evaluated 413 patients. They reported three deaths early in treatment due to acute tumor lysis syndrome, as well as 11 additional deaths related to toxicity of therapy. Two patients developed second malignancies with NHL.[29] Study BFM 95 looked at a total of 505 patients. There was one death due to acute tumor lysis syndrome in a patient with acute B cell leukemia, and ten deaths due to sepsis on therapy. Three patients developed second malignancies: two NHL and one case of malignant melanoma.[9] While it is a significant challenge in the management of Burkitt and Burkitt-like B cell lymphoma, acute tumor lysis syndrome is rare in DLBCL.

Study LMB 89 enrolled a total of 545 patients. They reported eight toxicity-related deaths. There were six events after 3 years: one myeloproliferative disorder and five second malignancies – Ewing sarcoma, NHL (two cases), anaplastic astrocytoma, and CNS primitive neuroectodermal tumor (PNET).[10]

Surgery

As noted above, stratification for risk group and therapy relies on extent of resection, especially in abdominal tumors. How important this is in DLBCL has never been looked at specifically, but with good outcomes, it seems appropriate to pursue complete resection when feasible.

Studies BFM 90 and SFOP 89 both used 'second-look' procedures to establish the nature of residual masses at previously known sites of disease.[10,29] The risk of an invasive procedure outweighs the benefit for the majority of patients in this setting. It is possible that new radiographic modalities such as PET will be useful as a less invasive way to evaluate such residual masses.

Radiation therapy

In pediatric lymphoma, therapy has focused on reducing exposure to radiation therapy. This has been fueled primarily by a desire to minimize late effects of therapy and associated risks for secondary malignancy in the radiation field. Recent results, as cited above, show excellent cure rates with minimal use of radiation therapy. Radiation has been limited to patients with CNS disease and those with an 'inadequate' response to chemotherapy.

FUTURE DIRECTIONS

In general, outcomes for DLBCL are excellent with current therapy. As noted above, historically DLBCL has been grouped with other NHL. In order to clarify prognostic features and fine-tune therapy, future efforts must focus on treating DLBCL as a separate entity and stratifying therapy within this diagnosis, potentially guided by molecular as well as clinical features. The significance of the clinical features used for stratification is unclear for DLBCL as it has represented a relatively small subset of patients within the larger mature B cell lymphoma group. Clearly there are significant differences between patients with DLBCL and the more common Burkitt and Burkitt-like lymphoma, both histologically and clinically. A significant difference in the incidence of CNS involvement, for example, may imply that therapy designed to optimize outcomes in Burkitt and Burkitt-like lymphoma may not be ideal for DLBCL. Patterns of failure are also distinct. In contrast to Burkitt and Burkitt-like lymphoma, in which the majority of relapses occur within 1 year, LMB 89/96 reported relapses as late as 54 months in DLBCL.[36] In the POG approach, there is a precedent to believe that anaplastic large cell lymphoma and other large cell lymphomas are not biologically similar enough to DLBCL to be treated and evaluated as a group. This is especially relevant when considering targeted therapies such as rituximab in B cell malignancies.

Targeted therapies have been used successfully with conventional chemotherapy in adult trials to improve outcome.[43] Whether rituximab will prove beneficial in pediatric DLBCL with a different chemotherapeutic backbone is currently under investigation. In addition, efforts are ongoing to identify other immunophenotypic targets for therapy in pediatric B cell NHL.[44]

It will be challenging to approach DLBCL in pediatrics, as the disease is rare. With collaborative efforts amongst pediatric groups, however, advances are feasible. In addition, forging collaborative relationships with adult oncology groups for patients in the late adolescent and young adult age group may be beneficial in this disease. As noted earlier, it is unclear whether DLBCL is biologically similar enough in children and adults to warrant a combined approach. However, investigating this further, especially with regard to molecular studies in pediatric cases, will provide a basis for future advances.

KEY POINTS

- Diffuse large B cell lymphoma accounts for 10–20 percent of non-Hodgkin lymphoma in children.
- Atypical Burkitt lymphoma and DLBCL may have a similar morphologic appearance and not be easily distinguishable by cell-surface features and cytogenetics. Gene expression profiling may help in classifying these difficult cases.
- The most common sites of presentation of DLBCL in children are intrathoracic and abdominal. Bone marrow and CNS involvement are rare in these patients.
- Primary mediastinal large B cell lymphoma is a distinct clinical and pathologic entity with a predilection for young females (age 16–30 years).
- Most recent pediatric oncology investigators have treated patients with DLBCL and Burkitt lymphoma on the same protocols.
- The cornerstone of treatment for this disease is chemotherapy.
  - For patients with limited stage disease (St. Jude stage 1 and 2), three cycles of CHOP chemotherapy without involved field radiation therapy has resulted in 5-year event-free survival (EFS) rates greater than 90 percent.
  - Children with advanced stage disease require more intensive chemotherapy, and have 5-year EFS rates of 70–90 percent with 6 months to 1 year of treatment.
  - Children with PMLBCL have a slightly worse outcome (EFS 65–70 percent) than other children with comparable-stage DLBCL.
- Further advances in therapy will require continued collaborative efforts between pediatric and adult oncology groups and identification of molecular features in childhood DLBCL as potential targets for novel therapies, such as rituximab.

REFERENCES

● = Key primary paper
◆ = Major review article

◆1. Sandlund JT, Downing JR, Crist WM. Non-Hodgkin's lymphoma in childhood. *N Engl J Med* 1996; **334**: 1238–48.

◆2. Raetz E, Perkins S, Davenport V, Cairo MS. B large-cell lymphoma in children and adolescents. *Cancer Treatment Rev* 2003; **29**: 91–8.

◆3. Harris NL, Jaffe ES, Stein H *et al.* A revised European-American classification of lymphoid neoplasms: a proposal from the international lymphoma study group. *Blood* 1994; **84**: 1361–92.

4. Rosenwald AG, Wright WC, Chan JM *et al.* The use of molecular profiling to predict survival after chemotherapy for diffuse large-B-cell lymphoma. *N Engl J Med* 2002; **346**: 1937–47.

5. Alizadeh AA, Eisen MB, Davis RE *et al.* Distinct types of diffuse large B-cell lymphoma identified by gene expression profiling. *Nature* 2000; **403**: 503–11.

6. Shipp MA, Ross KN, Tamayo P *et al.* Diffuse large B-cell lymphoma outcome prediction by gene-expression profiling and supervised machine learning. *Nat Med* 2002; **8**: 68–74.

◆7. Jemal A, Clegg LX, Ward E *et al.* Annual Report to the Nation on the Status of Cancer, 1975–2001, with a special feature regarding survival. *Cancer* 2004; **101**: 3–27.

8. Link MP, Devidas M, Murphy SB *et al.* Favorable treatment outcome of children with early stage large B-cell and anaplastic large cell lymphomas. *Proc Annu Meet Am Soc Clin Oncol* 2003; 04-AB-779 (abstract).

9. Woessmann W, Seidemann K, Mann G *et al.* The impact of the methotrexate administration schedule and dose in the treatment of children and adolescents with B-cell neoplasms: a report of the BFM Group Study NHL-BFM95. *Blood* 2005; **105**: 948–58.

10. Patte C, Auperin A, Michon J *et al.* The Société Francaise d'Oncologie Pédiatrique LMB89 protocol: highly effective multiagent chemotherapy tailored to the tumor burden and initial response in 561 unselected children with B-cell lymphomas and L3 leukemia. *Blood* 2001; **97**: 3370–9.

◆11. Percy CL, Smith MA, Linet M *et al.* Lymphomas and reticuloendothelial neoplasms. ICC II. SEER Pediatric Monograph. National Cancer Institute, 1999: 35–50.

◆12. Levine AM. Acquired immunodeficienty syndrome-related lymphoma. *Blood* 1992; **80**: 8–20.

13. Seidemann K, Tiemann M, Henze G *et al.* Therapy for non-Hodgkin lymphoma in children with primary immunodeficiency: analysis of 19 patients from the BFM trials. *Med Pediatr Oncol* 1999; **33**: 536–44.

14. Huang JZ, Weisenberger DD, Vose JM *et al.* Diffuse large B-cell lymphoma arising in nodular lymphocyte predominant Hodgkin lymphoma: a report of 21 cases from the Nebraska Lymphoma Study Group. *Leuk Lymphoma* 2004; **45**: 1551–7.

◆15. Demirer T, Dail DH, Aboulafia DM. Four varied cases of intravascular lymphomatosis and a literature review. *Cancer* 1994; **73**: 1738–45.

16. Oschlies I, Klapper W, Zimmerman M *et al.* Diffuse large B-cell lymphoma in pediatric patients belongs predominantly to the germinal-center type B-cell lymphomas: a clinicopathologic analysis of cases included in the German BFM (Berlin-Frankfurt-Munster) Multicenter Trial. *Blood* 2006; **107**: 4047–52.

17. Frost M, Newell J, Lones MA *et al.* Comparative immunohistochemical analysis of pediatric Burkitt lymphoma and diffuse large B-cell lymphoma. *Am J Clin Pathol* 2004; **121**: 384–92.

18. Heerema NA, Bernheim A, Lim MS *et al.* State of the Art and Future Needs in Cytogenetic/Molecular Genetics/Arrays in childhood lymphoma: summary report of workshop at the First International Symposium on childhood and adolescent non-Hodgkin lymphoma, April 9, 2003, New York City, NY. *Pediatr Blood Cancer* 2005; **45**: 616–22.

19. Dave BJ, Weisenberger DD, Higgins CM *et al.* Cytogenetics and fluorescence *in situ* hybridization studies of diffuse large B-cell lymphoma in children and young adults. *Cancer Genet Cytogenet* 2004; **153**: 115–21.

◆20. Le Beau MM, Rowley JD. Chromosomal abnormalities in leukemia and lymphoma: clinical and biological significance. *Adv Hum Genet* 1986; **15**: 1–54.

21. Cattoretti G, Pasqualucci L, Ballon G *et al.* Deregulated BCL6 expression recapitulates the pathogenesis of human diffuse large B cell lymphomas in mice. *Cancer Cell* 2005; **7**: 445–55.

22. Baron BW, Anastasi J, Montag A *et al.* The human BCL6 transgene promotes the development of lymphomas in the mouse. *Proc Natl Acad Sci U S A* 2004; **101**: 14198–203.

23. Kusam S, Vasanwala FH, Dent AL. Transcriptional repressor BCL-6 immortalizes germinal center-like B cells in the absence of p53 function. *Oncogene* 2004; **23**: 839–44.

24. Salzberg J, Burkhardt B, Zimmermann M *et al.* Prevalence, clinical pattern and outcome of CNS involvement in childhood and adolescent non-Hodgkin's lymphoma differ by non-Hodgkin's lymphoma subtype: a Berlin-Frankfurt-Munster Group Report. *J Clin Oncol* 2007; **25**: 3915–22.

25. Shamberger RC, Holzman RS, Griscom NT *et al.* Prospective evaluation by computed tomography and pulmonary function tests of children with mediastinal masses. *Surgery* 1995; **118**: 486–71.

26. Hermann S, Wormanns D, Pixberg M *et al.* Staging in childhood lymphoma. Differences between FDG-PET and CT. *Nuklearmedizin* 2005; **44**: 1–7.

◆27. Reske SN, Kotzerke J. FDG-PET for clinical use. Results of the 3rd German Interdisciplinary Consensus Conference, Onko-PET III, 21 July and 19 September 2000. *Eur J Nucl Med* 2001; **28**: 1707–23.

28. Laver JH, Kraveka JM, Hutchison RE *et al.* Advanced-stage large-cell lymphoma in children and adolescents: results of a randomized trial incorporating intermediate-dose methotrexate and high-dose cytarabine in the

maintenance phase of the APO regimen: a Pediatric Oncology Group Phase III Trial. *J Clin Oncol* 2005; **23**: 541–7.

29. Reiter A, Schrappe M, Tiemann M *et al.* Improved treatment results in childhood B-cell neoplasms with tailored intensification of therapy: a report of the Berlin-Frankfurt-Munster Group Trial NHL-BFM 90. *Blood* 1999; **94**: 3294–306.

30. Lones MA, Perkins SL, Sposto R *et al.* Non-Hodgkin's lymphoma arising in bone in children and adolescents is associated with an excellent outcome: a Children's Cancer Group Report. *J Clin Oncol* 2002; **20**: 2293–301.

31. Suryanarayan K, Shuster JJ, Donaldson SS *et al.* Treatment of localized primary non-Hodgkin's lymphoma of bone in children: a pediatric oncology group study. *J Clin Oncol* 1999; **17**: 456–9.

32. Seidemann K, Tiemann M, Lauterbach I *et al.* Primary mediastinal large B-cell lymphoma with sclerosis in pediatric and adolescent patients: treatment and results from three therapeutic studies of the Berlin-Frankfurt-Munster Group. *J Clin Oncol* 2003; **21**: 1782–9.

33. Lones MA, Perkins SL, Sposto R *et al.* Large-cell lymphoma arising in the mediastinum in children and adolescents is associated with an excellent outcome: a Children's Cancer Group Report. *J Clin Oncol* 2000; **18**: 3845–53.

34. Gerard M, Cairo M, Weston C *et al.* Results of the FAB international study in children and adolescents (C+A) with localized resected B cell lymphoma (large cell [LCL], Burkitt [BL] and Burkitt-like [BLL]). *Proc Am Soc Clin Oncol* 2003; **22**: 795 (abstract 3197).

35. Link MP, Shuster JJ, Donaldson SS *et al.* Treatment of children and young adults with early-stage non-Hodgkin's lymphoma. *N Engl J Med* 1997; **337**: 1259–66.

36. Patte C, Auperin A, Gerrard M *et al.* Results of the randomized international FAB/LMB96 trail for intermediate risk B-cell non-Hodgkin lymphoma in children and adolescents: it is possible to reduce treatment for the early responding patients. *Blood* 2007; **109**: 2773–80.

37. Miller JB, Variakojis D, Bitran JD *et al.* Diffuse histiocytic lymphoma with sclerosis: A clinicopathologic entity frequently causing superior venacaval obstruction. *Cancer* 1981; **47**: 748–56.

38. Addis BJ, Isaacson PG. Large cell lymphoma of the mediastinum: a B-cell tumour of probable thymic origin. *Histopathology* 1986; **10**: 379–90.

39. Savage KJ, Monti S, Kutok JL *et al.* The molecular signature of mediastinal large B-cell lymphoma differs from that of other diffuse large B-cell lymphomas and shares features with classical Hodgkin lymphoma. *Blood* 2003; **102**: 3871–9.

40. Mikhaeel NG, Hutchings M, Fields PA *et al.* FDG-PET after two to three cycles of chemotherapy predicts progression-free and overall survival in high-grade non-Hodgkin lymphoma. *Ann Oncol* 2005; **16**: 1514–23.

41. Kostakoglu L, Goldsmith SJ, Leonard JP *et al.* FDG-PET after 1 cycle of therapy predicts outcome in diffuse large cell lymphoma and classic Hodgkin disease. *Cancer* 2006; **107**: 2678–87.

42. Cairo MS, Gerrard M, Sposto R *et al.* Results of the randomized international FAB/LMB96 trial for intermediate risk B-cell non-Hodgkin lymphoma in children and adolescents: it is possible to reduce treatment for the early responding patients. *Blood* 2007; **109**: 2773–80.

43. Pfreundschuh M, Trumper L, Osterborg A et al. CHOP-like chemotherapy plus rituximab versus CHOP-like chemotherapy alone in young patients with good-prognosis diffuse large-B-cell lymphoma: a randomized controlled trial by the MabThera International Trial (MInT) Group. *Lancet Oncol* 2006; **7**: 379–91.

44. Miles RR, Cairo MS, Satwani P *et al.* Immunophenotypic identification of possible therapeutic targets in paediatric non-Hodgkin lymphomas: a Children's Oncology Group report. *Br J Haematol* 2007; **138**: 506–12.

45. Murphy SB. Classification, staging and end results of treatment of childhood non-Hodgkin's lymphomas: dissimilarities from lymphomas in adults. *Semin Oncol* 1980; **7**: 332–9.

71

Diffuse large B cell lymphoma in adults

BERTRAND COIFFIER AND GILLES SALLES

INTRODUCTION

Diffuse large B cell lymphoma (DLBCL) is the most frequent lymphoma worldwide, accounting for 30 percent to 40 percent of all lymphomas encountered in adults.[1–3] This lymphoma is described as aggressive since it has a poor outcome if inadequately treated or if primary treatment fails to induce a response. It is, however, a curable disease in a significant percentage of patients, depending on the initial characteristics of the disease.

The treatment of DLBCL has been completely modified in recent years by the combination of rituximab with chemotherapy, increasing the percentage of patients cured.[2,3] Although the combination of rituximab with CHOP chemotherapy (cyclophosphamide, doxorubicin, vincristine, and prednisone) has become the standard treatment for these patients, numerous questions remain, particularly for patients with the highest risk of failure.

Some of these patients will have had an indolent lymphoma originally, which was not diagnosed prior to transformation.[4] This entity is now more frequently diagnosed, even if the subtype of the indolent lymphoma is not individualized. *De novo* transformed lymphoma should be suspected in the presence of a small cell infiltrate as well as infiltration by large cells, or bone marrow infiltration with small cells.[5,6] These patients need to be treated as primary DLBCL and, in contrast to patients with secondary transformation, have a good outcome, not really different from that of primary DLBCL.

CLINICAL PRESENTATION

As for most lymphomas, the clinical presentation of DLBCL is very heterogeneous. In most cases, the first symptom is one or several lymph nodes rapidly increasing in volume. When these are situated in the thorax or abdomen, patients may present with symptoms secondary to compression of normal organs such as cough, pain, constipation, or diarrhea, or general symptoms like fever, weight loss, and fatigue. More than 30 percent of DLBCL occurs in extranodal sites like the stomach, skin, lung, and testis. In these locations, the tumor may have a typical aspect of lymphoma – for example, gastric or cutaneous DLBCL – or it may resemble a solid tumor of the organ. In fact, DLBCL may occur anywhere in the body, the only difference between sites being the frequency of such a location. Thus, initial staging comprises systematic examination and other investigations guided by the patients' symptoms.

INITIAL REQUIREMENTS FOR TREATMENT

Diagnosis and staging

The World Health Organization (WHO) lymphoma classification (described in another chapter of this book; see Chapter 18) recognizes different subtypes such as centroblastic, immunoblastic, T cell rich, and anaplastic cases, but treatment and outcome are not really different. In addition, although primary mediastinal large B cell lymphoma, intravascular lymphoma, or primary effusion lymphoma represent distinct clinical and pathologic entities, the management is similar to that of other DLBCL. A definitive diagnosis of lymphoma requires full characterization of the tumor. Biopsy of a large lymph node or of a part of an extranodal site is the only correct way to make the diagnosis. Pathologic examination comprises morphologic characterization including immunophenotyping, and additional analyses of fresh cells or cryopreserved specimens for obtaining or confirming the diagnosis in difficult cases and for establishing biological and molecular prognostic factors. Whenever possible, and in any questionable case, the diagnosis should be confirmed by one or several pathologists experienced in lymphoid malignancies. Image-guided core needle biopsies may be sufficient for confirming the diagnosis at relapse but not for the initial diagnosis.

In order to optimize care, the following parameters should be documented: clinical examination to evaluate the possibility of any unusual localization of the disease, performance status (PS) according to the Eastern Clinical Oncology Group (ECOG) or WHO scale, the presence or absence of B symptoms, and any underlying medical condition that may compromise the therapeutic strategy. Staging necessarily includes computed tomography (CT) scans of the neck, thoracic, abdominal, and pelvic regions, together with documentation of other specific lesions (Waldeyer's ring, bone, gastrointestinal tract, etc.), bone marrow biopsy, and cytologic examination of the spinal fluid. Tumor burden should be measured at different locations to aid in assessing the prognosis and to act as a baseline for assessment of response. Since functional imaging is gaining a wider use for response evaluation, it is recommended to perform a ^{18}F-fluorodeoxyglucose positron emission tomography (FDG-PET) scan prior to therapy. In addition to routine laboratory examinations (complete blood count, assessment of heart, kidney, and liver functions), serum lactate dehydrogenase (LDH) and serum β_2-microglobulin levels should be determined. Finally, hepatitis B virus (HBV), hepatitis C virus (HCV), and human immunodeficiency virus (HIV) serology are mandatory because of the clinical implications for treatment and because lymphoma may be the first manifestation of acquired immune deficiency syndrome (AIDS).

Prognostic factors

The International Prognostic Index (IPI) was developed for use in DLBCL and allocates individual patients into distinct risk groups with different 5-year outcomes.[7] The full index is based on age, stage, performance status, serum LDH level, and number of extranodal sites of disease. The simplified index includes only stage, LDH level, and performance status and is helpful in stratifying patients below or over the age of 60 years and is much more commonly used in clinical practice. The IPI, developed in 1993, has been shown to be robust in different series and is still valid within the era of monoclonal antibody therapy.

Many biological parameters directly related to the tumor have been identified as prognostic factors in DLBCL:[8] deregulated expression of several proteins (BCL2, BCL6),[9,10] mutations of TP53,[11] cytogenetic abnormalities,[12] and gene expression.[13] Other prognostic factors, such as circulating cytokine levels or cytokine gene polymorphisms, are probably determinants of the host tumor response.[14] More recently, gene expression arrays have been able to distinguish different subgroups of DLBCL with distinct outcomes.[15,16] Validation of these subgroups at the protein level has also been proposed. Although all of these factors, (described in other chapters of this book) represent an exciting field for the understanding of the disease and for the design of new therapeutic options, their practical impact in daily practice still remains investigational.

Response evaluation and clinical endpoints

Patients with DLBCL can experience long-term remissions and may be cured of their disease. The initial response to first-line treatment is a major prognostic determinant and achievement of a complete response is a prerequisite for long-term survival. International response criteria have been developed to homogenize assessment of response.[17] One of the pitfalls encountered by clinicians was the persistence of a residual mass after induction therapy, usually documented on CT scans, that led to the definition of 'unconfirmed complete response.' It has been previously suggested that, upon careful reevaluation of these lesions, such residual masses may not influence disease outcome. Recently, functional imaging has demonstrated its usefulness in further discriminating between active lymphoma and true fibronecrotic residual masses.[18] The predictive value of PET imaging is strong, whether performed at the end of treatment or early, after 2 or 3 cycles of chemotherapy.[18,19] It is, however, still unclear as to how this improvement in evaluating the *quality* of treatment response may help in modifying therapeutic strategy, either by reinforcing therapy in slowly responding patients or abbreviating/diminishing treatment intensity in patients who achieve a rapid metabolic response.

THERAPEUTIC OPTIONS IN DIFFUSE LARGE B CELL LYMPHOMA

Development of dose-dense and dose-intense regimens

In 1993, Fisher demonstrated that the CHOP regimen was associated with the same results in terms of complete remission (CR) rate, progression-free survival (PFS), and overall survival (OS) as more complicated regimens.[20] However, this regimen resulted in only 30 percent to 40 percent survival at 5 years without a plateau and around 30 percent of patients did not respond, with progression during treatment or just after. For this reason, various lymphoma research groups have investigated increasing doses (dose-intense regimens) and/or shorter intercycle times (dose-dense regimens) to try to improve the response rates (Fig. 71.1), or the use of high-dose therapy (HDT) with autologous transplant to decrease the relapse rates. Even outside of clinical trials, particularly in the USA, these regimens have demonstrated significantly better results.[21] Several phase II studies in the USA and randomized studies in Europe have shown an improvement over the standard CHOP regimen.[22–26] The benefit associated with these specific studies will be described later.

The rituximab effect

Following the demonstration of activity for rituximab in aggressive B cell lymphomas in two phase II studies[27,28] – one with rituximab alone in patients with recurrent disease and the other with R-CHOP (rituximab combined with the CHOP regimen) in untreated patients – several groups launched randomized studies in different settings to quantify the benefit of R-CHOP compared to CHOP alone (Table 71.1). The first report of a significant benefit for patients treated with R-CHOP was reported by the GELA (Groupe d'Etude des Lymphomes de l'Adulte) in 2000 (Table 71.2 and Fig. 71.1).[29] Since then, these results have been confirmed by three other randomized studies and one population-based study in DLBCL patients.[30–32] These studies have resulted in a new 'standard of care' for

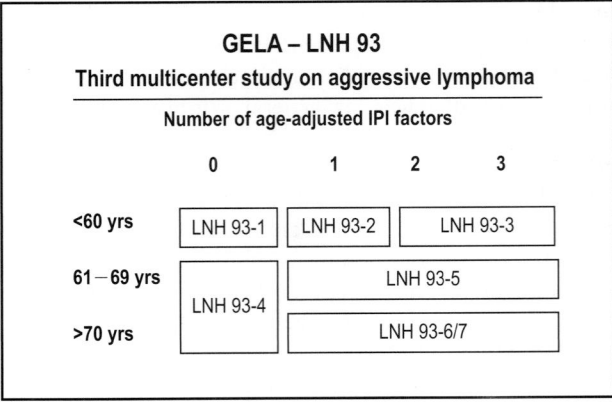

Figure 71.1 Example of study design for the successive randomized prospective studies run within the GELA (Groupe d'Etude des Lymphomes de l'Adulte) group for patients with aggressive lymphoma. Here the LNH 93 studies are presented, of which the 93-1, 93-3, and 93-5 have been published;[24,40,93] the other studies have as yet only been presented as abstracts. IPI, International Prognostic Index.

treating patients with DLBCL, namely, the combination of CHOP plus rituximab, or R-CHOP.[33–35]

The results from the GELA study are currently the most mature of all randomized studies, with a 5-year median follow-up.[36] The number of 'events' is clearly greater in the CHOP arm and at 5 years nearly half of the patients in the R-CHOP arm have not relapsed, compared to 28 percent in the CHOP arm (Table 71.2). Event-free survival (EFS), PFS, disease-free survival (DFS), and OS remain statistically significant in favor of the combination of CHOP plus rituximab with P values of 0.00002, <0.00001, 0.00031, and 0.0073, respectively (Fig. 71.2). Patients with low-risk or high-risk lymphoma according to the age-adjusted IPI (aaIPI) have longer survivals if treated with the combination of CHOP and rituximab (Fig. 71.3). No long-term toxicity appears to be associated with the R-CHOP combination. So, this represents a significant improvement in outcome for older patients with DLBCL, with significant survival benefit maintained over a 5-year follow-up.

Good-risk patients

Patients with a score of 0 or 1 in the aaIPI have either localized disease or disseminated disease with normal LDH level and good performance status. For those with localized disease, 3 cycles of CHOP followed by involved field radiation therapy became standard treatment after the study of the Southwest Oncology Group (SWOG).[37] However, the advantage of CHOP–radiation therapy disappeared with longer follow-up, with identical survival at 10 years.[38] The ECOG study evaluated 8 cycles of CHOP, with or without radiation therapy, in complete responders who presented with unfavorable stage I disease (bulky, mediastinal, or

Table 71.1 Results of different randomized studies comparing chemotherapy to rituximab plus chemotherapy in previously untreated patients with diffuse large B cell lymphoma

Study	Setting	CR rate	Median EFS	Median PFS	Median DFS	Median OS
GELA[29,36]	DLBCL	75%[b]	3.8 yr[c]	NR[c]	NR[c]	NR[b]
– R-CHOP	60–80 years, all IPI	63%	1.1 yr	1.5 yr	2.45 yr	3.1 yr
– CHOP	Intent-to-treat analysis					
Intergroup study[32]	DLBCL	NA	NA	At 3.5 yr	NA	NS
– R-CHOP	>60 years			53%[a]		
– CHOP	Not published		NA	46 %	NA	NS
				At 2 yr		
– R-CHOP + maintenance				79%[c]		
– R-CHOP w/o maintenance				77%		
– CHOP + maintenance				74%		
– CHOP w/o maintenance				45%		
MInT[31]	DLBCL		At 3 yr	At 3 yr	NA	At 3 yr
– R-Chemotherapy	<60 years, IPI score 0-1	86%[c]	79%[c]	85%[c]		93%[c]
– Chemotherapy	Intent-to-treat analysis	68%	59%	68%		84%
RICOVER[92]	DLBCL	NA	NA	At 2 yr	NA	NS
– R-CHOP-14	61–80 years, all IPI			$P < 0.001$		
– CHOP-14	Not published					

[a] P value <0.05; [b] P value <0.01; [c] P value <0.001; NS, not significantly different.
CR, complete remission; EFS, event-free survival; PFS, progression-free survival; DFS, disease-free survival; OS, overall survival; NR, not reached; NA, not available; yr, years; w/o, without; IPI, International Prognostic Index; CHOP: cyclophosphamide, doxorubicin, vincristine, and prednisone; R, rituximab; CHOP-14, CHOP regimen administered every two weeks.

Table 71.2 Number and type of events observed in both arms of the LNH 98.5 study with a median follow-up of 5 years[36]

Event	CHOP		R-CHOP	
	n	%	n	%
PD during treatment	44	22	19	9.5
New treatment	9	4.5	11	5.5
PD after SD	1	1	1	0.5
PD after PR	4	2	6	3
Relapse	67	34	40	20
Death during treatment	12	6	12	6
Death in CR	5	2.5	17	8
All events	**142**	**72**	**106**	**52.5**
No event	55	28	96	47.5
Total patients	**197**	**100**	**202**	**100**

CHOP: cyclophosphamide, doxorubicin, vincristine, and prednisone; R-CHOP, rituximab combined with CHOP regimen; PD, progressive disease; SD, stable disease; PR, partial response; CR, complete remission.

retroperitoneal) or stage IE, II, or IIE disease. In this study (which was underpowered), DFS at 6 years was greater for patients who received radiation therapy (73 percent vs 56 percent, two-sided $P = 0.05$) but differences in OS were not statistically significant.[39]

Another study from the GELA compared 3 cycles of CHOP plus involved field radiation therapy (the Miller regimen) or chemotherapy alone using the ACVBP regimen with sequential consolidation (Fig. 71.4) in previously untreated patients under 61 years of age with stage I–II aggressive lymphoma and no adverse prognostic factors.[40] With a median follow-up of 7.7 years, EFS and OS were significantly longer in the chemotherapy-alone group ($P < 0.001$ and $P = 0.001$, respectively). The 5-year estimates of EFS were 82 percent for patients receiving chemotherapy alone and 74 percent for patients treated with CHOP plus radiation therapy. The 5-year estimates of OS were 90 percent and 81 percent, respectively (Fig. 71.5). In a multivariate analysis, EFS and OS were affected by treatment arm, independently of stage and tumor bulk. This study demonstrated that chemotherapy alone with 3 cycles of ACVBP followed by sequential consolidation is superior to 3 cycles of CHOP plus radiation therapy for the treatment of low-risk, localized lymphoma in patients younger than 61 years. These results applied to patients with or without a large tumor mass.

The GELA has run another study in elderly patients also testing the benefit of radiation therapy. In this LNH 93.4 study, patients older than 60 years were randomized to either 4 cycles of CHOP or 4 cycles of CHOP plus involved field radiation therapy. Patients had localized stage I or II disease without any adverse prognostic factor according to the aaIPI. Preliminary results showed that complete response at the end of treatment and EFS and OS rates were similar in both groups.[41]

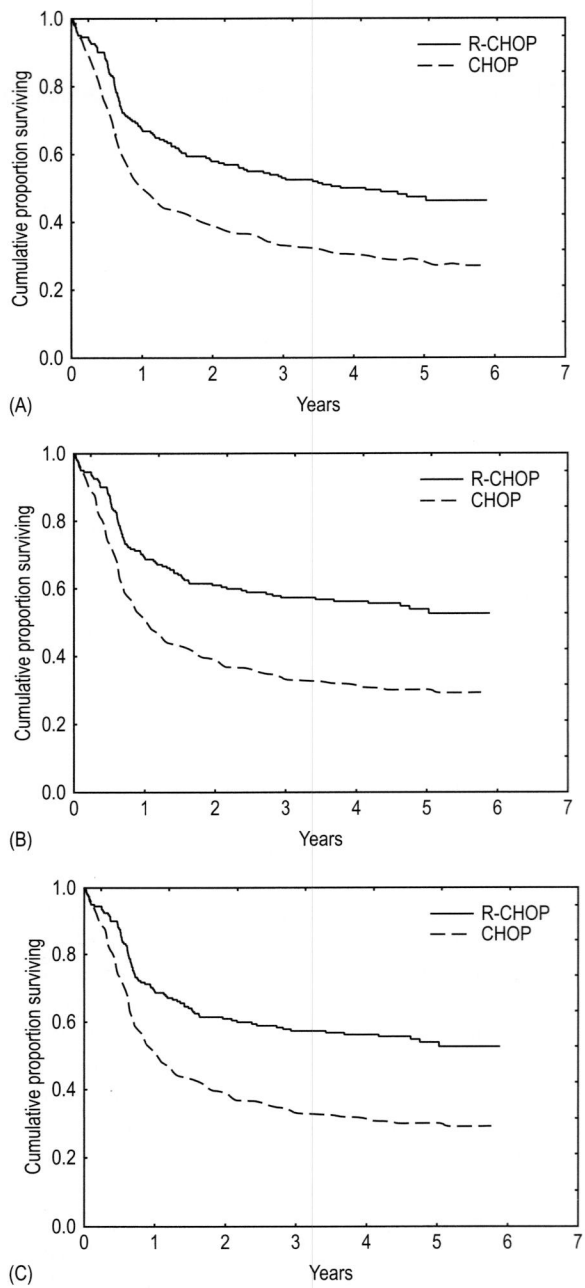

Figure 71.2 (A) Event-free survival, (B) progression-free survival, and (C) overall survival with a median follow-up of 5 years in CHOP and R-CHOP-treated patients in the LNH 98.5 study.[36] Log-rank test *P* values are 0.00002, <0.00001, and 0.0073, respectively. CHOP, cyclophosphamide, doxorubicin, vincristine, and prednisone; R-CHOP, rituximab combined with CHOP regimen.

These four randomized prospective studies allow the conclusion that radiation therapy does not add to chemotherapy *if the chemotherapy is sufficient*. In patients with stage II or bulky stage I disease, chemotherapy alone is probably better than the combination although no direct comparison has been made. In very limited disease (stage I),

both modalities will probably be equivalent. The burning question concerns the place of rituximab (if any) in these patients. Elderly patients treated with 4 cycles of CHOP, with or without radiation therapy, only have a 60 percent OS at 5 years, a figure lower than patients with more disseminated disease.[41] So, there is certainly room for improvement and the GELA currently recommend 6 cycles of R-CHOP for these patients. In younger patients, R-CHOP will probably not increase survival but might be less toxic than the regimen currently used by the GELA (ACVBP).

Two additional studies are pertinent to the discussion of good-risk patients. The German Non-Hodgkin's Lymphoma Study Group evaluated CHOP given on a 2- or 3-week schedule and the addition of etoposide (CHOEP), also on a 2- or 3-week schedule, in younger patients (18–60 years) with DLBCL and a normal LDH.[42] About two-thirds of the study group had an aaIPI of 0. In this study, which also included other histologic subtypes and some T cell lymphomas, the addition of etoposide resulted in superior response rates and EFS but similar overall survival at 5 years. Of note, the 2- or 3-week schedules showed similar results, not validating the finding of superiority for the CHOP regimen administered every 2 weeks ('CHOP-14') in younger patients. As noted below, CHOEP and CHOP have also been evaluated in combination with rituximab in the MInT trial, whereupon the differences in these regimens were no longer apparent.[31]

Some patients with a good-risk aaIPI score have disseminated disease, with good PS and normal LDH level. A better outcome was seen in these patients with the intensive regimens used in the older GELA studies (without rituximab). Here too, in future, 6–8 cycles of R-CHOP need to be compared with more toxic regimens. This is currently the objective of the LNH 03.2B study in the GELA.

Older patients with poor-risk diffuse large B cell lymphoma

Classically, older patients are defined by an age older than 60 years. They represent 50 percent of patients with aggressive lymphoma but patients older than 80 years will increasingly be seen in the future and the treatment strategy will probably need to be different from that currently considered as standard in older patients.

Two studies in older patients have demonstrated that the combination of rituximab with CHOP is clearly superior to CHOP alone.[29,32,36] The first was reported by the GELA and was described above (Table 71.2, Fig. 71.1, and Fig. 71.2). The second came from the intergroup study formed by ECOG, CALGB (Cancer and Leukemia Group B), and SWOG. The E4494 study compared CHOP versus R-CHOP, and then, for responding patients, maintenance with rituximab alone (four infusions every 6 months) for 2 years versus no further treatment. There are several differences between E4494 and the GELA study: in the former

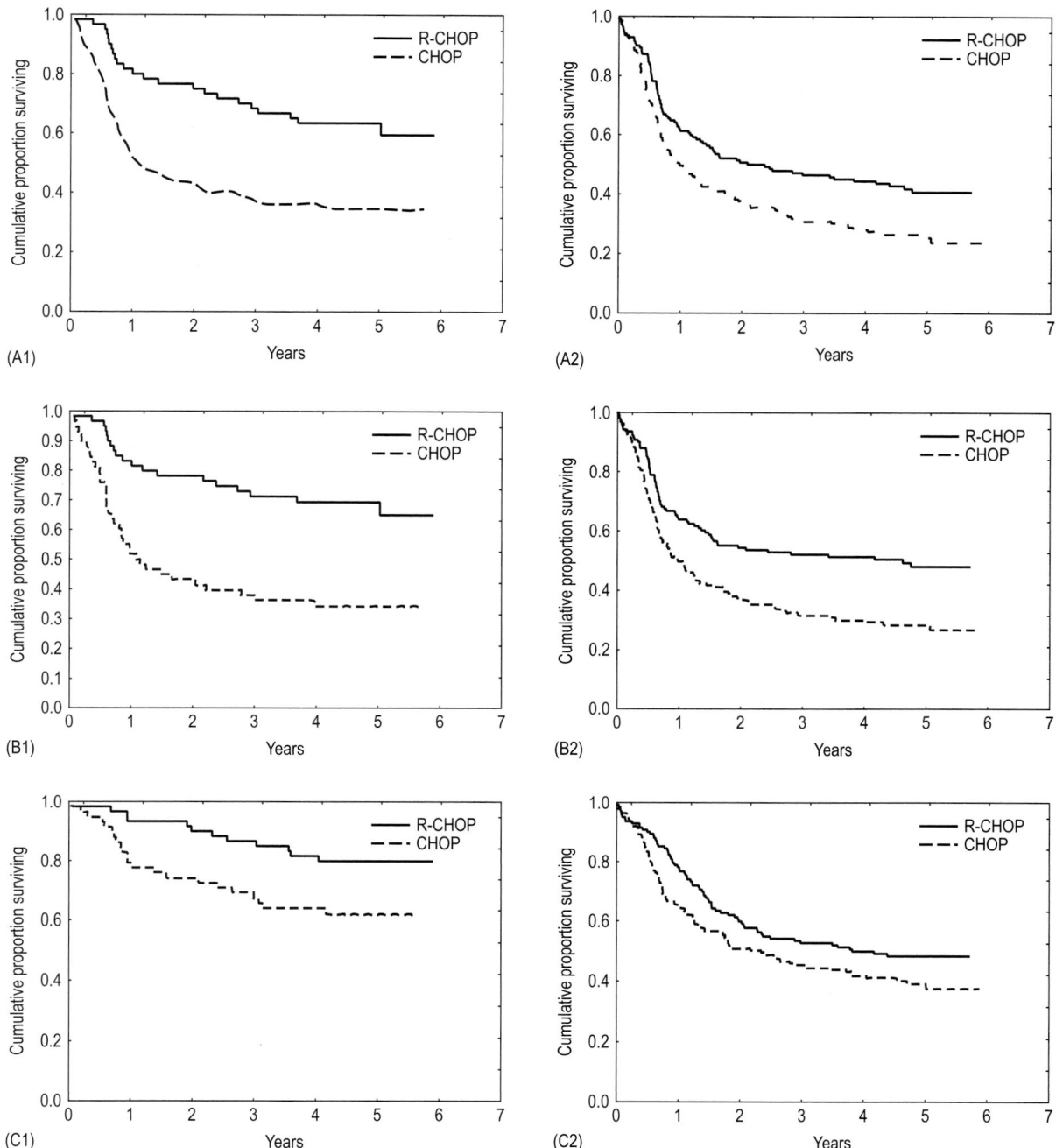

Figure 71.3 (A1, A2) Event-free survival, (B1, B2) progression-free survival, and (C1, C2) overall survival with a median follow-up of 5 years of patients treated with R-CHOP and CHOP in the LNH 98.5 study according to the age-adjusted International Prognostic Index score at diagnosis: (A1, B1, C1) low-risk patients (scores 0 and 1); (A2, B2, C2) high-risk patients (scores 2 and 3). All differences are statistically significant except for overall survival in high-risk patients: *P* values are 0.00085, 0.0037, 0.00013, 0.00078, 0.023, and 0.062, respectively.[36] CHOP, cyclophosphamide, doxorubicin, vincristine, and prednisone; R-CHOP, rituximab combined with CHOP regimen.

(1) rituximab was given only every 2 cycles of CHOP, so that patients received half the total amount of rituximab compared to GELA patients; (2) patients in CR at 4 cycles received a total of 6 cycles of CHOP and only 33 percent of patients received 7 or more cycles; and (3) half of responding patients received maintenance with rituximab.

The clinical characteristics of the patients were broadly similar to those of patients in the GELA study but only 50 percent had aaIPI scores >1 compared to 60 percent in the GELA study. The median follow-up was 3.5 years. In contrast to the GELA study, rituximab did not seem to influence response rate or early disease progression; the

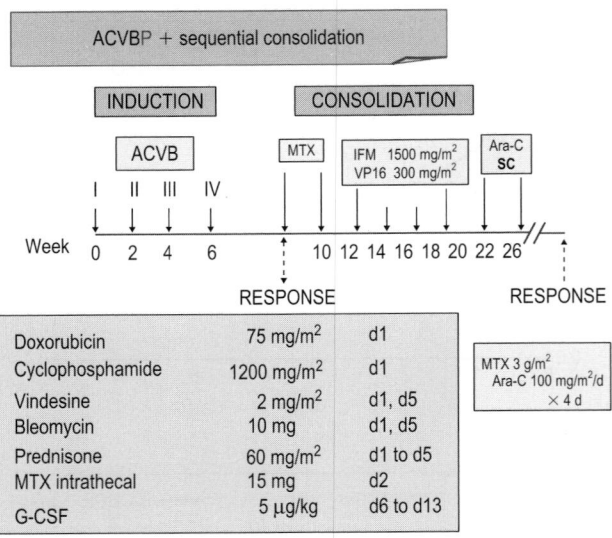

Figure 71.4 Description of the ACVBP regimen used since 1984 by the GELA (Groupe d'Etude des Lymphomes de l'Adulte) in different prospective studies.[94] The schema of this regimen has slightly changed during the years of the studies: for example, only 3 cycles of ACVBP were realized in patients with localized disease (LNH 93.1) or delays between cycles were 3 weeks or 2 weeks in elderly patients.[24,40] MTX, methotrexate; IFM, ifosfamide; VP16, etoposide; Ara-C; cytosine arabinoside; SC, subcutaneous; G-CSF, granulocyte colony-stimulating factor; d, day.

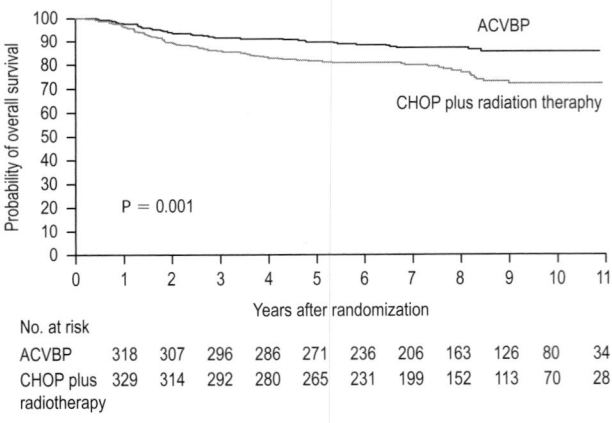

Figure 71.5 Overall survival among 647 patients assigned to chemotherapy alone with the ACVBP regimen (see Fig. 71.4) or to CHOP plus involved field radiatiion therapy in the LNH 93.1 study.[40] CHOP, cyclophosphamide, doxorubicin, vincristine, and prednisone.

lower total dose of rituximab in the intergroup study might have influenced these results. Time to treatment failure (TTF) was better with R-CHOP (53 percent at 3 years) than CHOP (46 percent at 3 years, $P = 0.04$). Maintenance rituximab significantly prolonged TTF ($P = 0.009$) overall, but only in patients who had received CHOP ($P = 0.0004$), not after R-CHOP ($P = 0.81$). There was no significant difference in OS according to induction therapy

($P = 0.18$). However, if the results are analyzed only in relation to initial therapy, an advantage for R-CHOP is observed for failure-free survival but not for OS.[32]

Other significant results have been demonstrated and may help us to design the best therapeutic options for these patients. 'Younger' elderly patients (60 to 65 years old) may benefit from dose-dense dose-intense regimens like younger patients.[24] In a study comparing 8 cycles of CHOP with ACVBP followed by sequential consolidation, 5-year EFS was 39 percent in the ACVBP group and 29 percent in the CHOP group ($P = 0.005$). Five-year OS was also significantly longer for patients treated with ACVBP: 46 percent compared with 38 percent with CHOP ($P = 0.036$). However, it appears that ACVBP cannot be used in patients over 65 years of age because of its toxicity. A German study has also shown an improvement over classical CHOP (CHOP given every 3 weeks or 'CHOP-21') when the CHOP regimen was administered every 2 weeks ('CHOP-14').[43] The conclusions of these two studies have to be reviewed in the era of rituximab therapy because the advantages of dose-intense or dose-dense regimens, which are potentially more toxic, might not be confirmed when rituximab is added to CHOP.

If the results achieved in 'good-risk' patients in the GELA study are satisfactory, this is not the case for 'poor-risk' patients and better therapies need to be found for them. Currently, the GELA is testing whether giving R-CHOP every 2 weeks might increase the response rate and prolong the response, particularly in patients with 'poor-risk' lymphoma. The feasibility of giving such dose-dense chemotherapy in elderly patients with a high aaIPI score and concomitant diseases is questioned but not known. The GELA is also testing whether treating and preventing anemia (that is, maintaining the hemoglobin level at 13 g/dL) in these patients may render them better able to tolerate a dose-dense regimen. New monoclonal antibodies and drugs interacting with signal transduction are currently in early development.

Young patients with intermediate-risk diffuse large B cell lymphoma

According to the aaIPI, these patients have one adverse prognostic factor, usually disseminated stage or a high LDH level. Such patients were previously usually treated with CHOP and are now treated with R-CHOP. The German lymphoma group has recently shown that the use of R-CHOP or R-'CHOP-like' regimens is associated with a better outcome than the same regimen given without rituximab (the MInT study).[31] Patients with aaIPI scores of 0 or 1 were entered into the latter study but 57 percent had a score of 1. After a median follow-up of 34 months, patients treated with R-CHOP-like regimens had a significantly longer TTF ($P < 0.00001$), with estimated 3-year TTF rates of 59 percent (CHOP-like) versus 79 percent (R-CHOP-like). Similarly, OS was significantly different

($P < 0.001$), with 3-year survival rates of 84 percent (CHOP-like) and 93 percent (R-CHOP-like), respectively. However, 3-year TTF with the R-CHOP-like regimen in patients with bulky disease and/or an aaIPI score of 1 was significantly worse ($P < 0.001$) than in patients with an aaIPI score of 0 and no bulk (71 percent vs 90 percent, respectively). Because of these results, outside of a clinical study, R-CHOP is the recommended regimen.

Is it possible to achieve survival better than 60–70 percent at 10 years in such patients? High-dose therapy with autologous stem cell transplantation has not shown any benefit in subgroup analyses of randomized trials in these intermediate-risk patients. To date, no prospective randomized study has concluded that a dose-dense or dose-intense regimen is better than CHOP or R-CHOP in this particular group of patients. Currently, the GELA is comparing R-CHOP to R-ACVBP for this group; however, the standard regimen remains R-CHOP-21. A study comparing R-CHOP-14 to R-CHOP-21 is currently in progress in the UK.

Young patients with poor-risk diffuse large B cell lymphoma

These patients, defined by an aaIPI score of 2 or 3 and age younger than 60 years, have the worst outcome. Around 30 percent of them are truly refractory to chemotherapy; that is, they progress during treatment or relapse early after the end of treatment. They also have a higher relapse rate than patients with lower aaIPI scores. So far, all attempts to modify the chemotherapy regimen in order to decrease the number of patients who progress whilst on treatment have failed and the best CR rate is currently around 65 percent. However, attempts to decrease the recurrence rate have been somewhat more successful. The GELA has conducted a study, LNH 87.2, comparing standard consolidation after 4 cycles of ACVBP with a CBV high-dose regimen (HDT) supported by autologous stem cell transplantation.[26] With a median follow-up of 8 years, HDT was superior to sequential chemotherapy, with DFS rates of 55 percent (95 percent confidence interval [CI] 46–64 percent) and 39 percent (95 percent CI 30–48 percent), respectively. The 8-year OS rate was also significantly superior in the HDT arm (64 percent) compared with the sequential chemotherapy arm (49 percent). A recent randomized study from another French group has confirmed these results.[44] Based on these data, HDT with autologous stem cell transplantation may be considered for selected patients who achieve CR with a dose-intense and/or dose-dense regimen.[21] However, the role of HDT and transplantation in this setting has been challenged by a recent metaanalysis.[31,45] The current US intergroup study (S9704), which is assessing the role of HDT and autologous stem cell transplantation after 5 cycles of R-CHOP versus completing 8 total cycles in younger patients with high-intermediate or high-risk disease, should further inform this debate.

To build on these results, the GELA is currently testing two hypotheses. The first one includes rituximab in the ACVBP regimen in order to decrease progression during treatment. The second tries to decrease the relapse rate further with the use of rituximab maintenance after HDT. Preliminary results of this latter study indicate a potential benefit of such rituximab maintenance in patients in CR after HDT.[46]

The recommended approach in these high-risk patients might combine everything that has proven efficacy: rituximab combined with a dose-dense and dose-intense chemotherapy, intensification with autologous stem cell transplantation, and maintenance with rituximab. If this approach does not succeed in improving outcome, success may only come from new drugs not yet available.

Very old patients with diffuse large B cell lymphoma

Patients aged over 80 years represent a growing group and more than 50 percent of those who develop lymphoma have DLBCL. Most of them are able to receive life-prolonging treatment but conventional therapies may not be feasible due to comorbid conditions, poor general health, or inadequate marrow reserve.[47] However, a not-negligible proportion may be alive in CR 2 years later, provided an active regimen is used.[48] Relatively few prospective studies have specifically addressed this group of patients. Single-agent chemotherapy is associated with a very poor outcome and standard chemotherapy should be tested, but classical CHOP is probably too toxic for most of these patients.[49,50] The addition of rituximab to chemotherapy will certainly increase the response to treatment without additional toxicity, as in younger patients, but the best chemotherapy regimen to be used remains unknown. The GELA is currently conducting a study with 'adapted' R-CHOP in these patients. 'Adapted' means that the doses of doxorubicin, cyclophosphamide, and vincristine are reduced for the first cycle (25 mg/m^2, 400 mg/m^2, and 1 mg/m^2, respectively) but may be increased in subsequent cycles if the tolerance is good. With the combination of rituximab, it seems possible that there will be a significant number of complete responses and that it will be possible to prolong the survival of these patients without harming them.

POSITRON EMISSION TOMOGRAPHY SCANS FOR EVALUATION OF RESPONSE AND MAKING TREATMENT DECISIONS

Positron emission tomography using ^{18}F-fluorodeoxyglucose is a powerful functional imaging tool for staging, restaging, and response assessment in DLBCL patients (see separate chapter in this book; see Chapter 45). The advantage of PET over conventional imaging techniques is its ability to distinguish between viable tumor and fibrosis in residual mass(es) often present following treatment. This information may have important clinical consequences: in a retrospective study of 56 patients with DLBCL, PET not only increased the number of documented CRs, but the term CRu (complete remission unconfirmed) was eliminated.[18] Such findings provided the rationale for incorporating FDG-PET into the revised criteria of the International Working Group on response evaluation.[51]

However, a number of issues with PET need to be considered before applying it to all patients and basing studies on its results. First, the technique for performing and interpreting PET is not yet standardized. There is variability among both readers and equipment. Positron emission tomography is also associated with false-positive findings due to non-lymphoma masses such as 'rebound' thymic hyperplasia, infectious or inflammatory changes, or 'brown fat.' Particularly important is the false positivity secondary to macrophage activation in large initial tumor masses. So, histologic confirmation is recommended before intensifying treatment as a consequence of FDG uptake on the PET scan. False negativity is rare in patients with DLBCL.

Currently, PET is strongly recommended prior to treatment for patients with DLBCL to better delineate the extent of disease. Positron emission tomography is essential for the posttreatment assessment of DLBCL, particularly if there are persistent masses on the CT scan. Numerous studies have also demonstrated that PET performed after 1–4 cycles of chemotherapy predicts patient outcome.[19,52,53] This may be the way to propose PET-driven studies where patients would receive a different treatment according to the PET response. However, there are as yet no data demonstrating any improvement in patient outcome by altering treatment based on this information.

SPECIAL LOCATIONS

It is widely believed that lymphomas may behave differently in certain sites, and this is certainly true with regard to initial manifestations of the disease and diagnostic procedures. However, no analysis has confirmed this peculiarity with respect to prognostic parameters, type of treatment required, or outcome. Whatever the initial site involved, treatment strategy is dictated by the histologic subtype of the lymphoma and the presence of adverse prognostic parameters, not by its location, with the exception of central nervous system (CNS) lymphomas.

Gastrointestinal tract lymphomas

One-half of gastrointestinal (GI) tract lymphomas are small cell 'MALT' (mucosal-associated lymphoid tissue) lymphomas, which are commonly localized and have a very good outcome; the other half are DLBCL or Burkitt lymphomas and are associated with a poorer prognosis, even if localized. However, a high proportion of gastric DLBCL may occur as a transformation of a 'MALT' lymphoma, as witnessed by the persistence of a small cell component. Today, there is no agreement on the percentage of large cells that need to be present for the diagnosis of transformation, nor on the prognostic importance of the presence of these large cells. Patients with less than 20 percent of large cells may be treated as 'small cell only' patients, using antibiotics, but patients presenting with a high proportion of large cells must be treated as for primary DLBCL.

Diagnosis of lymphoma in the stomach or colon is relatively easy with endoscopy, but laparotomy is often required for diagnosis of small bowel lymphomas. The latter are characterized by their insidious course and an acute revelation if intestinal obstruction occurs. In all cases, extensive surgical resection should be avoided. Patients with GI tract lymphomas are treated like patients with the same histologic subtype elsewhere. Patients with DLBCL may have localized disease and surgery is the only way to make the diagnosis. However, treatment should not be different from that for any other localized DLBCL.

Primary central nervous system lymphomas

Patients with primary CNS lymphoma usually have localized disease and a DLBCL subtype. Surgical resection provides little therapeutic benefit. Radiation therapy alone results in a median survival of 12 months and is rarely curative. Complete responses can be achieved with standard chemotherapy regimens containing high-dose methotrexate and intrathecal methotrexate.[54,55] Used in conjunction with radiation therapy, they result in a median survival of 30 months but there is a high local failure rate.

The most effective regimen and the need for radiation therapy have yet to be defined. Recent chemotherapy regimens which include high-dose methotrexate (but no irradiation) result in the same outcome as those using irradiation, but with less neurological toxicity.[55,56] Monoclonal antibodies seem to have the same advantage as in lymphomas at other sites.[57] Inclusion of such patients in prospective trials is mandatory.

Central nervous system relapse occurs as the only site of relapse in 5 percent of patients with DLBCL. Thus, CNS prophylaxis for all patients is certainly not needed. An initial cerebrospinal fluid (CSF) examination is mandatory, particularly in patients with bone marrow infiltration, head and neck location, elevated LDH level, or other adverse parameters, as evidenced by a high-risk IPI score.[58] There is no curative treatment for CNS relapse but high-dose methotrexate alone or combined with high-dose cytarabine yields some responses.

Skin lymphomas

Diffuse large B cell lymphoma may be localized to one site of the skin for a long period of time before disseminating. It is not known whether these patients may be treated with local radiation therapy alone or whether they also need chemotherapy. However, the majority of cutaneous lymphomas behave like other localized lymphomas, with the same outcome and prognostic factors.[59,60] The new WHO-EORTC (European Organization for Research and Treatment in Cancer) classification has determined subtypes associated with location and a good or worse response to treatment. However, the names given to these entities are somewhat misleading; for example, the 'leg type' has a poor outcome irrespective of where it is situated.[61]

Diffuse large B cell lymphomas of bone

Diffuse large B cell lymphoma of bone may be localized to one site, disseminated in several bony sites, or associated with other locations.[62] Primary lymphoma of bone is more frequent in children.[63] These patients should be treated with standard chemotherapy regimens.[64] The only special characteristic is the persistence of bone alterations long after the disappearance of the lymphoma cells, which makes it difficult to evaluate their response to treatment. Positron emission tomography scanning may have a role here.[65] The value of local radiation therapy has not been demonstrated although some retrospective studies have shown longer survival with combined modality therapy.

SPECIAL SITUATIONS

Post-transplant lymphoma and lymphoproliferative disorders

Post-transplant lymphoproliferative disorder (PTLD) includes a large group of lymphoid proliferations affecting solid organ and bone marrow transplant recipients. The wide spectrum of diseases ranges from reactive lymphoid hyperplasias, borderline proliferations, to malignant lymphomas. Post-transplant lymphoproliferative disorder develops in 1 percent to 10 percent of transplant recipients. The main etiologic factors of PTLD development are chronic infections, which because of permanent antigen stimulation cause proliferation, mainly of B lymphocytes. At first they have a reactive polyclonal character, but in the course of the disease they escape from the control of suppressor T lymphocytes and the proliferation becomes monoclonal and neoplastic. Epstein–Barr virus plays a principal role, especially in the development of the much more common lymphomas of the B cell phenotype. According to the newest WHO classification, PTLD is divided into four basic histologic types: (1) reactive early lesions of plasmacytic hyperplasia or infectious mononucleosis-like disease; (2) polymorphic PTLD; (3) monomorphic PTLD, which encompasses different lymphomas described in patients without immunologic deficiency; and (4) Hodgkin and Hodgkin-like lymphomas.

Post-transplant lymphoproliferative disorder may develop in children after allogeneic bone marrow transplant and in adults after organ transplant. In a recent series in 197 adults, extranodal disease including grafted organ involvement was present in 85 patients (80 percent) and the grafted organ was involved in 30 patients (28 percent).[66] At the time of these analyses, 62 patients (58 percent) had died and the median survival for the entire cohort was 31.5 months. In univariate analysis, poor prognostic parameters for overall survival from the time of PTLD diagnosis were poor PS, grafted organ involvement, presence of one or more extranodal sites, both nodal and extranodal disease, high IPI score, advanced stage, and elevated LDH.

Classically, treatment comprises a decrease in immunosuppressive treatment and chemotherapy has been associated with variable results. Recently, rituximab has demonstrated activity in post-transplant lymphomas: 44 percent of 43 patients responded, two-thirds of them remaining in continuous CR at 1 year, with a 56 percent 1-year survival.[67,68] For patients not responding to or progressing after rituximab, chemotherapy is indicated, but no standard exists regarding the regimen or its dose intensity and it is often considered toxic.[69,70]

Lymphoma during pregnancy

Coincidental lymphoma and pregnancy is a rare event, occurring in about 1 in 1000 deliveries. The number of pregnant women with newly diagnosed non-Hodgkin lymphoma (NHL) is undoubtedly less than with Hodgkin lymphoma. Pregnant women with NHL usually present with unusual manifestations, aggressive subtypes, advanced stage disease, and poor outcome. Both staging and treatment depend on the term of the pregnancy. A high incidence of breast, uterine, cervical, and ovarian involvement has been reported. Most of the lymphomas associated with pregnancy are disseminated. One likely explanation for this pattern is the frequent delay in diagnosis, some symptoms of pregnancy mimicking symptoms of lymphoma (asthenia, vomiting, weight loss, breast enlargement, colicky abdominal pain).[71]

Major toxicities for the fetus occur during the first trimester of pregnancy, so treatment should be avoided during this period. If the treatment cannot be delayed until the end of the first trimester, often the patient with aggressive NHL requires early chemotherapy, and a therapeutic abortion should be proposed. However, most of these women, especially those with Hodgkin lymphoma or DLCL in the second part of pregnancy, will be cured, remain fertile, and can potentially become pregnant again. Recent observations tend to demonstrate that if modern treatment modalities are applied early in the course of the lymphoma, during pregnancy, the response to treatment, failure, and progression rates are similar to those of nonpregnant women.[71,72] Standard treatment for DLBCL during pregnancy should be R-CHOP chemotherapy as for nonpregnant women.

Patients with transformed lymphoma at time of diagnosis

An unknown fraction of patients diagnosed with DLBCL are in fact those who have had undiagnosed small cell lymphoma for some weeks, months, or years prior to transformation into more aggressive lymphoma. This is evidenced by the presence of a small cell infiltrate in the tumor or in another part of the body, particularly bone marrow.[4–6] Sometimes, it is only the fact that the patient develops a small cell lymphoma at recurrence that allows one to retrospectively classify the case as a transformed lymphoma. Usually, the small cell proliferation is follicular or marginal zone lymphoma, but small lymphocytic lymphoma is possible, and sometimes the correct diagnosis is only made at the time of recurrence.

Few prospective studies exist for such de novo transformed lymphoma but the consensus among experts is that standard treatment, i.e., R-CHOP, is the best regimen.[73] Others consider these patients as having more aggressive disease and advocate HDT with autotransplant as part of first-line therapy.

NONRESPONDING PATIENTS

Refractory patients

Refractory patients are defined as those who progress during initial treatment and those who do not reach a partial or complete response at the end of planned chemotherapy. Sometimes, patients in whom a response has been achieved but who relapse very early (say, within 6 months) are included in this definition.

Refractoriness to a standard chemotherapy regimen is a major adverse prognostic parameter, with only a very small proportion of these patients responding to a salvage regimen and reaching the point of HDT with autologous transplant. No specific parameter has been described as being associated with refractoriness and if it is more frequent in patients with a high-risk IPI score, and it may also occur in patients with less aggressive disease. The use of dose-intense or dose-dense chemotherapy is associated with nearly the same percentage of refractory patients as that seen with CHOP or R-CHOP regimens.

No chemotherapy regimen results in a good response rate in such patients. EPOCH (etoposide, prednisone, vincristine, cyclophosphamide and doxorubicin) combined

with rituximab has been proposed.[74] Other classical salvage regimens may result in a response but the overall survival of these patients is usually very poor, with fewer than 5 percent alive 3 years after diagnosis.

Partial response

Partial response is not sufficient to ensure long life in DLBCL; all such patients usually progress within months of stopping treatment. Salvage chemotherapy may result in a 50 percent response rate but fewer than 30 percent CRs and all responders usually fail within 2 years.[75] High-dose therapy with autologous stem cell transplantation has been effective in some of these patients.[76] However, these studies were conducted at a time when PET scans were not available and probably few of these patients had proven persistent lymphoma. Nonetheless, HDT is currently the only possibility for cure.

TREATMENT AT RECURRENCE

Around 30 percent of patients with DLBCL in whom a complete response is achieved will subsequently relapse. Relapses usually occur during the first 2 years following completion of therapy. Duration of first response and response to the salvage chemotherapy are major prognostic factors, although prognostic parameters that influenced outcome at diagnosis are also predictive of outcome after relapse.

Numerous salvage regimens that incorporate drugs not used in first-line therapy have been proposed.[77] If 70 percent of the patients respond to salvage therapy, only 20–35 percent achieve a second complete response, and the median TTF is usually less than 1 year, with fewer than 10 percent of patients with recurrent disease experiencing long disease-free survival. Interpretation of clinical trials of salvage regimens is complicated because many patients with recurrent lymphoma die before receiving therapy or are not included in clinical trials. Although no randomized study has demonstrated a benefit for adding rituximab to chemotherapy, numerous phase II or retrospective analyses have shown better results when it is included than those achieved with the same regimen without the antibody.

HIGH-DOSE TREATMENT

The promising results of pilot series using HDT in recurrent DLCL lymphoma were confirmed by the results of the PARMA trial.[78] High-dose therapy with autologous stem cell transplantation is the only treatment that yields more than 5 percent long-term survival in patients with recurrent disease and it should be considered after first relapse in all patients younger than 65 years who respond to salvage chemotherapy.[79] The different high-dose therapy modalities that need to be explored and the questions that remain are:

- Whether it is necessary to 'purge' peripheral blood progenitor cells of residual, morphologically undetectable lymphoma cells and how to do it. No trial has as yet succeeded in showing a benefit for the *ex vivo* 'purge.' The use of rituximab prior to HDT has the advantage of also depleting (*in vivo*) blood and bone marrow of lymphoma cells.[80]
- The best conditioning regimen has still to be defined.[81]
- The advantage of incorporating radiolabeled monoclonal antibodies into the conditioning regimen is being investigated.[82]
- The possible advantage of maintenance therapy with rituximab in patients in whom CR has been achieved.[83]

High-dose therapy should be considered for all patients who relapse after chemotherapy, and then respond to salvage therapy, because lymphoma cells may acquire resistance with progression, and subsequent complete responses are rare and of short duration. For patients with recurrent disease who do not respond to salvage therapy, HDT is not helpful: it is estimated that fewer than 5 percent will benefit.[84] There is some evidence that late relapses are not associated with a better outcome than early relapses (manuscript in preparation) and thus HDT with auto-transplant should be proposed to all patients who are eligible for such therapy.

FUTURE DEVELOPMENTS AND PENDING QUESTIONS

Treatment for DLBCL is not yet standardized, and many questions remain to be answered in prospective trials. The most important ones concern: how to recognize and treat patients with refractory disease; the role of maintenance therapy after CR; the place of radiation therapy (if any) in the initial treatment of DLBCL; the importance of adding drug-resistance modulators to current regimens; and the exact role of oncogenes and antioncogenes in the development and treatment of lymphomas.

Immunotherapy

The use of rituximab in combination with chemotherapy is now established. However, the role of other interesting treatment modalities such as radioimmunotherapy or immunotoxins (as compared to naked monoclonal antibodies) is not well defined.[85,86] New monoclonal antibodies with different target antigens are currently being developed and their place in therapy is not known. In animal models, both clinical and immune responses have been documented in subjects with B cell lymphoma

using vaccines. Novel approaches to further enhance the immunologic and clinical activity of vaccines targeting patient-specific proteins are being studied.[87]

Radiation therapy

As described above, radiation therapy has been used as part of treatment for localized disease or in bulky disease in conjunction with chemotherapy. Late toxicity has been demonstrated in Hodgkin lymphoma and no randomized trials have demonstrated any benefit for combined modality therapy in DLBCL (see above). However, even in the absence of any evidence of benefit, it continues to be used routinely by some physicians.

Drug resistance

Several mechanisms of acquired resistance to anticancer drugs have been described but multiple drug resistance (MDR) is the best known. Although fewer than 5 percent of lymphoma cells are MDR+ at diagnosis, the percentage increases in patients progressing. Around 15 percent of DLBCL are refractory to initial treatment. Mechanisms other than MDR have a role but have not yet been completely explained.[88] The precise role of drug resistance is unknown but it may account for most of the observed failures; this needs to be analyzed in the future, as do inhibitors of the different mechanisms.[89]

Oncogene modulation and antioncogenes as lymphoma treatment

Oncogene activation or tumor-suppressor gene inhibition are responsible for lymphoma development and progression through numerous mechanisms, which are still only partially understood. Modulation of the activity of these genes could be a promising future challenge. Gene modulation may be attempted with cell-surface receptor stimulation or inhibition, antisense therapy, or genetic modulation. Few of these have as yet demonstrated efficacy and progressed to clinical application.

CONCLUSIONS

During the last 20 years, the outcome of patients with DLBCL has improved significantly. Major improvements were (1) the addition of rituximab to chemotherapy regimens, with higher response rates and lower relapse rates; (2) intensification with high-dose therapy for patients with poor-risk lymphoma in whom CR was achieved; and (3) the benefit associated with dose-dense and dose-intense regimens. However, more studies need to be conducted to improve the outcome of these patients, particularly those with truly refractory lymphoma and those older than 80 years.

Cure is usually obtained with first-line therapy, but high-dose therapy may be needed at recurrence and for patients in whom only a partial response is achieved. However, definitive strategies are still pending and entering patients into prospective trials is highly recommended.

Patients refractory to initial chemotherapy have a very poor prognosis and nothing in the current spectrum of antilymphoma drugs results in lasting responses in these patients. However, new agents with *in vitro* activity in lymphoma are in ongoing phase I or phase II studies.[90,91]

Better outcome may be observed in patients treated by physicians with extensive experience in this complicated disease, and physicians who treat fewer than 20 patients a year would be well advised to have regular contact with a referral center. Whatever the treatment and its results, patients with lymphoma should be followed up for years for detection of possible late adverse effects and late recurrences.

KEY POINTS

Key issues covered in this chapter:

- Diffuse large B cell lymphoma
- R-CHOP
- Rituximab
- Chemotherapy
- Relapse
- Autotransplant
- Cure

REFERENCES

● = Key primary paper
◆ = Major review article

◆1. Coiffier B. Current strategies for the treatment of diffuse large B cell lymphoma. *Curr Opin Hematol* 2005; **12**: 259–65.

◆2. Coiffier B. State-of-the-art therapeutics: diffuse large B-cell lymphoma. *J Clin Oncol* 2005; **23**: 6387–93.

3. Coiffier B, Reye F. Best treatment of aggressive non-Hodgkin's lymphoma: A French perspective. *Oncology* 2005; **18**(4 Suppl): 7–15.

4. Ghesquières H, Berger F, Felman P *et al.* Clinicopathological characteristics and outcome of diffuse large B-cell lymphomas presenting with an associated low-grade component at diagnosis. *J Clin Oncol* 2006; **24**: 5234–41.

5. Kim H. Composite lymphoma and related disorders. *Am J Clin Pathol* 1993; **99**: 445–51.

6. Conlan MG, Bast M, Armitage JO, Weisenburger DD. Bone marrow involvement by non-Hodgkin's lymphoma: the clinical significance of morphologic discordance between the lymph node and bone marrow. *J Clin Oncol* 1990; **8**: 1163–72.

●7. The International Non-Hodgkin's Lymphoma Prognostic Factors Project. A predictive model for aggressive non-Hodgkin's lymphoma. *N Engl J Med* 1993; **329**: 987–94.

8. Wu G, Keating A. Biomarkers of potential prognostic significance in diffuse large B-cell lymphoma. *Cancer* 2006; **106**: 247–57.

◆9. Shivakumar L, Armitage JO. Bcl-2 gene expression as a predictor of outcome in diffuse large B-cell lymphoma. *Clin Lymphoma Myeloma* 2006; **6**: 455–7.

10. Winter JN, Weller EA, Horning SJ *et al.* Prognostic significance of Bcl-6 protein expression in DLBCL treated with CHOP or R-CHOP: a prospective correlative study. *Blood* 2006; **107**: 4207–13.

11. Visco C, Canal F, Parolini C *et al.* The impact of P53 and P21waf1 expression on the survival of patients with the germinal center phenotype of diffuse large B-cell lymphoma. *Haematologia* 2006; **91**: 687–90.

◆12. Campbell LJ. Cytogenetics of lymphomas. *Pathology* 2005; **37**:493–507.

◆13. Dunphy CH. Gene expression profiling data in lymphoma and leukemia: review of the literature and extrapolation of pertinent clinical applications. *Arch Pathol Lab Med* 2006; **130**: 483–520.

14. Lech-Maranda E, Baseggio L, Bienvenu J *et al.* Interleukin-10 gene promoter polymorphisms influence the clinical outcome of diffuse large B-cell lymphoma. *Blood* 2004; **103**: 3529–34.

●15. Rosenwald A, Wright G, Chan WC *et al.* The use of molecular profiling to predict survival after chemotherapy for diffuse large-B-cell lymphoma. *N Engl J Med* 2002; **346**: 1937–47.

16. Hans CP, Weisenburger DD, Greiner TC *et al.* Confirmation of the molecular classification of diffuse large B-cell lymphoma by immunohistochemistry using a tissue microarray. *Blood* 2004; **103**: 275–82.

●17. Cheson BD, Horning SJ, Coiffier B *et al.* Report of an international workshop to standardize response criteria for non-Hodgkin's lymphomas. *J Clin Oncol* 1999; **17**: 1244–53.

●18. Juweid ME, Wiseman GA, Vose JM *et al.* Response assessment of aggressive non-Hodgkin's lymphoma by integrated International Workshop Criteria and fluorine-18-fluorodeoxyglucose positron emission tomography. *J Clin Oncol* 2005; **23**: 4652–61.

19. Haioun C, Itti E, Rahmouni A *et al.* [18F]fluoro-2-deoxy-D-glucose positron emission tomography (FDG-PET) in aggressive lymphoma: an early prognostic tool for predicting patient outcome. *Blood* 2005; **106**: 1376–81.

●20. Fisher RI, Gaynor ER, Dahlberg S *et al.* Comparison of a standard regimen (CHOP) with three intensive chemotherapy regimens for advanced non-Hodgkin's lymphoma. *N Engl J Med* 1993; **328**: 1002–6.

21. Coiffier B. Increasing chemotherapy intensity in aggressive lymphomas: A renewal? *J Clin Oncol* 2003; **21**: 2457–9.

22. Shipp MA, Neuberg D, Janicek M *et al.* High-dose CHOP as initial therapy for patients with poor-prognosis aggressive

non-Hodgkin's lymphoma: a dose-finding pilot study. *J Clin Oncol* 1995; **13**: 2916–23.

23. Blayney DW, LeBlanc ML, Grogan T *et al.* Dose-intense chemotherapy every 2 weeks with dose-intense cyclophosphamide, doxorubicin, vincristine, and prednisone may improve survival in intermediate- and high-grade lymphoma: a phase II study of the Southwest Oncology Group (SWOG 9349). *J Clin Oncol* 2003; **21**: 2466–73.

24. Tilly H, Lepage E, Coiffier B *et al.* Intensive conventional chemotherapy (ACVBP regimen) compared with standard CHOP for poor-prognosis aggressive non-Hodgkin lymphoma. *Blood* 2003; **102**: 4284–9.

25. Pfreundschuh M, Trumper L, Kloess M *et al.* Two-weekly or 3-weekly CHOP chemotherapy with or without etoposide for the treatment of elderly patients with aggressive lymphomas: Results of the NHL-B2 trial of the DSHNHL. *Blood* 2004; **104**: 634–41.

●26. Haioun C, Lepage E, Gisselbrecht C *et al.* Survival benefit of high-dose therapy in poor-risk aggressive non-Hodgkin's lymphoma: final analysis of the prospective LNH87-2 protocol – a Groupe d'Etude des Lymphomes de l'Adulte Study. *J Clin Oncol* 2000; **18**: 3025–30.

27. Coiffier B, Haioun C, Ketterer N *et al.* Rituximab (anti-CD20 monoclonal antibody) for the treatment of patients with relapsing or refractory aggressive lymphoma: a multicenter phase II study. *Blood* 1998; **92**: 1927–32.

28. Vose JM, Link BK, Grossbard ML *et al.* Phase II study of rituximab in combination with CHOP chemotherapy in patients with previously untreated, aggressive non-Hodgkin's lymphoma. *J Clin Oncol* 2001; **19**: 389–97.

●29. Coiffier B, Lepage E, Briere J *et al.* CHOP chemotherapy plus rituximab compared with CHOP alone in elderly patients with diffuse large-B-cell lymphoma. *N Engl J Med* 2002; **346**: 235–42.

30. Sehn LH, Donaldson J, Chhanabhai M *et al.* Introduction of combined CHOP plus rituximab therapy dramatically improved outcome of diffuse large B-cell lymphoma in British Columbia. *J Clin Oncol* 2005; **23**: 5027–33.

●31. Pfreundschuh M, Trumper L, Osterborg A *et al.* CHOP-like chemotherapy plus rituximab versus CHOP-like chemotherapy alone in young patients with good-prognosis diffuse large-B-cell lymphoma: a randomised controlled trial by the MabThera International Trial (MInT) Group. *Lancet Oncol* 2006; **7**: 379–91.

32. Habermann TM, Weller EA, Morrison VA *et al.* Rituximab-CHOP versus CHOP alone or with maintenance rituximab in older patients with diffuse large B-cell lymphoma. *J Clin Oncol* 2006; **24**: 3121–7.

33. Coiffier B. Treatment of Diffuse Large B-cell Lymphoma. *Curr Hematol Rep* 2005; **4**:7–14.

34. Coiffier B. Treatment of aggressive lymphomas: Disseminated cases. *ASCO 2003 Educational book* 2003; 606–11.

35. Pfreundschuh M, Schubert J, Ziepert M *et al.* Six versus eight cycles of bi-weekly CHOP-14 with or without rituximab in elderly patients with aggressive CD20+ B-cell lymphomas: a randomised controlled trial (RICOVER-60). *Lancet Oncol* 2008; **9**: 105–16.

●36. Feugier P, Van Hoof A, Sebban C *et al.* Long-term results of the R-CHOP study in the treatment of elderly patients with diffuse large B-cell lymphoma: a study by the Groupe d'Etude des Lymphomes de l'Adulte. *J Clin Oncol* 2005; **23**: 4117–26.

37. Miller TP, Dahlberg S, Cassady JR *et al.* Chemotherapy alone compared with chemotherapy plus radiotherapy for localized intermediate-and high-grade non-Hodgkin's lymphoma. *N Engl J Med* 1998; **339**: 21–6.

38. Miller TP, Leblanc M, Spier CM *et al.* CHOP alone compared to CHOP plus radiotherapy for early stage aggressive non-Hodgkin's lymphomas: update of the Southwest Oncology Group (SWOG) randomized trial. *Blood* 2001; **98**: 742a.

39. Horning SJ, Weller E, Kim K *et al.* Chemotherapy with or without radiotherapy in limited-stage diffuse aggressive non-Hodgkin's lymphoma: Eastern Cooperative Oncology Group study 1484. *J Clin Oncol* 2004; **22**: 3032–8.

●40. Reyes F, Lepage E, Ganem G *et al.* ACVBP versus CHOP plus radiotherapy for localized aggressive lymphoma. *N Engl J Med* 2005; **352**: 1197–205.

41. Bonnet C, Fillet G, Mounier N *et al.* CHOP alone versus CHOP plus radiotherapy for localized aggressive lymphoma in elderly patients. *J Clin Oncol* 2007; **25**: 787–92.

42. Pfreundschuh M, Trumper L, Kloess M *et al.* Two-weekly or 3-weekly CHOP chemotherapy with or without etoposide for the treatment of young patients with good-prognosis (normal LDH) aggressive lymphomas: results of the NHL-B1 trial of the DSHNHL. *Blood* 2004; **104**: 626–33.

43. Pfreundschuh M, Trumper L, Kloess M *et al.* Two-weekly or 3-weekly CHOP chemotherapy with or without etoposide for the treatment of elderly patients with aggressive lymphomas: results of the NHL-B2 trial of the DSHNHL. *Blood* 2004; **104**: 634–41.

44. Milpied N, Deconinck E, Gaillard F *et al.* Initial treatment of aggressive lymphoma with high-dose chemotherapy and autologous stem-cell support. *N Engl J Med* 2004; **350**: 1287–95.

45. Greb A, Schiefer DH, Bohlius J *et al.* High-dose chemotherapy with autologous stem cell support is not superior to conventional-dose chemotherapy in the first-line treatment of aggressive non-Hodgkin lymphoma: results of a comprehensive meta-analysis. *Blood* 2004; **104**: 263a.

46. Haioun C, Mounier N, Emile J *et al.* Rituximab compared to observation after high-dose consolidative first-line chemotherapy (HDC) with autologous stem cell transplantation in poor-risk diffuse large B-cell lymphoma: updated results of the LNH98-B3 GELA study. Proceedings of the American Soceity of Clinical Oncology Annual Meeting 2007: 8012 (abstract).

47. Thieblemont C, Coiffier B. Lymphoma in older patients. *J Clin Oncol* 2007; **25**: 1916–23.

48. Bairey O, Benjamini O, Blickstein D *et al.* Non-Hodgkin's lymphoma in patients 80 years of age or older. *Ann Oncol* 2006; **17**: 928–34.

49. Thieblemont C, Grossoeuvre A, Houot R *et al.* Lymphoma in very elderly patients more than 80 years old: a retrospective analysis. *Ann Oncol* 2005; **16**(Suppl 5): 102.

50. Thieblemont C, Grossoeuvre A, Houot R *et al.* Non-Hodgkin's lymphoma in very elderly patients over 80 years. A descriptive analysis of clinical presentation and outcome. *Ann Oncol* 2008; **19**: 774–9.

51. Cheson BD, Pfistner B, Juweid ME *et al.* Recommendations for revised response criteria for malignant lymphoma. *J Clin Oncol* 2006; **24**(Suppl): 18S.

52. Kostakoglu L, Coleman M, Leonard JP *et al.* PET predicts prognosis after 1 cycle of chemotherapy in aggressive lymphoma and Hodgkin's disease. *J Nucl Med* 2002; **43**: 1018–27.

53. Spaepen K, Stroobants S, Dupont P *et al.* Prognostic value of positron emission tomography (PET) with fluorine-18 fluorodeoxyglucose. *J Clin Oncol* 2001; **19**: 414–19.

54. Ferreri AJM, Abrey LE, Blay JY *et al.* Summary statement on primary central nervous system lymphomas from the Eighth International Conference on Malignant Lymphoma, Lugano, Switzerland, June 12 to 15, 2002. *J Clin Oncol* 2003; **21**: 2407–14.

55. Batchelor T, Loeffler JS. Primary CNS lymphoma. *J Clin Oncol* 2006; **24**: 1281–8.

56. Fliessbach K, Helmstaedter C, Urbach H *et al.* Neuropsychological outcome after chemotherapy for primary CNS lymphoma: a prospective study. *Neurology* 2005; **64**: 1184–8.

57. Wong ET. Management of central nervous system lymphomas using monoclonal antibodies: challenges and opportunities. *Clin Cancer Res* 2005; **11**: 7151s–7s.

58. McMillan A. Central nervous system-directed preventative therapy in adults with lymphoma. *Br J Haematol* 2005; **131**: 13–21.

59. Querfeld C, Guitart J, Kuzel T, Rosen S. Primary cutaneous lymphomas: a review with current treatment options. *Blood Rev* 2003; **17**: 131–42.

60. Zinzani PL, Quaglino P, Pimpinelli N *et al.* Prognostic factors in primary cutaneous B-cell lymphoma: the Italian Study Group for Cutaneous Lymphomas. *J Clin Oncol* 2006; **24**: 1376–82.

61. Willemze R, Jaffe ES, Burg G *et al.* WHO-EORTC classification for cutaneous lymphomas. *Blood* 2005; **105**: 3768–85.

62. Gill P, Wenger DE, Inwards DJ. Primary lymphomas of bone. *Clin Lymphoma Myeloma* 2005; **6**: 140–2.

63. Glotzbecker MP, Kersun LS, Choi JK *et al.* Primary non-Hodgkin's lymphoma of bone in children. *J Bone Joint Surg Am* 2006; **88**: 583–94.

64. Beal K, Allen L, Yahalom J. Primary bone lymphoma: treatment results and prognostic factors with long-term follow-up of 82 patients. *Cancer* 2006; **106**: 2652–6.

65. Park YH, Kim S, Choi SJ *et al.* Clinical impact of whole-body FDG-PET for evaluation of response and therapeutic decision-making of primary lymphoma of bone. *Ann Oncol* 2005; **16**: 1401–2.

66. Ghobrial IM, Habermann TM, Maurer MJ *et al.* Prognostic analysis for survival in adult solid organ transplant recipients with post-transplantation lymphoproliferative disorders. *J Clin Oncol* 2005; **23**: 7574–82.

67. Choquet S, Leblond V, Herbrecht R *et al.* Efficacy and safety of rituximab in B-cell post-transplantation lymphoproliferative disorders: results of a prospective multicenter phase 2 study. *Blood* 2006; **107**: 3053–7.

68. Svoboda J, Kotloff R, Tsai DE. Management of patients with post-transplant lymphoproliferative disorder: the role of rituximab. *Transpl Int* 2006; **19**: 259–69.

69. Elstrom RL, Andreadis C, Aqui NA *et al.* Treatment of PTLD with rituximab or chemotherapy. *Am J Transplant* 2006; **6**: 569–76.

70. Komrokji RS, Oliva JL, Zand M *et al.* Mini-BEAM and autologous hematopoietic stem-cell transplant for treatment of post-transplant lymphoproliferative disorders. *Am J Hematol* 2005; **79**: 211–15.

71. Traullé C, Coiffier B. Lymphoma and pregnancy. In: Canellos GP, Lister TA, Young B. (eds) *The lymphomas.* Philadelphia, PA: Saunders Elsevier, 2006: 536–41.

72. Pohlman B, Macklis RM. Lymphoma and pregnancy. *Semin Oncol* 2000; **27**: 657–66.

73. Ghesquieres H, Berger F, Felman P *et al.* Clinicopathologic characteristics and outcome of diffuse large B-cell lymphomas presenting with an associated low-grade component at diagnosis. *J Clin Oncol* 2006; **24**: 5234–41.

74. Jermann M, Jost LM, Taverna C *et al.* Rituximab-EPOCH, an effective salvage therapy for relapsed, refractory or transformed B-cell lymphomas: results of a phase II study. *Ann Oncol* 2004; **15**: 511–16.

75. Bosly A, Coiffier B, Gisselbrecht C *et al.* Bone marrow transplantation prolongs survival after relapse in aggressive lymphoma patients treated with the LNH-84 regimen. *J Clin Oncol* 1992; **10**: 1615–23.

76. Haioun C, Lepage E, Gisselbrecht C *et al.* High-dose therapy followed by stem cell transplantation in partial response after first-line induction therapy for aggressive non-Hodgkin's lymphoma. *Ann Oncol* 1998; **9**(Suppl 1): 5–8.

77. Salles G, Shipp MA, Coiffier B. Chemotherapy of non-Hodgkin's aggressive lymphomas. *Semin Hematol* 1994; **31**: 46–69.

78. Philip T, Guglielmi C, Hagenbeek A *et al.* Autologous bone marrow transplantation as compared with salvage chemotherapy in relapses of chemotherapy-sensitive non Hodgkin's lymphoma. *N Engl J Med* 1995; **333**: 1540–5.

79. Shipp MA, Abeloff MD, Antman KH *et al.* International consensus conference on high-dose therapy with hematopoietic stem-cell transplantation in aggressive non-Hodgkin's lymphomas: report of jury. *Ann Oncol* 1999; **10**: 13–19.

80. Arcaini L, Orlandi E, Alessandrino EP *et al.* A model of in vivo purging with Rituximab and high-dose AraC in follicular and mantle cell lymphoma. *Bone Marrow Transplant* 2004; **34**: 175–9.

◆81. Mounier N, Gisselbrecht C. Conditioning regimens before transplantation in patients with aggressive non-Hodgkin's lymphoma. *Ann Oncol* 1998; **9**(Suppl 1): 15–21.

82. Cilley J, Winter JN. Radioimmunotherapy and autologous stem cell transplantation for the treatment of B-cell lymphomas. *Haematologica* 2006; **91**: 113–20.

83. Lim SH, Zhang Y, Wang Z *et al.* Maintenance rituximab after autologous stem cell transplant for high-risk B-cell lymphoma induces prolonged and severe hypogammaglobulinemia. *Bone Marrow Transplant* 2005; **35**: 207–8.

●84. Vose JM, Zhang MJ, Rowlings PA *et al.* Autologous transplantation for diffuse aggressive non-Hodgkin's lymphoma in patients never achieving remission: a report from the Autologous Blood and Marrow Transplant Registry. *J Clin Oncol* 2001; **19**: 406–13.

◆85. Nowakowski GS, Witzig TE. Radioimmunotherapy for B-cell non-Hodgkin lymphoma. *Clin Adv Hematol Oncol* 2006; **4**: 225–31.

86. Frankel AE, Neville DM, Bugge TA *et al.* Immunotoxin therapy of hematologic malignancies. *Semin Oncol* 2003; **30**: 545–57.

87. Bendandi M. The role of idiotype vaccines in the treatment of human B-cell malignancies. *Expert Rev Vaccines* 2004; **3**: 163–70.

88. Carter TA, Wodicka LM, Shah NP *et al.* Inhibition of drug-resistant mutants of ABL, KIT, and EGF receptor kinases. *Proc Natl Acad Sci U S A* 2005; **102**: 11011–16.

89. Hersey P, Zhang XD. Overcoming resistance of cancer cells to apoptosis. *J Cell Physiol* 2003; **196**: 9–18.

90. Cheson BD. What is new in lymphoma? *CA Cancer J Clin* 2004; **54**: 260–72.

91. O'Connor A. Developing new drugs for the treatment of lymphoma. *Eur J Haematol* 2005; **75**(Suppl 66): 150–8.

92. Pfreundschuh M, Kloess M, Schmits R *et al.* Six, Not eight cycles of bi-weekly CHOP with rituximab (R-CHOP-14) is the preferred treatment for elderly patients with diffuse large B-cell lymphoma (DLBCL): results of the RICOVER-60 trial of the German High-Grade Non-Hodgkin Lymphoma Study Group (DSHNHL). *Am Soc Hematol Annu Meet Abstr* 2005; **106**: 13 (abstract).

93. Gisselbrecht C, Lepage E, Molina T *et al.* Shortened first-line high-dose chemotherapy for patients with poor-prognosis aggressive lymphoma. *J Clin Oncol* 2002; **20**: 2472–9.

94. Coiffier B. Fourteen years of high-dose CHOP (ACVB regimen): preliminary conclusions about the treatment of aggressive-lymphoma patients. *Ann Oncol* 1995; **6**: 211–17.

72

Hodgkin lymphoma in adults

BEATE KLIMM AND VOLKER DIEHL

INTRODUCTION

Hodgkin lymphoma (HL), belonging to the neoplastic diseases of the lymphatic tissue, is one of the few curable cancers in adults. Thomas Hodgkin first described the disease in 1832 in his historic paper entitled 'On Some Morbid Appearances of the Exorbant Glands and Spleen'.[1] About 70 years later, Carl Sternberg (1898) and Dorothy Reed (1902) contributed the first definitive microscopic descriptions of the pathognomonic Hodgkin and Reed-Sternberg (RS) cells.[2,3] At that time, Dorothy Reed wrote 'the treatment for this disease is dismal. All patients die within 3–4 years. Even if you resect the tumor totally, it will recur and grow even faster than before…'. Hodgkin already assumed an autonomous lymphatic process rather than an inflammatory condition or an infectious disease like tuberculosis. However, despite the evidence for the malignant nature of HL over the last century, the detection of the malignant clonal origin of RS cells as germinal center-derived B lymphocytes was demonstrated only recently.[4,5]

Since these first descriptions of HL, therapeutic strategies have developed remarkably from surgery, herbs, and arsenic acid to sophisticated stage- and risk-adapted treatment regimens including modern polychemotherapy and radiation therapy. To date, about 80 percent of patients achieve long-term disease-free survival, rendering this entity one of the most curable human cancers. It is therefore of pivotal importance to maintain the high standard of cure rates over all stages reached but at the same time to reduce toxicity.

Current strategies in first-line treatment aim at further improving outcome and thereby preventing therapy-induced complications, such as infertility, cardiopulmonary toxicity, and secondary malignancies. Ongoing trials for patients with early stage disease aim at finding the minimal necessary curative therapy, with the least acute and long-term toxicity. In recent years, there has been a trend to combine chemotherapy and radiation therapy. Recent studies have predominantly investigated lower radiation doses and smaller radiation fields and a possible reduction of chemotherapy in terms of the number of drugs or number of cycles given. For patients with advanced stage disease, newly designed scheduling of established drug combinations with higher dose density and intensity have been developed, which are currently being evaluated in clinical trials. Ongoing studies also utilize positron emission tomography (PET) with fluorodeoxyglucose to detect an early satisfactory response after chemotherapy, possibly rendering consolidation with radiation unnecessary. Approaches for relapsed HL consist of salvage radiation therapy, salvage chemotherapy, and high-dose chemotherapy followed by autologous stem cell transplantation. In recent years, the introduction of effective salvage high-dose therapy and a better understanding of prognostic factors have remarkably improved the management of relapsed HL. For multiply pretreated patients, antibody-based agents such as radioimmunoconjugates, monoclonal antibodies, and, lately, small molecules targeting signal transcription pathways have demonstrated some clinical efficacy; these efforts, however, are still purely experimental.

EPIDEMIOLOGY AND ETIOLOGY

Incidence, age, and histologic distribution

In Europe and the United States, the annual incidence of HL is about 2–3 per 100 000 persons at risk, and this has stayed almost constant over the last few decades.[6] As a result of remarkable clinical progress in recent years, the mortality rate has simultaneously dropped, particularly in the 1990s, from previous rates above 2 per 100 000 to a current mortality rate of about 0.5 per 100 000.[7]

Slightly more men than women develop HL (1.4:1). Four out of five male sufferers and three out of four females develop HL prior to the age of 60 years, which is very early compared to most other malignancies.[8] In industrialized countries, the age at onset of HL has historically shown two peaks, one in the third decade and a second peak for patients older than 50 years. However, in more recent analyses, the second peak seems to disappear, because some types of large B cell lymphomas of that age group were mistaken for the lymphocyte-depleted subtype of HL in the past.[9] There is a noteworthy difference in the onset of HL between developing and industrialized countries: in developing countries, the disorder usually appears during childhood and the incidence decreases with age, whereas in industrialized countries the first peak is seen in young adulthood. Furthermore, in economically developed countries the early occurrence of HL is often related to high maternal education, early birth order, low number of siblings and playmates, and single family dwellings.[10,11]

The incidence of HL by age also depends upon histologic subtype. Among the group of young adults, the most common subtype is nodular sclerosing (NS) HL, occurring at a higher frequency than the mixed-cellularity (MC) subtype. The frequency of MC HL increases with age, while

Table 72.1 World Health Organization classification of Hodgkin lymphoma

	Frequency
Classical Hodgkin lymphoma	
Nodular sclerosis Hodgkin lymphoma (grades 1 and 2)	60–70%
Mixed cellularity Hodgkin lymphoma	20–30%
Lymphocyte-rich classical Hodgkin lymphoma	3–5%
Lymphocyte-depleted Hodgkin lymphoma	0.8–1%
Nodular lymphocyte-predominant Hodgkin lymphoma	3–5%

Extracted and modified from Harris et al. 1999.[13]

NS subtypes reach a plateau in the group more than 30 years of age. According to the World Health Organization (WHO) classification, the subtypes of lymphocyte-rich classical HL (LRCHL), nodular lymphocyte-predominant HL (NLPHL), and lymphocyte-depleted HL (LDHL) are less commonly diagnosed (Table 72.1).[12,13]

Role of Epstein–Barr virus and genetic factors

Involvement of viral infections (e.g., Epstein–Barr virus [EBV]) in the pathogenesis of HL was suggested by several studies. Patients with a medical history of EBV-related mononucleosis have a two- to threefold increased risk of developing HL.[14] In about 50 percent of cases of classical HL in Western countries, EBV DNA is present in the RS cells, predominantly in the mixed-cellularity subtype.[15] In contrast, patients with low socioeconomic status as well as patients from developing countries show EBV-positive RS cells in about 90 percent of the cases.[16–18] However, since EBV is not present in the tumor cells of a substantial proportion of patients in the Western world, other viruses might be involved in the transformation process although their role is uncertain.

Genetic components seem to contribute to the appearance of HL. Family members of patients affected by HL are at a three- to ninefold increased risk of developing the disease.[19,20] Furthermore, the analysis of monozygotic twin pairs and the remarkable proportion in which both twins are affected strongly supports the idea of HL as a genetically imbalanced disorder.[21] However, no specific mechanism of inheritance or evidence for a genetic translocation unique to cases of familial HL have been identified so far and familial HL only appears to play a role in a small subset of patients.

Pathophysiology

For a long time HL was considered as an infectious disease, as indicated by its former name 'lymphogranulomatosis.' The giant mono- and multinucleated RS cells typically account for less than 1 percent of the affected tissue in classical HL, which made systematic analyses difficult in the past. Reed-Sternberg cells are derived from germinal center B cells in more than 90 percent of cases;[5] however, in a small group of patients the RS cells exhibit T cell characteristics.[22]

Hodgkin lymphoma can basically be distinguished from others types of malignant lymphoma by the presence of RS cells in a background of non-neoplastic cells such as lymphocytes, histiocytes, neutrophils, eosinophils, and monocytes. The histologic subclassification of HL (see Table 72.1) considers both the morphology and immunophenotype of the RS cells and the composition of the cellular background. The WHO differentiates between the classical form of HL with CD30-positive RS cells and the nodular lymphocyte-predominant form of HL (NLPHL) with CD20-positive lymphocytic and histiocytic (L&H) cells. In classical HL, immunophenotyping demonstrates that RS cells stain positive for CD15 in about 80 percent and for CD30 in about 90 percent of cases. The activation of B cell antigens has only been reported in a few cases.[23] In contrast, in NLPHL, the L&H cells are scattered within the nodular structures and are usually CD45 positive. They express B cell-associated antigens such as CD20 in 98 percent of the cases, but also express CD19, CD22, CD79a, and epithelial membrane antigen (EMA); however, they lack CD15 and CD30 expression.

Despite enormous efforts and progress in basic research, many key questions concerning transforming events and pathways, oncogenic viruses, and the exact mechanism(s) by which RS cells proliferate and resist apoptosis in the germinal center still remain unanswered. Some reports suggest that nuclear factor κB (NF-κB) is a central effector of malignant transformation in classical HL by downregulation of an antiapoptotic signaling network.[24] Also, *LMP-1*, as an EBV-encoded gene, may induce tumorigenesis by triggering NF-κB activation.[25]

DIAGNOSIS, STAGING, AND CHOICE OF TREATMENT

Clinical presentation

Usually, indolent swellings that are localized to the cervical or supraclavicular region (60–70 percent) are noticed, but axillary or inguinal lymph nodes are also often observed. Almost two-thirds of patients with newly diagnosed classical HL have radiographic evidence of intrathoracic involvement. Symptoms caused by a large mediastinal mass can include a feeling of pressure, cough, venous congestion, or even dyspnea owing to tracheal compression or pericardial or pleural effusions. Hepato- or splenomegaly can indicate hepatic or splenic involvement, but affected organs can also be of normal size. In advanced stages, adjacent regions such as lung, pericardium, chest wall, or bone can be invaded and patients sometimes suffer from bone pain or neurological or endocrinological symptoms. Compared

Table 72.2   Anatomic sites of disease involved in untreated patients with Hodgkin lymphoma

Anatomic site	Involvement (%)
Waldeyer's ring	1–2
Cervical nodes	60–70
Axillary nodes	30–35
Mediastinum	50–60
Hilar nodes	15–35
Paraaortic nodes	30–40
Iliac nodes	15–20
Mesenteric nodes	1–4
Inguinal nodes	8–15
Spleen	30–35
Liver	2–6
Bone marrow	1–4
Total extranodal	10–15

Modified from Gupta RK, Gospodarowicz MK, Lister TA. Clinical evaluation and staging of Hodgkin's disease. In: Mauch PM, Armitage JO, Diehl V *et al.* (eds) *Hodgkin's disease.* Philadelphia: Lippincott Williams and Wilkins, 1999: Chapter 15.

with non-Hodgkin lymphomas (NHLs), bulky infradiaphragmatic lesions with obstructive symptoms are rare in HL. Bone marrow involvement occurs in fewer than 10 percent of newly diagnosed patients. Details of organ involvement at diagnosis are given in Table 72.2.

About 40 percent of patients, especially those with initial abdominal involvement or advanced stage disease, demonstrate systemic symptoms – so-called 'B-symptoms' – which are defined as fever >38°C, drenching night sweats, or weight loss >10 percent within the previous 6 months (deliberate or not from other causes). Other symptoms comprise pain at the site of nodal involvement shortly after drinking alcohol, pruritus, or fatigue. Compared with classical HL, NLPHL normally begins as a localized, slowly growing and rather benign entity with participation of only one peripheral nodal region, mostly a cervical or axillary or inguinal lymph node.

Initial diagnostics

Excision biopsy of a suspicious lymph node should be performed to confirm the initial diagnosis. Assessment of the bone marrow is important for disease staging and for evaluation of normal bone marrow function prior to therapy. Accurate staging procedures and risk factor assessment are indispensable for an adequate allocation to treatment groups. However, clinical staging (CS) methods have become less invasive in recent years. They usually include chest x-ray, computed tomography (CT) scans of the neck, thorax, abdomen, and pelvis, bone marrow biopsy, and bone marrow or skeletal radionuclide imaging; abdominal ultrasound is not routinely used any more. In some cases, additional

Table 72.3   The Cotswolds staging classification for Hodgkin lymphoma

Stage	Definition
Stage I	Involvement of a single lymph node region or lymphoid structure (e.g., spleen, thymus, Waldeyer's ring) or involvement of a single extralymphatic site (IE)
Stage II	Involvement of two or more lymph node regions on the same side of the diaphragm; localized contiguous involvement of only one extranodal organ or site and lymph node region(s) on the same side of the diaphragm (IIE) The number of anatomic regions involved should be indicated by a subscript (e.g., II$_3$)
Stage III	Involvement of lymph node regions on both sides of the diaphragm (III), which may also be accompanied by involvement of the spleen (IIIS) or by localized contiguous involvement of only one extranodal organ site (IIIE) or both (IIISE) III$_1$: With or without involvement of splenic, hilar, celiac, or portal nodes III$_2$: With involvement of paraaortic, iliac, and mesenteric nodes
Stage IV	Diffuse or disseminated involvement of one or more extranodal organs or tissues, with or without associated lymph node involvement

Designations applicable to any disease stage

A	No symptoms
B	Fever (temperature >38°C), drenching night sweats, unexplained loss of 10% of body weight within the preceding 6 months
X	Bulky disease (a widening of the mediastinum by more than one-third or the presence of a nodal mass with a maximal dimension greater than 10 cm)
E	Involvement of a single extranodal site that is contiguous or proximal to the known nodal site
CS	Clinical stage
PS	Pathological stage (as determined by laparotomy)

Extracted and modified from Lister *et al.* 1989.[27]

procedures including magnetic resonance imaging (MRI), PET, or a liver biopsy may be indicated. Pathological staging (PS) procedures such as laparotomy or splenectomy to assess occult infradiaphragmatic disease are no longer used routinely. They are associated with possible side effects such as the overwhelming postsplenectomy infection (OPSI) syndrome. Furthermore, better imaging techniques and the introduction of systemic chemotherapy to the majority of patients in early stages have restricted invasive measures to a very few patients for whom the initial diagnostics give conflicting or unresolved results.

Staging classification

Patients with HL are usually treated according to stage and risk factors. The histologic subtype – except the lymphocyte-predominant type – does not influence the treatment decision. The stage of HL at diagnosis is ascribed according to the Ann Arbor classification.[26] The presence (B) or absence (A) of systemic symptoms further characterizes severity of disease. Clinical, biologic, and serologic (age, performance status, high erythrocyte sedimentation rate [ESR]) risk factors also influence the choice of treatment. The Cotswolds classification[27] (a modification of the Ann Arbor classification) includes information about prognostic factors such as mediastinal mass, other bulky nodal disease, extranodal extension of disease, and the extent of subdiaphragmatic disease (Table 72.3).

Prognostic factors and choice of treatment

Prognostic factors define the likely outcome of the disease for an individual patient and help in the selection of appropriate treatment. The two major determinants for dividing patients with HL according to a risk- or prognosis-adapted therapeutic approach are stage and B symptoms. A third clinically relevant factor is massive local tumor burden, e.g., bulk greater than 10 cm or a large mediastinal mass one-third or more of the thoracic diameter.

In North America, the Canada Clinical Trial Group (NCIC) and the ECOG (Eastern Cooperative Oncology Group) treat patients with HL according to the traditional separation into 'early stage' and 'advanced stage' disease. Patients with early stage (CS I–IIA) are further subdivided into a low- and high-risk group. The low-risk category comprises patients aged less than 40 years, with NLPHL or NS histology, with an ESR less than 50 mm/h, and involvement of three or fewer than three nodal sites, whereas the high-risk category includes all other stages I–IIA. Thus, not only patients with stage III–IV disease are considered as having 'advanced stage' as in European studies. Patients with stage CS I–II disease with B symptoms and all patients with CS I–II with bulky disease are included. With this strategy, more patients are included in the advanced stage group and receive more therapy. This must be considered when comparing the data. In Europe, the EORTC (European Organization for Research and Treatment of Cancer), the GELA (Groupe d'Etudes des Lymphomes de

Table 72.4   Definition of treatment groups according to the EORTC, GELA, and GHSG

Treatment groups	EORTC/GELA	GHSG
Early stage favorable	CS I–II without risk factors (supradiaphragmatic)	CS I–II without risk factors
Early stage unfavorable (intermediate)	CS I–II with ⩾1 risk factor (supradiaphragmatic)	CS I, CSIIA ⩾1 risk factor;
		CS IIB with C/D but without A/B
Advanced stage	CS III–IV	CS IIB with A/B
		CS III–IV
Risk factors	A: large mediastinal mass	A: large mediastinal mass
	B: age ⩾50 years	B: extranodal disease
	C: elevated ESR[a]	C: elevated ESR[a]
	D: ⩾4 involved regions	D: ⩾3 involved areas

[a]ESR (erythrocyte sedimentation rate) ⩾50 mm/h without or ⩾30 mm/h with B symptoms.
GHSG, German Hodgkin Lymphoma Study Group; EORTC, European Organization for Research and Treatment of Cancer; GELA, Groupe d'Etude des Lymphomes de l'Adulte; CS, clinical stage.

l'Adulte), and the GHSG (German Hodgkin Lymphoma Study Group) assign patients with early stage disease (I–II) to the favorable or to the unfavorable (intermediate) group depending on the risk factors listed in Table 72.4.[28–30]

In an attempt to define the 'risk' of patients with advanced HL more precisely, a variety of clinical and laboratory parameters were analyzed to construct a prognostic index. The International Prognostic Score (IPS) consists of seven factors that were significantly related to an unfavorable prognosis when present at initial diagnosis of HL: serum albumin <4 g/dL, hemoglobin <10.5 g/dL, male sex, age >45 years, stage IV disease, leukocytosis >15 000/mm^3, lymphocytopenia <600/mm^3, and/or <8 percent of white cells.[31]

FIRST-LINE TREATMENT

Early stage, 'favorable' Hodgkin lymphoma

In the treatment of early stage disease, extended field radiation therapy (EFRT) has been considered the standard treatment modality for a long time. The EFRT technique includes all initially involved and adjacent lymph node regions, leading to large irradiation fields compared with involved field radiation therapy (IFRT), which is restricted to initially involved lymph node regions only.

Together with the successful introduction of MOPP[32] (mechlorethamine, Oncovin [vincristine], procarbazine, and prednisone) and ABVD[33] (adriamycin [doxorubicin], bleomycin, vinblastine, and dacarbazine) chemotherapy for more advanced stage disease in the 1980s, the paradigm shift away from radiation alone to additional chemotherapy in early stage disease was accelerated by the realization of the long-term toxicity and mortality related to large radiation fields and radiation therapy doses. Longer follow-up of patients who underwent EFRT disclosed severe late effects as competing causes of death, including heart failure,[34] pulmonary dysfunction,[35] and secondary malignancies.[36–38] Furthermore, though complete remission was mostly

achieved, there was a high risk of relapse following EFRT alone.[39] Two different strategies evolved to try and prevent these relapses: application of even more intensive radiation therapy and the addition of chemotherapy to control occult lesions.[40] The latter strategy resulted in better outcomes and at the same time made it possible to reduce the amount of radiation therapy.

Today, most centers and groups in Europe and the USA have accepted combined modality treatment, consisting of 2–4 cycles of ABVD, followed by 20–30 Gy IFRT as the standard of care for early favorable stages. Several randomized studies have confirmed the superiority of combined modality treatment over radiation therapy alone.

Recent and ongoing trials are shown in Table 72.5. The Southwest Oncology Group (SWOG) demonstrated that patients treated with combined modality therapy consisting of 3 cycles of doxorubicin and vinblastine followed by subtotal lymphoid irradiation (STLI) had a markedly superior outcome in terms of freedom from treatment failure (FFTF) than those receiving STLI alone.[41] Studies from Milan and Stanford revealed that STLI can be effectively replaced by IFRT after short-duration chemotherapy, such as ABVD or Stanford-V (8 weeks), while maintaining progression-free and overall survival.[42,43] The EORTC and GELA studies demonstrated that combined modality therapy with either 6 cycles of EBVP (epirubicin, bleomycin, vinblastine, and prednisone) (H7F trial) or 3 cycles of MOPP/ABV (H8F trial) followed by IFRT yielded a significantly better event-free survival compared with subtotal nodal irradiation alone.[44,45] The aim of the H9F trial was to evaluate possible dose reduction of radiation therapy (36 Gy, 20 Gy, or no radiation therapy) after administering 6 cycles of EBVP. However, the arm without radiation therapy was closed prematurely due to a higher relapse rate than expected.[46,47] Furthermore, in another analysis that was recently published by the Canada Clinical Trials Group and the ECOG, freedom from progression was superior for a strategy including radiation therapy compared with ABVD alone for early 'favorable-risk' patients.[48]

Table 72.5   Selected trials for early stage favorable Hodgkin lymphoma

Trial	Therapy regimen	n	Outcome	Ref.
SWOG 9133	A. 3 (dox + vinbl) + STLI (36–40 Gy)	165	94% (FFTF); 98% (OS)	41
	B. STLI (36–40 Gy)	161	81% (FFTF); 96% (OS) [3 years]	
Milan 1990–1997	A. 4 ABVD + STLI	65	97% (FFP); 93% (OS)	42
	B. 4 ABVD + IFRT	68	97% (FFP); 93% (OS) [5 years]	
Stanford-V (CSI-IIA)	8 weeks of Stanford-V + modified IFRT (30 Gy)	65	94.6% (FFP); 96.6% (OS) [16 months; estimated for 3 years]	43
EORTC/GELA H7F	A. 6 EBVP + IFRT (36 Gy)	168	90% (RFS); 98% (OS)	44
	B. STNI	165	81% (RFS); 95% (OS) [5 years]	
EORTC/GELA H8F	A. 3 MOPP/ABV + IFRT (36 Gy)	271	99% (RFS); 99% (OS)	45
	B. STNI	272	80% (RFS); 95% (OS) [4 years]	
EORTC/GELA H9F	A. 6 EBVP + IFRT (36 Gy)	783	87% (EFS); 98% (OS)	47
	B. 6 EBVP + IFRT (20 Gy)		84% (EFS); 98% (OS) [4 years]	
	C. 6 EBVP		C closed because of high relapse rate;	
GHSG HD7	A. EFRT 30 Gy (40 Gy IF)	305	75% (FFTF); 94% (OS);	49
	B. 2 ABVD + EFRT 30 Gy (40 Gy IF)	312	91% (FFTF); 94% (OS) [5 years]	
GHSG HD10	A. 4 ABVD + IFRT (30 Gy)	847	Interim analysis [2 years]	50
	B. 4 ABVD + IFRT (20 Gy)		all pts	
	C. 2 ABVD + IFRT (30 Gy)		96.6%(FFTF)	
	D. 2 ABVD + IFRT (20 Gy)		98.5% (OS)	
GHSG HD13	A. 2 ABVD + IFRT (30 Gy)		Ongoing trial	
	B. 2 ABV + IFRT (30 Gy)			
	C. 2 AVD + IFRT (30 Gy)			
	D. 2 AV + IFRT (30 Gy)			

SWOG, Southwest Oncology Group; EORTC, European Organization for Research and Treatment of Cancer; GELA, Groupe d'Etude des Lymphomes de l'Adulte; GHSG, German Hodgkin Lymphoma Study Group; EF/IFRT, extended/involved field radiation therapy; STLI, subtotal lymphoid irradiation; STNI, subtotal nodal irradiation; FFTF, freedom from treatment failure; RFS, relapse-free survival; FFP, freedom from progression; EFS, event-free suvival; OS, overall survival; pts, patients; dox, doxorubicin; vinbl, vinblastine; ABVD: adriamycin (doxorubicin), bleomycin, vinblastine, dacarbazine; Stanford-V: mechlorethamine, adriamycin (doxorubicin), vinblastine, vincristine, bleomycin, etoposide, prednisone; EBVP: epirubicin, bleomycin, vinblastine, prednisone; MOPP: mechlorethamine, Oncovin (vincristine), procarbazine, prednisone.

Thus, the use of chemotherapy only in early stages should still be regarded as experimental.

In the GHSG study, a combined modality approach was established in the HD7 trial, in which 2 cycles of ABVD plus EFRT were shown to be superior to EFRT alone in terms of FFTF. Overall survival (OS) was equal in both arms due to effective salvage treatment.[49]

With respect to the excellent long-term survival rates, further improvement of treatment seems difficult. Thus, strategies to reduce drug dose and toxicity while maintaining efficacy are being pursued. In the subsequent HD10 trial of the GHSG, a possible reduction in chemotherapy from four to two cycles of ABVD and/or IFRT from 30 to 20 Gy was evaluated. After a median observation time of two years, FFTF and OS rates were 96.6 percent and 98.5 percent, respectively. So far, no significant differences in FFTF and OS have been detected between 4 × ABVD and 2 × ABVD, or between the different doses of radiation therapy (30 Gy vs 20 Gy).[50] The aim of the ongoing GHSG HD13 trial is to omit the presumably less effective but toxic drugs bleomycin or dacarbazine from ABVD. Patients are thus randomized between 2 cycles of ABVD, ABV, AVD, or AV followed by 30 Gy IFRT.

Early stage, 'unfavorable' (intermediate) Hodgkin lymphoma

Patients with early stage, 'unfavorable' (intermediate) HL generally qualify for combined modality treatment. However, the ideal chemotherapy and radiation regimens are not yet clearly defined. Attempts are being made to reduce both radiation dose and field size. Several trials seem to indicate that reduction of field size does not compromise efficacy: a cooperative study comparing 6 cycles of MOPP sandwiched around 40 Gy of radiation therapy (either IFRT or EFRT) indicated no difference in terms of disease-free survival or OS.[51] Another trial from Italy comparing STLI with IFRT after 4 cycles of ABVD in patients with early 'favorable' (see Table 72.5) and 'unfavorable' disease reported a similar treatment outcome in both arms.[42] In the H8U trial (EORTC) patients were randomized between 6 cycles of MOPP/ABV plus 36 Gy IFRT, 4 cycles of MOPP/ABV plus 36 Gy IFRT, and 4 cycles MOPP/ABV plus STLI. There was no difference in terms of response rates, failure-free survival, or overall survival.[52] The largest trial investigating radiation therapy reduction was conducted by the GHSG: in the HD8 trial, patients were randomized to two alternating cycles of COPP (cyclophosphamide, Oncovin [vincristine], procarbazine, and prednisone)/ABVD plus radiation therapy, either EFRT (arm A) or IFRT (arm B). Final results at 5 years did not disclose significant differences between the two arms in terms of FFTF and OS; however, more toxicity was reported in the patients who were treated with EFRT (Table 72.6).[53]

Efforts have also been made to improve the efficacy of chemotherapy by altering drugs and schedules as well as the number of cycles. In the past, alternation or hybridization of a MOPP-like regimen with ABVD did not produce better outcomes when compared with ABVD alone. Furthermore, studies in advanced stage HL indicated that ABVD alone is equally effective and less myelotoxic compared with alternating MOPP/ABVD, and both are superior to MOPP alone.[54] Thus, a combined modality treatment consisting of 4–6 cycles of ABVD followed by 30 Gy IFRT is considered standard for patients with early stage, 'unfavorable' HL. Despite the excellent initial remission rates obtained with ABVD and radiation therapy, approximately 15 percent of patients in early 'unfavorable' stage disease relapse within 5 years and about another 5 percent suffer from primary refractory disease. These outcome rates are comparable to those for patients with advanced stage disease, when treated with more intensive regimens.

Thus, regimens are currently being evaluated (Table 72.6) that were previously pioneered for the treatment of advanced stage HL. In the ongoing intergroup trial 2496, the ECOG and SWOG assess whether the Stanford-V regimen (12 weeks) is superior to 6 cycles of ABVD. In another

approach, a comparison between 4 cycles of ABVD and 4 of 'BEACOPP baseline' (bleomycin, etoposide, adriamycin [doxorubicin], cyclophosphamide, Oncovin [vincristine], procarbazine, and prednisone) is being conducted by the EORTC-GELA (H9U trial) as well as by the GHSG (HD11 trial). In addition, two large trials are addressing the question of whether 4 cycles of combined modality treatment are as effective as 6 cycles (EORTC H8U and H9U trials).

In the H9U trial that was recently presented by the EORTC and GELA, patients were randomly assigned to 6 cycles of ABVD or 4 cycles of ABVD or 4 cycles of 'BEACOPP baseline,' followed by 30 Gy of IFRT in all arms. After a median follow-up of 4 years, no significant difference was observed in event-free survival (EFS) or OS.[47] Interim results of the GHSG trial HD11 at 2 years demonstrated a FFTF of 89.9 percent and an OS of 97.4 percent for all patients. There was also no difference in outcome between ABVD and BEACOPP nor between 30 Gy and 20 Gy IFRT.[55] Taking into account that these were relatively early data, there is no evidence for changing treatment from 4 to 6 cycles of ABVD or for recommending 4 cycles of 'BEACOPP baseline' in this group of patients. However, the low FFTF in this risk group led the GHSG to a further intensification of treatment. In the ongoing HD14 trial for early 'unfavorable' stage disease, the 'BEACOPP escalated' regimen was introduced, which had shown high efficacy in the treatment of advanced HL.[56] Patients are currently being randomized to 2 × 'BEACOPP escalated' plus 2 × ABVD, or 4 × ABVD followed by 30 Gy IFRT.

Table 72.6 Selected trials for early stage 'unfavorable' Hodgkin lymphoma

Trial	Therapy regimen	n	Outcome	Ref.
EORTC/GELA H8U	A. 6 MOPP/ABV + IFRT (36 Gy)	335	94% (RFS); 90% (OS)	52
	B. 4 MOPP/ABV + IFRT (36 Gy)	333	95% (RFS); 95% (OS)	
	C. 4 MOPP/ABV + STNI	327	96% (RFS); 93% (OS) [4 years]	
GHSG HD8	A. 2 COPP + ABVD + EFRT (30 Gy) + Bulk (10 Gy)	532	86% (FFTF); 91% (OS)	53
	B. 2 COPP + ABVD + IFRT (30 Gy) + Bulk (10 Gy)	532	84% (FFTF); 92% (OS) [5 years]	
SWOG/ECOG 2496	A. 6 ABVD + IFRT (36 Gy) to bulk (>5 cm)		Ongoing trial	
	B. 12 weeks Stanford-V + IFRT (36 Gy) to bulk (>5 cm)			
EORTC/GELA H9U	A. 6 ABVD + IFRT	808	94% (EFS); 96% (OS)	47
	B. 4 ABVD + IFRT		89% (EFS); 95% (OS)	
	C. 4 BEACOPP bas.+ IFRT		91% (EFS); 93% (OS) [4 years]	
GHSG HD11	A. 4 ABVD + IFRT (30 Gy)	1047	Interim analysis [2 years]	55
	B. 4 ABVD + IFRT (20 Gy)		all pts	
	C. 4 BEACOPP bas. + IFRT (30 Gy)		97.4% (FFTF)	
	D. 4 BEACOPP bas. + IFRT (20 Gy)		89.9% (OS)	
GHSG HD14	A. 4 ABVD + IFRT (30 Gy)		Ongoing trial	
	B. 2 BEACOPP esc. + 2 ABVD + IFRT (30 Gy)			

SWOG, Southwest Oncology Group; EORTC, European Organization for Research and Treatment of Cancer; GELA, Groupe d'Etude des Lymphomes de l'Adulte; GHSG, German Hodgkin Lymphoma Study Group; ECOG, Eastern Cooperative Oncology Group; EF/IFRT, extended/involved field radiation therapy; STNI, subtotal nodal irradiation; FFTF, freedom from treatment failure; RFS, relapse-free survival; EFS, event-free suvival; OS, overall survival; pts, patients; bas., baseline; esc., escalated; ABVD: adriamycin (doxorubicin), bleomycin, vinblastine, dacarbazine; MOPP: mechlorethamine, Oncovin (vincristine), procarbazine, prednisone; Stanford-V: mechlorethamine, adriamycin (doxorubicin), vinblastine, vincristine, bleomycin, etoposide, prednisone; COPP: cyclophosphamide, Oncovin (vincristine), procarbazine, prednisone; BEACOPP: bleomycin, etoposide, adriamycin (doxorubicin), cyclophosphamide, Oncovin (vincristine), procarbazine, prednisone.

Advanced stage Hodgkin lymphoma

For advanced stage disease, MOPP has successfully been used for many years, producing long-term remission rates of nearly 50 percent.[32,57] This regimen was then replaced by ABVD, since large multicenter trials proved the superiority of ABVD and alternating MOPP/ABVD over MOPP alone.[58,59] Hybrid regimens such as MOPP/ABV were demonstrated to be only equally effective when compared with alternating MOPP/ABVD, and even rapidly alternating multidrug regimens such as COPP/ABV/IMEP (cyclophosphamide, vincristine, procarbazine, and prednisone/doxorubicin, bleomycin, and vinblastine/ifosfamide, methotrexate, and etoposide) did not result in better outcome.[60,61] However, more acute toxicity and a higher incidence of secondary leukemia were reported after MOPP/ABV hybrid compared with ABVD.[58] Thus far, ABVD is regarded as the current standard regimen against which all new combinations are tested. However, a long-term follow-up report of 123 patients who were treated with ABVD for advanced HL revealed a failure-free survival of only 47 percent and an overall survival of 59 percent after 14.1 years.[62]

Therefore, different study groups aimed at improving these results by developing new regimens using additional drugs and by increasing both dose intensity and density using colony-stimulating factors and modern antibiotics. These new approaches include multidrug regimens such as Stanford-V, MEC, VAPEC-B, ChlVPP/EVA, and BEACOPP (Table 72.7).[56,63–65]

The GHSG HD9 trial compared the three entities COPP/ABVD, 'BEACOPP baseline,' and 'BEACOPP escalated.' Results from 1195 patients demonstrated a clear superiority for the 'escalated BEACOPP' version. At 5 years, FFTF and OS rates were, respectively, 69 percent and 83 percent in the COPP/ABVD group, 76 percent and 88 percent in the 'BEACOPP baseline' group, and 87 percent and 91 percent in the 'BEACOPP escalated' group.[56] The follow-up data at 7 years clearly underline these results (Fig. 72.1 and Fig. 72.2).[66]

Table 72.7 Selected trials for advanced Hodgkin lymphoma

Trial	Therapy regimen	n	Outcome	Ref.
Stanford	Stanford-V (12 weeks) (+ RT to initial mediastinal bulk + hilar + supracl. nodes)	108	95% (OS) 83% (FFP) [CS III/IV; 12 years]	63, 119
Intergroup Italy	A. ABVD (6 cycles)	98	83% (FFS); 86% (FFP); 90% (OS)	64, 120
	B. Stanford-V (12 weeks)	89	67% (FFS); 76% (FFP); 83% (OS)	
	C. MEC hybrid (six courses) (+ RT initial bulk/residual mass)	88	85% (FFS); 93% (FFP); 90% (OS) [5 years]	
Intergroup	A. ChlVPP/EVA hybrid (6 cycles)	144	82% (FFP); 78% (EFS); 89% (OS)	65
GB and Italy	B. VAPEC-B (11 weeks) (± RT initial bulk/residual mass)	138	62% (FFP); 58% (EFS); 79% (OS) [5 years]	
GHSG HD9	A. COPP/ABVD (4 cycles)	260	67% (FFTF); 79% (OS)	66
	B. BEACOPP baseline (8 cycles)	469	75% (FFTF) 84% (OS)	
	C. BEACOPP escalated (8 cycles)	466	84% (FFTF); 90% (OS) [7years]	
GHSG HD12	A. 8 BEA esc.	348	4th interim analysis [2 years]	66
	B. 8 BEA esc.	345	all pts	
	C. 4 BEA esc. + 4 BEA baseline	351	88% (FFTF); 94% (OS)	
	D. 4 BEA esc. + 4 BEA baseline (A.+ C. + RT bulk/residual mass)	352		
GHSG HD15	A. 8 BEA esc.		Ongoing trial	
	B. 6 BEA esc.			
	C. 8 BEA-14 (+ RT to PET+ residual mass ≥2.5 cm)			
Intergroup 20012 EORTC	8 × ABVD 4 BEA esc. + 4 BEA baseline		Ongoing trial	

EORTC, European Organization for Research and Treatment of Cancer; GHSG, German Hodgkin Lymphoma Study Group; RT, radiation therapy; FFS, failure free survival; FFP, freedom from progression FFTF, freedom from treatment failure; EFS, event-free suvival; OS, overall survival; supracl., supraclavicular; esc., escalated; ABVD: adriamycin (doxorubicin), bleomycin, vinblastine, dacarbazine; Stanford-V: mechlorethamine, adriamycin (doxorubicin), vinblastine, vincristine, bleomycin, etoposide, prednisone; COPP: cyclophosphamide, Oncovin (vincristine), procarbazine, prednisone; BEACOPP: bleomycin, etoposide, adriamycin (doxorubicin), cyclophosphamide, Oncovin (vincristine), procarbazine, prednisone; MEC: mechlorethamine, Oncovin (vincristine), procarbazine, prednisone, epidoxorubicin, bleomycin, vinblastine, CCNU (lomustine), alkeran, vindesine; VAPEC-B: vincristine, adriamycin (doxorubicin), prednisolone, etoposide, cyclophosphamide, bleomycin; ChlVPP/EVA: chlorambucil, vinblastine, procarbazine, prednisolone, etoposide, vincristine, adriamycin (doxorubicin).

The subsequent GHSG HD12 trial aimed at de-escalating chemotherapy and radiation therapy by comparing eight courses of 'BEACOPP escalated' with four 'escalated' and four 'baseline' courses of BEACOPP, with or without

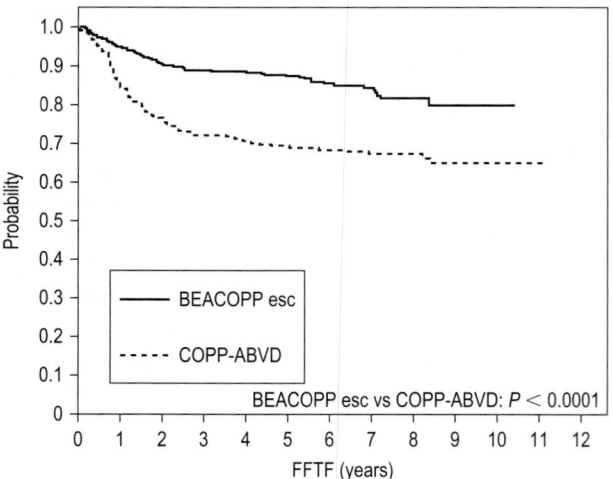

Figure 72.1 Follow-up data of the German Hodgkin Study Group (GHSG) HD9 trial at 7 years. Freedom from treatment failure (FFTF) 84% (BEACOPP esc) and 67% (COPP-ABVD). esc, escalated. BEACOPP esc, BEACOPP escalated (bleomycin, etoposide, adriamycin [doxorubicin], cyclophosphamide, Oncovin [vincristine], procarbazine, and prednisone); COPP-ABVD: cyclophosphamide, Oncovin (vincristine), procarbazine, and prednisone – adriamycin (doxorubicin), bleomycin, vinblastine, dacarbazine.

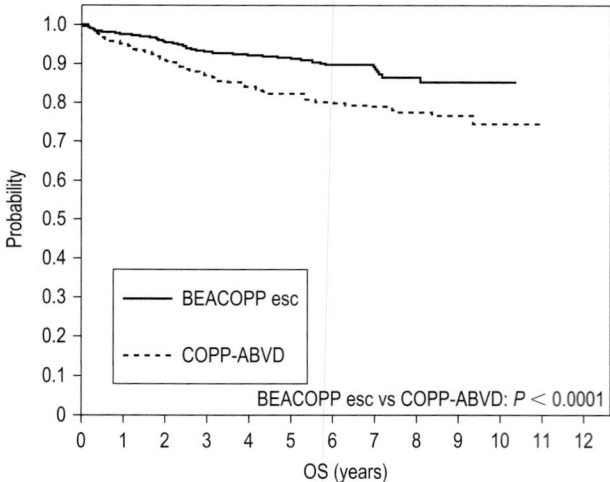

Figure 72.2 Follow-up data of German Hodgkin Study Group (GHSG) HD9 trial at 7 years. Overall survival (OS) 90% (BEACOPP esc) and 79% (COPP-ABVD). esc, escalated. BEACOPP esc, BEACOPP escalated (bleomycin, etoposide, adriamycin [doxorubicin], cyclophosphamide, Oncovin [vincristine], procarbazine, and prednisone); COPP-ABVD: cyclophosphamide, Oncovin (vincristine), procarbazine, and prednisone – adriamycin (doxorubicin), bleomycin, vinblastine, dacarbazine.

radiation to initial bulky and residual disease. In the last interim analysis of HD12, at a median follow-up of 30 months, the FFTF was 88 percent and OS 94 percent for the total cohort. There was no significant difference between the different study arms.[66]

In the ongoing HD15 trial, patients are randomized between 8 cycles of 'BEACOPP escalated,' 6 cycles of 'BEACOPP escalated,' or 8 cycles of 'BEACOPP-14,' which is a time-intensified 'BEACOPP baseline' variant. Additional radiation therapy is only applied to PET-positive residual lesions greater than 2.5 cm. The question as to whether 'escalated BEACOPP' is superior to ABVD alone in a randomized setting is currently being evaluated in an intergroup trial initiated by the EORTC (study 20012)[46] Here, 8 cycles of ABVD are being compared with 4 cycles of 'BEACOPP escalated' plus 4 cycles of 'BEACOPP baseline' (Table 72.7).

Further intensification of first-line therapy in high-risk patients by directly administering high-dose therapy and autologous stem cell transplantation after 4 instead of 8 cycles of ABVD did not improve outcome compared with conventional treatment.[67] BEACOPP is generally associated with higher hematological toxicity, sterility, and secondary leukemia when compared with ABVD. Nevertheless, cardiotoxicity and pulmonary side effects are similar with both regimens especially when combined with radiation therapy. A combination of gemcitabine and bleomycin in a 'BEACOPP variant' (BAGCOPP) resulted in severe pulmonary toxicity and should be avoided.[68]

ROLE OF RADIATION THERAPY IN ADVANCED STAGE DISEASE

The role of radiation therapy after effective chemotherapy in the treatment of patients with advanced HL is still the subject of controversy. A metaanalysis comparing combined modality approaches and chemotherapy alone reported equal tumor control and better overall survival in patients treated with chemotherapy alone.[69] Therefore, randomized trials are currently evaluating the impact of radiation therapy after effective chemotherapy. A study conducted by the EORTC recently indicated that IFRT as consolidation did not result in better outcome in patients who had already achieved a complete remission after 6–8 cycles of MOPP/ABV.[70] In the previously described GHSG HD12 trial, consolidating radiation to initial bulky and residual disease was randomly compared with no radiation therapy. In the last interim analysis, no difference was seen between the two study arms; however, patients with larger residual masses received radiation therapy irrespective of the initial randomization. Thus, radiation might become obsolete for patients with little or no residual disease after chemotherapy. However, longer follow-up of the recently terminated GHSG HD12 trial and the ongoing HD15 trial may help to define the role of radiation therapy for residual disease.

TREATMENT OF RELAPSED AND REFRACTORY HODGKIN LYMPHOMA

To date, the majority of patients achieve complete remission (CR) after first-line treatment. However, patients who relapse still have a chance for cure with adequate salvage treatment. Depending on first-line therapy, patients with recurrent and refractory HL have various treatment options; conventional chemotherapy is the treatment of choice for patients relapsing after initial radiation therapy. In contrast, options for those who relapse after chemotherapy include salvage radiation therapy for localized relapse in previously nonirradiated areas, salvage chemotherapy, or high-dose chemotherapy (HDT) with autologous stem cell transplantation (ASCT). Other options, such as allogeneic stem cell transplantation and experimental strategies, are being evaluated for multiply pretreated patients. Depending on the length of remission after first-line treatment, most study groups categorize failures into three subgroups: early and late relapses and primary progressive HL.

Salvage radiation therapy and salvage polychemotherapy

For a selected subset of patients with localized relapses in previously nonirradiated areas, salvage radiation therapy alone offers an effective treatment option. In a retrospective analysis from the GHSG database, including 624 patients with recurrent or refractory HL, the 5-year freedom from second failure (FF2F) and OS rates were 28 percent and 51 percent, respectively. Prognostic factors for OS were B symptoms, stage at relapse, performance status, and duration of first remission in limited stage relapse.[71]

Conventional chemotherapy is the treatment of choice for patients who relapse after initial radiation therapy for early stage disease. The survival of these patients is at least equal to that of patients with advanced stage HL initially treated with chemotherapy.[72]

However, the best treatment for recurrent HL after primary chemotherapy is less clear. A number of conventional salvage protocols have been developed during the last decade; however, follow-up is still short and most of the patients achieving CR and partial remission (PR) immediately proceeded to HDT/ASCT. Overall response rates to salvage therapy were high (60–80 percent) but only 20–35 percent of the patients achieved CR.

High-dose chemotherapy followed by autologous stem cell transplantation

Patients who relapse after initial chemotherapy are mostly treated with HDT and peripheral blood stem cell transplantation (PBSCT). This strategy has been shown to result in 30–65 percent long-term disease-free survival in selected patients with refractory and relapsed HL.[73,74] In addition, the reduction of early treatment-related mortality to less than 5 percent has led to widespread acceptance. Thus far, two randomized trials have demonstrated the superiority of HDT followed by ASCT over conventional chemotherapy. The British National Lymphoma Investigation (BNLI) reported that patients with relapsed or refractory HL receiving high-dose BEAM (BCNU [carmustine], etoposide, cytarabine [Ara-C], and melphalan) with ASCT fared significantly better than those treated with conventional-dose mini-BEAM, resulting in a 3-year event-free survival of 53 percent versus 10 percent.[75] In the HD-R1 trial of the GHSG, chemosensitive patients relapsing after initial chemotherapy were randomized between 4 cycles of Dexa-BEAM (BEAM plus dexamethasone) and 2 cycles of Dexa-BEAM followed by BEAM and ASCT. Final results demonstrated a higher FF2F in the transplanted group compared with the group receiving conventional salvage chemotherapy (55 percent vs 34 percent).[76] Even in the subgroup of patients with late relapse the FF2F was significantly better (75 percent vs 44 percent). For patients with early relapse, FF2F in the two groups was 41 percent and 12 percent, respectively. The OS did not differ significantly between the two treatment arms. This might at least in part be due to the fact that many patients relapsing after conventional salvage therapy finally received ASCT after further relapse. The follow-up data after 7 years confirm these results.

The success of high-dose chemotherapy followed by PBSCT does not only depend on obvious factors such as tumor burden or chemosensitivity. A prognostic score based on treatment outcome of patients with relapsed HL also identified time to relapse, the clinical stage at relapse, and the presence of anemia as independent risk factors.[77]

Sequential high-dose chemotherapy and the HD-R2 trial

Reduction of tumor volume prior to HDT followed by ASCT is an important variable affecting outcome. A brief tumor-reducing program with 2 cycles of DHAP (dexamethasone, Ara-C, and cisplatin) given at short intervals supported by granulocyte colony-stimulating factor (G-CSF) proved to be both effective and well tolerated in patients with relapsed and refractory HL.[78] Therefore this regimen was chosen for the HD-R2 study instead of the previously used regimen Dexa-BEAM, which was associated with severe treatment-related toxicity and mortality. Furthermore, the DHAP regimen can be used to successfully collect stem cells in more than 90 percent of HL patients.[79]

The strategy of sequential high-dose chemotherapy follows the Norton-Simon hypothesis: after initial cytoreduction, a few non-cross-resistant agents are given at short intervals. The use of peripheral blood stem cells and growth factors allows application of the most effective drugs at the highest possible doses at short intervals. The Cologne high-dose sequential trial conducted by the GHSG evaluated the feasibility and efficacy of this approach including a high-dose sequential chemotherapy program and a final myeloablative course in 102 patients with relapsed or refractory HL. Treatment consisted of 2 cycles of DHAP followed by sequential high-dose chemotherapy with cyclophosphamide, methotrexate plus vincristine, and etoposide. The final myeloablative course was BEAM followed by PBSCT. With a median follow-up of 30 months, FF2F and OS were 59 percent and 78 percent for all patients. Freedom from second failure and OS for patients with early relapse were 62 percent and 81 percent, for late relapse 65 percent and 81 percent, for progressive disease 41 percent and 48 percent, and for multiple relapse 39 percent and 48 percent, respectively.[80] In multivariate analysis, response after DHAP and duration of first remission were prognostic factors for FF2F and OS. Based on the promising results of this study, the GHSG together with the EORTC, the GEL/TAMO (Grupo Español de Linfomas/ Trasplante Autólogo de Médula Ósea; the Spanish Group for Lymphoma and Autologous Transplantation) and the EBMT (European Group for Blood and Marrow Transplantation) started a prospective European inter-group trial in 2001 (HD-R2) that is still open. The rationale is to compare the effectiveness of two courses of DHAP followed by BEAM with the intensified sequential strategy in a randomized setting. Patients with histologically confirmed early or late recurrent HL and patients in second relapse with no prior HDT are included.[81]

Primary progressive and refractory Hodgkin lymphoma

For patients with primary progressive disease during induction treatment (or within 3 months of completing first-line therapy), conventional salvage chemotherapy has given disappointing results. No response at all or only a very short response to salvage treatment resulted in an 8-year OS between 0 percent and 8 percent.[82,83]

To determine prognostic factors and treatment outcome of patients with primary progressive HL, the GHSG retrospectively analyzed 206 patients with progressive disease. The 5-year FF2F and OS for all patients were 17 percent and 26 percent, respectively. Freedom from second failure and OS for patients treated with HDCT were 31 percent and 43 percent, respectively. The low percentage of only 33 percent of patients who received HDT was due to rapidly fatal disease or life-threatening severe toxicity after salvage therapy. Other reasons for not proceeding to HDT were insufficient stem cell harvest, poor performance status, and older age. In multivariate analysis, low Karnofsky performance score at the time of progression, age above 50 years, and failure to attain a temporary remission with first-line treatment were significant adverse prognostic factors for OS.[84]

Allogeneic stem cell transplantation

Allogeneic stem cell transplantation (SCT) cannot yet be considered a standard treatment for patients with relapsed HL. So far, the advantages of a potential graft-versus-lymphoma effect have been offset by a very high transplant-related mortality (TRM) of more than 50 percent. Furthermore, donor availability and age constraints have limited the broader application of allogeneic SCT in patients with HL. As shown by matched-pair analysis, TRM might be significantly reduced by employing reduced-intensity conditioning (RIC).[85] Allogeneic SCT following RIC might thus become an appropriate strategy in selected subgroups of young, poor-risk patients, e.g., for those failing autologous transplantation, patients with primary refractory disease, or patients with early relapse and further risk factors.[86] However, to date, the number of patients treated is small and further clinical studies and information are required in order to define clear indications.

SPECIAL CONSIDERATIONS

Lymphocyte-predominant subtype of Hodgkin lymphoma

Patients with a primary diagnosis of nodular lymphocyte-predominant subtype of HL with clinical stage IA disease and no risk factors are usually not included in ongoing trials. On the basis of the very favorable prognosis of this subtype, the EORTC and the GHSG currently recommend treatment with 30 Gy IFRT only. While being less toxic, this strategy seems to produce similar responses to combined modality treatment.[87] The humanized monoclonal anti-CD20 antibody rituximab has given impressive results in relapsed lymphocyte-predominant HL[88,89] and will shortly be evaluated in a GHSG phase II study in selected patients with stage IA lymphocyte-predominant HL.

Elderly patients

Although elderly patients with HL vary greatly with respect to general health and physical condition, older age at diagnosis remains an unfavorable risk factor, particularly in advanced stages. In most groups, patients are considered 'elderly' if they are aged 60 years or older. Factors such as more aggressive disease, advanced stage, comorbidity, poor tolerance of treatment, failure to maintain dose intensity, shorter survival after relapse, and death due to other causes contribute to the poorer outcome of older patients.[90] In the HD9$_{elderly}$ trial of the GHSG, patients between 66 and 75 years of age with advanced stage HL were treated with either COPP/ABVD or 'BEACOPP baseline.' Tumor control appeared to be better with the BEACOPP regimen, but toxicity was higher, resulting in no differences in FFTF or OS.[91] In phase I/II trials of the

GHSG, two new regimens are currently being evaluated: PVAG (prednisone, vinblastine, doxorubicin, and gemcitabine) and BACOPP (bleomycin, doxorubicin, cyclophosphamide, vincristine, procarbazine, and prednisone).

Fertility

Based on the substantially improved long-term survival in young patients with HL undergoing chemotherapy, preservation of fertility has become an increasingly important issue. Regimens such as COPP, MOPP, or BEACOPP containing alkylating agents such as procarbazine or cyclophosphamide often lead to therapy-induced infertility, whereas ABVD is less gonadotoxic. For men, cryopreservation of semen prior to therapy is possible; however, strategies for women are less clear. A birth after ovarian cryopreservation and reimplantation has been reported.[92] Nevertheless, reproductive technologies – including ovarian cryopreservation with auto- or xenotransplantation as well as *in vitro* maturation of thawed primordial follicles, followed by fertilization and embryo transfer – are not yet successfully established.

Data on cotreatment preserving ovarian function are still scarce. A retrospective analysis of the GHSG demonstrates that the rate of therapy-induced amenorrhea is higher in women receiving 8 cycles of 'dose-escalated BEACOPP' compared to women treated with ABVD alone, COPP/ABVD, or standard BEACOPP. Moreover, amenorrhea after therapy was most pronounced in women with advanced stage HL, in those older than 30 years at treatment, and in women who did not take oral contraceptives during chemotherapy.[93] Both administration of oral contraceptives or gonadotropin-releasing hormone agonists (goserelin) during chemotherapy may achieve lower rates of ovarian failure.[94,95] An ongoing GHSG phase II study

(PROFE) for the first time compares both strategies in a randomized setting for females (aged 18–40 years) with advanced HL.

LONG-TERM MANAGEMENT

Palliative treatment

Depending on age, number and character of relapses, previous therapies, and presence of concomitant diseases, doctors should carefully evaluate whether a curative or a palliative approach is chosen. A palliative regimen can achieve satisfactory pain control, improve general health, and lead to partial, sometimes long-lasting, remissions. Drugs such as gemcitabine, vinorelbine, vinblastine, idarubicin, or etoposide are mostly given as single agents, which can be combined with corticosteroids. The most promising alternative is gemcitabine, which proved to be a suitable and well-tolerated substance, even for patients with multiple relapses of HL, in a phase II study.[96] Efforts are underway to incorporate gemcitabine into first-line treatment.

Follow-up and sequelae of treatment

During the follow-up period, attention should be paid to the fact that more than two-thirds of relapses occur within 2.5 years and more than 90 percent within 5 years of initial treatment. Thus, follow-up is essential (Table 72.8). Furthermore, a number of long-term toxic effects related to treatment can occur. These include endocrine dysfunction, long-term immunosuppression, and viral infections. More serious impairments consist of lung fibrosis from bleomycin and/or irradiation,[35,97,98] myocardial damage from anthracyclines and/or irradiation,[34,99] sterility,[94,100,101]

Table 72.8 Information for Hodgkin lymphoma patients concerning follow-up examinations

Examination time point	1st year Month 3	Month 6	Month 12	2nd–4th year Every 6 months	5th year onward Annually
Anamnesis	X	X	X	X	X
Physical examination	X	X	X	X	X
Laboratory tests					
Blood count and differential distribution	X	X	X	X	X
ESR, CRP	X	X	X	X	X
TSH	X	X	X	X	X
Computed tomography[a] (if PR)	X[a]		X		
Chest x-ray (if no CT)	X		X	X[b]	X
Lung function			X		
Abdominal ultrasound	X		X	X	X

[a]Further CT scans are recommended according to findings in final restaging and follow-up.
[b]Imaging examinations annually.
ESR, erythrocyte sedimentation rate; CRP, C-reactive protein; TSH, thyroid-stimulating hormone; CT, computed tomography; PR, partial remission.
Extracted and modified from the current GHSG trial protocol HD15 for advanced stage Hodgkin lymphoma.

growth abnormalities in children, opportunistic infections, psychological and psychosocial problems, and fatigue.[102] Potentially fatal effects include the OPSI-syndrome after splenectomy or splenic irradiation and secondary neoplasms. Secondary acute myeloid leukemia/myelodysplastic syndrome is mostly observed within the first 3–5 years and secondary non-Hodgkin lymphoma mainly at 5–15 years after initial treatment. Solid tumors, e.g., lung or breast cancer, can also occur decades after initial treatment and sometimes even as multiple tumors.[36–38,103]

EXPERIMENTAL THERAPIES

Data from HL and NHL cases suggest that small numbers of residual tumor cells remaining after first-line treatment can give rise to late relapses. Thus, eliminating residual malignant lymphoma cells after first-line treatment might further improve outcome in these diseases. In addition, a combined immunochemotherapy might help to reduce the amount of cytotoxic drugs needed, resulting in less toxicity. Experimental strategies in the treatment of HL include passive immunotherapy based on monoclonal antibodies to specifically target malignant cells and active immunotherapy with modulation of cellular response by cytokines, tumor vaccines, or gene transfer.

Hodgkin lymphoma seems to be an ideal target for antibody-based therapeutic approaches since RS cells express specific surface antigens such as CD25 and CD30 in large amounts. Approaches involving antibody-based agents have given promising results in experimental HL models and have demonstrated some clinical efficacy in patients with advanced refractory HL. Clinical phase I/II trials with so-called 'naked' humanized or human monoclonal antibodies (mAbs), bispecific constructs, immunotoxins, and radioimmunoconjugates have been conducted. However, it seems unlikely that patients with resistant disease and large tumor masses can be cured by these approaches. Future strategies aim at combining conventional chemotherapy and/or radiation therapy with experimental therapies with biologic agents to kill residual RS cells and thus prevent relapse.

Monoclonal antibodies

Since CD30 is expressed in high amounts on RS cells of classical HL, it is the most interesting antigen for immunotherapy in HL. Currently, clinical investigation includes two anti-CD30 antibodies: the humanized SGN-30 and the 'fully human' 5F11. SGN-30, a chimeric antibody, has demonstrated antitumor activity in preclinical models of HL and anaplastic large cell lymphoma (ALCL). In a phase I trial it showed minimal toxicity associated with doses of 1–15 mg/kg and antitumor activity was seen in two of 13 patients.[104] In a phase I/II dose-escalation study of six weekly intravenous (IV) infusions of SGN-30

at doses of 2–12 mg/kg per cohort, 24 patients were enrolled. The treatment was very well tolerated; adverse events have been typically mild.[105] Of the 21 patients with HL accrued to the phase I study, four patients had stable disease. Fifteen patients have been enrolled in a phase II multidose study using six weekly IV infusions of 6 mg/kg SGN-30. Of twelve evaluable patients, disease stabilization was reported in six.

MDX-060 is a fully human IgG1k antibody that recognizes CD30 and mediates killing of HL and ALCL cell lines *in vitro* and in xenograft tumor models. In a phase I/II open-label, dose-escalation study in patients with relapsed or refractory HL, ALCL, or other CD30-positive lymphomas, MDX-060 was administered intravenously at dose levels of 0.1–10 mg/kg weekly for 4 weeks without any dose-limiting toxicities. There were two drug-related serious adverse events (Grade 3 elevated liver transaminase and Grade 3 pneumonia/Grade 4 acute respiratory distress syndrome [ARDS]). In the ongoing phase II study, patients receive MDX-060 at 10 or 15 mg/kg.[106] To date, 48 patients including 40 with HL have been treated without significant infusion-related reactions. Objective clinical responses have been observed in three patients with HL (1 CR, 2 PR). These preliminary results indicate MDX-060 to be well tolerated and to have some clinical activity.

The anti-CD20 antibody rituximab has demonstrated clinical efficacy in lymphocyte-predominant HL in which RS cells express B cell antigens such as CD20. In a multicenter phase II trial, 11 patients with refractory HL with CD20-positive histology were treated at the standard dose ($4 \times 375 \, \text{mg/m}^2$, weekly).[88] Nine patients achieved CR and two PR. Ten patients were still in remission at the time of writing with a median response duration of 14 or more months. Similar results were seen in another trial involving 22 patients with recurrent lymphocyte-predominant HL with an overall response rate of 100 percent.[89] Treatment of classical HL with rituximab is less successful,[107] which is not surprising since only a small proportion of patients' tumors express CD20. Twenty-two patients with relapsed HL receiving $6 \times 375 \, \text{mg/m}^2$ were evaluable for response, with an overall response rate of 5/22, lasting for a median of 7.8 months. Response occurred irrespective of CD20 expression of RS cells, indicating a transient decrease in size of the lymph nodes due to elimination of CD20-positive B cells.

Radioimmunotherapy

Radiolabeled antibodies (RAbs) have been studied for both imaging and treatment of lymphoma. Most RAbs for therapeutic use consist of a specific antibody labeled with iodine-131 (^{131}I) or yttrium-90 (^{90}Y). A substantial advantage of RAbs is the ability to kill tumor cells adjacent to cells to which the radioimmunoconjugate is bound (the crossfire effect). Currently, both nonmyeloablative and myeloablative strategies involving RAbs are being pursued. Since HL is very sensitive to radiation therapy, radioimmunotherapeutic approaches have been studied using polyclonal antiferritin antibodies labeled with ^{131}I or ^{90}Y and using the anti-CD30 mAb Ki-4 labeled with [131]I.

In a trial using polyclonal ferritin-directed antibodies, 38 patients received ^{131}I-labeled polyclonal ferritin-directed antibodies delivering an activity of 50 mCi, resulting in 40 percent tumor regression.[108] In another trial, the use of fractionated (2×0.25 mCi/kg) or unfractionated (0.3–0.5 mCi/kg) ^{90}Y-labeled antiferritin RAbs in HL was evaluated.[109] Tumor response was dose related, varying from 22 percent to 86 percent. A total of 15/90 CRs and 29/90 PRs with a median duration of 6 months were observed. Another study included low-dose radioimmunotherapy using an anti-CD30 mAb. Twenty-two patients with relapsed or refractory CD30-positive HL were treated with ^{131}I-labeled Ki-4.[110] The best predictors of hematotoxicity were ESR and Karnofsky index reflecting advanced disease. Response included one CR, five PRs, and three minor responses.

A phase I/II study of high-dose ^{90}Y-labeled polyclonal antiferritin immunoglobulins and autologous bone marrow transplantation (ABMT) has been conducted in patients with refractory HL.[111] Nineteen patients received doses ranging from 20 to 50 mCi followed by ABMT, with an overall response rate (ORR) of 65 percent. Sixteen patients with bone marrow involvement or unsuccessful marrow harvest were treated with a reduced dose (20 mCi) achieving an ORR of 58 percent. In general, responses were better in patients with a smaller tumor burden, and when the ORRs were compared, 20 mCi ^{90}Y-labeled antiferritin was as effective as 40 mCi, while myelosuppression was reduced with the lower dose. An update of this trial including 39 patients reported ten CRs and ten PRs, with nine CRs occurring in patients who received more than one cycle of treatment.[112]

Another trial evaluated the feasibility of combining radioimmunotherapy with high-dose chemotherapy followed by ABMT.[113] Twelve patients received 20–30 mCi ^{90}Y-labeled antiferritin and high-dose cyclophosphamide, carmustine, and etoposide with bone marrow reinfusion. Four patients suffered early transplant-related mortality caused by infections, bleeding, and diffuse alveolar damage. Response of the remaining eight patients included one CR and three PRs. Based on these encouraging results, radioimmunotherapy appears to be a promising new option for patients with relapsed or refractory HL, either alone or in combination with chemotherapy and/or immunotherapy.

Bispecific monoclonal antibodies

The murine bispecific monoclonal antibody HRS-3/A9 has shown specific binding to the CD30 antigen (HRS-3) and the CD16 surface molecule (A9), triggering specific lysis of the CD30-positive Hodgkin-derived cell line L540Cy by natural killer cells *in vitro* and in mice. In a subsequent phase I/II study involving 15 patients with refractory HL, HRS-3/A9 was administered in doses of 1–64 mg/m^2 four

times every 3–4 days without reaching the maximum tolerated dose.[114] Toxicity was mild with fever and pain in affected lymph nodes; 60 percent of the patients developed human anti-(mouse immunoglobulin) antibodies. Responses included one CR and one PR lasting 3–6 months. In an additional trial, the effect of concomitant treatment with cytokines (interleukin-2 [IL-2], granulocyte macrophage colony-stimulating factor [GM-CSF]) was analyzed in 16 patients.[115] Response included one CR and three PRs.

More recently, a novel bispecific molecule consisting of F(ab') fragments derived from the murine anti-CD30 mAb Ki-4 and the humanized CD64-specific mAb H22 was developed.[116] Ten patients were enrolled and were evaluable for toxicity and response. Responses to the H22xKi-4 antibody included one CR, three PRs, and four with 'stable disease.' It was concluded that the H22xKi-4 antibody could be given safely and that it showed measurable activity in heavily pretreated patients with refractory HL, which warrants further clinical evaluation.

Cellular therapy

Modulation of EBV-directed T cell activity may be an immunotherapeutic option for the treatment of HL, because approximately one-half of HL cases are positive for EBV. Epstein–Barr virus-specific cytotoxic T lymphocytes (CTL) were developed for treatment of EBV-associated lymphoma after bone marrow transplantation.[117] This approach was adapted to EBV-positive cases of HL.[118] Nine patients with active relapsed HL and four who were in complete remission after first-line or subsequent therapy were treated with autologous EBV-specific CTLs. A 100-fold reduction of EBV-DNA was observed in all patients; in two of them B symptoms disappeared.

KEY POINTS

- Hodgkin lymphoma should always be proven by excisional biopsy, which is sent to an expert hematopathologist for initial diagnosis.
- Accurate staging procedures and risk factor assessment are indispensable.
- Patients with Hodgkin lymphoma should preferably be enrolled into clinical trials.
- In most centers, patients with early stage 'favorable' or early stage 'unfavorable' HL are treated with combined modality strategies including 2–6 cycles of chemotherapy (e.g., ABVD) followed by radiation therapy to the involved field. The treatment for advanced stages comprises more cycles or the use of a more intensive regimen, plus radiation therapy to possible residual masses.

- For patients relapsing after combined modality treatment or patients with primary progressive disease, high-dose chemotherapy with autologous stem cell transplantation still offers a definite chance of cure.
- With regard to the excellent cure rates, modern treatment strategies also aim at reducing therapy-induced acute and long-term toxicities without loss of efficacy.
- Potential future treatments may combine chemotherapy with experimental strategies.

ACKNOWLEDGMENTS

Our research is supported in parts by the German Cancer Aid (Deutsche Krebshilfe), the German Federal Ministry of Education and Research (Bundesministerium für Bildung und Forschung), and the Competence Network Malignant Lymphoma (Kompetenznetz Maligne Lymphome).

REFERENCES

● = Key primary paper
◆ = Major review article

●1. Hodgkin T. On some morbid appearances of the absorbent glands and spleen. *Medico-Churgical Trans* 1832; **17**: 68–97.

2. Sternberg C. Über eine eigenartige unter dem Bilde der Pseudoleukamie verlaufende Tuberkulose des lymphatischen Apparates. *Zeitschr Heilk* 1898; **19**: 21–90.

3. Reed DM. On the pathological changes in Hodgkin's disease, with special reference to its relation to tuberculosis. *Johns Hopkins Hosp Rep* 1902; **10**: 133–96.

4. Kuppers R, Rajewsky K. The origin of Hodgkin and Reed/Sternberg cells in Hodgkin's disease. *Annu Rev Immunol* 1998; **16**: 471–93.

5. Braeuninger A, Kuppers R, Strickler JG et al. Hodgkin and Reed-Sternberg cells in lymphocyte predominant Hodgkin disease represent clonal populations of germinal center-derived tumor B cells. *Proc Natl Acad Sci U S A* 1997; **94**: 9337–42.

6. Parkin DM, Muir CS. Cancer incidence in five continents. Comparability and quality of data. *IARC Sci Publ* 1992; **120**: 45–173.

7. EUCAN online database. Incidence and mortality data on Hodgkin's disease: 1998 estimates, version 5.0; www.dep.iarc.fr/eucan/eucan.htm

8. Krebs in Deutschland, Häufigkeiten und Trends. Arbeitsgemeinschaft Bevölkerungsbezogener Krebsregister in Deutschland, in Zusammenarbeit mit dem Robert-Koch-Institut. 4. überarbeitete, aktualisierte Ausgabe, Saarbrücken, 2004.

9. Miller T, LeBlanc M, Braziel R et al. Was the bimodal age incidence of Hodgkin's lymphoma a result of mistaken diagnoses of non-Hodgkin's lymphoma? *Proc Ann Meet Am Soc Hematol* 2002; **100**: 3048a.

10. Gutensohn N, Shapiro D. Social class risk factors among children with Hodgkin's disease. *Int J Cancer* 1982; **30**: 433–5.

11. Chang ET, Zheng T, Lennette ET et al. Heterogeneity of risk factors and antibody profiles in Epstein-Barr virus genome-positive and -negative Hodgkin lymphoma. *J Infect Dis* 2004; **189**: 2271–81.

12. Crowther D, Bonadonna G. Hodgkin's disease in adults. In: Peckham MPH, Veronesi U. (eds) *Oxford textbook of oncology*. New York: Oxford University Press, 1995: 1720–5.

◆13. Harris NL, Jaffe ES, Diebold J et al. The World Health Organization classification of neoplastic diseases of the hematopoietic and lymphoid tissues. Report of the Clinical Advisory Committee meeting, Airlie House, Virginia, November, 1997. *Ann Oncol* 1999; **10**: 1419–32.

14. Mueller N, Evans A, Harris NL et al. Hodgkin's disease and Epstein-Barr virus. Altered antibody pattern before diagnosis. *N Engl J Med* 1989; **320**: 689–95.

15. Weiss LM, Strickler JG, Warnke RA et al. Epstein-Barr viral DNA in tissues of Hodgkin's disease. *Am J Pathol* 1987; **129**: 86–91.

16. Glaser S, Lin R, Stewart S et al. Epstein-Barr virus-associated Hodgkin's disease: epidemiologic characteristics in international data. *Int J Cancer* 1997; **70**: 375–82.

17. Zarate-Osorno A, Roman L, Kingma D et al. Hodgkin's disease in Mexico. Prevalence of Epstein-Barr virus sequences and correlations with histologic subtype. *Cancer* 1995; **75**: 1360–6.

18. Jarrett RF, MacKenzie J. Epstein-Barr virus and other candidate viruses in the pathogenesis of Hodgkin's disease. *Semin Hematol* 1999; **36**: 260–9.

19. Haim N, Cohen Y, Robinson E. Malignant lymphoma in first-degree blood relatives. *Cancer* 1982; **49**: 2197–200.

20. Lindelof B, Eklund G. Analysis of hereditary component of cancer by use of a familial index by site. *Lancet* 2001; **358**: 1696–8.

21. Mack T, Cozen W, Shibata D et al. Concordance for Hodgkin's disease in identical twins suggesting genetic susceptibility to the young-adult form of the disease. *N Engl J Med* 1995; **332**: 413–18.

22. Muschen M, Rajewsky K, Brauninger A et al. Rare occurrence of classical Hodgkin's disease as a T cell lymphoma. *J Exp Med* 2000; **191**: 387–94.

23. Falini B, Stein H, Pileri S et al. Expression of lymphoid-associated antigens on Hodgkin's and Reed-Sternberg cells of Hodgkin's disease. An immunocytochemical study on lymph node cytospins using monoclonal antibodies. *Histopathology* 1987; **11**: 1229–42.

24. Bargou RC, Emmerich F, Krappmann D et al. Constitutive nuclear factor-kappaB-RelA activation is required for proliferation and survival of Hodgkin's disease tumor cells. *J Clin Invest* 1997; **100**: 2961–9.

25. Gires O, Zimber-Strobl U, Gonnella R *et al.* Latent membrane protein 1 of Epstein-Barr virus mimics a constitutively active receptor molecule. *EMBO J* 1997; **16**: 6131–40.

26. Rosenberg SA, Boiron M, DeVita VT Jr *et al.* Report of the Committee on Hodgkin's Disease Staging Procedures. *Cancer Res* 1971; **31**: 1862–3.

◆27. Lister TA, Crowther D, Sutcliffe SB *et al.* Report of a committee convened to discuss the evaluation and staging of patients with Hodgkin's disease: Cotswolds meeting. *J Clin Oncol* 1989; **7**: 1630–6.

28. Carde P, Burgers JM, Henry-Amar M *et al.* Clinical stages I and II Hodgkin's disease: a specifically tailored therapy according to prognostic factors. *J Clin Oncol* 1988; **6**: 239–52.

29. Loeffler M, Pfreundschuh M, Ruhl U *et al.* Risk factor adapted treatment of Hodgkin's lymphoma: strategies and perspectives. *Recent Results Cancer Res* 1989; **117**: 142–62.

◆30. Diehl V, Stein H, Hummel M *et al.* Hodgkin's lymphoma: biology and treatment strategies for primary, refractory, and relapsed disease. *Hematology* (*Am Soc Hematol Educ Program*) 2003; 225–472.

●31. Hasenclever D, Diehl V. A prognostic score for advanced Hodgkin's disease. International Prognostic Factors Project on Advanced Hodgkin's Disease. *N Engl J Med* 1998; **339**: 1506–14.

32. Longo DL, Young RC, Wesley M *et al.* Twenty years of MOPP chemotherapy for Hodgkin's disease. *J Clin Oncol* 1986; **4**: 1295–306.

●33. Bonadonna G, Zucali R, Monfardini S *et al.* Combination chemotherapy of Hodgkin's disease with adriamycin, bleomycin, vinblastine, and imidazole carboximide versus MOPP. *Cancer* 1975; **36**: 252–9.

34. Hancock SL, Tucker MA, Hoppe RT. Factors affecting late mortality from heart disease after treatment of Hodgkin's disease. *JAMA* 1993; **270**: 1949–55.

35. Dubray B, Henry-Amar M, Meerwaldt JH *et al.* Radiation-induced lung damage after thoracic irradiation for Hodgkin's disease: the role of fractionation. *Radiother Oncol* 1995; **36**: 211–17.

36. Ng AK, Bernardo MV, Weller E *et al.* Second malignancy after Hodgkin disease treated with radiation therapy with or without chemotherapy: long-term risks and risk factors. *Blood* 2002; **100**: 1989–96.

37. Bhatia S, Yasui Y, Robison LL *et al.* High risk of subsequent neoplasms continues with extended follow-up of childhood Hodgkin's disease: report from the Late Effects Study Group. *J Clin Oncol* 2003; **21**: 4386–94.

38. van Leeuwen FE, Klokman WJ, Stovall M *et al.* Roles of radiation dose, chemotherapy, and hormonal factors in breast cancer following Hodgkin's disease. *J Natl Cancer Inst* 2003; **95**: 971–80.

39. Horwich A, Specht L, Ashley S. Survival analysis of patients with clinical stages I or II Hodgkin's disease who have relapsed after initial treatment with radiotherapy alone. *Eur J Cancer* 1997; **33**: 848–53.

40. Specht L, Gray RG, Clarke MJ, Peto R. Influence of more extensive radiotherapy and adjuvant chemotherapy on long-term outcome of early-stage Hodgkin's disease: a meta-analysis of 23 randomized trials involving 3,888 patients. International Hodgkin's Disease Collaborative Group. *J Clin Oncol* 1998; **16**: 830–43.

41. Press OW, LeBlanc M, Lichter AS *et al.* Phase III randomized intergroup trial of subtotal lymphoid irradiation versus doxorubicin, vinblastine, and subtotal lymphoid irradiation for stage IA to IIA Hodgkin's disease. *J Clin Oncol* 2001; **19**: 4238–44.

42. Bonadonna G, Bonfante V, Viviani S *et al.* ABVD plus subtotal nodal versus involved-field radiotherapy in early-stage Hodgkin's disease: long-term results. *J Clin Oncol* 2004; **22**: 2835–41.

43. Horning SJ, Hoppe RT, Breslin S *et al.* Very brief (8 week) chemotherapy (CT) and low dose (30 Gy) radiotherapy (RT) for limited stage Hodgkin's disease (HD): preliminary results of the Stanford–Kaiser G4 Study of Stanford V + RT. *Blood* 1999; **94**: 1717a.

44. Carde P, Noordijk E, Hagenbeek A *et al.* Superiority of EBVP chemotherapy in combination with involved field irradiation over subtotal nodal irradiation in favorable clinical stage I-II Hodgkin's disease: The EORTC-GPMC H7F randomized trial. *Proc Am Soc Clin Oncol* 1997; **16**: 13.

45. Hagenbeek A, Eghbali H, Fermé C *et al.* Three cycles of MOPP/ABV hybrid and involved-field irradiation is more effective than subtotal nodal irradiation in favorable supradiaphragmatic clinical stages I-II Hodgkin's disease: Preliminary results of the EORTC-GELA H8F randomized trial in 543 patients. *Blood* 2000; **96**: 575a.

◆46. Raemaekers J, Kluin-Nelemans H, Teodorovic I *et al.* The achievements of the EORTC Lymphoma Group. European Organisation for Research and Treatment of Cancer. *Eur J Cancer* 2002; **38**: S107–13.

47. Noordijk EM, Thomas J, Fermé C *et al.* First results of the EORTC-GELA H9 randomized trials: the H9-F trial (comparing 3 radiation dose levels) and H9-U trial (comparing 3 chemotherapy schemes) in patients with favorable or unfavorable early stage Hodgkin's lymphoma (HL). *J Clin Oncol* 2005; **23**: 6505a.

●48. Meyer RM, Gospodarowicz MK, Connors JM *et al.* Randomized comparison of ABVD chemotherapy with a strategy that includes radiation therapy in patients with limited-stage Hodgkin's lymphoma: National Cancer Institute of Canada Clinical Trials Group and the Eastern Cooperative Oncology Group. *J Clin Oncol* 2005; **23**: 4634–42.

49. Sieber M, Franklin J, Tesch H *et al.* Two cycles ABVD plus extended field radiotherapy is superior to radiotherapy alone in early stage Hodgkin's disease: results of the German Hodgkin's Lymphoma Study Group (GHSG) trial HD7. *Blood* 2002; **100**: 341a.

50. Diehl V, Brillant C, Engert A *et al.* HD10: Investigating reduction of combined modality treatment intensity in early stage Hodgkin's lymphoma. Interim analysis of a

randomized trial of the German Hodgkin Study Group (GHSG). *J Clin Oncol* 2005; **23**: 6506a.

51. Zittoun R, Audebert A, Hoerni B *et al.* Extended versus involved fields irradiation combined with MOPP chemotherapy in early clinical stages of Hodgkin's disease. *J Clin Oncol* 1985; **3**: 207–14.

52. Fermé C, Eghbali H, Habenbeek A *et al.* MOPP/ABV (M/A) hybrid and irradiation in unfavorable supradiaphragmatic clinical stages I-II HD: Comparison of three treatment modalities, preliminary results of the EORTC-GELA H8-U randomized trial in 995 patients. *Blood* 2000; **96**: 576a.

●53. Engert A, Schiller P, Josting A *et al.* Involved-field radiotherapy is equally effective and less toxic compared with extended-field radiotherapy after four cycles of chemotherapy in patients with early-stage unfavorable Hodgkin's Lymphoma: Results of the HD8 trial of the German Hodgkin's Lymphoma Study Group. *J Clin Oncol* 2003; **21**: 3601–8.

●54. Canellos GP, Anderson JR, Propert KJ *et al.* Chemotherapy of advanced Hodgkin's disease with MOPP, ABVD, or MOPP alternating with ABVD. *N Engl J Med* 1992; **327**: 1478–84.

55. Klimm B, Engert A, Brillant C *et al.* Comparison of BEACOPP and ABVD chemotherapy in intermediate stage Hodgkin's lymphoma: results of the fourth interim analysis of the HD 11 trial of the GHSG. *J Clin Oncol* 2005; **23**: 6507a.

●56. Diehl V, Franklin J, Pfreundschuh M *et al.* Standard and increased-dose BEACOPP chemotherapy compared with COPP-ABVD for advanced Hodgkin's disease. *N Engl J Med* 2003; **348**: 2386–95.

57. Bonadonna G, Valagussa P, Santoro A. Alternating non-cross-resistant combination chemotherapy or MOPP in stage IV Hodgkin's disease. A report of 8-year results. *Ann Intern Med* 1986; **104**: 739–46.

●58. Duggan DB, Petroni GR, Johnson JL *et al.* Randomized comparison of ABVD and MOPP/ABV hybrid for the treatment of advanced Hodgkin's disease: report of an intergroup trial. *J Clin Oncol* 2003; **21**: 607–14.

59. Santoro A, Bonadonna G, Valagussa P *et al.* Long-term results of combined chemotherapy–radiotherapy approach in Hodgkin's disease: superiority of ABVD plus radiotherapy versus MOPP plus radiotherapy. *J Clin Oncol* 1987; **5**: 27–37.

60. Connors JM, Klimo P, Adams G *et al.* Treatment of advanced Hodgkin's disease with chemotherapy – comparison of MOPP/ABV hybrid regimen with alternating courses of MOPP and ABVD: A report from the National Cancer Institute of Canada Clinical Trials Group. *J Clin Oncol* 1997; **15**: 1638–45.

61. Sieber M, Tesch H, Pfistner B *et al.* Treatment of advanced Hodgkin's disease with COPP/ABV/IMEP versus COPP/ABVD and consolidating radiotherapy: final results of the German Hodgkin's Lymphoma Study Group HD6 trial. *Ann Oncol* 2004; **15**: 276–82.

62. Canellos GP, Niedzwiecki D. Long-term follow-up of Hodgkin's disease trial. *N Engl J Med* 2002; **346**: 1417–18.

●63. Horning SJ, Hoppe RT, Breslin S *et al.* Stanford V and radiotherapy for locally extensive and advanced Hodgkin's disease: mature results of a prospective clinical trial. *J Clin Oncol* 2002; **20**: 630–7.

●64. Chisesi T, Federico M, Levis A *et al.* ABVD versus Stanford V versus MEC in unfavourable Hodgkin's lymphoma: results of a randomised trial. *Ann Oncol* 2002; **13**: 102–6.

●65. Radford JA, Rohatiner AZ, Ryder WD *et al.* ChlVPP/EVA hybrid versus the weekly VAPEC-B regimen for previously untreated Hodgkin's disease. *J Clin Oncol* 2002; **20**: 2988–94.

66. Diehl V, Brillant C, Franklin J *et al.* BEACOPP chemotherapy for advanced Hodgkin's disease: results of further analyses of the HD9- and HD12-trials of the German Hodgkin Study Group (GHSG). *Blood* 2004; **104**: 307a.

67. Federico M, Bellei M, Brice P *et al.* High-dose therapy and autologous stem-cell transplantation versus conventional therapy for patients with advanced Hodgkin's lymphoma responding to front-line therapy. *J Clin Oncol* 2003; **21**: 2320–5.

68. Bredenfeld H, Franklin J, Nogova L *et al.* Severe pulmonary toxicity in patients with advanced-stage Hodgkin's disease treated with a modified bleomycin, doxorubicin, cyclophosphamide, vincristine, procarbazine, prednisone, and gemcitabine (BEACOPP) regimen is probably related to the combination of gemcitabine and bleomycin: a report of the German Hodgkin's Lymphoma Study Group. *J Clin Oncol* 2004; **22**: 2424–9.

69. Loeffler M, Brosteanu O, Hasenclever D *et al.* Meta-analysis of chemotherapy versus combined modality treatment trials in Hodgkin's disease. International Database on Hodgkin's Disease Overview Study Group. *J Clin Oncol* 1998; **16**: 818–29.

●70. Aleman BM, Raemaekers JM, Tirelli U *et al.* Involved-field radiotherapy for advanced Hodgkin's lymphoma. *N Engl J Med* 2003; **348**: 2396–406.

71. Josting A, Nogova L, Franklin J *et al.* Salvage radiotherapy in patients with relapsed and refractory Hodgkin's lymphoma: a retrospective analysis from the German Hodgkin Lymphoma Study Group. *J Clin Oncol* 2005; **23**: 1522–9.

72. Santoro A, Viviani S, Villarreal CJ *et al.* Salvage chemotherapy in Hodgkin's disease irradiation failures: superiority of doxorubicin-containing regimens over MOPP. *Cancer Treat Rep* 1986; **70**: 343–51.

73. Bierman PJ, Bagin RG, Jagannath S *et al.* High dose chemotherapy followed by autologous hematopoietic rescue in Hodgkin's disease: long-term follow-up in 128 patients. *Ann Oncol* 1993; **4**: 767–73.

74. Reece DE, Connors JM, Spinelli JJ *et al.* Intensive therapy with cyclophosphamide, carmustine, etoposide $\pm$ cisplatin, and autologous bone marrow transplantation for Hodgkin's disease in first relapse after combination chemotherapy. *Blood* 1994; **83**: 1193–9.

●75. Linch DC, Winfield D, Goldstone AH *et al.* Dose intensification with autologous bone-marrow transplantation in relapsed and resistant Hodgkin's disease: results of a BNLI randomised trial. *Lancet* 1993; **341**: 1051–4.

●76. Schmitz N, Pfistner B, Sextro M *et al.* Aggressive conventional chemotherapy compared with high-dose chemotherapy with autologous haemopoietic stem-cell transplantation for relapsed chemosensitive Hodgkin's disease: a randomised trial. *Lancet* 2002; **359**: 2065–71.

77. Josting A, Franklin J, May M *et al.* New prognostic score based on treatment outcome of patients with relapsed Hodgkin's lymphoma registered in the database of the German Hodgkin's lymphoma study group. *J Clin Oncol* 2002; **20**: 221–30.

78. Josting A, Rudolph C, Reiser M *et al.* Time-intensified dexamethasone/cisplatin/cytarabine: an effective salvage therapy with low toxicity in patients with relapsed and refractory Hodgkin's disease. *Ann Oncol* 2002; **13**: 1628–35.

79. Smardova L, Engert A, Haverkamp H *et al.* Successful mobilization of peripheral blood stem cells with the DHAP regimen (dexamethasone, cytarabine, cisplatinum) plus granulocyte colony-stimulating factor in patients with relapsed Hodgkin's disease. *Leuk Lymphoma* 2005; **46**: 1017–22.

80. Josting A, Rudolph C, Mapara M *et al.* Cologne high-dose sequential chemotherapy in relapsed and refractory Hodgkin lymphoma: results of a large multicenter study of the German Hodgkin Lymphoma Study Group (GHSG). *Ann Oncol* 2005; **16**: 116–23.

81. Glossmann JP, Josting A, Pfistner B *et al.* A randomized trial of chemotherapy with carmustine, etoposide, cytarabine, and melphalan (BEAM) plus peripheral stem cell transplantation (PBSCT) vs single-agent high-dose chemotherapy followed by BEAM plus PBSCT in patients with relapsed Hodgkin's disease (HD-R2). *Ann Hematol* 2002; **81**: 424–9.

82. Longo DL, Duffey PL, Young RC *et al.* Conventional-dose salvage combination chemotherapy in patients relapsing with Hodgkin's disease after combination chemotherapy: the low probability for cure. *J Clin Oncol* 1992; **10**: 210–18.

83. Bonfante V, Santoro A, Viviani S *et al.* Outcome of patients with Hodgkin's disease failing after primary MOPP/ABVD. *J Clin Oncol* 1997; **15**: 528–34.

●84. Josting A, Rueffer U, Franklin J *et al.* Prognostic factors and treatment outcome in primary progressive Hodgkin lymphoma: a report from the German Hodgkin Lymphoma Study Group. *Blood* 2000; **96**: 1280–6.

85. Sureda A, Robinson S, De Elvira CR *et al.* Allogeneic stem cell tranplantation significantly reduces transplant related mortality in comparison with conventional allogeneic transplantation in relapsed or refractory Hodgkin's disease: Results of the European Group for Blood and Marrow Transplantation. *Blood* 2003; **102**: 692a.

86. Schmitz N, Sureda A, Robinson S. Allogeneic transplantation of hematopoietic stem cells after nonmyeloablative conditioning for Hodgkin's disease: indications and results. *Semin Oncol* 2004; **31**: 27–32.

87. Nogová L, Reineke T, Eich HT *et al.* Extended field radiotherapy, combined modality treatment or involved field radiotherapy for patients with stage IA lymphocyte-predominant Hodgkin's lymphoma: a retrospective analysis from the German Hodgkin Study Group (GHSG). *Ann Oncol* 2005; **16**: 1683–7.

●88. Rehwald U, Schulz H, Reiser M *et al.* Treatment of relapsed CD20+ Hodgkin lymphoma with the monoclonal antibody rituximab is effective and well tolerated: results of a phase 2 trial of the German Hodgkin Lymphoma Study Group. *Blood* 2003; **101**: 420–4.

●89. Ekstrand BC, Lucas JB, Horwitz SM *et al.* Rituximab in lymphocyte-predominant Hodgkin disease: results of a phase 2 trial. *Blood* 2003; **101**: 4285–9.

90. Engert A, Ballova V, Haverkamp H *et al.* Hodgkin's lymphoma in elderly patients: a comprehensive retrospective analysis from the German Hodgkin's Study Group. *J Clin Oncol* 2005; **23**: 5052–60.

91. Ballova V, Ruffer JU, Haverkamp H *et al.* A prospectively randomized trial carried out by the German Hodgkin Study Group (GHSG) for elderly patients with advanced Hodgkin's disease comparing BEACOPP baseline and COPP-ABVD (study HD9elderly). *Ann Oncol* 2005; **16**: 124–31.

●92. Donnez J, Dolmans MM, Demylle D *et al.* Livebirth after orthotopic transplantation of cryopreserved ovarian tissue. *Lancet* 2004; **364**: 1405–10.

93. Behringer K, Breuer K, Reineke T *et al.* Secondary amenorrhoea after Hodgkin's disease is influenced by age at treatment, stage of disease, chemotherapy regimen, and the use of oral contraceptives during therapy: a report from the German Hodgkin Lymphoma Study Group (GHSG). *J Clin Oncol* 2005; **23**: 7555–64.

94. Kreuser ED, Felsenberg D, Behles C *et al.* Long-term gonadal dysfunction and its impact on bone mineralization in patients following COPP/ABVD chemotherapy for Hodgkin's disease. *Ann Oncol* 1992; **3**(Suppl 4): 105–10.

95. Blumenfeld Z, Dann E, Avivi I *et al.* Fertility after treatment for Hodgkin's disease. *Ann Oncol* 2002; **13**(Suppl 1): 138–47.

96. Santoro A, Bredenfeld H, Devizzi L *et al.* Gemcitabine in the treatment of refractory Hodgkin's disease: results of a multicenter phase II study. *J Clin Oncol* 2000; **18**: 2615–19.

97. Hirsch A, Vander Els N, Straus DJ *et al.* Effect of ABVD chemotherapy with and without mantle or mediastinal irradiation on pulmonary function and symptoms in early-stage Hodgkin's disease. *J Clin Oncol* 1996; **14**: 1297–305.

98. Horning SJ, Adhikari A, Rizk N *et al.* Effect of treatment for Hodgkin's disease on pulmonary function: results of a prospective study. *J Clin Oncol* 1994; **12**: 297–305.

99. Hull MC, Morris CG, Pepine CJ *et al.* Valvular dysfunction and carotid, subclavian, and coronary artery disease in

survivors of Hodgkin lymphoma treated with radiation therapy. *JAMA* 2003; **290**: 2831–7.

100.   Viviani S, Ragni G, Santoro A *et al.* Testicular dysfunction in Hodgkin's disease before and after treatment. *Eur J Cancer* 1991; **27**: 1389–92.

101.   Familiari G, Caggiati A, Nottola SA *et al.* Ultrastructure of human ovarian primordial follicles after combination chemotherapy for Hodgkin's disease. *Hum Reprod* 1993; **8**: 2080–7.

102.   Ruffer JU, Flechtner H, Tralls P *et al.* Fatigue in long-term survivors of Hodgkin's lymphoma; a report from the German Hodgkin Lymphoma Study Group (GHSG). *Eur J Cancer* 2003; **39**: 2179–86.

103.   Travis LB, Gospodarowicz M, Curtis RE *et al.* Lung cancer following chemotherapy and radiotherapy for Hodgkin's disease. *J Natl Cancer Inst* 2002; **94**: 182–92.

104.   Bartlett NL, Younes A, Carabasi MA *et al.* Phase I study of SGN-30, a chimeric monoclonal antibody (mAb), in patients with refractory or recurrent CD30+ hematologic malignancies. *Blood* 2002; **100**: 1403a (abstract).

105.   Leonard JP, Rosenblatt JD, Bartlett NL *et al.* Phase II study of SGN-30 (anti-CD30 monoclonal antibody) in patients with refractory or recurrent Hodgkin's disease. *Blood* 2004; **104**: 2635a.

106.   Ansell SM, Byrd JC, Horwitz SM *et al.* Phase I/II, ppen-label, dose-escalating study of MDX-060 administered weekly for 4 weeks in subjects with refractory/relapsed CD30 positive lymphoma. *Blood* 2004; **104**: 2636a.

107.   Younes A, Romaguera J, Hagemeister F *et al.* A pilot study of rituximab in patients with recurrent, classic Hodgkin disease. *Cancer* 2003; **98**: 310–14.

108.   Lenhard RE Jr, Order SE, Spunberg JJ *et al.* Isotopic immunoglobulin: a new systemic therapy for advanced Hodgkin's disease. *J Clin Oncol* 1985; **3**: 1296–300.

109.   Vriesendorp HM, Quadri SM, Wyllie CT *et al.* Fractionated radiolabeled antiferritin therapy for patients with recurrent Hodgkin's disease. *Clin Cancer Res* 1999; **5**: 3324s–9s.

•110.   Schnell R, Dietlein M, Staak JO *et al.* Treatment of refractory Hodgkin's lymphoma patients with an iodine-131-labeled murine anti-CD30 monoclonal antibody (131-I-Ki-4). *J Clin Oncol* 2005; **23**: 4669–78.

111.   Vriesendorp HM, Herpst JM, Germack MA *et al.* Phase I-II studies of yttrium-labeled antiferritin treatment for end-stage Hodgkin's disease, including Radiation Therapy Oncology Group 87-01. *J Clin Oncol* 1991; **9**: 918–28.

112.   Herpst JM, Klein JL, Leichner PK *et al.* Survival of patients with resistant Hodgkin's disease after polyclonal yttrium 90-labeled antiferritin treatment. *J Clin Oncol* 1995; **13**: 2394–400.

113.   Bierman PJ, Vose JM, Leichner PK *et al.* Yttrium 90-labeled antiferritin followed by high-dose chemotherapy and autologous bone marrow transplantation for poor-prognosis Hodgkin's disease. *J Clin Oncol* 1993; **11**: 698–703.

114.   Hartmann F, Renner C, Jung W *et al.* Treatment of refractory Hodgkin's disease with an anti-CD16/CD30 bispecific antibody. *Blood* 1997; **89**: 2042–7.

115.   Hartmann F, Renner C, Jung W *et al.* Anti-CD16/CD30 bispecific antibody treatment for Hodgkin's disease: role of infusion schedule and costimulation with cytokines. *Clin Cancer Res* 2001; **7**: 1873–81.

116.   Borchmann P, Schnell R, Fuss I *et al.* Phase 1 trial of the novel bispecific molecule H22xKi-4 in patients with refractory Hodgkin lymphoma. *Blood* 2002; **100**: 3101–7.

117.   Heslop HE, Ng CY, Li C *et al.* Long-term restoration of immunity against Epstein-Barr virus infection by adoptive transfer of gene-modified virus-specific T lymphocytes. *Nat Med* 1996; **2**: 551–5.

118.   Roskrow MA, Suzuki N, Gan Y *et al.* Epstein-Barr virus (EBV)-specific cytotoxic T lymphocytes for the treatment of patients with EBV-positive relapsed Hodgkin's disease. *Blood* 1998; **91**: 2925–34.

119.   Horning SJ, Hoppe RT, Advani R *et al.* Efficacy and late effects of Stanford V chemotherapy and radiotherapy in untreated Hodgkin's disease: mature data in early and advanced stage patients. *Blood* 2004; **104**: abstract 308.

120.   Federico M, Levis A, Luminari S *et al.* ABVD vs. STANFORD V (SV) vs. MOPP-EBV-CAD (MEC) in advanced Hodgkin's lymphoma. Final results of the IIL HD9601 randomized trial. *J Clin Oncol* 2004; **22**(Suppl 14): 6507 (abstract).

73

Hodgkin lymphoma in children

DEBRA L FRIEDMAN AND CINDY L SCHWARTZ

INTRODUCTION

The first description of Hodgkin lymphoma (HL) was anatomic in nature, in 1832, when Thomas Hodgkin described seven patients with enlarged lymph glands and spleen. This was followed, at the turn of the twentieth century, by histologic descriptions of the now-characteristic multinucleated giant cells by Sternberg in 1898[1] and Reed in 1902.[2] In the 1960s, the clonality of the Reed-Sternberg cell was established[3] and in the past decade attention has been focused on understanding the molecular biology of the disease, with respect to immunoglobulin genes, transcription factors, apoptotic pathways, and Epstein–Barr virus (EBV) incorporation.[4–7]

Therapeutic advances in HL began in 1902 when Pusey reported on the use of radiation therapy.[8] This was followed by the use of single-agent chemotherapy with mechlorethamine (nitrogen mustard) in 1946.[9] Over the next two decades, research was directed toward the use of combination chemotherapy, leading to the introduction of the four-drug MOPP protocol in 1964[10] and ABVD in the 1970s.[11] Donaldson and colleagues at Stanford introduced the concept of combined modality therapy for pediatric patients using the MOPP backbone and low-dose radiation therapy.[12] (See Table 73.4 for acronyms of treatment protocols.) This was followed both in the medical and pediatric oncology arenas by the rapid development of multimodality, risk-adapted therapies designed to balance efficacy with toxicity, as well as the study of adverse long-term outcomes related to the disease and its treatment.

EPIDEMIOLOGY

Incidence

The following information is based on the United States Surveillance, Epidemiology, and End Results (SEER) data.[13] Hodgkin lymphoma makes up 8.8 percent of all childhood cancer under the age of 20 years, but 17.7 percent of cancer in children between ages 15 and 17 years. The overall annual incidence rate in the United States is 12.1 per million for children under 20 years increasing to 32 per million when limiting the analysis to adolescents aged between 15 and 19 years.

Overall, there is a slight female predominance when considering all children less than 20 years old (male:female = 0.9) but a clear male predominance among children under 5 years of age (male:female = 5.3). The Caucasian:African American ratio is 1.3:1.[13]

Histology also differs by age and gender. Overall among children less than 20 years of age, the nodular sclerosing subtype accounts for 70 percent of cases, followed by mixed cellularity (16 percent), lymphocyte predominant (7 percent), lymphocyte depleted (less than 2 percent), and others not well specified (6 percent). However, under the age of 10 years, the mixed-cellularity subtype accounts for 32 percent of cases and, across all pediatric age groups, is more common in males. Similarly, the nodular sclerosing subtype is most prevalent among those 15–19 years of age (74 percent) and is more common in females across all pediatric age groups.[13]

Risk factors

There are several factors that are known to increase the risk of developing HL, which include family history of HL, EBV infections, socioeconomic status, and social contacts. For young adult disease (ages 16–44 years), there is a 99-fold increased risk among monozygotic twins and a 7-fold increased risk among other siblings.[14–16] The interaction between EBV and HL is quite fascinating with respect to epidemiology and biology (see below). Epstein–Barr virus-associated HL (EBV genome incorporated in tumor DNA) is most commonly reported with the mixed-cellularity histologic subtype, in children from underdeveloped and developing nations, and in young adult males. A history of infectious mononucleosis and high-titer antibodies to EBV are associated with young adult HL where, paradoxically, it is rare to see incorporation of the EBV genome in the tumor.[7,17–20] The association between HL and socioeconomic status, interestingly, also differs by age. In children under 10 years the disease is associated with lower socioeconomic status and large sibship.[21,22] In contrast, risk in young adult patients increases with higher socioeconomic status and with the related characteristics of small nuclear family, single family housing, and fewer siblings or childhood playmates. These findings may be related to an association with infections, where increased infections in early childhood may reduce the risk of young adult HL.[23,24] There are inconsistent data regarding clustering of young adult cases.[25,26] These epidemiologic data are summarized in Table 73.1.

Biology

The biology of HL has been difficult to elucidate since rare Reed–Sternberg (RS) cells are embedded within a reactive infiltrate of lymphocytes, macrophages, granulocytes, and eosinophils.[27] The RS cell is the hallmark of classical HL and is a binucleated or multinucleated giant cell that is often characterized by a bilobed nucleus, with two large nucleoli, giving the classically described 'owl's eye' appearance.[28]

The RS cell and its variants most commonly derive from a neoplastic clone originating from B lymphocytes in lymph node germinal centers. Molecular sequence analyses of RS cell clones reveal rearrangements of immunoglobulin variable-region genes that result in the lack of immunoglobulin production. Such cells should die from apoptosis, but it is thought that RS cells evade the apoptotic pathway, leading to the genesis of HL.[4,5] The B lymphoid cells from which RS cells arise have high levels of constitutive nuclear factor κB (NF-κB), a transcription factor known to mediate gene expression related to inflammatory and immune responses; deregulation of NF-κB has been postulated as a mechanism by which RS cells evade apoptosis.[6,29] Nuclear factor κB dimers are held in an inactive cytoplasmic complex with inhibitory proteins, the IκBs.[29] B cell stimulation by diverse signals results in rapid activation of the IκB kinase (IKK). The IKK complex phosphorylates two critical serine residues of IκBs,[30–32] thereby targeting them for rapid ubiquitin-mediated proteasomal degradation. Active NF-κB dimers are then released and translocated to the nucleus, where they activate gene transcription. Activation of NF-κB appears to be a final common effect of costimulatory interactions, genetic aberrations, or viral proteins that operate in HL.[33]

There are a number of determinants of RS cell survival. Reed–Sternberg cells express CD40, and CD40 ligand (CD40L) is expressed on inflammatory T cells and dendritic cells that surround them. CD40/CD40L interactions normally provide a second signal from activated helper T cells to normal B cells, resulting in activation of NF-κB. Nuclear factor κB in turn causes proliferation and induces expression of BCLX$_L$, which protects B cells from apoptosis.[34] Tumor necrosis factor receptor-associated factor 1 (TRAF-1) is overexpressed in EBV-transformed lymphoid cells and RS cells[35] and is associated with activation of NF-κB and protection of lymphoid cells from antigen-induced apoptosis. Activation of NF-κB, in turn, leads to expression of

Table 73.1 Etiologic risk factors for Hodgkin lymphoma

Risk factor	Associations
Epstein–Barr virus (EBV) exposure	Increased risk of young adult HL
Incorporation of EBV genome	Increased risk of mixed cellularity histology, disease in underdeveloped nations, and young adult males
High socioeconomic status	Increased risk of young adult disease
Low socioeconomic status	Increased risk in children age <10 years
Small nuclear family and single family housing, few early playmates	Increased risk of young adult disease
Early childhood infections	Decreased risk of young adult disease

HL, Hodgkin lymphoma.

TRAF-1, thereby establishing a positive feedback loop that maximizes NF-κB-dependent gene expression.[36] Epstein–Barr virus latent membrane protein 1 (LMP-1) interacts with TRAF-1, and tumors with TRAF-1–LMP-1 aggregates exhibit high NF-κB activity.[37,38] Latent membrane protein 1 activates NF-κB by promoting IκBα turnover.[39] Reed-Sternberg cells express CD30, and CD30 ligation promotes proliferation of HL-derived cells with constitutive activation of NF-κB.[40]

Epstein–Barr virus may play a role in the rescue and repair of RS cells, further aiding their evasion of apoptosis. Genome fragments can be found in approximately 30–50 percent of HL specimens.[7,41–43] Three latent viral antigens are expressed in EBV-positive HL in RS cells: Epstein–Barr nuclear antigen-1 (EBNA-1), required for viral episome maintenance; LMP-1 with transforming properties; and LMP-2, which is nontransforming.[44,45]

Histology

Hodgkin lymphoma can broadly be divided into two pathologic classes: classical Hodgkin lymphoma (CHL) and nodular lymphocyte-predominant Hodgkin lymphoma (NLPHL).[46,47] In turn, CHL can be further divided into four subtypes: lymphocyte rich (LRCHL), nodular sclerosis (NSHL), mixed cellularity (MCHL), and lymphocyte depleted (LDHL).

Tumor cells (RS cells) in CHL do not express B cell antigens such as CD45, CD19, and CD79A, but virtually all express CD30 and approximately 70 percent express CD15, while only 20–30 percent express CD20.[48] In comparison, the tumor cells of NLPHL do express B cell antigens such as CD19, CD20, CD22, and CD79A, may or may not express CD30, and do not express CD15.[49] In addition, the *OCT2* and *BOB1* oncogenes are downregulated in CHL but not in NLPHL, correlating with immunoglobulin transcription.[50]

CLINICAL CONSIDERATIONS

Presentation and staging

Eighty percent of patients present with painless adenopathy in a pattern that suggests contiguous lymph node spread. Mediastinal involvement is present in approximately 76 percent of adolescents compared with a much lower prevalence (33 percent) in children aged 10 years or younger. A large mediastinal mass with a maximum diameter that is greater than one-third of the chest diameter and/or a node or nodal aggregate greater than 10 cm occurs in about 20 percent of patients.[51,52] Approximately 20 percent of patients may also have associated B symptoms. B symptoms are defined as (1) unexplained loss of more than 10 percent of body weight in the 6 months preceding the diagnosis; (2) unexplained fever with temperatures

greater than 38 degrees Celsius for more than 3 days; or (3) drenching night sweats. Pruritus is also a systemic complaint, which may be associated with adverse outcome but is not considered a B symptom.[52–54] Employing a combination of physical examination and imaging studies, staging is now performed clinically, based on the Ann Arbor staging system[55] as revised in 1989.[53] Approximately 80–85 percent of children and adolescents with HL have involvement limited to or direct extension from the lymph nodes and/or the spleen (stages I–III), whereas 15–20 percent of patients have noncontiguous extranodal involvement involving the lung, bone marrow, bone, or liver.[55] While the staging definitions, B symptoms, and definition of extranodal extension are relatively standard, bulk disease and substaging has not been consistently applied across studies (Table 73.2).

Diagnostic evaluation

The diagnostic workup for HL is summarized in Table 73.3. A detailed history should be obtained to elicit the presence of B symptoms. A thorough physical evaluation should be performed, documenting the site and size of all adenopathy as well as splenic involvement or evidence of organ dysfunction. A surgical procedure should be performed to obtain a specimen for biopsy and an excisional lymph node biopsy is the recommended procedure. Fine-needle aspirations may provide specimens that are inadequate for full histologic evaluation, including appropriate immunophenotyping.

Computed tomography (CT) scans of the neck, thorax, abdomen, and pelvis should be performed. In addition, an upright chest radiograph (CXR) with posteroanterior (PA) and lateral views is required for documentation of a large mediastinal mass (bulk mediastinal disease), defined as tumor diameter greater than one-third the thoracic diameter (measured transversely at the level of the dome of the diaphragm on a six-foot upright PA CXR).[56]

Nuclear medicine imaging is also part of the diagnostic staging of HL and, together with CT, is useful in monitoring response to therapy. It is not uncommon for lesions of HL to have less than 100 percent regression; nuclear medicine imaging may help distinguish post-therapy active disease from scarring. Gallium-67 scintigraphy has been widely used and is particularly sensitive in the neck and mediastinum.[57] Due to limitations of gallium scintigraphy with respect to low resolution, physiologic biodistribution, need for delayed scanning, and problematic interpretation in disease below the diaphragm, fluorodeoxyglucose positron emission tomography (FDG-PET) is now being recognized as the nuclear imaging modality of choice. It is a 1-day procedure with higher resolution, better dosimetry, and less intestinal activity. In addition, with the advent of combined CT-PET scans, areas of disease can be evaluated simultaneously with both modalities in an overlapping fashion.[57–60] The role of response by FDG-PET is now

Table 73.2   Clinical and staging criteria for Hodgkin lymphoma

A. Stage grouping

Stage I: Involvement of single lymph node region (I) or localized involvement of a single extralymphatic organ or site (IE)

Stage II: Involvement of two or more lymph node regions on the same side of the diaphragm (II) or localized contiguous
                  involvement of a single extralymphatic organ or site and its regional lymph node(s) with involvement of one or
                  more lymph node regions on the same side of the diaphragm (IIE)

Stage III: Involvement of lymph node regions on both sides of the diaphragm (III), which may also be accompanied by
                  localized contiguous involvement of an extralymphatic organ or site (IIIE), by involvement of the spleen (IIIS),
                  or both (IIIE+S)

Stage IV: Disseminated (multifocal) involvement of one or more extralymphatic organs or tissues, with or without
                  associated lymph node involvement, or isolated extralymphatic organ involvement with distant (nonregional)
                  nodal involvement

B. Symptoms and presentations

A symptoms: Lack of 'B' symptoms

B symptoms: At least one of the following:
                  Unexplained weight loss >10% in the preceding 6 months
                  Unexplained recurrent fever >38°C
                  Drenching night sweats

X   Bulk disease (see C below)

E   Involvement of a single extranodal site that is contiguous or proximal to the known nodal site

C. Bulk disease

One or both of the following presentations are considered 'bulk' disease:

Large mediastinal mass:

Tumor diameter >1/3 the thoracic diameter (measured transversely at the level of the dome of the diaphragm on a 6-foot upright PA CXR). In the presence of hilar nodal disease the maximal mediastinal tumor measurement may be taken at the level of the hilus. This should be measured as the maximum mediastinal width (at a level containing tumor and any normal mediastinal structures at the level) over the maximum thoracic ratio

Large extramediastinal nodal aggregate:

A continuous aggregate of nodal tissue that measures >6 cm[a] in the longest transverse diameter in any nodal area

[a]Some studies use 10 cm for definition of extramediastinal bulk disease.
PA CXR, posteroanterior chest radiograph.

Table 73.3   Diagnostic workup and staging for Hodgkin lymphoma

Surgical
Excisional lymph node biopsy
Bilateral bone marrow biopsies

Imaging studies
CT scan of the neck, chest, abdomen, pelvis
Gallium-67 scintigraphy with SPECT or FDG-PET
Technetium-99 bone scintigraphy

Laboratory studies
Complete blood count
Blood chemistries for renal and hepatic function
Erythrocyte sedimentation rate

CT, computed tomography; SPECT, single photon emission CT; FDG-PET, fluorodeoxyglucose positron emission tomography.

being used in cooperative group trials. In the German Pediatric Oncology Hematology (GPOH) 2003 study, PET was used to change stage if CT or magnetic resonance imaging (MRI) results are inconclusive. An isolated focus of increased activity without a morphologic correlate will not upstage patients.[61] The Children's Oncology Group (COG) is assessing the role of FDG-PET for assessment of early response to chemotherapy and for definition of complete response. Children's Oncology Group trials are not recommending PET for the determination of stage without correlation with CT.

Recommendations for additional imaging studies are based on the likelihood of detected higher stage disease, the impact of such detection on therapy, or its use as a baseline for assessing therapeutic response. Technetium-99 bone scintigraphy should be performed in patients with bone pain or elevated alkaline phosphatase; positive findings may increase stage or extent of radiation fields. Bone marrow biopsy is recommended for all stage III and IV patients or patients with B symptoms. There are less consistent recommendations for lower stage patients without B symptoms; the utility of these tests is being evaluated in clinical trials.[62,63] Laboratory studies include a complete blood count, blood chemistries to evaluate hepatic and renal function, and acute phase reactants such as ferritin, erythrocyte sedimentation rate, and serum copper, which may be seen as nonspecific markers of tumor activity.

Prognostic factors

Adverse prognostic markers noted in clinical trials form the basis for modification of therapeutic algorithms. In sequential trials, these adverse prognostic markers of disease are then often abrogated by the therapy, which is often risk adapted. For example, in the German-Austrian Pediatric DAL-HD-90 trial, bulk disease was not an adverse prognostic factor, a likely result of boost doses of radiation therapy given to sites of post-chemotherapy residual disease.[64] Pretreatment factors that have been shown in several pediatric studies to be associated with adverse outcome include advanced stage, B symptoms, bulk disease, extranodal extension, male gender, and elevated erythrocyte sedimentation rate, and in some studies, hemoglobin $<11.0\,g/dL$ or white blood cell count $>11\,500/mm^3$, age 5–10 years, and increased number of sites of disease.[65–71] Patients with NLPHL appear to have an overall better prognosis than those with CHL, and amongst those with CHL, histologic subtype is not consistently associated with prognosis.[69,72] There is an evolving area of research surrounding intermediate serum markers that may confer adverse prognostic risk, such as soluble vascular adhesion molecule-1, tumor necrosis factor, soluble CD30, β_2-microglobulin, transferin, serum IL-10, and serum CD8 antigen.[73–78] High RS cell levels of caspase-3 may be associated with a more favorable outcome.[79]

Early response to treatment may also be an important prognostic factor, allowing titration of therapy to the individual.[70,80–82] Such therapeutic response to therapy is likely to reflect the underlying biology of the disease and of the host. Understanding the biologic correlates of such response will facilitate the implementation of tailored therapies and ultimately of biologically targeted therapies. Studies that examine biologic correlates of response require the large correlative studies that are feasible in cooperative group studies.

Initial treatment for pediatric Hodgkin lymphoma

COOPERATIVE GROUP PROTOCOLS

Hodgkin lymphoma is one of the few pediatric malignancies that shares aspects of its biology and natural history with the same cancer in adults. As a result, early treatment

Table 73.4   Common chemotherapy protocols and acronyms

Acronym	Chemotherapy agents
ABV	Doxorubicin, bleomycin, vinblastine
ABVD	Doxorubicin, bleomycin, vinblastine, dacarbazine (DTIC)
BEACOPP	Bleomycin, etoposide, doxorubicin, cyclophosphamide, vincristine, procarbazine, prednisone
CHOP	Cyclophosphamide, doxorubicin, vincristine, prednisone
COP (P)	Cyclophosphamide, vincristine, procarbazine, (prednisone)
D(A)BVE (PC)	Doxorubicin, bleomycin, vincristine, etoposide, (prednisone, cyclophosphamide)
MOPP	Mechlorethamine (nitrogen mustard), vincristine, procarbazine, prednisone
VAMP	Vincristine, doxorubicin, methotrexate, prednisone
VEPA	Vinblastine, etoposide, prednisone, doxorubicin
OEPA	Vincristine, etoposide, prednisone, doxorubicin
OPPA	Vincristine, procarbazine, prednisone, doxorubicin
ICE	Ifosfamide, carboplatin, etoposide
IV	Ifosfamide, vinorelbine
BEAM	Carmustine, etoposide, cytarabine, melphalan

approaches were modeled after those used in adults. While the cure rate was high, enthusiasm for this approach was quickly offset by the substantial morbidities that resulted from higher doses of radiation therapy and later from specific types of chemotherapy.[83] Contemporary standard approaches to pediatric HL evolved to include multiagent chemotherapy with low-dose involved field radiation therapy (IFRT). The volume of radiation therapy, the chemotherapeutic choice, intensity, and duration are now determined in a risk-adapted manner, using a combination of disease stage, symptoms, disease bulk, and other prognostic factors to assign risk stratification. In general terms, the overriding principles of these treatment regimens are to balance efficacy with both acute and, perhaps more importantly, long-term toxicities.[84–86] A summary of common protocols with acronyms is found in Table 73.4.

Since the initial use of MOPP in the 1960s, marked improvement in cure rate has taken place in pediatric Hodgkin lymphoma.[87] Donaldson and colleagues at Stanford introduced the concept of combined modality therapy for pediatric patients using the MOPP backbone and low-dose radiation therapy.[12] Subsequent therapies have built upon the MOPP backbone. ABVD was added as an alternative effective regimen in an attempt to improve survival and decrease long-term effects of treatment. Published complete remission rates with MOPP, MOPP/ABVD, and ABVD range from 69 percent to 92 percent, with the results for each regimen varying considerably from study to study.[88]

Between 1987 and 2001, the Children's Cancer Group (CCG), the Pediatric Oncology Group (POG), and the Dana Farber–Stanford–St. Jude Pediatric Hodgkin's Consortium (PHC) and the German pediatric cooperative groups (DAL and GPOH) have conducted the largest risk-adapted therapeutic studies for children and adolescents with Hodgkin lymphoma. These protocols evaluated a series of research questions designed to maximize cure while minimizing long-term adverse outcomes of therapy.

In an attempt to decrease alkylator therapy and potential cardiotoxicity, and provide dose-intensive treatment, the POG developed a series of studies built upon the ABVD backbone, substituting dacarbazine with etoposide. The use of vincristine instead of vinblastine allowed for escalation of doxorubicin and etoposide. POG 9226 piloted therapy with 4 cycles of DBVE followed by low-dose IFRT in patients with stages I, IIA, and IIIA; 5-year event-free survival (EFS) was 89 percent.[89] POG 9426 evaluated the same chemotherapy in a nonrandomized response-based manner. Those with a rapid response (60 percent tumor reduction, gallium scan negative) after 2 cycles proceeded to consolidative IFRT without further chemotherapy; slow responders continued to receive 4 cycles plus IFRT. In POG 9425 (for patients with advanced stage disease) prednisone and cyclophosphamide were added to the ABVE-PC backbone, with more rapid delivery of therapy to intensify the weekly therapeutic intensity. Response was assessed after 3 cycles (9 weeks). Those with rapid response did not receive the additional 2 cycles of chemotherapy. Overall 3-year EFS was 87 percent and overall survival (OS) 96 percent, with no difference in EFS between slow and rapid responders and a progressive disease rate of only 1 percent. All patients received consolidative regional low-dose (20 Gy) radiation therapy.[81,86] Both studies evaluated the efficacy of dexrazoxane in reducing cardiac and pulmonary toxicity. While it is still too early to know whether there was a significant benefit, dexrazoxane was associated with an increased risk of acute (hematologic/infectious) toxicities and development of second malignancies, mostly treatment-related leukemia.[90]

With the goal of continued excellent long-term survival and decreasing long-term effects of treatment, the POG and CCG have conducted trials to evaluate elimination of radiation therapy. In the CCG 521 study, patients were randomized between 12 cycles of alternating MOPP/AVBD and 6 cycles of AVBD plus low-dose regional chemotherapy. Event-free survival was only 77 percent for stage III and IV patients and there was excess pulmonary toxicity with ABVD.[91] POG 8725 compared 8 cycles of MOPP/AVBD with and without IFRT in stage IIB, III, and IV patients. There was no significant benefit for radiation therapy,[92] but the study used a large amount of chemotherapy, which is associated with potential significant long-term adverse outcomes including gonadal toxicity, cardiac toxicity, and secondary leukemia (see long-term outcomes

of therapy below). Response following 3 cycles was a strong prognostic factor, with a 94 percent EFS in the rapid early responders as opposed to a 78 percent EFS in those who did not respond quickly. There was no change in therapy for slow early responders and the comparison was made retrospectively.[92] CCG 5942 studied the elimination of radiation therapy in a randomized fashion in all patients who had a complete response following chemotherapy. Patients were treated with 4 cycles of COPP/ABV, 6 cycles of COPP/ABV, or 2 cycles each of COPP/ABV, cytarabine/etoposide, and CHOP, depending on stage of disease and presence of bulk disease. Of the 829 eligible patients, complete response was achieved in 83 percent and 501 were randomized to receive IFRT or no further therapy. Event-free survival for all stage II, III, and IV patients was 84.4 percent, 76 percent, and 81 percent at 4 years, respectively. In all groups the difference in EFS post-randomization was highly significant and overall EFS was 91 percent for the group who received IFRT and 86 percent for those who did not. Despite the differences in EFS, early evaluation of overall survival is not affected by the inclusion of IFRT.[65] A pilot study, CCG 59704, utilized the German Hodgkin Disease Group's BEACOPP backbone for patients with B symptoms or advanced stage disease. Overall the 3-year EFS was 95 percent with patients receiving 6–8 cycles of chemotherapy with or without radiation therapy on the basis of a gender-stratified, response-based therapeutic algorithm.[93]

The COG, representing the merger of POG and CCG, has since moved forward with design of studies to improve efficacy and decrease long-term adverse effects of treatment. Open studies evaluate the principles of risk-adapted therapy, where therapy is decreased for those at lowest risk and with favorable early responses to chemotherapy and augmented for those with more advanced disease or a slow response to initial chemotherapy. In this setting, the goal is to identify the likely small cohort of pediatric patients who require radiation therapy and to limit or avoid its use in others.

The Dana Farber-Stanford-St. Jude pediatric Hodgkin lymphoma consortium studies have focused efforts on reduction in alkylating agent, anthracycline, and radiation therapy doses. Low-risk patients have been treated with 4 cycles of an alkylator-free chemotherapy protocol, VAMP, with radiation therapy doses of 15 Gy or 25.5 Gy based upon response to the first 2 cycles of chemotherapy. This approach resulted in a 5-year EFS of 93 percent.[94] Current efforts are being directed toward determining whether a group of patients can be identified who can be effectively treated with the alkylator-free chemotherapeutic regimen (VAMP) without radiation therapy. For patients with higher-risk disease, two protocols have been evaluated – VAMP/COP and VEPA – both with IFRT. Results have been less acceptable with 5-year EFS of 74 percent and 68 percent, respectively.[95,96] The group is now evaluating the Stanford-V regimen[97] that has been successfully employed in adult patients.

In the same era, the German cooperative groups have built upon COPP chemotherapy in both pediatric and adult Hodgkin lymphoma. The DAL-HL-90 study used OEPA/COPP for males and OPPA/COPP for females, both followed by IFRT. Event-free survival for stages II, III, and IV were 92, 86, and 90 percent, respectively.[98] The GPOH-95 study was designed to assess elimination of radiation therapy for those with a complete response. It built on the OPPA/OEPA backbones by adding cycles of COPP for patients with more advanced disease. Radiation therapy dose was determined by the post-chemotherapy disease reduction. Complete response was defined as complete resolution of all disease (as opposed to 70 percent reduction in CCG 5942 and 59704). Only 22 percent of patients achieved a complete response. Fifty percent achieved between 75 percent and 95 percent disease reduction and were treated with 20 Gy radiation therapy, while 4 percent had less than a 75 percent reduction and were treated with 30 Gy. Twenty percent of patients had residual masses treated with boost doses to 35 Gy. Overall the EFS was 92 percent for those receiving radiation therapy compared with 88 percent in those treated with chemotherapy alone. This difference was largely influenced by patients with more advanced stage disease or B symptoms. For patients with IA, IB, and IIA disease, EFS was not different among those with a complete response to chemotherapy and no other therapy (97 percent) and those with a partial response subsequently treated with radiation therapy (94 percent). However, for all other patients the EFS was 79 percent for those treated with chemotherapy alone compared with 91 percent for those treated with combined modality therapy.[99] A summary of these protocols is found in Table 73.5.

Treatment for low-risk NLPHL patients requires specific comment, since some patients may be treated with surgery alone. There are multiple small reports in both adult and pediatric HL patients of successful treatment of completely resected stage I disease. For those who did relapse, salvage rates were encouraging and death from disease was very low.[100–103] This has prompted a study in the COG to formally evaluate surgery only in patients with involvement of a single, completely resected lymph node with NLPHL.

Based on the results of these studies, together with the many studies that have preceded them, effective therapies for HL are presented in Table 73.6.

RADIATION THERAPY FOR HODGKIN LYMPHOMA

It has been recognized since the 1950s that HL is an extremely radiosensitive disease. Initially this therapy was delivered using orthovoltage where limited fields could safely be treated to high doses. With the advent of the linear accelerator, Kaplan and colleagues at Stanford University developed techniques to safely and effectively treat large fields with high doses.[52] Initially all patients, regardless of age, were treated with common radiation therapy protocols, until the 1970s when pediatric-specific protocols were developed. At the present time, for children and adolescents with HL, radiation therapy is almost exclusively delivered in the context of multimodality therapy. Doses of 15–25 Gy are commonly used, and some experimental protocols are attempting to identify groups of patients for whom the exclusion of radiation therapy is possible without affecting disease-free survival.[104]

We briefly review some basic principles surrounding radiation therapy for HL, but refer the reader to the chapters specifically dedicated to radiation therapy in this text (see Chapter 51). In understanding these principles, it must be remembered that delivery of radiation therapy requires a large degree of judgment and careful assessment of the extent of disease. Considerations regarding the use and dose of radiation therapy include the age of the patient, tumor burden and location, and potential short- and long-term complications of the treatment.

Megavoltage energies are now the treatment of choice for pediatric HL. A 4–6-MeV linear accelerator should be used to treat supradiaphragmatic fields, whereas 8–15-MeV machines may be appropriate for treating paraaortic nodes. Distances of less than 80 cm are to be avoided as they will result in suboptimal depth-dosage. Although there are differences in treatment techniques among radiation oncologists and specific institutions, the general technical principles remain constant across centers.[105–107]

The fields of radiation therapy treatment must be meticulously and judiciously designed with the goal of delivering the optimum volume of radiation therapy for disease control while avoiding normal tissue damage. Involved fields typically include the entire lymph node region in which the diseased nodes are found, but may also include adjacent areas that are part of another lymph node region. For example, cervical nodes are treated if any abnormal node is found in this region, consistent with the anatomic node region. However, hila are treated when there is disease in the mediastinum, although they are parts of separate lymph node regions.[104] Guidelines for involved fields are found in Table 73.7.

Another important issue in the design of fields is to exclude uninvolved normal tissues, which can often be accomplished by careful positioning of the patient. Similarly, dosage calculations should take into account lack of homogeneity of tissues within a field. Such an example is a full mantle, which includes neck, axilla, and the mediastinum, each of which requires separate dosimetry calculations for best precision of dose. Field reductions, particularly in the mediastinum, may be appropriate based on the response to chemotherapy and the dose of radiation therapy. Customized shielding blocks should be utilized as appropriate to protect normal tissue. These may include posterior cervical spine, humeral head, laryngeal, occipital, lung, and cardiac blocks. Blocking the genitalia is of specific importance when pelvic fields are included. In females, while scattered and transmitted dose to the ovaries will be inevitable, medial or lateral transposition

Table 73.5 Selected completed cooperative group and consortium trials 1988–2001

Protocol (dates of accrual)	Study questions and treatment stratum	Survival: EFS/OS
POG 8625 (1986–1992) MOPP/ABVD ± IFRT POG 8725 (1987–1992) MOPP/ABVD ± TNRT	**Elimination of radiation therapy based on response** 3 chemotherapy cycles, no RT vs 2 chemotherapy cycles + 25 Gy IFRT 8 chemotherapy cycles; with CR, randomization ± 21 Gy TNRT	8-year: 86.9%/95.4% 8-year: 79%/92%
PHC (1990–1993) VEPA + IFRT	**Avoidance of alkylating agents and reduction in anthracycline dose** 6 chemotherapy cycles + 25.5 Gy IFRT	5-year: 67.8%/81.9%
PHC (1990–2000) VAMP + IFRT	**Avoidance of alkylating agents** **Reduction in radiation therapy doses** 4 chemotherapy cycles + 15 Gy IFRT for those who achieved a CR, or 25.5 Gy for those who achieved a PR following the first 2 cycles	5-year: 93%/93%
PHC (1990–) VAMP/COP + IFRT	**Reduction in alkylating agents and anthracycline dose** 6 chemotherapy cycles + 25.5 Gy IFRT	5-year: 74.2%/91.7%
CCG 5942 (1994–1998) COPP/ABV ± IFRT CHOP, COPP/ABV, ARA-C, VP16 ± IFRT	**Elimination of radiation therapy based on response** 4 or 6 chemotherapy cycles; with CR, randomization ± 21 Gy IFRT Novel hybrid chemotherapy; with CR, randomization ± 21 Gy IFRT	4-year: 85.4%/94.8%
POG 9426 (1996–2000) DBVE + IFRT ± DZR	**Reduction in chemotherapy based on rapid early response** **Elimination of procarbazine** **Feasibility/efficacy of dose-intensive therapy** **Dexrazoxane as cardioprotectant** RER after 2 chemotherapy cycles: 25 Gy IFRT SER after 2 chemotherapy cycles: 2 additional chemotherapy cycles + 25 IFRT ± DZR	3-year: 88.7%/97.7%
CCG 59704 (1997–2000) BEACOPP + IFRT BEACOPP/COPP ABV BEACOPP/ABVD + IFRT	**Elimination of radiation therapy for females with rapid early response** **Reduction of procarbazine for males with rapid early response** **Feasibility of dose-intensive therapy** 4 cycles of BEACOPP For female RER, 4 additional courses COPP/ABV: CR, no IFRT; <CR, 21 Gy IFRT For male RER, ABVD × 2 + 21 Gy IFRT SER, 8 cycles of BEACOPP + 21 Gy IFRT	3-year: 96%/98%
POG 9425 (1997–2001) DBVE-PC + IFRT ± DZR	**Reduction in chemotherapy based on rapid early response** **Elimination of procarbazine** **Feasibility/efficacy of dose-intensive therapy** **Dexrazoxane as cardioprotectant** RER after 2 chemotherapy cycles: 25 Gy IFRT SER after 2 chemotherapy cycles: 3 additional chemotherapy cycles + 25 IFRT ± DZR	3-year: 86.4%/96.8%
GPOH-95	**Chemotherapy based on stage and gender** **Radiation therapy dose based on response to chemotherapy** IA/IIA: OPPA × 2 or OEPA × 2 IIEA, IIB, IIIA: above + COPP × 2 IIEB, IIIEA, IIIB, IV: above + COPP × 4 IFRT post-chemotherapy CR: none (21.9%) >75%: 20 Gy (50%) <75%: 30 Gy (4.1%) Residual masses >50 mL boosted to 35 Gy (20.2%)	No IFRT 88%; IFRT 92% DFS

IFRT, involved field radiation therapy; TNRT, total nodal radiation therapy; RT, radiation therapy; CR, complete response; PR, partial response; EFS, event-free survival; OS, overall survival; RER, rapid early response; SER, slow early response; DZR, dexrazoxane; DFS, disease free survival.

Table 73.6 Recommendations for standard therapy in pediatric Hodgkin lymphoma

Risk group	Stage and presentation	Recommended therapy	Commonly accepted regimens
Low	IA, IIA <4 nodal regions without B symptoms, bulk disease, or extranodal extension	2–4 cycles of non-cross-resistant chemotherapy plus LD-IFRT	VAMP × 4 + LD-IFRT COPP/ABV hybrid × 4 + LD-IFRT DBVE × 4 + LD-IFRT OEPA or OPPA × 2 + LD-IFRT
Intermediate	IA, IIA with bulk disease, >3 nodal regions, or extranodal extension IIB[a], IIIA, IVA[a]	4–6 cycles of non-cross-resistant chemotherapy plus LD-IFRT	COPP/ABV × 6 + LD-IFRT DBVE-PC × 3–5 + LD-IFRT OPPA/OEPA × 2 + COPP × 2 + LD-IFRT
High	IIB[a], IIIB, IVB[a]	4–8 cycles of non-cross-resistant chemotherapy plus LD-IFRT	DBVE-PC × 3–5 + LD-IFRT BEACOPP × 8 (or BEACOPP × 4 + ABVD × 2 + LD-IFRT or + COPP/ABV × 4) ± LD-IFRT OPPA/OEPA × 2 + COPP × 4 + LD-IFRT

[a]It remains unclear whether IIB disease, particularly with bulk disease, is intermediate or high risk. Similarly some regimens treat all stage IV patients as high risk, although most studies show that patients with IVA disease have better outcomes than those with IVB.
LD-IFRT, low-dose involved field radiation therapy (15–25 Gy).

Table 73.7 Guidelines for involved field radiation

Involved nodes	Radiation therapy field
Cervical	Neck, supraclavicular/infraclavicular
Supraclavicular	Supraclavicular/infraclavicular, lower neck
Axillary	Axilla ± supraclavicular/infraclavicular
Mediastinum	Mediastinum, hila, and infraclavicular/supraclavicular
Hila	Hila, mediastinum
Spleen	Spleen ± paraaortic
Paraaortic	Paraaortic ± spleen
Iliac	Iliac, inguinal, femoral
Inguinal	External iliac, inguinal, femoral
Femoral	External iliac, inguinal, femoral

of the ovaries (oophoropexy) results in doses of 8–10 percent and 4–5 percent, respectively, of the pelvic dose,[108,109] which will be compatible with the preservation of fertility. For males, the greatest shielding to the testes is afforded by use of a frog-leg position together with an individually fitted shield, which will reduce the scatter to approximately 0.75 percent of the pelvic lymph node dose.[110]

Daily radiation therapy is delivered using equally weighted anterior and posterior fields, with fractional doses of 1.5–1.8 Gy daily, five times per week. It is imperative to design fields to minimize retreatment match-line problems if additional radiation therapy is needed to treat recurrence.[104]

Treatment for relapsed Hodgkin lymphoma

Hodgkin lymphoma may be cured even if it has recurred after initial treatment. Relapse usually occurs within the first 4 years following treatment. A spectrum of possible treatment options exists, and the choice is dependent upon factors including stage and burden of disease, site of relapse, previous chemotherapy/radiation therapy, time from initial treatment, and previous toxicities related to treatment. Potentially curative options include conventional chemotherapy/radiation therapy protocols for those with lower-risk relapses, radiation therapy alone for those relapsing in a limited nodal pattern, reinduction chemotherapy followed by autologous hematopoietic stem cell transplantation (HSCT), and experimental therapies such as immunotherapy.[111–118] Palliative care should always be considered for patients with refractory or recurrent disease when curative intent is not likely,[119] but care should be taken not to miss a potential curative opportunity.[120] Much of the data on relapsed HL come from studies that include both adult and pediatric patients. It remains unclear whether outcomes vary according to age.

There is no standard reinduction protocol. Chemotherapy agents are chosen, in part, dependent upon previous chemotherapy and radiation therapy exposures as well as planned additional therapy, such as the need for mobilization of stem cells and HSCT. Regardless of the salvage regimen, when HSCT is being considered, disease response to cytoreductive therapy prior to HSCT predicts overall survival. Hematopoietic stem cell transplantation is most effective for patients who enter with minimal or chemosensitive disease.[118,121,122] Two ifosfamide-based regimens have been used with good response rates – ICE[113,121] and, more recently, IV.[123] In addition, ICE has been used in the preparative regimen in a recently reported tandem transplant regimen.[124]

Patients with low stage disease (stage I, II), no B symptoms, and no bulk disease who were initially treated with non-dose-intensive chemotherapy and no radiation therapy may be salvaged with conventional chemotherapy and low-dose IFRT, or sometimes standard-dose radiation therapy alone.[114,125,126] However, B symptoms and extra-nodal disease at the time of relapse are poor prognostic factors,[127] as is shorter duration of initial remission.[128,129] For those who have previously been treated with chemotherapy/radiation therapy, particularly with standard radiation therapy or with newer dose-intensive regimens, recurrence within 12 months of completion of therapy results in overall survival rates of 10–30 percent with conventional chemotherapy regimens.[112,117,128,129] Relapses occurring at 12 months or later are more responsive to salvage chemotherapy, but overall survival rates remain low – 20–50 percent – with conventional chemotherapy.[128–130] Thus for patients with advanced stage disease, B symptoms, or bulk disease, or those previously treated with combined modality regimens that included dose-intensive chemotherapy or standard-dose radiation therapy, or those with a short period of remission, reinduction chemotherapy followed by HSCT and radiation therapy remains the treatment of choice, although survival rates range broadly from 25 to 80 percent.[111,118,120,131–139] An advantage of transplantation has been reported in two randomized trials, from the British National Lymphoma Investigation and the German Hodgkin's Lymphoma Study Group together with the European Group for Blood and Marrow Transplantation, where EFS was superior in the transplant arm compared to the conventional therapy arm, using a backbone of BEAM.[140,141]

Autologous HSCT is most commonly used for recurrent or refractory HD. However, an allogeneic effect has been observed, albeit offset by transplant-related morbidity and mortality.[135–137,142] This has led to research investigating reduced-intensity allogeneic approaches as well as immune modulation and induction of autologous graft-versus-host disease, in order to benefit from the allogeneic effect.[143–147]

LONG-TERM OUTCOMES OF HODGKIN LYMPHOMA AND ITS TREATMENT

Multimodality therapy for HL achieved a 5-year relative survival of 85.3 percent in the period from 1995 to 2001.[148] However, this survival is accompanied by adverse long-term health-related outcomes, which may include second malignant neoplasms, organ dysfunction, and psychosocial sequelae,[149] which are discussed in greater detail elsewhere in the text (see Chapter 61) and we refer the reader to that information. However, as treatment for HL is developed, in part, to avoid or reduce these adverse long-term outcomes, some discussion is warranted.

Second malignant neoplasms

Several large studies have examined the incidence and spectrum of second malignant neoplasms in HL survivors, with reports from large cohorts demonstrating a 7- to 18-times higher risk of subsequent malignancies compared with the general population. The risk of leukemia appears to plateau at 10–15 years post-therapy, while the risk of second solid malignancies, including sarcoma, melanoma, breast, lung, thyroid, and gastrointestinal cancer, rises with ongoing follow-up.[111,131,150–163] Compared with adults, children may be more prone to develop subsequent malignancy due to their growth potential and endogenous hormonal factors. Patterns of second solid tumors differ among pediatric and adult survivors, with breast cancer being more common following childhood HL and lung cancers following adult HL.[151,155,157,158,162,163]

Cardiac dysfunction

Hodgkin lymphoma survivors exposed to doxorubicin and thoracic radiation therapy are at risk for long-term cardiac toxicity,[164–171] which can increase non-relapse-related mortality.[172,173]

Late effects of radiation to the heart include the following: delayed pericarditis; pancarditis, which includes pericardial and myocardial fibrosis, with or without endocardial fibroelastosis; myopathy; coronary artery disease (CAD); functional valve injury; and conduction defects[111,164,166,174] However, with current techniques and reduced doses of radiation therapy, this is likely to change. Anthracycline-related cardiomyopathy is associated with female gender, cumulative doses greater than 200–300 mg/m^2, younger age at time of exposure, and increased time from exposure.[175,176]

Pulmonary dysfunction

Pulmonary fibrotic disease is seen as a late complication following radiation therapy. Acute pneumonitis, manifested by fever, congestion, cough, and dyspnea, can follow radiation therapy alone at doses of greater than 40 Gy to focal lung volumes, or after lower doses (15–20 Gy) when combined with chemotherapy and including generous or whole lung volumes.[177] Bleomycin-associated pulmonary fibrosis with decreased diffusion capacity is most commonly seen following doses greater than 200–400 units/m^2,[178–180] higher than those used in contemporary HL regimens.

Thyroid disease

Thyroid dysfunction, manifested by primary hypothyroidism, hyperthyroidism, goiter, or nodules, may be seen following radiation therapy to the neck for HL. The likelihood of thyroid dysfunction varies with the dose of radiation and the length of follow-up, while the detection depends on the biochemical criteria utilized to make the diagnosis.[181] For hypothyroidism, there is a clear dose response with a 20-year risk of 20 percent for those who had received less than 35 Gy, 30 percent following 35–44.9 Gy, and 50 percent following greater than 45 Gy to the thyroid gland. The risk for both hypo- and hyperthyroidism increases in the first 3–5 years since diagnosis, whereas that for nodules increases 10 and more years from diagnosis.[182]

Gonadal dysfunction and infertility

Spermatogenesis is highly sensitive to cyclophosphamide, procarbazine, and nitrogen mustard and thus infertility is a common complication of therapy following regimens that contain these agents, with azoospermia rates of up to 86 percent.[183–185] Males who receive less than 4 g/m^2 of cyclophosphamide, without testicular radiation or any other alkylating agent, are likely to retain their fertility. However, when combined with procarbazine, even lower doses of cyclophosphamide can result in sterility.[186] Cumulative doses of cyclophosphamide above 9 g/m^2 are likely to result in sterility.[111,185,187]

With respect to radiation therapy, the male germinal epithelium is damaged by much lower doses ($<$1 Gy) of radiation therapy than are Leydig cells (20–30 Gy). Doses less than 30 Gy are unlikely to affect endocrine function and boys can progress through puberty normally. Although temporary oligospermia can occur after these very low radiation doses, permanent azoospermia results from doses of greater

Table 73.8   General guidelines for radiation late effects assessment and management

System	Potential effects	Monitoring recommendations[a]
Cardiac	Cardiomyopathy Pericarditis Coronary artery disease Valvular disease	Electrocardiogram and echocardiogram
Pulmonary	Pulmonary fibrosis	Pulmonary function tests (including DLCO and spirometry)
Thyroid	Overt or compensated hypothyroidism Thyroid nodules or cancer Hyperthyroidism	Free T4; TSH
Gonadal (female)	Delayed/arrested puberty Early menopause Ovarian failure	FSH, LH, estradiol
Gonadal (male)	Germ cell failure Infertility/azoospermia Leydig cell dysfunction Hypogonadism Delayed/arrested puberty	FSH, LH, testosterone Semen analysis
Bone	**Osteopenia** Bone mineral density $\geqslant$1 and $<$2.5 SD below mean **Osteoporosis** Bone mineral density $\geqslant$2.5 SD below mean **Osteonecrosis** (avascular necrosis)	Bone density evaluation (DEXA or quantitative CT) MRI as clinically indicated by signs or symptoms suggestive of avascular necrosis
Second malignancies	Sarcomas CNS tumors Breast cancer Melanoma Non-melanoma skin cancer Thyroid cancer Other solid tumors	Routine cancer screening per general population guidelines Mammography to screen for female breast cancer at age 25 years or 10 years post-RT exposure, whichever is later

[a]Monitoring recommendations all include a risk-adapted health history and physical examination. The frequency with which diagnostic studies and laboratory tests should be performed is dependent on many factors including dose of radiation therapy, chemotherapy exposures, age at exposure, and other clinical parameters.
DLCO, carbon monoxide diffusing capacity; T4, thyroxine; TSH, thyroid-stimulating hormone; FSH, follicle-stimulating hormone; LH, luteinizing hormone; DEXA, dual energy x-ray absorptiometry; CT, computed tomography; MRI, magnetic resonance imaging; SD, standard deviation; CNS, central nervous system; RT, radiation therapy.

than 3–4 Gy. The potential for a return of spermatogenesis in the intermediate dose range of 1–3 Gy is variable.[188,189]

In females, the risk of menstrual irregularity, ovarian failure, and infertility increases with age at treatment.[190] Amenorrhea and premature ovarian failure occur more commonly in adult women treated with cyclophosphamide and other alkylating agents than in adolescents, with prepubertal females tolerating cumulative doses as high as 25 g/m^2.[191,192] Reviews of the changes in HL therapy over time indicate that the substitution of cyclophosphamide for mechlorethamine appears to have significantly reduced the risk of ovarian dysfunction, which is then further lessened by reduction in total dose of both agents.[85,193,194]

Psychosocial problems

Survivors of HL are also at risk for adverse psychologic outcomes. In the Childhood Cancer Survivor Study, 5.4 percent of 1843 HL survivors reported symptoms of depression and 15 percent reported somatic distress higher than that for other malignancies or from a sibling cohort. Female gender, lower household income, less than a high school education, and lack of current employment increased risk for depression and somatic distress symptoms, with older age also increasing risk for somatic distress.[195]

Monitoring for adverse long-term outcomes

The common potential long-term effects of radiation therapy and chemotherapy for HL are summarized, together with general monitoring recommendations, in Tables 73.8 and 73.9, respectively. To date, there do not exist uniformly effective long-term follow-up plans for survivors of childhood HL, as evidenced by published research over the past decade that documents a significant lost-to-follow-up rate, lack of knowledge on the part of HL and other childhood cancer survivors about their past treatment and potential for adverse health sequelae, inadequate provision of follow-up care, and poor utilization of available health services.[196–198] Various pediatric cooperative groups have addressed the problem with the development of long-term follow-up guidelines, which provide a foundation for what follow-up care should be delivered.[199,200] However, the recommendations are not completely consistent with one another and there is, at present, a lack of sufficient resources committed to ensure their implementation. Therefore, ongoing research is required to develop a uniform set of 'best practice' guidelines that can be utilized as an integral part of clinical care for survivors of childhood and adolescent HL.

Table 73.9 General guidelines for chemotherapy late effects assessment and management

System	Agents	Potential effects	Monitoring guidelines[a]
Cardiac	Anthracyclines	Cardiomyopathy Arrhythmias	Electrocardiogram and echocardiogram
Pulmonary	Bleomycin	Restrictive lung disease	PFTs (including DLCO and spirometry)
Gonadal (female)	Alkylating agents	Delayed/arrested puberty Early menopause Ovarian failure	FSH, LH, estradiol
Gonadal (male)	Alkylating agents	Germ cell failure Infertility/azoospermia Leydig cell dysfunction Hypogonadism Delayed/arrested puberty	FSH, LH, testosterone
Bone	Corticosteroids ± methotrexate	Osteopenia	Bone density evaluation (DEXA or quantitative CT)
	Alkylating agents (due to hypogonadism)	Bone mineral density ⩾1 and <2.5 SD below mean	MRI as clinically indicated by signs or symptoms suggestive of avascular necrosis
	Corticosteroids	Osteoporosis Bone mineral density ⩾2.5 SD below mean Osteonecrosis (avascular necrosis)	
Second malignancies	Alkylating agents: topoisomerase II inhibitors Cyclophosphamide	Leukemia	CBC/differential
		Transitional bladder carcinoma	Urinalysis

[a]Monitoring recommendations all include a risk-adapted health history and physical examination. The frequency with which diagnostic studies and laboratory tests should be performed is dependent on many factors including dose of chemotherapy, radiation therapy exposures, age at exposure, and other clinical parameters.

PFTs, pulmonary function tests; DLCO, carbon monoxide diffusing capacity; FSH, follicle-stimulating hormone; LH, luteinizing hormone; SD, standard deviation; DEXA, dual energy x-ray absorptiometry; CT, computed tomography; MRI, magnetic resonance imaging; CBC, complete blood count.

CONCLUSIONS

Hodgkin lymphoma is characterized by complex biology and epidemiology that require additional study to better understand how they interface with one another and affect disease presentation, response to therapy, and long-term outcomes. Cure rates remain one of the highest in pediatric oncology, but adverse long-term outcomes are similarly quite frequent in occurrence. Ongoing clinical trials thus seek to balance efficacy with both short- and long-term toxicity. For higher-risk initial disease and refractory and recurrent disease, the challenge remains increasing the cure rate and incorporating novel agents that may better target the underlying biology and pathophysiology.

KEY POINTS

- Hodgkin lymphoma is one of the most common malignancies in adolescents, accounting for close to 18 percent of all childhood cancer in the 15–17-year-old range.
- Epidemiologic risk factors include family history of lymphoma, exposure to Epstein–Barr virus, socioeconomic status, residence, and social contacts.
- Biology of HL is where Reed-Sternberg cells arise from B lymphoid cells that have high levels of constitutive nuclear NF-κB, a transcription factor known to mediate gene expression related to inflammatory and immune responses, and activation of NF-κB appears to be a final common effect of costimulatory interactions, genetic aberrations, or viral proteins that operate in HL.
- Hodgkin lymphoma can broadly be divided into two pathologic classes – classical Hodgkin lymphoma and nodular lymphocyte-predominant Hodgkin lymphoma – with differing cell-surface markers.
- Most patients present with painless adenopathy in a pattern that suggests contiguous lymph node spread. Patients may also have systemic symptoms of fever, weight loss, or night sweats (B symptoms) as well as pruritus.
- Standard initial treatment consists of risk-adapted chemotherapy with low-dose involved field radiation therapy.
- Treatment for recurrent disease includes both conventional chemotherapy/radiation therapy as well as hematopoietic stem cell transplantation.
- Potential adverse long-term toxicities include cardiopulmonary dysfunction, gonadal dysfunction and infertility, thyroid disease, psychosocial problems, and second malignant neoplasms.

REFERENCES

● = Key primary paper
◆ = Major review article

1. Sternberg C. Uber eind Eigenartige unter dem Bilde der Pseudoleuk mie verlaufende Turberculose des lymphatischen. *Apparates Z Heldk* 1898; **19**: 21.
2. Reed D. On the pathological changes in Hodgkin's disease, with special reference to its relation to its relation to tuberculosis. *Johns Hopkins Hosp Rep* 1902; **10**: 133.
3. Seif GS, Spriggs AI. Chromosome changes in Hodgkin's disease. *J Natl Cancer Inst* 1967; **39**: 557–70.
4. Jox A, Zander T, Diehl V *et al.* Clonal relapse in Hodgkin's disease. *N Engl J Med* 1997; **337**: 499.
5. Kanzler H, Kuppers R, Helmes S *et al.* Hodgkin and Reed-Sternberg-like cells in B-cell chronic lymphocytic leukemia represent the outgrowth of single germinal-center B-cell-derived clones: potential precursors of Hodgkin and Reed-Sternberg cells in Hodgkin's disease. *Blood* 2000; **95**: 1023–31.
6. Fiumara P, Snell V, Li Y *et al.* Functional expression of receptor activator of nuclear factor kappaB in Hodgkin disease cell lines. *Blood* 2001; **98**: 2784–90.
●7. Ambinder RF, Browning PJ, Lorenzana I *et al.* Epstein-Barr virus and childhood Hodgkin's disease in Honduras and the United States. *Blood* 1993; **81**: 462–7.
8. Pusey WA. Cases of sarcoma and Hodgkin's disease treated with exposures to x-rays: a preliminary report. *JAMA* 1902; **132**: 166.
9. Goodman LS, Wintrobe MM, Dameshek W *et al.* Nitrogen mustard therapy: use methyl bis(beta-chloroethyl)amine hydrochloride for Hodgkin's disease, lymphsarcoma, leukemia and certain allied and miscellaneous disorders. *JAMA* 1946; **132**: 126.
◆10. DeVita VT Jr, Canellos GP, Moxley JH. A decade of combination chemotherapy of advanced Hodgkin's disease. *Cancer* 1972; **30**: 1495–504.
●11. Santoro A, Bonadonna G, Valagussa P *et al.* Long-term results of combined chemotherapy-radiotherapy approach in Hodgkin's disease: superiority of ABVD plus radiotherapy versus MOPP plus radiotherapy. *J Clin Oncol* 1987; **5**: 27–37.
●12. Donaldson SS, Link MP. Combined modality treatment with low-dose radiation and MOPP chemotherapy for children with Hodgkin's disease. *J Clin Oncol* 1987; **5**: 742–9.
13. Percy CL, Smith MA, Linet M *et al. Lymphomas and reticuloendothelial neoplasms.* Bethesda, MD: National Cancer Institute, SEER program, 1999.
14. Mack TM, Cozen W, Shibata DK *et al.* Concordance for Hodgkin's disease in identical twins suggesting genetic susceptibility to the young-adult form of the disease. *N Engl J Med* 1995; **332**: 413–18.
15. Devesa SS, Blot WJ, Stone BJ *et al.* Recent cancer trends in the United States. *J Natl Cancer Inst* 1995; **87**: 175–82.

16. Kersey JH, Shapiro RS, Filipovich AH. Relationship of immunodeficiency to lymphoid malignancy. *Pediatr Infect Dis J* 1988; **7**(5 Suppl): S10–12.

17. Kusuda M, Toriyama K, Kamidigo NO *et al.* A comparison of epidemiologic, histologic, and virologic studies on Hodgkin's disease in western Kenya and Nagasaki, Japan. *Am J Trop Med Hyg* 1998; **59**: 801–7.

18. Armstrong AA, Alexander FE, Cartwright R *et al.* Epstein-Barr virus and Hodgkin's disease: further evidence for the three disease hypothesis. *Leukemia* 1998; **12**: 1272–6.

19. Glaser SL, Lin RJ, Stewart SL *et al.* Epstein-Barr virus-associated Hodgkin's disease: epidemiologic characteristics in international data. *Int J Cancer* 1997; **70**: 375–82.

20. Sleckman BG, Mauch PM, Ambinder RF *et al.* Epstein-Barr virus in Hodgkin's disease: correlation of risk factors and disease characteristics with molecular evidence of viral infection. *Cancer Epidemiol Biomarkers Prev* 1998; **7**: 1117–21.

21. Grufferman S, Delzell E. Epidemiology of Hodgkin's disease. *Epidemiol Rev* 1984; **6**: 76–106.

22. Stiller CA. What causes Hodgkin's disease in children? *Eur J Cancer* 1998; **34**: 523–8.

23. Gutensohn NM. Social class and age at diagnosis of Hodgkin's disease: new epidemiologic evidence for the "two-disease hypothesis". *Cancer Treat Rep* 1982; **66**: 689–95.

24. Grufferman S, Cole P, Smith PG *et al.* Hodgkin's disease in siblings. *N Engl J Med* 1977; **296**: 248–50.

25. Grufferman S, Cole P, Levitan TR. Evidence against transmission of Hodgkin's disease in high schools. *N Engl J Med* 1979; **300**: 1006–11.

26. Grufferman S. Is Hodgkin's disease infectious? *Eur J Cancer* 1995; **31A**: 1388–9.

27. Staudt LM. The molecular and cellular origins of Hodgkin's disease. *J Exp Med* 2000; **191**: 207–12.

28. Bräuninger A, Schmitz R, Bechtel D *et al.* Molecular biology of Hodgkin's and Reed/Sternberg cells in Hodgkin's lymphoma. *Int J Cancer* 2006; **118**: 1853–61.

29. Baeuerle PA, Baltimore D. NF-kappa B: ten years after. *Cell* 1996; **87**: 13–20.

30. Karin M, Delhase M. The I kappa B kinase (IKK) and NF-kappa B: key elements of proinflammatory signalling. *Semin Immunol* 2000; **12**: 85–98.

31. Delhase M, Hayakawa M, Chen Y *et al.* Positive and negative regulation of IkappaB kinase activity through IKKbeta subunit phosphorylation. *Science* 1999; **284**: 309–13.

32. Li ZW, Chu W, Hu Y *et al.* The IKKbeta subunit of IkappaB kinase (IKK) is essential for nuclear factor kappaB activation and prevention of apoptosis. *J Exp Med* 1999; **189**: 1839–45.

33. Bargou RC, Leng C, Krappmann D *et al.* High-level nuclear NF-kappa B and Oct-2 is a common feature of cultured Hodgkin/Reed-Sternberg cells. *Blood* 1996; **87**: 4340–7.

34. Ravi R, Bedi GC, Engstrom LW *et al.* Regulation of death receptor expression and TRAIL/Apo2L-induced apoptosis by NF-kappaB. *Nat Cell Biol* 2001; **3**: 409–16.

35. Durkop H, Foss HD, Demel G *et al.* Tumor necrosis factor receptor-associated factor 1 is overexpressed in Reed-Sternberg cells of Hodgkin's disease and Epstein-Barr virus-transformed lymphoid cells. *Blood* 1999; **93**: 617–23.

36. Wang CY, Mayo MW, Korneluk RG *et al.* NF-kappaB antiapoptosis: induction of TRAF1 and TRAF2 and c-IAP1 and c-IAP2 to suppress caspase-8 activation. *Science* 1998; **281**: 1680–3.

37. Mosialos G, Birkenbach M, Yalamanchili R *et al.* The Epstein-Barr virus transforming protein LMP1 engages signaling proteins for the tumor necrosis factor receptor family. *Cell* 1995; **80**: 389–99.

38. Devergne O, Hatzivassiliou E, Izumi KM *et al.* Association of TRAF1, TRAF2, and TRAF3 with an Epstein-Barr virus LMP1 domain important for B-lymphocyte transformation: role in NF-kappaB activation. *Mol Cell Biol* 1996; **16**: 7098–108.

39. Sylla BS, Hung SC, Davidson DM *et al.* Epstein-Barr virus-transforming protein latent infection membrane protein 1 activates transcription factor NF-kappaB through a pathway that includes the NF-kappaB-inducing kinase and the IkappaB kinases IKKalpha and IKKbeta. *Proc Natl Acad Sci U S A* 1998; **95**: 10106–11.

40. Mir SS, Richter BW, Duckett CS. Differential effects of CD30 activation in anaplastic large cell lymphoma and Hodgkin disease cells. *Blood* 2000; **96**: 4307–12.

41. Klein G. Epstein-Barr virus-carrying cells in Hodgkin's disease. *Blood* 1992; **80**: 299–301.

42. Weiss LM, Movahed LA, Warnke RA *et al.* Detection of Epstein-Barr viral genomes in Reed-Sternberg cells of Hodgkin's disease. *N Engl J Med* 1989; **320**: 502–6.

43. Weiss LM, Strickler JG, Warnke RA *et al.* Epstein-Barr viral DNA in tissues of Hodgkin's disease. *Am J Pathol* 1987; **129**: 86–91.

44. Khanna R, Burrows SR. Role of cytotoxic T lymphocytes in Epstein-Barr virus-associated diseases. *Annu Rev Microbiol* 2000; **54**: 19–48.

45. Yang J, Lemas VM, Flinn IW *et al.* Application of the ELISPOT assay to the characterization of CD8(+) responses to Epstein-Barr virus antigens. *Blood* 2000; **95**: 241–8.

46. Harris NL. Hodgkin's lymphomas: classification, diagnosis, and grading. *Semin Hematol* 1999; **36**: 220–32.

47. Pileri SA, Ascani S, Leoncini L *et al.* Hodgkin's lymphoma: the pathologist's viewpoint. *J Clin Pathol* 2002; **55**: 162–76.

48. Tzankov A, Zimpfer A, Pehrs AC *et al.* Expression of B-cell markers in classical Hodgkin lymphoma: a tissue microarray analysis of 330 cases. *Mod Pathol* 2003; **16**: 1141–7.

49. Anagnostopoulos I, Hansmann ML, Franssila K *et al.* European Task Force on Lymphoma project on lymphocyte predominance Hodgkin disease: histologic and immunohistologic analysis of submitted cases reveals 2 types of Hodgkin disease with a nodular growth pattern and abundant lymphocytes. *Blood* 2000; **96**: 1889–99.

50. Stein H, Marafioti T, Foss HD *et al.* Down-regulation of BOB.1/OBF.1 and Oct2 in classical Hodgkin disease but not in lymphocyte predominant Hodgkin disease correlates with immunoglobulin transcription. *Blood* 2001; **97**: 496–501.

51. Mauch PM, Kalish LA, Kadin M *et al.* Patterns of presentation of Hodgkin disease. Implications for etiology and pathogenesis. *Cancer* 1993; **71**: 2062–71.

52. Kaplan H. *Hodgkin's disease.* Cambridge, MA: Harvard University Press, 1980.

53. Lister TA, Crowther D, Sutcliffe SB *et al.* Report of a committee convened to discuss the evaluation and staging of patients with Hodgkin's disease: Cotswolds meeting. *J Clin Oncol* 1989; **7**: 1630–6.

●54. Lister TA, Crowther D. Staging for Hodgkin's disease. *Semin Oncol* 1990; **17**: 696–703.

55. Carbone PP, Kaplan HS, Musshoff K *et al.* Report of the Committee on Hodgkin's Disease Staging Classification. *Cancer Res* 1971; **31**: 1860–1.

56. Castellino RA, Blank N, Hoppe RT *et al.* Hodgkin disease: contributions of chest CT in the initial staging evaluation. *Radiology* 1986; **160**: 603–5.

57. Castellani MR, Cefalo G, Terenziani M *et al.* Gallium scan in adolescents and children with Hodgkin's disease (HD). Treatment response assessment and prognostic value. *Q J Nucl Med* 2003; **47**: 22–30.

58. Friedberg JW, Fischman A, Neuberg D *et al.* FDG-PET is superior to gallium scintigraphy in staging and more sensitive in the follow-up of patients with de novo Hodgkin lymphoma: a blinded comparison. *Leuk Lymphoma* 2004; **45**: 85–92.

59. Hudson MM, Krasin MJ, Kaste SC. PET imaging in pediatric Hodgkin's lymphoma. *Pediatr Radiol* 2004; **34**: 190–8.

60. Hueltenschmidt B, Sautter-Bihl ML, Lang O *et al.* Whole body positron emission tomography in the treatment of Hodgkin disease. *Cancer* 2001; **91**: 302–10.

61. Korholz D, Claviez A, Hasenclever D *et al.* The concept of the GPOH-HD 2003 therapy study for pediatric Hodgkin's disease: evolution in the tradition of the DAL/GPOH studies. *Klin Padiatr* 2004; **216**: 150–6.

62. Mahoney DH, Jr., Schreuders LC, Gresik MV *et al.* Role of staging bone marrow examination in children with Hodgkin disease. *Med Pediatr Oncol* 1998; **30**: 175–7.

63. Hanna SL, Fletcher BD, Boulden TF *et al.* MR imaging of infradiaphragmatic lymphadenopathy in children and adolescents with Hodgkin disease: comparison with lymphography and CT. *J Magn Reson Imaging* 1993; **3**: 461–70.

64. Dieckmann K, Potter R, Hofmann J *et al.* Does bulky disease at diagnosis influence outcome in childhood Hodgkin's disease and require higher radiation doses? Results from the German-Austrian Pediatric Multicenter Trial DAL-HD-90. *Int J Radiat Oncol Biol Phys* 2003; **56**: 644–52.

65. Nachman JB, Sposto R, Herzog P *et al.* Randomized comparison of low-dose involved-field radiotherapy and no radiotherapy for children with Hodgkin's disease who achieve a complete response to chemotherapy. *J Clin Oncol* 2002; **20**: 3765–71.

66. Ruhl U, Albrecht M, Dieckmann K *et al.* Response-adapted radiotherapy in the treatment of pediatric Hodgkin's disease: an interim report at 5 years of the German GPOH-HD 95 trial. *Int J Radiat Oncol Biol Phys* 2001; **51**: 1209–18.

67. Krasin MJ, Rai SN, Kun LE *et al.* Patterns of treatment failure in pediatric and young adult patients with Hodgkin's disease: local disease control with combined-modality therapy. *J Clin Oncol* 2005; **23**: 8406–13.

●68. Smith RS, Chen Q, Hudson MM *et al.* Prognostic factors for children with Hodgkin's disease treated with combined-modality therapy. *J Clin Oncol* 2003; **21**: 2026–33.

69. Shankar AG, Ashley S, Radford M *et al.* Does histology influence outcome in childhood Hodgkin's disease? Results from the United Kingdom Children's Cancer Study Group. *J Clin Oncol* 1997; **15**: 2622–30.

70. Landman-Parker J, Pacquement H, Leblanc T *et al.* Localized childhood Hodgkin's disease: response-adapted chemotherapy with etoposide, bleomycin, vinblastine, and prednisone before low-dose radiation therapy-results of the French Society of Pediatric Oncology Study MDH90. *J Clin Oncol* 2000; **18**: 1500–7.

◆71. Schwartz CL. Prognostic factors in pediatric Hodgkin disease. *Curr Oncol Rep* 2003; **5**: 498–504.

72. Mauch P, Tarbell N, Weinstein H *et al.* Stage IA and IIA supradiaphragmatic Hodgkin's disease: prognostic factors in surgically staged patients treated with mantle and paraaortic irradiation. *J Clin Oncol* 1988; **6**: 1576–83.

73. Bohlen H, Kessler M, Sextro M *et al.* Poor clinical outcome of patients with Hodgkin's disease and elevated interleukin-10 serum levels. Clinical significance of interleukin-10 serum levels for Hodgkin's disease. *Ann Hematol* 2000; **79**: 110–13.

74. Hann HW, Lange B, Stahlhut MW *et al.* Prognostic importance of serum transferrin and ferritin in childhood Hodgkin's disease. *Cancer* 1990; **66**: 313–16.

75. Chronowski GM, Wilder RB, Tucker SL *et al.* An elevated serum beta-2-microglobulin level is an adverse prognostic factor for overall survival in patients with early-stage Hodgkin disease. *Cancer* 2002; **95**: 2534–8.

76. Nadali G, Tavecchia L, Zanolin E *et al.* Serum level of the soluble form of the CD30 molecule identifies patients with Hodgkin's disease at high risk of unfavorable outcome. *Blood* 1998; **91**: 3011–16.

77. Warzocha K, Bienvenu J, Ribeiro P *et al.* Plasma levels of tumour necrosis factor and its soluble receptors correlate with clinical features and outcome of Hodgkin's disease patients. *Br J Cancer* 1998; **77**: 2357–62.

78. Christiansen I, Sundstrom C, Enblad G *et al.* Soluble vascular cell adhesion molecule-1 (sVCAM-1) is an independent prognostic marker in Hodgkin's disease. *Br J Haematol* 1998; **102**: 701–9.

79. Dukers DF, Meijer CJ, ten Berge RL *et al*. High numbers of active caspase 3-positive Reed-Sternberg cells in pretreatment biopsy specimens of patients with Hodgkin disease predict favorable clinical outcome. *Blood* 2002; **100**: 36–42.

80. Carde P, Koscielny S, Franklin J *et al*. Early response to chemotherapy: a surrogate for final outcome of Hodgkin's disease patients that should influence initial treatment length and intensity? *Ann Oncol* 2002; **13**(Suppl 1): 86–91.

81. Schwartz C, Constine L, London W *et al*. Intensive response-based therapy with or without dexrazoxane for intermediate/high-stage (I/HS) pediatric Hodgkin's disease (HD): a Pediatric Oncology Group (POG) Study. In: Polliack A, Armitage JO, Diehl V *et al*. (eds) *Fifth International Symposium on Hodgkin's Lymphoma*. Koln, Germany: Harwood Academic, 2001.

●82. Weiner MA, Leventhal BG, Marcus R *et al*. Intensive chemotherapy and low-dose radiotherapy for the treatment of advanced-stage Hodgkin's disease in pediatric patients: a Pediatric Oncology Group study. *J Clin Oncol* 1991; **9**: 1591–8.

◆83. Donaldson SS. Lessons from our children. *Int J Radiat Oncol Biol Phys* 1993; **26**: 739–49.

◆84. Donaldson SS. Pediatric Hodgkin's disease – up, up, and beyond. *Int J Radiat Oncol Biol Phys* 2002; **54**: 1–8.

◆85. Hudson MM. Pediatric Hodgkin's therapy: time for a paradigm shift. *J Clin Oncol* 2002; **20**: 3755–7.

◆86. Schwartz CL. Special issues in pediatric Hodgkin's disease. *Eur J Haematol Suppl* 2005; 55–62.

87. DeVita VT Jr. Is alternating cyclic chemotherapy better than standard four-drug chemotherapy for Hodgkin's disease? No. *Important Adv Oncol* 1993; 197–208.

88. Raney RB. Hodgkin's disease in childhood: a review. *J Pediatr Hematol Oncol* 1997; **19**: 502–9.

89. Tebbi CK, Mendenhall N, London WB *et al*. Treatment of stage I, IIA, IIIA(1) pediatric Hodgkin disease with doxorubicin, bleomycin, vincristine and etoposide (DBVE) and radiation: a Pediatric Oncology Group (POG) study. *Pediatr Blood Cancer* 2006; **46**: 198–202.

90. Schwartz C, Tebbi CK, London W *et al*. Enhanced toxicity in pediatric Hodgkin Disease (HD) patients treated with DBVE or DBVE-OPC and Dexrazoxane (DXR). *Blood* 2003; **102**: 493.

●91. Hutchinson RJ, Fryer CJ, Davis PC *et al*. MOPP or radiation in addition to ABVD in the treatment of pathologically staged advanced Hodgkin's disease in children: results of the Children's Cancer Group Phase III Trial. *J Clin Oncol* 1998; **16**: 897–906.

●92. Weiner MA, Leventhal B, Brecher ML *et al*. Randomized study of intensive MOPP-ABVD with or without low-dose total-nodal radiation therapy in the treatment of stages IIB, IIIA2, IIIB, and IV Hodgkin's disease in pediatric patients: a Pediatric Oncology Group study. *J Clin Oncol* 1997; **15**: 2769–79.

93. Kelly KM, Hutchinson RJ, Sposto R *et al*. Feasibility of upfront dose-intensive chemotherapy in children with advanced-stage Hodgkin's lymphoma: preliminary results from the Children's Cancer Group Study CCG-59704. *Ann Oncol* 2002; **13**(Suppl 1): 107–11.

●94. Donaldson SS, Hudson MM, Lamborn KR *et al*. VAMP and low-dose, involved-field radiation for children and adolescents with favorable, early-stage Hodgkin's disease: results of a prospective clinical trial. *J Clin Oncol* 2002; **20**: 3081–7.

95. Hudson MM, Krasin M, Link MP *et al*. Risk-adapted, combined-modality therapy with VAMP/COP and response-based, involved-field radiation for unfavorable pediatric Hodgkin's disease. *J Clin Oncol* 2004; **22**: 4541–50.

96. Friedmann AM, Hudson MM, Weinstein HJ *et al*. Treatment of unfavorable childhood Hodgkin's disease with VEPA and low-dose, involved-field radiation. *J Clin Oncol* 2002; **20**: 3088–94.

●97. Horning SJ, Hoppe RT, Breslin S *et al*. Stanford V and radiotherapy for locally extensive and advanced Hodgkin's disease: mature results of a prospective clinical trial. *J Clin Oncol* 2002; **20**: 630–7.

●98. Schellong G, Potter R, Bramswig J *et al*. High cure rates and reduced long-term toxicity in pediatric Hodgkin's disease: the German-Austrian multicenter trial DAL-HD-90. The German-Austrian Pediatric Hodgkin's Disease Study Group. *J Clin Oncol* 1999; **17**: 3736–44.

●99. Dorffel W, Luders H, Ruhl U *et al*. Preliminary results of the multicenter trial GPOH-HD 95 for the treatment of Hodgkin's disease in children and adolescents: analysis and outlook. *Klin Padiatr* 2003; **215**: 139–45.

100. Seyyedi S, Luders H, Marciniak H *et al*. Nodular lymphocyte predominant Hodgkin's disease (NLPHD) – results of the German multicenter trial GPOH-HD 95. *Leuk Lymphoma* 2001; **42**(Suppl 1): P-065, 43.

101. Sandoval C, Venkateswaran L, Billups C *et al*. Lymphocyte-predominant Hodgkin disease in children. *J Pediatr Hematol Oncol* 2002; **24**: 269–73.

102. Pellegrino B, Terrier-Lacombe MJ, Oberlin O *et al*. Lymphocyte-predominant Hodgkin's lymphoma in children: therapeutic abstention after initial lymph node resection – a Study of the French Society of Pediatric Oncology. *J Clin Oncol* 2003; **21**: 2948–52.

●103. Murphy SB, Morgan ER, Katzenstein HM *et al*. Results of little or no treatment for lymphocyte-predominant Hodgkin disease in children and adolescents. *J Pediatr Hematol Oncol* 2003; **25**: 684–7.

104. Hudson MM, Constine LS. Hodgkins' disease. In Halperin EC, Constine LS, Tarbell NJ *et al*. (eds) *Pediatric radiation oncology*, 4th Edn. Philadelphia, PA: Lippincott Williams and Wilkins, 2005; 223–60.

105. Prosnitz LR, Brizel DM, Light KL. Radiation techniques for the treatment of Hodgkin's disease with combined modality therapy or radiation alone. *Int J Radiat Oncol Biol Phys* 1997; **39**: 885–95.

106. Hoppe RT. Treatment planning in the radiation therapy of Hodgkin's disease. *Front Radiat Ther Oncol* 1987; **21**: 270–87.

107. Nautiyal J, Weichselbaum RR, Vijayakumar S. Radiation therapy techniques in the treatment of Hodgkin's disease. *Semin Radiat Oncol* 1996; **6**: 172–184.

108. Haie-Meder C, Mlika-Cabanne N, Michel G *et al.* Radiotherapy after ovarian transposition: ovarian function and fertility preservation. *Int J Radiat Oncol Biol Phys* 1993; **25**: 419–24.

109. Ortin TT, Shostak CA, Donaldson SS. Gonadal status and reproductive function following treatment for Hodgkin's disease in childhood: the Stanford experience. *Int J Radiat Oncol Biol Phys* 1990; **19**: 873–80.

110. Pedrick TJ, Hoppe RT. Recovery of spermatogenesis following pelvic irradiation for Hodgkin's disease. *Int J Radiat Oncol Biol Phys* 1986; **12**: 117–21.

111. Glossmann JP, Staak JO, Nogova L *et al.* Autologous tandem transplantation in patients with primary progressive or relapsed/refractory lymphoma. *Ann Hematol* 2005; **84**: 517–25.

112. Healey EA, Tarbell NJ, Kalish LA *et al.* Prognostic factors for patients with Hodgkin disease in first relapse. *Cancer* 1993; **71**: 2613–20.

113. Hertzberg MS, Crombie C, Benson W *et al.* Outpatient-based ifosfamide, carboplatin and etoposide (ICE) chemotherapy in transplant-eligible patients with non-Hodgkin's lymphoma and Hodgkin's disease. *Ann Oncol* 2003; **14**(Suppl 1): i11–16.

114. Josting A, Nogova L, Franklin J *et al.* Salvage radiotherapy in patients with relapsed and refractory Hodgkin's lymphoma: a retrospective analysis from the German Hodgkin Lymphoma Study Group. *J Clin Oncol* 2005; **23**: 1522–9.

115. Pfreundschuh MG, Rueffer U, Lathan B *et al.* Dexa-BEAM in patients with Hodgkin's disease refractory to multidrug chemotherapy regimens: a trial of the German Hodgkin's Disease Study Group. *J Clin Oncol* 1994; **12**: 580–6.

116. Ruffer JU, Ballova V, Glossmann J *et al.* BEACOPP and COPP/ABVD as salvage treatment after primary extended field radiation therapy of early stage Hodgkins disease – results of the German Hodgkin Study Group. *Leuk Lymphoma* 2005; **46**: 1561–7.

117. Yahalom J. Management of relapsed and refractory Hodgkin's disease. *Semin Radiat Oncol* 1996; **6**: 210–24.

●118. Yuen AR, Rosenberg SA, Hoppe RT *et al.* Comparison between conventional salvage therapy and high-dose therapy with autografting for recurrent or refractory Hodgkin's disease. *Blood* 1997; **89**: 814–22.

119. Friedman DL, Hilden JM, Powaski K. Issues and challenges in palliative care for children with cancer. *Curr Oncol Rep* 2004; **6**: 431–7.

120. Yahalom J. Do not miss a second (and possibly last) chance to cure Hodgkin's disease. *Int J Radiat Oncol Biol Phys* 1997; **39**: 595–7.

121. Moskowitz CH, Bertino JR, Glassman JR *et al.* Ifosfamide, carboplatin, and etoposide: a highly effective cytoreduction and peripheral-blood progenitor-cell mobilization regimen for transplant-eligible patients with non-Hodgkin's lymphoma. *J Clin Oncol* 1999; **17**: 3776–85.

122. Rapoport AP, Rowe JM, Kouides PA *et al.* One hundred autotransplants for relapsed or refractory Hodgkin's disease and lymphoma: value of pretransplant disease status for predicting outcome. *J Clin Oncol* 1993; **11**: 2351–61.

123. Bonfante V, Viviani S, Devizzi L *et al.* High-dose ifosfamide and vinorelbine as salvage therapy for relapsed or refractory Hodgkin's disease. *Eur J Haematol Suppl* 2001; **64**: 51–5.

124. Ahmed T, Rashid K, Waheed F *et al.* Long-term survival of patients with resistant lymphoma treated with tandem stem cell transplant. *Leuk Lymphoma* 2005; **46**: 405–14.

125. Enrici RM, Anselmo AP, Donato V *et al.* Relapse and late complications in early-stage Hodgkin's disease patients with mediastinal involvement treated with radiotherapy alone or plus one cycle of ABVD. *Haematologica* 1999; **84**: 917–23.

126. Wirth A, Corry J, Laidlaw C *et al.* Salvage radiotherapy for Hodgkin's disease following chemotherapy failure. *Int J Radiat Oncol Biol Phys* 1997; **39**: 599–607.

127. Moskowitz CH, Nimer SD, Zelenetz AD *et al.* A 2-step comprehensive high-dose chemoradiotherapy second-line program for relapsed and refractory Hodgkin disease: analysis by intent to treat and development of a prognostic model. *Blood* 2001; **97**: 616–23.

128. Viviani S, Santoro A, Negretti E *et al.* Salvage chemotherapy in Hodgkin's disease. Results in patients relapsing more than twelve months after first complete remission. *Ann Oncol* 1990; **1**: 123–7.

129. Longo DL, Duffey PL, Young RC *et al.* Conventional-dose salvage combination chemotherapy in patients relapsing with Hodgkin's disease after combination chemotherapy: the low probability for cure. *J Clin Oncol* 1992; **10**: 210–18.

130. Fisher RI, DeVita VT, Hubbard SP *et al.* Prolonged disease-free survival in Hodgkin's disease with MOPP reinduction after first relapse. *Ann Intern Med* 1979; **90**: 761–3.

131. Forrest DL, Hogge DE, Nevill TJ *et al.* High-dose therapy and autologous hematopoietic stem-cell transplantation does not increase the risk of second neoplasms for patients with Hodgkin's lymphoma: a comparison of conventional therapy alone versus conventional therapy followed by autologous hematopoietic stem-cell transplantation. *J Clin Oncol* 2005; **23**: 7994–8002.

132. Goldstone AH. The case for and against high-dose therapy with stem cell rescue for early poor prognosis Hodgkin's disease in first remission. *Ann Oncol* 1998; **9**(Suppl 5): S83–5.

133. Josting A, Sieniawski M, Glossmann JP *et al.* High-dose sequential chemotherapy followed by autologous stem cell transplantation in relapsed and refractory aggressive non-Hodgkin's lymphoma: results of a multicenter phase II study. *Ann Oncol* 2005; **16**: 1359–65.

◆134. Josting A. Autologous transplantation in relapsed and refractory Hodgkin's disease. *Eur J Haematol Suppl* 2005; 141–5.

◆135. Schmitz N, Sureda A. The role of allogeneic stem-cell transplantation in Hodgkin's disease. *Eur J Haematol Suppl* 2005; 146–9.

136. Claviez A, Klingebiel T, Beyer J et al. Allogeneic peripheral blood stem cell transplantation following fludarabine-based conditioning in six children with advanced Hodgkin's disease. Ann Hematol 2004; 83: 237–41.

137. Cooney JP, Stiff PJ, Toor AA et al. BEAM allogeneic transplantation for patients with Hodgkin's disease who relapse after autologous transplantation is safe and effective. Biol Blood Marrow Transplant 2003; 9: 177–82.

138. Lieskovsky YE, Donaldson SS, Torres MA et al. High-dose therapy and autologous hematopoietic stem-cell transplantation for recurrent or refractory pediatric Hodgkin's disease: results and prognostic indices. J Clin Oncol 2004; 22: 4532–40.

139. Baker KS, Gordon BG, Gross TG et al. Autologous hematopoietic stem-cell transplantation for relapsed or refractory Hodgkin's disease in children and adolescents. J Clin Oncol 1999; 17: 825–31.

140. Schmitz N, Sureda A, Robinson S. Allogeneic transplantation of hematopoietic stem cells after nonmyeloablative conditioning for Hodgkin's disease: indications and results. Semin Oncol 2004; 31: 27–32.

141. Linch DC, Winfield D, Goldstone AH et al. Dose intensification with autologous bone-marrow transplantation in relapsed and resistant Hodgkin's disease: results of a BNLI randomised trial. Lancet 1993; 341: 1051–4.

142. Anderson JE, Litzow MR, Appelbaum FR et al. Allogeneic, syngeneic, and autologous marrow transplantation for Hodgkin's disease: the 21-year Seattle experience. J Clin Oncol 1993; 11: 2342–50.

143. Peggs KS, Hunter A, Chopra R et al. Clinical evidence of a graft-versus-Hodgkin's-lymphoma effect after reduced-intensity allogeneic transplantation. Lancet 2005; 365: 1934–41.

144. Streetly M, Kazmi M, Radia D et al. Second autologous transplant with cyclosporin/interferon alpha-induced graft versus host disease for patients who have failed first-line consolidation. Bone Marrow Transplant 2004; 33: 1131–5.

145. Faulkner RD, Craddock C, Byrne JL et al. BEAM-alemtuzumab reduced-intensity allogeneic stem cell transplantation for lymphoproliferative diseases: GVHD, toxicity, and survival in 65 patients. Blood 2004; 103: 428–34.

146. Porter DL, Stadtmauer EA, Lazarus HM. 'GVHD': graft-versus-host disease or graft-versus-Hodgkin's disease? An old acronym with new meaning. Bone Marrow Transplant 2003; 31: 739–46.

147. Vogelsang G, Bitton R, Piantadosi S et al. Immune modulation in autologous bone marrow transplantation: cyclosporine and gamma-interferon trial. Bone Marrow Transplant 1999; 24: 637–40.

148. Reis LAG, Eisner MP, Hankey BF et al. SEER Cancer Statistics Review, 1975–2002. Bethesda, MD: National Cancer Institute.

◆149. Mauch P, Ng A, Aleman B et al. Report from the Rockefellar Foundation Sponsored International Workshop on reducing mortality and improving quality of life in long-term survivors of Hodgkin's disease: July 9–16, 2003, Bellagio, Italy. Eur J Haematol Suppl 2005; 68–76.

150. Baker KS, DeFor TE, Burns LJ et al. New malignancies after blood or marrow stem-cell transplantation in children and adults: incidence and risk factors. J Clin Oncol 2003; 21: 1352–8.

●151. Bhatia S, Robison L, Meadows A. High risk of second malignant neoplasms (SMN) continues with extended follow-up of childhood Hodgkin's disease (HD) cohort: report from the Late Effects Study Group (LESG). Blood 2001; 98: 768a.

152. Green DM, Hyland A, Barcos MP et al. Second malignant neoplasms after treatment for Hodgkin's disease in childhood or adolescence. J Clin Oncol 2000; 18: 1492–9.

153. Josting A, Wiedenmann S, Franklin J et al. Secondary myeloid leukemia and myelodysplastic syndromes in patients treated for Hodgkin's disease: a report from the German Hodgkin's Lymphoma Study Group. J Clin Oncol 2003; 21: 3440–6.

154. Kenney LB, Yasui Y, Inskip PD et al. Breast cancer after childhood cancer: a report from the Childhood Cancer Survivor Study. Ann Intern Med 2004; 141: 590–7.

●155. Metayer C, Lynch CF, Clarke EA et al. Second cancers among long-term survivors of Hodgkin's disease diagnosed in childhood and adolescence. J Clin Oncol 2000; 18: 2435–43.

●156. Metayer C, Curtis RE, Vose J et al. Myelodysplastic syndrome and acute myeloid leukemia after autotransplantation for lymphoma: a multicenter case-control study. Blood 2003; 101: 2015–23.

157. Neglia JP, Friedman DL, Yasui Y et al. Second malignant neoplasms in five-year survivors of childhood cancer: childhood cancer survivor study. J Natl Cancer Inst 2001; 93: 618–29.

158. Travis LB, Gospodarowicz M, Curtis RE et al. Lung cancer following chemotherapy and radiotherapy for Hodgkin's disease. J Natl Cancer Inst 2002; 94: 182–92.

159. Travis LB, Hill DA, Dores GM et al. Breast cancer following radiotherapy and chemotherapy among young women with Hodgkin disease. JAMA 2003; 290: 465–75.

●160. Travis LB, Hill D, Dores GM et al. Cumulative absolute breast cancer risk for young women treated for Hodgkin lymphoma. J Natl Cancer Inst 2005; 97: 1428–37.

●161. van Leeuwen FE, Klokman WJ, Veer MB et al. Long-term risk of second malignancy in survivors of Hodgkin's disease treated during adolescence or young adulthood. J Clin Oncol 2000; 18: 487–97.

162. Dores GM, Metayer C, Curtis RE et al. Second malignant neoplasms among long-term survivors of Hodgkin's disease: a population-based evaluation over 25 years. J Clin Oncol 2002; 20: 3484–94.

163. Swerdlow AJ, Barber JA, Hudson GV et al. Risk of second malignancy after Hodgkin's disease in a collaborative British cohort: the relation to age at treatment. J Clin Oncol 2000; 18: 498–509.

◆164. Adams MJ, Lipshultz SE, Schwartz C et al. Radiation-associated cardiovascular disease: manifestations and management. Semin Radiat Oncol 2003; 13: 346–56.

165. Adams MJ, Lipsitz SR, Colan SD et al. Cardiovascular status in long-term survivors of Hodgkin's disease treated with chest radiotherapy. J Clin Oncol 2004; 22: 3139–48.

166. Hancock SL, Donaldson SS, Hoppe RT. Cardiac disease following treatment of Hodgkin's disease in children and adolescents. J Clin Oncol 1993; 11: 1208–15.

167. King V, Constine LS, Clark D et al. Symptomatic coronary artery disease after mantle irradiation for Hodgkin's disease. Int J Radiat Oncol Biol Phys 1996; 36: 881–9.

168. Kremer LC, Caron HN. Anthracycline cardiotoxicity in children. N Engl J Med 2004; 351: 120–1.

169. Pein F, Sakiroglu O, Dahan M et al. Cardiac abnormalities 15 years and more after adriamycin therapy in 229 childhood survivors of a solid tumour at the Institut Gustave Roussy. Br J Cancer 2004; 91: 37–44.

170. Hull MC, Morris CG, Pepine CJ, Mendenhall NP. Valvular dysfunction and carotid, subclavian, and coronary artery disease in survivors of Hodgkin lymphoma treated with radiation therapy. JAMA 2003; 290: 2831–7.

171. Heidenreich PA, Hancock SL, Vagelos RH et al. Diastolic dysfunction after mediastinal irradiation. Am Heart J 2005; 150: 977–82.

172. Mertens AC, Yasui Y, Neglia J et al. Late mortality experience in five-year survivors of childhood and adolescent cancer: the Childhood Cancer Survivor Study. J Clin Oncol 2001; 19: 3163–72.

173. Moller TR, Garwicz S, Perfekt R et al. Late mortality among five-year survivors of cancer in childhood and adolescence. Acta Oncol 2004; 43: 711–18.

174. Heidenreich PA, Hancock SL, Vagelos RH et al. Diastolic dysfunction after mediastinal irradiation. Am Heart J 2005; 150: 977–82.

175. Sorensen K, Levitt GA, Bull C et al. Late anthracycline cardiotoxicity after childhood cancer: a prospective longitudinal study. Cancer 2003; 97: 1991–8.

●176. Lipshultz S, Lipsitz S, Sallan S. Chronic progressive left ventricular systolic dysfunction and afterload excess years after doxorubicin therapy for childhood acute lymphoblastic leukemia. Proc Annu Meet Am Soc Clin Oncol 2000; 580a.

177. Mah K, Van Dyk J, Keane T et al. Acute radiation-induced pulmonary damage: a clinical study on the response to fractionated radiation therapy. Int J Radiat Oncol Biol Phys 1987; 13: 179–88.

178. Kreisman H, Wolkove N. Pulmonary toxicity of antineoplastic therapy. Semin Oncol 1992; 19: 508–20.

179. Fryer CJ, Hutchinson RJ, Krailo M et al. Efficacy and toxicity of 12 courses of ABVD chemotherapy followed by low-dose regional radiation in advanced Hodgkin's disease in children: a report from the Children's Cancer Study Group. J Clin Oncol 1990; 8: 1971–80.

180. Bossi G, Cerveri I, Volpini E et al. Long-term pulmonary sequelae after treatment of childhood Hodgkin's disease. Ann Oncol 1997; 1: 19–24.

●181. Gleeson HK, Darzy K, Shalet SM. Late endocrine, metabolic and skeletal sequelae following treatment of childhood cancer. Best Pract Res Clin Endocrinol Metab 2002; 16: 335–48.

182. Sklar C, Whitton J, Mertens A et al. Abnormalities of the thyroid in survivors of Hodgkin's disease: data from the Childhood Cancer Survivor Study. J Clin Endocrinol Metab 2000; 85: 3227–32.

183. Ben Arush MW, Solt I, Lightman A et al. Male gonadal function in survivors of childhood Hodgkin and non-Hodgkin lymphoma. Pediatr Hematol Oncol 2000; 17: 239–45.

184. Kreuser ED, Felsenberg D, Behles C et al. Long-term gonadal dysfunction and its impact on bone mineralization in patients following COPP/ABVD chemotherapy for Hodgkin's disease. Ann Oncol 1992; 3(Suppl 4): 105–10.

185. Hill M, Milan S, Cunningham D et al. Evaluation of the efficacy of the VEEP regimen in adult Hodgkin's disease with assessment of gonadal and cardiac toxicity. J Clin Oncol 1995; 13: 387–95.

186. Hobbie WL, Ginsberg JP, Ogle SK et al. Fertility in males treated for Hodgkins disease with COPP/ABV hybrid. Pediatr Blood Cancer 2005; 44: 193–6.

187. Relander T, Cavallin-Stahl E, Garwicz S et al. Gonadal and sexual function in men treated for childhood cancer. Med Pediatr Oncol 2000; 35: 52–63.

188. Ash P. The influence of radiation on fertility in man. Br J Radiol 1980; 53: 271–8.

189. Lushbaugh CC, Casarett GW. The effects of gonadal irradiation in clinical radiation therapy: a review. Cancer 1976; 37: 1111–25.

190. Thompson EB, Smith JR, Bourgeois S et al. Glucocorticoid receptors in human leukemias and related diseases. Klin Wochenschr 1985; 63: 689–98.

191. Damewood MD, Grochow LB. Prospects for fertility after chemotherapy or radiation for neoplastic disease. Fertil Steril 1986; 45: 443–59.

192. Kreuser ED, Xiros N, Hetzel WD et al. Reproductive and endocrine gonadal capacity in patients treated with COPP chemotherapy for Hodgkin's disease. J Cancer Res Clin Oncol 1987; 113: 260–6.

193. Linch DC, Gosden RG, Tulandi T et al. Hodgkin's lymphoma: choice of therapy and late complcations. Am Soc Hematol Educ Program 2000; 205–21.

194. Schwartz CL. The management of Hodgkin disease in the young child. Curr Opin Pediatr 2003; 15: 10–6.

◆195. Zebrack BJ, Zeltzer LK, Whitton J et al. Psychological outcomes in long-term survivors of childhood leukemia, Hodgkin's disease, and non-Hodgkin's lymphoma: a report from the Childhood Cancer Survivor Study. Pediatrics 2002; 110: 42–52.

196. Kadan-Lottick NS, Robison LL, Gurney JG et al. Childhood cancer survivors' knowledge about their past diagnosis and treatment: Childhood Cancer Survivor Study. JAMA 2002; 287: 1832–9.

197. Oeffinger KC, Mertens AC, Hudson MM *et al.* Health care of young adult survivors of childhood cancer: a report from the Childhood Cancer Survivor Study. *Ann Fam Med* 2004; **2**: 61–70.

198. Taylor A, Hawkins M, Griffiths A *et al.* Long-term follow-up of survivors of childhood cancer in the UK. *Pediatr Blood Cancer* 2004; **42**: 161–8.

●199. Landier W, Bhatia S, Eshelman DA *et al.* Development of risk-based guidelines for pediatric cancer survivors: the Children's Oncology Group Long-Term Follow-Up Guidelines from the Children's Oncology Group Late Effects Committee and Nursing Discipline. *J Clin Oncol* 2004; **22**: 4979–90.

●200. Landier W, Wallace WHB, Hudson MM. Long-term follow-up of pediatric cancer survivors: education, surveillance and screening. *Pediatr Blood Cancer* 2006; **46**: 149–58.

74

Plasma cell neoplasms

G COOK AND J ASHCROFT

PLASMA CELL MYELOMA

INTRODUCTION

Plasma cell myeloma (PCM) is a plasma cell tumor with an incidence of 3–4 new cases per 100 000 population per annum, though this incidence demonstrates ethnic variation: the incidence is lowest in Chinese races at 1 per 100 000 and highest in European races at 4 per 100 000 and is commoner in Afro-American individuals with a male:female ratio of 3:2.[1] It accounts for approximately 10 percent of hematologic malignancies and is characterized by a monoclonal proliferation of plasma cells which produce a monoclonal immunoglobulin heavy and/or light chain (paraprotein, M-protein, or M-component). The patient-specific paraprotein is present in the serum in all but 1–2 percent of patients who have nonsecretory disease. The median age at diagnosis is 65–70 years and there is a higher incidence in Afro-Caribbean ethnic groups.[2]

Prior to the introduction of alkylating agents, the median survival of patients with PCM was less than one year.[3] Approximately 60 percent of patients will respond to conventional chemotherapy though the median survival without dose-escalated therapy remains at 3 years. Using conventional-dose chemotherapy, approximately 25 percent of patients will be alive at 5 years though less than 10 percent will be alive at 10 years. Over the last 10–15 years, the use of high-dose chemotherapy, either as a single treatment episode or as part of a cyclical high-dose therapeutic strategy, has improved the disease response rates and prolonged overall survival in patients with responsive disease. The support of such high-dose therapeutic strategies with autologous stem cells (peripheral blood derived more so than bone marrow derived) has become standard practice for those patients deemed fit to undergo such intensive therapy. The role of allogeneic stem cell transplantation (allo-SCT) in PCM, however, has still to be clarified as the pursuit of the putative graft-versus-myeloma (GvM) effect is complicated by significant therapy-related morbidity and mortality. A significant advance in assessing the role of high-dose chemotherapy strategies, including allo-SCT, has been the adoption of common response criteria, thus enabling clinicians to compare the outcomes of different trials and to decide their impact on patient disease-free and overall survival.[4]

The last 5 years have seen the successful development of novel biologic therapies and through clearly designed clinical intervention trials, the role of such new agents has been investigated, both as single agents and in combination with conventional therapy. As we learn more about the biology, the heterogeneity of the clinical manifestations, and the variability of response to therapy of patients with PCM, including study of the newer agents, the question that remains to be addressed is which patient would benefit from which agent or combination and in what sequence should these be used over the clinical course of the disease. The development of clinically applicable prognostic scoring systems and the attempts to identify *high-risk* patients based on biologic variables, including tumor cell gene expression profiles, is aimed at stratifying patients at presentation so that potentially tailor-made treatment strategies can be developed for individual patients.

CLINICAL FEATURES

Plasma cell myeloma was first reported by Dr Samuel Solly in his communication to the Royal Medical Chirugical Society in London[5] though Dr William MacIntyre is frequently credited with the first description when he reported a case of light chain PCM.[6] However, it was not until 1873 that the disease was referred to as *Multiple Myeloma* by Dr Rustizky, to indicate the multiple nature of the bone marrow tumors. In 1900, Dr Wright discovered that the homogeneous cellular infiltrate seen in the bone marrow of patients with PCM was in fact a tumor of plasma cells rather than myeloid cells (hence the previous name of myeloma).

The disease most commonly presents with an excess of a monoclonal antibody (~60 percent are immunoglobulin G [IgG] subclass, ~15 percent are IgA subclass, with IgM, IgD, and IgE accounting for fewer than 2 percent of patients) or monoclonal excess of light chains (~20 percent of patients have κ or λ light chains) though occasional patients (~1 percent) present without any serum or urinary evidence of excess antibody/light-chain production (nonsecretory myeloma).

In the 1960s, the disease presented most commonly with back pain, reported in up to 70 percent of patients. Owing to increased awareness of the disease and availability of rapid biochemical analysis, fewer than 40 percent of patients now present with symptomatic bone disease and at least 20 percent of patients are now diagnosed whilst totally asymptomatic.

Patients may present with renal dysfunction, anemia, hypercalcemia, recurrent bacterial infections, signs and symptoms of spinal cord compression, features suggestive of amyloidosis, or a persistently raised erythrocyte sedimentation rate (ESR), plasma viscosity, or serum paraprotein detectable on routine investigations. Fewer than 10 percent of patients present with symptoms of hyperviscosity syndrome, which is most likely to occur in patients with the IgA subclass variant. Bleeding defects also occur in approximately 15 percent of patients with the IgG subclass and 30 percent of patients with the IgA subclass, resulting from a combination of acquired coagulation factor inhibition by the paraprotein, microvessel thrombi generation, perivascular amyloid deposition, and anoxia.

Plasma cell myeloma is also associated with several defects in the host's immune system.[7] A characteristic feature of the disease is the associated hypogammaglobulinemia and the inability of patients with PCM to respond to vaccination against influenza, *Streptococcus pneumoniae*, and *Haemophilus influenza* type B. In addition, cell-mediated immunity is impaired, resulting in part from tumor-derived transforming growth factor β (TGFβ), a potent inhibitor of T cell function. Transforming growth factor β may also suppress B cell function and production of immunoglobulins and may be an important factor in myeloma-associated anemia.

Initial investigations of a patient suspected of suffering from PCM should include serum and concentrated urine electrophoresis, followed by immunofixation (IF) to confirm and type the monoclonal protein (paraprotein, M-protein). Quantification should be performed by electrophoretic densitometry of the monoclonal peak, though immunochemical measurement of total isotype level may be helpful for IgA and IgD subtypes. The quantification of the urinary light-chain excretion can be performed either on a 24-hour urinary collection or on a random urinary sample calibrated in relation to the urinary creatinine level (protein creatinine index [PCI]). More recently, the availability of assays to quantitate the serum free light chain excess production (sFLC assay) has been used as an alternative methodology in patients with light chain disease or those who have nonsecretory disease.[8] The use of the sFLC assay in patients with detectable paraprotein disease, in particular to determine response to and relapse from treatment, is currently under investigation.

Whilst a bone marrow aspiration for the examination of the marrow morphology can confirm the diagnosis of PCM (plasma cell infiltrate greater than 10 percent), the histologic examination of a trephine core biopsy can provide a more reliable assessment of plasma cell infiltrate

(Fig. 74.1). A trephine biopsy should be performed at diagnosis as it provides a suitable baseline measurement to determine response to therapy. Flow cytometry performed on the marrow aspirate may permit assessment of the plasma cell surface phenotype and confirm the clonality and determine the proportion of plasma cells in cell cycle (plasma cell labeling index). Malignant plasma cells can be differentiated from normal plasma cells by the surface phenotype CD19$^-$/CD45$^-$/CD56$^+$/CD138$^+$ (Fig. 74.2). The role of conventional metaphase cytogenetics or fluorescence *in situ* hybridization (FISH) to determine clonal genetic abnormalities is currently under investigation.

A skeletal survey of the axial skeleton using plain radiographs should be part of the initial staging process. This standard radiologic imaging technique will allow large areas to be examined for generalized bone density (to detect osteopenia/osteoporosis) and lytic lesions (Fig. 74.3) and to assess the threat of pathologic fracture in involved bones. The skeletal survey should include posteroanterior (PA) views of the chest and anteroposterior (AP) and lateral views of the cervical, thoracic, and lumbar spine with AP and lateral views of both humeri and femori. An AP and lateral view of the skull and AP view of the pelvis will complete the imaging of the axial skeleton. In addition, any area of bone-associated pain should be imaged for distal skeletal involvement. Computed tomography (CT) has a higher sensitivity than plain radiographs at detecting small lytic lesions and can accurately depict the presence and extent of associated soft tissue infiltration. Magnetic resonance imaging (MRI) is extremely useful for examining the extent and the nature of soft tissue involvement (Fig. 74.4), especially for the investigation of those presenting with neurologic symptoms, where it can provide an accurate assessment of the level and extent of cord or nerve root compression, the size of the tumor mass, and the degree to which it has extended into the epidural space.

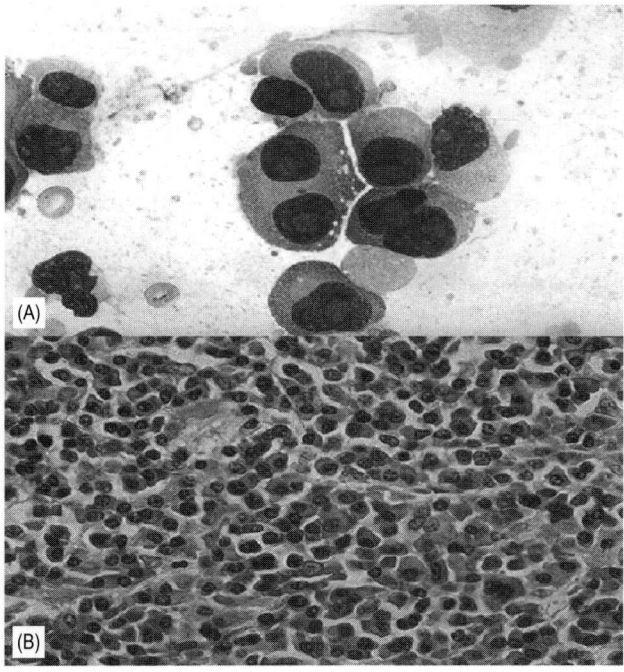

Figure 74.1   Bone marrow plasma cell infiltrate in plasma cell myeloma. (A) The morphology of bone marrow aspirate (Geimsa, ×400) and (B) histology of paraffin-embedded marrow trephine biopsy (hematoxylin and eosin, ×200) demonstrating atypical plasma cells.

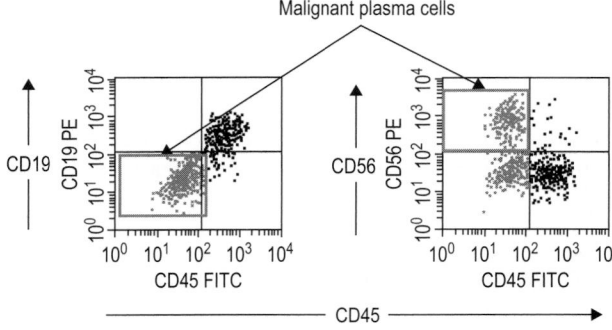

Figure 74.2   Flow cytometric determination of malignant plasma cells, as characterized as CD19$^-$/CD45$^-$/CD56$^+$.

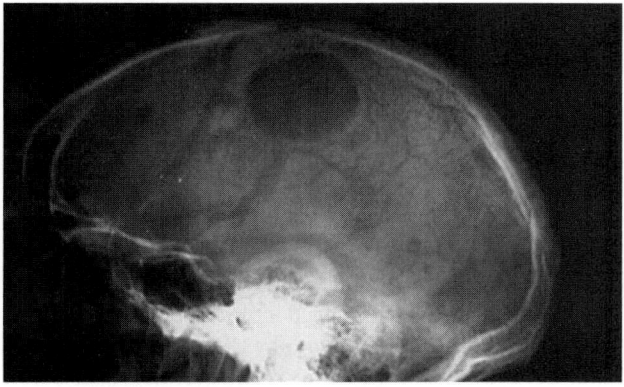

Figure 74.3   Plain radiograph of the skull demonstrating characteristic lytic lesions.

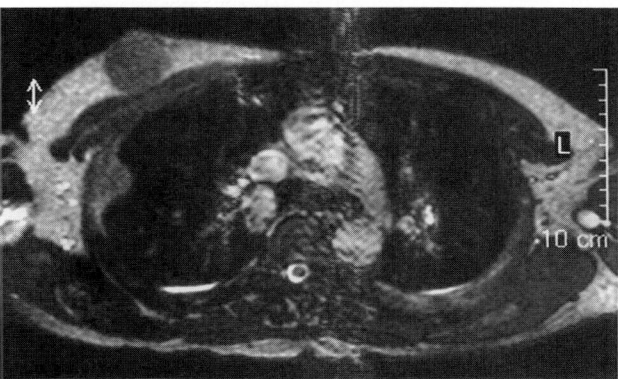

Figure 74.4   Magnetic resonance imaging of the upper thorax demonstrating extramedullary relapse (arrow) of plasma cell myeloma after high-dose therapy.

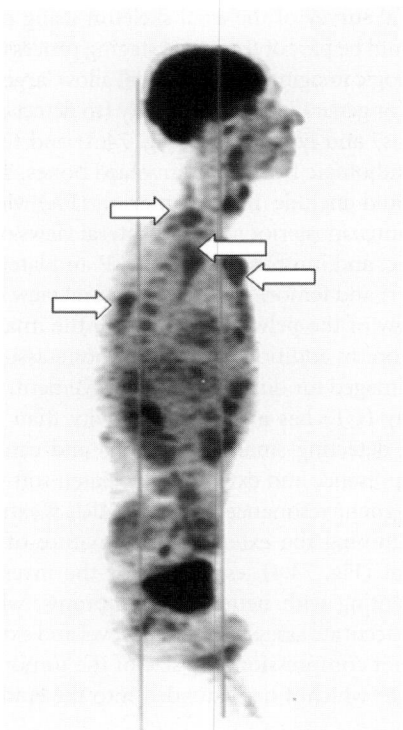

Figure 74.5 Positron emission tomography image of a patient with relapsed disease post-allogeneic stem cell transplantation. Sites of disease activity are indicated by arrows.

Magnetic resonance imaging of the whole spine should be performed in patients with solitary plasmacytomas, irrespective of the site of the primary, presenting lesion. When following up a patient after treatment, any new symptomatic skeletal event should first be imaged by plain radiography, with CT or MRI being employed if the radiographs are negative. Positron emission tomography (PET) has recently been reported as a useful imaging technique for assessing occult disease and soft tissue infiltration (Fig. 74.5), though due to availability of the technology, it is not used routinely.[9]

Bone scintigraphy has a low sensitivity in PCM as a result of the lack of osteoblastic activity, characteristic in the lytic lesions of PCM. As such, scintigraphy has no routine role in the diagnosis and follow-up assessment of patients with PCM. Dual energy x-ray absorptiometry scanning is a standard procedure for assessing osteopenia/osteoporosis, and lower lumbar spine bone density has been correlated with an inherent risk of vertebral body collapse, though preexisting lesions can give rise to interpretation difficulties and absorptiometry is not routinely performed.

Diagnostic criteria

The diagnosis is usually confirmed by demonstrating the presence of a monoclonal antibody in the serum and/or urine, lytic bone lesions (Fig. 74.3), and increased numbers of plasma cells infiltrating the bone marrow (Fig. 74.1). As

---

> **Myeloma-Related Organ and/or Tissue Impairment (*ROTI*) due to Plasma Cell Infiltrative Process: *CRAB***
>
> **C:**   Hypercalcemia >10 mg/L (0.25 mmol/L) above the upper limit of normal (ULN) or >110 mg/L (>2.75 mmol/L)
> **R:**   Renal insufficiency as demonstrated by a serum creatinine of >20 mg/L (>173 mmol/L)
> **A:**   Anemia >2 g/dL below the normal range or a Hb <10 g/dL
> **B:**   Bone lesions including osteolytic lesions or osteoporosis with compression fractures (demonstrated by CT or MRI)
>
> **Other:**   -symptomatic hyperviscosity
>   -amyloidosis
>   -recurrent bacterial infections (>2 per 12 months)

Figure 74.6 Definition of systemic effect of plasma cell myeloma. Hb, hemoglobin; CT, computed tomography; MRI, magnetic resonance imaging.

> **ASYMPTOMATIC MYELOMA** (Smoldering Myeloma)
> • M-protein level of ≥30 g/L
> • **or** bone marrow plasma cell infiltrate of ≥10%
> • No *ROTI*
>
> **SYMPTOMATIC MYELOMA**
> • M-protein in serum or urine
> • Bone marrow plasma cell infiltrate ≤10%* or plasmacytoma
> • Evidence of *ROTI*
> *If flow cytometry confirms >90% neoplastic phenotype
>
> **NONSECRETORY MYELOMA**
> • No M-protein or detectable light chain excess
> • Bone marrow plasma cell infiltrate of ≥10% or plasmacytoma
> • Evidence of *ROTI*

Figure 74.7 Definition of symptomatic/asymptomatic plasma cell myeloma. ROTI, related organ and/or tissue impairment.

monoclonal antibodies are detected in other plasma cell dyscrasias (monoclonal gammopathy of undetermined significance [MGUS], amyloid, solitary plasmacytomas), an international working group has developed a classification based on the level of paraprotein, percentage of marrow infiltration, and the presence or absence of myeloma-related organ and/or tissue impairment (*ROTI*, Fig. 74.6). The criteria define the classification of MGUS and asymptomatic and symptomatic myeloma (Fig. 74.7).[10] Asymptomatic myeloma encapsulates previously termed conditions such as *equivocal*, *indolent*, or *smoldering* myeloma and patients who do not have clinically overt symptom complexes may be classified as symptomatic myeloma due to the presence of *ROTI*. Patients with asymptomatic myeloma do not require treatment but do require intensive monitoring and follow-up.

Prognostic indicators

Due to the relative heterogeneity of the clinical presentation and response to therapy, there has always been an impetus to develop a prognostic scoring system to differentiate those

Stage	Criteria	Median survival (months)
I	Serum β_2-MG <3.5 mg/L and serum albumin >35 g/L	62
II	Neither I nor III Serum β_2-MG <3.5 mg/L and serum albumin <35 g/L *or* Serum β_2-MG 3.5–5.5 mg/L	45
III	Serum β_2-MG >5.5 mg/L	29

Figure 74.8 International Prognostic Staging System (Greipp *et al.* 2005[12]). β_2-MG, β_2-microglobulin.

patients who will benefit from conventional chemotherapy from those who will require dose-escalation therapy or novel agents (similar to the International Prognostic Scoring system used in managing patients with malignant lymphoma). The first clinically useful staging system utilizing a number of clinical prognostic indicators reflecting tumor burden was devised in the early 1980s, the Durie-Salmon clinical staging system.[11] This system, based on the presence of bone marrow failure, renal dysfunction, and the extent of lytic bone disease, could separate patients prognostically into early stage disease (low tumor burden) with a median survival of 5 years and those with advanced stage disease (high tumor burden) with a median survival of 15 months. The addition of biologic variables such as β_2-microglobulin (β_2-MG) and C reactive protein (CRP, surrogate indicator of interleukin-6 [IL-6] levels) and cytogenetic abnormalities may further refine this crude clinical staging system to allow the identification of those patients who will demonstrate the best response to conventional therapy. Abnormalities of chromosome 13 in PCM are associated with a poor prognosis. However, it is not clear whether the deletions of chromosome 13 are related to abnormalities of *RB1* (pRb), as the regions involved in the deletions are quite extensive and may involve other tumor suppressor genes. Mutations of oncogenes such as *NRAS* and *KRAS* and the tumor suppressor gene, *TP53*, have limited prognostic predictability as these events are most frequently encountered in advanced stages of disease and are relatively rare events at presentation.

Recently a working group has devised, tested, and validated an International Prognostic Index based on serum levels of β_2-MG and serum albumin, separating patients into three prognostic groups, irrespective of the therapy used (Fig. 74.8).[12] The β_2-MG level reflects not only the tumor mass but also the renal function, as an indicator of glomerular filtration rate, and may also reflect other as yet unknown factors. The specific role of decreased albumin in patients with PCM is uncertain and may represent the effect of cytokine production on organ dysfunction such as excessive IL-6 production or hepatic synthetic function. This system is simple and easily applied in clinical practice; however, it has not yet been adopted to direct patient-specific therapy.

MANAGEMENT

The aim of therapy in patients with PCM is to control the disease process, to maximize quality of life, and to prolong survival. This is provided through both tumor-specific therapy and directed supportive care, though the importance of tailoring the therapeutic approach to the specific needs of the individual patient needs to be met, especially in light of the disease heterogeneity. Whilst it is current practice for most patients, who are deemed fit enough, to proceed with a dose-intensification protocol including high-dose therapy and stem cell transplantation, the majority will not be suitable for such an approach. With the advent of novel, biologic therapies, many more patients will survive longer after initial presentation. However, the role of these therapies and, more specifically, the timing of administration of these newer agents are yet to be determined and ongoing clinical intervention studies hope to answer these questions.

Response criteria

There has been an expansion of therapeutic strategies and agents in the management of PCM. With this increased choice has come the need to clearly define response criteria, so that each of these new strategies and agents can be compared directly as to their efficacy and durability. In addition, for the practising clinician, the need arises to determine when a treatment strategy has (and perhaps more importantly has not) been efficacious, to allow alternative treatments to be implemented and to determine when best to withdraw therapy.

Response criteria were first developed by the Committee of the Chronic Leukemia and Myeloma TASK Force of the US National Cancer Institute in 1968, which were subsequently reviewed in 1973. The main parameter was a reduction in the paraprotein of at least 50 percent. In 1972, the Southwest Oncology Group (SWOG) advanced this definition to include *objective response*, which related to a more than 75 percent reduction in the serum paraprotein (including a greater than 90 percent reduction in urinary light-chain excretion) which was sustained for at least 2 months. However, with the development of high-dose therapy (see below), a definition of a *complete response* (CR) was required. Many investigators reported their results of high-dose therapy, both in nonrandomized and randomized studies, but uniformity in the definition of CR was lacking. In 1998, the Myeloma Subcommittee of the European Blood and Marrow Transplantation (EBMT) Chronic Leukemia Working Party in collaboration with the Myeloma Working Committee of the International Bone Marrow Transplant Registry (IBMTR), set out what has since been universally adopted as response criteria.[13] The main tenets are illustrated in Table 74.1. The published documents provide criteria for CR, partial response (PR), minimal response (MR), stable disease (SD), progressive disease (PD), plateau response, and relapse.

Table 74.1   European Group for Blood and Marrow Transplant (EBMT) Clinical Response Criteria (Blade *et al.* 1998[13])

Complete response (CR) requires all of the following:

1. Absence of the original monoclonal paraprotein in serum and urine by immunofixation, maintained for a minimum of 6 weeks. The presence of oligoclonal bands consistent with oligoclonal immune reconstitution does not exclude CR
2. <5% plasma cells in a bone marrow aspirate and also on trephine bone biopsy if biopsy is performed. If absence of monoclonal protein is sustained for 6 weeks it is not necessary to repeat the bone marrow, except in patients with nonsecretory myeloma where the marrow examination must be repeated after an interval of at least 6 weeks to confirm CR
3. No increase in size or number of lytic bone lesions (development of a compression fracture does not exclude response)
4. Disappearance of soft tissue plasmacytomas

Patients in whom some, but not all, of the criteria for CR are fulfilled are classified as PR, providing the remaining criteria satisfy the requirements for PR. This includes patients in whom routine electrophoresis is negative but in whom immunofixation has not been performed

Partial response (PR) requires all of the following:

1. ≥50% reduction in the level of the serum monoclonal paraprotein, maintained for a minimum of 6 weeks
2. Reduction in 24 h urinary light chain excretion either by ≥90% or to <200 mg, maintained for a minimum of 6 weeks
3. For patients with nonsecretory myeloma only, ≥50% reduction in plasma cells in a bone marrow aspirate and on trephine biopsy, if biopsy is performed, maintained for a minimum of 6 weeks
4. ≥50% reduction in the size of soft tissue plasmacytomas (by radiography or clinical examination)
5. No increase in size or number of lytic bone lesions (development of a compression fracture does not exclude response)

Patients in whom some, but not all, the criteria for PR are fulfilled are classified as MR, provided the remaining criteria satisfy the requirements for MR

Minimal response (MR) requires all of the following:

1. 25–49% reduction in the level of the serum monoclonal paraprotein maintained for a minimum of 6 weeks
2. 50–89% reduction in 24 h urinary light chain excretion, which still exceeds 200 mg/24 h, maintained for a minimum of 6 weeks
3. For patients with nonsecretory myeloma only, 25–49% reduction in plasma cells in a bone marrow aspirate and on trephine biopsy, if biopsy is performed, maintained for a minimum of 6 weeks
4. 25–49% reduction in the size of soft tissue plasmacytomas (by radiography or clinical examination)
5. No increase in the size or number of lytic bone lesions (development of a compression fracture does not exclude response).
   MR also includes patients in whom some, but not all, of the criteria for PR are fulfilled, provided the remaining criteria satisfy the requirements for MR

No change (NC)

1. Not meeting the criteria of either minimal response or progressive disease

Plateau

1. Stable values (within 25% above or below value at the time response is assessed) maintained for at least 3 months

Time point for assessing response

1. Response to the transplant procedure will be assessed by comparison with results immediately prior to conditioning
2. If transplant is part of a treatment program, response to the whole treatment program will be assessed by comparison with the results at the start of the program

Relapse from CR requires at least one of the following:

1. Reappearance of serum or urinary paraprotein on immunofixation or routine electrophoresis, confirmed by at least one further investigation and excluding oligoclonal immune reconstitution
2. ≥5% plasma cells in a bone marrow aspirate or on trephine bone biopsy
3. Development of new lytic bone lesions or soft tissue plasmacytomas or definite increase in the size of residual bone lesions (development of a compression fracture does not exclude continued response and may not indicate progression)
4. Development of hypercalcemia (corrected serum calcium >11.5 mg/dL or 2.8 mmol/L) not attributable to any other cause

Progressive disease (for patients not in CR) requires one or more of the following:

1. >25% increase in the level of the serum monoclonal paraprotein, which must also be an absolute increase of at least 5 g/L and confirmed by at least one repeated investigation
2. >25% increase in the 24 h urinary light chain excretion, which must also be an absolute increase of at least 200 mg/24 h and confirmed by at least one repeated investigation
3. >25% increase in plasma cells in a bone marrow aspirate or on trephine biopsy, which must also be an absolute increase of at least 10%
4. Definite increase in the size of existing bone lesions or soft tissue plasmacytomas
5. Development of new bone lesions or soft tissue plasmacytomas (development of a compression fracture does not exclude continued response and may not indicate progression)
6. Development of hypercalcemia (corrected serum calcium >11.5 mg/dL or 2.8 mmol/L) not attributable to any other cause

Induction therapy

Most newly diagnosed patients less than 65 years of age (or older if fit) are candidates for dose-escalation therapy including high-dose alkylating agent chemotherapy supported by autologous stem cell transplantation (ASCT) with cryopreserved peripheral blood stem cells. Following several larger clinical intervention studies,[14,15] such a strategy is now considered 'good standard care' and initial (induction) therapy must avoid agents with cumulative myelosuppressive side effects in order to permit collection of an adequate number of stem cells. Common pre-ASCT induction regimens have included high-dose dexamethasone (HDD) alone or in combination with infusional vincristine and adriamycin (VAD).[16] VAD results in PR in approximatley 50–60 percent of patients, with complete response (CR; as defined in Table 74.1) being observed in 5–10 percent of patients. VAD and VAD-hybrids achieve rapid, effective initial disease control[17] and the addition of weekly cyclophosphamide has improved response rates without compromising the stem cell compartment.[15] An oral alternative to these infusional approaches using the lipophilic anthracycline, idarubicin, with high-dose dexamethasone (Z–Dex) has demonstrated similar efficacy without compromising the stem cell pool, without the need for a central venous catheter and its associated morbidity, and with the convenience of outpatient administration.[18] The duration of induction therapy is usually 4–6 months, which achieves maximum response in the majority of patients who then can proceed with stem cell mobilization and ASCT. Induction regimens are illustrated in Table 74.2.

Thalidomide, developed in the 1950s as a sedative antiemetic, was found in the late 1990s to have antitumor activity. The demonstration of antimyeloma efficacy, particularly in the setting of advanced and refractory disease, was only the third independently active compound for treating myeloma.[19] In the setting of de novo/untreated disease, the combination of thalidomide and dexamethasone has been demonstrated to be efficacious (Table 74.2). Other investigators have added thalidomide to VAD-like regimens as initial therapy in ongoing trials. These regimens produce higher rates of CR or near CR (nCR) and do not compromise stem cell collection or ASCT. Thalidomide regimens, particularly when given early in the disease course and in combination with chemotherapeutic agents, are associated with increased toxicity, especially venous thromboembolic (VTE) events.[20] The precise mechanism of the thalidomide VTE event is unknown, as is the best method of prevention. Although some benefit of prophylactic aspirin or low-dose warfarin has been reported, the use of low-molecular-weight heparin (LMWH) or full doses of warfarin may be more effective and the results from ongoing clinical intervention studies are awaited.

Not all patients are potential candidates for dose-escalation programs, including ASCT, and the aim of therapy in those patients (usually older and less fit) who are unsuitable to progress through such a program is to achieve disease control with minimal side effects, inducing improved quality of life. Melphalan and prednisone (MP) has been the mainstay of treatment in such patients and yields partial remission in 50–55 percent, with only occasional CR.[21] Prednisone has been replaced with dexamethasone and directly compared to MP. The response rates were similar but there was considerably greater toxicity associated with dexamethasone.[22]

Cyclophosphamide is efficacious, especially when used in combination with steroids. Other combinations of alkylating agents, such as VBMCP (vincristine, carmustine, melphalan, cyclophosphamide, and prednisone), have been utilized and, more recently, thalidomide has been added to MP with improved response rates but increased toxicity.[23] The aim of MP therapy is to deliver maximum response followed by 3 months of therapy and to date no randomized study has shown a benefit to prolonging therapy beyond this timeframe. The introduction of thalidomide to MP (MPT) may alter this timeframe, especially the notion of following maximum response to MPT with thalidomide monotherapy as a maintenance strategy, and is currently under investigation.

High–dose therapy

AUTOLOGOUS STEM CELL TRANSPLANTATION

More than 20 years ago, the efficacy of high-dose alkylating-agent chemotherapy in the treatment of high-risk PCM and plasma cell leukemia was demonstrated, though associated with significant morbidity and mortality.[24] As a result, the use of stem cells (ASCT) to support hematopoietic reconstitution after high-dose melphalan ($140–200\,mg/m^2$) has become standard practice in the management of PCM. The stem cell support was initially provided in the mid-1980s by bone marrow harvests, though this was replaced by the late 1980s with growth factor-mobilized peripheral blood stem cells (PBSC). Three randomized clinical intervention studies have now demonstrated improved response rates and progression-free survival (PFS), though most patients received maintenance therapy in the form of interferon α (Table 74.2). A single ASCT after induction regimens typically results in CR in about 20–40 percent of patients, with a median PFS in the range of 2.5–4 years and overall survival (OS) of 4–5 years. Other studies in which high-dose treatment was deferred until relapse have also suggested similar OS, although post-ASCT remissions were shorter compared with those achieved with ASCT used earlier in the course of the illness.

Attempts to predict the outcome of ASCT and, in particular, to identify those patients who will not benefit from high-dose chemotherapy have, to date, centered around similar prognostic factors identified at diagnosis, such as a high β_2-MG level. In addition, detection of a deletion of

Table 74.2 Summary of selected therapeutic intervention studies in patients with plasma cell myeloma

Study	n	Response rate (CR/PR)	PFS (mo)	OS (mo)	Comment	Reference
Induction						
VAD vs Z-Dex	106	74% vs 58% (P = 0.075)	–	–	Infections more common in VAD group	Cook et al. 2004[18]
MP vs MPT		48% vs 73% (P = 0.006)	27% vs 54% at 3 years (P = 0.006)	70% vs 89% at 3 years (P = 0.03)		Palumbo et al. 2004[23]
Thalidomide/HDD vs HDD	207	58% vs 42%	–	–	Pre-ASCT induction	Rajkumar et al. 2008[169]
IFM95-01 MP vs MD vs HDD vs HDD/IFNα	488	42% vs 41% vs 73% vs 43% (P < 0.001)	22 vs 13 vs 22 vs 13 (P < 0.001)	–	Higher morbidity associated with HDD	Facon et al. 2006[170]
CC vs ASCT						
IFM90	200	CR: 14% vs 38% (P < 0.001)	18 vs 28	44 vs 57	Randomized at entry	Attal et al. 1996[14]
MRCVII	401	CR: 8% vs 44% (P < 0.001)	20 vs 32 (P < 0.001)	42 vs 54 (P = 0.04)	Randomized at entry	Child et al. 2003[15]
PETHEMA	164	CR: 11 vs 30 (P < 0.002)	34 vs 43	67 vs 65	Responders to induction randomized only	Bladé et al. 2005[171]
ASCT × 1 vs ASCT × 2						
IFM94 (Mel140/TBI vs Mel140 → Mel140/TBI)	399	CR: 42% vs 50 (P = 0.1)	10 vs 20 (P = 0.03)	21 vs 42 (P = 0.01)		Attal et al. 2003[32]
HOVON (Mel70 × 2 vs Mel70 × 2 → Cy/TBI)	303	13% vs 28% (P < 0.01)	20 vs 22	55 vs 50	Second ASCT more beneficial in high-risk PCM	Segeren et al. 2003[172]
ASCT × 2 vs ASCT/Allo-SCT						
IFM99-03/-04	284	51% vs 37.8%	30 vs 25 (P = 0.56)	41 vs 35 (P = 0.27)	High-risk disease	Garban et al. 2006[43]
Maintenance						
IFM99-02 (placebo vs bisphosphonate vs thalidomide/bisphosphonate)	780	–	39% vs 37% vs 50% (P < 0.02)	86% vs 78% vs 86% (P = NS)		Attal et al. 2006[173]
Relapsed disease						
Thalidomide + HDD	169	30%	5	–	Nonrandomized	Barlogie et al. 2001[174]
Thalidomide, cyclophosphamide + prednisone	71	55%	NYR	–	Nonrandomized	Garcia-Sanz et al. 2004[175]
Bortezomib/HDD vs HDD	202	18% vs 38%	6.2 vs 3.5	–		Richardson et al. 2005[45]
Lenalidomide/HDD vs HDD	353	61% vs 19.9%	11.1 vs 4.7	29.6 vs 20.2		Weber et al. 2007[176]

CR, complete response; PR, partial response; VAD: vincristine, adriamycin (doxorubicin), and dexamethasone; Z-Dex: idarubicin (doxorubicin) and dexamethasone; MP: melphalan and prednisone; MPT: MP and thalidomde; HDD, high-dose dexamethasone; CC, conventional dose chemotherapy; ASCT, high-dose therapy and autologous stem cell transplantation; PFS, progression-free survival; OS, overall survival; (mo), months; NYR, not yet reached; NS, not significant.

chromosome 13 (detected by conventional cytogenetics) may confer a particularly poor prognosis. Some investigators have reported that patients with t(4;14) and *TP53* deletions (17p13) have an inferior prognosis and outcome following ASCT.[25] Although the use of cytogenetic data does not routinely affect treatment decisions in individual patients at this time, risk-adapted approaches are under investigation in clinical trials.

Attempts to improve the outcome of ASCT, both in terms of response rates and PFS/OS, have centered around improving the conditioning regimen, including melphalan dose escalation, additional alkylating agents, and incorporation of total-body irradiation and the incorporation of novel agents into conditioning regimens. Tandem transplantation has also been evaluated as well as post-ASCT maintenance therapy. No benefit has been demonstrated for the incorporation of total-body irradiation in the conditioning regimen in terms of OS, despite improved event-free survival (EFS).[26] Increasing doses of melphalan have been explored by some investigators; up to $280\,mg/m^2$ has been administered in some studies where amifostine has been used as a mucosal protectant.[27] The incorporation of additional alkylating agents, in particular busulphan, into the conditioning regimen has been explored.[28,29] Whilst initial results are encouraging, as yet, definitive evidence for the routine addition of busulphan to high-dose melphalan is lacking. The IFM group (Intergroupe Francophone du Myélome) reported the results of their study in 219 high-risk patients (based on chromosome 13 deletion and high β_2-MG) where a second ASCT was conditioned with high-dose melphalan with or without an anti-IL-6 monoclonal antibody (BE-8). The study reports that the addition of this blocking antibody did not improve either progression-free or overall survival.[30]

The use of new drugs in conjunction with the pretransplant conditioning regimen has not been well studied. One preliminary report has assessed two doses of bortezomib prior to melphalan conditioning and preliminary results suggest an additive effect.[31]

In a further attempt to improve the outcome of ASCT, investigators turned to the sequential administration of high-dose chemotherapy and ASCT – so-called 'tandem transplantation.' Barlogie *et al.* at the University of Arkansas pioneered the use of tandem ASCT in the early management of PCM in their Total Therapy I program.[20] This program resulted in a CR rate of 41 percent and median overall survival of 79 months. The IFM94 trial was the first randomized study comparing single and tandem transplants, reporting improved EFS and OS in the tandem transplant group.[32] Though other randomized studies have been conducted, the data are not yet mature enough to definitively comment on the effectiveness of tandem procedures. However, in general, the data indicate that tandem ASCT improves PFS with a variable effect on overall survival and it has been suggested that the second procedure provides the most benefit in patients not achieving a CR, nCR, or very good PR (greater than 90 percent reduction

in serum monoclonal protein) after the first procedure.[32] Therefore, offering tandem ASCT to this subset of patients is a reasonable approach. An alternative strategy is to collect sufficient stem cells to support two transplants but to reserve the second for use only at the time of relapse, though the effectiveness of this approach remains to be proven.[33,34] Definitive recommendations regarding the optimal timing of second transplants are not clear at the current time, particularly in view of emerging information about the biologic subtypes of myeloma and the availability of more effective agents for recurrent disease.

In an attempt to improve the duration of response post-ASCT, maintenance strategies were developed. Continuing with pulsed conventional chemotherapy after ASCT has not been demonstrated to be useful in the setting of prevention of disease progression. Interferon α (IFNα) was shown to possess antimyeloma efficacy in several clinical interventional studies, both alone and in combination with corticosteroids and chemotherapy.[20] A number of studies were then designed to examine the role of IFNα in this setting. Overall, the data for IFNα as a maintenance therapy do not show significant benefit both in terms of prolonged disease response and overall survival. As a result, it is not routinely used due to the cost, toxicity, and limited efficacy. Corticosteroid maintenance has been shown to prolong remission after conventional therapy, but no data are available regarding its efficacy post-ASCT. The only study to examine the role of corticosteroids as maintenance compared alternate day oral prednisone at two different dose levels (10 mg vs 50 mg), with resulting prolongation of disease response and overall survival in patients receiving the higher dose of steroid.[35]

Newer approaches such as those based on thalidomide are under evaluation. The duration of thalidomide treatment is often limited by the development of side effects, including sedation, constipation, peripheral neuropathy, and thromboembolic disease (TED). The UK Myeloma Forum phase II study of thalidomide in the setting of maintenance therapy post-ASCT demonstrated that the majority of patients (77 percent) had to discontinue due to side effects though for those who were able to continue taking thalidomide for more than 12 months, there was a significantly improved EFS compared to those who did not.[36] The National Cancer Institute of Canada (NCIC) MY9 trial comparing maintenance with thalidomide 400 mg versus 200 mg daily revealed that, even with the lower dose, patient attrition was a considerable concern.[37] Encouraging results have been reported in the IFM99-02 trial. As an alternative to thalidomide, an ongoing CALGB 100104 phase III study compares lenalidomide with placebo after ASCT.

ALLOGENEIC STEM CELL TRANSPLANTATION

Myeloablative (allo-SCT) can result in cure in a small proportion of selected patients but is limited by lack of appropriate donors, age limitations, and significant risks of morbidity and mortality (transplant-related mortality [TRM]) due to graft-versus-host disease and other complications. Although the 5-year survival rates may be comparable to ASCT, relapses after this time are much less frequent in the allo-SCT treated patients. Full-intensity allo-SCT from an HLA-matched sibling donor may have a role in the management of younger patients, particularly when melphalan and 12 Gy fractionated total-body irradiation is utilized as the conditioning regimen.[38]

There has been an improvement in TRM over the last 10 years, reducing from 46 percent (2-year TRM) before 1994 to 30 percent after this time.[39] This may reflect the use of allo-SCT earlier in the disease process but may also be attributable to improved supportive care and use of PBSC with more rapid engraftment.

Several nonrandomized studies have demonstrated that allo-SCT in relapse/progressive disease is of limited benefit, whilst patients transplanted in first response demonstrate an approximately 60 percent CR rate.[40,41] Minimal residual disease (MRD) monitoring usually takes the form of observing immunofixation negativity reversing and aids the timing of immunotherapeutic intervention with donor lymphocyte infusions (DLI). The latter can induce disease responses in up to 50 percent of patients, almost a fifth of patients achieving an immunofixation-negative CR.

More recently, reduced-intensity conditioning (RIC) and nonmyeloablative regimens have been explored. This less intensive approach has been introduced in the setting of PCM to mitigate some of the TRM while maintaining the GvM of allo-SCT. Reduced-intensity conditioning allo-SCT has less early nonrelapse mortality, although late relapses and transplant-related deaths have become apparent.[20]

Several conditioning regimens have been explored from the minimally myelosuppressive fludarabine and low-dose total body irradiation (2 Gy) to more intensive regimens such as fludarabine and melphalan. Graft-versus-host disease prophylaxis is most commonly cyclosporine alone, though many centers add short-course methotrexate or *in vivo* T cell depletion (with antithymocyte globulin or alemtuzumab). With the latter, there is an associated increased need to use post-transplant DLI to deal with both residual disease and mixed lymphohemopoietic chimerism.

As GvM is most likely to be successful in the setting of MRD, the prevailing opinion is that RIC allo-SCT should be performed after ASCT as a consolidation measure. The preliminary results of two studies examining the use of such a tandem ASCT/allo-SCT approach have been reported, one of which is illustrated in Table 74.2.[42,43] Both studies demonstrate comparable OS and EFS, despite encouraging improved disease response rates, owing to the increased nonrelapse mortality (NRM) associated with the RIC allo-SCT arm of the study. More information will become available with longer follow-up of these and other trials.

The use of alternative or unrelated donors in allo-SCT for PCM is associated with significant TRM in the full-intensity setting. The use of RIC regimens when an unrelated donor is the source of the graft has been shown to be associated with a lower TRM.[20,41] Whilst there has been significant variability in the conditioning regimens used, some centers report up to 90 percent response rates with 50–55 percent OS at 2 years. The data are at present too immature to make recommendations on the use of unrelated donors in the setting of RIC allo-SCT.

New agents

BORTEZOMIB (VELCADE)

Bortezomib (formerly PS341) represents a novel class of agents that has established efficacy in relapsed and refractory PCM.[44,45] The proteasome is the final degradative enzyme involved in an important catabolic pathway for many intracellular regulatory proteins including IκB (inhibitor of nuclear factor κB [NF-κB])/NF-κB, TP53, and the cyclin-dependent kinase inhibitors p21 and p27. Bortezomib specifically, selectively, and reversibly inhibits the proteasome by binding tightly to the enzyme's active site. The antineoplastic effect of bortezomib may involve several distinct mechanisms, including inhibition of cell growth signaling pathways, induction of apoptosis, and inhibition of cellular adhesion molecule expression. A number of trials using this drug in combination with other agents, such as dexamethasone, anthracyclines, alkylating agents (melphalan), and thalidomide, have been activated in newly diagnosed patients.[20] Overall response rates have been impressive, ranging from 75 percent to 100 percent, with CR/nCR seen in 20–30 percent. So far, no detrimental effects on subsequent PBSC mobilization and ASCT have been observed. Side effects include diarrhea (controllable with mild antidiarrheal medication), hypotension, fatigue, and hematologic toxicity including mild to moderate neutropenia, lymphopenia, and thrombocytopenia. Similar to the neurotoxic limitations of thalidomide, bortezomib-related peripheral sensory neuropathy appears to resolve over a period of weeks after therapy is discontinued.

LENALIDOMIDE (REVLIMID)

Immunomodulatory drugs (IMiDs) have now been shown to block several pathways important for disease progression in multiple myeloma. First established as agents with antiangiogenic properties, IMiDs inhibit the production of IL-6, which is a growth factor for the proliferation of myeloma cells. In addition, they activate apoptotic pathways through caspase-8-mediated cell death.[46] At the mitochondrial level, they are responsible for c-Jun N-terminal kinase (JNK)-dependent release of cytochrome c and Smac into the cytosol of cells, where they regulate the activity of molecules that affect apoptosis. In addition, by activating T cells to produce IL-2, IMiDs alter natural killer (NK) cell numbers and function, thus augmenting the activity of NK-dependent cytotoxicity. Data delineating these events have been derived from *in vitro* experiments and as such the definitive mode of action *in vivo* remains speculative. Although thalidomide and IMiDs demonstrate similar biologic activities, IMiDs are more potent than thalidomide and achieve responses at lower doses.

CC-5013 (lenalidomide, Revlimid) is an IMiD that has also demonstrated efficacy, with a lower incidence of peripheral neuropathy, in relapsed/refractory myeloma patients.[47] A pilot study of dexamethasone plus lenalidomide has been initiated in newly diagnosed patients. Prophylactic aspirin has been added after thrombotic events were seen in the early phase of the trial. This combination is being studied in an ongoing randomized trial and, so far, there are no data available on the ability to collect PBSC after lenalidomide therapy. Lenalidomide is not yet approved by the US Food and Drug Administration (FDA) or other regulatory bodies.

Supportive care

Many patients present with anemia (hemoglobin [Hb] <10 g/dL; see above) either as a result of bone marrow infiltration or tumor-associated cytokine production, or associated with renal dysfunction or treatment, or a combination of these scenarios. Erythropoietin (EPO) therapy has been utilized in patients with PCM. Erythropoietin can induce a response, as defined by a rise in the Hb of >2 g/dL, in approximately 70 percent of patients, though results are best in those who have not been exposed to alkylating chemotherapeutic agents.[48] The current guidelines of the UK Myeloma Forum and Nordic Myeloma Study Group suggest that EPO not be used in newly diagnosed patients until initial response to chemotherapy has been determined, though a therapeutic trial in symptomatic patients can be tried.[2] High serum EPO (>200 IU/mL), a high transfusion requirement for packed red cells, and a low platelet count are negative prognostic indicators of response to EPO.

The risk of infection in patients with PCM at diagnosis or during treatment is not insignificant, resulting from a combination of both cellular and humoral immune defects and the direct immunosuppression and myelosuppression of the treatment strategies. The risk of infection is highest in the first 3 months after diagnosis but decreases with response to antimyeloma therapy. Prompt access to specialist medical assessment of febrile patients with PCM is recommended to promote rapid administration of appropriate antimicrobial therapy. Patients with PCM presenting with a febrile illness need to be treated with broad-spectrum antibiotics, especially intravenous antibiotics in the setting of severe disease. The prevention of infection in patients with PCM undergoing treatment has improved the overall outlook in such patients. The use of prophylactic immunoglobulin infusions (0.4 g/kg body weight) may be helpful, especially for those in plateau phase disease. Prophylactic antibiotics are not recommended except for the regular use of trimethoprim-sulphamethoxazole in the first 2–3 months from diagnosis. Vaccinations against influenza, *Streptococcus pneumoniae*, and *Haemophilus influenza* are recommended but the efficacy is likely to be limited given the established immune cell dysfunction associated with PCM.[2]

FOLLOW-UP

Almost all patients with PCM will relapse and therefore the management strategy for an individual should be based on this assumption and include plans to deal with disease progression. The usual approach to progressive disease has been the use of sequential regimens designed to control the disease with the best quality of life for as long as possible. Fortunately, the number of options available has increased. Patients who experience a remission lasting several years after a single, or even double, ASCT may derive benefit from another ASCT (see above), just as elderly patients with at least a 1-year remission may respond again to melphalan and prednisone. Alternative strategies are illustrated in Table 74.2.

Thalidomide has been extensively studied as a single agent or with corticosteroids in relapsed/refractory patients.[49] Although widely accepted as efficacious, no randomized data in this setting are available. Glasmacher and colleagues performed a systematic review of 42 clinical intervention studies involving 1642 patients. Thirty-two trials used a dose-escalation schedule with the target dose ranging from 200 to 800 mg/day orally (PO). The cumulative (on an intent-to-treat basis) overall (CR/PR) response rate was 29.4 percent (95 percent confidence interval [CI] 27–32 percent). The median overall survival from all studies was 14 months and severe side effects (World Health Organization [WHO] grade III–IV) were reported in 2–11 percent with VTE disease being reported in only 3 percent of patients. Combinations of thalidomide with either steroids alone or with steroids and cyclophosphamide are being evaluated in this setting. Weekly oral cyclophosphamide plus dexamethasone and thalidomide is effective in the setting of relapsed disease, and now represents one arm of first-line therapy in the Medical Research Council (MRC) Myeloma IX trial.

The APEX trial has demonstrated the superiority of bortezomib over HDD alone in terms of response rate and time to progression. The 1-year overall survival rates were 89 percent versus 72 percent, respectively. Patients with only one prior regimen had more favorable outcomes than those treated after two or three recurrences.[45] In patients who do not respond to bortezomib alone, the addition of dexamethasone has resulted in additional partial or minimal responses in 15–20 percent of patients in phase II trials.[44]

Several other potential avenues to deal with relapsed disease are being explored. Arsenic trioxide has been used in the management of relapsed PCM but with limited success to date, though it is the focus of continued study.[50] Double hemi-body irradiation can be utilized for palliation in patients with widespread bone disease or extramedullary plasmacytomas, though it is associated with significant myelosupression and may require support with PBSC.[51] New biologic agents that either target the clonal cell or its microenvironment are under development in preclinical studies. Such novel agents include CHIR-258, which inhibits fibroblast growth factor receptor 3; NVP-ADW742, which inhibits insulin-like growth factor receptor 1; and PTK787, which inhibits vascular endothelial growth factor (VEGF).[52] Undoubtedly, these agents will be first used in patients with relapsed or advanced disease and we await their future development.

MONOCLONAL GAMMOPATHY OF UNDETERMINED SIGNIFICANCE

INTRODUCTION

Monoclonal gammopathy of undetermined significance has two important characteristics: (1) a plasma immunoglobulin or urinary light chain with molecular features of a single clone; and (2) the absence of diagnostic criteria for a malignant condition such as multiple myeloma, Waldenstrom macroglobulinemia, or other lymphoproliferative disorder.[10]

During the mid-twentieth century with the evolving use of paper electrophoresis of plasma proteins, immunofixation techniques, and, more recently, using the serum free light chain (sFLC, Freelite®) assay, monoclonal plasma components or abnormal κ and λ light chain ratios have been found in the sera of apparently symptomless individuals. The incidence of this finding shows a progressive increase with age[53–55] and these abnormal monoclonal bands are often evident either in patients without associated disease or in those with nonlymphoid cancers, infections, and inflammatory disorders (Table 74.3). The great majority of patients with MGUS are initially entirely asymptomatic but, despite this, there is a low but definite risk of progression to clinically overt disease, which is estimated to be approximately 1 percent per annum.[56–64] It is these individuals, and those with associated autoimmune phenomena, who need to be identified to allow appropriate and timely interventions.

DIAGNOSTIC CRITERIA

The diagnosis of MGUS is essentially one of exclusion. Criteria have recently been revised by the International Myeloma Working Group and adopted by the British Committee for Standards in Haematology (Table 74.3). These guidelines clearly differentiate between MGUS, smoldering myeloma, and symptomatic myeloma, placing emphasis on related organ and/or tissue impairment (ROTI) to help define those with symptomatic disease (Fig. 74.6).

EPIDEMIOLOGY AND RISK FACTORS

Population-based studies have demonstrated the presence of monoclonal immunoglobulins in approximately 0.5 percent of adults. The incidence shows a progressive increase with age, with 1 percent of those aged 50 years and above and 3 percent of those aged over 70 years possessing monoclonal immunoglobulins in the serum.[53–55,65]

Both racial differences and a slight male predominance have been observed – the incidence of MGUS appears higher in black Americans than in age-matched whites and lower in Japan.[66–68] Despite these apparent racial differences MGUS has been widely described across most continents[53–57,59,60,66–71] but there are still no firm clear data on the influence of geography and ethnicity on the incidence of MGUS or its progression.

The cause of MGUS is unknown. Some epidemiologic studies have suggested a possible etiologic role for tobacco

Table 74.3 Diagnostic criteria for monoclonal gammopathy of undetermined significance (MGUS), asymptomatic myeloma, and symptomatic myeloma (International Myeloma Working Group, 2003[10])

MGUS	Asymptomatic myeloma	Symptomatic myeloma
M-protein in serum <30 g/L	M-protein in serum >30 g/L	M-protein in serum and/or urine
Bone marrow clonal plasma cells <10% and low level of plasma cell infiltration on trephine biopsy	and/or Bone marrow clonal plasma cells >10%	Bone marrow (clonal) plasma cells or biopsy-proven plasmacytoma
No myeloma-related organ or tissue impairment (including bone lesions) or symptoms	No myeloma-related organ or tissue impairment (including bone lesions) or symptoms	Myeloma-related organ or tissue impairment (including bone lesions)
No evidence of other B cell proliferative disorders or light-chain-associated amyloidosis or other light-chain, heavy-chain, or immunoglobulin-associated tissue damage		

smoking and occupational exposure to asbestos, fertilizers, mineral oils, petroleum, and radiation.[72] These studies have, however, generally been small and have lacked the statistical power to draw valid conclusions. There are also no known genetic risk factors for MGUS despite small numbers of familial cases being reported and as yet no candidate genes have been identified.[73,74]

PATHOPHYSIOLOGY

Over the last decade, there have been considerable advances in our understanding of the underlying biology of MGUS and this has largely occurred as a direct result of an improved understanding of the complex biology of multiple myeloma. It is now clear that the plasma cells of patients with IgG and IgA MGUS share many of the phenotypic and genotypic features seen in multiple myeloma plasma cells. Long-term epidemiologic studies have demonstrated a constant rate of progression from MGUS to multiple myeloma and it can be argued that these observations support the hypothesis of a 'two-hit' genetic model to explain the progression to malignancy; the risk of developing multiple myeloma is similar, regardless of the known duration of the MGUS clone, thus suggesting that a random second hit is responsible for progression.[56]

Despite these findings in IgA and IgG MGUS the underlying biology of IgM MGUS remains unclear, but available data suggest that it is likely to be very different. Immunoglobulin M MGUS rarely progresses to multiple myeloma and the characteristic chromosomal abnormalities seen in Waldenstrom macroglobulinemia (del 6q), the condition into which IgM MGUS may well evolve, are not accompanied by 14q32 and chromosome 13 deletions frequently seen in both multiple myeloma and IgA/IgG MGUS.[75–78] Discussion in the following sections concentrates to a greater extent on IgG and IgA MGUS cases, which have the propensity to progress toward multiple myeloma.

Genotypic studies and gene expression arrays

Conventional cytogenetic analysis is rarely if ever informative in MGUS. This is undoubtedly due to the low level of bone marrow infiltration and the low proliferative capacity of the clonal plasma cells. However, using FISH combined with immunofluorescence staining for cytoplasmic immunoglobulin, karyotypic assessment of even minimal numbers of plasma cells is possible. Such studies have shown that MGUS plasma cells do in fact possess complex karyotypic abnormalities with aneuploidy and hyperdiploidy being a common occurrence in up to 70 percent of patients at presentation.[79–82] Whole chromosome gains are also similar to those seen in multiple myeloma, with trisomies of chromosomes 3, 7, 9, and 11 being common.

Interestingly, the majority of chromosomal changes appear to be confined to those plasma cells with an aberrant phenotype.[82]

Translocations involving the immunoglobulin heavy chain (IGH) locus at 14q32 are common in MGUS and are also characteristically found in up to 60 percent of myeloma patient samples. These translocations are thought to arise due to errors in isotype switch recombination and are 'promiscuous,' involving a number of partner chromosomes including 4p16, 11q13, 16q23, and 6p25, which deregulate FGFR3, MAF, CCND1, and MUM1, respectively. Studies using FISH analysis have demonstrated that 14q32 translocations also occur in up to 50 percent of patients with MGUS and that the spectrum of translocations is similar to those seen in multiple myeloma.[78,83,84] Loss of chromosome 13 material (either large deletions or often loss of the whole chromosome) is a further common finding in both myeloma and MGUS, although the adverse outcome this confers in the former has not, as yet, been demonstrated in the latter.[85,86] It is worthy of note that the same patterns of chromosomal abnormalities have also been demonstrated in patients with primary amyloidosis,[87] which might suggest a common genetic basis for MGUS, primary amyloidosis, and multiple myeloma.

Further insights into the biology of MGUS have been gained with the use of gene expression profiling. Davies et al. demonstrated that the gene expression profile of MGUS plasma cells had a much greater resemblance to malignant than normal plasma cells. There did, however, remain marked differences between MGUS and multiple myeloma plasma cells, particularly in those genes influencing cell growth, signal transduction, and intracellular transport.[88] In the future, it is possible that these methods will help fathom the genetic events pivotal in the transformation of MGUS.

Immunophenotypic studies

Malignant and nonmalignant plasma cells possess characteristic immunophenotypic appearances. When analyzed using flow cytometry, malignant and nonmalignant cell populations differ in their scatter characteristics and expression profiles, malignant plasma cells being characterized by aberrant expression of CD56, CD117, and CD126, loss of CD19, and weaker expression of CD27, CD37, CD38, and CD45. These differences enable the identification of both normal and neoplastic plasma cell populations within the same specimen (Fig. 74.2). Using flow cytometric techniques, CD19 and CD56 are probably the most discriminatory markers, as normal plasma cells are consistently $CD19^+CD56^-$, while neoplastic plasma cells are in the main $CD19^-CD56^+$ (65 percent of cases), with a lesser proportion being $CD19^-CD56^-$ (30 percent of cases) or $CD19^+CD56^+$ (5 percent of cases). Neoplastic plasma cells can in fact be demonstrated in up to 90 percent of MGUS cases when analyzed by flow cytometric techniques. These neoplastic cells have been shown to be monoclonal and also aneuploid in a significant proportion of cases.[89–93]

CLINICAL FEATURES

The vast majority of MGUS patients will have no symptoms or clinical signs. A minority, however, can have clinical features, which are directly attributable to the presence of the monoclonal protein.

Autoimmune phenomena

In a proportion of patients, the monoclonal immunoglobulins (particularly IgM) have autoantibody specificity, which can result in a number of autoimmune phenomena.[94] Peripheral neuropathies occur in 5–10 percent of patients with IgM monoclonal proteins and are often associated with autoantibody activity directed against neural antigens, including myelin-associated glycoprotein (MAG). Peripheral neuropathies are also encountered in patients with IgG and IgA monoclonal proteins but a clear pathologic link is generally lacking and in many cases may simply represent coincidental findings in patients who might otherwise be diagnosed with chronic inflammatory demyelinating polyneuropathy (CIDP).[95,96] The related condition of POEMS syndrome is, however, often misdiagnosed as CIDP (due to the overriding symptom being peripheral neuropathy) or MGUS-associated peripheral neuropathy.

The POEMS syndrome usually presents between 50 and 70 years of age with a peripheral neuropathy which is primarily motor in nature (P), a monoclonal plasma cell population (M), and other features including organomegaly (O), endocrinopathy (E), skin lesions (S), papilledema, effusions and edema, thrombocytosis, and ascites. Alternative names for POEMs include osteosclerotic myeloma, Takatsuki syndrome, or Crow-Fukase syndrome. In patients suffering from this condition, there is a predominance of λ light chains to the degree that if the light chain component is κ, then the diagnosis should be carefully reconsidered (greater than 95 percent λ). Abnormal levels of a number of cytokines are found in patients with POEMS including IL-1β, TNFα, IL-6, and VEGF. Interestingly VEGF levels appear to fall in relation to treatment and, although this is not proven, may be directly involved in the pathobiology of the syndrome. The most common causes of death due to POEMS are cardiorespiratory failure, progressive disability, renal failure, capillary leak syndromes, and exhaustion leading to recurrent infections.[97,98] Survival figures vary quite widely from the original reports of between 12 and 33 months to median survivals of approximately 14 years in more recent patient groups.[98]

Other autoimmune manifestations of MGUS include conditions such as cold agglutinin disease, in which the monoclonal protein is almost invariably of IgM κ type and has autoantibody specificity directed against I or i blood group antigens. The affinity of the autoantibody is temperature dependent such that antibody binding seldom occurs at body temperature but only as the temperature falls. The classical clinical features are therefore Raynaud phenomenon, acrocyanosis, and episodic cold-induced hemolysis.

A range of other autoimmune disorders can also occur in patients with MGUS and may, or may not, be related to the monoclonal protein. Platelet antigen autoantibody specificity can result in immune thrombocytopenia, whilst specificity to the von Willebrand factor protein may induce a bleeding diathesis.[99,100] Acquired angioedema and myasthenia gravis have also been described in patients with monoclonal immunoglobulins but are relatively uncommon manifestations.[101,102]

Immunoglobulin deposition diseases

In some individuals, monoclonal immunoglobulins or, more commonly, fragments of monoclonal light chains have the propensity for tissue deposition. Primary amyloidosis is the commonest and best-characterized manifestation of this process. Patients may present with cardiac failure, nephrotic syndrome, malabsorption, carpal tunnel syndrome, and peripheral and autonomic neuropathies. These features occur as a result of the extracellular deposition of amyloid fibrils consisting of the amino termini of clonal immunoglobulin light chains in these tissues. The propensity for monoclonal proteins to form amyloid deposits and their tissue tropism appears to be determined by the immunoglobulin light chain genes (λ light chains predominate and specific λ variable-region genes associate with differing patterns of tissue deposition).[103] Primary AL amyloidosis is discussed in detail later in this chapter.

Nonamyloid immunoglobulin deposition is a rare complication of monoclonal gammopathy.[104–106] These deposits lack the structural and staining properties of amyloid in that they tend to form granular rather than fibrillar deposits, do not stain with Congo red, and can consist of monoclonal light chains or light chain fragments. These conditions are termed light chain deposition disease. In a minority of cases, deposits may consist of heavy chain (heavy chain deposition disease) or both light and heavy chain determinants (light and heavy chain deposition disease) and similar to AL amyloidosis, can present with renal, cardiac, hepatic, or peripheral nervous system involvement.

Adult acquired Fanconi syndrome, whose main clinical features include bone disease, renal dysfunction, and metabolic disturbances, also has features in common with light chain deposition disease; however, it is primarily associated with κ monoclonal light chains being deposited in the kidney.[107]

Cryoglobulins

Monoclonal immunoglobulins can also act as cryoglobulins (i.e., they precipitate at temperatures below 37°C and redissolve on warming). Type I cryoglobulins consist of monoclonal immunoglobulin only, while type II cryoglobulins generally consist of a complex of polyclonal IgG and a monoclonal immunoglobulin, usually IgM κ. Patients with type I cryoglobulins are frequently asymptomatic, while the presence of type II cryoglobulins is classically associated with skin purpura, arthralgia, Raynaud phenomenon, and vasculitis affecting the skin, kidneys, liver, and peripheral nerves.[108]

DIAGNOSIS AND DIFFERENTIAL DIAGNOSIS

Serum protein electrophoresis should be performed in all patients in whom multiple myeloma, primary amyloidosis, or a B cell lymphoproliferative disorder is suspected. Immunofixation is then required to determine both the heavy chain isotype and light chain class, whilst the sFLC assay, if available, is increasingly recognized as the best method to further define light chain production.

Patients with monoclonal immunoglobulins ideally should be referred for specialist assessment to identify those with an underlying malignant disorder but also the rare cases who have clinical features attributable to the properties of their monoclonal protein.

It is crucial to consider the heavy chain isotype when assessing patients with monoclonal gammopathy. Patients with IgG or IgA proteins may have underlying myeloma or occasionally primary amyloidosis, solitary plasmacytoma, or a B cell lymphoproliferative disorder. Immunoglobulin M-proteins are more commonly associated with an underlying lymphoproliferative disorder such as Waldenstrom macroglobulinemia/lymphoplasmacytic lymphoma, whilst primary amyloidosis is uncommon and IgM myeloma very rare.[109–111]

Laboratory assessment

Bone marrow examination should be performed in patients in whom there is a clinical suspicion of an underlying disorder. It is important to note that the presence of Bence-Jones proteinuria and immunoparesis does not necessarily mean a diagnosis of multiple myeloma, as both can be demonstrated in up to 40 percent of patients with MGUS.[109] The role of bone marrow examination in asymptomatic patients is more controversial. Some would suggest that bone marrow examination need only be performed in patients with monoclonal protein concentrations of 20 g/L or greater.[109] This approach is based upon the assumption that the monoclonal protein level is predictive of the underlying diagnosis. This is only partly valid, as although the concentration of monoclonal protein

rarely if ever exceeds 30 g/L in MGUS, patients with malignant disease can have much lower serum monoclonal components. The most striking example of this is Waldenstrom macroglobulinemia, where IgM levels can be much lower.[111]

Monoclonal gammopathy of undetermined significance can only be definitively diagnosed if the bone marrow shows no evidence of myeloma or a B cell lymphoproliferative disorder and there are no associated clinical symptoms or signs to suggest an alternative diagnosis. A more systematic approach to diagnosis would be the assessment of the majority of patients with a bone marrow aspirate and a trephine biopsy. Immunoglobulin G and IgA MGUS may be diagnosed if there are fewer than 10 percent plasma cells on an adequate marrow aspirate smear and minimal plasma cell infiltration on the trephine biopsy, with no other evidence of multiple myeloma and no evidence of a B cell lymphoproliferative disorder.[10] Immunoglobulin M MGUS may be diagnosed if there is no evidence of bone marrow infiltration by a B cell lymphoproliferative disorder.[112]

Flow cytometry is a useful adjunct to morphologic assessment in all MGUS cases to help assess neoplastic plasma cells and exclude other B cell lymphoproliferative disorders. Neoplastic plasma cells may be differentiated from their normal counterparts by virtue of the loss of CD19 and/or the expression of CD56 (normal plasma cells being consistently CD19$^+$ and CD56$^-$). Normal plasma cells are rarely if ever detected in patients with established myeloma but can be present in over 50 percent of patients with MGUS.[89–91,113] In approximately 40 percent of MGUS cases, neoplastic plasma cells are the exclusive cell population and careful assessment of the bone marrow trephine is required in these cases to help exclude multiple myeloma. The same depth of analysis should be applied to patients with IgM monoclonal proteins where B cell lymphoproliferative disorders are the main differential diagnosis.

TREATMENT

The vast majority of patients with MGUS do not require any specific therapeutic intervention. Those rare patients who present with clinical features attributable to their monoclonal protein often present difficult therapeutic challenges. There are, however, a number of key points to consider when assessing the treatment options for such patients. First, there is on the whole no relationship between the presence of an underlying lymphoproliferative disorder, concentration of monoclonal immunoglobulin, and symptomatology; indeed very significant symptoms can often occur with exceedingly low levels of monoclonal immunoglobulin. Second, a significant number of patients with these disorders may not require cytotoxic therapy and their symptoms can often be alleviated with other measures. Chemotherapy approaches may, in some individuals, be appropriate but it is essential to clarify the etiologic role of the monoclonal immunoglobulin before embarking upon such treatments.

Autoimmune phenomena

Patients with autoimmune phenomena can often benefit from symptomatic measures alone. Patients with cold agglutinin disease learn to avoid cold exposure, whilst those with peripheral neuropathies can gain relief from analgesics, amitriptyline, and gabapentin.[114] However, conditions such as acquired von Willebrand disease do often need active interventions and are typically treated with intravenous immunoglobulin factor replacement therapies such as recombinant Factor VIIa which are utilized if acute bleeding occurs.[115,116]

Cytotoxic treatment may be considered in a proportion of patients with IgM-associated demyelinating peripheral neuropathy. There are, however, only limited published data on the activity of alkylating agents, purine analogues, and rituximab in this setting and the results are generally disappointing.[114,117–119] Autologous stem cell transplantation has been utilized to achieve greater complete serologic response rates, hypothesizing that this increased depth of response may translate into better clinical outcome. Autologous transplantation may therefore have a role in selected patients.[120]

There are no published randomized trials in the treatment of POEMS syndrome and hence most data are retrospective. There is little evidence to support either intravenous immunoglobulins or plasmapheresis, which have classically been used to treat CIDP. The more effective treatments have developed from multiple myeloma-based regimens. Local radiation therapy to a single osteosclerotic lesion with associated POEMS can produce durable responses,[98] whilst up to 40 percent of patients will respond to melphalan and prednisone or combination chemotherapy regimens. The utilization of autologous transplantation may improve response rates further;[121] however, the use of novel agents such as thalidomide and bortezomib, although effective in multiple myeloma, may be limited due to concerns of exacerbating the neuropathy. Whether agents such as lenalidomide will offer an alternative approach is at present unclear. For the treatment of symptomatic cold agglutinin disease, options include rituximab, alkylating agents, and purine analogues.[122–124]

Immunoglobulin deposition diseases

Patients with nonamyloid monoclonal immunoglobulin deposition present considerable therapeutic challenges. It may, however, be appropriate to apply, with some qualifications, the treatment principles used in patients with primary amyloidosis (see section in this chapter) using myeloma-like therapy regimens.[125] There are, however, a proportion of patients who present with end-stage renal

or cardiac failure, and solid organ transplantation may be more applicable in this group, despite the inevitable deposition of immunoglobulin in the transplanted organs over time. Autologous stem cell transplantation is also an attractive approach that has been used in primary amyloidosis[126] and may be applicable to those patients with nonamyloid deposition diseases who have potentially reversible multisystem involvement.

Adult acquired Fanconi syndrome is one condition that should not be treated in this way. The prognosis is generally good and the disease is usually adequately controlled with supplements of calcium, phosphate, and vitamin D.

PROGNOSIS AND LONG-TERM MANAGEMENT

Progression risk

The risk of progression to symptomatic disease in MGUS is approximately 1 percent per annum and the vast majority of patients will die of unrelated causes. Given these statistics, it would seem appropriate that only those patients at high risk of progression would be appropriate for the testing of preventative strategies. To identify these individuals would both allow reassurance of those unlikely to ever need medical interventions and to target what will undoubtedly not be risk-free interventions at those who are most likely to become symptomatic and hence might benefit the most.

In probably the largest long-term study of MGUS yet published, 1384 patients from southeastern Minnesota were observed for a median of 15.4 years and a total of 11 009 person-years. The overall risk of progression was 12 percent, 25 percent, and 30 percent at 10, 20, and 30 years, respectively.[56]

In the Minnesota study, the most significant factor (out of 13 potential risk factors) associated with risk of progression was the concentration of monoclonal immunoglobulin and the subtype (IgA and IgM having greater risk). These data have been corroborated by other groups.[62] Several studies have also suggested that the presence of urinary free light chains and a reduction in normal polyclonal immunoglobulins are predictive of progression.[58,62] The prognostic relevance of cytogenetic abnormalities remains unclear.

Arguably the most significant recent risk factor identified to predict progression of MGUS to multiple myeloma is the presence of an abnormal serum free light chain (sFLC) ratio. The sFLC ratio may well be a surrogate marker for clonal evolution of the malignant plasma cell as it is most likely to reflect a loss of control of the ratio of heavy and light chains secreted.

Using the same cohort of patients as in previous studies from Minnesota, 1148 patient samples were analyzed using the sFLC assay (Freelite®). Using this method, the risk of progression in individuals with abnormal light chain ratios was significantly higher (hazard ratio 3.5, 95 percent

CI 2.3–5.5; $P < 0.001$).[127] The risk of developing multiple myeloma or a related B cell disorder at 10 years was increased from 5 percent to 17 percent and combined with established risk factors (type and size of serum monoclonal protein) allowed risk-stratification of patients.

Overall survival

The outcome of patients who develop myeloma, Waldenstrom macroglobulinemia, or other lymphoproliferative disorders following a diagnosis of MGUS is unclear, but the limited data available suggest that they are no different to those patients presenting with *de novo* disease. Indeed, survival from diagnosis may in fact be longer in the MGUS group due to a lower tumor burden.[58,128] As already outlined, the rate of progression is low; however, studies do exist demonstrating that overall survival in patients with MGUS is inferior to that of control populations[56,129] and this can, at least in part, be attributed to the excess mortality associated with the development of symptomatic disease. Hence the identification of individuals who are likely to become symptomatic is important.

Long-term management

The risk of progression to symptomatic disease requiring therapy is considered the main rationale for long-term follow-up in patients with MGUS.[56,109] Following the completion of initial staging investigations, most experts advocate review on at least an annual basis. It is assumed that such follow-up will allow earlier intervention with consequent reduction in morbidity and improvement in survival. However, a more systematic approach to risk assessment and follow-up is required as individuals can progress at markedly differing rates.[109,130] This is an area deserving of further work and the models outlined by Rajkumar *et al.*[127] utilizing the sFLC assay alongside the type and level of monoclonal immunoglobulin to identify high-risk individuals will undoubtedly be of great benefit in stratifying patients, modifying follow-up accordingly. Another potential approach to identifying patients at high risk of progression would be to identify those with occult evidence of end-organ impairment such as bone disease. It is evident that a proportion of MGUS patients do have markers of increased bone resorption but it remains to be seen whether these abnormalities predict progression.[131,132]

Alternative methods, identifying those patients in whom the risk of progression is negligible, are also worth consideration. These patients could be reassured and discharged from long-term follow-up whilst those remaining could be monitored in a more systematic and meaningful manner. Two stratification models to identify this group have been suggested utilizing combinations of the level of marrow disease, monoclonal immunoglobulin, urinary light chain excretion, and the presence of immunoparesis.[59,133] Flow cytometric methods could also have a role to play in this context, as persistence of normal plasma cells in the bone marrow appears to be associated with a negligible risk of progression.[134] Whether clonal karyotypic assessment will be helpful in predicting progression is at present unclear as the occurrence of either del(13q) or t(4;14) does not appear to result in the poor outcome seen in multiple myeloma. Possibly the most promising method to help identify the genetics that influence progression is that of gene expression profiling.[88] It is hoped that the results obtained from these techniques will allow the development of more systematic approaches to risk assessment which are clearly required.

PLASMACYTOMAS

INTRODUCTION

Solitary plasmacytomas are relatively rare and represent only 5 percent of patients with plasma cell dyscrasias. Solitary plasmacytomas may present either in the bone or as an extramedullary mass. Some will present with a painful/symptomatic lesion (Fig. 74.9) whilst others will be picked up during radiologic examination for either an unrelated disease or during the investigation of a monoclonal immunoglobulin.[135]

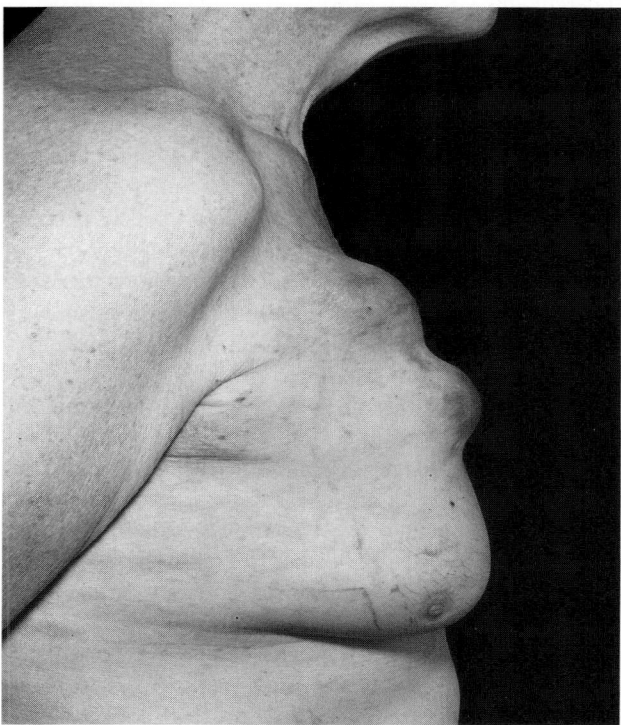

Figure 74.9 Extramedullary plasmacytoma in the subdermal plane of the anterior thorax.

Solitary bone plasmacytomas (SBP) have a high risk of progression to multiple myeloma and with the introduction of MRI scanning it is apparent that up to 25 percent of patients originally labeled as SBP will in fact have disease elsewhere.[136] Extramedullary plasmacytomas (EP) are in contrast almost always localized and have a high cure rate with radiation therapy.[137] The median age of presentation with plasmacytoma is in the mid-fifth decade, a little younger than multiple myeloma, and there is a male predominance.[138]

DIAGNOSIS AND INVESTIGATION

The diagnosis of plasmacytoma relies on histologic evidence of a mass lesion consisting of monoclonal plasma cells identified with appropriate immunohistochemical staining. Immunohistochemistry should, as a minimum, consist of assessment for CD138 and κ/λ staining to demonstrate monoclonal plasma cells, but other useful markers would include MUM1/IRF4, CD56, CD117, CD27, and cyclin D1.

To confidently diagnose a SBP there must be a single lytic lesion on skeletal survey and no evidence of systemic myeloma or related end-organ tissue damage (ROTI). Traditionally there should also be no evidence of plasma cell infiltrate in the bone marrow; however, more sensitive techniques are now demonstrating very low level infiltrates to be present in a proportion of cases. All patients should be fully assessed to exclude multiple myeloma.[139] Solitary bone plasmacytomas primarily affect the axial skeleton and vertebrae.[140] The role of sensitive imaging techniques is becoming apparent and MRI with or without CT of the spine to detect occult lesions not shown on plain radiography is certainly desirable and should be performed wherever possible.[2]

The monoclonal serum component is variable in patients with SBP but, depending on the series quoted, can occur in up to 72 percent of cases.[138] This is at odds with that seen in extramedullary plasmacytomas where the quoted incidence is much lower at less than 25 percent. The levels of serum monoclonal immunoglobulins do, however, tend to be lower than those seen in multiple myeloma and Bence-Jones proteinuria is less common.[139] This observation may be a reflection of both disease load and the differing biology of the conditions.

Extramedullary plasmacytomas occur more commonly in the respiratory sinuses and upper respiratory tract (more than 80 percent) alongside the gastrointestinal tract[141] but are seen in the skin, lymph nodes, thymus, and at almost any other site.[142–144] They are less common than those of bone and it is important to exclude bone destruction, occult disease at distant sites, and soft tissue spread of multiple myeloma before making the diagnosis. Added confusion may also occur in the diagnosis of plasmacytoma as most B cell lymphomas (e.g., MALToma and immunoblastic lymphoma[139]) can demonstrate a degree of plasma cell differentiation; this can occasionally predominate and mimic the diagnosis of plasmacytoma. Computed tomography or MRI scanning is certainly indicated to delineate the extent of the lesion but, at present, scanning of the spine and other areas has not yet been evaluated and is not considered essential. Patients should, however, be fully staged to exclude multiple myeloma.[139]

TREATMENT

Solitary plasmacytoma of bone

Local radiation therapy is the mainstay of treatment although there is no consensus in the literature for the most appropriate dosing schedule. Controversy also exists over the target volume of the radiation therapy but present guidance would suggest that a tumor margin of at least 2 cm and 40 Gy in 20 fractions for those lesions less than 5 cm and a higher dose of up to 50 Gy in 25 fractions should be considered for more bulky disease.[139] There is at present little evidence to back the use of bisphosphonates in the management of SBP and the use of other agents such as bortezomib and thalidomide has not yet found a place in routine management. Patients with more extensive disease should be treated as for multiple myeloma. The exception to this rule would be if the plasmacytoma was the only cause of symptoms, in which case to treat with radiation therapy and then defer cytotoxic treatment until there are signs of progression would be appropriate.[2]

Solitary extramedullary plasmacytoma

Radiation therapy should follow the same guidance as that for solitary plasmacytomas of bone. However, if cervical nodes are involved, as is the case in 10–40 percent of upper respiratory or upper gastrointestinal disease,[145,146] then these should be included in the radiation therapy field. Surgery is not generally recommended for the treatment of head and neck EP but should be considered at other sites if complete removal of the tumor is feasible. In the rare cases of relapsed/refractory/progressive disease, cytotoxic treatment should be considered.[139]

PROGNOSIS

Solitary plasmacytoma of bone, despite being extremely radiosensitive, will, in the majority of patients, progress to multiple myeloma after a median of 2–4 years; these individuals have a median overall survival of between 7 and 12 years. Between 15 percent and 45 percent of patients will, however, remain disease free at 10 years and this group is likely to be those in whom paraprotein concentrations become unrecordable within the first year posttreatment (implying the disease was fully eradicated with radiation therapy), rather than those with either persisting monoclonal immunoglobulins or nonsecretory disease.[143]

Extramedullary plasmacytoma is also very radiosensitive and local control is usually achieved in over 80 percent of patients, between 50 percent and 65 percent remaining disease free at 10 years. For those patients who do progress to multiple myeloma, this occurs after a median of 1.5–2.5 years and the prognosis at this point appears to be similar to those with *de novo* disease.

MONOCLONAL IMMUNOGLOBULIN DEPOSITION DISEASE

INTRODUCTION

The term *amyloidosis* describes a group of conditions characterized by the deposition of extracellular protein molecules in an ordered structure to make linear fibrils 7.5–10 nm wide, arranged in characteristic β-sheets. These β-sheets produce apple-green birefringence under polarized light when stained with Congo red. Amyloidosis was first reported in 1854 by Virchow and he coined the name due to the apparent affinity of the protein material for iodine, though the name was retained despite the proteinaceous nature of the fibrils.[147] The fibrillary nature of amyloid protein was first characterized by electron microscopy in 1959 by Cohen and Calkins.[148] Originally, the amyloidoses were classified as either primary (occurring in those with no underlying pathology) or secondary (occurring in those with chronic inflammation or infection). However, with the discovery that several different proteins could cause amyloidosis, the revised categorization is based on the protein precursor, as illustrated in Table 74.4. These

conditions are of particular interest to hemato-oncologists as one of the commonest varieties is AL amyloidosis, formerly known as primary amyloidosis, which is a protein conformation disorder associated with a clonal plasma cell dyscrasia.[149] Multiple organ disease results from the deposition of monoclonal immunoglobulin light chain fragments in insoluble fibrils which associate *in vivo* with the normal plasma protein serum amyloid P component (SAP), and this phenomenon is the basis for the use of SAP scintigraphy for imaging and monitoring amyloid deposits.[150] Accumulation of the fibrils progressively disrupts the normal tissue structure leading to organ dysfunction, e.g., of the kidneys, heart, and liver. Deposition of the amyloid fibrils evokes little or no local reaction in the tissues.

CLINICAL FEATURES

AL amyloidosis is a progressive and fatal disease, often (in about 80 percent of patients) within 2 years.[151] However, treatments that substantially reduce the supply of monoclonal immunoglobulin light chains frequently result in the stabilization or regression of existing amyloid deposits, and can be associated with improvement in end-organ function. AL amyloidosis may be associated with PCM or other B cell malignancies. A concurrent diagnosis of PCM or other B cell malignancy is made at diagnosis in patients with AL amyloidosis (see above) and coexistent AL amyloid deposits are identified either at presentation or at

Table 74.4 Nomenclature and classification of amyloid and amyloidoses

Amyloid type	Protein precursor	Protein type or variant	Associated clinical syndromes
AL	κ, λ	Aκ, Aλ	Primary amyloidosis, PCM, Waldenstrom macroglobulinemia
AH	IgG1	Aγ1	Heavy chain disease associated
AA	ApoSAA	AA	Reactive/secondary amyloidosis
			Familial Mediterranean fever
ATTR	Transthyretin		Hereditary amyloidosis:
		Met30	Familial amyloidotic polyneuropathies
		Met111	Familial amyloidotic cardiomyopathy
AApoAI	Apolipoprotein AI	Arg26	Familial amyloidotic polyneuropathy
		Arg60	Ostertag-type familial amyloidosis
AGel	Gelsolin	Asn187	Finnish-type familial amyloidosis
Aβ_2-m	β_2-microglobulin		Dialysis associated
Aβ	β-protein precursor	β A4 protein	Alzheimer disease, Down syndrome
	A4	Gln695	Hereditary cerebral hemorrhage with amyloid (Dutch)
ACys	Cystatin-C	Leu 68	Hereditary cerebral hemorrhage with amyloid (Icelandic)
AScr	PrP^c	PrP^c, PrP^{CJD}	Spongiform encephalopathies
ACal	(Pro)calcitonin	(Pro)calcitonin	Medullary carcinoma of thyroid
AANF	Atrial natriuretic factor	Atrial natriuretic factor	Isolated atrial amyloidosis
AIAPP	Islet-associated peptide	Islet-associated peptide	Amyloid of the islets, diabetes mellitus type II
A Lys	Lysozyme	Thr56	Hereditary nonneuropathic systemic amyloidosis
A Fib	Fibrinogen α chain	Leu554	Hereditary renal amyloidosis

Data from WHO-IUIS Nomenclature Subcommittee. Nomenclature of amyloid and amyloidosis. *Bull World Health Organ* 1993; **71**: 105–12.
PCM, plasma cell myeloma.

some time during the course of PCM in approximately 10–15 percent of patients and more rarely in Waldenstrom macroglobulinemia. AL amyloid deposits that are demonstrated histologically during the course of investigations in patients with these disorders may not be clinically significant but this can only be determined following comprehensive clinical and laboratory evaluation. It is rare for AL amyloidosis to progress to overt PCM presumably because of the short survival of patients with AL amyloidosis.

AL amyloid fibrils are derived from the N-terminal region of monoclonal immunoglobulin light chains and consist of the whole or part of the variable (V_L) domain. Intact light chains may rarely be found, and the molecular weight therefore varies between 8 kDa and 30 kDa. Monoclonal light chains that can form amyloid are able to exist in partly unfolded states, involving loss of tertiary or higher order structure. These readily aggregate with retention of β-sheet secondary structure into protofilaments and fibrils. Once the process has started, deposition may progress exponentially as expansion of the amyloid template 'captures' further precursor molecules. Only a small proportion of monoclonal light chains are *amyloidogenic*, but it is not possible to identify these from their class or abundance.

The age-adjusted incidence of AL amyloidosis in the United States is estimated to be between 5.1 and 12.8 per million persons per year,[152] which is equivalent to approximately 600 new cases per year in the United Kingdom. AL amyloidosis is estimated to be the cause of death in 1/1500 deaths in the UK. Approximately 60–70 percent of patients are aged between 50 and 70 years of age at diagnosis, with fewer than 10 percent being less than 50 years of age, and the male:female ratio is equal.

The most common clinical features at diagnosis are: (1) nephrotic syndrome with or without renal insufficiency; (2) congestive cardiomyopathy; (3) sensorimotor and/or autonomic peripheral neuropathy; and (4) hepatomegaly.[153] Whilst systemic symptoms of fatigue and weight loss may be common, they are rarely presenting features and patients generally present with one particular organ that is dysfunctional. Clinical characteristics are illustrated in Table 74.5.

DIAGNOSIS

AL amyloidosis should be considered in any patient who presents with nephrotic syndrome (with or without renal insufficiency), nondilated cardiomyopathy, peripheral neuropathy, hepatomegaly, or autonomic neuropathy, whether or not a paraprotein can be detected in the serum or urine. In particular, the diagnosis should be considered in patients with PCM with systemic symptoms. Confirmation of the diagnosis of amyloidosis is provided through tissue histology and should include serial investigations to determine the extent of disease. Amyloid deposits stain with Congo red and produce pathognomonic red-green birefringence

under cross-polarized light microscopy. Biopsy of an affected organ is usually diagnostic but less-invasive alternatives are possible. Abdominal fat aspirate and rectal and labial salivary gland biopsies yield positive results in up to 80 percent of cases in reported studies,[154,155] but are nondiagnostic in up to 50 percent of patients in routine clinical practice. Bone marrow biopsy should also be stained with Congo red, involvement being strongly suggestive of AL type. DNA analysis is principally used to distinguish AL amyloidosis from hereditary forms of amyloid. Amyloid fibril protein sequencing can be performed on tissue biopsy samples and the amino acid sequence determined. This method identifies the type of amyloidosis when other methods have failed.

Full investigation to determine the presence of a monoclonal plasma cell dyscrasia should be undertaken, as described in the PCM section above. A paraprotein is detectable in the serum or urine by routine electrophoresis in approximately 50 percent of patients, though it is less than 10 g/L in 30 percent of patients. As such, immunofixation is recommended to increase sensitivity of detection. As described above, serum free light chains can now be detected and quantitated in 98 percent of patients.[156,157]

Serum amyloid P component scintigraphy can be useful in determining the systemic extent of amyloid deposition but the availability of this type of imaging is somewhat limited. Radiolabeled SAP component localizes rapidly and specifically to amyloid deposits in proportion to the quantity of amyloid present. This enables the diagnosis and quantification of deposits by whole-body scintigraphy, although cardiac amyloid is poorly visualized.[158] In the latter case, electrocardiogram and echocardiography can demonstrate low-voltage changes, concentrically thickened ventricles, thickened valves, and dilated atria, with Doppler flow studies identifying diastolic dysfunction. Cardiac involvement can be graded according to the WHO criteria (Fig. 74.10). The chest x-ray may demonstrate reticulonodular shadowing. Nerve conduction studies and biopsy may be indicated in patients with primary neurological symptomatology. These may be required where neuropathy is the dominant presenting symptom.

MANAGEMENT

Prognosis is poor in patients with AL amyloidosis; the natural history varies with the extent and nature of organ involvement but fewer than 5 percent of all AL amyloidosis patients survive 10 or more years from the time of diagnosis.[151] A poor prognosis is associated with cardiac involvement, widespread deposition as determined by SAP scintigraphy, autonomic neuropathy, and hepatic involvement.

As yet, there is no specific therapy to augment the removal of amyloid fibrils and therefore treatment strategies are aimed at reducing or even stopping amyloid production, whilst providing supportive care for organ

Table 74.5 Clinical features of amyloidosis

Organ system	Frequency	Histopathology	Clinical features and symptoms
Kidney	~33%	Glomerular lesion causing marked proteinuria and nephrotic syndrome	Mild renal dysfunction is frequent, progressive renal failure is uncommon Ankle swelling, fatigue, and loss of energy Body cavity effusions (pericardial, pleural, peritoneal) Orthostatic hypotension
Cardiac	~20%	Amyloid deposition resulting in restrictive cardiomyopathy	Abnormalities on a 12-lead electrocardiogram, low-voltage changes Clinical signs of right-sided heart failure or those associated with a low cardiac output Orthostatic hypotension Arial thrombi and atrial fibrillation Restrictive cardiomyopathy
Nervous system	~20%	Amyloid deposition resulting in nerve conduction defects	Polyneuropathy may give rise to parasthesiae and muscle weakness Sensory neuropathy is usually symmetrical, affecting the lower extremities, and may be painful Motor neuropathy is rare Carpal tunnel syndrome is common Autonomic neuropathy giving rise to postural hypotension, impotence, and disturbed GI motility Postural hypotension (fall in systolic blood pressure of at least 20 mm Hg when a patient has been standing for 3–5 min after spending at least 5 min supine)
GI tract	10–25%	Mucosal/submucosal amyloid deposition	Focal or diffuse with symptoms relating to the site of involvement Macroglossia and occasionally obstructive airways symptoms and sleep apnea Diarrhea, chronic nausea, malabsorption, and weight loss GI perforation or hemorrhage Hepatomegaly
Hemostatic	~33–50%	Endothelial amyloid deposition distorting vessel contractibility	Hemostatic screen abnormalities Commonest manifestation of bleeding is purpura, e.g., periorbital purpura ('raccoon eyes') Life-threatening bleeding potential, particularly GI
Localized		Focal infiltrate of clonal lymphoplasmacytoid cells	Upper respiratory (vocal cords) and pulmonary infiltration Musculoskeletal (arthopathy) Urogenital Adrenal and thyroid glands GI tract Skin Localized disease is not usually associated with measurable paraprotein or serum free light chains

GI, gastrointestinal.

dysfunction. Chemotherapy regimens used in AL amyloidosis are based on those that have proved to be effective in patients with PCM. Clinical benefit from chemotherapy typically does not occur for many months after the underlying plasma cell dyscrasia has been adequately suppressed. Whilst slow-acting regimens may not impact the disease process given the limited overall survival, high-dose therapy regimens are associated with a high procedural risk compared to patients with PCM, as a result of multiorgan involvement.

For those patients deemed not suitable for intensive therapy, single-agent melphalan or cyclophosphamide (with or without prednisone) is appropriate, where symptomatic benefit can be seen in about 20–30 percent of patients, though only after a median of 12 months' treatment. In those deemed suitable, intermediate-dose therapy may be more appropriate. Monthly courses of VAD (vincristine, adriamycin, dexamethasone) and similar regimens, or intravenous intermediate-dose melphalan 25 mg/m^2, with or without dexamethasone, have been used. Whilst

WHO staging system for cardiac amyloid
1 NO symptomatic or occult cardiac amyloid by biopsy or noninvasive resting.
2 Asymptomatic cardiac involvement by biopsy or noninvasive testing, e.g., wall thickness >1.1 cm in the absence of prior hypertension or valvular disease, unexplained low-voltage electrocardiogram (ECG).
3 Compensated symptomatic cardiac involvement.
4 Uncompensated cardiomyopathy.

Figure 74.10 World Health Organization (WHO) criteria for diagnosing cardiac involvement with amyloid.

several advantages for using VAD and its hybrids exist, some specific cautions need to be observed in patients with amyloidosis such as the cardiotoxicity of adriamycin and exacerbation of peripheral and autonomic neuropathy by vincristine. High-dose dexamethasone can cause severe fluid retention causing problems in patients with renal or cardiac amyloidosis, and can lead to bone fractures and vertebral collapse in those with bone involvement. There have been anecdotal reports of good responses to VAD in AL amyloidosis,[159,160] although the regimen has not been assessed in a randomized controlled trial. However, VAD should be considered as first-line therapy in patients under the age of 70 years who do not have symptomatic cardiac failure, autonomic neuropathy, or peripheral neuropathy and requires careful monitoring in those who do demonstrate clinically significant end-organ damage. Dexamethasone alone in PCM has similar efficacy to VAD in terms of initial response and, when used alone, high-dose pulsed dexamethasone (HDD) has demonstrated a response in 12–16 percent of patients with amyloidosis.[161]

The variable absorption of melphalan from the gastrointestinal tract led Schey et al.[162] to investigate the use of intravenous intermediate-dose melphalan 25 mg/m^2 and oral dexamethasone in patients with PCM. However, more recently the IFM group have reported on their randomized study of high-dose melphalan and ASCT compared with standard-dose melphalan with dexamethasone, suggesting a trend to improved survival with standard-dose melphalan, especially in low-risk disease (OS at 3 years 58 percent in ASCT group compared with 80 percent in standard-dose melphalan group, $P = 0.13$).[163] Intermediate-dose melphalan may be considered in patients who are fit for intravenous therapy but in whom VAD is contraindicated or has produced an inadequate response.

Thalidomide is an effective therapy for PCM, though it is associated with a characteristic side-effect profile (see above). A preliminary analysis of a phase I/II trial in 12 patients with AL amyloidosis (without peripheral neuropathy) demonstrated that the maximum tolerated dose was 500 mg and all patients experienced side effects.[164] Four patients stopped treatment early because of side effects. Five of 11 patients had a limited hematologic response. Thalidomide therefore appears to have some activity in AL amyloidosis but further information regarding efficacy and toxicity is required.

There are no data at present on the use of thalidomide in combination with dexamethasone. Standard- and intermediate-dose colchicine may be effective in the treatment of AA amyloidosis complicating familial Mediterranean fever by suppressing the underlying inflammatory disease, but it has no role in AL amyloidosis.

Autologous stem cell transplantation with intravenous high-dose melphalan (100–200 mg/m^2) in patients with AL amyloidosis was first reported in 1996, and a series of 25 patients was reported shortly afterwards.[126] High-dose therapy and PBSC transplantation can result in reversal of the clinical manifestations of AL amyloidosis in up to 60 percent of patients who survive the procedure. This is associated with regression of AL deposits on SAP scanning, reduction or elimination of the causative clonal plasma cell disorder, and improved performance status and quality of life. However, the procedural-related mortality has been consistently and substantially higher in amyloidosis patients than those with PCM, ranging up to 40 percent in some studies.[165–168] This reflects compromised function of multiple organ systems and patient selection is pivotal to improve the TRM whilst allowing those who will benefit the most to proceed. The causes of death include cardiac arrhythmias, intractable hypotension, multiorgan failure, and gastrointestinal bleeding. Patients with poor renal function and those who are already dialysis-dependent fare particularly badly.[126] There is also a significant risk, including death, associated with stem cell mobilization in patients with AL amyloidosis, even when granulocyte colony-stimulating factor (G-CSF) is used alone.[126] Complications have included sudden onset of pulmonary edema and/or an unexplained syndrome of progressive hypoxia and hypotension, which may occur in patients without cardiac amyloid. It is therefore recommended that patients receive twice-daily dosing of G-CSF; collections may need to be interrupted because of worsening hypoxia or edema. Measures that can reduce morbidity and mortality during the PBSC transplantation procedure itself include avoidance of substantial prehydration, administering the melphalan in two divided doses, using a dose of $>5 \times 10^6$ CD34$^+$ cells/kg, and avoiding G-CSF support.[126] The role of PBSC transplantation therefore remains unclear and because of its special problems in AL amyloidosis, it is recommended that such patients be treated in units with expertise of this particular disease. It seems reasonable to restrict PBSC transplantation to younger patients with one or two involved organs who have not had previous amyloid-related gastrointestinal bleeding and who do not have severe cardiomyopathy or advanced renal failure or are dialysis-dependent.

The first successful allo-SCT for AL amyloidosis was reported in 1998 and was associated with complete clinical recovery at 3 years post-transplantation.[166] A small proportion of patients may derive significant clinical benefit from the procedure but at present it remains experimental and is likely to be associated with extremely high TRM. There are currently no data on the use of reduced-intensity conditioning in AL amyloidosis.

In addition to chemotherapy approaches, given the multiorgan system involvement in patients with AL amyloidosis, a multidisciplinary approach to supportive care needs to be developed. Patients with end-stage renal failure should be considered for dialysis and renal transplantation may be a suitable option for selected patients. In patients with cardiac involvement, congestive cardiac failure should be treated predominantly with diuretics; angiotensin-converting enzyme (ACE) inhibitors should be used with caution, and calcium-channel blockers and β-blockers are best avoided. Digoxin is generally contraindicated in patients with cardiac involvement, and in patients where cardiac manifestations are the predominant or only signs/symptoms of amyloidosis, cardiac transplantation may be considered but this procedure should be followed by chemotherapy treatment to prevent reaccumulation of amyloid in the transplanted heart. In patients who experience orthostatic hypotension, the use of support stockings coupled with modest doses of fludrocortisone can be effective in selected patients. Midodrine is the most effective drug for orthostatic hypotension in patients with amyloidosis, but can cause supine hypertension and should be used with caution.

KEY POINTS

Plasma cell myeloma

- Plasma cell myeloma (PCM) is a clonal B cell malignancy characterized by the production of either a monoclonal antibody (paraprotein) or light chain, in association with a plasmacytic bone marrow infiltration and lytic bone disease.
- PCM typically demonstrates a relapsing/responding course, though ultimately leads to an accelerated phase characterizing the terminal stages of the disease.
- PCM is subcharacterized as either symptomatic or asymptomatic myeloma, determined by the presence of related organ and/or tissue impairment (ROTI) including hypercalcemia, anemia, renal dysfunction, bone disease, or frequent bacterial infections.
- PCM is staged according to the level of serum albumin and β_2-microglobulin at diagnosis. The International Staging System categorizes disease in to stages I, II, and III, which confer decreasing overall survival.
- Chromosomal abnormalities can be detected in PCM but considerable heterogeneity is evident. Abnormalities of chromosome 13 confer a poor prognosis.
- Pain control is important in the clinical management of patients with PCM. Use of nonsteroidal anti-inflammatory drugs, opiate derivatives, and fractionated radiation therapy to lytic bone lesions are key to the pain management.
- Many patients present with anemia as a result of disease infiltration or tumor-associated cytokine production, associated with renal dysfunction or with treatment, or a combination of these scenarios. Erythropoietin therapy may be beneficial.
- The risk of infection in patients with PCM at diagnosis or during treatment is not insignificant and is highest in the first 3 months after diagnosis. The prevention of infection in patients using prophylactic immunoglobulin infusions and vaccination strategies can be helpful but prophylactic antibiotics are not recommended.
- Almost all patients with PCM will relapse after initial disease control and therefore the management strategy for individual patients should aim to treat the relapsing/remitting course of the disease.

Monoclonal gammopathy of undetermined significance

- Patients with a monoclonal immunoglobulin should be reviewed at a specialist center to exclude the presence of underlying pathology.
- The mechanisms underlying the transformation from MGUS to multiple myeloma or B lymphoproliferative disease remain unclear. The development of gene expression profiling is likely to provide future insight into the critical steps of progression and provide a more systematic approach to define those patients at a high risk of progression.
- As robust stratification techniques become available, thorough evaluation of all patients should allow the identification of both 'high-risk' MGUS and 'low-risk' MGUS. The identification of both groups is important and should allow the development of targeted interventions for the former and also prevent the worry and possible unnecessary use of resources in protracted follow-up of the latter, who are likely to have minimal risk of progression.
- Therapies available for the treatment of MGUS-related syndromes are primarily based on multiple myeloma-like treatment regimens and are at best only partially effective. The use of stem cell transplantation in selected groups has improved success rates but trials of agents such as thalidomide, Revlimid, and novel agents such as the proteasome inhibitors (bortezomib) may well prove to be useful in MGUS-related syndromes and as new agents appear in the treatment of 'high-risk' MGUS.

Monoclonal immunoglobulin deposition disease

- Amyloidosis describes a group of conditions characterized by the deposition of extracellular protein molecules in an ordered structure to make linear fibrils 7.5–10 nm wide arranged in characteristic β-sheets.
- It is a disease that involves multiple organ systems and symptomatology reflects the specific tissue infiltrations.
- Median survival for the majority of patient is less than 2 years.
- Patients most commonly present with renal involvement, usually with proteinuria or nephritic syndrome; cardiac involvement, usually with dysrhythmias and restrictive cardiomyopathy; and nervous system involvement, with peripheral neuropathy or autonomic neuropathy.
- Treatment takes a form similar to that used in treating PCM, as stopping the production of the amyloid protein rather than augmenting its removal is the treatment aim.
- Therapeutic strategies employed to treat amyloidosis are modified to take into account the multisystem dysfunction often present, though high-dose chemotherapy and autologous stem cell transplantation have been used successfully to modify the natural disease course.

REFERENCES

- = Key primary paper
◆ = Major review article

1. Reidel DA. Epidemiology of multiple myeloma. In: Wiernik PH, Kyle R, Schiffer CA. (eds) *Neoplastic diseases of the blood*, 2nd Edn. Churchill Livingstone, 1991: 347–73.
◆2. Smith A, Wisloff F, Samson D. Guidelines on the diagnosis and management of multiple myeloma 2005. *Br J Haematol* 2006; **132**: 410–51.
3. Korst DR, Clifford GO, Fowler WM *et al*. Multiple myeloma. II. Analysis of cyclophosphamide therapy in 165 patients. *JAMA* 1964; **189**: 758–62.
●4. Blade J, Esteve J, Rives S *et al*. High-dose therapy autotransplantation/intensification vs continued standard chemotherapy in multiple myeloma in first remission. Results of a non-randomized study from a single institution. *Bone Marrow Transplant* 2000; **26**: 845–9.
5. Solly S. Remarks on the pathology of mollities osseum. With cases. *Med Chir Soc Trans* 1844; **27**: 435–561.
6. MacIntyre W. Case of mollities and fragilitas ossium. *Med Chir Soc Trans* 1850; **33**: 211–32.
7. Harrison SJ, Cook G. Immunotherapy in multiple myeloma – possibility or probability? *Br J Haematol* 2005; **130**: 344–62.
8. Bradwell AR, Carr-Smith HD, Mead GP *et al*. Serum test for assessment of patients with Bence Jones myeloma. *Lancet* 2003; **361**: 489–91.
9. Mileshkin L, Blum R, Seymour JF *et al*. A comparison of fluorine-18 fluoro-deoxyglucose PET and technetium-99m sestamibi in assessing patients with multiple myeloma. *Eur J Haematol* 2004; **72**: 32–7.
◆10. International Myeloma Working Group. Criteria for the classification of monoclonal gammopathies, multiple myeloma and related disorders: a report of the International Myeloma Working Group. *Br J Haematol* 2003; **121**: 749–57.
●11. Durie BG, Salmon SE, Moon TE. Pretreatment tumor mass, cell kinetics, and prognosis in multiple myeloma. *Blood* 1980; **55**: 364–72.
12. Greipp PR, San Miguel J, Durie BG *et al*. International staging system for multiple myeloma. *J Clin Oncol* 2005; **23**: 3412–20.
●13. Blade J, Samson D, Reece D *et al*. Criteria for evaluating disease response and progression in patients with multiple myeloma treated by high-dose therapy and haemopoietic stem cell transplantation. Myeloma Subcommittee of the EBMT. European Group for Blood and Marrow *Transplant*. *Br J Haematol* 1998; 102: 1115–23.
●14. Attal M, Harousseau JL, Stoppa AM *et al*. A prospective, randomized trial of autologous bone marrow transplantation and chemotherapy in multiple myeloma. Intergroupe Francais du Myelome. *N Engl J Med* 1996; **335**: 91–7.
●15. Child JA, Morgan GJ, Davies FE *et al*. High-dose chemotherapy with hematopoietic stem-cell rescue for multiple myeloma. *N Engl J Med* 2003; **348**: 1875–83.
16. Barlogie B, Smith L, Alexanian R. Effective treatment of advanced multiple myeloma refractory to alkylating agents. *N Engl J Med* 1984; **310**: 1353–6.
17. Samson D, Gaminara E, Newland A *et al*. Infusion of vincristine and doxorubicin with oral dexamethasone as first-line therapy for multiple myeloma. *Lancet* 1989; **2**: 882–5.
18. Cook G, Clark RE, Morris TC *et al*. A randomized study (WOS MM1) comparing the oral regime Z-Dex (idarubicin and dexamethasone) with vincristine, adriamycin and dexamethasone as induction therapy for newly diagnosed patients with multiple myeloma. *Br J Haematol* 2004; **126**: 792–8.
●19. Singhal S, Mehta J, Desikan R *et al*. Antitumor activity of thalidomide in refractory multiple myeloma. *N Engl J Med* 1999; **341**: 1565–71.
20. Barlogie B, Shaughnessy J, Tricot G *et al*. Treatment of multiple myeloma. *Blood* 2004; **103**: 20–32.
◆21. Combination chemotherapy versus melphalan plus prednisone as treatment for multiple myeloma: an overview of 6,633 patients from 27 randomized trials. Myeloma Trialists' Collaborative Group. *J Clin Oncol* 1998; **16**: 3832–42.

22. Hernandez JM, Garcia-Sanz R, Golvano E *et al.* Randomized comparison of dexamethasone combined with melphalan versus melphalan with prednisone in the treatment of elderly patients with multiple myeloma. *Br J Haematol* 2004; **127**: 159–64.

●23. Palumbo A, Bringhen S, Musto P *et al.* A prospective randomized trial of oral melphalan, prednisolone, thalidomide (MPT) vs. oral melphalan, prednisolone (MP): an interim analysis. *Blood* 2004; **106**: 63a.

24. McElwain TJ, Powles RL. High-dose intravenous melphalan for plasma-cell leukaemia and myeloma. *Lancet* 1983; **2**: 822–4.

25. Chang H, Qi XY, Samiee S *et al.* Genetic risk identifies multiple myeloma patients who do not benefit from autologous stem cell transplantation. *Bone Marrow Transplant* 2005; **36**: 793–6.

26. Moreau P, Facon T, Attal M *et al.* Comparison of 200 mg/m(2) melphalan and 8 Gy total body irradiation plus 140 mg/m(2) melphalan as conditioning regimens for peripheral blood stem cell transplantation in patients with newly diagnosed multiple myeloma: final analysis of the Intergroupe Francophone du Myelome 9502 randomized trial. *Blood* 2002; **99**: 731–5.

27. Reece D, Vesole D, Flomenberg N *et al.* Intensive therapy with high-dose melphalan (MEL) 280 g/m^2 plus amifostine cytoprotection and ASCT as part of initial therapy in patients with multiple meloma. *Blood* 2002; **100**: 432a.

28. Lahuerta JJ, Grande C, Blade J *et al.* Myeloablative treatments for multiple myeloma: update of a comparative study of different regimens used in patients from the Spanish registry for transplantation in multiple myeloma. *Leuk Lymphoma* 2002; **43**: 67–74.

29. Clark AD, Douglas KW, Mitchell LD *et al.* Dose escalation therapy in previously untreated patients with multiple myeloma following Z-Dex induction treatment. *Br J Haematol* 2002; **117**: 605–12.

30. Moreau P, Hullin C, Garban F *et al.* Tandem autologous stem cell transplantation in high-risk de novo multiple myeloma: final results of the prospective and randomized IFM 99-04 protocol. *Blood* 2006; **107**: 397–403.

31. Hollmig K, Stover J, Talamo G *et al.* Addition of bortezomib (Velcade) to high dose melphalan (Vel-Mel) as an effective conditioning regimen with autologous stem cell support in multiple myeloma (MM). *Blood* 2004; **104**: 266a.

●32. Attal M, Harousseau JL, Facon T *et al.* Single versus double autologous stem-cell transplantation for multiple myeloma. *N Engl J Med* 2003; **349**: 2495–502.

33. Tricot G, Jagannath S, Vesole DH *et al.* Relapse of multiple myeloma after autologous transplantation: survival after salvage therapy. *Bone Marrow Transplant* 1995; **16**: 7–11.

34. Morris C, Iacobelli S, Brand R *et al.* Benefit and timing of second transplantations in multiple myeloma: clinical findings and methodological limitations in a European Group for Blood and Marrow Transplantation registry study. *J Clin Oncol* 2004; **22**: 1674–81.

35. Berenson JR, Crowley JJ, Grogan TM *et al.* Maintenance therapy with alternate-day prednisone improves survival in multiple myeloma patients. *Blood* 2002; **99**: 3163–8.

36. Feyler S, Rawstron A, Jackson GH *et al.* Thalidomide maintenance following high dose therapy in multiple myeloma: A UK. Myeloma Forum Phase II study. *Blood* 2005; **106**: 641.

37. Stewart AK, Chen CI, Howson-Jan K *et al.* Results of a multicenter randomized phase II trial of thalidomide and prednisone maintenance therapy for multiple myeloma after autologous stem cell transplant. *Clin Cancer Res* 2004; **10**: 8170–6.

38. Hunter HM, Peggs K, Powles R *et al.* Analysis of outcome following allogeneic haemopoietic stem cell transplantation for myeloma using myeloablative conditioning – evidence for a superior outcome using melphalan combined with total body irradiation. *Br J Haematol* 2005; **128**: 496–502.

◆39. Gahrton G, Svensson H, Cavo M *et al.* Progress in allogenic bone marrow and peripheral blood stem cell transplantation for multiple myeloma: a comparison between transplants performed 1983–93 and 1994–8 at European Group for Blood and Marrow Transplantation centres. *Br J Haematol* 2001; **113**: 209–16.

40. Corradini P, Cavo M, Lokhorst H *et al.* Molecular remission after myeloablative allogeneic stem cell transplantation predicts a better relapse-free survival in patients with multiple myeloma. *Blood* 2003; **102**: 1927–9.

41. Kroger N, Pérez-Simón JA, Myint H *et al.* Relapse to prior autograft and chronic graft-versus-host disease are the strongest prognostic factors for outcome of melphalan/fludarabine-based dose-reduced allogeneic stem cell transplantation in patients with multiple myeloma. *Biol Blood Marrow Transplant* 2004; **10**: 698–708.

42. Rosinol L, Pérez-Simón JA, Sureda A *et al.* Feasibility and efficacy of a planned second transplant ('auto' or 'miniallo') intensification in patients with multiple myeloma not achieving complete remission (CR) or near-CR with a first autologous transplant; results from a Spanish PETHEMA/GEM study. *Haematologica* 2005; **90**(Suppl 1): 50a.

43. Garban F, Attal M, Michallet M *et al.* Prospective comparison of autologous stem cell transplantation followed by dose-reduced allograft (IFM99-03 trial) with tandem autologous stem cell transplantation (IFM99-04 trial) in high-risk de novo multiple myeloma. *Blood* 2006; **107**: 3474–80.

44. Richardson PG, Barlogie B, Berenson J *et al.* A phase 2 study of bortezomib in relapsed, refractory myeloma. *N Engl J Med* 2003; **348**: 2609–17.

●45. Richardson PG, Sonneveld P, Schuster MW *et al.* Bortezomib or high-dose dexamethasone for relapsed multiple myeloma. *N Engl J Med* 2005; **352**: 2487–98.

◆46. Anderson KC. Lenalidomide and thalidomide: mechanisms of action – similarities and differences. *Semin Hematol* 2005; **42**(4 Suppl 4): S3–8.

●47. Richardson PG, Jagannath S, Schlossman R et al. A multicenter, randomized, phase II study to evaluate the efficacy and safety of 2 CDC-5013 dose regimens when used alone or in combination with dexamethasone (Dex) for the treatment of relapsed or refractory multiple myeloma. Blood 2003; 102: 235a.

48. Cazzola M, Beguin Y, Kloczko J et al. Once-weekly epoetin beta is highly effective in treating anaemic patients with lymphoproliferative malignancy and defective endogenous erythropoietin production. Br J Haematol 2003; 122: 386–93.

◆49. Glasmacher A, Hahn C, Hoffmann F et al. A systematic review of phase-II trials of thalidomide monotherapy in patients with relapsed or refractory multiple myeloma. Br J Haematol 2006; 132: 584–93.

50. Rousselot P, Larghero J, Arnulf B et al. A clinical and pharmacological study of arsenic trioxide in advanced multiple myeloma patients. Leukemia 2004; 18: 1518–21.

51. Miszczyk L, Sasiadek W. The evaluation of the effectiveness of half-body irradiation as palliative treatment in patients with multiple bone metastases. Przegl Lek 2001; 58: 431–4.

52. Morgan GJ, Krishnan B, Jenner M, Davies FE. Advances in oral therapy for multiple myeloma. Lancet Oncol 2006; 7: 316–25.

53. Axelsson U, Bachmann R, Hallen J. Frequency of pathological proteins (M-components) om 6,995 sera from an adult population. Acta Med Scand 1966; 179: 235–47.

54. Kyle RA, Finkelstein S, Elveback LR, Kurland LT. Incidence of monoclonal proteins in a Minnesota community with a cluster of multiple myeloma. Blood 1972; 40: 719–24.

55. Saleun JP, Vicariot M, Deroff P, Morin JF. Monoclonal gammopathies in the adult population of Finistere, France. J Clin Pathol 1982; 35: 63–8.

56. Kyle RA, Therneau TM, Rajkumar SV et al. A long-term study of prognosis in monoclonal gammopathy of undetermined significance. N Engl J Med 2002; 346: 564–9.

57. Kyle RA, Therneau TM, Rajkumar SV et al. Long-term follow-up of IgM monoclonal gammopathy of undetermined significance. Blood 2003; 102: 3759–64.

58. Cesana C, Klersy C, Barbarano L et al. Prognostic factors for malignant transformation in monoclonal gammopathy of undetermined significance and smoldering multiple myeloma. J Clin Oncol 2002; 20: 1625–34.

59. Van De Donk N, De Weerdt O, Eurelings M et al. Malignant transformation of monoclonal gammopathy of undetermined significance: cumulative incidence and prognostic factors. Leuk Lymphoma 2001; 42: 609–18.

60. Blade J, Lopez-Guillermo A, Rozman C et al. Malignant transformation and life expectancy in monoclonal gammopathy of undetermined significance. Br J Haematol 1992; 81: 391–4.

61. Giraldo MP, Rubio-Felix D, Perella M et al. Monoclonal gammopathies of undetermined significance. Clinical course and biological aspects of 397 cases. Sangre (Barc) 1991; 36: 377–82.

62. Gregersen H, Mellemkjaer L, Ibsen JS et al. The impact of M-component type and immunoglobulin concentration on the risk of malignant transformation in patients with monoclonal gammopathy of undetermined significance. Haematologica 2001; 86: 1172–9.

63. Ogmundsdottir HM, Haraldsdottir V, Johannesson M et al. Monoclonal gammopathy in Iceland: a population-based registry and follow-up. Br J Haematol 2002; 118: 166–73.

64. Morra E, Cesana C, Klersy C et al. Predictive variables for malignant transformation in 452 patients with asymptomatic IgM monoclonal gammopathy. Semin Oncol 2003; 30: 172–7.

65. Ligthart GJ, Radl J, Corberand JX et al. Monoclonal gammopathies in human aging: increased occurrence with age and correlation with health status. Mech Ageing Dev 1990; 52: 235–43.

66. Cohen HJ, Crawford J, Rao MK et al. Racial differences in the prevalence of monoclonal gammopathy in a community-based sample of the elderly. Am J Med 1998; 104: 439–44.

67. Bowden M, Crawford J, Cohen HJ, Noyama O. A comparative study of monoclonal gammopathies and immunoglobulin levels in Japanese and United States elderly. J Am Geriatr Soc 1993; 41: 11–14.

68. Kurihara Y, Shiba K, Fukumura Y et al. Occurrence of serum M-protein species in Japanese patients older than 50 years based on relative mobility in cellulose acetate membrane electrophoresis. J Clin Lab Anal 2000; 14: 64–9.

69. van de Poel MH, Coebergh JW, Hillen HF. Malignant transformation of monoclonal gammopathy of undetermined significance among out-patients of a community hospital in southeastern Netherlands. Br J Haematol 1995; 91: 121–5.

70. Anagnostopoulos A, Evangelopoulou A, Sotou D et al. Incidence and evolution of monoclonal gammopathy of undetermined significance (MGUS) in Greece. Ann Hematol 2002; 81: 357–61.

71. Pasqualetti P, Festuccia V, Collacciani A, Casale R. The natural history of monoclonal gammopathy of undetermined significance. A 5- to 20-year follow-up of 263 cases. Acta Haematol 1997; 97: 174–9.

72. Pasqualetti P, Collacciani A, Casale R. Risk of monoclonal gammopathy of undetermined significance: a case-referent study. Am J Hematol 1996; 52: 217–20.

73. Bizzaro N, Pasini P. Familial occurrence of multiple myeloma and monoclonal gammopathy of undetermined significance in 5 siblings. Haematologica 1990; 75: 58–63.

74. Lynch HT, Sanger WG, Pirruccello S et al. Familial multiple myeloma: a family study and review of the literature. J Natl Cancer Inst 2001; 93: 1479–83.

75. Schop RF, Jalal SM, Van Wier SA et al. Deletions of 17p13.1 and 13q14 are uncommon in Waldenstrom macroglobulinemia clonal cells and mostly seen at the time of disease progression. Cancer Genet Cytogenet 2002; 132: 55–60.

76. Schop RF, Kuehl WM, Van Wier SA et al. Waldenstrom macroglobulinemia neoplastic cells lack immunoglobulin heavy chain locus translocations but have frequent 6q deletions. *Blood* 2002; **100**: 2996–3001.

77. Avet-Loiseau H, Garand R, Lode L et al. 14q32 Translocations discriminate IgM multiple myeloma from Waldenstrom's macroglobulinemia. *Semin Oncol* 2003; **30**: 153–5.

78. Avet-Loiseau H, Li JY, Morineau N et al. Monosomy 13 is associated with the transition of monoclonal gammopathy of undetermined significance to multiple myeloma. Intergroupe Francophone du Myelome. *Blood* 1999; **94**: 2583–9.

79. Drach J, Angerler J, Schuster J et al. Interphase fluorescence in situ hybridization identifies chromosomal abnormalities in plasma cells from patients with monoclonal gammopathy of undetermined significance. *Blood* 1995; **86**: 3915–21.

80. Ahmann GJ, Jalal SM, Juneau AL et al. A novel three-color, clone-specific fluorescence in situ hybridization procedure for monoclonal gammopathies. *Cancer Genet Cytogenet* 1998; **101**: 7–11.

81. Zandecki M, Obein V, Bernardi F et al. Monoclonal gammopathy of undetermined significance: chromosome changes are a common finding within bone marrow plasma cells. *Br J Haematol* 1995; **90**: 693–6.

82. Rasillo A, Tabernero MD, Sanchez ML et al. Fluorescence in situ hybridization analysis of aneuploidization patterns in monoclonal gammopathy of undetermined significance versus multiple myeloma and plasma cell leukemia. *Cancer* 2003; **97**: 601–9.

83. Avet-Loiseau H, Facon T, Daviet A et al. 14q32 translocations and monosomy 13 observed in monoclonal gammopathy of undetermined significance delineate a multistep process for the oncogenesis of multiple myeloma. Intergroupe Francophone du Myelome. *Cancer Res* 1999; **59**: 4546–50.

84. Fonseca R, Bailey RJ, Ahmann GJ et al. Genomic abnormalities in monoclonal gammopathy of undetermined significance. *Blood* 2002; **100**: 1417–24.

85. Fonseca R, Blood E, Rue M et al. Clinical and biologic implications of recurrent genomic aberrations in myeloma. *Blood* 2003; **101**: 4569–75.

86. Avet-Louseau H, Daviet A, Sauner S, Bataille R. Chromosome 13 abnormalities in multiple myeloma are mostly monosomy 13. *Br J Haematol* 2000; **111**: 1116–7.

87. Harrison CJ, Mazzullo H, Ross FM et al. Translocations of 14q32 and deletions of 13q14 are common chromosomal abnormalities in systemic amyloidosis. *Br J Haematol* 2002; **117**: 427–35.

88. Davies FE, Dring AM, Li C et al. Insights into the multistep transformation of MGUS to myeloma using microarray expression analysis. *Blood* 2003; **102**: 4504–11.

89. Rawstron AC, Fenton JA, Ashcroft J et al. The interleukin-6 receptor alpha-chain (CD126) is expressed by neoplastic but not normal plasma cells. *Blood* 2000; **96**: 3880–6.

90. Ocqueteau M, Orfao A, Almeida J et al. Immunophenotypic characterization of plasma cells from monoclonal gammopathy of undetermined significance patients. Implications for the differential diagnosis between MGUS and multiple myeloma. *Am J Pathol* 1998; **152**: 1655–65.

91. Rawstron AC, Owen RG, Davies FE et al. Circulating plasma cells in multiple myeloma: characterization and correlation with disease stage. *Br J Haematol* 1997; **97**: 46–55.

92. Harada H, Kawano MM, Huang N et al. Phenotypic difference of normal plasma cells from mature myeloma cells. *Blood* 1993; **81**: 2658–63.

93. Ocqueteau M, Orfao A, Garcia-Sanz R et al. Expression of the CD117 antigen (c-Kit) on normal and myelomatous plasma cells. *Br J Haematol* 1996; **95**: 489–93.

94. Stone MJ, McElroy YG, Pestronk A et al. Human monoclonal macroglobulins with antibody activity. *Semin Oncol* 2003; **30**: 318–24.

95. Nobile-Orazio E, Casellato C, Di Troia A. Neuropathies associated with IgG and IgA monoclonal gammopathy. *Rev Neurol (Paris)* 2002; **158**: 979–87.

96. Hughes RA. Systematic reviews of treatment for chronic inflammatory demyelinating neuropathy. *Rev Neurol (Paris)* 2002; **158**: S32–6.

97. Nakanishi T, Sobue I, Toyokura Y et al. The Crow-Fukase syndrome: a study of 102 cases in Japan. *Neurology* 1984; **34**: 712–20.

98. Dispenzieri A, Kyle RA, Lacy MQ et al. POEMS syndrome: definitions and long-term outcome. *Blood* 2003; **101**: 2496–506.

99. Rinder MR, Richard RE, Rinder HM. Acquired von Willebrand's disease: a concise review. *Am J Hematol* 1997; **54**: 139–45.

100. Michiels JJ, Budde U, van der Planken M et al. Acquired von Willebrand syndromes: clinical features, aetiology, pathophysiology, classification and management. *Best Pract Res Clin Haematol* 2001; **14**: 401–36.

101. Dimopoulos MA, Panayiotidis P, Moulopoulos LA et al. Waldenstrom's macroglobulinemia: clinical features, complications, and management. *J Clin Oncol* 2000; **18**: 214–26.

102. Ahlberg RE, Lefvert AK. Monoclonal gammopathy and antibody activity against the acetylcholine receptor. *Am J Hematol* 1988; **29**: 49–51.

103. Comenzo RL, Zhang Y, Martinez C et al. The tropism of organ involvement in primary systemic amyloidosis: contributions of Ig V(L) germ line gene use and clonal plasma cell burden. *Blood* 2001; **98**: 714–20.

104. Ronco PM, Alyanakian MA, Mougenot B, Aucouturier P. Light chain deposition disease: a model of glomerulosclerosis defined at the molecular level. *J Am Soc Nephrol* 2001; **12**: 1558–65.

105. Buxbaum JN, Genega EM, Lazowski P et al. Infiltrative nonamyloidotic monoclonal immunoglobulin light chain cardiomyopathy: an underappreciated manifestation of plasma cell dyscrasias. *Cardiology* 2000; **93**: 220–8.

106. Kambham N, Markowitz GS, Appel GB et al. Heavy chain deposition disease: the disease spectrum. Am J Kidney Dis 1999; 33: 954–62.

107. Ma CX, Lacy MQ, Rompala JF et al. Acquired Fanconi syndrome is an indolent disorder in the absence of overt multiple myeloma. Blood 2004; 104: 40–42.

108. Ferri C, Zignego AL, Pileri SA. Cryoglobulins. J Clin Pathol 2002; 55: 4–13.

◆109. Kyle RA, Rajkumar SV. Monoclonal gammopathies of undetermined significance: a review. Immunol Rev 2003; 194: 112–39.

110. Gertz MA, Kyle RA, Noel P. Primary systemic amyloidosis: a rare complication of immunoglobulin M monoclonal gammopathies and Waldenstrom's macroglobulinemia. J Clin Oncol 1993; 11: 914–20.

111. Owen RG, Parapia LA, Higginson J et al. Clinicopathological correlates of IgM paraproteinemias. Clin Lymphoma 2000; 1: 39–43; discussion 44–5.

112. Owen RG, Treon SP, Al-Katib A et al. Clinicopathological definition of Waldenstrom's macroglobulinemia: consensus panel recommendations from the Second International Workshop on Waldenstrom's Macroglobulinemia. Semin Oncol 2003; 30: 110–5.

113. Sezer O, Heider U, Zavrski I, Possinger K. Differentiation of monoclonal gammopathy of undetermined significance and multiple myeloma using flow cytometric characteristics of plasma cells. Haematologica 2001; 86: 837–43.

114. Wicklund MP, Kissel JT. Paraproteinemic neuropathy. Curr Treat Options Neurol 2001; 3: 147–156.

115. Friederich PW, Wever PC, Briet E et al. Successful treatment with recombinant factor VIIa of therapy-resistant severe bleeding in a patient with acquired von Willebrand disease. Am J Hematol 2001; 66: 292–4.

116. Lamboley V, Zabraniecki L, Sie P et al. Myeloma and monoclonal gammopathy of uncertain significance associated with acquired von Willebrand's syndrome. Seven new cases with a literature review. Joint Bone Spine 2002; 69: 62–7.

117. Wilson HC, Lunn MP, Schey S, Hughes RA. Successful treatment of IgM paraproteinaemic neuropathy with fludarabine. J Neurol Neurosurg Psychiatry 1999; 66: 575–80.

118. Pestronk A, Florence J, Miller T et al. Treatment of IgM antibody associated polyneuropathies using rituximab. J Neurol Neurosurg Psychiatry 2003; 74: 485–9.

119. Gorson KC, Ropper AH, Weinberg DH, Weinstein R. Treatment experience in patients with anti-myelin-associated glycoprotein neuropathy. Muscle Nerve 2001; 24: 778–86.

120. Rudnicki SA, Harik SI, Dhodapkar M, et al. Nervous system dysfunction in Waldenstrom's macroglobulinemia: response to treatment. Neurology 1998; 51: 1210–3.

121. Jaccard A, Royer B, Bordessoule D et al. High-dose therapy and autologous blood stem cell transplantation in POEMS syndrome. Blood 2002; 99: 3057–9.

122. Berentsen S, Ulvestad E, Gjertsen BT et al. Rituximab for primary chronic cold agglutinin disease: a prospective study of 37 courses of therapy in 27 patients. Blood 2004; 103: 2925–8.

123. Nakagawa M, Miyagishima T, Kamata T et al. Refractory idiopathic cold agglutinin disease successfully treated with intermittent high-dose cyclophosphamide. Rinsho Ketsueki 2001; 42: 713–5.

124. Jacobs A. Cold agglutinin hemolysis responding to fludarabine therapy. Am J Hematol 1996; 53: 279–80.

125. Sanders PW. Management of paraproteinemic renal disease. Curr Opin Nephrol Hypertens 2005; 14: 97–103.

126. Comenzo RL, Gertz MA. Autologous stem cell transplantation for primary systemic amyloidosis. Blood 2002; 99: 4276–82.

127. Rajkumar SV, Kyle RA, Therneau TM et al. Serum free light chain ratio is an independent risk factor for progression in monoclonal gammopathy of undetermined significance. Blood 2005; 106: 812–7.

128. Patriarca F, Fanin R, Silvestri F et al. Clinical features and outcome of multiple myeloma arising from the transformation of a monoclonal gammapathy of undetermined significance. Leuk Lymphoma 1999; 34: 591–6.

129. Gregersen H, Ibsen J, Mellemkjoer L et al. Mortality and causes of death in patients with monoclonal gammopathy of undetermined significance. Br J Haematol 2001; 112: 353–7.

130. Salgado C, Blade J, Lopez-Guillermo A et al. Multiple myeloma after monoclonal gammopathy of uncertain significance. Study of 10 patients. Sangre (Barc) 1993; 38: 371–4.

131. Politou M, Terpos E, Anagnostopoulos A et al. Role of receptor activator of nuclear factor-kappa B ligand (RANKL), osteoprotegerin and macrophage protein 1-alpha (MIP-1a) in monoclonal gammopathy of undetermined significance (MGUS). Br J Haematol 2004; 126: 686–9.

132. Pecherstorfer M, Seibel MJ, Woitge HW et al. Bone resorption in multiple myeloma and in monoclonal gammopathy of undetermined significance: quantification by urinary pyridinium cross-links of collagen. Blood 1997; 90: 3743–50.

133. Baldini L, Guffanti A, Cesana BM et al. Role of different hematologic variables in defining the risk of malignant transformation in monoclonal gammopathy. Blood 1996; 87: 912–8.

134. Rawstron AC, Orfao A, Beksac M et al. Report of the European Myeloma Network on multiparametric flow cytometry in multiple myeloma and related disorders. Haematologica 2008; 93: 431–8.

◆135. Kyle RA. Monoclonal gammopathy of undetermined significance and solitary plasmacytoma. Implications for progression to overt multiple myeloma. Hematol Oncol Clin North Am 1997; 11: 71–87.

136. Moulopoulos LA, Dimopoulos MA, Weber D et al. Magnetic resonance imaging in the staging of solitary plasmacytoma of bone. J Clin Oncol 1993; 11: 1311–5.

137. Dimopoulos MA, Kiamouris C, Moulopoulos LA. Solitary plasmacytoma of bone and extramedullary plasmacytoma. *Hematol Oncol Clin North Am* 1999; **13**: 1249–57.

138. Dimopoulos MA, Moulopoulos LA, Maniatis A, Alexanian R. Solitary plasmacytoma of bone and asymptomatic multiple myeloma. *Blood* 2000; **96**: 2037–44.

♦139. Soutar R, Lucraft H, Jackson G *et al*. Guidelines on the diagnosis and management of solitary plasmacytoma of bone and solitary extramedullary plasmacytoma. *Br J Haematol* 2004; **124**: 717–26.

140. Chang MY, Shih LY, Dunn P *et al*. Solitary plasmacytoma of bone. *J Formos Med Assoc* 1994; **93**: 397–402.

141. Kyle RA. Multiple myeloma and other plasma cell disorders. In: Hoffman R. (ed.) *Hematology: basic principles and practice*, 2nd Edn. New York: Churchill Livingstone, 1995.

142. Liebross RH, Ha CS, Cox JD *et al*. Clinical course of solitary extramedullary plasmacytoma. *Radiother Oncol* 1999; **52**: 245–9.

143. Wilder RB, Ha CS, Cox JD *et al*. Persistence of myeloma protein for more than one year after radiotherapy is an adverse prognostic factor in solitary plasmacytoma of bone. *Cancer* 2002; **94**: 1532–7.

144. Dimopoulos MA, Hamilos G. Solitary bone plasmacytoma and extramedullary plasmacytoma. *Curr Treat Options Oncol* 2002; **3**: 255–9.

145. Susnerwala SS, Shanks JH, Banerjee SS *et al*. Extramedullary plasmacytoma of the head and neck region: clinicopathological correlation in 25 cases. *Br J Cancer* 1997; **75**: 921–7.

146. Hu K, Yahalom J. Radiotherapy in the management of plasma cell tumors. *Oncology (Williston Park)* 2000; **14**: 101–8, 111; discussion 111–2, 115.

147. Friedrich N, Kekulé A. Zur Amyloidfrage. *Virchows Arch Path Anat Klin Med* 1859; **16**: 50–65.

148. Cohen AS, Calkins E. Electron microscopic observations on a fibrous component in amyloid of diverse origins. *Nature* 1959; **183**: 1202–3.

149. Falk RH, Comenzo RL, Skinner M. The systemic amyloidoses. *N Engl J Med* 1997; **337**: 898–909.

150. Hawkins PN, Lavender JP, Pepys MB. Evaluation of systemic amyloidosis by scintigraphy with 123I-labeled serum amyloid P component. *N Engl J Med* 1990; **323**: 508–13.

151. Kyle RA, Gertz MA, Greipp PR *et al*. Long-term survival (10 years or more) in 30 patients with primary amyloidosis. *Blood* 1999; **93**: 1062–6.

152. Kyle RA, Linos A, Beard CM *et al*. Incidence and natural history of primary systemic amyloidosis in Olmsted County, Minnesota, 1950 through 1989. *Blood* 1992; **79**: 1817–22.

153. Kyle RA, Gertz MA. Primary systemic amyloidosis: clinical and laboratory features in 474 cases. *Semin Hematol* 1995; **32**: 45–59.

154. Libbey CA, Skinner M, Cohen AS. Use of abdominal fat tissue aspirate in the diagnosis of systemic amyloidosis. *Arch Intern Med* 1983; **143**: 1549–52.

155. Duston MA, Skinner M, Shirahama T, Cohen AS. Diagnosis of amyloidosis by abdominal fat aspiration. Analysis of four years' experience. *Am J Med* 1987; **82**: 412–4.

156. Bradwell AR, Carr-Smith HD, Mead GP *et al*. Highly sensitive, automated immunoassay for immunoglobulin free light chains in serum and urine. *Clin Chem* 2001; **47**: 673–80.

157. Lachmann HJ, Gallimore R, Gillmore JD *et al*. Outcome in systemic AL amyloidosis in relation to changes in concentration of circulating free immunoglobulin light chains following chemotherapy. *Br J Haematol* 2003; **122**: 78–84.

158. Hawkins PN. Serum amyloid P component scintigraphy for diagnosis and monitoring amyloidosis. *Curr Opin Nephrol Hypertens* 2002; **11**: 649–55.

159. Wardley AM, Jayson GC, Goldsmith DJ *et al*. The treatment of nephrotic syndrome caused by primary (light chain) amyloid with vincristine, doxorubicin and dexamethasone. *Br J Cancer* 1998; **78**: 774–6.

160. Sezer O, Schmid P, Shweigert M *et al*. Rapid reversal of nephrotic syndrome due to primary systemic AL amyloidosis after VAD and subsequent high-dose chemotherapy with autologous stem cell support. *Bone Marrow Transplant* 1999; **23**: 967–9.

161. Gertz MA, Lacy MQ, Lust JA *et al*. Phase II trial of high-dose dexamethasone for untreated patients with primary systemic amyloidosis. *Med Oncol* 1999; **16**: 104–9.

162. Schey SA, Kazmi M, Ireland R, Lakhani A. The use of intravenous intermediate dose melphalan and dexamethasone as induction treatment in the management of de novo multiple myeloma. *Eur J Haematol* 1998; **61**: 306–10.

163. Jaccard A, Moreau P, Leblond V *et al*. High-dose melphalan versus melphalan plus dexamethasone for AL amyloidosis. *N Engl J Med* 2007; **357**: 1083–93.

164. Seldin DC, Choufani E, Skinner M *et al*. A phase I/II trial of thalidomide for patients with AL Amyloidosis. *Blood* 2001; **98**: 164a (abstract 691).

165. Moreau P, Leblond V, Bourquelot P *et al*. Prognostic factors for survival and response after high-dose therapy and autologous stem cell transplantation in systemic AL amyloidosis: a report on 21 patients. *Br J Haematol* 1998; **101**: 766–9.

166. Gillmore JD, Davies J, Iqbal A *et al*. Allogeneic bone marrow transplantation for systemic AL amyloidosis. *Br J Haematol* 1998; **100**: 226–8.

167. Gertz MA, Lacy MQ, Gastineau DA *et al*. Blood stem cell transplantation as therapy for primary systemic amyloidosis (AL). *Bone Marrow Transplant* 2000; **26**: 963–9.

168. Sanchorawala V, Wright DG, Seldin DC *et al*. An overview of the use of high-dose melphalan with autologous stem cell transplantation for the treatment of AL amyloidosis. *Bone Marrow Transplant* 2001; **28**: 637–42.

169. Rajkumar SV, Rosinol L, Hussein M *et al*. Multicenter, randomized, double-blind, placebo-controlled study of thalidomide plus dexamethasone compared with dexamethasone as initial therapy for newly diagnosed multiple myeloma. *J Clin Oncol* 2008; **26**: 2171–7.

170. Facon T, Mary JY, Pégourie B et al. Dexamethasone-based regimens versus melphalan-prednisone for elderly multiple myeloma patients ineligible for high-dose therapy. Blood 2006; **107**: 1292–8.

171. Bladé J, Rosinol L, Sureda A et al. High-dose therapy intensification compared with continued standard chemotherapy in multiple myeloma patients responding to the initial chemotherapy: long-term results from a prospective randomized trial from the Spanish cooperative group PETHEMA. Blood 2005; **106**: 3755–9.

172. Segeren CM, Sonneveld P, van der Holt B et al. Overall and event-free survival are not improved by the use of myeloablative therapy following intensified chemotherapy in previously untreated patients with multiple myeloma: a prospective randomized phase 3 study. Blood 2003; **101**: 2144–51.

173. Attal M, Harousseau JL, Leyvraz S et al. Maintenance therapy with thalidomide improves survival in patients with multiple myeloma. Blood 2006; **108**: 3289–94.

174. Barlogie B, Desikan R, Eddlemon P et al. Extended survival in advanced and refractory multiple myeloma after single-agent thalidomide: identification of prognostic factors in a phase 2 study of 169 patients. Blood 2001; **98**: 492–4.

175. García-Sanz R, González-Porras JR, Hernández JM et al. The oral combination of thalidomide, cyclophosphamide and dexamethasone (ThaCyDex) is effective in relapsed/refractory multiple myeloma. Leukemia 2004; **18**: 856–63.

176. Weber DM, Chen C, Niesvizky R et al. Lenalidomide plus dexamethasone for relapsed multiple myeloma in North America. N Engl J Med 2007; **357**: 2133–42.

75

The management of natural killer cell malignancies

YOK-LAM KWONG AND RAYMOND H LIANG

INTRODUCTION

Natural killer (NK) cells are cytolytic cells capable of killing a variety of target cells, including tumor cells and cells infected with bacteria and viruses.[1] Morphologically, NK cells are lymphocytes showing pale cytoplasm with azurophilic granules. Immunophenotypically, NK cells express variably the T lineage-associated antigens, such as CD2, CD7, and CD8. They are typically negative for surface CD3, but they do express the cytoplasmic CD3 epsilon (ε) chain. Natural killer cells also express a number of 'NK-associated' markers, including CD16, CD56, and CD57.[2] Of these, CD56 is the most consistently expressed, and has been designated as a marker for NK cells. However, CD56 is not entirely specific for NK cells, and can also be found on NK-like T cells, neural and neuroendocrine tissues, and sometimes on skeletal muscles.[3]

The bone marrow is the main site for NK cell development. Although NK cells represent a separate lineage of lymphocytes distinct from T cells, these two lineages are developmentally related.[1] There exists a bipotential T/NK progenitor, which can either commit to the NK cell lineage (without rearrangement of the T cell receptor [TCR] genes), or alternatively develop into the T cell lineage (with rearrangement of the TCR genes).

HISTORICAL PERSPECTIVES

For a long time, certain midline facial destructive lesions of unknown origin had been noticed. For want of a better clinicopathologic description, the term 'lethal midline granuloma' had been used.[4] Most of these lesions had been described to deteriorate progressively, leading to destruction of the hard palate, nose, and even part of the face. These disorders were clinically malignant, although whether they were actually neoplastic could not be determined.

With the development of better histopathologic investigations and facilities, it became clear that some of these 'lethal midline granulomas' in Caucasian patients were in fact nonneoplastic disorders.[5] When Wegener granulomatosis and sarcoidosis are excluded, the majority of the lesions are either carcinomas or conventional sinonasal B cell lymphomas.[6]

In Asian and South American populations, however, a different disease entity would emerge.[7] Histopathologic examination of these lesions showed atypical lymphoid cells together with a polymorphic background of inflammatory cells, including polymorphs, eosinophils, and plasma cells. As the lymphoid cells showed nuclear atypia and pleomorphism, and the disease often ran a fatal course even if treated, these lesions were regarded as malignant. However, to distinguish them from the monomorphic lymphoid infiltrates characteristic of conventional lymphomas, the lesion was termed 'polymorphic reticulosis.'[8]

With the advent of monoclonal antibodies, immunohistochemical analysis showed that the neoplastic lymphoid cells expressed the T cell marker CD3. Therefore, polymorphic reticulosis became classified as T cell lymphomas.[9] Furthermore, as polymorphic reticulosis became better recognized, the lesions were found to demonstrate angiocentricity and angiodestruction, leading to their classification as angiocentric T cell lymphomas in the Revised European-American Lymphoma (REAL) classification scheme.[10]

NATURAL KILLER CELL LYMPHOMAS

The concept that neoplastic disorders might arise from NK cells owes much to the widespread availability of anti-CD56 antibodies. When anti-CD56 antibodies were used in immunophenotyping, a subset of lymphomas that occurred mostly in the nose and the upper aerodigestive tract were found on immunophenotyping to express the antigen.[11,12] Yet the NK cell nature of the lymphoma was not initially recognized, as the neoplastic cells also expressed CD3 on immunohistochemical analysis. Therefore, these lymphomas were considered to be CD56-expressing T cell lymphomas. The problem was ultimately resolved when it was realized that because T cells and NK cells shared the same ontogeny, they both expressed $CD3\varepsilon$.[13,14] However, T cells also express surface CD3, whereas NK cells do not. Hence, when immunohistochemical analysis is performed on formalin-fixed paraffin-embedded sections with a polyclonal anti-CD3 antibody, which stains surface CD3 and cytoplasmic $CD3\varepsilon$, both T cell and NK cell lymphomas will appear positive. On the other hand, when immunophenotyping is performed by flow cytometry or on cryostat sections with a monoclonal anti-CD3 antibody, which stains surface CD3 but not cytoplasmic $CD3\varepsilon$, only T cells and not NK cells are positive. When NK cells can be more confidently distinguished from T cell lymphomas, it becomes evident that most nasal T cell lymphomas, or angiocentric T cell lymphomas, are in fact NK cell lymphomas. For this reason, in the World Health Organization (WHO) classification system, these lymphomas were for the first time referred to as NK/T cell lymphomas.[15] This improvement in diagnosis

is the main reason for a decrease in the incidence of T cell lymphomas, particularly in Asian populations where NK cell lymphomas are prevalent. T cell lymphomas were previously thought to account for up to 25 percent of non-Hodgkin lymphomas in Asian populations. A recent study that adhered strictly to the WHO classification criteria showed that in a Chinese population, T cell lymphomas only accounted for about 10 percent of all non-Hodgkin lymphomas, similar to the incidence in the West, whereas the incidence of NK cell lymphomas was about 7 percent.[16] Therefore, the decline in the incidence of T cell lymphomas is due to better diagnosis and recognition of NK cell lymphomas as a distinct clinicopathological entity.

EPSTEIN–BARR VIRUS INFECTION OF NATURAL KILLER LYMPHOMA CELLS

The pathogenetic mechanisms leading to malignant transformation of NK cells remain undefined. However, an almost invariable observation is the presence of Epstein–Barr virus (EBV) in the NK lymphoma cells obtained from Asian, European, and South American patients.[17–25] Analysis of the terminal repeat region of the EBV genome shows that the virus is present in a clonal episomal form. In addition to providing an indirect proof of the clonal nature of the NK cell proliferation, it also implies that EBV may play an important etiologic role and is not just a bystander. The selective strong association with EBV in NK cell lymphomas, but not in T cell and B cell lymphomas, in the nasal cavity provides additional evidence of the important role of EBV in NK cell lymphomagenesis.[25]

The consistent presence of EBV infection in NK cell lymphoma has important clinical implications. *In situ* hybridization (ISH) for the EBV encoded early small RNA (EBER) provides an accurate means of identifying NK lymphoma cells in histopathologic specimens.[26] *In situ* hybridization for EBER is particularly useful in anatomic sites where EBV is usually absent, such as the liver and bone marrow. Accordingly, the finding of EBER-positive cells in liver or marrow biopsies in a patient with NK cell lymphoma is strong evidence of disease involvement.[26]

CLINICAL FEATURES OF NATURAL KILLER CELL LYMPHOMAS

The WHO classification divides NK cell lymphomas into two histologic types: NK/T cell lymphoma, nasal type,[15] and aggressive NK cell leukemia.[27,28] This is a pathologic classification. In clinical practice, NK cell lymphomas can be classified into three categories: nasal, non-nasal, and aggressive lymphoma/leukemia subtypes (Table 75.1).[29] It is important to note that NK cell lymphomas are predominantly extranodal, and involvement of lymph nodes, either at presentation or subsequently, is uncommon.[30]

Table 75.1 Clinical features and treatment of nasal natural killer (NK) cell lymphoma, non-nasal NK cell lymphoma, and aggressive NK cell lymphoma/leukemia

	Nasal NK cell lymphoma	Non-nasal NK cell lymphoma	Aggressive NK cell lymphoma/leukemia
Gender	Male > Female	Male > Female	Male = Female
Median age	50–60 years	50–60 years	30–40 years
Main sites of involvement	Nasal cavities and paranasal sinuses, upper aerodigestive tract	Skin, gastrointestinal tract, testis, salivary glands, other organs and soft tissues	Disseminated, liver, spleen, bone marrow, lymph nodes
Treatment	Stage I: radiation therapy Stage II: radiation therapy ± chemotherapy Stage III/IV: chemotherapy	Chemotherapy	Chemotherapy
Outcome	Aggressive, median survival <12 months	Highly aggressive, median survival <4 months	Extremely rapid fatal course, median survival <2 months

Nasal natural killer cell lymphoma

Nasal NK cell lymphomas refer in general to tumors that occur in the nose and the upper aerodigestive tract.[31–35] The median age of presentation is in the fifth decade, with a male to female ratio of approximately 3:1. Natural killer cell lymphoma is the commonest lymphoma type among primary lymphomas of the nasal cavity in Asian populations. Structures that may be the initial sites of involvement include the nasal cavity, nasopharynx, paranasal sinuses, tonsils, hypopharynx, and larynx. Patients present with a mass lesion, facial swelling, nasal obstruction, and bleeding (Fig. 75.1A). Occasionally, when the lymphoma arises from the hypopharynx and larynx, hoarseness of voice, pain, and difficulty in swallowing may also occur. The lymphoma is locally invasive. Extension of nasal lymphoma into the paranasal sinuses leads to nasal obstruction, local swelling, and intractable bloody nasal discharge. Upward extension of the lymphoma into the orbits may lead to proptosis and impairment of extraocular movement. The vision may also be threatened. Downward extension of the lymphoma results in erosion of the floor of the nasal cavity, sometimes leading to destruction of the hard palate and the formation of the characteristic midline perforation, from which the term 'lethal midline granuloma' was originally derived (Fig. 75.1B). The perforated hard palate makes it difficult to eat and drink, gravely affecting the nutrition of the patients. Furthermore, the lesion leads to a constant discharge and severe halitosis, thereby seriously impairing the quality of life of the patients. Lymphomas in the tonsils, hypopharynx, and larynx may invade the epiglottis and esophagus, resulting in airway obstruction, hoarseness of voice, aphonia, and dysphagia. Lesions in these areas, in contrast to the nasal counterparts, may give excruciating pain.

Non-nasal natural killer cell lymphomas

Non-nasal NK cell lymphomas may involve any part of the body.[36,37] The median age of presentation is in the fifth decade, with a male to female ratio of approximately 2.5:1. The common primary sites include the skin,[38,39] gastrointestinal tract,[40,41] salivary glands,[42] spleen,[43] and testis.[44] Occasional cases of muscle[45] and uterine[46] involvement have also been reported. Isolated nodal involvement is highly unusual, and such cases must be carefully evaluated to exclude involvement by other CD56-expressing hematolymphoid malignancies.[47] Most cases present with involvement of more than one anatomic site. Clinical manifestations are protean. In the skin, the lymphoma may appear as erythematous lesions, nodules, or an ulcerating mass (Fig. 75.1C and Fig. 75.1D). When the gastrointestinal tract is involved, perforation is the most frequent presentation, which is different from other lymphomas where a mass lesion causing pain and intestinal obstruction is the commonest problem. Interestingly, primary sites of non-nasal NK cell lymphomas are also the areas where nasal NK cell lymphomas may disseminate to terminally. This phenomenon may be attributable to the expression of CD56 on cells of these tissues as well as the neoplastic NK cells, as CD56 is a homotypic molecule that facilitates cellular adhesion.[3] For this reason, the diagnosis of non-nasal NK cell lymphoma requires the exclusion of nasal involvement at presentation. Practically, for all patients who present with NK cell lymphomas involving sites other than the upper aerodigestive tract, a nasal panendoscopy with random biopsies should be performed to exclude an occult nasal tumor.

Aggressive natural killer cell leukemia/lymphoma

Aggressive NK cell leukemia/lymphoma is a catastrophic disease.[25,28,48,49] The median age of presentation is in the third decade, which is earlier than nasal and non-nasal NK cell lymphomas. Men and women are equally affected. On presentation to the physician, patients will have been unwell for no more than a few weeks. Typically, the patient is very ill with significant weight loss, jaundice, and a high swinging fever. Lymphadenopathy is commonly found, which is different from other subtypes of NK cell lymphomas where

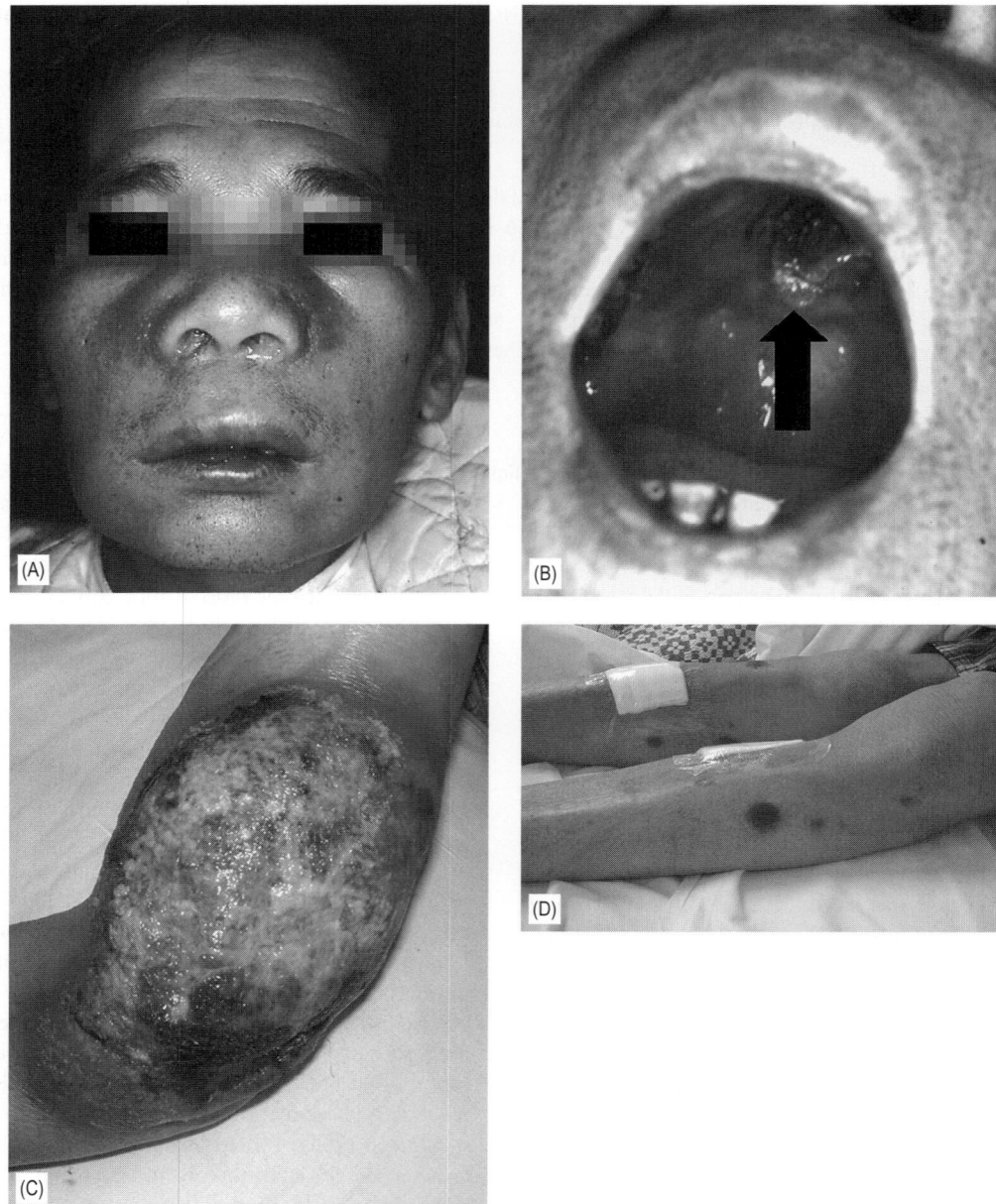

Figure 75.1   Clinical manifestations of nasal and non-nasal natural killer (NK) cell lymphomas. (A) Nasal NK cell lymphoma involving the nasal cavity and maxillary sinuses. Note the facial swelling and nasal discharge. (B) Nasal NK cell lymphoma with downward invasion and perforation of the hard palate (arrow). (C) Non-nasal NK cell lymphoma of the elbow, presenting as a huge ulcerating mass. (D) Non-nasal NK cell lymphoma of the skin in the legs, presenting as purplish subcutaneous lesions, one of which was biopsied.

lymph node involvement is unusual. Gross hepato-splenomegaly may also be present. There may be skin infiltration. Severe anemia and thrombocytopenia are common. The cytopenias may be due to marrow infiltration, or very active hemophagocytosis, which is a common concomitant occurrence in these patients. Occasionally, hemophagocytosis may be found in the peripheral blood.[25] The white cell count is more variable, and can be depressed or increased. Circulating neoplastic cells, varying between large granular lymphocytes to frank blasts in morphology, may be present and should be sought by careful examination of the peripheral

blood film and the buffy coat. Involvement of the marrow ranges from patchy to diffuse infiltration. The liver function is impaired, with increase in bilirubin and alkaline phosphatase. Hepatitis with increases in transaminases is more unusual and may indicate other underlying disorders. As the disease progresses, derangement of coagulation and features of disseminated intravascular coagulopathy appear. The clinical course is relentless in spite of treatment. Aggressive NK cell leukemia/lymphoma is one of the most malignant tumors known, with the survival measured often just in days to weeks.

Patterns of dissemination of natural killer cell lymphomas

Nasal NK cell lymphomas are locally malignant. About 30 percent of patients have disease confined solely to the nasal cavity.[50] Extension into the paranasal sinuses occurs in about 60–70 percent of patients, with the alveolar bones, hard palate, and subcutaneous tissues of the nasal ala, cheek, and buccinator spaces involved in 30–50 percent of them. Extension into the superior nasal cavity with involvement of the adjacent orbital, ethmoidal, and maxillary sinus occurs less frequently. Extension into the infratemporal spaces and nasopharyngeal involvement may also be found. Bone involvement is frequent. Erosion of the medial maxillary wall is present in about one-third of the patients with maxillary antrum involvement. As the disease progresses, most of the midline facial soft tissues and bones can be destroyed.

At presentation, distant organ involvement is uncommon, occurring in about 10 percent of patients. Fewer than 10 percent of patients will have marrow infiltration.[51] The tumor metastasizes terminally, with about 60–70 percent of cases showing systemic dissemination. The usual sites of metastases are areas that are commonly primary sites of non-nasal NK cell lymphomas. The central nervous system is, however, involved in fewer than 5 percent of cases, even terminally.[34,52]

In contrast to nasal NK cell lymphomas, non-nasal NK cell lymphomas tend to disseminate early. Sites of dissemination are similar to those of nasal NK cell lymphomas. Interestingly, non-nasal NK cell lymphomas rarely disseminate to the nasal area if the site is not initially involved.[36,37] This argues against non-nasal NK cell lymphoma being simply a disseminated form of nasal NK cell lymphomas.

Aggressive NK cell lymphoma/leukemia is disseminated at presentation. It is readily separated from a rare terminal leukemic form of nasal/non-nasal NK cell lymphoma by the absence of a previous history of NK cell malignancies, a much shorter history, a younger age at presentation, and a very aggressive clinical course. However, aggressive NK cell lymphoma/leukemia is pathologically indistinguishable from the leukemic form of nasal/non-nasal NK cell lymphomas.

Peripheral blood and marrow involvement in nasal and non–nasal natural killer cell lymphomas

At presentation, pancytopenia may be found in about 10–15 percent of cases of nasal and non-nasal NK cell lymphomas. Many of these cases are not due to marrow infiltration. In fact, a careful examination of the peripheral blood will usually not show abnormal lymphoid cells. On the other hand, examination of the marrow shows active hemophagocytosis. The phagocytic cells are bland looking, and probably represent activated cells of the reticuloendothelial system. Immunohistochemical staining for CD56 may be helpful in

excluding infiltration by neoplastic NK cells. However, CD56 may occasionally be 'shed.'[47] Therefore, staining for CD56 cannot be relied on solely for the exclusion of neoplastic infiltration. A more sensitive and specific test is ISH for EBER, which identifies accurately neoplastic cells in the marrow. Therefore, in nasal and non-nasal NK cell lymphomas at diagnosis, morphologic examination of the marrow must also be supplemented by ISH for EBER in order to confidently diagnose or exclude marrow infiltration.[51] On the other hand, in rare circumstances occurring in less than 5 percent of terminal cases, a true leukemic form may develop. There may be a leukocytosis, and examination of the peripheral blood film shows the presence of neoplastic NK cells. Rarely, hemophagocytosis by the neoplastic cells in the peripheral blood may also be seen.[25] The marrow shows heavy infiltration by neoplastic NK cells with active hemophagocytosis. Immunohistochemical and ISH studies show an abundance of CD56[+] and EBER-positive cells. As in patients with aggressive NK cell lymphoma/leukemia, marrow involvement in nasal/non-nasal NK cell lymphomas heralds a grave prognosis.

STAGING AND ASSESSMENT OF NATURAL KILLER CELL LYMPHOMAS

Staging of natural killer cell lymphomas

Certain characteristics of NK cell lymphomas affect the way in which they are staged. Natural killer cell lymphomas are almost exclusively extranodal. Involvement of lymph nodes, either at presentation or subsequently, is uncommon, except in aggressive NK cell lymphoma/leukemia.[30] Therefore, the Ann Arbor staging system, based on the concept of contiguous lymphatic spread and devised mainly for Hodgkin lymphoma, may not always be applicable to all NK cell lymphomas. In many previous studies of nasal NK cell lymphoma, the involvement of adjacent anatomical structures (including the nasal cavity, the neighboring paranasal sinuses, and nasopharynx) was regarded as stage I$_E$ disease.[25,31,34,52–59] As the majority of the tumors are locally invasive, most patients will have stage I disease by this criterion. However, as is true in other non-Hodgkin lymphomas, the Ann Arbor staging does not take into account the tumor burden, and has not been found to correlate well with prognosis.

A staging system devised mainly for conventional sinonasal B cell lymphomas has been proposed.[60] This tumor (T) staging comprises: T1, tumor confined to the nasal cavity; T2, extension of the tumor to the maxillary antra, anterior ethmoid sinus, or hard palate; T3, extension to the posterior ethmoid sinus, sphenoidal sinus, orbit, superior alveolar bones, cheeks, or superior buccinator space; and T4, involvement of the inferior alveolar bone, inferior buccinator space, infratemporal fossa, nasopharynx, or cranial fossa. This staging system has been tested in nasal NK cell lymphoma. Initial results showed that patients with stage T1/T2 disease had a superior outcome compared with patients with stage T3/T4.[50] However, whether the T staging may be an independent prognostic factor remains to be tested in a larger number of patients.

The International Prognostic Index (IPI), which takes into account not only stage but also the age, performance status, and the lactate dehydrogenase (LDH) level, has been shown to be prognostically relevant in a variety of non-Hodgkin lymphomas.[61] The IPI has been tested retrospectively in patients with nasal NK cell lymphoma and found to be prognostically relevant.[35] Current studies are ongoing to test prospectively if a combination of the Ann Arbor stage, IPI, and local tumor staging may be a more accurate stratification system that may correlate with disease extent, response to treatment, and prognosis.

For non-nasal NK cell lymphomas, which are again exclusively extranodal in their distribution, the Ann Arbor staging system also has obvious limitations. Again, the size of the primary lesion may have more significant impact on the treatment results. Lymphomas that show widespread tissue involvement have an unfavorable outcome and tend to disseminate systemically in a short period of time.[36,37]

Initial assessment of nasal natural killer cell lymphoma

A thorough initial assessment of the patient is required before a suitable strategy of treatment can be devised. The medical history should be taken in detail. It is not unusual to find a history of prolonged sinonasal infection and obstruction in these patients. Symptoms referable to organs commonly involved in disease dissemination, such as the skin, gastrointestinal tract, salivary glands, and testicles, must be carefully sought. Any relevant symptom should be actively investigated. A careful physical examination is necessary. Special attention should again be paid to areas that may be involved in disseminated diseases.

The nasal tumor should be evaluated by an experienced otolaryngologist. A nasal panendoscopy is mandatory. Any involved or suspicious areas should be biopsied. A number of precautions should be observed with the biopsies. Marked tumor zonal necrosis is a characteristic of NK cell lymphomas.[15] This means that the biopsies should be as large as possible to avoid including just the necrotic areas. The biopsies should not be immersed in formalin, but instead sent fresh to the pathology laboratory so that cryostat sections or flow cytometric analysis may be performed. This is to enable the detection of surface CD3 expression, which distinguishes between NK cell and T cell lymphomas. Finally, the histopathologists should be alerted beforehand, so that the appropriate investigations can be arranged. However, if fresh tumor biopsies are not available, the distinction between NK cell and T cell lymphomas can be achieved by molecular analysis of the TCR genes. In NK cell lymphomas the TCR genes are typically in germ-line configuration, whereas in T cell lymphoma the TCR genes are clonally rearranged.[15,25,29,30]

Radiologic imaging of the primary tumor is an essential initial evaluation. Computerized tomographic (CT) scan is a traditional imaging technique in lymphoma, but its use in nasal NK cell lymphoma is surpassed by magnetic resonance imaging (MRI), which has several distinct advantages.[50] In general, MRI gives images of superior quality and resolution (Fig. 75.2). Furthermore, soft tissue involvement is best defined by MRI. This is particularly important because the lymphoma frequently obstructs the

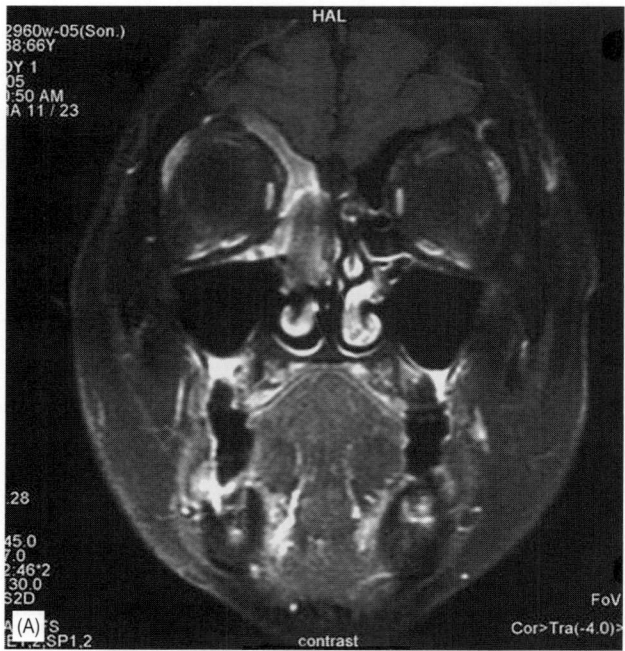

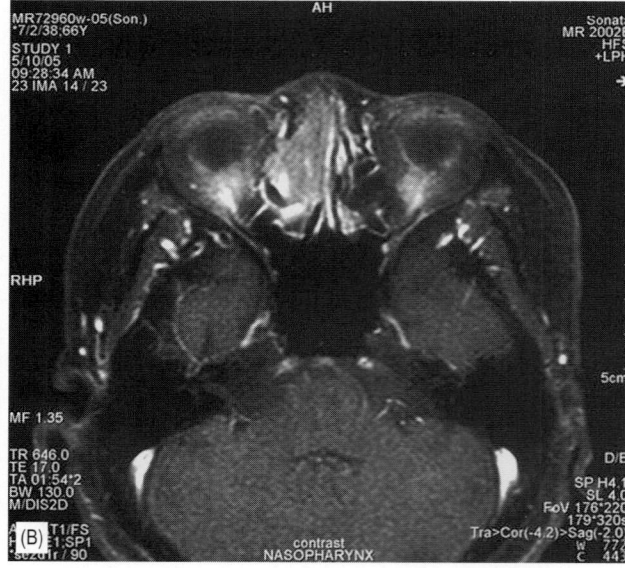

Figure 75.2 Magnetic resonance imaging of a nasal natural killer cell lymphoma. Note the soft tissue mass that had completely obliterated the right nasal cavity, with deviation and partial destruction of the nasal septum. (A) Coronal section, (B) Sagittal section.

nasal sinuses, giving rise to chronic sinusitis and fluid retention. These changes cannot be reliably differentiated from direct tumor infiltration on CT scanning, but may be distinguishable by MRI. On MRI, fluid is nonenhancing and markedly 'hyperintense' when compared to muscle on T2-weighted images, and mucosal thickening is homogeneously 'hyperintense' to muscle on T2-weighted images with homogeneous enhancement. However, lymphomatous infiltration is 'isointense' to normal muscle on T1-weighted sequences, and mild to moderate 'hyperintense' to muscle with heterogeneous enhancement on T2-weighted sequences.

The exact definition of the extent of the lesion is crucial for the planning of radiation therapy. Significant infection of the paranasal areas is present in the majority of patients at presentation, and the accurate distinction of this from lymphomatous infiltration can greatly limit the field and hence the morbidity of irradiation. Magnetic resonance imaging is also useful in the follow-up of patients after treatment, as mucosal infection often continues after successful treatment, making it sometimes difficult on clinical grounds to evaluate if there is persistence of lymphoma. The use of other radiologic imaging techniques, such as positron emission tomography (PET), has not been formally appraised. The use of PET scan, or PET in conjunction with CT scan, has been shown to be more accurate in the staging and assessment of response to treatment in Hodgkin lymphoma and other types of aggressive lymphoma.[62] In nasal NK cell lymphoma, however, PET scan may not be expected to give additional information, as mucosal infection cannot be reliably differentiated from lymphomatous infiltration.

Because the majority of patients with nasal NK cell lymphoma have stage I/II disease at presentation, the apparent clinical or radiologic involvement of distant sites should not be assumed to be lymphomatous, and should always be confirmed by appropriate histologic examination if feasible. This pertains particularly to involvement of remote lymph nodes. In addition to achieving an accurate staging, this approach also helps to disclose other possible concomitant pathologies. Assessment of the extent of systemic involvement should include a careful morphologic evaluation of the peripheral blood and marrow, supplemented with immunophenotyping or ISH for EBER if necessary. Imaging of the thorax and abdomen with CT scan is necessary. In about 10 percent of patients, there may be derangement of liver function tests at presentation.[25] The pattern is mainly cholestatic, with increase in bilirubin and alkaline phosphatase. Liver biopsy is necessary to exclude hepatic involvement. However, the commonest histopathologic change of the liver biopsy is the presence of hemophagocytosis. Liver infiltration at presentation is unusual, occurring in fewer than 5 percent of cases. Involvement of the spleen is uncommon, with splenomegaly indicating almost certainly dissemination of disease. Dissemination to the regional lymph nodes is unusual, and to distant lymph nodes exceptionally rare. Therefore, any enlarged lymph nodes should be biopsied to exclude the presence of other concomitant pathologies. Finally, central nervous system involvement is uncommon, and routine lumbar puncture should not be considered as part of the initial assessment.

Initial assessment of non-nasal natural killer cell lymphomas and aggressive natural killer cell lymphoma/leukemia

The evaluation of non-nasal NK cell lymphomas and aggressive NK cell lymphoma/leukemia is similar to that for nasal NK cell lymphomas. In patients with disease presenting at non-nasal sites, the nasal area and the upper aerodigestive tract must be examined to exclude occult involvement. In some centers, random biopsies are taken from the nose or nasal areas even if the examination is normal. If occult nasal involvement is shown, the case is reclassified as nasal NK cell lymphoma with systemic spread. This distinction affects the staging and hence the treatment of the lymphoma. In aggressive NK cell lymphoma/leukemia, the disease is disseminated at presentation.

Quantification of circulating plasma Epstein–Barr virus DNA

The prototype of EBV-associated lymphoid malignancy is the post-transplantation lymphoproliferative diseases (PTLD). In the absence of an effective immunologic response, EBV-infected lymphoid cells proliferate opportunistically. Furthermore, there is also an increase in circulating plasma EBV DNA. The increase in EBV DNA is attributed to possible lytic EBV reactivation, which occurs as a result of the severe immunosuppression that has led to the PTLD.

In EBV-associated lymphoid malignancies occurring in immunocompetent hosts, early studies have also shown an increase in circulating EBV DNA.[63] A possible mechanism is tumor release of EBV DNA into the circulation, mediated through apoptosis of proliferating tumor cells.[64] This implies that the quantification of circulating plasma EBV DNA may be a potential surrogate tumor marker.

Serial studies of circulating plasma EBV DNA have indeed shown it to correlate with the disease status of the patient.[65] Quantification of EBV DNA is achieved by real-time quantitative polymerase chain reaction (Q-PCR), with EBV DNA sequences cloned in plasmids as the standard for enumeration of DNA copy numbers. Several significant findings are observed. In patients with lymphomas unrelated to EBV, there is no increase in EBV DNA, even during chemotherapy. This means that the immunosuppression associated with lymphoma and the subsequent standard chemotherapy will not give rise to reactivation of latent EBV. Furthermore, circulating EBV DNA is increased invariably in patients with NK cell malignancies before treatment, at a range of 10^5 to 10^{10} copies/mL. The presentation EBV DNA correlates with clinical stage and the LDH level, indicating that this is a useful surrogate marker of tumor load. If facilities for Q-PCR are available, quantification of circulating EBV DNA is a useful investigation to be included in the initial evaluation of NK cell malignancies.

TREATMENT OF NATURAL KILLER CELL LYMPHOMA

Radiation therapy

Radiation therapy has been conventionally used as the initial treatment for patients with lethal midline granuloma and polymorphic reticulosis. The response rate was high, and 5-year overall survival might be as high as 60 percent.[66,67] Although the exact histopathology of these lesions was uncertain, the results showed that at least a subset of patients with nasal lymphomas responded well to radiation therapy alone.

With the advent of immunophenotyping, many of these cases were reclassified as angiocentric T cell lymphoma according to the REAL classification. The use of radiation therapy for nasal angiocentric lymphoma at stage I/II disease had again been reported to be highly efficacious, with the overall response (OR) rate ranging from 60 percent to 80 percent, complete remission (CR) rate 40–80 percent, and 5-year overall survival (OS) 40–59 percent.[34,53–56,59,68]

The results of radiation therapy for stage I/II nasal NK cell lymphomas diagnosed according to the WHO classification scheme have not been well reported. The results are, however, similar to those reported for nasal angiocentric lymphomas, with an OR rate of about 80 percent and a CR rate of 70 percent.[58,59]

Typically, a total dose of 30–60 Gy of radiation therapy will be delivered, with the median at about 50 Gy. The fractional dose will be 1.5–2.5 Gy. The target volume usually includes the nasal cavities and the nasopharynx, at 1–2 cm beyond the tumor margin. Computerized tomographic scan or MRI should be used to determine the target volumes. When a nasal sinus is involved, the whole of the sinus will be covered. The field is extended to cover the cervical regions if cervical lymph nodes are involved. The planning of radiation therapy should also take into account the organs that may be affected. The eye should be spared if possible, in view of the favorable long-term outcome of some patients. In patients who have widespread local involvement, the initial use of chemotherapy to shrink the tumor in order to decrease the field of radiation therapy should be considered.

Radiation therapy is in general well tolerated. Successful results are quickly obtained and often dramatic. Radiation dermatitis, oral and nasal mucosal damage, and transient loss of taste are the commonest side effects. Because of the destructive and obstructive nature of the primary lesion, many patients have persistent nasal symptoms, including nasal discharge and bleeding, for some years after radiation therapy.

Although the initial efficacy of radiation therapy is high, a significant number of patients relapse after radiation therapy. The exact proportion of patients relapsing after radiotherapy varies in different studies, with around 50 percent being the most usual frequency,[34,52] although relapse rates as low as 17 percent[58] or as high as 77 percent[59] have been reported. The patterns of radiation therapy failure can be divided into 'in field' failures, margin failures, and systemic recurrence. Several points are worthy of note in the consideration of local failures. First, the dose of radiation therapy for NK cell lymphoma may have to be higher than that for conventional sinonasal B cell lymphomas.[30] A radiation therapy dose of less than 45 Gy was found to predict for local relapse in one study,[59] and less than 50 Gy was similarly predictive in another study.[52] Although with the probability of local recurrence as the endpoint, the dose-response curve was found to plateau at 54 Gy;[59] additional boosting of radiation therapy to 60–70 Gy has also been shown to be effective in about one-half of the patients with residual disease after the planned dosage.[52] Second, meticulous image-assisted planning of radiation therapy is needed; patients not having imaging studies before radiation therapy suffer a higher chance of local relapse.[52] Therefore, to increase the efficacy of radiation therapy for local lymphoma control, adequate dosage and careful planning are crucial. Finally, it is currently unclear as to whether the concomitant administration of radiosensitizers may improve outcome. Most failures happen within the first year of treatment, and local recurrences after 2 years are very uncommon.[34,52]

Systemic failure has been reported to occur in 25–30 percent of patients with stage I/II disease treated with radiation therapy alone.[34,52,58,59] In more than half of these cases, the systemic relapse was not associated with local recurrence. This implies that a significant proportion of apparently stage I/II patients at presentation have in fact more disseminated disease. It appears logical that the use of systemic chemotherapy in such patients may increase the chance of success. However, none of the studies reported so far have been able to identify risk factors that can predict the occurrence of systemic relapse. A continued search for better disease indicators, such as the tumor volume as defined by MRI and innovative molecular or surrogate tumor markers, will be needed to improve the staging of patients and stratification of treatment.

The role of radiation therapy in non-nasal NK cell lymphoma has not been formally evaluated. Similar to nasal tumors, non-nasal NK cell lymphomas are very sensitive to radiation therapy. However, since non-nasal NK cell lymphomas tend to be advanced in stage at presentation, and early stage disease disseminates quite rapidly, radiation therapy is seldom considered suitable as the initial therapy. Therefore, radiation therapy is usually confined to adjuvant or palliative situations. Radiation therapy is indicated in the palliative treatment of symptomatic and localized lesions in aggressive NK cell lymphoma/leukemia.

Chemotherapy

Chemotherapy plays an important role in the treatment of patients with stage III/IV nasal NK cell lymphoma. However, since the relapse rate is also high in patients with early stage disease treated by radiation therapy alone, chemotherapy has been advocated as part of the treatment regimen of stage I/II disease. Therefore, in most treatment centers, medically fit patients with nasal NK cell lymphoma at any clinical stage will receive chemotherapy as part of their treatment.

The choice of chemotherapy depends on many factors, with age being the most important consideration. Although there is no indication that anthracyclines are an essential component of chemotherapy, most studies have in fact utilized anthracycline-containing regimens. The intended chemotherapy varies from three to six monthly cycles. For patients with nasal NK cell lymphoma and stage I/II disease, primary chemotherapy results in a CR rate of 40–60 percent.[25,52,57,58] Two observations are important. First, disease progression during chemotherapy occurs in 30–40 percent of patients,[52,57] necessitating the use of salvage radiation therapy. An alternative chemotherapeutic regimen in patients with disease progression during primary chemotherapy is ineffective. Second, a high relapse rate, reaching 30–40 percent, is seen in patients in CR after chemotherapy. Therefore, the overall failure rate of chemotherapy reaches 67 percent.[30,52] There is no evidence that any of the more complicated regimens, such as BACOP, m-BACOD, or ProMACE-CytaBOM, are superior to CHOP in treatment outcome.

Chemotherapy has not been compared formally with radiation therapy. The relative rarity of the disease even in populations where NK cell lymphomas are considered common has precluded randomized trials. Furthermore, the choice of the initial therapy is often affected by the local extent of the disease, which can differ widely in stage I/II patients. These limitations notwithstanding, radiation therapy has consistently been shown to be superior to chemotherapy alone in the treatment of patients with stage I/II disease.[52,58,59] Furthermore, nasal NK cell lymphomas that have not responded to chemotherapy can be salvaged by radiation therapy in about 50 percent of cases. On the contrary, patients in whom radiation therapy has failed respond minimally to salvage chemotherapy.[52] Finally, the addition of consolidation chemotherapy to treatment for patients with stage I disease achieving CR after primary radiation therapy confers no additional survival advantage.[52,58,59]

The high failure rate of chemotherapy has been attributed to the expression of the multidrug resistance (MDR) gene (P-glycoprotein) in the lymphoma cells. Actually, of all myeloid and lymphoid cells, NK cells express the highest level of P-glycoprotein.[69] The MDR phenotype is recapitulated in neoplastic NK cells, where P-glycoprotein expression has been frequently found to be at high levels in nasal NK lymphoma cells.[70] Furthermore, drug penetration is often compromised by tissue necrosis in the tumor.

For stage III/IV nasal tumors, non-nasal tumors at any stage, and aggressive lymphoma/leukemia, chemotherapy remains the only choice of treatment. However, the results are poor. Complete remission rates for chemotherapy of stage III/IV nasal and non-nasal tumors are less than 15 percent.[25,37] Conventional chemotherapy for aggressive NK cell lymphoma/leukemia results in few if any remissions.

Therefore, for nasal NK cell lymphoma, primary chemotherapy alone is not the ideal treatment for patients with stage I/II disease. Chemotherapy should not be routinely added to radiation therapy in patients with stage I disease. However, the role of additional chemotherapy after radiation therapy in patients with stage II disease requires further studies. For nasal NK cell lymphomas in advanced stages, as well as other forms of NK cell lymphomas, conventional chemotherapy gives unsatisfactory results, implying that innovative therapeutic regimens should be devised for these patients.

Combined chemotherapy and radiation therapy

The high frequency of systemic failure of patients treated with radiation therapy, and the low efficacy of chemotherapy, makes combined chemotherapy and radiation therapy an attractive option in patients with stage I/II nasal lymphomas. However, in any strategy that utilizes the combination, radiation therapy should be administered early, owing to its high efficacy. The combination of 6 cycles of chemotherapy, with sandwiched radiation therapy after three courses, has also been tested in early stage nasal NK cell lymphomas.[71] Preliminary results suggest that this is a feasible approach, although the long-term treatment outcome remains to be determined.

Prognostic factors of natural killer cell lymphomas

Of the three clinical subtypes, aggressive NK cell lymphoma/leukemia has the most dismal prognosis. No survival has been reported with conventional chemotherapy.[25,30] The early use of allogeneic hematopoietic stem cell transplantation has been described to result in remission in a few cases of aggressive NK cell lymphoma/leukemia, although whether this had led to long-term survival is unknown.[72,73] The outlook of non-nasal NK cell lymphomas is marginally better, with long-term remission reported in fewer than 10 percent of cases.[30,37]

On the other hand, a potential cure may be achieved with radiation therapy and conventional chemotherapy in some cases of nasal NK cell lymphoma. Therefore, the prognostication of patients for the identification of those who may respond to conventional treatment, and those who may require additional or innovative therapy, becomes an important issue. The IPI has been shown to be applicable to diffuse large B cell lymphomas and T cell lymphomas. In nasal NK cell lymphoma, the IPI has been shown to be useful in predicting treatment outcome. In a study of 67 patients,[35] irrespective of whether radiation therapy or chemotherapy was the initial treatment, patients with an IPI score of ≤1 were superior to those with IPI score ≥2 for 20-year OS. Subgroup analysis of patients treated with intensive chemotherapy followed by involved field radiation therapy also showed that patients with IPI score ≤1 were superior to those with IPI score ≥2 in terms of CR rate and 10-year OS. These results show that the IPI score may be useful in stratifying patients for different treatment regimens. A recent study incorporating the IPI and other clinical parameters has shown similar results.[74]

The use of circulating EBV DNA as a surrogate tumor marker for prognostication has also been explored.[65] In a study of 23 patients with various forms of NK cell lymphoma treated primarily with chemotherapy and supplemented by involved field radiation therapy, multivariate analysis, taking into account the presentation EBV load, stage, age, and LDH level, showed that presentation EBV DNA was the only significant factor, with a load of $>6.1 \times 10^7$ copies/mL negatively impacting on disease-free survival (DFS).

Prognostication of early stage nasal NK cell lymphoma remains an important issue. Prospective studies are required to investigate whether a combination of local tumor staging, IPI score, and plasma EBV DNA load may provide a better guide to treatment and for predicting the outcome.

Patient monitoring after treatment

There are several special problems in the monitoring of patients with NK cell lymphomas. Many patients with nasal NK cell lymphomas have chronic infection of the nasal sinuses. This may be related to the obstruction of the sinuses due to the primary tumor, and further compounded by the mucosal damage resulting from irradiation. Consequently, nasal obstruction and discharge often persist after adequate treatment has been given. Furthermore, on radiologic imaging, the lining of the nasal cavity and paranasal sinuses is commonly thickened, making assessment of resolution of disease difficult. Therefore, frequent otolaryngoscopic examination with biopsies of thickened mucosa is necessary to define disease status. In these biopsies, the detection of small numbers of tumor cells by morphologic analysis may not be accurate, and immunohistochemical analyses for CD56 and ISH for EBER-positive cells are needed.

As NK cells lack a clonal marker, molecular analysis for residual disease is difficult. This is different from the situation in conventional B cell and in T cell lymphomas, where rearrangement of the immunoglobulin heavy chain gene and T cell receptor genes can be used as a clonal marker. So far, molecular pathologic studies of NK cell lymphomas have failed to identify specific genetic lesions.[75–78]

However, frequent aberrant promoter methylation leading to transcriptional repression and gene silencing has been found in NK cell lymphomas.[77] The genes implicated are usually tumor suppressor genes, and have included *TP73*, *retinoic acid receptor β*, and *death associated protein kinase*. Although the genes involved in epigenetic methylation are not specific to any particular tumor, they are nevertheless only methylated in tumor cells. Therefore, when the gene methylation pattern is known in the primary tumor, detection of aberrant methylation serves as a surrogate tumor marker. With the methylation-specific polymerase chain reaction, which has a sensitivity of 10^{-3} of detecting the methylated allele, aberrant gene methylation has been found to be more sensitive than morphologic or immunophenotypic examination for the detection of minimal residual lymphoma in biopsies.[79] If this strategy is adopted, a panel of genes should be tested for aberrant methylation in the primary tumor. When a biopsy is subsequently taken from a suspicious lesion, the methylation-specific polymerase chain reaction can be employed to detect aberrant methylation, which serves as a surrogate tumor marker.

Two circulating markers have also been reported to reflect the lymphoma load. First, it has been found that soluble Fas-ligand is secreted by NK cells, and that increased circulating soluble Fas-ligand may be found in neoplastic proliferations of NK cells.[80] The level of soluble Fas-ligand was found to be significantly increased in aggressive NK cell lymphoma/leukemia, but undetectable in patients in remission.[81] However, an enzyme-linked immunosorbent assay for Fas-ligand is not widely available, so these results have not been extensively validated.

Second, dynamic studies of circulating EBV DNA have also been shown to be useful in the monitoring of patients (Fig. 75.3).[65] During treatment, a decrease in circulating EBV DNA occurs in a proportion of patients. This correlates with clinical control of the lymphoma, and CR is associated with a fall of EBV DNA to undetectable levels. Accordingly, patients who during any stage of their disease show a rise of EBV DNA to levels exceeding those at presentation, which indicates progression of the lymphoma, or who fail to achieve a fall of EBV DNA to undetectable levels, which signifies inability to reach a CR, have a much inferior prognosis. The test is especially valuable in deciding whether patients who have reached a clinical remission should receive extra treatment. Patients in apparent CR who have high levels of circulating EBV DNA will almost invariably relapse, and are therefore candidates for additional or innovative therapy.

High–dose chemotherapy and hematopoietic stem cell transplantation in natural killer cell lymphomas

Despite combined treatment with chemotherapy and radiation therapy, an overall 50–70 percent of patients with

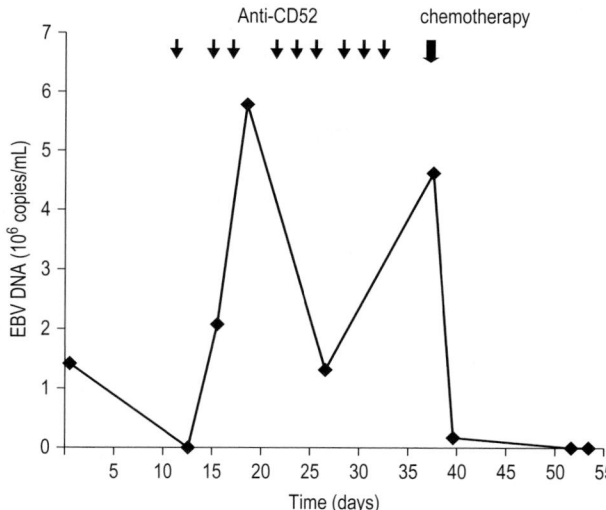

Figure 75.3 Monitoring of circulating plasma Epstein–Barr virus (EBV) DNA during the course of treatment of a case of relapsed nasal natural killer cell lymphoma. The patient showed no response to conventional chemotherapy at relapse. Anti-CD52 antibody (alemtuzumab) was administered, which resulted initially in a clinical response with a fall of EBV DNA. However, a complete response was not obtained. Combination chemotherapy incorporating L-asparaginase resulted in a complete remission of the nasal lymphoma and reduction of plasma EBV DNA to undetectable levels.

NK cell lymphoma will still relapse.[30] Treatment results of relapsed NK cell lymphomas are poor. Based on these observations, the use of high-dose chemotherapy and hematopoietic stem cell transplantation (HSCT) has been explored in NK cell lymphomas.

As involvement of the marrow is uncommon, autologous HSCT (auto-HSCT) is potentially applicable to most patients. Patients who may be suitable candidates include those with stage I/II disease in first complete remission (CR1), relapsed patients in second CR (CR2) or with chemotherapy-sensitive disease, and primary or secondary refractory patients with uninvolved marrow. Some issues are conceptually important in assessing the role of auto-HSCT. For patients with stage I/II disease achieving CR1 after radiation therapy and/or chemotherapy, about 30 percent of them are potentially cured. Although several important prognostic factors have been established, none has been evaluated in identifying patients who may require HSCT in order to achieve durable remission. Therefore, there is currently a lack of data to define which population of patients with stage I/II disease in CR1 may benefit from HSCT.

Patients in first relapse have different clinical patterns of disease. These include local or systemic relapses after radiation therapy, chemotherapy, or combined radiation therapy and chemotherapy. The optimal salvage therapy for each of these categories has not been defined, since NK cell lymphomas may be relatively chemotherapy resistant. Accordingly, whether a single conditioning regimen will fit all these different categories of patients is unclear.

These issues are reflected in the variable efficacy of auto-HSCT in NK cell lymphoma patients. About sixty patients with NK cell malignancies have undergone high-dose chemotherapy and auto-HSCT.[82–89] The median age at HSCT was 42 (16–67) years. There was a predominance of nasal NK cell lymphomas (89 percent). At initial diagnosis, 63 percent of patients had early stage (stage I/II) disease, whereas 37 percent had late stage (stage III/IV) disease. At the time of HSCT, 56 percent of patients were without active disease (CR1: 18/57, 31.5 percent; CR2: 14/57, 24.5 percent), whereas 44 percent had persistent disease (in partial remission [PR], refractory disease, or untreated relapses 1 or 2). At the time of reporting of these studies, about 50 percent of patients were still in remission after HSCT. Other patients had either relapsed and were still living (16 percent) or had died of disease relapse or progression (33 percent). Multivariate regression analysis showed that the status at HSCT was the only factor significantly related to overall survival, with stage I/II patients faring significantly better than stage III/IV patients. However, none of these studies was controlled, and the results of auto-HSCT did not appear to be superior to historical controls of chemotherapy- or radiation therapy-treated patients. Therefore, with a definite therapeutic advantage not established, auto-HSCT for stage I/II NK cell lymphomas at CR1 should not be routinely offered outside the context of a clinical trial. The use of auto-HSCT in patients beyond CR1 is associated with poor results.[82–89] Patients auto-transplanted at CR2, chemotherapy-sensitive in first relapse not yet reaching CR2, or with uncontrolled primary disease or relapse had uniformly poor outcomes and virtually no long-term survival. Failure in these patients was usually attributable to disease progression at the sites involved before HSCT, implying that the conditioning regimen was ineffective. Hence, before an optimal conditioning regimen can be defined, patients in these situations are unlikely to benefit from auto-HSCT and should be offered experimental or innovative therapy.

With the role of auto-HSCT undefined, allogeneic HSCT becomes an attractive option. The only theoretical advantage of allogeneic over autologous HSCT in NK cell lymphoma is the potential graft-versus-lymphoma effect. This may be particularly relevant, as the NK lymphoma cells express EBV antigens, which may be additional alloreactive targets. Fewer than forty patients undergoing allogeneic HSCT from HLA-identical siblings or HLA-matched unrelated donors have been reported.[72,73,83,90–93] At the time of transplantation, ten patients were in apparent remission, whereas the other patients had residual or refractory disease. There were more female patients, and the median age of presentation was in the third decade. All but five patients received myeloablative conditioning regimens. At the time of reporting of these studies, about one-half of the patients were alive, a quarter having died from treatment-related mortality, and the other quarter dead from disease progression. Although the results appeared to be encouraging, there may be a reporting bias toward successful cases. Consequently, more patients have to be studied to define the role of allogeneic HSCT in NK cell lymphomas.

Additional treatment options for refractory natural killer cell lymphomas

The possibility of multidrug resistance in NK cell lymphoma has prompted the investigation of agents that are not affected by P-glycoprotein.[94] The drug L-asparaginase has been reported to be effective in refractory cases of NK cell lymphomas.[95–97] L-asparaginase works by depletion of asparagine. As lymphoid cells lack L-asparagine synthetase, they are susceptible to L-asparaginase-induced inhibition of synthesis of protein, DNA, and RNA. Experiments *in vitro* have also demonstrated a specific action of L-asparaginase on NK lymphoma cells.[98] As a single agent (6000 units/day for 7 days), L-asparaginase induced a complete remission in one case of relapsed non-nasal NK cell lymphoma.[97] Used together with vincristine and steroids, L-asparaginase (4000–6000 units/day for 7 days) was reported to lead to CR in 56 percent of patients with nasal NK cell lymphoma.[96] A recent pilot study of the combination of L-asparaginase with prednisone, methotrexate, ifosfamide, and etoposide has also shown promising results in patients with advanced stage or refractory NK cell malignancies.[99] Common side effects included allergic rashes, derangement of liver function, and hyperglycemia, and neutropenia when L-asparaginase was used in combination chemotherapy. However, the long-term outcome of patients treated with L-asparaginase has not been reported. Therefore, the role of L-asparaginase in the management of NK cell malignancies remains to be defined.

Management of local problems in nasal natural killer cell lymphomas

Perforation of the hard palate is a unique problem. This may be the presenting problem or a complication of treatment. The latter situation occurs when the lymphoma has extensively eroded but not yet perforated the hard palate. After chemotherapy or radiation therapy, destruction of the lymphoma weakens the hard palate and may result in its perforation. A communication between the oral and nasal cavity causes a major problem in eating and drinking, as well as predisposing to persistent nasal infection. As a temporary means to overcome this problem, an obdurator can be constructed (Fig. 75.4). After the primary lymphoma has been treated and a remission confirmed, definitive surgical reconstruction can be performed.

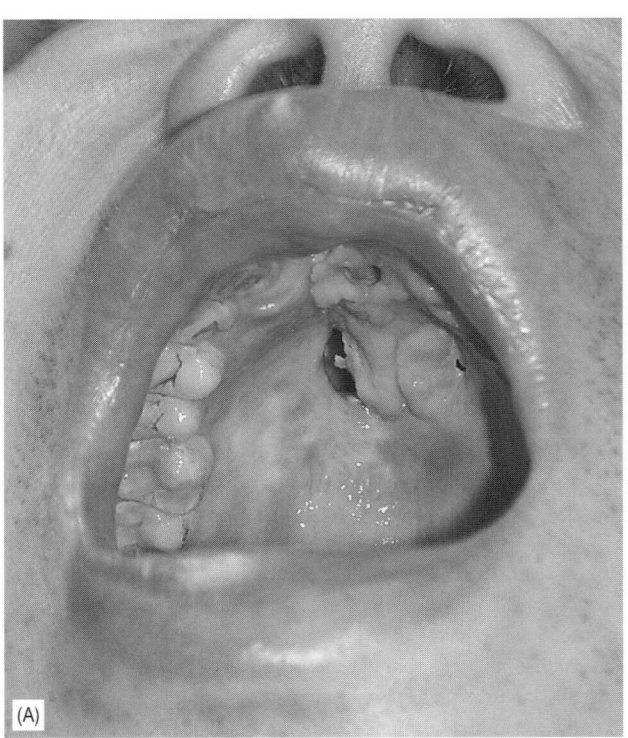

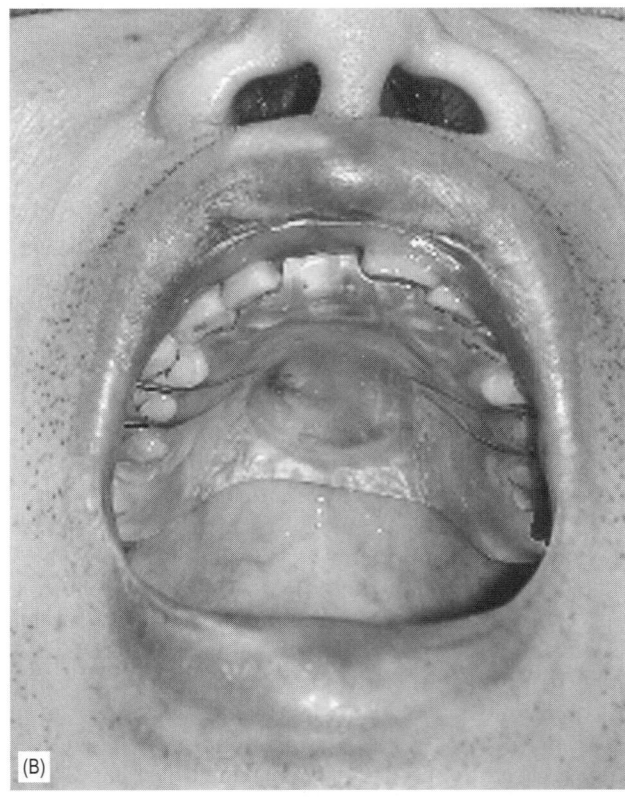

Figure 75.4 Nasal natural killer cell lymphoma with destruction of the hard palate, leading to a characteristic communication between the nasal and oral cavity. (A) Note the perforation of the hard palate in three different sites, with necrotic tissue preventing a total communication. (B) The communications could be completely obliterated by a suitably constructed obdurator.

POST–TRANSPLANTATION LYMPHOPROLIFERATIVE DISEASES OF NATURAL KILLER CELL LINEAGE

Rare cases of PTLD of NK cell lineage have been described after organ allografting.[100–102] It is uncertain if these cases reflect chance occurrence or the opportunistic neoplastic proliferation of EBV-infected NK cells. All reported cases of NK-PTLD pursued an aggressive clinical course and showed no response to the withdrawal of immunosuppression. Therefore, NK-PTLD should be treated with strategies similar to *de novo* NK cell lymphomas.

CHRONIC ACTIVE EPSTEIN–BARR VIRUS INFECTION

Chronic active EBV infection is an uncommon condition, characterized by high circulating EBV DNA loads and abnormal proliferation of EBV-infected T cells and NK cells.[103] With analysis of EBV terminal repeats, some of these patients have been shown to have a clonal proliferation of T and NK cells. Transformation to a frankly malignant NK cell lymphoma may occur.[104] Treatment with autologous EBV-specific cytotoxic T cells may be effective before transformation.[105] When NK cell lymphoma develops, the prognosis is poor. Occasional success has been reported with the use of allogeneic HSCT.[106]

BLASTIC NATURAL KILLER CELL LYMPHOMA

Blastic NK cell lymphoma has been regarded by the WHO classification as a distinct disease entity.[107] However, this lymphoma is clearly different from other subtypes of NK cell malignancies. There is no racial predilection, and to date no association with EBV has been described. In fact, the neoplastic cells are now considered to be derived from plasmacytoid dendritic cells, and the neoplasm more accurately classified as a CD4+CD56+ hematodermic neoplasm.[108] The optimal therapy is unclear, although treatment with protocols designed for acute leukemia appeared to be associated with better responses than those designed for lymphomas.[109]

FUTURE PERSPECTIVES

Natural killer cell lymphomas have a predominant predilection for Asian and South American peoples and are extremely uncommon in other populations. Part of the underlying cause is therefore likely to be genetic. The definition of this predisposition may have important implications in treatment. Although NK cell lymphomas are considered prevalent in Asian countries, they only account for 6–7 percent of all non-Hodgkin lymphomas in these populations.[16] In order to advance the knowledge of this interesting malignancy, patients should be referred to experienced centers in countries where they are available. International collaborative studies are required to define the optimal treatment regimens.

KEY POINTS

- Epidemiology: Natural killer (NK) cell lymphomas show a predilection for Asian and South American populations and are rare in Western populations. Epstein–Barr virus (EBV) infection of the lymphoma cells is a consistent observation.
- Diagnosis: NK cell lymphomas are often confused with peripheral T cell lymphomas. Most nasal lymphomas in Asian populations are NK cell lymphomas and T cell lymphomas are uncommon. NK cell lymphomas express cytoplasmic but not surface CD3, whereas T cell lymphomas express surface CD3. The typical phenotype of NK cell lymphoma is CD2+, CD3ε+, CD56+, cytotoxic molecules+, and EBV+.
- Clinical features: Clinically, NK cell lymphomas can be divided into nasal, non-nasal, and aggressive lymphoma/leukemia subtypes. They have different clinical behaviors, treatment approaches, and therapeutic outcome.
- Prognostication: The International Prognostic Index is of prognostic relevance. Other potential prognostic indicators include tumor size and the amount of plasma EBV DNA load, a surrogate tumor biomarker.
- Treatment: For stage I/II nasal NK cell lymphomas, radiation therapy is an important therapeutic component. Chemotherapy is the mainstay of treatment for late stage nasal NK cell lymphomas and for other subtypes of NK cell lymphomas.
- Monitoring after treatment: Quantification of plasma EBV DNA load is useful in the monitoring of patients after treatment.
- Treatment outcome: Stage I/II nasal NK cell lymphomas have a better prognosis. However, stage III/IV nasal NK cell lymphomas and other subtypes of NK cell lymphomas are all associated with a poor prognosis. Innovative treatment strategies are needed.

REFERENCES

● = Key primary paper
◆ = Major review article

◆1. Spits H, Lanier LL, Phillips JH. Development of human T and natural killer cells. *Blood* 1995; **85**: 2654–70.

2. Lanier LL. NK cell receptors. *Annu Rev Immunol* 1998; **16**: 359–93.

3. Lanier LL, Testi R, Bindl J, Phillips JH. Identity of Leu-19 (CD56) leukocyte differentiation antigen and neural cell adhesion molecule. *J Exp Med* 1989; **169**: 2233–8.

4. Feder BH, Shramek JH, Ikeda TS. Large-field radiotherapy in lethal midline granuloma. *Radiology* 1963; **81**: 293–9.

5. Byrd LJ, Shearn MA, Tu WH. Relationship of lethal midline granuloma to Wegener's granulomatosis. *Arthritis Rheum* 1969; **12**: 247–53.

6. Batsakis JG, Luna MA. Midfacial necrotizing lesions. *Semin Diagn Pathol* 1987; **4**: 90–116.

7. Aozasa K, Ohsawa M, Tajima K *et al.* Nationwide study of lethal mid-line granuloma in Japan: frequencies of Wegener's granulomatosis, polymorphic reticulosis, malignant lymphoma and other related conditions. *Int J Cancer* 1989; **44**: 63–6.

8. Eichel BS, Harrison EG Jr, Devine KD *et al.* Primary lymphoma of the nose including a relationship to lethal midline granuloma. *Am J Surg* 1966; **112**: 597–605.

9. Strickler JG, Meneses MF, Habermann TM *et al.* Polymorphic reticulosis: a reappraisal. *Hum Pathol* 1994; **25**: 659–65.

10. Harris NL, Jaffe ES, Stein H *et al.* A revised European-American classification of lymphoid neoplasms: a proposal from the International Lymphoma Study Group. *Blood* 1994; **84**: 1361–92.

11. Wong KF, Chan JK, Ng CS *et al.* CD56 (NKH1)-positive hematolymphoid malignancies: an aggressive neoplasm featuring frequent cutaneous/mucosal involvement, cytoplasmic azurophilic granules, and angiocentricity. *Hum Pathol* 1992; **23**: 798–804.

●12. Kern WF, Spier CM, Hanneman EH *et al.* Neural cell adhesion molecule-positive peripheral T-cell lymphoma: a rare variant with a propensity for unusual sites of involvement. *Blood* 1992; **79**: 2432–7.

●13. Chan JK, Tsang WY, Ng CS. Clarification of CD3 immunoreactivity in nasal T/natural killer cell lymphomas: the neoplastic cells are often CD3 epsilon+. *Blood* 1996; **87**: 839–41.

14. Emile JF, Boulland ML, Haioun C *et al.* CD5-CD56+ T-cell receptor silent peripheral T-cell lymphomas are natural killer cell lymphomas. *Blood* 1996; **87**: 1466–73.

◆15. Chan JK, Jaffe ES, Ralfkiaer E. Extranodal NK/T-cell lymphoma, nasal type. In: Jaffe ES, Harris NL, Stein H, Vardiman JW. (eds) *Tumours of haematopoietic and lymphoid tissues. World Health Organization classification of tumours.* Lyon: IARC Press, 2001: 204–7.

●16. Au WY, Ma SY, Chim CS *et al.* Clinicopathologic features and treatment outcome of mature T-cell and natural killer-cell lymphomas diagnosed according to the World Health Organization classification scheme: a single center experience of 10 years. *Ann Oncol* 2005; **16**: 206–14.

17. Kawa-Ha K, Ishihara S, Ninomiya T *et al.* CD3-negative lymphoproliferative disease of granular lymphocytes containing Epstein-Barr viral DNA. *J Clin Invest* 1989; **84**: 51–5.

18. Medeiros LJ, Peiper SC, Elwood L *et al.* Angiocentric immunoproliferative lesions: a molecular analysis of eight cases. *Hum Pathol* 1991; **22**: 1150–7.

19. Hart DN, Baker BW, Inglis MJ *et al.* Epstein-Barr viral DNA in acute large granular lymphocyte (natural killer) leukemic cells. *Blood* 1992; **79**: 2116–23.

20. Arber DA, Weiss LM, Albujar PF *et al.* Nasal lymphomas in Peru. High incidence of T-cell immunophenotype and Epstein-Barr virus infection. *Am J Surg Pathol* 1993; **17**: 392–9.

21. Minarovits J, Hu LF, Imai S *et al.* Clonality, expression and methylation patterns of the Epstein-Barr virus genomes in lethal midline granulomas classified as peripheral angiocentric T cell lymphomas. *J Gen Virol* 1994; **75**: 77–84.

22. Tao Q, Ho FC, Loke SL, Srivastava G. Epstein-Barr virus is localized in the tumour cells of nasal lymphomas of NK, T or B cell type. *Int J Cancer* 1995; **60**: 315–20.

23. Elenitoba-Johnson KS, Zarate-Osorno A, Meneses A *et al.* Cytotoxic granular protein expression, Epstein-Barr virus strain type, and latent membrane protein-1 oncogene deletions in nasal T-lymphocyte/natural killer cell lymphomas from Mexico. *Mod Pathol* 1998; **11**: 754–61.

◆24. Siu LL, Chan JK, Kwong YL. Natural killer cell malignancies: clinicopathologic and molecular features. *Histol Histopathol* 2002; **17**: 539–54.

25. Kwong YL, Chan AC, Liang R *et al.* CD56+ NK lymphomas: clinicopathological features and prognosis. *Br J Haematol* 1997; **97**: 821–9.

26. Chan JK, Yip TT, Tsang WY *et al.* Detection of Epstein-Barr viral RNA in malignant lymphomas of the upper aerodigestive tract. *Am J Surg Pathol* 1994; **18**: 938–46.

◆27. Chan JK, Wong KF, Jaffe ES, Ralfkiaer E. Aggressive NK-cell leukaemia. In: Jaffe ES, Harris NL, Stein H, Vardiman JW. (eds) *Tumours of haematopoietic and lymphoid tissues. World Health Organization classification of tumours.* Lyon: IARC Press, 2001: 198–200.

●28. Suzuki R, Suzumiya J, Nakamura S *et al.* Aggressive natural killer-cell leukemia revisited: large granular lymphocyte leukemia of cytotoxic NK cells. *Leukemia* 2004; **18**: 763–70.

29. Kwong YL, Chan AC, Liang RH. Natural killer cell lymphoma/leukemia: pathology and treatment. *Hematol Oncol* 1997; **15**: 71–9.

◆30. Cheung MM, Chan JK, Wong KF. Natural killer cell neoplasms: a distinctive group of highly aggressive lymphomas/leukemias. *Semin Hematol* 2003; **40**: 221–32.

●31. Cheung MM, Chan JK, Lau WH *et al.* Primary non-Hodgkin's lymphoma of the nose and nasopharynx: clinical features, tumor immunophenotype, and treatment outcome in 113 patients. *J Clin Oncol* 1998; **16**: 70–7.

32. Cuadra-Garcia I, Proulx GM, Wu CL *et al.* Sinonasal lymphoma: a clinicopathologic analysis of 58 cases from the Massachusetts General Hospital. *Am J Surg Pathol* 1999; **23**: 1356–69.

33. Gaal K, Sun NC, Hernandez AM, Arber DA. Sinonasal NK/T-cell lymphomas in the United States. *Am J Surg Pathol* 2000; **24**: 1511–7.

●34. Kim GE, Cho JH, Yang WI *et al*. Angiocentric lymphoma of the head and neck: patterns of systemic failure after radiation treatment. *J Clin Oncol* 2000; **18**: 54–63.

●35. Chim CS, Ma SY, Au WY *et al*. Primary nasal natural killer cell lymphoma: long-term treatment outcome and relationship with the International Prognostic Index. *Blood* 2004; **103**: 216–21.

36. Nakamura S, Suchi T, Koshikawa T *et al*. Clinicopathologic study of CD56 (NCAM)-positive angiocentric lymphoma occurring in sites other than the upper and lower respiratory tract. *Am J Surg Pathol* 1995; **19**: 284–96.

●37. Chan JK, Sin VC, Wong KF *et al*. Nonnasal lymphoma expressing the natural killer cell marker CD56: a clinicopathologic study of 49 cases of an uncommon aggressive neoplasm. *Blood* 1997; **89**: 4501–13.

38. Mraz-Gernhard S, Natkunam Y, Hoppe RT *et al*. Natural killer/natural killer-like T-cell lymphoma, CD56+, presenting in the skin: an increasingly recognized entity with an aggressive course. *J Clin Oncol* 2001; **19**: 2179–88.

39. Tse E, Yeung CK, Trendell-Smith N, Kwong YL. A cutaneous sore with black eschar in a cowhide worker. *Lancet* 2002; **360**: 306.

40. Martin AR, Chan WC, Perry DA *et al*. Aggressive natural killer cell lymphoma of the small intestine. *Mod Pathol* 1995; **8**: 467–72.

41. Chim CS, Au WY, Shek TW *et al*. Primary CD56 positive lymphomas of the gastrointestinal tract. *Cancer* 2001; **91**: 525–33.

42. Chan JK, Tsang WY, Hui PK *et al*. T- and T/natural killer-cell lymphomas of the salivary gland: a clinicopathologic, immunohistochemical and molecular study of six cases. *Hum Pathol* 1997; **28**: 238–45.

43. Chan JK. Splenic involvement by peripheral T-cell and NK-cell neoplasms. *Semin Diagn Pathol* 2003; **20**: 105–20.

44. Chan JK, Tsang WY, Lau WH *et al*. Aggressive T/natural killer cell lymphoma presenting as testicular tumor. *Cancer* 1996; **77**: 1198–205.

45. Chim CS, Au WY, Poon C *et al*. Primary natural killer cell lymphoma of skeletal muscle. *Histopathology* 2002; **41**: 371–4.

46. Chim CS, Choy C, Liang R, Kwong YL. Isolated uterine relapse of nasal T/NK cell lymphoma. *Leuk Lymphoma* 1999; **34**: 629–32.

47. Chim CS, Ma ES, Loong F, Kwong YL. Diagnostic cues for natural killer cell lymphoma: primary nodal presentation and the role of in situ hybridisation for Epstein-Barr virus encoded early small RNA in detecting occult bone marrow involvement. *J Clin Pathol* 2005; **58**: 443–5.

48. Imamura N, Kusunoki Y, Kawa-Ha K *et al*. Aggressive natural killer cell leukaemia/lymphoma: report of four cases and review of the literature. Possible existence of a new clinical entity originating from the third lineage of lymphoid cells. *Br J Haematol* 1990; **75**: 49–59.

49. Gelb AB, van de Rijn M, Regula DP Jr *et al*. Epstein-Barr virus-associated natural killer-large granular lymphocyte leukemia. *Hum Pathol* 1994; **25**: 953–60.

50. Ooi GC, Chim CS, Liang R *et al*. Nasal T-cell/natural killer cell lymphoma: CT and MR imaging features of a new clinicopathologic entity. *AJR Am J Roentgenol* 2000; **174**: 1141–5.

51. Wong KF, Chan JK, Cheung MM, So JC. Bone marrow involvement by nasal NK cell lymphoma at diagnosis is uncommon. *Am J Clin Pathol* 2001; **115**: 266–70.

52. Cheung MM, Chan JK, Lau WH *et al*. Early stage nasal NK/T-cell lymphoma: clinical outcome, prognostic factors, and the effect of treatment modality. *Int J Radiat Oncol Biol Phys* 2002; 54: 182–90.

53. Sakata K, Hareyama M, Ohuchi A *et al*. Treatment of lethal midline granuloma type nasal T-cell lymphoma. *Acta Oncol* 1997; **36**: 307–11.

54. Shikama N, Izuno I, Oguchi M *et al*. Clinical stage IE primary lymphoma of the nasal cavity: radiation therapy and chemotherapy. *Radiology* 1997; **204**: 467–70.

55. Li YX, Coucke PA, Li JY *et al*. Primary non-Hodgkin's lymphoma of the nasal cavity: prognostic significance of paranasal extension and the role of radiotherapy and chemotherapy. *Cancer* 1998; **83**: 449–56.

56. Lei KI, Suen JJ, Hui P *et al*. Primary nasal and nasopharyngeal lymphomas: a comparative study of clinical presentation and treatment outcome. *Clin Oncol (R Coll Radiol)* 1999; **11**: 379–87.

57. Kim WS, Song SY, Ahn YC *et al*. CHOP followed by involved field radiation: is it optimal for localized nasal natural killer/T-cell lymphoma? *Ann Oncol* 2001; **12**: 349–52.

58. You JY, Chi KH, Yang MH *et al*. Radiation therapy versus chemotherapy as initial treatment for localized nasal natural killer (NK)/T-cell lymphoma: a single institute survey in Taiwan. *Ann Oncol* 2004; **15**: 618–25.

59. Koom WS, Chung EJ, Yang WI *et al*. Angiocentric T-cell and NK/T-cell lymphomas: radiotherapeutic viewpoints. *Int J Radiat Oncol Biol Phys* 2004; **59**: 1127–37.

60. Robbins KT, Fuller LM, Vlasak M *et al*. Primary lymphomas of the nasal cavity and paranasal sinuses. *Cancer* 1985; **56**: 814–9.

61. A predictive model for aggressive non-Hodgkin's lymphoma. The International Non-Hodgkin's Lymphoma Prognostic Factors Project. *N Engl J Med* 1993; **329**: 987–94.

62. Juweid ME, Cheson BD. Role of positron emission tomography in lymphoma. *J Clin Oncol* 2005; **23**: 4577–80.

63. Lei KI, Chan LY, Chan WY *et al*. Diagnostic and prognostic implications of circulating cell-free Epstein-Barr virus DNA in natural killer/T-cell lymphoma. *Clin Cancer Res* 2002; **8**: 29–34.

64. Chan KC, Zhang J, Chan AT *et al*. Molecular characterization of circulating EBV DNA in the plasma of nasopharyngeal carcinoma and lymphoma patients. *Cancer Res* 2003; **63**: 2028–32.

●65. Au WY, Pang A, Choy C *et al*. Quantification of circulating Epstein-Barr virus (EBV) DNA in the diagnosis and monitoring of natural killer cell and EBV-positive lymphomas in immunocompetent patients. *Blood* 2004; **104**: 243–9.

66. Halperin EC, Dosoretz DE, Goodman M, Wang CC. Radiotherapy of polymorphic reticulosis. *Br J Radiol* 1982; **55**: 645–9.

67. Itami J, Itami M, Mikata A *et al.* Non-Hodgkin's lymphoma confined to the nasal cavity: its relationship to the polymorphic reticulosis and results of radiation therapy. *Int J Radiat Oncol Biol Phys* 1991; **20**: 797–802.

68. Ribrag V, Ell Hajj M, Janot F *et al.* Early locoregional high-dose radiotherapy is associated with long-term disease control in localized primary angiocentric lymphoma of the nose and nasopharynx. *Leukemia* 2001; **15**: 1123–6.

69. Egashira M, Kawamata N, Sugimoto K *et al.* P-glycoprotein expression on normal and abnormally expanded natural killer cells and inhibition of P-glycoprotein function by cyclosporin A and its analogue, PSC833. *Blood* 1999; **93**: 599–606.

70. Yamaguchi M, Kita K, Miwa H *et al.* Frequent expression of P-glycoprotein/MDR1 by nasal T-cell lymphoma cells. *Cancer* 1995; **76**: 2351–6.

71. Cheung MM, Chan JK, Wong KH. Early stage nasal NK/T-cell lymphoma: preliminary results of intensifying treatment with concurrent chemo-radiation and high dose chemotherapy. *Ann Oncol* 2002; **12**(Suppl 2): 82 (abstract).

72. Ebihara Y, Manabe A, Tanaka R *et al.* Successful treatment of natural killer (NK) cell leukemia following a long-standing chronic active Epstein-Barr virus (CAEBV) infection with allogeneic bone marrow transplantation. *Bone Marrow Transplant* 2003; **31**: 1169–71.

73. Okamura T, Kishimoto T, Inoue M *et al.* Unrelated bone marrow transplantation for Epstein-Barr virus-associated T/NK-cell lymphoproliferative disease. *Bone Marrow Transplant* 2003; **31**: 105–11.

74. Lee J, Suh C, Park YH *et al.* Extranodal natural killer T-cell lymphoma, nasal-type: a prognostic model from a retrospective multicenter study. *J Clin Oncol* 2006; **24**: 612–8.

75. Siu LL, Wong KF, Chan JK, Kwong YL. Comparative genomic hybridization analysis of natural killer cell lymphoma/leukemia. Recognition of consistent patterns of genetic alterations. *Am J Pathol* 1999; **155**: 1419–25.

76. Siu LL, Chan V, Chan JK *et al.* Consistent patterns of allelic loss in natural killer cell lymphoma. *Am J Pathol* 2000; **157**: 1803–9.

77. Siu LL, Chan JK, Wong KF, Kwong YL. Specific patterns of gene methylation in natural killer cell lymphomas: p73 is consistently involved. *Am J Pathol* 2002; **160**: 59–66.

78. Shen L, Liang AC, Lu L *et al.* Frequent deletion of Fas gene sequences encoding death and transmembrane domains in nasal natural killer/T-cell lymphoma. *Am J Pathol* 2002; **161**: 2123–31.

79. Siu LL, Chan JK, Wong KF *et al.* Aberrant promoter CpG methylation as a molecular marker for disease monitoring in natural killer cell lymphomas. *Br J Haematol* 2003; **122**: 70–7.

80. Tanaka M, Suda T, Haze K *et al.* Fas ligand in human serum. *Nat Med* 1996; **2**: 317–22.

81. Kato K, Ohshima K, Ishihara S *et al.* Elevated serum soluble Fas ligand in natural killer cell proliferative disorders. *Br J Haematol* 1998; **103**: 1164–6.

82. Nawa Y, Takenaka K, Shinagawa K *et al.* Successful treatment of advanced natural killer cell lymphoma with high-dose chemotherapy and syngeneic peripheral blood stem cell transplantation. *Bone Marrow Transplant* 1999; 23: 1321–2.

83. Takenaka K, Shinagawa K, Maeda Y *et al.* High-dose chemotherapy with hematopoietic stem cell transplantation is effective for nasal and nasal-type CD56+ natural killer cell lymphomas. *Leuk Lymphoma* 2001; **42**: 1297–303.

84. Nagafuji K, Fujisaki T, Arima F, Ohshima K. L-asparaginase induced durable remission of relapsed nasal NK/T-cell lymphoma after autologous peripheral blood stem cell transplantation. *Int J Hematol* 2001; **74**: 447–50.

85. Sanda T, Lida S, Ito M *et al.* Successful treatment of nasal T-cell lymphoma with a combination of local irradiation and high-dose chemotherapy. *Int J Hematol* 2002; **75**: 195–200.

●86. Au WY, Lie AK, Liang R *et al.* Autologous stem cell transplantation for nasal NK/T-cell lymphoma: a progress report on its value. *Ann Oncol* 2003; **14**: 1673–6.

87. Koizumi K, Fujimoto K, Haseyama Y *et al.* Effective high-dose chemotherapy combined with CD34+-selected peripheral blood stem cell transplantation in a patient with cutaneous involvement of nasal NK/T-cell lymphoma. *Eur J Haematol* 2004; **72**: 140–4.

●88. Suzuki R, Suzumiya J, Nakamura S *et al.* Hematopoietic stem cell transplantation for natural killer-cell lineage neoplasms. *Bone Marrow Transplant* 2006; **37**: 425–31.

●89. Kim HJ, Bang SM, Lee J *et al.* High-dose chemotherapy with autologous stem cell transplantation in extranodal NK/T-cell lymphoma: a retrospective comparison with non-transplantation cases. *Bone Marrow Transplant* 2006; **37**: 819–24.

90. Teshima T, Miyaji R, Fukuda M, Ohshima K. Bone-marrow transplantation for Epstein-Barr-virus-associated natural killer cell-large granular lymphocyte leukaemia. *Lancet* 1996; **347**: 1124.

91. Takami A, Nakao S, Yachie A *et al.* Successful treatment of Epstein-Barr virus-associated natural killer cell large granular lymphocytic leukaemia using allogeneic peripheral blood stem cell transplantation. *Bone Marrow Transplant* 1998; **21**: 1279–82.

92. Makita M, Maeda Y, Takenaka K *et al.* Successful treatment of progressive NK cell lymphoma with allogeneic peripheral stem cell transplantation followed by early cyclosporine tapering and donor leukocyte infusions. *Int J Hematol* 2002; **76**: 94–7.

●93. Murashige N, Kami M, Kishi Y *et al.* Allogeneic haematopoietic stem cell transplantation as a promising treatment for natural killer-cell neoplasms. *Br J Haematol* 2005; **130**: 561–7.

94. Charamella LJ, Meyer C, Thompson GE, Dimitrov NV. Chemotherapeutic agents and modulation of natural

killer cell activity in vitro. *J Immunopharmacol* 1985; **7**: 53–65.

95. Obama K, Tara M, Niina K. L-asparaginase-Based induction therapy for advanced extranodal NK/T-cell lymphoma. *Int J Hematol* 2003; **78**: 248–50.

96. Yong W, Zheng W, Zhang Y *et al.* L-asparaginase-based regimen in the treatment of refractory midline nasal/nasal-type T/NK-cell lymphoma. *Int J Hematol* 2003; **78**: 163–7.

97. Matsumoto Y, Nomura K, Kanda-Akano Y *et al.* Successful treatment with Erwinia L-asparaginase for recurrent natural killer/T cell lymphoma. *Leuk Lymphoma* 2003; **44**: 879–82.

●98. Ando M, Sugimoto K, Kitoh T *et al.* Selective apoptosis of natural killer-cell tumours by L-asparaginase. *Br J Haematol* 2005; **130**: 860–8.

99. Yamaguchi M, Suzuki R, Kwong YL *et al.* Phase I study of dexamethasone, methotrexate, ifosfamide, L-asparaginase, and etoposide (SMILE) chemotherapy for advanced-stage, relapsed or refractory extranodal natural killer (NK)/T-cell lymphoma and leukemia. *Cancer Sci* 2008; **99**: 1016–20.

100. Hsi ED, Picken MM, Alkan S. Post-transplantation lymphoproliferative disorder of the NK-cell type: a case report and review of the literature. *Mod Pathol* 1998; **11**: 479–84.

101. Kwong YL, Lam CC, Chan TM. Post-transplantation lymphoproliferative disease of natural killer cell lineage: a clinicopathological and molecular analysis. *Br J Haematol* 2000; **110**: 197–202.

102. Tsao L, Draoua HY, Mansukhani M *et al.* EBV-associated, extranodal NK-cell lymphoma, nasal type of the breast, after heart transplantation. *Mod Pathol* 2004; **17**: 125–30.

103. Kimura H, Hoshino Y, Kanegane H *et al.* Clinical and virologic characteristics of chronic active Epstein-Barr virus infection. *Blood* 2001; **98**: 280–6.

104. Kanno H, Onodera H, Endo M *et al.* Vascular lesion in a patient of chronic active Epstein-Barr virus infection with hypersensitivity to mosquito bites: vasculitis induced by mosquito bite with the infiltration of nonneoplastic Epstein-Barr virus-positive cells and subsequent development of natural killer/T-cell lymphoma with angiodestruction. *Hum Pathol* 2005; **36**: 212–8.

105. Savoldo B, Huls MH, Liu Z *et al.* Autologous Epstein-Barr virus (EBV)-specific cytotoxic T cells for the treatment of persistent active EBV infection. *Blood* 2002; **100**: 4059–66.

106. Ebihara Y, Manabe A, Tanaka R *et al.* Successful treatment of natural killer (NK) cell leukemia following a long-standing chronic active Epstein-Barr virus (CAEBV) infection with allogeneic bone marrow transplantation. *Bone Marrow Transplant* 2003; **31**: 1169–71.

107. Chan JK, Jaffe ES, Ralfkiaer E. Blastic NK-cell lymphoma. In: Jaffe ES, Harris NL, Stein H, Vardiman JW. (eds) *Tumours of haematopoietic and lymphoid tissues. World Health Organization classification of tumours.* Lyon: IARC Press, 2001: 214–5.

108. Willemze R, Jaffe ES, Burg G *et al.* WHO-EORTC classification for cutaneous lymphomas. *Blood* 2005; **105**: 3768–85.

109. Bekkenk MW, Jansen PM, Meijer CJ, Willemze R. CD56+ hematological neoplasms presenting in the skin: a retrospective analysis of 23 new cases and 130 cases from the literature. *Ann Oncol* 2004; **15**: 1097–108.

76

Anaplastic large cell lymphoma in adults

HERVÉ TILLY

BACKGROUND

Anaplastic large cell lymphoma (ALCL) was first described 20 years ago as a novel entity characterized by a cohesive growth pattern of neoplastic lymphoid cells with anaplastic features and constant expression of the Ki-1/CD30 antigen.[1] It rapidly became apparent that ALCL had numerous cytomorphologic variants, a heterogeneous immunophenotype, and variable clinical features.

In the 1980s, the translocation t(2;5)(p23;q35)[2,3] was found to be associated with some ALCL leading to the cloning of the *NPM-ALK* (nucleophosmin–anaplastic lymphoma kinase) fusion gene in 1994.[4] The molecular mechanisms leading to the constitutive expression of ALK,[5,6] supposed to be the primary oncogenic event, were then characterized.[7] Expression of ALK appeared to be the prominent characteristic of the most typical form of systemic ALCL. However, some lymphomas with morphologic and immunophenotypic features of ALCL may lack ALK expression.[8] The evolving definition of ALCL during these years explains the heterogeneity of the cases included in clinical series. Only a few, relatively recent reports relate to the present definition of ALCL.

GENERAL DESCRIPTION

Anaplastic large cell lymphoma is recognized as a category of mature T cell neoplasm in the World Health Organization (WHO) classification[9] and accounts for 2–3 percent of adult non-Hodgkin lymphomas.[10] It is now recognized that what was once considered to be B cell ALCL is in fact a morphologic and phenotypic variant of diffuse large B cell lymphoma (DLBCL).[6]

Apart from the common form of ALCL (70 percent of cases; see Chapter 76), two cytomorphologic variants are recognized in the WHO classification: lymphohistiocytic (10 percent) and small cell (5–10 percent), but neither appears at the present time to have different phenotypic, molecular, or clinical features.

Expression of CD30 is contained in the definition of ALCL. Some variants, however, may only be weakly positive.[11] ALK expression is found in 50–60 percent of adult cases where it defines the most typical form of systemic ALCL. The vast majority of patients express one or more T cell antigens, especially CD3, CD2, and CD4. Some cases do not and have an apparent null-cell phenotype. These latter cases probably belong to the T cell type because they express cytotoxic antigens and show clonal rearrangement of the T cell receptor.[12]

The translocation t(2;5)(p23;q35) is present in 70–80 percent of ALK-positive ALCL[9], and causes fusion of the *ALK* gene to the *NPM* gene resulting in the synthesis of a NPM-ALK fusion protein. This can form homodimers which lead to the constitutive activation of the catalytic domain of ALK. Numerous experimental findings suggest that deregulated activation of ALK could play a major role in lymphomagenesis.[7,13] Several variant translocations have also been described producing variant ALK fusion proteins.[14] Thus far, no etiologic factor has been identified.

CLINICAL FEATURES

Most series of ALCL in adults[10,15–18] were collected in the 1990s and interpretation of the data could be limited by inclusion of cases that are no longer recognized as ALCL (Hodgkin-like ALCL, B cell ALCL) or were not studied for ALK expression, which is now considered to be the major distinctive feature.[6] However, the high proportion of young adults with T cell or null-cell phenotype suggests that these series contained a significant number of ALK-positive ALCL.[6]

ALK-positive and ALK-negative anaplastic large cell lymphoma

The importance of ALK expression in determining clinical presentation and outcome was first reported by Shiota et al.[8] and confirmed in three large series.[19–21] ALK-positive ALCL mostly occurs in children and young adults. A male predominance is seen, especially in young adults, with a male/female ratio of 6.5 in the study from Falini et al.[19] Most cases present with disseminated stage III/IV disease and systemic symptoms, especially fever.[18–20,22,23] Nodal involvement is nearly constant and extranodal involvement is detected in the majority of the cases, skin, lung, bone, soft tissue, and muscle being the most frequently affected sites.[8,16,19] Bone marrow involvement is found in 10–15 percent of the cases when studied by conventional morphology.[16,19] However, this proportion increases to 40 percent when bone marrow is studied with anti-CD30 and anti-EMA (epithelial membrane antigen) immunostaining,[24] and to 60 percent when NPM-ALK-positive cases are studied by polymerase chain reaction (PCR).[25] Peripheral blood involvement is unusual but some cases with a leukemic phase at presentation have been described and may raise the differential diagnosis with other forms of leukemias.[26–28] This occurrence is more frequent in the small cell variant[29,30] and is associated with a poor prognosis.[28] Very rare cases of ALCL of the central nervous system have been described,[31] half of which were ALK positive. Most of these tumors had involvement of the dura or leptomeninges. In these cases, young age and ALK positivity were associated with a better

outcome.[31] Bone lesions are rare but can be solitary or multiple osteolytic lesions expressing T cell markers and ALK.[32]

ALK-negative systemic ALCL affects older patients and has a poorer clinical outcome (Table 76.1). This heterogeneous entity is frequently characterized by unfavorable clinical features and a high International Prognostic Index (IPI) score.[33] Its prognosis is closer to those of other peripheral T cell lymphomas than to that of ALK-positive ALCL.[21]

Outcome

Most investigators report high response rates to chemotherapy, with complete remission (CR) rates ranging from 70 percent to 90 percent.[10,15–18,22,23,34–37] Anaplastic large cell lymphoma is also considered to have a relatively favorable survival,[15,17,18] especially when compared to DLBCL or peripheral T cell lymphomas.[10,16] When ALK immunostaining became available it appeared that ALK expression was a major prognostic factor. As shown in Table 76.1, 5-year overall survival was significantly better for ALK-positive ALCL, being 71 percent compared to 30–40 percent for ALK-negative ALCL.

Prognostic factors

Several prognostic factors previously recognized in diffuse large cell lymphoma, such as age, Ann Arbor stage, B symptoms, performance status, and lactate dehydrogenase (LDH) level, have been identified in ALCL. The IPI,[38] designed for aggressive lymphoma, has been shown to be predictive in ALCL.[16,39] In ALK-positive ALCL, the 5-year survival reaches 94 percent for the low/low-intermediate group versus 41 percent for the high/high-intermediate group.[19]

At the present time, there is no firm correlation between morphologic subtypes or variant translocations and prognosis.[6,20] Cases of ALK-positive lymphoma that express fusion proteins other than ALK-NPM appear to share immunophenotypic features, clinical presentation, and a favorable outcome with typical ALK-NPM-positive ALCL.[40]

Table 76.1 Differences in presentation and outcome in ALK-positive and ALK-negative anaplastic large cell lymphomas

	Median age (years)		IPI (% HI–H)		CR rate (%)		5-year survival	
	ALK+	ALK−	ALK+	ALK−	ALK+	ALK−	ALK+	ALK−
Shiota et al.[8]	16	51	–	–	–	–	80	33
Falini et al.[19]	22	–	47	28	77	56	71	30
Gascoyne et al.[20]	30	61	–	–	–	–	93	37
ten Berge et al.[21]	23	54	8	36	92	68	90	40

IPI, International Prognostic Index; HI-H, high-intermediate–high; CR, complete remission.

Many biological markers have been associated with clinical presentation and outcome. For instance, serum levels of soluble CD30 (sCD30) are increased in most ALCL cases at diagnosis.[41,42] A high pretreatment sCD30 level has been reported to correlate with treatment failure and shorter survival.[42] CD30 belongs to the tumor necrosis factor (TNF) receptor superfamily whose members are involved in signal transduction events that can mediate apoptosis. It has been hypothesized that sCD30 could block CD30 ligand biologic activity and protect CD30-positive tumor cells from CD30 ligand-induced apoptosis.[43] Serum level of soluble interleukin-2, which is considered a marker of disease activity in CD25-positive malignancies, has been reported to correlate with sCD30 level in patients with ALK-positive ALCL.[44]

MUC-1 (also known as epithelial membrane antigen), is a transmembrane glycoprotein frequently expressed on cells from systemic forms of ALCL.[45–47] MUC-1 expression, as detected by immunohistochemistry, has been reported to be more commonly or exclusively found in ALK-positive ALCL.[47,48] It has been found to correlate with a favorable outcome, especially in ALK-negative ALCL.[48]

A number of other proteins also involved in apoptosis have been related to response to chemotherapy and outcome. ALK-positive lymphomas usually have a higher apoptotic rate (as determined by a modified TUNEL assay) compared with ALK-negative tumors.[49] ALK-positive and ALK-negative ALCL show marked differences in expression of the BCL2 family of proteins.[49,50] It has been shown that high expression of the antiapoptotic protein BCL2 is never found in ALK-positive ALCLs as compared with half of ALK-negative lymphomas.[49,50] However, as observed in DLBCL,[51] BCL2 expression strongly correlates with worse survival.[50] In the same way, the proapoptotic proteins BAX and $BCLX_S$ are more commonly expressed in ALK-positive lymphomas and the antiapoptotic protein $BCLX_L$ is more commonly expressed in ALK-negative tumors.[49] Furthermore, the level of caspase-3 activation has been reported to correlate to ALK status.[50] It could reflect the proper functioning of a major apoptotic pathway and be related to chemotherapy sensitivity, as suggested by the excellent outcome of patients with more than 5 percent of tumor cells expressing active caspase-3.[50]

Survivin is a protein that strongly inhibits apoptosis and its expression correlates with a poor survival in DLBCL.[52] Schlette et al.[53] have shown that survivin expression is a strong indicator of poor survival regardless of ALK status and IPI score.[53] The level of survivin expression also correlates with STAT3, a transcription factor activated by NPM-ALK in vitro.[54] An association between STAT3 activation and poor survival in ALK-positive and ALK-negative ALCL has also been observed by the MD Anderson Cancer Center group.[55]

Tumor suppressor genes may likewise play an important role in the prognosis of ALCL. The retinoblastoma protein (Rb) expression in lymphoma cells significantly correlates with an unfavorable outcome in both ALK-positive and ALK-negative ALCL.[56] Whereas the TP53 tumor suppressor gene is rarely mutated in ALCL, TP53 protein expression appears to be quite common in both ALK-positive and ALK-negative lymphomas.[57]

CD56, a neural cell adhesion molecule that is expressed in various lymphoid malignancies and is a marker of natural killer (NK) cells, has been found to be expressed in 25 out of 140 cases of ALCL.[58] In both ALK-positive and ALK-negative groups, CD56 expression predicted an unfavorable outcome.[58] A high percentage of activated cytotoxic T lymphocytes has also been shown to be an unfavorable prognostic marker in ALCL, but only in ALK-negative cases.[59]

Primary cutaneous anaplastic large cell lymphoma

Cutaneous ALCL is now included in the primary CD30+ lymphoproliferative disorders of the WHO-EORTC (European Organization for Research and Treatment in Cancer) classification of cutaneous lymphomas.[60] This classification considers cutaneous ALCL and lymphomatoid papulosis to be the extremes of a spectrum of diseases containing 'borderline cases.' Histologic and immunophenotypic characteristics are often not sufficient to distinguish between ALCL and lymphomatoid papulosis. Clinical appearance and outcome are often required to differentiate between the entities.

Primary cutaneous ALCL accounts for approximately 8 percent of cutaneous lymphomas.[60] It affects mainly adults, with a male predominance.[61] The most frequent form is a solitary nodule with superficial ulceration (Plate 133, see plate section) but multiple nodules in a limited area or multifocal tumors can occur.[62] As in lymphomatoid papulosis, spontaneous partial or complete regression of the skin tumors may occur. Extracutaneous dissemination of the disease, mainly to regional lymph nodes, is described in 10 percent of cases.[60]

By contrast, lymphomatoid papulosis generally presents as disseminated papules with a necrotic center.[62] The most typical characteristic is spontaneous regression of individual skin lesions within 3 to 12 weeks with frequent relapses.[60] The histologic features of lymphomatoid papulosis are variable but can be indistinguishable from those of ALCL. In these cases, the clinical course of the disease is important to differentiate between the entities. Primary cutaneous ALCL generally expresses the cutaneous lymphocyte antigen (CLA) but does not express EMA and ALK.[60] Translocations involving the ALK gene are usually not found.[63]

MANAGEMENT

Systemic anaplastic large cell lymphoma

Given the low frequency of ALCL in adults, no large prospective clinical trial has been published so far. The largest series have included up to a hundred patients and are either retrospective studies or subgroup analyses of large prospective trials in 'aggressive' lymphoma. Most of these studies were focused on description of prognostic factors, rather than evaluation of different treatments. Furthermore, the majority include patients with CD30-positive DLBCL or Hodgkin-like ALCL and do not distinguish between ALK-positive and ALK-negative ALCL.

Systemic ALCL is usually treated as an 'aggressive' lymphoma with a doxorubicin-containing chemotherapy regimen, e.g., CHOP, m-BACOD, MACOP-B, or ACVBP.[16–18,64,65] With such treatment, ALCL has a relatively favorable prognosis, at least when compared with DLBCL or other T cell lymphomas, with CR rates ranging from 70 percent to 80 percent and a 3-year survival of more than 65 percent (Table 76.2).

High-dose treatment (HDT) with autologous stem cell transplantation has been proposed for patients with ALCL but the superiority of this approach over conventional chemotherapy remains to be prospectively assessed. Early reports, in patients treated in first remission, gave impressive results, with 100 percent CR rates and absence of relapse after a median follow-up of 3 years.[66] Further studies confirmed that HDT as consolidation of first remission could provide a high CR rate and an event-free survival of more than 70 percent.[37,67] A report of the European Group for Blood and Bone Marrow Transplant also showed that HDT was able to induce prolonged remission in patients with relapsed or refractory disease.[68] However, it has been shown more recently that HDT failed to achieve long-term disease-free survival in patients with chemotherapy-sensitive, recurrent ALK-negative ALCL.[69]

Cutaneous anaplastic large cell lymphoma

Surgical excision or electron beam therapy, sometimes used in combination, are the treatments of choice for solitary or localized disease.[60] Some authors recommend a period of observation initially in order to allow for possible spontaneous regression.[70]

Several treatments have been proposed for multifocal cutaneous ALCL. Radiation therapy could be used in cases with limited regional extension. Systemic therapy with low-dose oral methotrexate has been proposed, as in lymphomatoid papulosis, leading to prolonged remissions.[71] Anthracycline-based chemotherapy has been considered as the classical treatment for multifocal cutaneous lesions.[62,72] However, there is strong evidence that most patients treated in this way experience further relapse in the skin. This approach is still recommended in patients with rapidly progressing cutaneous disease or with extracutaneous involvement.[60] Complete remissions in patients with cutaneous ALCL treated with 13-cis retinoic acid,[73] bexacarotene, and interferon α[74] or with anti-CD30[75] have also been described.

Targeted therapies

As is already the case for B cell lymphomas, it is likely that targeted treatments will have an important place in the future management of adult ALCL.

ANTI–CD30 THERAPIES

As CD30 is selectively overexpressed on anaplastic lymphoma cells, it represents a promising target for

Table 76.2   Outcome characteristics in the largest series of adult anaplastic large cell lymphomas

	n	Number null/T cell	Median age	Chemotherapy	CR rate	FFP %	Survival %
Shulman et al.[18]	31	21	44	CHOP m-BACOD ProMACE-CytaBOM	81	48 (3 yr)	70 (3 yr)
Zinzani et al.[17]	47	35	47	MACOP-B F-MACHOP	70	68 (3 yr)	60 (3 yr)
Clavio et al.[65]	53	44	–	Various regimens	78	–	70 (3 yr)
Tilly et al.[16]	146	82	–	ACVBP m-BACOD Various regimens	75	–	66 (5 yr)
Longo et al.[64]	36	26	42	MOPP/EBV/CAD	78	–	69 (3 yr)

ACVBP: doxorubicin, cyclophosphamide, vincristine, bleomycin, prednisone; CAD: lomustine, doxorubicin, vindesine; CHOP: cyclophosphamide, doxorubicin, vincristine, prednisone; CR, complete remission; EBV: epidoxirubicin, bleomycin, vinblastine; FFP, freedom from progression; F-MACHOP: vincristine, cyclophosphamide, fluorouracil, cytarabine, doxorubicin, methotrexate with leucovorin, prednisone; MACOP-B: methotrexate with leucovorin, doxorubicin, cyclophosphamide, vincristine, bleomycin, prednisone; m-BACOD: methotrexate, bleomycin, cyclophosphamide, doxorubicin, vincristine, dexamethasone; MOPP: L-asparaginase and mechlorethamine, vincristine, prednisone, procarbazine; ProMACE-CytaBOM: cyclophosphamide, doxorubicin, etoposide cytozar, bleomycin, vincristine, methotrexate; yr, year.

immunotherapy.[76] Two monoclonal antibodies, humanized SGN030 and human 5F11, have been generated to target CD30-positive cells in Hodgkin lymphoma and ALCL. Phase II studies in cutaneous and systemic ALCL are ongoing but promising clinical responses have already been reported.[75,77,78] As described for rituximab in DLBCL, anti-CD30 could sensitize lymphoma cells to cytotoxic agents.[79,80]

Several different approaches to enhance the efficacy of monoclonal antibodies have been developed: combination to bortezomib in order to increase apoptosis,[81] combination of the antibody with a toxin[82,83] or cytotoxic drug,[84] radiolabeling,[85] and bispecific constructs.[86]

ALK–TARGETED THERAPIES

The constitutive expression of ALK, induced by chromosomal translocations, in ALK-positive ALCL appears to play a crucial role in cell proliferation and survival.[87] It is conceivable that inhibition of ALK tyrosine kinase activity would lead to biologic changes capable of inhibiting cell growth or inducing apoptosis. *In vitro* attempts to silence the expression of ALK have been described recently using RNA interference[88] or 'small hairpin RNA.'[89] This latter approach has been shown to induce apoptosis and inhibition of tumor growth in ALCL cells.[89] In the same way, targeting the transcription factor STAT3, an important substrate of ALK activity, with antisense oligonucleotide, could inhibit the growth of human NPM-ALK tumors *in vivo*.[90]

ALK protein could also be considered to be a lymphoma-associated antigen[91] which could induce a T cell response and lead to anti-ALK vaccination strategies.[92]

KEY POINTS

- Anaplastic large cell lymphoma (ALCL) accounts for 2–3 percent of adult non-Hodgkin lymphomas.
- Only tumors of T cell or null-cell phenotype are recognized as ALCL in the WHO classification.
- ALK expression determines clinical presentation and outcome.
- Systemic ALK-positive ALCL has a rather favorable outcome but the prognosis of ALK-negative ALCL is comparable to that of other T cell lymphomas.
- Cutaneous ALCL could be indistinguishable from lymphomatoid papulosis.
- Currently, treatment of systemic ALCL is chemotherapy but development of targeted therapies is in progress.

REFERENCES

● = Key primary paper
◆ = Major review article

●1. Stein H, Mason DY, Gerdes J et al. The expression of the Hodgkin's disease associated antigen Ki-1 in reactive and neoplastic lymphoid tissue: evidence that Reed-Sternberg cells and histiocytic malignancies are derived from activated lymphoid cells. *Blood* 1985; **66**: 848–58.

2. Rimokh R, Magaud JP, Berger F et al. A translocation involving a specific breakpoint (q35) on chromosome 5 is characteristic of anaplastic large cell lymphoma ('Ki-1 lymphoma'). *Br J Haematol* 1989; **71**: 31–6.

3. Kaneko E, Frizzera G, Edamura S et al. A novel translocation, t(2;5)(p23;q35), in childhood phagocytic large T-cell lymphoma mimicking malignant histiocytosis. *Blood* 1989; **73**: 806–13.

●4. Morris SW, Kirstein MN, Valentine MB et al. Fusion of a kinase gene, ALK, to a nucleolar protein gene, NPM, in non-Hodgkin's lymphoma. *Science* 1994; **263**: 1281–4.

◆5. Stein H. CD30+ anaplastic large cell lymphoma: a review of its histopathologic, genetic, and clinical features. *Blood* 2000; **96**: 3681–95.

6. Falini B. Anaplastic large cell lymphoma: pathological, molecular and clinical features. *Br J Haematol* 2001; **114**: 741–60.

7. Pulford K, Lamant L, Espinos E et al. The emerging normal and disease-related roles of anaplastic lymphoma kinase. *Cell Mol Life Sci* 2004; **61**: 2939–53.

8. Shiota M, Nakamura S, Ichinohasama R et al. Anaplastic large cell lymphomas expressing the novel chimeric protein p80NPM/ALK: a distinct clinicopathologic entity. *Blood* 1995; **86**: 1954–60.

◆9. Delsol G, Ralfkiaer E, Stein H et al. *Anaplastic large cell lymphoma*. Lyon: IARC Press, 2001.

10. The Non-Hodgkin's Lymphoma Classification P. A Clinical Evaluation of the International Lymphoma Study Group Classification of Non-Hodgkin's Lymphoma. *Blood* 1997; **89**: 3909–18.

11. Benharroch D, Meguerian-Bedoyan Z, Lamant L et al. ALK-positive lymphoma: a single disease with a broad spectrum of morphology. *Blood* 1998; **91**: 2076–84.

12. Foss HD, Anagnostopoulos I, Araujo I et al. Anaplastic large cell lymphomas of T-cell and null-cell phenotype express cytotoxic molecule. *Blood* 1996; **88**: 4005–11.

●13. Kutok JL, Aster JC. Molecular biology of anaplastic lymphoma kinase-positive anaplastic large-cell lymphoma. *J Clin Oncol* 2002; **20**: 3691–702.

14. Duyster J, Bai RY, Morris SW. Translocations involving anaplastic lymphoma kinase (ALK). *Oncogene* 2001; **20**: 5623–37.

15. Greer JP, Kinney MC, Collins RD et al. Clinical features of 31 patients with Ki-1 anaplastic large-cell lymphoma. *J Clin Oncol* 1991; **9**: 539–47.

16. Tilly H, Gaulard P, Lepage E *et al.* Primary anaplastic large-cell lymphoma in adults: clinical presentation, immunophenotype, and outcome. *Blood* 1997; **90**: 3727–34.

17. Zinzani PL, Bendandi M, Martelli M *et al.* Anaplastic large-cell lymphoma: clinical and prognostic evaluation of 90 adult patients. *J Clin Oncol* 1996; **14**: 955–62.

18. Shulman LN, Frisard B, Antin JH *et al.* Primary Ki-1 anaplastic large-cell lymphoma in adults: clinical characteristics and therapeutic outcome. *J Clin Oncol* 1993; **11**: 937–42.

●19. Falini B, Pileri S, Zinzani PL *et al.* ALK+ lymphoma: clinico-pathological findings and outcome. *Blood* 1999; **93**: 2697–706.

20. Gascoyne RD, Aoun P, Wu D *et al.* Prognostic significance of anaplastic lymphoma kinase (ALK) protein expression in adults with anaplastic large cell lymphoma. *Blood* 1999; **93**: 3913–21.

21. ten Berge RL, de Bruin PC, Oudejans JJ *et al.* ALK-negative anaplastic large-cell lymphoma demonstrates similar poor prognosis to peripheral T-cell lymphoma, unspecified. *Histopathology* 2003; **43**: 462–9.

22. Chott A, Kaserer K, Augustin I *et al.* Ki-1 positive large-cell lymphoma. A clinicopathologic study of 41 cases. *Am J Surg Pathol* 1990; **14**: 439–48.

23. Pileri S, Bocchia M, Baroni CD *et al.* Anaplastic large cell lymphoma (CD30+/Ki-1+): results of a prospective clinico-pathological study of 69 cases. *Br J Haematol* 1994; **86**: 513–23.

24. Fraga M, Brousset P, Schlaifer D *et al.* Bone marrow involvement in anaplastic large cell lymphoma. Immunohistochemical detection of minimal disease and its prognostic significance. *Am J Clin Pathol* 1995; **103**: 82–9.

25. Mussolin L, Pillon M, d'Amore E *et al.* Prevalence and clinical implications of bone marrow involvement in pediatric anaplastic large cell lymphoma. *Leukemia* 2005; **19**: 1643–7.

26. Anderson MM, Ross CW, Singleton TP *et al.* Ki-1 anaplastic large cell lymphoma with a prominent leukemic phase. *Hum Pathol* 1996; **27**: 1093–5.

27. Villamor N, Rozman M, Esteve J *et al.* Anaplastic large-cell lymphoma with rapid evolution to leukemic phase. *Ann Hematol* 1999; **78**: 478–82.

28. Onciu M, Behm F, Raimondi SC *et al.* ALK-positive anaplastic large-cell lymphoma with leukemic peripheral blood involvement is a clinicopathologic entity with an unfavorable prognosis. *Am J Clin Pathol* 2003; **120**: 617–25.

29. Kinney MC, Collins RD, Greer JP *et al.* A small-cell-predominant variant of primary Ki-1 (CD30)+ T-cell lymphoma. *Am J Surg Pathol* 1993; **17**: 859–68.

30. Awaya N, Mori S, Takeuchi H *et al.* CD30 and the NPM-ALK fusion protein (p80) are differentially expressed between peripheral blood and bone marrow in primary small cell variant of anaplastic large cell lymphoma. *Am J Hematol* 2002; **69**: 200–4.

31. George DH, Scheithauer BW, Aker FV *et al.* Primary anaplastic large cell lymphoma of the central nervous system: prognostic effect of ALK-1 expression. *Am J Surg Pathol* 2003; **27**: 487–93.

32. Nagasaka T, Nakamura S, Medeiros LJ *et al.* Anaplastic large cell lymphomas presented as bone lesions: a clinicopathologic study of six cases and review of the literature. *Mod Pathol* 2000; **13**: 1143–9.

33. ten Berge RL, Oudejans JJ, Ossenkoppele GJ, Meijer CJ. ALK-negative systemic anaplastic large cell lymphoma: differential diagnostic and prognostic aspects – a review. *J Pathol* 2003; **200**: 4–15.

34. Nakamura S, Shiota M, Nakagawa A *et al.* Anaplastic large cell lymphoma: a distinct molecular pathologic entity: a reappraisal with special reference to p80(NPM/ALK) expression. *Am J Surg Pathol* 1997; **21**: 1420–32.

35. Romaguera JE, Manning JT Jr, Tornos CS *et al.* Long-term prognostic importance of primary Ki-1 (CD30) antigen expression and anaplastic morphology in adult patients with diffuse large-cell lymphoma. *Ann Oncol* 1994; **5**: 317–22.

36. Tirelli U, Vaccher E, Zagonel V *et al.* CD30 (Ki-1)-positive anaplastic large-cell lymphomas in 13 patients with and 27 patients without human immunodeficiency virus infection: the first comparative clinicopathologic study from a single institution that also includes 80 patients with other human immunodeficiency virus-related systemic lymphomas. *J Clin Oncol* 1995; **13**: 373–80.

37. Fanin R, Sperotto A, Silvestri F *et al.* The therapy of primary adult systemic CD30-positive anaplastic large cell lymphoma: results of 40 cases treated in a single center. *Leuk Lymphoma* 1999; **35**: 159–69.

38. The International Non-Hodgkin's Lymphoma Prognostic Factors Project. A predictive model for aggressive non-Hodgkin's lymphoma. *N Engl J Med* 1993; **329**: 987–94.

39. Lee SC, Kueh YK, Lehnert M *et al.* Characteristics and prognosis of KI-1 positive anaplastic large cell lymphoma in Asians. *Aust N Z J Med* 1998; **28**: 790–4.

●40. Falini B, Pulford K, Pucciarini A *et al.* Lymphomas expressing ALK fusion protein(s) other than NPM-ALK. *Blood* 1999; **94**: 3509–15.

41. Nadali G, Vinante F, Stein H *et al.* Serum levels of the soluble form of CD30 molecule as a tumor marker in CD30+ anaplastic large-cell lymphoma. *J Clin Oncol* 1995; **13**: 1355–60.

42. Zinzani PL, Pileri S, Bendandi M *et al.* Clinical implications of serum levels of soluble CD30 in 70 adult anaplastic large-cell lymphoma patients. *J Clin Oncol* 1998; **16**: 1532–7.

43. Younes A, Consoli U, Snell V *et al.* CD30 ligand in lymphoma patients with CD30+ tumors. *J Clin Oncol* 1997; **15**: 3355–62.

44. Janik JE, Morris JC, Pittaluga S *et al.* Elevated serum-soluble interleukin-2 receptor levels in patients with anaplastic large cell lymphoma. *Blood* 2004; **104**: 3355–7.

45. Delsol G, Al Saati T, Gatter KC et al. Coexpression of epithelial membrane antigen (EMA), Ki-1, and interleukin-2 receptor by anaplastic large cell lymphomas. Diagnostic value in so-called malignant histiocytosis. Am J Pathol 1988; 130: 59–70.

46. de Bruin PC, Beljaards RC, van Heerde P et al. Differences in clinical behaviour and immunophenotype between primary cutaneous and primary nodal anaplastic large cell lymphoma of T-cell or null cell phenotype. Histopathology 1993; 23: 127–35.

47. ten Berge RL, Oudejans JJ, Dukers DF et al. Percentage of activated cytotoxic T-lymphocytes in anaplastic large cell lymphoma and Hodgkin's disease: an independent biological prognostic marker. Leukemia 2001; 15: 458–64.

48. Rassidakis GZ, Goy A, Medeiros LJ et al. Prognostic significance of MUC-1 expression in systemic anaplastic large cell lymphoma. Clin Cancer Res 2003; 9: 2213–20.

49. Rassidakis GZ, Sarris AH, Herling M et al. Differential expression of BCL-2 family proteins in ALK-positive and ALK-negative anaplastic large cell lymphoma of T/null-cell lineage. Am J Pathol 2001; 159: 527–35.

50. ten Berge RL, Meijer CJ, Dukers DF et al. Expression levels of apoptosis-related proteins predict clinical outcome in anaplastic large cell lymphoma. Blood 2002; 99: 4540–6.

51. Hermine O, Haioun C, Lepage E et al. Prognostic significance of bcl-2 protein expression in aggressive non-Hodgkin's lymphoma. Groupe d'Etude des Lymphomes de l'Adulte (GELA). Blood 1996; 87: 265–72.

52. Adida C, Haioun C, Gaulard P et al. Prognostic significance of survivin expression in diffuse large B-cell lymphomas. Blood 2000; 96: 1921–5.

53. Schlette EJ, Medeiros LJ, Goy A et al. Survivin expression predicts poorer prognosis in anaplastic large-cell lymphoma. J Clin Oncol 2004; 22: 1682–8.

54. Zamolo G, Gruber F, Bosner A et al. CD30-positive cutaneous anaplastic large cell lymphoma with ichthyosis acquisita. Tumori 1999; 85: 71–4.

55. Khoury JD, Medeiros LJ, Rassidakis GZ et al. Differential expression and clinical significance of tyrosine-phosphorylated STAT3 in ALK+ and ALK- anaplastic large cell lymphoma. Clin Cancer Res 2003; 9: 3692–9.

56. Rassidakis GZ, Lai R, Herling M et al. Retinoblastoma protein is frequently absent or phosphorylated in anaplastic large-cell lymphoma. Am J Pathol 2004; 164: 2259–67.

57. Rassidakis GZ, Thomaides A, Wang S et al. p53 gene mutations are uncommon but p53 is commonly expressed in anaplastic large cell lymphoma. Leukemia 2005; 19: 1663–9.

58. Suzuki R, Kagami Y, Takeuchi K et al. Prognostic significance of CD56 expression for ALK-positive and ALK-negative anaplastic large-cell lymphoma of T/null cell phenotype. Blood 2000; 96: 2993–3000.

59. ten Berge RL, Dukers DF, Oudejans JJ et al. Adverse effects of activated cytotoxic T lymphocytes on the clinical outcome of nodal anaplastic large cell lymphoma. Blood 1999; 93: 2688–96.

◆60. Willemze R, Jaffe ES, Burg G et al. WHO-EORTC classification for cutaneous lymphomas. Blood 2005; 105: 3768–85.

61. Willemze R, Meijer CJ. Primary cutaneous CD30-positive lymphoproliferative disorders. Hematol Oncol Clin North Am 2003; 17: 1319–32, vii–viii.

62. Paulli M, Berti E, Rosso R et al. CD30/Ki-1-positive lymphoproliferative disorders of the skin – clinicopathologic correlation and statistical analysis of 86 cases: a multicentric study from the European Organization for Research and Treatment of Cancer Cutaneous Lymphoma Project Group. J Clin Oncol 1995; 13: 1343–54.

63. DeCoteau JF, Butmarc JR, Kinney MC, Kadin ME. The t(2;5) chromosomal translocation is not a common feature of primary cutaneous CD30+ lymphoproliferative disorders: comparison with anaplastic large-cell lymphoma of nodal origin. Blood 1996; 87: 3437–41.

64. Longo G, Fiorani C, Sacchi S et al. Clinical characteristics, treatment outcome and survival of 36 adult patients with primary anaplastic large cell lymphoma. Gruppo Italiano per lo Studio dei Linfomi (GISL). Haematologica 1999; 84: 425–30.

65. Clavio M, Rossi E, Truini M et al. Anaplastic large cell lymphoma: a clinicopathologic study of 53 patients. Leuk Lymphoma 1996; 22: 319–27.

66. Fanin R, Silvestri F, Geromin A et al. Primary systemic CD30 (Ki-1)-positive anaplastic large cell lymphoma of the adult: sequential intensive treatment with the F-MACHOP regimen (+/− radiotherapy) and autologous bone marrow transplantation. Blood 1996; 87: 1243–8.

67. Deconinck E, Lamy T, Foussard C et al. Autologous stem cell transplantation for anaplastic large-cell lymphomas: results of a prospective trial. Br J Haematol 2000; 109: 736–42.

68. Fanin R, Ruiz de Elvira MC, Sperotto A et al. Autologous stem cell transplantation for T and null cell CD30-positive anaplastic large cell lymphoma: analysis of 64 adult and paediatric cases reported to the European Group for Blood and Marrow Transplantation (EBMT). Bone Marrow Transplant 1999; 23: 437–42.

69. Zamkoff KW, Matulis MD, Mehta AD et al. High-dose therapy and autologous stem cell transplant does not result in long-term disease-free survival in patients with recurrent chemotherapy-sensitive ALK-negative anaplastic large-cell lymphoma. Bone Marrow Transplant 2004; 33: 635–8.

70. Bekkenk MW, Geelen FAMJ, Van Voorst Vader PC et al. Primary and secondary cutaneous CD30+ lymphoproliferative disorders: a report of the Dutch Cutaneous Lymphoma Group on the long-term follow-up data of 219 patients and guidelines for diagnosis and treatment. Blood 2000; 95: 3653–61.

71. Vonderheid EC, Sajjadian A, Kadin ME. Methotrexate is effective therapy for lymphomatoid papulosis and other primary cutaneous CD30-positive lymphoproliferative disorders. J Am Acad Dermatol 1996; 34: 470–81.

72. Willemze R, Beljaards RC. Spectrum of primary cutaneous CD30 (Ki-1) positive lymphoproliferative disorders; a proposal for classification and guidelines for management and treatment. J Am Acad Dermatol 1993; 28: 973–86.

73. Chou WC, Su IJ, Tien HF *et al.* Clinicopathologic, cytogenetic, and molecular studies of 13 Chinese patients with Ki-1 anaplastic large cell lymphoma. Special emphasis on the tumor response to 13-cis retinoic acid. *Cancer* 1996; **78**: 1805–12.

74. French LE, Shapiro M, Junkins-Hopkins JM *et al.* Regression of multifocal, skin-restricted, CD30 positive large T-cell lymphoma with interferon alfa and bexarotene therapy. *J Am Acad Dermatol* 2001; **45**: 914–18.

75. Shehan JM, Kalaaji AN, Markovic SN, Ahmed I. Management of multifocal primary cutaneous CD30 anaplastic large cell lymphoma. *J Am Acad Dermatol* 2004; **51**: 103–10.

76. Tian ZG, Longo DL, Funakoshi S *et al.* In vivo antitumor effects of unconjugated CD30 monoclonal antibodies on human anaplastic large-cell lymphoma xenografts. *Cancer Res* 1995; **55**: 5335–41.

77. Duvic M, Kunishige J, Kim YH *et al.* Preliminary phase II results of SGN-30 (anti-CD30 monoclonal antibody) in patients with cutaneous anaplastic large cell lymphoma (ALCL). *Blood* 2005; **106**: 4802 (abstract).

78. Forero-Torres A, Bernstein SH, Gopal AK *et al.* SGN-30 (anti-CD30 monoclonal antibody) is active and well tolerated in patients with refractory or recurrent systemic anaplastic large cell lymphoma (ALCL). *Blood* 2005; **106**: 3356 (abstract).

79. Heuck F, Ellermann J, Borchmann P *et al.* Combination of the human anti-CD30 antibody 5F11 with cytostatic drugs enhances its antitumor activity against Hodgkin and anplastic large cell lymphoma cell lines. *J Immunother* 2004; **27**: 347–53.

80. Cerveny CG, Law CL, McCormick RS *et al.* Signaling via the anti-CD30 mAb SGN-30 sensitizes Hodgkin's disease cells to conventional chemotherapeutics. *Leukemia* 2005; **19**: 1648–55.

81. Boll B, Hansen H, Heuck F *et al.* The fully human anti-CD30 antibody 5F11 activates NF-kappaB and sensitizes lymphoma cells to bortezomib-induced apoptosis. *Blood* 2005; **106**: 1839–42.

82. Pasqualucci L, Wasik M, Teicher BA *et al.* Antitumor activity of anti-CD30 immunotoxin (Ber-H2/saporin) in vitro and in severe combined immunodeficiency disease mice xenografted with human CD30+ anaplastic large-cell lymphoma. *Blood* 1995; **85**: 2139–46.

83. Schnell R, Staak O, Borchmann P *et al.* A phase I study with an anti-CD30 ricin A-chain immunotoxin (Ki-4.dgA) in patients with refractory CD30+ Hodgkin's and non-Hodgkin's lymphoma. *Clin Cancer Res* 2002; **8**: 1779–86.

●84. Francisco JA, Cerveny CG, Meyer DL *et al.* cAC10-vcMMAE, an anti-CD30-monomethyl auristatin E conjugate with potent and selective antitumor activity. *Blood* 2003; **102**: 1458–65.

85. Schnell R, Dietlein M, Staak JO *et al.* Treatment of refractory Hodgkin's lymphoma patients with an Iodine-131-labeled murine anti-CD30 monoclonal antibody. *J Clin Oncol* 2005; **23**: 4669–78.

86. Hartmann F, Renner C, Jung W *et al.* Treatment of refractory Hodgkin's disease with an anti-CD16/CD30 bispecific antibody. *Blood* 1997; **89**: 2042–7.

87. Wan W, Albom MS, Lu L *et al.* Anaplastic lymphoma kinase activity is essential for the proliferation and survival of anaplastic large-cell lymphoma cells. *Blood* 2006; **107**: 1617–23.

88. Ritter U, Damm-Welk C, Fuchs U *et al.* Design and evaluation of chemically synthesized siRNA targeting the NPM-ALK fusion site in anaplastic large cell lymphoma (ALCL). *Oligonucleotides* 2003; **13**: 365–73.

●89. Piva R, Chiarle R, Manazza AD *et al.* Ablation of oncogenic ALK is a viable therapeutic approach for anaplastic large-cell lymphomas. *Blood* 2006; **107**: 689–97.

●90. Chiarle R, Simmons WJ, Cai H *et al.* Stat3 is required for ALK mediated lymphomagenesis and provides a possible therapeutic target. *Nat Med* 2005; **11**: 623–9.

91. Passoni L, Scardino A, Bertazzoli C *et al.* ALK as a novel lymphoma-associated tumor antigen: identification of 2 HLA-A2.1-restricted CD8+ T-cell epitopes. *Blood* 2002; **99**: 2100–6.

92. Passoni L, Gallo B, Biganzoli E *et al.* In vivo T-cell immune response against anaplastic lymphoma kinase in patients with anaplastic large cell lymphomas. *Haematologica* 2006; **91**: 48–55.

77

Anaplastic large cell lymphoma in children

ANGELO ROSOLEN

INTRODUCTION

Anaplastic large cell lymphoma (ALCL) as reported in the World Health Organization (WHO) classification[1] was first described by Stein et al.[2] in 1985 as a separate entity, defined by a frequently cohesive proliferation of large pleomorphic blasts and a constant expression of the CD30/Ki-1 antigen on the tumor cells.[3]

More recently, the reciprocal chromosomal translocation t(2;5)(p23;q35)[4,5] was described in the majority of cases and was later found to result in juxtaposition of the nucleophosmin (NPM) and the anaplastic lymphoma kinase (ALK) genes.[6,7] The chimeric protein resulting from the fusion gene can be identified by standard immunohistochemical techniques making this marker of great diagnostic value.[8–10]

Morphologically, several forms of anaplastic large cell lymphoma have been described.[11] The common type is the most frequent variant, representing about 70 percent of cases, followed by the small cell, lymphohistiocytic, giant cell, and mixed variants.[12–16] All of these forms are recognized in routine histologic diagnosis, but only the small cell and the lymphohistiocytic types are recognized in the WHO classification.[1]

Although ALCL is a rather recently described entity, a great deal of biological knowledge has been gained in this malignancy. It is not completely clear how the disease differs in children compared to adults in terms of histopathologic, clinical, and therapeutic features.

EPIDEMIOLOGY OF PEDIATRIC ANAPLASTIC LARGE CELL LYMPHOMA

Anaplastic large cell lymphoma accounts for approximately 10–15 percent of all non-Hodgkin lymphomas (NHL) in childhood[17–19] and corresponds to an incidence of 1.2–1.5 per million individuals younger than 15 years of age.[19] These figures may vary in different geographic areas, but little information is available and has mostly been obtained from relatively small patient populations.[20–22]

Although it was suggested that the incidence of ALCL may be higher in East- and Southeast-Asian children,[19] this was not confirmed in other studies.[23,24] The incidence of ALCL in Asia appears to be similar to that in Europe and North America, although some uncertainty remains over the incidence in Japan[25] and only occasional single-institution reports have been published concerning prevalence and incidence of ALCL in South America and Africa. Overall, there is insufficient information to demonstrate relevant differences in incidence worldwide.

BIOLOGY

Anaplastic lymphoma kinase

The most significant biological characteristic of ALCL is the expression of the anaplastic lymphoma kinase (ALK), a member of the insulin receptor superfamily of receptor tyrosine kinases[26] that can interfere with different biological activities including cell growth and proliferation, apoptosis, and specific gene transcription.[27,28] The kinase activity originates from a chimeric protein in which several partner proteins may be fused with the intracellular domain of ALK. These proteins characteristically possess oligomerization domains that are maintained in the chimeric protein. The product of the fusion gene NPM-ALK, originating from the chromosomal translocation t(2;5)(p23;q35), through its oligomerization domain brings together two ALK moieties which, as dimers, are active in several biological pathways and can ultimately express transforming activity.[29–31] Interestingly, the ALK chimeric protein localizes to different cell compartments, depending on the molecular characteristics of the partner protein: in the case of NPM, the fusion protein can be detected in the nucleus and in the cytoplasm. Nucleophosmin is a ubiquitously expressed nuclear protein associated with the nucleolus, whose major function is to shuttle continuously between the nucleolus and the cytoplasm carrying newly synthesized ribonuclear complexes, thereby playing a role in ribosome assembly.[32,33] The NPM-ALK fusion transcript encodes a chimeric polypeptide of 80 kDa (p80) consisting of the N-terminal portion of NPM and the C-terminal portion of ALK, which includes the entire ALK intracellular domain.[7,34] The NPM-ALK fusion proteins are also heavily phosphorylated on tyrosine residues, consistent with constitutive activation of the ALK kinase.[35] Alternative fusion partners for ALK include the clathrin heavy polypeptide-like gene (CLTC),[36] the non-muscle tropomyosin 3 and 4 genes (TPM3,[37] TPM4[38]), moesin (MSN),[39] Trk fusion gene (TFG),[40] the non-muscle myosin heavy chain gene (MYH9),[41] and 5-aminoimidazole-4-carboxamide-1-beta-D-ribonucleotide transformylase/IMP cyclohydrolase gene (ATIC).[42] The lack of nuclear localization signal in all identified ALK-variant fusion proteins accounts for their cytoplasmic-restricted expression, while their specific intracellular localization can influence the immunohistochemical staining pattern of anti-ALK antibody. The NPM-ALK fusion protein can be detected with high sensitivity by immunohistochemistry using anti-ALK antibodies whereas, occasionally and limited to variant fusion proteins, this approach fails to demonstrate an ALK-containing protein in cells where fluorescence in situ hybridization (FISH) or reverse transcription polymerase chain reaction (RT-PCR) can identify an ALK rearrangement.[27,28]

Although the majority of ALCL are positive for ALK rearrangements, the percentage varies between adult and pediatric cases, ALK positivity being detected in 60–70 percent of ALCL in adults[8,9] and as many as 90–95 percent of childhood ALCL.[43] The NPM-ALK is the commonest chimeric protein expressed in ALCL, independent of patient age, and accounts for approximately 85 percent of all ALK-positive cases.[12,44,45]

Among the ALK-negative ALCL, primary cutaneous and ALK-negative ALCL are rare entities in childhood.[46]

Functional activity of ALK in anaplastic large cell lymphoma cells

Dimerization of ALK is a prerequisite for autophosphorylation and constitutive activation of the ALK tyrosine kinase. Activated ALK binds several adapter proteins including phospholipase Cγ (PLCγ), phosphatidylinositol 3-kinase (PI3K)/Akt, signal transducer and activator of transcription 3 (STAT3), insulin receptor substrate 1 (IRS1), growth factor receptor-bound protein 2 (Grb2), and sarcoma gene (SRC). When bound to adapter proteins, NPM-ALK can activate different signaling pathways involved in cell proliferation, survival, inhibition of apoptosis, and transformation.[27,47–49] As to the transforming activity of NPM-ALK, it was recently demonstrated that transduction of the fusion gene has the ability to induce tumors in mice after a variable latency, partially related to the mouse model used.[31,50] Furthermore, it was demonstrated that very low levels of NPM-ALK transcript can be detected in blood and lymphoid tissues of healthy individuals.[51,52] These and other findings suggest that, despite the presence of the NPM-ALK fusion gene, additional genetic alterations are required to result in complete transformation, such as the activation and overexpression of the Myc protooncogene.[53] Given the involvement of NPM-ALK in both proliferation and antiapoptotic functions, this fusion product as well as its adapter proteins represent targets against which to develop specific therapeutic approaches.

In addition to ALK's direct involvement in signal transduction and in a number of cell functions related to the tumor phenotype, ALK overexpression can elicit a host immune reaction giving rise to autologous anti-ALK antibodies in patients with ALK-positive ALCL.[9,54] This may in part explain the apparently favorable prognosis of ALK-positive ALCL patients, but may also represent the basis for a possible vaccination approach to this tumor.[55]

CLINICAL PRESENTATION

Primary systemic ALCL represents approximately 3–8 percent of all lymphomas and accounts for 10–15 percent of NHL in childhood. The median age of ALCL patients is lower compared to most other NHL subtypes. Age distribution is bimodal with a large peak in the second and third decades and a second, smaller peak in the sixth and seventh decades.[56–59] A male predominance is usually observed with a male/female ratio of 1.5–2:1 in most patient series reported in the literature.[60–64]

Anaplastic large cell lymphoma usually presents with enlarged peripheral and abdominal lymph nodes[16,65] and this is also the case for children, in whom lymph node involvement occurs in 70–90 percent of the cases.[60–63,66] Mediastinal involvement, although less frequent than in Hodgkin lymphoma, is reported in 30–40 percent of children. Extranodal involvement is observed in approximately 60 percent of cases:[61,63,64] frequent sites of disease are spleen (10–20 percent of cases), liver (15–25 percent), lung (10–15 percent), bone (10–15 percent), and skin (15–30 percent) (Table 77.1). The prevalence of extranodal disease varies in different patient series and this may be due in part to the different methods of assessment used (Table 77.1). In particular, liver and spleen involvement is considered positive in a portion of cases based on significant organ enlargement in the absence of nodular lesions, whereas histologic assessment is not usually required. Bone marrow (BM) can also be involved, but significantly less frequently than in other NHL subtypes, accounting for approximately 10 percent of the patients. Because ALCL cells are difficult to distinguish in a bone marrow smear based on the sole morphologic analysis, prevalence of BM involvement increases as immunocytochemical studies are carried out using anti-CD30 and/or anti-ALK antibodies. In such conditions as many as 30 percent of patients were found to have microscopic BM infiltration.[67] If other high-sensitivity methods are used, such as RT-PCR, for the identification of *NPM-ALK* transcript, the prevalence of BM involvement can be as high as 60 percent.[68]

A leukemic presentation is also possible but very uncommon[69–72] and is usually characterized by a very aggressive clinical course and poor prognosis. It is often associated with the small cell variant.[70–72]

The central nervous system (CNS) is not an elective site of disease and its infrequent involvement is confirmed by the patient series published so far,[60–64] with only occasional case reports of primary CNS ALCL.[73–75] This has practical implications for CNS prophylaxis in ALCL.

B symptoms, including fever, weight loss, and night sweats as defined for Hodgkin lymphoma,[76] are present at diagnosis in approximately two-thirds of the cases.[61–64] Pruritus has also been reported in pediatric ALCL and occasionally may be one of the first symptoms.[77]

Overall, all the signs and symptoms described above refer to systemic ALCL of childhood, which are in the great majority ALK positive, but they are similar in terms of prevalence and quality in adults with ALK-positive ALCL. These findings suggest that ALK-positive ALCL may have a very similar clinical presentation independent of patient age.

Besides the more common systemic ALCL, a second distinct clinical form of primary ALCL is that limited to the skin.[78] This is different from the ALCL cases where lymph node or extranodal sites are combined with skin lesions at diagnosis.[79]

Isolated CD30-positive lesions of the skin appear as a different clinical entity both in terms of the histopathologic characteristics and for their prognosis. CD30-positive cutaneous lymphoproliferative disorders cover a wide spectrum of lesions ranging from primary cutaneous ALCL to lymphomatoid papulosis, including the so called 'borderline lesions'; that is, lesions that cannot

Table 77.1   Anaplastic large cell lymphoma in childhood: clinical characteristics

Study	n	Age (years)	M/F	Stage I–II/ III–IV[a]	High LDH (%)	B symptoms (%)	Skin involvement (%)	BM involvement (%)	Mediastinum involvement (%)
Vecchi *et al.* 1993[109]	13	3–12	1.2	8/5	9	0	0	0	15
Sandlund *et al.* 1994[122]	18	2–20	2.6	4/14	5		27	5	33
Reiter *et al.* 1994[61]	62	0.8–17.6	2	26/36	na	42	21	0	29
Brugières *et al.* 1998[63]	82	1.5–17	0.6	23/59	18	68	33	16	39
Massimino *et al.* 1995[105]	27	2.6–16.7[c]	2	11/16	na	65	40	0	15
Seidemann *et al.* 2001[62]	89	0.8–17.3	2.3	28/61	10	52	18	6	32
Williams *et al.* 2002[64]	72	1.1–16.4	1.3	15/57	na	50	25	1	40
Mora *et al.* 2000[124]	19	5–19	na	0/19	na	na	5	0	42
Laver *et al.* 2005[121]	86	1–19	na	0/86[b]	45	47	11	na	61
Rosolen *et al.* 2005[66]	34	4.2–14.9	1.1	10/24	36	na	12	6	47

[a]St. Jude stage; [b]Patient series including only advanced stage disease.
[c]Age range was evaluated on the entire series of 32 anaplastic large cell lymphoma (ALCL) patients, including 5 nonevaluable children.
M/F, male/female; LDH, lactate dehydrogenase; N, normal; BM, bone marrow; na, not available.

clearly be assigned to the first two categories at their onset,[80,81] although a wait-and-see approach will often clarify their nature as ALCL or lymphomatoid papulosis. Characteristically, isolated CD30-positive skin lesions tend to occur in older patients (median age in the seventh decade), with a male predominance.[82,83] Approximately 20 percent of patients experience spontaneous regression of the primary lesion. However, more than half of the patients experience recurrences, often in the same anatomic site as the initial lesion, whereas 20–25 percent eventually develop systemic lymphoma. These clinical features are typical also of the infrequent isolated CD30-positive skin lesions in children. In addition, isolated CD30-positive skin lesions are almost invariably ALK negative both in adults and in children,[84–86] although occasional pediatric cases have been reported harboring the t(2;5) translocation in their genome.[87] Overall, patients with primary cutaneous ALCL have a better prognosis compared to those with systemic ALCL and this, along with the tendency to spontaneous regression, should be considered in order to decide the best therapeutic approach for this specific clinical entity.[88]

Secondary ALCL occurs mostly in the elderly and results from malignant transformation of other lymphomas, including Hodgkin lymphoma, mycosis fungoides, peripheral T cell lymphomas, or isolated CD30-positive skin lesions and lymphomatoid papulosis.[12,28,89] They are usually ALK negative and have a poor prognosis.[9]

Anaplastic large cell lymphoma has been reported in patients with acquired immunodeficiency syndrome[90–92] but these lymphomas are rare, particularly in childhood, and mostly ALK negative. Similarly, post-transplant lymphomas are rarely of the ALCL subtype, although exceptionally ALK-positive ALCL can occur.[93,94]

DIAGNOSIS

Diagnosis of ALCL rests mostly on standard morphologic and immunohistochemical analyses. Some clinical characteristics at presentation may, however, suggest the hypothesis of a possible ALCL. The presence of lymph node enlargement that can partially spontaneously regress, with or without B symptoms and/or mediastinum, liver, lung, or skin involvement, are suggestive clinical features of ALCL at disease onset, although, except for skin involvement, these signs and symptoms are more common in Hodgkin lymphoma. As to the lymphadenopathy, the inguinal localization is more typical of ALCL and infrequent in Hodgkin lymphoma.[95]

Independently from the WHO-recognized variants, several morphologic subtypes of ALCL have been described.[28] A notable diagnostic feature of ALCL is the frequent partial involvement of the lymph node and the propensity of tumor cells to invade the lymph node sinuses.[2]

Histologically, the common type represents about 70 percent of all ALCL and is characterized by pleomorphic, large tumor cells with abundant cytoplasm and horseshoe- or kidney-shaped nuclei (Fig. 77.1). Cells with such cytologic features are often referred to as hallmark cells[13] and can be detected in all morphologic variants of ALCL. Erythrophagocytosis can also be found.

Immunophenotype determination is mandatory for a correct diagnosis of ALCL and to differentiate ALCL from other diseases such as Hodgkin lymphoma or other forms of large cell lymphomas. Among the mandatory antibodies to be used for the diagnosis, there are anti-B cell and anti-T cell antibodies and antibodies to CD30, CD15, EMA (epithelial membrane antigen), ALK, and LMP-1 (latent membrane protein 1 of Epstein–Barr virus) or EBER (EBV encoded early small RNA) (Table 77.2). These markers are relevant not only for the initial diagnosis of ALCL – that is, characteristically of T or null-cell phenotype and CD30 positive – but are critical in the differential diagnosis between ALCL and Hodgkin lymphoma. The latter is also CD30 positive, but in most instances is CD15 positive and EMA negative, whereas ALCL is usually EMA positive and CD15 negative.

Other markers used for better diagnostic and prognostic characterization of ALCL include T cell markers and antibodies recognizing proteins associated with cytotoxic granules (perforin, granzyme), proliferation-associated antigens, and BNH-9 (Table 77.2).

Certainly the most relevant tool now available for the diagnosis of ALCL is the ALK-1 (or other anti-ALK) antibody (Fig. 77.1). By this means we can identify the presence of chimeric proteins containing ALK sequences

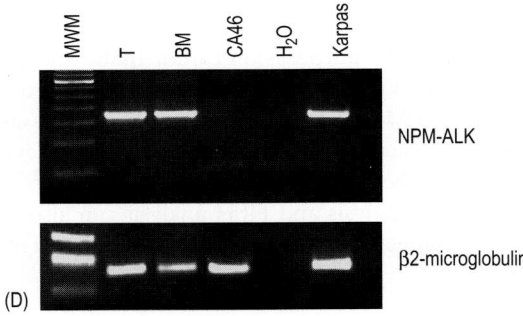

Figure 77.1 Histologic and molecular analysis of anaplastic large cell lymphoma (ALCL). (A) Plate 134. (B) Plate 134. (C) Plate 134. (D) Reverse transcription polymerase chain reaction (RT-PCR) analysis of *NPM-ALK* transcript derived from the t(2;5) chromosomal translocation in a case of pediatric ALCL. The tumor (T) expressed the chimeric transcript that was used for the study of minimal disseminated disease in the bone marrow (BM), which was also positive. The CA46 Burkitt cell line and water (H_2O) were used as negative controls. MWM, molecular weight marker; Karpas, ALCL cell line used as a positive control. Histologic figures provided courtesy of Dr ES d'Amore.

Table 77.2 Immunophenotypic markers for anaplastic large cell lymphoma diagnosis

Mandatory antibodies	Optional antibodies
B cell: CD79a, CD20	T cell: CD2, CD4, CD5, CD7, CD8
T cell: CD3, CD43	perforin, TIA1, granzyme
CD30	Mib1 or Ki-67
CD15	clusterin
EMA	BNH-9
ALK-1	
LMP-1 and/or EBER	

Table summarizes the targets that need to be determined by immunohistochemical technique using the minimal required panel (mandatory) or an extended panel of antibodies (mandatory and optional antibodies) for the diagnosis of anaplastic large cell lymphoma (ALCL). Together with morphologic features they allow the diagnosis of ALCL and the differentiation between ALCL and Hodgkin lymphoma.

Table 77.3 Definition of therapeutic groups (EICNHL)

Therapeutic groups	Definition/comments
Isolated skin lesions	No lymph node or organ involvement
Low-risk group	Stage I, completely resected
Standard-risk group	No skin, mediastinum, liver, spleen, lung involvement
High-risk group	Biopsy-proven skin involvement[a] or mediastinum or liver, spleen, lung involvement
CNS involvement	Intracerebral/spinal lesion, blasts in CSF, fusion transcript-positive CSF, cranial nerve palsy not otherwise explained

[a]Involvement of the skin overlaying a positive lymph node should not be considered as skin involvement.
EICNHL, European Intergroup for Childhood non-Hodgkin's Lymphoma; CNS, central nervous system; CSF, cerebrospinal fluid.

derived from the classic t(2;5) chromosomal translocation and the variant fusion proteins derived from other *ALK* gene rearrangements. ALK positivity, together with the intracellular localization of ALK-1 reactivity (cytoplasm; cytoplasm and nuclear) and the staining pattern (granular vs finely dispersed), can be useful in defining whether the tumor cells harbor the classic NPM-ALK fusion protein or specific variant fusion products.[28,41,96] In this regard, it needs to be pointed out that other pediatric tumors, besides ALCL, can express ALK chimeric proteins, including myofibroblastic tumors[97,98] and the rare plasmablastic variant of large B cell lymphomas expressing the CLTC-ALK protein.[99–101]

Because the great majority of pediatric ALCL are ALK positive and more than 90 percent of them harbor the NPM-ALK fusion product, RT-PCR analysis based on NPM- and ALK-specific primers is a relevant approach both for diagnostic purposes on tumor tissue and for the study of minimal residual disease in the bone marrow.[43,68] Considering *NPM-ALK* fusion transcript as a tumor-specific marker, some caution must be used as very low levels of expression may be found in reactive lymph nodes.[52]

Cytogenetic analysis and FISH analysis can also detect the *ALK* fusion genes and may be helpful in the diagnostic workup.[43]

STAGING

Staging of pediatric ALCL is usually based on the St. Jude classification[102] and on the Ann Arbor staging system for Hodgkin lymphoma.[103] Given the peculiar biology and clinical features of ALCL though, neither of the staging systems appear to be as predictive of prognosis as in other lymphomas. Several studies have reported that statistical analysis of outcome in relation to extent of disease often fails to demonstrate significant differences in outcome of localized versus disseminated disease (stage I–II vs III–IV)

treated with short-pulse chemotherapy protocols,[62,64,104,105] with few exceptions and only in the setting of univariate analysis.[63] This does not appear to depend on the treatment strategy used, given that even using leukemia-like treatments, lasting up to 24 months, stage apparently does not significantly associate with prognosis.[66] This is not only the case for pediatric ALCL, but occurs also in adults.[65,106]

Evaluation of prognostic factors in ALCL has instead demonstrated that factors other than stage bear a relevant prognostic value. Among them, specific organ involvement and some biological characteristics may better relate to prognosis. For this reason, as in B cell non-Hodgkin lymphomas, in recent international trials a grouping of patients based on risk categories has been devised and used to allocate children to different treatment categories. In the ongoing international trial of the European Intergroup for Childhood non-Hodgkin's Lymphomas (EICNHL), children are divided into standard and high-risk groups, based on organ involvement (Table 77.3). Special localization such as isolated skin lesions and the rare CNS-positive ALCL are still considered special disease categories. Only a large prospective trial will eventually make it possible to establish the optimal staging approach for ALCL.

Obviously, the change in perspective from the standard staging system to the identification of risk groups implies a somewhat different approach to the definition of disease extension and site involvement, particularly relevant with regard to the assessment of visceral and skin involvement. A detailed clinical examination should be carried out with special attention to performance status, fever, weight loss, lymph node enlargement, and skin lesions. Skin lesions may vary from a few pink macular papules to numerous brownish lesions: skin localization must be biopsy proven.

Chest x-ray and computed tomography (CT) scans of the abdomen, pelvis, and chest must be performed in order to determine extent of disease. Abdominal ultrasound scan should also be performed. Cranial/spinal magnetic resonance imaging (MRI) is compulsory in cases with neurological signs or if the cerebrospinal fluid (CSF) contains blasts. Bilateral BM aspirates and trephines for morphologic and immunohistochemical analyses, and CSF microscopic examination and cytopreps are to be performed. Bone scan with x-ray of any suspicious areas are also recommended to determine possible bone localizations. Standard blood chemical analysis including lactate dehydrogenase (LDH) should be performed in the initial diagnostic workup. Cytogenetic and molecular analyses on tumor tissue and BM/CSF are strongly recommended (Fig. 77.1D).

PROGNOSTIC FACTORS

As pointed out above, systemic ALCL in children and young adults clinically resemble ALK-positive ALCL of adults. Because pediatric ALCL cases are in the vast majority ALK-positive, the clinical behavior of systemic ALCL may relate to the expression of the chimeric product derived from the *ALK* gene rearrangements. While the prognostic impact of ALK expression has not been clearly established yet in the pediatric patient population and may be rather difficult to determine due to the limited number of ALK-negative cases, a significant prognostic difference between ALK-positive and ALK-negative ALCL, as determined by immunohistochemical analysis, was reported initially by Shiota et al.[107] In their study, the authors reported a 5-year survival rate of 79.8 percent for ALK-positive patients versus only 32.9 percent for the ALK-negative group. Similar results were confirmed in other, more recent series[16,65] where ALK expression was also determined by immunohistochemical analysis on tumor biopsies. When comparing NPM-ALK-expressing ALCL versus those with variant fusion proteins, no significant difference in outcome was observed,[45] thus suggesting that ALK-positive ALCL cases have a similar prognosis independent of the specific *ALK* rearrangement. The reason for the better prognosis of ALK-positive ALCL is not clear yet, but it may depend on the ability of patients to generate an immune response against ALK protein,[54] or on the higher proliferation rate of tumor cells that may influence response to chemotherapy.[108]

Histology has also been considered to be related to prognosis. It was at one time suggested that the provisional entity defined as Hodgkin-like ALCL (which is not recognized in the recent WHO classification and is now believed to represent true Hodgkin lymphoma) and B cell lymphoma with anaplastic morphology (that now belongs in the large B cell NHL category) may be associated with different clinical behavior and prognosis compared to common type ALCL; however, no clear evidence of a differential prognosis associated with specific histologic subtypes has been obtained. This is the case both for pediatric and adult ALCL patients.

If analysis of prognostic factors is confined to children[23,61,63,64,109] and young adults[106,110] where the prevalence of ALK positivity is very high, ALK expression appears to be associated with a favorable prognosis.

Considering the largest pediatric series of ALCL published so far, multivariate analysis pointed out several negative prognostic factors. An evaluation of 82 children treated in the French group, SFCE, demonstrated in multivariate analysis that mediastinal involvement, visceral involvement, and high LDH level (above 800 IU/L) had a negative prognostic impact.[63] A first report from the German BFM (Berlin-Frankfurt-Munster) group on 62 children demonstrated a significant impact on prognosis only for skin involvement[61] by Cox analysis, although univariate analysis also identified splenomegaly as a risk factor. A subsequent series of 89 children from the same group revealed lung involvement, splenomegaly, and B symptoms to be risk factors in univariate analysis, but only B symptoms maintained a significant negative prognostic impact when analyzed by the Cox regression model.[62] The United Kingdom experience of 72 patients confirmed in multivariate analysis the increased risk of failure in cases with visceral or mediastinal involvement.[64]

A retrospective analysis of prognostic factors conducted by the EICNHL in 225 children with ALCL treated with similar short-pulse chemotherapy protocols in Germany, France, and the UK (BFM, SFCE, and the United Kingdom Children's Cancer Study Group [UKCCSG], respectively) has identified several factors associated with a higher risk of failure in univariate analysis. B symptoms, mediastinal involvement, skin lesions (except for isolated skin lesions), visceral involvement, high stage according to the St. Jude or Ann Arbor classification, and elevated LDH had a significantly negative impact on prognosis, whereas patients with bone lesions seemed to fare better than the overall patient population. On multivariate analysis,[111] three poor prognostic factors were identified: mediastinal involvement (relative risk of failure 2.1, $P = 0.004$); visceral involvement defined as lung, liver, or spleen involvement (relative risk of failure 2.1, $P = 0.006$); and skin lesions in the presence of other disease localizations (relative risk of failure 1.9, $P = 0.02$). Based on these findings, two major prognostic groups of ALCL could be identified: a good prognostic group without skin, mediastinal, or visceral involvement and a 5-year progression-free survival (PFS) of 89 percent and overall survival (OS) of 94 percent; and a poor prognostic group characterized by skin and/or mediastinal and/or visceral involvement that showed a 5-year PFS of 61 percent and OS of 73 percent.

Stage according to the St. Jude or Ann Arbor classifications has a rather limited prognostic impact in pediatric ALCL, suggesting that those staging systems may indeed be not useful for ALCL in children.[66]

Other parameters have also been evaluated as prognostic indicators in adults, but their role in children has to be defined. The International Prognostic Index (IPI),[112,113] based on age, LDH level, performance status, stage, and involvement of extranodal sites, is applicable to young adults.[16,65] Some of the parameters considered in the IPI have also been found to have a prognostic impact in children.

Less clear is the role of biological variables. A high serum level of CD30 at diagnosis was an indicator of poor prognosis and was associated to advanced stage and bulky disease.[114] A study from Japan in 143 patients suggested that CD56 expression identifies a poor prognostic group, independently from other factors including IPI score and ALK expression.[115] The presence of activated cytotoxic T lymphocytes (defined as T cells expressing granzyme B) in the tumor biopsy has also been reported as a possible indicator of poor prognosis in patients with nodal ALCL,[116] but these findings need further confirmation on a larger patient series. A later study in 64 patients with nodal ALCL suggested that the presence of Bcl-2 and granzyme B-specific protease inhibitor 9 (PI-9) is a strong predictor of poor outcome, whereas the presence of high numbers of caspase-3-positive cells indicates a good prognosis in systemic ALCL,[117] thus implying that apoptosis-related proteins may be involved in the clinical course of the disease.

Survivin, a member of the inhibitor of apoptosis family that is expressed during embryonic and fetal development but not in adult tissues, can be expressed in a variety of human cancers. An immunohistochemical analysis on 62 ALCL biopsies showed that survivin expression is an independent negative prognostic factor in ALCL, both in terms of failure-free survival and overall survival.[118]

MUC-1, also known as epithelial membrane antigen (EMA), has also been reported to correlate with prognosis,[119] in that its expression has a negative impact on survival in ALCL, particularly in ALK-negative ALCL. These results need to be confirmed in the pediatric setting where ALK positivity is far more frequent than in adult series and where, possibly, MUC-1 expression may differ from adults.

Recently, a prospective evaluation of minimal bone marrow infiltration by tumor cells has suggested that BM positivity as defined by molecular techniques has a negative impact on event-free and overall survival.[68] The negative prognostic impact of minimal bone marrow and peripheral blood disease was confirmed by quantitative analysis.[120] These findings need to be evaluated further in the context of a large prospective trial and the predictive value defined by multivariate analysis.

Special mention should be given to the isolated skin localization of ALCL that, although more frequent in the elderly, can also be found in childhood. These lymphomas are usually CD30 positive and almost invariably ALK negative[88] and may regress spontaneously or progress to systemic ALCL. Overall, patients with localized ALCL have a better prognosis than other groups of ALCL and, given the frequent 'wax-and-wane' clinical behavior, should be subjected to strict monitoring in order to decide whether, and eventually when, treatment should be started.

TREATMENT OF ANAPLASTIC LARGE CELL LYMPHOMA

Clinical trials

Since the 1990s in most European studies, ALCL has been considered as a separate entity and treated with intensive chemotherapy as used for B cell NHL[62–64] or, less frequently, with longer, leukemia-like treatments in use for T cell NHL (Table 77.4).[66,105,109] In North America, children with ALCL have for a long time been treated in the context of trials for large cell lymphomas, regardless of the immunologic subtype.[121–124]

Treatment has been ascribed on the basis of stage (using the St. Jude staging system, as in the BFM protocol and to some extent in the UKCCSG and Italian Association of Pediatric Hematology and Oncology [AIEOP] studies) or independent of stage, as in the French Society of Pediatric Oncology group study. In the BFM treatment study, after 5 days of cytoreductive therapy, patients were stratified into three groups of different treatment intensity: K1, K2, and K3 (Fig. 77.2). Patients with stage I or II (completely resected) disease were treated in arm K1 of the study and received 3 5-day cycles comprising methotrexate (MTX) $(0.5\,g/m^2)$, dexamethasone, ifosfamide/cyclophosphamide, etoposide, and cytarabine/doxorubicin and intrathecal chemotherapy. Patients in arm K2 (stage II nonresected and stage III) received 6 cycles of chemotherapy. Children in arm K3 (stage IV or multifocal bone disease) were treated with 6 intensified cycles including MTX $5.0\,g/m^2$ and high-dose cytarabine/etoposide. The Kaplan-Meier estimated 5-year EFS was 76 percent overall and 100 percent, 73 percent, and 79 percent for K1, K2, and K3 groups, respectively.[62] Relapses occurred most frequently at the site of the primary tumor. These results are in keeping with those of an earlier study from the BFM group in 62 patients treated according to the same strategy.[61] In the BFM studies, duration of treatment was relatively short, ranging from 2 months to 5 months, whereas in other trials duration of treatment ranges from 10 months to 2 years. In addition, the cumulative dose of critical drugs was comparatively low with a maximum of $3.4\,g/m^2$ cyclophosphamide, $12\,g/m^2$ ifosfamide, $150\,mg/m^2$ anthracyclines, and $0.6–1.3\,g/m^2$ of etoposide. The other major differences between the BFM 90 protocol and other published regimens for pediatric ALCL[63,122,125] are the use of dexamethasone instead of prednisone, the use of ifosfamide, and infusion of MTX over a period of 24 hours, with a 'late' leucovorin rescue and the use of intrathecal therapy.

In the French Society of Pediatric Oncology study, treatment consisted of two COPADM cycles (MTX, cyclophosphamide, doxorubicin, vincristine, and prednisone) and maintenance therapy for 5–7 months,[63] independent of stage and other parameters. No intrathecal therapy was administered. The probability of survival and EFS at 3 years was 83 percent and 66 percent, respectively. On multivariate

Table 77.4 Characteristics and treatment results of pediatric anaplastic large cell lymphoma reported patient series

Study	n	Treatment regimen	Radiation therapy on primary site[a]	CNS prophylaxis	CR rate (%)	Overall survival (%)	Event–free survival (%)	Treatment duration (months)
Vecchi et al. 1993[109]	13	Modified LSA$_2$-L$_2$	Yes	Yes	100	100 (4-yr)	62.9 (4-yr)	24
Sandlund et al. 1994[122]	18	CHOP or MACOP-B ± maintenance	Yes	na	na	84 (5-yr)	57 (5-yr)	
Reiter et al. 1994[61]	62	BFM 83, 86, 90	No	Yes	93	83 (9-yr)	81 (9-yr)	2–5
Brugières et al. 1998[63]	82	COP-COPADM	No	No	95	83 (3-yr)	66 (3-yr)	7–8
Massimino et al. 1995[105]	27	Institutional protocol for lymphoblastic NHL	Yes	No	100	84 (8-yr)	72 (8-yr)	8–24
Seidemann et al. 2001[62]	89	BFM 90	No	Yes	na	na	76 (5-yr)	2–5
Williams et al. 2002[64]	72	COP-COPADM	No	Yes	82	65 (5-yr)	59 (5-yr)	5
Mora et al. 2000[124]	19	LSA$_2$-L$_2$	Yes	Yes	na	84 (5-yr)	56 (5-yr)	24
Laver et al. 2005[121]	86	APO + maintenance	Yes	Yes	na	88 (4-yr)	72 (4-yr)	12
Rosolen et al. 2005[66]	34	Modified LSA$_2$-L$_2$	Yes	Yes	88	85 (10-yr)	65 (10-yr)	24

[a]Criteria for administration of radiation therapy varied for some series based on the enrolment period, on disease extension, or on response to induction therapy.
CNS, central nervous system; CR, complete remission; NHL, non-Hodgkin lymphoma; yr, year; na, not available.

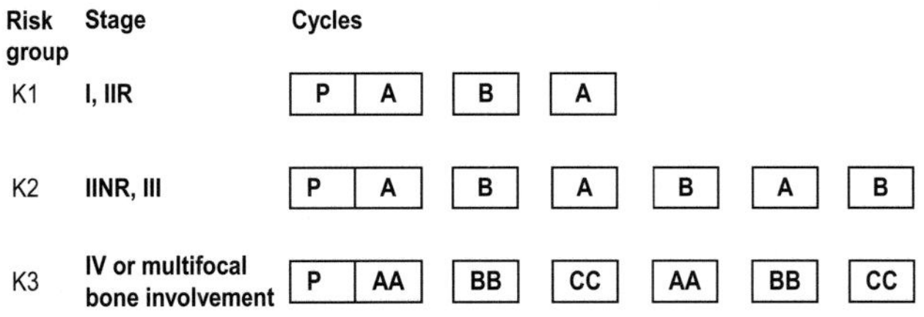

Figure 77.2 Treatment strategy for anaplastic large cell lymphoma (ALCL) in the non-Hodgkin lymphoma BFM 90 trial. Therapy intensity was stratified according to three patient risk groups (K1, K2, and K3) based on stage (St. Jude staging system). After a 5-day cytoreductive prephase (P), 3–6 5-day alternating chemotherapy cycles were administered. For more details see Seidemann et al. 2001.[62]

analysis, mediastinal involvement, visceral involvement (lung, liver, spleen), and LDH >800 IU/L were found to be predictive of a higher risk of failure. Based on these parameters, two groups of patients were identified: a 'low-risk' group with none of these risk factors, with 3-year EFS of 95 percent; and a 'high-risk' group, with at least one risk factor, with a 3-year EFS of 47 percent. Stage (I–II versus III–IV) was a significant predictor of prognosis only on univariate analysis.

Another recent report is from the UKCCSG in 72 children with ALCL.[64] Therapy varied according to stage and was based on chemotherapy cycles similar to the French group's protocol. The complete remission (CR) rate was lower compared to the French and BFM results (82 percent versus 95 percent). Overall survival and EFS at 5 years were 65 percent and 59 percent, respectively. The reasons for this worse outcome are not clear, although in part they

may depend on the different patient distribution in relationship to risk factors.

The experience of the St. Jude Children's Hospital is based mostly on the use of the CHOP regimen (cyclophosphamide, vincristine, doxorubicin, and prednisone) to treat 18 patients diagnosed between 1975 and 1990 with CD30-positive large cell NHL.[122] Six cycles were given to patients with stage III and IV ALCL, but additional maintenance treatment and/or radiation therapy was also administered depending on the enrolment period. The 5-year EFS was 75 percent and 57 percent for localized and extensive disease, respectively. Results were better for CD30-positive lymphoma compared to large B cell NHL in the case of extensive disease, but due to the relatively small number of patients and the different treatments used, any comparison with other series is difficult.

A recent report on advanced stage large cell lymphoma from the Pediatric Oncology Group included 86 patients with ALCL.[121] They were treated with an initial chemotherapy regimen containing doxorubicin, vincristine, and prednisone (APO induction) and later randomized to receive maintenance treatment composed of short cycles of the same drugs with the addition of 6-mercaptopurine (APO maintenance), or alternating with MTX and cytarabine, to complete a total of 12 months of chemotherapy treatment. All patients received intrathecal MTX as CNS prophylaxis. The 4-year EFS and OS for all ALCL patients (n = 86) were 71.8 percent and 88.1 percent, respectively. No significant difference in EFS between the two treatments was found.

Another small series of patients was reported by Mora et al.[124] Of the 78 patients with large cell NHL enrolled in two consecutive protocols at the Memorial Sloan-Kettering

Cancer Center, 19 cases were retrospectively classified as ALCL on the basis of morphology and CD30 positivity. Patients were treated with the LSA_2-L_2 chemotherapy regimen[126] and achieved a 5-year OS of 84 percent and an EFS of 56 percent. Radiation therapy, ranging from 20 to 55 Gy depending on the enrolment period, was administered to all patients with bulky disease (larger than 5 cm) at the primary tumor site. Five children developed recurrent lymphoma but were all reinduced into remission with the same protocol. A series of 32 children with Ki-1-positive NHL were treated at the Istituto Nazionale dei Tumori in Milan according to the institutional protocol for T lymphoblastic lymphoma with a total duration of 24 months for disseminated disease and 8–12 months for single-nodal or single-extranodal disease, without CNS prophylaxis.[127] Radiation therapy (25–40 Gy) was administered in all patients who did not achieved a CR after the first 4 weeks of treatment. All of the 27 evaluable patients reached a CR by the end of induction therapy and seven relapsed in a median time of 7 months. Five-year OS was 84 percent and EFS 72 percent.

Recently, the results of the AIEOP study were reported in a series of 34 children with ALCL treated with a modified LSA_2-L_2 therapy lasting 2 years independent of disease stage.[66] In the context of that leukemia-like regimen, radiation therapy (25 Gy) was only delivered to patients ($n = 3$) with residual mass larger than 5 cm at the end of the consolidation phase. Results showed a 10-year OS of 85 percent and EFS of 65 percent. Treatment was well tolerated but long-term toxicity is a concern in long therapy protocols such as those based on the acute lymphoblastic leukemia/lymphoma strategies.

Thus, it appears that this disease group has been treated with short, intensive chemotherapy or with more protracted, leukemia-like regimens. Overall, the former seems to be preferable, both because of its superiority in terms of outcome and for the shorter duration and lower cumulative doses of critically toxic drugs. The optimal therapeutic approach is, however, yet to be defined, including the role of radiation therapy and of antitumor drugs that are currently under evaluation as part of first-line therapy for ALCL, such as vinblastine.

There is less information on the optimal treatment for ALCL in adults. A number of studies were based on the CHOP regimen, but MACOP-B or similar regimens have also been used: this was the case in the study where 40 patients with Hodgkin-like ALCL were randomly treated with MACOP-B or with ABVD[128] and showed comparable results. The same group reported a series of 90 patients treated with F-MACHOP or MACOP-B with a 5-year OS of 60 percent and 63 percent for classic type ALCL and Hodgkin-like ALCL, respectively.[110]

Radiation therapy

In some clinical trials, irradiation has been used as part of first-line therapy for bulky tumors, independently of response to treatment,[124] or for residual tumor masses[127] or at later stages of treatment.[66] Radiation therapy as part of first-line treatment has mostly been combined with conventional, leukemia-like therapy but not with short, high-intensity chemotherapy.[62–64] As mentioned above, the latter approach has generally resulted in better outcome. Although no randomized study on the role of radiation therapy in ALCL has been conducted, this observation, together with the high prevalence of disease relapse at sites different from those involved at diagnosis, would suggest that radiation therapy may not be beneficial in the context of front-line therapy of childhood ALCL, even in patients with a slow clinical response to chemotherapy.

Bone marrow transplantation

The role of bone marrow transplantation (BMT) as part of first-line treatment for ALCL has not been completely clarified. Although intensification of therapy with BMT is considered in resistant disease, there is no definitive evidence to support its use for consolidation of first-line therapy. This is in part due to the relatively high 'rescue' rate for patients with ALCL at recurrence and by the impossibility of identifying a subpopulation of ALCL in whom standard-dose second-line chemotherapy will fail.

In the adult setting, there are a few reports suggesting that autologous BMT used to intensify first-line therapy may improve outcome,[129,130] but these are based on small numbers of patients and need to be evaluated in larger prospective randomized trials.

Central nervous system disease and CNS prophylaxis

Central nervous system involvement in primary ALCL is a rare event, both in adults and children.[131] In contrast to adults, several clinical trials for pediatric ALCL have included intrathecal chemotherapy as CNS prophylaxis. However, CNS relapse appears to be a very infrequent event in pediatric ALCL, regardless of whether the first-line treatment included CNS prophylaxis in the form of intrathecal chemotherapy[61,62,64] or the use of systemic high-dose MTX infusion (3 g/m² in 3 hours).[63] Central nervous system relapse is also rare in patients treated with chemotherapy protocols as used in lymphoblastic lymphoma, with[66,124] or without CNS prophylaxis.[105]

Isolated skin lesions

Primary cutaneous CD30-positive T cell lymphoproliferative disorders (LPDs) are a rare group of diseases that encompass several distinct entities ranging from lymphomatoid papulosis (LyP) to primary cutaneous ALCL (C-ALCL) with borderline lesions in between.[2,132] They are usually of T cell phenotype, ALK negative, and often EMA negative.[86]

They are very rare in the pediatric population; in a large series of patients younger than 20 years, they were only present in 12/219 individuals with LPDs[88] and are mostly represented by LyP. As in LyP, which is characterized by a relapsing/remitting clinical behavior, C-ALCL often show spontaneous remission. Thus, it is of great relevance to distinguish between C-ALCL and systemic ALCL with cutaneous involvement. The first is a disease that can spontaneously regress and does not appear to benefit from systemic chemotherapy (given that it frequently recurs after treatment).[46,86] Skin involvement in a case of systemic ALCL warrants chemotherapy, as skin localization seems to be associated with a worse prognosis.[111] Consequently, every effort must be made to assess whether any other sites of disease exist in children with apparently isolated skin involvement by LPDs.

Treatment at recurrence

Anaplastic large cell lymphoma is a disease which tends to recur. The site of relapse often includes,[62,64] but is not restricted to, the initial area of involvement.[61,63] Relapses mostly occur within the first 12–15 months from diagnosis, although occasionally occur as late as 5 years.[62] It is not clear whether these late events are indeed recurrences or the development of a second ALCL. In patients treated with chemotherapy protocols of long duration, recurrences tend to occur later compared to short chemotherapy protocols.[66,124]

Despite the tendency for disease to recur, most ALCL patients can obtain a second or further long-lasting CR when treated with therapy similar to that used originally, or with different and generally more intensive chemotherapy. In the BFM experience, a second CR could be achieved with the administration of the same chemotherapy as used in first-line therapy, followed (or not) by BMT.[61] The French Society of Pediatric Oncology group showed a probability of achieving a second remission of 88 percent on the basis of a series of 41 patients with recurrent ALCL.[133] In this cohort of patients, 25/35 children who reached a second CR were treated with CCNU, vinblastine, cytarabine (Ara-C), and bleomycin. The final outcome, taking into account the fact that 15 children underwent autologous BMT in second CR, was an OS of 69 percent and EFS of 44 percent at 3 years. It is worth noting that 12 patients in this series were treated with weekly vinblastine for 6–18 months at the first or further relapse, including six relapses which occurred after high-dose chemotherapy and autologous BMT.

As to the role of BMT in recurrent ALCL, little information is available. Furthermore, no definitive information on risk factors that would suggest the need for an intensified treatment with BMT rescue is available, although early relapse (less than 12 months from diagnosis) appears to have a negative impact on outcome.[63,64] Thus, there is a need to evaluate the role of BMT in treatment of relapsed ALCL based on risk factor analysis of a large patient population. A further step would be the definition of a BMT approach that is the most beneficial for a selected subgroup of relapsed ALCL, including allogeneic BMT, that has been used in children with high-risk features and that may improve outcome in selected patient subgroups.[134,135] Of course, great caution should be paid to this specific issue, in the light of the relatively high probability of achieving a second CR in relapsed ALCL with chemotherapy alone and of the treatment-related toxicity that BMT implies.

FUTURE DIRECTIONS

Much progress has been made during the past 10 years in terms of both diagnosis and management of ALCL of childhood. A more detailed immunohistochemical definition of ALCL subtypes and developments in the biology of the disease have been achieved. In parallel, from relatively large pediatric ALCL patient series, a therapeutic approach has been identified that can cure more than three-quarters of the patients and will serve as the backbone on which to build further improvement.

Several questions remain to be answered, including the optimal duration and intensity of therapy, the role of specific drugs (i.e., vinblastine), treatment of relapse, and the role of BMT. To solve these and other open questions, large collaborative prospective studies such as those activated in the context of the EICNHL are warranted.

It will also be important to look at novel therapeutic approaches, such as the use of anti-CD30 or a vaccination strategy based on the NPM-ALK tumor-associated antigens. The use of drugs inhibiting the NPM-ALK kinase activity or interfering with the downstream signaling pathways may also play a role in the treatment of ALCL.

KEY POINTS

- ALCL in childhood accounts for 10–15 percent of all non-Hodgkin lymphomas, thus representing the third most frequent lymphoma. In more than 90 percent of cases, ALCL harbor the oncogenic fusion gene *NPM-ALK* (or other less frequent *ALK*-containing fusion genes).
- Extranodal involvement, including spleen, liver, lung, and skin, is present in the majority of pediatric ALCL at diagnosis. The central nervous system is rarely involved at disease onset.
- Isolated CD30-positive skin lesions, usually ALK negative, should be considered as separate entities that need not be treated in the absence of signs of systemic ALCL. Among these, lymphomatoid papulosis represents a premalignant condition that may evolve, but not necessarily, into systemic ALCL.
- Diagnosis of ALCL relies on histologic and immunohistochemical analyses. Among mandatory markers, CD30, CD15, EMA, ALK,

CD3, CD43, CD20, and CD79a are included. They are necessary also for differential diagnosis with Hodgkin lymphoma.

- The most frequently used treatment for systemic ALCL is based on sequential short-duration chemotherapy cycles. Radiation therapy is not routinely used.
- Specific histologic subtypes, mediastinum, spleen, liver, lung, and skin involvement, and, more recently, minimal disseminated disease, appear to have significant impact on prognosis in pediatric ALCL. However, stage of disease does not seem to have a relevant prognostic role.
- Future therapeutic approaches may include, together with chemotherapy, the use of anti-CD30 antibodies and kinase inhibitors of NPM-ALK activity. Vaccination therapy may also be explored in the clinical setting.

REFERENCES

● = Key primary paper
◆ = Major review article

1. Anderson J, Armitage J, Weisenburger D. Epidemiology of the non-Hodgkin's lymphomas: distributions of the major subtypes differ by geographic locations. Non-Hodgkin's Lymphoma Classification Project. *Ann Oncol* 1998; **9**: 717–20.
●2. Stein H, Mason DY, Gerdes J *et al.* The expression of the Hodgkin's disease associated antigen Ki-1 in reactive and neoplastic lymphoid tissue: evidence that Reed-Sternberg cells and histiocytic malignancies are derived from activated lymphoid cells. *Blood* 1985; **66**: 848–58.
3. Schwab U, Stein H, Gerdes J *et al.* Production of a monoclonal antibody specific for Hodgkin and Sternberg-Reed cells of Hodgkin's and subset of normal lymphoid cells. *Nature* 1982; **2**: 65–7.
4. Rimokh R, Magaud JP, Berger F *et al.* A translocation involving a specific breakpoint (q35) on chromosome 5 is characteristic of anaplastic large cell lymphoma ('Ki-1 lymphoma'). *Br J Haematol* 1989; **71**: 31–6.
5. Mason DY, Pulford KA, Bischof D *et al.* Nucleolar localization of the nucleophosmin-anaplastic lymphoma kinase is not required for malignant transformation. *Cancer Res* 1998; **58**: 1057–62.
6. Robinson D, Halperin N, Agar G *et al.* Shoulder girdle neoplasms mimicking frozen shoulder syndrome. *J Shoulder Elbow Surg* 2003; **12**: 451–5.
●7. Morris SW, Kirstein MN, Valentine MB *et al.* Fusion of a kinase gene, ALK, to a nucleolar protein gene, NPM, in non-Hodgkin's lymphoma. *Science* 1994; **263**: 1281–4.

●8. Falini B, Bigerna B, Fizzotti M *et al.* ALK expression defines a distinct group of T/null lymphomas ('ALK lymphomas') with a wide morphological spectrum. *Am J Pathol* 1998; **153**: 875–86.
9. Pulford K, Lamant L, Morris SW *et al.* Detection of anaplastic lymphoma kinase (ALK) and nucleolar protein nucleophosmin (NPM)-ALK proteins in normal and neoplastic cells with the monoclonal antibody ALK1. *Blood* 1997; **89**: 1394–404.
10. Hutchison RE, Banki K, Shuster JJ *et al.* Use of an anti-ALK antibody in the characterization of anaplastic large-cell lymphoma of childhood. *Ann Oncol* 1997; **8**(Suppl 1): 37–42.
11. Kadin ME. Anaplastic large cell lymphoma and its morphological variants. *Cancer Surv* 1997; **30**: 77–86.
12. Stein H, Foss HD, Durkop H *et al.* CD30(+) anaplastic large cell lymphoma: a review of its histopathologic, genetic, and clinical features. *Blood* 2000; **96**: 3681–95.
13. Benharroch D, Meguerian-Bedoyan Z, Lamant L *et al.* ALK-positive lymphoma: a single disease with a broad spectrum of morphology. *Blood* 1998; **91**: 2076–84.
14. Kinney MC, Collins RD, Greer JP *et al.* A small-cell-predominant variant of primary Ki-1 (CD30)+ T-cell lymphoma. *Am J Surg Pathol* 1993; **17**: 859–68.
15. Pileri S, Falini B, Delsol G *et al.* Lymphohistiocytic T-cell lymphoma (anaplastic large cell lymphoma CD30+/Ki-1+ with a high content of reactive histiocytes). *Histopathology* 1990; **16**: 383–91.
16. Falini B, Pileri S, Zinzani PL *et al.* ALK+ lymphoma: clinico-pathological findings and outcome. *Blood* 1999; **93**: 2697–706.
17. Murphy SB. Pediatric lymphomas: recent advances and commentary on Ki-1-positive anaplastic large-cell lymphomas of childhood. *Ann Oncol* 1994; **5**(Suppl 1): 31–3.
18. Wright D, McKeever P, Carter R. Childhood non-Hodgkin lymphomas in the United Kingdom: findings from the UK Children's Cancer Study Group. *J Clin Pathol* 1997; **50**: 128–34.
19. Alessandri AJ, Pritchard SL, Schultz KR, Massing BG. A population-based study of pediatric anaplastic large cell lymphoma. *Cancer* 2002; **94**: 1830–5.
20. Samuelsson BO, Ridell B, Rockert L *et al.* Non-Hodgkin lymphoma in children: a 20-year population-based epidemiologic study in western Sweden. *J Pediatr Hematol Oncol* 1999; **21**: 103–10.
21. Lin CN, Hou CC, Hwang WS, Chuang SS. Anaplastic large cell lymphoma – a rare disorder in southern Taiwan. *Leuk Lymphoma* 2003; **44**: 1727–31.
22. Noorali S, Pervez S, Yaqoob N *et al.* Prevalence and characterization of anaplastic large cell lymphoma and its association with Epstein-Barr virus in Pakistani patients. *Pathol Res Pract* 2004; **200**: 669–79.
23. Sandlund JT, Pui CH, Roberts WM *et al.* Clinicopathologic features and treatment outcome of children with large-cell lymphoma and the t(2;5)(p23;q35). *Blood* 1994; **84**: 2467–71.

24. Morra J, Filippa DA, Thaler HT *et al.* Large cell non-Hodgkin lymphoma of childhood: analysis of 78 consecutive patients enrolled in 2 prospective protocols at the Memorial Sloan-Kettering Cancer Center. *Cancer* 2000; **88**: 186–97.

25. Shih LY, Liang DC. Non-Hodgkin's lymphoma in Asia. *Hematol Oncol Clin North Am* 1991; **5**: 983–1001.

26. Iwahara T, Fujimoto J, Wen D *et al.* Molecular characterization of ALK, a receptor tyrosine kinase expressed specifically in the nervous system. *Oncogene* 1997; **14**: 439–49.

27. Drexler HG, Gignac SM, von Wasielewski R *et al.* Pathobiology of NPM-ALK and variant fusion genes in anaplastic large cell lymphoma and other lymphomas. *Leukemia* 2000; **14**: 1533–59.

◆28. Falini B. Anaplastic large cell lymphoma: pathological, molecular and clinical features. *Br J Haematol* 2001; **114**: 741–60.

29. Fujimoto J, Shiota M, Iwahara T *et al.* Characterization of the transforming activity of p80, a hyperphosphorylated protein in a Ki-1 lymphoma cell line with chromosomal translocation t(2;5). *Proc Natl Acad Sci U S A* 1996; **93**: 4181–6.

30. Bai RY, Dieter P, Peschel C *et al.* Nucleophosmin-anaplastic lymphoma kinase of large-cell anaplastic lymphoma is a constitutively active tyrosine kinase that utilizes phospholipase C-gamma to mediate its mitogenicity. *Mol Cell Biol* 1998; **18**: 6951–61.

31. Kuefer MU, Look AT, Pulford K *et al.* Retrovirus-mediated gene transfer of NPM-ALK causes lymphoid malignancy in mice. *Blood* 1997; **90**: 2901–10.

32. Borer RA, Lehner CF, Eppenberger HM, Nigg EA. Major nucleolar proteins shuttle between nucleus and cytoplasm. *Cell* 1989; **56**: 379–90.

33. Chan WY, Liu QR, Borjigin J *et al.* Characterization of the cDNA encoding human nucleophosmin and studies of its role in normal and abnormal growth. *Biochemistry* 1989; **28**: 1033–9.

34. Bischof D, Pulford K, Mason DY, Morris SW. Role of the nucleophosmin (NPM) portion of the non-Hodgkin's lymphoma-associated NPM-anaplastic lymphoma kinase fusion protein in oncogenesis. *Mol Cell Biol* 1997; **17**: 2312–25.

35. Pulford K, Morris SW, Turturro F. Anaplastic lymphoma kinase proteins in growth control and cancer. *J Cell Physiol* 2004; **199**: 330–58.

36. Bridge JA, Kanamori M, Ma Z *et al.* Fusion of the ALK gene to the clathrin heavy chain gene, CLTC, in inflammatory myofibroblastic tumor. *Am J Pathol* 2001; **159**: 411–15.

37. Lamant L, Dastugue N, Pulford K *et al.* A new fusion gene TPM3-ALK in anaplastic large cell lymphoma created by a (1;2)(q25;p23) translocation. *Blood* 1999; **93**: 3088–95.

38. Meech SJ, McGavran L, Odom LF *et al.* Unusual childhood extramedullary hematologic malignancy with natural killer cell properties that contains tropomyosin 4-anaplastic lymphoma kinase gene fusion. *Blood* 2001; **98**: 1209–16.

39. Tort F, Pinyol M, Pulford K *et al.* Molecular characterization of a new ALK translocation involving moesin (MSN-ALK) in anaplastic large cell lymphoma. *Lab Invest* 2001; **81**: 419–26.

40. Hernandez L, Pinyol M, Hernandez S *et al.* TRK-fused gene (TFG) is a new partner of ALK in anaplastic large cell lymphoma producing two structurally different TFG-ALK translocations. *Blood* 1999; **94**: 3265–8.

41. Lamant L, Gascoyne RD, Duplantier MM *et al.* Non-muscle myosin heavy chain (MYH9): a new partner fused to ALK in anaplastic large cell lymphoma. *Genes Chromosomes Cancer* 2003; **37**: 427–32.

42. Ma Z, Cools J, Marynen P *et al.* Inv(2)(p23q35) in anaplastic large-cell lymphoma induces constitutive anaplastic lymphoma kinase (ALK) tyrosine kinase activation by fusion to ATIC, an enzyme involved in purine nucleotide biosynthesis. *Blood* 2000; **95**: 2144–9.

43. Liang X, Meech SJ, Odom LF *et al.* Assessment of t(2;5)(p23;q35) translocation and variants in pediatric ALK+ anaplastic large cell lymphoma. *Am J Clin Pathol* 2004; **121**: 496–506.

44. Falini B, Mason DY. Proteins encoded by genes involved in chromosomal alterations in lymphoma and leukemia: clinical value of their detection by immunocytochemistry. *Blood* 2002; **99**: 409–26.

45. Falini B, Pulford K, Pucciarini A *et al.* Lymphomas expressing ALK fusion protein(s) other than NPM-ALK. *Blood* 1999; **94**: 3509–15.

46. Tomaszewski MM, Moad JC, Lupton GP. Primary cutaneous Ki-1(CD30) positive anaplastic large cell lymphoma in childhood. *J Am Acad Dermatol* 1999; **40**: 857–61.

47. Pulford K, Morris SW, Mason DY. Anaplastic lymphoma kinase proteins and malignancy. *Curr Opin Hematol* 2001; **8**: 231–6.

48. Nieborowska-Skorska M, Slupianek A, Xue L *et al.* Role of signal transducer and activator of transcription 5 in nucleophosmin/anaplastic lymphoma kinase-mediated malignant transformation of lymphoid cells. *Cancer Res* 2001; **61**: 6517–23.

49. Slupianek A, Nieborowska-Skorska M, Hoser G *et al.* Role of phosphatidylinositol 3-kinase-Akt pathway in nucleophosmin/anaplastic lymphoma kinase-mediated lymphomagenesis. *Cancer Res* 2001; **61**: 2194–9.

50. Chiarle R, Gong JZ, Guasparri I *et al.* NPM-ALK transgenic mice spontaneously develop T-cell lymphomas and plasma cell tumors. *Blood* 2003; **101**: 1919–27.

51. Trumper L, Pfreundschuh M, Bonin FV, Daus H. Detection of the t(2;5)-associated NPM/ALK fusion cDNA in peripheral blood cells of healthy individuals. *Br J Haematol* 1998; **103**: 1138–44.

52. Maes B, Vanhentenrijk V, Wlodarska I *et al.* The NPM-ALK and the ATIC-ALK fusion genes can be detected in non-neoplastic cells. *Am J Pathol* 2001; **158**: 2185–93.

53. Inghirami G, Macri L, Cesarman E *et al.* Molecular characterization of CD30+ anaplastic large-cell

lymphoma: high frequency of c-myc proto-oncogene activation. *Blood* 1994; **83**: 3581–90.

54. Pulford K, Falini B, Banham AH *et al.* Immune response to the ALK oncogenic tyrosine kinase in patients with anaplastic large-cell lymphoma. *Blood* 2000; **96**: 1605–7.

55. Passoni L, Gambacorti-Passerini C. ALK a novel lymphoma-associated tumor antigen for vaccination strategies. *Leuk Lymphoma* 2003; **44**: 1675–81.

56. Delsol G, Al Saati T, Gatter KC *et al.* Coexpression of epithelial membrane antigen (EMA), Ki-1, and interleukin-2 receptor by anaplastic large cell lymphomas. Diagnostic value in so-called malignant histiocytosis. *Am J Pathol* 1988; **130**: 59–70.

57. Nakamura S, Takagi N, Kojima M *et al.* Clinicopathologic study of large cell anaplastic lymphoma (Ki-1-positive large cell lymphoma) among the Japanese. *Cancer* 1991; **68**: 118–29.

58. Greer JP, Kinney MC, Collins RD *et al.* Clinical features of 31 patients with Ki-1 anaplastic large-cell lymphoma. *J Clin Oncol* 1991; **9**: 539–47.

59. Skinnider BF, Connors JM, Sutcliffe SB, Gascoyne RD. Anaplastic large cell lymphoma: a clinicopathologic analysis. *Hematol Oncol* 1999; **17**: 137–48.

60. Massimino M, Spreafico F, Luksch R, Giardini R. Prognostic significance of p80 and visceral involvement in childhood CD30 anaplastic large cell lymphoma (ALCL). *Med Pediatr Oncol* 2001; **37**: 97–102.

61. Reiter A, Schrappe M, Tiemann M *et al.* Successful treatment strategy for Ki-1 anaplastic large-cell lymphoma of childhood: a prospective analysis of 62 patients enrolled in three consecutive Berlin-Frankfurt-Munster group studies. *J Clin Oncol* 1994; **12**: 899–908.

●62. Seidemann K, Tiemann M, Schrappe M *et al.* Short-pulse B-non-Hodgkin lymphoma-type chemotherapy is efficacious treatment for pediatric anaplastic large cell lymphoma: a report of the Berlin-Frankfurt-Munster Group Trial NHL-BFM 90. *Blood* 2001; **97**: 3699–706.

●63. Brugières L, Deley MC, Pacquement H *et al.* CD30(+) anaplastic large-cell lymphoma in children: analysis of 82 patients enrolled in two consecutive studies of the French Society of Pediatric Oncology. *Blood* 1998; **92**: 3591–8.

●64. Williams DM, Hobson R, Imeson J *et al.* Anaplastic large cell lymphoma in childhood: analysis of 72 patients treated on The United Kingdom Children's Cancer Study Group chemotherapy regimens. *Br J Haematol* 2002; **117**: 812–20.

65. Gascoyne RD, Aoun P, Wu D *et al.* Prognostic significance of anaplastic lymphoma kinase (ALK) protein expression in adults with anaplastic large cell lymphoma. *Blood* 1999; **93**: 3913–21.

66. Rosolen A, Pillon M, Garaventa A *et al.* Anaplastic large cell lymphoma (ALCL) treated with a leukemia-like therapy: report of the Italian Association of Pediatric Hematology and Oncology (AIEOP) LNH-92 protocol. *Cancer* 2005; **104**: 2133–40.

67. Fraga M, Brousset P, Schlaifer D *et al.* Bone marrow involvement in anaplastic large cell lymphoma.

Immunohistochemical detection of minimal disease and its prognostic significance. *Am J Clin Pathol* 1995; **103**: 82–9.

68. Mussolin L, Pillon M, d'Amore ES *et al.* Prevalence and clinical implications of bone marrow involvement in pediatric anaplastic large cell lymphoma. *Leukemia* 2005; **19**: 1643–7.

69. Chhanabhai M, Britten C, Klasa R, Gascoyne RD. t(2;5) positive lymphoma with peripheral blood involvement. *Leuk Lymphoma* 1998; **28**: 415–22.

70. Bayle C, Charpentier A, Duchayne E *et al.* Leukaemic presentation of small cell variant anaplastic large cell lymphoma: report of four cases. *Br J Haematol* 1999; **104**: 680–8.

71. Villamor N, Rozman M, Esteve J *et al.* Anaplastic large-cell lymphoma with rapid evolution to leukemic phase. *Ann Hematol* 1999; **78**: 478–82.

72. Onciu M, Behm FG, Raimondi SC *et al.* ALK-positive anaplastic large cell lymphoma with leukemic peripheral blood involvement is a clinicopathologic entity with an unfavorable prognosis. Report of three cases and review of the literature. *Am J Clin Pathol* 2003; **120**: 617–25.

73. Armstrong G, Szallasi A, Biegel JA *et al.* Early molecular detection of central nervous system relapse in a child with systemic anaplastic large cell lymphoma: case report and review of the literature. *Pediatr Blood Cancer* 2005; **44**: 400–6.

74. Abdulkader I, Cameselle-Teijeiro J, Fraga M *et al.* Primary anaplastic large cell lymphoma of the central nervous system. Hum Pathol 1999; **30**: 978–81.

75. Buxton N, Punt J, Hewitt M. Primary Ki-1-positive T-cell lymphoma of the brain in a child. *Pediatr Neurosurg* 1998; **29**: 250–2.

76. Lister TA, Crowther SB, Sutcliffe SB *et al.* Report of a committee convened to discuss the evaluation and staging of patinets with Hodgkin's doisease: Cotswolds meeting. *J Clin Oncol* 1989; **7**: 1630–6.

77. Vecsei A, Attarbaschi A, Krammer U *et al.* Pruritus in pediatric non-Hodgkin's lymphoma. *Leuk Lymphoma* 2002; **43**: 1885–7.

78. Harris NL, Jaffe ES, Diebold J *et al.* World Health Organization classification of neoplastic diseases of the hematopoietic and lymphoid tissues: report of the clinical advisory committee meeting-Airlie House,Virginia, November 1997. *J Clin Oncol* 1999; **17**: 3835–49.

79. Kadin ME, Sako D, Berliner N *et al.* Childhood Ki-1 lymphoma presenting with skin lesions and peripheral lymphadenopathy. *Blood* 1986; **68**: 1042–9.

80. Jaffe ES, Harris NL, Stein H, Vardiman J. Pathology and genetics of tumours of haematopoietic and lymphoid tissues. *World Health Organization classification of tumours.* Lyon: IARC Press, 2001.

81. Willemze R, Jaffe ES, Burg G *et al.* WHO-EORTC classification for cutaneous lymphomas. *Blood* 2005; **105**: 3768–85.

82. de Bruin PC, Beljaards RC, van Heerde P *et al.* Differences in clinical behaviour and immunophenotype between

primary cutaneous and primary nodal anaplastic large cell lymphoma of T-cell or null cell phenotype. *Histopathology* 1993; **23**: 127–35.

●83. Paulli M, Berti E, Rosso R *et al.* CD30/Ki-1-positive lymphoproliferative disorders of the skin – clinicopathologic correlation and statistical analysis of 86 cases: a multicentric study from the European Organization for Research and Treatment of Cancer Cutaneous Lymphoma Project Group. *J Clin Oncol* 1995; **13**: 1343–54.

84. ten Berge RL, de Bruin PC, Oudejans JJ *et al.* ALK-negative anaplastic large-cell lymphoma demonstrates similar poor prognosis to peripheral T-cell lymphoma, unspecified. *Histopathology* 2003; **43**: 462–9.

85. Kadin ME, Morris SW. The t(2;5) in human lymphomas. *Leuk Lymphoma* 1998; **29**: 249–56.

86. Kumar S, Pittaluga S, Raffeld M *et al.* Primary cutaneous CD30-positive anaplastic large cell lymphoma in childhood: report of 4 cases and review of the literature. *Pediatr Dev Pathol* 2005; **8**: 52–60.

87. Hinshaw M, Trowers AB, Kodish E *et al.* Three children with CD30 cutaneous anaplastic large cell lymphomas bearing the t(2;5)(p23;q35) translocation. *Pediatr Dermatol* 2004; **21**: 212–17.

●88. Bekkenk MW, Geelen FA, van Voorst Vader PC *et al.* Primary and secondary cutaneous CD30(+) lymphoproliferative disorders: a report from the Dutch Cutaneous Lymphoma Group on the long-term follow-up data of 219 patients and guidelines for diagnosis and treatment. *Blood* 2000; **95**: 3653–61.

89. Salhany KE, Cousar JB, Greer J *et al.* Transformation of cutaneous T cell lymphoma to large cell lymphoma. A clinicopathologic and immunologic study. *Am J Pathol* 1988; **132**: 265–77.

90. Nosari A, Cantoni S, Oreste P *et al.* Anaplastic large cell (CD30/Ki-1+) lymphoma in HIV+ patients: clinical and pathological findings in a group of ten patients. *Br J Haematol* 1996; **95**: 508–12.

91. Tirelli U, Vaccher E, Zagonel V *et al.* CD30 (Ki-1)-positive anaplastic large-cell lymphomas in 13 patients with and 27 patients without human immunodeficiency virus infection: the first comparative clinicopathologic study from a single institution that also includes 80 patients with other human immunodeficiency virus-related systemic lymphomas. *J Clin Oncol* 1995; **13**: 373–80.

92. Funkhouser AW, Katzman PJ, Sickel JZ, Lambert JS. CD30-positive anaplastic large cell lymphoma (ALCL) of T-cell lineage in a 14-month-old infant with perinatally acquired HIV-1 infection. *J Pediatr Hematol Oncol* 1998; **20**: 556–9.

93. Sebire NJ, Malone M, Ramsay AD. Posttransplant lymphoproliferative disorder presenting as CD30+, ALK+, anaplastic large cell lymphoma in a child. *Pediatr Dev Pathol* 2004; **7**: 290–3.

94. Costes-Martineau V, Delfour C, Obled S *et al.* Anaplastic lymphoma kinase (ALK) protein expressing lymphoma after liver transplantation: case report and literature review. *J Clin Pathol* 2002; **55**: 868–71.

95. Kadin ME. Primary Ki-1-positive anaplastic large-cell lymphoma: a distinct clinicopathologic entity. *Ann Oncol* 1994; **5**(Suppl 1): 25–30.

96. Jaffe ES. Anaplastic large cell lymphoma: the shifting sands of diagnostic hematopathology. *Mod Pathol* 2001; **14**: 219–28.

97. Coffin CM, Patel A, Perkins S *et al.* ALK1 and p80 expression and chromosomal rearrangements involving 2p23 in inflammatory myofibroblastic tumor. *Mod Pathol* 2001; **14**: 569–76.

98. Chun YS, Wang L, Nascimento AG *et al.* Pediatric inflammatory myofibroblastic tumor: anaplastic lymphoma kinase (ALK) expression and prognosis. *Pediatr Blood Cancer* 2005; **45**: 796–801.

99. De Paepe P, Baens M, van Krieken H *et al.* ALK activation by the CLTC-ALK fusion is a recurrent event in large B-cell lymphoma. *Blood* 2003; **102**: 2638–41.

100. Bubala H, Maldyk J, Wlodarska I *et al.* ALK-positive diffuse large B-cell lymphoma. *Pediatr Blood Cancer* 2006; **46**: 649–53.

101. Isimbaldi G, Bandiera L, d'Amore ES *et al.* ALK-positive plasmablastic B-cell lymphoma with the Clathrin-ALK gene rearrangement. *Pediatr Blood Cancer* 2006; **46**: 390–1.

102. Murphy SB. Classification, staging and end results of treatment of childhood non-Hodgkin's lymphomas: dissimilarities from lymphomas in adults. *Semin Oncol* 1980; **7**: 332–9.

103. Carbone PP, Kaplan HS, Musshoff K *et al.* Report of the committee on Hodgkin's disease staging classification. *Cancer Res* 1971; **31**: 1860–1.

104. Reiter A, Tiemann M, Ludwig WD *et al.* NHL-BFM 90 therapy study in treatment of malignant non-Hodgkin's lymphomas in children and adolescents. Part 1: Classification and allocation to strategic therapy groups. BIF study group. *Klin Padiatr* 1994; **206**: 222–33.

105. Massimino M, Gasparini M, Giardini R. Ki-1 (CD30) anaplastic large-cell lymphoma in children. *Ann Oncol* 1995; **6**: 915–20.

106. Tilly H, Gaulard P, Lepage E *et al.* Primary anaplastic large-cell lymphoma in adults: clinical presentation, immunophenotype, and outcome. *Blood* 1997; **90**: 3727–34.

●107. Shiota M, Nakamura S, Ichinohasama R *et al.* Anaplastic large cell lymphomas expressing the novel chimeric protein p80NPM/ALK: a distinct clinicopathologic entity. *Blood* 1995; **86**: 1954–60.

108. Leoncini L, Lazzi S, Scano D *et al.* Expression of the ALK protein by anaplastic large-cell lymphomas correlates with high proliferative activity. *Int J Cancer* 2000; **86**: 777–81.

109. Vecchi V, Burnelli R, Pileri S *et al.* Anaplastic large cell lymphoma (Ki-1+/CD30+) in childhood. *Med Pediatr Oncol* 1993; **21**: 402–10.

110. Zinzani PL, Bendandi M, Martelli M et al. Anaplastic large-cell lymphoma: clinical and prognostic evaluation of 90 adult patients. J Clin Oncol 1996; 14: 955–62.

111. Le Deley MC, Reiter A, Williams DE et al. Prognostic factors in childhood anaplastic large cell lymphoma: results of a large European Intergroup Study. Blood 2008; 11: 1560–66.

112. Shipp MA, Harrington DP, Anderson JR et al. A predictive model for aggressive NHL: the International non-Hodgkin's Lymphoma Prognostic Factors Project. N Engl J Med 1993; 329: 987–94.

113. Shipp MA. Prognostic factors in aggressive non-Hodgkin's lymphoma: who has high-risk disease? Blood 1994; 83: 1165–73.

114. Zinzani PL, Pileri S, Bendandi M et al. Clinical implications of serum levels of soluble CD30 in 70 adult anaplastic large-cell lymphoma patients. J Clin Oncol 1998; 16: 1532–7.

115. Suzuki R, Kagami Y, Takeuchi K et al. Prognostic significance of CD56 expression for ALK-positive and ALK-negative anaplastic large-cell lymphoma of T/null cell phenotype. Blood 2000; 96: 2993–3000.

116. ten Berge RL, Dukers DF, Oudejans JJ et al. Adverse effects of activated cytotoxic T lymphocytes on the clinical outcome of nodal anaplastic large cell lymphoma. Blood 1999; 93: 2688–96.

117. ten Berge RL, Meijer CJ, Dukers DF et al. Expression levels of apoptosis-related proteins predict clinical outcome in anaplastic large cell lymphoma. Blood 2002; 99: 4540–6.

118. Schlette EJ, Medeiros LJ, Goy A et al. Survivin expression predicts poorer prognosis in anaplastic large-cell lymphoma. J Clin Oncol 2004; 22: 1682–8.

119. Rassidakis GZ, Goy A, Medeiros LJ et al. Prognostic significance of MUC-1 expression in systemic anaplastic large cell lymphoma. Clin Cancer Res 2003; 9: 2213–20.

120. Damm-Welk C, Busch K, Burkhardt B et al. Prognostic significance of circulating tumor cells in bone marrow or peripheral blood as detected by qualitative and quantitative PCR in pediatric NPM-ALK-positive anaplastic large-cell lymphoma. Blood 2007; 110: 670–77.

●121. Laver JH, Kraveka JM, Hutchison RE et al. Advanced-stage large-cell lymphoma in children and adolescents: results of a randomized trial incorporating intermediate-dose methotrexate and high-dose cytarabine in the maintenance phase of the APO regimen: a Pediatric Oncology Group phase III trial. J Clin Oncol 2005; 23: 541–7.

122. Sandlund JT, Pui CH, Santana VM et al. Clinical features and treatment outcome for children with CD30+ large-cell non-Hodgkin's lymphoma. J Clin Oncol 1994; 12: 895–8.

123. Anderson JR, Jenkin RD, Wilson JF et al. Long-term follow-up of patients treated with COMP or LSA2L2 therapy for childhood non-Hodgkin's lymphoma: a report of CCG-551 from the Childrens Cancer Group. J Clin Oncol 1993; 11: 1024–32.

124. Mora J, Filippa DA, Thaler HT et al. Large cell non-Hodgkin lymphoma of childhood: analysis of 78 consecutive patients enrolled in 2 consecutive protocols at the Memorial Sloan-Kettering Cancer Center. Cancer 2000; 88: 186–97.

125. Hutchison RE, Berard CW, Shuster JJ et al. B-cell lineage confers a favorable outcome among children and adolescents with large-cell lymphoma: a Pediatric Oncology Group study. J Clin Oncol 1995; 13: 2023–32.

126. Wollner N, Burchenal JH, Lieberman PH et al. Non-Hodgkin's lymphoma in children. A comparative study of two modalities of treatment. Cancer 1976; 37: 123–34.

127. Gasparini M, Lombardi F, Bellani FF et al. Childhood non-Hodgkin's lymphoma: long-term results of an intensive chemotherapy regimen. Cancer 1981; 48: 1508–12.

128. Zinzani PL, Martelli M, Magagnoli M et al. Anaplastic large cell lymphoma Hodgkin's-like: a randomized trial of ABVD versus MACOP-B with and without radiation therapy. Blood 1998; 92: 790–4.

129. Fanin R, Silvestri F, Geromin A et al. Primary systemic CD30 (Ki-1)-positive anaplastic large cell lymphoma of the adult: sequential intensive treatment with the F-MACHOP regimen (± radiotherapy) and autologous bone marrow transplantation. Blood 1996; 87: 1243–8.

130. Deconinck E, Lamy T, Foussard C et al. Autologous stem cell transplantation for anaplastic large-cell lymphomas: results of a prospective trial. Br J Haematol 2000; 109: 736–42.

131. George DH, Scheithauer BW, Aker FV et al. Primary anaplastic large cell lymphoma of the central nervous system: prognostic effect of ALK-1 expression. Am J Surg Pathol 2003; 27: 487–93.

132. Kadin ME. Ki-1/CD30+ (anaplastic) large-cell lymphoma: maturation of a clinicopathologic entity with prospects of effective therapy. J Clin Oncol 1994; 12: 884–7.

133. Brugières L, Quartier P, Le Deley MC et al. Relapses of childhood anaplastic large-cell lymphoma: treatment results in a series of 41 children – a report from the French Society of Pediatric Oncology. Ann Oncol 2000; 11: 53–8.

134. Cesaro S, Pillon M, Visintin G et al. Unrelated bone marrow transplantation for high-risk anaplastic large cell lymphoma in pediatric patients: a single center case series. Eur J Haematol 2005; 75: 22–6.

135. Chakravarti V, Kamani NR, Bayever E et al. Bone marrow transplantation for childhood Ki-1 lymphoma. J Clin Oncol 1990; 8: 657–60.

78

Mycosis fungoides and Sézary syndrome

YOUN H KIM, RANJANA ADVANI AND RICHARD T HOPPE

GENERAL DESCRIPTION

Cutaneous T cell lymphomas (CTCL) collectively describe T cell non-Hodgkin lymphomas (NHL) that have primary cutaneous involvement. Mycosis fungoides and Sézary syndrome constitute major subsets of CTCL and are distinct clinical entities from primary cutaneous lymphomas in the new World Health Organization–European Organization for Research and Treatment in Cancer (WHO-EORTC) classification.[1] With advances in immunohistochemical and molecular characterization, other distinct clinicopathologic subsets of CTCL have been established.

Mycosis fungoides (MF) is distinguished from other CTCL by its unique clinical and histopathologic features,[2–4] typically presenting as an indolent cutaneous eruption with erythematous scaly patches or plaques. The diagnosis of MF is often preceded by a 'premycotic' period which may range from several months to several years or longer. Patients in this 'premycotic' phase frequently have nonspecific scaly skin eruptions and nondiagnostic skin biopsies. The histologic hallmark of MF is 'Pautrier microabscesses,' which are clusters of tumor cells in the epidermis.

Sézary syndrome (SS) is considered a distinct subtype of CTCL, which usually presents without the indolent phase and is characterized by generalized erythroderma, lymphadenopathy, and circulating neoplastic T cells, i.e., Sézary cells, in the peripheral blood. Patients may present initially with all components of SS or with only one component, e.g., generalized erythroderma, and subsequently progress to develop other clinical features of SS. With progression of the disease, SS patients may develop infiltrating tumors of the skin and extracutaneous sites.

A diagnosis of MF/SS is based on close integration of clinical and pathologic findings. Particularly in early MF or in erythroderma, a definitive histopathologic diagnosis by light miscroscopy alone may be difficult. Thus, the International Society for Cutaneous Lymphomas proposed a diagnostic algorithm for early MF, which utilizes a point-based system.[5] There are multiple clinical and histologic subtypes or variants of MF, including folliculotropic/follicular MF, Woringer-Kolopp disease, granulomatous MF, granulomatous slack skin disease, hypopigmented/vitiliginous MF, bullous MF, interstitial MF, and pigmented purpuric MF.[1,3]

Epidemiology

Although MF and SS are uncommon forms of NHL, they are the most common lymphomas with primary involvement of the skin. The annual incidence in the United States is estimated at 0.36 cases per 100 000.[6] Mycosis fungoides and SS are diseases of older adults with a median age at diagnosis between 55 and 60 years. Both occur in individuals of less than 30 years, although essentially never in children.[7] There is 2:1 male predominance and black patients have a twofold greater risk for developing MF/SS than white.

The etiology of MF and SS remains undetermined. Various studies and case reports have suggested an association with genetic factors, environmental exposure, or an infectious etiology, but none has confirmed such causal association. Many chromosomal abnormalities have been described in MF; however, persistent, MF-specific chromosomal translocations have not been identified.[1] Chromosomal loss at 10q and abnormalities in *p15, p16*, and *TP*53 tumor suppressor genes are commonly found in patients with MF.[8] Several studies have shown an identical pattern of chromosomal abnormalities in SS as identified in MF, suggesting that both conditions have similar pathogenesis and represent spectrums of the same disease process.[9] The significance of these chromosomal abnormalities is unclear.

Recent studies have shown that the malignant T cells display widespread promoter hypermethylation associated with inactivation of several tumor suppressor genes involved in DNA repair, cell cycle, and apoptosis signaling pathways.[10] Nuclear factor κB (NF-κB) may play a key role in the resistance to apoptosis in MF and SS. Downregulation of the constitutive activation of NF-κB induces apoptosis in CTCL cells.[11]

The immunopathogenesis has been a focus of much research in the last decade. It is now well accepted that the malignant T cells in MF express the skin-homing receptors CLA and CCR4. The CD4$^+$ malignant cells are associated with a skewed profile of increased T helper type 2 (TH2) and reduced TH1 cytokine production.[3] The source or trigger of T cell activation and subsequent clonal expansion of these malignant cells in the skin remains unclear.

Chronic antigenic stimulation has been proposed by some investigators as an etiologic factor for clonal T cell expansion.[12,13] Prolonged exposure to contact allergens, for example, has been postulated as affecting the host immune response in some way, such that the development of MF and SS is more likely.[14] A subsequent case-controlled study did not, however, support this hypothesis since patients with MF do not appear to have an altered immune response to skin allergens.[15] Toxic environmental exposures, such as industrial chemicals, pesticides, and herbicides, have been implicated as potential oncogenic factors.[16,17] However, well-designed, case-controlled studies have failed to support this possibility.

A search for a viral etiology of MF and SS has been pursued for many years,[18,19] with particular focus on human T cell lymphotrophic virus 1 (HTLV-1), a virus that was initially isolated from a patient erroneously believed to have SS. However, extensive testing of patient blood and tissues for HTLV-1 has not provided clear evidence for the involvement of this virus in the pathogenesis of MF and SS.[20,21]

CLINICAL FEATURES

Mycosis fungoides is characterized by heterogeneous cutaneous manifestations.[1–3] The initial cutaneous presentation of MF can be as patches, plaques, tumors, or generalized erythroderma. A patient may present with more than one morphologic type of skin disease or the disease may evolve from one morphologic type to another in the course of time. The most common initial presentation is with patch and plaque disease. Patches or plaques in MF are often localized, typically in a 'bathing trunk' distribution, although any area of the body can be involved. However, the skin involvement can be much more extensive and sometimes may progress to tumors or generalized erythroderma involving essentially the entire skin surface. In the more generalized presentations, the palms and soles are frequently involved, nails may be dystrophic, and scalp involvement can result in alopecia. Pruritus is the most common symptom in these patients and may prompt a visit to the dermatologist. Patches and plaques often resemble the lesions of psoriasis and eczematous dermatitis, leading to delay in establishing the correct diagnosis.

Less frequently, the initial skin manifestation of MF is tumor-like (the so-called *d'emblée* presentation) or consists of generalized erythroderma. Many of the previously described patients with *d'emblée* presentation may be better classified into primary cutaneous, CD4$^+$ small/medium pleomorphic T cell lymphoma or peripheral T cell lymphoma, unspecified, in the updated WHO-EORTC classification.[1] Extensive involvement of the face with indurated plaques or tumors can result in 'leonine facies' reminiscent of the facies observed in patients with lepromatous leprosy.

The risk and extent of extracutaneous disease tend to correlate with the extent and type of skin involvement, which, in MF, is subdivided into a T (tumor) classification.[22–24] Extracutaneous involvement at presentation is exceedingly rare in patients with T1 disease, infrequent in patients with T2 disease (2 percent), and most likely in patients with T3 (13 percent) or T4 (24 percent) disease.[23,24] Patients who present with limited cutaneous involvement (T1) only may never progress to more advanced T classification, especially when appropriate treatment is administered. Although MF may be a systemic disease from the outset, the clinical behavior is such that extracutaneous involvement is usually preceded by progression of skin involvement. Any visceral sites can be involved with MF, although many are detected only at autopsy. The most common sites of involvement detected premortum include the lungs, bone marrow, gastrointestinal tract, liver, and central nervous system. Involvement of the oral cavity may occur when the disease is advanced and is associated with a poor prognosis.[25]

Staging and prognosis

The standard clinical staging system for MF is based on the TNMB classification, which is in turn based on the extent and type of skin involvement (T classification), the presence of lymph node (N classification) or visceral disease (M classification), and the detection of abnormal (Sézary) cells in the peripheral blood (B classification).[26]

The original classification and staging system for MF and SS established in 1979 has been recently revised.[27] Tables 78.1 and 78.2 summarize the revised TNMB classification and the overall clinical staging systems. Sézary syndrome is defined as a level of blood involvement by Sézary cells that meets the criteria of Sézary significance either by morphology, flow cytometry, or molecular analysis.[27,28] Accurate staging is important because therapeutic approaches in MF are largely based on the clinical stage of the disease.

The recommendations for staging evaluation in MF and SS are clearly outlined in the National Comprehensive Cancer Network (NCCN) Practice Guidelines[29] and in the revised staging document.[27] In general, the initial evaluation of newly diagnosed patients with MF includes a comprehensive physical examination, a chemistry panel and complete blood count, flow cytometry for examination of circulating Sézary (malignant) cells, and a chest x-ray. Whole body imaging studies in patients with early stages of MF are unproductive.[30] If the patient has palpable lymphadenopathy

Table 78.1   TNMB classification for mycosis fungoides

TNMB stages		
T (Skin)	T1	Limited patches,[a] papules, and/or plaques[b] covering <10% of the skin surface. May further stratify into T1a (patch only) vs T1b (plaque ± patch)
	T2	Patches, papules, or plaques covering ≥10% of the skin surface. May further stratify into T2a (patch only) vs T2b (plaque ± patch)
	T3	One or more tumors[c] (≥1 cm diameter)
	T4	Confluence of erythema covering ≥80% body surface area
N (Node)	N0	No clinically abnormal peripheral lymph nodes[d]; biopsy not required
	N1	Clinically abnormal peripheral lymph nodes; histopathology Dutch grade 1 or NCI LN0–2
	N1a	Clone negative[g]
	N1b	Clone positive[g]
	N2	Clinically abnormal peripheral lymph nodes; histopathology Dutch grade 2 or NCI LN3
	N2a	Clone negative[g]
	N2b	Clone positive[g]
	N3	Clinically abnormal peripheral lymph nodes; histopathology Dutch grades 3–4 or NCI LN4; clone positive or negative
	NX	Clinically abnormal peripheral lymph nodes; no histologic confirmation
M (Visceral)	M0	No visceral organ involvement
	M1	Visceral involvement (must have pathology confirmation[e] and organ involved should be specified)
B (Blood)	B0	Absence of significant blood involvement: ≤5% of peripheral blood lymphocytes are atypical (Sézary) cells[f]
	B0a	Clone negative[g]
	B0b	Clone positive[g]
	B1	Low blood tumor burden: >5% of peripheral blood lymphocytes are atypical (Sézary) cells but does not meet the criteria of B2
	B1a	Clone negative[g]
	B1b	Clone positive[g]
	B2	High blood tumor burden: ≥1000/μL Sézary cells[f] with positive clone[g]

[a]For skin, patch indicates any size skin lesion without significant elevation or induration. Presence/absence of hypo- or hyperpigmentation, scale, crusting, and/or poikiloderma should be noted.

[b]For skin, plaque indicates any size skin lesion that is elevated or indurated. Presence or absence of scale, crusting, and/or poikiloderma should be noted. Histologic features such as folliculotropism or large-cell transformation (>25% large cells), CD30$^+$ or CD30$^-$, and clinical features such as ulceration are important to document.

[c]For skin, tumor indicates at least one 1 cm diameter solid or nodular lesion with evidence of depth and/or vertical growth. Note total number of lesions, total volume of lesions, largest size lesion, and region of body involved. Also note if histologic evidence of large-cell transformation has occurred. Phenotyping for CD30 is encouraged.

[d]For node, abnormal peripheral lymph node(s) indicates any palpable peripheral node that on physical examination is firm, irregular, clustered, fixed or 1.5 cm or larger in diameter. Node groups examined on physical examination include cervical, supraclavicular, epitrochlear, axillary, and inguinal. Central nodes, which are not generally amenable to pathologic assessment, are not currently considered in the nodal classification unless used to establish N3 histopathologically.

[e]For viscera, spleen and liver may be diagnosed by imaging criteria.

[f]For blood, Sézary cells are defined as lymphocytes with hyperconvoluted cerebriform nuclei. If Sézary cells are not able to be used to determine tumor burden for B2, then one of the following modified ISCL criteria along with a positive clonal rearrangement of the TCR may be used instead: (1) expanded CD4$^+$ or CD3$^+$ cells with CD4/CD8 ratio of 10 or more, (2) expanded CD4$^+$ cells with abnormal immunophenotype including loss of CD7 or CD26.

[g]A T cell clone is defined by PCR or Southern blot analysis of the T cell receptor gene.

Table 78.2 Clinical staging system for mycosis fungoides and Sézary syndrome

Clinical stages	TNMB classification			
IA	T1	N0	M0	B0–1
IB	T2	N0	M0	B0–1
II	T1–2	N1–2	M0	B0–1
IIB	T3	N0–2	M0	B0–1
III	T4	N0–2	M0	B0–1
IIIA	T4	N0–2	M0	B0
IIIB	T4	N0–2	M0	B1
IVA_1	T1–4	N0–2	M0	B2
IVA_2	T1–4	N3	M0	B0–2
IVB	T1–4	N0–3	M1	B0–2

or presents with advanced skin involvement (T3 or T4), or has other bad prognostic features (folliculocentric or large cell transformed disease), appropriate imaging studies (computed tomography [CT] of chest, abdomen, and pelvis or integrated positron emission tomography [PET]/CT scan) should be obtained to further assess the extracutaneous sites. If the clinical suspicion of lymph node involvement is confirmed by imaging, a lymph node biopsy should be performed to determine the N classification. Patients with extensive skin involvement may often have dermatopathic or reactive lymphadenopathy, rather than involvement of the node by lymphoma. Integrated PET/CT scanners can provide simultaneous anatomical and metabolic information[31] that may help detect and select the most informative lymph node region for biopsy, resulting in improved staging accuracy in MF and SS.[32]

Suspected sites of visceral involvement must be confirmed by appropriate imaging studies and histologic evaluation when possible. Significant bone marrow involvement is extremely rare in patients with limited skin disease[33] and is most often present in patients who meet the clinical criteria for SS. Significant bone marrow disease is usually reflected by the presence of readily detectable Sézary cells in the peripheral blood. Therefore, bone marrow biopsy is not routinely employed as part of the initial staging procedure for MF patients.[27,29]

Patients with MF and SS have varying risks for disease progression or death. The most important clinical predictive factors for survival include age, T classification, and the presence of extracutaneous disease.[23,34] The risk for disease progression to a more advanced TNMB classification, worse clinical stage, or death due to MF correlates with the initial T classification. The risk for development of extracutaneous disease also correlates with T classification. It is extremely rare to have T1 disease at the time that extracutaneous disease is detected.[24] In addition to clinical predictive factors, there are histologic factors such as large cell transformation[35,36] and folliculocentric histologic presentations[37] that have been shown to correlate with worse outcome and may lead to more aggressive management.

TREATMENT APPROACHES

GENERAL

There are multiple therapeutic options for MF and SS (Table 78.3). Selection of a specific treatment plan is based on the clinical stage, prognostic factors, acute/cumulative toxicities of the treatment options, the accessibility of different treatment approaches, the patient's age and other social and medical problems, and the cost–benefit ratio. The most important factor in designing a treatment plan is the clinical stage. In general, the treatment options in MF/SS are categorized into primarily skin-directed treatments, systemic biologic therapies, and systemic cytotoxic chemotherapies (Table 78.3). Combination treatment strategies may include multiple skin-directed therapies, a combination of skin-directed with systemic therapy options, or a combination of systemic therapies. In recent years, major consensus treatment guidelines for MF and SS have become available, including the NCCN Practice Guidelines in Oncology[29] and the EORTC consensus documentation.[38]

For patients with T1 and T2 disease without extracutaneous involvement (stages IA–IIA), the primary treatment plan will usually be limited to skin-directed therapies unless these have failed or the patient presents with either large cell transformation or folliculotropic features, when a more intensive regimen may be indicated. Patients with cutaneous tumor disease (stage IIB) often have coexistent patch/plaque and tumor lesions; thus, their treatment plan depends on the extent of the tumor lesions. If the tumor lesions are minimal, the treatment options for stage IA–IIA would be considered and limited areas of tumor lesion(s) can be dealt with by local radiation therapy. If the tumor lesions are extensive, total skin electron beam therapy or combination therapies may be considered. The affected skin in patients with erythroderma (T4) is very sensitive; thus, the patients often cannot tolerate intensive skin-directed measures such as topical chemotherapy, phototherapy, or radiation therapy. The ideal primary therapy for patients with erythroderma is the use of systemic biologic response modifiers such as photopheresis, oral retinoids/rexinoids, interferons, or denileukin diftitox (fusion toxin), alone, or in a combination regimen. When biologic therapies fail in T4 patients, single-agent chemotherapy such as methotrexate, gemcitabine, or PEGylated liposomal doxorubicin can be considered.

Combination chemotherapy is reserved for those patients with lymph node or visceral disease and has little value for control of skin disease in MF. Patients with advanced disease in whom primary treatment fails are candidates for potential allogeneic stem cell transplantation. There is no evidence that early aggressive systemic therapy is preferable to conservative therapy in the management of limited disease. Despite decades of experience in the treatment of MF and SS, well-designed, prospective, controlled clinical studies comparing the efficacy of various therapies, whether traditional, newer or investigative, are lacking.

Table 78.3 Treatment alternatives in mycosis fungoides and Sézary syndrome

Skin-directed (topical) therapy
  Topical steroid, topical chemotherapy (nitrogen mustard, BCNU), topical retinoid/rexinoid (Targretin®), phototherapy (NB-UVB, PUVA), electron beam therapy

Systemic therapy
  Biologicals
    Photopheresis, interferon, retinoid/rexinoid (Targretin®), fusion protein/toxin (Ontak®), alemtuzumab
  HDAC inhibitors
  Vorinostat (Zolinza®)
  Cytotoxic chemotherapy
    Methotrexate, liposomal doxorubicin, gemcitabine, pentostatin, chlorambucil, etoposide, cyclophosphamide, temozolomide, combination chemotherapy regimens

Combined modality therapy
  Skin-directed + skin-directed, skin-directed + systemic, systemic + systemic

Investigative therapy
  Monoclonal antibodies (e.g., CD4, CD30)
  HDAC inhibitors (e.g., depsipeptide, PXD101, LBH589)
  PNP inhibitors
  Recombinant cytokines (e.g., rhIL-12)
  TLR agonists (e.g., CpG ODNs)
  PKC-b inhibitor (enzastaurin)
  Newer chemotherapy agents (sapacitabine, pralatrexate)
  Allo-HSC transplantation

BCNU, carmustine; NB-UVB, narrowband UVB; PUVA, psoralen and UVA treatment; HDAC, histone deacetylase; PNP, purine nucleoside phosphorylase; rhIL-12, human recombinant interleukin-12; TLR, Toll-like receptor; ODN, oligodeoxynucleotide; PKC, protein kinase C; Allo-HSC, allogeneic hematopoietic stem cell.

Nonspecific, symptomatic treatment of MF and SS patients is an integral component of the overall therapeutic regimen. Pruritus and xerosis, either as a result of the disease or therapy, can be severe in these patients, and thus supportive measures such as aggressive emolliation, topical steroids, and oral antipruritics should be utilized as necessary. Patients with erythroderma (T4) have compromised skin barrier function and are especially susceptible to infections with common skin pathogens. Thus, there should be a low threshold for initiating antibiotic therapy, especially in addressing Gram-positive organisms. In patients with SS, the pruritus can be very severe and life altering. In these unrelenting chronic diseases, it is essential to consider the patients' altered quality of life due to severe pruritus or cumulative toxicities, in addition to improving their survival.

SKIN-DIRECTED THERAPIES

Despite advances in treatment for MF and SS, traditional skin-directed therapies are still used as the primary therapeutic modality in the majority of patients with stage I–IIA (patch/plaque, T1–2) disease. In patients in whom initial skin-directed therapy has failed or in those with severely symptomatic disease, the skin-directed therapies can be combined with systemic treatments, or the patients may be referred for experimental therapy.

Topical corticosteroid therapy

Topical steroids can be used either as primary treatment in patients with limited patch or thin plaque disease, or combined with other skin-directed treatments for added symptomatic control. For patients with very limited skin involvement, this can be a very cost-effective option for disease control. In a clinical study of 79 patients with T1 or T2 disease, overall response rates of 94 percent were observed in T1 patients with limited disease and 82 percent in patients with T2 disease.[39] Long-term use of topical steroids may lead to epidermal atrophy and other topical steroid-associated toxicities.

Topical chemotherapy

Topical nitrogen mustard (mechlorethamine hydrochloride, HN2) is the major form of topical chemotherapy used for MF and SS.[40] Topical carmustine (BCNU) has also been used.[41] These topical agents are indicated as initial primary therapy for patients with stage IA disease with limited patches or plaques or with less infiltrated, generalized patch/plaque disease of stage IB.[42] Topical chemotherapy is an alternative for those patients who are candidates for psoralen with ultraviolet A (PUVA) therapy, but topical therapy is often selected in preference to PUVA because of the convenience of home application and avoidance of photodamage.

Topical HN2 is the most widely utilized topical chemotherapeutic agent for MF because of its well-demonstrated efficacy, safety, and ease of application.[43–45] There is no evidence of significant systemic absorption so that, in contrast to BCNU, hematologic monitoring is unnecessary. The mechanism of action of topical HN2 in MF is unclear and may not be related simply to its alkylating agent properties. Its activity may be mediated by immune mechanisms (e.g., immune stimulation) or by interaction with the epidermal cell–Langerhans cell–T cell axis.

Topical HN2 is formulated as either an aqueous or ointment base.[40,42] For aqueous preparation, the patients dissolve 10–20 mg of HN2 powder in 50–100 mL of water in order to achieve a final concentration of 10–20 mg/dL or a 10–20 mg% (w/v) solution of HN2. The ointment form should be prepared by a pharmacist and is formulated by dissolving the powdered HN2 in aquaphor, a common ointment base, to achieve a similar 10–20 mg% (w/w) concentration of HN2 for initial application. The aqueous form of HN2 must be prepared daily, whereas the HN2 in ointment base remains stable for several months.

Either form of the topical HN2 preparation is applied to the skin once-daily as initial therapy. If the disease is very localized, the application field may be limited to the regional area of involvement. The face, scalp, intertriginous, and genital areas are not usually included in the initial treatment unless there is evidence of active disease. In order to accelerate the response, the concentration of the HN2 may be increased to 30–40 mg% or the frequency of application may be increased to twice a day. If complete skin clearing is achieved with topical HN2, a maintenance regimen of some kind is usually instituted. The duration of maintenance regimens used has varied between 1–2 months and 2 years.[42] There is no evidence that more prolonged maintenance is beneficial.

Several large patient series have been reported in which the efficacy of topical HN2 has been evaluated.[43–45] Most patients treated with topical HN2 experience some skin clearing with therapy. In patients with T1 disease, the overall and complete response rates are 90–95 percent and 65–75 percent, respectively, and in T2 patients are 70–80 percent and 30–50 percent, respectively. The degree of response is dependent on the extent and type (T classification) of skin involvement. Patients with refractory plaques or tumors often receive supplemental local radiation therapy to their lesions. The average time to achieve complete skin clearing is approximately 6 months, with a range of 3–12 months. Despite the high rate of complete response with topical HN2, most patients will relapse after discontinuation of therapy, although the duration of remission is highly variable.

Both acute and chronic complications have been associated with topical HN2 therapy. One frequently observed acute complication is the development of immediate or delayed cutaneous hypersensitivity reactions. This may occur in as many as 60 percent of patients with the aqueous preparation and in fewer than 10 percent of patients with the ointment-base preparation of HN2. Patients experiencing hypersensitivity reactions can be desensitized with a variety of topical or systemic desensitizing regimens.[40,42] The development of dry skin is also a more frequent problem when the aqueous formulation is used. For these reasons, either heavy emolliation or the ointment preparation of HN2 is recommended for those patients who have significant skin dryness.

Chronic use of topical HN2 as monotherapy is not associated with increased risk of secondary cutaneous malignancies.[45] However, in patients who have used topical HN2 in combination or sequentially with other skin-damaging therapies (e.g., ultraviolet [UV] phototherapy, radiation therapy) there is an increased risk for non-melanoma skin cancers.[43,46] Application of HN2 in the genital areas should be avoided at all times since genital application has been linked with development of secondary skin cancers. Topical HN2 can be used safely in the pediatric age group and studies have not shown worse adverse effects in children.[42,45]

Topical retinoid therapy

Bexarotene (Targretin) 1 percent gel, a selective synthetic retinoid, is the most commonly used topical retinoid for treating MF. Bexarotene gel is applied with a thin application to the patches or plaques and is most effective and best tolerated when used twice daily.[47] Due to the irritant effect of the retinoids, it is only feasible to use this agent when there is a discrete number of patches or plaques. It is not intended for generalized application. An early trial reported an overall response rate of 63 percent with a complete response rate of 21 percent.[48] A phase III trial included 50 patients with refractory or persistent early stage disease (stages IA–IIA).[49] Responses were seen in 62 percent of patients with stage IA and 50 percent of patients with stage IB disease. Three patients with stage IIA or IIB disease did not respond. The most common toxicity of bexarotene gel is irritation at the sites of application, which occurs in the majority of patients. Because of the erythema from the irritant reaction, it may be necessary to withhold therapy for a few weeks to assess disease activity.

Phototherapy

Phototherapy involves using UV radiation in the form of UVA or UVB wavelengths, which can be used alone, together, or with psoralen, a photosensitizing agent. The long-wave UVA has the advantage over UVB in its greater depth of penetration into the dermal infiltrates of MF. For early limited disease, UVB alone[50] or home UV phototherapy (UVA + UVB)[51] has been shown to be effective.

More recently, narrowband UVB (NB-UVB, 311 nm) phototherapy has been shown to be more effective than the traditional broadband UVB. Narrowband UVB is considered to have less toxicity than broadband UVB or PUVA. Several published studies using NB-UVB in MF[52,53] have shown clinical efficacy that is superior to broadband UVB; however, it is not more effective than PUVA.[54]

Psoralen with UVA is also referred to as photochemotherapy. PUVA therapy was initially developed for treatment of psoriasis and is widely used in dermatology for various dermatoses. PUVA is indicated as primary therapy in generalized plaque-type MF and erythrodermic MF without evidence of extracutaneous disease. It is also given as palliative therapy in patients with advanced disease, often in combination with other treatment. The efficacy of PUVA in MF has been demonstrated by many investigators.[54–57]

Initially, PUVA treatments are given 2–3 times per week, with a minimum of 48 hours between treatments to monitor the delayed erythema reaction (the reaction observed with UVB is more immediate).[55] The initial dose of UVA and the rate at which the dose is increased is dependent upon the skin type and additional factors that are relevant to photosensitivity. Erythrodermic patients tend to require very low starting doses with very small dose increments. After a maximal steady-state response has been achieved, the frequency of PUVA treatments is decreased to a maintenance level. Refractory lesions can be supplemented with local measures such as radiation therapy or topical chemotherapy.

In a study of 82 patients treated with PUVA therapy, complete response was observed in 88 percent of patients with limited plaque (T1) disease and 52 percent with generalized plaque (T2) disease.[58] A smaller number of patients with erythrodermic (T4) MF had excellent responses but most relapsed when the treatments were decreased to a maintenance level. Patients with tumor stage T3 disease in this study had only partial responses. A recent long-term follow-up study of 66 patients with MF stages IA–IB/IIA who achieved a complete response (median follow-up time of nearly 8 years) reported that PUVA can induce long-term remissions.[57] The disease-free survival rates at 5 and 10 years for stage IA were 56 percent and 30 percent, respectively, and for stage IB/IIA were 74 percent and 50 percent, respectively. However, one-third of these patients developed signs of chronic photodamage and secondary cutaneous malignancies.

Psoralens intercalate between pyrimidines within DNA and, upon UVA irradiation, form photoadducts and DNA crosslinks.[59,60] This process results in direct cytotoxic and antiproliferative effects, as well as possibly immunomodulatory effects, through either a direct effect on T cells or an indirect effect by modulating cytokine production. The optimal time for UVA irradiation is 1.5–2.0 hours after oral ingestion of psoralen when the peak serum level is attained. The most widely used and tolerated psoralen is Oxsoralen-Ultra, a rapidly absorbed formulation of 8-methoxypsoralen.

Both acute and chronic adverse effects can be observed with PUVA therapy.[55] Nausea from psoralen ingestion is observed in 10–20 percent of patients and can be managed by ingesting the drug with food or milk, or with appropriate antiemetics.[60] Acute toxicities include phototoxic reactions ranging from erythema to the development of bullae. Ultraviolet-opaque goggles must be worn during the UVA irradiation. After each PUVA treatment, appropriate photoprotection, including application of sunscreens, protective clothing, and UV-shielding glasses, should be used for a minimum of 24 hours. Long-term PUVA therapy with high cumulative doses has been linked to an increased risk for the development of squamous cell carcinomas,[57,61] pigmented macules,[62] and cataract formation.[60]

Radiation therapy

Mycosis fungoides is an extremely radiosensitive neoplasm. Individual plaques or tumors of MF may be treated with electron beam therapy (EBT) to total doses of 24–36 Gy, with a high likelihood of achieving long-term local control.

Techniques have been developed to treat the entire skin surface with electrons (total skin EBT or TSEBT).[63]

Conventional linear accelerators may be modified to treat patients in the standing position at an extended distance. By having the patients assume multiple positions, the entire skin surface may be irradiated. The most common treatment technique uses a six-field technique (anterior, posterior, and four opposed oblique fields). Treatment is administered four times a week to a total dose of 30–36 Gy. Supplementary treatment is required for the soles of the feet, the perineum, and inframammary areas. Only the eyes are shielded routinely, but other areas may be shielded during part of the treatment to help control localized skin reactions.

The complications of TSEBT include acute erythema, desquamation, and temporary loss of fingernails and toenails, as well as an impaired ability to perspire for up to 12 months. There is an increased risk of secondary squamous cell and basal cell carcinomas of the skin, but the risk is greatest in those who have received protracted treatment with a variety of skin-damaging therapies including PUVA and UVB.[46]

Several centers have developed expertise in the use of TSEBT.[64,65] Overall response rates are nearly 100 percent with complete response rates ranging from 40 percent to 98 percent depending on the extent and severity of skin involvement. As many as 50 percent of patients with limited plaque (T1) disease may remain disease free for more than 5 years after completion of a single course of EBT. Although the curative potential of this treatment remains disputed, there is no doubt that it provides important palliative benefit, especially for patients with extensive or severely symptomatic disease. Often, when disease recurs, it is in a more limited distribution and may be controlled more readily with localized skin-directed therapies. The use of TSEBT is often indicated as primary or secondary management of patients with generalized plaque or tumor involvement of the skin. After complete skin clearance, adjuvant therapy with topical HN2 with or without systemic biologic therapy may be utilized. Repeat courses of TSEBT may be administered in selected situations.[66]

In patients who have lymph node involvement, traditional megavoltage (4–15 MeV) photon irradiation may be helpful in providing important additional palliation. Doses of 30–36 Gy in 3–4 weeks are often sufficient to achieve local control of lymph node or other extracutaneous disease.[67]

SYSTEMIC THERAPIES

Systemic therapies are indicated in those patients in whom skin-directed primary therapies fail or those who present with aggressive or advanced MF disease. Patients with significant circulating Sézary cells should also have a systemic therapy as part of their treatment regimen. Traditionally, cytotoxic systemic chemotherapy has not resulted in durable remissions in MF/SS. As a consequence, emerging therapeutic efforts have focused on targeted biologic agents that promote tumor cell apoptosis and/or manipulate the host immune response using multimodality, combination therapy approaches. Combining biologic agents may result in improved clinical responses by a synergistic mechanism and/or a reduction in toxicity by allowing the use of lower doses of each therapy. Whenever appropriate, skin-directed therapies should be combined with systemic therapy to maximize symptomatic control of disease.

Biologic therapies

EXTRACORPOREAL PHOTOPHERESIS

Also known as extracorporeal or 'systemic' photochemotherapy, extracorporeal photopheresis (ECP) is considered by some investigators to be the treatment of choice for erythrodermic (T4) MF and SS.[3,68] Since its introduction in the mid-1980s,[69] the efficacy of ECP has been demonstrated mostly in erythrodermic (T4) MF and SS patients and its effectiveness in T1, T2, and T3 disease remains undetermined. A large study of patients with erythrodermic MF/SS[68] revealed that the majority (83 percent) experienced some level of response to ECP. The complete response rate was lower (20 percent), but 41 percent of patients experienced at least 50 percent improvement in their skin disease. The best responders were erythrodermic (T4) patients with disease limited to the skin and a lower CD4/CD8 ratio, less Sézary burden, and increased CD8$^+$ T cells and natural killer (NK) cells in the peripheral blood at the start of therapy.[3]

Extracorporeal photopheresis is a method of delivering PUVA systemically by utilizing an extracorporeal technique.[70] The white blood cells are collected (leukapheresis) and exposed to a photoactivating agent (8-methoxypsoralen) in the leukapheresed bag, which is then irradiated with UVA. The irradiated cells are returned to the patient in a closed system. The ECP instrument performs the leukapheresis and delivers the UVA treatment. A standard complete ECP regimen for CTCL consists of two consecutive days of therapy. The 2-day ECP treatment is usually repeated at 2–4-week intervals, the frequency of administration being adjusted according to disease severity and/or clinical response. After maximal, stable response has been achieved, the frequency of treatments is gradually decreased, then stopped completely, unless the disease relapses or flares during the weaning process, or when maintenance therapy is given. Maintenance therapy is given every 4–6 weeks; a repeat attempt at weaning can be made at a later time. If an adequate response is not attained with ECP monotherapy, or if patients have a SS level of circulating Sézary cells, additional biologic agents should be added, such as interferon or systemic retinoid. A minimum of 4–6 months of treatment should be given before ECP is considered a failure.

The mechanism of action of ECP involves induction of malignant T cell apoptosis with psoralen plus UVA, accompanied by enhancement of a tumor-specific immune response. Extracorporeal photopheresis induces monocytes to differentiate into dendritic cells capable of phagocytosing and processing the apoptotic tumor cell antigens.[3,71]

One of the greatest advantages of ECP is that the adverse effects are minimal.[70] There may be mild fatigue associated with leukapheresis and fluid shifts. Peripheral intravenous access for treatment is preferable to central access to minimize complications. There are no significant side effects in terms of any laboratory parameters. Patients who receive psoralen, thus need to protect their eyes and skin from UV exposure for 24 hours after treatment.

INTERFERON α

Interferon α (IFNα) therapy is indicated for refractory or advanced disease and is often combined with other skin-directed or systemic therapies. Interferon α has been shown in several small clinical trials to be effective as a primary therapeutic agent for MF and SS.[72,73] The reported overall response rates when used as monotherapy are 53–74 percent, with complete response rates of 21–35 percent. Administration of IFNα for MF and SS is initiated usually at a low dose of 3–5 million units (MU) subcutaneously three times a week and is gradually increased, depending on the clinical response and the severity of adverse effects. Intralesional administration of IFNα has also been reported to result in complete or partial clearing of skin lesions.[74,75]

The clinical response and response duration appear to be better with the combined regimen of PUVA and IFNα as compared with either treatment alone, with complete response rates of 75–80 percent in stage IB/IIA.[58] When a patient's skin clears completely, IFNα is stopped and maintenance therapy with PUVA at a reduced frequency is begun.

Interferon α induces a variety of immunologic effects that may lead to clinical response.[3] It directly enhances cell-mediated cytotoxicity by CD8$^+$ T cells and NK cells which augments antitumor response. Interferon α also suppresses TH2 cytokine production by malignant T cells, which can lead to enhanced immunomodulation.

RETINOIDS

Systemic retinoids are indicated primarily in patients with refractory or advanced disease and can be used as monotherapy or, more effectively, as part of combination regimens with skin-directed or other biologic therapies. The most commonly used systemic retinoid is a retinoid X receptor (RXR) agonist, bexarotene; however, retinoic acid receptor (RAR) agonists, such as isotretinoin, acitretin, or all-trans retinoic acid, are available as alternative agents.[76] The initial dose of oral bexarotene is 100–300 mg/m^2/day, which can be adjusted according to the clinical response and the severity of adverse effects, especially hyperlipidemia. The overall response rate as monotherapy is 45–60 percent, with a complete response rate of 10–20 percent depending on the dose of bexarotene used and the severity of disease.[77,78]

When systemic retinoids were used in combination with PUVA, responses were obtained with fewer PUVA treatments and with a lower cumulative UVA dose, thus with less skin toxicity when compared with PUVA alone. Retinoids can be combined with other systemic agents including IFNα, ECP, or denileukin diftitox therapy, often with better efficacy and safety profiles compared with using individual biologic agents alone.[3,79–81]

There is a common toxicity profile for the different forms of retinoids and many of these adverse effects are dose dependent. Most commonly, patients experience photosensitivity and dryness of the skin and mucous membranes. Other adverse effects include myalgia, arthralgia, and fatigue, and less commonly, headaches, which on rare occasions are due to pseudotumor cerebri.

The well-known teratogenic effects of retinoids must be carefully addressed in female patients of childbearing age. Because of their potential hepatotoxic and hyperlipidemic effects, liver function and serum lipid levels (triglycerides/cholesterol) should be monitored during treatment. Potential long-term, cumulative toxicity of retinoids includes the development of bony changes such as hyperostosis. Bexarotene has unique effects on the pituitary–thyroid axis, which results in hypothyroidism with low free thyroxine (FT4) and low thyroid-stimulating hormone (TSH) levels. It also has more profound effects on serum lipid levels, especially hypertriglyceridemia, than any other retinoid. Thus, it is conventional to have the patients on lipid-lowering agents and thyroid supplements during bexarotene therapy. Gemfibrizol is contraindicated with bexarotene and the preferred lipid-lowering drugs are of the statin or finofibrate class of agents.[82] Most toxicities associated with systemic retinoids are reversible upon cessation of therapy.

RECOMBINANT FUSION PROTEINS

Therapy with recombinant fusion proteins, such as the interleukin-2 (IL-2)–diphtheria toxin fusion protein (denileukin diftitox), involves the use of fusion toxins designed specifically to kill defined neoplastic cell populations. Denileukin diftitox has undergone a multicenter phase III trial in patients with IL-2 receptor (CD25$^+$)-expressing MF.[83] The overall response rate was 30 percent with a complete response rate of 10 percent in patients in whom multiple prior therapies had failed. The major toxicities include a 'capillary leak' syndrome, which may be ameliorated by pre- and posttreatment hydration, and a hypersensitivity reaction, which can be countered with premedication with corticosteroids. Denileukin diftitox has been approved by the US Food and Drug Administration (FDA) for patients with CTCL who have persistent or recurrent disease.

HISTONE DEACETYLASE INHIBITORS

Histone deacetylase inhibitors (HDACi) are a novel class of agents that address epigenetic defects in cancer, and lead to transcriptional activation of multiple genes involved in the induction of tumor cell growth arrest, differentiation, or apoptosis.[84] There are multiple HDACi in development for various malignancies including CTCL. Vorinostat (suberoylanilide hydroxamic acid [SAHA]; Zolinza®) is an oral agent and the first HDACi to undergo a phase IIB pivotal trial in patients with MF/SS. In the earlier trials in CTCL, vorinostat showed clinical activity, with a response rate of 30 percent as monotherapy.[85] Vorinostat also demonstrated a potent effect in control of pruritus, even in patients who did not meet objective response criteria. Vorinostat became the most recent drug to receive FDA approval (October 2006) for patients with CTCL. There are several other HDACi in clinical development.

MONOCLONAL ANTIBODY THERAPY

The safety and efficacy of alemtuzumab, a chimeric monoclonal antibody against CD52, was tested in 22 previously treated patients, most of whom had stage III or IV disease, reduced performance status, and severe pruritus.[86] Complete and partial responses were noted in 32 percent and 23 percent, respectively, with a median time to treatment failure of 1 year. Serious infections (cytomegalovirus, generalized herpes simplex virus, fatal fungal and mycobacterial infections) were noted. Thus, alemtuzumab should be reserved for those patients with advanced disease in whom other, traditional therapies have failed, and the patients should be followed closely for development of serious infections and cardiac toxicity. Additional studies have confirmed the clinical efficacy of alemtuzumab, especially in those with erythrodermic MF or SS, with an acceptable safety profile.[87]

Systemic chemotherapy

Systemic chemotherapy is appropriate for patients with recalcitrant tumor (T3) disease or extracutaneous involvement (stage IV); however, most chemotherapy regimens result in only temporary palliative responses. Virtually all drugs that are effective as single agents or in combination therapy in the treatment of patients with non-Hodgkin lymphomas have been tested in MF/SS.

For single-agent chemotherapy, no particular drug is clearly superior and no large, randomized studies comparing agents have been reported. In 526 patients reported in single-agent chemotherapy trials, the response rate was 20–80 percent and the median duration of responses ranged from 3 to 22 months.[88] The most data exist for methotrexate, which has activity in many doses and schedules. It is not clear that high-dose methotrexate is superior to lower doses. With low-dose methotrexate, the overall response rate ranges from 33 percent to 58 percent, and the time to treatment failure is 15–32 months, depending upon the extent of prior therapy.[89] Another common single agent has been chlorambucil[90] administered daily in 2 mg doses titrating the dose according to hematologic

Table 78.4 Results of chemotherapy treatment in mycosis fungoides

Study	Therapy	Patients	ORR n (%)	CR n (%)	Median duration of response (months)
Single-agent chemotherapy					
Bunn et al.[88]	Single-agent chemotherapy	528	329 (62)	91 (33)	3–32
Zackheim et al.[89]	Low-dose methotrexate	69	20 (33)	13 (22)	15
Holmes et al.[90]	Chlorambucil + prednisone	21	11 (57)	3 (14)	Not reported
Tsimberidau et al.[91]	Pentostatin	32	13 (54.8)	6 (14)	4.3
Saven et al.[92]	2-CdA	15	7 (47)	3 (20)	5
Kuzel et al.[93]	2-CdA	21	6 (28)	3 (14)	2–16
Zinzani et al.[94]	Gemcitabine	30	21 (70)	5 (11)	6–22
Wollina et al.[96]	Liposomal doxorubicin	6	5 (83)	4/6	Not reported
Combination chemotherapy					
Bunn et al.[88]	Combination	331	(81)	(38)	5–41
Kaye et al.[103]	CAVE	52	47 (90)	20 (38)	Not reported
Fierro et al.[101]	VICOB-P	25	(80)	(36)	8–7

ORR, overall response rate; CR, complete remission; 2-CdA, cladribine.

toxicity. Prednisone has been given at 20 mg/day initially with a taper as palliation is achieved. Some newer drugs have shown encouraging single-agent activity in early clinical trials and are summarized in Table 78.4.

The purine analogues are a class of drugs that have demonstrated activity in MF and a variety of other non-Hodgkin lymphomas. T cells have a high level of adenosine deaminase (ADA), a key enzyme in the purine degradation pathway. The purine analogues pentostatin (deoxycoformycin), fludarabine, and cladribine (2-CdA) are a group of structurally similar agents which were developed to target ADA. They have different interactions with ADA but all result in DNA damage. The largest overall experience has been reported with pentostatin, although each individual study is small. The response rates vary from 14 percent to 70 percent.[91] Cladribine[92,93] and fludarabine have also been used with response rates of 20–40 percent. Hematologic toxicity and opportunistic infections are the most common complications associated with this class of drugs. Prophylactic antibiotics against *Pneumocystis carinii* and antivirals to prevent herpesvirus infection are routinely indicated. Combinations of purine analogues with interferon have also been utilized in small studies and show an increased response rate compared with series using these agents alone.

Gemcitabine (2′2′-difluorodeoxycytidine), a novel nucleoside analogue, is a deoxycytidine analogue with excellent antitumor activity against a number of solid tumors and lymphoproliferative disorders. Gemcitabine must be activated by deoxycytidine kinase and other kinases to its triphosphate form, gemcitabine triphosphate, which can then be incorporated into RNA and DNA. The latter action causes masked chain termination and inhibition of DNA repair and is considered to be responsible for its antitumor effect. Response rates as high as 70 percent have been reported,[94] but the complete remission rate is low. Recently this agent has also been used as front-line therapy with a

median duration of complete remission of 10 months (range 4–22 months).[95]

PEGylated liposomes are stable, long-circulating carriers useful for delivering doxorubicin to tumor sites with a lower toxicity than the free drug. In a study of patients who had refractory or relapsed CTCL, PEGylated doxorubicin (Doxil) was given as 20 mg/m² every month until a complete response was achieved, or a total dose of 400 mg.[96] An overall response rate of 80 percent and response duration of 15 months were reported. The most frequent side effects were mild anemia and lymphopenia. Another significant toxicity with this class of drugs is palmoplantar erythrodysesthesia.

Another new cytotoxic agent is temozolomide, which showed encouraging activity in MF in phase I studies and needs prospective further testing. Its mechanism of action is similar to that of other alkylating agents. It induces DNA damage by crosslinking and resistance has been associated with high levels of the scavenger protein O6-alkylguanine-DNA alkyltransferase in tumor cells. Response rates of 26–33 percent have been reported in patients with relapsed stage IB–IVA disease.[97,98]

There are no randomized trials comparing combination chemotherapy with single-agent regimens. The largest experience is with combinations that include cyclophosphamide, vincristine, and prednisone, with or without doxorubicin.[99,100] Complete response rates are generally about 25 percent (range 11–57 percent) and response duration is 3–20 months. Most of the patients treated with combination chemotherapy have advanced disease (IIB–IV), although a few patients with early stage disease (IA–IIA) who had a complete response were disease free (with short follow-up) at the time of the reports.

Intensive chemotherapy using VICOB-P (etoposide, idarubicin, cyclophosphamide, vincristine, prednisone, and bleomycin) has been used as front-line therapy.[101] Administered weekly for 12 weeks, it resulted in a response rate of 80 percent (complete response rate 36 percent). The median duration of response was 6–7 months, similar to that reported for CHOP (cyclophosphamide, doxorubicin, vincristine, and prednisone) chemotherapy. No response was seen in patients with Sézary syndrome. Another intense salvage regimen, ESHAP (etoposide, high-dose cytarabine, and methylprednisone), has also been used without significant durable remissions and poor tolerance due to prolonged myelosuppression and infectious complications.[102]

At one time, based on uncontrolled studies, combined modality therapy with combination chemotherapy and total skin irradiation was proposed as a preferred treatment. This concept was then tested in a prospective randomized trial at the National Cancer Institute (NCI), which compared an aggressive program of combination chemotherapy (cyclophosphamide, doxorubin, vincristine, and etoposide) and total skin electron beam irradiation with sequential conservative therapies.[103] The objective response rates (90 percent vs 65 percent) and complete response rates (38 percent vs 18 percent) were higher with the combined therapy. However, there was no difference in overall survival and considerably greater toxicity in the combination therapy group. There are several reports of combining chemotherapy with biologic agents, such as targeted toxins and immunomodulating agents, which appear encouraging and need to be confirmed in large prospective studies.[104]

HIGH-DOSE CHEMOTHERAPY WITH HEMATOPOIETIC STEM CELL TRANSPLANTATION

Recent interest has been shown in using high-dose chemotherapy followed by peripheral stem cell support (autologous or allogeneic) in MF. Given the small number of patients treated thus far, there are no well-defined prognostic factors to identify patients suitable for this therapy.

Bigler and associates[105] reported that five of six patients achieved a complete response with an autologous transplant. Three of the responses lasted less than 100 days and two patients were disease free at 1 year. In another study,[106] eight of nine patients achieved a complete response of brief duration: 2 months in four of the patients, but three others were disease free at 11 months. All of the patients in these studies ultimately relapsed, suggesting that autologous transplantation is not a curative approach.

The concept of allogeneic hematopoietic stem cell transplantation (HSCT) is provocative, since even in the absence of a complete response, an allogeneic graft-versus-tumor effect may provide an immune mechanism to control the malignant T cell process. In a report by Guitart and associates,[107] three patients received an allograft from human leukocyte antigen (HLA)-matched siblings. Complete and sustained clinical and histologic remissions were achieved in two patients that continued for longer than 4.5 years and longer than 15 months. The third patient was in complete response for 9 months followed by a limited cutaneous recurrence. Molina and associates reported a complete response in all eight patients transplanted for refractory MF or SS. Two patients died from transplantation-related complications: graft-versus-host disease (GVHD; $n = 1$) and acute infection ($n = 1$). With a median follow-up of 56 months, six patients remained alive and without evidence of lymphoma.[108] Mild acute and chronic GVHD developed in all patients who survived. A nonmyeloablative approach has also been reported.[109] All three patients achieved a durable complete response but there was a high incidence of infection.

Thus it appears that compared to autologous HSCT, allogeneic HSCT may result in durable long-term remissions. With better understanding of the disease biology and with newer molecular characteristics, it may be possible to identify patients and develop prognostic factors, so that these aggressive approaches can be offered to suitable patients. Larger studies will be required to identify the best conditioning regimen, efficacy, safety, and impact on quality of life.

NOVEL OR INVESTIGATIVE THERAPIES

Knowledge of the immunopathogenesis of MF/SS and its incurability, especially in the advanced stages, has led to the development of a variety of experimental therapies. The efficacy of anti-T cell antibodies has been studied in CTCL. Early trials with mouse monoclonal antibodies were unsuccessful due to the development of human antimouse antibodies. More recently, strategies employing chimeric, humanized, or fully human antibodies have been developed for targeted therapy. The T cell targets that have been explored in MF or SS include CD3, CD4,[110,111] CD25, CD30, and CD52. The phase II trial of fully human anti-CD4 antibody (zanolumumab) in MF and SS demonstrated promising clinical responses, especially in patients with refractory tumor disease.[111] Despite a reduction in CD4 counts, patients did not have a significantly increased risk of life-threatening infections. The mechanism of action of these targeted antibody therapies is not fully understood, but many of them lead to malignant T cell apoptosis, growth arrest, or tumor destruction by antibody-dependent cell cytotoxicity (zanolimumab)

Various Toll-like receptor (TLR) agonists – potent stimulators of the human immune system – are under development for cancer therapy.[112] CpG oligodeoxynucleotide (CpG ODN) is a TLR9 agonist and is being tested for its antitumor activity in solid and hematolymphoid malignancies. CpG 7909 is a potent activator of B cells and plasmacytoid dendritic cells, leading to increased cytokine production, expression of critical immune accessory molecules, and enhanced tumor-specific cytotoxicity. In the initial phase I/II study of CpG 7909 in patients with MF/SS, CpG 7909 had activity and complete responses were seen.[113] CpG ODNs can be used alone or in combination with other anticancer agents such as chemotherapy, radiation, monoclonal antibodies, or vaccine therapy.

Profound suppression of T cell immunity is seen in patients with an inherited deficiency of purine nucleoside phosphorylase (PNP) inhibitor. These children have a very selective T cell deficiency with an associated increase in the levels of deoxyguanosine (dGUO) and deoxyguanosine triphosphate (dGTP). The accumulation of dGTP leads to alteration in the deoxynucleotide pools resulting in T cell apoptosis. Forodesine hydrochloride is a potent, selective transition-state analogue inhibitor of human PNP.[114] In the initial clinical trial in CTCL patients, forodesine hydrochloride showed clinical activity, including complete responses in those who received the drug intravenously. Subsequently, a phase I/II multicenter trial with forodesine hydrochloride given orally confirmed clinical activity of this novel PNP inhibitor in MF and SS.[115] A pivotal phase II multicenter study is currently ongoing in patients with heavily treated, refractory MF and SS.

KEY POINTS

- Cutaneous presentation as patches, plaques, tumors, or generalized erythroderma.
- Key clinical prognostic factors are patient age, T classification, and presence of extracutaneous disease.
- Most important factor in treatment selection is clinical stage.
- Skin-directed therapies are the primary modality in stage I.
- Successful use of systemic biologic therapies is key to management of recalcitrant or advanced disease.
- Use of combinations of skin-directed and/or systemic therapies to improve response and reduce individual toxicity is essential.
- Chemotherapy has only a palliative role.
- Allogeneic hematopoietic stem cell transplantation may result in durable remission.
- Promising investigative therapies are in development.

REFERENCES

● = Key primary paper
◆ = Major review article

◆1.   Willemze R, Jaffe ES, Burg G et al. WHO-EORTC classification for cutaneous lymphomas. *Blood* 2005; **105**: 3768–85.

◆2.   Hoppe R, Kim Y. Treatment of mycosis fungoides and Sezary syndrome. In: *UpToDate in non-Hodgkin's lymphoma (CD-ROM)*. Waltham, MA: UpToDate Inc., 2006.

◆3.   Kim E, Hess S, Richardson S et al. Immunopathogenesis and therapy of cutaneous T-cell lymphoma. *J Clin Invest* 2005; **115**: 798–812.

◆4.   Girardi M, Heald P, Wilson L. The pathogenesis of mycosis fungoides. *N Engl J Med* 2004; **350**: 1978–88.

●5.   Pimpinelli N, Olsen E, Santucci M et al. Defining early mycosis fungoides. *J Am Acad Dermatol* 2005; **53**: 1053–63.

●6.   Weinstock M, Gardstein B. Twenty-year trends in the reported incidence of mycosis fungoides and associated mortality. *Am J Public Health* 1999; **89**: 1240–4.

●7.   Crowley J, Nikko A, Varghese A et al. Mycosis fungoides in young patients: clinical characteristics and outcome. *J Am Acad Dermatol* 1998; **38**: 696–701.

◆8.   Smoller B, Santucci M, Wood GS, Whittaker S. Histopathology and genetics of cutaneous T-cell lymphoma. *Hematol Oncol Clin North Am* 2003; **17**: 1277–311.

●9.   Mao X, Lillington D, Scarisbrick J et al. Molecular cytogenetic analysis of cutaneous T-cell lymphomas: identification of common genetic alterations in Sezary syndrome and mycosis fungoides. *Br J Dermatol* 2002; **147**: 464–75.

10.   van Doorn R, Zoutman W, Dijkman R et al. Epigenetic profiling of cutaneous T-cell lymphoma: promoter hypermethylation of multiple tumor suppressor genes including BCL7a, PTPRG, and p73. *J Clin Oncol* 2005; **23**: 3886–96.

11.   Sors A, Jean-Louis F, Pellet C et al. Down-regulating constitutive activation of the NF-kB canonical pathway overcomes the resistance of cutaneous T-cell lymphoma to apoptosis. *Blood* 2006; **107**: 2354–63.

◆12.   Thiers B. Controversies in mycosis fungoides. *J Am Acad Dermatol* 1982; **7**: 1–16.

●13.   Wood G. Lymphocyte activation in cutaneous T-cell lymphoma. *J Invest Dermatol* 1995; **105**(Suppl 1): 105S–9S.

●14.   Tan R, Butterworth C, McLaughlin H et al. Mycosis fungoides – a disease of antigen persistence. *Br J Dermatol* 1974; **91**: 607–16.

●15.   Whittemore AS, Holly EA, Lee IM et al. Mycosis fungoides in relation to environmental exposures and immune response: a case-control study. *J Natl Cancer Inst* 1989; **81**: 1560–7.

●16.   Cohen S, Stenn K, Braverman I, Beck G. Mycosis fungoides: clinicopathologic relationships, survival, and therapy in 59 patients with observations on occupation as a new prognostic factor. *Cancer* 1980; **46**: 2654–66.

●17.   Tuyp E, Burgoyne A, Aitchison T, MacKie R. A case-control study of possible causative factors in mycosis fungoides. *Arch Dermatol* 1987; **123**: 196–200.

●18.   Wantzin G, Thomsen K, Nissen N et al. Occurrence of human T cell lymphotrophic virus (type I) antibodies in cutaneous T cell lymphoma. *J Am Acad Dermatol* 1986; **15**: 598–602.

●19.   Hall W, Liu C, Schneewind O et al. Deleted HTLV-I provirus in blood and cutaneous lesions of patients with mycosis fungoides. *Science* 1991; **253**: 317–20.

●20. Wood G, Salvekar A, Schaffer J et al. Evidence against a role for HTLV-I in the pathogenesis of American cutaneous T-cell lymphoma. J Invest Dermatol 1996; **107**: 301–7.

●21. Wood G, Schaffer J, Boni R et al. No evidence of HTLV-I proviral integration in lymphoproliferative disorders associated with cutaneous T-cell lymphoma. Am J Pathol 1997; **150**: 667–73.

●22. Zackheim H, Amin S, Kashani-Sabet M, McMillan A. Prognosis in cutaneous T-cell lymphoma by skin stage: long-term survival in 489 patients. J Am Acad Dermatol 1999; **40**: 418–25.

●23. Kim Y, Liu H, Mraz-Gernhard S et al. Long-term outcome of 525 patients with mycosis fungoides and Sezary syndrome. Arch Dermatol 2003; **139**: 857–66.

●24. de Coninck E, Kim Y, Varghese A, Hoppe R. Clinical characteristics and outcome of patients with extracutaneous mycosis fungoides. J Clin Oncol 2001; **19**: 779–84.

●25. Sirois D, Miller A, Harwick R, Vonderheid E. Oral manifestations of cutaneous T-cell lymphoma. A report of eight cases. Oral Surg Oral Med Oral Pathol 1993; **75**: 700–5.

●26. Bunn PJ, Lamberg S. Report of the committee on staging and classification of cutaneous T-cell lymphomas. Cancer Treat Rep 1979; **63**: 725–8.

27. Olsen A, Vonderheid E, Pimpinelli N et al. Revisions to the staging and classification of mycosis fungoides and Sezary syndrome: a proposal of the International Society for Cutaneous Lymphomas (ISCL) and the cutaneous lymphoma task force of the European Organization of Research and Treatment of Cancer (EORTC). Blood 2007; **110**: 1713–22.

●28. Vonderheid E, Bernengo M, Burg G et al. Update on erythrodermic cutaneous T-cell lymphoma: report of the International Society for Cutaneous Lymphomas. J Am Acad Dermatol 2002; **46**: 95–106.

29. NCCN Practice Guidelines in Oncology – v.1.2008. Mycosis fungoides/Sézary syndrome of the cutaneous T-cell lymphomas. www.nccn.org

●30. Kulin P, Marglin S, Shuman W et al. Diagnostic imaging in the initial staging of mycosis fungoides and Sezary syndrome. Arch Dermatol 1990; **126**: 914–18.

◆31. Juweid M, Cheson B. Role of positron emission tomography in lymphoma. J Clin Oncol 2005; **23**: 4577–80.

●32. Tsai E, Taur A, Espinosa L et al. Staging accuracy in mycosis fungoides/Sezary syndrome using integrated positron emission tomography and computed tomography. Arch Dermatol 2006; **142**: 577–84.

●33. Salhany K, Greer J, Cousar J, Collins R. Marrow involvement in cutaneous T-cell lymphoma. A clinicopathologic study of 60 cases. Am J Clin Pathol 1989; **92**: 747–54.

●34. van Doorn R, Van Haselen C, van Voorst Vader P et al. Mycosis fungoides: disease evolution and prognosis of 309 Dutch patients. Arch Dermatol 2000; **136**: 504–10.

●35. Vergier B, de Muret A, Beylot-Barry M et al. Transformation of mycosis fungoides: clinicopathological and prognostic features of 45 cases. Blood 2000; **95**: 2212–18.

●36. Diamandidou E, Colome-Grimmer M, Fayad L et al. Transformation of mycosis fungoides/Sezary syndrome: clinical characteristics and prognosis. Blood 1998; **92**: 1150–9.

●37. van Doorn R, Scheffer E, Willemze R. Follicular mycosis fungoides, a distinct disease entity with or without associated follicular mucinosis: a clinicopathologic and follow-up study of 51 patients. Arch Dermatol 2002; **138**: 191–8.

38. Trautinger F, Knobler R, Willemze R. EORTC consensus recommendations for the treatment of mycosis fungoides/Sezary syndrome. Eur J Cancer 2006; **42**: 1014–30.

●39. Zackheim H, Kashani-Sabet M, Amin S. Topical corticosteroids for mycosis fungoides. Experience in 79 patients. Arch Dermatol 1998; **134**: 949–54.

◆40. Ramsay D, Meller J, Zackheim H. Topical treatment of early cutaneous T-cell lymphoma. Hematol Oncol Clin North Am 1995; **9**: 1031–56.

●41. Zackheim H, Epstein E, Crain W. Topical carmustine (BCNU) for cutaneous T cell lymphoma: a 15-year experience in 143 patients. J Am Acad Dermatol 1990; **22**: 802–10.

◆42. Kim Y. Management with topical nitrogen mustard in mycosis fungoides. In: Tharp M. (ed.) Dermatologic therapy. Blakewell Sciences, 2003: 288–98.

●43. Vonderheid E, Tan E, Kantor A et al. Long-term efficacy, curative potential, and carcinogenicity of topical mechlorethamine chemotherapy in cutaneous T cell lymphoma. J Am Acad Dermatol 1989; **20**: 416–28.

●44. Ramsay D, Halperin P, Zeleniuch-Jacquotte A. Topical mechlorethamine therapy for early stage mycosis fungoides. J Am Acad Dermatol 1988; **19**: 684–91.

●45. Kim Y, Martinez G, Varghese A, Hoppe R. Topical nitrogen mustard in the management of mycosis fungoides. Arch Dermatol 2003; **139**: 165–73.

●46. Smoller B, Marcus R. Risk of secondary cutaneous malignancies in patients with long-standing mycosis fungoides. J Am Acad Dermatol 1994; **30**: 201–4.

●47. Liu H, Kim Y. Bexarotene gel: a food and drug administration-approved skin-directed therapy for early-stage cutaneous T-cell lymphoma. Arch Dermatol 2002; **138**: 398–9.

●48. Breneman D, Duvic M, Kuzel T et al. Phase 1 and 2 trial of bexarotene gel for skin-directed treatment of patients with cutaneous T-cell lymphoma. Arch Dermatol 2002; **138**: 325–32.

●49. Heald P, Mehlmauer M, Martin A et al. Topical bexarotene therapy for patients with refractory or persistent early-stage cutaneous T-cell lymphoma: results of the phase III clinical trial. J Am Acad Dermatol 2003; **49**: 801–15.

●50. Ramsay D, Lish K, Yalowitz C, Soter N. Ultraviolet-B phototherapy for early-stage cutaneous T-cell lymphoma. Arch Dermatol 1992; **128**: 931–3.

●51. Resnik K, Vonderheid E. Home UV phototherapy of early mycosis fungoides: long-term follow-up observations in thirty-one patients. J Am Acad Dermatol 1993; **29**: 73–7.

●52. Gathers R, Scherschun L, Malick F et al. Narrowband UVB phototherapy for early-stage mycosis fungoides. J Am Acad Dermatol 2002; **47**: 191–7.

●53. Boztepe G, Sahin S, Ayhan M et al. Narrowband ultraviolet B phototherapy to clear and maintain clearance in patients with mycosis fungoides. J Am Acad Dermatol 2005; **53**: 242–6.

●54. Diederen P, van Weelden H, Sanders C et al. Narrowband UVB and psoralen-UVA in the treatment of early-stage mycosis fungoides: a retrospective study. J Am Acad Dermatol 2003; **48**: 215–19.

◆55. Herrmann J, Roenigk HJ, Honigsmann H. Ultraviolet radiation for treatment of cutaneous T-cell lymphoma. Hematol Oncol Clin North Am 1995; **9**: 1077–88.

●56. Herrmann J, Roenigk H, Hurria A et al. Treatment of mycosis fungoides with photochemotherapy (PUVA): long-term follow-up. J Am Acad Dermatol 1995; **33**: 234–42.

●57. Querfeld C, Rosen S, Kuzel T et al. Long-term follow-up of patients with early-stage cutaneous T-cell lymphoma who achieved complete remisson with psoralen plus UV-A monotherapy. Arch Dermatol 2005; **141**: 305–11.

●58. Roenigk H, Kuzel T, Skoutelis A et al. Photochemotherapy alone or combined with interferon alpha-2a in the treatment of cutneous T-cell lymphoma. J Invest Dermatol 1990; **95**: 198S–205S.

◆59. Edelson R. Light-activated drugs. Sci Am 1988; **259**: 68–75.

◆60. Gupta A, Anderson T. Psoralen photochemotherapy. J Am Acad Dermatol 1987; **17**: 703–34.

●61. Stern R, Laird N, Melski J et al. Cutaneous squamous cell carcinoma in patients treated with PUVA. N Engl J Med 1984; **310**: 1156–61.

●62. Rhodes A, Harrist T, Momtaz T. The PUVA-induced pigmented macule: a lentiginous proliferation of large, sometimes cytologically atypical, melanocytes. J Am Acad Dermatol 1983; **9**: 47–58.

◆63. Jones G, Hoppe R, Glatstein E. Electron beam treatment for cutaneous T-cell lymphoma. Hematol Oncol Clin North Am 1995; **9**: 1057–76.

◆64. Hoppe R. Total skin electron beam therapy in the management of mycosis fungoides. Front Radiat Ther Oncol 1991; **25**: 80–9.

●65. Jones G, Tadros A, Hodson D et al. Prognosis with newly diagnosed mycosis fungoides after total skin electron radiation of 30 or 35 Gy. Int J Radiat Oncol Biol Phys 1994; **28**: 839–45.

●66. Becker M, Hoppe R, Knox S. Multiple courses of high-dose total skin electron beam therapy in the management of mycosis fungoides. Int J Radiat Oncol Biol Phys 1995; **32**: 1445–9.

◆67. Hoppe R. Mycosis fungoides: radiation therapy. Dermatol Ther 2003; **16**: 347–54.

●68. Heald P, Rook A, Perez M et al. Treatment of erythrodermic cutaneous T-cell lymphoma with extracorporeal photochemotherapy. J Am Acad Dermatol 1992; **27**: 427–33.

●69. Edelson R, Berger C, Gasparro F et al. Treatment of cutaneous T-cell lymphoma by extracorporeal photochemotherapy. N Engl J Med 1987; **316**: 297–303.

◆70. Knobler R, Jantschitsch C. Extracorporeal photochemoimmunotherapy in cutaneous T-cell lymphoma. Transfus Apher Sci 2003; **28**: 81–9.

●71. Edelson R. Cutaneous T-cell lymphoma: the helping hand of dendritic cells. Ann N Y Acad Sci 2001; **941**: 1–11.

●72. Olsen E, Rosen S, Vollmer R et al. Interferon alfa-2a in the treatment of cutaneous T-cell lymphoma. J Am Acad Dermatol 1989; **20**: 395–407.

●73. Vegna ML, Papa G, Defazio D et al. Interferon alpha-2a in cutaneous T-cell lymphoma. Eur J Haematol 1990; **52**(suppl): 32–5.

●74. Wolff JM, Zitelli J, Rabin B et al. Intralesional interferon in the treatment of early mycosis fungoides. J Am Acad Dermatol 1985; **13**: 604–12.

●75. Vonderheid E, Thompson R, Smiles K, Lattanand A. Recombinant interferon alfa-2b in plaque-phase mycosis fungoides. Arch Dermatol 1987; **123**: 757–63.

●76. Querfeld C, Rosen S, Guitart J et al. Comparison of selective retinoic acid receptor- and retinoic X receptor-mediated efficacy, tolerance, and survival in cutaneous T-cell lymphoma. J Am Acad Dermatol 2004; **51**: 25–32.

●77. Duvic M, Martin A, Kim Y et al. Phase 2 and 3 clinical trial of oral bexarotene (Targretin Capsules) for the treatment of refractory or persistent early-stage cutaneous T-cell lymphoma. Arch Dermatol 2001; **137**: 581–93.

●78. Duvic M, Hymes K, Heald P et al. Bexarotene is effective and safe for treatment of refractory advanced-stage cutaneous T-cell lymphoma: multinational phase II–III trial results. J Clin Oncol 2001; **19**: 2456–71.

●79. Knobler R, Trautinger F, Radaszkiewicz T et al. Treatment of cutaneous T-cell lymphoma with a combination of low-dose interferon alpha-2b and retinoids. J Am Acad Dermatol 1991; **24**: 247–52.

●80. Suchin K, Cucchiara A, Gottleib S et al. Treatment of cutaneous T-cell lymphoma with combined immunomodulatory therapy: a 14-year experience at a single institution. Arch Dermatol 2002; **138**: 1054–60.

●81. Foss F, Demierre M, DiVenuti G. A phase I trial of bexarotene and denileukin diftitox in patients with relapsed or refractory cutaneous T-cell lymphoma. Blood 2005; **106**: 454–7.

●82. Talpur R, Ward S, Apisamthanarax N et al. Optimizing bexarotene therapy for cutaneous T-cell lymphoma. J Am Acad Dermatol 2002; **47**: 672–84.

●83. Olsen E, Duvic M, Frankel A et al. Pivotal phase III trial of two dose levels of denileukin diftitox for the treatment of cutaneous T-cell lymphoma. J Clin Oncol 2001; **19**: 376–88.

◆84. Bhalla K. Epigenetic and chromatin modifiers as targeted therapy of hematologic malignancies. J Clin Oncol 2005; **23**: 3971–93.

85. Olsen E, Kim Y, Kuzel T et al. A phase IIb multicenter trial of vorinostat (suberoylanilide hyrosamic acid, SAHA) in patients with persistent, progressive or treatment refractory

mycosis fungoides or Sezay syndrome subtypes of cutaneous T-cell lymphoma. *J Clin Oncol* 2007; **25**: 3109–15

●86. Lundin J, Hagberg H, Repp R *et al.* Phase 2 study of alemtuzumab (anti-CD52 monclonal antibody) in patients with advanced mycosis fungoides/Sezary syndrome. *Blood* 2003; **101**: 4267–72.

87. Bernengo M, Quaglino P, Comessatti A *et al.* Low-dose intermittent alemtuzumab in the treatment of Sezary syndrome: clinical and immunologic findings in 14 patients. *Haematologica* 2007; **92**: 784–94.

◆88. Bunn PJ, Hoffman S, Norris D *et al.* Systemic therapy of cutaneous T-cell lymphoma (mycosis fungoides and the Sezary syndrome). *Ann Intern Med* 1994; **121**: 592–602.

●89. Zackheim H, Kashani-Sabet M, McMillan A. Low-dose methotrexate to treat mycosis fungoides: a retrospective study in 69 patients. *J Am Acad Dermatol* 2003; **49**: 873–8.

●90. Holmes R, McGibbon D, Black M. Mycosis fungoides: progression towards Sezary syndrome reversed with chlorambucil. *Clin Exp Dermatol* 1983; **8**: 429–35.

●91. Tsimberidou A, Giles F, Duvic M *et al.* Phase II study of pentostatin in advanced T-cell lymphoid malignancies: update of an MD Anderson Cancer Center series. *Cancer* 2004; **100**: 342–9.

●92. Saven A, Carrera C, Carson D *et al.* 2-chlorodeoxyadenosine: an active agent in the treatment of cutaneous T-cell lymphoma. *Blood* 1992; **80**: 587–92.

●93. Kuzel T, Hurria A, Samuelson E *et al.* Phase II trial of 2-chlorodeoxyadenosine for the treatment of cutaneous T-cell lymphoma. *Blood* 1996; **87**: 906–11.

●94. Zinzani P, Baliva G, Magagnoli M *et al.* Gemcitabine treatment in pretreated cutaneous T-cell lymphoma: experience in 44 patients. *J Clin Oncol* 2000; **18**: 2603–6.

●95. Marchi E, Alinari L, Tani M *et al.* Gemcitabine as frontline treatment for cutaneous T-cell lymphoma: phase II study of 32 patients. *Cancer* 2005; **104**: 2437–41.

●96. Wollina U, Graefe T, Karte K. Treatment of relapsing or recalcitrant cutaneous T-cell lymphoma with pegylated liposomal doxorubicin. *J Am Acad Dermatol* 2000; **42**: 40–6.

●97. Kuzel T, Guitart J, Martone B *et al.* Phase II trial of temozolomide for treatment of mycosis fungoides/Sezary syndrome. *Proc Am Soc Clin Oncol* 2002; **21**: 286A.

●98. Tani M, Fina M, Alinari L *et al.* Phase II trial of temozolomide in patients with pretreated cutaneous T-cell lymphoma. *Hematologica* 2005; **90**: 1283–4.

●99. Molin L, Thomsen K, Volden G *et al.* Combination chemotherapy in the tumor stage of mycosis fungoides with cyclophosphamide, vincristine, VP-16, adriamycin, and prednisolone (COP, CHOP, CAVOP): a report from the Scandinavian Mycosis Fungoides Study Group. *Acta Derm Venereol* 1980; **60**: 542–4.

●100. Tirelli U, Carbone A, Zagonel V *et al.* Staging and treatment with cyclophosphamide, vincristine, and prednisone (CVP) in advanced cutaneous T-cell lymphoma. *Hematol Oncol* 1986; **4**: 83–90.

●101. Fierro M, Doveil GC, Quaglino P *et al.* Combination of etoposide, idarubicin, cyclophosphamide, vincristine,

prednisone and bleomycin (VICOP-B) in the treatment of advanced cutaneous T-cell lymphoma. *Dermatology* 1997; **194**: 268–72.

●102. Mebazaa A, Dupuy A, Rybojad M *et al.* ESHAP for primary cutaneous T-cell lymphomas: efficacy and tolerance in 11 patients. *Hematol J* 2005; **5**: 553–8.

●103. Kaye F, Bunn P, Steinberg S *et al.* A randomized trial comparing combination electron-beam radiation and chemotherapy with topical therapy in the initial treatment of mycosis fungoides. *N Engl J Med* 1989; **321**: 1784–90.

●104. Duvic M, Apisamthanarax N, Cohen D *et al.* Analysis of long-term outcomes of combined modality therapy for cutaneous T-cell lymphoma. *J Am Acad Dermatol* 2003; **49**: 35–49.

●105. Bigler R, Crilley P, Micaily B *et al.* Autologous bone marrow transplantation for advanced stage mycosis fungoides. *Bone Marrow Transplant* 1991; **7**: 133–7.

●106. Russell-Jones R, Child F, Olavarria E *et al.* Autologous peripheral blood stem cell transplantation in tumor-stage mycosis fungoides: predictors of disease-free survival. *Ann N Y Acad Sci* 2001; **941**: 147–54.

●107. Guitart J, Wickless S, Oyama Y *et al.* Long-term remission after allogeneic hematopoietic stem cell transplantation for refractory cutaneous T-cell lymphoma. *Arch Dermatol* 2002; **138**: 1359–65.

●108. Molina A, Zain J, Arber D *et al.* Durable clinical, cytogenetic, and molecular remissions after allogeneic hematopoietic cell transplantation for refractory Sezary syndrome and mycosis fungoides. *J Clin Oncol* 2005; **23**: 6163–71.

●109. Soligo D, Ibatici A, Berti E *et al.* Treatment of advanced mycosis fungoides by allogeneic stem-cell transplantation with a nonmyeloablative regimen. *Bone Marrow Transplant* 2003; **31**: 663–6.

●110. Knox S, Levy R, Hodgkinson S *et al.* Observations on the effect of chimeric anti-CD4 monoclonal antibody in patients with mycosis fungoides. *Blood* 1991; **77**: 20–30.

●111. Kim YH, Duvic M, Obitz E *et al.* Clinical efficacy of zanolimumab (HuMax-CD4): two phase 2 studies in refractory cutaneous T-cell lymphoma. *Blood* 2007; **109**: 4655–62.

◆112. Krieg A. Antitumor applications of stimulating toll-like receptor 9 with CpG oligodeoxynucleotide. *Curr Oncol Rep* 2004; **6**: 88–95.

●113. Kim Y, Girardi M, Duvic M *et al.* TLR9 agonist immunomodulator treatment of cutaneous T-cell lymphoma (CTCL) with CPG7909. *Blood* 2004; **104**: 743.

●114. Gandhi V, Kilpatrick J, Plunkett W *et al.* A proof-of-principle pharmacokinetic, pharmacodynamic, and clinical study with purine nucleoside phosphorylase inhibitor immucillin-H (BCX-1777, forodesine). *Blood* 2005; **106**: 4253–60.

115. Duvic M, Forero-Torres A, Foss F *et al.* Response to oral forodesine in refractory cutaneous T-cell lymphoma: interim results of a phaseI/II study. *Blood* 2007; **110**: 122 (abstract).

79

Adult T cell leukemia/lymphoma

TAKAYUKI ISHIKAWA AND KAZUNORI IMADA

GENERAL DESCRIPTION

Historical perspective

The development of immunologic techniques to classify lymphocytes into T cells and B cells revealed that the frequency of T cell leukemia was considerably higher in Japan than in Western countries. As many Japanese with T cell leukemia shared characteristic clinical features which were previously undescribed and, surprisingly, the birthplace of these patients clustered in southwestern Japan, it was proposed that adult T cell leukemia (ATL) is a distinct clinical entity.[1] The patients described in the original report had acute or chronic leukemia with rapidly progressive terminal phases. Subsequently, sera from these patients were shown to contain antibodies against ATL-associated antigens which were found in a cell line derived from a patient with ATL.[2] The introduction of an assay which easily detected the presence of antibodies against ATL-associated antigens expanded the disease spectrum of ATL. Sera from a significant proportion of Japanese patients with T cell lymphoma tested positive. In addition, histologic features of lymph nodes derived from patients with ATL and most of the seropositive T cell lymphomas were shown to be identical.[3] The clinical course was frequently characterized by leukemic transformation and, at that point, a distinction

from classical ATL could not be made. The term lymphoma-type ATL was given.

A nationwide sero-epidemiologic study revealed a high incidence (6–37 percent) of antibody-positive donors in several regions of Japan.[4] It was noticed that small proportions of seropositive individuals showed low percentages of ATL cells in their peripheral blood. Some of them with long-lasting skin or lung diseases were reported to develop aggressive ATL after long periods of indolent disease. A proposal for 'smoldering' ATL was postulated for such a prodromal phase.[5] Such heterogeneity produced considerable confusion in the early days; however, the discovery of human T cell lymphotrophic virus type 1 (HTLV-1) as the etiologic agent of ATL has made it possible not only to make a definitive diagnosis by using molecular studies,[6] but also to clearly define the disease entity of ATL as a T cell neoplasm caused by HTLV-1 infection.[7]

HTLV-1 and its role in leukemogenesis

Human T cell lymphotrophic virus type 1 was the first retrovirus discovered in humans[6,8] and belongs to the family of deltaretroviruses. Based on the finding that the HTLV-1 proviral genome was clonally integrated in ATL cells, HTLV-1 was demonstrated to be the causative agent of ATL.[9] The HTLV-1 proviral genome contains *gag*, *pol*, and *env* genes, which are common in retroviruses. Although HTLV-1 causes leukemia, it has no typical oncogene contained in leukemia viruses of animal origin. Instead, a unique structure, called pX, is present between the *env* gene and the 3′ long terminal repeat (LTR). Accordingly, HTLV-1 viral products encoded by the pX region, including Tax, Rex, p12, and others, have been intensively studied, leading to the notion that these viral products, especially Tax, play an important role in immortalizing primary T cells and promoting cell proliferation.[10] However, ATL develops after a long latent period and viral gene expression is usually undetectable or at a very low level in fresh ATL cells,[11,12] indicating that additional events are required for leukemogenesis. Indeed, it has been suggested from analysis of the age-specific occurrence of ATL that the accumulation of five independent events is required for the development of ATL,[13] supporting the concept of multistep leukemogenesis.

Epidemiology

ADULT T CELL LEUKEMIA PATIENTS AND HTLV-1 CARRIERS

As described, by screening sera from adult donors for anti-HTLV-1 antibody, a nationwide sero-epidemiologic survey in Japan showed that there were at least seven endemic regions, one in northern Japan and the others in southwestern regions.[4] The distribution of anti-HTLV-1 antibody-endemic areas corresponded to that of ATL-endemic areas. It was estimated that there were one to two million people infected with HTLV-1 in Japan. In contrast, another nationwide survey estimated the annual incidence of ATL as 500–1000 patients, which clearly demonstrated that only a small proportion of HTLV-1 carriers will develop ATL in their lifetime.[14] In fact, the cumulative risk for developing ATL from 30 to 79 years of age among HTLV-1 carriers was estimated to be 2–6 percent.[15]

Endemic areas of HTLV-1 infection are not restricted to Japan but are distributed, in several geographic clusters, all over the world: the Caribbean islands, intertropical Africa, the Middle East, and elsewhere. A serological survey carried out in Jamaica revealed that 6.1 percent of residents were seropositive for HTLV-1.[16] It is estimated that twenty to thirty million individuals worldwide are infected with this virus.[17] As for the incidence of ATL in the general population, all the reports from endemic areas such as southwestern Japan, Caribbean islands, and French Guiana are similar; the estimated crude incidence rate of ATL is around 2–5/100 000 persons per year.

AGE AND GENDER DIFFERENCE

Soon after the advent of serological surveys, it was noticed that the positive rate of anti-HTLV-1 antibody increased with age, especially in females. An evaluation in HTLV-1-endemic areas in Japan demonstrated that there is no gender difference in the prevalence of HTLV-1 positivity among those under the age of 20 years. The ratio of HTLV-1 carriers increased with age in men and women, but seroprevalence was significantly higher in women, when ages were adjusted in both genders.[15] In contrast, the incidence of ATL was higher in men than women, and so the crude annual incidence of ATL among HTLV-1 carriers was 1.5 times higher in men than women.

The age-specific incidence of ATL increased steeply after the age of 50 years. The annual incidence of ATL among men in their thirties was estimated to be 0.04 percent, increasing to 0.25 percent for men in their seventies.[15] In Japan, the median age of onset of ATL is around 60 years old.

The findings that HTLV-1 seroprevalence was strongly associated with age and gender were also confirmed in the Jamaican study, as well as in the study in Guyana. However, outside Japan, the median age of onset of ATL was reported to be significantly lower (the fourth decade).

ROUTES OF TRANSMISSION

Human T cell lymphotrophic virus type 1 has been shown to be present only in lymphocytes, mainly in CD4$^+$ T cells, *in vivo*. In addition, close cell-to-cell contact is required for transmission of this virus (Table 79.1).[18] Unlike the situation with another human T cell trophic retrovirus, human immunodeficiency virus, exposure to serum is insufficient for viral transmission, and the invasion of cellular components into the host is necessary.

The findings that the prevalence of HTLV-1 carriers increases from the second decade of life in both genders and is higher in women suggested horizontal transmission.[4,19] From the survey of HTLV-1-endemic small islands in Japan, the possibility of HTLV-1 transmission from husband to wife is estimated to be 60.8 percent, and that from wife to husband to be 0.4 percent over a 10-year period.[20] Another report from Jamaica also confirmed a

Table 79.1 Routes of transmission, risk for developing disease, and prevention

Route	Risk of disease manifestation		Prevention
	ATL	HAM/TSP	
Sexually transmitted	Rare	+	Not done
Blood transfusion	Rare	++	Screening
Organ transplantation	Rare	++	Screening
Mother-to-child	+	+	Refrain from breast feeding

+, infrequent; ++, slightly more frequent than '+.'
ATL, adult T cell leukemia; HAM/TSP, human T cell lymphotrophic virus type 1-associated myelopathy/tropical spastic paraparesis.

male-to-female predominance in the transmission of HTLV-1, and the presence of a sexually transmitted disease was proven to be a risk factor for male-to-female as well as female-to-male transmission.

In addition, the serological screening of pregnant women and their offspring clearly demonstrated the presence of mother-to-child transmission.[19] As for the route of mother-to-child transmission, breast milk was regarded to be the main channel, because HTLV-1 infection was more prevalent among breast-fed than bottle-fed children,[21,22] and common marmosets were shown to be infected with HTLV-1 by oral inoculation of fresh milk derived from an HTLV-1 carrier.[23]

The third route of transmission is direct contact with blood or tissue derived from an HTLV-1 carrier; namely, by way of blood transfusion, organ transplantation, and needles that are infected with contaminated blood.

PREVENTION OF ADULT T CELL LEUKEMIA

Human T cell lymphotrophic virus type 1 causes not only ATL but also several inflammatory diseases, such as HTLV-1-associated myelopathy/tropical spastic paraparesis (HAM/TSP),[24] or HTLV-1-associated uveitis.[25] Several reports demonstrated that the latent periods for the development of HAM/TSP tended to be short (several years) when transmission of HTLV-1 occurred through organ transplantation or blood transfusion from asymptomatic carriers.[26,27] In contrast, ATL developing in HTLV-1 carriers who were infected after adolescence by way of sexual intercourse or blood transfusion is rare. A long latency period (40–60 years) is believed to be required for the development of ATL after infection with HTLV-1. The vast majority of patients with ATL are believed to be infected with HTLV-1 during their early childhood. As the most common route of transmission in this period is through breast milk from the carrier mother, programs to test for anti-HTLV-1 antibody in pregnant women and recommendations for carrier mothers to refrain from breast feeding, or to shorten the breast-feeding period (less than 6 months), started in the mid-1980s. Twenty years after the introduction of this program, a survey done in Okinawa, one of the endemic regions in Japan, revealed a significant decrease in the prevalence of HTLV-1 carriers among healthy residents less than 20 years old (from 4.6 percent to 0.1 percent).[28] This striking decrease appeared to be mainly attributable to the program of surveys and recommendations. In the future, the incidence of ATL in Japan should be greatly reduced.

Subtypes

At the time that this disease entity was proposed, a diverse clinical course was regarded as one of the characteristics of ATL. To determine the natural history, treatment strategy, and leukemogenesis of ATL, appropriate classification systems are mandatory.[5,29,30] Shimoyama and members of the Lymphoma Study Group in Japan reviewed clinical data for 854 cases of ATL registered between 1984 and 1987 during the nationwide surveys and, according to the prognosis on the basis of survival data, they postulated diagnostic criteria for clinical subtypes of ATL in 1991.[31] Their classification included four clinical subtypes of ATL: smoldering, chronic, lymphoma, and acute. By definition, patients with smoldering ATL show 5 percent or more leukemic cells in their blood without lymphocytosis. Patients may complain of skin lesions and sometimes show an abnormal shadow on their chest x-ray. They do not have lymphadenopathy or hepatosplenomegaly. Chronic ATL is characterized by lymphocytosis ($4 \times 10^3/\mu L$ or more), with more than $3.5 \times 10^3/\mu L$ T cells. Patients may complain of enlarged lymph nodes, hepatomegaly, splenomegaly, and cutaneous and pulmonary lesions. However, no signs or symptoms of excessive tumor growth are present. The serum lactate dehydrogenase (LDH) level should not exceed twice the upper limit of normal and the corrected serum calcium must be normal. Patients with tumorous lesions in the central nervous system, bone, gastrointestinal tract, or body cavities (presence of pleural effusion and/or ascites) are considered not to have chronic ATL. Lymphoma-type ATL patients present with histologically proven lymphadenopathy, with no lymphocytosis and less than 1 percent of abnormal T cells on their blood films. The presence of extranodal lesions is permitted. Acute ATL was defined as the remaining cases, most of which presented with leukemic manifestations.

The criteria have several practical advantages; clinical features and conventional laboratory data are sufficient for classification even at the time of diagnosis, and patients categorized as having aggressive types of ATL (acute and lymphoma) are generally regarded to be candidates for immediate therapy. In the meantime, as abnormal cells are defined mainly by morphologic examination, the distinction between the smoldering type and a carrier not diagnosable as having ATL, or between the lymphoma and acute type, is sometimes difficult to make and not consistent among physicians. In addition, the prognosis for chronic ATL shows considerable heterogeneity. After the introduction of novel therapeutic strategies, this classification system will require substantial refinement.

Diagnostic evaluation

To make a diagnosis of ATL, the first step is examination of a peripheral blood smear or lymph node (Table 79.2). In acute ATL, neoplastic cells show nuclear polymorphism: blast-like to multilobulated cells which are designated as 'flower cells.' In chronic and smoldering ATL, leukemic cells tend to be small in size, and careful examination will also reveal 'flower cells.' In lymphoma-type cases, tumor cells in lymph nodes show nuclear irregularity and pleomorphism.

The second step involves analysis of cell-surface antigens on the pathological cells. Adult T cell leukemia cells express mature T cell antigens, such as CD2 and CD3, but CD7 is usually absent. In the majority of patients

Table 79.2 Shimoyama's diagnostic criteria for clinical subtype of adult T cell leukemia

	Smoldering	Chronic	Lymphoma	Acute
Anti-HTLV-1 antibody	Essential	Essential	Essential	Essential
Total peripheral lymphocytes ($\times 10^3/\mu$L)	<4	≥4[a]	<4	Any
Abnormal T cell	≥5%	Essential[b]	≤1%	Essential[b]
Flower cells of T cell marker	Occassionally	Occassionally	No	Essential
LDH	≤1.5 N	≤2 N	Any	Any
Corrected serum calcium (mmol/L)	<2.74	<2.74	Any	Any
Histology-proven lymph node lesion	No	Any	Essential	Any
Tumor lesion				
Skin, lung	Any	Any	Any	Any
Lymph node	No	Any	Essential	Any
Liver, spleen	No	Any	Any	Any
CNS, bone, GI tract	No	No	Any	Any
Ascites, pleural effusion	No	No	Any	Any

[a]T cell count must exceed $3.5 \times 10^9/\mu$L.
[b]In case abnormal T cells are less than 5% in peripheral blood, histology-proven tumor lesion is required.
HTLV-1, human T cell lymphotrophic virus type 1; LDH, lactate dehydrogenase; CNS, central nervous system; GI, gastrointestinal; N, normal.

(80–90 percent), leukemic cells also express CD4. CD8 is sometimes accompanied by CD4. In the remainder, the phenotype of CD4$^-$ CD8$^+$ or CD4$^-$ CD8$^-$ is observed.[32] The expression of activation phenotypes including CD25 is commonly observed.[33] In endemic areas, the possibility of having ATL in patients with T cell malignancies or abnormal T cells in the peripheral blood should be ruled out. In nonendemic areas, the presence of unexplained hypercalcemia or opportunistic infections raises the possibility of ATL. In such instances, the birthplace of these patients and their mothers may be important information.

Patients suspected of having ATL are subjected to a serological test for HTLV-1. If they test positive, the final step in making a definitive diagnosis is the demonstration of clonality of HTLV-1 proviral DNA in tumor cells. Southern blotting or an inverse polymerase chain reaction (PCR) is used for this purpose.[34] This final step is indispensable because a retrospective analysis showed that, among T cell lymphomas arising in ATL-endemic areas, clonal integration of HTLV-1 proviral DNA in lymph node cells was not documented in 66 of 313 patients who tested positive for anti-HTLV-1 antibody in the serum. In this survey, although there are suspected to be some false-negative results due to insufficient lymph node samples, it should be recognized that there are patients with T cell lymphomas other than ATL which had coincidently occurred in HTLV-1 carriers.[35]

CLINICAL FEATURES

In the first report on ATL, 16 patients with subacute or chronic leukemia were described.[1] After the introduction of a serological diagnostic approach, it became apparent that patients with ATL display diverse clinical features and

at least four subtypes of ATL were proposed. To better understand ATL, the symptoms, signs, and laboratory findings which are observed in many subtypes, and those which are restricted to specific subtypes, should be described separately.

Clinical features commonly observed in adult T cell leukemia

Except in cases of smoldering ATL, the majority (up to 80 percent) of patients with ATL present with painless lymphadenopathy. Bulky lymph nodes are not common. Autopsy findings reveal that tumorous lesions are evenly distributed throughout the lymph node regions and lymphoid tissues except in the cortex of the thymus.[36] Lack of a mediastinal mass in spite of T cell origin has been regarded as a distinguishable feature of ATL. Skin lesions such as papules, erythema, and nodules are frequently observed in all subtypes; at presentation, about one-half of patients exhibit such lesions and, in the course of their illness, more patients complain of skin lesions. Histologically, individual skin lesions have various degrees of tumor cell infiltration from the epidermis (as Pautrier microabscess) into the subcutaneous adipose tissue.[37] Pulmonary complications are also frequent. Patients may complain of productive or nonproductive coughing, dyspnea, and chest pain, and about 40 percent of patients have been reported to have significant findings on chest x-ray films, such as reticulonodular shadows, patchy consolidation, pleural thickening, and pleural effusions at the time of diagnosis.[38] For many patients with abnormal chest x-rays, a transbronchial lung biopsy (TBLB) reveals tumor cell infiltration with interstitial fibrosis to some degree, even in patients with smoldering and chronic ATL.[39]

In cases of these indolent subtypes of ATL, patients may be diagnosed as having chronic lung disease before the diagnosis of ATL is made.

In addition to the clinical features directly attributable to tumor cell infiltration, patients with ATL show a profound immunosuppressive status and sometimes complain of opportunistic infections despite having an adequate neutrophil count. Transbronchial lung biopsy of affected tissues frequently reveals not only a tumorous infiltration but also concurrent pneumonia caused by various pathogens, such as *Pneumocystis carinii*, *Cryptococcus spp.*, and cytomegalovirus. Opportunistic infection may be the first symptom of smoldering ATL. Strongyloidiasis is also frequent in endemic areas. The risk of opportunistic infection rises steeply as the disease progresses, and opportunistic infections can be fatal especially among patients who have received chemotherapy.[40]

Laboratory features commonly observed in cases of adult T cell leukemia

As ATL is a neoplasm derived from mature lymphocytes, the characteristics of the peripheral blood count show several similarities to those of B cell chronic lymphocytic leukemia. The white blood cell (WBC) count ranges from normal to highly elevated (up to $500 \times 10^3/\mu L$). In patients with an elevated WBC count, lymphocytosis is predominant but sometimes accompanied by neutrophilia. Neutropenia is rare at presentation even in cases of acute ATL. Eosinophilia is frequently observed as well as in other T cell malignancies. Anemia (hemoglobin less than 10 g/dL) and thrombocytopenia (platelet count less than $100 \times 10^9/\mu L$) are not common; fewer than 20 percent of patients with acute ATL show anemia or thrombocytopenia, and the frequency is lower in other types.

In acute ATL, neoplastic cells in the peripheral blood are medium sized to large, with nuclear polymorphisms.[41] The nuclear features are variable from blast-like cells to cells with many nuclear lobules. In chronic and smoldering ATL, tumor cells are small with condensed chromatin. Nuclei also show a convoluted or multilobulated appearance. The histologic findings of lymph nodes are also heterogeneous. Some tumors are dominated by small cells, but many are composed of large cells with lobulated nuclei. Giant cells, which closely resemble Hodgkin cells, are frequently observed. Although less frequent, lymph nodes closely resembling Hodgkin lymphoma or anaplastic large cell lymphoma are encountered.

Bone marrow biopsy usually reveals scattered foci of ATL cells; however, a dense infiltration of tumor cells into the bone marrow spaces is not common at presentation. The number of osteoclasts may be increased even in the absence of leukemic cells.

Several laboratory parameters have been shown to be useful in assessing and monitoring tumor load and disease activity. Serum levels of β_2-microglobulin and LDH reflect the extent of disease. In addition, as ATL cells inevitably express CD25, the α chain of the interleukin-2 receptor (IL-2R), the serum level of soluble IL-2R is an extremely sensitive indicator of tumor load.[42] By using flow cytometry, ATL cells are characterized as $CD3^+ CD25^+$ and, in most instances, $CD4^+$. As the intensity of CD3 antigen is low on ATL cells compared with nonleukemic T cells, $CD3^{low} CD4^+ CD25^+$ cells are regarded as ATL cells. The monitoring of cells with such a phenotype is also useful in assessing tumor activity and response to treatment.

Clinical and laboratory findings restricted to specific subtypes

CLINICAL FEATURES OF INDOLENT DISEASE (SMOLDERING AND CHRONIC ATL)

Although most patients with smoldering and chronic ATL do not complain of any symptoms, they are at risk of developing opportunistic infections and more aggressive diseases. Opportunistic infections are not uncommon in patients with indolent ATL or HTLV-1 carriers. In fact, even in cases of HAM/TSP (another HTLV-1-associated disease) there have been several reports of the occurrence of *Pneumocystis cariini* pneumonia, cytomegalovirus infection, and intractable strongyloidiasis. Although the mechanism underlying the impaired immunity is not well understood, it is estimated that the presence of HTLV-1 itself would disrupt the function of thymic or dendritic cells, leading to a decreased number of newly produced T cells and impaired antigen-presenting functions.[43,44] In addition, some ATL cells may behave as regulatory T cells, which affect immunosuppressive status.[45] Patients with indolent ATL frequently suffer from oral candidiasis, stomatitis, and keratitis caused by reactivated herpes simplex virus and herpes zoster. In some patients, cutaneous or pulmonary involvement by ATL causes unpleasant symptoms, which need topical or systematic treatment.

CLINICAL FEATURES OF AGGRESSIVE DISEASE (ACUTE AND LYMPHOMA–TYPE ATL)

Clinical features of aggressive ATL are brought about by widespread infiltration of various organs and tissues, metabolic problems derived from tumor cells, and a profoundly suppressed immune status.

Acute ATL displays a highly aggressive clinical course. Tumor cell infiltration of the skin, lung, bone, liver, gastrointestinal tract, and central nervous system results in widely heterogeneous signs and symptoms, such as skin rash, dyspnea, bone pain, jaundice, abdominal fullness, and motor weakness. Marked leukocytosis with morphologically characteristic leukemic cells, a high serum LDH level, and a markedly elevated soluble IL-2R level are consistent findings. However, in comparison to acute leukemia other than ATL, the symptoms and signs which reflect reduced bone marrow function are not conspicuous.

Lymphoma-type ATL is also aggressive. A vast majority of patients with this tumor present with advanced stage according to the Ann Arbor staging classification. Although the predominant feature of lymphoma-type ATL is lymph node swelling, the patients have many clinical characteristics of acute ATL.

Since the leukemic cells of aggressive ATL produce several kinds of cytokines and chemokines and express molecules which influence metabolism, patients frequently complain of unexplained fever, hypercalcemia, and, in some cases, hypoglycemia. In particular, hypercalcemia is one of the most frequent and serious complications. The frequency as well as severity of hypercalcemia is remarkably high compared with other hematologic malignancies. In patients with ATL, it is evident that in over 50 percent of acute cases and around 15 percent of lymphoma-type cases at presentation, and, during the entire clinical course, 70 percent of patients develop this condition. Hypercalcemia develops rapidly, and sometimes results in acute renal failure or coma within a few days. The accumulation of morphologically active osteoclasts is demonstrated by pathologic analysis and supposedly induces marked bone resorption and hypercalcemia. Such increased activity of osteoclasts is shown to be mediated by the overproduction of the receptor activator of nuclear factor κB ligand (RANKL) and parathyroid hormone-related protein produced by ATL cells.[46,47]

Immunity against several pathogens is more profoundly impaired than in indolent diseases. Opportunistic infections including *Pneumocystis carinii* pneumonia and a generalized cryptococcosis may accompany the disease even at presentation.

MANAGEMENT

Therapeutic principles for indolent disease

Many patients with smoldering ATL are asymptomatic and diagnosed by chance. A major proportion of patients with smoldering ATL show a stable clinical course, although the rate of transformation is high compared with that of HTLV-1 carriers not diagnosed with ATL. A recent retrospective survey carried out in Kyushu and Okinawa, endemic areas in Japan, revealed that the median survival of 136 patients with smoldering ATL was 5.2 years. In this survey, the early introduction of antineoplastic therapy did not result in any improvement in terms of survival.[48] In fact, there have been no documented approaches for delaying or preventing the progression to aggressive ATL. As cytotoxic therapy sometimes results in an overwhelming opportunistic infection by way of profound immune suppression, no cytotoxic therapy is warranted for patients with smoldering ATL. For patients with persistent cutaneous lesions, a topical steroid ointment, psoralen plus ultraviolet A irradiation (PUVA), or electron beam therapy may be applied.

In contrast, the prognosis of patients with chronic ATL is far from reassuring. Although some patients live a long time without progression of the disease, the median survival of patients with chronic ATL is reported to be 3.6 years.[48] The Japan Clinical Oncology Group (JCOG) postulated that chronic ATL should be subdivided into favorable and unfavorable types, because the median survival of unfavorable chronic ATL (defined as having at least one of three unfavorable prognostic factors, i.e., low serum albumin level, elevated serum LDH level, or high concentration of blood urea nitrogen) was similar to that of aggressive ATL, and, for this reason, unfavorable chronic ATL was included in clinical trials using intensive combination chemotherapy.[49,50] Although the numbers of patients with unfavorable chronic ATL included in these studies were small, there is no clear difference in median survival between unfavorable chronic ATL and aggressive ATL, leaving the significance of intensive chemotherapy for chronic ATL undefined. Several reports have demonstrated that the expression of multidrug-resistant protein and lung-resistant protein, by which tumor cells would acquire drug resistance, was as extensive in chronic ATL as in acute ATL, and significantly higher than in lymphoma-type ATL.[51,52] These reports are consistent with the clinical experience that it is difficult to induce durable remission of chronic ATL with combination chemotherapy. In addition, the spontaneous regression of chronic ATL into smoldering ATL is not uncommon.[48] Taking all this into account, it is advisable to withhold multiagent chemotherapy for chronic ATL until signs or symptoms attributable to disease progression develop. Low-dose, single-agent chemotherapies, such as the oral administration of etoposide, have been used as systemic treatment for symptomatic chronic ATL with slow growth. However, whether these therapies extend survival is not clear. Allogeneic stem cell transplantation may be one therapeutic option for patients with unfavorable or symptomatic chronic ATL. In cases where skin involvement causes disturbing pain or itching, PUVA or local skin irradiation should be considered.[53]

Therapeutic approaches for patients critically debilitated at presentation

At presentation, many patients with acute ATL and a proportion of those with lymphoma-type ATL are critically debilitated because they show simultaneous medical emergencies; severe organ dysfunction due to fulminating tumor infiltration, metabolic emergencies such as hypercalcemia, and simultaneous opportunistic infections. Poor performance status (grade 2 or more) was reported in 68 percent of acute-type cases and 45 percent of lymphoma-type cases, and this report also found that the incidence of performance status grade 4 reached 24 percent in acute ATL.[31] Although immediate chemotherapy is mandatory for organ dysfunction caused by leukemic infiltration, the correction of hypercalcemia, if present, has therapeutic precedence. Immediate extracellular volume expansion with intravenous saline and subsequent use of furosemide should be started. In addition, administration of calcitonin and corticosteroid would be required, especially for patients who could not tolerate a sufficient volume load because of impaired renal or cardiac functions. Immediate hemodialysis is also a therapy of choice for patients with renal failure. Bisphosphonate compounds are quite useful in the continuous control of the serum calcium level, although a few days are required for maximal effects. Chemotherapy is also effective in reducing the serum calcium level, and should be given after the general condition of the patient has stabilized.

In cases where an opportunistic infection is suspected, treatment for the infection should take precedence. However, if the ATL is life threatening and urgent antitumor therapy is required to save the patient, simultaneous administration of anticancer drugs and antibiotics, such as sulphamethoxazole/trimethoprim and/or ganciclovir, may be necessary.

When urgent chemotherapy is indicated before the condition of the patient has improved, the schedule of chemotherapy should be adjusted individually according to organ functions and the medical situation. The goal of the initial therapy should be to improve the patient's general condition as well as organ function. After the initial chemotherapy, programmed therapy aimed at remission of the ATL can be conducted.

Therapeutic principles for aggressive disease

For a definitive diagnosis of ATL, confirmation of a monoclonally integrated HTLV-1 provirus in tumor cells is necessary. However, in many cases of acute ATL, there is not enough time to wait for a definitive diagnosis. If all the following criteria are met – namely, the characteristic morphology of leukemic cells, the presence of hypercalcemia or a severely immunocompromised status, immunophenotypes of mature and activated T cells, and the presence of anti-HTLV-1 antibody – the probability of ATL is exceedingly high. If immediate treatment is indicated, chemotherapy designed for ATL should be initiated. Fortunately, lymphoma-type ATL is generally not as aggressive as acute ATL. In most patients, chemotherapy can be started after the diagnosis has been established.

Although the use of antiviral agents has been reported to be effective as initial therapy against ATL, the initial experience in Japan with interferon and zidovudine for ATL was discouraging, and this combination has been seldom tried in routine practice.[54] We regard cytotoxic chemotherapy as the treatment of choice for newly diagnosed patients with aggressive ATL.

COMBINATION CHEMOTHERAPY

As ATL is a neoplasm of mature T cells, combination chemotherapy regimens for aggressive non-Hodgkin lymphoma were initially utilized (Table 79.3). Between 1981 and 1983, 54 patients with aggressive ATL and 28 with HTLV-1-negative peripheral T cell lymphoma were treated with VEPA (vincristine, cyclophosphamide, prednisone, and doxorubicin) or VEPA-M (VEPA plus methotrexate).[55] Although the distribution of each subtype of ATL in this study is not known (criteria for classifying ATL had not been established at that time), most of the patients in this study were thought to have the lymphoma type because patients with lymphomatous presentations were mainly enrolled. The complete remission (CR) rate and 4-year survival rate were reported to be 28 percent and 8 percent, respectively, which were significantly lower than those of patients with HTLV-1-negative peripheral T cell lymphomas.[55]

Nationwide surveys of ATL conducted between 1984 and 1987 revealed that survival curves of patients with lymphoma-type and acute ATL were almost identical. The 4-year survival rate was shown to be only 5.0 percent for acute ATL and 5.4 percent for lymphoma-type ATL.[31] Retrospective analysis revealed unique properties of patients treated with chemotherapy;[56] long-term therapy with increased use of doxorubicin was effective in increasing the number of long-term survivors, but fatal infectious complications were frequently observed, even in remission. Recognition of an extremely poor prognosis for patients with aggressive ATL, irrespective of subtype, prompted the exploitation of new treatment regimens exclusively designed for aggressive ATL. Characteristics common to these regimens were weekly or bi-weekly administration of cytotoxic drugs, an extended therapy period, and reinforced prophylaxis for opportunistic infections. Repetitive intrathecal chemotherapies were also included in some studies because meningeal recurrence had been frequently encountered. A response-oriented cyclic multidrug protocol, in which 11 drugs were combined with the aim of weekly administration of non-cross-resistant drugs,[57] and utilization of long-term maintenance chemotherapy[58] were unsuccessful in improving the CR rate and extending median survival. More intensive combination chemotherapy regimens supported by granulocyte colony-stimulating factor (G-CSF) were marginally effective in elevating the CR rate, but median survival time did not exceed 1 year.[59] Until now, the most successful reported regimen of combination chemotherapy was LSG15,[50] which comprises three regimens: VCAP (vincristine, cyclophosphamide, doxorubicin, and prednisone), AMP (doxorubicin, ranimustine, and prednisone), and VECP (vindesine, etoposide, carboplatin, and prednisone). VCAP, AMP, and VECP were administered on days 1, 8, and 15–17, respectively, and the next cycle was started on day 29. Therapy was continued for 7 cycles, unless disease progression or toxic complications were observed. Granulocyte colony-stimulating factor support in the neutropenic period was included because profound myelosuppression was expected. A total of 96 patients with ATL (58 with acute, 28 with lymphoma-type, and 10 with unfavorable chronic ATL) were enrolled.

Table 79.3 Multiagent chemotherapy in the treatment of adult T cell leukemia

Author, year	n	Regimen	Response	Median survival time (months)	Survival
Shimoyama et al. 1988[55]	54, mainly lymphoma type	VCR 1 mg/m^2: day 1, 8, 15, 22, 29, 35; CPM 350 mg/m^2: day 1, 8, 15, 22, 29, 35; ADR 40 mg/m^2: day 1, 22; PSL 40 mg/m^2: day 1–3, 8–10, 15–17, 22–24, 29–31, 35–37; ± MTX 30 mg/m^2: day 1, 22. Repeat 2 cycles	CR 28%	Not described	2-year survival 8%
Uozumi et al. 1995[57]	43 (acute 28)	CPM 500 mg/m^2: day 1, 8, 15, 22; PSL 40 mg/m^2: day 1, 8, 15, 22; VDS 2 mg/m^2: day 1; MCNU 70 mg/m^2: day 1; MTX 40 mg/m^2: day 8; THP 40 mg/m^2: day 8; ETP 70 mg/m^2: day 15; PEP 7 mg/m^2: day 15; Ara-C 40 mg/m^2: day 15; MMC 2 mg/m^2: day 22; ADR 40 mg/m^2: day 22. Repeat 5-week interval until progression	CR 20.9%, PR 65.1%	Acute 5.0, lymphoma 6.0	Not described
Taguchi et al. 1996[59]	83 (acute 44)	VCR 1 mg/m^2: day 1; ADR 40 mg/m^2: day 1; CPM 400 mg/m^2: day 1; PSL 40 mg/m^2: day 1–3, 8–10; ETP 35 mg/m^2: day 1–8; VDS 2 mg/m^2: day 8; MCNU 50 mg/m^2: day 8; MIT 7 mg/m^2: day 8; G-CSF 50 μg/m^2: day 9–21. Repeat 3-week interval for 2–4 cycles	CR 35.8%, PR 38.3%	8.5	3-year survival 13.5%
Matsushita et al. 1999[58]	87 (acute 51)	VCR 0.7 mg/m^2 (or MTX 14 mg/m^2) day 1; ETP 70 mg/m^2: day 1; CPM 200 mg/m^2: day 1; PSL 20 mg/m^2: day 1. Repeat weekly until progression	CR 31.0%, PR 58.6%	7.1	Not described
Yamada et al. 2001[50]	96 (acute 58)	VCR 1 mg/m^2: day 1; ADR 40 mg/m^2: day 1; 30 mg/m^2: day 8; CPM 350 mg/m^2: day 1; PSL 40 mg/m^2: day 1, 8, 15–17; MCNU 60 mg/m^2: day 8; ETP 100 mg/m^2: day 15–17; VDS 2.4 mg/m^2: day 15; CBDCA 250 mg/m^2: day 15; G-CSF 50 μg/m^2: day 2–7, 9–13, 18–27. Repeat 4-week interval for 7 cycles	CR 35.5%, PR 45.2%	13.0	2-year survival 31.3%
Tsukasaki et al. 2003[49]	62 (acute 34)	VCR 1 mg/m^2: day 1, 8; ADR 40 mg/m^2: day 1; ETP 100 mg/m^2: day 1–3; PSL 40 mg/m^2: day 1–2; DCF 5 mg/m^2: day 8, 15, 22. Repeat 4-week interval for 10 cycles	CR 28%, PR 23%	7.4	2-year survival 15.5%

CR, complete remission; PR, partial remission; VCR, vincristine; CPM, cyclophosphamide; ADR, adriamycin (doxorubicin); PSL, prednisone; MTX, methotrexate; VDS, vindesine; MCNU, ranimustine; THP, pirarubicin; ETP, etoposide; PEP, pepleomycin; Ara-C, cytarabine; MMC, mitomicin-C; MIT, mitoxantrone; CBDCA, carboplatin; G-CSF, granulocyte colony-stimulating factor; DCF, deoxycoformycin (pentostatin).

Seventy-five patients responded, with 33 obtaining complete responses. The median survival was 13 months and overall survival at 2 years was estimated to be 31.3 percent. Notably, better responses for lymphoma-type ATL were observed, with a CR rate of 66.7 percent, a median survival of 19.7 months, and a 2-year survival around 40 percent. Although the outcome reported using LSG15 was excellent compared to previous studies, several issues remain. First, hematologic toxicity was severe, with 30 patients experiencing more than grade 2 infections, and 16 patients were unable to complete the study, mainly due to prolonged bone marrow suppression. Among the remaining patients, long-term hospitalization was usually required. Second, therapeutic responses in acute ATL were poor; CR rate was 19.6 percent, median survival 10.9 months, and 2-year survival around 20 percent. Treatment was stopped due to progressive disease or recurrence of ATL in 41 patients, in whom acute ATL was predominant. Last, the exclusion criteria prevented the enrollment of patients with highly aggressive acute ATL who comprise a significant proportion of patients with this disease and generally show inferior outcomes.

It is expected that chemotherapy could further improve the outcome of lymphoma-type ATL. In contrast, the incorporation of new drugs or another strategy will be required for obtaining better outcomes in acute ATL.

OTHER CYTOTOXIC AGENTS

To overcome the limitations of conventional chemotherapy, new cytotoxic drugs have also been tested. As deoxycoformycin (DCF; pentostatin), a purine analogue and potent inhibitor of adenosine deaminase, has shown activity against hairy cell leukemia and T cell prolymphocytic leukemia, it was used for the treatment of recurrent or resistant ATL.[60] Three independent studies involving a total of 29 patients showed that a partial response was obtained in six patients by single-agent chemotherapy. As the antitumor activity of DCF differs from that of conventional cytotoxic drugs, a trial of multiagent chemotherapy consisting of vincristine, doxorubicin, etoposide, prednisone, and DCF was conducted for previously untreated patients with ATL.[49] This trial, however, did not produce promising results: the CR rate was reported to be 28 percent, the median survival 7.4 months, and the 2-year survival rate 15.5 percent. The combined use of DCF and cytotoxic drugs seemed to be too toxic and offset any beneficial effects in many patients. Cladribine, another purine analogue, has also been tried as a single agent for relapsed and refractory aggressive ATL.[61] One out of fifteen eligible patients was reported to show an objective response.

Irinotecan hydrochloride (CPT-11), an inhibitor of topoisomerase I, has been reported to be active against doxorubicin-resistant leukemia. A phase II study of CPT-11 was therefore conducted to evaluate its efficacy in 13 patients with refractory ATL.[62] One CR, which lasted 10 weeks, and four partial responses were reported. The efficacy of combination therapy including CTP-11 for patients with ATL has not been demonstrated.

HIGH-DOSE THERAPY AND AUTOLOGOUS STEM CELL RESCUE

Myeloablative therapy followed by autologous stem cell transplantation (ASCT) has been shown to prolong survival, when compared to conventional therapies, for patients with recurrent but chemosensitive aggressive lymphoma. As for ASCT in cases of ATL, there have been only a few reports.[63] In fact, opportunities for collecting stem cells are rarely encountered because of the aggressive clinical course and chemoresistant nature of ATL. In the selected patients for whom stem cells could be prepared for ASCT, the clinical outcomes reported were accompanied by early recurrence and fatal infections. At present, ASCT is thought to have little, if any, role in the therapy of ATL.

ANTIVIRAL DRUGS AND INTERFERON

In 1995, two reports were independently published on the effectiveness of the combination of interferon alpha (IFNα) and zidovudine (AZT) as a novel therapeutic approach to ATL. Hermine et al. reported that four patients with acute ATL and one with smoldering ATL obtained durable remission with a combination of IFNα and AZT.[64] Gill et al. also showed that IFNα/AZT induced five CR and six partial responses in 19 ATL patients, seven of whom had either relapsed or showed refractory disease after combination chemotherapy.[65] They also reported that the median period required for a clinical response was 33 days (range 5–168) and two patients with a Karnofsky score of less than 30 entered remission. The median survival of responders was 13 months. The efficacy of this combination was confirmed in several recent reports but response rates have varied substantially (Table 79.4). A report from the UK described 15 patients with acute ATL and lymphoma-type ATL, 12 of whom had received prior chemotherapy. Responses to IFNα/AZT were seen in 10 patients with a median duration of 10 months.[66] A prospective study in France and Lebanon demonstrated that treatment with IFNα/AZT resulted in a CR rate of 58 percent and partial response rate of 33 percent among 14 patients with aggressive ATL who received IFNα/AZT as initial treatment. However, most patients relapsed within a year and the median survival was reported to be 11 months.[67] A North American study reported that a response to IFNα/AZT was observed in only three out of 18 patients, many of whom had been heavily pretreated, but that two patients continued in remission for more than 20 months.[68] The heterogeneous nature of the patients' backgrounds makes interpretation of these results difficult. Bazarbachi and Hermine reported that good responses were observed in patients with newly diagnosed acute ATL, and that the use of high doses of both agents (IFNα at 9 million units per day

Table 79.4 Use of interferon α and zidovudine in the treatment of adult T cell leukemia

Author, year	n	Regimen	Response	Median survival time	Survival
Hermine et al. 1995[64]	5	AZT: 500–1000 mg, daily; IFNα: 500–900 $\times$ 10^4 IU, daily	2 CR, 3 PR	Not described	4 pts alive at 12–27 months
Gill et al. 1995[65]	19	AZT: 1000 mg, daily; IFNα: 500–1000 $\times$ 10^4 IU, daily	CR 26%	Not described	6 pts survived more than 12 months
White et al. 2001[68]	18	AZT 250–1000 mg, daily; IFNα: 250–1000 $\times$ 10^4 IU, daily	1 CR, 2 PR	6 months for 17 patients who died	2 pts continued response more than 20 months
Matutes et al. 2001[66]	15	AZT 1000 mg, daily; IFNα: 300–500 $\times$ 10^4 IU, daily	10 responders	18 months	3 pts alive at 2 years
Hermine et al. 2002[67]	19	AZT 1000 mg, daily; IFNα: 900 $\times$ 10^4 IU, daily	CR 53%, PR 23.5%	11 months	2-year survival around 20%

CR, complete remission; PR, partial remission; AZT, zidovudine; IFN, interferon; pts, patients.

and AZT at 1 g per day) was required for a successful response, at least in the initial phase of therapy.[69] As the combination of IFNα/AZT is suggested to have a good safety profile, it may be an alternative treatment approach, especially for patients with acute ATL. However, sustained remission of ATL with IFNα/AZT is exceptional, and additional therapy to prevent relapse is mandatory. At present, the precise role of IFNα/AZT in the treatment of ATL remains unclear.

MONOCLONAL ANTIBODIES

As ATL cells highly express CD25 and expression of CD25 in normal tissues is restricted to activated lymphocytes, CD25 is regarded as an ideal target for immunologic intervention in ATL. Using an unconjugated murine antibody against CD25, anti-Tac, Waldmann et al. achieved partial response or CR in seven out of 19 ATL patients.[70] For the patients who responded, remission was associated with correction of hypercalcemia or of the immunodeficient state accompanying ATL. Long-lasting remission was, unfortunately, exceptional. To intensify the therapeutic effect of anti-Tac an approach in which this antibody is used as a carrier for cytotoxic substances has been investigated. Eighteen patients with ATL were treated with yttrium-90-labeled anti-Tac antibody.[71] Six out of nine responders survived 1 year without progression. Several other monoclonal antibodies, including humanized anti-Tac, anti-CD2, and anti-CCR4, are now being investigated in preclinical or clinical studies.

ALLOGENEIC STEM CELL TRANSPLANTATION

Until recently, allogeneic stem cell transplantation (allo-SCT) was not regarded as an appropriate treatment for ATL because of the poor chemosensitivity, immunologic

fragility, and advanced age of onset of this disease. There were also concerns that the use of immunosuppressants might result in a markedly suppressed immune status in patients with ATL for an extended period after allo-SCT, which might result in uncontrollable opportunistic infections. In addition, HTLV-1, which can reside anywhere within the patient, might cause HTLV-1-associated diseases after allo-SCT.

Recent improvements in prophylaxis for graft-versus-host disease (GVHD), in the management of opportunistic infections, and in supportive care have decreased the early mortality after allo-SCT. In the hope of a potential immune-mediated eradication of tumor cells, allo-SCT is now being attempted in patients with ATL.[72] To date, three retrospective surveys have been reported[73–75] in which clinical data for over 50 patients were analyzed (Table 79.5). The majority of patients received a myeloablative conditioning regimen and the 3-year overall survival was reported to be around 40 percent. Although patients who were in partial remission or those with resistant disease achieved complete remission after allo-SCT, the latter group had an inferior outcome, as with allo-SCT for other hematologic malignancies. The clinical outcome of allo-SCT for ATL is thus comparable to that for acute lymphoblastic and acute myelogenous leukemia. Early concerns regarding the possibility of serious opportunistic infections were shown to be unfounded, as most of the episodes of opportunistic infection were successfully controlled.

According to a report by Fukushima et al.,[75] although relapse was one of the major causes of transplant failure, over half of the deaths were attributable to transplant-related toxicity, such as thrombotic microangiopathy, GVHD, and fungal infections. They also reported that the frequency of acute GVHD (grade II to IV) was 45 percent and the presence of any grade of acute GVHD correlated negatively with overall survival.

Table 79.5   Allogeneic stem cell transplantation for adult T cell leukemia

Author, year	n	Median age (range)	Disease status before SCT	Donors	Conditioning regimens	Non-relapse mortality	Relapse	Survival
Utsunomiya et al. 2001[73]	10	43 (33–51)	4 CR, 5 PR, 1 NR	9 MSD, 1 URD	TBI-containing myeloablative regimens	3/10	2/10	6 pts alive (median 30+ months)
Kami et al. 2003[74]	11	46 (15–59)	6 CR, 1 PR, 3 PD, 1 Rel	9 MSD, 1 URD, 1 PMRD	9 myeloablative (8 TBI-containing), 2 reduced intensity	5/11	2/11	4 pts alive (median 25+ months)
Fukushima et al. 2005[75]	40[a]	44 (28–53)	15 CR, 13 PR, 3 NR, 9 PD	27 MSD, 8 URD, 5 PMRD	39 myeloablative (22 TBI-containing), 1 reduced intensity	16/40	10/40	3-year overall survival 45.3%
Okamura et al. 2005[76]	16	56 (51–67)	15 CR or PR, 1 PD	16 MSD	16 reduced intensity	3/15	9/15	5 pts alive (median 38+ months)

[a]This study included four patients reported by Utsunomiya et al.
SCT, stem cell transplantation; CR, complete remission; PR, partial remission; NR, no response; PD, progressive disease; Rel, relapsed; MSD, matched sibling donor; URD, unrelated donor; PMRD, partially matched related donor; TBI, total-body irradiation; pts, patients.

Although multivariate analysis did not show any benefit for GVHD in preventing relapse, these studies have shed light on the potential presence of a graft-versus-ATL effect in a proportion of patients with ATL. A substantial number of patients who relapsed after allo-SCT achieved subsequent remission with discontinuation of immunosuppressive therapy or infusion of donor lymphocytes. Unfortunately, rapid tapering of the immunosuppressant or administration of donor lymphocyte infusions was frequently accompanied by severe and fatal GVHD, but there have been some long-term survivors.

Since more than two-thirds of patients with ATL are older than 50 years and cannot therefore safely receive conventional allo-SCT, the advent of reduced-intensity allografting (RIA) provides new possibilities. A phase I trial of RIA for ATL was conducted by Okamura et al.[76] Sixteen patients with acute and lymphoma-type ATL, aged over 50 years, and in complete or partial remission were treated using a human leukocyte antigen (HLA)-matched sibling donor after a reduced-intensity conditioning regimen comprising fludarabine, busulfan, and antithymocyte globulin. Patients were required to be in complete or partial remission at the time of registration. The treatment was well tolerated and no grade IV nonhematologic toxicity was reported. However, nine patients developed recurrent disease, six within 3 months. Interestingly, three patients who relapsed were reported to achieve subsequent remission by rapid tapering of the immunosuppressant, and two were alive 2 years later. It has been suggested that the rapid growth of tumor cells, in the absence of myeloablative conditioning, may exceed the rate of tumor killing by an immunologic effect in cases of aggressive malignancies such as ATL. Reduced-intensity conditioning is not indicated for patients with refractory ATL.

As for the potential risk of HTLV-1-associated diseases developing after allo-SCT, this has not occurred thus far. However, to clarify this issue, further studies in large numbers of patients with longer follow-up are necessary.

INVESTIGATIONAL DRUGS

New approaches that target specific molecules have been developed for many cancers including leukemia and lymphoma. Although clinical data for such approaches in ATL are limited, several promising drugs are worth mentioning.

All-trans retinoic acid (ATRA), which is active against acute promyelocytic leukemia (APL), is reported to have an antiproliferative and apoptosis-inducible effect on ATL cells in vitro.[77] All-trans retinoic acid has been used for one patient with chronic and one with chemotherapy-resistant acute ATL.[78,79] In both reports, ATRA significantly reduced the number of ATL cells without inducing adverse events. Although HTLV-1-infected cells are reported to sometimes lack the retinoic acid receptor-alpha, ATRA may be a promising approach, at least for patients whose leukemic cells show sensitivity to ATRA in vitro.

Arsenic trioxide, another effective drug for APL, is also known to have significant activity in inducing apoptosis of ATL cells, probably by way of inhibiting the nuclear factor κB (NF-κB) pathway.[80] Four out of seven patients with relapsed or refractory ATL were reported to be responsive to the combination of arsenic trioxide and IFNα. Although this treatment was accompanied by substantial toxicity and early relapse, the fact that one patient remained disease free at 32 months is worthy of further study.[81]

Other drugs targeting NF-κB, such as bortezomib and Bay 11-7082, also show antiproliferative and apoptosis-inducing activity against ATL cells in vitro. Unfortunately, no clinical data have been reported.

FOLLOW-UP

Indolent types (smoldering and chronic ATL)

GENERAL COMMENTS

As described previously, patients with smoldering and chronic ATL are at risk of developing more aggressive disease and opportunistic infections. A prospective follow-up study of HTLV-1 carriers with ATL cells detectable at the molecular level and patients with smoldering and chronic ATL revealed that 10-year survival and transition to aggressive ATL were closely associated with initial leukocyte counts. Individuals with a normal leukocyte count (less than $9 \times 10^3/\mu L$) had a 10-year survival rate of 90 percent, and the annual incidence of developing acute ATL was 2.5 percent. In contrast, individuals with an elevated leukocyte count showed a 10-year survival rate of only 39.4 percent, mostly attributable to the increased rate of developing aggressive ATL.[82] The serum level of soluble IL-2R is reported to be proportional to tumor burden, and there are several reports describing that elevation of soluble IL-2R level in patients with smoldering or chronic ATL is associated with transition into aggressive ATL.[83,84]

Recent studies have demonstrated that the impaired immunity of patients with ATL is a consequence of both decreased numbers of uninfected T cells and direct dysregulation of innate and adoptive immunity induced by HTLV-1 itself. A survey of HTLV-1 carriers, in which a direct relationship between the presence of strongyloidiasis and high circulating proviral load was shown,[85] supports this hypothesis. Therefore, measurement of HTLV-1 proviral load using quantitative PCR would provide information useful for finding high-risk patients who are likely to develop opportunistic infections, especially amongst those with smoldering ATL. Prophylactic use of trimethoprim/sulphamethoxazole and fluconazole may be indicated for these patients.

SMOLDERING ADULT T CELL LEUKEMIA

Evolution into a more aggressive form of ATL is a major concern for patients with smoldering ATL. Serial measurements of WBC or peripheral T cell counts as well as serum soluble IL-2R level are useful in predicting the risk of disease progression. Although it is not possible to decrease the risk of disease progression for high-risk patients, close observation enables one to initiate appropriate treatment before serious organ and metabolic dysfunctions develop.

The impaired immunity of patients with smoldering ATL may also increase the risk of developing malignancies other than ATL. However, a follow-up study in such patients revealed that this happened rarely, probably because the development of aggressive ATL preceded the occurrence of other malignancies.

CHRONIC ADULT T CELL LEUKEMIA

Chronic ATL encompasses a wide disease spectrum in terms of survival and disease progression. Many patients may have stable disease for several years, whereas some develop aggressive disease within a few months. According to a retrospective analysis done by the JCOG, a low serum albumin, high serum LDH, and raised blood urea nitrogen are poor prognostic factors.[49] Other studies have demonstrated that an elevated peripheral WBC count, unusual morphology of peripheral leukemic cells,[86] increasing serum IL-2R value, and a high percentage of Ki-67-positive cells[87] are associated with disease progression. In brief, a steady increase in tumor load and the acquisition by tumor cells of an invasive nature are predictive of progression to aggressive ATL.

In accordance with the deterioration in the clinical course, the frequency, the refractoriness, and severity of opportunistic infections increase. Attention to the medical history, physical examination, and investigations for early detection of *Pneumocystis carinii* pneumonia, visceral mycosis, and cytomegalovirus infection are required.

Spontaneous regression without any cytotoxic drugs has been reported in chronic ATL with acute exacerbation.[88] Cases where patients diagnosed with chronic ATL have regressed into smoldering ATL have also been documented, although this is rare.

Aggressive types (lymphoma and acute ATL)

Although patients are critically debilitated at presentation, chemotherapy usually improves their physical condition by reducing tumor burden and normalizing the serum calcium. However, they are still prone to suffer from overwhelming opportunistic infections. Serial monitoring of serum metabolites, antigens, and nucleic acids derived from fungi or viruses makes it possible to treat such infections early.

In lymphoma-type ATL, recent chemotherapy approaches have improved long-term survival from less than 10 percent to 20 percent. In acute ATL, however, the improved response rate has not resulted in improved long-term survival, which remains less than 10 percent at 5 years. Serum soluble IL-2R values are quite sensitive for evaluating treatment response as well as predicting disease recurrence. An insufficient decrease or progressive increase after normalization of the soluble IL-2R level indicates approaching exacerbation of disease.

Evaluation of therapeutic response is sometimes confused by the presence of residual, atypical lymphocytes in the peripheral blood. Molecular analysis reveals that HTLV-1-infected T cells, which are polyclonal and not identical to the original leukemic clone, may remain in the circulation even after effective chemotherapy. Although flow cytometric analysis can estimate the proportion of ATL cells, simple methods to distinguish ATL cells from nonleukemic cells have not been established. In most clinical trials, the criteria for complete remission include normalization of the absolute lymphocyte count with less than 5 percent of morphologically atypical cells. The significance of residual ATL cells to the subsequent clinical course has not been elucidated.

KEY POINTS

- HTLV-1 transmission occurs from mother to child largely by way of breast feeding; via sexual intercourse, especially from men to women; and via blood transfusion, organ transplantation, and needle use. In all cases, HAM/TSP may develop; however, ATL exclusively develops in patients who were infected with HTLV-1 in early childhood.
- Patients with indolent ATL (smoldering and chronic) should be managed in a watchful-waiting manner, protected from opportunistic infections, and treated if symptoms develop.
- Multiagent chemotherapy in the treatment of aggressive ATL is less effective compared with other HTLV-1-negative T cell malignancies; is less active in acute ATL than lymphoma-type ATL; and may provide extended survival for selected patients, most of whom have lymphoma-type ATL.
- Antiviral treatment for ATL is not enough by itself because of the short duration of responses. It may be an alternative to multiagent chemotherapy, especially in the initial treatment of acute ATL. It has not been extensively investigated, and its role in the treatment of ATL is undetermined.

REFERENCES

● = Key primary paper
◆ = Major review article

●1. Uchiyama T, Yodoi J, Sagawa K *et al.* Adult T-cell leukemia: clinical and hematologic features of 16 cases. *Blood* 1977; **50**: 481–92.

2. Hinuma Y, Nagata K, Hanaoka M *et al.* Adult T-cell leukemia: antigen in an ATL cell line and detection of antibodies to the antigen in human sera. *Proc Natl Acad Sci U S A* 1981; **78**: 6476–80.

3. Hanaoka M, Sasaki M, Matsumoto H *et al.* Adult T cell leukemia. Histological classification and characteristics. *Acta Pathol Jpn* 1979; **29**: 723–38.

●4. Hinuma Y, Komoda H, Chosa T *et al.* Antibodies to adult T-cell leukemia-virus-associated antigen (ATLA) in sera from patients with ATL and controls in Japan: a nation-wide sero-epidemiologic study. *Int J Cancer* 1982; **29**: 631–5.

5. Yamaguchi K, Nishimura H, Kohrogi H *et al.* A proposal for smoldering adult T-cell leukemia: a clinicopathologic study of five cases. *Blood* 1983; **62**: 758–66.

6. Yoshida M, Miyoshi I, Hinuma Y. Isolation and characterization of retro-virus from cell lines of human adult T-cell leukemia and its implication in the disease. *Proc Natl Acad Sci U S A* 1982; **79**: 2031–5.

◆7. Uchiyama T. Human T cell leukemia virus type I (HTLV-I) and human diseases. *Annu Rev Immunol* 1997; **15**: 15–37.

8. Poiesz BJ, Ruscetti FW, Gazdar AF *et al.* Detection and isolation of type C retrovirus particles from fresh and cultured lymphocytes of a patient with cutaneous T-cell lymphoma. *Proc Natl Acad Sci U S A* 1980; **77**: 7415–19.

9. Yoshida M, Seiki M, Yamaguchi K, Takatsuki K. Monoclonal integration of human T-cell leukemia provirus in all primary tumors of adult T-cell leukemia suggests causative role of human T-cell leukemia virus in the disease. *Proc Natl Acad Sci U S A* 1984; **81**: 2534–7.

10. Yoshida M. Multiple viral strategies of HTLV-1 for dysregulation of cell growth control. *Annu Rev Immunol* 2001; **19**: 475–96.

11. Franchini G, Wong-Staal F, Gallo RC. Human T-cell leukemia virus (HTLV-I) transcripts in fresh and cultured cells of patients with adult T-cell leukemia. *Proc Natl Acad Sci U S A* 1984; **81**: 6207–11.

12. Kinoshita T, Shimoyama M, Tobinai K *et al.* Detection of mRNA for the tax1/rex1 gene of human T-cell leukemia virus type I in fresh peripheral blood mononuclear cells of adult T-cell leukemia patients and viral carriers by using the polymerase chain reaction. *Proc Natl Acad Sci U S A* 1989; **86**: 5620–4.

13. Okamoto T, Ohno Y, Tsugane S *et al.* Multi-step carcinogenesis model for adult T-cell leukemia. *Jpn J Cancer Res* 1989; **80**: 191–5.

●14. Tajima K. The 4th nation-wide study of adult T-cell leukemia/lymphoma (ATL) in Japan: estimates of risk of ATL and its geographical and clinical features. The T- and B-cell Malignancy Study Group. *Int J Cancer* 1990; **45**: 237–43.

●15. Arisawa K, Soda M, Endo S *et al.* Evaluation of adult T-cell leukemia/lymphoma incidence and its impact on non-Hodgkin lymphoma incidence in southwestern Japan. *Int J Cancer* 2000; **85**: 319–24.

16. Murphy EL, Figueroa JP, Gibbs WN *et al.* Human T-lymphotropic virus type I (HTLV-I) seroprevalence in Jamaica. I. Demographic determinants. *Am J Epidemiol* 1991; **133**: 1114–24.

17. Edlich RF, Arnette JA, Williams FM. Global epidemic of human T-cell lymphotropic virus type-1 (HTLV-1). *J Emerg Med* 2000; **18**: 109–19.

18. Igakura T, Stinchcombe JC, Goon PK *et al.* Spread of HTLV-I between lymphocytes by virus-induced polarization of the cytoskeleton. *Science* 2003; **299**: 1713–16.

19. Tajima K, Tominaga S, Suchi T *et al.* Epidemiological analysis of the distribution of antibody to adult T-cell leukemia-virus-associated antigen: possible horizontal transmission of adult T-cell leukemia virus. *Gann* 1982; **73**: 893–901.

20. Kajiyama W, Kashiwagi S, Ikematsu H *et al.* Intrafamilial transmission of adult T cell leukemia virus. *J Infect Dis* 1986; **154**: 851–7.

21. Hino S, Yamaguchi K, Katamine S *et al.* Mother-to-child transmission of human T-cell leukemia virus type-I. *Jpn J Cancer Res* 1985; **76**: 474–80.

22. Hino S, Sugiyama H, Doi H *et al.* Breaking the cycle of HTLV-I transmission via carrier mothers' milk. *Lancet* 1987; **2**: 158–9.

23. Yamanouchi K, Kinoshita K, Moriuchi R *et al.* Oral transmission of human T-cell leukemia virus type-I into a common marmoset (Callithrix jacchus) as an experimental model for milk-borne transmission. *Jpn J Cancer Res* 1985; **76**: 481–7.

24. Osame M, Usuku K, Izumo S *et al.* HTLV-I associated myelopathy, a new clinical entity. *Lancet* 1986; **1**: 1031–2.

25. Mochizuki M, Watanabe T, Yamaguchi K *et al.* HTLV-I uveitis: a distinct clinical entity caused by HTLV-I. *Jpn J Cancer Res* 1992; **83**: 236–9.

26. Gout O, Baulac M, Gessain A *et al.* Rapid development of myelopathy after HTLV-I infection acquired by transfusion during cardiac transplantation. *N Engl J Med* 1990; **322**: 383–8.

27. Osame M, Janssen R, Kubota H *et al.* Nationwide survey of HTLV-I-associated myelopathy in Japan: association with blood transfusion. *Ann Neurol* 1990; **28**: 50–6.

●28. Kashiwagi K, Furusyo N, Nakashima H *et al.* A decrease in mother-to-child transmission of human T lymphotropic virus type I (HTLV-I) in Okinawa, Japan. *Am J Trop Med Hyg* 2004; **70**: 158–63.

29. Kawano F, Yamaguchi K, Nishimura H *et al.* Variation in the clinical courses of adult T-cell leukemia. *Cancer* 1985; **55**: 851–6.

30. Kinoshita K, Amagasaki T, Ikeda S *et al.* Preleukemic state of adult T cell leukemia: abnormal T lymphocytosis induced by human adult T cell leukemia-lymphoma virus. *Blood* 1985; **66**: 120–7.

●31. Shimoyama M. Diagnostic criteria and classification of clinical subtypes of adult T-cell leukaemia-lymphoma. A report from the Lymphoma Study Group (1984–87). *Br J Haematol* 1991; **79**: 428–37.

32. Hattori T, Uchiyama T, Toibana T *et al.* Surface phenotype of Japanese adult T-cell leukemia cells characterized by monoclonal antibodies. *Blood* 1981; **58**: 645–7.

33. Uchiyama T, Hori T, Tsudo M *et al.* Interleukin-2 receptor (Tac antigen) expressed on adult T cell leukemia cells. *J Clin Invest* 1985; **76**: 446–53.

34. Takemoto S, Matsuoka M, Yamaguchi K, Takatsuki K. A novel diagnostic method of adult T-cell leukemia: monoclonal integration of human T-cell lymphotropic virus type I provirus DNA detected by inverse polymerase chain reaction. *Blood* 1994; **84**: 3080–5.

●35. Ohshima K, Suzumiya J, Sato K *et al.* Nodal T-cell lymphoma in an HTLV-I-endemic area: proviral HTLV-I DNA, histological classification and clinical evaluation. *Br J Haematol* 1998; **101**: 703–11.

◆36. Hanaoka M. Progress in adult T cell leukemia research. *Acta Pathol Jpn* 1982; **32**(Suppl 1): 171–85.

37. Setoyama M, Katahira Y, Kanzaki T. Clinicopathologic analysis of 124 cases of adult T-cell leukemia/lymphoma with cutaneous manifestations: the smouldering type with skin manifestations has a poorer prognosis than previously thought. *J Dermatol* 1999; **26**: 785–90.

38. Tamura K, Yokota T, Mashita R, Tamura S. Pulmonary manifestations in adult T-cell leukemia at the time of diagnosis. *Respiration* 1993; **60**: 115–19.

●39. Yoshioka R, Yamaguchi K, Yoshinaga T, Takatsuki K. Pulmonary complications in patients with adult T-cell leukemia. *Cancer* 1985; **55**: 2491–4.

40. Suzumiya J, Marutsuka K, Nabeshima K *et al.* Autopsy findings in 47 cases of adult T-cell leukemia/lymphoma in Miyazaki prefecture, Japan. *Leuk Lymphoma* 1993; **11**: 281–6.

◆41. Kikuchi M, Jaffe ES, Ralfkiaer E. Adult T-cell leukemia/lymphoma. In: Jaffe ES, Harris NL, Stein H, Vardiman JW. (eds) *Pathology and genetics of tumors of haematopoietic and lymphoid tissues.* Lyon: IARC Press, 2001: 200–3.

42. Motoi T, Uchiyama T, Uchino H *et al.* Serum soluble interleukin-2 receptor levels in patients with adult T-cell leukemia and human T-cell leukemia/lymphoma virus type-I seropositive healthy carriers. *Jpn J Cancer Res* 1988; **79**: 593–9.

43. Yasunaga Ji, Sakai T, Nosaka K *et al.* Impaired production of naive T lymphocytes in human T-cell leukemia virus type I-infected individuals: its implications in the immunodeficient state. *Blood* 2001; **97**: 3177–83.

44. Hishizawa M, Imada K, Kitawaki T *et al.* Depletion and impaired interferon-alpha-producing capacity of blood plasmacytoid dendritic cells in human T-cell leukaemia virus type I-infected individuals. *Br J Haematol* 2004; **125**: 568–75.

45. Yagi H, Nomura T, Nakamura K *et al.* Crucial role of FOXP3 in the development and function of human CD25+CD4+ regulatory T cells. *Int Immunol* 2004; **16**: 1643–56.

46. Takaori-Kondo A, Imada K, Yamamoto I *et al.* Parathyroid hormone-related protein-induced hypercalcemia in SCID mice engrafted with adult T-cell leukemia cells. *Blood* 1998; **91**: 4747–51.

●47. Nosaka K, Miyamoto T, Sakai T *et al.* Mechanism of hypercalcemia in adult T-cell leukemia: overexpression of receptor activator of nuclear factor kappaB ligand on adult T-cell leukemia cells. *Blood* 2002; **99**: 634–40.

◆48. Yamada Y, Tomonaga M. The current status of therapy for adult T-cell leukaemia-lymphoma in Japan. *Leuk Lymphoma* 2003; **44**: 611–18.

49. Tsukasaki K, Tobinai K, Shimoyama M *et al.* Deoxycoformycin-containing combination chemotherapy for adult T-cell leukemia-lymphoma: Japan Clinical Oncology Group Study (JCOG9109). *Int J Hematol* 2003; **77**: 164–70.

●50. Yamada Y, Tomonaga M, Fukuda H *et al.* A new G-CSF-supported combination chemotherapy, LSG15, for adult

T-cell leukaemia-lymphoma: Japan Clinical Oncology Group Study 9303. *Br J Haematol* 2001; **113**: 375–82.

51. Ikeda K, Oka M, Yamada Y *et al.* Adult T-cell leukemia cells over-express the multidrug-resistance-protein (MRP) and lung-resistance-protein (LRP) genes. *Int J Cancer* 1999; **82**: 599–604.

52. Ohno N, Tani A, Uozumi K *et al.* Expression of functional lung resistance-related protein predicts poor outcome in adult T-cell leukemia. *Blood* 2001; **98**: 1160–5.

53. Baba Y, Arakawa A, Furusawa M *et al.* Radiation therapy of adult T-cell leukemia. *Acta Oncol* 1994; **33**: 667–70.

54. Tobinai K, Kobayashi Y, Shimoyama M. Interferon alfa and zidovudine in adult T-cell leukemia-lymphoma. Lymphoma Study Group of the Japan Clinical Oncology Group. *N Engl J Med* 1995; **333**: 1285.

●55. Shimoyama M, Ota K, Kikuchi M *et al.* Major prognostic factors of adult patients with advanced T-cell lymphoma/leukemia. *J Clin Oncol* 1988; **6**: 1088–97.

●56. Tsukasaki K, Ikeda S, Murata K *et al.* Characteristics of chemotherapy-induced clinical remission in long survivors with aggressive adult T-cell leukemia/lymphoma. *Leuk Res* 1993; **17**: 157–66.

57. Uozumi K, Hanada S, Ohno N *et al.* Combination chemotherapy (RCM protocol: response-oriented cyclic multidrug protocol) for the acute or lymphoma type adult T-cell leukemia. *Leuk Lymphoma* 1995; **18**: 317–23.

58. Matsushita K, Matsumoto T, Ohtsubo H *et al.* Long-term maintenance combination chemotherapy with OPEC/MPEC (vincristine or methotrexate, prednisolone, etoposide and cyclophosphamide) or with daily oral etoposide and prednisolone can improve survival and quality of life in adult T-cell leukemia/lymphoma. *Leuk Lymphoma* 1999; **36**: 67–75.

59. Taguchi H, Kinoshita KI, Takatsuki K *et al.* An intensive chemotherapy of adult T-cell leukemia/lymphoma: CHOP followed by etoposide, vindesine, ranimustine, and mitoxantrone with granulocyte colony-stimulating factor support. *J Acquir Immune Defic Syndr Hum Retrovirol* 1996; **12**: 182–6.

60. Daenen S, Rojer RA, Smit JW *et al.* Successful chemotherapy with deoxycoformycin in adult T-cell lymphoma-leukaemia. *Br J Haematol* 1984; **58**: 723–7.

61. Tobinai K, Uike N, Saburi Y *et al.* Phase II study of cladribine (2-chlorodeoxyadenosine) in relapsed or refractory adult T-cell leukemia-lymphoma. *Int J Hematol* 2003; **77**: 512–17.

62. Tsuda H, Takatsuki K, Ohno R *et al.* Treatment of adult T-cell leukaemia-lymphoma with irinotecan hydrochloride (CPT-11). CPT-11 Study Group on Hematological Malignancy. *Br J Cancer* 1994; **70**: 771–4.

63. Tsukasaki K, Maeda T, Arimura K *et al.* Poor outcome of autologous stem cell transplantation for adult T cell leukemia/lymphoma: a case report and review of the literature. *Bone Marrow Transplant* 1999; **23**: 87–9.

●64. Hermine O, Bouscary D, Gessain A *et al.* Treatment of adult T-cell leukemia-lymphoma with zidovudine and interferon alfa. *N Engl J Med* 1995; **332**: 1749–51.

●65. Gill PS, Harrington W Jr, Kaplan MH *et al.* Treatment of adult T-cell leukemia-lymphoma with a combination of interferon alfa and zidovudine. *N Engl J Med* 1995; **332**: 1744–8.

66. Matutes E, Taylor GP, Cavenagh J *et al.* Interferon alpha and zidovudine therapy in adult T-cell leukaemia lymphoma: response and outcome in 15 patients. *Br J Haematol* 2001; **113**: 779–84.

67. Hermine O, Allard I, Levy V *et al.* A prospective phase II clinical trial with the use of zidovudine and interferon-alpha in the acute and lymphoma forms of adult T-cell leukaemia/lymphoma. *Hematol J* 2002; **3**: 276–82.

68. White JD, Wharfe G, Stewart DM *et al.* The combination of zidovudine and interferon alpha-2B in the treatment of adult T-cell leukemia/lymphoma. *Leuk Lymphoma* 2001; **40**: 287–94.

◆69. Bazarbachi A, Hermine O. Treatment of adult T-cell leukaemia/lymphoma: current strategy and future perspectives. *Virus Res* 2001; **78**: 79–92.

●70. Waldmann TA, White JD, Goldman CK *et al.* The interleukin-2 receptor: a target for monoclonal antibody treatment of human T-cell lymphotrophic virus I-induced adult T-cell leukemia. *Blood* 1993; **82**: 1701–12.

71. Waldmann TA, White JD, Carrasquillo JA *et al.* Radioimmunotherapy of interleukin-2R alpha-expressing adult T-cell leukemia with Yttrium-90-labeled anti-Tac. *Blood* 1995; **86**: 4063–75.

◆72. Ishikawa T. Current status of therapeutic approaches to adult T-cell leukemia. *Int. J. Hematol* 2003; **78**: 304–11.

●73. Utsunomiya A, Miyazaki Y, Takatsuka Y *et al.* Improved outcome of adult T cell leukemia/lymphoma with allogeneic hematopoietic stem cell transplantation. *Bone Marrow Transplant* 2001; **27**: 15–20.

●74. Kami M, Hamaki T, Miyakoshi S *et al.* Allogeneic haematopoietic stem cell transplantation for the treatment of adult T-cell leukaemia/lymphoma. *Br J Haematol* 2003; **120**: 304–9.

●75. Fukushima T, Miyazaki Y, Honda S *et al.* Allogeneic hematopoietic stem cell transplantation provides sustained long-term survival for patients with adult T-cell leukemia/lymphoma. *Leukemia* 2005; **19**: 829–34.

●76. Okamura J, Utsunomiya A, Tanosaki R *et al.* Allogeneic stem-cell transplantation with reduced conditioning intensity as a novel immunotherapy and antiviral therapy for adult T-cell leukemia/lymphoma. *Blood* 2005; **105**: 4143–5.

77. Miyatake JI, Maeda Y. Inhibition of proliferation and CD25 down-regulation by retinoic acid in human adult T cell leukemia cells. *Leukemia* 1997; **11**: 401–7.

78. Maeda Y, Naiki Y, Sono H *et al.* Clinical application of all-trans retinoic acid (tretinoin) for adult T-cell leukaemia. *Br J Haematol* 2000; **109**: 677–8.

79. Toshima M, Nagai T, Izumi T *et al.* All-trans-retinoic acid treatment for chemotherapy-resistant acute adult T-cell leukemia. *Int J Hematol* 2000; **72**: 343–5.

80. Nasr R, Rosenwald A, El-Sabban ME *et al.* Arsenic/ interferon specifically reverses 2 distinct gene networks

critical for the survival of HTLV-1-infected leukemic cells. *Blood* 2003; **101**: 4576–82.

81. Hermine O, Dombret H, Poupon J *et al.* Phase II trial of arsenic trioxide and alpha interferon in patients with relapsed/refractory adult T-cell leukemia/lymphoma. *Hematol J* 2004; **5**: 130–4.

●82. Ikeda S, Momita S, Kinoshita K *et al.* Clinical course of human T-lymphotropic virus type I carriers with molecularly detectable monoclonal proliferation of T lymphocytes: defining a low- and high-risk population. *Blood* 1993; **82**: 2017–24.

83. Kamihira S, Atogami S, Sohda H *et al.* Significance of soluble interleukin-2 receptor levels for evaluation of the progression of adult T-cell leukaemia. *Cancer* 1994; **73**: 2753–8.

84. Araki K, Harada K, Nakamoto K *et al.* Clinical significance of serum soluble IL-2R levels in patients with adult T cell leukaemia (ATL) and HTLV-1 carriers. *Clin Exp Immunol* 2000; **119**: 259–63.

85. Gabet AS, Mortreux F, Talarmin A *et al.* High circulating proviral load with oligoclonal expansion of HTLV-1 bearing T cells in HTLV-1 carriers with strongyloidiasis. *Oncogene* 2000; **19**: 4954–60.

86. Tsukasaki K, Imaizumi Y, Tawara M *et al.* Diversity of leukaemic cell morphology in ATL correlates with prognostic factors, aberrant immunophenotype and defective HTLV-1 genotype. *Br J Haematol* 1999; **105**: 369–75.

87. Shirono K, Hattori T, Takatsuki K. A new classification of clinical stages of adult T-cell leukemia based on prognosis of the disease. *Leukemia* 1994; **8**: 1834–7.

88. Murakawa M, Shibuya T, Teshima T *et al.* Spontaneous remission from acute exacerbation of chronic adult T-cell leukemia. *Blut* 1990; **61**: 346–9.

80

Other peripheral T cell lymphomas

STEFANO LUMINARI AND MASSIMO FEDERICO

INTRODUCTION

Peripheral T cell lymphomas (PTCLs) comprise a heterogeneous group of neoplasms that are derived from post-thymic lymphoid cells at different stages of differentiation with different morphologic patterns, phenotypes, and clinical presentations.[1] Peripheral T cell lymphomas are highly diverse, reflecting the diverse cells from which they originate. These include different types of T cells ($\alpha\beta$ or $\gamma\delta$) and may have features of cytotoxic, helper, or suppressor lymphocytes, or they may present an aberrant phenotype.[1–6]

Notwithstanding progress in pathology, biology, and genetics, PTCLs remain difficult to classify for several reasons. Not only is the group as a whole rare, but it is divided into multiple subtypes, so that some of these neoplasms represent less than 1 percent of non-Hodgkin lymphomas (NHLs). Moreover, PTCLs lack a phenotypic marker of clonality, are morphologically heterogeneous, and show poor correlation between morphology and prognosis. Finally, the lack of diagnostic consensus has limited our knowledge of therapeutic experience, and PTCL overall and failure-free survival rates (OS and FFS) are still among the lowest of NHLs.[7]

Mature T cell lymphomas are currently subclassified according to their clinical features, using World Health Organization (WHO) criteria, into leukemic, cutaneous, other extranodal, and nodal (Table 80.1). The clinical subtypes of PTCL can be further divided into well-defined and not well-defined clinical entities based on the presence of distinguishing clinico-biologic features.[1] Real entities, which include mycosis fungoides (MF), anaplastic large cell lymphoma (ALCL), and adult T cell leukemia/lymphoma

Table 80.1 Clinical classification of mature T cell and natural killer (NK) cell neoplasms (World Health Organization[1])

Nodal
Peripheral T cell lymphoma, unspecified
Angioimmunoblastic T cell lymphoma
Anaplastic large cell lymphoma

Leukemic or disseminated
T cell prolymphocytic leukemia
T cell granular lymphocytic leukemia
Aggressive NK cell leukemia
Adult T cell lymphoma/leukemia

Cutaneous
Blastic NK cell lymphoma[a]
Mycosis fungoides/Sézary syndrome
Primary cutaneous anaplastic large cell lymphoma

Extranodal
Extranodal NK/T cell lymphoma, nasal type
Enteropathy-type T cell lymphoma
Hepatosplenic T cell lymphoma
Subcutaneous panniculitis-like T cell lymphoma

[a]Neoplasm of uncertain lineage and stage of differentiation.

(ATLL), along with natural killer (NK) cell-derived lymphomas, are described elsewhere in this book (see Chapters 75–79). This chapter will focus on nodal PTCL (i.e., PTCL, unspecified and angioimmunoblastic T cell lymphoma) together with all the other extranodal PTCLs (i.e., enteropathy-type T cell lymphoma, hepatosplenic γδ T cell lymphoma, and subcutaneous panniculitis-like T cell lymphoma). Peripheral T cell lymphoma will be described with a special emphasis on epidemiology, clinical features, and principles of management.

GENERAL DESCRIPTION

The origin from T lymphocytes of one subset of lymphomas became apparent during the 1970s, when the immune system began to be subdivided into B and T cell lineages.[8–10] Prior to the identification of T cell lymphomas as distinct from B cell lymphomas, PTCLs were considered within major histologic subtypes and only poorly described according to growth pattern.[11] Even with the subsequent Working Formulation (WF) classification, the difficulty of differential diagnosis, the rarity of the diseases, and the behavior of T cell lymphomas as 'aggressive' neoplasms led to the inclusion of PTCL in that wide and heterogeneous group of 'aggressive' diseases where the phenotype was not considered in the clinical setting.[12]

In the 1980s and 1990s, PTCLs were treated with the same regimens developed for other 'aggressive' lymphomas. However, retrospective analyses evaluating the role of phenotype showed that T cell lymphomas were characterized by worse outcomes than B cell-derived lymphoproliferative disorders. It was therefore suggested that different treatment modalities were required for PTCL.[13] The role of immunophenotype in distinguishing disease entities was affirmed by the Revised European–American Lymphoma (REAL) classification published in 1994 and confirmed by the more recent WHO project.[1,14] In the latter classification, PTCLs are classified using a multiparametric approach integrating morphologic, immunophenotypic, genetic, and clinical features; the simple distinctions between clinical groups in the WF classification have been definitively abandoned (Table 80.2).[1,12,14,15]

Peripheral T cell lymphomas, unspecified (PTCL-U) are the largest group, accounting for approximately half of PTCLs seen in Western countries. The term 'unspecified' is used to emphasize the fact that these cases cannot be included in one of the better-defined entities.[1,14] Peripheral T cell lymphomas, unspecified correspond to several morphologic subtypes that are distinguished in other classification systems mainly on the basis of cytology, which, due to concerns about reproducibility, is now considered less relevant than formerly.[14,16–19] According to the WHO classification, PTCL-U also includes the entity previously defined as lymphoepithelioid lymphoma or Lennert Lymphoma (LeL). The use of genomic analysis to investigate the biologic basis of the differences among lymphoproliferative diseases will probably be of value for identifying more reproducible, distinctive features of PTCL-U.

Table 80.2   Nodal and other extranodal peripheral T cell lymphomas according to different classification systems

WHO[1]	REAL[14]	Kiel updated[15]	Working formulation[12]
Peripheral T cell lymphoma, unspecified (PTCL-U)	Peripheral T cell lymphoma, unspecified (provisional cytologic categories: large cell, medium-sized cell, mixed)	T-zone lymphoma, lymphoepithelioid cell (Lennert) lymphoma, pleomorphic T cell lymphoma small, medium-sized, and large cell types, T immunoblastic lymphoma	Diffuse small cleaved cell, diffuse mixed small and large cell, diffuse large cell, immunoblastic
Angioimmunoblastic T cell lymphoma (AITL)	Angioimmunoblastic T cell lymphoma	AILD type (lymphogranulomatosis X) T cell lymphoma	Diffuse mixed small and large cell, diffuse large cell, immunoblastic, atypical hyperplasia
Enteropathy-type T cell lymphoma (ETL)	Intestinal T cell lymphoma (with and without entheropathy)	Not listed (pleomorphic T cell lymphoma, medium and large cell)	Not listed (diffuse large cell, immunoblastic)
Hepatosplenic T cell lymphoma (HSTCL)	Hepatosplenic γδ T cell lymphoma	Not listed (pleomorphic T cell lymphoma, small cell, medium-sized cell)	Not listed (diffuse small cleaved cell)
Subcutaneous panniculitis T cell lymphoma (SPTCL)	Subcutaneous panniculitis T cell lymphoma	Not listed (pleomorphic T cell lymphoma, small, medium-sized, mixed or large cell, immunoblastic T cell lymphoma)	Diffuse small cleaved cell, diffuse mixed small and large cell, diffuse large cell, immunoblastic

WHO, World Health Organization; REAL, Revised European–American Lymphoma; AILD, angioimmunoblastic lymphadenopathy.

The clinical course of PTCL-U is aggressive; with current therapeutic approaches, only 40–50 percent of patients achieve complete remission and fewer than 30 percent are long-term survivors. As an example, the survival curve for patients with PTCL-U treated by the Gruppo Italiano Studio Linfomi (GISL) centers between 1988 and 2005 is given in Figure 80.1.

Among the other PTCL entities, angioimmunoblastic T cell lymphoma (AITL) was the first to be described in 1974 as a distinct clinicopathological entity, characterized by generalized lymphadenopathy, hepatosplenomegaly, anemia, and hypergammaglobulinemia.[20,21] Angioimmunoblastic T cell lymphoma was initially designated by a variety of terms, including 'immunoblastic lymphadenopathy,' 'lymphogranulomatosis X,' and 'lymphadenopathy with dysprotidemia,' mainly because the histologic features of malignancy were not easily recognizable.[22] Angioimmunoblastic T cell lymphoma typically follows an aggressive clinical course. Treatment with systemic chemotherapy results in complete remission rates of 50–70 percent although, as with PTCL-U, only 10–30 percent of patients survive long term.[23,24] Enteropathy-type T cell lymphoma (ETL) was defined in 1985 by Isaacson et al.,[25] who identified a rearrangement of the T cell receptor in the disease formerly defined by the same group as 'malignant hystiocytosis of the intestine.'[26] The disease has also been defined as 'entheropathy-associated T cell lymphoma' by O'Farrely et al. in 1986,[27] as 'intestinal T cell lymphoma' (with or without enteropathy) in the REAL classification,[14] and as ETL in the recent WHO classification.[1] Enteropathy-type T cell lymphoma is a clinical entity distinct from non-enteropathy-associated T cell lymphoma, which should be considered a peripheral T cell NHL with intestinal localization.[1] Although the two forms of intestinal T cell lymphoma (ITL) share particular symptoms and clinical features that result when the intestine is the primary site of involvement, only ETL is typically characterized by association with celiac disease, and has distinct immunologic and molecular features.[28–30] The outcome of the disease is poor, due partly to the poor nutritional status of patients, surgical emergencies at presentation, and low sensitivity to commonly used chemotherapy regimens. As a result, about one-half of patients do not complete their initial treatment and reported 5-year OS and disease-free survival (DFS) are around 20 percent and 3 percent, respectively.[31]

Hepatosplenic T cell lymphoma (HSTCL) was recognized as a distinct entity in 1990 on the basis of its typical clinical presentation (hepatosplenomegaly, anemia, thrombocytopenia, neutropenia, and lymphocytosis), pattern of histologic involvement (resulting from the sinusal/sinusoidal tropism of neoplastic cells), and the typical association with isochromosome 7q and trisomy 8.[32,33] Although rearrangement of $\gamma\delta$ T cell receptors is a characteristic feature of the disease, some cases expressing the $\alpha\beta$ receptor have been reported[34] and are to be considered an immunophenotypic variant of the same disease. The clinical course of HSTCL is commonly 'aggressive' despite multiagent chemotherapy; the median survival time is 12–14 months.[35]

Subcutaneous panniculitis-like T cell lymphoma (SPTCL) is an uncommon T cell lymphoma originating from cytotoxic T cells and was originally described by Gonzalez et al. in 1991 as 'cytophagic histiocytic panniculitis.'[36] More recently, some authors have suggested that at least two subtypes of SPTCL can be recognized. This distinction has also been confirmed in the recent WHO-EORTC (European Organization for the Research and Treatment of Cancer) classification for cutaneous lymphomas.[37] Cases with an $\alpha\beta$ T cell phenotype, which are usually CD8$^+$, are characterized by an indolent course and are restricted to the subcutaneous tissue, without dermal and epidermal involvement.[38–40] In contrast, a smaller group of SPTCLs, representing about 25 percent of cases, has a $\gamma\delta$ phenotype, is typically CD4$^-$ and CD8$^-$, coexpresses CD56, can infiltrate the dermis or epidermis, and has a very 'aggressive' behavior.[38–42] The latter group is considered a distinct category of $\gamma\delta$ cutaneous lymphomas. In the WHO-EORTC system, the term 'SPTCL' is used only for the $\alpha\beta^+$ cases. Gamma/delta cases can sometimes be misdiagnosed as NK cutaneous lymphomas; in these cases, the search for T cell receptor rearrangement should be performed to reach a correct diagnosis.[43]

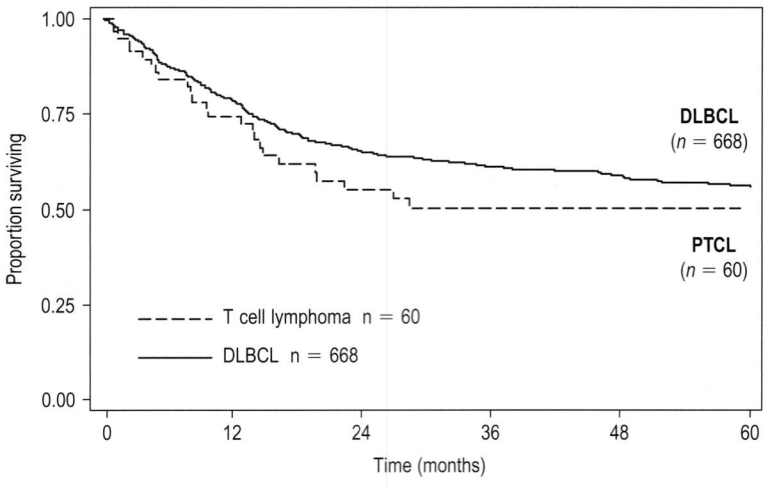

Figure 80.1 Overall survival curve of peripheral T cell lymphoma (PTCL) cases compared with patients with diffuse large B cell lymphoma (DLBCL). Reported patients were diagnosed from 1988 to 2005 and enrolled into clinical trials performed by the Gruppo Italiano Studio Linfomi (GISL). All patients received anthracycline-based chemotherapy. DLBCL and PTCL were comparable in terms of clinical features.

EPIDEMIOLOGY AND RISK FACTORS

Peripheral T cell lymphomas account for 5–10 percent of all lymphoproliferative disorders in the Western hemisphere,[19,44] with an overall incidence of 0.5–2 per 100 000 per year,[45] and have a striking epidemiologic distribution, with a higher incidence in Asia.[46] This may result from both a real higher incidence and the relatively lower frequency in Asia of many B cell lymphomas such as follicular lymphoma. In a large, population-based study performed in the United States, total lymphoid neoplasms were 70 percent higher for whites than for Asians; the difference was mostly due to a higher rate in whites of chronic lymphocytic leukemia/small lymphocytic lymphoma (CLL/SLL), follicular lymphoma, mantle cell lymphoma, and hairy cell leukemia, while the incidence rate ratios for T cell neoplasms for whites and Asians were comparable.[47] In addition to race-linked factors, a possible cause of geographic variation is the higher incidence of NK- and human T cell lymphotrophic virus type 1 (HTLV-1)-related lymphomas in Asian countries (due, for the latter subtype, to the high prevalence of HTLV-1 infection in those countries). When only PTCL-U and rarer subtypes are considered, the geographic incidence variation is less evident.[47] A study performed by the International Lymphoma Study Group to evaluate the distribution of the major lymphoma subtypes in different geographic regions found higher incidences of PTCL-U in London (8 percent), Cape Town (8 percent), and Hong Kong (10 percent) and lower incidences in Vancouver, Omaha, Wurzburg/Gottingen, Lyon, and Locarno (1–6 percent).[48] More recent data from the International Peripheral T Cell and NK/T cell Lymphoma Study group documented additional geographic variations among PTCL subtypes, with increased frequency of AITL and ETL in Europe compared to Asia and North America (JM Vose, personal communication).

Overall, PTCL-U is the most frequent subtype, accounting for 27–55 percent of PTCL cases. It is followed by AITL, which accounts for approximately 4–24 percent of cases. The other subtypes are rare and account for the remaining 1–7 percent of PTCLs (Table 80.3).[7,16–18,49–51] No consistent risk factors and no etiologic agent for the development of the disease have been reported to date, although patients usually share some sort of underlying immunologic disorder and frequent bacterial, fungal, and viral infections have been described in patients with PTCL.[52,53]

A significant proportion of subjects with AITL have a medication history, particularly antibiotics, but this is more likely to be a consequence of systemic illness clinically mimicking an infectious process rather than the primary cause of the disease.[22] Further, 10–20 percent of HSTCL cases arise in immunocompromised patients, predominantly in the solid-organ transplant setting,[54,55] and a strong association has been found between ETL and adult-onset celiac disease (CD). A relationship between malabsorption and lymphoma was first described in 1855 by Sir William Gull,[56] but it was not until 1962 that it was suggested that intestinal lymphoma was a consequence of adult CD.[57] Enteropathy-type T cell lymphoma typically occurs in patients with a history of adult-onset CD and is rarer with cases of childhood-onset disease. A strict relationship between ETL and celiac disease is supported by the observation that the tumor margins are always surrounded by villous atrophy and crypt hyperplasia, typical of CD.[31] For patients with newly diagnosed adult CD, the risk of developing ETL is approximately 1 in 20 after 4 years of follow-up; for patients over 50 years of age with newly diagnosed adult CD, the risk is 1 in 10.[28] The underlying mechanism which leads to the development of ETL in patients with CD is not clear. Unlike CD patients without ETL, CD patients with developing ETL are characterized by a low titer of systemic anti-gliadin antibodies not modified by a gluten-free diet. This suggests that either the ETL cases are immunocompromised – possibly due to lymphoma – or are not hypersensitive to gluten and therefore have a different type of enteropathy.[27,58] On the other hand, Holmes et al. showed that treatment of enteropathy with a gluten-free diet for over 5 years reduces the risk of developing lymphoma to that of the general population.[29]

A role for infectious agents (in particular, lymphotrophic viruses) in the pathogenesis of PTCL has long been suggested on the basis of the 30 percent positivity rate of Epstein–Barr virus (EBV) infection for PTCL cases and by the four- to fivefold higher frequency of EBV infection in PTCL cases compared with B-NHL. Further, EBV positivity is confined to a subset of T-NHL subtypes (AITL, Lennert lymphoma, ETL, and PTCL-U) whereas low-grade cutaneous, lymphoblastic, and anaplastic large cell lymphoma are consistently EBV negative.[59] A difference in the EBV positivity rate for ETL cases has also been documented in different geographic areas, suggesting significant epidemiologic differences.[60]

The role of EBV has been particularly studied in AITL, which has the highest frequency of EBV infection among other PTCLs. Interestingly, when infection is present in these cases, EBV-positive cells are mainly B lymphocytes, not T cells, supporting the concept that the infection is unlikely to have a direct role in lymphomagenesis. Infections by other viruses such as human herpes virus 6 (HHV6), HHV8, human immunodeficiency virus (HIV),

Table 80.3   Frequency of other peripheral T cell lymphomas[16–18,49–51]

WHO classification	%	
	NHL	T_{NK}–NHL
Peripheral T cell lymphoma, unspecified	4–6	27–55
Angioimmunoblastic T cell lymphoma	1–2	4–24
Enteropathy-type T cell lymphoma	<1	1–7
Hepatosplenic T cell lymphoma	<1	1–7
Subcutaneous panniculitis T cell lymphoma	<1	1–7

WHO, World Health Organization; NHL, non-Hodgkin lymphoma; NK, natural killer.

and hepatitis C virus (HCV) have also been described in patients with AITL,[61–64] but, as already described for EBV, the infected cells are B cells and the role of such agents in the pathogenesis of AITL remains dubious.

CLINICAL FEATURES

The clinical features of PTCL are extremely heterogeneous. Peripheral T cell lymphomas express even more clinical diversity than B cell NHLs, and there is a close, though not absolute, relationship between some unusual clinical features and certain histologic subtypes. Based on clinical presentation, PTCLs can be considered predominantly leukemic, nodal, extranodal, or cutaneous (Table 80.1).

Median age at presentation is 55–60 years. However, younger ages of presentation have been described for patients with HSTCL, and occasional cases of SPTCL have been reported in children. Peripheral T cell lymphoma, unspecified usually shows a slight predominance in males (overall male:female [M:F] ratio of 3:2). Among specific subtypes, male predominance is evident for ETL (M:F ratio of 3:1) and HSTCL (M:F ratio of 2.5:1).[31,65,66]

Peripheral T cell lymphoma, unspecified

Peripheral T cell lymphomas, unspecified are included among the 'nodal' PTCLs. Lymphadenopathy may be present in 80 percent of cases, being the most common presenting sign. Exclusively nodal disease, however, is uncommon, accounting for only about 15 percent of cases. When compared to B cell lymphomas, PTCL-U patients usually present with more advanced disease, more extranodal disease, a higher frequency of systemic symptoms, and spleen involvement. In some instances, lymphadenopathies may wax and wane for several weeks or months before diagnosis. Bulky masses with diameters greater than 10 cm are less frequent than in B cell NHL. Lymphadenopathies usually occur on both sides of the diaphragm, with a slight prevalence of subdiaphragmatic disease when only one side is involved. Mediastinal and abdominal lymphadenopathies are reported in 15–30 percent and 60 percent of cases, respectively.[46,67–70] The distribution of nodal disease in a series of consecutive cases of PTCL referred to GISL centers over the last 17 years (1988–2005) is shown in Figure 80.2. Superior vena caval obstruction may occasionally occur as a consequence of bulky and compressive masses, as encountered in T-lymphoblastic lymphomas.[69,70] The spleen is involved in about one-third of cases, and some PTCLs may present with predominant splenomegaly;[69–71] however, when splenic involvement is documented, differential diagnosis with HSTCL should be considered.[32] Tonsillar involvement is rare and has been associated more specifically with lymphoepithelioid lymphoma.[72]

The bone marrow is involved in approximately one-third of cases[73] and sometimes may be the only source of tissue

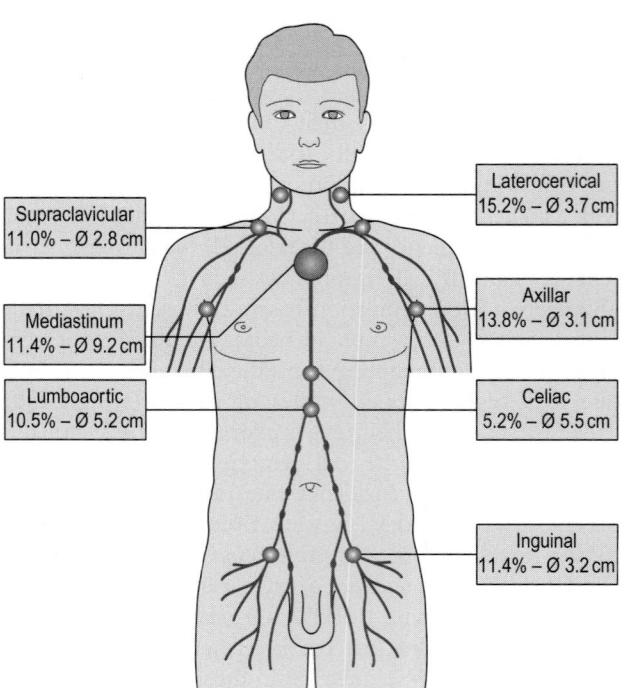

Figure 80.2 Pattern of lymph node involvement in nodal peripheral T cell lymphoma (PTCL). For each nodal region, frequency of involvement is provided with the median length of the maximum transverse diameter of enlarged nodes. Data are calculated for patients with PTCL enrolled into clinical trials performed by Gruppo Italiano Studio Linfomi (GISL) from 1988 to 2005 (n = 60).

for diagnosis (Table 80.4). The interpretation of bone marrow histology may be difficult, however, because histologic features are subtle and overlap with a variety of reactive T cell proliferations and other malignant processes. Moreover, PTCL frequently induces secondary changes in the marrow microenvironment, including hemophagocytosis,[74,75] granulocytic hyperplasia, eosinophilia, plasmacytosis, granulomatous inflammation, vascular proliferation, and myelofibrosis,[76,77] all of which may obscure the neoplastic infiltrate. Extranodal involvement is present in 65–82 percent of patients, while primary extranodal disease accounts for 27–45 percent of cases.[18,19,46,65,78–81] When the disease arises at extranodal sites it is usually more difficult to diagnose and can be confused with reactive processes. The more commonly involved extranodal sites are skin (12–18 percent), liver (9–13 percent), soft tissue (10 percent), intestine (9 percent), head and neck area (6 percent), central nervous system (4 percent), and lung and pleura (3 percent).[18,65]

Cases of cutaneous PTCL-U are rare and represent 3 percent of primary cutaneous T cell lymphomas.[37] Along with cases of cutaneous PTCL-U, rare cases of primary cutaneous $\gamma\delta$ lymphoma, CD8$^+$ cytotoxic T cell lymphoma, and primary cutaneous small-medium CD4$^+$ T cell lymphoma have also been described. These are now being considered as provisional entities by the recent

Table 80.4 Clinical characteristics of peripheral T cell lymphoma, unspecified

	Zaja[81] n = 23	Armitage[46] n = 76	Lopez-Guillermo[18] n = 95	Rudiger[19] n = 53	Kim[78] n = 31	Kojima[80] n = 36	Savage[65] n = 117	Gallamini[79] n = 385
Median age (years)	55	61	52[a]	59	54	68	64	54
Male	70	55	61	44	65	58	61	65
Stage III–IV	83	80	79	60[b]	71	83	67	76
B symptoms	43	50	57	41	52	47	38	45
Elevated LDH	47	64	53	65	52	72	43	45
ECOG PS ≥2	43	68	24	28	32	39	36	28
Tumor bulk ≥10 cm	30[c]	12	NA	9	NA	NA	NA	15
Extranodal involvement	69	82	65	79	NA	76	78	73
Bone marrow involvement	30	36	41	NA	32	50	26	31
IPI score ≥2	65	83	72	60[d]	68	83	69	45[e]

Values are % patients, with exception of median age (years).
[a]% of patients older than 60 years; [b]only stage IV; [c]diameter not defined; [d]IPI score 3/5; [e]IPI score 3/4.
ECOG, Eastern Cooperative Oncology Group; IPI, International Prognostic Index; LDH, lactate dehydrogenase; NA, not assessed; PS, performance status.

WHO-EORTC classification of cutaneous lymphomas.[37] In all cases, a diagnosis of MF should be ruled out. Skin lesions may present as solitary, localized, or disseminated nodules or tumors[1,82–84] on the face, neck, or upper trunk as in CD4+ small to medium-sized PTCL; they may also present as ulcerated, necrotic, or hyperkeratotic nodules, patches, and plaques, as in CD8+ cytotoxic PTCL or primary cutaneous γδ lymphoma. The two latter entities are usually associated with a poorer outcome; disease spread to visceral organs is common.[39,85,86]

Central nervous system (CNS) involvement is rather rare, whether at presentation or during the course of the disease, suggesting that mature T cell malignancies exhibit less neurotropism than precursor T cell neoplasias. T cell primary central nervous system lymphomas (T-PCNSLs) account for 2–8 percent of CNS lymphoma, but a higher frequency (16.7 percent) has been reported in one series from South Korea.[87–89] T-PCNSLs usually show a helper/inducer T cell phenotype, but cases with cytotoxic/suppressor phenotype have also been described.[90] The pattern of CNS involvement has recently been evaluated in a retrospective series of 45 patients and is not dissimilar from that in B-PCNSL, with 60 percent of patients presenting with lesions of the cerebral hemisphere and the remaining 40 percent with lesions in deeper sites. Involvement of the cerebrospinal fluid is present in 20 percent of cases. The course of the disease is very aggressive, with 2- and 5-year disease-specific survival rates of 51 percent and 17 percent, respectively.[91]

Intestinal involvement may occur in about 10 percent of cases; restriction of involvement to the intestine defines the group of primary intestinal T cell lymphomas (PITCLs). Primary intestinal PTCL-U represents 20 percent of PITCLs, ETL being the most frequent histologic subtype. As a consequence of the typical site of involvement, intestinal PTCL-U and ETL share common clinical features and a poor prognosis; however, according to the WHO classification, they should be considered distinct entities.[1] Patients with PTCL usually show some degree of immune deficiency, which may also help the differential diagnosis. The most typical accompanying clinical feature is hemophagocytic syndrome (HPS), which is sometimes the major determinant of clinical presentation. Hemophagocytic syndrome is characterized by pronounced systemic manifestations such as high fever, jaundice, marked hepatosplenomegaly, severe pancytopenia, abnormal liver function tests, blood coagulation disorders with prolonged prothrombin and activated partial thromboplastin times, hypofibrinogenemia, and hypertriglyceridemia.[74,92] As described for other PTCLs,[93] many of the clinical manifestations of HPS can be related to the expression by the neoplastic cells of cytokines and chemokines such as interferon gamma (IFNγ), interleukin-1 (IL-1), or tumor necrosis factor (TNF).[94,95]

A role for EBV infection in inducing HPS has been postulated.[45] The diagnosis of HPS is based on the finding of benign-looking hemophagocytizing histiocytes in the bone marrow. Histologic features of HPS may also be found in the spleen or lymph nodes and may overwhelm the lymphomatous component.[74] Hemophagocytic syndrome may occur at any time during the clinical course of the disease, whether at initial presentation, accompanying relapse, or even during apparent complete remission.[92]

Unusual presentations such as neuropathy,[96] predominant liver disease,[32,97] vasculitis and hypereosinophilia,[98,99] and primary leptomeningeal[100] or adrenal involvement[101] have also been reported in PTCL.

Blood counts are usually unremarkable, although mild anemia and/or thrombocytopenia may be observed. Hypereosinophilia is sometimes the predominant laboratory feature[98,102,103] and has been observed in as many as 29 percent of patients.[104] A leukemic phase is rare but may eventually develop.

Angioimmunoblastic T cell lymphoma

Angioimmunoblastic T cell lymphoma is a nodal PTCL characterized by fever, weight loss, generalized lymphadenopathy, liver enlargement, splenomegaly, pulmonary infiltrates, and bone marrow involvement. The clinical syndrome of AITL overlaps with a variety of inflammatory and neoplastic processes, and changes seen in peripheral blood and on bone marrow examination may be nonspecific. The diagnosis of AITL can only be confirmed by biopsy and histologic examination of one of the enlarged lymph nodes. In a large retrospective study performed by the Kiel Lymphoma Study Group, in which 62 consecutive patients were evaluated, 90 percent of patients presented with stage III or IV disease and systemic symptoms were observed in 68 percent (Table 80.5). Patients presented with a skin rash (49 percent), pruritus (32 percent), edema (38 percent), pleural effusion (37 percent), arthritis (18 percent), or ascites (23 percent). Furthermore, they exhibited autoimmune phenomena such as cold agglutinins, circulating immune complexes, a positive Coombs test, smooth-muscle antibodies, rheumatoid factors, immune hemolysis, a paraprotein, antinuclear antibodies, and cryoglobulins.[24] Skin rash, often with pruritus, is frequently present and may be associated with a history of drug hypersensitivity.[24,105] Autoimmune disorders and an increased risk of infection are frequently present at the onset of disease. Laboratory findings include the presence of circulating immune complexes, cold agglutinins with hemolytic anemia, positive rheumatoid factor, and anti-smooth-muscle antibodies. Rarely, a serum monoclonal component can be detected.[20–22,72]

Most AITL cases carry a rearrangement of the T cell receptor beta chain gene, although in some instances it is not possible to demonstrate clonality or rearrangement of immunoglobulin genes.[106–111] This absence of clonality has been interpreted by some authors as a sign of a benign or premalignant lesion. The presence of a B cell receptor gene rearrangement in a significant minority of cases has been interpreted as a consequence of continuous immune stimulation by viral agents, rather than as evidence of coexisting B cell lymphoma. A subset of AITL patients do develop diffuse large B cell,[21,112,113] Burkitt,[114] or Hodgkin lymphoma.[115]

The clinical course of AITL is aggressive, with a median survival of less than 3 years.[24,116] Infections are the direct cause of death in most cases, mainly in patients who have achieved only partial remission or whose disease is progressing rapidly.[112]

Enteropathy-type T cell lymphoma

Eighty percent of primary intestinal T cell lymphomas are ETLs. Intestinal involvement in ETL is not only the pathognomonic feature of the disease but a major determinant of its poor outcome. Enteropathy-type T cell lymphoma usually involves the duodenum and the first part of the jejunum, with diffuse or focal segmental lesions showing extensive mucosal ulceration. The disease is typically associated with weight loss, abdominal pain, and diarrhea. Fever and night sweats can be present in about one-third of cases (Table 80.6).

Patients may also present with small-bowel obstruction or perforation. The length of the preclinical phase may vary from weeks to years, but the onset of the disease can represent a medical emergency requiring surgical intervention.[31] Patients usually have a history of symptomatic CD, and in some cases ETL may arise after CD has become refractory to a gluten-free diet. Cases of *de novo* ETL have also been described; however, in some of these cases the diagnosis of

Table 80.5 Clinical characteristics of angioimmunoblastic T cell lymphoma

	Lopez–Guillermo[18] n = 22	Rudiger[19] n = 17	Savage[65] n = 10
Median age (years)	59[a]	65	66
Male	68	53	40
Stage III–IV	95	83[b]	100
B symptoms	64	65	80
Elevated LDH	56	60	100
ECOG PS ⩾2	45	38	60
Extranodal involvement	50	88	70
Bone marrow involvement	32	NA	30
IPI score ⩾2	72	86[c]	100

Values are % patients, with exception of median age (years).
[a]% of patients older than 60 years; [b]only stage IV; [c]IPI score 3/5.
ECOG, Eastern Cooperative Oncology Group; IPI, International Prognostic Index; LDH, lactate dehydrogenase; NA, not assessed; PS, performance status.

Table 80.6 Clinical characteristics of enteropathy-type T cell lymphoma

	Lopez–Guillermo[18] n = 12	Gale[31] n = 31	Savage[65] n = 9
Median age (years)	33[a]	50	61
Male	33	74	67
Stage III–IV	83	23	67
B symptoms	67	29	78
Elevated LDH	33	25	75
ECOG PS ⩾2	75	72	67
Extranodal involvement	100	100	100
Bone marrow involvement	8	8	0
IPI score ⩾2	70	NA	100

Values are % patients, with exception of median age (years).
[a]% of patients older than 60 years.
ECOG, Eastern Cooperative Oncology Group; IPI, International Prognostic Index; LDH, lactate dehydrogenase; NA, not assessed; PS, performance status.

CD is made at the same time as the lymphoma is discovered. Latency between CD and ETL varies from months to years, with a median of 3–10 years.[117,118]

The typical intestinal localization of the disease usually requires a double-contrast barium enema examination. Findings are similar to those of inflammatory bowel disease and different from colorectal lymphoma of the B cell phenotype.[119] Fluorine-18-fluorodeoxyglucose positron emission tomography (^{18}F-FDG-PET) may be a useful technique for staging and follow-up of ETL, as demonstrated in a recent study on a small but significant series of patients. The results showed that unlike other PTCLs, for which PET positivity is reported in 40 percent of cases, ETL cases are always PET positive. In the same study, a series of uncomplicated CD was also included, which did not result in PET positivity; ^{18}F-FDG-PET can therefore be used for early diagnosis of ETL, even in the context of long-standing CD.[120]

Hepatosplenic γδ T cell lymphoma

Patients with HSTCL are usually referred to the hemato-oncologist due to enlargement of the spleen or cytopenia. Presenting features may also include B symptoms and abdominal pain. The onset of the disease is aggressive, with a short time from the appearance of symptoms to the first visit. Splenomegaly is always present and is typically a homogeneous enlargement without evidence of nodules or hilar lymph nodes; however, splenectomy is always associated with evidence of tumor infiltration. Spleen weight can range from 700 to 6000 g. Splenic architecture is preserved, but with marked hyperplasia of the red pulp and atrophy of the white pulp. Liver enlargement is frequently (but not always) present; if enlargement is not present, the hepatic infiltrate can be documented by biopsy. The hepatic infiltrate typically involves the sinusoids and shares the immunologic findings of HSTCL.

Table 80.7 Clinical characteristics of hepatosplenic T cell lymphoma

	Weidmann[35] n = 41	Belhadj[66] n = 21
Median age (years)	29	34
Male	83	71
Stage III–IV	100	100
B symptoms	NA	67
Elevated LDH	62	55
ECOG PS ⩾2	NA	33
Extranodal involvement	100	100
Bone marrow involvement	72	100
IPI score ⩾2	NA	100

Values are % patients, with exception of median age (years).
ECOG, Eastern Cooperative Oncology Group; IPI, International Prognostic Index; LDH, lactate dehydrogenase; NA, not assessed; PS, performance status.

Lymph node involvement has not been documented in HSTCL (Table 80.7).[32,35,66] Laboratory features include anemia and leukopenia in approximately two-thirds of cases. In rare cases, leukocytosis with atypical circulating cells can be documented; approximately one-half of cases without leukocytosis show atypical cells when a blood smear is performed. Monocyte counts can be high (above 1000 cells/mm^3); this feature should be considered for differential diagnosis with myelomonocytic leukemia. An increase in liver enzymes is often present, with slight elevations of both aminotransferases and alkaline phosphatases. Lactate dehydrogenase (LDH) levels can be increased in one-half of cases. Serologic tests are negative for HTLV-1, HIV, and hepatitis B and C viruses. Hemophagocytic syndrome can be present at diagnosis.[6,32,35,66,121,122]

Hepatosplenic T cell lymphoma is typically associated with isochromosome 7q and trisomy 8, but the functional role of these changes has yet to be determined.[35] The bone marrow is invariably involved in HSTCL, but involvement is often subtle and requires accurate immunostaining to avoid false-negative results. Typical bone marrow findings include hypercellularity and (less often) monocytosis. Given the consistent and typical marrow involvement, splenectomy can be avoided in most cases and is supported by the fact that patients have a similar outcome irrespective of whether a splenectomy is performed.[35]

The differential diagnosis of HSTCL should include large granular lymphocyte leukemia, which usually occurs in older patients having a history of rheumatologic disease. Large granular lymphocyte leukemia has an indolent course and most often arises from CD57$^+$ rather than CD56$^+$ T cells.[123,124] Hepatosplenomegaly may also be the presenting feature of aggressive NK leukemia; these cases exhibit more blastic cell morphology and express all cytolytic proteins, whereas HSTCL expresses TIA-1 only and lacks granzyme B and perforin.[125–130] Finally, HSTCL may mimic CD8$^+$ T cell CLL, but usually bone marrow involvement is more prominent in HSTCL and cytolytic granules and NK cell-associated antigens are not present.[131]

Subcutaneous panniculitis–like T cell lymphoma

In subcutaneous panniculitis-like T cell lymphoma, the disease is typically localized to the subcutaneous tissue (with epidermal sparing) and is associated with multiple or solitary nodules or plaques. Lesions are erythematous to deep-seated violaceous. The most common sites of localization are the lower extremities, followed by the trunk, arms, and face.[132,133] Lesions may be small (diameter approximately 5 mm) but sometimes can reach 10 cm or more. Ulceration of subcutaneous nodules occurs in 20 percent of cases and is more frequent in the presence of larger nodules.[42,43] Lymph node and extracutaneous involvement are rare (Table 80.8). The disease is often associated with systemic HPS. The clinical course of SPTCL is variable, ranging from indolent

Table 80.8 Clinical characteristics of subcutaneous panniculitis-like T cell lymphoma

	Hoque[133] n = 6	Savage[65] n = 4
Median age (years)	48	49
Male	0	50
Stage III–IV	100	100
B symptoms	50	50
Elevated LDH	NA	50
ECOG PS ⩾2	NA	25
Extranodal site	100	100
Bone marrow involvement	0	25
IPI score ⩾2	NA	NA

Values are % patients, with exception of median age (years).
ECOG, Eastern Cooperative Oncology Group; IPI, International Prognostic Index; LDH, lactate dehydrogenase; NA, not assessed; PS, performance status.

to rapidly fatal. The presence of HPS indicates a grave prognosis and patients do poorly regardless of treatment modality.[38,132] Hemophagocytic syndrome is usually more frequent in γδ cases, which, however, also express NK markers and are considered a distinct entity in the recent WHO-EORTC classification of cutaneous lymphomas.[37]

Due to its typical cutaneous involvement, differential diagnosis of SPTCL should include lupus profundus, erythema nodosum, erythema induratum, and cytophagic histiocytic panniculitis (CHP).[134] The latter is a controversial entity and is thought to represent a reactive proliferation of cytophagic histiocytes as a result of an abnormal or exaggerated T cell immune response. However, SPTCL cases with a protracted CHP-like phase have been described. Distinguishing between the two is often very difficult. When carefully reviewed, some cases of CHP can be reclassified as SPTCL.[135]

PROGNOSTIC FACTORS

Despite efforts to translate the most recent advances in the treatment of B cell lymphomas to patients with T cell lymphomas, the prognosis of patients with PTCL is still poor. The complete response rate is low, ranging from 40 percent to 50 percent, with a median relapse-free survival (RFS) of 2–3 years. As a consequence of the aggressiveness of the disease and of the low efficacy of available salvage treatments, OS is also short and the long-term survival rate is less than 10 percent in many series.

Based on this discouraging outcome, several authors have tried to assess if the T cell phenotype itself could represent an adverse prognostic factor for cases falling into the broad class of 'aggressive' lymphomas. However, studies aimed at comparing the outcomes of T and B cell lymphomas have yielded contradictory results. Several investigators have found the T cell phenotype to be an independent prognostic factor,[13,44] but others have been unable to

confirm these findings.[136–140] However, several studies performed in the 1980s and 1990s were biased by the lack of a consensus on therapy of PTCL and, more importantly, did not correctly classify individual subtypes of peripheral T cell lymphomas. In a large study published by the Groupe d'Etude des Lymphomes de l'Adulte (GELA) in 1998, patients with PTCL more frequently had adverse clinical prognostic factors and lower complete remission rates than those with B cell lymphoma; also, the 5-year OS rates and event-free survival (EFS) rates were significantly shorter for PTCL. Comparison of the different histologic subtypes of lymphoma showed that the 5-year OS rate for T-ALCL (64 percent) was superior to that of other PTCLs (35 percent) as well as of diffuse large B cell NHL (53 percent).[16] These data, along with those of other recently published studies, suggest that the natural history of PTCL may in fact differ from that of diffuse large B cell lymphoma (DLBCL). Overall, patients with PTCL have a less favorable clinical outcome. This is only partially attributable to the immunophenotype itself; it is mostly due to different prevalence of adverse prognostic factors in the PTCL group.[16,44,141]

Several studies have been performed to assess the contribution of a number of clinical and biological factors to the prognosis of PTCL.[17–19,65,79,81,142] In most of them, adverse prognostic features such as poor performance status, advanced stage, presence of extranodal sites, bulky disease, and high LDH levels were significantly correlated with shorter OS (Table 80.9). The usefulness of the International Prognostic Index (IPI) for PTCL-U has also been investigated and confirmed by several authors. However, compared to DLBCL, many patients with PTCL-U have a poor outcome, even those in the low-risk IPI category. In contrast with PTCL-U, the IPI is not helpful in recognizing cases of ETL and HSTCL with different prognoses.

To better define the clinical outcome of PTCL-U, the Intergruppo Italiano Linfomi (IIL) performed a large study on 385 patients diagnosed and treated in the 1990s and defined a prognostic model specifically devised for patients with this uncommon disease. Among different clinical parameters assessed at time of diagnosis, age (less than 60 years), performance status (Eastern Cooperative Oncology Group [ECOG] performance status 2 or higher), high LDH level, and bone marrow involvement were independent predictors of OS (Table 80.10). Because the relative risks associated with the four factors were comparable, the authors constructed a new prognostic score, called PIT (Prognostic Index for peripheral T cell lymphomas), combining variables as follows: group 1, no risk factors; group 2, one risk factor; group 3, two risk factors; and group 4, three or four risk factors (Fig. 80.3). Patients were more or less evenly distributed among the four risk groups (20 percent, 34 percent, 26 percent, and 20 percent, respectively, in groups 1, 2, 3, and 4); OS differences were significant, with 5-year OS rates of 62 percent, 53 percent, 33 percent, and 18 percent, respectively, for groups 1, 2, 3, and 4 (P < 0.0001; log rank 66.79). Interestingly, in a simplified two-group model in which groups 1 and 2 and groups 3 and

Table 80.9 Prognostic factors univariate and multivariate analysis

Author	Year	n	Prognostic factors (OS) Univariate	Multivariate	Annotation
Ascani[17]	1997	168	Bulky disease, PTCL subtype, advanced clinical stage	NA	Both ALCL and PTCL-U cases included
Ansell[142]	1997	78	IPI, liver, BM involvement	IPI	Single institution; both ALCL and PTCL-U cases included
Zaja[81]	1997	23	IPI	NA	Single institution
Lopez-Guillermo[18]	1998	174	Age, PS, B symptoms, extranodal involvement, BM involvement, clinical stage, LDH level, β_2-microglobulin level, IPI	IPI	Both ALCL and PTCL-U cases included
Rudiger[19]	2002	96	PS, IPI	NA	Cases from NHL classification project
Gallamini[79]	2004	385	Age, PS, LDH level, BM involvement, clinical stage, IPI, response to therapy	Age, PS, LDH level, BM involvement	Definition of the Prognostic Index for PTCL-U patients (PIT) score
Savage[65]	2004	199	PTCL subtype, IPI	NA	Single institution; all PTCL subtypes included

BM, bone marrow; IPI, International Prognostic Index; LDH, lactate dehydrogenase; NA, not assessed; NHL, non-Hodgkin lymphoma; PS, performance status; PTCL, peripheral T cell lymphoma; PTCL-U, PTCL, unspecified; ALCL, anaplastic large cell lymphoma.

Table 80.10 Clinical parameters influencing survival in multivariate analysis. From: Gallamini A, Stelitano C, Calvi R et al. Peripheral T-cell lymphoma unspecified (PTCL-U): a new prognostic model from a retrospective multicentric clinical study. Blood 2004; 103: 2474–2479. Copyright American Society of Hematology, used with permission.

Parameter	Significance, P	Relative risk (exp. B)	95% CI Low	High
Age	<0.0001	1.732	1.300	2.309
PS	<0.0001	1.719	1.269	2.327
LDH level	<0.0001	1.905	1.415	2.564
BM attainment	0.026	1.424	1.405	2.023

BM, bone marrow; LDH, lactate dehydrogenase; PS, performance status; CI, confidence interval.

4 were merged, the entire body of patients could be split into two parts, each containing around 50 percent of cases and characterized by consistent and clinically useful differences in survival (5-year OS of 58 percent and 27 percent for the low- and high-risk group, respectively). The fact that many patients with PTCL-U fall into the high-risk categories with poor survival emphasizes the urgent need for better therapies. In comparison with the IPI score, the authors found that the PIT score had superior predictive capacity and that the difference was mainly due to a better discriminatory power for the intermediate-risk groups (PIT groups 2 and 3 vs IPI groups intermediate-low and intermediate-high).

Interestingly, in contrast to the IPI, stage and extranodal disease were not among the independent prognostic factors; this has been explained by differences in the natural history and clinical features of PTCL-U, which more frequently than DLBCL has extranodal involvement or is diagnosed at an advanced stage.[79] In addition to defining a prognostic model specifically devised for PTCL-U, the IIL study confirms the relevance of research on series of clearly defined cases in order to aid the development of rationally designed and potentially more efficacious treatment modalities.

Cytology of the neoplastic cell has long been debated as a prognostic factor, and in the updated Kiel classification system, PTCL is categorized into various subtypes and, according to cell size-related criteria, stratified into two major prognostic groups, high grade and low grade.[15] However, even if cell size may have some prognostic significance, the WHO classification no longer considers it a prognostic tool, mainly due to concerns regarding reproducibility.[1,19]

Infectious agents may also play a role in determining patient outcome, as has been clearly demonstrated for EBV in a large study on 520 NHL cases of both B and T cell origin.[59] The study documented the presence of EBV encoded early small RNA (EBER) in 31 percent of PTCL (mainly AITL [85 percent] and other PTCL-U cases [36 percent to 71 percent]), 7 percent of B-NHL, and 0 percent of MF or ALCL. In a multivariate analysis for T-NHL, EBER positivity was one of the three most significant factors recognized by the final prognostic model – surpassed only by performance status >1 and older age – and was a more powerful predictor than B symptoms, elevated LDH, or disseminated disease. Why EBV infection should confer a poorer prognosis for infected patients is unclear; however, some authors have observed that EBV-positive T-NHLs are more frequently associated with constitutional symptoms and aggressive features of the disease than noninfected cases, and express multidrug resistance markers.[59,143]

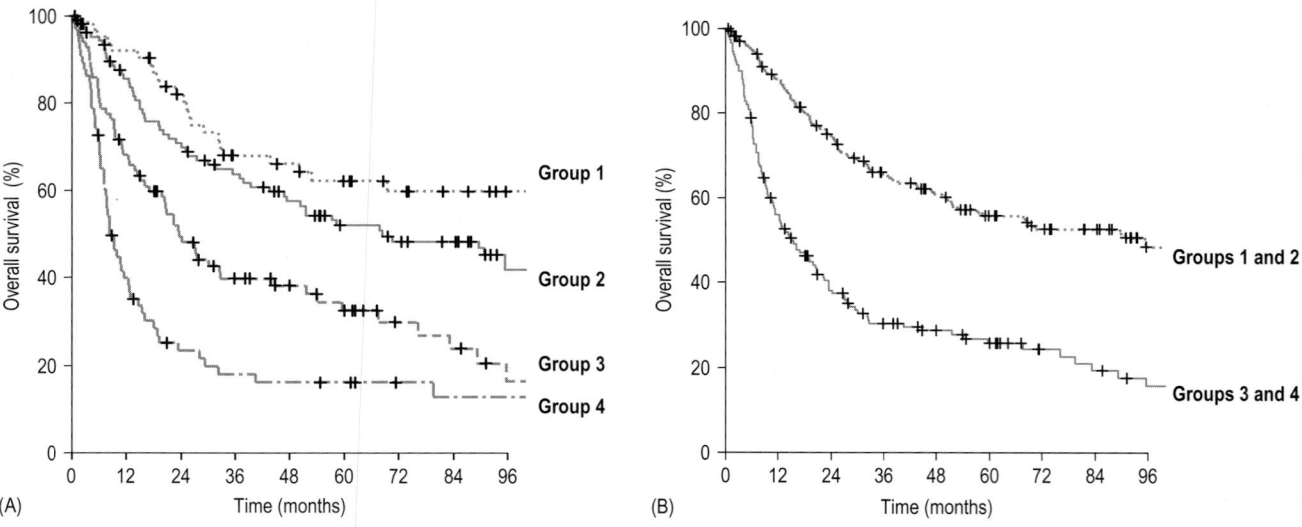

Figure 80.3 (A) Overall survival (OS) according to the proposed Prognostic Index for PTCL-U patients (PIT). (B) Overall survival according to two-class, simplified PIT. Groups were defined as follows: group 1, no risk factors; group 2, one risk factor; group 3, two risk factors; and group 4, three or four risk factors. In the simplified two-group model, groups 1 and 2 and groups 3 and 4 were merged. From: Gallamini A, Stelitano C, Calvi R et al. Peripheral T-cell lymphoma unspecified (PTCL-U): a new prognostic model from a retrospective multicentric clinical study. *Blood* 2004; 103: 2474–2479. Copyright American Society of Hematology, used with permission.

More recently, the role of biological features of the disease is emerging as an important issue not only for understanding its pathogenesis but also for prognosis and for addressing specific biologic targets. The expression of T helper 1 (TH1)- or TH2-associated antigens or of the activated T cell receptor, for example, has been recently evaluated in a series of T-NHLs. The pattern of expression of such antigens correlated with the specific subtype of nodal T cell lymphoma (AITL, ALCL, and PTCL-U) and allowed the identification of subgroups of PTCL-U patients with different probabilities of survival.[144] In particular, patients with PTCL-U expressing one of the TH1 or TH2 antigens tended to show a favorable prognosis compared with cases not expressing TH1 or TH2 antigens.

Significant progress in the prognosis of PTCL can be expected from the novel, sophisticated, and powerful technologies of genomics and proteomics, which will allow more reliable subtyping of PTCL into distinct clinical groups characterized by different patterns of survival, as already demonstrated for some B-NHLs.[145]

TREATMENT

Unfortunately, the optimal therapy for PTCL is still unknown. The unfavorable prognosis in the majority of patients with PTCL, the rarity of the disease, the variable clinical course, the lack of data from large, randomized trials, and, probably, uncertainty in how to manage the individual patient have all contributed to prevent the establishment of treatment standards to improve outcome.

Current concepts about treatment of patients with PTCL are derived from studies investigating the role of anthracycline-based combination chemotherapy in larger trials including patients with aggressive T and B cell lymphomas. In these studies, patients were treated with CHOP (cyclophosphamide, doxorubicin, vincristine, and prednisone) alone, CHOP alternating with DHAP (dexamethasone, cisplatin, and cytarabine), m-BACOD (methotrexate, bleomycin, doxorubicin, cyclophosphamide, vincristine, and dexamethasone), ProMACE-CytaBOM (cyclophosphamide, vincristine, doxorubicin, bleomycin, etoposide, cytarabine, methotrexate, and prednisone), ACVBP (doxorubicin, cyclophosphamide, vindesine, bleomycin, and prednisone), VIM3 (mitoxantrone, ifosfamide, mitoguazone, teniposide, prednisone, and methotrexate), CHOP with etoposide, and COPBLAM (cyclophosphamide, vincristine, prednisone, bleomycin, doxorubicin and procarbazine).[16,44,146,147] On the basis of published data, it can be assumed that PTCL almost always requires systemic therapy and that no available regimen is superior to anthracycline-containing combination regimens as an initial standard approach for individual patients.

Subset analysis of the GELA trials LNH-84 and LNH-87 showed that, with the exception of ALCL cases, T cell phenotype was associated with worse outcome than B cell phenotype. Patients with PTCL treated with intensive regimens used in the LNH-87 study achieved a 5-year survival rate of 41 percent, comparable to that reported by other groups,[13,24,136,140,148] with no difference among PTCL subtypes. However, the 5-year OS rate of 23 percent for patients with PTCL with three or more IPI adverse prognostic factors clearly shows the limits of conventional chemotherapy and cries out for new strategies.

In some phase II trials, higher doses of drugs than those given in CHOP have been used, but the number of patients with PTCL is too small to assess the impact of dose intensity on disease control.[136,149] Trials investigating the role of high-dose purine analogues or of platinum-based regimens are currently ongoing but preliminary results seem to confirm that neither of these regimens improves outcome when compared to CHOP.[150]

Several other therapeutic agents have been tested in small series of patients with relapsed or refractory PTCL and have shown different degrees of activity. These include purine and pyrimidine antimetabolite agents (nucleoside analogues and gemcitabine, respectively), denileukin diftitox, and retinoic acid combined with interferon α.

Nucleoside analogues such as 2′-deoxicoformycin (pentostatin), fludarabine, and 2′-chlorodeoxyadenosine (cladribine) have been tested, mostly in patients with cutaneous NHL, although several investigators have reported satisfactory results in the treatment of different types of relapsed or refractory PTCL.[151–156] In particular, data suggest that pentostatin has significant antitumor activity in PTCL patients, with response rates ranging from 33 percent to over 70 percent. Approximately one-third of the responses were complete, and some prolonged remissions were achieved; however, most responses were of short duration. These observations suggest that further exploration of this agent in combination with other drugs active in T cell lymphomas is warranted.[157] Gemcitabine has shown activity in relapsed PTCLs as a single agent[154] but has not been explored with other agents.

Denileukin diftitox is a novel recombinant fusion protein consisting of peptide sequences for the enzymatically active and membrane translocation domains of diphtheria toxin combined with human interleukin-2 (IL-2). The drug, which has been designed to target the cytocidal action of diphtheria toxin to cells that express the IL-2 receptor, has demonstrated clinical activity in patients with pretreated cutaneous T cell NHL.[158] Some reports have also described clinical benefit in other types of PTCL.[159,160]

Huang et al. studied 17 patients with refractory/relapsed PTCL using cis-retinoic acid (cRA) with IFNα. Treatment included oral administration of 13-cRA 1 mg/kg/day, divided into three doses, and intramuscular injection of IFNα2a 4.5 MU/m², three times per week. A response was documented in one of seven patients with PTCL-U and in four of six patients with ALCL, although duration of response was short (2.5 months) and median survival for the entire group was only 3.6 months.[161]

Notwithstanding the variable number of previous treatments and the conflicting results in term of durable remission, the action of these drugs needs further investigation, both to evaluate their activity in naïve patients and to define their role in combination therapies.

Antibody treatment of peripheral T cell lymphomas

So far, several antigens that are characteristically expressed by PTCL have been studied as targets for immunologic treatments. Monoclonal antibodies have been developed against the CD3 antigen and the IL-2 receptor CD25, CD30, and CD7; however, research in monoclonal antibody therapy in the subset of PTCL has failed to achieve therapeutic responses as a consequence of the remarkable variation in stage of T cell differentiation and thus antigen expression. For example, the IL-2 receptor CD25 or CD30 markers are expressed only in a limited number of T cell tumors. Also, anti-CD3 antibodies are not reactive in all PTCL but show a degree of activity in some T cell lymphoblastic leukemia cases. In addition, clinical experience with such antibodies, though limited, has shown that even low doses are likely to be associated with severe side effects.[162–165]

More promising results have been obtained in the treatment of PTCL with antibodies directed against the CD4 and CD52 antigens. Zanolimumab (HuMax-CD4) is a fully human anti-CD4 monoclonal antibody isolated from transgenic mice as a hybridoma clone and subsequently expressed in Chinese hamster ovary cells. The antibody is specific for the CD4 receptor expressed on most T lymphocytes and to a lesser extent on macrophages. The antibody prevents interaction between the CD4 receptor and the major histocompatibility complex class II molecule and thereby interferes with T cell activation. Further, in vitro data demonstrate cell killing via antibody-dependent cellular cytotoxicity (ADCC). Zanolimumab does not induce complement-dependent cytotoxicity (CDC) when bound to the cell surface in vitro.[166] The clinical activity has been tested in phase II studies in patients with therapy-resistant cutaneous T cell lymphoma of CD4+ MF and Sézary syndrome subtypes. Zanolimumab showed marked efficacy both in early and advanced stage MF in the highest-dose groups (56 percent overall response rate) and was well tolerated with no dose-related toxicity.[167] Given its promising activity in CD4-positive lymphomas, zanolimumab is currently being investigated in combination with CHOP in the initial treatment of PTCL-U.

Alemtuzumab (Campath) is a humanized immunoglobulin G1 (IgG1) anti-CD52 monoclonal antibody that binds to the cell membrane of more than 95 percent of all normal human blood lymphocytes as well as to most B and T cell lymphomas.[168] In addition to its documented activity in B cell CLL,[169,170] alemtuzumab has shown promising clinical activity in patients with mature T cell lymphomas.[171] Malignant T cells appear to express extraordinarily high numbers of CD52 cell-surface molecules.[172] Thus, T cell lymphomas, including PTCL, may be particularly suitable for therapy with alemtuzumab. The typical schedule of administration of 30 mg three times weekly for up to 12 weeks produced a promising complete remission (CR) rate of 60 percent in patients with T prolymphocytic leukemia; however, patients ultimately relapse and alemtuzumab cannot be considered curative.[173] Alemtuzumab was also tested in patients with relapsed or refractory PTCL;[174] the overall response rate was 36 percent, with a 21 percent CR rate, but all patients in complete remission relapsed within 1 year. The study demonstrated clinical efficacy of the drug but also confirmed that treatment was associated with significant hematologic toxicity and infectious complications (mainly cytomegalovirus reactivation).

The promising results of a phase II trial investigating the clinical activity of a C-CHOP regimen combining CHOP with concomitant alemtuzumab as first-line treatment of PTCL were recently published; twenty-five patients were enrolled and 17 achieved CR (71 percent). After a median follow-up of 16 months, the 2-year OS was 53 percent. The regimen was well tolerated and associated with manageable infectious episodes.[175] Several trials investigating concomitant or sequential use of anthracycline- or fludarabine-containing regimens with alemtuzumab are ongoing and mature results are needed to support the efficacy of such strategies.

High–dose therapy

The exact role of high-dose therapy (HDT) followed by autologous stem cell transplantation (HDT-ASCT) or allogeneic stem cell transplantation (allo-SCT) in patients with PTCL is still unknown.

Based on the results of the PARMA trial, HDT-ASCT is an accepted therapeutic approach for patients with aggressive lymphoma in first relapse responding to additional platinum-based chemotherapy, regardless of whether the lymphoma is of B or T cell origin.[176] However, the PARMA trial was not specifically designed to address the role of HDT in patients with PTCL, and results from randomized trials comparing salvage chemotherapy alone to chemotherapy with autologous hematopoietic stem cell transplantation for relapsed PTCL are not yet available. As a consequence, evaluation of HDT efficacy in PTCL can only be based on the results of retrospective analyses.

In a first study in 36 patients with PTCL who received HDT-ASCT due to disease recurrence after prior conventional chemotherapy, Rodriguez et al.[177] reported a 3-year OS of 36 percent and progression-free survival (PFS) of 28 percent. This suggests that the activity of HDT-ASCT in patients with relapsed PTCL is similar to that observed in patients with relapsed DLBCL and seems to confirm the results of the PARMA trial.

The issue of HDT in patients with PTCL never achieving complete remission after conventional chemotherapy was addressed by the GEL-TAMO group. In a retrospective analysis of 35 patients,[178] a CR rate of 66 percent and 5-year OS, freedom from progression, and DFS rates of 37 percent, 36 percent, and 55 percent, respectively, were observed. These results were considered promising, and the authors concluded that patients with PTCL failing to respond to front-line chemotherapy could be 'rescued' with HDT-ASCT, similar to patients with aggressive B cell lymphoma.

Discordant results, however, were obtained by Song et al., who compared the outcome of 35 patients with relapsed or refractory ALCL and PTCL with those of 97 patients with DLBCL who received HDT-ASCT in the same institution over the same period of time (1987–2001).[179] Patients' baseline characteristics and overall treatment results were similar for the groups of B- and T-NHL, but when only the 20 patients with PTCL-U were analyzed, these cases showed inferior event-free survival compared with that of patients with DLBCL and ALCL. The authors concluded that patients with PTCL-U in whom primary treatment fails should be offered experimental treatment modalities. Similar conclusions were drawn in a matched-control analysis conducted by GELA researchers by pooling data on patients enrolled in the LNH-87 and LNH-93 trials.[180] This study evaluated the outcome of 330 patients who received ASCT after responding to front-line ACVBP chemotherapy; for the 29 patients with PTCL-U histology, HDT-ASCT did not result in superior survival as compared with additional chemotherapy, either in terms of 5-year OS (49 percent vs 44 percent for ASCT and chemotherapy, respectively; $P = 0.87$) or DFS (45 percent vs 38 percent, respectively; $P = 0.89$).

Given the dismal prognosis of HDT used in the salvage setting, transplantation has more recently been employed as part of the upfront treatment following induction therapy. In a recent phase II study, 74 patients with PTCL underwent high-dose chemotherapy and ASCT in first partial and complete remissions; with a median follow-up of 67 months, the 5-year OS was 68 percent and PFS was 63 percent.[181]

In conclusion, based on published data, HDT followed by ASCT is a promising but still experimental approach and should be used exclusively in the context of controlled clinical trials. In particular, further study of the biology and prognosis of the disease and larger clinical trials specifically devised for patients with PTCL are warranted in order to define which subset of patients can do better with intensive treatments. The same is true for allo-SCT. Case series and reports (mostly small) considering both B and T cell lymphomas have emphasized the feasibility of allo-SCT, but the efficacy of this procedure is still overshadowed by a high treatment-related mortality.[177,182,183] The reduced-intensity conditioning (RIC) regimens, which allow engraftment of allogeneic stem cells with limited organ toxicity, seem to offer new opportunities, including for patients with refractory PTCL. The RIC regimen, consisting of thiotepa, cyclophosphamide, and fludarabine, has been prospectively evaluated in a series of 17 patients with refractory or relapsed PTCL (nine patients with PTCL-U, four with AITL, and four with ALK-negative ALCL). All received a debulking treatment with DHAP regimen prior to RIC. Three patients died, two from disease progression and one due to acute graft-versus-host disease. Three-year OS and PFS were 81 percent and 64 percent, respectively; two patients had a second remission following donor lymphocyte infusion after disease progression, thus demonstrating the existence of a graft-versus-lymphoma effect.[184]

Radiation therapy

The role of radiation therapy (RT) for PTCL is still uncertain and the literature provides little information on outcomes of patients treated with or without radiation therapy for early stage disease. The role of RT alone has not been investigated so far for subtypes of PTCL other than limited stage NK lymphomas, for which first-line radiation therapy seems to give favorable results when administered prior to chemotherapy.[185]

Although RT may exert some local effect, its exclusive use should be discouraged. Radiation therapy can be given at the end of chemotherapy to sites of previous bulky disease or to sites which responded slowly or partially to chemotherapy, although this approach is mainly derived from experience with treatment of aggressive B cell lymphomas and information on patients with PTCL is limited.

Treatment of specific entities

ANGIOIMMUNOBLASTIC T CELL LYMPHOMA

The most difficult objective in AITL is the induction of long-lasting remission. Treatment options for AITL range from steroid use to combination chemotherapy to more intensive regimens. The use of anthracycline-based combination chemotherapy results in CR rates of 50–70 percent, although only 10–30 percent are long-term survivors. In a prospective, nonrandomized, multicenter study, Siegert et al. treated newly diagnosed patients with stable AITL with single-agent prednisone and used COPBLAM/IMVP combination chemotherapy (cyclophosphamide, vincristine, prednisone, bleomycin, doxorubicin, procarbazine, ifosfamide, methotrexate, and etoposide) initially if life-threatening disease was present at diagnosis or as salvage treatment for relapsing and refractory patients.[186] The CR rate with single-agent prednisone was 29 percent, whereas the CR rates for relapsed and refractory patients and patients treated initially with combination chemotherapy were 56 percent and 64 percent, respectively. The observed OS and DFS rates were 41 percent and 32 percent, respectively; median OS was 15 months. The poor results obtained with conventional therapy suggest that novel approaches to the treatment of AITL patients are warranted.

The role of HDT-ASCT in patients with AITL has been investigated in some clinical trials. It has been shown that this strategy may prolong survival in patients with recurrent disease, but confirmatory results are needed in patients who receive front-line high-dose treatment.[150]

Anecdotal reports also showed that patients with relapsed AITL may respond to immunosuppressive therapy (e.g., low-dose methotrexate/prednisone) and to purine analogue treatments.[187,188] Finally Piccaluga et al. recently found that vascular endothelial growth factor (VEGF) was expressed by AITL neoplastic cells, suggesting that VEGF could represent a possible target for treatment with antiangiogenesis agents.[189]

ENTEROPATHY–TYPE T CELL LYMPHOMA

Treatment results for patients with ETL are discouraging, as fewer than 50 percent complete their planned chemotherapy due to treatment-related toxicity effects such as gastrointestinal bleeding or perforation.[31] Other major determinants of poor outcome are late diagnosis and deterioration in performance status at the time of diagnosis; moreover, malabsorption and malnutrition make tolerance of chemotherapy difficult. In a recent retrospective analysis of 31 patients,[31] 77 percent received chemotherapy, mainly with anthracycline-containing regimens; response to treatment was observed in 58 percent of cases, but 79 percent of patients relapsed within 5 years. Finally, nutritional support with parenteral or enteral nutrition should always be considered for patients with ETL.

HEPATOSPLENIC T CELL LYMPHOMA

Patients with HSTCL usually respond to initial treatment but eventually die due to early relapse or progression despite the use of intensive salvage treatment. As a consequence, the median OS is 12–14 months.[6,35] Moreover, 10–20 percent of patients with a history of organ transplant or immunosuppression do not respond to reduction in immunosuppression alone and survival time is measured in weeks to months regardless of treatment.[190] Interesting results have been obtained with the use of purine analogues, e.g., 2′-chlorodeoxyadenosine (cladribine) and pentostatin.[156] The latter showed a selective cytotoxic effect on tumoral T cells in vitro and an ability to induce complete responses in some HSTCL cases.[193]

SUBCUTANEOUS PANNICULITIS-LIKE T CELL LYMPHOMA

The clinical course of SPTCL is variable, ranging from indolent disease to rapidly fatal lymphoma with fulminant hemophagocytosis. When treatment is warranted, most patients respond to systemic combination chemotherapy or to local radiation therapy. The $\gamma\delta$ cutaneous lymphomas with panniculitis-like lesions have an aggressive behavior; in these cases, the disease is usually resistant to chemotherapy or radiation and the median survival is less than 2 years. In contrast, based on the few reports in which $\alpha\beta$ SPTCL is correctly identified, the 5-year survival of such patients is around 80 percent. Patients with $\alpha\beta$ SPTCL are usually treated with doxorubicin-containing chemotherapy or radiation therapy, but some evidence suggests that the disease can also be controlled with steroids.[36,38–41,132,133] In these cases, the clinical course is protracted, with recurrent subcutaneous lesions without extracutaneous dissemination or development of HPS.[40,133]

REFERENCES

● = Key primary paper
◆ = Major review article

●1. Harris NL, Jaffe ES, Diebold J et al. World Health Organization classification of neoplastic diseases of the hematopoietic and lymphoid tissues: report of the Clinical Advisory Committee meeting-Airlie House, Virginia, November 1997. J Clin Oncol 1999; 17: 3835–49.

◆2. Delves PJ, Roitt IM. The immune system. First of two parts. N Engl J Med 2000; 343: 37–49.

◆3. Delves PJ, Roitt IM. The immune system. Second of two parts. N Engl J Med 2000; 343: 108–17.

4. Jones D, O'Hara C, Kraus MD et al. Expression pattern of T-cell-associated chemokine receptors and their chemokines correlates with specific subtypes of T-cell non-Hodgkin lymphoma. Blood 2000; 96: 685–90.

5. Picker LJ, Weiss LM, Medeiros LJ et al. Immunophenotypic criteria for the diagnosis of non-Hodgkin's lymphoma. Am J Pathol 1987; 128: 181–201.

6. Cooke CB, Krenacs L, Stetler-Stevenson M et al. Hepatosplenic T-cell lymphoma: a distinct clinicopathologic entity of cytotoxic gamma delta T-cell origin. Blood 1996; 88: 4265–74.

●7. A clinical evaluation of the International Lymphoma Study Group classification of non-Hodgkin's lymphoma. The Non-Hodgkin's Lymphoma Classification Project. Blood 1997; 89: 3909–18.

8. Lennert K, Mohri N. Malignant lymphoma, lymphocytic T-zone type (T-zone lymphoma). In: Malignant lymphomas other than Hodgkin's disease. Berlin: Springer Verlag, 1978: 196–209.

9. Knowles DM. Immunophenotypic and antigen receptor gene rearrangement analysis in T cell neoplasia. Am J Pathol 1989; 134: 761–85.

10. Pinkus GS, Said JW, Hargreaves H. Malignant lymphoma, T-cell type. A distinct morphologic variant with large multilobated nuclei, with a report of four cases. Am J Clin Pathol 1979; 72: 540–50.

11. Rappaport H. Tumors of the hematopoietic system. Washington DC: Armed Forces Institute of Pathology, 1966.

●12. National Cancer Institute sponsored study of classifications of non-Hodgkin's lymphomas: summary and description of a working formulation for clinical usage. The Non-Hodgkin's Lymphoma Pathologic Classification Project. Cancer 1982; 49: 2112–35.

13. Coiffier B, Brousse N, Peuchmaur M et al. Peripheral T-cell lymphomas have a worse prognosis than B-cell lymphomas: a prospective study of 361 immunophenotyped patients treated with the LNH-84 regimen. The GELA (Groupe d'Etude des Lymphomes Agressives). Ann Oncol 1990; 1: 45–50.

●14. Harris NL, Jaffe ES, Stein H et al. A revised European-American classification of lymphoid neoplasms: a proposal from the International Lymphoma Study Group. Blood 1994; 84: 1361–92.

15. Richards MA, Stansfeld AG. Updated Kiel classification. Lancet 1988; 1: 937.

●16. Gisselbrecht C, Gaulard P, Lepage E et al. Prognostic significance of T-cell phenotype in aggressive non-Hodgkin's lymphomas. Groupe d'Etudes des Lymphomes de l'Adulte (GELA). Blood 1998; 92: 76–82.

17. Ascani S, Zinzani PL, Gherlinzoni F et al. Peripheral T-cell lymphomas. Clinico-pathologic study of 168 cases diagnosed according to the R.E.A.L. Classification. Ann Oncol 1997; 8: 583–92.

●18. Lopez-Guillermo A, Cid J, Salar A et al. Peripheral T-cell lymphomas: initial features, natural history, and prognostic factors in a series of 174 patients diagnosed according to the R.E.A.L. Classification. Ann Oncol 1998; 9: 849–55.

●19. Rudiger T, Weisenburger DD, Anderson JR et al. Peripheral T-cell lymphoma (excluding anaplastic large-cell lymphoma): results from the Non-Hodgkin's Lymphoma Classification Project. Ann Oncol 2002; 13: 140–9.

20. Frizzera G, Moran EM, Rappaport H. Angio-immunoblastic lymphadenopathy with dysproteinaemia. Lancet 1974; 1: 1070–3.

21. Knecht H, Schwarze EW, Lennert K. Histological, immunohistological and autopsy findings in lymphogranulomatosis X (including angio-immunoblastic lymphadenopathy). Virchows Arch A Pathol Anat Histopathol 1985; 406: 105–24.

◆22. Dogan A, Attygalle AD, Kyriakou C. Angioimmunoblastic T-cell lymphoma. Br J Haematol 2003; 121: 681–91.

23. Sallah S, Gagnon GA. Angioimmunoblastic lymphadenopathy with dysproteinemia: emphasis on pathogenesis and treatment. Acta Haematol 1998; 99: 57–64.

24. Siegert W, Nerl C, Agthe A et al. Angioimmunoblastic lymphadenopathy (AILD)-type T-cell lymphoma: prognostic impact of clinical observations and laboratory findings at presentation. The Kiel Lymphoma Study Group. Ann Oncol 1995; 6: 659–64.

25. Isaacson PG, O'Connor NT, Spencer J et al. Malignant histiocytosis of the intestine: a T-cell lymphoma. Lancet 1985; 2: 688–91.

26. Isaacson P, Wright DH. Intestinal lymphoma associated with malabsorption. *Lancet* 1978; **1**: 67–70.

27. O'Farrelly C, Feighery C, O'Briain DS *et al.* Humoral response to wheat protein in patients with coeliac disease and enteropathy associated T cell lymphoma. *Br Med J (Clin Res Ed)* 1986; **293**: 908–10.

28. Holmes GK, Stokes PL, Sorahan TM *et al.* Coeliac disease, gluten-free diet, and malignancy. *Gut* 1976; **17**: 612–19.

29. Holmes GK, Prior P, Lane MR *et al.* Malignancy in coeliac disease – effect of a gluten free diet. *Gut* 1989; **30**: 333–8.

30. Chott A, Haedicke W, Mosberger I *et al.* Most CD56+ intestinal lymphomas are CD8+CD5-T-cell lymphomas of monomorphic small to medium size histology. *Am J Pathol* 1998; **153**: 1483–90.

31. Gale J, Simmonds PD, Mead GM *et al.* Enteropathy-type intestinal T-cell lymphoma: clinical features and treatment of 31 patients in a single center. *J Clin Oncol* 2000; **18**: 795–803.

●32. Farcet JP, Gaulard P, Marolleau JP *et al.* Hepatosplenic T-cell lymphoma: sinusal/sinusoidal localization of malignant cells expressing the T-cell receptor gamma delta. *Blood* 1990; **75**: 2213–19.

33. Salhany KE, Feldman M, Kahn MJ *et al.* Hepatosplenic gammadelta T-cell lymphoma: ultrastructural, immunophenotypic, and functional evidence for cytotoxic T lymphocyte differentiation. *Hum Pathol* 1997; **28**: 674–85.

34. Macon WR, Levy NB, Kurtin PJ *et al.* Hepatosplenic alphabeta T-cell lymphomas: a report of 14 cases and comparison with hepatosplenic gammadelta T-cell lymphomas. *Am J Surg Pathol* 2001; **25**: 285–96.

35. Weidmann E. Hepatosplenic T cell lymphoma. A review on 45 cases since the first report describing the disease as a distinct lymphoma entity in 1990. *Leukemia* 2000; **14**: 991–7.

36. Gonzalez CL, Medeiros LJ, Braziel RM, Jaffe ES. T-cell lymphoma involving subcutaneous tissue. A clinicopathologic entity commonly associated with hemophagocytic syndrome. *Am J Surg Pathol* 1991; **15**: 17–27.

●37. Willemze R, Jaffe ES, Burg G *et al.* WHO-EORTC classification for cutaneous lymphomas. *Blood* 2005; **105**: 3768–85.

38. Salhany KE, Macon WR, Choi JK *et al.* Subcutaneous panniculitis-like T-cell lymphoma: clinicopathologic, immunophenotypic, and genotypic analysis of alpha/beta and gamma/delta subtypes. *Am J Surg Pathol* 1998; **22**: 881–93.

39. Santucci M, Pimpinelli N, Massi D *et al.* Cytotoxic/natural killer cell cutaneous lymphomas. Report of EORTC Cutaneous Lymphoma Task Force Workshop. *Cancer* 2003; **97**: 610–27.

40. Massone C, Chott A, Metze D *et al.* Subcutaneous, blastic natural killer (NK), NK/T-cell, and other cytotoxic lymphomas of the skin: a morphologic, immunophenotypic, and molecular study of 50 patients. *Am J Surg Pathol* 2004; **28**: 719–35.

41. Burg G, Dummer R, Wilhelm M *et al.* A subcutaneous delta-positive T-cell lymphoma that produces interferon gamma. *N Engl J Med* 1991; **325**: 1078–81.

42. Marzano AV, Berti E, Paulli M, Caputo R. Cytophagic histiocytic panniculitis and subcutaneous panniculitis-like T-cell lymphoma: report of 7 cases. *Arch Dermatol* 2000; **136**: 889–96.

43. Kumar S, Krenacs L, Medeiros J *et al.* Subcutaneous panniculitic T-cell lymphoma is a tumor of cytotoxic T lymphocytes. *Hum Pathol* 1998; **29**: 397–403.

44. Melnyk A, Rodriguez A, Pugh WC, Cabannillas F. Evaluation of the revised European-American lymphoma classification confirms the clinical relevance of immunophenotype in 560 cases of aggressive non-Hodgkin's lymphoma. *Blood* 1997; **89**: 4514–20.

◆45. Delmer A, Zittoun R. Other peripheral T-cell Lymphomas. In: Magrath, IT. (ed) *The non-Hodgkin's lymphomas*. 2nd Edn. London: Hodder Arnold, 1996.

●46. Armitage JO, Weisenburger DD. New approach to classifying non-Hodgkin's lymphomas: clinical features of the major histologic subtypes. Non-Hodgkin's Lymphoma Classification Project. *J Clin Oncol* 1998; **16**: 2780–95.

47. Morton L, Wang SS, Devesa SS *et al.* Lymphoma incidence patterns by WHO subtype in the United States, 1992–2001. *Blood* 2006; **107**: 265–76.

48. Anderson JR, Armitage JO, Weisenburger DD. Epidemiology of the non-Hodgkin's lymphomas: distributions of the major subtypes differ by geographic locations. Non-Hodgkin's Lymphoma Classification Project. *Ann Oncol* 1998; **9**: 717–20.

49. Arrowsmith ER, Macon WR, Kinney MC *et al.* Peripheral T-cell lymphomas: clinical features and prognostic factors of 92 cases defined by the revised European American lymphoma classification. *Leuk Lymphoma* 2003; **44**: 241–9.

50. Lee SS, Cho KJ, Kim CW, Kang YK. Clinicopathological analysis of 501 non-Hodgkin's lymphomas in Korea according to the revised European-American classification of lymphoid neoplasms. *Histopathology* 1999; **35**: 345–54.

51. The world health organization classification of malignant lymphomas in japan: incidence of recently recognized entities. Lymphoma Study Group of Japanese Pathologists. *Pathol Int* 2000; **50**: 696–702.

52. Rho R, Laddis T, McQuain C *et al.* Miliary tuberculosis in a patient with Epstein-Barr virus-associated angioimmunoblastic lymphadenopathy. *Ann Hematol* 1996; **72**: 333–5.

53. Konig M, Grunder K, Nilles M, Schill WB. Cutaneous cryptococcosis as the first symptom of a disseminated cryptococcosis in a patient with lymphogranulomatosis X. *Mycoses* 1991; **34**: 309–11.

54. Kraus MD, Crawford DF, Kaleem Z *et al.* T gamma/delta hepatosplenic lymphoma in a heart transplant patient after an Epstein-Barr virus positive lymphoproliferative disorder: a case report. *Cancer* 1998; **82**: 983–92.

55. Wu H, Wasik MA, Przybylski G et al. Hepatosplenic gamma-delta T-cell lymphoma as a late-onset posttransplant lymphoproliferative disorder in renal transplant recipients. Am J Clin Pathol 2000; 113: 487–96.

56. Gull W. Fatty stools from disease of the mesenteric glands. Guys Hosp Rep 1855; 1: 369.

57. Gough KR, Read AE, Naish JM. Intestinal reticulosis as a complication of idiopathic steatorrhoea. Gut 1962; 3: 232–9.

58. Ilyas M, Niedobitek G, Agathanggelou A et al. Non-Hodgkin's lymphoma, coeliac disease, and Epstein-Barr virus: a study of 13 cases of enteropathy-associated T- and B-cell lymphoma. J Pathol 1995; 177: 115–22.

●59. d'Amore F, Johansen P, Houmand A et al. Epstein-Barr virus genome in non-Hodgkin's lymphomas occurring in immunocompetent patients: highest prevalence in nonlymphoblastic T-cell lymphoma and correlation with a poor prognosis. Danish Lymphoma Study Group, LYFO. Blood 1996; 87: 1045–55.

60. Quintanilla-Martinez L, Lome-Maldonado C, Ott G et al. Primary non-Hodgkin's lymphoma of the intestine: high prevalence of Epstein-Barr virus in Mexican lymphomas as compared with European cases. Blood 1997; 89: 644–51.

61. Luppi M, Marasca R, Barozzi P et al. Frequent detection of human herpesvirus-6 sequences by polymerase chain reaction in paraffin-embedded lymph nodes from patients with angioimmunoblastic lymphadenopathy and angioimmunoblastic lymphadenopathy-like lymphoma. Leuk Res 1993; 17: 1003–11.

62. Luppi M, Torelli G. The new lymphotropic herpesviruses (HHV-6, HHV-7, HHV-8) and hepatitis C virus (HCV) in human lymphoproliferative diseases: an overview. Haematologica 1996; 81: 265–81.

63. Luppi M, Torelli G. Human herpesvirus 8 and interstitial pneumonitis in an HIV-negative patient. N Engl J Med 1996; 335: 351–2.

64. Helm TN, Steck WD, Proffitt MR et al. Kaposi's sarcoma, angioimmunoblastic lymphadenopathy, and antibody to HIV-1 p24 antigen in a patient nonreactive for HIV-1 with use of ELISA. J Am Acad Dermatol 1990; 23: 317–18.

●65. Savage KJ, Chhanabhai M, Gascoyne RD, Connors JM. Characterization of peripheral T-cell lymphomas in a single North American institution by the WHO classification. Ann Oncol 2004; 15: 1467–75.

66. Belhadj K, Reyes F, Farcet JP et al. Hepatosplenic gammadelta T-cell lymphoma is a rare clinicopathologic entity with poor outcome: report on a series of 21 patients. Blood 2003; 102: 4261–9.

67. Armitage JO, Greer JP, Levine AM et al. Peripheral T-cell lymphoma. Cancer 1989; 63: 158–63.

68. Coiffier B, Berger F, Bryon PA, Magaud JP. T-cell lymphomas: immunologic, histologic, clinical, and therapeutic analysis of 63 cases. J Clin Oncol 1988; 6: 1584–9.

69. Pinkus GS, O'Hara CJ, Said JW. Peripheral/post-thymic T-cell lymphomas: a spectrum of disease. Clinical, pathologic, and immunologic features of 78 cases. Cancer 1990; 65: 971–98.

70. Delmer A, Caulet S, Bryard F et al. Peripheral T-cell malignant lymphomas. Clinical, morphologic and developmental features in 22 cases. Presse Med 1990; 19: 851–5.

71. Stroup RM, Burke JS, Sheibani K et al. Splenic involvement by aggressive malignant lymphomas of B-cell and T-cell types. A morphologic and immunophenotypic study. Cancer 1992; 69: 413–20.

72. Nakamura S, Suchi T. A clinicopathologic study of node-based, low-grade, peripheral T-cell lymphoma. Angioimmunoblastic lymphoma, T-zone lymphoma, and lymphoepithelioid lymphoma. Cancer 1991; 67: 2566–78.

73. Dogan A, Morice WG. Bone marrow histopathology in peripheral T-cell lymphomas. Br J Haematol 2004; 127: 140–54.

74. Falini B, Pileri S, De Solas I et al. Peripheral T-cell lymphoma associated with hemophagocytic syndrome. Blood 1990; 75: 434–44.

75. Linn YC, Tien SL, Lim LC et al. Haemophagocytosis in bone marrow aspirate – a review of the clinical course of 10 cases. Acta Haematol 1995; 94: 182–91.

76. Rao SA, Gottesman SR, Nguyen MC, Braverman AS. T cell lymphoma associated with myelofibrosis. Leuk Lymphoma 2003; 44: 715–18.

77. Uehara E, Tasaka T, Matsuhashi Y et al. Peripheral T-cell lymphoma presenting with rapidly progressing myelofibrosis. Leuk Lymphoma 2003; 44: 361–3.

78. Kim K, Kim WS, Jung CW et al. Clinical features of peripheral T-cell lymphomas in 78 patients diagnosed according to the Revised European-American lymphoma (REAL) classification. Eur J Cancer 2002; 38: 75–81.

●79. Gallamini A, Stelitano C, Calvi R et al. Peripheral T-cell lymphoma unspecified (PTCL-U): a new prognostic model from a retrospective multicentric clinical study. Blood 2004; 103: 2474–9.

80. Kojima H, Hasegawa Y, Suzukawa K et al. Clinicopathological features and prognostic factors of Japanese patients with 'peripheral T-cell lymphoma, unspecified' diagnosed according to the WHO classification. Leuk Res 2004; 28: 1287–92.

81. Zaja F, Russo D, Silvestri F et al. Retrospective analysis of 23 cases with peripheral T-cell lymphoma, unspecified: clinical characteristics and outcome. Haematologica 1997; 82: 171–7.

82. Grange F, Hedelin G, Joly P et al. Prognostic factors in primary cutaneous lymphomas other than mycosis fungoides and the Sezary syndrome. The French Study Group on Cutaneous Lymphomas. Blood 1999; 93: 3637–42.

83. Beljaards RC, Meijer CJ, Van der Putte SC et al. Primary cutaneous T-cell lymphoma: clinicopathological features and prognostic parameters of 35 cases other than mycosis fungoides and CD30-positive large cell lymphoma. J Pathol 1994; 172: 53–60.

84. Bekkenk MW, Vermeer MH, Jansen PM *et al.* Peripheral T-cell lymphomas unspecified presenting in the skin: analysis of prognostic factors in a group of 82 patients. *Blood* 2003; **102**: 2213–19.

85. Berti E, Tomasini D, Vermeer MH *et al.* Primary cutaneous CD8-positive epidermotropic cytotoxic T cell lymphomas. A distinct clinicopathological entity with an aggressive clinical behavior. *Am J Pathol* 1999; **155**: 483–92.

86. Berti E, Cerri A, Cavicchini S *et al.* Primary cutaneous gamma/delta T-cell lymphoma presenting as disseminated pagetoid reticulosis. *J Invest Dermatol* 1991; **96**: 718–23.

87. Hayabuchi N, Shibamoto Y, Onizuka Y. Primary central nervous system lymphoma in Japan: a nationwide survey. *Int J Radiat Oncol Biol Phys* 1999; **44**: 265–72.

88. Choi JS, Nam DH, Ko YH *et al.* Primary central nervous system lymphoma in Korea: comparison of B- and T-cell lymphomas. *Am J Surg Pathol* 2003; **27**: 919–28.

89. Bataille B, Delwail V, Menet E *et al.* Primary intracerebral malignant lymphoma: report of 248 cases. *J Neurosurg* 2000; **92**: 261–6.

90. Liu D, Schelper RL, Carter DA *et al.* Primary central nervous system cytotoxic/suppressor T-cell lymphoma: report of a unique case and review of the literature. *Am J Surg Pathol* 2003; **27**: 682–8.

●91. Shenkier TN, Blay JY, O'Neill BP *et al.* Primary CNS lymphoma of T-cell origin: a descriptive analysis from the international primary CNS lymphoma collaborative group. *J Clin Oncol* 2005; **23**: 2233–9.

92. Yao M, Cheng AL, Su IJ *et al.* Clinicopathological spectrum of haemophagocytic syndrome in Epstein-Barr virus-associated peripheral T-cell lymphoma. *Br J Haematol* 1994; **87**: 535–43.

93. Wano Y, Hattori T, Matsuoka M *et al.* Interleukin 1 gene expression in adult T cell leukemia. *J Clin Invest* 1987; **80**: 911–6.

94. Lay JD, Tsao CJ, Chen JY *et al.* Upregulation of tumor necrosis factor-alpha gene by Epstein-Barr virus and activation of macrophages in Epstein-Barr virus-infected T cells in the pathogenesis of hemophagocytic syndrome. *J Clin Invest* 1997; **100**: 1969–79.

95. Teruya-Feldstein J, Setsuda J, Yao X *et al.* MIP-1alpha expression in tissues from patients with hemophagocytic syndrome. *Lab Invest* 1999; **79**: 1583–90.

96. Gherardi R, Gaulard P, Prost C *et al.* T-cell lymphoma revealed by a peripheral neuropathy. A report of two cases with an immunohistologic study on lymph node and nerve biopsies. *Cancer* 1986; **58**: 2710–16.

97. Gaulard P, Zafrani ES, Mavier P *et al.* Peripheral T-cell lymphoma presenting as predominant liver disease: a report of three cases. *Hepatology* 1986; **6**: 864–8.

98. O'Shea JJ, Jaffe ES, Lane HC *et al.* Peripheral T cell lymphoma presenting as hypereosinophilia with vasculitis. Clinical, pathologic, and immunologic features. *Am J Med* 1987; **82**: 539–45.

99. Diez-Martin JL, Lust JA, Witzig TE *et al.* Unusual presentation of extranodal peripheral T-cell lymphomas with multiple paraneoplastic features. *Cancer* 1991; **68**: 834–41.

100. Marsh WL Jr, Stevenson DR, Long HJ 3rd. Primary leptomeningeal presentation of T-cell lymphoma. Report of a patient and review of the literature. *Cancer* 1983; **51**: 1125–31.

101. Schnitzer B, Smid D, Lloyd RV. Primary T-cell lymphoma of the adrenal glands with adrenal insufficiency. *Hum Pathol* 1986; **17**: 634–6.

102. Caulet S, Delmer A, Audouin J *et al.* Histopathological study of bone marrow biopsies in 30 cases of T-cell lymphoma with clinical, biological and survival correlations. *Hematol Oncol* 1990; **8**: 155–68.

103. Delmer A, Audoin J, Rio B *et al.* Peripheral T-cell lymphoma presenting as hypereosinophilia with vasculitis. *Am J Med* 1988; **84**: 565–6.

104. Greer JP, York JC, Cousar JB *et al.* Peripheral T-cell lymphoma: a clinicopathologic study of 42 cases. *J Clin Oncol* 1984; **2**: 788–98.

105. Jaffe ES. Angioimmunoblastic T-cell lymphoma: new insights, but the clinical challenge remains. *Ann Oncol* 1995; **6**: 631–2.

106. Feller AC, Griesser H, Schilling CV *et al.* Clonal gene rearrangement patterns correlate with immunophenotype and clinical parameters in patients with angioimmunoblastic lymphadenopathy. *Am J Pathol* 1988; **133**: 549–56.

107. Smith JL, Hodges E, Quin CT *et al.* Frequent T and B cell oligoclones in histologically and immunophenotypically characterized angioimmunoblastic lymphadenopathy. *Am J Pathol* 2000; **156**: 661–9.

108. Weiss LM, Strickler JG, Dorfman RF *et al.* Clonal T-cell populations in angioimmunoblastic lymphadenopathy and angioimmunoblastic lymphadenopathy-like lymphoma. *Am J Pathol* 1986; **122**: 392–7.

109. Tobinai K, Minato K, Ohtsu T *et al.* Clinicopathologic, immunophenotypic, and immunogenotypic analyses of immunoblastic lymphadenopathy-like T-cell lymphoma. *Blood* 1988; **72**: 1000–6.

110. Lipford EH, Smith HR, Pittaluga S *et al.* Clonality of angioimmunoblastic lymphadenopathy and implications for its evolution to malignant lymphoma. *J Clin Invest* 1987; **79**: 637–42.

111. Ree HJ, Kadin ME, Kikuchi M *et al.* Angioimmunoblastic lymphoma (AILD-type T-cell lymphoma) with hyperplastic germinal centers. *Am J Surg Pathol* 1998; **22**: 643–55.

112. Nathwani BN, Rappaport H, Moran EM *et al.* Malignant lymphoma arising in angioimmunoblastic lymphadenopathy. *Cancer* 1978; **41**: 578–606.

113. Abruzzo LV, Schmidt K, Weiss LM *et al.* B-cell lymphoma after angioimmunoblastic lymphadenopathy: a case with oligoclonal gene rearrangements associated with Epstein-Barr virus. *Blood* 1993; **82**: 241–6.

114. Mazur EM, Lovett DH, Enriquez RE *et al.* Angioimmunoblastic lymphadenopathy evolution to a Burkitt-like lymphoma. *Am J Med* 1979; **67**: 317–24.

115. Nakamura S, Sasajima Y, Koshikawa T *et al.* Angioimmunoblastic T-cell lymphoma (angioimmunoblastic lymphadenopathy with dysproteinemia [AILD]-type T-cell lymphoma) followed by Hodgkin's disease associated with Epstein-Barr virus. *Pathol Int* 1995; **45**: 958–64.

116. Pautier P, Devidas A, Delmer A *et al.* Angioimmunoblastic-like T-cell non Hodgkin's lymphoma: outcome after chemotherapy in 33 patients and review of the literature. *Leuk Lymphoma* 1999; **32**: 545–52.

117. Brandt L, Hagander B, Norden A, Stenstam M. Lymphoma of the small intestine in adult coeliac disease. *Acta Med Scand* 1978; **204**: 467–70.

118. Cooper BT, Holmes GK, Ferguson R, Cooke WT. Celiac disease and malignancy. *Medicine* (*Baltimore*) 1980; **59**: 249–61.

119. Lee HJ, Im JG, Goo JM *et al.* Peripheral T-cell lymphoma: spectrum of imaging findings with clinical and pathologic features. *Radiographics* 2003; **23**: 7–26; discussion 26–8.

120. Hoffmann M, Vogelsang H, Kletter K *et al.* 18F-fluoro-deoxy-glucose positron emission tomography (18F-FDG-PET) for assessment of enteropathy-type T cell lymphoma. *Gut* 2003; **52**: 347–51.

121. Yao M, Tien HF, Lin MT *et al.* Clinical and hematological characteristics of hepatosplenic T gamma/delta lymphoma with isochromosome for long arm of chromosome 7. *Leuk Lymphoma* 1996; **22**: 495–500.

122. Saito T, Matsuno Y, Tanosaki R *et al.* Gamma delta T-cell neoplasms: a clinicopathological study of 11 cases. *Ann Oncol* 2002; **13**: 1792–8.

123. Agnarsson BA, Loughran TP Jr, Starkebaum G, Kadin ME. The pathology of large granular lymphocyte leukemia. *Hum Pathol* 1989; **20**: 643–51.

124. Loughran TP Jr. Clonal diseases of large granular lymphocytes. *Blood* 1993; **82**: 1–14.

125. Chan JK, Sin VC, Wong KF *et al.* Nonnasal lymphoma expressing the natural killer cell marker CD56: a clinicopathologic study of 49 cases of an uncommon aggressive neoplasm. *Blood* 1997; **89**: 4501–13.

126. Quintanilla-Martinez L, Jaffe ES. Commentary: aggressive NK cell lymphomas: insights into the spectrum of NK cell derived malignancies. *Histopathology* 2000; **37**: 372–4.

127. Imamura N, Kusunoki Y, Kawa-Ha K *et al.* Aggressive natural killer cell leukaemia/lymphoma: report of four cases and review of the literature. Possible existence of a new clinical entity originating from the third lineage of lymphoid cells. *Br J Haematol* 1990; **75**: 49–59.

128. Mori N, Yamashita Y, Tsuzuki T *et al.* Lymphomatous features of aggressive NK cell leukaemia/lymphoma with massive necrosis, haemophagocytosis and EB virus infection. *Histopathology* 2000; **37**: 363–71.

129. Sun T, Brody J, Susin M *et al.* Aggressive natural killer cell lymphoma/leukemia. A recently recognized clinicopathologic entity. *Am J Surg Pathol* 1993; **17**: 1289–99.

130. Kwong YL, Chan AC, Liang RH. Natural killer cell lymphoma/leukemia: pathology and treatment. *Hematol Oncol* 1997; **15**: 71–9.

131. Ascani S, Leoni P, Fraternali Orcioni G *et al.* T-cell prolymphocytic leukaemia: does the expression of CD8$^+$ phenotype justify the identification of a new subtype? Description of two cases and review of the literature. *Ann Oncol* 1999; **10**: 649–53.

132. Weenig RH, Ng CS, Perniciaro C. Subcutaneous panniculitis-like T-cell lymphoma: an elusive case presenting as lipomembranous panniculitis and a review of 72 cases in the literature. *Am J Dermatopathol* 2001; **23**: 206–15.

133. Hoque SR, Child FJ, Whittaker SJ *et al.* Subcutaneous panniculitis-like T-cell lymphoma: a clinicopathological, immunophenotypic and molecular analysis of six patients. *Br J Dermatol* 2003; **148**: 516–25.

134. Perniciaro C. Unusual cutaneous lymphomas. *Dermatol Surg* 1996; **22**: 288–92.

135. Craig AJ, Cualing H, Thomas G *et al.* Cytophagic histiocytic panniculitis – a syndrome associated with benign and malignant panniculitis: case comparison and review of the literature. *J Am Acad Dermatol* 1998; **39**: 721–36.

136. Karakas T, Bergmann L, Stutte HJ *et al.* Peripheral T-cell lymphomas respond well to vincristine, adriamycin, cyclophosphamide, prednisone and etoposide (VACPE) and have a similar outcome as high-grade B-cell lymphomas. *Leuk Lymphoma* 1996; **24**: 121–9.

137. Lippman SM, Miller TP, Spier CM *et al.* The prognostic significance of the immunotype in diffuse large-cell lymphoma: a comparative study of the T-cell and B-cell phenotype. *Blood* 1988; **72**: 436–41.

138. Cheng AL, Chen YC, Wang CH *et al.* Direct comparisons of peripheral T-cell lymphoma with diffuse B-cell lymphoma of comparable histological grades—should peripheral T-cell lymphoma be considered separately? *J Clin Oncol* 1989; **7**: 725–31.

139. Montalban C, Obeso G, Gallego A *et al.* Peripheral T-cell lymphoma: a clinicopathological study of 41 cases and evaluation of the prognostic significance of the updated Kiel classification. *Histopathology* 1993; **22**: 303–10.

140. Kwak LW, Wilson M, Weiss LM *et al.* Similar outcome of treatment of B-cell and T-cell diffuse large-cell lymphomas: the Stanford experience. *J Clin Oncol* 1991; **9**: 1426–31.

141. Morabito F, Gallamini A, Stelitano C *et al.* Clinical relevance of immunophenotype in a retrospective comparative study of 297 peripheral T-cell lymphomas, unspecified, and 496 diffuse large B-cell lymphomas: experience of the Intergruppo Italiano Linformi. *Cancer* 2004; **101**: 1601–8.

142. Ansell SM, Habermann TM, Kurtin PJ *et al.* Predictive capacity of the International Prognostic Factor Index in patients with peripheral T-cell lymphoma. *J Clin Oncol* 1997; **15**: 2296–301.

143. Cheng AL, Su IJ, Chen YC *et al.* Expression of P-glycoprotein and glutathione-S-transferase in recurrent lymphomas: the possible role of Epstein-Barr virus, immunophenotypes, and other predisposing factors. *J Clin Oncol* 1993; **11**: 109–15.

144. Tsuchiya T, Ohshima K, Karube K *et al*. Th1, Th2, and activated T-cell marker and clinical prognosis in peripheral T-cell lymphoma, unspecified: comparison with AILD, ALCL, lymphoblastic lymphoma, and ATLL. *Blood* 2004; **103**: 236–41.

●145. Rosenwald A, Wright G, Chan WC *et al*. The use of molecular profiling to predict survival after chemotherapy for diffuse large-B-cell lymphoma. *N Engl J Med* 2002; **346**: 1937–47.

146. Reiser M, Josting A, Soltani M *et al*. T-cell non-Hodgkin's lymphoma in adults: clinicopathological characteristics, response to treatment and prognostic factors. *Leuk Lymphoma* 2002; **43**: 805–11.

●147. Fisher RI, Gaynor ER, Dahlberg S *et al*. A phase III comparison of CHOP vs. m-BACOD vs. ProMACE-CytaBOM vs. MACOP-B in patients with intermediate- or high-grade non-Hodgkin's lymphoma: results of SWOG-8516 (Intergroup 0067), the National High-Priority Lymphoma Study. *Ann Oncol* 1994; **5**(Suppl 2): 91–5.

148. Armitage JO, Vose JM, Linder J *et al*. Clinical significance of immunophenotype in diffuse aggressive non-Hodgkin's lymphoma. *J Clin Oncol* 1989; **7**: 1783–90.

149. Waits TM, Greco FA, Greer JP *et al*. Effective therapy for poor-prognosis non-Hodgkin's lymphoma with 8 weeks of high-dose-intensity combination chemotherapy. *J Clin Oncol* 1993; **11**: 943–9.

150. Weidmann E, Gramatzki M, Wilhelm M, Mitrou PS. Diagnosis and actual therapy strategies in peripheral T-cell lymphomas: summary of an international meeting. *Ann Oncol* 2004; **15**: 369–74.

151. Ho AD, Suciu S, Stryckmans P *et al*. Pentostatin in T-cell malignancies – a phase II trial of the EORTC. Leukemia Cooperative Group. *Ann Oncol* 1999; **10**: 1493–8.

152. Lorand-Metze I, Oliveira GB, Aranha FJ. Treatment of prolymphocytic leukemia with cladribine. *Ann Hematol* 1998; **76**: 85–6.

153. Sallah S, Wehbie R, Lepera P *et al*. The role of 2-chlorodeoxyadenosine in the treatment of patients with refractory angioimmunoblastic lymphadenopathy with dysproteinemia. *Br J Haematol* 1999; **104**: 163–5.

154. Sallah S, Wan JY, Nguyen NP. Treatment of refractory T-cell malignancies using gemcitabine. *Br J Haematol* 2001; **113**: 185–7.

155. Zinzani PL, Magagnoli M, Bendandi M *et al*. Therapy with gemcitabine in pretreated peripheral T-cell lymphoma patients. *Ann Oncol* 1998; **9**: 1351–3.

156. Iannitto E, Barbera V, Quintini G *et al*. Hepatosplenic gammadelta T-cell lymphoma: complete response induced by treatment with pentostatin. *Br J Haematol* 2002; **117**: 995–6.

157. Kurzrock R. Therapy of T cell lymphomas with pentostatin. *Ann N Y Acad Sci* 2001; **941**: 200–5.

158. Olsen E, Duvic M, Frankel A *et al*. Pivotal phase III trial of two dose levels of denileukin diftitox for the treatment of cutaneous T-cell lymphoma. *J Clin Oncol* 2001; **19**: 376–88.

159. LeMaistre CF, Saleh MN, Kuzel TM *et al*. Phase I trial of a ligand fusion-protein (DAB389IL-2) in lymphomas expressing the receptor for interleukin-2. *Blood* 1998; **91**: 399–405.

160. Talpur R, Apisarnthanarax N, Ward S, Duvic M. Treatment of refractory peripheral T-cell lymphoma with denileukin diftitox (ONTAK). *Leuk Lymphoma* 2002; **43**: 121–6.

161. Huang CL, Lin ZZ, Su IJ *et al*. Combination of 13-cis retinoic acid and interferon-alpha in the treatment of recurrent or refractory peripheral T-cell lymphoma. *Leuk Lymphoma* 2002; **43**: 1415–20.

162. Gramatzki M, Burger R, Strobel G *et al*. Therapy with OKT3 monoclonal antibody in refractory T cell acute lymphoblastic leukemia induces interleukin-2 responsiveness. *Leukemia* 1995; **9**: 382–90.

163. Baum W, Steininger H, Bair HJ *et al*. Therapy with CD7 monoclonal antibody TH-69 is highly effective for xenografted human T-cell ALL. *Br J Haematol* 1996; **95**: 327–38.

164. Leca G, Vita N, Maiza H *et al*. A monoclonal antibody to the Hodgkin's disease-associated antigen CD30 induces activation and long-term growth of human autoreactive gamma delta T cell clone. *Cell Immunol* 1994; **156**: 230–9.

165. Frankel AE, Laver JH, Willingham MC *et al*. Therapy of patients with T-cell lymphomas and leukemias using an anti-CD7 monoclonal antibody-ricin A chain immunotoxin. *Leuk Lymphoma* 1997; **26**: 287–98.

166. Rider DA, Havenith CE, de Ridder R *et al*. A human CD4 monoclonal antibody for the treatment of T-cell lymphoma combines inhibition of T-cell signaling by a dual mechanism with potent Fc-dependent effector activity. *Cancer Res* 2007; **67**: 9945–53.

167. Kim YH, Duvic M, Obitz E *et al*. Clinical efficacy of zanolimumab (HuMax-CD4): two phase 2 studies in refractory cutaneous T-cell lymphoma. *Blood* 2007; **109**: 4655–62.

168. Salisbury JR, Rapson NT, Codd JD *et al*. Immunohistochemical analysis of CDw52 antigen expression in non-Hodgkin's lymphomas. *J Clin Pathol* 1994; **47**: 313–17.

169. Lundin J, Kimby E, Bjorkholm M *et al*. Phase II trial of subcutaneous anti-CD52 monoclonal antibody alemtuzumab (Campath-1H) as first-line treatment for patients with B-cell chronic lymphocytic leukemia (B-CLL). *Blood* 2002; **100**: 768–73.

170. Keating MJ, Flinn I, Jain V *et al*. Therapeutic role of alemtuzumab (Campath-1H) in patients who have failed fludarabine: results of a large international study. *Blood* 2002; **99**: 3554–61.

171. Lundin J, Hagberg H, Repp R *et al*. Phase 2 study of alemtuzumab (anti-CD52 monoclonal antibody) in patients with advanced mycosis fungoides/Sezary syndrome. *Blood* 2003; **101**: 4267–72.

172. Ginaldi L, De Martinis M, Matutes E *et al*. Levels of expression of CD52 in normal and leukemic B and T cells: correlation with in vivo therapeutic responses to Campath-1H. *Leuk Res* 1998; **22**: 185–91.

173. Pawson R, Dyer MJ, Barge R *et al*. Treatment of T-cell prolymphocytic leukemia with human CD52 antibody. *J Clin Oncol* 1997; **15**: 2667–72.

●174. Enblad G, Hagberg H, Erlanson M *et al*. A pilot study of alemtuzumab (anti-CD52 monoclonal antibody) therapy for patients with relapsed or chemotherapy-refractory peripheral T-cell lymphomas. *Blood* 2004; **103**: 2920–4.

175. Gallamini A, Zaja F, Patti C *et al*. Alemtuzumab (Campath-1H) and CHOP chemotherapy as first-line treatment of peripheral T-cell lymphoma: results of a GITIL (Gruppo Italiano Terapie Innovative nei Linfomi) prospective multicenter trial. *Blood* 2007; **110**: 2316–23.

●176. Philip T, Guglielmi C, Hagenbeek A *et al*. Autologous bone marrow transplantation as compared with salvage chemotherapy in relapses of chemotherapy-sensitive non-Hodgkin's lymphoma. *N Engl J Med* 1995; **333**: 1540–5.

177. Rodriguez J, Munsell M, Yazji S *et al*. Impact of high-dose chemotherapy on peripheral T-cell lymphomas. *J Clin Oncol* 2001; **19**: 3766–70.

178. Rodriguez J, Caballero MD, Gutierrez A *et al*. High dose chemotherapy and autologous stem cell transplantation in patients with peripheral T-cell lymphoma not achieving complete response after induction chemotherapy. The GEL-TAMO experience. *Haematologica* 2003; **88**: 1372–7.

179. Song KW, Mollee P, Keating A, Crump M. Autologous stem cell transplant for relapsed and refractory peripheral T-cell lymphoma: variable outcome according to pathological subtype. *Br J Haematol* 2003; **120**: 978–85.

●180. Mounier N, Gisselbrecht C, Briere J *et al*. All aggressive lymphoma subtypes do not share similar outcome after front-line autotransplantation: a matched-control analysis by the Groupe d'Etude des Lymphomes de l'Adulte (GELA). *Ann Oncol* 2004; **15**: 1790–7.

181. Rodriguez J, Conde E, Gutierrez A *et al*. The results of consolidation with autologous stem-cell transplantation in patients with peripheral T-cell lymphoma (PTCL) in first complete remission: the Spanish Lymphoma and Autologous Transplantation Group experience. *Ann Oncol* 2007; **18**: 652–7.

182. Kahl C, Leithauser M, Wolff D *et al*. Treatment of peripheral T-cell lymphomas (PTCL) with high-dose chemotherapy and autologous or allogeneic hematopoietic transplantation. *Ann Hematol* 2002; **81**: 646–50.

183. Okamura T, Kishimoto T, Inoue M *et al*. Unrelated bone marrow transplantation for Epstein-Barr virus-associated T/NK-cell lymphoproliferative disease. *Bone Marrow Transplant* 2003; **31**: 105–11.

184. Corradini P, Dodero A, Zallio F *et al*. Graft-versus-lymphoma effect in relapsed peripheral T-cell non-Hodgkin's lymphomas after reduced-intensity conditioning followed by allogeneic transplantation of hematopoietic cells. *J Clin Oncol* 2004; **22**: 2172–6.

185. Cheung MM, Chan JK, Lau WH *et al*. Primary non-Hodgkin's lymphoma of the nose and nasopharynx: clinical features, tumor immunophenotype, and treatment outcome in 113 patients. *J Clin Oncol* 1998; **16**: 70–7.

186. Siegert W, Agthe A, Griesser H *et al*. Treatment of angioimmunoblastic lymphadenopathy (AILD)-type T-cell lymphoma using prednisone with or without the COPBLAM/IMVP-16 regimen. A multicenter study. Kiel Lymphoma Study Group. *Ann Intern Med* 1992; **117**: 364–70.

187. Quintini G, Iannitto E, Barbera V *et al*. Response to low-dose oral methotrexate and prednisone in two patients with angio-immunoblastic lymphadenopathy-type T-cell lymphoma. *Hematol J* 2001; **2**: 393–5.

188. Tsatalas C, Margaritis D, Kaloutsi V *et al*. Successful treatment of angioimmunoblastic lymphadenopathy with dysproteinemia-type T-cell lymphoma with fludarabine. *Acta Haematol* 2001; **105**: 106–8.

189. Piccaluga PP, Agostinelli C, Califano A *et al*. Gene expression analysis of angioimmunoblastic lymphoma indicates derivation from T follicular helper cells and vascular endothelial growth factor deregulation. *Cancer Res* 2007; **67**: 10703–10.

190. Hanson MN, Morrison VA, Peterson BA *et al*. Posttransplant T-cell lymphoproliferative disorders – an aggressive, late complication of solid-organ transplantation. *Blood* 1996; **88**: 3626–33.

191. Gopcsa L, Banyai A, Tamaska J *et al*. Hepatosplenic gamma delta T-cell lymphoma with leukemic phase successfully treated with 2-chlorodeoxyadenosine. *Haematologia* 2002; **32**: 519–27.

192. Corazzelli G, Capobianco G, Russo F *et al*. Pentostatin (2′-deoxycoformycin) for the treatment of hepatosplenic gammadelta T-cell lymphomas. *Haematologica* 2005; **90**: ECR14.

193. Aldinucci D, Poletto D, Zagonel V *et al*. In vitro and in vivo effects of 2′-deoxycoformycin (Pentostatin) on tumour cells from human gammadelta+ T-cell malignancies. *Br J Haematol* 2000; **110**: 188–96.

194. Grigg AP. 2′-Deoxycoformycin for hepatosplenic gammadelta T-cell lymphoma. *Leuk Lymphoma* 2001; **42**: 797–9.

81

HIV-associated lymphoid neoplasms

KIERON DUNLEAVY AND WYNDHAM H WILSON

INTRODUCTION

Human immunodeficiency virus (HIV) infection continues to be a pandemic of unrelenting and unprecedented pervasiveness. Lymphoid neoplasms are an important complication of HIV infection where they occur with increased frequency and are a significant cause of morbidity and mortality. While most lymphoma subtypes principally occur in immunocompetent patients, for example, diffuse large B cell lymphoma (DLBCL), others are primarily associated with HIV infection, such as primary effusion lymphoma (PEL) and plasmablastic lymphoma (PBL) of the oral cavity. Overall, HIV-associated lymphoid neoplasms are both histologically and clinically aggressive. With the ever-increasing prevalence of HIV infection, these disorders are becoming more widely diagnosed. It is fortunate that HAART (highly active antiretroviral therapy) has reduced the incidence and improved the outcome of acquired immune deficiency syndrome (AIDS)-related lymphomas (ARL), in large measure due to better control of HIV replication and enhanced immune function. Sadly though, affected populations in continents with the highest prevalence of HIV, such as sub-Saharan Africa, have little access to HAART and this should be kept in mind when considering the benefits achieved in HIV-associated lymphoid diseases.

EPIDEMIOLOGY

In the setting of HIV infection, several distinct subtypes of non-Hodgkin lymphoma (NHL) are encountered with varying frequencies. While the overall increased risk of NHL is greater than 100-fold, the incidence of primary central nervous system lymphoma (PCNSL) is increased 3600-fold and Burkitt lymphoma 1000-fold when compared to HIV-negative populations.[1–4] Though not AIDS-defining illnesses, the relative risk of other lymphoid neoplasms such as Hodgkin lymphoma (HL), extranodal marginal zone lymphoma, and certain T cell lymphomas also appears increased in the setting of HIV infection.[5–8]

Several studies have investigated the impact of HAART on the incidence of ARL. The results of these studies have been somewhat confusing. A few studies found no change in the incidence of ARL in the post-HAART era but it is likely that these studies suffered from inadequate design.[9,10] They compared the incidence of ARL in different time periods but did not examine or compare factors such as population demographics, CD4 cell number, access to and compliance with HAART therapy, or patterns of HIV-drug resistance within populations; factors that potentially impact the incidence of ARL. Other studies, however, have shown a decline in the overall incidence of lymphomas in the HAART era.[11,12] This was demonstrated in a large international study of 47 936 HIV-positive patients from 23 prospective studies.[11] When all data were combined, the adjusted incidence rate per 1000 person-years of NHL declined from 6.2 to 3.6 over the periods of 1992–1996 and 1997–1999, respectively. Other studies have also confirmed this decline.[13–15] Interestingly, when analyzed by lymphoma subtype, a decline was observed in PCNSL and immunoblastic DLBCL, which are more common in patients with low CD4 cell counts. No decline was observed in Burkitt lymphoma, which is more common in patients with higher CD4 cell counts (Fig. 81.1A). This observation is not inconsistent with results from a large European study. In this study, the overall incidence of ARL dropped from 86 to 42.9 between the pre- and post-HAART eras, while PCNSL incidence fell from 27.8 to 9.7 per 10 000 person-years (Fig. 81.1B).[12] However, when the authors compared the incidence of ARL and PCNSL within CD4 cell count strata, they found no differences. This suggests that the decline is due to a reduced proportion of patients with lower CD4 counts in whom the incidence of lymphoma is highest (Fig. 81.1B). The incidence of Hodgkin lymphoma does not appear to have changed since the use of HAART.[11,13] It is important to recognize, however, that the overall beneficial effects of HAART on immune function seen over the past several years may decline as HIV resistance emerges, resulting in a rise in the overall incidence of HIV-associated lymphomas.

ETIOLOGY AND PATHOGENESIS

The pathogenesis of ARL involves a complex interplay of factors and mechanisms. Among these are CD4-dependent immunodeficiency, chronic antigen stimulation, coinfecting oncogenic viruses such as Epstein–Barr virus (EBV) and human herpes virus 8 (HHV-8; also known as Kaposi sarcoma herpes virus [KSHV]), cytokine dysregulation, and genetic abnormalities. Most ARLs are of B cell lineage and, being monoclonal, harbor clonal rearrangement of immunoglobulin genes. Occasional T cell lymphomas are observed and would have T cell receptor gene rearrangements.[4,16]

The risk of developing systemic and primary CNS lymphoma in HIV infection is closely associated with the CD4 cell count.[12] In one study, the incidence of systemic ARL rose from 15.6 to 253.8 per 10 000 person-years and PCNSL from 2 to 93.9 per 10 000 person-years when comparing patients with a CD4 cell count of greater than 350 cells/μL versus less than 50 cells/μL, respectively.[12] In addition, the incidence of various systemic lymphoma subtypes is associated with CD4 cell count. Patients with severe CD4 cell depletion tend to develop the immunoblastic and plasmablastic subtypes, which have a poor prognosis, whereas patients with higher CD4 cell counts tend to develop centroblastic DLBCL and Burkitt lymphomas.[4,17–19] Hence, the decline in patients with low CD4 cell counts in

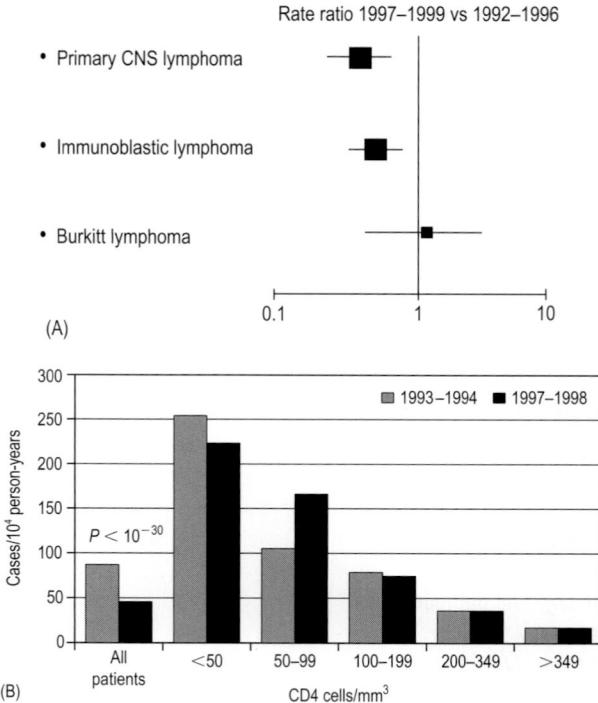

Figure 81.1   Incidence of human immunodeficiency virus (HIV)-associated lymphomas during the pre- and post-HAART (highly active antiretroviral therapy) eras. (A) Incidence rate ratios of three lymphoma types during 1992–1996 and 1997–1999 are shown for cancer incidence data from 23 prospective studies.[11] The incidence rate of primary central nervous system and immunoblastic lymphomas declined in the post-HAART era with rate ratios of 0.42 and 0.57, respectively, whereas Burkitt lymphoma remained unchanged with a rate ratio of 1.18. Figure reproduced by permission of the publisher. (B) Incidence rates for all patients and stratified by CD4 cell count during 1993–1994 and 1997–1998 are shown for a population of HIV-infected patients in the French Hospital Database.[12] Whereas the incidence of lymphoma for all patients significantly declined in the post-HAART era, there was no significant change when analyzed by CD4 count strata.

the post-HAART era is likely to lead to a shift in histologic subtypes.[12,19–21]

The mechanisms underlying the association of immune deficiency with lymphomagenesis in HIV patients are multifactorial but ultimately lead to the acquisition of genetic mutations leading to malignant transformation. Diminished immune surveillance is often postulated as a central mechanism leading to increased survival of 'abnormal' lymphocytes and a more permissive environment for oncogenic viruses such as KSHV/HHV-8 and EBV. Other factors are also likely to impact. Chronic antigen stimulation, which is associated with HIV infection, can lead to polyclonal B cell expansion and likely promotes the emergence of monoclonal B cells. Such events are presumably both time and microenvironment dependent and therefore more common

Table 81.1 Viral and genetic abnormalities in human immunodeficiency virus (HIV)-associated lymphomas

Histologic subtype	EBV⁺	KSHV/HHV–8⁺	Recurring chromosomal abnormalities
Diffuse large B cell lymphoma			*MYC* (20%); *BCL6* (20% of centroblastic DLBCL)[38,39]
Centroblastic	30%[25–27]	0	*TP53* (40%)[29,35]
Immunoblastic	90%[25–27]	0	
Plasmablastic lymphoma	>50%[70]	40%[149]	None
Primary effusion lymphoma	Common[135]	100%[30]	*BCL6* (60%)[37]
Burkitt lymphoma	30–70%[4,28]	0	*MYC* (100%)[34]; *TP53* (50–60%)[29,35]
Primary CNS lymphoma	100%[25]	0	None
Polymorphic lymphoid proliferations	Common[29]	0	None
Hodgkin lymphoma	100%[4]	0	

EBV, Epstein–Barr virus; KSHV/HHV-8, Kaposi sarcoma herpes virus/human herpes virus 8; CNS, central nervous system; DLBCL, diffuse large B cell lymphoma.

in patients with low CD4 cell counts. Indeed, the role of chronic antigen stimulation in lymphomagenesis is well illustrated in lymphoma subtypes such as gastric mucosal-associated lymphoid tissue (MALT) lymphomas, where *Helicobacter pylori*-specific T cells stimulate B cells, and marginal zone lymphomas, where hepatitis C virus and Sjögren syndrome drive monoclonal B cell expansion.[22–24]

Oncogenic viruses also appear to play an important role in HIV-associated lymphomas. Among these, EBV is most commonly seen (Table 81.1). Epstein–Barr virus is present in most immunoblastic (90 percent) but usually absent in centroblastic DLBCL lymphomas.[25–27] In Burkitt lymphoma, EBV is found in 30 percent to 70 percent of tumors, similar to HIV-negative cases, and nearly all cases of HL and PCNSL are EBV positive.[4,28] In plasmablastic lymphoma of the oral cavity, EBV is present in over 50 percent of cases, and polymorphic lymphoid proliferations resembling post-transplant-associated lymphoproliferative disease are sometimes EBV positive.[29] Virtually all cases of PEL harbor KSHV/HHV-8 and many are also EBV positive.[30] EBV-positive ARLs frequently express the EBV-encoded transforming antigen latent membrane protein 1 (LMP-1).[31] LMP-1 activates cellular proliferation through the activation of the nuclear factor κB (NF-κB) pathway and may induce *BCL2* overexpression, hence promoting B cell survival and lymphomagenesis.[32,33]

There are several distinct, well-defined genetic abnormalities in ARL (Table 81.1). Burkitt lymphoma (BL) is associated with activation of the *MYC* gene and resembles sporadic rather than endemic BL, which is similar to HIV-negative cases.[34] Mutations and deletions of the *TP53* tumor suppressor gene are found in 50–60 percent of BL and 40 percent of DLBCL cases.[29,35] Interestingly, 20 percent of DLBCLs harbor a *MYC* translocation, which raises the question of whether some of these cases may actually be atypical Burkitt lymphomas, as recently described in HIV-negative patients.[36] Mutations of the *BCL6* protooncogene are found in approximately 20 percent of AIDS-related centroblastic DLBCL lymphomas, and mutations in the 5′ non-coding region of *BCL6* are common in primary

effusion lymphoma.[37–39] For plasmablastic lymphoma of the oral cavity, no recurring genetic abnormalities have been described thus far. *RAS* protooncogene mutations have also been described in some 15 percent of HIV-associated lymphomas.[40,41]

Cytokine and chemokine dysregulation, such as of interleukins (IL) 6, 10, and 13, probably also play an important and permissive role in lymphomagenesis.[42,43] Interestingly, the AIDS-protective chemokine receptor variant CCR5-Δ32 is highly protective against the development of ARL, suggesting a role for this receptor pathway in lymphomagenesis.[44]

A significant understanding of the pathobiology of ARL can be gleaned from studies of similar lymphoma subtypes in HIV-negative patients. While it is important to recognize that HIV infection, with its attendant effects on immune suppression and stimulation, will confound the application of such results to ARL, some findings appear to be basic. Diffuse large B cell lymphoma is recognized as more than one disease in the World Health Organization (WHO) classification, but it has been difficult to readily subdivide it into distinct disease entities because of overlapping morphology and variable pathogenetic features.[4] Large-scale genomic profiling, however, has the potential to recognize new subtypes of DLBCL and to relate them to treatment outcome.

Initial microarray studies compared DLBCL cases from untreated patients to normal lymphocyte subsets and other lymphoma subtypes. Genes associated with cellular proliferation show a clear distinction with DLBCL generally showing higher expression compared to other lymphoma subtypes, a finding that corresponds to the relatively high tumor proliferation index as measured by Ki-67/MIB-1 antibodies found in DLBCL.[45] The proliferation signature genes are a diverse group and include cell-cycle control and check-point genes, DNA synthesis and replication genes, as well as the Ki-67 gene. Another prominent feature of DLBCL is a group of genes that define a 'lymph node' signature that appears to reflect nonmalignant cells in the biopsy samples. Genes that distinguish germinal center B cells (GCB) from other stages of B cell differentiation are also differentially expressed in the

DLBCL cases and have been used to define different subsets.[46,47] Such analyses indicate that DLBCL can be divided into two major groups defined by expression of genes associated with normal GCB, termed germinal center B cell-like (GCB) DLBCL, and genes associated with post-germinal center B cells, termed activated B cell-like (ABC) DLBCL (Plate 135, see plate section). Genes associated with GCB DLBCL include known markers of germinal center differentiation such as CD10 and the *BCL6* gene, which may be translocated or somatically mutated in DLBCL, as found in some HIV-associated lymphomas (Table 81.1; Plate 136, see plate section).[48] In contrast, most genes that define ABC DLBCL are not expressed by normal GCB cells, but instead are induced during *in vitro* activation of peripheral B cells, such as cyclin D2 and CD44. The ABC DLBCL signature also includes the interferon regulatory factor 4 (*IRF4* [*MUM1*]) gene that is transiently induced during normal lymphocyte activation and is necessary for antigen receptor-driven B cell proliferation.[49,50] A noteworthy feature of ABC DLBCL is the expression of *BCL2*, a prominent antiapoptotic gene that is induced over 30-fold during peripheral B cell activation.[51] Indeed, most ABC DLBCL have a greater than fourfold higher *BCL2* expression than GCB DLBCL and there are no associated *BCL2* translocations.[47] Interestingly, there were significant histological differences among the subgroups, with centroblastic histology more common in the GCB subtype and immunoblastic histologies more common in the ABC subtypes (Plate 136).[52]

If the new taxonomy defines true DLBCL subtypes, one would also predict that it should have clinical prognostic value. To assess this, gene array results were correlated with overall survival of the patients, all of whom had received doxorubicin-based chemotherapy.[46,47,52] This analysis revealed a statistically significant difference in overall survival at 5 years of 59 percent in GCB and 31 percent in ABC subtypes of DLBCL. These findings led to a larger study in which samples from 240 patients with DLBCL were analyzed by molecular profiling and for the presence of genomic abnormalities.[52] This larger study reconfirmed the validity of the ABC and GCB taxonomy and led to the development of a molecular prognostic predictor for DLBCL.[52] Although the applicability of this prognostic model to HIV-associated DLBCL is uncertain given the adverse effects of immune depletion on outcome in ARL, the adverse prognostic effect of the ABC subtype remains relevant.[19–21]

Gene expression profiling has also been applied to PEL to help define its relationship with other B cell lymphoma subtypes and normal B cells.[53,54] In one study, PEL had a profile distinct from BL and DLBCL, including the centroblastic type of HIV-associated DLBCL.[53] Overall, PEL showed a profile most similar to the immunoblastic type of HIV-associated DLBCL, but with features intermediate between immunoblasts and plasma cells, supporting a plasmablastic derivation. Gene expression analysis was also used to assess the impact of KSHV/HHV-8 and EBV infection on the pathogenesis of PEL.[54] A comparison of KSHV/HHV-8-positive to KSHV/HHV-8-negative but EBV-positive lymphomatous effusions revealed some 500 differentially expressed genes, which included genes encoding transcriptional factors, apoptosis regulators, and cell cycle signal transducers. Within KSHV/HHV-8-positive PEL cases, two subtypes could be distinguished according to their EBV infection status. Such results suggest that KSHV/HHV-8 plays an important role in the pathogenesis of PEL while the effect of EBV is more subtle.

Insights into the molecular pathogenesis of aggressive B cell lymphomas, including subtypes that principally occur in immunosuppressed patients, can be applied to the development of a histogenetic model of HIV-associated lymphomas. Such a model was recently proposed by Carbone and Gloghini based on the premise that different clinicopathologic categories of ARL derive from distinct B cell subsets and their associated pathogenetic pathways and that the level of immune deficiency selects the type of ARL.[19] An expanded view of this model would incorporate the microarray taxonomy proposed by Alizadeh *et al.* whereby DLBCL can be separated into GCB and ABC subtypes, which generally correspond to the centroblastic and immunoblastic histologic subtypes, respectively (Fig. 81.2).[47,52] Whereas these histologic subtypes occur in both HIV-negative and HIV-positive patients, there are important differences, particularly regarding the frequency of EBV, where its presence in most HIV-associated immunoblastic lymphomas suggests a prominent role in lymphomagenesis (Table 81.1). In contrast, EBV involvement in BL appears similar in HIV-positive and HIV-negative patients, suggesting similar pathways of lymphomagenesis. Epidemiologic studies indicate the degree of HIV immune suppression significantly impacts the histogenesis of HIV-associated lymphomas, with a significant increase in EBV-positive and KSHV/HHV-8-positive lymphomas among patients with severe immunodeficiency. These lymphomas are more frequently derived from post-germinal center B cells, and have immunoblastic or plasmacytic features (Plate 136). It is interesting that HIV patients with relatively intact immunity are more likely to develop Burkitt and centroblastic lymphomas, which are derived from germinal center B cells. Although EBV can be present in these lymphomas, its frequency appears similar to HIV-negative cases, raising the possibility that HIV does not significantly alter the mechanisms of lymphomagenesis in this setting.[4,19,55]

Tumor immunophenotype is useful for identification of a tumor's histogenesis and generally reflects the antigen expression of its normal B cell counterpart.[21,56] Like normal germinal center B cells, Burkitt and centroblastic lymphomas typically express CD10 and *BCL6* but not MUM1/IRF4 or CD138/syndecan-1, which are expressed by post-germinal center activated B cells and plasma cells (Plates 135, 136, and Fig. 81.2). MUM1/IRF4 is more broadly expressed by post-germinal center B cells, and is found on both immunoblastic and plasmacytic lymphomas, whereas CD138/syndecan-1 expression is restricted to plasma cells and is primarily found on PEL and plasmablastic lymphomas. CD20 expression also tracks with their normal B cell counterparts with some exceptions. Germinal center-derived lymphomas strongly

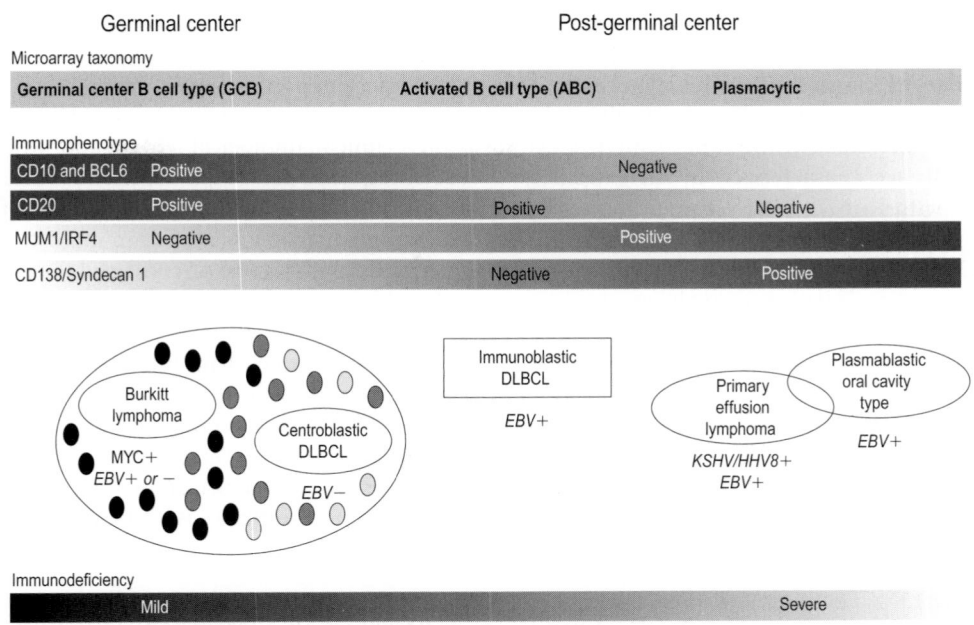

Figure 81.2   A model for the histogenesis of human immunodeficiency virus (HIV)-associated lymphomas, showing molecular and viral pathogenesis, and diffuse large B cell lymphoma (DLBCL) molecular taxonomy.[19,52]

express CD20 while plasmacytic lymphomas, like normal plasma cells, are usually CD20 negative. Expression of CD20 on immunoblastic lymphomas can be more variable. While activated B cells, the putative cell of origin of many immunoblastic DLBCLs, typically express CD20, EBV may downregulate CD20 expression and promote plasmacytic differentiation. Indeed, it is worth noting that differentiating DLBCL with plasmacytic differentiation from a 'true' plasmablastic lymphoma using immunophenotype and histology can be quite difficult in the setting of HIV infection.[57,58]

PATHOLOGY

The WHO classification of tumors of hematopoietic and lymphoid tissues divides HIV-associated lymphomas into three separate categories (Table 81.2).[4] While DLBCL and BL are subtypes commonly encountered in immunocompetent patients (Category I), PEL and plasmablastic lymphoma of the oral cavity occur more specifically in HIV-positive individuals (Category II). Because HL, peripheral T cell lymphoma, and extranodal marginal zone B cell lymphoma of MALT type are only slightly more frequent in HIV patients, they are considered within category I. Lymphomas occurring in other immunodeficiency states are also considered (Category III).

Category I lymphomas

BURKITT LYMPHOMA

Histologically, HIV-associated BL is divided into three separate entities.[4] The classical type accounts for

Table 81.2   World Health Organization classification of human immunodeficiency virus (HIV)-associated lymphomas

Category I. Lymphomas also occurring in immunocompetent patients

    Burkitt lymphoma
        Classical
        With plasmacytoid differentiation
        Atypical
    Diffuse large B cell lymphoma
        Centroblastic
        Immunoblastic
    Extranodal marginal zone B cell lymphoma of MALT type
    Peripheral T cell lymphoma
    Classical Hodgkin lymphoma

Category II. Lymphomas occurring more specifically in HIV⁺ patients

    Primary effusion lymphoma
    Plasmablastic lymphoma of the oral cavity

Category III. Lymphomas also occurring in other immunodeficiency states

    Polymorphic B cell lymphoma

MALT, mucosal-associated lymphoid tissue.

approximately 30 percent of all HIV-associated lymphomas and morphologically resembles classical BL encountered in HIV-negative patients. Burkitt lymphoma with plasmacytoid differentiation, which accounts for 20 percent of ARL, is characterized by medium-sized cells. Cells have abundant cytoplasm, a central nucleus, and usually a centrally located nucleolus. In addition, cytoplasmic immunoglobulin is often present. Atypical Burkitt/Burkitt-like type is characterized by a morphologic appearance similar to classical BL. This type exhibits greater pleomorphism in the size and shape of cells and is less frequently encountered than the other subtypes. All three entities of BL are characterized by an extremely high mitotic rate, with Ki-67/MIB-1 scores in the region of 100 percent. Regarding immunophenotypic features, CD19, CD20, CD79a, and CD10 are expressed whereas BCL2 is negative. Epstein–Barr virus involvement ranges from 30 percent in the classical type to 50–70 percent in BL with plasmacytoid differentiation.[16,28,59]

DIFFUSE LARGE B CELL LYMPHOMA

Human immunodeficiency virus-associated DLBCL is divided into centroblastic and immunoblastic variants. The centroblastic type is characterized by diffuse sheets of large lymphoid cells with round or oval nuclei and fairly prominent nucleoli (Plate 136). These tumors often express germinal center-associated markers such as CD10 and BCL6, and are virtually always CD20 positive (Plate 136).[4,34,60] The immunoblastic variant refers to those cases containing more than 90 percent immunoblasts and often exhibits features of plasmacytoid differentiation which may confound the distinction from plasmablastic lymphoma.[4,57,58] These tumors are CD10 negative, being of post-germinal center derivation, and frequently positive for MUM1/IRF4 and CD138/syndecan-1, markers associated with plasma cell derivation.[4,34] These tumors have frequent mitoses with high Ki-67/MIB-1 scores.[21] The centroblastic type represents approximately 25 percent of HIV-associated lymphomas whereas the immunoblastic type represents about 10 percent. In immunoblastic lymphoma, tumor cells may lose CD20 expression due to coexpression of EBV. Markers associated with activation such as CD30, CD38, and CD71 are often expressed in immunoblastic types.[4,34]

HODGKIN LYMPHOMA AND OTHER TYPES

Most cases of HIV-associated HL are of mixed cellularity type, with lymphocyte depleted and nodular sclerosis histologies also frequently encountered.[61] In contrast to HL in HIV-negative patients, almost all HIV-associated cases are EBV positive. Other lymphoid neoplasms that appear to occur with an increased frequency in HIV infection include T cell lymphomas such as peripheral T cell lymphoma, anaplastic large cell lymphoma, and mycosis fungoides as well as extranodal marginal zone lymphomas.[62–64]

Category II lymphomas

PRIMARY EFFUSION LYMPHOMA

Primary effusion lymphoma accounts for up to 5 percent of ARL cases and is rarely encountered in the absence of HIV infection.[65] This lymphoma has a predilection for body cavities where it takes on the form of lymphomatous effusions of the pleura or peritoneum, and there is usually an absence of nodal disease. Very rarely it presents outside cavities in nodal or extranodal sites.[19,66] It represents a distinct clinicopathological entity and KSHV/HHV-8 has been implicated in its pathogenesis.[53] The KSHV/HHV-8 virus, whose presence can usually be confirmed by polymerase chain reaction or by immunohistochemistry, is also associated with Kaposi sarcoma and the plasma cell variant of multicentric Castleman disease.[53] The neoplastic cells in PEL range in appearance from large immunoblastic to anaplastic large cell lymphoma-type cells. The cells have large nuclei and prominent nucleoli. They can resemble Reed-Sternberg cells but are CD15 negative. Though this tumor is of B cell origin, surface B cell antigens such as CD20 or CD79a are usually not expressed. CD45 (leukocyte common antigen) is usually positive as are CD30, CD38, and CD138. Epstein–Barr virus may be present.[53,67]

PLASMABLASTIC LYMPHOMA

These rare lymphomas typically occur in the oral cavity or jaw but may occur at other sites and are almost always associated with HIV. They are characterized by large tumor cells with an eccentric blast-like nucleus and prominent central nucleoli, surrounded by plasmacytoid cytoplasm. CD38, CD138, and MUM1/IRF4 are usually positive with CD45 and CD20 staining being negative (Plate 136).[58] Epstein–Barr virus is present in greater than 50 percent of cases and is best detected by EBV encoded small RNA (EBER) *in situ* hybridization.[68] These tumors appear to biologically overlap with PEL.[53]

Category III lymphomas

Polymorphic B cell lymphomas resembling post-transplant lymphoproliferative disorder (PTLD), although encountered less frequently than in the post-transplant setting, are occasionally associated with HIV infection. They are composed of a polymorphic lymphoid cell population with cells ranging from small cells, often with plasmacytoid features, to atypical immunoblasts.[4,69] Epstein–Barr virus is frequently positive.[69]

CLINICAL PRESENTATION

Patients with ARL commonly present with advanced stage disease and constitutional (B) symptoms.[21] Approximately 60 percent of patients present with stage IV disease. These lymphomas have a very high propensity to involve extranodal sites that include the bone marrow, gastrointestinal tract, CNS, and liver. Often unusual sites of involvement are seen such as the oral cavity and jaw and other body cavities. Bone marrow involvement is seen in approximately

20 percent of patients at initial diagnosis.[70] Central nervous system involvement occurs in approximately 20 percent of patients.[21,71] While these figures specifically apply to non-Hodgkin lymphomas, HL in the setting of AIDS is also associated with advanced stage disease, and extranodal sites and an aggressive clinical course.[71,72]

In ARL, there are distinct clinical presentations and characteristics that are associated with certain histopathologic subtypes. Primary effusion lymphoma, for example, is typically characterized by a lack of nodal involvement and involves the pleural, pericardial, and peritoneal cavities typically.[73] It tends to present in older males and is associated with severe immunosuppression. Due to a common etiologic link with KSHV/HHV-8, approximately one-third of patients also have Kaposi sarcoma.[30] In this setting, Kaposi sarcoma usually presents with involvement of just one of these body cavities and can occasionally involve extranodal sites such as the gastrointestinal tract.[74] Occasionally, disease in cavities can extend to involve adjacent structures. Plasmablastic lymphoma of the oral cavity is another unique lymphoma type that usually involves the oral cavity or jaw but can present in nodal or extranodal sites.[57,75]

DIAGNOSTIC EVALUATION

A thorough examination of the patient's HIV history is required at initial assessment including detailed history of symptoms, prior opportunistic infections, and HAART therapy. A detailed physical examination should include a careful assessment of all lymph node regions to assess the extent of peripheral lymphadenopathy. Evaluation of the chest wall and an abdominal examination to detect hepatosplenomegaly are important. As is the case with other lymphomas, the single most useful diagnostic test for a patient with suspected ARL is a technically adequate and properly evaluated excisional biopsy of abnormal tissue. A fine needle aspiration biopsy is usually inadequate for a definitive diagnosis, although a core needle biopsy may be acceptable. The pathologic evaluation should be performed by an expert hematopathologist who is experienced in the diagnosis of lymphomas.

Important laboratory studies include a complete blood count, chemistry profile, and lactate dehydrogenase and uric acid levels. T lymphocyte subset analysis with determination of CD4 cell count and HIV viral load should be determined. These both have been found to correlate with prognosis. A bone marrow aspirate and biopsy should be performed at initial diagnosis as bone marrow involvement by lymphoma is found in up to 20 percent of patients.[70] A lumbar puncture should be performed and cerebrospinal fluid evaluated by cytology and flow cytometry.[76]

Imaging studies for the initial evaluation of ARL should include computed tomography (CT) scanning of the chest, abdomen, and pelvis. Radiographic evaluation of the head should also be performed with either magnetic resonance imaging (MRI) or CT scanning. Gallium-67 scanning is not routinely performed in the initial evaluation of ARL but has been a useful adjunct to CT. In particular circumstances, such as differentiating lymphoma from Kaposi sarcoma, opportunistic infections, or reactive hyperplasia, it may have a role.[77,78] Fluorodeoxyglucose positron emission tomography (FDG-PET), based on the finding that malignant cells have a higher rate of metabolism and glucose uptake than normal cells, is a newer imaging modality that has largely replaced gallium-67 scanning in non-AIDS-related lymphoma. FDG-PET has a greater sensitivity and appears to have a high predictive value for treatment failure in HIV-negative patients with residual masses after treatment of aggressive lymphomas.[79–81] It has not been well studied in ARL and, in the absence of effective salvage treatment, may have limited utility. Indeed, a small and preliminary study in ARL suggested that early FDG-PET scans may not predict outcome with the dose-adjusted (DA) EPOCH-R (etoposide, prednisone, vincristine, cyclophosphamide, doxorubicin and rituximab) regimen.[82]

CLINICAL AND MOLECULAR PROGNOSTIC FACTORS

Clinical factors continue to be the mainstay for prognostic assessment in lymphomas. The most widely applied method is the International Prognostic Index (IPI), which was initially developed and validated in HIV-negative aggressive non-Hodgkin lymphomas but has proven useful in ARL.[71,83–85] Other clinical factors such as involvement of the CNS occur with higher frequency in HIV-positive aggressive lymphomas and assume a relevant prognostic role in ARL.[21] It is also important to consider the effects of the immune environment on the risks associated with infection and tumor biology. While these prognostic risks may be globally captured by the CD4 cell count, where values under 100 cells/μL are associated with worse outcome, it is important to consider the individual components.[21,27,86] The adverse effect of immune deficiency on ARL outcome has often been ascribed to infection risk, both during and after chemotherapy, and has led to the testing of lower-dose chemotherapy.[87] Based on recent clinical studies, however, it has been suggested that the salutary effect of HAART on immune restoration improves ARL treatment response, though no mechanism has been proposed.[88] In another study, a positive virologic response to HAART, which may be a marker for better immune function, was associated with improved ARL survival.[89] While one cannot discount the impact of immune deficiency on non-lymphoma-related deaths, it is difficult to understand how it would directly modulate chemotherapy response. We believe it more likely, and consistent with recent epidemiologic trends, that tumor pathobiology underlies much of the effect of immune status and HAART treatment on the outcome of ARL.[12,19,21,52,55]

Molecular indices of tumor pathobiology have emerged as important and independent prognostic biomarkers in HIV-negative lymphomas.[52,90,91] Similarly, tumor immunophenotype is a relevant prognostic factor in HIV-associated lymphomas. Recently, Hoffmann and colleagues correlated prognosis of HIV-associated DLBCL with immunophenotypic profile and found that the immunophenotype representing post-germinal center differentiation (BCL6 and CD10 negative; MUM1/IRF4 and/or CD138/syndecan-1 positive) was associated with a worse prognosis.[20] This finding is not inconsistent with the observation that immunoblastic DLBCL, which is associated with the ABC subtype, is more likely to occur in the setting of advanced immunosuppression and have a poor outcome. On the other side, Little *et al.* also showed that the progression-free survival of BCL2-negative DLBCL, which occurs more commonly in germinal center-derived lymphomas, is similar in HIV-positive or HIV-negative patients, highlighting the importance of tumor biology on the favorable prognosis of this group.[21,52] One also cannot dismiss the importance of tumor histology and treatment selection on outcome. It is well established in HIV-negative patients that CHOP-based treatments, which are the mainstay of treatment in ARL, have a poor outcome in Burkitt lymphoma; a finding that appears relevant to HIV-associated Burkitt lymphoma as well.[36,92]

Such results raise the hypothesis that the improved outcome of ARL in the post-HAART era is driven in large measure by tumor pathobiology and not the direct effect of immune function on tumor control.[20,21] Such results suggest that patients with low CD4 cell counts are more likely to have chemotherapy-resistant lymphomas, such as the immunoblastic and plasmablastic subtypes, and highlight the importance of obtaining molecular indices of outcome.

TREATMENT

The pre–HAART era

The treatment and outcome of ARL has changed significantly over the past 30 years. To understand how current treatment standards have emerged and treatment controversies have arisen, it is worthwhile reviewing the history of ARL therapy from inception and following its course from the pre- to post-HAART eras (Table 81.3). Early experience with chemotherapy in ARL, prior to the availability of HAART, demonstrated very poor outcomes with median survival of only 5 or 6 months. This was demonstrated in one early study by Kaplan and colleagues in which survival was shorter among patients who received higher compared to standard doses of cyclophosphamide.[93] These patients were very immunosuppressed and thus highly susceptible to developing opportunistic infections to which they frequently succumbed. In an attempt to reduce deaths from infection and toxicity, trials were begun to explore lower-dose chemotherapy.[87,94]

In the most important of these trials, the AIDS Clinical Trials Group randomly assigned 192 patients with previously untreated AIDS lymphoma to receive standard-dose m-BACOD (methotrexate, bleomycin, doxorubicin, cyclophosphamide, vincristine, and dexamethasone) with granulocyte macrophage colony-stimulating factor (GM-CSF) support or low-dose m-BACOD without GM-CSF in an effort to reduce the toxicity of chemotherapy.[87] The study showed that compared to full-dose therapy, reduced-dose treatment had a similar response rate (52 percent versus 41 percent, respectively) and median survival (6.8 versus 7.7 months, respectively), but lower hematologic toxicity. The authors concluded that lower-dose chemotherapy was preferable in ARL. Although the authors controlled for the absolute CD4 cell count in the analysis of survival, the primary end point, the study did not have sufficient patients with high CD4 cell counts. A calculation of the power to detect a difference (two-tailed = 0.05) in survival from 6 to 9 months, as the authors proposed, yields a power of only 50 percent in the subgroup with CD4 cell count of greater than 100 cells/μL.[95] Thus, the study could not support a definitive recommendation for this group, which would likely benefit most from chemotherapy for several reasons. Foremost is that dose intensity is an important prognostic factor in HIV-negative aggressive lymphomas, and there is no reason to suggest this should be altered by HIV status.[96] What is different in HIV-positive lymphomas is that the antitumor effects of chemotherapy must be balanced against its effect on immune function. In this regard, patients with high CD4 cell counts are most likely to benefit from the curative potential of chemotherapy and least likely to die from chemotherapy-induced immunodeficiency, compared to patients with low CD4 cell counts.[21] Importantly, before this trial was even completed, an intergroup randomized, multicenter study in HIV-negative aggressive NHL compared m-BACOD to CHOP (cyclophosphamide, doxorubicin, vincristine, and prednisone) and showed CHOP to be equally effective and less toxic (Table 81.4).[97] Questions surrounding the efficacy of low-dose m-BACOD in ARL and the better therapeutic index of CHOP led to its being embraced as a standard treatment for ARL.[27]

The HAART era

The introduction of HAART in the mid-1990s had a dramatic and positive impact on the outcome of ARL. A comparison of median survival of the pre- and post-HAART eras showed a significant increase from 6.3 to 21.2 months (Fig. 81.3). While the reasons for this are multifaceted, they can be ultimately attributed to salutary effects on CD4 cell counts. It was thus clinically predictable that the overall rise in CD4 cell count would improve ARL outcome based on the well-established association between poor outcome and low CD4 cell count.[21,27] Of course, patients with better immune function have a lower risk of infectious complications, thereby enabling chemotherapy administration and reducing infectious deaths. Perhaps most important, however, is the more favorable biology associated with

Table 81.3 Pivotal trials in human immunodeficiency virus (HIV)-associated lymphomas

Study	Study type	Study design	Main findings
Kaplan et al.[87]	Prospective multicenter randomized phase III (n = 192)	Randomization to standard-dose m-BACOD with GM-CSF versus low-dose m-BACOD without GM-CSF. Patients did not receive HAART	Similar efficacy of both regimens but less hematologic toxicity with low-dose m-BACOD
Ratner et al.[98]	Prospective multicenter sequential phase II (n = 65)	First 40 patients received modified-dose (m)CHOP (50% cyclophosphamide and doxorubicin) and the next 25 patients received standard-dose CHOP. HAART was administered	CR higher with full-dose CHOP compared to mCHOP (48% vs 30%). Authors concluded that concomitant HAART was safe. Unable to conclude if one regimen was better
Sparano et al.[101]	Prospective multicenter sequential phase II (n = 98)	First 43 patients received didanosine and the next 55 patients received HAART with CDE	At 2 years, FFS and OS were 36% and 43%. Patients receiving concomitant HAART had better survival and less hematologic and nonhematologic toxicity
Little et al.[21]	Prospective single center phase II (n = 39)	All patients received DA-EPOCH and G-CSF with antiretroviral suspension	CR was 74%. At 53 months, DFS and OS were 92% and 60%. Patients in remission achieved CD4 cell recovery and HIV control posttreatment. Conclusion that antiretroviral suspension with EPOCH is highly effective
Kaplan et al.[111]	Prospective multicenter randomized phase III (n = 150)	Randomization (2:1) to R-CHOP versus CHOP with concomitant HAART. Some patients received maintenance rituximab	CR higher with R-CHOP compared to CHOP (57.6% vs 47%). Increased infectious deaths with R-CHOP (14% vs 2%), mostly in patients with low CD4 cell counts. Conclusion that rituximab does not improve clinical outcome
Spina et al.[110]	Retrospective analysis of 3 phase II trials (n = 74)	Pooled results from 3 trials of CDE with rituximab	CR rate was 70%. At 2 years, FFS and OS were 59% and 64%. Conclusion that R-CDE is effective but rituximab may increase infections

GM-CSF, granulocyte macrophage colony-stimulating factor; G-CSF, granulocyte colony stimulating factor; HAART, highly active antiretroviral therapy; CR, complete remission; FFS, failure-free survival; OS, overall survival; DFS, disease-free survival; m-BACOD, methotrexate, bleomycin, doxorubicin, cyclophosphamide, vincristine, and dexamethasone; CHOP, cyclophosphamide, doxorubicin, vincristine, and prednisone; R, rituximab; CDE, cyclophosphamide, doxorubicin, and etoposide; EPOCH, etoposide, prednisone, vincristine, cyclophosphamide, and doxorubicin; DA, dose adjusted.

lymphomas that occur in patients with higher CD4 cell counts.[19,21]

These findings led to the assumption that HAART during chemotherapy would be beneficial. One of the first trials to investigate the concomitant use of HAART with chemotherapy was performed by the AIDS Malignancy Consortium (AMC) in which patients received either modified (m) dose (50 percent lower cyclophosphamide and doxorubicin) or standard CHOP chemotherapy (Table 81.3).[98] This was not randomized, as the initial 40 patients received mCHOP and the subsequent 25 patients received CHOP (Table 81.4). All patients received a HAART regimen consisting of stavudine, lamivudine, and indinavir. In this study, mCHOP and CHOP had similar toxicity and both were reasonably well tolerated, providing some assurance for the safety of HAART with CHOP chemotherapy. Perhaps not unexpectedly, patients who received CHOP had a somewhat better outcome compared to those who received mCHOP, but in the absence of a randomized design, the authors could only conclude that the regimens were active and tolerable. A potentially important finding of the study comes from the pharmacokinetic (PK) analysis, which showed that cyclophosphamide clearance was reduced 1.5-fold but doxorubicin clearance was unchanged compared to historical controls. While it is reassuring that the doxorubicin PK was unaffected, as found in other studies, the reduced clearance of cyclophosphamide, an inactive prodrug, will likely result in a reduction of active metabolites and potentially compromise efficacy.[99]

The safety and efficacy of CHOP with HAART was also assessed in comparison to a historical matched control group treated with CHOP alone.[100] Interestingly, anemia and autonomic neurotoxicity were significantly greater in the CHOP-HAART group but other toxicities were similar. Patients who received CHOP-HAART had significantly

Table 81.4   Standard regimens in human immunodeficiency virus (HIV)-associated lymphomas

Regimen	Dose and schedule	Notes
CDE[101]	Cyclophosphamide 200 mg/m^2/day CIV × 4 Doxorubicin 12.5 mg/m^2/day CIV × 4 Etoposide 60 mg/m^2/day CIV × 4 G-CSF: day 5 until ANC recovery	Cycles every 28 days. Maximum 8 cycles with 2 cycles beyond CR R-CDE:[110] same doses plus rituximab 375 mg/m^2 day 1
DA-EPOCH[21]	Etoposide 50 mg/m^2/day CIV × 4 Vincristine 0.4 mg/m^2/day CIV × 4 Doxorubicin 10 mg/ m^2/day CIV × prednisone 60 mg/m^2/day PO day 1–5 Cyclophosphamide IV day 5 of cycle 1 based on CD4 count (187 or 375 mg/m^2 for CD4 < or ≥100 cells/μL, respectively). G-CSF: day 5 until ANC recovery Suspend antiretrovirals	Cycles every 21 days for 6 cycles. Cyclophosphamide dose increased or decreased by 187 mg/m^2 if nadir ANC ≥ or <500 cells/μL, respectively, to 750 mg/m^2 maximum dose Short-course EPOCH-R:[82] same doses except cyclophosphamide 750 mg/m^2 cycle 1. Rituximab 375 mg/m^2 day 1 and 5 of each cycle. Administer SC EPOCH-R for 1 cycle beyond maximum response for minimum 3 and maximum 6 cycles
CHOP[98]	Cyclophosphamide 750 mg/m^2 IV day 1 Doxorubicin 50 mg/m^2 IV day 1 Vincristine 1.4 mg/m^2 (2 mg cap) IV day 1 Prednisone 100 mg PO day 1–5 G-CSF: day 4 to day 13 or ANC >10 000 cells/μL	Cycles every 21 days. Stage I and non-bulky stage II disease receive 3 cycles and involved field RT. Other stages receive 6 cycles R-CHOP:[113] same doses plus rituximab 375 mg/m^2 day 1. Patients in CR or PR received rituximab maintenance every 3 months

CIV, continuous intravenous; G-CSF, granulocyte colony-stimulating factor; ANC, absolute neutrophil count; CR, complete remission; PR, partial remission; RT, radiation therapy.

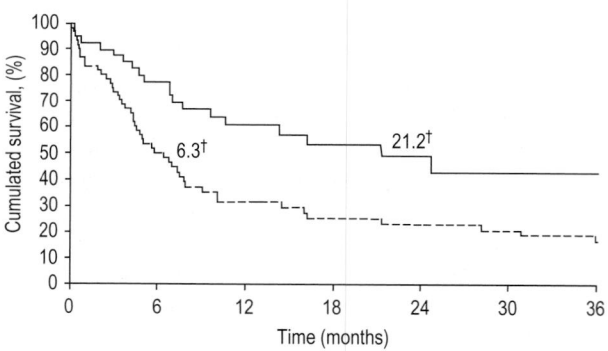

Figure 81.3   Kaplan-Meier estimate of survival of patients with systemic acquired immune deficiency syndrome (AIDS)-related lymphoma (ARL) between 1993–1994 (*n* = 63) and 1997–1998 (*n* = 42), corresponding to the pre- and post-HAART (highly active antiretroviral therapy) eras, respectively, in three French hospitals.[12] Median survival(†) increased significantly from 6.3 to 21.2 months, respectively (*P* = 0.004 by Log-rank test). Reproduced by permission.

fewer opportunistic infections and longer survival, leading the authors to conclude that CHOP-HAART was feasible.

The combination of HAART and infusional CDE (cyclophosphamide, doxorubicin, and etoposide) therapy has also been assessed.[101] Sparano and colleagues evaluated CDE in 43 patients who received concurrent didanosine and 55 patients who received concurrent HAART

(Table 81.3 and Table 81.4).[101] Hematologic and non-hematologic toxicity were lower and overall survival was higher in the CDE-HAART group, providing additional evidence for the safety of HAART and chemotherapy treatment. Of note, in a prior study, Sparano *et al.* had shown that compared to CDE alone, the administration of concurrent didanosine resulted in an 11 percent to 38 percent reduction in mean steady-state plasma etoposide concentrations and lower hematologic toxicity.[102]

HAART suspension during chemotherapy

It is prudent to carefully consider the role of concomitant HAART during chemotherapy treatment. While studies show that HAART does not excessively increase the toxicity of chemotherapy, there is no direct evidence that it improves outcome. The argument that control of HIV viral replication by HAART during chemotherapy benefits immune function is sound but should be considered in light of several factors. Perhaps of foremost concern is the potential for adverse PK and pharmacodynamic interactions related to hepatic metabolism and/or the multidrug resistant (mdr) pumps.[103] HAART drugs may decrease active cyclophosphamide metabolites and etoposide, which could compromise outcome. This is particularly worrisome for infusional-based regimens such as CDE and EPOCH where threshold concentrations are of importance.[104] Furthermore, HAART drugs may inhibit mdr and increase hematologic toxicity and decrease dose intensity, while conferring no benefit on tumor sensitivity.[105] Effects of HAART drugs on hematologic and nonhematologic toxicities may also conspire to reduce chemotherapy dose intensity.[100,106] Of unknown significance are the inhibitory effects of some antiretroviral drugs on lymphoid cell apoptosis, which theoretically could antagonize chemotherapy effects.[107,108] It is also possible that HAART compliance could be compromised by chemotherapy and promote the emergence of HIV viral mutations.

Based on such considerations, the National Cancer Institute investigated the effects of suspension of antiretroviral treatment during DA-EPOCH therapy with immediate reinstitution on chemotherapy completion (Table 81.3 and Table 81.4).[21] In this study of 39 patients with newly diagnosed ARL, pretreatment antiretroviral therapy included HAART in 46 percent, single or dual agents in 26 percent, and 23 percent were treatment naïve. Following antiretroviral suspension during DA-EPOCH, the viral loads increased a median of 0.83 $\log_{10}$ with a plateau between cycles 4 and 6, and at 3 months after restarting antiretroviral treatment, the viral loads declined −0.61 $\log_{10}$, below baseline (Fig. 81.4A). A similar pattern was observed in seven of eight patients with resistant HIV. CD4 cells declined during chemotherapy treatment by a median of 189 cells/μL but recovered to baseline by 6 to 12 months following reinstitution of antiretroviral therapy (Fig. 81.4B). New opportunistic infections were only observed in five patients, all following DA-EPOCH completion. The treatment strategy appeared quite effective with complete remissions in 74 percent of patients, and at a median follow-up time of 53 months, disease-free and overall survivals were 92 percent and 60 percent, respectively. These results are among the best reported to date and raise the question of whether they were benefited by suspension of antiretroviral therapy.[27] Indeed, the salutary effects of HAART on immune function have led to the belief that this benefit exceeds any potential adverse effects on tumor control. Unfortunately, prospective studies have yet to address this potentially important question.

The role of rituximab in AIDS-related lymphoma

The finding that the addition of rituximab to CHOP chemotherapy significantly improves the survival of HIV-negative patients with DLBCL led to its testing in untreated ARL.[109] Pooled results from three phase II studies of rituximab and CDE in ARL have been recently reported (Table 81.3).[110] In this study of 74 patients, 70 percent achieved complete remission and at the median follow-up of approximately 2 years, the estimated failure-free and overall survivals were 59 percent and 64 percent, respectively. New opportunistic infections during or within 3 months of treatment occurred in 14 percent of

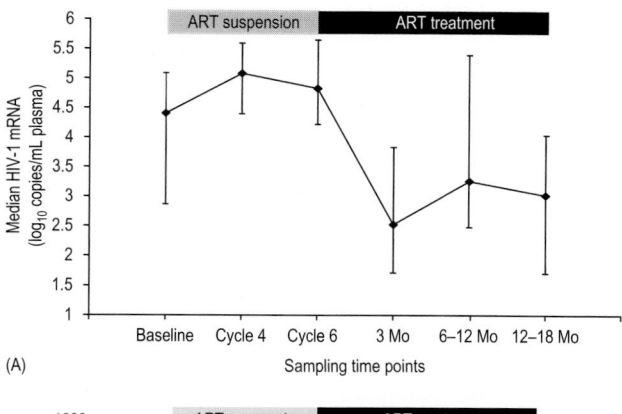

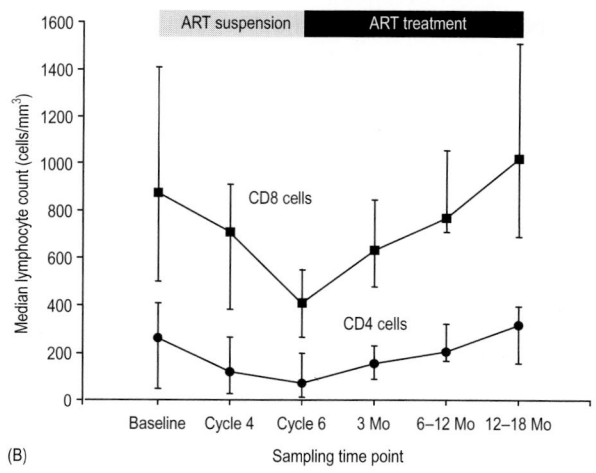

Figure 81.4   Dynamics of human immunodeficiency virus (HIV) viral load and T cell subsets in 30 patients receiving dose-adjusted (DA) EPOCH with temporary suspension of antiretroviral treatment for untreated acquired immune deficiency syndrome (AIDS)-related lymphoma (ARL). (A) Mean change in plasma mRNA HIV viral load during and following DA-EPOCH. (B) Mean change in CD4+ and CD8 T cells measured during and following DA-EPOCH. Vertical bars indicate interquartile range (25th–75th percentile). EPOCH: etoposide, prednisone, vincristine, cyclophosphamide, and doxorubicin.

patients and death from infection occurred in 8 percent of patients. While the good survival outcomes suggest that rituximab conferred a benefit compared to CDE alone, the favorable effects on survival associated with the post-HAART era cannot be discounted.[101]

To help address the role of rituximab, Kaplan *et al.* performed a multicenter randomized (2:1) phase III trial of CHOP with or without rituximab in untreated ARL patients with concomitant HAART administration (Table 81.3).[111] In this trial of 150 patients, disease control was significantly better in patients receiving R-CHOP with lower progression on treatment ($P_2 = 0.02$; Chi-squared test) and reduced death due to lymphoma ($P_2 = 0.02$; Chi-squared test).[112] However, because there was no difference in overall or event-free survival, due to increased infectious deaths in patients receiving R-CHOP, the authors concluded that rituximab does not improve clinical outcome in ARL. It should not escape attention that most treatment-related infectious deaths occurred in patients with low CD4 cell numbers, a group enriched with tumors of ABC type and most likely to benefit from rituximab.[19,21,90] It is also important to note that the administration of maintenance rituximab after chemotherapy, which has not been shown to be necessary in HIV-negative DLBCL, may have contributed to the infection-related fatalities.[113] Indeed, rituximab has recently been linked to the development of late-onset neutropenia (LON) and the administration of maintenance rituximab in ARL could increase the incidence of LON that could be complicated by infectious sequelae.[114]

Employing a somewhat different strategy, the National Cancer Institute is investigating the outcome of a short course (SC) of EPOCH with dose-dense rituximab (375 mg/m^2 days 1 and 5) (SC-EPOCH-R) to reduce treatment-related toxicity. In this study, patients with untreated ARL receive one cycle beyond maximum response, with a minimum of three cycles, compared to six cycles with DA-EPOCH alone.[21,82] Preliminary results in 26 patients reveal a progression-free and overall survival of 79 percent and 74 percent, respectively, at the 29 month median follow-up. Notably, patients received a median of three treatment cycles, compared to six cycles on the prior DA-EPOCH trial. SC-EPOCH-R may also be associated with less CD4 cell loss, with a median decrement of 42 CD4 cells/μL (range +271 to −320) compared to DA-EPOCH, which had a median loss of 189 CD4 cells/μL (range +19 to −973).[21,82]

While the role of rituximab requires further investigation, the aforementioned trials suggest that rituximab is of benefit in ARL. To help further define the role of rituximab, the AMC is currently performing a randomized phase II trial comparing DA-EPOCH-R to DA-EPOCH alone followed by sequential rituximab in responding patients. At the current time, however, we believe it unwise to omit rituximab from the treatment of ARL and hasten to add that while treatment-related infectious deaths can be ameliorated with careful medical attention, disease progression cannot.

Burkitt lymphoma in the HAART era

While there has been an improvement in the collective outcome of HIV-associated lymphomas since HAART, a recent study indicates no improvement in the Burkitt lymphoma subtype.[88,89,92] Lim and colleagues retrospectively analyzed the clinical characteristics and outcome of HIV-associated DLBCL and BL diagnosed between 1982 and 2003 from their institution.[92] In this study, the outcome of BL in the pre- and post-HAART era was similar with complete remission rates of 32 percent and 35 percent and median survivals of 6.4 and 5.7 months, respectively.

This contrasts with the outcome of DLBCL during these periods, which revealed an improvement in complete remission rate from 32 percent to 57 percent and median survival from 8.3 to 43.2 months, respectively. Importantly, the groups had no significant differences in clinical characteristics.

These results raise the possibility that the overall improvement in outcome of HIV-associated lymphomas in the HAART era may be primarily attributable to the better outcome of DLBCL, the most common histologic subtype. Indeed, these findings are not inconsistent with our premise that the higher median CD4 cell counts associated with HAART have increased the proportion of DLBCL with more favorable pathobiology.[19] This does not seem to be the case in BL, which occurs at a high median CD4 cell count and has not shown widely variable pathobiology.[36] As the authors suggest, the relatively poor outcome of HIV-associated BL may be due to the use of CHOP-based regimens, which are known to have a poor outcome in this disease.[36,115] Dose-intense regimens like hyper-CVAD (hyperfractionated cyclophosphamide, vincristine, doxorubicin, and dexamethasone alternating with high-dose methotrexate and cytarabine) have shown encouraging results in HIV-associated BL with a complete remission rate of 92 percent but are often quite toxic.[116] Involvement of the CNS by BL may also contribute to reduced survival and highlights the need for CNS prophylaxis.[21]

Burkitt lymphoma, as an important example, highlights the necessity to balance treatment efficacy and toxicity in patients with HIV infection. Dose-intense 'Burkitt lymphoma' regimens have been considered too toxic to warrant their general use in HIV-positive patients. This has led to the use of CHOP-based treatment with an associated relatively poor outcome. It is worth noting, in this regard, that we are studying the DA-EPOCH-R regimen in BL based on its good activity in highly proliferative DLBCL.[91] Among 15 HIV-negative untreated patients with BL treated with DA-EPOCH-R, we have observed a complete remission rate and overall survival of 100 percent at the median follow-up of 31 months (unpublished observations). Such results suggest that DA-EPOCH-R may be an excellent and well-tolerated alternative to dose-intense regimens for BL in HIV-positive patients.

Treatment at recurrence

Relapsed ARL is associated with a very poor prognosis even in the era of HAART and median survivals tend to be less than 1 year. Therapy options for this group of patients are extremely limited. In the pre-HAART era, an Italian group treated 21 relapsed patients with a combination of etoposide, mitoxantrone, and predmustine. The results were very poor with an overall median survival of just 2 months.[117] Unfortunately, results in the HAART era for salvage therapy in ARL have not shown major improvement. The ESHAP regimen (etoposide, methylprednisone, cytarabine, and cisplatin) has been tested in 13 patients with refractory or relapsed ARL.[118] Although an overall response rate of 54 percent is reported by the authors, the median survival was a mere 7.1 months. Infusional CDE has also been tested in 40 patients with resistant or recurrent ARL. Similar to the above studies, results were discouraging with an overall median survival of only 4 months.[119] Recently, autologous stem cell transplantation has been evaluated in patients with relapsed ARL. Early results suggest that stem cell transplantation may be useful in some relapsed patients but small patient numbers limit any definitive conclusions.[120]

OTHER HIV-ASSOCIATED LYMPHOPROLIFERATIVE DISEASES

Hodgkin lymphoma

Hodgkin lymphoma occurring in the setting of HIV infection is characterized by an aggressive presentation, with a greater likelihood of an unfavorable histology and more advanced disease compared to HL in HIV-negative patients. Principles of therapy should take this into consideration. Because of the high incidence of advanced disease, it is almost always treated with systemic chemotherapy and localized radiation therapy is rarely used. Historically, in the pre-HAART era, patients with HIV-associated HL did poorly with median survivals of 12 to 18 months.[121,122] As in non-Hodgkin lymphoma, the advent of HAART has significantly improved the outcome of HL.[123–125] Few studies have evaluated different regimens in HIV-associated HL, particularly since the advent of HAART, and studies that do exist are too small to make definitive recommendations about regimen efficacy.[123] Thus, ABVD chemotherapy (doxorubicin, bleomycin, vinblastine, and dacarbazine), the standard in HIV-negative patients, should also be considered a standard in HIV-associated HL. The role of concomitant HAART remains controversial, although most specialists would recommend its use.

Primary central nervous system lymphoma

Primary CNS lymphoma associated with HIV typically presents in advanced immunosuppression with median CD4 counts below 50 cells/μL.[126] The incidence of PCNSL has dramatically decreased since the advent of HAART, due to fewer patients with low CD4 cell counts. However, it remains incurable in most patients with an associated short life expectancy.

Primary CNS lymphoma in HIV-positive patients is almost always of DLBCL subtype similar to HIV-negative patients. However, unlike HIV-negative patients, PCNSL in HIV patients is EBV positive.[4] Interestingly, these tumors typically display an immunophenotypic pattern of the GCB type, a favorable biological characteristic in HIV-negative systemic DLBCL.[52,127] Patients frequently present with changes in mental status or focal neurological symptoms and signs and, unlike HIV-negative PCNSL, patients tend to have multiple brain lesions at diagnosis. While CT and MRI are useful imaging modalities, they tend to be nonspecific. With the degree of immunosuppression present in these patients, intracranial opportunistic infections must be considered in the differential diagnoses, and FDG-PET scanning can be useful in this regard.[128]

Unlike HIV-negative PCNSL, where high-dose methotrexate and, more recently, combination chemotherapy regimens are effective, total brain irradiation remains standard in HIV-positive patients.[128] In the pre-HAART era, most studies reported a median survival of approximately 3 months, with half of patients unable to complete therapy.[129] Increased survival to greater than 1.5 years in patients responding to HAART has been reported following effective radiation therapy.[130] One small study looked at using high-dose methotrexate and reported an improvement on this.[131] However, the role of systemic chemotherapy remains undefined in this disease. Novel approaches using rituximab and antiviral therapy against EBV have been reported with some interesting outcomes.[132] Hydroxyurea, again as an anti-EBV therapy, has been reported anecdotally to have promising results.[133]

Primary effusion and plasmablastic lymphoma

The outcome for patients who develop PEL is very poor despite treatment and median survival for this group of patients does not exceed 6 months.[134] Unlike other systemic ARL subtypes, HAART does not seem to have had a dramatic impact on survival of these patients. At this time, the optimal therapy of PEL remains to be defined, but regimens such as CHOP, CDE, or EPOCH are appropriate.[65] Other approaches including the use of high-dose methotrexate with CHOP and parenteral zidovudine (AZT) with interferon alpha have been studied but as yet have demonstrated limited efficacy.[135,136] Patients with PEL should be considered for referral to a clinical trial.

The prognosis of plasmablastic lymphoma in the setting of HIV is poor with median survival of 6 months.[68] Immunologic and virologic control of HIV infection may be important in improving clinical outcome of this disease and anecdotal reports indicate that the prognosis may be better in the era of HAART.[137]

Castleman disease

Castleman disease is a rare clinicopathological entity, originally described in 1954.[138,139] It is typically separated into localized or unicentric Castleman disease (which usually presents with localized lymphadenopathy) and multicentric Castleman disease (MCD), which can present with diffuse lymphadenopathy and multiorgan involvement. A plasmablastic variant of MCD has also been described.[140]

In the setting of HIV, MCD is not infrequently encountered. An association between MCD and AIDS-associated Kaposi sarcoma was first observed in the 1980s.[141] Kaposi sarcoma herpes virus/HHV-8 was subsequently etiologically linked to MCD in the setting of HIV.[142] Evidence suggests that IL-6, expressed by the KSHV/HHV-8 genome, is important in the pathogenesis of MCD.[139] Histologically, MCD is characterized by the plasma cell variant in contrast to the hyalinized vascular type which is found in 90 percent of cases of localized disease. In the plasma cell variant, affected lymph nodes show no evidence of hyalinization. Concentric sheets of plasma cells occupy the germinal centers and interfollicular areas of nodes. The intense vascular proliferation seen with the hyalinized vascular type is absent.

Patients with HIV-associated MCD often present with constitutional symptoms including fevers, night sweats, and weight loss. Multiple lymphadenopathy and hepatosplenomegaly are common. Edema and pleural and pericardial effusions can be present and pulmonary complications of the disease are frequently encountered in the setting of HIV. There are limited data on the impact of HAART on the course of MCD. Some small series suggest an improved survival in the HAART era but reports are few and it is difficult to make any meaningful conclusions.[143] Several therapies for MCD have been reported including immune modulators like interferon alpha and thalidomide, monoclonal antibodies against CD20 (rituximab) and IL-6, antiviral therapy, and systemic chemotherapy.[140,144–147] Though some of these approaches are promising, the long-term prognosis for most patients remains poor.

CONCLUSIONS

Over recent years, significant progress has been made in the understanding and management of HIV-associated lymphoid neoplasms. Having once been a usually fatal complication of HIV infection, the development of novel chemotherapeutic strategies and HAART treatment has made ARL a curable complication. Significant controversies remain such as the role of concomitant HAART during chemotherapy and the role of the monoclonal antibody rituximab. Hopefully, the results of ongoing clinical trials will help address some of these controversies. Nevertheless, it is clear that the new treatment frontiers need to focus on patients with severe immune suppression and the poor prognosis histologic subtypes which are more common in this setting.

KEY POINTS

Key issues covered in this chapter:

- Evolving epidemiology of HIV-associated lymphoid neoplasms and impact of HAART.
- Etiology, pathogenesis, and pathobiology of HIV-associated lymphoid neoplasms.
- Clinical, diagnostic, and prognostic (molecular and clinical) features of HIV-associated lymphoid neoplasms.
- Therapy of AIDS-related lymphoma and impact of histology, pathobiology, and HAART on outcome.
- Impact of molecular pathobiology on new therapeutic approaches.

REFERENCES

● = Key primary paper

◆ = Major review article

1. Goedert JJ, Cote TR, Virgo P et al. Spectrum of AIDS-associated malignant disorders. *Lancet* 1998; **351**: 1833–9.
2. Beral V, Peterman T, Berkelman R, Jaffe H. AIDS-associated non-Hodgkin lymphoma. *Lancet* 1991; **337**: 805–9.
3. Cote TR, Biggar RJ, Rosenberg PS et al. Non-Hodgkin's lymphoma among people with AIDS: incidence, presentation and public health burden. AIDS/Cancer Study Group. *Int J Cancer* 1997; **73**: 645–50.
4. Jaffe ES, Harris NL, Stein H, Vardiman JW. *World Health Organization classification of tumours. Pathology and genetics of tumours of hematopoietic and lymphoid tissues.* Lyon: IARC Press, 2001.
5. Frisch M, Biggar RJ, Engels EA, Goedert JJ. Association of cancer with AIDS-related immunosuppression in adults. *JAMA* 2001; **285**: 1736–45.
6. Navarro WH, Kaplan LD. AIDS-related lymphoproliferative disease. *Blood* 2006; **107**: 13–20.
7. Grulich AE, Wan X, Law MG et al. Risk of cancer in people with AIDS. *AIDS* 1999; **13**: 839–43.
8. Mbulaiteye SM, Katabira ET, Wabinga H et al. Spectrum of cancers among HIV-infected persons in Africa: The Uganda AIDS-Cancer Registry Match Study. *Int J Cancer* 2006; **118**: 985–90.
9. Ledergerber B, Telenti A, Egger M. Risk of HIV related Kaposi's sarcoma and non-Hodgkin's lymphoma with potent antiretroviral therapy: prospective cohort study. Swiss HIV Cohort Study. *BMJ* 1999; **319**: 23–4.
10. Cooper IA, Wolf MM, Robertson TI et al. Randomized comparison of MACOP-B with CHOP in patients with intermediate-grade non-Hodgkin's lymphoma. The

Australian and New Zealand Lymphoma Group.
J Clin Oncol 1994; **12**: 769–78.

11. Highly active antiretroviral therapy and incidence of cancer in human immunodeficiency virus-infected adults. *J Natl Cancer Inst* 2000; **92**: 1823–30.

●12. Besson C, Goubar A, Gabarre J *et al.* Changes in AIDS-related lymphoma since the era of highly active antiretroviral therapy. *Blood* 2001; **98**: 2339–44.

13. Clifford GM, Polesel J, Rickenbach M *et al.* Cancer risk in the Swiss HIV Cohort Study: associations with immunodeficiency, smoking, and highly active antiretroviral therapy. *J Natl Cancer Inst* 2005; **97**: 425–32.

14. Grulich AE, Li Y, McDonald AM *et al.* Decreasing rates of Kaposi's sarcoma and non-Hodgkin's lymphoma in the era of potent combination anti-retroviral therapy. *AIDS* 2001; **15**: 629–33.

15. Kirk O, Pedersen C, Cozzi-Lepri A *et al.* Non-Hodgkin lymphoma in HIV-infected patients in the era of highly active antiretroviral therapy. *Blood* 2001; **98**: 3406–12.

16. Raphael MM, Audouin J, Lamine M *et al.* Immunophenotypic and genotypic analysis of acquired immunodeficiency syndrome-related non-Hodgkin's lymphomas. Correlation with histologic features in 36 cases. French Study Group of Pathology for HIV-Associated Tumors. *Am J Clin Pathol* 1994; **101**: 773–82.

◆17. Little RF, Wilson WH. Update on the pathogenesis, diagnosis, and therapy of AIDS-related lymphoma. *Curr Infect Dis Rep* 2003; **5**: 176–84.

18. Kalter SP, Riggs SA, Cabanillas F *et al.* Aggressive non-Hodgkin's lymphomas in immunocompromised homosexual males. *Blood* 1985; **66**: 655–9.

◆19. Carbone A, Gloghini A. AIDS-related lymphomas: from pathogenesis to pathology. *Br J Haematol* 2005; **130**: 662–70.

20. Hoffmann C, Tiemann M, Schrader C *et al.* AIDS-related B-cell lymphoma (ARL): correlation of prognosis with differentiation profiles assessed by immunophenotyping. *Blood* 2005; **106**: 1762–9.

●21. Little RF, Pittaluga S, Grant N *et al.* Highly effective treatment of acquired immunodeficiency syndrome-related lymphoma with dose-adjusted EPOCH: impact of antiretroviral therapy suspension and tumor biology. *Blood* 2003; **101**: 4653–9.

22. Carbonari M, Caprini E, Tedesco T *et al.* Hepatitis C virus drives the unconstrained monoclonal expansion of VH1-69-expressing memory B cells in type II cryoglobulinemia: a model of infection-driven lymphomagenesis. *J Immunol* 2005; **174**: 6532–9.

23. Isaacson PG, Du MQ. Gastrointestinal lymphoma: where morphology meets molecular biology. *J Pathol* 2005; **205**: 255–74.

24. Hussell T, Isaacson PG, Crabtree JE, Spencer J. The response of cells from low-grade B-cell gastric lymphomas of mucosa-associated lymphoid tissue to Helicobacter pylori. *Lancet* 1993; **342**: 571–4.

25. Ambinder RF. Epstein-Barr virus associated lymphoproliferations in the AIDS setting. *Eur J Cancer* 2001; **37**: 1209–16.

26. Carbone A, Tirelli U, Gloghini A *et al.* Human immunodeficiency virus-associated systemic lymphomas may be subdivided into two main groups according to Epstein-Barr viral latent gene expression. *J Clin Oncol* 1993; **11**: 1674–81.

27. Lim ST, Levine AM. Recent advances in acquired immunodeficiency syndrome (AIDS)-related lymphoma. *CA Cancer J Clin* 2005; **55**: 229–41, 260–1, 264.

28. Davi F, Delecluse HJ, Guiet P *et al.* Burkitt-like lymphomas in AIDS patients: characterization within a series of 103 human immunodeficiency virus-associated non-Hodgkin's lymphomas. Burkitt's Lymphoma Study Group. *J Clin Oncol* 1998; **16**: 3788–95.

29. Martin A, Flaman JM, Frebourg T *et al.* Functional analysis of the p53 protein in AIDS-related non-Hodgkin's lymphomas and polymorphic lymphoproliferations. *Br J Haematol* 1998; **101**: 311–17.

●30. Nador RG, Cesarman E, Chadburn A *et al.* Primary effusion lymphoma: a distinct clinicopathologic entity associated with the Kaposi's sarcoma-associated herpes virus. *Blood* 1996; **88**: 645–56.

31. Gaidano G, Capello D, Carbone A. The molecular basis of acquired immunodeficiency syndrome-related lymphomagenesis. *Semin Oncol* 2000; **27**: 431–41.

32. Henderson S, Rowe M, Gregory C *et al.* Induction of bcl-2 expression by Epstein-Barr virus latent membrane protein 1 protects infected B cells from programmed cell death. *Cell* 1991; **65**: 1107–15.

33. Rothe M, Sarma V, Dixit VM, Goeddel DV. TRAF2-mediated activation of NF-kappa B by TNF receptor 2 and CD40. *Science* 1995; **269**: 1424–7.

◆34. Carbone A. Emerging pathways in the development of AIDS-related lymphomas. *Lancet Oncol* 2003; **4**: 22–9.

35. Gaidano G, Carbone A. AIDS-related lymphomas: from pathogenesis to pathology. *Br J Haematol* 1995; **90**: 235–43.

36. Dave SS, Fu K, Wright G *et al.* Gene expression distinguishes Burkitt lymphoma from other aggressive lymphomas and identifies patients who are highly curable with intensive chemotherapeutic regimens. *Blood* 2005; **106**: 415.

37. Gaidano G, Capello D, Cilia AM *et al.* Genetic characterization of HHV-8/KSHV-positive primary effusion lymphoma reveals frequent mutations of BCL6: implications for disease pathogenesis and histogenesis. *Genes Chromosomes Cancer* 1999; **24**: 16–23.

38. Gaidano G, Carbone A, Pastore C *et al.* Frequent mutation of the 5′ noncoding region of the BCL-6 gene in acquired immunodeficiency syndrome-related non-Hodgkin's lymphomas. *Blood* 1997; **89**: 3755–62.

39. Gaidano G, Lo Coco F, Ye BH *et al.* Rearrangements of the BCL-6 gene in acquired immunodeficiency syndrome-associated non-Hodgkin's lymphoma: association with diffuse large-cell subtype. *Blood* 1994; **84**: 397–402.

40. Ballerini P, Gaidano G, Gong JZ et al. Multiple genetic lesions in acquired immunodeficiency syndrome-related non-Hodgkin's lymphoma. Blood 1993; 81: 166–76.

41. Gaidano G, Pastore C, Lanza C et al. Molecular pathology of AIDS-related lymphomas. Biologic aspects and clinicopathologic heterogeneity. Ann Hematol 1994; 69: 281–90.

42. Breen EC, Boscardin WJ, Detels R et al. Non-Hodgkin's B cell lymphoma in persons with acquired immunodeficiency syndrome is associated with increased serum levels of IL10, or the IL10 promoter -592 C/C genotype. Clin Immunol 2003; 109: 119–29.

43. Emilie D, Zou W, Fior R et al. Production and roles of IL-6, IL-10, and IL-13 in B-lymphocyte malignancies and in B-lymphocyte hyperactivity of HIV infection and autoimmunity. Methods 1997; 11: 133–42.

44. Rabkin CS, Yang Q, Goedert JJ et al. Chemokine and chemokine receptor gene variants and risk of non-Hodgkin's lymphoma in human immunodeficiency virus-1-infected individuals. Blood 1999; 93: 1838–42.

45. Wilson WH, Teruya-Feldstein J, Fest T et al. Relationship of p53, bcl-2, and tumor proliferation to clinical drug resistance in non-Hodgkin's lymphomas. Blood 1997; 89: 601–9.

46. Wiestner A, Staudt, LM. Towards a molecular diagnosis and targeted therapy of lymphoid malignancies. Semin Hematol 2003; 40: 296–307.

47. Alizadeh AA, Eisen MB, Davis RE et al. Distinct types of diffuse large B-cell lymphoma identified by gene expression profiling. Nature 2000; 403: 503–11.

48. Dalla-Favera R, Migliazza A, Chang CC et al. Molecular pathogenesis of B cell malignancy: the role of BCL-6. Curr Top Microbiol Immunol 1999; 246: 257–63, discussion 263–5.

49. Matsuyama T, Grossman A, Mittrucker HW et al. Molecular cloning of LSIRF, a lymphoid-specific member of the interferon regulatory factor family that binds the interferon-stimulated response element (ISRE). Nucleic Acids Res 1995; 23: 2127–36.

50. Mittrucker HW, Matsuyama T, Grossman A et al. Requirement for the transcription factor LSIRF/IRF4 for mature B and T lymphocyte function. Science 1997; 275: 540–43.

51. Tschopp J, Irmler M, Thome M. Inhibition of fas death signals by FLIPs. Curr Opin Immunol 1998; 10: 552–8.

52. Rosenwald A, Wright G, Chan WC et al. The use of molecular profiling to predict survival after chemotherapy for diffuse large-B-cell lymphoma. N Engl J Med 2002; 346: 1937–47.

●53. Klein U, Gloghini A, Gaidano G et al. Gene expression profile analysis of AIDS-related primary effusion lymphoma (PEL) suggests a plasmablastic derivation and identifies PEL-specific transcripts. Blood 2003; 101: 4115–21.

●54. Fan W, Bubman D, Chadburn A et al. Distinct subsets of primary effusion lymphoma can be identified based on their cellular gene expression profile and viral association. J Virol 2005; 79: 1244–51.

●55. Carbone A, Gloghini A, Larocca LM et al. Expression profile of MUM1/IRF4, BCL-6, and CD138/syndecan-1 defines novel histogenetic subsets of human immunodeficiency virus-related lymphomas. Blood 2001; 97: 744–51.

56. Hans CP, Weisenburger DD, Greiner TC et al. Confirmation of the molecular classification of diffuse large B-cell lymphoma by immunohistochemistry using a tissue microarray. Blood 2004; 103: 275–82.

57. Colomo L, Loong F, Rives S et al. Diffuse large B-cell lymphomas with plasmablastic differentiation represent a heterogeneous group of disease entities. Am J Surg Pathol 2004; 28: 736–47.

58. Vega F, Chang CC, Medeiros LJ et al. Plasmablastic lymphomas and plasmablastic plasma cell myelomas have nearly identical immunophenotypic profiles. Mod Pathol 2005; 18: 806–15.

59. Raphael M, Gentilhomme O, Tulliez M et al. Histopathologic features of high-grade non-Hodgkin's lymphomas in acquired immunodeficiency syndrome. The French Study Group of Pathology for Human Immunodeficiency Virus-Associated Tumors. Arch Pathol Lab Med 1991; 115: 15–20.

60. Jaffe ES, Harris NL, Diebold J, Muller-Hermelink HK. World Health Organization classification of neoplastic diseases of the hematopoietic and lymphoid tissues. A progress report. Am J Clin Pathol 1999; 111: S8–12.

61. Thompson LD, Fisher SI, Chu WS et al. HIV-associated Hodgkin lymphoma: a clinicopathologic and immunophenotypic study of 45 cases. Am J Clin Pathol 2004; 121: 727–38.

62. Biggar RJ, Engels EA, Frisch M, Goedert JJ. Risk of T-cell lymphomas in persons with AIDS. J Acquir Immune Defic Syndr 2001; 26: 371–6.

63. McClain KL, Leach CT, Jenson HB et al. Molecular and virologic characteristics of lymphoid malignancies in children with AIDS. J Acquir Immune Defic Syndr 2000; 23: 152–9.

64. Teruya-Feldstein J, Temeck BK, Sloas MM et al. Pulmonary malignant lymphoma of mucosa-associated lymphoid tissue (MALT) arising in a pediatric HIV-positive patient. Am J Surg Pathol 1995; 19: 357–63.

65. Simonelli C, Spina M, Cinelli R et al. Clinical features and outcome of primary effusion lymphoma in HIV-infected patients: a single-institution study. J Clin Oncol 2003; 21: 3948–54.

66. Chadburn A, Hyjek E, Mathew S et al. KSHV-positive solid lymphomas represent an extra-cavitary variant of primary effusion lymphoma. Am J Surg Pathol 2004; 28: 1401–16.

67. Hamoudi R, Diss TC, Oksenhendler E et al. Distinct cellular origins of primary effusion lymphoma with and without EBV infection. Leuk Res 2004; 28: 333–8.

●68. Delecluse HJ, Anagnostopoulos I, Dallenbach F et al. Plasmablastic lymphomas of the oral cavity: a new entity associated with the human immunodeficiency virus infection. Blood 1997; 89: 1413–20.

69. Nador RG, Chadburn A, Gundappa G et al. Human immunodeficiency virus (HIV)-associated polymorphic

lymphoproliferative disorders. *Am J Surg Pathol* 2003; **27**: 293–302.

70. Seneviratne L, Espina BM, Nathwani BN *et al.* Clinical, immunologic, and pathologic correlates of bone marrow involvement in 291 patients with acquired immunodeficiency syndrome-related lymphoma. *Blood* 2001; **98**: 2358–63.

71. Bower M, Gazzard B, Mandalia S *et al.* A prognostic index for systemic AIDS-related non-Hodgkin lymphoma treated in the era of highly active antiretroviral therapy. *Ann Intern Med* 2005; **143**: 265–73.

72. Ames ED, Conjalka MS, Goldberg AF *et al.* Hodgkin's disease and AIDS. Twenty-three new cases and a review of the literature. *Hematol Oncol Clin North Am* 1991; **5**: 343–56.

73. Gaidano G, Carbone A. Primary effusion lymphoma: a liquid phase lymphoma of fluid-filled body cavities. *Adv Cancer Res* 2001; **80**: 115–46.

74. Huang Q, Chang KL, Gaal K, Arber DA. Primary effusion lymphoma with subsequent development of a small bowel mass in an HIV-seropositive patient: a case report and literature review. *Am J Surg Pathol* 2002; **26**: 1363–7.

75. Chetty R, Hlatswayo N, Muc R *et al.* Plasmablastic lymphoma in HIV+ patients: an expanding spectrum. *Histopathology* 2003; **42**: 605–9.

●76. Hegde U, Filie A, Little RF *et al.* High incidence of occult leptomeningeal disease detected by flow cytometry in newly diagnosed aggressive B-cell lymphomas at risk for central nervous system involvement: the role of flow cytometry versus cytology. *Blood* 2005; **105**: 496–502.

77. Turoglu HT, Akisik MF, Naddaf SY *et al.* Tumor and infection localization in AIDS patients: Ga-67 and Tl-201 findings. *Clin Nucl Med* 1998; **23**: 446–59.

78. Podzamczer D, Ricart I, Bolao F *et al.* Gallium-67 scan for distinguishing follicular hyperplasia from other AIDS-associated diseases in lymph nodes. *AIDS* 1990; **4**: 683–5.

79. Foo SS, Mitchell PL, Berlangieri SU *et al.* Positron emission tomography scanning in the assessment of patients with lymphoma. *Intern Med J* 2004; **34**: 388–97.

80. Stumpe KD, Urbinelli M, Steinert HC *et al.* Whole-body positron emission tomography using fluorodeoxyglucose for staging of lymphoma: effectiveness and comparison with computed tomography. *Eur J Nucl Med* 1998; **25**: 721–8.

81. Burton C, Ell P, Linch D. The role of PET imaging in lymphoma. *Br J Haematol* 2004; **126**: 772–84.

82. Dunleavy K, Wayne A, Little R *et al.* The addition of rituximab to dose-adjusted EPOCH with HAART suspension is highly effective and tolerable in AIDS-related lymphoma (ARL) and allows the delivery of abbreviated chemotherapy. *Blood* 2005; **106**: 930.

83. A predictive model for aggressive non-Hodgkin's lymphoma. The International Non-Hodgkin's Lymphoma Prognostic Factors Project. *N Engl J Med* 1993; **329**: 987–94.

84. Rossi G, Donisi A, Casari S *et al.* The International Prognostic Index can be used as a guide to treatment decisions regarding patients with human immunodeficiency virus-related systemic non-Hodgkin lymphoma. *Cancer* 1999; **86**: 2391–7.

85. Vaccher E, Tirelli U, Spina M *et al.* Age and serum lactate dehydrogenase level are independent prognostic factors in human immunodeficiency virus-related non-Hodgkin's lymphomas: a single-institute study of 96 patients. *J Clin Oncol* 1996; **14**: 2217–23.

86. Straus DJ, Huang J, Testa MA *et al.* Prognostic factors in the treatment of human immunodeficiency virus-associated non-Hodgkin's lymphoma: analysis of AIDS Clinical Trials Group protocol 142 – low-dose versus standard-dose m-BACOD plus granulocyte-macrophage colony-stimulating factor. National Institute of Allergy and Infectious Diseases. *J Clin Oncol* 1998; **16**: 3601–6.

87. Kaplan LD, Straus DJ, Testa MA *et al.* Low-dose compared with standard-dose m-BACOD chemotherapy for non-Hodgkin's lymphoma associated with human immunodeficiency virus infection. National Institute of Allergy and Infectious Diseases AIDS Clinical Trials Group. *N Engl J Med* 1997; **336**: 1641–8.

88. Lascaux AS, Hemery F, Goujard C *et al.* Beneficial effect of highly active antiretroviral therapy on the prognosis of AIDS-related systemic non-Hodgkin lymphomas. *AIDS Res Hum Retroviruses* 2005; **21**: 214–20.

89. Wolf T, Brodt HR, Fichtlscherer S *et al.* Changing incidence and prognostic factors of survival in AIDS-related non-Hodgkin's lymphoma in the era of highly active antiretroviral therapy (HAART). *Leuk Lymphoma* 2005; **46**: 207–15.

90. Wilson WH, Dunleavy K, Pittaluga S *et al.* Dose-adjusted EPOCH-rituximab is highly effective in the GCB and ABC subtypes of untreated diffuse large B-cell lymphoma. *Blood* 2004; **104**: 159.

91. Wilson WH, Grossbard ML, Pittaluga S *et al.* Dose-adjusted EPOCH chemotherapy for untreated large B-cell lymphomas: a pharmacodynamic approach with high efficacy. *Blood* 2002; **99**: 2685–93.

●92. Lim ST, Karim R, Nathwani BN *et al.* AIDS-related Burkitt's lymphoma versus diffuse large-cell lymphoma in the pre-highly active antiretroviral therapy (HAART) and HAART eras: significant differences in survival with standard chemotherapy. *J Clin Oncol* 2005; **23**: 4430–38.

93. Kaplan LD, Abrams DI, Feigal E *et al.* AIDS-associated non-Hodgkin's lymphoma in San Francisco. *JAMA* 1989; **261**: 719–24.

94. Levine AM, Wernz JC, Kaplan L *et al.* Low-dose chemotherapy with central nervous system prophylaxis and zidovudine maintenance in AIDS-related lymphoma. A prospective multi-institutional trial. *JAMA* 1991; **266**: 84–8.

95. Wilson WH. Chemotherapy for AIDS-related lymphomas. *N Engl J Med* 1997; **337**: 1172–3; author reply 1173–4.

96. Kwak LW, Halpern J, Olshen RA, Horning SJ. Prognostic significance of actual dose intensity in diffuse large-cell lymphoma: results of a tree-structured survival analysis. *J Clin Oncol* 1990; **8**: 963–77.

97. Fisher RI, Gaynor ER, Dahlberg S et al. Comparison of a standard regimen (CHOP) with three intensive chemotherapy regimens for advanced non-Hodgkin's lymphoma. N Engl J Med 1993; **328**: 1002–6.

●98. Ratner L, Lee J, Tang S et al. Chemotherapy for human immunodeficiency virus-associated non-Hodgkin's lymphoma in combination with highly active antiretroviral therapy. J Clin Oncol 2001; **19**: 2171–8.

●99. Toffoli G, Corona G, Cattarossi G et al. Effect of highly active antiretroviral therapy (HAART) on pharmacokinetics and pharmacodynamics of doxorubicin in patients with HIV-associated non-Hodgkin's lymphoma. Ann Oncol 2004; **15**: 1805–9.

100. Vaccher E, Spina M, di Gennaro G et al. Concomitant cyclophosphamide, doxorubicin, vincristine, and prednisone chemotherapy plus highly active antiretroviral therapy in patients with human immunodeficiency virus-related, non-Hodgkin lymphoma. Cancer 2001; **91**: 155–63.

101. Sparano JA, Lee S, Chen MG et al. Phase II trial of infusional cyclophosphamide, doxorubicin, and etoposide in patients with HIV-associated non-Hodgkin's lymphoma: an Eastern Cooperative Oncology Group Trial (E1494). J Clin Oncol 2004; **22**: 1491–500.

102. Sparano J, Wiernik P, Hu X et al. Pilot trial of infusional cyclophosphamide, doxorubicin, and etoposide plus didanosine and filgrastim in patients with human immunodeficiency virus-associated non-Hodgkin's lymphoma. J Clin Oncol 1996; **14**: 3026–35.

103. Tulpule A, Sherrod A, Dharmapala D et al. Multidrug resistance (MDR-1) expression in aids-related lymphomas. Leuk Res 2002; **26**: 121–7.

104. Lynch A, Harvey J, Aylott M et al. Investigations into the concept of a threshold for topoisomerase inhibitor-induced clastogenicity. Mutagenesis 2003; **18**: 345–53.

105. Wilson WH, Bates SE, Fojo A et al. Controlled trial of dexverapamil, a modulator of multidrug resistance, in lymphomas refractory to EPOCH chemotherapy. J Clin Oncol 1995; **13**: 1995–2004.

106. Sparano JA, Wiernik PH, Hu X et al. Saquinavir enhances the mucosal toxicity of infusional cyclophosphamide, doxorubicin, and etoposide in patients with HIV-associated non-Hodgkin's lymphoma. Med Oncol 1998; **15**: 50–57.

107. Phenix BN, Cooper C, Owen C, Badley AD. Modulation of apoptosis by HIV protease inhibitors. Apoptosis 2002; **7**: 295–312.

108. Phenix BN, Lum JJ, Nie Z et al. Antiapoptotic mechanism of HIV protease inhibitors: preventing mitochondrial transmembrane potential loss. Blood 2001; **98**: 1078–85.

109. Coiffier B, Lepage E, Briere J et al. CHOP chemotherapy plus rituximab compared with CHOP alone in elderly patients with diffuse large-B-cell lymphoma. N Engl J Med 2002; **346**: 235–42.

●110. Spina M, Jaeger U, Sparano JA et al. Rituximab plus infusional cyclophosphamide, doxorubicin, and etoposide in HIV-associated non-Hodgkin lymphoma: pooled results from 3 phase 2 trials. Blood 2005; **105**: 1891–7.

●111. Kaplan LD, Lee JY, Ambinder RF et al. Rituximab does not improve clinical outcome in a randomized phase 3 trial of CHOP with or without rituximab in patients with HIV-associated non-Hodgkin lymphoma: AIDS-Malignancies Consortium Trial 010. Blood 2005; **106**: 1538–43.

112. Dunleavy K, Wilson WH, Kaplan LD. The case for rituximab in AIDS-related lymphoma. Blood 2006; **107**: 3014–15.

113. Habermann TM, Weller E, Morrison VA et al. Rituximab-CHOP versus CHOP with or without maintenance rituximab in patients 60 years of age or older with diffuse large B-cell lymphoma (DLBCL): an update. Blood 2004; **104**: 127.

●114. Dunleavy K, Hakim F, Kim HK et al. B-cell recovery following rituximab-based therapy is associated with perturbations in stromal derived factor-1 and granulocyte homeostasis. Blood 2005; **106**: 795–802.

115. Bishop PC, Rao VK, Wilson WH. Burkitt's lymphoma: molecular pathogenesis and treatment. Cancer Invest 2000; **18**: 574–83.

116. Cortes J, Thomas D, Rios A et al. Hyperfractionated cyclophosphamide, vincristine, doxorubicin, and dexamethasone and highly active antiretroviral therapy for patients with acquired immunodeficiency syndrome-related Burkitt lymphoma/leukemia. Cancer 2002; **94**: 1492–9.

117. Tirelli U, Errante D, Spina M et al. Second-line chemotherapy in human immunodeficiency virus-related non-Hodgkin's lymphoma: evidence of activity of a combination of etoposide, mitoxantrone, and prednimustine in relapsed patients. Cancer 1996; **77**: 2127–31.

118. Bi J, Espina BM, Tulpule A et al. High-dose cytosine-arabinoside and cisplatin regimens as salvage therapy for refractory or relapsed AIDS-related non-Hodgkin's lymphoma. J Acquir Immune Defic Syndr 2001; **28**: 416–21.

119. Spina M, Vaccher E, Juzbasic S et al. Human immunodeficiency virus-related non-Hodgkin lymphoma: activity of infusional cyclophosphamide, doxorubicin, and etoposide as second-line chemotherapy in 40 patients. Cancer 2001; **92**: 200–6.

120. Krishnan A, Molina A, Zaia J et al. Durable remissions with autologous stem cell transplantation for high-risk HIV-associated lymphomas. Blood 2005; **105**: 874–8.

121. Hartmann P, Rehwald U, Salzberger B et al. Current treatment strategies for patients with Hodgkin's lymphoma and HIV infection. Expert Rev Anticancer Ther 2004;**4**: 401–10.

122. Levine AM, Li P, Cheung T et al. Chemotherapy consisting of doxorubicin, bleomycin, vinblastine, and dacarbazine with granulocyte-colony-stimulating factor in HIV-infected patients with newly diagnosed Hodgkin's disease: a prospective, multi-institutional AIDS clinical trials group

study (ACTG 149). *J Acquir Immune Defic Syndr* 2000; **24**: 444–50.

123. Hartmann P, Rehwald U, Salzberger B *et al.* BEACOPP therapeutic regimen for patients with Hodgkin's disease and HIV infection. *Ann Oncol* 2003; **14**: 1562–9.

124. Hoffmann C, Chow KU, Wolf E *et al.* Strong impact of highly active antiretroviral therapy on survival in patients with human immunodeficiency virus-associated Hodgkin's disease. *Br J Haematol* 2004; **125**: 455–62.

125. Gerard L, Galicier L, Boulanger E *et al.* Improved survival in HIV-related Hodgkin's lymphoma since the introduction of highly active antiretroviral therapy. *AIDS* 2003; **17**: 81–7.

126. Levine AM. Acquired immunodeficiency syndrome-related lymphoma: clinical aspects. *Semin Oncol* 2000; **27**: 442–53.

●127. Montesinos-Rongen M, Kuppers R, Schluter D *et al.* Primary central nervous system lymphomas are derived from germinal-center B cells and show a preferential usage of the V4-34 gene segment. *Am J Pathol* 1999; **155**: 2077–86.

128. Heald AE, Hoffman JM, Bartlett JA, Waskin HA. Differentiation of central nervous system lesions in AIDS patients using positron emission tomography (PET). *Int J STD AIDS* 1996; **7**: 337–46.

129. Ling SM, Roach M 3rd, Larson DA, Wara WM. Radiotherapy of primary central nervous system lymphoma in patients with and without human immunodeficiency virus. Ten years of treatment experience at the University of California San Francisco. *Cancer* 1994; **73**: 2570–82.

130. Hoffmann C, Tabrizian S, Wolf E *et al.* Survival of AIDS patients with primary central nervous system lymphoma is dramatically improved by HAART-induced immune recovery. *AIDS* 2001; **15**: 2119–27.

131. Jacomet C, Girard PM, Lebrette MG *et al.* Intravenous methotrexate for primary central nervous system non-Hodgkin's lymphoma in AIDS. *AIDS* 1997; **11**: 1725–30.

132. Hanel M, Fiedler F, Thorns C. Anti-CD20 monoclonal antibody (Rituximab) and Cidofovir as successful treatment of an EBV-associated lymphoma with CNS involvement. *Onkologie* 2001; **24**: 491–4.

133. Slobod KS, Taylor GH, Sandlund JT *et al.* Epstein-Barr virus-targeted therapy for AIDS-related primary lymphoma of the central nervous system. *Lancet* 2000; **356**: 1493–4.

134. Boulanger E, Gerard L, Gabarre J *et al.* Prognostic factors and outcome of human herpesvirus 8-associated primary

effusion lymphoma in patients with AIDS. *J Clin Oncol* 2005; **23**: 4372–80.

135. Boulanger E, Daniel MT, Agbalika F, Oksenhendler E. Combined chemotherapy including high-dose methotrexate in KSHV/HHV8-associated primary effusion lymphoma. *Am J Hematol* 2003; **73**: 143–8.

●136. Ghosh SK, Wood C, Boise LH *et al.* Potentiation of TRAIL-induced apoptosis in primary effusion lymphoma through azidothymidine-mediated inhibition of NF-kappa B. *Blood* 2003; **101**: 2321–7.

137. Lester R, Li C, Phillips P *et al.* Improved outcome of human immunodeficiency virus-associated plasmablastic lymphoma of the oral cavity in the era of highly active antiretroviral therapy: a report of two cases. *Leuk Lymphoma* 2004; **45**: 1881–5.

138. Castleman B, Towne VW. Case records of the Massachusetts General Hospital: Case No. 40231. *N Engl J Med* 1954; **250**: 1001–5.

139. Waterston A, Bower M. Fifty years of multicentric Castleman's disease. *Acta Oncol* 2004; **43**: 698–704.

◆140. Casper C. The aetiology and management of Castleman disease at 50 years: translating pathophysiology to patient care. *Br J Haematol* 2005; **129**: 3–17.

141. Chen KT. Multicentric Castleman's disease and Kaposi's sarcoma. *Am J Surg Pathol* 1984; **8**: 287–93.

●142. Soulier J, Grollet L, Oksenhendler E *et al.* Kaposi's sarcoma-associated herpesvirus-like DNA sequences in multicentric Castleman's disease. *Blood* 1995; **86**: 1276–80.

143. Aaron L, Lidove O, Yousry C *et al.* Human herpesvirus 8-positive Castleman disease in human immunodeficiency virus-infected patients: the impact of highly active antiretroviral therapy. *Clin Infect Dis* 2002; **35**: 880–82.

144. Jung CP, Emmerich B, Goebel FD, Bogner JR. Successful treatment of a patient with HIV-associated multicentric Castleman disease (MCD) with thalidomide. *Am J Hematol* 2004; **75**: 176–7.

145. Kumari P, Schechter GP, Saini N, Benator DA. Successful treatment of human immunodeficiency virus-related Castleman's disease with interferon-alpha. *Clin Infect Dis* 2000; **31**: 602–4.

146. Marcelin AG, Aaron L, Mateus C *et al.* Rituximab therapy for HIV-associated Castleman disease. *Blood* 2003; **102**: 2786–8.

147. Nishimoto N, Sasai M, Shima Y *et al.* Improvement in Castleman's disease by humanized anti-interleukin-6 receptor antibody therapy. *Blood* 2000; **95**: 56–61.

82

Lymphoid neoplasms in immunodeficiency, immunosuppression and autoimmunity

PL AMLOT

INTRODUCTION

Impaired immunity resulting from acquired or primary immune deficiency (PID), immunosuppression (IS), or autoimmunity (AI) predisposes to infection and malignancy. Infection and chronic antigenic stimulation are important etiologic factors for malignancies arising in immunodeficiency (ID) and the malignancies are not the same as those seen in the general population. Lymphomas are the most common neoplasms seen in ID. The commonest infective agent in ID causing cancer is the oncogenic Epstein–Barr virus (EBV or human herpes virus 4 [HHV-4]) present in diffuse large B cell lymphoma (DLBCL), Burkitt lymphoma (BL), Hodgkin disease (HD), and lymphomatoid granulomatosis (LyG). Less commonly involved is the Kaposi sarcoma herpes virus (KSHV or HHV-8) in some DLBCL and primary effusion lymphoma (PEL) or *Helicobacter pylori* predisposing to marginal zone (MZ) or mucosal-associated lymphoid tissue (MALT) lymphomas.

The nature of the immune deficiency and environmental factors can influence the risk of lymphomagenesis. There are certain common features about lymphomas arising in ID. These are summarized below and followed by descriptions of the distinguishing features of the different types of ID.

1. Increased malignancy in PID was described nearly four decades ago[1] but as PID consists of rare diseases, a full documentation of the incidence, relative risk, and appropriate therapy is still not established. The rarity of all forms of ID means that there are few, if any, studies on sufficient numbers of patients to make evidence-based decisions about optimal clinical management. To date there are no controlled comparative therapeutic trials on lymphomas in ID.

2. The age at which ID arises is important because exposure to different infectious organisms may result in immunity, possibly protecting against lymphomas. The variety of infectious organisms an individual has met is lowest at birth and progressively increases with age. Primary infection with EBV while immunodeficient or immunosuppressed increases the risk of EBV-related lymphomas. In general, PID, with the exception of common variable immunodeficiency (CVID), affects predominantly a pediatric population and is commoner in males because of frequent X-linkage in PID.

3. The severity of ID will determine the ability to respond to infectious agents and the time to development of lymphoma. Patients with severe combined immune deficiency (SCID) are at great

risk of dying early in life from pathogenic bacterial or viral disease and only if exposure to oncogenic viruses occurs early will lymphomas appear. With milder forms of ID there is a much longer exposure to a wider variety of infections giving rise to more varied types of lymphomas arising later in life. Assessment of the underlying immune disorder is important not only for lymphomagenesis but also in determining appropriate treatment.

4. Deficiency in cell-mediated immunity (CMI) is more important than deficiency in antibody-mediated immunity for lymphomagenesis. For example, increased susceptibility to lymphoma in CVID characterized by low immunoglobulin levels but with a significant CMI defect does not affect X-linked agammaglobulinemia, a pure antibody deficiency.

5. Chronic antigen stimulation in the presence of abnormal or impaired immune responses may contribute to the lymphomas found in AI disease, in certain forms of PID and transplantation, due to auto-, infection-related, and transplant antigens, respectively.

6. The risk of lymphoma in ID is compounded by those syndromes which also have defective DNA repair such as ataxia telangiectasia (AT) or Nijmegen breakage syndrome (NBS). Lymphomas are more common in the defective DNA repair syndromes than those purely due to ID.

7. Clinical presentation is similar to lymphomas arising in the general population but usually disease is more advanced at presentation and response to and tolerance of therapy is much worse. There is a much higher risk of sepsis and treatment-related mortality. Sometimes the clinical presentation of the lymphoma may be the first sign of the underlying PID, particularly in X-linked lymphoproliferative disease (XLP).

NOTES ON HISTOPATHOLOGY AND IMMUNOHISTOLOGY

The comments that follow are restricted to specific differences between ID-related lymphomas and sporadic cases. General aspects of herpes viruses and lymphoma diagnosis are dealt with in Chapters 7, 18, and 19, respectively. Histopathological diagnosis and classification of lymphoma are made difficult in ID because they rely on changes in normal lymphoid structure and cells. In ID there is often no normal lymphoid structure and the lymphomas are commonly extranodal and by definition lack lymphoid structure. Lymphoid hyperplasia may precede lymphoma in autoimmune lymphoproliferative syndrome (ALPS), CVID, and Wiskott–Aldrich syndrome (WAS) and this complicates the differentiation between benign and malignant processes. Furthermore, neither monoclonal gammopathy[2,3] nor monoclonal gene rearrangement which may be detected in ID[4] is diagnostic of lymphoma even though the presence of clonality is helpful as a guide.[5] In ID most lymphomas are of B cell lineage but in EBV-positive (EBV[+]) types of malignant lymphoma (ML), pan B cell antigens (CD20, CD19, and CD79a) may be absent and cells often lack surface membrane immunoglobulin.

The types of lymphoma found in excess in ID are shown in Table 82.1. The table is based on the World Health Organization (WHO) classification of lymphomas in PTLD[6] with the addition of types found in other ID diseases. The early lesions listed for PTLD are not truly lymphomas but represent primary infectious mononucleosis (IM) or lymphoid hyperplasia that occurs in some forms of ID. However, these nonlymphomatous forms of lymphoproliferation in the face of severe ID may lead to explosive and lethal disease that is called fulminant infectious mononucleosis (FIM). Distinguishing polymorphic from monomorphic forms of lymphoma (Plate 137 A and B, see

Table 82.1 Modified WHO classification of PTLD lymphomas to include all immunodeficiency

Morphology	Cell	Infection	Most prevalent	Classification
Early lesions	B	EBV+	PTLD	Reactive plasmacytic hyperplasia
	B	?	CVID, ALPS	Lymphoid hyperplasia, granuloma
Polymorphic	B	EBV+	All	DLBCL
	B	EBV+	WAS	Lymphomatoid granulomatosis
	N	EBV+	ALPS, SLE	Hodgkin disease; Hodgkin-like
Monomorphic	B	EBV±	All	DLBCL
	B	HCV+	EMC	DLBCL
	B	EBV±	All	Burkitt or Burkitt-like
	B	EBV+	PTLD, SLE	Plasma cell myeloma
	B	H. pylori±	CVID, SS	Marginal zone – MALToma
	T	EBV±	AT, CD	Peripheral T cell

Infection, associated lymphomagenic agent; +, agent almost invariably found; ±, agent found in some cases; Most prevalent, commonest form of immunodeficiency in which the type of malignant lymphoma is seen.
WHO, World Health Organization; PTLD, post-transplant lymphoproliferative disease; EBV, Epstein–Barr virus; HCV, hepatitis C virus; CVID, common variable immunodeficiency; ALPS, autoimmune lymphoproliferative syndrome; WAS, Wiskott–Aldrich syndrome; SLE, systemic lupus erythematosus; EMC, essential mixed cryoglobulinemia type II; SS, Sjögren syndrome; AT, ataxia telangiectasia; CD, celiac disease; DLBCL, diffuse large B cell lymphoma; MALT, mucosal-associated lymphoid tissue; NBS, Nijmegen breakage syndrome.

plate section) is important in that only about 50–60 percent of the polymorphic DLBCL show monoclonality (compared to 100 percent of monomorphic forms), they arise earlier than monomorphic, are almost invariably EBV$^+$, and respond therapeutically to modulation of immunity, where this is possible.

To detect EBV expression unequivocally in conventionally fixed tissue requires staining for EBV encoded small nuclear RNA (EBER) or, on fresh frozen tissue, for Epstein–Barr nuclear antigen 1 (EBNA-1)[7] or with the monoclonal antibody RFD3[8] (Plate 137 C and D). Staining for EBER is helpful in determining the total EBV expression and therefore the proportion of EBV$^+$ lymphoma cells within tissues. This helps to distinguish between EBV$^+$ lymphomas, in which malignant cells form the majority of the infiltrate, and HD in which a minority are EBV$^+$, correlating with CD15 or CD30 expression (Plate 137 C, D, E, and F). Detection of EBV antigens by staining for latent membrane protein (LMP) or EBNA-2 always underestimates the proportion of EBV$^+$ cells and may be completely negative in the presence of EBER or EBNA-1 positivity. In EBV$^+$ lymphomas, analysis of the terminal repeat sequence (EBV-TR) may be used to determine clonality.

PRIMARY IMMUNODEFICIENCY DISEASE

There are now more than 120 distinct genetic defects accounting for over 150 different types of PID.[9] Despite different underlying genetic defects the types of PID can be grouped according to similar clinical presentations and outcome. For example, SCID arises from at least 13 different genetic defects but these have similar clinical courses. The main groups of PID susceptible to ML are given below and, to orient the reader, a brief description of the features of each group will be followed by the types of ML and when treatment or outcome differs from conventional therapy.

The understanding of incidence and prevalence of different types of lymphomas has been complicated by the rarity of the underlying PID, the acquisition of data in the Immunodeficiency Cancer Registry without knowledge about the PID cohort from which these patients accrued that did not develop ML, and the successive changes that have occurred with lymphoma classification. A literature search for PID lymphomas diagnosed by Revised European–American Lymphoma (REAL) or WHO classification generated 385 cases and is used to give an idea of lymphoma prevalence in different forms of PID (Table 82.2). The demography of all forms of ID is shown in Table 82.3 grouped by PID, PTLD, and AI and sorted according to the mean time from the presentation of the ID to development of ML, and shows that the sooner ML develops the more likely it is to be EBV$^+$, except for AI patients.

Table 82.2 Prevalence (%) of lymphomas seen in primary immunodeficiency (PID) compared to sporadic malignant lymphoma (ML)

Type n	ML	ALPS 20	AT 104	CVID 100	SCID 60	WAS 43	XLP 58
ALCL	1.8		1.0	1.0			
B-ALL	0.2		8.7^a	1.0			
BL	1.8	10.0	1.9	1.0	3.3	4.7	22.4
DLBCL	22.3	30.0	32.7	47.0	90.0	76.7	74.1
FCL	16.1	5.0		3.0			
LPC	0.9			2.0			
LyG					7.0		
MCL	4.4						
MM	24.0						
MZ	6.9	5.0		21.0			
SLL	4.9			3.0			
ML-T	5.5	10.0	20.2^b	7.0		2.3	1.7
T-ALL	1.2		20.2				
HD	10.0	40.0	15.4	13.0	6.7	9.3	1.7
PEL				1.0			

n = total number of cases.
^{a}1 B-ALL and 4 Null-ALL.
^{b}6 T-CLL, 8 T-PLL, and 6 nodal.
ALCL, anaplastic large cell lymphoma; ALL, acute lymphoblastic leukemia; ALPS, autoimmune lymphoproliferative syndrome; AT, ataxia telangiectasia; B-ALL, B cell ALL; BL, Burkitt lymphoma; CVID, common variable immunodeficiency; DLBCL, diffuse large B cell lymphoma; FCL, follicular cell lymphoma; HD, Hodgkin disease; LPC, lymphoplasmacytic lymphoma; LyG, lymphomatoid granulomatosis; MCL, mantle cell lymphoma; ML-T, peripheral T cell lymphoma; MM, multiple myeloma; MZ, marginal zone lymphoma; PEL, primary effusion lymphoma; SCID, severe combined immunodeficiency; SLL, small lymphocytic lymphoma; T-ALL, T cell ALL; WAS, Wiskott–Aldrich syndrome; XLP, X-linked lymphoproliferative disease.

X-linked lymphoproliferative syndrome

X-linked lymphoproliferative syndrome is a rare genetic defect affecting males (Table 82.3) and has a variety of clinical outcomes. In a report on 161 patients from 44 kindred, 57 percent died of FIM, 17 percent with aplastic anemia or agranulocytosis, 29 percent developed chronic hypogammaglobulinemia, and 24 percent had ML.[10] Fulminant infectious mononucleosis is triggered upon primary infection by EBV and usually involves a virus-associated hemophagocytic syndrome. In some cases, EBV infection may lead to chronic IM. Hypogammaglobulinemia occurring in XLP patients arose before, after, or unrelated to IM in 16, 26, and 58 percent of cases, respectively. Hypogammaglobulinemia is due to inefficient interaction between B cells and signaling lymphocytic activation molecule (SLAM)-associated protein (SAP)-deficient T cells that were unable to upgrade inducible costimulator (ICOS) or produce interleukin-10 (IL-10).[11] Seventy percent of the XLP patients die by 10 years old and none survived beyond 40 years, with

Table 82.3 Demography of PID, PTLD, or AI and lymphoma incidence

Disease	Prevalence $\times 10^6$	Diagnosis[a]	ML %[b]	RR or SIR	Yr to ML	EBV$^+$ML %
XLP	1	6	30		0	88
SCID	11	<1			0.5	78
WAS	4	1	2	100	5	75
AT	10	1	12	37	8	75
ALPS	<0.001	2	1	14, 51[c]	15	50
CVID	20	30	5	12	16	50
BM/SCT	10–100		1	54	0.5	92
SOT-PTLD	10–60		1–15	12–240	4	70
SS	3700	45	4	13	12	5
CD	1000	3	0.5	2, 51[d]	15	7
EMC	10	47	4	35	15	0
SLE	150–500	30	0.5	5	18	75
RA	8000	50	0.2	3	20	27

Blank cells indicate the data are either not available or not appropriate.

EBV$^+$, % of reported cases with EBV$^+$ ML with appropriate EBV staining.

[a]Median age at diagnosis of immunodeficiency in years.

[b]% of patients developing a lymphoma.

[c]ML and HD, respectively

[d]ML and ETL, respectively

PID, primary immunodeficiency; PTLD, post-transplant lymphoproliferative disease; AI, autoimmunity; ML, malignant lymphoma; RR, relative risk; SIR, standardized incidence ratio; EBV, Epstein–Barr virus; EMC, essential mixed cryoglobulinemia type II; WAS, Wiskott–Aldrich syndrome; XLP, X-linked lymphoproliferative disease; ALPS, autoimmune lymphoproliferative syndrome; SCID, severe combined immunodeficiency; AT, ataxia telangiectasia; CVID, common variable immunodeficiency; BM/SCT, bone marrow or stem cell transplantation; SOT-PTLD, solid organ transplantation–post-transplant lymphoproliferative disease; SS, Sjögren syndrome; CD, celiac disease; SLE, systemic lupus erythematosus; RA, rheumatoid arthritis; HD, Hodgkin disease; ETL, enteropathy-type T cell lymphoma.

the longer-term survivors being those developing hypo-gammaglobulinemia or treated ML. Malignant lymphomas arising in XLP are almost exclusively BL or DLBCL (Fig. 82.1) with a surprisingly high proportion involving the terminal ileum (74 percent).

In XLP, two forms of genetic defect are described affecting *SH2D1A* (XLP 1) and *X1AP* (XLP 2). *SH2D1A* (Src homology 2 domain-containing gene 1A) encodes the SLAM-associated protein (SAP) and *X1AP* encodes for an inhibitor of apoptosis.[12] About 60 percent of all XLP patients have a detectable mutation at *SH2D1A* and there is evidence that the remaining patients without *SH2D1A* mutations may have undetectable SAP for other reasons.[13] SLAM-associated protein is expressed on T cells, natural killer (NK) cells, and NK-T cells, where it binds to the cytoplasmic domain of the surface receptor SLAM and related receptors CD244, CD84, CD229 antigen, and CD2-like receptor activating cytotoxic T cells. These interactions prevent recruitment of SHP-2 (SH2 domain-containing protein tyrosine phosphatase 2) to the cytoplasmic domains of these receptors and result in a failure to initiate cytotoxicity[14] or downregulation of the immune response.

Examination of patients developing severe or fatal IM showed mutations in the *SH2D1A* gene in patients without a family history of XLP, suggesting that FIM in the general population may represent sporadic cases of XLP.[15] Epstein–Barr virus was thought to be the only virus

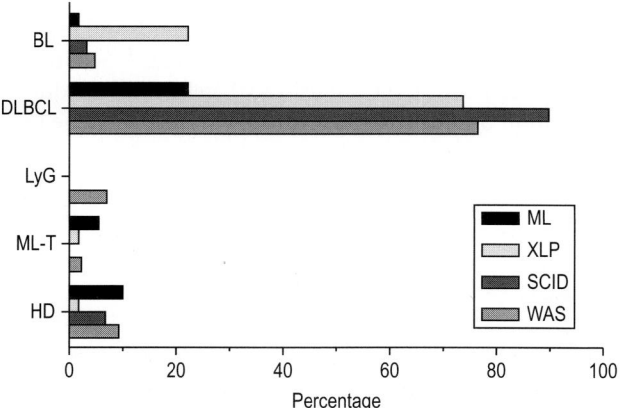

Figure 82.1 Prevalence of different types of lymphoma in primary immunodeficiency. ML gives prevalence for sporadic cases in the general population. BL, Burkitt lymphoma; DLBCL, diffuse large B cell lymphoma; LyG, lymphomatoid granulomatosis; ML-T, peripheral T cell lymphoma; HD, Hodgkin disease; ML, malignant lymphoma; XLP, X-linked lymphoproliferative disease; SCID, severe combined immunodeficiency; WAS, Wiskott–Aldrich syndrome.

triggering the XLP syndrome but there is increasing evidence that EBV is not always involved in XLP-related illness; in 38/304 (12.5 percent) symptomatic males in the XLP registry there was no evidence of EBV infection.[16] X-linked lymphoproliferative syndrome forms not triggered by EBV may express novel mutations of the *SH2D1A* gene.[17]

Conventional therapy is used to treat ML arising in XLP, with similar outcomes, except for a higher risk of infection associated with hypogammaglobulinemia. Treatment of FIM with cytotoxic chemotherapy has no value but CD20 antibody therapy may reduce morbidity and mortality by removing B cells.[18] Identification of XLP families and prophylactic therapy by allogeneic bone marrow/stem cell transplantation (BM/SCT) is recommended for newborn XLP probands prior to EBV exposure.[19]

Severe combined immunodeficiency

There are 13 different genetic forms of SCID giving rise to severe deficiency in both T and B lymphocyte lineages or their function.[9] About half of the forms of SCID have neither T nor B cells. In the remainder, severe T cell deficiency impairs B cell function, causing low immunoglobulin and antibody levels, but B cells are present. The types of SCID that have B cells are susceptible to lymphoma (Table 82.2 and Fig. 82.1). All forms of SCID are life threatening from birth and require urgent allogeneic BM/SCT, gene therapy, or replacement therapy. It is not surprising that following BM/SCT or epithelial transplantation the children are at high risk of developing EBV⁺ PTLD because of young age and immunodeficiency.[20] Furthermore, SCID patients with adenosine deaminase deficiency receiving PEG-ADA (PEGylated adenosine deaminase) replacement therapy, which partially corrects the immune deficiency and restores B cells, become susceptible to lymphoma.[21] Separately, gene therapy for SCID can lead to T cell leukemia due to integration of the retroviral vector into the oncogene promoter region.[22]

Treatment of the lymphomas in SCID carries a very high morbidity and mortality due to infectious complications.

Wiskott–Aldrich syndrome

Wiskott–Aldrich syndrome is an X-linked syndrome consisting of eczema, recurrent pyogenic infection, thrombocytopenia with decreased platelet volume, and immunodeficiency. Wiskott–Aldrich syndrome is caused by mutations in a protein (WASP) defined by the condition, leading to a cytoskeletal defect affecting hematopoietic stem cell derivatives. Wiskott–Aldrich syndrome patients can be grouped on the basis of WASP levels expressed on blood mononuclear cells, platelets, or EBV cell lines. Patients with WASP-positive T cells but negative B cells are particularly prone to develop lymphomas.[23] Improvements in management have led to survival of WAS patients into their second and third decades. Immunodeficiency in the presence of normal B cells means susceptibility to lymphomas (Table 82.2) but the prolonged survival exposes patients to late-arising ML such as HD (Fig. 82.1). Diagnosis of ML needs a degree of caution because WAS may show atypical

lymphoproliferation that can regress spontaneously[24] or monoclonality while following a benign or indolent course.[3,25] Preemptive BM/SCT is the treatment of choice[26] but transplantation of any form carries a high risk of PTLD, particularly where antilymphocyte globulin (ALG) or antithymocyte globulin (ATG) therapy is used.[27]

Ataxia telangiectasia and DNA repair defects

DNA repair deficiency syndromes include AT, NBS, and the Bloom syndrome. Ataxia telangiectasia is the commonest of these and will be used as an example (Tables 82.2 and 82.3). Ataxia telangiectasia is a rare multisystem, autosomal recessive disease characterized by progressive neuronal degeneration, genome instability, variable immunodeficiency, oculocutaneous telangiectasia, impaired organ maturation, and an increased risk of cancer. Although rare, the incidence of heterozygosity is 1.8 percent. Median survival in AT is about 20 years. Diffuse large B cell lymphoma is the commonest lymphoma arising in AT but with the later onset of ML and DNA repair deficiency, there is a striking increase in other forms of lymphoproliferative disease including lymphoid leukemia (Fig. 82.2). The very few NBS cases differed from AT in that 8/9 tumors in NBS were lymphomas not leukemia.[28]

Patients with DNA repair deficiencies are extremely sensitive to ionizing radiation and certain cytotoxic drugs. Treatment by x-irradiation or bleomycin must be avoided because they lead to destruction of normal tissues and lethal pulmonary disease, respectively. Occasionally, MLs arise before the diagnosis of AT is recognized and the severe tissue destruction following irradiation reveals the diagnosis. Protection of the bladder is advisable when

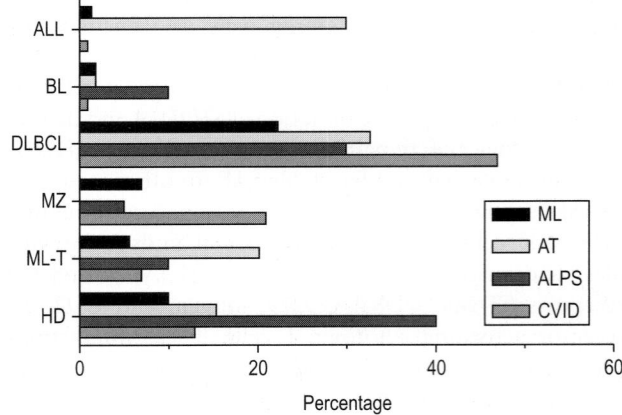

Figure 82.2 Prevalence of different types of lymphoma in primary immunodeficiency. ALL, acute lymphoblastic leukemia; BL, Burkitt lymphoma; DLBCL, diffuse large B cell lymphoma; MZ, marginal zone lymphoma; ML-T, peripheral T cell lymphoma; HD, Hodgkin disease; ML, malignant lymphoma; AT, ataxia telangiectasia; ALPS, autoimmune lymphoproliferative syndrome; CVID, common variable immunodeficiency.

treating with cyclophosphamide. Despite these restrictions, full-dosage chemotherapy is needed for effective treatment, wherever possible. Response to treatment of HD is poor and this is also seen in all other ID groups.

Autoimmune lymphoproliferative syndrome

Autoimmune lymphoproliferative syndrome is characterized by autoimmunity, chronic nonmalignant lymphadenopathy, and splenomegaly with high levels of $CD4^-CD8^-$ T cells of $\alpha\beta$ lineage (double negative T cells). The underlying defect is in the Fas/CD95-mediated apoptotic pathway and abnormal immune regulation with persistence of autoreactive T cells. Autoimmune lymphoproliferative syndrome has been subdivided according to the genetic defect: ALPS type I is due to mutations of the *TNFRSF6* gene, which encodes Fas; ALPS type II has alterations in the caspase-10 gene encoding for a protease which acts downstream from Fas; ALPS type IIb has a mutation of caspase-8, but lack of autoimmunity differentiates this from classic ALPS; ALPS type III encompasses patients whose genetic defect has not been identified. The commonest expressions of autoimmunity are thrombocytopenia and hemolytic anemia. Family studies strongly suggest the contribution of one or more additional factors to the pathogenesis of ALPS. This may pertain to defective immunoregulation by an altered IL-2/IL-2 receptor system, reflected in the specific loss of $CD4^+/CD25^+$ T cells, and/or by the highly increased IL-10 levels. There are interesting combinations of defects that may lead to probands developing ALPS, whereby parents with similar Fas defects may live healthy lives because they lack a contributory defective gene.[29]

The incidence of lymphoma is difficult to assess because only 200 cases have been described over the 15 years since the original description of the syndrome.[30] The long time from diagnosis to ML appearance is consistent with the wider range of ML types seen, but HD is particularly prominent in ALPS (Table 82.3 and Fig. 82.2). Caution about ML diagnosis is necessary because of difficulty interpreting lymph node histopathology and because even in the presence of monoclonal expansion it may resolve spontaneously. A careful watch-and-wait policy is recommended and caution in the long-term use of immunosuppressive drugs. A claim that pyrimethamine is effective for ALPS has not been substantiated. Autoimmune lymphoproliferative syndrome can be corrected by bone marrow transplantation.[31] Tolerance of cytotoxic therapy is normal.

Common variable immunodeficiency and immunoglobulin disorders

There is no susceptibility to lymphoma in the eight different forms of congenital hypogammaglobulinemia with absent B cells. On the other hand, CVID is a heterogeneous group of diseases with hypogammaglobulinemia affecting immunoglobulin G (IgG) most severely (less than 4 g/L) but which can include all Ig subclasses. B cell numbers may be normal or decreased. By definition, the onset of CVID is not until after the second year of life and peaks in the fifth decade (Table 82.3). It is associated with autoimmune and granulomatous disease and variable T cell deficiency. A number of patients diagnosed as CVID have subsequently been shown to have Fas defects and overlap with ALPS,[29] or lack expression of SAP and overlap with those patients with XLP who develop hypogammaglobulinemia.[13,32–34]

Common variable immunodeficiency patients develop lymphomas much later than other PID cases, largely due to the late onset of disease and the prolonged exposure to lymphomagenic triggers combined with a relatively mild T cell deficiency. Diffuse large B cell lymphoma is still the commonest form of ML; about one-half of cases are EBV^+ and rare $HHV-8^+$ forms are seen.[35] Prevalence of marginal zone lymphomas, with or without *H. pylori*, is increased (Fig. 82.2). A proportion of patients develop lymphoid hyperplasia of the lung and gastrointestinal tract[5] and lymphomas arising in this setting make diagnosis difficult. Treatment with radiation therapy or cytotoxic chemotherapy is conventional but there is a higher risk of sepsis necessitating careful attention to IgG levels by intravenous immunoglobulin (IVIG) and granulocyte colony-stimulating factor (G-CSF) support.

HYPER IGM AND HYPER IGE (JOB SYNDROME) SYNDROMES

Prevalence of malignant lymphomas is also increased in patients with the dysgammaglobulinemia syndromes hyper IgM and hyper IgE (Job syndrome). A very high relative risk (RR) of 259 has been calculated for the latter.[36] In hyper IgM there is an increase in IgM^+IgD^+ B cells. Germinal centers are absent but there are extensive IgM-producing plasma cells extranodally, found in the gastrointestinal tract, liver, and gallbladder. These can be so extensive that they may be fatal without the development of lymphoma.

POST-TRANSPLANT LYMPHOPROLIFERATIVE DISEASE

Modulation of immunity is usually not feasible in ML arising in PID patients. However, the ML arising in PTLD, most of which are EBV^+, form a group in which modulation of immunosuppression can be achieved by reducing immunosuppression. Post-transplant lymphoproliferative diseases also raise significant questions about the EBV latency commonly attributed to them (Chapter 7).

Bone marrow or stem cell transplantation

Post-transplant lymphoproliferative disease arising in allogeneic BM/SCT is almost invariably donor derived and of polymorphic EBV$^+$ type (DLBCLp$^+$), similar to SCID patients (Table 82.3). The prevalence overall of PTLD is about 1 percent after 10 years follow-up.[37] The similarity with SCID and the early onset is due to the severe ID induced by conditioning regimens preceding BM/SCT. The conditioning regimens (see Chapter 56) aim to eradicate minimal residual disease in cases of previous malignancy and obliterate the patient's lymphoid system in order to facilitate colonization of the donor's tissue. Bone marrow or stem cell transplant recipients are at risk of PTLD during the first 5–6 months post-transplant, because during this time the donor's bone marrow or stem cell transplant has to regenerate the immune repertoire and the capability to respond to EBV and other infections. The risk of PTLD is increased if donor (D)/recipient (R) EBV status is D$^-$R$^+$ or D$^+$R$^+$, and by major histocompatibility complex (MHC) mismatch, intensity of IS, and selective T cell depletion of the donor's bone marrow or stem cells, as this removes any passively transferred CMI. Lymphocyte depletion affecting both T and B cells (Campath-1, CDw52) is less likely to predispose to PTLD. The risk factor for a relatively low number of late-onset PTLD cases is extensive chronic graft-verus-host disease (GVHD), combining ID with chronic alloantigen stimulation.[37]

Treatment of PTLD in BM/SCT is complicated by the status of the regenerating bone marrow. Early use of cytotoxic drugs may cause bone marrow failure and death from sepsis. The poor outcome with cytotoxic chemotherapy led to a search for alternative forms of treatment. Infusion of donor-derived lymphocytes provides a ready means of restoring EBV immunity passively and successfully leads to resolution of the PTLD. Unfortunately, with the restoration of immunity, alloreactivity to recipient MHC antigens often leads to severe GVHD. The high incidence of PTLD (20–25 percent) in children receiving T cell-depleted BM/SCT prompted the generation of EBV-specific cytotoxic T lymphocytes (CTL) from each donor. These CTL clones were administered preemptively in children undergoing BM/SCT and protected completely against the development of PTLD[38] and induced a complete response in two of three patients with established PTLD. The procedure is costly in terms of technical effort, the potential risk of transferring infection, and redundancy (more than 75 percent of patients in this instance will not require the CTL generated).

An alternative approach to prevent PTLD has used monitoring of the EBV viral load in the blood of BM/SCT patients post-transplant, with or without monitoring for EBV-specific T cells, to predict those patients at risk of PTLD. Patients with a progressively rising EBV load, or where a cutoff value is exceeded, were treated with rituximab to eliminate B cells. This has been very successful in preventing PTLD but is not effective once PTLD is established.[39] The simplicity and ready availability of this technique has largely replaced efforts to use CTL for prevention of PTLD in BM/SCT.

Solid organ transplantation

In contrast to BM/SCT patients, PTLD following solid organ transplantation (SOT) is overwhelmingly recipient derived. Rare exceptions may be seen when large amounts of lymphoid tissue are transplanted with the organ (e.g., lung or bowel). The risk of PTLD is determined by the intensity of IS, which is linked to the type of organ transplant and the individual patient sensitivity to IS (Table 82.4). Risk factors for PTLD include the type and dosage of IS, the use of lymphocyte-depleting antibodies, infections inducing IS (particularly viruses such as cytomegalovirus [CMV] or the polyomavirus, BK), patient age, degree of MHC mismatch between donor and recipient, and EBV-naïve status. The highest levels of IS drugs are given during the first year post-transplant and this is when the incidence of PTLD is highest, ranging from 0.3 percent to 20 percent (Table 82.4). After the first year the incidence is 5–10-fold less than during the first year but still higher than in the general population. Introduction of new and more potent IS drugs is often followed by an increase in PTLD as clinicians gain experience on the optimal use of the new drug. The introduction of cyclosporine A was followed by a marked rise in PTLD but this fell to the same level as for previously used IS as clinical experience was gained.[40] The lymphocyte-depleting antibodies OKT3 and ATG/ALG have been consistently associated with a twofold increase in PTLD during the first post-transplant year. Nondepleting antibodies, such as the IL-2 receptor-blocking monoclonal antibodies, have no effect upon PTLD incidence. Tacrolimus has persisted in causing a twofold increase in PTLD even though clinical experience with this drug is now mature.[40] The twofold higher incidence of PTLD seen in the USA compared to Europe corresponds to the widespread use of OKT3 or ATG/ALG for induction, as well as the more uniform use of tacrolimus. The effect of age on PTLD is due to the protective effect of previous exposure and acquisition of EBV immunity. Epstein–Barr virus is ubiquitous and exposure starts shortly after birth, to affect

Table 82.4 Incidence of post-transplant lymphoproliferative disease in different organ transplants[40,66,67]

Organ (n)	1 year	RR	5 years	RR	5-year survival
Kidney (145 104)	0.3%	24	0.8%	13	34%
Pancreas (4081)	0.5%	31	1.4%	35	
Liver (15 631)	0.8%	90	1.7%	30	30%
Heart (25 485)	1.0%	130	2.8%	28	26%
Lung (4415)	2.0%	300	3.1%	59	
Heart/lung (1222)	4.3%	520	5.6%	240	
Small bowel (96)	20%	2000			

n = number of patients evaluated for post-transplant lymphoproliferative disease.

RR, relative risk.

about 90 percent of the population by adulthood. The risk of PTLD is therefore greatest in children with an EBV-naïve status and a lack of EBV-specific CMI. The very high incidence of PTLD in small bowel transplantation (Table 82.4) is due to a predominantly pediatric population and the need for intense IS. Although most marked in small bowel transplantation, the greater risk in young transplant recipients is seen for all organs when the RR is calculated on the basis of age. Overall, EBV⁻ recipients have a 20-fold higher incidence of PTLD than EBV⁺ recipients.

Because SOT is an elective procedure, there is time to estimate the risk of PTLD, similarly to that described above for BM/SCT. Pre-transplantation EBV serology should be done to define the EBV status of recipients and donors. The EBV R⁻D⁺ combination places recipients at greatest risk and post-transplantation requires at least monthly monitoring for EBV serology and viral load in the blood, plus careful questioning for symptoms of IM and physical examination. With the onset of EBV infection, laboratory evaluation of the cellular anti-EBV immune response can be made.[41] If the cellular immune response is inappropriate or negative, reduction of IS may enable an effective anti-EBV response to appear and greatly reduce the risk of PTLD. At least 70 percent of EBV-naïve transplant recipients make an asymptomatic EBV seroconversion

without PTLD. In the remaining 30 percent, a mixture of IM and PTLD occurs, with only the latter normally requiring therapy.

Diagnosis of PTLD, just like conventional ML, requires biopsy confirmation and accurate classification. The types of ML, cellular lineage, and EBV tumor status are given for a series of PTLD patients monitored at the Royal Free Hospital, London (Table 82.5 and Fig. 82.3). Though there is no comparably large histopathological series, it is consistent with compiled reports from the literature, except for a relatively low number of ML-T. Reports of the percentage of ML-T types of PTLD have ranged between 1.6 percent and 11.6 percent[42,43] with a mean of 7.8 percent from seven studies, each including 20 or more patients, with a total of 318 patients. There is a distinct order in time from transplantation to the onset of the different types of PTLD. Polymorphic EBV⁺ DLBCL arise first, followed by BL, monomorphic EBV⁺ DLBCL, and EBV⁻ DLBCL or HD last (Fig. 82.4). It is tempting to speculate that the appearance of different types of PTLD in the transplant setting may represent the interaction between the oncogenic properties of EBV and the host's immunity. Thus EBV-naïve patients or those unable to mount a response to EBV during heavy immunosuppression are likely to develop polymorphic DLBCL expressing full EBV latency type III

Table 82.5 Prevalence (%) of lymphomas seen in PTLD and autoimmunity compared to sporadic malignant lymphoma

	C	TP	Autoimmunity				
Type	ML	PTLD	CD	SLE	RA	SS	EMC
n		260	155	82	526	181	58
ALCL	1.8	1.9	0.6	1.2	2.3	0.6	1.7
B-ALL	0.2			1.2	0.2	0.6	
BL	1.8	5.4	1.3	3.7	0.8		1.7
DLBCL	22.3	75.8	8.4	39.0	55.5	19.9	51.7
FCL	16.1	0.4		3.7	6.3	5.0	22.4
LPC	0.9	0.4		1.2	2.3	0.6	3.4
LyG				1.2		1.1	
MCL	4.4				1.0	1.1	1.7
MM	24.0	3.5		12.2	8.4	7.2	
MZ	6.9	2.3	1.3	2.4	3.0	53.6	8.6
SLL	4.9			7.3	6.8		8.6
ML-T	5.5	1.2	87.8	4.9	5.3	7.8	
T-ALL	1.2				0.2		
HD	10.0	9.2	0.6	22.0	8.6	2.8	

ALCL, anaplastic large cell lymphoma; B-ALL, B cell ALL; BL, Burkitt lymphoma; CD, celiac disease; DLBCL, diffuse large B cell lymphoma; FCL, follicular cell lymphoma; HD, Hodgkin disease; LPC, lymphoplasmacytic lymphoma; LyG, lymphomatoid granulomatosis; MCL, mantle cell lymphoma; ML-T, peripheral T cell lymphoma; MM, multiple myeloma; MZ, marginal zone lymphoma; SLL, small lymphocytic lymphoma; T-ALL, T cell ALL; PTLD, post-transplant lymphoproliferative disease; ML, malignant lymphoma; SS, Sjögren syndrome; SLE, systemic lupus erythematosus; RA, rheumatoid arthritis; EMC, essential mixed cryoglobulinemia type II; TP, transplant; C, control.

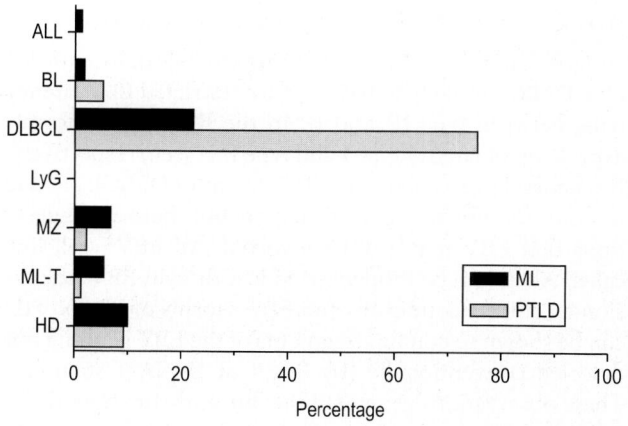

Figure 82.3 Prevalence of different types of lymphoma in post-transplant lymphoproliferative disease (PTLD). Two hundred sixty of 341 patients with PTLD, whose histology was reviewed and classified according to World Health Organization (WHO) classification,[6] consisted of 7 bone marrow, 7 cardiac, 34 hepatic (including 5 combined small bowel), 1 lung, and 211 renal (including 2 combined pancreas) transplants. Overall, Epstein–Barr virus (EBV) was positive in 72 percent of PTLD. This included 1/3 (33 percent) ALCL, 8/10 (80 percent) BL, 117/158 (74 percent) DLBCL, 20/22 (91 percent) HD, and 7/8 (87 percent) MM. EBV was negative in FCL, LPC, and MZ types. Two T-rich B cell lymphomas included in the DLBCL group were EBV negative. Three of 5 (60 percent) ALCL, 8/21 (38 percent) HD, and all BL (14/14), DLBCL (180/180), FCL (1/1), LCL (1/1), MM (9/9), and MZ (6/6) lymphomas were B cell lineage. Male to female ratio was 2.5:1 (244:96). The ratio of DLBCL characterized as polymorphic compared to monomorphic was 1.4:1 (63:46).

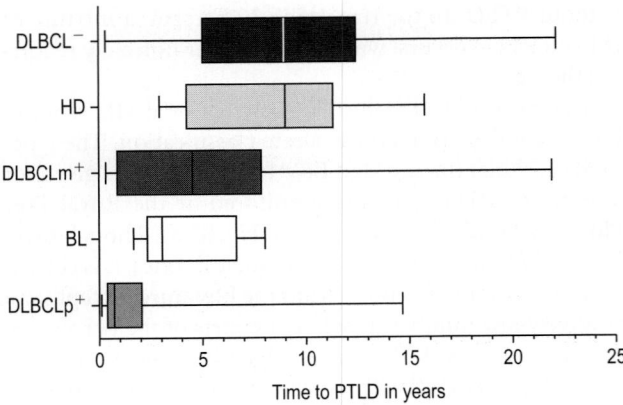

Figure 82.4 Box and whisker graph of median time (± 95 percent confidence interval) to onset of post-transplant lymphoproliferative disease (PTLD). Values given are the median (25–75 percent in box) and range by error bars. Median time is 0.74, 3.07, 4.55, 9.05, and 8.99 years for DLBCLp+, BL, DLBCLm+, DLBCL−, and HD, respectively, with highly significant differences between the groups (P = 0.002 by ANOVA). DLBCLp+, Epstein–Barr virus+ (EBV+) polymorphic diffuse large B cell lymphoma (n = 54); BL, Burkitt lymphoma (9/12 EBV+); DLBCLm+, EBV+ monomorphic diffuse large B cell lymphoma (n = 39); HD, Hodgkin disease (19/21 EBV+); DLBCL−, EBV− diffuse large B cell lymphoma (n = 34).

antigens, similar to IM. The later appearance of monomorphic DLBCL is likely to have a more restricted EBV latency lying between type III and II. In the BL and HD forms, expression of latency type I and type II is seen, respectively. It is generally assumed that EBV− forms of DLBCL are due to other unknown oncogenic factors but there are suggestions that EBV may still be involved. An EBV+ cell line called Akata can be influenced to lose or gain EBV expression by culture conditions and EBV− forms of BL and HD can be shown to contain fragments of the EBV genome not detected conventionally (by EBER or EBNA-1 staining). These observations generated the 'hit-and-run' hypothesis of EBV induction of tumors.[44]

Management of patients who develop PTLD requires close collaboration between the transplant clinician and oncologist. Generally, PTLD still carries a poor prognosis compared to sporadic lymphomas but in the 1970s it was exceptionally poor, when abysmal responses to cytotoxic chemotherapy were common, with deaths mostly due to neutropenic sepsis. The treatment options for PTLD are antiviral drugs, reduction of immunosuppression (RIS), rituximab (anti-CD20), radiation therapy (RT) or surgery, cytotoxic chemotherapy (CT), and experimental protocols. Poor prognostic factors for the outcome of PTLD treatment have been identified as poor performance status, more than one system site involved, CNS involvement, EBV− tumors, T cell PTLD, high lactate dehydrogenase (LDH), and treatment with chemotherapy.[45–47] The value of poor prognostic features for 'PTLD' as an entity is moot

because the types of lymphoma arising in PTLD are very different. For example, in the list above, high LDH is associated with BL and that carries a worse prognosis than DLBCL in sporadic lymphomas. Only when sufficiently large numbers of patients are examined will effective prognostic factors be established for the individual types of PTLD. In a study of 135 patients with PTLD, the 5-year survival was 83 percent, 61 percent, 53 percent, 37 percent, and 35 percent for DLBCLp+, DLBCLm+, DLBCL−, BL, and HD, respectively.[48]

ANTIVIRAL DRUGS

There is no convincing clinical or theoretical evidence that thymidine kinase inhibitors, such as acyclovir, have any beneficial effect in PTLD. These drugs interfere with the replication of the linear form of EBV but not the circular episomal form found in the nuclei of PTLD tumors. Much more potent anti-EBV drugs, such as cidofovir or foscarnet, have not been evaluated because of the concerns over toxicity, particularly interstitial nephritis. Despite the lack of evidence-based medicine for the use of thymidine kinase inhibitors, their lack of toxicity and familiarity to the transplant community means that they are commonly used in PTLD.

A novel approach has used arginine butyrate, which induces thymidine kinase transcription by EBV-transformed cell lines. When arginine butyrate is used in conjunction with ganciclovir there is a synergism leading to suppression of proliferation and cell death. In a phase I/II study, four of six patients resistant to conventional therapy achieved a complete response (CR).[49]

IMMUNOMODULATION: REDUCTION OF IMMUNOSUPPRESSION OR PASSIVE CYTOTOXIC T LYMPHOCYTES

The seminal observation that RIS could lead to resolution of PTLD was made in 1984[50] and since then RIS has become the *de facto* standard first line of therapy. The risk that abrupt RIS can lead to transplant rejection creates concerns about its use in organs essential for life lacking any form of replacement therapy (heart, heart/lung, liver, and small bowel transplantation). Although RIS has been used for over two decades there has been little change in the rapid withdrawal procedure and short evaluation time (2 weeks) before deciding if there is no benefit and instituting other therapies. Withdrawal of IS for reasons other than PTLD had shown that gradual reduction over 3 months was much less likely to cause rejection than more rapid withdrawal. On the basis of this experience, a gradual RIS protocol was introduced for treatment of PTLD (Table 82.6). Immunosuppression in SOT consists of a combination of two to four drugs. The mainstay of all regimens has been the calcineurin inhibitors, cyclosporine or tacrolimus, with added azathioprine, prednisone, methylprednisolone, mycophenolate mofetil, sirolimus, or anti-lymphocyte

Table 82.6   Gradual reduction of immunosuppression protocol

Week	% of the starting immunosuppressive dose at PTLD diagnosis		
	Stable[a]	Progressive[b]	Life threatening[c]
0	90	90	60
1		75	
2	75	60	30
3		45	
4	60	30	0
5		15	
6	45	0	
7			
8	30		
9			
10	15		
11			
12	0		

[a]Stable PTLD is where there is no change in the size of measurable PTLD masses.
[b]Progressive disease is where there has been a 25% increase in the size of measurable masses.
[c]Life threatening is where vital organs (lungs, heart, circulatory system, or graft) are threatened by the PTLD and clinical assessment is that death would be imminent if not treated rapidly.
PTLD, post-transplant lymphoproliferative disease.

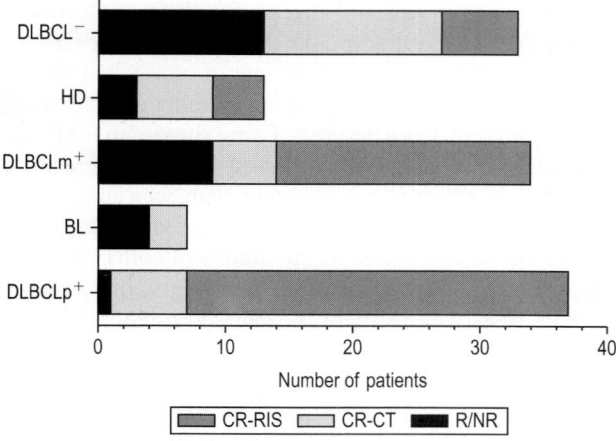

Figure 82.5   Post-transplant lymphoproliferative disease response to reduction of immunosuppression (RIS) or cytotoxic chemotherapy in renal transplant patients. All patients with DLBCLp+ and DLBCLm+ were treated by RIS as primary therapy. Only 1 BL, 8 HD, and 10 DLBCL− patients were treated with RIS. Complete response (CR) was achieved in 81.1 percent, 58.8 percent, 0 percent, 50 percent, and 60 percent of patients treated with RIS only in DLBCLp+, DLBCLm+, BL, HD, and DLBCL− patients, respectively. CR-RIS, patients achieving CR with RIS alone; CR-CT, patients needing cytotoxic chemotherapy to achieve CR; R/NR, relapsed patients or no response. DLBCLp+, Epstein–Barr virus+ (EBV+) polymorphic diffuse large B cell lymphoma; BL, Burkitt lymphoma; DLBCLm+, EBV+ monomorphic diffuse large B cell lymphoma; HD, Hodgkin disease; DLBCL−, EBV− diffuse large B cell lymphoma.

antibodies. Because RIS may fail to achieve a response and necessitate treatment with CT, any myelotoxic drug (azathioprine, mycophenolate, and sirolimus) is stopped abruptly (unless it is the major IS) and only the major IS drug reduced gradually (usually cyclosporine or tacrolimus). The longer that myelotoxic drugs are suspended, the less the risk of neutropenia with subsequent CT. The result of RIS in a series of renal transplant patients[48] is shown in Figure 82.5. The outcome confirmed that early, polymorphic DLBCL could respond well to RIS, but not expected were the good responses seen in late and monomorphic forms of DLBCL. It is difficult to judge the apparently good responses seen in HD and DLBCL− patients because only small numbers and selected patients were treated by RIS. The mean reduction of the main IS drug was to 30 percent of the pre-PTLD levels, taking an average of 2 months to achieve the final dosage, when either a significant clinical response was seen or an anti-EBV immune response was detected. The time to achieve CR (mean of 20 weeks) was much longer than the short observation times quoted in the literature before switching to other forms of therapy. Relapses were infrequent after achieving CR with RIS, but for relapses, partial response, and no response to RIS there was the possibility of salvage with CT. Importantly, there was a low incidence of acute rejection episodes, with 1-year graft survival of 95 percent post-PTLD in gradual RIS compared to 60 percent in standard rapid RIS. Epstein–Barr virus+ PTLD at all sites was responsive to RIS. Of

particular note, 60 percent of cases with CNS involvement by DLBCL achieved CR with RIS alone.

When assessing treatment by RIS, all factors affecting IS should be reviewed. Cytomegalovirus infection induces IS that will not be alleviated unless effective anti-CMV therapy is used. Recent treatment with lymphocyte-depleting antibodies (up to 3 months after treatment) may make RIS impracticable.

Passive provision of EBV-specific CTL used in BM/SCT has also been used in SOT. Raising individual CTL from transplant recipients is even more daunting because of the enormous redundancy of the system, with 80–99 percent of patients never needing to use their CTL. To circumvent this, a panel of CTL was generated from healthy blood donors and the best MHC match between allogeneic CTL and recipient was used to treat PTLD. The allogeneic CTL tended to be very short lived in the recipient but, nonetheless, CR was seen in 43 percent of 33 patients.[51]

RITUXIMAB (ANTI-CD20)

Early studies with murine monoclonal antibodies suggested that PTLD may respond to serotherapy.[52] Since the introduction of the chimeric anti-CD20 monoclonal antibody, rituximab, there have been several uncontrolled studies in PTLD and widespread use. Immunohistology is advisable before using rituximab therapy because CD20 is absent on PTLD in about 20 percent of cases when BL and HD are included. Most multiple myeloma and about 10 percent of DLBCL are negative. Using rituximab for PTLD treatment, a CR has been achieved in 28–57 percent of patients,[53,54] which is much higher than seen in sporadic DLBCL (approximately 6 percent). The difficulty interpreting the results is due to the unknown contribution of RIS, which precedes or accompanies the use of rituximab in most cases. Unless there is a marked biological difference between sporadic and PTLD forms of DLBCL, it raises the question as to the role of immunity and RIS in the responses seen. In the RIS study described above,[48] no durable response was seen using rituximab after patients had conclusively failed to respond to RIS.

RADIATION THERAPY AND SURGERY

These modalities are reserved for localized PTLD and are infrequently used. There is anecdotal evidence of successful outcome by removing isolated skin or gum lesions.

CYTOTOXIC CHEMOTHERAPY

Cytotoxic chemotherapy (CT) regimens must be matched to the type of PTLD and not a 'one version fits all' approach. R-CHOP (rituximab, cyclophosphamide, doxorubicin, vincristine, and prednisone) is standard for DLBCL, and ABVD (doxorubicin, bleomycin, vinblastine, and dacarbazine) for HD, but caution is necessary in using doxorubicin on heart transplant patients. Their tolerance to doxorubicin may be as low as 10 percent of normal. Burkitt lymphoma-specific regimens using high-dose methotrexate require caution or omission in renal transplant patients but care is also required in other SOT because most patients receive calcineurin inhibitors that cause greater or lesser degrees of renal impairment. The risk of neutropenic sepsis is high, particularly in patients receiving myelotoxic IS drugs and when CT is instituted rapidly after suspending those drugs. The use of G-CSF should be standard and, for the first course of CT, a 50 percent reduction of myelotoxic cytotoxic drugs should be considered.

Responses to CT have been very variable. In early studies the 5-year survival ranged between 24 percent and 34 percent using CHOP or other combination therapies and was only 5 percent using single agents.[43,55] Recent studies have achieved CR in 30–60 percent of patients and a mean 5-year survival of 43 percent.

AUTOIMMUNE DISEASE: CHRONIC IMMUNOSTIMULATION AND IMMUNOSUPPRESSIVE THERAPY

The demographics of PID, PTLD, and AI are sorted by years to onset of ML in Table 82.3. Both PID and PTLD show an inverse relationship between time to onset of ML and EBV[+]

disease, but this does not occur in autoimmune diseases, which generally have a much longer time between onset of AI and appearance of ML. Immunodeficiency in PID and immunosuppression in PTLD are dominant factors in lymphomagenesis but these play a secondary and debatable role in AI-related ML, where organ-specific antigenic stimulation determines the organ in which the ML arises.[56]

Sjögren syndrome

Sjögren syndrome (SS) is a chronic organ-specific autoimmune disease characterized by lymphocytic infiltration into the salivary and lachrymal glands, with one-half of cases progressing to systemic disease. Three stages can be defined: stage I is restricted to the sicca syndrome in about 50 percent of cases; stage II involves lymphocytic organ damage affecting pulmonary, renal, hepatic, hematologic, and/or skin tissues; and stage III defines patients developing ML (Table 82.3). The malignant lymphomas are characterized by lymphoepithelial lesions in which there are close interactions among epithelial, T, and B cells. The B cells in the lesions become activated through the interaction between CD40 ligand (CD40L) and CD40. The progression from polyclonal to monoclonal lymphoproliferation, to mucosal-associated lymphoid tissue (MALT) lymphoma, and finally to high-grade malignant lymphoma is regarded as a multistep process. Antigenic activation of B cells, together with oncogenic events including *TP53* inactivation and BCL2 activation, are important transforming events. The rheumatoid factor clone is regarded as a candidate B cell clone that undergoes transformation. Risk factors for ML development are palpable skin purpura or vasculitis, enlarged parotid glands, low C3 or C4 components of complement, and CD4[+] T cell lymphocytopenia. Two chromosomal aberrations involving the *MALT1* gene, t(11;18)(q21;q21) and t(14;18)(q32;q21) translocations, have been reported as genetic events specific for MALT lymphoma.[57] *MALT1* rearrangement is low in extra-gastrointestinal lymphoma but high in gastric MALT lymphoma associated with SS, and may help identify patients responsive to *H. pylori* eradication therapy. Salivary gland involvement and MZ/MALT types of ML are strikingly increased in SS (Table 82.5 and Fig. 82.6).

Therapy of ML and outcome in SS is conventional but it should be noted that treatment with anti-CD20 antibody frequently leads to human anti-chimeric antibody response severe enough to cause serum sickness.[58]

Celiac disease

Presumed chronic antigenic stimulation from the bowels of patients with resistant celiac disease (CD) renders them susceptible to enteropathy-type T cell lymphoma (ETL). In resistant CD the jejunum contains premalignant intraepithelial lymphocytes (IEL) with the same clonality as the

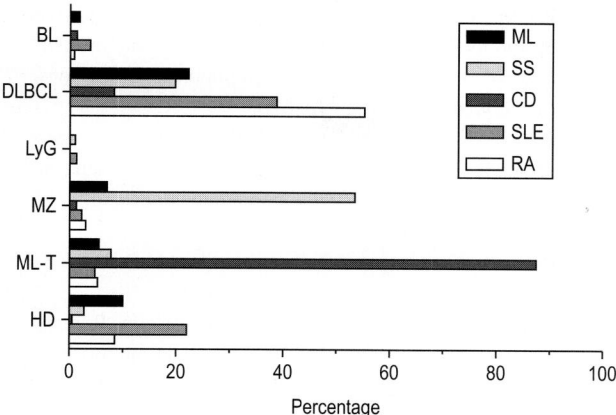

Figure 82.6 Prevalence of different types of lymphoma in autoimmunity. BL, Burkitt lymphoma; DLBCL, diffuse large B cell lymphoma; LyG, lymphomatoid granulomatosis; MZ, marginal zone lymphoma; ML-T, peripheral T cell lymphoma; HD, Hodgkin disease; ML, malignant lymphoma; SS, Sjögren syndrome; CD, celiac disease; SLE, systemic lupus erythematosus; RA, rheumatoid arthritis.

subsequent ETL. The phenotype of the aberrant monoclonal IEL is mostly CD3$^+$ and CD8$^-$ and can be detected in the blood of about 25 percent of patients. The ETL pleomorphic T cell lymphomas rarely express CD8 or CD56. Loss of heterozygosity at chromosome 9p21 is frequent in large-celled ETL. This chromosome area encodes for tumor suppressor genes *p14/ARF*, *p15/INK4b*, and *p16/INK4a*; 17p13, where *TP53* is located, may play a role in ETL progression.[59] Enteropathy-type T cell lymphoma is the predominant form of ML in CD (Table 82.5, Fig. 82.6). In patients with dermatitis herpetiformis without CD, most ML are diffuse large cell lymphomas of B lineage.

Resistant CD (RCD) is categorized as RCD I or II according to responsiveness or lack of response to azathioprine, respectively. RCD I patients are free from ETL, while over half of RCD II patients develop ETL. RCD II has an overall 5-year survival of 58 percent but this falls to 8 percent in those developing ETL.[60] There is a poor outlook for ETL patients with RCD, most dying from progressive disease, with 1- and 5-year survival rates of 30 percent and 10 percent, respectively. Problems with cytotoxic chemotherapy include gastrointestinal hemorrhage, poor patient status related to nutrition, and poor tumor response.

Systemic lupus erythematosus

Systemic lupus erythematosus (SLE) has a relatively small excess of lymphoma unrelated to immunosuppressive therapy. Many arise in the brain. Despite the long time to appearance of malignant lymphomas, they are frequently EBV$^+$, which goes against the trend seen in PID and PTLD. However, the wide variety of ML types seen in SLE is consistent with the long delay from diagnosis (Table 82.5). Treatment of ML in SLE is conventional.

Rheumatoid arthritis

Rheumatoid arthritis (RA) is the commonest autoimmune disease, with a female predominance (2.5:1) that is reversed in those developing ML (1:1.2). There is a definite association between the use of immunosuppressive drugs and the risk of ML (Table 82.3), with evidence that the risk is greater with more potent immunosuppression. The median time to onset of ML in RA treated with methotrexate was 11 years compared to 20 years in those without methotrexate. Analysis of cohort studies gave a RR of 2.5 for patients treated conventionally and 10 for those treated with immunosuppressive therapy. Subset analysis of RA patients showed that those treated with conventional therapy or cytotoxic or biological agents had standardized incidence ratios of 2.5, 5.1, and 11.5, respectively.[61] The data supporting a role of increasing immunosuppression in lymphomagenesis are strong but the strongest correlation between RA and ML has been the intensity of cumulative RA disease activity that leads to increasing intensity of immunosuppression.[62] Although the identity of the antigen in RA is unknown, the correlation between disease activity and ML suggests that, as for other autoimmune diseases, antigenic stimulation may underlie the susceptibility to ML. The diverse forms of ML in RA are consistent with the long delay between onset of RA and ML and the relatively low proportion of EBV$^+$ types.

Withdrawal of immunosuppression can lead to a complete response of the ML in about 25 percent of cases. Five-year survival is worse than in sporadic ML and patients developing HD (RR of 8) fare particularly badly, with only 40 percent surviving to 3 years.[63] This is consistent with the experience of HD in SOT. The recommendation in RA is to withdraw cytotoxic immunosuppression (e.g., methotrexate) with close supervision for 2–3 months, especially in EBV$^+$ cases, before proceeding to cytotoxic therapy if necessary.[64]

Essential mixed cryoglobulinemia type II

Essential mixed cryoglobulinemia (EMC) type II is distinguished from other types because the cryoglobulin consists of an immune complex composed of a monoclonal IgM rheumatoid factor binding to polyclonal IgG. About 15 percent of patients with ML are hepatitis C virus (HCV) positive.[65] When subsets of ML patients were analyzed, 50 percent, 70 percent, and 5 percent of lymphomas arising in EMC$^+$, immunocytomas, and non-EMC cases, respectively, were HCV positive. Hepatitis C virus infects liver and salivary glands and these are involved by ML arising in HCV-positive patients. The chronicity of HCV infection provides yet another example of chronic antigen stimulation in patients with autoimmune disease.

KEY POINTS

- Immunodeficiency and immunosuppression markedly increase the risk of developing lymphomas.
- Lymphomas arising in immunodeficiency and immunosuppression are commonly associated with oncogenic viruses; the most frequent is EBV.
- The time from immunodeficiency diagnosis or use of immunosuppressive drugs to onset of lymphoma is earlier in severe and later in milder forms of immunodeficiency/immunosuppression.
- Diffuse large B cell lymphomas (DLBCL) overwhelmingly dominate the early onset types of immunodeficiency-related lymphoma. Lymphoma types become more varied with later onset, although DLBCL continues to dominate.
- In immunodeficiency, lymphomas expressing viral antigens or associated with infectious agents may regress completely if the immunodeficiency can be reversed. The most reversible form of immunodeficiency is immunosuppressive drug therapy used in transplantation or autoimmune disease.

REFERENCES

● = Key primary paper
◆ = Major review article

1. Gatti RA, Good RA. Occurrence of malignancy in immunodeficiency diseases. A literature review. *Cancer* 1971; **28**: 89–98.
2. Laszewski MJ, Kemp JD, Goeken JA *et al.* Clonal immunoglobulin gene rearrangement in nodular lymphoid hyperplasia of the gastrointestinal tract associated with common variable immunodeficiency. *Am J Clin Pathol* 1990; **94**: 338–43.
3. Bruce RM, Blaese RM. Monoclonal gammopathy in the Wiskott-Aldrich syndrome. *J Pediatr* 1974; **85**: 204–7.
4. Gompels MM, Hodges E, Lock RJ *et al.* Lymphoproliferative disease in antibody deficiency: a multi-centre study. *Clin Exp Immunol* 2003; **134**: 314–20.
5. Sander CA, Medeiros LJ, Weiss LM *et al.* Lymphoproliferative lesions in patients with common variable immunodeficiency syndrome. *Am J Surg Pathol* 1992; **16**: 1170–82.
◆6. Jaffe ES, Harris NL, Stein H, Vardiman JW. Posttransplant lymphoproliferative disease. *World Health Organization classification of tumours: pathology and genetics of tumours of haematopoietic and lymphoid tissues.* Lyon, France: IARC Press, 2001: 264–71.

7. Reedman BM, Klein G. Cellular localization of an Epstein-Barr virus (EBV)-associated complement-fixing antigen in producer and non-producer lymphoblastoid cell lines. *Int J Cancer* 1973; **11**: 499–520.
8. Pokrovska T, Guppy A, Bunn C, Amlot PL. The monoclonal antibody RFD3 detects nuclear staining for all stages of Epstein-Barr virus latency in human cell lines and lymphoma tissues. Unpublished work, 2008.
◆9. Geha RS, Notarangelo LD, Casanova JL *et al.* Primary immunodeficiency diseases: an update from the International Union of Immunological Societies Primary Immunodeficiency Diseases Classification Committee. *J Allergy Clin Immunol* 2007; **120**: 776–94.
10. Grierson H, Purtilo DT. Epstein-Barr virus infections in males with the X-linked lymphoproliferative syndrome. *Ann Intern Med* 1987; **106**: 538–45.
11. Ma CS, Hare NJ, Nichols KE *et al.* Impaired humoral immunity in X-linked lymphoproliferative disease is associated with defective IL-10 production by CD4$^+$ T cells. *J Clin Invest* 2005; **115**: 1049–59.
12. Rigaud S, Fondaneche MC, Lambert N *et al.* XIAP deficiency in humans causes an X-linked lymphoproliferative syndrome. *Nature* 2006; **444**: 110–4.
13. Gilmour KC, Cranston T, Jones A *et al.* Diagnosis of X-linked lymphoproliferative disease by analysis of SLAM-associated protein expression. *Eur J Immunol* 2000; **30**: 1691–7.
14. Tangye SG, Phillips JH, Lanier LL, Nichols KE. Functional requirement for SAP in 2B4-mediated activation of human natural killer cells as revealed by the X-linked lymphoproliferative syndrome. *J Immunol* 2000; **165**: 2932–6.
15. Parolini O, Kagerbauer B, Simonitsch-Klupp I *et al.* Analysis of SH2D1A mutations in patients with severe Epstein-Barr virus infections, Burkitt's lymphoma, and Hodgkin's lymphoma. *Ann Hematol* 2002; **81**: 441–7.
16. Sumegi J, Huang D, Lanyi A *et al.* Correlation of mutations of the SH2D1A gene and Epstein-Barr virus infection with clinical phenotype and outcome in X-linked lymphoproliferative disease. *Blood* 2000; **96**: 3118–25.
17. Brandau O, Schuster V, Weiss M *et al.* Epstein-Barr virus-negative boys with non-Hodgkin lymphoma are mutated in the SH2D1A gene, as are patients with X-linked lymphoproliferative disease (XLP). *Hum Mol Genet* 1999; **8**: 2407–13.
18. Milone MC, Tsai DE, Hodinka RL *et al.* Treatment of primary Epstein-Barr virus infection in patients with X-linked lymphoproliferative disease using B-cell-directed therapy. *Blood* 2005; **105**: 994–6.
19. Lankester AC, Visser LF, Hartwig NG *et al.* Allogeneic stem cell transplantation in X-linked lymphoproliferative disease: two cases in one family and review of the literature. *Bone Marrow Transplant* 2005; **36**: 99–105.
20. Shearer WT, Ritz J, Finegold MJ *et al.* Epstein-Barr virus-associated B-cell proliferations of diverse clonal origins after bone marrow transplantation in a 12-year-old patient with severe combined immunodeficiency. *N Engl J Med* 1985; **312**: 1151–9.

21. Husain M, Grunebaum E, Naqvi A *et al.* Burkitt's lymphoma in a patient with adenosine deaminase deficiency-severe combined immunodeficiency treated with polyethylene glycol-adenosine deaminase. *J Pediatr* 2007; **151**: 93–5.

22. Hacein-Bey-Abina S, Von KC, Schmidt M *et al.* LMO2-associated clonal T cell proliferation in two patients after gene therapy for SCID-X1. *Science* 2003; **302**: 415–9.

23. Shcherbina A, Rosen FS, Remold-O'Donnell E. WASP levels in platelets and lymphocytes of Wiskott-Aldrich syndrome patients correlate with cell dysfunction. *J Immunol* 1999; **163**: 6314–20.

24. Ma YC, Shyur SD, Ho TY *et al.* Wiskott-Aldrich syndrome complicated by an atypical lymphoproliferative disorder: a case report. *J Microbiol Immunol Infect* 2005; **38**: 289–92.

◆25. Elenitoba-Johnson KS, Jaffe ES. Lymphoproliferative disorders associated with congenital immunodeficiencies. *Semin Diagn Pathol* 1997; **14**: 35–47.

26. Filipovich AH, Stone JV, Tomany SC *et al.* Impact of donor type on outcome of bone marrow transplantation for Wiskott-Aldrich syndrome: collaborative study of the International Bone Marrow Transplant Registry and the National Marrow Donor Program. *Blood* 2001; **97**: 1598–1603.

27. Ozsahin H, Le Deist F, Benkerrou M *et al.* Bone marrow transplantation in 26 patients with Wiskott-Aldrich syndrome from a single center. *J Pediatr* 1996; **129**: 238–44.

28. Kobayashi N, Naitoh K, Kudo H *et al.* Primary immunodeficiency syndromes and malignant neoplasms. *Gan No Rinsho* [*Japanese Journal of Cancer Clinics*] 1987; **33**: 495–500.

29. Campagnoli MF, Garbarini L, Quarello P *et al.* The broad spectrum of autoimmune lymphoproliferative disease: molecular bases, clinical features and long-term follow-up in 31 patients. *Haematologica* 2006; **91**: 538–41.

30. Straus SE, Jaffe ES, Puck JM *et al.* The development of lymphomas in families with autoimmune lymphopro-liferative syndrome with germline Fas mutations and defective lymphocyte apoptosis. *Blood* 2001; **98**: 194–200.

31. Sleight BJ, Prasad VS, DeLaat C *et al.* Correction of autoimmune lymphoproliferative syndrome by bone marrow transplantation. *Bone Marrow Transplant* 1998; **22**: 375–80.

32. Nistala K, Gilmour KC, Cranston T *et al.* X-linked lymphoproliferative disease: three atypical cases. *Clin Exp Immunol* 2001; **126**: 126–30.

33. Morra M, Silander O, Calpe S *et al.* Alterations of the X-linked lymphoproliferative disease gene SH2D1A in common variable immunodeficiency syndrome. *Blood* 2001; **98**: 1321–5.

34. Soresina A, Lougaris V, Giliani S *et al.* Mutations of the X-linked lymphoproliferative disease gene SH2D1A mimicking common variable immunodeficiency. *Eur J Pediatr* 2002; **161**: 656–9.

35. Wheat WH, Cool CD, Morimoto Y *et al.* Possible role of human herpesvirus 8 in the lymphoproliferative disorders in common variable immunodeficiency. *J Exp Med* 2005; **202**: 479–84.

36. Leonard GD, Posadas E, Herrmann PC *et al.* Non-Hodgkin's lymphoma in Job's syndrome: a case report and literature review. *Leuk Lymphoma* 2004; **45**: 2521–5.

●37. Curtis RE, Travis LB, Rowlings PA *et al.* Risk of lymphoproliferative disorders after bone marrow transplantation: a multi-institutional study. *Blood* 1999; **94**: 2208–16.

38. Rooney CM, Smith CA, Ng CYC *et al.* Infusion of cytotoxic T cells for the prevention and treatment of Epstein-Barr virus-induced lymphoma in allogeneic transplant recipients. *Blood* 1998; **92**: 1549–55.

●39. Clave E, Agbalika F, Bajzik V *et al.* Epstein-Barr virus (EBV) reactivation in allogeneic stem-cell transplantation: relationship between viral load, EBV-specific T-cell reconstitution and rituximab therapy. *Transplantation* 2004; **77**: 76–84.

●40. Opelz G, Dohler B. Lymphomas after solid organ transplantation: a collaborative transplant study report. *Am J Transplant* 2004; **4**: 222–30.

41. Guppy AE, Rawlings E, Madrigal JA *et al.* A quantitative assay for Epstein-Barr Virus-specific immunity shows interferon-gamma producing CD8$^+$ T cells increase during immunosuppression reduction to treat posttransplant lymphoproliferative disease. *Transplantation* 2007; **84**: 1534–9.

42. Dockrell DH, Strickler JG, Paya CV. Epstein-Barr virus-induced T cell lymphoma in solid organ transplant recipients. *Clin Infect Dis* 1998; **26**: 180–2.

43. Allen U, Hebert D, Moore D *et al.* Epstein-Barr virus-related post-transplant lymphoproliferative disease in solid organ transplant recipients, 1988–97: a Canadian multi-centre experience. *Pediatr Transplant* 2001; **5**: 198–203.

44. Ambinder RF. Gammaherpesviruses and "Hit-and-Run" oncogenesis. *Am J Pathol* 2000; **156**: 1–3.

45. Leblond V, Dhedin N, Mamzer Bruneel MF *et al.* Identification of prognostic factors in 61 patients with posttransplantation lymphoproliferative disorders. *J Clin Oncol* 2001; **19**: 772–8.

46. Muti G, Cantoni S, Oreste P *et al.* Post-transplant lymphoproliferative disorders: improved outcome after clinico-pathologically tailored treatment. *Haematologica* 2002; **87**: 67–77.

47. Ghobrial IM, Habermann TM, Maurer MJ *et al.* Prognostic analysis for survival in adult solid organ transplant recipients with post-transplantation lymphoproliferative disorders. *J Clin Oncol* 2005; **23**: 7574–82.

48. Amlot PL, Tahami F, Venkat-Raman G *et al.* Reduction of immunosuppression (RIS) in treatment of post transplant lymphoproliferative disease (PTLD) revisited. *N Engl J Med* (submitted).

49. Mentzer SJ, Perrine SP, Faller DV. Epstein–Barr virus post-transplant lymphoproliferative disease and virus-specific therapy: pharmacological re-activation of viral target genes with arginine butyrate. *Transpl Infect Dis* 2001; **3**: 177–85.

50. Starzl TE, Nalesnik MA, Porter KA *et al.* Reversibility of lymphomas and lymphoproliferative lesions developing under cyclosporin-steroid therapy. *Lancet* 1984; **1**: 583–7.

51. Haque T, Wilkie GM, Jones MM *et al.* Allogeneic cytotoxic T-cell therapy for EBV-positive posttransplantation lymphoproliferative disease: results of a phase 2 multicenter clinical trial. *Blood* 2007; **110**: 1123–31.

52. Benkerrou M, Jais JP, Leblond V *et al.* Anti-B-cell monoclonal antibody treatment of severe posttransplant B- lymphoproliferative disorder: prognostic factors and long-term outcome. *Blood* 1998; **92**: 3137–47.

●53. Choquet S, Leblond V, Herbrecht R *et al.* Efficacy and safety of rituximab in B-cell post-transplantation lymphoproliferative disorders: results of a prospective multicenter phase 2 study. *Blood* 2006; **107**: 3053–7.

54. Milpied N, Vasseur B, Parquet N *et al.* Humanized anti-CD20 monoclonal antibody (Rituximab) in post transplant B-lymphoproliferative disorder: a retrospective analysis on 32 patients. *Ann Oncol* 2000; **11**(Suppl 1): 113–6.

55. Buell JF, Gross TG, Hanaway MJ *et al.* Chemotherapy for posttransplant lymphoproliferative disorder: the Israel Penn International Transplant Tumor Registry experience. *Transplant Proc* 2005; **37**: 956–7.

◆56. Smedby KE, Baecklund E, Askling J. Malignant lymphomas in autoimmunity and inflammation: a review of risks, risk factors, and lymphoma characteristics. *Cancer Epidemiol Biomarkers Prev* 2006; **15**: 2069–77.

57. Streubel B, Huber D, Wohrer S *et al.* Frequency of chromosomal aberrations involving MALT1 in mucosa-associated lymphoid tissue lymphoma in patients with Sjogren's syndrome. *Clin Cancer Res* 2004; **10**: 476–80.

58. Pijpe J, van Imhoff GW, Spijkervet FK *et al.* Rituximab treatment in patients with primary Sjogren's syndrome: an open-label phase II study. *Arthritis Rheum* 2005; **52**: 2740–50.

59. Obermann EC, Diss TC, Hamoudi RA *et al.* Loss of heterozygosity at chromosome 9p21 is a frequent finding in enteropathy-type T-cell lymphoma. *J Pathol* 2004; **202**: 252–62.

60. Al-Toma A, Verbeek WH, Hadithi M *et al.* Survival in refractory coeliac disease and enteropathy-associated T-cell lymphoma: retrospective evaluation of single-centre experience. *Gut* 2007; **56**: 1373–8.

61. Zintzaras E, Voulgarelis M, Moutsopoulos HM. The risk of lymphoma development in autoimmune diseases: a meta-analysis. *Arch Intern Med* 2005; **165**: 2337–44.

●62. Baecklund E, Iliadou A, Askling J *et al.* Association of chronic inflammation, not its treatment, with increased lymphoma risk in rheumatoid arthritis. *Arthritis Rheum* 2006; **54**: 692–701.

63. Mariette X, Cazals-Hatem D, Warszawki J *et al.* Lymphomas in rheumatoid arthritis patients treated with methotrexate: a 3-year prospective study in France. *Blood* 2002; **99**: 3909–15.

64. Salloum E, Cooper DL, Howe G *et al.* Spontaneous regression of lymphoproliferative disorders in patients treated with methotrexate for rheumatoid arthritis and other rheumatic diseases. *J Clin Oncol* 1996; **14**: 1943–9.

65. Silvestri F, Pipan C, Barillari G *et al.* Prevalence of hepatitis C virus infection in patients with lymphoproliferative disorders. *Blood* 1996; **87**: 4296–301.

66. Finn L, Reyes J, Bueno J, Yunis E. Epstein-Barr virus infections in children after transplantation of the small intestine. *Am J Surg Pathol* 1998; **22**: 299–309.

67. Reyes J, Bueno J, Kocoshis S *et al.* Current status of intestinal transplantation in children. *J Pediatr Surg* 1998; **33**: 243–54.

83

Uncommon histologic subtypes of non-Hodgkin lymphoma in children

JOHN T SANDLUND

INTRODUCTION

One of the largest series of uncommon histologic subtypes of non-Hodgkin lymphoma (NHL) occurring in children was reported by Ribeiro et al.[1] approximately 15 years ago. Patients were classified according to the National Cancer Institute (NCI) Working Formulaton.[2] An uncommon histologic subtype was identified in 36 of 1336 cases (2.7 percent) of newly diagnosed NHL in children treated at either St. Jude Children's Research Hospital or at a participating Pediatric Oncology Group institution.[1] Among these 36 cases, 17 were identified as having follicular histology and 19 were classified as having diffuse histology of low or intermediate grade. Among the 17 follicular cases, six were described as mixed small and large cell, nine as large cell, and two as small noncleaved cell. Among the 19 cases with diffuse histology, 18 were described as mixed small cell and large cell and one as small cell lymphocytic.

There were distinct differences in the clinical features and treatment outcome between those with follicular as compared to diffuse histology. Those with follicular histology were generally associated with limited stage disease involving lymph nodes or tonsils and had an excellent treatment outcome as reflected in the actuarial 5-year event-free survival of 94 percent. In contrast, those with diffuse histology tended to have more advanced stage disease, and had a somewhat poorer treatment outcome with only 74 percent alive in continuous complete remission at 5 years (actuarial 5-year event-free survival of 70 percent). Thus, those with diffuse histology had an outcome similar to that of children treated for 'high-grade' histology. There are, however, limitations with the NCI Working Formulation[2] in the description of the clinico-biologic features of the uncommon histologic subtypes of pediatric non-Hodgkin lymphomas, particularly for those of diffuse histology.

The World Health Organization (WHO) classification system for hematopoeitic malignancies incorporates morphologic, biologic (i.e., immunophenotypic and cytogenetic), and clinical features (Table 83.1).[3] According to this system, the most common subtypes of non-Hodgkin lymphomas in children are Burkitt lymphoma, lymphoblastic lymphoma (usually precursor T cell), diffuse large B cell lymphoma, and anaplastic large cell lymphoma. Although more than 90 percent of NHL subtypes fall into these four categories,[4] a small percentage of very unusual NHL subtypes are encountered in children. They fall under both the mature B cell and mature T cell neoplasm categories (Table 83.2) and are discussed in this chapter. Each section includes a brief summary of the clinico-biologic features associated with the histologic subtype, followed by additional published data regarding treatment, including that which pertains specifically to children.

Table 83.1   Non-Hodgkin lymphoma subtypes according to WHO classification system[3]

A. B cell neoplasms
1. Precursor B cell
2. Mature B cell

B. T cell neoplasms
1. Precursor T cell
2. Mature and NK/T cell malignancies

WHO, World Health Organization; NK, natural killer.

Table 83.2   Uncommon pediatric non-Hodgkin lymphoma subtypes according to WHO classification system[3]

A. Mature B cell neoplasms
1. Follicular lymphoma
2. Extranodal marginal zone B cell lymphoma of mucosal-associated lymphoid tissue (MALT)
3. Nodal marginal zone B cell lymphoma

B. Mature T cell neoplasms
1. Hepatosplenic T cell lymphoma
2. Subcutaneous panniculitis-like T cell lymphoma
3. Extranodal NK/T cell lymphoma, nasal type
4. Mycosis fungoides
5. T cell large granular lymphocytic leukemia

WHO, World Health Organization; NK, natural killer.

MATURE B CELL NEOPLASMS

Follicular lymphoma

The WHO system specifies that follicular lymphomas feature nodal infiltration by centrocytes and centroblasts.[3] Centrocytes are small to medium-sized cells, with cleaved nuclei and scant pale cytoplasm, whereas centroblasts are large transformed cells with round nuclei, one to three peripheral nucleoli, and a narrow rim of basophilic cytoplasm. These tumors are graded from 1 to 3 based on the number of centroblasts per high power field (0–1/HPF, 6–15/HPF, and >15/HPF, respectively). The histologic pattern is designated on the basis of percentage of follicular component, and includes follicular (more than 75 percent follicular), follicular and diffuse (25–75 percent follicular), and focally follicular (less than 25 percent follicular). There are various cytogenetic abnormalities that may be identified including t(14;18)(q32;q21) in 80 percent of cases, +7 in 20 percent, +18 in 20 percent, 3q27-28 in 15 percent, 6q23-26 in 15 percent, and 17p in 15 percent.[3] Oncogene abnormalities include the *BCL2* and *BCL6* rearrangements and *BCL6* 5′ mutation in 80 percent, 15 percent, and 40 percent of cases, respectively.[3] The treatment of adults with follicular lymphoma varies with stage and relapse status (for example, CHOP, fludarabine, involved field irradiation, rituximab, and hematopoietic stem cell transplantation).[5–7]

Lorsbach *et al.*[8] reported their findings of a retrospective study of 23 children with follicular lymphoma. The median age was 11 years. Among the 19 with available presenting clinical features, the majority were found to have limited stage disease and were designated as stage I (*n* = 15), stage II (*n* = 1), and stage III/IV (*n* = 3). The treatment included CHOP-based (cyclophosphamide, doxorubicin, vincristine, and prednisone) chemotherapy in most patients, and involved field irradiation in four patients. With respect to histopathology, all cases had follicular architecture, with 74 percent of cases designated as grade 2 or 3. CD20 and BCL6 expression was identified in all cases, whereas BCL2 expression was identified in only five of 16 cases studied. Of interest, all BCL2-negative cases were stage I, achieved a complete remission (CR), and never relapsed. In contrast, the BCL2-positive cases were associated with either stage III or IV disease, or had refractory disease. Thus, in this review, the majority of pediatric follicular lymphomas were biologically different from those occurring in adults.

In a retrospective study of the UK NHL registry, performed by Atra *et al.*,[9] seven of 447 children with NHL were reported to have follicular lymphoma. The median age was 7.5 years and all had localized disease (stage I, *n* = 4; stage II, *n* = 3). Disease sites included cervical lymph nodes and tonsils (*n* = 5), ileum (*n* = 1), and parotid gland (*n* = 1). The treatment regimen varied and included complete surgical resection only (*n* = 3), or complete surgical resection (*n* = 1) or incomplete resection (*n* = 3) followed by multiagent chemotherapy given over 23 weeks. Among these children, six remained in complete continuous remission (including three who received no chemotherapy) and one expired with recurrent lymphoma.

Thus, the role of chemotherapy in follicular lymphomas of childhood remains somewhat controversial, particularly for those with completely resected disease that is BCL2 negative.

Extranodal marginal zone B cell lymphoma of mucosal–associated lymphoid tissue (MALT) and nodal marginal zone B cell lymphomas

According to the WHO system, extranodal marginal zone B cell lymphomas of mucosal-associated lymphoid tissue (MALT) are characterized histologically by a marginal zone distribution, with small to medium-sized B cells containing irregular nuclei and inconspicuous nucleoli.[3] The WHO system specifies that plasmacytic differentiation may be identified in up to one-third of gastric MALT tumors and is a very prominent characteristic of most thyroid MALT and IPSID (immunoproliferative small intestinal disease) tumors. Cytogenetic features include trisomy 3 in approximately 60 percent of cases, and t(11;18) in 25–50 percent of cases. Among adults, 50 percent occur in the gastrointestinal tract (stomach, 85 percent; small intestine in IPSID tumors occurring in the Middle East).

Risk factors include *Helicobacter pylori* infection for gastric MALTs, chronic intestinal infection (IPSID tumors), and autoimmune disorders (e.g., Hashimoto thyroiditis). These tumors are generally slow to disseminate.[3]

A recent review of IPSID tumors by Al-Saleem and Al-Mondhiry identified *Campylobacter jejuni* infection as an associated risk factor for developing this lymphoma; they described presenting clinical features consistent with proximal small bowel involvement including malabsorption, abdominal pain, and diarrhea.[10] They also noted that IPSID tumors are characterized by excessive plasma cell differentiation, producing truncated alpha heavy chain proteins which lack light chains; also reported was an associated t(9;14) translocation involving the *PAX5* gene. In this review, antibiotic therapy resulted in a 30–70 percent complete response rate among early stage patients.

The WHO classification indicates that in nodal marginal zone B cell lymphomas, both the interfollicular and marginal zone regions of the lymph node are characterized by infiltration by centrocyte-like marginal zone B cells, small lymphocytes (B cell), and monocytoid B cells. It also describes two subtypes: those that are similar in appearance to splenic marginal zone lymphoma and those whose morphology is similar to nodal involvement by MALT.[3]

Taddesse-Heath *et al.* published a retrospective review of marginal zone B cell lymphomas (MZL) in children and young adults ranging in age from 2 to 29 years.[11] Fifty-two percent of the patients in this review were less than 18 years of age. Two types of presentations were identified, which included both nodal ($n = 32$, 67 percent) and extranodal ($n = 16$, 33 percent) types. Among the nodal cases, there was a male predominance (5.4:1) and no preexisting autoimmune or underlying disease. They generally presented with localized lymph node involvement (stage I, 90 percent) and had an excellent outcome, with relapses occurring infrequently. Among the extranodal cases, sites of involvement included ocular adnexa (31 percent), salivary glands (25 percent), and skin (19 percent). A male predominance was reported (1.2:1) as well as preexisting autoimmune disease in 19 percent. They generally presented with localized disease (stage I, 73 percent) and also had an excellent outcome. The treatment approaches were variable for both the nodal and extranodal tumors. Treatment for the 32 nodal tumors included excision alone ($n = 19$), involved field irradiation ($n = 5$), chemotherapy ($n = 3$), and involved field irradiation plus chemotherapy ($n = 1$); type of treatment was not available for four patients. Among these cases there was only one relapse, which occurred in a patient treated with excision alone. Treatment for the 16 extranodal tumors included excision alone ($n = 2$), involved field irradiation ($n = 5$), and chemotherapy ($n = 2$); type of treatment was not stated for seven patients. Among these there was only one relapse, which occurred in a patient treated with excision alone.

Thus, the optimal therapeutic approach for this rare NHL subtype is also somewhat controversial.

MATURE T CELL NEOPLASMS

Hepatosplenic T cell lymphoma

According to the WHO classification system, this subtype is characterized by medium-sized cells with a rim of pale cytoplasm, and marked sinusoidal infiltration of the liver and spleen.[3] Sinusoidal infiltration of the bone marrow may also be identified. These lymphomas are usually $\gamma\delta$ positive; however, $\alpha\beta$ variants have been described. Lymph nodes are usually not involved. The prognosis is generally poor. Immunocompromised hosts may be at increased risk for developing these lymphomas – in separate reports by Khan *et al.*[12] and Wu *et al.*,[13] this lymphoma was identified in renal transplant recipients. Cytogenetic abnormalities identified by Weidmann in a retrospective study of 45 cases of hepatosplenic T cell lymphoma included i(7)(q10), trisomy 8, and loss of sex chromosomes.[14]

The treatment outcome for the 45 patients, who were treated with a spectrum of multiagent chemotherapy regimens including autologous or allogeneic hematopoietic stem cell transplantation in some cases, was generally very poor. Among the 39 for whom follow-up data were available, there were only five survivors. In a subsequent review by Belhadj *et al.*, among 21 patients with hepatosplenic $\gamma\delta$ T cell lymphoma there were only two survivors.[15] Many of the patients were responsive to initial CHOP-like induction therapy; however, most subsequently relapsed even if autologous hematopoietic stem cell transplantation was implemented as consolidation. There are very few published data on the clinical presentation and treatment of this lymphoma occurring in children. Moleti *et al.* reported the successful treatment with chemotherapy alone of a 19-year-old male.[16] His treatment included 4 cycles of IEV (ifosfamide, epirubicin, and etoposide), followed by an 8-week course of modified MACOP-B (etoposide instead of adriamycin). Additional data on the management of this lymphoma in children are required.

Subcutaneous panniculitis–like T cell lymphoma

Morphologic examination of this tumor reveals a cell size ranging from small to large transformed, with rimming of neoplastic cells around fat cells.[3] There is subcutaneous infiltration by tumor, which is usually $\alpha\beta$ positive. Immunophenotype studies usually demonstrate expression of CD8, as well as that of various cytotoxic molecules including granzyme B and perforin.[3] This tumor typically arises in the subcutaneous fat, and disseminates to lymph nodes late in the disease course.[3] There are two subsets of this lymphoma type: those derived from $\alpha\beta$ T cells, which usually have a protracted course, and those derived from $\gamma\delta$ T cells (associated with CD56 expression), which have a much more aggressive course.[17]

Most of what is understood about treatment strategies and outcomes for these patients comes from the experiences reported in managing adults with this disorder. The treatment outcome is variable, although most report a fair to poor outcome. Adverse prognostic factors include the $\gamma\delta$ T cell phenotype and hemophagocytic syndrome at diagnosis.[18] Various treatment approaches have been studied. Prednisone alone generally results in infrequent durable remissions.[18] In a review by Go and Wester, it was concluded that anthracycline-based regimens had been used most commonly and appeared to be the most effective, resulting in long term CR rates of ≈ 30 percent.[18] High-dose chemotherapy followed by hematopoietic stem cell transplantation has been used for refractory disease, with a median response duration of greater than 14 months in one study.[18]

There has been very little published on the subcutaneous panniculitis-like T cell lymphomas (SPTCL) occurring in children. Thomson et al. reported a case occurring in a 3-year-old male as well as a review of the six prior cases reported in the literature.[19] Their patient, whose lymphoma arose in the head and neck area and expressed both CD8 and CD56, was successfully treated with a multiagent intensive regimen, including vincristine, doxorubicin, prednisone, methotrexate, cytarabine, thioguanine, and etoposide, and remained in remission at 2 years. Clinical data were available for four of six patients in their review of the literature; they received various treatments, ranging from prednisone alone to CHOP (cyclophosphamide, doxorubicin, vincristine, and prednisone). Among these four, one treated with prednisone alone was in remission at 3 years, two died of infection, and one treated with prednisone and cyclosporine A died of hemophagocytic syndrome. Shani-Adir et al. reported the activity of cyclosporine in two adolescent boys with SPTCL, and suggested an approach that features the early introduction of cyclosporine along with multiagent chemotherapy for children presenting with SPTCL.[20] There is clearly a need for additional data to make formal treatment guidelines for children with this neoplasm.

Extranodal natural killer/T cell lymphoma, nasal type

These lymphomas are characterized histologically by an angiocentric infiltrate of small to large cells, which are CD2$^+$, CD56$^+$, surface CD3$^-$, cytoplasmic CD3$^+$, granzyme$^+$, perforin$^+$, and usually negative for all other T and natural killer (NK) cell antigens.[3] Epstein–Barr virus (EBV) is characteristically detected. The two most frequently identified cytogenetic abnormalities include del(6)(q21q25) and i(6)(p10). The typical sites of involvement include the nasal cavity, palate, and nasopharynx.[3] The prognosis is generally considered to be fair to poor.

Prognostic factors included the presence of B symptoms and stage in one study,[21] and the IPI (International Prognositic Index) score in another.[22] Kim et al. reported a 3-year overall survival rate of 59 percent with a regimen consisting of CHOP and involved field irradiation, and concluded that further improvement in treatment was needed.[21] In this regard, Chim et al. are currently examining a regimen which comprises multiagent chemotherapy and involved field irradiation with a randomization for incorporation of hematopoietic stem cell transplantation in high-risk IPI score cases.[22] Both Kim et al.[21] and Chim et al.[22] suggest that the early use of involved field irradiation may be of benefit. There does appear to be a biphasic disease-free survival curve, with late failures being described.[22]

Chim et al. reviewed the various anthracycline- and non-anthracycline-containing regimens that have been implemented in these patients.[22] It is not clear which if any regimen is optimal. An L-asparaginase-based regimen (L-asparaginase, vincristine, and prednisone) described by Obama et al. was shown to be active in a 70-year-old male.[23] The optimal treatment approach in children has yet to be elucidated; however, insights from the adult experience are providing the basis for treatment approaches in children.

Mycosis fungoides

The tumor cells are characterized by irregular (cerebriform) nuclei, forming Pautrier microabscesses within the epidermis.[3] Tumor cells are typically CD2$^+$, CD3$^+$, T cell receptor β^+, CD5$^+$, CD4$^+$, and CD8$^-$. Clonal T cell receptor gene rearrangements are identified in most cases.[3] Various treatment approaches have been used, including involved field irradiation, topical nitrogen mustard, and PUVA (psoralen with ultraviolet light A). Systemic modalities include cytotoxic chemotherapy (cyclophosphamide, adriamycin, etoposide, vincristine, 2-deoxycoformycin, fludarabine, 2-chlorodeoxyadenosine, gemcitabine, and temozolamide), chromatin remodeling agents such as depsipeptide, and biologics such as interferon α and denileukin diftitox (interleukin-2–diphtheria toxin fusion protein).[24–26]

Mycosis fungoides is rarely encountered in children, and when it does occur is associated with heterogeneous clinical, histologic, and immunopathologic features.[27] In adults, cutaneous involvement may spread to lymph nodes, and ultimately bone marrow, liver, spleen, lung, and peripheral blood (Sézary syndrome). Adults with mycosis fungoides are also at risk for the development of other lymphomas including Hodgkin lymphoma.[27] The small number of reported cases of mycosis fungoides in children precludes making a meaningful comparison of the natural history of the disease in children with that reported in adults. However, in a review of five children with mycosis fungoides by Peters et al., three were found to have extracutaneous involvement, leading authors to suggest that the prognosis may be poorer in younger patients with this neoplasm.[27] Additionally, Hodgkin lymphoma subsequently developed in two of these five patients. Additional data are needed regarding the clinical presentation, treatment, and outcome for children with mycosis fungoides.

T cell large granular lymphocytic leukemia

The large granular lymphocytic leukemia (LGL) cells are characterized by abundant cytoplasm and contain either fine or coarse azurophilic granules. The tumor cells typically have a mature T cell immunophenotype (CD3$^+$, TCR α/β^+, CD4$^-$, and CD8$^+$).[3]

The clinical course is generally indolent with the development of moderate splenomegaly.[3] Recurrent bacterial infections, splenomegaly, and cytopenias may occur in up to two-thirds of patients.[28] The prognosis is variable.[3,28] Treatment approaches have included cyclosporine A, methotrexate, cyclophosphamide, and steroids.[3] These immunosuppressive measures are not curative, but may control cytopenias and symptoms in over 50 percent of patients.[28] This is primarily a disorder occurring in adults, with little experience in children, although rare cases have been reported.[29]

KEY POINTS

- Follicular lymphomas can generally be managed with conservative treatment; BCL2 expression identifies a higher risk group.
- Hepatosplenic T cell lymphomas have a poor prognosis; novel strategies are needed.
- Prospective studies of the clinical and biological features of the rare lymphomas of childhood are needed.

ACKNOWLEDGMENTS

Supported in part by a Grant from the National Cancer Institute (CA 21765), by a Center of Excellence grant from the State of Tennessee, and by the American Lebanese Syrian Associated Charities (ALSAC).

REFERENCES

● = Key primary paper
◆ = Major review article

● 1. Ribeiro RC, Pui CH, Murphy SB et al. Childhood malignant non-Hodgkin lymphomas of uncommon histology. Leukemia 1992; 6: 761–5.
2. National Cancer Institute sponsored study of classifications of non-Hodgkin's lymphomas: summary and description of a working formulation for clinical usage. The Non-Hodgkin's Lymphoma Pathologic Classification Project. Cancer 1982; 49: 2112–35.
3. Jaffe ES, Harris N, Stein H et al. Pathology and genetics of tumours of haematopoietic and lymphoid tissues. In: Kleihues P, Sobin LH (eds). World Health Organization classification of tumours. Lyon: IARC Press, 2001.
◆4. Murphy SB, Fairclough DL, Hutchison RE, Berard CW. Non-Hodgkin's lymphomas of childhood: an analysis of the histology, staging, and response to treatment of 338 cases at a single institution. J Clin Oncol 1989; 7: 186–93.
5. Ganti AK, Bociek RG, Bierman PJ et al. Follicular lymphoma: expanding therapeutic options. Oncology (Williston Park) 2005; 19: 213–28; discussion 228, 233–6, 239.
6. Fisher RI, LeBlanc M, Press OW et al. New treatment options have changed the survival of patients with follicular lymphoma. J Clin Oncol 2005; 23: 8447–52.
●7. Zinzani PL, Pulsoni A, Perrotti A et al. Fludarabine plus mitoxantrone with and without rituximab versus CHOP with and without rituximab as front-line treatment for patients with follicular lymphoma. J Clin Oncol 2004; 22: 2654–61.
●8. Lorsbach RB, Shay-Seymore D, Moore J et al. Clinicopathologic analysis of follicular lymphoma occurring in children. Blood 2002; 99: 1959–64.
●9. Atra A, Meller ST, Stevens RS et al. Conservative management of follicular non-Hodgkin's lymphoma in childhood. Br J Haematol 1998; 103: 220–3.
10. Al-Saleem T, Al-Mondhiry H. Immunoproliferative small intestinal disease (IPSID): a model for mature B-cell neoplasms. Blood 2005; 105: 2274–80.
●11. Taddesse-Heath L, Pittaluga S, Sorbara L et al. Marginal zone B-cell lymphoma in children and young adults. Am J Surg Pathol 2003; 27: 522–31.
12. Khan WA, Yu L, Eisenbrey AB et al. Hepatosplenic gamma/delta T-cell lymphoma in immunocompromised patients. Report of two cases and review of literature. Am J Clin Pathol 2001; 116: 41–50.
13. Wu H, Wasik MA, Przybylski G et al. Hepatosplenic gamma-delta T-cell lymphoma as a late-onset posttransplant lymphoproliferative disorder in renal transplant recipients. Am J Clin Pathol 2000; 113: 487–96.
●14. Weidmann E. Hepatosplenic T cell lymphoma. A review on 45 cases since the first report describing the disease as a distinct lymphoma entity in 1990. Leukemia 2000; 14: 991–7.
●15. Belhadj K, Reyes F, Farcet JP et al. Hepatosplenic gammadelta T-cell lymphoma is a rare clinicopathologic entity with poor outcome: report on a series of 21 patients. Blood 2003; 102: 4261–9.
16. Moleti ML, Testi AM, Giona F et al. Gamma-delta hepatosplenic T-cell lymphoma. Description of a case with immunophenotypic and molecular follow-up successfully treated with chemotherapy alone. Leuk Lymphoma 2006; 47: 333–6.
17. Hoque SR, Child FJ, Whittaker SJ et al. Subcutaneous panniculitis-like T-cell lymphoma: a clinicopathological, immunophenotypic and molecular analysis of six patients. Br J Dermatol 2003; 148: 516–25.

●18. Go RS, Wester SM. Immunophenotypic and molecular features, clinical outcomes, treatments, and prognostic factors associated with subcutaneous panniculitis-like T-cell lymphoma: a systematic analysis of 156 patients reported in the literature. *Cancer* 2004; **101**: 1404–13.

19. Thomson AB, McKenzie KJ, Jackson R, Wallace WH. Subcutaneous panniculitic T-cell lymphoma in childhood: successful response to chemotherapy. *Med Pediatr Oncol* 2001; **37**: 549–52.

20. Shani-Adir A, Lucky AW, Prendiville J *et al*. Subcutaneous panniculitic T-cell lymphoma in children: response to combination therapy with cyclosporine and chemotherapy. *J Am Acad Dermatol* 2004; **50**(2 Suppl): S18–22.

●21. Kim WS, Song SY, Ahn YC *et al*. CHOP followed by involved field radiation: is it optimal for localized nasal natural killer/T-cell lymphoma? *Ann Oncol* 2001; **12**: 349–52.

●22. Chim CS, Ma SY, Au WY *et al*. Primary nasal natural killer cell lymphoma: long-term treatment outcome and relationship with the International Prognostic Index. *Blood* 2004; **103**: 216–21.

23. Obama K, Tara M, Niina K. L-asparaginase-Based induction therapy for advanced extranodal NK/T-cell lymphoma. *Int J Hematol* 2003; **78**: 248–50.

24. Foss F. Mycosis fungoides and the Sezary syndrome. *Curr Opin Oncol* 2004; **16**: 421–8.

25. Lundin J, Hagberg H, Repp R *et al*. Phase 2 study of alemtuzumab (anti-CD52 monoclonal antibody) in patients with advanced mycosis fungoides/Sezary syndrome. *Blood* 2003; **101**: 4267–72.

26. Olsen E, Duvic M, Frankel A *et al*. Pivotal phase III trial of two dose levels of denileukin diftitox for the treatment of cutaneous T-cell lymphoma. *J Clin Oncol* 2001; **19**: 376–88.

27. Peters MS, Thibodeau SN, White JW Jr, Winkelmann RK. Mycosis fungoides in children and adolescents. *J Am Acad Dermatol* 1990; **22**: 1011–18.

28. Sokol L, Loughran TP Jr. Large granular lymphocyte leukemia. *Oncologist* 2006; **11**: 263–73.

29. Boeckx N, Uyttebroeck A, Langerak AW *et al*. Clonal proliferation of T-Cell large granular lymphocytes. *Pediatr Blood Cancer* 2004; **42**: 275–7.

FUTURE DIRECTIONS IN DIAGNOSIS AND TREATMENT

84

Molecular profiling and lymphoma diagnosis

WING C CHAN AND KISHOR BHATIA

HISTORIC PERSPECTIVE

In the past two decades, there have been major advances in our understanding of the pathogenesis and biology of lymphoid malignancies.[1,2] Translocation breakpoints associated with many types of lymphomas[3–5] have been cloned and their mechanisms of action are being elucidated. Many genetic abnormalities or markers with significant diagnostic or prognostic importance have also been identified. One excellent example is the translocations involving the *MALT1* gene in extranodal marginal zone lymphoma (EMZL).[6,7] In gastric EMZL, the presence of this translocation indicates that the tumor is no longer responsive to antibiotic therapy directed against *Helicobacter pylori*.[8] In addition, these tumors have a spectrum of genetic abnormalities different from ones present in tumors without the translocation and, interestingly, they rarely progress to a diffuse large B cell lymphoma (DLBCL).[9] Inactivation of tumor suppressor genes such as *TP53*, *p16*^{INK4a}, and *p27* and abnormalities in the apoptotic pathways have been associated with poorer survival or tumor progression in a number of lymphomas.[10–16] Molecular diagnostics should not only serve as an aid to render a diagnosis, but also should measure parameters that are relevant to the biologic and clinical behavior of a tumor.

Traditionally, the investigation and measurement of genetic parameters have been performed individually, rather than globally. With the development of DNA microarray technology for large-scale gene expression profiling, it is now possible to obtain a comprehensive genome-wide picture of gene expression alterations associated with normal or disease processes.[17–20] Recognizing the potential of this technology when coupled with a large tumor/clinical resource, a number of groups have explored the use of gene expression profiling in lymphoma diagnosis and outcome prediction. The application of this technology has, in the past few years, led to the discovery of unique gene expression signatures for the major groups of B cell non-Hodgkin lymphoma (NHL) including some novel subtypes,[21–23] the construction of molecular prognosticators,[22,24–26] and insight into the molecular mechanisms that determine the behavior of a tumor.[26,27]

In addition to structural abnormalities at the genomic level that render tumor suppressor genes and apoptotic pathways inactive, changes at the epigenomic level have also been defined which result in the loss of expression of critical genes controlling cell growth or promoting cell death. There is increasing evidence supporting the postulate that lymphomagenesis is as much a result of a deregulated epigenome as it is a consequence of changes at the genomic level.[28] Available evidence derived from studies in specific hematologic malignancies[29,30] further suggest that epigenetic changes complement and cooperate with genetic lesions in the pathogenesis and evolution of these cancers. Analyses of DNA methylation in lymphoid neoplasms have provided a strategy complementary to genome-wide expression analyses in the discovery of biomarkers that can be utilized to aid detection and diagnosis of lymphomas[31] and, in preliminary studies, appear to be of value in the prognosis and monitoring of lymphoma[32,33] and may guide the choice of therapeutic regimens.

MOLECULAR PROFILING: TECHNICAL AND ANALYTICAL CONSIDERATIONS

Gene expression profiling has great potential but at the same time provides unique challenges. Because of the large number of parameters studied in each experiment, the number of samples that are available for study is invariably far from ideal, introducing a large discrepancy in dimensionality. While a sophisticated analytical program can be helpful, it is difficult to draw meaningful conclusions from studying a few cases. Therefore, it is essential to include as many cases as possible, often requiring the collaborative efforts from multiple institutions, especially for rarer entities. It is also desirable to have samples collected and processed uniformly to facilitate analysis but this is frequently not possible in retrospective studies, especially when samples are collected from different institutions. It should also be noted that for solid tumors, tumor cells are generally not separated from stromal elements when RNA is extracted. This complicates subsequent analysis but on the other hand, it also provides useful information pertaining to host–tumor interaction.

Due to the significant challenges encountered in the analysis of microarray experiments, it is imperative that significant findings or conclusions be validated. Validation can be directed at experimental data, data analysis, or conclusions and can be performed in a variety of ways. The expression levels of selected genes can be measured independently by techniques such as real-time quantitative reverse transcription polymerase chain reaction (RT-PCR) or by in situ hybridization if one wants to determine the distribution of the markers. Immunohistochemical assay can also be employed if there is a correlation between mRNA and protein level, provided that the appropriate antibody is available. Validation of data analysis and conclusions can be computational by using different analytical programs and by introducing perturbations to test the robustness of the analysis. Other approaches include the correlation with independent data sets such as clinical data, pathologic data/classification, genetic data, and known biological variables. It is also important to examine if different studies come up with similar findings and conclusions. This effort will be facilitated if experimental data are accessible and experimental methods and analytical approaches are presented in sufficient detail and in a standard format that allow independent analysis by other laboratories. Certain standards in data submission have been drawn up and many large data sets have been deposited by laboratories engaged in microarray analysis. Even though the use of different platforms by different laboratories presents significant problems in the comparison of data across the board, these large databases provide valuable resources for discovery and validation. Recently, a large multi-institution Microarray Quality Control (MAQC) project[34] was conducted to examine a variety of microarray-based and alternative technology platforms. This study shows a significant degree of intra- and inter-platform

concordance suggesting that carefully performed microarray studies can provide reliable and verifiable data.

CURRENT STATUS OF GENE EXPRESSION PROFILING IN LYMPHOMA DIAGNOSIS

Diffuse large B cell lymphoma is the most frequent lymphoma, accounting for 30–40 percent of all cases. There is good evidence for considerable clinical and biological heterogeneity within this entity but it is difficult for pathologists to reproducibly subclassify DLBCL into different subgroups. In one of the early gene expression profiling studies, two distinct subgroups of DLBCL were identified: one shows expression of a set of genes that are characteristic of germinal center (GC) B cells: the GC B cell-like (GCB) DLBCL. The other subset does not express this GC B cell signature but instead overexpresses a group of genes upregulated in peripheral blood B cells activated by mitogenic stimuli in vitro, the activated B cell-like (ABC) DLBCL.[21] Survival of patients with GCB DLBCL appears to be significantly better than that of the other subset.[21] These initial findings were subsequently validated in a study of 240 cases and, in addition, a small subset of cases that cannot be assigned into either one of these categories – the unclassified DLBCL (previously termed type III) – was identified (Plate 138, see plate section).[22,35] This set of cases shows low expression of both the GCB and ABC signatures. In about half of the cases, this is due to the low number of tumor B cells in the specimen. However, in the other half, abundant tumor B cells are present and the expression profile reflects the profile of the tumor cells. This subset of cases is being further studied to determine if it represents a unique third subset of DLBCL.

An uncommon form of DLBCL with prominent stromal fibrosis occurs in the anterior mediastinum and tends to affect young females. There has been much debate on whether this is a distinct entity. Recent studies from two groups[23,36] have identified a unique gene expression profile that can distinguish primary mediastinal DLBCL (PMBL) from other DLBCLs that happen to occur in the anterior mediastinum (Plate 139, see plate section). The PMBL profile is characterized by downregulated expression of a number of B cell receptor components and its downstream signaling molecules (B lymphocyte-specific tyrosine kinase [BLK], B cell linker protein [BLNK], protein kinase C β1 [PKC β1], nuclear factor of activated T cells c [NFATc], and CD22). Several functional groups of genes were upregulated such as genes in several cytokine pathways (interleukin-13 receptor α1 [IL-13Rα1], Janus kinase 2 [JAK2], signal transducer and activator of transcription 1 [STAT1], nuclear factor, interleukin-3 regulated [NFIL3], RANTES [CCL5], and interferon γ-inducible protein 10 [IP10]), tumor necrosis factor (TNF) family members and induced proteins (OX40 ligand, CD95, TNF receptor-associated factor 1 [TRAF-1], and TNFα-induced protein 3), and the extracellular

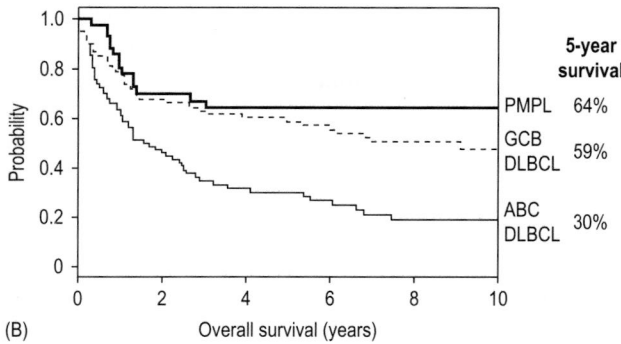

(B)

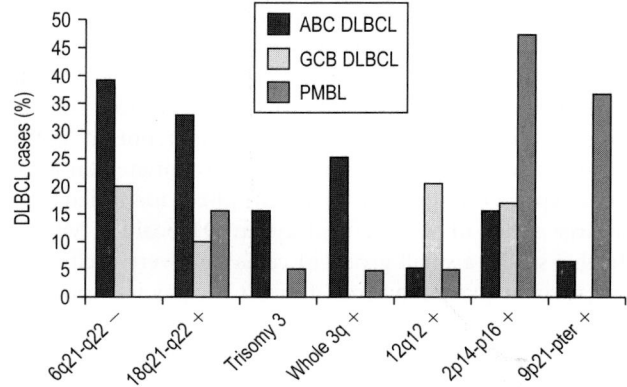

Figure 84.1 (A) Plate 139, see plate section. (B) Primary mediastinal large cell lymphoma has a similar survival to the germinal center B cell (GCB) type DLBCL, which is significantly better than the activated B cell (ABC) type of DLBCL. Reprinted with permission: Rosenwald A *et al. J Exp Med* 2003; **198**: 851–62, Figure 2A and Figure 3A.

Figure 84.2 Gene expression profile-defined subgroups of diffuse large B cell lymphoma (DLBCL) have distinctive patterns of genetic abnormalities. PMBL, primary mediastinal large B cell lymphoma; GCB, germinal center B cell; ABC, activated B cell. Reprinted with permission: Bea S *et al. Blood* 2005; **106**: 3183–90, Figure 1D.

matrix element tissue inhibitor of metalloproteinases 1 (TIMP-1). On reanalyzing the previously profiled cases of DLBCL,[22] 12 of the cases previously classified in the GCB group have the molecular profile of PMBL. Patients diagnosed with PMBL by the predictor were younger, had preferential involvement of thoracic structures, and had better 5-year survival than ABC DLBCL (64 percent vs 30 percent) (Fig. 84.1B). Interestingly, this gene expression profile bears significant similarity to that observed in Hodgkin lymphoma (HL)-derived cell lines[23,36] suggesting shared pathobiologic characteristics between PMBL and HL. In support of the validity of the gene expression-based subclassification of DLBCL, it has been demonstrated that distinct patterns of genetic abnormalities are associated with the different DLBCL subsets: BCL2 translocation in GCB DLBCL;[22,37,38] frequent gains of 9p24 (involving JAK2, PDL1, PDL2, and SMARCA2 genes) and 2p14-16 in PMBL;[23,36] and frequent gains in regions of chromosome 3, 18q21-22, and loss of 6q21-23 in ABC DLBCL (Fig. 84.2).[39]

It is interesting to note that several mutations that may be important in the pathogenesis of DLBCL are associated with unique gene expression profiling-defined categories. Thus, deleterious mutations of PRDM1 are found in the ABC subtype of DLBCL,[40,41] while SOCS1 mutations are associated with PMBL.[42]

Burkitt lymphoma (BL) is a highly aggressive, rapidly proliferating lymphoma with a characteristic morphology and translocation of the MYC oncogene. While the diagnosis is readily made in typical cases, cases with atypical morphology and/or immunophenotype may be difficult to differentiate from DLBCL with some features of BL. Two recent studies have used typical cases of BL to help construct a diagnostic signature for BL and then use this signature to examine the atypical cases and DLBCL.[43,44] It was found that the gene expression profiling-derived signatures are very useful in identifying BL among these cases.

Dave and colleagues found that BLs are characterized molecularly by the high expression of MYC target genes and a subset of the GC B cell signature. On the other hand, major histocompatibility complex (MHC) class I genes and nuclear factor κB (NF-κB) target genes are expressed at a much lower level compared with DLBCL (Plate 140, see plate section). Burkitt lymphomas from children and adults are characterized by the same diagnostic signature. With appropriate high-intensity chemotherapy, BL, especially in children, has good overall survival and it is, therefore, important not to miss these cases.

Gene expression profiling studies on a few less common or less well recognized DLBCL such as primary effusion lymphoma (PEL) and CD5+ DLBCL have been reported.[45–47]

Primary effusion lymphoma is characterized by a 'plasmoblastic' gene expression profile, having features of both immunoblasts and plasma cells. Further heterogeneity is seen based on the viral status of Kaposi sarcoma herpes virus (KSHV) and Epstein–Barr virus (EBV) with a more prominent influence of the former on the gene expression profile.[48] A small subset of DLBCL expresses surface CD5 and these cases have been reported to have a more aggressive clinical behavior with poorer survival.[48] Gene expression profiling on a small series identified a signature for these CD5+ cases that was also able to identify some cases that were CD5 negative. Genetic studies also suggest that this may be a distinct entity.[49,50]

Mantle cell lymphoma (MCL) accounts for 3–10 percent of NHL in the USA and Europe. It predominantly occurs in older adults (median age ~60 years) with a marked male predominance. Mantle cell lymphoma is an aggressive lymphoma with moderate chemosensitivity and a median survival of 3–5 years.[51] Mantle cell lymphoma cells typically bear surface immunoglobulin M (IgM) and IgD and are CD5 positive.[51] The cardinal feature of MCL is the t(11;14)(q13;q32) translocation in which the cyclin D1 locus is brought into proximity of the immunoglobulin heavy chain gene enhancers, leading to its overexpression. The existence of cyclin D1-negative MCL has been controversial. Without solid objective evidence, reported 'cyclin D1-negative MCLs' are difficult to substantiate. An MCL gene expression signature has recently been identified from a large series of well-defined cyclin D1-positive MCL.[25] In this study, a small group of cases that were cyclin D1-negative by quantitative real-time PCR assay was found to express this MCL signature. The MCL signature and diagnostic algorithm have been further refined and cases with the morphology of MCL and the typical molecular signature but lacking the characteristic translocation and cyclin D1 expression can indeed be identified (Plate 141, see plate section).[52] Using this signature, it is now possible to identify these *cyclin D1/BCL1* translocation-negative lymphomas to further evaluate their clinical features and biological relationship to typical MCL and to determine if they share similar pathogenetic mechanisms.

Follicular lymphoma (FL) is a GC B cell-derived malignancy, and t(14;18)(q32;q21) is a common genetic alteration occurring in up to 90 percent of cases. This translocation leads to the overexpression of the antiapoptotic protein BCL2 resulting in accumulation of follicle center cells. Additional genes have been described to be overexpressed in FL compared to normal splenic GC B cells in a gene expression profiling study using cDNA microarrays with 588 gene probes.[53] The authors found 32 genes to be differentially expressed, including transcription factors/regulators like PAX5 and ID2, TNF, IL-2Rγ, and IL-4Rα. Tumor necrosis factor is important for the establishment and maintenance of the structure of lymphoid tissues including GCs.[54] A monoclonal antibody directed at the B cell antigen CD20, rituximab, is now widely used in the treatment for FL. In a study that investigated the correlation between gene expression patterns and response to rituximab,[55] rituximab nonresponders clustered within the subgroup exhibiting a gene expression pattern more similar to nonmalignant spleen and tonsil. These results suggest a biological diversity in FL at the time of diagnosis identifiable by gene expression profiling and can be used to predict outcome to rituximab treatment. However, this study was carried out with only 24 FL patients and a larger, independent series of patients is required for validation. Clinical response to rituximab may be influenced by pharmacokinetics of the administered antibody and the genotype of the Fc receptor, FcγR.[56] The eight genes encoding three classes and several subclasses of FcγR display functional allotypes that may influence antibody-dependent cytotoxicity. These issues need to be taken into consideration in future studies.

In 25–60 percent of FL there is transformation to an aggressive lymphoma associated with a rapidly progressive clinical course and short survival.[57] A variety of genetic changes have been reported with this transformation such as *MYC* rearrangement,[58] *TP53* mutation,[12] mutations in the 5′ untranslated region of the *BCL6* gene, mutations of the translocated *BCL2* gene,[59] or *p15* or *p16* alterations including deletion, mutation, and hypermethylation.[60,61] However, it is not certain if these changes are directly associated with transformation and some may just represent interval changes that occurred between the initial biopsy and the transformation. More studies are needed to characterize all the genetic aberrations that are critical for transformation. In a recent cDNA microarray study,[62] two different gene expression profiles were observed to be associated with the transformation of FL to DLBCL; only one of these showed increased expression of *MYC* and its target genes. In an extended study using the same cases, array comparative genomic hybridization (aCGH) was performed,[63] with the expectation that the combination of aCGH and gene expression profiling would be synergistic in elucidating the mechanisms of transformation. aCGH demonstrated previously described genomic imbalances as well as imbalances not generally associated with FL: (1) gains of 9p23-p24, which are common in PMBL and classical Hodgkin lymphoma; (2) gains of 6p12-p21 that may involve oncogenes such as *PIM1* and *CCDN3*; and (3) gains of 17q21.33, containing the *NEM1* gene, a transcription factor and nucleoside diphosphate kinase that is upregulated by *MYC* and has a role in the transcriptional regulation of *MYC* expression. None of the transformed cases had elevated copy numbers of the *MYC* gene.[62] Thus, the observed overexpression of *MYC*, in up to 50 percent of transformed cases, was not due to gene amplification. The authors suggested that one of the possible mechanisms could be changes in *MYC* promoter methylation. It was also noted that several of the *MYC* target genes like *NME1* in 17q21, *JTV1* in 7p22, *CYP51* and *CUTL1* in 7q22, *CDK2* and *CDK4* in 12q, and *AHCY* in 20q11 were located in genomic areas that are often involved in transformation and genomic imbalances and may therefore contribute to differential expression of *MYC* target genes in some of the cases.

In another study of FL transformation, 12 matched pairs of FL and the corresponding DLBCL were examined. All the DLBCL exhibited a GCB-like profile[64] and 113 genes were identified as a classifier that distinguished the FL from their transformed counterparts. Several members of the *RAS* family, growth factors and cytokine receptors with known growth-promoting activity (*MET*, *FGFR3*, *LTB*R, and *PDGFRB*), and *p38MAPK* were found to have high expression levels in DLBCL. From this classifier, a three-gene predictor (*PLA2*, *PDGFRB*, and *RAB6*) was proposed. The authors also showed that inhibition of *p38MAPK* blocked the growth of t(14;18)-positive lymphoma cell lines, and inactivation of *p38MAPK* inhibited the growth of transplanted tumors in nonobese diabetic severe combined immunodeficient (NOD-SCID) mice, suggesting that pharmacologic targeting of *p38MAPK* may be an effective strategy against transformed FL. In a more recent report involving 20 paired FL and transformed FL samples,[65] it was also found that the transformed tumors had a GCB-DLBCL profile, and two different profiles regarding proliferation were observed similar to what was described by Lossos and coworkers.[62] Interestingly, genetic abnormalities involving *TP53*, *REL*, and *CDKN2A* were mostly associated with the group with high proliferation.[65]

Several uncommon types of lymphomas have been examined by gene expression profiling. In a recent study by Thieblemont and colleagues,[66] small lymphocytic lymphoma and splenic marginal zone B cell lymphoma (MZL) were reported to be distinguishable by gene expression profiling. There are still many questions regarding the relationship between nodal, extranodal, and splenic MZL and the heterogeneity within and among these entities. Development of accurate and biologically relevant class predictors may in the future improve the classification of this group of lymphomas. However, MZL is difficult to study due to its relatively low incidence of cases, the frequent small biopsy size, the large admixture of normal reactive immune cells, and manifestation at many different extranodal sites.

Recently, a few studies on the much less frequent T cell lymphomas have been reported.[67–69] It is not surprising that T lymphoblastic lymphoma, anaplastic large cell lymphoma (ALCL), and peripheral T cell lymphoma (PTCL) can be readily separated. The angioimmunoblastic type (AITL) of PTCL forms a unique cluster quite readily separable from other cases. The reader is referred to a more recent article.[70] The further classification of the remaining PTCL is more challenging. Three clusters of cases were identified by Ballester and coworkers (PTCL-U1, U2, and U3) (Fig. 84.3).[69] The U1 cluster tends to have fewer reactive cells and cytokine/chemokine gene expression is not prominent. It expresses some genes known to be associated with aggressive tumor behavior or unfavorable outcome. The U2 cluster is characterized by transcripts involved in protein translation and signal transduction. The authors also emphasized the activation of the NF-κB pathway and overexpression of BCL2 in this cluster. The U3 cluster appears to be dominated by the macrophage signature that corresponds to the 'histocyte-rich' histology of these tumors. In a study examining the expression of NF-κB pathway genes in T cell lymphoma,[67] it was found that T lymphoblastic lymphoma and ALCL had low expression of this group of genes while most of the PTCLs had high expression. As normal lymphoid cells and stromal cells may also express many of these genes, cases with a large amount of reactive components included in the NF-κB-positive group. It was also reported that there was good correlation between immunohistochemically demonstrated expression of p65 in tumor cells and the expression of the NF-κB signature gene.[67] However, it is not always easy to distinguish tumor from reactive elements in PTCL. It is likely that cases with low NF-κB target gene expression indeed have neoplastic T cells with low NF-κB activation, and it is interesting that this group of cases had poorer survival compared with the NF-κB-positive group. It is possible that the former group overlap with the U1 subtype reported by Ballester *et al.*[69] Thompson and coworkers[68] examined the gene expression

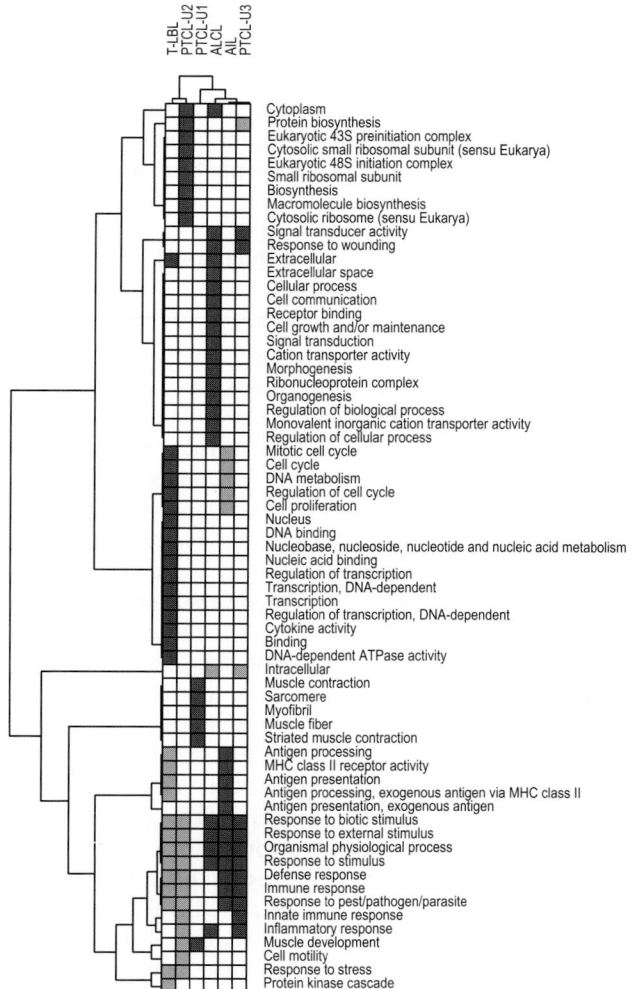

Figure 84.3 T lymphoblastic lymphoma (T-LBL), anaplastic large cell lymphoma (ALCL), and peripheral T cell lymphoma (PTCL) can be readily distinguished from one another. Among the PTCLs, the angioimmunoblastic type (AIL) forms a relatively distinct group different from the other PTCLs that can again be roughly divided into three subgroups with different gene expression signatures (intensity of shading indicates level of expression). PTCL-U, PTCL, unspecified. Modified with permission: Ballester B *et al. Oncogene* 2006; **25**: 1560–70, Figure 4.

profile of anaplastic lymphoma kinase (ALK) positive (ALK⁺) and ALK⁻ ALCL in an attempt to find common as well as unique pathogenetic mechanisms for these two groups. They observed that several genes encoding signal transduction molecules were overexpressed while a number of transcription factors were underexpressed in the ALK⁺ group. Cyclin D3 is upregulated at the mRNA and protein level in many ALK⁺ cases and may be significant in its pathogenesis. However, no dominant and common pathogenetic pathway has been found.

These studies provided some interesting information but also highlighted some major hurdles in studying PTCL, which include the variable presence of large amounts of reactive elements that make interpretation of the findings difficult. The difficulty of obtaining a large number of high-quality frozen tissues for study is another impediment. Furthermore, the classification of these cases is not straightforward and so the 'gold standard' for comparison with a gene expression profiling study may not be that reliable.

GENE EXPRESSION PROFILING AND PREDICTION OF OUTCOME

The possibility of predicting clinical outcome from gene expression profiles of the initial biopsy specimens has also been examined. In DLBCL, molecular predictors that have prognostic value independent of the International Prognostic Index (IPI)[71] have been described.[22,24] In these studies, survival data were used to guide the discovery process (supervised approach). Shipp and coworkers analyzed 58 cases of DLBCL on oligonucleotide microarrays with 6817 genes.[24] They divided the DLBCL into cured versus fatal or refractory disease groups, and generated a 13-gene predictor. Three of the genes in the predictor were also observed to correlate well with outcome in a previous study by Alizadeh,[21] namely neuron-derived orphan receptor (NOR1), phosphodiesterase (PDE) 4B and PKCβ2. The latter two genes are highly expressed in the ABC DLBCL that is associated with poor outcome. A list of predictor genes was also generated by Rosenwald and coworkers in a study including 240 de novo cases of DLBCL using the Lymphochip.[22] Seventeen genes were selected and a predictor generated by Cox proportional-hazards model. Sixteen of the 17 genes chosen represented four different gene expression signatures: GCB differentiation, proliferation, MHC class II, and lymph node stroma (Fig. 84.4). One additional gene (BMP6) was found to have added predictive value but this finding was not confirmed in analysis with another platform (unpublished data). High expression of the GCB signature (represented by BCL6, GCET1, and GCET2) and gene expression indicating an active stromal reaction (alpha actinin, collagen type III alpha I, connective tissue growth factor, fibronectin, urokinase, plasminogen activator) were predictive of good outcome. Overexpression of the proliferation signature (represented by MYC, E21G3, and NPM3) and low expression of MHC class II genes (represented by HLA-DPα, HLA-DQα, HLA-DRα, and HLA-DRβ) were found to correlate with poor prognosis. The correlation of poor survival with low MHC class II gene expression has been confirmed for DLBCL in general and also in PMBL using immunostaining for HLA-DR.[72,73]

An analysis of 92 MCL cases revealed a 48-gene signature whose expression correlated with overall survival.[25] A subset of these genes was associated with cellular proliferation – the proliferation signature (Plate 142, see plate section). The proliferation signature average was inversely correlated with survival with high significance ($P = 7.44 \times 10^{-5}$), and the addition of other genes from the original set of 48 did not significantly improve the predictive value.

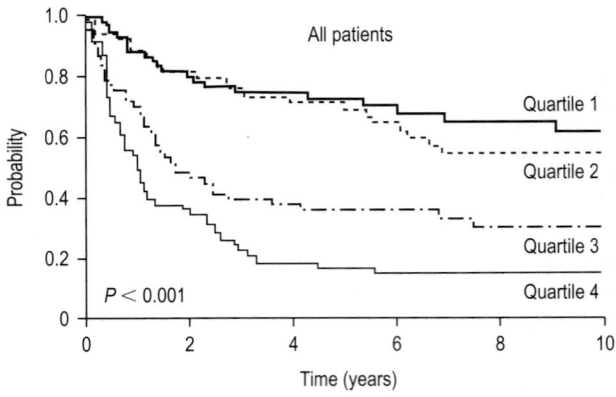

Figure 84.4　Using a 17-gene signature to construct a prognosticator, diffuse large B cell lymphoma is then divided into four quartiles according to the prognostic scores. A significant difference in survival among the cases can be demonstrated using this prognosticator. Reprinted with permission: Rosenwald A *et al. N Engl J Med* 2002; **346**: 1937–47, Figure 2C.

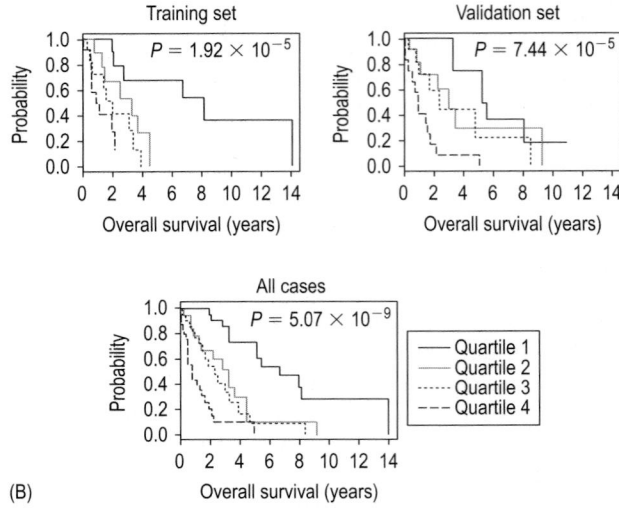

Figure 84.5　(A) Plate 142, see plate section. (B) The proliferation signature score is highly predictive of survival. Patients with low scores have markedly better survival than patients with high proliferation scores. Reprinted with permission: Rosenwald A *et al. Cancer Cell* 2002; **3**: 185–97, Figure 2A and Figure 2B.

Proliferation signature was also a better predictor of survival than the morphologic classification ($P = 5.07 \times 10^{-9}$). The quartile of patients with the highest proliferation-signature average had a median survival of 0.8 year, whereas the quartile with the lowest level had a median survival of 6.7 years (Fig. 84.5B). The study also examined the relationship between deletion of tumor suppressor genes and proliferation rate and overall survival in MCL. Deletion of the INK4a/ARF locus encoding p16$^{\text{INK4a}}$ and p14^{ARF} was detected in 21 percent of the cases and these cases had a poor prognosis. The p16$^{\text{INK4a}}$ protein controls G1 to S transition in the cell cycle by inhibiting the cyclin D-dependent kinases CDK4 and CDK6, thereby preventing phosphorylation of the retinoblastoma protein (RB).[72] The p14^{ARF} protein sequesters HDM2, which is a negative regulator of TP53, thereby allowing TP53 to mediate apoptosis and cell cycle arrest in the proper setting. Deletion of the *INK4a/ARF* locus in MCL may thus compromise both the RB and TP53 pathways.[74] Also noteworthy was the observation that overexpression of BMI1, a transcription repressor of *p16^{INK4a}* and *p14^{ARF}*,[75] was present only in MCL cases without deletion of the *INK4a/ARF* locus.[25] The level of cyclin D1 also correlated positively with the proliferation index that appears to represent an integrator of a number of different signals that adversely affect survival in MCL, including the deletion of the *INK4a/ARF* locus and the high expression of cyclin D1.[25]

Gene expression profiling has also identified a molecular predictor of prognosis for FL.[26] One hundred ninety one samples obtained from patients with newly diagnosed FL were profiled using Affymetrix U133 chips. The samples were divided into two groups – a training set of 91 cases for developing the molecular prognosticator and an independent set of 100 cases for validation of the model. Two gene signatures were noted to be highly synergistic in predicting survival, and these signatures were combined to form a molecular prognosticator for FL (Plate 143, see plate section).

The immune response-1 gene signature contains several genes that are known T cell markers including CD7, CD8B, and IL-2-inducible T cell kinase (ITK). The genes from the immune response-2 signature appear to be derived from the myeloid and monocytic lineage, as suggested by the presence of genes such as *FCGR1A* (CD64), Toll-like receptor 5 (*TLR5*), and scavenger receptor B2 (*SCARB2*). Thus, both gene signatures appear to be derived from the nonmalignant, tumor-infiltrating immune cells. This was confirmed by additional molecular studies using flow cytometry-sorted FL cells. This finding points to an important interaction between the host immune system and the malignant cells. This prognosticator also strongly predicts survival in the validation set of patients. The molecular predictor of survival was independent of the International Prognostic Index. Thus, gene expression profiling of FL has improved our understanding of the molecular determinants of long-term survival and provided new insights into the role of stromal immune-response cells, and tumor–host interactions. These findings may allow the risk-stratification of patients who will most likely benefit from experimental treatments in this generally indolent but currently incurable disease.[26]

The determinants of survival differ significantly in the three types of lymphomas studied, but in both DLBCL and FL significant components of the prognosticators reflect tumor–host interaction. This observation indicates that it is essential to obtain the stromal signature in tumors in the evaluation of outcome predictors. The discovery of these predictors indicates that gene expression profiling can provide us with a new and more biologically relevant approach to predict survival. While this represents a major advance in outcome prediction, the current prognosticators need to be validated and further refined. There are likely to be determinants of prognosis that were not included in the original expression profiles due either to technical or analytical limitations. It is also likely that certain biologic variables are not readily measurable by gene expression profiling alone. In addition, these prognosticators were constructed from cases treated before the advent of treatment regimens including anti-CD20. A reevaluation of the prognosticator on patients treated with current therapeutic regimens is certainly relevant. The reader is referred to a recent publication by Lenz *et al.*[76]

EPIGENETIC MODULATION IN LYMPHOMAS

Epigenetic changes modulate the inheritance of genetic information in daughter cells, rather than directly modifying the sequence of bases that constitute this genetic information. Epigenetic changes are thus defined as mitotically heritable changes in gene expression that result without a direct alteration in the primary DNA sequence.[77–81] Aberrant epigenetic lesions, unlike other genomic alterations, are potentially reversible. Variation in the accessibility of the transcriptional machinery to selected regions of the DNA template is the central process through which the perturbations in the epigenome of the tumor influence the biological and the clinical behavior of the tumor. This accessibility is controlled by reversible changes in chromatin structure and/or changes in DNA methylation.[82–85] Alterations in chromatin structure result from covalent modifications of the N-terminal histone tails, or from an active remodeling of the nucleosomes.[88–90] An additional epigenetic mechanism that appears to alter the genomic expression profile of human cancer cells is the transcriptional and/or the post-transcriptional silencing of genes induced by the novel family of transcripts, the microRNAs.[91,92] The more widely studied and more frequently observed epigenetic modification in human malignancies is aberrant DNA hypermethylation at CpG islands in promoter or regulatory regions of genes. Aberrant DNA methylation has been detected in a wide spectrum of human lymphoid neoplasia and other malignancies.[93,94]

While hypermethylation is clearly linked to oncogenic processes, it is important to note that both genome-wide hypomethylation as well as region-specific and local hypermethylation may together contribute to these processes. Clues to the involvement of DNA hypomethylation come from studies in mice, using DNA methylation inhibitors and methyl-deficient diet. Global DNA hypomethylation resulting from such treatments appears to cause tumors, by hypomethylating the genome and thereby activating protooncogenes.[95] Since mutations in DNA methylating enzyme DNMT3b are causally linked to genomic instability, resulting in the rare syndrome that exhibits immunodeficiency and chromosome instability,[96] it is possible that hypomethylation induces destabilization of the genome and thereby contributes to tumorigenesis. Indeed, T cell lymphomas have been shown to occur in mice with substantially reduced activity of the DNA methylating enzyme DNMT1.[97]

This section of the chapter will review various areas of epigenetic alterations in lymphoid neoplasia with an emphasis on aberrant DNA methylation patterns. Challenges and opportunities associated in fully realizing the clinical potential of the knowledge from epigenetics of lymphomas will also be discussed.

Profiles of aberrant promoter CpG methylation in human lymphoid neoplasia

A profile of CpG island hypermethylation likely exists for each tumor type; this unique pattern and panel of genes affected by hypermethylation has been termed as the 'methylotype' in analogy with the term 'genotype.' Methylotypes for several hematologic malignancies have been described including both leukemia and lymphoma. Indeed, methylotypes of leukemia have been shown to predict class distinction between myeloid and lymphoid leukemia. While the majority of the available data are based upon analysis of hypermethylation using candidate gene approaches, these data are nonetheless indicative that differences between methylated loci exist among various human cancers. Several tumor suppressor genes frequently hypermethylated in epithelial tumors are not similarly methylated in hematologic malignancies; examples of these include frequent methylation of BRCA1 and p14 in epithelial tumors but lack of methylation in leukemia and lymphoma. Furthermore, not all tumor suppressor genes that are subject to deletion and/or inactivation by mutations are candidates for silencing by methylation; thus there is very little evidence that the expression of the DNA damage responsive genes, TP53 and CHK2, is repressed epigenetically. A comparison of the most commonly hypermethylated tumor suppressor genes demonstrates notable differences in the pattern, spectrum, and frequency even between human leukemia and lymphomas, indicating the distinct pathogenic correlations between disease entities and the methylotype of the tumors. It is likely, however, that as the panel of candidate genes examined for the status of CpG island methylation increases and as methylation profiles of additional lymphoma subtypes are analyzed, general relationships between methylation profiles and disease subtypes will change and become clearer. For example, it was generally believed that methylation of the cell cycle inhibitors p15 and p16 correlated with leukemic nature of hematologic malignancy. Hypermethylation of p15 was generally associated with various leukemias. In contrast, p16 was associated more often with lymphomas rather than leukemia. Exceptions to the exclusivity of the aberrant methylation of either p15 or p16 have now been described in natural killer (NK) cell lymphomas and mucosal-associated lymphoid tissue (MALT) lymphomas.

Studies that have analyzed concurrent methylation of multiple genes demonstrate varying frequencies of methylation of the candidate genes. At least in part, these studies may indicate that the methylation status at affected loci is dependent upon the progressive evolution of hematologic malignancies. Some genes, such as DAPK in lymphoma, may be methylated early during lymphomagenesis whereas for others, such as TP73 in BL, methylation may occur later in the progression of these tumors. Methylation of p16 may be an early event in MALT lymphomas and maintained throughout the progression of the tumor.[98]

Similar to the genomic instability subtypes in tumors, a hypermethylated subtype called the CpG island methylator phenotype has also been described in some human malignancies and the level of methylation, denoted as the methylation index, has been shown to associate with tumor progression and in some cases with clinical outcome.[99,100]

It is likely that even small changes in a single gene's expression can significantly impact the biological behavior of the tumor. Since changes in CpG island methylation affect not only the number of genes that are methylated but may also influence the density of methylation in a given gene, studies that correlate density of methylation with clinical behavior may reveal epigenotype and phenotype correlations influenced by the level of methylation and thus the level of attenuation in the expression of these genes.[101]

The clinical application of methylation studies ranges from the use of methylated loci as biomarkers in disease monitoring to establishing the rationale for targeted therapies using demethylating agents. These applications are, however, based upon the premise that the involved loci are not extensively methylated in normal cells. Since methylation is also involved in the regulation of gene expression during development and differentiation, tissue-specific and development-specific genes can be methylated in subsets of normal hematopoietic cells; thus, methylation mechanisms ensure that the expression of myeloperoxidase is restricted to more mature myeloid cells.[102] At least some of the genes that have been detected to be aberrantly methylated in lymphomas and leukemias may also be methylated in subsets of normal cells during differentiation and development. In hematologic malignancies, one of the most intensively studied of genes that are epigenetically regulated is the cell cycle regulatory gene p15. P15 inhibits the cyclin-dependent kinase CDK4 and thereby controls progression from G1 to S phase of the cell cycle. P15 has been shown to be methylated in myeloid as well as lymphoid leukemias. Whereas demethylation of p15 is observed in normal human CD34-positive progenitor cells, methylation of p15 occurs during the proliferative phase of CD34-positive cells. The epigenetic regulation of p15 may thus be associated with stem cell expansion,[103] although additional studies are needed to understand better the contributions of epigenetic regulation of p15 in normal and neoplastic myeloid cells.[104] Epigenetic changes are also seen during maturation of lymphoid cells, and the repression of CD4 in double negative T cells and in T cells selected to be CD8 positive may also be regulated through epigenetic changes. The process of differential expression of either maternal- or paternal-derived genes, termed genome imprinting, is also under epigenetic control and deregulation of this genome-imprinting process has been associated with leukemogenesis. Thus loss of imprinting of the insulin-like growth factor 2 (*IGF2*) gene is associated with acute lymphoblastic leukemia (ALL) and acute myeloid leukemia (AML). Present data indicate a significant role played by epigenetic mechanisms beyond methylation, such as histone modification, in the regulation of this locus.[105] Furthermore, progressive changes in methylation have also been detected with age. These considerations are important in developing assays that use hypermethylation of specific genes as biomarkers either in disease diagnosis or in monitoring disease.

Epigenetic analysis of human leukemia has demonstrated distinct patterns associated with acute myeloid and lymphoid leukemia. Such epigenetic changes in AML and ALL are nonrandom and independent of chromosomal translocations associated with these leukemias. Methylation of multiple genes has been demonstrated in ALL. Methylation of *CDH1* appears to be frequent in ALL. Different methylation patterns between adult and pediatric leukemia and between molecularly distinct subclasses of leukemia have also been reported. Methylation of cell cycle inhibitors such as p57 and p27 has been correlated with clinical outcome. Although disparate results have been reported for methylation associated at the *p21* locus, the cell cycle regulators p14, p21, and TP53 are only infrequently downregulated by aberrant hypermethylation. In one study, methylation of *FHIT* was found to be associated with hyperdiploid ALL and more likely to occur in the subgroup of pediatric precursor B cell leukemia characterized by absence of the common translocations observed in these malignancies.[106]

In a large study, concurrent methylation of a notably comprehensive panel of genes was used to correlate extent of hypermethylated genes either with the presence and the type of translocations in pediatric ALL or with clinical outcome. Using a panel of seven genes, Gutierrez, Siraj *et al.*[107] demonstrated that ALL with translocations involving chromosome 11 was more likely to incur extensive hypermethylation, while the more mature B cell leukemia associated with the t(1:19) infrequently demonstrated hypermethylation of any of these seven genes examined. Furthermore, differences in the extent and pattern of methylation between T and B cell ALL were also noted. More recently, Taylor *et al.*[108] used CpG island microarray analysis to develop a global profile of DNA methylation in ALL and identified specific chromosomal methylation hotspots associated with ALL. Methylation of specific loci such as *DDX51* differed between T cell and B cell ALL. Epigenetic regulation of noncoding transcripts such as the microRNAs has also been reported in ALL[109] and appears to correlate with clinical outcome. In addition to methylation of individual genes, coordinated repression through epigenetic modulation such as through the Polycomb group of repressors can regulate expression of the entire *INK4b-ARF-INK4a* locus.[110]

Restriction landmark genomic scanning was used to compare genome-wide methylation patterns associated with chronic lymphocytic leukemia (CLL) to those in normal CD19 B cells.[111] An average of 4.8 percent of 3000 CpG islands were nonrandomly methylated in CLL. A key prognostic marker in CLL identified using gene expression array studies is ZAP70. Corcoran and colleagues[112] noted a high concordance between the loss of expression of ZAP70 and the methylation status of CpG sites between intron 1 and exon 2 of the *ZAP70* gene in over 90 percent of CLL cases, suggesting that methylation status of this gene could be a useful marker of risk assessment in CLL.

To date, investigations indicate that aberrant promoter methylation of at least some genes can be detected in most of the major lymphoma subtypes defined in the World Health Organization (WHO) classification.

The WHO classification of hematolymphoid neoplasms recognized NK cell tumors as a distinct entity. The diagnosis of the disease at presentation is aided by distinct clinical presentation and by distinct histologic and immunophenotypic characteristics associated with the tumor. Relapsed or residual disease is, however, more difficult to ascertain, because the germ-line status of the immunoglobulin and the T cell receptor genes in NK cells cannot be used as biomarkers in aiding clinicopathological analysis. Using a candidate gene approach demonstrated the frequent methylation of *TP73*, *p16*, *p15*, *hMLH1*, and *RARb* genes in NK cell lymphomas.[113] Methylation of *TP73* is detected in the majority of NK cell lymphomas, while methylation of *p15* is detected in about 48 percent of the tumors. These methylated loci were further evaluated as surrogate molecular markers for disease monitoring. By comparing clinicopathological findings with status of methylation of the CpG islands of *TP73*, *p16*, *hMLH1*, *RARb*, and *p15*, methylation markers were found to be of value in disease monitoring. The knowledge of methylation status of the panel of genes frequently modified at presentation in the original tumor can therefore be clinically used in disease monitoring and in the detection of occult disease and disease recurrence.

Among B cell lymphomas, methylation studies have identified distinct extents and patterns of methylation suggesting that methylation of candidate genes is not randomly distributed in these B cell malignancies and that such methylation correlates with the etiopathogenesis and/or the molecular subclasses of these lymphomas. An example of this correlation is seen in *Helicobacter pylori*-dependent and *H. pylori*-independent MALT lymphomas. Kaneko and colleagues[114] examined the methylation status of eight genes in *H. pylori*-dependent and *H. pylori*-independent MALT lymphomas and demonstrated that *H. pylori*-independent MALT lymphomas associated with the translocation t(11;18), which results in the expression of the fusion product of the antiapoptotic gene *AP12* with that of the *MALT1* gene, are less likely to incur aberrant methylation than lymphomas that are *H. pylori* dependent.

Similarly, primary cutaneous large B cell lymphomas (PCLBCL) classified as either primary cutaneous follicular center lymphoma or PCLBCL of the leg type, demonstrate in addition to different genetic alterations, differences in methylation pattern and thus the expression of cell cycle genes. Methylation of *p16* is detected preferentially in PCLBCL leg type lymphomas, but not in primary cutaneous follicular center lymphomas. Loss of p16 expression in these lymphomas is associated with disease progression and with adverse prognosis. Methylation of *p16* is also rarely seen in mantle cell lymphomas, and the inactivation of this gene occurs more because of genetic rather than epigenetic alteration in these tumors.[115]

Rossi *et al.*[116] reported methylation patterns associated with multiple genes including death-associated protein kinase (*DAPK*), methylguanine methyltransferase (*MGMT*), glutathione S-transferase pi 1 (*GSTP1*), caspase-8, and TP73 in a large panel of B cell lymphomas and correlated these patterns with the clinicopathological spectrum of these lymphomas. Aberrant methylation was evident both in precursor B cell neoplasms as well as in mature B cell malignancies, although the candidate genes involved in methylation differ; for example, methylation of *TP73* was more common in precursor B cell malignancies rather than in mature B cell lymphomas. Methylation of *DAPK* is frequently evident all across the spectrum of B cell lymphomas with a particularly higher fraction in follicular lymphomas. Similarly, methylation of *GSTP1* was more often associated with hairy cell leukemia, followed by follicular lymphomas and Burkitt lymphoma. Caspase-8 was rarely methylated in any of these lymphomas. Agrelo *et al.*[117] reported that inactivation of expression of the lamin A/C gene by hypermethylation occurs in nodal diffuse B cell lymphoma and infrequently in Burkitt lymphoma and that such methylation was associated with a decrease in failure-free survival in the diffuse large B cell lymphomas. The methylation and consequent loss of expression of the DNA repair gene O^6-methylguanine methytransferase (*MGMT*), which has been reported to occur frequently in diffuse large B cell lymphomas, is also a useful marker for predicting outcome following multidrug regimen therapy which includes cyclophosphamide. Inactivation of expression of the tumor suppressor gene *FHIT* occurs in about one-third of Burkitt lymphomas and is less likely to associate with acquired immune deficiency syndrome BL but more likely to associate with Epstein–Barr virus-positive BL.

Methylation of B cell-specific genes contributes to the loss of B cell identity in Hodgkin disease. Such methylation downregulates expression of a spectrum of B cell-specific genes. Gene expression array studies have been a crucial component in demonstrating the loss of expression or downregulation of such genes as *CD19*, *CD20*, *CD79a*, *CD79b*, *SYK*, *LCK*, and *BCMA*.[118] This coordinated pathway-specific downregulation is achieved by epigenetic alteration in the promoter regions of key transcriptional factors that govern the expression of the B cell identity genes including transcription factors SPT1 (PU.1) and POU2AF1 (BOB1). Inhibition of immunoglobulin transcription in

Hodgkin lymphomas is mediated to some extent by hypermethylation. Additionally, promoter and regulatory regions of several genes that were identified to be downregulated by expression array studies were found to be hypermethylated in Hodgkin lymphomas. These include *CD19*, *CD20*, *CD79a*, *CD79b*, *SYK*, *LCK*, and *BCMA*,[119] It is likely that epigenetic-mediated downregulation of these genes is pathogenetically relevant to oncogenic pathways leading to the development of Hodgkin lymphoma, since several of these genes are involved in pathway decisions of survival versus apoptosis in B cells following B cell receptor activation. In addition to such hypermethylation-mediated loss of B cell identity in Hodgkin lymphomas, hypermethylation of regulators of cell cycle, such as *p15* and *p16*, and of other tumor suppressor genes including *SOCS1* and *RASSF1* has also been reported. Comparative studies to assess promoter methylation of RASSF1 in Hodgkin versus non-Hodgkin lymphomas support preferential inactivation of RASSF1 by methylation in Hodgkin lymphoma. Interestingly, loss of expression of the p18 gene by promoter hypermethylation also appears to be preferentially associated with Hodgkin lymphoma and correlates with clinical outcome.[120]

Aberrant methylation has also been reported in several T cell neoplasms, including pediatric and adult T cell ALL and mature T cell lymphomas. Yasunaga *et al.*[121] explored genome-wide differences in genes methylated in adult T cell leukemia/lymphoma (ATLL) versus activated normal T cells and identified as many as 53 differentially hypermethylated DNA fragments. Expression analysis conducted for a subset of 13 of the involved genes demonstrated that multiple genes normally expressed in activated T cells are silenced by methylation in ATLL; several of these are involved in blocking apoptosis. Furthermore, some genes were specifically shown to incur progressive methylation with disease progression. Similarly, Nosaka *et al.*[122] demonstrated that the *CDKN2A* gene was more frequently methylated in cases of acute ATLL or lymphoma-type ATLL than in those with chronic ATLL, supporting the concept that methylation is critical both to lymphomagenesis and to determining clinical course. Van Doorn *et al.*[123] assessed the epigenetic profile of mature T cell lymphomas using both a candidate gene and a differential methylation hybridization analysis that provides for a genome-wide approach to identification of methylation pattern. The methylation profile of cutaneous T cell lymphomas (CTCL) showed a frequent involvement of the tumor suppressor gene *BCL7a* in aggressive versus indolent CTCLs. In addition, methylation of the cell cycle inhibitor, *TP73*, and *p16* was also frequently identified, although *p15* was only occasionally inactivated by methylation.

FUTURE DIRECTIONS

Gene expression profiling studies over the last 5 years have provided sufficient information to construct reliable expression signatures for the major subtypes of B cell lymphoma: DLBCL, BL/atypical BL, FL, MCL, and CLL/small lymphocytic lymphoma (SLL). The less common B cell NHLs and most of the non-B cell lymphoid malignancies, accounting for fewer than 15 percent of the cases, do not have robust diagnostic expression signatures defined yet. Studies in the next 5–10 years may address the following questions to utilize more fully gene expression profiling in the clinical setting.

1. How reliable are the previously defined gene expression signatures in classifying new lymphoma cases in the clinical setting and can they be further refined?
2. Can unique gene expression signatures be identified and validated for additional, uncommon NHL categories?
3. Can we validate and refine prognosticators for the major groups of lymphomas?
4. In what way will the findings from gene expression profiling be best utilized in clinical practice?

Currently, all the known diagnostic signatures on NHLs as well as the published prognosticators can be represented by a relatively small number of genes. The entire list can be easily accommodated on a small diagnostic array and possibly, with some modifications, on other platforms. The platform is open and will allow addition and deletion of features to refine existing diagnostic and prognostic algorithms as additional series of cases with relevant clinical and biologic information are examined. The signatures of the uncommon subtypes of lymphoma can be added as specific gene expression signatures are identified and validated. This diagnostic array, once established, will supply a large amount of clinically relevant information in a single platform. It should be able to identify lymphoma subtypes that are not possible to diagnose confidently with traditional methodology and provide accurate prognostic information that is important in the treatment of individual patients as well as in conducting future clinical trials.

DNA microarray assays require well-preserved RNA, which is generally obtained from fresh or fresh-frozen materials. There is some concern whether the requirement of well-preserved RNA would be a major impediment to the clinical application of this technology. This would require a widespread acceptance of submitting tissue biopsies in the fresh state with a representative sample reserved for microarray analysis. The reproducibility of the assay performed at different sites and the influence of tissue handling, transportation, and processing on assay performance will have to be assessed and specific performance guidelines drawn up for reference.

It may be difficult to change the traditional pattern of tissue handling in many institutions and fresh tissue may not be available due to financial, organizational, or infrastructural limitations. There are also occasions where it is desirable to study a large series of archival cases for validation of expression/prognostication signatures or other related retrospective investigations. It is, therefore, important to explore adapation of the established gene expression signatures to platforms suitable for archival tissues. While current gene expression signatures frequently contain a substantial number of genes, it has been shown in a number of studies[124,125] that this number can be substantially reduced without significantly compromising the discriminatory power of the original signature (Fig. 84.6).

For a gene expression parameter to be successfully transferred to an immunohistochemical platform, the following conditions must be met: (1) there is a correlation between the level of the transcript and protein expression; (2) a suitable antibody for immunohistochemistry is available; (3) the epitope recognized by the antibody is stable and retrievable for antibody binding; and (4) the reaction is robust and readily quantifiable. A number of antibodies, including antibodies to B cell transcription factors, receptor signaling pathways, MHC class II molecules, and lymph node stroma, are available for immunohistochemistry.[124,126–131] Additional antibodies will likely be identified or developed in the future. Novel technologies that will significantly enhance our ability to quantitate immunohistochemistry will be of great interest as quantitation may be necessary for certain parameters.

An alternative approach is to develop a platform utilizing quantitative RT-PCR. The quantitation of well-preserved mRNA by real-time RT-PCR[132] is currently well established and the application of this technology to RNA from paraffin-embedded tissue has also been reported by multiple groups.[133–139] A recent comprehensive study by Cronin and coworkers[140] has clearly demonstrated that it is a viable approach for archival tissues and can be performed as a moderately high throughput assay.

A comparative genomic hybridization (CGH) study on a series of DLBCL that were gene expression profiled[39] has provided evidence that the gene expression-defined subgroups of DLBCL have distinct but overlapping patterns of genetic abnormalities. Furthermore, certain genetic abnormalities such as +3q are associated with poorer survival independent of gene expression-defined prognosticators. Based on these preliminary data, it would be of interest to obtain more comprehensive/high-resolution CGH data using the array CGH technology to validate and extend the traditional CGH data that have been obtained.[141] It is highly likely that the incorporation of relevant genetic data will lead to a superior prognostic model as well as better understanding of the mechanistic basis underlying the predictor. As genetic alterations may be caused by changes such as methylation or mutations that are not detectable by methods such as CGH, this information should ideally be obtained for a more complete evaluation of parameters that will affect survival. It may be possible to identify gene expression signatures that represent the genetic parameters of interest and hence incorporate the information into one platform. The successful completion of this endeavor will provide a robust, comprehensive system for accurate diagnostic and prognostic applications for the vast majority of NHLs. Alternative platforms based on immunohistochemistry or quantitative RT-PCR that can be more readily

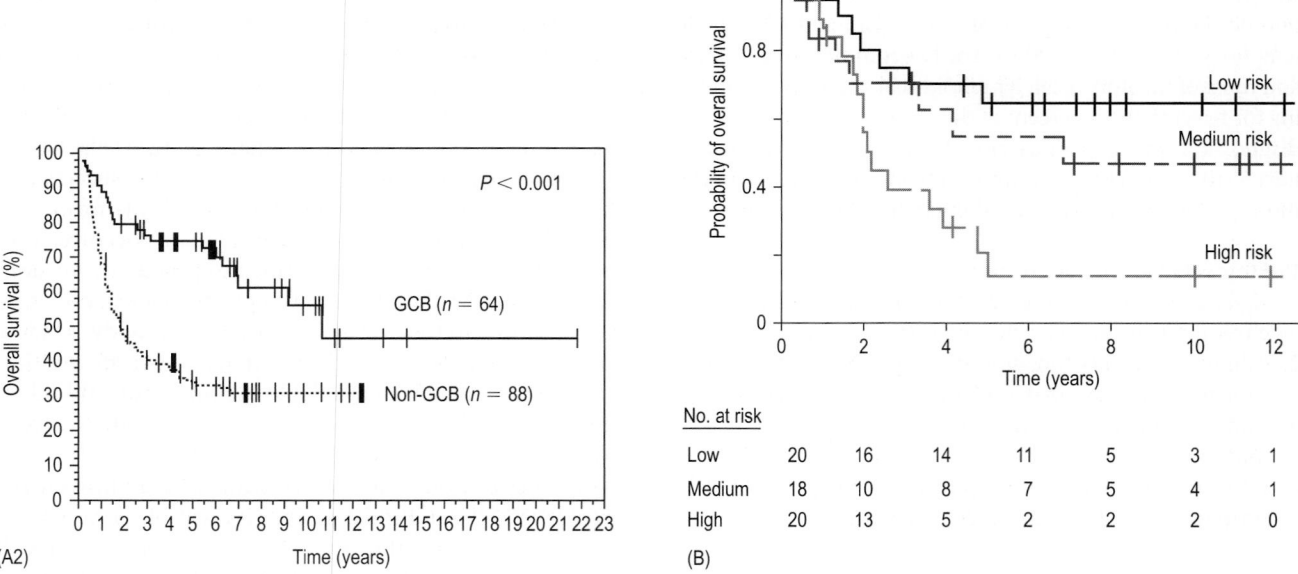

Figure 84.6 (A1) Plate 144, see plate section (A2) Using antibodies to stain for CD10, BCL6, and MUM1, Hans and coworkers derived an algorithm that is useful in distinguishing germinal center B cell type diffuse large B cell lymphoma (GCB DLBCL) from non-GCB DLBCL in archival tissues. Reprinted with permission: Hans CP *et al. Blood* 2004; **103**: 275–82, Figure 2 and Figure 3A. (B) The weighted score of the expression level of six selected genes as measured by quantitative reverse transcription polymerase chain reaction (RT-PCR) can also segregate diffuse large B cell lymphoma (DLBCL) into low, medium, and high risk groups. These studies indicated that gene expression profiling information can be substantially captured using a relatively small number of parameters. Reprinted with permission: Lossos IS *et al. N Engl J Med* 2004; **350**: 1828–37, Figure 2B.

applied to paraffin-embedded tissue can also be developed to capture the essential information of the microarray platform. This will expand the application of the new knowledge obtained from these global investigations in both investigative and diagnostic arenas. As prognosticators may change with the availability of more effective treatments, reevaluation of predictive models in patients treated with new regimens needs to be performed. The addition of CD20 antibody to multiagent chemotherapy can significantly improve overall survival in patients with DLBCL and antibody therapy is now being expanded to other lymphoma subtypes.[142,143] Prognosticators obtained in the pre-rituximab era must be redefined. It is important to point out that mechanistic insights will also be obtained from these studies in addition to defining classifiers and prognosticators. Activation of the NF-κB pathway[144] and overexpression of PKCβ[24] in ABC DLBCL, the striking influence of the stromal signature and MHC class II expression on survival in DLBCL,[22,126] the critical role of tumor–host interaction in the prognosis of patients with FL, and the dominant role of the proliferation signature in the survival of MCL patients are just some examples. Observed changes in prognosticators for patients treated with new therapies may similarly illuminate mechanisms behind responsiveness and resistance to novel approaches. It is anticipated that insight into molecular mechanisms will lead to the identification of important targets, both in the tumor cells and in the tumor microenvironment, for novel therapeutic intervention.

Targeting epigenetic pathways: therapeutic approaches

Understanding of specific epigenetic pathways deregulated in hematologic malignancies provides opportunities for using this information to guide therapy as well as to develop novel approaches for treatment.

Methylation of the *p21* gene, for example, is associated with poor clinical outcome in ALL. Differences in the methylation of cell cycle genes *p21*, *p57*, *p73*, and *p15* have been observed between adult and pediatric ALL. *P57* is frequently methylated in adult ALL and, when associated with hypermethylation of *p15* and *TP73*, predicts poor prognosis in Philadelphia chromosome (Ph)-negative adult ALL. Methylation and resulting silencing of expression of the O[6]-methylguanine DNA methyltransferase in diffuse large B cell lymphomas correlates with clinical outcome in patients treated with drug regimens that include an alkylating agent. Similarly, resistance to methotrexate in primary central nervous system lymphomas may result from loss of expression of the reduced folate carrier gene, which in turn may be mediated by aberrant methylation of its promoter.[145]

The framework for exploiting epigenetic pathways to develop antilymphoma therapies is based upon the consideration that major epigenetic mechanisms contributing to sustaining the lymphoma phenotype – histone modification and methylation – act by transcriptional repression and thus silencing of target genes. Frequently these genes are tumor suppressor genes and the silencing of transcription of these genes provides growth advantage or a block to differentiation and maturation to the lymphoid cell. Inhibiting enzymes involved in methylation or blocking methylation in newly replicated DNA and blocking histone deacetylation results in reexpression of such repressed genes, inducing differentiation or apoptosis in malignant lymphocytes. However, each of these epigenetic mechanisms, including histone modifications, CpG methylation, and chromatin remodeling proteins such as SW1, control transcriptional regulation of a wide array of genes; inhibition of such transcriptional regulation is thus theoretically likely to perturb the expression of a broad spectrum of genes, diminishing the specificity of such therapy while providing the inhibitors of epigenetic mechanisms with a broader spectrum of activity.

Much of the available knowledge pertaining to the clinical utility of epigenetic pathway inhibitors comes from studies utilizing drugs that antagonize either the histone deacetylase or the hypermethylation mechanisms. There is limited availability of compounds that inhibit other mechanisms. Recently inhibitors of the chromatin remodeling complex protein SW1 have also been reported.

Inhibitors of the histone deacetylases include compounds that contain hydroxamic acid, such as trichostatin A and suberoylanilide hydroxamic acid. Phase I and II studies with suberoylanilide hydroxamic acid demonstrated manageable toxicity with some clinical activity in T cell lymphomas. Additionally compounds such as butyrate and valproic acid have also been shown to block the activity of these enzymes. Nicotinamide is another molecule that has the ability to inhibit histone deacetylases. A novel small molecule inhibitor of the sirtuin histone deacetylase, splitomicin, was reported by Grozinger et al.[146]

Although the rationale that such compounds will act through reactivating tumor suppressor genes in mediating their antitumor effects has been the basis of considering the clinical application of such agents, it is important to note that several of these drugs influence other biological pathways in addition to chromatin-directed regulation of transcription. Valproic acid for instance activates protein kinases. Furthermore, experiments conducted to assess the impact of these drugs on gene expression demonstrate that these compounds cause both reactivation as well as repression of gene transcription. In addition to permitting the acetylation of histones, inhibitors of histone deacetylation have also been shown to promote acetylation of other proteins including transcription factors.

Much of the clinical experience in therapeutic approaches toward targeting epigenetic pathways comes from the use of inhibitors of DNA methyltransferases. The reversal of gene repression caused by hypermethylation can be achieved by the nucleoside analogues 5-aza-cytidine and decitabine. Zebularine is another analogue that is also capable of inhibiting DNA methyltransferases and was demonstrated to inhibit the development of T cell lymphomas in a murine model.[147] Treatment with DNA methyltransferase-inhibiting agents has been shown to have some clinical efficacy in ALL. These DNA methyltransferase inhibitors have been shown to reactivate the expression of tumor suppressor genes including p21, p15, and p16 and cause growth arrest, differentiation, and/or apoptosis. Because of limited activity and specificity, the use of such agents in combination with other drugs is being considered. Additional novel compounds that target DNA hypermethylation through binding with methyl CpG binding proteins are also being explored.

The complex interactions between the epigenetic regulatory pathways and the genetic lesions in human lymphomas clearly present opportunities to develop therapeutic and diagnostic approaches in the management of lymphomas. The limited experience so far in utilizing methylation patterns as signatures for clinical behavior of lymphomas and preliminary clinical data in the use of agents that modify epigenetic pathways indicate that this is a promising approach. It is quite likely the use of DNA methyltransferase inhibitors or the histone deacetylase inhibitors in combination with each other or in combination with standard cytotoxic agents will yield better results. Examples of added benefits of such combinations are evident from the use of histone deacetylase inhibitors with all-trans retinoic acid in acute promyelocytic leukemia and AML. The use of biomarkers, such as assessments of reactivation of gene expression, in evaluating the clinical efficacy of new agents will be essential to successful development of these novel therapeutic approaches.

KEY POINTS

- Gene expression profiling has proven to be useful in providing robust molecular classifiers for lymphomas, in identifying new subtypes of disease and in defining prognosticators.
- Gene expression profiling may extend to non-coding RNA including microRNA, am improtant family and small regulatory RNA.
- The optimal platform to utilize the information in clinical practice has not been defined.
- High resolution aCGH studies provide complementary information and are synergistic for gene expression analysis and vice versa.
- Epigenetic aberrations including DNA methylation and histone modification are integral parts of the cancer genome landscape.
- These epigenetics changes may lead to aberrant activation of oncogenes or inactivation of tumor suppressor genes or alterations in the differentiation program.
- All the above studies will help to identify novel targets for therapy.
- The ability to define the key molecular aberrations and oncogenic pathways of a lymphoma will help to direct therapy for individualized treatment.

REFERENCES

● = Key primary paper
◆ = Major review article

1. Willis TG, Dyer MJ. The role of immunoglobulin translocations in the pathogenesis of B-cell malignancies. *Blood* 2000; **96**: 808–22.
2. Jaffe ES, Harris NL, Stein H, Vardiman JW. *World Health Organization classification of tumours. Pathology and genetics of tumours of haemotopoietic and lymphoid tissues.* Lyon: IARC Press, 2001.
3. Morris SW, Kirstein MN, Valentine MB *et al.* Fusion of a kinase gene, ALK, to a nucleolar protein gene, NPM, in non-Hodgkin's lymphoma. *Science* 1995; **263**: 1281–4.
4. Dierlamm J, Baens M, Wlodaraka I *et al.* The apoptosis inhibitor gene API2 and a novel 18q gene, MLT, are recurrently rearranged in the t(11;18)(q21;q21)p6 associated with mucosa-associated lymphoid tissue lymphomas. *Blood* 1999; **93**: 3601–9.
5. Willis TG, Jadayel DM, Du MQ *et al.* Bcl10 is involved in t(1;14)(p22;q32) of MALT B cell lymphoma and mutated in multiple tumor types. *Cell* 1999; **96**: 35–45.
6. Auer IA, Gascoyne RD, Connors JM *et al.* t(11;18)(q21;q21) is the most common translocation in MALT lymphomas. *Ann Oncol* 1997; **8**: 979–85.
7. Streubel B, Lamprecht A, Dierlamm J *et al.* T(14;18)(q32;q21) involving IGH and MALT1 is a frequent chromosomal aberration in MALT lymphoma. *Blood* 2003; **101**: 2335–9.
8. Liu H, Ye H, Dogan A *et al.* T(11;18)(q21;q21) is associated with advanced mucosa-associated lymphoid tissue lymphoma that expresses nuclear BCL10. *Blood* 2001; **98**: 1182–7.
9. Starostik P, Patzner J, Greiner A *et al.* Gastric marginal zone B-cell lymphomas of MALT type develop along 2 distinct pathogenetic pathways. *Blood* 2002; **99**: 3–9.
10. Ichikawa A, Hotta T, Takagi N *et al.* Mutations of p53 gene and their relation to disease progression in B-cell lymphoma. *Blood* 1992; **79**: 2701–7.
11. Lo Coco F, Gaidano G, Louie DC *et al.* p53 mutations are associated with histologic transformation of follicular lymphoma. *Blood* 1993; **82**: 2289–95.
12. Sander CA, Yano T, Clark HM *et al.* p53 mutation is associated with progression in follicular lymphomas. *Blood* 1993; **82**: 1994–2004.
13. Greiner TC, Moynihan MJ, Chan WC *et al.* p53 mutations in mantle cell lymphoma are associated with variant cytology and predict a poor prognosis. *Blood* 1996; **87**: 4302–10.
14. Pinyol M, Hernandez L, Cazorla M *et al.* Deletions and loss of expression of p16INK4a and p21Waf1 genes are associated with aggressive variants of mantle cell lymphomas. *Blood* 1997; **89**: 272–80.
15. Gronbaek K, de Nully Brown P, Møller MB *et al.* Concurrent disruption of p16INK4a and the ARF-p53 pathway predicts poor prognosis in aggressive non-Hodgkin's lymphoma. *Leukemia* 2000; **14**: 1727–35.

16. Sanchez-Beato M, Saez AI, Navas IC *et al.* Overall survival in aggressive B-cell lymphomas is dependent on the accumulation of alterations in p53, p16, and p27. *Am J Pathol* 2001; **159**: 205–13.
17. Alizadeh A, Eisen M, Davis RE *et al.* The lymphochip: a specialized cDNA microarray for the genomic-scale analysis of gene expression in normal and malignant lymphocytes. *Cold Spring Harb Symp Quant Biol* 1999; **64**: 71–8.
18. Brown PO, Botstein D. Exploring the new world of the genome with DNA microarrays. *Nat Genet* 1999; **21**: 33–7.
19. Eisen MB, Brown PO. DNA arrays for analysis of gene expression. *Methods Enzymol* 1999; **303**: 179–205.
20. Staudt LM, Brown PO. Genomic views of the immune system*. *Annu Rev Immunol* 2000; **18**: 829–59.
21. Alizadeh AA, Eisen MB, Davis RE *et al.* Distinct types of diffuse large B-cell lymphoma identified by gene expression profiling. *Nature* 2000; **403**: 503–11.
22. Rosenwald A, Wright G, Chan WC *et al.* The use of molecular profiling to predict survival after chemotherapy for diffuse large-B-cell lymphoma. *N Engl J Med* 2002; **346**: 1937–47.
23. Rosenwald A, Wright G, Leroy K *et al.* Molecular diagnosis of primary mediastinal B cell lymphoma identifies a clinically favorable subgroup of diffuse large B cell lymphoma related to Hodgkin lymphoma. *J Exp Med* 2003; **198**: 851–62.
24. Shipp MA, Ross KN, Tamayo P *et al.* Diffuse large B-cell lymphoma outcome prediction by gene-expression profiling and supervised machine learning. *Nat Med* 2002; **8**: 68–74.
25. Rosenwald A, Wright G, Weistner A *et al.* The proliferation gene expression signature is a quantitative integrator of oncogenic events that predicts survival in mantle cell lymphoma. *Cancer Cell* 2003; **3**: 185–97.
26. Dave SS, Wright G, Tan B *et al.* Prediction of survival in follicular lymphoma based on molecular features of tumor-infiltrating immune cells. *N Engl J Med* 2004; **351**: 2159–69.
27. Davis RE, Brown KD, Siebenlist U, Staudt LM. Constitutive nuclear factor kappaB activity is required for survival of activated B cell-like diffuse large B cell lymphoma cells. *J Exp Med* 2001; **194**: 1861–74.
28. Ting AH, McGarvey KM, Baylin SB. The cancer epigenome-components and function correlates. *Genes Dev* 2006; **20**: 3215–31.
29. Esteller M. Profiling aberrant DNA methylation in hematologic neoplasms: a view from the tip of the iceberg. *Clin Immunol* 2003; **109**: 80–8.
30. Lehmann U, Brakensiek K, Kreipe H. Role of epigenetic changes in hematological malignancies. *Ann Hematol* 2004; **83**: 137–52.
31. Wagner PD, Verma M, Srivastava S. Challenges for biomarkers in cancer detection. *Ann N Y Acad Sci* 2004; **1022**: 9–16.
32. Esteller M, Gaidano G, Goodman SN *et al.* Hypermethylation of the DNA repair gene O(6)-methylguanine DNA

methyltransferase and survial of patients with diffuse large B-cell lymphoma. *J Natl Cancer Inst* 2002; **94**: 26–32.

33. Shen L, Toyota M, Kondo Y *et al.* Aberrant DNA methylation of p57KIP2 identifies a cell-cycle regulatory path way with prognostic impact in adult acute lymphocytic leukemia. *Blood* 2003; **101**: 4131–6.

34. MAQC Consortium, Shi L, Reid LH *et al.* The MicroArray Quality Control (MAQC) project shows inter- and intraplatform reproducibility of gene expression measurements. *Nat Biotechnol* 2006; **24**: 1151–61.

35. Wright G, Tan B, Rosenwald A *et al.* A gene expression-based method to diagnose clinically distinct subgroups of diffuse large B cell lymphoma. *Proc Natl Acad Sci U S A* 2003; **100**: 9991–6.

36. Savage KJ, Monti S, Kutok JL *et al.* The molecular signature of mediastinal large B-cell lymphoma differs from that of other diffuse large B-cell lymphomas and shares features with classical Hodgkin lymphoma. *Blood* 2003; **102**: 3871–9.

37. Huang JZ, Sanger WG, Greiner TC *et al.* The t(14;18) defines a unique subset of diffuse large B-cell lymphoma with a germinal center B-cell gene expression profile. *Blood* 2002; **99**: 2285–90.

38. Iqbal J, Sanger WG, Horsman DE *et al.* BCL2 Translocation Defines a Unique Tumor Subset within the Germinal Center B-Cell-Like Diffuse Large B-Cell Lymphoma. *Am J Pathol* 2004; **165**: 159–66.

39. Bea S, Zettl A, Wright G *et al.* Diffuse large B-cell lymphoma subgroups have distinct genetic profiles that influence tumor biology and improve gene-expression-based survival prediction. *Blood* 2005; **106**: 3183–90.

40. Pasqualucci L, Compagno M, Houldsworth J *et al.* Inactivation of the PRDM1/BLIMP1 gene in diffuse large B cell lymphoma. *J Exp Med* 2006; **203**: 311–17.

41. Tam W, Gomez M, Chadburn A *et al.* Mutational analysis of PRDM1 indicates a tumor-suppressor role in diffuse large B-cell lymphomas. *Blood* 2006; **107**: 4090–100.

42. Melzner I, Bucur AJ, Brüderlein S *et al.* Biallelic mutation of SOCS-1 impairs JAK2 degradation and sustains phospho-JAK2 action in the MedB-1 mediastinal lymphoma line. *Blood* 2005; **105**: 2535–42.

43. Dave SS, Fu K, Wright GW *et al.* Molecular diagnosis of Burkitt's lymphoma. *N Engl J Med* 2006; **354**: 2431–42.

44. Hummel M, Bentink S, Berger H *et al.* A biologic definition of Burkitt's lymphoma from transcriptional and genomic profiling. *N Engl J Med* 2006; **354**: 2419–30.

45. Klein U, Gloghini A, Gaidano G *et al.* Gene expression profile analysis of AIDS-related primary effusion lymphoma (PEL) suggests a plasmablastic derivation and identifies PEL-specific transcripts. *Blood* 2003; **101**: 4115–21.

46. Fan W, Bubman D, Chadburn A *et al.* Distinct subsets of primary effusion lymphoma can be identified based on their cellular gene expression profile and viral association. *J Virol* 2005; **79**: 1244–51.

47. Suguro M, Tagawa H, Kagami Y *et al.* Expression profiling analysis of the CD5+ diffuse large B-cell lymphoma

48. Yamaguchi M, Seto M, Okamoto M *et al.* De novo CD5+ diffuse large B-cell lymphoma: a clinicopathologic study of 109 patients. *Blood* 2002; **99**: 815–21.

49. Tagawa H, Tsuzuki S, Suzuki R *et al.* Genome-wide array-based comparative genomic hybridization of diffuse large B-cell lymphoma: comparison between CD5-positive and CD5-negative cases. *Cancer Res* 2004; **64**: 5948–55.

50. Yoshioka T, Miura I, Kume M *et al.* Cytogenetic features of de novo CD5-positive diffuse large B-cell lymphoma: chromosome aberrations affecting 8p21 and 11q13 constitute major subgroups with different overall survival. *Genes Chromosomes Cancer* 2005; **42**: 149–57.

51. Swerdlow SH, Berger F, Isaacson PG *et al.* Mantle cell lymphoma. In: Jaffe ES, Harris NL, Stein H, Vardiman JW. (eds) *World health organization classification of tumours pathology and genetics of tumours of haematopoietic and lymphoid tissues.* Lyon: IARC Press 2001: 168–70.

52. Fu K, Weisenburger DD, Greiner TC *et al.* Cyclin D1-negative mantle cell lymphoma: a clinicopathologic study based on gene expression profiling. *Blood* 2005; **106**: 4315–21.

53. Husson H, Carideo EG, Neuberg D *et al.* Gene expression profiling of follicular lymphoma and normal germinal center B cells using cDNA arrays. *Blood* 2002; **99**: 282–9.

54. Ruuls SR, Hoek RM, Ngo VN *et al.* Membrane-bound TNF supports secondary lymphoid organ structure but is subservient to secreted TNF in driving autoimmune inflammation. *Immunity* 2001; **15**: 533–43.

55. Bohen SP, Troyanskaya OG, Alter O *et al.* Variation in gene expression patterns in follicular lymphoma and the response to rituximab. *Proc Natl Acad Sci U S A* 2003; **100**: 1926–30.

56. Cartron G, Dacheux L, Salles G *et al.* Therapeutic activity of humanized anti-CD20 monoclonal antibody and polymorphism in IgG Fc receptor FcgammaRIIIa gene. *Blood* 2002; **99**: 754–8.

57. Horning SJ, Rosenberg SA. The natural history of initially untreated low-grade non-Hodgkin's lymphomas. *N Engl J Med* 1984; **311**: 1471–5.

58. Yano T, Jaffe ES, Longo DL, Roffeld M. MYC rearrangements in histologically progressed follicular lymphomas. *Blood* 1992; **80**: 758–67.

59. Matolcsy A, Casali P, Warnke RA, Knowles DM. Morphologic transformation of follicular lymphoma is associated with somatic mutation of the translocated Bcl-2 gene. *Blood* 1996; **88**: 3937–44.

60. Elenitoba-Johnson KS, Gascoyne RD, Lims MS *et al.* Homozygous deletions at chromosome 9p21 involving p16 and p15 are associated with histologic progression in follicle center lymphoma. *Blood* 1998; **91**: 4677–85.

61. Pinyol M, Cobo F, Bea S *et al.* p16(INK4a) gene inactivation by deletions, mutations, and hypermethylation is associated with transformed and aggressive variants of non-Hodgkin's lymphomas. *Blood* 1998; **91**: 2977–84.

subgroup: development of a CD5 signature. *Cancer Sci* 2006; **97**: 868–74.

62. Lossos IS, Alizadeh AA, Diehn M et al. Transformation of follicular lymphoma to diffuse large-cell lymphoma: alternative patterns with increased or decreased expression of c-myc and its regulated genes. Proc Natl Acad Sci U S A 2002; 99: 8886–91.

63. Martinez-Climent JA, Alizadeh AA, Segraves R et al. Transformation of follicular lymphoma to diffuse large cell lymphoma is associated with a heterogeneous set of DNA copy number and gene expression alterations. Blood 2003; 101: 3109–17.

64. Elenitoba-Johnson KS, Jenson SD, Abbott RT et al. Involvement of multiple signaling pathways in follicular lymphoma transformation: p38-mitogen-activated protein kinase as a target for therapy. Proc Natl Acad Sci U S A 2003; 100: 7259–64.

65. Davies AJ. Transformation of follicular lymphoma to diffuse large B-cell lymphoma proceeds by distinct oncogenic mechanisms. Br J Haematol 2006; 136: 286–93.

66. Thieblemont C, Nasser V, Felman P et al. Small lymphocytic lymphoma, marginal zone B-cell lymphoma, and mantle cell lymphoma exhibit distinct gene-expression profiles allowing molecular diagnosis. Blood 2004; 103: 2727–37.

67. Martinez-Delgado B, Cuadros M, Honrado D et al. Differential expression of NF-kappaB pathway genes among peripheral T-cell lymphomas. Leukemia 2005; 19: 2254–63.

68. Thompson MA, Stumph J, Henrickson SE et al. Differential gene expression in anaplastic lymphoma kinase-positive and anaplastic lymphoma kinase-negative anaplastic large cell lymphomas. Hum Pathol 2005; 36: 494–504.

69. Ballester B, Ramuz O, Gisselbrecht C et al. Gene expression profiling identifies molecular subgroups among nodal peripheral T-cell lymphomas. Oncogene 2006; 25: 1560–70.

70. de Leval L, Rickman DS, Thielen C et al. The gene expression profile of nodal peripheral T-cell lymphoma demonstrates a molecular link between angioimmunoblastic T-cell lymphoma (AITL) and follicular helper T (TFH) cells. Blood 2007; 109: 4952–63.

71. Shipp MA. Prognostic factors in aggressive non-Hodgkin's lymphoma: who has 'high-risk' disease? Blood 1994; 83: 1165–73.

72. Rimsza LM, Roberts RA, Campo E et al. Loss of major histocompatibility class II expression in non-immune-privileged site diffuse large B-cell lymphoma is highly coordinated and not due to chromosomal deletions. Blood 2006; 107: 1101–7.

73. Roberts RA, Wright G, Rosenwald AR et al. Loss of major histocompatibility class II gene and protein expression in primary mediastinal large B-cell lymphoma is highly coordinated and related to poor patient survival. Blood 2006; 108: 311–18.

74. Sherr CJ, McCormick F. The RB and p53 pathways in cancer. Cancer Cell 2002; 2: 103–12.

75. Bea S, Tort F, Pinyol M et al. BMI-1 gene amplification and overexpression in hematological malignancies occur mainly in mantle cell lymphomas. Cancer Res 2001; 61: 2409–12.

76. Lenz G, Wright G, Dave SS et al. Stromal gene signatures in large-B-cell lymphomas. N Engl J Med 2008; 339: 2313–23.

77. Feinberg AP, Tycko B. The history of cancer epigenetics. Nat Rev Cancer 2004; 4: 143–53.

78. Jones PA. DNA methylation and cancer. Oncogene 2002; 21: 5358–60.

79. Baylin SB, Herman JG, Graff JR, Verfino PM, Issa JP. Alterations in DNA methylation: a fundamental aspect of neoplasia. Adv Cancer Res 1998; 72: 141–96.

80. Lengauer C, Issa JP. The role of epigenetics in cancer. DNA Methylation, Imprinting and the Epigenetics of Cancer – an American Association for Cancer Research Special Conference, Las Croabas, Puerto Rico, 12–16 December 1997. Mol Med Today 1998; 4: 102–3

81. Jones PA, Laird PW. Cancer epigenetics comes of age. Nat Genet 1999; 21: 163–7.

82. Cameron EE, Bachman KE, Myöhänen S et al. Synergy of demethylation and histone deacetylase inhibition in the re-expression of genes silenced in cancer. Nat Genet 1999; 21: 103–7.

83. Li E. Chromatin modification and epigenetic reprogramming in mammalian development. Nat Rev Genet 2002; 3: 662–73.

84. Robertson KD. DNA methylation and chromation – unraveling the tangled web. Oncogene 2002; 21: 5361–79.

85. Reik W, Walter J. Evolution of imprinting mechanisms: the battle of the sexes begins in the zygote. Nat Genet 2001; 27: 255–6.

86. Sleutels F, Barlow DP. The origins of genomic imprinting in mammals. Adv Genet 2002; 46: 119–63.

87. Campanero MR, Armstrong MI, Flemington EK. CpG methylation as a mechanism for the regulation of E2F activity. Proc Natl Acad Sci U S A 2000; 97: 6481–6.

88. Lee TI, Yong RA. Transcription of eukaryotic protein-coding genes. Annu Rev Genet 2000; 34: 77–137.

89. Fishle W, Wang Y, Allis CD. Histone and chromatin cross-talk. Curr Opin Cell Biol 2003; 15: 172–83.

90. Sims RJ 3rd, Nishioka K, Reinberg D. Histone lysine methylation: a signature for chromatin function. Trends Genet 2003; 19: 629–39.

91. Shi Y. Mammalian RNAi for the masses. Trends Genet 2003; 19: 9–12.

92. Downward J. RNA interference. Br Med J 2004; 328: 1245–8.

93. Issa JP. CpG island methylator phenotype in cancer Nat Rev Cancer 2004; 4: 988–93.

94. Herman JG, Baylin SB. Gene silencing in cancer in association with promoter hypermethylation. N Engl J Med 2003; 349: 2042–54.

95. Ehrlich M. Cancer-linked DNA hypomethylation and its relationship to hypermethylation. Curr Top Microbiol Immunol 2006; 310: 251–74.

96. Xu GL, Bestor TH, Bourc'his D et al. Chromosome instability and immunodeficiency syndrome caused by mutations in a DNA methyltransferase gene. Nature 1999; 402: 187–91.

97. Gaudet F, Hodgson JG, Eden A et al. Induction of tumors in mice by genomic hypomethylation. Science 2003; 300: 489–2.

98. Takino H, Okabe M, Li C *et al.* p16/INK4a gene methylation is a frequent finding in pulmonary MALT lymphomas at diagnosis. *Mod Pathol* 2005; **18**: 1187–92.

99. Roman-Gomez J, Jimenez-Velasco A *et al.* Lack of CpG island methlylator phenotype defines a clinical subtype of T-cell acute lymphoblastic leukemia associated with good prognosis. *J Clin Oncol* 2005; **23**: 7043–9.

100. Roman-Gomez J, Jimenez-Velasco A *et al.* CpG island methylator phenotype redefines the prognostic effect of t(12;21) in childhood acute lymphoblastic leukemia. *Clin Cancer Res* 2006; **12**: 4845–50.

101. Matsuno N, Hoshino K, Nanri T *et al.* p15 mRNA expression detected by real-time quantitative reverse transcriptase-polymerase chain reaction correlates with the methylation density of the gene in adult acute leukemia. *Leuk Res* 2005; **29**: 557–64.

102. Lübbert M, Miller CW, Koeffler HP. Changes of DNA methylation and chromatin structure in the human myeloperoxidase gene during myeloid differentiation. *Blood* 1991; **78**: 345–56.

103. Milhem M, Mahmud N, Lavelle D *et al.* Modification of hematopoietic stem cell fate by 5aza 2′deoxycytidine and trichostatin A. *Blood* 2004; **103**: 4102–10.

104. Guo Y, Engelhardt M, Wider D *et al.* Effects of 5-aza-2′-deoxycytidine on proliferation, differentiation and p15/INK4b regulation of human hematopoietic progenitor cells. *Leukemia* 2006; **20**: 115–21.

105. Vu TH, Li T, Hoffman AR. Promoter-restricted histone code, not the differentially methylated DNA regions or antisense transcripts, marks the imprinting status of IGF2R in human and mouse. *Hum Mol Genet* 2004; **13**: 2233–45.

106. Zheng S, Ma X, Zhang L *et al.* Hypermethylation of the 5′ CpG island of the FHIT gene is associated with hyperdiploid and translocation-negative subtypes of pediatric leukemia. *Cancer Res* 2004; **64**: 2000–6.

107. Gutierrez MI, Siraj AK, Bhargava M. Concurrent methylation of multiple genes in childhood ALL: correlation with phenotype and molecular subgroup. *Leukemia* 2003; **17**: 1845–50.

108. Taylor KH, Pena-Hernandez KE, Davis JW. Large-scale CpG methylation analysis identifies novel candidate genes and reveals methylation hotspots in acute lymphoblastic leukemia. *Cancer Res* 2007; **67**: 2617–25.

109. Roman Gomez J, Agirre-X, Jimnez-Velasoc A *et al.* Epigenetic regulation of microRNAs in acute lymphoblastic leukemia. *J Clin Oncol* 2009; **27**: 1318–22.

110. Gil J, Peters G. Regulation of the INK4b-ARF-INK4a tumour suppressor locus: all for one or one for all. *Nat Rev Mol Cell Biol* 2006; **7**: 677–77.

111. Rush LJ, Raval A, Funchain P. Epigenetic profiling in chronic lymphocytic leukemia reveals novel methylation targets. *Cancer Res* 2004; **64**: 2424–33.

112. Corcoran M, Parker A, Orchard J *et al.* Zap-70 methylation status is associated with ZAP-70 expression status in chronic lymphocytic leukemia *Haematologica* 2005; **90**: 1078–88.

113. Siu LL, Chan JK, Wong KF *et al.* Aberrant promoter CpG methylation as a molecular marker for disease monitoring in natural killer cell lymphomas. *Br J Haematol* 2003; **122**: 70–7.

114. Kaneko Y, Sakurai S, Hironaka M *et al.* Distinct methylated profiles in *Helicobacter pylori* dependent and independent gastric MALT lymphomas. *Gut* 2003; **52**: 641–6.

115. Hutter G, Scheubner M, Zimmerman Y *et al.* Differential effect of epigenetic alterations and genomic deletions of CDK inhibitors [p16(INK4a), p15(INK4b). p14(ARF)] in mantle cell lymphoma. *Genes Chromosomes Cancer* 2006; **45**: 203–10.

116. Rossi D, Capello D, Gloghini A *et al.* Aberrant promoter methylation of multiple genes throughout the clinico-pathologic spectrum of B-cell neoplasia. *Haematologica* 2004; **89**: 154–64.

117. Agrelo R, Setien F, Espada J *et al.* Inactivation of the lamin A/C gene by CpG island promoter hypermethylation in hematologic malignancies, and its association with poor survival in nodal diffuse large B-cell lymphoma. *J Clin Oncol* 2005; **23**; 3940–7.

118. Schwering I, Bräuninger A, Klein U *et al.* Loss of the B-lineage-specific gene expression program in Hodgkin and Reed-Sternberg cells of Hodgkin lymphoma. *Blood* 2003; **101**: 1505–12.

119. Ushmorov A, Leithäuser F, Sakk O *et al.* Epigenetic processes play a major role in B-cell-specific gene silencing in classical Hodgkin lymphoma. *Blood* 2006; **107**: 2493–500.

120. Sanchez-Aguilera A, Delgado J, Camacho FI *et al.* Silencing of the p18INK4c gene by promoter hypermethylation in Reed-Sternberg cells in Hodgkin lymphomas. *Blood* 2004; **103**: 2351–7.

121. Yasunaga J, Taniguchi Y, Nosaka K *et al.* Identification of aberrantly methylated genes in association with adult T-cell leukemia. *Cancer Res* 2004; **64**: 6002–9.

122. Nosaka K, Maeda M, Tamiya S *et al.* Increasing methylation of the CDKN2A gene is associated with the progression of adult T-cell leukemia. *Cancer Res* 2000; **60**: 1043–8.

123. van Doorn R, Zoutman WH, Dijkman R *et al.* Epigenetic profiling of cutaneous T-cell lymphoma: promoter hypermethylation of multiple tumor suppressor genes including BCL7a, PTPRG, and p73. *J Clin Oncol* 2005; **23**: 3886–96.

124. Hans CP, Weisenburger DD, Greiner TC *et al.* Confirmation of the molecular classification of diffuse large B-cell lymphoma by immunohistochemistry using a tissue microarray. *Blood* 2004; **103**: 275–82.

125. Lossos IS, Czerwinski DK, Alizadeh AA *et al.* Prediction of survival in diffuse large-B-cell lymphoma based on the expression of six genes. *N Engl J Med* 2004; **350**: 1828–37.

126. Rimsza LM, Roberts RA, Miller TP *et al.* Loss of MHC class II gene and protein expression in diffuse large B-cell lymphoma is related to decreased tumor immunosurveillance and poor patient survival regardless of other prognostic factors: a follow-up study from the Leukemia and Lymphoma Molecular Profiling Project. *Blood* 2004; **103**: 4251–8.

127. Banham AH, Beasley N, Campo E *et al.* The FOXP1 winged helix transcription factor is a novel candidate tumor suppressor gene on chromosome 3p. *Cancer Res* 2001; **61**: 8820–9.

128. Loddenkemper C, Anagnostopoulos I, Hummel M *et al.* Differential Emu enhancer activity and expression of BOB.1/OBF.1, Oct2, PU.1, and immunoglobulin in reactive B-cell populations, B-cell non-Hodgkin lymphomas, and Hodgkin lymphomas. *J Pathol* 2004; **202**: 60–9.

129. Marafioti T, Mancini C, Ascani S *et al.* Leukocyte-specific phosphoprotein-1 and PU.1: two useful markers for distinguishing T-cell-rich B-cell lymphoma from lymphocyte-predominant Hodgkin's disease. *Haematologica* 2004; **89**: 957–64.

130. Marafioti T, Pozzobon M, Hansmann ML *et al.* Expression of intracellular signaling molecules in classical and lymphocyte predominance Hodgkin disease. *Blood* 2004; **103**: 188–93.

131. Pozzobon M, Marafioti T, Hansmann ML *et al.* Intracellular signalling molecules as immunohistochemical markers of normal and neoplastic human leucocytes in routine biopsy samples. *Br J Haematol* 2004; **124**: 519–33.

132. Heid CA, Stevens J, Livak KJ, Williams PM. Real time quantitative PCR. *Genome Res* 1996; **6**: 986–94.

133. Sheils OM, Sweeney EC. TSH receptor status of thyroid neoplasms–TaqMan RT-PCR analysis of archival material. *J Pathol* 1999; **188**: 87–92.

134. Godfrey TE, Kim SH, Chavira M *et al.* Quantitative mRNA expression analysis from formalin-fixed, paraffin-embedded tissues using 5′ nuclease quantitative reverse transcription-polymerase chain reaction. *J Mol Diagn* 2000; **2**: 84–91.

135. Specht K, Kremer M, Müller U *et al.* Identification of cyclin D1 mRNA overexpression in B-cell neoplasias by real-time reverse transcription-PCR of microdissected paraffin sections. *Clin Cancer Res* 2002; **8**: 2902–11.

136. Abrahamsen HN, Steiniche T, Nexo E *et al.* Towards quantitative mRNA analysis in paraffin-embedded tissues using real-time reverse transcriptase-polymerase chain reaction: a methodological study on lymph nodes from melanoma patients. *J Mol Diagn* 2003; **5**: 34–41.

137. Koopmans M, Monroe SS, Coffield LM, Zaki SR. Optimization of extraction and PCR amplification of RNA extracts from paraffin-embedded tissue in different fixatives. *J Virol Methods* 1993; **43**: 189–204.

138. D'Orazio D, Stumm M, Sieber C *et al.* Accurate gene expression measurement in formalin-fixed and paraffin-embedded tumor tissue. *Am J Pathol* 2002; **160**: 383–4.

139. Thomazy VA, Luthra R, Uthman MO *et al.* Determination of cyclin D1 and CD20 mRNA levels by real-time quantitative RT-PCR from archival tissue sections of mantle cell lymphoma and other non-Hodgkin's lymphomas. *J Mol Diagn* 2002; **4**: 201–8.

140. Cronin M, Pho M, Dutta D *et al.* Measurement of gene expression in archival paraffin-embedded tissues: development and performance of a 92-gene reverse transcriptase-polymerase chain reaction assay. *Am J Pathol* 2004; **164**: 35–42.

141. Ishkanian AS, Malloff CA, Watson SK *et al.* A tiling resolution DNA microarray with complete coverage of the human genome. *Nat Genet* 2004; **36**: 299–303.

142. Coiffier B, Lepage E, Briere J *et al.* CHOP chemotherapy plus rituximab compared with CHOP alone in elderly patients with diffuse large-B-cell lymphoma. *N Engl J Med* 2002; **346**: 235–42.

143. Sehn LH, Donaldson J, Chanabhai M *et al.* Introduction of Combined CHIP-Rituximab Therapy Dramatically Improved Outcome of Diffuse Large B-cell lymphoma (DLBC) in Britis Columbia (BC). *Blood* 2003; **102**: 29a.

144. Davis JE, Smyth MJ, Trapani JA *et al.* Granzyme A and B-deficient killer lymphocytes are defective in eliciting DNA fragmentation but retain potent in vivo anti-tumor capacity. *Eur J Immunol* 2001; **31**: 39–47.

145. Ferreri AJ, Dell'Oro S, Capello D *et al.* Aberrant methylation in the promoter region of the reduced folate carrier gene is a potential mechanism of resistance to methotrexate in primary central nervous system lymphomas. *Br J Haematol* 2004; **126**: 657–64.

146. Grozinger CM, Schreiber SL. Deacetylase enzymes: biological functions and the use of small-molecule inhibitors. *Chem Biol* 2002; **9**: 3–16.

147. Fraga MF, Herranz M, Espada J *et al.* A mouse skin multistage carcinogenesis model reflects the aberrant DNA methylation patterns of human tumors. *Cancer Res* 2004; **64**: 5527–34.

85

New therapies for lymphoid neoplasms

JASMINE ZAIN, YUKIKO KITAGAWA, MATKO KALAC, LUCA PAOLUZZI AND OWEN A O'CONNOR

The lymphoid neoplasms represent some of the most heterogeneous and diverse malignancies known to medicine. The spectrum of clinical diseases ranges from rapidly growing diseases like Burkitt and lymphoblastic lymphoma to some of the slowest and most indolent cancers known to science, like small lymphocytic lymphoma and follicular lymphoma. This diversity in clinical behavior reflects the molecular heterogeneity that often defines these complex neoplasms which, based on the World Health Organization (WHO) classification, can be subdivided into at least 40 different subtypes.[1] Important advances in immunohistochemistry and cytogenetics, coupled with our historical skills in basic morphology, have now allowed the delineation of each non-Hodgkin lymphoma (NHL) subtype as a distinct clinical entity – each with its own unique clinical behavior and treatment paradigms. Recent advances in gene expression profiling (GEP) have led to an entirely new way to think about lymphoma classification based on individual gene clusters that correlate with prognosis and clinical behavior. These types of classification models offer an opportunity to think about designing rational and specific therapeutic regimens targeted against the unique biological basis of the disease. Chapter 84 provides a more extensive update on gene expression profiling of lymphomas.

For example, Alizadeh et al.[2] reported the application of GEP on tissue from patients with diffuse large B cell lymphoma (DLBCL), and proposed a molecular classification that divided DLBCL into subtypes based on the cell of origin. These included categorizing DLBCL into a germinal center (GC) subtype and an activated B cell (ABC) or post-germinal center subtype, with a favorable outcome seen in lymphomas arising from the GC. Shipp et al.[3] applied similar approaches in gene profiling and classified DLBCL based on clustering of consensus genes into three groups, including: (1) those with genes over-representing metabolic pathways involved in oxidative phosphorylation (i.e., the Ox Phos phenotype); (2) those with genes over-represented in the B cell receptor signaling pathway (i.e., the BCR phenotype); and (3) those with genes over-representing the host response. The BCR large B cell lymphomas have increased expression of the BCR signaling cascade and B cell transcription factors including BCL6. Interestingly, these tumors exhibit tonic BCR signaling and have been found to be sensitive to targeted inhibition of the BCR signaling pathway by blocking SYK (spleen tyrosine kinase). These important observations have now led to the identification of a completely new class of drugs (SYK inhibitors) targeting this specific biology.[4] The Ox Phos clusters show increased expression of genes regulating mitochondrial function, electron transport, and proteasomes. The histiocyte-rich (HR) DLBCLs exhibit a robust host immune response and have a prominent inflammatory infiltrate as part of their nodal architecture. Gene expression profiling is now being applied to nearly all lymphoma subtypes and will likely be reflected in the upcoming classifications of lymphoma, as well as in future prognostic models. More importantly, this information is being used to better understand the molecular pathogenesis of these diseases, which is creating a new platform for thinking about a new generation of targeted therapies for all forms of lymphoma.

Standard therapies for both NHL and Hodgkin lymphoma (HL) have incorporated the principles of combination cytotoxic chemotherapy developed in the 1970s through the 1980s. These strategies relied on exploiting the most efficacious agents with nonoverlapping toxicities that could be administered to patients in a convenient schedule. Decades of studies had led to the observation that many different types of drugs were active in the treatment of NHL, including alkylating agents (mechlorethamine, cyclophosphamide, ifosfamide), antimetabolites (methotrexate, cytarabine, fludarabine, 2-chlorodeoxyadenosine [2-CDA]), mitotic spindle poisons (vinblastine, vincristine), topoisomerase inhibitors (doxorubicin, etoposide), and even steroids (prednisone, dexamethasone). One of the great challenges during this time was trying to determine the best way to combine these many active agents into a program that was both effective and tolerable. As a result, many treatment programs emerged, some with purportedly better activity and safety than others. It wasn't until the results of the intergroup trial[5] that CHOP (cyclophosphamide, adriamycin [doxorubicin], vincristine, and prednisone) chemotherapy administered every 3 weeks emerged as the gold standard, based mostly on the fact that it exhibited the most favorable toxicity profile with effectiveness comparable to other multidrug regimens. Similarly for HL, it was established that combination chemotherapy regimens like ABVD (adriamycin [doxorubicin], bleomycin, vinblastine, and dacarbazine) and MOPP (mechlorethamine, vincristine, procarbazine, and prednisone) produced similar efficacy with response rates in the range of 80–90 percent and a freedom-from-relapse rate in the range of 60–65 percent. However, ABVD was associated with a significantly lower risk of secondary malignancies and infertility[6] and thus emerged as the gold standard for patients with this unusual form of lymphoma. The recent approval of the CD20-directed chimeric antibody rituximab has improved the response rates of all types of B cell lymphomas, including follicular lymphoma and DLBCL.[7]

Despite these advances and successes, we are still far from being able to offer all patients a treatment modality that offers the promise of cure or long-term disease control. In the last decade, a plethora of new treatment alternatives have emerged for the treatment of many different forms of cancer, but especially in the treatment of lymphoma. These drugs are not merely new derivatives of old favorites, but represent major advances in molecular

pharmacology. These advances included agents that target new aspects of cancer biology, including novel drugs targeting gene transcription (histone deacetylase inhibitors and hypomethylating agents), the proteasome (bortezomib), and immunomodulatory pathways (thalidomide and lenalidomide) and new generations of bifunctional agents that are intended to hybridize the functional aspects of different cytotoxic agents in ways that generate novel chemical platforms (bendamustine). Table 85.1 presents some of these agents and the novel targets they affect. While it is beyond the scope of this chapter to cover all these agents, we will focus on a few of the major drugs or new drug classes that have firmly established themselves in the treatment of lymphoma. Given the enormous plethora of new agents, the chapter will largely focus on those drug already approved by the United States Food and Drug Administration (FDA).

TARGETING THE UBIQUITIN PROTEASOME PATHWAY: BORTEZOMIB

Over the past decade, one truly novel class of drugs that has moved rapidly from the laboratory to the clinic is the proteasome inhibitors. These drugs, originally developed to counteract the effects of protein wasting and cachexia syndromes associated with advanced cancer, have been found to possess important antineoplastic activity in both preclinical and clinical settings. Over a very short period of time, these drugs have had a major impact on the management of several hematologic malignancies, including multiple myeloma and mantle cell lymphoma (MCL). This therapeutic opportunity has grown from our understanding of the complex biology underlying the ubiquitin-proteasome pathway (UPP) in normal cells, now leading to the identification of several agents capable of selectively inhibiting proteolytic degradation in the 26S proteasome. Intuitively, one would not necessarily anticipate that inhibiting such an important and ubiquitous aspect of cellular biology would lead to a novel therapeutic agent. Though clearly, as both a therapy and a tool, these drugs are now helping patients and teaching us much about cancer biology.

The proteasome is in fact a component of the larger UPP, the major means of degrading and eliminating intracellular proteins.[8] The proteasome itself is a complex structure consisting of many proteins, some of which play a structural role, others of which are specific proteases. The UPP plays a critical role in regulating the balance of essential regulatory proteins involved in growth and survival. Bortezomib (formerly known as PS-341, also known as Velcade), is a potent and selective inhibitor of the chymotryptic-like enzymatic function residing in the 26S proteasome.[9] Inhibition of this enzyme has been associated with a remarkable number of different biological effects, including inhibition of nuclear factor κB (NF-κB) through the stabilization of inhibitor of NF-κB (IκB); cell cycle arrest mediated through the accumulation of cell cycle regulatory

Table 85.1   Emerging novel targets and agents for the treatment of lymphoma

Mechanism	Drugs	Rationale
Inhibition of antiapoptotic BCL2 family members and survivin	ABT-737/263 AT-101 GX015- Oblimersen	Silence the antiapoptotic influence of BCL2, BCLX$_L$, BCLW, and MCL1
Proteasome inhibitors	Bortezomib Carfilzomib	Pleotropic drugs capable of inhibiting NF-κB, inducing cell cycle arrest by inhibiting degradation of p27 and p21, and inducing apoptosis by shifting the balance of proapoptotic and antiapoptotic BCL2 family members
Epigenetic agents – histone deacetylase inhibitors	Vorinostat Depsipeptide LBH589 Belinostat	Pleotropic drugs capable of affecting the transcriptional state of chromatin and affecting the post-translational state of many non-histone proteins like BCL6 and TP53
Immunomodulatory agents (IMiDs)	Thalidomide Lenalidomide	Known to inhibit TNF, to be antiangiogenic, and to activate NK cells in addition to many other biological effects
New derivatives of established agents	Bendamustine Pralatrexate Clofarabine Nelarabine	These drugs appear to be non-cross-resistant to other conventional alkylating agents and antifols. In addition, they may be able to induce effects in cell division or lymphocyte activation pathways that may distinguish them
Inhibition of selective cell cycle–dependent kinases	PD-0332991 (CDK4/6) CINK4 (CDK4/6) Seliciclib (CDK2/1) BMS-387032 (CDK2/1) PNU-252808 (CDK2/1) PNU-252808 (CDK2/1) NU6102, NU6140 (CDK2/1)	Inhibit specific phase transitions of cell cycle progression
mTOR/AKT inhibitors	Temsirolimus Rapamycin Perifosine	Associated with broad effects on cancer cell biology, including protein translation, NF-κB, transcription factors, and apoptosis

NF-κB, nuclear factor κB; TNF, tumor necrosis factor; CDK, cyclin-dependent kinase.

proteins like p21 and p27; and induction of apoptosis mediated by effects on BH3-only mimetics and proapoptotic BCL2 family members.[8] Inhibiting the chymotryptic function of the proteasome has also been associated with impressive clinical activity, as validated by the approval of a first-in-class proteasome inhibitor bortezomib in the treatment of multiple myeloma and MCL.

Biological effects of proteasome inhibition

While targeting the proteasome has proven to be an important new approach for the treatment of several hematologic cancers, proteasome inhibition is associated with innumerable cellular effects (Fig. 85.1). At present, it is not entirely clear precisely how proteasome inhibitors affect tumor cells, though a multitude of theories abound. One line of evidence has shown that inhibition of the proteasome leads to the accumulation of several cell cycle regulatory proteins. It has been well established that inhibition of the 26S proteasome leads to accumulation of a host of different cell cycle regulators including the cyclins

and cyclin-dependent kinase (CDK) inhibitors like p21 and p27.[10–13] This mechanism could produce cell cycle arrest, or even lead to the induction of apoptosis through other indirect pathways. Another potentially important mechanism pertains to the influence of bortezomib on BCL2 family members. It is also well established that proteasome inhibitors can cause accumulation of select BH3-only proteins like NOXA, which serve to shift the balance of a cell toward apoptosis. Similarly, multiple reports have demonstrated that proteasome inhibition can increase the quantity of proapoptotic proteins like BAX and BIK.[14–17]

Perhaps the most widely proclaimed mechanism of action of bortezomib revolves around its ability to inhibit the degradation of IκB, which is the natural cognate inhibitor of NF-κB. Inhibition of NF-κB leads to downregulation of NF-κB-dependent genes, which has been shown to kill lymphomas which are intrinsically addicted to NF-κB (22–27).[18–23] In normally quiescent cells, NF-κB exists in an inactivated form bound to IκB. In malignant cells, and in cells stimulated or stressed through exposure to various cytokines, cytotoxic drugs, viruses, oxidative triggers, or other mitogenic factors, IκB is phosphorylated by IκB

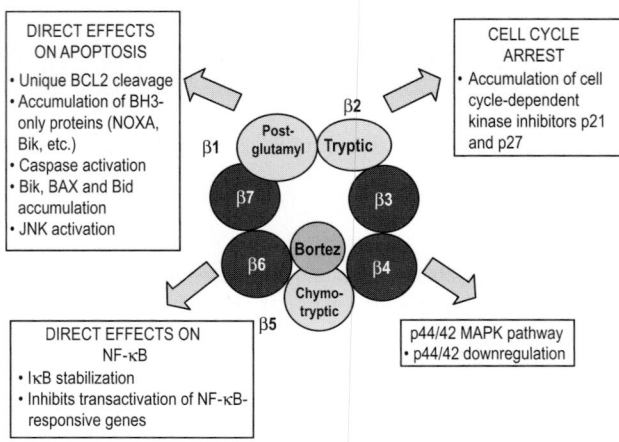

Figure 85.1 Cellular effects of proteasome inhibition. Beta subunits shown as $\beta1–\beta7$. Bortez, bortezomib; NF-κB, nuclear factor κB; IκB, inhibitor of NK-κB; MAPK, mitogen-activated protein kinase.

kinase and then ubiquitinated, leading to its eventual degradation and liberation of active free NF-κB. Subsequently, NF-κB is translocated to the nucleus where it binds to very specific DNA sequences on the promoters of specific target genes. The products of these genes include proteins that play an important role in suppressing the induction of apoptosis, the activation of cell proliferation, the induction of cytokine production, and release of angiogenic factors facilitating angiogenesis.[24] Collectively, many of these biological processes contribute to the malignant phenotype, favoring the uncontrolled growth and metastasis of tumor cells.[22,23] Inhibition of the NF-κB influence could, at least theoretically, mitigate some of the malignant behaviors associated with transformed cells. Additionally, there are now multiple lines of evidence to suggest that inhibition of the proteasome can sensitize cells to a host of conventional and experimental drugs in a fashion that is at least additive, and more often than not, synergistic.

Evidence for important clinical activity in the lymphoproliferative malignancies

The phase I study of bortezomib in patients with hematologic malignancies initially reported activity of the drug in three diseases: multiple myeloma, MCL, and follicular lymphoma.[25] To date, based on the Summit trial, bortezomib has gained approval for the treatment of relapsed or refractory multiple myeloma.[26] In the lymphoproliferative malignancies, the activity in MCL, confirmed in a registration-directed study (PINNACLE), has led to approval of this drug in MCL.[27] Other subtypes of NHL where activity has been reported include follicular lymphoma and marginal zone lymphoma.

The first experience with bortezomib in lymphoma reported a response rate of 77 percent (in nine assessable

Table 85.2 Bortezomib exhibits selective activity across the spectrum of lymphoma[2,20–23,28–33]

Disease	Total number of patients (n)	CR	PR	ORR
Mantle cell NHL	259	8–15%	21–46%	30–45%
Follicular NHL	36	0–22%	0–28%	0–50%
Marginal zone NHL	23	3	6	39%
CLL/SLL	7	0 of 7	1 of 7	NA
Hodgkin disease	44	0%	0%	0%
Diffuse large B cell NHL	12	0 of 12	1 of 12	0%
T cell lymphoma	15	2	6	67%

CR, complete remission; PR, partial remission; ORR, overall response rate; NHL, non-Hodgkin lymphoma; CLL/SLL, chronic lymphocytic leukemia/small lymphocytic lymphoma.

patients, including two complete remissions [CR]) in patients with follicular lymphoma, and 50 percent in ten assessable patients with MCL. While the numbers were small, activity was also appreciated in two patients with marginal zone NHL.[9] Subsequent studies of bortezomib by other investigators in lymphoma confirmed marked activity in MCL, with little to no activity in patients with chronic lymphocytic leukemia, HL, and DLBCL.[28–30] Despite the realization that bortezomib was not universally active across all subtypes of lymphoma (Table 85.2), there was enthusiasm around the consistency of observations generated in MCL (Table 85.3). This reproducible activity across several phase II studies led to a registration-directed phase II study (the PINNACLE study) in 155 patients with relapsed or refractory MCL.[27] A recent update of these data reported an overall response rate of 32 percent, including a complete remission rate of 8 percent. What was even more interesting was the duration of response among these patients. The time to progression and overall survival for all patients was 6.7 and 23.5 months, respectively. However, for those patients attaining a response, the time to progression and overall survival were 12.4 and 35.4 months, respectively. Even in patients whose lymphoma was refractory to their prior line of chemotherapy, the overall response rate and duration of that response were remarkably similar to those patients who had relapsed disease.[31] These data from the PINNACLE trial formed the basis of the regulatory approval of bortezomib in MCL, establishing it as the first drug ever approved for the treatment of this disease.

Despite the rapidly emerging experience with bortezomib in MCL, there is also a significant interest in combining this agent with conventional chemotherapy regimens. Recent data, exploring the substitution of bortezomib for vincristine in standard R-CVP, have established that even in patients frankly resistant to prior chemotherapy, the bortezomib-containing regimen is capable of overcoming the prior intrinsic and acquired drug resistance.[32] Recent reports of two phase I studies have evaluated the safety and efficacy of

Table 85.3   Single-agent activity of bortezomib in mantle cell lymphoma

Study	Bortezomib regimen	Evaluable patients(n)	CR/CRu	PR	OR
O'Connor (ICML 2005)	1.5 mg/m^2 days 1, 4, 8, 11; 21-day cycle	37	13%	27%	40%
Goy (JCO 2005)	1.5 mg/m^2 days 1, 4, 8, 11; 21-day cycle	29	21%	21%	41%
Strauss/Lister (IMCL 2005)	1.3 mg/m^2 days 1, 4, 8, 11; 21-day cycle	24	255	4$	29%
Belch (ASH 2004)	1.3 mg/m^2 days 1, 4, 8, 11; 21-day cycle	13 untreated	0%	46%	46%
		15 treated	7%	40%	47%
PINNACLE (ASCO 2005)	1.3 mg/m^2 days 1, 4, 8, 11; 21-day cycle	141	8%	26%	33%

CR, complete remission; CRu, complete remission, unconfirmed; PR, partial remission; OR, overall response.

a weekly and twice-weekly regimen, establishing that the substitution is safe and associated with response rates of 57 percent and 72 percent in patients with follicular or mantle cell lymphoma, respectively. Based on these data, international studies now aimed at exploring the merits of substituting bortezomib for vincristine in R-CVP and R-CHOP are underway. The single-agent activity of bortezomib in follicular lymphoma also remains an interesting prospect. One experience has established that the duration of exposure may be one of the more critical determinants of bortezomib activity in this patient population.[9] Select experiences by some investigators have suggested little to no activity in follicular lymphoma, especially in studies where the duration of drug treatment was limited to one or two cycles.[28,29] Interestingly, the largest experience which allowed for protracted treatment found that the median time to response was approximately 12 weeks, compared to approximately 4 to 5 weeks for patients with MCL. Many of these patients continued to respond during the first 3 to 6 months off therapy, and nearly all have had very durable remissions. These data raise the interesting prospect that bortezomib may be functioning as an immunomodulatory agent in this setting, and that protracted treatment with the drug is a critical determinant of response.

Future directions

At present, there are a host of different trials beginning to explore the merits of integrating bortezomib into conventional chemotherapy regimens for the treatment of nearly all NHL subtypes. These studies will be exploring the use of the drug as both a sensitizer to conventional chemotherapy approaches as well as a maintenance strategy in MCL. While bortezomib's activity in lymphoma matures, newer proteasome inhibitors have taken slightly different pharmacodynamic approaches: one being designed to be a more selective inhibitor of the chymotryptic proteasome (carfilzomib),[33] as others tout the therapeutic merits of a more pan-proteasome protease inhibitor approach

(Salinosporamide A; NPI-0052).[34] While it is too early to comment on these agents, it is clear that targeting the proteasome is a bona fide therapeutic target for the treatment of lymphoma. What remains challenging is the process of trying to identify the specific subtypes of lymphoma where bortezomib is active, and to elucidate precisely how it works across the broad spectrum of lymphoproliferative malignancies.

TARGETING EPIGENETIC PATHWAYS IN THE TREATMENT OF LYMPHOMA: VORINOSTAT

The linear representation of the DNA molecule is a highly simplified graphical model for explaining the mechanisms of DNA composition and function. In fact, DNA is a complex molecule with a complicated three-dimensional structure that interacts with numerous proteins forming what is known as the chromatin. In eukaryotic cells, the major structural proteins around which the more than two meters of DNA is organized are called histones. These are small low-molecular-weight proteins containing a large proportion of positively charged amino acids, mostly lysine and arginine. There are five types of histones (H1, H2A, H2B, H3, and H4) of which four of them (H2A, H2B, H3, and H4) form an octamer (containing two of each histone type) around which the DNA is tightly supercoiled, forming the fundamental unit of chromatin called the nucleosome. The H1 histone serves as a linker protein, bridging the DNA between two separate nucleosomes.[35,36] The post-translational modification of histones through a variety of different biochemical reactions, including acetylation, sumoylation, phosphorylation, and methylation, plays a pivotal role in determining the transcriptional state of DNA. While there is bound to be a host of other biochemical modifications that will lead to changes in the transcriptional state of DNA, the effects of acetylation and methylation are probably the best studied to date. Further information on epigenetic modulation in lymphomas is also provided in Chapter 84.

Table 85.4   Classes of histone deacetylases

Class I	Class II	Class III	Class IV
HDAC 1, 2, 3, and 8	HDAC 4, 5, 6, 7, and 9	Sirtuins 1–7	Class 11
Require Zn ion for their enzymatic activity. Crystallographic analysis of the interaction between TSA or vorinostat with HDACs from these classes shows inhibition at this active center		Require NAD$^+$ for their activity. Broad class I/II HDACi do not affect these enzymes	Contains both catalytic residues contained in Class I and II HDACs, also requires Zn ion

HDAC, histone deacetylase; HDACi, histone deacetylase inhibitor; TSA, trichostatin A.

Acetylation typically occurs on the terminal epsilon (ε) amino moieties of the lysine residues and is catalyzed by two sets of enzymes – histone acetyltransferases (HATs) which add acetyl groups to histones, and histone deacetylases (HDACs) which remove them.[37] Positively charged lysine residues bind strongly to the negatively charged DNA, causing chromatin condensation which makes it inaccessible to transcription factors and thus transcriptionally silent. The addition of the acetyl groups neutralizes the positive charge, consequently moving the DNA away from the histones, inducing chromatin decondensation, making the chromatin structure more relaxed and transcriptionally active. These balanced reactions set the stage for transcriptional control. Methylation is a process that primarily occurs on cytosine bases usually located 5′ to a guanine base, resulting in repression of transcription. Genome-wide hypermethylation has been found in all types of human neoplasms and has been recognized as an important epigenetic process in the malignant transformation of cells as well as an important therapeutic target.[38]

To date, approximately 18 different HDACs have been discovered in human cells, and are broadly divided into four major classes based on their homology to yeast HDACs (Table 85.4). The smaller-sized histones, including HDAC 1, 2, 3, and 8, are grouped into class I, while the larger proteins[39] including HDAC 4, 5, 6, 7, and 9 are grouped into class II (Table 85.4). Both class I and II HDACs, taken together with class IV enzymes represented by HDAC 11, contain highly conserved residues in the catalytic core regions and require a zinc ion for their activity. On the other hand, class III HDACs, also called the sirtuins, contain seven enzymes (SIRT 1–7) that require nicotinamide adenine dinucleotide (NAD$^+$) for their activity. This difference in the catalytic core implies that there will also be a difference in the compounds capable of blocking HDACs. In addition, beyond merely histones, it is clear HATs and HDACs can affect a host of other cytosolic and nuclear proteins including BCL6, TP53, and heat shock proteins (HSP90). As our understanding of these drugs emerges, it is becoming increasingly clear that the effects on these non-histone-related proteins may play a pivotal role in understanding the mechanism of action of these agents.

Histone deacetylases and oncogenesis

Disruption of histone acetylation is a common feature of many different types of cancer cells, and there is a rapidly emerging body of evidence describing mutations in HATs and HDACs as important mediators of cellular transformation. Mutations in HAT genes leading to cancer have been well established. For example, Rubenstein-Taybi syndrome, characterized by mental and growth retardation, dysmorphology, and an increased incidence of neoplasia, is caused by mutations in *CREBBP* and *EP300*, which are genes encoding histone acetyltransferases.[40] The MYST family of HATs play an important role in the of acetylation of TP53,[41] inducing apoptosis after DNA damage.[42] The gene for KAT5, a histone acetyltransferase, is a frequent target for monoallelic loss in human lymphomas.[43] Gorrini *et al.*[43] reported that loss of KAT5 could synergize with mutations in *TP53* and contribute to tumor progression. Mutations of HDAC genes have also been described. Ropero *et al.*[44] have described mutations in the gene encoding HDAC 2 in colorectal and endometrial cancer cell lines. They found that cell lines with HDAC 2 mutations were resistant to the effects of trichostatin A (a potent laboratory HDAC inhibitor) including resulting in hyperacetylation of histones and blockade of cell cycle and apoptosis.[44] In addition to these pathways, there is now clear evidence that many viruses, including adenoviruses, human immunodeficiency virus, and Epstein–Barr virus, synthesize proteins that bind HATs, which can lead to cellular transformation.[45–47] These data point to the recognition that mutations in epigenetic genes can themselves be oncogenic and should be considered as oncogenes.

Histone deacetylase inhibitors

To date, there may be more HDAC inhibitors in development than any other class of antineoplastic agents. Broadly, there are considered to be four major chemical classes of HDAC inhibitors, including: (1) hydroxamic acids like vorinostat, LBH589, and belinostat; (2) aliphatic acids like phenylbutyric acid and valproic acid; (3) benzamides including agents like MS-275 and MGCD0103; and (4) the cyclic peptides including agents like depsipeptide (Table 85.5). While these agents all share the ability to

Table 85.5   Classes of histone deacetylase inhibitors

HDAC inhibitor class (potency *in vitro* [IC_{50}])	Compounds	Representative chemical structure	Pharmacologic profile
Short-chain fatty acids (millimolar)	Valproic acid, phenylbutyrate	Valproic acid	Short plasma half-life, rapid metabolism, nonspecific mode of action
Hydroxamic acids (nanomolar)	Trichostatin A, vorinostat (SAHA), PXD-101 (belinostat), LBH589 (panobinostat), ITF2357, pyroxamide, oxamflatin, scriptaid	Vorinostat (SAHA)	Potent HDAC I/II/IV inhibitors, also called pan-HDAC inhibitors
Benzamides (micromolar)	MGCD0103, MS-275, CI-994, SK-7041	MGCD0103	MGCD0103 is a class I-specific HDAC inhibitor
Cyclic peptides (nanomolar)	Romidepsin (depsipeptide)		Very potent HDAC inhibitor with IC_{50} in low nanomolar range
Class III HDAC inhibitors (millimolar)	Niacinamide, sirtinol	Niacinamide	Class II-specific HDAC inhibitors

HDAC, histone deacetylase; IC_{50}, concentration required for 50 percent maximum inhibition; SAHA, suberoylanilide hydroxamic acid.

inhibit histone deacetylases, there are still many questions regarding the differences between these agents, especially with regard to the specific HDAC enzymes they affect, the differences in gene expression they influence, and the non-histone proteins they affect from a post-translational perspective.

The bulk of the clinical experience with these compounds has focused on the pan-HDAC inhibitors; that is, those inhibiting both class I and II enzymes. These drugs represent a very broad group of diverse chemical structures, associated with a wide range of effective concentrations (from low nanomolar to high millimolar). The first HDAC inhibitors noted to have activity were the aliphatic acids valproate and butyrate. Their activity, however, was found to be weak, with IC_{50} (concentration required for 50 percent maximum inhibition) values in the millimolar range. Crystallographic analyses of potent HDAC inhibitors, like trichostatin A (TSA) and suberoylanilide hydroxamic acid (SAHA, vorinostat), and their interaction with their target enzymes shed light on the nature of how these drugs interface with their protein target. For example, both TSA and vorinostat are known to contain three distinct structural components important in their biological activity: (1) a hydroxamic acid residue that binds to the zinc ion on the HDAC; (2) a hydrophobic spacer that aids in spanning the entire active center of the enzyme pocket; and (3) a hydrophobic cap that covers the active center.[47] It was the early clarification of trichostatin's mechanism of action that eventually led to the development of the hydroxamic acid-based HDAC inhibitors, the best known of which is vorinostat (SAHA). All the HDAC inhibitors that inhibit the zinc-containing enzymes (class I, II, and IV) have no effect on the class III HDACs. Recently, some intriguing experiments in mammalian cells have established that the inhibition of class III HDACs (also called the sirtuins) may play a role in transcriptional regulation, but may also play an even bigger role in regulating the activity of *TP53*. It has been shown that the site of local DNA damage and activation of PARP1 leads to depletion of local NAD^+ molecules and synthesis of niacinamide, a class III HDAC inhibitor that binds to and inhibits the NAD^+-containing site of sirtuins leading to a change in chromatin accessibility.[2] Niacinamide, which does not affect class I, II, and IV HDACs, has been shown to have cytotoxic effects in tumor cell lines in high, millimolar concentrations, and it is currently being assessed for its synergistic effects with radiation therapy in solid tumors and with pan-class I/II HDAC inhibitors.

Clinical activity of histone deacetylase inhibitors

Although a number of HDAC inhibitors are currently in clinical trials (Table 85.6), only suberoylanilide hydroxamic acid (vorinostat), commercially known as Zolinza, is approved by the FDA for clinical use in cutaneous T cell lymphomas. Vorinostat is a hydroxymate with the ability to induce differentiation and apoptosis in a number of cell lines and cause the accumulation of acetylated histones.[48,49] In phase I clinical trials in patients with both solid tumors and hematologic malignancies, both oral and intravenous (IV) formulations were shown to be very well tolerated and active.[49] These studies demonstrated a favorable pharmacokinetic profile[50] and promising activity in T cell lymphoma, which led to the initiation of a phase II study in patients with cutaneous T cell lymphoma (CTCL). This phase II experience, reported by Duvic et al.,[51] enrolled 33 patients with advanced heavily pretreated CTCL. Three different orally administered dosages and schedules were sequentially evaluated. Group 1 received 400 mg of drug daily; group 2 received 300 mg twice daily for 3 days followed by 4 days of rest; and group 3 received 300 mg twice daily for 14 days with a week of rest followed by 200 mg twice daily. Treatment was continued until the patients showed signs of progression or intolerable toxicity was encountered. The overall response rate (ORR) was 24.2 percent with eight patients having a partial remission (PR) including four patients with Sézary syndrome. More importantly, 14 of the 33 patients (42 percent) reported significant pruritus relief. The median time to response was 11.9 weeks, while the median duration of response was 15.1 weeks. The major side effects included fatigue, thrombocytopenia, and gastrointestinal symptoms (predominantly diarrhea and nausea). Most of the responses were seen in groups 1 and 3, thus the 400 mg per day dosage was established as having the best safety profile and was approved for use. This was the maximum tolerated dose (MTD) identified in the earlier phase I studies in patients with hematologic malignancies. Subsequently, a registration-directed phase II study reported by Olsen et al. included 74 patients with CTCL and showed an ORR of 29.7 percent, with one patient achieving CR.[52] Clinical activity of vorinostat has also been seen in other lymphomas. Kirschbaum et al.[53] presented the interim analysis of a phase II study of vorinostat in relapsed or refractory indolent NHL including mantle cell lymphomas. Seventeen patients who were refractory or had progressed on chemotherapy (including rituximab) were enrolled in the study at a dose of 200 mg twice a day for 14 days followed by a 1-week rest. Of the 17 patients enrolled, there were four complete remissions and two partial remissions as defined by the recent Cheson criteria. The major toxicities were thrombocytopenia, anemia, and fatigue, all well-established effects of vorinostat. SWOG 0517 is a phase II trial of vorinostat in patients with relapsed or refractory Hodgkin disease. Phase I data suggested that vorinostat could effect responses and prolong disease stabilization in patients with heavily treated Hodgkin disease. These data led to the initiation of a multicenter phase II trial in relapsed or refractory Hodgkin disease. The dosing schedule consisted of 200 mg twice a day for 14 days on a 21-day cycle. With 27 patients being accrued to the study, only a single partial remission was observed, though there was

Table 85.6   Clinical status of various HDAC inhibitors in development

HDAC inhibitor	Class	Route of administration	Clinical trial	Comments
Valproic acid	Aliphatic acids	Oral	As a single agent – case report: a CR seen in heavily pretreated patient with NHL	
			Phase II trials when used in combination with 5-azacytidine in AML and MDS patients	ORR 42%, CR 22%
AN-9	Aliphatic acids	Intravenous	Phase II in non-small-cell lung carcinoma (NSCLC)	ORR 7.3% No CR
Savicol	Aliphatic acids		Phase II in colon adenocarcinoma	
SAHA (vorinostat)	Hydroxamates	Oral, intravenous	FDA approval for the treatment of cutaneous T cell lymphoma (CTCL) which has progressed on the conventional treatment	ORR 24.2%, No CR ORR 29.7%, CR 1.3% (1 patient)
			Ongoing trials in patients with multiple myeloma, AML, MDS, CML, various solid tumors	
PXD101 (belinostat)	Hydroxamates	Intravenous	Phase II trials in patients with peripheral or cutaneous T cell lymphoma	ORR 22.2%, CR 11.1% (3 patients)
			Phase II trials in multiple myeloma patients	Stabilization of the disease
LBH589 (panobinostat)	Hydroxamates	Oral	Phase I in various hematologic and solid tumors	
			Phase II in CTCL	ORR 45%, CR 18% (2 patients)
ITF2357	Hydroxamates		Currently in phase I and II for refractory lymphoma and chronic myeloproliferative diseases	Interesting finding that ITF2357 targets JAK-2 V617F mutation
MS-275	Benzamide	Oral	Phase I in AML	
			Phase II in combination with azacytidine in patients with AML, MDS, and chronic myelomonocytic leukemia	ORR 22%, CR 7% (2 patients)
			Phase II in melanoma	No responses observed
MGCD0103	Benzamide	Oral	Phase II in combination with azacytidine in patients with AML and MDS	ORR 29%, CR 12.5% (3 patients), CR_p 12.5%
Depsipeptide (romidepsin)	Cyclic peptides	Intravenous	Phase II in patients with CTCL and PTCL	ORR 35%, CR 10% (3 patients)

HDAC, histone deacetylase; CR, complete remission; NHL, non-Hodgkin lymphoma; MDS, myelodysplastic syndrome; AML, acute myeloid leukemia; ORR, overall response rate; SAHA, suberoylyanilide hydroxamic acid; FDA, United States Food and Drug Administration; CML, chronic myeloid leukemia; PTCL, peripheral T cell lymphoma; CR_p, complete response with low platelets.

stabilization of disease in four patients for up to 16 months. While this result was not encouraging, it raises the issue regarding the role of dose and schedule. Given the earlier observations at the higher dose, it is conceivable that alternative schedules could be associated with greater efficacy.

Valproic acid (VPA; Depakote) is a commonly used anticonvulsant with HDAC inhibitory activity. It belongs to the class of aliphatic acids along with phenylbutyrate, which are well-recognized pan-class I/II HDAC inhibitors. Because these agents are considerably less potent than many of the newer-generation HDAC inhibitors, relatively high millimolar concentrations are required to see effects

on histones and cytotoxicity. To date, the bulk of the clinical experience comes from trials in patients with solid tumors, as well as studies exploring combinations of VPA with conventional cytotoxic therapy or hypomethylating agents. Recently, Zain et al. reported a complete remission in a patient with DLBCL refractory to previous lines of therapy following monotherapy with VPA.[54] Patients ($n = 53$) with acute myeloid leukemia (AML) and high risk myelodysplastic syndrome (MDS) have been evaluated in a phase II clinical trial combining 5-azacytidine and VPA, with an ORR of 42 percent and with 22 percent of these patients attaining a complete remission.[55]

Depsipeptide (Romidepsin, FK228) is a cyclic peptide originally isolated from the broth culture of *Chromobacterium violaceum*.[56] Depsipeptide was in fact the first HDAC inhibitor reported to demonstrate activity in chemotherapy-resistant CTCL.[57] This experience from the National Cancer Institute was initially focused on patients with refractory or relapsed solid tumors, where the dose-limiting toxicity was found to be nausea, vomiting, thrombocytopenia, and neutropenia.[58] Expansion of this initial trial in the phase II study,[59] and most recently in a second international registration-directed experience reported by Kim et al.,[60] further established the considerable activity of depsipeptide in patients with CTCL. In addition, the agent has also shown promising activity in peripheral T cell lymphomas with response rates of 23 percent, including two complete remissions and two partial remissions[59] in heavily pretreated patients. Encouragingly, the duration of response was ongoing at 8–19 months. The established dosing of depsipeptide is $14\,mg/m^2$ given intravenously on days 1, 8, and 15 every 28 days. This agent is currently in trial for a number of solid tumors and hematologic tumors.[60]

Future directions

The prospect of targeting transcription, or the transcriptional state of a tumor cell, represents one of the most exciting breakthroughs in the area of novel drug development. The proof of principle has emerged, and now, with a plethora of new HDAC inhibitors becoming available, the major challenge will be trying to understand the differences between these widely divergent drugs, the particular disease setting where each is likely to work, and precisely how we believe these agents are facilitating tumor cell death. Discriminating the lethal events mediated through changes in the chromatin structure versus the post-translational effects on key regulatory proteins will not be a simple task, but could offer new insights for tailoring the treatment to very specific NHL subtypes. While some of these HDAC inhibitors may find an indication as monotherapy, as in the case of vorinostat, and possibly with depsipeptide in rare lymphomas, it is likely these agents will couple favorably with new and older drugs alike. The likelihood that these agents will rely on the right partnership with other antineoplastic agents raises the important fact that we will need to try and optimize the best of these partnerships in the most appropriate preclinical models. Validation of the optimal combination strategies in this setting will streamline early and later-phase clinical development. Today, HDAC inhibitors seem to function additively or better in combination with hypomethylating agents, proteasome inhibitors, BCL2-targeted drugs, and select conventional cytotoxic agents like topoisomerase inhibitors. At present, a number of clinical trials are exploring these possible combinations and, over the years to come, will better define the best approach for using these drugs in lymphoma.

TARGETING IMMUNOMODULATORY PATHWAYS: THALIDOMIDE AND LENALIDOMIDE (REVLIMID®)

Thalidomide is a synthetic glutamic acid derivative with a phthaloyl ring that was synthesized initially as a sedative and antiemetic agent in the 1950s. This drug was used extensively in pregnant women in over 40 countries, except the USA. Following this experience, approximately 10 000 children were born with severe structural malformations including phocomelia (a defect in limb bud development), leading to the withdrawal of thalidomide from the market.[61,62] The drug remained dormant until approximately 1965 when, quite serendipitously, it was shown to improve the inflammatory symptoms in a patient with erythema nodosum leprosum by downregulating the production of tumor necrosis factor α (TNFα).[63] This observation led to further evaluation of thalidomide as an immunomodulatory, anti-inflammatory, and antiangiogenic agent. Presently, the drug is approved for the treatment of multiple myeloma[64] and the cutaneous manifestations of erythema nodosum leprosum. In addition it has been recognized to have activity in rheumatoid arthritis, systemic lupus erythematosus,[65] metastatic melanoma,[66] and prostate cancer.[67]

Lenalidomide (CC-5013; Revlimid), a second-generation analogue of thalidomide (Fig. 85.2), is an immunomodulatory agent (IMiD) with potent anticancer properties.[68] It was synthesized as an analogue of thalidomide, the first IMiD, by adding an amino moiety at position 4 of the phthaloyl ring and by removing one of the carbonyl groups. This resulted in a more potent drug with a more favorable side-effect profile as compared to thalidomide.[61]

Lenalidomide (Revlimid™)

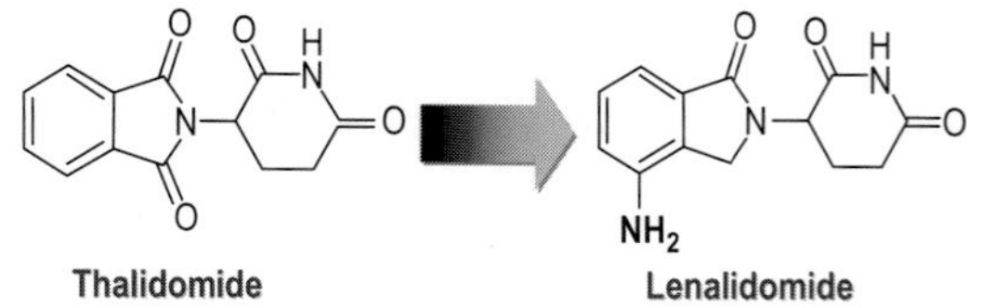

Thalidomide   Lenalidomide

- 10–1000 times more potent
- Safety profile: non-neurotoxic, non-teratogenic, non-sedating

Figure 85.2 Pharmacologic evolution of lenalidomide (CC-5013, Revlimid®). Lenalidomide is a 4-amino-glutamyl analogue of thalidomide that is up to 1000 times more potent at inhibiting tumor necrosis factor α compared with the parent compound. The IMiDs, including lenalidomide, are far more potent than thalidomide with respect to costimulating T cells and inhibiting angiogenesis. Clinical trials have shown that treatment with lenalidomide is not associated with neuropathy and sedation, which may be associated with thalidomide treatment. Lenalidomide was nonteratogenic in a rabbit toxicology model that is traditionally used to detect drug teratogenicity.[61,106]

Preclinical evidence of antilymphoma activity for lenalidomide

The IMiDs have been found to possess many common biological effects, including: activation of natural killer (NK) cells and T cells; modulation of various cytokines such as TNFα, interleukin (IL)-12, and interferon gamma (IFNγ) in the tumor microenvironment; and inhibition of angiogenesis.[61] They have also been shown to have direct antitumor activity by causing growth arrest and caspase-dependent apoptosis of tumor cells.(1) Based on these preclinical observations, and an extension of the observation that thalidomide is a potent agent in the treatment of multiple myeloma, a number of studies have begun to demonstrate remarkable activity of these agents across a broad spectrum of different NHL subtypes.

The direct effects of lenalidomide (CC-5013), and even new-generation IMiDs like CC-4047, on malignant B cell proliferation have been demonstrated by various groups.[69] These data suggest that these agents lead to an upregulation of Sacrated Protein Acidic and Rich in Cysteine (SPARC) and p21, and inhibit the cyclin-dependent kinases including CDK2, CDK4, and CDK6, inducing cell cycle arrest and apoptosis. SPARC is a matrix-associated protein that influences the synthesis of extracellular matrix. These observations have been corroborated in murine xenograft models by Lentzsch et al.,[70] who demonstrated that IMiDs have a direct antitumor effect on B cell malignancies in immunocompromised mouse models, establishing in vivo activity. In this setting, lenalidomide and CC-4047 were more potent than thalidomide in suppressing tumor growth and extending survival, while also demonstrating significantly better antiangiogenic properties as demonstrated by tumor microvascular density. The mechanistic effects of IMiDs are considered to be quite pleotropic, extending well beyond the direct effects on cancer cells, and include effects on immune effector and stromal cells: stimulation of cytotoxic T cells, activation of dendritic cells,[71] and induction of NK cell activity by increasing levels of cytokines like IL-2, TNFα, and IFNγ. While the role of angiogenesis in lymphoma remains to be clarified, these agents appear to have the unique capability to produce significant anti-vascular endothelial growth factor (anti-VEGF) activity, which appears to be independent of the antiproliferative effects.

Although still primarily confined to laboratory investigation, it is now clear that the IMiDs appear to complement the activity of a host of other drugs known to be active in the treatment of lymphomas. For example, the rationale for combining the immunologic effects of an IMiD and a monoclonal antibody is being tested both in the preclinical and clinical setting. Rituximab, an immunoglobulin G1 (IgG1) chimeric monoclonal antibody targeting CD20, and IMiDs like lenalidomide have been shown to produce at least additive benefit in preclinical studies in severe combined immunodeficiency (SCID) mouse models.[72] These effects appear to be mediated by immunomodulation leading to increased NK cell activity, modification of the cytokine environment, and even an augmented rituximab-associated antibody-dependent cellular toxicity.[73] Furthermore, in vitro data have also demonstrated that the IMiDs have differential effects on normal and malignant cells, which may provide them with a favorable therapeutic window, and have been shown to stimulate the proliferation of CD34+ cells,[73] an effect that was enhanced when lenalidomide was combined with an HDAC inhibitor (i.e., valproic acid).

Current clinical studies of lenalidomide in non–Hodgkin lymphoma

Lenalidomide is currently approved for the treatment of relapsed multiple myeloma and myelodysplastic syndrome. Promising preclinical data have led to several phase II clinical trials of lenalidomide as a single agent in NHL. All trials have used the standard dose of 25 mg once a day on days 1–21 every 28 days. The most commonly seen toxicities were hematologic, as expected, but the results were very impressive across a broad array of different histologic subtypes of B cell NHL.

Witzig et al.[74] were among the first to report an experience with lenalidomide in lymphoma. They conducted a single-agent phase II study of lenalidomide monotherapy in 43 patients with relapsed or refractory indolent NHL. All patients had failed a median of three prior therapies. Eleven of the 43 patients (26 percent) experienced an objective response with a median time to response of 3.6 months. This included two complete remissions, one complete remission unconfirmed, as well as eight partial remissions. The progression-free survival, an important clinical endpoint in indolent lymphomas, was 7.7 months in responding patients. The study demonstrated that, overall, the lenalidomide had a reasonable level of activity in a diverse population of patients with relapsed indolent lymphoma and was well tolerated, with the most common toxicity being hematologic.

Subsequent to the Mayo Clinic experience, Wiernik and colleagues[75] reported the results of a large multicenter phase II study of lenalidomide in 49 patients with relapsed or refractory aggressive lymphomas, including DLBCL ($n = 26$), follicular lymphoma grade III ($n = 5$), MCL ($n = 15$), and transformed disease ($n = 3$). These patients were also considered to be heavily treated, having received a median of four prior therapies, with more than 60 percent of the patients being characterized as rituximab refractory. Of the original 49 patients, 17 patients experienced an objective response, producing an overall response rate of 35 percent (6 CR and 11 PR). In the largest subgroup of patients, including 26 patients with DLBCL, there were three CR, two PR, and seven patients with stabilization of disease. Interestingly, in a subsequent multivariate analysis, response to lenalidomide was associated with low tumor burden (less than $50\,cm^2$) and being more than 230 days from the last rituximab treatment. Patients with favorable features for both of these factors ($n = 24$) had an overall response rate of 67 percent compared to 4 percent in the alternative subgroup. In addition, patients with the favorable risk features experienced a progression-free survival of 7.4 months compared to only 1.9 months. While the sensitivity to rituximab did not correlate with response to lenalidomide, these data clearly illustrate the many difficulties in developing drugs for the treatment of lymphoma. Table 85.7 provides a summary of the collective experience with lenalidomide in NHL to date.

Combination studies of lenalidomide have been conducted with rituximab. Wang et al.[76] have reported the results of the first phase I/II clinical study of lenalidomide in combination with rituximab for patients with relapsed or refractory MCL. In cohorts of three patients, lenalidomide was dosed from 10 mg to 25 mg, given once daily on days 1–21 of a 28-day cycle, and rituximab was administered at 375 mg/m² weekly for 4 weeks only during the first cycle. The phase I study defined an MTD of 20 mg orally every day in combination with rituximab. The major dose-limiting toxicities included grade 3 hypercalcemia and grade 4 non-neutropenic fever. The MTD has been defined at 20 mg a day. Common adverse events included fatigue, pruritus, myalgia, and rash. Encouraging signs of activity were appreciated in this heavily treated patient population, including in seven out of ten patients who achieved objective responses (three complete remissions and four partial remissions). The study has now been expanded into the phase II arm and is actively accruing patients. The Cancer and Leukemia Group B cooperative group (CALGB) is also conducting a multicenter phase II clinical trial to investigate the combination of bortezomib and lenalidomide (CALGB-50501)(25).

T cell lymphoma

In addition to the dramatic activity seen in B cell lymphoma, there are encouraging data with IMiDs in the treatment of T cell lymphomas, though these experiences are still quite limited to date. Querfeld et al.[77] reported the first ten patients enrolled in a phase II trial of lenalidomide for cutaneous T cell lymphoma. Three of eight patients

Table 85.7 Summary of clinical trials of lenalidomide in lymphoma

Author	Histology	Number of patients (n)	ORR and CR	Duration of response and PFS	Comments/toxicity
Khan and Cheson[100]	CLL	45	ORR 57%, CR 18%	NA	First study to demonstrate activity in CLL
Czuczman et al.[101]	Relapsed/refractory aggressive NHL	46	ORR 40–50%	NA	Response to lenalidomide associated with >230 days from last rituximab treatment and tumor burden <50 cm²; hematologic toxicity
Ferrajoli et al.[102]	CLL	44	ORR 32%	NA	NA
Lossos et al.[103]	Relapsed/refractory DLBCL	26	ORR 19%	Median PFS 3 months	Response best if >230 days from last rituximab and tumor burden <50 cm²; hematologic toxicity
Tuscano et al.[104]	Relapsed/refractory mantle cell lymphoma	15	ORR 53%	NA	Response best if >230 days from last rituximab and tumor burden <50 cm²; hematologic toxicity
Vose et al.[105]	Relapsed and refractory NHL with prior stem cell transplant	14	ORR 50%	Response seen up to 11 months in 2 patients	Hematologic toxicity
Wiernik et al.[75]	Relapsed/refractory aggressive NHL	49	ORR 35%	Median duration of response 6.2 months	Response to lenalidomide associated with >230 days from last rituximab treatment and tumor burden <50 cm²; hematologic toxicity
Witzig et al.[74]	Relapsed/refractory indolent NHL	43	ORR 26%, FCC 32%, SLL 22%	Ongoing at >10 months	Hematologic toxicity and thrombocytopenia

ORR, overall response rate; CR, complete remission; PFS, progression-free survival; CLL, chronic lymphocytic leukemia; NA, not assessed; NHL, non-Hodgkin lymphoma; DLBCL, diffuse large B cell lymphoma; FCC, follicular center cell lymphoma; SLL, small lymphocytic lymphoma.

who were evaluable for response demonstrated objective responses while four patients achieved a minor response, including improvement in skin-based disease and regression of lymphoadenopathy (26). A phase II trial of lenalidomide in peripheral T cell lymphoma was reported by Reiman et al.[78] Again, though early data, four of ten patients treated experienced a major response. Similar to the B cell lymphomas, the biological heterogeneity of the T cell lymphomas raises the potentially challenging situation where drugs like lenalidomide may exhibit very restricted patterns of activity across the diversity of disease defining T cell lymphoma. Clearly, over time, our experience with lenalidomide will need to establish its activity in the many subtypes of T cell lymphoma, even the very rare ones, and will need to define how best to integrate this agent into the present standards of care.

Adverse effects profile of the immunomodulatory agents

While generally considered to be a well-tolerated drug, lenalidomide is associated with a number of unique toxicities. Myelosuppression[79] is a major side effect of lenalidomide and has been seen in almost all trials in lymphoma(17)(21)(22)(24). Nonhematologic toxicities including fatigue, pruritus, and rash have also been noted, but in contrast to thalidomide, the incidence of somnolence, constipation, and neuropathy appears to be significantly less frequent. Deep vein thrombosis is rarely reported in trials where lenalidomide is used as a monotherapy. Palumbo et al.[80] reported that lenalidomide alone does not induce a high risk of venous thromboembolism and thromboprophylaxis is not suggested when it is used as a single agent in multiple myeloma therapy.(29) However, in one MCL study, Tuscano et al. reported grade 4 thromboembolism which occurred in 13 percent of evaluable patients receiving lenalidomide monotherapy (23). Moreover, when lenalidomide was combined with dexamethasone, the incidence of venous thromboembolism became higher in myeloma directed trials. As a result, the FDA recommends prophylactic anticoagulation during lenalidomide treatment.

Future directions

Although lenalidomide has made a major impact in the treatment of patients with lymphoma so far, clinical experiences are still limited, and additional trials to evaluate the applicability of this agent to other lymphoproliferative malignancies need to be performed. Lenalidomide's unique pharmacologic properties could make it an attractive compound to incorporate in combination regimens with other drugs. In addition to bortezomib and rituximab, which have already been studied in clinical trials, several additional compounds have emerged as potentially complementary agents to lenalidomide. The HDAC inhibitor valproic acid appears to synergize with lenalidomide in lymphoma cell line panels in vitro.(14) Galiximab, an anti-CD80 monoclonal antibody,[71] has also demonstrated antilymphoma activity with lenalidomide in a synergistic manner in vivo. Moreover, in myeloma cell line panels, lenalidomide has synergized with rapamycin[81] (an mTOR inhibitor) and enzastaurin,[82] a protein kinase $C\beta$ inhibitor. As these compounds are known to be effective in lymphoma, further combination studies are planned, which will hopefully lead to promising therapies for the lymphoproliferative malignancies.

MULTIFUNCTIONAL ALKYLATING AGENTS: BENDAMUSTINE

Bendamustine (4-5-[bis(2-chloroethyl)amino]-1-methyl-2-benzimidazole butyric acid hydrochloride) is designed to possess the properties of both a purine analogue and an alkylating agent.[83,84] Bendamustine has demonstrated significant clinical activity in many human cancers including NHL, chronic lymphocytic leukemia (CLL), multiple myeloma, breast cancer, and small cell lung cancer. The drug was recently approved (in March 2008) in the United States for the treatment of chronic lymphocytic leukemia.[85]

Bendamustine was originally developed in East Germany in the 1960s from a nitrogen mustard backbone.[86] The drug has significant DNA alkylating effects and produces an active metabolite. Interestingly, unlike most other predominantly alkylating-type drugs, bendamustine exhibits activity in cell lines that are refractory to more conventional alkylating agents. Structurally, it contains three basic features: a 2-chloroethylamine alkylating group shared by other alkylators; a butyric acid side chain shared by chlorambucil; and a benzimidazole ring that gives the drug its unique antimetabolite properties similar to purine analogues. The drug has been marketed and used as a single agent in Germany for many years in patients with NHL, CLL, multiple myeloma, breast cancer, and other solid tumors such as lung cancer.

The mechanism of action of bendamustine is thought to involve two distinct pathways: induction of apoptosis and mitotic catastrophe. The alkylating properties of the drug result in crosslinkage of both single and double strands of DNA resulting in strand breakage, which appears more extensive and less amenable to DNA repair than that induced by other alkylating agents. Leoni et al.[87] demonstrated that bendamustine resulted in the initiation of the TP53-dependent stress pathway and activation of the intrinsic apoptotic pathways. Again, this effect was stronger and more rapid compared to equitoxic doses of chlorambucil. In addition, bendamustine exposure resulted in inhibition of several mitotic checkpoints, allowing cells to enter mitosis with extensive DNA damage. The accumulation of DNA damage and loss of checkpoint control led to the initiation of a unique form of cell death referred to as mitotic catastrophe. This particular cellular process occurs during metaphase and is distinct from apoptosis. Mitotic checkpoints are designed to halt the cell cycle if there is DNA damage to allow DNA repair mechanisms to be activated, preempting the accumulation of damaged DNA. If cells continue to proceed through mitosis with extensive DNA damage, then mitotic catastrophe results. The hallmark of this event is chromatin condensation with multinucleation and micronucleation in cells. This alternative mechanism of cell death is thought to distinguish this agent from other alkylating agents, and is felt to potentially explain the efficacy of bendamustine in tumor cells that have become resistant to apoptosis following preexposure to conventional alkylating agents. In addition, the activity of bendamustine appears to be enhanced by the inhibition of base excision repair mechanisms indicating that it may rely on this pathway for its activity. While these insights into the potential mechanistic differences between bendamustine and other alkylating agents is intriguing, it is also clear that there are many unanswered questions regarding the drug's significant activity across a broad panoply of different NHL subtypes and precisely how it evades the cross-resistance with other conventional alkylating agents.

Clinical activity – chronic lymphocytic leukemia

The pivotal study that led to the FDA approval of bendamustine in the United States was reported in late 2007. Knauf et al.[88] presented the results of a multicenter phase III clinical trial performed in patients with CLL, Rai stage I–IV. Patients were randomized between two arms: (1) bendamustine administered at a dose of $100 \, \text{mg/m}^2$ on days 1 and 2, or (2) chlorambucil at standard dosing. In total, 305 patients were treated on the study, which demonstrated a clear advantage in overall response (68 percent vs 39 percent) and progression-free survival (21.7 months vs 9.3 months) for bendamustine compared to chlorambucil. The most common side effects were hematologic toxicity, nausea, fatigue, and diarrhea.

Non–Hodgkin lymphomas

Based on the promising data from Germany,[89] and the pivotal study in CLL, a number of investigators have begun exploring the activity of bendamustine in other subtypes of NHL and in combination therapy. Rummel et al.[90] reported on the efficacy of the combination of bendamustine and rituximab in patients with indolent and mantle cell lymphoma who had relapsed or were refractory to the previous therapy, including rituximab. This study used a dosing schedule of $90 \, \text{mg/m}^2$ of bendamustine on days 1 and 2 and rituximab at a dose of $375 \, \text{mg/m}^2$ weekly for 4 weeks. The overall response rate was 90 percent with a CR rate of 60 percent, while the median progression-free

survival was 24 months. In 16 patients with MCL, this combination showed a response rate of 75 percent with a CR rate of 50 percent.

More recently, a multicenter US and Canadian trial published by Friedberg et al.[91] evaluated bendamustine as a single agent in 67 patients with indolent or mantle cell lymphoma who had failed prior chemotherapy. Thirty-seven percent of these patients had also failed rituximab. In this study, the dose of bendamustine was $120 \, \text{mg/m}^2$ given on days 1 and 2 and given every 3 weeks. The results were promising, revealing an overall response rate of 77 percent with 34 percent complete responses. The median duration of response was 6.7 months with 36 percent of these responses lasting more than a year.

In an effort to see if bendamustine could substitute for other conventional alkylating agents in more traditional lymphoma regimens, the German group conducted a randomized trial comparing BOP[92] (bendamustine, oncovin, and prednisone) to COP (cyclophosphamide, oncovin, and prednisone) in 164 patients with indolent NHL or MCL. While the toxicities and overall response rates were similar in both regimens, the 5-year survival was superior in those patients receiving BOP (61 percent) compared to COP (46 percent). Toxicity was acceptable in both study arms.

Conclusion and future directions

Bendamustine has been shown to have activity in B cell lymphomas and is currently in several clinical trials, mostly in combination[93,94] with other cytotoxic agents and as a replacement for cyclophosphamide both for standard-dose and high-dose chemotherapy in the setting of stem cell transplantation. As a conditioning agent it remains particularly attractive for low-grade lymphomas that utilize nucleoside analogues as a therapeutic modality.

NOVEL ANTIFOL DERIVATIVES: PRALATREXATE

While at first new derivatives of old drugs may not seem like the most exciting of new developments in the treatment of cancer, occasionally one of those new derivatives displays a pattern of activity that is not only unqiue, but dramatic. Antifols have been the cornerstone of many historical lymphoma treatment paradigms, and still to this day are major components of many regimens used for the treatment of lymphoma. For example, high-dose methotrexate treatment protocols remain one of the most commonly employed approaches for the treatment of primary central nervous system (CNS) lymphoma and even CNS relapses. Methotrexate is also used commonly in many acute lymphoblastic leukemia (ALL) treatment protocols where it is used as a maintenance therapy. This includes a regimen known as hyper-CVAD, which has now become a commonly used treatment of MCL. The interposition of methotrexate and cytarabine following cytoreduction with a fractionated cyclophosphamide regimen appeals to our knowledge of tumor growth kinetics. And, of course, methotrexate remains one of our most important intrathecal agents for patients with CNS involvement.

Pralatrexate, a propargyl aminopterin designed after methotrexate, was not designed to be a better substrate for dihydrofolate reductase, the target of methotrexate, but to be a high-affinity substrate for the reduced folate carrier (RFC).[95–97] The rationale for the drug revolves around the fact that RFC is recognized as an oncofetal protein known to be highly expressed on highly proliferating tissues, such as those found in embryonic and malignant tissues. This biology gives the drug a potentially valuable therapeutic window. The second rationale revolves around the fact that targeting a transporter found on malignant tissue would result in significant bioaccumulation of the drug in tumor cells, potentially overcoming other well-known determinants of antifol activity.

Early clinical trials demonstrated that pralatrexate produced significant mucositis, which was related to high area-under-the-curve exposures and poor nutritional states, as reflected by marked elevations in homocysteine and methylmalonic acid.[98] Correction of the nutritional state with vitamin B12 and folic acid repletion and conversion to low-dose weekly schedules markedly shifted the mucositis risk from predominantly high grade 3–4 to essentially grade 0–1. Subsequent phase II studies in patients with lymphoma revealed marked activity in patients with T cell lymphomas, with the overwhelming number of patients achieving durable complete remissions. In fact, the overall response rate in the entire 42 patient population was 28 percent, but when analyzed by lineage, the ORR in B cell lymphomas was 10 percent and in T cell lymphomas 54 percent, with the majority of these responses (nine out of ten) actually being either complete remissions or negative on positron emission tomography (PET) scan. Even more encouraging were the durations of response. Most responding patients in fact had disease refractory to their prior line of chemotherapy, and achieved durable remission in the range of 3 to 26 months. In almost all these cases, the response to pralatrexate exceeded the response to the line of therapy prior to study enrolment.[98]

Based on preclinical data demonstrating a synergistic interaction between pralatrexate and gemcitabine, subsequent combination phase I studies have been launched.[99] While it is too early to comment on the results of these trials, there is a very clear intent among physicians familiar with T cell lymphoma to think about new, non-CHOP-based chemotherapy approaches for the upfront treatment of T cell lymphoma. To date, the standard regimens for treating these diseases have been primarily CHOP based, a regimen largely established for the treatment of B cell lymphomas. Presently, the emergence of a plethora of new drugs with clear-cut activity in T cell lymphoma, including agents like the HDAC inhibitors, gemcitabine, clofarabine, pralatrexate, bortezomib, and new monoclonal antibodies directed against T cell antigens, has raised the expectation that improving outcomes for patients with T cell lymphoma may not be that far off into the future. Clearly, identifying and understanding the many new classes of agents with more T cell-centric activity could pave the way for more effective upfront treatment programs, which should be a major priority for this disease.

KEY POINTS

- There are several new classes of agents currently available for treating lymphoid neoplasms.
- The new therapeutic agents target specific pathogenic pathways thus differentiating them from conventional chemotherapy agents.
- The most promising agents to date consist of proteosome inhibitors, HDAC inhibitors, the novel antifolate Pralaltrexate and the IMIDS.
- Rational combinations of these agents based on sound preclinical work and biological correlates of activity are likely to be the basis of future therapies.

REFERENCES

● = Key primary paper
◆ = Major review article

1. Harris NL, Jaffe ES, Diebold J et al. The World Health Organization classification of neoplastic diseases of the hematopoietic and lymphoid tissues. Report of the Clinical Advisory Committee meeting, Airlie House, Virginia, November, 1997. Ann Oncol 1999; 10: 1419.

2. Alizadeh AA, Eisen MB, Davis RE et al. Distinct types of diffuse large B-cell lymphoma identified by gene expression profiling. Nature 2000; 403: 503.

3. Shipp MA, Ross KN, Tamayo P et al. Diffuse large B-cell lymphoma outcome prediction by gene-expression profiling and supervised machine learning. Nat Med 2002; 8: 68.

4. Chen L, Monti S, Juszczynski P et al. SYK-dependent tonic B-cell receptor signaling is a rational treatment target in diffuse large B-cell lymphoma. Blood 2008; 111: 2230.

5. Fisher RI, Gaynor ER, Dahlberg S et al. Comparison of a standard regimen (CHOP) with three intensive chemotherapy regimens for advanced non-Hodgkin's lymphoma. N Engl J Med 1993; 328: 1002.

6. Somers R, Carde P, Henry-Amar M *et al.* A randomized study in stage IIIB and IV Hodgkin's disease comparing eight courses of MOPP versus an alteration of MOPP with ABVD: a European Organization for Research and Treatment of Cancer Lymphoma Cooperative Group and Groupe Pierre-et-Marie-Curie controlled clinical trial. *J Clin Oncol* 1994; **12**: 279.

7. Coiffier B, Lepage E, Briere J *et al.* CHOP chemotherapy plus rituximab compared with CHOP alone in elderly patients with diffuse large-B-cell lymphoma. *N Engl J Med* 2002; **346**: 235.

8. Paoluzzi L, O'Connor OA. Mechanistic rationale and clinical evidence for the efficacy of proteasome inhibitors against indolent and mantle cell lymphomas. *BioDrugs* 2006; **20**: 13.

9. O'Connor OA, Wright J, Moskowitz C *et al.* Phase II clinical experience with the novel proteasome inhibitor bortezomib in patients with indolent non-Hodgkin's lymphoma and mantle cell lymphoma. *J Clin Oncol* 2005; **23**: 676.

10. Pagano M, Tam SW, Theodoras AM *et al.* Role of the ubiquitin-proteasome pathway in regulating abundance of the cyclin-dependent kinase inhibitor p27. *Science* 1995; **269**: 682.

11. Blagosklonny MV, Wu GS, Omura S *et al.* Proteasome-dependent regulation of p21WAF1/CIP1 expression. *Biochem Biophys Res Commun* 1996; **227**: 564.

12. King RW, Deshaies RJ, Peters JM *et al.* How proteolysis drives the cell cycle. *Science* 1996; **274**: 1652.

13. Machiels BM, Henfling ME, Gerards WL *et al.* Detailed analysis of cell cycle kinetics upon proteasome inhibition. *Cytometry* 1997; **28**: 243.

14. Ling YH, Liebes L, Jiang JD *et al.* Mechanisms of proteasome inhibitor PS-341-induced G(2)-M-phase arrest and apoptosis in human non-small cell lung cancer cell lines. *Clin Cancer Res* 2003; **9**: 1145.

15. Marshansky V, Wang X, Bertrand R *et al.* Proteasomes modulate balance among proapoptotic and antiapoptotic Bcl-2 family members and compromise functioning of the electron transport chain in leukemic cells. *J Immunol* 2001; **166**: 3130.

16. Ling YH, Liebes L, Ng B *et al.* PS-341, a novel proteasome inhibitor, induces Bcl-2 phosphorylation and cleavage in association with G2-M phase arrest and apoptosis. *Mol Cancer Ther* 2002; **1**: 841.

17. Perez-Soler R, Kemp B, Wu QP *et al.* Response and determinants of sensitivity to paclitaxel in human non-small cell lung cancer tumors heterotransplanted in nude mice. *Clin Cancer Res* 2000; **6**: 4932-8.

18. Palombella VJ, Conner EM, Fuseler JW *et al.* Role of the proteasome and NF-kappaB in streptococcal cell wall-induced polyarthritis. *Proc Natl Acad Sci U S A* 1998; **95**: 15671.

19. Bellas RE, FitzGerald MJ, Fausto N *et al.* Inhibition of NF-kappa B activity induces apoptosis in murine hepatocytes. *Am J Pathol* 1997; **151**: 891.

20. Baldwin AS Jr. The NF-kappa B and I kappa B proteins: new discoveries and insights. *Annu Rev Immunol* 1996; **14**: 649.

21. Thanos D, Maniatis T. NF-kappa B: a lesson in family values. *Cell* 1995; **80**: 529.

22. Grilli M, Chiu JJ, Lenardo MJ. NF-kappa B and Rel: participants in a multiform transcriptional regulatory system. *Int Rev Cytol* 1993; **143**: 1.

23. Baeuerle PA, Baltimore D. NF-kappa B: ten years after. *Cell* 1996; **87**: 13.

24. Beg AA, Baltimore D. An essential role for NF-kappaB in preventing TNF-alpha-induced cell death. *Science* 1996; **274**: 782.

25. Orlowski RZ, Stinchcombe TE, Mitchell BS *et al.* Phase I trial of the proteasome inhibitor PS-341 in patients with refractory hematologic malignancies. *J Clin Oncol* 2002; **20**: 4420.

26. Richardson PG, Barlogie B, Berenson J *et al.* A phase 2 study of bortezomib in relapsed, refractory myeloma. *N Engl J Med* 2003; **348**: 2609.

27. Fisher RI, Bernstein SH, Kahl BS *et al.* Multicenter phase II study of bortezomib in patients with relapsed or refractory mantle cell lymphoma. *J Clin Oncol* 2006; **24**: 4867.

28. Goy A, Younes A, McLaughlin P *et al.* Phase II study of proteasome inhibitor bortezomib in relapsed or refractory B-cell non-Hodgkin's lymphoma. *J Clin Oncol* 2005; **23**: 667.

29. Strauss SJ, Maharaj L, Hoare S *et al.* Bortezomib therapy in patients with relapsed or refractory lymphoma: potential correlation of in vitro sensitivity and tumor necrosis factor alpha response with clinical activity. *J Clin Oncol* 2006; **24**: 2105.

30. Belch A, Kouroukis T, Crump M *et al.* Phase II Trial of Bortezomib in Mantle Cell Lymphoma. *Blood* 2004; **104**: Abstract 608.

31. O'Connor OA, Portlock C, Moskowitz C *et al.* A multicentre phase II clinical experience with the novel aza-epothilone Ixabepilone (BMS247550) in patients with relapsed or refractory indolent non-Hodgkin lymphoma and mantle cell lymphoma. *Br J Haematol* 2008; **143**: 201–9.

32. Gerecitano J, Portlock C, Hamlin *et al. Annals of Oncology* 2008; **19**: Abstract 443.

33. Kuhn DJ, Chen Q, Voorhees PM *et al.* Potent activity of carfilzomib, a novel, irreversible inhibitor of the ubiquitin-proteasome pathway, against preclinical models of multiple myeloma. *Blood* 2007; **110**: 3281.

34. Chauhan D, Singh A, Brahmandam M *et al.* Combination of proteasome inhibitors bortezomib and NPI-0052 trigger in vivo synergistic cytotoxicity in multiple myeloma. *Blood* 2008; **111**: 1654.

35. Xu WS, Parmigiani RB, Marks PA. Histone deacetylase inhibitors: molecular mechanisms of action. *Oncogene* 2007; **26**: 5541.

36. Kruszewski M, Szumiel I. Sirtuins (histone deacetylases III) in the cellular response to DNA damage—facts and hypotheses. *DNA Repair (Amst)* 2005; **4**: 1306.

37. O'Connor OA. *Oncology* (2006).

38. Oki Y, Aoki E, Issa JP. Decitabine—bedside to bench. *Crit Rev Oncol Hematol* 2007; **61**: 140.

39. Marks PA, Dokmanovic M. Histone deacetylase inhibitors: discovery and development as anticancer agents. *Expert Opin Investig Drugs* 2005; **14**: 1497.

40. Roelfsema JH, Peters DJ. Rubinstein-Taybi syndrome: clinical and molecular overview. *Expert Rev Mol Med* 2007; **9**: 1.

41. Sykes SM, Mellert HS, Holbert MA et al. *Mol Cell* 2006; **24**: 841.

42. Tyteca S, Legube G, Trouche D. *Mol Cell* 2006; **24**: 807.

43. Gorrini C, Squatrito M, Luise C et al. Tip60 is a haplo-insufficient tumour suppressor required for an oncogene-induced DNA damage response. *Nature* 2007; **448**: 1063.

44. Ropero S, Fraga MF, Ballestar E et al. A truncating mutation of HDAC2 in human cancers confers resistance to histone deacetylase inhibition. *Nat Genet* 2006; **38**: 566.

45. Fax P, Lehmkuhler O, Kuhn C et al. E1A12S-mediated activation of the adenovirus type 12 E2 promoter depends on the histone acetyltransferase activity of p300/CBP. *J Biol Chem* 2000; **275**: 40554.

46. Deng L, Wang D, de la Fuente C et al. Enhancement of the p300 HAT activity by HIV-1 Tat on chromatin DNA. *Virology* 2001; **289**: 312.

47. Marks PA, Richon VM, Rifkind RA. Histone deacetylase inhibitors: inducers of differentiation or apoptosis of transformed cells. *J Natl Cancer Inst* 2000; **92**: 1210.

48. Butler LM, Agus DB, Scher HI et al. Suberoylanilide hydroxamic acid, an inhibitor of histone deacetylase, suppresses the growth of prostate cancer cells in vitro and in vivo. *Cancer Res* 2000; **60**: 5165.

49. Richon VM, Webb Y, Merger R et al. Second generation hybrid polar compounds are potent inducers of transformed cell differentiation. *Proc Natl Acad Sci U S A* 1996; **93**: 5705.

50. Kelly WK, O'Connor OA, Krug LM et al. Phase I study of an oral histone deacetylase inhibitor, suberoylanilide hydroxamic acid, in patients with advanced cancer. *J Clin Oncol* 2005; **23**: 3923.

51. Duvic M, Talpur R, Ni X et al. Phase 2 trial of oral vorinostat (suberoylanilide hydroxamic acid, SAHA) for refractory cutaneous T-cell lymphoma (CTCL). *Blood* 2007; **109**: 31.

52. Olsen EA, Kim YH, Kuzel TM et al. Phase IIb multicenter trial of vorinostat in patients with persistent, progressive, or treatment refractory cutaneous T-cell lymphoma. *J Clin Oncol* 2007; **25**: 3109.

53. Kirschbaum MH, Stein AS, Tuscano J et al. A Phase I Study of the Farnesyltransferase Inhibitor Tipifarnib in a Week-On Week-Off Dose Schedule in Acute Myelogenous Leukemia. *Blood* 2007; **110**: Abstract 891.

54. Zain J, Rotter A, Weiss L et al. Valproic acid monotherapy leads to CR in a patient with refractory diffuse large B cell lymphoma. *Leuk Lymphoma* 2007; **48**: 1216.

55. Soriano AO, Yang H, Faderl S et al. Safety and clinical activity of the combination of 5-azacytidine, valproic acid, and all-trans retinoic acid in acute myeloid leukemia and myelodysplastic syndrome. *Blood* 2007; **110**: 2302.

56. Ueda H, Nakajima H, Hori Y et al. Action of FR901228, a novel antitumor bicyclic depsipeptide produced by Chromobacterium violaceum no. 968, on Ha-ras transformed NIH3T3 cells. *Biosci Biotechnol Biochem* 1994; **58**: 1579.

57. Piekarz RL, Robey R, Sandor V et al. Inhibitor of histone deacetylation, depsipeptide (FR901228), in the treatment of peripheral and cutaneous T-cell lymphoma: a case report. *Blood* 2001; **98**: 2865.

58. Sandor V, Bakke S, Robey RW et al. Phase I trial of the histone deacetylase inhibitor, depsipeptide (FR901228, NSC 630176), in patients with refractory neoplasms. *Clin Cancer Res* 2002; **8**: 718.

59. Piekarz RL, Robey RW, Zhan Z et al. T-cell lymphoma as a model for the use of histone deacetylase inhibitors in cancer therapy: impact of depsipeptide on molecular markers, therapeutic targets, and mechanisms of resistance. *Blood* 2004; **103**: 4636.

60. Kim YH, Reddy S, Kim EJ et al. *Blood* 2007; **110**: Abstract 123.

61. Bartlett JB, Dredge K, Dalgleish AG. The evolution of thalidomide and its IMiD derivatives as anticancer agents. *Nat Rev Cancer* 2004; **4**: 314.

62. Marriott JB, Muller G, Dalgleish AG. Thalidomide as an emerging immunotherapeutic agent. *Immunol Today* 1999; **20**: 538.

63. Sheskin J. Thalidomide in the treatment of lepra reactions. *Clin Pharmacol Ther* 1965; **6**: 303.

64. Singhal S, Mehta J, Desikan R et al. Antitumor activity of thalidomide in refractory multiple myeloma. *N Engl J Med* 1999; **341**: 1565.

65. Atra E, Sato EI. Treatment of the cutaneous lesions of systemic lupus erythematosus with thalidomide. *Clin Exp Rheumatol* 1993; **11**: 487.

66. Eisen T, Boshoff C, Mak I et al. Continuous low dose Thalidomide: a phase II study in advanced melanoma, renal cell, ovarian and breast cancer. *Br J Cancer* 2000; **82**: 812.

67. Macpherson GR, Franks M, Tomoaia-Cotisel A et al. Current status of thalidomide and its role in the treatment of metastatic prostate cancer. *Crit Rev Oncol Hematol* 2003; **46**(Suppl): S49.

68. Crane E, List A. Immunomodulatory drugs. *Cancer Invest* 2005; **23**: 625.

69. Verhelle D, Corral LG, Wong K et al. Lenalidomide and CC-4047 inhibit the proliferation of malignant B cells while expanding normal CD34+ progenitor cells. *Cancer Res* 2007; **67**: 746.

70. Lentzsch S, LeBlanc R, Podar K et al. Immunomodulatory analogs of thalidomide inhibit growth of Hs Sultan cells and angiogenesis in vivo. *Leukemia* 2003; **17**: 41.

71. Reddy N, Hernandez-Ilizaliturri FJ, Knight J, Myron CS. Lenalidomide enhances the biological activity of galiximab against non-Hogkin's lymphoma *in vitro* and *in vivo*. (Intr. by Myron S. Czuczman), *Blood* 2007; **110**: Abstract 2353.

72. Hernandez-Ilizaliturri FJ, Reddy N, Holkova B et al. Immunomodulatory drug CC-5013 or CC-4047 and rituximab enhance antitumor activity in a severe combined

immunodeficient mouse lymphoma model. *Clin Cancer Res* 2005; **11**: 5984.

73. Reddy N, Hernandez-Ilizaliturri FJ, Deeb G *et al.* Immunomodulatory drugs stimulate natural killer-cell function, alter cytokine production by dendritic cells, and inhibit angiogenesis enhancing the anti-tumour activity of rituximab in vivo. *Br J Haematol* 2008; **140**: 36.

74. Witzig TE, Reeder CB, Polikoff J *et al.* Initial Results from an International Study in Relapsed/Refractory Aggressive Non-Hodgkin's Lymphoma To Confirm the Activity, Safety and Criteria for Predicting Response to Lenalidomide Monotherapy. *Blood* 2007; **110**: Abstract 2572.

75. Wiernik PH, Lossos IS, Tuscano JM *et al.* Lenalidomide Response in Relapsed/Refractory Aggressive Non-Hodgkin's Lymphoma is Related to Tumor Burden and Time from Rituximab Treatment. *Blood* 2007; **110**: Abstract 2565.

76. Wang M, Fayad L, Hagemeister F, *et al.* Lenalidomide (Len) in Combination with Rituximab (R) Demonstrated Early Evidence of Efficacy in a Phase I/II Study in Relapsed/Refractory Mantle Cell Lymphoma (MCL). *Blood* (ASH Annual Meeting Abstracts) 2007; **110**: 2562.

77. Querfeld C, Kuzel TM, Guitart J, Rosen ST. Preliminary Results of a Phase II Study of CC-5013 (Lenalidomide, Revlimid®) in Patients with Cutaneous T-Cell Lymphoma. *Blood* (ASH Annual Meeting Abstracts) 2005; **106**: 3351.

78. Reiman T, Finch D, Chua N *et al.* First Report of a Phase II Clinical Trial of Lenalidomide Oral Therapy for Peripheral T-Cell Lymphoma. *Blood* (ASH Annual Meeting Abstracts); 2007; **110**: 2579.

79. Richardson PG, Schlossman RL, Weller E *et al.* Immunomodulatory drug CC-5013 overcomes drug resistance and is well tolerated in patients with relapsed multiple myeloma. *Blood* 2002; **100**: 3063.

80. Palumbo A, Rajkumar SV, Dimopoulos MA *et al.* Prevention of thalidomide- and lenalidomide-associated thrombosis in myeloma. *Leukemia* 2008; **22**: 414.

81. Chumsri S, Zhao M, Garofalo M *et al.* Inhibition of the mammalian target of rapamycin (mTOR) in a case of refractory primary cutaneous anaplastic large cell lymphoma. *Leuk Lymphoma* 2008; **49**: 359.

82. Morschhauser F, Seymour JF, Kluin-Nelemans HC *et al.* A phase II study of enzastaurin, a protein kinase C beta inhibitor, in patients with relapsed or refractory mantle cell lymphoma. *Ann Oncol* 2008; **19**: 247.

83. Apostolopoulos C, Castellano L, Stebbing J, Giamas G. Bendamustine as a model for the activity of alkylating agents. *Future Oncol* 2008; **4**: 323.

84. Keating MJ, Bach C, Yasothan U, Kirkpatrik P. Bendamustine. *Nat Rev Drug Discov* 2008; **7**: 473.

85. Traynor K. Treanda approved for chronic lymphocytic leukemia. *Am J Health Syst Pharm* 2008; **65**: 793.

86. Forero-Torres A, Saleh MN. Bendamustine in non-Hodgkin lymphoma: the double-agent that came from the Cold War. *Clin Lymphoma Myeloma* 2007; **8**(Suppl 1): S13.

87. Leoni LM, Bailey B, Reifert J *et al.* Bendamustine (Treanda) displays a distinct pattern of cytotoxicity and unique

88. mechanistic features compared with other alkylating agents. *Clin Cancer Res* 2008; **14**: 309.

89. Knauf W, Lissichkov T, Aldaoud A *et al.* Bendamustine Versus Chlorambucil in Treatment-Naive Patients with B-Cell Chronic Lymphocytic Leukemia (B-CLL): Results of an International Phase III Study. *Blood* (ASH Annual Meeting Abstracts); 2007; **110**: 2043.

89. Bergmann MA, Goebeler ME, Herold M *et al.* Efficacy of bendamustine in patients with relapsed or refractory chronic lymphocytic leukemia: results of a phase I/II study of the German CLL Study Group. *Haematologica* 2005; **90**: 1357.

90. Rummel MJ, Al-Batran SE, Kim SZ *et al.* Bendamustine plus rituximab is effective and has a favorable toxicity profile in the treatment of mantle cell and low-grade non-Hodgkin's lymphoma. *J Clin Oncol* 2005; **23**: 3383.

91. Friedberg JW, Cohen P, Chen L *et al.* Bendamustine in patients with rituximab-refractory indolent and transformed non-Hodgkin's lymphoma: results from a phase II multicenter, single-agent study. *J Clin Oncol* 2008; **26**: 204.

92. Herold M, Schulze A, Niederwieser D *et al.* Bendamustine, vincristine and prednisone (BOP) versus cyclophosphamide, vincristine and prednisone (COP) in advanced indolent non-Hodgkin's lymphoma and mantle cell lymphoma: results of a randomised phase III trial (OSHO# 19). *J Cancer Res Clin Oncol* 2006; **132**: 105.

93. Bertoni F, Zucca E. Bendamustine in lymphomas: more to combine? *Leuk Lymphoma* 2007; **48**: 1264.

94. Weide R, Hess G, Koppler H *et al.* High anti-lymphoma activity of bendamustine/mitoxantrone/rituximab in rituximab pretreated relapsed or refractory indolent lymphomas and mantle cell lymphomas. A multicenter phase II study of the German Low Grade Lymphoma Study Group (GLSG). *Leuk Lymphoma* 2007; **48**: 1299.

95. Schmid FA, Sirotnak FM, Otter GM, Degraw JI. New folate analogs of the 10-deaza-aminopterin series: markedly increased antitumor activity of the 10-ethyl analog compared to the parent compound and methotrexate against some human tumor xenografts in nude mice. *Cancer Treat Rep* 1985; **69**: 551.

96. Sirotnak FM, DeGraw JI, Moccio DM *et al.* New folate analogs of the 10-deaza-aminopterin series. Basis for structural design and biochemical and pharmacologic properties. *Cancer Chemother Pharmacol* 1984; **12**: 18.

97. Sirotnak FM, DeGraw JI, Schmid FA *et al.* New folate analogs of the 10-deaza-aminopterin series. Further evidence for markedly increased antitumor efficacy compared with methotrexate in ascitic and solid murine tumor models. *Cancer Chemother Pharmacol* 1984; **12**: 26.

98. O'Connor OA, Hamlin P, Moskowitz C *et al.* Pralatrexate (pdx) produces a high and durable complete response rate in patients with chemotherapy resistant t-cell lymphomas. *Annals of Oncology* 2008; **19** (Suppl 4): Abstract 138.

99. Toner LE, Vrhovac R, Smith EA *et al.* The schedule-dependent effects of the novel antifolate pralatrexate and gemcitabine are superior to methotrexate and cytarabine

in models of human non-Hodgkin's lymphoma. *Clin Cancer Res* 2006; **12**: 924.

100. Khan C, Cheson B. Lenalidomide for the treatment of B cell malignanices. *J Clin Oncol* 2008; **26**: 1544.

101. Czuczman M *et al. Blood* 2007; **110**: [Abstract 2572]

102. Ferrajoli A, O'Brien S. Therapy with lenalidomide in patients with chronic lymphocytic leukemia. *Leuk Lymphoma* 2007; **48**: 160.

103. Lossos IS, Wiernik PH, Justice G. Lenalidomide response in relapsed/refractory diffuse large B-cell non-Hodgkin's lymphoma. *Blood* (ASH Annual Meeting Abstracts) 2007; **110**: 2564.

104. Tuscano JM, Lossos IS, Justice G. Lenalidomide oral monotherapy produces a 53 percent response rate in patients with relapsed/refractory mantle-cell non-Hodgkin's lymphoma. *Blood* (ASH Annual Meeting Abstracts) 2007; **110**: 2563.

105. Vose JM, Tuscano JM, Justice G. High response rate to lenalidomide in relapsed/refractory aggressive non-Hodgkin's lymphoma with prior stem cell transplant. *Blood* (ASH Annual Meeting Abstracts) 2007; **110**: 2570.

106. Stirling D. Thalidomide: a novel template for anticancer drugs. *Semin Oncol* 2001; **28**: 602.

86

Monoclonal antibody therapy for lymphomas and leukemias

PUJA SAPRA, ZHENGXING QU AND IVAN D HORAK

Excellent target specificity and a favorable safety profile have been major underpinnings behind over three decades of intensive effort to add immunotherapy and radioimmunotherapy (RIT), novel treatments, to the cancer armamentarium. Since the introduction of the first therapeutic mouse-derived antibody in 1986, there have been major advances in the understanding of mechanism of action and safety profile of monoclonal antibodies (mAbs). In the first advancement, 'chimerization' and 'humanization' have improved safety profiles and efficacy. Development of commercial production made the antibody a serious contender in the therapeutic arena. Monoclonal antibodies, either in their native form or conjugated to therapeutic agents, have wide utilities in managing lymphoid malignancies largely because these agents have favorable pharmacokinetics (PK) in humans, are often very specific to certain cell types, and have an excellent safety profile that permits combination with a broad range of chemotherapeutics to suit various clinical settings.

Until the early 1990s, treatment options for patients with lymphoid neoplasms were limited to cytotoxic agents and radiation therapy. The effectiveness of anticancer agents (drugs or radioisotopes) is limited by toxicities to normal cells because they indiscriminately kill malignant proliferating cells as well as normal tissue cells. Monoclonal antibodies that recognize specific markers on the surface of tumor cells can be conjugated with drugs, prodrugs, or radioisotopes, and offer an effective modality that is tumor specific and thus less toxic. For example, iodine-131 (^{131}I)-labeled tositumomab (Bexxar®) and yttrium-90-labeled ibritumomab tiuxetan (Zevaline®), both radioimmunoconjugates directed against CD20, exhibit significant antitumor activity[1] and have been approved for use in patients with low-grade non-Hodgkin lymphoma (NHL). In addition,

Table 86.1   Monoclonal antibodies approved by the FDA for lymphoid malignancies

Date of approval	Generic name	Trade name	Isotype and format	Target	Indication	Sponsor
26-Nov-1997	Rituximab	Rituxan®	Chimeric IgG1	CD20	Relapsed or refractory, low-grade or follicular, CD20-positive, B cell NHL	Genentech, Biogen IDEC
10-Feb-2006					Diffuse large B cell, CD20-positive NHL in combination with CHOP or other anthracycline-based chemotherapy	
29-Sep-2006					Follicular, CD20-positive, B cell NHL in combination with CVP chemotherapy	
7-May-2001	Alemtuzumab	Campath®	Humanized IgG1	CD52	B cell chronic lymphocytic leukemia (B-CLL) in patients who have been treated with alkylating agents and who have failed fludarabine therapy	ILEX, Genzyme
19-Feb-2002	Ibritumomab tiuxetan	Zevalin®	^{90}Y-labeled murine IgG1	CD20	Relapsed or refractory low-grade, follicular, or transformed B cell NHL, including patients with rituximab-refractory follicular NHL	Biogen IDEC, Schering AG
27-Jun-2003	Tositumomab and ^{131}I-tositumomab	Bexxar®	^{131}I-labeled murine IgG2a	CD20	CD20-positive NHL with and without transformation in patients whose disease is refractory to rituximab and has relapsed following chemotherapy	Corixa, GlaxoSmithKline

FDA, United States Food and Drug Administration; IgG, immunoglobulin G; NHL, non-Hodgkin lymphoma; CHOP: cyclophosphamide, doxorubicin, vincristine, and prednisone; CVP: cyclophosphamide, vincristine, and prednisolone; ^{90}Y, yttrium-90; ^{131}I, iodine-131.

gemtuzumab ozogamicin (Mylotarg®), an anti-CD33 antibody conjugated to the drug calicheamicin, has been approved for use in patients with refractory acute myeloid leukemia (AML).[2]

Some antibodies themselves are potent cytotoxic agents, which are more attractive for clinical oncology. An ideal therapeutic mAb would achieve clinical responses by specifically binding to tumor cells, and then recruiting other humoral and cellular immune defense components of the host to attack the target cells (antibody-dependent cell-mediated cytotoxicity [ADCC] and complement-dependent cytotoxicity [CDC]), as well as inducing cytotoxic effects, such as apoptosis, or intracellular negative signaling to cell-cycle arrest or growth inhibition. Yet, some mAbs can act as sensitizing agents to improve the efficacy of radioisotopes or cytotoxic drugs against cancer.

Development of the first chimeric antibody, rituximab, began in the early 1990s. In 1997, approval of rituximab for the therapy of relapsed and refractory indolent NHL further rekindled the effort to advance immunotherapy and radiation therapy in the treatment of cancer. Since 1997, the United States Food and Drug Administration (FDA) has approved five antibodies for hematologic

malignancies; four of these antibodies have been approved for lymphoid malignancies (Table 86.1). Approval of rituximab for cancer treatment revolutionized treatment of lymphoid malignancies. In addition, more than 100 mAbs are being tested currently in clinical trials for various indications. Most of these antibodies were raised initially in mice and reengineered to suit human use and pharmaceutical production. In this chapter, the development of antibody-based therapy and the utilization of naked and conjugated antibodies in the therapy of lymphoid neoplasms will be discussed.

REENGINEERED AND FULLY HUMAN MONOCLONAL ANTIBODIES GENERATED BY RECOMBINANT DNA TECHNIQUES – BETTER SUITED FOR HUMANS

The immunogenicity of murine mAbs in humans has been a major obstacle limiting their clinical use (**h**uman **a**nti-**m**ouse **a**ntibodies [HAMA]). Therefore, over the last two decades, major effort was focused to modify murine antibodies into antibodies that are physically or functionally more like human immunoglobulin (Ig), mainly chimeric or

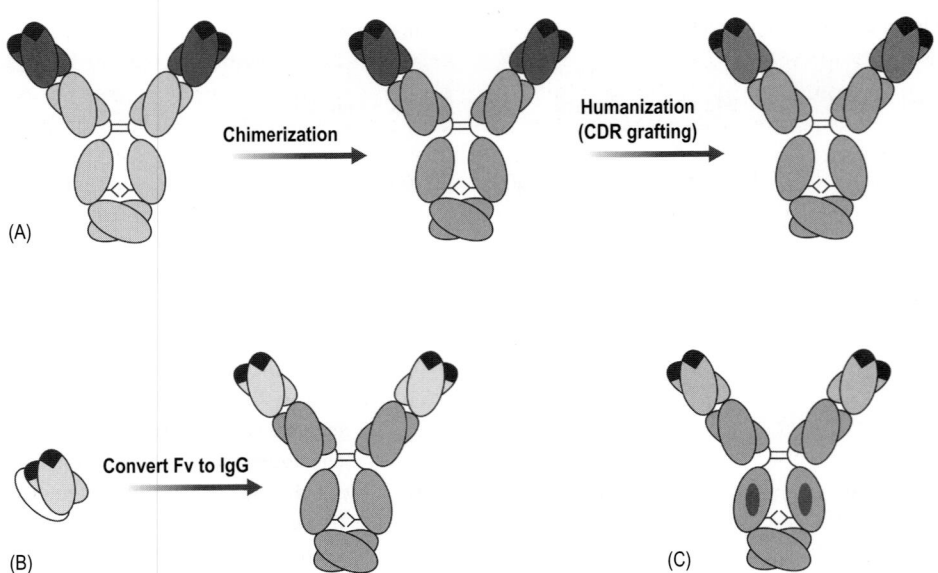

Figure 86.1   Reengineering of monoclonal antibodies. (A) Mouse monoclonal antibody (mAb), immunoglobulin G (IgG), is composed of constant and variable regions. The antigen-binding site is a part of the variable region. A chimeric antibody is constructed by simple fusion of the variable region to the constant region of a human IgG. In a humanized antibody, the variable region is constructed by grafting the antigen-binding region sequence to the variable region of a human antibody. (B) Single-chain Fv (scFv) or Fv fragment selected from a human antibody library can be converted to a human monoclonal IgG molecule. (C) Humanized antibody can be further modified in the CH2 region for an enhanced Fc function. CDR, complementarity-determining region.

humanized mAb (Fig. 86.1A). A chimeric antibody is constructed by simply fusing the light and heavy chain variable regions (VL and VH, respectively) of a murine mAb to the corresponding human constant regions using recombinant deoxyribonucleic acid (DNA) technology. Approximately 70 percent of the structure of a chimeric antibody is of human origin. Chimeric antibodies couple the specific antigen binding characteristics of the parent mouse antibody to the immune system, eliciting immune responses of a human antibody. However, while chimeric antibodies solve the problem of efficient interaction with the human immune system, these antibodies, which still have about 30 percent mouse protein sequence, can still elicit a HACA (**h**uman **a**nti-chimeric **a**ntibody) response against the rodent part.

To address immunogenicity of chimeric antibodies, Greg Winter and colleagues[3] at the University of Cambridge developed the recombinant DNA technique of antibody humanization. In this technique, the VL and VH domains of the original murine mAb are further engineered so that only the complementarity-determining regions (CDRs), which are amino acid fragments directly involved in antigen binding, are transplanted onto the scaffolds of corresponding human V region frameworks (FRs), termed CDR grafting (Fig. 86.1A). An optimal humanized antibody will contain the fewest number of rodent amino acids required to reproduce the binding strength and specificity of the original mouse antibody (usually 5 percent to 10 percent of the total), and will possess attributes essential to enhanced clinical utility, i.e., decreased immunogenicity, longer serum half-life in humans, and the ability to recruit effector

functions (CDC and ADCC) of the immune system. The efficacy and safety of humanized antibodies is exemplified by those already on the market (alemtuzumab, trastuzumab, and bevacizumab), as well as the many currently in clinical trials worldwide.

Conventional hybridoma technology is insufficient in generating a large quantity of human mAbs for clinical use. New technologies have created clones of transgenic and transchromosomal mice producing purely human antibody repertoires, which can be immunized to raise human antibodies with desired specificities and, combined with conventional hybridoma technology, to produce fully human mAbs. Antibodies of human origin also can be selected *ex vivo* by screening natural or synthetic human antibody libraries. This is commonly achieved by the phage-display technology or the yeast two-hybrid system, resulting in Fv fragments, the smallest antibody unit with desired antigen-binding activity.[4–7] The Fv fragment can then be reengineered to a fully human IgG antibody (Fig. 86.1B).

TECHNOLOGIES MIMICKING SOMATIC HYPERMUTATION – POTENTIAL IMPROVEMENT IN THE ANTIGEN–BINDING AFFINITY OF MONOCLONAL ANTIBODIES

Antibodies generated from mice or display libraries typically have an antigen-binding dissociation constant (K_d) in the range of 10^{-7} to 10^{-9} M. It is generally believed that high-affinity antibodies bind more efficiently to the antigenic targets and are more useful in broad clinical applications. To improve antibody affinity, various *in vitro* strategies have been developed to mimic the mammalian *in vivo* process of somatic hypermutation and selection. These approaches include site-specific mutagenesis based on structural information, combinatorial mutagenesis of CDRs, and random mutagenesis of the entire gene or chain shuffling.[8–12]

MODIFYING THE FC PORTION OF MONOCLONAL ANTIBODIES – POTENTIAL IMPROVEMENT IN PHARMACOKINETICS AND THERAPEUTIC EFFICACY

Most of the effective unconjugated antibodies possess the backbone of human IgG1, the most effective antibody isotype that elicits three main effector functions in humans: ADCC, CDC, and phagocytosis. Antibody-dependent cell-mediated cytotoxicity and phagocytosis are mediated through interaction of tumor cell-bound mAbs with the Fc receptors for IgG (FcγRs) on the surface of effector cells.[13] Complement-dependent cytotoxicity is mediated by the interaction of tumor cell-bound mAbs with the complement system. In addition, the PK of a mAb *in vivo* are affected by the interaction of its Fc portion with the neonatal Fc receptor (FcRn). FcγRs play a critical role in linking other antibody-mediated immune responses with cellular effector functions, such as release of inflammatory mediators, endocytosis of immune complexes, and regulation of immune system cell activation. Several new strategies incorporate additional Fc domain modifications to enhance effector function of antibodies.

Three types of FcγRs have been identified and characterized on immune system effector cells: FcγRI (CD64), FcγRII (CD32), and FcγRIII (CD16). In humans, variants of the latter two types are FcγRIIa and FcγRIIb, and FcγRIIIa and FcγRIIIb. The complexity of the human FcγR system is amplified by the presence of polymorphic forms of the receptors. FcγRIIa has two isoforms, Arg-131 and His-131, which differ in the binding of IgG2.[14] FcγRIIIa has polymorphism at positions 48 (Leu/His/Arg) and 158 (Phe/Val).[15,16] FcγRIIIb polymorphic forms NA1 and NA2 differ in four amino acid residues.[17] The binding sites on human IgG1 for human FcγRI, FcγRIIa, FcγRIIb, FcγRIIIa, FcγRIIIb, FcγRn, and C1q have been mapped by site-directed mutagenesis. All solvent-exposed residues in human IgG1 Fc were individually altered to Ala (alanine scanning mutagenesis) and each variant tested for binding to the different receptors. Residues affecting the binding were identified. In another strategy, Fc variants made to randomize all the contact residues in FcR and/or C1q interaction were screened for the binding to all FcγRs, FcRn, and C1q. A database is being built to include the properties of all possible variants. With this information, it is possible to engineer a variant Fc with desired FcγR, FcRn, and C1q binding properties into therapeutic antibodies and to

evaluate whether the resulting antibody has improved potency in clinical applications and in patients with a particular genotype. A new generation of antibodies with the Fc portion tailored for specific affinity to FcγR is in the clinic, exploring the opportunity to enhance efficacy in patients with lymphoid neoplasms.

NEXT GENERATION OF MONOCLONAL ANTIBODIES

As effective as mAbs have become, these agents still suffer from some major drawbacks – namely size, delivery, and cost. The large size of a mAb often limits deep tumor penetration and homogenous distribution, and sometimes inhibits the ability of the mAb to effectively bind to antigen cavities or receptor clefts. Human and murine mAbs can be enzymatically digested to smaller antigen-binding fragments, F(ab')$_2$ or Fab (Fig. 86.2). Using recombinant DNA technology, even smaller fragments containing only the VH and VL domains of the IgG, namely single chain Fv (scFv), can be constructed (Fig. 86.2). These fragments should have the same antigen-binding specificity and affinity as the intact IgG, but their PK and biodistribution profiles would be different from each other and from that of the intact IgG. Therefore, it is possible to design and modify mAb drugs based on desired profiles to improve safety and efficacy.

Novel mAbs varying in size or antigen-binding valency, with or without the Fc fragment, also can be made by combining IgG and the fragments. A few examples are illustrated in Figure 86.2. Furthermore, by combining the fragments of different mAbs, bispecific or multispecific mAbs can be produced.

Unconventional antibodies consisting of homodimer heavy chains, which are found in camelids[22] and sharks,[23] have only VH for antigen recognition and binding and are known as single-domain (antigen-binding) antibodies (sdAb). The VH of shark sdAb, NAR (new antigen receptor), has only two CDRs and four conserved FRs, making it the smallest antigen-binding unit with immunoglobulin-like scaffolds, approximately 12 kDa (Fig. 86.2). Due to their small size, sdAbs may be able to access antigen epitopes not generally recognized by conventional antibodies.[24] Several biotechnology companies are striving to develop the next generation of mAb platforms based on sdAbs. Nanobodies derived from these sdAb are the smallest functional fragment of naturally occurring antibodies.[25] These novel formats provide several advantages: the ability to slip into receptor cavities, the ability to recognize hidden epitopes, improved biodistribution and tumor penetration, and low immunogenic potential. Pharmaceutical properties of these novel structures may be enhanced via PEGylation or by attaching an anti-serum albumin molecule. In the near future, it is likely that antibody will be specifically tailored (e.g., glycosylation pattern) to optimize performance of the molecule.

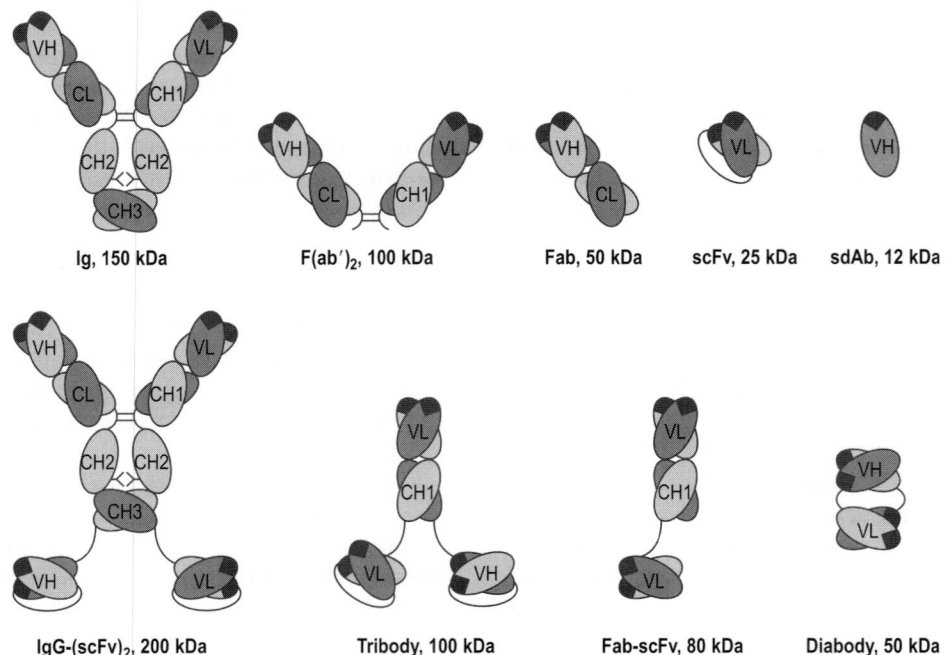

Figure 86.2 Tailoring second-generation therapeutic antibodies. F(ab')$_2$ and Fab are the products of enzymatic digestion of immunoglobulin G (IgG). A single-chain Fv (scFv) is the smallest binding unit of a conventional IgG.[18] Tetravalent and bivalent bispecific antibodies were constructed by fusion of scFv to the C-terminus of CH3 or C-terminus of CH1.[19] Trivalent antibodies (triAb) were constructed by fusion of a scFv to the C-terminus of CH1 and a scFv to the C-terminus of CL.[20] A diabody is composed of two crosswise paired scFv.[21] A single-domain antibody (sdAb) is the smallest antigen-binding unit with Ig-like scaffolds.

UNCONJUGATED MONOCLONAL ANTIBODIES

Anti–CD20 (rituximab)

CD20 was one of many lymphocyte-specific surface antigens identified in the 1970s. The prototype antigen, B1, was found to be B cell specific and distinct from other B cell antigens. CD20, a 33–37 kDa membrane phosphoprotein, is expressed on virtually all normal B cells, starting at the pre-B cell stage, and expression is lost upon differentiation to the plasma cells stage. Cell-surface CD20 is absent on stem cells. The density of CD20 on the cell surface varies among different B cell neoplasms. Only about half of childhood B cell acute lymphoblastic leukemias (ALLs) are CD20 positive. Among the mature B cell malignancies, the lowest level of CD20 expression is found in chronic lymphocytic leukemia (CLL) and small lymphocytic lymphoma (SLL).[26,27] A very high level of CD20 expression is seen in hairy cell leukemia (HCL). Abundant expression is seen in most mature B cell malignancies but not in multiple myeloma (MM).[28] CD20 is not modulated or shed upon ligation and does not internalize, or internalizes very slowly, upon antibody binding. Circulating CD20 (cCD20) has been documented in patients with CLL and NHL, and appears to be an indicator of adverse prognosis.[29]

Since its first use in humans in the early 1990s, rituximab has become an essential component of treatment of almost all types of B cell NHLs and has been tested in B cell ALL as well. Despite its widespread use, the optimal dose and schedule of rituximab, either alone or in combination with other modalities, is not completely defined. Remarkable single-agent activity, an excellent safety profile, and a lack of overlapping toxicity with chemotherapy have contributed to the broad use of rituximab in patients with CD20-positive neoplasms. Rituximab has many proposed mechanisms of action, some of which depend on the activation of complement (CDC) and the host immune system (antibody-dependent cytotoxicity) and possibly a vaccinal effect. In addition, rituximab has been shown to induce apoptosis and to sensitize chemoresistant human lymphoma cell lines.[30]

Rituximab (Rituxan®; BiogenIDEC and Genentech, Inc.) is a chimeric mouse-human anti-CD20 mAb (human IgG and kappa constant regions) approved by the FDA in 1997 for the treatment of relapsed or refractory, CD20-positive, B cell, low-grade or follicular NHL at the schedule of 375 mg/m^2 weekly for 4 consecutive weeks. The clinical activity of rituximab leading to FDA approval was reported in a multicenter nonrandomized pivotal trial in which 166 patients with relapsed or refractory low-grade lymphoma were treated with 4 weekly doses of 375 mg/m^2 rituximab.[31] The overall response rate was 48 percent, with a 6 percent complete remission (CR) rate and a median time to progression (TTP) of 13 months.

Dose and schedule: In the original phase I study of rituximab, no dose-limiting toxicity (DLT) was determined; the dose of 375 mg/m^2 was selected based on the drug availability for the phase II study. Only a limited number of studies investigated lower and higher dosages (CLL – up to 2250 mg/m^2, and diffuse large B cell lymphoma [DLBCL] – up to 500 mg/m^2). Response to rituximab can appear rapidly, but usually the time to maximum response is measured in months. Although the response rate after 4 weeks of rituximab treatment provided a satisfactory response rate, it soon became evident that the response duration was shorter than that observed with chemotherapy. In an effort to improve upon these results, various investigators tried to extend the duration of treatment to 6 or 8 weeks.[32,33] The PK analysis in the first pivotal study of rituximab indicated that patients maintaining a higher and more prolonged blood level of rituximab had an increased chance of responding,[34] an observation which led to the investigation of extended treatment duration beyond the standard 4 weeks. Hainsworth *et al.* piloted a retreatment consisting of 4 weeks of rituximab therapy every 6 months, for a total of 4 cycles. In nonrandomized studies in patients with follicular lymphoma (FL) and CLL, the duration of response was much higher than that expected using a standard treatment regimen.[35,36] A randomized phase II study of scheduled retreatment compared to retreatment at relapse did not confirm overall clinical benefit.[37] A different approach was used by the Swiss Group for Clinical Cancer Research (SAKK), where patients with FL or mantle cell lymphoma (MCL) received the standard rituximab induction regimen followed by one infusion of rituximab every 2 months for 4 cycles. Response duration for patients with FL was doubled with maintenance therapy.[38,39]

It is clear that resistance to rituximab may be present at the time of initial therapy or may develop following rituximab exposure. In most cases, the mechanism of resistance to rituximab is poorly understood. Loss of the CD20 antigen, impaired CD20-mediated signaling, or acquired resistance to the immune effector functions may play an important role.[40] Innate resistance to rituximab has been observed in certain settings of FL. The polymorphism that encodes FcγRIIIa with either a phenylalanine (F) or a valine at amino acid position 158 results in a higher affinity for human IgG1, and increased ADCC when V is the allotype. In one study, patients with the 158V genotype had a median event-free survival (EFS) of 41 months compared with only 9 months for the FF genotype.[38] Since ADCC appears to play an important role in the response to rituximab, several approaches to stimulate effector cell function have been evaluated in a clinical setting. Several clinical studies have evaluated the role of cytokines in combination with rituximab (interleukin [IL]-2, IL-12, granulocyte colony-stimulating factor [G-CSF], interferon α [IFNα], and CpG).[41–46] One ongoing randomized study is evaluating the role of IFN with rituximab. Rituximab has been safely combined with IL-2 and IL-12,[41–43] but the clinical benefit will have to be confirmed in large, prospective, randomized studies.

FOLLICULAR LYMPHOMA

Rituximab single-agent therapy

The development of antibody-based therapeutic strategies clearly has changed the standard clinical approach to treating patients with advanced FL. In addition to activity in relapsed or refractory indolent lymphomas, rituximab monotherapy also has proven highly effective as first-line treatment of indolent lymphomas, with response rates of 47 percent to 73 percent and CR rates of 7 percent to 20 percent.[47] With only four extra injections of rituximab every 2 months, the TTP was doubled from 19 months to 36 months. Thus, rituximab maintenance strategies seem promising.[48–50] Confirmatory data from a large, prospective, randomized study are needed before this approach can be generally recommended. At present, patients should be enrolled in clinical trials evaluating the role of maintenance rituximab therapy in various post-induction settings. Today, only minimal infusion-related toxicity has been associated with rituximab therapy. Rituximab therapy has been associated with reactivation/progression of some chronic infections such as hepatitis B and progressive multifocal leukoencephalopathy, which may be fatal (black box warning).[51,52] In addition, infections with cytomegalovirus (CMV) and varicella-zoster virus (VZV) have been documented following rituximab therapy.[53] Thus, additional data are needed to quantify the long-term risks of hypogammaglobulinemia, neutropenia, and serious infections associated with extended B cell depletion.

Rituximab in combination with chemotherapy

Due to the favorable toxicity profile of rituximab, its combination with conventional chemotherapy represents an attractive approach to enhance efficacy. The safety and efficacy of rituximab in combination with various chemotherapy regimens have been evaluated in phase II studies. In one of the first of these phase II trials, the combination of CHOP (cyclophosphamide, doxorubicin, vincristine, and prednisone) with rituximab induced responses in all evaluable patients, with a CR rate of 63 percent.[54] A recent update of this study reported an impressive median TTP and response duration of 82 months and 83.5 months, respectively, with 16 of 38 patients still in ongoing remission 6 to 9 years after treatment.[55] Since this trial, a number of studies have described the combination of rituximab with other chemotherapeutics such as fludarabine, mitoxantrone, and cyclophosphamide.[56] The clinical benefit of rituximab in combination with chemotherapy has been tested in several phase III studies. The German Low-grade Lymphoma Study Group (GLSG) randomized patients with previously untreated advanced FL to either 6 to 8 cycles of rituximab plus CHOP (R-CHOP) or CHOP alone.[57] Although the impact of post-remission therapy cannot be excluded, R-CHOP was superior regarding overall response rate (96 percent versus 90 percent, respectively; $P = 0.011$), time to treatment failure ($P < 0.0001$), and duration of response ($P < 0.0006$). There was a trend toward improved overall survival within the first 3 years; the advantage was evident for younger and older patients and for patients with a low and high International Prognostic Index (IPI) score. In the second large phase III trial, Marcus *et al.* also demonstrated the advantage of rituximab in combination with CVP (cyclophosphamide, vincristine, and prednisolone) in previously untreated patients with advanced FL.[58] Based on the outcome of these large randomized studies, rituximab in combination with CHOP or CVP should be considered the new paradigm for patients with advanced FL. Rituximab has been approved as the first-line treatment of follicular, CD20-positive, B cell NHL in combination with CVP chemotherapy. Various prospective studies are testing the role of rituximab maintenance therapy after completion of chemotherapy or immunochemotherapy.[59–61] In patients who have not received rituximab as part of induction, maintenance rituximab therapy seems to be beneficial. In patients with relapsed disease, the benefits of maintenance therapy are well established.[62] The applicability of maintenance therapy for patients undergoing first-line rituximab-based induction therapy should be clarified by the recently completed PRIMA trial (The European Primary Rituximab and Maintenance study). In this study, after completion of induction chemoimmunotherapy (rituximab combined with CHOP, CVP, FCM [fludarabine, cyclophosphamide, and mitoxantrone], or MCP [mitoxantrone, cyclophosphamide, and prednisone]), patients were randomized to observation or a single dose of rituximab every 2 months for 24 months.

The efficacy of rituximab in SLL is not well known, as conflicting results have been reported.[63] Response rates were lower in patients with CLL/SLL (10 percent to 15 percent) than in those with relapsed or refractory FL. Lower response rate has been attributed to the low density of CD20 expression. Response rates are significantly higher when rituximab is used in previously untreated patients with CLL/SLL. Neither increasing the dose nor dose density of administration of rituximab has improved the benefit of rituximab in patients with CLL. More encouraging results have been obtained with the combination of rituximab and chemotherapy. Concurrent administration of fludarabine and rituximab induced a 90 percent response rate with 47 percent CR; myelosuppression was more profound with immunochemotherapy.[64] The combination of alemtuzumab and rituximab has been evaluated in patients with relapsed and refractory lymphoid malignancies; overall, this was a well-tolerated combination for patients with relapsed CLL. Efficacy of rituximab in patients with marginal zone lymphoma seems comparable to the efficacy in FL. Several phase II studies have shown a good response rate in patients with Waldenström macroglobulinemia. In the largest study, a response was achieved in 44 percent of the patients with a median TTP of 16 months.[65] The German CLL study group conducted a phase III trial (ClinicalTrials.gov NCT00281918 – CLL8) evaluating combined immunochemotherapy with fludarabine,

cyclophosphamide, and rituximab (FC-R) versus chemotherapy with fludarabine and cyclophosphamide (FC) alone in patients with previously untreated CLL. A total of 817 patients were randomized. According to a recent press release, this study met the primary endpoint of a significant increase in progression-free survival (PFS) of FC-R versus chemotherapy.

DIFFUSE LARGE B CELL LYMPHOMA

For the past three decades, chemotherapy with CHOP has been the standard treatment for patients with DLBCL. The treatment of DLBCL has completely changed in recent years with the combination of rituximab and chemotherapy. The significant benefit for elderly patients treated with R-CHOP was first reported by the Groupe d'Etudes des Lymphomes de l'Adulte (GELA) in 2002.[66] Since then, the results have been confirmed by two other randomized studies.[67] With a 5-year median follow-up, EFS, PFS, disease-free survival, and overall survival remained statistically in favor of the R-CHOP.[68] The 5-year EFS was 47 percent in patients treated with R-CHOP compared with 29 percent in patients treated with chemotherapy only. Both patients with low-risk and high-risk lymphoma had longer survival if treated with immunochemotherapy. No long-term toxicity appeared to be associated with the R-CHOP regimen. The German Lymphoma Study Group studied the role of immunochemotherapy in young patients with good-prognosis stage II to IV and bulky stage I DLBCL (the MInT study).[69] A total of 413 patients were assigned to rituximab and CHOP-like chemotherapy, and 411 patients received CHOP-like chemotherapy alone. After a median follow-up of 34 months, patients who received immunochemotherapy had a 3-year EFS of 79 percent versus 59 percent for the chemotherapy-treated group ($P < 0.0001$); overall survival was 93 percent versus 84 percent, respectively ($P = 0.001$). Immunochemotherapy was well tolerated. Therefore, outside of a clinical study, R-CHOP might be the recommended regimen for elderly patients with DLBCL and for young patients with low- and intermediate-risk disease. R-CHOP has been approved by the FDA as chemoimmunotherapy for elderly patients.[70] The role of rituximab in the management of young patients with poor-risk diseases has been tested in prospective studies.

MANTLE CELL LYMPHOMA

Rituximab has single-agent activity in MCL, with a response rate of approximately 30 percent and response duration of 6–12 months. The GLSG initiated a randomized trial comparing R-CHOP with CHOP alone as first-line therapy for patients with advanced MCL.[71] One hundred twenty-two previously untreated patients with advanced stage MCL were randomly assigned to receive 6 cycles of CHOP ($n = 60$) or R-CHOP ($n = 62$). The immunochemotherapy with R-CHOP resulted in a significantly higher response rate (94 percent versus 75 percent; $P = 0.0054$), higher complete remission rate (34 percent versus 7 percent; $P = 0.00024$), and a prolongation of the time to treatment failure (21 months versus 14 months; $P = 0.0131$) as compared with chemotherapy alone. Toxicity was acceptable with no major differences between the two therapeutic groups. Hyper-CVAD (fractionated cyclophosphamide, vincristine, doxorubicin, and dexamethasone) plus rituximab was studied in 97 patients.[72] The overall response rate was 97 percent, including an 87 percent CR. The 3-year failure-free survival rate was 64 percent, and the overall survival rate was 82 percent with a median follow-up of 40 months. As expected, the main toxicity was hematologic. Hence, R-CHOP or hyper-CVAD may serve as a new baseline regimen for advanced stage MCL, but needs to be further improved by novel strategies in induction and remission.[73]

ACUTE LYMPHOBLASTIC LEUKEMIA

Acute lymphoblastic leukemia blast cells express a variety of specific antigens which may serve as targets, e.g., CD19, CD20, CD22, CD33, and CD52. Anti-CD20 (rituximab) has been the most studied antibody in patients with this malignancy. In ALL, rituximab is combined with chemotherapy mainly in mature B-ALL and Burkitt lymphoma, and interim results are very promising. Studies with rituximab also have been recently initiated in B-precursor ALL. Rituximab has been evaluated with the hyper-CVAD chemotherapy in 31 adult patients with newly diagnosed B cell lymphoma or leukemia.[74] Addition of antibody did not increase toxicity compared with chemotherapy alone, and clinical outcome was improved, especially in the elderly. All 14 patients with B cell ALL achieved CR, with an overall 3-year survival rate of 74 percent.

Although minimal pediatric data have been published, results have been reported recently for 19 children with mature B cell lymphoma/B-ALL who received rituximab, alone or in combination with chemotherapy, as salvage therapy after failure of intensive chemotherapy.[75] Fifteen of 19 patients (79 percent) responded, and 12 (63 percent) remained alive in continuous CR at 5+ to 48+ months of follow-up. Monotherapy with antibody in relapsed ALL also has occasionally resulted in responses, but greater effects can be expected from combination with chemotherapy and treatment in the state of minimal residual disease (MRD). Prospective well-defined studies (e.g., level of antigen expression, timing, schedule, dose, and stage of disease) will determine the role of rituximab in the management of CD20-positive ALL.[76]

Central nervous system (CNS) dissemination of NHL is an important cause of morbidity and death in patients with high-grade disease.[77] Most CNS lymphomas are CD20-positive DLBCL. New therapies are needed to prevent and treat CNS dissemination. Cerebrospinal fluid (CSF) levels of rituximab after intravenous (IV) administration are only approximately 0.1 percent of matched serum levels. In the phase I study, 25 mg was determined to be the maximum tolerated dose (MTD) of rituximab.[78] Cytologic responses were detected in six of ten patients, with four CRs. These results suggest that intrathecal rituximab is feasible and effective treatment for patients with CNS lymphomas.

Second-generation anti-CD20 antibodies

Anti-CD20 therapy has had a truly dramatic impact on the treatment of NHL, but most responses to single-agent rituximab are incomplete, and all patients with FL will experience disease progression at some point following rituximab therapy. There are multiple potential approaches to overcoming rituximab resistance, including engineered antibodies that are optimized for their ability to mediate ADCC or CDC. In addition, human or humanized structures have also been employed to potentially improve PK and immunogenicity.

Humax-CD20 (ofatumumab, Genmab A/S) is a fully human IgG1 mAb developed using human immunoglobulin transgenic mice. Humax-CD20 seems to bind to a slightly different CD20 epitope than rituximab. In preclinical studies, the antibody was shown to be exceptionally active in CDC, being able to lyse a range of rituximab-resistant targets, such as CD20-low CLL, presumably due to slower 'off rates' of the mAb.[79] The full human nature of the mAb should also favor the immunogenicity and PK profile. HuMax-CD20 is in clinical development for the treatment of NHL and CLL. Phase I data suggest that this agent is well tolerated and is associated with meaningful clinical activity. HuMax-CD20 has been granted 'Fast Track Product' status by the FDA for development as a therapy for patients with CLL who have failed fludarabine-containing therapy. The pivotal nonrandomized study started in 2006. In the phase I/II studies that support further development of this agent, 13 of 26 evaluable patients (50 percent) who received the highest ofatumumab dose had an objective response (OR), with median TTP of 23 weeks (range 20 to 31 weeks). Ofatumumab is also being tested in a phase II study in combination with fludarabine and cyclophosphamide for the first-line treatment of patients with CLL as well as in a phase III study of rituximab-refractory NHL. The efficacy of ofatumumab has not yet been directly compared with that of rituximab in clinical trials, but *in vitro* and preclinical data suggest that ofatumumab is more effective at killing CD20-expressing cells, even when CD20 expression levels are very low. Moreover, ofatumumab is effective at killing cells resistant to rituximab.[79]

Genentech Inc. in collaboration with Hoffman La Roche and Biogen Idec Inc. is developing a second generation of a humanized IgG1 anti-CD20 antibody (ocrelizumab), which differs in the Fc region by two amino acid sequences, resulting in slightly increased ADCC and slightly decreased CDC compared with rituximab. Preclinical studies in cynomolgus monkeys have demonstrated B cell depletion in peripheral blood and significantly reduced B cells in lymphoid tissues after treatment with PRO70769 (ocrelizumab) on days 1 and 15.[80] After recovery, B cell subsets were reconstituted to normal levels. Although this agent currently is being developed for autoimmune indications, it may have a role in hematologic malignancies.

Another humanized anti-CD20 antibody (IMMU-106) is being developed by Immunomedics, Inc. IMMU-106 shares the same human IgG framework as epratuzumab (anti-CD22 antibody) and the mechanisms of action are similar to rituximab, namely direct apoptosis, antibody-dependent cellular cytotoxicity, and complement-mediated cytotoxicity.[81] Additionally, treatment of Raji-bearing severe combined immunodeficiency (SCID) mice with IMMU-106 gave a survival advantage compared with control mice.[81] Clinical trials are ongoing in patients with B cell NHL, and objective responses (including CRs) have been observed. In a recent case study, IMMU-106 produced response in a patient with severe resistant systemic lupus erythematosus (SLE) in the presence of anti-chimeric antibody against rituximab due to prior rituximab therapy.[82] Similarly, IMMU-106 may yield clinical benefit in patients with lymphoma for whom rituximab may be contraindicated. In addition, IMMU-106 has been developed for subcutaneous application.

AME-133 (LY-2469298) is another humanized and optimized mAb version of rituximab under development by Applied Molecular Evolution (AME; Lilly) for the treatment of NHL.

TRU-015 is a small modular immunopharmaceutical (SMIP™) drug candidate designed to target and deplete B cells. *In vitro*, TRU-015 binds to CD20 and elicits ADCC and induces apoptosis. TRU-015 is in phase IIa trials for rheumatoid arthritis, and the phase I/II trial in NHL has been initiated.

Alemtuzumab

Alemtuzumab (Campath®) was the first mAb approved by the FDA for the treatment of patients who have been treated with alkylating agents and who have failed fludarabine therapy.[83] Alemtuzumab is a humanized antibody that targets the CD52 antigen. CD52 is expressed on virtually all B and T lymphocytes, as well as monocytes, macrophages, and eosinophils. Although the highest levels of expression of CD52 appear to be on T prolymphocytic leukemia cells, significant expression is observed on B-CLL, with only low levels on normal B cells. Alemtuzumab mediates cell killing via a variety of mechanisms including CDC, ADCC, and induction of apoptosis. The optimal dose and route of administration of alemtuzumab remain to be defined. In trials that led to the registration of alemtuzumab, responses were observed in 42 percent of patients with CLL refractory to alkylating agents and in 33 percent of patients with CLL refractory to fludarabine therapy. The median TTP for responders was 9.5 months; clinical

benefit was noted in both responders and those with stable disease. The median survival was 16 months overall and 32 months for responders. Responses with alemtuzumab therapy are often limited to the peripheral blood, bone marrow, and spleen with lower responses in bulky lymph nodes. Finally, in CLL, the efficacy of alemtuzumab does not appear to be affected by Fc receptor polymorphisms.[84] Adverse events associated with alemtuzumab therapy include infusion-related events, infections (severe in 55 percent of patients, life threatening in 25 percent), hematologic toxicity, and opportunistic infections due to depletion of normal B and T cells. Therefore, prophylactic antibiotic therapy is required.[85]

In a phase II trial of subcutaneous injection of alemtuzumab as first-line treatment for B-CLL, infusion-related toxicities were rare; an objective response rate (ORR) of 87 percent was obtained with 19 percent CR rate.[86] Also, alemtuzumab may be effective in clearing leukemia cells that lack TP53 function.[87] In addition, alemtuzumab currently is being evaluated in combination with other cytotoxic drugs or rituximab. Potential synergy between fludarabine and alemtuzumab was first suggested by a small trial. The FluCam regimen consists of fludarabine 30 mg/m^2 immediately followed by alemtuzumab 30 mg IV, both given on days 1 through 3 of each 4-week course, for a total of six courses.[87] This regimen has been evaluated in previously treated patients; the ORR was 83 percent (11 CRs, 19 partial responses [PRs], one stable disease, and five progressive disease).[88] Alemtuzumab has been studied in combination with chemotherapy and rituximab. Furthermore, alemtuzumab has been studied in patients who have residual disease after purine analogue-based therapy to primarily eliminate residual bone marrow disease.[89] Responses in refractory T cell prolymphocytic leukemia also have been achieved with alemtuzumab treatment.[90]

In Western countries, peripheral T cell lymphomas (PTCL) account for 15 percent to 20 percent of aggressive NHL and 7 percent to 10 percent of all NHL. The natural history of PTCL seems to be unaffected by second and third generations of chemotherapy regimens. The feasibility and clinical efficacy of the combination of CHOP regimen with alemtuzumab were evaluated in a multicenter study in patients with PTCL. Alemtuzumab 30 mg was administered subcutaneously on day −1. Results for 24 patients have been reported.[91] Complete remission was achieved in 17 (71 percent) patients, and one PR was reported. Grade 4 neutropenia and CMV reactivation were the most common side effects. Thirteen patients were disease free, with an overall median duration of response of 11 months. A prospective multicenter study is evaluating the role of CHOP in combination with alemtuzumab for patients with PTCL.

There is limited experience with alemtuzumab in ALL. An ongoing phase II study in adult patients with ALL will evaluate efficacy of alemtuzumab in eradicating MRD.[92] In a pediatric trial of children with relapsed CD52-positive ALL, alemtuzumab will be tested as a single agent for

1 month and then will be tested in combination with mercaptopurine and methotrexate.

Anti-CD22 (epratuzumab)

NON-HODGKIN LYMPHOMA

Despite the significant impact of rituximab on the long-term outcome of FL and DLBCL, a significant portion of patients failed therapy and, therefore, new targets for therapeutic intervention need to be explored. Epratuzumab (hLL2) is a humanized IgG1 mAb derived from the murine IgG2a, LL2. Epratuzumab targets the CD22 antigen, a 135 kDa B lymphocyte restricted type I transmembrane sialoglycoprotein that is expressed in the cytoplasm of early pre-B cells and on the surface of mature B cells. CD22 is lost before differentiation to plasma cells. In B cell malignancies, CD22 has been observed in more than 60 percent to 80 percent of samples evaluated. Phase I and II studies with hLL2 have demonstrated durable responses in patients with indolent and aggressive NHL with acceptable toxicities.[93] Additionally, in a more recent phase II trial, full-dose combination of epratuzumab with rituximab was well tolerated and had significant clinical activity in NHL with 67 percent OR, including 60 percent CRs (including unconfirmed CRs [CRu]).[94] Four of six patients with DLBCL achieved an OR, including three CRs. Median TTP for all patients with indolent NHL was 17.8 months.

A pilot study of epratuzumab in combination with R-CHOP (ER-CHOP) was conducted in previously untreated patients with DLBCL.[95] This chemoimmunotherapy was well tolerated. Overall, 13 of 15 patients (87 percent) had an OR; the CR rate was 67 percent. At a median follow up of 30 months, only three of 15 patients had shown disease progression. A larger, multicenter, phase II study exploring safety and efficacy of ER-CHOP is currently underway.

ACUTE LYMPHOBLASTIC LEUKEMIA

While combination chemotherapy provides cure rates approaching 80 percent to 90 percent in pediatric patients with ALL, long-term outcome of pediatric patients with relapsed disease and adult patients with ALL is limited. The CD22 antigen is expressed on leukemic cells by most patients with ALL.[96] In the initial phase I study conducted by the Children's Oncology Group (COG), 12 patients were first treated with epratuzumab for 14 days, followed by a combination of chemotherapy and epratuzumab.[97] This study confirmed that epratuzumab in combination with standard chemotherapy is feasible and well tolerated in children with relapsed ALL, producing favorable responses in most patients. The COG has initiated a phase II trial (NCT00098839) which will evaluate the safety and efficacy of epratuzumab together with combination chemotherapy in young patients with relapsed ALL.

Anti-CD23

An anti-CD23 (IDEC-152; lumiliximab) is a primatized mAb, with strong similarity to the human antibody and no mouse component. CD23 is a low-affinity FcεRII that binds to IgE and is a characteristic feature of CLL cells. Anti-CD23 binds complement and mediates ADCC by binding FcγRI and RII and also induces apoptosis in vitro. Anti-CD23 currently is being evaluated in phase I/II trials for the treatment of B-CLL (clinicaltrials.gov).

Anti-CD80

Galiximab is a chimeric, anti-CD80 mAb with human constant regions and primate (cynomolgus monkey) variable regions. CD80 (B7.1) is a membrane-bound costimulatory molecule that regulates T cell activity by B cells and dendritic cells. Although CD80 is transiently expressed on the surface of activated B cells, antigen-presenting cells, and T cells, it is constitutively expressed on a variety of NHLs, including FL, making it an attractive target for lymphoma therapy. Preclinical studies have evaluated galiximab as a targeted therapy for lymphoma with promising results.[98] A recent phase I/II trial of galiximab in combination with rituximab in relapsed or refractory FL demonstrated that galiximab can be safely combined with a standard course of rituximab.[99] A phase III randomized study (NCT00363636) has been initiated to compare the clinical benefit of galiximab when given in combination with rituximab as compared with rituximab alone (given with a placebo) in follicular NHL. Safety and PK also will be evaluated.

Anti-CD74

Efficacy in SCID xenograft models of NHL was demonstrated with a humanized anti-CD74 mAb (hLL1). CD74 (invariant chain, Ii) is a type II transmembrane glycoprotein of 216 amino acids that associates with the MHC class II α and β chains and directs the transport of class II molecules to lysosomal and endosomal compartments, where the invariant chain is degraded.[100] The invariant chain-free MHC class II chains subsequently can bind antigenic peptides and appear on the cell surface for presentation to CD4-positive T lymphocytes. The anti-CD74 mAb LL1 has been humanized (hLL1 [milatuzumab] or IMMU-115) and can provide the basis for novel therapeutic approaches to B cell malignancies, particularly because this antibody shows rapid internalization into CD74-positive malignant cells (Table 86.2). As with rituximab, in most human lymphoma or MM cell lines, hLL1 alone does not show a direct cytotoxic effect in vitro. However, in the presence of an appropriate crosslinking agent, hLL1 causes inhibition of cell proliferation and induces apoptosis. Unlike rituximab, hLL1 induces little or no ADCC or CDC. In vivo, therapeutic efficacy of hLL1 was shown in SCID mice using NHL

Table 86.2 Selected immunoconjugates in late preclinical and clinical development

Name	Targeting mAb	Chemotherapeutic	Indication	Status	Sponsor	Reference(s)
Drug immunoconjugate						
CMC-544	Humanized anti-CD22	Calicheamicin	NHL, B cell NHL	1/2	Wyeth-Ayerst	(101–103)
SGN-35	Humanized anti-CD30	Monomethyl auristatin E (MMAE)	Relapsed or refractory Hodgkin lymphoma or other CD30-positive hematologic malignancies	1	Seattle Genetics	(104)
SAR3419	Humanized anti-CD19	Maytansinoid (DM4)	NHL, B cell NHL	1	Sanofi Aventis, Immunogen	(105)
hLL1-DOX (IMMU-110)	Humanized anti-CD74	Doxorubicin	NHL, multiple myeloma	Preclinical	Immuno-medics	(106)
Immunotoxin						
BL22	Murine anti-CD22 dsFv	Truncated PE38	Hairy cell leukemia, B cell CLL, prolymphocytic leukemia, lymphomas	1/2	NCI	(107,108)
LMB-2	Murine anti-CD25 scFv	Truncated PE38	Hairy cell leukemia, CLL, Hodgkin disease, prolymphocytic leukemia, cutaneous T cell lymphoma	1/2	NCI	(109,110)
LL2-onconase; epratuzumab	Humanized anti-CD22	Onconase®	NHL, lymphomas, B cell malignancies	Preclinical	NCI, Immuno-medics	(111)
LL1-onconase	Humanized anti-CD74	Onconase®/RNase	B cell NHL	Preclinical	Immuno-medics	(112)
Bispecific mAb						
MT103/MEDI-538	Rabbit anti-CD19scFv	scFv of murine anti-CD3	NHL, CLL, MCL	1/2	Micromet, Medimmune	(113,114)
Immunoliposome						
anti-CD19-doxorubicin/vincristine	Murine anti-CD19 (IgG or Fab' fragment)	Doxorubicin/vincristine	NHL	Preclinical	University of Alberta	(115)

mAb, monoclonal antibody; NHL, non-Hodgkin lymphoma; dsFv, disulfide-stabilized Fv; scFv, single-chain Fv; NCI, National Cancer Institute; CLL, chronic lymphocytic leukemia; MCL, mantle cell lymphoma; IgG, immunoglobulin G.

and MM cell lines. In the human Burkitt lymphoma xenografts, Daudi and Raji, median survival was extended significantly; a 45 percent increase was obtained in Raji-bearing mice, and a 19 percent increase was obtained in Daudi-bearing SCID mice given lower doses of hLL1.[116]

hLL1 currently is being evaluated in a phase I trial in patients with recurrent NHL and CLL who have failed at least one prior standard systemic treatment; hLL1 is being administered on days 1 and 4 for 6 weeks.

Anti–HLA-DR

Another humanized mAb, Hu1D10, reacts with a polymorphism on the HLA-DR beta chain. However, disappointing results and toxicities have been noted in initial clinical trials.[117]

Anti–CD30

At least two anti-CD30 antibodies (MDX-060 and SGN-30) are in clinical development for treatment of Hodgkin disease, certain forms of NHL, leukemia, and immunologic diseases such as multiple sclerosis and SLE. CD30 is a type II 120 kDa transmembrane glycoprotein and a member of the tumor necrosis factor receptor (TNFR) superfamily. CD30 is highly expressed on Reed-Sternberg cells in Hodgkin disease, on anaplastic large cell lymphoma (ALCL), and on subsets of NHLs as well as on some solid tumors. In preclinical studies, the chimeric SGN-30 antibody induced growth arrest and apoptosis of Hodgkin disease cell lines and improved survival of mice containing Hodgkin disease xenografts.[118] Another antibody targeting CD30 is iratumumab (MDX-060), a fully human antibody being developed by Medarex for the treatment of CD30-positive lymphomas, including Hodgkin disease and ALCL.

SGN-30 recently was evaluated in patients with relapsed Hodgkin disease or ALCL.[119] Twenty-four patients were treated with escalating doses ranging from 1 to 12 mg/kg by weekly infusion for 6 consecutive weeks. Early results showed one CR.

Iratumumab (MDX-060) is a fully human anti-CD30 IgG1 antibody that binds to CD30 with nanomolar avidity. Twenty-one patients with Hodgkin disease, three patients with anaplastic lymphoma, and two patients with CD30-positive T cell lymphoma were treated with escalating doses ranging from 0.1 to 15 mg/kg administered weekly for 4 weeks.[120] In the phase II portion of this study, an additional 51 patients, 47 with Hodgkin disease and four with large cell lymphoma, were treated at four doses. MDX-060 was well tolerated, and an MTD has not been identified. Clinical responses were observed in six patients.

Anti–CD40

CD40 is expressed by normal B cells, monocytes, and dendritic cells. B and T cell lymphomas and Hodgkin disease

cells express CD40 antigen. Two antibodies targeting CD40 (SGN-40 and HCD 122) currently are being evaluated in clinical trials. SGN-40 is a humanized IgG1 anti-CD40 antibody. *In vitro* studies suggest apoptosis induction due to caspase-3 activation and ADCC are key mechanisms underlying the antitumor activity of SGN-40. In mouse studies, SGN-40 showed potent antitumor activity comparable with that of rituximab against xenograft lymphomas.[121] SGN-40 is being evaluated in phase I clinical trials for patients with MM or NHL and in a phase I/II clinical trial for CLL.

HCD 122 is a humanized IgG1 anti-CD40 antibody that has demonstrated *in vitro* activity in various human B cell lymphoma cell lines.[122] HCD 122 currently is being investigated in a phase I/II trial of patients with Hodgkin lymphoma or NHL (NCT00670592) and in a phase I trial of patients with MM (NCT00231166).

Anti–CD19

CD19 is a critical signal transduction molecule that regulates B lymphocyte development, activation, and differentiation. On the surface of B cells, CD19 forms a protein complex with CD21 (complement receptor type 2), CD81 (TAPA-1; a target for antiproliferation antibody), Leu-13, and other unidentified proteins.[123,124] Engagement of CD19 by mAbs leads to tyrosine phosphorylation of cytoplasmic and cell-surface proteins including CD19, activation of phospholipase C (PLC), inositol phospholipid turnover, intracellular calcium mobilization, stimulation of serine-specific protein kinases including protein kinase C, and activation of nuclear factor κB.[125,126] Several unconjugated anti-CD19 antibodies currently are being developed and are mostly in preclinical stages, the primary ones being XmAb-5574, a humanized version, under development by Xencor; MDX-1342, a fully human antibody developed by Medarex; and MEDI-551, being developed by MedImmune (AstraZeneca).

Anti–CD2

CD2 is a transmembrane glycoprotein with an important role in both T and natural killer (NK) cell functions. CD2 antigen is a rational target for treatment of T cell lymphoma. Siplizumab (MEDI-507) is a humanized IgG1 mAb that binds to human CD2. Preclinical studies demonstrated that siplizumab kills target cells by ADCC. This antibody currently is being evaluated in a phase I study in patients with adult T cell leukemia and peripheral T cell lymphoma.

Anti–CD4

Zanolimumab is a human IgG1 mAb against CD4 that is in clinical development for the treatment of cutaneous and nodal T cell lymphomas. Merck Serono SA, under license from Genmab A/S and Medarex Inc., is developing zanolimumab for the potential treatment of cutaneous (CTCL) and noncutaneous (NCTCL) T cell lymphomas. Zanolimumab currently is being investigated in phase III clinical trials for CTCL and phase II clinical trials for NCTCL.[127] Zanolimumab was found to inhibit CD4-positive T cells by combining signaling inhibition with the potent Fc-dependent lysis of CD4-positive T cells.[128] The efficacy and safety of zanolimumab in patients with refractory CTCL have been assessed in two phase II, multicenter, prospective, open-label, uncontrolled clinical studies.[129] Patients with treatment-refractory CD4-positive CTCL (mycosis fungoides [MF], $n = 38$; Sézary syndrome [SS], $n = 9$) received 17 weekly infusions of zanolimumab (early stage patients, 280 and 560 mg; advanced stage patients, 280 and 980 mg). The primary endpoint was OR, as assessed by composite assessment of index lesion disease activity score. Secondary endpoints included physician's global assessment (PGA), time to response, response duration, and TTP. Objective responses were recorded for patients in both CTCL types (MF, 13 ORs; SS, 2 ORs). In the high-dose groups (560 mg and 980 mg dose groups), a response rate of 56 percent was obtained, with a median response of 81 weeks. Adverse events reported most frequently included low-grade infections and eczematous dermatitis. Zanolimumab showed marked clinical efficacy in the treatment of patients with refractory MF, with early onset of response, high response rate, and durable responses. The treatment was well tolerated with no dose-related toxicity other than the targeted depletion of peripheral T cells. Based on these findings, a pivotal study (NCT00127881) has been initiated to determine the efficacy of the drug, HuMax-CD4, in patients with MF and SS who are intolerant to or do not respond to treatment with Targretin® (bexarotene) and one other standard therapy.

Anti–vascular endothelial growth factor

Increased angiogenesis has been documented in patients with all types of lymphoma, but is more prominent in those with aggressive histologies. The anti-vascular endothelial growth factor (anti-VEGF) antibody bevacizumab has been investigated in a phase II trial for treatment of patients with advanced stage aggressive NHL in first and second relapse.[130] Patients received bevacizumab 10 mg/kg every 2 weeks. Of 52 patients, two achieved PR and eight had stable disease. A Southwest Oncology Group (SWOG) study (#S0515) is currently evaluating the combination of bevacizumab with CHOP for patients with advanced stage DLBCL, and another study is evaluating bevacizumab and rituximab for the treatment of patients with relapsed DLBCL and MCL.

Anti–CD47

Chugai Pharmaceutical (Roche) is developing a monoclonal disulfide-stabilized dimer of a single-chain antibody

against CD47 as a therapy for CLL and other lymphoid malignancies. The integrin-associated protein IAP/CD47 is a 50 kDa cell-surface protein that is physically associated with $\alpha_v\beta_3$ integrins in various cells and acts as a transducer element modulating cell activation mediated via integrins. Ligation of CD47 with mAbs can induce rapid cell death in T cells and CLL B cells in a caspase-independent manner.[131] The company developed the mAb, MABL, against the extracellular domain of human CD47 (hCD47). The F(ab')$_2$ fragment of MABL induced cell death in hCD47-positive CLL cell lines, CCRF-CEM and JOK-1, but not in vitro in CD34-positive hematopoietic progenitor cells; MABL also induced hemoagglutination in erythrocytes, which were also CD47 positive.[132] In SCID mice, the F(ab')$_2$ fragment of MABL, given at 30 mg/kg/day × 5, markedly prolonged the survival of mice inoculated with JOK-1.[132] To develop MABL for leukemic therapy, single-chain Fv (scFv) of MABL was constructed. The scFv dimers of MABL induced apoptosis in a human CD47-transfected mouse lymphoid leukemia cell line in a dose-dependent manner, without hemoagglutination.[133,134]

BISPECIFIC ANTIBODIES

Bispecific antibodies are either full IgG or fragments, such as F(ab')$_2$ or scFv, which bind to two different epitopes commonly on different antigens. As a result, bispecific antibodies have been exploited to enhance immune effector mechanisms by crosslinking tumor cells with effector cells. Several studies have shown retargeting of cytotoxic T lymphocytes through binding to the T cell coreceptor molecule CD3. One such bispecific scFv molecule (MT103) directed against CD19 and CD3 is being investigated in a phase I trial for the treatment of NHL or B cell lymphoma and in a phase II study for B-precursor ALL (Table 86.2). This construct was shown to be very potent in destroying CD19-expressing tumor cells in vitro and in vivo in a T cell costimulation-independent way.[113,114] Natural killer cells also have been retargeted with recombinant bispecific antibodies directed against FcγRIII (CD16). In a phase I/II trial in refractory Hodgkin disease evaluating HRS-3/A9 (murine anti-CD16/CD30, which binds with one arm to the CD30 antigen and second arm to FcγRIII or CD16), one CR, three PRs, and four responses of stable disease were reported.[135] Several preclinical studies in xenograft models have evaluated combinations of bispecific antibodies or combination of bispecific antibodies with other chemotherapeutics. Some studies included coapplication of anti-CD19 × anti-CD3 and anti-CD19 × anti-CD16 bispecific diabodies targeting and activating two different effector cell types and the coapplication of an anti-CD19 × anti-CD16 bispecific diabody together with thalidomide as chemotherapeutic drug.[136] These studies described synergistic effects between the different compounds.

CONJUGATED MONOCLONAL ANTIBODIES

An approach to increase the efficacy of mAbs involves conjugation of the mAbs to cytotoxic agents. The concept of mAb–drug conjugates for treatment of malignant diseases can be traced back to the early 1900s, when Ehrlich suggested the use of an antibody conjugated to diphtheria toxin.[137] These cytotoxic agents include but are not limited to small-molecule anticancer drugs, toxins, and radionuclides. A different strategy to deliver payload to tumor is via targeted drug delivery involving encapsulating cytotoxic agents in liposomes and nanoparticles coated with mAbs. Ideally, conjugated antibodies should be designed such that they remain nontoxic in circulation *in vivo* until they reach the target site. After binding to the target cell, the conjugate is internalized by a process called receptor-mediated endocytosis. After the drug or toxin is released intracellularly, it can then act on the target site(s). An understanding of the trafficking of the conjugates following internalization and the controlled release of the drug within the desired intracellular compartment is critical to successful drug delivery.

Radioimmunotherapeutics

Conjugates of mAbs and radioisotopes (radioimmunotherapies [RITs]) have been widely researched since the 1960s, initially as tumor detection and imaging agents and later as agents for delivering cytotoxic radiation to tumors. Yttrium-90-labeled ibritumomab tiuxetan (Zevalin®; Biogen IDEC Pharmaceuticals Corporation) and ^{131}I-labeled tositumomab (Bexxar®; Corixa and GlaxoSmithKline) currently are the only two FDA-approved radiolabeled mAbs, and the first one has been registered recently in Europe. Both mAbs are murine in origin, target CD20 antigen, and are indicated for the treatment of recurrent or refractory indolent B cell lymphoma and related conditions, but few studies have been done outside this indication. The main therapeutic effect of radiolabeled antibodies resides in their ability to deliver radiation. The advantage of radiolabeled over unconjugated antibodies is that there is no need to target every cell to achieve an antitumor effect. The choice of antibody and radioisotopes is critical for the success of RIT. The murine nature of the mAb results in a short half-life and, therefore, limited radiation exposure. The characteristics and the specificity of each of these compounds are determined by the physical properties of the radioisotope attached to the antibody. Yttrium-90, a pure β-emitter with a half-life of 2.7 days, is linked to the antibody by a chelator (tiuxetan). The long β-path length of yttrium-90 is potentially advantageous in patients with bulky disease.[138] Thus, yttrium-90 cannot be used for imaging, and indium-11 has to be used as a surrogate for imaging purposes. Iodine-131 is an α- and a β-emitter with a half-life of 8 days, and can be used directly for imaging. Ibritumomab is the murine mAb that was humanized to

obtain rituximab, so direct comparisons between them are informative. In a randomized, controlled multicenter trial, involving 143 rituximab-naïve patients with relapsed or refractory indolent or transformed NHL, the ibritumomab tiuxetan group benefited with overall response rates of 80 percent (CR/CRu 34 percent and PR 45 percent) compared to 56 percent (CR/CRu 20 percent and PR 36 percent) for rituximab.[139] Despite a high overall response rate, therapy with ibritumomab tiuxetan did not provide survival benefit or significant improvement in TTP (12.6 months versus 10.2 months; $P = 0.062$). Ibritumomab tiuxetan should not be administered to patients with low platelet count (less than $100\,000/mm^3$) or to patients with bone marrow involvement of more than 25 percent because of possible hematologic toxicity. The maximum allowable radiation dose is 32 mCi, independent of weight or body surface area. The major toxicity of yttrium-90-labeled ibritumomab tiuxetan is myelosuppression. Grade 3 or 4 neutropenia and thrombocytopenia were observed in 60 percent and 63 percent of patients, respectively. Median duration of grade 3 or 4 bone marrow toxicity was 23 days and 28 days, respectively. Approximately 1 percent of patients developed myelodysplastic syndrome. The safety and efficacy of ibritumomab tiuxetan in the treatment of B cell NHL other than FL is not well known and warrants further evaluation.

[131]I-tositumomab (the murine anti-CD20 antibody, originally designated as B1, labeled with ^{131}I) has been studied for more than 10 years. It has been used as a part of a nonmyeloablative or a myeloablative regimen. Based on the dosimetry calculated before drug administration, the desired dose of radiation for patients with well-preserved bone marrow function is 75 cGy, and 65 cGy for patients with platelet count between 100 000 and $149\,000/mm^3$. In a pivotal study of ^{131}I-labeled tositumomab, 60 patients with chemorefractory indolent or transformed CD20-positive B cell NHL received a standard dose of RIT.[140] The ORR was 65 percent (CR 20 percent and PR 45 percent), with a median response duration of 6.5 months. ^{131}I-tositumomab also has been studied in 76 patients with untreated FL, with an ORR of 97 percent (CR 34 percent and PR 63 percent) and a 3-year PFS of 68 percent.[141] As with yttrium-90-labeled ibritumomab, myelosuppression is an important side effect, but only a small portion of patients developed grade 4 cytopenias. The median time for nadir blood count is between 5 weeks and 7 weeks. A phase II trial enrolled 90 patients with previously untreated advanced stage FL.[142] Four to 8 weeks after completion of 6 cycles of CHOP, patients received ^{131}I-tositumomab. Treatment was well tolerated. The overall response rate was 90 percent, with a 67 percent CR and a 23 percent PR. At a median follow-up of 2.3 years, the PFS was 81 percent and overall survival was 97 percent. Randomized trials currently are underway to further evaluate the role of chemotherapy in combination with RIT in patients with advanced FL.

Radioimmunotherapy with anti-CD20-based agents also has been tried in other types of NHL, including DLBCL and MCL. In a recent study in MCL, an ORR of 75 percent (all CR) was obtained with sequential treatment with ^{131}I-tositumomab followed by CHOP chemotherapy. Other RITs that have shown promising results in clinical trials of NHL include ^{131}I-rituximab (i.e., with chimeric anti-CD20) and yttrium-90-labeled epratuzumab (anti-CD22) and Lym-1 (murine anti-HLA-DR10β). For all of these compounds, only limited clinical data are available, and therefore it is impossible to determine the importance of these compounds in the future. Radiolabeled mAbs are an important and promising new class of agents, but only well-designed clinical trials will be able to determine optimal use of RIT in the management of patients with NHL.

Pretargeting radioimmunotherapy

An attractive alternative to direct radiolabeling of mAbs is a pretargeting approach that separates antibody targeting from radionuclide delivery and thus increases the tumor-to-background ratios. In this two-step approach, a mAb conjugate that binds to tumor-associated antigen is given as the first injection. At the time of maximal tumor accretion and circulatory clearance, a low-molecular-weight radioactive ligand that binds to the localized mAb is given as the second injection. The radioactive ligand binds to the recognition site of the tumor-localizing antibody, whereas unbound ligand is cleared from the circulation, thus achieving high tumor-to-blood and tumor-to-normal tissue ratios. This procedure can utilize bifunctional mAbs with dual specificity for tumor-associated antigens and radionuclide carriers or biotinylated antibodies or streptavidin-conjugated antibodies that have high affinity for biotin-conjugated radionuclides. In one such approach, preclinical and clinical efficacy in patients with NHL was shown using streptavidin-conjugated anti-CD20 as the first step, followed by ^{90}Y-DOTA (1,4,7,10-tetraazacyclododecane-tetraacetic acid)–biotin. As chemical conjugates of streptavidin and mAbs are difficult to manufacture, single-chain anti-CD20–streptavidin fusion proteins have been constructed as the targeting moiety. In a phase I trial with this construct in patients with NHL, there were two CRs and one PR with encouraging dosimetry, safety, and efficacy.[143]

Drug immunoconjugates

Conjugates of mAbs with small-molecule anticancer drugs have been investigated for many years as a potential approach to delivering these drugs specifically to cancers. In these immunoconjugates, a cytotoxic drug is attached via a linker, which ideally should be stable in circulation but should efficiently cleave in the tumor tissue to release the drug. The drug, mAb, and linker play important roles in the successful design of potent and efficient immunoconjugates. The cytotoxic agents used in the immunoconjugates should be highly potent because only a limited number of molecules can be loaded on each mAb without diminishing the binding affinity of the mAb moiety. The most frequently used linkers are hydrazone, peptides, and disulfide linkers. Selection of an appropriate linker will depend on the cancer type, mAb, and cytotoxic agent; thus, no linker is universal.

To date, only one drug immunoconjugate, gemtuzumab ozogamicin (Mylotarg®, Wyeth/Celltech group), has been approved for the treatment of AML in elderly patients (at least 60 years of age) in first relapse who are not candidates for other therapies.[144,145] Gemtuzumab ozogamicin is a conjugate of humanized anti-CD33 mAb, hP67.6, linked via an acid-labile linker to a derivative of the potent cytotoxic agent, calicheamicin.[146,147] Calicheamicin belongs to a family of highly cytotoxic enediyne-based agents that bind DNA in the minor groove and cause double-strand DNA breaks, leading to cell death.

A similar calicheamicin conjugate, CMC-544 (Wyeth), currently is being evaluated in clinical trials in patients with NHL (Table 86.2). CMC-544 is composed of calicheamicin conjugated to an internalizing humanized IgG4 anti-CD22 mAb. CMC-544 has shown excellent therapeutic responses in preclinical models of human B cell lymphoma.[101–103]

Other immunoconjugates that have utilized highly potent drugs include SGN-35 (Seattle Genetics) (Table 86.2), an immunoconjugate of monomethyl auristatin E (MMAE) and cAC10 (anti-CD30 mAb). MMAE is a synthetic analogue of a natural product dolastatin 10 that works via inhibition of tubulin polymerization. MMAE linked via an enzyme-cleavable protease-sensitive diapeptide (valine-citrulline) linker to cAC10 demonstrated potent and selective cytotoxicity against CD30-positive tumor lines. Release of MMAE into the cytosol induced G2/M-phase growth arrest and cell death through the induction of apoptosis. *In vivo* efficacy of cAC10-vcMMAE was demonstrated in SCID mouse xenograft models of ALCL or Hodgkin disease.[148] SGN-35 currently is being evaluated in phase I trials of patients with relapsed Hodgkin lymphoma or other CD30-positive hematologic malignancies. Maytansinoids are highly potent tubulin polymerization inhibitors that have been conjugated to a humanized anti-CD19 mAb, to yield SAR3419 (Immunogen and Sanofi Aventis). SAR3419 is being investigated in phase I trials in patients with relapsed or refractory B cell NHL (Table 86.2).[105]

An approach to delivering moderately potent drugs such as anthracyclines is to use mAbs that bind rapidly internalizing antigens and thus internalize large quantities of drugs inside the cells. One such immunoconjugate, hLL1-DOX (IMMU-110; Immunomedics, Inc.), composed of doxorubicin conjugated to a rapidly internalizing humanized mAb, anti-CD74, using an acid-labile hydrazone linker, has demonstrated excellent preclinical results in xenograft models of human B cell lymphoma and MM (Table 86.2).[106,149] CD74 is a type II transmembrane chaperone molecule that associates with HLA-DR and can internalize up to 8×10^6 anti-CD74 molecules per cell per day. In xenograft mouse models of NHL (Raji) and MM (MC/CAR), treatment with a single dose of hLL1-DOX as low as 2.5 mg/kg or 5.8 mg/kg protein-equivalent dose, respectively, 5 days after injection of cells, resulted in a cure of most mice.[106,149] In CD74-positive cynomolgus monkeys, the conjugate was well tolerated up to a dose of 30 mg/kg, thus demonstrating a good therapeutic window of the conjugate in preclinical studies. The clinical significance of this immunoconjugate remains to be evaluated.[106]

Immunotoxins

Immunotoxins are antibody–toxin chimeric molecules that kill cancer cells via binding to a surface antigen, with internalization and delivery of the toxin moiety to the cell cytosol. In the cytosol, toxins kill cells by inactivating protein synthesis, resulting in cell death. The toxins are derived from plants or bacteria, and some commonly used toxins are *Pseudomonas* exotoxin, ricin, or diphtheria. These toxins are extremely potent; in most cases, a single molecule in the appropriate compartment inside the cell is sufficient to kill the cell. Toxins generally are modified to improve their selectivity for target cancer cells and are often deglycosylated to avoid rapid clearance by hepatocytes expressing mannose receptors.

Conventional immunotoxins contained mAbs chemically conjugated to a mutated or modified toxin. Examples of such immunotoxins included anti-CD19 or anti-CD22 antibodies conjugated to ricin A-chain (RTA) or gelonin and saporin. Although these agents demonstrated impressive preclinical results, and in some cases were able to induce responses in patients, their application was compromised due to DLT including vascular leak syndrome, thrombocytopenia, hepatic damage, and immunogenicity.[150,151] To circumvent some of these issues, more recent immunotoxins are made of recombinant ligands fused to truncated toxin units. Two examples of such immunotoxins used in hematologic cancers include RFB4(dsFv)-PE38 (BL22) and anti-Tac(Fv)-PE38 (LMB-2), targeting CD22 and CD25, respectively, in which Fvs of mAbs targeting these antigens are fused to truncated *Pseudomonas* exotoxin.[152]

BL22 (RFB4[dsFV]-PE38) is composed of the variable domains of the anti-CD22 mAb, RFB4, fused to a 38 kDa portion of toxin *Pseudomonas* exotoxin (PE38) (Table 86.2).[153] Following internalization, the adenosine diphosphate-ribosylating domain of PE38 separates from the antibody subunit and inhibits elongation factor 2 and protein synthesis, eventually leading to tumor cell killing. BL22 currently is being evaluated for the treatment of B cell lymphomas, HCL, and promyelocytic leukemia. In a recent phase I trial, BL22 was active in HCL in 31 patients, with 19 CRs (61 percent) and six PRs (19 percent).[107]

Lower but significant activity also occurred in CLL. Results from a US phase II trial of Cambridge Antibody Technologies' CAT-3888 (BL22) were presented at the 43rd Annual Meeting of the American Society of Clinical Oncology.[108] During this study, 35 patients with chemoresistant HCL were treated with CAT-3888. Eligible patients had relapsed HCL less than 4 years after prior cladribine (CdA) therapy. The activity of CAT-3888 in CdA-resistant HCL was confirmed with high CR and OR rates. CAT-3888 response was higher in patients without splenectomy and with mild–moderate splenomegaly. The only serious toxicity was completely reversible grade 3 hemolytic uremic syndrome (not requiring plasmapheresis) in one patient.

LMB-2 is composed of variable light and heavy chains of anti-CD25 mAb, anti-Tac, fused to PE38 (Table 86.2). LMB-2 was tested in patients with CD25-positive, chemotherapy-resistant lymphoid malignancies.[109] Objective responses were obtained in chemotherapy-resistant patients with HCL, CLL, Hodgkin disease, and CTCL. Phase II trials are ongoing in patients with CD25-positive CLL and CTCL.[110]

Members of the pancreatic ribonuclease family also have been explored as an alternative to bacterial and plant toxins. A unique member of this family, Onconase® (ranpirnase), was isolated from *Rana pipiens* oocytes. Once internalized into the cytosol, Onconase® selectively degrades transfer ribonucleic acid (tRNA), inducing inhibition of protein synthesis and induction of apoptosis. Immunotoxins made by chemically conjugating Onconase® and anti-CD22 were demonstrated to be potent and specific in cell culture and efficacious in SCID mice containing disseminated Daudi B cell lymphoma.[111] In another study, CD74-targeted recombinant immunotoxin containing two molecules of ranpirnase was shown to have curative therapeutic effects at doses as low as 5 μg/mouse in animal models of human B cell lymphoma.[112] Although Onconase® is an amphibian protein, no immunogenicity-related problems associated with repeated administration in humans have been reported.[154]

IMMUNOLIPOSOMES

Targeting via immunoliposomes relies on encapsulating chemotherapeutics or gene therapeutics into liposomes and targeting via mAbs attached at the liposome surface or to the terminus of polymers such as polyethylene glycol (PEG) that are attached at the liposome surface. The mAbs promote the selective binding of the liposomes to tumor-associated antigens or receptors, the liposome drug package is internalized intracellularly, and the drug is released. Up to several thousand drug molecules can be entrapped in a single liposome, and this drug-liposome package can be delivered to target cells via only a few antibody molecules. Immunoliposomal doxorubicin and vincristine targeted against the B cell antigens CD19 and CD20 have demonstrated efficacy in xenograft models of human B cell lymphoma (Table 86.2).[155,156] In these models, immunoliposomal drugs were shown to have better efficacy than nontargeted liposomes, free drugs, or naked mAbs. In these studies, targeting against internalizing epitopes was better than against noninternalizing epitopes for schedule-independent drugs having slow release rate from liposomes (e.g., doxorubicin).[157] For immunoliposomes containing the high-potency, cell cycle-dependent drug, vincristine, targeting to either internalizing or noninternalizing epitopes appeared to be equally efficacious. In other reports, immunoliposomal doxorubicin, targeted via an anti-idiotype antibody to murine B cell lymphoma, also prolonged survival in mice compared to nontargeted liposomes or free doxorubicin.[158] In another study, anti-CD19-targeted liposomes containing imatinib (Gleevac®) were demonstrated to be superior to free imatinib in primary ALL cells from four patients.[159] Immunoliposomal anticancer drugs have yet to be evaluated in a clinical setting.

CONCLUSIONS

Modern immunological-based therapies such as mAbs, RIT, and drug immunoconjugates have the potential to alter the natural history of lymphoid neoplasms. Recent results from phase III trials in patients with NHL show improvements in PFS and overall survival for patients treated with combinations of the anti-CD20 antibody, rituximab, compared to chemotherapy alone. The role of maintenance rituximab in the management of NHL is still unclear. It remains to be seen if the new generation of specifically tailored anti-CD20 antibodies (e.g., modified ADCC and CDC functions) have an improved therapeutic index. Clinically meaningful activities have been determined targeting various receptors on B and T cells. Only prospective clinical trials will define the role of combination of anti-CD20 antibodies and antibodies directed at other targets (e.g., CD22 or CD80) in the management of lymphoid neoplasms (lymphomas and leukemias). Ongoing clinical trials should define the role of RIT in the management of FL. Since the approval of the first immunodrug conjugate, there has been significant progress in designing novel linkers to improve safety and efficacy of this novel therapeutic. After almost two decades of incremental improvement in the natural history of NHL, there is a significant opportunity for advancement. A search of clinicaltrials.gov revealed approximately 50 ongoing phase III trials of mAbs (rituximab, gemtuzumab ozogamicin, alemtuzumab, and ibritumomab tiuxetan) in patients with lymphomas and leukemias. Therefore, it is critical that investigators continue enrolling patients into definitive clinical trials to further clarify the role of immunotherapeutics in the management of lymphoid neoplasms.

KEY POINTS

- Monoclonal antibodies (mAbs) have broad uses in managing lymphoid malignancies.
- Monoclonal antibodies that recognize specific markers on the surface of tumor cells can be conjugated with drugs, prodrugs, or radioisotopes, and offer an effective modality that is tumor specific and less toxic than traditional cytotoxic agents.
- Second-generation mAbs are tailored to specific needs based on the modification of size and portion critical for recruiting the immune system.
- Rituximab is a critical component of multiagent front-line therapy for patients with follicular lymphoma and diffuse large B cell lymphoma. Thus, the role of postinduction use of rituximab in patients with non-Hodgkin lymphoma (NHL) has to be determined.
- Ongoing pivotal studies will determine the role of radioimmunotherapy in the management of NHLs.
- Participation in well-defined pivotal studies is critical for future advances in therapy of lymphoid neoplasms.

REFERENCES

● = Key primary paper
◆ = Major review article

1. Macklis RM. Radioimmunotherapy as a therapeutic option for non-Hodgkin's lymphoma. *Semin Radiat Oncol* 2007; **17**: 176–83.
◆2. Abutalib SA, Tallman MS. Monoclonal antibodies for the treatment of acute myeloid leukemia. *Curr Pharm Biotechnol* 2006; **7**: 343–69.
3. Glennie MJ, van de Winkel JG. Renaissance of cancer therapeutic antibodies. *Drug Discov Today* 2003; **8**: 503–10.
4. Fishwild DM, O'Donnell SL, Bengoechea T *et al.* High-avidity human IgG kappa monoclonal antibodies from a novel strain of minilocus transgenic mice. *Nat Biotechnol* 1996; **14**: 845–51.
5. Kretzschmar T, von Rüden T. Antibody discovery: phage display. *Curr Opin Biotechnol* 2002; **13**: 598–602.
6. Mendez MJ, Green LL, Corvalan JR *et al.* Functional transplant of megabase human immunoglobulin loci recapitulates human antibody response in mice. *Nat Genet* 1997; **15**: 146–56.
7. Tomizuka K, Shinohara T, Yoshida H *et al.* Double trans-chromosomic mice: maintenance of two individual human chromosome fragments containing Ig heavy and kappa loci and expression of fully human antibodies. *Proc Natl Acad Sci U S A* 2000; **97**: 722–7.

8. Cumbers SJ, Williams GT, Davies SL *et al.* Generation and iterative affinity maturation of antibodies *in vitro* using hypermutating B-cell lines. *Nat Biotechnol* 2002; **20**: 1129–34.

9. Gram H, Marconi LA, Barbas CF 3rd *et al.* In vitro selection and affinity maturation of antibodies from a naive combinatorial immunoglobulin library. *Proc Natl Acad Sci U S A* 1992; **89**: 3576–80.

10. Griffiths AD, Malmqvist M, Marks JD *et al.* Human anti-self antibodies with high specificity from phage display libraries. *EMBO J* 1993; **12**: 725–34.

11. Ho M, Kreitman RJ, Onda M, Pastan I. In vitro antibody evolution targeting germline hot spots to increase activity of an anti-CD22 immunotoxin. *J Biol Chem* 2005; **280**: 607–17.

12. Yoon SO, Lee TS, Kim SJ *et al.* Construction, affinity maturation, and biological characterization of an anti-tumor-associated glycoprotein-72 humanized antibody. *J Biol Chem* 2006; **281**: 6985–92.

13. Vidarsson G, Stemerding AM, Stapleton NM *et al.* FcRn: an IgG receptor on phagocytes with a novel role in phagocytosis. *Blood* 2006; **108**: 3573–9.

14. Warmerdam PA, Parren PW, Vlug A *et al.* Polymorphism of the human Fc gamma receptor II (CD32): molecular basis and functional aspects. *Immunobiology* 1992; **185**: 175–82.

15. Koene HR, Kleijer M, Algra J *et al.* Fc gammaRIIIa-158V/F polymorphism influences the binding of IgG by natural killer cell Fc gammaRIIIa, independently of the Fc gammaRIIIa-48L/R/H phenotype. *Blood* 1997; **90**: 1109–14.

16. Wu J, Edberg JC, Redecha PB *et al.* A novel polymorphism of FcgammaRIIIa (CD16) alters receptor function and predisposes to autoimmune disease. *J Clin Invest* 1997; **100**: 1059–70.

17. Ory PA, Goldstein IM, Kwoh EE, Clarkson SB. Characterization of polymorphic forms of Fc receptor III on human neutrophils. *J Clin Invest* 1989; **83**: 1676–81.

18. Bird RE, Hardman KD, Jacobson JW *et al.* Single-chain antigen-binding proteins. *Science* 1988; **242**: 423–6.

19. Coloma MJ, Morrison SL. Design and production of novel tetravalent bispecific antibodies. *Nat Biotechnol* 1997; **15**: 159–63.

20. Müller KM, Arndt KM, Strittmatter W, Plückthun A. The first constant domain (C(H)1 and C(L)) of an antibody used as heterodimerization domain for bispecific miniantibodies. *FEBS Lett* 1998; **422**: 259–64.

21. Holliger P, Prospero T, Winter G. 'Diabodies': small bivalent and bispecific antibody fragments. *Proc Natl Acad Sci U S A* 1993; **90**: 6444–8.

22. Hamers-Casterman C, Atarhouch T, Muyldermans S *et al.* Naturally occurring antibodies devoid of light chains. *Nature* 1993; **363**: 446–8.

23. Greenberg AS, Avila D, Hughes M *et al.* A new antigen receptor gene family that undergoes rearrangement and extensive somatic diversification in sharks. *Nature* 1995; **374**: 168–73.

24. Nuttall SD, Irving RA, Hudson PJ. Immunoglobulin VH domains and beyond: design and selection of single-domain binding and targeting reagents. *Curr Pharm Biotechnol* 2000; **1**: 253–63.

25. Cortez-Retamozo V, Backmann N, Senter PD *et al.* Efficient cancer therapy with a nanobody-based conjugate. *Cancer Res* 2004; **64**: 2853–7.

26. Almasri NM, Duque RE, Iturraspe J *et al.* Reduced expression of CD20 antigen as a characteristic marker for chronic lymphocytic leukemia. *Am J Hematol* 1992; **40**: 259–63.

27. Ginaldi L, De Martinis M, Matutes E *et al.* Levels of expression of CD19 and CD20 in chronic B cell leukaemias. *J Clin Pathol* 1998; **51**: 364–9.

28. Anderson KC, Bates MP, Slaughenhoupt BL *et al.* Expression of human B cell-associated antigens on leukemias and lymphomas: a model of human B cell differentiation. *Blood* 1984; **63**: 1424–33.

29. Manshouri T, Do KA, Wang X *et al.* Circulating CD20 is detectable in the plasma of patients with chronic lymphocytic leukemia and is of prognostic significance. *Blood* 2002; **101**: 2507–13.

30. Demidem A, Lam T, Alas S *et al.* Chimeric anti-CD20 (IDEC-C2B8) monoclonal antibody sensitizes a B cell lymphoma cell line to cell killing by cytotoxic drugs. *Cancer Biother Radiopharm* 1997; **12**: 177–86.

●31. McLaughlin P, Grillo-López AJ, Link BK *et al.* Rituximab chimeric anti-CD20 monoclonal antibody therapy for relapsed indolent lymphoma: half of patients respond to a four-dose treatment program. *J Clin Oncol* 1998; **16**: 2825–33.

32. Bremer K. Semi-extended, six weekly rituximab infusions in pre-treated advanced low-grade B cell non-Hodgkin's lymphoma: a phase II study. *Anticancer Drugs* 2003; **14**: 809–15.

33. Piro LD, White CA, Grillo-López AJ *et al.* Extended rituximab (anti-CD20 monoclonal antibody) therapy for relapsed or refractory low-grade or follicular non-Hodgkin's lymphoma. *Ann Oncol* 1999; **10**: 655–61.

34. Berinstein NL, Grillo-López AJ, White CA *et al.* Association of serum rituximab (IDEC-C2B8) concentration and anti-tumor response in the treatment of recurrent low-grade or follicular non-Hodgkin's lymphoma. *Ann Oncol* 1998; **9**: 995–1001.

35. Hainsworth JD, Litchy S, Burris HA 3rd *et al.* Rituximab as first-line and maintenance therapy for patients with indolent non-Hodgkin's lymphoma. *J Clin Oncol* 2002; **20**: 4261–7.

36. Hainsworth JD, Litchy S, Barton JH *et al.* Single-agent rituximab as first-line and maintenance treatment for patients with chronic lymphocytic leukemia or small lymphocytic lymphoma: a phase II trial of the Minnie Pearl Cancer Research Network. *J Clin Oncol* 2003; **21**: 1746–51.

37. Hainsworth JD, Litchy S, Shaffer DW *et al.* Maximizing therapeutic benefit of rituximab: maintenance therapy versus re-treatment at progression in patients with

indolent non-Hodgkin's lymphoma – a randomized phase II trial of the Minnie Pearl Cancer Research Network. *J Clin Oncol* 2005; **23**: 1088–95.

38.   Ghielmini M, Rufibach K, Salles G *et al.* Single agent rituximab in patients with follicular or mantle cell lymphoma: clinical and biological factors that are predictive of response and event-free survival as well as the effect of rituximab on the immune system: a study of the Swiss Group for Clinical Cancer Research (SAKK). *Ann Oncol* 2005; **16**: 1675–82.

39.   Ghielmini M, Schmitz SF, Cogliatti SB *et al.* Prolonged treatment with rituximab in patients with follicular lymphoma significantly increases event-free survival and response duration compared with the standard weekly x 4 schedule. *Blood* 2004; **103**: 4416–23.

●40.   Jazirehi AR, Vega MI, Bonavida B. Development of rituximab-resistant lymphoma clones with altered cell signaling and cross-resistance to chemotherapy. *Cancer Res* 2007; **67**: 1270–81.

41.   Ansell SM, Witzig TE, Kurtin PJ *et al.* Phase 1 study of interleukin-12 in combination with rituximab in patients with B-cell non-Hodgkin lymphoma. *Blood* 2002; **99**: 67–74.

42.   Ansell SM, Geyer SM, Maurer MJ *et al.* Randomized phase II study of interleukin-12 in combination with rituximab in previously treated non-Hodgkin's lymphoma patients. *Clin Cancer Res* 2006; **12**: 6056–63.

43.   Friedberg JW, Neuberg D, Gribben JG *et al.* Combination immunotherapy with rituximab and interleukin 2 in patients with relapsed or refractory follicular non-Hodgkin's lymphoma. *Br J Haematol* 2002; **117**: 828–34.

44.   Friedberg JW, Kim H, McCauley M *et al.* Combination immunotherapy with a CpG oligonucleotide (1018 ISS) and rituximab in patients with non-Hodgkin lymphoma: increased interferon-α/β-inducible gene expression, without significant toxicity. *Blood* 2005; **105**: 489–95.

45.   Kimby E, Jurlander J, Geisler C *et al.* Long-term molecular remissions in patients with indolent lymphoma treated with rituximab as a single agent or in combination with interferon alpha-2a: A randomized phase II study from the Nordic Lymphoma Group. *Leuk Lymphoma* 2008; **49**: 102–12.

46.   van der Kolk LE, Grillo-López AJ, Baars JW, van Oers MH. Treatment of relapsed B-cell non-Hodgkin's lymphoma with a combination of chimeric anti-CD20 monoclonal antibodies (rituximab) and G-CSF: final report on safety and efficacy. *Leukemia* 2003; **17**: 1658–64.

◆47.   Buske C, Weigert O, Dreyling M *et al.* Current status and perspective of antibody therapy in follicular lymphoma. *Haematologica* 2006; **91**: 104–12.

48.   Coiffier B. Unanswered questions in follicular lymphoma. *Oncology* 2008; **22**: 33–4.

49.   Hainsworth JD. Critical questions about rituximab maintenance in lymphoma patients. *Oncology* 2008; **22**; 26–9.

50.   Maloney DG. What is the role of maintenance rituximab in follicular NHL? *Oncology* 2008; **22**; 20–6.

51.   Freim Wahl SG, Folvik MR, Torp SH. Progressive multifocal leukoencephalopathy in a lymphoma patient with complete remission after treatment with cytostatics and rituximab: case report and review of the literature. *Clin Neuropathol* 2007; **26**: 68–73.

52.   Perceau G, Diris N, Estines O *et al.* Late lethal hepatitis B virus reactivation after rituximab treatment of low-grade cutaneous B-cell lymphoma. *Br J Dermatol* 2006; **155**: 1053–6.

53.   Aksoy S, Harputluoglu H, Kilickap S *et al.* Rituximab-related viral infections in lymphoma patients. *Leuk Lymphoma* 2007; **48**: 1307–12.

54.   Czuczman MS, Grillo-López AJ, White CA *et al.* Treatment of patients with low-grade B-cell lymphoma with the combination of chimeric anti-CD20 monoclonal antibody and CHOP chemotherapy. *J Clin Oncol* 1999; **17**: 268–76.

●55.   Czuczman MS, Weaver R, Alkuzweny B *et al.* Prolonged clinical and molecular remission in patients with low-grade or follicular non-Hodgkin's lymphoma treated with rituximab plus CHOP chemotherapy: 9-year follow-up. *J Clin Oncol* 2004; **22**: 4711–6.

56.   Herold M, Haas A, Srock S *et al.* Rituximab added to first-line mitoxantrone, chlorambucil, and prednisolone chemotherapy followed by interferon maintenance prolongs survival in patients with advanced follicular lymphoma: an East German Study Group Hematology and Oncology Study. *J Clin Oncol* 2007; **25**: 1986–92.

57.   Hiddemann W, Kneba M, Dreyling M *et al.* Frontline therapy with rituximab added to the combination of cyclophosphamide, doxorubicin, vincristine, and prednisone (CHOP) significantly improves the outcome for patients with advanced-stage follicular lymphoma compared with therapy with CHOP alone: results of a prospective randomized study of the German Low-Grade Lymphoma Study Group. *Blood* 2005; **106**: 3725–32.

58.   Marcus R, Imrie K, Belch A *et al.* CVP chemotherapy plus rituximab compared with CVP as first-line treatment for advanced follicular lymphoma. *Blood* 2005; **105**: 1417–23.

59.   Forstpointner R, Dreyling M, Repp R *et al.* The addition of rituximab to a combination of fludarabine, cyclophosphamide, mitoxantrone (FCM) significantly increases the response rate and prolongs survival as compared with FCM alone in patients with relapsed and refractory follicular and mantle cell lymphomas: results of a prospective randomized study of the German Low-Grade Lymphoma Study Group. *Blood* 2004; **104**: 3064–71.

60.   Hochster H, Weller E, Gascovne RD *et al.* Maintenance rituximab after cyclophosphamide, vincristine, and prednisone prolongs progression-free survival in advanced indolent lymphoma: results of the randomized phase III ECOG1496 Study. *J Clin Oncol* 2009; **27**: 1607–14.

61.   van Oers MH, Klasa R, Marcus RE *et al.* Rituximab maintenance improves clinical outcome of relapsed/resistant follicular non-Hodgkin lymphoma

in patients both with and without rituximab during induction: results of a prospective randomized phase 3 intergroup trial. *Blood* 2006; **108**: 3295–301.

62. Marcus R, Hagenbeek A. The therapeutic use of rituximab in non-Hodgkin's lymphoma. *Eur J Haematol* 2007; **78**(Suppl 67): 5–14.

63. Coiffier B. Monoclonal antibodies in the treatment of indolent lymphomas. *Best Pract Res Clin Haematol* 2005; **18**: 69–80.

64. Cheson BD. Monoclonal antibody therapy of chronic lymphocytic leukemia. *Cancer Immunol Immunother* 2006; **55**: 188–96.

65. Dimopoulos MA, Zervas C, Zomas A *et al.* Treatment of Waldenström's macroglobulinemia with rituximab. *J Clin Oncol* 2002; **20**: 2327–33.

66. Coiffier B, Lepage E, Briere J *et al.* CHOP chemotherapy plus rituximab compared with CHOP alone in elderly patients with diffuse large-B-cell lymphoma. *N Engl J Med* 2002; **346**: 235–42.

◆67. Coiffier B. Current strategies for the treatment of diffuse large B cell lymphoma. *Curr Opin Hematol* 2005; **12**: 259–65.

68. Feugier P, Van Hoof A, Sebban C *et al.* Long-term results of the R-CHOP study in the treatment of elderly patients with diffuse large B-cell lymphoma: a study by the Groupe d'Etude des Lymphomes de l'Adulte. *J Clin Oncol* 2005; **23**: 4117–26.

69. Pfreundschuh M, Trümper L, Osterborg A *et al.* CHOP-like chemotherapy plus rituximab versus CHOP-like chemotherapy alone in young patients with good-prognosis diffuse large-B-cell lymphoma: a randomised controlled trial by the MabThera International Trial (MInT) Group. *Lancet Oncol* 2006; **7**: 379–91.

70. Habermann TM, Weller EA, Morrison VA *et al.* Rituximab-CHOP versus CHOP alone or with maintenance rituximab in older patients with diffuse large-B-cell lymphoma. *J Clin Oncol* 2006; **24**: 3121–7.

●71. Lenz G, Dreyling M, Hoster E *et al.* Immunochemotherapy with rituximab and cyclophosphamide, doxorubicin, vincristine, and prednisone significantly improves response and time to treatment failure, but not long-term outcome in patients with previously untreated mantle cell lymphoma: results of a prospective randomized trial of the German Low Grade Lymphoma Study Group (GLSG). *J Clin Oncol* 2005; **23**: 1984–92.

72. Romaguera JE, Fayad L, Rodriguez MA *et al.* High rate of durable remissions after treatment of newly diagnosed aggressive mantle-cell lymphoma with rituximab plus hyper-CVAD alternating with rituximab plus high-dose methotrexate and cytarabine. *J Clin Oncol* 2005; **23**: 7013–23.

73. Goy A. Mantle cell lymphoma: evolving novel options. *Curr Oncol Rep* 2007; **9**: 391–8.

74. Thomas DA, Faderl S, O'Brien S *et al.* Chemoimmunotherapy with hyper-CVAD plus rituximab for the treatment of adult Burkitt and Burkitt-type lymphoma or acute lymphoblastic leukemia. *Cancer* 2006; **106**: 1569–80.

75. Attias D, Weitzman S. The efficacy of rituximab in high-grade pediatric B-cell lymphoma/leukemia: a review of available evidence. *Curr Opin Pediatr* 2008; **20**: 17–22.

76. Gökbuget N, Hoelzer D. Novel antibody-based therapy for acute lymphoblastic leukaemia. *Best Pract Res Clin Haematol* 2006; **19**: 701–13.

77. van Besien K, Ha CS, Murphy S *et al.* Risk factors, treatment, and outcome of central nervous system recurrence in adults with intermediate-grade and immunoblastic lymphoma. *Blood* 1998; **91**: 1178–84.

78. Rubenstein JL, Fridlyand J, Abrey L *et al.* Phase I study of intraventricular administration of rituximab in patients with recurrent CNS and intraocular lymphoma. *J Clin Oncol* 2007; **25**: 1350–6.

●79. Teeling JL, French RR, Cragg MS *et al.* Characterization of new human CD20 monoclonal antibodies with potent cytolytic activity against non-Hodgkin lymphomas. *Blood* 2004; **104**: 1793–800.

●80. Vugmeyster Y, Beyer J, Howell K *et al.* Depletion of B cells by a humanized anti-CD20 antibody PRO70769 in Macaca fascicularis. *J Immunother* 2005; **28**: 212–19.

●81. Stein R, Qu Z, Chen S *et al.* Characterization of a new humanized anti-CD20 monoclonal antibody, IMMU-106, and Its use in combination with the humanized anti-CD22 antibody, epratuzumab, for the therapy of non-Hodgkin's lymphoma. *Clin Cancer Res* 2004; **10**: 2868–78.

82. Tahir H, Rohrer J, Bhatia A *et al.* Humanized anti-CD20 monoclonal antibody in the treatment of severe resistant systemic lupus erythematosus in a patient with antibodies against rituximab. *Rheumatology (Oxford)* 2005; **44**: 561–2.

●83. Keating MJ, Flinn I, Jain V *et al.* Therapeutic role of alemtuzumab (Campath-1H) in patients who have failed fludarabine: results of a large international study. *Blood* 2002; **99**: 3554–61.

84. Lin TS, Flinn IW, Modali R *et al.* FCGR3A and FCGR2A polymorphisms may not correlate with response to alemtuzumab in chronic lymphocytic leukemia. *Blood* 2005; **105**: 289–91.

85. Ravandi F, O'Brien S. Alemtuzumab in CLL and other lymphoid neoplasms. *Cancer Invest* 2006; **24**: 718–25.

86. Lundin J, Kimby E, Björkholm M *et al.* Phase II trial of subcutaneous anti-CD52 monoclonal antibody alemtuzumab (Campath-1H) as first-line treatment for patients with B-cell chronic lymphocytic leukemia (B-CLL). *Blood* 2002; **100**: 768–73.

●87. Wierda WG, Kipps TJ, Keating MJ. Novel immune-based treatment strategies for chronic lymphocytic leukemia. *J Clin Oncol* 2005; **23**: 6325–32.

88. Elter T, Borchmann P, Schulz H *et al.* Fludarabine in combination with alemtuzumab is effective and feasible in patients with relapsed or refractory B-cell chronic lymphocytic leukemia: results of a phase II trial. *J Clin Oncol* 2005; **23**: 7024–31.

89. Montillo M, Tedeschi A, Miqueleiz S *et al.* Alemtuzumab as consolidation after a response to fludarabine is effective in purging residual disease in patients with

chronic lymphocytic leukemia. *J Clin Oncol* 2006; **24**: 2337–42.

90. Dearden C. The role of alemtuzumab in the management of T-cell malignancies. *Semin Oncol* 2006; **33**(2 Suppl 5): S44–52.

●91. Gallamini A, Zaja F, Patti C *et al.* Alemtuzumab (Campath-1H) and CHOP chemotherapy as first-line treatment of peripheral T-cell lymphoma: results of a GITIL (Gruppo Italiano Terapie Innovative nei Linfomi) prospective multicenter trial. *Blood* 2007; **110**: 2316–23.

92. Stock W, Yu D, Sanford B *et al.* Incorporation of alemtuzumab into frontline therapy adult acute lymphoblastic leukemia (ALL) is feasible: a phase I/II study from the Cancer and Leukemia Group B (CALGB 10102). *Blood* 2005; **106**: 145 (abstract).

●93. Leonard JP, Coleman M, Ketas JC *et al.* Epratuzumab, a humanized anti-CD22 antibody, in aggressive non-Hodgkin's lymphoma: phase I/II clinical trial results. *Clin Cancer Res* 2004; **10**: 5327–34.

94. Leonard JP, Coleman M, Ketas J *et al.* Combination antibody therapy with epratuzumab and rituximab in relapsed or refractory non-Hodgkin's lymphoma. *J Clin Oncol* 2005; **23**: 5044–51.

95. Micallef IN, Kahl BS, Maurer MJ *et al.* A pilot study of epratuzumab and rituximab in combination with cyclophosphamide, doxorubicin, vincristine, and prednisone chemotherapy in patients with previously untreated, diffuse large B-cell lymphoma. *Cancer* 2006; **107**: 2826–32.

96. Béné MC. Immunophenotyping of acute leukaemias. *Immunol Lett* 2005; **98**: 9–21.

97. Raetz EA, Cairo MS, Borowitz MJ *et al.* Chemoimmunotherapy reinduction with epratuzumab in children with acute lymphoblastic leukemia in marrow relapse: a Children's Oncology Group Pilot Study. *J Clin Oncol* 2008; **26**: 3756–62.

98. Suvas S, Singh V, Sahdev S *et al.* Distinct role of CD80 and CD86 in the regulation of the activation of B cell and B cell lymphoma. *J Biol Chem* 2002; **277**: 7766–75.

99. Leonard JP, Friedberg JW, Younes A *et al.* A phase I/II study of galiximab (an anti-CD80 monoclonal antibody) in combination with rituximab for relapsed or refractory, follicular lymphoma. *Ann Oncol* 2007; **18**: 1216–23.

100. Cresswell P. Assembly, transport, and function of MHC class II molecules. *Annu Rev Immunol* 1994; **12**: 259–93.

101. DiJoseph JF, Dougher MM, Kalyandrug LB *et al.* Antitumor efficacy of a combination of CMC-544 (inotuzumab ozogamicin), a CD22-targeted cytotoxic immunoconjugate of calicheamicin, and rituximab against non-Hodgkin's B-cell lymphoma. *Clin Cancer Res* 2006; **12**: 242–9.

102. DiJoseph JF, Goad ME, Dougher MM *et al.* Potent and specific antitumor efficacy of CMC-544, a CD22-targeted immunoconjugate of calicheamicin, against systemically disseminated B-cell lymphoma. *Clin Cancer Res* 2004; **10**: 8620–9.

103. DiJoseph JF, Popplewell A, Tickle S *et al.* Antibody-targeted chemotherapy of B-cell lymphoma using calicheamicin conjugated to murine or humanized antibody against CD22. *Cancer Immunol Immunother* 2005; **54**: 11–24.

104. Younes A, Forero-Torres A, Bartlett N *et al.* Multiple complete responses in a phase 1 dose-escalation study of the antibody-drug conjugate, SGN-35 in patients with relapsed or refractory CD30-positive lymphomas. *Blood* 2008; **112**: 370a (abstract 1006).

105. Aboukameel A, Goustin A, Mohammad R *et al.* Superior anti-tumor activity of the CD19-directed immunotoxin, SAR3419 to rituximab in non-Hodgkin's xenograft animal models: preclinical evaluation. *Blood* 2007; **110**: 2339 (abstract).

106. Sapra P, Stein R, Pickett J *et al.* Anti-CD74 antibody-doxorubicin conjugate, IMMU-110, in a human multiple myeloma xenograft and in monkeys. *Clin Cancer Res* 2005; **11**: 5257–64.

107. Kreitman RJ, Squires DR, Stetler-Stevenson M *et al.* Phase I trial of recombinant immunotoxin RFB4(dsFv)-PE38 (BL22) in patients with B-cell malignancies. *J Clin Oncol* 2005; **23**: 6719–29.

108. Kreitman RJ, Wilson WH, Stetler-Stevenson M *et al.* Phase II trial of CAT-3888 (BL22) in chemo-resistant hairy cell leukemia. *J Clin Oncol* 2007; **25**: 7095 (abstract).

109. Kreitman RJ, Wilson WH, White JD *et al.* Phase I trial of recombinant immunotoxin anti-Tac(Fv)-PE38 (LMB-2) in patients with hematologic malignancies. *J Clin Oncol* 2000; **18**: 1622–36.

110. Kreitman RJ, Pastan I. Immunotoxins in the treatment of hematologic malignancies. *Curr Drug Targets* 2006; **7**: 1301–11.

111. Newton DL, Hansen HJ, Mikulski SM *et al.* Potent and specific antitumor effects of an anti-CD22-targeted cytotoxic ribonuclease: potential for the treatment of non-Hodgkin lymphoma. *Blood* 2001; **97**: 528–35.

112. Chang CH, Sapra P, Vanama SS *et al.* Effective therapy of human lymphoma xenografts with a novel recombinant ribonuclease/anti-CD74 humanized IgG4 antibody immunotoxin. *Blood* 2005; **106**: 4308–14.

113. Mølhøj M, Crommer S, Brischwein K *et al.* CD19-/CD3-bispecific antibody of the BiTE class is far superior to tandem diabody with respect to redirected tumor cell lysis. *Mol Immunol* 2007; **44**: 1935–43.

114. Schlereth B, Quadt C, Dreier T *et al.* T-cell activation and B-cell depletion in chimpanzees treated with a bispecific anti-CD19/anti-CD3 single-chain antibody construct. *Cancer Immunol Immunother* 2006; **55**: 503–14.

115. Cheng WW, Allen TM. Targeted delivery of anti-CD19 liposomal doxorubicin in B-cell lymphoma: A comparison of whole monoclonal antibody, Fab' fragments and single chain Fv. *J Control Release* 2008; **126**: 50–8.

116. Stein R, Mattes MJ, Cardillo TM *et al.* CD74: a new candidate target for the immunotherapy of B-cell neoplasms. *Clin Cancer Res* 2007; **13**(18 Pt 2): 5556s–63s.

117. Rech J, Repp R, Rech D *et al.* A humanized HLA-DR antibody (hu1D10, apolizumab) in combination with granulocyte colony-stimulating factor (filgrastim) for the

treatment of non-Hodgkin's lymphoma: a pilot study. *Leuk Lymphoma* 2006; **47**: 2147–54.

118. Wahl AF, Klussman K, Thompson JD *et al.* The anti-CD30 monoclonal antibody SGN-30 promotes growth arrest and DNA fragmentation in vitro and affects antitumor activity in models of Hodgkin's disease. *Cancer Res* 2002; **62**: 3736–42.

119. Bartlett NL, Younes A, Carabisi MH *et al.* A phase 1 multidose study of SGN-30 immunotherapy in patients with refractory or recurrent CD30+ hematologic malignancies, *Blood* 2008; **111**: 1848–54.

120. Ansell SM, Horwitz SM, Engert A *et al.* Phase I/II study of an anti-CD30 monoclonal antibody (MDX-060) in Hodgkin's lymphoma and anaplastic large-cell lymphoma. *J Clin Oncol* 2007; **25**: 2764–9.

121. Law CL, Gordon KA, Collier J *et al.* Preclinical antilymphoma activity of a humanized anti-CD40 monoclonal antibody, SGN-40. *Cancer Res* 2005; **65**: 8331–8.

122. Luqman M, Klabunde S, Lin K *et al.* The antileukemia activity of a human anti-CD40 antagonist antibody, HCD122, on human chronic lymphocytic leukemia cells. *Blood* 2008; **112**: 711–20.

123. Ghetie MA, Ghetie V, Vitetta ES. Anti-CD19 antibodies inhibit the function of the P-gp pump in multidrug-resistant B lymphoma cells. *Clin Cancer Res* 1999; **5**: 3920–7.

124. Matsumoto AK, Kopicky-Burd J, Carter RH *et al.* Intersection of the complement and immune systems: a signal transduction complex of the B lymphocyte-containing complement receptor type 2 and CD19. *J Exp Med* 1991; **173**: 55–64.

125. Tedder TF, Inaoki M, Sato S. The CD19-CD21 complex regulates signal transduction thresholds governing humoral immunity and autoimmunity. *Immunity* 1997; **6**: 107–18.

126. Tedder TF, Zhou LJ, Engel P. The CD19/CD21 signal transduction complex of B lymphocytes. *Immunol Today* 1994; **15**: 437–42.

127. Assaf C, Sterry W. Drug evaluation: zanolimumab, a human monoclonal antibody targeted against CD4. *Curr Opin Mol Ther* 2007; **9**: 197–203.

128. Rider DA, Havenith CE, de Ridder R *et al.* A human CD4 monoclonal antibody for the treatment of T-cell lymphoma combines inhibition of T-cell signaling by a dual mechanism with potent Fc-dependent effector activity. *Cancer Res* 2007; **67**: 9945–53.

129. Kim YH, Duvic M, Obitz E *et al.* Clinical efficacy of zanolimumab (HuMax-CD4): two phase 2 studies in refractory cutaneous T-cell lymphoma. *Blood* 2007; **109**: 4655–62.

130. Stopeck AT, Unger JM, Rimsza LM *et al.* A phase II trial of single agent bevacizumab in patients with relapsed, aggressive non-Hodgkin lymphoma: Southwest oncology group study S0108. *Leuk Lymphoma* 2009; **50**: 728–35.

131. Mateo V, Lagneaux L, Bron D *et al.* CD47 ligation induces caspase-independent cell death in chronic lymphocytic leukemia. *Nat Med* 1999; **5**: 1277–84.

132. Uno S, Kinoshita Y, Azuma Y *et al.* Antitumor activity of a monoclonal antibody against CD47 in xenograft models of human leukemia. *Oncol Rep* 2007; **17**: 1189–94.

133. Kikuchi Y, Uno S, Kinoshita Y *et al.* Apoptosis inducing bivalent single-chain antibody fragments against CD47 showed antitumor potency for multiple myeloma. *Leuk Res* 2005; **29**: 445–50.

134. Kikuchi Y, Uno S, Yoshimura Y *et al.* A bivalent single-chain Fv fragment against CD47 induces apoptosis for leukemic cells. *Biochem Biophys Res Commun* 2004; **315**: 912–8.

135. Hartmann F, Renner C, Jung W *et al.* Anti-CD16/CD30 bispecific antibody treatment for Hodgkin's disease: role of infusion schedule and costimulation with cytokines. *Clin Cancer Res* 2001; **7**: 1873–81.

136. Schlenzka J, Moehler TM, Kipriyanov SM *et al.* Combined effect of recombinant CD19 × CD16 diabody and thalidomide in a preclinical model of human B cell lymphoma. *Anticancer Drugs* 2004; **15**: 915–9.

137. Ehrlich P. A general review of the recent work in Immunity. In: Himmelweit F, Marquardt M, Dale H. (eds) *Immunology and cancer research*, Vol. 2. London: Pergamon, 1956: 442–7.

138. Witzig TE, Gordon LI, Cabanillas F *et al.* Randomized controlled trial of yttrium-90-labeled ibritumomab tiuxetan radioimmunotherapy versus rituximab immunotherapy for patients with relapsed or refractory low-grade, follicular, or transformed B-cell non-Hodgkin's lymphoma. *J Clin Oncol* 2002; **20**: 2453–63.

139. Witzig TE, Flinn IW, Gordon LI *et al.* Treatment with ibritumomab tiuxetan radioimmunotherapy in patients with rituximab-refractory follicular non-Hodgkin's lymphoma. *J Clin Oncol* 2002; **20**: 3262–9.

140. Kaminski MS, Zelenetz AD, Press OW *et al.* Pivotal study of iodine I 131 tositumomab for chemotherapy-refractory low-grade or transformed low-grade B-cell non-Hodgkin's lymphomas. *J Clin Oncol* 2001; **19**: 3918–28.

141. Kaminski MS, Tuck M, Estes J *et al.* 131I-tositumomab therapy as initial treatment for follicular lymphoma. *N Engl J Med* 2005; **352**: 441–9.

142. Press OW, Unger JM, Braziel RM *et al.* A phase 2 trial of CHOP chemotherapy followed by tositumomab/iodine I 131 tositumomab for previously untreated follicular non-Hodgkin lymphoma: Southwest Oncology Group Protocol S9911. *Blood* 2003; **102**: 1606–12.

143. Forero A, Weiden PL, Vose JM *et al.* Phase 1 trial of a novel anti-CD20 fusion protein in pretargeted radioimmunotherapy for B-cell non-Hodgkin lymphoma. *Blood* 2004; **104**: 227–36.

144. Bross PF, Beitz J, Chen G *et al.* Approval summary: gemtuzumab ozogamicin in relapsed acute myeloid leukemia. *Clin Cancer Res* 2001; **7**: 1490–6.

145. Mylotarg™ (gemtuzumab ozogamicin for Injection) package insert, 2006. Available at: http://www.fda.gov/cder/foi/label/2006/021174s020lbl.pdf

146. Hamann PR, Hinman LM, Beyer CF *et al.* An anti-CD33 antibody-calicheamicin conjugate for treatment of acute myeloid leukemia. Choice of linker. *Bioconjug Chem* 2002; **13**: 40–6.

147. Hamann PR, Hinman LM, Hollander I *et al.* Gemtuzumab ozogamicin, a potent and selective anti-CD33 antibody-calicheamicin conjugate for treatment of acute myeloid leukemia. *Bioconjug Chem* 2002; **13**: 47–58.

148. Francisco JA, Cerveny CG, Meyer DL *et al.* cAC10-vcMMAE, an anti-CD30-monomethyl auristatin E conjugate with potent and selective antitumor activity. *Blood* 2003; **102**: 1458–65.

149. Griffiths GL, Mattes MJ, Stein R *et al.* Cure of SCID mice bearing human B-lymphoma xenografts by an anti-CD74 antibody-anthracycline drug conjugate. *Clin Cancer Res* 2003; **9**: 6567–71.

150. Sausville EA, Headlee D, Stetler-Stevenson M *et al.* Continuous infusion of the anti-CD22 immunotoxin IgG-RFB4-SMPT-dgA in patients with B-cell lymphoma: a phase I study. *Blood* 1995; **85**: 3457–65.

151. Vitetta ES, Stone M, Amlot P *et al.* Phase I immunotoxin trial in patients with B-cell lymphoma. *Cancer Res* 1991; **51**: 4052–8.

152. Kreitman RJ. Toxin-labeled monoclonal antibodies. *Curr Pharm Biotechnol* 2001; **2**: 313–25.

153. Mansfield E, Amlot P, Pastan I, FitzGerald DJ. Recombinant RFB4 immunotoxins exhibit potent cytotoxic activity for CD22-bearing cells and tumors. *Blood* 1997; **90**: 2020–6.

154. Mikulski SM, Costanzi JJ, Vogelzang NJ *et al.* Phase II trial of a single weekly intravenous dose of ranpirnase in patients with unresectable malignant mesothelioma. *J Clin Oncol* 2002; **20**: 274–81.

155. Lopes de Menezes DE, Pilarski LM, Allen TM. In vitro and in vivo targeting of immunoliposomal doxorubicin to human B-cell lymphoma. *Cancer Res* 1998; **58**: 3320–30.

156. Sapra P, Moase EH, Ma J, Allen TM. Improved therapeutic responses in a xenograft model of human B lymphoma (Namalwa) for liposomal vincristine versus liposomal doxorubicin targeted via anti-CD19 IgG2a or Fab' fragments. *Clin Cancer Res* 2004; **10**: 1100–11.

157. Sapra P, Tyagi P, Allen TM. Ligand-targeted liposomes for cancer treatment. *Curr Drug Deliv* 2005; **2**: 369–81.

158. Tseng YL, Hong RL, Tao MH, Chang FH. Sterically stabilized anti-idiotype immunoliposomes improve the therapeutic efficacy of doxorubicin in a murine B-cell lymphoma model. *Int J Cancer* 1999; **80**: 723–30.

159. Harata M, Soda Y, Tani K *et al.* CD19-targeting liposomes containing imatinib efficiently kill Philadelphia chromosome-positive acute lymphoblastic leukemia cells. *Blood* 2004; **104**: 1442–9.

87

Cellular therapies for lymphoma

CATHERINE M BOLLARD, CLIONA M ROONEY AND HELEN E HESLOP

INTRODUCTION

Adoptive immunotherapy approaches have a defined clinical role in treating relapse of certain malignancies and some types of infection after allogeneic hematopoietic stem cell (HSC) transplantation.[1–5] Because of the success of this approach in this scenario a number of studies are investigating whether immunotherapy approaches may be of benefit in the therapy of lymphoma. This modality of treatment is attractive because patients with lymphoma who do not enter remission or who subsequently relapse are rarely cured using therapy at conventional doses.[6,7] Moreover, nonfatal sequelae of therapy, such as altered somatic growth, infertility, and restrictive lung disease, can seriously affect the quality of life of survivors.[8] It would therefore be desirable to develop novel therapies that could improve disease-free survival in relapsed/refractory patients and might ultimately reduce the incidence of long-term treatment-related complications in all patients. This chapter therefore reviews the current status of adoptive immunotherapy strategies for lymphoma.

TARGETS FOR IMMUNOTHERAPY

A prerequisite for developing immunotherapy approaches is to identify antigens on the tumor cells that might be targets. Advances in genomics have simplified the identification of putative tumor antigens through the use of technologies such as serological analysis of recombinant cDNA expression libraries (SEREX) and new informatics tools to deduce epitopes from candidate genes, which allows screening of candidate peptides. The identification of candidate tumor antigens and the mapping of specific epitopes recognized by $CD4^+$ and $CD8^+$ T cells have facilitated the development of strategies designed to augment tumor antigen-specific T cell responses. If a tumor is to be a target it must not only contain unique proteins capable of providing epitopes for specific immune responses, but also present candidate peptides frequently enough and for sufficient duration to engage responder T cells. In addition, either the tumor cell or a specialized antigen-presenting cell through the process of cross priming must express major histocompatibility complex (MHC) antigens and express costimulatory molecules such as CD28 to induce

Table 87.1 Potential targets for immunotherapy of lymphoma

Target	Examples	Malignancies
Viral antigens	EBV	Non-Hodgkin lymphoma[68]
		Hodgkin disease[84]
	SV40	Non-Hodgkin lymphoma[15]
Differentiation antigen	CD19 or CD20	Non-Hodgkin lymphoma[105]
	CD30	Hodgkin disease[137]
Cancer-testis antigens	MAGE 1	Testicular and many
	NY-ESO	hematologic malignancies[13]
Minor antigens	HA1, HA2	Post-transplant[138]
Tumor-specific antigens	Telomerase	Many types of malignancies[19]
	Idiotype	Non-Hodgkin lymphoma[18,126]

EBV, Epstein–Barr virus; SV40, simian virus 40.

T cell activation. The T cell response is therefore influenced by the type of antigen-presenting cell, which determines if there is effector and memory T cell generation or development of T cell tolerance.[9] CD4 cells also play an important role in providing help for cytotoxic T lymphocytes (CTL) and in the development of memory.[10] There are a number of potential inhibitory factors which may also interfere with the generation of a CTL response *in vivo*[11] and these can potentially be circumvented if CTL are cultured *ex vivo*. However, the adoptively transferred T cell response may not be maintained *in vivo* in the presence of inhibitory factors and cell populations.

Potential antigens for targeting on lymphoma cells fall into several major categories (Table 87.1).

Viral antigens

Many lymphomas are associated with viruses, which will present unique epitopes that are usually highly immunogenic as targets for a T cell response. Latent Epstein–Barr virus (EBV) infection is associated with a heterogeneous group of non-Hodgkin lymphoma (NHL), including Burkitt lymphoma, natural killer (NK)-T lymphomas, and lymphoproliferative disease (LPD) as well as with a subset of Hodgkin disease (HD).[4,12,13] The role of EBV in contributing to lymphomagenesis is well established in the EBV lymphoproliferative diseases that arise in immunosuppressed individuals but it is less well defined in other EBV-associated lymphomas, whether EBV is a contributing factor to oncogenesis or a passenger virus. Nevertheless, the presence of EBV in tumor cells offers a target for immunotherapy approaches. Human herpes virus 8 (HHV-8) is primarily associated with primary effusion lymphoma in patients with acquired immune deficiency syndrome (AIDS) but is also found in some solid lymphomas.[14] Simian virus 40 has also been reported to be detectable in some types of NHL.[15] Unlike most malignant cells, which probably express small

quantities of a single modified peptide as a CTL target, virus-transformed cells may express a range of viral antigens that can be presented for CTL recognition. These cells are therefore potentially much more susceptible to T lymphocyte-mediated immunotherapy than tumor cells transformed by other mechanisms.

Lineage–specific antigens

Another category of targets is differentiation antigens that are selectively expressed in tumor cells. B-lineage antigens such as CD19 and CD20 have been successfully targeted with antibody therapy and preclinical studies have identified peptides that may be targets for T cell recognition.[16] CD30 is highly expressed on Reed-Sternberg cells and anaplastic large cell lymphoma and so is another potential target. Epitopes expressed on membrane-bound but not soluble CD30 have been identified.[17] The presence of immunoglobulin on B cells also provides a potential target and human immunoglobulin-derived peptides derived from framework regions of the variable regions of the immunoglobulin capable of inducing cytotoxic T lymphocyte responses have been identified.[18]

Universal antigens

Several antigens have been identified that are overexpressed in a number of different tumor cells including telomerase and cytochrome P450 1B1.[19,20] Perhaps the most promising target would be an antigen that was also crucial for tumor cell function such as CDC27 or other cell cycle genes.[21]

Cancer-testis antigens

Cancer-testis antigens (CTAs), which are proteins with restricted expression among tumor cells and germinal tissues, are also overexpressed in some cases of lymphoma and have potential to be used as a target for many cancer immunotherapies.[22–25] For example NY-ESO-1 is frequently expressed in poor prognosis B cell malignancies and is capable of eliciting spontaneous humoral and T cell immunity.[26] However, it remains a challenge to expand CTL specific for such tumor antigens *in vitro* to the numbers required for clinical use.

Alloantigens

In the setting of allogeneic bone marrow transplantation (BMT), alloantigens that differ between donor and recipient are targets for T cell recognition. Alloantigens include MHC molecules when donor and recipient are mismatched and minor histocompatibility antigens, which are naturally processed peptides derived from normal cellular proteins where different polymorphisms are present in donor and recipient. A number of minor histocompatibility antigens have been identified, and recent data showing that responses to donor lymphocyte infusions (DLI) correlate with increase in immune responses directed against these antigens confirm their importance.[27,28] In many of these cases, alloreactivity results in graft-versus-host disease (GVHD) as well as graft-versus-leukemia reactions. However, the pattern of tissue expression of minor antigens varies, and those selectively expressed on hemopoietic cells or on particular lineages would provide specific targets for recognition.

TYPES OF ADOPTIVE IMMUNOTHERAPY FOR LYMPHOMA

Cellular immune responses have significant therapeutic potential as evidenced by the graft-versus-lymphoma effect following allogeneic stem cell transplantation for lymphoma which has resulted in reduced relapse rates.[29–32] Minor histocompatibility antigen disparities are presumably important targets of donor T cells with antilymphoma activity in the allogeneic setting, but there may also be a component that is not associated with alloreactivity. Immunotherapy approaches have therefore been evaluated in both the autologous and allogeneic setting.

Autologous nonspecifically expanded T cells

Over the past few years, several studies have correlated faster recovery of lymphocyte counts with improved outcome after autologous transplant for both NHL and HD.[33,34] One group has therefore recently assessed the administration of T cells expanded *ex vivo* using anti-CD3 and anti-CD28 antibodies.[35] These CD3/28 expanded T cells were administered in a dose-escalation study to patients with refractory or relapsed NHL 14 days following high-dose chemotherapy and CD34-selected autologous rescue. Prior to T cell infusion, all patients had severe lymphopenia and T cell dysfunction but, in general, the T cells expanded *ex vivo* had normal function and cytokine secretion profile.[35] Dose-dependent inflammatory-related infusion toxicities were observed. Although a rapid reconstitution of lymphocytes was observed, there were persistent defects in CD4 T cells. Clinical responses included five patients with a complete response, seven patients with a partial response, and four patients with stable disease. At a median follow-up of 33 months, five patients were alive with stable or relapsed disease and three patients remained in complete remission suggesting that the adoptive transfer of autologous CD3/28 stimulated T cells is feasible and relatively safe in heavily pretreated patients with advanced NHL and this approach warrants further study to better assess *in vivo* efficacy.[35]

Expanded cells have also been used in the autologous setting to treat relapse or to augment T cell function

against minimal residual disease. Cytokine-induced killer (CIK) cells are a unique population of CTL with a characteristic $CD3^+CD56^+$ phenotype. In a clinical study, nine patients with advanced HD and NHL were treated with escalating doses of CIK cells. No significant toxicity was seen and there were two partial responses and two patients with stabilization of disease.[36] As these were heavily pretreated patients who had all relapsed post-transplantation, this approach may have greater activity in a setting of minimal residual disease.

Infusion of functional subsets

Another approach to overcome the problem of GVHD is to administer subsets of lymphocytes in the hope that graft-versus-lymphoma (GvL) and GVHD may be separated. In animal models, the culture of functionally defined T cell subsets, such as T cytotoxic 2 (Tc2) or T helper 2 (TH2) cells, has allowed antitumor effects to be produced in the absence of alloreactivity. A trial at the National Institutes of Health (NIH) is currently evaluating the feasibility of infusing donor $CD4^+$ TH2 cells that are generated *in vitro* via CD3/CD28 costimulation in the presence of interleukin (IL)-4 post-transplantation.[37]

Unmanipulated allogeneic T cells (donor lymphocyte infusion)

The ability of DLI to effect antitumor responses was initially described in patients with chronic myeloid leukemia (CML) in hematologic relapse post-allogeneic stem cell transplantation[5] but lymphomas and HD are also sensitive to the effects of DLI.[38–40] In general, response rates are higher in patients with HD or low-grade lymphoma than in those with high-grade lymphoma.[39–41] This modality of therapy is limited by potentially fatal complications that arise from alloreactive T cells also present in the lymphocyte infusion.[5]

The initial reports of successful DLI in the therapy of lymphoma were in patients who developed EBV-associated post-transplant lymphoma (Table 87.2). Investigators from Memorial Sloan-Kettering Cancer Center administered donor lymphocytes to HSC transplant recipients with established EBV-associated lymphoproliferative disease (EBV-LPD).[1] The rationale for this strategy was that this malignancy only occurs in immunosuppressed patients and is normally controlled by an EBV-specific T cell response. Most EBV-seropositive individuals have a high frequency of EBV-specific precursors, so that transfer of unmanipulated donor lymphocyte populations should be able to restore the immune response to EBV. In the Sloan-Kettering experience, the overall response rate was high with 20 of 22 patients attaining complete remissions.[42] Other centers have seen lower response rates to donor leukocyte infusions,[43] which may reflect different patient

Table 87.2   Donor lymphocyte infusion for treatment of PTLD or relapsed lymphoma after HSCT

Study	Number of patients	Type of lymphoma	Product	Results
O'Reilly et al.[42]	22	PTLD	Unmanipulated donor T cells	20 patients responded
Heslop et al.[139]	1	PTLD	Unmanipulated donor T cells	1 patient attained CR
Porter et al.[140]	1	PTLD	Unmanipulated donor T cells	1 patient attained CR
Lucas et al.[43]	12	PTLD	Unmanipulated donor T cells	3 patients attained CR
Sasahara et al.[141]	1	PTLD	Unmanipulated donor T cells	1 patient attained CR
Gross et al.[142]	1	PTLD	Unmanipulated donor T cells	No response
Bonini et al.[50]	2	PTLD	Tk-transduced T cells	1 patient attained CR
Tiberghien et al.[143]	12	PTLD	Tk-transduced T cells	3 of 12 patients treated prophylactically developed PTLD
Peggs et al.[38]	16	Hodgkin disease	Unmanipulated donor T cells	8 CR and 1 PR
Anderlini et al.[144]	9	Hodgkin disease	Unmanipulated donor T cells	4 responses
Marks et al.[40]	13	NHL low grade	Unmanipulated donor T cells	8 of 13 with follicular lymphoma attained CR
Robinson et al.[145]	14	NHL	Unmanipulated donor T cells	10 of 14 responses
Morris et al.[39]	14	NHL	Unmanipulated donor T cells	High grade 2 of 7 responses Low grade 4 of 7 responses Mantle cell 1 of 2 responses
Russell et al.[41]	14	NHL	Unmanipulated donor T cells	High grade 0/5 attained CR Mantle cell 4/4 attained CR Low grade 3/4 attainedCR
Mandigers et al.[46]	7	NHL low grade	Unmanipulated donor T cells	6/7 responses (6 CR, 2 PR)

PTLD, post-transplant lymphoproliferative disease; HSCT, hematopoietic stem cell transplantation; CR, complete remission; PR, partial response; Tk, thymidine kinase; NHL, non-Hodgkin lymphoma.

populations with more advanced disease or suboptimal EBV-specific immune responses in donors.

There have also been several groups who have used DLI for the treatment of residual or recurrent lymphoma following allogeneic stem cell transplantation.[39–41,44,45] Response rates of over 60 percent have been seen in patients with low-grade lymphoma but the response rate in patients with high-grade lymphoma has been low.[39,40,45,46] The existence of significant graft-versus-Hodgkin lymphoma activity following allogeneic transplantation has proven difficult to establish and is probably hindered by the particularly high treatment-related mortality rates in this heavily pretreated patient population. There is evidence from transplant registry-based studies that relapse rates are lower in HD patients who develop GVHD post-allogeneic stem cell transplantation versus those who do not.[47,48] More recently, a study has been reported where 49 patients with relapsed HD were treated with an allogeneic stem cell transplant using a reduced-intensity conditioning regimen, followed by DLI in 16 patients who had residual disease or disease progression post-transplant. Of the 16 patients, six developed severe GVHD (grade III–IV) and five developed chronic GVHD. Nine showed disease responses including eight complete responses.[38] Further investigation of allogeneic approaches in HD as well as NHL are therefore clearly warranted. However, the development of strategies to maximize efficacy and minimize the toxicity of these T cell therapies for the treatment of lymphoma is critical.

T cells transduced with suicide genes

As discussed above, the infusion of an unmanipulated T cell product will contain alloreactive cells, which can induce GVHD. One means of reducing this risk is to transduce the donor T cells with a suicide gene that can be activated if the recipient develops GVHD. The most commonly used suicide gene is herpes simplex virus thymidine kinase (HSV-tk) that renders transduced T cells sensitive to the cytotoxic effects of ganciclovir. HSV-tk-transduced T cells have been evaluated in several clinical trials[49–52] and the preliminary results suggest that GVHD can be effectively controlled by ganciclovir-induced elimination of the transduced T cells. One drawback is that the thymidine kinase suicide gene is virus derived and therefore CTL-mediated immune responses against the genetically modified cells can lead to selective elimination of these cells.[53] In a recent study, seven of 23 patients developed an immune response with detectable thymidine kinase (TK)-specific CD8[+] T cells.[54] To overcome this problem, new nonimmunogenic suicide genes based on inducible Fas and caspase-9 have been developed. These molecules are involved in T cell apoptosis and their activation is dependent on a dimerization process[55-57] that can be activated by a non-toxic chemical inducer of dimerization (CID). Fas and caspase-9 molecules have been fused to a human FK506 binding protein (FKBP) to allow conditional dimerization and in both *in vitro* and *in vivo* studies T cells stably transduced with a retroviral vector coding for the dimerizable gene can be selectively eliminated after the exposure to the CID.[55,57]

A second concern with suicide gene approaches is that the *ex vivo* culture techniques used for transduction may reduce the immune function of the gene-modified T cells.[58] In a phase I study of 12 patients who received donor T cells transduced with the TK gene early post-transplantation, three developed EBV-LPD likely due to impaired EBV reactivity in the product.[58] Current studies are addressing if this defect can be overcome by using CD3 and CD28 costimulation and modifying culture conditions.

Allodepleted T cells

An alternative approach to the problem of alloreactivity is to selectively deplete the T cell product of alloreactive cells expressing activation markers in response to alloantigen. Alloreactive cells express activation markers after exposure to alloantigen, including CD69, CD147, and the IL-2 receptor CD25, which is expressed within the first 24 hours of T cell activation. In a study using a CD25 immunotoxin to deplete alloreactive T cells *ex vivo*, the residual T cells were able to respond in a third party mixed lymphocyte reaction or to viral or myeloid leukemia-associated antigens.[59] Several groups are now initiating clinical trials using this strategy and three studies have been published.[60-62] All studies used a CD25 immunotoxin to selectively deplete cells responding to alloantigen in recipients of haploidentical CD34-selected grafts or HLA-identical sibling transplants.[60-62] The approach was able to promote immune reconstitution and recovery of virus-specific immunity without significant GVHD but it is not yet clear whether there was an antitumor effect.

Antigen-specific T cell therapies

The use of antigen-specific CTL may overcome the problems of alloreactivity and a low frequency of such immune cells in any situation where an antigen recognized by the cytotoxic lymphocytes is known. To generate these cells *ex vivo* requires an antigen-presenting cell that can effectively present the antigen to T cells and a defined antigen. It is therefore a significant challenge to generate T cells specific for tumor antigens in clinical settings where the malignant cell presents antigen poorly, and the putative target antigens are weak. For this reason, initial studies were undertaken targeting type 3 latency EBV antigens where the antigen is highly immunogenic and an excellent antigen-presenting cell is readily available.

T cell therapies targeting Epstein–Barr virus

All EBV-associated malignancies are associated with the virus' latent cycle, and three distinct types of EBV latency have been characterized.[63,64] All are EBV-encoded small RNA (EBER) positive, but the EBV latent protein expression varies. Latency type III is expressed in lymphoblastoid cell lines (LCL), which can be readily produced by infecting B cells *in vitro* with EBV, and is characterized by expression of the entire array of nine EBV latency proteins: EBV nuclear antigens (EBNAs) 1, 2, 3A, 3B, 3C, LP, BARF0, and the two viral membrane proteins latent membrane protein 1 (LMP1) and LMP2. This pattern of EBV gene expression characterizes the EBV-LPDs that occur in individuals severely immunocompromised by solid organ or stem cell transplantation, congenital immunodeficiency, or human immunodeficiency virus (HIV) infection. Latency type II is the hallmark of EBV-positive Hodgkin disease and peripheral T/NK cell lymphomas where a more restricted array of proteins including EBNA1, LMP1, and LMP2 are expressed. In latency type I, found in EBV-positive Burkitt lymphoma, only EBNA1 is expressed. As EBNA1 is not well processed by the class I processing machinery,[65] lymphomas expressing type 1 latency may not be a good target for immunotherapy approaches, although CD4 epitopes have been described in EBNA1 and in a murine model EBNA1-specific CD4 T cells can suppress tumorigenesis.[66] However, immunotherapy approaches targeting EBV antigens do have potential for treating type II and type III latency EBV lymphomas.

EBV-ASSOCIATED LYMPHOMA POSTHEMATOPOIETIC STEM CELL TRANSPLANTATION

Post-transplant LPD is a serious, life-threatening disease and encompasses a heterogeneous group of lymphoproliferative disorders ranging from reactive, polyclonal hyperplasias to aggressive non-Hodgkin lymphomas. Risk factors include the degree of mismatch between donor and recipient, manipulation of the graft to deplete T cells, and the degree of immunosuppression used to prevent GVHD.[4] Epstein–Barr virus-associated lymphoma arising after bone marrow transplantation is an ideal model to evaluate EBV-specific CTL, as the tumor cells are highly immunogenic, expressing all nine latent cycle EBV antigens including the immunodominant EBNA3 antigens. Furthermore, the outgrowing EBV-infected B cell tumors have the same phenotype and pattern of EBV gene expression as do LCL, which are an excellent antigen-presenting cell.

Our group therefore developed a CTL generation methodology where donor lymphocytes are infected with a laboratory strain of EBV to initiate an LCL that can be used as antigen-presenting cells of viral antigens. Then, irradiated LCLs are used to stimulate peripheral blood mononuclear cells (PBMC) and expand EBV-specific CTL

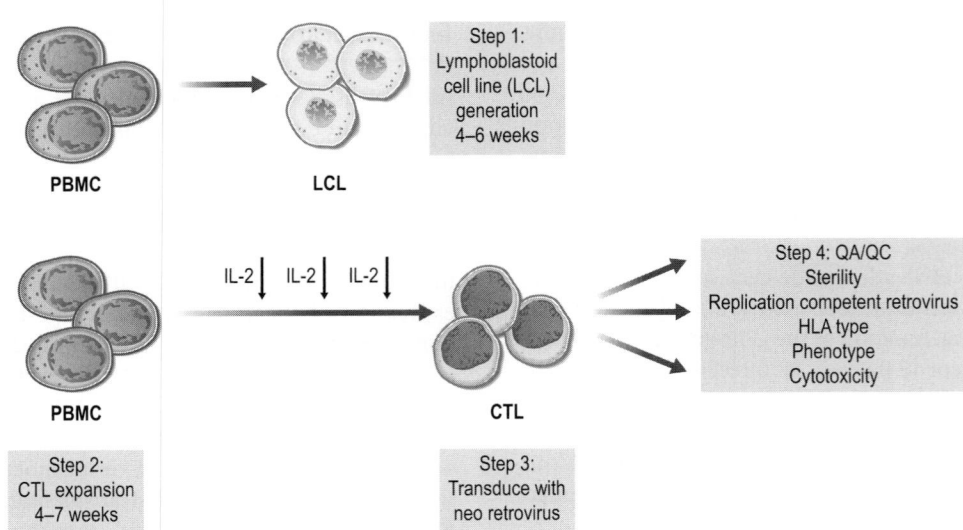

Figure 87.1   Generation of Epstein–Barr virus (EBV)-specific cytotoxic T lymphocytes (CTL). Step 1: First, peripheral blood mononuclear cells (PBMC) are infected with a laboratory strain of EBV to generate an EBV-transformed B lymphoblastoid cell line (LCL) (4–6 weeks). Step 2: Irradiated LCL are then used as antigen-presenting cells to stimulate EBV-specific CTL. The EBV-specific CTL are stimulated weekly with irradiated LCL and interleukin-2 (IL-2) to generate sufficient cell numbers (4–7 weeks). Step 3: In some protocols the CTL are genetically marked by transduction with the G1Na or LNSJ1 retroviral vectors, which contain the *Escherichia coli*-derived neomycin resistance gene (*neo*). After transduction, the CTL are returned to their regular growth schedule. Step 4: Finally, extensive testing including HLA typing, phenotyping, cytotoxicity assay, sterility testing, and replication competent retrovirus (RCR) testing is performed before the EBV-specific CTL are released and can be used for adoptive immunotherapy. QA/QC, quality assurance/quality control.

(Fig. 87.1). We have used donor-derived EBV-specific T cell lines as prophylaxis for EBV-induced lymphoma in over 60 patients posthematopoietic stem cell transplantation (HSCT) who received a T cell-depleted HSCT or who were transplanted for an EBV-associated malignancy.[4,67,68] None of the patients treated with this approach developed post-transplant LPD, compared with an incidence of 11.5 percent in a historical nontreated control group.[68] Gene marking of donor CTL allowed us to show persistence of infused CTL for as long as 7 years.[69] Furthermore, high EBV genome loads that existed prior to CTL administration rapidly decreased to normal levels with an increase of EBV-specific cytotoxicity.[67] Similar results were seen by another group who treated six T cell-depleted allogeneic BMT recipients prophylactically with EBV-specific CTL. One patient, who received a T cell line lacking a major EBV-specific component, progressed to fatal EBV-positive lymphoma. However, in the other five patients treatment resulted in reduction of the viral load thereby confirming the efficacy of this approach (Table 87.3).[70]

Immunotherapy using EBV-CTL was also used to treat six patients with overt lymphoma; in five patients treatment was successful and gene-marked CTL accumulated at sites of disease.[68] One of the responders required temporary mechanical ventilation due to airway compromise from the inflammatory response at the disease site. The sixth patient who received CTL as treatment died with progressive disease 24 days after infusion.[71] In this patient,

the cytolytic activity of the generated CTL line was directed mainly against two HLA-11 restricted epitopes in the EBNA3b gene. However, after CTL infusion, only virus with an EBNA3b deletion could be detected, allowing the tumor to evade the immune response.[71] This experience illustrates a means by which tumors may evade the immune response if a CTL line with restricted specificity is infused and argues for the use of a product with broad specificity. Again, other groups have also confirmed that EBV-CTL can successfully treat overt lymphoma, including tumors resistant to rituximab (Table 87.3).[72,73]

EBV–ASSOCIATED LYMPHOMA POSTSOLID ORGAN TRANSPLANTATION

In recipients of solid organ transplants (SOT), the severe impairment of T cell function as a result of the required immunosuppressive regimen post-transplantation also places these patients at risk for the development of post-transplant lymphoproliferative disease (PTLD) with incidence dependent on the type of organ transplanted and the degree of immunosuppression. As reducing immunosuppression can often control LPD, administration of EBV-specific CTL might be an alternate means of restoring the immune response. There are some different issues with generating EBV-specific CTL in this clinical scenario, as the SOT donor is not HLA matched. Moreover, whereas PTLD is usually donor derived in the HSCT setting, in SOT recipients the tumor arises from recipient lymphocytes.

Table 87.3 Clinical trials on use of EBV–cytotoxic T cells as prophylaxis or treatment for post–transplant lymphoproliferative disease (PTLD) postbone marrow transplantation (BMT) or solid organ transplantation (SOT)

Study	Patient number	Type of transplant	Pathologic evidence of PTLD	Cytotoxic T cell (CTL) lines	Results
Rooney et al.[68] Hale et al.[69]	59	T-depleted HSCT (mismatch related donor or matched unrelated donor)	No – prophylaxis study	Allogeneic (donor-derived) EBV-CTL	No patients developed PTLD compared with 11.5% controls
Rooney et al.[68] Gottschalk et al.[4]	6	T-depleted HSCT	Yes	Allogeneic (donor-derived) EBV-CTL	5 complete remission, 1 died (no response to CTL secondary to tumor mutation resistant to CTL)
Gustafsson et al.[70]	6	T-depleted HSCT or unmanipulated HSCT with ATG/OKT3	No – treatment based on ↑ EBV DNA levels	Allogeneic (donor-derived) EBV-CTL	5 patients had ↓ EBV DNA levels; 1 patient subsequently died of PTLD
Lucas et al.[43]	1	T-depleted HSCT	Yes	Allogeneic (donor-derived) EBV-CTL	Patient attained CR
Imashuku et al.[146]	1	Mismatched HSCT with ATG	Yes	Allogeneic (donor-derived) EBV-CTL	Patient failed to respond
O'Reilly et al.[73]	17	T-depleted HSCT (14) and SOT (3)	Therapy	Allogeneic (donor-derived) EBV-CTL	11 attained CR
					2 long-term disease stabilization
Comoli et al.[76]	7	SOT	Prophylaxis	Autologous EBV-specific CTL	No patient developed PTLD
Haque et al.[147]	3	SOT	Prophylaxis	Autologous EBV-specific CTL	No patient developed PTLD
Khanna et al.[74]	1	SOT	Yes	Autologous EBV-specific CTL	Significant regression
Sherrit et al.[148]	1	SOT	Yes	Autologous EBV-specific CTL	Complete remission
Comoli et al.[78]	5	SOT	Yes	Autologous EBV-specific CTL	Complete remission (used as adjuvant after chemotherapy and rituxan)
Savoldo et al.[77]	12	SOT	Prophylaxis and therapy	Autologous EBV-specific CTL	No patient developed PTLD 2/2 with PTLD attained CR
Sun et al.[82]	2	SOT	Yes	Closely matched allogeneic EBV-specifc CTL	2 attained CR
Haque et al.[81]	5	SOT	Yes	Closely matched allogeneic EBV-specifc CTL	3 attained CR; 2 did not respond
Haque et al.[83]	33	SOT and HSCT	Therapy	Closely matched allogeneic EBV-specific CTL	14 attained CR, 3 had PR and 16 had no response at 6 months
Gandhi et al.[149]	3	SOT	Therapy	Closely matched allogeneic EBV-specific CTL	2 attained CRs

EBV, Epstein–Barr virus; CTL, cytotoxic T cells; HSCT, hematopoietic stem cell transplantation; CR, complete remission; PR, partial response.

Most studies in SOT recipients have therefore used autologous CTL generated from peripheral blood of SOT recipients.[74–77] The results of these studies are summarized in Table 87.3. In patients with high viral load, infusion of EBV-specific CTL resulted in a reduction of EBV-DNA viral load and an increase, albeit transient, in EBV-specific CTL precursor frequency was detected.[76–79] In addition, Khanna et al. treated one patient with established PTLD with multiple infusions of ex vivo expanded autologous EBV-specific CTL. The PTLD regressed and the frequency of EBV-specific precursors increased, without signs of graft rejection.[74] However, the patient developed a secondary PTLD and died, despite further CTL infusions. A second patient who received a cardiac transplant and developed multiple subcutaneous nodules required six doses of CTL to achieve remission.[80] Thus, initial concerns that EBV-specific CTL might have alloreactivity and cause graft rejection have been allayed and the results obtained so far confirm that EBV-specific immunity can at least be temporarily restored in these patients. However, the persistence of CTL appears to be less than that observed post-HSCT suggesting that the long-term immunosuppressive therapy these patients receive might compromise CTL persistence and function. Another issue with autologous CTL is the time required for product generation and two groups have circumvented this by using banked allogeneic EBV-specific CTL (Table 87.3).[81–83] In a recent phase II study, HSCT and SOT recipients who had failed to respond to conventional PTLD therapy received the most closely matched cell line from such a bank and the response rate was 64 percent and 52 percent at 5 weeks and 6 months, respectively.[83] Patients with closer HLA-matching donors showed better responses at 6 months.

EBV–ASSOCIATED TYPE II LATENCY LYMPHOMA

Adapting immunotherapy approaches that have proved successful in type III latency EBV tumors to type II latency tumors provides a challenge, as a more restricted array of subdominant EBV antigens is expressed and the frequency of clones recognizing the LMP1 or LMP2 antigens expressed on these tumors is low in a polyclonal EBV-CTL line generated using LCL as the antigen-presenting cell.[84] Epstein–Barr virus-associated HD and NHL which develop in the immune-competent host show type II latency where viral gene expression is limited to the immunosubdominant latent membrane proteins LMP1 and LMP2, EBNA1, and EBERs.[85–86] This expression of a minimal subset of genes, which are weak targets for CTL activity, therefore allows the malignant cells to evade the immune system.[87] Nevertheless, the subdominant EBV antigens EBNA1, LMP1, and LMP2 may serve as targets for immunotherapy approaches (Table 87.4). In a phase I dose-escalation study, we evaluated the use of autologous EBV-specific CTL for patients with EBV-positive HD.[84] We treated 14 patients with relapsed HD with two infusions (2×10^7 cells/m^2–1.2×10^8 cells/m^2) of EBV-specific CTL. In seven of these patients the CTL were retrovirally marked. We used a combination of gene-marking, tetramer, and functional analyses to track the fate and assess the activity

Table 87.4 Clinical trials on use of EBV-cytotoxic T cells as treatment for EBV-positive Hodgkin disease or non-Hodgkin lymphoma

Study	Number of patients	Type of disease	Cytotoxic T cell (CTL) lines and dose	Results
Sun et al.[82]	4	EBV+ve HD and NHL (including 1 HIV associated and 2 patients postsolid organ transplant)	Allogeneic (2 partially HLA matched and 2 from HLA-matched siblings) EBV-CTL; 5×10^6/kg	1 CR, 1 CRu, 1 PR, and 1 NR
Lucas et al.[89]	6	Relapsed EBV+ve HD	Allogeneic (partially HLA matched) EBV-CTL; 1.5×10^7/kg ± pretreatment with fludarabine	1 CR, 4 PR, 1 NR (although ? effect of fludarabine)
Bollard et al.[84]	14	Relapsed EBV+ve HD – either as adjuvant treatment after SCT or for treatment of active disease	Autologous EBV-CTL; 4×10^7/m^2–1.2×10^8/m^2	5 CR (includes 2 with active disease), 1 PR, 5 SD, 3 NR
Cho et al.[150]	3	Extranodal NK/T cell lymphoma, nasal type	Autologous EBV-CTL in 1, allogeneic (HLA-matched siblings) EBV-CTL in 2	2/3 disease stablization for over 3 years
Bollard et al.[100]	16	Relapsed EBV+ve HD or NHL – either as adjuvant treatment after SCT/chemo or for treatment of active disease	Autologous LMP2–CTL; 4×10^7/m^2–3×10^8/m^2	13 CR (includes 4 with active disease), 1 PR, 2 NR

EBV, Epstein–Barr virus; HD, Hodgkin disease; NHL, non-Hodgkin lymphoma; HIV, human immunodeficiency virus; SCT, stem cell transplantation; CR, complete remission; CRu, complete remission unconfirmed; PR, partial response; NR, no response; SD, stabilized disease; LMP2, latent membrane protein 2; NK, natural killer; +ve, positive.

of the CTL *in vivo*. Viral load decreased, demonstrating the biologic activity of the infused CTL. Gene-marking studies showed that infused effector cells could further expand by several logs *in vivo* (persisting up to 12 months) as well as traffic to tumor sites. Tetramer and functional analyses showed that T cells reactive with the tumor-associated antigen LMP2 were present in the infused lines, expanded in peripheral blood following infusion, and could also track to sites of disease. Clinically, EBV-CTL were well tolerated, could control type B symptoms (fever, night sweats, weight loss), and had antitumor activity. Following CTL infusion, five patients were in complete remission at up to 40 months, two of whom had clearly measurable tumor at the time of treatment. One additional patient had a partial response, and five had stable disease.[84]

One of the difficulties with the use of CTL therapy for heavily pretreated patients with relapsed HD is the expansion of the autologous CTL to the numbers required for a clinical trial.[88] One strategy is therefore to use allogeneic CTL. In a phase I study, EBV-CTL were expanded from partially HLA-matched normal donors and infused into patients with relapsed EBV-positive HD, with one cohort receiving CTL therapy and a second cohort of patients preconditioned with fludarabine prior to receiving CTL.[89] Five out of six patients had reductions in measurable disease and the maximum duration of response was 22 months. However, donor EBV-specific CTL could not be detected *in vivo* in either of the patient groups and, as in the SOT setting, this approach may be limited by the short-term persistence of the allogeneic cells.[89]

Although these results using EBV-specific CTL in type II latency tumors have shown some activity (Table 87.4), the response rate is less impressive than that seen in EBV-LPD post-HSCT. Moreover, apart from the patients with relatively low tumor burden who have demonstrated durable responses, the majority of the antitumor responses have been transient, and no patient with aggressive, bulky relapsed HD has been cured by CTL therapy alone. This may be due to a lack of specificity of the EBV-specific CTL for the immunosubdominant LMP1 and LMP2 antigens present on the Hodgkin tumor. In addition, the tumor produces inhibitory factors such as tumor growth factor-β, thymus- and activation-regulated chemokine (TARC), galectin, IL-10, and IL-13, which affect CTL and antigen-presenting cell activity.[11,90–94]

Current studies are evaluating whether there is increased activity if CTL lines are biased toward the LMP2 antigens expressed in these tumors. Our group and others have hypothesized that expanding CTL specifically targeting type II viral latency antigens might result in greater activity in these patients.[95–98] Strategies to expand LMP2-specific CTL *in vitro* have included retroviral transduction of the T cell receptor (TCR) from a LMP2 peptide-specific CTL clone[98] or transfecting autologous dendritic cells (DC) with LMP2a RNA to use as antigen-presenting cells to stimulate and expand LMP2-specific CTL.[97] We have shown that LMP-CTL could be generated from normal

donors using DC genetically modified with a recombinant adenovirus encoding LMP (Ad5LMP).[95] However, this approach required the generation of large numbers of DC to expand LMP-CTL and was not practical in these heavily pretreated patients.[99] We therefore modified the generation protocol to use DC for the initial stimulation, followed by stimulation with LCL that had been genetically modified to overexpress LMP2a by transduction with an Ad5f35LMP2a vector (Fig. 87.2).[99]

In a clinical trial we have generated LMP2-specific CTL lines in patients with EBV-positive HD or EBV-positive B cell or T/NK cell NHL.[100] Using LMP2-specific tetramers, a significantly increased number of LMP2-specific CTL were detected in the LMP2-CTL lines compared to EBV-CTL lines generated with genetically unmodified LCL from the same patients. Patients have received doses of 4×10^7 CTL/m^2 to 1.2×10^8 CTL/m^2. No immediate toxicity has been observed and nine of ten patients without radiological evidence of disease who received CTL as adjuvant therapy post-HSCT or chemotherapy remain in remission; five of

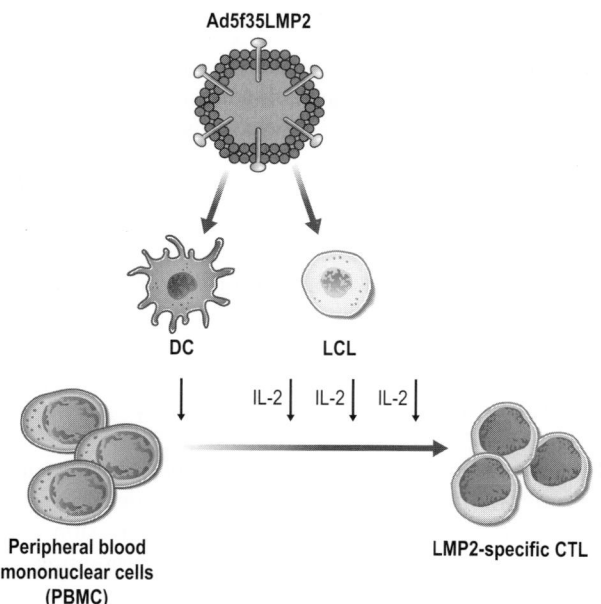

Figure 87.2   Generation of latent membrane protein 2 (LMP2)-specific cytotoxic T lymphocytes (CTL) with LMP2-transduced dendritic cells and lymphoblastoid cell line (LCL) stimulations. A recombinant adenovirus Ad5f35LMP2A for the transduction of dendritic cells (DC) and LCL was generated as previously described.[72] Peripheral blood mononuclear cells (PBMCs) are then stimulated with Ad5f35LMP2A-transduced autologous DC on day 0 and then cultures are restimulated on day 10 with irradiated Ad5f35LMP2A-transduced LCL at a responder-to-stimulator ratio of 4:1 and after that weekly with irradiated autologous Ad5f35LMP2A-transduced LCL at a responder-to-stimulator ratio of 4:1. Interleukin-2 (IL-2, 50–100 U/ml, Proleukin; Chiron, Emeryville, CA) is added 3 days after the second stimulation and added twice weekly.

six patients with active relapsed disease had a tumor response, which was complete in four cases.[100] Immunotherapy with autologous LMP2-CTL was well tolerated in patients with relapsed EBV-positive HD/NHL and infused LMP2-CTL cells accumulated at tumor sites and induced clinical responses. In a follow-up study we are now targeting LMP1 as well as LMP2.

Immunotherapy for human immunodeficiency virus

Patients with HIV infection may also develop EBV-associated lymphomas and the risk appears to correlate with increasing viral load in the absence of an EBV-specific immune response.[101] This observation implies that these complications may be prevented if the EBV-specific T cell response could be augmented. However, this would present logistic challenges, as cells would have to be obtained early in the patient's clinical course for potential later use. In addition, the protection offered by infused virus-specific T cells is likely to be short lived as they will be susceptible to HIV if infection is not controlled. For these reasons, immunotherapy approaches have not been extensively explored although there is one report of a patient with an EBV-positive B cell lymphoma that regressed after treatment with EBV-specific CTL generated from archived autologous PBMC.[102] Human herpesvirus 8 is also expressed in primary effusion lymphoma and would be a potential target for immunotherapy approaches.[103] Preclinical studies have described methodology for generating HHV-8-specific CTL although the proposed application was in Kaposi sarcoma rather than HHV-8-associated lymphoma.[104]

Chimeric antigen–transduced T cells

The generation of tumor-specific T cells either *ex vivo* or by immunization is limited by poor antigenicity of most tumors and also by the requirement for expression of an appropriate antigen by an effective antigen-presenting cell. One means of circumventing this problem is the transduction of T cells with chimeric surface proteins that transmit TCR signals in response to target cells. Such proteins are composed of an extracellular domain (ectodomain) usually derived from immunoglobulin variable chains, which recognizes and binds target antigen. This is attached via a spacer to an intracytoplasmic signaling domain (endodomain), usually the cytoplasmic segment of TCR-ζ chain, which transmits an activation signal to the T cell. Genetic engineering of CTL for redirected CD30-, CD20-, and CD19-specific target cell recognition has been achieved and these CTL are capable of mediating a variety of CD30-, CD20-, and CD19-specific antilymphoma effector functions including cytolytic activity against lymphoma cells, secretion of TH1 cytokines, and CTL proliferation in the presence of stimulating tumor cells.[105–109] Clinical trials are underway with strategies targeting CD20 and CD19. In the

one study reported so far, patients with indolent B cell lymphoma or mantle cell lymphoma and active disease received autologous T cells genetically modified with a CD20-specific chimeric T cell receptor. The transferred cells persisted only up to 3 weeks in the first three patients who received clones but persisted up to 8 weeks in the next three patients who received polyclonal lines.[110]

However, chimeric receptor signaling produces only limited activation of the T cells, and clinical trials in patients with solid tumors have shown that T cells expressing transgenic antigen-specific chimeric receptors have limited therapeutic activity, in part because engagement of the chimeric receptor alone is insufficient to sustain T cell growth and activation. One means of solving this problem is to transduce antigen-specific T cells rather than nonspecifically activated cells and take advantage of the costimulation provided to the native TCR by antigen.[111] Our group has evaluated this strategy using transduced EBV-specific T cells with chimeric receptor genes. We showed *in vitro* that these could be expanded and maintained long term in the presence of EBV-infected B cells. While they recognize EBV-infected targets through their conventional T cell receptor and thereby become activated, they are also able to recognize and lyse tumor targets through their chimeric receptors.[112] The strategy of using an endogenous virus-specific receptor has also been explored using cytomegalovirus (CMV)-specific T cells reprogrammed into leukemia-reactive T cells by transferring a T cell receptor specific for the minor histocompatibility antigen HA2, and influenza-specific T cells transduced with a CD19 chimeric antigen receptor.[113,114] An alternate strategy is to provide additional costimulatory signals, and the signaling domain of the TCR has been combined with specific endodomains derived from different costimulatory molecules including CD28, 4-1BB, or OX40.[111,115,116] T cells expressing these new constructs, after the binding with the specific target, exhibit antitumor activity and secrete significant amounts of IL-2, enhancing their persistence *in vivo*.[117]

Natural killer cells

Natural killer cells are defined by the absence of the TCR and by the expression of CD56 or CD19. Their mode of cytolytic killing is mediated in MHC-unrestricted fashion. In the bone marrow transplant setting, NK cell alloreactivity is a result of a mismatch between donor NK clones, carrying specific inhibitory receptors for self-MHC class I molecules, and ligands on recipient cells. When allogeneic targets are mismatched, these donor NK clones therefore mediate alloreactions and transplantation from NK-alloreactive haploidentical donors may control relapse and improve engraftment without causing GVHD.[118] The biological effects of the adoptive transfer of related-donor haploidentical NK cells to patients with HD, melanoma, renal cell carcinoma, and acute myeloid leukemia (AML) have been assessed.[119] Patients received immune-suppression regimens prior to infusion of NK cells that were expanded after CD3 depletion of a pheresis product in high-dose IL-2. All patients received subcutaneous IL-2 after NK cell infusions. Patients who received lower-intensity regimens showed transient persistence but no expansion of donor cells *in vivo*. In contrast, patients who received NK cell infusions after the more intense conditioning regimen had a significant expansion of donor NK cells *in vivo*, and complete hematologic remissions were seen in five of 19 poor-prognosis patients with AML.[119] These findings therefore suggest that haploidentical NK cells can expand and may have antitumor efficacy *in vivo*. However, the utility of NK cell therapy for the treatment of lymphoma is at this stage speculative and warrants further study.

IMPROVING CELLULAR IMMUNOTHERAPY APPROACHES

Improving *ex vivo* generation

One of the limitations of adoptive immunotherapy is the lack of a convenient source of the antigen-presenting cells necessary to generate antigen-specific CTL. A number of artificial antigen-presenting cells have been evaluated where ligands for the T cell receptor and costimulatory surface molecules are grafted onto mouse fibroblasts or beads.[120–122] An alternative approach is to modify tumor cells to express costimulatory molecules. For example, mantle cell lymphoma cells that have been modified so that CD40 is ligated function as effective antigen-presenting cells and stimulate CD8-positive CTL lines that can lyse primary mantle cell lymphoma cells.[123] There has also been much recent effort to identify the optimum phenotype of infused T cells. It seems likely that for optimum persistence, a product containing both CD4 and CD8 cells and both effector and memory cells will be required.[124] A recent study in a primate model showed that only antigen-specific CD8 T cells derived from central memory T cells could persist long term *in vivo* and revert to the memory pool.[125]

Genetic modification of antigen-presenting cells may influence the T cell product generated; for example, fusing idiotype to a lysosomal-associated membrane protein enables processing through both the class I and class II processing pathways and produces a CTL line containing both CD8$^+$ and CD4$^+$ clones specific for idiotype that may be useful therapeutically in NHL.[126] It will therefore be important to correlate *in vivo* function with the type of product generated using different sources of antigen-presenting cells.

Genetic modification of T cells to overcome tumor evasion mechanisms

Tumor cells may evade a transferred T cell response by a number of mechanisms such as downregulation of MHC and costimulatory molecules and secretion of inhibitory cytokines by the Hodgkin Reed-Sternberg or lymphoma cells. Studies in HD have shown that outcome can be predicted by the types of T cell populations in the tumor.[127] The cytokine that has the most devastating effects on CTL proliferation and function is transforming growth factor β (TGFβ).[91,128] This cytokine is secreted by a wide variety of tumors as a powerful mechanism by which the tumor cells can escape the immune response. To overcome this inhibition, we have evaluated if transduction with a retrovirus vector expressing the dominant-negative TGFβ type II receptor (DNRII) that prevents the formation of the functional tetrameric receptor[129] can render T cells resistant to this inhibitory cytokine. Studies *in vitro* showed that DNR-transduced CTLs were resistant to the antiproliferative effects of recombinant TGFβ. In addition, while transduced CTLs were protected from the negative effects of TGFβ, long-term expression of this construct had no deleterious effects on the function, phenotype, or growth characteristics of the transduced-CTL lines.[129] Additional support for this approach comes from murine models where transgenic mice genetically engineered so that all of their T cells are insensitive to TGF signaling were able to eradicate tumors[130] and adoptive transfer of TGFβ-DNR-transduced T cells resulted in eradication of tumor cells.[131] Cytotoxic T lymphocytes expressing the DNR may therefore have a selective advantage *in vivo* in patients with TGFβ-secreting tumors such as HD.

Many tumors have also been reported to aberrantly express Fas ligand (FasL) and induce a premature apoptosis of effector T cells expressing the death receptor Fas. In a recent report, T cells were transduced with small interfering RNA (siRNA) to downmodulate the Fas receptor resulting in a significant reduction of their susceptibility to Fas/FasL-mediated apoptosis.[132] All these genetic modifications improve the functionality of antigen-specific CTLs without any modification of their antigen specificity, suggesting that they may increase the antitumor effect of adoptively transferred CTLs *in vivo*, although this still remains to be tested.

Lymphodepletion to improve expansion of T cells *in vivo*

Another limitation of clinical studies of adoptive immunotherapy outside the setting of HSCT has been poor lymphocyte survival or function. Several groups have evaluated strategies to induce a proliferative environment by administering lymphodepleting chemotherapy such as fludarabine or monoclonal antibodies to deplete the lymphoid compartment prior to T cell infusion.[133,134] This strategy may potentiate the function of infused T cells in two ways. First, it may deplete not only intratumoral TH2 and T regulatory cells that function to inhibit the entry, activity, and characteristics of TH1 tumor-specific T cells, but also peripheral T regulatory cells. In HD in particular, the Hodgkin Reed-Sternberg cells accumulate in their environment a large proportion of T cells that are of T regulatory phenotype and function (CD25$^+$CD4$^+$FOXP3^{high}).[135] Second, it would create a deficit in the T lymphoid compartment that would promote the homeostatic expansion of infused, activated CTL lines. Clinical studies have already shown expansion of T cells specific for antigens expressed on solid tumors after lymphodepletion[136] and studies in patients with HD and lymphoma are underway.

CONCLUSIONS

T cell therapies have produced definitive benefits in the treatment of relapsed low-grade lymphoma after transplantation and EBV-associated malignancy. However, clinical studies have also identified limitations of such therapies including inadequate persistence or expansion. With increased knowledge of the optimum methodology for generation of T cell products, identification of additional antigen targets, and optimization of gene therapy approaches to enhance the function of adoptively transferred T cells, adoptive immunotherapy strategies may find a defined role in the therapy of lymphoma.

KEY POINTS

- Targets for immunotherapy in lymphoma include lineage-specific antigens, viral antigens, and cancer-testis antigens.
- In the postallogeneic transplant setting minor antigens differing between donor and recipient may also be a target.
- Autologous nonspecifically expanded T cells have hastened immune recovery postautologous transplant in patients with lymphoma.
- Antigen-specific CTL targeting EBV antigens have had activity in phase I studies in patients with EBV-associated lymphomas.
- The presence of a graft-versus-lymphoma effect in some types of lymphoma is supported by the efficacy of DLI in low-grade lymphoma and Hodgkin disease.
- Genetic modification of T cells with chimeric antigen receptors targeting CD19 or CD20 is currently being evaluated in the clinic.

REFERENCES

● = Key primary paper
◆ = Major review article

●1. Papadopoulos EB, Ladanyi M, Emanuel D et al. Infusions of donor leukocytes to treat Epstein-Barr virus-associated lymphoproliferative disorders after allogeneic bone marrow transplantation. N Engl J Med 1994; 330: 1185–91.

2. Walter EA, Greenberg PD, Gilbert MJ et al. Reconstitution of cellular immunity against cytomegalovirus in recipients of allogeneic bone marrow by transfer of T-cell clones from the donor. N Engl J Med 1995; 333: 1038–44.

◆3. Porter DL, Antin JH. The graft-versus-leukemia effects of allogeneic cell therapy. Annu Rev Med 1999; 50: 369–86.

◆4. Gottschalk S, Rooney CM, Heslop HE. Post-transplant lymphoproliferative disorders. Annu Rev Med 2005; 56: 29–44.

◆5. Kolb HJ, Schmid C, Barrett AJ, Schendel DJ. Graft-versus-leukemia reactions in allogeneic chimeras. Blood 2004; 103: 767–76.

6. Baker KS, Gordon BG, Gross TG et al. Autologous hematopoietic stem-cell transplantation for relapsed or refractory Hodgkin's disease in children and adolescents. J Clin Oncol 1999; 17: 825–31.

7. Ladenstein R, Pearce R, Hartmann O et al. High-dose chemotherapy with autologous bone marrow rescue in children with poor-risk Burkitt's lymphoma: a report from the European Lymphoma Bone Marrow Transplantation Registry. Blood 1997; 90: 2921–30.

8. Aisenberg AC. Problems in Hodgkin's disease management. Blood 1999; 93: 761–79.

9. Lanzavecchia A, Sallusto F. Antigen decoding by T lymphocytes: from synapses to fate determination. Nat Immunol 2001; 2: 487–92.

10. Morris EC, Tsallios A, Bendle GM et al. A critical role of T cell antigen receptor-transduced MHC class I-restricted helper T cells in tumor protection. Proc Natl Acad Sci U S A 2005; 102: 7934–9.

11. Zou W. Immunosuppressive networks in the tumour environment and their therapeutic relevance. Nat Rev Cancer 2005; 5: 263–74.

◆12. Young LS, Rickinson AB. Epstein-Barr virus: 40 years on. Nat Rev Cancer 2004; 4: 757–768.

◆13. Cohen JI. Benign and malignant Epstein-Barr virus-associated B-cell lymphoproliferative diseases. Semin Hematol 2003; 40: 116–23.

14. Chadburn A, Hyjek E, Mathew S et al. KSHV-positive solid lymphomas represent an extra-cavitary variant of primary effusion lymphoma. Am J Surg Pathol 2004; 28: 1401–16.

15. Vilchez RA, Madden CR, Kozinetz CA et al. Association between simian virus 40 and non-Hodgkin lymphoma. Lancet 2002; 359: 817–23.

16. Bae J, Martinson JA, Klingemann HG. Identification of CD19 and CD20 peptides for induction of antigen-specific CTLs against B-cell malignancies. Clin Cancer Res 2005; 11: 1629–38.

17. Nagata S, Ise T, Onda M et al. Cell membrane-specific epitopes on CD30: Potentially superior targets for immunotherapy. Proc Natl Acad Sci U S A 2005; 102: 7946–51.

18. Trojan A, Schultze JL, Witzens M et al. Immunoglobulin framework-derived peptides function as cytotoxic T-cell epitopes commonly expressed in B-cell malignancies. Nat Med 2000; 6: 667–72.

19. Vonderheide RH. Telomerase as a universal tumor-associated antigen for cancer immunotherapy. Oncogene 2002; 21: 674–9.

20. McFadyen MC, Melvin WT, Murray GI. Cytochrome P450 enzymes: novel options for cancer therapeutics. Mol Cancer Ther 2004; 3: 363–71.

21. Wang RF, Wang X, Atwood AC *et al.* Cloning genes encoding MHC class II-restricted antigens: mutated CDC27 as a tumor antigen. *Science* 1999; **284**: 1351–4.

22. Zendman AJ, Ruiter DJ, Van Muijen GN. Cancer/testis-associated genes: identification, expression profile, and putative function. *J Cell Physiol* 2003; **194**: 272–88.

23. Liggins AP, Guinn BA, Banham AH. Identification of lymphoma-associated antigens using SEREX. *Methods Mol Med* 2005; **115**: 109–28.

24. Haffner AC, Tassis A, Zepter K *et al.* Expression of cancer/testis antigens in cutaneous T cell lymphomas. *Int J Cancer* 2002; **97**: 668–70.

25. Liggins AP, Brown PJ, Asker K *et al.* A novel diffuse large B-cell lymphoma-associated cancer testis antigen encoding a PAS domain protein. *Br J Cancer* 2004; **91**: 141–9.

26. van Rhee F, Szmania SM, Zhan F *et al.* NY-ESO-1 is highly expressed in poor-prognosis multiple myeloma and induces spontaneous humoral and cellular immune responses. *Blood* 2005; **105**: 3939–44.

27. Marijt WA, Heemskerk MH, Kloosterboer FM *et al.* Hematopoiesis-restricted minor histocompatibility antigens HA-1- or HA-2-specific T cells can induce complete remissions of relapsed leukemia. *Proc Natl Acad Sci U S A* 2003; **100**: 2742–7.

28. Kloosterboer FM, Luxemburg-Heijs SA, van Soest RA *et al.* Minor histocompatibility antigen-specific T cells with multiple distinct specificities can be isolated by direct cloning of IFNgamma-secreting T cells from patients with relapsed leukemia responding to donor lymphocyte infusion. *Leukemia* 2005; **19**: 83–90.

29. Jones RJ, Ambinder RF, Piantadosi S, Santos GW. Evidence of a graft-versus-lymphoma effect associated with allogeneic bone marrow transplantation. *Blood* 1991; **77**: 649–53.

30. Peniket AJ, Ruiz De Elvira MC, Taghipour G *et al.* An EBMT registry matched study of allogeneic stem cell transplants for lymphoma: allogeneic transplantation is associated with a lower relapse rate but a higher procedure-related mortality rate than autologous transplantation. *Bone Marrow Transplant* 2003; **31**: 667–78.

31. Herbert KE, Spencer A, Grigg A *et al.* Graft-versus-lymphoma effect in refractory cutaneous T-cell lymphoma after reduced-intensity HLA-matched sibling allogeneic stem cell transplantation. *Bone Marrow Transplant* 2004; **34**: 521–5.

32. Khouri IF, Keating M, Korbling M *et al.* Transplant-lite: induction of graft-versus-malignancy using fludarabine-based nonablative chemotherapy and allogeneic blood progenitor-cell transplantation as treatment for lymphoid malignancies. *J Clin Oncol* 1998; **16**: 2817–24.

33. Porrata LF, Inwards DJ, Micallef IN *et al.* Early lymphocyte recovery post-autologous haematopoietic stem cell transplantation is associated with better survival in Hodgkin's disease. *Br J Haematol* 2002; **117**: 629–33.

34. Porrata LF, Gertz MA, Inwards DJ *et al.* Early lymphocyte recovery predicts superior survival after autologous hematopoietic stem cell transplantation in multiple myeloma or non-Hodgkin lymphoma. *Blood* 2001; **98**: 579–85.

●35. Laport GG, Levine BL, Stadtmauer EA *et al.* Adoptive transfer of costimulated T cells induces lymphocytosis in patients with relapsed/refractory non-Hodgkin's lymphoma following CD34-selected hematopoietic cell transplantation. *Blood* 2003; **102**: 2004–13.

36. Leemhuis T, Wells S, Scheffold C *et al.* A phase I trial of autologous cytokine-induced killer cells for the treatment of relapsed Hodgkin disease and non-Hodgkin lymphoma. *Biol Blood Marrow Transplant* 2005; **11**: 181–7.

37. Fowler DH, Bishop MR, Gress RE. Immunoablative reduced-intensity stem cell transplantation: potential role of donor Th2 and Tc2 cells. *Semin Oncol* 2004; **31**: 56–67.

●38. Peggs KS, Hunter A, Chopra R *et al.* Clinical evidence of a graft-versus-Hodgkin's-lymphoma effect after reduced-intensity allogeneic transplantation. *Lancet* 2005; **365**: 1934–41.

39. Morris E, Thomson K, Craddock C *et al.* Outcomes after alemtuzumab-containing reduced-intensity allogeneic transplantation regimen for relapsed and refractory non-Hodgkin lymphoma. *Blood* 2004; **104**: 3865–71.

40. Marks DI, Lush R, Cavenagh J *et al.* The toxicity and efficacy of donor lymphocyte infusions given after reduced-intensity conditioning allogeneic stem cell transplantation. *Blood* 2002; **100**: 3108–14.

41. Russell NH, Byrne JL, Faulkner RD *et al.* Donor lymphocyte infusions can result in sustained remissions in patients with residual or relapsed lymphoid malignancy following allogeneic haemopoietic stem cell transplantation. *Bone Marrow Transplant* 2005; **36**: 437–41.

42. O'Reilly RJ, Small TN, Papadopoulos E *et al.* Adoptive immunotherapy for Epstein-Barr virus-associated lymphoproliferative disorders complicating marrow allografts. *Springer Semin Immunopathol* 1998; **20**: 455–91.

43. Lucas KG, Burton RL, Zimmerman SE *et al.* Semiquantitative Epstein-Barr virus (EBV) polymerase chain reaction for the determination of patients at risk for EBV-induced lymphoproliferative disease after stem cell transplantation. *Blood* 1998; **91**: 3654–61.

44. Mandigers CM, Meijerink JP, Raemaekers JM *et al.* Graft-versus-lymphoma effect of donor leucocyte infusion shown by real-time quantitative PCR analysis of t(14;18). *Lancet* 1998; **352**: 1522–3.

45. Bloor AJ, Thomson K, Chowdhry N *et al.* High response rate to donor lymphocyte infusion after allogeneic stem cell transplantation for indolent non-Hodgkin lymphoma. *Biol Blood Marrow Transplant* 2008; **14**: 50–58.

46. Mandigers CM, Verdonck LF, Meijerink JP *et al.* Graft-versus-lymphoma effect of donor lymphocyte infusion in indolent lymphomas relapsed after allogeneic stem cell transplantation. *Bone Marrow Transplant* 2003; **32**: 1159–63.

47. Gajewski JL, Phillips GL, Sobocinski KA *et al.* Bone marrow transplants from HLA-identical siblings in advanced Hodgkin's disease. *J Clin Oncol* 1996; **14**: 572–8.

48. Milpied N, Fielding AK, Pearce RM *et al.* Allogeneic bone marrow transplant is not better than autologous transplant for patients with relapsed Hodgkin's disease. European Group for Blood and Bone Marrow Transplantation. *J Clin Oncol* 1996; **14**: 1291–6.

49. Bonini C, Ciceri F, Apperley J, Slavin S. Hsv-Tk engineered donor lymphocytes provides early immune reconstitution and control of GvDH aftre haplo-identical hemopoietic stem cell transplantation. *Blood* 2003; **102**: 155a (abstract).

50. Bonini C, Ferrari G, Verzeletti S *et al.* HSV-TK gene transfer into donor lymphocytes for control of allogeneic graft versus leukemia. *Science* 1997; **276**: 1719–24.

51. Tiberghien P. Use of suicide gene-expressing donor T-cells to control alloreactivity after haematopoietic stem cell transplantation. *J Intern Med* 2001; **249**: 369–77.

52. Ciceri F, Bonini C, Marktel S *et al.* Antitumor effects of HSV-TK-engineered donor lymphocytes after allogeneic stem-cell transplantation. *Blood* 2007; **109**: 4698–707.

53. Riddell SR, Elliot M, Lewinsohn DA *et al.* T-cell mediated rejection of gene-modified HIV-specific cytotoxic T lymphocytes in HIV-infected patients. *Nat Med* 1996; **2**: 216–23.

●54. Traversari C, Marktel S, Magnani Z *et al.* The potential immunogenicity of the TK suicide gene does not prevent full clinical benefit associated with the use of TK-transduced donor lymphocytes in HSCT for hematologic malignancies. *Blood* 2007; **109**: 4708–15.

55. Berger C, Blau CA, Huang ML *et al.* Pharmacologically regulated Fas-mediated death of adoptively transferred T cells in a nonhuman primate model. *Blood* 2004; **103**: 1261–9.

56. Marktel S, Magnani Z, Ciceri F *et al.* Immunologic potential of donor lymphocytes expressing a suicide gene for early immune reconstitution after hematopoietic T-cell-depleted stem cell transplantation. *Blood* 2003; **101**: 1290–98.

57. Straathof KC, Pule M, Yotnda P *et al.* An inducible caspase 9 safety switch for T-cell therapy. *Blood* 2005; **105**: 4247–54.

58. Sauce D, Bodinier M, Garin M *et al.* Retrovirus-mediated gene transfer in primary T lymphocytes impairs their anti-Epstein-Barr virus potential through both culture-dependent and selection process-dependent mechanisms. *Blood* 2002; **99**: 1165–73.

59. Montagna D, Yvon E, Calcaterra V *et al.* Depletion of alloreactive T cells by a specific anti-interleukin-2 receptor p55 chain immunotoxin does not impair in vitro antileukemia and antiviral activity. *Blood* 1999; **93**: 3550–57.

60. Andre-Schmutz I, Le Deist F, Hacein-Bey-Abina S *et al.* Immune reconstitution without graft-versus-host disease after haemopoietic stem-cell transplantation: a phase 1/2 study. *Lancet* 2002; **360**: 130–37.

61. Solomon SR, Mielke S, Savani BN *et al.* Selective depletion of alloreactive donor lymphocytes: a novel method to reduce the severity of graft-versus-host disease in older patients undergoing matched sibling donor stem cell transplantation. *Blood* 2005; **106**: 1123–9.

62. Amrolia PJ, Muccioli-Casadei G, Huls H *et al.* Adoptive immunotherapy with allodepleted donor T-cells improves immune reconstitution after haploidentical stem cell transplantation. *Blood* 2006; **108**: 1797–808.

63. Young LS, Dawson CW, Eliopoulos AG. The expression and function of Epstein-Barr virus encoded latent genes. *Mol Pathol* 2000; **53**: 238–47.

64. Hsu JL, Glaser SL. Epstein-barr virus-associated malignancies: epidemiologic patterns and etiologic implications. *Crit Rev Oncol Hematol* 2000; **34**: 27–53.

65. Levitskaya J, Coram M, Levitsky V *et al.* Inhibition of antigen processing by the internal repeat region of the Epstein-Barr virus nuclear antigen-1. *Nature* 1995; **375**: 685–8.

66. Fu T, Voo KS, Wang RF. Critical role of EBNA1-specific CD4+ T cells in the control of mouse Burkitt lymphoma in vivo. *J Clin Invest* 2004; **114**: 542–50.

●67. Heslop HE, Ng CYC, Li C *et al.* Long-term restoration of immunity against Epstein-Barr virus infection by adoptive transfer of gene-modified virus-specific T lymphocytes. *Nat Med* 1996; **2**: 551–5.

●68. Rooney CM, Smith CA, Ng CYC *et al.* Infusion of cytotoxic T cells for the prevention and treatment of Epstein-Barr virus-induced lymphoma in allogeneic transplant recipients. *Blood* 1998; **92**: 1549–55.

69. Hale GA, Pule M, Amrolia PJ *et al.* Long-term follow-up of administration of donord EBV-specific CTLs to prevent and treat EBV lymphoma after hemopoietic stem cell transplant. *Biol Blood Marrow Transplant* 2008; **14**: 3 (abstract).

70. Gustafsson A, Levitsky V, Zou JZ *et al.* Epstein-Barr virus (EBV) load in bone marrow transplant recipients at risk to develop posttransplant lymphoproliferative disease: prophylactic infusion of EBV-specific cytotoxic T cells. *Blood* 2000; **95**: 807–14.

71. Gottschalk S, Ng CYC, Smith CA *et al.* An Epstein-Barr virus deletion mutant that causes fatal lymphoproliferative disease unresponsive to virus-specific T cell therapy. *Blood* 2001; **97**: 835–43.

72. Comoli P, Basso S, Zecca M *et al.* Preemptive therapy of EBV-related lymphoproliferative disease after pediatric haploidentical stem cell transplantation. *Am J Transplant* 2007; **7**: 1648–55.

73. O'Reilly RJ, Doubrovina E, Trivedi D *et al.* Adoptive transfer of antigen-specific T-cells of donor type for immunotherapy of viral infections following allogeneic hematopoietic cell transplants. *Immunol Res* 2007; **38**: 237–50.

74. Khanna R, Bell S, Sherritt M *et al.* Activation and adoptive transfer of Epstein-Barr virus-specific cytotoxic T cells in solid organ transplant patients with posttransplant lymphoproliferative disease. *Proc Natl Acad Sci U S A* 1999; **96**: 10391–6.

75. Savoldo B, Goss J, Liu Z *et al.* Generation of autologous Epstein Barr virus (EBV)-specific cytotoxic T cells (CTL) for adoptive immunotherapy in solid organ transplant recipients. *Transplantation* 2001; **72**: 1078–86.

76. Comoli P, Labirio M, Basso S *et al.* Infusion of autologous Epstein-Barr virus (EBV)-specific cytotoxic T cells for prevention of EBV-related lymphoproliferative disorder in solid organ transplant recipients with evidence of active virus replication. *Blood* 2002; **99**: 2592–8.

77. Savoldo B, Goss JA, Hammer MM *et al.* Treatment of solid organ transplant recipients with autologous Epstein Barr virus-specific cytotoxic T lymphocytes (CTLs). *Blood* 2006; **108**: 2942–9.

78. Comoli P, Maccario R, Locatelli F *et al.* Treatment of EBV-related post-renal transplant lymphoproliferative disease with a tailored regimen including EBV-specific T cells. *Am J Transplant* 2005; **5**: 1415–22.

79. Haque T, Taylor C, Wilkie GM *et al.* Complete regression of posttransplant lymphoproliferative disease using partially HLA-matched Epstein Barr virus-specific cytotoxic T cells. *Transplantation* 2001; **72**: 1399–402.

80. Sherritt MA, Bharadwaj M, Burrows JM *et al.* Reconstitution of the latent T-lymphocyte response to Epstein-Barr virus is coincident with long-term recovery from posttransplant lymphoma after adoptive immunotherapy. *Transplantation* 2003; **75**: 1556–60.

● 81. Haque T, Wilkie GM, Taylor C *et al.* Treatment of Epstein-Barr-virus-positive post-transplantation lymphoproliferative disease with partly HLA-matched allogeneic cytotoxic T cells. *Lancet* 2002; **360**: 436–42.

82. Sun Q, Burton R, Reddy V, Lucas KG. Safety of allogeneic Epstein-Barr virus (EBV)-specific cytotoxic T lymphocytes for patients with refractory EBV-related lymphoma. *Br J Haematol* 2002; **118**: 799–808.

● 83. Haque T, Wilkie GM, Jones MM *et al.* Allogeneic cytotoxic T-cell therapy for EBV-positive posttransplantation lymphoproliferative disease: results of a phase 2 multicenter clinical trial. *Blood* 2007; **110**: 1123–31.

● 84. Bollard CM, Aguilar L, Straathof KC *et al.* Cytotoxic T lymphocyte therapy for Epstein-Barr Virus+ Hodgkin's disease. *J Exp Med* 2004; **200**: 1623–33.

85. Qu L, Rowe DT. Epstein-Barr virus latent gene expression in uncultured peripheral blood lymphocytes. *J Virol* 1992; **66**: 3715–24.

86. Tierney RJ, Steven N, Young LS, Rickinson AB. Epstein-Barr virus latency in blood mononuclear cells: analysis of viral gene transcription during primary infection and in the carrier state. *J Virol* 1994; **68**: 7374–85.

87. Deacon EM, Pallesen G, Niedobitek G *et al.* Epstein-Barr virus and Hodgkin's disease: transcriptional analysis of virus latency in the malignant cells. *J Exp Med* 1993; **177**(2): 339–49.

88. Roskrow MA, Suzuki N, Gan Y-J *et al.* EBV-specific cytotoxic T lymphocytes for the treatment of patients with EBV positive relapsed Hodgkin's disease. *Blood* 1998; **91**: 2925–34.

89. Lucas KG, Salzman D, Garcia A, Sun Q. Adoptive immunotherapy with allogeneic Epstein-Barr virus (EBV)-specific cytotoxic T-lymphocytes for recurrent, EBV-positive Hodgkin disease. *Cancer* 2004; **100**: 1892–901.

90. Newcom SR, Gu L. Transforming growth factor beta 1 messenger RNA in Reed-Sternberg cells in nodular sclerosing Hodgkin's disease. *J Clin Pathol* 1995; **48**: 160–63.

91. Poppema S, Potters M, Visser L, van den Berg AM. Immune escape mechanisms in Hodgkin's disease. *Ann Oncol* 1998; **9**(Suppl 5): S21–4.

92. Skinnider BF, Elia AJ, Gascoyne RD *et al.* Interleukin 13 and interleukin 13 receptor are frequently expressed by Hodgkin and Reed-Sternberg cells of Hodgkin lymphoma. *Blood* 2001; **97**: 250–55.

93. van den Berg A, Visser L, Poppema S. High expression of the CC chemokine TARC in Reed-Sternberg cells. A possible explanation for the characteristic T-cell infiltrate in Hodgkin's lymphoma. *Am J Pathol* 1999; **154**: 1685–91.

94. Juszczynski P, Ouyang J, Monti S *et al.* The AP1-dependent secretion of galectin-1 by Reed Sternberg cells fosters immune privilege in classical Hodgkin lymphoma. *Proc Natl Acad Sci U S A* 2007; **104**: 13134–9.

95. Gahn B, Siller-Lopez F, Pirooz AD *et al.* Adenoviral gene transfer into dendritic cells efficiently amplifies the immune response to the LMP2A-antigen: a potential treatment strategy for Epstein-Barr virus-positive Hodgkin's lymphoma. *Int J Cancer* 2001; **93**: 706–13.

96. Gottschalk S, Edwards OL, Sili U *et al.* Generating CTL against the subdominant Epstein-Barr virus LMP1 antigen for the adoptive immunotherapy of EBV-associated malignancies. *Blood* 2003; **101**: 1905–12.

97. Su Z, Peluso MV, Raffegerst SH *et al.* The generation of LMP2a-specific cytotoxic T lymphocytes for the treatment of patients with Epstein-Barr virus-positive Hodgkin disease. *Eur J Immunol* 2001; **31**: 947–58.

98. Orentas RJ, Roskopf SJ, Nolan GP, Nishimura MI. Retroviral transduction of a T cell receptor specific for an Epstein-Barr virus-encoded peptide. *Clin Immunol* 2001; **98**: 220–28.

99. Bollard CM, Straathof KC, Huls MH *et al.* The generation and characterization of LMP2-specific CTLs for use as adoptive transfer from patients with relapsed EBV-positive Hodgkin disease. *J Immunother* 2004; **27**: 317–27.

● 100. Bollard CM, Gottschalk S, Leen AM *et al.* Complete responses of relapsed lymphoma following genetic modification of tumor-antigen presenting cells and T-lymphocyte transfer. *Blood* 2007; **110**: 2838–45.

101. van Baarle D, Hovenkamp E, Callan MF *et al.* Dysfunctional Epstein-Barr virus (EBV)-specific CD8(+) T lymphocytes and increased EBV load in HIV-1 infected individuals progressing to AIDS-related non-Hodgkin lymphoma. *Blood* 2001; **98**: 146–55.

102. Wheatley HG, McKinnon K, Lilly S et al. Adoptive immunotherapy using autologous EBV-specific CTL in a HIV infected patient with refractory Epstein Barr virus expressing B cell Lymphoma. J Acquir Immune Defic Syndr Hum Retrovirol 1997; **14**: A53.

103. Ambinder RF. Viruses as potential targets for therapy in HIV-associated malignancies. Hematol Oncol Clin North Am 2003; **17**: 697–702, v–vi.

104. Stebbing J, Gazzard B, Patterson S et al. Simplified one-step antibody-HLA directed expansion of HIV-specific cytotoxic T lymphocytes: a system suited for use in vivo. AIDS 2004; **18**: 2099–101.

105. Cooper LJ, Topp MS, Serrano LM et al. T-cell clones can be rendered specific for CD19: toward the selective augmentation of the graft-versus-B-lineage leukemia effect. Blood 2003; **101**: 1637–44.

106. Jensen MC. Targeting malignant B cells of lymphoma and leukemia with genetically engineered T-cell clones. Cytotherapy 2002; **4**: 443–4.

107. Jensen M, Cooper L, Wu A et al. Engineered CD20-specific primary human cytotoxic T lymphocytes for targeting B-cell malignancy. Cytotherapy 2003; **5**: 131–8.

108. Wang J, Press OW, Lindgren CG et al. Cellular immunotherapy for follicular lymphoma using genetically modified CD20-specific CD8+ cytotoxic T lymphocytes. Mol Ther 2004; **9**: 577–86.

109. Savoldo B, Rooney CM, Di SA et al. Epstein Barr virus specific cytotoxic T lymphocytes expressing the anti-CD30zeta artificial chimeric T-cell receptor for immunotherapy of Hodgkin disease. Blood 2007; **110**: 2620–30.

●110. Till BG, Jensen MC, Wang J et al. Adoptive immunotherapy for indolent non-Hodgkin lymphoma and mantle cell lymphoma using genetically modified autologous CD20-specific T cells. Blood 2008; **112**: 2261–71.

111. Maher J, Brentjens RJ, Gunset G et al. Human T-lymphocyte cytotoxicity and proliferation directed by a single chimeric TCRzeta /CD28 receptor. Nat Biotechnol 2002; **20**: 70–75.

112. Rossig C, Bollard CM, Nuchtern JG et al. Epstein-Barr virus-specific human T lymphocytes expressing antitumor chimeric T-cell receptors: potential for improved immunotherapy. Blood 2002; **99**: 2009–16.

113. Heemskerk MH, Hoogeboom M, Hagedoorn R et al. Reprogramming of virus-specific T cells into leukemia-reactive T cells using T cell receptor gene transfer. J Exp Med 2004; **199**: 885–94.

114. Cooper LJ, Al Kadhimi Z, Serrano LM et al. Enhanced antilymphoma efficacy of CD19-redirected influenza MP1-specific CTLs by cotransfer of T cells modified to present influenza MP1. Blood 2005; **105**: 1622–31.

115. Pule MA, Straathof KC, Dotti G et al. A chimeric T cell antigen receptor that augments cytokine release and supports clonal expansion of primary human T cells. Mol Ther 2005; **12**: 933–41.

116. Imai C, Mihara K, Andreansky M et al. Chimeric receptors with 4-1BB signaling capacity provoke potent cytotoxicity against acute lymphoblastic leukemia. Leukemia 2004; **18**: 676–84.

●117. Brentjens RJ, Latouche JB, Santos E et al. Eradication of systemic B-cell tumors by genetically targeted human T lymphocytes co-stimulated by CD80 and interleukin-15. Nat Med 2003; **9**: 279–86.

118. Ruggeri L, Capanni M, Urbani E et al. Effectiveness of donor natural killer cell alloreactivity in mismatched hematopoietic transplants. Science 2002; **295**: 2097–100.

119. Miller JS, Soignier Y, Panoskaltsis-Mortari A et al. Successful adoptive transfer and in vivo expansion of human haploidentical NK cells in patients with cancer. Blood 2005; **105**: 3051–7.

120. Maus MV, Thomas AK, Leonard DG et al. Ex vivo expansion of polyclonal and antigen-specific cytotoxic T lymphocytes by artificial APCs expressing ligands for the T-cell receptor, CD28 and 4-1BB. Nat Biotechnol 2002; **20**: 143–8.

121. Latouche JB, Sadelain M. Induction of human cytotoxic T lymphocytes by artificial antigen-presenting cells. Nat Biotechnol 2000; **18**: 405–9.

122. Oelke M, Maus MV, Didiano D et al. Ex vivo induction and expansion of antigen-specific cytotoxic T cells by HLA-Ig-coated artificial antigen-presenting cells. Nat Med 2003; **9**: 619–25.

123. Hoogendoorn M, Olde WJ, Smit WM et al. Primary allogeneic T-cell responses against mantle cell lymphoma antigen-presenting cells for adoptive immunotherapy after stem cell transplantation. Clin Cancer Res 2005; **11**: 5310–18.

124. Sallusto F, Geginat J, Lanzavecchia A. Central memory and effector memory T cell subsets: function, generation, and maintenance. Annu Rev Immunol 2004; **22**: 745–63.

●125. Berger C, Jensen MC, Lansdorp PM et al. Adoptive transfer of effector CD8+ T cells derived from central memory cells establishes persistent T cell memory in primates. J Clin Invest 2008; **118**: 294–305.

126. Muraro S, Bondanza A, Bellone M et al. Molecular modification of idiotypes from B-cell lymphomas for expression in mature dendritic cells as a strategy to induce tumor-reactive CD4+ and CD8+ T-cell responses. Blood 2005; **105**: 3596–604.

127. Alvaro T, Lejeune M, Salvado MT et al. Outcome in Hodgkin's lymphoma can be predicted from the presence of accompanying cytotoxic and regulatory T cells. Clin Cancer Res 2005; **11**: 1467–73.

128. Dukers DF, Jaspars LH, Vos W et al. Quantitative immunohistochemical analysis of cytokine profiles in Epstein-Barr virus-positive and -negative cases of Hodgkin's disease. J Pathol 2000; **190**: 143–9.

129. Bollard CM, Rössig C, Calonge MJ et al. Adapting a transforming growth factor beta-related tumor protection strategy to enhance antitumor immunity. Blood 2002; **99**: 3179–87.

130. Gorelik L, Flavell RA. Immune-mediated eradication of tumors through the blockade of transforming growth factor-beta signaling in T cells. Nat Med 2001; **7**: 1118–22.

131. Zhang Q, Yang X, Pins M *et al.* Adoptive transfer of tumor-reactive transforming growth factor-beta-insensitive CD8+ T cells: eradication of autologous mouse prostate cancer. *Cancer Res* 2005; **65**: 1761–9.

132. Dotti G, Savoldo B, Pule M *et al.* Human cytotoxic T lymphocytes with reduced sensitivity to Fas-induced apoptosis. *Blood* 2005; **105**: 4677–84.

133. Klebanoff CA, Khong HT, Antony PA *et al.* Sinks, suppressors and antigen presenters: how lymphodepletion enhances T cell-mediated tumor immunotherapy. *Trends Immunol* 2005; **26**: 111–7.

◆134. Dudley ME, Rosenberg SA. Adoptive-cell-transfer therapy for the treatment of patients with cancer. *Nat Rev Cancer* 2003; **3**: 666–75.

135. Marshall NA, Christie LE, Munro LR *et al.* Immunosuppressive regulatory T cells are abundant in the reactive lymphocytes of Hodgkin lymphoma. *Blood* 2004; **103**: 1755–62.

136. Dudley ME, Wunderlich JR, Robbins PF *et al.* Cancer regression and autoimmunity in patients after clonal repopulation with antitumor lymphocytes. *Science* 2002; **298**: 850–54.

137. Hombach A, Heuser C, Sircar R *et al.* An anti-CD30 chimeric receptor that mediates CD3-zeta-independent T-cell activation against Hodgkin's lymphoma cells in the presence of soluble CD30. *Cancer Res* 1998; **58**: 1116–9.

138. Hambach L, Goulmy E. Immunotherapy of cancer through targeting of minor histocompatibility antigens. *Curr Opin Immunol* 2005; **17**: 202–10.

139. Heslop HE, Brenner MK, Rooney CM. Donor T cells to treat EBV-associated lymphoma. *N Engl J Med* 1994; **331**: 679–80.

140. Porter DL, Orloff GJ, Antin JH. Donor mononuclear cell infusions as therapy for B-cell lymphoproliferative disorder following allogeneic bone marrow transplant. *Transplant Sci* 1994; **4**: 12–14.

141. Sasahara Y, Kawai S, Itano M *et al.* Epstein-Barr virus-associated lymphoproliferative disorder after unrelated bone marrow transplantation in a young child with Wiskott-Aldrich syndrome. *Pediatr Hematol Oncol* 1998; **15**: 347–52.

142. Gross TG, Steinbuch M, DeFor T *et al.* B cell lymphoproliferative disorders following hematopoietic stem cell transplantation: risk factors, treatment and outcome. *Bone Marrow Transplant* 1999; **23**: 251–8.

143. Tiberghien P, Ferrand C, Lioure B *et al.* Administration of herpes simplex-thymidine kinase-expressing donor T cells with a T-cell-depleted allogeneic marrow graft. *Blood* 2001; **97**: 63–72.

144. Anderlini P, Acholonu SA, Okoroji GJ *et al.* Donor leukocyte infusions in relapsed Hodgkin's lymphoma following allogeneic stem cell transplantation: CD3+ cell dose, GVHD and disease response. *Bone Marrow Transplant* 2004; **34**: 511–4.

145. Robinson SP, Goldstone AH, Mackinnon S *et al.* Chemoresistant or aggressive lymphoma predicts for a poor outcome following reduced-intensity allogeneic progenitor cell transplantation: an analysis from the Lymphoma Working Party of the European Group for Blood and Bone Marrow Transplantation. *Blood* 2002; **100**: 4310–16.

146. Imashuku S, Goto T, Matsumura T *et al.* Unsuccessful CTL transfusion in a case of post-BMT Epstein-Barr virus-associated lymphoproliferative disorder (EBV-LPD). *Bone Marrow Transplant* 1998; **20**: 337–40.

147. Haque T, Amlot PL, Helling N *et al.* Reconstitution of EBV-specific T cell immunity in solid organ transplant recipients. *J Immunol* 1998; **160**: 6204–9.

148. Sherritt MA, Bharadwaj M, Burrows JM *et al.* Reconstitution of the latent T-lymphocyte response to Epstein-Barr virus is coincident with long-term recovery from posttransplant lymphoma after adoptive immunotherapy. *Transplantation* 2003; **75**: 1556–60.

149. Gandhi MK, Wilkie GM, Dua U *et al.* Immunity, homing and efficacy of allogeneic adoptive immunotherapy for posttransplant lymphoproliferative disorders. *Am J Transplant* 2007; **7**: 1293–9.

150. Cho HI, Hong YS, Lee MA *et al.* Adoptive transfer of Epstein-Barr virus-specific cytotoxic T-lymphocytes for the treatment of angiocentric lymphomas. *Int J Hematol* 2006; **83**: 66–73.

88

Vaccine therapies

H QIN, SS NEELAPU, A WOO, SC CHA AND LW KWAK

IMMUNOGLOBULIN IDIOTYPE ANTIGEN VACCINES

The development of therapeutic vaccines against human malignancies has been a long-sought goal. Many efforts toward this end have been frustrated by the lack of identified, tumor-specific antigens that would allow tumor cells to be distinguished from normal cells. Conceptually, such an antigen could be used as an immunogen to activate host antitumor immunity.

B cell malignancies in humans are composed of clonal proliferations of cells arising at various stages of normal B cell differentiation, each synthesizing a single rearranged immunoglobulin gene product with unique variable regions. For example, most cases of acute lymphocytic leukemia are the neoplastic counterparts of precursor B cells, which fail to express either immunoglobulin or cytoplasmic μ chains. In contrast, B cell lymphomas are neoplasms of mature, resting, and reactive lymphocytes, which generally express immunoglobulin on the cell surface. To complete the spectrum of stages of B cell development, multiple myeloma is a neoplasm of terminally differentiated plasma cells. The variable region of immunoglobulin receptor molecules contains unique determinants, termed idiotypes, which can themselves be recognized as antigens. The idiotypic determinants of the surface immunoglobulin of a B cell lymphoma can thus serve as tumor-specific markers for the malignant clone and can serve as targets for therapeutic approaches. The use of idiotype as a form of active immunotherapy – immunization of a human host with

human tumor antigen – should be distinguished from original studies of passive immunotherapy, in which murine antibodies with specificity for idiotype were used as the immunotherapeutic agent. Active immunization might produce both humoral and cellular immunity against tumor cells bearing the unique idiotype antigen. These responses would be of host origin and might therefore be long lasting. Because active immunization with immunoglobulin idiotype should result in the induction of a polyclonal immune response directed against multiple idiotypic determinants on the molecule, this strategy may overcome the problem of tumor heterogeneity with the emergence of tumor cell variants. Previously, mutated surface immunoglobulins limited the success of anti-idiotype antibody therapy.

The discoveries providing the rationale for this approach were initially made in the 1970s when Sirisinha and Eisen observed that inbred mice could be induced to make antibodies against idiotypic determinants on myeloma proteins from mice of the same strain (syngeneic).[1] Soon thereafter, Lynch *et al.* showed that immunization of syngeneic mice against a myeloma protein resulted in protection from subsequent lethal challenge with myeloma cells from which the protein had been derived.[2] Subsequent studies in a number of syngeneic experimental tumor models confirmed that active immunization against idiotypic determinants on malignant B cells produced resistance to tumor growth, as well as specific antitumor therapy against established tumors.[3–13] At least in one model, optimal immunization of lymphoma-derived idiotype required conjugation of the protein to an immunogenic protein carrier, keyhole limpet hemocyanin (KLH), and emulsification in an adjuvant.[14]

KLH–CONJUGATED IDIOTYPE PROTEIN VACCINES

Production of human idiotype vaccines and phase I/II clinical trials in follicular lymphoma

The initial strategy used to isolate immunoglobulin from the surface of human B cell lymphoma involves the formation of a somatic cell hybrid between the lymphoma cell and a modified mouse myeloma cell that grows *in vitro* and has the cellular machinery to synthesize and secrete large quantities of immunoglobulin.[15] Murine myeloma fusion partners have been engineered so that they are unable to secrete immunoglobulin of their own; therefore, the secreted immunoglobulin is purely derived from the human tumor.

Production of idiotype protein begins with the isolation of malignant cells from tumor biopsy specimens, most commonly from lymph nodes. However, tumor cells can also be isolated from peripheral blood, bone marrow, or spleen. Starting material is a minimum of about 10 to 15 million tumor cells. Lymphoma cells are fused with a hypoxanthine-aminopterin-thymidine (HAT)-sensitive fusion partner, and heteromyelomas are selected from HAT medium. Identity of fusions and follicular lymphoma was determined by comparing immunoglobulin heavy-chain variable region (V_H) CD3 sequences. Heteromyelomas identified in this way are expanded, and idiotype protein is then purified from collected culture supernatants by affinity chromatography using Sepharose–anti-human IgM or Sepharose–Protein A, depending on the isotype of the lymphoma immunoglobulin. Finally, each idiotype is conjugated to KLH, which is used to immunize the patient from whose tumor the idiotype protein was originally isolated.

Working in Levy's laboratory, Kwak pioneered an initial pilot study of autologous idiotype immunization in nine patients with B cell lymphoma using idiotype isolated as described.[14] This first experience in approximately 40 patients demonstrated primarily humoral idiotype-specific immune response.[16] Building on these results, the Kwak laboratory designed a phase II clinical trial, focusing on developing a therapeutic vaccine formulation that was more effective in activating the cellular arm of the immune system.[17] Individuals recruited in this phase II trial were previously untreated patients with follicular lymphoma. After initial lymph node harvest for individualized vaccine production, all patients were cytoreduced with a uniform chemotherapy regimen (prednisone, doxorubicin, cyclophosphamide, and etoposide; PACE) to complete remission (CR) by standard clinical criteria. This produced a homogeneous group of patients, all in first CR, who were then given vaccine treatment. A 6-month rest period between chemotherapy and vaccination allowed recovery from the immunosuppressive effects of this combination chemotherapy. This vaccine formulation consisted of idiotype-KLH conjugate physically mixed with soluble granulocyte macrophage colony-stimulating factor

(GM-CSF). This choice of vaccine formulation was important and was a direct translation of prior preclinical studies in a murine lymphoma model screening several promising immunological adjuvants for their ability to enhance the response to idiotype-KLH immunization.[18] In this study, GM-CSF emerged as the most promising cytokine, which was consistent with the results of earlier gene therapy studies by other investigators.[19,20] Furthermore, these studies showed a minimal effect of GM-CSF on antibody levels, while T cell subset depletion experiments demonstrated the requirement for CD8+ T cells in the effector phase of protective immunity. Thus, the addition of GM-CSF met the study's criteria for a vaccine formulation that was both more potent and more effective in the induction of CD8+ T cells compared to the prototype vaccine alone.

The entire vaccine formulation was injected subcutaneously as five monthly doses. Twenty patients who were in CR completed the vaccination protocol. Cell targets were carefully selected to measure both B and T cell responses, with the objective to demonstrate immune responses that could neutralize autologous tumor cells. Of primary interest, peripheral blood mononuclear cells (PBMC) from immunized patients were incubated *in vitro* with autologous tumor (lymph node biopsy cells, specifically enriched for tumor in some cases) and 5 days later cytokine responses (tumor necrosis factor α [TNFα], interferon γ [IFNγ], and GM-CSF) were measured. Overall, 19 of 20 patients (95 percent) had tumor-specific T cell responses. Importantly, significant levels of HLA class I-restricted killing of autologous tumor targets were also detected in the vast majority of patients. Nonneoplastic, normal B cells from the same patients were not killed, indicating specificity of this response. Furthermore, when CD8+ T cells were fractionated from PBMC, this subpopulation of cells reproduced the response seen with the bulk PBMC. Thus, vaccination against idiotype with GM-CSF provided the first substantial evidence for eliciting CD8+ T cells specific for autologous lymphoma. Peptide mapping studies identified several defined HLA II idiotype epitopes.[21]

Using a molecular end point, the study was able to monitor potential antitumor effects of immunization. The t(14;18) chromosomal translocation has been proposed as a minimal residual disease marker for follicular lymphoma.[22] Approximately 50 percent to 60 percent of follicular lymphomas have a translocation that can be amplified using polymerase chain reaction (PCR). Of the 20 patients in this study, 11 were found to have PCR-positive breakpoints in their tumors and were evaluable for this molecular analysis. Given the natural history of inevitable relapse of this disease, it was not an unexpected finding that all 11 patients had tumor cells in the blood detectable by PCR, even though they were in a CR at the time of vaccination. In eight of these 11 patients, this signal was no longer detectable in postvaccine samples and in subsequent follow-up samples, suggesting a conversion from PCR positivity to negativity associated with the vaccine. In the three other patients, the PCR positivity seen before vaccination was also seen after vaccination and in follow-up samples. Demonstration of clinical benefit was more difficult, because the vaccine was given as an adjuvant to induction chemotherapy to patients who were already in CR. However, analysis of time-to-relapse may also provide an independent indication of clinical benefit. After a median follow-up period of 7 years after the completion of induction chemotherapy, one-half of the patients in this trial remain in continuous first clinical CR. Thus, this disease-free survival outcome is encouraging; however, without a concurrent control group of patients, results cannot be regarded as definitive evidence for clinical benefit.

This phase II study overcame two limitations of previous idiotype vaccine studies: (1) the induction of tumor-specific, CD8+ T cells and (2) the demonstration of antitumor effects in a homogeneous group of patients. In addition, although not generally feasible for solid tumors, this study also established the killing of autologous tumor targets as a standard for future vaccine studies in lymphoma. The important, broader questions of identifying the precise mechanisms of tumor eradication and the immunologic assays that correlate with antitumor effects will ultimately require larger numbers of patients treated with this or other effective cancer vaccines. However, the observation that at least three patients achieved molecular remissions without a detectable antibody response indicates that a humoral response may not be required. Finally, this study established GM-CSF as an essential component of this vaccine, since the earlier study using the same immunogen administered without GM-CSF showed humoral but no CD8+ T cell responses.[14] GM-CSF likely works by recruiting antigen-presenting cells (APC), including dendritic cells (DC), which may activate pathways of antigen processing that allow exogenous proteins to be presented by class I molecules.[23]

Idiotype vaccine following rituximab therapy in mantle cell lymphoma

This idiotype protein vaccine was also tested in a homogeneous group of mantle cell lymphoma (MCL) patients in first remission after a rituximab-containing chemotherapy regimen.[24] Twenty-six previously untreated MCL patients received 6 cycles of dose-adjusted EPOCH-R (rituximab, etoposide, vincristine, doxorubicin, cyclophosphamide, prednisone),[25] followed 12 weeks later by five monthly cycles of autologous, tumor-derived idiotype-KLH + GM-CSF vaccine. Following EPOCH-R, CR/complete remission, unconfirmed (CRu) was achieved in 92 percent and partial response in 8 percent of patients. With a median potential follow-up of 46 months, overall survival probability is 89 percent, median event-free survival is 22 months, and five patients remain in continuous first complete remission.

Following EPOCH-R, peripheral blood B cells were completely depleted in all patients, began to recover at approximately 6 months, and returned to baseline levels by 1 year in most patients. In contrast, CD4+ T cell numbers decreased only slightly after EPOCH-R and recovered by the start of vaccination with a median time of 3 months, and CD8+ T cell numbers did not change substantially. Unexpectedly, antibodies to KLH and Id were detected in 17 out of 23 (74 percent) patients and in seven out of 23 (30 percent) patients, respectively, usually after the fourth or fifth vaccination, and correlated with peripheral blood B cell recovery. Tumor-specific T cell responses were observed in 20 out of 23 (87 percent) patients, and were detectable after the third vaccination, at which time peripheral blood B cells were essentially undetectable. Thus, this study demonstrated for the first time that tumor-specific CD4+ and CD8+ T cells could be induced in humans despite severe B cell depletion by rituximab. Although most patients relapsed, the overall survival of 89 percent at 46 months raises the intriguing possibility that idiotype vaccination modified the natural history of mantle cell lymphoma. This study is especially relevant for vaccine development in lymphoma patients since rituximab is increasingly being used for the treatment of lymphoma.[26] However, because the relative role of cellular versus humoral immunity for lymphoma vaccine efficacy is uncertain, it may be advisable to administer booster vaccinations following B cell recovery to optimize humoral responses.

Phase III study design

Based on promising results of the phase II trial,[17] the National Cancer Institute (NCI) opened a controlled phase III study in January 2000.[27] The principal objective of this multicenter double-blinded randomized trial is to answer the question of clinical efficacy of idiotype-KLH vaccine combined with GM-CSF using disease-free survival as the primary end point (Fig. 88.1). The design of the study follows the protocol used in the phase II trial.[17] In brief, the study focuses on previously untreated patients with follicular non-Hodgkin lymphoma and with a peripheral lymph node greater or equal to 2 cm in diameter for biopsy and harvest for vaccine preparation. Before vaccination, treatment with PACE chemotherapy is administered to attain minimal residual disease. Patients achieving a clinical CR or CRu provide a homogeneous population for randomization of vaccine treatment (specific versus nonspecific). Patients in the control group in this study receive KLH and GM-CSF (nonspecific vaccine). Both reagents have potential antitumor effects when used alone. Moreover, two-thirds of the patients are randomized to receive the specific vaccine treatment, instead of 50 percent, which is customary. The study aims at recruiting a total of 563 patients to randomize a total of 375 patients. This number is required to allow approximately 80 percent power to detect a difference between disease-free survival curves with initial hazard of 1.0 for the first 8 months (when treatments are expected to be the same in both randomized arms) and then an intended hazard ratio of 2.0 after the first

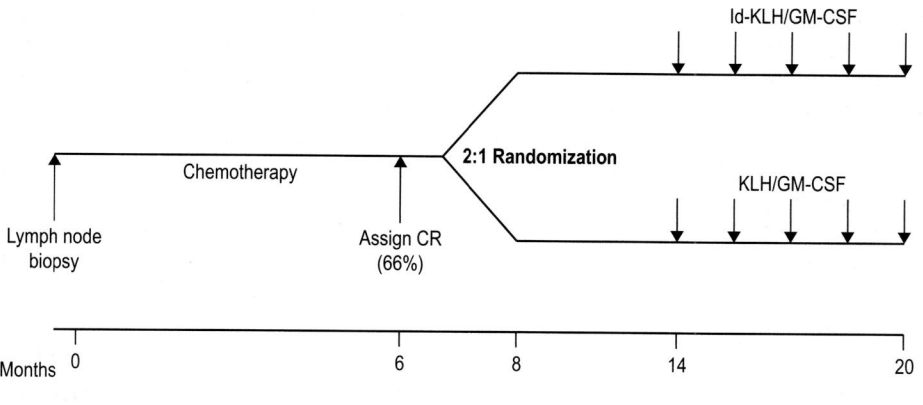

Figure 88.1 Phase III clinical trial of lymphoma idiotype vaccine (National Cancer Institute). Id-KLH, idiotype-keyhole limpet hemocyanin conjugate; GM-CSF, granulocyte macrophage colony-stimulating factor; CR, complete remission.

8 months. At the present time, approximately 180 patients have been enrolled in the study. Sponsorship of this phase III trial was transferred to a commercial partner in 2005. Subsequently, two other commercially sponsored phase III trials of recombinant idiotype protein vaccines, both using GM-CSF as the immunological adjuvant, have been initiated.

OTHER LYMPHOMA VACCINES

In addition to the idiotype vaccine for B cell lymphoma, other strategies have been tested as potential vaccines for lymphoid malignancies. Several novel strategies are summarized in Table 88.1. The first tumor vaccine attempted to use irradiated tumor cells to activate the immune system to recognize and eventually eliminate tumor cells. However, early studies using this approach failed to elicit antitumor immunity. A variety of modified vaccine formulations have been tested to improve tumor cell-based vaccines. The GM-CSF-transduced and CD40 ligand (CD40L)-transduced tumor cell vaccines and tumor cell lysate-pulsed DC vaccine effectively induced T cell-mediated tumor protection against B cell and T cell lymphomas, respectively.[28,29] Another formulation using whole cell membrane protein derived from autologous B lymphoma cells, coadministered with interleukin-2 (IL-2), has moved to phase I clinical trial.[30]

Tumor-derived heat shock protein (HSP) peptide complexes represent another potential category of lymphoma vaccine, which was consistently able to elicit tumor-specific immune responses and antitumor effects in preclinical studies.[31,32] The simplicity of isolating HSP from autologous tumor facilitates the development of HSP vaccines for cancer patients. Indeed, the safety and immunogenicity of HSP vaccines have been confirmed by several independent phase I studies.[33,34] The clinical efficacy of HSP vaccines in non-Hodgkin lymphoma was under investigation in a completed phase II trial.[35]

Vaccines targeting T cell lymphoma using T cell receptor (TCR) as a tumor antigen have been described. Like the

Table 88.1 Additional novel strategies for lymphoma vaccines

Vaccine	Clinical phase of testing	Reference
GM-CSF-transduced tumor cells	Phase I	[29]
CD40L-transduced tumor cells	Phase I	[89]
Tumor cell lysate-pulsed DC	Phase I	[28]
Membrane protein + IL-2	Phase I	Unpublished
Heat shock protein	Phase II	[35]
T cell receptor	Preclinical	[36]
ALK	Preclinical	[37]
Survivin	Preclinical	[38]
Cytochrome P450 1B1	Phase I	[39]

GM-CSF, granulocyte macrophage colony-stimulating factor; CD40L, CD40 ligand; DC, dendritic cells; IL-2, interleukin-2; ALK, anaplastic lymphoma kinase.

immunoglobulin idiotype on B cells, TCR is also a unique antigen due to its variable region generated by V(D)J recombination. Vaccination of TCR proteins derived from a murine T cell lymphoma induced antibody-based tumor protection,[36] which highlights the feasibility of translational development of TCR vaccines for T cell malignancies.

Lastly, peptide vaccines derived from several recently identified, tumor-associated antigens are being developed and tested for their antitumor effects using preclinical tumor models.[37–39]

SECOND-GENERATION LYMPHOMA IDIOTYPE VACCINES

Other vaccine carriers and delivery systems have been investigated to improve the therapeutic potency of idiotype vaccines by enhancing CD8$^+$ T cell-mediated antitumor immunity. This section is devoted to an in-depth discussion of the development of second-generation vaccines, liposomal-formulated vaccines (OncoVAX-idiotype/IL-2) and chemokine-fused single-chain DNA vaccines.

Liposomal–formulated idiotype vaccine

Liposomes have been widely accepted as effective carriers for vaccines for reasons that include the following: (1) encapsulating antigens with liposomes facilitates APC uptake of antigens; (2) antigens and immune adjuvants or mediators can be easily co-loaded on the same vehicle; and (3) while the majority of the endocytosed liposome-encapsulated antigens are processed in lysosomes, a small portion of antigens could be released into the cytosol to access the MHC class I pathway. As a result, both CD4+ and CD8+ T cell priming occurs.[40,41] A preclinical study was designed to test the potential of liposome-encapsulated idiotype.[42] The vaccine was formulated to combine idiotype proteins with IL-2, which serves as an immune adjuvant to boost both innate and adaptive immune responses. Using a murine lymphoma model, significant, prolonged survival was observed after a single dose of liposome-encapsulated idiotype/IL-2 vaccine given by intraperitoneal injection. The potency of vaccine-induced antitumor immunity was dose dependent. At a dosage of 40 μg, the liposome-encapsulated idiotype/IL-2 protein vaccine was notably more effective at inducing tumor protection when compared to an optimal dose of idiotype-KLH prototype vaccine containing 50 μg of idiotype protein. Further experiments supported the finding that improved tumor protection of the idiotype/IL-2 liposomal vaccine was mainly due to the activation of T cell-mediated immunity. Depletion of either CD4+ or CD8+ T cells considerably abrogated the ability of the vaccine to induce protection against tumor challenge, demonstrating the necessary role of T cells in the immune response.

Liposome-encapsulated idiotype/IL-2 vaccine enhanced tumor protection and induced tumor-specific T cell immunity, providing the rationale to translate this vaccine to clinical study. Neelapu et al. designed a phase I clinical trial at the NCI to evaluate the safety and immunogenicity of this liposomal vaccine formulated with 2 mg patient-specific, tumor-derived idiotype protein, 4×10^6 international units (IU) IL-2, and 160 mg dimyristoylphosphatidylcholine (all amounts per milliliter) to generate liposomes (OncoVAX, Biomira USA, Cranberry, NJ).[43] The trial included ten previously untreated patients, all of whom had stage II–IV follicular lymphoma grade 1 or 2. A lymph node biopsy was harvested for vaccine preparation before the chemotherapy was initiated. A uniform PACE chemotherapy regimen was administered to all patients for a minimum of 6 cycles to achieve minimal residual disease status, which was comprehensively assessed by physical examination, computerized tomography scans, lymphoangiograms, and bilateral bone marrow biopsies. Thus, a homogeneous population was generated with a complete clinical response in nine patients and a partial response in one patient following chemotherapy. The vaccination began 6 months after completion of chemotherapy. All patients received five doses of the vaccine at months 0, 1, 2, 3, and 5.

The vaccine was well tolerated with no evidence of adverse events greater than grade 2. Minor inflammation was observed in all patients at the site of injection, lasting up to 1 week. Consistent with observations from the preclinical study, liposomal idiotype vaccine induced tumor-specific cellular immunity in all patients. Postvaccine, but not prevaccine, PBMC responded to autologous tumor cells by producing type I cytokines including IFNγ, GM-CSF, and TNFα. The same PBMC, however, failed to react to autologous normal B cells, confirming the specificity of the immune response. Additional studies demonstrated that the cellular immune responses were HLA class I and II associated, suggesting that both CD4+ and CD8+ T cell responses were involved in the antitumor immune response. Using autologous idiotype proteins for stimulation, an antigen-specific cellular response was observed in nine of ten patients.[43] Interestingly, only four patients had antibody-mediated immunity against autologous idiotype proteins. Thus, this trial demonstrated that liposomal idiotype/IL-2 vaccine is a safe formulation for clinical purpose, and the vaccine favors a tumor-specific T cell response. Although the number of patients from this single-arm study is too limited to evaluate clinical efficacy, patients experienced favorable outcomes. Six patients remained in continuous first complete remission after a median follow-up of 50 months. Three other patients had evidence of progressive disease at the end of the vaccination, while another developed secondary acute myeloid leukemia. A randomized phase II trial is needed to directly compare the immunogenicity and clinical efficacy of this liposomal idiotype vaccine with the prototype Id-KLH + GM-CSF vaccine.

Chemokine–idiotype single–chain fusion DNA vaccines

Given that the lymphoma idiotype is an individualized, patient-specific antigen, current hybridoma approaches for vaccine preparation are time consuming and laborious. An easy and convenient method is necessary to make idiotype vaccine therapy more practical. The specificity of an immunoglobulin is determined by the genetic information embedded in the variable regions of both light and heavy chains. Advances in antibody engineering now facilitate identification and cloning of these variable regions and assembly into a single-chain (sFv) format that encodes a single polypeptide consisting solely of V_H and V_L genes linked together in-frame with a short, 15 amino acid linker. In vivo expression of foreign genes encoding the tumor antigen by DNA vaccination requires the gene to be cloned under regulatory elements of eukaryotic or viral elements into an expression cassette, which is then either injected in solution via intramuscular or intradermal routes or delivered into the epidermis by particle-mediated bombardment of DNA-coated gold particles (gene gun). The host's cellular machinery carries out protein translation, which avoids many technical problems such as post-translational modification and protein folding, concerns when expressing proteins by nonmammalian cell systems. The simplicity and ease of vaccine generation therefore gives DNA vaccines tremendous potential for streamlining the production of individualized idiotype vaccines.[44]

Initial studies revealed that the sFv DNA vaccine itself was nonimmunogenic unless conjugated with an adjuvant.[45–48] Fortunately, the single-chain format considerably reduced the molecular size of idiotypic antigen and thus paved the way for genetic modification of the tumor antigen. This strategy was used to generate a second-generation idiotype vaccine where idiotype sFv was engineered to target APC, thus activating the cellular immune response to an otherwise nonimmunogenic lymphoma idiotype. Among all APC subtypes, DC draw the most attention due to their exclusive ability of priming naïve T cells, essential in initiating and maintaining a T cell immune response against malignant cells. Accordingly, the potency of inducing T cell immunity and the clinical efficacy of a tumor vaccine might be dependent on the ability of DC to capture tumor antigens. For this purpose, a novel strategy of fusing idiotype sFv with chemotactic cytokines, termed chemokines, was employed for *in vivo* targeting of DC for tumor antigens.[49]

Chemokines are a group of secreted polypeptides (7–15 kDa) that induce inflammatory responses by orchestrating the selective migration, diapedesis, and activation of blood-borne leukocytes. Chemokines bind to specific, cell-surface heptahelical G-protein-coupled receptors and are internalized upon ligand binding.[50–53] Given that numerous chemokine receptors, including CCR1, CCR2, CCR5, CXCR1, and CXCR3, have been identified on DC,[54,55] physically linking idiotype sFv with chemokines improves the likelihood that DC capturing tumor antigens will be generated.

This novel strategy targets DC for chemokine receptor-mediated uptake of tumor antigen, which in turn leads to antigen processing and presentation. By this proposed mechanism, the binding of chimeric chemokine-sFv fusions with chemokine receptors on DC is essential to inducing antitumor immunity. In initial characterization studies, idiotype sFv was generated from two different murine B cell lymphoma models, 38C and A20, which express surface IgM and IgG2a, respectively, and was fused to proinflammatory chemokine genes monocyte chemotactic protein 3 (MCP-3) or macrophage inflammatory protein 3α (MIP-3α). The genetic chemokine-sFv chimeric proteins retained their critical biological activities, particularly receptor-binding properties, as compared with control unmodified chemokines. For example, the recombinant

fusion proteins, produced as insoluble inclusion bodies in *Escherichia coli*, bound and induced chemotaxis of cells that either endogenously expressed or were engineered to express corresponding chemokine receptors.[49,56] For the vaccine formulation used in preclinical studies, chemokine fusions were designed as a DNA vaccine that encodes secreted soluble proteins. This was done by incorporation of a secretion signal sequence of the IP-10 inducible protein into the fusion cassette.

Biragyn *et al.* demonstrated that MCP-3-fused or MIP-3α-fused sFv DNA vaccines induced tumor protection in both A20 and 38C models. Antitumor effects were observed in prophylactic studies where mice were immunized followed by tumor challenge, as well as in therapeutic experiments where vaccines were given to eliminate the minimal preexisting tumors.[49,56] In comparison with the prototype idiotype-KLH conjugated protein vaccine, chemokine-sFv fusion DNA vaccines induced equivalent tumor protection in the 38C model and superior antitumor effects in the A20 model. The activation of cellular tumor-specific immunity, especially a CD8+ T cell response, was evident. Depletion of either CD8+ or CD4+ T cells dramatically inhibited vaccine-induced tumor protection, suggesting that T cell-mediated immunity plays a dominant role in protecting animals from tumor challenge. These features of chemokine-sFv fusions distinguish them from other reported DNA idiotype vaccines. In particular, the generation of CD8+ T cell immunity distinguishes these fusions from previously reported fusions of lymphoma idiotype with GM-CSF, which exclusively elicited an antibody response,[45] and from a DNA vaccine encoding sFv with fragment C of tetanus toxin, which elicited a CD4+ T cell-mediated protective immune response.[48,57] The finding that chemokine-sFv fusions induced a CD8+ T cell response, leading to an antitumor effect comparable to that of idiotype-KLH vaccine, thus provided the rationale for the translational development of chemokine-fused idiotype vaccine for clinical trials. A similar strategy was also applied to generate a human immunodeficiency virus (HIV) vaccine by linking HIV envelope protein gp120 antigen with MCP-3. Vaccination of mice with this DNA vaccine activated CD8+ T cell-based systemic and mucosal immunity against gp120 antigens, highlighting the potential of chemokine fusions as a general strategy for therapeutic vaccine design.[58]

Mechanistic experiments suggest that the induction of tumor-specific T cell immunity required physically linking chemokines with sFv. Using a well-established CD4+ T cell clone that specifically recognizes an MHC class II molecule-binding idiotypic peptide derived from plasmacytoma MOPC315 immunoglobulin, chemokine receptor-mediated endocytosis loaded idiotype sFv into the MHC class II pathway, which in turn activated antigen-specific CD4+ T cells.[59] T cell stimulation optimally required chemokine receptor engagement because DC or splenocytes incubated with an unlinked mixture of free sFv with chemokine stimulated T cells only weakly. Moreover, fusion proteins containing mutated chemokines, which were unable to bind their respective receptors, failed to activate T cells. *In vitro* T cell activation was abrogated by blocking endoplasmic reticulum–Golgi transport or lysosomal activity, but not by inhibiting proteasomal degradation, thus suggesting that chemoattractant receptors on APC can efficiently internalize chemokine-fused antigens, which are then processed through the early/late endocytic compartments in the MHC class II presentation pathway. Similarly, APC capable of stimulating the idiotype-specific T cell clone were isolated from draining lymph nodes from mice previously immunized with chemokine fusion, but not with sFv protein alone. The observation was further confirmed using human fusion proteins; specifically, chemokine fusion proteins facilitated the uptake and presentation of a human lymphoma sFv and stimulated idiotype-specific CD4[+] T cells from the same patient.[59] This stimulation was greater than DC treated with sFv alone or a fusion containing the same chemokine fused with an irrelevant murine sFv. *In vivo* evidence linking receptor-mediated antigen uptake to the activation of effector T cells included the following results: (1) antitumor effects were not observed in mice immunized with sFv plasmid DNA alone or with a mixture of free, unlinked chemokine and sFv on a different plasmid; (2) secretion of *de novo* synthesized fusion proteins was required, since deletion of the secretion leader from fusion constructs abrogated vaccine-induced tumor protection; and (3) a fusion containing sFv with a mutant MCP-3, where a genetic mutation was introduced to disrupt the chemokine receptor binding, failed to protect mice from tumor challenge. Thus, both *in vitro* and *in vivo* results highlight a potential mechanism by which the chemokine fusions induce tumor protection. Specifically, fusion of sFv with proinflammatory chemokines targets APC for the tumor antigen, which leads to the conversion of the nonimmunogenic lymphoma idiotype to a potent tumor-rejection antigen.

Although targeting antigen delivery to receptors on APC was shown to be the principal mechanism to stimulate vaccine-induced tumor protection, chemokine-antigen fusions may also work by delivering maturation signals to APC. Constructs incorporating additional chemokine and chemokine-like molecules (defensins) were designed and tested to explore these other mechanisms *in vivo*. Defensins are a family of cationic antimicrobial, chemoattractant proteins stored in the cytoplasmic granules of neutrophils for release into the extracellular milieu in the process of degranulation in response to microbes, including bacteria. Furthermore, although defensin peptides have long been regarded as an essential component of innate immunity, a recent publication reported that human β-defensin 2 could induce chemotaxis of DC via the CCR6 receptor.[60] Murine β-defensin 2 from the skin of BALB/c mice was cloned for this purpose. Surprisingly, murine bone marrow-derived immature DC incubated with purified defensin-sFv fusion proteins (95 percent purity, less than 0.5 units endotoxin), but not

functionally inactive pro-defensin, expressed higher levels of MHC class II and B7[+]/CD40[+] cells. This direct effect of β-defensin 2 on DC maturation was mediated by Toll-like receptor 4, rather than CCR6.[61]

Since chemokines are among the key effector molecules regulating the trafficking of DC selectively through peripheral tissues to reach lymph nodes,[62,63] studies investigated whether chemotaxis also accounts for vaccine-induced tumor protection. Several chemokines, MCP-3, MIP-1α, macrophage-derived chemokine (MDC), and stromal cell-derived factor (SDF)-1, have been reported to be chemotactic for DC.[50,64,65] Use of chemokines as immune adjuvants has drawn much recent attention. In a HIV vaccine study, coadministration of plasmids encoding HIV envelope protein gp120 and MIP-1α significantly improved the potency of viral-specific immunity and antiviral effects.[66] The proinflammatory chemokine MIP-1α recruited DC to vaccination sites, resulting in a synergistic antiviral effect. However, the same strategy, when applied to nonimmunogenic idiotype antigen, failed to elicit protective antitumor immunity.[49] A chemokine receptor antagonist would help to elucidate whether induction of immune cell recruitment is necessary for chemokine fusion-elicited immunity. Viral chemokines are used by viruses to suppress infiltration and inflammation or to preferentially attract specific subsets of immune cells, thus modulating the immune response.[67] Several chemokines have been identified to have antagonistic activities upon binding to chemokine receptors. For example, the molluscum contagiosum virus (MCV) chemokine MC148, a highly selective viral ligand of chemokine receptor CCR8 expressed on monocytes/macrophages,[68–70] acts as a receptor antagonist and fails to induce chemotaxis.[71,72] Based on receptor antagonistic activity of MC148, Ruffini *et al.* generated a chemotaxis-deficient genetic fusion containing MC148 and sFv derived from the 38C lymphoma model.[73] This DNA vaccine was compared with another plasmid encoding the same sFv but fused to a highly selective CCR8 agonist, the herpes simplex virus-derived chemokine macrophage inflammatory protein 1 (vMIP-1),[71,74] for the ability to protect against lethal tumor challenge. Surprisingly, no significant difference was found in long-term survival between mice immunized with MC148 or vMIP-1 fusions, suggesting that chemokine receptor-mediated delivery of idiotype antigen to APC is sufficient to elicit protective immunity even in the absence of chemotaxis. Targeting of MC148 fusion vaccines to chemokine receptors *in vivo* was further evidenced when potency of the vaccine was suppressed by coinjecting a competing construct that expressed wild-type MC148 or by abrogating the receptor-binding property of MC148 fusion.[73] However, it is tempting to speculate that vaccine-induced chemotaxis may still be advantageous to initiate a local inflammatory response by recruiting immune cells expressing the relevant chemokine receptor. For example, binding of the MC148 fusion protein may induce expression of costimulatory molecules and production of proinflammatory

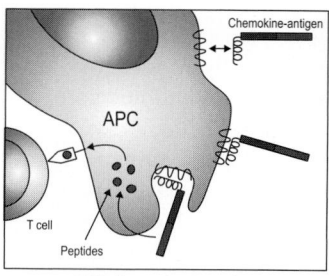
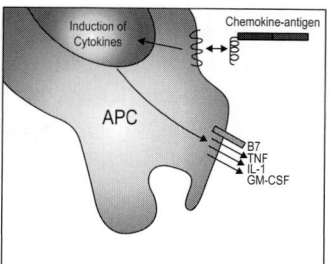
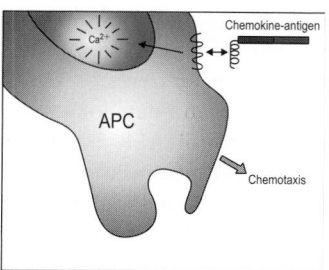

APC Receptor targeting   APC Maturation/Activation   Chemotaxis of APC and other cells

Figure 88.2 Possible modes of action of chemokine-antigen fusions *in vivo*. APC, antigen-presenting cell; TNF, tumor necrosis factor; IL-1, interleukin-1; GM-CSF, granulocyte macrophage colony-stimulating factor.

cytokines by various subsets of immature DC *in vivo*; thus, the possibility of a 'secondary' *in vivo* recruitment of immune cells at the site of vaccine administration cannot be formally excluded.

Taken together, these results suggest that chemokine-sFv fusion DNA vaccines may engage antigen-presenting cells by multiple mechanisms to trigger type 1 idiotype-specific T cell immunity. Indeed, the best vaccine delivery platform may need to work by all three mechanisms, namely (a) APC receptor targeting for antigen delivery, (b) APC maturation/activation, and (c) chemotaxis (recruitment) of APC and other cells (Fig. 88.2).

SUMMARY AND FUTURE DIRECTIONS

Lymphoma idiotype is unique for its exclusive expression on tumor cells, which makes it an ideal immunotherapeutic target for B cell malignancies. However, its inherent drawbacks, including weak immunogenicity and individualized, patient-specific nature, present challenges to developing an idiotype vaccine with significant clinical efficacy. From the KLH-conjugated prototype protein vaccine to the newly developed chemokine-sFv fusion DNA vaccine, a variety of strategies have been tested to overcome these limitations of idiotype antigens. KLH-conjugated idiotype protein coadministered with GM-CSF was the first formulation that elicited CD8$^+$ T cell immunity and was associated with clinical benefits, including molecular remission and long-term disease-free survival. If the clinical benefit is confirmed in phase III clinical trials it may move idiotype vaccine closer to clinical use. A second promising vaccine formulation is liposome-encapsulated idiotype, for which a pilot trial confirmed safety and the ability to induce tumor-specific CD8$^+$ immunity. A phase II trial is needed to further evaluate the clinical efficacy of this formulation.

Chemokine-fused sFv DNA vaccines appear to be a promising second-generation idiotype vaccine. In comparison with the current lymphoma idiotype vaccines used in clinical trials, several improvements were incorporated to this vaccine. First, the single-chain format was introduced for substitution of idiotype immunoglobulin. This feature, together with the simplicity of DNA formation, makes it feasible to streamline the production of these individualized vaccines. Second, *in vivo* targeting of APC with tumor antigens was achieved by genetic fusion of sFv with chemokines or chemokine-like molecules. Third, T cell immunity, which is required for optimal therapeutic efficacy, accounts for the principal mechanism of tumor protection with this formulation. Based on these findings, future studies will focus on the translational development of chemokine-fused sFv DNA vaccine. Specifically, it is essential to identify the chemokine or chemokine-like molecules which induce the most favorable T cell-mediated antitumor immunity when fused with sFv antigen. An ideal chemotactic leader should optimize the following functions: APC receptor targeting for antigen delivery, activating APC, and recruiting APC by chemotaxis. Another developmental goal is to optimize potency of antitumor immunity. Enhanced efficiency of antigen presentation by APC is a prerequisite for T cell activation. However, the potency of antitumor T cell responses depends on multiple factors. T cell activation is frequently undermined by negative regulators such as cytotoxic T lymphocyte-associated antigen 4 (CTLA-4) and programmed death-1 (PD-1), tumor-released inhibitory cytokines, and regulatory T cells.[75–79] Hence, a combined strategy of chemokine-sFv DNA vaccine with molecular adjuvants boosting T cell activity might be advantageous. For example, blocking antibodies to CTLA-4 and PD-1 have demonstrated both preclinical and clinical benefit in cancer immunotherapy.[80–82] Proof-of-principle studies revealed that inhibition of STAT3 signaling in tumor cells ameliorated the immunosuppressive tumor microenvironment, and that activation of Toll-like receptor signals overcame regulatory CD8$^+$ T cell-mediated tolerance.[83,84] Together, these studies support the rationale of improving vaccine-induced T cell immunity by combined therapy aimed at reversing immune suppression. Eventually a phase I trial will be required to evaluate clinical safety and immunogenicity of the optimized DNA vaccine.

With efforts to translate idiotype vaccine to clinical application, concurrent attempts are being made to seek shared lymphoma antigens for vaccines. Anaplastic lymphoma kinase (ALK) may be one example of a lymphoma-associated antigen. In adults, this receptor tyrosine kinase is exclusively found in specific regions of the nervous system. The aberrant expression of ALK in lymphoid cells is due to a chromosomal translocation, which results in the formation of oncogenic ALK fusion proteins.[85] These unique features make ALK a potential candidate for a lymphoma vaccine. The immunogenicity of ALK has been confirmed by the generation of epitope-specific CD8[+] T cell lines.[37] Other promising antigens include survivin and cytochrome P450 1B1 (CYP1B1). Although not lymphoma specific, their overexpression has been widely identified in a variety of tumors, including lymphoma. In tumor cells, upregulation of survivin, a member of the family of inhibitors of apoptosis proteins, has been regarded as a potential mechanism that tumor cells use to escape immune attack. CYP1B1, a drug-metabolizing extrahepatic enzyme, has enzymatic activities that are proposed to activate carcinogens such as polycyclic aromatic hydrocarbons. Immunogenic epitopes derived from both of these antigens have been identified.[38,86] Results from the first reported trial showed potent antigen-specific T cell responses in melanoma patients who received survivin epitope-pulsed DC vaccines.[87]

Finally, in addition to these well-characterized tumor-associated antigens, finding novel lymphoma antigens is another future direction for vaccine studies. Using autologous prevaccine and postvaccine sera to screen a phage library generated from a patient who had follicular lymphoma and received idiotype-KLH + GM-CSF vaccines, two B cell epitopes recognized by postvaccine but not prevaccine sera were identified. After careful screening, the possibility that these epitopes were derived from the patient's idiotype protein was excluded (Cha, unpublished data). Likewise, a tumor-specific T cell line established using postvaccine PBMC from a mantle cell lymphoma patient who was given the same vaccine failed to respond to the patient's idiotype antigen (Neelapu et al., unpublished data). These results suggest that idiotype vaccine potentially elicits responses to other immunogenic lymphoma antigens by a phenomenon called 'epitope spreading.'[88] Identification of such lymphoma shared antigens will potentially yield candidates for other novel lymphoma vaccines.

KEY POINTS

- The idiotype of the immunoglobulin receptor expressed on malignant B cells is a clonal marker that can be used as a tumor-specific antigen for active immunotherapy.
- In a phase II clinical trial, immunization of follicular lymphoma patients with KLH-conjugated idiotype protein plus GM-CSF induced tumor-specific T cell immunity and molecular remission, and was associated with prolonged disease-free survival.
- A multicenter randomized phase III clinical trial is being performed to definitively evaluate the clinical benefit of idiotype vaccine in follicular lymphoma patients.
- Administration of KLH-conjugated idiotype vaccine with GM-CSF elicited tumor-specific T cell immunity despite severe B cell depletion induced by rituximab in mantle cell lymphoma patients.
- Second-generation vaccine formulations such as DNA vaccines encoding novel idiotype-chemokine fusions are easier and less costly to produce than protein vaccines, and could potentially enhance the efficacy by *in vivo* targeting of dendritic cells.
- An overview is provided on the development of new lymphoma vaccine strategies other than idiotype vaccines.

REFERENCES

● = Key primary paper
◆ = Major review article

1. Sirisinha S, Eisen HN. Autoimmune-like antibodies to the ligand-binding sites of myeloma proteins. *Proc Natl Acad Sci U S A* 1971; **68**: 3130–35.
2. Lynch RG, Graff RJ, Sirisinha S et al. Myeloma proteins as tumor-specific transplantation antigens. *Proc Natl Acad Sci U S A* 1972; **69**: 1540–44.
3. Jorgensen T, Gaudernack G, Hannestad K. Immunization with the light chain and the VL domain of the isologous myeloma protein 315 inhibits growth of mouse plasmacytoma MOPC315. *Scand J Immunol* 1980; **11**: 29–35.
4. Daley MJ, Gebel HM, Lynch RG. Idiotype-specific transplantation resistance to MOPC-315: abrogation by post-immunization thymectomy. *J Immunol* 1978; **120**: 1620–24.
5. Bridges SH, Participation of the humoral immune system in the myeloma-specific transplantation resistance. *J Immunol* 1978; **121**: 479–83.
6. Freedman PM, Autry JR, Tokuda S, Williams RC Jr. Tumor immunity induced by preimmunization with BALB/c mouse myeloma protein. *J Natl Cancer Inst* 1976; **56**: 735–40.
7. Sugai S, Palmer DW, Talal N, Witz IP. Protective and cellular immune responses to idiotypic determinants on cells from a spontaneous lymphoma of NZB-NZW F1 mice. *J Exp Med* 1974; **140**: 1547–58.
8. Stevenson FK, Gordon J. Immunization with idiotypic immunoglobulin protects against development of B lymphocytic leukemia, but emerging tumor cells can evade antibody attack by modulation. *J Immunol* 1983; **130**: 970–73.
9. George AJ, Tutt AL, Stevenson FK. Anti-idiotypic mechanisms involved in suppression of a mouse B cell lymphoma, BCL1. *J Immunol* 1987; **138**: 628–34.

10. Kaminski MS, Kitamura K, Maloney DG, Levy R. Idiotype vaccination against murine B cell lymphoma. Inhibition of tumor immunity by free idiotype protein. *J Immunol* 1987; **138**: 1289–96.

11. Campbell MJ, Esserman L, Byars NE *et al.* Idiotype vaccination against murine B cell lymphoma. Humoral and cellular requirements for the full expression of antitumor immunity. *J Immunol* 1990; **145**: 1029–36.

12. George AJ, Folkard SG, Hamblin TJ, Stevenson FK. Idiotypic vaccination as a treatment for a B cell lymphoma. *J Immunol* 1988; **141**: 2168–74.

13. Campbell MJ, Esserman L, Levy R. Immunotherapy of established murine B cell lymphoma. Combination of idiotype immunization and cyclophosphamide. *J Immunol* 1988; **141**: 3227–33.

14. Kwak LW, Campbell MJ, Czerwinski DK *et al.* Induction of immune responses in patients with B-cell lymphoma against the surface-immunoglobulin idiotype expressed by their tumors. *N Engl J Med* 1992; **327**: 1209–15.

15. Carroll WL, Thielemans K, Dilley J, Levy R. Mouse × human heterohybridomas as fusion partners with human B cell tumors. *J Immunol Methods* 1986; **89**: 61–72.

16. Hsu FJ, Caspar CB, Czerwinski D *et al.* Tumor-specific idiotype vaccines in the treatment of patients with B-cell lymphoma – long-term results of a clinical trial. *Blood* 1997; **89**: 3129–35.

●17. Bendandi M, Gocke CD, Kobrin CB *et al.* Complete molecular remissions induced by patient-specific vaccination plus granulocyte-monocyte colony-stimulating factor against lymphoma. *Nat Med* 1999; **5**: 1171–7.

18. Kwak LW, Young HA, Pennington RW, Weeks SD. Vaccination with syngeneic, lymphoma-derived immunoglobulin idiotype combined with granulocyte/macrophage colony-stimulating factor primes mice for a protective T-cell response. *Proc Natl Acad Sci U S A* 1996; **93**: 10972–7.

19. Dranoff G, Jaffee E, Lazenby A *et al.* Vaccination with irradiated tumor cells engineered to secrete murine granulocyte-macrophage colony-stimulating factor stimulates potent, specific, and long-lasting anti-tumor immunity. *Proc Natl Acad Sci U S A* 1993; **90**: 3539–43.

20. Disis ML, Bernhard H, Shiota FM *et al.* Granulocyte-macrophage colony-stimulating factor: an effective adjuvant for protein and peptide-based vaccines. *Blood* 1996; **88**: 202–10.

21. Baskar S, Kobrin CB, Kwak LW. Autologous lymphoma vaccines induce human T cell responses against multiple, unique epitopes. *J Clin Invest* 2004; **113**: 1498–510.

22. Gribben JG, Freedman A, Woo SD *et al.* All advanced stage non-Hodgkin's lymphomas with a polymerase chain reaction amplifiable breakpoint of bcl-2 have residual cells containing the bcl-2 rearrangement at evaluation and after treatment. *Blood* 1991; **78**: 3275–80.

23. Grabbe S, Beissert S, Schwarz T, Granstein RD. Dendritic cells as initiators of tumor immune responses: a possible strategy for tumor immunotherapy? *Immunol Today* 1995; **16**: 117–21.

24. Neelapu SS, Kwak LW, Kobrin CB *et al.* Vaccine-induced tumor-specific immunity despite severe B-cell depletion in mantle cell lymphoma. *Nat Med* 2005; **11**: 986–91.

25. Baris D, Kwak LW, Rothman N *et al.* Blood levels of organochlorines before and after chemotherapy among non-Hodgkin's lymphoma patients. *Cancer Epidemiol Biomarkers Prev* 2000; **9**: 193–7.

26. Hennessy BT, Hanrahan EO, Daly PA. Non-Hodgkin lymphoma: an update. *Lancet Oncol* 2004; **5**: 341–53.

27. Neelapu SS, Gause BL, Nikcevich DA. *et al.* Phase III randomized trial of patient-specific vaccination for previously untreated patients with follicularl in first complete remission: protocol summary and interim report. *Clin Lymphoma* 2005; **6**: 61–4.

28. Gatza E, Okada CY. Tumor cell lysate-pulsed dendritic cells are more effective than TCR Id protein vaccines for active immunotherapy of T cell lymphoma. *J Immunol* 2002; **169**: 5227–35.

29. Borrello I, Sotomayor EM, Rattis FM *et al.* Sustaining the graft-versus-tumor effect through posttransplant immunization with granulocyte-macrophage colony-stimulating factor (GM-CSF)-producing tumor vaccines. *Blood* 2000; **95**: 3011–19.

30. Neelapu SS, Gause BL, Harvey L *et al.* Human autologous tumor-specific T-cell responses induced by liposome encapsulated lymphoma membrane proteins. *Blood* 2004; **104**: 749 (abstract).

31. Udono H, Srivastava PK. Heat shock protein 70-associated peptides elicit specific cancer immunity. *J Exp Med* 1993; **178**: 1391–6.

32. Tamura Y, Peng P, Liu K *et al.* Immunotherapy of tumors with autologous tumor-derived heat shock protein preparations. *Science*, 1997; **278**: 117–20.

33. Belli F, Testori A, Rivoltini L *et al.* Vaccination of metastatic melanoma patients with autologous tumor-derived heat shock protein gp96-peptide complexes: clinical and immunologic findings. *J Clin Oncol* 2002; **20**: 4169–80.

34. Mazzaferro V, Coppa J, Carrabba MG *et al.* Vaccination with autologous tumor-derived heat-shock protein gp96 after liver resection for metastatic colorectal cancer. *Clin Cancer Res* 2003; **9**: 3235–45.

35. Younes A. A phase II study of heat shock protein-peptide complex-96 vaccine therapy in patients with indolent non-Hodgkin's lymphoma. *Clin Lymphoma* 2003; **4**: 183–5.

36. Lambert SL, Okada CY, Levy R. TCR vaccines against a murine T cell lymphoma: a primary role for antibodies of the IgG2c class in tumor protection. *J Immunol* 2004; **172**: 929–36.

37. Passoni L, Scardino A, Bertazzoli C *et al.* ALK as a novel lymphoma-associated tumor antigen: identification of 2 HLA-A2.1-restricted CD8+ T-cell epitopes. *Blood* 2002; **99**: 2100–6.

38. Schmitz M, Diestelkoetter P, Weigle B *et al.* Generation of survivin-specific CD8+ T effector cells by dendritic cells pulsed with protein or selected peptides. *Cancer Res* 2000; **60**: 4845–9.

39. Gribben JG, Ryan DP, Boyajian R *et al.* Unexpected association between induction of immunity to the universal

tumor antigen CYP1B1 and response to next therapy. *Clin Cancer Res* 2005; **11**: 4430–36.

40. Harding CV, Collins DS, Slot JW *et al.* Liposome-encapsulated antigens are processed in lysosomes, recycled, and presented to T cells. *Cell* 1991; **64**: 393–401.

41. Harding CV, Collins DS, Kanagawa O, Unanue ER. Liposome-encapsulated antigens engender lysosomal processing for class II MHC presentation and cytosolic processing for class I presentation. *J Immunol* 1991; **147**: 2860–63.

42. Kwak LW, Pennington R, Boni L *et al.* Liposomal formulation of a self lymphoma antigen induces potent protective antitumor immunity. *J Immunol* 1998; **160**: 3637–41.

43. Neelapu SS, Baskar S, Gause BL *et al.* Human autologous tumor-specific T-cell responses induced by liposomal delivery of a lymphoma antigen. *Clin Cancer Res* 2004; **10**: 8309–17.

♦44. Ruffini PA, Neelapu SS, Kwak LW, Biragyn A. Idiotypic vaccination for B-cell malignancies as a model for therapeutic cancer vaccines: from prototype protein to second generation vaccines. *Haematologica* 2002; **87**: 989–1001.

45. Syrengelas AD, Chen TT, Levy R. DNA immunization induces protective immunity against B-cell lymphoma. *Nat Med* 1996; **2**: 1038–41.

46. Hakim I, Levy S, Levy R. A nine-amino acid peptide from IL-1beta augments antitumor immune responses induced by protein and DNA vaccines. *J Immunol* 1996; **157**: 5503–11.

47. Spellerberg MB, Zhu D, Thompsett A *et al.* DNA vaccines against lymphoma: promotion of anti-idiotypic antibody responses induced by single chain Fv genes by fusion to tetanus toxin fragment C. *J Immunol* 1997; **159**: 1885–92.

48. King CA, Spellerberg MB, Zhu D *et al.* DNA vaccines with single-chain Fv fused to fragment C of tetanus toxin induce protective immunity against lymphoma and myeloma. *Nat Med* 1998; **4**: 1281–6.

49. Biragyn A, Tani K, Grimm MC *et al.* Genetic fusion of chemokines to a self tumor antigen induces protective, T-cell dependent antitumor immunity. *Nat Biotechnol* 1999; **17**: 253–8.

50. Yanagihara S, Komura E, Nagafune J *et al.* EBI1/CCR7 is a new member of dendritic cell chemokine receptor that is up-regulated upon maturation. *J Immunol* 1998; **161**: 3096–102.

51. Solari R, Offord RE, Remy S *et al.* Receptor-mediated endocytosis of CC-chemokines. *J Biol Chem* 1997; **272**: 9617–20.

52. Prado GN, Suzuki H, Wilkinson N *et al.* Role of the C terminus of the interleukin 8 receptor in signal transduction and internalization. *J Biol Chem* 1996; **271**: 19186–90.

53. Signoret N, Oldridge J, Pelchen-Matthews A *et al.* Phorbol esters and SDF-1 induce rapid endocytosis and down modulation of the chemokine receptor CXCR4. *J Cell Biol* 1997; **139**: 651–64.

54. Sallusto F, Schaerli P, Loetscher P *et al.* Rapid and coordinated switch in chemokine receptor expression during dendritic cell maturation. *Eur J Immunol* 1998; **28**: 2760–69.

55. Cella M, Jarrossay D, Facchetti F *et al.* Plasmacytoid monocytes migrate to inflamed lymph nodes and produce large amounts of type I interferon. *Nat Med* 1999; **5**: 919–23.

56. Biragyn A, Surenhu M, Yang D *et al.* Mediators of innate immunity that target immature, but not mature, dendritic cells induce antitumor immunity when genetically fused with nonimmunogenic tumor antigens. *J Immunol* 2001; **167**: 6644–53.

57. McCarthy H, Ottensmeier CH, Hamblin TJ, Stevenson FK. Anti-idiotype vaccines. *Br J Haematol* 2003; **123**: 770–81.

58. Biragyn A, Belyakov IM, Chow YH *et al.* DNA vaccines encoding human immunodeficiency virus-1 glycoprotein 120 fusions with proinflammatory chemoattractants induce systemic and mucosal immune responses. *Blood* 2002; **100**: 1153–9.

59. Biragyn A, Ruffini PA, Coscia M *et al.* Chemokine receptor-mediated delivery directs self-tumor antigen efficiently into the class II processing pathway in vitro and induces protective immunity in vivo. *Blood* 2004; **104**: 1961–9.

60. Yang D, Chertov O, Bykovskaia SN *et al.* Beta-defensins: linking innate and adaptive immunity through dendritic and T cell CCR6. *Science* 1999; **286**: 525–8.

61. Biragyn A, Ruffini PA, Leifer CA *et al.* Toll-like receptor 4-dependent activation of dendritic cells by beta-defensin 2. *Science* 2002; **298**: 1025–9.

62. Rollins BJ, Chemokines. *Blood* 1997; **90**: 909–28.

63. Luster AD, Chemokines – chemotactic cytokines that mediate inflammation. *N Engl J Med* 1998; **338**: 436–45.

64. Sozzani S, Sallusto F, Luini W *et al.* Migration of dendritic cells in response to formyl peptides, C5a, and a distinct set of chemokines. *J Immunol* 1995; **155**: 3292–5.

65. Xu LL, Warren MK, Rose WL *et al.* Human recombinant monocyte chemotactic protein and other C-C chemokines bind and induce directional migration of dendritic cells in vitro. *J Leukoc Biol* 1996; **60**: 365–71.

66. Sumida SM, McKay PF, Truitt DM *et al.* Recruitment and expansion of dendritic cells in vivo potentiate the immunogenicity of plasmid DNA vaccines. *J Clin Invest* 2004; **114**: 1334–42.

67. Murphy PM. Viral exploitation and subversion of the immune system through chemokine mimicry. *Nat Immunol* 2001; **2**: 116–22.

68. Luo Y, Dorf ME. Beta-chemokine TCA3 binds to mesangial cells and induces adhesion, chemotaxis, and proliferation. *J Immunol* 1996; **156**: 742–8.

69. Tiffany HL, Lautens LL, Gao JL *et al.* Identification of CCR8: a human monocyte and thymus receptor for the CC chemokine I-309. *J Exp Med* 1997; **186**: 165–70.

70. Trebst C, Staugaitis SM, Kivisakk P *et al.* CC chemokine receptor 8 in the central nervous system is associated with phagocytic macrophages. *Am J Pathol* 2003; **162**: 427–38.

71. Dairaghi DJ, Fan RA, McMaster BE *et al.* HHV8-encoded vMIP-I selectively engages chemokine receptor CCR8. Agonist and antagonist profiles of viral chemokines. *J Biol Chem* 1999; **274**: 21569–74.

72. Luttichau HR, Stine J, Boesen TP *et al.* A highly selective CC chemokine receptor (CCR)8 antagonist encoded by the poxvirus molluscum contagiosum. *J Exp Med* 2000; **191**: 171–80.

73. Ruffini PA, Biragyn A, Coscia M *et al.* Genetic fusions with viral chemokines target delivery of nonimmunogenic antigen to trigger antitumor immunity independent of chemotaxis. *J Leukoc Biol* 2004; **76**: 77–85.

74. Endres MJ, Garlisi CG, Xiao H *et al.* The Kaposi's sarcoma-related herpesvirus (KSHV)-encoded chemokine vMIP-I is a specific agonist for the CC chemokine receptor (CCR)8. *J Exp Med* 1999; **189**: 1993–8.

75. Krummel MF, Allison JP. CTLA-4 engagement inhibits IL-2 accumulation and cell cycle progression upon activation of resting T cells. *J Exp Med* 1996; **183**: 2533–40.

76. Iwai Y, Ishida M, Tanaka Y *et al.* Involvement of PD-L1 on tumor cells in the escape from host immune system and tumor immunotherapy by PD-L1 blockade. *Proc Natl Acad Sci U S A* 2002; **99**: 12293–7.

77. Nakashima M, Sonoda K, Watanabe T. Inhibition of cell growth and induction of apoptotic cell death by the human tumor-associated antigen RCAS1. *Nat Med* 1999; **5**: 938–42.

78. Mellado M, de Ana AM, Moreno MC *et al.* A potential immune escape mechanism by melanoma cells through the activation of chemokine-induced T cell death. *Curr Biol* 2001; **11**: 691–6.

79. Casares N, Arribillaga L, Sarobe P *et al.* CD4+/CD25+ regulatory cells inhibit activation of tumor-primed CD4+ T cells with IFN-gamma-dependent antiangiogenic activity, as well as long-lasting tumor immunity elicited by peptide vaccination. *J Immunol* 2003; **171**: 5931–9.

80. Hirano F, Kaneko K, Tamura H *et al.* Blockade of B7-H1 and PD-1 by monoclonal antibodies potentiates cancer therapeutic immunity. *Cancer Res* 2005; **65**: 1089–96.

81. Phan GQ, Yang JC, Sherry RM *et al.* Cancer regression and autoimmunity induced by cytotoxic T lymphocyte-associated antigen 4 blockade in patients with metastatic melanoma. *Proc Natl Acad Sci U S A* 2003; **100**: 8372–7.

82. Hodi FS, Mihm MC, Soiffer RJ *et al.* Biologic activity of cytotoxic T lymphocyte-associated antigen 4 antibody blockade in previously vaccinated metastatic melanoma and ovarian carcinoma patients. *Proc Natl Acad Sci U S A* 2003; **100**: 4712–7.

83. Yang Y, Huang CT, Huang X, Pardoll DM. Persistent Toll-like receptor signals are required for reversal of regulatory T cell-mediated CD8 tolerance. *Nat Immunol* 2004; **5**: 508–15.

84. Wang T, Niu G, Kortylewski M *et al.* Regulation of the innate and adaptive immune responses by Stat-3 signaling in tumor cells. *Nat Med* 2004; **10**: 48–54.

85. Passoni L, Gambacorti-Passerini C. ALK a novel lymphoma-associated tumor antigen for vaccination strategies. *Leuk Lymphoma* 2003; **44**: 1675–81.

86. Maecker B, Sherr DH, Vonderheide RH *et al.* The shared tumor-associated antigen cytochrome P450 1B1 is recognized by specific cytotoxic T cells. *Blood* 2003; **102**: 3287–94.

87. Otto K, Andersen MH, Eggert A *et al.* Lack of toxicity of therapy-induced T cell responses against the universal tumour antigen survivin. *Vaccine* 2005; **23**: 884–9.

88. Vanderlugt CL, Miller SD. Epitope spreading in immune-mediated diseases: implications for immunotherapy. *Nat Rev Immunol* 2002; **2**: 85–95.

89. Wierda WG, Cantwell MJ, Woods SJ *et al.* CD40-ligand (CD154) gene therapy for chronic lymphocytic leukemia. *Blood* 2000; **96**: 2917–24.

89

Lymphoma microenvironment

B HERREROS, A SANCHEZ-AGUILERA AND MA PIRIS

INTRODUCTION

The growth of lymphoma cells may depend not only on the accumulation of genetic alterations but also on signals derived from the milieu that drive cell proliferation or inhibit apoptosis. The relevance of the microenvironment to lymphoma pathogenesis has been highlighted by the observations linking specific microbial and viral pathogens to specific types of lymphoproliferative syndromes. However, it has also become apparent that lymphoma development is dependent on a particular stromal microenvironment that conditions the nature of the developed neoplasms.

In this chapter we review the status of our knowledge and summarize the main features of the interaction between stroma and tumoral cells. It is divided into three sections, dealing in turn with the roles of inflammatory and autoimmune disorders, chemokines, and non-tumoral cells.

ROLE OF INFLAMMATORY AND AUTOIMMUNE DISORDERS IN THE PATHOGENESIS OF LYMPHOPROLIFERATIVE DISORDERS

Much evidence has accumulated to support the idea that neoplasms, including those of a lymphoproliferative nature,

are influenced by their environment. This evidence has come from a range of conditions such as inflammation, bacterial and viral infection, endemic diseases, and autoantigen stimulation of the immune system. In this section we describe several lymphoproliferative diseases that are paradigms of this environmental influence (for an overview, see Table 89.1).

MALT-type marginal zone lymphoma in extranodal tissues: *Helicobacter pylori* and MALT lymphoma

To date, the most instructive example of the dependence of tumoral cell survival on the presence of microbial or viral pathogens has been provided by observations of mucosa-associated lymphoid tissue-type (MALT-type) gastric marginal zone lymphoma (MZL) and *Helicobacter pylori*.[1] A body of evidence supports the hypothesis that the bacterium *H. pylori* can provide the antigenic stimulus for promoting and sustaining the growth of MZL in the stomach. The microorganism can be found in the gastric mucosa in nearly all instances of gastric MALT lymphoma, where it causes acute and chronic gastritis, and a close association has been reported in epidemiological studies

Table 89.1 Autoimmune/inflammatory disorders associated with lymphoma development

Associated lymphoproliferative neoplasm	Predisposing condition	Etiologic agent	Response to alternative therapies	References
Gastric MZL, MALT	Gastritis	*Helicobacter pylori*	Yes	1–6
IPSID	Jejunitis	*Campylobacter jejuni*	Yes	7–9
Cutaneous B cell lymphoma	Lyme disease	*Borrelia burgdorferi*	Some cases	10–13
Ocular adnexal lymphoma	*Chlamydia psittaci* infection	*Chlamydia psittaci*	Yes	14–17
MZL, MALT in the salivary gland	Sjögren syndrome	Autoantigen	Uncertain	18,19
SMZL	Malaria, HCV, autoimmune disorders	*Plasmodium falciparum*, HCV, autoantigen	Yes for HCV	20–25
CLL	Autoimmune disorders	Autoantigen	Uncertain	18,26–28
Intestinal T cell lymphoma	Celiac disease	Environmental antigen (gluten)	Uncertain	29,30
Pyothorax-associated lymphoma	Tuberculosis (chronic inflammation), EBV infection	*Mycobacterium tuberculosis*, EBV	Uncertain	31
Hodgkin lymphoma	Infectious mononucleosis	EBV	Uncertain	32
Endemic Burkitt lymphoma	Infectious mononucleosis	EBV	Uncertain	32–34
Plasmablastic lymphoma (oral mucosa)	Infectious mononucleosis	EBV	Uncertain	35
T/NK lymphoma (nasal type)	Infectious mononucleosis	EBV	Uncertain	36
Primary effusion lymphoma	Herpes infection	Kaposi sarcoma, herpesvirus	Uncertain	37

Many lymphoma types develop in the setting of previous inflammatory or autoimmune disorders that create a favorable environment for the development of the lymphoproliferative disease, promoting selection of specific B cell or T cell clones, proliferation, and/or preventing apoptosis. MZL, marginal zone lymphoma; IPSID, immunoproliferative small intestinal disease; MALT, mucosal-associated lymphoid tissue; SMZL, splenic marginal zone lymphoma; CLL, chronic lymphocytic leukemia; HCV, hepatitis C virus; EBV, Epstein-Barr virus; NK, natural killer.

between *H. pylori* infection and gastric lymphoma,[2] in addition to gastric cancer. *In vitro* experiments have demonstrated that the neoplastic cells of low-grade gastric MALT lymphomas proliferate in a strain-specific response to *H. pylori* and that this response is dependent on T cell activation by the microorganism.[3] A potential oncogenic role may also be expected in the inflammatory background that accompanies *H. pylori* infection.

Based on these findings, it has been proposed that T and B cells are recruited *de novo* in the gastric mucosa as part of the immune response to *H. pylori*. Thus, B cell proliferation is induced by the combined action of reactive T cells and through the B cell nuclear factor κB (NF-κB) activation caused by *H. pylori* and the associated inflammation.[4] It is not known whether T cell activation requires *H. pylori* as a continuous source of antigenic stimuli or if it is related to an indirect autoimmune mechanism. In fact, neoplastic B cells often show antibody specificity for autoantigens and need contact-dependent help from intratumoral T cells (mediated by CD40 and CD40 ligand [CD40L] interactions) to proliferate. The role of mucosal T cells and

H. pylori in regulating lymphoma-cell survival may explain the difficulty that low-grade MALT lymphomas lacking other cytogenetic abnormalities have in spreading beyond the stomach.

With respect to the treatment of gastric MZL, antibiotic therapy in MALT-type has been validated in multiple studies, and approximately 75 percent of gastric MALT lymphomas regress after the eradication of *H. pylori*. Tumors that are unresponsive to antibiotics either carry a chromosomal translocation involving the MALT1 gene or others leading to NF-κB constitutive activation, or are diagnosed at advanced stages.[5] However, recent studies incorporating polymerase chain reaction (PCR) analysis have shown that histologic and endoscopic remission are not necessarily associated with complete healing of gastric MZL. In fact, the long-term persistence of monoclonal B cells after histologic regression of the lymphoma has been reported in about half of the cases, suggesting that *H. pylori* eradication plays a complementary role and that other, currently unknown antigens or genetic events may participate in the tumorigenesis.[6]

Immunoproliferative small intestinal disease

Although the incidence of immunoproliferative small intestinal disease (IPSID) is decreasing dramatically, in association with improvement in public health in Middle Eastern countries,[7] this disease is a paradigm of the role of microenvironment in lymphoma pathogenesis. Geographically, it is most prevalent in the Middle East and has previously been linked with the incidence of *Vibrio cholerae* infection.[8] It is a variant of the B cell MZL, MALT-type, which mainly involves the proximal small intestine and results in malabsorption, diarrhea, and abdominal pain. IPSID lymphomas show the mixture of cell types characteristic of other MALT lymphomas, but with massive plasma-cell differentiation producing truncated α heavy chain proteins that lack the light chains as well as the first constant domain. Recently, Lecuit *et al.*[9] have demonstrated the presence of *Campylobacter jejuni* in the intestinal tissue obtained from a patient with IPSID who had a dramatic response to antibiotics. A follow-up retrospective analysis of archival intestinal biopsy specimens using fluorescent *in situ* hybridization (FISH) and immunohistochemical techniques disclosed *Campylobacter* species in four of six additional IPSID patients. It therefore seems that *C. jejuni* infection is very likely to be an agent in the pathogenesis of IPSID, participating in a process that involves chronic antigenic stimulation within the gut that leads to the proliferation of immunoglobulin A (IgA) plasma cells in the intestine, possibly double-stranded DNA breaks induced by the *C. jejuni* toxin, and additional ongoing events including generation of truncated α heavy chain immunoglobulin and mutational events involving *PAX5* or other oncogenes. These may finally lead to neoplastic progression to lymphoplasmacytic and immunoblastic lymphoma and to the full-blown lymphomatous phase of IPSID.[10]

Skin marginal zone lymphoma and *Borrelia*

A related disorder, marginal zone lymphoma of the skin, has been linked with *Borrelia* infection,[11] although this association does not seem to be universal. Thus, Garbe *et al.* described four cases of cutaneous B cell lymphoma (CBCL) in patients with positive serology for *Borrelia*. However, these reported links may still have been circumstantial, as the cases came from areas where *Borrelia* was endemic.[12] Goodlad *et al.* found *Borrelia*-specific flagellin gene DNA by PCR amplification in six out of 19 cases (32 percent) of CBCL from the Highlands of Scotland.[13] Cerroni *et al.* found *Borrelia*-specific genomic DNA by PCR and Southern blot analysis in nine out of 50 cases (18 percent) of CBCL.[14] Some of the *Borrelia*-infected cases responded to antibiotic treatment, thus confirming the role that *Borrelia* plays in a relatively rare subset of these tumors.[15]

Ocular adnexa lymphoma

Ocular adnexa lymphoma is characterized by its indolent course, and is constituted by marginal zone B cells with a strong presence of infiltrating reactive T cells. Several lines of evidence have established an association between *Chlamydia psittaci* infection and this lymphoma type. In fact, it has been reported that *C. psittaci* DNA can be detected in up to 80 percent of ocular adnexal lymphoma patients.[16] Chronic persistence of the infectious agent may cause prolonged antigen stimulation, thus playing an important role in the clonal expansion of these lymphomas. The presence of somatic hypermutations in clonally rearranged immunoglobulin heavy-chain variable genes (*IGHV*) in this type of marginal zone B cell lymphoma shows a molecular similarity with the normal properties of B cells positively selected by a cognate antigen within the germinal center. Confirming the involvement of infection in the etiology of the disease, *C. psittaci*-eradicating antibiotic therapy with doxycycline is followed by objective response in patients with ocular adnexa lymphoma.[16–18] Nevertheless, *C. psittaci* infection is far from being a universal finding in ocular adnexa lymphoma, and the prevalence of *C. psittaci* infection in MALT lymphoma has been shown to vary among the geographic regions examined. A variable frequency has been found ranging from 0 percent to 47 percent.[19,20]

MALT–type marginal zone lymphoma in the salivary gland and Sjögren syndrome

A dramatic increase in the incidence of marginal zone lymphomas has been noticed in patients with Sjögren syndrome, also followed by a striking increase in the proportion of diffuse large B cell lymphomas.[21] This effect was found to be independent of the use of immunosuppressants. Indeed, the presence of lymphoepithelial lesions is a cardinal feature of both diseases, marginal zone lymphoma involving the salivary gland and Sjögren syndrome.[22]

Splenic marginal zone lymphoma

The role of viral and bacterial antigens in the pathogenesis of splenic marginal zone lymphoma (SMZL) is suggested from the findings of several studies:

- *IGHV*-biased selection. *IGHV* mutational studies have demonstrated that roughly one-half of SMZL cases use *IGHV1-2*, which contrasts with the use of this *IGHV* gene in normal B cells, since only around 1 percent of normal peripheral blood B cells use this gene.[23]
- Association with malaria and idiopathic splenomegaly.[24–27] Two different lymphoproliferative disorders – tropical splenic lymphoma, characterized by splenomegaly and circulating naïve CD5-negative

villous B lymphocytes, and hyperreactive malarial splenomegaly – have been described in malaria-endemic areas. Although no relation has been found with other B-lymphotropic viruses, patients with tropical splenic lymphoma have been found to exhibit raised Epstein–Barr virus (EBV) antibody levels.

- Hepatitis C virus (HCV) infection in SMZL patients is known to be more prevalent than average in specific places and studies, and even regression of splenic lymphoma with villous lymphocytes (SLVL) has been described in patients with HCV infection after antiviral treatment, thereby demonstrating a direct role of HCV in lymphomagenesis.[28] Interestingly, symptomatic mixed cryoglobulinemia was a common feature in these cases.[29]

Chronic lymphocytic leukemia and autoimmune disorders

Several lines of evidence suggest a role for antigens in the survival of B chronic lymphocytic leukemia (CLL) tumoral cells:

- Patients with rheumatoid arthritis have an increase of $CD5^+$ cells in the peripheral blood.[30]
- There is a greater incidence of CLL (and other B cell lymphomas) in patients with autoimmune disorders.[21]
- Structural similarities of the B cell receptors ($V_H DJ_H$, V_L, and J_L genes) of CLL cells from different patients suggest that the antigens identified by these receptors must be similar and thus relevant to the pathogenesis of CLL.[31]
- B-CLL cell survival depends on the interaction of the tumoral cells with nurse-like cells (NLCs).[32]

Celiac disease and intestinal T cell lymphoma

Celiac disease (CD) is a genetically determined chronic inflammatory intestinal disease induced by gluten, an environmental precipitant. Intraepithelial lymphocytosis is one of the hallmarks of CD and its importance is underlined by the appearance of major complications of the disease such as enteropathy-associated T cell lymphoma (EATL). Indeed, surgical EATL samples frequently exhibit increased intraepithelial lymphocytosis, villous atrophy, or both.

A nearly 20-fold greater risk of T cell lymphoma, frequently involving the gastrointestinal tract, and a nearly threefold increased risk of diffuse large B cell lymphoma have been observed in CD patients. This is consistent with results showing the presence of an immunophenotypically aberrant clonal intraepithelial T cell population (similar to that of most cases of EATL) in up to 75 percent of patients with refractory celiac sprue, thus suggesting that refractory sprue associated with an aberrant clonal EATL may be the missing link between CD and T cell lymphoma.[33]

However, Smedby et al.[34] have recently shown that CD is associated with a far greater variety of malignant lymphoma types than had previously been appreciated. Indeed, nonintestinal B cell and T cell non-Hodgkin lymphoma (NHL) together constituted most celiac disease-associated malignant lymphomas in their prospectively identified population-based cohort.

Pyothorax-associated lymphoma

Pyothorax-associated lymphoma (PAL) is a B cell NHL that develops in the pleural cavity of patients after a long history of pyothorax resulting from an artificial pneumothorax for the treatment of pulmonary tuberculosis or tuberculous pleuritis.[35] Virtually all PAL cases are EBV-positive, with expression of EBV latent genes such as EBV nuclear antigen 2 (EBNA2) and latent membrane protein 1 (LMP1), together with EBNA1.

Hodgkin lymphoma and Epstein–Barr virus

Epstein–Barr virus is detected in Hodgkin and Reed–Sternberg (H-RS) lymphoma cells in approximately 40 percent of Hodgkin lymphoma (HL) cases. This association is even stronger in Latin America, where nearly all cases of children with HL are EBV positive, probably reflecting early EBV exposure. The H-RS cells containing the EBV genome are monoclonal, implying that the virus plays a role in the transformation and rescue of preapoptotic B cells from the germinal center. LMP-1 seems to be the key factor in this process, in which it functions by mimicking CD40 stimulation of the B cells.[36]

Endemic Burkitt lymphoma, Epstein–Barr virus, and dentinogenesis

Association of cofactors such as malaria, EBV, and local inflammatory conditions, such as those associated with dentinogenesis, could explain the geographic distribution and anatomically selective localization of endemic Burkitt lymphoma (BL). The possibility that dentinogenesis could represent a microenvironment with an increased risk of BL development is supported by Wright's observation that jaw involvement was the main presenting clinical feature in all 3-year-old Ugandan BL children, while its incidence was only 16 percent in 16-year-old patients.[37]

In its endemic form, nearly all cases of BL are EBV positive. The tumor also occurs as a rare, sporadic lymphoma outside endemic areas, with an association with EBV in 20–30 percent of cases. The mechanisms of EBV B cell transformation in BL have been extensively reviewed by Küppers.[36]

The potential role of other environmental agents, such as arboviruses and plants, in the pathogenesis of endemic BL has been reviewed by van den Bosch.[38]

Less frequent tumours

Plasmablastic B cell lymphomas with aberrant immunophenotype and EBV presence occurring in human immunodeficiency virus (HIV)-positive patients and showing very frequent involvement of the oral cavity or gastrointestinal tract have recently been reviewed by Dong *et al.*[39] All cases were positive for EBV-encoded RNA (EBER) but lacked EBV late membrane proteins (LMPs). All patients had extramedullary tumors and most of them had an extranodal tumor at initial presentation, with rare bone marrow involvement. The most commonly involved location was the oral cavity (6 of 13 cases), followed by bone and soft tissue (4 of 13), and the gastrointestinal tract (3 of 13).[39] These tumors represent an interesting example of risk accumulation associated with different lymphotropic viruses, and of how the interaction between foreign antigens and the immune system determines the selective localization of specific tumor types in discrete microenvironments.

The same principle, whereby one or a combination of several lymphotropic viruses transforms B or T cells in specific microenvironments, applies to other tumors, such as **nasal type T/natural killer (NK) lymphoma**, a tumor of CD56-positive cells that is EBV positive in all cases;[40] **primary effusion lymphoma** (PEL), a tumor that led to the confirmation of the lymphoma oncogenic role of Kaposi sarcoma herpes virus (KSHV);[41] and **adult T cell leukemia/lymphoma** (ATLL),[42] a tumor related with human T cell lymphotrophic virus 1 (HTLV-1). The latter clearly demonstrates another striking feature of these tumors – their selective localization in specific geographic areas.

CHEMOKINES

Introduction

Cytokines are secreted proteins that regulate the nature of immune responses. They are involved in nearly every aspect of immunity and inflammation, from induction of the innate immune response to the generation of cytotoxic T cells and the development of antibodies. Typically, cytokines can act either in a paracrine or an autocrine manner, regulating the cells that produce them. The combination of cytokines produced in response to a specific stimulus determines which arm of the immune system will be activated. Among cytokines, chemokines are now of great interest because of their relevance in tumorigenesis and tumor prognosis.

Chemokines consist of a family of over 40 small (8 kDa) related proteins whose function is to move cells along a chemotactic gradient, either organizing cells within an organ, facilitating the movement of leukocytes around the body, or recruiting them to inflammatory sites. They are classified into four highly conserved groups – CXC, CC, C, and CX3C – on the basis of the position of the first two cysteine residues adjacent to the amino terminus. Chemokines exert their effects by binding to seven-transmembrane-domain G protein-coupled receptors. However, this structure-based division of chemokines into the four groups does little to illustrate any differences in their function. In fact, there is redundancy in the system whereby each receptor can respond to more than one chemokine, most chemokines can use more than one receptor, and each leukocyte subset may express several receptors. Chemokines can be also classified as inducible or constitutively expressed.[43] Those inducible are typically expressed in response to an inflammatory stimulus to attract neutrophils, eosinophils, monocytes, and lymphocytes; the constitutively expressed types are involved in embryogenesis and maintenance of normal trafficking of immune cells toward specific lymphoid and nonlymphoid organs. There is now considerable evidence that the differential expression of chemokine receptors enables trafficking and homing of neoplastic cells into lymphoid organs.[44,45]

Since signals from the tumor microenvironment critically contribute to the progression of lymphoid malignancies, increasing emphasis is being placed on the analysis and eventual therapeutic targeting of the tumor-cell microenvironment.

Although here we thoroughly discuss only HL and CLL as examples of the role of chemokines in lymphoma survival, the importance of chemokines in other disorders is noted throughout the chapter and in Table 89.2.

Role of chemokines in specific lymphoma types

HODGKIN LYMPHOMA

Classical Hodgkin lymphoma (CHL) is a lymphoid neoplasia in which the malignant cells (H-RS cells) constitute only a minor population within the affected tissue, which mainly consists of a heterogeneous infiltrate of T and B lymphocytes, histiocytes, macrophages, plasma cells, neutrophils, eosinophils, and fibroblasts. A complex network of cytokine- and cell-contact-mediated interactions between tumor and inflammatory cells is thought to regulate the proliferation of H-RS cells and may also rescue these cells from the proapoptotic state arising from their characteristic B cell receptor deficiency by providing alternative survival signals. We will discuss the relevance of these interactions in this section and of others elsewhere in this chapter.

High levels of expression of several chemokines in HL may cause an influx of reactive cells into the lymphoid tissue and thereby the formation of the characteristic non-neoplastic infiltrate. H-RS cells express a complex pattern of chemokines. CCL17 is involved in trafficking and activation of mature T cells and is strongly expressed in H-RS cells in most cases. Its receptor, CCR4, is expressed in a high proportion of lymphocytes surrounding H-RS cells,

Table 89.2 Significance of chemokines in lymphoma development

Chemokine	Produced by	Receptors	Cells affected	Effects	Relevant in	References
CXCL9	H-RS, macrophages	CXCR3	T cells (CD4$^+$)	Trafficking, activation, and proliferation of CD4$^+$ cells	HL	43
CXCL10	H-RS, macrophages	CXCR3	T cells (CD4$^+$)	Trafficking, activation, and proliferation of CD4$^+$ cells	HL	43
CXCL12 (SDF-1)	Stromal cells, NLC	CXCR4	Naïve T cells, progenitor B cells, CLL B-cells, H-RS	B cell development, lymphocyte or H-RS homing	CLL, HL, FL	28,43,45,62
CXCL13	Follicular dendritic cells	CXCR5	B cells	Lymphocyte homing (B cell follicles)	AITL, FL	66,72,73
CCL17	H-RS	CCR4	T cells (CD4$^+$)	Trafficking, activation, and proliferation of CD4$^+$ cells	HL	43
CCL19 (MIP-3β)	Stromal cells, dendritic cells	CCR7	Activated B cells, T cells, H-RS	T cell localization; directing B cells to the interface with the T cell zone; H-RS homing in the interfollicular region	CLL, HL	44,46
CCL21 (SLE)	Stromal cells	CCR7	Activated B cells, T cells, dendritic cells, H-RS	T cell and dendritic cell localization in secondary lymphoid tissues; directing B cells to the interface with the T cell zone	CLL, HL	44,46

Several studies have shown the importance of chemokines in normal and tumoral lymphoid development. They are produced by different cell populations, such as stroma cells or follicular dendritic cells, to direct lymphoid or tumoral cells to secondary lymphoid organs and to favor contacts with T cells. Other chemokines are involved in T cell trafficking (i.e., those secreted by macrophages or H-RS cells) or in B cell development (i.e., those secreted by nurse-like-cells [NLC] in CLL). H-RS, Hodgkin Reed–Sternberg cell; HL, Hodgkin lymphoma; CLL, chronic lymphocytic leukemia; FL, follicular lymphoma; AITL, angioimmunoblastic T cell lymphoma.

especially T helper type 2 (TH2) cells. H-RS cells also express CCL22, which has a similar effect to CCL17.

The TH1 chemokines CXCL9, CXCL10, CCL3 (MIP-1α), CCL4 (MIP-1β), and CCL5 (RANTES) are expressed more strongly in CHL than in benign lymphoid tissue and are expressed by inflammatory cells (mainly macrophages and, for CCL5, also T cells) but also, for CXCL9/10 and probably CCL5, by H-RS cells. Receptors for these chemokines (CCR5 [receptor for CCL3/4] and CXCR3 [receptor for CXCL9/10]) are expressed by a fraction of reactive cells, especially CD4+ lymphocytes.[46] These chemokines induce T cell migration, proliferation, and interleukin-2 (IL-2) production, and CCL5 also attracts monocytes.

Conversely, chemokines could regulate the homing and adhesion of tumor cells to nodal microenvironments. H-RS cells show strong and frequent expression of the chemokine receptors CCR7 and CXCR4 and moderate CXCR5 expression, whereas the respective ligands (CCL19/CCL21, CXCL12, and CXCL13) are markedly expressed by infiltrating cells. This is consistent with the frequent homing of H-RS cells to the interfollicular zone and their absence from germinal centers (in parallel with the expression of the ligands).[47]

CHRONIC LYMPHOCYTIC LEUKEMIA

Although little is known about the mechanisms determining lymph node or bone marrow infiltration in CLL, this process involves a complex set of steps including malignant cell movement into, and within, nodes or bone marrow, local survival signaling, and enhanced accumulation. In normal lymphoid tissues, these processes are controlled by lymphocyte responses to distinct chemokines, stromal cells, and extracellular matrix, and by maturation-induced changes in the cells' response to these microenvironmental signals. An increasing number of studies also show that signaling through chemokines plays an important role in the development and maintenance of CLL.

CD4+ T cells gather in pseudofollicles and acquire the expression of CD40L, providing stimuli that may influence the proliferation of the CLL cell population (and of circulating CLL cells). Interactions between CLL cells and T cells lead to production of several cytokines, such as IL-10, interferon (IFN) α and IFNγ, that inhibit CLL cell apoptosis. However, it seems that activated T cells give only short-term support to the leukemic cells since they have the potential to limit the progressive expansion of B cells (by CD95–CD95L interactions). Interestingly, it has been shown that a subset of blood mononuclear cells from CLL patients can differentiate into NLCs and sustain CLL culture *in vitro*. In fact, it is believed that these NLCs may also play an important role *in vivo* because cells with these characteristics have been found in the secondary lymphoid organs of patients with CLL.[48] Significant levels of the tumor necrosis factor (TNF) family members BAFF and APRIL and chemokine CXCL12 (SDF-1), a survival factor produced by stromal cells, are expressed by NLCs

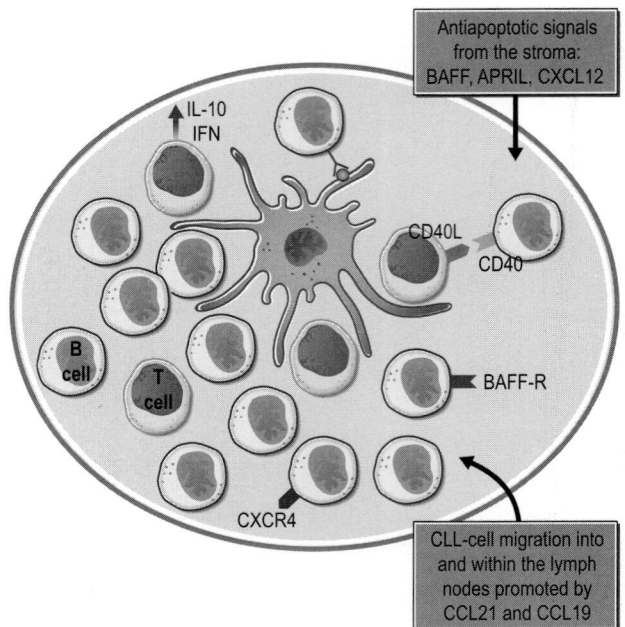

Figure 89.1 Microenvironment in chronic lymphocytic leukemia (CLL). One of the features that characterize CLL is the accumulation of B cell clones with biased immunoglobulin heavy-chain variable gene (*IGHV*) selection, indicating the possible role of autoantigens in their selection. B cell–T cell interactions may provide additional survival signaling for the tumoral cells. Other factors secreted by stroma cells (BAFF, APRIL, and chemokine CXCL12) provide further survival signaling. CCL19 and CCL21 are involved in B CLL-cell trafficking into the lymph nodes from the peripheral blood. Tumoral B cells are shown in violet, proliferation center dendritic cells in yellow, and T cells in green. IFN, interferon; IL-10, interleukin-10.

(Fig. 89.1). BAFF and APRIL induce activation of the NF-κB transcription factors, enhancing the expression of the antiapoptotic Mcl-1 protein, while CXCL12 exerts its action by phosphorylation of the ERK1/2 mitogen-activated kinase and attracting CLL cells to supporting microenvironments.[32] CLL cells express high levels of CXCR4, the chemokine receptor for CXCL12, which directs leukemia-cell chemotaxis. Other chemokine receptors, such as CCR7 (the receptor of CCL19 and CCL21 chemokines), that are expressed by CLL B cells have been shown to be important for the migration of leukemic cells into lymph nodes.[49]

The CLL proliferating compartment in the lymph node and bone marrow is represented by proliferation centers, or pseudofollicles, which are vaguely nodular areas without mantles that represent the histopathological hallmark of CLL. Pseudofollicles are not only a collection of proliferating cells but they also host non-tumoral bystander cells, including CD4+ cells in close contact with CLL proliferating cells, fibroblastic reticulum cells, and rare follicular dendritic cells.[50] These fibroblastic reticulum cells could represent the tissue counterpart of the NLCs.

Therefore, the CXCR4–CXCL12 interaction is being studied as a potential therapeutic target in CLL.[48,51,52] Recent work has evaluated the activity of some CXCR4-specific antagonists: T140, TC14012, and TN14003.[52] These inhibit actin polymerization, chemotaxis, and migration of CLL cells beneath stromal cells. They also abolish CXCL12-induced phosphorylation of ERK1/2 and STAT3, a signal transducer and activator of transcription. In fact, these compounds are able to antagonize the antiapoptotic effect of synthetic CXCL12 and stromal cell-mediated protection of CLL cells. As stromal cells are believed to protect CLL cells from chemotherapy-induced apoptosis via CXCL12, treatment with CXCR4 antagonists induces apoptosis in fludarabine-treated CLL cells even when co-cultured with stromal cells. In summary, not only can CXCR4 antagonists inhibit CXCL12-dependent migration and signaling in CLL cells, but they are also able to abolish the stromal protection from spontaneous or fludarabine-induced apoptosis.

NON–TUMORAL CELL POPULATIONS

Introduction

Increasing attention is being paid to the role of non-tumoral cell populations attracting neoplastic lymphoid cells to specific niches, conveying survival signaling, and/or regulating immune response.

Hodgkin lymphoma

A hallmark of HL is the presence of a large number of inflammatory cells. There is mounting evidence that the infiltrating cells may support proliferation and rescue H-RS cells from apoptosis. Here we describe briefly how these interactions between H-RS cells and other tumor-infiltrating cells take place.

T cells, which are predominantly CD4$^+$, make up a significant component of the HL infiltrate. These cells are not necessarily the result of the specific recognition of tumor-specific antigens by T cells, and may be recruited non-specifically by chemoattractants such as CCL17, CCL22, and CCL11 produced by HL tissues.

It has been widely believed that the inflammatory infiltrate of HL comprises mainly activated TH2-like lymphocytes, but this is not fully consistent with their unusual phenotype: most HL-infiltrating lymphocytes do not produce the TH2 cytokines IL-4 or IL-13, fail to express functional IL-2 receptor (they can express CD25 but lack the β chain), and express CTLA-4 (a costimulatory molecule expressed in regulatory T cells). Moreover, HL-infiltrating lymphocytes are anergic (hyporesponsive to stimulation with mitogens or antigens) and can inhibit TH cell responses. These data suggest that HL-infiltrating lymphocytes are highly enriched in regulatory T cells (Plate 145, see plate section), which create a profoundly immunosuppressive environment.[53] This explains the lack of an effective antitumor response to antigens expressed by H-RS cells (for example, EBV proteins).[54]

Regulatory T cells (Tregs) are a specific subset of T cells with the capacity to inhibit effector immune responses, which are important in the control of responses to foreign antigens and as protectors against autoimmune disease. Regulatory T cells were initially characterized by the surface expression of CD25, which is the α chain of the IL-2 receptor and is expressed by virtually all activated T cells (Treg cells express CD25 owing to the continued engagement of the T cell receptor [TCR] by self-antigens in the periphery). However, CD25 is also expressed in recently activated T cells, which have no suppressive capacity. In addition, some CD4$^+$CD25$^-$ T cells have a regulatory capacity, as has been shown by different studies. The transcription factor FOXP3, a member of the forkhead family of DNA-binding transcription factors,[55] has been found to be strongly expressed in CD4$^+$ regulatory T cells. Mutations in the *FOXP3* gene cause the fatal autoimmune and inflammatory disorder of scurfy in mice and the clinical and molecular features of the immune dysregulation, polyendocrinopathy, enteropathy, X-linked (IPEX) syndrome in humans. Mice with scurfy and patients with the IPEX syndrome both have defects in T cell activation and low frequencies and impaired suppressor functions of CD4$^+$CD25$^+$ T cells. As FOXP3 is both necessary and sufficient for regulatory function, it is now used for the definitive detection of Tregs.[56,57]

A subset of Tregs develops in the thymus and requires strong self-antigen stimulation through the TCR as well as costimulatory signals through CD28-CD80/86. Another subset of Treg cells is known to be generated from peripheral mature T cells or from Treg cells produced in the thymus under certain conditions of antigenic stimulation (infection and organ transplantation, among others). Their development might be triggered by low-affinity antigen stimulation and seems to be dependent on cytokine signaling and independent of CD28. Regulatory T cells can mediate their effects by producing immunosuppressive cytokines such as IL-10 or transforming growth factor β (TGFβ), or by a mechanism involving direct interactions with responding T cells or antigen-presenting cells.[58]

CD8$^+$ cells make up a small proportion of the T cell infiltrate and are typically not in close contact with H-RS cells. They do not appear to be directed against a common antigen. Although the number of CD8$^+$ cells is higher in EBV-positive cases, and EBV-specific cytotoxic T lymphocytes (CTLs) can be detected in the peripheral blood of patients with EBV-positive CHL, no CTLs targeting EBV proteins expressed by H-RS cells can be identified within the tumors. Moreover, the presence of a high percentage of activated CTLs (granzyme B$^+$) in the affected tissue is an unfavorable prognostic marker, associated with shorter progression-free survival.[59,60] These data suggest that CTLs that could potentially target the H-RS cells either fail to penetrate the tumor site or fail to function within the tumor microenvironment. This could be the final

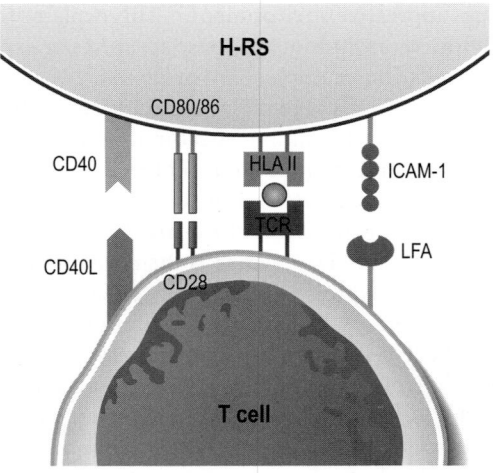

Figure 89.2   Crosstalk between T cells and Hodgkin Reed–Sternberg (H-RS) cells in Hodgkin lymphoma (HL). A significant proportion of the non-tumoral infiltrate in HL is made up of T cells. Interactions between them and H-RS cells take place through several receptors: CD40, CD70, HLA II, CD80/86, and ICAM-1. TCR, T cell receptor; ICAM, intracellular adhesion molecule.

consequence of changes in the HL cells, such as downregulation of major histocompatibility complex (MHC) class I in H-RS cells,[61] or induction of local T cell anergy by IL-10 or TGFβ, expression of perforin-neutralizing proteins, and induction of apoptosis in CTLs by H-RS cells via CD95L.

A functional exploration of the macrophage and T cell subsets present in HL tissue is still pending. Meanwhile, initial findings are proving to be interesting. For instance, the composition of the T cell infiltrate (CTLs vs Tregs) has been found to be a predictive factor of clinical outcome in HL. A small number of FOXP3$^+$ (Treg) cells and high infiltration of TIA-1$^+$ cells (CTLs, NK cells, neutrophils, and macrophages) represent an independent prognostic factor of unfavorable outcome (event-free and disease-free survival).[53] Another interesting observation is the presence of STAT1-activated **macrophages** surrounding HL cells (Fig. 89.2), associated with unfavorable prognosis,[60] which could be associated with the immunosuppressive capacity of these STAT1-activated macrophages.[62]

It is also important to consider that T lymphocytes in HL express ligands for a number of molecules that are strongly expressed in H-RS cells – CD40L (for CD40), CD27 (for CD70), CD4 (for HLA-II), CD28/CTLA-4 (for CD80/86), and LFA-1 (for ICAM-1, binding to lymphocytes in an antigen-independent way)[63] – which underlines the presence of crosstalk between HL cells and T cells (Fig. 89.2).

Mast cells are present in virtually all HLs, express functional CD30L, and are the predominant CD30L$^+$ cells in HL. *In vitro*, a mast cell line stimulated CD30L-mediated proliferation of H-RS cell lines. It has been observed that a high degree of mast-cell infiltration is associated with nodular sclerosis histology and poorer relapse-free survival.[64]

Lymph nodes involved in CHL typically show heavy infiltration by eosinophils. Cytokines and chemokines may contribute to this eosinophilia both by increasing the production/activation of eosinophils and stimulating their recruitment to the site of CHL involvement (via IL-5, CCL28, and CCL11 secreted by H-RS cells themselves or by fibroblasts and macrophages). Eosinophils express ligands for CD30 and CD40 (receptors expressed by H-RS), providing proliferative and antiapoptotic signals for H-RS cells. Furthermore, eosinophils produce TGFβ and may therefore be involved in fibroblast activation and fibrosis. A high eosinophil content was found to be related to poor prognosis,[65] although this has not been confirmed in other studies.[66]

Many **fibroblast**-like cells can be detected, often in association with H-RS cells, especially in the nodular sclerosis subtype. Three crucial mechanisms have been proposed as being involved in the generation of fibrosis: (1) unbalanced production of TH2 over TH1 cytokines causing an abnormal reaction to tissue damage (e.g., fibroblasts express IL-13R, especially in the nodular sclerosis subtype, and can be activated by IL-13 secreted by H-RS cells); (2) the increased production of TGFβ and basic fibroblast growth factor (b-FGF) by H-RS and reactive cells (potent stimulators of fibroblast proliferation and extracellular matrix [ECM] protein synthesis); and (3) the engagement of CD40, expressed by fibroblasts, by CD40L (expressed by activated T cells, mast cells, and eosinophils). Primary fibroblasts from HL also produce growth factors for H-RS cells, such as IL-6 and IL-7.[67,68]

Angioimmunoblastic T cell lymphoma

Angioimmunoblastic T cell lymphoma (AITL) is the paradigmatic neoplasm of the interaction of T cells with the stroma and B cells. Findings from recent studies suggest that it is derived from **follicular B helper T cells** (T$_{FH}$).[69–71] These T$_{FH}$ have a characteristic cell-surface phenotype and gene expression profile that are distinct from any other T cell population. It is still unclear whether T$_{FH}$ differentiate as a third, separate lineage at the time of T cell priming or whether they emerge at a later stage from nonpolarized, primed T cells or even from polarized TH2 or TH1 cells. It has been shown that, after activation, T$_{FH}$ express OX14 (CD134) and induce upregulation of CD40L and activation-induced cytidine deaminase (AID) expression in B cells, promoting germinal center B cell survival and differentiation and allowing immunoglobulin class switching and somatic hypermutation.[70] They also upregulate the expression of CXCR5, the receptor for CXCL13, a chemokine produced by follicular dendritic cells that promotes B cell entry into the germinal center and therefore B cell–T cell contacts.

In early lymph node involvement by AITL, the neoplastic T cells preferentially occupy the B cell follicles and the immediate perifollicular area, sometimes mimicking a follicular lymphoma of B cell origin or a follicular hyperplasia. This observation suggests that the germinal center microenvironment must be critical for tumor development. CXCL13 promotes proliferation of follicular dendritic cells and B cell recruitment and activation leading to a marked immune deregulation that characterizes AITL, rather than aggressive tumor growth.

It is a characteristic finding that AITL cases display a striking hyperplasia of CD30-positive large B cells.[72] Monoclonal expansion of these EBV-positive B cells has even been observed in some AITL cases.[73] In spite of this, the progression to an open B cell lymphoma is only a rare finding in AITL cases, even in those displaying monoclonal Ig rearrangements. This suggests that the presence of B cells in AITL could constitute a virally induced reversible lymphoproliferative process, promoted through the combined action of EBV and the continued survival stimulus received from the neoplastic T_{FH} cells. This EBV-driven B cell hyperplasia, which occasionally includes H-RS-like cells, can be observed in other peripheral T cell lymphomas, although at a lower frequency.[74]

These observations identify the T cell–B cell crosstalk and the molecules involved in this process (ICOS, CD84, SAP, IL-21, and CXCR5) as being potential targets for therapeutic intervention in AITL patients.[70]

This phenomenon is the opposite of that observed in **T cell-rich B cell lymphoma**, an aggressive B cell lymphoma in which a minority of germinal center-derived neoplastic B cells persist within a background of reactive T cells and histiocytes.[75] The nature of the interaction between the neoplastic large B cells and the accompanying histiocytes and reactive T cells requires further study.

Follicular lymphoma

In follicular lymphoma (FL), the tumor cells grow in a follicular pattern and the same cellular components are found as those present in normal germinal centers (helper T cells, follicular dendritic cells, and macrophages), suggesting that these cellular interactions are similar to those in normal germinal centers. The dependency of FL cells on their microenvironment is supported by the fact that these cells are very difficult to grow *in vitro* in the absence of stromal cells and without stimulation of the CD40 receptor, which is a main signaling pathway for interactions between B cells and T cells.[76] In fact, it has been shown that chemokines CXCL12 and CXCL13, among others, enhance the migration of FL B cells to specific localization in lymph nodes.[77,78] Interestingly, Dave and colleagues[79] identified two signatures that together represented the best predictor of survival for follicular lymphoma patients, dividing them into quartiles based on survival time. The genes that best defined both signatures were expressed primarily by T cells, macrophages, or dendritic cells, but not by the tumor cells themselves. This dominant influence of the cellular microenvironment on the prognosis of follicular lymphoma is further evidence of the participation of immune cells in the biology and pathogenesis of this type of tumor.

More recently, Farinha et al.[80] have shown that **lymphoma-associated macrophages** (LAMs) are an independent predictor of survival, while Carreras et al. have shown that high Treg numbers predict improved survival of follicular lymphoma patients,[81] thus confirming the important role of microenvironment in follicular lymphoma.

Considering their heterogeneity, cells of the monocyte–macrophage lineage are very versatile in their response to very different microenvironmental signals. Macrophages associated with tumors belong to the polarized M2 macrophage population, which is usually induced by IL-10, IL-4, IL-13, glucocorticoid hormones, and vitamin D3. Tumor-associated macrophages (TAMs) suppress T cell activation and proliferation by secreting IL-10 and TGFβ. As they release a variety of growth factors such as epidermal growth factor (EGF), factors of the fibroblast growth factor (FGF) family, some chemokines, and vascular endothelial growth factor (VEGF) and proangiogenic factors such as hypoxia-inducible factor 2α (HIF2α) and HIF1, tumoral growth and angiogenesis are enhanced. Finally, another recognized role of TAMs in cancer is the promotion of metastasis through extracellular matrix (ECM) digestion by matrix metalloproteinases.[82]

The identification of the critical components of the interactions between tumoral and non-tumoral cells could give rise to new treatment options directed at interfering with the specific growth-promoting actions of the inflammatory cells in particular environments. As a recent example of the potential utility of this approach, Staudt and coworkers have demonstrated that survival after R-CHOP treatment of diffuse large B cell lymphoma is influenced by differences in immune cells, fibrosis, and angiogenesis in the tumor microenvironment,[83] thus bringing new prognostic parameters and potential therapeutic targets derived from the tumoral environment.

KEY POINTS

- During recent decades the classical view of cancer biology has focused on genetic lesions and altered signaling pathways within tumoral cells. As a consequence, most current cancer therapies aim at targeting the neoplastic cell population. However, new findings have shown that the tumor microenvironment may also play an important role in the genesis and progression of the disease.
- Increasing attention is being paid to the role of the microenvironment in early phases of lymphoproliferative disorders. Here we provide different examples of lymphoproliferative diseases in which inflammatory processes related to viral or bacterial infections and autoimmune disorders could drive tumorigenesis.

- Much evidence has shown that chemokines, a subset of cytokines that regulate migration of leukocytes along a chemical gradient, contribute to the development of lymphomas. In fact, differential expression of chemokine receptors in neoplastic cells determines their trafficking and homing into lymphoid organs.
- Interactions with non-tumoral cells via chemokines or direct interactions attract tumoral cells to specific niches, where they are supported by different survival stimuli.
- New cancer therapies targeting the tumor cell microenvironment could be developed. Some of these, such as chemokine receptor antagonists, are being evaluated in preclinical studies or clinical trials.

REFERENCES

● = Key primary paper
◆ = Major review article

1. Wotherspoon AC, Doglioni C, Diss TC et al. Regression of primary low-grade B-cell gastric lymphoma of mucosa-associated lymphoid tissue type after eradication of Helicobacter pylori. Lancet 1993; **342**: 575–7.
●2. Parsonnet J, Hansen S, Rodriguez L et al. Helicobacter pylori infection and gastric lymphoma. N Engl J Med 1994; **330**: 1267–71.
3. Hussell T, Isaacson PG, Crabtree JE, Spencer J. Helicobacter pylori-specific tumour-infiltrating T cells provide contact dependent help for the growth of malignant B cells in low-grade gastric lymphoma of mucosa-associated lymphoid tissue. J Pathol 1996; **178**: 122–7.
4. Ohmae T, Hirata Y, Maeda S et al. Helicobacter pylori activates NF-kappaB via the alternative pathway in B lymphocytes. J Immunol 2005; **175**: 7162–9.
5. Parsonnet J, Isaacson PG. Bacterial infection and MALT lymphoma. N Engl J Med 2004; **350**: 213–15.
6. Zucca E, Bertoni F, Roggero E, Cavalli F. The gastric marginal zone B-cell lymphoma of MALT type. Blood 2000; **96**: 410–19.
7. Lankarani KB, Masoompour SM, Masoompour MB et al. Changing epidemiology of IPSID in Southern Iran. Gut 2005; **54**: 311–2.
●8. Al-Saleem TI. Evidence of acquired immune deficiencies in Mediterranean lymphoma. A possible aetiological link. Lancet 1978; **2**: 709–12.
9. Lecuit M, Abachin E, Martin A et al. Immunoproliferative small intestinal disease associated with Campylobacter jejuni. N Engl J Med 2004; **350**: 239–48.
10. Al-Saleem T, Al-Mondhiry H. Immunoproliferative small intestinal disease (IPSID): a model for mature B-cell neoplasms. Blood 2005; **105**: 2274–80.
11. Roggero E, Zucca E, Mainetti C et al. Eradication of Borrelia burgdorferi infection in primary marginal zone B-cell lymphoma of the skin. Hum Pathol 2000; **31**: 263–8.
12. Garbe C, Stein H, Gollnick H et al. Cutaneous B cell lymphoma in chronic Borrelia burgdorferi infection. Report of 2 cases and a review of the literature. Hautarzt 1988; **39**: 717–26.
13. Goodlad JR, Davidson MM, Hollowood K et al. Primary cutaneous B-cell lymphoma and Borrelia burgdorferi infection in patients from the Highlands of Scotland. Am J Surg Pathol 2000; **24**: 1279–85.
14. Cerroni L, Zochling N, Putz B, Kerl H. Infection by Borrelia burgdorferi and cutaneous B-cell lymphoma. J Cutan Pathol 1997; **24**: 457–61.
15. Kutting B, Bonsmann G, Metze D et al. Borrelia burgdorferi-associated primary cutaneous B cell lymphoma: complete clearing of skin lesions after antibiotic pulse therapy or intralesional injection of interferon alfa-2a. J Am Acad Dermatol 1997; **36**: 311–14.
16. Ferreri AJ, Guidoboni M, Ponzoni M et al. Evidence for an association between Chlamydia psittaci and ocular adnexal lymphomas. J Natl Cancer Inst 2004; **96**: 586–94.
17. Ferreri AJ, Ponzoni M, Viale E et al. Association between Helicobacter pylori infection and MALT-type lymphoma of the ocular adnexa: clinical and therapeutic implications. Hematol Oncol 2005; **24**: 33–7.
●18. Ferreri AJ, Ponzoni M, Guidoboni M et al. Regression of ocular adnexal lymphoma after Chlamydia psittaci-eradicating antibiotic therapy. J Clin Oncol 2005; **23**: 5067–73.
19. Rosado MF, Byrne GE Jr, Ding F et al. Ocular adnexal lymphoma: a clinicopathologic study of a large cohort of patients with no evidence for an association with Chlamydia psittaci. Blood 2006; **107**: 467–72.
20. Chanudet E, Zhou Y, Bacon C et al. Chlamydia psittaci is variably associated with ocular adnexal MALT lymphoma in different geographical regions. J Pathol 2006; **209**: 344–51.
21. Smedby KE, Hjalgrim H, Askling J et al. Autoimmune and chronic inflammatory disorders and risk of non-Hodgkin lymphoma by subtype. J Natl Cancer Inst 2006; **98**: 51–60.
22. Martin T, Weber JC, Levallois H et al. Salivary gland lymphomas in patients with Sjogren's syndrome may frequently develop from rheumatoid factor B cells. Arthritis Rheum 2000; **43**: 908–16.
23. Algara P, Mateo MS, Sanchez-Beato M et al. Analysis of the IgV(H) somatic mutations in splenic marginal zone lymphoma defines a group of unmutated cases with frequent 7q deletion and adverse clinical course. Blood 2002; **99**: 1299–304.
24. Bidegain F, Berry A, Alvarez M et al. Acute Plasmodium falciparum malaria following splenectomy for suspected lymphoma in 2 patients. Clin Infect Dis 2005; **40**: e97–100.
25. Bates I, Bedu-Addo G. Chronic malaria and splenic lymphoma: clues to understanding lymphoma evolution. Leukemia 1997; **11**: 2162–7.
26. Wallace S, Bedu-Addo G, Rutherford TR, Bates I. Serological similarities between hyperreactive malarial

splenomegaly and splenic lymphoma in west Africa. *Trans R Soc Trop Med Hyg* 1998; **92**: 463–7.

27. Bates I, Bedu-Addo G, Jarrett RF *et al.* B-lymphotropic viruses in a novel tropical splenic lymphoma. *Br J Haematol* 2001; **112**: 161–6.

◆28. Hermine O, Lefrere F, Bronowicki JP *et al.* Regression of splenic lymphoma with villous lymphocytes after treatment of hepatitis C virus infection. *N Engl J Med* 2002; **347**: 89–94.

●29. Saadoun D, Suarez F, Lefrere F *et al.* Splenic lymphoma with villous lymphocytes, associated with type II cryoglobulinemia and HCV infection: a new entity? *Blood* 2005; **105**: 74–6.

30. Plater-Zyberk C, Maini RN, Lam K *et al.* A rheumatoid arthritis B cell subset expresses a phenotype similar to that in chronic lymphocytic leukemia. *Arthritis Rheum* 1985; **28**: 971–6.

31. Chiorazzi N, Rai KR, Ferrarini M. Chronic lymphocytic leukemia. *N Engl J Med* 2005; **352**: 804–15.

32. Nishio M, Endo T, Tsukada N *et al.* Nurselike cells express BAFF and APRIL, which can promote survival of chronic lymphocytic leukemia cells via a paracrine pathway distinct from that of SDF-1alpha. *Blood* 2005; **106**: 1012–20.

◆33. Cellier C, Delabesse E, Helmer C *et al.* Refractory sprue, coeliac disease, and enteropathy-associated T-cell lymphoma. French Coeliac Disease Study Group. *Lancet* 2000; **356**: 203–8.

34. Smedby KE, Akerman M, Hildebrand H *et al.* Malignant lymphomas in coeliac disease: evidence of increased risks for lymphoma types other than enteropathy-type T cell lymphoma. *Gut* 2005; **54**: 54–9.

35. Aozasa K, Takakuwa T, Nakatsuka S. Pyothorax-associated lymphoma: a lymphoma developing in chronic inflammation. *Adv Anat Pathol* 2005; **12**: 324–31.

36. Küppers R. B cells under influence: transformation of B cells by Epstein-Barr virus. *Nat Rev Immunol* 2003; **3**: 801–12.

37. Wright DH. Burkitt's lymphoma: a review of the pathology, immunology, and possible etiologic factors. *Pathol Annu* 1971; **6**: 337–63.

38. van den Bosch CA. Is endemic Burkitt's lymphoma an alliance between three infections and a tumour promoter? *Lancet Oncol* 2004; **5**: 738–46.

39. Dong HY, Scadden DT, de Leval L *et al.* Plasmablastic lymphoma in HIV-positive patients: an aggressive Epstein-Barr virus-associated extramedullary plasmacytic neoplasm. *Am J Surg Pathol* 2005; **29**: 1633–41.

40. Jaffe ES, Krenacs L, Kumar S *et al.* Extranodal peripheral T-cell and NK-cell neoplasms. *Am J Clin Pathol* 1999; **111**: S46–55.

◆41. Schulz TF. The pleiotropic effects of Kaposi's sarcoma herpesvirus. *J Pathol* 2006; **208**: 187–98.

42. Taylor GP, Matsuoka M. Natural history of adult T-cell leukemia/lymphoma and approaches to therapy. *Oncogene* 2005; **24**: 6047–57.

43. Balkwill F. Cancer and the chemokine network. *Nat Rev Cancer* 2004; **4**: 540–50.

44. Laurence AD. Location, movement and survival: the role of chemokines in haematopoiesis and malignancy. *Br J Haematol* 2006; **132**: 255–67.

45. Stein JV, Nombela-Arrieta C. Chemokine control of lymphocyte trafficking: a general overview. *Immunology* 2005; **116**: 1–12.

46. Maggio E, van den Berg A, Diepstra A *et al.* Chemokines, cytokines and their receptors in Hodgkin's lymphoma cell lines and tissues. *Ann Oncol* 2002; **13**(Suppl 1): 52–6.

47. Hopken UE, Foss HD, Meyer D *et al.* Up-regulation of the chemokine receptor CCR7 in classical but not in lymphocyte-predominant Hodgkin disease correlates with distinct dissemination of neoplastic cells in lymphoid organs. *Blood* 2002; **99**: 1109–16.

◆48. Ghia P, Circosta P, Scielzo C *et al.* Differential effects on CLL cell survival exerted by different microenvironmental elements. *Curr Top Microbiol Immunol* 2005; **294**: 135–45.

49. Till KJ, Lin K, Zuzel M, Cawley JC. The chemokine receptor CCR7 and alpha4 integrin are important for migration of chronic lymphocytic leukemia cells into lymph nodes. *Blood* 2002; **99**: 2977–84.

●50. Stevenson FK, Caligaris-Cappio F. Chronic lymphocytic leukemia: revelations from the B-cell receptor. *Blood* 2004; **103**: 4389–95.

51. Burger JA, Kipps TJ. CXCR4: a key receptor in the crosstalk between tumor cells and their microenvironment. *Blood* 2006; **107**: 1761–7.

52. Burger M, Hartmann T, Krome M *et al.* Small peptide inhibitors of the CXCR4 chemokine receptor (CD184) antagonize the activation, migration, and antiapoptotic responses of CXCL12 in chronic lymphocytic leukemia B cells. *Blood* 2005; **106**: 1824–30.

53. Alvaro T, Lejeune M, Salvado MT *et al.* Outcome in Hodgkin's lymphoma can be predicted from the presence of accompanying cytotoxic and regulatory T cells. *Clin Cancer Res* 2005; **11**: 1467–73.

◆54. Marshall NA, Christie LE, Munro LR *et al.* Immunosuppressive regulatory T cells are abundant in the reactive lymphocytes of Hodgkin lymphoma. *Blood* 2004; **103**: 1755–62.

55. Schubert LA, Jeffery E, Zhang Y *et al.* Scurfin (FOXP3) acts as a repressor of transcription and regulates T cell activation. *J Biol Chem* 2001; **276**: 37672–9.

●56. Hori S, Nomura T, Sakaguchi S. Control of regulatory T cell development by the transcription factor Foxp3. *Science* 2003; **299**: 1057–61.

57. Fontenot JD, Rasmussen JP, Williams LM *et al.* Regulatory T cell lineage specification by the forkhead transcription factor foxp3. *Immunity* 2005; **22**: 329–41.

58. Bluestone JA, Abbas AK. Natural versus adaptive regulatory T cells. *Nat Rev Immunol* 2003; **3**: 253–7.

59. Oudejans JJ, Jiwa NM, Kummer JA *et al.* Activated cytotoxic T cells as prognostic marker in Hodgkin's disease. *Blood* 1997; **89**: 1376–82.

60. Sanchez-Aguilera A, Montalban C, de la Cueva P *et al.* Tumor microenvironment and mitotic checkpoint are key

factors in the outcome of classic Hodgkin lymphoma. *Blood* 2006; **108**: 662–8.

61. Poppema S, Visser L. Absence of HLA class I expression by Reed-Sternberg cells. *Am J Pathol* 1994; **145**: 37–41.

62. Kusmartsev S, Gabrilovich DI. STAT1 signaling regulates tumor-associated macrophage-mediated T cell deletion. *J Immunol* 2005; **174**: 4880–91.

63. Poppema S, van den Berg A. Interaction between host T cells and Reed-Sternberg cells in Hodgkin lymphomas. *Semin Cancer Biol* 2000; **10**: 345–50.

64. Molin D, Edstrom A, Glimelius I *et al*. Mast cell infiltration correlates with poor prognosis in Hodgkin's lymphoma. *Br J Haematol* 2002; **119**: 122–4.

65. von Wasielewski R, Seth S, Franklin J *et al*. Tissue eosinophilia correlates strongly with poor prognosis in nodular sclerosing Hodgkin's disease, allowing for known prognostic factors. *Blood* 2000; **95**: 1207–13.

66. Axdorph U, Porwit-MacDonald A, Grimfors G, Bjorkholm M. Tissue eosinophilia in relation to immunopathological and clinical characteristics in Hodgkin's disease. *Leuk Lymphoma* 2001; **42**: 1055–65.

◆67. Aldinucci D, Lorenzon D, Olivo K *et al*. Interactions between tissue fibroblasts in lymph nodes and Hodgkin/Reed-Sternberg cells. *Leuk Lymphoma* 2004; **45**: 1731–9.

68. Khnykin D, Troen G, Berner JM, Delabie J. The expression of fibroblast growth factors and their receptors in Hodgkin's lymphoma. *J Pathol* 2006; **208**: 431–8.

69. Grogg KL, Attygalle AD, Macon WR *et al*. Angioimmunoblastic T-cell lymphoma: a neoplasm of germinal-center T-helper cells? *Blood* 2005; **106**: 1501–2.

70. Vinuesa CG, Tangye SG, Moser B, Mackay CR. Follicular B helper T cells in antibody responses and autoimmunity. *Nat Rev Immunol* 2005; **5**: 853–65.

71. de Leval L, Rickman DS, Thielen C *et al*. The gene expression profile of nodal peripheral T-cell lymphoma demonstrates a molecular link between angioimmunoblastic T-cell lymphoma (AITL) and follicular helper T (TFH) cells. *Blood* 2007; **109**: 4952–63.

72. Korbjuhn P, Anagnostopoulos I, Hummel M *et al*. Frequent latent Epstein-Barr virus infection of neoplastic T cells and bystander B cells in human immunodeficiency virus-negative European peripheral pleomorphic T-cell lymphomas. *Blood* 1993; **82**: 217–23.

73. Brauninger A, Spieker T, Willenbrock K *et al*. Survival and clonal expansion of mutating "forbidden" (immunoglobulin receptor-deficient) Epstein-Barr virus-infected B cells in angioimmunoblastic T cell lymphoma. *J Exp Med* 2001; **194**: 927–40.

74. Quintanilla-Martinez L, Fend F, Moguel LR *et al*. Peripheral T-cell lymphoma with Reed-Sternberg-like cells of B-cell phenotype and genotype associated with Epstein-Barr virus infection. *Am J Surg Pathol* 1999; **23**: 1233–40.

75. Abramson JS. T-cell/histiocyte-rich B-cell lymphoma: biology, diagnosis, and management. *Oncologist* 2006; **11**: 384–92.

●76. Eray M, Postila V, Eeva J *et al*. Follicular lymphoma cell lines, an in vitro model for antigenic selection and cytokine-mediated growth regulation of germinal centre B cells. *Scand J Immunol* 2003; **57**: 545–55.

77. Corcione A, Ottonello L, Tortolina G *et al*. Stromal cell-derived factor-1 as a chemoattractant for follicular center lymphoma B cells. *J Natl Cancer Inst* 2000; **92**: 628–35.

78. Husson H, Freedman AS, Cardoso AA *et al*. CXCL13 (BCA-1) is produced by follicular lymphoma cells: role in the accumulation of malignant B cells. *Br J Haematol* 2002; **119**: 492–5.

79. Dave SS, Wright G, Tan B *et al*. Prediction of survival in follicular lymphoma based on molecular features of tumor-infiltrating immune cells. *N Engl J Med* 2004; **351**: 2159–69.

80. Farinha P, Masoudi H, Skinnider BF *et al*. Analysis of multiple biomarkers shows that lymphoma-associated macrophage (LAM) content is an independent predictor of survival in follicular lymphoma (FL). *Blood* 2005; **106**: 2169–74.

81. Carreras J, Lopez-Guillermo A, Fox BC *et al*. High numbers of tumor-infiltrating FOXP3-positive regulatory T cells are associated with improved overall survival in follicular lymphoma. *Blood* 2006; **108**: 2957–64.

82. Mantovani A, Sozzani S, Locati M *et al*. Macrophage polarization: tumor-associated macrophages as a paradigm for polarized M2 mononuclear phagocytes. *Trends Immunol* 2002; **23**: 549–55.

83. Lenz G, Wright G, Dave SS *et al*. Stromal gene signatures in large-B-cell lymphomas. *N Engl J Med* 2008; **359**: 2313–23.

90

Molecular pathway therapy for non-Hodgkin lymphomas

FINBARR E COTTER AND REBECCA L AUER

Therapy for lymphomas has entered a promising and potentially beneficial era. The understanding, development, and optimal application of such treatment are pivotal if we are to exploit it to the full benefit of patients with lymphoma. Rituximab has led the way but much more can be achieved by new agents, either alone or in logical combinations, based on the biological pathways of lymphoma cells. These pathways are often aberrantly activated by the altered molecular genetics of the lymphoma cell. Molecular therapy being developed is largely aimed at silencing these overexpressed pathways at either the DNA or RNA level, although quenching the protein product is also possible. All this builds logically on our greater understanding of the molecular and cellular biology of lymphoma and differs for each individual subtype of lymphoma. Primarily the new molecular therapies involve the apoptosis, cell cycle, angiogenesis, and proteasome pathways. Earlier new molecules such as antisense oligonucleotides showed that the paradigm for gene silencing was effective but not as beneficial as hoped, probably due to poor application and some naïvety of understanding for the molecule. In this chapter we will approach the new therapies available on a pathways-directed basis. The current emphasis is to modify lymphoma cell biology by pathway-silencing molecules, rendering them more sensitive to the application of conventional DNA-damaging treatment such as chemotherapy and radiation therapy. However, it is envisaged that in the future the combination of molecular therapies can be used in a more sophisticated manner as individualized medicine. This requires not only the therapeutic molecules, but also greater improvements in cellular diagnostics and biomarkers of response, which can be blamed in part for holding back the field. Recent technological developments will advance our application of the therapy outlined.

APOPTOSIS PATHWAYS

BCL2

Cloning of the *BCL2* gene from the t(14;18) translocation, a signature genetic marker for follicular lymphoma, in 1984, its resultant deregulated overexpression, and an awareness of its pivotal antiapoptotic effects, made this one of the first and favorite molecular targets for lymphoma therapy.[1,2] The antisense oligonucleotide approach was taken and to date remains possibly the most successful for lymphoma.[2–5] Other small-molecule approaches include BH3 mimetics that prevent homodimerization of BCL2 which is essential for its antiapoptotic function, and direct mitochondrial transition pore agents.[6] The caspase-9 mitochondrial pathway remains the target for these molecules and all aim to induce the release of cytochrome C with subsequent induction of apoptosis via the intrinsic apoptotic pathway.[1,2]

BCL2 antisense (G3139, Genasense®)

The Genasense® BCL2 antisense molecule is a synthetically manufactured single-strand 18 base oligonucleotide that has been chemically modified by changing the linking molecule from oxygen to sulphur (a phosphorothioate).[7] This confers resistance to the nuclease enzyme and thus prolongs its half-life from minutes to days. The sequence is complementary to the start codon of *BCL2* mRNA and has been demonstrated to bind to *BCL2* mRNA resulting in reduced levels of BCL2 protein.[2,4]

Preclinical studies, both *in vitro* and *in vivo* in severe combined immune deficiency/nonobese diabetic (SCID/NOD) mouse models, are extensive and reveal a wealth of potential applications for Genasense®. These include, in the lymphoma field, single-agent activity in follicular lymphoma models,[8] sensitization to chemotherapy, including rituximab,[9] and combinations with the proteasome inhibitor bortezomib and cyclophosphamide for diffuse large B cell lymphomas (DLBCL).[5,10] However, these have not translated to clinical trials in most cases. Three studies have been reported to date. The first and pivotal phase I study showed objective responses, including a prolonged complete remission in nearly half of the 21 heavily pretreated patients with an indolent B cell lymphoma background.[3,4] The patients were treated with a single 2-week subcutaneous infusion of Genasense®. It was well tolerated and, most importantly, showed that responses were found in those whose BCL2 protein levels were reduced by Genasense®.[3] Further phase II and III studies were then conducted in melanoma,[11] chronic lymphocytic leukemia (CLL),[12] and myeloma[13] with less impressive results, but not lymphoma. It is worth noting that the majority of the lymphoma patients treated had the t(14;18) translocation within their lymphoma cells. Since then two other studies have been reported. One is in relapsed mantle cell lymphoma (MCL), which is noted for high levels of BCL2, and Genasense® was combined with rituximab and CHOP chemotherapy. Seven responses were observed from 16 patients, including one complete remission.[14] The other clinical study was from the MD Anderson Cancer Center[15] (Lugano 2005) and demonstrated responses in previous rituximab failures when retreated with rituximab in combination with Genasense®, revealing the ability of the BCL2 antisense to overcome rituximab resistance. Many of these lymphomas contained the t(14;18) translocation. This was in keeping with the preclinical study. In summary, Genasense® has shown activity in B cell lymphomas particularly when bearing the t(14;18) translocation and where BCL2 was significantly reduced by the molecule. The numbers are small and definitive registration

Table 90.1 Apoptosis-targeting small molecules in development with potential for lymphoma therapy

Agent	Company	Stage
GX015-070 (BH3 binding, anti-MCL1/BCL2)[16]	GeminX	Phase I
BCL2 inhibitor[6]	Ascenta Therapeutics	Phase I
ABT-737 (BCL2 inhibitor)[6]	Abbott Laboratories	Preclinical
BCL2 inhibitor[6]	Infinity Pharma	Preclinical
Amplimexon (mitochondria thiol-binding agent)[6]	AmpliMed	Phase I
Small molecule XIAP antagonist[17]	Burnham Institute	Preclinical

XIAP, X-linked inhibitor of apoptosis protein

studies have not been performed, making this a disappointingly unfulfilled therapeutic molecule despite the extensive preclinical studies. However, BCL2 antisense has indicated that BCL2 and the apoptotic machinery are a valid target for molecular therapy in B cell lymphomas[2,3] and this has led to the development of a number of other small molecules targeting BCL2 and other antiapoptosis genes that are overexpressed in some forms of lymphoma.

Apoptosis-targeting small molecules

The majority of apoptosis-targeting small molecules are aimed at the BCL2 molecule and are summarized in Table 90.1. While some have been reported to have preclinical activity in B cell lymphomas it remains to be seen if this translates into clinical activity. Some clinical phase I studies are underway.

Conclusions for apoptosis-targeting therapy

Apoptosis-targeting therapy is an area where there is a rich promise of success but a failure to apply this solidly to the field of lymphoma. Antisense oligonucleotides have been shown to have efficacy but need to be validated in large studies. It is clear that BCL2 is a good target for molecular therapy in some cases of B cell lymphoma and the presence of the t(14;18) translocation is probably a good indicator for treatment. It also would appear from preclinical studies that combinations with rituximab and/or bortezomib would make the basis of good therapy.

CYCLIN INHIBITION

Cell cycle dysregulation

Progression through the cell cycle (Fig. 90.1) is a highly regulated process dependent on the activity of the cyclin-dependent kinases (CDK)-cyclin complexes which in turn

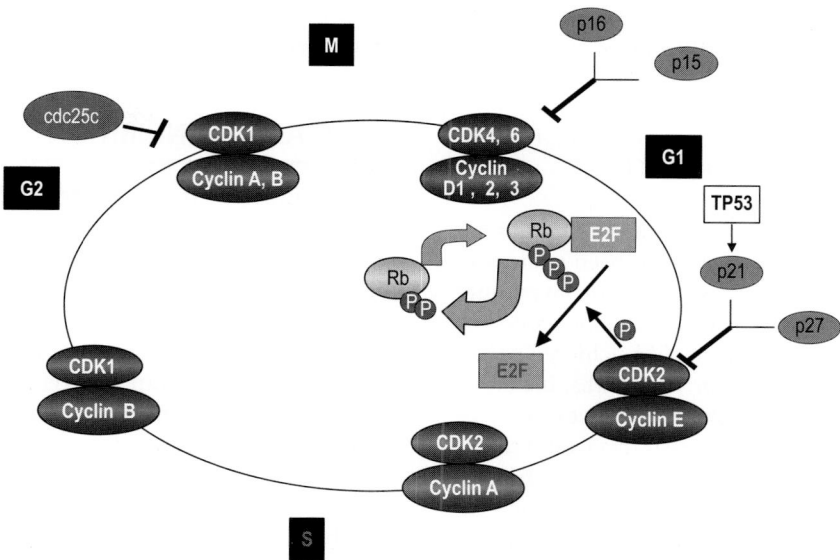

Figure 90.1 Cell cycle control. Cell cycle division consists of S phase (DNA synthesis) when chromosomes are replicated once, M phase (mitosis) when chromosomes segregate to produce two genetically identical daughter cells, and G1 and G2 (gap phases), intervals of growth and reorganization. When cells stop cycling they enter a state of quiescence, G0. Progress through the cell cycle is controlled by the activity of the cyclin–dependent kinase (CDK)/cyclin complexes and various checkpoints.

are controlled by a complex network of events including induction and degradation of the cyclin subunit, phosphorylation and dephosphorylation of the CDK subunit, and binding of CDK inhibitors to the CDK-cyclin complex.[18,19] These inhibitors include the INK4 family of p16, p15, p18, and p19 and the Cip/Kip family of p21 and p27.[20,21] Malignant transformation is associated with an overexpression of cyclins and progressive loss of CDK inhibitors, leading to proliferation through cell cycle dysregulation.

Mantle cell lymphoma is the paradigm for a disease of cell cycle dysregulation with the t(11;14) genetic hallmark, present in virtually all cases, resulting in deregulation and upregulation of cyclin D1, an important regulator of the G1 phase of the cell cycle. In MCL there are a number of additional alterations that all lead to dysregulation of cell cycle machinery, the common element being to upregulate cyclin D1 and increase the protein drive on cell cycling and proliferation. These include genomic amplification of cyclin-dependent kinase 4 (*CDK4*), deletion of cyclin-dependent kinase inhibitor 2A/p16 (*CDKN2A*), and overexpression of *BMI1*, a transcriptional repressor of p16,[22] all adding fuel to the fire by enhancing progression of cell cycling and, along with *TP53* deletions, are usually found in blastoid variants with poorer outcomes.[23] Loss of cyclin-dependent kinases p21 and p27 which normally inhibit cyclin D1 also occurs and removes a 'brake' to the G1-S checkpoint in MCL. Deletions on the long arm of chromosome 11q22-23 are found in nearly half of MCLs involving the *ATM* gene[24] which is commonly mutated.[25] *ATM* is an important response gene to DNA damage, setting in motion a cascade of genes within the DNA repair

pathways for which *TP53* is also a central participant. Their activation in response to DNA damage leads to suppression of cell cycling predominantly at the G1-S checkpoint. Thus, in addition to the cyclin D1 drive, inactivation of *ATM* in MCL removes a brake on the G1-S checkpoint further promoting cell cycling. The overexpression of cyclin D1, intrinsic to MCL biology, makes this a suitable target for molecular directed therapy.

Targeting the cyclin–dependent kinases: flavopiridol – a CDK inhibitor

The active site of the CDK-cyclin complexes was identified as an ATP-binding region,[26] thus opening the way for a potential target for cancer therapy. Flavopiridol was identified as a specific inhibitor[27] leading to direct inhibition of CDK activity and growth arrest at the G1 and G2 phases of the cell cycle.[28] This has translated into suppression of tumor growth in leukemia and lymphoma cell lines and xenograft models.[29] Since flavopiridol was first recognized as inducing cell cycle arrest through inhibition of the CDKs, multiple additional mechanisms of action have been identified:

1. Suppression of cyclin D1, directly through transcriptional repression of the cyclin D1 promoter[30] and indirectly through inhibition of nuclear factor κB (NF-κB).[31]
2. Inhibition of positive elongation factor B,[32] leading to transcription 'halt,' affecting proapoptotic proteins such as MCL1 and XIAP.[33]

3. Modulation of extracellular signaling pathways: activation of p38 MAP kinase with suppression of ERK activity[34] and inhibition of phosphatidylinositol 3-kinase (PI3K)/AKT[35] pathways.
4. Antiangiogenesis, downregulating expression of vascular endothelial growth factor (VEGF).[36,37]

Despite the *in vitro* promise of flavopiridol, this has not been borne out *in vivo*. Most progress has been made with CLL, adopting a novel dosing strategy for maximum effect.[38] Using *in vitro*-derived pharmacokinetic modeling, 45 percent of patients with refractory CLL achieved partial responses which lasted longer than 12 months, including patients with genetically high-risk disease. Because of its effects on cyclin D1, there was hope that this would reflect as an effective agent for MCL. There have been two trials of flavopiridol in MCL using different dosing schedules. In the earlier study, a 72-hour infusion was administered every 14 days to ten patients with refractory disease but no clinical response occurred despite a tolerable side-effect profile.[39] In their study, the National Cancer Institute of Canada Clinical Trials Group treated 28 patients with previously untreated or relapsed (the majority) MCL at a dose of 50 mg/m^2 over 1 hour daily for 3 days every 3 weeks. Only three patients achieved partial remission with no complete remissions but 11 patients had stable disease suggesting the 1-hour schedule has activity rather than the longer infusion.[40]

Targeting cyclin D1 translation – mTOR inhibitors

The translation of cyclin D1 is largely regulated by mammalian target of rapamycin (mTOR) activity, a downstream target of the PI3K/AKT signaling pathway. mTOR is a large and highly conserved kinase that regulates mRNA translation by phosphorylation of two critical substrates, namely eukaryotic translation initiation factor 4E (eIF4E) binding proteins (4E-BPs) and ribosomal p70 S6 kinase (p70S6K). These phosphorylation events enhance translation of cyclin D1 mRNA into the protein.[41–43] mTOR can be inhibited by rapamycin analogues, such as temsirolimus (CCI-779), prompting development for lymphoma treatment for which there is additional rationale for their use. The mTOR pathway mediates the oncogenic effects of PI3K/AKT, activated by chimeric nucleophosmin-anaplastic lymphoma kinase (ALK) aberrantly expressed as a result of the t(2;5)(p23;q35) in ALK-positive anaplastic large cell lymphoma.[44,45] Constitutive activation of the PI3K/AKT pathway also occurs in MCL and preferentially in blastoid variants.[46] There are *in vitro* data to support activity of this class of drug in DLBCL.[47] Additional effects of the mTOR inhibitors include suppression of angiogenesis[48–50] and inhibition of NF-κB activity.[51] Early clinical trials in MCL show substantial tumor responses in heavily pretreated patients.[52] An oral derivative of rapamycin, everolimus

(RAD001, Novartis), has been developed but with no responses to date in patients with MCL.[53]

PROTEASOME INHIBITION

The ubiquitin proteasome system

The ubiquitin proteasome system is now recognized as the major protein-degradation pathway whereby ubiquitin is conjugated to protein substrates in a multistep process. This degradation of intracellular proteins is involved in the regulation of a wide range of cellular processes, including cell cycle and division and transcription factor regulation, and assures cellular quality control. The attachment of ubiquitin to proteins to form polyubiquitin conjugates mostly results in ATP-dependent proteolytic degradation by a complex cellular structure, the proteasome. The proteasome is a large, 26S, multicatalytic protease that degrades polyubiquinated proteins to small peptides. It is composed of two subcomplexes: a 20S core particle (CP) that carries the catalytic activity and a 19S regulatory particle (RP). The 20S CP is barrel shaped and composed of four stacked rings, two identical outer α rings and two identical inner β rings. The α and β rings are each composed of seven distinct subunits. The catalytic sites are localized to the $\beta1$, $\beta2$, and $\beta5$ subunits with enzymatic activities described as chymotryptic-like, tryptic-like, and post-glutamyl peptidyl hydrolytic-like. The 19S RP contains multiple ATPases and a binding site for ubiquitin concatemers. One important function of the 19S RP is to recognize ubiquinated proteins and other potential substrates for the proteasome. A second function is to open an orifice in the ring to allow entry of the substrate into the proteolytic chamber.[54,55]

A number of important transcription factors are affected by phosphorylation-dependent ubiquitination, in particular NF-κB. Normally, NF-κB, a key transcription factor affecting cell growth and survival, is transcriptionally inactive in the cytoplasm of most cells because it is bound to its cytoplasmic inhibitor IκBα. Activation follows phosphorylation and ubiquitination of its inhibitory chaperone IκBα, stimulated by proinflammatory cytokines such as tumor necrosis factor α (TNFα) or interleukin-1 (IL-1), allowing NF-κB to translocate into the nucleus and subsequently activate the expression of important target genes, for example *BCL2*.[56] Nuclear factor κB activity is critical for normal B cell development and survival, and distinct NF-κB heterodimers participate in different stages of B cell differentiation and activation.[57] In addition, mature B cells require acute increases in NF-κB activity in order to proliferate and survive. As in many other cancers, NF-κB is constitutively activated in a number of lymphomas. Cell lines from DLBCL tumors with an activated B cell-like (ABC) phenotype (associated with an inferior prognosis[58]) have high nuclear NF-κB DNA binding activity, constitutive IκB kinase (IKK) activity, and rapid IκBα

degradation that is not seen in cell lines representing the other DLBCL subtype, germinal center B-like (GCB). Moreover, dominant interference with the NF-κB pathway by retroviral transduction of a super-repressor form of IκBα or dominant negative forms of IKKβ was toxic to ABC DLBCL cells, but not to GCB DLBCL cells, thus validating NF-κB and its upstream activating pathways as a molecular target for certain types of DLBCL.[59] Lymphoma cells with the t(14;18) translocation show high levels of nuclear NF-κB proteins and this decreases when IκBα super-repressor is expressed in the cells.[60] In mantle cell lymphoma, NF-κB is constitutively activated and inhibition leads to cell cycle arrest in G1 and rapid induction of apoptosis.[61] These data all highlight a pivotal role for NF-κB in promoting malignant B cell survival and the NF-κB pathway represents a rational therapeutic target.

Proteasome inhibition – bortezomib

The principle behind the development of proteasome inhibitors as suitable antitumor agents is that proteasome inhibition (Fig. 90.2) can cause cellular apoptosis by affecting the levels of various short-lived proteins, essentially (1) inhibition of NF-κB activity through the stabilization of

its inhibitor, IκBα, (2) increased activity of TP53 and Bax proteins, and (3) accumulation of cyclin-dependent kinase inhibitors p27 and p21,[62,63] all key targets for molecular directed lymphoma therapy. Numerous proteasome inhibitors have been developed and the boronic acid dipeptide, bortezomib, led the way as the first in this class of drugs by reversibly inhibiting the chymotryptic-like activity of the 20S proteasome very efficiently and specifically.[62]

Aside from the effects on the NF-κB signaling pathways, bortezomib, by slowing down degradation of p21 and p27, can significantly increase the inhibitory effects against cyclin D1, thus reintroducing the G1-S cell cycle checkpoint. However, as prominent targets of the ubiquitin-proteasome pathway, their half-lives can be short allowing progression through the G1-S transition. In the presence of high cyclin D1 protein levels, rapid degradation of p21 and p27 leads to reduced inhibition of cyclin D1. Loss of the p21[64,65] and p27[66,67] proteins is a common finding in lymphomas and appears to be particularly intrinsic to mantle cell lymphomagenesis where it is also linked to poor survival.[68,69] Proteasome inhibition with the specific inhibitor lactacystin induces apoptosis and cell cycle arrest in MCL cells accompanied by accumulation of p21.[70] In MCL, *CDKNIB* (*P27KIP1*) RNA levels are normal but p27 protein degradation activity is increased via the proteasome

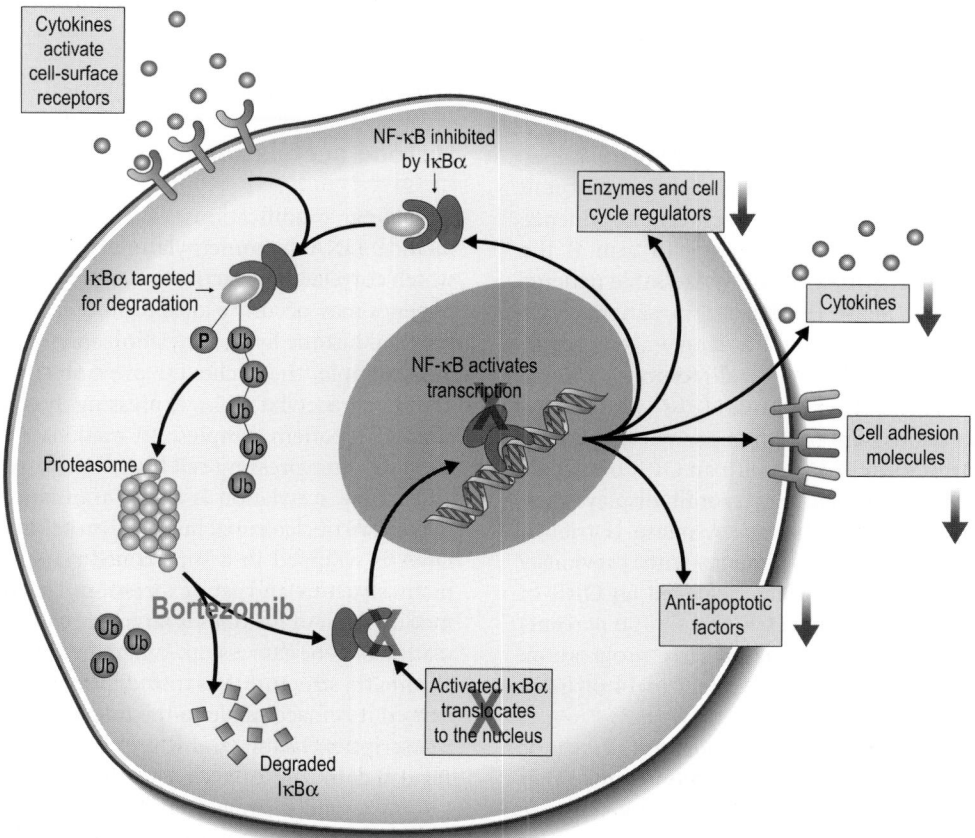

Figure 90.2 The effects of bortezomib. NF-κB, nuclear factor κB; IκBα, inhibitor of NF-κB.

pathway.[69] There are several explanations for the loss of p27 in MCL, including sequestration by cyclin D1[71] and cyclin D3[72] and increased levels of Skp2 which occur with increasing grade of non-Hodgkin lymphoma (NHL).[67] In blastic MCL and other aggressive B cell lymphomas, high Skp2 levels are associated with low p27 levels and may be indicative of ubiquitin-mediated degradation of this protein. Skp2 is a member of the substrate-recognition subunit of Skp1-Cul1-F-box (SCF) ubiquitin ligase complex and has been implicated in targeting p27 for degradation.[73] Thus, the loss of p21 and p27 in MCL further exacerbates the constitutive expression of cyclin D1 which is integral to the biology of this disease.

Perhaps not surprisingly therefore, MCL appears to be particularly sensitive to bortezomib and this has led to United States Food and Drug Administration (FDA) approval in patients who have received at least one prior therapy. Four pivotal trials of bortezomib in lymphoma have demonstrated activity in MCL as well as some of the other B cell lymphomas.[74–77] O'Connor et al. treated 26 patients with MCL and indolent lymphomas (follicular, marginal zone, small lymphocytic lymphoma [SLL]). An overall response rate of 58 percent was achieved, with one complete remission (CR), one unconfirmed CR (CRu), and four partial remissions (PR) among patients with follicular lymphoma. One patient with MCL achieved a CRu, four achieved PR, and four had stable disease. Both patients with marginal zone lymphoma achieved PR and all responses were durable. Patients with SLL had not responded at the time of publication.[74] Phase II data from the MD Anderson Cancer Center comprised 33 patients with MCL (group A) and 27 patients with a variety of B cell lymphoma subtypes (group B). In arm A, 12 of 29 assessable patients responded (six CR and six PR) for an overall response rate (ORR) of 41 percent (95 percent confidence interval [CI] 24 percent to 61 percent). In arm B the response rate was lower with four of 21 assessable patients responding.[75] Further phase II data in 155 patients with relapsed MCL confirm the activity of single-agent bortezomib in this disease, with an overall response rate of around 30 percent.[76] Data from Strauss et al.,[77] who treated 51 patients with various lymphoid malignancies, reinforce the activity of bortezomib in MCL with an ORR of 24 percent despite heavy pretreatment. Bortezomib displays antitumor activity in T cell lymphomas. A phase II trial of single-agent bortezomib in 12 patients with previously treated cutaneous T cell lymphoma achieved an ORR of 67 percent, with two (17 percent) CR and six (50 percent) PR. The remaining four patients had disease progression. The responses were durable, lasting from 7 to 14 or more months.[78]

In vitro data suggest, however, that bortezomib will be most effective when given in combination with either chemotherapy or other biologic agents. When given in vitro with cyclophosphamide and rituximab (BRC) to MCL cell lines and primary tumor cells, apoptosis was significantly enhanced compared with single-agent treatment.

Furthermore, in vivo studies with MCL-bearing SCID mice showed that BRC eradicated subcutaneous tumors and significantly prolonged the long-term event-free survival in 70 percent of the mice.[79] Recent in vitro data have shown that synergistic cytotoxic effects can also be achieved in MCL cell lines in combination with the histone deacetylase inhibitor (HDACi), suberoylanilide hydroxamic acid (SAHA). As well as targeting the proteasome and histone acetylation, respectively, both drugs cause a reduction in NF-κB activity.[80] This sensitization effect of bortezomib is seen again in mice xenograft models bearing DLBCL cells when given together with BCL2 antisense and cyclophosphamide.[10]

A second generation of drugs targeting the proteasome is now emerging. These drugs include salinosporamide A (NPI-0052), a highly potent and selective 20S proteasome inhibitor with irreversible activity against all three catalytic sites. In preclinical studies, NPI-0052 has been shown to outperform bortezomib, with activity against myeloma cells resistant to bortezomib, steroids, and thalidomide, and with less toxicity to normal cells.[81] A phase I trial has recently begun in the USA in patients with solid tumors and lymphomas. A synthetic analogue of epoxomicin, PR-171, irreversibly inhibits the chymotryptic site with equal potency but greater selectivity than bortezomib. In cell culture, PR-171 is more cytotoxic than bortezomib and has antitumor activity in human tumor xenograft models.[82] Phase I trials are underway in patients with multiple myeloma and NHL.

TARGETING HISTONES

Histone acetylation

Epigenetic modifications of eukaryotic gene promoters include DNA hypomethylation and histone acetylation, which correlate with activation of transcription. Activation of genes may occur by local promoter DNA hypomethylation and histone hyperacetylation and the converse is true.[83] For example, the cyclin D1 promoter is hypomethylated and hyperacetylated in expressing lymphoma cell lines and MCL patient samples, yet methylated and hypoacetylated in nonexpressing cell lines.[84]

Histone acetylation is a post-translational modification of the core nucleosomal histones, proteins around which the DNA is wrapped in a supercoiled state, that affects chromatin structure and gene expression. This post-translational modification of histones is an important process in the regulation of gene expression. When the DNA exists in an open chromatin structure, it is transcriptionally active; when condensed it is inaccessible to the transcriptional machinery of transcription factors and RNA polymerase. This process is regulated by the opposing action of histone deacetylases (HDACs) and histone acetyltransferases (HATs), enzymes that regulate chromatin structure and function through the removal (favoring chromatin condensation) and addition (favoring an open chromatin structure), respectively, of the acetyl group from the lysine residues of the core nucleosomal histones. Histone deacetylases are classified into three main families (classes I–III) depending on the homology with the transcriptional control sequence in yeast. Histone deacetylases have many protein targets whose structure and function are altered by acetylation, including histones and the non-histone component of transcription factors controlling gene expression and proteins that regulate cell proliferation, migration, and death.[63]

One of the best examples of how important acetylation is in regulating gene function is for that of BCL6. BCL6 is selectively expressed in mature B cells within germinal centers and is required for the formation of germinal centers, where it is thought to repress genes involved in the control of lymphocyte activation, differentiation, and apoptosis.[85-89] Thus, downregulation of BCL6 is required for normal B cells to exit germinal centers, yet in the majority of lymphomas, BCL6 is constitutively expressed.[85,86] Acetylation regulates the function of BCL6, occurs physiologically in germinal center B cells, and leads to its inactivation by preventing the recruitment of complexes containing HDACs, an essential component of its transcription-repressing function.[90] BCL6 acetylation is controlled by two of the deacetylation pathways and this represents an attractive therapeutic target. Furthermore, pharmacological inhibition of these pathways leads to the accumulation of the inactive acetylated BCL6 and to cell cycle arrest and apoptosis in B cell lymphoma cells.[90]

Histone deacetylase inhibition

A large number of natural and synthetic HDACi exist, extremely heterogeneous in their biochemistry, their principle mechanism of action being to bind to and block the catalytic site of the HDAC enzymes. In this way the transcription of genes involved in cell growth, maturation, survival, and apoptosis is altered. However, the mechanism of action is not entirely clear; this is not the only target of HDACi and how HDACi induce cell death in tumor cells remains unresolved. Multiple mechanisms of action promoting apoptosis are proposed including disruption of corepressor complexes, induction of oxidative injury, upregulation of the expression of death receptors, generation of lipid second messengers such as ceramide, interference with the function of chaperone proteins, modulation of NF-κB activity, and inhibition of angiogenesis.[91] There are at least four main classes of HDACi: the hydroxamic acid derivatives such as trichostatin A (TSA) and SAHA; the short-chain fatty acids such as 4-phenylbutyrate and valproic acid; the cyclic tetrapeptides such as depsipeptide; and the benzamides such as MS-275.[92] Malignant cells appear more sensitive to the proapoptotic effects of HDACi, although normal cells are also affected, reflected in the toxicity profile of this novel class of agent.

Treatment with HDACi will restore the function of important tumor suppressor and cell cycle regulatory

genes silenced in malignant cells, by inducing hyperacetylation. One of the best examples is for that of CDKN1A which encodes p21, the inhibitor of cyclin E-CDK2 and cyclin A-CDK. p21 is transcriptionally inactivated through recruitment of HDAC-containing repressor complexes to an Sp 1 binding site in its promoter and similarly for p16.[93] Treatment of lymphoid cancer cells with various HDACi – SAHA, sodium butyrate, valproic acid, and FK228 (depsipeptide) – can restore the expression of p21 and p27[94-96] with an increase in the level of acetylated histones associated with the p21 promoter.[94,96] Likewise, p21 is strongly upregulated with inhibition of proliferation of lymphoma cell lines by a novel hydroxamate-based HDACi, R306465, which exhibits class I HDAC isotype selectivity.[97] In addition, cyclin D1 and D2 are downregulated with overall inhibition of proliferation and induction of apoptosis.[94,95] Duan et al.[98] have demonstrated the potential for these agents in follicular lymphoma. They showed in vitro that two structurally different HDACi, TSA and sodium butyrate, repress both endogenous BCL2 expression and BCL2 promoter activity, inducing cell cycle arrest and apoptosis in two lymphoma cell lines bearing the t(14;18) translocation. Repression of BCL2 occurred at the transcriptional level and this correlated with localized histone deacetylation of the BCL2 promoters and decreased binding of transcription factors.[98] These effects on some of the key pathways that promote lymphomagenesis all suggest promising in vivo potential for this class of agent.

There are now a number of novel HDACi on the market and at various stages of clinical trial. One such agent, SAHA (vorinostat/Zolinza®), is approved by the FDA for the treatment of cutaneous manifestations of cutaneous T cell lymphoma (CTCL) in patients with progressive, persistent, or recurrent disease on or following two systemic therapies. The pivotal study supporting approval was a single-arm open-label phase II trial that enrolled 74 patients.[99] The objective response rate was 30 percent with an estimated median response duration of 168 days, and median time to tumor progression of 202 days. The most common side effects were diarrhea (49 percent), fatigue (46 percent), nausea (43 percent), and anorexia (26 percent) which were mostly grade 2 or lower. Grade 3 or higher toxicities occurred in a minority of patients and included fatigue (5 percent), pulmonary embolism (5 percent), thrombocytopenia (5 percent), and nausea (4 percent). In a phase I study of patients with refractory hematologic malignancies, including various subtypes of aggressive lymphoma, SAHA was safely administered with accumulation of acetylated histones in peripheral blood mononuclear cells and an objective response in two of 12 patients.[100]

ANGIOGENESIS

Lymphomas have a higher microvessel density (MVD), a frequently used parameter of angiogenesis, than reactive lymph nodes, increasing with clinically more aggressive lymphoma subtypes and advanced stage disease.[101–103] Angiogenesis is a tightly regulated physiological process with VEGF being the most important proangiogenic factor. The VEGF family comprises five structurally related members, VEGF-A, -B, -C, and -D, and placenta growth factor (PlGF), and their effects are mediated through three structurally homologous tyrosine kinase receptors: VEGFR-1, VEGFR-2, and VEGFR-3. Although the main stimulus for VEGF expression is hypoxia, cytokines, including those secreted by tumors, and oncogenes will upregulate expression. Of the angiogenic factors, VEGF has been most extensively investigated in lymphoma. Diffuse large B cell lymphomas, central nervous system (CNS) lymphomas, transformed indolent lymphomas, and MCL all portray significantly raised levels of VEGF protein and mRNA.[104] Prognostically, several large studies have demonstrated high levels of VEGF correspond to significantly shorter survival, independent of all other risk factors for the aggressive lymphomas.[105–108] No such relationship can be demonstrated for the indolent subtypes.[109] Likewise, high serum levels of basic fibroblast growth factor (b-FGF) have independent poor prognostic value,[110,111] the highest prognostic power being obtained when VEGF and b-FGF were examined as a combination.[107] Of the other angiogenic factors that have been analyzed, endostatin, an inhibitor of angiogenesis, is increased in the serum of lymphoma patients and high levels are associated with a poor outcome in patients with aggressive but not indolent lymphomas.[112] Aside from the angiogenic factors, also of interest are the findings of a recent study in B cell lymphomas showing that endothelial cells of tumor vessels harbor lymphoma-specific chromosome translocations and numerical chromosomal aberrations.[113]

Targeting angiogenesis for therapy should provide a positive treatment modality and data from mouse models of lymphoma demonstrate that inhibiting angiogenesis results in tumor regression. Exogenous administration of the antiangiogenic drug endostatin to NOD/SCID mice transplanted with Namalwa cells (derived from Epstein–Barr virus-positive Burkitt NHL) given after chemotherapy or immunotherapy effectively induced tumor stabilization.[114] Using species-specific monoclonal antibodies against human and mouse VEGF receptors to treat NOD/SCID mice engrafted with human DLBCL, Wang et al. suppressed the growth of established DLBCL tumors and confirmed the importance of VEGF/VEGFR-mediated pathways in lymphoma growth.[115] The combination of vasostatin, a direct and specific inhibitor of new vessel formation that inhibits proliferating endothelial cells, and IL-12, which inhibits angiogenesis indirectly through downstream interferon gamma (IFNγ)-inducible mediators, reduced tumor growth in athymic nude mice inoculated with human Burkitt lymphoma cells.[116] A novel derivative of thalidomide, S-3-[3-amino-phthalimido]-glutarimide (S-3APG), has similar in vivo antitumor effects.[117] In a mouse model of T cell lymphoma the angiogenesis inhibitor TNP-470 was able to reduce tumor load significantly.[118]

Inhibitors of angiogenesis

Antiangiogenesis therapy for lymphoma is novel and currently under investigation. Four classes of inhibitors of angiogenesis are currently available for clinical use: immunomodulatory drugs (IMiDs), VEGF inhibitors, cyclooxygenase 2 (COX-2) inhibitors, and therapy directed at the tumor stroma.

IMMUNOMODULATORY DRUGS

Thalidomide and the newer thalidomide derivatives possess multiple mechanisms of action, among them being potent inhibition of angiogenesis, although the mechanism is not entirely clear. Amongst the lymphomas, it is in MCL that most progress with thalidomide has been demonstrated, although clinical usage is still very much in its infancy. Efficacy has been observed alone[119] and in combination with rituximab.[120] Whilst these patients had relapsed or refractory disease, results are encouraging with objective responses observed in over 80 percent of patients and complete remissions in around one-third.[120] Response rates in indolent lymphomas are poor[121] whilst there are anecdotal reports of efficacy in angioimmunoblastic T cell lymphoma.[122–124] The newer IMiDs, lenalidomide and actimid, are more potent analogues of thalidomide with a safer toxicity profile. Lenalidomide has recently entered clinical trial for patients with relapsed lymphoproliferative disorders. In vivo studies of both agents in human lymphoma SCID mouse models are promising, with the ability to enhance the activity of rituximab when used in combination.[125] Not only did these agents have significant effects on the MVD of murine tumors, but significant antilymphoma effects occurred through modulation of the murine immune system with recruitment of natural killer (NK) cells through stimulation of dendritic cells and alteration of cytokine production.[125,126] In addition, effects of lenalidomide and actimid on upregulation of p21 expression and cell cycle arrest could potentially translate in MCL into clinical effect.[127] Further evaluation of IMiDs plus rituximab in patients with B cell lymphoma is required.

VASCULAR ENDOTHELIAL GROWTH FACTOR INHIBITORS

Vascular endothelial growth factor inhibitors are currently under investigation and are a logical target for therapy. Two such agents have reached clinical trial: bevacizumab, a monoclonal antibody against VEGF, and VEGF antisense (VEGF-AS), an antisense oligonucleotide. Other molecular therapies such as the HDACi[95] and flavopiridol[36,37] can, amongst their multiple mechanisms of action, suppress VEGF production. Bevacizumab followed by rituximab and CHOP has been given to 13 patients with newly diagnosed DLBCL with an overall response rate of 85 percent and complete response rate of 38 percent. All tumors showed high levels of VEGF expression. There were no episodes of the previously documented toxicity of proteinuria, heart failure, or hemorrhage.[128] In a phase I study, VEGF-AS has been safely given to 51 patients with advanced malignancies with a mixed but dramatic response in one patient with cutaneous T cell lymphoma.[129]

CYCLOOXYGENASE 2 INHIBITORS

Cyclooxygenase 2 inhibitors are more selective inhibitors of angiogenesis[130] and can reduce the incidence of neoplastic lesions in familial adenomatous polyposis.[131] For reasons that are unclear, the blood vessels supplying tumors, including lymphomas, are rich in COX2[132–134] which is thought to stimulate angiogenesis through the production of proangiogenic factors including VEGF, b-FGF, platelet-derived growth factor, transforming growth factor-β1, and endothelin-1, suggesting that a selective COX2 inhibitor would be efficacious.[130] In addition, *in vitro* data from various lymphoma cell lines demonstrate that the COX2 inhibitor, etodolac, can induce apoptosis through a COX2-independent, BCL2-regulated pathway.[135] In a phase II trial the COX2 inhibitor celecoxib given in high doses with low-dose continuous cyclophosphamide resulted in a response rate of 37.5 percent in a group of heavily pretreated patients with aggressive histology lymphoma; 25 percent of the patients were refractory to their preceding conventional-dose therapy. Moreover, an overall response of 37 percent was achieved in the 11 patients who had progressed after high-dose therapy. Median response duration was 8.2 months.[136]

THERAPY DIRECTED AT THE TUMOR STROMA

The extracellular matrix protein component tenascin-C is contained in the microvessel membrane and in the membrane-bound reticular stromal network. In lymphoma, expression is increased and correlates with angiogenesis, vessel immaturity, and aggressiveness.[137] This enhanced expression prompted the evaluation of iodine-131 (^{131}I)-labeled anti-tenascin chimeric 81C6, a radiolabeled chimeric antibody directed at this stromal component, in nine patients with relapsed or refractory NHL. Despite hematologic toxicity in two patients requiring stem cell infusion, one of nine patients achieved a complete remission and one a partial remission.[138]

SUMMARY

Logical pathway-specific therapies are bringing about real improvements in mortality and morbidity of patients with lymphoma. We are in the early days of their development and, as such, the full potential of combination molecular therapy has not yet been achieved. Improvements in molecular and cellular diagnostics have a role in realizing these benefits. One of the great advantages of the new agents is that they do not have the major myelotoxicity profiles associated with conventional DNA-damaging therapy and, as such, can be added to current treatment without increasing the adverse effects and may even facilitate the reduction of myelosuppressive treatment while potentiating a greater antitumor effect. All of the pathways discussed in this chapter have interactions and thus there is considerable overlap in the new biological agents. It is from this arena of improved understanding and innovative molecular pathways therapy that the lymphoma patient will see real improvements in their survival and care.

KEY POINTS

- Anti-apoptotic protein BCL2 is over-expressed in B cell malignancies and has been successfully inhibited *in vivo* with antisense therapy.
- The genes encoding cyclin dependent kinases (CDKs) involved in G1-S progression are often amplified in B cell malignancies. CDK inhibitors, for example flavopiridol, have the potential to induce growth arrest and apoptosis in cancer cells. Flavopiridol has demonstrated activity in clinical trials for B cell malignancies.
- The transcription factor NFKB is constitutively active in a number of lymphomas and promotes cell growth and survival. By stabilizing its inhibitor IKBα, proteasome inhibitors reduce activity of NFKB. Bortezomib is one such agent and is approved for treating multiple myeloma and mantle cell lymphoma.
- Histone acetylation is an important post-translational modification and the germinal centre protein BCL6 is regulated in this way. Reversible acetylation is mediated by histone deacetylase (HDAC) and inhibitors de-repress genes that subsequently result in growth inhibition, differentiation and apoptosis of cancer cells. A number of HDAC inhibitors are in development with vorinostat/SAHA approved for the treatment of cutaneous T cell lymphoma.
- Expression of VEGF is increased in lymphomas and high levels have been shown to correlate with reduced survival. Monoclonal antibodies targeting VEGF are in development. The immunomodulatory drugs, thalidomide and lenalidomide, have potent anti-angiogenic activity and are effective in inducing responses in patients with relapsed lymphoma.

REFERENCES

● = Key primary paper
◆ = Major review article

◆1. Cotter FE. Antisense therapy of hematologic malignancies. *Semin Hematol* 1999; **36**: 9–14.

2. Cotter FE, Waters J, Cunningham D. Human Bcl-2 antisense therapy for lymphomas. *Biochim Biophys Acta* 1999; **1489**: 97–106.

3. Waters JS, Webb A, Cunningham D *et al*. Phase I clinical and pharmacokinetic study of bcl-2 antisense oligonucleotide therapy in patients with non-Hodgkin's lymphoma. *J Clin Oncol* 2000; **18**: 1812–23.

●4. Webb A, Cunningham D, Cotter F *et al*. BCL-2 antisense therapy in patients with non-Hodgkin lymphoma. *Lancet* 1997; **349**: 1137–41.

5. Chanan-Khan A. Bcl-2 antisense therapy in B-cell malignancies. *Blood Rev* 2005; **19**: 213–21.

◆6. Garber K. Targeting mitochondria emerges as therapeutic strategy. *J Natl Cancer Inst* 2005; **97**: 1800–1.

7. Iversen P. In vivo studies with phosphorothioate oligonucleotides: pharmacokinetics prologue. *Anticancer Drug Des* 1991; **6**: 531–8.

8. Cotter FE, Johnson P, Hall P *et al*. Antisense oligonucleotides suppress B-cell lymphoma growth in a SCID-hu mouse model. *Oncogene* 1994; **9**: 3049–55.

9. Ramanarayanan J, Hernandez-Ilizaliturri FJ, Chanan-Khan A, Czuczman MS. Pro-apoptotic therapy with the oligonucleotide Genasense (oblimersen sodium) targeting Bcl-2 protein expression enhances the biological anti-tumour activity of rituximab. *Br J Haematol* 2004; **127**: 519–30.

10. O'Connor OA, Smith EA, Toner LE *et al*. The combination of the proteasome inhibitor bortezomib and the bcl-2 antisense molecule oblimersen sensitizes human B-cell lymphomas to cyclophosphamide. *Clin Cancer Res* 2006; **12**: 2902–11.

11. Bedikian AY, Millward M, Pehamberger H *et al*. Bcl-2 antisense (oblimersen sodium) plus dacarbazine in patients with advanced melanoma: the Oblimersen Melanoma Study Group. *J Clin Oncol* 2006; **24**: 4738–45.

●12. O'Brien S, Moore JO, Boyd TE *et al*. Randomized phase III trial of fludarabine plus cyclophosphamide with or without oblimersen sodium (Bcl-2 antisense) in patients with relapsed or refractory chronic lymphocytic leukemia. *J Clin Oncol* 2007; **25**: 1114–20.

13. Badros AZ, Goloubeva O, Rapoport AP *et al*. Phase II study of G3139, a Bcl-2 antisense oligonucleotide, in combination with dexamethasone and thalidomide in relapsed multiple myeloma patients. *J Clin Oncol* 2005; **23**: 4089–99.

14. Leonard JP, Coleman M, Vose J *et al*. Phase II study of oblimersen sodium (G3139) alone and with R-CHOP in mantle cell lymphoma (MCL). *Proc Am Soc Clin Oncol* 2003: 227.

15. Pro B, Leber B, Smith M *et al*. Phase II multicenter study of oblimersen sodium, a Bcl-2 antisense oligonucleotide, in combination with rituximab in patients with recurrent B-cell non-Hodgkin lymphoma. *Br J Haematol* 2008; **143**: 355–60. Epub 2008 Sep 1.

16. Nguyen M, Marcellus RC, Roulston A *et al*. Small molecule obatoclax (GX15-070) antagonizes MCL-1 and overcomes MCL-1-mediated resistance to apoptosis. *Proc Natl Acad Sci U S A* 2007; **104**: 19512–17.

17. Cillessen SA, Reed JC, Welsh K *et al*. Small-molecule XIAP antagonist restores caspase-9 mediated apoptosis in XIAP-positive diffuse large B-cell lymphoma cells. *Blood* 2008; **111**: 369–75.

18. Collins K, Jacks T, Pavletich NP. The cell cycle and cancer. *Proc Natl Acad Sci U S A* 1997; **94**: 2776–8.

19. Funk JO. Cancer cell cycle control. *Anticancer Res* 1999; **19**: 4772–80.

20. Guan KL, Jenkins CW, Li Y *et al*. Isolation and characterization of p19INK4d, a p16-related inhibitor specific to CDK6 and CDK4. *Mol Biol Cell* 1996; **7**: 57–70.

●21. Hall M, Bates S, Peters G. Evidence for different modes of action of cyclin-dependent kinase inhibitors: p15 and p16 bind to kinases, p21 and p27 bind to cyclins. *Oncogene* 1995; **11**: 1581–8.

22. Fernandez V, Hartmann E, Ott G *et al*. Pathogenesis of mantle-cell lymphoma: all oncogenic roads lead to dysregulation of cell cycle and DNA damage response pathways. *J Clin Oncol* 2005; **23**: 6364–9.

23. Rubio-Moscardo F, Climent J, Siebert R *et al*. Mantle-cell lymphoma genotypes identified with CGH to BAC microarrays define a leukemic subgroup of disease and predict patient outcome. *Blood* 2005; **105**: 4445–54.

24. Stilgenbauer S, Winkler D, Ott G *et al*. Molecular characterization of 11q deletions points to a pathogenic role of the ATM gene in mantle cell lymphoma. *Blood* 1999; **94**: 3262–4.

25. Schaffner C, Idler I, Stilgenbauer S *et al*. Mantle cell lymphoma is characterized by inactivation of the ATM gene. *Proc Natl Acad Sci U S A* 2000; **97**: 2773–8.

●26. Jeffrey PD, Russo AA, Polyak K *et al*. Mechanism of CDK activation revealed by the structure of a cyclinA-CDK2 complex. *Nature* 1995; **376**: 313–20.

27. De Azevedo WF Jr, Mueller-Dieckmann HJ, Schulze-Gahmen U *et al*. Structural basis for specificity and potency of a flavonoid inhibitor of human CDK2, a cell cycle kinase. *Proc Natl Acad Sci U S A* 1996; **93**: 2735–40.

28. Kaur G, Stetler-Stevenson M, Sebers S *et al*. Growth inhibition with reversible cell cycle arrest of carcinoma cells by flavone L86-8275. *J Natl Cancer Inst* 1992; **84**: 1736–40.

29. Arguello F, Alexander M, Sterry JA *et al*. Flavopiridol induces apoptosis of normal lymphoid cells, causes immunosuppression, and has potent antitumor activity In vivo against human leukemia and lymphoma xenografts. *Blood* 1998; **91**: 2482–90.

30. Carlson B, Lahusen T, Singh S *et al*. Down-regulation of cyclin D1 by transcriptional repression in MCF-7 human breast carcinoma cells induced by flavopiridol. *Cancer Res* 1999; **59**: 4634–41.

31. Takada Y, Aggarwal BB. Flavopiridol inhibits NF-kappaB activation induced by various carcinogens and inflammatory agents through inhibition of IkappaBalpha kinase and p65 phosphorylation: abrogation of cyclin D1, cyclooxygenase-2, and matrix metalloprotease-9. *J Biol Chem* 2004; **279**: 4750–9.

32. Chao SH, Price DH. Flavopiridol inactivates P-TEFb and blocks most RNA polymerase II transcription in vivo. *J Biol Chem* 2001; **276**: 31793–9.

33. Rosato RR, Almenara JA, Kolla SS *et al.* Mechanism and functional role of XIAP and Mcl-1 down-regulation in flavopiridol/vorinostat antileukemic interactions. *Mol Cancer Ther* 2007; **6**: 692–702.

34. Pepper C, Thomas A, Fegan C *et al.* Flavopiridol induces apoptosis in B-cell chronic lymphocytic leukaemia cells through a p38 and ERK MAP kinase-dependent mechanism. *Leuk Lymphoma* 2003; **44**: 337–42.

35. Yu C, Rahmani M, Dai Y *et al.* The lethal effects of pharmacological cyclin-dependent kinase inhibitors in human leukemia cells proceed through a phosphatidylinositol 3-kinase/Akt-dependent process. *Cancer Res* 2003; **63**: 1822–33.

36. Melillo G, Sausville EA, Cloud K *et al.* Flavopiridol, a protein kinase inhibitor, down-regulates hypoxic induction of vascular endothelial growth factor expression in human monocytes. *Cancer Res* 1999; **59**: 5433–7.

37. Rapella A, Negrioli A, Melillo G *et al.* Flavopiridol inhibits vascular endothelial growth factor production induced by hypoxia or picolinic acid in human neuroblastoma. Int J Cancer. 2002; **99**: 658–64.

38. Byrd JC, Lin TS, Dalton JT *et al.* Flavopiridol administered using a pharmacologically derived schedule is associated with marked clinical efficacy in refractory, genetically high-risk chronic lymphocytic leukemia. *Blood* 2007; **109**: 399–404.

39. Lin TS, Howard OM, Neuberg DS *et al.* Seventy-two hour continuous infusion flavopiridol in relapsed and refractory mantle cell lymphoma. *Leuk Lymphoma* 2002; **43**: 793–7.

40. Kouroukis CT, Belch A, Crump M *et al.* Flavopiridol in untreated or relapsed mantle-cell lymphoma: results of a phase II study of the National Cancer Institute of Canada Clinical Trials Group. *J Clin Oncol* 2003; **21**: 1740–5.

♦41. Bjornsti MA, Houghton PJ. The TOR pathway: a target for cancer therapy. *Nat Rev Cancer* 2004; **4**: 335–48.

42. Sawyers CL. Will mTOR inhibitors make it as cancer drugs? *Cancer Cell* 2003; **4**: 343–8.

43. Hay N, Sonenberg N. Upstream and downstream of mTOR. *Genes Dev* 2004; **18**: 1926–45.

44. Vega F, Medeiros LJ, Leventaki V *et al.* Activation of mammalian target of rapamycin signaling pathway contributes to tumor cell survival in anaplastic lymphoma kinase-positive anaplastic large cell lymphoma. *Cancer Res* 2006; **66**: 6589–97.

45. Marzec M, Kasprzycka M, Liu X *et al.* Oncogenic tyrosine kinase NPM/ALK induces activation of the rapamycin-sensitive mTOR signaling pathway. *Oncogene* 2007; **26**: 5606–14.

46. Rudelius M, Pittaluga S, Nishizuka S *et al.* Constitutive activation of Akt contributes to the pathogenesis and survival of mantle cell lymphoma. *Blood* 2006; **108**: 1668–76.

47. Wanner K, Hipp S, Oelsner M *et al.* Mammalian target of rapamycin inhibition induces cell cycle arrest in diffuse large B cell lymphoma (DLBCL) cells and sensitises DLBCL cells to rituximab. *Br J Haematol* 2006; **134**: 475–84.

48. Majumder PK, Febbo PG, Bikoff R *et al.* mTOR inhibition reverses Akt-dependent prostate intraepithelial neoplasia through regulation of apoptotic and HIF-1-dependent pathways. *Nat Med* 2004; **10**: 594–601.

49. Guba M, Yezhelyev M, Eichhorn ME *et al.* Rapamycin induces tumor-specific thrombosis via tissue factor in the presence of VEGF. *Blood* 2005; **105**: 4463–9.

50. Costa LF, Balcells M, Edelman ER *et al.* Proangiogenic stimulation of bone marrow endothelium engages mTOR and is inhibited by simultaneous blockade of mTOR and NF-kappaB. *Blood* 2006; **107**: 285–92.

51. Jundt F, Raetzel N, Muller C *et al.* A rapamycin derivative (everolimus) controls proliferation through down-regulation of truncated CCAAT enhancer binding protein {beta} and NF-{kappa}B activity in Hodgkin and anaplastic large cell lymphomas. *Blood* 2005; **106**: 1801–7.

●52. Witzig TE, Geyer SM, Ghobrial I *et al.* Phase II trial of single-agent temsirolimus (CCI-779) for relapsed mantle cell lymphoma. *J Clin Oncol* 2005; **23**: 5347–56.

53. Yee KW, Zeng Z, Konopleva M *et al.* Phase I/II study of the mammalian target of rapamycin inhibitor everolimus (RAD001) in patients with relapsed or refractory hematologic malignancies. *Clin Cancer Res* 2006; **12**: 5165–73.

54. Mani A, Gelmann EP. The ubiquitin-proteasome pathway and its role in cancer. *J Clin Oncol* 2005; **23**: 4776–89.

55. Ciechanover A. Intracellular protein degradation: from a vague idea thru the lysosome and the ubiquitin-proteasome system and onto human diseases and drug targeting. *Hematology Am Soc Hematol Educ Program* 2006: 1–12, 505–6.

56. Feng Z, Porter AG. NF-kappaB/Rel proteins are required for neuronal differentiation of SH-SY5Y neuroblastoma cells. *J Biol Chem* 1999; **274**: 30341–4.

♦57. Gugasyan R, Grumont R, Grossmann M *et al.* Rel/NF-kappaB transcription factors: key mediators of B-cell activation. *Immunol Rev* 2000; **176**: 134–40.

●58. Alizadeh AA, Eisen MB, Davis RE *et al.* Distinct types of diffuse large B-cell lymphoma identified by gene expression profiling. *Nature* 2000; **403**: 503–11.

●59. Davis RE, Brown KD, Siebenlist U, Staudt LM. Constitutive nuclear factor kappaB activity is required for survival of activated B cell-like diffuse large B cell lymphoma cells. *J Exp Med* 2001; **194**: 1861–74.

60. Heckman CA, Mehew JW, Boxer LM. NF-kappaB activates Bcl-2 expression in t(14;18) lymphoma cells. *Oncogene* 2002; **21**: 3898–908.

61. Pham LV, Tamayo AT, Yoshimura LC *et al.* Inhibition of constitutive NF-kappa B activation in mantle cell lymphoma B cells leads to induction of cell cycle arrest and apoptosis. *J Immunol* 2003; **171**: 88–95.

◆62. Rajkumar SV, Richardson PG, Hideshima T, Anderson KC. Proteasome inhibition as a novel therapeutic target in human cancer. *J Clin Oncol* 2005; **23**: 630–9.

◆63. O'Connor OA. Targeting histones and proteasomes: new strategies for the treatment of lymphoma. *J Clin Oncol* 2005; **23**: 6429–36.

64. Stefanaki K, Tzardi M, Kouvidou C *et al.* Expression of p53, p21, mdm2, Rb, bax and Ki67 proteins in lymphomas of the mucosa-associated lymphoid (MALT) tissue. *Anticancer Res* 1998; **18**: 2403–8.

65. Sanchez E, Chacon I, Plaza MM *et al.* Clinical outcome in diffuse large B-cell lymphoma is dependent on the relationship between different cell-cycle regulator proteins. *J Clin Oncol* 1998; **16**: 1931–9.

66. Quintanilla-Martinez L, Thieblemont C, Fend F *et al.* Mantle cell lymphomas lack expression of p27Kip1, a cyclin-dependent kinase inhibitor. *Am J Pathol* 1998; **153**: 175–82.

●67. Lim MS, Adamson A, Lin Z *et al.* Expression of Skp2, a p27(Kip1) ubiquitin ligase, in malignant lymphoma: correlation with p27(Kip1) and proliferation index. *Blood* 2002; **100**: 2950–6.

68. Letestu R, Ugo V, Valensi F *et al.* Prognostic impact of p27KIP1 expression in cyclin D1 positive lymphoproliferative disorders. *Leukemia* 2004; **18**: 953–61.

69. Chiarle R, Budel LM, Skolnik J *et al.* Increased proteasome degradation of cyclin-dependent kinase inhibitor p27 is associated with a decreased overall survival in mantle cell lymphoma. *Blood* 2000; **95**: 619–26.

70. Bogner C, Ringshausen I, Schneller F *et al.* Inhibition of the proteasome induces cell cycle arrest and apoptosis in mantle cell lymphoma cells. *Br J Haematol* 2003; **122**: 260–8.

71. Quintanilla-Martinez L, Davies-Hill T, Fend F *et al.* Sequestration of p27Kip1 protein by cyclin D1 in typical and blastic variants of mantle cell lymphoma (MCL): implications for pathogenesis. *Blood* 2003; **101**: 3181–7.

72. Sanchez-Beato M, Camacho FI, Martinez-Montero JC *et al.* Anomalous high p27/KIP1 expression in a subset of aggressive B-cell lymphomas is associated with cyclin D3 overexpression. p27/KIP1-cyclin D3 colocalization in tumor cells. *Blood* 1999; **94**: 765–72.

73. Tsvetkov LM, Yeh KH, Lee SJ *et al.* p27(Kip1) ubiquitination and degradation is regulated by the SCF(Skp2) complex through phosphorylated Thr187 in p27. *Curr Biol* 1999; **9**: 661–4.

74. O'Connor OA, Wright J, Moskowitz C *et al.* Phase II clinical experience with the novel proteasome inhibitor bortezomib in patients with indolent non-Hodgkin's lymphoma and mantle cell lymphoma. *J Clin Oncol* 2005; **23**: 676–84.

75. Goy A, Younes A, McLaughlin P *et al.* Phase II study of proteasome inhibitor bortezomib in relapsed or refractory B-cell non-Hodgkin's lymphoma. *J Clin Oncol* 2005; **23**: 667–75.

●76. Fisher RI, Bernstein SH, Kahl BS *et al.* Multicenter phase II study of bortezomib in patients with relapsed or refractory mantle cell lymphoma. *J Clin Oncol* 2006; **24**: 4867–74.

77. Strauss SJ, Maharaj L, Hoare S *et al.* Bortezomib therapy in patients with relapsed or refractory lymphoma: potential correlation of in vitro sensitivity and tumor necrosis factor alpha response with clinical activity. *J Clin Oncol* 2006; **24**: 2105–12.

78. Zinzani PL, Musuraca G, Tani M *et al.* Phase II trial of proteasome inhibitor bortezomib in patients with relapsed or refractory cutaneous T-cell lymphoma. *J Clin Oncol* 2007; **25**: 4293–7.

79. Wang M, Han XH, Zhang L *et al.* Bortezomib is synergistic with rituximab and cyclophosphamide in inducing apoptosis of mantle cell lymphoma cells in vitro and in vivo. *Leukemia* 2008; **22**: 179–85.

80. Heider U, von Metzler I, Kaiser M *et al.* Synergistic interaction of the histone deacetylase inhibitor SAHA with the proteasome inhibitor bortezomib in mantle cell lymphoma. *Eur J Haematol* 2008; **80**: 133–42.

81. Chauhan D, Catley L, Li G *et al.* A novel orally active proteasome inhibitor induces apoptosis in multiple myeloma cells with mechanisms distinct from Bortezomib. *Cancer Cell* 2005; **8**: 407–19.

82. Demo SD, Kirk CJ, Aujay MA *et al.* Antitumor activity of PR-171, a novel irreversible inhibitor of the proteasome. *Cancer Res* 2007; **67**: 6383–91.

◆83. Herman JG, Baylin SB. Gene silencing in cancer in association with promoter hypermethylation. *N Engl J Med* 2003; **349**: 2042–54.

84. Liu H, Wang J, Epner EM. Cyclin D1 activation in B-cell malignancy: association with changes in histone acetylation, DNA methylation, and RNA polymerase II binding to both promoter and distal sequences. *Blood* 2004; **104**: 2505–13.

85. Cattoretti G, Chang CC, Cechova K *et al.* BCL-6 protein is expressed in germinal-center B cells. *Blood* 1995; **86**: 45–53.

86. Onizuka T, Moriyama M, Yamochi T *et al.* BCL-6 gene product, a 92- to 98-kD nuclear phosphoprotein, is highly expressed in germinal center B cells and their neoplastic counterparts. *Blood* 1995; **86**: 28–37.

●87. Ye BH, Cattoretti G, Shen Q *et al.* The BCL-6 proto-oncogene controls germinal-centre formation and Th2-type inflammation. *Nat Genet* 1997; **16**: 161–70.

●88. Dent AL, Shaffer AL, Yu X *et al.* Control of inflammation, cytokine expression, and germinal center formation by BCL-6. *Science* 1997; **276**: 589–92.

89. Shaffer AL, Yu X, He Y *et al.* BCL-6 represses genes that function in lymphocyte differentiation, inflammation, and cell cycle control. *Immunity* 2000; **13**: 199–212.

●90. Bereshchenko OR, Gu W, Dalla-Favera R. Acetylation inactivates the transcriptional repressor BCL6. *Nat Genet* 2002; **32**: 606–13.

91. Rosato RR, Grant S. Histone deacetylase inhibitors: insights into mechanisms of lethality. *Expert Opin Ther Targets* 2005; **9**: 809–24.

◆92. Marks P, Rifkind RA, Richon VM *et al.* Histone deacetylases and cancer: causes and therapies. *Nat Rev Cancer* 2001; **1**: 194–202.

93. Magdinier F, Wolffe AP. Selective association of the methyl-CpG binding protein MBD2 with the silent p14/p16 locus in human neoplasia. *Proc Natl Acad Sci U S A* 2001; **98**: 4990–5.

94. Sakajiri S, Kumagai T, Kawamata N *et al.* Histone deacetylase inhibitors profoundly decrease proliferation of human lymphoid cancer cell lines. *Exp Hematol* 2005; **33**: 53–61.

95. Heider U, Kaiser M, Sterz J *et al.* Histone deacetylase inhibitors reduce VEGF production and induce growth suppression and apoptosis in human mantle cell lymphoma. *Eur J Haematol* 2006; **76**: 42–50.

96. Sasakawa Y, Naoe Y, Inoue T *et al.* Effects of FK228, a novel histone deacetylase inhibitor, on human lymphoma U-937 cells in vitro and in vivo. *Biochem Pharmacol* 2002; **64**: 1079–90.

97. Arts J, Angibaud P, Marien A *et al.* R306465 is a novel potent inhibitor of class I histone deacetylases with broad-spectrum antitumoral activity against solid and haematological malignancies. *Br J Cancer* 2007; **97**: 1344–53.

98. Duan H, Heckman CA, Boxer LM. Histone deacetylase inhibitors down-regulate bcl-2 expression and induce apoptosis in t(14; 18) lymphomas. *Mol Cell Biol* 2005; **25**: 1608–19.

●99. Olsen EA, Kim YH, Kuzel TM *et al.* Phase IIb multicenter trial of vorinostat in patients with persistent, progressive, or treatment refractory cutaneous T-cell lymphoma. *J Clin Oncol* 2007; **25**: 3109–15.

100. Kelly WK, Richon VM, O'Connor O *et al.* Phase I clinical trial of histone deacetylase inhibitor: suberoylanilide hydroxamic acid administered intravenously. *Clin Cancer Res* 2003; **9**: 3578–88.

101. Ribatti D, Vacca A, Nico B *et al.* Angiogenesis spectrum in the stroma of B-cell non-Hodgkin's lymphomas. An immunohistochemical and ultrastructural study. *Eur J Haematol* 1996; **56**: 45–53.

102. Vacca A, Ribatti D, Ruco L *et al.* Angiogenesis extent and macrophage density increase simultaneously with pathological progression in B-cell non-Hodgkin's lymphomas. *Br J Cancer* 1999; **79**: 965–70.

103. Jorgensen JM, Sorensen FB, Bendix K *et al.* Angiogenesis in non-Hodgkin's lymphoma: clinico-pathological correlations and prognostic significance in specific subtypes. *Leuk Lymphoma* 2007; **48**: 584–95.

104. Koster A, Raemaekers JM. Angiogenesis in malignant lymphoma. *Curr Opin Oncol* 2005; **17**: 611–16.

105. Salven P, Teerenhovi L, Joensuu H. A high pretreatment serum vascular endothelial growth factor concentration is associated with poor outcome in non-Hodgkin's lymphoma. *Blood* 1997; **90**: 3167–72.

106. Bertolini F, Paolucci M, Peccatori F *et al.* Angiogenic growth factors and endostatin in non-Hodgkin's lymphoma. *Br J Haematol* 1999; **106**: 504–9.

107. Salven P, Orpana A, Teerenhovi L, Joensuu H. Simultaneous elevation in the serum concentrations of the angiogenic growth factors VEGF and bFGF is an independent predictor of poor prognosis in non-Hodgkin lymphoma: a single-institution study of 200 patients. *Blood* 2000; **96**: 3712–18.

108. Zhao WL, Mourah S, Mounier N *et al.* Vascular endothelial growth factor-A is expressed both on lymphoma cells and endothelial cells in angioimmunoblastic T-cell lymphoma and related to lymphoma progression. *Lab Invest* 2004; **84**: 1512–19.

109. Koster A, van Krieken JH, Mackenzie MA *et al.* Increased vascularization predicts favorable outcome in follicular lymphoma. *Clin Cancer Res* 2005; **11**: 154–61.

110. Salven P, Teerenhovi L, Joensuu H. A high pretreatment serum basic fibroblast growth factor concentration is an independent predictor of poor prognosis in non-Hodgkin's lymphoma. *Blood* 1999; **94**: 3334–9.

111. Pazgal I, Zimra Y, Tzabar C *et al.* Expression of basic fibroblast growth factor is associated with poor outcome in non-Hodgkin's lymphoma. *Br J Cancer* 2002; **86**: 1770–5.

112. Bono P, Teerenhovi L, Joensuu H. Elevated serum endostatin is associated with poor outcome in patients with non-Hodgkin lymphoma. *Cancer* 2003; **97**: 2767–75.

113. Streubel B, Chott A, Huber D *et al.* Lymphoma-specific genetic aberrations in microvascular endothelial cells in B-cell lymphomas. *N Engl J Med* 2004; **351**: 250–9.

114. Bertolini F, Fusetti L, Mancuso P *et al.* Endostatin, an antiangiogenic drug, induces tumor stabilization after chemotherapy or anti-CD20 therapy in a NOD/SCID mouse model of human high-grade non-Hodgkin lymphoma. *Blood* 2000; **96**: 282–7.

115. Wang ES, Teruya-Feldstein J, Wu Y *et al.* Targeting autocrine and paracrine VEGF receptor pathways inhibits human lymphoma xenografts in vivo. *Blood* 2004; **104**: 2893–902.

116. Yao L, Pike SE, Setsuda J *et al.* Effective targeting of tumor vasculature by the angiogenesis inhibitors vasostatin and interleukin-12. *Blood* 2000; **96**: 1900–5.

117. Lentzsch S, Rogers MS, LeBlanc R *et al.* S-3-Amino-phthalimido-glutaramide inhibits angiogenesis and growth of B-cell neoplasias in mice. *Cancer Res* 2002; **62**: 2300–5.

118. Noren-Nystrom U, Eriksson M, Eriksson B *et al.* Antitumor activity of the angiogenesis inhibitor TNP-470 on murine lymphoma/leukemia cells in vivo and in vitro. *Exp Hematol* 2003; **31**: 143–9.

119. Damaj G, Lefrere F, Delarue R *et al.* Thalidomide therapy induces response in relapsed mantle cell lymphoma. *Leukemia* 2003; **17**: 1914–15.

120. Kaufmann H, Raderer M, Wohrer S *et al.* Antitumor activity of rituximab plus thalidomide in patients with relapsed/refractory mantle cell lymphoma. *Blood* 2004; **104**: 2269–71.

121. Smith SM, Grinblatt D, Johnson JL *et al.* Thalidomide has limited single-agent activity in relapsed or refractory indolent non-Hodgkin lymphomas: a phase II trial of the Cancer and Leukemia Group B. *Br J Haematol* 2008; **140**: 313–19.

122. Damaj G, Bouabdallah R, Vey N *et al.* Single-agent thalidomide induces response in T-cell lymphoma. *Eur J Haematol* 2005; **74**: 169–71.

123. Dogan A, Ngu LS, Ng SH, Cervi PL. Pathology and clinical features of angioimmunoblastic T-cell lymphoma after successful treatment with thalidomide. *Leukemia* 2005; **19**: 873–5.

124. Strupp C, Aivado M, Germing U *et al.* Angioimmunoblastic lymphadenopathy (AILD) may respond to thalidomide treatment: two case reports. *Leuk Lymphoma* 2002; **43**: 133–7.

125. Hernandez-Ilizaliturri FJ, Reddy N, Holkova B *et al.* Immunomodulatory drug CC-5013 or CC-4047 and rituximab enhance antitumor activity in a severe combined immunodeficient mouse lymphoma model. *Clin Cancer Res* 2005; **11**: 5984–92.

126. Reddy N, Hernandez-Ilizaliturri FJ, Deeb G *et al.* Immunomodulatory drugs stimulate natural killer-cell function, alter cytokine production by dendritic cells, and inhibit angiogenesis enhancing the anti-tumour activity of rituximab in vivo. *Br J Haematol* 2008; **140**: 36–45.

127. Verhelle D, Corral LG, Wong K *et al.* Lenalidomide and CC-4047 inhibit the proliferation of malignant B cells while expanding normal CD34+ progenitor cells. *Cancer Res* 2007; **67**: 746–55.

128. Ganjoo KN, An CS, Robertson MJ *et al.* Rituximab, bevacizumab and CHOP (RA-CHOP) in untreated diffuse large B-cell lymphoma: safety, biomarker and pharmacokinetic analysis. *Leuk Lymphoma* 2006; **47**: 998–1005.

129. Levine AM, Tulpule A, Quinn DI *et al.* Phase I study of antisense oligonucleotide against vascular endothelial growth factor: decrease in plasma vascular endothelial growth factor with potential clinical efficacy. *J Clin Oncol* 2006; **24**: 1712–19.

130. Horrobin DF. A low toxicity maintenance regime, using eicosapentaenoic acid and readily available drugs, for mantle cell lymphoma and other malignancies with excess cyclin D1 levels. *Med Hypotheses* 2003; **60**: 615–23.

131. Steinbach G, Lynch PM, Phillips RK *et al.* The effect of celecoxib, a cyclooxygenase-2 inhibitor, in familial adenomatous polyposis. *N Engl J Med* 2000; **342**: 1946–52.

132. Hazar B, Ergin M, Seyrek E *et al.* Cyclooxygenase-2 (Cox-2) expression in lymphomas. *Leuk Lymphoma* 2004; **45**: 1395–9.

133. Li HL, Sun BZ, Ma FC. Expression of COX-2, iNOS, p53 and Ki-67 in gastric mucosa-associated lymphoid tissue lymphoma. *World J Gastroenterol* 2004; **10**: 1862–6.

134. Wun T, McKnight H, Tuscano JM. Increased cyclooxygenase-2 (COX-2): a potential role in the pathogenesis of lymphoma. *Leuk Res* 2004; **28**: 179–90.

135. Kobayashi M, Nakamura S, Shibata K *et al.* Etodolac inhibits EBER expression and induces Bcl-2-regulated apoptosis in Burkitt's lymphoma cells. *Eur J Haematol* 2005; **75**: 212–20.

136. Buckstein R, Kerbel RS, Shaked Y *et al.* High-dose celecoxib and metronomic 'low-dose' cyclophosphamide is an effective and safe therapy in patients with relapsed and refractory aggressive histology non-Hodgkin's lymphoma. *Clin Cancer Res* 2006; **12**: 5190–8.

137. Vacca A, Ribatti D, Fanelli M *et al.* Expression of tenascin is related to histologic malignancy and angiogenesis in b-cell non-Hodgkin's lymphomas. *Leuk Lymphoma* 1996; **22**: 473–81.

138. Rizzieri DA, Akabani G, Zalutsky MR *et al.* Phase 1 trial study of 131I-labeled chimeric 81C6 monoclonal antibody for the treatment of patients with non-Hodgkin lymphoma. *Blood* 2004; **104**: 642–8.

91

Therapeutic strategies employing viral-associated targets

MARINA I GUTIERREZ AND KISHOR BHATIA

SUMMARY

The association of viruses with several human tumors has now clearly been established. The most common viruses associated with lymphomas are the herpesviruses. Epstein–Barr virus (EBV), a gammaherpesvirus, is widely distributed in all human populations and persists in the individuals as a lifelong, asymptomatic infection of B cells. Apart from this ubiquity, EBV is causative and/or associated with a growing number of benign and malignant lymphoid and epithelial diseases. These include infectious mononucleosis, oral hairy leukoplakia, post-transplant B cell proliferations, Burkitt lymphoma, nasopharyngeal carcinomas, Hodgkin lymphomas, and others. Epstein–Barr virus adopts different forms of latent infection, defined by the restricted pattern of genes expressed (latency I, II, III) in different tumor types and reflecting the complex interaction between the virus and the host cell. Regardless of the role of the virus in the pathogenesis of these diseases (which remains to be completely elucidated), the virus itself represents a target par excellence for designing tumor-selective therapeutic approaches. The presence of the EBV genome in virtually all tumor cells stands in contrast to the rare infection of normal cells, ensuring that EBV-targeted therapeutic approaches will have a high specificity and a low toxicity. In this chapter we review all developing strategies that use EBV as a target to mediate tumor cell death in EBV-associated malignancies. Several pharmacologic and immunotherapeutic approaches to treat or prevent EBV-associated tumors are at varying levels of clinical studies. These strategies are all based on altering viral gene expression to render the EBV-positive tumor cells sensitive to antiviral drugs, and commit to initiate the replicative cycle, utilizing its own lytic potential to kill the host tumor cell or, alternatively, the altered gene expression allows the tumor cells to bypass immune evasion strategies of the virus and become a target that is on the radar of the host cellular immune system.

INTRODUCTION

Studies as far back as the early 1900s sought to define etiologic links between viruses and cancers. The association of viruses with several human tumors has now clearly been established and the hunt for new viral links with other human malignancies continues. While there is much to be learnt about the exact role and the processes whereby some of these viruses transform the normal cell, sustain the malignant phenotype, and contribute to the clinical behavior of the tumor, associations of specific viruses with a specific tumor such as papilloma virus with cervical cancer,[1] hepatitis C virus with hepatocellular carcinoma,[2] or herpes virus 8 with Kaposi sarcoma[3] are no longer controversial. Cancers linked to an infectious etiology remain a significant fraction of the overall global cancer burden, with as

Table 91.1 Viral associations with lymphoproliferative diseases

Virus	Pathology	Association
EBV/HHV-4	Burkitt lymphoma, Hodgkin lymphoma, T/NK cell lymphoma, PTLD, primary effusion lymphoma, CNS lymphoma, AIDS-associated NHL	Confirmed
KSHV/HHV-8	Primary effusion lymphoma	Confirmed
HTLV-1	Adult T cell leukemia	Confirmed
HCV	B cell NHL, mantle cell lymphoma	Confirmed
HTLV-2	Hairy cell leukemia	Few studies
SV40	NHL	Controversial
HHV-6	B cell NHL	Controversial

HHV, human herpesvirus; PTLD, post-transplant lymphoproliferative disease; CNS, central nervous system; NHL, non-Hodgkin lymphoma; KSHV, Kaposi sarcoma herpesvirus; HTLV: human T cell lymphotrophic virus; HCV, hepatitis C virus; NK, natural killer; AIDS, acquired immune deficiency syndrome.

many as 1.8 million cases worldwide. Included among these are human lymphoid neoplasms, mostly associated with herpesviruses.[4] Classical examples are the association of EBV with Burkitt lymphoma and Hodgkin lymphoma[5,6] or herpesvirus 8 with primary effusion lymphoma (PEL).[7] Other viral associations (polyomaviruses, retroviruses) with lymphoproliferative diseases have been more recently described[8–11] or are debatable.[12–16] Table 91.1 summarizes the current knowledge of virus-associated lymphoproliferative diseases. This chapter will focus on EBV as a model of viral-targeted therapies since it is the most studied and used in therapeutic approaches.

Epstein–Barr virus (EBV/human herpesvirus 4 [HHV-4]) is a large DNA virus that infects more than 90 percent of the human population. Epstein–Barr virus is one of the most successful human viruses due to its ability to establish a lifelong nonsymptomatic association with the host. Following primary infection, which can occasionally cause infectious mononucleosis, this virus continues to persist for life in the infected individual, most likely in a B cell reservoir.[17–20] The virus also assures its maintenance in the human species by occasional reactivation in cells in the oropharyngeal region and transmission via saliva to other noninfected individuals.

Epstein–Barr virus consists of a 172 kilobase (kb) linear, double-stranded DNA coding for about 90 open reading frames (ORF) and containing 4–12 terminal repeats of 500 base pairs (bp) each. Although the infective particles carry linear genomes, in latently infected cells the viral genomes form circular episomes in the nucleus. Unlike retroviruses, the complete viral genome becomes part of the cell as extrachromosomal episomes, while integration into human chromosomes is rare and random.[21]

In addition to causing infectious mononucleosis following the primary acquisition of the virus during adolescence, EBV is causally associated with other nonmalignant and malignant diseases; examples of the former are chronic active EBV infection (CAEBV), oral hairy leukoplakia, and hemophagocytic lymphocytosis.[22,23] Human cancers attributable in some way to EBV infection include Burkitt lymphoma, nasopharyngeal carcinomas, Hodgkin lymphoma, post-transplant lymphoproliferative disorders (PTLD), nasal lymphomas, peripheral T cell lymphomas, gastric and breast carcinomas, and smooth muscle tumors such as leiomyosarcoma.[24–28] It is not clear yet what factors play a role in whether an infected individual will succumb to an EBV-associated malignancy, but it is likely that multiple factors including environment, age of infection, host, and possibly genetic variation within the viral strains contribute. Whether EBV plays a direct pathogenetic role or an indirect promoting role, or is a mere passenger, is likely to vary with the histologic type of cancer it is associated with and a single mechanism to explain its role in all malignancies may not necessarily exist. Nonetheless, EBV has been classified as a class I carcinogen by the International Agency for Research on Cancer (IARC).[29]

The mechanism of viral tumorigenesis aside, when associated with a tumor, EBV is frequently present in all the tumor cells, while at the same time only a small number of normal cells containing EBV constitute the EBV reservoir in the individual. This fact therefore provides an excellent tumor-specific target that can be exploited as a therapeutic tool. Indeed, several strategies have been developed (Table 91.2).

EPSTEIN–BARR VIRUS–BASED THERAPEUTIC APPROACHES

All viral-targeted therapeutic strategies directly or indirectly have their basis in modulating the expression of the viral genome or in some way harnessing the regulation that governs this expression in the infected cells. Viral gene expression *in vivo* is limited to a few (1–6 genes) latency genes, a mechanism clearly employed by the virus to avoid immune surveillance.[17–20] Several EBV-targeted therapeutic strategies have been designed and they are in different stages of development. For example, the immunotherapeutic approaches have now been clinically adapted with promising success. The spectrum of approaches utilizing EBV as a target for therapy includes:

1. Immunotherapies (EBV-specific cytotoxic T lymphocyte [CTL] infusion)
2. EBV vaccination
3. Inhibition of viral transforming genes
4. Elimination of EBV episomes
5. Modulation of epigenetic targets
6. EBV-dependent expression of toxic/apoptotic genes
7. EBV-dependent induction of the lytic cycle

Table 91.2   Epstein–Barr virus-targeted therapeutic approaches

Strategy	EBV target	Studies
Enhancement of immune response:		
CTL infusion	EBNA3A, -3B, -3C, EBNA2, LMP1, LMP2	Phase II/III
Vaccine	gp350, gp85, LPRA, LMP1, EBNA1	Phase I/II
Modulation of viral gene expression:		
Inhibition of transforming genes	LMP1, EBNA1	Preclinical
Elimination of episomes	Episome, OriP?	Preclinical, few patients
Epigenetic changes	Latency program, immediate-early promoters, thymidine kinase	Preclinical, phase I
Gene therapy:		
Toxic/apoptotic genes	Exogenous genes	Preclinical
Viral immediate-early genes	Exogenous BZLF1/BRLF1	Preclinical
Pharmacological induction lytic cycle	BZLF1/BRLF1 promoters	Preclinical, phase I/II

EBV, Epstein–Barr virus; CTL, cytotoxic T lymphocyte; EBNA, EBV nuclear antigen; LMP, latent membrane protein; OriP, EBV origin of replication; gp, glycoprotein.

Table 91.2 summarizes some of these approaches, which are described in greater detail below.

ENHANCEMENT OF THE IMMUNE RESPONSE TO VIRAL PROTEINS

Since EBV-infected tumor cells express viral antigens, strategies based upon enhancement of the host immune response to viral proteins are actively pursued and have already proven promising for treatment of certain types of tumors, like post-transplant lymphoproliferative diseases.[30,31] This approach is based on immune reconstitution with *ex vivo* expanded EBV-specific CTLs.

Normal CTL responses are classic virus-specific responses (CD8+, class I restricted) and are mostly directed against the immunogenic EBV nuclear antigens (EBNA) EBNA3 (3A, 3B, and 3C) and, to a lesser extent, EBNA2, latent membrane protein 1 (LMP1), and LMP2. Therefore, this approach is likely to benefit those EBV-associated tumors that express latency III. This method has been refined by the infusion of EBV-specific CTLs expanded *in vitro* from donor cells. However, donor cells are not always available and the risk of tumors originating from the recipient's cells (normally in solid organ tumor recipients) needs to be considered. To overcome these hurdles, CTLs have been generated from the patient's own cells before receiving immunosuppressive therapy. Alternatively, a CTL bank can be created from healthy donors and HLA-matched CTLs can be selected for infusion in a given patient.[32,33] More importantly, there is some evidence that infused allogeneic CTLs can access the central nervous system (CNS) and dramatically reduce an EBV-positive primary CNS lymphoma.[34]

The adoptive transfer of virus-specific CTLs has been used prophylactically as well as to control PTLD. Since the first use of this strategy[35] other groups have treated hematopoietic stem cell transplant patients, with demonstration of a reduction of the plasma EBV load and clinical remissions.[36,37] In PTLD patients following solid organ transplants, infusion of autologous CTLs confirms that EBV-specific immunity can at least be temporarily restored.[38,39] In spite of these advances in prevention and treatment of PTLD, cases of tumor resistance to infused CTLs due to mutations of the EBV epitopes recognized by the CTLs have been described.[40]

Clinical trials in Hodgkin lymphoma (HL) and nasopharyngeal carcinoma (NPC)[41] utilizing a similar strategy are also ongoing. Since these EBV-positive tumors express a more restricted array of viral genes (latency II), and possess active immune evasion strategies, autologous EBV-specific CTLs have shown less impressive clinical responses. It is believed that tumor paracrine effects, for example secretion of interleukin-10 (IL-10) by the Reed-Sternberg cells, may limit the applicability of this approach for these patients with intact CTL function. However, antiviral activity and immune effects are possible. For example, Roskrow et al.[42] have successfully generated EBV-specific CTLs in patients with EBV-positive HL. After infusion, these CTLs homed to the tumor sites, persisted in the circulation for more than 9 months, and produced clinical benefits. However, this benefit was only transient, due in part to the fact that lymphoblastoid cell line (LCL) cells were used as EBV antigen-presenting cells. Lymphoblastoid cell line cells activated polyclonal CTL populations that were preferentially directed against the immunodominant EBNA3A, -3B, and -3C, which are not expressed in HL cells.

Thus, several studies are being evaluated to improve the efficacy of adoptive immunotherapy and outcome of patients. The most compelling EBV antigen targets for HL and NPC would include LMP1 and LMP2. Latent membrane protein 1-specific CTLs are very rare in EBV-seropositive individuals while most donors have a low but measurable frequency of circulating LMP2A-specific CTLs that can be activated and expanded *in vitro*. Furthermore, LMP2A-specific CTLs generated *in vitro* can be amplified by culturing with recombinant IL-12 (rIL-12) or rIL-15[43] or enriched based on interferon gamma (IFNγ) production.[44]

A study in HL in children and young adults nicely demonstrated that it is possible to generate polyclonal EBV-specific CTL lines with an effector-memory phenotype containing clones specific for the subdominant tumor antigen LMP2 expressed by the Reed-Sternberg cells.[45] The infused cells further expanded *in vivo* and persisted for up to 1 year after infusion, trafficking to tumor sites. EBV-CTLs were safe and some tumor responses were observed, including complete remissions. While the study provided promising evidence supporting the principle of such approaches, more than half of the patients did not respond and died of disease. These limitations precluded further clinical adaptation and have prompted further refinement of these strategies.

An alternative strategy is based on the production of CTLs by genetically modified dendritic cells (DC) that direct the CTL response to virally transduced genes. This approach allows expression of the whole protein, leading to presentation of multiple, undefined antigen epitopes. Recombinant adenoviruses encoding the entire LMP2A were transduced into DC that were used as antigen-presenting cells facilitating stimulation of LMP2A-specific CTLs.[46] Preliminary results of a clinical trial have been recently published.[47]

Although LMP2 epitopes have been identified for only a limited number of HLA alleles, very recently, T cell responses to 1–5 LMP2 epitopes were found in 84 percent of cell lines from patients screened using an LMP2 peptide library.[48,49] These newly identified LMP2 epitopes broaden the diversity of HLA alleles with available epitopes proving a valuable tool for immune monitoring.

The other potential target epitope for CTL therapy in latency II EBV-associated tumors is LMP1. However, LMP1-specific CTLs, if present, have a very low frequency. Gottschalk *et al.*[50] have constructed a mutant inactive LMP1 (DeltaLMP1) that could be expressed in DC without the toxic effect of LMP1, enabling activation and expansion of polyclonal LMP1-specific CTLs. This tool may prove to be very useful in improving the efficacy of adoptive therapy in HL.

EPSTEIN–BARR VIRUS VACCINATION

The enhancement of the host immune response toward viral antigens, referred to as vaccination, is another strategy that has been explored. Such approaches include both preventive and therapeutic vaccines. A preventive EBV vaccine could protect against the acquisition of primary infection and, therefore, eradicate EBV infection in the human population and thereby reduce the incidence of tumors in which the virus is believed to play a pathogenetic role. The success of a preventive vaccine program is dependent upon both the long-term efficacy of the vaccine as well as an efficient care-delivery system such that a large population is protected with the vaccine. However, if the vaccine were to be effective only in delaying primary infection, rather than preventing infection, it is likely to increase the burden of infectious mononucleosis since primary infection in young children is normally asymptomatic while primary infection in young adults can more easily cause infectious mononucleosis. Indeed, the socio-economic benefits of such vaccination are still a matter of debate.

A therapeutic vaccine, on the other hand, is directed to intervene in individuals already infected with EBV. Such an EBV vaccine could contribute to the treatment of patients with an EBV-associated neoplasm by boosting the host immunity. An efficient EBV vaccine with a limited indication, such as one that will allow organ donor recipients to be immunized prior to transplantation, may be a first step toward the incorporation of vaccine approaches in targeting post-transplantation lymphomas.

Several vaccines aimed at both preventing primary infection and generating a CTL response in a virus-associated cancer patient have been tested in phase I or II clinical trials.[51] Vaccination with a recombinant vaccinia virus expressing an EBV glycoprotein could protect and/or delay EBV infection by the natural route in naïve infants.[52] However, use of live vaccinia virus vaccines may be unacceptable. Interestingly, CTLs from acute infectious mononucleosis patients display strong *ex vivo* reactivity against structural antigens (glycoprotein 350 [gp350] and gp85). Long-term follow-up studies on infectious mononucleosis-recovered individuals showed that these individuals maintain gp350- and gp85-specific memory CTL, albeit at low levels, in the peripheral blood.[53] Direct injection of a plasmid containing the gp350 gene has also been tested and appeared to be useful for both prophylactic and therapeutic vaccinations since it effectively induced humoral and cellular immune responses.[54] An ongoing phase II, randomized, double-blind, placebo-controlled trial using gp350 in an aluminum-based adjuvant is aimed at determining the efficacy of this EBV vaccine to prevent infectious mononucleosis.[55]

Generation of a peptide-based vaccine against persistent viral infections, such as EBV, requires identification of immunodominant epitopes recognized by antiviral cytotoxic T cells. Results of a phase I study were recently published.[56] However, it should be considered that multiple infections are possible.[57] A more recent approach for an EBV vaccine that could be potentially active against primary infection identified a novel immunodominant epitope, termed LPRA, from an EBV helicase-primase-associated protein. Cytotoxic and proliferative CTL responses to the LPRA peptide were readily demonstrated *ex vivo*.[58]

A preclinical trial used a recombinant poxvirus vaccine that encodes a polyepitope protein comprising six HLA-A2-restricted epitopes from LMP1.[59] Immunization of HLA-A2/K mice with this vaccine consistently generated strong LMP1-specific CTL responses and, furthermore, it reversed the outgrowth of LMP1-expressing tumors in mice. However, the high degree of genetic variation in LMP1 has been considered a major impediment for its use as a potential immunotherapeutic target. Duraiswamy *et al.*[60] have conducted an extensive sequence analysis of LMP1 and revealed that the majority of the T cell epitopes are highly conserved in EBV isolates from Caucasian, Papua New Guinean, African, and Southeast Asian populations. It is important that these conserved regions are considered in designing epitope-based immunotherapeutic strategies in different ethnic populations.

Another preclinical study has recently identified a cocktail of six peptides containing highly promiscuous MHC class II epitopes derived from the EBV latency II antigens (three from EBNA1, one from LMP1, and two from LMP2). Not only was this cocktail immunogenic in HLA-DR transgenic mice, leading to a specific cellular and humoral response, but it incited recognition responses from CD4[+] T cells from healthy individuals and HL patients.[61]

Laboratory-engineered epitopes have also been tested as potential tools in developing an EBV vaccine. For example, a modified vaccinia virus Ankara recombinant, MVA-EL, included the C-terminal domain of EBNA1 fused to full-length LMP2. The endogenously expressed fusion protein EL was efficiently processed via the HLA class I pathway, and MVA-EL-infected dendritic cells selectively reactivated LMP2-specific CD8[+] memory T cell responses from immune donors *in vitro*.[62] Surprisingly, endogenously expressed EL also directly accesses the HLA class II presentation pathway and, unlike endogenously expressed EBNA1 itself, efficiently reactivated CD4[+] memory T cell responses *in vitro*.

These studies are ongoing and further research is required before an active and entirely safe EBV vaccine can be produced. Large clinical trials are expected.

INHIBITION OF EPSTEIN–BARR VIRUS TRANSFORMING GENES

This approach is based on the hypothesis that inhibition of EBV genes required for B cell transformation *in vitro* (*LMP1*) or EBV genes that appear to be indispensable (*EBNA1*) may reverse the malignant phenotype of some EBV-associated tumors. The use of antisense RNA directed toward *LMP1*, an oncogenic viral gene, can bring about the inhibition of expression of LMP1. Indeed, antisense *LMP1* reduced the expression of *LMP1* and downstream target genes such as *BCL2*. This effect resulted in an increased apoptosis and sensitivity to chemotherapeutic drugs.[63,64] Although these results *in vitro* are encouraging, the clinical application of antisense oligonucleotides delivered to tumor cells remains challenging.

In more recent years a novel tool for inhibition of gene expression has been widely developed and consists of the use of small double-stranded RNA molecules (small interfering RNA [siRNA]) homologous to the target gene to cause degradation of the corresponding messenger RNA (mRNA). Since EBNA1 is required for replication and persistence of the EBV episome, it is universally expressed in all EBV-associated tumor cells. EBNA1 thus presents as a master target, the inhibition of which will almost certainly lead to loss of EBV genomes during subsequent cell divisions. Furthermore, EBNA1 may have additional lymphomagenic functions including the modulation of transcription of translocated Myc as well as acting as an antiapoptotic factor. EBNA-1-specific siRNAs can inhibit EBNA1 expression and function. Small interfering RNAs were generated against three target sites in the EBNA1 mRNA, and two of these were found to inhibit EBNA1 expression, suppressing the episomal maintenance function and inhibiting tumor cell growth/survival.[65] Suppression of EBNA1 by siRNA was also associated with downregulation of the EBV oncogene *EBNA2*, a decreased proliferating cell nuclear antigen (PCNA) labeling index, and increased G0/G1 fraction in cell cycle analysis in EBV-positive lymphoma cells.[66]

These observations highlight the potential therapeutic applications for antisense or siRNA delivery to control EBV-associated malignant disorders. Although these studies point out the effectiveness of this approach to inhibit EBV latent gene expression *in vitro*, clinical use will require the development of efficient delivery methods to tumor cells *in vivo* as well as the need to overcome other challenges associated with using antisense or siRNA.

Since the transforming genes of the virus are critically dependent upon interaction with cellular pathways to enable the oncogenic influence of the virus, an alternative approach is to target the downstream proteins of these pathways and thereby prevent the biological influence of these viral genes. For example, targeting the nuclear factor κB (NF-κB) pathway through the use of a nondegradable mutant of the inhibitor of NF-κB (IκBα mutant) can abrogate the effects of LMP1 in EBV-associated tumors that express LMP1. Expression of such a mutant has been shown to inhibit the NF-κB pathway and drive the tumor cells to apoptosis.[67] One advantage of this approach is the ability to exploit the repertoire of pharmacologic compounds that are being continuously designed to intervene and block cellular pathways involved in nonviral oncogenic processes. However, this advantage to some extent compromises the specificity inherent in targeting the upstream viral targets.

ELIMINATION OF EPSTEIN–BARR VIRUS EPISOMES

Since EBV is present in the tumor cells of the EBV-positive malignancies, it is highly likely that the virus contributes, at least transiently, to the development of such tumors. It is also possible that the viral elements are necessary for the sustenance of the tumor phenotype. Therefore, therapies designed to induce loss of the EBV genome are theoretically capable of controlling EBV-associated malignancies.

Hydroxyurea (HU) is an inhibitor of ribonucleotide reductase and has been used in the treatment of malignancies, especially of myeloid origin. Chronic exposure of EBV-positive lymphoid cells *in vitro* to low-dose hydroxyurea has been shown to result in loss of viral episomes from such cells.[68] When the EBV genome of virus-associated lymphoid cells grown as xenografts in severe combined immune deficiency (SCID) mice was targeted with HU treatment, it resulted in retardation and/or inhibition of growth and decreased tumorigenicity in these mice. Pan *et al.*[69] have recently shown that HU reduces the original level of EBV genomes to approximately two-thirds and dramatically suppresses the expression of EBV lytic genes.

On the basis of these observations, low-dose HU was used to treat two patients with acquired immune deficiency syndrome (AIDS)-related CNS lymphomas.[70] Both patients showed clinical improvement and an extended survival. More recently, a patient who received an unrelated hematopoietic stem cell transplant and developed multiple CNS lymphoproliferative disorder lesions was also treated with oral low-dose HU and responded satisfactorily.[71]

The benefit and limited toxicity of HU therapy merit its further consideration as treatment for EBV-related malignancies. However, larger clinical studies are still required to confirm the utility of this drug in different types of tumors. For example, *in vitro*, the EBV genome is more easily lost from Burkitt lymphoma cell lines than from epithelioid cell lines when cultured in the presence of HU.[72] However, it was observed that HU enhanced the antitumor effect of acyclic nucleoside phosphonate analogues, like cidofovir, in EBV-transformed epithelial cells derived from NPC.[73] The effect is due to an enhancement of apoptosis through the caspase cascade causing enhanced cell toxicity and growth inhibition of NPC grown in athymic mice.

On the other hand, chronic treatment with HU can cause resistance, which can be overcome by gemcitabine, another inhibitor of ribonucleotide reductase. This observation suggests that targeting the viral genome may also require chemotherapeutic combination of relevant agents.[74]

It is well known that multiagent treatments are more effective than single agents in many types of tumors. In this regard, another appealing combination for the treatment of EBV-associated Burkitt lymphoma is a regimen based on HU and azidothymidine (AZT). In EBV-positive Burkitt lymphoma AZT induces apoptosis through inhibition of the NF-κB pathway with a consequent upregulation of EBV gene expression, including thymidine kinase. Phosphorylation of AZT to the monophosphate form, as well as apoptosis, was markedly enhanced in the presence of HU.[75] Azidothymidine has also been shown to induce apoptosis in HHV-8-positive/EBV-negative PEL cells in culture, by induction of a tumor necrosis factor-related apoptosis-inducing ligand (TRAIL)-mediated suicide program, and significantly increase survival in animal models of these lymphomas.[76]

More recent observations may lead to another potential strategy to evict episomal EBV DNA from EBV-positive cells. The EBV origin of replication (OriP) uses the cellular licensing machinery to regulate replication during latent infection. The minimal replicator sequence of OriP, flanked by nucleosomes, is subjected to cell cycle-dependent chromatin remodeling and histone modifications. Remarkably, histone H3 acetylation of the OriP nucleosomes decreased during late G1, coinciding with nucleosome remodeling and preceding the onset of DNA replication.[77] Therefore, drugs that target the chromatin structure (see below) around OriP may eventually lead to viral episomal loss. The possibility of specific agents derived from peptidomic analysis that may bind OriP and inhibit the recruitment of replication and/or modification proteins to this site is another strategy that could allow the loss of EBV in daughter cells.

EPIGENETIC TARGETS

It is now widely recognized that cancer is a result of not only genetic defects but also epigenetic abnormalities, and both types of alterations cooperate to produce and maintain the malignant phenotype.[78] Two epigenetic changes for which there are sufficient data particularly in the context of targeting the epigenome for clinical applications in malignancies are DNA methylation and histone deacetylation. Viruses, including EBV, are capable of inducing both genetic and epigenetic changes in the infected cells.[79] DNA methylation, in general, suppresses the viral gene expression; yet, methylation of distinct sets of gene promoters in EBV signifies different latency stages (I–III), which is essential for EBV to establish persistent infection and helps the virus to evade the host immune system. At the same time, viruses use similar strategies to alter the epigenetic information of their host cell. For example, viral proteins can directly or indirectly activate DNA methyltransferases (DNMTs), especially *DNMT3B*, a gene required for *de novo* DNA methylation. DNA methyltransferases are key enzymes to inactivate transcription by DNA hypermethylation and to ensure proper gene repression. Latent membrane protein 1 is capable of activating DNMTs via the AP-1/JNK signaling pathway.[80] This activation causes hypermethylation of E-cadherin and possibly other tumor suppressor genes, thus contributing to tumor development and/or maintenance. Since epigenetic changes are reversible, therapeutically targeting DNA methylation may restore multiple gene functions at the same time. To date, many chemical agents have been discovered that selectively inhibit either DNMTs or histone deacetylases. Histone deacetylases participate in the remodeling of chromatin structure by removing acetyl groups from lysine residues in the amino-terminal region of histones.[81] Histone deacetylation stabilizes chromatin structure and represses transcription. Therefore, histone deacetylase inhibitors cause differentiation, apoptosis, and/or cell cycle arrest in several cancer and lymphoblastoid cell lines.[82,83]

Demethylating agents, such as 5-azacytidine, or agents that cause histone acetylation, such as butyrates, are able to induce the EBV lytic cycle in latently infected cell lines, another theoretically possible therapeutic option for EBV-associated malignancies (see below). Moore et al.[84] have tested a combination of azacytidine and ganciclovir (GCV) to induce viral lytic expression, including the viral thymidine kinase, and render the host cells sensitive to GCV. 5-Azacytidine has been clinically used in the treatment of leukemias, myelodysplasias, and hemoglobinopathies for more than two decades. While such an approach may necessitate the use of higher doses of GCV, the regimen is likely to result in manageable myelotoxicity, since GCV will be required only during a short period.

A preclinical study was developed to evaluate the effect of a histone deacetylase inhibitor, depsipeptide, on EBV-lymphoid cell lines in a mouse model.[85] Preclinical data demonstrated that depsipeptide has anticancer activity and induces apoptosis via caspase-dependent and caspase-independent pathways in EBV latency III but not in EBV latency I cells. This observation warrants design of clinical trials for latency III EBV-associated tumors, especially considering that the depsipeptide doses required in mouse models are achievable in humans and this drug has a proven safety record in phase I trials.[86,87]

EPSTEIN–BARR VIRUS-DEPENDENT EXPRESSION OF TOXIC/APOPTOTIC GENES

Several approaches to gene therapy are feasible and can be potentially effective for EBV-containing tumors. However, therapeutic genes need to be delivered with high efficiency to the tumor cells. Gene therapy efforts in the context of lymphoid cancer have been hampered by the lack of suitable vectors that can achieve high levels of transgene expression. Attempts with a replication-defective herpes simplex virus 1 (HSV-1) vector indicated some advantages, including the infectivity of a broad spectrum of cells (even CD34$^+$ hematopoietic progenitor cells), the low multiplicity of infection required, and the large exogenous gene (up to 30 kb) that can be inserted.[88] Such a vector containing the thymidine kinase (TK) gene was able to transduce EBV-transformed lymphocytes with efficiencies of more than 20 percent and achieved significant tumor cell killing upon GCV treatment.

Regardless of the delivery system used, which goes beyond the scope of this chapter, an exciting notion is to achieve an efficient EBV-dependent expression of suicide genes. Thus, this strategy would be specifically targeted to EBV-containing cells and therefore safe and virtually tumor-directed, since very few memory B cells carry EBV in seropositive individuals (about one in a million). Multiple studies have explored this approach and we mention some examples below.

Franken et al.[89] constructed a vector with the TK gene under the control of the Cp promoter. Following treatment with GCV, EBNA2-expressing cells were selectively killed. Since all EBV-associated malignant cells express EBNA1, several groups have developed vectors that express toxins under the control of OriP, which is activated by EBNA1. Indeed, the family of repeats (FR) region of OriP constitutes the highest affinity binding site for EBNA1 in the EBV genome. Therefore, binding of EBNA1 to the FR region of OriP transcriptionally activates the juxtaposed gene. One suicide gene utilized first by Judde et al.[90] and later by Kenney et al.[91] is cytosine deaminase, which converts 5-fluorocytosine into 5-fluorouracil. Transfection of this vector causes death in EBV-positive lymphoma cells following treatment with 5-fluorocytosine (5-FC) due to endogenous EBNA1 activation of cytosine deaminase. Similarly, Hirai et al.[92] constructed an OriP-HSV-TK vector sensitizing EBV-positive cells to GCV. All these reports demonstrate the specificity of this approach by which EBV-negative cells are not significantly affected. However, depending on the suicide gene used, bystander effects to neighboring cells have been observed.[90]

Using a similar approach, it was demonstrated that the use of a replication-deficient adenoviral vector containing the TP53 tumor suppressor gene under the direction of EBNA1 has greater efficacy in epithelial EBV-positive than in EBV-negative cells.[93] The resulting tumor cytotoxicity was shown to be mediated by apoptosis, and could be further enhanced by ionizing radiation. Since adenoviral vectors infect normal lymphocytes (EBV reservoir) poorly, this approach is likely to be more relevant in treating EBV-positive epithelial neoplasia.

Although promising, all these approaches would require improvement in delivery systems for gene therapy before being widely used in the clinic.

INDUCTION OF THE LYTIC CYCLE

The activation of the lytic phase of EBV is not conducive to the maintenance of the malignant phenotype since it will result in cell death. However, it is important to note that some level of EBV reactivation does occur in tumors[94] suggesting that the tumor cells are permissive for activating viral replication and thus the lytic cycle. This lytic potential of the virus can be harnessed to use the virus as an effective oncolytic agent.

Two immediate-early genes, *BZLF1* and *BRLF1*, are necessary and sufficient to mediate the switch from latent to lytic EBV infection.[95] These genes encode transcription factors that activate the entire lytic cascade and, once initiated, infective virions are produced and the host cell is destroyed. Consequently, *BZLF1/Zta/Zebra* and *BRLF1/Rta* are genes that are tightly controlled through positive and negative regulation. Discrete regions in the promoters control expression of these master lytic inducers through interactions with multiple factors, including the positive regulators SP1, CREB, ATF1, ATF2/c-jun, and MEF2D and the negative regulators YY1 and ZEB. In addition, epigenetic mechanisms also contribute and are critical in regulating the expression of Zta and Rta. The chromatin around the immediate-early promoters is in the unacetylated form and the DNA is hypermethylated. These promoters are thus maintained to remain inactive in latently infected cells. Pharmacologically active agents, such as the phorbol ester 12-O-tetradecanoylphorbol-13-acetate (TPA), butyrates, and calcium ionophores, and other stimuli such as the engagement of the B cell receptor, as well as demethylating agents and inhibitors of histone deacetylases, have been shown to reverse this inactivation.[96] Indeed, pharmacologic induction of the lytic cycle in latently infected tumor cells with 5-azacytidine is a potential therapeutic option[97,98] that has been explored.

Since the induction of the lytic cycle in tumor cells ends with production of infective particles, one concern would be the effect of this massive virion release, with a high probability of infection and even transformation of new host cells. However, proof-of-concept studies demonstrated that this concern could be mitigated with concomitant treatment with an antiviral drug that blocks replication of the viral genome, without inhibiting the actual pathways that mediate lysis of the host cells. Indeed, we demonstrated that once the lytic cycle is triggered by expression of *BZLF1*, acyclovir precluded virion formation without altering the cell death process of the lytic cascade.[99]

Two strategies are possible to purposely induce the lytic cycle of EBV, and both have been explored in experimental trials:

- Gene-therapy approaches using vectors containing *BZLF1* and/or *BRLF1* under the control of a heterologous promoter;
- Pharmacologic induction of the endogenous EBV with agents that will directly or indirectly activate *BZLF1* and/or *BRLF1* promoters.

Forced expression of immediate-early genes in tumor cells has the advantage of bypassing the tight regulation of these genes and the disadvantage of being dependent on delivery systems that are still not optimal. Forced expression of *BZLF1/BRLF1* requires the presence of endogenous EBV genomes to induce the lytic cascade. Indeed,

this gene-therapy system is more cytotoxic to EBV-containing cells than to EBV-negative cells. However, some nonspecific toxicity because of high level of expression in EBV-negative cells can occur, especially if *BRLF1* is used.[100] To improve this and target the gene-therapy system to EBV-containing cells, we constructed an EBV-dependent vector in which *BZLF1* expression is under the control of OriP sequences.[99] Therefore, there are two levels of specificity: endogenous EBNA1 is required for transcription of the exogenous *BZLF1* and the entire endogenous EBV genome is required to complete the lytic cascade by transactivation of genes. In this system, EBV provides both the target and the executor for mediating tumor-specific cell death, markedly increasing the specificity of this potential therapy. No bystander effect was observed in mixed EBV-positive and EBV-negative cell cultures.

Another group has demonstrated similar proof-of-concept results in epithelial EBV-associated tumors using adenoviral vectors expressing *BZLF1* or *BRLF1*.[100] This system induced preferential killing of EBV-positive gastric carcinoma cells *in vitro*. Furthermore, injection of this adenoviral vector in NPC tumors grown in nude mice also significantly inhibited tumor growth.

Pharmacologic reactivation of the endogenous EBV by drugs and small molecules that are able to activate BZLF1/BRLF1 expression has the advantage of easy delivery but requires more knowledge of viral gene regulation and consideration of the pleiotropic effects of the drugs. Some chemotherapeutic drugs, including but not limited to doxorubicin, cis-platinum, and 5-fluorouracil (5-FU),[101,102] are able to induce lytic EBV. This effect appears to be cell-type specific, since 5-FU, for example, is active in gastric carcinoma cells but not in lymphoid cells. Drug actions are mediated by simultaneous engagement of several signal transduction pathways, including mitogen-activated protein (MAP) kinases, phosphatidylinositol 3-kinase (PI3K), and protein kinase C.

Arginine butyrate has long been known to induce EBV reactivation. In a phase I/II trial for PTLD therapy, Mentzer *et al.*[103] have used arginine butyrate combined with GCV to induce EBV lytic expression, including the TK gene and sensitizing cells to GCV. Complete or partial responses have been observed.

It was recently shown that methotrexate (MTX), a widely used drug for treatment of hematologic malignancies, induces reactivation of EBV and virion production from latently infected lymphoma and gastric carcinoma cells.[104] Similar to other agents, this effect is caused by activation of BZLF1 and BRLF1 and the same transcription factor binding motifs are required for MTX-mediated EBV reactivation.

Natural products can also induce EBV lytic cycle, like terpenes from *Euphorbia* spp. or bryostatin.[105,106] It is likely that among the vast variety of herbal and botanic products, drugs with similar properties but even more effective and less toxic can be identified.

KEY POINTS

- An increasing list of tumors is associated with viruses. Lymphomas are mostly associated with herpesviruses.
- EBV, a widespread and successful human herpesvirus that persists throughout the life of the infected individual, is associated with malignant and benign diseases that involve lymphoid and epithelial tissues.
- The pathogenetic role of EBV is not completely understood. However, the virus itself can be the target for therapies against tumor cells.
- Like other tumor-targeted therapies, approaches targeting EBV are tumor-specific (high specificity), causing very little damage to normal cells (low toxicity).
- All EBV-directed therapies affect directly viral gene expression or the virus–host interaction.
- Several strategies are at different stages of development, from preclinical experimental studies to phase III clinical studies.
- EBV-targeted therapies include immunotherapies (infusion of EBV-specific CTLs), prophylactic or therapeutic vaccines, inhibition of transforming genes or the entire episome, epigenetic modulation of viral gene expression, EBV-dependent expression of suicide genes, and induction of the lytic cycle.

REFERENCES

● = Key primary paper
◆ = Major review article

◆1. Snijders PJ, Steenbergen RD, Heideman DA, Meijer CJ. HPV-mediated cervical carcinogenesis: concepts and clinical implications. *J Pathol* 2006; **208**: 152–64.

◆2. Liang TJ, Heller T. Pathogenesis of hepatitis C-associated hepatocellular carcinoma. *Gastroenterology* 2004; **127**(5 Suppl 1): S62–71.

◆3. Ablashi DV, Chatlynne LG, Whitman Jr JE, Cesarman E. Spectrum of Kaposi's sarcoma-associated herpesvirus, or human herpesvirus 8, diseases. *Clin Microbiol Rev* 2002; **15**: 439–64.

◆4. Jarret RF. Viruses and lymphoma/leukaemia. *J Pathol* 2006; **208**: 176–86.

◆5. Young LS, Rickinson AB. Epstein-Barr virus: 40 years on. *Nat Rev Cancer* 2004; **4**: 757–68.

◆6. Lopes V, Young LS, Murray PG. Epstein–Barr Virus-associated cancers: Aetiology and treatment. Epstein-Barr Virus-associated cancers. *Herpes* 2003; **10**: 78–82.

7. Carbone A, Gloghini A, Vaccher E *et al.* Kaposi's sarcoma-associated herpesvirus DNA sequences in AIDS-related and AIDS-unrelated lymphomatous effusions. *Br J Haematol* 1996; **94**: 533–43.

◆8. Libra M, Gasparotto D, Gloghini A *et al.* Hepatitis C virus (HCV) infection and lymphoproliferative disorders. *Front Biosci* 2005; **10**: 2460–71.

9. Sansonno D, Tucci FA, De Re V *et al.* HCV-associated B cell clonalities in the liver do not carry the t(14; 18) chromosomal translocation. *Hepatology* 2005; **42**: 1019–27.

10. Besson C, Canioni D, Lepage E *et al.* Characteristics and outcome of diffuse large B-cell lymphoma in hepatitis C virus-positive patients in LNH 93 and LNH 98 Groupe d'Etude des Lymphomes de l'Adulte programs. *J Clin Oncol* 2006; **24**: 953–60.

◆11. Feuer G, Green PL. Comparative biology of human T-cell lymphotropic virus type 1 (HTLV-1) and HTLV-2. *Oncogene* 2005; **24**: 5996–6004.

12. Shivapurkar N, Harada K, Reddy J *et al.* Presence of simian virus 40 DNA sequences in human lymphomas. *Lancet* 2002; **359**: 851–2.

13. Capello D, Rossi D, Gaudino G *et al.* Simian virus 40 infection in lymphoproliferative disorders. *Lancet* 2003; **361**: 88–9.

14. Schuler F, Dolken SC, Hirt C *et al.* No evidence for simian virus 40 DNA sequences in malignant non-Hodgkin lymphomas. *Int J Cancer* 2006; **118**: 498–504.

15. Shah KV. SV40 and human cancer: a review of recent data. *Int J Cancer* 2007; **120**: 215–23.

16. Hernandez-Losa J, Fedele CG, Pozo F *et al.* Lack of association of poliomavirus and herpesvirus types 6 and 7 in human lymphomas. *Cancer* 2005; **103**: 293–8.

●17. Cohen JI. Epstein–Barr virus infection. *N Engl J Med* 2000; **343**: 481–92.

◆18. Faulkner GC, Krajewski AS, Crawford DH. The ins and outs of EBV infection. *Trends Microbiol* 2000; **8**: 185–9.

◆19. William H, Crawford DH. Epstein-Barr virus: the impact of scientific advances on clinical practice. *Blood* 2006; **107**: 862–9.

◆20. Murray PG, Young LS. Epstein–Barr virus infection: basis of malignancy and potential for therapy. *Expert Rev Mol Med* 2001; **3**: 1–20. http://www-ermm.cbcu.cam.ac.uk/01003842h.htm

21. Gulley ML, Raphael M, Lutz CT *et al.* Epstein-Barr virus integration in human lymphomas and lymphoid cell lines. *Cancer* 1992; **70**: 185–91.

22. Okano M, Kawa K, Kimura H *et al.* Proposed guidelines for diagnosing chronic active Epstein-Barr virus infection. *Am J Hematol* 2005; **80**: 64–9.

23. Niedobitek G, Agathanggelou A, Steven N, Young LS. Epstein-Barr virus (EBV) in infectious mononucleosis: detection of the virus in tonsillar B lymphocytes but not in desquamated oropharyngeal epithelial cells. *Mol Pathol* 2000; **53**: 37–42.

24. Koriyama C, Akiba S, Minakami Y, Eizuru Y. Environmental factors related to Epstein-Barr virus-associated gastric cancer in Japan. *J Exp Clin Cancer Res* 2005; **24**: 547–53.

25. Magrath I, Bhatia K. Breast cancer: a new Epstein-Barr virus-associated disease? *J Natl Cancer Inst* 1999; **91**: 1349–50.

26. Jenson HB, Montalvo EA, McClain KL *et al.* Characterization of natural Epstein-Barr virus infection and replication in smooth muscle cells from a leiomyosarcoma. *J Med Virol* 1999; **57**: 36–46.

27. Chan AT, Teo PM, Huang DP. Pathogenesis and treatment of nasopharyngeal carcinoma. *Semin Oncol* 2004; **31**: 794–801.

◆28. Israel BF, Kenney SC. Virally targeted therapies for EBV-associated malignancies. *Oncogene* 2003; **22**: 5122–30.

29. International Agency for Research on Cancer (IARC). Epstein-Barr virus and Kaposi's sarcoma herpesvirus/human herpesvirus 8. *IARC Monogr Eval Carcinogenic Risks Humans* 1997; **70**.

◆30. Khanna R, Moss D, Gandhi M. Technology insight: Applications of emerging immunotherapeutic strategies for Epstein-Barr virus-associated malignancies. *Nat Clin Pract Oncol* 2005; **2**: 138–49.

◆31. Straathof KCM, Bollard CM, Rooney CM, Heslop HE. Immunotherapy for Epstein-Barr virus-associated cancers in children. *Oncologist* 2003; **8**: 83–98.

32. Haque T, Wilkie GM, Taylor C *et al.* Treatment of Epstein-Barr virus-positive post-transplantation lymphoproliferative disease with partly HLA-matched allogeneic cytotoxic T cells. *Lancet* 2002; **360**: 436–41.

●33. Wilkie GM, Taylor C, Jones MM *et al.* Establishment and characterization of a bank of cytotoxic T lymphocytes for immunotherapy of Epstein-Barr virus-associated diseases. *J Immunother* 2004; **27**: 309–16.

34. Wynn RF, Arkwright PD, Haque T *et al.* Treatment of Epstein-Barr virus-associated primary CNS B cell lymphoma with allogeneic T cell immunotherapy and stem-cell transplantation. *Lancet Oncol* 2005; **6**: 344–6.

●35. Papadopoulos EB, Ladanyi M, Emanuel D *et al.* Infusions of donor leukocytes to treat Epstein-Barr virus-associated lymphoproliferative disorders after allogeneic bone marrow transplantation. *N Engl J Med* 1994; **330**: 1185–91.

36. Nolte A, Buhmann R, Straka C *et al.* Assessment and characterization of the cytolytic T lymphocyte response against Epstein-Barr virus in patients with non-Hodgkin's lymphoma after autologous peripheral blood stem cell transplantation. *Bone Marrow Transplant* 1998; **21**: 909–16.

◆37. Gottschalk S, Heslop SE, Rooney CM. Adoptive immunotherapy for EBV-associated malignancies. *Leuk Lymphoma* 2005; **46**: 1–10.

38. Khanna R, Bell S, Sherritt M *et al.* Activation and adoptive transfer of Epstein-Barr virus-specific cytotoxic T cells in solid organ transplant patients with posttransplant lymphoproliferative disease. *Proc Natl Acad Sci U S A* 1999; **96**: 10391–6.

39. Comoli P, Maccario R, Locatelli F *et al.* Treatment of EBV-related post-renal transplant lymphoproliferative disease with a tailored regimen including EBV-specific T cells. *Am J Transplant* 2005; **5**: 1415–22.

40. Gottschalk S, Ng CY, Perez M *et al.* An Epstein-Barr virus deletion mutant associated with fatal lymphoproliferative disease unresponsive to therapy with virus-specific CTLs. *Blood* 2001; **97**: 835–43.

41. Chua D, Huang J, Zheng B *et al.* Adoptive transfer of autologous Epstein-Barr virus-specific cytotoxic T cells for nasopharyngeal carcinoma. *Int J Cancer* 2001; **94**: 73–80.

42. Roskrow MA, Suzuki N, Gan Y *et al.* Epstein-Barr virus (EBV)-specific cytotoxic T lymphocytes for the treatment of patients with EBV-positive relapsed Hodgkin's disease. *Blood* 1998; **91**: 2925–34.

43. Wagner HJ, Sili U, Gahn B *et al.* Expansion of EBV latent membrane protein 2 specific cytotoxic T cells for the adoptive immunotherapy of EBV latency type 2 malignancies: influence of recombinant IL12 and IL15. *Cytotherapy* 2003; **5**: 231–40.

44. Sun Q, Brewer N, Dunham K *et al.* Interferon-gamma expressing EBV LMP2A-specific T cells for cellular immunotherapy. *Cell Immunol* 2007; **246**: 81–91.

●45. Bollard CM, Aguilar L, Straathof KC *et al.* Cytotoxic T lymphocyte therapy for Epstein-Barr virus-Hodgkin's disease. *J Exp Med* 2004; **200**: 1623–33.

46. Gahn B, Siller-Lopez F, Pirooz AD *et al.* Adenoviral gene transfer into dendritic cells efficiently amplifies the immune response to LMP2A antigen: A potential treatment strategy for Epstein-Barr Virus–positive Hodgkin's lymphoma. *Int J Cancer* 2001; **93**: 706–13.

47. Bollard CM, Gottschalk S, Leen AM *et al.* Complete responses of relapsed lymphoma following genetic modification of tumor-antigen presenting cells and T-lymphocyte transfer. *Blood* 2007; **110**: 2838–45.

48. Straathof KC, Leen AM, Buza EL *et al.* Characterization of latent membrane protein 2 specificity in CTL lines from patients with EBV-positive nasopharyngeal carcinoma and lymphoma. *J Immunol* 2005; **176**: 4137–47.

49. Provenzano M, Selleri S, Jin P *et al.* Comprehensive epitope mapping of the Epstein-Barr virus latent membrane protein-2 in normal, non tumor-bearing individuals. *Cancer Immunol Immunother* 2007; **56**: 1047–63.

50. Gottschalk S, Edwards OL, Sili U *et al.* Generating CTLs against the subdominant Epstein-Barr virus LMP1 antigen for the adoptive immunotherapy of EBV-associated malignancies. *Blood* 2003; **101**: 1905–12.

51. Jackman WT, Mann KA, Hoffmann HJ, Spaete RR. Expression of Epstein-Barr virus gp350 as a single chain glycoprotein for an EBV subunit vaccine. *Vaccine* 1999; **17**: 660–68.

●52. Gu SY, Huang TM, Ruan L *et al.* First EBV vaccine trial in humans using recombinant vaccinia virus expressing the major membrane antigen. *Dev Biol Stand* 1995; **84**: 171–7.

53. Khanna R, Sherritt M, Burrows SR. EBV structural antigens, gp350 and gp85, as targets for ex vivo virus-specific CTL during acute infectious mononucleosis: potential use of gp350/gp85 CTL epitopes for vaccine design. *J Immunol* 1999; **162**: 3063–9.

54. Jung S, Chung YK, Chang SH *et al*. DNA-mediated immunization of glycoprotein 350 of Epstein-Barr virus induces the effective humoral and cellular immune responses against the antigen. *Mol Cells* 2001; **12**: 41–9.

55. Sokal EM, Hoppenbrouwers K, Vandermeulen C *et al*. Recombinant gp350 vaccine for infectious mononucleosis: a phase 2, randomized, double-blind, placebo-controlled trial to evaluate the safety, immunogenicity, and efficacy of an Epstein-Barr virus vaccine in healthy young adults. *J Infect Dis* 2007; **196**: 1749–53.

56. Elliott SL, Suhrbier A, Miles JJ *et al*. Phase I trial of a CD8+ T-cell peptide epitope-based vaccine for infectious mononucleosis. *J Virol* 2008; **82**: 1448–57.

57. Walling DM, Brown AL, Etinne W *et al*. Multiple Epstein-Barr virus infections in healthy individuals. *J Virol* 2003; **77**: 6546–50.

58. Turcanova V, Hollsberg P. Sustained CD8+ T-cell immune response to a novel immunodominant HLA-B*0702-associated epitope derived from an Epstein-Barr virus helicase-primase-associated protein. *J Med Virol* 2004; **72**: 635–45.

59. Duraiswamy J, Sherritt M, Thomson S *et al*. Therapeutic LMP1 polyepitope vaccine for EBV-associated Hodgkin's disease and nasopharyngeal carcinoma. *Blood* 2003; **101**: 3150–56.

60. Duraiswamy J, Burrows JM, Bharadwaj M *et al*. Ex vivo analysis of T-cell responses to Epstein-Barr virus-encoded oncogene latent membrane protein 1 reveals highly conserved epitope sequences in virus isolates from diverse geographic regions. *J Virol* 2003; **77**: 7401–10.

61. Depil S, Morales O, Maillere B *et al*. Determination of a HLA II promiscuous peptide cocktail as potential vaccine against EBV latency II malignances. *Blood* 2005; **106**: 1478 (abstract).

62. Taylor GS, Haigh TA, Gudgeon NH *et al*. Dual stimulation of Epstein-Barr Virus (EBV)-specific CD4+- and CD8+- T-cell responses by a chimeric antigen construct: potential therapeutic vaccine for EBV-positive nasopharyngeal carcinoma. *J Virol* 2004; **78**: 768–78.

63. Kenney JL, Guinness ME, Curiel T, Lacy J. Antisense to the Epstein-Barr virus (EBV)-encoded latent membrane protein 1 (LMP-1) suppresses LMP-1 and bcl-2 expression and promotes apoptosis in EBV-immortalized B cells. *Blood* 1998; **92**: 1721–7.

64. Chen JJ, Raab-Traub N, Yao QY *et al*. Inhibiting target gene expression and controlling growth of Epstein-Barr virus transformed cells by antisense RNA transcripts. *Ai Zheng* 2002; **21**: 16–20.

●65. Yin Q, Flemington EK. siRNAs against the Epstein Barr virus latency replication factor, EBNA1, inhibit its function and growth of EBV-dependent tumor cells. *Virology* 2006; **346**: 385–93.

66. Hong M, Murai Y, Kutsuna T *et al*. Suppression of Epstein-Barr nuclear antigen 1 (EBNA1) by RNA interference inhibits proliferation of EBV-positive Burkitt's lymphoma cells. *J Cancer Res Clin Oncol* 2006; **132**: 1–8.

67. Cahir-McFarland ED, Davidson DM, Schauer SL *et al*. NF-kappa B inhibition causes spontaneous apoptosis in Epstein-Barr virus-transformed lymphoblastoid cells. *Proc Natl Acad Sci U S A* 2000; **97**: 6055–60.

68. Chodosh J, Holder VP, Gan YJ *et al*. Eradication of latent Epstein-Barr virus by hydroxyurea alters the growth-transformed cell phenotype. *J Infect Dis* 1998; **177**: 1194–201.

69. Pan YR, Fang CY, Chang YS, Chang HY. Analysis of Epstein-Barr virus gene expression upon phorbol ester and hydroxyurea treatment by real-time quantitative PCR. *Arch Virol* 2005; **150**: 755–70.

●70. Slobod KS, Taylor GH, Sandlund JT *et al*. Epstein-Barr virus-targeted therapy for AIDS-related primary lymphoma of the central nervous system. *Lancet* 2000; **356**: 1493–4.

71. Pakakasama S, Eames GM, Morriss MC *et al*. Treatment of Epstein-Barr virus lymphoproliferative disease after hematopoietic stem-cell transplantation with hydroxyurea and cytotoxic T-cell lymphocytes. *Transplantation* 2004; **78**: 755–7.

●72. Jiang R, Kanamori M, Satoh Y *et al*. Contrasting effects of hydroxyurea on cell growth and reduction in Epstein-Barr virus genomes in EBV-infected epithelioid cell lines vs Burkitt's lymphoma cell lines. *J Med Virol* 2003; **70**: 244–52.

73. Wakisaka N, Yoshizaki T, Raab-Traub N, Pagano JS. Ribonucleotide reductase inhibitors enhance cidofovir-induced apoptosis in EBV-positive nasopharyngeal carcinoma xenografts. *Int J Cancer* 2005; **116**: 640–45.

●74. Jiang R, Zhang JL, Satoh Y, Sairenji T. Mechanism for induction of hydroxyurea resistance and loss of latent EBV genome in hydroxyurea-treated Burkitt's lymphoma cell line Raji. *J Med Virol* 2004; **73**: 589–95.

75. Kurokawa M, Ghosh SK, Ramos JC *et al*. Azidothymidine inhibits NF-kappaB and induces Epstein-Barr virus gene expression in Burkitt lymphoma. *Blood* 2005; **106**: 235–40.

76. Wu W, Rochford R, Toomey L *et al*. Inhibition of HHV-8/KSHV infected primary effusion lymphomas in NOD/SCID mice by azidothymidine and interferon-alpha. *Leuk Res* 2005; **29**: 545–55.

77. Zhou J, Chau CM, Deng Z *et al*. Cell cycle regulation of chromatin at an origin of DNA replication. *EMBO J* 2005; **24**: 1406–17.

◆78. Jones PA. Overview of cancer epigenetics. *Semin Hematol* 2005; **42** (Suppl 2): S3–8.

79. Li HP, Leu YW, Chang YS. Epigenetic changes in virus-associated human cancers. *Cell Res* 2005; **15**: 262–71.

◆80. Tsai CN, Tsai CL, Tse KP *et al*. The Epstein-Barr virus oncogene product, latent membrane protein 1, induces the downregulation of E-cadherin gene expression via activation of DNA methyltransferases. *Proc Natl Acad Sci U S A* 2002; **99**: 10084–9.

◆81. Goodsell DS. The molecular perspective: Histone deacetylase. *Oncologist* 2003; **8**: 389–91.

82. Seo JS, Cho NY, Kim HR *et al.* Cell cycle arrest and lytic induction of EBV-transformed B lymphoblastoid cells by a histone deacetylase inhibitor, Trichostatin A. *Oncol Rep* 2008; **19**: 93–8.

83. Ye J, Gradoville L, Daigle D, Miller G. De novo protein synthesis is required for lytic cycle reactivation of Epstein-Barr virus, but not Kaposi's sarcoma-associated herpesvirus, in response to histone deacetylase inhibitors and protein kinase C agonists. *J Virol* 2007; **81**: 9279–91.

●84. Moore SM, Cannon JS, Tanheco YC *et al.* Induction of Epstein-Barr virus kinases to sensitize tumor cells to nucleoside analogues. Antimicrob Agents *Chemother* 2001; **45**: 2082–91.

85. Roychowdhury S, Baiocchi RA, Vourganti S *et al.* Selective efficacy of depsipeptide in a xenograft model of Epstein-Barr virus–positive lymphoproliferative disorder. *J Natl Cancer Inst* 2004; **96**: 1447–57.

●86. Sandor V, Bakke S, Robey RW *et al.* Phase I trial of the histone deacetylase inhibitor, depsipeptide (FR901228, NSC 630176), in patients with refractory neoplasms. *Clin Cancer Res* 2002; **8**: 718–28.

87. Piekarz RL, Robey R, Sandor V *et al.* Inhibitor of histone deacetylation, depsipeptide (FR901228), in the treatment of peripheral and cutaneous T-cell lymphoma: a case report. *Blood* 2001; **98**: 2865–8.

88. Suzuki T, Piche A, Kasono K *et al.* Efficient gene delivery into Epstein-Barr virus (EBV)-transformed human B cells mediated by replication-defective herpes simplex virus-1 (HSV-1): A gene therapy model for EBV-related B cell malignancy. *Biochem Biophys Res Comm* 1998; **252**: 686–90.

●89. Franken M, Estabrooks A, Cavacini L *et al.* Epstein-Barr virus driven gene therapy for EBV-related lymphomas. *Nat Med* 1996; **2**: 1379–82.

90. Judde JG, Spangler G, Magrath I, Bhatia K. Use of Epstein-Barr virus nuclear antigen-1 in targeted therapy of EBV-associated neoplasia. *Hum Gene Ther* 1996; **7**: 647–53.

●91. Kenney S, Ge JQ, Westphal EM, Olsen J. Gene therapy strategies for treating Epstein-Barr virus-associated lymphomas: comparison of two different Epstein-Barr virus-based vectors. *Hum Gene Ther* 1998; **9**: 1131–41.

92. Hirai H, Satoh E, Osawa M *et al.* Use of EBV-based Vector/HVJ-liposome complex vector for targeted gene therapy of EBV-associated neoplasms. *Biochem Biophys Res Comm* 1997; **241**: 112–18.

93. Li J-H, Chia M, Shi W *et al.* Tumor-targeted gene therapy for nasopharyngeal carcinoma. *Cancer Res* 2002; **62**: 171–8.

94. Gutiérrez MI, Bhatia K, Magrath IT. Replicative viral DNA in Epstein-Barr virus associated Burkitt's lymphoma biopsies. *Leukemia Res* 1993; **17**: 285–9.

●95. Miller G. The switch between latency and replication of Epstein-Barr virus. *J Infect Dis* 1990; **161**: 833–44.

◆96. Amon W, Farrel PJ. Reactivation of Epstein-Barr virus from latency. *Rev Med Virol* 2005; **15**: 149–56.

●97. Robertson KD, Barletta J, Samid D, Ambinder RF. Pharmacologic activation of expression of immunodominant viral antigens: a new strategy for the treatment of Epstein-Barr-virus-associated malignancies. *Curr Top Microbiol Immunol* 1995; **194**: 145–54.

98. Westphal EM, Blackstock W, Feng WH *et al.* Activation of lytic Epstein-Barr virus (EBV) infection by radiation and sodium butyrate in vitro and in vivo: a potential method for treating EBV-positive malignancies. *Cancer Res* 2000; **60**: 5781–8.

●99. Gutiérrez MI, Judde J-G, Magrath IT, Bhatia KG. Switching viral latency to viral lysis: A novel therapeutic approach for Epstein-Barr virus-associated neoplasia. *Cancer Res* 1996; **56**: 969–72.

●100. Feng WH, Westphal E, Mauser A *et al.* Use of adenovirus vectors expressing Epstein-Barr virus (EBV) immediate-early protein BZLF1 or BRLF1 to treat EBV-positive tumors. *J Virol* 2002; **76**: 10951–9.

101. Feng WH, Israel B, Raab-Traub N *et al.* Chemotherapy induces lytic EBV replication and confers ganciclovir susceptibility to EBV-positive tumors. *Cancer Res* 2002; **62**: 1920–26.

102. Feng WH, Hong G, Delecluse HJ, Kenney SC. Lytic induction therapy for Epstein-Barr virus-positive B-cell lymphomas. *J Virol* 2004; **78**: 1893–902.

◆103. Mentzer SJ, Perrine SP, Faller DV. Epstein-Barr virus post-transplant lymphoproliferative disease and virus-specific therapy: pharmacological re-activation of viral target genes with arginine butyrate. *Transpl Infect Dis* 2001; **3**: 177–85.

●104. Feng WH, Cohen JI, Fischer S *et al.* Reactivation of latent Epstein–Barr virus by methotrexate: A potential contributor to methotrexate-associated lymphomas. *J Natl Cancer Inst* 2004; **96**:1691–702.

105. MacNeil A, Sumba OP, Lutzke ML *et al.* Activation of the Epstein-Barr virus lytic cycle by the latex of the plant Euphorbia tirucalli. *Br J Cancer* 2003; **88**: 1566–9.

106. Stewart JP, McGown AT, Prendiville J *et al.* Bryostatin 1 induces productive Epstein-Barr virus replication in latently infected cells: implications for use in immunocompromised patients. *Cancer Chemother Pharmacol* 1993; **33**: 89–91.

Index